Robbins and Cotran Pathologic Basis of Disease

ROBBINS AND COTRAN

Pathologic Basis of Disease

NINTH EDITION

Vinay Kumar, MBBS, MD, FRCPath
Donald N. Pritzker Professor
and Chairman, Department of Pathology
Biologic Sciences Division and
The Pritzker School of Medicine
The University of Chicago
Chicago, Illinois

Abul K. Abbas, MBBS
Distinguished Professor and Chair
Department of Pathology
University of California San Francisco
San Francisco, California

Jon C. Aster, MD, PhD
Professor of Pathology
Harvard Medical School
Brigham and Women's Hospital
Boston, Massachusetts

WITH ILLUSTRATIONS BY
James A. Perkins, MS, MFA

Get more from this publication online 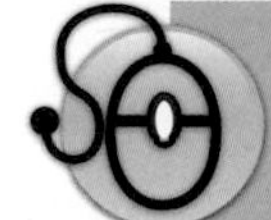

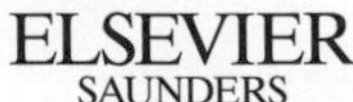

ELSEVIER
SAUNDERS

1600 John F. Kennedy Blvd.
Ste 1800
Philadelphia, PA 19103-2899

ROBBINS AND COTRAN PATHOLOGIC BASIS OF DISEASE, Ninth Edition ISBN: 978-1-4557-2613-4
International edition ISBN: 978-0-8089-2450-0
Professional Edition ISBN: 978-0-323-26616-1

Notices

Knowledge and best practice in this field are constantly changing. As new research and experience broaden our understanding, changes in research methods, professional practices, or medical treatment may become necessary.

Practitioners and researchers must always rely on their own experience and knowledge in evaluating and using any information, methods, compounds, or experiments described herein. In using such information or methods they should be mindful of their own safety and the safety of others, including parties for whom they have a professional responsibility.

With respect to any drug or pharmaceutical products identified, readers are advised to check the most current information provided (i) on procedures featured or (ii) by the manufacturer of each product to be administered, to verify the recommended dose or formula, the method and duration of administration, and contraindications. It is the responsibility of practitioners, relying on their own experience and knowledge of their patients, to make diagnoses, to determine dosages and the best treatment for each individual patient, and to take all appropriate safety precautions.

To the fullest extent of the law, neither the Publisher nor the authors, contributors, or editors assume any liability for any injury and/or damage to persons or property as a matter of products liability, negligence or otherwise, or from any use or operation of any methods, products, instructions, or ideas contained in the material herein.

Library of Congress Cataloging-in-Publication Data
Robbins and Cotran pathologic basis of disease / [edited by] Vinay Kumar, Abul K. Abbas, Jon C. Aster ; with illustrations by James A. Perkins. — Ninth edition.
p. ; cm.
Pathologic basis of disease
Includes bibliographical references and index.
ISBN 978-1-4557-2613-4 (hardback : alk. paper) — ISBN 978-0-8089-2450-0 (international edition : alk. paper) — ISBN 978-0-323-26616-1 (professional edition : alk. paper)
I. Kumar, Vinay, 1944- editor. II. Abbas, Abul K., editor. III. Aster, Jon C., editor. IV. Title: Pathologic basis of disease.
[DNLM: 1. Pathologic Processes. QZ 140]
RB111
616.07 — dc23

2014017443

Executive Content Strategist: William Schmitt
Manager, Content Development: Rebecca Gruliow
Publishing Services Manager: Anne Altepeter
Project Manager: Jennifer Nemec
Design Direction: Lou Forgione

Printed in Canada

Last digit is the print number: 9 8 7 6 5 4 3 2 1

DEDICATION

To
Our teachers
For inspiring us

To
Our students
For constantly challenging us

To our spouses
Raminder Kumar
Ann Abbas
Erin Malone
For their unconditional support

Contributors

Charles E. Alpers, MD
Professor and Vice-Chair
Department of Pathology
University of Washington School of Medicine
Pathologist
University of Washington Medical Center
Seattle, Washington
The Kidney

Douglas C. Anthony, MD, PhD
Professor
Pathology and Laboratory Medicine
Warren Alpert Medical School of Brown University
Chief of Pathology
Lifespan Academic Medical Center
Providence, Rhode Island
The Central Nervous System; Peripheral Nerves and Skeletal Muscles

Anthony Chang, MD
Associate Professor of Pathology
Director of Renal Pathology
Department of Pathology
The University of Chicago
Chicago, Illinois
The Kidney

Umberto De Girolami, MD
Professor of Pathology
Harvard Medical School
Director of Neuropathology
Brigham and Women's Hospital
Boston, Massachusetts
The Central Nervous System

Lora Hedrick Ellenson, MD
Professor and Director of Gynecologic Pathology
Department of Pathology and Laboratory Medicine
New York Presbyterian Hospital-Weill Cornell Medical College
Attending Pathologist
New York Presbyterian Hospital
New York, New York
The Female Genital Tract

Jonathan I. Epstein, MD
Professor of Pathology, Urology, and Oncology
The Reinhard Professor of Urologic Pathology
The Johns Hopkins University School of Medicine
Director of Surgical Pathology
The Johns Hopkins Hospital
Baltimore, Maryland
The Lower Urinary Tract and Male Genital System

Robert Folberg, MD
Founding Dean and Professor of Biomedical Sciences, Pathology, and Ophthalmology
Oakland University William Beaumont School of Medicine
Rochester, Michigan
Chief Academic Officer
Beaumont Hospitals
Royal Oak, Michigan
The Eye

Matthew P. Frosch, MD, PhD
Lawrence J. Henderson Associate Professor of Pathology and Health Sciences and Technology
Harvard Medical School
Director
Neuropathology Core
Massachusetts General Hospital
Boston, Massachusetts
The Central Nervous System

Andrew Horvai, MD, PhD
Professor
Department of Pathology
Associate Director of Surgical Pathology
University of California San Francisco
San Francisco, California
Bones, Joints, and Soft Tissue Tumors

Ralph H. Hruban, MD
Professor of Pathology and Oncology
Director of the Sol Goldman Pancreatic Cancer Research Center
The Johns Hopkins University School of Medicine
Baltimore, Maryland
The Pancreas

Aliya N. Husain, MBBS
Professor
Department of Pathology, Director of Pulmonary, Pediatric and Cardiac Pathology
Pritzker School of Medicine
The University of Chicago
Chicago, Illinois
The Lung

Christine A. Iacobuzio-Donahue, MD, PhD
Attending Physician
Department of Pathology
Associate Director for Translational Research
Center for Pancreatic Cancer Research
Memorial Sloan Kettering Cancer Center
New York, New York
The Pancreas

Alexander J.F. Lazar, MD, PhD
Associate Professor
Departments of Pathology and Dermatology
Sarcoma Research Center
University of Texas M.D. Anderson Cancer Center
Houston, Texas
The Skin

Susan C. Lester, MD, PhD
Assistant Professor of Pathology
Harvard Medical School
Chief, Breast Pathology
Brigham and Women's Hospital
Boston, Massachusetts
The Breast

Mark W. Lingen, DDS, PhD, PRCPath
Professor
Department of Pathology, Director of Oral Pathology
Pritzker School of Medicine
The University of Chicago
Chicago, Illinois
Head and Neck

Tamara L. Lotan, MD
Associate Professor of Pathology and Oncology
The Johns Hopkins Hospital
Baltimore, Maryland
The Lower Urinary Tract and Male Genital System

Anirban Maitra, MBBS
Professor of Pathology and Translational Molecular Pathology
University of Texas M.D. Anderson Cancer Center
Houston, Texas
Diseases of Infancy and Childhood; The Endocrine System

Alexander J. McAdam, MD, PhD
Vice Chair
Department of Laboratory Medicine
Medical Director
Infectious Diseases Diagnostic Laboratory
Boston Children's Hospital
Associate Professor of Pathology
Harvard Medical School
Boston, Massachusetts
Infectious Diseases

Danny A. Milner, MD, MSc, FCAP
Assistant Professor of Pathology
Assistant Medical Director, Microbiology
Harvard Medical School
Boston, Massachusetts
Infectious Diseases

Richard N. Mitchell, MD, PhD
Lawrence J. Henderson Professor of Pathology and Health Sciences and Technology
Department of Pathology
Harvard Medical School
Staff Pathologist
Brigham and Women's Hospital
Boston, Massachusetts
The Cell as a Unit of Health and Disease; Blood Vessels; The Heart

George F. Murphy, MD
Professor of Pathology
Harvard Medical School
Director of Dermatopathology
Brigham and Women's Hospital
Boston, Massachusetts
The Skin

Edyta C. Pirog, MD
Associate Professor of Clinical Pathology and Laboratory Medicine
New York Presbyterian Hospital-Weil Medical College of Cornell University
Associate Attending Pathologist
New York Presbyterian Hospital
New York, New York
The Female Genital Tract

Peter Pytel, MD
Associate Professor, Director of Neuropathology
Department of Pathology
The University of Chicago Medicine
Chicago, Illinois
Peripheral Nerves and Skeletal Muscles

Frederick J. Schoen, MD, PhD
Professor of Pathology and Health Sciences and Technology
Harvard Medical School
Director
Cardiac Pathology
Executive Vice Chairman
Department of Pathology
Brigham and Women's Hospital
Boston, Massachusetts
The Heart

Arlene H. Sharpe, MD, PhD
Professor of Pathology
Co-Director of Harvard Institute of Translational Immunology
Harvard Medical School
Department of Pathology
Brigham and Women's Hospital
Boston, Massachusetts
Infectious Diseases

Neil Theise, MD
Professor, Pathology and Medicine
Division of Digestive Diseases
Beth Israel Medical Center—Albert Einstein College of Medicine
New York, New York
The Liver and Gallbladder

Jerrold R. Turner, MD, PhD
Sara and Harold Lincoln Thompson Professor
Associate Chair
Department of Pathology
Pritzker School of Medicine
The University of Chicago
Chicago, Illinois
The Gastrointestinal Tract

Raminder Kumar, MBBS, MD
Chicago, Illinois
Clinical Editor for Diseases of the Heart, Lung, Gastrointestinal Tract, Liver, and Kidneys

Preface: A New Chapter

As we launch the ninth edition of *Pathologic Basis of Disease* we look to the future of pathology as a discipline and how this textbook can remain most useful to readers in the twenty-first century. It is obvious that an understanding of disease mechanisms is based more than ever on a strong foundation of basic science. We have always woven the relevant basic cell and molecular biology into the sections on pathophysiology in various chapters. *In this edition we go one step further and introduce a new chapter at the very beginning of the book titled "The Cell as a Unit of Health and Disease."* In this chapter we have attempted to encapsulate aspects of cell and molecular biology that we believe are helpful in preparing readers for the more detailed discussions of specific diseases. We would like to remind readers that the last time a new chapter was added to this book was in 1967 when Stanley Robbins, at that time the sole author, decided to add a chapter on genetic diseases, one of many farsighted decisions by Dr. Robbins. We hope that the new chapter will be in keeping with his legacy.

In the preface of the very first edition (1957), Stanley Robbins wrote:

"The pathologist is interested not only in the recognition of structural alterations, but also in their significance, i.e., *the effects of these changes on cellular and tissue function* and ultimately the effect of these changes on the patient. It is not a discipline isolated from the living patient, but rather *a basic approach to a better understanding of disease and therefore a foundation of sound clinical medicine.*"

We hope we continue to illustrate the principles of pathology that Dr. Robbins enunciated with such elegance and clarity over half a century ago.

This edition, like all previous ones, has been extensively revised, and some areas have been completely rewritten. A few examples of significant changes are as follows:

- A feature new to this edition is the introduction of Key Concepts boxes, scattered in each chapter to summarize "take home" messages relating to major topics covered in each disease or disease group.
- Chapter 2 has been updated to include novel pathways of cell death beyond the long-established pathways of necrosis and apoptosis. Indeed, the distinction between these two is being blurred. Autophagy, which has begun to take center stage in diseases ranging from aging to cancer and neurodegeneration, has been revised, as have the possible molecular mechanisms of aging.
- Chapter 3 now combines the discussion of inflammation with repair, since these two processes run concurrently and share common mediators.
- Chapter 5 includes a completely rewritten section on molecular diagnosis that reflects rapid advances in DNA sequencing technology.
- Chapter 7 has been extensively revised to incorporate knowledge and concepts of tumor biology gleaned from deep sequencing of cancers.
- The ongoing revolution in "genomic medicine" has provided the impetus for extensive updates of many disease entities associated with newly described germline or somatic genetic alterations. Throughout, we have taken pains to try to only emphasize the lesions that are most common and most informative in terms of disease pathogenesis.
- Chapter 18, covering diseases of the liver, has been reorganized and extensively revised to include discussion of the molecular basis of hepatic fibrosis and its regression.
- Chapter 27, covering diseases of nerves and muscles, also has a fresh look. The diseases are now organized anatomically, starting from neurons and going to muscles, with diseases of neuromuscular junction bridging the two.
- In addition to the revision and reorganization of the text, many new photographs and schematics have been added and a large number of the older "gems" have been enhanced by digital technology.

Despite the changes highlighted above, our goals remain the same as those articulated by Robbins and Cotran over the past many years.

- To integrate into the discussion of pathologic processes and disorders the newest established information available—morphologic as well as molecular.
- To organize information into logical and uniform presentations, facilitating readability, comprehension, and learning.
- To maintain the book at a reasonable size and yet provide adequate discussion of the significant lesions, processes, and disorders. Indeed, despite the addition of a new 30-page chapter and Key Concepts, we have kept the overall length of the book unchanged. One of our most challenging tasks is to decide what to eliminate to make room for new findings.
- To place great emphasis on clarity of writing and proper use of language in the recognition that struggling to comprehend is time-consuming and wearisome and gets in the way of the learning process.
- To make this first and foremost a student text—used by students throughout all years of medical school and into their residencies—but, at the same time, to provide sufficient detail and depth to meet the needs of more advanced readers.

We have repeatedly been told by readers that up-to-datedness is a special feature that makes this book very valuable. We have strived to remain current by providing new information from the recent literature, some from 2014, the current year. We have removed the references from the text and aggregated the most useful review articles in our lists of suggested readings.

We are now into the digital age, and so the text will be available online to those who own the print version. Such access gives the reader the ability to search across the entire text, bookmark passages, add personal notes, use PubMed to view references, and exploit many other exciting features. In addition, also available online are case studies developed by one of us (VK) in collaboration with Herb Hagler, PhD, and Nancy Schneider, MD, PhD, at the University of Texas Southwestern Medical School in Dallas. The cases are designed to enhance and reinforce learning by challenging students to apply their knowledge to solve clinical cases. To assist in the classroom, we have also made the images available for instructors on the Evolve website. Instructors may register at https://evolve.elsevier.com/ to gain access to the images for teaching purposes.

All three of us have reviewed, critiqued, and edited each chapter to ensure the uniformity of style and flow that have been the hallmarks of the book. Together, we hope that we have succeeded in equipping the readers with the scientific basis for the practice of medicine and in whetting their appetite for learning beyond what can be offered in any textbook.

Vinay Kumar
Abul K. Abbas
Jon C. Aster

Acknowledgments

First and foremost we wish to express our respects and deep gratitude to the late Dr. Nelson Fausto for having been the coeditor of the last two editions of this book. Many of his words are retained in this edition and will continue to benefit future readers. He shall be greatly missed.

All three of us offer thanks to our contributing authors for their commitment to this textbook. Many are veterans of previous editions; others are new to the ninth edition. All are acknowledged in the table of contents. Their names lend authority to this book, for which we are grateful. As in previous editions, the three of us have chosen not to add our own names to the chapters we have been responsible for writing, in part or whole.

Many colleagues have enhanced the text by reading various chapters and providing helpful critiques in their area of expertise. They include Drs. Seungmin Hwang, Kay McLeod, Megan McNerney, Ivan Moskovitz, Jeremy Segal, Humaira Syed, Helen Te, and Shu-Yuan Xiao at the University of Chicago; Marcus Peter at Northwestern University, Chicago; Dr Meenakshi Jolly at Rush University, Chicago; Drs. Kimberley Evason, Kuang-Yu Jen, Richard Jordan, Marta Margeta, and Zoltan Laszik at the University of California, San Francisco; Dr. Antony Rosen at Johns Hopkins University; Dr. Lundy Braun at Brown University; Dr. Peter Byers at the University of Washington; Drs. Frank Bunn, Glenn Dranoff, and John Luckey at Harvard Medical School; Dr. Richard H. Aster at the Milwaukee Blood Center and Medical College of Wisconsin; and Dr. Richard C. Aster at Colorado State University. Special thanks are due to Dr. Raminder Kumar for updating clinical information and extensive proofreading of many chapters in addition to her role as consulting clinical editor for several chapters. Many colleagues provided photographic gems from their collections. They are individually acknowledged in the text.

Our administrative staff needs special mention since they maintain order in the chaotic lives of the authors and have willingly chipped in when needed for multiple tasks relating to the text. At the University of Chicago, they include Ms. Nhu Trinh and Ms. Garcia Wilson; at the University of California at San Francisco, Ms. Ana Narvaez; and at the Brigham and Women's Hospital, Muriel Goutas. All of the graphic art in this book was created by Mr. James Perkins, Professor of Medical Illustration at Rochester Institute of Technology. His ability to convert complex ideas into simple and aesthetically pleasing sketches has considerably enhanced this book.

Many individuals associated with our publisher, Elsevier (under the imprint of WB Saunders), need our special thanks. Outstanding among them is Jennifer Nemec, Project Manager, and our partner in the production of this book. Her understanding of the needs of the authors, promptness in responding to requests (both reasonable and unreasonable), and cheerful demeanor went a long way in reducing our stress and making our lives less complicated. Mr. William (Bill) Schmitt, Publishing Director of Medical Textbooks, has always been our cheerleader and is now a dear friend. Our thanks also go to Managing Editor Rebecca Gruliow and Design Manager Lou Forgione at Elsevier. Undoubtedly there are many others who may have been left out unwittingly—to them we say "thank you" and tender apologies for not acknowledging you individually.

Efforts of this magnitude take a toll on the families of the authors. We thank our spouses, Raminder Kumar, Ann Abbas, and Erin Malone for their patience, love, and support of this venture, and for their tolerance of our absences.

Vinay Kumar
Abul K. Abbas
Jon C. Aster

Contents

General Pathology

Systemic Pathology: Diseases of Organ Systems

Chapters without listed contributors were written by the editors. To gain access to the images for teaching purposes, instructors may register at https://evolve.elsevier.com/.

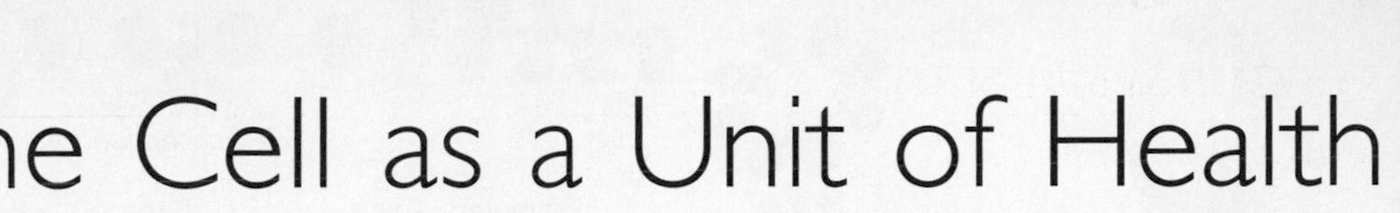

CHAPTER 1

The Cell as a Unit of Health and Disease

Richard N. Mitchell

CHAPTER CONTENTS

Pathology literally translates to the study of *suffering* (Greek *pathos* = suffering, *logos* = study); more prosaically, the term *pathology* is invoked to represent the study of *disease.* Germane to this opening chapter, Virchow coined the term *cellular pathology* to emphasize the basic tenet that all diseases originate at the cellular level. Thus, modern pathology is basically the study of *cellular* abnormalities. Therefore, diseases and the underlying mechanisms are best understood in the context of *normal* cellular structure and function.

It is unrealistic (and even undesirable) to condense the vast and fascinating field of cell biology into a single chapter. Moreover, students of biology are likely quite familiar with many of the broader concepts of cell structure and function. Consequently, rather than attempting a comprehensive review, our goal is to survey some basic principles and highlight some recent advances that are relevant to the pathologic basis of disease that is emphasized throughout the text. We hope this chapter will be useful to review key topics in normal cell biology as they apply to the areas of Pathology that are covered from Chapter 2 onwards.

The Genome

The sequencing of the human genome represented a landmark achievement of biomedical science. Published in draft form in 2001 and more completely detailed in 2003, the information has already led to remarkable advances in science and medicine. Since then there has been an exponential decrease in the cost of sequencing and an exponential increase in data accrual; this new information, now literally at our fingertips, promises to revolutionize our understanding of health and disease. However, the sheer volume of the data is formidable, and there is a dawning realization that we have only begun to scratch the surface of its complexity; uncovering the relevance to disease and then developing new therapies remain challenges that both excite and inspire scientists and the lay public alike.

Noncoding DNA

The human genome contains roughly 3.2 billion DNA base pairs. Within the genome there are about 20,000 protein-encoding genes, comprising only about 1.5% of the genome. These proteins variously function as enzymes, structural components, and signaling molecules and are used to assemble and maintain all of the cells in the body. Although 20,000 is an underestimation of the number of proteins encoded in the human genome (given that many genes produce multiple RNA transcripts encoding different protein isoforms), it is nevertheless startling to realize that worms composed of fewer than 1000 cells—with genomes of only about 0.1 billion DNA base pairs—are also assembled using about 20,000 genes to produce proteins. Even more surprising is that many of these proteins are recognizable homologs of molecules expressed in humans. What then separates humans from worms?

The answer is not completely known, but the weight of current evidence suggests that much of the difference

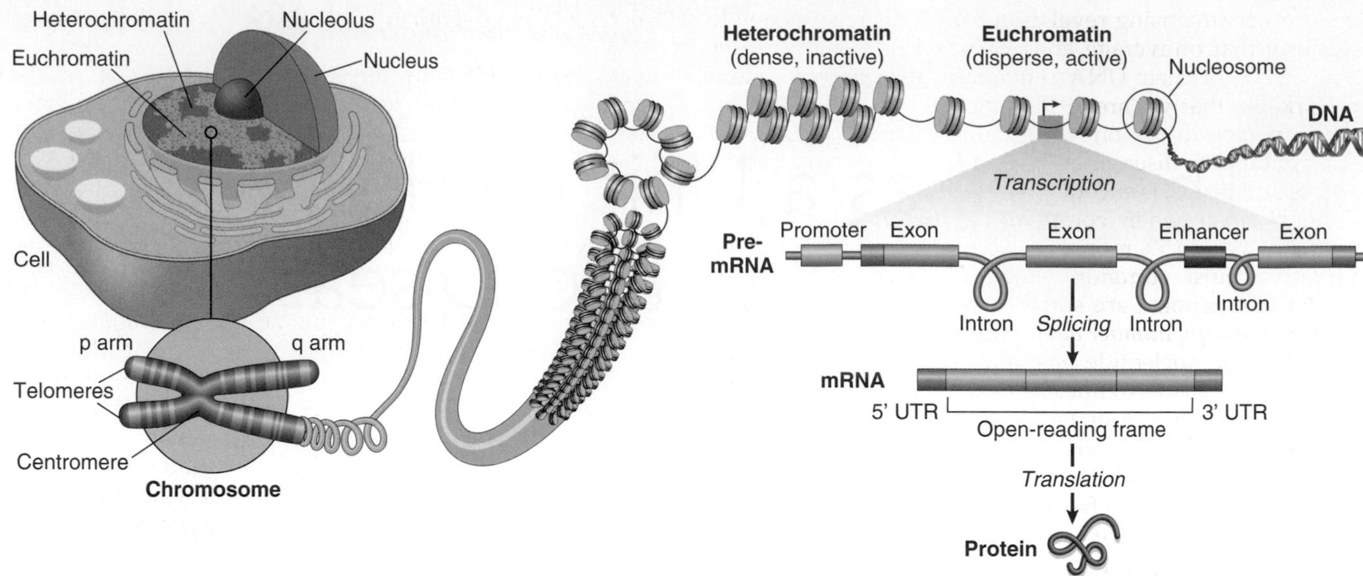

Figure 1-1 The organization of nuclear DNA. At the light microscopic level, the nuclear genetic material is organized into dispersed, transcriptionally active *euchromatin* or densely packed, transcriptionally inactive *heterochromatin*; chromatin can also be mechanically connected with the nuclear membrane, and nuclear membrane perturbation can thus influence transcription. Chromosomes (as shown) can only be visualized by light microscopy during cell division. During mitosis, they are organized into paired chromatids connected at *centromeres*; the centromeres act as the locus for the formation of a *kinetochore* protein complex that regulates chromosome segregation at metaphase. The *telomeres* are repetitive nucleotide sequences that cap the termini of chromatids and permit repeated chromosomal replication without loss of DNA at the chromosome ends. The chromatids are organized into short "P" (*"petite"*) and long "Q" (*"next letter in the alphabet"*) arms. The characteristic banding pattern of chromatids has been attributed to relative GC content (less GC content in bands relative to interbands), with genes tending to localize to interband regions. Individual chromatin fibers are comprised of a string of nucleosomes—DNA wound around octameric histone cores—with the nucleosomes connected via DNA linkers. Promoters are noncoding regions of DNA that initiate gene transcription; they are on the same strand and upstream of their associated gene. Enhancers are regulatory elements that can modulate gene expression over distances of 100 kB or more by looping back onto promoters and recruiting additional factors that are needed to drive the expression of pre-mRNA species. The intronic sequences are subsequently spliced out of the pre-mRNA to produce the definitive message that is translated into protein—without the 3′- and 5′-untranslated regions (UTR). In addition to the enhancer, promoter, and UTR sequences, noncoding elements are found throughout the genome; these include short repeats, regulatory factor binding regions, noncoding regulatory RNAs, and transposons.

lies in the 98.5% of the human genome that does not encode proteins. It has been known for some time that protein-coding genes in higher organisms are separated by long stretches of DNA whose function has been obscure for many years—sometime denoted as "dark matter" of the genome. That viewpoint has subsequently been modified, driven by the multinational ENCODE (Encyclopedia of DNA Elements) project that set out in 2007 to identify all regions of the genome that could be ascribed some function. The striking conclusion is that as much as **80% of the human genome either binds proteins, implying it is involved in regulating gene expression, or can be assigned some functional activity, mostly related to the regulation of gene expression, often in a cell-type specific fashion.** It follows that while proteins provide the building blocks and machinery required for assembling cells, tissues and organisms, it is the noncoding regions of the genome that provide the critical "architectural planning." Practically stated, the difference between worms and humans apparently lies more in the genomic "blueprints" than in the construction materials.

The major classes of functional non–protein-coding sequences found in the human genome are the following (Fig. 1-1):

- *Promoter* and *enhancer* regions that provide binding sites for transcription factors
- Binding sites for factors that organize and maintain higher order *chromatin structures*
- *Noncoding regulatory RNAs.* More than 60% of the genome is transcribed into RNAs that are never translated into protein, but which nevertheless can regulate gene expression through a variety of mechanisms. The two best-studied varieties—micro-RNAs and long noncoding RNAs—are described later.
- *Mobile genetic elements* (e.g., *transposons*). Remarkably, more than one third of the human genome is composed of these elements, popularly denoted as "jumping genes." These segments can move around the genome, exhibiting wide variation in number and positioning even amongst closely related species (i.e., humans and other primates). They are implicated in gene regulation and chromatin organization, but their function is still not well established.
- Special structural regions of DNA, in particular *telomeres* (chromosome ends) and *centromeres* (chromosome "tethers")

One of the reasons these findings have generated so much interest is that many, and perhaps most, of the genetic variations (*polymorphisms*) associated with diseases are located in non–protein-coding regions of the genome. Thus, variation in gene regulation may prove to be more important in disease causation than structural changes in specific proteins.

Another surprising revelation from the recent genomic studies is that, on average, any two individuals share greater than 99.5% of their DNA sequences. It is perhaps more remarkable that we are 99% identical with chimpanzees! Thus, person-to-person variation, including differential susceptibility to diseases and in response to environmental agents and drugs, is encoded in less than 0.5% of our DNA. Though small when compared to the total nucleotide sequences, this 0.5% represents about 15 million base pairs. **The two most common forms of DNA variation in the human genome are *single-nucleotide polymorphisms (SNPs) and copy number variations (CNVs)*.** SNPs are variants at single nucleotide positions and are almost always biallelic (i.e., only two choices exist at a given site within the population, such as A or T). Much effort has been devoted to mapping common SNPs in human populations. Over 6 million human SNPs have been identified, many of which show wide variation in frequency in different populations. SNPs occur across the genome—within exons, introns, intergenic regions, and coding regions. Overall, about 1% of SNPs occur in coding regions, which is about what would be expected by chance, since coding regions comprise about 1.5% of the genome. SNPs located in non-coding regions may fall in regulatory elements in the genome, thereby altering gene expression; in such instances the SNP may have a direct influence on disease susceptibility. In other instances, the SNP may be a "neutral" variant that has no effect on gene function or carrier phenotype. However, even "neutral" SNPs may be useful markers if they happen to be co-inherited with a disease-associated gene as a result of physical proximity. In other words, the SNP and the causative genetic factor are in *linkage disequilibrium.* There is hope that groups of SNPs may serve as markers of risk for multigenic complex diseases such as type II diabetes and hypertension. However, the effect of most SNPs on disease susceptibility is weak, and it remains to be seen if identification of such variants, alone or in combination, can be used to develop effective strategies for disease prevention.

CNVs are a more recently identified form of genetic variation consisting of different numbers of large contiguous stretches of DNA from 1000 base pairs to millions of base pairs. In some instances these loci are, like SNPs, biallelic and simply duplicated or deleted in a subset of the population. In other instances there are complex rearrangements of genomic material, with multiple alleles in the human population. Current estimates are that CNVs are responsible for between 5 and 24 million base pairs of sequence difference between any two individuals. Approximately 50% of CNVs involve gene-coding sequences; thus, CNVs may underlie a large portion of human phenotypic diversity. We currently know much less about CNVs than SNPs, therefore their influence on disease susceptibility is less established.

It should be pointed out that despite all these advances in the understanding of human genetic variation, it is clear that alterations in DNA sequence cannot by themselves explain the diversity of phenotypes in human populations. Nor can classic genetics explain how monozygotic twins can have differing phenotypes. The answer may lie in *epigenetics,* which is defined as heritable changes in gene expression that are not caused by alterations in DNA sequence. The molecular basis of epigenetic changes will be discussed next.

Histone Organization

Even though virtually all cells in the body contain the same genetic material, terminally differentiated cells have distinct structures and functions. Clearly, different cell types are distinguished by lineage-specific programs of gene expression. Such cell type-specific differences in DNA transcription and translation depend on *epigenetic factors* (literally, factors that are "above genetics") that can be conceptualized as follows (Fig. 1-2):

- *Histones and histone modifying factors. Nucleosomes* consist of DNA segments 147 base pairs long that are wrapped around a central core structure of highly conserved low molecular weight proteins called *histones.* The resulting DNA-histone complex resembles a series of beads joined by short DNA linkers and is generically called *chromatin.* The naked DNA of a human cell is about 1.8 meters long, but wound around histones like spools, DNA can be packed into a nucleus as small as 7 to 8 micrometers in diameter—the width of a resting lymphocyte. In most cases, DNA is not *uniformly* and compactly wound. Thus, at the light microscopic level, nuclear chromatin exists in two basic forms: (1) cytochemically dense and transcriptionally inactive *heterochromatin* and (2) cytochemically dispersed and transcriptionally active *euchromatin* (Fig. 1-1). Moreover, which portion of the nuclear chromatin is "unwound" regulates gene expression and thereby dictates cellular identity and activity.

  Histones are not static, but rather are highly dynamic structures regulated by a host of nuclear proteins and chemical modifications. Thus, *chromatin remodeling complexes* can reposition nucleosomes on DNA, exposing (or obscuring) gene regulatory elements such as promoters. *"Chromatin writer" complexes,* on the other hand, carry out more than 70 different histone modifications generically denoted as *marks.* Such covalent alterations include methylation, acetylation, or phosphorylation of specific amino acid residues on the histones.

  Actively transcribed genes in euchromatin are associated with histone marks that make the DNA accessible to RNA polymerases. In contrast, inactive genes have histone marks that enable DNA compaction into heterochromatin. Histone marks are reversible through the activity of *"chromatin erasers."* Still other proteins function as *"chromatin readers,"* binding histones that bear particular marks and thereby regulating gene expression.
- *Histone methylation.* Both lysines and arginines can be methylated by specific writer enzymes; in particular, methylation of lysine residues in histones may be associated with either transcriptional activation or repression, depending on the histone residue that is "marked".
- *Histone acetylation.* Lysine residues are acetylated by histone acetyl transferases (HAT), whose modifications tend to open up the chromatin and increase transcription. In turn, these changes can be reversed by histone deacetylases (HDAC), leading to chromatin condensation.
- *Histone phosphorylation.* Serine residues can be modified by phosphorylation; depending on the specific residue,

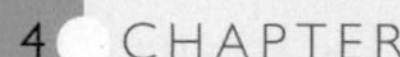

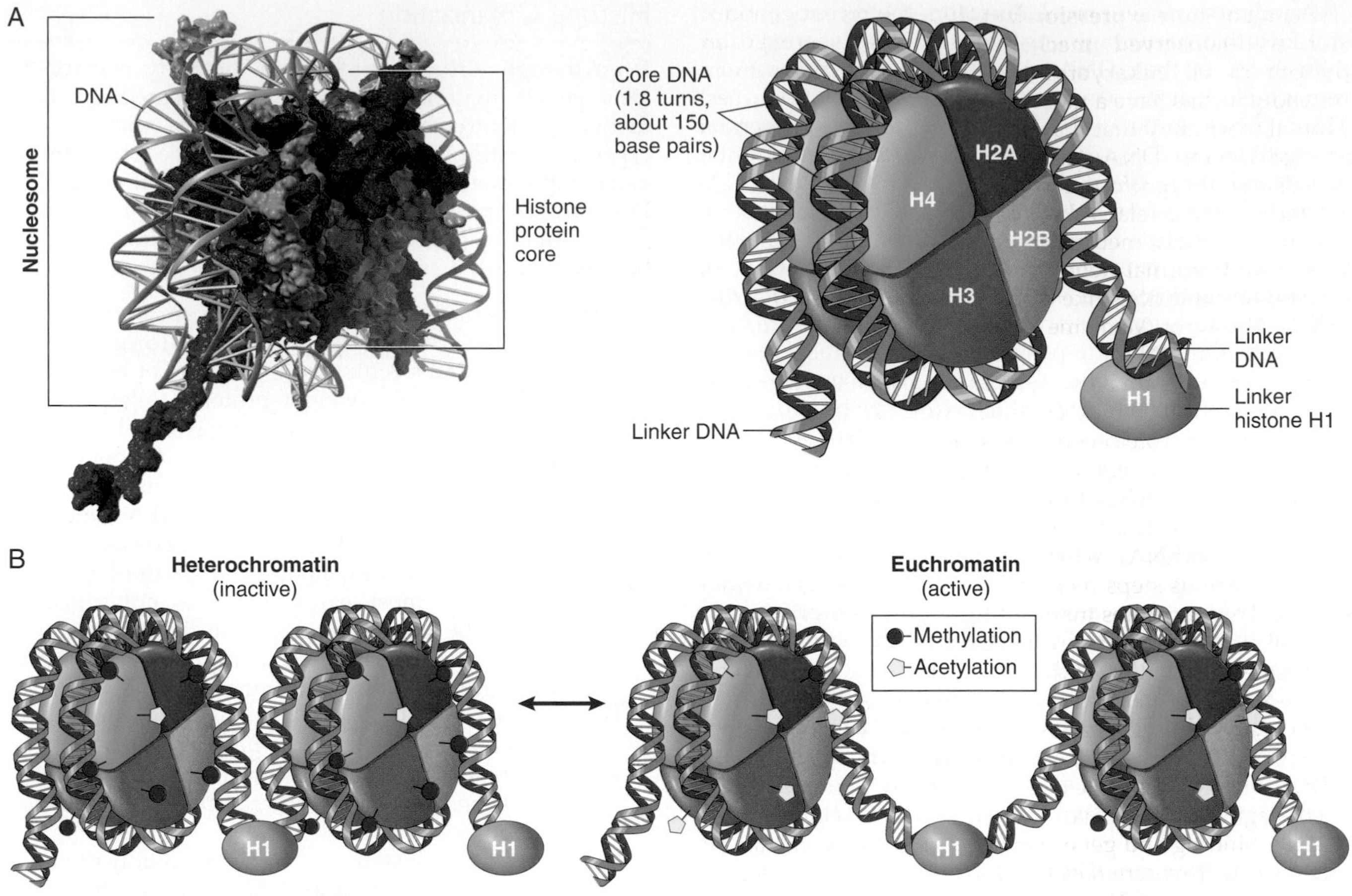

Figure 1-2 Histone organization. **A,** Nucleosomes are comprised of octamers of histone proteins (two each of histone subunits H2A, H2B, H3, and H4) encircled by 1.8 loops of 147 base pairs of DNA; histone H1 sits on the 20-80 nucleotide linker DNA between nucleosomes and helps stabilizes the overall chromatin architecture. The histone subunits are positively charged, thus allowing the compaction of the negatively charged DNA. **B,** The relative state of DNA unwinding (and thus access for transcription factors) is regulated by histone modification, for example, by acetylation, methylation, and/or phosphorylation (so-called "marks"); marks are dynamically written and erased. Certain marks such as histone acetylation "open up" the chromatin structure, whereas others, such as methylation of particular histone residues, tends to condense the DNA and leads to gene silencing. DNA itself can also be also be methylated, a modification that is associated with transcriptional inactivation.

the DNA may be opened up for transcription or condensed to become inactive.

- *DNA methylation.* High levels of DNA methylation in gene regulatory elements typically result in transcriptional silencing. Like histone modifications, DNA methylation is tightly regulated by methyltransferases, demethylating enzymes, and methylated-DNA-binding proteins.
- *Chromatin organizing factors.* Much less is known about these proteins, which are believed to bind to noncoding regions and control long-range looping of DNA, which is important in regulating the spatial relationships between gene enhancers and promoters that control gene expression.

Deciphering the mechanisms that allow epigenetic factors to control genomic organization and gene expression in a cell-type-specific fashion is an extraordinarily complex proposition. Despite the intricacies, there is already ample evidence that dysregulation of the "epigenome" has a central role in malignancy (Chapter 7), and there is growing evidence that many other diseases are associated with inherited or acquired epigenetic alterations. Another reason for excitement is that—unlike genetic changes—many epigenetic alterations (e.g., histone acetylation and DNA methylation) are reversible and are amenable to therapeutic intervention; thus, HDAC inhibitors and DNA methylation inhibitors are already being tested in the treatment of various forms of cancer.

Micro-RNA and Long Noncoding RNA

Another mechanism of gene regulation depends on the functions of noncoding RNAs. As the name implies, these are encoded by genes that are transcribed but not translated. Although many distinct families of noncoding RNAs exist, we will only discuss two examples here: small RNA molecules called *microRNAs,* and *long noncoding RNAs* >200 nucleotides in length.

Micro-RNA (miRNA)

The miRNAs do not encode proteins; instead, they function primarily to modulate the translation of target mRNAs into their corresponding proteins. **Posttranscriptional**

silencing of gene expression by miRNA is a fundamental and well-conserved mechanism of gene regulation present in all eukaryotes (plants and animals). Even microorganisms have a more primitive version of the same general machinery that they can use to protect themselves against foreign DNA (e.g., from phages and viruses). Because of the profound influence of miRNAs on gene regulation, these relatively short RNAs (22 nucleotides on average) have assumed central importance in the illumination of both normal developmental pathways, as well as pathologic conditions like cancer. Indeed, the Nobel Prize in Physiology or Medicine in 2006 was awarded for the discovery of miRNAs.

By current estimates, the human genome encodes approximately 1000 miRNA genes, some 20-fold less than the number of protein-coding genes. However, individual miRNAs appear to regulate multiple protein-coding genes, allowing each miRNA to co-regulate entire programs of gene expression. Transcription of miRNA genes produces a primary miRNA, which is progressively processed through various steps including trimming by the enzyme *DICER*. This generates mature single-stranded miRNAs of 21 to 30 nucleotides that are associated with a multiprotein aggregate called RNA-induced silencing complex (RISC; Fig. 1-3). Subsequent base pairing between the miRNA strand and its target mRNA directs the RISC to either induce mRNA cleavage or repress its translation. All mRNAs contain a so-called *seed sequence* in their 3′ untranslated region (UTR) that determines the specificity of miRNA binding and gene silencing. In this way, the target mRNA is *posttranscriptionally silenced*.

Small interfering RNAs (siRNAs) are short RNA sequences that can be introduced experimentally into cells. These serves as substrates for Dicer and interact with the RISC complex in a mannaer analogous to endogenous miRNAs. Synthetic siRNAs targeted against specific mRNA species have become useful laboratory tools to study gene function (so-called *knockdown* technology); they are also being developed as possible therapeutic agents to silence pathogenic genes, such as oncogenes involved in neoplastic transformation.

Long Noncoding RNA (lncRNA)

Recent studies have further identified an untapped universe of lncRNAs—by some calculations, the number of lncRNAs may exceed coding mRNAs by 10- to 20-fold. **lncRNAs modulate gene expression in many ways** (Fig. 1-4); for example, they can bind to regions of chromatin, restricting RNA polymerase access to coding genes within the region. The best known example of a repressive function involves XIST, which is transcribed from the X chromosome and plays an essential role in physiologic X chromosome inactivation. XIST itself escapes X inactivation, but forms a repressive "cloak" on the X chromosome from which it is transcribed, resulting in gene silencing. Conversely, it has recently been appreciated that many enhancers are sites of lncRNA synthesis, and these lncRNAs appear to often increase transcription from gene promoters through a variety of mechanisms (Fig. 1-4). Emerging studies are exploring the roles of lncRNAs in various human diseases, from atherosclerosis to cancer.

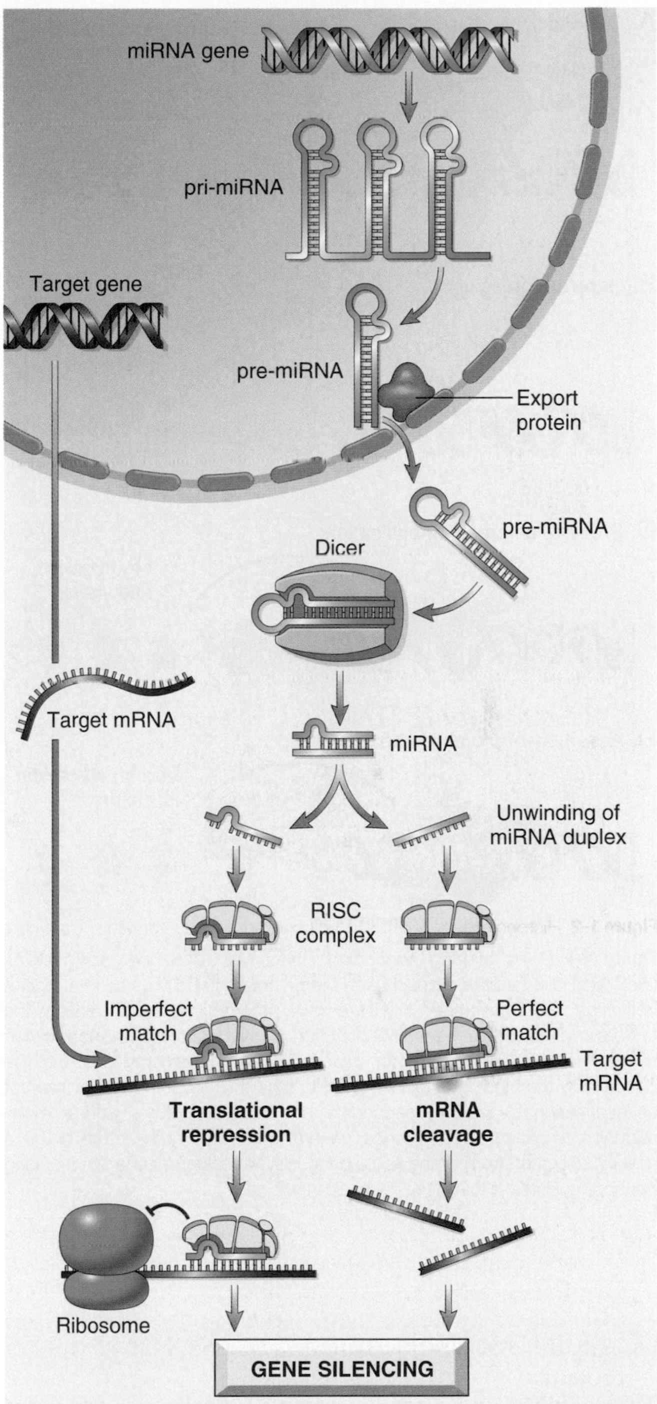

Figure 1-3 Generation of microRNAs (miRNA) and their mode of action in regulating gene function. miRNA genes are transcribed to produce a primary miRNA (*pri-miRNA*), which is processed within the nucleus to form *pre-miRNA* composed of a single RNA strand with secondary hairpin loop structures that form stretches of double-stranded RNA. After this pre-miRNA is exported out of the nucleus via specific transporter proteins, the cytoplasmic *Dicer enzyme* trims the pre-miRNA to generate mature double-stranded miRNAs of 21 to 30 nucleotides. The miRNA subsequently unwinds, and the resulting single strands are incorporated into the multiprotein *RNA-induced silencing complex (RISC)*. Base pairing between the single-stranded miRNA and its target mRNA directs RISC to either cleave the mRNA target or repress its translation. In either case, the target mRNA gene is silenced posttranscriptionally.

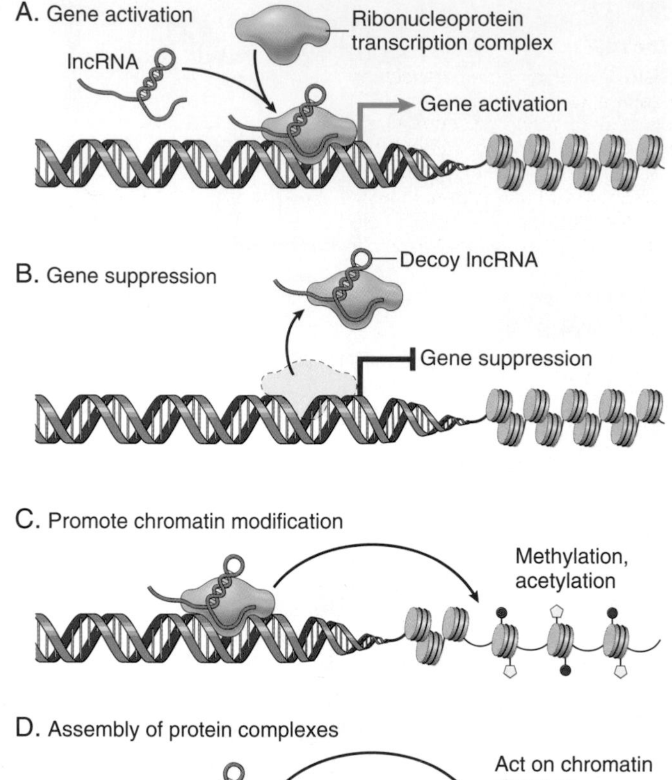

Figure 1-4 Roles of long noncoding RNAs. **A,** Long non-coding RNAs (lncRNAs) can facilitate transcription factor binding and thus promote gene activation. **B,** Conversely, lncRNAs can preemptively bind transcription factors and thus prevent gene transcription. **C,** Histone and DNA modification by acetylases or methylases (or deacetylases and demethylases) may be directed by the binding of lncRNAs. **D,** In other instances, lncRNAs may act as scaffolding to stabilize secondary or tertiary structures and/or multi-subunit complexes that influence general chromatin architecture or gene activity. (Adapted from Wang KC, Chang HY: Molecular mechanisms of long noncoding RNAs. Mol Cell 43:904, 2011.)

Cellular Housekeeping

The viability and normal activity of cells depend on a variety of fundamental housekeeping functions that all differentiated cells must perform. These functions include *protection from the environment, nutrient acquisition, communication, movement, renewal of senescent molecules, molecular catabolism,* and *energy generation.*

Many normal housekeeping functions are compartmentalized within membrane-bound intracellular organelles (Fig. 1-5). By isolating certain cellular functions within distinct compartments, functionally important, potentially injurious degradative enzymes or reactive metabolites can be concentrated or stored at high concentrations in specific organelles without risking damage to other cellular constituents. Moreover, compartmentalization allows the creation of unique intracellular environments (e.g., low pH or high calcium) that may then selectively regulate the function of enzymes or metabolic pathways.

New proteins destined for the plasma membrane or points beyond are synthesized in the *rough endoplasmic reticulum (RER)* and physically assembled in the *Golgi apparatus;* proteins intended for the cytosol are synthesized on free ribosomes. *Smooth endoplasmic reticulum (SER)* may be abundant in certain cell types such as gonads and liver where it is used for steroid hormone and lipoprotein synthesis, as well as for the modification of hydrophobic compounds (for example, drugs) into water-soluble molecules for export.

Proteins and organelles must also be broken down if they become damaged, as must proteins and other molecules that are taken up into the cell by endocytosis. Catabolism of these constituents takes place at three different sites and serves different functions. *Lysosomes* are intracellular organelles that contain degradative enzymes that permit the digestion of a wide-range of macromolecules, including proteins, polysaccharides, lipids, and nucleic acids. *Proteasomes,* on the other hand are a specialized type of "grinder" that selectively chews up denatured proteins, releasing peptides. In some cases the peptides so generated can be presented in the context of class I major histocompatibility molecules (Chapter 6). In other cases signaling molecules trigger the proteasomal degradation of negative regulatory proteins, leading to activation of pathways that alter transcription. These are described in more detail later in the chapter. *Peroxisomes* play a specialized role in the breakdown of fatty acids, generating hydrogen peroxide in this process.

The contents and position of cellular organelles are also subject to regulation. *Endosomal vesicles* shuttle internalized material to the appropriate intracellular sites or direct newly synthesized materials to the cell surface or targeted organelle. Cell movement—both organelles and proteins *within* the cell, as well as movement of the cell in its environment—is accomplished through the *cytoskeleton.* These structural proteins also maintain basic cellular shape and intracellular organization, requisites for maintaining *cell polarity.* This is particularly critical in epithelium, in which the top of the cell (*apical*) and the bottom and side of the cell (*basolateral*) are often exposed to different environments and have distinct functions. Most of the ATP that powers cells is made through oxidative phosphorylation in the *mitochondria.* However, mitochondria also serve as an important source of metabolic intermediates that are needed for anabolic metabolism; they are sites of synthesis of certain macromolecules (e.g., heme), and contain important sensors of cell damage that can initiate and regulate the process of programmed cell death.

Cell growth and maintenance require a constant supply of both energy and the building blocks that are needed for synthesis of macromolecules. In growing and dividing cells, all of these organelles have to be replicated (*organellar biogenesis*) and correctly apportioned in daughter cells following mitosis. Moreover, because the macromolecules and organelles have finite lifespans (mitochondria, for example, last only about 10 days), mechanisms must also exist that allow for the recognition and degradation of "worn out" cellular components.

With this as a primer, we now move on to discuss cellular components and their function in greater detail.

Relative volumes of intracellular organelles (hepatocyte)

Compartment	% total volume	number/cell	role in the cell
Cytosol	54%	1	metabolism, transport, protein translation
Mitochondria	22%	1700	energy generation, apoptosis
Rough ER	9%	1*	synthesis of membrane and secreted proteins
Smooth ER, Golgi	6%	1*	protein modification, sorting, catabolism
Nucleus	6%	1	cell regulation, proliferation, DNA transcription
Endosomes	1%	200	intracellular transport and export, ingestion of extracellular substances
Lysosomes	1%	300	cellular catabolism
Peroxisomes	1%	400	very long-chain fatty acid metabolism

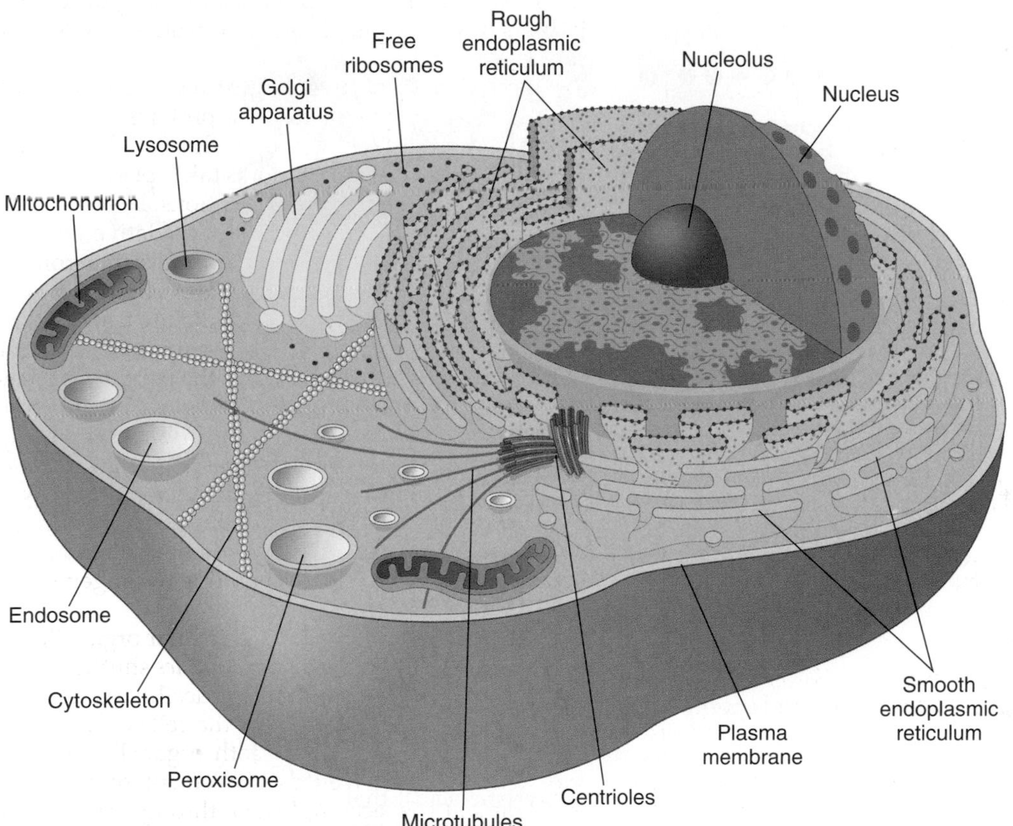

Figure 1-5 Basic subcellular constituents of cells. The table presents the number of the various organelles within a typical hepatocyte, as well as their volume within the cell. The figure shows geographic relationships but is not intended to be accurate to scale. (Adapted from Weibel ER, Stäubli W, Gnägi HR, et al: Correlated morphometric and biochemical studies on the liver cell. I. Morphometric model, stereologic methods, and normal morphometric data for rat liver. J Cell Biol 42:68, 1969.)

Plasma Membrane: Protection and Nutrient Acquisition

Plasma membranes (and all other organellar membranes) are more than just static lipid sheaths. Rather, they are fluid bilayers of amphipathic phospholipids with hydrophilic head groups that face the aqueous environment and hydrophobic lipid tails that interact with each other to form a barrier to passive diffusion of large or charged molecules (Fig. 1-6). The bilayer is composed of a heterogeneous collection of different phospholipids, which are distributed asymmetrically—for example, certain membrane lipids preferentially associate with extracellular or cytosolic faces. Proper organization of phospholipids is important for cell health, as specific phospholipids interact with particular membrane proteins, influencing their distribution and function. In addition, asymmetric partitioning of phospholipids is important in several other cellular processes, as follows:

- *Phosphatidylinositol* on the inner membrane leaflet can be phosphorylated, serving as an electrostatic scaffold for intracellular proteins; alternatively, polyphosphoinositides can be hydrolyzed by phospholipase C to generate intracellular second signals like diacylglycerol and inositol trisphosphate.
- *Phosphatidylserine* is normally restricted to the inner face where it confers a negative charge involved in electrostatic protein interactions; however, when it flips to the extracellular face, which happens in cells undergoing apoptosis (programmed cell death), it becomes an "eat me" signal for phagocytes. In the special case of platelets, it serves as a cofactor in the clotting of blood.
- *Glycolipids* and *sphingomyelin* are preferentially expressed on the extracellular face; glycolipids (and particularly gangliosides, with complex sugar linkages and terminal sialic acids that confer negative charges) are important in cell-cell and cell-matrix interactions,

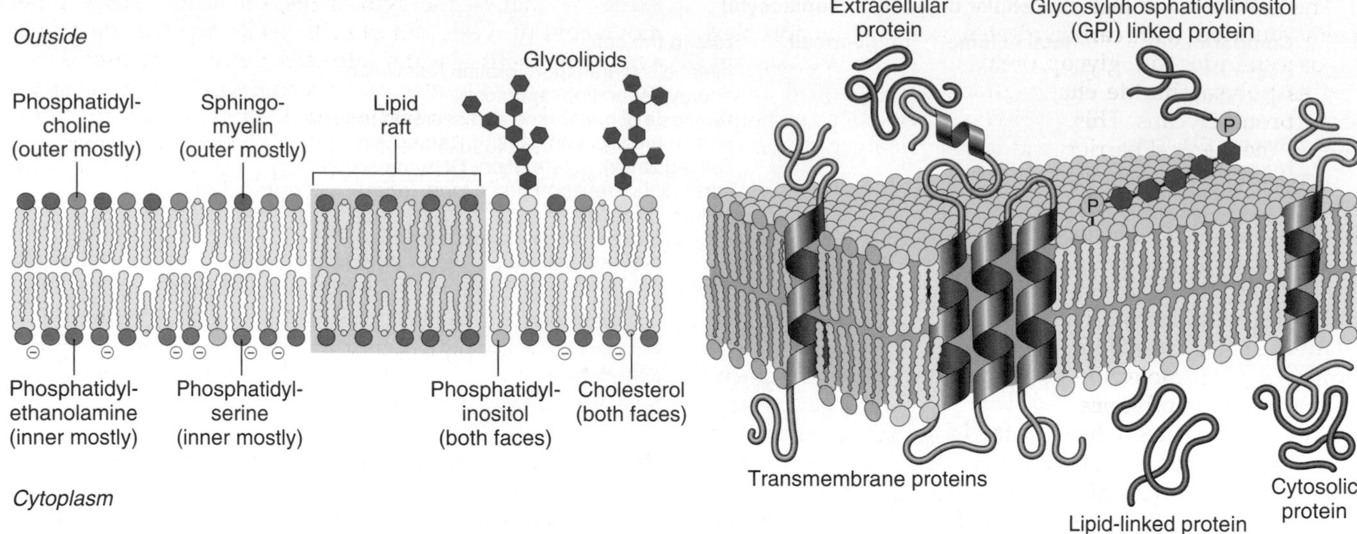

Figure 1-6 Plasma membrane organization and asymmetry. The plasma membrane is a bilayer of phospholipids, cholesterol, and associated proteins. The phospholipid distribution within the membrane is asymmetric due to the activity of *flippases*; *phosphatidylcholine* and *sphingomyelin* are overrepresented in the outer leaflet, and *phosphatidylserine* (negative charge) and *phosphatidylethanolamine* are predominantly found on the inner leaflet; glycolipids occur only on the outer face where they contribute to the extracellular glycocalyx. Although the membrane is laterally fluid and the various constituents can diffuse randomly, specific domains—*lipid rafts*—can also stably develop. Membrane-associated proteins may traverse the membrane (singly or multiply) via α-helical hydrophobic amino acid sequences; depending on the membrane lipid content and the hydrophobicity of protein domains, such proteins may have non-random distributions within the membrane. Proteins on the cytosolic face may associate with membranes through post-translational modifications, e.g., farnesylation, or addition of palmitic acid. Proteins on the extracytoplasmic face may associate with the membrane via glycosyl phosphatidyl inositol linkages. Besides protein-protein interactions within the membrane, membrane proteins can also associate with extracellular and/or intracytoplasmic proteins to generate large, relatively stable complexes (e.g., the *focal adhesion complex*). Transmembrane proteins can translate mechanical forces (e.g., from the cytoskeleton or extracellular matrix) as well as chemical signals across the membrane. It is worth remembering that a similar organization of lipids and associated proteins also occurs within the various organellar membranes.

including inflammatory cell recruitment and sperm-egg interactions.

Moreover, certain membrane components have a predilection for association through horizontal interactions in the bilayer, which leads to the creation of distinct lipid domains known as *"lipid rafts."* Since inserted membrane proteins have different intrinsic solubilities in various lipid domains, they tend to accumulate in certain regions of the membrane and to become depleted from others. As might be imagined the nonrandom distribution of lipids and membrane proteins has important effects on cell-cell and cell-matrix interactions, as well as in intracellular signaling and the generation of specialized membrane regions involved in secretory or endocytic pathways.

The plasma membrane is liberally studded with a variety of proteins and glycoproteins involved in (1) ion and metabolite transport, (2) fluid-phase and receptor-mediated uptake of macromolecules, and (3) cell-ligand, cell-matrix, and cell-cell interactions. Proteins associate with the lipid bilayer by one of four general arrangements; how they integrate into the membrane informs function.

- Most proteins are integral or transmembrane proteins, having one or more relatively hydrophobic α-helical segments that traverse the lipid bilayer. Integral membrane proteins typically contain positively charged aminoacids in their cytoplasmic domains, which anchor the proteins to the negatively charged head groups of membrane phospholipids.
- Proteins may be synthesized in the cytosol and post-translationally attached to prenyl groups (e.g., farnesyl, related to cholesterol) or fatty acids (e.g., palmitic or myristic acid), that insert into the cytosolic side of the plasma membrane.
- Insertion into the membrane may occur through glycosylphosphatidylinositol (GPI) anchors on the extracellular face of the membrane.
- Peripheral membrane proteins may noncovalently associate with true transmembrane proteins.

Many plasma membrane proteins function together as large complexes; these may either be aggregated under the control of chaperone molecules in the RER or by lateral diffusion in the plasma membrane followed by complex formation in situ. The latter mechanism is characteristic of many protein receptors (e.g., cytokine receptors) that dimerize or trimerize in the presence of ligand to form functional signaling units. Although lipid bilayers are fluid in the two-dimensional plane of the membrane, membrane components can also be confined to discrete domains. This may be achieved through localization to lipid rafts, already discussed, or through intercellular protein-protein interactions (e.g., at *tight junctions*) that establish discrete boundaries; indeed, this strategy is used to maintain *cell polarity* (e.g., top/apical vs bottom/basolateral) in epithelial layers. Alternatively, unique membrane domains can be generated by the interaction of proteins with cytoskeletal molecules or extracellular matrix.

The extracellular face of the plasma membrane is diffusely studded with carbohydrates, not only as complex oligosaccharides on glycoproteins and glycolipids, but also as polysaccharide chains attached to integral membrane proteoglycans. This *glycocalyx* functions as a chemical and mechanical barrier, and is also involved in *cell-cell* and *cell-matrix interactions*.

Passive Membrane Diffusion. Small, nonpolar molecules like O_2 and CO_2 readily dissolve in lipid bilayers and therefore rapidly diffuse across them; in addition, hydrophobic molecules (e.g., steroid-based molecules like estradiol or vitamin D) also cross lipid bilayers with relative impunity. Similarly, polar molecules smaller than 75 daltons in mass readily cross membranes (e.g., water, ethanol, and urea). However, in tissues where water is transported in large volumes (e.g., renal tubular epithelium), special integral membrane proteins called *aquaporins* augment passive water transport. In contrast, the lipid bilayer is an effective barrier to the passage of polar molecules of greater than 75 daltons in mass, even those that are only slightly larger, such as glucose. Lipid bilayers are also impermeant to ions, no matter how small, due to their charge and high degree of hydration. We will discuss next specialized mechanisms that regulate traffic across plasma membranes.

Carriers and Channels. For each of the larger polar molecules that must cross membranes to support normal cellular functions (e.g., for nutrient uptake and waste disposal), a unique plasma membrane protein is typically required. For low molecular weight species (ions and small molecules up to approximately 1000 daltons), *channel proteins* and *carrier proteins* may be used (although this discussion focuses on plasma membranes, it should be noted that similar pores and channels are needed for transport across organellar membranes). Each transported molecule (e.g., ion, sugar, nucleotide) requires a transporter, which are often highly specific for a select molecule in each class (e.g., glucose but not galactose):

- *Channel proteins* create hydrophilic pores, which, when open, permit rapid movement of solutes (usually restricted by size and charge, Fig. 1-7).
- *Carrier proteins* bind their specific solute and undergo a series of conformational changes to transfer the ligand across the membrane; their transport is relatively slow.

In most cases, a concentration and/or electrical gradient between the inside and outside of the cell drives solute movement via *passive transport* (virtually all plasma membranes have an electrical potential difference across them, with the inside negative relative to the outside). In some cases, *active transport* of certain solutes *against* a concentration gradient is accomplished by carrier molecules (not channels) using energy released by ATP hydrolysis or a coupled ion gradient. Transporter ATPases also include the infamous *multidrug resistance (MDR) protein*, which pumps polar compounds (e.g., chemotherapeutic drugs) out of cells and may render cancer cells resistant to treatment.

Because plasma membranes are freely permeable to water, it moves into and out of cells by osmosis, depending on relative solute concentrations. Thus, extracellular salt in excess of that in the cytosol (*hypertonicity*) causes a net movement of water out of cells, while *hypotonicity* causes a net movement of water into cells. Since the cytosol is rich in charged metabolites and protein species that attract a large number of counterions that tend to increase the intracellular osmolarity, cells need to constantly pump out small inorganic ions (e.g., Na^+ and Cl^-), typically through the activity of the membrane sodium-potassium ATPase, lest they become overhydrated. Loss of the ability to generate energy (e.g., in a cell injured by toxins or ischemia) therefore results in osmotic swelling and eventual rupture of cells. Similar transport mechanisms also regulate intracellular and intraorganellar pH; most cytosolic enzymes prefer to work at pH 7.4 whereas lysosomal enzymes function best at pH 5 or less.

Receptor-mediated and fluid-phase uptake (Fig. 1-7). Uptake of fluids or macromolecules by the cell, called *endocytosis*, occurs by two fundamental mechanisms. Certain small molecules—including some vitamins—are taken up by invaginations of the plasma membrane called *caveolae*. For bigger molecules, uptake occurs after binding to specific cell-surface receptors; internalization occurs through a membrane invagination process driven by an intracellular coat of *clathrin* proteins. Clathrin is a hexamer of proteins that spontaneously assembles into a basket-like lattice to drive the invagination process. We shall come back to these later.

The process by which large molecules are exported from cells is called *exocytosis*; In this process, proteins synthesized and packaged within the RER and Golgi apparatus are concentrated in secretory vesicles, which then fuse with the plasma membrane and expel their contents.

Transcytosis is the movement of endocytosed vesicles between the apical and basolateral compartments of cells; this is a mechanism for transferring large amounts of intact proteins across epithelial barriers (e.g., ingested antibodies in maternal milk across intestinal epithelia) or for the rapid movement of large volumes of solute. In fact, increased transcytosis probably plays a role in the increased vascular wall permeability seen in healing wounds and in tumors.

We now return to the two forms of endocytosis mentioned earlier

- *Caveolae-mediated endocytosis.* Caveolae ("little caves") are *noncoated* plasma membrane invaginations associated with GPI-linked molecules, cyclic adenosine monophosphate (cAMP) binding proteins, SRC-family kinases, and the folate receptor. Caveolin is the major structural protein of caveole. Internalization of caveolae with any bound molecules and associated extracellular fluid is sometimes called *potocytosis*—literally "cellular sipping." Although caveolae likely participate in the transmembrane delivery of some molecules (e.g., folate), they are increasingly implicated in the regulation of transmembrane signaling and/or cellular adhesion via the internalization of receptors and integrins.
- *Pinocytosis and receptor-mediated endocytosis* (Fig. 1-7). *Pinocytosis* ("cellular drinking") describes a fluid-phase process during which the plasma membrane invaginates and is pinched off to form a cytoplasmic vesicle. Endocytosed vesicles may recycle back to the plasma

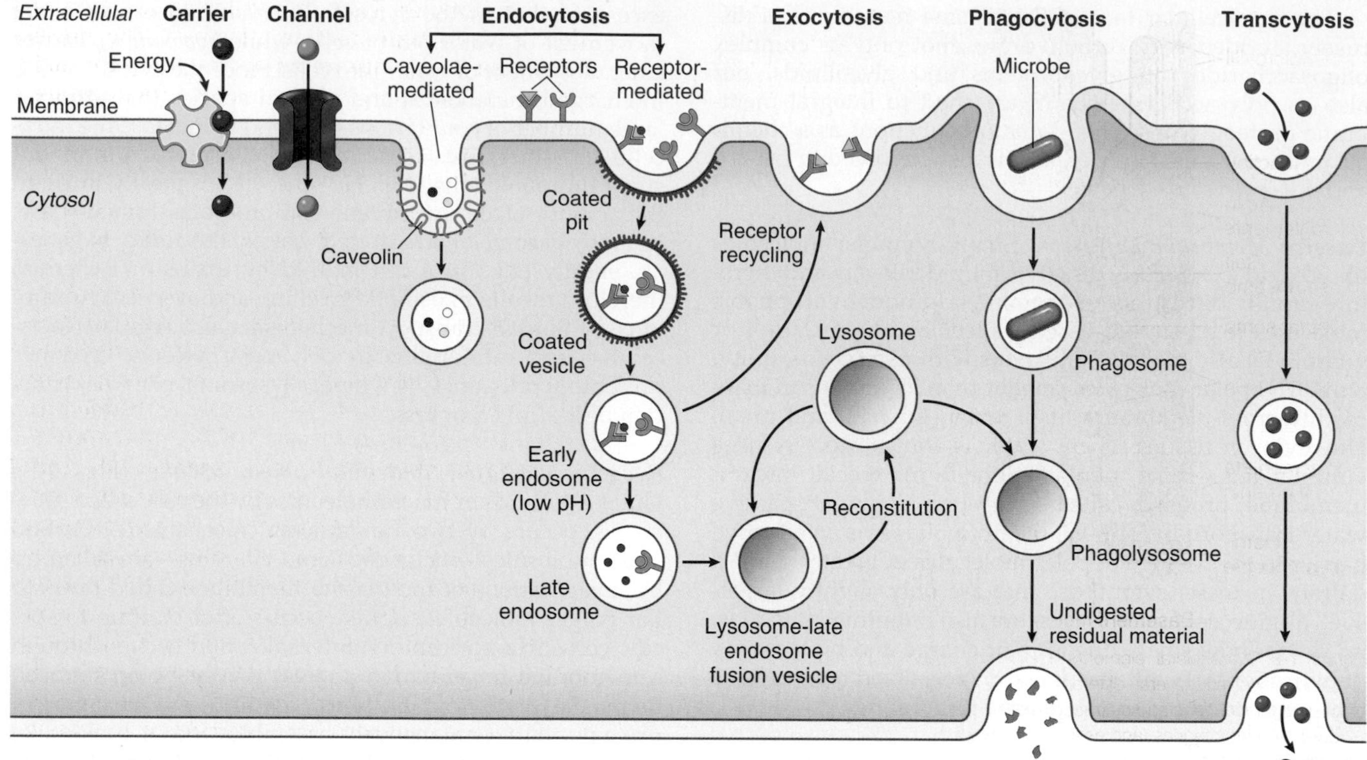

Figure 1-7 Movement of small molecules and larger structures across membranes. The lipid bilayer is relatively impermeable to all but the smallest and/or most hydrophobic molecules. Thus, the import or export of charged species requires specific transmembrane transporter proteins; the internalization or externalization of large proteins, complex particles, or even cells requires encircling them with segments of the membrane.

Small charged solutes can move across the membrane using either channels or carriers; in general, each molecule requires a unique transporter. *Channels* are used when concentration gradients can drive the solute movement. *Carriers* are required when solute is moved *against* a concentration gradient.

Receptor-mediated and fluid-phase uptake of material involves membrane bound vacuoles. *Caveolae* endocytose extracellular fluid, membrane proteins, and some receptor bound molecules (e.g., folate) in a process driven by caveolin proteins concentrated within lipid rafts (*potocytosis*). *Pinocytosis* of extracellular fluid and most surface receptor-ligand pairs involves *clathrin-coated pits and vesicles*. After internalization, the clathrin dissociates and can be re-used, while the resulting vesicle progressively matures and acidifies. In the early and/or late endosome, ligand can be released from its receptor (e.g., iron released from transferrin bound to the transferrin receptor) with receptor recycling to the cell surface for another round. Alternatively, receptor and ligand within endosomes can be targeted to fuse with lysosomes (e.g., epidermal growth factor bound to its receptor); after complete degradation, the late endosome-lysosome fusion vesicle can regenerate lysosomes. *Phagocytosis* involves the non-clathrin-mediated membrane invagination of large particles—typically by specialized phagocytes (e.g., macrophages or neutrophils). The resulting phagosomes eventually fuse with lysosomes to facilitate the degradation of the internalized material. *Transcytosis* involves the transcellular endocytotic transport of solute and/or bound ligand from one face of a cell to another. *Exocytosis* is the process by which membrane-bound vesicles fuse with the plasma membrane and discharge their contents to the extracellular space.

membrane (*exocytosis*) for another round of ingestion. Endocytosis and exocytosis must be tightly coupled since a cell will typically pinocytose 10% to 20% of its own cell volume each hour, or about 1% to 2% of its plasma membrane each minute. Pinocytosis and receptor-mediated endocytosis begin at a specialized region of the plasma membrane called the *clathrin-coated pit,* which rapidly invaginates and pinches off to form a *clathrin-coated vesicle;* trapped within the vesicle is a gulp of the extracellular milieu and in some cases receptor bound macromolecules described below. The vesicles then rapidly uncoat and fuse with an acidic intracellular structure called the *early endosome* where they discharge their contents for digestion and further passage to the lysosome.

Receptor-mediated endocytosis is the major uptake mechanism for certain macromolecules, as exemplified by transferrin and low-density lipoprotein (LDL). These macromolecules bind to receptors that are localized in clathrin coated pits. After binding to their specific receptors, LDL and transferrin are endocytosed in vesicles that fuse with lysosomes. In the acidic environment of the lysosome, LDL and transferrin release their cargo (cholesterol and iron, respectively), which is subsequently taken up into the cytoplasm. Remarkably, the LDL receptor and the transferrin receptor are resistant to the harsh environment of the lysosome, allowing them to be recycled back to the plasma membrane. Defects in receptor-mediated transport of LDL are responsible for familial hypercholesterolemia, as described in Chapter 5.

Cytoskeleton and Cell-Cell Interactions

The ability of cells to adopt a particular shape, maintain polarity, organize the relationship of intracellular organelles, and move about depends on the intracellular scaffolding of proteins called the *cytoskeleton* (Fig. 1-8). In eukaryotic cells, there are three major classes of cytoskeletal proteins:

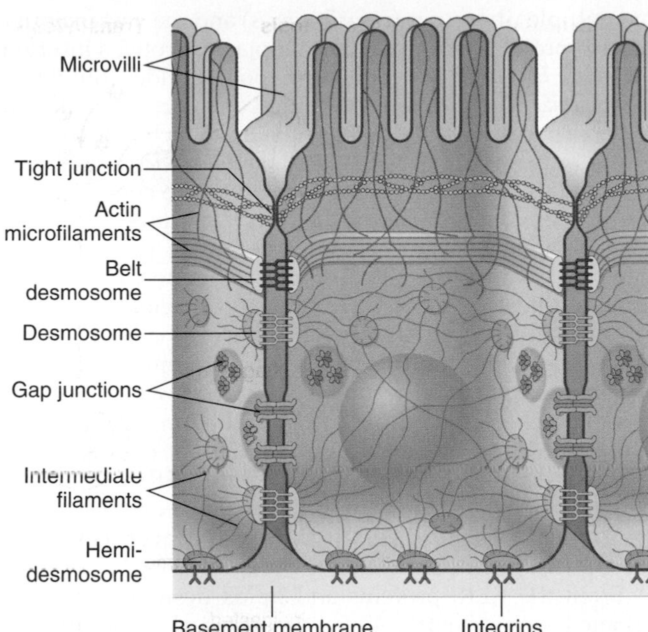

Figure 1-8 Cytoskeletal elements and cell-cell interactions. Interepithelial adhesion involves several different surface protein interactions, including through *tight junctions* and *desmosomes*; adhesion to the extracellular matrix involves cellular integrins (and associated proteins) within *hemidesmosomes*. See text for details.

- *Actin microfilaments* are 5- to 9-nm diameter fibrils formed from the **g**lobular protein actin (**G**-actin), the most abundant cytosolic protein in cells. The G-actin monomers noncovalently polymerize into long **f**ilaments (**F**-actin) that intertwine to form double-stranded helices with a defined polarity; new globular subunits are added (or lost) at the "positive" end of the strand. In muscle cells, the filamentous protein *myosin* binds to actin, and moves along it, driven by ATP hydrolysis (the basis of muscle contraction). In non-muscle cells, F-actin assembles via an assortment of actin-binding proteins into well-organized bundles and networks that control cell shape and movement.
- *Intermediate filaments* are 10-nm diameter fibrils that comprise a large and heterogeneous family. Individual types have characteristic tissue-specific patterns of expression that can be useful for assigning a cell of origin for poorly differentiated tumors.
  - *Lamin A, B, and C:* nuclear lamina of all cells
  - *Vimentin:* mesenchymal cells (fibroblasts, endothelium)
  - *Desmin:* muscle cells, forming the scaffold on which actin and myosin contract
  - *Neurofilaments:* axons of neurons, imparting strength and rigidity
  - *Glial fibrillary acidic protein:* glial cells around neurons
  - *Cytokeratins:* at least 30 distinct varieties, subdivided into acidic (type I) and neutral/basic (type II); different types present in different cells, hence can be used as cell markers

  These ropelike *intermediate filament* fibers are found predominantly in a polymerized form within cells and do not usually actively reorganize like actin and microtubules. They impart tensile strength and allow cells to bear mechanical stress. The nuclear membrane lamins are important not only for maintaining nuclear morphology but also for regulating normal nuclear transcription. The importance of lamins is seen in rare but fascinating disorders caused by lamin mutations, which range from certain froms of muscular dystrophy to progeria, a disease of premature aging. Intermediate filaments also form the major structural proteins of skin and hair.
- *Microtubules* are 25-nm-thick fibrils composed of noncovalently polymerized dimers of α- and β-tubulin arrayed in constantly elongating or shrinking hollow tubes with a defined polarity; the ends are designated "+" or "−". The "−" end is typically embedded in a *microtubule organizing center (MTOC or centrosome)* near the nucleus where it is associated with paired *centrioles*; the "+" end elongates or recedes in response to various stimuli by the addition or subtraction of tubulin dimers. Within cells, microtubules can serve as connecting cables for "molecular motor" proteins that use ATP to move vesicles, organelles, or other molecules around cells along microtubules. There are two varieties of these motor proteins: *kinesins*, for anterograde (− to +) transport, and *dyneins*, for retrograde (+ to −) transport; they also participate in sister chromatid separation during mitosis. Notably, microtubules (and their associated motors) have been adapted to form motile cilia (e.g., in bronchial epithelium) or flagella (in sperm).

Cell-Cell Interactions. **Cells interact and communicate with one another by forming junctions that provide mechanical links and enable surface receptors to recognize ligands on other cells.** *Cell junctions* are organized into three basic types (Fig. 1-8):

- *Occluding junctions (tight junctions)* seal adjacent cells together to create a continuous barrier that restricts the paracellular (between cells) movement of ions and other molecules. Viewed en face, occluding junctions form a tight meshlike network of macromolecular contacts between neighboring cells. The complexes that mediate the cell-cell interactions are composed of multiple transmembrane proteins, including *occludin, claudin, zonulin,* and *catenin*. Besides forming a high-resistance barrier to solute movement, this zone also represents the boundary that allows the segregation of apical and basolateral domains of cells, helping to maintain cellular polarity. Nevertheless, these junctions (as well as the desmosomes described later) are dynamic structures that can dissociate and reform as required to facilitate epithelial proliferation or inflammatory cell migration.
- *Anchoring junctions (desmosomes)* mechanically attach cells—and their intracellular cytoskeletons—to other cells or to the extracellular matrix (ECM). When the adhesion focus is between cells, and is small and rivet-like, it is designated a *spot desmosome* or *macula adherens*. When such a focus attaches the cell to the ECM, it is called a *hemidesmosome*. Similar adhesion domains can also occur as broad bands between cells, where they are denoted as *belt desmosomes*.

Cell-cell desmosomal junctions are formed by homotypic association of transmembrane glycoproteins called *cadherins*. In spot desmosomes, the cadherins are called *desmogleins* and *desmocollins*; they are linked to intracellular intermediate filaments and allow extracellular forces to be mechanically communicated (and dissipated) over multiple cells. In belt desmosomes, the transmembrane adhesion molecules are called *E-cadherins* and are associated with intracellular actin microfilaments, by which they can influence cell shape and/or motility. In hemidesmosomes, the transmembrane connector proteins are called *integrins*; like cadherins, these attach to intracellular intermediate filaments, and thus functionally link the cytoskeleton to the extracellular matrix. *Focal adhesion complexes* are large (>100 proteins) macromolecular complexes that can be localized at hemidesmosomes, and include proteins that can generate intracellular signals when cells are subjected to increased shear stress, such as endothelium in the bloodstream, or cardiac myocytes in a failing heart.

- *Communicating junctions (gap junctions)* mediate the passage of chemical or electrical signals from one cell to another. The junction consists of a dense planar array of 1.5- to 2-nm pores (called *connexons*) formed by hexamers of transmembrane proteins called *connexins*. These pores permit the passage of ions, nucleotides, sugars, amino acids, vitamins, and other small molecules; the permeability of the junction is rapidly reduced by lowered intracellular pH or increased intracellular calcium. Gap junctions play a critical role in cell-cell communication; in cardiac myocytes, for example, cell-to-cell calcium fluxes through gap junctions allow the myocardium to behave like a functional syncytium capable of coordinated waves of contraction—the beating of the heart.

Biosynthetic Machinery: Endoplasmic Reticulum and Golgi

The structural proteins and enzymes of the cell are constantly renewed by ongoing synthesis tightly balanced with intracellular degradation. The endoplasmic reticulum (ER) is the site for synthesis of all the transmembrane proteins and lipids for plasma membrane and cellular organelles, including ER itself. It is also the initial site for the synthesis of all molecules destined for export out of the cell. The ER is organized into a meshlike interconnected maze of branching tubes and flattened lamellae forming a continuous sheet around a single lumen that is topologically equivalent to the extracellular environment. The ER is composed of contiguous but distinct domains, distinguished by the *presence* (rough ER or RER) or *absence* (smooth ER or SER) of ribosomes (Fig. 1-5).

Membrane-bound ribosomes on the cytosolic face of RER translate mRNA into proteins that are extruded into the ER lumen or become integrated into the ER membrane. This process is directed by specific *signal sequences* on the N-termini of nascent proteins. For proteins lacking a signal sequence, translation occurs on free ribosomes in the cytosol. Typically, such transcripts are read simultaneously by multiple ribosomes (*polyribosomes*) and the vast majority of such proteins remain in the cytoplasm. Proteins inserted into the ER fold and can form polypeptide complexes (*oligomerize*); in addition, disulfide bonds are formed, and *N-linked oligosaccharides* (sugar moieties attached to asparagine residues) are added. *Chaperone molecules* retain proteins in the ER until these modifications are complete and the proper conformation is achieved. If a protein fails to appropriately fold or oligomerize, it is retained and degraded within the ER. The most common pathogenic mutation involving the CFTR protein, a membrane transporter that is defective in cystic fibrosis (Chapter 5), illustrates this quality control mechanism. This mutation causes the absence of a single amino acid (phe_{508}), which leads to misfolding, ER retention, and degradation of the CFTR protein. Moreover, excess accumulation of misfolded proteins—exceeding the capacity of the ER to edit and degrade them—leads to the *ER stress response* (also called the *unfolded protein response* or *UPR*) that triggers cell death through *apoptosis* (Chapter 2).

From the RER, proteins and lipids destined for other organelles or for extracellular export are shuttled into the *Golgi apparatus*. This organelle consists of stacked cisternae that progressively modify proteins in an orderly fashion from *cis* (near the ER) to *trans* (near the plasma membrane); macromolecules are shuttled between the various cisternae within membrane-bound vesicles. As molecules move from *cis* to *trans*, the *N-linked oligosaccharides* originally added to proteins in the ER are pruned and further modified in a step-wise fashion; *O-linked oligosaccharides* (sugar moieties linked to serine or threonine) are also appended. Some of this glycosylation is important in directing molecules to lysosomes (via the *mannose-6-phosphate receptor*, Chapter 5); other glycosylation adducts may be important for cell-cell or cell-matrix interactions, or for clearing senescent cells (e.g., platelets and red cells). In addition to the stepwise glycosylation of lipids and proteins, the *cis Golgi network* can recycle proteins back to the ER; the *trans Golgi network* sorts proteins and lipids and dispatches them to other organelles (including the plasma membrane), or to secretory vesicles destined for extracellular release. The Golgi complex is especially prominent in cells specialized for secretion, including goblet cells of the intestine, bronchial epithelium (secreting large amounts of polysaccharide-rich mucus), and plasma cells (secreting large quantities of antibodies).

The SER in most cells is relatively sparse and primarily exists as the transition zone from RER to transport vesicles moving to the Golgi. However, in cells that synthesize steroid hormones (e.g., in the gonads or adrenals), or that catabolize lipid-soluble molecules (e.g., in the liver), the SER may be particularly conspicuous. Indeed, repeated exposure to compounds that are metabolized by the SER (e.g., phenobarbital catabolism by the cytochrome P-450 system), can lead to a reactive SER hyperplasia. The SER is also responsible for sequestering intracellular calcium; subsequent release from the SER into the cytosol can mediate a number of responses to extracellular signals (including apoptotic cell death). In addition, in muscle cells, specialized SER called *sarcoplasmic reticulum* is responsible for the cyclical release and sequestration of calcium ions that regulates muscle contraction and relaxation, respectively.

Waste Disposal: Lysosomes and Proteasomes

As already mentioned in brief, **cellular waste disposal depends on the activities of lysosomes and proteasomes** (Fig. 1-9).

- **Lysosomes** are membrane-bound organelles containing roughly 40 different acid hydrolases (i.e., enzymes that function best in acidic pH ≤ 5); these hydrolases include proteases, nucleases, lipases, glycosidases, phosphatases, and sulfatases. Lysosomal enzymes are initially synthesized in the ER lumen and then tagged with a mannose-6-phosphate (M6P) residue within the Golgi apparatus. Such M6P-modified proteins are subsequently delivered to lysosomes through trans-Golgi vesicles that express M6P receptors. The other

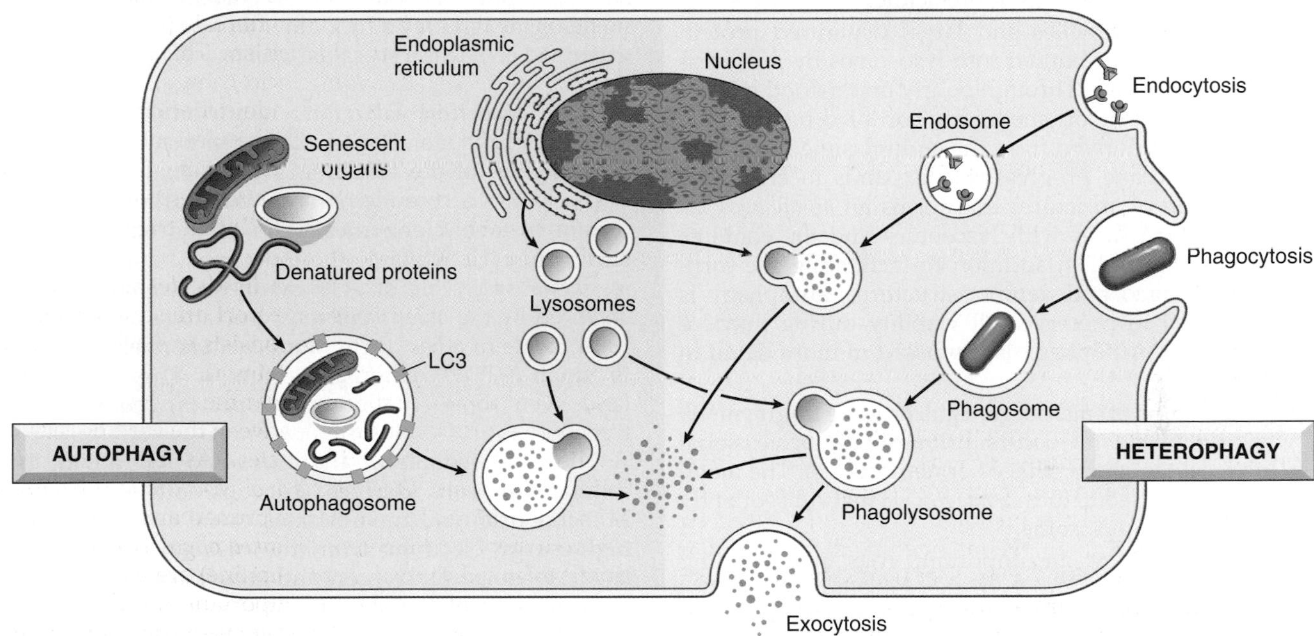

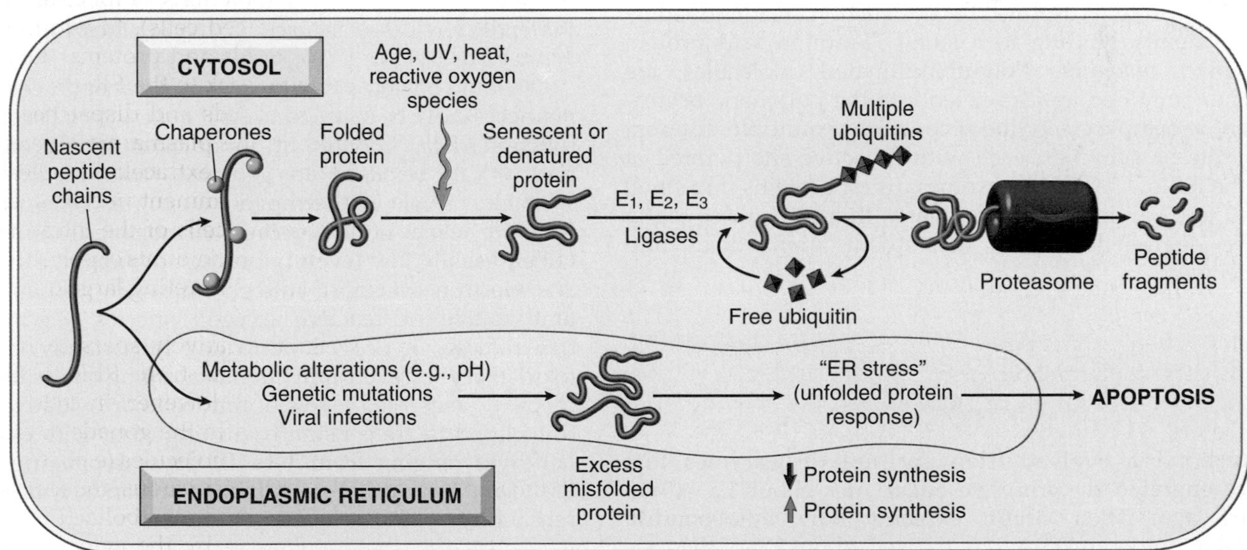

Figure 1-9 Intracellular catabolism. **A,** Lysosomal degradation. In *heterophagy* (right side), lysosomes fuse with endosomes or phagosomes to facilitate the degradation of their internalized contents (see Fig. 1-7). The end-products may be released into the cytosol for nutrition or discharged into the extracellular space (*exocytosis*). In *autophagy* (left side), senescent organelles or denatured proteins are targeted for lysosome-driven degradation by encircling them with a double membrane derived from the endoplasmic reticulum and marked by LC3 proteins (microtubule-associated protein 1A/1B-light chain 3). Cell stressors such as nutrient depletion or certain intracellular infections can also activate the autophagocytic pathway. **B,** Proteasome degradation. Cytosolic proteins destined for turnover (e.g., transcription factors or regulatory proteins), senescent proteins, or proteins that have become denatured due to extrinsic mechanical or chemical stresses can be tagged by multiple ubiquitin molecules (through the activity of E_1, E_2, and E_3 ubiquitin ligases). This marks the proteins for degradation by proteasomes, cytosolic multi-subunit complexes that degrade proteins to small peptide fragments. High levels of misfolded proteins within the endoplasmic reticulum (ER) trigger a protective *unfolded protein response*—engendering a broad reduction in protein synthesis, but specific increases in chaperone proteins that can facilitate protein refolding. If this is inadequate to cope with the levels of misfolded proteins, apoptosis is induced.

macromolecules destined for catabolism in the lysosomes arrive by one of three other pathways (Fig. 1-9):

- Material internalized by *fluid-phase pinocytosis* or *receptor-mediated endocytosis* passes from plasma membrane to early endosome to late endosome, and ultimately into the lysosome. The early endosome is the first acidic compartment encountered, while proteolytic enzymes only begin significant digestion in the late endosome; late endosomes mature into lysosomes. During the maturation process, the organelle becomes progressively more acidic.
- Senescent organelles and large, denatured protein complexes are shuttled into lysosomes by a process called *autophagy*. Through poorly understood mechanisms, obsolete organelles are corralled by a double membrane derived from the endoplasmic reticulum; the membrane progressively expands to encircle a collection of structures and forms an *autophagosome* which then fuses with lysosomes and the contents are catabolized. In addition to facilitating the turnover of aged and defunct structures, autophagy is also used to preserve cell viability during nutrient depletion. Autophagy is discussed in more detail in Chapter 2.
- *Phagocytosis* of microorganisms or large fragments of matrix or debris occurs primarily in professional phagocytes (macrophages or neutrophils). The material is engulfed to form a *phagosome* that subsequently fuses with a lysosome.

- **Proteasomes** play an important role in degrading cytosolic proteins (Fig. 1-9); these include denatured or misfolded proteins (akin to what occurs within the ER), as well as any other macromolecule whose lifespan needs to be regulated (e.g., transcription factors). Many proteins destined for destruction are identified by covalently binding to a small 76–amino acid protein called *ubiquitin*. Poly-ubiquitinated molecules are then unfolded and funneled into the polymeric proteasome complex, a cylinder containing multiple different protease activities, each with its active site pointed at the hollow core. Proteasomes digest proteins into small (6 to 12 amino acids) fragments that can subsequently be degraded to their constituent amino acids and recycled.

Cellular Metabolism and Mitochondrial Function

Mitochondria evolved from ancestral prokaryotes that were engulfed by primitive eukaryotes about 1.5 billion years ago. Their origin explains why mitochondria contain their own DNA (circularized, about 1% of the total cellular DNA), encoding roughly 1% of the total cellular proteins and approximately 20% of the proteins involved in *oxidative phosphorylation*. Although their genomes are small, mitochondria can nevertheless carry out all the steps of DNA replication, transcription, and translation. Interestingly, the mitochondrial machinery is similar to present-day bacteria; for example, mitochondria initiate protein synthesis with N-formylmethionine and are sensitive to antibacterial antibiotics. Moreover, since the ovum contributes the vast majority of cytoplasmic organelles to the fertilized zygote, mitochondrial DNA is virtually entirely *maternally inherited*. Nevertheless, because the protein constituents of mitochondria derive from both nuclear and mitochondrial genetic transcription, mitochondrial disorders may be X-linked, autosomal, or maternally inherited.

Mitochondria provide the enzymatic machinery for oxidative phosphorylation (and thus the relatively efficient generation of energy from glucose and fatty acid substrates). They also have an important role in anabolic metabolism and play a fundamental role in regulating programmed cell death, so-called *apoptosis* (Fig. 1-10).

Energy Generation. Each mitochondrion has two separate and specialized membranes. The inner membrane contains the enzymes of the respiratory chain folded into *cristae*. This encloses a core *matrix space* that harbors the bulk of certain metabolic enzymes, such as the enzymes of the citric acid cycle. Outside the inner membrane is the *intermembrane space*, site of ATP synthesis, which is, in turn, enclosed by the *outer membrane*; the latter is studded with *porin* proteins that form aqueous channels permeable to small (<5000 daltons) molecules. Larger molecules (and even some smaller polar species) require specific transporters.

The major source of the energy to run all the basic cellular functions derives from oxidative metabolism. Mitochondria oxidize substrates to CO_2, transferring the high-energy electrons from the original molecule (e.g., sugar) to molecular oxygen, and generating the low-energy electrons of water. The oxidation of various metabolites drives *hydrogen ion (proton) pumps* that transfer H^+ from the core matrix into the intermembrane space. As the H^+ ions flow back down their electrochemical gradient, the energy released is used in the synthesis of *adenosine triphosphate (ATP)*.

It should be noted that the electron transport chain need not necessarily be coupled to ATP generation. Through the function of *thermogenin*, an inner membrane protein, the energy can be used to generate heat. Hence tissues with high levels of thermogenin, such as brown fat, can generate heat by non-shivering thermogenesis. As a natural (albeit usually low-level) byproduct of substrate oxidation and electron transport, mitochondria are also an important source of reactive oxygen species (e.g., oxygen free radicals, hydrogen peroxide); importantly, hypoxia, toxic injury, or even mitochondrial aging can lead to significantly increased levels of intracellular oxidative stress. Mitochondria are constantly turning over, with estimated half-lives ranging from 1 to 10 days, depending on the tissue, nutritional status, metabolic demands, and intercurrent injury.

Intermediate metabolism. As described in Chapter 7, pure oxidative phosphorylation produces abundant ATP, but also "burns" glucose to CO_2 and H_2O, leaving no carbon moieties suitable for use as building blocks for lipids or proteins. For this reason, rapidly growing cells (both benign and malignant) upregulate glucose and glutamine uptake and decrease their production of ATP per glucose molecule, a phenomenon called the Warburg effect. Both glucose and glutamine provide carbon moieties that prime

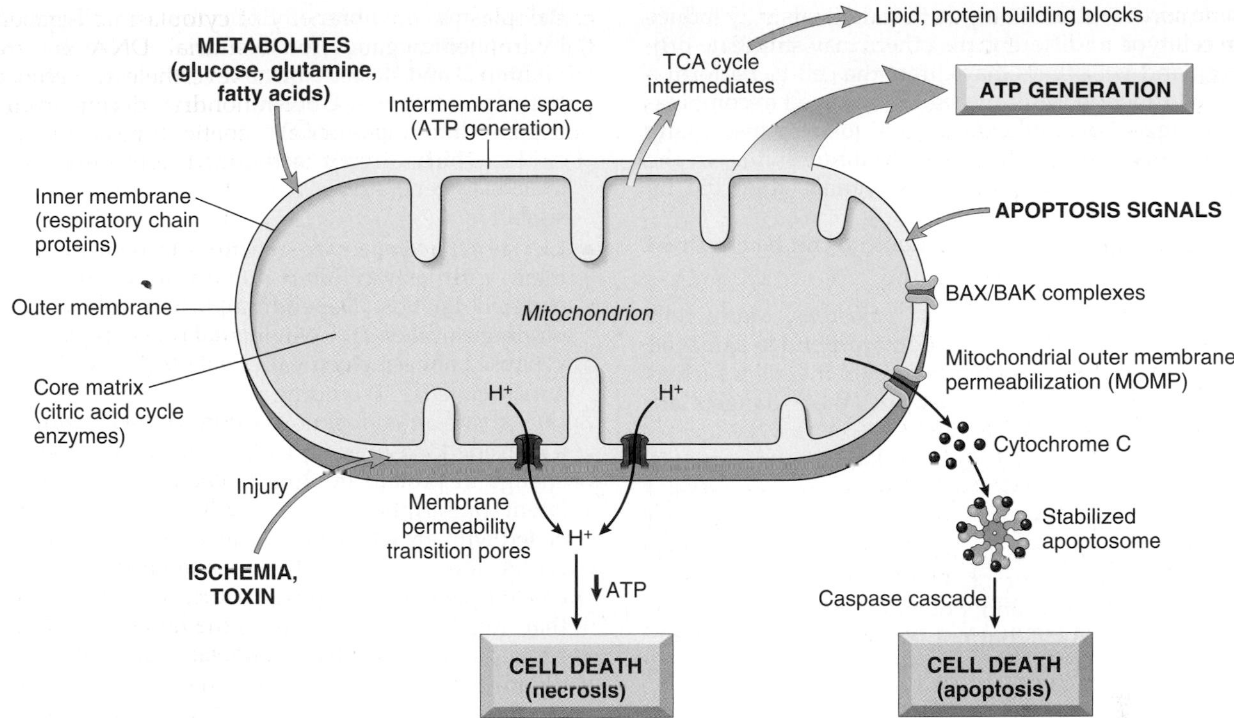

Figure 1-10 Roles of the mitochondria. Besides the efficient generation of ATP from carbohydrate and fatty acid substrates, mitochondria have an important role in intermediary metabolism, serving as the source of molecules used to synthesize lipids and proteins, and are also are centrally involved in cell life-and-death decisions.

the mitochondrial TCA cycle, but instead of being used to make ATP, intermediates are "spun-off" to make lipids, nucleic acids, and proteins . Thus, depending on the growth state of the cell, mitochondrial metabolism can be modulated to support either cellular maintenance or cellular growth. Ultimately, these metabolic decisions are governed by growth factors, nutrient and oxygen supplies, and cellular signaling pathways and sensors that respond to these exogenous factors.

Cell Death. In addition to providing ATP and metabolites that enable the bulk of cellular activity, mitochondria also regulate the balance of cell survival and death. There are two major pathways of cell death (Chapter 2):

- *Necrosis*: External cellular injury (toxin, ischemia, trauma) can damage mitochondria, inducing the formation of mitochondrial permeability transition pores in the outer membrane. These channels allow the dissipation of the proton potential so that mitochondrial ATP generation fails and the cell dies.
- *Apoptosis*: Programmed cell death is a central feature of normal tissue development and turnover and can be triggered by extrinsic signals (including cytotoxic T cells and inflammatory cytokines), or intrinsic pathways (including DNA damage and intracellular stress). Mitochondria play a central role in the intrinsic pathway of apoptosis. If mitochondria are damaged (a sign of irreversible cell injury or stress) or the cell cannot synthesize adequate amounts of survival proteins (because of deficient growth signals), mitochondria become leaky. Cytochrome c, which is normally sequestered inside the mitochondria, leaks into the cytosol, where it forms a complex with other proteins that ultimately activate caspases, the enzymes that induce apoptosis. This process is described in more detail in Chapter 2. Failure of apoptosis can contribute to malignancy (Chapter 7) and too much apoptosis can lead to premature cell death, as occurs in some neurodegenerative disorders (Chapter 28).

Although mitochondria were discovered well over 100 years ago, the secrets of their functions continue to be unraveled.

Cellular Activation

Cell communication is critical in multicellular organisms. At the most basic level, extracellular signals determine whether a cell lives or dies, or whether it remains quiescent or is stimulated to perform its specific function. Intercellular signaling is clearly important in the developing embryo, and in maintaining tissue organization; it is also important in the intact organism, assuring that tissues respond in an adaptive and effective fashion to various threats, such as local tissue trauma or a systemic infection. Loss of cellular communication and the "social controls" that maintain normal relationships of cells can variously lead to unregulated growth (cancer) or an ineffective response to an extrinsic stress (as in shock).

Cell Signaling

An individual cell is chronically exposed to a remarkable variety of signals, which it must sort through and integrate into some sort of rational output. Some signals may induce a given cell type to differentiate, others may stimulate proliferation, and yet others may direct the cell to perform a specialized function. Multiple signals received in combination may trigger yet another totally unique response. Many cells require certain inputs just to continue living; in the absence of appropriate exogenous signals, they die by apoptosis.

The signals that most cells respond to can be classified into several groups:

- *Damage to neighboring cells and pathogens.* Many cells have an innate capacity to sense and respond to damaged cells (*danger signals*), as well as foreign invaders such as microbes. The receptors that detect these dangers are discussed in Chapters 3 and 6.
- *Contact with neighboring cells,* mediated through adhesion molecules and/or gap junctions. As mentioned previously, *gap junction signaling* is accomplished between adjacent cells via hydrophilic connexons that permit the movement of small ions (e.g., calcium), various metabolites, and potential second messenger molecules like cAMP, but not larger macromolecules.
- *Contact with ECM,* mediated through integrins, which are discussed in the context of leukocyte attachment to other cells during inflammation in Chapter 3.
- *Secreted molecules.* The most important secreted molecules include *growth factors,* discussed later; *cytokines,* a term reserved for mediators of inflammation and immune responses (also discussed in Chapters 3 and 6); and *hormones,* which are secreted by endocrine organs and act on different cell types (Chapter 24).

Extracellular cell-cell signaling pathways are classified into different types, based on the distance over which the signal functions:

- *Paracrine signaling.* Cells in just the immediate vicinity are affected. To accomplish this, there can be only minimal diffusion, with the signal being rapidly degraded, taken up by other cells, or trapped in the ECM.
- *Autocrine signaling* occurs when molecules secreted by a cell affect that same cell. This can be a means to entrain groups of cells undergoing synchronous differentiation during development, or can be used to amplify a response or for its feedback inhibition.
- *Synaptic signaling.* Activated neurons secrete *neurotransmitters* at specialized cell junctions (*synapses*) onto target cells.
- *Endocrine signaling.* A mediator is released into the bloodstream and acts on target cells at a distance.

Regardless of the nature of an extracellular stimulus (paracrine, synaptic, or endocrine), the signal it conveys is transmitted to the cell via a specific *receptor* protein. Signaling molecules (*ligands*) bind their respective receptors and initiate a cascade of intracellular events culminating in the desired cellular response. Ligands usually have high affinities for receptors and at physiologic concentrations bind receptors with exquisite specificity. Receptors may be present on the cell surface or located within the cell (Fig. 1-11):

- *Intracellular receptors* are transcription factors that are activated by lipid-soluble ligands that can easily cross the plasma membrane. Examples of cell-permeable, hydrophobic ligands for this class of receptor include vitamin D and steroid hormones, which activate nuclear hormone receptors. Uncommonly, the signaling ligand diffuses into adjacent cells; this is the case with nitric oxide, which directly activates the enzyme guanylyl cyclase to generate cyclic GMP, an intracellular second signal.
- *Cell-surface receptors* are generally transmembrane proteins with extracellular domains that bind soluble secreted ligands. Depending on the receptor, ligand binding can then (1) open ion channels (typically at the synapse between electrically excitable cells), (2) activate an associated GTP-binding regulatory protein (*G protein*), (3) activate an endogenous or associated enzyme, often a tyrosine kinase; or (4) trigger a proteolytic event or a change in protein binding or stability that activates a latent transcription factor. Activities (2) and (3) are associated with growth factor signaling pathways that drive cell proliferation, while activity (4) is a common feature of multiple pathways (e.g., Notch, Wnt, and Hedgehog) that regulate normal development. Understandably, signals transduced by cell surface receptors are often deranged in developmental disorders and in cancers.

Signal Transduction Pathways

Binding of a ligand to a cell surface receptor mediates signaling by inducing clustering of the receptor *(receptor cross-linking)* or other types of physcial perturbations (Fig. 1-11). The common theme is that all of these perturbations cause a change in the physical state of the intracellular domain of the receptor, which then triggers additional biochemical events that lead to signal transduction.

Cellular receptors are grouped into several types based on the signaling mechanisms they use and the intracellular biochemical pathways they activate (Fig. 1-11). Receptor signaling typically leads to the formation or modification of biochemical intermediates and/or activation of enzymes, and ultimately to the generation of active transcription factors that enter the nucleus and alter gene expression:

- *Receptors associated with kinase activity.* Downstream phosphorylation is a common pathway (but not the only one) by which these signals are transduced. Thus, alterations in receptor geometry can elicit intrinsic receptor *protein kinase* activity or promote the enzymatic activity of recruited intracellular kinases—resulting in the addition of charged phosphate residues to target molecules. *Tyrosine kinases* phosphorylate specific tyrosine residues, whereas *serine/threonine kinases* add phosphates to distinct serine or threonine residues, and *lipid kinases* phosphorylate lipid substrates. For every phosphorylation event, there is also a *phosphatase,* an enzyme that can remove the phosphate residue and thus modulate signaling; usually, phosphatases play an inhibitory role in signal transduction.
  - *Receptor tyrosine kinases (RTKs)* are integral membrane proteins (e.g., receptors for insulin, epidermal growth factor, and platelet derived growth factor); ligand-induced cross-linking activates intrinsic

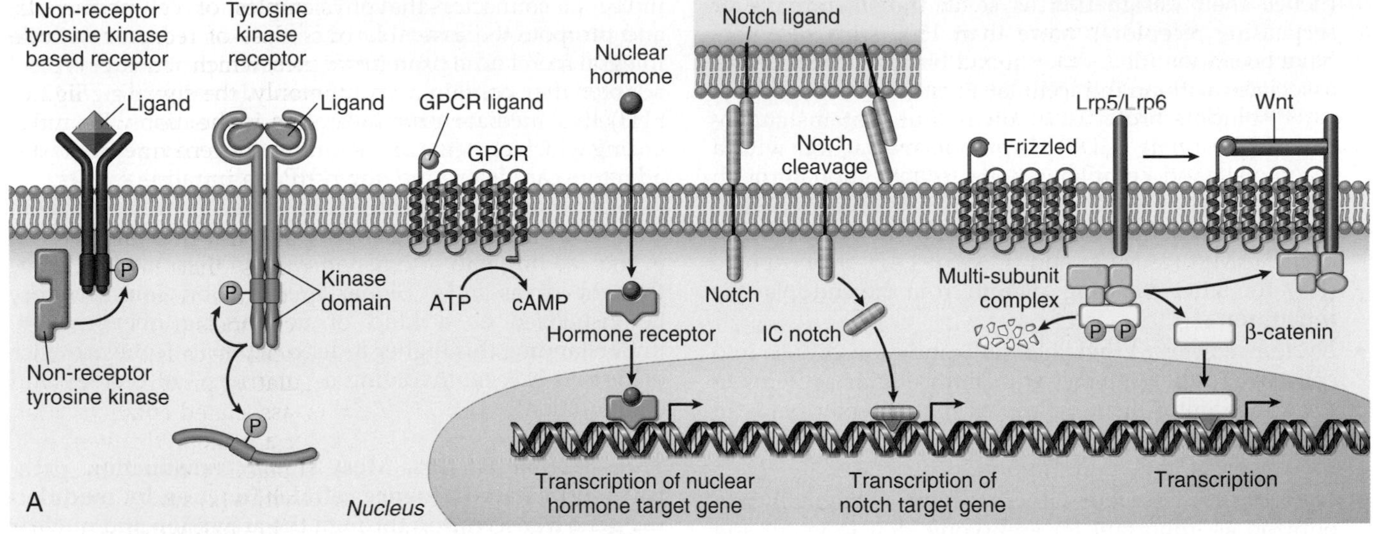

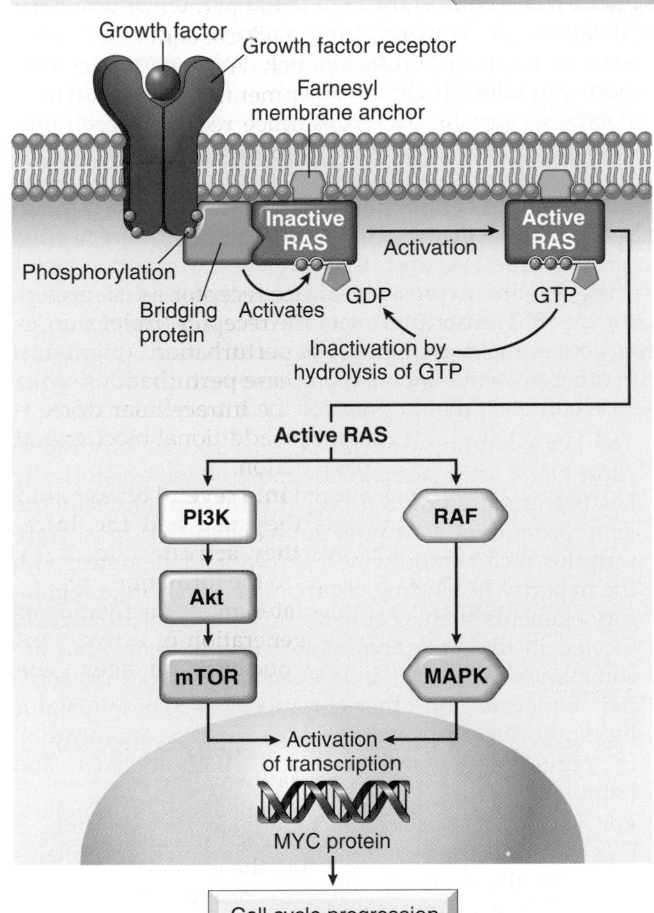

Figure 1-11 Receptor-mediated signaling. **A,** Categories of signaling receptors, including receptors that utilize a nonreceptor tyrosine kinase; a receptor tyrosine kinase; a nuclear receptor that binds its ligand and can then influence transcription; a seven-transmembrane receptor linked to heterotrimeric G proteins; Notch, which recognizes a ligand on a distinct cell and is cleaved yielding an intracellular fragment that can enter the nucleus and influence transcription of specific target genes; and the Wnt/Frizzled pathway where activation releases intracellular β-catenin from a protein complex that normally drives its constitutive degradation. The released β-catenin can then migrate to the nucleus and act as a transcription factor. Lrp5/Lrp6, low-density-lipoprotein (LDL) receptor related proteins 5 and 6, are highly homologous and act as co-receptors in Wnt/Frizzled signaling. **B,** Signaling from a tyrosine kinase-based receptor. Binding of the growth factor (ligand) causes receptor dimerization and autophosphorylation of tyrosine residues. Attachment of adapter (or bridging) proteins couples the receptor to inactive, GDP-bound RAS, allowing the GDP to be displaced in favor of GTP and yielding activated RAS. Activated RAS interacts with and activates RAF (also known as *MAP kinase kinase kinase)*. This kinase then phosphorylates MAPK (mitogen-activated protein kinase) and activated MAP kinase phosphorylates other cytoplasmic proteins and nuclear transcription factors, generating cellular responses. The phosphorylated tyrosine kinase receptor can also bind other components, such as phosphatidyl 3-kinase (PI3 kinase), which activates other signaling systems. The cascade is turned off when the activated RAS eventually hydrolyzes GTP to GDP converting RAS to its inactive form. Mutations in RAS that lead to delayed GTP hydrolysis can thus lead to augmented proliferative signaling. GDP, Guanosine diphosphate; GTP, guanosine triphosphate; mTOR, mammalian target of rapamycin.

tyrosine kinase domains located in their cytoplasmic tails.

- Several kinds of receptors have no intrinsic catalytic activity (e.g., immune receptors, some cytokine receptors, and integrins). For these, a separate intracellular protein—known as a *nonreceptor tyrosine kinase*—phosphorylates specific motifs on the receptor or other proteins. The cellular homolog of the transforming protein of the Rous sarcoma virus, called SRC, is the prototype for an important family of such nonreceptor tyrosine kinases (*Src-family kinases*). SRC contains unique functional regions, such as *Src-homology 2* (SH2) and *Src-homology 3* (SH3) domains. SH2 domains typically bind to receptors phosphorylated by another kinase, allowing the aggregation of multiple enzymes. SH3 domains mediate other protein-protein interactions, often involving proline-rich domains.
- *G-protein coupled receptors* are polypeptides that characteristically traverse the plasma membrane seven times

(hence their designation as seven-transmembrane or serpentine receptors); more than 1500 such receptors have been identified. After ligand binding, the receptor associates with an intracellular guanosine triphosphate (GTP)-binding protein (G protein) that contains guanosine diphosphate (GDP). G-protein interaction with a receptor-ligand complex results in activation through the exchange of GDP for GTP. Downstream receptor-mediated signaling events result in the generation of cyclic AMP (cAMP), and inositol-1,4,5,-triphosphate (IP_3), the latter releasing calcium from the endoplasmic reticulum.

- *Nuclear receptors*. Lipid-soluble ligands can diffuse into cells where they interact with intracellular proteins to form a receptor-ligand complex that directly binds to nuclear DNA; the results can be either activation or repression of gene transcription.
- *Other classes of receptors*. Other receptors—originally recognized as important for embryonic development and cell fate determination—have since been shown to participate in the functions of mature cells, particularly within the immune system.
  - Receptor proteins of the *Notch* family fall in this category; ligand binding to Notch receptors leads to proteolytic cleavage of the receptor and subsequent nuclear translocation of the cytoplasmic piece (intracellular Notch) to form a transcription complex.
  - *Wnt* protein ligands can also influence cell development through a pathway involving transmembrane *Frizzled* family receptors, which regulate the intracellular levels of β-catenin. Normally, β-catenin is constantly targeted for ubiquitin-directed proteasome degradation. However, Wnt binding to Frizzled (and other co-receptors) recruits yet another intracellular protein (*Disheveled*) that leads to disruption of the degradation-targeting complex. The stabilized pool of β-catenin molecules then translocates to the nucleus, where β-catenin forms a transcriptional complex.

Modular Signaling Proteins, Hubs, and Nodes. The traditional *linear* view of signaling—that receptor activation triggers an orderly sequence of biochemical intermediates that ultimately leads to changes in gene expression and the desired biological response—is almost certainly oversimplified. Instead, it is increasingly clear that any initial signal results in multiple diverging effects, each of which contributes in varying degrees to the final outcome. For example, specific phosphorylation of any given protein can allow it to associate with a host of other molecules, resulting in multiple effects such as:

- Enzyme activation (or inactivation)
- Nuclear (or cytoplasmic) localization of transcription factors (see later)
- Transcription factor activation (or inactivation)
- Actin polymerization (or depolymerization)
- Protein degradation (or stabilization)
- Activation of feedback inhibitory (or stimulatory) loops

Adaptor proteins play a key role in organizing intracellular signaling pathways. These proteins function as molecular connectors that physically link different enzymes and promote the assembly of complexes; adaptors can be integral membrane proteins or cytosolic proteins. A typical adaptor may contain a few specific domains (e.g., SH2 or SH3) that mediate protein-protein interactions. By influencing which proteins are recruited to signaling complexes, adaptors can determine downstream signaling events.

By analogy with computer networks, the protein-protein complexes can be considered *nodes* and the biochemical events feeding into or emanating from these nodes can be thought of as *hubs*. Signal transduction can therefore be visualized as a kind of networking phenomenon; understanding this higher order complexity is the province of *systems biology*, involving a "marriage" of biology and computation.

Transcription Factors. **Most signal transduction pathways ultimately influence cellular function by modulating gene transcription through the activation and nuclear localization of transcription factors.** Conformational changes of transcription factors (e.g., following phosphorylation) can allow their translocation into the nucleus or can expose specific DNA or protein binding motifs. Transcription factors may drive the expression of a relatively limited set of genes or may have much more widespread effects on gene expression. Among the transcription factors that regulate the expression of genes that are needed for growth are MYC and JUN, while a transcription factor that triggers the expression of genes that lead to growth arrest is p53. Transcription factors have a modular design, often containing domains that bind DNA and that interact with other proteins, such as components of the RNA polymerase complex, that are needed to drive transcription.

- The DNA-binding domain permits specific binding to short DNA sequences. While most interest historically has been focused on binding of transcription factors to gene promoters, it is now appreciated that most transcription factors bind widely throughout genomes, with the majority of binding occurring in long-range regulatory elements such as enhancers. Enhancers are usually located in the "neighborhood" close to genes, but are sometimes far away; it is even suspected that some may be located on other chromosomes! These insights highlight the importance of chromatin organization in regulating gene expression, both normal and pathologic.
- For a transcription factor to induce transcription, it must also possess protein:protein interaction domains that directly or indirectly recruit histone modifying enzymes, chromatin remodeling complexes, and (most importantly) RNA polymerase—the large multiprotein enzymatic complex that is responsible for RNA synthesis.

Growth Factors and Receptors

A major role of growth factors is to stimulate the activity of genes that are required for cell growth and cell division. Growth factor activity is mediated through binding to specific receptors, ultimately influencing the expression of genes that can:

- Promote entry of cells into the cell cycle
- Relieve blocks on cell cycle progression (thus promoting replication)
- Prevent apoptosis
- Enhance biosynthesis of cellular components (nucleic acids, proteins, lipids, carbohydrates) required for a mother cell to give rise to two daughter cells

Although growth factors are characteristically thought of as proteins that stimulate cell proliferation and/or survival, it is important to remember that they can also drive a host of nongrowth activities, including migration, differentiation, and synthetic capacity.

Growth factors are involved in the proliferation of cells at steady state as well as after injury, when irreversibly damaged cells must be replaced. Uncontrolled proliferation can result when the growth factor activity is dysregulated, or when growth factor signaling pathways are altered to become constitutively active. Thus, many growth factor pathway genes are *proto-oncogenes;* gain-of-function mutations in these genes can convert them into oncogenes capable of driving unfettered cell proliferation and tumor formation. Table 1-1 (and the following discussion) summarizes selected growth factors that are involved in two important proliferative processes, tissue repair and tumor development. Although the growth factors described here all involve receptors with intrinsic kinase activity, other growth factors may signal through each of the various pathways shown in Figure 1-11.

Epidermal Growth Factor and Transforming Growth Factor-α. Both of these factors belong to the EGF family and bind to the same receptors, which explains why they share many biologic activities. EGF and TGF-α are produced by macrophages and a variety of epithelial cells, and are mitogenic for hepatocytes, fibroblasts, and a host of epithelial cells. The "EGF receptor family" includes four membrane receptors with intrinsic tyrosine kinase activity; the best-characterized is EGFR1, also known as ERB-B1, or simply EGFR. EGFR1 mutations and/or amplification frequently occur in a number of cancers including those of the lung, head and neck, breast, and brain. The *ERBB2 receptor* (also known as *HER2*) is overexpressed in a subset of breast cancers. Many of these receptors have been successfully targeted by antibodies and small molecule antagonists.

Hepatocyte Growth Factor. Hepatocyte growth factor (HGF; also known as scatter factor) has mitogenic effects on hepatocytes and most epithelial cells, including biliary, pulmonary, renal, mammary,and epidermal. HGF acts as a *morphogen* in embryonic development (i.e., it influences the pattern of tissue differentiation), promotes cell migration (hence its designation as *scatter factor*), and enhances hepatocyte survival. HGF is produced by fibroblasts and most mesenchymal cells, as well as endothelium and non-hepatocyte liver cells. It is synthesized as an inactive precursor (pro-HGF) that is proteolytically activated by serine proteases released at sites of injury. MET is the receptor for HGF, it has intrinsic tyrosine kinase activity and is frequently overexpressed or mutated in tumors, particularly renal and thyroid papillary carcinomas. Consequently, MET inhibitors may be of value for cancer therapy.

Platelet-Derived Growth Factor. Platelet-derived growth factor (PDGF) is a family of several closely related proteins, each consisting of two chains (designated by pairs of letters). Three isoforms of PDGF (AA, AB, and BB) are constitutively active; PDGF-CC and PDGF-DD must be activated by proteolytic cleavage. PDGF is stored in platelet granules and is released on platelet activation. Although originally isolated from platelets (hence the name), it is also produced by many other cells, including activated macrophages, endothelium, smooth muscle cells, and a variety of tumors. All PDGF isoforms exert their effects by binding to two cell surface receptors (PDGFR α and β), both having intrinsic tyrosine kinase activity. PDGF induces fibroblast, endothelial, and smooth muscle cell proliferation and matrix synthesis, and is chemotactic for these cells (and

Table 1-1 Growth Factors Involved in Regeneration and Repair

Growth Factor	Sources	Functions
Epidermal growth factor (EGF)	Activated macrophages, salivary glands, keratinocytes, and many other cells	Mitogenic for keratinocytes and fibroblasts; stimulates keratinocyte migration; stimulates formation of granulation tissue
Transforming growth factor-α (TGF-α)	Activated macrophages, keratinocytes, many other cell types	Stimulates proliferation of hepatocytes and many other epithelial cells
Hepatocyte growth factor (HGF) (scatter factor)	Fibroblasts, stromal cells in the liver, endothelial cells	Enhances proliferation of hepatocytes and other epithelial cells; increases cell motility
Vascular endothelial growth factor (VEGF)	Mesenchymal cells	Stimulates proliferation of endothelial cells; increases vascular permeability
Platelet-derived growth factor (PDGF)	Platelets, macrophages, endothelial cells, smooth muscle cells, keratinocytes	Chemotactic for neutrophils, macrophages, fibroblasts, and smooth muscle cells; activates and stimulates proliferation of fibroblasts, endothelial, and other cells; stimulates ECM protein synthesis
Fibroblast growth factors (FGFs), including acidic (FGF-1) and basic (FGF-2)	Macrophages, mast cells, endothelial cells, many other cell types	Chemotactic and mitogenic for fibroblasts; stimulates angiogenesis and ECM protein synthesis
Transforming growth factor-β (TGF-β)	Platelets, T lymphocytes, macrophages, endothelial cells, keratinocytes, smooth muscle cells, fibroblasts	Chemotactic for leukocytes and fibroblasts; stimulates ECM protein synthesis; suppresses acute inflammation
Keratinocyte growth factor (KGF) (i.e., FGF-7)	Fibroblasts	Stimulates keratinocyte migration, proliferation, and differentiation

ECM, Extracellular membrane.

inflammatory cells), thus promoting recruitment of the cells into areas of inflammation and tissue injury.

Vascular Endothelial Growth Factor. Vascular endothelial growth factors (VEGFs)—VEGF-A, -B, -C, and -D, and PIGF (placental growth factor)—are a family of homodimeric proteins. VEGF-A is generally referred to simply as VEGF; it is the major *angiogenic* factor (inducing blood vessel development) after injury and in tumors. In comparison, VEGF-B and PlGF are involved in embryonic vessel development, and VEGF-C and -D stimulate both angiogenesis and lymphatic development (*lymphangiogenesis*). VEGFs are also involved in the maintenance of normal adult endothelium (i.e., not involved in angiogenesis), with the highest expression in epithelial cells adjacent to fenestrated epithelium (e.g., podocytes in the kidney, pigment epithelium in the retina, and choroid plexus in the brain). VEGF induces angiogenesis by promoting endothelial cell migration, proliferation (capillary sprouting), and formation of the vascular lumen. VEGFs also induce vascular dilation and increased vascular permeability. As might be anticipated, hypoxia is the most important inducer of VEGF production, through pathways that involve intracellular hypoxia-inducible factor (HIF-1). Other VEGF inducers—produced at sites of inflammation or wound healing—include PDGF and TGF-α.

VEGFs bind to a family of receptor tyrosine kinases (VEGFR-1, -2, and -3); VEGFR-2 is highly expressed in endothelium and is the most important for angiogenesis. Antibodies against VEGF are approved for the treatment of several tumors such as renal and colon cancers since they require angiogenesis for their spread and growth. Anti-VEGF antibodies are also being used for a number of ophthalmic diseases including "wet" age-related macular degeneration (AMD is a disorder of inappropriate angiogenesis and vascular permeability that causes adult-onset blindness); the angiogenesis associated with retinopathy of prematurity; and the leaky vessels that lead to diabetic macular edema. Finally, increased levels of soluble versions of VEGFR-1 (s-FLT-1) in pregnant women may cause preeclampsia (hypertension and proteinuria) by "sopping up" the free VEGF required for maintaining normal endothelium.

Fibroblast Growth Factor. Fibroblast growth factor (FGF) is a family of growth factors with of more than 20 members. Acidic FGF (aFGF, or FGF-1) and basic FGF (bFGF, or FGF-2) are the best characterized; FGF-7 is also referred to as keratinocyte growth factor (KGF). Released FGFs associate with heparan sulfate in the extracellular matrix, which serves as a reservoir for inactive factors that can be subsequently released by proteolysis (e.g., at sites of wound healing). FGFs transduce signals through four tyrosine kinase receptors (FGFR 1-4). FGFs contribute to wound healing responses, hematopoiesis, and development; bFGF has all the activities necessary for angiogenesis as well.

Transforming Growth Factor-β. TGF-β, which is distinct from TGF-α, has three isoforms (TGF-β1, TGF-β2, TGF-β3), each belonging to a family of about 30 members that includes bone morphogenetic proteins (BMPs), activins, inhibins, and müllerian inhibiting substance. TGF-β1 has the most widespread distribution, and is more commonly referred to as TGF-β. It is a homodimeric protein produced by multiple cell types, including platelets, endothelium, and mononuclear inflammatory cells; TGF-β is secreted as a precursor that requires proteolysis to yield the biologically active protein. There are two TGF-β receptors (types I and II), both with serine/threonine kinase activity that induce the phosphorylation of a variety of downstream cytoplasmic transcription factors called *Smads*. Phosphorylated Smads form heterodimers with Smad4, allowing nuclear translocation and association with other DNA-binding proteins to activate or inhibit gene transcription. TGF-β has multiple and often opposing effects depending on the tissue and concurrent signals. Agents with such multiplicity of effects are called *pleiotropic*. Because of the bewildering diversity of TGF-β effects (see later), this growth factor is said to be "pleiotropic with a vengeance." Primarily, however, TGF-β drives scar formation, and applies brakes on the inflammation that accompanies wound healing.

- TGF-β stimulates the production of collagen, fibronectin, and proteoglycans, and it inhibits collagen degradation by both decreasing matrix metalloproteinase (MMP) activity and increasing the activity of tissue inhibitors of proteinases (TIMPs; discussed later). TGF-β is involved not only in scar formation after injury, but also drives fibrosis in lung, liver, and kidneys in the setting of chronic inflammation.
- TGF-β is an antiinflammatory cytokine that serves to limit and terminate inflammatory responses. It does this by inhibiting lymphocyte proliferation and the activity of other leukocytes. Animal models lacking TGF-β have widespread and persistent inflammation.

Interaction with the Extracellular Matrix

Extracellular matrix (ECM) is a network of interstitial proteins that constitutes a significant proportion of any tissue. **Cell interactions with ECM are critical for development and healing, as well as for maintaining normal tissue architecture** (Fig. 1-12). Much more than a simple "space filler" around cells, ECM serves several key functions:

- *Mechanical support* for cell anchorage and cell migration, and maintenance of cell polarity
- *Control of cell proliferation,* by binding and displaying growth factors and by signaling through cellular receptors of the integrin family. As discussed earlier, the ECM provides a depot for a variety of latent growth factors that can be activated within foci of injury or inflammation.
- *Scaffolding for tissue renewal.* Because maintenance of normal tissue structure requires a basement membrane or stromal scaffold, the integrity of the basement membrane or the stroma of parenchymal cells is critical for the organized regeneration of tissues. Thus, ECM disruption results in defective tissue regeneration and repair, as occurs in the development of liver cirrhosis following injury to the liver cells and the collapse of the hepatic stroma.
- *Establishment of tissue microenvironments.* Basement membrane acts as a boundary between epithelium and

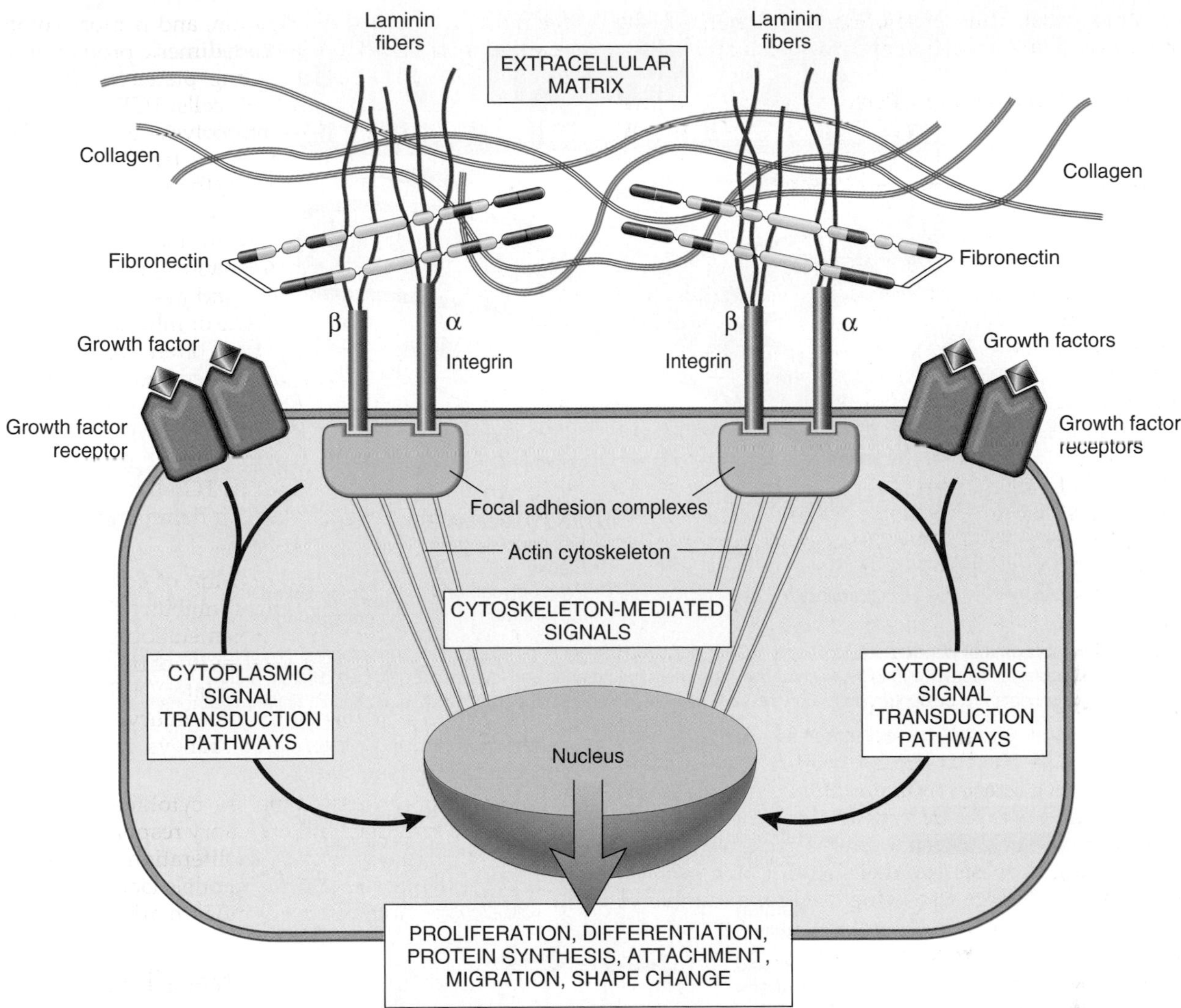

Figure 1-12 Interactions of extracellular matrix (ECM) and growth factors mediated cell signaling. Cell surface integrins interact with the cytoskeleton at focal adhesion complexes (protein aggregates that include vinculin, α-actinin, and talin; see Fig. 1-16C). This can initiate the production of intracellular messengers or can directly transduce signals to the nucleus. Cell surface receptors for growth factors can activate signal transduction pathways that overlap with those mediated through integrins. Signals from ECM components and growth factors can be integrated by the cells to produce a given response, including changes in proliferation, locomotion, and/or differentiation.

underlying connective tissue; it does not just provide support to the epithelium but is also functional. For example, in the kidney, it forms part of the filtration apparatus.

The ECM is constantly being remodeled; its synthesis and degradation accompany morphogenesis, tissue regeneration and repair, chronic fibrosis, and tumor invasion and metastasis. The appreciation of the structure and functions of the ECM has led to many recent attempts to create "artificial organs" by growing epithelia on various ECM substrates. This is a potential approach for replacing damaged tissues and organs.

ECM occurs in two basic forms: interstitial matrix and basement membrane (Fig. 1-13).

- *Interstitial matrix* is present in the spaces between cells in connective tissue, and between parenchymal epithelium and the underlying supportive vascular and smooth muscle structures. Interstitial matrix is synthesized by mesenchymal cells (e.g., fibroblasts), forming a three-dimensional, relatively amorphous gel. Its major constituents are fibrillar and nonfibrillar collagens, as well as fibronectin, elastin, proteoglycans, hyaluronate, and other constituents (see later).
- *Basement membrane.* The seemingly random array of interstitial matrix in connective tissues becomes highly organized around epithelial cells, endothelial cells, and smooth muscle cells, forming the specialized basement membrane. The basement membrane is synthesized by contributions from the overlying epithelium and underlying mesenchymal cells, forming a flat lamellar "chicken wire" mesh (although labeled as a *membrane*, it is quite porous). The major constituents are amorphous nonfibrillar type IV collagen and laminin.

Components of the Extracellular Matrix. The components of ECM fall into three groups of proteins (Fig. 1-14):

- *Fibrous structural proteins* such as collagens and elastins that confer tensile strength and recoil

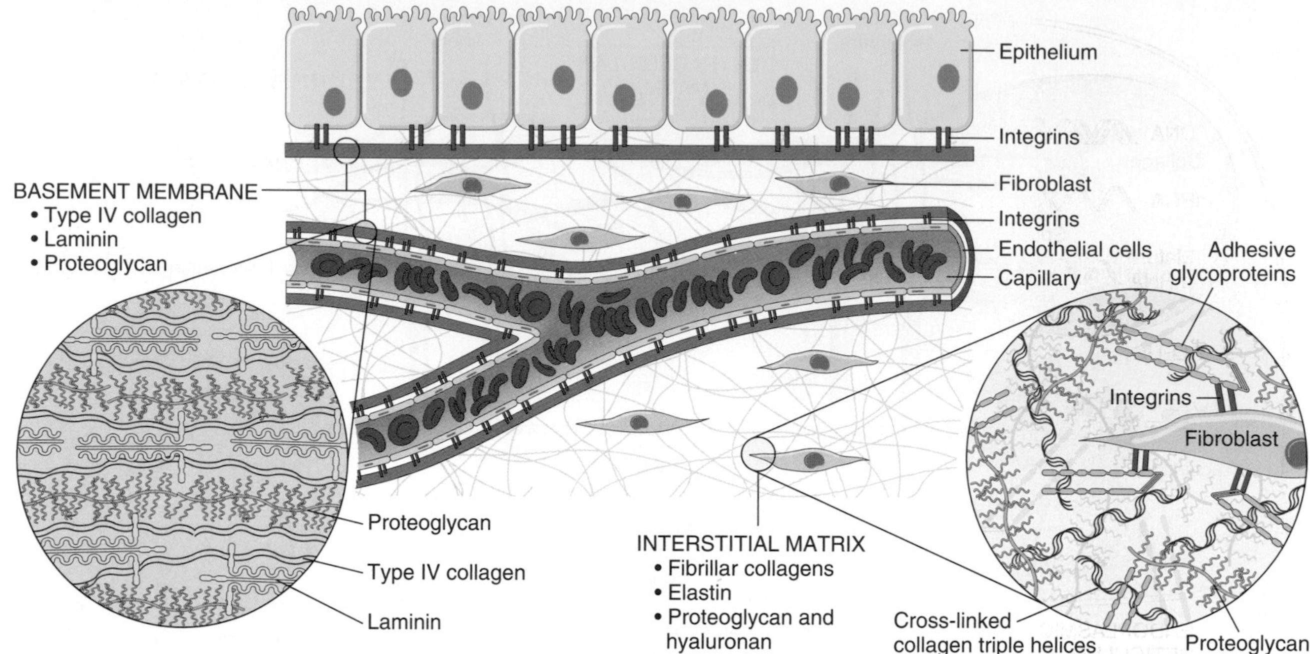

Figure 1-13 Main components of the extracellular matrix (ECM), including collagens, proteoglycans, and adhesive glycoproteins. Both epithelial and mesenchymal cells (e.g., fibroblasts) interact with ECM via integrins. Basement membranes and interstitial ECM have different architecture and general composition, although certain components are present in both. For the sake of clarity, many ECM components (e.g., elastin, fibrillin, hyaluronan, and syndecan) are not included.

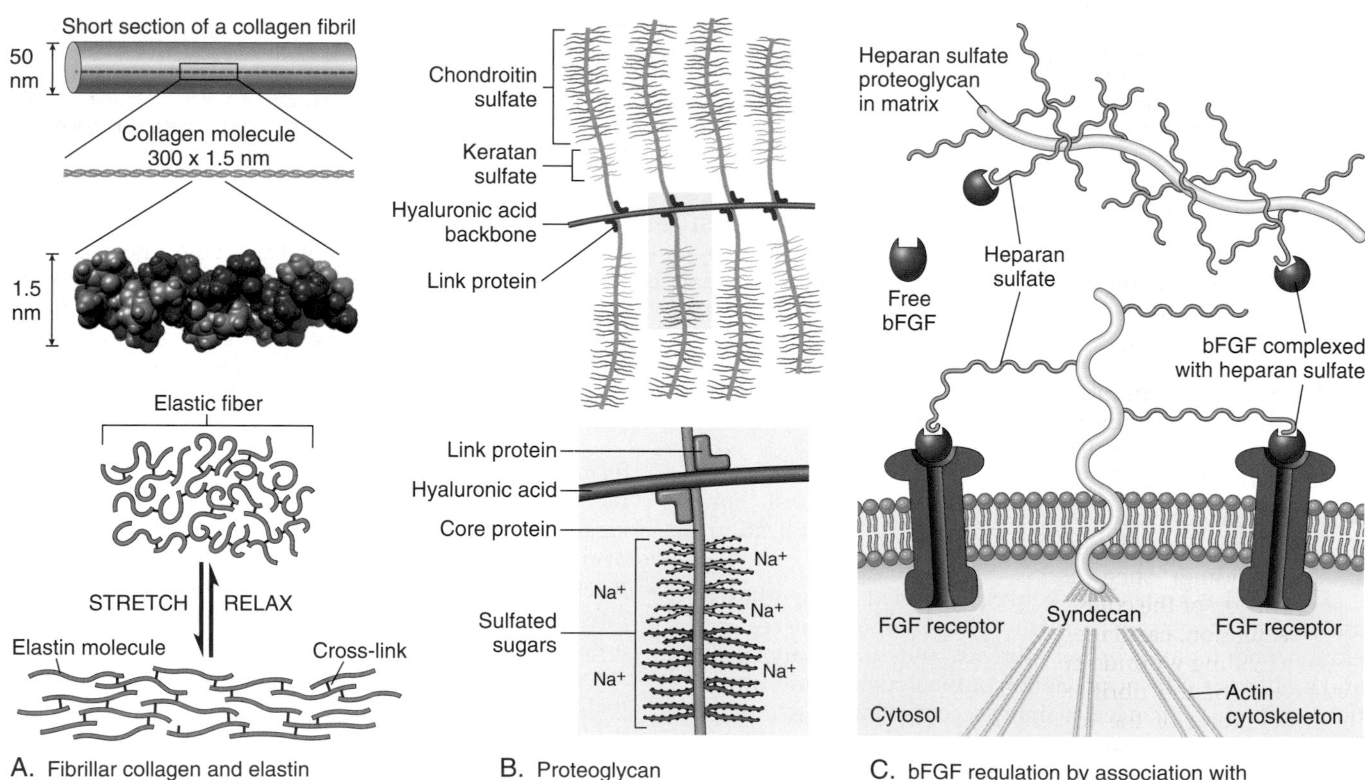

Figure 1-14 Extracellular matrix (ECM) components. **A,** Fibrillar collagen, and elastic tissue structures. Due to rodlike fibril stacking and extensive lateral cross-linking (through the activity of lysyl oxidase), collagen fibers have marked tensile strength but do not have much elasticity. Elastin is also massively cross-linked through lysyl oxidase activity but differs in having large hydrophobic segments that form a dense globular configuration at rest. As stretch is exerted, the hydrophobic domains are pulled open, but the cross-links keep the tissue intact; release of the stretch tension allows the hydrophobic domains of the proteins to refold. **B,** Proteoglycan structure. The highly negatively charged sulfated sugars on the proteoglycan "bristles" recruit sodium and water to generate a viscous, but compressible matrix. **C,** Regulation of basic fibroblast growth factor (bFGF, FGF-2) activity by ECM and cellular proteoglycans. Heparan sulfate binds bFGF secreted in the ECM. Syndecan is a cell surface proteoglycan with a transmembrane core protein and extracellular glycosaminoglycan side chains that can bind bFGF, with a cytoplasmic tail that interacts with the intracellular actin cytoskeleton. Syndecan side chains bind bFGF released from damaged ECM, thus facilitating a concentrated interaction with cell surface receptors.

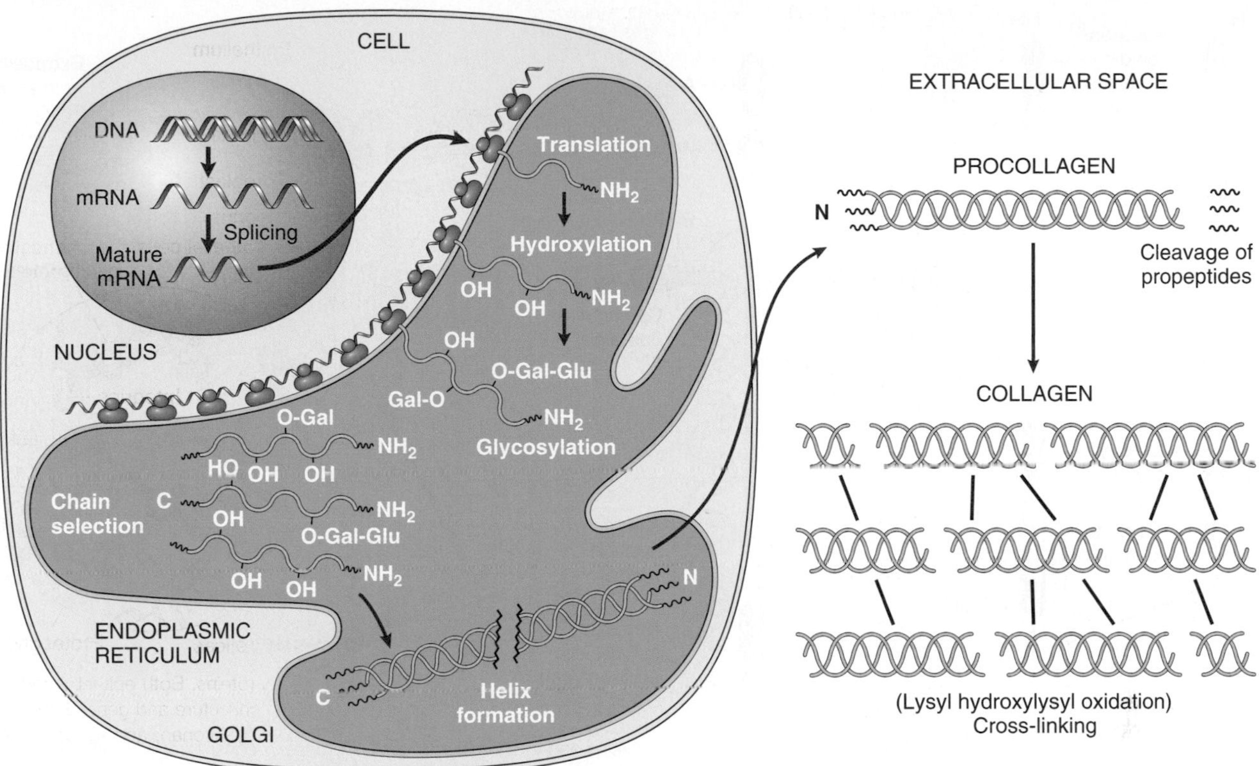

Figure 1-15 Collagen biosynthetic pathway. The α-chains that make up a fibrillar collagen molecule are synthesized as precursor pro-α-chains, with large globular polypeptide regions flanking the central triple-helical domain. After proline and lysine hydroxylation and lysine glycosylation within the endoplasmic reticulum, three procollagen chains align to form a triple helix. For all the fibrillar collagens, the C-propeptide is completely removed by endoproteinase activity after secretion, and the resulting triple-helical rod-like domains polymerize in a staggered fashion into fibrillar arrays. After secretion, the collagen achieves lateral stability though collagen cross-linking involving lysyl oxidase and the previously hydroxylated residues. Defects in primary sequence, procollagen endopeptidase processing, hydroxylation, or cross-linking can all lead to weak connective tissues. The specific tissues affected (e.g., blood vessels, skin, bone, ligaments) by such disorders is based on the type of collagen that predominates in that tissue.

- *Water-hydrated gels* such as proteoglycans and hyaluronan that permit compressive resistance and lubrication
- *Adhesive glycoproteins* that connect ECM elements to one another and to cells

Collagens. Collagens are typically composed of three separate polypeptide chains braided into a ropelike triple helix (Fig. 1-15). About 30 collagen types have been identified, some of which are unique to specific cells and tissues.

- Some collagen types (e.g., types I, II, III, and V collagens) form linear fibrils stabilized by interchain hydrogen bonding; such *fibrillar collagens* form a major proportion of the connective tissue in structures such as bone, tendon, cartilage, blood vessels, and skin, as well as in healing wounds and particularly scars. The tensile strength of the fibrillar collagens derives from lateral cross-linking of the triple helices, formed by covalent bonds facilitated by the activity of lysyl oxidase. Since this process is dependent on vitamin C, children with ascorbate deficiency have skeletal deformities, and people of any age with vitamin C deficiency bleed easily because of weak vascular wall basement membrane, and heal poorly. Genetic defects in collagens cause diseases such as *osteogenesis imperfecta* and certain forms of *Ehlers-Danlos syndrome* (Chapter 5).
- *Non-fibrillar* collagens may contribute to the structures of planar basement membranes (type IV collagen); help regulate collagen fibril diameters or collagen-collagen interactions via so-called **f**ibril-**a**ssociated **c**ollagen with **i**nterrupted **t**riple helices (FACITs, such as type IX collagen in cartilage); or provide anchoring fibrils to basement membrane beneath stratified squamous epithelium (type VII collagen).

Elastin. The ability of tissues to recoil and recover their shape after physical deformation is conferred by elastin (Fig. 1-14). This is especially important in cardiac valves and for large blood vessels (that must accommodate recurrent pulsatile flow), as well as in the uterus, skin, and ligaments. Morphologically, elastic fibers consist of a central core of elastin with an associated meshlike network composed of fibrillin. The latter relationship partially explains why fibrillin synthetic defects lead to skeletal abnormalities and weakened aortic walls, as in individuals with Marfan sydrome (Chapter 5).

Proteoglycans and hyaluronan (Fig. 1-14). Proteoglycans form highly hydrated compressible gels that confer resistance to compressive forces; in joint cartilage, proteoglycans also provide a layer of lubrication between adjacent boney surfaces. Proteoglycans consist of long polysaccharides, called *glycosaminoglycans* (examples are keratan sulfate and chondroitin sulfate) attached to a core protein; these are then linked to a long hyaluronic acid polymer

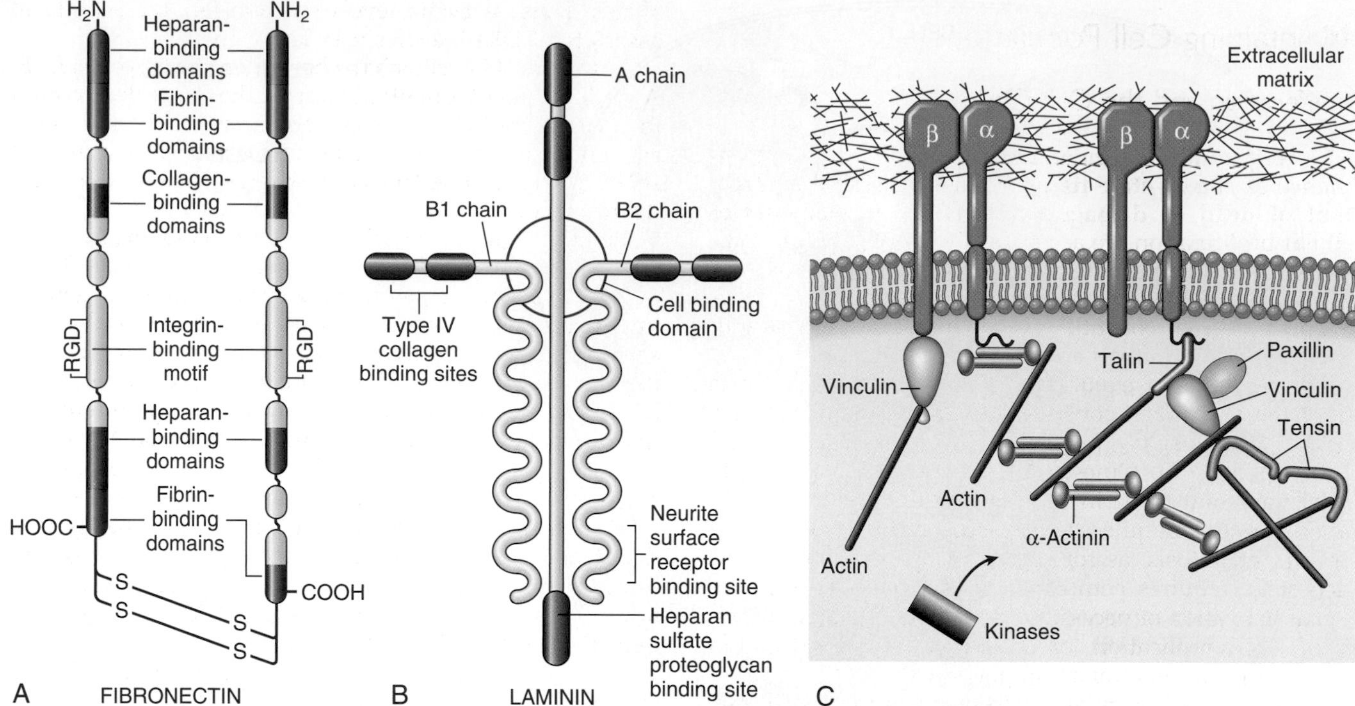

Figure 1-16 Cell and extracellular matrix (ECM) interactions: adhesive glycoproteins and integrin signaling. **A,** *Fibronectin* consists of a disulfide-linked dimer, with several distinct domains that allow binding to ECM and to integrins, the latter through arginine-glycine-aspartic acid (RGD) motifs. **B,** The cross-shaped *laminin* molecule is one of the major components of basement membranes; its multi-domain structure allows interactions between type IV collagen, other ECM components, and cell-surface receptors. **C,** Integrins and integrin-mediated signaling events at focal adhesion complexes. Each α-β heterodimeric integrin receptor is a transmembrane dimer that links ECM and intracellular cytoskeleton. It is also associated with a complex of linking molecules (e.g., vinculin, and talin) that can recruit and activate kinases that ultimately trigger downstream signaling cascades.

called *hyaluronan,* in a manner reminiscent of the bristles on a test tube brush. The highly negatively charged nature of the densely packed sulfated sugars pulls in cations (mostly sodium) that, in turn, osmotically attract water; the result is a viscous, gelatin-like matrix. Besides providing compressibility to tissues, proteoglycans also serve as reservoirs for growth factors secreted into the ECM (e.g., FGF and HGF). Some proteoglycans are integral cell membrane proteins that have roles in cell proliferation, migration, and adhesion, for example, by binding growth factors and chemokines and providing high local concentrations of these mediators (Fig. 1-14).

Adhesive glycoproteins and adhesion receptors are structurally diverse molecules variously involved in cell-to-cell adhesion, linking cells to the ECM, and the interactions between ECM components (Fig. 1-16). Prototypical adhesive glycoproteins include *fibronectin* (a major component of the interstitial ECM) and *laminin* (a major constituent of basement membrane). *Integrins* are representative of the adhesion receptors, also known as cell adhesion molecules (CAMs); the CAMs also include immunoglobulins, cadherins, and selectins.

- *Fibronectin* is a large (450 kD) disulfide-linked heterodimer that exists in tissue and plasma forms; it is synthesized by a variety of cells, including fibroblasts, monocytes, and endothelium. Fibronectin has specific domains that can bind to distinct ECM components (e.g., collagen, fibrin, heparin, and proteoglycans), as well as integrins (Fig. 1-16). In healing wounds, tissue and plasma fibronectin provide the scaffolding for subsequent ECM deposition, angiogenesis, and reepithelialization.
- *Laminin* is the most abundant glycoprotein in basement membrane. It is an 820-kD cross-shaped heterotrimer that connects cells to underlying ECM components such as type IV collagen and heparan sulfate (Fig. 1-16). Besides mediating attachment to basement membrane, laminin can also modulate cell proliferation, differentiation, and motility.
- *Integrins* are a large family of transmembrane heterodimeric glycoproteins (composed of α- and β-subunits) that allow cells to attach to ECM constituents such as laminin and fibronectin, thus functionally and structurally linking the intracellular cytoskeleton with the outside world. Integrins on the surface of leukocytes are also essential in mediating firm adhesion and transmigration across endothelium at sites of inflammation (Chapter 3), and they play a critical role in platelet aggregation (Chapter 4). Integrins attach to ECM components via a tripeptide arginine-glycine-aspartic acid motif (abbreviated RGD). Besides providing focal attachment to underlying substrates, binding through the integrin receptors can also trigger signaling cascades that can influence cell locomotion, proliferation, shape, and differentiation (Fig. 1-16).

Maintaining Cell Populations

Proliferation and the Cell Cycle

Cell proliferation is fundamental to development, maintenance of steady-state tissue homeostasis, and replacement of dead or damaged cells. The key elements of cellular proliferation are accurate DNA replication accompanied by the coordinated synthesis of all other cellular constituents, followed by equal apportionment of DNA and other cellular constituents (e.g., organelles) to daughter cells through mitosis and cytokinesis.

The sequence of events that results in cell division is called the *cell cycle;* it consists of G_1 (presynthetic *growth*), S (DNA *synthesis*), G_2 (premitotic *growth*), and M (*mitotic*) phases (Fig. 1-17). Quiescent cells that are not actively cycling are said to be in the G_0 state. Cells can enter G_1 either from the G_0 quiescent cell pool, or after completing a round of mitosis, as for continuously replicating cells. Each stage requires completion of the previous step, as well as activation of necessary factors (see later); nonfidelity of DNA replication, or cofactor deficiency result in arrest at the various transition points.

The cell cycle is regulated by activators and inhibitors. Cell cycle progression is driven by proteins called *cyclins*—named for the cyclic nature of their production and degradation—and cyclin-associated enzymes called *cyclin-dependent kinases* (CDKs) (Fig. 1-18). CDKs acquire the ability to phosphorylate protein substrates (i.e., kinase activity) by forming complexes with the relevant cyclins. Transiently increased synthesis of a particular cyclin leads to increased kinase activity of the appropriate CDK binding partner; as the CDK completes its round of phosphorylation, the associated cyclin is degraded and the CDK activity abates. Thus, as cyclin levels rise and fall, the activity of associated CDKs likewise wax and wane.

More than 15 cyclins have been identified; cyclins D, E, A, and B appear sequentially during the cell cycle and bind to one or more CDKs. The cell cycle can thus be conceived as a relay race in which each leg is regulated by a distinct set of cyclins: as one collection of cyclins leaves the track, the next set takes over.

Embedded in the cell cycle are surveillance mechanisms primed to sense DNA or chromosomal damage. These quality control *checkpoints* ensure that cells with genetic imperfections do not complete replication. Thus, the G_1-S checkpoint monitors the integrity of DNA before irreversibly committing cellular resources to DNA replication. Later in the cell cycle, the G_2-M restriction point ensures that there has been accurate genetic replication before the cell actually divides. When cells do detect DNA irregularities, checkpoint activation delays cell cycle progression and triggers DNA repair mechanisms. If the genetic derangement is too severe to be repaired, the cells will undergo apoptosis; alternatively, they may enter a nonreplicative state called *senescence*—primarily through p53-dependent mechanisms (see later).

Enforcing the cell cycle checkpoints is the job of *CDK inhibitors (CDKIs);* they accomplish this by modulating CDK-cyclin complex activity. There are several different CDKIs:

- One family—composed of three proteins called *p21* (CDKN1A), *p27* (CDKN1B), and *p57* (CDKN1C)—broadly inhibits multiple CDKs.
- The other family of CDKI proteins has selective effects on cyclin CDK4 and cyclin CDK6; these proteins are called *p15* (CDKN2B), *p16* (CDKN2A), *p18* (CDKN2C), and *p19* (CDKN2D).

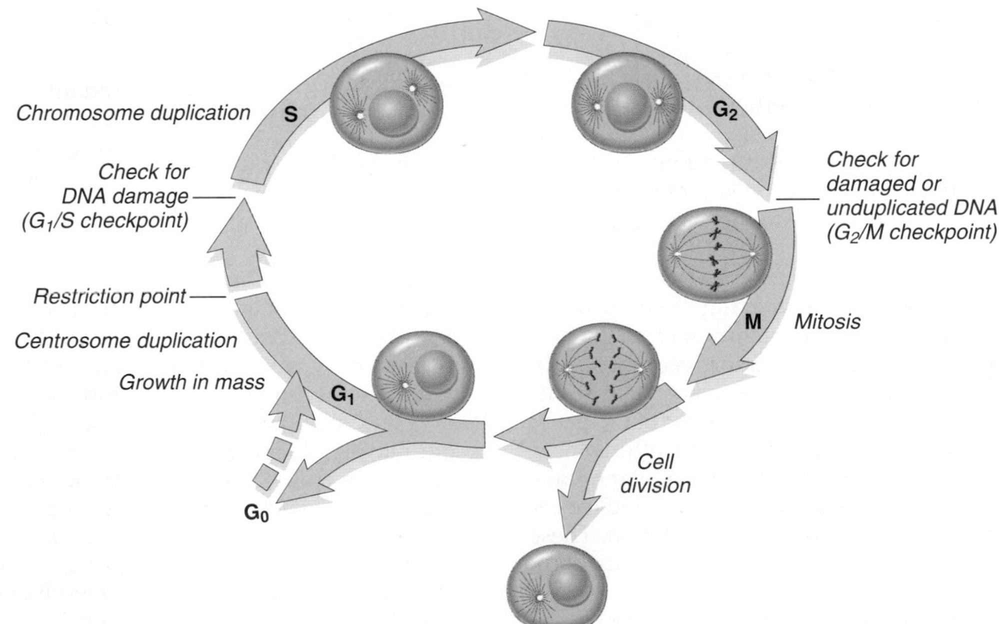

Figure 1-17 Cell cycle landmarks. The figure shows the cell cycle phases (G_0, G_1, G_2, S, and M), the location of the G_1 restriction point, and the G_1/S and G_2/M cell cycle checkpoints. Cells from labile tissues such as the epidermis and the GI tract may cycle continuously; stable cells such as hepatocytes are quiescent but can enter the cell cycle; permanent cells such as neurons and cardiac myocytes have lost the capacity to proliferate. (Modified from Pollard TD, Earnshaw WC: Cell Biology. Philadelphia, Saunders, 2002.)

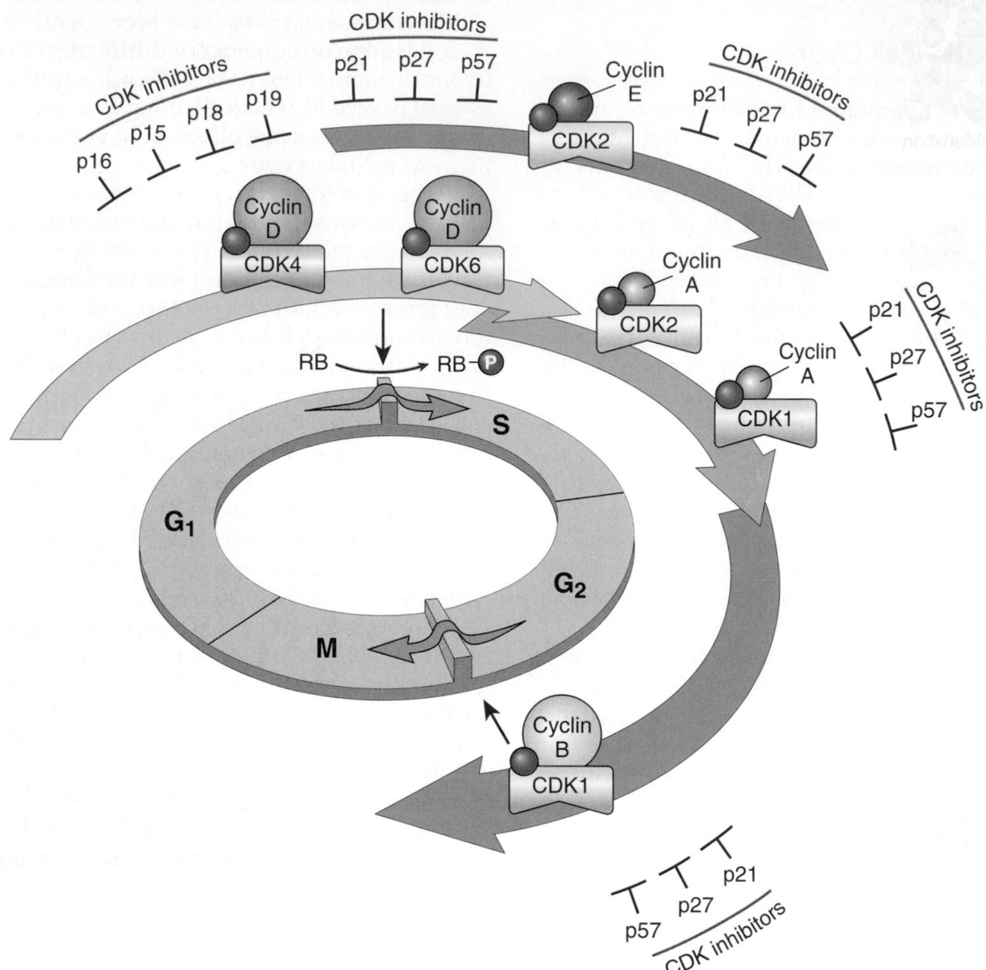

Figure 1-18 Role of cyclins, cyclin-dependent kinases (CDKs), and CDK inhibitors in regulating the cell cycle. The *shaded arrows* represent the phases of the cell cycle during which specific cyclin-CDK complexes are active. As illustrated, cyclin D-CDK4, cyclin D-CDK6, and cyclin E-CDK2 regulate the G_1-to-S transition by phosphorylating the Rb protein (pRb). Cyclin A-CDK2 and cyclin A-CDK1 are active in the S phase. Cyclin B-CDK1 is essential for the G_2-to-M transition. Two families of CDK inhibitors can block activity of CDKs and progression through the cell cycle. The so-called INK4 inhibitors, composed of p16, p15, p18, and p19, act on cyclin D-CDK4 and cyclin D-CDK6. The other family of three inhibitors, p21, p27, and p57, can inhibit all CDKs.

Defective CDKI checkpoint proteins allow cells with damaged DNA to divide, resulting in mutated daughter cells with the potential of developing into malignant tumors.

An equally important aspect of cell growth and division is the biosynthesis of other cellular components needed to make two daughter cells, such as membranes and organelles. At the same time that growth factor receptor signaling stimulates cell cycle progression, it also activates events that promote changes in cellular metabolism that support growth. Chief among these is the Warburg effect, mentioned earlier, which is marked by increased cellular uptake of glucose and glutamine, increased glycolysis, and (counter-intuitively) decreased oxidative phoshorylation. These changes become fixed in cancer cells and are discussed in greater detail in Chapter 7.

Stem Cells

During development, stem cells give rise to all the various differentiated tissues; in the adult organism, stem cells replace damaged cells and maintain tissue populations as individual cells within them undergo replicative senescence due to attrition of telomeres (described in chapter 2). There is a homeostatic equilibrium between the replication, self-renewal, and differentiation of stem cells and the death of the mature, fully differentiated cells (Fig. 1-19). The dynamic relationship between stem cells and terminally differentiated parenchyma is particularly evident in the continuously dividing epithelium of the skin. Thus, stem cells at the basal layer of the epithelium progressively differentiate as they migrate to the upper layers of the epithelium before dying and being shed.

Stem cells are characterized by two important properties:

- *Self-renewal*, which permits stem cells to maintain their numbers.
- *Asymmetric division,* in which one daughter cell enters a differentiation pathway and gives rise to mature cells, while the other remains undifferentiated and retains its self-renewal capacity.

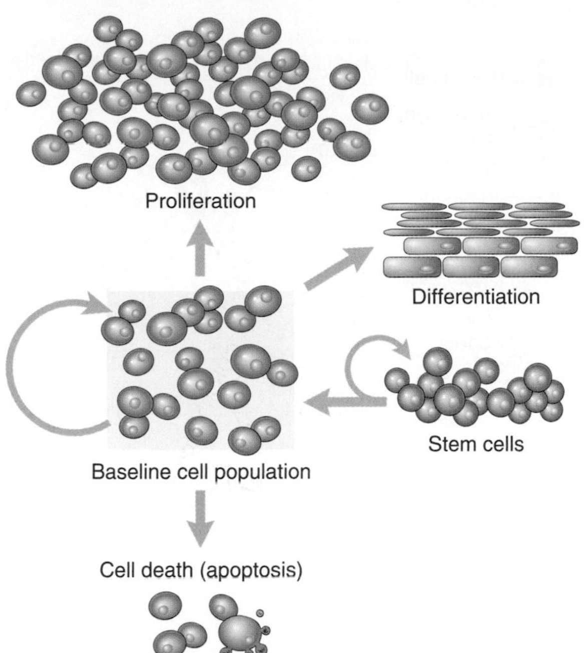

Figure 1-19 Mechanisms regulating cell populations. Cell numbers can be altered by increased or decreased rates of stem cell input, cell death due to apoptosis, or changes in the rates of proliferation or differentiation. (Modified from McCarthy NJ, et al: Apoptosis in the development of the immune system: growth factors, clonal selection and bcl-2. Cancer Metastasis Rev 11:157, 1992.)

Although there is a tendency in the scientific literature to partition stem cells into several different subsets, fundamentally there are only two varieties:

- *Embryonic stem cells (ES cells)* are the most undifferentiated. They are present in the inner cell mass of the blastocyst, have virtually limitless cell renewal capacity, and can give rise to every cell in the body; they are thus said to be *totipotent* (Fig. 1-20). While ES cells can be maintained for extended periods without differentiating, they can be induced under appropriate culture conditions to form specialized cells of all three germ cell layers, including neurons, cardiac muscle, liver cells, and pancreatic islet cells.
- *Tissue stem cells* (also called *adult stem cells*) are found in intimate association with the differentiated cells of a given tissue. They are normally protected within specialized tissue microenvironments called *stem cell niches*. Such niches have been demonstrated in many organs—including the brain, where neural stem cells inhabit the subventricular zone and dentate gyrus. Skin stem cells are found in the bulge region of the hair follicle, and in the cornea they are found at the limbus. Soluble factors and other cells within the niches keep the stem cells quiescent until there is a need for expansion and differentiation of the precursor pool (Fig. 1-21). Adult stem cells have a limited repertoire of differentiated cells that they can generate. Thus, although adult stem cells can maintain tissues with high (e.g., skin, and gastrointestinal tract) or low (e.g., heart and brain) cell turnover, the adult stem cells in any given tissue can usually only produce cells that are normal constituents of that tissue.

The most extensively studied of the tissue stem cells are the hematopoietic stem cells that continuously replenish all the cellular elements of the blood as they are consumed. Hematopoietic stem cells may be isolated directly from bone marrow, as well as from the peripheral blood after administration of certain colony stimulating factors (CSF) that induce their release from bone marrow niches. Although rare, hematopoietic stem cells can be purified to virtual homogeneity based on cell surface markers and ability to give rise to blood cell of lineages. Clinically, these stem cells can be used to repopulate marrows depleted

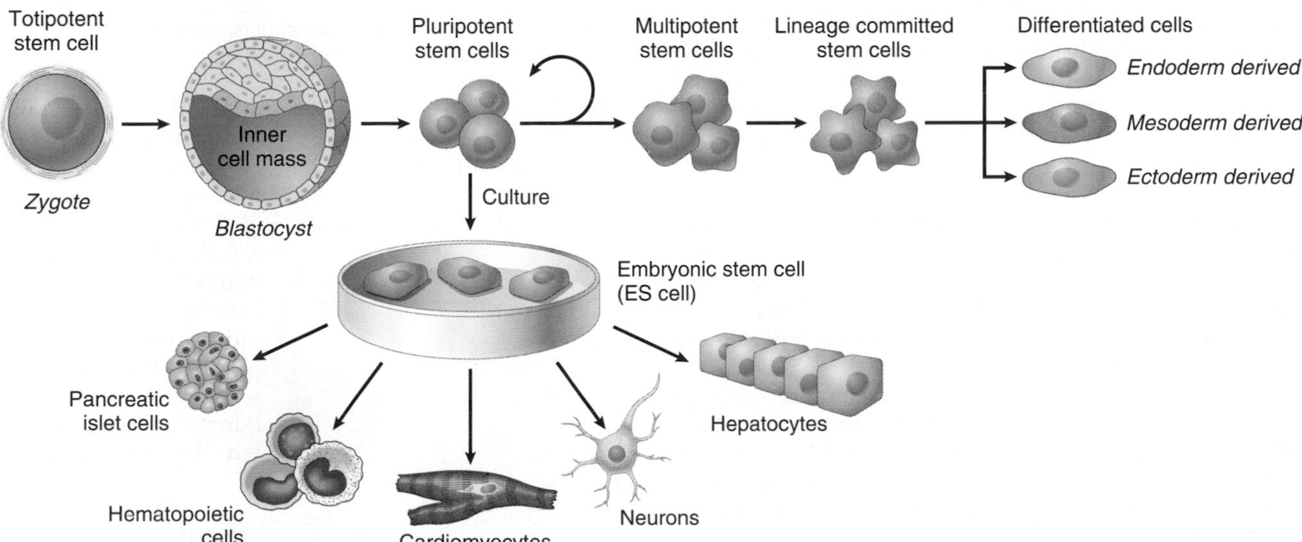

Figure 1-20 Embryonal stem cells. The zygote, formed by the union of sperm and egg, divides to form blastocysts, and the inner cell mass of the blastocyst generates the embryo. The pluripotent cells of the inner cell mass, known as embryonic stem (ES) cells, can be induced to differentiate into cells of multiple lineages. In the embryo, pluripotent stem cells can asymmetrically divide to yield a residual stable pool of ES cells in addition to generating populations that have progressively more restricted developmental capacity, eventually generating stem cells that are committed to just specific lineages. ES cells can be cultured in vitro and be induced to give rise to cells of all three lineages.

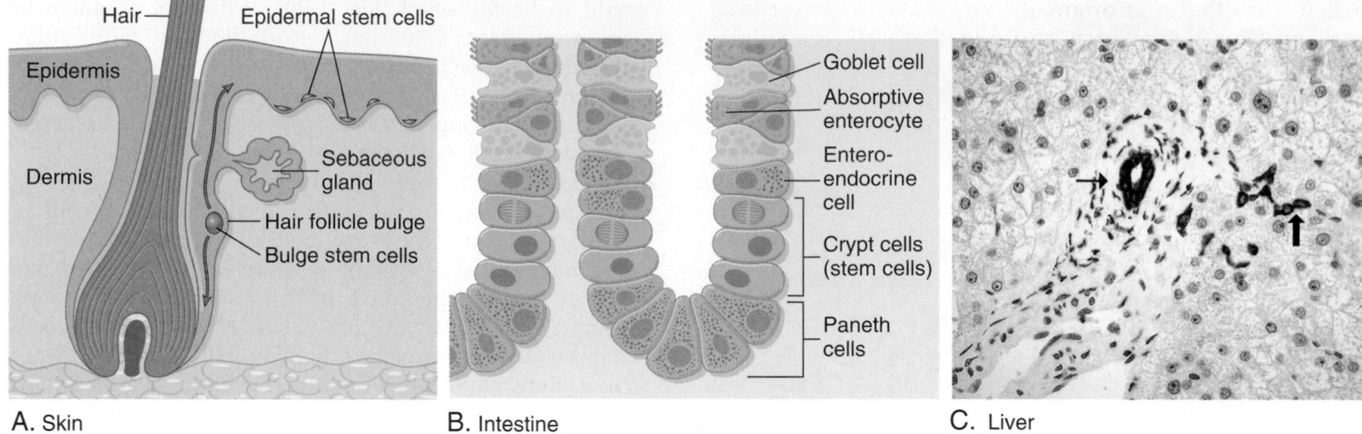

Figure 1-21 Stem cell niches in various tissues. **A,** Skin stem cells are located in the bulge area of the hair follicle, in sebaceous glands, and in the lower layer of the epidermis. **B,** Small intestine stem cells are located near the base of the crypt, above Paneth cells. **C,** Liver stem cells (*oval cells*) are located in the canals of Hering (*thick arrow*), structures that connect bile ductules (*thin arrow*) to parenchymal hepatocytes. Bile duct cells and canals of Hering are stained here with an immunohistochemical stain for cytokeratin 7. (**C,** Courtesy Tania Roskams, MD, University of Leuven, Belgium).

after chemotherapy (e.g., for leukemia), or to provide normal precursors to correct various blood cell defects (e.g., sickle cell disease, Chapter 14).

Besides hematopoietic stem cells, the bone marrow (and notably, other tissues such as fat) also contains a population of *mesenchymal stem cells*. These are multipotent cells that can differentiate into a variety of stromal cells including chondrocytes (cartilage), osteocytes (bone), adipocytes (fat), and myocytes (muscle). Because these cells can be expanded to large numbers, and can also generate a locally immunosuppressive microenvironment (thus potentially evading rejection), they may represent a ready means of manufacturing the stromal cellular scaffolding for tissue regeneration.

Regenerative Medicine

The ability to identify, isolate, expand, and transplant stem cells has given birth to the new field of regenerative medicine. Theoretically, the differentiated progeny of ES or adult stem cells can be used to repopulate damaged tissues, or to construct entire organs for replacement. In particular, there is considerable excitement about the therapeutic opportunities for restoring damaged tissues that have low intrinsic regenerative capacity, such as myocardium after a myocardial infarct or neurons after a stroke. Unfortunately, despite an improving ability to purify and expand stem cell populations, much of the initial enthusiasm has been tempered by difficulties encountered in introducing and *functionally integrating* the replacement cells into sites of damage.

Another potential problem is the immunogenecity of most stem cells; although mesenchymal stem cells may be weakly immunogenic, most other adult stem cells, as well as ES cells (from fertilized blastocysts), express histocompatibility (HLA) molecules of the sperm and egg donors that provoke immunologic rejection by the host (Chapter 6). Hence, considerable effort has been expended to generate cells that are totipotential like ES cells but are derived from the patient into whom they will be implanted. To accomplish this, a handful of genes have been identified whose products can—remarkably—reprogram somatic cells to achieve the "stem-ness" of ES cells. When such genes are introduced into fully differentiated cells (e.g., fibroblasts), *induced pluripotent stem cells (iPS cells)* are generated (Fig. 1-22). Since these cells are derived from the patient, their differentiated progeny (e.g., insulin-secreting β-cells in a patient with diabetes) can be engrafted without eliciting a rejection reaction. Another exciting recent development is genomic editing, a process using a nuclease

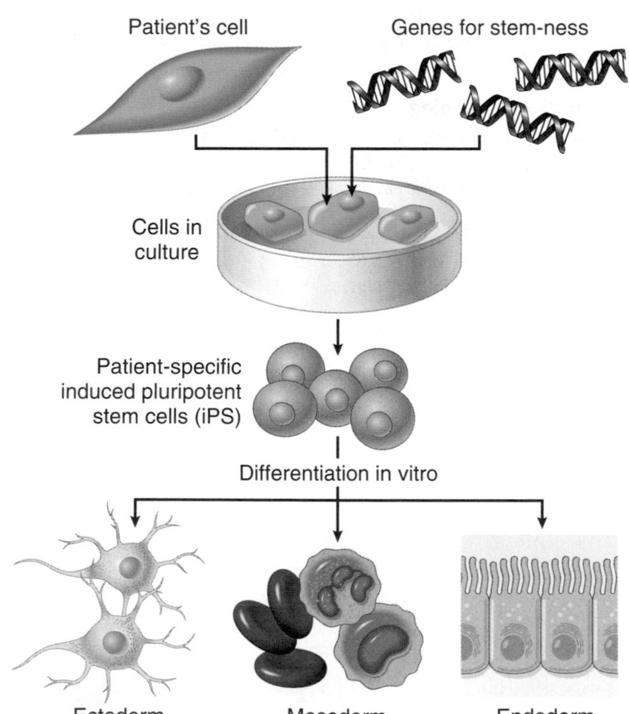

Figure 1-22 The production of induced pluripotent stem cells (iPS cells). Genes that confer stem cell properties are introduced into a patient's differentiated cells, giving rise to stem cells that can be induced to differentiate into various lineages. (Modified from Hochedlinger K, Jaenisch R: Nuclear transplantation, embryonic stem cells, and the potential for cell therapy. N Engl J Med 349:275-286, 2003.)

called Cas9 that was originally identified in prokaryotes that can be used together with guide RNAs called CRISPRs to selectively alter or correct DNA sequences, such as disease-causing mutations. While iPS cells and Cas9 technology hold considerable promise, whether they are the Holy Grail of tissue regeneration remains to be seen.

Concluding Remarks. This survey of selected topics in cell biology will serve as a basis for our later discussions of pathology, and we will refer back to it throughout the book. Students should, however, remember that this summary is intentionally brief, and more information about some of the fascinating topics reviewed here can be readily found in textbooks devoted to cell and molecular biology.

SUGGESTED READINGS

Genetics and Epigenetics

Cech TR, Steitz JA: The noncoding RNA revolution—trashing old rules to forge new ones. *Cell* 157:77, 2014. [*An excellent review of the roles played by non- coding RNAs.*]

Hübner MR, Eckersley-Maslin MA, Spector DL: Chromatin organization and transcriptional regulation. *Curr Opin Genet Dev* 23:89, 2013. [*Nice discussion of genome organization and chromatin structure-function relationships that regulate cell type-specific nuclear transcription.*]

Jarovcevski M, Akbarian S: Epigenetic mechanisms in neurologic disease. *Nat Med* 18:1194, 2012. [*A well-written overview of genomic organization and transcriptional regulation, with a specific focus on neurologic disease.*]

Teperino R, Lempradl A, Pospisilik JA: Bridging epigenomics and complex disease: the basics. *Cell Mol Life Sci* 70:1609, 2013. [*An introductory review of the epigenetic basis for human disease.*]

Wang KC, Chang HY: Molecular mechanisms of long noncoding RNAs. *Mol Cell* 43:904, 2011. [*Excellent review examining the rapidly expanding universe of long non-coding RNA species, with discussion of their form and function, and roles as signal transducers.*]

Cellular Housekeeping

Andersson ER: The role of endocytosis in activating and regulating signal transduction. *Cell Mol Life Sci* 69:1755, 2011. [*Overview of endocytosis with specific emphasis on its role in modulating intracellular signaling.*]

Choi AM, Ryter SW, Levine B: Autophagy in human health and disease. *N Eng J Med* 368:651, 2013. [*Superb review concerning the physiologic and pathophysiologic aspects of autophagy.*]

English AR, Zurek N, Voeltz GK: Peripheral ER structure and function. *Curr Opin Cell Biol* 21:596, 2009. [*Overview of the structural and functional organization of the endoplasmic reticulum and its relationship to other cellular organelles.*]

Guillot C, Lecuit T: Mechanics of epithelial tissue homeostasis and morphogenesis. *Science* 340:1185, 2013. [*Topical discussion about cellular interactions and the mechanical basis of tissue maintenance.*]

Simons K, Sampaio JL: Membrane organization and lipid rafts. *Cold Spring Harb Perspect Biol* 3:1, 2013. [*Nice review of the general principles of membrane architecture and emphasizing domain organization.*]

Wong E, Cuervo AM: Integration of clearance mechanisms: the proteasome and autophagy. *Cold Spring Harb Perspect Biol* 2:1, 2010. [*Overview of intracellular degradation pathways, specifically focusing on the elimination of aberrant or abnormal constituents.*]

Cellular Metabolism and Mitochondrial Function

Dang CV: Links between metabolism and cancer. *Genes Dev* 26:877, 2012. [*An excellent review on metabolic functions of mitochondria.*]

Kushnareva Y, Newmeyer DD: Bioenergetics and cell death. *Ann NY Acad Sci* 1201:50, 2010. [*Overview of the mitochondrial outer membrane permeabilization and its role in apoptosis and bioenergetics*].

Tait SW, Green DR: Mitochondria and cell death: outer membrane permeabilization and beyond. *Nat Rev Mol Cell Biol* 11:621, 2010. [*Review of the role of mitochondria in cell death pathways.*]

Cellular Activation

Deupi X, Kobilka B: Activation of G protein-coupled receptors. *Adv Protein Chem* 74:137, 2007. [*Good overview of the fundamental mechanisms of the activation of these receptors.*]

Duronio RJ, Xiong Y: Signaling pathways that control cell proliferation. *Cold Spring Harb Perspect Biol* 5:1, 2013. [*Excellent overall review of cell signaling and proliferation.*]

Morrison DK: MAP kinase pathways. *Cold Spring Harb Perspect Biol* 4:1, 2012. [*Review of mitogen-activated kinase signaling pathways.*]

Perona R: Cell signalling: growth factors and tyrosine kinase receptors. *Clin Transl Oncol* 8:77, 2011. [*Update on signaling pathways with an emphasis on how these become dysregulated in malignancy.*]

Maintaining Cell Populations

Alvarado AS, Yamanaka S: Rethinking differentiation: stem cells, regeneration, and plasticity. *Cell* 157:110, 2014.

Fuchs E, Chen T: A matter of life and death: self-renewal in stem cells. *EMBO Rep* 14:39, 2013. [*Scholarly review on the conceptual framework and experimental underpinnings of our understanding regarding stem cell renewal, using cutaneous stem cells as a paradigm.*]

Li M, Liu GH, Izpisua-Belmonte JC: Navigating the epigenetic landscape of pluripotent stem cells. *Nat Rev Mol Cell Biol* 13:524, 2012. [*Good discussion of the epigenetic regulation of stem cell proliferation and subsequent differentiation.*]

See TARGETED THERAPY available online at www.studentconsult.com

CHAPTER 2

Cellular Responses to Stress and Toxic Insults: Adaptation, Injury, and Death

CHAPTER CONTENTS

Introduction to Pathology

Pathology is devoted to the study of the structural, biochemical, and functional changes in cells, tissues, and organs that underlie disease. By the use of molecular, microbiologic, immunologic, and morphologic techniques, pathology attempts to explain the whys and wherefores of the signs and symptoms manifested by patients while providing a rational basis for clinical care and therapy. It thus serves as the bridge between the basic sciences and clinical medicine, and is the scientific foundation for all of medicine. In chapter 1 we examined the cellular and molecular mechanisms that "define" healthy cells. In this chapter we will build upon that knowledge to discuss the fundamental mechanisms that underlie various forms of cell injury and death.

Traditionally the study of pathology is divided into general pathology and systemic pathology. General pathology is concerned with the common reactions of cells and tissues to injurious stimuli. Such reactions are often not tissue specific: thus acute inflammation in response to bacterial infections produces a very similar reaction in most tissues. On the other hand, systemic pathology examines the alterations and underlying mechanisms in organ specific diseases such as ischemic heart disease. In this book we first cover the principles of general pathology and then proceed to specific disease processes as they affect particular organs or systems.

The four aspects of a disease process that form the core of pathology are its cause *(etiology)*, the biochemical and molecular mechanisms of its development *(pathogenesis)*, the structural alterations induced in the cells and organs of the body *(morphologic changes)*, and the functional consequences of these changes *(clinical manifestations)*.

Etiology or ***Cause.*** Although there are myriads of factors that cause disease, they can all be grouped into two classes: genetic (e.g., inherited mutations and disease-associated gene variants, or polymorphisms) and acquired (e.g., infectious, nutritional, chemical, physical). The idea that one etiologic agent is the cause of one disease—developed from the study of infections and inherited disorders caused by single genes—is not applicable to the majority of diseases. In fact, most of our common afflictions, such as atherosclerosis and cancer, are multifactorial and arise from the effects of various external triggers on a genetically susceptible individual. The relative contribution of inherited susceptibility and external influences varies in different diseases.

***Pathogenesis. Pathogenesis* refers to the sequence of cellular, biochemical, and molecular events that follow the exposure of cells or tissues to an injurious agent.** The study of pathogenesis remains one of the main domains of pathology. Even when the initial cause is known (e.g., infection or mutation), it is many steps removed from the expression of the disease. For example, to understand cystic fibrosis it is essential to know not only the defective gene and gene product, but also the biochemical and morphologic events leading to the formation of cysts and fibrosis in the lungs, pancreas, and other organs. Indeed, as we shall see throughout the book, the mutated genes underlying a great number of diseases have been identified, but the functions of the encoded proteins and how mutations induce disease—the pathogenesis—are still not fully understood. With more research into clinical genomics it may become feasible to link specific molecular abnormalities to disease manifestations and to possibly use this knowledge to design new therapeutic approaches. For these reasons, the study of pathogenesis has never been more exciting scientifically or more relevant to medicine.

***Morphologic Changes.* Morphologic changes refer to the structural alterations in cells or tissues that are either characteristic of a disease or diagnostic of an etiologic process.** Traditionally, the practice of diagnostic pathology has used morphology to determine the nature of disease and to follow its progression. Although morphology remains a diagnostic cornerstone, its limitations have been evident for many years. For example, morphologically identical lesions may arise by distinct molecular mechanisms. Nowhere is this more striking than in the study of tumors; breast cancers that are indistinguishable morphologically may have widely different courses, therapeutic responses, and prognosis. Molecular analysis by techniques such as next generation sequencing (Chapter 5) has begun to reveal genetic differences that predict the behavior of the tumors as well as their responsiveness to different therapies. Increasingly, targeted therapies based on molecular alterations are being used for the treatment of cancers. Hence the field of diagnostic pathology has expanded to include molecular biologic and proteomic approaches for analyzing disease states.

Functional Derangements and Clinical Manifestations. The end results of genetic, biochemical, and structural changes in cells and tissues are functional abnormalities, which lead to the clinical manifestations (symptoms and signs) of disease, as well as its progress (clinical course and outcome). Hence, clinicopathologic correlations are very important in the study of disease.

Virtually all forms of disease start with molecular or structural alterations in cells. This concept of the cellular basis of disease was first put forth in the nineteenth century by Rudolf Virchow, known as the father of modern pathology. We therefore begin our consideration of pathology with the study of the causes, mechanisms, and morphologic and biochemical correlates of *cell injury*. Injury to cells and to extracellular matrix ultimately leads to *tissue and organ injury*, which determines the morphologic and clinical patterns of disease.

Overview: Cellular Responses to Stress and Noxious Stimuli

The normal cell is confined to a fairly narrow range of function and structure by its state of metabolism, differentiation, and specialization; by constraints of neighboring cells; and by the availability of metabolic substrates. It is nevertheless able to handle physiologic demands, maintaining a steady state called *homeostasis*. *Adaptations* are reversible functional and structural responses to changes

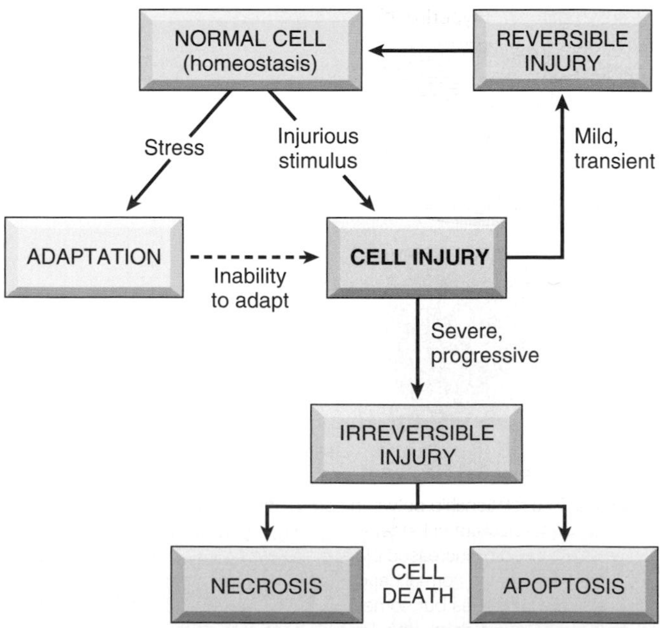

Figure 2-1 Stages of the cellular response to stress and injurious stimuli.

Table 2-1 Cellular Responses to Injury

Nature of Injurious Stimulus	Cellular Response
Altered physiologic stimuli; some nonlethal injurious stimuli	Cellular adaptations
Increased demand, increased stimulation (e.g., by growth factors, hormones)	Hyperplasia, hypertrophy
Decreased nutrients, decreased stimulation	Atrophy
Chronic irritation (physical or chemical)	Metaplasia
Reduced oxygen supply; chemical injury; microbial infection	Cell injury
Acute and transient	Acute reversible injury Cellular swelling fatty change
Progressive and severe (including DNA damage)	Irreversible injury → cell death Necrosis Apoptosis
Metabolic alterations, genetic or acquired; chronic injury	Intracellular accumulations; calcification
Cumulative sublethal injury over long life span	Cellular aging

in physiologic states (e.g., pregnancy) and some pathologic stimuli, during which new but altered steady states are achieved, allowing the cell to survive and continue to function (Fig. 2-1 and Table 2-1). The adaptive response may consist of an increase in the size of cells (hypertrophy) and functional activity, an increase in their number (hyperplasia), a decrease in the size and metabolic activity of cells (atrophy), or a change in the phenotype of cells (metaplasia). When the stress is eliminated the cell can recover to its original state without having suffered any harmful consequences.

If the limits of adaptive responses are exceeded or if cells are exposed to injurious agents or stress, deprived of essential nutrients, or become compromised by mutations that affect essential cellular constituents, a sequence of events follows that is termed cell injury (Fig. 2-1). Cell injury is *reversible* up to a certain point, but if the stimulus persists or is severe enough from the beginning, the cell suffers *irreversible injury* and ultimately undergoes *cell death. Adaptation, reversible injury,* and *cell death* may be stages of progressive impairment following different types of insults. For instance, in response to increased hemodynamic loads, the heart muscle becomes enlarged, a form of adaptation, and can then become injured. If the blood supply to the myocardium is compromised or inadequate, the muscle first suffers reversible injury, manifested by certain cytoplasmic changes (described later). Eventually, the cells suffer irreversible injury and die (Fig. 2-2).

Cell death, the end result of progressive cell injury, is one of the most crucial events in the evolution of disease in any tissue or organ. It results from diverse causes, including ischemia (reduced blood flow), infection, and toxins. Cell death is also a normal and essential process in embryogenesis, the development of organs, and the maintenance of

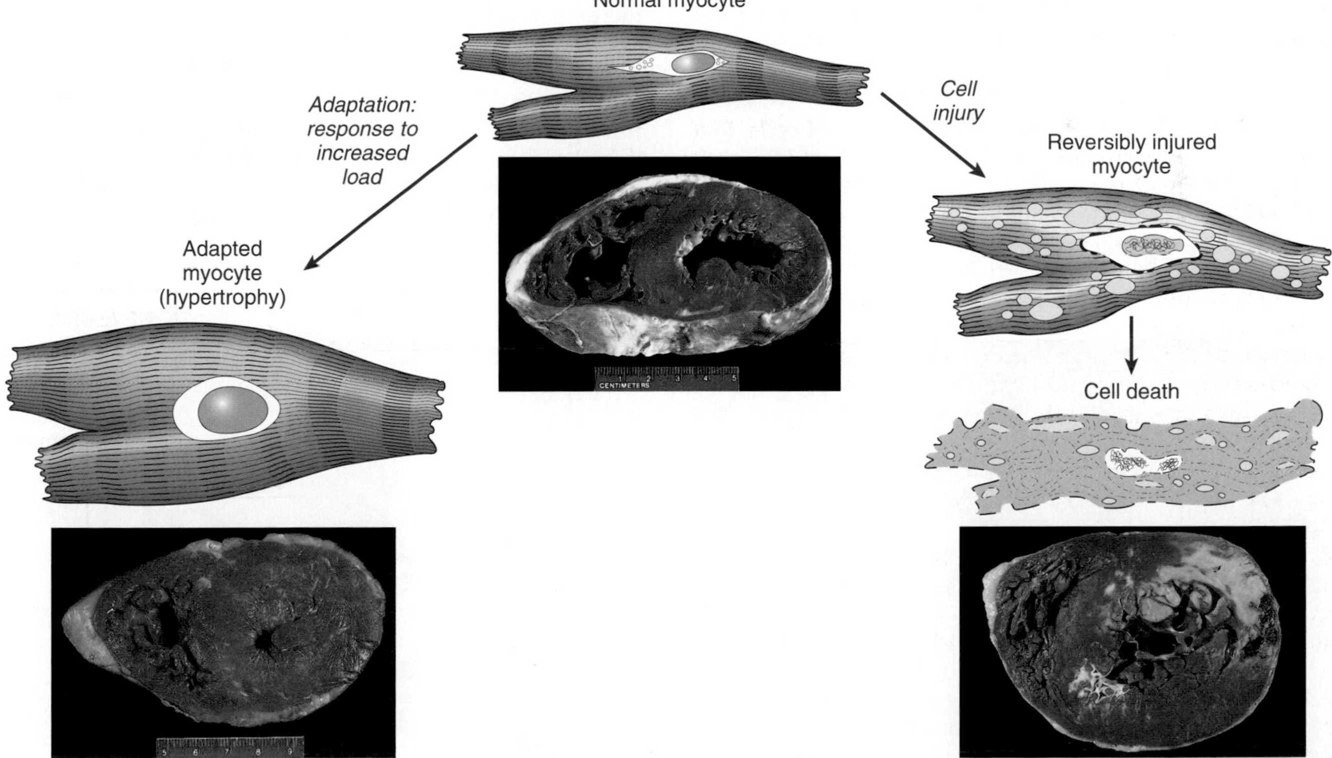

Figure 2-2 The relationship between normal, adapted, reversibly injured, and dead myocardial cells. All three transverse sections of the heart have been stained with triphenyltetrazolium chloride, an enzyme substrate that colors viable myocardium magenta. The cellular adaptation shown here is myocardial hypertrophy *(lower left)*, caused by increased blood pressure requiring greater mechanical effort by myocardial cells. This adaptation leads to thickening of the left ventricular wall (compare with the normal heart). In reversibly injured myocardium (illustrated schematically, *right*), there are functional alterations, usually without any gross or microscopic changes but sometimes with cytoplasmic changes such as cellular swelling and fat accumulation. In the specimen showing necrosis, a form of cell death *(lower right)*, the light area in the posterolateral left ventricle represents an acute myocardial infarction caused by reduced blood flow (ischemia).

homeostasis. There are two principal pathways of cell death, *necrosis* and *apoptosis*. Nutrient deprivation triggers an adaptive cellular response called *autophagy* that may also culminate in cell death. A detailed discussion of these pathways of cell death follows later in the chapter.

Stresses of different types may induce changes in cells and tissues other than typical adaptations, cell injury, and death (Table 2-1). Metabolic derangements in cells and sublethal, chronic injury may be associated with *intracellular accumulations* of a number of substances, including proteins, lipids, and carbohydrates. Calcium is often deposited at sites of cell death, resulting in *pathologic calcification*. Finally, the normal process of *aging* is accompanied by characteristic morphologic and functional changes in cells.

This chapter discusses first how cells adapt to stresses, and then the causes, mechanisms, and consequences of the various forms of acute cell damage, including reversible cell injury, and cell death. We conclude with three other processes that affect cells and tissues: intracellular accumulations, pathologic calcification, and cell aging.

Adaptations of Cellular Growth and Differentiation

Adaptations are reversible changes in the size, number, phenotype, metabolic activity, or functions of cells in response to changes in their environment. Such adaptations may take several distinct forms.

Hypertrophy

Hypertrophy refers to an increase in the size of cells, that results in an increase in the size of the affected organ. The hypertrophied organ has no new cells, just larger cells. The increased size of the cells is due to the synthesis and assembly of additional intracellular structural components. Cells capable of division may respond to stress by undergoing both hyperplasia (described later) and hypertrophy, whereas in non dividing (e.g., myocardial fibers) increased tissue mass is due to hypertrophy. In many organs hypertrophy and hyperplasia may coexist and contribute to increased size.

Hypertrophy can be *physiologic* or *pathologic;* the former is caused by increased functional demand or by stimulation by hormones and growth factors. The striated muscle cells in the heart and skeletal muscles have only a limited capacity for division, and respond to increased metabolic demands mainly by undergoing hypertrophy. *The most common stimulus for hypertrophy of muscle is increased workload.* For example, the bulging muscles of bodybuilders engaged in "pumping iron" result from enlargement of individual muscle fibers in response to increased demand. In the heart, the stimulus for hypertrophy is usually chronic hemodynamic overload, resulting from either hypertension or faulty valves (Fig. 2-2). In both tissue types the muscle cells synthesize more proteins and the number of myofilaments increases. This increases the amount of force each myocyte can generate, and thus increases the strength and work capacity of the muscle as a whole.

The massive physiologic growth of the uterus during pregnancy is a good example of hormone-induced enlargement an organ that results mainly from hypertrophy of muscle fibers (Fig. 2-3). Uterine hypertrophy is stimulated by estrogenic hormones acting on smooth muscle through estrogen receptors, eventually resulting in increased synthesis of smooth muscle proteins and an increase in cell size.

Mechanisms of Hypertrophy

Hypertrophy is the result of increased production of cellular proteins. Much of our understanding of hypertrophy is based on studies of the heart. There is great interest in defining the molecular basis of hypertrophy since beyond a certain point, hypertrophy of the heart becomes maladaptive and can lead to heart failure, arrhythmias and

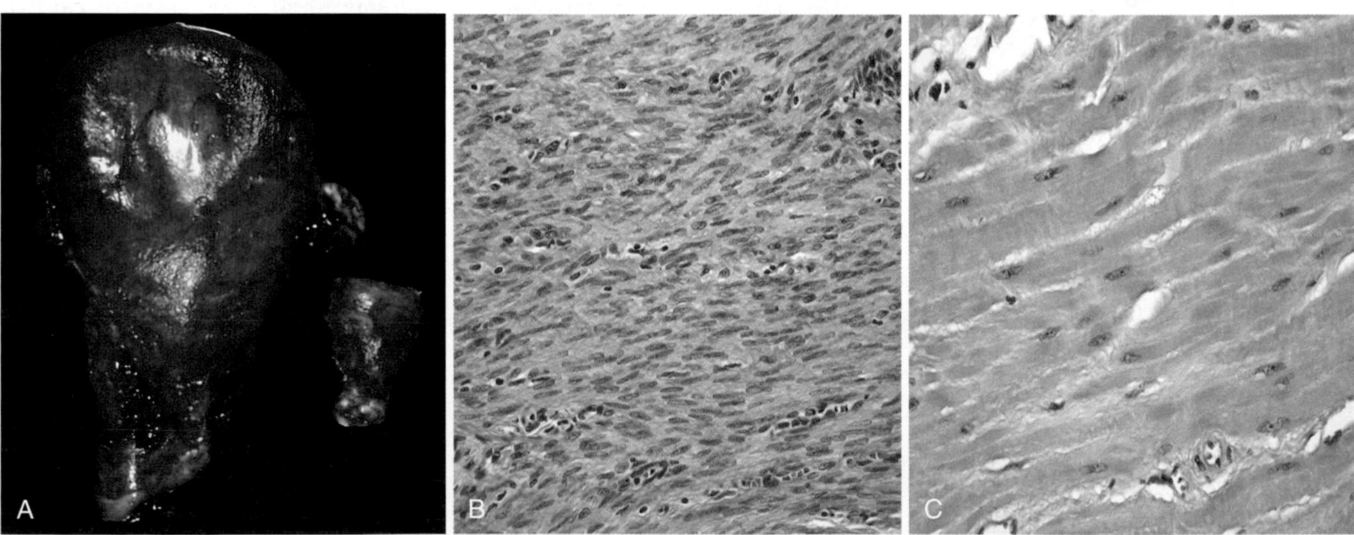

Figure 2-3 Physiologic hypertrophy of the uterus during pregnancy. **A,** Gross appearance of a normal uterus *(right)* and a gravid uterus (removed for postpartum bleeding) *(left)*. **B,** Small spindle-shaped uterine smooth muscle cells from a normal uterus, compared with **C,** large plump cells from the gravid uterus, at the same magnification.

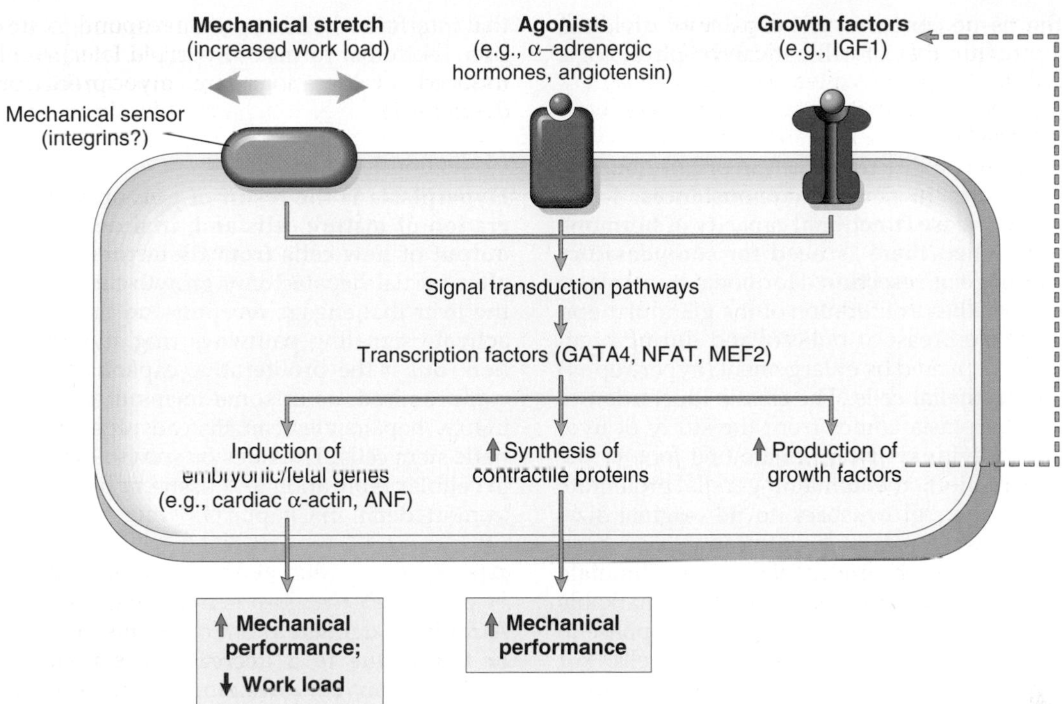

Figure 2-4 Biochemical mechanisms of myocardial hypertrophy. The major known signaling pathways and their functional effects are shown. Mechanical sensors appear to be the major triggers for physiologic hypertrophy, and agonists and growth factors may be more important in pathologic states. ANF, Atrial natriuretic factor; GATA4, transcription factor that binds to DNA sequence GATA; IGF1, insulin-like growth factor; NFAT, nuclear factor activated T cells; MEF2, myocardial enhancing factor 2.

sudden death (Chapter 11). There are three basic steps in the molecular pathogenesis of cardiac hypertrophy:

- The integrated actions of mechanical sensors (that are triggered by increased workload), growth factors (including TGF-β, insulin-like growth factor 1 [IGF1], fibroblast growth factor), and vasoactive agents (e.g., α-adrenergic agonists, endothelin-1, and angiotensin II). Indeed, mechanical sensors themselves induce production of growth factors and agonists (Fig. 2-4).
- These signals originating in the cell membrane activate a complex web of signal transduction pathways. Two such biochemical pathways involved in muscle hypertrophy are the phosphoinositide 3-kinase (PI3K)/AKT pathway (postulated to be most important in physiologic, e.g., exercise-induced, hypertrophy) and signaling downstream of G-protein–coupled receptors (induced by many growth factors and vasoactive agents, and thought to be more important in pathologic hypertrophy).
- These signaling pathways activate a set of transcription factors such as GATA4, nuclear factor of activated T cells (NFAT), and myocyte enhancer factor 2 (MEF2). These transcription factors work coordinately to increase the synthesis of muscle proteins that are responsible for hypertrophy.

Hypertrophy is also associated with a switch of contractile proteins from adult to fetal or neonatal forms. For example, during muscle hypertrophy, the α isoform of myosin heavy chain is replaced by the β isoform, which has a slower, more energetically economical contraction. In addition, some genes that are expressed only during early development are reexpressed in hypertrophic cells, and the products of these genes participate in the cellular response to stress. For example, the gene for atrial natriuretic factor is expressed in both the atrium and the ventricle in the embryonic heart, but it is down-regulated after birth. Cardiac hypertrophy is associated with increased atrial natriuretic factor gene expression. Atrial natriuretic factor is a peptide hormone that causes salt secretion by the kidney, decreases blood volume and pressure, and therefore serves to reduce hemodynamic load.

Whatever the exact cause and mechanism of cardiac hypertrophy, it eventually reaches a limit beyond which enlargement of muscle mass is no longer able to cope with the increased burden. At this stage several regressive changes occur in the myocardial fibers, of which the most important are lysis and loss of myofibrillar contractile elements. In extreme cases myocyte death can occur. The net result of these changes is cardiac failure, a sequence of events that illustrates how an adaptation to stress can progress to functionally significant cell injury if the stress is not relieved.

To prevent such consequences, several drugs that inhibit key signaling pathways involving *NFAT, GATA4,* and *MEF2* genes are in phase 1 or 2 clinical trials.

Hyperplasia

Hyperplasia is defined as an increase in the number of cells in an organ or tissue in response to a stimulus. Although hyperplasia and hypertrophy are distinct processes, they frequently occur together, and may be triggered by the same external stimulus. Hyperplasia can only take place if the tissue contains cells capable of dividing; thus increasing the number of cells. It can be physiologic or pathologic.

Physiologic Hyperplasia

Physiologic hyperplasia due to the action of hormones or growth factors occurs in several circumstances: when there is a need to increase functional capacity of hormone sensitive organs; when there is need for compensatory increase after damage or resection. Hormonal hyperplasia is well illustrated by the proliferation of the glandular epithelium of the female breast at puberty and during pregnancy, usually accompanied by enlargement (hypertrophy) of the glandular epithelial cells. The classic illustration of compensatory hyperplasia comes from the study of liver regeneration. In individuals who donate one lobe of the liver for transplantation, the remaining cells proliferate so that the organ soon grows back to its original size. Experimental models of partial hepatectomy have been very useful for defining the mechanisms that stimulate regeneration of the liver (Chapter 3). Marrow is remarkable in its capacity to undergo rapid hyperplasia in response to a deficiency of terminally differentiated blood cells. For example, in the setting of an acute bleed or premature breakdown of red cells (hemolysis), feedback loops involving the growth factor erythropoietin are activated that stimulate the growth of red cell progenitors, allowing red cell production to increase as much as 8-fold. The regulation of hematopoiesis is discussed further in Chapter 13.

Pathologic Hyperplasia

Most forms of pathologic hyperplasia are caused by excessive or inappropriate actions of hormones or growth factors acting on target cells. Endometrial hyperplasia is an example of abnormal hormone-induced hyperplasia. Normally, after a menstrual period there is a rapid burst of proliferative activity in the endometrium that is stimulated by pituitary hormones and ovarian estrogen. It is brought to a halt by the rising levels of progesterone, usually about 10 to 14 days before the end of the menstrual period. In some instances, however, the balance between estrogen and progesterone is disturbed, resulting in absolute or relative increases in the amount of estrogen, with consequent hyperplasia of the endometrial glands. This form of pathologic hyperplasia is a common cause of abnormal menstrual bleeding. Benign prostatic hyperplasia is another common example of pathologic hyperplasia induced in responses to hormonal stimulation by androgens. Although these forms of pathologic hyperplasias are abnormal, the process remains controlled and the hyperplasia regresses if the hormonal stimulation is eliminated. As is discussed in Chapter 7, in cancer the growth control mechanisms become deregulated or ineffective because of genetic aberrations, that drive unrestrained proliferation. *Thus, while hyperplasia is distinct from cancer, pathologic hyperplasia constitutes a fertile soil in which cancerous proliferations may eventually arise.* For instance, patients with hyperplasia of the endometrium are at increased risk for developing endometrial cancer (Chapter 22).

Hyperplasia is a characteristic response to certain *viral infections*, such as papillomaviruses, which cause skin warts and several mucosal lesions composed of masses of hyperplastic epithelium. Here, the viruses make factors that interfere with host proteins that regulate cell proliferation. Like other forms of hyperplasia, some of these virally induced proliferations are also precursors to cancer (Chapter 7).

Mechanisms of Hyperplasia

Hyperplasia is the result of growth factor-driven proliferation of mature cells and, in some cases, by increased output of new cells from tissue stem cells. For instance, after partial hepatectomy growth factors are produced in the liver that engage receptors on the surviving cells and activate signaling pathways that stimulate cell proliferation. But if the proliferative capacity of the liver cells is compromised, as in some forms of hepatitis causing cell injury, hepatocytes can instead regenerate from intrahepatic stem cells. The roles of growth factors and stem cells in cellular replication and tissue hyperplasia are discussed in more detail in Chapter 3.

Atrophy

Atrophy is defined as a reduction in the size of an organ or tissue due to a decrease in cell size and number. Atrophy can be physiologic or pathologic. *Physiologic atrophy* is common during normal development. Some embryonic structures, such as the notochord and thyroglossal duct, undergo atrophy during fetal development. The decrease in the size of the uterus that occurs shortly after parturition is another form of physiologic atrophy.

Pathologic atrophy has several causes and it can be local or generalized. The common causes of atrophy are the following:

- *Decreased workload (atrophy of disuse).* When a fractured bone is immobilized in a plaster cast or when a patient is restricted to complete bed rest, skeletal muscle atrophy rapidly ensues. The initial decrease in cell size is reversible once activity is resumed. With more prolonged disuse, skeletal muscle fibers decrease in number (due to apoptosis) as well as in size; muscle atrophy can be accompanied by increased bone resorption, leading to osteoporosis of disuse.
- *Loss of innervation (denervation atrophy).* The normal metabolism and function of skeletal muscle are dependent on its nerve supply. Damage to the nerves leads to atrophy of the muscle fibers supplied by those nerves (Chapter 27).
- *Diminished blood supply.* A gradual decrease in blood supply (ischemia) to a tissue as a result of slowly developing arterial occlusive disease results in atrophy of the tissue. In late adult life, the brain may undergo progressive atrophy, mainly because of reduced blood supply as a result of atherosclerosis (Fig. 2-5). This is called *senile atrophy,* which also affects the heart.
- *Inadequate nutrition.* Profound protein-calorie malnutrition (marasmus) is associated with the utilization of skeletal muscle proteins as a source of energy after other reserves such as adipose stores have been depleted. This results in marked muscle wasting *(cachexia;* Chapter 9). Cachexia is also seen in patients with chronic inflammatory diseases and cancer. In the former, chronic overproduction of the inflammatory cytokine tumor necrosis factor (TNF) is thought to be responsible for appetite

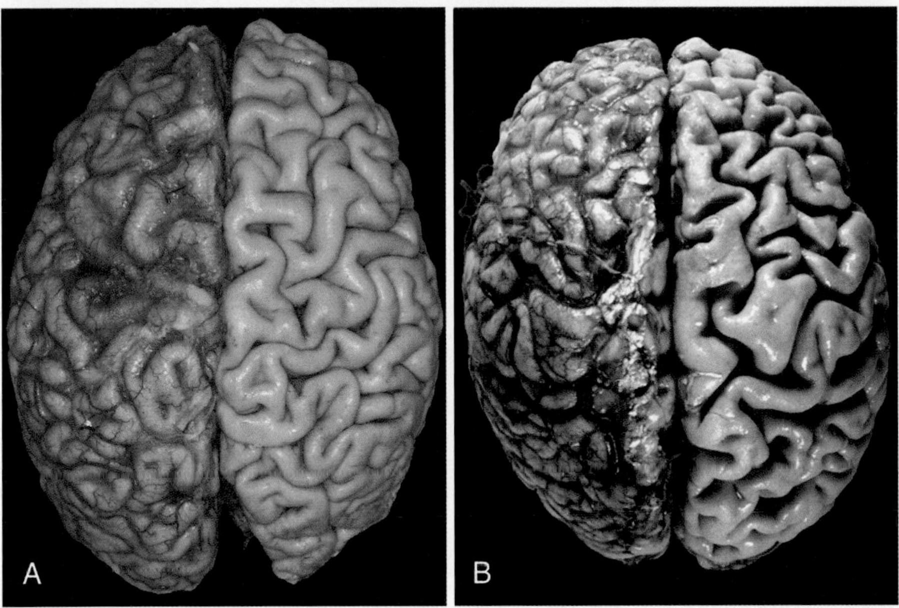

Figure 2-5 Atrophy. **A,** Normal brain of a young adult. **B,** Atrophy of the brain in an 82-year-old man with atherosclerotic cerebrovascular disease, resulting in reduced blood supply. Note that loss of brain substance narrows the gyri and widens the sulci. The meninges have been stripped from the right half of each specimen to reveal the surface of the brain.

suppression and lipid depletion, culminating in muscle atrophy.

- *Loss of endocrine stimulation.* Many hormone-responsive tissues, such as the breast and reproductive organs, are dependent on endocrine stimulation for normal metabolism and function. The loss of estrogen stimulation after menopause results in physiologic atrophy of the endometrium, vaginal epithelium, and breast.
- *Pressure.* Tissue compression for any length of time can cause atrophy. An enlarging benign tumor can cause atrophy in the surrounding uninvolved tissues. Atrophy in this setting is probably the result of ischemic changes caused by compromise of the blood supply by the pressure exerted by the expanding mass.

The fundamental cellular changes associated with atrophy are identical in all of these settings. The initial response is a decrease in cell size and organelles, which may reduce the metabolic needs of the cell sufficiently to permit its survival. In atrophic muscle, the cells contain fewer mitochondria and myofilaments and a reduced amount of rough endoplasmic reticulum (RER). By bringing into balance the cell's metabolic demands and the lower levels of blood supply, nutrition, or trophic stimulation, a new equilibrium is achieved. *Early in the process atrophic cells and tissues have diminished function, but cell death is minimal.* However, atrophy caused by gradually reduced blood supply may progress to the point at which cells are irreversibly injured and die, often by apoptosis. Cell death by apoptosis also contributes to the atrophy of endocrine organs after hormone withdrawal.

Mechanisms of Atrophy

Atrophy results from decreased protein synthesis and increased protein degradation in cells. Protein synthesis decreases because of reduced metabolic activity.

The degradation of cellular proteins occurs mainly by the ubiquitin-proteasome pathway. Nutrient deficiency and disuse may activate ubiquitin ligases, which attach the small peptide ubiquitin to cellular proteins and target these proteins for degradation in *proteasomes.* This pathway is also thought to be responsible for the accelerated proteolysis seen in a variety of catabolic conditions, including cancer cachexia. In many situations, atrophy is also accompanied by increased *autophagy,* marked by the appearance of increased numbers of *autophagic vacuoles.* Autophagy ("self-eating") is the process in which the starved cell eats its own components in an attempt to reduce nutrient demand to match the supply. Some of the cell debris within the autophagic vacuoles may resist digestion and persist in the cytoplasm as membrane-bound *residual bodies.* An example of residual bodies is *lipofuscin granules,* discussed later in the chapter. When present in sufficient amounts, they impart a brown discoloration to the tissue *(brown atrophy).* Autophagy is associated with various types of cell injury, and we will discuss it in more detail later.

Metaplasia

Metaplasia is a reversible change in which one differentiated cell type (epithelial or mesenchymal) is replaced by another cell type. It often represents an adaptive response in which one cell type that is sensitive to a particular stress is replaced by another cell type that is better able to withstand the adverse environment.

The most common epithelial metaplasia is *columnar to squamous* (Fig. 2-6), as occurs in the respiratory tract in response to chronic irritation. In the habitual cigarette smoker, the normal ciliated columnar epithelial cells of the trachea and bronchi are often replaced by stratified squamous epithelial cells. Stones in the excretory ducts of the salivary glands, pancreas, or bile ducts, which are normally lined by secretory columnar epithelium, may also lead to squamous metaplasia by stratified squamous epithelium. A deficiency of vitamin A (retinoic acid) induces squamous metaplasia in the respiratory epithelium (Chapter 9). In all

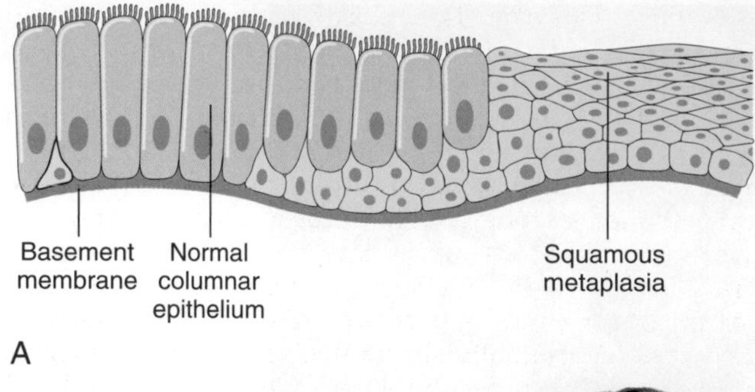

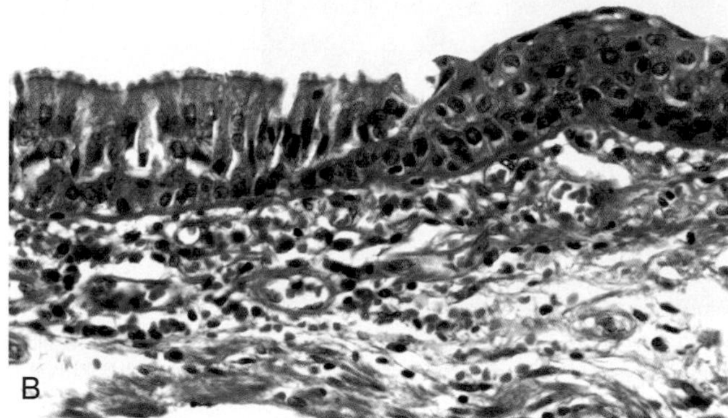

Figure 2-6 Metaplasia of columnar to squamous epithelium. **A,** Schematic diagram. **B,** Metaplasia of columnar epithelium *(left)* to squamous epithelium *(right)* in a bronchus.

these instances the more rugged stratified squamous epithelium is able to survive under circumstances in which the more fragile specialized columnar epithelium might have succumbed. However, the change to metaplastic squamous cells comes with a price. In the respiratory tract, for example, although the epithelial lining becomes tough, important mechanisms of protection against infection—mucus secretion and the ciliary action of the columnar epithelium—are lost. Thus, epithelial metaplasia is a double-edged sword and, in most circumstances, represents an undesirable change. Moreover, *the influences that predispose to metaplasia, if persistent, can initiate malignant transformation in metaplastic epithelium.* Thus, a common form of cancer in the respiratory tract is composed of squamous cells, which can arise in areas where the normal columnar epithelium has been replaced by squamous epithelium.

Metaplasia from squamous to columnar type may also occur, as in *Barrett esophagus*, in which the esophageal squamous epithelium is replaced by intestinal-like columnar cells under the influence of refluxed gastric acid. Cancers may arise in these areas; these are typically glandular (adenocarcinomas) (Chapter 17).

Connective tissue metaplasia is the formation of cartilage, bone, or adipose tissue (mesenchymal tissues) in tissues that normally do not contain these elements. For example, bone formation in muscle, designated *myositis ossificans*, occasionally occurs after intramuscular hemorrhage. This type of metaplasia is less clearly seen as an adaptive response, and may be a result of cell or tissue injury.

Mechanisms of Metaplasia

Metaplasia does not result from a change in the phenotype of an already differentiated cell type; instead it is the result of a reprogramming of stem cells that are known to exist in normal tissues, or of undifferentiated mesenchymal cells present in connective tissue. In a metaplastic change, these precursor cells differentiate along a new pathway. The differentiation of stem cells to a particular lineage is brought about by signals generated by cytokines, growth factors, and extracellular matrix components in the cells' environment. These external stimuli promote the expression of genes that drive cells toward a specific differentiation pathway. A direct link between transcription factor dysregulation and metaplasia is seen with vitamin A (retinoic acid) deficiency or excess, both of which may cause metaplasia. Retinoic acid regulates gene transcription directly through nuclear retinoid receptors (Chapter 9), which can influence the differentiation of progenitors derived from tissue stem cells. How other external stresses cause metaplasia is unknown, but it is clear that they too somehow alter the activity of transcription factors that regulate differentiation.

KEY CONCEPTS

Cellular Adaptations to Stress

- **Hypertrophy**: increased cell and organ size, often in response to increased workload; induced by growth factors produced in response to mechanical stress or other stimuli; occurs in tissues incapable of cell division
- **Hyperplasia**: increased cell numbers in response to hormones and other growth factors; occurs in tissues whose cells are able to divide or contain abundant tissue stem cells
- **Atrophy**: decreased cell and organ size, as a result of decreased nutrient supply or disuse; associated with decreased synthesis of cellular building blocks and increased breakdown of cellular organelles
- **Metaplasia**: change in phenotype of differentiated cells, often in response to chronic irritation, that makes cells better able to withstand the stress; usually induced by altered differentiation pathway of tissue stem cells; may result in reduced functions or increased propensity for malignant transformation

Overview of Cell Injury and Cell Death

As stated at the beginning of the chapter, cell injury results when cells are stressed so severely that they are no longer able to adapt or when cells are exposed to inherently damaging agents or suffer from intrinsic abnormalities. Injury may progress through a reversible stage and culminate in cell death (Fig. 2-1).

- *Reversible cell injury.* In early stages or mild forms of injury, the functional and morphologic changes are reversible if the damaging stimulus is removed. The hallmarks of reversible injury are reduced oxidative phosphorylation with resultant depletion of energy stores in the form of adenosine triphosphate (ATP), and cellular swelling caused by changes in ion concentrations and water influx. In addition, various intracellular organelles, such as mitochondria and the cytoskeleton, may show alterations.

- *Cell death.* With continuing damage the injury becomes irreversible, at which time the cell cannot recover and it dies. *Historically, two principal types of cell death, necrosis and apoptosis, which differ in their morphology, mechanisms, and roles in physiology and disease,* have been recognized.
  - Necrosis has been considered an "accidental" and unregulated form of cell death resulting from damage to cell membranes and loss of ion homeostasis. When damage to membranes is severe, lysosomal enzymes enter the cytoplasm and digest the cell giving rise to a set of morphologic changes described as necrosis. Cellular contents also leak through the damaged plasma membrane into the extracellular space, where they elicit a host reaction (inflammation). Necrosis is the pathway of cell death in many commonly encountered injuries, such as those resulting from ischemia, exposure to toxins, various infections, and trauma.
  - In contrast to necrosis, when the cell's DNA or proteins are damaged beyond repair, the cell kills itself by *apoptosis*, a form of cell death that is characterized by nuclear dissolution, fragmentation of the cell without complete loss of membrane integrity, and rapid removal of the cellular debris. Because cellular contents do not leak out, unlike in necrosis, there is no inflammatory reaction. Mechanistically, apoptosis is known to be a highly regulated process driven by a series of genetic pathways. It is hence also sometimes called "programmed cell death."
  - *Whereas necrosis is always a pathologic process, apoptosis serves many normal functions and is not necessarily associated with cell injury.* Despite the distinctive morphologic manifestations of necrosis and apoptosis, it is now clear that the mechanistic distinction between necrosis and apoptosis is not as clear cut as previously imagined. In some cases necrosis is also regulated by a series of signaling pathways, albeit largely distinct from those that are involved in apoptosis. In other words, in some cases necrosis, like apoptosis, is also a form of programmed cell death. In recognition of this similarity, this form of necrosis has been called *necroptosis* as will be discussed later. Despite some potential overlap of mechanisms, it is still useful to discuss necrosis and apoptosis, the two principal pathways of cell death, separately because of the differing circumstances in which they develop.

The morphologic features, mechanisms, and significance of these death pathways are discussed in more detail later in the chapter. We will discuss first the causes of cell injury.

Causes of Cell Injury

The causes of cell injury range from the physical violence of an automobile accident to subtle cellular abnormalities, such as a mutation causing lack of a vital enzyme that impairs normal metabolic function. Most injurious stimuli can be grouped into the following broad categories.

Oxygen Deprivation. *Hypoxia* is a deficiency of oxygen, which causes cell injury by reducing aerobic oxidative respiration. Hypoxia is an extremely important and common cause of cell injury and cell death. *Causes of hypoxia* include reduced blood flow (*ischemia*), inadequate oxygenation of the blood due to cardiorespiratory failure, and decreased oxygen-carrying capacity of the blood, as in anemia or carbon monoxide poisoning (producing a stable carbon monoxyhemoglobin that blocks oxygen carriage) or after severe blood loss. Depending on the severity of the hypoxic state, cells may adapt, undergo injury, or die. For example, if an artery is narrowed, the tissue supplied by that vessel may initially shrink in size (atrophy), whereas more severe or sudden hypoxia induces injury and cell death.

Physical Agents. Physical agents capable of causing cell injury include mechanical trauma, extremes of temperature (burns and deep cold), sudden changes in atmospheric pressure, radiation, and electric shock (Chapter 9).

Chemical Agents and Drugs. The list of chemicals that may produce cell injury defies compilation. Simple chemicals such as glucose or salt in hypertonic concentrations may cause cell injury directly or by deranging electrolyte balance in cells. Even oxygen at high concentrations is toxic. Trace amounts of *poisons*, such as arsenic, cyanide, or mercuric salts, may damage sufficient numbers of cells within minutes or hours to cause death. Other potentially injurious substances are our daily companions: environmental and air pollutants, insecticides, and herbicides; industrial and occupational hazards, such as carbon monoxide and asbestos; recreational drugs such as alcohol; and the ever-increasing variety of therapeutic drugs. Many of these are discussed further in Chapter 9.

Infectious Agents. These agents range from the submicroscopic viruses to tapeworms several feet in length. In between are the rickettsiae, bacteria, fungi, and higher forms of parasites. The ways by which these biologic agents cause injury are diverse (Chapter 8).

Immunologic Reactions. The immune system serves an essential function in defense against infectious pathogens, but immune reactions may also cause cell injury. Injurious reactions to endogenous self antigens are responsible for several autoimmune diseases (Chapter 6). Immune reactions to many external agents, such as viruses and environmental substances, are also important causes of cell and tissue injury (Chapters 3 and 6).

Genetic Derangements. As described in Chapter 5, genetic abnormalities as obvious as an extra chromosome, as in Down syndrome, or as subtle as a single base pair substitution leading to an amino acid substitution, as in sickle cell anemia, may produce highly characteristic clinical phenotypes ranging from congenital malformations to anemias. Genetic defects may cause cell injury because of deficiency of functional proteins, such as enzyme defects in inborn errors of metabolism, or accumulation of damaged DNA or misfolded proteins, both of which trigger cell death when they are beyond repair. DNA sequence variants that are common in human populations (polymorphisms) can also influence the susceptibility of cells to injury by chemicals and other environmental insults.

Nutritional Imbalances. Nutritional imbalances continue to be major causes of cell injury. Protein-calorie deficiencies cause an appalling number of deaths, chiefly among underprivileged populations. Deficiencies of specific vitamins are found throughout the world (Chapter 9). Nutritional problems can be self-imposed, as in anorexia nervosa (self-induced starvation). Ironically, nutritional excesses have also become important causes of cell injury. Excess of cholesterol predisposes to atherosclerosis; obesity is associated with increased incidence of several important diseases, such as diabetes and cancer. Atherosclerosis is virtually endemic in the United States, and obesity is rampant. In addition to the problems of undernutrition and overnutrition, the composition of the diet makes a significant contribution to a number of diseases.

Table 2-2 Features of Necrosis and Apoptosis

Feature	Necrosis	Apoptosis
Cell size	Enlarged (swelling)	Reduced (shrinkage)
Nucleus	Pyknosis → karyorrhexis → karyolysis	Fragmentation into nucleosome-size fragments
Plasma membrane	Disrupted	Intact; altered structure, especially orientation of lipids
Cellular contents	Enzymatic digestion; may leak out of cell	Intact; may be released in apoptotic bodies
Adjacent inflammation	Frequent	No
Physiologic or pathologic role	Invariably pathologic (culmination of irreversible cell injury)	Often physiologic, means of eliminating unwanted cells; may be pathologic after some forms of cell injury, especially DNA damage

Morphologic Alterations in Cell Injury

It is useful to describe the basic alterations that occur in damaged cells before discussing the biochemical mechanisms that bring about these changes. All stresses and noxious influences exert their effects first at the molecular or biochemical level. There is a time lag between the stress and the morphologic changes of cell injury or death; the duration of this delay may vary with the sensitivity of the methods used to detect these changes (Fig. 2-7). With histochemical or ultrastructural techniques, changes may be seen in minutes to hours after injury; however, it may take considerably longer (hours to days) before changes can be seen by light microscopy or on gross examination. As would be expected, the morphologic manifestations of necrosis take more time to develop than those of reversible damage. For example, in ischemia of the myocardium, cell swelling is a reversible morphologic change that may occur in a matter of minutes, and may progress to irreversibility within an hour or two. Unmistakable light microscopic changes of cell death, however, may not be seen until 4 to 12 hours after onset of ischemia.

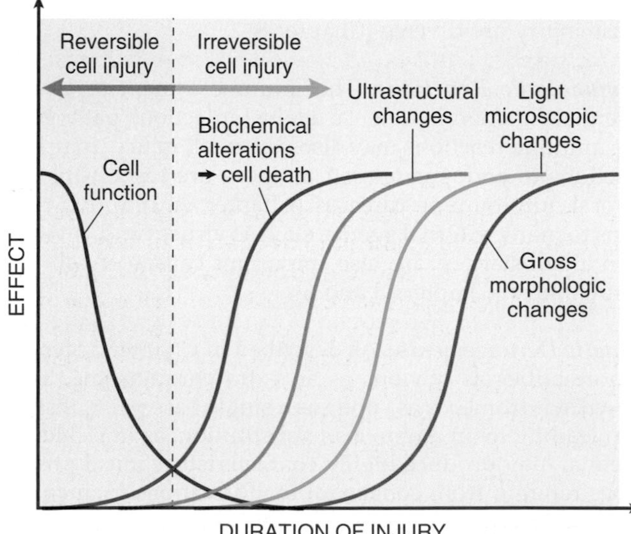

Figure 2-7 Sequential development of biochemical and morphologic changes in cell injury. Cells may become rapidly nonfunctional after the onset of injury, although they may still be viable, with potentially reversible damage; a longer duration of injury may lead to irreversible injury and cell death. Note that irreversible biochemical alterations may cause cell death, and typically this precedes ultrastructural, light microscopic, and grossly visible morphologic changes.

The sequential morphologic changes in cell injury progressing to cell death are illustrated in Figure 2-8. Reversible injury is characterized by generalized swelling of the cell and its organelles, blebbing of the plasma membrane, detachment of ribosomes from the ER, and clumping of nuclear chromatin. These morphologic changes are associated with decreased generation of ATP, loss of cell membrane integrity, defects in protein synthesis, cytoskeletal damage, and DNA damage. Within limits, the cell can repair these derangements and, if the injurious stimulus abates, will return to normalcy. Persistent or excessive injury, however, causes cells to pass the rather nebulous "point of no return" into irreversible injury and *cell death*. Different injurious stimuli may induce death by necrosis or apoptosis (Fig. 2-8 and Table 2-2). Severe mitochondrial damage with depletion of ATP and rupture of lysosomal and plasma membranes are typically associated with necrosis. Necrosis occurs in many commonly encountered injuries, such as those following ischemia, exposure to toxins, various infections, and trauma. Apoptosis has many unique features (see later).

Reversible Injury

Two features of reversible cell injury can be recognized under the light microscope: *cellular swelling* and *fatty change*. Cellular swelling appears whenever cells are incapable of maintaining ionic and fluid homeostasis and is the result of failure of energy-dependent ion pumps in the plasma membrane. Fatty change occurs in hypoxic injury and various forms of toxic or metabolic injury. It is manifested by the appearance of lipid vacuoles in the cytoplasm. It is seen mainly in cells involved in and dependent on fat metabolism, such as hepatocytes and myocardial cells. The mechanisms of fatty change are discussed later in the chapter.

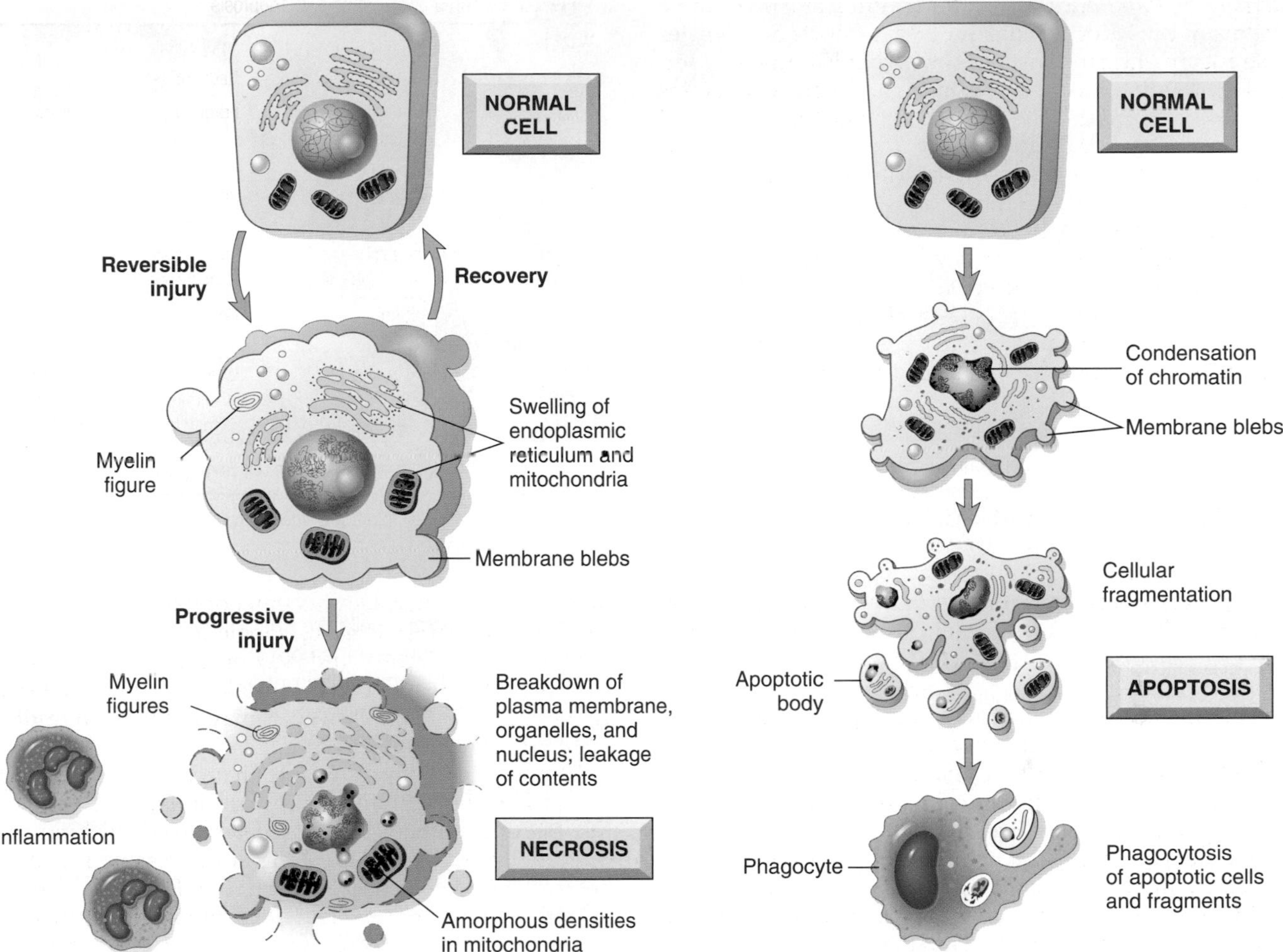

Figure 2-8 Schematic illustration of the morphologic changes in cell injury culminating in necrosis or apoptosis.

MORPHOLOGY

Cellular swelling is the first manifestation of almost all forms of injury to cells (Fig. 2-9*B*). It is a difficult morphologic change to appreciate with the light microscope; it may be more apparent at the level of the whole organ. When it affects many cells, it causes some pallor, increased turgor, and increase in weight of the organ. On microscopic examination, small clear vacuoles may be seen within the cytoplasm; these represent distended and pinched-off segments of the ER. This pattern of nonlethal injury is sometimes called **hydropic change** or **vacuolar degeneration**. Swelling of cells is reversible. Cells may also show increased eosinophilic staining, which becomes much more pronounced with progression to necrosis (described later).

The ultrastructural changes of reversible cell injury (Fig. 2-10*B*) include:

1. **Plasma membrane alterations,** such as blebbing, blunting, and loss of microvilli
2. **Mitochondrial changes,** including swelling and the appearance of small amorphous densities
3. **Dilation** of the **ER,** with detachment of polysomes; intracytoplasmic myelin figures may be present (see later)
4. **Nuclear alterations,** with disaggregation of granular and fibrillar elements

Necrosis

The morphologic appearance of necrosis as well as necroptosis is the result of denaturation of intracellular proteins and enzymatic digestion of the lethally injured cell. Necrotic cells are unable to maintain membrane integrity and their contents often leak out, a process that may elicit inflammation in the surrounding tissue. The enzymes that digest the necrotic cell are derived from the lysosomes of the dying cells themselves and from the lysosomes of leukocytes that are called in as part of the inflammatory reaction. Digestion of cellular contents and the host response may take hours to develop, and so there would be no detectable changes in cells if, for example, a myocardial infarct caused sudden death. The earliest histologic evidence of myocardial necrosis does not become apparent until 4 to 12 hours later. However, because of the loss of plasma membrane integrity, cardiac-specific enzymes and proteins are rapidly released from necrotic muscle and can be detected in the blood as early as 2 hours after myocardial cell necrosis (Chapter 12).

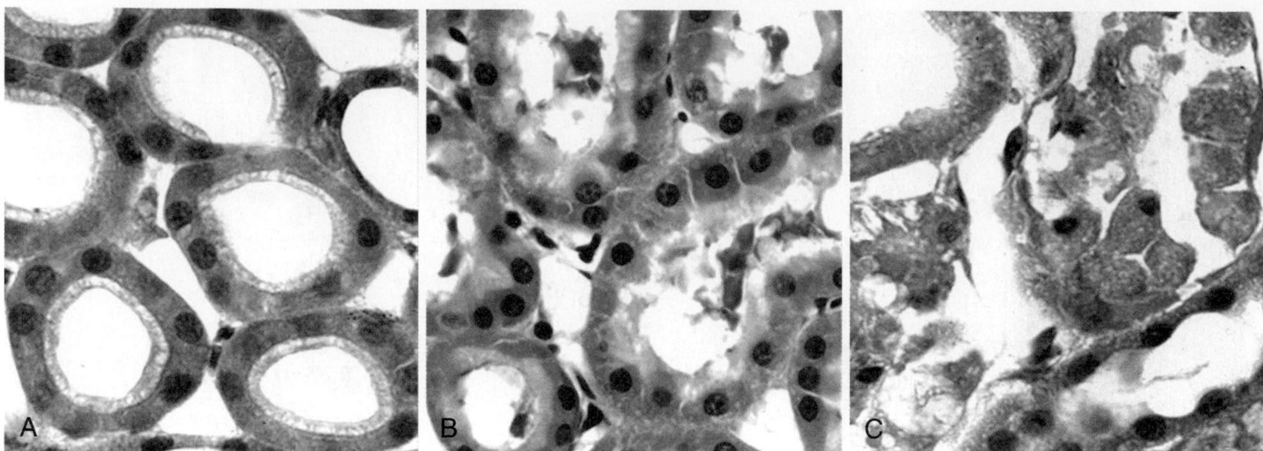

Figure 2-9 Morphologic changes in reversible cell injury and necrosis. **A,** Normal kidney tubules with viable epithelial cells. **B,** Early (reversible) ischemic injury showing surface blebs, increased eosinophilia of cytoplasm, and swelling of occasional cells. **C,** Necrosis (irreversible injury) of epithelial cells, with loss of nuclei, fragmentation of cells, and leakage of contents. The ultrastructural features of these stages of cell injury are shown in Fig. 2-10. (Courtesy Drs. Neal Pinckard and M. A. Venkatachalam, University of Texas Health Sciences Center, San Antonio, Texas.)

MORPHOLOGY

Necrotic cells show **increased eosinophilia** in hematoxylin and eosin (H & E) stains, attributable in part to the loss of cytoplasmic RNA (which binds the blue dye, hematoxylin) and in part to denatured cytoplasmic proteins (which bind the red dye, eosin). The necrotic cell may have a more glassy homogeneous appearance than do normal cells, mainly as a result of the loss of glycogen particles (Fig. 2-9*C*). When enzymes have digested the cytoplasmic organelles, the cytoplasm becomes vacuolated and appears moth-eaten. Dead cells may be replaced by large, whorled phospholipid masses called **myelin figures** that are derived from damaged cell membranes. These phospholipid precipitates are then either phagocytosed by other cells or further degraded into fatty acids; calcification of such fatty acid residues results in the generation of calcium soaps. Thus, the dead cells may ultimately become calcified. By electron microscopy, necrotic cells are characterized by discontinuities in plasma and organelle membranes, marked dilation of mitochondria with the appearance of large amorphous densities, intracytoplasmic myelin figures, amorphous debris, and aggregates of fluffy material probably representing denatured protein (Fig. 2-10*C*).

Nuclear changes appear in one of three patterns, all due to nonspecific breakdown of DNA (Fig. 2-9*C*). The basophilia of the chromatin may fade **(karyolysis)**, a change that presumably reflects loss of DNA because of enzymatic degradation by endonucleases. A second pattern (which is also seen in apoptotic cell death) is **pyknosis**, characterized by nuclear shrinkage and increased basophilia. Here the chromatin condenses into a solid, shrunken basophilic mass. In the third pattern, known as **karyorrhexis**, the pyknotic nucleus undergoes fragmentation. With the passage of time (a day or two), the nucleus in the necrotic cell totally disappears.

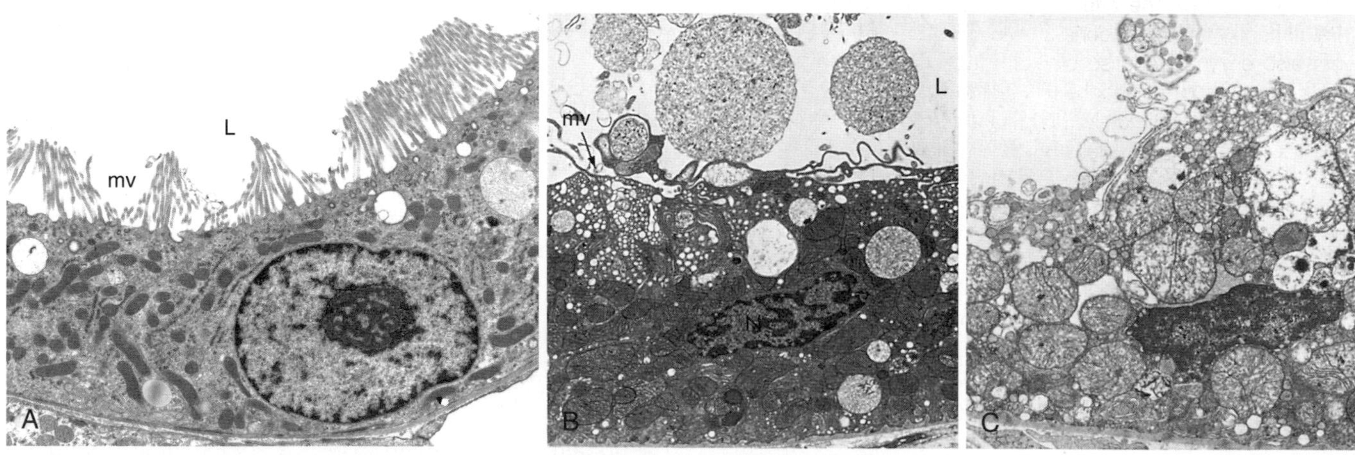

Figure 2-10 Ultrastructural features of reversible and irreversible cell injury (necrosis) in a rabbit kidney. **A,** Electron micrograph of a normal epithelial cell of the proximal kidney tubule. Note abundant microvilli (mv) lining the luminal surface (L). **B,** Epithelial cell of the proximal tubule showing early cell injury resulting from reperfusion following ischemia. The microvilli are lost and have been incorporated in apical cytoplasm; blebs have formed and are extruded in the lumen. Mitochondria would have been swollen during ischemia; with reperfusion, they rapidly undergo condensation and become electron-dense. **C,** Proximal tubular cell showing late injury, expected to be irreversible. Note the markedly swollen mitochondria containing electron-dense deposits, expected to contain precipitated calcium and proteins. Higher magnification micrographs of the cell would show disrupted plasma membrane and swelling and fragmentation of organelles. (**A,** Courtesy Dr. Brigitte Kaisslin, Institute of Anatomy, University of Zurich, Switzerland. **B, C,** Courtesy Dr. M. A. Venkatachalam, University of Texas Health Sciences Center, San Antonio, Texas.)

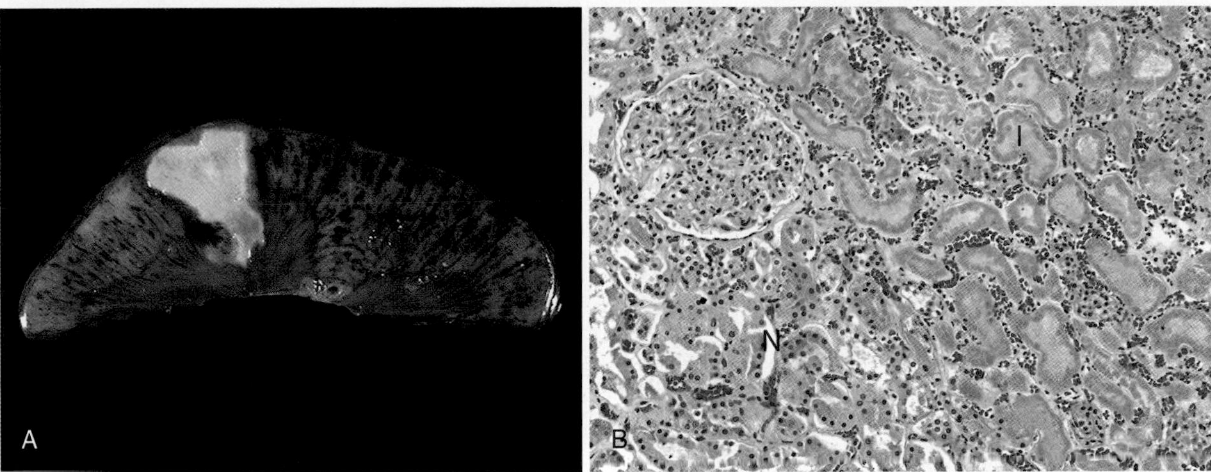

Figure 2-11 Coagulative necrosis. **A,** A wedge-shaped kidney infarct (yellow). **B,** Microscopic view of the edge of the infarct, with normal kidney (N) and necrotic cells in the infarct (I) showing preserved cellular outlines with loss of nuclei and an inflammatory infiltrate (seen as nuclei of inflammatory cells in between necrotic tubules).

Patterns of Tissue Necrosis

The discussion of necrosis has focused so far on changes in individual cells. When large numbers of cells die the tissue or organ is said to be necrotic; thus, a myocardial infarct is necrosis of a portion of the heart caused by death of many myocardial cells. Necrosis of tissues has several morphologically distinct patterns, which are important to recognize because they may provide clues about the underlying cause. Although the terms that describe these patterns are somewhat outdated, they are used often and their implications are understood by pathologists and clinicians.

MORPHOLOGY

Coagulative necrosis is a form of necrosis in which the architecture of dead tissues is preserved for a span of at least some days (Fig. 2-11). The affected tissues exhibit a firm texture. Presumably, the injury denatures not only structural proteins but also enzymes and so blocks the proteolysis of the dead cells; as a result, eosinophilic, anucleate cells may persist for days or weeks. Ultimately the necrotic cells are removed by phagocytosis of the cellular debris by infiltrating leukocytes and by digestion of the dead cells by the action of lysosomal enzymes of the leukocytes. Ischemia caused by obstruction in a vessel may lead to coagulative necrosis of the supplied tissue in all organs except the brain. A localized area of coagulative necrosis is called an **infarct**.

Liquefactive necrosis, in contrast to coagulative necrosis, is characterized by digestion of the dead cells, resulting in transformation of the tissue into a liquid viscous mass. It is seen in focal bacterial or, occasionally, fungal infections, because microbes stimulate the accumulation of leukocytes and the liberation of enzymes from these cells. The necrotic material is frequently creamy yellow because of the presence of dead leukocytes and is called **pus**. For unknown reasons, hypoxic death of cells within the central nervous system often manifests as liquefactive necrosis (Fig. 2-12).

Gangrenous necrosis is not a specific pattern of cell death, but the term is commonly used in clinical practice. It is usually applied to a limb, generally the lower leg, that has lost its blood supply and has undergone necrosis (typically coagulative necrosis) involving multiple tissue planes. When bacterial infection is superimposed there is more liquefactive necrosis because of the actions of degradative enzymes in the bacteria and the attracted leukocytes (giving rise to so-called **wet gangrene**).

Caseous necrosis is encountered most often in foci of tuberculous infection (Chapter 8). The term "caseous" (cheese-like) is derived from the friable white appearance of the area of necrosis (Fig. 2-13). On microscopic examination, the necrotic area appears as a structureless collection of fragmented or lysed cells and amorphous granular debris enclosed within a distinctive inflammatory border; this appearance is characteristic of a focus of inflammation known as a **granuloma** (Chapter 3).

Fat necrosis is a term that is entrenched in medical parlance but does not in reality denote a specific pattern of necrosis. Rather, it refers to focal areas of fat destruction, typically

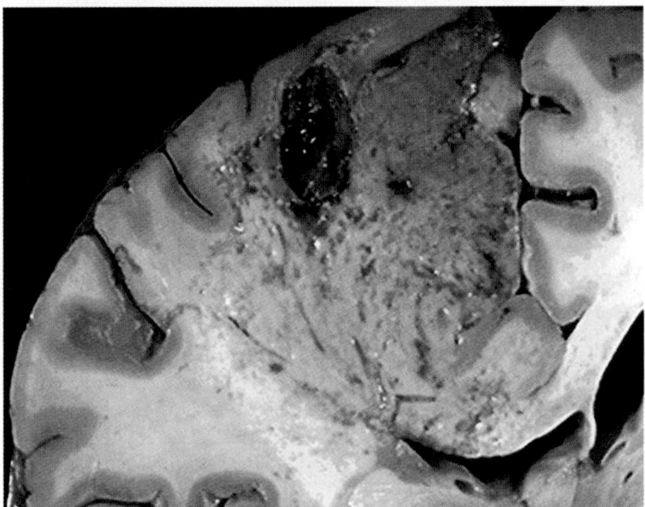

Figure 2-12 Liquefactive necrosis. An infarct in the brain, showing dissolution of the tissue.

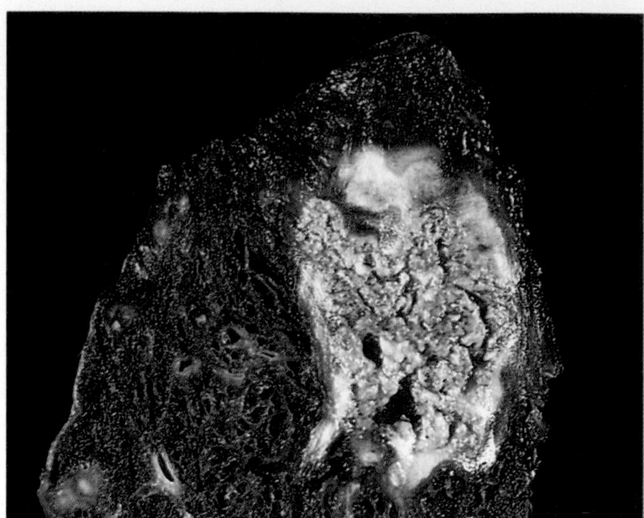

Figure 2-13 Caseous necrosis. Tuberculosis of the lung, with a large area of caseous necrosis containing yellow-white and cheesy debris.

resulting from release of activated pancreatic lipases into the substance of the pancreas and the peritoneal cavity. This occurs in the calamitous abdominal emergency known as acute pancreatitis (Chapter 19). In this disorder pancreatic enzymes leak out of acinar cells and liquefy the membranes of fat cells in the peritoneum. The released lipases split the triglyceride esters contained within fat cells. The fatty acids, so derived, combine with calcium to produce grossly visible chalky-white areas (fat saponification), which enable the surgeon and the pathologist to identify the lesions (Fig. 2-14). On histologic examination the necrosis takes the form of foci of shadowy outlines of necrotic fat cells, with basophilic calcium deposits, surrounded by an inflammatory reaction.

Fibrinoid necrosis is a special form of necrosis usually seen in immune reactions involving blood vessels. This pattern of necrosis typically occurs when complexes of antigens and antibodies are deposited in the walls of arteries. Deposits of these "immune complexes," together with fibrin that has leaked out of vessels, result in a bright pink and amorphous appearance in H&E stains, called "fibrinoid" (fibrin-like) by pathologists (Fig. 2-15). The immunologically mediated vasculitis syndromes in which this type of necrosis is seen are described in Chapter 11.

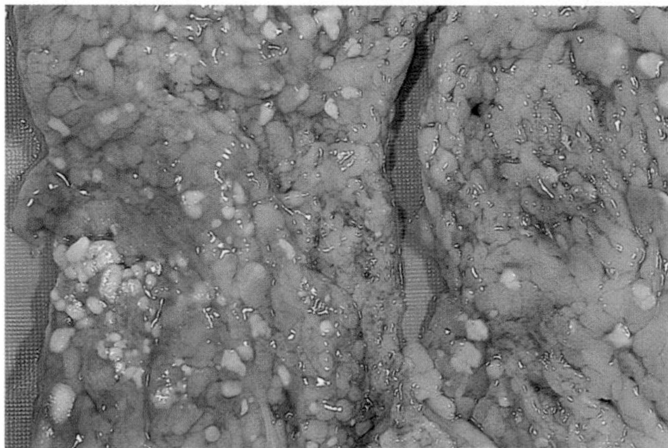

Figure 2-14 Fat necrosis. The areas of white chalky deposits represent foci of fat necrosis with calcium soap formation (saponification) at sites of lipid breakdown in the mesentery.

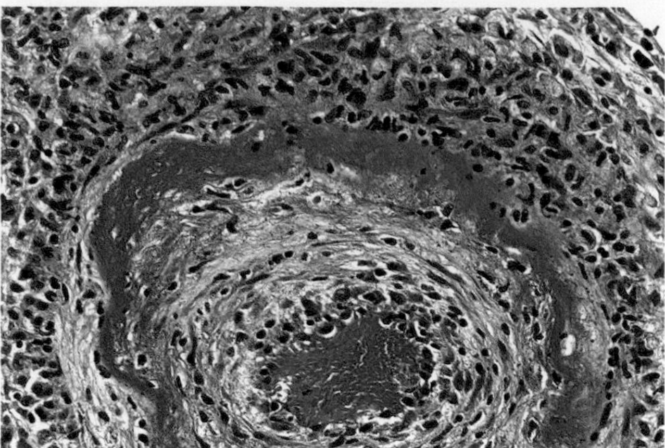

Figure 2-15 Fibrinoid necrosis in an artery. The wall of the artery shows a circumferential bright pink area of necrosis with inflammation (neutrophils with dark nuclei).

Ultimately, in the living patient most necrotic cells and their contents disappear due to enzymatic digestion and phagocytosis of the debris by leukocytes. If necrotic cells and cellular debris are not promptly destroyed and reabsorbed, they provide a nidus for the deposition of calcium salts and other minerals and thus tend to become calcified. This phenomenon, called *dystrophic calcification*, is considered later in the chapter.

KEY CONCEPTS

Morphologic Alterations in Injured Cells and Tissues

- **Reversible cell injury:** Cellular swelling, fatty change, plasma membrane blebbing and loss of microvilli, mitochondrial swelling, dilation of the ER, eosinophilia (due to decreased cytoplasmic RNA)
- **Necrosis:** Increased eosinophilia; nuclear shrinkage, fragmentation, and dissolution; breakdown of plasma membrane and organellar membranes; abundant myelin figures; leakage and enzymatic digestion of cellular contents
- **Patterns of tissue necrosis:** Under different conditions, necrosis in tissues may assume specific patterns: coagulative, liquefactive, gangrenous, caseous, fat, and fibrinoid

Mechanisms of Cell Injury

The discussion of the cellular pathology of cell injury and necrosis sets the stage for a consideration of the mechanisms and biochemical pathways of cell injury. The molecular pathways that lead to cell injury are complex and are best understood in the context of normal cell biology (Chapter 1). There are, however, several principles that are relevant to most forms of cell injury:

- **The cellular response to injurious stimuli depends on the nature of the injury, its duration, and its severity.** Small doses of a chemical toxin or brief periods of ischemia may induce reversible injury, whereas large doses of the same toxin or more prolonged ischemia might

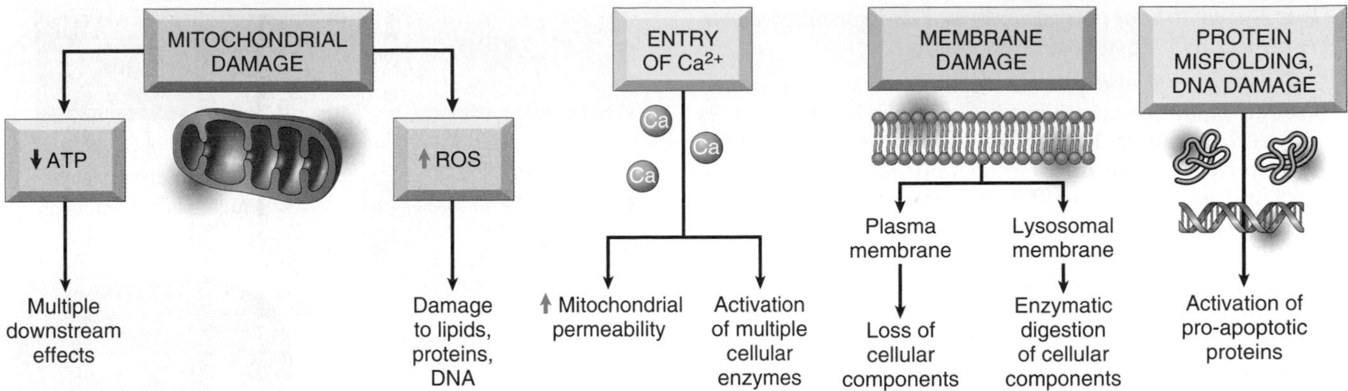

Figure 2-16 The principal biochemical mechanisms and sites of damage in cell injury. ATP, Adenosine triphosphate; ROS, reactive oxygen species.

result either in instantaneous cell death or in slow, irreversible injury leading in time to cell death.

- **The consequences of cell injury depend on the type, state, and adaptability of the injured cell.** The cell's nutritional and hormonal status and its metabolic needs are important in its response to injury. How vulnerable is a cell, for example, to loss of blood supply and hypoxia? When the striated muscle cell in the leg is deprived of its blood supply, it can be placed at rest and preserved; not so the striated muscle of the heart. Exposure of two individuals to identical concentrations of a toxin, such as carbon tetrachloride, may produce no effect in one and cell death in the other. This may be due to polymorphisms in genes encoding hepatic enzymes that metabolize carbon tetrachloride (CCl_4) to toxic by-products (Chapter 9). With the complete mapping of the human genome, there is great interest in identifying genetic polymorphisms that affect the responses of different individuals to various injurious agents.
- **Cell injury results from different biochemical mechanisms acting on several essential cellular components** (Fig. 2-16). These mechanisms are described individually in subsequent paragraphs. The cellular components that are most frequently damaged by injurious stimuli include mitochondria, cell membranes, the machinery of protein synthesis and packaging, and DNA. Any injurious stimulus may simultaneously trigger multiple interconnected mechanisms that damage cells. This is one reason why it is difficult to ascribe cell injury in a particular situation to a single or even dominant biochemical derangement.

The following section describes the biochemical mechanisms that may be activated by different injurious stimuli and that contribute to cell injury and necrosis. Apoptosis is described next, and finally necroptosis, which shares features with necrosis and apoptosis, is discussed.

Depletion of ATP

Reduction in ATP levels is fundamental cause of necrotic cell death. ATP depletion and decreased ATP synthesis are frequently associated with both hypoxic and chemical (toxic) injury (Fig. 2-17). ATP is produced in two ways. The major pathway in mammalian cells is oxidative phosphorylation of adenosine diphosphate, in a reaction that results in reduction of oxygen by the electron transfer system of mitochondria. The second is the glycolytic pathway, which can generate ATP in the absence of oxygen using glucose derived either from body fluids or from the hydrolysis of glycogen. *The major causes of ATP depletion are reduced supply of oxygen and nutrients, mitochondrial damage, and the actions of some toxins (e.g., cyanide).*

High-energy phosphate in the form of ATP is required for virtually all synthetic and degradative processes within the cell. These include membrane transport, protein synthesis, lipogenesis, and the deacylation-reacylation reactions necessary for phospholipid turnover. *Depletion of*

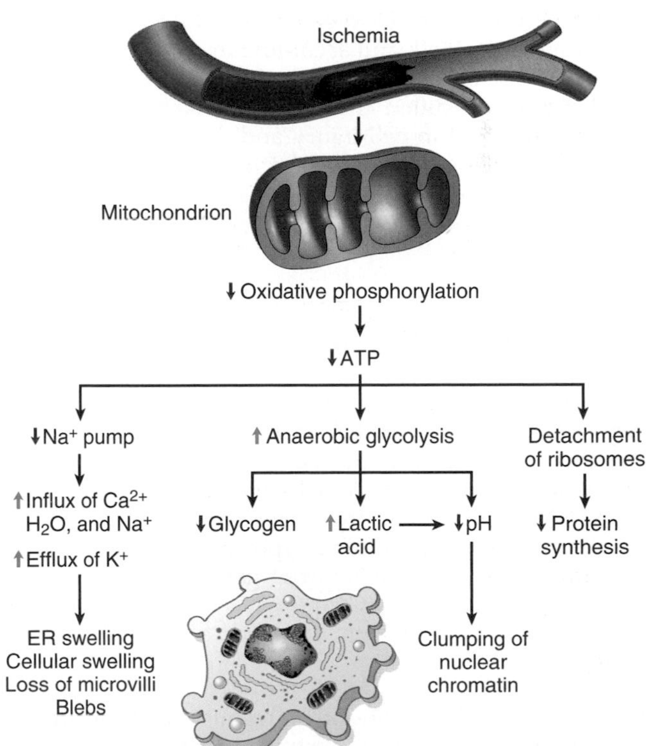

Figure 2-17 Functional and morphologic consequences of decreased intracellular adenosine triphosphate (ATP) during cell injury. The morphologic changes shown here are indicative of reversible cell injury. Further depletion of ATP results in cell death, typically by necrosis. ER, Endoplasmic reticulum.

ATP to 5% to 10% of normal levels has widespread effects on many critical cellular systems:

- The activity of the *plasma membrane energy-dependent sodium pump* (ouabain-sensitive Na^+, K^+-ATPase) is reduced (Chapter 1). Failure of this active transport system causes sodium to enter and accumulate inside cells and potassium to diffuse out. The net gain of solute is accompanied by isosmotic gain of water, causing *cell swelling*, and dilation of the ER.
- *Cellular energy metabolism is altered.* If the supply of oxygen to cells is reduced, as in ischemia, oxidative phosphorylation ceases, resulting in a decrease in cellular ATP and associated increase in adenosine monophosphate. These changes stimulate phosphofructokinase and phosphorylase activities, leading to an increased rate of *anaerobic glycolysis*, which is designed to maintain the cell's energy sources by generating ATP through metabolism of glucose derived from glycogen. As a consequence *glycogen stores are rapidly depleted.* Anaerobic glycolysis results in the accumulation of *lactic acid* and inorganic phosphates from the hydrolysis of phosphate esters. This reduces the intracellular pH, resulting in decreased activity of many cellular enzymes.
- Failure of the Ca^{2+} pump leads to influx of Ca^{2+}, with damaging effects on numerous cellular components, described later.
- With prolonged or worsening depletion of ATP, structural disruption of the protein synthetic apparatus occurs, manifested as detachment of ribosomes from the rough ER and dissociation of polysomes, with a consequent *reduction in protein synthesis.*
- In cells deprived of oxygen or glucose, proteins may become misfolded, and accumulation of misfolded proteins in the endoplasmic reticulum (ER) triggers a cellular reaction called the *unfolded protein response* that may culminate in cell injury and even death (Chapter 1). This process is described further later in this chapter.
- Ultimately, there is irreversible damage to mitochondrial and lysosomal membranes, and the cell undergoes *necrosis.*

Mitochondrial Damage

Mitochondria are critical players in cell injury and cell death by all pathways. This should be expected because they supply life-sustaining energy by producing ATP. Mitochondria can be damaged by increases of cytosolic Ca^{2+}, reactive oxygen species (discussed later), and oxygen deprivation, and so they are sensitive to virtually all types of injurious stimuli, including hypoxia and toxins. In addition, mutations in mitochondrial genes are the cause of some inherited diseases (Chapter 5).

There are three major *consequences of mitochondrial damage.*

- Mitochondrial damage often results in the formation of a high-conductance channel in the mitochondrial membrane, called the *mitochondrial permeability transition pore* (Fig. 2-18). The opening of this conductance channel leads to the loss of mitochondrial membrane potential, resulting in failure of oxidative phosphorylation and progressive depletion of ATP, culminating in necrosis of the cell. One of the structural components of the mitochondrial permeability transition pore is the protein cyclophilin D, which is one of several cyclophilins that are targeted by the immunosuppressive drug cyclosporine (used to prevent graft rejection). In some experimental models of ischemia, cyclosporine reduces injury by preventing opening of the mitochondrial permeability transition pore—an interesting example of molecularly targeted therapy for cell injury. The role of cyclosporine in reducing ischemic myocardial injury in humans is under investigation.
- Abnormal oxidative phosphorylation also leads to the formation of *reactive oxygen species,* which have many deleterious effects, described later.
- The mitochondria sequester between their outer and inner membranes several proteins that are capable of activating apoptotic pathways; these include cytochrome c and proteins that indirectly activate apoptosis-inducing enzymes called *caspases*. Increased permeability of the outer mitochondrial membrane may result in leakage of these proteins into the cytosol and death by apoptosis (discussed later).

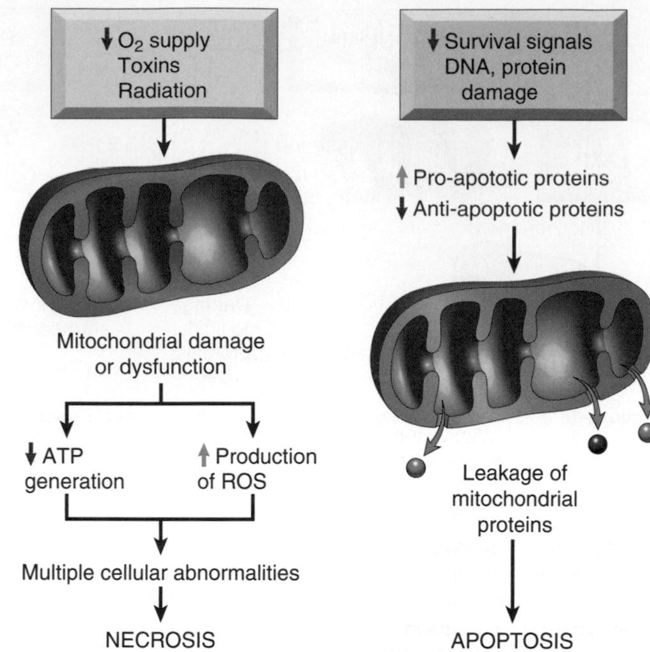

Figure 2-18 Role of mitochondria in cell injury and death. Mitochondria are affected by a variety of injurious stimuli and their abnormalities lead to necrosis or apoptosis. ATP, Adenosine triphosphate; ROS, reactive oxygen species.

Influx of Calcium and Loss of Calcium Homeostasis

Calcium ions are important mediators of cell injury. In keeping with this, depleting calcium protects cells from injury induced by a variety of harmful stimuli. Cytosolic free calcium is normally maintained at very low concentrations (~0.1 μmol) compared with extracellular levels of 1.3 mmol, and most intracellular calcium is sequestered in mitochondria and the ER. Ischemia and certain toxins cause an increase in cytosolic calcium concentration, initially because of release of Ca^{2+} from intracellular stores,

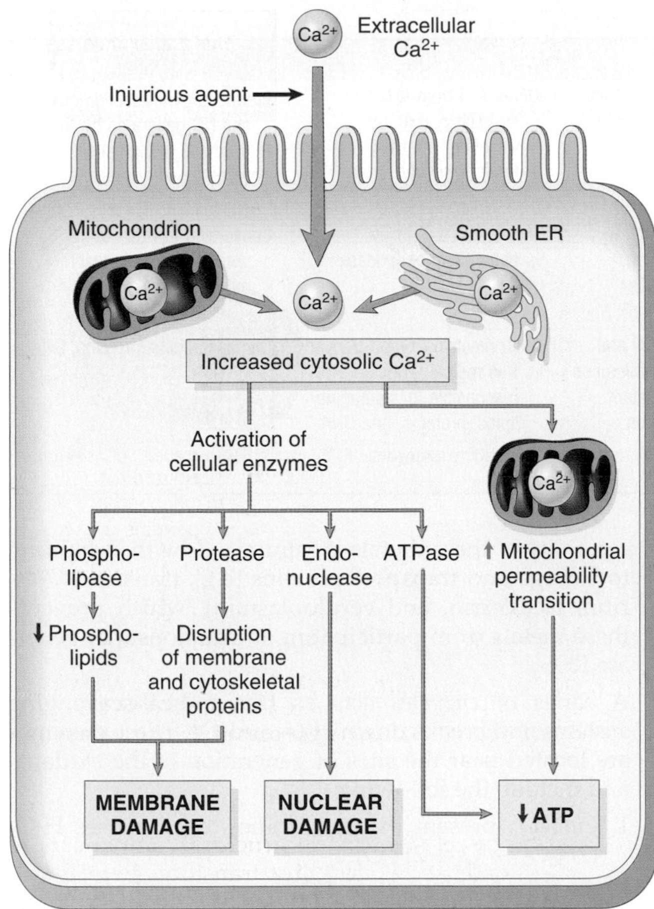

Figure 2-19 The role of increased cytosolic calcium in cell injury. ER, Endoplasmic reticulum.

and later due to increased influx across the plasma membrane (Fig. 2-19). Increased intracellular Ca^{2+} causes cell injury by several mechanisms.

- The accumulation of Ca^{2+} in mitochondria results in opening of the mitochondrial permeability transition pore and, as described earlier, failure of ATP generation.
- Increased cytosolic Ca^{2+} activates a number of enzymes with potentially deleterious effects on cells. These enzymes include *phospholipases* (which cause membrane damage), *proteases* (which break down both membrane and cytoskeletal proteins), *endonucleases* (which are responsible for DNA and chromatin fragmentation), and *ATPases* (thereby hastening ATP depletion).
- Increased intracellular Ca^{2+} levels also result in the induction of apoptosis, by direct activation of caspases and by increasing mitochondrial permeability.

Accumulation of Oxygen-Derived Free Radicals (Oxidative Stress)

Cell injury induced by free radicals, particularly reactive oxygen species, is an important mechanism of cell damage in many pathologic conditions, such as chemical and radiation injury, ischemia-reperfusion injury (induced by restoration of blood flow in ischemic tissue), cellular aging, and microbial killing by phagocytes. *Free radicals* are chemical species that have a single unpaired electron in an outer orbit. Unpaired electrons are highly reactive and "attack" and modify adjacent molecules, such as inorganic or organic chemicals—proteins, lipids, carbohydrates, nucleic acids—many of which are key components of cell membranes and nuclei. Some of these reactions are autocatalytic, whereby molecules that react with free radicals are themselves converted into free radicals, thus propagating the chain of damage.

Reactive oxygen species (ROS) are a type of oxygen-derived free radical whose role in cell injury is well established. ROS are produced normally in cells during mitochondrial respiration and energy generation, but they are degraded and removed by cellular defense systems. Thus, cells are able to maintain a steady state in which free radicals may be present transiently at low concentrations but do not cause damage. Increased production or decreased scavenging of ROS may lead to an excess of these free radicals, a condition called *oxidative stress.* Oxidative stress has been implicated in a wide variety of pathologic processes, including cell injury, cancer, aging, and some degenerative diseases such as Alzheimer disease. ROS are also produced in large amounts by activated leukocytes, particularly neutrophils and macrophages, during inflammatory reactions aimed at destroying microbes and cleaning up dead cells and other unwanted substances (Chapter 3).

The following section discusses the generation and removal of ROS, and how they contribute to cell injury. The properties of some of the most important free radicals are summarized in Table 2-3.

Generation of Free Radicals. Free radicals may be generated within cells in several ways (Fig. 2-20):

- *The reduction-oxidation reactions that occur during normal metabolic processes.* As a part of normal respiration, molecular O_2 is reduced by the transfer of four electrons to H_2 to generate two water molecules. This conversion is catalyzed by oxidative enzymes in the ER, cytosol, mitochondria, peroxisomes, and lysosomes. During this process small amounts of partially reduced intermediates are produced in which different numbers of electrons have been transferred from O_2; these include superoxide anion ($O_2^{\bar{\cdot}}$, one electron), hydrogen peroxide (H_2O_2, two electrons), and hydroxyl ions ($^{\bullet}OH$, three electrons).
- *Absorption of radiant energy* (e.g., ultraviolet light, x-rays). For example, ionizing radiation can hydrolyze water into $^{\bullet}OH$ and hydrogen (H) free radicals.
- Rapid bursts of ROS are produced in activated leukocytes during *inflammation.* This occurs in a precisely controlled reaction carried out by a plasma membrane multiprotein complex that uses NADPH oxidase for the redox reaction (Chapter 3). In addition, some intracellular oxidases (e.g., xanthine oxidase) generate $O_2^{\bar{\cdot}}$.
- *Enzymatic metabolism of exogenous chemicals or drugs* can generate free radicals that are not ROS but have similar effects (e.g., CCl_4 can generate $^{\bullet}CCl_3$, described later in the chapter).
- *Transition metals* such as iron and copper donate or accept free electrons during intracellular reactions and catalyze free radical formation, as in the Fenton reaction

Table 2-3 Properties of the Principal Free Radicals Involved in Cell Injury

Properties	$O_2^{\bar{\bullet}}$	H_2O_2	$^{\bullet}OH$	$ONOO^-$
Mechanisms of production	Incomplete reduction of O_2 during oxidative phosphorylation; by phagocyte oxidase in leukocytes	Generated by SOD from $O_2^{\bar{\bullet}}$ and by oxidases in peroxisomes	Generated from H_2O by hydrolysis, e.g., by radiation; from H_2O_2 by Fenton reaction; from $O_2^{\bar{\bullet}}$	Produced by interaction of $O_2^{\bar{\bullet}}$ and NO generated by NO synthase in many cell types (endothelial cells, leukocytes, neurons, others)
Mechanisms of inactivation	Conversion to H_2O_2 and O_2 by SOD	Conversion to H_2O and O_2 by catalase (peroxisomes), glutathione peroxidase (cytosol, mitochondria)	Conversion to H_2O by glutathione peroxidase	Conversion to HNO_2 by peroxiredoxins (cytosol, mitochondria)
Pathologic effects	Stimulates production of degradative enzymes in leukocytes and other cells; may directly damage lipids, proteins, DNA; acts close to site of production	Can be converted to $^{\bullet}OH$ and OCl^-, which destroy microbes and cells; can act distant from site of production	Most reactive oxygen-derived free radical; principal ROS responsible for damaging lipids, proteins, and DNA	Damages lipids, proteins, DNA

HNO_2, nitrite; H_2O_2, hydrogen peroxide; NO, nitric oxide; $O_2^{\bar{\bullet}}$, superoxide anion; OCl^-, hypochlorite; $^{\bullet}OH$, hydroxyl radical; $ONOO^-$, peroxynitrite; ROS, reactive oxygen species; SOD, superoxide dismutase.

($H_2O_2 + Fe^{2+} \rightarrow Fe^{3+} + {}^{\bullet}OH + OH^-$). Because most of the intracellular free iron is in the ferric (Fe^{3+}) state, it must be reduced to the ferrous (Fe^{2+}) form to participate in the Fenton reaction. This reduction can be enhanced by $O_2^{\bar{\bullet}}$, and thus sources of iron and $O_2^{\bar{\bullet}}$ may cooperate in oxidative cell damage.

- *Nitric oxide (NO)*, an important chemical mediator generated by endothelial cells, macrophages, neurons, and other cell types (Chapter 3), can act as a free radical and can also be converted to highly reactive peroxynitrite anion ($ONOO^-$) as well as NO_2 and NO_3^-.

Removal of Free Radicals. Free radicals are inherently unstable and generally decay spontaneously. $O_2^{\bar{\bullet}}$, for example, is unstable and decays (dismutates) spontaneously to O_2 and H_2O_2 in the presence of water. In addition, cells have developed multiple nonenzymatic and enzymatic mechanisms to remove free radicals and thereby minimize injury (Fig. 2-20). These include the following:

- *Antioxidants* either block free radical formation or inactivate (e.g., scavenge) free radicals. Examples are the lipid-soluble vitamins E and A as well as ascorbic acid and glutathione in the cytosol.
- As we have seen, free *iron* and *copper* can catalyze the formation of ROS. Under normal circumstances, the reactivity of these metals is minimized by their binding to storage and transport proteins (e.g., transferrin, ferritin, lactoferrin, and ceruloplasmin), which prevents these metals from participating in reactions that generate ROS.
- A series of *enzymes* acts as free radical-scavenging systems and breaks down H_2O_2 and $O_2^{\bar{\bullet}}$. These enzymes are located near the sites of generation of the oxidants and include the following:
  1. *Catalase,* present in peroxisomes, decomposes H_2O_2 ($2H_2O_2 \rightarrow O_2 + 2H_2O$).
  2. *Superoxidase dismutases* (SODs) are found in many cell types and convert $O_2^{\bar{\bullet}}$ to H_2O_2 ($2O_2^{\bar{\bullet}} + 2H \rightarrow H_2O_2 + O_2$). This group of enzymes includes both manganese-SOD, which is localized in mitochondria, and copper-zinc-SOD, which is found in the cytosol.
  3. *Glutathione peroxidase* also protects against injury by catalyzing free radical breakdown (H_2O_2 + 2GSH $\rightarrow$ GSSG [glutathione homodimer] + $2H_2O$, or $2^{\bullet}OH$ + 2GSH $\rightarrow$ GSSG + $2H_2O$). The intracellular ratio of oxidized glutathione (GSSG) to reduced glutathione (GSH) is a reflection of the oxidative state of the cell and is an important indicator of the cell's ability to detoxify ROS.

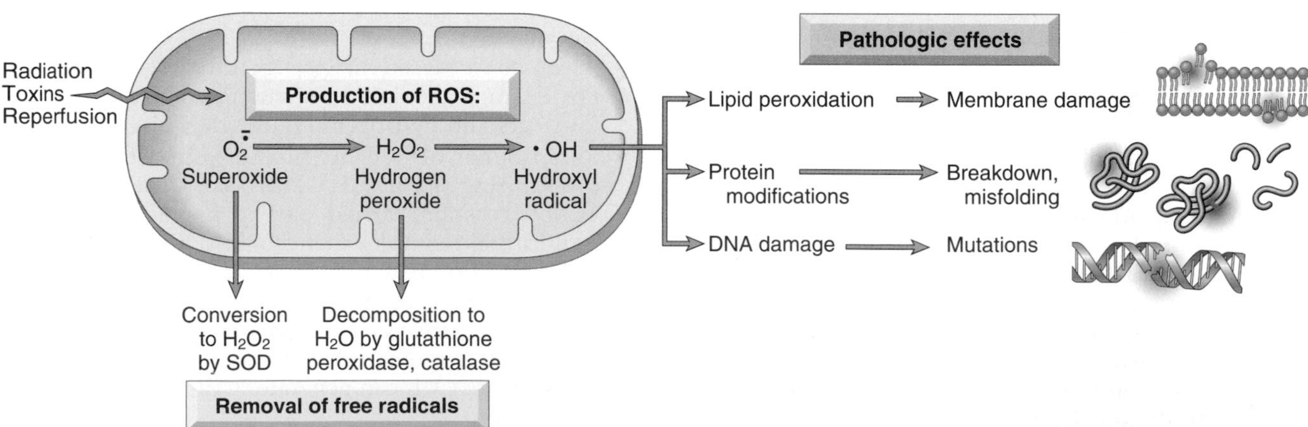

Figure 2-20 The generation, removal, and role of reactive oxygen species (ROS) in cell injury. The production of ROS is increased by many injurious stimuli. These free radicals are removed by spontaneous decay and by specialized enzymatic systems. Excessive production or inadequate removal leads to accumulation of free radicals in cells, which may damage lipids (by peroxidation), proteins, and deoxyribonucleic acid (DNA), resulting in cell injury.

Pathologic Effects of Free Radicals. The effects of ROS and other free radicals are wide-ranging, but three reactions are particularly relevant to cell injury (Fig. 2-20):

- *Lipid peroxidation in membranes*. In the presence of O_2, free radicals may cause peroxidation of lipids within plasma and organellar membranes. Oxidative damage is initiated when the double bonds in unsaturated fatty acids of membrane lipids are attacked by O_2-derived free radicals, particularly by $^{\bullet}OH$. The lipid-free radical interactions yield peroxides, which are themselves unstable and reactive, and an autocatalytic chain reaction ensues (called *propagation*) that can result in extensive membrane damage.
- *Oxidative modification of proteins*. Free radicals promote oxidation of amino acid side chains, formation of covalent protein-protein cross-lins (e.g., disulfide bonds), and oxidation of the protein backbone. Oxidative modification of proteins may damage the active sites of enzymes, disrupt the conformation of structural proteins, and enhance proteasomal degradation of unfolded or misfolded proteins, raising havoc throughout the cell.
- *Lesions in DNA*. Free radicals are capable of causing single- and double-strand breaks in DNA, cross-linking of DNA strands, and formation of adducts. Oxidative DNA damage has been implicated in cell aging (discussed later in this chapter) and in malignant transformation of cells (Chapter 7).

The traditional thinking about free radicals was that they cause cell injury and death by necrosis, and, in fact, the production of ROS is a frequent prelude to necrosis. However, it is now clear that free radicals can trigger apoptosis as well. Recent studies have also revealed a role of ROS in signaling by a variety of cellular receptors and biochemical intermediates. In fact, according to one hypothesis, the major actions of $O_2^{\bar{\bullet}}$ stem from its ability to stimulate the production of degradative enzymes rather than direct damage of macromolecules. It is also possible that these potentially deadly molecules, when produced under physiologic conditions in the "right" dose, serve important physiologic functions.

Defects in Membrane Permeability

Early loss of selective membrane permeability, leading ultimately to overt membrane damage, is a consistent feature of most forms of cell injury (except apoptosis). Membrane damage may affect the functions and integrity of all cellular membranes. The following paragraphs discuss the mechanisms and pathologic consequences of membrane damage.

Mechanisms of Membrane Damage. In ischemic cells, membrane defects may be the result of ATP depletion and calcium-mediated activation of phospholipases. The plasma membrane can also be damaged directly by various bacterial toxins, viral proteins, lytic complement components, and a variety of physical and chemical agents. Several biochemical mechanisms may contribute to membrane damage (Fig. 2-21):

- *Reactive oxygen species*. Oxygen free radicals cause injury to cell membranes by lipid peroxidation, discussed earlier.

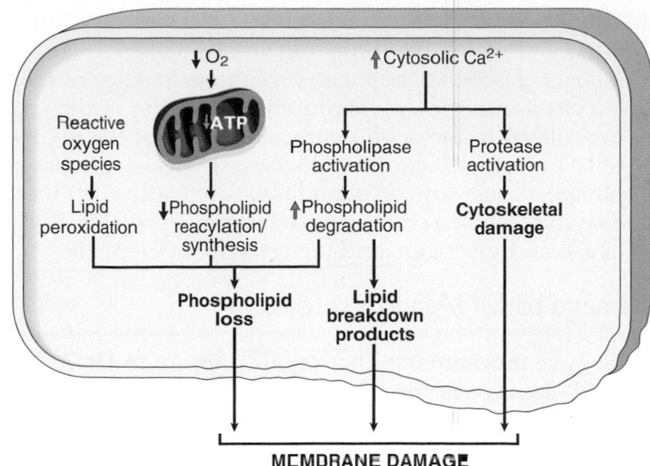

Figure 2-21 Mechanisms of membrane damage in cell injury. Decreased O_2 and increased cytosolic Ca^{2+} are typically seen in ischemia but may accompany other forms of cell injury. Reactive oxygen species, which are often produced on reperfusion of ischemic tissues, also cause membrane damage (not shown).

- *Decreased phospholipid synthesis*. The production of phospholipids in cells may be reduced as a consequence of defective mitochondrial function or hypoxia, both of which decrease the production of ATP and thus affect energy-dependent biosynthetic pathways. The decreased phospholipid synthesis may affect all cellular membranes, including the mitochondria themselves.
- *Increased phospholipid breakdown*. Severe cell injury is associated with increased degradation of membrane phospholipids, probably due to activation of calcium-dependent phospholipases by increased levels of cytosolic and mitochondrial $Ca2^+$. Phospholipid breakdown leads to the accumulation of *lipid breakdown products*, including unesterified free fatty acids, acyl carnitine, and lysophospholipids, which have a detergent effect on membranes. They may also either insert into the lipid bilayer of the membrane or exchange with membrane phospholipids, potentially causing changes in permeability and electrophysiologic alterations.
- *Cytoskeletal abnormalities*. Cytoskeletal filaments serve as anchors connecting the plasma membrane to the cell interior. Activation of proteases by increased cytosolic calcium may cause damage to elements of the cytoskeleton. In the presence of cell swelling, this damage results, particularly in myocardial cells, in detachment of the cell membrane from the cytoskeleton, rendering it susceptible to stretching and rupture.

Consequences of Membrane Damage. The most important sites of membrane damage during cell injury are the mitochondrial membrane, the plasma membrane, and membranes of lysosomes.

- *Mitochondrial membrane damage*. As discussed earlier, damage to mitochondrial membranes results in opening of the mitochondrial permeability transition pore, leading to decreased ATP generation and release of proteins that trigger apoptotic death.
- *Plasma membrane damage*. Plasma membrane damage results in loss of osmotic balance and influx of fluids and ions, as well as loss of cellular contents. The cells may

also leak metabolites that are vital for the reconstitution of ATP, thus further depleting energy stores.

- *Injury to lysosomal membranes* results in leakage of their enzymes into the cytoplasm and activation of the acid hydrolases in the acidic intracellular pH of the injured cell. Lysosomes contain RNases, DNases, proteases, phosphatases, and glucosidases. Activation of these enzymes leads to enzymatic digestion of proteins, RNA, DNA, and glycogen, and the cells die by necrosis.

Damage to DNA and Proteins

Cells have mechanisms that repair damage to DNA, but if DNA damage is too severe to be corrected (e.g., after exposure to DNA damaging drugs, radiation, or oxidative stress), the cell initiates a suicide program that results in death by apoptosis. A similar reaction is triggered by improperly folded proteins, which may be the result of inherited mutations or acquired triggers such as free radicals. Because these mechanisms of cell injury typically cause apoptosis, they are discussed later in the chapter.

Reversible vs Irreversible Injury. Before concluding the discussion of the mechanisms of cell injury, it is useful to consider the possible events that determine when reversible injury becomes irreversible and progresses to cell death. The clinical relevance of this question is obvious—if we can answer it, we may be able to devise strategies for preventing cell injury from having permanent deleterious consequences. However, the molecular mechanisms connecting most forms of cell injury to ultimate cell death have proved elusive, for several reasons. The "point of no return," at which the damage becomes irreversible, is still largely undefined, and there are no reliable morphologic or biochemical correlates of irreversibility. *Two phenomena consistently characterize irreversibility—the inability to reverse mitochondrial dysfunction* (lack of oxidative phosphorylation and ATP generation) even after resolution of the original injury, and *profound disturbances in membrane function.* As mentioned earlier, injury to lysosomal membranes results in the enzymatic dissolution of the injured cell that is characteristic of necrosis.

Leakage of intracellular proteins through the damaged cell membrane and ultimately into the circulation provides a means of detecting tissue-specific cellular injury and necrosis using blood serum samples. Cardiac muscle, for example, contains a specific isoform of the enzyme creatine kinase and of the contractile protein troponin; liver (and specifically bile duct epithelium) contains an isoform of the enzyme alkaline phosphatase; and hepatocytes contain transaminases. Irreversible injury and cell death in these tissues are reflected in increased levels of such proteins in the blood, and measurement of these biomarkers is used clinically to assess damage to these tissues.

KEY CONCEPTS

Mechanisms of Cell Injury

- ATP depletion: failure of energy-dependent functions → reversible injury → necrosis
- Mitochondrial damage: ATP depletion → failure of energy-dependent cellular functions → ultimately, necrosis; under some conditions, leakage of mitochondrial proteins that cause apoptosis
- Influx of calcium: activation of enzymes that damage cellular components and may also trigger apoptosis
- Accumulation of reactive oxygen species: covalent modification of cellular proteins, lipids, nucleic acids
- Increased permeability of cellular membranes: may affect plasma membrane, lysosomal membranes, mitochondrial membranes; typically culminates in necrosis
- Accumulation of damaged DNA and misfolded proteins: triggers apoptosis

Clinicopathologic Correlations: Selected Examples of Cell Injury and Necrosis

Having briefly reviewed the causes, morphology, and mechanisms of cell injury and necrotic cell death, we now describe some common and clinically significant forms of cell injury that typically culminate in necrosis. These examples illustrate many of the mechanisms and sequence of events in cell injury described earlier.

Ischemic and Hypoxic Injury

Ischemia is the most common type of cell injury in clinical medicine and it results from hypoxia induced by reduced blood flow, most commonly due to a mechanical arterial obstruction. It can also be caused by reduced venous drainage. In contrast to hypoxia, during which energy production by anaerobic glycolysis can continue, ischemia compromises the delivery of substrates for glycolysis. Thus, in ischemic tissues, not only is aerobic metabolism compromised but anaerobic energy generation also stops after glycolytic substrates are exhausted, or glycolysis is inhibited by the accumulation of metabolites that would otherwise be washed out by flowing blood. For this reason, *ischemia tends to cause more rapid and severe cell and tissue injury than does hypoxia in the absence of ischemia.*

Mechanisms of Ischemic Cell Injury

The sequence of events following hypoxia or ischemia reflects many of the biochemical alterations in cell injury described earlier and summarized here. As the oxygen tension within the cell falls, there is loss of oxidative phosphorylation and decreased generation of ATP. The depletion of ATP results in failure of the sodium pump, leading to efflux of potassium, influx of sodium and water, and cell swelling. There is also influx of $Ca2^{+}$, with its many deleterious effects. There is progressive loss of glycogen and decreased protein synthesis. The functional consequences may be severe at this stage. For instance, heart muscle ceases to contract within 60 seconds of coronary artery occlusion. Note, however, that loss of contractility does not mean cell death. If hypoxia continues, worsening ATP depletion causes further deterioration. The cytoskeleton disperses, resulting in the loss of ultrastructural features such as microvilli and the formation of "blebs" at the cell surface (Figs. 2-9 and 2-10). "Myelin figures," derived from degenerating cellular membranes, may be seen within the cytoplasm (in autophagic vacuoles) or extracellularly. They are thought to result from unmasking of phosphatide groups, promoting the uptake and intercalation of water between the lamellar stacks of membranes. At this time the mitochondria are usually swollen, as a result of loss of volume control in these organelles; the ER remains dilated; and the entire cell is markedly swollen, with increased concentrations of water, sodium, and chloride and a decreased concentration of potassium. *If oxygen is restored, all of these disturbances are reversible.*

If ischemia persists, irreversible injury and necrosis ensue. Irreversible injury is associated morphologically with severe swelling of mitochondria, extensive damage to plasma membranes (giving rise to myelin figures) and swelling of lysosomes (Fig. 2-10C). Large, flocculent, amorphous densities develop in the mitochondrial matrix. In the myocardium, these are indications of irreversible injury and can be seen as early as 30 to 40 minutes after ischemia. Massive influx of calcium into the cell then occurs, particularly if the ischemic zone is reperfused. Death is mainly by necrosis, but apoptosis also contributes; the apoptotic pathway is probably activated by release of pro-apoptotic molecules from leaky mitochondria. The cell's components are progressively degraded, and there is widespread leakage of cellular enzymes into the extracellular space and, conversely, entry of extracellular macromolecules from the interstitial space into the dying cells. Finally, the dead cells may become replaced by large masses composed of phospholipids in the form of myelin figures. These are then either phagocytosed by leukocytes or degraded further into fatty acids. Calcification of such fatty acid residues may occur, with the formation of calcium soaps.

As mentioned before, leakage of intracellular enzymes and other proteins across the abnormally permeable plasma membrane and into the blood provides important clinical indicators of cell death. For example, elevated serum levels of cardiac muscle creatine kinase MB and troponin are early signs of myocardial infarction, and may be seen before the infarct is detectable morphologically (Chapter 12).

Mammalian cells have developed protective responses to deal with hypoxic stress. The best-defined of these is induction of a transcription factor called *hypoxia-inducible factor-1*, which promotes new blood vessel formation, stimulates cell survival pathways, and enhances anaerobic glycolysis. It remains to be seen if understanding of such oxygen-sensing mechanisms will lead to new strategies for preventing or treating ischemic and hypoxic cell injury.

Despite many investigations in experimental models there are still no reliable therapeutic approaches for reducing the injurious consequences of ischemia in clinical situations. The strategy that is perhaps the most useful in ischemic (and traumatic) brain and spinal cord injury is the transient induction of hypothermia (reducing the core body temperature to 92°F). This treatment reduces the metabolic demands of the stressed cells, decreases cell swelling, suppresses the formation of free radicals, and inhibits the host inflammatory response. All of these may contribute to decreased cell and tissue injury.

Ischemia-Reperfusion Injury

Restoration of blood flow to ischemic tissues can promote recovery of cells if they are reversibly injured, but can also paradoxically exacerbate the injury and cause cell death. As a consequence, reperfused tissues may sustain loss of cells in addition to the cells that are irreversibly damaged at the end of ischemia. This process, called *ischemia-reperfusion injury*, is clinically important because it contributes to tissue damage during myocardial and cerebral infarction and following therapies to restore blood flow (Chapters 12 and 28).

How does reperfusion injury occur? The likely answer is that new damaging processes are set in motion during reperfusion, causing the death of cells that might have recovered otherwise. Several mechanisms have been proposed:

- *Oxidative stress.* New damage may be initiated during reoxygenation by increased generation of *reactive oxygen and nitrogen species*. These free radicals may be produced in reperfused tissue as a result of incomplete reduction of oxygen by damaged mitochondria, or because of the action of oxidases in leukocytes, endothelial cells, or parenchymal cells. Cellular antioxidant defense mechanisms may be compromised by ischemia, favoring the accumulation of free radicals.
- *Intracellular calcium overload.* As mentioned earlier, intracellular and mitochondrial calcium overload begins during acute ischemia; it is exacerbated during reperfusion due to influx of calcium resulting from cell membrane damage and ROS mediated injury to sarcoplasmic reticulum. Calcium overload favors opening of the mitochondrial permeability transition pore with resultant depletion of ATP. This in turn causes further cell injury.
- *Inflammation.* Ischemic injury is associated with inflammation as a result of "dangers signals" released from dead cells, cytokines secreted by resident immune cells such as macrophages, and increased expression of adhesion molecules by hypoxic parenchymal and endothelial cells, all of which act to recruit circulating neutrophils to reperfused tissue. The inflammation causes additional tissue injury (Chapter 3). The importance of neutrophil influx in reperfusion injury has been demonstrated experimentally by the salutary effects of treatment with antibodies that block cytokines or adhesion molecules and thereby reduce neutrophil extravasation.
- Activation of the *complement system* may contribute to ischemia-reperfusion injury. Some IgM antibodies have a propensity to deposit in ischemic tissues, for unknown reasons, and when blood flow is resumed, complement proteins bind to the deposited antibodies, are activated, and cause more cell injury and inflammation.

Chemical (Toxic) Injury

Chemical injury remains a frequent problem in clinical medicine and is a major limitation to drug therapy. Because many drugs are metabolized in the liver, this organ is a frequent target of drug toxicity. In fact, toxic liver injury is perhaps the most frequent reason for terminating the therapeutic use or development of a drug. The mechanisms by which chemicals, certain drugs, and toxins produce injury are described in greater detail in Chapter 9 in the discussion of environmental diseases. Here the major pathways of chemically induced injury with selected examples are described.

Chemicals induce cell injury by one of two general mechanisms:

- *Direct toxicity.* Some chemicals can injure cells directly by combining with critical molecular components. For example, in mercuric chloride poisoning, mercury binds to the sulfhydryl groups of cell membrane proteins, causing increased membrane permeability and inhibition of ion transport. In such instances, the greatest damage is usually to the cells that use, absorb, excrete, or concentrate the chemicals—in the case of mercuric chloride, the cells of the gastrointestinal tract and kidney (Chapter 9). *Cyanide* poisons mitochondrial cytochrome oxidase and thus inhibits oxidative phosphorylation. Many antineoplastic chemotherapeutic agents and antibiotics also induce cell damage by direct cytotoxic effects.
- *Conversion to toxic metabolites.* Most toxic chemicals are not biologically active in their native form but must be converted to reactive toxic metabolites, which then act on target molecules. This modification is usually accomplished by the cytochrome P-450 mixed-function oxidases in the smooth ER of the liver and other organs. The toxic metabolites cause membrane damage and cell injury mainly by formation of *free radicals* and subsequent lipid peroxidation; direct covalent binding to membrane proteins and lipids may also contribute. For instance, CCl_4, which was once widely used in the dry cleaning industry, is converted by cytochrome P-450 to the highly reactive free radical $^{\bullet}CCl_3$, which causes lipid peroxidation and damages many cellular structures. Acetaminophen, an analgesic drug, is also converted to a toxic product during detoxification in the liver, leading to cell injury. These and other examples of chemical injury are described in Chapter 9.

KEY CONCEPTS

Ischemic and Toxic Injury

- Mild Ischemia: Reduced oxidative phosphorylation →. reduced ATP generation → failure of Na pump → influx of sodium and water → organelle and cellular swelling (reversible)
- Severe/prolonged ischemia: severe swelling of mitochondria, calcium influx into mitochondria and into the cell with rupture of lysosomes and plasma membrane. Death by necrosis and apoptosis due the release of cytochrome c from mitochondria
- Reperfusions injury follows blood flow into ischemic area is caused by oxidative stress due to release of free radicals from leukocytes and endothelial cells. Blood brings calcium that overloads reversibly injured cells with consequent mitochondrial injury. Influx of leukocytes generates free radicals and cytokines. Local activation of complement by IgM antibodies deposited in ischemic tissues.
- Chemicals may cause injury directly or by conversion into toxic metabolites. The organs chiefly affected are those involved in absorption or excretion of chemicals or others such as liver where the chemicals are converted to toxic metabolites. Direct injury to critical organelles such as mitochondria or indirect injury from free radicals generated from the chemicals/toxins is involved.

Apoptosis

Apoptosis is a pathway of cell death that is induced by a tightly regulated suicide program in which cells destined to die activate intrinsic enzymes that degrade the cells' own nuclear DNA and nuclear and cytoplasmic proteins. Apoptotic cells break up into fragments, called *apoptotic bodies,* which contain portions of the cytoplasm and nucleus. The plasma membrane of the apoptotic cell and bodies remains intact, but its structure is altered in such a way that these become "tasty" targets for phagocytes. The dead cell and its fragments are rapidly devoured, before the contents have leaked out, and therefore cell death by this pathway does not elicit an inflammatory reaction in the host. The process was recognized in 1972 by the distinctive morphologic appearance of membrane-bound fragments derived from cells, and named after the Greek designation for "falling off." It was quickly appreciated that apoptosis was a unique mechanism of cell death, distinct from necrosis, which is characterized by loss of membrane integrity, enzymatic digestion of cells, leakage of cellular contents, and frequently a host reaction (Fig. 2-8 and Table 2-2). Because it is genetically regulated, apoptosis is sometimes referred to as *programmed cell death.* As already alluded to, certain forms of necrosis, called *necroptosis,* are also genetically programmed, but by a distinct set of genes.

Causes of Apoptosis

Apoptosis occurs normally both during development and throughout adulthood, and serves to remove unwanted, aged, or potentially harmful cells. It is also a pathologic event when diseased cells become damaged beyond repair and are eliminated.

Apoptosis in Physiologic Situations

Death by apoptosis is a normal phenomenon that serves to eliminate cells that are no longer needed, and to maintain a steady number of various cell populations in tissues. It is important in the following physiologic situations:

- *The destruction of cells during embryogenesis,* including implantation, organogenesis, developmental involution, and metamorphosis. The term *programmed cell death* was originally coined to denote death of specific cell types that was precisely regulated and occurred at defined times during the development of multicellular organisms. Apoptosis is a generic term for this pattern of cell death, regardless of the context, but it is often used interchangeably with programmed cell death. However, it is best to avoid this term to denote apoptosis, since in some cases necrosis may also be a form of programmed cell death
- *Involution of hormone-dependent tissues upon hormone withdrawal,* such as endometrial cell breakdown during the menstrual cycle, ovarian follicular atresia in menopause, the regression of the lactating breast after weaning, and prostatic atrophy after castration.
- *Cell loss in proliferating cell populations,* such as immature lymphocytes in the bone marrow and thymus and B

lymphocytes in germinal centers that fail to express useful antigen receptors (Chapter 6), and epithelial cells in intestinal crypts, so as to maintain a constant number *(homeostasis)*.

- *Elimination of potentially harmful self-reactive lymphocytes,* either before or after they have completed their maturation, so as to prevent reactions against one's own tissues (Chapter 6).
- Death of host cells that have served their useful purpose, such as neutrophils in an *acute inflammatory response,* and lymphocytes at the end of an *immune response.* In these situations cells undergo apoptosis because they are deprived of necessary survival signals, such as growth factors.

Apoptosis in Pathologic Conditions

Apoptosis eliminates cells that are injured beyond repair without eliciting a host reaction, thus limiting collateral tissue damage. Death by apoptosis is responsible for loss of cells in a variety of pathologic states:

- *DNA damage.* Radiation, cytotoxic anticancer drugs, and hypoxia can damage DNA, either directly or via production of free radicals. If repair mechanisms cannot cope with the injury, the cell triggers intrinsic mechanisms that induce apoptosis. In these situations elimination of the cell may be a better alternative than risking mutations in the damaged DNA, which may result in malignant transformation.
- *Accumulation of misfolded proteins.* Improperly folded proteins may arise because of mutations in the genes encoding these proteins or because of extrinsic factors, such as damage caused by free radicals. Excessive accumulation of these proteins in the ER leads to a condition called *ER stress,* which culminates in apoptotic cell death. Apoptosis caused by the accumulation of misfolded proteins has been invoked as the basis of several degenerative diseases of the central nervous system and other organs.
- *Cell death in certain infections,* particularly viral infections, in which loss of infected cells is largely due to apoptosis that may be induced by the virus (as in adenovirus and HIV infections) or by the host immune response (as in viral hepatitis). An important host response to viruses consists of cytotoxic T lymphocytes specific for viral proteins, which induce apoptosis of infected cells in an attempt to eliminate reservoirs of infection. During this process there can be significant tissue damage. The same T-cell–mediated mechanism is responsible for cell death in *tumors* and cellular rejection of *transplants.*
- *Pathologic atrophy in parenchymal organs after duct obstruction,* such as occurs in the pancreas, parotid gland, and kidney.

Morphologic and Biochemical Changes in Apoptosis

Before discussing the mechanisms of apoptosis, the morphologic and biochemical characteristics of this process are described.

MORPHOLOGY

The following morphologic features, some best seen with the electron microscope, characterize cells undergoing apoptosis (Fig. 2-22, and see Fig. 2-8).

Cell shrinkage. The cell is smaller in size, the cytoplasm is dense (Fig. 2-22*A*), and the organelles, although relatively normal, are more tightly packed. (Recall that in other forms of cell injury, an early feature is cell swelling, not shrinkage.)

Chromatin condensation. This is the most characteristic feature of apoptosis. The chromatin aggregates peripherally, under the nuclear membrane, into dense masses of various shapes and sizes (Fig. 2-22*B*). The nucleus itself may break up, producing two or more fragments.

Formation of cytoplasmic blebs and apoptotic bodies. The apoptotic cell first shows extensive surface blebbing, then undergoes fragmentation into membrane-bound apoptotic bodies composed of cytoplasm and tightly packed organelles, with or without nuclear fragments (Fig. 2-22*C*).

Phagocytosis of apoptotic cells or cell bodies, usually by macrophages. The apoptotic bodies are rapidly ingested by phagocytes and degraded by the phagocyte's lysosomal enzymes.

Plasma membranes are thought to remain intact during apoptosis, until the last stages, when they become permeable to normally retained solutes.

On histologic examination, in tissues stained with hematoxylin and eosin, the apoptotic cell appears as a round or oval mass of intensely eosinophilic cytoplasm with fragments of dense nuclear chromatin (Fig. 2-22*A*). Because the cell shrinkage and formation of apoptotic bodies are rapid and the pieces are quickly phagocytosed, considerable apoptosis may occur in tissues before it becomes apparent in histologic sections. In addition, apoptosis—in contrast to necrosis—does not elicit inflammation, making it more difficult to detect histologically.

Mechanisms of Apoptosis

Apoptosis results from the activation of enzymes called *caspases* (so named because they are cysteine proteases that cleave proteins after aspartic residues). Like many proteases, caspases exist as inactive proenzymes, or zymogens, and must undergo enzymatic cleavage to become active. The presence of cleaved, active caspases is a marker for cells undergoing apoptosis (Fig. 2-22*C*). The process of apoptosis may be divided into an *initiation phase,* during which some caspases become catalytically active, and an *execution phase,* during which other caspases trigger the degradation of critical cellular components. The activation of caspases depends on a finely tuned balance between production of pro-apoptotic and anti-apoptotic proteins.

Two distinct pathways converge on caspase activation: the mitochondrial pathway and the death receptor pathway (Fig 2-23). Although these pathways can intersect, they are generally induced under different conditions, involve different molecules, and serve distinct roles in physiology and disease.

The Intrinsic (Mitochondrial) Pathway of Apoptosis

The mitochondrial pathway is the major mechanism of apoptosis in all mammalian cells. It results from increased permeability of the mitochondrial outer membrane with consequent release of death-inducing (pro-apoptotic)

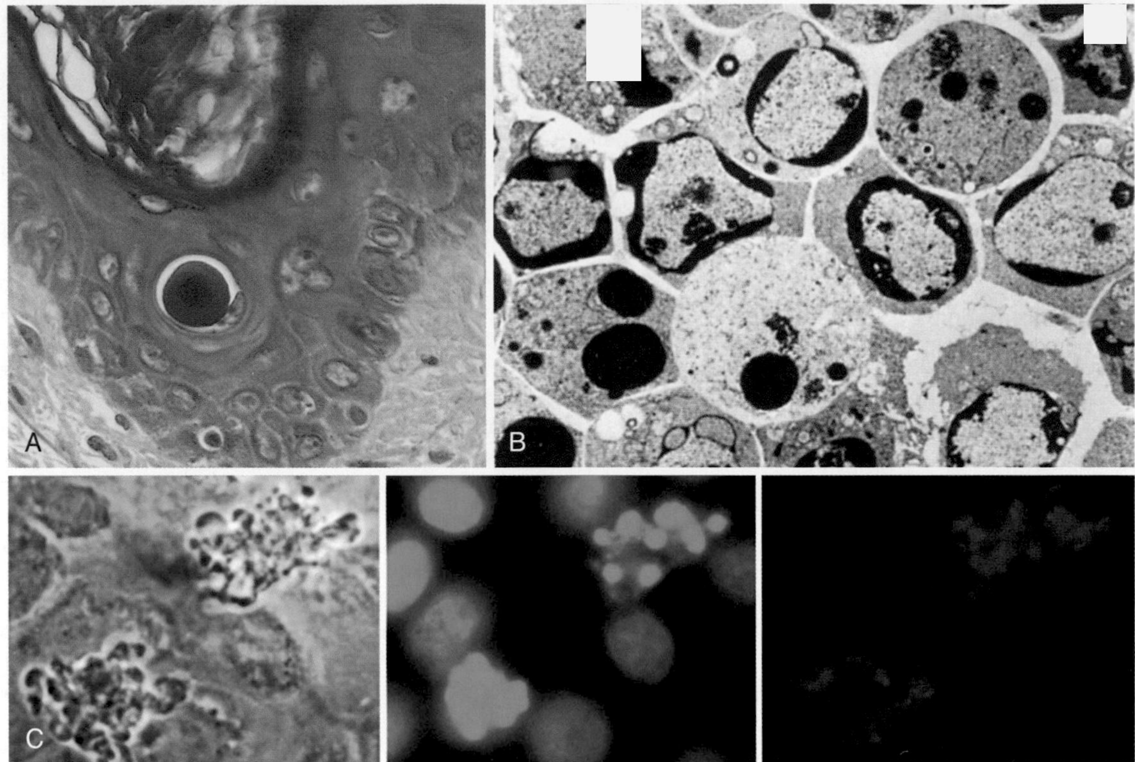

Figure 2-22 Morphologic features of apoptosis. **A,** Apoptosis of an epidermal cell in an immune reaction. The cell is reduced in size and contains brightly eosinophilic cytoplasm and a condensed nucleus. **B,** This electron micrograph of cultured cells undergoing apoptosis shows some nuclei with peripheral crescents of compacted chromatin, and others that are uniformly dense or fragmented. **C,** These images of cultured cells undergoing apoptosis show blebbing and formation of apoptotic bodies (*left panel*, phase contrast micrograph), a stain for DNA showing nuclear fragmentation (*middle panel*), and activation of caspase-3 (*right panel*, immunofluorescence stain with an antibody specific for the active form of caspase-3, revealed as red color). (**B,** From Kerr JFR, Harmon BV: Definition and incidence of apoptosis: a historical perspective. In Tomei LD, Cope FO (eds): Apoptosis: The Molecular Basis of Cell Death. Cold Spring Harbor, NY, Cold Spring Harbor Laboratory Press, 1991, pp 5-29; **C,** Courtesy Dr. Zheng Dong, Medical College of Georgia, Augusta, Ga.)

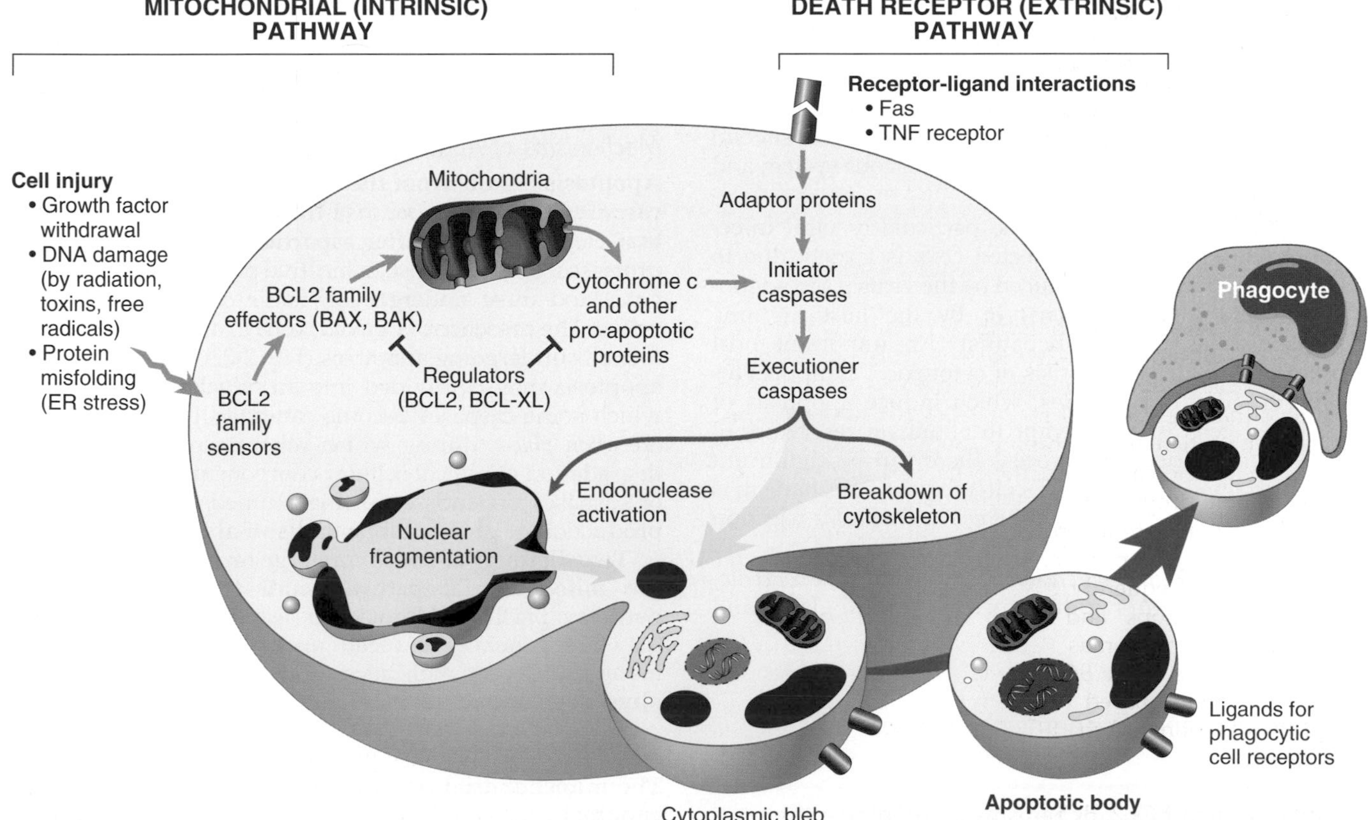

Figure 2-23 Mechanisms of apoptosis. The two pathways of apoptosis differ in their induction and regulation, and both culminate in the activation of caspases. In the mitochondrial pathway, proteins of the BCL2 family, which regulate mitochondrial permeability, become imbalanced and leakage of various substances from mitochondria leads to caspase activation. In death receptor pathway, signals from plasma membrane receptors lead to the assembly of adaptor proteins into a "death-including signaling complex," which activates caspases, and the end result is the same.

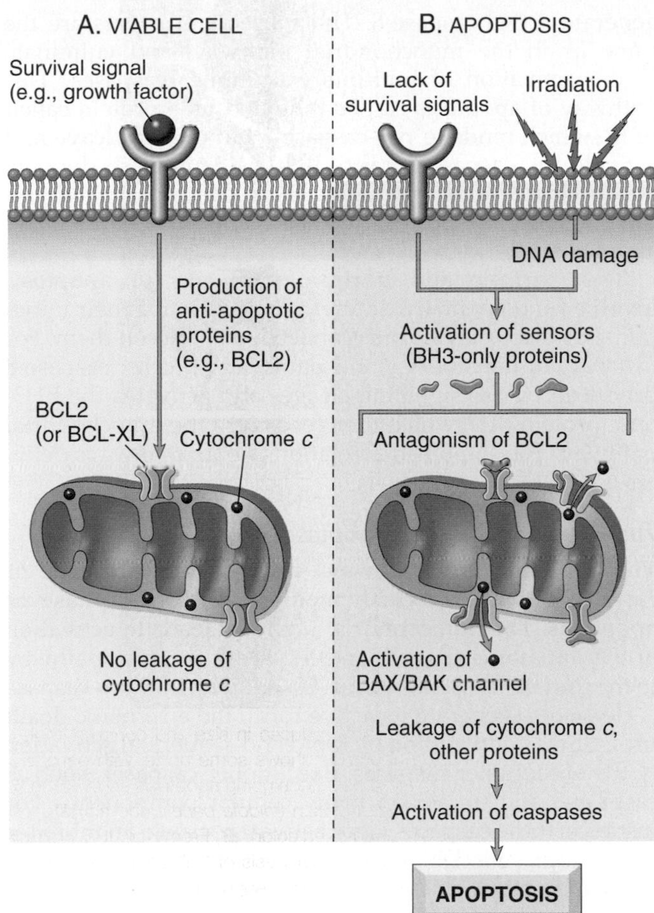

Figure 2-24 The intrinsic (mitochondrial) pathway of apoptosis. **A,** Cell viability is maintained by the induction of anti-apoptotic proteins such as BCL2 by survival signals. These proteins maintain the integrity of mitochondrial membranes and prevent leakage of mitochondrial proteins. **B,** Loss of survival signals, DNA damage, and other insults activate sensors that antagonize the anti-apoptotic proteins and activate the pro-apoptotic proteins BAX and BAK, which form channels in the mitochondrial membrane. The subsequent leakage of cytochrome c (and other proteins, not shown) leads to caspase activation and apoptosis.

molecules from the mitochondrial intermembrane space into the cytoplasm (Fig. 2-24). Mitochondria are remarkable organelles in that they contain proteins such as cytochrome c that are essential for life, but some of the same proteins, in particular cytochrome c, when released into the cytoplasm (an indication that the cell is not healthy), initiate the suicide program of apoptosis. The release of mitochondrial pro-apoptotic proteins is tightly controlled by the BCL2 family of proteins This family is named after *BCL2*, which is frequently overexpressed due to chromosomal translocations and resulting rearrangements in certain B cell lymphomas (Chapter 13). There are more than 20 members of the *BCL* family, which can be divided into three groups based on their pro-apoptotic or anti-apoptotic function and the BCL2 homology (BH) domains they possess.

- *Anti-apoptotic.* BCL2, BCL-XL, and MCL1 are the principal members of this group; they possess four BH domains (called BH1-4). These proteins reside in the outer mitochondrial membranes as well as the cytosol and ER membranes. By keeping the mitochondrial outer membrane impermeable they prevent leakage of cytochrome c and other death-inducing proteins into the cytosol (Fig. 2-24*A*).
- *Pro-apoptotic.* BAX and BAK are the two prototypic members of this group. Like their anti-apoptotic cousins they also have four BH domains. Upon activation, BAX and BAK oligomerize within the outer mitochondrial protein and promote mitochondrial outer membrane permeability. The precise mechanism by which Bax-Bak permeabilize membranes is not settled. According to one model illustrated in Fig 2-24*B*, they form a channel in the outer mitochondrial membrane, allowing leakage of cytochrome c from the intermembranous space.
- *Sensors.* Members of this group, including BAD, BIM, BID, Puma, and Noxa, contain only one BH domain, the third of the four BH domains, and hence are sometimes called BH3-only proteins. BH3-only proteins act as sensors of cellular stress and damage, and regulate the balance between the other two groups, thus acting as arbiters of apoptosis.

Growth factors and other survival signals stimulate the production of anti-apoptotic proteins such as BCL2, thus preventing the leakage of death-inducing proteins from the outer mitochondrial membrane. When cells are deprived of survival signals or their DNA is damaged, or misfolded proteins induce ER stress, the BH3-only proteins "sense" such damage and are activated. These sensors in turn activate the two critical (pro-apoptotic) effectors, BAX and BAK, which form oligomers that insert into the mitochondrial membrane and allow proteins from the inner mitochondrial membrane to leak out into the cytoplasm. BH3-only proteins may also bind to and block the function of BCL2 and BCL-XL. At the same time, the synthesis of BCL2 and BCL-XL may decline because of the relative deficiency of survival signals. The net result of BAX-BAK activation coupled with loss of the protective functions of the anti-apoptotic BCL2 family members is the release into the cytoplasm of several mitochondrial proteins that can activate the caspase cascade (Fig. 2-24). As already mentioned, one of these proteins is cytochrome c, well known for its role in mitochondrial respiration.

Once released into the cytosol, cytochrome c binds to a protein called APAF-1 (apoptosis-activating factor-1), which forms a wheel-like hexamer that has been called the *apoptosome*. This complex is able to bind caspase-9, the critical initiator caspase of the mitochondrial pathway, and the enzyme cleaves adjacent caspase-9 molecules, thus setting up an autoamplification process. Cleavage activates caspase-9, which triggers a cascade of caspase activation by cleaving and thereby activating other pro-caspases, and the active enzymes mediate the execution phase of apoptosis (discussed later). Other mitochondrial proteins, with arcane names like Smac/Diablo, enter the cytoplasm, where they bind to and neutralize cytoplasmic proteins that function as physiologic inhibitors of apoptosis (called IAPs). The normal function of the IAPs is to block the activation of caspases, including executioners like caspase-3, and keep cells alive. Thus, the neutralization of these IAPs permits the initiation of a caspase cascade.

The Extrinsic (Death Receptor-Initiated) Pathway of Apoptosis

This pathway is initiated by engagement of plasma membrane death receptors on a variety of cells. Death receptors are members of the TNF receptor family that contain a cytoplasmic domain involved in protein-protein interactions that is called the *death domain* because it is essential for delivering apoptotic signals. (Some TNF receptor family members do not contain cytoplasmic death domains; their function is to activate inflammatory cascades [Chapter 3], and their role in triggering apoptosis is much less established.) The best known death receptors are the type 1 TNF receptor (TNFR1) and a related protein called Fas (CD95), but several others have been described. The mechanism of apoptosis induced by these death receptors is well illustrated by Fas, a death receptor expressed on many cell types (Fig. 2-25). The ligand for Fas is called Fas ligand (FasL). FasL is expressed on T cells that recognize self antigens (and functions to eliminate self-reactive lymphocytes), and on some cytotoxic T lymphocytes (which kill virus-infected and tumor cells). When FasL binds to Fas, three or more molecules of Fas are brought together, and their cytoplasmic death domains form a binding site for an adaptor protein that also contains a death domain and is called FADD (*F*as-*a*ssociated *d*eath *d*omain). FADD that is attached to the death receptors in turn binds an inactive form of caspase-8 (and, in humans, caspase-10), again via a death domain. Multiple pro-caspase-8 molecules are thus brought into proximity, and they cleave one another to generate active caspase-8. The subsequent events are the same as in the mitochondrial pathway, and culminate in the activation of multiple executioner caspases. This pathway of apoptosis can be inhibited by a protein called FLIP, which binds to pro-caspase-8 but cannot cleave and activate the caspase because it lacks a protease domain. Some viruses and normal cells produce FLIP and use this inhibitor to protect themselves from Fas-mediated apoptosis.

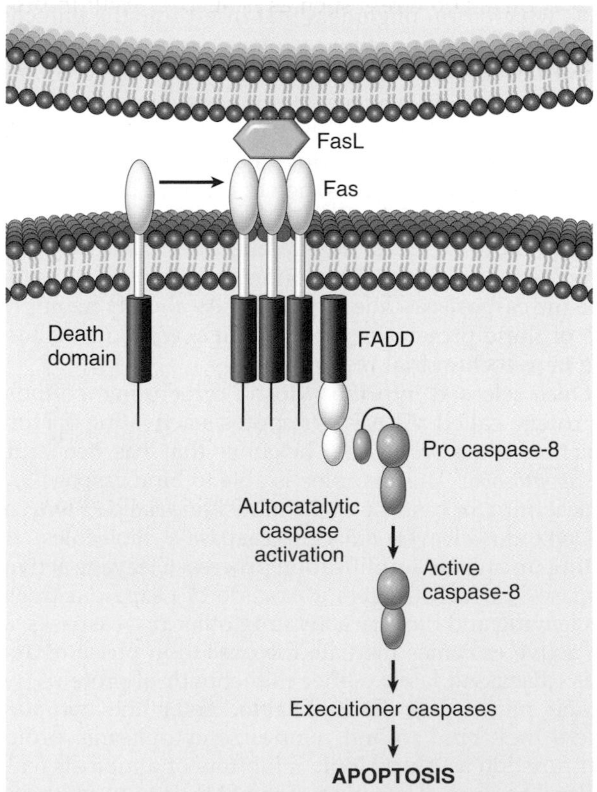

Figure 2-25 The extrinsic (death receptor initiated) pathway of apoptosis, illustrated by the events following Fas engagement. FAAD, Fas-associated death domain; FasL, Fas ligand.

The extrinsic and intrinsic pathways of apoptosis involve fundamentally different molecules for their initiation, but there may be interconnections between them. For instance, in hepatocytes and pancreatic β cells, caspase-8 produced by Fas signaling cleaves and activates the BH3-only protein BID, which then feeds into the mitochondrial pathway. The combined activation of both pathways delivers a fatal blow to the cells.

The Execution Phase of Apoptosis

The two initiating pathways converge to a cascade of caspase activation, which mediates the final phase of apoptosis. The mitochondrial pathway leads to activation of the initiator caspase-9, and the death receptor pathway to the initiator caspases-8 and -10. After an initiator caspase is cleaved to generate its active form, the enzymatic death program is set in motion by rapid and sequential activation of the executioner caspases. Executioner caspases, such as caspase-3 and -6, act on many cellular components. For instance, these caspases, once activated, cleave an inhibitor of a cytoplasmic DNase and thus make the DNase enzymatically active; this enzyme induces cleavage of DNA. Caspases also degrade structural components of the nuclear matrix and thus promote fragmentation of nuclei. Some of the steps in apoptosis are not fully defined. For instance, we do not know how the structure of the plasma membrane is changed in apoptotic cells, or how membrane blebs and apoptotic bodies are formed.

Removal of Dead Cells

The formation of apoptotic bodies breaks cells up into "bite-sized" fragments that are edible for phagocytes. Apoptotic cells and their fragments also undergo several changes in their membranes that actively promote their phagocytosis so they are most often cleared before they undergo secondary necrosis and release their cellular contents (which can result in injurious inflammation). In healthy cells, phosphatidylserine is present on the inner leaflet of the plasma membrane, but in apoptotic cells this phospholipid "flips" out and is expressed on the outer layer of the membrane, where it is recognized by several macrophage receptors. Cells that are dying by apoptosis secrete soluble factors that recruit phagocytes. Some apoptotic bodies are coated by thrombospondin, an adhesive glycoprotein that is recognized by phagocytes, and macrophages themselves may produce proteins that bind to apoptotic cells (but not to live cells) and thus target the dead cells for engulfment. Apoptotic bodies may also become coated with natural antibodies and proteins of the complement system, notably C1q, which are recognized by phagocytes. Thus, numerous receptors on phagocytes and ligands induced on apoptotic cells serve as "eat me" signals and are involved in the binding and engulfment of these cells. This process of phagocytosis of apoptotic cells is so efficient that dead cells disappear, often within minutes, without leaving a trace, and inflammation is absent even in the face of extensive apoptosis.

Clinicopathologic Correlations: Apoptosis in Health and Disease

Examples of Apoptosis

Cell death in many situations is known to be caused by apoptosis, and the selected examples listed illustrate the role of this death pathway in normal physiology and in disease.

Growth Factor Deprivation. Hormone-sensitive cells deprived of the relevant hormone, lymphocytes that are not stimulated by antigens and cytokines, and neurons deprived of nerve growth factor die by apoptosis. In all these situations, apoptosis is triggered by the intrinsic (mitochondrial) pathway and is attributable to decreased synthesis of BCL2 and BCL-XL and activation of BIM and other pro-apoptotic members of the BCL2 family.

DNA Damage. Exposure of cells to radiation or chemotherapeutic agents induces apoptosis by a mechanism that is initiated by DNA damage (genotoxic stress) and that involves the tumor-suppressor gene *TP53*. p53 protein accumulates in cells when DNA is damaged, and it arrests the cell cycle (at the G_1 phase) to allow time for repair (Chapter 7). However, if the damage is too great to be repaired successfully, p53 triggers apoptosis. When *TP53* is mutated or absent (as it is in many cancers), cells with damaged DNA fail to undergo p53-mediated apoptosis and instead survive. In such cells, the DNA damage may result in mutations of various types that lead to neoplastic transformation (Chapter 7). Thus, p53 serves as a critical "life or death" switch following genotoxic stress. The mechanism by which p53 triggers the distal death effector machinery—the caspases—is complex but seems to involve its function as a DNA-binding transcription factor. Among the proteins whose production is stimulated by p53 are several pro-apoptotic members of the BCL2 family, notably BAX, BAK and some BH3-only proteins, mentioned earlier.

Protein Misfolding. Chaperones in the ER control the proper folding of newly synthesized proteins, and misfolded polypeptides are ubiquitinated and targeted for proteolysis in proteasomes (Chapter 1). If, however, unfolded or misfolded proteins accumulate in the ER because of inherited mutations or stresses, they trigger a number of cellular responses, collectively called the *unfolded protein response*. The unfolded protein response activates signaling pathways that increase the production of chaperones, enhance proteasomal degradation of abnormal proteins, and slow protein translation, thus reducing the load of misfolded proteins in the cell (Fig. 2-26). However, if this cytoprotective response is unable to cope with the accumulation of misfolded proteins, the cell activates caspases and induces apoptosis. This process is called *ER stress*. Intracellular accumulation of abnormally folded proteins, caused by genetic mutations, aging, or unknown environmental factors, is now recognized as a feature of a number of neurodegenerative diseases, including Alzheimer, Huntington, and Parkinson diseases (Chapter 28), and possibly type 2 diabetes. Deprivation of glucose and oxygen, and stress such as heat, also result in protein

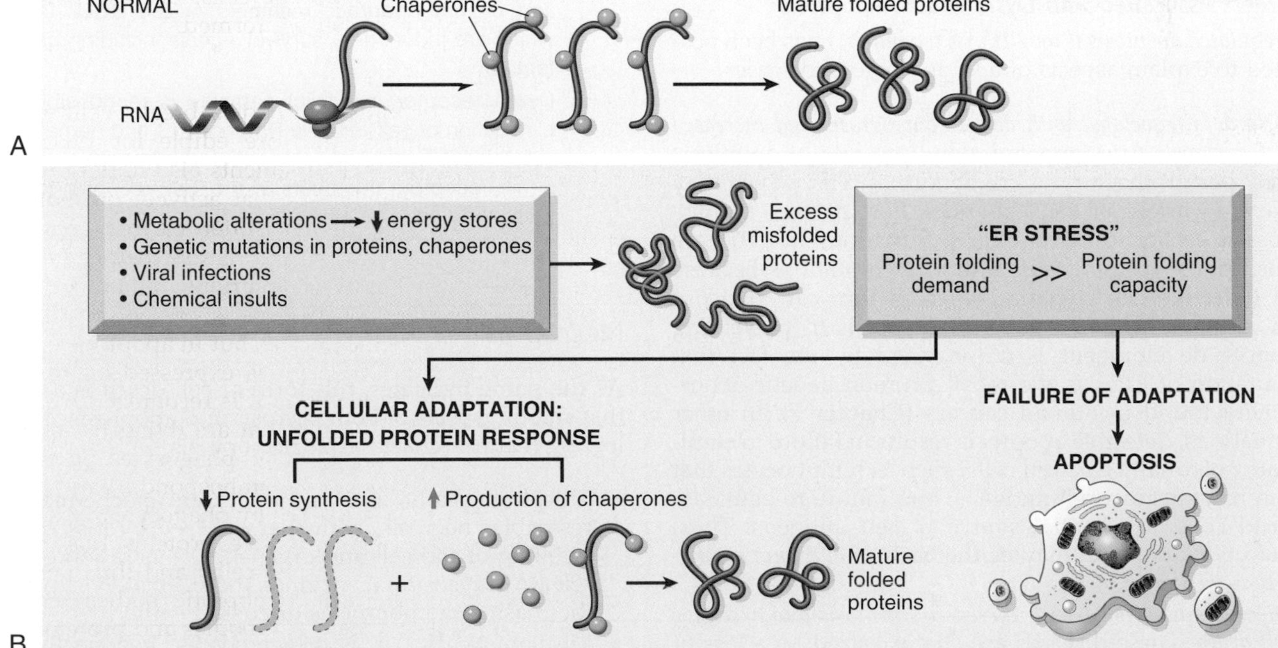

Figure 2-26 The unfolded protein response and endoplasmic reticulum (ER) stress. **A,** In healthy cells, newly synthesized proteins are folded with the help of chaperones and are then incorporated into the cell or secreted. **B,** Various external stresses or mutations induce a state called ER stress, in which the cell is unable to cope with the load of misfolded proteins. Accumulation of these proteins in the ER triggers the unfolded protein response, which tries to restore protein homeostasis; if this response is inadequate, the cell dies by apoptosis.

Table 2-4 Selected Examples of Diseases Caused by Misfolding of Proteins

Disease	Affected Protein	Pathogenesis
Cystic fibrosis	Cystic fibrosis transmembrane conductance regulator (CFTR)	Loss of CFTR leads to defects in chloride transport
Familial hypercholesterolemia	LDL receptor	Loss of LDL receptor leading to hypercholesterolemia
Tay-Sachs disease	Hexosaminidase β subunit	Lack of the lysosomal enzyme leads to storage of GM_2 gangliosides in neurons
Alpha-1-antitrypsin deficiency	α_1-antitrypsin	Storage of nonfunctional protein in hepatocytes causes apoptosis; absence of enzymatic activity in lungs causes destruction of elastic tissue giving rise to emphysema
Creutzfeldt-Jacob disease	Prions	Abnormal folding of PrPsc causes neuronal cell death
Alzheimer disease	Aβ peptide	Abnormal folding of Aβ peptides causes aggregation within neurons and apoptosis

misfolding, culminating in cell injury and death. A list of diseases associated with protein misfolding is provided in Table 2-4).

Apoptosis Induced by the TNF Receptor Family. FasL on T cells binds to Fas on the same or neighboring lymphocytes. This interaction plays a role in the elimination of lymphocytes that recognize self antigens, and mutations affecting Fas or FasL result in autoimmune diseases in humans and mice (Chapter 6).

Cytotoxic T Lymphocyte-Mediated Apoptosis. Cytotoxic T lymphocytes (CTLs) recognize foreign antigens presented on the surface of infected host cells (Chapter 6). Upon activation, CTLs secrete *perforin*, a transmembrane pore-forming molecule, which promotes entry of the CTL granule serine proteases called *granzymes*. Granzymes cleave proteins at aspartate residues and thus activate a variety of cellular caspases. In this way the CTL kills target cells by directly inducing the effector phase of apoptosis.

Disorders Associated with Dysregulated Apoptosis

Dysregulated apoptosis ("too little or too much") has been postulated to explain aspects of a wide range of diseases.

- *Disorders associated with defective apoptosis and increased cell survival.* An inappropriately low rate of apoptosis may permit the survival of abnormal cells, which may have a variety of consequences. For instance, as discussed earlier, cells that carry mutations in *TP53* are susceptible to the accumulation of mutations because of defective DNA repair, which in turn can give rise to cancer. The importance of apoptosis in preventing cancer development is emphasized by the fact that mutation of *TP53* is the most common genetic abnormality found in human cancers (Chapter 7). In other situations, defective apoptosis results in failure to eliminate potentially harmful cells, such as lymphocytes that can react against self antigens, and failure to eliminate dead cells, a potential source of self antigens. Thus, defective apoptosis may be the basis of *autoimmune disorders* (Chapter 6).
- *Disorders associated with increased apoptosis and excessive cell death.* These diseases are characterized by a loss of cells and include (1) *neurodegenerative diseases*, manifested by loss of specific sets of neurons, in which apoptosis is caused by mutations and misfolded proteins (Chapter 28); (2) *ischemic injury*, as in myocardial infarction (Chapter 12) and stroke (Chapter 28); and (3) *death of virus-infected cells* in many viral infections (Chapter 8).

KEY CONCEPTS

Apoptosis

- Regulated mechanism of cell death that serves to eliminate unwanted and irreparably damaged cells, with the least possible host reaction
- Characterized by enzymatic degradation of proteins and DNA, initiated by caspases; and by recognition and removal of dead cells by phagocytes
- Initiated by two major pathways:
  - Mitochondrial (intrinsic) pathway is triggered by loss of survival signals, DNA damage, and accumulation of misfolded proteins (ER stress); associated with leakage of pro-apoptotic proteins from mitochondrial membrane into the cytoplasm, where they activate caspases; inhibited by anti-apoptotic members of the BCL2 family, which are induced by survival signals including growth factors
  - Death receptor (extrinsic) pathway is responsible for elimination of self-reactive lymphocytes and damage by cytotoxic T lymphocytes; is initiated by engagement of death receptors (members of the TNF receptor family) by ligands on adjacent cells.

Necroptosis

As the name indicates, this form of cell death is a hybrid that shares aspects of both necrosis and apoptosis. The following features characterize necroptosis:

- Morphologically, and to some extent biochemically, it resembles necrosis, both characterized by loss of ATP, swelling of the cell and organelles, generation of ROS, release of lysosomal enzymes and ultimately rupture of the plasma membrane as discussed earlier.
- Mechanistically, it is triggered by genetically programmed signal transduction events that culminate in cell death. In this respect it resembles programmed cell death, which is considered the hallmark of apoptosis.

Because of the duality of these features, necroptosis is sometimes called *programmed necrosis* to distinguish it from the more usual forms of necrosis driven passively by toxic or anoxic injury to the cell. *In sharp contrast to apoptosis, the genetic program that drives necroptosis does not result in caspase activation* and hence it is also sometimes referred to as "caspase-independent" programmed cell death.

The process of necroptosis starts in a manner similar to that of the extrinsic form of apoptosis, that is, by ligation of a receptor by its ligand. While ligation of TNFR1 is the most widely studied model of necroptosis, many other signals, including ligation of Fas, and yet to be identified sensors of viral DNA and RNA, as well as genotoxic agents, can also trigger necroptosis. Since TNF can cause both apoptosis and necroptosis, the mechanisms underlying these effects of TNF are especially illustrative (Fig. 2-27).

While the entire set of signaling molecules and their interactions is not known, necroptosis involves two unique kinases called receptor associated kinase 1 and 3 (RIP1 and RIP3). As indicated in Fig. 2-27, ligation of TNFR1 recruits RIP1 and RIP3 into a multiprotein complex that also contains caspase-8. While events downstream of RIP1 and RIP3 kinase activation are still murky, it is clear that unlike in apoptosis, caspases are not activated and as in necrosis the terminal events include permeabilization of lysosomal membranes, generation of ROS, damage to the mitochondria, and reduction of ATP levels. *This explains the morphologic similarity of necroptosis with necrosis initiated by other injuries.*

Necroptosis is being recognized as an important death pathway both in physiologic and pathologic conditions. For example, necroptosis occurs during the formation of the mammalian bone growth plate; it is associated with cell death in steatohepatitis, acute pancreatitis, reperfusion injury, and neurodegenerative diseases such as Parkinson disease. Necroptosis also acts as a backup mechanism in host defense against certain viruses that encode caspase inhibitors (e.g., cytomegalovirus).

Before closing this discussion, we should briefly mention another form of programmed cell death called *pyroptosis,* so called because it is accompanied by the release of fever inducing cytokine IL-1 and because it bears some biochemical similarities with apoptosis.

As is well known, microbial products that enter the cytoplasm of infected cells are recognized by cytoplasmic innate immune receptors and can activate the multiprotein complex called the *inflammasome* (Chapter 6). The function of the inflammasome is to activate caspase-1, (also known as interleukin-1β converting enzyme) which cleaves a precursor form of IL-1 and releases its biologically active form. IL-1 is a mediator of many aspects of inflammation, including leukocyte recruitment and fever (Chapter 3). Caspase-1 and, more importantly, the closely related caspase-11 also induce death of the cells. Unlike classical apoptosis, this pathway of cell death is characterized by swelling of cells, loss of plasma membrane integrity, and release of inflammatory mediators. Pyroptosis results in the death of some microbes that gain access to the cytosol and promotes the release of inflammasome-generated IL-1.

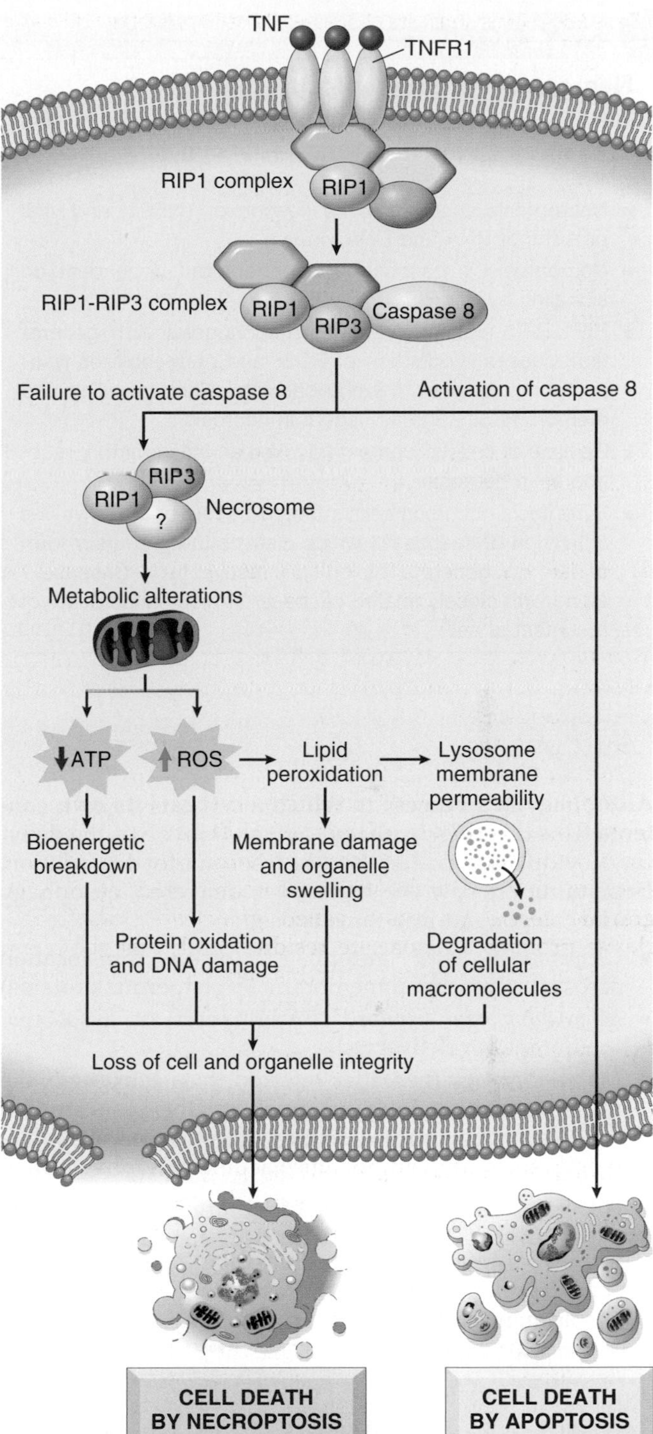

Figure 2-27 Molecular mechanism of TNF-mediated necroptosis. Cross-linking of TNFR1 by TNF causes recruitment of RIP1 and RIP3 along with caspase 8. Activation of the caspase leads to apoptosis as described in the text. Inhibition of caspase 8, as may occur in some viral infections, allows RIP1 and RIP3 to initiate signals that affect mitochondrial generation of ATP and ROS. This is followed by events typical of necrosis. (Adapted from Galluzi L, et al: Programmed necrosis from molecules to health and disease. Int Rev Cell Molec Biol 289:1, 2011.)

KEY CONCEPTS

Necroptosis and Pyroptosis

- Necroptosis resembles necrosis morphologically and apoptosis mechanistically as a form of programmed cell death.
- Necroptosis is triggered by ligation of TNFR1, and viral proteins of RNA and DNA viruses.
- Necroptosis is caspase-independent but dependent on signaling by the RIP1 and RIP3 complex.
- RIP1-RIP3 signaling reduces mitochondrial ATP generation, causes production of ROS, and permeabilizes lysosomal membranes, thereby causing cellular swelling and membrane damage as occurs in necrosis.
- Release of cellular contents evokes an inflammatory reaction as in necrosis.
- Pyroptosis occurs in cells infected by microbes.It involves activation of caspase-1 which cleaves the precursor form of IL-1 to generate biologically active IL-1. Caspase-1 along with closely related caspase-11 also cause death of the infected cell.

Autophagy

Autophagy is a process in which a cell eats its own contents *(Greek:* **auto,** *self;* **phagy,** *eating).* It involves the delivery of cytoplasmic materials to the lysosome for degradation. Depending on how the material is delivered, autophagy can be categorized into three types:

- *Chaperone-mediated* autophagy (direct translocation across the lysosomal membrane by chaperone proteins)
- *Microautophagy* (inward invagination of lysosomal membrane for delivery)
- *Macroautophagy* (hereafter referred to as *autophagy*), the major form of autophagy involving the sequestration and transportation of portions of cytosol in a double-membrane bound autophagic vacuole (autophagosome)

Autophagy is seen in single-celled organisms as well as mammalian cells. It is an evolutionarily conserved survival mechanism whereby, in states of nutrient deprivation, the starved cell lives by cannibalizing itself and recycling the digested contents. Autophagy is implicated in many physiologic states (e.g., aging and exercise) and pathologic processes. It proceeds through several steps (Fig. 2-28):

- Formation of an isolation membrane, also called phagophore, and its nucleation; the isolation membrane is believed to be derived from the ER
- Elongation of the vesicle
- Maturation of the autophagosome, its fusion with lysosomes, and eventual degradation of the contents

In recent years, more than a dozen "autophagy-related genes" called *Atgs* have been identified whose products are required for the creation of the autophagosome. While the details of the process are still not fully understood, its outlines have been defined. In a simple model, environmental cues like starvation or depletion of growth factors activate an initiation complex of four proteins that stimulates the assembly of a nucleation complex. This in turn promotes the nucleation of the autophagosomal membrane. The autophagosomal membrane elongates further, surrounds and captures its cytosolic cargo, and closes to form the autophagosome. The elongation and closure of the autophagosomal membrane requires the coordinated action of several ubiquitin-like conjugation systems, including the microtubule-associated protein light chain 3 (LC3). The synthesis of LC3 is augmented during autophagy and it is therefore a useful marker for identifying cells in which autophagy is occurring. The newly formed autophagosome fuses with endosomes and then finally with lysosomes to form an autophagolysosome. In the terminal step, the inner membrane and enclosed cytosolic cargoes are degraded by lysosomal enzymes. There is some evidence that autophagy is not a random process that engulfs cytosolic contents indiscriminately. Instead, it appears that the loading of cargo into the autophagosome is "selective" and that one of the functions of the LC3 system is to "target" protein aggregates and effete organelles.

Autophagy functions as a survival mechanism under various stress conditions, maintaining the integrity of cells by recycling essential metabolites and clearing cellular debris. It is therefore prominent in atrophic cells, which are

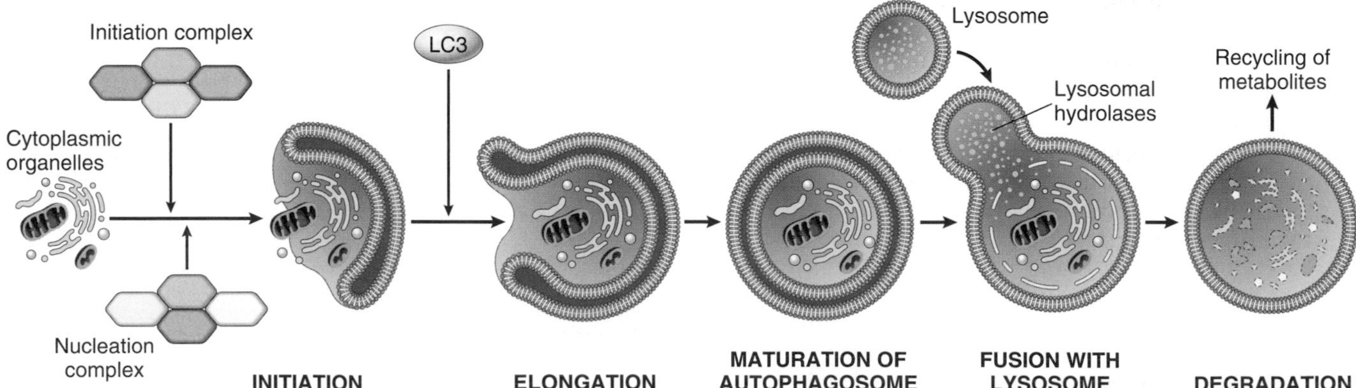

Figure 2-28 Autophagy. Cellular stresses, such as nutrient deprivation, activate an autophagy pathway that proceeds through several phases (initiation, nucleation, and elongation of isolation membrane) and eventually creates double-membrane-bound vacuoles (autophagosome) in which cytoplasmic materials including organelles are sequestered and then degraded following fusion of the vesicles with lysosomes. In the final stage, the digested materials are released for recycling of metabolites. See text for details. (Modified from Choi, AMK, Ryter S, Levine B: Autophagy in human health and disease. N Engl J Med 368:651, 2013.)

exposed to severe nutrient deprivation. Autophagy is also involved in the turnover of organelles like ER, mitochondria, and lysosomes and the clearance of intracellular aggregates that accumulate during aging, stress and various other diseases states. Autophagy can trigger cell death if it is inadequate to cope with the stress imposed on the cell. This pathway of cell death is distinct from necrosis and apoptosis, but the mechanism is unknown. Furthermore, it is not clear whether cell death is caused by autophagy or by the stress that triggered autophagy. Nevertheless, autophagic vacuolization often precedes or accompanies cell death.

There is increasing evidence that autophagy plays a role in human diseases. Some examples are listed:

- *Cancer:* This is an area of active investigation and as discussed in Chapter 7, autophagy can both promote cancer growth and act as a defense against cancers.
- *Neurodegenerative disorders*: Many neurodegenerative disorders are associated with dysregulation of autophagy. In Alzheimer disease, formation of autophagosomes is accelerated and in mouse models genetic defects in autophagy accelerate neurodegeneration. In Huntington disease, mutant huntingtin impairs autophagy.
- *Infectious diseases*: Many pathogens are degraded by autophagy; these include mycobacteria, *Shigella* spp., and HSV-1. This is one way by which microbial proteins are digested and delivered to antigen presentation pathways. Macrophage-specific deletion of Atg5 increases susceptibility to tuberculosis.
- *Inflammatory bowel diseases*: Genome-wide association studies have linked both Crohn disease and ulcerative colitis to SNPs in autophagy related genes.

KEY CONCEPTS

Autophagy

- Autophagy involves sequestration of cellular organelles into cytoplasmic autophagic vacuoles (autophagosomes) that fuse with lysosomes and digest the enclosed material.
- Autophagy is an adaptive response that is enhanced during nutrient deprivation, allowing the cell to cannibalize itself to survive.
- Autophagosome formation is regulated by more than a dozen proteins that act in a coordinated and sequential manner.
- Dysregulation of autophagy occurs in many disease states including cancers, inflammatory bowel diseases, and neurodegenerative disorders. Autophagy plays a role in host defense against certain microbes.

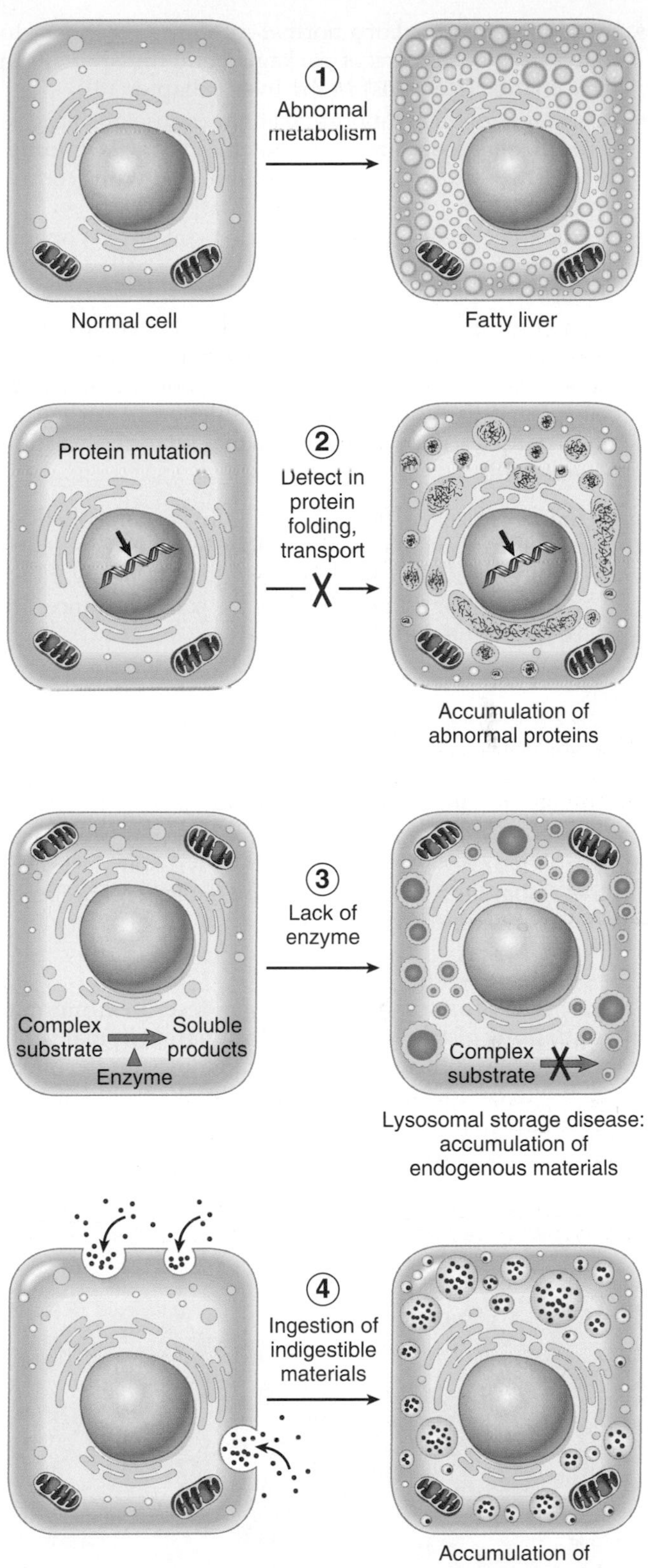

Figure 2-29 Mechanisms of intracellular accumulations discussed in the text.

Intracellular Accumulations

One of the manifestations of metabolic derangements in cells is the intracellular accumulation of abnormal amounts of various substances that may be harmless or associated with varying degrees of injury. The substance may be located in the cytoplasm, within organelles (typically lysosomes), or in the nucleus, and it may be synthesized by the affected cells or may be produced elsewhere.

There are four main pathways of abnormal intracellular accumulations (Fig. 2-29):

- Inadequate removal of a normal substance secondary to defects in mechanisms of packaging and transport, as in fatty change (steatosis) in the liver (Chapter 18)
- Accumulation of an abnormal endogenous substance as a result of genetic or acquired defects in its folding, packaging, transport, or secretion, as with certain mutated forms of α_1-antitrypsin (Chapter 15)
- Failure to degrade a metabolite due to inherited enzyme deficiencies. The resulting disorders are called *storage diseases* (Chapter 5).
- Deposition and accumulation of an abnormal exogenous substance when the cell has neither the enzymatic machinery to degrade the substance nor the ability to transport it to other sites. Accumulation of carbon or silica particles is an example of this type of alteration (Chapter 15).

In many cases, if the overload can be controlled or stopped, the accumulation is reversible. In inherited storage diseases, accumulation is progressive, and the overload may cause cellular injury, leading in some instances to death of the tissue and the patient.

Lipids

All major classes of lipids can accumulate in cells: triglycerides, cholesterol/cholesterol esters, and phospholipids. Phospholipids are components of the myelin figures found in necrotic cells. In addition, abnormal complexes of lipids and carbohydrates accumulate in the lysosomal storage diseases (Chapter 5). Triglyceride and cholesterol accumulations are discussed here.

Steatosis (Fatty Change)

The terms steatosis and fatty change describe abnormal accumulations of triglycerides within parenchymal cells. Fatty change is often seen in the liver because it is the major organ involved in fat metabolism (Fig. 2-30), but it also occurs in heart, muscle, and kidney. The causes of steatosis include toxins, protein malnutrition, diabetes mellitus, obesity, and anoxia. *In developed nations, the most common causes of significant fatty change in the liver (fatty liver) are alcohol abuse and nonalcoholic fatty liver disease, which is often associated with diabetes and obesity.* Fatty liver is discussed in more detail in Chapter 18.

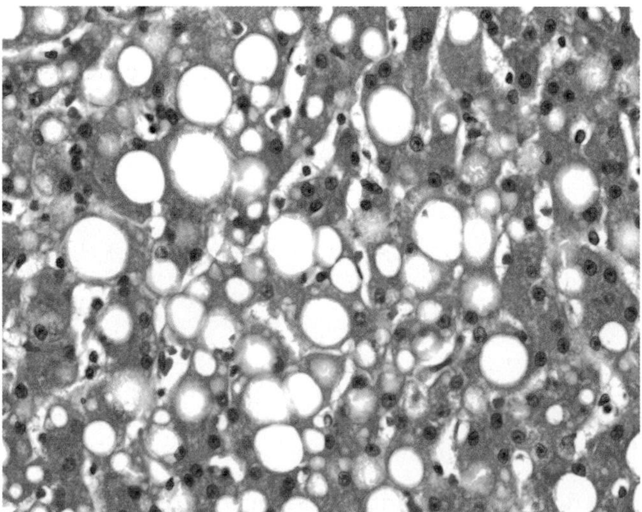

Figure 2-30 Fatty liver. High-power detail of fatty change of the liver. In most cells the well-preserved nucleus is squeezed into the displaced rim of cytoplasm about the fat vacuole. (Courtesy Dr. James Crawford, Department of Pathology, University of Florida School of Medicine, Gainesville, Fla.)

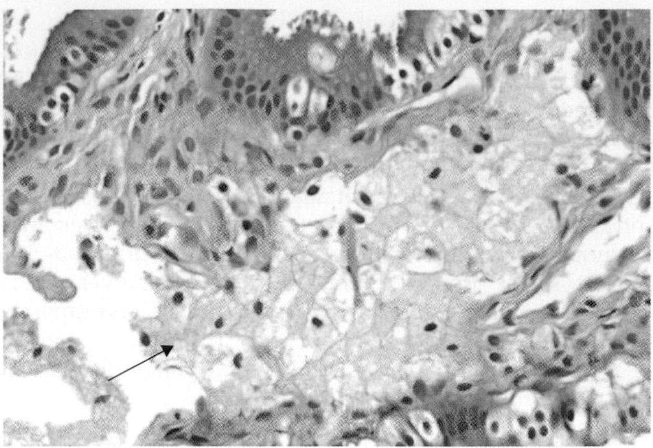

Figure 2-31 Cholesterolosis. Cholesterol-laden macrophages (foam cells, *arrow*) in a focus of gallbladder cholesterolosis. (Courtesy Dr. Matthew Yeh, Department of Pathology, University of Washington, Seattle, Wash.)

Cholesterol and Cholesterol Esters

The cellular metabolism of cholesterol (Chapter 5) is tightly regulated such that most cells use cholesterol for the synthesis of cell membranes without intracellular accumulation of cholesterol or cholesterol esters. Accumulations manifested histologically by intracellular vacuoles are seen in several pathologic processes.

- *Atherosclerosis.* **In atherosclerotic plaques, smooth muscle cells and macrophages within the intimal layer of the aorta and large arteries are filled with lipid vacuoles, most of which are made up of cholesterol and cholesterol esters.** Such cells have a foamy appearance (foam cells), and aggregates of them in the intima produce the yellow cholesterol-laden atheromas characteristic of this serious disorder. Some of these fat-laden cells may rupture, releasing lipids into the extracellular space. The mechanisms of cholesterol accumulation in atherosclerosis are discussed in detail in Chapter 11. The extracellular cholesterol esters may crystallize in the shape of long needles, producing quite distinctive clefts in tissue sections.
- *Xanthomas.* **Intracellular accumulation of cholesterol within macrophages is also characteristic of acquired and hereditary hyperlipidemic states.** Clusters of foamy cells are found in the subepithelial connective tissue of the skin and in tendons, producing tumorous masses known as xanthomas.
- *Cholesterolosis.* This refers to the focal accumulations of cholesterol-laden macrophages in the lamina propria of the gallbladder (Fig. 2-31). The mechanism of accumulation is unknown.
- *Niemann-Pick disease, type C.* This lysosomal storage disease is caused by mutations affecting an enzyme involved in cholesterol trafficking, resulting in cholesterol accumulation in multiple organs (Chapter 5).

Proteins

Intracellular accumulations of proteins usually appear as rounded, eosinophilic droplets, vacuoles, or aggregates in the cytoplasm. By electron microscopy they can be amorphous, fibrillar, or crystalline in appearance. In some disorders, such as certain forms of amyloidosis, abnormal proteins deposit primarily in extracellular spaces (Chapter 6).

Excesses of proteins within the cells sufficient to cause morphologically visible accumulation have diverse causes.

- *Reabsorption droplets in proximal renal tubules* are seen in renal diseases associated with protein loss in the urine (proteinuria). In the kidney small amounts of protein filtered through the glomerulus are normally reabsorbed by pinocytosis in the proximal tubule. In disorders with heavy protein leakage across the glomerular filter there is increased reabsorption of the protein into vesicles, and the protein appears as pink hyaline droplets within the cytoplasm of the tubular cell (Fig. 2-32). The process is reversible; if the proteinuria diminishes, the protein droplets are metabolized and disappear.
- The proteins that accumulate may be normal secreted proteins that are produced in excessive amounts, as occurs in certain plasma cells engaged in active synthesis of immunoglobulins. The ER becomes hugely distended, producing large, homogeneous eosinophilic inclusions called *Russell bodies.*
- *Defective intracellular transport and secretion of critical proteins.* In α_1-antitrypsin deficiency, mutations in the protein significantly slow folding, resulting in the buildup of partially folded intermediates, which aggregate in the ER of the liver and are not secreted. The resultant deficiency of the circulating enzyme causes emphysema (Chapter 15). In many of these diseases the pathology results not only from loss of protein function but also ER stress caused by the misfolded proteins, culminating in apoptotic death of cells (discussed earlier).
- *Accumulation of cytoskeletal proteins.* There are several types of cytoskeletal proteins, including microtubules (20 to 25 nm in diameter), thin actin filaments (6 to 8 nm), thick myosin filaments (15 nm), and intermediate filaments (10 nm). Intermediate filaments, which provide a flexible intracellular scaffold that organizes the cytoplasm and resists forces applied to the cell, are divided into five classes: keratin filaments (characteristic of epithelial cells), neurofilaments (neurons), desmin filaments (muscle cells), vimentin filaments (connective tissue cells), and glial filaments (astrocytes). Accumulations of keratin filaments and neurofilaments are associated with certain types of cell injury. Alcoholic hyaline is an eosinophilic cytoplasmic inclusion in liver cells that is characteristic of alcoholic liver disease, and is composed predominantly of *keratin* intermediate filaments (Chapter 18). The *neurofibrillary tangle* found in the brain in Alzheimer disease contains neurofilaments and other proteins (Chapter 28).
- *Aggregation of abnormal proteins.* Abnormal or misfolded proteins may deposit in tissues and interfere with normal functions. The deposits can be intracellular, extracellular, or both, and the aggregates may either directly or indirectly cause the pathologic changes. Certain forms of *amyloidosis* (Chapter 6) fall in this category of diseases. These disorders are sometimes called *proteinopathies* or *protein-aggregation diseases.*

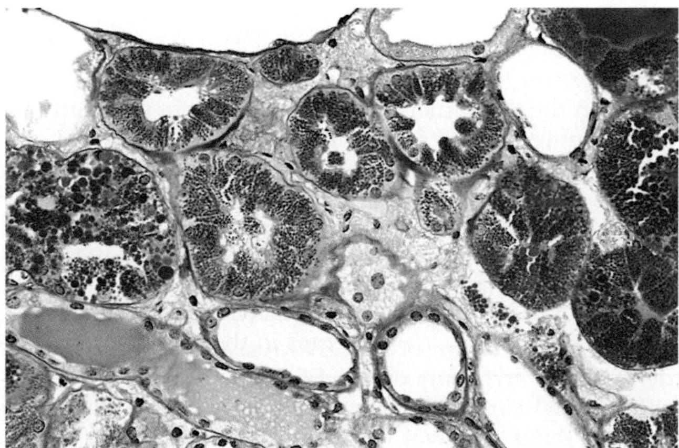

Figure 2-32 Protein reabsorption droplets in the renal tubular epithelium. (Courtesy Dr. Helmut Rennke, Department of Pathology, Brigham and Women's Hospital, Boston, Mass.)

Hyaline Change

The term hyaline usually refers to an alteration within cells or in the extracellular space that gives a homogeneous, glassy, pink appearance in routine histologic sections stained with hematoxylin and eosin. It is widely used as a descriptive histologic term rather than a specific marker for cell injury. This morphologic change is produced by a variety of alterations and does not represent a specific pattern of accumulation. Intracellular accumulations of protein, described earlier (reabsorption droplets, Russell bodies, alcoholic hyaline), are examples of intracellular hyaline deposits.

Extracellular hyaline has been more difficult to analyze. Collagenous fibrous tissue in old scars may appear hyalinized, but the biochemical basis of this change is not clear. In long-standing hypertension and diabetes mellitus, the walls of arterioles, especially in the kidney, become hyalinized, resulting from extravasated plasma protein and deposition of basement membrane material.

Glycogen

Glycogen is a readily available energy source stored in the cytoplasm of healthy cells. Excessive intracellular deposits of glycogen are seen in patients with an abnormality in either glucose or glycogen metabolism. Whatever the clinical setting, the glycogen masses appear as clear vacuoles within the cytoplasm. Glycogen dissolves in aqueous fixatives; thus, it is most readily identified when tissues are fixed in absolute alcohol. Staining with Best carmine or the PAS reaction imparts a rose-to-violet color to the glycogen, and diastase digestion of a parallel section before staining serves as a further control by hydrolyzing the glycogen.

Diabetes mellitus is the prime example of a disorder of glucose metabolism. In this disease glycogen is found

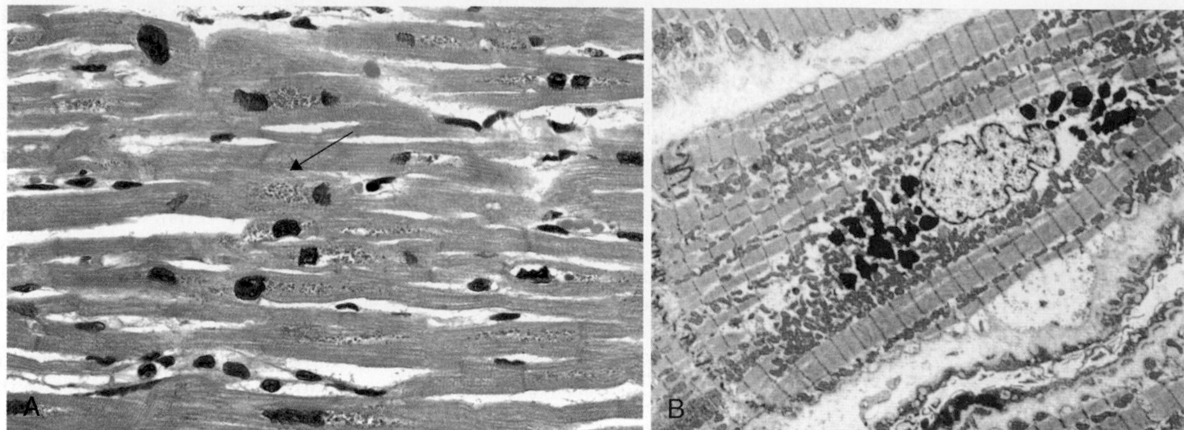

Figure 2-33 Lipofuscin granules in a cardiac myocyte shown by **(A)** light microscopy (deposits indicated by *arrows*), and **(B)** electron microscopy (note the perinuclear, intralysosomal location).

in renal tubular epithelial cells, as well as within liver cells, β cells of the islets of Langerhans, and heart muscle cells.

Glycogen accumulates within the cells in a group of related genetic disorders that are collectively referred to as the *glycogen storage diseases*, or *glycogenoses* (Chapter 5). In these diseases enzymatic defects in the synthesis or breakdown of glycogen result in massive accumulation, causing cell injury and cell death.

Pigments

Pigments are colored substances, some of which are normal constituents of cells (e.g., melanin), whereas others are abnormal and accumulate in cells only under special circumstances. Pigments can be exogenous, coming from outside the body, or endogenous, synthesized within the body itself.

Exogenous Pigments

The most common exogenous pigment is carbon (coal dust), a ubiquitous air pollutant in urban areas. When inhaled it is picked up by macrophages within the alveoli and is then transported through lymphatic channels to the regional lymph nodes in the tracheobronchial region. Accumulations of this pigment blacken the tissues of the lungs *(anthracosis)* and the involved lymph nodes. In coal miners the aggregates of carbon dust may induce a fibroblastic reaction or even emphysema and thus cause a serious lung disease known as *coal worker's pneumoconiosis* (Chapter 15). *Tattooing* is a form of localized, exogenous pigmentation of the skin. The pigments inoculated are phagocytosed by dermal macrophages, in which they reside for the remainder of the life of the embellished (sometimes with embarrassing consequences for the bearer of the tattoo when proposing to Mary while the tattoo says Valerie!). The pigments do not usually evoke any inflammatory response.

Endogenous Pigments

Lipofuscin is an insoluble pigment, also known as lipochrome or wear-and-tear pigment. Lipofuscin is composed of polymers of lipids and phospholipids in complex with protein, suggesting that it is derived through lipid peroxidation of polyunsaturated lipids of subcellular membranes. Lipofuscin is not injurious to the cell or its functions. Its importance lies in its being a telltale sign of free radical injury and lipid peroxidation. The term is derived from the Latin (*fuscus*, brown), referring to brown lipid. In tissue sections it appears as a yellow-brown, finely granular cytoplasmic, often perinuclear, pigment (Fig. 2-33). It is seen in cells undergoing slow, regressive changes and is particularly prominent in the liver and heart of aging patients or patients with severe malnutrition and cancer cachexia.

Melanin, derived from the Greek (*melas*, black), is an endogenous, brown-black, pigment formed when the enzyme tyrosinase catalyzes the oxidation of tyrosine to dihydroxyphenylalanine in melanocytes. It is discussed further in Chapter 25. For practical purposes melanin is the *only endogenous brown-black pigment*. The only other that could be considered in this category is homogentisic acid, a black pigment that occurs in patients with *alkaptonuria*, a rare metabolic disease. Here the pigment is deposited in the skin, connective tissue, and cartilage, and the pigmentation is known as *ochronosis*.

Hemosiderin, a hemoglobin-derived, golden yellow-to-brown, granular or crystalline pigment is one of the major storage forms of iron. Iron metabolism and hemosiderin are considered in detail in Chapters 14 and 18. Iron is normally carried by specific transport protein called transferrin. In cells, it is stored in association with a protein, apoferritin, to form ferritin micelles. Ferritin is a constituent of most cell types. *When there is a local or systemic excess of iron, ferritin forms hemosiderin granules*, which are easily seen with the light microscope. Hemosiderin pigment represents aggregates of ferritin micelles. Under normal conditions small amounts of hemosiderin can be seen in the mononuclear phagocytes of the bone marrow, spleen, and liver, which are actively engaged in red cell breakdown.

Local or systemic excesses of iron cause hemosiderin to accumulate within cells. *Local excesses* result from hemorrhages in tissues. The best example of localized hemosiderosis is the common bruise. Extravasated red cells at the site of injury are phagocytosed over several days by macrophages, which break down the hemoglobin and recover the iron. After removal of iron, the heme moiety is converted first to biliverdin ("green bile") and then to bilirubin ("red bile"). In parallel, the iron released from heme is incorporated into ferritin and eventually hemosiderin.

These conversions account for the often dramatic play of colors seen in a healing bruise, which typically changes from red-blue to green-blue to golden-yellow before it is resolved.

When there is *systemic overload of iron* hemosiderin may be deposited in many organs and tissues, a condition called *hemosiderosis*. The main causes of hemosiderosis are (1) increased absorption of dietary iron due to an inborn error of metabolism called hemochromatosis, (2) hemolytic anemias, in which premature lysis of red cells leads to release of abnormal quantities of iron, and (3) repeated blood transfusions, because transfused red cells constitute an exogenous load of iron. These conditions are discussed in Chapters 14 and 18.

Pathologic Calcification

Pathologic calcification is the abnormal tissue deposition of calcium salts, together with smaller amounts of iron, magnesium, and other mineral salts. There are two forms of pathologic calcification. When the deposition occurs locally in dying tissues it is known as *dystrophic calcification;* it occurs despite normal serum levels of calcium and in the absence of derangements in calcium metabolism. In contrast, the deposition of calcium salts in otherwise normal tissues is known as *metastatic calcification*, and it almost always results from hypercalcemia secondary to some disturbance in calcium metabolism.

Dystrophic Calcification

Dystrophic calcification is encountered in areas of necrosis, whether they are of coagulative, caseous, or liquefactive type, and in foci of enzymatic necrosis of fat. Calcification is almost always present in the atheromas of advanced atherosclerosis. It also commonly develops in aging or damaged heart valves, further hampering their function (Fig. 2-34). Whatever the site of deposition, the calcium salts appear macroscopically as fine, white granules or clumps, often felt as gritty deposits. Sometimes a tuberculous lymph node is virtually converted to stone.

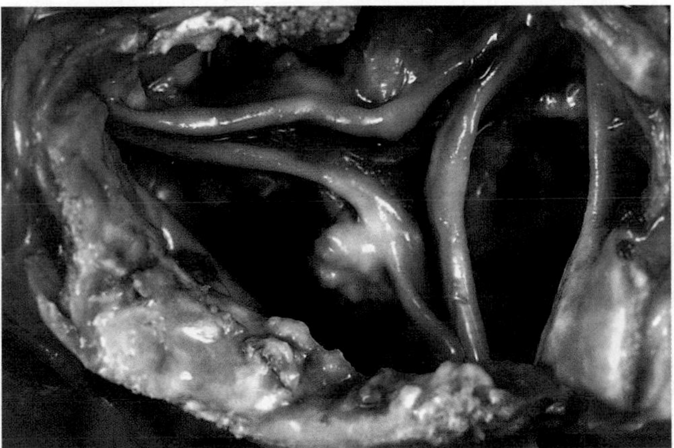

Figure 2-34 Dystrophic calcification of the aortic valve. View looking down onto the unopened aortic valve in a heart with calcific aortic stenosis. It is markedly narrowed (stenosis). The semilunar cusps are thickened and fibrotic, and behind each cusp are irregular masses of piled-up dystrophic calcification.

MORPHOLOGY

Histologically, with the usual hematoxylin and eosin stain, calcium salts have a basophilic, amorphous granular, sometimes clumped appearance. They can be intracellular, extracellular, or in both locations. In the course of time, **heterotopic** bone may be formed in the focus of calcification. On occasion single necrotic cells may constitute seed crystals that become encrusted by the mineral deposits. The progressive acquisition of outer layers may create lamellated configurations, called **psammoma bodies** because of their resemblance to grains of sand. Some types of papillary cancers (e.g., thyroid) are apt to develop psammoma bodies. In asbestosis, calcium and iron salts gather about long slender spicules of asbestos in the lung, creating exotic, beaded dumbbell forms (Chapter 15).

Although dystrophic calcification may simply be a telltale sign of previous cell injury, it is often a cause of organ dysfunction. Such is the case in calcific valvular disease and atherosclerosis, as will become clear in further discussion of these diseases. Serum calcium is normal in dystrophic calcification.

Metastatic Calcification

Metastatic calcification may occur in normal tissues whenever there is hypercalcemia. Hypercalcemia also accentuates dystrophic calcification. There are four principal causes of hypercalcemia: (1) increased secretion of parathyroid hormone (PTH) with subsequent bone resorption, as in *hyperparathyroidism* due to parathyroid tumors, and ectopic secretion of PTH-related protein by malignant tumors (Chapter 7); (2) *resorption of bone tissue*, secondary to primary tumors of bone marrow (e.g., multiple myeloma, leukemia) or diffuse skeletal metastasis (e.g., breast cancer), accelerated bone turnover (e.g., Paget disease), or immobilization; (3) *vitamin D–related disorders*, including vitamin D intoxication, sarcoidosis (in which macrophages activate a vitamin D precursor), and idiopathic hypercalcemia of infancy (Williams syndrome), characterized by abnormal sensitivity to vitamin D; and (4) *renal failure*, which causes retention of phosphate, leading to secondary hyperparathyroidism. Less common causes include aluminum intoxication, which occurs in patients on chronic renal dialysis, and milk-alkali syndrome, which is due to excessive ingestion of calcium and absorbable antacids such as milk or calcium carbonate.

Metastatic calcification may occur widely throughout the body but principally affects the interstitial tissues of the gastric mucosa, kidneys, lungs, systemic arteries, and pulmonary veins. Although quite different in location, all of these tissues excrete acid and therefore have an internal alkaline compartment that predisposes them to metastatic calcification. In all these sites, the calcium salts morphologically resemble those described in dystrophic calcification. Thus, they may occur as noncrystalline amorphous deposits or, at other times, as hydroxyapatite crystals.

Usually the mineral salts cause no clinical dysfunction, but on occasion massive involvement of the lungs produces remarkable x-ray images and respiratory compromise. Massive deposits in the kidney (nephrocalcinosis) may in time cause renal damage (Chapter 20).

KEY CONCEPTS

Abnormal Intracellular Depositions and Calcifications

Abnormal deposits of materials in cells and tissues are the result of excessive intake or defective transport or catabolism.

- **Deposition of lipids**
  - Fatty change: Accumulation of free triglycerides in cells, resulting from excessive intake or defective transport (often because of defects in synthesis of transport proteins); manifestation of reversible cell injury
  - Cholesterol deposition: Result of defective catabolism and excessive intake; in macrophages and smooth muscle cells of vessel walls in atherosclerosis
- **Deposition of proteins:** Reabsorbed proteins in kidney tubules; immunoglobulins in plasma cells
- **Deposition of glycogen:** In macrophages of patients with defects in lysosomal enzymes that break down glycogen (glycogen storage diseases)
- **Deposition of pigments:** Typically indigestible pigments, such as carbon, lipofuscin (breakdown product of lipid peroxidation), or iron (usually due to overload, as in hemosiderosis)
- **Pathologic calcifications**
  - Dystrophic calcification: Deposition of calcium at sites of cell injury and necrosis
  - Metastatic calcification: Deposition of calcium in normal tissues, caused by hypercalcemia (usually a consequence of parathyroid hormone excess)

Cellular Aging

Mankind has pursued immortality from time immemorial. Toth and Hermes, two Egyptian and Greek deities, are said to have discovered the elixir of youth and become immortal. Sadly, despite intense search, that elixir is nowhere to be found. Shakespeare probably characterized aging best in his elegant description of the seven ages of man. It begins at the moment of conception, involves the differentiation and maturation of the organism and its cells, at some variable point in time leads to the progressive loss of functional capacity characteristic of senescence, and ends in death.

Individuals age because their cells age. Although public attention on the aging process has traditionally focused on its cosmetic manifestations, aging has important health consequences, because age is one of the strongest independent risk factors for many chronic diseases, such as cancer, Alzheimer disease, and ischemic heart disease. Perhaps one of the most striking discoveries about cellular aging is that it is not simply a consequence of cells "running out of steam," but in fact is regulated by genes that are evolutionarily conserved from yeast to worms to mammals.

Cellular aging is the result of a progressive decline in cellular function and viability caused by genetic abnormalities and the accumulation of cellular and molecular damage due to the effects of exposure to exogenous influences (Fig. 2-35). Studies in model systems have clearly established that aging is influenced by a limited number of genes, and genetic anomalies underlie syndromes resembling premature aging in humans as well. Such findings suggest that aging is associated with definable mechanistic alterations. Several mechanisms, some cell intrinsic and others environmentally induced, are believed to play a role in aging.

DNA Damage. A variety of exogenous (physical, chemical, and biologic) agents and endogenous factors such as ROS threaten the integrity of nuclear and mitochondrial DNA. Although most DNA damage is repaired by DNA repair enzymes, some persists and accumulates as cells age. Several lines of evidence point to the importance of DNA repair in the aging process. Next generation DNA sequencing studies have shown that the average hematopoieitic stem cell suffers 14 new mutations per year, and it is likely that this accumulating damage explains why, like most cancers, the most common hematologic malignancies are diseases of the aged. Patients with *Werner syndrome* show premature aging, and the defective gene product is a DNA helicase, a protein involved in DNA replication and repair and other functions requiring DNA unwinding. A defect in this enzyme causes rapid accumulation of chromosomal damage that may mimic the injury that normally accumulates during cellular aging. Genetic instability in somatic

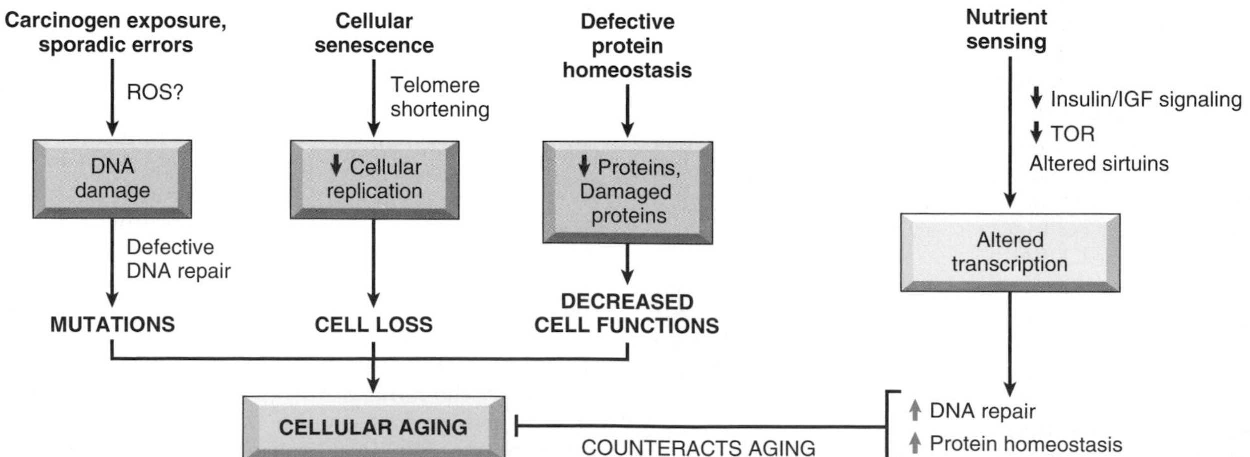

Figure 2-35 Mechanisms that cause and counteract cellular aging. DNA damage, replicative senescence, and decreased and misfolded proteins are among the best described mechanisms of cellular aging. Nutrient sensing exemplified by calorie restriction, counteracts aging by activating various signaling pathways and transcription factors. IG, Insulin-like growth factor; TOR, target of rapamycin.

cells is also characteristic of other disorders in which patients display some of the manifestations of aging at an increased rate, such as *Bloom syndrome* and *ataxia-telangiectasia,* in which the mutated genes encode a proteins involved in repairing double-strand breaks in DNA (Chapter 7).

Cellular Senescence. **All normal cells have a limited capacity for replication, and after a fixed number of divisions cells become arrested in a terminally nondividing state,** known as replicative *senescence.* Aging is associated with progressive replicative senescence of cells. Cells from children have the capacity to undergo more rounds of replication than do cells from older people. Two mechanisms are believed to underlie cellular senescence:

- *Telomere attrition.* **One mechanism of replicative senescence involves progressive shortening of telomeres, which ultimately results in cell cycle arrest.** *Telomeres* are short repeated sequences of DNA present at the ends of linear chromosomes that are important for ensuring the complete replication of chromosome ends and for protecting the ends from fusion and degradation. When somatic cells replicate, a small section of the telomere is not duplicated and telomeres become progressively shortened. As the telomeres become shorter, the ends of chromosomes cannot be protected and are seen as broken DNA, which signals cell cycle arrest. Telomere length is maintained by nucleotide addition mediated by an enzyme called *telomerase.* Telomerase is a specialized RNA-protein complex that uses its own RNA as a template for adding nucleotides to the ends of chromosomes. Telomerase activity is expressed in germ cells and is present at low levels in stem cells, but it is absent in most somatic tissues (Fig. 2-36) Therefore, as most somatic cells age, their telomeres become shorter and they exit the cell cycle, resulting in an inability to generate new cells to replace damaged ones. Conversely, in immortalized cancer cells, telomerase is usually reactivated and telomere length is stabilized, allowing the cells to proliferate indefinitely. This is discussed more fully in Chapter 7. The causal links between telomere length and cellular senescence have been established in mouse models. Genetically engineered mice with shortened telomeres exhibit reduced life spans that can be restored to normal by telomere activation. As discussed in other chapters, telomere shortening has also been associated with premature development of diseases, such as pulmonary fibrosis (Chapter 15) and aplastic anemia (Chapter 14).
- *Activation of tumor suppressor genes.* In addition to telomere attrition, activation of certain tumor suppressor genes, particularly those encoded by the *CDKN2A* locus, also seems to be involved in controlling replicative senescence. The CDKN2A locus encodes two tumor suppressor proteins, expression of one of which, known as p16 or INK4a, is correlated with chronologic age in virtually all human and mouse tissues examined. By controlling G1 to S phase progression during the cell cycle (Chapter 1), p16 protects the cells from uncontrolled mitogenic signals and pushes cells along the senescence pathway. This is discussed further in Chapter 7.

Defective Protein Homeostasis. Protein homeostasis involves two mechanisms: those that maintain proteins in

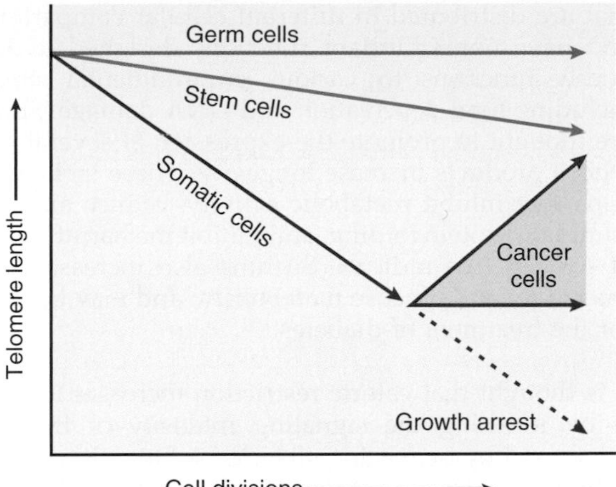

Figure 2-36 The role of telomeres and telomerase in replicative senescence of cells. Telomere length is plotted against the number of cell divisions. In most somatic cells there is no telomerase activity and telomeres progressively shorten with increasing cell divisions until growth arrest or until senescence occurs. Germ cells and stem cells both contain telomerase, but only germ cells have sufficient levels of the enzyme to stabilize telomere length completely. In cancer cells, telomerase is often reactivated. (Data from Holt SE, et al: Refining the telomere-telomerase hypothesis of aging and cancer. Nat Biotechnol 14:836, 1996, MacMillan Publishers Ltd.)

there correctly folded conformations (mediated by chaperones) and others that degrade misfolded proteins by the autophagy-lysosome system and ubiquitin-proteasome system. There is evidence that both normal folding and degradation of misfolded proteins are impaired with aging. Mutant mice deficient in chaperones of the heat shock protein family age rapidly, and conversely, those that overexpress such chaperones are long-lived. Similar data exist for the role of autophagy and proteasomal degradation of proteins. Of interest, administration of rapamycin, which inhibits the mTOR pathway, increases the life span of middle aged mice. Rapamycin has multiple effects including promotion of autophagy. Abnormal protein homeostasis can have many effects on cell survival, replication, and functions. In addition, it may lead to accumulation of misfolded proteins, which can trigger pathways of apoptosis.

Deregulated Nutrient Sensing. Paradoxical though it may seem, eating less increases longevity. Caloric restriction increases life span in all eukaryotic species in which it has been tested, with encouraging results even in nonhuman primates and a few usually disciplined people who are the envy of others! Because of these observations, there has been much interest in deciphering the role of nutrient sensing in aging. The following paragraphs review two major neurohormonal circuits that regulate metabolism.

- *Insulin and insulin-like growth factor 1 (IGF-1) signaling pathway.* IGF-1 is produced in many cell types in response to growth hormone secretion by the pituitary. IGF-1, as indicated by its name, mimics intracellular signaling by insulin and thereby informs the cells of the availability of glucose, promoting an anabolic state as well as cell growth and replication. IGF-1 signaling has multiple downstream targets; relevant to this discussion are two kinases: AKT and its downstream target, mTOR (mammalian target of rapamycin), which, as the name implies, is inhibited by rapamycin.
- *Sirtuins.* Sirtuins are a family of NAD-dependent protein deacetylases. There are at least seven types of sirtuins

that are distributed in different cellular compartments and have nonredundant functions designed to adapt bodily functions to various environmental stresses, including food deprivation and DNA damage. Sirtuins are thought to promote the expression of several genes whose products increase longevity. These include proteins that inhibit metabolic activity, reduce apoptosis, stimulate protein folding, and inhibit the harmful effects of oxygen free radicals. Sirtuins also increase insulin sensitivity and glucose metabolism, and may be targets for the treatment of diabetes.

It is thought that caloric restriction increases longevity both by reducing the signaling intensity of the IGF-1 pathway and by increasing sirtuins. Attenuation of IGF-1 signaling leads to lower rates of cell growth and metabolism and possibly reduced cellular damage. This effect can be mimicked by rapamycin. An increase in sirtuins, particularly sirtuin-6, serves dual functions: the sirtuins (1) contribute to metabolic adaptations of caloric restriction and (2) promote genomic integrity by activating DNA repair enzymes through deacylation. Although the antiaging effects of sirtuins have been widely publicized, much remains to be known before sirtuin-activating pills will be available to increase longevity. Nevertheless, optimistic wine-lovers have been delighted to hear that a constituent of red wine may activate sirtuins and thus increase life span!

The various forms of cellular derangements and adaptations described in this chapter cover a wide spectrum, ranging from adaptations in cell size, growth, and function; to the reversible and irreversible forms of acute cell injury; to the regulated type of cell death represented by apoptosis; to the pathologic alterations in cell organelles; to the less ominous forms of intracellular accumulations, including pigmentations. Reference is made to all these alterations throughout this book, because all organ injury and ultimately all clinical disease arise from derangements in cell structure and function.

KEY CONCEPTS

Cellular Aging

- Cellular aging results from a combination of accumulating cellular damage (e.g., by free radicals), reduced capacity to divide (replicative senescence), reduced ability to repair damaged DNA, and defective protein homeostasis
  - **Accumulation of DNA damage:** Defective DNA repair mechanisms; conversely, caloric restriction activates DNA repair and is known to prolong aging in model organisms
  - **Replicative senescence:** Reduced capacity of cells to divide secondary to progressive shortening of chromosomal ends (telomeres)
  - **Defective protein homeostasis:** Resulting from impaired chaperone and proteasome functions.
  - **Nutrient sensing system:** Caloric restriction increases longevity. Mediators may be reduced IGF-1 signaling and increases in sirtuins.

SUGGESTED READINGS

Hypertrophy

Frohlich ED, Susic D: Pressure overload. *Heart Failure Clin* 8:21, 2012. *[A succinct discussion of the pathophysiology of myocardial hypertrophy.]*

van Berlo JH, Maillet M, Molkentin JD: Signaling effectors underlying pathologic growth and remodeling of the heart. *J Clin Invest* 123:37, 2013. *[A review of the cellular and molecular mechanisms of cardiac muscle hypertrophy.]*

Cell Death

Galluzzi L, Kepp O, Trojel-Hansen C, et al: Mitochondrial control of cellular life, stress, and death. *Circ Res* 111:1198, 2012. *[Role of mitochondrial in cellular response to stress.]*

Galluzzi L, Vitale I, Abrams JM, et al: Molecular definitions of cell death subroutines: recommendations of the nomenclature committee on cell death 2012. *Cell Death Differ* 19:107, 2011. *[A summary of molecular definitions of different forms of cell death by an international group of experts.]*

Hausenloy DJ, Yellon DM: Myocardial ischemia-reperfusion injury: a neglected therapeutic target. *J Clin Invest* 123:92, 2013.*[Molecular basis of reperfusion injury and possible therapeutic targets.]*

Nikoletopoulou V, Markaki M, Palikaras K: Crosstalk between apoptosis, necrosis and autophagy. *Biochim Biophys Acta* 2013. *[A general review of different forms of cell death.]*

Apoptosis

Andersen J, Kornbluth S: The Tangled circuitry of metabolism and apoptosis. *Mol Cell* 49:399, 2013. *[A review of the linkage between metabolism and cell death pathways regulated by Bcl-2.]*

Chipuk J, Moldoveanu T, Llambi F, et al: The BCL-2 family reunion. *Mol Cell* 37, 2010. *[Discussion of the role played by BCL-2 family in regulating cell death.]*

Kaufmann T, Strasser A, Jost PJ: Fas death receptor signaling: roles of Bid and XIAP. *Cell Death Differ* 19:42, 2012. *[A discussion of extrinsic apoptosis and its linkages to other forms of cell death.]*

Martinou JC, Youle RJ: Mitochondria in apoptosis: BCL-2 family members and mitochondrial dynamics. *Developmental Cell* 21, 2011. *[A discussion of the molecular mechanisms of intrinsic apoptosis pathway.]*

Necroptosis

Han J, Zhong C, Zhang D: Programmed necrosis: backup to and competitor with apoptosis in the immune system. *Nat Immunol* 12:1143, 2011. *[An excellent discussion of the functional and molecular connection between apoptosis and necroptosis.]*

Kaczmarek A, Vandenabeele P, Krysko DV: Necroptosis: the release of damage-associated molecular patterns and its physiological relevance. *Immunity* 38:209, 2013. *[A discussion of the role of RIP1 and RIP3 in necroptosis.]*

Vanden Berghe T, Linkermann A, Jouan-Lanhouet S, et al: Regulated necrosis: the expanding network of non-apoptotic cell death pathways. *Nat Rev Mol Cell Biol* 15:135, 2014. *[A current review of various forms of programmed non apoptotic pathways of cell death.]*

Autophagy

Choi AMK, Ryter S, Levine B: Autophagy in human health and disease. *N Engl J Med* 368:7, 2013. *[An excellent discussion of the mechanisms and significance of autophagy.]*

Nixon R: The role of autophagy in neurodegenerative disease. *Nat Med* 8:983, 2013. *[An in depth discussion of autophagy and neurodegenerative disorders.]*

Aging

Guarente L: Sirtuins, aging, and medicine. *N Engl J Med* 364:23, 2011. *[The role of sirturins in aging in a clinical context.]*

Lopez-Otin C, Blasco MA, Partridge L, et al: The hallmarks of aging. *Cell* 153:1194, 2013. *[A landmark review that suggest nine hallmarks of aging and directions for future research.]*

Newgard CB, Sharpless NE: Coming of age: molecular drivers of aging and therapeutic opportunities. *J Clin Invest* 3:946, 2013. *[A summary of key molecular pathways in aging.]*

See TARGETED THERAPY available online at www.studentconsult.com

CHAPTER 3

Inflammation and Repair

CHAPTER CONTENTS

Overview of Inflammation: Definitions and General Features

Inflammation is a response of vascularized tissues to infections and damaged tissues that brings cells and molecules of host defense from the circulation to the sites where they are needed, in order to eliminate the offending agents. Although in common medical and lay parlance, inflammation suggests a harmful reaction, it is actually a protective response that is essential for survival. It serves to rid the host of both the initial cause of cell injury (e.g., microbes, toxins) and the consequences of such injury (e.g., necrotic cells and tissues). The mediators of defense include phagocytic leukocytes, antibodies, and complement proteins. Most of these normally circulate in the blood, from which they can be rapidly recruited to any site in the body; some of the cells also reside in tissues. The process of inflammation delivers these cells and proteins to damaged or necrotic tissues and foreign invaders, such as microbes, and activates the recruited cells and molecules, which then function to get rid of the harmful or unwanted substances. Without inflammation, infections would go unchecked, wounds would never heal, and injured tissues might remain permanent festering sores. In addition to inflammatory cells, components of innate immunity include other cells, such as natural killer cells, dendritic cells, and epithelial cells, as well as soluble factors such as the proteins of the complement system. Together, these components of innate immunity serve as the first responders to infection. They also function to eliminate damaged cells and foreign bodies.

The typical inflammatory reaction develops through a series of sequential steps:

- The offending agent, which is located in extravascular tissues, is recognized by host cells and molecules.
- Leukocytes and plasma proteins are recruited from the circulation to the site where the offending agent is located.
- The leukocytes and proteins are activated and work together to destroy and eliminate the offending substance.
- The reaction is controlled and terminated.
- The damaged tissue is repaired.

Before discussing the mechanisms, functions, and pathology of the inflammatory response, it is useful to review some of its fundamental properties.

- **Components of the inflammatory response.** The major participants in the inflammatory reaction in tissues are blood vessels and leukocytes (Fig. 3-1). As will be discussed in more detail later, blood vessels dilate to slow down blood flow, and by increasing their permeability, they enable selected circulating proteins to enter the site of infection or tissue damage. Characteristics of the endothelium lining blood vessels also change, such that circulating leukocytes first come to a halt and then migrate into the tissues. Leukocytes, once recruited, are activated and acquire the ability to ingest and destroy microbes and dead cells, as well as foreign bodies and other unwanted materials in the tissues.
- **Harmful consequences of inflammation.** Protective inflammatory reactions to infections are often accompanied by local tissue damage and its associated signs and symptoms (e.g., pain and functional impairment). Typically, however, these harmful consequences are self-limited and resolve as the inflammation abates, leaving little or no permanent damage. In contrast, there are many diseases in which the inflammatory reaction is misdirected (e.g., against self tissues in autoimmune diseases), occurs against normally harmless environmental substances (e.g., in allergies), or is inadequately controlled. In these cases, the normally protective inflammatory reaction becomes the cause of the disease, and the damage it causes is the dominant feature. In clinical medicine, great attention is given to the injurious consequences of inflammation (Table 3-1). Inflammatory reactions underlie common chronic diseases, such as rheumatoid arthritis, atherosclerosis, and lung fibrosis, as well as life-threatening hypersensitivity reactions to insect bites, drugs, and toxins. For this reason our pharmacies abound with antiinflammatory drugs, which ideally would control the harmful sequelae of inflammation yet not interfere with its beneficial effects. In fact, inflammation may contribute to a variety of diseases that are thought to be primarily metabolic, degenerative, or genetic disorders, such as type 2 diabetes, Alzheimer disease, and cancer. In recognition of the wide-ranging harmful consequences of inflammation, the lay press has rather melodramatically referred to it as "the silent killer."
- **Local and systemic inflammation.** Much of this discussion of inflammation focuses on the tissue reaction that is a local response to an infection or to localized damage. Although even such local reactions can have some systemic manifestations (e.g., fever in the setting of bacterial or viral pharyngitis), the reaction is largely confined to the site of infection or damage. In rare situations, such as some disseminated bacterial infections, the inflammatory reaction is systemic and causes widespread pathologic abnormalities. This reaction has been called *sepsis,* which is one form of the *systemic inflammatory response syndrome*. This serious disorder is discussed in Chapter 4.
- **Mediators of inflammation.** The vascular and cellular reactions of inflammation are triggered by soluble factors that are produced by various cells or derived from plasma proteins and are generated or activated

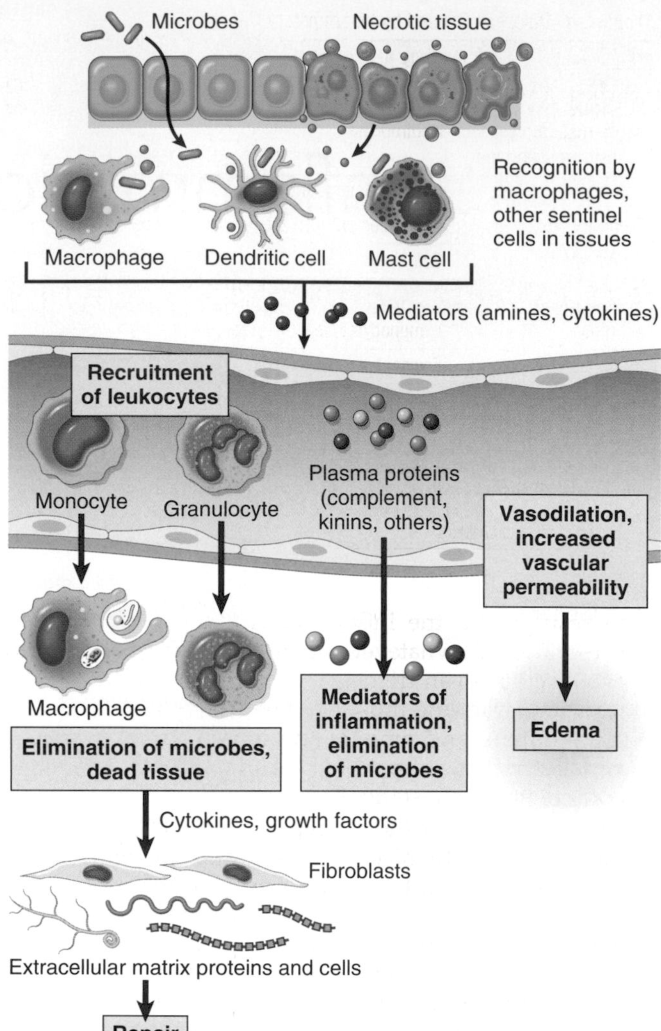

Figure 3-1 Sequence of events in an inflammatory reaction. Macrophages and other cells in tissues recognize microbes and damaged cells and liberate mediators, which trigger the vascular and cellular reactions of inflammation.

Table 3-1 Diseases Caused by Inflammatory Reactions

Disorders	Cells and Molecules Involved in Injury
Acute	
Acute respiratory distress syndrome	Neutrophils
Asthma	Eosinophils; IgE antibodies
Glomerulonephritis	Antibodies and complement; neutrophils, monocytes
Septic shock	Cytokines
Chronic	
Arthritis	Lymphocytes, macrophages; antibodies?
Asthma	Eosinophils; IgE antibodies
Atherosclerosis	Macrophages; lymphocytes
Pulmonary fibrosis	Macrophages; fibroblasts

Listed are selected examples of diseases in which the inflammatory response plays a significant role in tissue injury. Some, such as asthma, can present with acute inflammation or a chronic illness with repeated bouts of acute exacerbation. These diseases and their pathogenesis are discussed in relevant chapters.

in response to the inflammatory stimulus. Microbes, necrotic cells (whatever the cause of cell death), and even hypoxia can trigger the elaboration of inflammatory mediators and thus elicit inflammation. Such mediators initiate and amplify the inflammatory response and determine its pattern, severity, and clinical and pathologic manifestations.

- **Acute and chronic inflammation** (Table 3-2). The initial, rapid response to infections and tissue damage is called *acute inflammation*. It typically develops within minutes or hours and is of short duration, lasting for several hours or a few days; its main characteristics are the exudation of fluid and plasma proteins (edema) and the emigration of leukocytes, predominantly neutrophils (also called polymorphonuclear leukocytes). When acute inflammation achieves its desired goal of eliminating the offenders, the reaction subsides, but if the response fails to clear the stimulus, the reaction can progress to a protracted phase that is called *chronic inflammation*. Chronic inflammation is of longer duration and is associated with more tissue destruction, the presence of lymphocytes and macrophages, the proliferation of blood vessels, and the deposition of connective tissue. Chronic inflammation is discussed later in this chapter. Acute inflammation is one of the reactions of the type of host defense known as *innate immunity*, and chronic inflammation is more prominent in the reactions of *adaptive immunity* (Chapter 6).
- **Termination of inflammation and initiation of tissue repair.** Inflammation is terminated when the offending agent is eliminated. The reaction resolves because mediators are broken down and dissipated, and leukocytes have short life spans in tissues. In addition, antiinflammatory mechanisms are activated, serving to control the response and prevent it from causing excessive damage to the host. Once inflammation has achieved its goal of eliminating the offending agents, it also sets into motion the process of *tissue repair*. Repair consists of a series of events that heal damaged tissue. In this process, the injured tissue is replaced through *regeneration* of surviving cells and filling of residual defects with connective tissue *(scarring)*.

Table 3-2 Features of Acute and Chronic Inflammation

Feature	Acute	Chronic
Onset	Fast: minutes or hours	Slow: days
Cellular infiltrate	Mainly neutrophils	Monocytes/macrophages and lymphocytes
Tissue injury, fibrosis	Usually mild and self-limited	Often severe and progressive
Local and systemic signs	Prominent	Less

This chapter describes the causes (etiology) of and stimuli for inflammation, and then the sequence of events, mediators, and morphologic patterns of acute inflammation. This is followed by a discussion of chronic inflammation, and then the process of tissue repair. The study of inflammation has a rich history, and we first touch on past work that paved the way for our current understanding of this fascinating process.

Historical Highlights

Although clinical features of inflammation were described in an Egyptian papyrus dated around 3000 BC, Celsus, a Roman writer of the first century AD, first listed the four cardinal signs of inflammation: *rubor* (redness), *tumor* (swelling), *calor* (heat), and *dolor* (pain). These signs are hallmarks of acute inflammation. A fifth clinical sign, loss of function *(functio laesa)*, was added by Rudolf Virchow in the 19th century. In 1793, the Scottish surgeon John Hunter noted what is now considered an obvious fact: inflammation is not a disease but a stereotypic response that has a salutary effect on its host. In the 1880s, Russian biologist Elie Metchnikoff discovered the process of *phagocytosis* by observing the ingestion of rose thorns by amebocytes of starfish larvae and of bacteria by mammalian leukocytes. He concluded that the purpose of inflammation was to bring phagocytic cells to the injured area to engulf invading bacteria. This concept was satirized by George Bernard Shaw in his play "The Doctor's Dilemma," in which one physician's cure-all is to "stimulate the phagocytes!" Sir Thomas Lewis, studying the inflammatory response in skin, established the concept that *chemical substances, such as histamine (produced locally in response to injury), mediate the vascular changes of inflammation.* This fundamental concept underlies the important discoveries of chemical mediators of inflammation and the use of antiinflammatory drugs in clinical medicine.

Causes of Inflammation

Inflammatory reactions may be triggered by a variety of stimuli:

- **Infections** (bacterial, viral, fungal, parasitic) and microbial toxins are among the most common and medically important causes of inflammation. Different infectious pathogens elicit varied inflammatory responses, from mild acute inflammation that causes little or no lasting damage and successfully eradicates the infection, to severe systemic reactions that can be fatal, to prolonged chronic reactions that cause extensive tissue injury. The outcomes are determined largely by the type of pathogen and, to some extent, by characteristics of the host that remain poorly defined.

- **Tissue necrosis** elicits inflammation regardless of the cause of cell death, which may include *ischemia* (reduced blood flow, the cause of myocardial infarction), *trauma*, and *physical and chemical injury* (e.g., thermal injury, as in burns or frostbite; irradiation; exposure to some environmental chemicals). Several molecules released from necrotic cells are known to trigger inflammation; some of these are described below.
- **Foreign bodies** (splinters, dirt, sutures) may elicit inflammation by themselves or because they cause traumatic tissue injury or carry microbes. Even some endogenous substances can be considered potentially harmful if large amounts are deposited in tissues; such substances include urate crystals (in the disease gout), cholesterol crystals (in atherosclerosis), and lipids (in obesity-associated metabolic syndrome).
- **Immune reactions** (also called *hypersensitivity*) are reactions in which the normally protective immune system damages the individual's own tissues. The injurious immune responses may be directed against self antigens, causing *autoimmune diseases*, or may be inappropriate reactions against environmental substances, as in *allergies*, or against microbes. Inflammation is a major cause of tissue injury in these diseases (Chapter 6). Because the stimuli for the inflammatory responses (e.g., self and environmental antigens) cannot be eliminated, autoimmune and allergic reactions tend to be persistent and difficult to cure, are often associated with chronic inflammation, and are important causes of morbidity and mortality. The inflammation is induced by cytokines produced by T lymphocytes and other cells of the immune system (Chapter 6).

Recognition of Microbes and Damaged Cells

Recognition of offending agents is the first step in all inflammatory reactions. The cells and receptors that perform this function of recognizing invaders evolved as adaptation of multicellular organisms to the presence of microbes in the environment, and the responses they trigger are critical for the survival of the organisms. Several cellular receptors and circulating proteins are capable of recognizing microbes and products of cell damage and triggering inflammation.

- **Cellular receptors for microbes.** Cells express receptors in the plasma membrane (for extracellular microbes), the endosomes (for ingested microbes), and the cytosol (for intracellular microbes) that enable the cells to sense the presence of foreign invaders in any cellular compartment. The best defined of these receptors belong to the family of *Toll-like receptors (TLRs)*; these and other cellular receptors of innate immunity are described in Chapter 6. The receptors are expressed on many cell types, including epithelial cells (through which microbes enter from the external environment), dendritic cells, macrophages, and other leukocytes (which may encounter microbes in various tissues). Engagement of these receptors triggers production of molecules involved in inflammation, including adhesion molecules on endothelial cells, cytokines, and other mediators.
- **Sensors of cell damage.** All cells have cytosolic receptors that recognize a diverse set of molecules that are liberated or altered as a consequence of cell damage. These molecules include uric acid (a product of DNA breakdown), ATP (released from damaged mitochondria), reduced intracellular K+ concentrations (reflecting loss of ions because of plasma membrane injury), even DNA when it is released into the cytoplasm and not sequestered in nuclei, as it should be normally, and many others. These receptors activate a multiprotein cytosolic complex called the *inflammasome* (Chapter 6), which induces the production of the cytokine interleukin-1 (IL-1). IL-1 recruits leukocytes and thus induces inflammation (see later). Gain-of-function mutations in the sensor are the cause of rare diseases known as *autoinflammatory syndromes* that are characterized by spontaneous inflammation; IL-1 antagonists are effective treatments for these disorders. The inflammasome has also been implicated in inflammatory reactions to urate crystals (the cause of *gout*), lipids (in metabolic syndrome), cholesterol crystals (in atherosclerosis), and even amyloid deposits in the brain (in Alzheimer disease). These disorders are discussed later in this and other chapters.
- **Other cellular receptors involved in inflammation.** In addition to directly recognizing microbes, many leukocytes express receptors for the Fc tails of antibodies and for complement proteins. These receptors recognize microbes coated with antibodies and complement (the coating process is called *opsonization*) and promote ingestion and destruction of the microbes as well as inflammation.
- **Circulating proteins.** The *complement system* reacts against microbes and produces mediators of inflammation (discussed later). A circulating protein called *mannose-binding lectin* recognizes microbial sugars and promotes ingestion of the microbes and the activation of the complement system. Other proteins called *collectins* also bind to and combat microbes.

KEY CONCEPTS

General Features and Causes of Inflammation

- Inflammation is a beneficial host response to foreign invaders and necrotic tissue, but it may also cause tissue damage.
- The main components of inflammation are a vascular reaction and a cellular response; both are activated by mediators that are derived from plasma proteins and various cells.
- The steps of the inflammatory response can be remembered as the five Rs: (1) recognition of the injurious agent, (2) recruitment of leukocytes, (3) removal of the agent, (4) regulation (control) of the response, and (5) resolution (repair).
- The causes of inflammation include infections, tissue necrosis, foreign bodies, trauma, and immune responses.

- Epithelial cells, tissue macrophages and dendritic cells, leukocytes, and other cell types express receptors that sense the presence of microbes and damage. Circulating proteins recognize microbes that have entered the blood.
- The outcome of acute inflammation is either elimination of the noxious stimulus followed by decline of the reaction and repair of the damaged tissue, or persistent injury resulting in chronic inflammation.

Acute Inflammation

Acute inflammation has three major components: (1) dilation of small vessels leading to an increase in blood flow, (2) increased permeability of the microvasculature enabling plasma proteins and leukocytes to leave the circulation, and (3) emigration of the leukocytes from the microcirculation, their accumulation in the focus of injury, and their activation to eliminate the offending agent (Fig. 3-1). When an individual encounters an injurious agent, such as an infectious microbe or dead cells, phagocytes that reside in all tissues try to eliminate these agents. At the same time, phagocytes and other sentinel cells in the tissues recognize the presence of the foreign or abnormal substance and react by liberating cytokines, lipid messengers, and other mediators of inflammation. Some of these mediators act on small blood vessels in the vicinity and promote the efflux of plasma and the recruitment of circulating leukocytes to the site where the offending agent is located.

Reactions of Blood Vessels in Acute Inflammation

The vascular reactions of acute inflammation consist of changes in the flow of blood and the permeability of vessels, both designed to maximize the movement of plasma proteins and leukocytes out of the circulation and into the site of infection or injury. The escape of fluid, proteins, and blood cells from the vascular system into the interstitial tissue or body cavities is known as *exudation* (Fig. 3-2). An *exudate* is an extravascular fluid that has a high protein concentration and contains cellular debris. Its presence implies that there is an increase in the permeability of small blood vessels triggered by some sort of tissue injury and an ongoing inflammatory reaction. In contrast, a *transudate* is a fluid with low protein content (most of which is albumin), little or no cellular material, and low specific gravity. It is essentially an ultrafiltrate of blood plasma that is produced as a result of osmotic or hydrostatic imbalance across the vessel wall without an increase in vascular permeability (Chapter 4). *Edema* denotes an excess of fluid in the interstitial tissue or serous cavities; it can be either an exudate or a transudate. *Pus*, a *purulent* exudate, is an inflammatory exudate rich in leukocytes (mostly neutrophils), the debris of dead cells and, in many cases, microbes.

Changes in Vascular Flow and Caliber

Changes in vascular flow and caliber begin early after injury and consist of the following.

- **Vasodilation is induced by the action of several mediators, notably histamine, on vascular smooth muscle.**

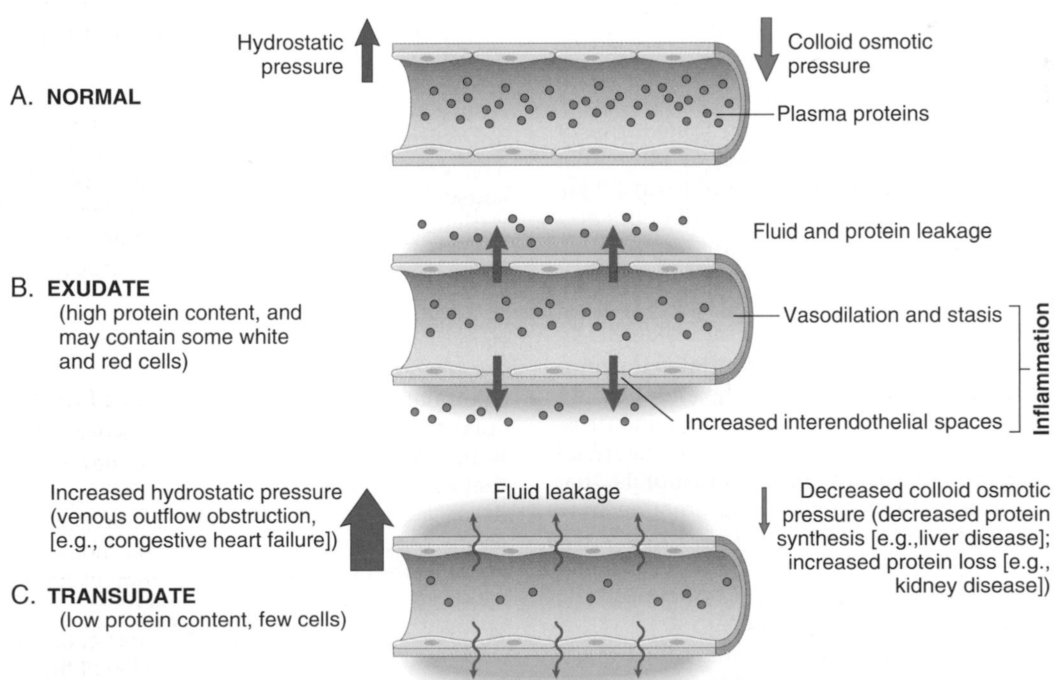

Figure 3-2 Formation of exudates and transudates. **A,** Normal hydrostatic pressure *(blue arrow)* is about 32 mm Hg at the arterial end of a capillary bed and 12 mm Hg at the venous end; the mean colloid osmotic pressure of tissues is approximately 25 mm Hg *(green arrow)*, which is equal to the mean capillary pressure. Therefore, the net flow of fluid across the vascular bed is almost nil. **B,** An exudate is formed in inflammation, because vascular permeability increases as a result of increased interendothelial spaces. **C,** A transudate is formed when fluid leaks out because of increased hydrostatic pressure or decreased osmotic pressure.

It is one of the earliest manifestations of acute inflammation. Vasodilation first involves the arterioles and then leads to opening of new capillary beds in the area. The result is *increased blood flow*, which is the cause of heat and redness *(erythema)* at the site of inflammation.

- Vasodilation is quickly followed by **increased permeability of the microvasculature**, with the outpouring of protein-rich fluid into the extravascular tissues; this process is described in detail below.
- The loss of fluid and increased vessel diameter lead to slower blood flow, concentration of red cells in small vessels, and increased viscosity of the blood. These changes result in **engorgement of small vessels with slowly moving red cells, a condition termed *stasis*,** which is seen as *vascular congestion* and localized redness of the involved tissue.
- As stasis develops, **blood leukocytes, principally neutrophils, accumulate along the vascular endothelium.** At the same time endothelial cells are activated by mediators produced at sites of infection and tissue damage, and express increased levels of adhesion molecules. Leukocytes then adhere to the endothelium, and soon afterward they migrate through the vascular wall into the interstitial tissue, in a sequence that is described later.

Increased Vascular Permeability (Vascular Leakage)

Several mechanisms are responsible for the increased permeability of postcapillary venules, a hallmark of acute inflammation (Fig. 3-3):

- **Contraction of endothelial cells resulting in increased interendothelial spaces is the most common mechanism of vascular leakage**. It is elicited by histamine, bradykinin, leukotrienes, and other chemical mediators. It is called the *immediate transient response* because it occurs rapidly after exposure to the mediator and is usually short-lived (15 to 30 minutes). In some forms of mild injury (e.g., after burns, irradiation or ultraviolet radiation, and exposure to certain bacterial toxins), vascular leakage begins after a delay of 2 to 12 hours and lasts for several hours or even days; this *delayed prolonged leakage* may be caused by contraction of endothelial cells or mild endothelial damage. Late-appearing sunburn is a good example of this type of leakage.
- **Endothelial injury, resulting in endothelial cell necrosis and detachment.** Direct damage to the endothelium is encountered in severe injuries, for example, in burns, or is induced by the actions of microbes and microbial toxins that target endothelial cells. Neutrophils that adhere to the endothelium during inflammation may also injure the endothelial cells and thus amplify the reaction. In most instances leakage starts immediately after injury and is sustained for several hours until the damaged vessels are thrombosed or repaired.
- Increased transport of fluids and proteins, called *transcytosis*, through the endothelial cell. This process may involve intracellular channels that may be stimulated by certain factors, such as vascular endothelial growth factor (VEGF), that promote vascular leakage. However, the contribution of this process to the vascular permeability of acute inflammation is uncertain.

A. NORMAL
Leukocytes
Plasma proteins
Endothelium
Vessel lumen
Tissues

B. RETRACTION OF ENDOTHELIAL CELLS
• Induced by histamine, other mediators
• Rapid and short-lived (minutes)

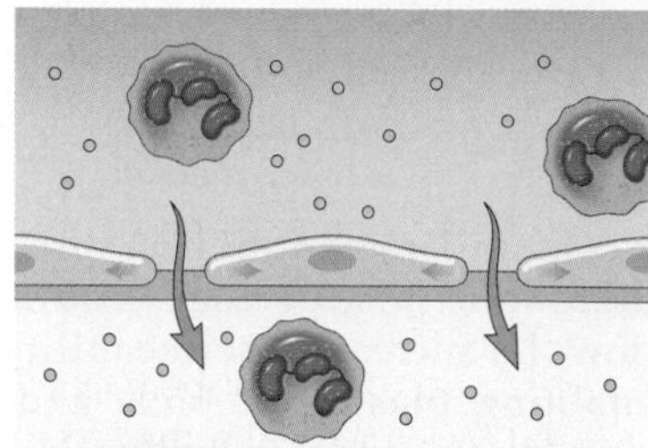

C. ENDOTHELIAL INJURY
• Caused by burns, some microbial toxins
• Rapid; may be long-lived (hours to days)

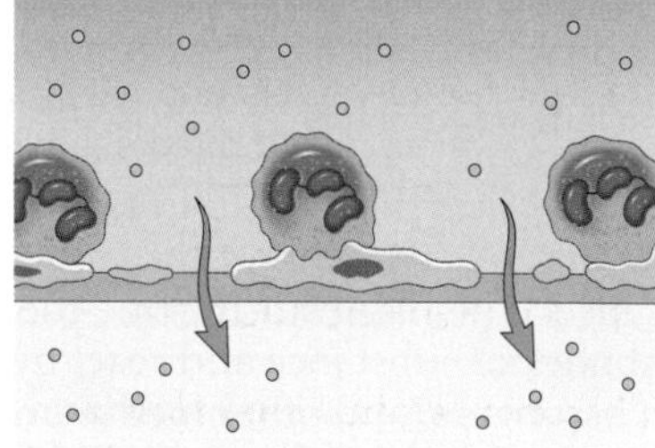

Figure 3-3 Principal mechanisms of increased vascular permeability in inflammation and their features and underlying causes.

Although these mechanisms of increased vascular permeability are described separately, all probably contribute in varying degrees in responses to most stimuli. For example, at different stages of a thermal burn, leakage results from chemically mediated endothelial contraction and direct and leukocyte-dependent endothelial injury. The vascular leakage induced by these mechanisms can cause life-threatening loss of fluid in severely burned patients.

Responses of Lymphatic Vessels and Lymph Nodes

In addition to blood vessels, lymphatic vessels also participate in acute inflammation. The system of lymphatics and lymph nodes filters and polices the extravascular fluids. Lymphatics normally drain the small amount of extravascular fluid that has seeped out of capillaries. In inflammation, lymph flow is increased and helps drain edema fluid that accumulates because of increased vascular permeability. In addition to fluid, leukocytes and cell debris, as well as microbes, may find their way into lymph. Lymphatic vessels, like blood vessels, proliferate during inflammatory reactions to handle the increased load. The lymphatics may become secondarily inflamed *(lymphangitis)*, as may the draining lymph nodes *(lymphadenitis)*. Inflamed lymph nodes are often enlarged because of hyperplasia of the lymphoid follicles and increased numbers of lymphocytes and macrophages. This constellation of pathologic changes is termed *reactive*, or *inflammatory, lymphadenitis* (Chapter 13). For clinicians the presence of red streaks near a skin wound is a telltale sign of an infection in the wound. This streaking follows the course of the lymphatic channels and is diagnostic of lymphangitis; it may be accompanied by painful enlargement of the draining lymph nodes, indicating lymphadenitis.

KEY CONCEPTS

Vascular Reactions in Acute Inflammation

- Vasodilation is induced by chemical mediators such as histamine (described later), and is the cause of erythema and stasis of blood flow.
- Increased vascular permeability is induced by histamine, kinins, and other mediators that produce gaps between endothelial cells, by direct or leukocyte-induced endothelial injury, and by increased passage of fluids through the endothelium.
- Increased vascular permeability allows plasma proteins and leukocytes, the mediators of host defense, to enter sites of infection or tissue damage. Fluid leak from blood vessels results in edema.
- Lymphatic vessels and lymph nodes are also involved in inflammation, and often show redness and swelling.

Leukocyte Recruitment to Sites of Inflammation

The changes in blood flow and vascular permeability are quickly followed by an influx of leukocytes into the tissue. These leukocytes perform the key function of eliminating the offending agents. The most important leukocytes in typical inflammatory reactions are the ones capable of phagocytosis, namely neutrophils and macrophages. These leukocytes ingest and destroy bacteria and other microbes, as well as necrotic tissue and foreign substances. Leukocytes also produce growth factors that aid in repair. A price that is paid for the defensive potency of leukocytes is that, when strongly activated, they may induce tissue damage and prolong inflammation, because the leukocyte products that destroy microbes and help "clean up" necrotic tissues can also injure normal bystander host tissues.

The journey of leukocytes from the vessel lumen to the tissue is a multistep process that is mediated and controlled by adhesion molecules and cytokines called chemokines. This process can be divided into sequential phases (Fig. 3-4):

1. In the lumen: *margination, rolling, and adhesion to endothelium.* Vascular endothelium in its normal, unactivated state does not bind circulating cells or impede their passage. In inflammation, the endothelium is activated and can bind leukocytes as a prelude to their exit from the blood vessels.
2. Migration across the endothelium and vessel wall
3. Migration in the tissues toward a chemotactic stimulus

Leukocyte Adhesion to Endothelium

In normally flowing blood in venules, red cells are confined to a central axial column, displacing the leukocytes toward the wall of the vessel. Because blood flow slows early in inflammation (stasis), hemodynamic conditions change (wall shear stress decreases), and more white cells assume a peripheral position along the endothelial surface. This process of leukocyte redistribution is called *margination.* Subsequently, leukocytes adhere transiently to the

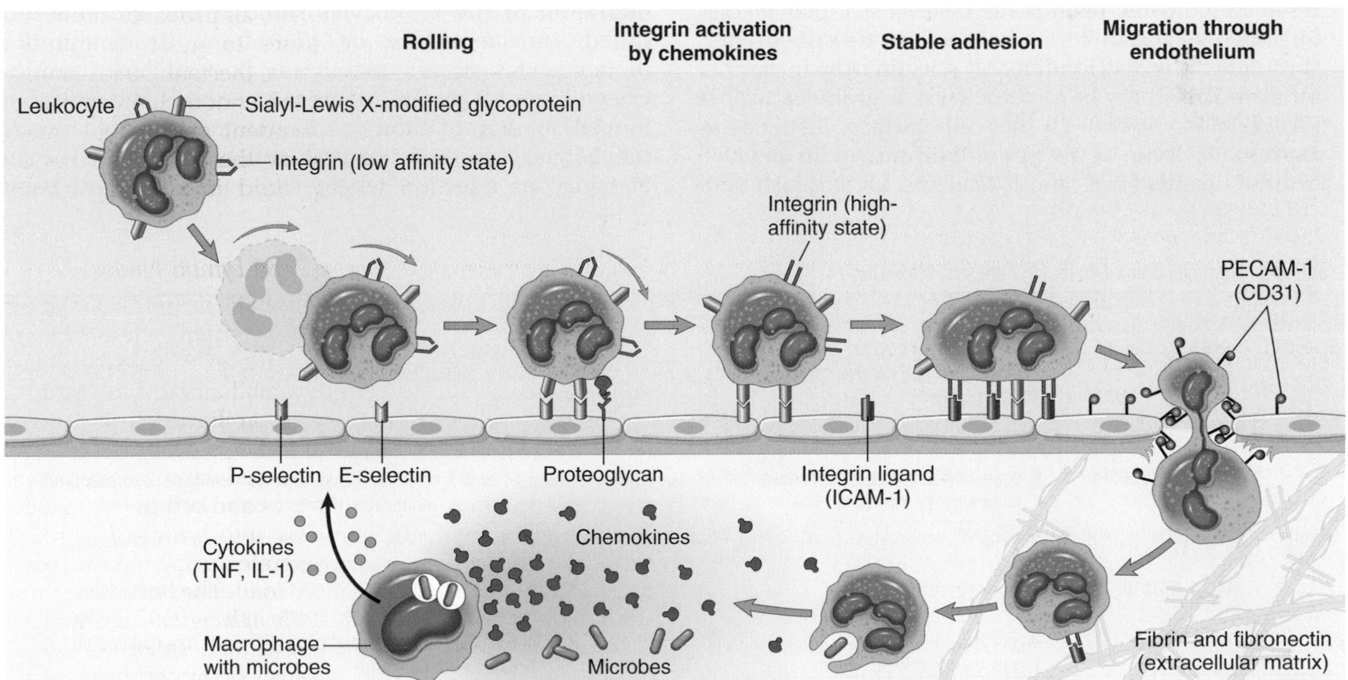

Figure 3-4 The multistep process of leukocyte migration through blood vessels, shown here for neutrophils. The leukocytes first roll, then become activated and adhere to endothelium, then transmigrate across the endothelium, pierce the basement membrane, and migrate toward chemoattractants emanating from the source of injury. Different molecules play predominant roles in different steps of this process: selectins in rolling; chemokines (usually displayed bound to proteoglycans) in activating the neutrophils to increase avidity of integrins; integrins in firm adhesion; and CD31 (PECAM-1) in transmigration. ICAM-1, Intercellular adhesion molecule 1; PECAM-1 (CD31), platelet endothelial cell adhesion molecule-1; TNF, tumor necrosis factor.

endothelium, detach and bind again, thus *rolling* on the vessel wall. The cells finally come to rest at some point where they *adhere* firmly (resembling pebbles over which a stream runs without disturbing them).

The attachment of leukocytes to endothelial cells is mediated by complementary adhesion molecules on the two cell types whose expression is enhanced by cytokines. Cytokines are secreted by sentinel cells in tissues in response to microbes and other injurious agents, thus ensuring that leukocytes are recruited to the tissues where these stimuli are present.

The two major families of molecules involved in leukocyte adhesion and migration are the selectins and integrins, and their ligands. They are expressed on leukocytes and endothelial cells.

- The initial rolling interactions are mediated by a family of proteins called *selectins* (Table 3-3). There are three types of selectins: one expressed on leukocytes (L-selectin), one on endothelium (E-selectin), and one in platelets and on endothelium (P-selectin). The ligands for selectins are sialylated oligosaccharides bound to mucin-like glycoprotein backbones. The expression of selectins and their ligands is regulated by cytokines produced in response to infection and injury. Tissue macrophages, mast cells, and endothelial cells that encounter microbes and dead tissues respond by secreting several cytokines, including tumor necrosis factor (TNF), IL-1, and chemokines (*chemo*attractant cyto*kines*). (Cytokines are described in more detail later and in Chapter 6.) TNF and IL-1 act on the endothelial cells of postcapillary venules adjacent to the infection and induce the coordinate expression of numerous adhesion molecules. Within 1 to 2 hours the endothelial cells begin to express E-selectin and the ligands for L-selectin. Other mediators such as histamine and thrombin, described later, stimulate the redistribution of P-selectin from its normal intracellular stores in endothelial cell granules (called *Weibel-Palade bodies*) to the cell surface. Leukocytes express L-selectin at the tips of their microvilli and also express ligands for E- and P-selectins, all of which bind to the complementary molecules on the endothelial cells. These are low-affinity interactions with a fast off-rate, and they are easily disrupted by the flowing blood. As a result, the bound leukocytes bind, detach, and bind again, and thus begin to roll along the endothelial surface.
- These weak rolling interactions slow down the leukocytes and give them the opportunity to bind more firmly to the endothelium. Firm adhesion is mediated by a family of heterodimeric leukocyte surface proteins called *integrins* (Table 3-3). TNF and IL-1 induce endothelial expression of ligands for integrins, mainly vascular cell adhesion molecule 1 (VCAM-1, the ligand for the β1 integrin VLA-4) and intercellular adhesion molecule-1 (ICAM-1, the ligand for the β2 integrins LFA-1 and Mac-1). Leukocytes normally express integrins in a low-affinity state. Chemokines that were produced at the site of injury bind to endothelial cell proteoglycans, and are displayed at high concentrations on the endothelial surface. These chemokines bind to and activate the rolling leukocytes. One of the consequences of activation is the conversion of VLA-4 and LFA-1 integrins on the leukocytes to a high-affinity state. The combination of cytokine-induced expression of integrin ligands on the endothelium and increased integrin affinity on the leukocytes results in firm integrin-mediated binding of the leukocytes to the endothelium at the site of inflammation. The leukocytes stop rolling, their cytoskeleton is reorganized, and they spread out on the endothelial surface.

Leukocyte Migration Through Endothelium

The next step in the process of leukocyte recruitment is migration of the leukocytes through the endothelium, called *transmigration* or *diapedesis*. Transmigration of leukocytes occurs mainly in postcapillary venules. Chemokines act on the adherent leukocytes and stimulate the cells to migrate through interendothelial spaces toward the chemical concentration gradient, that is, toward the site of injury or infection where the chemokines are being

Table 3-3 Endothelial and Leukocyte Adhesion Molecules

Family	Molecule	Distribution	Ligand
Selectin	L-selectin (CD62L)	Neutrophils, monocytes T cells (naïve and central memory) B cells (naïve)	Sialyl-Lewis X/PNAd on GlyCAM-1, CD34, MAdCAM-1, others; expressed on endothelium (HEV)
	E-selectin (CD62E)	Endothelium activated by cytokines (TNF, IL-1)	Sialyl-Lewis X (e.g., CLA) on glycoproteins; expressed on neutrophils, monocytes, T cells (effector, memory)
	P-selectin (CD62P)	Endothelium activated by cytokines (TNF, IL-1), histamine, or thrombin	Sialyl-Lewis X on PSGL-1 and other glycoproteins; expressed on neutrophils, monocytes, T cells (effector, memory)
Integrin	LFA-1 (CD11aCD18)	Neutrophils, monocytes, T cells (naïve, effector, memory)	ICAM-1 (CD54), ICAM-2 (CD102); expressed on endothelium (upregulated on activated endothelium)
	MAC-1 (CD11bCD18)	Monocytes, DCs	ICAM-1 (CD54), ICAM-2 (CD102); expressed on endothelium (upregulated on activated endothelium)
	VLA-4 (CD49aCD29)	Monocytes T cells (naïve, effector, memory)	VCAM-1 (CD106); expressed on endothelium (upregulated on activated endothelium)
	α4β7 (CD49DCD29)	Monocytes T cells (gut homing naïve effector, memory)	VCAM-1 (CD106), MAdCAM-1; expressed on endothelium in gut and gut-associated lymphoid tissues
Ig	CD31	Endothelial cells, leukocytes	CD31 (homotypic interaction)

CLA, Cutaneous lymphocyte antigen-1; GlyCAM-1, glycan-bearing cell adhesion molecule-1; HEV, high endothelial venule; Ig, immunoglobulin; IL-1, interleukin-1; ICAM, intercellular adhesion molecule; MAdCAM-1, mucosal adhesion cell adhesion molecule-1; PSGL-1, P-selectin glycoprotein ligand-1; TNF, tumor necrosis factor; VCAM, vascular cell adhesion molecule.

produced. Several adhesion molecules present in the intercellular junctions between endothelial cells are involved in the migration of leukocytes. These molecules include a member of the immunoglobulin superfamily called *CD31* or *PECAM-1* (platelet endothelial cell adhesion molecule). After traversing the endothelium, leukocytes pierce the basement membrane, probably by secreting collagenases, and enter the extravascular tissue. The cells then migrate toward the chemotactic gradient created by chemokines and other chemoattractants and accumulate in the extravascular site.

The most telling proof of the importance of leukocyte adhesion molecules is the existence of genetic deficiencies in these molecules that result in recurrent bacterial infections as a consequence of impaired leukocyte adhesion and defective inflammation. These leukocyte adhesion deficiencies are described in Chapter 6.

Chemotaxis of Leukocytes

After exiting the circulation, leukocytes move in the tissues toward the site of injury by a process called *chemotaxis*, which is defined as locomotion along a chemical gradient. Both exogenous and endogenous substances can act as chemoattractants. The most common exogenous agents are *bacterial products,* including peptides that possess an *N*-formylmethionine terminal amino acid and some lipids. Endogenous chemoattractants include several chemical mediators (described later): (1) *cytokines,* particularly those of the chemokine family (e.g., IL-8); (2) *components of the complement system, particularly C5a;* and (3) *arachidonic acid (AA) metabolites, mainly leukotriene* B_4 *(*LTB_4*).* All these chemotactic agents bind to specific seven-transmembrane G protein-coupled receptors on the surface of leukocytes. Signals initiated from these receptors result in activation of second messengers that increase cytosolic calcium and activate small guanosine triphosphatases of the Rac/Rho/cdc42 family as well as numerous kinases. These signals induce polymerization of actin, resulting in increased amounts of polymerized actin at the leading edge of the cell and localization of myosin filaments at the back. The leukocyte moves by extending filopodia that pull the back of the cell in the direction of extension, much as an automobile with front-wheel drive is pulled by the wheels in front (Fig. 3-5). The net result is that leukocytes migrate toward the inflammatory stimulus in the direction of the locally produced chemoattractants.

The nature of the leukocyte infiltrate varies with the age of the inflammatory response and the type of stimulus. In most forms of acute inflammation neutrophils predominate in the inflammatory infiltrate during the first 6 to 24 hours and are replaced by monocytes in 24 to 48 hours (Fig. 3-6). There are several reasons for the early preponderance of neutrophils: they are more numerous in the blood than other leukocytes, they respond more rapidly to chemokines, and they may attach more firmly to the adhesion molecules that are rapidly induced on endothelial cells, such as P- and E-selectins. After entering tissues, neutrophils are short-lived; they undergo apoptosis and disappear within 24 to 48 hours. Monocytes not only survive longer but may also proliferate in the tissues, and thus they become the dominant population in prolonged inflammatory reactions. There are, however, exceptions to this stereotypic pattern of cellular infiltration.

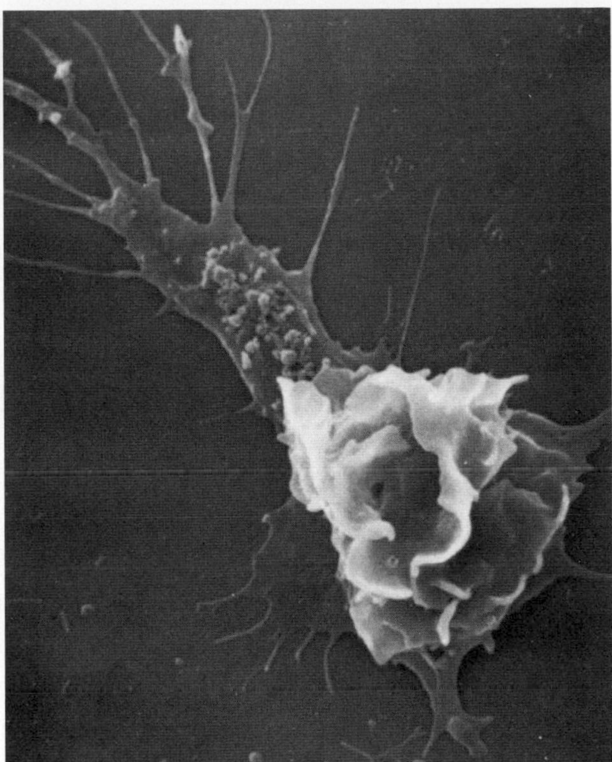

Figure 3-5 Scanning electron micrograph of a moving leukocyte in culture showing a filopodium *(upper left)* and a trailing tail. (Courtesy Dr. Morris J. Karnovsky, Harvard Medical School, Boston, Mass.)

In certain infections—for example, those produced by *Pseudomonas* bacteria—the cellular infiltrate is dominated by continuously recruited neutrophils for several days; in viral infections, lymphocytes may be the first cells to arrive; some hypersensitivity reactions are dominated by activated lymphocytes, macrophages, and plasma cells (reflecting the immune response); and in allergic reactions, eosinophils may be the main cell type.

The molecular understanding of leukocyte recruitment and migration has provided a large number of potential therapeutic targets for controlling harmful inflammation. Agents that block TNF, one of the major cytokines in leukocyte recruitment, are among the most successful therapeutics ever developed for chronic inflammatory diseases, and antagonists of leukocyte integrins are approved for inflammatory diseases or are being tested in clinical trials. Predictably, these antagonists not only have the desired effect of controlling the inflammation but can also compromise the ability of treated patients to defend themselves against microbes, which, of course, is the physiologic function of the inflammatory response.

KEY CONCEPTS

Leukocyte Recruitment to Sites of Inflammation

- Leukocytes are recruited from the blood into the extravascular tissue where infectious pathogens or damaged tissues may be located, migrate to the site of infection or tissue injury, and are activated to perform their functions.
- Leukocyte recruitment is a multistep process consisting of loose attachment to and rolling on endothelium (mediated

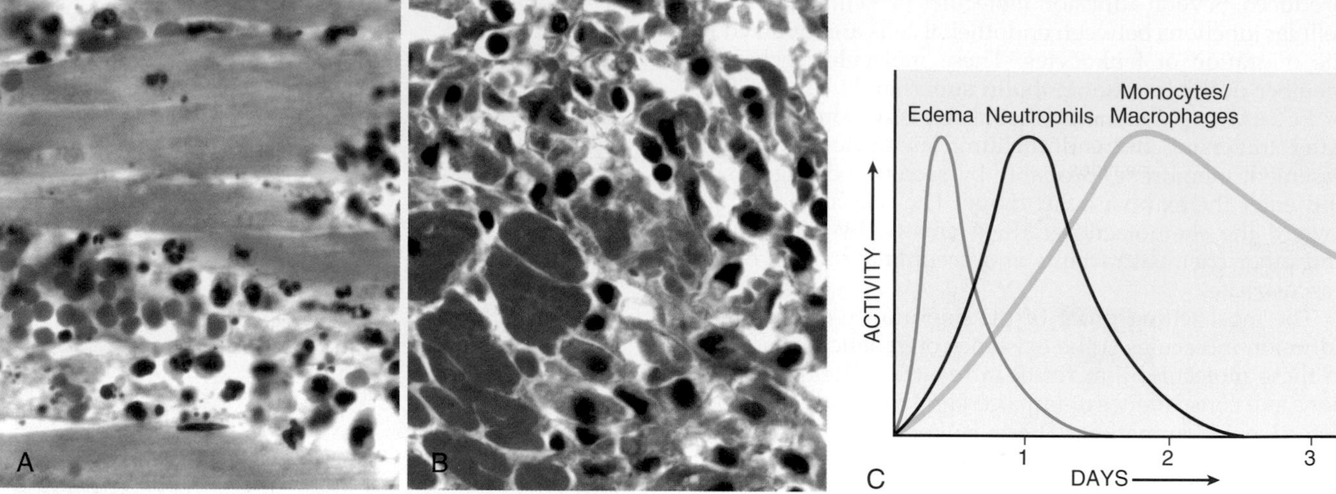

Figure 3-6 Nature of leukocyte infiltrates in inflammatory reactions. The photomicrographs show an inflammatory reaction in the myocardium after ischemic necrosis (infarction). **A,** Early (neutrophilic) infiltrates and congested blood vessels. **B,** Later (mononuclear) cellular infiltrates. **C,** The approximate kinetics of edema and cellular infiltration. For simplicity, edema is shown as an acute transient response, although secondary waves of delayed edema and neutrophil infiltration can also occur.

by selectins); firm attachment to endothelium (mediated by integrins); and migration through interendothelial spaces.

- Various cytokines promote expression of selectins and integrin ligands on endothelium (TNF, IL-1), increase the avidity of integrins for their ligands (chemokines), and promote directional migration of leukocytes (also chemokines); many of these cytokines are produced by tissue macrophages and other cells responding to the pathogens or damaged tissues.
- Neutrophils predominate in the early inflammatory infiltrate and are later replaced by monocytes and macrophages.

Once leukocytes (particularly neutrophils and monocytes) have been recruited to a site of infection or cell death, they must be activated to perform their functions. The responses of these leukocytes consist of (1) recognition of the offending agents by TLRs and other receptors, described earlier, which deliver signals that (2) activate the leukocytes to phagocytose and destroy the offending agents.

Phagocytosis and Clearance of the Offending Agent

Recognition of microbes or dead cells induces several responses in leukocytes that are collectively called *leukocyte activation* (Fig. 3-7). Activation results from signaling pathways that are triggered in leukocytes, resulting in increases in cytosolic Ca^{2+} and activation of enzymes such as protein kinase C and phospholipase A_2. The functional responses that are most important for destruction of microbes and other offenders are phagocytosis and intracellular killing. Several other responses aid in the defensive functions of inflammation and may contribute to its injurious consequences.

Phagocytosis

Phagocytosis involves three sequential steps (Fig. 3-8): (1) *recognition* and *attachment* of the particle to be ingested by the leukocyte; (2) *engulfment*, with subsequent formation of a phagocytic vacuole; and (3) *killing* or *degradation* of the ingested material.

Phagocytic Receptors. **Mannose receptors, scavenger receptors, and receptors for various opsonins bind and ingest microbes.** The macrophage *mannose receptor* is a lectin that binds terminal mannose and fucose residues of glycoproteins and glycolipids. These sugars are typically part of molecules found on microbial cell walls, whereas mammalian glycoproteins and glycolipids contain terminal sialic acid or *N*-acetylgalactosamine. Therefore, the mannose receptor recognizes microbes and not host cells. *Scavenger receptors* were originally defined as molecules that bind and mediate endocytosis of oxidized or acetylated low-density lipoprotein (LDL) particles that can no longer interact with the conventional LDL receptor. Macrophage scavenger receptors bind a variety of microbes in addition to modified LDL particles. Macrophage integrins, notably Mac-1 (CD11b/CD18), may also bind microbes for phagocytosis. The efficiency of phagocytosis is greatly enhanced when microbes are opsonized by specific proteins (opsonins) for which the phagocytes express high-affinity receptors. The major opsonins are IgG antibodies, the C3b breakdown product of complement, and certain plasma lectins, notably mannose-binding lectin, all of which are recognized by specific receptors on leukocytes.

Engulfment. After a particle is bound to phagocyte receptors, extensions of the cytoplasm (pseudopods) flow around it, and the plasma membrane pinches off to form a vesicle (phagosome) that encloses the particle. The phagosome then fuses with a lysosomal granule, resulting in discharge of the granule's contents into the phagolysosome (Fig. 3-8). During this process the phagocyte may also release granule contents into the extracellular space.

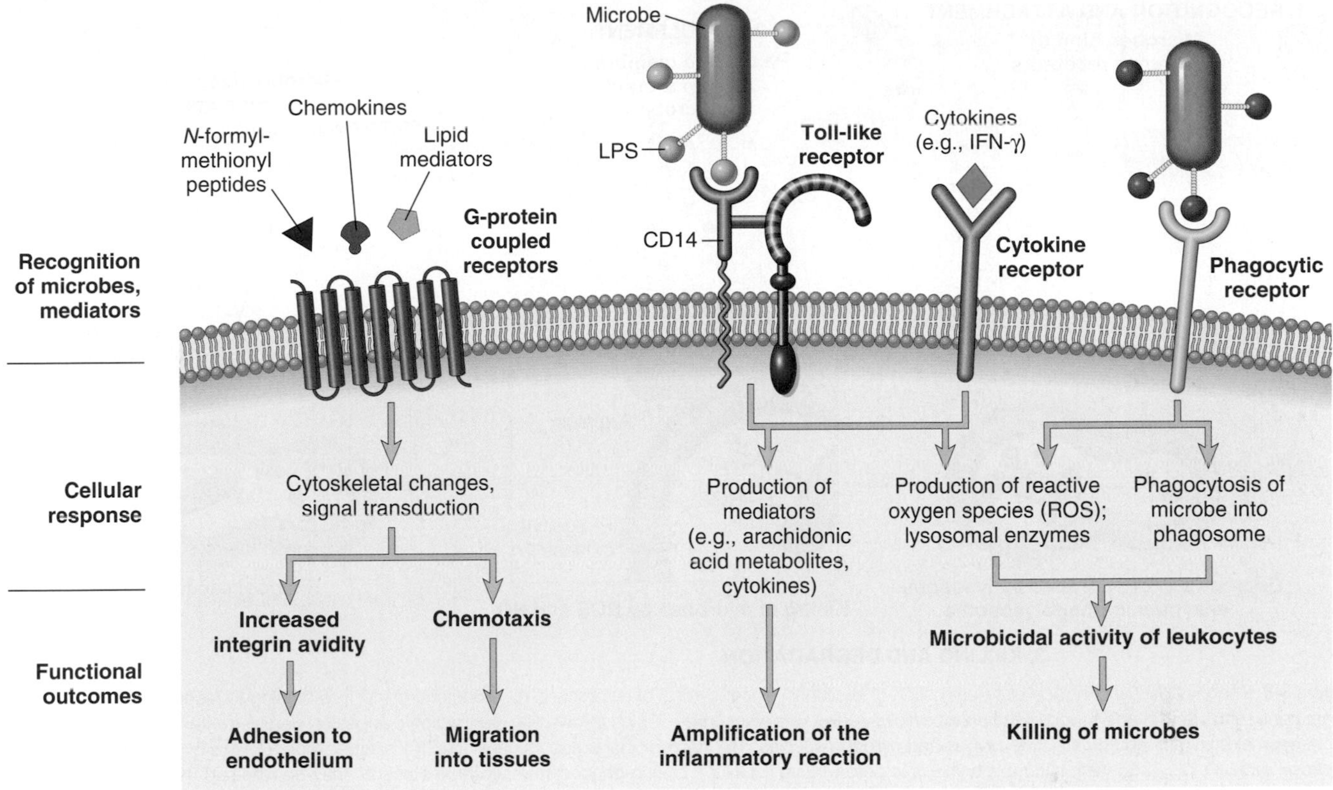

Figure 3-7 Leukocyte activation. Different classes of cell surface receptors of leukocytes recognize different stimuli. The receptors initiate responses that mediate the functions of the leukocytes. Only some receptors are depicted (see text for details). LPS first binds to a circulating LPS-binding protein (not shown). IFN-γ, Interferon-γ; LPS, lipopolysaccharide.

The process of phagocytosis is complex and involves the integration of many receptor-initiated signals that lead to membrane remodeling and cytoskeletal changes. Phagocytosis is dependent on polymerization of actin filaments; it is, therefore, not surprising that the signals that trigger phagocytosis are many of the same that are involved in chemotaxis.

Intracellular Destruction of Microbes and Debris

Killing of microbes is accomplished by reactive oxygen species (ROS, also called *reactive oxygen intermediates*) and reactive nitrogen species, mainly derived from nitric oxide (NO), and these as well as lysosomal enzymes destroy phagocytosed debris (Fig. 3-8). This is the final step in the elimination of infectious agents and necrotic cells. The killing and degradation of microbes and dead cell debris within neutrophils and macrophages occur most efficiently after activation of the phagocytes. All these killing mechanisms are normally sequestered in lysosomes, to which phagocytosed materials are brought. Thus, potentially harmful substances are segregated from the cell's cytoplasm and nucleus to avoid damage to the phagocyte while it is performing its normal function.

Reactive Oxygen Species. ROS are produced by the rapid assembly and activation of a multicomponent oxidase, NADPH oxidase (also called phagocyte oxidase), which oxidizes NADPH (reduced nicotinamide-adenine dinucleotide phosphate) and, in the process, reduces oxygen to superoxide anion ($O_2^{\bullet}$). In neutrophils, this oxidative reaction is triggered by activating signals and accompanies phagocytosis, and is called the *respiratory burst*. Phagocyte oxidase is an enzyme complex consisting of at least seven proteins. In resting neutrophils, different components of the enzyme are located in the plasma membrane and the cytoplasm. In response to activating stimuli, the cytosolic protein components translocate to the phagosomal membrane, where they assemble and form the functional enzyme complex. Thus, the *ROS are produced within the lysosome and phagolysosome*, where they can act on ingested particles without damaging the host cell. $O_2^{\bullet}$ is then converted into hydrogen peroxide (H_2O_2), mostly by spontaneous dismutation. H_2O_2 is not able to efficiently kill microbes by itself. However, the azurophilic granules of neutrophils contain the enzyme *myeloperoxidase* (MPO), which, in the presence of a halide such as Cl^-, converts H_2O_2 to hypochlorite (OCl_2^-, the active ingredient in household bleach). The latter is a potent antimicrobial agent that destroys microbes by *halogenation* (in which the halide is bound covalently to cellular constituents) or by *oxidation* of proteins and lipids (lipid peroxidation). The H_2O_2-MPO-halide system is the most efficient bactericidal system of neutrophils. Nevertheless, inherited deficiency of MPO by itself leads to minimal increase in susceptibility to infection, emphasizing the redundancy of microbicidal mechanisms in leukocytes. H_2O_2 is also converted to hydroxyl radical (^{-}OH), another powerful destructive agent. As discussed in Chapter 2, these oxygen-derived free radicals bind to and modify cellular lipids, proteins, and nucleic acids, and thus destroy cells such as microbes.

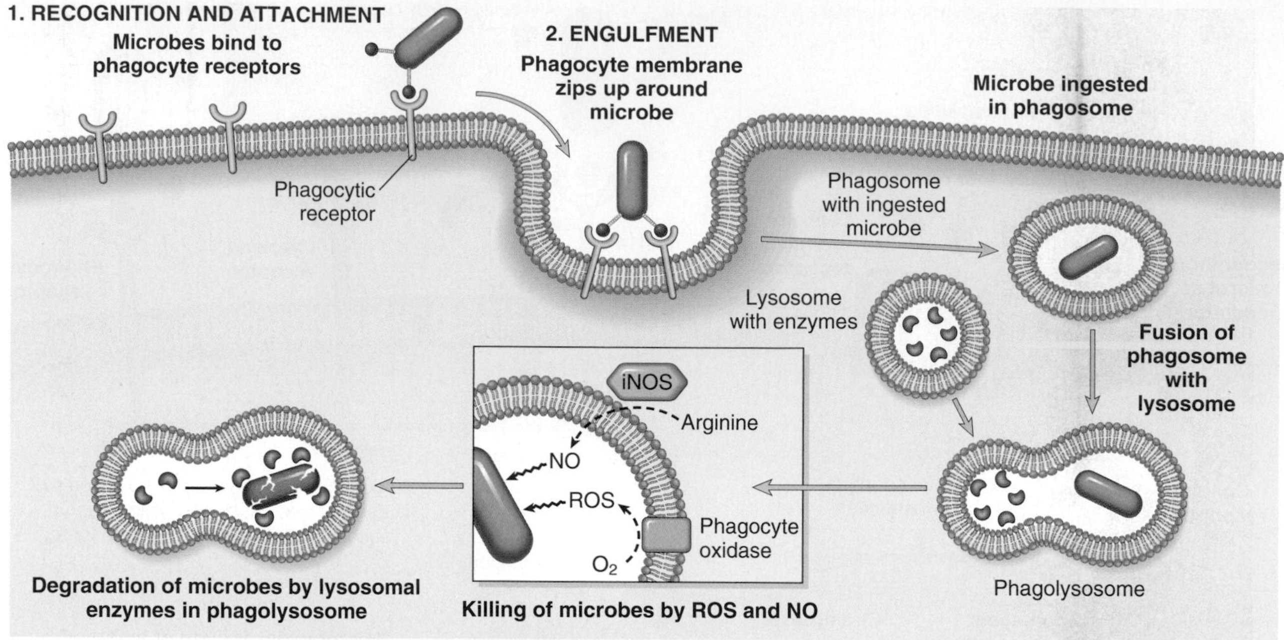

Figure 3-8 Phagocytosis and intracellular destruction of microbes. Phagocytosis of a particle (e.g., a bacterium) involves binding to receptors on the leukocyte membrane, engulfment, and fusion of the phagocytic vacuoles with lysosomes. This is followed by destruction of ingested particles within the phagolysosomes by lysosomal enzymes and by reactive oxygen and nitrogen species. The microbicidal products generated from superoxide (O_2^-) are hypochlorite ($HOCl^-$) and hydroxyl radical (^-OH), and from nitric oxide (NO) it is peroxynitrite ($OONO^-$). During phagocytosis, granule contents may be released into extracellular tissues (not shown). MPO, Myeloperoxidase; iNOS, inducible NO synthase; ROS, reactive oxygen species.

Oxygen-derived radicals may be released extracellularly from leukocytes after exposure to microbes, chemokines, and antigen-antibody complexes, or following a phagocytic challenge. These ROS are implicated in tissue damage accompanying inflammation.

Serum, tissue fluids, and host cells possess *antioxidant mechanisms* that protect against these potentially harmful oxygen-derived radicals. These antioxidants are discussed in Chapter 2; they include (1) the enzyme *superoxide dismutase*, which is found in or can be activated in a variety of cell types; (2) the enzyme *catalase*, which detoxifies H_2O_2; (3) *glutathione peroxidase*, another powerful H_2O_2 detoxifier; (4) the copper-containing serum protein *ceruloplasmin*; and (5) the iron-free fraction of serum *transferrin*. Thus, the influence of oxygen-derived free radicals in any given inflammatory reaction depends on the balance between production and inactivation of these metabolites by cells and tissues.

Nitric Oxide. NO, a soluble gas produced from arginine by the action of nitric oxide synthase (NOS), also participates in microbial killing. There are three different types of NOS: endothelial (eNOS), neuronal (nNOS), and inducible (iNOS). eNOS and nNOS are constitutively expressed at low levels and the NO they generate functions to maintain vascular tone and as a neurotransmitter, respectively. iNOS, the type that is involved in microbial killing, is induced when macrophages and neutrophils are activated by cytokines (e.g., IFN-γ) or microbial products. In macrophages, NO reacts with superoxide ($O_2^{\bullet}$) to generate the highly reactive free radical peroxynitrite ($ONOO^-$). These nitrogen-derived free radicals, similar to ROS, attack and damage the lipids, proteins, and nucleic acids of microbes and host cells (Chapter 2). Reactive oxygen and nitrogen species have overlapping actions, as shown by the observation that knockout mice lacking either phagocyte oxidase or iNOS are only mildly susceptible to infections but mice lacking both succumb rapidly to disseminated infections by normally harmless commensal bacteria.

In addition to its role as a microbicidal substance, NO relaxes vascular smooth muscle and promotes vasodilation. It is not clear if this action of NO plays an important role in the vascular reactions of acute inflammation.

Lysosomal Enzymes and Other Lysosomal Proteins. Neutrophils and monocytes contain lysosomal granules that contribute to microbial killing and, when released, may contribute to tissue damage. Neutrophils have two main types of granules. The smaller *specific* (or secondary) granules contain lysozyme, collagenase, gelatinase, lactoferrin, plasminogen activator, histaminase, and alkaline phosphatase. The larger *azurophil* (or primary) granules contain myeloperoxidase, bactericidal factors (lysozyme, defensins), acid hydrolases, and a variety of neutral proteases (elastase, cathepsin G, nonspecific collagenases, proteinase 3). Both types of granules can fuse with phagocytic vacuoles containing engulfed material, or the granule contents can be released into the extracellular space.

Different granule enzymes serve different functions. *Acid proteases* degrade bacteria and debris within the phagolysosomes, which are acidified by membrane-bound proton pumps. *Neutral proteases* are capable of degrading various extracellular components, such as collagen, basement membrane, fibrin, elastin, and cartilage, resulting in the tissue destruction that accompanies inflammatory processes. Neutral proteases can also cleave C3 and C5

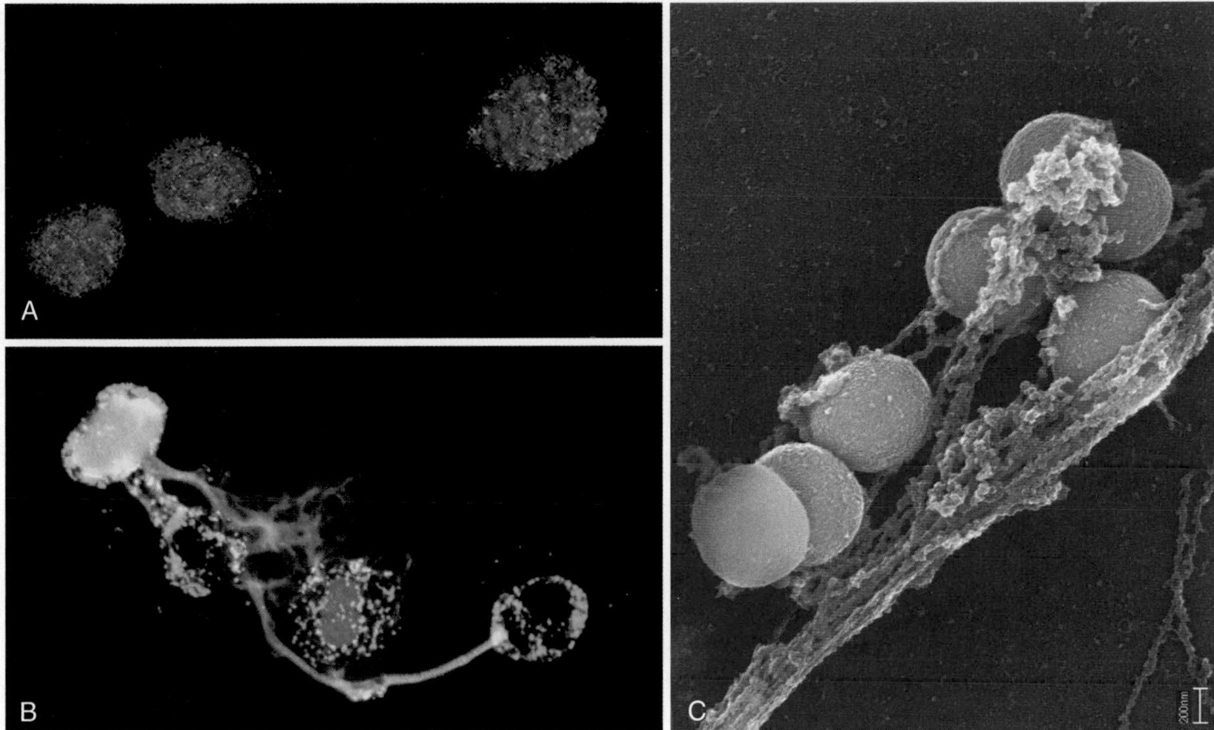

Figure 3-9 Neutrophil extracellular traps (NETs). **A,** Healthy neutrophils with nuclei stained red and cytoplasm green. **B,** Release of nuclear material from neutrophils (note that two have lost their nuclei), forming extracellular traps. **C,** An electron micrograph of bacteria (staphylococci) trapped in NETs. (From Brinkmann V, Zychlinsky A. Beneficial suicide: why neutrophils die to make NETs. Nat Rev Microbiol 2007;5:577, with permission.)

complement proteins directly, yielding anaphylatoxins, and release a kinin-like peptide from kininogen. Neutrophil elastase has been shown to degrade virulence factors of bacteria and thus combat bacterial infections. Macrophages also contain acid hydrolases, collagenase, elastase, phospholipase, and plasminogen activator.

Because of the destructive effects of lysosomal enzymes, the initial leukocytic infiltration, if unchecked, can potentiate further inflammation by damaging tissues. These harmful proteases, however, are normally controlled by a system of *antiproteases* in the serum and tissue fluids. Foremost among these is α_1-antitrypsin, which is the major inhibitor of neutrophil elastase. A deficiency of these inhibitors may lead to sustained action of leukocyte proteases, as is the case in patients with α_1-antitrypsin deficiency (Chapter 15). α_2-Macroglobulin is another antiprotease found in serum and various secretions.

Other microbicidal granule contents include *defensins*, cationic arginine-rich granule peptides that are toxic to microbes; *cathelicidins*, antimicrobial proteins found in neutrophils and other cells; *lysozyme*, which hydrolyzes the muramic acid-*N*-acetylglucosamine bond, found in the glycopeptide coat of all bacteria; *lactoferrin*, an iron-binding protein present in specific granules; and *major basic protein*, a cationic protein of eosinophils, which has limited bactericidal activity but is cytotoxic to many parasites.

Neutrophil Extracellular Traps

Neutrophil extracellular traps (NETs) are extracellular fibrillar networks that provide a high concentration of antimicrobial substances at sites of infection and prevent the spread of the microbes by trapping them in the fibrils. They are produced by neutrophils in response to infectious pathogens (mainly bacteria and fungi) and inflammatory mediators (e.g., chemokines, cytokines [mainly interferons], complement proteins, and ROS). The extracellular traps consist of a viscous meshwork of of nuclear chromatin that binds and concentrates granule proteins such as antimicrobial peptides and enzymes (Fig. 3-9). In the process of NET formation, the nuclei of the neutrophils are lost, leading to death of the cells. NETs have also been detected in the blood during sepsis, and it is believed that their formation in the circulation is dependent on platelet activation. The nuclear chromatin in the NETs, which includes histones and associated DNA, has been postulated to be a source of nuclear antigens in systemic autoimmune diseases, particularly lupus, in which individuals react against their own DNA and nucleoproteins (Chapter 6).

Leukocyte-Mediated Tissue Injury

Leukocytes are important causes of injury to normal cells and tissues under several circumstances:

- As part of a normal defense reaction against infectious microbes, when adjacent tissues suffer collateral damage. In some infections that are difficult to eradicate, such as tuberculosis and certain viral diseases, the prolonged host response contributes more to the pathology than does the microbe itself.
- When the inflammatory response is inappropriately directed against host tissues, as in certain autoimmune diseases.
- When the host reacts excessively against usually harmless environmental substances, as in allergic diseases, including asthma.

In all these situations, **the mechanisms by which leukocytes damage normal tissues are the same as the mechanisms involved in antimicrobial defense**, because once the leukocytes are activated, their effector mechanisms do not distinguish between offender and host. During activation and phagocytosis, neutrophils and macrophages produce microbicidal substances (ROS, NO, and lysosomal enzymes) within the phagolysosome; these substances are also released into the extracellular space. These released substances are capable of damaging normal cells and vascular endothelium, and may thus amplify the effects of the initial injurious agent. If unchecked or inappropriately directed against host tissues, the leukocyte infiltrate itself becomes the offender, and indeed leukocyte-dependent tissue injury underlies many acute and chronic human diseases (Table 3-1). This fact becomes evident in the discussion of specific disorders throughout the book.

The contents of lysosomal granules are secreted by leukocytes into the extracellular milieu by several mechanisms. Controlled secretion of granule contents is a normal response of activated leukocytes. If phagocytes encounter materials that cannot be easily ingested, such as immune complexes deposited on immovable flat surfaces (e.g., glomerular basement membrane), the inability of the leukocytes to surround and ingest these substances *(frustrated phagocytosis)* triggers strong activation, and the release of large amounts of lysosomal enzymes into the extracellular environment. Some phagocytosed substances, such as urate crystals, may damage the membrane of the phagolysosome and also lead to the release of lysosomal granule contents.

Other Functional Responses of Activated Leukocytes

In addition to eliminating microbes and dead cells, activated leukocytes play several other roles in host defense. Importantly, these cells, especially macrophages, produce cytokines that can either amplify or limit inflammatory reactions, growth factors that stimulate the proliferation of endothelial cells and fibroblasts and the synthesis of collagen, and enzymes that remodel connective tissues. Because of these activities, macrophages are also critical cells of chronic inflammation and tissue repair, after the inflammation has subsided. These functions of macrophages are discussed later in the chapter.

In this discussion of acute inflammation, we emphasize the importance of neutrophils and macrophages. However, it has recently become clear that some T lymphocytes, which are cells of adaptive immunity, also contribute to acute inflammation. The most important of these cells are those that produce the cytokine IL-17 (so-called T_H17 cells), which are discussed in more detail in Chapter 6. IL-17 induces the secretion of chemokines that recruit other leukocytes. In the absence of effective T_H17 responses, individuals are susceptible to fungal and bacterial infections, and the skin abscesses that develop are "cold abscesses," lacking the classic features of acute inflammation, such as warmth and redness.

Termination of the Acute Inflammatory Response

Such a powerful system of host defense, with its inherent capacity to cause tissue injury, needs tight controls to minimize damage. In part, inflammation declines after the offending agents are removed simply because the mediators of inflammation are produced in rapid bursts, only as long as the stimulus persists, have short half-lives, and are degraded after their release. Neutrophils also have short half-lives in tissues and die by apoptosis within a few hours after leaving the blood. In addition, as inflammation develops, the process itself triggers a variety of stop signals that actively terminate the reaction. These active termination mechanisms include a switch in the type of arachidonic acid metabolite produced, from proinflammatory leukotrienes to antiinflammatory lipoxins (described later), and the liberation of antiinflammatory cytokines, including transforming growth factor-β (TGF-β) and IL-10, from macrophages and other cells. Other control mechanisms that have been demonstrated experimentally include neural impulses (cholinergic discharge) that inhibit the production of TNF in macrophages.

> **KEY CONCEPTS**
>
> **Leukocyte Activation and Removal of Offending Agents**
>
> - Leukocytes can eliminate microbes and dead cells by phagocytosis, followed by their destruction in phagolysosomes.
> - Destruction is caused by free radicals (ROS, NO) generated in activated leukocytes and lysosomal enzymes.
> - Neutrophils can extrude their nuclear contents to form extracellular nets that trap and destroy microbes.
> - Enzymes and ROS may be released into the extracellular environment.
> - The mechanisms that function to eliminate microbes and dead cells (the physiologic role of inflammation) are also capable of damaging normal tissues (the pathologic consequences of inflammation).
> - Antiinflammatory mediators terminate the acute inflammatory reaction when it is no longer needed.

Mediators of Inflammation

The mediators of inflammation are the substances that initiate and regulate inflammatory reactions. Many mediators have been identified and targeted therapeutically to limit inflammation. In this discussion, we review their shared properties and the general principles of their production and actions.

- **The most important mediators of acute inflammation are vasoactive amines, lipid products (prostaglandins and leukotrienes), cytokines (including chemokines), and products of complement activation** (Table 3-4). These mediators induce various components of the inflammatory response typically by distinct mechanisms, which is why inhibiting each has been therapeutically beneficial. However, there is also some overlap (redundancy) in the actions of the mediators.
- **Mediators are either secreted by cells or generated from plasma proteins.** *Cell-derived mediators* are normally sequestered in intracellular granules and can be rapidly secreted by granule exocytosis (e.g., histamine in mast cell granules) or are synthesized de novo (e.g., prostaglandins and leukotrienes, cytokines) in response

Table 3-4 Principal Mediators of Inflammation

Mediator	Source	Action
Histamine	Mast cells, basophils, platelets	Vasodilation, increased vascular permeability, endothelial activation
Prostaglandins	Mast cells, leukocytes	Vasodilation, pain, fever
Leukotrienes	Mast cells, leukocytes	Increased vascular permeability, chemotaxis, leukocyte adhesion, and activation
Cytokines (TNF, IL-1, IL-6)	Macrophages, endothelial cells, mast cells	Local: endothelial activation (expression of adhesion molecules). Systemic: fever, metabolic abnormalities, hypotension (shock)
Chemokines	Leukocytes, activated macrophages	Chemotaxis, leukocyte activation
Platelet-activating factor	Leukocytes, mast cells	Vasodilation, increased vascular permeability, leukocyte adhesion, chemotaxis, degranulation, oxidative burst
Complement	Plasma (produced in liver)	Leukocyte chemotaxis and activation, direct target killing (membrane attack complex), vasodilation (mast cell stimulation)
Kinins	Plasma (produced in liver)	Increased vascular permeability, smooth muscle contraction, vasodilation, pain

to a stimulus. **The major cell types that produce mediators of acute inflammation are the sentinels that detect invaders and damage in tissues, that is, macrophages, dendritic cells, and mast cells,** but platelets, neutrophils, endothelial cells, and most epithelia can also be induced to elaborate some of the mediators. *Plasma-derived mediators* (e.g., complement proteins) are produced mainly in the liver and are present in the circulation as inactive precursors that must be activated, usually by a series of proteolytic cleavages, to acquire their biologic properties.

- **Active mediators are produced only in response to various stimuli.** These stimuli include microbial products and substances released from necrotic cells. Some of the stimuli trigger well-defined receptors and signaling pathways, described earlier, but we still do not know how other stimuli induce the secretion of mediators (e.g., from mast cells in response to cell injury or mechanical irritation). The usual requirement for microbes or dead tissues as the initiating stimulus ensures that inflammation is normally triggered only when and where it is needed.
- **Most of the mediators are short-lived.** They quickly decay, or are inactivated by enzymes, or they are otherwise scavenged or inhibited. There is thus a system of checks and balances that regulates mediator actions. These built-in control mechanisms are discussed with each class of mediator.
- **One mediator can stimulate the release of other mediators.** For instance, products of complement activation stimulate the release of histamine, and the cytokine TNF acts on endothelial cells to stimulate the production of another cytokine, IL-1, and many chemokines. The secondary mediators may have the same actions as the initial mediators but may also have different and even opposing activities. Such cascades provide mechanisms for amplifying—or, in certain instances, counteracting—the initial action of a mediator.

We next discuss the more important mediators of acute inflammation, focusing on their mechanisms of action and roles in acute inflammation.

Vasoactive Amines: Histamine and Serotonin

The two major vasoactive amines, so named because they have important actions on blood vessels, are *histamine* and *serotonin*. They are stored as preformed molecules in cells and are therefore among the first mediators to be released during inflammation. The richest sources of histamine are the mast cells that are normally present in the connective tissue adjacent to blood vessels. It is also found in blood basophils and platelets. Histamine is stored in mast cell granules and is released by mast cell degranulation in response to a variety of stimuli, including (1) physical injury, such as trauma, cold, or heat, by unknown mechanisms; (2) binding of antibodies to mast cells, which underlies immediate hypersensitivity (allergic) reactions (Chapter 6); and (3) products of complement called *anaphylatoxins* (C3a and C5a), described later. Antibodies and complement products bind to specific receptors on mast cells and trigger signaling pathways that induce rapid degranulation. In addition, leukocytes are thought to secrete some histamine-releasing proteins but these have not been characterized. Neuropeptides (e.g., substance P) and cytokines (IL-1, IL-8) may also trigger release of histamine.

Histamine causes dilation of arterioles and increases the permeability of venules. Histamine is considered to be the principal mediator of the immediate transient phase of increased vascular permeability, producing interendothelial gaps in venules, as discussed earlier. Its vasoactive effects are mediated mainly via binding to receptors, called H_1 receptors, on microvascular endothelial cells. The antihistamine drugs that are commonly used to treat some inflammatory reactions, such as allergies, are H_1 receptor antagonists that bind to and block the receptor. Histamine also causes contraction of some smooth muscles.

Serotonin (5-hydroxytryptamine) is a preformed vasoactive mediator present in platelets and certain neuroendocrine cells, such as in the gastrointestinal tract, and in mast cells in rodents but not humans. Its primary function is as a neurotransmitter in the gastrointestinal tract. It is also a vasoconstrictor, but the importance of this action in inflammation is unclear.

Arachidonic Acid Metabolites

The lipid mediators *prostaglandins* and *leukotrienes* are produced from arachidonic acid (AA) present in membrane phospholipids, and stimulate vascular and cellular reactions in acute inflammation. AA is a 20-carbon polyunsaturated fatty acid (5,8,11,14-eicosatetraenoic acid) that is derived from dietary sources or by conversion from the

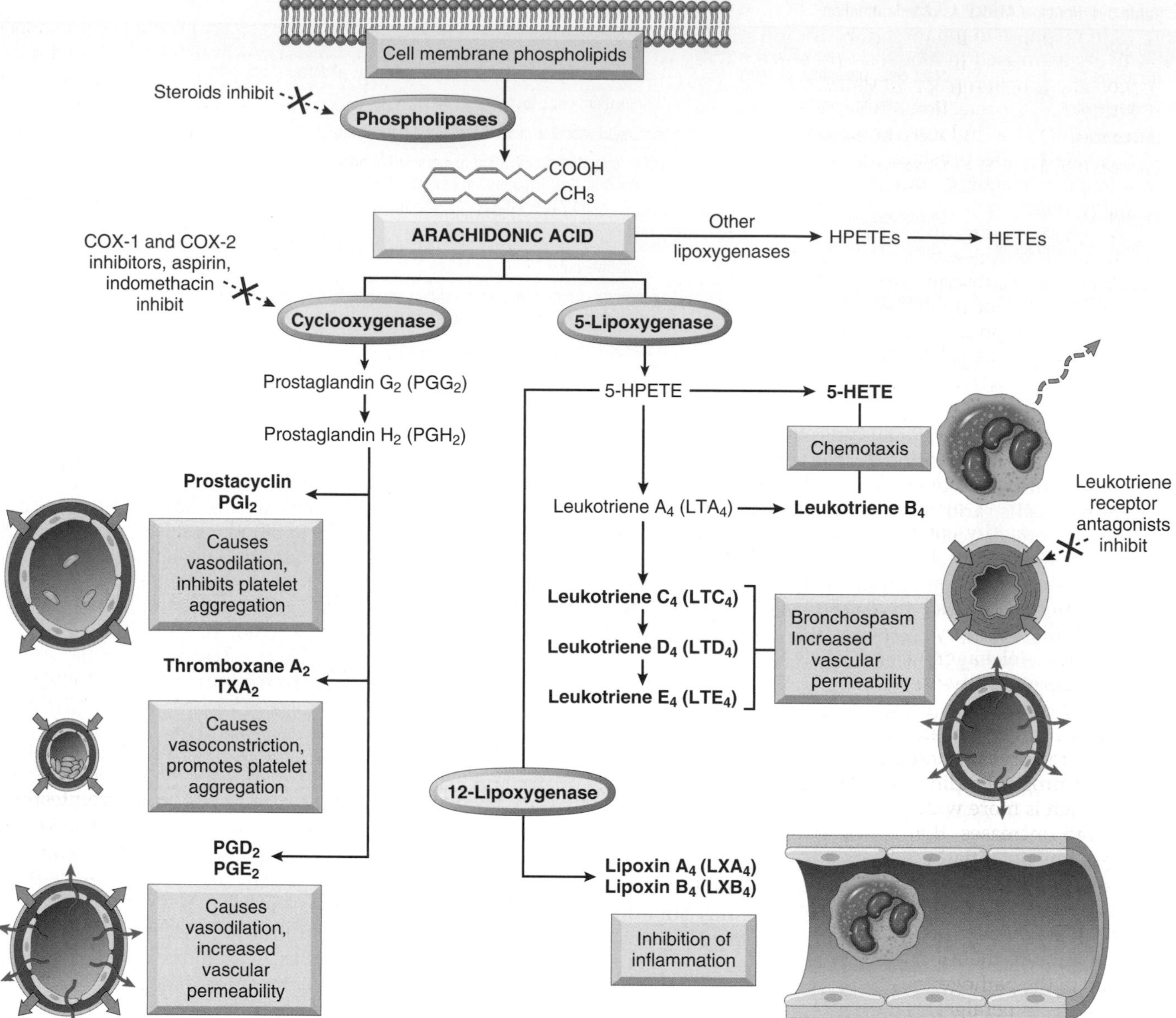

Figure 3-10 Production of arachidonic acid metabolites and their roles in inflammation. Note the enzymatic activities whose inhibition through pharmacologic intervention blocks major pathways (denoted with a red X). COX-1, COX-2, Cyclooxygenase 1 and 2; HETE, hydroxyeicosatetraenoic acid; HPETE, hydroperoxyeicosatetraenoic acid.

essential fatty acid linoleic acid. It does not occur free in the cell but is normally esterified in membrane phospholipids. Mechanical, chemical, and physical stimuli or other mediators (e.g., C5a) release AA from membrane phospholipids through the action of cellular phospholipases, mainly phospholipase A_2. The biochemical signals involved in the activation of phospholipase A_2 include an increase in cytoplasmic Ca^{2+} and activation of various kinases in response to external stimuli. AA-derived mediators, also called *eicosanoids* (because they are derived from 20-carbon fatty acids; Greek *eicosa* = 20), are synthesized by two major classes of enzymes: cyclooxygenases (which generate prostaglandins) and lipoxygenases (which produce leukotrienes and lipoxins) (Fig. 3-10). Eicosanoids bind to G protein-coupled receptors on many cell types and can mediate virtually every step of inflammation (Table 3-5).

Prostaglandins

Prostaglandins **(PGs) are produced by mast cells, macrophages, endothelial cells, and many other cell types, and are involved in the vascular and systemic reactions of inflammation.** They are generated by the actions of two

Table 3-5 Principal Actions of Arachidonic Acid Metabolites in Inflammation

Action	Eicosanoid
Vasodilation	Prostaglandins PGI_2 (prostacyclin), PGE_1, PGE_2, PGD_2
Vasoconstriction	Thromboxane A_2, leukotrienes C_4, D_4, E_4
Increased vascular permeability	Leukotrienes C_4, D_4, E_4
Chemotaxis, leukocyte adhesion	Leukotrienes B_4, HETE

HETE, Hydroxyeicosatetraenoic acid.

cyclooxgenases, called COX-1 and COX-2. COX-1 is produced in response to inflammatory stimuli and is also constitutively expressed in most tissues, where it may serve a homeostatic function (e.g., fluid and electrolyte balance in the kidneys, cytoprotection in the gastrointestinal tract). In contrast, COX-2 is induced by inflammatory stimuli and thus generates the prostaglandins that are involved in inflammatory reactions, but it is low or absent in most normal tissues.

Prostaglandins are divided into series based on structural features as coded by a letter (PGD, PGE, PGF, PGG, and PGH) and a subscript numeral (e.g., 1, 2), which indicates the number of double bonds in the compound. The most important ones in inflammation are PGE_2, PGD_2, PGF_{2a}, PGI_2 (prostacyclin), and TxA_2 (thromboxane A2), each of which is derived by the action of a specific enzyme on an intermediate in the pathway. Some of these enzymes have restricted tissue distribution. For example, platelets contain the enzyme thromboxane synthase, and hence TxA_2 is the major product in these cells. TxA_2, a potent platelet-aggregating agent and vasoconstrictor, is itself unstable and rapidly converted to its inactive form TxB_2. Vascular endothelium lacks thromboxane synthase but possesses prostacyclin synthase, which is responsible for the formation of prostacyclin (PGI_2) and its stable end product PGF_{1a}. Prostacyclin is a vasodilator and a potent inhibitor of platelet aggregation, and also markedly potentiates the permeability-increasing and chemotactic effects of other mediators. A thromboxane-prostacyclin imbalance has been implicated as an early event in thrombus formation in coronary and cerebral blood vessels. PGD_2 is the major prostaglandin made by mast cells; along with PGE_2 (which is more widely distributed), it causes vasodilation and increases the permeability of postcapillary venules, thus potentiating edema formation. PGF_{2a} stimulates the contraction of uterine and bronchial smooth muscle and small arterioles, and PGD_2 is a chemoattractant for neutrophils.

In addition to their local effects, the prostaglandins are involved in the pathogenesis of *pain* and *fever* in inflammation. PGE_2 is hyperalgesic and makes the skin hypersensitive to painful stimuli, such as intradermal injection of suboptimal concentrations of histamine and bradykinin. It is involved in cytokine-induced fever during infections (described later).

Leukotrienes

***Leukotrienes* are produced by leukocytes and mast cells by the action of lipoxygenase and are involved in vascular and smooth muscle reactions and leukocyte recruitment.** There are three different lipoxygenases, 5-lipoxygenase being the predominant one in neutrophils. This enzyme converts AA to 5-hydroxyeicosatetraenoic acid, which is chemotactic for neutrophils, and is the precursor of the leukotrienes. LTB_4 is a potent chemotactic agent and activator of neutrophils, causing aggregation and adhesion of the cells to venular endothelium, generation of ROS, and release of lysosomal enzymes. The cysteinyl-containing leukotrienes LTC_4, LTD_4, and LTE_4 cause intense vasoconstriction, bronchospasm (important in asthma), and increased permeability of venules. Leukotrienes are more potent than is histamine in increasing vascular permeability and causing bronchospasm.

Lipoxins

***Lipoxins* are also generated from AA by the lipoxygenase pathway, but unlike prostaglandins and leukotrienes, the lipoxins suppress inflammation by inhibiting the recruitment of leukocytes.** They inhibit neutrophil chemotaxis and adhesion to endothelium. They are also unusual in that two cell populations are required for the transcellular biosynthesis of these mediators. Leukocytes, particularly neutrophils, produce intermediates in lipoxin synthesis, and these are converted to lipoxins by platelets interacting with the leukocytes.

Pharmacologic Inhibitors of Prostaglandins and Leukotrienes

The importance of eicosanoids in inflammation has driven attempts to develop drugs that inhibit their production or actions and thus suppress inflammation. These anti-inflammatory drugs include the following.

- **Cyclooxygenase inhibitors** include aspirin and other nonsteroidal anti-inflammatory drugs (NSAIDs), such as ibuprofen. They inhibit both COX-1 and COX-2 and thus inhibit prostaglandin synthesis (hence their efficacy in treating pain and fever); aspirin does this by irreversibly acetylating and inactivating cyclooxygenases. Selective COX-2 inhibitors are a newer class of these drugs; they are 200-300 fold more potent in blocking COX-2 than COX-1. There has been great interest in COX-2 as a therapeutic target because of the possibility that COX-1 is responsible for the production of prostaglandins that are involved in both inflammation and homeostatic functions (e.g., fluid and electrolyte balance in the kidneys, cytoprotection in the gastrointestinal tract), whereas COX-2 generates prostaglandins that are involved only in inflammatory reactions. If this idea is correct, the selective COX-2 inhibitors should be anti-inflammatory without having the toxicities of the nonselective inhibitors, such as gastric ulceration. However, these distinctions are not absolute, as COX-2 also seems to play a role in normal homeostasis. Furthermore, selective COX-2 inhibitors may increase the risk of cardiovascular and cerebrovascular events, possibly because they impair endothelial cell production of prostacyclin (PGI_2), a vasodilator and inhibitor of platelet aggregation, but leave intact the COX-1-mediated production by platelets of thromboxane A_2 (TxA_2), an important mediator of platelet aggregation and vasoconstriction. Thus, selective COX-2 inhibition may tilt the balance towards thromboxane and promote vascular thrombosis, especially in individuals with other factors that increase the risk of thrombosis. Nevertheless, these drugs are still used in individuals who do not have risk factors for cardiovascular disease when their benefits outweigh their risks.
- **Lipoxygenase inhibitors.** 5-lipoxygenase is not affected by NSAIDs, and many new inhibitors of this enzyme pathway have been developed. Pharmacologic agents that inhibit leukotriene production (e.g., Zileuton) are useful in the treatment of asthma.
- **Corticosteroids** are broad-spectrum antiinflammatory agents that reduce the transcription of genes encoding COX-2, phospholipase A_2, proinflammatory cytokines (e.g., IL-1 and TNF), and iNOS.

- **Leukotriene receptor antagonists** block leukotriene receptors and prevent the actions of the leukotrienes. These drugs (e.g., Montelukast) are useful in the treatment of asthma.
- Another approach to manipulating inflammatory responses has been to modify the intake and content of dietary lipids by increasing the consumption of fish oil. The proposed explanation for the effectiveness of this approach is that the polyunsaturated fatty acids in fish oil are poor substrates for conversion to active metabolites by the cyclooxygenase and lipoxygenase pathways but are better substrates for the production of antiinflammatory lipid products.

Cytokines and Chemokines

***Cytokines* are proteins produced by many cell types (principally activated lymphocytes, macrophages, and dendritic cells, but also endothelial, epithelial, and connective tissue cells) that mediate and regulate immune and inflammatory reactions.** By convention, growth factors that act on epithelial and mesenchymal cells are not grouped under cytokines. The general properties and functions of cytokines are discussed in Chapter 6. Here the cytokines involved in acute inflammation are reviewed (Table 3-6).

Tumor Necrosis Factor (TNF) and Interleukin-1 (IL-1)

TNF and IL-1 serve critical roles in leukocyte recruitment by promoting adhesion of leukocytes to endothelium and their migration through vessels. These cytokines are produced mainly by activated macrophages and dendritic cells; TNF is also produced by T lymphocytes and mast cells, and IL-1 is produced by some epithelial cells as well. The secretion of TNF and IL-1 can be stimulated by microbial products, immune complexes, foreign bodies, physical injury, and a variety of other inflammatory stimuli. The production of TNF is induced by signals through TLRs and other microbial sensors, and the synthesis of IL-1 is stimulated by the same signals but the generation of the biologically active form of this cytokine is dependent on the inflammasome, described earlier.

The actions of TNF and IL-1 contribute to the local and systemic reactions of inflammation (Fig. 3-11). The most important roles of these cytokines in inflammation are the following.

- **Endothelial activation.** Both TNF and IL-1 act on endothelium to induce a spectrum of changes referred to as *endothelial activation*. These changes include increased expression of endothelial adhesion molecules, mostly E- and P-selectins and ligands for leukocyte integrins; increased production of various mediators, including other cytokines and chemokines, growth factors, and eicosanoids; and increased procoagulant activity of the endothelium.
- **Activation of leukocytes and other cells.** TNF augments responses of neutrophils to other stimuli such as bacterial endotoxin and stimulates the microbicidal activity of macrophages, in part by inducing production of NO. IL-1 activates fibroblasts to synthesize collagen and stimulates proliferation of synovial and other mesenchymal cells. IL-1 also stimulates T_H17 responses, which in turn induce acute inflammation.
- **Systemic acute-phase response.** IL-1 and TNF (as well as IL-6) induce the systemic acute-phase responses associated with infection or injury, including *fever* (described later in the chapter). They are also implicated in the syndrome of *sepsis,* resulting from disseminated bacterial infection. TNF regulates energy balance by promoting lipid and protein mobilization and by suppressing appetite. Therefore, sustained production of TNF contributes to *cachexia*, a pathologic state characterized by weight loss and anorexia that accompanies some chronic infections and neoplastic diseases.

TNF antagonists have been remarkably effective in the treatment of chronic inflammatory diseases, particularly rheumatoid arthritis and also psoriasis and some types of inflammatory bowel disease. One of the complications of this therapy is that patients become susceptible to mycobacterial infection, reflecting the reduced ability of macrophages to kill intracellular microbes. Although many of the actions of TNF and IL-1 seem overlapping, IL-1 antagonists are not as effective, for reasons that remain

Table 3-6 Cytokines in Inflammation

Cytokine	Principal Sources	Principal Actions in Inflammation
In Acute Inflammation		
TNF	Macrophages, mast cells, T lymphocytes	Stimulates expression of endothelial adhesion molecules and secretion of other cytokines; systemic effects
IL-1	Macrophages, endothelial cells, some epithelial cells	Similar to TNF; greater role in fever
IL-6	Macrophages, other cells	Systemic effects (acute phase response)
Chemokines	Macrophages, endothelial cells, T lymphocytes, mast cells, other cell types	Recruitment of leukocytes to sites of inflammation; migration of cells in normal tissues
IL-17	T lymphocytes	Recruitment of neutrophils and monocytes
In Chronic Inflammation		
IL-12	Dendritic cells, macrophages	Increased production of IFN-γ
IFN-γ	T lymphocytes, NK cells	Activation of macrophages (increased ability to kill microbes and tumor cells)
IL-17	T lymphocytes	Recruitment of neutrophils and monocytes

IFN-γ, Interferon-γ; IL-1, interleukin-1; NK cells, natural killer cells; TNF, tumor necrosis factor.
The most important cytokines involved in inflammatory reactions are listed. Many other cytokines may play lesser roles in inflammation. There is also considerable overlap between the cytokines involved in acute and chronic inflammation. Specifically, all the cytokines listed under acute inflammation may also contribute to chronic inflammatory reactions.

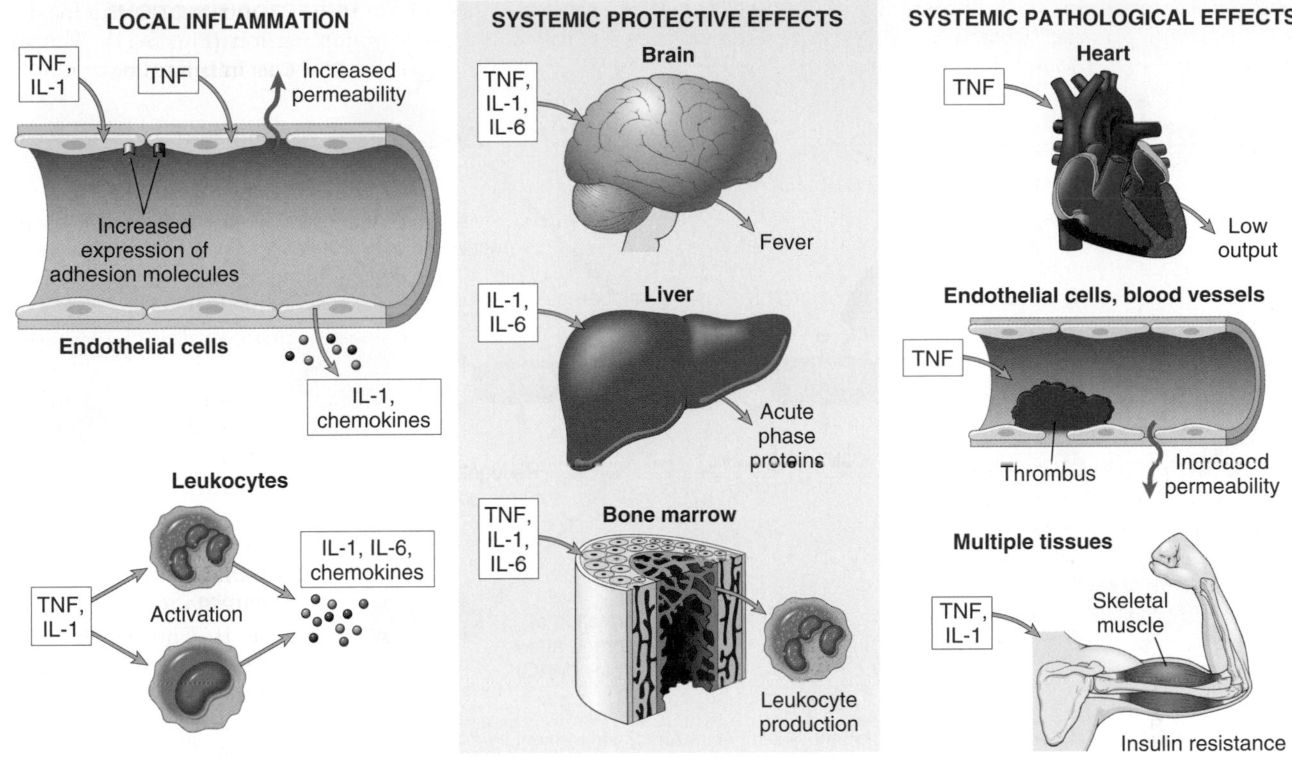

Figure 3-11 Major roles of cytokines in acute inflammation. PDGF, Platelet-derived growth factor; PGE, prostaglandin E; PGI, prostaglandin I.

obscure. Also, blocking either cytokine has no effect on the outcome of sepsis, perhaps because other cytokines contribute to this serious systemic inflammatory reaction.

Chemokines

Chemokines are a family of small (8 to 10 kD) proteins that act primarily as chemoattractants for specific types of leukocytes. About 40 different chemokines and 20 different receptors for chemokines have been identified. They are classified into four major groups, according to the arrangement of cysteine (C) residues in the proteins:

- *C-X-C chemokines* have one amino acid residue separating the first two of the four conserved cysteine residues. These chemokines act primarily on neutrophils. IL-8 is typical of this group. It is secreted by activated macrophages, endothelial cells, and other cell types, and causes activation and chemotaxis of neutrophils, with limited activity on monocytes and eosinophils. Its most important inducers are microbial products and other cytokines, mainly IL-1 and TNF.
- *C-C chemokines* have the first two conserved cysteine residues adjacent. The C-C chemokines, which include monocyte chemoattractant protein (MCP-1), eotaxin, macrophage inflammatory protein-1α (MIP-1α), and RANTES (regulated and normal T-cell expressed and secreted), generally attract monocytes, eosinophils, basophils and lymphocytes, but are not as potent chemoattractants for neutrophils. Although most of the chemokines in this class have overlapping actions, eotaxin selectively recruits eosinophils.
- *C chemokines* lack the first and third of the four conserved cysteines. The C chemokines (e.g., lymphotactin) are relatively specific for lymphocytes.
- *CX_3C chemokines* contain three amino acids between the two cysteines. The only known member of this class is called *fractalkine.* This chemokine exists in two forms: a cell surface-bound protein induced on endothelial cells by inflammatory cytokines that promotes strong adhesion of monocytes and T cells, and a soluble form, derived by proteolysis of the membrane-bound protein, that has potent chemoattractant activity for the same cells.

Chemokines mediate their activities by binding to seven-transmembrane G protein–coupled receptors. These receptors (called *CXCR* or *CCR*, for C-X-C or C-C chemokine receptors) usually exhibit overlapping ligand specificities, and leukocytes generally express more than one receptor type. As discussed in Chapter 6, certain chemokine receptors (CXCR-4, CCR-5) act as coreceptors for a viral envelope glycoprotein of human immunodeficiency virus (HIV), the cause of AIDS, and are thus involved in binding and entry of the virus into cells.

Chemokines may be displayed at high concentrations attached to proteoglycans on the surface of endothelial cells and in the extracellular matrix. They have two main functions:

- **In acute inflammation.** *Inflammatory chemokines* are the ones whose production is induced by microbes and other stimuli. These chemokines stimulate leukocyte attachment to endothelium by acting on leukocytes to increase the affinity of integrins, and they stimulate migration (chemotaxis) of leukocytes in tissues to the site of infection or tissue damage.
- **Maintenance of tissue architecture.** Some chemokines are produced constitutively in tissues and are sometimes called *homeostatic chemokines.* These organize

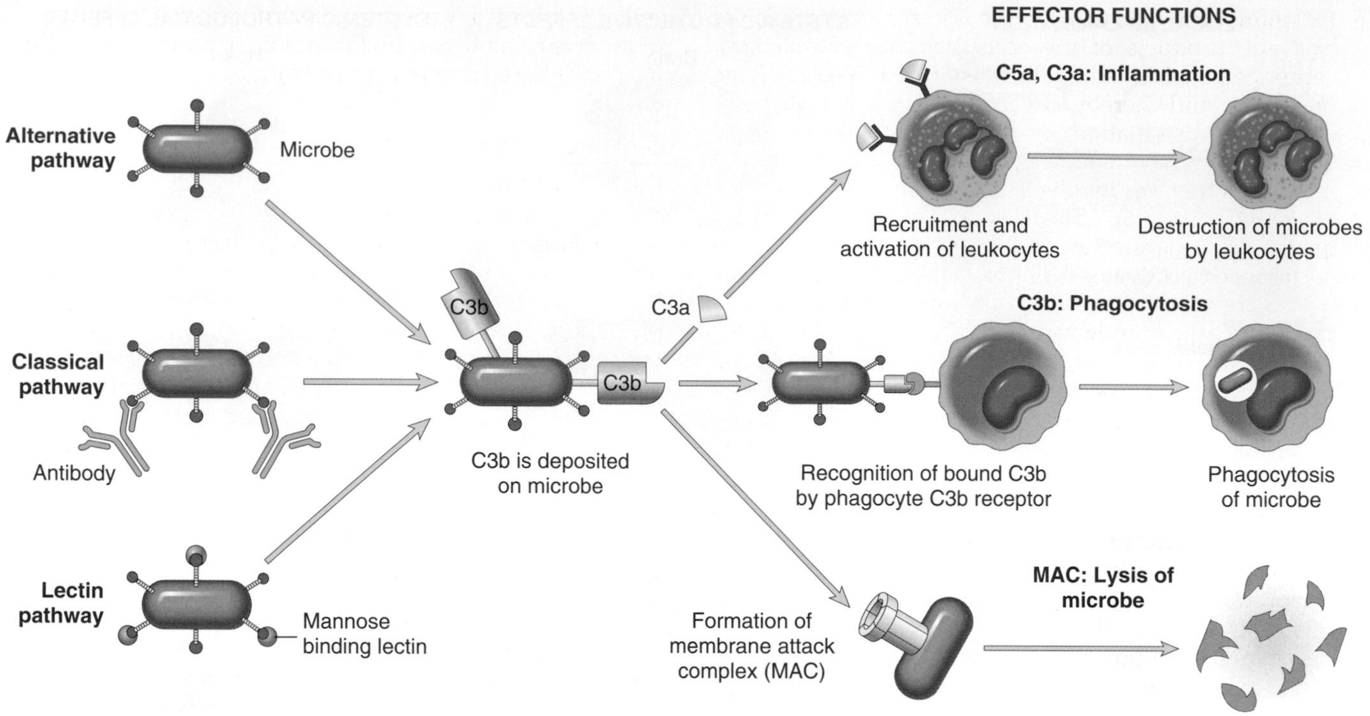

Figure 3-12 The activation and functions of the complement system. Activation of complement by different pathways leads to cleavage of C3. The functions of the complement system are mediated by breakdown products of C3 and other complement proteins, and by the membrane attack complex (MAC).

various cell types in different anatomic regions of the tissues, such as T and B lymphocytes in discrete areas of the spleen and lymph nodes (Chapter 6).

Although the role of chemokines in inflammation is well established, it has proved difficult to develop antagonists that block the activities of these proteins.

Other Cytokines in Acute Inflammation

The list of cytokines implicated in inflammation is huge and constantly growing. In addition to the ones described earlier, two that have received considerable recent interest are IL-6, made by macrophages and other cells, which is involved in local and systemic reactions, and IL-17, produced mainly by T lymphocytes, which promotes neutrophil recruitment. Antagonists against both are approved or have shown impressive efficacy in the treatment of inflammatory diseases. Type I interferons, whose normal function is to inhibit viral replication, contribute to some of the systemic manifestations of inflammation. Cytokines also play key roles in chronic inflammation; these are described later in the chapter.

Complement System

The complement system is a collection of soluble proteins and membrane receptors that function mainly in host defense against microbes and in pathologic inflammatory reactions. The system consists of more than 20 proteins, some of which are numbered C1 through C9. This system functions in both innate and adaptive immunity for defense against microbial pathogens. In the process of complement activation, several cleavage products of complement proteins are elaborated that cause increased vascular permeability, chemotaxis, and opsonization. The activation and functions of complement are outlined in Figure 3-12.

Complement proteins are present in inactive forms in the plasma, and many of them are activated to become proteolytic enzymes that degrade other complement proteins, thus forming an enzymatic cascade capable of tremendous amplification. The critical step in complement activation is the proteolysis of the third (and most abundant) component, C3. **Cleavage of C3 can occur by one of three pathways**:

- The *classical pathway*, which is triggered by fixation of C1 to antibody (IgM or IgG) that has combined with antigen
- The *alternative pathway*, which can be triggered by microbial surface molecules (e.g., endotoxin, or LPS), complex polysaccharides, cobra venom, and other substances, in the absence of antibody
- The *lectin pathway*, in which plasma mannose-binding lectin binds to carbohydrates on microbes and directly activates C1.

All three pathways of complement activation lead to the formation of an active enzyme called the *C3 convertase*, which splits C3 into two functionally distinct fragments, C3a and C3b. C3a is released, and C3b becomes covalently attached to the cell or molecule where complement is being activated. More C3b then binds to the previously generated fragments to form *C5 convertase*, which cleaves C5 to release C5a and leave C5b attached to the cell surface. C5b binds the late components (C6-C9), culminating in the formation of the membrane attack complex (MAC, composed of multiple C9 molecules).

The complement system has three main functions (Fig. 3-12):

- **Inflammation.** *C3a*, *C5a*, and, to a lesser extent, *C4a* are cleavage products of the corresponding complement components that stimulate histamine release from mast cells and thereby increase vascular permeability and cause vasodilation. They are called *anaphylatoxins* because they have effects similar to those of mast cell mediators that are involved in the reaction called *anaphylaxis* (Chapter 6). C5a is also a chemotactic agent for neutrophils, monocytes, eosinophils, and basophils. In addition, C5a activates the lipoxygenase pathway of AA metabolism in neutrophils and monocytes, causing further release of inflammatory mediators.
- **Opsonization and phagocytosis.** *C3b* and its cleavage product *iC3b* (inactive C3b), when fixed to a microbial cell wall, act as opsonins and promote phagocytosis by neutrophils and macrophages, which bear cell surface receptors for the complement fragments.
- **Cell lysis.** The deposition of the MAC on cells makes these cells permeable to water and ions and results in death (lysis) of the cells. This role of complement is important mainly for the killing of microbes with thin cell walls, such as *Neisseria* bacteria, and deficiency of the terminal components of complement predisposes to *Neisseria* infections.

The activation of complement is tightly controlled by cell-associated and circulating regulatory proteins. Different regulatory proteins inhibit the production of active complement fragments or remove fragments that deposit on cells. These regulators are expressed on normal host cells and are thus designed to prevent healthy tissues from being injured at sites of complement activation. Regulatory proteins can be overwhelmed when large amounts of complement are deposited on host cells and in tissues, as happens in autoimmune diseases, in which individuals produce complement-fixing antibodies against their own cell and tissue antigens (Chapter 6). The most important of these regulatory proteins are the following:

- **C1 inhibitor (C1 INH)** blocks the activation of C1, the first protein of the classical complement pathway. Inherited deficiency of this inhibitor is the cause of *hereditary angioedema*.
- **Decay accelerating factor (DAF)** and **CD59** are two proteins that are linked to plasma membranes by a glycophosphatidyl (GPI) anchor. DAF prevents formation of C3 convertases and CD59 inhibits formation of the membrane attack complex. An acquired deficiency of the enzyme that creates GPI anchors leads to deficiency of these regulators and excessive complement activation and lysis of red cells (which are sensitive to complement-mediated cell lysis) in the disease called *paroxysmal nocturnal hemoglobinuria (PNH)* (Chapter 14).
- Other complement regulatory proteins proteolytically cleave active complement components.

The complement system contributes to disease in several ways. The activation of complement by antibodies or antigen-antibody complexes deposited on host cells and tissues is an important mechanism of cell and tissue injury (Chapter 6). Inherited deficiencies of complement proteins cause increased susceptibility to infections (Chapter 6), and, as mentioned earlier, deficiencies of regulatory proteins cause a variety of disorders, such as macular degeneration and hemolytic uremic syndrome, resulting from excessive complement activation.

Other Mediators of Inflammation

Platelet-Activating Factor (PAF)

PAF is a phospholipid-derived mediator that was discovered as a factor that caused platelet aggregation, but it is now known to have multiple inflammatory effects. A variety of cell types, including platelets themselves, basophils, mast cells, neutrophils, macrophages, and endothelial cells, can elaborate PAF, in both secreted and cell-bound forms. In addition to platelet aggregation, PAF causes vasoconstriction and bronchoconstriction, and at low concentrations it induces vasodilation and increased venular permeability. In the 1990s there was great interest in PAF as a mediator of inflammation, but trials of PAF antagonists in various inflammatory diseases have been disappointing.

Products of Coagulation

Studies done more than 50 years ago suggested that inhibiting coagulation reduced the inflammatory reaction to some microbes, leading to the idea that coagulation and inflammation are linked processes. This concept was supported by the discovery of protease-activated receptors (PARs), which are activated by thrombin (the protease that cleaves fibrinogen to produce fibrin, which forms the clot), and are expressed on platelets and leukocytes. It is, however, likely that the major role of the PARs is in platelet activation during clotting (Chapter 4). In fact, it is difficult to dissociate clotting and inflammation, since virtually all forms of tissue injury that lead to clotting also induce inflammation, and inflammation causes changes in endothelial cells that increase the likelihood of abnormal clotting (thrombosis, described in Chapter 4). However, whether the products of coagulation, per se, have a key role in stimulating inflammation is still not established.

Kinins

Kinins are vasoactive peptides derived from plasma proteins, called *kininogens*, by the action of specific proteases called kallikreins. The enzyme kallikrein cleaves a plasma glycoprotein precursor, high-molecular-weight kininogen, to produce *bradykinin*. **Bradykinin increases vascular permeability and causes contraction of smooth muscle, dilation of blood vessels, and pain when injected into the skin.** These effects are similar to those of histamine. The action of bradykinin is short-lived, because it is quickly inactivated by an enzyme called kininase. Bradykinin has been implicated as a mediator in some forms of allergic reaction, such as anaphylaxis (Chapter 6).

Neuropeptides

Neuropeptides are secreted by sensory nerves and various leukocytes, and may play a role in the initiation and regulation of inflammatory responses. These small peptides, such as substance P and neurokinin A, are produced in the central and peripheral nervous systems. Nerve fibers containing substance P are prominent in the lung and gastrointestinal tract. Substance P has many biologic functions, including the transmission of pain signals, regulation of

Table 3-7 Role of Mediators in Different Reactions of Inflammation

Reaction of Inflammation	Principal Mediators
Vasodilation	Histamine Prostaglandins
Increased vascular permeability	Histamine and serotonin C3a and C5a (by liberating vasoactive amines from mast cells, other cells) Leukotrienes C_4, D_4, E_4
Chemotaxis, leukocyte recruitment and activation	TNF, IL-1 Chemokines C3a, C5a Leukotriene B_4
Fever	IL-1, TNF Prostaglandins
Pain	Prostaglandins Bradykinin
Tissue damage	Lysosomal enzymes of leukocytes Reactive oxygen species

blood pressure, stimulation of hormone secretion by endocrine cells, and increasing vascular permeability.

When Lewis discovered the role of histamine in inflammation, one mediator was thought to be enough. Now, we are wallowing in them! Yet, from this large compendium, it is likely that a few mediators are most important for the reactions of acute inflammation in vivo, and these are summarized in Table 3-7. The redundancy of the mediators and their actions ensures that this protective response remains robust and is not readily subverted.

KEY CONCEPTS

Actions of the Principal Mediators of Inflammation

- Vasoactive amines, mainly histamine: vasodilation and increased vascular permeability
- Arachidonic acid metabolites (prostaglandins and leukotrienes): several forms exist and are involved in vascular reactions, leukocyte chemotaxis, and other reactions of inflammation; antagonized by lipoxins
- Cytokines: proteins produced by many cell types; usually act at short range; mediate multiple effects, mainly in leukocyte recruitment and migration; principal ones in acute inflammation are TNF, IL-1, and chemokines
- Complement proteins: Activation of the complement system by microbes or antibodies leads to the generation of multiple breakdown products, which are responsible for leukocyte chemotaxis, opsonization, and phagocytosis of microbes and other particles, and cell killing
- Kinins: produced by proteolytic cleavage of precursors; mediate vascular reaction, pain

Morphologic Patterns of Acute Inflammation

The morphologic hallmarks of acute inflammatory reactions are dilation of small blood vessels and accumulation of leukocytes and fluid in the extravascular tissue. However, special morphologic patterns are often superimposed on these general features, depending on the severity of the reaction, its specific cause, and the particular tissue and site involved. The importance of recognizing the gross and microscopic patterns is that they often provide valuable clues about the underlying cause.

Serous Inflammation

Serous inflammation is marked by the exudation of cell-poor fluid into spaces created by cell injury or into body cavities lined by the peritoneum, pleura, or pericardium. Typically, the fluid in serous inflammation is not infected by destructive organisms and does not contain large numbers of leukocytes (which tend to produce purulent inflammation, described later). In body cavities the fluid may be derived from the plasma (as a result of increased vascular permeability) or from the secretions of mesothelial cells (as a result of local irritation); accumulation of fluid in these cavities is called an *effusion.* (Effusions also occur in noninflammatory conditions, such as reduced blood outflow in heart failure, or reduced plasma protein levels in some kidney and liver diseases.) The skin blister resulting from a burn or viral infection represents accumulation of serous fluid within or immediately beneath the damaged epidermis of the skin (Fig. 3-13).

Fibrinous Inflammation

With greater increase in vascular permeability, large molecules such as fibrinogen pass out of the blood, and fibrin is formed and deposited in the extracellular space. **A fibrinous exudate develops when the vascular leaks are large or there is a local procoagulant stimulus** (e.g., cancer cells). A fibrinous exudate is characteristic of inflammation in the lining of body cavities, such as the meninges, pericardium (Fig. 3-14*A*), and pleura. Histologically, fibrin appears as an eosinophilic meshwork of threads or sometimes as an amorphous coagulum (Fig. 3-14B). Fibrinous exudates may be dissolved by fibrinolysis and cleared by macrophages. If the fibrin is not removed, over time it may stimulate the ingrowth of fibroblasts and blood vessels and thus lead to scarring. Conversion of the fibrinous exudate to scar tissue *(organization)* within the pericardial sac leads to opaque fibrous thickening of the pericardium and

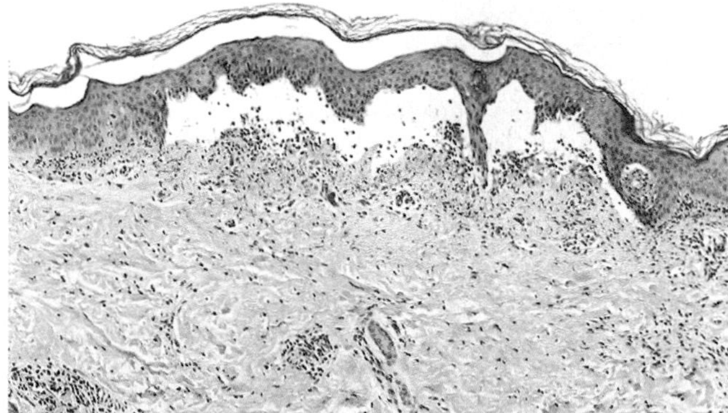

Figure 3-13 Serous inflammation. Low-power view of a cross-section of a skin blister showing the epidermis separated from the dermis by a focal collection of serous effusion.

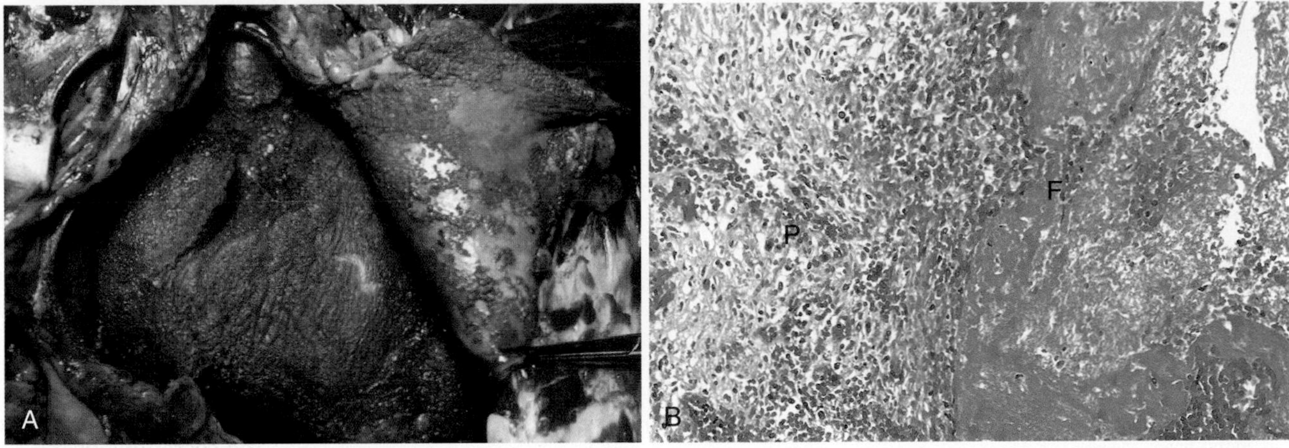

Figure 3-14 Fibrinous pericarditis. **A,** Deposits of fibrin on the pericardium. **B,** A pink meshwork of fibrin exudate (F) overlies the pericardial surface (P).

epicardium in the area of exudation and, if the fibrosis is extensive, obliteration of the pericardial space.

Purulent (Suppurative) Inflammation, Abscess

Purulent inflammation is characterized by the production of pus, an exudate consisting of neutrophils, the liquefied debris of necrotic cells, and edema fluid. The most frequent cause of purulent (also called *suppurative*) inflammation is infection with bacteria that cause liquefactive tissue necrosis, such as staphylococci; these pathogens are referred to as *pyogenic* (pus-producing) bacteria. A common example of an acute suppurative inflammation is acute appendicitis. ***Abscesses* are localized collections of purulent inflammatory tissue** caused by suppuration buried in a tissue, an organ, or a confined space. They are produced by seeding of pyogenic bacteria into a tissue (Fig. 3-15). Abscesses have a central region that appears as a mass of necrotic leukocytes and tissue cells. There is usually a zone of preserved neutrophils around this necrotic focus, and outside this region there may be vascular dilation and parenchymal and fibroblastic proliferation, indicating chronic inflammation and repair. In time the abscess may become walled off and ultimately replaced by connective tissue.

Ulcers

An ulcer is a local defect, or excavation, of the surface of an organ or tissue that is produced by the sloughing (shedding) of inflamed necrotic tissue (Fig. 3-16). Ulceration can occur only when tissue necrosis and resultant inflammation exist on or near a surface. It is most commonly encountered in (1) the mucosa of the mouth, stomach, intestines, or genitourinary tract, and (2) the skin and subcutaneous tissue of the lower extremities in older persons who have circulatory disturbances that predispose to extensive ischemic necrosis.

Ulcerations are best exemplified by peptic ulcer of the stomach or duodenum, in which acute and chronic inflammation coexist. During the acute stage there is intense polymorphonuclear infiltration and vascular dilation in the margins of the defect. With chronicity, the margins and base of the ulcer develop fibroblastic proliferation, scarring, and the accumulation of lymphocytes, macrophages, and plasma cells.

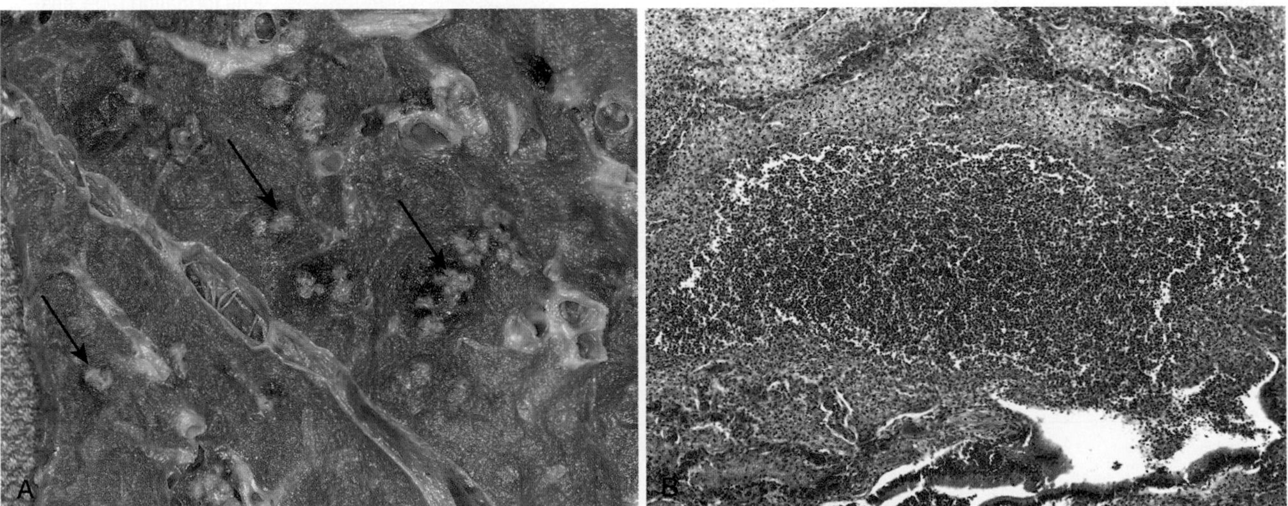

Figure 3-15 Purulent inflammation. **A,** Multiple bacterial abscesses (arrows) in the lung in a case of bronchopneumonia. **B,** The abscess contains neutrophils and cellular debris, and is surrounded by congested blood vessels.

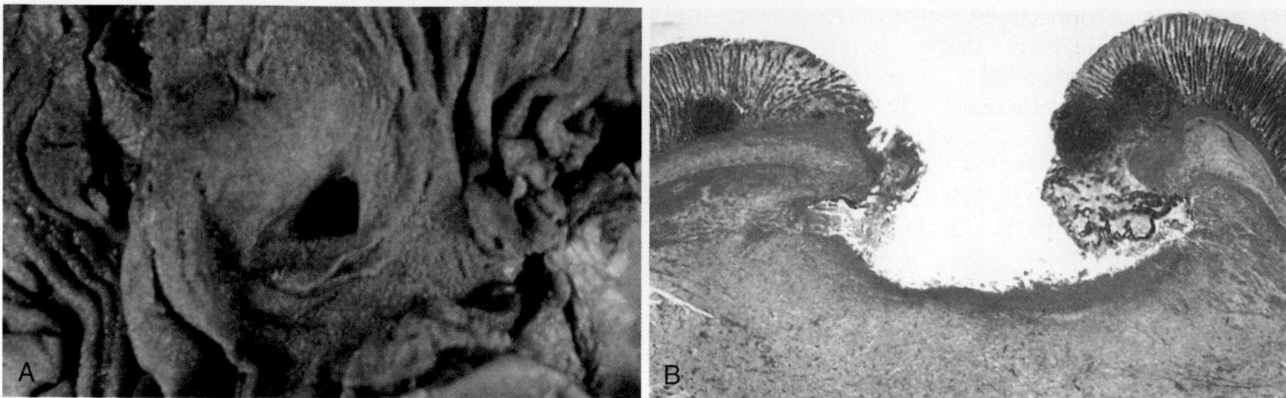

Figure 3-16 The morphology of an ulcer. **A,** A chronic duodenal ulcer. **B,** Low-power cross-section view of a duodenal ulcer crater with an acute inflammatory exudate in the base.

Outcomes of Acute Inflammation

Although, as might be expected, many variables may modify the basic process of inflammation, including the nature and intensity of the injury, the site and tissue affected, and the responsiveness of the host, **all acute inflammatory reactions typically have one of three outcomes** (Fig. 3-17):

- **Complete resolution.** In a perfect world, all inflammatory reactions, once they have succeeded in eliminating the offending agent, should end with restoration of the site of acute inflammation to normal. This is called *resolution* and is the usual outcome when the injury is limited or short-lived or when there has been little tissue destruction and the damaged parenchymal cells can regenerate. Resolution involves removal of cellular debris and microbes by macrophages, and resorption of edema fluid by lymphatics.
- **Healing by connective tissue replacement (scarring, or fibrosis).** This occurs after substantial tissue destruction, when the inflammatory injury involves tissues that are incapable of regeneration, or when there is abundant fibrin exudation in tissue or in serous cavities (pleura, peritoneum) that cannot be adequately cleared. In all

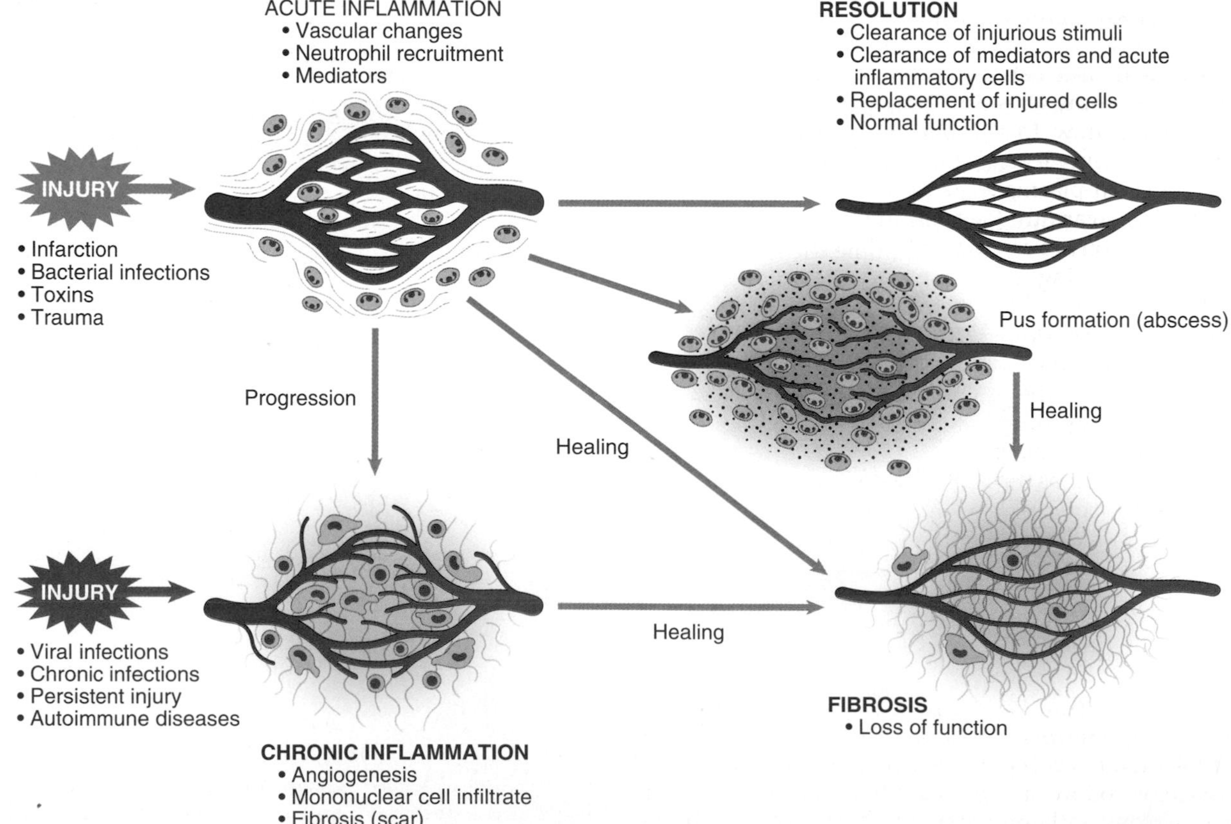

Figure 3-17 Outcomes of acute inflammation: resolution, healing by fibrosis, or chronic inflammation. The components of the various reactions and their functional outcomes are listed.

these situations, connective tissue grows into the area of damage or exudate, converting it into a mass of fibrous tissue, a process also called *organization.*

- Progression of the response to **chronic inflammation** (discussed later). Acute to chronic transition occurs when the acute inflammatory response cannot be resolved, as a result of either the persistence of the injurious agent or some interference with the normal process of healing.

Summary of Acute Inflammation

Now that we have described the components, mediators, and pathologic manifestations of acute inflammatory responses, it is useful to summarize the main features of a typical response of this type. When a host encounters an injurious agent, such as an infectious microbe or dead cells, phagocytes that reside in all tissues try to eliminate these agents. At the same time, phagocytes and other host cells react to the presence of the foreign or abnormal substance by liberating cytokines, lipid messengers, and other mediators of inflammation. Some of these mediators act on small blood vessels in the vicinity and promote the efflux of plasma and the recruitment of circulating leukocytes to the site where the offending agent is located. The recruited leukocytes are activated by the injurious agent and by locally produced mediators, and the activated leukocytes try to remove the offending agent by phagocytosis. As the injurious agent is eliminated and anti-inflammatory mechanisms become active, the process subsides and the host returns to a normal state of health. If the injurious agent cannot be quickly eliminated, the result may be chronic inflammation.

The vascular and cellular reactions account for the signs and symptoms of the inflammatory response. The increased blood flow to the injured area and increased vascular permeability lead to the accumulation of extravascular fluid rich in plasma proteins, known as *edema*. The redness *(rubor)*, warmth *(calor)*, and swelling *(tumor)* of acute inflammation are caused by the increased blood flow and edema. Circulating leukocytes, initially predominantly neutrophils, adhere to the endothelium via adhesion molecules, traverse the endothelium, and migrate to the site of injury under the influence of chemotactic agents. Leukocytes that are activated by the offending agent and by endogenous mediators may release toxic metabolites and proteases extracellularly, causing tissue damage. During the damage, and in part as a result of the liberation of prostaglandins, neuropeptides, and cytokines, one of the local symptoms is pain *(dolor)*.

Chronic Inflammation

Chronic inflammation is a response of prolonged duration (weeks or months) in which inflammation, tissue injury and attempts at repair coexist, in varying combinations. It may follow acute inflammation, as described earlier, or chronic inflammation may begin insidiously, as a low-grade, smoldering response without any manifestations of a preceding acute reaction.

Causes of Chronic Inflammation

Chronic inflammation arises in the following settings:

- **Persistent infections** by microorganisms that are difficult to eradicate, such as mycobacteria and certain viruses, fungi, and parasites. These organisms often evoke an immune reaction called *delayed-type hypersensitivity* (Chapter 6). The inflammatory response sometimes takes a specific pattern called a *granulomatous reaction* (discussed later). In other cases, an unresolved acute inflammation may evolve into chronic inflammation, as may occur in acute bacterial infection of the lung that progresses to a chronic lung abscess.
- **Hypersensitivity diseases.** Chronic inflammation plays an important role in a group of diseases that are caused by excessive and inappropriate activation of the immune system. Under certain conditions immune reactions develop against the individual's own tissues, leading to *autoimmune diseases* (Chapter 6). In these diseases, autoantigens evoke a self-perpetuating immune reaction that results in chronic tissue damage and inflammation; examples of such diseases are rheumatoid arthritis and multiple sclerosis. In other cases, chronic inflammation is the result of unregulated immune responses against microbes, as in inflammatory bowel disease. Immune responses against common environmental substances are the cause of *allergic diseases*, such as bronchial asthma (Chapter 6). Because these autoimmune and allergic reactions are inappropriately triggered against antigens that are normally harmless, the reactions serve no useful purpose and only cause disease. Such diseases may show morphologic patterns of mixed acute and chronic inflammation because they are characterized by repeated bouts of inflammation. Fibrosis may dominate the late stages.
- **Prolonged exposure to potentially toxic agents, either exogenous or endogenous.** An example of an exogenous agent is particulate silica, a nondegradable inanimate material that, when inhaled for prolonged periods, results in an inflammatory lung disease called *silicosis* (Chapter 15). *Atherosclerosis* (Chapter 11) is thought to be a chronic inflammatory process of the arterial wall induced, at least in part, by excessive production and tissue deposition of endogenous cholesterol and other lipids.
- Some forms of chronic inflammation may be important in the pathogenesis of diseases that are not conventionally thought of as inflammatory disorders. These include neurodegenerative diseases such as Alzheimer disease, metabolic syndrome and the associated type 2 diabetes, and certain cancers in which inflammatory reactions promote tumor development. The role of inflammation in these conditions is discussed in the relevant chapters.

Morphologic Features

In contrast to acute inflammation, which is manifested by vascular changes, edema, and predominantly neutrophilic infiltration, **chronic inflammation is characterized by:**

- **Infiltration with mononuclear cells,** which include macrophages, lymphocytes, and plasma cells (Fig. 3-18)

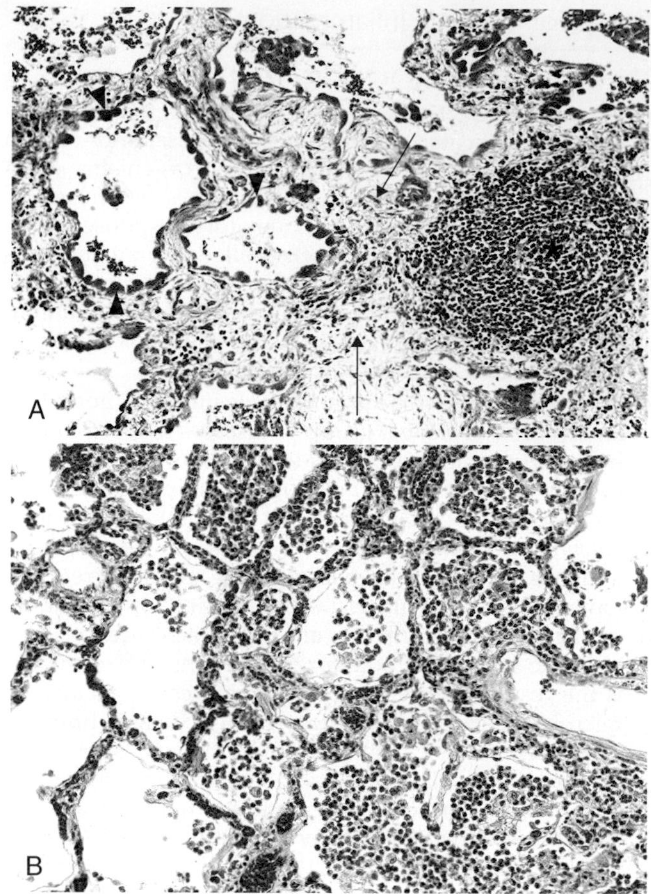

Figure 3-18 **A,** Chronic inflammation in the lung, showing all three characteristic histologic features: (1) collection of chronic inflammatory cells (*), (2) destruction of parenchyma (normal alveoli are replaced by spaces lined by cuboidal epithelium, *arrowheads*), and (3) replacement by connective tissue (fibrosis, *arrows*). **B,** In contrast, in acute inflammation of the lung (acute bronchopneumonia), neutrophils fill the alveolar spaces and blood vessels are congested.

- **Tissue destruction,** induced by the persistent offending agent or by the inflammatory cells
- **Attempts at healing** by connective tissue replacement of damaged tissue, accomplished by *angiogenesis* (proliferation of small blood vessels) and, in particular, *fibrosis*

Because angiogenesis and fibrosis are also components of wound healing and repair, they are discussed later, in the context of tissue repair.

Cells and Mediators of Chronic Inflammation

The combination of leukocyte infiltration, tissue damage, and fibrosis that characterize chronic inflammation is the result of the local activation of several cell types and the production of mediators.

Role of Macrophages

The dominant cells in most chronic inflammatory reactions are macrophages, which contribute to the reaction by secreting cytokines and growth factors that act on various cells, by destroying foreign invaders and tissues, and by activating other cells, notably T lymphocytes. Macrophages are professional phagocytes that act as filters for particulate matter, microbes, and senescent cells. They also function as effector cells that eliminate microbes in cellular and humoral immune responses (Chapter 6). But they serve many other roles in inflammation and repair. Here we review the basic biology of macrophages, including their development and functional responses.

Macrophages are tissue cells derived from hematopoietic stem cells in the bone marrow and from progenitors in the embryonic yolk sac and fetal liver during early development (Fig. 3-19). Circulating cells of this lineage are known as *monocytes*. Macrophages are normally diffusely scattered in most connective tissues. In addition, they are found in specific locations in organs such as the liver (where they are called Kupffer cells), spleen and lymph nodes (called sinus histiocytes), central nervous system (microglial cells), and lungs (alveolar macrophages). Together these cells comprise the *mononuclear phagocyte system*, also known by the older (and inaccurate) name of reticuloendothelial system.

Committed progenitors in the bone marrow give rise to monocytes, which enter the blood, migrate into various tissues and differentiate into macrophages. This is typical of macrophages at sites of inflammation and in some tissues such as the skin and intestinal tract. The half-life of blood monocytes is about 1 day, whereas the life span of tissue macrophages is several months or years. Most tissue resident macrophages, such as microglia, Kupffer cells, alveolar macrophages and macrophages in the spleen and connective tissues, may arise from yolk sac or fetal liver very early in embryogenesis, populate the tissues, stay for long periods in the steady state, and are replenished mainly by proliferation of resident cells. As discussed earlier, in inflammatory reactions, monocytes begin to emigrate into extravascular tissues quite early, and within 48 hours they may constitute the predominant cell type. Extravasation of monocytes is governed by the same factors that are involved in neutrophil emigration, that is, adhesion molecules and chemical mediators with chemotactic and activating properties.

There are two major pathways of macrophage activation, called *classical* and *alternative* (Fig. 3-20). The stimuli that activate macrophages by these pathways, and the functions of the activated cells, are quite different.

- **Classical macrophage activation** may be induced by microbial products such as endotoxin, which engage TLRs and other sensors; by T cell–derived signals, importantly the cytokine IFN-γ, in immune responses; or by foreign substances including crystals and particulate matter. Classically activated (also called M1) macrophages produce NO and ROS and upregulate lysosomal enzymes, all of which enhance their ability to kill ingested organisms, and secrete cytokines that stimulate inflammation. These macrophages are important in host defense against microbes and in many inflammatory reactions. As discussed earlier in the context of acute inflammation and leukocyte activation, the same activated cells are capable of injuring normal tissues.
- **Alternative macrophage activation** is induced by cytokines other than IFN-γ, such as IL-4 and IL-13, produced by T lymphocytes and other cells. These macrophages

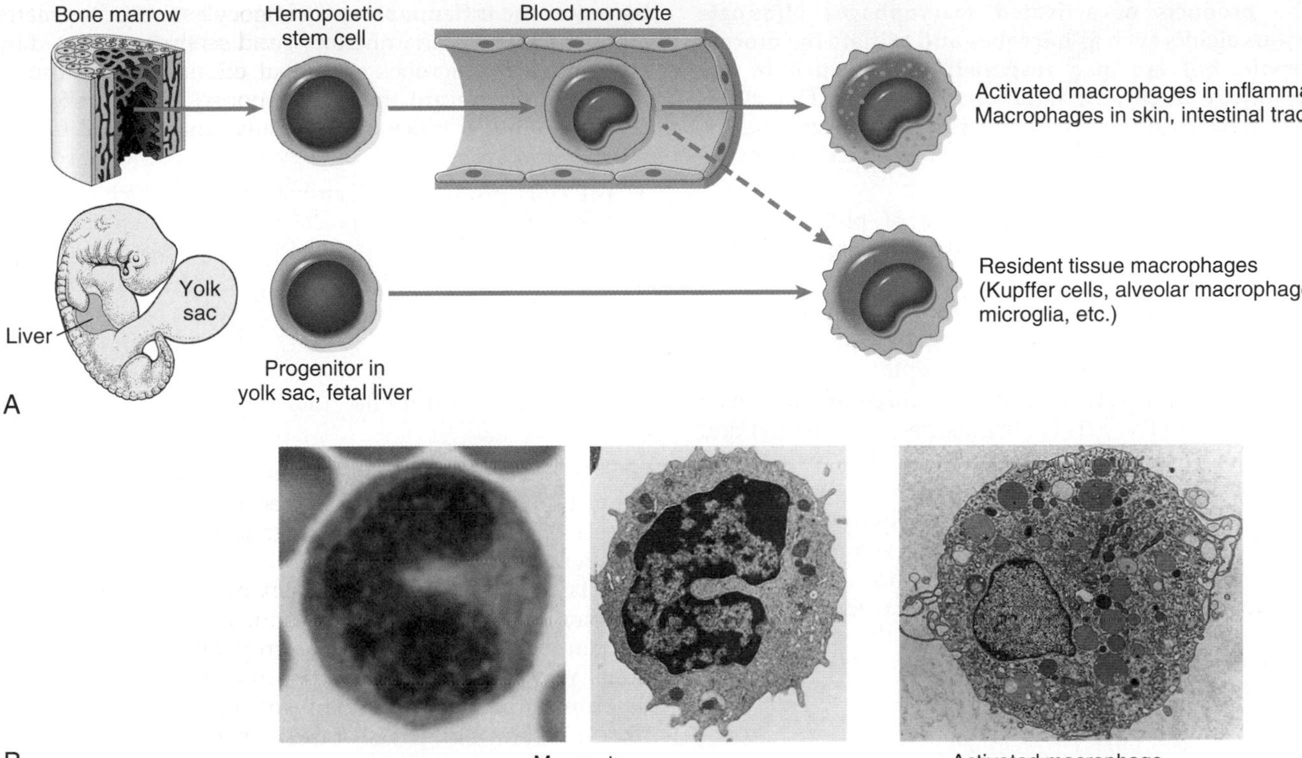

Figure 3-19 Maturation of mononuclear phagocytes. **A,** In the steady state, some tissue macrophages, including microglia and alveolar macrophages, may be derived from embryonic precursors and populate the tissues. The development of macrophages from hematopoietic precursors and monocytes may be more prominent when tissue macrophages need to be increased or replenished, as after injury and during inflammation. **B,** The morphology of a monocyte and activated macrophage.

are not actively microbicidal and the cytokines may actually inhibit the classical activation pathway; instead, the principal function of alternatively activated (M2) macrophages is in tissue repair. They secrete growth factors that promote angiogenesis, activate fibroblasts, and stimulate collagen synthesis. It seems plausible that in response to most injurious stimuli, the first activation pathway is the classical one, designed to destroy the offending agents, and this is followed by alternative activation, which initiates tissue repair. However, such a precise sequence is not well documented in most inflammatory reactions.

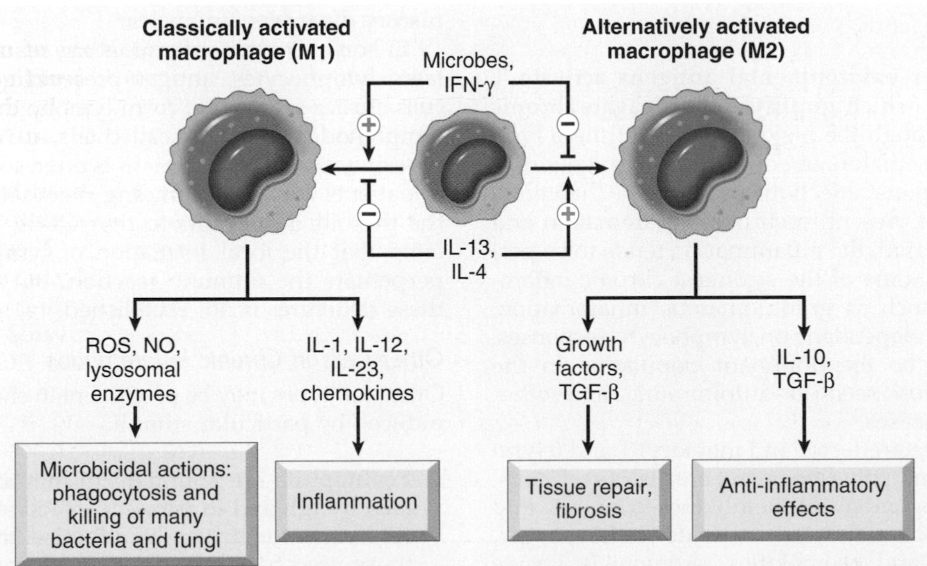

Figure 3-20 Classical and alternative macrophage activation. Different stimuli activate monocytes/macrophages to develop into functionally distinct populations. Classically activated macrophages are induced by microbial products and cytokines, particularly IFN-γ. They phagocytose and destroy microbes and dead tissues and can potentiate inflammatory reactions. Alternatively activated macrophages are induced by other cytokines and are important in tissue repair and the resolution of inflammation.

The products of activated macrophages eliminate injurious agents such as microbes and initiate the process of repair, but are also responsible for much of the tissue injury in chronic inflammation. Several functions of macrophages are central to the development and persistence of chronic inflammation and the accompanying tissue injury.

- Macrophages, like the other type of phagocyte, the neutrophils, **ingest and eliminate microbes and dead tissues.**
- Macrophages **initiate the process of tissue repair** and are involved in scar formation and fibrosis. These processes are discussed later in the chapter.
- Macrophages **secrete mediators of inflammation,** such as cytokines (TNF, IL-1, chemokines, and others) and eicosanoids. Thus, macrophages are central to the initiation and propagation of inflammatory reactions.
- Macrophages **display antigens to T lymphocytes and respond to signals from T cells,** thus setting up a feedback loop that is essential for defense against many microbes by cell-mediated immune responses. These interactions are described further in the discussion of the role of lymphocytes in chronic inflammation, below, and in more detail in Chapter 6 where cell-mediated immunity is considered.

Their impressive arsenal of mediators makes macrophages powerful allies in the body's defense against unwanted invaders, but the same weaponry can also induce considerable tissue destruction when macrophages are inappropriately or excessively activated. It is because of these activities of macrophages that tissue destruction is one of the hallmarks of chronic inflammation.

In some instances, if the irritant is eliminated, macrophages eventually disappear (either dying off or making their way into the lymphatics and lymph nodes). In others, macrophage accumulation persists, as a result of continuous recruitment from the circulation and local proliferation at the site of inflammation.

Role of Lymphocytes

Microbes and other environmental antigens activate T and B lymphocytes, which amplify and propagate chronic inflammation. Although the major function of these lymphocytes is as the mediators of adaptive immunity, which provides defense against infectious pathogens (Chapter 6), these cells are often present in chronic inflammation and when they are activated, the inflammation tends to be persistent and severe. Some of the strongest chronic inflammatory reactions, such as granulomatous inflammation, described later, are dependent on lymphocyte responses. Lymphocytes may be the dominant population in the chronic inflammation seen in autoimmune and other hypersensitivity diseases.

Antigen-stimulated (effector and memory) T and B lymphocytes use various adhesion molecule pairs (selectins, integrins and their ligands) and chemokines to migrate into inflammatory sites. Cytokines from activated macrophages, mainly TNF, IL-1, and chemokines, promote leukocyte recruitment, setting the stage for persistence of the inflammatory response.

By virtue of their ability to secrete cytokines, CD4+ T lymphocytes promote inflammation and influence the nature of the inflammatory reaction. These T cells greatly amplify the early inflammatory reaction that is induced by recognition of microbes and dead cells as part of innate immunity. There are three subsets of CD4+ T cells that secrete different types of cytokines and elicit different types of inflammation.

- T_H1 cells produce the cytokine IFN-γ, which activates macrophages by the classical pathway.
- T_H2 cells secrete IL-4, IL-5, and IL-13, which recruit and activate eosinophils and are responsible for the alternative pathway of macrophage activation.
- T_H17 cells secrete IL-17 and other cytokines, which induce the secretion of chemokines responsible for recruiting neutrophils (and monocytes) into the reaction.

Both T_H1 and T_H17 cells are involved in defense against many types of bacteria and viruses and in autoimmune diseases. T_H2 cells are important in defense against helminthic parasites and in allergic inflammation. These T cell subsets and their functions are described in more detail in Chapter 6.

Lymphocytes and macrophages interact in a bidirectional way, and these interactions play an important role in propagating chronic inflammation (Fig. 3-21). Macrophages display antigens to T cells, express membrane molecules (called costimulators), and produce cytokines (IL-12 and others) that stimulate T-cell responses (Chapter 6). Activated T lymphocytes, in turn, produce cytokines, described earlier, which recruit and activate macrophages, promoting more antigen presentation and cytokine secretion. The result is a cycle of cellular reactions that fuel and sustain chronic inflammation.

Activated B lymphocytes and antibody-producing plasma cells are often present at sites of chronic inflammation. The antibodies may be specific for persistent foreign or self antigens in the inflammatory site or against altered tissue components. However, the specificity and even the importance of antibodies in most chronic inflammatory disorders are unclear.

In some chronic inflammatory reactions, the accumulated lymphocytes, antigen-presenting cells, and plasma cells cluster together to form lymphoid tissues resembling lymph nodes. These are called *tertiary lymphoid organs;* this type of *lymphoid organogenesis* is often seen in the synovium of patients with long-standing rheumatoid arthritis and in the thyroid in Hashimoto thyroiditis. It has been postulated that the local formation of lymphoid organs may perpetuate the immune reaction, but the significance of these structures is not established.

Other Cells in Chronic Inflammation

Other cell types may be prominent in chronic inflammation induced by particular stimuli.

- **Eosinophils** are abundant in immune reactions mediated by IgE and in parasitic infections (Fig. 3-22). Their recruitment is driven by adhesion molecules similar to those used by neutrophils, and by specific chemokines (e.g., eotaxin) derived from leukocytes and epithelial cells. Eosinophils have granules that contain *major basic protein*, a highly cationic protein that is toxic to parasites but also causes lysis of mammalian epithelial cells. This

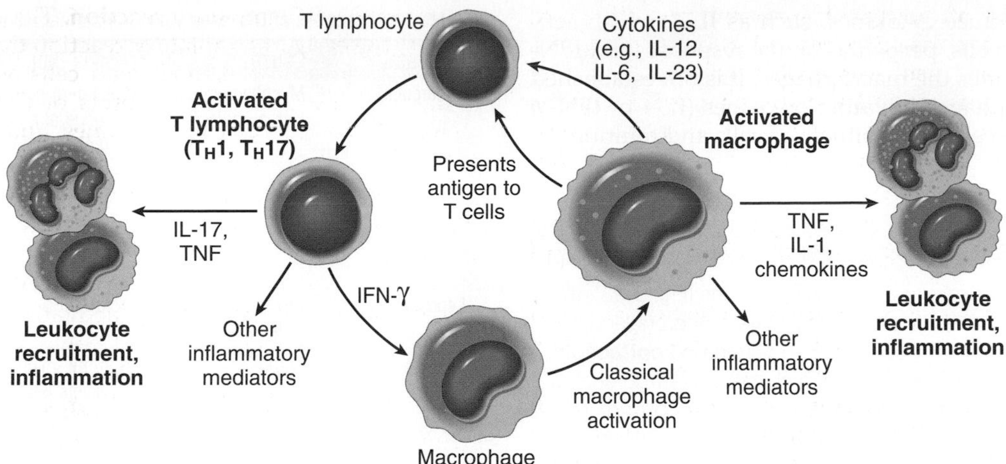

Figure 3-21 Macrophage-lymphocyte interactions in chronic inflammation. Activated T cells produce cytokines that recruit macrophages (TNF, IL-17, chemokines) and others that activate macrophages (IFN-γ). Activated macrophages in turn stimulate T cells by presenting antigens and via cytokines such as IL-12.

is why eosinophils are of benefit in controlling parasitic infections, yet they also contribute to tissue damage in immune reactions such as allergies (Chapter 6).

- **Mast cells** are widely distributed in connective tissues and participate in both acute and chronic inflammatory reactions. Mast cells express on their surface the receptor (FcεRI) that binds the Fc portion of IgE antibody. In immediate hypersensitivity reactions, IgE antibodies bound to the cells' Fc receptors specifically recognize antigen, and the cells degranulate and release mediators, such as histamine and prostaglandins (Chapter 6). This type of response occurs during allergic reactions to foods, insect venom, or drugs, sometimes with catastrophic results (e.g., anaphylactic shock). Mast cells are also present in chronic inflammatory reactions, and because they secrete a plethora of cytokines, they may promote inflammatory reactions in different situations.
- Although **neutrophils** are characteristic of acute inflammation, many forms of chronic inflammation, lasting for months, continue to show large numbers of neutrophils, induced either by persistent microbes or by mediators produced by activated macrophages and T lymphocytes. In chronic bacterial infection of bone (osteomyelitis), a neutrophilic exudate can persist for many months. Neutrophils are also important in the chronic damage induced in lungs by smoking and other irritant stimuli (Chapter 15). This pattern of inflammation has been called *acute on chronic*.

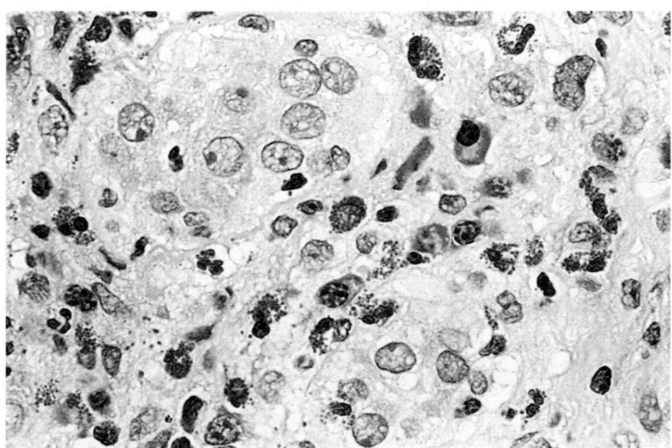

Figure 3-22 A focus of inflammation containing numerous eosinophils.

Granulomatous Inflammation

Granulomatous inflammation is a form of chronic inflammation characterized by collections of activated macrophages, often with T lymphocytes, and sometimes associated with central necrosis. Granuloma formation is a cellular attempt to contain an offending agent that is difficult to eradicate. In this attempt there is often strong activation of T lymphocytes leading to macrophage activation, which can cause injury to normal tissues. The activated macrophages may develop abundant cytoplasm and begin to resemble epithelial cells, and are called *epithelioid cells*. Some activated macrophages may fuse, forming multinucleate *giant cells*.

There are two types of granulomas, which differ in their pathogenesis.

- **Foreign body granulomas** are incited by relatively inert foreign bodies, in the absence of T cell–mediated immune responses. Typically, foreign body granulomas form around materials such as talc (associated with intravenous drug abuse) (Chapter 9), sutures, or other fibers that are large enough to preclude phagocytosis by a macrophage and do not incite any specific inflammatory or immune response. Epithelioid cells and giant cells are apposed to the surface of the foreign body. The foreign material can usually be identified in the center of the granuloma, particularly if viewed with polarized light, in which it appears refractile.
- **Immune granulomas** are caused by a variety of agents that are capable of inducing a persistent T cell–mediated immune response. This type of immune response produces granulomas usually when the inciting agent is difficult to eradicate, such as a persistent microbe or a self antigen. In such responses, macrophages activate

T cells to produce cytokines, such as IL-2, which activates other T cells, perpetuating the response, and IFN-γ, which activates the macrophages. It is not established which macrophage-activating cytokines (IL-4 or IFN-γ) transform the cells into epithelioid cells and multinucleate giant cells.

MORPHOLOGY

In the usual hematoxylin and eosin preparations (Fig. 3-23), the activated macrophages in granulomas have pink granular cytoplasm with indistinct cell boundaries and are called **epithelioid cells** because of their resemblance to epithelia. The aggregates of epithelioid macrophages are surrounded by a collar of lymphocytes. Older granulomas may have a rim of fibroblasts and connective tissue. Frequently, but not invariably, multinucleated **giant cells** 40 to 50 μm in diameter are found in granulomas; these are called Langhans giant cells. They consist of a large mass of cytoplasm and many nuclei, and they derive from the fusion of multiple activated macrophages. In granulomas associated with certain infectious organisms (most classically *Mycobacterium tuberculosis*), a combination of hypoxia and free radical–mediated injury leads to a central zone of necrosis. Grossly, this has a granular, cheesy appearance and is therefore called **caseous necrosis.** Microscopically, this necrotic material appears as amorphous, structureless, eosinophilic, granular debris, with complete loss of cellular details. The granulomas in Crohn disease, sarcoidosis, and foreign body reactions tend to not have necrotic centers and are said to be *noncaseating*. Healing of granulomas is accompanied by fibrosis that may be extensive.

Granulomas are encountered in certain specific pathologic states; recognition of the granulomatous pattern is important because of the limited number of conditions (some life-threatening) that cause it (Table 3-8). In the setting of persistent T-cell responses to certain microbes (e.g., *M. tuberculosis*, *Treponema pallidum*, or fungi), T cell–derived cytokines are responsible for chronic macrophage activation and granuloma formation. Granulomas may also develop in some immune-mediated inflammatory diseases, notably Crohn disease, which is one type of inflammatory bowel disease and an important cause of granulomatous inflammation in the United States, and in a disease of unknown etiology called *sarcoidosis.* **Tuberculosis is the prototype of a granulomatous disease caused by infection and should always be excluded as the cause when granulomas are identified.** In this disease the granuloma is referred to as a *tubercle.* The morphologic patterns in the various granulomatous diseases may be sufficiently different to allow reasonably accurate diagnosis by an experienced pathologist (see Table 3-8); however, there are so many atypical presentations that it is always necessary to identify the specific etiologic agent by special stains for organisms (e.g., acid-fast stains for tubercle bacilli), by culture methods (e.g., in tuberculosis and fungal diseases), by molecular techniques (e.g., the polymerase chain reaction in tuberculosis), and by serologic studies (e.g., in syphilis).

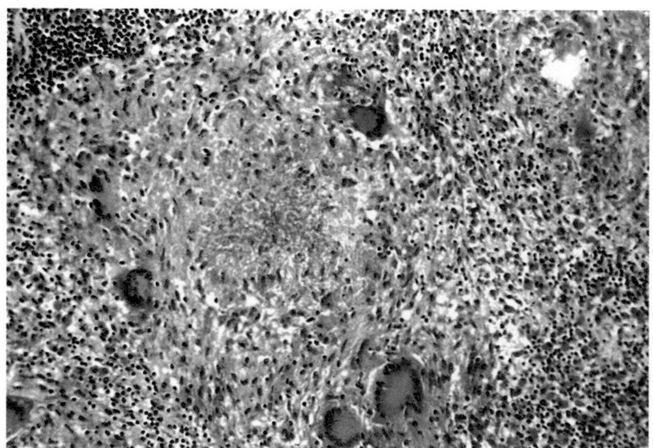

Figure 3-23 Typical tuberculous granuloma showing an area of central necrosis surrounded by multiple Langhans-type giant cells, epithelioid cells, and lymphocytes.

Table 3-8 Examples of Diseases with Granulomatous Inflammation

Disease	Cause	Tissue Reaction
Tuberculosis	*Mycobacterium tuberculosis*	Caseating granuloma (tubercle): focus of activated macrophages (epithelioid cells), rimmed by fibroblasts, lymphocytes, histiocytes, occasional Langhans giant cells; central necrosis with amorphous granular debris; acid-fast bacilli
Leprosy	*Mycobacterium leprae*	Acid-fast bacilli in macrophages; noncaseating granulomas
Syphilis	*Treponema pallidum*	Gumma: microscopic to grossly visible lesion, enclosing wall of histiocytes; plasma cell infiltrate; central cells are necrotic without loss of cellular outline
Cat-scratch disease	Gram-negative bacillus	Rounded or stellate granuloma containing central granular debris and recognizable neutrophils; giant cells uncommon
Sarcoidosis	Unknown etiology	Noncaseating granulomas with abundant activated macrophages
Crohn disease (inflammatory bowel disease)	Immune reaction against intestinal bacteria, possibly self antigens	Occasional noncaseating granulomas in the wall of the intestine, with dense chronic inflammatory infiltrate

KEY CONCEPTS

Chronic Inflammation

- Chronic inflammation is a prolonged host response to persistent stimuli.
- It is caused by microbes that resist elimination, immune responses against self and environmental antigens, and some toxic substances (e.g., silica); underlies many medically important diseases.
- It is characterized by coexisting inflammation, tissue injury, attempted repair by scarring, and immune response.

- The cellular infiltrate consists of macrophages, lymphocytes, plasma cells, and other leukocytes.
- It is mediated by cytokines produced by macrophages and lymphocytes (notably T lymphocytes); bidirectional interactions between these cells tend to amplify and prolong the inflammatory reaction.
- Granulomatous inflammation is a pattern of chronic inflammation induced by T cell and macrophage activation in response to an agent that is resistant to eradication.

Systemic Effects of Inflammation

Inflammation, even if it is localized, is associated with cytokine-induced systemic reactions that are collectively called the *acute-phase response*. Anyone who has suffered through a severe bout of a viral illness (e.g.., influenza) has experienced the systemic manifestations of acute inflammation. These changes are reactions to cytokines whose production is stimulated by bacterial products such as LPS and by other inflammatory stimuli. **The cytokines TNF, IL-1, and IL-6 are important mediators of the acute-phase reaction; other cytokines, notably type I interferons, also contribute to the reaction.**

The acute-phase response consists of several clinical and pathologic changes:

- **Fever,** characterized by an elevation of body temperature, usually by 1° to 4°C, is one of the most prominent manifestations of the acute-phase response, especially when inflammation is associated with infection. Substances that induce fever are called *pyrogens.* The increase in body temperature is caused by prostaglandins that are produced in the vascular and perivascular cells of the hypothalamus. Bacterial products, such as LPS (called *exogenous pyrogens*), stimulate leukocytes to release cytokines such as IL-1 and TNF (called *endogenous pyrogens*) that increase the enzymes (cyclooxygenases) that convert AA into prostaglandins. In the hypothalamus, the prostaglandins, especially PGE_2, stimulate the production of neurotransmitters that reset the temperature set point at a higher level. NSAIDs, including aspirin, reduce fever by inhibiting prostaglandin synthesis. An elevated body temperature has been shown to help amphibians ward off microbial infections, and it is assumed that fever is a protective host response in mammals as well, although the mechanism is unknown. One hypothesis is that fever may induce heat shock proteins that enhance lymphocyte responses to microbial antigens.
- **Acute-phase proteins** are plasma proteins, mostly synthesized in the liver, whose plasma concentrations may increase several hundred-fold as part of the response to inflammatory stimuli. Three of the best-known of these proteins are C-reactive protein (CRP), fibrinogen, and serum amyloid A (SAA) protein. Synthesis of these molecules in hepatocytes is stimulated by cytokines, especially IL-6 (for CRP and fibrinogen) and IL-1 or TNF (for SAA). Many acute-phase proteins, such as CRP and SAA, bind to microbial cell walls, and they may act as opsonins and fix complement. They also bind chromatin, possibly aiding in clearing necrotic cell nuclei. Fibrinogen binds to red cells and causes them to form stacks (rouleaux) that sediment more rapidly at unit gravity than do individual red cells. This is the basis for measuring the *erythrocyte sedimentation rate* as a simple test for an inflammatory response caused by any stimulus. Acute-phase proteins have beneficial effects during acute inflammation, but prolonged production of these proteins (especially SAA) in states of chronic inflammation causes *secondary amyloidosis* (Chapter 6). Elevated serum levels of CRP have been proposed as a marker for increased risk of myocardial infarction in patients with coronary artery disease. It is postulated that inflammation involving atherosclerotic plaques in the coronary arteries may predispose to thrombosis and subsequent infarction. Another peptide whose production is increased in the acute-phase response is the iron-regulating peptide *hepcidin*. Chronically elevated plasma concentrations of hepcidin reduce the availability of iron and are responsible for the *anemia* associated with chronic inflammation (Chapter 14).
- **Leukocytosis** is a common feature of inflammatory reactions, especially those induced by bacterial infections. The leukocyte count usually climbs to 15,000 or 20,000 cells/mL, but sometimes it may reach extraordinarily high levels of 40,000 to 100,000 cells/mL. These extreme elevations are referred to as *leukemoid reactions,* because they are similar to the white cell counts observed in leukemia and have to be distinguished from leukemia. The leukocytosis occurs initially because of accelerated release of cells from the bone marrow postmitotic reserve pool (caused by cytokines, including TNF and IL-1) and is therefore associated with a rise in the number of more immature neutrophils in the blood, referred to as a *left shift*. Prolonged infection also induces proliferation of precursors in the bone marrow, caused by increased production of colony-stimulating factors. Thus, the bone marrow output of leukocytes is increased to compensate for the loss of these cells in the inflammatory reaction. (See also the discussion of leukocytosis in Chapter 13.) Most bacterial infections induce an increase in the blood neutrophil count, called *neutrophilia*. Viral infections, such as infectious mononucleosis, mumps, and German measles, cause an absolute increase in the number of lymphocytes *(lymphocytosis)*. In some allergies and parasitic infestations, there is an increase in the absolute number of eosinophils, creating an *eosinophilia*. Certain infections (typhoid fever and infections caused by some viruses, rickettsiae, and certain protozoa) are associated with a decreased number of circulating white cells *(leukopenia)*.
- Other manifestations of the acute-phase response include increased pulse and blood pressure; decreased sweating, mainly because of redirection of blood flow from cutaneous to deep vascular beds, to minimize heat loss through the skin; rigors (shivering), chills (search for warmth), anorexia, somnolence, and malaise, probably because of the actions of cytokines on brain cells.
- In severe bacterial infections *(sepsis),* the large amounts of bacteria and their products in the blood stimulate the production of enormous quantities of several cytokines, notably TNF and IL-1. High blood levels of cytokines cause various widespread clinical manifestations such

as disseminated intravascular coagulation, hypotensive shock, and metabolic disturbances including insulin resistance and hyperglycemia. This clinical triad is known as *septic shock;* it is discussed in more detail in Chapter 4.

KEY CONCEPTS

Systemic Effects of Inflammation

- Fever: cytokines (TNF, IL-1) stimulate production of prostaglandins in hypothalamus
- Production of acute-phase proteins: C-reactive protein, others; synthesis stimulated by cytokines (IL-6, others) acting on liver cells
- Leukocytosis: cytokines (colony-stimulating factors) stimulate production of leukocytes from precursors in the bone marrow
- In some severe infections, septic shock: fall in blood pressure, disseminated intravascular coagulation, metabolic abnormalities; induced by high levels of TNF and other cytokines

Excessive inflammation is the underlying cause of many human diseases, described throughout this book. Conversely, defective inflammation is responsible for increased susceptibility to infections. The most common cause of defective inflammation is leukocyte deficiency resulting from replacement of the bone marrow by leukemias and metastatic tumors, and suppression of the marrow by therapies for cancer and graft rejection. Inherited genetic abnormalities of leukocyte adhesion and microbicidal function are rare but very informative; these are described in Chapter 6, in the context of immunodeficiency diseases. Deficiencies of the complement system are mentioned earlier and are described further in Chapter 6.

We next consider the process of *repair,* which is a healing response to tissue destruction caused by inflammatory or non-inflammatory causes.

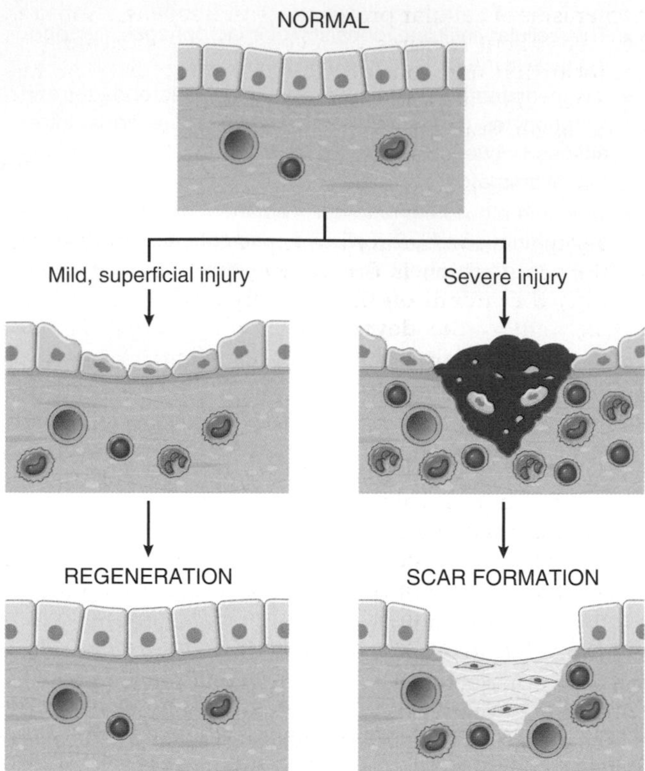

Figure 3-24 Mechanisms of tissue repair: regeneration and scar formation. Following mild injury, which damages the epithelium but not the underlying tissue, resolution occurs by regeneration, but after more severe injury with damage to the connective tissue, repair is by scar formation.

Tissue Repair

Overview of Tissue Repair

Repair, sometimes called healing, refers to the restoration of tissue architecture and function after an injury. (By convention, the term *repair* is often used for parenchymal and connective tissues and *healing* for surface epithelia, but these distinctions are not based on biology and we use the terms interchangeably.) Critical to the survival of an organism is the ability to repair the damage caused by toxic insults and inflammation. Hence, the inflammatory response to microbes and injured tissues not only serves to eliminate these dangers but also sets into motion the process of repair.

Repair of damaged tissues occurs by two types of reactions: regeneration by proliferation of residual (uninjured) cells and maturation of tissue stem cells, and the deposition of connective tissue to form a scar (Fig. 3-24).

- **Regeneration.** Some tissues are able to replace the damaged components and essentially return to a normal state; this process is called *regeneration.* Regeneration occurs by proliferation of cells that survive the injury and retain the capacity to proliferate, for example, in the rapidly dividing epithelia of the skin and intestines, and in some parenchymal organs, notably the liver. In other cases, tissue stem cells may contribute to the restoration of damaged tissues. However, mammals have a limited capacity to regenerate damaged tissues and organs, and only some components of most tissues are able to fully restore themselves.
- **Connective tissue deposition (scar formation).** If the injured tissues are incapable of complete restitution, or if the supporting structures of the tissue are severely damaged, repair occurs by the laying down of connective (fibrous) tissue, a process that may result in scar formation. Although the fibrous scar is not normal, it provides enough structural stability that the injured tissue is usually able to function. The term *fibrosis* is most often used to describe the extensive deposition of collagen that occurs in the lungs, liver, kidney, and other organs as a consequence of chronic inflammation, or in the myocardium after extensive ischemic necrosis (infarction). If fibrosis develops in a tissue space occupied by an inflammatory exudate, it is called *organization* (as in organizing pneumonia affecting the lung).

After many common types of injury, both regeneration and scar formation contribute in varying degrees to the ultimate repair. Both processes involve the proliferation of various cells, and close interactions between cells and the extracellular matrix (ECM). We first discuss the general mechanisms of cellular proliferation and regeneration, and then the salient features of regeneration and healing by scar formation, and conclude with a description of cutaneous wound healing and fibrosis (scarring) in parenchymal organs as illustrations of the repair process.

Cell and Tissue Regeneration

The regeneration of injured cells and tissues involves cell proliferation, which is driven by growth factors and is critically dependent on the integrity of the extracellular matrix, and by the development of mature cells from stem cells. Before describing examples of repair by regeneration, the general principles of cell proliferation are discussed.

Cell Proliferation: Signals and Control Mechanisms

Several cell types proliferate during tissue repair. These include the remnants of the injured tissue (which attempt to restore normal structure), vascular endothelial cells (to create new vessels that provide the nutrients needed for the repair process), and fibroblasts (the source of the fibrous tissue that forms the scar to fill defects that cannot be corrected by regeneration).

The ability of tissues to repair themselves is determined, in part, by their intrinsic proliferative capacity. Based on this criterion, the tissues of the body are divided into three groups.

- **Labile (continuously dividing) tissues.** Cells of these tissues are continuously being lost and replaced by maturation from tissue stem cells and by proliferation of mature cells. Labile cells include hematopoietic cells in the bone marrow and the majority of surface epithelia, such as the stratified squamous epithelia of the skin, oral cavity, vagina, and cervix; the cuboidal epithelia of the ducts draining exocrine organs (e.g., salivary glands, pancreas, biliary tract); the columnar epithelium of the gastrointestinal tract, uterus, and fallopian tubes; and the transitional epithelium of the urinary tract. These tissues can readily regenerate after injury as long as the pool of stem cells is preserved.
- **Stable tissues.** Cells of these tissues are quiescent (in the G_0 stage of the cell cycle) and have only minimal proliferative activity in their normal state. However, these cells are capable of dividing in response to injury or loss of tissue mass. Stable cells constitute the parenchyma of most solid tissues, such as liver, kidney, and pancreas. They also include endothelial cells, fibroblasts, and smooth muscle cells; the proliferation of these cells is particularly important in wound healing. With the exception of liver, stable tissues have a limited capacity to regenerate after injury.
- **Permanent tissues.** The cells of these tissues are considered to be terminally differentiated and nonproliferative in postnatal life. The majority of neurons and cardiac muscle cells belong to this category. Thus, injury to the brain or heart is irreversible and results in a scar, because neurons and cardiac myocytes cannot regenerate. Limited stem cell replication and differentiation occur in some areas of the adult brain, and there is some evidence that heart muscle cells may proliferate after myocardial necrosis. Nevertheless, whatever proliferative capacity may exist in these tissues, it is insufficient to produce tissue regeneration after injury. Skeletal muscle is usually classified as a permanent tissue, but satellite cells attached to the endomysial sheath provide some regenerative capacity for muscle. In permanent tissues, repair is typically dominated by scar formation.

Although it is believed that most mature tissues contain variable proportions of continuously dividing cells, quiescent cells that can return to the cell cycle, and nondividing cells, it is actually difficult to quantify the proportions of these cells in any tissue. Also, we now realize that cell proliferation is only one pathway of regeneration and that stem cells contribute to this process in important ways.

Cell proliferation is driven by signals provided by growth factors and from the extracellular matrix. Many different growth factors have been described; some act on multiple cell types and others are cell-selective (Chapter 1, Table 1-1). Growth factors are typically produced by cells near the site of damage. The most important sources of these growth factors are macrophages that are activated by the tissue injury, but epithelial and stromal cells also produce some of these factors. Several growth factors bind to ECM proteins and are displayed at high concentrations. All growth factors activate signaling pathways that ultimately induce the production of proteins that are involved in driving cells through the cell cycle and other proteins that release blocks on the cell cycle (checkpoints) (Chapter 1). In addition to responding to growth factors, cells use integrins to bind to ECM proteins, and signals from the integrins can also stimulate cell proliferation.

In the process of regeneration, proliferation of residual cells is supplemented by development of mature cells from stem cells. In Chapter 1 we introduced the major types of stem cells. In adults, the most important stem cells for regeneration after injury are tissue stem cells. These stem cells live in specialized niches, and it is believed that injury triggers signals in these niches that activate quiescent stem cells to proliferate and differentiate into mature cells that repopulate the injured tissue.

Mechanisms of Tissue Regeneration

The importance of regeneration in the replacement of injured tissues varies in different types of tissues and with the severity of injury.

- In labile tissues, such as the epithelia of the intestinal tract and skin, injured cells are rapidly replaced by proliferation of residual cells and differentiation of tissue stem cells provided the underlying basement membrane is intact. The growth factors involved in these processes are not defined. Loss of blood cells is corrected by proliferation of hematopoietic stem cells in the bone marrow and other tissues, driven by growth factors called colony-stimulating factors (CSFs), which are produced in response to the reduced numbers of blood cells.
- Tissue regeneration can occur in parenchymal organs with stable cell populations, but with the exception of the liver, this is usually a limited process. Pancreas, adrenal, thyroid, and lung have some regenerative capacity. The surgical removal of a kidney elicits in the remaining kidney a compensatory response that

consists of both hypertrophy and hyperplasia of proximal duct cells. The mechanisms underlying this response are not understood, but likely involve local production of growth factors and interactions of cells with the ECM. The extraordinary capacity of the liver to regenerate has made it a valuable model for studying this process, as described below.

Restoration of normal tissue structure can occur only if the residual tissue is structurally intact, as after partial surgical resection. By contrast, if the entire tissue is damaged by infection or inflammation, regeneration is incomplete and is accompanied by scarring. For example, extensive destruction of the liver with collapse of the reticulin framework, as occurs in a liver abscess, leads to scar formation even though the remaining liver cells have the capacity to regenerate.

Liver Regeneration

The human liver has a remarkable capacity to regenerate, as demonstrated by its growth after partial hepatectomy, which may be performed for tumor resection or for living-donor hepatic transplantation. The mythologic image of liver regeneration is the regrowth of the liver of Prometheus, which was eaten every day by an eagle sent by Zeus as punishment for stealing the secret of fire, and grew back overnight. The reality, although less dramatic, is still quite impressive.

Regeneration of the liver occurs by two major mechanisms: proliferation of remaining hepatocytes and repopulation from progenitor cells. Which mechanism plays the dominant role depends on the nature of the injury.

- **Proliferation of hepatocytes following partial hepatectomy.** In humans, resection of up to 90% of the liver can be corrected by proliferation of the residual hepatocytes. This classic model of tissue regeneration has been used experimentally to study the initiation and control of the process.

  Hepatocyte proliferation in the regenerating liver is triggered by the combined actions of cytokines and polypeptide growth factors. The process occurs in distinct stages (Fig. 3-25). In the first, or *priming,* phase, cytokines such as IL-6 are produced mainly by Kupffer cells and act on hepatocytes to make the parenchymal cells competent to receive and respond to growth factor signals. In the second, or *growth factor,* phase, growth factors such as HGF and TGF-α, produced by many cell types, act on primed hepatocytes to stimulate cell metabolism and entry of the cells into the cell cycle. Because hepatocytes are quiescent cells, it takes them several hours to enter the cell cycle, progress from G_0 to G_1, and reach the S phase of DNA replication. Almost all hepatocytes replicate during liver regeneration after partial hepatectomy. The wave of hepatocyte replication is followed by replication of nonparenchymal cells (Kupffer cells, endothelial cells, and stellate cells). During the phase of hepatocyte replication, more than 70 genes are activated; these include genes encoding transcription factors, cell cycle regulators, regulators of energy metabolism, and many others. In the final, *termination,* phase, hepatocytes return to quiescence. The nature of the stop signals is poorly understood; antiproliferative cytokines of the TGF-β family are likely involved.

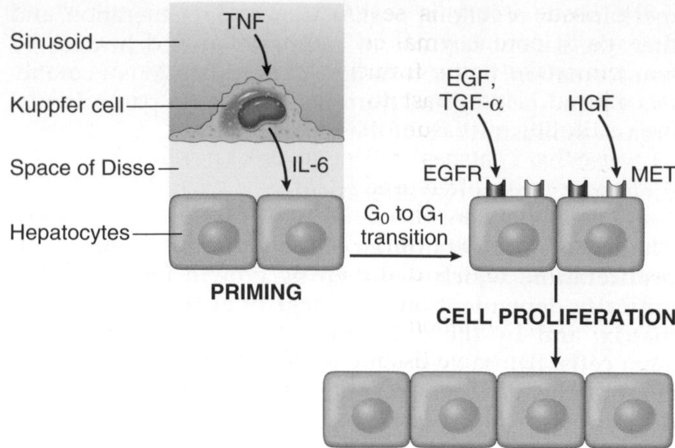

Figure 3-25 Liver regeneration by proliferation of hepatocytes. Following partial hepatectomy, the liver regenerates by proliferation of surviving cells. The process occurs in stages, including priming, followed by growth factor-induced proliferation. The main signals involved in these steps are shown. Once the mass of the liver is restored, the proliferation is terminated (not shown).

- **Liver regeneration from progenitor cells.** In situations where the proliferative capacity of hepatocytes is impaired, such as after chronic liver injury or inflammation, progenitor cells in the liver contribute to repopulation. In rodents, these progenitor cells have been called *oval cells* because of the shape of their nuclei. Some of these progenitor cells reside in specialized niches called *canals of Hering,* where bile canaliculi connect with larger bile ducts. The signals that drive proliferation of progenitor cells and their differentiation into mature hepatocytes are topics of active investigation.

KEY CONCEPTS

Repair by Regeneration

- Tissues are classified as labile, stable, and permanent, according to the proliferative capacity of their cells.
- Continuously dividing tissues (labile tissues) contain stem cells that differentiate to replenish lost cells and maintain tissue homeostasis.
- Cell proliferation is controlled by the cell cycle, and is stimulated by growth factors and interactions of cells with the extracellular matrix.
- Regeneration of the liver is a classic example of repair by regeneration. It is triggered by cytokines and growth factors produced in response to loss of liver mass and inflammation. In different situations, regeneration may occur by proliferation of surviving hepatocytes or repopulation from progenitor cells.

Repair by Connective Tissue Deposition

If repair cannot be accomplished by regeneration alone it occurs by replacement of the injured cells with connective tissue, leading to the formation of a scar, or by a combination of regeneration of some residual cells and scar formation. As discussed earlier, scarring may happen if the tissue injury is severe or chronic and results in damage to parenchymal cells and epithelia as well as to the connective tissue framework, or if nondividing cells are injured. In contrast to regeneration, which involves the restitution of tissue components, scar formation is a response that "patches" rather than restores the tissue. The term *scar* is most often used in connection to *wound healing* in the skin, but may also be used to describe the replacement of parenchymal cells in any tissue by collagen, as in the heart after myocardial infarction.

Steps in Scar Formation

Repair by connective tissue deposition consists of sequential processes that follow tissue injury and the inflammatory response (Fig. 3-26):

- **Angiogenesis** is the formation of new blood vessels, which supply nutrients and oxygen needed to support the repair process. Newly formed vessels are leaky because of incomplete interendothelial junctions and because VEGF, the growth factor that drives angiogenesis, increases vascular permeability. This leakiness accounts in part for the edema that may persist in healing wounds long after the acute inflammatory response has resolved.
- **Formation of granulation tissue.** Migration and proliferation of fibroblasts and deposition of loose connective tissue, together with the vessels and interspersed leukocytes, form *granulation tissue*. The term *granulation tissue* derives from its pink, soft, granular gross appearance, such as that seen beneath the scab of a skin wound. Its histologic appearance is characterized by proliferation of fibroblasts and new thin-walled, delicate capillaries (angiogenesis), in a loose extracellular matrix, often with admixed inflammatory cells, mainly macrophages (Fig. 3-27*A*). Granulation tissue progressively invades the site of injury; the amount of granulation tissue that is formed depends on the size of the tissue deficit created by the wound and the intensity of inflammation.
- **Remodeling of connective tissue.** Maturation and reorganization of the connective tissue (remodeling) produce the stable fibrous *scar*. The amount of connective tissue increases in the granulation tissue, eventually resulting

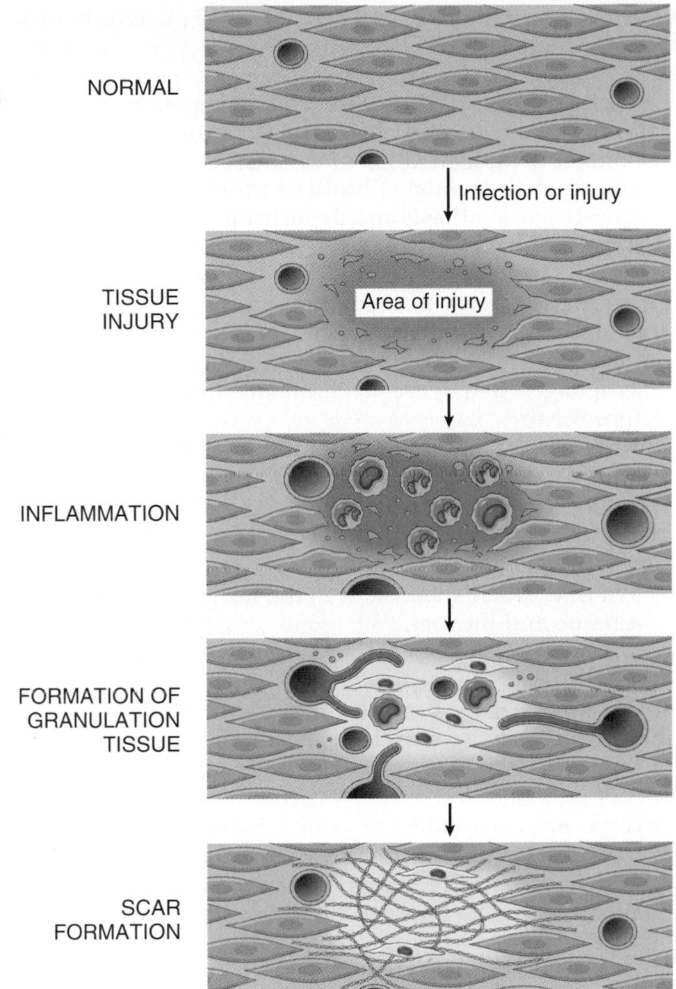

Figure 3-26 Steps in repair by scar formation. Injury to a tissue, such as muscle (which has limited regenerative capacity), first induces inflammation, which clears dead cells and microbes, if any. This is followed by the formation of vascularized granulation tissue and then the deposition of extracellular matrix to form the scar.

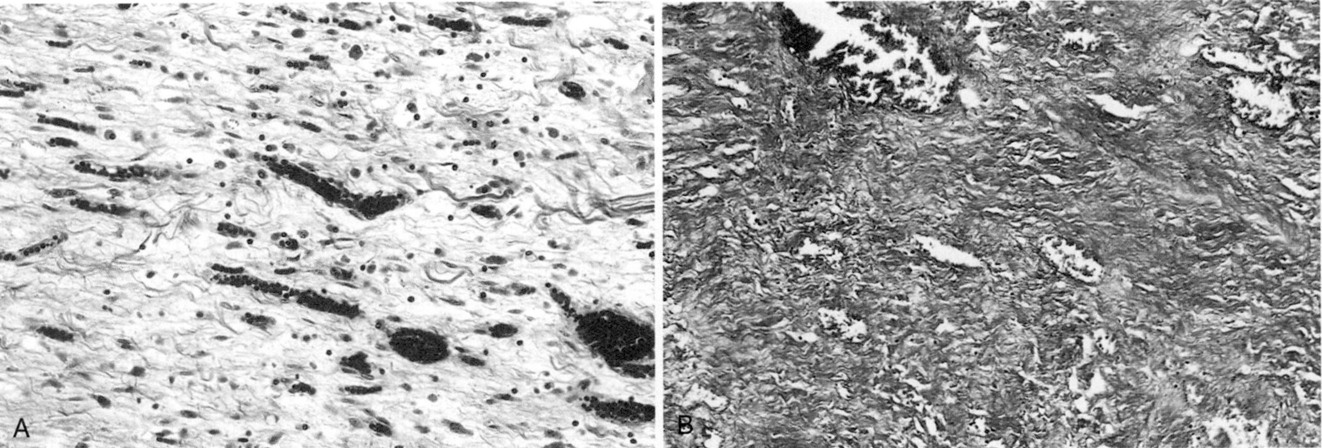

Figure 3-27 A, Granulation tissue showing numerous blood vessels, edema, and a loose extracellular matrix containing occasional inflammatory cells. Collagen is stained blue by the trichrome stain; minimal mature collagen can be seen at this point. **B,** Trichrome stain of mature scar, showing dense collagen, with only scattered vascular channels.

in the formation of a scar (Fig. 3-27*B*), which may remodel over time.

Macrophages play a central role in repair by clearing offending agents and dead tissue, providing growth factors for the proliferation of various cells, and secreting cytokines that stimulate fibroblast proliferation and connective tissue synthesis and deposition. The macrophages that are involved in repair are mostly of the alternatively activated (M2) type. It is not clear how the classically activated macrophages that dominate during inflammation, and are involved in getting rid of microbes and dead tissues, are gradually replaced by alternatively activated macrophages that serve to terminate inflammation and induce repair.

Repair begins within 24 hours of injury by the emigration of fibroblasts and the induction of fibroblast and endothelial cell proliferation. By 3 to 5 days, the specialized granulation tissue that is characteristic of healing is apparent.

We next describe the steps in the formation of granulation tissue and the scar.

Angiogenesis

Angiogenesis is the process of new blood vessel development from existing vessels. It is critical in healing at sites of injury, in the development of collateral circulations at sites of ischemia, and in allowing tumors to increase in size beyond the constraints of their original blood supply. Much work has been done to understand the mechanisms underlying angiogenesis, and therapies to either augment the process (e.g., to improve blood flow to a heart ravaged by coronary atherosclerosis) or inhibit it (to frustrate tumor growth or block pathologic vessel growth such as in diabetic retinopathy) are being developed.

Angiogenesis involves sprouting of new vessels from existing ones, and consists of the following steps (Fig. 3-28):

- Vasodilation in response to nitric oxide and increased permeability induced by vascular endothelial growth factor (VEGF)
- Separation of pericytes from the abluminal surface and breakdown of the basement membrane to allow formation of a vessel sprout
- Migration of endothelial cells toward the area of tissue injury
- Proliferation of endothelial cells just behind the leading front ("tip") of migrating cells
- Remodeling into capillary tubes
- Recruitment of periendothelial cells (pericytes for small capillaries and smooth muscle cells for larger vessels) to form the mature vessel
- Suppression of endothelial proliferation and migration and deposition of the basement membrane.

The process of angiogenesis involves several signaling pathways, cell-cell interactions, ECM proteins, and tissue enzymes.

- **Growth factors.** *Vascular endothelial growth factors (VEGFs)*, mainly VEGF-A (Chapter 1), stimulates both migration and proliferation of endothelial cells, thus initiating the process of capillary sprouting in angiogenesis. It promotes vasodilation by stimulating the production of NO and contributes to the formation of the vascular lumen. *Fibroblast growth factors (FGFs)*, mainly FGF-2, stimulates the proliferation of endothelial cells. It also promotes the migration of macrophages and fibroblasts to the damaged area, and stimulates epithelial cell migration to cover epidermal wounds. *Angiopoietins 1 and 2 (Ang 1 and Ang 2)* are growth factors that play a role in angiogenesis and the structural maturation of new vessels. Newly formed vessels need to be stabilized by the recruitment of pericytes and smooth muscle cells and by the deposition of connective tissue. Ang1 interacts with a tyrosine kinase receptor on endothelial cells called Tie2. The growth factors PDGF and TGF-β also participate in the stabilization process: PDGF recruits smooth muscle cells and TGF-β suppresses endothelial proliferation and migration, and enhances the production of ECM proteins.
- **Notch signaling.** Through "cross-talk" with VEGF, the Notch signaling pathway regulates the sprouting and branching of new vessels and thus ensures that the new vessels that are formed have the proper spacing to effectively supply the healing tissue with blood.

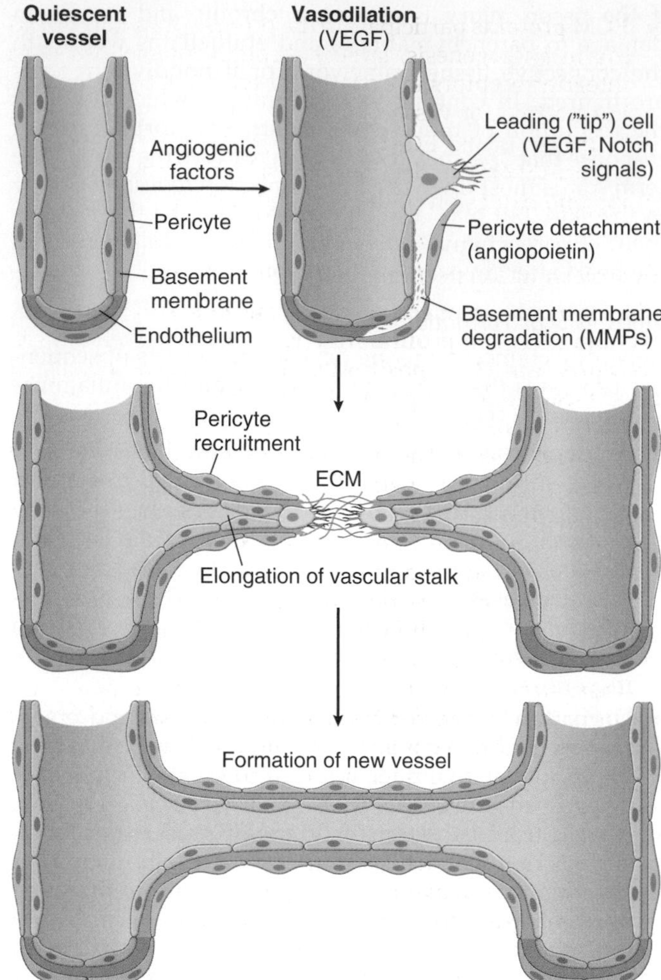

Figure 3-28 Angiogenesis. In tissue repair, angiogenesis occurs mainly by sprouting of new vessels. The steps in the process, and the major signals involved, are illustrated. The newly formed vessel joins up with other vessels (not shown) to form the new vascular bed.

- **ECM proteins** participate in the process of vessel sprouting in angiogenesis, largely through interactions with integrin receptors in endothelial cells and by providing the scaffold for vessel growth.
- **Enzymes** in the ECM, notably the matrix metalloproteinases (MMPs), degrade the ECM to permit remodeling and extension of the vascular tube.

Deposition of Connective Tissue

The laying down of connective tissue occurs in two steps: (1) migration and proliferation of fibroblasts into the site of injury and (2) deposition of ECM proteins produced by these cells. These processes are orchestrated by locally produced cytokines and growth factors, including PDGF, FGF-2, and TGF-β. The major sources of these factors are inflammatory cells, particularly alternatively activated (M2) macrophages, which are present at sites of injury and in granulation tissue. Sites of inflammation are also rich in mast cells, and in the appropriate chemotactic milieu lymphocytes may also be present. Each of these can secrete cytokines and growth factors that contribute to fibroblast proliferation and activation.

***Transforming growth factor-β (TGF-β)* is the most important cytokine for the synthesis and deposition of connective tissue proteins.** It is produced by most of the cells in granulation tissue, including alternatively activated macrophages. The levels of TGF-β in tissues are primarily regulated not by the transcription of the gene but by the posttranscriptional activation of latent TGF-β, the rate of secretion of the active molecule, and factors in the ECM, notably integrins, that enhance or diminish TGF-β activity. TGF-β stimulates fibroblast migration and proliferation, increased synthesis of collagen and fibronectin, and decreased degradation of ECM due to inhibition of metalloproteinases. TGF-β is involved not only in scar formation after injury but also in the development of fibrosis in lung, liver, and kidneys that follows chronic inflammation. TGF-β is also an antiinflammatory cytokine that serves to limit and terminate inflammatory responses. It does this by inhibiting lymphocyte proliferation and the activity of other leukocytes.

As healing progresses, the number of proliferating fibroblasts and new vessels decreases; however, the fibroblasts progressively assume a more synthetic phenotype, and hence there is increased deposition of ECM. Collagen synthesis, in particular, is critical to the development of strength in a healing wound site. As described later, collagen synthesis by fibroblasts begins early in wound healing (days 3 to 5) and continues for several weeks, depending on the size of the wound. Net collagen accumulation, however, depends not only on increased synthesis but also on diminished collagen degradation (discussed later). Ultimately, the granulation tissue evolves into a scar composed of largely inactive, spindle-shaped fibroblasts, dense collagen, fragments of elastic tissue, and other ECM components (Fig. 3-27*B*). As the scar matures, there is progressive vascular regression, which eventually transforms the highly vascularized granulation tissue into a pale, largely avascular scar. Some of the fibroblasts also acquire features of smooth muscle cells, including the presence of actin filaments, and are called *myofibroblasts*. These cells contribute to the contraction of the scar over time.

Remodeling of Connective Tissue

The outcome of the repair process is influenced by a balance between synthesis and degradation of ECM proteins. After its deposition, the connective tissue in the scar continues to be modified and remodeled. The degradation of collagens and other ECM components is accomplished by a family of *matrix metalloproteinases (MMPs)*, so called because they are dependent on metal ions (e.g., zinc) for their activity. MMPs should be distinguished from neutrophil elastase, cathepsin G, plasmin, and other serine proteinases that can also degrade ECM but are not metalloenzymes. MMPs include interstitial collagenases, which cleave fibrillar collagen (MMP-1, -2 and -3); gelatinases (MMP-2 and 9), which degrade amorphous collagen and fibronectin; and stromelysins (MMP-3, -10, and -11), which degrade a variety of ECM constituents, including proteoglycans, laminin, fibronectin, and amorphous collagen.

MMPs are produced by a variety of cell types (fibroblasts, macrophages, neutrophils, synovial cells, and some epithelial cells), and their synthesis and secretion are regulated by growth factors, cytokines, and other agents. The activity of the MMPs is tightly controlled. They are produced as inactive precursors (zymogens) that must be first activated; this is accomplished by proteases (e.g., plasmin) likely to be present only at sites of injury. In addition, activated collagenases can be rapidly inhibited by specific tissue inhibitors of metalloproteinases (TIMPs), produced by most mesenchymal cells. Thus, during scar formation, MMPs are activated to remodel the deposited ECM and then their activity is shut down by the TIMPs.

A family of enzymes related to MMPs is called ADAM (a disintegrin and metalloproteinase). ADAMs are anchored to the plasma membrane and cleave and release extracellular domains of cell-associated cytokines and growth factors, such as TNF, TGF-β, and members of the EGF family.

KEY CONCEPTS

Repair by Scar Formation

- Tissues are repaired by replacement with connective tissue and scar formation if the injured tissue is not capable of proliferation or if the structural framework is damaged and cannot support regeneration.
- The main components of connective tissue repair are angiogenesis, migration and proliferation of fibroblasts, collagen synthesis, and connective tissue remodeling.
- Repair by connective tissue starts with the formation of granulation tissue and culminates in the laying down of fibrous tissue.
- Multiple growth factors stimulate the proliferation of the cell types involved in repair.
- TGF-β is a potent fibrogenic agent; ECM deposition depends on the balance between fibrogenic agents, metalloproteinases (MMPs) that digest ECM, and the tissue inhibitors of MMPs (TIMPs).

Factors That Influence Tissue Repair

Tissue repair may be altered by a variety of influences, frequently reducing the quality or adequacy of the reparative process. Variables that modify healing may be extrinsic (e.g., infection) or intrinsic to the injured tissue, and systemic or local:

- **Infection** is clinically one of the most important causes of delay in healing; it prolongs inflammation and potentially increases the local tissue injury.
- **Diabetes** is a metabolic disease that compromises tissue repair for many reasons (Chapter 24), and is one of the most important systemic causes of abnormal wound healing.
- **Nutritional status** has profound effects on repair; protein deficiency, for example, and particularly vitamin C deficiency, inhibits collagen synthesis and retards healing.
- **Glucocorticoids (steroids)** have well-documented anti-inflammatory effects, and their administration may result in weakness of the scar due to inhibition of TGF-β production and diminished fibrosis. In some instances, however, the anti-inflammatory effects of glucocorticoids are desirable. For example, in corneal infections, glucocorticoids are sometimes prescribed (along with antibiotics) to reduce the likelihood of opacity that may result from collagen deposition.
- **Mechanical factors** such as increased local pressure or torsion may cause wounds to pull apart, or dehisce.
- **Poor perfusion,** due either to arteriosclerosis and diabetes or to obstructed venous drainage (e.g., in varicose veins), also impairs healing.
- **Foreign bodies** such as fragments of steel, glass, or even bone impede healing.
- **The type and extent of tissue injury** affects the subsequent repair. Complete restoration can occur only in tissues composed of stable and labile cells; even then, extensive injury will probably result in incomplete tissue regeneration and at least partial loss of function. Injury to tissues composed of permanent cells must inevitably result in scarring with, at most, attempts at functional compensation by the remaining viable elements. Such is the case with healing of a myocardial infarct.
- The **location of the injury** and the character of the tissue in which the injury occurs are also important. For example, inflammation arising in tissue spaces (e.g., pleural, peritoneal, synovial cavities) develops extensive exudates. Subsequent repair may occur by digestion of the exudate, initiated by the proteolytic enzymes of leukocytes and resorption of the liquefied exudate. This is called *resolution*, and in the absence of cellular necrosis, normal tissue architecture is generally restored. However, in the setting of larger accumulations, the exudate undergoes organization: granulation tissue grows into the exudate, and a fibrous scar ultimately forms.

Selected Clinical Examples of Tissue Repair and Fibrosis

So far, we have discussed the general principles and mechanisms of repair by regeneration and scar formation. In this section we describe two clinically significant types of repair—the healing of skin wounds (cutaneous wound healing) and fibrosis in injured parenchymal organs.

Healing of Skin Wounds

This is a process that involves both epithelial regeneration and the formation of connective tissue scar and is thus illustrative of the general principles that apply to healing in all tissues.

Based on the nature and size of the wound, the healing of skin wounds is said to occur by first or second intention.

Healing by First Intention

When the injury involves only the epithelial layer, the principal mechanism of repair is epithelial regeneration, also called *primary union* or *healing by first intention.* One of the simplest examples of this type of wound repair is the healing of a clean, uninfected surgical incision approximated by surgical sutures (Fig. 3-29). The incision causes only focal disruption of epithelial basement membrane continuity and death of relatively few epithelial and connective tissue cells. The repair consists of three connected processes: *inflammation*, *proliferation* of epithelial and other cells, and *maturation* of the connective tissue scar.

- Wounding causes the rapid activation of coagulation pathways, which results in the formation of a blood clot on the wound surface (Chapter 4). In addition to entrapped red cells, the clot contains fibrin, fibronectin, and complement proteins. The clot serves to stop bleeding and acts as a scaffold for migrating cells, which are attracted by growth factors, cytokines, and chemokines released into the area. Release of VEGF leads to increased vessel permeability and edema. As dehydration occurs at the external surface of the clot, a scab covering the wound is formed.
- Within 24 hours, neutrophils are seen at the incision margin, migrating toward the fibrin clot. They release proteolytic enzymes that begin to clear the debris. Basal cells at the cut edge of the epidermis begin to show increased mitotic activity. Within 24 to 48 hours, epithelial cells from both edges have begun to migrate and proliferate along the dermis, depositing basement membrane components as they progress. The cells meet in the midline beneath the surface scab, yielding a thin but continuous epithelial layer that closes the wound.
- By day 3, neutrophils have been largely replaced by macrophages, and granulation tissue progressively invades the incision space. As mentioned earlier, macrophages are key cellular constituents of tissue repair, clearing extracellular debris, fibrin, and other foreign material, and promoting angiogenesis and ECM deposition. Collagen fibers are now evident at the incision margins. Epithelial cell proliferation continues, forming a covering approaching the normal thickness of the epidermis.
- By day 5, neovascularization reaches its peak as granulation tissue fills the incisional space. These new vessels are leaky, allowing the passage of plasma proteins and fluid into the extravascular space. Thus, new granulation tissue is often edematous. Migration of fibroblasts to the site of injury is driven by chemokines, TNF, PDGF, TGF-β, and FGF. Their subsequent proliferation is triggered by multiple growth factors, including PDGF, EGF, TGF-β, and FGF, and the cytokines IL-1 and

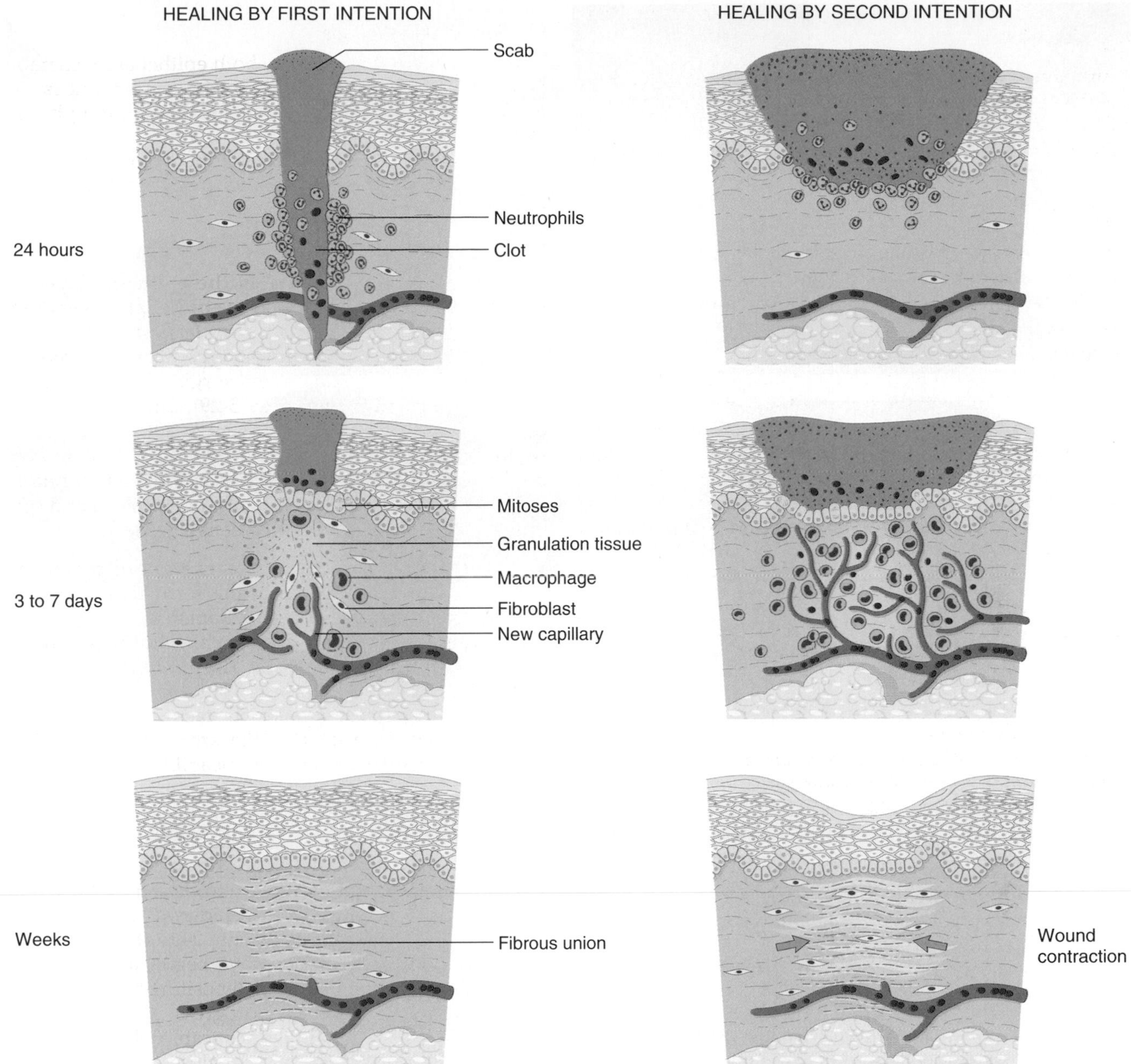

Figure 3-29 Steps in wound healing by first intention (left) and second intention (right). In the latter, note the large amount of granulation tissue and wound contraction.

TNF. Macrophages are the main source for these factors, although other inflammatory cells and platelets may also produce them. The fibroblasts produce ECM proteins, and collagen fibrils become more abundant and begin to bridge the incision. The epidermis recovers its normal thickness as differentiation of surface cells yields a mature epidermal architecture with surface keratinization.

- During the second week, there is continued collagen accumulation and fibroblast proliferation. The leukocyte infiltrate, edema, and increased vascularity are substantially diminished. The process of "blanching" begins, accomplished by increasing collagen deposition within the incisional scar and the regression of vascular channels.
- By the end of the first month, the scar comprises a cellular connective tissue largely devoid of inflammatory cells and covered by an essentially normal epidermis. However, the dermal appendages destroyed in the line of the incision are permanently lost. The tensile strength of the wound increases with time, as described later.

Healing by Second Intention

When cell or tissue loss is more extensive, such as in large wounds, abscesses, ulceration, and ischemic necrosis (infarction) in parenchymal organs, the repair process involves a combination of regeneration and scarring. In healing of skin wounds by *second intention*, also known as healing by *secondary union* (Figs. 3-29 and 3-30), the

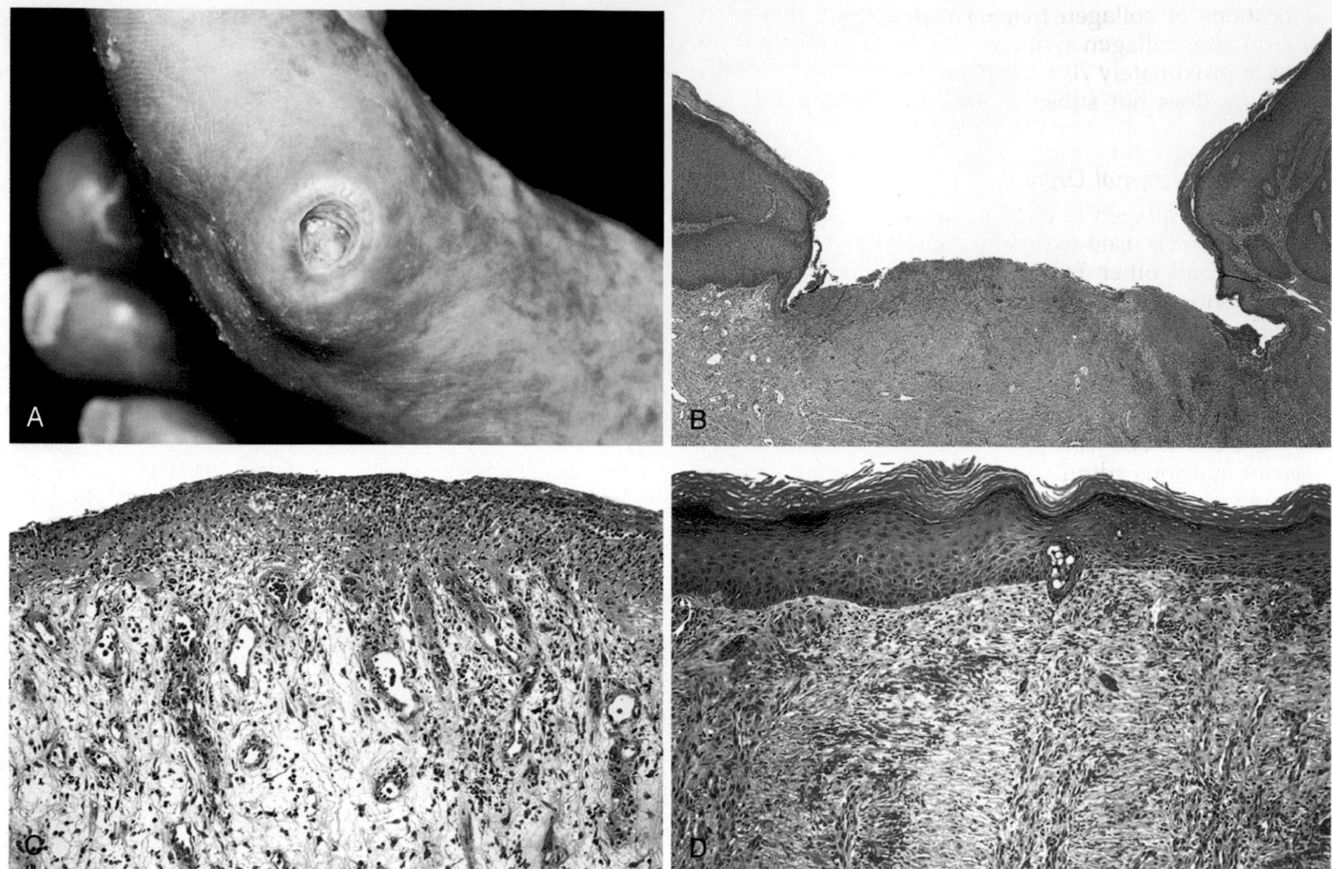

Figure 3-30 Healing of skin ulcers. **A,** Pressure ulcer of the skin, commonly found in diabetic patients. The histologic slides show a skin ulcer with a large gap between the edges of the lesion **(B),** a thin layer of epidermal reepithelialization and extensive granulation tissue formation in the dermis **(C),** and continuing reepithelialization of the epidermis and wound contraction **(D).** (Courtesy Z. Argenyi, MD, University of Washington, Seattle, Wash.)

inflammatory reaction is more intense, there is development of abundant granulation tissue, accumulation of ECM and formation of a large scar, and wound contraction by the action of myofibroblasts.

Secondary healing differs from primary healing in several respects:

- In wounds causing large tissue deficits, the fibrin clot is larger, and there is more exudate and necrotic debris in the wounded area. Inflammation is more intense because large tissue defects have a greater volume of necrotic debris, exudate, and fibrin that must be removed. Consequently, large defects have a greater potential for secondary, inflammation-mediated, injury.
- Much larger amounts of granulation tissue are formed. Larger defects require a greater volume of granulation tissue to fill in the gaps and provide the underlying framework for the regrowth of tissue epithelium. A greater volume of granulation tissue generally results in a greater mass of scar tissue.
- At first a provisional matrix containing fibrin, plasma fibronectin, and type III collagen is formed, but in about 2 weeks this is replaced by a matrix composed primarily of type I collagen. Ultimately, the original granulation tissue scaffold is converted into a pale, avascular scar, composed of spindle-shaped fibroblasts, dense collagen, fragments of elastic tissue, and other ECM components. The dermal appendages that have been destroyed in the line of the incision are permanently lost. The epidermis recovers its normal thickness and architecture. By the end of the first month, the scar is made up of acellular connective tissue devoid of inflammatory infiltrate, covered by intact epidermis.
- Wound contraction generally occurs in large surface wounds. The contraction helps to close the wound by decreasing the gap between its dermal edges and by reducing the wound surface area. Hence, it is an important feature in healing by secondary union. The initial steps of wound contraction involve the formation, at the edge of the wound, of a network of *myofibroblasts*, which are modified fibroblasts exhibiting many of the ultrastructural and functional features of contractile smooth muscle cells. Within 6 weeks, large skin defects may be reduced to 5% to 10% of their original size, largely by contraction.

Wound Strength

Carefully sutured wounds have approximately 70% of the strength of normal skin, largely because of the placement of sutures. When sutures are removed, usually at 1 week, wound strength is approximately 10% of that of unwounded skin, but this increases rapidly over the next 4 weeks. The recovery of tensile strength results from the excess of collagen synthesis over collagen degradation during the first 2 months of healing, and, at later times, from structural modifications of collagen fibers (cross-linking, increased fiber size) after collagen synthesis ceases. Wound strength reaches approximately 70% to 80% of normal by 3 months but usually does not substantially improve beyond that point.

Fibrosis in Parenchymal Organs

Deposition of collagen is part of normal wound healing. The term *fibrosis* is used to denote the excessive deposition of collagen and other ECM components in a tissue. As already mentioned, the terms *scar* and *fibrosis* are used interchangeably, but *fibrosis* most often refers to the abnormal deposition of collagen that occurs in internal organs in chronic diseases. The basic mechanisms of fibrosis are the same as those of scar formation in the skin during tissue repair. Fibrosis is a pathologic process induced by persistent injurious stimuli such as chronic infections and immunologic reactions, and is typically associated with loss of tissue (Fig. 3-31). It may be responsible for substantial organ dysfunction and even organ failure.

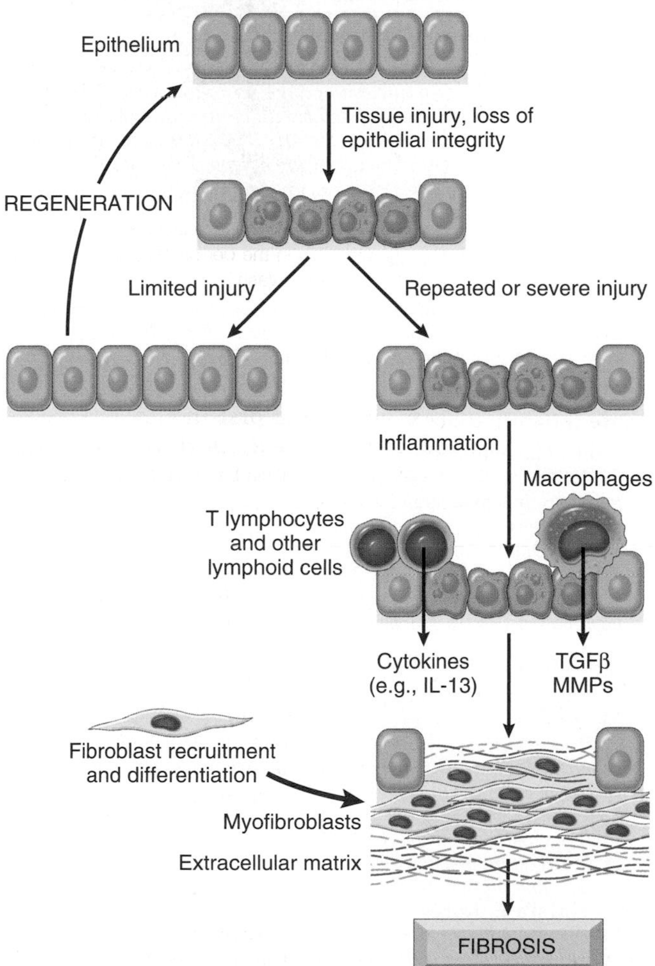

Figure 3-31 Mechanisms of fibrosis. Persistent tissue injury leads to chronic inflammation and loss of tissue architecture. Cytokines produced by macrophages and other leukocytes stimulate the migration and proliferation of fibroblasts and myofibroblasts and the deposition of collagen and other extracellular matrix proteins. The net result is replacement of normal tissue by fibrosis.

As discussed earlier, the major cytokine involved in fibrosis is TGF-β. The mechanisms that lead to the activation of TGF-β in fibrosis are not precisely known, but cell death by necrosis or apoptosis and the production of reactive oxygen species seem to be important triggers of the activation, regardless of the tissue. Similarly, the cells that produce collagen under TGF-β stimulation may vary depending on the tissue. In most organs, such as in lung and kidney, myofibroblasts are the main source of collagen, but stellate cells are the major collagen producers in liver cirrhosis.

Fibrotic disorders include diverse chronic and debilitating diseases such as liver cirrhosis, systemic sclerosis (scleroderma), fibrosing diseases of the lung (idiopathic pulmonary fibrosis, pneumoconioses, and drug-, radiation-induced pulmonary fibrosis), end-stage kidney disease, and constrictive pericarditis. These conditions are discussed in the appropriate chapters throughout the book. Because of the tremendous functional impairment caused by fibrosis in these conditions, there is great interest in the development of antifibrotic drugs.

Abnormalities in Tissue Repair

Complications in tissue repair can arise from abnormalities in any of the basic components of the process, including deficient scar formation, excessive formation of the repair components, and formation of contractures.

- **Inadequate formation of granulation tissue or formation of a scar can lead to two types of complications: wound dehiscence and ulceration.** Dehiscence or rupture of a wound, although not common, occurs most frequently after abdominal surgery and is due to increased abdominal pressure. Vomiting, coughing, or ileus can generate mechanical stress on the abdominal wound. Wounds can ulcerate because of inadequate vascularization during healing. For example, lower extremity wounds in individuals with atherosclerotic peripheral vascular disease typically ulcerate (Chapter 11). Nonhealing wounds also form in areas devoid of sensation. These neuropathic ulcers are occasionally seen in patients with diabetic peripheral neuropathy (Chapters 24 and 27).
- **Excessive formation of the components of the repair process can give rise to hypertrophic scars and keloids.** The accumulation of excessive amounts of collagen may give rise to a raised scar known as a *hypertrophic scar*; if the scar tissue grows beyond the boundaries of the original wound and does not regress, it is called a *keloid* (Fig. 3-32). Keloid formation seems to be an individual predisposition, and for unknown reasons this aberration is somewhat more common in African Americans. Hypertrophic scars generally develop after thermal or traumatic injury that involves the deep layers of the dermis.
- **Exuberant granulation** is another deviation in wound healing consisting of the formation of excessive amounts of granulation tissue, which protrudes above the level of the surrounding skin and blocks reepithelialization (this process has been called, with more literary fervor, *proud flesh*). Excessive granulation must be removed by cautery or surgical excision to permit restoration of the

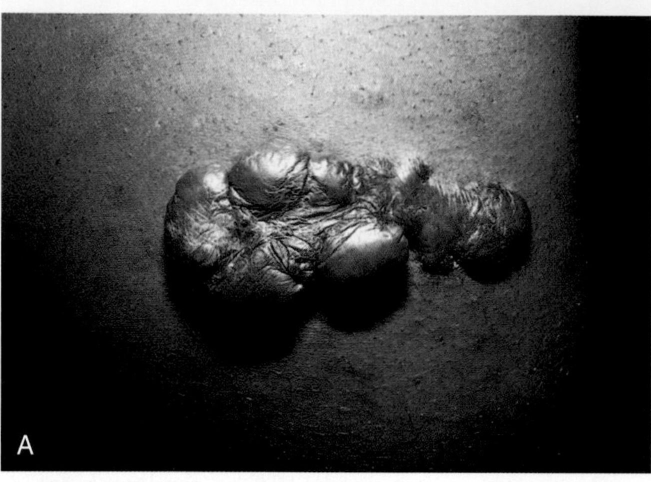

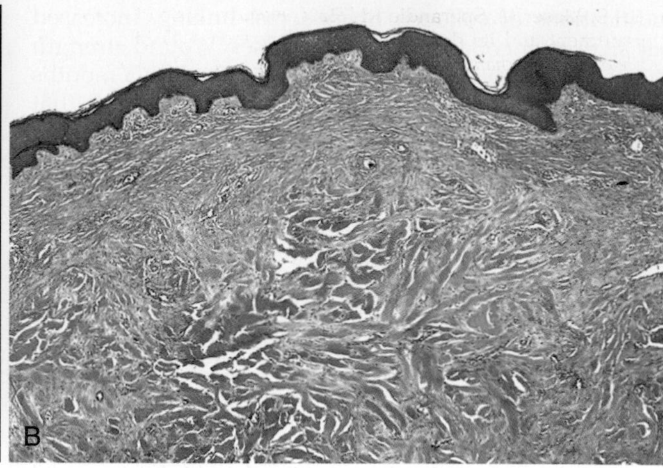

Figure 3-32 Keloid. **A,** Excess collagen deposition in the skin forming a raised scar known as *keloid*. **B,** Note the thick connective tissue deposition in the dermis. (**A,** From Murphy GF, Herzberg AJ: Atlas of Dermatopathology. Philadelphia, WB Saunders, 1996, p 219; **B,** Courtesy Z. Argenyi, MD, University of Washington, Seattle, Wash.)

continuity of the epithelium. Fortunately rarely, incisional scars or traumatic injuries may be followed by exuberant proliferation of fibroblasts and other connective tissue elements that may, in fact, recur after excision. Called *desmoids*, or *aggressive fibromatoses*, these neoplasms lie in the interface between benign and malignant (though low-grade) tumors.

- *Contraction* in the size of a wound is an important part of the normal healing process. An exaggeration of this process gives rise to contracture and results in deformities of the wound and the surrounding tissues. Contractures are particularly prone to develop on the palms, the soles, and the anterior aspect of the thorax. Contractures are commonly seen after serious burns and can compromise the movement of joints.

KEY CONCEPTS

Cutaneous Wound Healing and Pathologic Aspects of Repair

- The main phases of cutaneous wound healing are inflammation, formation of granulation tissue, and ECM remodeling.
- Cutaneous wounds can heal by primary union (first intention) or secondary union (secondary intention); secondary healing involves more extensive scarring and wound contraction.
- Wound healing can be altered by many conditions, particularly infection and diabetes; the type, volume, and location of the injury are important factors that influence the healing process.
- Excessive production of ECM can cause keloids in the skin.
- Persistent stimulation of collagen synthesis in chronic inflammatory diseases leads to fibrosis of the tissue, often with extensive loss of the tissue and functional impairment.

SUGGESTED READINGS

General Mechanisms of Inflammation

Okin D, Medzhitov R: Evolution of inflammatory diseases. *Curr Biol* 22:R733–40, 2012. *[An interesting conceptual discussion of the balance between the high potential cost and benefit of the inflammatory response and how this balance may be disturbed by environmental changes, accounting for the association between inflammation and many of the diseases of the modern world.]*

Rock KL, Latz E, Ontiveros F, et al: The sterile inflammatory response. *Annu Rev Immunol* 28:321–42, 2010. *[An excellent discussion of how the immune system recognizes necrotic cells and other noninfectious harmful agents.]*

Takeuchi O, Akira S: Pattern recognition receptors and inflammation. *Cell* 140:805, 2010. *[An excellent overview of Toll-like receptors and other pattern recognition receptor families, and their roles in host defense and inflammation.]*

Acute Inflammation: Vascular Reactions

Alitalo K: The lymphatic vasculature in disease. *Nat Med* 17:1371–80, 2011. *[An excellent review of the cell biology of lymphatic vessels, their functions in immune and inflammatory reactions, and their roles in inflammatory, neoplastic and other diseases.]*

Vestweber D: Relevance of endothelial junctions in leukocyte extravasation and vascular permeability. *Ann N Y Acad Sci* 1257:184–92, 2012. *[A good review of the basic processes of vascular permeability and how interendothelial junctions are regulated.]*

Acute Inflammation: Role of Leukocytes

Amulic B, Cazalet C, Hayes GL, et al: Neutrophil Function: From Mechanisms to Disease. *Annu Rev Immunol* 30:459–89, 2012. *[An excellent review on neutrophils – their recruitment, activation, functions in microbe elimination, and interactions with other cells of the immune system.]*

Flannagan RS, Jaumouillé V, Grinstein S: The Cell Biology of Phagocytosis. *Annu Rev Pathol* 7:61–98, 2012. *[A modern discussion of the receptors involved in phagocytosis, the molecular control of the process, and the biology and functions of phagosomes.]*

Kolaczkowska E, Kubes P: Neutrophil recruitment and function in health and inflammation. *Nat Rev Immunol* 13:159–75, 2013. *[An excellent review of neutrophil generation, recruitment, functions and fates, and their roles in different types of inflammatory reactions.]*

Muller WA: Mechanisms of leukocyte transendothelial migration. *Annu Rev Pathol* 6:323, 2011. *[A thoughtful review of the mechanisms by which leukocytes traverse the endothelium.]*

Papayannapoulos V, Zychlinsky A: NETs: a new strategy for using old weapons. *Trends Immunol* 30:513, 2009. *[A review of a newly discovered mechanism by which neutrophils destroy microbes.]*

Schmidt S, Moser M, Sperandio M: The molecular basis of leukocyte recruitment and its deficiencies. *Mol Immunol* 55:49–58, 2013. *[A review of the mechanisms of leukocyte recruitment and leukocyte adhesion deficiencies.]*

Williams MR, Azcutia V, Newton G, et al: Emerging mechanisms of neutrophil recruitment across endothelium. *Trends Immunol* 32:461–9, 2011. *[A review of the stimuli for leukocyte migration through blood vessels and the signaling pathways activated in leukocytes in response to these stimuli.]*

Mediators of Inflammation

Andersson U, Tracey KJ: Neural reflexes in inflammation and immunity. *J Exp Med* 209:1057–68, 2012. *[A thoughtful review that explores the mechanisms by which neural reflexes may influence inflammatory reactions.]*

Charo IF, Ransohoff RM: The many roles of chemokines and chemokine receptors in inflammation. *N Engl J Med* 354:610, 2006. *[An overview of the functions of chemokines in inflammation.]*

Di Gennaro A, Haeggström JZ: The leukotrienes: immune-modulating lipid mediators of disease. *Adv Immunol* 116:51–92, 2012. *[A comprehensive review of the biochemistry of leukotrienes and their receptors, and the roles of these mediators in various diseases.]*

Gabay C, Lamacchia C, Palmer G: IL-1 pathways in inflammation and human diseases. *Nat Rev Rheumatol* 6:232, 2010. *[An excellent review of the biology of IL-1 and the therapeutic targeting of this cytokine in inflammatory diseases.]*

Keystone EC, Ware CF: Tumor necrosis factor and anti-tumor necrosis factor therapies. *J Rheumatol Suppl* 85:27–39, 2010. *[An excellent review of TNF and its receptors, and the development and clinical efficacy of TNF inhibitors.]*

Khanapure SP, Garvey DS, Janero DR, et al: Eicosanoids in inflammation: biosynthesis, pharmacology, and therapeutic frontiers. *Curr Top Med Chem* 7:311, 2007. *[A summary of the properties of this important class of inflammatory mediators.]*

Nathan C, Cunningham-Bussel A: Beyond oxidative stress: an immunologist's guide to reactive oxygen species. *Nat Rev Immunol* 13:349–61, 2013. *[An excellent modern review of the production, catabolism, targets and actions of reactive oxygen species, and their roles in inflammation.]*

Ricklin D, Lambris JD: Complement in immune and inflammatory disorders. *J Immunol* 190:3831–8, *3839–47*, 2013. *[Two companion articles on the biochemistry and biology of the complement system, and the development of therapeutic agents to alter complement activity in disease.]*

Zlotnik A, Yoshie O: The chemokine superfamily revisited. *Immunity* 36:705–16, 2012. *[An excellent update on the classification, functions, and clinical relevance of chemokines and their receptors.]*

Chronic Inflammation: Role of Macrophages and Other Cells

Caielli S, Banchereau J, Pascual V: Neutrophils come of age in chronic inflammation. *Curr Opin Immunol* 24:671–7, 2012. *[A discussion of the underappreciated role of neutrophils in disorders characterized by chronic inflammation.]*

Nagy JA, Dvorak AM, Dvorak HF: VEGF-A and the induction of pathological angiogenesis. *Annu Rev Pathol* 2:251, 2007. *[A review of the VEGF family of growth factors and their role in angiogenesis in cancer, inflammation, and various disease states.]*

Nathan C, Ding A: Nonresolving inflammation. *Cell* 140:871, 2010. *[A discussion of the abnormalities that lead to chronic inflammation.]*

Sica A, Mantovani A: Macrophage plasticity and polarization: in vivo veritas. *J Clin Invest* 122:787–95, 2012. *[An excellent review of macrophage subpopulations, their generation, and their roles in inflammation, infections, cancer, and metabolic disorders.]*

Sepsis

Aziz M, Jacob A, Yang WL, et al: Current trends in inflammatory and immunomodulatory mediators in sepsis. *J Leukoc Biol* 93:329–42, 2013. *[A comprehensive review of the roles of cytokines and other mediators in the development and resolution of the systemic inflammatory response syndrome.]*

Stearns-Kurosawa DJ, Osuchowski MF, Valentine C, et al: The pathogenesis of sepsis. *Annu Rev Pathol* 6:19–48, 2011. *[An excellent review of the pathogenesis of sepsis, focusing on the cells involved, the importance of cell death, the links between inflammation and coagulation, the utility of biomarkers, and therapeutic approaches.]*

Tissue Repair: Regeneration and Fibrosis

Daley GQ: The promise and perils of stem cell therapeutics. *Cell Stem Cell* 10:740–9, 2012. *[An excellent summary of the challenges in the development of stem cell based therapies, and the potential of such treatments.]*

Friedman SL, Sheppard D, Duffield JS, et al: Therapy for fibrotic diseases: nearing the starting line. *Sci Transl Med* 5:167sr1, 2013. *[An excellent review of the current concepts of the pathogenesis of fibrosis, emphasizing the roles of different cell populations and the extracellular matrix, and the potential for translating basic knowledge to the development of new therapies.]*

Grompe M: Tissue stem cells: new tools and functional diversity. *Cell Stem Cell* 10:685–9, 2012. *[A brief overview of the properties and identification of stem cells in different tissues.]*

Gurtner GC, Werner S, Barrandon Y, et al: Wound repair and regeneration. *Nature* 453:314–21, 2008. *[A thoughtful discussion of the mechanisms of repair after tissue damage in mammals.]*

Hernandez-Gea V, Friedman SL: Pathogenesis of liver fibrosis. *Annu Rev Pathol* 6:425–56, 2011. *[A comprehensive discussion of the mechanisms of fibrosis in the liver, emphasizing the roles of different cells and matrix proteins and the molecular control of the process.]*

Hubmacher D, Apte SS: The biology of the extracellular matrix: novel insights. *Curr Opin Rheumatol* 25:65–70, 2013. *[A brief review of the structural and biochemical properties of the ECM.]*

Klingberg F, Hinz B, White ES: The myofibroblast matrix: implications for tissue repair and fibrosis. *J Pathol* 229:298–309, 2013. *[An excellent review of the properties of myofibroblasts and ECM proteins, and their roles in tissue repair and fibrosis.]*

Mantovani A, Biswas SK, Galdiero MR, et al: Macrophage plasticity and polarization in tissue repair and remodelling. *J Pathol* 229: 176–85, 2013. *[An excellent review comparing macrophage subsets and the role of these cells in the resolution of inflammation and tissue repair.]*

Murawala P, Tanaka EM, Currie JD: Regeneration: the ultimate example of wound healing. *Semin Cell Dev Biol* 23:954–62, 2012. *[A thoughtful discussion of the process of regeneration in amphibians and how and why it is different in mammals.]*

Novak ML, Koh TJ: Macrophage phenotypes during tissue repair. *J Leukoc Biol* 93:875–81, 2013. *[A review of macrophage phenotypes and how they change during inflammation and tissue repair, emphasizing the concept that these phenotypes are plastic and dynamic and may not represent committed lineages.]*

Okita K, Yamanaka S: Induced pluripotent stem cells: opportunities and challenges. *Philos Trans R Soc Lond B Biol Sci* 366:2198–207, 2011. *[A review of the exciting technology for generating iPS cells for regenerative medicine.]*

Page-McCaw A, Ewald AJ, Werb Z: Matrix metalloproteinases and the regulation of tissue remodelling. *Nat Rev Mol Cell Biol* 8:221, 2007. *[A review of the function of matrix modifying enzymes in tissue repair.]*

Van Dyken SJ, Locksley RM: Interleukin-4- and interleukin-13-mediated alternatively activated macrophages: roles in homeostasis and disease. *Annu Rev Immunol* 31:317–43, 2013. *[An excellent review of the generation and functions of alternatively activated macrophages.]*

Wick G, Grundtman C, Mayerl C, et al: The immunology of fibrosis. *Annu Rev Immunol* 31:107–35, 2013. *[An excellent review of the role of the immune system in fibrosis during tissue repair and in chronic diseases, including autoimmune disorders, atherosclerosis, fibrotic disorders of different organs, and cancer.]*

Wynn TA, Ramalingam TR: Mechanisms of fibrosis: therapeutic translation for fibrotic disease. *Nat Med* 18:1028–40, 2012. *[An excellent review of the mechanisms of tissue fibrosis and the antifibrotic therapeutic strategies being developed.]*

See TARGETED THERAPY available online at www.studentconsult.com

CHAPTER 4

Hemodynamic Disorders, Thromboembolic Disease, and Shock

CHAPTER CONTENTS

Cardiovascular disease is the most important cause of morbidity and mortality in Western society. In 2008, it was estimated that 83 million people in the United States had one or more forms of cardiovascular disease, accounting for 35% to 40% of deaths. These diseases primarily affect one of the three major components of the cardiovascular system: the heart, the blood vessels, and the blood itself, which is composed of water, salts, a wide variety of proteins, elements that regulate clotting (the coagulation factors and platelets), and other formed elements (red cells and white cells). For simplicity, disorders that affect each component of the cardiovascular system are considered separately, recognizing that disturbances affecting one component often lead to adaptations and abnormalities involving others. Herein, we focus on disorders of hemodynamics (edema, effusions, congestion, and shock), provide an overview of disorders of abnormal bleeding and clotting (thrombosis), and discuss the various forms of embolism. Diseases that primarily affect the blood vessels and the heart are discussed in Chapters 11 and 12, respectively, while specific bleeding disorders are covered in greater detail in Chapter 14.

Edema and Effusions

Disorders that perturb cardiovascular, renal, or hepatic function are often marked by the accumulation of fluid in tissues (edema) or body cavities (effusions). Under normal circumstances, the tendency of vascular hydrostatic pressure to push water and salts out of capillaries into the interstitial space is nearly balanced by the tendency of plasma colloid osmotic pressure to pull water and salts back into vessels. There is usually a small net movement of fluid into the interstitium, but this drains into lymphatic vessels and ultimately returns to the bloodstream via the thoracic duct, keeping the tissues "dry" (Fig. 4-1). **Elevated hydrostatic pressure or diminished colloid osmotic pressure disrupts this balance and results in increased movement of fluid out of vessels.** If the net rate of fluid movement exceeds the rate of lymphatic drainage, fluid accumulates. Within tissues the result is *edema*, and if a serosal surface is involved, fluid may accumulate within the adjacent body cavity as an *effusion*.

Edema fluids and effusions may be *inflammatory* or *noninflammatory* (Table 4-1). Inflammation-related edema and effusions are discussed in detail in Chapter 3. These protein-rich *exudates* accumulate due to increases in vascular permeability caused by inflammatory mediators. Usually, inflammation-associated edema is localized to one or a few tissues, but in systemic inflammatory states, such as sepsis, that produce widespread endothelial injury and dysfunction, generalized edema may appear, often with severe consequences (discussed later). In contrast, noninflammatory edema and effusions are protein-poor fluids called *transudates*. Noninflammatory edema and effusions are common in many diseases, including heart failure, liver failure, renal disease, and severe nutritional disorders (Fig. 4-2). We will now discuss the various causes of edema.

The contributions of Dr. Richard N Mitchell to this chapter over the past many editions are gratefully acknowledged.

Increased Hydrostatic Pressure

Increases in hydrostatic pressure are mainly caused by disorders that impair venous return. If the impairment is localized (e.g., a deep venous thrombosis [DVT] in a lower extremity), then the resulting edema is confined to the affected part. Conditions leading to systemic increases in venous pressure (e.g., *congestive heart failure*, Chapter 12) are understandably associated with more widespread edema.

Reduced Plasma Osmotic Pressure

Under normal circumstances albumin accounts for almost half of the total plasma protein; it follows that conditions leading to inadequate synthesis or increased loss of albumin from the circulation are common causes of reduced plasma oncotic pressure. Reduced albumin synthesis occurs mainly in severe liver diseases (e.g., end-stage cirrhosis, Chapter 18) and protein malnutrition (Chapter 9). An important cause of albumin loss is the *nephrotic syndrome* (Chapter 20), in which albumin leaks into the urine through abnormally permeable glomerular capillaries. Regardless of cause, reduced plasma osmotic pressure leads in a stepwise fashion to edema, reduced intravascular volume, renal hypoperfusion, and secondary hyperaldosteronism. Not only does the ensuing salt and water retention by the kidney fail to correct the plasma volume deficit, but it also exacerbates the edema, because the primary defect—a low plasma protein level—persists.

Table 4-1 Pathophysiologic Categories of Edema

Increased Hydrostatic Pressure
Impaired Venous Return
Congestive heart failure
Constrictive pericarditis
Ascites (liver cirrhosis)
Venous obstruction or compression
Thrombosis
External pressure (e.g., mass)
Lower extremity inactivity with prolonged dependency
Arteriolar Dilation
Heat
Neurohumoral dysregulation
Reduced Plasma Osmotic Pressure (Hypoproteinemia)
Protein-losing glomerulopathies (nephrotic syndrome)
Liver cirrhosis (ascites)
Malnutrition
Protein-losing gastroenteropathy
Lymphatic Obstruction
Inflammatory
Neoplastic
Postsurgical
Postirradiation
Sodium Retention
Excessive salt intake with renal insufficiency
Increased tubular reabsorption of sodium
Renal hypoperfusion
Increased renin-angiotensin-aldosterone secretion
Inflammation
Acute inflammation
Chronic inflammation
Angiogenesis

Modified from Leaf A, Cotran RS. Renal pathophysiology, 3rd ed. New York, Oxford University Press, 1985, p 146.

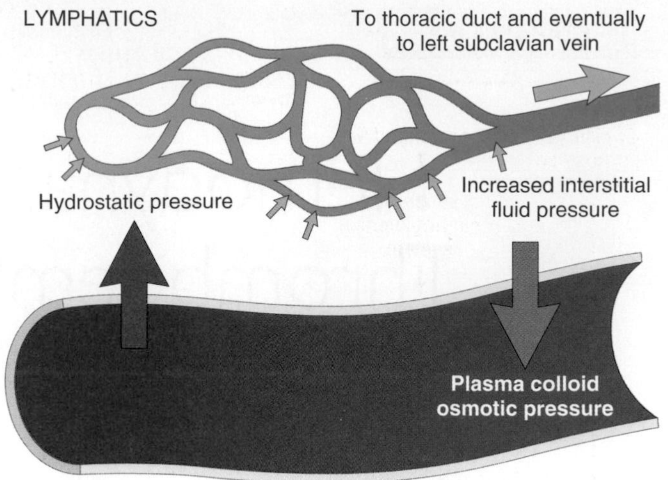

Figure 4-1 Factors influencing fluid movement across capillary walls. Normally, hydrostatic and osmotic forces are nearly balanced so that there is little net movement of fluid out of vessels. Many different pathologic disorders (Table 4-1) are associated with increases in capillary hydrostatic pressure or decreases in plasma osmotic pressure that lead to the extravasation of fluid into tissues. Lymphatic vessels remove much of the excess fluid, but if the capacity for lymphatic drainage is exceeded, tissue edema results.

Sodium and Water Retention

Increased salt retention—with obligate retention of associated water—causes both increased hydrostatic pressure (due to intravascular fluid volume expansion) and diminished vascular colloid osmotic pressure (due to dilution). Salt retention occurs whenever renal function is compromised, such as in primary kidney disorders and in cardiovascular disorders that decrease renal perfusion. One of the most important causes of renal hypoperfusion is congestive heart failure, which (like hypoproteinemia) results in the activation of the renin-angiotensin-aldosterone axis. In early heart failure, this response is beneficial, as the retention of sodium and water and other adaptations, including increased vascular tone and elevated levels of antidiuretic hormone, improve cardiac output and restore normal renal perfusion. However, as heart failure worsens and cardiac output diminishes, the retained fluid merely increases the hydrostatic pressure, leading to edema and effusions.

Lymphatic Obstruction

Trauma, fibrosis, invasive tumors, and infectious agents can all disrupt lymphatic vessels and impair the clearance of interstitial fluid, resulting in *lymphedema* in the affected part of the body. A dramatic example is seen in parasitic *filariasis,* in which the organism induces obstructive fibrosis of lymphatic channels and lymph nodes. This may result in edema of the external genitalia and lower limbs that is so massive as to earn the appellation *elephantiasis.* Severe edema of the upper extremity may also complicate surgical removal and/or irradiation of the breast and associated axillary lymph nodes in patients with breast cancer.

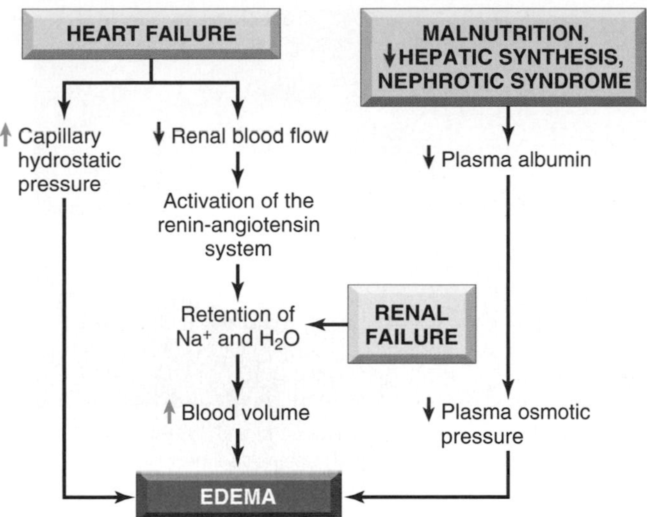

Figure 4-2 Mechanisms of systemic edema in heart failure, renal failure, malnutrition, hepatic failure, and nephrotic syndrome.

MORPHOLOGY

Edema is easily recognized grossly; microscopically, it is appreciated as clearing and separation of the extracellular matrix and subtle cell swelling. Any organ or tissue can be involved, but edema is most commonly seen in subcutaneous tissues, the lungs, and the brain. **Subcutaneous edema** can be diffuse or more conspicuous in regions with high hydrostatic pressures. Its distribution is often influenced by gravity (e.g., it appears in the legs when standing and the sacrum when recumbent), a feature termed **dependent edema**. Finger pressure over markedly edematous subcutaneous tissue displaces the interstitial fluid and leaves a depression, a sign called **pitting edema**.

Edema resulting from **renal dysfunction** often appears initially in parts of the body containing loose connective tissue, such as the eyelids; **periorbital edema** is thus a characteristic finding in severe renal disease. With **pulmonary edema,** the lungs are often two to three times their normal weight, and sectioning yields frothy, blood-tinged fluid—a mixture of air, edema, and extravasated red cells. **Brain edema** can be localized or generalized depending on the nature and extent of the pathologic process or injury. The swollen brain exhibits narrowed sulci and distended gyri, which are compressed by the unyielding skull (Chapter 28).

Effusions involving the pleural cavity (**hydrothorax**), the pericardial cavity (**hydropericardium**), or the peritoneal cavity (**hydroperitoneum** or **ascites**) are common in a wide range of clinical settings. Transudative effusions are typically protein-poor, translucent and straw colored; an exception are peritoneal effusions caused by lymphatic blockage (chylous effusion), which may be milky due to the presence of lipids absorbed from the gut. In contrast, exudative effusions are protein-rich and often cloudy due to the presence of white cells.

Clinical Features

The consequences of edema range from merely annoying to rapidly fatal. *Subcutaneous edema* is important primarily because it signals potential underlying cardiac or renal disease; however, when significant, it can also impair wound healing or the clearance of infections. *Pulmonary edema* is a common clinical problem that is most frequently seen in the setting of left ventricular failure; it can also occur with renal failure, acute respiratory distress syndrome (Chapter 15), and pulmonary inflammation or infection. Not only does fluid collect in the alveolar septa around capillaries and impede oxygen diffusion, but edema fluid in the alveolar spaces also creates a favorable environment for bacterial infection. *Pulmonary effusions* often accompany edema in the lungs and can further compromise gas exchange by compressing the underlying pulmonary parenchyma. *Peritoneal effusions* (*ascites*) resulting most commonly from portal hypertension are prone to seeding by bacteria, leading to serious and sometimes fatal infections. *Brain edema* is life threatening; if severe, brain substance can *herniate* (extrude) through the foramen magnum, or the brain stem vascular supply can be compressed. Either condition can injure the medullary centers and cause death (Chapter 28).

KEY CONCEPTS

Edema

Edema is the result of the movement of fluid from the vasculature into the interstitial spaces; the fluid may be protein-poor (*transudate*) or protein-rich (*exudate*).

Edema may be caused by:

- Increased hydrostatic pressure (e.g., heart failure)
- Decreased colloid osmotic pressure caused by reduced plasma albumin, either due to decreased synthesis (e.g., liver disease, protein malnutrition) or to increased loss (e.g., nephrotic syndrome)
- Increased vascular permeability (e.g., inflammation), which is usually localized but may occur throughout the body in severe systemic inflammatory states such as sepsis
- Lymphatic obstruction (e.g., infection or neoplasia)
- Sodium and water retention (e.g., renal failure)

Hyperemia and Congestion

Hyperemia and congestion both stem from increased blood volumes within tissues, but have different underlying mechanisms and consequences. *Hyperemia* is an active process in which arteriolar dilation (e.g., at sites of inflammation or in skeletal muscle during exercise) leads to increased blood flow. Affected tissues turn red (*erythema*) because of increased delivery of oxygenated blood. *Congestion* is a passive process resulting from reduced outflow of blood from a tissue. It can be systemic, as in cardiac failure, or localized, as in isolated venous obstruction.

As a result of increased hydrostatic pressures, congestion commonly leads to edema. In long-standing *chronic passive congestion,* the associated chronic hypoxia may result in ischemic tissue injury and scarring. In chronically congested tissues, capillary rupture can also produce small hemorrhagic foci; subsequent catabolism of extravasated red cells can leave residual telltale clusters of hemosiderin-laden macrophages.

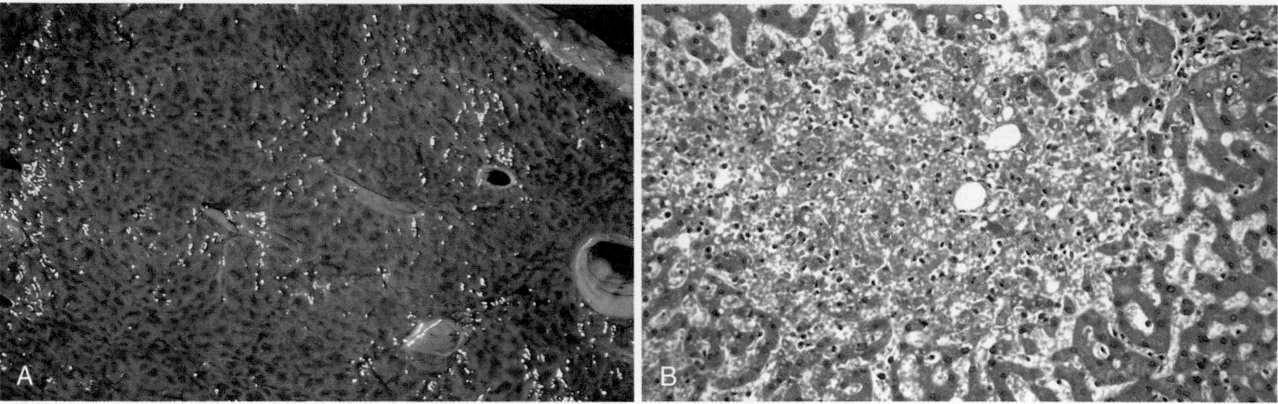

Figure 4-3 Liver with chronic passive congestion and hemorrhagic necrosis. **A,** Central areas are red and slightly depressed compared with the surrounding tan viable parenchyma, forming a "nutmeg liver" pattern (so-called because it resembles the cut surface of a nutmeg). **B,** Centrilobular necrosis with degenerating hepatocytes and hemorrhage. (Courtesy Dr. James Crawford, Department of Pathology, University of Florida, Gainesville, Fla.)

MORPHOLOGY

Congested tissues take on a dusky reddish-blue color (*cyanosis*) due to red cell stasis and the presence of deoxygenated hemoglobin. Microscopically, **acute pulmonary congestion** exhibits engorged alveolar capillaries, alveolar septal edema, and focal intraalveolar hemorrhage. In **chronic pulmonary congestion**, which is often caused by congestive heart failure, the septa are thickened and fibrotic, and the alveoli often contain numerous hemosiderin-laden macrophages called **heart failure cells**. In **acute hepatic congestion**, the central vein and sinusoids are distended. Because the centrilobular area is at the distal end of the hepatic blood supply, centrilobular hepatocytes may undergo ischemic necrosis while the periportal hepatocytes—better oxygenated because of proximity to hepatic arterioles—may only develop fatty change. In **chronic passive hepatic congestion**, the centrilobular regions are grossly red-brown and slightly depressed (because of cell death) and are accentuated against the surrounding zones of uncongested tan liver (**nutmeg liver**) (Fig. 4-3*A*). Microscopically, there is centrilobular hemorrhage, hemosiderin-laden macrophages, and variable degrees of hepatocyte dropout and necrosis (Fig. 4-3*B*).

Hemostasis, Hemorrhagic Disorders, and Thrombosis

Hemostasis can be defined simply as the process by which blood clots form at sites of vascular injury. Hemostasis is essential for life and is deranged to varying degrees in a broad range of disorders, which can be divided into two groups. In *hemorrhagic disorders,* characterized by excessive bleeding, hemostatic mechanisms are either blunted or insufficient to prevent abnormal blood loss. By contrast, in *thrombotic disorders* blood clots (often referred to as *thrombi*) form within intact blood vessels or within the chambers of the heart. As is discussed in Chapters 11 and 12, thrombosis has a central role in the most common and clinically important forms of cardiovascular disease.

While useful, it must be recognized that this division between bleeding and thrombotic disorders sometimes breaks down, in that generalized activation of clotting sometimes paradoxically produces bleeding due to the consumption of coagulation factors, as in *disseminated intravascular coagulation (DIC).* To provide context for understanding disorders of bleeding and clotting, this discussion begins with normal hemostasis, focusing on the contribution of platelets, coagulation factors, and endothelium.

Hemostasis

Hemostasis is a precisely orchestrated process involving platelets, clotting factors, and endothelium that occurs at the site of vascular injury and culminates in the formation of a blood clot, which serves to prevent or limit the extent of bleeding. The general sequence of events leading to hemostasis at a site of vascular injury is shown in Figure 4-4.

- *Arteriolar vasoconstriction* occurs immediately and markedly reduces blood flow to the injured area (Fig. 4-4*A*). It is mediated by reflex neurogenic mechanisms and augmented by the local secretion of factors such as *endothelin,* a potent endothelium-derived vasoconstrictor. This effect is transient, however, and bleeding would resume if not for activation of platelets and coagulation factors.
- *Primary hemostasis: the formation of the platelet plug.* Disruption of the endothelium exposes subendothelial von Willebrand factor (vWF) and collagen, which promote platelet adherence and activation. Activation of platelets results in a dramatic shape change (from small rounded discs to flat plates with spiky protrusions that markedly increased surface area), as well as the release of secretory granules. Within minutes the secreted products recruit additional platelets, which undergo *aggregation* to form a *primary hemostatic plug* (Fig. 4-4*B*).
- *Secondary hemostasis: deposition of fibrin. Tissue factor* is also exposed at the site of injury. Tissue factor is a membrane-bound procoagulant glycoprotein that is normally expressed by subendothelial cells in the vessel wall, such as smooth muscle cells and fibroblasts. Tissue factor binds and activates factor VII (see later), setting in motion a cascade of reactions that culiminates in *thrombin* generation. Thrombin cleaves circulating fibrinogen into insoluble *fibrin,* creating a fibrin meshwork, and also is a potent activator of platelets, leading to additional platelet aggregation at the site of injury. This sequence, referred to as *secondary hemostasis,* consolidates the initial platelet plug (Fig. 4-4C).
- *Clot stabilization and resorption.* Polymerized fibrin and platelet aggregates undergo contraction to form a solid,

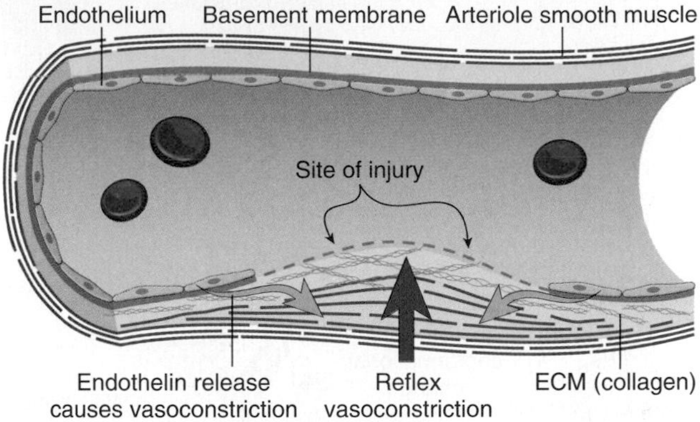

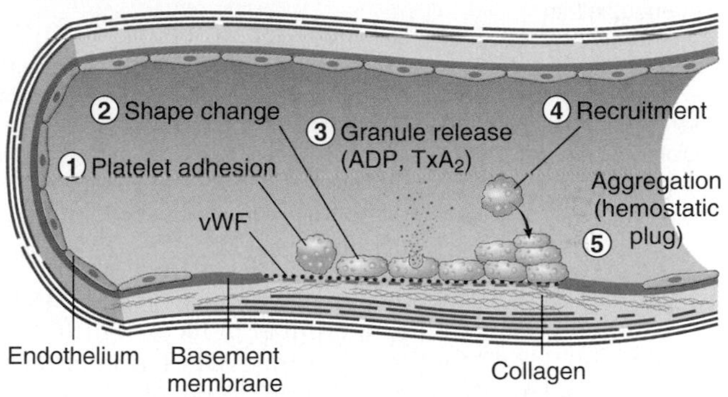

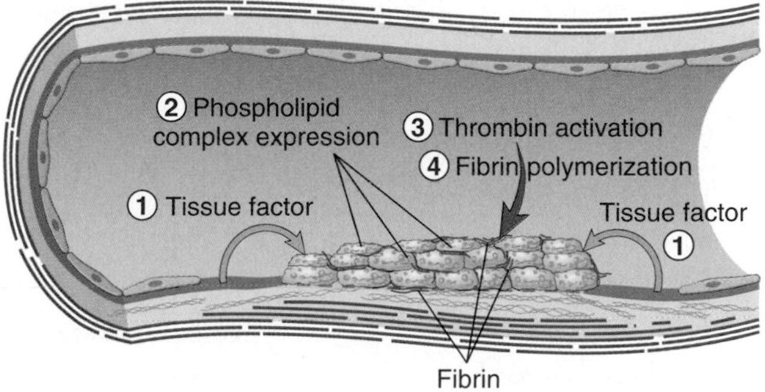

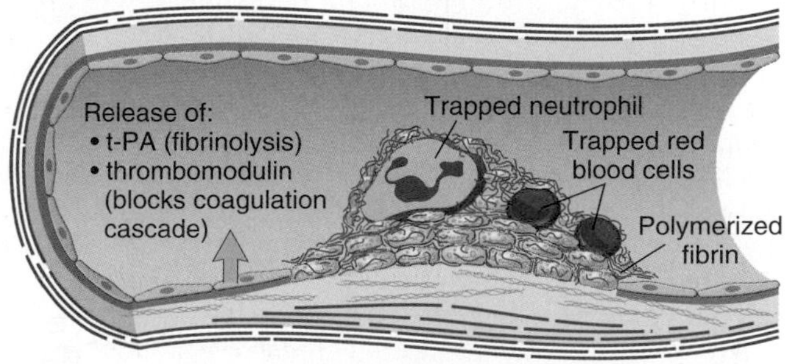

Figure 4-4 Normal hemostasis. **A,** After vascular injury, local neurohumoral factors induce a transient vasoconstriction. **B,** Platelets bind via glycoprotein Ib (GpIb) receptors to von Willebrand factor (vWF) on exposed extracellular matrix (ECM) and are activated, undergoing a shape change and granule release. Released adenosine diphosphate (ADP) and thromboxane A_2 (TxA_2) induce additional platelet aggregation through platelet GpIIb-IIIa receptor binding to fibrinogen, and form the *primary* hemostatic plug. **C,** Local activation of the coagulation cascade (involving tissue factor and platelet phospholipids) results in fibrin polymerization, "cementing" the platelets into a definitive *secondary* hemostatic plug. **D,** Counterregulatory mechanisms, mediated by tissue plasminogen activator (t-PA, a fibrinolytic product) and thrombomodulin, confine the hemostatic process to the site of injury.

permanent plug that prevents further hemorrhage. At this stage, counterregulatory mechanisms (e.g., *tissue plasminogen activator, t-PA*) are set into motion that limit clotting to the site of injury (Fig. 4-4*D*) and eventually lead to clot resorption and tissue repair.

The following sections discuss the roles of the platelets, coagulation factors, and endothelium in hemostasis in greater detail.

Platelets

Platelets play a critical role in hemostasis by forming the primary plug that initially seals vascular defects and by providing a surface that binds and concentrates activated coagulation factors. Platelets are disc-shaped anucleate cell fragments that are shed from megakaryocytes in the bone marrow into the bloodstream. Their function depends on several glycoprotein receptors, a contractile cytoskeleton, and two types of cytoplasmic granules. *α-Granules* have the adhesion molecule P-selectin on their membranes (Chapter 3) and contain proteins involved in coagulation, such as fibrinogen, coagulation factor V, and vWF, as well as protein factors that may be involved in wound healing, such as fibronectin, platelet factor 4 (a heparin-binding chemokine), platelet-derived growth factor (PDGF), and transforming growth factor-β. *Dense* (or δ) *granules* contain adenosine diphosphate (ADP) and adenosine triphosphate, ionized calcium, serotonin, and epinephrine.

After a traumatic vascular injury, platelets encounter constituents of the subendothelial connective tissue, such as vWF and collagen. On contact with these proteins, platelets undergo a sequence of reactions that culminate in the formation of a platelet plug (Fig. 4-4*B*).

- *Platelet adhesion* is mediated largely via interactions with vWF, which acts as a bridge between the platelet surface receptor glycoprotein Ib (GpIb) and exposed collagen (Fig. 4-5). Notably, genetic deficiencies of vWF (von Willebrand disease, Chapter 14) or GpIb (Bernard-Soulier syndrome) result in bleeding disorders, attesting to the importance of these factors.
- *Platelets rapidly change shape* following adhesion, being converted from smooth discs to spiky "sea urchins" with greatly increased surface area. This change is accompanied by alterations in *glycoprotein IIb/IIIa* that increase its affinity for fibrinogen (see later), and by the translocation of *negatively charged phospholipids* (particularly phosphatidylserine) to the platelet surface. These phospholipids bind calcium and serve as nucleation sites for the assembly of coagulation factor complexes.
- *Secretion (release reaction) of granule contents* occurs along with changes in shape; these two events are

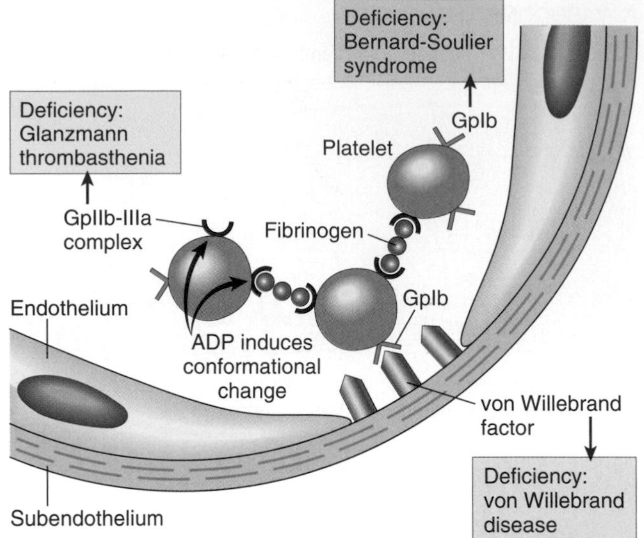

Figure 4-5 Platelet adhesion and aggregation. Von Willebrand factor functions as an adhesion bridge between subendothelial collagen and the glycoprotein Ib (GpIb) platelet receptor. Aggregation is accomplished by fibrinogen bridging GpIIb-IIIa receptors on different platelets. Congenital deficiencies in the various receptors or bridging molecules lead to the diseases indicated in the colored boxes. ADP, adenosine diphosphate.

often referred to together as *platelet activation*. Platelet activation is triggered by a number of factors, including he coagulation factor thrombin and ADP. Thrombin activates platelets through a special type of G-protein–coupled receptor referred to as a *protease-activated receptor* (PAR), which is switched on by a proteolytic cleavage carried out by thrombin. ADP is a component of dense-body granules; thus, platelet activation and ADP release begets additional rounds of platelet activation, a phenomenon referred to as *recruitment*. Activated platelets also produce the prostaglandin *thromboxane* A_2 (TxA_2), a potent inducer of platelet aggregation. *Aspirin* inhibits platelet aggregation and produces a mild bleeding defect by inhibiting cyclooxygenase, a platelet enzyme that is required for TxA_2 synthesis. Although the phenomenon is less well characterized, it is also suspected that growth factors released from platelets contribute to the repair of the vessel wall following injury.

- *Platelet aggregation* follows their activation. The conformational change in glycoprotein IIb/IIIa that occurs with platelet activation allows binding of fibrinogen, a large bivalent plasma polypeptide that forms bridges between adjacent platelets, leading to their aggregation. Predictably, inherited deficiency of GpIIb-IIIa results in a bleeding disorder called *Glanzmann thrombasthenia)*. The initial wave of aggregation is reversible, but concurrent activation of thrombin stabilizes the platelet plug by causing further platelet activation and aggregation, and by promoting irreversible *platelet contraction*. Platelet contraction is dependent on the cytoskeleton and consolidates the aggregated platelets. In parallel, thrombin also converts fibrinogen into insoluble *fibrin*, cementing the platelets in place and creating the definitive *secondary hemostatic plug*. Entrapped red cells and leukocytes are also found in hemostatic plugs, in part due to adherence of leukocytes to P-selectin expressed on activated platelets.

Coagulation Cascade

The coagulation cascade is series of amplifying enzymatic reactions that leads to the deposition of an insoluble fibrin clot. As discussed later, the dependency of clot formation on various factors differs in the laboratory in the laboratory test tube and in blood vessels in vivo (Fig. 4-6).

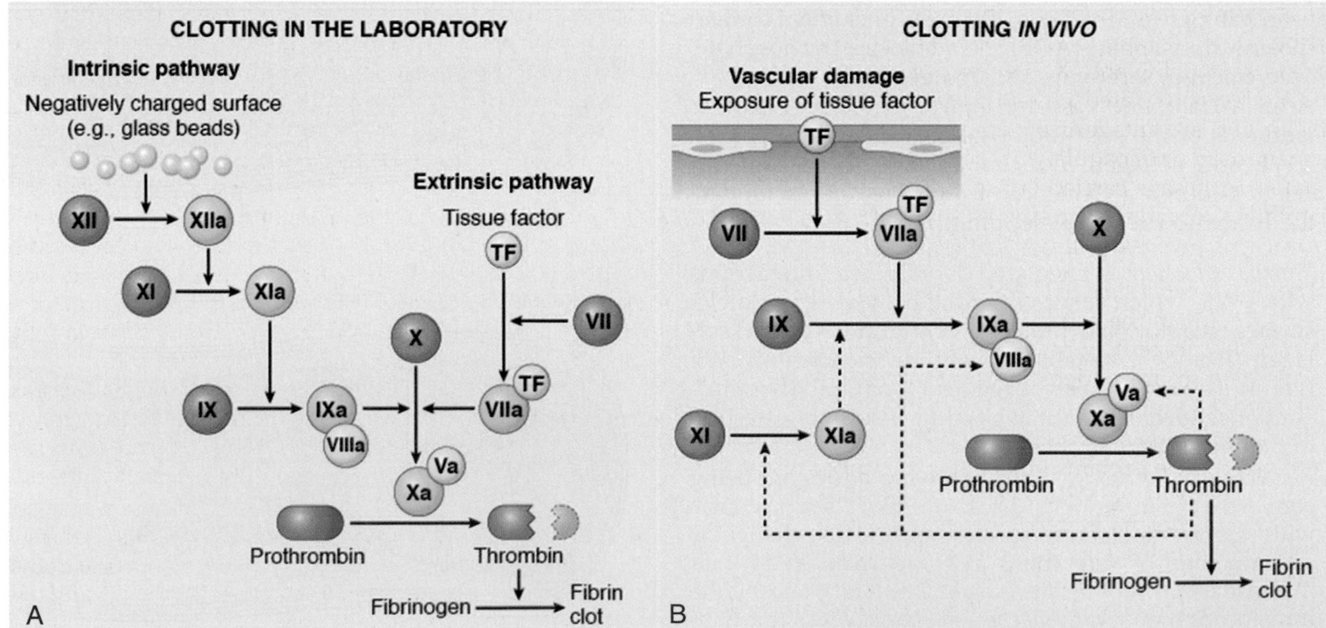

Figure 4-6 The coagulation cascade in the laboratory and in vivo. **A,** Clotting is initiated in the laboratory by adding phospholipids, calcium, and either a negative charged substance such as glass beads (intrinsic pathway) or a source of tissue factor (extrinsic pathway). **B,** In vivo, tissue factor is the major initiator of coagulation, which is amplified by feedback loops involving thrombin *(dotted lines)*. The red polypeptides are inactive factors, the dark green polypeptides are active factors, while the light green polypeptides correspond to cofactors..

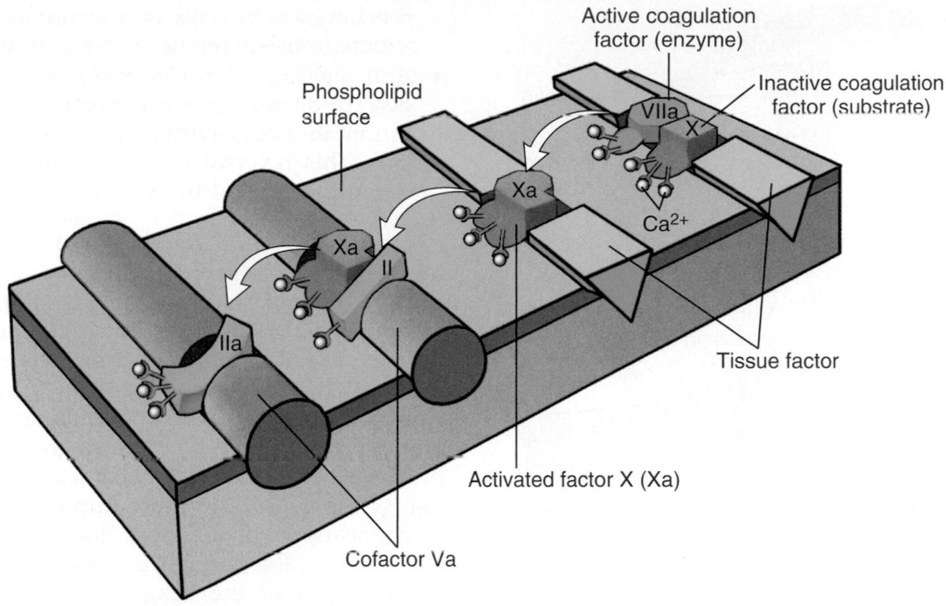

Figure 4-7 Schematic illustration of the conversion of factor X to factor Xa via the extrinsic pathway, which in turn converts factor II (prothrombin) to factor IIa (thrombin). The initial reaction complex consists of a proteolytic enzyme (factor VIIa), a substrate (factor X), and a reaction accelerator (tissue factor), all assembled on a platelet phospholipid surface. Calcium ions hold the assembled components together and are essential for the reaction. Activated factor Xa becomes the protease for the second adjacent complex in the coagulation cascade, converting prothrombin substrate (II) to thrombin (IIa) using factor Va as the reaction accelerator.

However, clotting in vitro and in vivo both follow the same general principles, as follows.

The cascade of reactions in the pathway can be likened to a "dance," in which coagulation factors are passed from one partner to the next (Fig. 4-7). Each reaction step involves an enzyme (an activated coagulation factor), a substrate (an inactive proenzyme form of a coagulation factor), and a cofactor (a reaction accelerator). These components are assembled on a negatively charged phospholipid surface, which is provided by activated platelets. Assembly of reaction complexes also depends on calcium, which binds to γ-carboxylated glutamic acid residues that are present in factors II, VII, IX, and X. The enzymatic reactions that produce γ-carboxylated glutamic acid use vitamin K as a cofactor and are antagonized by drugs such as coumadin, a widely used anticoagulant.

Based on assays carried out in clinical laboratories, the coagulation cascade has traditionally been divided into the *extrinsic* and *intrinsic* pathways (Fig. 4-6*A*).

- The *prothrombin time* (PT) assay assesses the function of the proteins in the extrinsic pathway (factors VII, X, V, II, and fibrinogen). In brief, tissue factor, phospholipids, and calcium are added to plasma and the time for a fibrin clot to form is recorded.
- The *partial thromboplastin time* (PTT) assay screens the function of the proteins in the intrinsic pathway (factors XII, XI, IX, VIII, X, V, II, and fibrinogen). In this assay, clotting of plasma is initiated by addition of negative-charged particles (e.g., ground glass) that activate factor XII (Hageman factor) together with phospholipids and calcium, and the time to fibrin clot formation is recorded.

While the PT and PTT assays are of great utility in evaluating coagulation factor function in patients, they fail to recapitulate the events that lead to coagulation in vivo. This point is most clearly made by considering the clinical effects of deficiencies of various coagulation factors. Deficiencies of factors V, VII, VIII, IX, and X are associated with moderate to severe bleeding disorders, and prothrombin deficiency is likely incompatible with life. In contrast, factor XI deficiency is only associated with mild bleeding, and individuals with factor XII deficiency do not bleed and in fact may be susceptible to thrombosis. The paradoxical effect of factor XII deficiency may be explained by involvement of factor XII in the fibrinolysis pathway (discussed later); while there is also some evidence from experimental models suggesting that factor XII may promote thrombosis under certain circumstances, the relevance of these observations to human thrombotic disease remains to be determined.

Based on the effects of various factor deficiencies in humans, it is believed that, in vivo, factor VIIa/tissue factor complex is the most important activator of factor IX and that factor IXa/factor VIIIa complex is the most important activator of factor X (Fig. 4-6*B*). The mild bleeding tendency seen in patients with factor XI deficiency is likely explained by the ability of thrombin to activate factor XI (as well as factors V and VIII), a feedback mechanism that amplifies the coagulation cascade.

Among the coagulation factors, thrombin is the most important, in that its various enzymatic activities control diverse aspects of hemostasis and link clotting to inflammation and repair. Among thrombin's most important activities are the following:

- *Conversion of fibrinogen into crosslinked fibrin.* Thrombin directly converts soluble fibrinogen into fibrin monomers that polymerize into an insoluble clot, and also amplifies the coagulation process, not only by activating factor XI, but also be activating two critical co-factors, factors V and VIII. It also stabilizes the secondary hemostatic plug by activating factor XIII, which covalently cross-links fibrin.

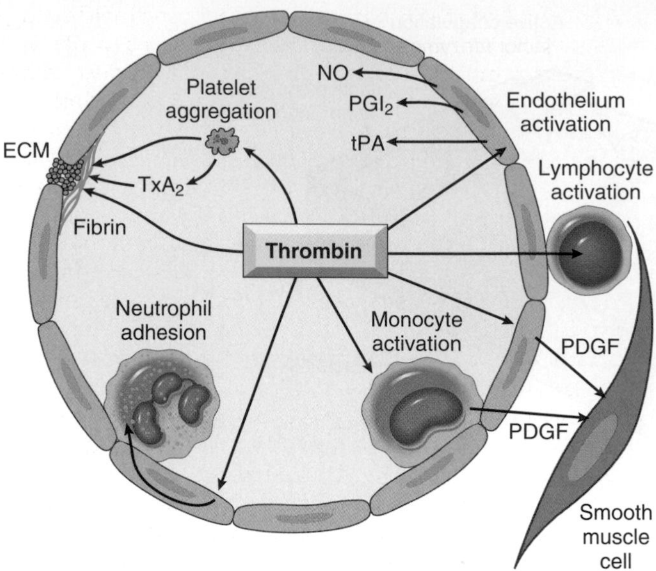

Figure 4-8 Role of thrombin in hemostasis and cellular activation. Thrombin plays a critical role in generating cross-linked fibrin (by cleaving fibrinogen to fibrin and by activating factor XIII), as well as activating several other coagulation factors (see Fig. 4-6*B*). Through protease-activated receptors (PARs, see text), thrombin also modulates several cellular activities. It directly induces platelet aggregation and TxA_2 production, and activates endothelial cells, which respond by expressing adhesion molecules and a variety of fibrinolytic (t-PA), vasoactive (NO, PGI_2), and cytokine mediators (e.g., PDGF). Thrombin also directly activates leukocytes. ECM, extracellular matrix; NO, nitric oxide; PDGF, platelet-derived growth factor; PGI_2, prostacyclin; TxA_2, thromboxane A_2; t-PA, tissue plasminogen activator. See Figure 4-10 for additional anticoagulant activities mediated by thrombin. (Courtesy Shaun Coughlin, MD, PhD, Cardiovascular Research Institute, University of California at San Francisco; modified with permission.)

- *Platelet activation.* Thrombin is a potent inducer of platelet activation and aggregation through its ability to activate PARs, thereby linking platelet function to coagulation.
- *Pro-inflammatory effects.* PARs are also expressed on inflammatory cells, endothelium, and other cell types (Fig. 4-8), and activation of these receptors by thrombin is believed to mediate proinflammatory effects that contribute to tissue repair and angiogenesis.
- *Anticoagulant effects.* Remarkably, through mechanisms described later, upon encountering normal endothelium thrombin changes from a procoagulant to an anticoagulant. This reversal in function prevents clotting from extending beyond the site of the vascular injury.

Factors That Limit Coagulation. Once initiated, coagulation must be restricted to the site of vascular injury to prevent deleterious consequences. One limiting factor is simple dilution; blood flowing past the site of injury washes out activated coagulation factors, which are rapidly removed by the liver. A second is the requirement for negatively charged phospholipids, which, as mentioned, are mainly provided by platelets that have been activated by contact with subendothelial matrix at sites of vascular injury. However, the most important counterregulatory mechanisms involve factors that are expressed by intact endothelium adjacent to the site of injury (described later).

Activation of the coagulation cascade also sets into motion a *fibrinolytic cascade* that limits the size of the clot and contributes to its later dissolution (Fig. 4-9). Fibrinolysis is largely accomplished through the enzymatic activity of *plasmin*, which breaks down fibrin and interferes with its polymerization. An elevated level of breakdown products of fibrinogen (often called fibrin split products), most notably fibrin-derived *D-dimers*, are a useful clinical markers of several thrombotic states (described later). Plasmin is generated by enzymatic catabolism of the inactive circulating precursor *plasminogen*, either by a factor XII–dependent pathway (possibly explaining the association of factor XII deficiency and thrombosis) or by plasminogen activators. The most important plasminogen activator is t-PA; it is synthesized principally by endothelium and is most active when bound to fibrin. This characteristic makes t-PA a useful therapeutic agent, since its fibrinolytic activity is largely confined to sites of recent thrombosis. Once activated, plasmin is in turn tightly controlled by counterregulatory factors such as α_2-plasmin inhibitor, a plasma protein that binds and rapidly inhibits free plasmin.

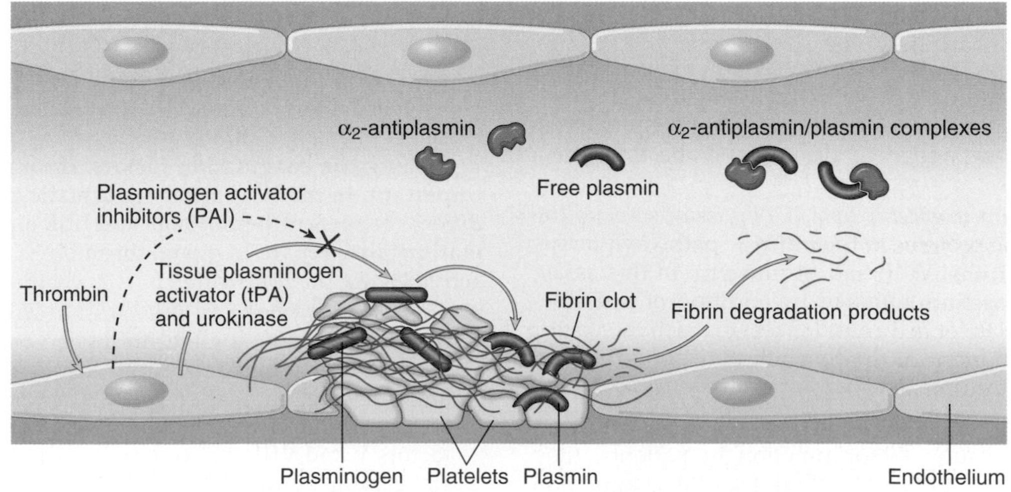

Figure 4-9 The fibrinolytic system, illustrating various plasminogen activators and inhibitors (see text).

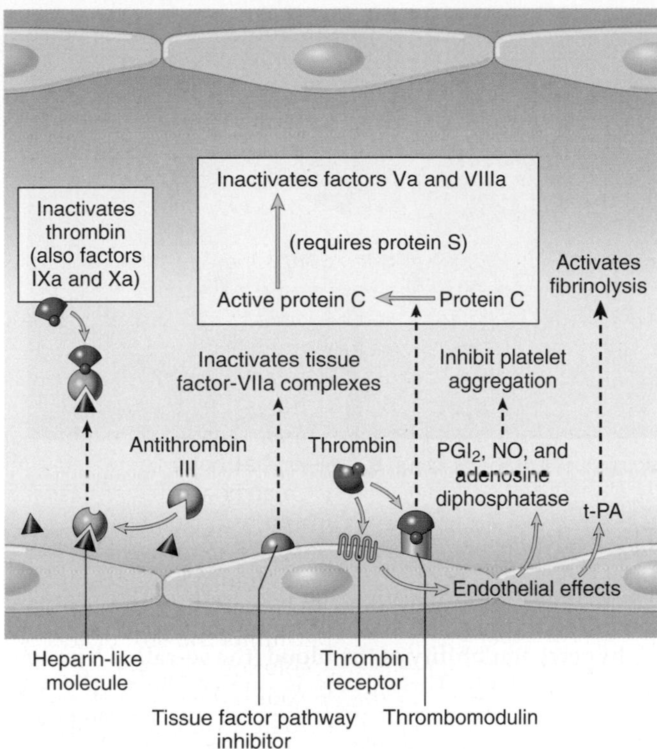

Figure 4-10 Anticoagulant activities of normal endothelium. NO, nitric oxide; PGI_2, prostacyclin; t-PA, tissue plasminogen activator; vWF, von Willebrand factor. The thrombin receptor is also called a protease-activated receptor (PAR).

Endothelium

The balance between the anticoagulant and procoagulant activities of endothelium often determines whether clot formation, propagation, or dissolution occurs. As alluded to earlier, normal endothelial cells express a multitude of factors that inhibit the procoagulant activities of platelets and coagulation factors and that augment fibrinolysis (Fig. 4-10). These factors act in concert to prevent thrombosis and to limit clotting to sites of vascular damage. However, if injured or exposed to proinflammatory factors, endothelial cells lose many of their antithrombotic properties. Here, we complete the discussion of hemostasis by focusing on the antithrombotic activities of normal endothelium; we return to the "dark side" of endothelial cells later when discussing thrombosis.

The antithrombotic properties of endothelium can be divided into activities directed at platelets, coagulation factors, and fibrinolysis.

- *Platelet inhibitory effects.* An obvious effect of intact endothelium is to serve as a barrier that shields platelets from subendothelial vWF and collagen. However, normal endothelium also releases a number of factors that inhibit platelet activation and aggregation. Among the most important are *prostacyclin (PGI_2), nitric oxide (NO),* and *adenosine diphosphatase;* the latter degrades ADP, already discussed as a potent activator of platelet aggregation. Finally, endothelial cells bind and alter the activity of thrombin, which is one of the most potent activators of platelets.
- *Anticoagulant effects.* Normal endothelium shields coagulation factors from tissue factor in vessel walls and expresses multiple factors that actively oppose coagulation, most notably thrombomodulin, endothelial protein C receptor, heparin-like molecules, and tissue factor pathway inhibitor. *Thrombomodulin* and *endothelial protein C receptor* bind thrombin and protein C, respectively, in a complex on the endothelial cell surface. When bound in this complex, thrombin loses its ability to activate coagulation factors and platelets, and instead cleaves and activates *protein C,* a vitamin K–dependent protease that requires a cofactor, protein S. Activated protein C/protein S complex is a potent inhibitor of coagulation factors Va and VIIIa. *Heparin-like molecules* on the surface of endothelium bind and activate antithrombin III, which then inhibits thrombin and factors IXa, Xa, XIa, and XIIa. The clinical utility of heparin and related drugs is based on their ability to stimulate antithrombin III activity. *Tissue factor pathway inhibitor* (TFPI), like protein C, requires protein S as a cofactor and, as the name implies, binds and inhibits tissue factor/factor VIIa complexes.
- *Fibrinolytic effects.* Normal endothelial cells synthesize t-PA, already discussed, as a key component of the fibrinolytic pathway.

Hemorrhagic Disorders

Disorders associated with abnormal bleeding inevitably stem from primary or secondary defects in vessel walls, platelets, or coagulation factors, all of which must function properly to ensure hemostasis. The presentation of abnormal bleeding varies widely. At one end of the spectrum are massive bleeds associated with ruptures of large vessels such as the aorta or of the heart; these catastrophic events simply overwhelm hemostatic mechanisms and are often fatal. Diseases associated with sudden, massive hemorrhage include aortic dissection in the setting of Marfan syndrome (Chapter 5), and aortic abdominal aneurysm (Chapter 11) and myocardial infarction (Chapter 12) complicated by rupture of the aorta or the heart. At the other end of the spectrum are subtle defects in clotting that only become evident under conditions of hemostatic stress, such as surgery, childbirth, dental procedures, menstruation, or trauma. Among the most common causes of mild bleeding tendencies are inherited defects in von Willebrand factor (Chapter 14), aspirin consumption, and uremia (renal failure); the latter alters platelet function through uncertain mechanisms. Between these extremes lie deficiencies of coagulation factors (the hemophilias, Chapter 14), which are usually inherited and lead to severe bleeding disorders if untreated.

Additional specific examples of disorders associated with abnormal bleeding are discussed throughout the book. The following are general principles related to abnormal bleeding and its consequences.

- *Defects of primary hemostasis (platelet defects or von Willebrand disease)* often present with small bleeds in skin or mucosal membranes. These bleeds typically take the form of petechiae, minute 1- to 2-mm hemorrhages (Fig. 4-11*A*), or *purpura,* which are slightly larger

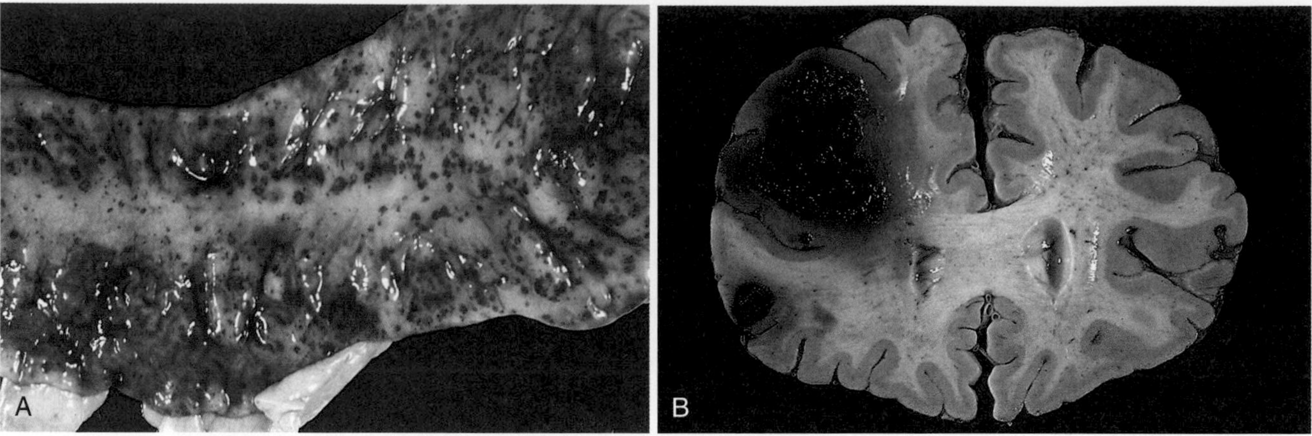

Figure 4-11 **A,** Punctate petechial hemorrhages of the colonic mucosa, a consequence of thrombocytopenia. **B,** Fatal intracerebral bleed.

(≥3 mm) than petechiae. It is believed that the capillaries of the mucosa and skin are particularly prone to rupture following minor trauma and that under normal circumstances platelets seal these defects virtually immediately. Mucosal bleeding associated with defects in primary hemostasis may also take the form of epistaxis (nosebleeds), gastrointestinal bleeding, or excessive menstruation (menorrhagia). A feared complication of very low platelet counts (*thrombocytopenia*) is intracerebral hemorrhage, which may be fatal.

- *Defects of secondary hemostasis (coagulation factor defects)* often present with bleeds into soft tissues (e.g., muscle) or joints. Bleeding into joints (*hemarthrosis*) following minor trauma is particularly characteristic of hemophilia (Chapter 14). It is unknown why severe defects in secondary hemostasis present with this peculiar pattern of bleeding; as with severe platelet defects, intracranial hemorrhage, sometimes fatal, may also occur.
- *Generalized defects involving small vessels* often present with "palpable purpura" and ecchymoses. *Ecchymoses* (sometimes simply called bruises) are hemorrhages of 1 to 2 cm in size. In both purpura and ecchymoses, the volume of extravasated blood is sufficient to create a palpable mass of blood known as a *hematoma*. Purpura and ecchymoses are particularly characteristic of systemic disorders that disrupt small blood vessels (e.g., vasculitis, Chapter 11) or that lead to blood vessel fragility (e.g., amyloidosis, Chapter 6; scurvy, Chapter 9).

The clinical significance of hemorrhage depends on the volume of the bleed, the rate at which it occurs, and its location. Rapid loss of up to 20% of the blood volume may have little impact in healthy adults; greater losses, however, can cause *hemorrhagic (hypovolemic) shock* (discussed later). Bleeding that is trivial in the subcutaneous tissues can cause death if located in the brain (Fig. 4-11*B*); because the skull is unyielding, intracranial hemorrhage may increase intracranial pressure to a level that compromises the blood supply or causes herniation of the brainstem (Chapter 28). Finally, chronic or recurrent external blood loss (e.g., peptic ulcer or menstrual bleeding) causes iron loss and can lead to an iron deficiency anemia. In contrast, when red cells are retained (e.g., hemorrhage into body cavities or tissues), iron is recovered and recycled for use in the synthesis of hemoglobin.

Thrombosis

The primary abnormalities that lead to thrombosis are (1) endothelial injury, (2) stasis or turbulent blood flow, and (3) hypercoagulability of the blood (the so-called Virchow triad) (Fig. 4-12). Thrombosis is one of the scourges of modern man, because it underlies the most serious and common forms of cardiovascular disease. Here, the focus is on its causes and consequences; its role in cardiovascular disorders is discussed in detail in Chapters 11 and 12.

Endothelial Injury

Endothelial injury leading to platelet activation almost inevitably underlies thrombus formation in the heart and the arterial circulation, where the high rates of blood flow impede clot formation. Notably, cardiac and arterial clots are typically rich in platelets, and it is believed that platelet adherence and activation is a necessary prerequisite for thrombus formation under high shear stress, such as exists

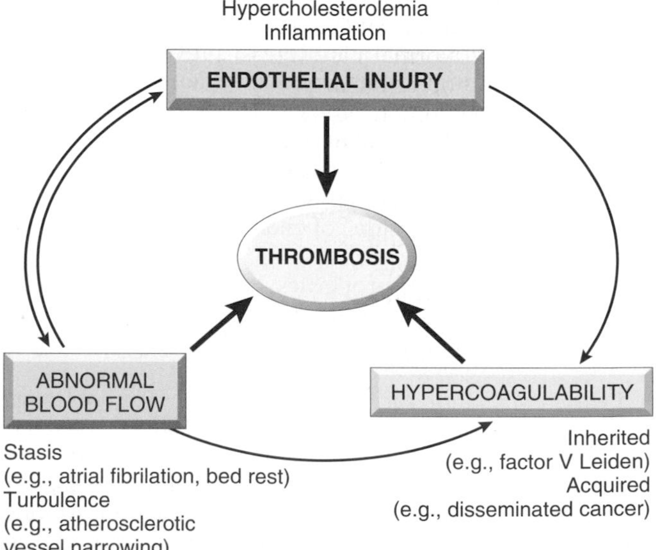

Figure 4-12 The Virchow triad in thrombosis. Endothelial integrity is the most important factor. Injury to endothelial cells can alter local blood flow and affect coagulability. Abnormal blood flow (stasis or turbulence), in turn, can cause endothelial injury. These factors may promote thrombosis independently or in combination.

in arteries. This insight provides part of the reasoning behind the use of aspirin and other platelet inhibitors in coronary artery disease and acute myocardial infarction.

Obviously, severe endothelial injury may trigger thrombosis by exposing vWF and tissue factor. However, inflammation and other noxious stimuli also promote thrombosis by shifting the pattern of gene expression in endothelium to one that is "prothrombotic." This change is sometimes referred to as *endothelial activation* or *dysfunction* and can be produced by diverse exposures, including physical injury, infectious agents, abnormal blood flow, inflammatory mediators, metabolic abnormalities, such as hypercholesterolemia or homocystinemia, and toxins absorbed from cigarette smoke. Endothelial activation is believed to have an important role in triggering arterial thrombotic events.

The role of endothelial cell activation and dysfunction in arterial thrombosis is discussed in detail in Chapters 11 and 12. Here it suffices to mention several of the major prothrombotic alterations:

- *Procoagulant changes.* Endothelial cells activated by cytokines downregulate the expression of *thrombomodulin,* already described as a key modulator of thrombin activity. This may result in sustained activation of thrombin, which can in turn stimulate platelets and augment inflammation through PARs expressed on platelets and inflammatory cells. In addition, inflamed endothelium also downregulates the expression of other anticoagulants, such as protein C and tissue factor protein inhibitor, changes that further promote a procoagulant state.
- *Antifibrinolytic effects.* Activated endothelial cells secrete *plasminogen activator inhibitors* (PAIs), which limit fibrinolysis, and downregulate the expression of t-PA, alterations that also favor the development of thrombi.

Alternations in Normal Blood Flow

Turbulence contributes to arterial and cardiac thrombosis by causing endothelial injury or dysfunction, as well as by forming countercurrents that contribute to local pockets of stasis. *Stasis* is a major contributor in the development of venous thrombi. Normal blood flow is *laminar* such that the platelets (and other blood cellular elements) flow centrally in the vessel lumen, separated from endothelium by a slower moving layer of plasma. Stasis and turbulence therefore:

- Promote endothelial activation, enhancing procoagulant activity and leukocyte adhesion, in part through flow-induced changes in the expression of adhesion molecules and pro-inflammatory factors
- Disrupt laminar flow and bring platelets into contact with the endothelium
- Prevent washout and dilution of activated clotting factors by fresh flowing blood and the inflow of clotting factor inhibitors

Altered blood flow contributes to thrombosis in several clinical settings. Ulcerated atherosclerotic plaques not only expose subendothelial vWF and tissue factor but also cause turbulence. Aortic and arterial dilations called *aneurysms* result in local stasis and are therefore fertile sites for thrombosis (Chapter 11). Acute myocardial infarctions result in areas of noncontractile myocardium and sometimes in cardiac aneurysms; both are associated with stasis and flow abnormalities that promote the formation of cardiac mural thrombi (Chapter 12). Rheumatic mitral valve stenosis results in left atrial dilation; in conjunction with atrial fibrillation, a dilated atrium is a site of profound stasis and a prime location for thrombosis (Chapter 12). *Hyperviscosity* (such as is seen with polycythemia vera; Chapter 13) increases resistance to flow and causes small vessel stasis, and the deformed red cells in *sickle cell anemia* (Chapter 14) impede blood flow through small vessels, with the resulting stasis also predisposing to thrombosis.

Hypercoagulability

Hypercoagulability (also called thrombophilia) can be loosely defined as any disorder of the blood that predisposes to thrombosis. Hypercoagulability has a particularly important role in venous thrombosis and can be divided into *primary* (genetic) and *secondary* (acquired) disorders (Table 4-2). Of the inherited causes of hypercoagulability, point mutations in the factor V gene and prothrombin gene are the most common.

- Approximately 2% to 15% of Caucasians carry a single-nucleotide mutation in factor V that is called the *factor V Leiden,* after the city in The Netherlands where it was discovered. Among individuals with recurrent DVT, the frequency of this mutation is considerably higher, approaching 60%. The mutation results in a glutamine

Table 4-2 Hypercoagulable States

Primary (Genetic)
Common
Factor V mutation (Arg to Glu substitution in amino acid residue 506 leading to resistance to activated protein C; factor V Leiden)
Prothrombin mutation (G20210A noncoding sequence variant leading to increased prothrombin levels)
Increased levels of factors VIII, IX, XI, or fibrinogen (genetics unknown)
Rare
Antithrombin III deficiency
Protein C deficiency
Protein S deficiency
Very Rare
Fibrinolysis defects
Homozygous homocystinuria (deficiency of cystathione β-synthetase)
Secondary (Acquired)
High Risk for Thrombosis
Prolonged bed rest or immobilization
Myocardial infarction
Atrial fibrillation
Tissue injury (surgery, fracture, burn)
Cancer
Prosthetic cardiac valves
Disseminated intravascular coagulation
Heparin-induced thrombocytopenia
Antiphospholipid antibody syndrome
Lower Risk for Thrombosis
Cardiomyopathy
Nephrotic syndrome
Hyperestrogenic states (pregnancy and postpartum)
Oral contraceptive use
Sickle cell anemia
Smoking

to arginine substitution at amino acid residue 506 that renders factor V resistant to cleavage and inactivation by protein C. As a result, an important antithrombotic counterregulatory pathway is lost (Fig. 4-10). Indeed, heterozygotes have a five-fold increased relative risk of venous thrombosis, and homozygotes have a 50-fold increase.

- A single nucleotide change (G20210A) in the 3′-untranslated region of the *prothrombin gene* is another common mutation (1% to 2% of the population) associated with hypercoagulability. It leads to elevated prothrombin levels and an almost three-fold increased risk of venous thrombosis.
- Elevated levels of *homocysteine* contribute to arterial and venous thrombosis, as well as the development of atherosclerosis (Chapter 11). The prothrombotic effects of homocysteine may be due to thioester linkages formed between homocysteine metabolites and a variety of proteins, including fibrinogen. Marked elevations of homocysteine may be caused by an inherited deficiency of cystathione β-synthetase.
- Rare inherited causes of primary hypercoagulability include deficiencies of anticoagulants such as antithrombin III, protein C, or protein S; affected individuals typically present with venous thrombosis and recurrent thromboembolism beginning in adolescence or early adulthood.

The most common thrombophilic genotypes found in various populations (heterozygosity for factor V Leiden and heterozygosity for the prothrombin G20210A variant) impart only a moderately increased risk of thrombosis; most individuals with these genotypes, when otherwise healthy, are free of thrombotic complications. However, factor V and prothrombin mutations are frequent enough that homozygosity and compound heterozygosity are not rare, and such genotypes are associated with greater risk. Moreover, individuals with such mutations have a significantly increased frequency of venous thrombosis in the setting of other acquired risk factors (e.g., pregnancy or prolonged bed rest). Thus, factor V Leiden heterozygosity may trigger DVT when combined with enforced inactivity, such as during prolonged airplane travel. Consequently, **inherited causes of hypercoagulability must be considered in patients younger than age 50 years who present with thrombosis—even when acquired risk factors are present.**

Unlike hereditary disorders, the pathogenesis of *acquired thrombophilia* is frequently multifactorial (Table 4-2). In some cases (e.g., cardiac failure or trauma), stasis or vascular injury may be most important. Hypercoagulability due to oral contraceptive use or the hyperestrogenic state of pregnancy is probably caused by increased hepatic synthesis of coagulation factors and reduced anticoagulant synthesis. In disseminated cancers, release of various procoagulants from tumors predisposes to thrombosis. The hypercoagulability seen with advancing age may be due to reduced endothelial PGI_2 production. Smoking and obesity promote hypercoagulability by unknown mechanisms.

Among the acquired thrombophilic states, the heparin-induced thrombocytopenia and the antiphospholipid antibody syndromes are particularly important clinical problems that deserve special mention.

Heparin-Induced Thrombocytopenia (HIT) Syndrome

HIT occurs following the administration of *unfractionated heparin*, which may induce the appearance of antibodies that recognize complexes of heparin and platelet factor 4 on the surface of platelets (Chapter 14), as well as complexes of heparin-like molecules and platelet factor 4-like proteins on endothelial cells. Binding of these antibodies to platelets results in their activation, aggregation, and consumption (hence the *thrombocytopenia* in the syndrome name). This effect on platelets and endothelial damage induced by antibody binding combine to produce a *prothrombotic state*, even in the face of heparin administration and low platelet counts. Low-molecular-weight heparin preparations induce HIT less frequently, and other classes of anticoagulants such as direct inhibitors of factor X and thrombin may also obviate the risk.

Antiphospholipid Antibody Syndrome

This syndrome (previously called the lupus anticoagulant syndrome) has protean clinical manifestations, including recurrent thromboses, repeated miscarriages, cardiac valve vegetations, and thrombocytopenia. Depending on the vascular bed involved, the clinical presentations can include pulmonary embolism (PE) (following lower extremity venous thrombosis), pulmonary hypertension (from recurrent subclinical pulmonary emboli), stroke, bowel infarction, or renovascular hypertension. Fetal loss does not appear to be explained by thrombosis, but rather seems to stem from antibody-mediated interference with the growth and differentiation of trophoblasts, leading to a failure of placentation. Antiphospholipid antibody syndrome is also a cause of renal microangiopathy, resulting in renal failure associated with multiple capillary and arterial thromboses (Chapter 20).

The name antiphospholipid antibody syndrome is misleading, as it is believed that the most important pathologic effects are mediated through binding of the antibodies to epitopes on proteins that are somehow induced or "unveiled" by phospholipids. Transfer of antiphospholipid antibodies to rodents can induce thrombosis, clearly indicating their pathogenicity, but the precise mechanisms remain uncertain. Suspected antibody targets include β2-glycoprotein I, a plasma protein that associates with the surfaces of endothelial cells and trophoblasts, and thrombin. In vivo, it is suspected that these antibodies bind to these and perhaps other proteins, thereby inducing a hypercoagulable state through uncertain mechanisms. However, in vitro, the antibodies interfere with phospholipids and thus inhibit coagulation. The antibodies also frequently give a false-positive serologic test for syphilis because the antigen in the standard assay is embedded in cardiolipin.

Antiphospholipid antibody syndrome has primary and secondary forms. Individuals with a well-defined autoimmune disease, such as systemic lupus erythematosus (Chapter 6), are designated as having *secondary antiphospholipid syndrome* (hence the earlier term *lupus anticoagulant syndrome*). In *primary antiphospholipid syndrome*, patients exhibit only the manifestations of a hypercoagulable state and lack evidence of other autoimmune disorders; occasionally, it appears following exposure to certain drugs or infections. Therapy involves anticoagulation and immunosuppression. Although antiphospholipid antibodies are clearly associated with thrombotic diatheses, they have also been identified in 5% to 15% of apparently normal individuals, implying that they are necessary but not sufficient to cause the full-blown syndrome.

MORPHOLOGY

Thrombi can develop anywhere in the cardiovascular system and vary in size and shape depending on the involved site and the underlying cause. Arterial or cardiac thrombi usually begin at sites of turbulence or endothelial injury, whereas venous thrombi characteristically occur at sites of stasis. Thrombi are focally attached to the underlying vascular surface, particularly at the point of initiation. From here, arterial thrombi tend to grow retrograde, while venous thrombi extend in the direction of blood flow; thus both propagate toward the heart. The propagating portion of a thrombus is often poorly attached and therefore prone to fragmentation and embolization.

Thrombi often have grossly and microscopically apparent laminations called **lines of Zahn,** which are pale platelet and fibrin deposits alternating with darker red cell–rich layers. Such laminations signify that a thrombus has formed in flowing blood; their presence can therefore distinguish antemortem clots from the bland nonlaminated clots that occur postmortem (see later).

Thrombi occurring in heart chambers or in the aortic lumen are designated **mural thrombi.** Abnormal myocardial contraction (arrhythmias, dilated cardiomyopathy, or myocardial infarction) or endomyocardial injury (myocarditis or catheter trauma) promotes cardiac mural thrombi (Fig. 4-13*A*), while ulcerated atherosclerotic plaque and aneurysmal dilation are the precursors of aortic thrombi (Fig. 4-13*B*).

Arterial thrombi are frequently **occlusive**; the most common sites in decreasing order of frequency are the coronary, cerebral, and femoral arteries. They typically consist of a friable meshwork of platelets, fibrin, red cells, and degenerating leukocytes. Although these are usually superimposed on a ruptured atherosclerotic plaque, other vascular injuries (vasculitis, trauma) may be the underlying cause.

Venous thrombosis (phlebothrombosis) is almost invariably occlusive, with the thrombus forming a long luminal cast. Because these thrombi form in the sluggish venous circulation, they tend to contain more enmeshed red cells (and relatively few platelets) and are therefore known as **red,** or **stasis, thrombi.** Venous thrombi are firm, are focally attached to the vessel wall, and contain lines of Zahn, features that help distinguish them from postmortem clots (see later). The veins of the lower extremities are most commonly involved (90% of cases); however, upper extremities, periprostatic plexus, or the ovarian and periuterine veins can also develop venous thrombi. Under special circumstances, they can also occur in the dural sinuses, portal vein, or hepatic vein.

Postmortem clots can sometimes be mistaken for antemortem venous thrombi. However, clots that form after death are gelatinous and have a dark red dependent portion where red cells have settled by gravity and a yellow "chicken fat" upper portion, and are usually not attached to the underlying vessel wall.

Thrombi on heart valves are called **vegetations**. Bloodborne bacteria or fungi can adhere to previously damaged valves (e.g., due to rheumatic heart disease) or can directly cause valve damage; in either case, endothelial injury and disturbed blood flow can induce the formation of large thrombotic masses (**infective endocarditis**; Chapter 12). Sterile vegetations can also develop on noninfected valves in persons with hypercoagulable states, so-called **nonbacterial thrombotic endocarditis** (Chapter 12). Less commonly, sterile verrucous endocarditis (**Libman-Sacks endocarditis**) can occur in the setting of systemic lupus erythematosus (Chapter 6).

Fate of the Thrombus

If a patient survives the initial thrombosis, in the ensuing days to weeks thrombi undergo some combination of the following four events:

- *Propagation.* Thrombi accumulate additional platelets and fibrin (discussed earlier).
- *Embolization.* Thrombi dislodge and travel to other sites in the vasculature (discussed later).
- *Dissolution.* Dissolution is the result of fibrinolysis, which can lead to the rapid shrinkage and total disappearance of recent thrombi. In contrast, the extensive fibrin deposition and cross-linking in older thrombi renders them more resistant to lysis. This distinction explains why therapeutic administration of fibrinolytic

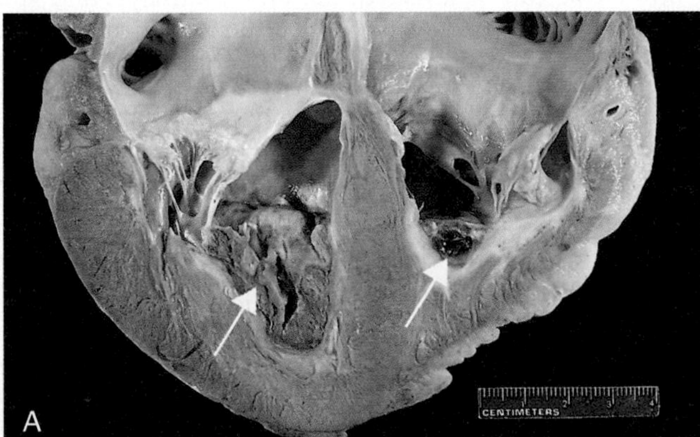

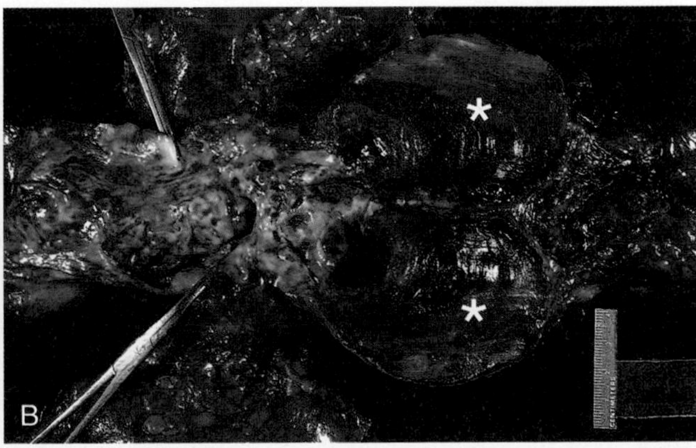

Figure 4-13 Mural thrombi. **A,** Thrombus in the left and right ventricular apices (arrows), overlying white fibrous scar. **B,** Laminated thrombus in a dilated abdominal aortic aneurysm (denoted by asterisks). Numerous friable mural thrombi are also superimposed on advanced atherosclerotic lesions of the more proximal aorta *(left side of picture).*

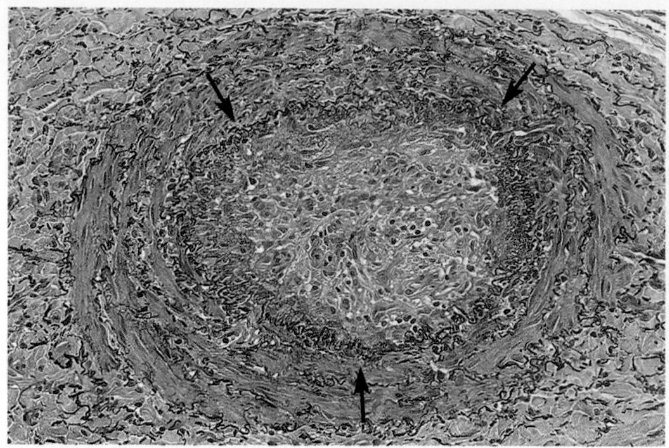

Figure 4-14 Low-power view of a thrombosed artery stained for elastic tissue. The original lumen is delineated by the internal elastic lamina *(arrows)* and is totally filled with organized thrombus, now punctuated by several recanalized endothelium-lined channels (white spaces).

agents such as t-PA (e.g., in the setting of acute coronary thrombosis) is generally effective only when given during the first few hours of a thrombotic event.

- *Organization and recanalization.* Older thrombi become organized by the ingrowth of endothelial cells, smooth muscle cells, and fibroblasts (Fig. 4-14). Capillary channels eventually form that reestablish the continuity of the original lumen, albeit to a variable degree. Continued recanalization may convert a thrombus into a smaller mass of connective tissue that becomes incorporated into the vessel wall. Eventually, with remodeling and contraction of the mesenchymal elements, only a fibrous lump may remain to mark the original thrombus.

Occasionally the centers of thrombi undergo enzymatic digestion, presumably as a result of the release of lysosomal enzymes from trapped leukocytes and platelets. In the setting of bacteremia, such thrombi may become infected, producing an inflammatory mass that erodes and weakens the vessel wall. If unchecked, this may result in a mycotic aneurysm (Chapter 11).

Clinical Features

Thrombi come to clinical attention when they obstruct arteries or veins, or give rise to emboli. The clinical presentation depends on the involved site. Venous thrombi can cause painful congestion and edema distal to an obstruction, but are mainly of concern due to their tendency to embolize to the lungs (see later). Conversely, although arterial thrombi can also embolize and cause downstream infarctions, the chief clinical problem is more often related to occlusion of a critical vessel (e.g., a coronary or cerebral artery), which can have serious or fatal consequences.

Venous Thrombosis (Phlebothrombosis). Most venous thrombi occur in the superficial or deep veins of the leg. Superficial venous thrombi typically occur in the saphenous veins in the setting of varicosities. Such thrombi can cause local congestion, swelling, pain, and tenderness, but rarely embolize. Nevertheless, the associated edema and impaired venous drainage predispose the overlying skin to the development of infections and ulcers (*varicose ulcers*). Deep venous thrombosis (DVT) involving one of the large leg veins—at or above the knee (e.g., the popliteal, femoral, and iliac veins)—is more serious because such thrombi more often embolize to the lungs and give rise to pulmonary infarction (see later and Chapter 15). Although DVTs may cause local pain and edema due to venous obstruction, these symptoms are often absent due the opening of venous collateral channels. Consequently, DVTs are asymptomatic in approximately 50% of affected individuals and are recognized only in retrospect after embolization.

Lower extremity DVTs are often associated with hypercoagulable states, as described earlier (Table 4-2). Common predisposing factors include bed rest and immobilization (because they reduce the milking action of the leg muscles, resulting in stasis), and congestive heart failure (also a cause of impaired venous return). Trauma, surgery, and burns not only immobilize a person but are also associated with vascular insults, procoagulant release from injured tissues, increased hepatic synthesis of coagulation factors, and decreased t-PA production. Many elements contribute to the thrombotic diathesis of pregnancy, including decreased venous return from leg veins and systemic hypercoagulability associated with the hormonal changes of late pregnancy and the postpartum period. Tumor-associated inflammation and coagulation factors (tissue factor, factor VIII), as well as procoagulants (e.g., mucin) released from tumor cells, all contribute to the increased risk of thromboembolism in disseminated cancers, so-called *migratory thrombophlebitis* or *Trousseau syndrome.* Regardless of the specific clinical setting, advanced age also increases the risk of DVT.

Arterial and Cardiac Thrombosis. *Atherosclerosis* is a major cause of arterial thromboses because it is associated with loss of endothelial integrity and with abnormal blood flow (Fig. 4-13*B*). Myocardial infarction can predispose to cardiac mural thrombi by causing dyskinetic myocardial contraction and endocardial injury (Fig. 4-13*A*), and rheumatic heart disease may engender atrial mural thrombi by causing atrial dilation and fibrillation. Both cardiac and aortic mural thrombi are prone to embolization. Although any tissue can be affected, the brain, kidneys, and spleen are particularly likely targets because of their rich blood supply.

KEY CONCEPTS

Thrombosis

- Thrombus development usually is related to one or more components of the Virchow triad:
  - Endothelial injury (e.g., by toxins, hypertension, inflammation, or metabolic products) associated with endothelial activation and changes in endothelial gene expression that favor coagulation
  - Abnormal blood flow—stasis or turbulence (e.g., due to aneurysms, atherosclerotic plaque)

- Hypercoagulability, either primary (e.g., factor V Leiden, increased prothrombin synthesis, antithrombin III deficiency) or secondary (e.g., bed rest, tissue damage, malignancy, or development of antiphospholipid antibodies [antiphospholipid antibody syndrome]) or antibodies against platelet factor IV/heparin complexes [heparin-induced thrombocytopenia])
- Thrombi may propagate, resolve, become organized, or embolize.
- Thrombosis causes tissue injury by local vascular occlusion or by distal embolization.

Disseminated Intravascular Coagulation

DIC is not a specific disease but rather a complication of a large number of conditions associated with systemic activation of thrombin. Disorders ranging from obstetric complications to advanced malignancy can be complicated by DIC, which leads to widespread formation of thrombi in the microcirculation. These microvascular thrombi can cause diffuse circulatory insufficiency and organ dysfunction, particularly of the brain, lungs, heart, and kidneys. To complicate matters, the runaway thrombosis "uses up" platelets and coagulation factors (hence the synonym *consumptive coagulopathy*) and often activates fibrinolytic mechanisms. Thus, symptoms initially related to thrombosis can evolve into a bleeding catastrophe, such as hemorrhagic stroke or hypovolemic shock. DIC is discussed in greater detail along with other bleeding diatheses in Chapter 14.

Embolism

An embolus is a detached intravascular solid, liquid, or gaseous mass that is carried by the blood from its point of origin to a distant site, where it often causes tissue dysfunction or infarction. The vast majority of emboli are dislodged thrombi, hence the term *thromboembolism*. Other rare emboli are composed of fat droplets, nitrogen bubbles, atherosclerotic debris *(cholesterol emboli)*, tumor fragments, bone marrow, or even foreign bodies. Emboli travel through the blood until they encounter vessels too small to permit further passage, causing partial or complete vascular occlusion. Depending on where they originate, emboli can lodge anywhere in the vascular tree; as discussed later, the clinical consequences vary widely depending on the size and the position of the lodged embolus, as well as the vascular bed that is impacted.

Pulmonary Embolism

Pulmonary emboli originate from deep venous thromboses and are the most common form of thromboembolic disease. Pulmonary embolism (PE) has had a fairly stable incidence since the 1970s of roughly 2 to 4 per 1000 hospitalized patients in the United States, although the numbers vary depending on the mix of patient age and diagnosis (i.e., surgery, pregnancy, and malignancy all increase the risk). PE causes about 100,000 deaths per year in the United States. In more than 95% of cases, PEs originate from leg DVTs.

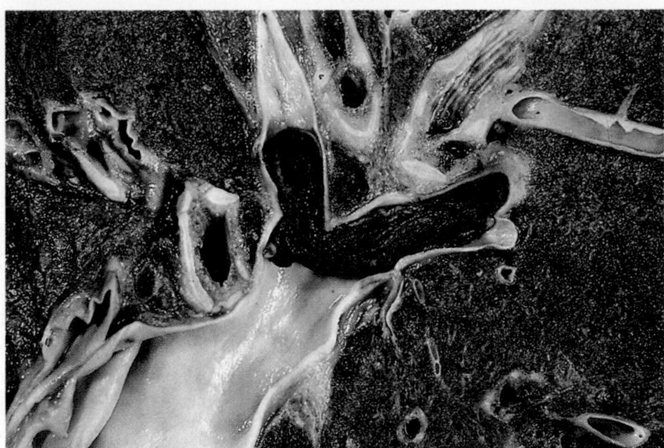

Figure 4-15 Embolus from a lower extremity deep venous thrombosis, lodged at a pulmonary artery branchpoint.

Fragmented thrombi from DVTs are carried through progressively larger veins and the right side of the heart before slamming into the pulmonary arterial vasculature. Depending on the size of the embolus, it can occlude the main pulmonary artery, straddle the pulmonary artery bifurcation *(saddle embolus)*, or pass out into the smaller, branching arteries (Fig. 4-15). Frequently there are multiple emboli, occurring either sequentially or simultaneously as a shower of smaller emboli from a single large mass; in general, **the patient who has had one PE is at high risk for more.** Rarely, a venous embolus passes through an interatrial or interventricular defect and gains access to the systemic arterial circulation *(paradoxical embolism)*. A more complete discussion of PEs is presented in Chapter 15; the following is an overview of the major functional consequences of pulmonary emboli.

- Most pulmonary emboli (60% to 80%) are clinically silent because they are small. With time they become organized and are incorporated into the vascular wall; in some cases organization of the thromboembolus leaves behind a delicate, bridging fibrous *web*.
- Sudden death, right heart failure *(cor pulmonale)*, or cardiovascular collapse occurs when emboli obstruct 60% or more of the pulmonary circulation.
- Embolic obstruction of medium-sized arteries with subsequent vascular rupture can result in pulmonary hemorrhage but usually does not cause pulmonary infarction. This is because the lung is supplied by both the pulmonary arteries and the bronchial arteries, and the intact bronchial circulation is usually sufficient to perfuse the affected area. Understandably, if the bronchial arterial flow is compromised (e.g., by left-sided cardiac failure), infarction may occur.
- Embolic obstruction of small end-arteriolar pulmonary branches often does produce hemorrhage or infarction.
- Multiple emboli over time may cause pulmonary hypertension and right ventricular failure.

Systemic Thromboembolism

Most systemic emboli (80%) arise from intracardiac mural thrombi, two thirds of which are associated with left ventricular wall infarcts and another one fourth with left atrial dilation and fibrillation. The remainder originates from aortic aneurysms, atherosclerotic plaques, valvular vegetations, or venous thrombi (paradoxical emboli); 10% to 15% are of unknown origin. In contrast to venous emboli, the vast majority of which lodge in the lung, arterial emboli can travel to a wide variety of sites; the point of arrest depends on the source and the relative amount of blood flow that downstream tissues receive. Most come to rest in the lower extremities (75%) or the brain (10%), but other tissues, including the intestines, kidneys, spleen, and upper extremities, may be involved on occasion. The consequences of systemic emboli depend on the vulnerability of the affected tissues to ischemia, the caliber of the occluded vessel, and whether a collateral blood supply exists; in general, however, the outcome is tissue infarction.

Fat and Marrow Embolism

Microscopic fat globules—sometimes with associated hematopoietic bone marrow—can be found in the pulmonary vasculature after fractures of long bones or, rarely, in the setting of soft tissue trauma and burns. Presumably these injuries rupture vascular sinusoids in the marrow or small venules, allowing marrow or adipose tissue to herniate into the vascular space and travel to the lung. Fat and marrow emboli are very common incidental findings after vigorous cardiopulmonary resuscitation and are probably of no clinical consequence. Indeed, fat embolism occurs in some 90% of individuals with severe skeletal injuries (Fig. 4-16), but less than 10% of such patients have any clinical findings.

Fat embolism syndrome is the term applied to the minority of patients who become symptomatic. It is characterized by pulmonary insufficiency, neurologic symptoms, anemia, and thrombocytopenia, and is fatal in about 5% to 15% of cases. Typically, 1 to 3 days after injury there is a sudden onset of tachypnea, dyspnea, and tachycardia; irritability and restlessness can progress to delirium or coma. Thrombocytopenia is attributed to platelet adhesion to fat globules and subsequent aggregation or splenic sequestration; anemia can result from similar red cell aggregation and/or hemolysis. A diffuse petechial rash (seen in 20% to 50% of cases) is related to rapid onset of thrombocytopenia and can be a useful diagnostic feature.

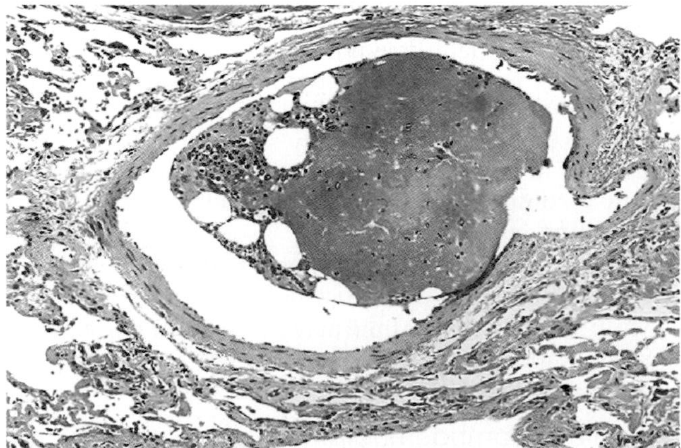

Figure 4-16 Bone marrow embolus in the pulmonary circulation. The cellular elements on the left side of the embolus are hematopoietic cells, while the cleared vacuoles represent marrow fat. The relatively uniform red area on the right of the embolus is an early organizing thrombus.

The pathogenesis of fat emboli syndrome probably involves both mechanical obstruction and biochemical injury. Fat microemboli and associated red cell and platelet aggregates can occlude the pulmonary and cerebral microvasculature. Release of free fatty acids from the fat globules exacerbates the situation by causing local toxic injury to endothelium, and platelet activation and granulocyte recruitment (with free radical, protease, and eicosanoid release) complete the vascular assault. Because lipids are dissolved out of tissue preparations by the solvents routinely used in paraffin embedding, the microscopic demonstration of fat microglobules typically requires specialized techniques, including frozen sections and stains for fat.

Air Embolism

Gas bubbles within the circulation can coalesce to form frothy masses that obstruct vascular flow and cause distal ischemic injury. For example, a very small volume of air trapped in a coronary artery during bypass surgery, or introduced into the cerebral circulation by neurosurgery in the "sitting position," can occlude flow with dire consequences. A larger volume of air, generally more than 100 cc, is necessary to produce a clinical effect in the pulmonary circulation; unless care is taken, this volume of air can be inadvertently introduced during obstetric or laparoscopic procedures, or as a consequence of chest wall injury.

A particular form of gas embolism, called *decompression sickness,* occurs when individuals experience sudden decreases in atmospheric pressure. Scuba and deep sea divers, underwater construction workers, and individuals in unpressurized aircraft in rapid ascent are all at risk. When air is breathed at high pressure (e.g., during a deep sea dive), increased amounts of gas (particularly nitrogen) are dissolved in the blood and tissues. If the diver then ascends (depressurizes) too rapidly, the nitrogen comes out of solution in the tissues and the blood.

The rapid formation of gas bubbles within skeletal muscles and supporting tissues in and about joints is responsible for the painful condition called *the bends* (so named in the 1880s because it was noted that those afflicted characteristically arched their backs in a manner reminiscent of a then-popular women's fashion pose called the Grecian bend). In the lungs, gas bubbles in the vasculature cause edema, hemorrhage, and focal atelectasis or emphysema, leading to a form of respiratory distress called the *chokes.* A more chronic form of decompression sickness is called *caisson disease* (named for the pressurized vessels used in bridge construction; workers in these vessels suffered both acute and chronic forms of decompression sickness). In caisson disease, persistence of gas emboli in the skeletal system leads to multiple foci of ischemic necrosis; the more common sites are the femoral heads, tibia, and humeri.

Individuals affected by acute decompression sickness are treated by being placed in a chamber under sufficiently high pressure to force the gas bubbles back into solution. Subsequent slow decompression permits gradual resorption and exhalation of the gases, which prevents the obstructive bubbles from reforming.

Amniotic Fluid Embolism

Amniotic fluid embolism is the fifth most common cause of maternal mortality worldwide; it accounts for roughly 10% of maternal deaths in the United States and results in permanent neurologic deficit in as many as 85% of survivors. Amniotic fluid embolism is an ominous complication of labor and the immediate postpartum period. Although the incidence is only approximately 1 in 40,000 deliveries, the mortality rate is up to 80%. The onset is characterized by sudden severe dyspnea, cyanosis, and shock, followed by neurologic impairment ranging from headache to seizures and coma. If the patient survives the initial crisis, pulmonary edema typically develops, frequently accompanied by disseminated intravascular coagulation. Note that these features differ from those observed with pulmonary embolism from a deep venous thrombosis; in fact, much of the morbidity and mortality in amniotic fluid embolism may stem from the biochemical activation of coagulation factors and components of the innate immune system by substances in the amniotic fluid, rather than the mechanical obstruction of pulmonary vessels by amniotic debris.

The underlying cause is the infusion of amniotic fluid or fetal tissue into the maternal circulation via a tear in the placental membranes or rupture of uterine veins. Classic findings at autopsy include the presence of squamous cells shed from fetal skin, lanugo hair, fat from vernix caseosa, and mucin derived from the fetal respiratory or gastrointestinal tract in the maternal pulmonary microvasculature (Fig. 4-17). Other findings include marked pulmonary edema, *diffuse alveolar damage* (Chapter 15), and the presence of fibrin thrombi in many vascular beds due to disseminated intravascular coagulation.

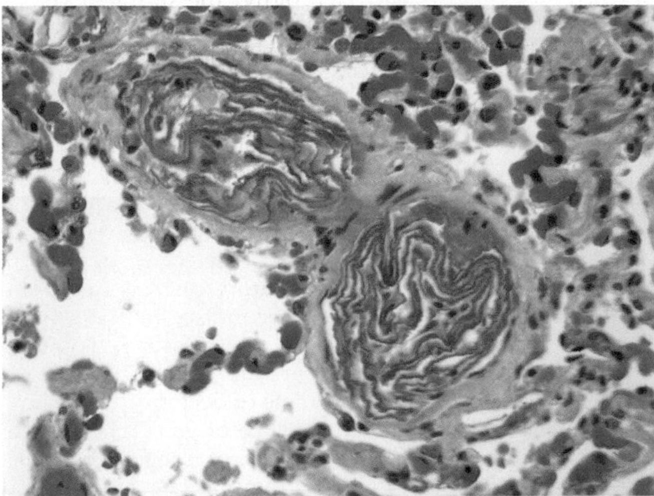

Figure 4-17 Amniotic fluid embolism. Two small pulmonary arterioles are packed with laminated swirls of fetal squamous cells. There is marked edema and congestion. Elsewhere the lung contained small organizing thrombi consistent with disseminated intravascular coagulation. (Courtesy Dr. Beth Schwartz, Baltimore, Md.)

KEY CONCEPTS

Embolism

- An embolus is a solid, liquid, or gaseous mass carried by the blood to a site distant from its origin; most are dislodged thrombi.
- Pulmonary emboli derive primarily from lower extremity deep vein thrombi; their effects depend mainly on the size of the embolus and the location in which it lodges. Consequences may include right-sided heart failure, pulmonary hemorrhage, pulmonary infarction, or sudden death.
- Systemic emboli derive primarily from cardiac mural or valvular thrombi, aortic aneurysms, or atherosclerotic plaques; whether an embolus causes tissue infarction depends on the site of embolization and the presence or absence of collateral circulation.

Infarction

An infarct is an area of ischemic necrosis caused by occlusion of either the arterial supply or the venous drainage. Tissue infarction is a common and extremely important cause of clinical illness. Roughly 40% of all deaths in the United States are caused by cardiovascular disease, and most of these are attributable to myocardial or cerebral infarction. Pulmonary infarction is also a common complication in many clinical settings, bowel infarction is frequently fatal, and ischemic necrosis of the extremities *(gangrene)* is a serious problem in the diabetic population.

Arterial thrombosis or arterial embolism underlies the vast majority of infarctions. Less common causes of arterial obstruction leading to infarction include local vasospasm, hemorrhage into an atheromatous plaque, or extrinsic vessel compression (e.g., by tumor). Other uncommon causes of tissue infarction include torsion of a vessel (e.g., in testicular torsion or bowel volvulus), traumatic vascular rupture, or vascular compromise by edema (e.g., *anterior compartment syndrome*) or by entrapment in a hernia sac. Although venous thrombosis can cause infarction, the more common outcome is just congestion; in this setting, bypass channels rapidly open and permit vascular outflow, which then improves arterial inflow. Infarcts caused by venous thrombosis are thus more likely in organs with a single efferent vein (e.g., testis and ovary).

MORPHOLOGY

Infarcts are classified according to color and the presence or absence of infection; they are either red (hemorrhagic) or white (anemic) and may be septic or bland.

- **Red infarcts** (Fig. 4-18*A*) occur (1) with venous occlusions (e.g., testicular torsion, Chapter 19), (2) in loose, spongy tissues (e.g., lung) where blood can collect in the infarcted zone, (3) in tissues with dual circulations (e.g., lung and small intestine) that allow blood to flow from an unobstructed parallel supply into a necrotic zone, (4) in tissues previously

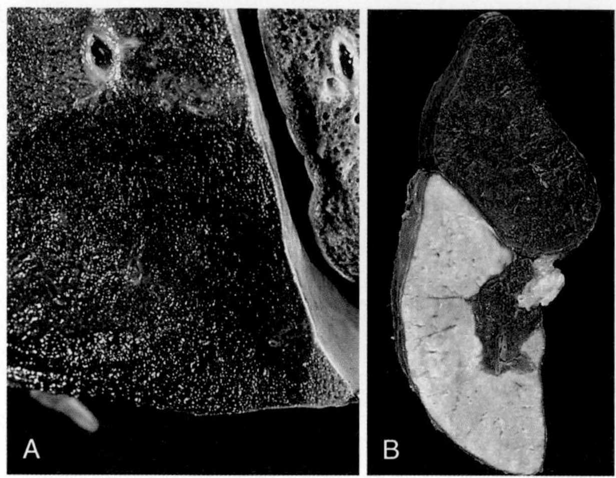

Figure 4-18 Red and white infarcts. **A,** Hemorrhagic, roughly wedge-shaped pulmonary *red infarct*. **B,** Sharply demarcated *white infarct* in the spleen.

congested by sluggish venous outflow, and (5) when flow is reestablished to a site of previous arterial occlusion and necrosis (e.g., following angioplasty of an arterial obstruction).

- **White infarcts** (Fig. 4-18*B*) occur with arterial occlusions in solid organs with end-arterial circulation (e.g., heart, spleen, and kidney), and where tissue density limits the seepage of blood from adjoining capillary beds into the necrotic area.

Infarcts tend to be wedge-shaped, with the occluded vessel at the apex and the periphery of the organ forming the base (Fig. 4-18); when the base is a serosal surface there may be an overlying fibrinous exudate resulting from an acute inflammatory response to mediators release from injured and necrotic cells. Fresh infarcts are poorly defined and slightly hemorrhagic, but over a few days the margins tend to become better defined by a narrow rim of congestion attributable to inflammation. With further passage of time, infarcts resulting from arterial occlusions in organs without a dual blood supply typically become progressively paler and more sharply defined (Fig. 4-18*B*). In comparison, in the lung hemorrhagic infarcts are the rule (Fig. 4-18*A*). Extravasated red cells in hemorrhagic infarcts are phagocytosed by macrophages, which convert heme iron into hemosiderin; small amounts do not grossly impart any appreciable color to the tissue, but extensive hemorrhage can leave a firm, brown hemosiderin-rich residuum.

The dominant histologic characteristic of infarction is **ischemic coagulative necrosis** (Chapter 2). Importantly, if the vascular occlusion has occurred shortly (minutes to hours) before the death of the person, histologic changes may be absent; it takes 4 to 12 hours for the dead tissue to show microscopic evidence of frank necrosis. Acute inflammation is present along the margins of infarcts within a few hours and is usually well defined within 1 to 2 days. Eventually a reparative response begins in the preserved margins (Chapter 3). In stable or labile tissues, parenchymal regeneration can occur at the periphery where underlying stromal architecture is preserved. However, most infarcts are ultimately replaced by *scar* (Fig. 4-19). The brain is an exception to these generalizations, in that central nervous system infarction results in **liquefactive necrosis** (Chapter 2).

Septic infarctions occur when infected cardiac valve vegetations embolize or when microbes seed necrotic tissue. In these cases the infarct is converted into an *abscess*, with a correspondingly greater inflammatory response (Chapter 3). The eventual sequence of organization, however, follows the pattern already described.

Factors That Influence Development of an Infarct. A vascular occlusion can cause effects ranging from virtually nothing to tissue dysfunction and necrosis sufficient to result in death. The variables that influence the outcome of vascular occlusion are the following:

- *Anatomy of the vascular supply.* The availability of an alternative blood supply is the most important determinant of whether vessel occlusion will cause tissue damage. As mentioned, the lungs have a dual pulmonary and bronchial artery blood supply that protects against thromboembolism-induced infarction. Similarly, the liver, with its dual hepatic artery and portal vein circulation, and the hand and forearm, with their dual radial and ulnar arterial supply, are all relatively resistant to infarction. In contrast, renal and splenic circulations are end-arterial, and vascular obstruction generally causes tissue death.
- *Rate of occlusion.* Slowly developing occlusions are less likely to cause infarction, because they provide time for development of collateral pathways of perfusion. For example, small interarteriolar anastomoses—normally with minimal functional flow—interconnect the three major coronary arteries in the heart. If one of the coronaries is occluded slowly (i.e., by an encroaching atherosclerotic plaque), flow within this *collateral circulation* may increase sufficiently to prevent infarction, even though the larger coronary artery is eventually occluded.
- *Tissue vulnerability to hypoxia.* Neurons undergo irreversible damage when deprived of their blood supply for only 3 to 4 minutes. Myocardial cells, although hardier than neurons, are also quite sensitive and die after only 20 to 30 minutes of ischemia (although, as mentioned, changes in the appearance of the dead cells take 4-12 hours to develop). In contrast, fibroblasts within myocardium remain viable even after many hours of ischemia (Chapter 12).

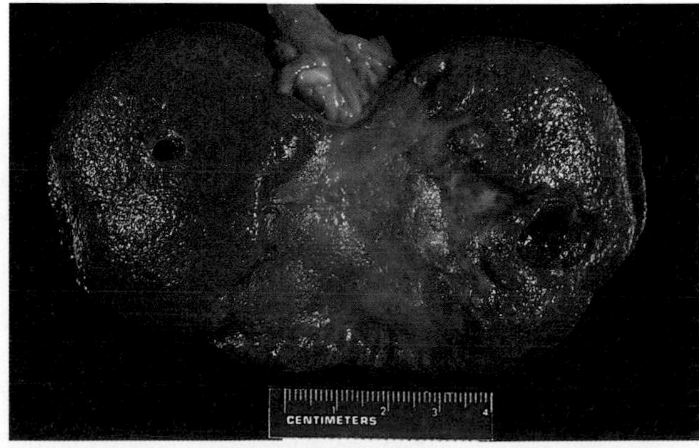

Figure 4-19 Remote kidney infarct replaced by a large fibrotic scar.

- *Hypoxemia.* Understandably, abnormally low blood O_2 content (regardless of cause) increases both the likelihood and extent of infarction.

KEY CONCEPTS

Infarction

- Infarcts are areas of ischemic necrosis most commonly caused by arterial occlusion (typically due to thrombosis or embolization); venous outflow obstruction is a less frequent cause.
- Infarcts caused by venous occlusion or occurring in spongy tissues with dual blood supply and where blood can collect typically are hemorrhagic (red); those caused by arterial occlusion in compact tissues typically are pale (white).
- Whether or not vascular occlusion causes tissue infarction is influenced by collateral blood supplies, the rate at which an obstruction develops, intrinsic tissue susceptibility to ischemic injury, and blood oxygenation.

Shock

Shock is a state in which diminished cardiac output or reduced effective circulating blood volume impairs tissue perfusion and leads to cellular hypoxia. At the outset the cellular injury is reversible; however, prolonged shock eventually leads to irreversible tissue injury and is often fatal. Shock may complicate severe hemorrhage, extensive trauma or burns, myocardial infarction, pulmonary embolism, and microbial sepsis. Its causes fall into three general categories (Table 4-3):

- *Cardiogenic shock* results from low cardiac output due to myocardial pump failure. This can be due to intrinsic myocardial damage (infarction), ventricular arrhythmias, extrinsic compression (cardiac tamponade; Chapter 11), or outflow obstruction (e.g., pulmonary embolism).
- *Hypovolemic shock* results from low cardiac output due to low blood volume, such as can occur with massive hemorrhage or fluid loss from severe burns.
- *Shock associated with systemic inflammation* may be triggered by a variety of insults, particularly microbial infections, burns, trauma, and or pancreatitis. The common pathogenic feature is a massive outpouring of inflammatory mediators from innate and adaptive immune cells that produce arterial vasodilation, vascular leakage, and venous blood pooling. These cardiovascular abnormalities result in tissue hypoperfusion, cellular hypoxia, and metabolic derangements that lead to organ dysfunction and, if severe and persistent, organ failure and death. It should be noted that diverse triggers of shock (microbial and non-microbial) associated with inflammation produce a similar set of clinical findings, which are referred to as the *systemic inflammatory response syndrome*. The pathogenesis of shock caused by microbial infection *(septic shock)* is discussed in detail below.

Less commonly, shock can occur in the setting of an anesthetic accident or a spinal cord injury *(neurogenic shock)*, or an IgE–mediated hypersensitivity reaction (*anaphylactic shock*, Chapter 6). In both of these forms of shock, acute vasodilation leads to hypotension and tissue hypoperfusion.

Pathogenesis of Septic Shock

With a mortality rate exceeding 20%, septic shock ranks first among the causes of death in intensive care units and accounts for over 200,000 lost lives each year in the United States. Its incidence is rising, ironically due to improvements in life support for critically ill patients, as well as the growing ranks of immunocompromised hosts (due to chemotherapy, immunosuppression, advanced age or HIV infection) and the increasing prevalence of multidrug resistant organisms in the hospital setting. Septic shock is most frequently triggered by gram-positive bacterial infections, followed by gram-negative bacteria and fungi. Hence, an older synonym, "endotoxic shock", is no longer appropriate.

The ability of diverse microorganisms to cause septic shock is consistent with the idea that a variety of microbial constituents can trigger the process. As you will recall from Chapter 3, macrophages, neutrophils, dendritic cells, endothelial cells, and soluble components of the innate immune system (e.g., complement) recognize and are activated by several substances derived from microorganisms. Once activated, these cells and factors initiate a number of inflammatory responses that interact in a complex, incompletely understood fashion to produce septic shock and multiorgan dysfunction (Fig. 4-20).

Factors believed to play major roles in the pathophysiology of septic shock include the following:

- *Inflammatory and counter-inflammatory responses.* In sepsis, various microbial cell wall constituents engage receptors on cells of the innate immune system,

Table 4-3 Three Major Types of Shock

Type of Shock	Clinical Example	Principal Mechanisms
Cardiogenic	Myocardial infarction Ventricular rupture Arrhythmia Cardiac tamponade Pulmonary embolism	Failure of myocardial pump resulting from intrinsic myocardial damage, extrinsic compression, or obstruction to outflow
Hypovolemic	Fluid loss (e.g., hemorrhage, vomiting, diarrhea, burns, or trauma)	Inadequate blood or plasma volume
Shock associated with systemic inflammation	Overwhelming microbial infections (bacterial and fungal) Superantigens (e.g., toxic shock syndrome) Trauma, burns, pancreatitis	Activation of cytokine cascades; peripheral vasodilation and pooling of blood; endothelial activation/injury; leukocyte-induced damage, disseminated intravascular coagulation

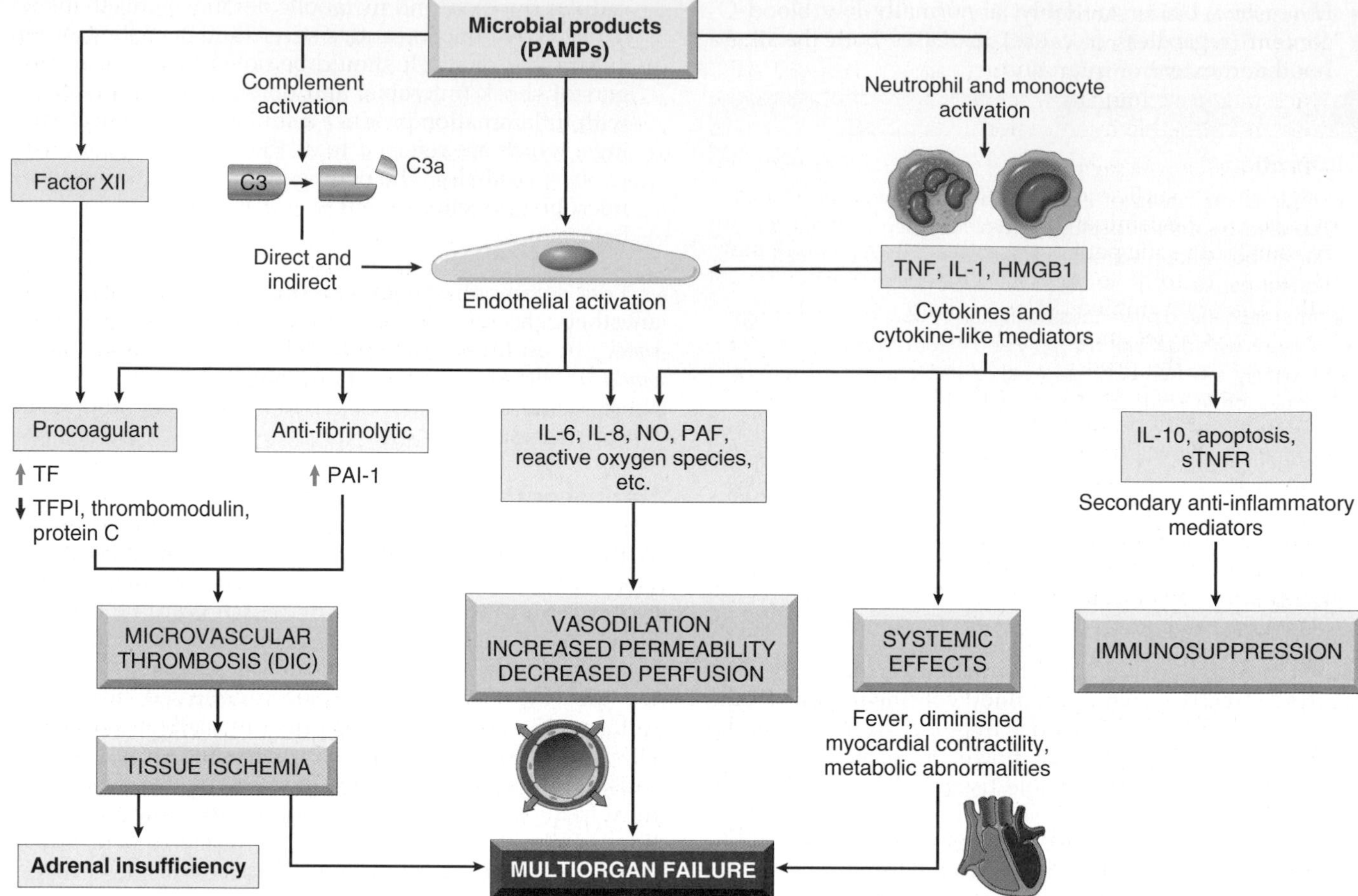

Figure 4-20 Major pathogenic pathways in septic shock. Microbial products (PAMPs, or pathogen-associated molecular patterns) activate endothelial cells and cellular and humoral elements of the innate immune system, initiating a cascade of events that lead to end-stage multiorgan failure. Additional details are given in the text. DIC, Disseminated vascular coagulation; HMGB1, high mobility group box 1 protein; NO, nitric oxide; PAF, platelet activating factor; PAI-1, plasminogen activator inhibitor 1; TF, tissue factor; TFPI, tissue factor pathway inhibitor.

triggering pro-inflammatory responses. Likely initiators of inflammation in sepsis are signaling pathways that lie downstream of *Toll-like receptors* (TLRs, Chapter 3), which you will recall recognize a host of microbe-derived substances containing so-called pathogen-associated molecular patterns (PAMPs), as well as G-protein coupled receptors that detect bacterial peptides, and nucleotide oligomerization domain proteins 1 and 2 [NOD1, NOD2]). Upon activation, innate immune cells produce TNF, IL-1, IFN-γ, IL-12, and IL-18, as well as other inflammatory mediators such as high mobility group box 1 protein (HMGB1). Reactive oxygen species and lipid mediators such as prostaglandins and platelet activating factor (PAF) are also elaborated. These effector molecules induce endothelial cells (and other cell types) to upregulate adhesion molecule expression and further stimulate cytokine and chemokine production. The *complement cascade* is also activated by microbial components, both directly and through the proteolytic activity of plasmin (Chapter 3), resulting in the production of anaphylotoxins (C3a, C5a), chemotactic fragments (C5a), and opsonins (C3b), all of which contribute to the pro-inflammatory state. In addition, microbial components can activate coagulation directly through factor XII and indirectly through altered endothelial function (discussed below). The accompanying widespread activation of thrombin may further augment inflammation by triggering protease-activated receptors (PARs) on inflammatory cells.

The hyperinflammatory state initiated by sepsis also activates counter-regulatory immunosuppressive mechanisms, which may involve both innate and adaptive immune cells. As a result, septic patients may oscillate between hyperinflammatory and immunosuppressed states during their clinical course. Proposed mechanisms for the immune suppression include a shift from pro-inflammatory (T_H1) to anti-inflammatory (T_H2) cytokines (Chapter 6), production of anti-inflammatory mediators (e.g., soluble TNF receptor, IL-1 receptor antagonist, and IL-10), lymphocyte apoptosis, the immunosuppressive effects of apoptotic cells, and the induction of cellular anergy.

- *Endothelial activation and injury*. The pro-inflammatory state and endothelial cell activation associated with sepsis leads to widespread vascular leakage and tissue edema, which have deleterious effects on both nutrient delivery and waste removal. One effect of inflammatory cytokines is to loosen endothelial cell tight junctions, making vessels leaky and resulting in the accumulation of protein-rich edema throughout the body. This alteration impedes tissue perfusion and may be exacerbated by attempts to support the patient with intravenous fluids. Activated endothelium also upregulates production of nitric oxide (NO) and other vasoactive inflammatory mediators (e.g., C3a, C5a, and PAF), which may contribute to vascular smooth muscle relaxation and systemic hypotension.

- *Induction of a procoagulant state.* The derangement in coagulation is sufficient to produce the formidable complication of disseminated intravascular coagulation in up to half of septic patients. Sepsis alters the expression of many factors so as to favor coagulation. Pro-inflammatory cytokines increase tissue factor production by monocytes and possibly endothelial cells as well, and decrease the production of endothelial anti-coagulant factors, such as tissue factor pathway inhibitor, thrombomodulin, and protein C (see Fig. 4-6 and Fig. 4-8). They also dampen fibrinolysis by increasing plasminogen activator inhibitor-1 expression (see Fig. 4-6*B* and Fig. 4-8). The vascular leak and tissue edema decrease blood flow at the level of small vessels, producing stasis and diminishing the washout of activated coagulation factors. Acting in concert, these effects lead to systemic activation of thrombin and the deposition of fibrin-rich thrombi in small vessels, often throughout the body, further compromising tissue perfusion. In full-blown disseminated intravascular coagulation, the consumption of coagulation factors and platelets is so great that deficiencies of these factors appear, leading to concomitant bleeding and hemorrhage (Chapter 14).
- *Metabolic abnormalities.* Septic patients exhibit insulin resistance and hyperglycemia. Cytokines such as TNF and IL-1, stress-induced hormones (such as glucagon, growth hormone, and glucocorticoids), and catecholamines all drive gluconeogenesis. At the same time, the pro-inflammatory cytokines suppress insulin release while simultaneously promoting insulin resistance in the liver and other tissues, likely by impairing the surface expression of GLUT-4, a glucose transporter. Hyperglycemia decreases neutrophil function—thereby suppressing bactericidal activity—and causes increased adhesion molecule expression on endothelial cells. Although sepsis is initially associated with an acute surge in glucocorticoid production, this phase may be followed by adrenal insufficiency and a functional deficit of glucocorticoids. This may stem from depression of the synthetic capacity of intact adrenal glands or frank adrenal necrosis due to disseminated intravascular dissemination (*Waterhouse-Friderichsen syndrome*, Chapter 25). Finally, cellular hypoxia and diminished oxidative phosphorylation leads to increased lactate production and lactic acidosis.
- *Organ dysfunction.* Systemic hypotension, interstitial edema, and small vessel thrombosis all decrease the delivery of oxygen and nutrients to the tissues, which fail to properly utilize those nutrients that are delivered due to cellular hypoxia. High levels of cytokines and secondary mediators diminish myocardial contractility and cardiac output, and increased vascular permeability and endothelial injury can lead to the *acute respiratory distress syndrome* (Chapter 15). Ultimately, these factors may conspire to cause the failure of multiple organs, particularly the kidneys, liver, lungs, and heart, culminating in death.

The severity and outcome of septic shock are likely dependent upon the extent and virulence of the infection; the immune status of the host; the presence of other co-morbid conditions; and the pattern and level of mediator production. The multiplicity of factors and the complexity of the interactions that underlie sepsis explain why most attempts to intervene therapeutically with antagonists of specific mediators have failed to be effective and may even have had deleterious effects in some cases. The standard of care remains antibiotics to treat the underlying infection and intravenous fluids, pressors and supplemental oxygen to maintain blood pressure and limit tissue hypoxia. Suffice it to say that even in the best of clinical centers, septic shock remains an obstinate clinical challenge.

It is worth mentioning here that an additional group of secreted bacterial proteins called *superantigens* also cause a syndrome similar to septic shock (e.g., *toxic shock syndrome*). Superantigens are polyclonal T-lymphocyte activators that induce the release of high levels of cytokines that result in a variety of clinical manifestations, ranging from a diffuse rash to vasodilation, hypotension, shock, and death.

Stages of Shock

Shock is a progressive disorder that, if uncorrected, leads to death. The exact mechanism(s) of death from sepsis are still unclear; aside from increased lymphocyte and enterocyte apoptosis there is only minimal cell death, and patients rarely have refractory hypotension, suggesting that organ failure secondary to edema and the attendant tissue hypoxia has a central role. For hypovolemic and cardiogenic shock, however, the pathways to death are reasonably well understood. Unless the insult is massive and rapidly lethal (e.g., a massive hemorrhage from a ruptured aortic aneurysm), shock in those settings tends to evolve through three general (albeit somewhat artificial) phases:

- An initial *nonprogressive phase* during which reflex compensatory mechanisms are activated and perfusion of vital organs is maintained
- A *progressive stage* characterized by tissue hypoperfusion and onset of worsening circulatory and metabolic imbalances, including lactic acidosis
- An *irreversible stage* that sets in after the body has incurred cellular and tissue injury so severe that even if the hemodynamic defects are corrected, survival is not possible

In the early nonprogressive phase of shock, a variety of *neurohumoral mechanisms* help to maintain cardiac output and blood pressure. These include baroreceptor reflexes, catecholamine release, activation of the renin-angiotensin axis, ADH release, and generalized sympathetic stimulation. The net effect is *tachycardia, peripheral vasoconstriction, and renal conservation of fluid.* Cutaneous vasoconstriction, for example, is responsible for the characteristic coolness and pallor of the skin in well-developed shock (although septic shock can initially cause cutaneous *vasodilation* and thus present with warm, flushed skin). Coronary and cerebral vessels are less sensitive to the sympathetic response and thus maintain relatively normal caliber, blood flow, and oxygen delivery.

If the underlying causes are not corrected, shock passes imperceptibly to the progressive phase, during which there is widespread tissue hypoxia. In the setting of persistent oxygen deficit, intracellular aerobic respiration is replaced by anaerobic glycolysis with excessive production of lactic acid. The resulting lactic acidosis lowers the tissue pH and blunts the vasomotor response; arterioles dilate, and blood begins to pool in the microcirculation. Peripheral pooling not only worsens the cardiac output, but also puts endothelial cells at risk for developing anoxic injury with subsequent disseminated intravascular coagulation. With widespread tissue hypoxia, vital organs are affected and begin to fail.

In severe cases, the process eventually enters an irreversible stage. Widespread cell injury is reflected in lysosomal enzyme leakage, further aggravating the shock state. If ischemic bowel allows intestinal flora to enter the circulation, bacteremic septic shock may be superimposed. At this point the patient may develop anuria as a result of acute tubular necrosis and renal failure (Chapter 20), and despite heroic measures the downward clinical spiral almost inevitably culminates in death.

MORPHOLOGY

The cellular and tissue changes induced by cardiogenic or hypovolemic shock are essentially those of hypoxic injury (Chapter 2); changes can manifest in any tissue although they are particularly evident in brain, heart, lungs, kidneys, adrenals, and gastrointestinal tract. The **adrenal** changes in shock are those seen in all forms of stress; essentially there is cortical cell lipid depletion. This does not reflect adrenal exhaustion but rather conversion of the relatively inactive vacuolated cells to metabolically active cells that utilize stored lipids for the synthesis of steroids. The **kidneys** typically exhibit acute tubular necrosis (Chapter 20). The **lungs** are seldom affected in pure hypovolemic shock, because they are somewhat resistant to hypoxic injury. However, when shock is caused by sepsis or trauma, **diffuse alveolar damage** (Chapter 15) may develop, the so-called shock lung**.** In septic shock, the development of disseminated intravascular coagulation leads to widespread deposition of fibrin-rich microthrombi, particularly in the brain, heart, lungs, kidney, adrenal glands, and gastrointestinal tract. The consumption of platelets and coagulation factors also often leads to the appearance of petechial hemorrhages on serosal surface and the skin.

With the exception of neuronal and myocyte ischemic loss, virtually all of these tissues may revert to normal if the individual survives. Unfortunately, most patients with irreversible changes due to severe shock die before the tissues can recover.

Clinical Consequences. The clinical manifestations of shock depend on the precipitating insult. In hypovolemic and cardiogenic shock the patient presents with hypotension; a weak, rapid pulse; tachypnea; and cool, clammy, cyanotic skin. In septic shock the skin may initially be warm and flushed because of peripheral vasodilation. The initial threat to life stems from the underlying catastrophe that precipitated the shock (e.g., myocardial infarct, severe hemorrhage, or sepsis). Rapidly, however, shock begets cardiac, cerebral, and pulmonary dysfunction, and eventually electrolyte disturbances and metabolic acidosis exacerbate the dire state of the patient further. Individuals who survive the initial complications may enter a second phase dominated by renal insufficiency and marked by a progressive fall in urine output as well as severe fluid and electrolyte imbalances. Coagulopathy frequently complicates shock, particularly when the cause is sepsis or trauma, and can have serious or even fatal consequences, particularly in patients with severe disseminated intravascular coagulation.

The prognosis varies with the origin of shock and its duration. Thus, greater than 90% of young, otherwise healthy patients with hypovolemic shock survive with appropriate management; in comparison, septic shock, or cardiogenic shock associated with extensive myocardial infarction, are associated with substantially worse mortality rates, even with state-of-the-art care.

KEY CONCEPTS

Shock

- Shock is defined as a state of systemic tissue hypoperfusion due to reduced cardiac output and/or reduced effective circulating blood volume.
- The major types of shock are cardiogenic (e.g., myocardial infarction), hypovolemic (e.g., blood loss), and shock associated with systemic inflammatory responses (e.g., in the setting of severe infections); acute spinal or brain injuries and severe hypersensitivity reactions can also cause neurogenic and anaphylactic shock, respectively
- Shock of any form can lead to hypoxic tissue injury if not corrected.
- Septic shock is caused by the host response to bacterial, viral or fungal infections; it is a systemic inflammatory condition characterized by endothelial cell activation, tissue edema, disseminated intravascular coagulation, and metabolic derangements that often lead to organ failure and death.

SUGGESTED READINGS

Fluid Dynamics

Chen H, Schrier R: Pathophysiology of volume overload in acute heart failure syndromes. *Am J Med* 119:S11, 2006. *[Older but still useful review of heart failure and fluid overload.]*

Hemostasis and Bleeding

Crawley J, Zanardelli S, Chion CK, Lane DA: The central role of thrombin in hemostasis. *J Thromb Haemost* 5(Suppl 1):95, 2007. *[Review of the various pathways impacted by thrombin activation.]*

Crawley J, Lane D: The haemostatic role of tissue factor pathway inhibitor. *Arterioscler Thromb Vasc Biol* 28:233, 2008. *[Summary of the physiologic roles of tissue factor pathway inhibitor.]*

De Candia E: Mechanisms of platelet activation by thrombin: a short history. *Thromb Res* 129:250–6, 2012. *[Review focused on platelet activation by PARs via thrombin, but also touching on other emerging points of possible crosstalk.]*

Kwaan HC, Samama MM: The significance of endothelial heterogeneity in thrombosis and hemostasis. *Semin Thromb Hemost* 36:286, 2010. *[Review focused on the influence of endothelium on hemostasis and thrombosis.]*

Mackman N, Tilley RE, Key NS: Role of the extrinsic pathway of blood coagulation in hemostasis and thrombosis. *Arterioscler Thromb Vasc Biol* 27:1687, 2007. *[General overview of fundamental pathways in coagulation.]*

Renne T, Schmaier AH, Nickel KF, et al: In vivo roles of factor XII. *Blood* 120:4296–303, 2012. *[A review summarizing new insights into the still uncertain in vivo functions of factor XII in thrombosis and vascular biology.]*

Rijken DC, Lijnen HR: New insights into the molecular mechanisms of the fibrinolytic system. *J Thromb Haemost* 7:4, 2009. *[Review of fibrinolytic pathways.]*

Thrombosis and Thromboembolism

Castoldi E, Rosing J: APC resistance: biological basis and acquired influences. *J Thromb Haemost* 8:445–53, 2010. *[Reviews the multifactorial etiology of activated protein C resistance (e.g., factor V Leiden) and discusses its clinical implications.]*

Cushman M: Epidemiology and risk factors for venous thrombosis. *Semin Hematol* 44:62, 2007. *[Overview of the risk factors and pathophysiology of DVT.]*

Donati MB, Lorenzet R: Thrombosis and cancer: 40 years of research. *Thromb Res* 129:348–52, 2012. *[A historical perspective on questions pertaining to cancer and thrombosis stretching from the era of Trousseau to the present.]*

Esmon CT, Esmon NL: The link between vascular features and thrombosis. *Annu Rev Physiol* 2011. *[Review of the interactions of endothelium, blood flow, and hemostasis/thrombosis.]*

Goldhaber SZ, Bounameaux H: Pulmonary embolism and deep vein thrombosis. *Lancet* 379:1835–46, 2012. *[A guide to the recognition and therapy of pulmonary embolism and DVT.]*

Hannaford PC: Epidemiology of the contraceptive pill and venous thromboembolism. *Thromb Res* 127(Suppl 3):S30–4, 2011. *[Discussion of risk for DVT in women using various forms of hormonal contraception.]*

Holy EW, Tanner FC: Tissue factor in cardiovascular disease pathophysiology and pharmacological intervention. *Adv Pharmacol* 59:259, 2010. *[Review of the roles of tissue factor in hemostasis and possible strategies to prevent thrombosis.]*

Hong MS, Amanullah AM: Heparin-induced thrombocytopenia: a practical review. *Rev Cardiovasc Med* 11:13, 2010. *[Review of HIT mechanisms and therapies.]*

Jennings LK: Mechanisms of platelet activation: need for new strategies to protect against platelet-mediated atherothrombosis. *Thromb Haemost* 102:248, 2009. *[Review of the roles played by platelets in thrombosis and inflammation, with an eye towards therapeutic intervention.]*

Kelton JG, Arnold DM, Bates SM: Nonheparin anticoagulants for heparin-induced thrombocytopenia. *N Eng J Med* 368:737, 2013. *[Discussion of heparin-induced thrombocytopenia and management of affected patients with non-heparin anticoagulants.]*

Montagnana M, Franchi M, Danese E, et al: Disseminated intravascular coagulation in obstetric and gynecologic disorders. *Semin Thromb Hemost* 36:404, 2010. *[Review of the mechanisms of DIC in the setting of pregnancy and gynecologic conditions.]*

Osinbowale O, Ali L, Chi YW: Venous thromboembolism: a clinical review. *Postgrad Med* 122:54, 2010. *[Basic review at a medical student/house officer level.]*

Ruiz-Irastorza G, Crowther M, Branch W, et al: Antiphospholipid syndrome. *Lancet* 376:1498, 2010. *[Summary of the anti-phospholipid syndrome that emphases diagnosis and therapy.]*

Watson HG, Baglin TP: Guidelines on travel-related venous thrombosis. *Br J Haematol* 152:31–4, 2011. *[Epidemilogy of travel-related DVT and clinical recommendations.]*

Willis R, Harris EN, Pierangeli SS: Pathogenesis of the antiphospholipid syndrome. *Semin Thromb Hemost* 38:305–21, 2012. *[Highlights possible mechanisms that contribute to the development and to the action of pathogenic anti-phospholipid antibodies.]*

Wu KK, Matijevic-Aleksic N: Molecular aspects of thrombosis and antithrombotic drugs. *Crit Rev Clin Lab Sci* 42:249, 2005. *[Thorough overview of the mechanisms of thrombus formation.]*

Zwicker J, Furie BC, Furie B: Cancer-associated thrombosis. *Crit Rev Oncol Hematol* 62:126, 2007. *[Review of the mechanisms underlying the hypercoagulable state of malignancy.]*

Unusual Forms of Embolic Disease

Akhtar S: Fat embolism. *Anesthesiol Clin* 27:533, 2009. *[Overview of the pathogenesis and clinical features of fat embolism syndrome.]*

Benson MD: Current concepts of immunology and diagnosis in amniotic fluid embolism. *Clin Dev Immunol* 2012:946576, 2012. *[Discussion of the pathophysiology of amniotic fluid embolism.]*

Septic Shock

Brosnahan AJ, Schlievert PM: Gram-positive bacterial superantigen outside-in signaling causes toxic shock syndrome. *FEBS J* 278:4649–67, 2011. *[A review of molecular mechanisms of toxic shock induced by bacterial components that act as superantigens.]*

Hotchkiss R, Karl I: The pathophysiology and treatment of sepsis. *N Engl J Med* 348:138, 2003. *[An older paper that lays a solid pathogenic foundation for understanding sepsis.]*

Lee WL, Slutsky AS: Sepsis and endothelial permeability. *N Engl J Med* 363:689–91, 2010. *[A brief review of the role of endothelial leakiness in the pathogenesis of sepsis.]*

Munford RS: Severe sepsis and septic shock: the role of gram-negative bacteremia. *Annu Rev Pathol* 1:467, 2006. *[A review of the role of gram-negative bacteria in septic shock.]*

Stearns-Kurosawa DJ, Osuchowski MF, Valentine C, et al: The pathogenesis of sepsis. *Ann Rev Pathol Mech Dis* 6:19, 2011. *[Update on approaches to understanding and treating sepsis.]*

See TARGETED THERAPY available online at www.studentconsult.com 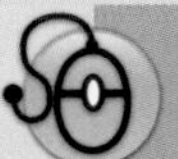

CHAPTER 5

Genetic Disorders

CHAPTER CONTENTS

Genes and Human Diseases

In chapter 1 we discussed the architecture of the normal human genome. Here we build upon that knowledge to discuss the genetic basis of human diseases.

Genetic disorders are far more common than is widely appreciated. The lifetime frequency of genetic diseases is estimated to be 670 per 1000. Furthermore, the genetic diseases encountered in medical practice represent only the tip of the iceberg, that is, those with less extreme genotypic errors that permit full embryonic development and live birth. It is estimated that 50% of spontaneous abortuses during the early months of gestation have a demonstrable chromosomal abnormality; there are, in addition, numerous smaller detectable errors and many other genetic lesions that are only now coming into view thanks to advances in DNA sequencing. About 1% of all newborn infants possess a gross chromosomal abnormality, and serious disease with a significant genetic component develops in approximately 5% of individuals younger than age 25 years. How many more mutations remain hidden?

Before discussing specific aberrations that may cause genetic diseases, it is useful to summarize the genetic contribution to human disease. Human genetic disorders can be broadly classified into three categories:

- *Disorders related to mutations in single genes with large effects.* These mutations cause the disease or predispose to the disease and with some exceptions, like hemoglobinopathies, are typically not present in normal population. Such mutations and their associated disorders are highly penetrant, meaning that the presence of the mutation is associated with the disease in a large proportion of individuals. Because these diseases are caused by single gene mutations, they usually follow the classic Mendelian pattern of inheritance and are also referred to as Mendelian disorders. A few important exceptions to this rule are noted later.

  Study of single genes and mutations with large effects has been extremely informative in medicine since a great deal of what is known about several physiologic pathways (e.g., cholesterol transport, chloride secretion) has been learned from analysis of single gene disorders. Although informative, these disorders are generally rare unless they are maintained in a population by strong selective forces (e.g., sickle cell anemia in areas where malaria is endemic, Chapter 14).
- *Chromosomal disorders.* These arise from structural or numerical alteration in the autosomes and sex chromosomes. Like monogenic disease they are uncommon but associated with high penetrance.
- *Complex multigenic disorders.* These are far more common than diseases in the previous two categories. They are caused by interactions between multiple variant forms of genes and environmental factors. Such variations in genes are common within the population and are also called *polymorphisms.* Each such variant gene confers a small increase in disease risk, and no single susceptibility gene is necessary or sufficient to produce the disease. It is only when several such polymorphisms are present in an individual that disease occurs, hence the term *multigenic* or *polygenic.* Thus, unlike mutant genes with large effects that are highly penetrant and give rise to Mendelian disorders, each polymorphism has a small effect and is of low penetrance. Since environmental interactions are important in the pathogenesis of these diseases, they are also called multifactorial disorders. In this category are some of the most common diseases that afflict humans, including atherosclerosis, diabetes mellitus, hypertension, and autoimmune diseases. Even normal traits such as height and weight are governed by polymorphisms in several genes.

The following discussion describes mutations that affect single genes, which underlie Mendelian disorders, followed by transmission patterns and selected samples of single gene disorders.

Mutations

A *mutation* is defined as a permanent change in the DNA. Mutations that affect germ cells are transmitted to the progeny and can give rise to inherited diseases. Mutations that arise in somatic cells understandably do not cause hereditary diseases but are important in the genesis of cancers and some congenital malformations.

General principles relating to the effects of gene mutations follow.

- ***Point mutations within coding sequences.*** A point mutation is a change in which a single base is substituted with a different base. It may alter the code in a triplet of bases and lead to the replacement of one amino acid by another in the gene product. Because these mutations alter the meaning of the sequence of the encoded protein, they are often termed *missense mutations.* If the substituted amino acid is biochemically similar to the original, typically it causes little change in the function of the protein and the mutation is called a "conservative" missense mutation. On the other hand, a "nonconservative" missense mutation replaces the normal amino acid with a biochemically different one. An excellent example of this type is the sickle mutation affecting the β-globin chain of hemoglobin (Chapter 14). Here the nucleotide triplet CTC (or GAG in mRNA), which encodes glutamic acid, is changed to CAC (or GUG in mRNA), which encodes valine. This single amino acid substitution alters the physicochemical properties of hemoglobin, giving rise to sickle cell anemia. Besides producing an amino acid substitution, a point mutation may change an amino acid codon to a chain terminator, or *stop codon (nonsense mutation).* Taking again the example of β-globin, a point mutation affecting the codon for glutamine (CAG) creates a stop codon (UAG) if U is substituted for C (Fig. 5-1). This change leads to premature termination of β-globin gene translation, and the short peptide that is produced is rapidly degraded. The resulting deficiency of β-globin chains can give rise to a severe form of anemia called β^0-thalassemia (Chapter 14).
- ***Mutations within noncoding sequences.*** Deleterious effects may also result from mutations that do not involve the exons. Recall that transcription of DNA is initiated and regulated by promoter and enhancer sequences (Chapter 1). Point mutations or deletions involving these regulatory sequences may interfere with binding of transcription factors and thus lead to a marked reduction in or total lack of transcription. Such is the case in certain forms of hereditary anemias called thalassemias (Chapter 14). In addition, point mutations within introns may lead to defective splicing of intervening sequences. This, in turn, interferes with normal processing of the initial mRNA transcripts and results in a failure to form mature mRNA. Therefore, translation cannot take place, and the gene product is not synthesized.

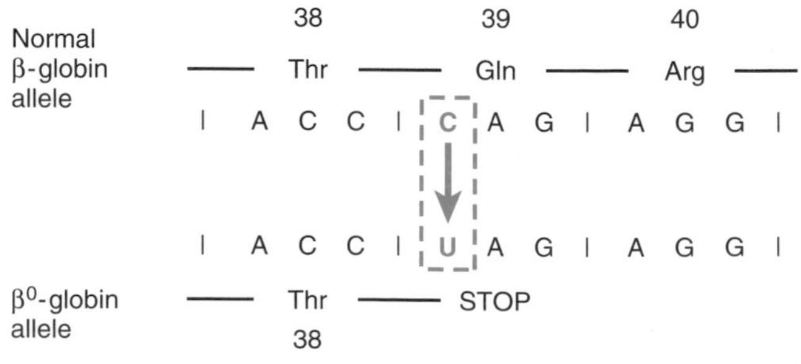

Figure 5-1 Nonsense mutation leading to premature chain termination. Partial mRNA sequence of the β-globin chain of hemoglobin showing codons for amino acids 38 to 40. A point mutation (C → U) in codon 39 changes a glutamine (Gln) codon to a stop codon, and hence protein synthesis stops at amino acid 38.

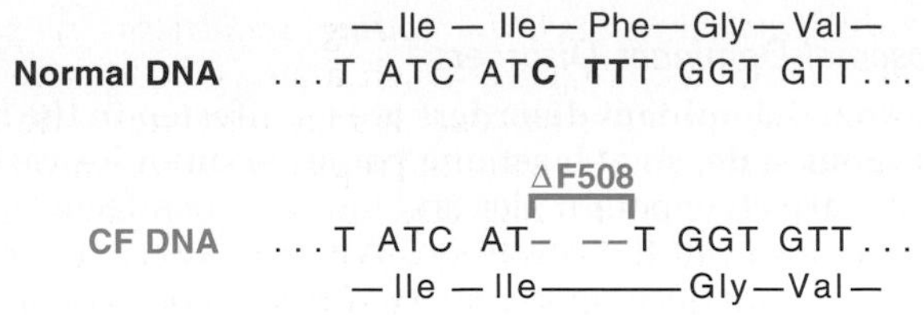

— Ile — Ile — Phe — Gly — Val —
Normal DNA ...T ATC ATC TTT GGT GTT...

ΔF508

CF DNA ...T ATC AT– ––T GGT GTT...
— Ile — Ile ——— Gly — Val —

Figure 5-2 Three-base deletion in the common cystic fibrosis (CF) allele results in synthesis of a protein that lacks amino acid 508 (phenylalanine). Because the deletion is a multiple of three, this is not a frameshift mutation. (From Thompson MW, et al: Thompson and Thompson Genetics in Medicine, 5th ed. Philadelphia, WB Saunders, 1991, p 135.)

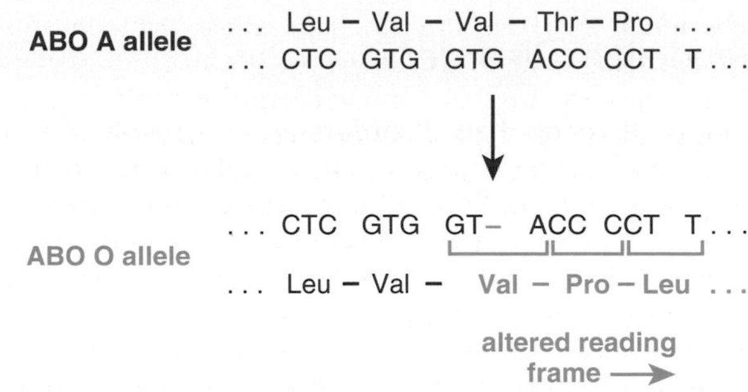

Figure 5-3 Single-base deletion at the ABO (glycosyltransferase) locus, leading to a frameshift mutation responsible for the O allele. (From Thompson MW, et al. Thompson and Thompson Genetics in Medicine, 5th ed. Philadelphia, WB Saunders, 1991, p 134.)

- ***Deletions and insertions.*** Small deletions or insertions involving the coding sequence can have two possible effects on the encoded protein. If the number of base pairs involved is three or a multiple of three, the reading frame will remain intact, and an abnormal protein lacking or gaining one or more amino acids will be synthesized (Fig. 5-2). If the number of affected coding bases is not a multiple of three, this will result in an alteration of the reading frame of the DNA strand, producing what is referred to as a frameshift mutation (Figs. 5-3 and 5-4). Typically, the result is the incorporation of a variable number of incorrect amino acids followed by truncation resulting from a premature stop codon.
- ***Trinucleotide-repeat mutations.*** Trinucleotide-repeat mutations belong to a special category of genetic anomaly. These mutations are characterized by amplification of a sequence of three nucleotides. Although the specific nucleotide sequence that undergoes amplification differs in various disorders, almost all affected sequences share the nucleotides guanine (G) and cytosine (C). For example, in fragile X syndrome, prototypical of this category of disorders, there are 250 to 4000 tandem repeats of the sequence CGG within a gene called *familial mental retardation 1 (FMR1).* In normal populations the number of repeats is small, averaging 29. Such expansions of the trinucleotide sequences prevent normal expression of the *FMR1* gene, thus giving rise to mental retardation. Another *distinguishing feature of trinucleotide-repeat mutations is that they are dynamic* (i.e., the degree of amplification increases during gametogenesis). These features, discussed in greater detail later, influence the pattern of inheritance and the phenotypic manifestations of the diseases caused by this class of mutation.

To summarize, mutations can interfere with gene expression at various levels. Transcription may be suppressed by gene deletions and point mutations involving promoter sequences. Abnormal mRNA processing may result from mutations affecting introns or splice junctions or both. Translation is affected if a nonsense mutation creates a stop codon (chain termination mutation) within an exon. Finally, some pathogenic point mutations may lead to expression of normal amounts of a dysfunctional protein.

Against this background, we now turn our attention to the three major categories of genetic disorders: (1) disorders related to mutant genes of large effect, (2) diseases with multifactorial inheritance, and (3) chromosomal disorders. To these three well-known categories must be added a heterogeneous group of *single-gene disorders with nonclassic patterns of inheritance.* This group includes disorders resulting from triplet-repeat mutations, those arising from mutations in mitochondrial DNA (mtDNA), and those in which the transmission is influenced by genomic imprinting or gonadal mosaicism. Diseases within this group are caused by mutations in single genes, but they do not follow the Mendelian pattern of inheritance. These are discussed later in this chapter.

It is beyond the scope of this book to review normal human genetics. Some fundamentals of DNA structure and regulation of gene expressions were described in Chapter 1. It is important here to clarify several commonly used terms—*hereditary, familial,* and *congenital.* Hereditary disorders, by definition, are derived from one's parents and are transmitted in the germ line through the generations and therefore are familial. The term *congenital* simply implies "born with." Some congenital diseases are not genetic; for example, congenital syphilis. Not all genetic diseases are congenital; individuals with Huntington disease, for example, begin to manifest their condition only after their 20s or 30s.

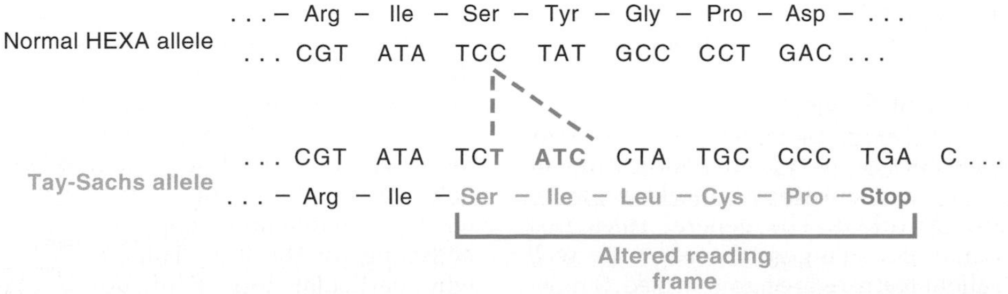

Normal HEXA allele
...– Arg – Ile – Ser – Tyr – Gly – Pro – Asp – ...
... CGT ATA TCC TAT GCC CCT GAC ...

Tay-Sachs allele
... CGT ATA TCT ATC CTA TGC CCC TGA C...
...– Arg – Ile – Ser – Ile – Leu – Cys – Pro – Stop

Altered reading frame

Figure 5-4 Four-base insertion in the hexosaminidase A gene, leading to a frameshift mutation. This mutation is the major cause of Tay-Sachs disease in Ashkenazi Jews. (From Nussbaum RL, et al: Thompson and Thompson Genetics in Medicine, 6th ed. Philadelphia, WB Saunders, 2001, p 212.)

Mendelian Disorders

Virtually all Mendelian disorders are the result of mutations in single genes that have large effects. It is not necessary to detail Mendel's laws here, since every student in biology, and possibly every garden pea, has learned about them at an early age. Only some comments of medical relevance are made.

It is estimated that every individual is a carrier of five to eight deleterious genes, a number originally estimated from studies of populations that appears to be borne out by genomic sequencing of normal individuals. Most of these are recessive and therefore do not have serious phenotypic effects. About 80% to 85% of these mutations are familial. The remainder represents new mutations acquired de novo by an affected individual.

Some autosomal mutations produce partial expression in the heterozygote and full expression in the homozygote. Sickle cell anemia is caused by substitution of normal hemoglobin (HbA) by hemoglobin S (HbS). When an individual is homozygous for the mutant gene, all the hemoglobin is of the abnormal, HbS, type, and even with normal saturation of oxygen the disorder is fully expressed (i.e., sickling deformity of all red cells and hemolytic anemia). In the heterozygote, only a proportion of the hemoglobin is HbS (the remainder being HbA), and therefore red cell sickling occurs only under unusual circumstances, such as exposure to lowered oxygen tension. This is referred to as the *sickle cell trait* to differentiate it from full-blown sickle cell anemia.

Although Mendelian traits are usually described as dominant or recessive, in some cases both of the alleles of a gene pair contribute to the phenotype—a condition called *codominance.* Histocompatibility and blood group antigens are good examples of codominant inheritance.

A single mutant gene may lead to many end effects, termed *pleiotropism;* conversely, mutations at several genetic loci may produce the same trait *(genetic heterogeneity).* Sickle cell anemia is an example of pleiotropism. In this hereditary disorder not only does the point mutation in the gene give rise to HbS, which predisposes the red cells to hemolysis, but also the abnormal red cells tend to cause a logjam in small vessels, inducing, for example, splenic fibrosis, organ infarcts, and bone changes. The numerous differing end-organ derangements are all related to the primary defect in hemoglobin synthesis. On the other hand, profound childhood deafness, an apparently homogeneous clinical entity, results from many different types of autosomal recessive mutations. Recognition of genetic heterogeneity not only is important in genetic counseling but also is relevant in the understanding of the pathogenesis of some common disorders, such as diabetes mellitus.

Transmission Patterns of Single-Gene Disorders

Mutations involving single genes typically follow one of three patterns of inheritance: autosomal dominant, autosomal recessive, and X-linked. The general rules that govern the transmission of single-gene disorders are well known; only a few salient features are summarized. Single-gene disorders with nonclassic patterns of inheritance are described later.

Autosomal Dominant Disorders

Autosomal dominant disorders are manifested in the heterozygous state, so at least one parent of an index case is usually affected; both males and females are affected, and both can transmit the condition. When an affected person marries an unaffected one, every child has one chance in two of having the disease. In addition to these basic rules, autosomal dominant conditions are characterized by the following:

- *With every autosomal dominant disorder, some proportion of patients do not have affected parents.* Such patients owe their disorder to new mutations involving either the egg or the sperm from which they were derived. Their siblings are neither affected nor at increased risk for disease development. The proportion of patients who develop the disease as a result of a new mutation is related to the effect of the disease on reproductive capability. If a disease markedly reduces reproductive fitness, most cases would be expected to result from new mutations. Many new mutations seem to occur in germ cells of relatively older fathers.
- *Clinical features can be modified by variations in penetrance and expressivity.* Some individuals inherit the mutant gene but are phenotypically normal. This is referred to as *incomplete penetrance.* Penetrance is expressed in mathematical terms. Thus, 50% penetrance indicates that 50% of those who carry the gene express the trait. In contrast to penetrance, if a trait is seen in all individuals carrying the mutant gene but is expressed differently among individuals, the phenomenon is called *variable expressivity.* For example, manifestations of neurofibromatosis type 1 range from brownish spots on the skin to multiple skin tumors and skeletal deformities. The mechanisms underlying incomplete penetrance and variable expressivity are not fully understood, but they most likely result from effects of other genes or environmental factors that modify the phenotypic expression of the mutant allele. For example, the phenotype of a patient with sickle cell anemia (resulting from mutation at the β-globin locus) is influenced by the genotype at the α-globin locus, because the latter influences the total amount of hemoglobin made (Chapter 14). The influence of environmental factors is exemplified by individuals heterozygous for familial hypercholesterolemia. The expression of the disease in the form of atherosclerosis is conditioned by the dietary intake of lipids.
- In many conditions the age at onset is delayed; symptoms and signs may not appear until adulthood (as in Huntington disease).

The biochemical mechanisms of autosomal dominant disorders depend upon the nature of the mutation and the type of protein affected. Most mutations lead to the reduced production of a gene product or give rise to a dysfunctional or inactive protein. Whether such a mutation gives rise to dominant or recessive disease depends on whether the remaining copy of the gene is capable of compensating for the loss. Thus, understanding the reasons why particular loss-of-function mutations give rise to dominant vs. recessive disease patterns requires an understanding of the biology. Many autosomal dominant diseases arising from deleterious mutations fall into one of a few familiar patterns:

1. *Those involved in regulation of complex metabolic pathways that are subject to feedback inhibition.* Membrane receptors such as the low-density lipoprotein (LDL) receptor provide one such example; in familial hypercholesterolemia, discussed later, a 50% loss of LDL receptors results in a secondary elevation of cholesterol that, in turn, predisposes to atherosclerosis in affected heterozygotes.
2. *Key structural proteins, such as collagen and cytoskeletal elements of the red cell membrane* (e.g., spectrin). The biochemical mechanisms by which a 50% reduction in the amounts of such proteins results in an abnormal phenotype are not fully understood. In some cases, especially when the gene encodes one subunit of a multimeric protein, the product of the mutant allele can interfere with the assembly of a functionally normal multimer. For example, the collagen molecule is a trimer in which the three collagen chains are arranged in a helical configuration. Each of the three collagen chains in the helix must be normal for the assembly and stability of the collagen molecule. Even with a single mutant collagen chain, normal collagen trimers cannot be formed, and hence there is a marked deficiency of collagen. In this instance the mutant allele is called *dominant negative,* because it impairs the function of a normal allele. This effect is illustrated by some forms of osteogenesis imperfecta, characterized by marked deficiency of collagen and severe skeletal abnormalities (Chapter 26).

Less common than loss-of-function mutations are *gain-of-function* mutations, which can take two forms. Some mutations result in an increase in a protein's normal function, for example, excessive enzymatic activity. In other cases, mutations impart a wholly new activity completely unrelated to the affected protein's normal function. The transmission of disorders produced by gain-of-function mutations is almost always autosomal dominant, as illustrated by Huntington disease (Chapter 28). In this disease the trinucleotide-repeat mutation affecting the Huntington gene (see later) gives rise to an abnormal protein, called *huntingtin,* that is toxic to neurons, and hence even heterozygotes develop a neurologic deficit.

Table 5-1 lists common autosomal dominant disorders. Many are discussed more logically in other chapters. A few conditions not considered elsewhere are discussed later in this chapter to illustrate important principles.

Table 5-1 Autosomal Dominant Disorders

System	Disorder
Nervous	Huntington disease Neurofibromatosis Myotonic dystrophy Tuberous sclerosis
Urinary	Polycystic kidney disease
Gastrointestinal	Familial polyposis coli
Hematopoietic	Hereditary spherocytosis von Willebrand disease
Skeletal	Marfan syndrome* Ehlers-Danlos syndrome (some variants)* Osteogenesis imperfecta Achondroplasia
Metabolic	Familial hypercholesterolemia* Acute intermittent porphyria

*Discussed in this chapter. Other disorders listed are discussed in appropriate chapters in the book.

Autosomal Recessive Disorders

Autosomal recessive traits make up the largest category of Mendelian disorders. They occur when both alleles at a given gene locus are mutated. These disorders are characterized by the following features: (1) The trait does not usually affect the parents of the affected individual, but siblings may show the disease; (2) siblings have one chance in four of having the trait (i.e., the recurrence risk is 25% for each birth); and (3) if the mutant gene occurs with a low frequency in the population, there is a strong likelihood that the affected individual (proband) is the product of a consanguineous marriage. The following features generally apply to most autosomal recessive disorders and distinguish them from autosomal dominant diseases:

- The expression of the defect tends to be more uniform than in autosomal dominant disorders.
- Complete penetrance is common.
- Onset is frequently early in life.
- Although new mutations associated with recessive disorders do occur, they are rarely detected clinically. Since the individual with a new mutation is an asymptomatic heterozygote, several generations may pass before the descendants of such a person mate with other heterozygotes and produce affected offspring.
- Many of the mutated genes encode enzymes. In heterozygotes, equal amounts of normal and defective enzyme are synthesized. Usually the natural "margin of safety" ensures that cells with half the usual complement of the enzyme function normally.

Autosomal recessive disorders include almost all inborn errors of metabolism. The various consequences of enzyme deficiencies are discussed later. The more common of these conditions are listed in Table 5-2. Most are presented elsewhere; a few prototypes are discussed later in this chapter.

Table 5-2 Autosomal Recessive Disorders

System	Disorder
Metabolic	Cystic fibrosis Phenylketonuria Galactosemia Homocystinuria Lysosomal storage diseases* α_1-Antitrypsin deficiency Wilson disease Hemochromatosis Glycogen storage diseases*
Hematopoietic	Sickle cell anemia Thalassemias
Endocrine	Congenital adrenal hyperplasia
Skeletal	Ehlers-Danlos syndrome (some variants)* Alkaptonuria*
Nervous	Neurogenic muscular atrophies Friedreich ataxia Spinal muscular atrophy

*Discussed in this chapter. Many others are discussed elsewhere in the text.

X-Linked Disorders

All sex-linked disorders are X-linked, and almost all are recessive. Several genes are located in the "male-specific region of Y"; all of these are related to spermatogenesis. *Males with mutations affecting the Y-linked genes are usually infertile, and hence there is no Y-linked inheritance.* As discussed later, a few additional genes with homologues on the X chromosome have been mapped to the Y chromosome, but only a few rare disorders resulting from mutations in such genes have been described.

X-linked recessive inheritance accounts for a small number of well-defined clinical conditions. The Y chromosome, for the most part, is not homologous to the X, and so mutant genes on the X do not have corresponding alleles on the Y. Thus, the male is said to be *hemizygous* for X-linked mutant genes, so these disorders are expressed in the male. Other features that characterize these disorders are as follows:

- An affected male does not transmit the disorder to his sons, but all daughters are carriers. Sons of heterozygous women have, of course, one chance in two of receiving the mutant gene.
- The heterozygous female usually does not express the full phenotypic change because of the paired normal allele. Because of the random inactivation of one of the X chromosomes in the female, however, females have a variable proportion of cells in which the mutant X chromosome is active. Thus, it is remotely possible for the normal allele to be inactivated in most cells, permitting full expression of heterozygous X-linked conditions in the female. Much more commonly, the normal allele is inactivated in only some of the cells, and thus the heterozygous female expresses the disorder partially. An illustrative condition is *glucose-6-phosphate dehydrogenase (G6PD) deficiency*. Transmitted on the X chromosome, this enzyme deficiency, which predisposes to red cell hemolysis in patients receiving certain types of drugs (Chapter 14), is expressed principally in males. In the female, a proportion of the red cells may be derived from precursors with inactivation of the normal allele. Such red cells are at the same risk for undergoing hemolysis as are the red cells in the hemizygous male. Thus, the female is not only a carrier of this trait but also is susceptible to drug-induced hemolytic reactions. Because the proportion of defective red cells in heterozygous females depends on the random inactivation of one of the X chromosomes, however, the severity of the hemolytic reaction is almost always less in heterozygous women than in hemizygous men. Most of the X-linked conditions listed in Table 5-3 are covered elsewhere in the text.

There are only a few *X-linked dominant* conditions. They are caused by dominant disease-associated alleles on the X chromosome. These disorders are transmitted by an affected heterozygous female to half her sons and half her daughters and by an affected male parent to all his daughters but none of his sons, if the female parent is unaffected. Vitamin D–resistant rickets is an example of this type of inheritance.

Table 5-3 X-Linked Recessive Disorders

System	Disease
Musculoskeletal	Duchenne muscular dystrophy
Blood	Hemophilia A and B Chronic granulomatous disease Glucose-6-phosphate dehydrogenase deficiency
Immune	Agammaglobulinemia Wiskott-Aldrich syndrome
Metabolic	Diabetes insipidus Lesch-Nyhan syndrome
Nervous	Fragile X syndrome*

*Discussed in this chapter. Others are discussed in appropriate chapters in the text.

KEY CONCEPTS

Transmission Patterns of Single-Gene Disorders

- **Autosomal dominant disorders** are characterized by expression in heterozygous state; they affect males and females equally, and both sexes can transmit the disorder.
- Enzyme proteins are not affected in autosomal dominant disorders; instead, receptors and structural proteins are involved.
- **Autosomal recessive diseases** occur when both copies of a gene are mutated; enzyme proteins are frequently involved. Males and females are affected equally.
- **X-linked disorders** are transmitted by heterozygous females to their sons, who manifest the disease. Female carriers usually are protected because of random inactivation of one X chromosome.

Biochemical and Molecular Basis of Single-Gene (Mendelian) Disorders

Mendelian disorders result from alterations involving single genes. The genetic defect may lead to the formation of an abnormal protein or a reduction in the output of the gene product. Virtually any type of protein may be affected in single-gene disorders and by a variety of mechanisms (Table 5-4). To some extent the pattern of inheritance of the disease is related to the kind of protein affected by the mutation. For this discussion, the mechanisms involved in single-gene disorders can be classified into four categories: (1) *enzyme defects and their consequences;* (2) *defects in membrane receptors and transport systems;* (3) *alterations in the structure, function, or quantity of nonenzyme proteins;* and (4) *mutations resulting in unusual reactions to drugs.*

Enzyme Defects and Their Consequences

Mutations may result in the synthesis of an enzyme with reduced activity or a reduced amount of a normal enzyme. In either case, the consequence is a metabolic block. Figure 5-5 provides an example of an enzyme reaction in which the substrate is converted by intracellular enzymes, denoted as 1, 2, and 3, into an end product through intermediates 1 and 2. In this model the final product exerts feedback control on enzyme 1. A minor pathway producing small quantities of M1 and M2 also exists. The biochemical

Table 5-4 Biochemical and Molecular Basis of Some Mendelian Disorders

Protein Type/ Function	Example	Molecular Lesion	Disease
Enzyme	Phenylalanine hydroxylase	Splice-site mutation: reduced amount	Phenylketonuria
	Hexosaminidase	Splice-site mutation or frameshift mutation with stop codon: reduced amount	Tay-Sachs disease
	Adenosine deaminase	Point mutations: abnormal protein with reduced activity	Severe combined immunodeficiency
Enzyme inhibitor	α_1-Antitrypsin	Missense mutations: impaired secretion from liver to serum	Emphysema and liver disease
Receptor	Low-density lipoprotein receptor	Deletions, point mutations: reduction of synthesis, transport to cell surface, or binding to low-density lipoprotein	Familial hypercholesterolemia
	Vitamin D receptor	Point mutations: failure of normal signaling	Vitamin D–resistant rickets
Transport			
Oxygen	Hemoglobin	Deletions: reduced amount	α-Thalassemia
		Defective mRNA processing: reduced amount	β-Thalassemia
		Point mutations: abnormal structure	Sickle cell anemia
Ion channels	Cystic fibrosis transmembrane conductance regulator	Deletions and other mutations: nonfunctional or misfolded proteins	Cystic fibrosis
Structural			
Extracellular	Collagen	Deletions or point mutations cause reduced amount of normal collagen or normal amounts of defective collagen	Osteogenesis imperfecta; Ehlers-Danlos syndromes
	Fibrillin	Missense mutations	Marfan syndrome
Cell membrane	Dystrophin	Deletion with reduced synthesis	Duchenne/Becker muscular dystrophy
	Spectrin, ankyrin, or protein 4.1	Heterogeneous	Hereditary spherocytosis
Hemostasis	Factor VIII	Deletions, insertions, nonsense mutations, and others: reduced synthesis or abnormal factor VIII	Hemophilia A
Growth regulation	Rb protein	Deletions	Hereditary retinoblastoma
	Neurofibromin	Heterogeneous	Neurofibromatosis type 1

consequences of an enzyme defect in such a reaction may lead to three major consequences:

- *Accumulation of the substrate*, depending on the site of block, may be accompanied by accumulation of one or both intermediates. Moreover, an increased concentration of intermediate 2 may stimulate the minor pathway and thus lead to an excess of M1 and M2. Under these conditions tissue injury may result if the precursor, the intermediates, or the products of alternative minor pathways are toxic in high concentrations. For example, in galactosemia, the deficiency of galactose-1-phosphate uridyltransferase (Chapter 10) leads to the accumulation of galactose and consequent tissue damage. Excessive accumulation of complex substrates within the lysosomes as a result of deficiency of degradative enzymes is responsible for a group of diseases generally referred to as *lysosomal storage diseases.*

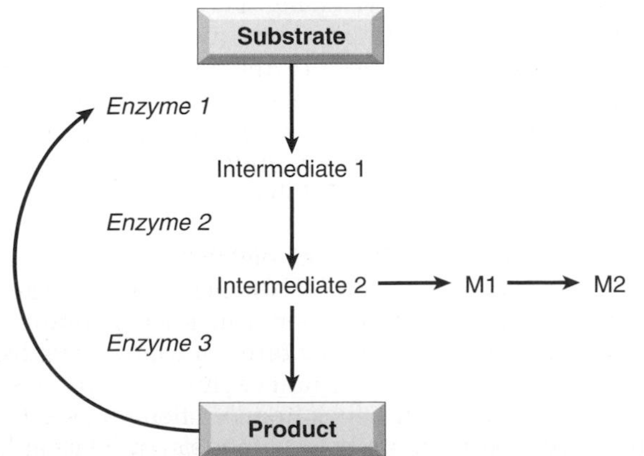

Figure 5-5 A possible metabolic pathway in which a substrate is converted to an end product by a series of enzyme reactions. M1, M2, products of a minor pathway.

- *An enzyme defect can lead to a metabolic block and a decreased amount of end product* that may be necessary for normal function. For example, a deficiency of melanin may result from lack of tyrosinase, which is necessary for the biosynthesis of melanin from its precursor, tyrosine, resulting in the clinical condition called *albinism.* If the end product is a feedback inhibitor of the enzymes involved in the early reactions (in Fig. 5-5 it is shown that the product inhibits enzyme 1), the deficiency of the end product may permit overproduction of intermediates and their catabolic products, some of which may be injurious at high concentrations. A prime example of a disease with such an underlying mechanism is the Lesch-Nyhan syndrome (Chapter 26).
- *Failure to inactivate a tissue-damaging substrate* is best exemplified by α_1-antitrypsin deficiency. Individuals who have an inherited deficiency of serum α_1-antitrypsin are unable to inactivate neutrophil elastase in their lungs. Unchecked activity of this protease leads to destruction of elastin in the walls of lung alveoli, leading eventually to pulmonary emphysema (Chapter 15).

Defects in Receptors and Transport Systems

As we discussed in chapter 1, biologically active substances have to be actively transported across the cell membrane. In some cases transport is achieved by receptor-mediated endocytosis. A genetic defect in a receptor-mediated transport system is exemplified by familial hypercholesterolemia, in which reduced synthesis or function of LDL receptors leads to defective transport of LDL into the cells and secondarily to excessive cholesterol synthesis by complex intermediary mechanisms. In cystic fibrosis the transport system for chloride ions in exocrine glands, sweat ducts, lungs, and pancreas is defective. By mechanisms not fully understood, impaired chloride transport leads to serious injury to the lungs and pancreas (Chapter 10).

Alterations in Structure, Function, or Quantity of Nonenzyme Proteins

Genetic defects resulting in alterations of nonenzyme proteins often have widespread secondary effects, as exemplified by sickle cell disease. The hemoglobinopathies, sickle cell disease being one, all of which are characterized by defects in the structure of the globin molecule, best exemplify this category. In contrast to the hemoglobinopathies, the thalassemias result from mutations in globin genes that affect the amount of globin chains synthesized. Thalassemias are associated with reduced amounts of structurally normal α-globin or β-globin chains (Chapter 14). Other examples of genetic disorders involving defective structural proteins include collagen, spectrin, and dystrophin, giving rise to osteogenesis imperfecta (Chapter 26), hereditary spherocytosis (Chapter 14), and muscular dystrophies (Chapter 27), respectively.

Genetically Determined Adverse Reactions to Drugs

Certain genetically determined enzyme deficiencies are unmasked only after exposure of the affected individual to certain drugs. This special area of genetics, called *pharmacogenetics,* is of considerable clinical importance. The classic example of drug-induced injury in the genetically susceptible individual is associated with a deficiency of the enzyme G6PD. Under normal conditions glucose-6 phosphate-dehydrogenase (G6PD) deficiency does not result in disease, but on administration, for example, of the antimalarial drug primaquine, a severe hemolytic anemia results (Chapter 14). In recent years an increasing number of polymorphisms of genes encoding drug-metabolizing enzymes, transporters, and receptors have been identified. In some cases these genetic factors have major impact on drug sensitivity and adverse reactions. It is hoped that advances in pharmacogenetics will lead to patient-tailored therapy, an example of "personalized medicine."

With this overview of the biochemical basis of single-gene disorders, we now consider selected examples grouped according to the underlying defect.

Disorders Associated with Defects in Structural Proteins

Several diseases caused by mutations in genes that encode structural proteins are listed in Table 5-4. Many are discussed elsewhere in the text. Only Marfan syndrome and Ehlers-Danlos syndromes (EDSs) are discussed here, because they affect connective tissue and hence involve multiple organ systems.

Marfan Syndrome

Marfan syndrome is a disorder of connective tissues, manifested principally by changes in the skeleton, eyes, and cardiovascular system. Its prevalence is estimated to be 1 in 5000. Approximately 70% to 85% of cases are familial and transmitted by autosomal dominant inheritance. The remainder are sporadic and arise from new mutations.

Pathogenesis. **Marfan syndrome results from an inherited defect in an extracellular glycoprotein called *fibrillin-1*.** There are two fundamental mechanisms by which loss of fibrillin leads to the clinical manifestations of Marfan syndrome: loss of structural support in microfibril rich connective tissue and excessive activation of TGF-β signaling. Each of these is discussed below.

- Fibrillin is the major component of microfibrils found in the extracellular matrix (Chapter 1). These fibrils provide a scaffolding on which tropoelastin is deposited to form elastic fibers. Although microfibrils are widely distributed in the body, they are particularly abundant in the aorta, ligaments, and the ciliary zonules that support the lens; these tissues are prominently affected in Marfan syndrome. Fibrillin occurs in two homologous forms, fibrillin-1 and fibrillin-2, encoded by two separate genes, *FBN1* and *FBN2,* mapped on chromosomes 15q21.1 and 5q23.31, respectively. Mutations of *FBN1* underlie Marfan syndrome; mutations of the related *FBN2* gene are less common, and they give rise to *congenital contractural arachnodactyly,* an autosomal dominant disorder characterized by skeletal abnormalities. Mutational analysis has revealed more than 600 distinct mutations of the *FBN1* gene in individuals with Marfan syndrome. Most of these are missense mutations that give rise to abnormal fibrillin-1. These can inhibit polymerization of fibrillin fibers (dominant negative effect). Alternatively, the reduction of fibrillin content below a certain threshold weakens the connective tissue (haploinsufficiency).
- While many clinical manifestations of Marfan syndrome can be explained by changes in the mechanical properties of the extracellular matrix resulting from abnormalities of fibrillin, several others such as bone overgrowth and myxoid changes in mitral valves cannot be attributed to changes in tissue elasticity. Recent studies indicate that loss of microfibrils gives rise to abnormal and excessive activation of transforming growth factor-β (TGF-β), since normal microfibrils sequester TGF-β and thus control the bioavailability of this cytokine. Excessive TGF-β signaling has deleterious effects on vascular smooth muscle development and it also increases the activity of metalloproteases, causing loss of extracellular matrix. This schema is supported by two sets of observations. First, in a small number of individuals with clinical features of Marfan syndrome (MFS2), there are no mutations in *FBN1* but instead gain-of-function mutations in genes that encode TGF-β receptors. Second, in mouse models of Marfan syndrome generated by mutations in *Fbn1*, administration of antibodies to TGF-β prevents alterations in the aorta and mitral valves.

MORPHOLOGY

Skeletal abnormalities are the most striking feature of Marfan syndrome. Typically the patient is unusually tall with exceptionally long extremities and long, tapering fingers and toes. The joint ligaments in the hands and feet are lax, suggesting that the patient is double-jointed; typically the thumb can be hyperextended back to the wrist. The head is commonly dolichocephalic (long-headed) with bossing of the frontal eminences and prominent supraorbital ridges. A variety of spinal deformities may appear, including kyphosis, scoliosis, or rotation or slipping of the dorsal or lumbar vertebrae. The chest is classically deformed, presenting either pectus excavatum (deeply depressed sternum) or a pigeon-breast deformity.

The **ocular changes** take many forms. Most characteristic is bilateral subluxation or dislocation (usually outward and upward) of the lens, referred to as ectopia lentis. This abnormality is so uncommon in persons who do not have this disease that the finding of bilateral ectopia lentis should raise the suspicion of Marfan syndrome.

Cardiovascular lesions are the most life-threatening features of this disorder. The two most common lesions are mitral valve prolapse and, of greater importance, dilation of the ascending aorta due to cystic medionecrosis. Histologically the changes in the media are virtually identical to those found in cystic medionecrosis not related to Marfan syndrome (Chapter 12). Loss of medial support results in progressive dilation of the aortic valve ring and the root of the aorta, giving rise to severe aortic incompetence. In addition, excessive TGF-β signaling in the adventitia may also contribute to aortic dilation. Weakening of the media predisposes to an intimal tear, which may initiate an intramural hematoma that cleaves the layers of the media to produce **aortic dissection.** After cleaving the aortic layers for considerable distances, sometimes back to the root of the aorta or down to the iliac arteries, the hemorrhage often ruptures through the aortic wall. Such a calamity is the cause of death in 30% to 45% of these individuals.

Clinical Features. Although mitral valve lesions are more frequent, they are clinically less important than aortic lesions. Loss of connective tissue support in the mitral valve leaflets makes them soft and billowy, creating a so-called floppy valve (Chapter 12). Valvular lesions, along with lengthening of the chordae tendineae, frequently give rise to mitral regurgitation. Similar changes may affect the tricuspid and, rarely, the aortic valves. Echocardiography greatly enhances the ability to detect the cardiovascular abnormalities and is therefore extremely valuable in the diagnosis of Marfan syndrome. The great majority of deaths are caused by rupture of aortic dissections, followed in importance by cardiac failure.

While the lesions just described typify Marfan syndrome, it must be emphasized that there is great variation in the clinical expression of this genetic disorder. Patients with prominent eye or cardiovascular changes may have few skeletal abnormalities, whereas others with striking changes in body habitus have no eye changes. Although variability in clinical expression may be seen within a family, interfamilial variability is much more common and extensive. Because of such variations, the clinical diagnosis of Marfan syndrome is currently based on the so called "revised Ghent criteria." These take into account family history, cardinal clinical signs in the absence of family history, and presence or absence of fibrillin mutation. In general, major involvement of two of the four organ systems (skeletal, cardiovascular, ocular, and skin) and minor involvement of another organ is required for diagnosis.

The variable expression of the Marfan defect is best explained on the basis of of the many different mutations that affect the fibrillin locus, which number more than 600. This genetic heterogeneity also poses formidable challenges in the diagnosis of Marfan syndrome. The evolving high throughput sequencing technologies discussed later in this chapter may overcome this problem in the future.

The mainstay of the medical treatment is administration of β blockers which likely act by reducing heart rate and aortic wall stress. In animal models inhibition of TGF-β action by use of specific antibodies has been found useful. Since lifelong use of such antibodies in humans is not feasible, other strategies to block TGF-β signaling are being tested. Blockade of angiotensin type 2 receptors accomplishes this effect in humans and several preliminary studies are very promising.

Ehlers-Danlos Syndromes (EDS)

EDSs comprise a clinically and genetically heterogeneous group of disorders that result from some defect in the synthesis or structure of fibrillar collagen. Other disorders resulting from mutations affecting collagen synthesis include osteogenesis imperfecta (Chapter 26), Alport syndrome (Chapter 20), and epidermolysis bullosa (Chapter 25).

Biosynthesis of collagen is a complex process (Chapter 1) that can be disturbed by genetic errors that may affect any one of the numerous structural collagen genes or enzymes necessary for posttranscriptional modifications of collagen. Hence, the mode of inheritance of EDS encompasses all three Mendelian patterns. On the basis of clinical and molecular characteristics, six variants of EDS have been recognized. These are listed in Table 5-5. It is beyond the scope of this book to discuss each variant individually; instead, the important clinical features common to most

Table 5-5 Classification of Ehlers-Danlos Syndromes

EDS Type*	Clinical Findings	Inheritance	Gene Defects
Classic (I/II)	Skin and joint hypermobility, atrophic scars, easy bruising	Autosomal dominant	*COL5A1, COL5A2*
Hypermobility (III)	Joint hypermobility, pain, dislocations	Autosomal dominant	Unknown
Vascular (IV)	Thin skin, arterial or uterine rupture, bruising, small joint hyperextensibility	Autosomal dominant	*COL3A1*
Kyphoscoliosis (VI)	Hypotonia, joint laxity, congenital scoliosis, ocular fragility	Autosomal recessive	Lysyl hydroxylase
Arthrochalasia (VIIa,b)	Severe joint hypermobility, skin changes (mild), scoliosis, bruising	Autosomal dominant	*COL1A1, COL1A2*
Dermatosparaxis (VIIc)	Severe skin fragility, cutis laxa, bruising	Autosomal recessive	Procollagen *N*-peptidase

*EDS types were previously classified by Roman numerals. Parentheses show previous numerical equivalents.

variants are summarized and clinical manifestations are correlated with the underlying molecular defects in collagen synthesis or structure.

As might be expected, tissues rich in collagen, such as skin, ligaments, and joints, are frequently involved in most variants of EDS. Because the abnormal collagen fibers lack adequate tensile strength, *skin is hyperextensible, and the joints are hypermobile.* These features permit grotesque contortions, such as bending the thumb backward to touch the forearm and bending the knee forward to create almost a right angle. It is believed that most contortionists have one of the EDSs. A predisposition to joint dislocation, however, is one of the prices paid for this virtuosity. *The skin is extraordinarily stretchable, extremely fragile, and vulnerable to trauma.* Minor injuries produce gaping defects, and surgical repair or intervention is accomplished with great difficulty because of the lack of normal tensile strength. *The basic defect in connective tissue may lead to serious internal complications.* These include rupture of the colon and large arteries (vascular EDS), ocular fragility with rupture of cornea and retinal detachment (kyphoscoliosis EDS), and diaphragmatic hernia (classic EDS).

The biochemical and molecular bases of these abnormalities are known in several forms of EDS. These are described briefly, because they offer some insights into the perplexing clinical heterogeneity of EDS. Perhaps the best characterized is the *kyphoscoliosis type, the most common autosomal recessive form of EDS.* It results from mutations in the gene encoding lysyl hydroxylase, an enzyme necessary for hydroxylation of lysine residues during collagen synthesis. Affected patients have markedly reduced levels of this enzyme. Because hydroxylysine is essential for the cross-linking of collagen fibers, a deficiency of lysyl hydroxylase results in the synthesis of collagen that lacks normal structural stability.

The *vascular type of EDS results from abnormalities of type III collagen.* This form is genetically heterogeneous, because at least three distinct types of mutations affecting the *COL3A1* gene encoding collagen type III can give rise to this variant. Some affect the rate of synthesis of pro-α1 (III) chains, others affect the secretion of type III procollagen, and still others lead to the synthesis of structurally abnormal type III collagen. Some mutant alleles behave as dominant negatives (see discussion under "Autosomal Dominant Disorders") and thus produce severe phenotypic effects. These molecular studies provide a rational basis for the pattern of transmission and clinical features that are characteristic of this variant. First, because vascular-type EDS results from mutations involving a structural protein (rather than an enzyme protein), an autosomal dominant pattern of inheritance would be expected. Second, because blood vessels and intestines are known to be rich in collagen type III, an abnormality of this collagen is consistent with severe structural defects (e.g., vulnerability to spontaneous rupture) in these organs.

In two forms of EDS—arthrochalasia type and dermatosparaxis type—the fundamental defect is in the conversion of type I procollagen to collagen. This step in collagen synthesis involves cleavage of noncollagen peptides at the N terminus and C terminus of the procollagen molecule. This is accomplished by N-terminal–specific and C-terminal–specific peptidases. The defect in the conversion of procollagen to collagen in the arthrochalasia type has been traced to mutations that affect one of the two type I collagen genes, COL1A1 and COL1A2. As a result, structurally abnormal pro-α 1 (I) or pro-α2 (I) chains that resist cleavage of N-terminal peptides are formed. In patients with a single mutant allele, only 50% of the type I collagen chains are abnormal, but because these chains interfere with the formation of normal collagen helices, heterozygotes manifest the disease. In contrast, the related dermatosparaxis type is caused by mutations in the procollagen-N-peptidase genes, essential for the cleavage of collagens. Because in this case the disease is caused by an enzyme deficiency, it follows an autosomal recessive form of inheritance.

Finally, in *classic type of EDS,* molecular analysis suggests that genes other than those that encode collagen may also be involved. In 30% to 50% of these cases, mutations in the genes for type V collagen (*COL5A1* and *COL5A2*) have been detected. Surprisingly, in the remaining cases, no other collagen gene abnormalities have been found despite clinical features typical of EDS. It is suspected that in some cases genetic defects that affect the biosynthesis of other extracellular matrix molecules that influence collagen synthesis indirectly may be involved. One example is an EDS-like condition caused by mutation in tenascin-X, a large multimeric protein, that affects the synthesis and fibril formation of type VI and type I collagens.

To summarize, the common thread in EDS is some abnormality of collagen. These disorders, however, are extremely heterogeneous. At the molecular level, a variety of defects, varying from mutations involving structural genes for collagen to those involving enzymes that are responsible for posttranscriptional modifications of mRNA, have been detected. Such molecular heterogeneity results in the expression of EDS as a clinically variable disorder with several patterns of inheritance.

KEY CONCEPTS

Marfan Syndrome

- Marfan syndrome is caused by a mutation in the *FBN1* gene encoding fibrillin, which is required for structural integrity of connective tissues and regulation of TGF-β signaling.
- The major tissues affected are the skeleton, eyes, and cardiovascular system.
- Clinical features may include tall stature, long fingers, bilateral subluxation of lens, mitral valve prolapse, aortic aneurysm, and aortic dissection.
- Clinical trials with drugs that inhibit TGF-β signaling such as angiotensin receptor blockers are ongoing, as these have been shown to improve aortic and cardiac function in mouse models.

Ehlers-Danlos Syndromes

- There are six variants of Ehlers-Danlos syndromes, all characterized by defects in collagen synthesis or assembly. Each of the variants is caused by a distinct mutation involving one of several collagen genes or genes that encode other ECM proteins like tenascin-X.
- Clinical features may include fragile, hyperextensible skin vulnerable to trauma, hypermobile joints, and ruptures involving colon, cornea, or large arteries. Wound healing is poor.

Disorders Associated with Defects in Receptor Proteins

Familial Hypercholesterolemia

Familial hypercholesterolemia is a "receptor disease" that is the consequence of a mutation in the gene encoding the receptor for LDL, which is involved in the transport and metabolism of cholesterol. As a consequence of receptor abnormalities there is a loss of feedback control and elevated levels of cholesterol that induce premature atherosclerosis, leading to a greatly increased risk of myocardial infarction.

Familial hypercholesterolemia is one of the most frequently occurring Mendelian disorders. Heterozygotes with one mutant gene, representing about 1 in 500 individuals, have from birth a two-fold to three-fold elevation of plasma cholesterol level, leading to tendinous xanthomas and premature atherosclerosis in adult life (Chapter 11). Homozygotes, having a double dose of the mutant gene, are much more severely affected and may have five-fold to six-fold elevations in plasma cholesterol levels. Skin xanthomas and coronary, cerebral, and peripheral vascular atherosclerosis may develop in these individuals at an early age. Myocardial infarction may occur before age 20 years. Large-scale studies have found that familial hypercholesterolemia is present in 3% to 6% of survivors of myocardial infarction.

Normal Process of Cholesterol Metabolism and Transport

Approximately 7% of the body's cholesterol circulates in the plasma, predominantly in the form of LDL. As might be expected, the amount of plasma cholesterol is influenced by its synthesis and catabolism, and the liver plays a crucial role in both these processes (Fig. 5-6). The first step in this complex sequence is the secretion of very-low-density lipoproteins (VLDLs) by the liver into the bloodstream. VLDL particles are rich in triglycerides, but they contain lesser amounts of cholesteryl esters. When a VLDL particle reaches the capillaries of adipose tissue or muscle, it is cleaved by lipoprotein lipase, a process that extracts most of the triglycerides. The resulting molecule, called *intermediate-density lipoprotein (IDL)*, is reduced in triglyceride content and enriched in cholesteryl esters, but it retains two of the three apoproteins (B-100 and E) present in the parent VLDL particle (Fig. 5-6). After release from the capillary endothelium, the IDL particles have one of two fates. Approximately 50% of newly formed IDL is rapidly taken up by the liver by receptor-mediated transport. The receptor responsible for the binding of IDL to the liver cell membrane recognizes both apoprotein B-100 and apoprotein E. It is called the *LDL receptor*, however, because it is also involved in the hepatic clearance of LDL (described later). In the liver cells, IDL is recycled to generate VLDL. The IDL particles not taken up by the liver are subjected to further metabolic processing that removes most of the remaining triglycerides and apoprotein E, yielding cholesterol-rich LDL particles. *IDL is the immediate and major source of plasma LDL.* There seem to be two mechanisms for removal of LDL from plasma, one mediated by an LDL receptor and the other by a receptor for oxidized LDL (scavenger receptor), described later.

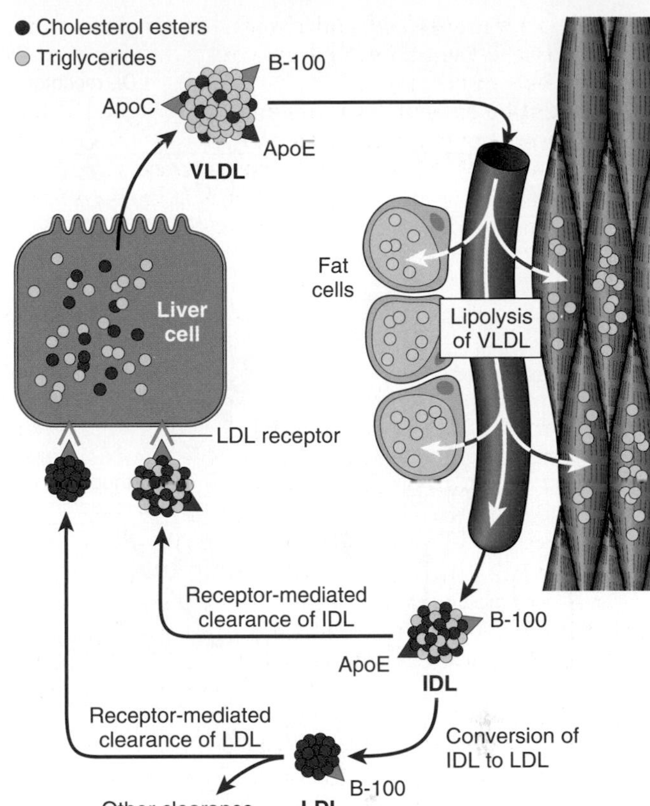

Figure 5-6 Low-density lipoprotein (LDL) metabolism and the role of the liver in its synthesis and clearance. Lipolysis of very-low-density lipoprotein (VLDL) by lipoprotein lipase in the capillaries releases triglycerides, which are then stored in fat cells and used as a source of energy in skeletal muscles. See text for explanation of abbreviations used.

Although many cell types, including fibroblasts, lymphocytes, smooth muscle cells, hepatocytes, and adrenocortical cells, possess high-affinity LDL receptors, approximately 70% of the plasma LDL is cleared by the liver, using a quite sophisticated transport process (Fig. 5-7). The first step involves binding of LDL to cell surface receptors, which are clustered in specialized regions of the plasma membrane called *coated pits* (Chapter 1). After binding, the coated pits containing the receptor-bound LDL are internalized by invagination to form coated vesicles, after which they migrate within the cell to fuse with the lysosomes. Here the LDL dissociates from the receptor, which is recycled to the surface. In the lysosomes the LDL molecule is enzymatically degraded; the apoprotein part is hydrolyzed to amino acids, whereas the cholesteryl esters are broken down to free cholesterol. This free cholesterol, in turn, crosses the lysosomal membrane to enter the cytoplasm, where it is used for membrane synthesis and as a regulator of cholesterol homeostasis. The exit of cholesterol from the lysosomes requires the action of two proteins, called NPC1 and NPC2 (see "Niemann-Pick Disease Type C"). Three separate processes are affected by the released intracellular cholesterol, as follows:

- Cholesterol *suppresses* cholesterol synthesis within the cell by inhibiting the activity of the enzyme 3-hydroxy-3-methylglutaryl coenzyme A (HMG CoA) reductase,

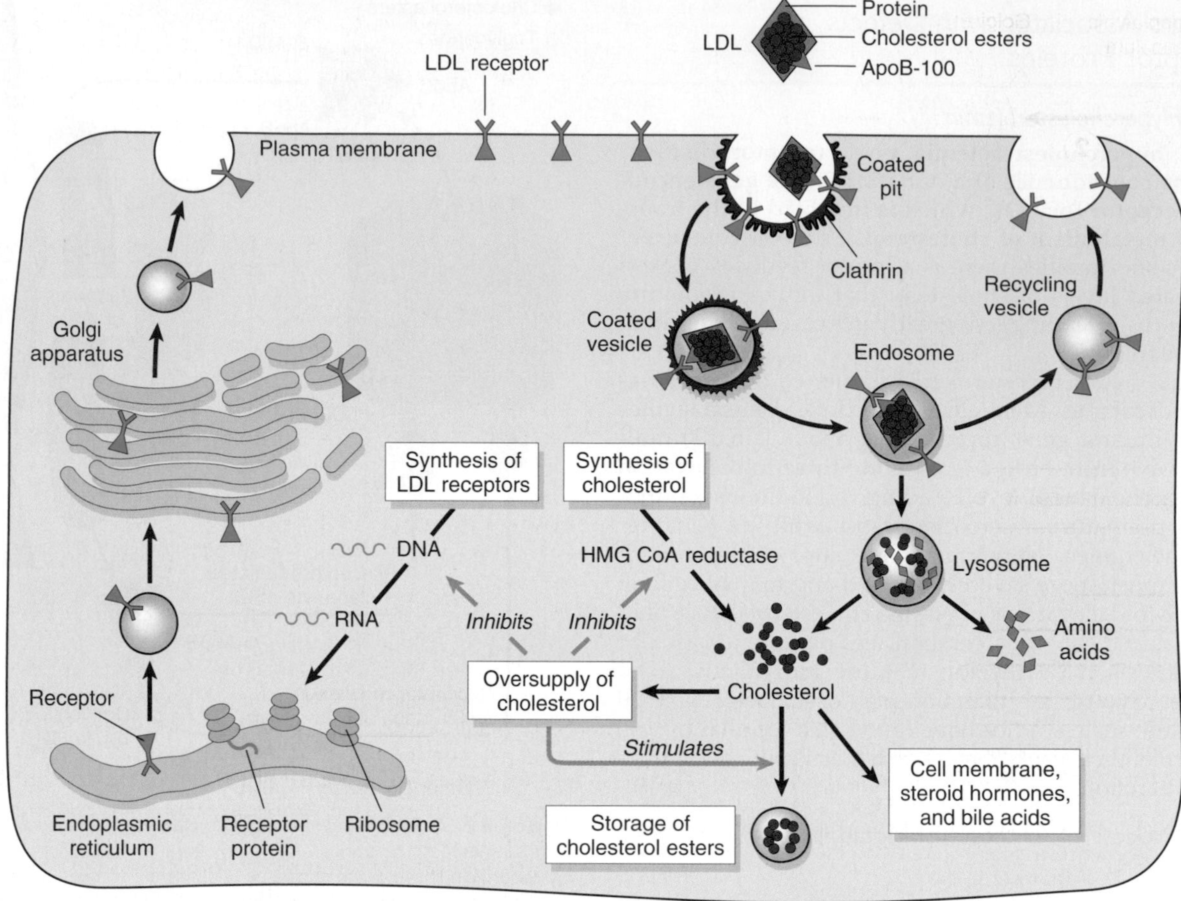

Figure 5-7 The LDL receptor pathway and regulation of cholesterol metabolism.

which is the rate-limiting enzyme in the synthetic pathway.

- Cholesterol *activates* the enzyme acyl-coenzyme A: cholesterol acyltransferase, favoring esterification and storage of excess cholesterol.
- Cholesterol *suppresses* the synthesis of LDL receptors, thus protecting the cells from excessive accumulation of cholesterol.

As mentioned earlier, familial hypercholesterolemia results from mutations in the gene encoding the receptor for LDL. Heterozygotes with familial hypercholesterolemia possess only 50% of the normal number of high-affinity LDL receptors, because they have only one normal gene. As a result of this defect in transport, the catabolism of LDL by the receptor-dependent pathways is impaired, and the plasma level of LDL increases approximately twofold. Homozygotes have virtually no normal LDL receptors in their cells and have much higher levels of circulating LDL. In addition to defective LDL clearance, both the homozygotes and heterozygotes have increased synthesis of LDL. The mechanism of increased synthesis that contributes to hypercholesterolemia also results from a lack of LDL receptors (Fig. 5-6). IDL, the immediate precursor of plasma LDL, also uses hepatic LDL receptors (apoprotein B-100 and E receptors) for its transport into the liver. In familial hypercholesterolemia, impaired IDL transport into the liver secondarily diverts a greater proportion of plasma IDL into the precursor pool for plasma LDL.

The transport of LDL via the scavenger receptor seems to occur at least in part into the cells of the mononuclear phagocyte system. Monocytes and macrophages have receptors for chemically altered (e.g., acetylated or oxidized) LDL. Normally the amount of LDL transported along this scavenger receptor pathway is less than that mediated by the LDL receptor-dependent mechanisms. In the face of hypercholesterolemia, however, there is a marked increase in the scavenger receptor-mediated traffic of LDL cholesterol into the cells of the mononuclear phagocyte system and possibly the vascular walls (Chapter 11). This increase is responsible for the appearance of xanthomas and contributes to the pathogenesis of premature atherosclerosis.

The molecular genetics of familial hypercholesterolemia is extremely complex. More than 900 mutations involving the LDL receptor gene, including insertions, deletions, and missense and nonsense mutations, have been identified. These can be classified into five groups (Fig. 5-8): *Class I mutations* are relatively uncommon and lead to a complete failure of synthesis of the receptor protein (null allele). *Class II mutations* are fairly common; they encode receptor proteins that accumulate in the endoplasmic reticulum because their folding defects make it impossible for them to be transported to the Golgi complex. *Class III mutations* affect the LDL-binding domain of the receptor; the encoded proteins reach the cell surface but fail to bind LDL or do so poorly. *Class IV mutations* encode proteins that are synthesized and transported to the cell surface efficiently.

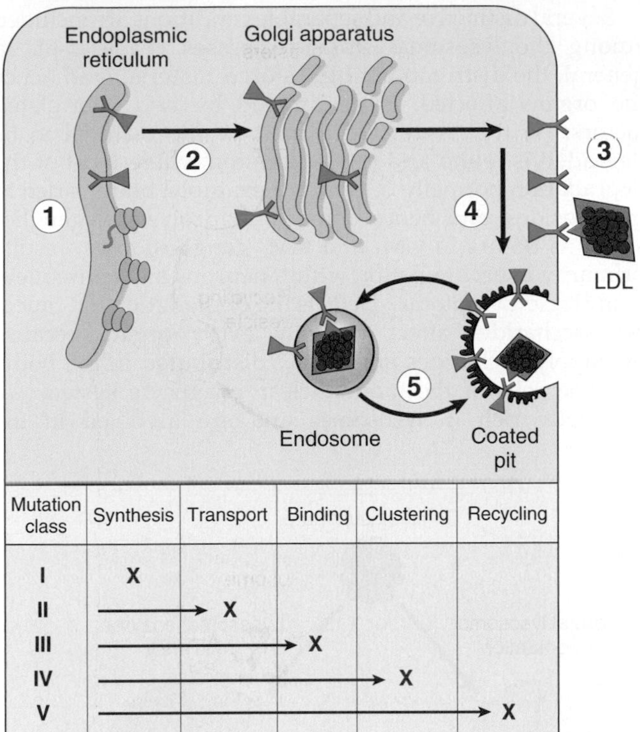

Mutation class	Synthesis	Transport	Binding	Clustering	Recycling
I	X				
II	→	X			
III	→	→	X		
IV	→	→	→	X	
V	→	→	→	→	X

Figure 5-8 Classification of LDL receptor mutations based on abnormal function of the mutant protein. These mutations disrupt the receptor's synthesis in the endoplasmic reticulum, transport to the Golgi complex, binding of apoprotein ligands, clustering in coated pits, and recycling in endosomes. Each class is heterogeneous at the DNA level.(Modified with permission from Hobbs HH, et al: The LDL receptor locus in familial hypercholesterolemia: mutational analysis of a membrane protein. Annu Rev Genet 24:133-170, 1990. © 1990 by Annual Reviews.)

They bind LDL normally, but they fail to localize in coated pits, and hence the bound LDL is not internalized. *Class V mutations* encode proteins that are expressed on the cell surface, can bind LDL, and can be internalized; however, the pH-dependent dissociation of the receptor and the bound LDL fails to occur. Such receptors are trapped in the endosome, where they are degraded, and hence they fail to recycle to the cell surface.

The discovery of the critical role of LDL receptors in cholesterol homeostasis has led to the rational design of drugs that lower plasma cholesterol by increasing the number of LDL receptors. One strategy is based on the ability of certain drugs (statins) to suppress intracellular cholesterol synthesis by inhibiting the enzyme HMG CoA reductase. This, in turn, allows greater synthesis of LDL receptors (Fig. 5-8). Statins have been widely and successfully used for secondary prevention of ischemic heart disease. They exemplify rational design of drugs based on an understanding of pathophysiology.

KEY CONCEPTS

Familial Hypercholesterolemia

- Familial hypercholesterolemia is an autosomal dominant disorder caused by mutations in the gene encoding the LDL receptor.
- Patients develop hypercholesterolemia as a consequence of impaired transport of LDL into the cells.
- In heterozygotes, elevated serum cholesterol greatly increases the risk of atherosclerosis and resultant coronary artery disease; homozygotes have an even greater increase in serum cholesterol and a higher frequency of ischemic heart disease. Cholesterol also deposits along tendon sheaths to produce xanthomas.

Disorders Associated with Defects in Enzymes

Lysosomal Storage Diseases

Lysosomes are key components of the "intracellular digestive tract." They contain a battery of hydrolytic enzymes, which have two special properties. First, they function in the acidic milieu of the lysosomes. Second, these enzymes constitute a special category of secretory proteins that are destined not for the extracellular fluids but for intracellular organelles. This latter characteristic requires special processing within the Golgi apparatus, which merits brief discussion.

Similar to all other secretory proteins, lysosomal enzymes (or *acid hydrolases*, as they are sometimes called) are synthesized in the endoplasmic reticulum and transported to the Golgi apparatus. Within the Golgi complex they undergo a variety of posttranslational modifications including the attachment of terminal mannose-6-phosphate groups to some of the oligosaccharide side chains. The phosphorylated mannose residues serve as an "address label" that is recognized by specific receptors found on the inner surface of the Golgi membrane. Lysosomal enzymes bind these receptors and are thereby segregated from the numerous other secretory proteins within the Golgi. Subsequently, small transport vesicles containing the receptor-bound enzymes are pinched off from the Golgi and proceed to fuse with the lysosomes. Thus, the enzymes are targeted to their intracellular abode, and the vesicles are shuttled back to the Golgi (Fig. 5-9). As indicated later, genetically determined errors in this remarkable sorting mechanism may give rise to one form of lysosomal storage disease.

The lysosomal enzymes catalyze the breakdown of a variety of complex macromolecules. These large molecules may be derived from the metabolic turnover of intracellular organelles (autophagy), or they may be acquired from outside the cells by phagocytosis (heterophagy). An inherited deficiency of a functional lysosomal enzyme gives rise to two pathologic consequences (Fig. 5-10):

- Catabolism of the substrate of the missing enzyme remains incomplete, leading to the accumulation of the partially degraded insoluble metabolite within the lysosomes. This is called "primary accumulation". Stuffed with incompletely digested macromolecules, lysosomes become large and numerous enough to interfere with normal cell functions.
- Since lysosomal function is also essential for autophagy, impaired autophagy gives rise to "secondary accumulation" of autophagic substrates such as polyubiquinated proteins and old and effete mitochondria. The absence of this quality control mechanism causes accumulation of dysfunctional mitochondria with poor calcium buffering capacity and altered membrane potentials. This can trigger generation of free radicals and apoptosis.

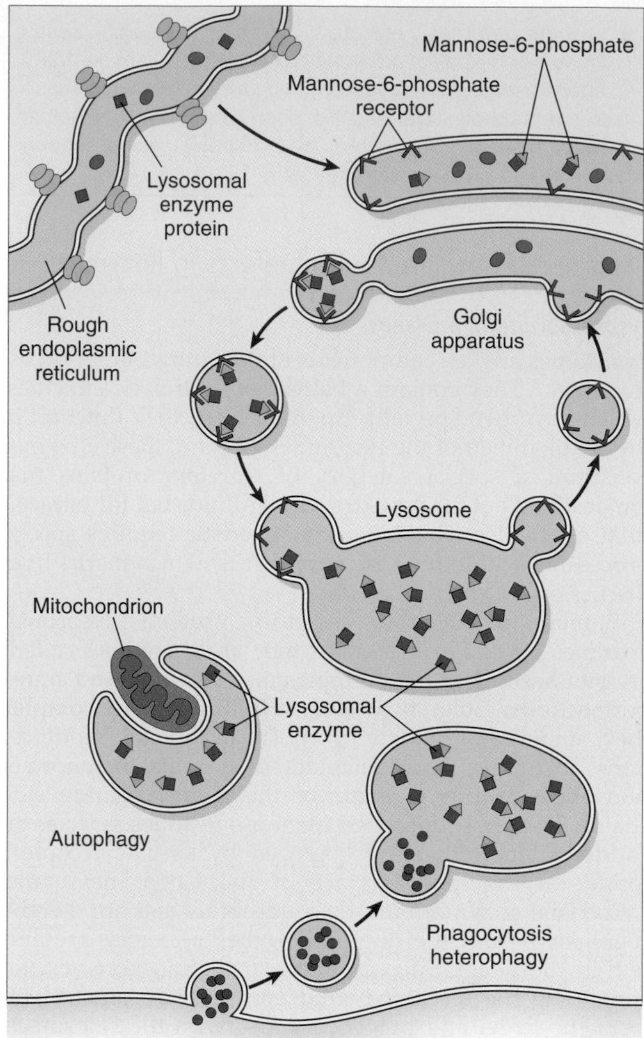

Figure 5-9 Synthesis and intracellular transport of lysosomal enzymes.

Several distinctive and separable conditions are included among the lysosomal storage diseases (Table 5-6). In general, the distribution of the stored material, and hence the organs affected, is determined by two interrelated factors: (1) the tissue where most of the material to be degraded is found and (2) the location where most of the degradation normally occurs. For example, brain is rich in gangliosides, and hence defective hydrolysis of gangliosides, as occurs in GM_1 and GM_2 gangliosidoses, results primarily in accumulation within neurons and consequent neurologic symptoms. Defects in degradation of mucopolysaccharides affect virtually every organ, because mucopolysaccharides are widely distributed in the body. Because cells of the mononuclear phagocyte system are especially rich in lysosomes and are involved in the

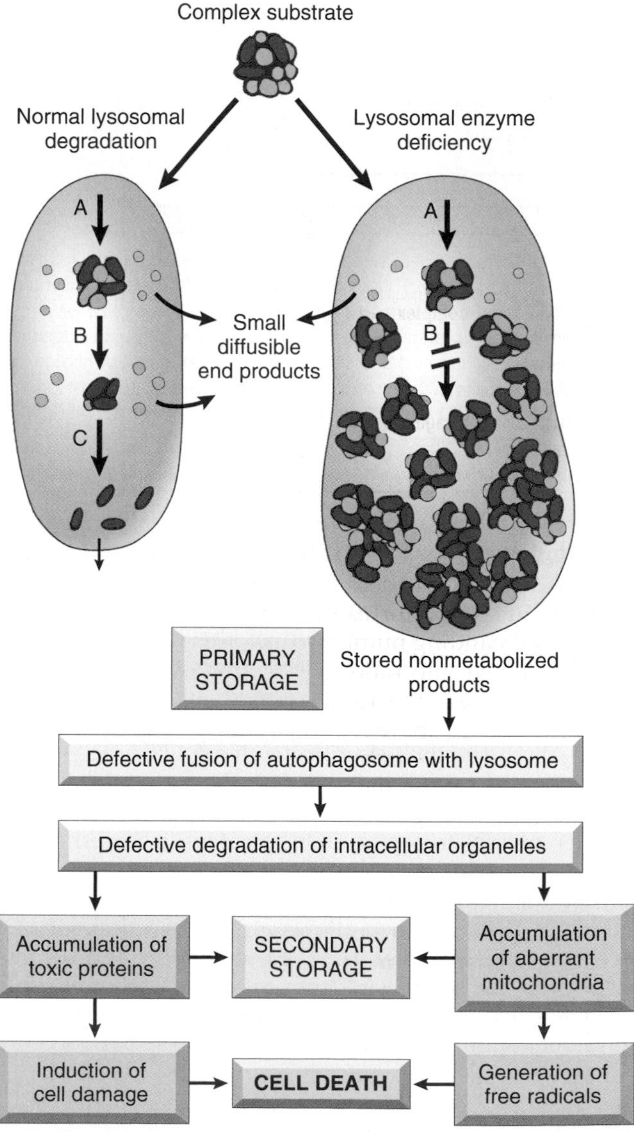

Figure 5-10 Pathogenesis of lysosomal storage diseases. In the example shown, a complex substrate is normally degraded by a series of lysosomal enzymes (A, B, and C) into soluble end products. If there is a deficiency or malfunction of one of the enzymes (e.g., B), catabolism is incomplete and insoluble intermediates accumulate in the lysosomes. In addition to this primary storage, secondary storage and toxic effects result from defective autophagy.

While details are still lacking it is clear that defects in autophagy are common in lysosomal storage diseases and play an important role in tissue damage.

There are three general approaches to the treatment of lysosomal storage diseases. The most obvious is enzyme replacement therapy, currently in use for several of these diseases. Another approach, the "substrate reduction therapy," is based on the premise that if the substrate to be degraded by the lysosomal enzyme can be reduced, the residual enzyme activity may be sufficient to catabolize it and prevent accumulation. A more recent strategy is based on the understanding of the molecular basis of enzyme deficiency. In many disorders, exemplified by Gaucher disease, the enzyme activity is low because the mutant proteins are unstable and prone to misfolding, and hence degraded in the endoplasmic reticulum. In such diseases an exogenous competitive inhibitor of the enzyme can, paradoxically, bind to the mutant enzyme and act as the "folding template" that assists proper folding of the enzyme and thus prevents its degradation. Such *molecular chaperone therapy* is under active investigation.

Table 5-6 Lysosomal Storage Diseases

Disease	Enzyme Deficiency	Major Accumulating Metabolites
Glycogenosis	Type 2—Pompe disease α-1,4-Glucosidase (lysosomal glucosidase)	Glycogen
Sphingolipidoses		
G_{M1} gangliosidosis Type 1—infantile, generalized Type 2—juvenile	G_{M1} ganglioside β-galactosidase	G_{M1} ganglioside, galactose-containing oligosaccharides
G_{M2} gangliosidosis		
Tay-Sachs disease	Hexosaminidase, α subunit	G_{M2} ganglioside
Sandhoff disease	Hexosaminidase, β subunit	G_{M2} ganglioside, globoside
G_{M2} gangliosidosis variant AB	Ganglioside activator protein	G_{M2} ganglioside
Sulfatidoses		
Metachromatic leukodystrophy	Arylsulfatase A	Sulfatide
Multiple sulfatase deficiency	Arylsulfatase A, B, C; steroid sulfatase; iduronate sulfatase; heparan *N*-sulfatase	Sulfatide, steroid sulfate, heparan sulfate, dermatan sulfate
Krabbe disease	Galactosylceramidase	Galactocerebroside
Fabry disease	α-Galactosidase A	Ceramide trihexoside
Gaucher disease	Glucocerebrosidase	Glucocerebroside
Niemann-Pick disease: types A and B	Sphingomyelinase	Sphingomyelin
Mucopolysaccharidoses (MPSs)		
MPS I H (Hurler)	α-L-Iduronidase	Dermatan sulfate, heparan sulfate
MPS II (Hunter)	L-Iduronosulfate sulfatase	
Mucolipidoses (MLs)		
I-cell disease (ML II) and pseudo-Hurler polydystrophy	Deficiency of phosphorylating enzymes essential for the formation of mannose-6-phosphate recognition marker; acid hydrolases lacking the recognition marker cannot be targeted to the lysosomes but are secreted extracellularly	Mucopolysaccharide, glycolipid
Other diseases of complex carbohydrates		
Fucosidosis	α-Fucosidase	Fucose-containing sphingolipids and glycoprotein fragments
Mannosidosis	α-Mannosidase	Mannose-containing oligosaccharides
Aspartylglycosaminuria	Aspartylglycosamine amide hydrolase	Aspartyl-2-deoxy-2-acetamido-glycosylamine
Other lysosomal storage diseases		
Wolman disease	Acid lipase	Cholesterol esters, triglycerides
Acid phosphate deficiency	Lysosomal acid phosphatase	Phosphate esters

degradation of a variety of substrates, organs rich in phagocytic cells, such as the spleen and liver, are frequently enlarged in several forms of lysosomal storage disorders. The ever-expanding number of lysosomal storage diseases can be divided into rational categories based on the biochemical nature of the accumulated metabolite, thus creating such subgroups as the *glycogenoses*, *sphingolipidoses (lipidoses)*, *mucopolysaccharidoses (MPSs)*, and *mucolipidoses* (Table 5-6). Only the most common disorders are considered here.

Tay-Sachs Disease (G_{M2} Gangliosidosis: Hexosaminidase α-Subunit Deficiency)

G_{M2} gangliosidoses are a group of three lysosomal storage diseases caused by an inability to catabolize G_{M2} gangliosides. Degradation of G_{M2} gangliosides requires three polypeptides encoded by three distinct genes. The phenotypic effects of mutations affecting these genes are fairly similar, because they result from accumulation of G_{M2} gangliosides. The underlying enzyme defect, however, is different for each. Tay-Sachs disease, the most common form of G_{M2} gangliosidosis, results from mutations in the α-subunit locus on chromosome 15 that cause a severe deficiency of hexosaminidase A. This disease is especially prevalent among Jews, particularly among those of Eastern European (Ashkenazic) origin, in whom a carrier rate of 1 in 30 has been reported.

MORPHOLOGY

The hexosaminidase A is absent from virtually all the tissues, so G_{M2} ganglioside accumulates in many tissues (e.g., heart, liver, spleen, nervous system), but the **involvement of neurons in the central and autonomic nervous systems and retina dominates the clinical picture.** On histologic examination, the neurons are ballooned with cytoplasmic vacuoles, each representing a markedly distended lysosome filled with gangliosides (Fig. 5-11*A*). Stains for fat such as oil red O and Sudan black B are positive. With the electron microscope, several types of **cytoplasmic inclusions** can be visualized, the most prominent being whorled configurations within lysosomes composed of onion-skin layers of membranes (Fig. 5-11*B*). In time there is progressive destruction of neurons, proliferation of microglia, and accumulation of complex lipids in phagocytes within the brain substance. A similar process occurs in the cerebellum as well as in neurons throughout the basal ganglia, brain stem, spinal cord, and dorsal root ganglia and in the neurons of the autonomic nervous system. The ganglion cells in the retina are similarly swollen with G_{M2} ganglioside, particularly at the margins of the macula. A **cherry-red spot thus appears in the macula,** representing accentuation of the normal color of the macular choroid contrasted with the pallor produced by the swollen ganglion cells in the remainder of the retina (Chapter 29). This finding is characteristic of Tay-Sachs disease and other storage disorders affecting the neurons.

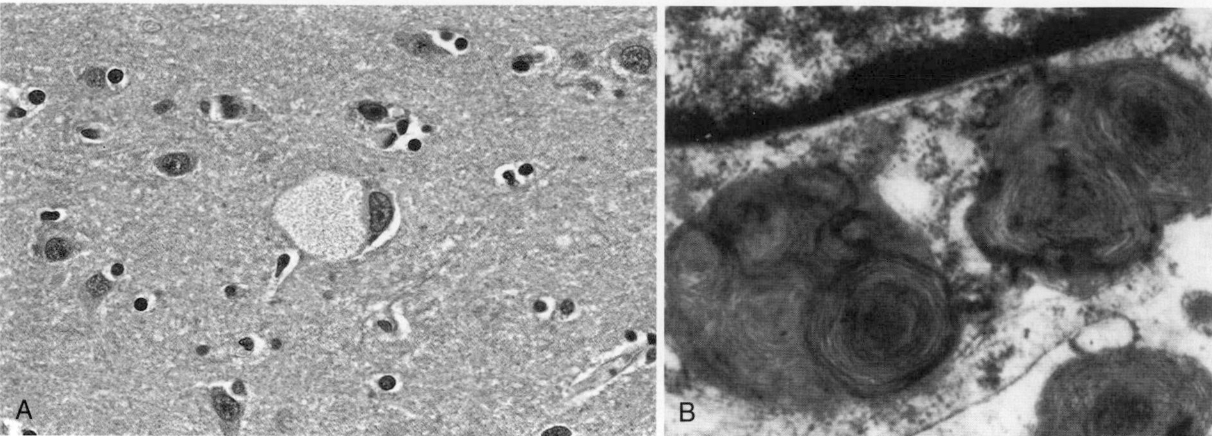

Figure 5-11 Ganglion cells in Tay-Sachs disease. **A,** Under the light microscope, a large neuron has obvious lipid vacuolation. **B,** A portion of a neuron under the electron microscope shows prominent lysosomes with whorled configurations. Part of the nucleus is shown above. (**A,** Courtesy of Dr. Arthur Weinberg, Department of Pathology, University of Texas Southwestern Medical Center, Dallas, TX. **B,** Electron micrograph courtesy of Dr. Joe Rutledge, University of Texas Southwestern Medical Center, Dallas, TX.)

Clinical Features. The affected infants appear normal at birth but begin to manifest signs and symptoms at about age 6 months. There is relentless motor and mental deterioration, beginning with motor incoordination, mental obtundation leading to muscular flaccidity, blindness, and increasing dementia. Sometime during the early course of the disease, the characteristic, but not pathognomonic, cherry-red spot appears in the macula of the eye in almost all patients. Over the span of 1 or 2 years a complete vegetative state is reached, followed by death at age 2 to 3 years. More than 100 mutations have been described in the α-subunit gene; most affect protein folding. Such misfolded proteins trigger the "unfolded protein" response (Chapter 1) leading to apoptosis. These findings have given rise to the possibility of chaperone therapy of Tay-Sachs disease.

Antenatal diagnosis and carrier detection are possible by enzyme assays and DNA-based analysis. The clinical features of the two other forms of G_{M2} gangliosidosis, Sandhoff disease, resulting from β-subunit defect, and G_{M2} activator deficiency, are similar to those of Tay-Sachs disease.

Niemann-Pick Disease Types A and B

Niemann-Pick disease types A and B are two related disorders that are characterized by lysosomal accumulation of sphingomyelin due to an inherited deficiency of sphingomyelinase. Type A is a severe infantile form with extensive neurologic involvement, marked visceral accumulations of sphingomyelin, and progressive wasting and early death within the first 3 years of life. In contrast, type B disease patients have organomegaly but generally no central nervous system involvement. They usually survive into adulthood. As with Tay-Sachs disease, Niemann-Pick disease types A and B are common in Ashkenazi Jews. The gene for acid sphingomyelinase maps to chromosome 11p15.4 and is one of the imprinted genes that is preferentially expressed from the maternal chromosome as a result of epigenetic silencing of the paternal gene (discussed later). Although, this disease is typically inherited as an autosomal recessive, those heterozygotes who inherit the mutant allele from the mother can develop Nieman Pick Disease. More than 100 mutations have been found in the acid sphingomyelinase gene and there seems to be a correlation between the type of mutation, the severity of enzyme deficiency, and the phenotype.

MORPHOLOGY

In the classic infantile type A variant, a missense mutation causes almost complete deficiency of sphingomyelinase. Sphingomyelin is a ubiquitous component of cellular (including organellar) membranes, and so the enzyme deficiency blocks degradation of the lipid, resulting in its progressive accumulation within lysosomes, particularly within cells of the mononuclear phagocyte system. **Affected cells become enlarged, sometimes to 90 μm in diameter, due to the distention of lysosomes with sphingomyelin and cholesterol.** Innumerable small vacuoles of relatively uniform size are created, imparting foaminess to the cytoplasm (Fig. 5-12). In frozen sections of fresh tissue, the vacuoles stain for fat. Electron microscopy confirms that the vacuoles are engorged secondary lysosomes that often contain membranous cytoplasmic bodies resembling concentric lamellated myelin figures, sometimes called "zebra" bodies.

The lipid-laden phagocytic foam cells are widely distributed in the spleen, liver, lymph nodes, bone marrow, tonsils, gastrointestinal tract, and lungs. **The involvement of the spleen generally produces massive enlargement**, sometimes to ten times its normal weight, but the hepatomegaly is usually not quite so striking. The lymph nodes are generally moderately to markedly enlarged throughout the body.

Involvement of the brain and eye deserves special mention. In the brain, the gyri are shrunken and the sulci widened. The neuronal involvement is diffuse, affecting all parts of the nervous system. **Vacuolation and ballooning of neurons** constitute the dominant histologic change, which in time leads to cell death and loss of brain substance. A **retinal cherry-red spot** similar to that seen in Tay-Sachs disease is present in about one third to one half of affected individuals.

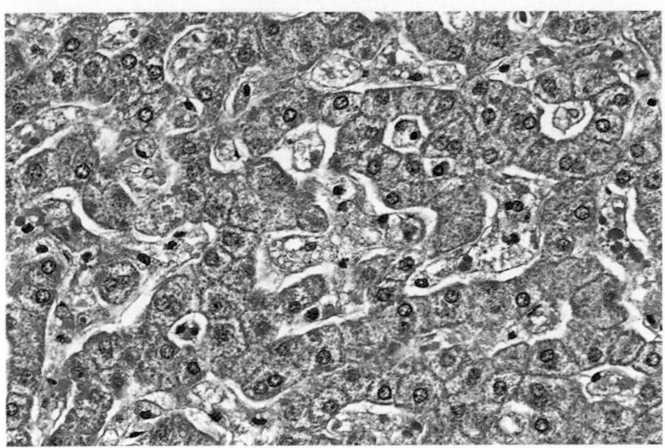

Figure 5-12 Niemann-Pick disease in liver. The hepatocytes and Kupffer cells have a foamy, vacuolated appearance due to deposition of lipids. (Courtesy of Dr. Arthur Weinberg, Department of Pathology, University of Texas Southwestern Medical Center, Dallas, TX.)

Clinical manifestations in type A disease may be present at birth and almost invariably become evident by age 6 months. Infants typically have a protuberant abdomen because of the hepatosplenomegaly. Once the manifestations appear, they are followed by progressive failure to thrive, vomiting, fever, and generalized lymphadenopathy as well as progressive deterioration of psychomotor function. Death comes, usually within the first or second year of life.

The diagnosis is established by biochemical assays for sphingomyelinase activity in liver or bone marrow biopsy. Individuals affected with types A and B as well as carriers can be detected by DNA analysis.

Niemann-Pick Disease Type C

Although previously considered to be related to types A and B, Niemann-Pick disease type C (NPC) is distinct at the biochemical and genetic levels and is more common than types A and B combined. Mutations in two related genes, *NPC1* and *NPC2*, can give rise to NPC, with *NPC1* being responsible for 95% of cases. Unlike most other storage diseases, NPC is due to a primary defect in nonenzymatic lipid transport. NPC1 is membrane bound whereas NPC2 is soluble. Both are involved in the transport of free cholesterol from the lysosomes to the cytoplasm. NPC is clinically heterogeneous. It may present as hydrops fetalis and stillbirth, as neonatal hepatitis, or, most commonly, as a chronic form characterized by progressive neurologic damage. The latter presents in childhood and is marked by ataxia, vertical supranuclear gaze palsy, dystonia, dysarthria, and psychomotor regression.

Gaucher Disease

Gaucher disease refers to a cluster of autosomal recessive disorders resulting from mutations in the gene encoding glucocerebrosidase. It is the most common lysosomal storage disorder. The affected gene encodes glucocerebrosidase, an enzyme that normally cleaves the glucose residue from ceramide. As a result of the enzyme defect, glucocerebroside accumulates principally in phagocytes but in some subtypes also in the central nervous system. Glucocerebrosides are continually formed from the catabolism of glycolipids derived mainly from the cell membranes of senescent leukocytes and red cells. It is clear now that the pathologic changes in Gaucher disease are caused not just by the burden of storage material but also by activation of macrophages and the consequent secretion of cytokines such as IL-1, IL-6, and tumor necrosis factor (TNF).

Three clinical subtypes of Gaucher disease have been distinguished.

- The most common, accounting for 99% of cases, is called type I, or the chronic nonneuronopathic form. In this type, storage of glucocerebrosides is limited to the mononuclear phagocytes throughout the body without involving the brain. Splenic and skeletal involvements dominate this pattern of the disease. It is found principally in Jews of European stock. Individuals with this disorder have reduced but detectable levels of glucocerebrosidase activity. Longevity is shortened but not markedly.
- Type II, or acute neuronopathic Gaucher disease, is the infantile acute cerebral pattern. This form has no predilection for Jews. In these patients there is virtually no detectable glucocerebrosidase activity in the tissues. Hepatosplenomegaly is also seen in this form of Gaucher disease, but the clinical picture is dominated by progressive central nervous system involvement, leading to death at an early age.
- A third pattern, type III, is intermediate between types I and II. These patients have the systemic involvement characteristic of type I but have progressive central nervous system disease that usually begins in adolescence or early adulthood.

MORPHOLOGY

Glucocerebrosides accumulate in massive amounts within phagocytic cells throughout the body in all forms of Gaucher disease. The **distended phagocytic cells, known as Gaucher cells, are found in the spleen, liver, bone marrow, lymph nodes, tonsils, thymus, and Peyer patches.** Similar cells may be found in both the alveolar septa and the air spaces in the lung. In contrast to other lipid storage diseases, Gaucher cells rarely appear vacuolated but instead have a fibrillary type of cytoplasm likened to crumpled tissue paper (Fig. 5-13). Gaucher cells are often enlarged, sometimes up to 100 μm in diameter, and have one or more dark, eccentrically placed nuclei. Periodic acid–Schiff staining is usually intensely positive. With the electron microscope **the fibrillary cytoplasm can be resolved as elongated, distended lysosomes,** containing the stored lipid in stacks of bilayers.

In type I disease, the **spleen is enlarged, sometimes up to 10 kg.** The lymphadenopathy is mild to moderate and is body-wide. The accumulation of Gaucher cells in the bone marrow occurs in 70% to 100% of cases of type I Gaucher disease. It produces areas of **bone erosion** that are sometimes small but in other cases sufficiently large to give rise to pathologic fractures. Bone destruction occurs due to the secretion of cytokines by activated macrophages. In patients with cerebral involvement, Gaucher cells are seen in the Virchow-Robin spaces, and arterioles are surrounded by swollen adventitial cells. There is no storage of lipids in the neurons, yet

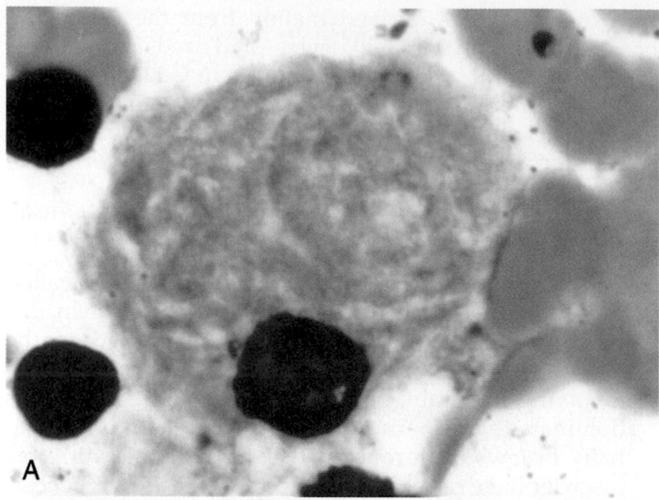

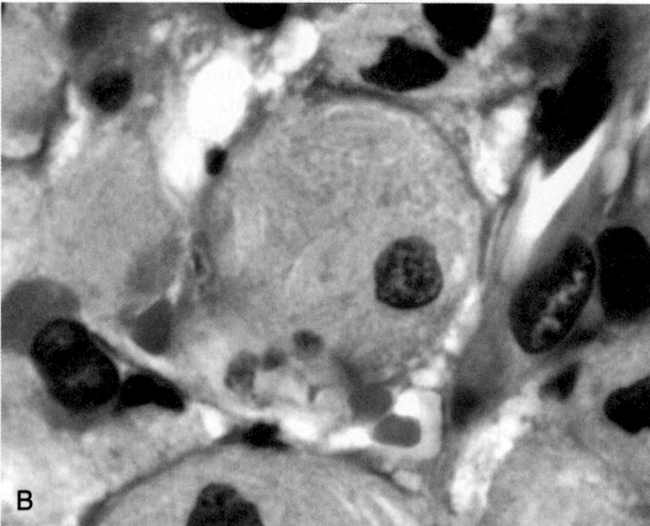

Figure 5-13 Gaucher disease involving the bone marrow. Gaucher cells (**A,** Wright stain; **B,** Hematoxylin and eosin) are plump macrophages that characteristically have the appearance in the cytoplasm of crumpled tissue paper due to accumulation of glucocerebroside. (Courtesy of Dr. John Anastasi, Department of Pathology, University of Chicago, Chicago, IL.)

neurons appear shriveled and are progressively destroyed. It is suspected that the lipids that accumulate in the phagocytic cells around blood vessels secrete cytokines that damage nearby neurons.

Clinical Features. The clinical course of Gaucher disease depends on the clinical subtype. In type I, symptoms and signs first appear in adult life and are related to splenomegaly or bone involvement. Most commonly there is pancytopenia or thrombocytopenia secondary to hypersplenism. Pathologic fractures and bone pain occur if there has been extensive expansion of the marrow space. Although the disease is progressive in the adult, it is compatible with long life. In types II and III, central nervous system dysfunction, convulsions, and progressive mental deterioration dominate, although organs such as the liver, spleen, and lymph nodes are also affected. The diagnosis of homozygotes can be made by measurement of glucocerebrosidase activity in peripheral blood leukocytes or in extracts of cultured skin fibroblasts. In principle, heterozygotes can be identified by detection of mutations. However, because more than 150 mutations in the glucocerebroside gene can cause Gaucher disease, currently it is not possible to use a single genetic test. However, with rapid advances in next generation sequencing (discussed later), it is likely that a comprehensive molecular diagnostic test for carriers will soon be developed.

Replacement therapy with recombinant enzymes is the mainstay for treatment of Gaucher disease; it is effective, and those with type I disease can expect normal life expectancy with this form of treatment. However, such therapy is extremely expensive. Because the fundamental defect resides in mononuclear phagocytic cells originating from marrow stem cells, allogeneic hematopoietic stem cell transplantation can be curative. Other work is directed toward correction of the enzyme defect by transfer of the normal glucocerebrosidase gene into the patient's hematopoietic stem cells. Substrate reduction therapy with inhibitors of glucosylceramide synthetase is also being evaluated.

Mucopolysaccharidoses (MPS)

The MPSs are a group of closely related syndromes that result from genetically determined deficiencies of enzymes involved in the degradation of mucopolysaccharides (glycosaminoglycans). Chemically, mucopolysaccharides are long-chain complex carbohydrates that are linked with proteins to form proteoglycans. They are abundant in the ground substance of connective tissue. The glycosaminoglycans that accumulate in MPSs are dermatan sulfate, heparan sulfate, keratan sulfate, and chondroitin sulfate. The enzymes involved in the degradation of these molecules cleave terminal sugars from the polysaccharide chains disposed along a polypeptide or core protein. In the absence of enzymes, these chains accumulate within lysosomes in various tissues and organs of the body.

Several clinical variants of MPS, classified numerically from MPS I to MPS VII, have been described, each resulting from the deficiency of one specific enzyme. All the MPSs except one are inherited as autosomal recessive traits; the exception, *Hunter syndrome*, is an X-linked recessive trait. Within a given group (e.g., MPS I, characterized by a deficiency of α-l-iduronidase), subgroups exist that result from different mutant alleles at the same genetic locus. Thus, the severity of enzyme deficiency and the clinical picture even within subgroups are often different.

In general, MPSs are progressive disorders, characterized by *coarse facial features, clouding of the cornea, joint stiffness*, and *mental retardation*. Urinary excretion of the accumulated mucopolysaccharides is often increased.

MORPHOLOGY

The accumulated **mucopolysaccharides are generally found in mononuclear phagocytic cells, endothelial cells, intimal smooth muscle cells, and fibroblasts** throughout the body. Common sites of involvement are thus the spleen, liver, bone marrow, lymph nodes, blood vessels, and heart.

Microscopically, affected cells are distended and have apparent clearing of the cytoplasm to create so-called balloon cells.

Under the electron microscope, the clear cytoplasm can be resolved as numerous minute vacuoles. These are swollen lysosomes containing a finely granular periodic acid–Schiff–positive material that can be identified biochemically as mucopolysaccharide. Similar lysosomal changes are found in the neurons of those syndromes characterized by central nervous system involvement. In addition, however, some of the lysosomes in neurons are replaced by lamellated zebra bodies similar to those seen in Niemann-Pick disease. **Hepatosplenomegaly, skeletal deformities, valvular lesions, and subendothelial arterial deposits, particularly in the coronary arteries, and lesions in the brain are common threads that run through all of the MPSs.** In many of the more protracted syndromes, coronary subendothelial lesions lead to myocardial ischemia. Thus, myocardial infarction and cardiac decompensation are important causes of death.

Clinical Features. Of the seven recognized variants, only two well-characterized syndromes are described briefly here. *Hurler syndrome,* also called MPS I-H, results from a deficiency of α-l-iduronidase. It is one of the most severe forms of MPS. Affected children appear normal at birth but develop hepatosplenomegaly by age 6 to 24 months. Their growth is retarded, and, as in other forms of MPS, they develop coarse facial features and skeletal deformities. Death occurs by age 6 to 10 years and is often due to cardiovascular complications. *Hunter syndrome,* also called MPS II, differs from Hurler syndrome in mode of inheritance (X-linked), absence of corneal clouding, and milder clinical course.

KEY CONCEPTS

Lysosomal Storage Diseases

Inherited mutations leading to defective lysosomal enzyme functions gives rise to accumulation and storage of complex substrates in the lysosomes and defects in autophagy resulting in cellular injury.

- **Tay-Sachs disease** is caused by an inability to metabolize G_{M2} gangliosides due to lack of the α subunit of lysosomal hexosaminidase. G_{M2} gangliosides accumulate in the central nervous system and cause severe mental retardation, blindness, motor weakness, and death by 2 to 3 years of age.
- **Niemann-Pick disease types A and B** are caused by a deficiency of sphingomyelinase. In the more severe type A variant, accumulation of sphingomyelin in the nervous system results in neuronal damage. Lipid also is stored in phagocytes within the liver, spleen, bone marrow, and lymph nodes, causing their enlargement. In type B, neuronal damage is not present.
- **Niemann-Pick disease type C** is caused by a defect in cholesterol transport and resultant accumulation of cholesterol and gangliosides in the nervous system. Affected children most commonly exhibit ataxia, dysarthria, and psychomotor regression.
- **Gaucher disease** results from lack of the lysosomal enzyme glucocerebrosidase and accumulation of glucocerebroside in mononuclear phagocytic cells. In the most common, type I variant, affected phagocytes become enlarged (Gaucher cells) and accumulate in liver, spleen, and bone marrow, causing hepatosplenomegaly and bone erosion. Types II and III are characterized by variable neuronal involvement.
- **Mucopolysaccharidoses** result in accumulation of mucopolysaccharides in many tissues including liver, spleen, heart, blood vessels, brain, cornea, and joints. Affected patients in all forms have coarse facial features. Manifestations of Hurler syndrome include corneal clouding, coronary arterial and valvular deposits, and death in childhood. Hunter syndrome is associated with a milder clinical course.

Glycogen Storage Diseases (Glycogenoses)

The glycogen storage diseases result from a hereditary deficiency of one of the enzymes involved in the synthesis or sequential degradation of glycogen. Depending on the tissue or organ distribution of the specific enzyme in the normal state, glycogen storage in these disorders may be limited to a few tissues, may be more widespread while not affecting all tissues, or may be systemic in distribution.

The significance of a specific enzyme deficiency is best understood from the perspective of the normal metabolism of glycogen (Fig. 5-14). Glycogen is a storage form of glucose. Glycogen synthesis begins with the conversion of glucose to glucose-6-phosphate by the action of a hexokinase (glucokinase). A phosphoglucomutase then transforms the glucose-6-phosphate to glucose-1-phosphate, which, in turn, is converted to uridine diphosphoglucose. A highly branched, large polymer is then built (molecular weight as high as 100 million), containing as many as 10,000 glucose molecules linked together by α-1,4-glucoside bonds. The glycogen chain and branches continue to be elongated by the addition of glucose molecules mediated by glycogen synthetases. During degradation, distinct phosphorylases in the liver and muscle split glucose-1-phosphate from the glycogen until about four glucose residues remain on each branch, leaving a branched oligosaccharide called *limit dextrin.* This can be further degraded only by the debranching enzyme. In addition to these major pathways, glycogen is also degraded in the lysosomes by acid maltase. If the lysosomes are deficient in this enzyme, the glycogen contained within them is not accessible to degradation by cytoplasmic enzymes such as phosphorylases.

On the basis of specific enzyme deficiencies and the resultant clinical pictures, glycogenoses have traditionally been divided into a dozen or so syndromes designated by roman numerals, and the list continues to grow. On the basis of pathophysiology glycogenoses can be divided into three major subgroups (Table 5-7):

- *Hepatic forms.* The liver is a key player in glycogen metabolism. It contains enzymes that synthesize glycogen for storage and ultimately break it down into free glucose, which is then released into the blood. An inherited deficiency of hepatic enzymes that are involved in glycogen degradation therefore leads not only to the storage of glycogen in the liver but also to a reduction in blood glucose concentrations (hypoglycemia) (Fig. 5-15). Deficiency of the enzyme glucose-6-phosphatase

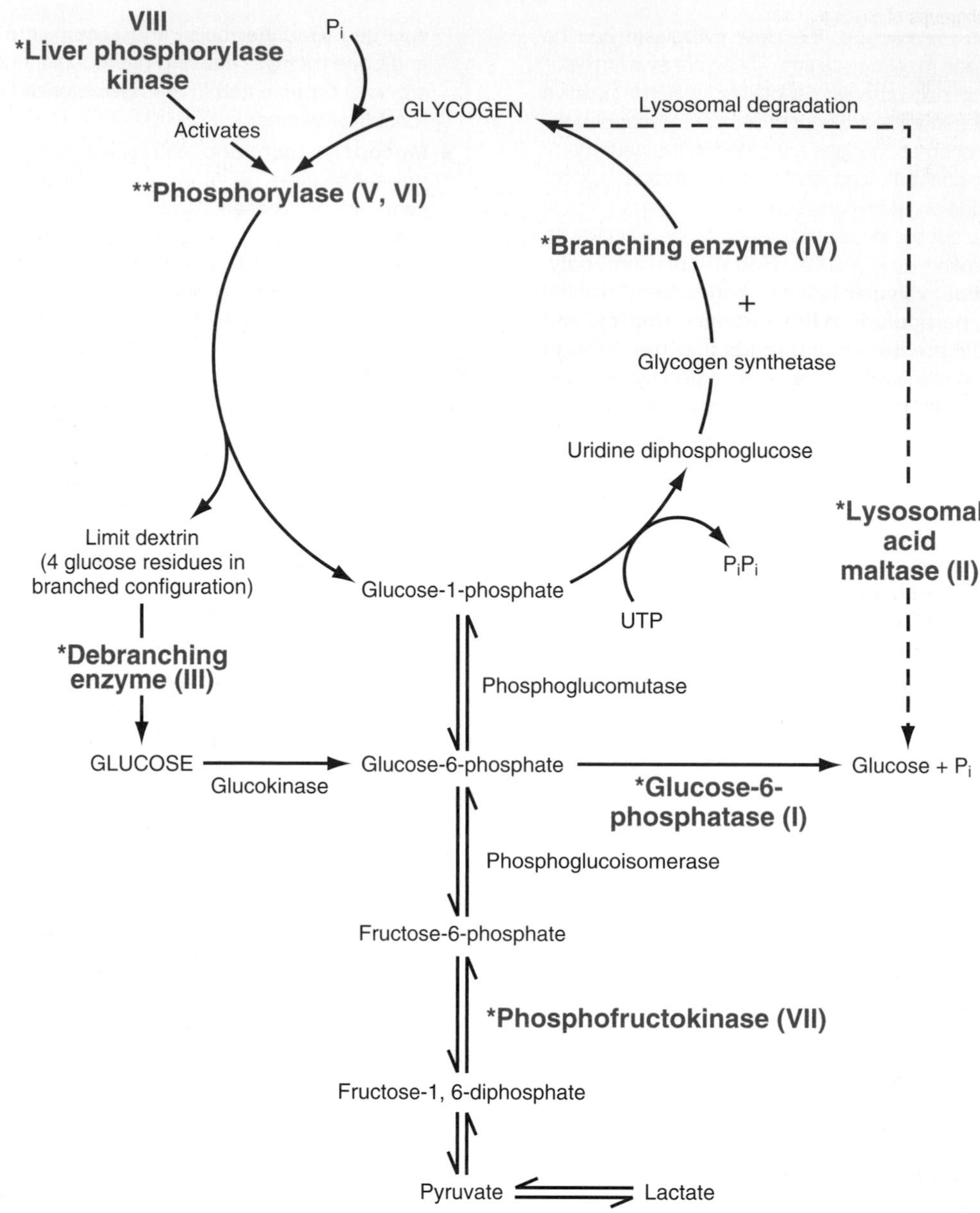

Figure 5-14 Pathways of glycogen metabolism. Asterisks mark the enzyme deficiencies associated with glycogen storage diseases. Roman numerals indicate the type of glycogen storage disease associated with the given enzyme deficiency. Types V and VI result from deficiencies of muscle and liver phosphorylases, respectively. (Modified from Hers H, et al: Glycogen storage diseases. In Scriver CR, et al [eds]: The Metabolic Basis of Inherited Disease, 6th ed. New York, McGraw-Hill, 1989, p 425.)

(von Gierke disease, or type I glycogenosis) is a prime example of the hepatic-hypoglycemic form of glycogen storage disease (Table 5-7). Other examples include deficiencies of liver phosphorylase and debranching enzyme, both involved in the breakdown of glycogen (Fig. 5-15). In all these disorders glycogen is stored in many organs, but *hepatic enlargement and hypoglycemia dominate the clinical picture.*

- *Myopathic forms.* In the skeletal muscles, as opposed to the liver, glycogen is used predominantly as a source of energy during physical activity. ATP is generated by glycolysis, which leads ultimately to the formation of lactate (Fig. 5-16). If the enzymes that fuel the glycolytic pathway are deficient, glycogen storage occurs in the muscles and is associated with muscular weakness due to impaired energy production. Examples in this category include deficiencies of muscle phosphorylase (McArdle disease, or type V glycogenosis), muscle phosphofructokinase (type VII glycogen storage disease), and several others. *Typically, individuals with the myopathic forms present with muscle cramps after exercise and lactate levels in the blood fail to rise after exercise due to a block in glycolysis.*
- *Glycogen storage diseases associated with (1) deficiency of α-glucosidase (acid maltase) and (2) lack of branching enzyme* do not fit into the hepatic or myopathic categories. They are associated with glycogen storage in many organs and death early in life. Acid maltase is a lysosomal enzyme, and hence its deficiency leads to lysosomal storage of glycogen (type II glycogenosis, or *Pompe disease*) in all organs, but *cardiomegaly is the most prominent feature* (Fig. 5-16).

Table 5-7 Principal Subgroups of Glycogenoses

Clinicopathologic Category	Specific Type	Enzyme Deficiency	Morphologic Changes	Clinical Features
Hepatic type	Hepatorenal—von Gierke disease (type I)	Glucose-6-phosphatase	Hepatomegaly—intracytoplasmic accumulations of glycogen and small amounts of lipid; intranuclear glycogen Renomegaly—intracytoplasmic accumulations of glycogen in cortical tubular epithelial cells	In untreated patients: failure to thrive, stunted growth, hepatomegaly, and renomegaly Hypoglycemia due to failure of glucose mobilization, often leading to convulsions Hyperlipidemia and hyperuricemia resulting from deranged glucose metabolism; many patients develop gout and skin xanthomas Bleeding tendency due to platelet dysfunction With treatment: Most survive and develop late complications (e.g., hepatic adenomas)
Myopathic type	McArdle disease (type V)	Muscle phosphorylase	Skeletal muscle only—accumulations of glycogen predominant in subsarcolemmal location	Painful cramps associated with strenuous exercise; myoglobinuria occurs in 50% of cases; onset in adulthood (>20 years); muscular exercise fails to raise lactate level in venous blood; serum creatine kinase always elevated; compatible with normal longevity
Miscellaneous types	Generalized glycogenosis—Pompe disease (type II)	Lysosomal glucosidase (acid maltase)	Mild hepatomegaly—ballooning of lysosomes with glycogen, creating lacy cytoplasmic pattern Cardiomegaly—glycogen within sarcoplasm as well as membrane-bound Skeletal muscle—similar to changes in heart	Massive cardiomegaly, muscle hypotonia, and cardiorespiratory failure within 2 years; a milder adult form with only skeletal muscle involvement, presenting with chronic myopathy; enzyme replacement therapy available

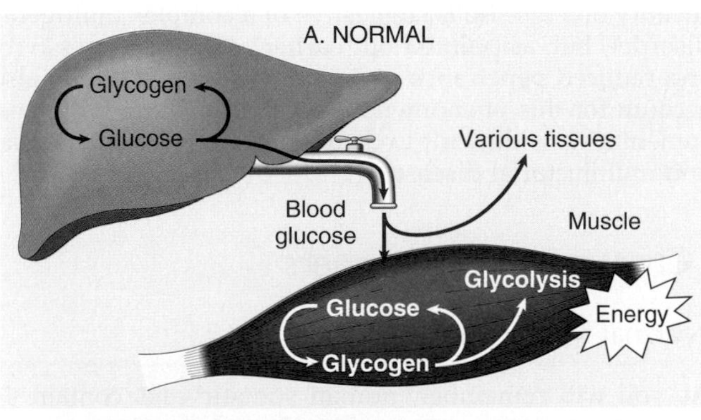

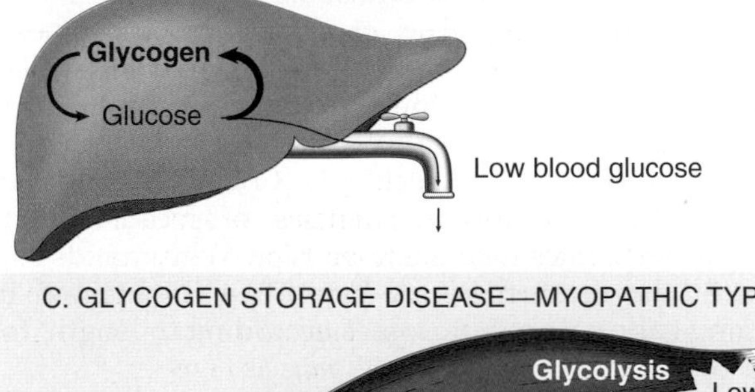

Figure 5-15 **A,** Normal glycogen metabolism in the liver and skeletal muscles. **B,** Effects of an inherited deficiency of hepatic enzymes involved in glycogen metabolism. **C,** Consequences of a genetic deficiency in the enzymes that metabolize glycogen in skeletal muscles.

KEY CONCEPTS

Glycogen Storage Diseases

- Inherited deficiency of enzymes involved in glycogen metabolism can result in storage of normal or abnormal forms of glycogen, predominantly in liver or muscles, but also in other tissues as well.
- In the **hepatic form** (von Gierke disease), liver cells store glycogen because of a lack of hepatic glucose-6-phosphatase. There are several **myopathic forms**, including McArdle disease, in which muscle phosphorylase lack gives rise to storage in skeletal muscles and cramps after exercise. In **Pompe disease** there is lack of lysosomal acid maltase, and all organs are affected, but heart involvement is predominant.

Disorders Associated with Defects in Proteins That Regulate Cell Growth

Normal growth and differentiation of cells are regulated by two classes of genes; proto-oncogenes and tumor suppressor genes, whose products promote or restrain cell growth (Chapter 7). It is now well established that mutations in these two classes of genes are important in the pathogenesis of tumors. In the vast majority of cases, cancer-causing mutations affect somatic cells and hence are not passed in the germ line. In approximately 5% of all cancers, however, mutations transmitted through the germ line contribute to the development of cancer. Most familial cancers are inherited in an autosomal dominant fashion, but a few recessive disorders have also been described. This subject is discussed in Chapter 7. Specific forms of familial tumors are described in various chapters.

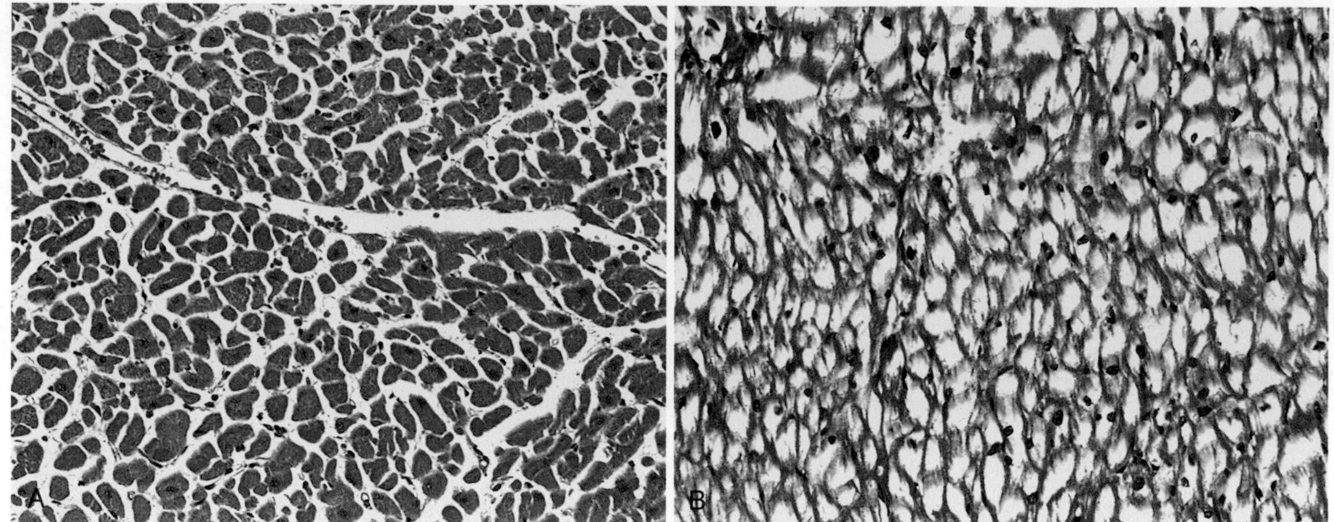

Figure 5-16 Pompe disease (glycogen storage disease type II). **A,** Normal myocardium with abundant eosinophilic cytoplasm. **B,** Patient with Pompe disease (same magnification) showing the myocardial fibers full of glycogen seen as clear spaces. (Courtesy of Dr. Trace Worrell, Department of Pathology, University of Texas Southwestern Medical Center, Dallas, TX.)

Complex Multigenic Disorders

As discussed previously, such disorders are caused by interactions between variant forms of genes and environmental factors. A gene that has at least two alleles, each of which occurs at a frequency of at least 1% in the population, is polymorphic, and each variant allele is referred to as a polymorphism. According to the common disease/common variant hypothesis, complex genetic disorders occur when many polymorphisms, each with a modest effect and low penetrance, are co-inherited. Two additional facts that have emerged from studies of common complex disorders, such as type 1 diabetes, are:

- While complex disorders result from the collective inheritance of many polymorphisms, different polymorphisms vary in significance. For example, of the 20 to 30 genes implicated in type 1 diabetes, six to seven are most important, and a few HLA-alleles contribute more than 50% of the risk (Chapter 24).
- Some polymorphisms are common to multiple diseases of the same type, while others are disease specific. This is best illustrated in immune-mediated inflammatory diseases (Chapter 6).

Several normal phenotypic characteristics are governed by multifactorial inheritance, such as hair color, eye color, skin color, height, and intelligence. These characteristics show a continuous variation in population groups, producing the standard bell-shaped curve of distribution. Environmental influences, however, significantly modify the phenotypic expression of complex traits. For example, type 2 diabetes mellitus has many of the features of a multifactorial disorder. It is well recognized that individuals often first manifest this disease after weight gain. Thus, obesity as well as other environmental influences unmasks the diabetic genetic trait. Nutritional influences may cause even monozygous twins to achieve different heights. The culturally deprived child cannot achieve his or her full intellectual capacity.

Assigning a disease to this mode of inheritance must be done with caution. It depends on many factors but first on familial clustering and the exclusion of Mendelian and chromosomal modes of transmission. A range of levels of severity of a disease is suggestive of a complex multigenic disorder, but, as pointed out earlier, variable expressivity and reduced penetrance of single mutant genes may also account for this phenomenon. Because of these problems, sometimes it is difficult to distinguish between Mendelian and multifactorial disease.

Chromosomal Disorders

Normal Karyotype

As you will remember, human somatic cells contain 46 chromosomes; these comprise 22 homologous pairs of autosomes and two sex chromosomes, XX in the female and XY in the male. The study of chromosomes—*karyotyping*—is the basic tool of the cytogeneticist. The usual procedure to examine chromosomes is to arrest dividing cells in metaphase with mitotic spindle inhibitors (e.g., *N*-diacetyl-*N*-methylcolchicine [Colcemid]) and then to stain the chromosomes. In a metaphase spread, the individual chromosomes take the form of two chromatids connected at the centromere. A karyotype is obtained by arranging each pair of autosomes according to length, followed by sex chromosomes.

A variety of staining methods have been developed that allow identification of individual chromosomes on the basis of a distinctive and reliable pattern of alternating light and dark bands. The one most commonly used involves a Giemsa stain and is hence called *G banding*. A normal male karyotype with G banding is illustrated in Figure 5-17. With standard G banding, approximately 400 to 800 bands per haploid set can be detected. The resolution obtained by banding can be markedly improved by obtaining the cells in prophase. The individual chromosomes appear markedly elongated, and as many as 1500 bands

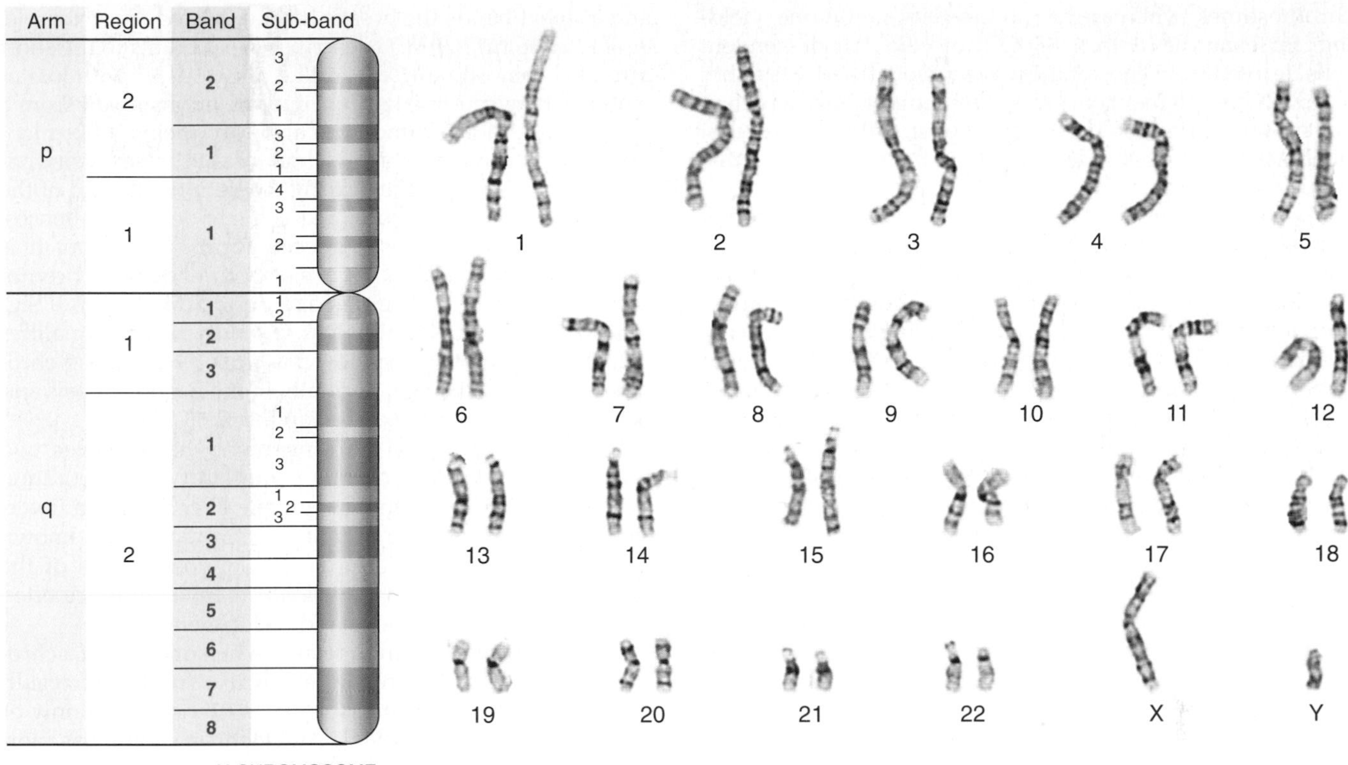

Figure 5-17 G-banded karyotype from a normal male (46,XY). Also shown is the banding pattern of the X-chromosome with nomenclature of arms, regions, bands, and sub-bands. (Courtesy of Dr. Stuart Schwartz, Department of Pathology, University of Chicago, Chicago, IL.)

per karyotype can be recognized. The use of these banding techniques permits certain identification of each chromosome and roughly delineates breakpoints and other gross alterations (described later).

Commonly Used Cytogenetic Terminology

Karyotypes are usually described using a shorthand system of notations in the following order: total number of chromosomes is given first, followed by the sex chromosome complement, and finally the description of abnormalities in ascending numerical order. For example, a male with trisomy 21 is designated *47,XY,+21*. Notations denoting structural alterations of chromosomes and their corresponding abnormalities are described later.

The short arm of a chromosome is designated *p* (for petit), and the long arm is referred to as *q* (the next letter of the alphabet). In a banded karyotype, each arm of the chromosome is divided into two or more regions bordered by prominent bands. The regions are numbered (e.g., 1, 2, 3) from the centromere outward. Each region is further subdivided into bands and sub-bands, and these are ordered numerically as well (Fig. 5-17). Thus, the notation *Xp21.2* refers to a chromosomal segment located on the short arm of the X chromosome, in region 2, band 1, and sub-band 2.

Structural Abnormalities of Chromosomes

The aberrations underlying cytogenetic disorders may take the form of an abnormal number of chromosomes or alterations in the structure of one or more chromosomes. The normal chromosome complement is expressed as 46,XX for the female and 46,XY for the male. Any exact multiple of the haploid number of chromosomes (23) is called *euploid.* If an error occurs in meiosis or mitosis and a cell acquires a chromosome complement that is not an exact multiple of 23, it is referred to as *aneuploidy.* The usual causes for aneuploidy are *nondisjunction* and *anaphase lag.* When nondisjunction occurs during gametogenesis, the gametes formed have either an extra chromosome (n + 1) or one less chromosome (n − 1). Fertilization of such gametes by normal gametes results in two types of zygotes—trisomic (2n + 1) or monosomic (2n − 1). In anaphase lag, one homologous chromosome in meiosis or one chromatid in mitosis lags behind and is left out of the cell nucleus. The result is one normal cell and one cell with monosomy. As seen subsequently, monosomy or trisomy involving the sex chromosomes, or even more bizarre aberrations, are compatible with life and are usually associated with variable degrees of phenotypic abnormalities. **Monosomy involving an autosome generally causes loss of too much genetic information to permit live birth or even embryogenesis, but several autosomal trisomies do permit survival.** With the exception of trisomy 21, all yield severely handicapped infants who almost invariably die at an early age.

Occasionally, *mitotic errors in early development give rise to two or more populations of cells with different chromosomal complement, in the same individual,* a condition referred to as *mosaicism.* Mosaicism can result from mitotic errors during the cleavage of the fertilized ovum or in somatic cells. Mosaicism affecting the sex chromosomes is relatively common. In the division of the fertilized ovum, an error may lead to one of the daughter cells receiving three sex chromosomes, whereas the other receives only one, yielding, for example, a 45,X/47,XXX mosaic. All descendent cells derived from each of these precursors thus have either a 47,XXX complement or a 45,X complement. Such a patient is a mosaic variant of Turner syndrome, with the extent of phenotypic expression dependent on the number and distribution of the 45,X cells.

Autosomal mosaicism seems to be much less common than that involving the sex chromosomes. An error in an early mitotic division affecting the autosomes usually leads to a nonviable mosaic due to autosomal monosomy. Rarely, the nonviable cell population is lost during embryogenesis, yielding a viable mosaic (e.g., 46,XY/47,XY,+21). Such a patient is a trisomy 21 mosaic with variable expression of Down syndrome, depending on the proportion of cells containing the trisomy.

A second category of chromosomal aberrations is associated with changes in the structure of chromosomes. To be visible by routine banding techniques, a fairly large amount of DNA (approximately 2 to 4 million base pairs), containing many genes, must be involved. The resolution is much higher with fluorescence in situ hybridization (FISH), which can detect changes as small as kilobases. Structural changes in chromosomes usually result from chromosome breakage followed by loss or rearrangement of material. In the next section the more common forms of alterations in chromosome structure and the notations used to signify them are reviewed.

Deletion refers to loss of a portion of a chromosome (Fig. 5-18). Most deletions are interstitial, but rarely terminal deletions may occur. Interstitial deletions occur when there are two breaks within a chromosome arm, followed by loss of the chromosomal material between the breaks and fusion of the broken ends. One can specify in which regions and at what bands the breaks have occurred. For example, *46,XY,del(16)(p11.2p13.1)* describes breakpoints in the short arm of chromosome 16 at 16p11.2 and 16p13.1 with loss of material between breaks. Terminal deletions result from a single break in a chromosome arm, producing a fragment with no centromere, which is then lost at the next cell division, and a chromosome bearing a deletion. The end of the chromosome is protected by acquiring telomeric sequences.

A *ring chromosome* is a special form of deletion. It is produced when a break occurs at both ends of a chromosome with fusion of the damaged ends (Fig. 5-18). If significant genetic material is lost, phenotypic abnormalities result. This might be expressed as *46,XY,r(14)*. Ring chromosomes do not behave normally in meiosis or mitosis and usually result in serious consequences.

Inversion refers to a rearrangement that involves two breaks within a single chromosome with reincorporation of the inverted, intervening segment (Fig. 5-18). An inversion involving only one arm of the chromosome is known as *paracentric*. If the breaks are on opposite sides of the centromere, it is known as *pericentric*. Inversions are often fully compatible with normal development.

Isochromosome formation results when one arm of a chromosome is lost and the remaining arm is duplicated, resulting in a chromosome consisting of two short arms only or of two long arms (Fig. 5-18). An isochromosome has morphologically identical genetic information in both arms. The most common isochromosome present in live births involves the long arm of the X and is designated *i(X)(q10)*. The Xq isochromosome is associated with monosomy for genes on the short arm of X and with trisomy for genes on the long arm of X.

In a *translocation*, a segment of one chromosome is transferred to another (Fig. 5-18). In one form, called *balanced*

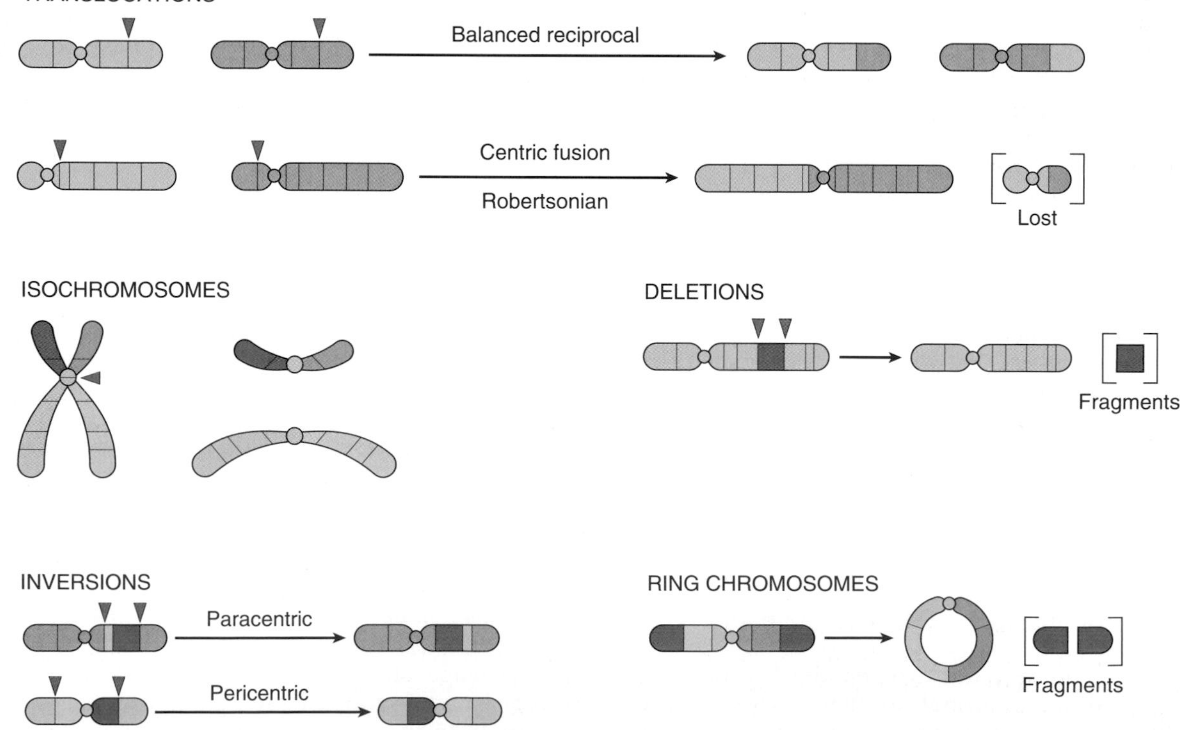

Figure 5-18 Types of chromosomal rearrangements.

reciprocal translocation, there are single breaks in each of two chromosomes, with exchange of material. A balanced reciprocal translocation between the long arm of chromosome 2 and the short arm of chromosome 5 would be written *46,XX,t(2;5)(q31;p14)*. This individual has 46 chromosomes with altered morphology of one of the chromosomes 2 and one of the chromosomes 5. Because there has been no loss of genetic material, the individual is likely to be phenotypically normal. A balanced translocation carrier, however, is at increased risk for producing abnormal gametes. For example, in the case cited earlier, a gamete containing one normal chromosome 2 and a translocated chromosome 5 may be formed. Such a gamete would be unbalanced because it would not contain the normal complement of genetic material. Subsequent fertilization by a normal gamete would lead to the formation of an abnormal (unbalanced) zygote, resulting in spontaneous abortion or birth of a malformed child. The other important pattern of translocation is called a *robertsonian translocation* (or centric fusion), a translocation between two acrocentric chromosomes. Typically the breaks occur close to the centromeres of each chromosome. Transfer of the segments then leads to one very large chromosome and one extremely small one. Usually the small product is lost (Fig. 5-18); however, because it carries only highly redundant genes (e.g., ribosomal RNA genes), this loss is compatible with a normal phenotype. Robertsonian translocation between two chromosomes is encountered in 1 in 1000 apparently normal individuals. The significance of this form of translocation also lies in the production of abnormal progeny, as discussed later with Down syndrome.

Many more numerical and structural chromosomal aberrations are described in specialized texts, and more and more abnormal karyotypes are being identified in disease. As pointed out earlier, the clinically detected chromosome disorders represent only the "tip of the iceberg." It is estimated that approximately 7.5% of all conceptions have a chromosomal abnormality, most of which are not compatible with survival or live birth. Even in live-born infants the frequency is approximately 0.5% to 1.0%. It is beyond the scope of this book to discuss most of the clinically recognizable chromosomal disorders. Hence, we focus attention on those few that are most common.

Cytogenetic Disorders Involving Autosomes

Trisomy 21 (Down Syndrome)

Down syndrome is the most common of the chromosomal disorders and is a major cause of mental retardation. In the United States the incidence in newborns is about 1 in 700. Approximately 95% of affected individuals have trisomy 21, so their chromosome count is 47. FISH with chromosome 21–specific probes reveals the extra copy of chromosome 21 in such cases (Fig. 5-19). Most others have normal chromosome numbers, but the extra chromosomal material is present as a translocation. As mentioned earlier, the most common cause of trisomy and therefore of Down syndrome is meiotic nondisjunction. The parents of such children have a normal karyotype and are normal in all respects.

Maternal age has a strong influence on the incidence of trisomy 21. It occurs once in 1550 live births in women under age 20, in contrast to 1 in 25 live births for mothers older than age 45. The correlation with maternal age suggested that most cases the meiotic nondisjunction of chromosome 21 occurs in the ovum. Indeed, studies in which DNA polymorphisms were used to trace the parental origin of chromosome 21 have revealed that in 95% of the cases with trisomy 21 the extra chromosome is of maternal origin. Although many hypotheses have been advanced, the reason for the increased susceptibility of the ovum to nondisjunction remains unknown.

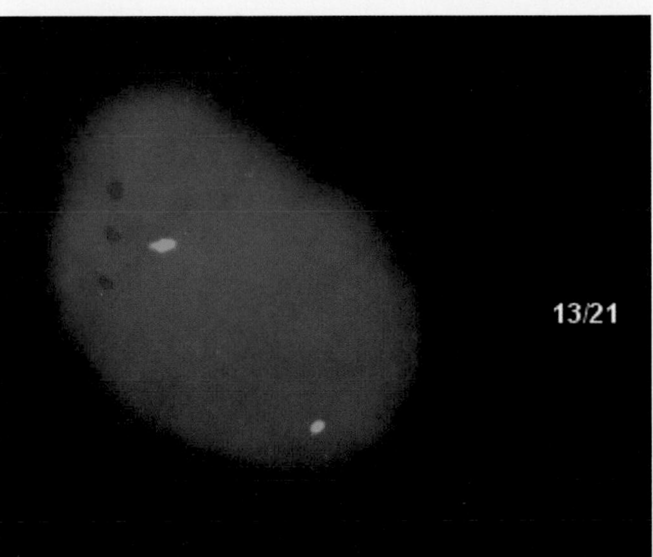

Figure 5-19 Fluorescence in situ hybridization analysis of an interphase nucleus using locus-specific probes to chromosome 13 (green) and chromosome 21 (red), revealing three red signals consistent with trisomy 21. (Courtesy of Dr. Stuart Schwartz, Department of Pathology, University of Chicago, Chicago, IL.)

In about 4% of cases of Down syndrome, the extra chromosomal material derives from the presence of a robertsonian translocation of the long arm of chromosome 21 to another acrocentric chromosome (e.g., 22 or 14). Because the fertilized ovum already possesses two normal autosomes 21, the translocated material provides the same triple gene dosage as in trisomy 21. Such cases are frequently (but not always) familial, and the translocated chromosome is inherited from one of the parents (usually the mother), who is a carrier of a robertsonian translocation, for example, a mother with karyotype 45,XX,der(14;21)(q10;q10). In cells with robertsonian translocations, the genetic material normally found on two pairs of chromosomes is distributed among only three chromosomes. This affects chromosome pairing during meiosis, and as a result the gametes have a high probability of being aneuploid.

Approximately 1% of Down syndrome patients are mosaics, having a mixture of cells with 46 or 47 chromosomes. This mosaicism results from mitotic nondisjunction of chromosome 21 during an early stage of embryogenesis. Symptoms in such cases are variable and milder, depending on the proportion of abnormal cells. Clearly, in cases of translocation or mosaic Down syndrome, maternal age is of no importance.

The diagnostic clinical features of this condition—flat facial profile, oblique palpebral fissures, and epicanthic folds (Fig. 5-20)**—are usually readily evident, even at**

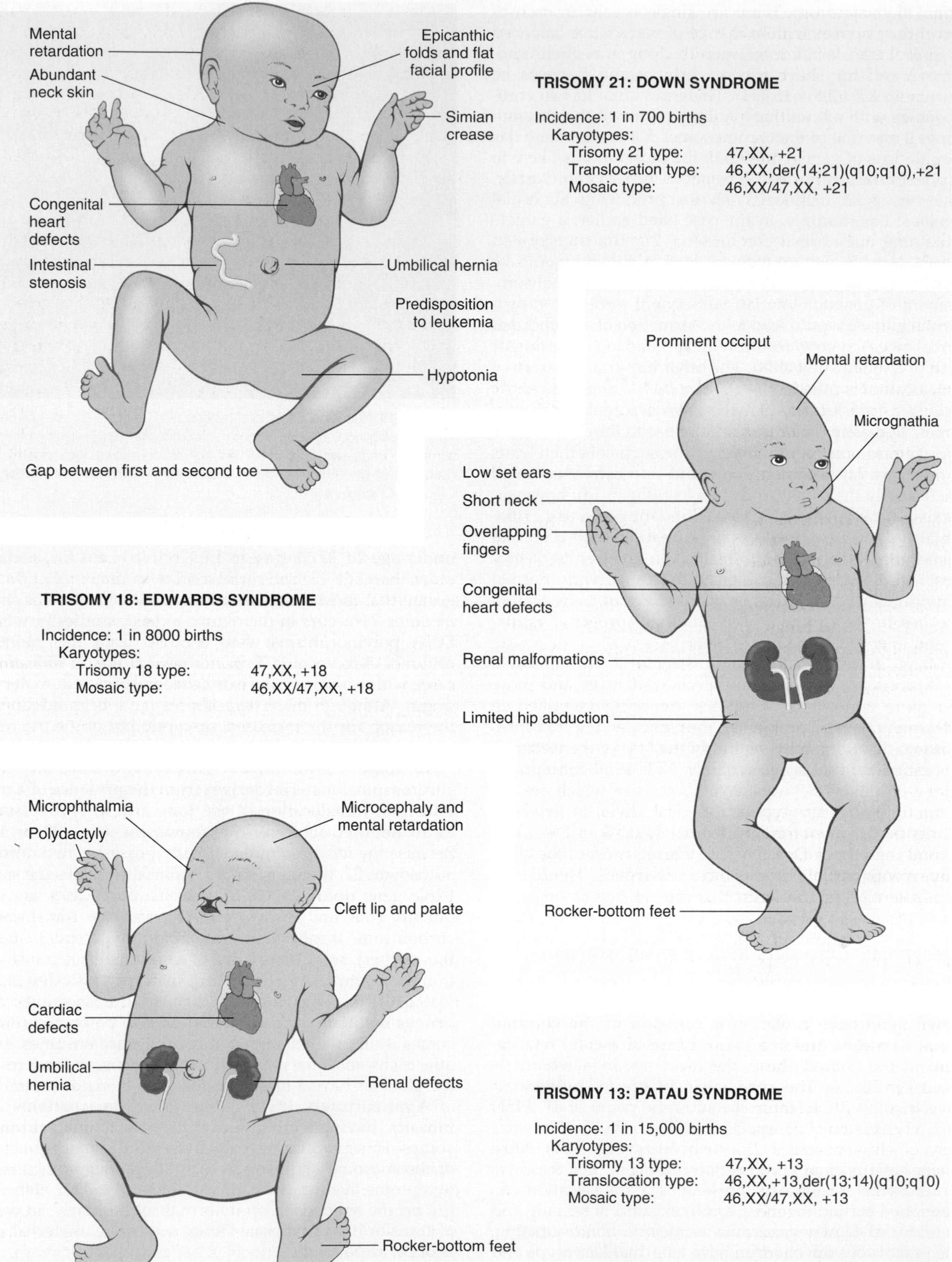

Figure 5-20 Clinical features and karyotypes of selected autosomal trisomies.

birth. Down syndrome is a leading cause of severe mental retardation; approximately 80% of those afflicted have an IQ of 25 to 50. While intellectually disadvantaged, these children typically have a gentle, shy manner and often seem more content with life than their normal siblings. It should be pointed out that some mosaics with Down syndrome have mild phenotypic changes and may even have normal or near-normal intelligence. In addition to the phenotypic abnormalities and the mental retardation already noted, some other clinical features are worthy of note.

- *Approximately 40% of the patients have congenital heart disease,* most commonly defects of the endocardial cushion, including ostium primum, atrial septal defects, atrioventricular valve malformations, and ventricular septal defects. Cardiac problems are responsible for the majority of the deaths in infancy and early childhood. Several other congenital malformations, including atresias of the esophagus and small bowel, are also common.
- *Children with trisomy 21 have a 10-fold to 20-fold increased risk of developing acute leukemia.* Both acute lymphoblastic leukemias and acute myeloid leukemias occur. The latter, most commonly, is acute megakaryoblastic leukemia.
- Virtually all patients with trisomy 21 older than age 40 develop *neuropathologic changes* characteristic of Alzheimer disease, a degenerative disorder of the brain.
- Patients with Down syndrome have *abnormal immune responses that predispose them to serious infections,* particularly of the lungs, and to thyroid autoimmunity. Although several abnormalities, affecting mainly T-cell functions, have been reported, the basis of immunologic disturbances is not clear.

Despite all these problems, improved medical care has increased the longevity of individuals with trisomy 21. Currently the median age at death is 47 years (up from 25 years in 1983).

Although the karyotype and clinical features of trisomy 21 have been known for decades, little is known about the molecular basis of Down syndrome. Based on study of humans with partial trisomy of chromosome 21 and mouse models of trisomy, the critical region of human chromosome 21 that is involved in the pathogenesis has been identified. Based on these studies, several gene clusters, each of which is predicted to participate in the same biologic pathway, have been implicated. For example, 16 genes are involved in the mitochondrial energy pathway; several are likely to influence central nervous system development and one group is involved in folate metabolism. It is not known how each of these groups of genes is related to Down syndrome. The gene dosage hypothesis assumes that the phenotypic features of the trisomy 21 are related to overexpression of genes. In reality only about 37% of the genes on chromosomes 21 are overexpressed by 150%, whereas others have variable degrees of changes in expression. Further complexity in defining the specific genes involved in the pathogenesis of Down syndrome is related to the presence of several miRNA genes on chromosome 21 that can shut down translation of genes that map elsewhere in the genome. Thus, despite the availability of the gene map of chromosome 21, the progress in understanding the molecular basis of Down syndrome remains slow.

Much progress is being made in the molecular diagnosis of Down syndrome prenatally. Approximately 5% to 10% of the total cell free DNA in maternal blood is derived from the fetus and can be identified by polymorphic genetic markers. By using next generation sequencing the gene dosage of chromosome 21 linked genes in fetal DNA can be determined with great precision. This is emerging as a powerful noninvasive method for prenatal diagnosis of trisomy 21 as well as other trisomies.

Other Trisomies

A variety of other trisomies involving chromosomes 8, 9, 13, 18, and 22 have been described. Only trisomy 18 (Edwards syndrome) and trisomy 13 (Patau syndrome) are common enough to merit brief mention here. As noted in Figure 5-20, they share several karyotypic and clinical features with trisomy 21. Thus, most cases result from meiotic nondisjunction and therefore carry a complete extra copy of chromosome 13 or 18. As in Down syndrome, an association with increased maternal age is also noted. In contrast to trisomy 21, however, the malformations are much more severe and wide ranging. As a result, only rarely do infants survive beyond the first year of life. Most succumb within a few weeks to months.

Chromosome 22q11.2 Deletion Syndrome

Chromosome 22q11.2 deletion syndrome encompasses a spectrum of disorders that result from a small deletion of band q11.2 on the long arm of chromosome 22. The syndrome is fairly common, occurring in as many as 1 in 4000 births, but it is often missed because of variable clinical features. These include *congenital heart defects, abnormalities of the palate, facial dysmorphism, developmental delay, and variable degrees of T-cell immunodeficiency and hypocalcemia.* Previously, these clinical features were considered to represent two different disorders—*DiGeorge syndrome* and *velocardiofacial syndrome.*

Patients with DiGeorge syndrome have thymic hypoplasia, with resultant T-cell immunodeficiency (Chapter 6), parathyroid hypoplasia giving rise to hypocalcemia, a variety of cardiac malformations affecting the outflow tract, and mild facial anomalies. The clinical features of the so-called velocardiofacial syndrome include facial dysmorphism (prominent nose, retrognathia), cleft palate, cardiovascular anomalies, and learning disabilities. Less frequently, these patients also have immunodeficiency.

Until recently the overlapping clinical features of these two conditions (e.g., cardiac malformations, facial dysmorphology) were not appreciated; it was only after these two apparently unrelated syndromes were found to be associated with a similar cytogenetic abnormality that the clinical overlap came into focus. Recent studies indicate that, in addition to the numerous structural malformations, individuals with the 22q11.2 deletion syndrome are at a particularly high risk for psychotic illnesses, such as *schizophrenia and bipolar disorders. In fact, it is estimated that schizophrenia develops in approximately 25% of adults with this syndrome.* Conversely, deletions of the region can be found in 2% to 3% of individuals with childhood-onset schizophrenia. In addition, attention deficit hyperactivity disorder is seen in 30% to 35% of affected children.

The diagnosis of this condition may be suspected on clinical grounds but can be established only by detection

Figure 5-21 Fluorescence in situ hybridization of both metaphase chromosomes and an interphase cell from a patient with DiGeorge syndrome demonstrating the deletion of a probe that maps to chromosome 22q11.2. The 22q11.2 probe is in red, and the control probe, localized to 22q, is in green. The metaphase spread shows one chromosome 22 with both a green signal (control probe) and a red signal (from the 22q11.2 probe). The other chromosome 22 shows only hybridization with the control probe (green), but no red 22q11.2 signal since there is a deletion on this chromosome. The interphase cell also shows a hybridization pattern consistent with a deletion of chromosome 22q11.2. (Courtesy of Dr. Stuart Schwartz, Department of Pathology, University of Chicago, Chicago, IL.)

of the deletion by FISH (Fig. 5-21). By this test, approximately 90% of those previously diagnosed as having DiGeorge syndrome and 80% of those with the velocardiofacial syndrome have a deletion of 22q11.2. Thirty percent of individuals with conotruncal cardiac defects but no other features of this syndrome also reveal deletions of the same chromosomal region.

The molecular basis of this syndrome is not fully understood. The deleted region is large (approximately 1.5 megabases) and includes many genes. The clinical heterogeneity, with predominant immunodeficiency in some cases (DiGeorge syndrome) and predominant dysmorphology and cardiac malformations in other cases, probably reflects the variable position and size of the deleted segment from this genetic region. Approximately 30 candidate genes have been mapped to the deleted region. Among these, *TBX1*, a T-box transcription factor is most closely associated with the phenotypic features of this syndrome. This gene is expressed in the pharyngeal mesenchyme and endodermal pouch from which facial structures, thymus, and parathyroid are derived. The targets of *TBX1* include *PAX9*, a gene that controls the development of the palate, parathyroids, and thymus. Clearly there are other genes that contribute to the behavioral and psychiatric disorders that remain to be identified.

KEY CONCEPTS

Cytogenetic Disorders Involving Autosomes

- **Down syndrome** is associated with an extra copy of genes on chromosome 21, most commonly due to trisomy 21 and less frequently from translocation of extra chromosomal material from chromosome 21 to other chromosomes or from mosaicism.
- Patients with Down syndrome have severe mental retardation, flat facial profile, epicanthic folds, cardiac malformations, higher risk of leukemia and infections, and premature development of Alzheimer disease.
- Deletion of genes at chromosomal locus 22q11.2 gives rise to malformations affecting the face, heart, thymus, and parathyroids. The resulting disorders are recognized as
  - **DiGeorge syndrome** (thymic hypoplasia with diminished T-cell immunity and parathyroid hypoplasia with hypocalcemia) and
  - **Velocardiofacial** syndrome (congenital heart disease involving outflow tracts, facial dysmorphism, and developmental delay).

Cytogenetic Disorders Involving Sex Chromosomes

Genetic diseases associated with changes involving the sex chromosomes are far more common than those related to autosomal aberrations. Furthermore, imbalances (excess or loss) of sex chromosomes are much better tolerated than are similar imbalances of autosomes. In large part, this latitude relates to two factors that are peculiar to the sex chromosomes: (1) lyonization or inactivation of all but one X chromosome and (2) the modest amount of genetic material carried by the Y chromosome. These features are discussed briefly in relation to sex chromosomal disorders.

In 1961, Lyon outlined the idea of X-inactivation, now commonly known as the Lyon hypothesis. It states that *(1) only one of the X chromosomes is genetically active, (2) the other X of either maternal or paternal origin undergoes heteropyknosis and is rendered inactive, (3) inactivation of either the maternal or paternal X occurs at random among all the cells of the blastocyst on or about day 5.5 of embryonic life, and (4) inactivation of the same X chromosome persists in all the cells derived from each precursor cell.* Thus, the great preponderance of normal females are in reality mosaics and have two populations of cells, one with an inactivated maternal X and the other with an inactivated paternal X. Herein lies the explanation of why females have the same dosage of X-linked active genes as have males. The inactive X can be seen in the interphase nucleus as a darkly staining small mass in contact with the nuclear membrane known as the Barr body, or X chromatin. The molecular basis of X inactivation involves a unique gene called *XIST*, whose product is a long noncoding RNA (Chapter 1) that is retained in the nucleus, where it "coats" the X chromosome that it is transcribed from and initiates a gene-silencing process by chromatin modification and DNA methylation. The *XIST* allele is switched off in the active X.

Although it was initially thought that all the genes on the inactive X are "switched off," more recent studies have revealed that many genes escape X inactivation. Molecular studies suggest that 21% of genes on Xp, and a smaller number (3%) on Xq escape X inactivation. At least some of the genes that are expressed from both X chromosomes are important for normal growth and development. This notion is supported by the fact that patients with monosomy of the X chromosome (Turner syndrome: 45,X) have severe somatic and gonadal abnormalities. If a single dose of X-linked genes were sufficient, no detrimental effect would be expected in such cases. Furthermore, although one X chromosome is inactivated in all cells during embryogenesis, it is selectively reactivated in oogonia before the first meiotic division. Thus, it seems that both X chromosomes are required for normal oogenesis.

With respect to the Y chromosome, it is well known that this chromosome is both necessary and sufficient for male development. **Regardless of the number of X chromosomes, the presence of a single Y determines the male sex.** The gene that dictates testicular development (*SRY*: sex-determining region Y gene) is located on its distal short arm. For quite some time this was considered to be the only gene of significance on the Y chromosome. Recent studies of the Y chromosome, however, have yielded a rich harvest of gene families in the so-called "male-specific Y," or MSY region encoding at least 75 protein coding genes All of these are believed to be testes-specific and are involved in spermatogenesis. In keeping with this, all Y chromosome deletions are associated with azoospermia. The following features are common to all sex chromosome disorders.

- In general, sex chromosome disorders cause subtle, chronic problems relating to sexual development and fertility.
- Sex chromosome disorders are often difficult to diagnose at birth, and many are first recognized at the time of puberty.
- In general, the greater the number of X chromosomes, in both male and female, the greater the likelihood of mental retardation.

The two most important disorders arising in aberrations of sex chromosomes are described briefly here.

Klinefelter Syndrome

Klinefelter syndrome is best defined as male hypogonadism that occurs when there are two or more X chromosomes and one or more Y chromosomes. It is one of the most frequent forms of genetic disease involving the sex chromosomes as well as one of the most common causes of hypogonadism in the male. The incidence of this condition is approximately 1 in 660 live male births.

Klinefelter syndrome can rarely be diagnosed before puberty, particularly because the testicular abnormality does not develop before early puberty. Most patients have a distinctive body habitus with an increase in length between the soles and the pubic bone, which creates the appearance of an elongated body. Also characteristic are eunuchoid body habitus with abnormally long legs; small atrophic testes often associated with a small penis; and lack of such secondary male characteristics as deep voice, beard, and male distribution of pubic hair. Gynecomastia may be present. The mean IQ is somewhat lower than normal, but mental retardation is uncommon. There is increased incidence of type 2 diabetes and the metabolic syndrome that gives rise to insulin resistance. Curiously, mitral valve prolapse is seen in about 50% of adults with Klinefelter syndrome. There is also an increased incidence of osteoporosis and fractures due to sex hormonal imbalance.

It should be evident that the clinical features of this condition are variable, the only consistent finding being hypogonadism. Plasma gonadotropin concentrations, particularly follicle-stimulating hormone, are consistently elevated, whereas testosterone levels are variably reduced. Mean plasma estradiol levels are elevated by an as yet unknown mechanism. The ratio of estrogens and testosterone determines the degree of feminization in individual cases.

Klinefelter syndrome is an important genetic cause of reduced spermatogenesis and male infertility. In some patients the testicular tubules are totally atrophied and replaced by pink, hyaline, collagenous ghosts. In others, apparently normal tubules are interspersed with atrophic tubules. In some patients all tubules are primitive and appear embryonic, consisting of cords of cells that never developed a lumen or progressed to mature spermatogenesis. Leydig cells appear prominent, as a result of the atrophy and crowding of the tubules and elevation of gonadotropin concentrations.

Patients with Klinefelter syndrome have a higher risk for breast cancer (20 times more common than in normal males), extragonadal germ cell tumors, and autoimmune diseases such as systemic lupus erythematosus.

The classic pattern of Klinefelter syndrome is associated with a 47,XXY karyotype (90% of cases). This complement of chromosomes results from nondisjunction during the meiotic divisions in the germ cells of one of the parents. Maternal and paternal nondisjunction at the first meiotic division are roughly equally involved. There is no phenotypic difference between those who receive the extra X chromosome from their father and those who receive it from their mother. Maternal age is increased in the cases associated with errors in oogenesis. In addition to this classic karyotype, approximately 15% of patients with Klinefelter syndrome have been found to have a variety of mosaic patterns, most of them being 46,XY/47,XXY. Other patterns are 47,XXY/48,XXXY and variations on this theme.

As is the case with normal females, all but one X chromosome undergoes inactivation in patients with Klinefelter syndrome. Why then, do the patients with this disorder have hypogonadism and associated features? The explanation for this lies in genes on the X chromosome that escape lyonization and in the pattern of X inactivation.

- One pathogenic mechanism is related to uneven dosage compensation during X-inactivation. In some cases about 15% of the X-linked genes escape inactivation. Thus, there is an extra dose of these genes compared to normal males in whom only one copy of X is active, and it appears that "overexpression" of one or more of these genes leads to hypogonadism.
- A second mechanism involves the gene encoding the androgen receptor, through which testosterone mediates its effects. The androgen receptor gene maps to the X chromosome and contains highly polymorphic CAG (trinucleotide) repeats. The functional response of the receptor to any particular dose of androgen is dictated, in part, by the number of CAG repeats, as receptors with shorter CAG repeats are more sensitive to androgens than those with long CAG repeats. In persons with Klinefelter syndrome, the X chromosome bearing the androgen receptor allele with the shortest CAG repeat is preferentially inactivated. In XXY males with low testosterone levels, expression of androgen receptors with long CAG repeats exacerbates the hypogonadism and

appears to account for certain aspects of the phenotype, such as small penis size.

Turner Syndrome

Turner syndrome results from complete or partial monosomy of the X chromosome and is characterized primarily by hypogonadism in phenotypic females. It is the most common sex chromosome abnormality in females, affecting about 1 in 2500 live-born females.

With routine cytogenetic methods, three types of karyotypic abnormalities are seen in individuals with Turner syndrome.

- *Approximately 57% are missing an entire X chromosome, resulting in a 45,X karyotype.* Of the remaining 43%, approximately one third (approximately 14%) have structural abnormalities of the X chromosomes, and two thirds (approximately 29%) are mosaics.
- *The common feature of the structural abnormalities is to produce partial monosomy of the X chromosome.* In order of frequency, the structural abnormalities of the X chromosome include (1) an isochromosome of the long arm, 46,X,i(X)(q10) resulting in the loss of the short arm; (2) deletion of portions of both long and short arms, resulting in the formation of a ring chromosome, 46,X,r(X); and (3) deletion of portions of the short or long arm, 46X,del(Xq) or 46X,del(Xp).
- *The mosaic patients have a 45,X cell population along with one or more karyotypically normal or abnormal cell types.* Examples of karyotypes that mosaic Turner females may have are the following: (1) 45,X/46,XX; (2) 45,X/46,XY; (3) 45,X/47,XXX; or (4) 45,X/46,X,i(X)(q10). Studies suggest that the prevalence of mosaicism in Turner syndrome may be much higher than the 30% detected by conventional cytogenetic studies. With the use of more sensitive techniques, the prevalence of mosaic Turner syndrome increases to 75%. Because 99% of conceptuses with an apparent 45,X karyotype are nonviable, many authorities believe that there are no truly nonmosaic Turner syndrome patients. While this issue remains controversial, it is important to appreciate the karyotypic heterogeneity associated with Turner syndrome, because it is responsible for significant variations in phenotype. In patients in whom the proportion of 45,X cells is high, the phenotypic changes are more severe than in those who have readily detectable mosaicism. The latter may have an almost normal appearance and may present only with primary amenorrhea.

Five percent to 10% of patients with Turner syndrome have Y chromosome sequences either as a complete Y chromosome (e.g., 45,X/46,XY karyotype) or as fragments of Y chromosomes translocated on other chromosomes. These patients are at a higher risk for development of a gonadal tumor (gonadoblastoma).

The most severely affected patients generally present during infancy with edema of the dorsum of the hand and foot due to lymph stasis, and sometimes *swelling of the nape of the neck.* The latter is related to markedly distended lymphatic channels, producing a so-called cystic hygroma (Chapter 10). As these infants develop, the swellings subside but often leave bilateral *neck webbing* and persistent looseness of skin on the back of the neck. *Congenital heart disease* is also common, affecting 25% to 50% of patients. Left-sided cardiovascular abnormalities, particularly preductal coarctation of the aorta and bicuspid aortic valve, are seen most frequently. *Cardiovascular abnormalities are the most important cause of increased mortality in children* with Turner syndrome.

The principal clinical features in the adolescent and adult are illustrated in Figure 5-22. At puberty there is *failure to develop normal secondary sex characteristics.* The genitalia remain infantile, breast development is inadequate, and there is little pubic hair. The mental status of these patients is usually normal, but subtle defects in nonverbal, visual-spatial information processing have been noted. Of particular importance in establishing the diagnosis in the adult is the shortness of stature (rarely exceeding 150 cm in height) and amenorrhea. *Turner syndrome is the single most important cause of primary amenorrhea,* accounting for approximately one third of the cases. For reasons not clear, approximately 50% of patients develop autoantibodies that react with the thyroid gland, and up to half of these develop clinically manifest hypothyroidism. Equally mysterious is the presence of glucose intolerance, obesity, and insulin resistance in a minority of patients. The last mentioned is significant, because therapy with growth hormone, commonly used in these patients, worsens insulin resistance.

The molecular pathogenesis of Turner syndrome is not completely understood, but studies have begun to shed some light. In approximately 75% of cases the X- chromosome is maternal in origin, thus suggesting that there is an abnormality in paternal gametogenesis. As mentioned earlier, both X chromosomes are active during oogenesis and are essential for normal development of the ovaries. During normal fetal development, ovaries contain as many as 7 million oocytes. The oocytes gradually disappear so that by menarche their numbers have dwindled to a mere 400,000, and when menopause occurs fewer than 10,000 remain. In Turner syndrome, fetal ovaries develop normally early in embryogenesis, but the absence of the second X chromosome leads to an accelerated loss of oocytes, which is complete by age 2 years. In a sense, therefore, "menopause occurs before menarche," and the ovaries are reduced to atrophic fibrous strands, devoid of ova and follicles *(streak ovaries).* Because patients with Turner syndrome also have other (nongonadal) abnormalities, it follows that some genes for normal growth and development of somatic tissues must also reside on the X chromosome. Among the genes involved in the Turner phenotype is the short stature homeobox (*SHOX*) gene at Xp22.33. This is one of several genes that remain active in both X chromosomes and has an active homologue on the short arm of the Y chromosome. Thus, both normal males and females have two copies of this gene. Haploinsufficiency of *SHOX* gives rise to short stature. Indeed, deletions of the *SHOX* gene are noted in 2% to 5% of otherwise normal children with short stature. In keeping with its role as a critical regulator of growth, the *SHOX* gene is expressed during fetal life in the growth plates of several long bones including the radius, ulna, tibia, and fibula. It is also expressed in the first and second pharyngeal arches. Just as the loss of *SHOX* is always associated with short stature, excess copies of this gene are associated with tall stature. Whereas haploinsufficiency of *SHOX* can explain growth deficit in Turner syndrome, it cannot explain other clinical

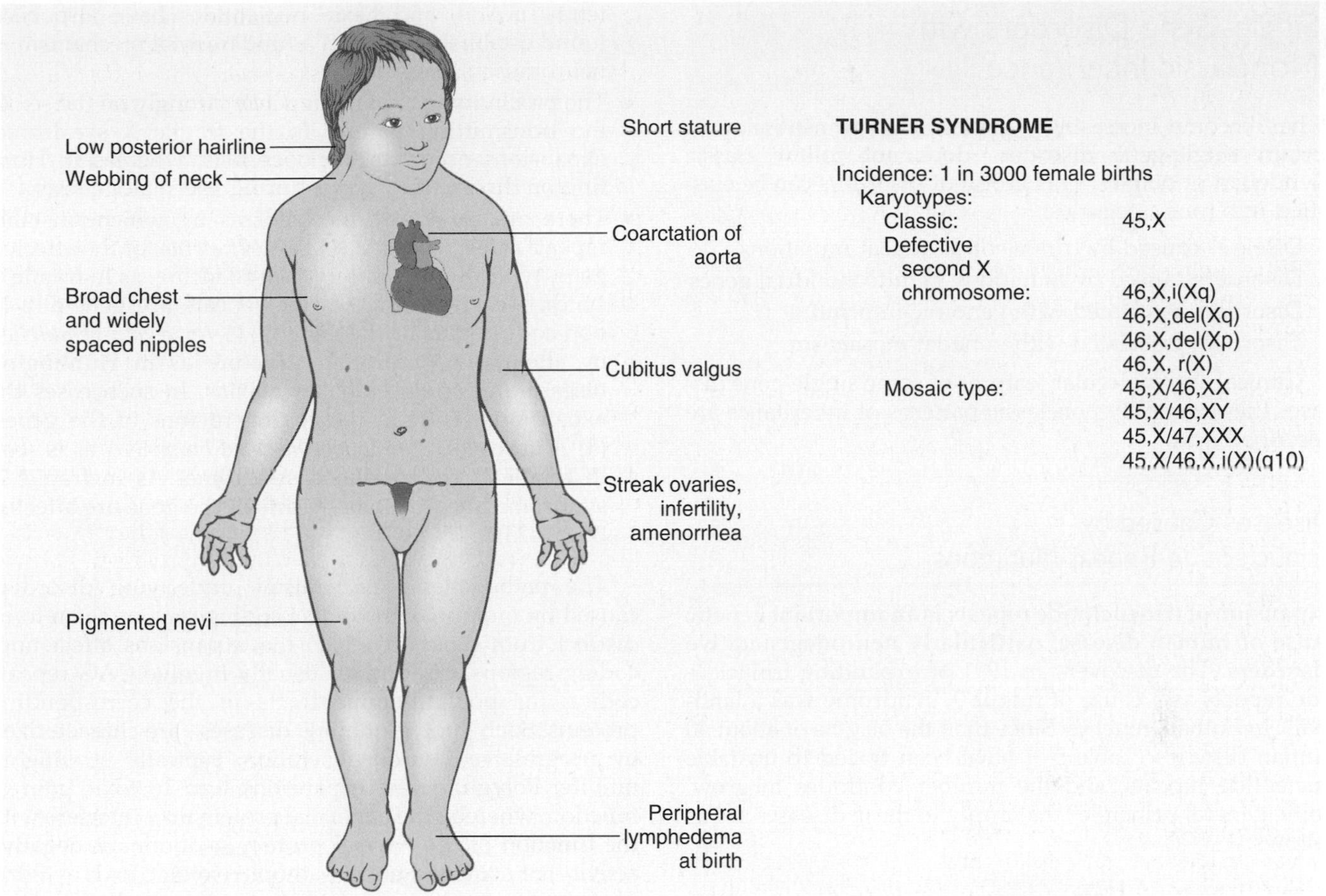

Short stature

Low posterior hairline

Webbing of neck

Coarctation of aorta

Broad chest and widely spaced nipples

Cubitus valgus

Streak ovaries, infertility, amenorrhea

Pigmented nevi

Peripheral lymphedema at birth

TURNER SYNDROME

Incidence: 1 in 3000 female births

Karyotypes:

Classic:	45,X
Defective second X chromosome:	46,X,i(Xq)
	46,X,del(Xq)
	46,X,del(Xp)
	46,X, r(X)
Mosaic type:	45,X/46,XX
	45,X/46,XY
	45,X/47,XXX
	45,X/46,X,i(X)(q10)

Figure 5-22 Clinical features and karyotypes of Turner syndrome.

features such as cardiac malformations and endocrine abnormalities. Clearly several other genes located on the X chromosome are also involved.

Hermaphroditism and Pseudohermaphroditism

The problem of sexual ambiguity is exceedingly complex, and only limited observations are possible here; for more details, reference should be made to specialized sources. It will be no surprise to medical students that the sex of an individual can be defined on several levels. *Genetic sex* is determined by the presence or absence of a Y chromosome. No matter how many X chromosomes are present, a single Y chromosome dictates testicular development and the genetic male gender. The initially indifferent gonads of both the male and the female embryos have an inherent tendency to feminize, unless influenced by Y chromosome-dependent masculinizing factors. *Gonadal sex* is based on the histologic characteristics of the gonads. *Ductal sex* depends on the presence of derivatives of the müllerian or wolffian ducts. *Phenotypic*, or *genital, sex* is based on the appearance of the external genitalia. Sexual ambiguity is present whenever there is disagreement among these various criteria for determining sex.

The term true *hermaphrodite* implies the presence of both ovarian and testicular tissue. In contrast, a pseudohermaphrodite represents a disagreement between the phenotypic and gonadal sex (i.e., a female pseudohermaphrodite has ovaries but male external genitalia; a male pseudohermaphrodite has testicular tissue but female-type genitalia). The genetic bases of these conditions are quite variable and beyond the scope of our discussion here.

KEY CONCEPTS

Cytogenetic Disorders Involving Sex Chromosomes

- In females, one X chromosome, maternal or paternal, is randomly inactivated during development (Lyon hypothesis).
- In **Klinefelter syndrome,** there are two or more X chromosomes with one Y chromosome as a result of nondisjunction of sex chromosomes. Patients have testicular atrophy, sterility, reduced body hair, gynecomastia, and eunuchoid body habitus. It is the most common cause of male sterility.
- In **Turner syndrome,** there is partial or complete monosomy of genes on the short arm of the X chromosome, most commonly due to absence of one X chromosome (45,X) and less commonly from mosaicism, or from deletions involving the short arm of the X chromosome. Short stature, webbing of the neck, cubitus valgus, cardiovascular malformations, amenorrhea, lack of secondary sex characteristics, and fibrotic ovaries are typical clinical features.

Single-Gene Disorders with Nonclassic Inheritance

It has become increasingly evident that transmission of certain single-gene disorders does not follow classic Mendelian principles. This group of disorders can be classified into four categories:

- Diseases caused by trinucleotide-repeat mutations
- Disorders caused by mutations in mitochondrial genes
- Disorders associated with genomic imprinting
- Disorders associated with gonadal mosaicism

Clinical and molecular features of some single-gene diseases that exemplify nonclassic patterns of inheritance are described next.

Diseases Caused by Trinucleotide-Repeat Mutations

Expansion of trineuclotide repeats is an important genetic cause of human disease, particularly neurodegenerative disorders. The discovery in 1991 of expanding trinucleotide repeats as a cause of fragile X syndrome was a landmark in human genetics. Since then the origins of about 40 human diseases (Table 5-8) have been traced to unstable nucleotide repeats, and the number continues to grow. Some general principles that apply to these diseases are as follows:

- The causative mutations are associated with the expansion of a stretch of trinucleotides that usually share the nucleotides G and C. In all cases the DNA is unstable, and an expansion of the repeats above a certain threshold impairs gene function in various ways, discussed later. In recent years diseases associated with unstable tetra-, penta-, and hexa- nucleotides have also been found establishing this as a fundamental mechanism of neuromuscular diseases.
- The proclivity to expand depends strongly on the sex of the transmitting parent. In the fragile X syndrome, expansions occur during oogenesis, whereas in Huntington disease they occur during spermatogenesis.
- There are three key mechanisms by which unstable repeats cause diseases: (1) *Loss of function* of the affected gene, typically by transcription silencing, as in fragile X syndrome. In such cases the repeats are generally in non-coding part of the gene (2) *A toxic gain of function* by alterations of protein structure as in Huntington disease and spinocerebellar ataxias. In such cases the expansions occur in the coding regions of the genes. (3) *A toxic gain of function mediated by mRNA* as is seen in fragile X tremor-ataxia syndrome. As in fragile X syndrome, the noncoding parts of the gene are affected (Fig. 5-23).

The pathogenetic mechanisms underlying disorders caused by mutations that affect coding regions seem to be distinct from those in which the expansions affect noncoding regions. The former usually involve CAG repeats coding for polyglutamine tracts in the corresponding proteins. Such "polyglutamine diseases" are characterized by progressive neurodegeneration, typically striking in midlife. Polyglutamine expansions lead to toxic gain of function, whereby the abnormal protein may interfere with the function of the normal protein (a dominant negative activity) or acquire a novel pathophysiologic toxic activity. The precise mechanisms by which expanded polyglutamine proteins cause disease is not fully understood. In most cases the proteins are misfolded and tend to aggregate; the aggregates may suppress transcription of other genes, cause mitochondrial dysfunction, or trigger the unfolded-protein stress response and apoptosis (Chapter 1). *A*

Table 5-8 Examples of Trinucleotide-Repeat Disorders

Disease	Gene	Locus	Protein	Repeat	No. of Repeats: Normal	No. of Repeats: Disease
Expansions Affecting Noncoding Regions						
Fragile X syndrome	*FMRI (FRAXA)*	Xq27.3	FMR-1 protein (FMRP)	CGG	6-55	55-200 (pre); >230 (full)
Friedreich ataxia	*FXN*	9q21.1	Frataxin	GAA	7-34	34-80 (pre); >100 (full)
Myotonic dystrophy	*DMPK*	19q13.3	Myotonic dystrophy protein kinase (DMPK)	CTG	5-37	34-80 (pre); >100 (full)
Expansions Affecting Coding Regions						
Spinobulbar muscular atrophy (Kennedy disease)	*AR*	Xq12	Androgen receptor (AR)	CAG	9-36	38-62
Huntington disease	*HTT*	4p16.3	Huntingtin	CAG	6-35	36-121
Dentatorubral-pallidoluysian atrophy (Haw River syndrome)	*ATNL*	12p13.31	Atrophin-1	CAG	6-35	49-88
Spinocerebellar ataxia type 1	*ATXN1*	6p23	Ataxin-1	CAG	6-44	39-82
Spinocerebellar ataxia type 2	*ATXN2*	12q24.1	Ataxin-2	CAG	15-31	36-63
Spinocerebellar ataxia type 3 (Machado-Joseph disease)	*ATXN3*	14q21	Ataxin-3	CAG	12-40	55-84
Spinocerebellar ataxia type 6	*CACNA2A*	19p13.3	α_{1A}-Voltage-dependent calcium channel subunit	CAG	4-18	21-33
Spinocerebellar ataxia type 7	*ATXN7*	3p14.1	Ataxin-7	CAG	4-35	37-306

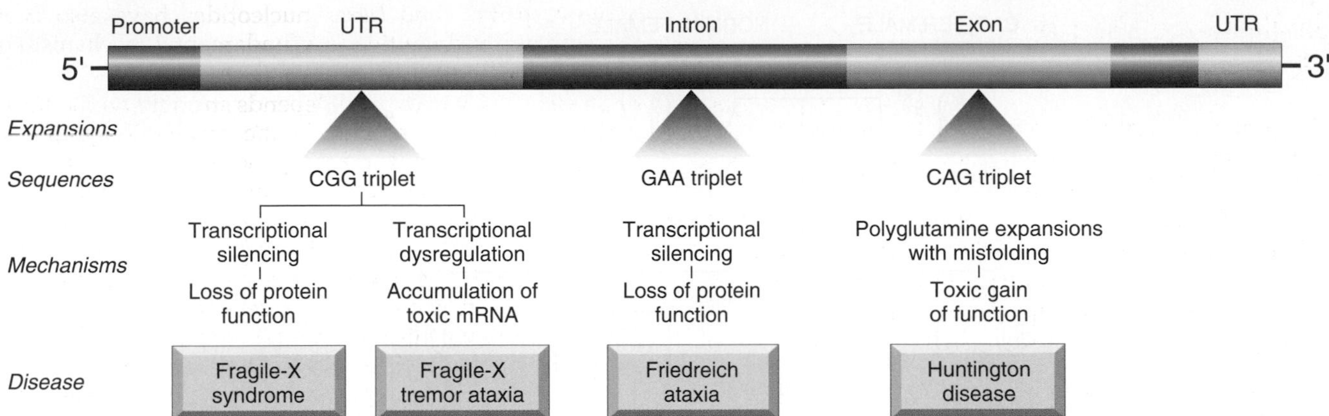

Figure 5-23 Sites of expansion and the affected sequence in selected diseases caused by nucleotide-repeat mutations. UTR, Untranslated region.

morphologic hallmark of these diseases is the accumulation of aggregated mutant proteins in large intranuclear inclusions. While formation of aggregates is common to many "polyglutamine disease," evidence of a direct toxic role of aggregates is not universal. In fact some observers believe that aggregation may be protective by sequestration of the misfolded protein. Other models of pathogenicity implicate downstream effects mediated by proteolytic fragments of the polyglutamine fragment. Much more needs to be learned before therapeutic strategies can be developed.

Fragile X Syndrome and Fragile X Tremor/Ataxia

Fragile X syndrome is the prototype of diseases in which the mutation is characterized by a long repeating sequence of three nucleotides. Although the specific nucleotide sequence that undergoes amplification differs in the 20 or so disorders included in this group, in most cases the affected sequences share the nucleotides guanine (G) and cytosine (C). The ensuing discussion considers the clinical features and inheritance pattern of the fragile-X syndrome, followed by the causative molecular lesion. The remaining disorders in this group are discussed elsewhere in this text. Although distinct diseases, fragile X syndrome and fragile X tremor/ataxia share common features and so are discussed together.

Fragile X syndrome is the second most common genetic cause of mental retardation after Down syndrome. It is caused by a trinucleotide mutation in the familial mental retardation-1 (FMR1) ***gene.*** Fragile-X-syndrome has a frequency of 1 in 1550 for affected males and 1 in 8000 for affected females and is characterized by an inducible cytogenetic abnormality in the X chromosome within which the *FMR1* gene maps. The cytogenetic alteration was discovered as a discontinuity of staining or as a constriction in the long arm of the X chromosome when cells are cultured in a folate-deficient medium. Because it appears that the chromosome is "broken" at this locale, it was named as a *fragile site* (Fig. 5-24). There are more than 100 "fragile sites" in the human genome of unknown significance; many are present in normal individuals.

In fragile X syndrome, the affected males are *mentally retarded,* with an IQ in the range of 20 to 60. They express a characteristic physical phenotype that includes a *long face with a large mandible, large everted ears,* and *large testicles (macro-orchidism).* Hyperextensible joints, a high arched palate, and mitral valve prolapse noted in some patients mimic a connective tissue disorder. These and other physical abnormalities described in this condition, however, are not always present and, in some cases, are quite subtle. *The most distinctive feature is macro-orchidism, which is observed in at least 90% of affected postpubertal males.*

As with all X-linked diseases, fragile X syndrome affects males. Analysis of several pedigrees, however, reveals some patterns of transmission not typically associated with other X-linked recessive disorders (Fig. 5-25). These include the following:

- *Carrier males:* Approximately 20% of males who, by pedigree analysis and by molecular tests, are known to carry a fragile X mutation are clinically and cytogenetically normal. Because carrier males transmit the trait through all their phenotypically normal daughters to affected grandchildren, they are called *normal transmitting males.*
- *Affected females:* 30% to 50% of carrier females are affected (i.e., mentally retarded), a number much higher than that in other X-linked recessive disorders.
- *Risk of phenotypic effects:* Risk depends on the position of the individual in the pedigree. For example, brothers of transmitting males are at a 9% risk of having mental retardation, whereas grandsons of transmitting males incur a 40% risk.
- *Anticipation:* This refers to the observation that clinical features of fragile X syndrome worsen with each successive generation, as if the mutation becomes increasingly deleterious as it is transmitted from a man to his grandsons and great-grandsons.

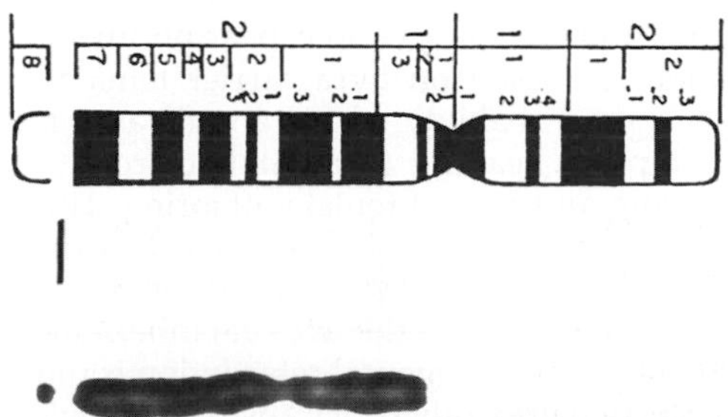

Figure 5-24 Fragile X seen as discontinuity of staining. (Courtesy of Dr. Patricia Howard-Peebles, University of Texas Southwestern Medical Center, Dallas, TX.)

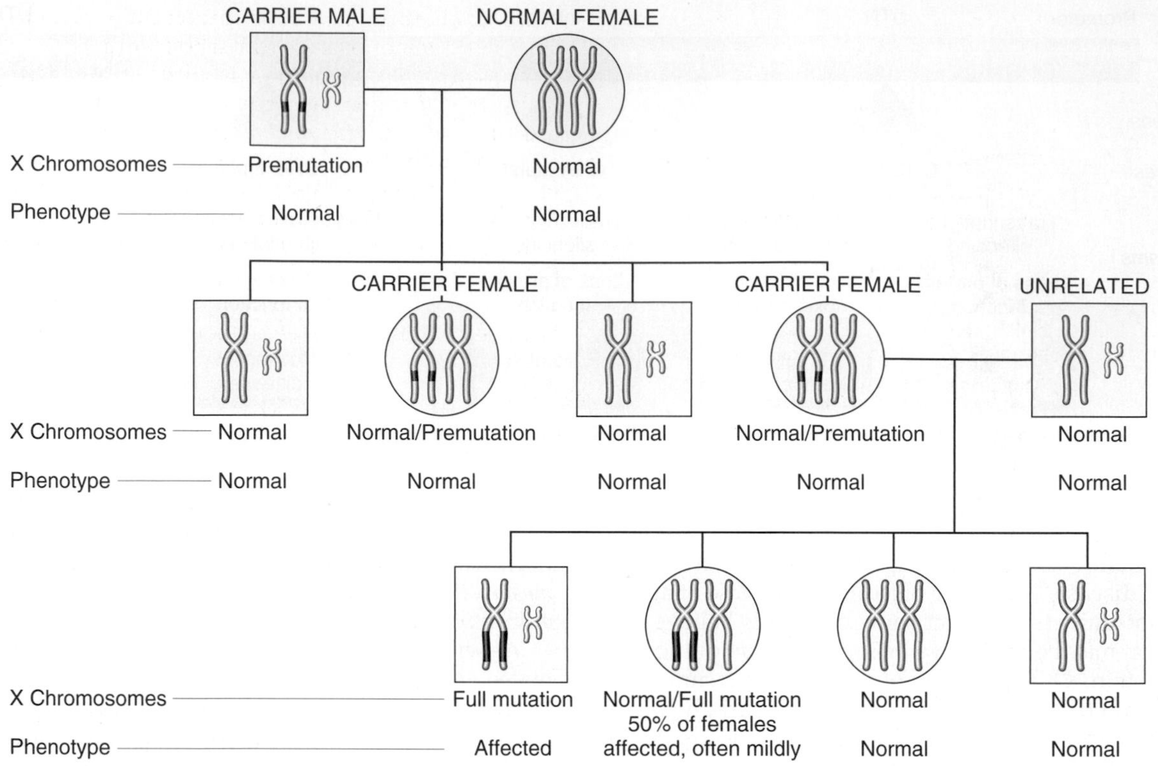

Figure 5-25 Fragile X pedigree. Note that in the first generation all sons are normal and all females are carriers. During oogenesis in the carrier female, premutation expands to full mutation; hence, in the next generation all males who inherit the X with full mutation are affected. However, only 50% of females who inherit the full mutation are affected, and only mildly. (Courtesy of Dr. Nancy Schneider, Department of Pathology, University of Texas Southwestern Medical Center, Dallas, TX.)

The first breakthrough in resolving these perplexing observations came when linkage studies localized the mutation responsible for this disease to Xq27.3, within the cytogenetically abnormal region. Within this region lies the *FMR1* gene, characterized by multiple tandem repeats of the nucleotide sequence CGG in its 5′ untranslated region. In the normal population, the number of CGG repeats is small, ranging from 6 to 55 (average, 29). The presence of clinical symptoms and a cytogenetically detectable fragile site is related to the amplification of the CGG repeats. Thus, normal transmitting males and carrier females carry 55 to 200 CGG repeats. Expansions of this size are called *premutations.* In contrast, affected individuals have an extremely large expansion of the repeat region (200 to 4000 repeats, or *full mutations*). Full mutations are believed to arise by further amplification of the CGG repeats seen in premutations. How this process takes place is quite peculiar. Carrier males transmit the repeats to their progeny with small changes in repeat number. When the premutation is passed on by a carrier female, however, there is a high probability of a dramatic amplification of the CGG repeats, leading to mental retardation in most male offspring and 50% of female offspring. Thus, *it seems that during the process of oogenesis, but not spermatogenesis, premutations can be converted to mutations by triplet-repeat amplification*. This explains the unusual inheritance pattern; that is, the likelihood of mental retardation is much higher in grandsons than in brothers of transmitting males because grandsons incur the risk of inheriting a premutation from their grandfather that is amplified to a "full mutation" in their mothers' ova. By comparison, brothers of transmitting males, being "higher up" in the pedigree, are less likely to have a full mutation. These molecular details also provide a satisfactory explanation of anticipation—a phenomenon observed by clinical geneticists but not believed by molecular geneticists until triplet-repeat mutations were identified. Why only 50% of the females with the full mutation are clinically affected is not clear. Presumably in those that are clinically affected there is unfavorable lyonization (i.e., there is a higher frequency of cells in which the X chromosome carrying the mutation is active).

The molecular basis of mental retardation and other somatic changes is related to a loss of function of the familial mental retardation protein (FMRP). As mentioned earlier, the normal *FMR1* gene contains up to 55 CGG repeats in its 5′ untranslated region. When the trinucleotide repeats in the *FMR1* gene exceed approximately 230, the DNA of the entire 5′ region of the gene becomes abnormally methylated. Methylation also extends upstream into the promoter region of the gene, resulting in transcriptional suppression of *FMR1.* The resulting absence of FMRP is believed to cause the phenotypic changes.

FMRP is a widely expressed cytoplasmic protein, most abundant in the brain and testis, the two organs most affected in this disease. Its proposed functions are the following:

- *FMRP selectively binds mRNAs associated with polysomes and regulates their intracellular transport to dendrites.* FMRP binds to approximately 4% of mammalian brain mRNAs. Unlike other cells, in neurons protein synthesis

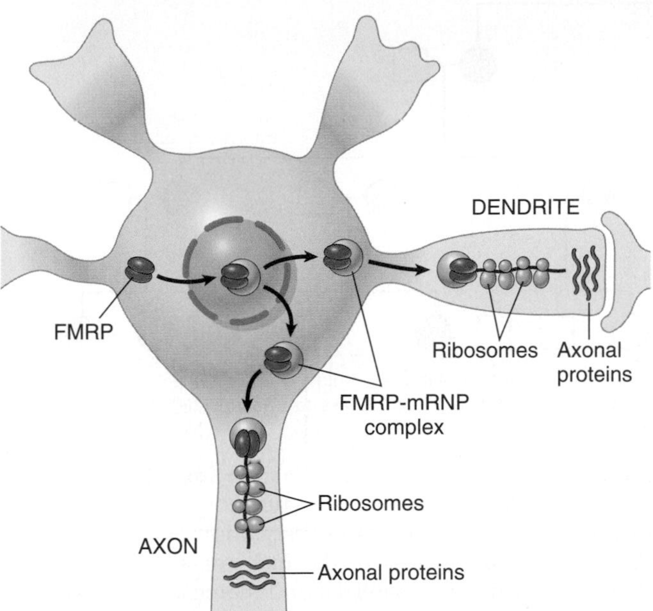

Figure 5-26 A model for the action of familial mental retardation protein (FMRP) in neurons. (Adapted from Hin P, Warren ST: New insights into fragile X syndrome: from molecules to neurobehavior. Trends Biochem Sci 28:152, 2003.)

occurs both in the perinuclear cytoplasm and in dendritic spines. Newly made FMRP translocates to the nucleus, where it assembles into a complex containing specific mRNA transcripts. The FRMP-mRNA complexes are then exported to the cytoplasm, from where they are trafficked to dendrites near neuronal synapses (Fig. 5-26). As would be anticipated, only mRNAs encoding proteins that regulate synaptic function are subject to shuttling by FMRP.
- *FRMP is a translation regulator.* At synaptic junctions FMRP suppresses protein synthesis from the bound mRNAs in response to signaling through group I metabotropic glutamate receptors (mGlu-R). Thus a reduction in FMRP in the fragile X syndrome results in increased translation of the bound mRNAs at the synaptic junctions. Such imbalance in turn causes permanent changes in synaptic activity and ultimately mental retardation.

Although demonstration of an abnormal karyotype led to the identification of this disorder, PCR-based detection of the repeats is now the method of choice for diagnosis.

Fragile X Tremor/Ataxia. **Although initially assumed to be innocuous, CGG premutations in the *FMR1* gene can cause a disease that is phenotypically different from fragile X syndrome through a distinct mechanism involving a toxic "gain-of-function".** A decade after the discovery that CGG repeat expansions cause fragile X syndrome, it became clear that approximately 20% of females carrying the premutation (carrier females) have premature ovarian failure (before the age of 40 years), and more than 50% of premutation-carrying males (transmitting males) exhibit a progressive neurodegenerative syndrome starting in their sixth decade. This syndrome, referred to as *fragile X tremor/ataxia,* is characterized by intention tremors and cerebellar ataxia and may progress to parkinsonism.

How do premutations cause disease? In these patients, the *FMR1* gene instead of being methylated and silenced continues to be transcribed. CGG-containing *FMR1* mRNAs so formed are "toxic." They accumulate in the nucleus and form intranuclear inclusions. In this process the aggregated mRNA recruits RNA-binding proteins. Perhaps sequestration of these proteins at abnormal locations leads to events that are toxic to the cell. In recent years, abnormal RNAs with toxic gain of function as a mechanism of tissue injury have also been implicated in certain myotoic muscular dystrophies.

KEY CONCEPTS

Fragile X Syndrome

- Pathologic amplification of trinucleotide repeats causes loss-of-function (fragile X syndrome) or gain-of-function mutations (Huntington disease). Most such mutations produce neurodegenerative disorders.
- Fragile X syndrome results from loss of FMR1 gene function and is characterized by mental retardation, macroorchidism, and abnormal facial features.
- In the normal population, there are about 29–55 CGG repeats in the *FMR1* gene. The genomes of carrier males and females contain premutations with 55 to 200 CGG repeats that can expand to 4000 repeats (full mutations) during oogenesis. When full mutations are transmitted to progeny, fragile X syndrome occurs.
- Fragile X tremor/ataxia due to expression of a *FMR1* gene bearing a premutation develops in some males and females. The accumulation of corresponding mRNA in the nucleus binds and sequesters certain proteins that are essential for normal neuronal functions.

Mutations in Mitochondrial Genes—Leber Hereditary Optic Neuropathy

The vast majority of genes are located on chromosomes in the cell nucleus and are inherited in classical Mendelian fashion. There exist several mitochondrial genes, however, that are inherited in quite a different manner. *A feature unique to mtDNA is maternal inheritance.* This peculiarity exists because ova contain numerous mitochondria within their abundant cytoplasm, whereas spermatozoa contain few, if any. Hence, the mtDNA complement of the zygote is derived entirely from the ovum. Thus, mothers transmit mtDNA to all their offspring, male and female; however, daughters but not sons transmit the DNA further to their progeny (Fig. 5-27). Several other features apply to mitochondrial inheritance. They are as follows:

- Human mtDNA contains 37 genes, of which 22 are transcribed into transfer RNAs and two into ribosomal RNAs. The remaining 13 genes encode subunits of the respiratory chain enzymes. Because mtDNA encodes enzymes involved in oxidative phosphorylation, mutations affecting these genes exert their deleterious effects primarily on the organs most dependent on oxidative phosphorylation such as the central nervous system, skeletal muscle, cardiac muscle, liver, and kidneys.

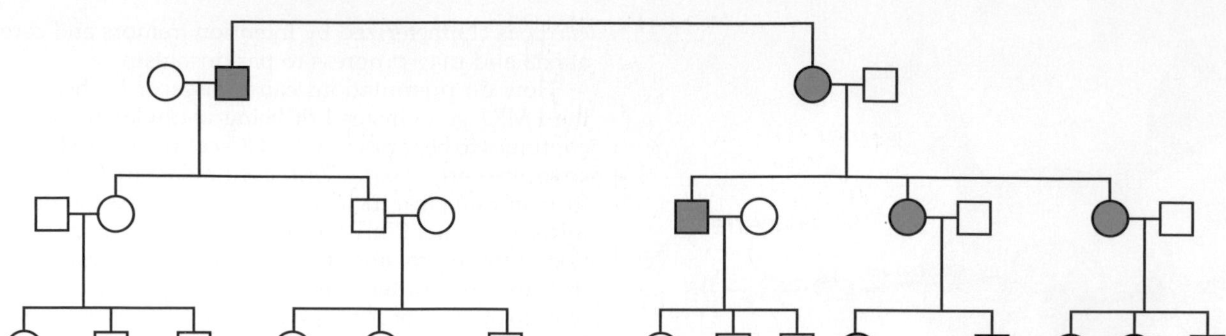

Figure 5-27 Pedigree of Leber hereditary optic neuropathy, a disorder caused by mutation in mitochondrial DNA. Note that all progeny of an affected male (shaded squares) are normal, but all children, male and female, of the affected female (shaded circles) manifest disease to a variable degree as discussed in the text.

- Each mitochondrion contains thousands of copies of mtDNA, and, typically, deleterious mutations of mtDNA affect some but not all of these copies. Thus, tissues and, indeed, individuals may harbor both wild-type and mutant mtDNA, a situation called *heteroplasmy*. A minimum number of mutant mtDNA must be present in a cell or tissue before oxidative dysfunction gives rise to disease. This is called the "threshold effect." Not surprisingly, the threshold is reached most easily in the metabolically active tissues listed earlier.
- During cell division, mitochondria and their contained DNA are randomly distributed to the daughter cells. Thus, when a cell containing normal and mutant mtDNA divides, the proportion of the normal and mutant mtDNA in daughter cells is extremely variable. Therefore, the expression of disorders resulting from mutations in mtDNA is quite variable.

Diseases associated with mitochondrial inheritance are rare and, as mentioned earlier, many of them affect the neuromuscular system. *Leber hereditary optic neuropathy* is a prototype of this type of disorder. It is a neurodegenerative disease that manifests as a progressive bilateral loss of central vision. Visual impairment is first noted between ages 15 and 35, leading eventually to blindness. Cardiac conduction defects and minor neurologic manifestations have also been observed in some families.

Genomic Imprinting

We all inherit two copies of each autosomal gene, carried on homologous maternal and paternal chromosomes. In the past, it had been assumed that there is no functional difference between the alleles derived from the mother or the father. Studies over the past two decades have provided definite evidence that, at least with respect to some genes, important functional differences exist between the paternal allele and the maternal allele. These differences result from an epigenetic process called *imprinting*. In most cases, imprinting selectively inactivates either the maternal or paternal allele. Thus, *maternal imprinting* refers to transcriptional silencing of the maternal allele, whereas *paternal imprinting* implies that the paternal allele is inactivated.

Imprinting occurs in the ovum or the sperm, before fertilization, and then is stably transmitted to all somatic cells through mitosis. As with other instances of epigenetic regulation, imprinting is associated with differential patterns of DNA methylation at CG nucleotides. Other mechanisms include histone H4 deacetylation and methylation (Chapter 1). Regardless of the mechanism, it is believed that such marking of paternal and maternal chromosomes occurs during gametogenesis, and thus it seems that from the moment of conception some chromosomes remember where they came from. The exact number of imprinted genes is not known; estimates range from 200 to 600. Although imprinted genes may occur in isolation, more commonly they are found in groups that are regulated by common *cis*-acting elements called imprinting control regions. Genomic imprinting is best illustrated by considering two uncommon genetic disorders: Prader-Willi syndrome and Angelman syndrome which were originally believed to be unrelated until the genetic lesions responsible for them were mapped to the very same location. They are described next.

Prader-Willi Syndrome and Angelman Syndrome

Prader-Willi syndrome is characterized by mental retardation, short stature, hypotonia, profound hyperphagia, obesity, small hands and feet, and hypogonadism. In 65% to 70% of cases, an interstitial deletion of band q12 in the long arm of chromosome 15, del(15)(q11.2q13), can be detected. In most cases the breakpoints are the same, causing a 5-Mb deletion. *It is striking that in all cases the deletion affects the paternally derived chromosome 15.* In contrast with the Prader-Willi syndrome, patients with the phenotypically distinct Angelman syndrome are *born with a deletion of the same chromosomal region derived from their mothers.* **Patients with Angelman syndrome are also mentally retarded, but in addition they present with ataxic gait, seizures, and inappropriate laughter.** Because of their laughter and ataxia, they have been referred to as "happy puppets." A comparison of these two syndromes clearly demonstrates the *parent-of-origin* effects on gene function.

The molecular basis of these two syndromes lies in the genomic imprinting (Fig. 5-28). Three mechanisms are involved:

- *Deletions.* It is known that a gene or set of genes on maternal chromosome 15q12 is imprinted (and hence silenced), and thus the only functional allele(s) are provided by the paternal chromosome. When these are lost as a result of a deletion, the person develops

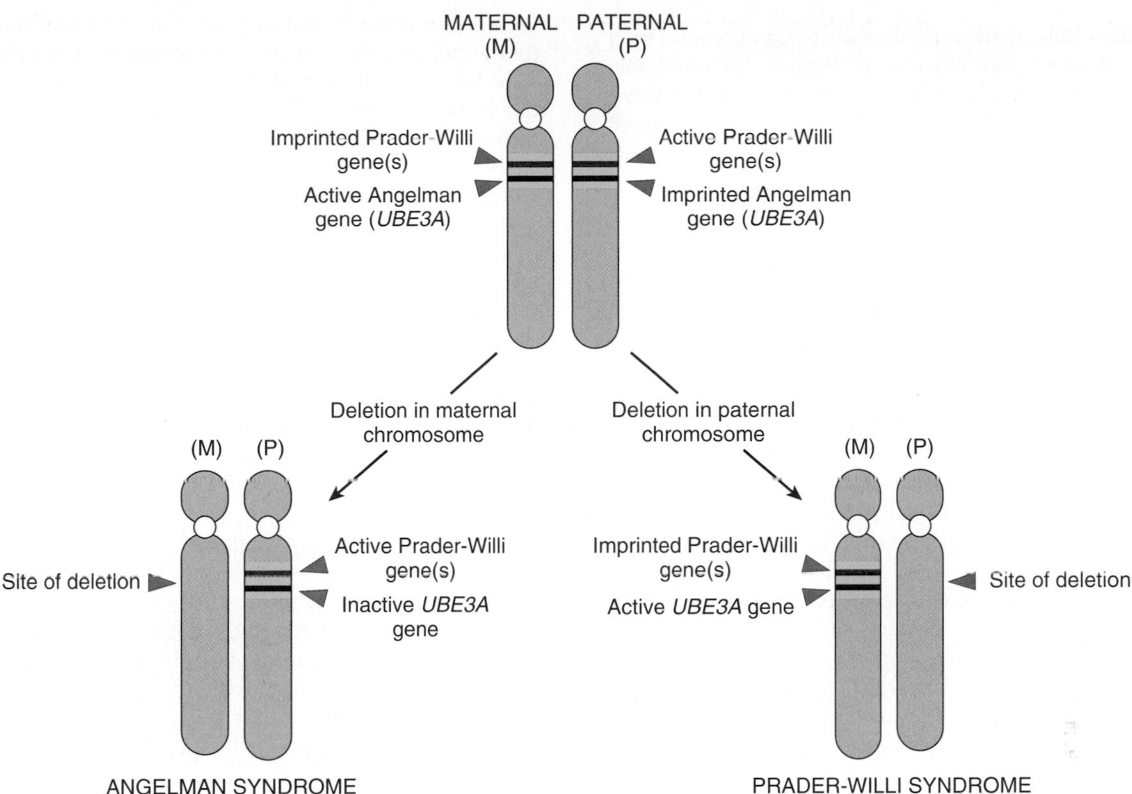

Figure 5-28 Diagrammatic representation of Prader-Willi and Angelman syndromes.

Prader-Willi syndrome. Conversely, a distinct gene that also maps to the same region of chromosome 15 is imprinted on the paternal chromosome. Only the maternally derived allele of this gene is normally active. Deletion of this maternal gene on chromosome 15 gives rise to the Angelman syndrome. Deletions account for about 70% cases.

- *Uniparental disomy.* Molecular studies of cytogenetically normal patients with the Prader-Willi syndrome (i.e., those without the deletion) have revealed that they have two maternal copies of chromosome 15. Inheritance of both chromosomes of a pair from one parent is called *uniparental disomy.* The net effect is the same (i.e., the person does not have a functional set of genes from the [nonimprinted] paternal chromosomes 15). Angelman syndrome, as might be expected, can also result from uniparental disomy of paternal chromosome 15. This is the second most common mechanism responsible for 20% to 25% cases.
- *Defective imprinting.* In a small minority of patients (1% to 4%), there is an imprinting defect. In some patients with Prader-Willi syndrome, the paternal chromosome carries the maternal imprint and conversely in Angelman syndrome the maternal chromosome carries the paternal imprint (hence there are no functional alleles).

The genetic basis of these two imprinting disorders is now being unraveled.

- In the Angelman syndrome, the affected gene is a ubiquitin ligase that is involved in catalyzing the transfer of activated ubiquitin to target protein substrates. The gene, called *UBE3A,* maps within the 15q12 region, is imprinted on the paternal chromosome, and is expressed from the maternal allele primarily in specific regions of the brain. The imprinting is tissue-specific in that *UBE3A* is expressed from both alleles in most tissues.
- In contrast to Angelman syndrome, no single gene has been implicated in Prader-Willi syndrome. Instead, a series of genes located in the 15q11.2-q13 interval (which are imprinted on the maternal chromosome and expressed from the paternal chromosome) are believed to be involved. These include the SNORP family of genes that encode small nucleolar RNAs which are involved in modifications of ribosomal RNAs. Loss of SNORP functions is believed to contribute to Prader-Willi syndrome.

Molecular diagnosis of these syndromes is based on assessment of methylation status of marker genes and FISH. The importance of imprinting is not restricted to rare chromosomal disorders. Parent-of-origin effects have been identified in a variety of inherited diseases, such as Huntington disease and myotonic dystrophy and in tumorigenesis.

KEY CONCEPTS

Genomic Imprinting

- Imprinting involves transcriptional silencing of the paternal or maternal copies of certain genes during gametogenesis. For such genes, only one functional copy exists in the individual. Loss of the functional (not imprinted) allele by deletion gives rise to diseases.

- In **Prader- Willi syndrome,** deletion of band q12 on long arm of paternal chromosome 15 occurs. Genes in this region of maternal chromosome 15 are imprinted so there is complete loss of their functions. Patients have mental retardation, short stature, hypotonia, hyperphagia, small hands and feet, and hypogonadism.
- In **Angelman syndrome** there is deletion of the same region from the maternal chromosome. Since genes on the corresponding region of paternal chromosome 15 are imprinted, these patients have mental retardation, ataxia, seizures, and inappropriate laughter.

Gonadal Mosaicism

It was mentioned earlier that with every autosomal dominant disorder some patients do not have affected parents. In such patients the disorder results from a new mutation in the egg or the sperm from which they were derived; as such, their siblings are neither affected nor at increased risk for development of the disease. This is not always the case, however. *In some autosomal dominant disorders, exemplified by osteogenesis imperfecta, phenotypically normal parents have more than one affected child.* This clearly violates the laws of Mendelian inheritance. Studies indicate that gonadal mosaicism may be responsible for such unusual pedigrees. Such mosaicism results from a mutation that occurs postzygotically during early (embryonic) development. If the mutation affects only cells destined to form the gonads, the gametes carry the mutation, but the somatic cells of the individual are completely normal. A phenotypically normal parent who has gonadal mosaicism can transmit the disease-causing mutation to the offspring through their mutated gametes. Because the progenitor cells of the gametes carry the mutation, there is a possibility that more than one child of such a parent would be affected. Obviously the likelihood of such an occurrence depends on the proportion of germ cells carrying the mutation.

Molecular Genetic Diagnosis

The nascent field of molecular diagnostics emerged in the latter half of the twentieth century, with the application of low throughput approaches such as conventional karyotyping for recognition of cytogenetic disorders (e.g., Down syndrome) and DNA-based assays such as Southern blotting for the diagnosis of Huntington disease. Over time, a steady stream of technologic breakthroughs has led to ever-increasing capabilities, including notably the development of Sanger DNA sequencing in 1977 and polymerase chain reaction (PCR) in 1983. Used together, these two techniques allowed the routine sequencing of any known segment of DNA, both rapidly accelerating research and providing a straightforward avenue for targeted diagnostics development.

Today, with the completion of the Human Genome Project and with newer and more powerful techniques for genetic and genomic analysis, nucleic acid–based testing is beginning to take a central role in the diagnosis and management of many diseases. Molecular diagnostic techniques have found application in virtually all areas of medicine, and their adoption continues to accelerate.

While an exhaustive discussion of molecular diagnostics is beyond the scope of this book, many of the better known approaches are highlighted in the ensuing sections. It is important to emphasize that, regardless of the technique used, human genetic markers can be either constitutional (i.e., present in each and every cell of the affected person, as with a *CFTR* mutation in a patient with cystic fibrosis) or somatic (i.e., restricted to specific tissue types or lesions, as with mutations in the *KRAS* gene in a variety of human cancers). In suspected infections, the goal is to detect and quantify nucleic acids that are specific to the infectious agent, which may be confined to particular cells or body sites. These considerations determine the nature of the sample used for the assay (e.g., peripheral blood cells, tumor tissue, nasopharyngeal swab).

Diagnostic Methods and Indications for Testing

There are a truly dizzying number of both techniques and indications for performing molecular genetic diagnostic tests on patient specimens, both for inherited and acquired genetic anomalies. The burden of choice can often be problematic, both for molecular pathologists who design tests as well as for clinicians who need to choose the optimal test for their patients.

Laboratory Considerations

On the laboratory side, pathologists focus on the sensitivity, specificity, accuracy, and reproducibility of different methods, as well as practical factors like cost, labor, reliability, and turn-around time. To choose the appropriate diagnostic technique, it is critical to first understand the spectrum of genetic anomalies that are responsible for the disease in the patient population under study. Disease-causing genetic anomalies range in size from single base substitutions up to gains or losses of entire chromosomes, and may vary widely in frequency among ethnic groups. Proper test design requires careful consideration of these factors. For example, standard cystic fibrosis testing for the 23 most common point mutations and small deletions (≤3 base pairs) in the *CFTR* gene has a sensitivity of 94% in Ashkenazi Jews, but identifies less than 50% of affected patients in Asian populations. In cases with negative standard test results and a high clinical suspicion, further tests are needed, such as extensive sequencing that covers all 27 exons of the *CFTR* gene. But even sequencing assays may miss large (kilobase scale) deletions involving one or more exons, which require a different test methodology. Issues like this arise quite frequently in genetic testing, and close communication between primary care clinicians, medical genetics specialists, and diagnosticians is often required in order to select the optimal test strategy in difficult cases.

Indications for Analysis of Inherited Genetic Alterations

Testing for inherited alterations may be required at any age, depending on clinical presentation, although in general most testing is performed during the prenatal or postnatal/childhood periods. Mendelian disorders that have been linked to specific genes number in the thousands, and definitive diagnosis for most of them is possible by direct sequencing. Some disorders, most with recessive inheritance, are associated with a limited number of recurrent mutations. Many others, especially those with dominant inheritance, are caused by mutations scattered throughout the responsible gene and represent a considerable diagnostic challenge.

Prenatal testing should be offered for all fetuses at risk for a cytogenetic abnormality. Possible indications include:

- Advanced maternal age
- A parent known to carry a balanced chromosomal rearrangement (because these greatly increase the frequency of abnormal chromosome segregation during meiosis and the risk of aneuploidy in the fertilized ovum)
- Fetal anomalies observed on ultrasound
- Routine maternal blood screening, indicating an increased risk of Down syndrome or another trisomy

Prenatal testing may also be considered for children at known risk for many other genetic disorders (e.g., cystic fibrosis, spinal muscular atrophy) using targeted analysis based on familial mutations or family history. At present it is usually performed on cells obtained by amniocentesis, chorionic villus biopsy, or umbilical cord blood. However, as much as 10% of the free DNA in a pregnant mother's blood is of fetal origin, and new technologies are opening the door to an era of noninvasive prenatal diagnostics utilizing this source of DNA.

Beyond prenatal testing, parents known to be at risk for having a child with a genetic disorder can choose to have genetic testing performed on embryos created in vitro prior to uterine implantation, eliminating the chance of generational transmission of a familial disease.

Following birth, testing is ideally done as soon as the possibility of constitutional genetic disease arises. It is most commonly performed on peripheral blood DNA and is targeted based on clinical suspicion. In newborns or children, indications may be as follows:

- Multiple congenital anomalies
- Suspicion of a metabolic syndrome
- Unexplained mental retardation and/or developmental delay
- Suspected aneuploidy (e.g., features of Down syndrome) or other syndromic chromosomal abnormality (e.g., deletions, inversions)
- Suspected monogenic disease, whether previously described or unknown

In older patients, testing logically becomes more focused toward genetic diseases that manifest at later stages of life. Again, the possibilities are vast, but the more common indications include:

- Inherited cancer syndromes (triggered by either family history or an unusual cancer presentation)
- Atypically mild monogenic disease (e.g., attenuated cystic fibrosis)
- Neurodegenerative disorders (e.g., familial Alzheimer disease, Huntington disease)

Indications for Analysis of Acquired Genetic Alterations

In this era of molecularly targeted therapies it is becoming increasingly important to identify nucleic acid sequences or aberrations that are specific for acquired diseases (e.g., cancer and infectious disease). The technical approaches are the same as those used for germ line Mendelian disorders, and the common indications include:

- Diagnosis and management of cancer (see also Chapter 7)
  - Detection of tumor-specific acquired mutations and cytogenetic alterations that are the hallmarks of specific tumors (e.g., *BCR-ABL* fusion genes in chronic myelogenous leukemia, or CML)
  - Determination of clonality as an indicator of a neoplastic condition
  - The identification of specific genetic alterations that can direct therapeutic choices (e.g., HER2 [official name *ERBB2*] amplification in breast cancer or EGFR [official name *ERBB1*] mutations in lung cancer)
  - Determination of treatment efficacy (e.g., minimal residual disease detection of *BCR-ABL* by PCR in CML)
  - Detection of drug-resistant secondary mutations in malignancies treated with genetically tailored therapeutics
- Diagnosis and management of infectious disease (see also Chapter 8)
  - Detection of microorganism-specific genetic material for definitive diagnosis (e.g., HIV, mycobacteria, human papillomavirus, herpesvirus in central nervous system)
  - The identification of specific genetic alterations in the genomes of microbes that are associated with drug resistance
  - Determination of treatment efficacy (e.g., assessment of viral loads in HIV, Epstein-Barr virus, and hepatitis C virus infection)

PCR and Detection of DNA Sequence Alterations

PCR analysis, which involves the synthesis of relatively short DNA fragments from a DNA template, has been a mainstay of molecular diagnostics for the last few decades. By using appropriate heat-stable DNA polymerases and thermal cycling, the target DNA (usually less than 1000 base pairs) lying between designed primer sites is exponentially amplified from as little as one original copy, greatly simplifying secondary sequence analysis. Many options exist for subsequent analysis, each with different strengths and weaknesses:

- *Sanger sequencing*. Here, the amplified DNA is mixed with a DNA polymerase, a DNA primer, nucleotides, and four dead-end (di-deoxy terminator) nucleotides (A, T, G, and C) labeled with different fluorescent tags. The ensuing reaction produces a series of DNA molecules of all possible lengths up to a kilobase or so, each labeled with a tag that corresponds to the base at which the reaction stopped due to incorporation of one of the terminator nucleotides. After size separation by capillary electrophoresis, the exact sequence can be "read" and compared with the normal sequence to detect the presence of mutations. Many applications of Sanger sequencing (and other PCR-based approaches) are starting to give way to next generation sequencing (discussed later), particularly when analysis of large genes or multiple genes is required. Still, 36 years after its Nobel-worthy invention by Frederick Sanger, Sanger sequencing is still considered the "gold standard" for sequence determination.

- *Pyrosequencing*: This approach takes advantage of the release of pyrophosphate when a nucleotide is incorporated into a growing DNA strand. Like Sanger sequencing, it is performed on PCR products using a single sequencing primer, but instead of terminator nucleotides it involves cycling individual nucleotides (A, C, T, or G) one at a time into the reaction. If one or more nucleotides are incorporated into the growing strand of DNA, pyrophosphate is released and participates in a secondary reaction involving luciferase that produces light, which is measured by a photo detector. Pyrosequencing is most often used when testing for particular sequence variants and is more sensitive than Sanger sequencing, allowing for detection of as little as 5% mutated alleles in a background of normal alleles. For this reason, it may be used to analyze DNA obtained from cancer biopsies, in which tumor cells are often "contaminated" with large numbers of admixed stromal cells.
- *Single-base primer extension.* This is a useful approach for identifying mutations at a specific nucleotide position (e.g., an oncogenic mutation in codon 600 of the *BRAF* gene). An interrogating sequencing primer is added to the PCR product, which binds just one base upstream of the target. Differently colored terminator fluorescent nucleotides are also added (corresponding to the normal and variant bases), and a single base polymerase extension is performed. The relative amounts of normal/variant fluorescence are then detected (Fig. 5-29). Like pyrosequencing, this technique is very sensitive, down to approximately 1% to 2% mutated alleles, with the obvious disadvantage of only producing one base pair of sequence data.
- *Restriction fragment length analysis.* This simple approach takes advantage of the digestion of DNA with endonucleases known as restriction enzymes that recognize and cut DNA at specific sequences. If the specific mutation is known to affect a restriction site, then the amplified PCR product may be digested, and the normal and mutant PCR products will yield fragments of different sizes. These can be identified as different bands following electrophoresis. Needless to say, this approach is considerably less comprehensive than direct sequencing but remains useful for molecular diagnosis when the causal mutation always occurs at an invariant nucleotide position.
- *Amplicon length analysis.* Mutations that affect the length of DNA (e.g., deletions or expansions) can be easily detected by PCR. As discussed earlier, several diseases, such as the fragile X syndrome, are associated with alterations in trinucleotide repeats. Figure 5-30 reveals how PCR analysis can be used to detect this mutation. Two primers that flank the region containing the trinucleotide repeats at the 5′ end of the *FMR1* gene are used to amplify the intervening sequences. Because there are large differences in the number of repeats, the size of the PCR products obtained from the DNA of normal individuals, or those with a premutation, is quite different and can be easily distinguished by gel electrophoresis. An important caveat is that this technique will fail if a trinucleotide repeat expansion is so large that it is beyond the amplification capacity of conventional PCR, a situation that is commonly seen in some trinucleotide repeat disorders. In such a case, Southern blot analysis of genomic DNA must be performed (see "Southern Blotting").
- *Real-time PCR.* A variety of PCR-based technologies that use fluorophore indicators can detect and quantify the presence of particular nucleic acid sequences in "real time" (i.e., during the exponential phase of DNA amplification rather than post-PCR). It is most often used to monitor the frequency of cancer cells bearing characteristic genetic lesions in the blood or in tissues (e.g., the level of *BCR-ABL* fusion gene sequences in patients with CML), or the infectious load of certain viruses (e.g., HIV, EBV). It can also be used to detect somatic point mutations in oncogenes such as KRAS and BRAF, an approach that has the advantage of avoiding the need for post-PCR analysis.

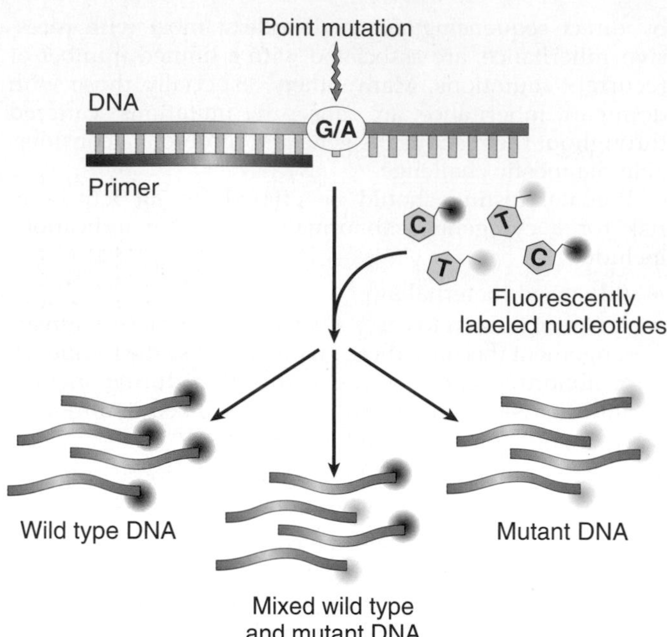

Figure 5-29 Single-base extension analysis of a PCR product, using a primer to interrogate a single base position. Nucleotides complementary to the mutant and wild-type bases at the queried position are labeled with different fluorophores, such that incorporation yields fluorescent signals of varying intensity based on the ratio of mutant to wild-type DNA present.

Molecular Analysis of Genomic Alterations

A significant number of genetic lesions involve large deletions, duplications, or more complex rearrangements that are not easily assayed using standard PCR methods. Such genomic-scale alterations can be studied using a variety of hybridization-based techniques.

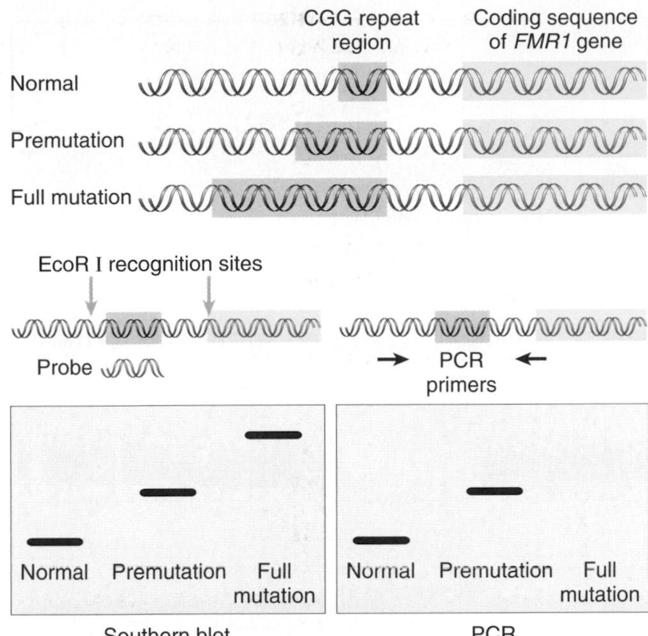

Figure 5-30 Diagnostic application of PCR and Southern blot analysis in fragile X syndrome. With PCR the differences in the size of CGG repeats between normal and premutation give rise to products of different sizes and mobility. With a full mutation, the region between the primers is too large to be amplified by conventional PCR. In Southern blot analysis the DNA is cut by enzymes that flank the CGG repeat region, and is then probed with a complementary DNA that binds to the affected part of the gene. A single small band is seen in normal males, a band of higher molecular weight in males with premutation, and a very large (usually diffuse) band in those with the full mutation.

Fluorescence in Situ Hybridization (FISH)

FISH uses DNA probes that recognize sequences specific to particular chromosomal regions. As part of the Human Genome Project, large libraries of bacterial artificial chromosomes that span the entire human genome were created. The human DNA inserts in these clones are on the order of 100,000-200,000 base pairs. These DNA clones are labeled with fluorescent dyes and applied to metaphase chromosome spreads or interphase nuclei that are pretreated so as to "melt" the genomic DNA. The probe hybridizes to its homologous genomic sequence and thus labels a specific chromosomal region that can be visualized under a fluorescent microscope. The ability of FISH to circumvent the need for dividing cells is invaluable when a rapid diagnosis is warranted (e.g., when deciding to treat a patient with acute myeloid leukemia with retinoic acid, which is only effective in a particular subtype with a chromosomal translocation involving the retinoic acid receptor gene [Chapter 13]). FISH can be performed on prenatal samples, peripheral blood cells, touch preparations from cancer biopsies, and even fixed archival tissue sections. FISH is used to detect numeric abnormalities of chromosomes (aneuploidy) (Fig. 5-19); subtle microdeletions (Fig. 5-20) or complex translocations that are not demonstrable by routine karyotyping; and gene amplification (e.g., *HER2* in breast cancer or *NMYC* amplification in neuroblastomas). Chromosome painting is an extension of FISH, whereby probes are prepared that span entire chromosomes. The number of chromosomes that can be detected simultaneously by chromosome painting is limited by the availability of fluorescent dyes that emit different wavelengths of visible light. This limitation has been overcome by the introduction of spectral karyotyping (also called multicolor FISH). Use of different mixtures of five fluorochromes in probes that are specific for each chromosome permits visualization of entire human genome. So powerful is spectral karyotyping that it might well be called "spectacular karyotyping."

Multiplex Ligation-Dependent Probe Amplification (MLPA)

MLPA blends DNA hybridization, DNA ligation, and PCR amplification to detect deletions and duplications of any size, including anomalies that are too large to be detected by PCR and too small to be identified by FISH. Briefly, each MLPA reaction uses a pair of probes that can hybridize side-by-side to one strand of the target DNA. Once bound, the probes are covalently joined via a ligase reaction. In addition to the target sequence, the probes also contain additional sequences at their ends that can be used as primer sequences in a PCR. The ligated probes thus create a template that can then be amplified by PCR. Quantification of the amplified DNA yields highly accurate information regarding the original amount of genetic starting material at the particular probe location (e.g., a probe at the site of a heterozygous deletion will produce only a 50% signal). Because it involves PCR amplification, MLPA can be performed on very small amounts of genomic DNA, and because each probe-set can be designed with identical primer sequences, many probe-sets can be applied and amplified in one reaction tube. Looking back to the cystic fibrosis example presented earlier, an MLPA probe-set covering the genomic coordinates corresponding to each of the 27 exons of the *CFTR* gene can readily detect deletions affecting one or more exons that would escape identification by PCR and conventional DNA sequencing.

Southern Blotting

Changes in the structure of specific loci can be detected by Southern blotting, which involves hybridization of radiolabeled sequence-specific probes to genomic DNA that has been first digested with a restriction enzyme and separated by gel electrophoresis. The probe usually detects one germ line band in normal individuals, and a different size band depending on the genetic anomaly. With the advent of FISH, MLPA, and microarray technology, Southern blotting is rarely used but remains useful in the detection of certain large-trinucleotide-expansion diseases, including the fragile X syndrome (Fig. 5-30).

Cytogenomic Array Technology

FISH requires prior knowledge of the one or few specific chromosomal regions suspected of being altered in the test sample. However, **genomic abnormalities can also be detected without prior knowledge by using microarray technology to perform a global genomic survey.** First generation platforms were designed for comparative genomic hybridization (CGH), while newer platforms incorporate SNP genotyping approaches, offering multiple benefits.

Array-Based Comparative Genomic Hybridization (Array CGH). In array CGH, the test DNA and a reference

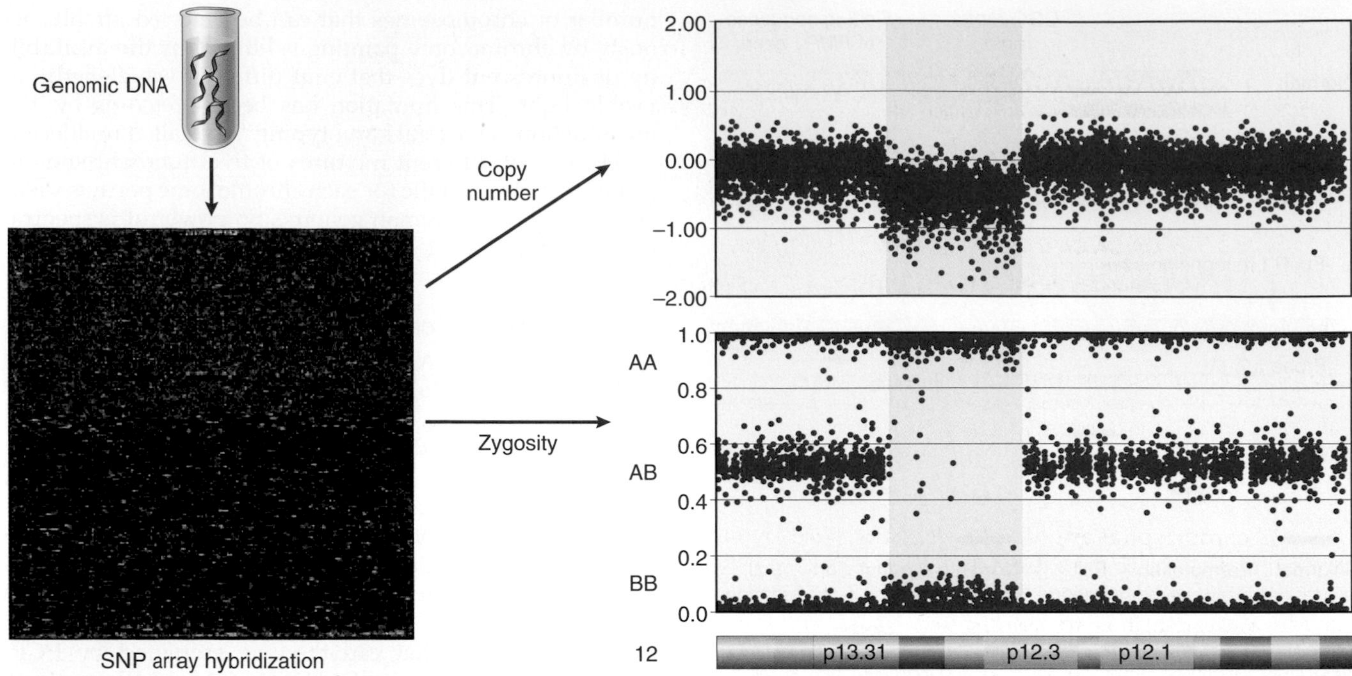

Figure 5-31 Analysis of copy number variation via SNP cytogenomic array. Genomic DNA is labeled and hybridized to an array containing potentially millions of probe spots. Copy number is determined by overall intensity and genotype is determined by allelic ratio. The example shown is the p arm of chromosome 12 in a pediatric leukemia. Here, the normal areas (green) show neutral (diploid) DNA content and the zygosity plot shows the expected ratio of AA, AB, and BB SNP genotypes. The anomalous area (red) shows decreased overall intensity, and the zygosity plot shows absence of the mixed AB genotype, indicating a full heterozygous deletion. (Modified from Paulsson K, et al: Genetic landscape of high hyperdiploid childhood acute lymphoblastic leukemia. PNAS 107(50):21719-24, 2010.)

(normal) DNA are labeled with two different fluorescent dyes. The differentially labeled samples are then co-hybridized to an array spotted with DNA probes that span the human genome at regularly spaced intervals, and usually cover all 22 autosomes and the sex chromosomes. At each chromosomal probe location, the binding of the labeled DNA from the two samples is compared. If the two samples are equal (i.e., the test sample is diploid), then all spots on the array will fluoresce yellow (the result of an equal admixture of green and red dyes). In contrast, if the test sample shows even a focal deletion or duplication, the probe spots corresponding to it will show skewing toward red or green (depending on gain or loss of material), allowing highly accurate determinations of copy number variants across the genome.

SNP Genotyping Arrays. Newer types of genomic arrays are based on a similar concept, but some or all of the probes are designed to identify single nucleotide polymorphism (SNP) sites genome-wide, which provides a number of advantages. As discussed earlier in Chapter 1, SNPs are the most common type of DNA polymorphism, occurring approximately every 1000 nucleotides throughout the genome (e.g., in exons, introns, and regulatory sequences). SNPs serve as both a physical landmark within the genome and as a genetic marker whose transmission can be followed from parent to child.

There are several testing platforms using different methodologies that allow SNPs to be analyzed genome-wide on arrays; details of these methods are beyond the scope of this discussion. Like CGH probes, these methods involving SNPs can be used to make copy number variations (CNV) calls, but by discriminating between SNP alleles at each particular location they also provide zygosity data (Fig. 5-31). The current generation of SNP arrays is quite comprehensive, with the largest containing greater than 4 million SNP probes. As a result, this technology is the mainstay of genome wide association studies (GWAS, described later).

In the clinical laboratory, SNP arrays are routinely used to uncover copy number abnormalities in pediatric patients when the karyotype is normal but a structural chromosomal abnormality is still suspected. Common indications include congenital abnormalities, dysmorphic features, developmental delay and autism. Here, the SNP data also proves useful. Typically, in areas of normal diploid copy number, the SNP results are roughly evenly split between homozygous and heterozygous calls. However, in anomalies such as uniparental disomy (e.g., in certain cases of Prader-Willi/Angelman syndromes), despite diploid copy number, the SNP calls in the affected region are all homozygous. SNP data can also help uncover other anomalies, such as mosaicism, which produces complex but distinctive skewing of zygosity plots.

Polymorphic Markers and Molecular Diagnosis

Clinical detection of disease-specific mutations is possible only if the gene responsible for the disorder is known and its sequence has been identified. If the exact nature of the genetic aberration is not known, or if testing for the primary defect is technically challenging or unfeasible, diagnostic labs can take advantage of the phenomenon of *linkage*. In humans, two DNA loci even 100,000 base pairs apart on

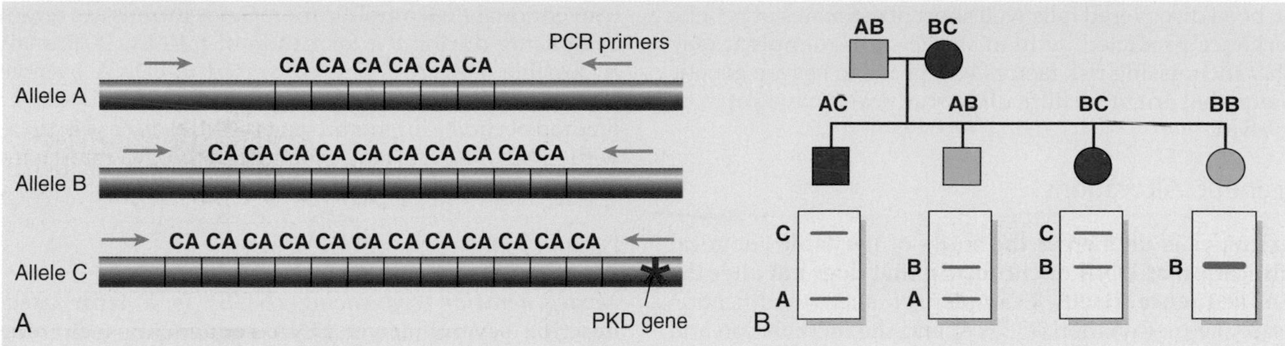

Figure 5-32 DNA polymorphisms resulting from a variable number of CA repeats. The three alleles produce PCR products of different sizes, thus identifying their origins from specific chromosomes. In the example depicted, allele C is linked to a mutation responsible for autosomal dominant polycystic kidney disease (PKD). Application of this to detect progeny carrying the disease-related gene (red symbols) is illustrated in one hypothetical pedigree. Males (squares); females (circles).

the same chromosome are almost certain to cosegregate during meiosis, due to the extremely low chance of a crossover event happening between them. Thus, the closer two loci are, the safer it is to assume that they will travel together in family pedigrees. In the event of a challenging or unknown pathogenic allele, a diagnostics lab can instead choose simply to examine nearby marker loci in the context of the family pedigree, as a surrogate approach. **The two types of genetic polymorphisms most useful for linkage analysis are SNPs (described earlier) and repeat-length polymorphisms known as minisatellite and microsatellite repeats.**

Human DNA contains short repetitive sequences of DNA giving rise to what are called repeat-length polymorphisms. These polymorphisms are often subdivided on the basis of their length into microsatellite repeats and minisatellite repeats. Microsatellites are usually less than 1 kilobase and are characterized by a repeat size of 2 to 6 base pairs. Minisatellite repeats, by comparison, are larger (1 to 3 kilobases), and the repeat motif is usually 15 to 70 base pairs. It is important to recall that the number of repeats, both in microsatellites and minisatellites, is extremely variable within a given population, and hence these stretches of DNA can be used quite effectively to establish genetic identity for linkage analysis. Microsatellites and the smaller minisatellites can be readily distinguished by using PCR primers that flank the repeat region. Figure 5-32 depicts the application of microsatellite linkage analysis to the *PKD1* gene (historically very difficult to sequence) for the familial diagnosis of adult polycystic kidney disease. It can be seen that the longest microsatellite allele is linked in the family to the disease allele and can be used to track transmission.

Assays to detect genetic polymorphisms are also important in many other areas of medicine, including in the determination of relatedness and identity in transplantation, cancer genetics, paternity testing, and forensic medicine. Since microsatellite markers are scattered throughout the human genome and have such a high level of polymorphism, they are ideal for differentiating between two individuals and to follow transmission of the marker from parent to child. Panels of microsatellite marker PCR assays have been extensively validated and are now routinely used for determining paternity and for criminal investigations. Since PCR can be performed even with highly degraded biologic samples, DNA technology is critical in forensic identifications. The same assays are regularly applied to the detection and quantification of transplant chimerism in allogeneic hematopoietic stem cell transplant patients, by looking for relative amounts of both donor- and host-specific microsatellite markers in host blood and blood cell subsets.

Polymorphisms and Genome-Wide Analyses

Beyond the clinic, linkage-based analysis has a long and storied history as a critical tool for discovery in the research laboratory. Many Mendelian diseases (including cystic fibrosis) were originally localized to candidate chromosomal locations using family pedigrees, testing a variety of candidate marker loci in a search for linkage disequilibrium, followed by subsequent refinement and testing of new nearby markers. Linkage studies have been similarly invaluable for identifying genes responsible for various phenotypes in laboratory animal models. However, similar analyses of complex (multifactorial) disorders have been unsuccessful since conventional linkage studies lack the statistical power to detect variants with small effects and low penetrance, which are thought to contribute to complex disorders.

To address this problem, researchers have utilized SNP genotyping array technology to perform large-scale linkage studies of complex diseases (e.g., type 2 diabetes, hypertension), which are termed genome wide association studies (GWAS). **In GWAS, large cohorts of patients with and without a disease (rather than families) are examined across the entire genome for common genetic variants or polymorphisms that are overrepresented in patients with the disease.** This identifies regions of the genome that contain a variant gene or genes that confer disease susceptibility and provides a springboard for further targeted research to find the true causative factor.

In addition to polygenic diseases, GWASs also have led to the identification of genetic loci that modulate common quantitative traits in humans, such as height, body mass, hair and eye color, and bone density. There has been much dispute about the value of GWAS studies, with criticisms often focusing on their underlying hypothesis that common disease risk could be explained by examining associations with common genetic variants. In support of that criticism, the combined relative risk from the associated variants that have been discovered falls well short of estimates of genetic inheritance predicted by twin studies, for example it may be that the missing risk factors will prove to be rare genetic variants that are more difficult to study, and have yet to be identified.

Epigenetic Alterations

Epigenetics is defined as the study of heritable chemical modification of DNA or chromatin that does not alter the DNA sequence itself. Examples of such modification include the methylation of DNA, and the methylation and acetylation of histones (Chapter 1). Our understanding of these types of molecular alterations is rapidly growing, and it is clear that epigenetic modifications are critical for normal human development—including the regulation of tissue-specific gene expression, X chromosome inactivation, and imprinting, as well as for understanding of the cellular perturbations in the aging and cancer.

Gene expression frequently correlates with the level of methylation of DNA, usually of cytosines specifically in CG dinucleotide-rich promoter regions known as CpG islands. As discussed earlier in the section on genomic imprinting, increased methylation of these loci is associated with decreased gene expression and is accompanied by concomitant specific patterns of histone methylation and acetylation. An ever increasing number of disease states warrant analysis of promoter methylation—for example, in the diagnosis of fragile X syndrome, in which hypermethylation results in *FMR1* silencing. Methylation analysis is also essential in the diagnosis of Prader-Willi and Angelman syndromes.

Since traditional Sanger sequencing alone cannot detect DNA methylation, other techniques have been developed to uncover these chemical modifications. One common approach is to treat genomic DNA with sodium bisulfite, a chemical that converts unmethylated cytosine to uracil, which acts like thymine in downstream reactions. Methylated cytosines are protected from modification and remain unchanged. After treatment, it is then straightforward to discriminate the unmethylated (modified) DNA from the methylated (unmodified) DNA on the basis of sequence analysis.

RNA Analysis

Because DNA exerts its effects on the cell through RNA expression and mature mRNA contains the coding sequences of all expressed genes, RNA can substitute for DNA in a wide range of diagnostic applications. From a practical standpoint, however, DNA-based diagnosis is usually preferred, since DNA is much more stable. Nonetheless, RNA analysis is critical in several areas of molecular diagnostics. The most important application is the detection and quantification of RNA viruses such as HIV and hepatitis C virus. Furthermore, mRNA expression profiling (described for breast cancer in Chapter 23) is emerging as an important tool for molecular stratification of tumors. In some instances cancer cells bearing particular chromosomal translocations are detected with greater sensitivity by analyzing mRNA (e.g., the *BCR-ABL* fusion transcript in CML). The principal reason for this is that most translocations occur in scattered locations within particular introns, which can be very large, beyond the capacity of conventional PCR amplification. Since introns are removed by splicing during the formation of mRNA, PCR analysis is possible if RNA is first converted to cDNA by reverse transcriptase. Real-time PCR performed on cDNA is the method of choice for monitoring residual disease in patients with CML and certain other hematologic malignancies (Chapter 13).

Next-Generation Sequencing

***Next-generation sequencing* (NGS) is a term used to describe several newer DNA sequencing technologies that are capable of producing large amounts of sequence data in a massively parallel manner.** These technologies, developed over the past decade, have already revolutionized biomedical research, and they are now beginning to have a similar impact on molecular diagnostics. The factors propelling rapid adoption of NGS are both price and performance: NGS allows us to perform previously impossible analyses at extremely low relative cost.

The fundamental factor that sets NGS apart from traditional Sanger sequencing is its input sample requirements. Whereas Sanger sequencing requires a single, simple, homogenous template DNA (usually either a specific PCR product or prepared plasmid), NGS has no such requirement: any DNA from almost any source can be used. Because Sanger sequencing essentially provides an "average" result for a DNA sample, samples with extreme sequence heterogeneity amongst input DNA molecules produce uninterpretable results. NGS instruments, in contrast, are well suited to heterogeneous DNA samples due to the application of these common basic processes (Fig. 5-33):

- *Spatial separation.* At the beginning of the procedure, individual input DNA molecules are physically isolated from each other in space. The specifics of this process are platform-dependent.
- *Local amplification.* After separation, the individual DNA molecules are amplified in situ using a limited number of PCR cycles. Amplification is necessary so that sufficient signal can be generated to ensure detection and accuracy.
- *Parallel sequencing.* The amplified DNA molecules are simultaneously sequenced by the addition of polymerases and other reagents, with each spatially separated and amplified original molecule yielding a "read" corresponding to its sequence. Sequence reads from NGS instruments are generally short, approximately less than 500 bp.

Bioinformatics

NGS instruments can generate a staggering amount of sequence data. For example one newer instrument is capable of analyzing over 500 million individual DNA clusters and producing 180 billion base pairs or more of sequence in a little more than a day. This is enough to produce a high-quality sequence spanning an entire human genome. The downstream analysis necessary to make sense of these enormous data sets is sufficiently complex that specialized training in bioinformatics is frequently needed to ensure its proper interpretation.

Bioinformatic computational pipelines can vary tremendously based on particular applications and sample types,

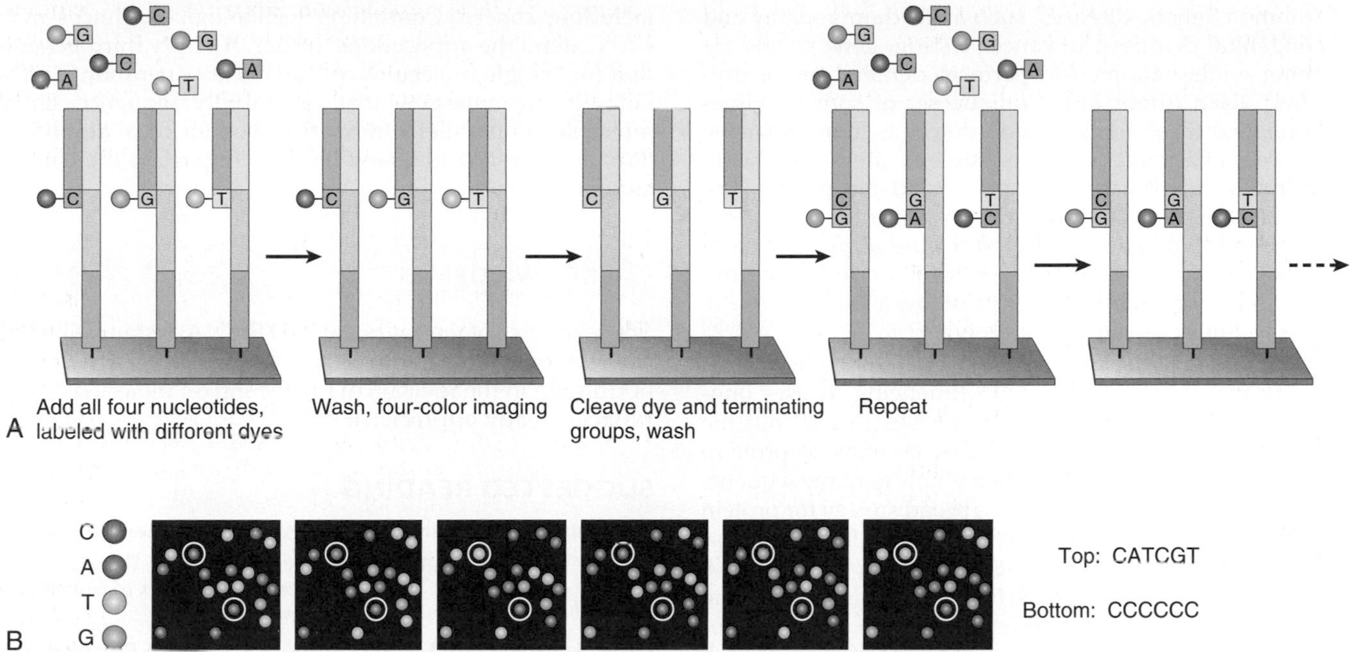

Figure 5-33 Principle of next-generation sequencing. Several alternative approaches currently are available for "NextGen" sequencing, and one of the more commonly used platforms is illustrated. **A**, Short fragments of genomic DNA ("template") between 100 and 500 base pairs in length are immobilized on a solid phase platform such as a glass slide, using universal capture primers that are complementary to adapters that have previously been added to ends of the template fragments. The addition of fluorescently labeled complementary nucleotides, one per template DNA per cycle, occurs in a "massively parallel" fashion, at millions of templates immobilized on the solid phase at the same time. A four-color imaging camera captures the fluorescence emanating from each template location (corresponding to the specific incorporated nucleotide), following which the fluorescent dye is cleaved and washed away, and the entire cycle is repeated. **B**, Powerful computational programs can decipher the images to generate sequences complementary to the template DNA at the end of one "run," and these sequences are then mapped back to the reference genomic sequence in order to identify alterations. (Reproduced with permission from Metzker M: Sequencing technologies—the next generation. Nat Rev Genet 11:31-46, 2010, © Nature Publishing Group.)

and a detailed discussion is beyond the scope of this text. However, it is worth describing the basic steps necessary to process this type of data in a generic human DNA context:

- *Alignment.* Alignment is the process by which the sequencing reads from a sample (which are individually uninformative) are mapped onto the appropriate reference genome, where they can be viewed and interpreted in context.
- *Variant calling.* This process involves "walking" across the reference genome and evaluating all of the sequence data that mapped to each position and comparing it with the reference sequence. The more reads that cover a particular location (sequencing depth), the more likely that a variant will be detected if present. If a locus shows sufficient evidence of a difference from the reference sequence, a variant call will be made.
- *Variant annotation and interpretation.* Called variants can be annotated with various sources of information (e.g., gene names, coding changes and protein effects predictions, SNP IDs, information from databases of both benign and pathogenic variants, clinical information). In the clinical laboratory the data may then be ready for interpretation and reporting.

Clinical Applications of NGS DNA Sequencing

As discussed, any DNA sample can be analyzed by NGS. However, the DNA needs to first be prepared for sequencing, and the choice of technique determines what data will be collected. In order to allow for binding and focal amplification on the instrument, input DNA must be in the form of small segments (<500 bp) with instrument-compatible linker oligonucleotide sequences incorporated at the ends. For whole genome sequencing this often involves automated genomic DNA fragmentation followed by ligation of adapter oligonucleotides. The final product is termed a *library*. There are many methods for NGS library preparation from genomic DNA, depending on the question and desired result. Currently in the clinical labs, most applications of NGS are targeted toward constitutional genetic disease and cancer diagnostics, using a few different basic approaches:

- *Targeted sequencing.* Most clinical laboratory NGS tests today fall in this category. With targeted sequencing just one gene or a panel of genes minimizes sequencing costs as well as the time and expense required for manual interpretation and clinical reporting. Sample preparation can be performed either by subselecting relevant clones from a whole genome library via custom complementary probes or by alternate preparations from genomic DNA, such as multiplex PCR. Single gene assays are more common for constitutional testing, and many laboratories that previously performed costly whole gene analyses by Sanger sequencing (i.e., comprehensive *CFTR* sequencing) are now moving those assays to NGS platforms. Analysis of large panels of genes (up to 100 or more) was previously unfeasible, but is now a commonplace approach for children with common genetic diseases, such as cardiomyopathy and congenital deafness. In cancer testing, gene panels are being widely adopted to perform detailed tumor profiling. Each tumor has a unique set of somatic mutations, and these assays aim to detect as many treatable or prognostic mutations as possible to offer individually tailored patient care. Currently available panels vary widely in size, from a few dozen genes up to nearly a thousand. For cancer, targeted testing allows for high-depth sequencing at low cost, helpful for detecting clinically relevant mutations present at low allelic percentage due to tumor or sample heterogeneity.

- *Whole exome sequencing (WES).* Exome sequencing is really just a type of targeted sequencing. It uses hundreds of thousands of custom probes to pull out the roughly 1.5% of the genome that consists of protein-encoding exons. At a time when whole genome sequencing is still costly, WES enables a broad survey for protein coding mutations (which are responsible for as much as 80% of Mendelian disease) at significantly reduced cost. This has led to some wonderful success stories, allowing physicians to deliver answers and even therapies for children with orphan diseases who had suffered through prolonged and unsuccessful diagnostic odysseys. WES is also used in oncology to perform a very broad analysis, mostly in the research setting but also in some clinical laboratories.
- *Whole genome sequencing (WGS).* Whole genome sequencing is the most comprehensive type of DNA analysis that can be performed on an individual. However, current costs and informatic challenges still preclude its routine use in clinical practice. Indications for use in medical genetics are mostly limited to cases where exome sequencing has failed to provide an answer but the clinical suspicion of genetic disease remains high. For cancer applications, WGS is the only NGS application that can detect novel structural rearrangements (e.g., insertions, deletions, translocations) that may be clinically relevant. Because of associated costs, WGS is generally performed to lower sequencing depth than either targeted panels or exomes, and may suffer from a lack of statistical power to detect low percentage mutations in heterogeneous tumor samples.

The choice of approach is mainly a function of sequencing cost and interpretive workload. Interpreting NGS clinical assays can be laborious, with considerable effort required to research the potential relevance of novel, suspicious variants. These interpretive challenges should lessen over time with improvements to variant databases.

Future Applications

Because NGS can be used to detect genetic anomalies of essentially any size scale, from SNPs to very large rearrangements and even aneuploidy, almost all of today's genetic diagnostic tests could in principle be supplanted by NGS. This includes RNA analysis, because NGS-based analysis of the transcriptome (RNA-seq) is straightforward. As costs continue to drop, it is reasonable to expect NGS to occupy an increasingly prominent place in the diagnostics lab. Additionally, NGS holds promise for application into novel areas, including microbiome analysis and blood screening for early markers of diseases, including cancer. Continuing technologic advances may even extend the applications further. Already third generation (or "single molecule" or "next next generation") technologies are emerging that can rapidly sequence single molecules in parallel without the need for focal amplification, and these could soon have an impact in the clinical laboratory.

Acknowledgment

The assistance of Jeremy Segal, MD PhD, Assistant Director, Division of Genomic and Molecular Pathology, University of Chicago in the revision of the section on molecular diagnosis is greatly appreciated.

SUGGESTED READING

Molecular Basis of Single Gene Disorders—General

Dietz HC: New Therapeutic Approaches to Mendelian Disorders. *New Engl J Med* 363:852, 2010. *[An excellent discussion of treatment of genetic disorders based on molecular pathogenesis.]*

Disorders Associated with Defects in Structural Proteins

De Paepe A, Malfait F: The Ehlers-Danlos syndrome, a disorder with many faces. *Clin Genet* 82:1, 2012. *[A modern appraisal of the molecular defects in this disorder of collagen.]*

Jondeau G, Michel JB, Boileau C: The translational science of Marfan syndrome. *Heart* 97:1206, 2011. *[An excellent review of the pathogenesis of Marfan syndrome.]*

Disorders Associated with Defects in Receptor Proteins

Faiz F, Hooper AJ, van Bockxmeer FM: Molecular pathology of familial hypercholesterolemia, related dyslipidemias and therapies beyond the statins. *Crit Rev Clin Lab Sci* 49:1, 2012. *[An update on molecular pathology of familial hypercholesterolemia.]*

Disorders Associated with Defects in Enzymes

Lieberman AP, Puertollano R, Raben N, et al: Autophagy in lysosomal storage disorders. *Autophagy* 8:719, 2012. *[Discussion of the emerging role of autophagy in lysosomal storage disorders.]*

Platt FM, Boland B, van der Spoel AC: Lysosomal storage disorders: The cellular impact of lysosomal dysfunction. *J Cell Biol* 199:723, 2012. *[A review of the multiple mechanisms that underline lysosomal disorders.]*

Cytogenetic Disorders Affecting Autosomes

Karayiorgou M, Simon TJ, Gogos JA: 2q11.2 microdeletions: linking DNA structural variation to brain dysfunction and schizophrenia. *Nat Rev Neurosci* 11:402, 2010. *[Discussion of molecular basis of neurologic deficits in 22q11.2.]*

Lana-Elola E, Watson-Scales SD, Fisher E M, et al: Down syndrome: searching for the genetic culprits. *Dis Model Mech* 4:586, 2011. *[Review of candidate genes involved in pathogenesis of Trisomy 21.]*

Simpson JL: Cell-free fetal DNA and maternal serum analytes for monitoring embryonic and fetal status. *Fertil Steril Inc* 99:1124, 2013. *[Recent advances in the diagnosis of cytogenetic disorders by analysis of fetal DNA in maternal serum.]*

Cytogenetic Disorders Affecting Sex Chromosomes

Groth KA, Skakkebaek A, Host C, et al: Klinefelter syndrome—A Clinical Update. *J Clin Endocrinol Metab* 98:20, 2013. *[A comprehensive discussion of clinical and genetic features of Klinefelter syndrome.]*

Heard E, Turner J: Function of the Sex Chromosomes in Mammalian Fertility. *CSH Perspectives Biol* 3:a002675, 2011. *[A review of the basic biology of sex chromosomes and their abnormalities.]*

Oliveira CS, Alves C: The role of the *SHOX* gene in the pathophysiology of Turner syndrome. *Endocrinol Nutr* 58:433, 2011. *[Discussion of molecular basis of Turner syndrome.]*

Pinsker JE: Turner Syndrome: Updating the Paradigm of Clinical Care. *J Clin Endocrinol Metab* 97:E994, 2012. *[A clinical review of Turner syndrome]*

Zhong Q, Layman LC: Genetic considerations in the patient with Turner syndrome—45, X with or without mosaicism. *Fertil Steril Inc* 98:775, 2012. *[An update on the genotype—phenotype correlation in Turner syndrome.]*

Diseases Caused by Trinucleotide Mutations

Bhakar AL, Dolen G, Bear MF: The Pathophysiology of Fragile X (and What It Teaches Us about Synapses). *Annu Rev Neurosci* 35:417, 2012. *[An excellent discussion of the pathogenesis of Fragile X syndrome.]*

Martelli A, Napierala M, Puccio H: Understanding the genetic and molecular pathogenesis of Friedreich's ataxia through animal and cellular models. *Dis Model Mech* 5:165, 2012. [*Molecular pathogenesis of Trinucleotide repeat mutation caused by loss of function.*]

Nelson DL, Orr HT, Warren ST: The Unstable Repeats—Three Evolving Faces of Neurological Disease. *Neuron* 5:825, 2013. *[An excellent review of how trinucleotide mutations give rise to disease.]*

Diseases Caused by Genomic Imprinting

Buiting K: Prader-Willi Syndrome and Angelman Syndrome. *Am J Med Genet Part C Semin* 154C:365, 2010. *[A succinct account of the two most common heritable diseases associated with genomic imprinting.]*

See TARGETED THERAPY available online at www.studentconsult.com 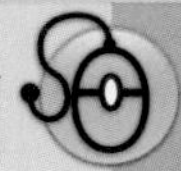

CHAPTER 6

Diseases of the Immune System

CHAPTER CONTENTS

The immune system is vital for survival, because it protects us from infectious pathogens that abound in the environment. Predictably, immune deficiencies render individuals easy prey to infections. But the immune system is itself capable of causing tissue injury and disease. Examples of disorders caused by immune responses include *allergies* and reactions against an individual's own tissues and cells *(autoimmunity)*.

This chapter is devoted to diseases caused by too little immunity or too much immunologic reactivity. We also consider amyloidosis, a disease in which an abnormal protein, derived in some cases from fragments of immunoglobulins, is deposited in tissues. First, we review some of the important features of normal immune responses, to provide a foundation for understanding the abnormalities that give rise to immunologic diseases.

The Normal Immune Response

The classic definition of *immunity* is protection from infectious pathogens, and the normal immune response is best understood in this context. The mechanisms of defense against microbes fall into two broad categories (Fig. 6-1). *Innate immunity* (also called natural, or native, immunity) refers to the mechanisms that are ready to react to infections even before they occur, and that have evolved to specifically recognize and combat microbes. *Adaptive immunity* (also called acquired, or specific, immunity) consists of mechanisms that are stimulated by ("adapt to") microbes and are capable of recognizing microbial and nonmicrobial substances. Innate immunity is the first line of defense. It is mediated by cells and molecules that recognize products of microbes and dead cells and induce rapid protective host reactions. Adaptive immunity develops later, after exposure to microbes and other foreign substances, and is even more powerful than innate immunity in combating infections. By convention, the term *immune response* usually refers to adaptive immunity.

Innate Immunity

Innate immunity is always present, ready to provide defense against microbes and to eliminate damaged cells. The receptors and components of innate immunity have evolved to serve these purposes. Innate immunity functions in stages: recognition of microbes and damaged cells, activation of various mechanisms, and elimination of the unwanted substances.

Components of Innate Immunity

The major components of innate immunity are epithelial barriers that block entry of microbes, phagocytic cells (mainly neutrophils and macrophages), dendritic cells, natural killer (NK) cells, and several plasma proteins, including the proteins of the complement system.

- *Epithelia* of the skin and gastrointestinal and respiratory tracts provide mechanical barriers to the entry of microbes from the external environment. Epithelial cells also produce antimicrobial molecules such as defensins, and lymphocytes located in the epithelia combat microbes at these sites. If microbes do breach epithelial boundaries, other defense mechanisms are called in.

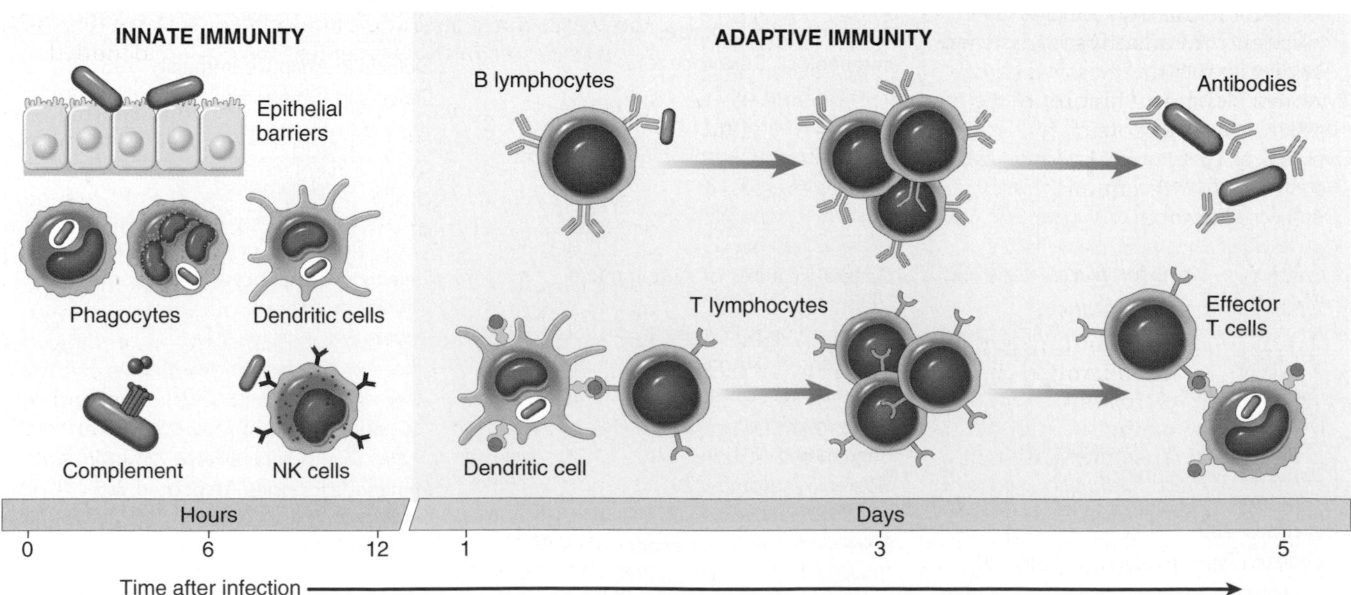

Figure 6-1 The principal mechanisms of innate immunity and adaptive immunity. NK cells, Natural killer cells.

- *Monocytes* and *neutrophils* are phagocytes in the blood that can rapidly be recruited to any site of infection; monocytes that enter the tissues and mature are called *macrophages*. All tissues contain resident macrophages, the professional phagocytes of the body. These cells not only sense the presence of microbes and other offending agents, but also ingest (phagocytose) these invaders and destroy them. Because macrophages are the dominant cells of chronic inflammation, we described them in more detail in Chapter 3 in the discussion of chronic inflammation.
- *Dendritic cells* are a specialized cell population present in epithelia, lymphoid organs, and most tissues. They capture protein antigens and display peptides for recognition by T lymphocytes. In addition to their antigen presenting function, dendritic cells are endowed with a rich collection of receptors that sense microbes and cell damage and stimulate the secretion of cytokines, mediators that play critical roles in inflammation and anti-viral defense. Thus, dendritic cells are involved in the initiation of innate immune responses, but, unlike macrophages, they are not key participants in the destruction of microbes and other offending agents.
- *Natural killer cells* provide early protection against many viruses and intracellular bacteria; their properties and functions are described later.
- Several other cell types can sense and react to microbes. These include *mast cells*, which are capable of producing many mediators of inflammation (discussed later), and even epithelial and endothelial cells.
- It has recently been recognized that cells with the appearance of lymphocytes but with features more like the cells of innate immunity may contribute to the early defense against microbes. These *innate lymphoid cells* are described later, when the properties and functions of lymphocytes are discussed.
- In addition to these cells, several soluble proteins play important roles in innate immunity. The proteins of the *complement system*, which were described in Chapter 3, are plasma proteins that are activated by microbes using the alternative and lectin pathways in innate immune responses; in adaptive immunity it is activated by antibodies using the classical pathway. Other circulating proteins of innate immunity are mannose-binding lectin and C-reactive protein, both of which coat microbes and promote phagocytosis. Lung surfactant is also a component of innate immunity, providing protection against inhaled microbes.

Cellular Receptors for Microbes, Products of Damaged Cells, and Foreign Substances

Cells that participate in innate immunity are capable of recognizing certain microbial components that are shared among related microbes and are often essential for infectivity (and thus cannot be mutated to allow the microbes to evade the defense mechanisms). These microbial structures are called *pathogen-associated molecular patterns.* Leukocytes also recognize molecules released by injured and necrotic cells, which are called *damage-associated molecular patterns.* Collectively, the cellular receptors that recognize these molecules are often called *pattern recognition receptors.*

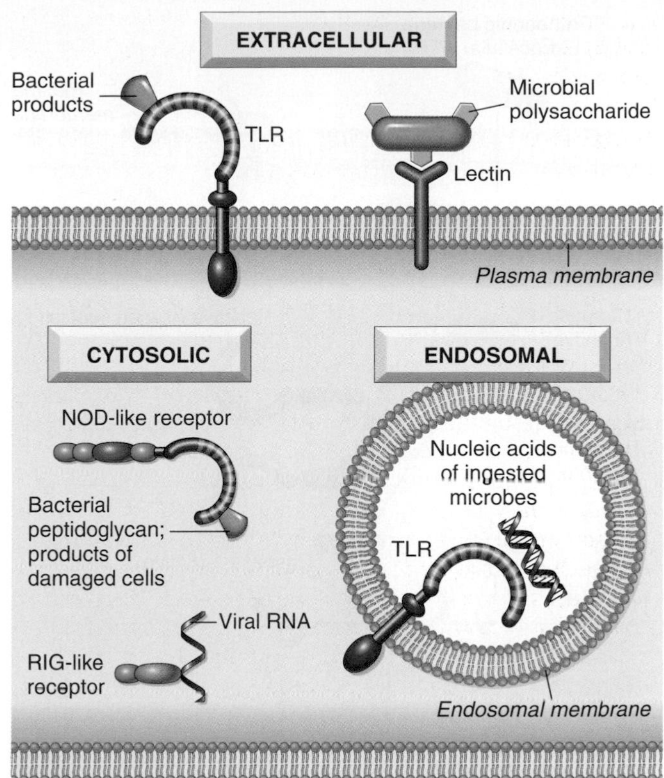

Figure 6-2 Cellular receptors for microbes and products of cell injury. Phagocytes, dendritic cells, and many types of epithelial cells express different classes of receptors that sense the presence of microbes and dead cells. Toll-like receptors (TLRs) located in different cellular compartments, as well as other cytoplasmic and plasma membrane receptors, recognize products of different classes of microbes. The four major classes of innate immune receptors are TLRs, NOD-like receptors in the cytosol (NLRs), C-type lectin receptors (CLRs), and RIG-like receptors for viral nucleic acids (RLRs).

Pattern recognition receptors are located in all the cellular compartments where microbes may be present: plasma membrane receptors detect extracellular microbes, endosomal receptors detect ingested microbes, and cytosolic receptors detect microbes in the cytoplasm (Fig. 6-2). Several classes of these receptors have been identified.

Toll-Like Receptors. The best known of the pattern recognition receptors are the Toll-like receptors (TLRs), whose founding member, *Toll,* was discovered in *Drosophila.* A family of related proteins was later shown to be essential for host defense against microbes. There are 10 TLRs in mammals, and each recognizes a different set of microbial molecules. The TLRs are present in the plasma membrane and endosomal vesicles (Fig. 6-2). All these receptors signal by a common pathway that culminates in the activation of two sets of transcription factors: (1) *NF-κB,* which stimulates the synthesis and secretion of cytokines and the expression of adhesion molecules, both of which are critical for the recruitment and activation of leukocytes (Chapter 3), and (2) *interferon regulatory factors (IRFs),* which stimulate the production of the antiviral cytokines, type I interferons. Germline loss-of-function mutations affecting TLRs and their signaling pathways are associated with rare but serious immunodeficiency syndromes, described later in the chapter.

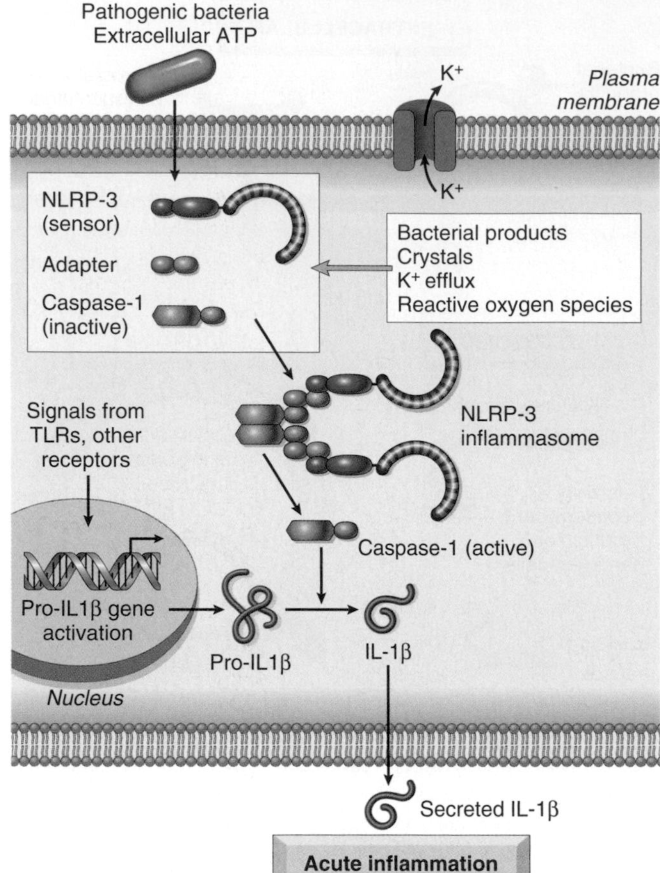

Figure 6-3 The inflammasome. The inflammasome is a protein complex that recognizes products of dead cells and some microbes and induces the secretion of biologically active interleukin 1. The inflammasome consists of a sensor protein (a leucine-rich protein called NLRP3), an adapter, and the enzyme caspase-1, which is converted from an inactive to an active form.

NOD-Like Receptors and the Inflammasome. NOD-like receptors (NLRs) are cytosolic receptors named after the founding member NOD-2. They recognize a wide variety of substances, including products of necrotic cells (e.g., uric acid and released ATP), ion disturbances (e.g., loss of K^+), and some microbial products. How this family of sensors is capable of detecting so many, quite diverse, signs of danger or damage is not known. Several of the NLRs signal via a cytosolic multiprotein complex called the *inflammasome*, which activates an enzyme (caspase-1) that cleaves a precursor form of the cytokine interleukin-1 (IL-1) to generate the biologically active form (Fig. 6-3). As is discussed later, IL-1 is a mediator of inflammation that recruits leukocytes and induces fever. Gain-of-function mutations in one of the NLRs result in periodic fever syndromes, called *autoinflammatory syndromes* (to be distinguished from autoimmune diseases, which result from T and B lymphocyte reactions against self antigens). The autoinflammatory syndromes respond very well to treatment with IL-1 antagonists. The NLR-inflammasome pathway may also play a role in many common disorders. For example, recognition of urate crystals by a class of NLRs underlies the inflammation associated with gout. These receptors may also be capable of detecting lipids and cholesterol crystals that are deposited in abnormally large amounts in tissues, and the resulting inflammation may contribute to obesity-associated type 2 diabetes and atherosclerosis, respectively.

Other Receptors for Microbial Products. *C-type lectin receptors* (CLRs) expressed on the plasma membrane of macrophages and dendritic cells detect fungal glycans and elicit inflammatory reactions to fungi. *RIG-like receptors* (RLRs), named after the founding member RIG-I, are located in the cytosol of most cell types and detect nucleic acids of viruses that replicate in the cytoplasm of infected cells. These receptors stimulate the production of antiviral cytokines. *G protein–coupled receptors* on neutrophils, macrophages, and most other types of leukocytes recognize short bacterial peptides containing *N*-formylmethionyl residues. Because all bacterial proteins and few mammalian proteins (only those synthesized within mitochondria) are initiated by *N*-formylmethionine, this receptor enables neutrophils to detect bacterial proteins and stimulate chemotactic responses of the cells. *Mannose receptors* recognize microbial sugars (which often contain terminal mannose residues, unlike mammalian glycoproteins) and induce phagocytosis of the microbes.

Reactions of Innate Immunity

The innate immune system provides host defense by two main reactions.

- *Inflammation*. Cytokines and products of complement activation, as well as other mediators, are produced during innate immune reactions and trigger the vascular and cellular components of inflammation. The recruited leukocytes destroy microbes and ingest and eliminate damaged cells. This reaction is described in Chapter 3.
- *Antiviral defense.* Type I interferons produced in response to viruses act on infected and uninfected cells and activate enzymes that degrade viral nucleic acids and inhibit viral replication, inducing what has been called an *antiviral state.*
- In addition to these defensive functions, innate immunity provides the danger signals that stimulate the subsequent more powerful adaptive immune response. The nature of some of these signals is described later.

Innate immunity, unlike adaptive immunity, does not have memory or fine antigen specificity. It is estimated that innate immunity uses about 100 different receptors to recognize 1,000 molecular patterns. In contrast, adaptive immunity uses two types of receptors (antibodies and T-cell receptors, described later), each with millions of variations, to recognize millions of antigens.

Adaptive Immunity

The adaptive immune system consists of lymphocytes and their products, including antibodies. The lymphocytes of adaptive immunity use highly diverse receptors to recognize a vast array of foreign substances. In the remainder of this introductory section we focus on lymphocytes and the reactions of the adaptive immune system.

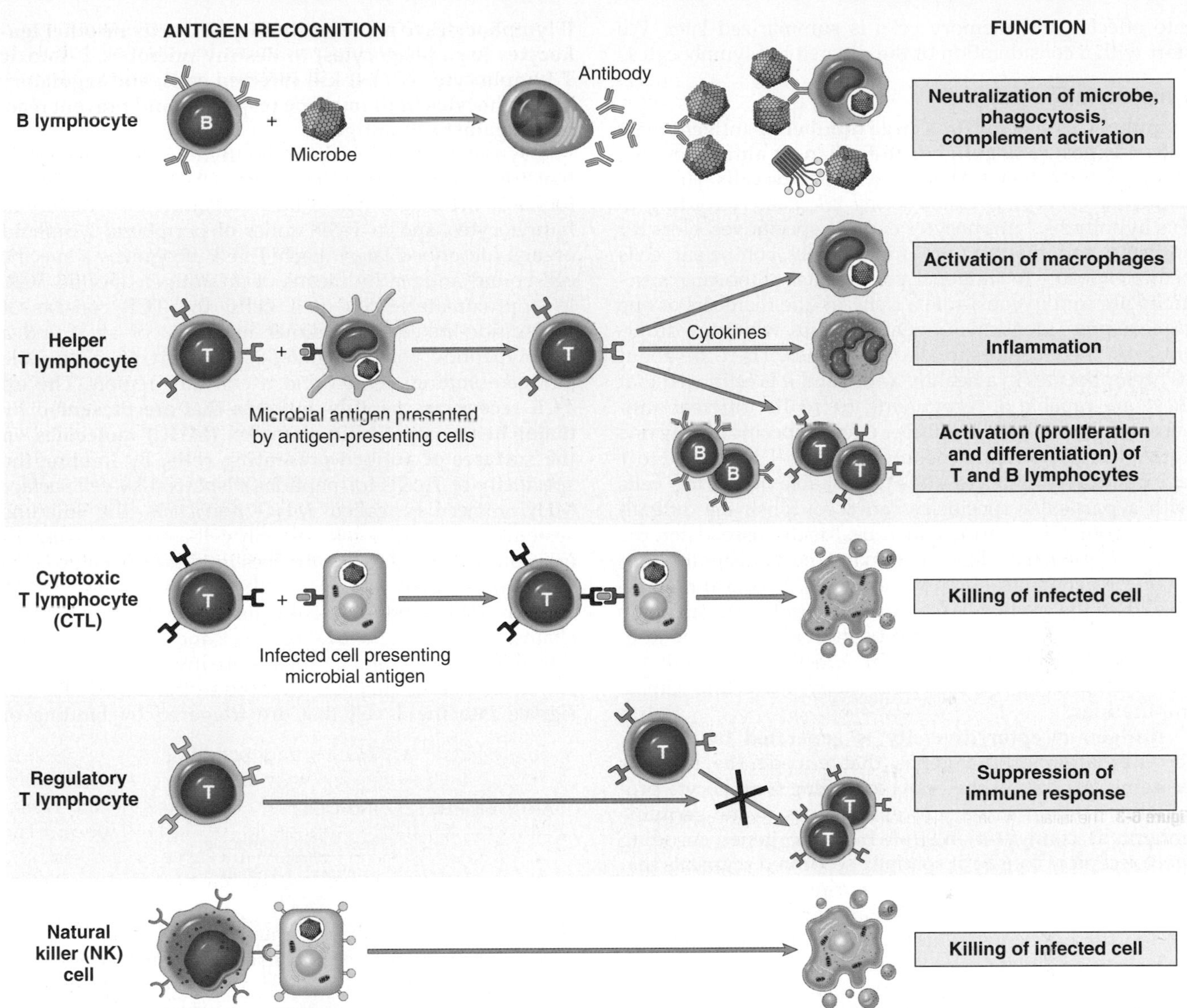

Figure 6-4 The principal classes of lymphocytes and their functions. B and T lymphocytes are cells of adaptive immunity and natural killer (NK) cells are cells of innate immunity. Several more classes of lymphocytes have been identified, including NK-T cells and so-called innate lymphoid cells (ILCs); the functions of these cells are not established.

There are two types of adaptive immunity: ***humoral immunity,*** **which protects against extracellular microbes and their toxins, and** ***cell-mediated*** **(or** ***cellular)*** ***immunity,*** **which is responsible for defense against intracellular microbes.** Humoral immunity is mediated by B (bone marrow–derived) lymphocytes and their secreted products, *antibodies* (also called *immunoglobulins,* Ig), and cellular immunity is mediated by T (thymus-derived) lymphocytes. Both classes of lymphocytes express highly specific receptors for a wide variety of substances, which are called *antigens.*

Cells of the Immune System

Although T and B lymphocytes and their subsets are morphologically unimpressive and appear quite similar to one another, they are actually remarkably heterogeneous and specialized in molecular properties and functions. The major classes of lymphocytes and their functions are illustrated in Figure 6-4. Lymphocytes and other cells involved in immune responses are not fixed in particular tissues (as are cells in most of the organs of the body) but constantly circulate among lymphoid and other tissues via the blood and the lymphatic circulation. This feature promotes immune surveillance by allowing lymphocytes to home to any site of infection. In lymphoid organs, different classes of lymphocytes are anatomically segregated in such a way that they interact with one another only when stimulated to do so by encounters with antigens and other stimuli. Mature lymphocytes that have not encountered the antigen for which they are specific are said to be *naive* (immunologically inexperienced). After they are activated by recognition of antigens and other signals described later, lymphocytes differentiate into *effector cells,* which perform the function of eliminating microbes, and *memory cells,* which live in a state of heightened awareness and are able to react rapidly and strongly to combat the microbe in case it returns. The process of lymphocyte differentiation into effector and memory cells is summarized later. We start with a consideration of the diversity of lymphocytes.

Lymphocyte Diversity

Lymphocytes specific for a large number of antigens exist before exposure to antigen, and when an antigen enters, it selectively activates the antigen-specific cells. This fundamental concept is called *clonal selection*. According to this hypothesis, lymphocytes express specific receptors for antigens and mature into functionally competent cells before exposure to antigen. Lymphocytes of the same specificity are said to constitute a *clone*; all the members of one clone express identical antigen receptors, which are different from the receptors in all other clones. There are about 10^{12} lymphocytes in a healthy adult, and it is estimated that these are capable of recognizing 10^7 to 10^9 different antigens. It follows that the number of cells specific for any one antigen is very small, probably less than 1 in 100,000 to 1 in 1 million lymphocytes. It is remarkable that so few cells with a particular specificity can accomplish the difficult task of combating various microbes; as discussed later, the immune system has developed many mechanisms for optimizing reactions to microbial antigens. It is also remarkable that the system is capable of producing so many receptors, far more than could be individually encoded in the genome. The mechanisms by which this happens are now well understood, and have many interesting clinical implications.

Antigen receptor diversity is generated by somatic recombination of the genes that encode the receptor proteins. All cells of the body, including lymphocyte progenitors, contain antigen receptor genes in the germline (inherited) configuration, in which the genes encoding these receptors consist of spatially separated segments that cannot be expressed as proteins. During lymphocyte maturation (in the thymus for T cells and the bone marrow for B cells), these gene segments recombine in random sets and variations are introduced at the sites of recombination, forming many different genes that can be transcribed and translated into functional antigen receptors. The enzyme in developing lymphocytes that mediates recombination of these gene segments is the product of *RAG-1* and *RAG-2* (recombination activating genes); inherited defects in RAG proteins result in a failure to generate mature lymphocytes. It is important to note that germline antigen receptor genes are present in all cells in the body, but only T and B cells contain recombined (also called rearranged) antigen receptor genes (the T-cell receptor [TCR] in T cells and immunoglobulin [Ig] in B cells). Hence, the presence of recombined TCR or Ig genes, which can be demonstrated by molecular analysis, is a marker of T- or B-lineage cells. Furthermore, because each T or B cell and its clonal progeny have a unique DNA rearrangement (and hence a unique antigen receptor), it is possible to distinguish polyclonal (nonneoplastic) lymphocyte proliferations from monoclonal (neoplastic) lymphoid tumors. Thus, **analysis of antigen receptor gene rearrangements is a valuable assay for detecting tumors derived from lymphocytes** (Chapter 13).

T Lymphocytes

There are three major populations of T cells, which serve distinct functions. **Helper T lymphocytes stimulate B lymphocytes to make antibodies and activate other leukocytes (e.g., phagocytes) to destroy microbes; cytotoxic T lymphocytes (CTLs) kill infected cells; and regulatory T lymphocytes limit immune responses and prevent reactions against self antigens.**

T lymphocytes develop in the thymus from precursors that arise from hematopoietic stem cells. Mature T cells are found in the blood, where they constitute 60% to 70% of lymphocytes, and in T-cell zones of peripheral lymphoid organs (described later). Each T cell recognizes a specific cell-bound antigen by means of an antigen-specific TCR. In approximately 95% of T cells, the TCR consists of a disulfide-linked heterodimer made up of an α and a β polypeptide chain (Fig. 6-5), each having a variable (antigen-binding) region and a constant region. **The αβ TCR recognizes peptide antigens that are presented by major histocompatibility complex (MHC) molecules on the surfaces of antigen-presenting cells.** By limiting the specificity of T cells for peptides displayed by cell surface MHC molecules, called *MHC restriction*, the immune system ensures that T cells see only cell-associated antigens (e.g., those derived from microbes in cells or from proteins ingested by cells).

Each TCR is noncovalently linked to six polypeptide chains, which form the CD3 complex and the ζ chain dimer (Fig. 6-5). The CD3 and ζ proteins are invariant (i.e., identical) in all T cells. They are involved in the transduction of signals into the T cell that are triggered by binding of

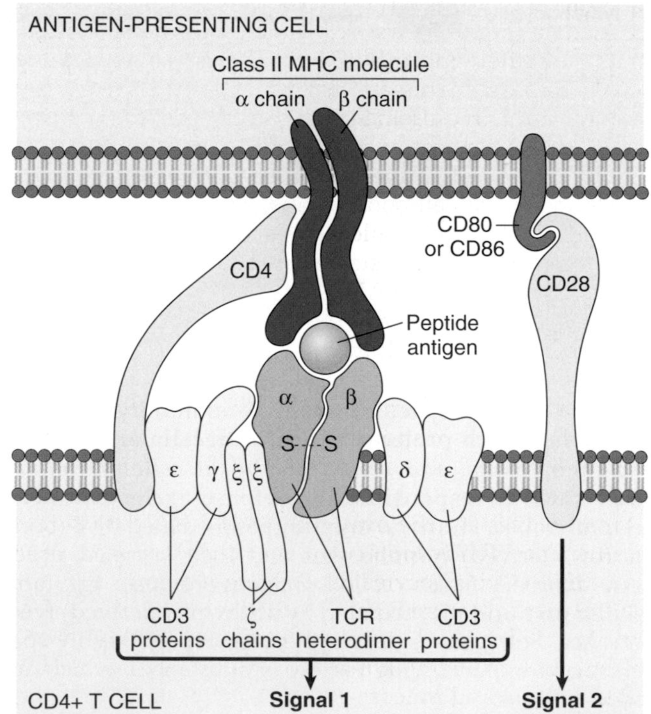

Figure 6-5 The T-cell receptor (TCR) complex and other molecules involved in T-cell activation. The TCR heterodimer, consisting of an α and a β chain, recognizes antigen (in the form of peptide-MHC complexes expressed on antigen-presenting cells, or APCs), and the linked CD3 complex and ζ chains initiate activating signals. CD4 and CD28 are also involved in T-cell activation. (Note that some T cells express CD8 and not CD4; these molecules serve analogous roles.) The sizes of the molecules are not drawn to scale. MHC, Major histocompatibility complex.

antigen to the TCR. Together with the TCR, these proteins form the *TCR complex*.

A small population of mature T cells expresses another type of TCR composed of γ and δ polypeptide chains. The γδ TCR recognizes peptides, lipids, and small molecules, without a requirement for display by MHC proteins. γδ T cells tend to aggregate at epithelial surfaces, such as the skin and mucosa of the gastrointestinal and urogenital tracts, suggesting that these cells are sentinels that protect against microbes that try to enter through epithelia. However, the functions of γδ T cells are not established. Another small subset of T cells expresses markers that are also found on NK cells; these cells are called NK-T cells. NK-T cells express a very limited diversity of TCRs, and they recognize glycolipids that are displayed by the MHC-like molecule CD1. The functions of NK-T cells are also not well defined.

In addition to CD3 and ζ proteins, T cells express several other proteins that assist the TCR complex in functional responses. These include CD4, CD8, CD28, and integrins. CD4 and CD8 are expressed on two mutually exclusive subsets of αβ T cells. Approximately 60% of mature T cells are CD4+ and about 30% are CD8+. Most CD4+ T cells function as cytokine-secreting helper cells that assist macrophages and B lymphocytes to combat infections. Most CD8+ cells function as cytotoxic (killer) T lymphocytes (CTLs) to destroy host cells harboring microbes. CD4 and CD8 serve as *coreceptors* in T-cell activation, so called because they recognize a part of the same ligand that the antigen receptor sees. During antigen recognition, CD4 molecules bind to class II MHC molecules that are displaying antigen (Fig. 6-5), and CD8 molecules bind to class I MHC molecules, and the CD4 or CD8 coreceptor initiates signals that are necessary for activation of the T cells. Because of this requirement for coreceptors, CD4+ helper T cells can recognize and respond to antigen displayed only by class II MHC molecules, whereas CD8+ cytotoxic T cells recognize cell-bound antigens only in association with class I MHC molecules; this segregation is described later. Integrins are adhesion molecules that promote the attachment of T-cells to APCs.

To respond, T cells have to recognize not only antigen-MHC complexes but additional signals provided by antigen-presenting cells. This process, in which CD28 plays an important role, is described later, when the steps in cell-mediated immune responses are summarized.

B Lymphocytes

B lymphocytes are the only cells in the body capable of producing antibody molecules, the mediators of humoral immunity. B lymphocytes develop from precursors in the bone marrow. Mature B cells constitute 10% to 20% of the circulating peripheral lymphocyte population and are also present in peripheral lymphoid tissues such as lymph nodes, spleen, and mucosa-associated lymphoid tissues. B cells recognize antigen via the B-cell antigen receptor complex. Membrane-bound antibodies of the IgM and IgD isotypes, present on the surface of all mature, naive B cells, are the antigen-binding component of the B-cell receptor complex (Fig. 6-6). After stimulation by antigen and other signals (described later), B cells develop into *plasma cells*, veritable protein factories for antibodies. It is estimated that a single plasma cell can secrete hundreds to thousands

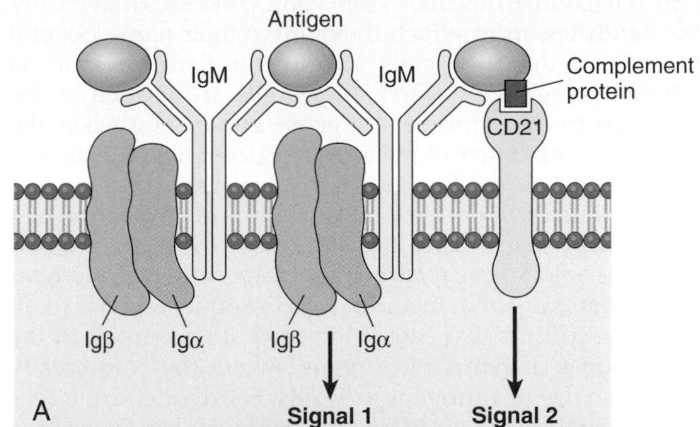

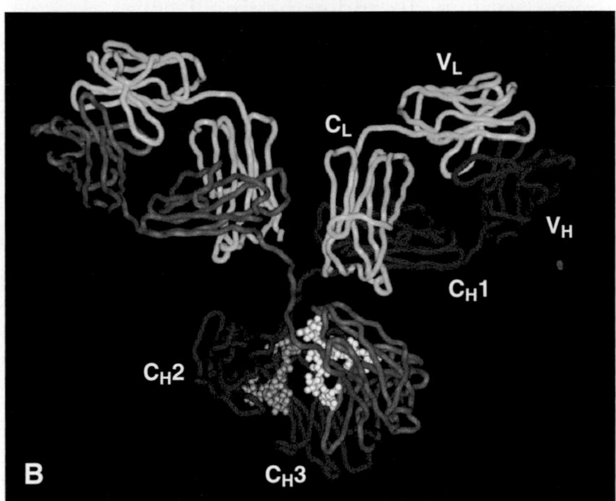

Figure 6-6 Structure of antibodies and the B-cell antigen receptor. **A,** The B-cell antigen receptor complex is composed of membrane immunoglobulin M (IgM; or IgD, not shown), which recognizes antigens, and the associated signaling proteins Igα and Igβ. CD21 is a receptor for a complement component that also promotes B-cell activation. **B,** Crystal structure of a secreted IgG molecule, showing the arrangement of the variable (V) and constant (C) regions of the heavy (H) and light (L) chains. (Courtesy Dr. Alex McPherson, University of California, Irvine, Calif.)

of antibody molecules per second, a remarkable measure of the power of the immune response for combating pathogens. Antibody-secreting cells are also detected in human peripheral blood; these are called *plasmablasts*.

In addition to membrane Ig, the B-cell antigen receptor complex contains a heterodimer of two invariant proteins called Igα and Igβ. Similar to the CD3 and ζ proteins of the TCR complex, Igα (CD79a) and Igβ (CD79b) are essential for signal transduction through the antigen receptor. B cells also express several other molecules that are essential for their responses. These include the type 2 complement receptor (CR2, or CD21), which recognizes complement products generated during innate immune responses to microbes, and CD40, which receives signals from helper T cells. CR2 is also used by the Epstein-Barr virus (EBV) as a receptor to enter and infect B cells.

Dendritic Cells

Dendritic cells (sometimes called *interdigitating dendritic cells*) **are the most important antigen-presenting cells for initiating T-cell responses against protein antigens.** These cells have numerous fine cytoplasmic processes that resemble dendrites, from which they derive their name. Several features of dendritic cells account for their key role in antigen presentation. First, these cells are located at the right place to capture antigens—under epithelia, the common site of entry of microbes and foreign antigens, and in the interstitia of all tissues, where antigens may be produced. Immature dendritic cells within the epidermis are called *Langerhans cells*. Second, dendritic cells express many receptors for capturing and responding to microbes (and other antigens), including TLRs and lectins. Third, in response to microbes, dendritic cells are recruited to the T-cell zones of lymphoid organs, where they are ideally located to present antigens to T cells. Fourth, dendritic cells express high levels of MHC and other molecules needed for presenting antigens to and activating T cells.

A second type of cell with dendritic morphology is present in the germinal centers of lymphoid follicles in the spleen and lymph nodes and is called the *follicular dendritic cell*. These cells bear Fc receptors for IgG and receptors for C3b and can trap antigen bound to antibodies or complement proteins. Such cells play a role in humoral immune responses by presenting antigens to B cells and selecting the B cells that have the highest affinity for the antigen, thus improving the quality of the antibody produced.

Macrophages

Macrophages are a part of the mononuclear phagocyte system; their origin, differentiation, and role in inflammation are discussed in Chapter 3. Here, their important functions in the induction and effector phases of adaptive immune responses are discussed.

- Macrophages that have phagocytosed microbes and protein antigens process the antigens and present peptide fragments to T cells. Thus, macrophages function as antigen-presenting cells in T-cell activation.
- Macrophages are key effector cells in certain forms of cell-mediated immunity, the reaction that serves to eliminate intracellular microbes. In this type of response, T cells activate macrophages and enhance their ability to kill ingested microbes (discussed later).
- Macrophages also participate in the effector phase of humoral immunity. As discussed in Chapter 3, macrophages efficiently phagocytose and destroy microbes that are opsonized (coated) by IgG or C3b.

Natural Killer Cells

The function of NK cells is to destroy irreversibly stressed and abnormal cells, such as virus-infected cells and tumor cells. NK cells make up approximately 5% to 10% of peripheral blood lymphocytes. They do not express TCRs or Ig. Morphologically, NK cells are somewhat larger than small lymphocytes, and they contain abundant azurophilic granules. NK cells are endowed with the ability to kill a variety of virus-infected cells and tumor cells, without prior exposure to or activation by these microbes or tumors. This ability makes NK cells an early line of defense against viral infections and, perhaps, some tumors. Two cell surface molecules, CD16 and CD56, are commonly used to identify NK cells. CD16 is an Fc receptor for IgG, and it confers on NK cells the ability to lyse IgG-coated target cells. This phenomenon is known as *antibody-dependent cell-mediated cytotoxicity (ADCC)*. The function of CD56 is not known.

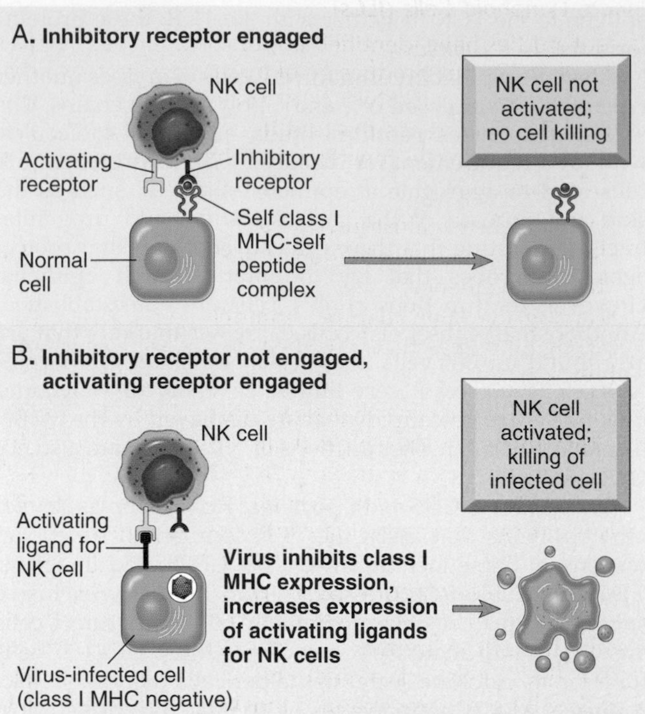

Figure 6-7 Activating and inhibitory receptors of natural killer (NK) cells. **A,** Healthy cells express self class I MHC molecules, which are recognized by inhibitory receptors, thus ensuring that NK cells do not attack normal cells. Note that healthy cells may express ligands for activating receptors (not shown) or may not express such ligands (as shown), but they do not activate NK cells because they engage the inhibitory receptors. **B,** In infected and stressed cells, class I MHC expression is reduced so that the inhibitory receptors are not engaged, and ligands for activating receptors are expressed. The result is that NK cells are activated and the infected cells are killed.

The functional activity of NK cells is regulated by a balance between signals from activating and inhibitory receptors (Fig. 6-7). There are many types of activating receptors, of which the NKG2D family is the best characterized. The NKG2D receptors recognize surface molecules that are induced by various kinds of stress, such as infection and DNA damage. NK cell inhibitory receptors recognize self class I MHC molecules, which are expressed on all healthy cells. The inhibitory receptors prevent NK cells from killing normal cells. Virus infection or neoplastic transformation often enhances expression of ligands for activating receptors and at the same time reduces the expression of class I MHC molecules. As a result the balance is tilted toward activation, and the infected or tumor cell is killed.

NK cells also secrete cytokines such as interferon-γ (IFN-γ), which activates macrophages to destroy ingested microbes, and thus NK cells provide early defense against intracellular microbial infections. The activity of NK cells is regulated by many cytokines, including the interleukins IL-2, IL-15, and IL-12. IL-2 and IL-15 stimulate proliferation of NK cells, whereas IL-12 activates killing and secretion of IFN-γ.

Innate Lymphoid Cells (ILCs)

Recent studies have identified populations of lymphocytes that lack TCRs but produce cytokines similar to those that are made by T cells. NK cells are considered the first defined ILC. Different subsets of ILCs produce IFN-γ, IL-5, IL-17, and IL-22. The functions that have been attributed to ILCs include:

- Early defense against infections
- Recognition and elimination of stressed cells (so-called stress surveillance)
- Shaping the later adaptive immune response, by providing cytokines that influence the differentiation of T lymphocytes.

Interest in these cells has been spurred by the hypothesis that they are early participants in inflammatory diseases, primarily as a source of cytokines. However, much remains to be learned about the functions and roles of these cells in normal and pathologic immune responses.

Tissues of the Immune System

The tissues of the immune system consist of the *generative* (also called *primary*, or *central*) lymphoid organs, in which T and B lymphocytes mature and become competent to respond to antigens, and the *peripheral* (or *secondary*) lymphoid organs, in which adaptive immune responses to microbes are initiated.

Generative Lymphoid Organs

The principal generative lymphoid organs are the thymus, where T cells develop, and the bone marrow, the site of production of all blood cells and where B lymphocytes mature. These organs are described in Chapter 13.

Peripheral Lymphoid Organs

The peripheral lymphoid organs—lymph nodes, spleen, and the mucosal and cutaneous lymphoid tissues—are organized to concentrate antigens, antigen-presenting cells, and lymphocytes in a way that optimizes interactions among these cells and the development of adaptive immune responses.

- *Lymph nodes* are nodular aggregates of lymphoid tissues located along lymphatic channels throughout the body (Fig. 6-8). As lymph slowly suffuses through lymph nodes, antigen-presenting cells in the nodes are able to sample the antigens of microbes that may enter through epithelia into tissues and are carried in the lymph. In addition, dendritic cells pick up and transport antigens of microbes from epithelia and tissues via lymphatic vessels to the lymph nodes. Thus, the antigens of microbes that enter through epithelia or colonize tissues become concentrated in draining lymph nodes.
- The *spleen* is an abdominal organ that serves the same role in immune responses to bloodborne antigen as the lymph nodes do in responses to lymph-borne antigens. Blood entering the spleen flows through a network of sinusoids. Bloodborne antigens are trapped by dendritic cells and macrophages in the spleen.
- The cutaneous and mucosal lymphoid systems are located under the epithelia of the skin and the gastrointestinal and respiratory tracts, respectively. They

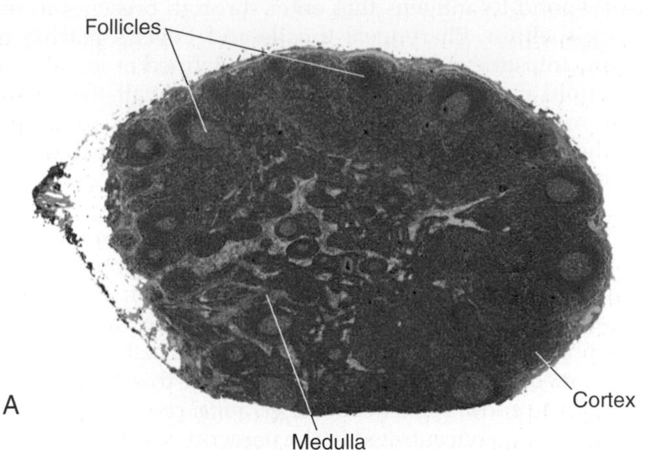

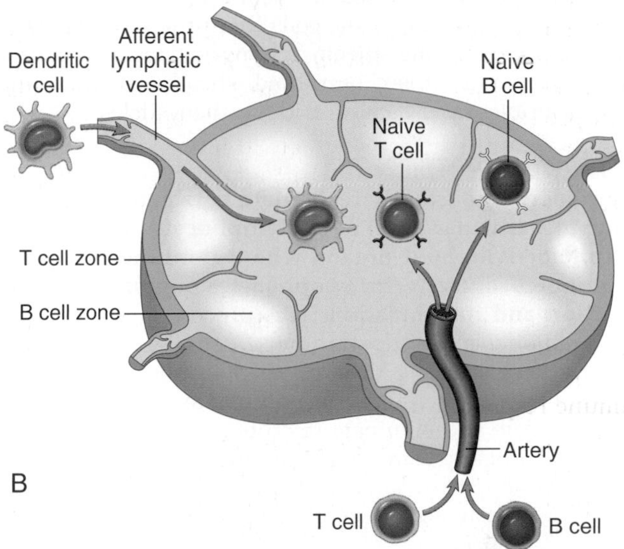

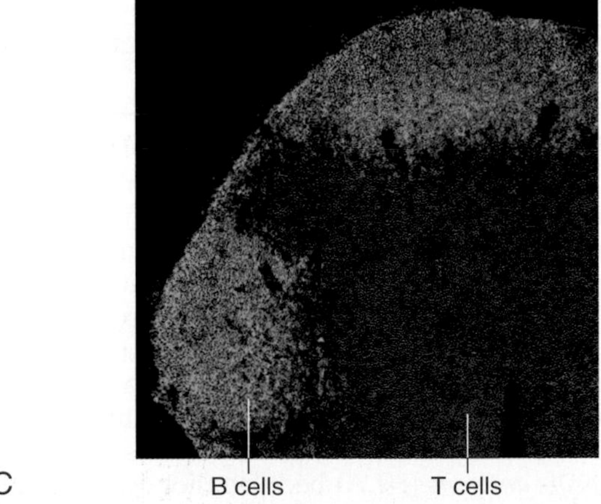

Figure 6-8 Morphology of a lymph node. **A,** The histology of a lymph node, with an outer cortex containing follicles and an inner medulla. **B,** The segregation of B cells and T cells in different regions of the lymph node, illustrated schematically. **C,** The location of B cells (stained green, using the immunofluorescence technique) and T cells (stained red) in a lymph node. (Courtesy Drs. Kathryn Pape and Jennifer Walter, University of Minnesota School of Medicine, Minneapolis, Minn.)

respond to antigens that enter through breaches in the epithelium. Pharyngeal tonsils and Peyer's patches of the intestine are two anatomically defined mucosal lymphoid tissues. At any time, more than half the body's lymphocytes are in the mucosal tissues (reflecting the large size of these tissues), and many of these are memory cells.

Within the peripheral lymphoid organs, T lymphocytes and B lymphocytes are segregated into different regions (Fig. 6-8). In lymph nodes the B cells are concentrated in discrete structures, called *follicles,* located around the periphery, or cortex, of each node. If the B cells in a follicle have recently responded to an antigen, this follicle may contain a central region called a *germinal center*. The T lymphocytes are concentrated in the paracortex, adjacent to the follicles. The follicles contain the follicular dendritic cells that are involved in the activation of B cells, and the paracortex contains the dendritic cells that present antigens to T lymphocytes. In the spleen, T lymphocytes are concentrated in periarteriolar lymphoid sheaths surrounding small arterioles, and B cells reside in the follicles.

Lymphocyte Recirculation

Lymphocytes constantly recirculate between tissues and home to particular sites; naive lymphocytes traverse the peripheral lymphoid organs where immune responses are initiated, and effector lymphocytes migrate to sites of infection and inflammation. This process of lymphocyte recirculation is most important for T cells, because naïve T cells have to circulate through the peripheral lymphoid organs where antigens are concentrated and effector T cells have to locate and eliminate microbes at any site of infection. In contrast, plasma cells remain in lymphoid organs and the bone marrow and do not need to migrate to sites of infection because they secrete antibodies that are carried to distant tissues.

Major Histocompatibility Complex (MHC) Molecules: The Peptide Display System of Adaptive Immunity

The function of MHC molecules is to display peptide fragments of protein antigens for recognition by antigen-specific T cells. Because MHC molecules are fundamental to the recognition of antigens by T cells and are linked to many autoimmune diseases, it is important to briefly review the structure and function of these molecules. MHC molecules were discovered as products of genes that evoke rejection of transplanted organs, and their name derives from their role in determining tissue compatibility between individuals. In humans the MHC molecules are called *human leukocyte antigens* (HLA) because they were initially detected on leukocytes by the binding of antibodies. The genes encoding HLA molecules are clustered on a small segment of chromosome 6 (Fig. 6-9). The HLA system is highly polymorphic, meaning that there are many alleles of MHC genes (in the thousands) in humans and each individual's HLA alleles differ from those inherited by most other individuals in the population. This, as we see subsequently, constitutes a formidable barrier in organ transplantation.

On the basis of their structure, cellular distribution and function, MHC gene products are classified into two major classes.

- *Class I MHC molecules* are expressed on all nucleated cells and platelets. They are heterodimers consisting of a polymorphic α, or heavy, chain (44-kD) linked noncovalently to a smaller (12-kD) nonpolymorphic protein called β_2-microglobulin. The α chains are encoded by three genes, designated *HLA-A, HLA-B,* and *HLA-C,* that lie close to one another in the MHC locus (Fig. 6-9). The extracellular region of the α chain is divided into three domains: α_1, α_2, and α_3. The α_1 and α_2 domains form a cleft, or groove, where peptides bind. The polymorphic amino acid residues line the sides and the base of the peptide-binding groove, explaining why different class I alleles bind different peptides.

  Class I MHC molecules display peptides that are derived from proteins, such as viral and tumor antigens, that are located in the cytoplasm and usually produced in the cell, and class I–associated peptides are recognized by CD8+ T lymphocytes. Cytoplasmic proteins are degraded in proteasomes and peptides are transported into the endoplasmic reticulum (ER) where the peptides bind to newly synthesized class I molecules. Peptide-loaded MHC molecules associate with β_2-microglobulin to form a stable trimer that is transported to the cell surface. The nonpolymorphic α_3 domain of class I MHC molecules has a binding site for CD8, and therefore the peptide-class I complexes are recognized by CD8+ T cells, which function as CTLs. In this interaction, the TCR recognizes the MHC-peptide complex, and the CD8 molecule, acting as a coreceptor, binds to the class I heavy chain. Since CD8+ T cells recognize peptides only if presented as a complex with class I MHC molecules, CD8+ T cells are said to be *class I MHC-restricted.* Because one of the important functions of CD8+ CTLs is to eliminate viruses, which may infect any nucleated cell, and tumors, which may arise from any nucleated cell, it makes good sense that all nucleated cells express class I HLA molecules and can be surveyed by CD8+ T cells.
- *Class II MHC molecule*s are encoded in a region called *HLA-D,* which has three subregions: *HLA-DP, HLA-DQ,* and *HLA-DR.* Each class II molecule is a heterodimer consisting of a noncovalently associated α chain and β chain, both of which are polymorphic. The extracellular portions of the α and β chains both have two domains designated α_1 and α_2, and β_1 and β_2. Crystal structure of class II molecules has revealed that, similar to class I molecules, they have peptide-binding clefts facing outward (Fig. 6-9). This cleft is formed by an interaction of the α_1 and β_1 domains, and it is in this portion that most class II alleles differ. Thus, as with class I molecules, polymorphism of class II molecules is associated with differential binding of antigenic peptides.

  Class II MHC molecules present antigens that are internalized into vesicles, and are typically derived from extracellular microbes and soluble proteins. The internalized proteins are proteolytically digested in endosomes or lysosomes. Peptides resulting from proteolytic cleavage then associate with class II heterodimers in the vesicles, and the stable peptide-MHC

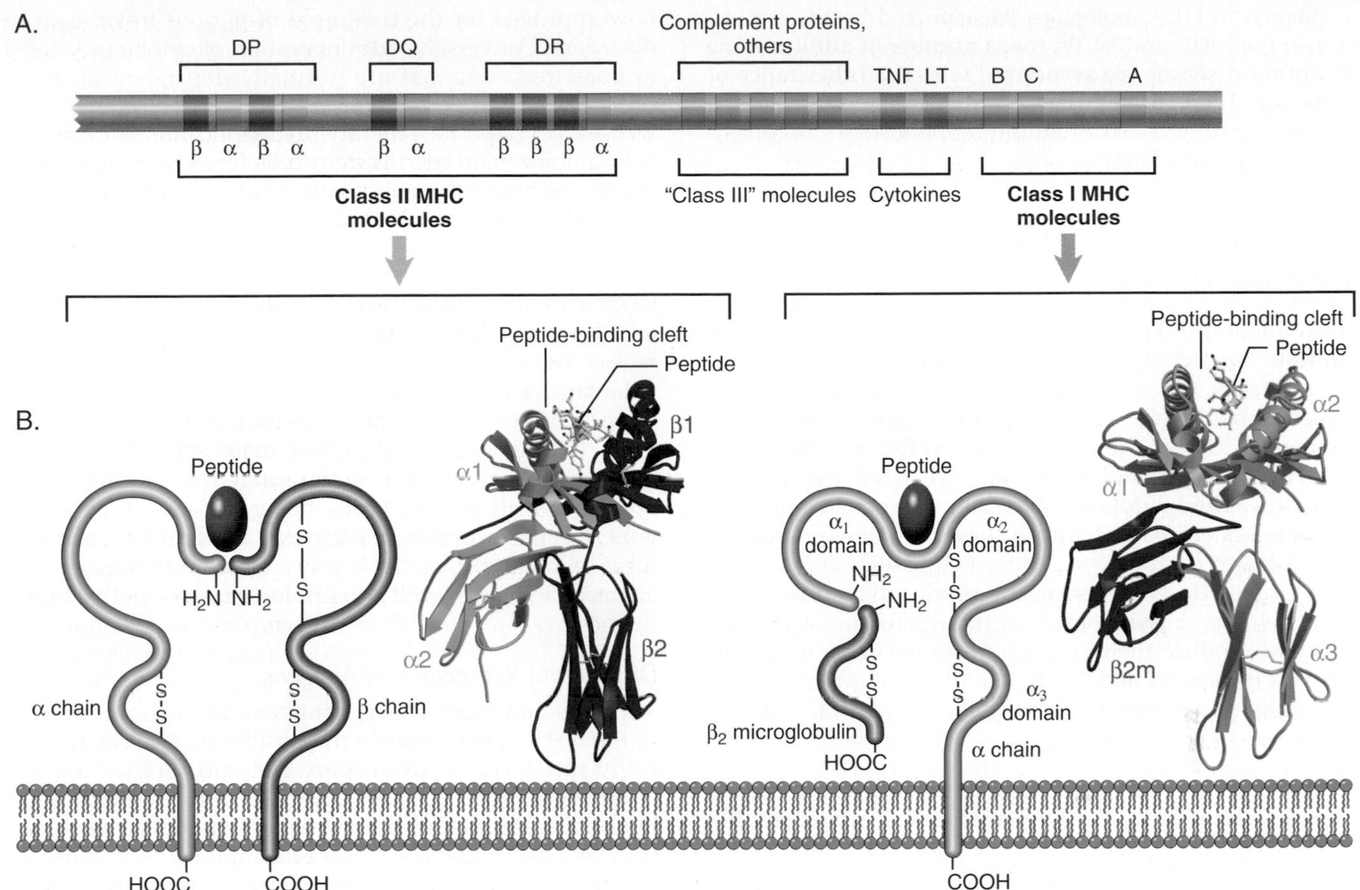

Figure 6-9 The human leukocyte antigen (HLA) complex and the structure of HLA molecules. **A,** The location of genes in the HLA complex. The relative locations, sizes, and distances between genes are not to scale. Genes that encode several proteins involved in antigen processing (the TAP transporter, components of the proteasome, and HLA-DM) are located in the class II region (not shown). **B,** Schematic diagrams and crystal structures of class I and class II HLA molecules. (Crystal structures are courtesy Dr. P. Bjorkman, California Institute of Technology, Pasadena, Calif.)

complexes are transported to the cell surface. The class II β_2 domain has a binding site for CD4, and therefore, the class II-peptide complex is recognized by CD4+ T cells, which function as helper cells. In this interaction, the CD4 molecule acts as the coreceptor. Because CD4+ T cells can recognize antigens only in the context of self class II molecules, they are referred to as *class II MHC-restricted*. In contrast to class I molecules, class II MHC molecules are mainly expressed on cells that present ingested antigens and respond to T-cell help (macrophages, B lymphocytes, and dendritic cells).

- The MHC locus also contains genes that encode some complement components and the cytokines tumor necrosis factor (TNF) and lymphotoxin, as well as some proteins that have no apparent role in the immune system.

The combination of HLA alleles in each individual is called the *HLA haplotype*. Any given individual inherits one set of HLA genes from each parent and thus typically expresses two different molecules for every locus. Because of the polymorphism of the HLA genes, virtually innumerable combinations of molecules exist in the population, and each individual expresses an MHC profile on his or her cell surface that is different from the haplotypes of most other individuals. It is believed that this polymorphism evolved to ensure that at least some individuals in a species would be able to display any microbial peptide and thus provide protection against any infection. This polymorphism also means that no two individuals (other than identical twins) are likely to express the same MHC molecules, and therefore grafts exchanged between these individuals are recognized as foreign and attacked by the immune system.

MHC molecules play several key roles in regulating T cell–mediated immune responses. First, because different antigenic peptides bind to different MHC molecules, it follows that an individual mounts an immune response against a protein antigen only if he or she inherits the genes for those MHC molecules that can bind peptides derived from the antigen and present it to T cells. The consequences of inheriting a given MHC (e.g., class II) gene depend on the nature of the antigen bound by the class II molecule. For example, if the antigen is a peptide from ragweed pollen, the individual who expresses class II molecules capable of binding the antigen would be genetically prone to allergic reactions against pollen. In contrast, an inherited capacity to bind a bacterial peptide may provide resistance to the infection by evoking a protective antibody response. Second, by segregating cytoplasmic and internalized antigens, MHC molecules ensure that the correct immune response is mounted against different microbes—CTL-mediated killing of cells harboring cytoplasmic microbes, and helper T cell–mediated antibody and macrophage activation to combat extracellular microbes.

Interest in HLA molecules was spurred by the realization, in the 1960s and 1970s, that **a number of autoimmune and other diseases are associated with the inheritance of particular HLA alleles.** These associations are discussed when the pathogenesis of autoimmune diseases is considered later in the chapter.

Cytokines: Messenger Molecules of the Immune System

The induction and regulation of immune responses involve multiple interactions among lymphocytes, dendritic cells, macrophages, other inflammatory cells (e.g., neutrophils), and endothelial cells. Some of these interactions depend on cell-to-cell contact; however, **many cellular interactions and functions of leukocytes are mediated by secreted proteins called *cytokines.*** Molecularly defined cytokines are called *interleukins*, because they mediate communications between leukocytes. Most cytokines have a wide spectrum of effects, and some are produced by several different cell types. The majority of these cytokines act on the cells that produce them (*autocrine* actions) or on neighboring cells (*paracrine*) and rarely at a distance (*endocrine*).

Cytokines contribute to different types of immune responses.

- In innate immune responses, cytokines are produced rapidly after encounter with microbes and other stimuli, and function to induce inflammation and inhibit virus replication. These cytokines include TNF, IL-1, IL-12, type I IFNs, IFN-γ, and chemokines (Chapter 3). Their major sources are macrophages, dendritic cells, and NK cells, but endothelial and epithelial cells can also produce them.
- In adaptive immune responses, cytokines are produced principally by CD4+ T lymphocytes activated by antigen and other signals, and function to promote lymphocyte proliferation and differentiation and to activate effector cells. The main ones in this group are IL-2, IL-4, IL-5, IL-17, and IFN-γ; their roles in immune responses are described later. Some cytokines serve mainly to limit and terminate immune responses; these include TGF-β and IL-10.
- Some cytokines stimulate hematopoiesis and are called *colony-stimulating factors* because they are assayed by their ability to stimulate formation of blood cell colonies from bone marrow progenitors (Chapter 13). Their functions are to increase leukocyte numbers during immune and inflammatory responses, and to replace leukocytes that are consumed during such responses. They are produced by marrow stromal cells, T lymphocytes, macrophages, and other cells. Examples include the colony-stimulating factors (CSFs) such as GM-CSF, and IL-7.

The knowledge gained about cytokines has numerous practical therapeutic applications. Inhibiting cytokine production or actions is an approach for controlling the harmful effects of inflammation and tissue-damaging immune reactions. Patients with rheumatoid arthritis often show dramatic responses to TNF antagonists, an elegant example of rationally designed and molecularly targeted therapy. Many other cytokine antagonists are now approved for the treatment of various inflammatory disorders. Conversely, administration of cytokines is used to boost reactions that are normally dependent on these proteins, such as hematopoiesis and defense against some viruses. An important therapeutic application of cytokines is to mobilize and recruit stem cells from bone marrow to peripheral blood; the cells are then collected from the blood for stem cell transplantation.

Overview of Lymphocyte Activation and Immune Responses

All adaptive immune responses develop in steps, consisting of: antigen recognition, activation of specific lymphocytes to proliferate and differentiate into effector and memory cells, elimination of the antigen, and decline of the response, with memory cells being the long-lived survivors. The major events in each step are summarized later; these general principles apply to protective responses against microbes as well as pathologic responses that injure the host.

Display and Recognition of Antigens

Microbes and other foreign antigens can enter anywhere in the body. It is obviously impossible for lymphocytes of every specificity to patrol every possible portal of antigen entry. In fact, antigens are captured and concentrated in lymphoid organs through which lymphocytes circulate, thus increasing the likelihood of lymphocytes finding the antigen they recognize. Microbes and their protein antigens are captured by dendritic cells that are resident in epithelia and tissues. These cells carry their antigenic cargo to draining lymph nodes (Fig. 6-10). Here the antigens are processed and displayed complexed with MHC molecules on the cell surface, where the antigens are recognized by T cells.

B lymphocytes use their antigen receptors (membrane-bound antibody molecules) to recognize antigens of many different chemical types, including proteins, polysaccharides, and lipids.

Even before the antigens of a microbe are recognized by T and B lymphocytes, the microbe elicits an innate immune response through recognition by pattern recognition receptors; this encounter is the first line of defense and also serves to activate adaptive immunity. In the case of immunization with a protein antigen, microbial mimics, called *adjuvants*, are given with the antigen and these stimulate innate immune responses. During the innate response the microbe or adjuvant activates antigen-presenting cells to express molecules called *costimulators* and to secrete cytokines that stimulate the proliferation and differentiation of T lymphocytes. The principal costimulators for T cells are the B7 proteins (CD80 and CD86) that are expressed on antigen-presenting cells and are recognized by the CD28 receptor on naive T cells. Thus, antigen ("signal 1") and costimulatory molecules produced during innate immune responses to microbes ("signal 2") function cooperatively to activate antigen-specific lymphocytes (Fig. 6-5). The requirement for microbe-triggered signal 2 ensures that the adaptive immune response is induced by microbes and not by harmless substances. In immune responses to tumors and transplants, "signal 2" may be provided by substances

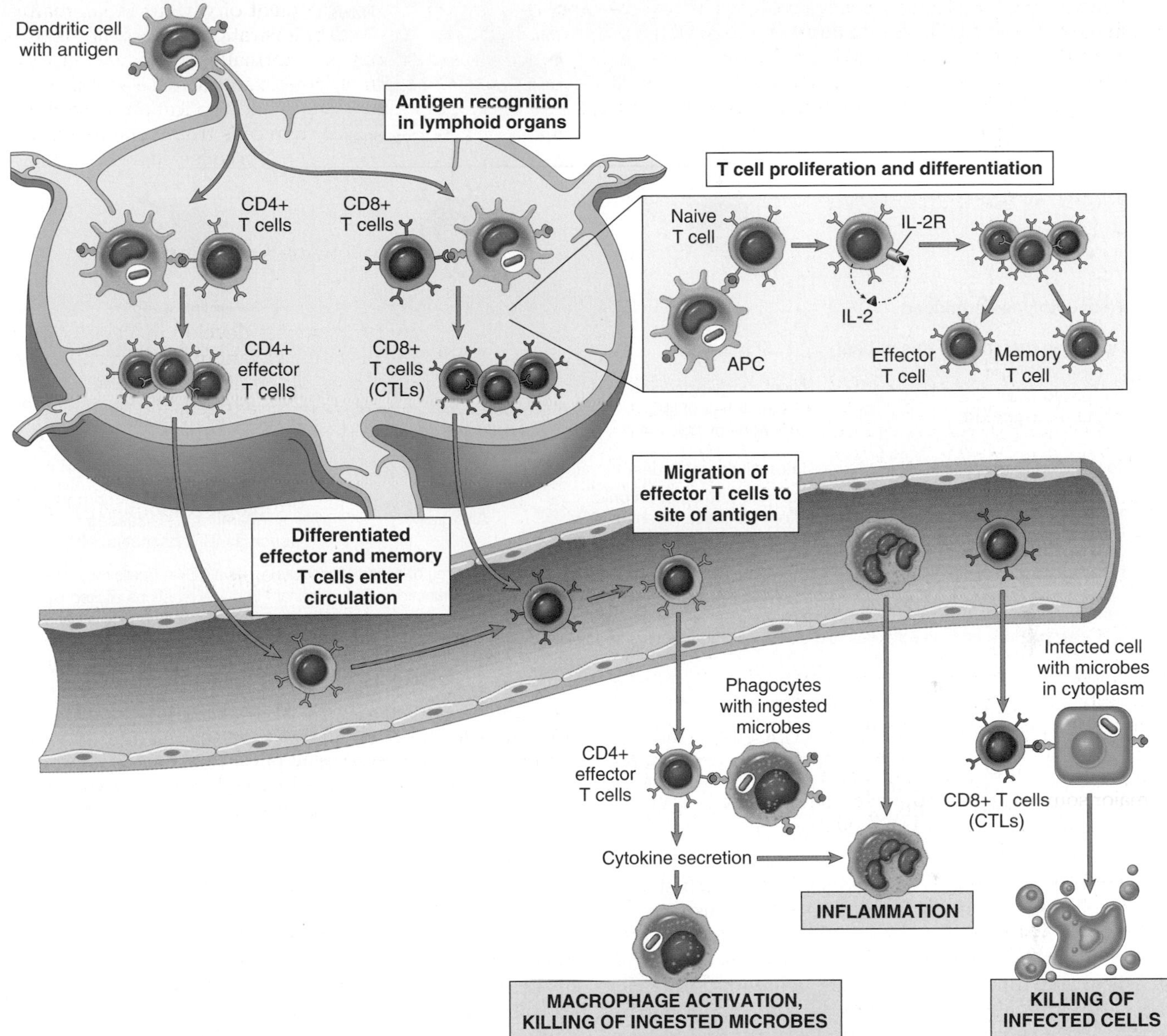

Figure 6-10 Cell-mediated immunity. Dendritic cells (DCs) capture microbial antigens from epithelia and tissues and transport the antigens to lymph nodes. During this process, the DCs mature, and express high levels of MHC molecules and costimulators. Naive T cells recognize MHC-associated peptide antigens displayed on DCs. The T cells are activated to proliferate and to differentiate into effector and memory cells, which migrate to sites of infection and serve various functions in cell-mediated immunity. CD4+ effector T cells of the T_H1 subset recognize the antigens of microbes ingested by phagocytes, and activate the phagocytes to kill the microbes; other subsets of effector cells enhance leukocyte recruitment and stimulate different types of immune responses. CD8+ cytotoxic T lymphocytes (CTLs) kill infected cells harboring microbes in the cytoplasm. Some activated T cells remain in the lymphoid organs and help B cells to produce antibodies, and some T cells differentiate into long-lived memory cells (not shown). APC, Antigen-presenting cell.

released from necrotic cells (the "damage-associated molecular patterns" mentioned earlier).

The reactions and functions of T and B lymphocytes differ in important ways and are best considered separately.

Cell-Mediated Immunity: Activation of T Lymphocytes and Elimination of Intracellular Microbes

Naive T lymphocytes are activated by antigen and costimulators in peripheral lymphoid organs, and proliferate and differentiate into effector cells that migrate to any site where the antigen (microbe) is present (Fig. 6-10). One of the earliest responses of CD4+ helper T cells is secretion of the cytokine IL-2 and expression of high-affinity receptors for IL-2. IL-2 is a growth factor that acts on these T lymphocytes and stimulates their proliferation, leading to an increase in the number of antigen-specific lymphocytes. The functions of helper T cells are mediated by the combined actions of CD40-ligand (CD40L) and cytokines. When CD4+ helper T cells recognize antigens being displayed by macrophages or B lymphocytes, the T cells express CD40L, which engages CD40 on the macrophages or B cells and activates these cells.

Some of the activated CD4+ T cells differentiate into effector cells that secrete different sets of cytokines and

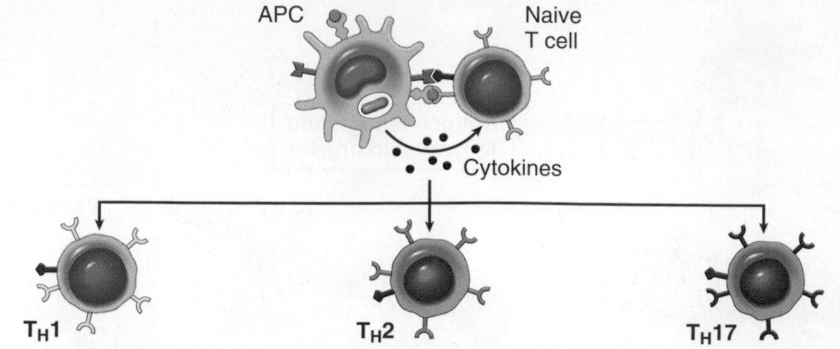

APC

Naive T cell

Cytokines

	T_H1	T_H2	T_H17
Major cytokines produced	IFN-γ	IL-4, IL-5, IL-13	IL-17, IL-22
Cytokines that induce this subset	IFN-γ, IL-12	IL-4	TGF-β, IL-6, IL-1, IL-23
Immunological reactions triggered	Macrophage activation, stimulation of IgG antibody production	Stimulation of IgE production, activation of mast cells and eosinophils	Recruitment of neutrophils, monocytes
Host defense against	Intracellular microbes	Helminthic parasites	Extracellular bacteria, fungi
Role in disease	Autoimmune and other chronic inflammatory diseases (such as IBD, psoriasis, granulomatous inflammation)	Allergies	Autoimmune and other chronic inflammatory diseases (such as IBD, psoriasis, MS)

Figure 6-11 Subsets of helper T (T_H) cells. In response to stimuli (mainly cytokines) present at the time of antigen recognition, naive CD4+ T cells may differentiate into populations of effector cells that produce distinct sets of cytokines and perform different functions. The dominant immune reactions elicited by each subset, and its role in host defense and immunologic diseases, are summarized. These populations may be capable of converting from one to another. Some activated T cells produce multiple cytokines and do not fall into a distinct subset. IBD, inflammatory bowel disease; MS, multiple sclerosis.

perform different functions (Fig. 6-11). Cells of the T_H1 subset secrete the cytokine IFN-γ, which is a potent macrophage activator. The combination of CD40- and IFN-γ-mediated activation results in "classical" macrophage activation (Chapter 3), leading to the induction of microbicidal substances in macrophages and the destruction of ingested microbes. T_H2 cells produce IL-4, which stimulates B cells to differentiate into IgE-secreting plasma cells, and IL-5, which activates eosinophils. Eosinophils and mast cells bind to IgE-coated microbes such as helminthic parasites, and function to eliminate helminths. T_H2 cells also induce the "alternative" pathway of macrophage activation, which is associated with tissue repair and fibrosis (Chapter 3). T_H17 cells, so called because the signature cytokine of these cells is IL-17, recruit neutrophils and monocytes, which destroy some extracellular bacteria and fungi and are involved in some inflammatory diseases.

Activated CD8+ T lymphocytes differentiate into CTLs that kill cells harboring microbes in the cytoplasm. By destroying the infected cells, CTLs eliminate the reservoirs of infection.

Humoral Immunity: Activation of B Lymphocytes and Elimination of Extracellular Microbes

Upon activation, B lymphocytes proliferate and then differentiate into plasma cells that secrete different classes of antibodies with distinct functions (Fig. 6-12). Antibody responses to most protein antigens require T cell help and are said to be *T-dependent*. In these responses, B cells ingest protein antigens into vesicles, degrade them, and display peptides bound to class II MHC molecules for recognition by helper T cells. The helper T cells are activated and express CD40L and secrete cytokines, which work together to stimulate the B cells. Many polysaccharide and lipid antigens cannot be recognized by T cells but have multiple identical antigenic determinants (epitopes) that are able to engage many antigen receptor molecules on each B cell and initiate the process of B-cell activation; these responses are said to be *T-independent*. T-independent responses are relatively simple, whereas T-dependent responses show features such as immunoglobulin isotype switching and affinity maturation (described below), which require T cell help and make the responses more varied and sophisticated.

Each plasma cell is derived from an antigen-stimulated B cell and secretes antibodies that recognize the same antigen that was bound to the BCR and initiated the response. Polysaccharides and lipids stimulate secretion mainly of IgM antibody. Protein antigens, by virtue of CD40L- and cytokine-mediated helper T-cell actions, induce the production of antibodies of different classes, or isotypes (IgG, IgA, IgE). *Isotype switching* is induced by cytokines including IFN-γ and IL-4. Helper T cells also stimulate the production of antibodies with high affinities for the antigen. This process, called *affinity maturation*, improves the quality of the humoral immune response. Isotype switching and affinity maturation occur mainly in germinal centers, which are formed by proliferating B cells, especially in helper T cell-dependent responses to protein antigens. Some activated B cells migrate into follicles and form germinal centers, which are the major sites of isotype switching and affinity maturation. The helper T-cells that stimulate these processes in B lymphocytes migrate to and reside in the germinal centers and are called *follicular helper T cells* (T_{FH}).

The humoral immune response combats microbes in many ways (Fig. 6-12). Antibodies bind to microbes and prevent them from infecting cells, thus neutralizing the

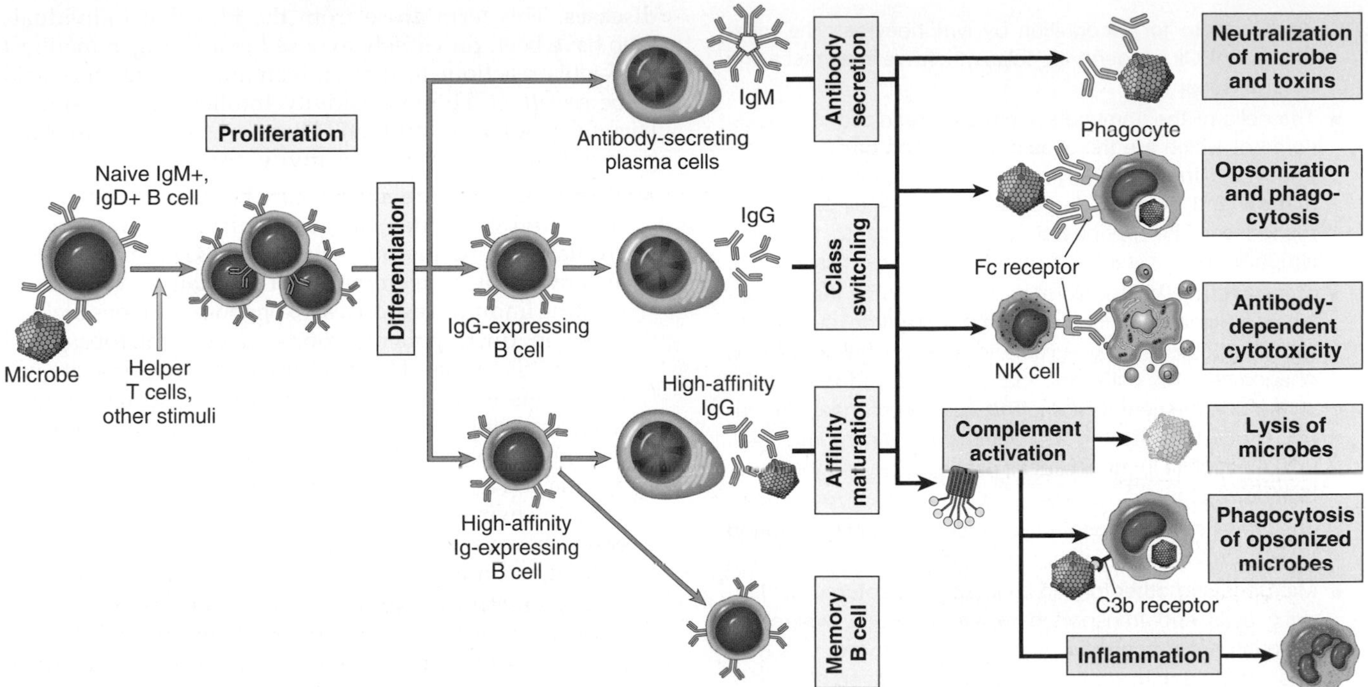

Figure 6-12 Humoral immunity. Naive B lymphocytes recognize antigens, and under the influence of T_H cells and other stimuli (not shown), the B cells are activated to proliferate and to differentiate into antibody-secreting plasma cells. Some of the activated B cells undergo heavy-chain class switching and affinity maturation, and some become long-lived memory cells. Antibodies of different heavy-chain classes (isotypes) perform different effector functions, shown on the right. Note that the antibodies shown are IgG; these and IgM activate complement; and the specialized functions of IgA (mucosal immunity) and IgE (mast cell and eosinophil activation) are not shown.

microbes. IgG antibodies coat (*opsonize*) microbes and target them for phagocytosis, since phagocytes (neutrophils and macrophages) express receptors for the Fc tails of IgG. IgG and IgM activate the complement system by the classical pathway, and complement products promote phagocytosis and destruction of microbes. Some antibodies serve special roles at particular anatomic sites. IgA is secreted from mucosal epithelia and neutralizes microbes in the lumens of the respiratory and gastrointestinal tracts (and other mucosal tissues). IgG is actively transported across the placenta and protects the newborn until the immune system becomes mature. IgE and eosinophils cooperate to kill parasites, mainly by release of eosinophil granule contents that are toxic to the worms. As mentioned above, T_H2 cytokines stimulate the production of IgE and activate eosinophils, and thus the response to helminths is orchestrated by T_H2 cells.

Most circulating IgG antibodies have half-lives of about 3 weeks. Some antibody-secreting plasma cells, particularly those that are generated in germinal centers, migrate to the bone marrow and live for months or even years, continuously producing antibodies during this time.

Decline of Immune Responses and Immunologic Memory

The majority of effector lymphocytes induced by an infectious pathogen die by apoptosis after the microbe is eliminated, thus returning the immune system to its resting state. The initial activation of lymphocytes also generates long-lived *memory cells,* which may survive for years after the infection. Memory cells are an expanded pool of antigen-specific lymphocytes (more numerous than the naive cells specific for any antigen that are present before encounter with that antigen), and they respond faster and more effectively when reexposed to the antigen than do naive cells. This is why the generation of memory cells is an important goal of vaccination.

KEY CONCEPTS

The Normal Immune Response: Cells, Tissues, Receptors, Mediators, and Overview

- The innate immune system uses several families of receptors, notably the Toll-like receptors, to recognize molecules present in various types of microbes and produced by damaged cells.
- Lymphocytes are the mediators of adaptive immunity and the only cells that produce specific and diverse receptors for antigens.
- T (thymus-derived) lymphocytes express antigen receptors called T cell receptors (TCRs) that recognize peptide fragments of protein antigens that are displayed by MHC molecules on the surface of antigen-presenting cells.
- B (bone marrow–derived) lymphocytes express membrane-bound antibodies that recognize a wide variety of antigens. B cells are activated to become plasma cells, which secrete antibodies.
- Natural killer (NK) cells kill cells that are infected by some microbes, or are stressed and damaged beyond repair. NK cells express inhibitory receptors that recognize MHC molecules that are normally expressed on healthy cells, and are thus prevented from killing normal cells.
- Antigen-presenting cells (APCs) capture microbes and other antigens, transport them to lymphoid organs, and

display them for recognition by lymphocytes. The most efficient APCs are dendritic cells, which live in epithelia and most tissues.

- The cells of the immune system are organized in tissues, some of which are the sites of production of mature lymphocytes (the generative lymphoid organs, the bone marrow and thymus), and others are the sites of immune responses (the peripheral lymphoid organs, including lymph nodes, spleen, and mucosal lymphoid tissues).
- The early reaction to microbes is mediated by the mechanisms of innate immunity, which are ready to respond to microbes. These mechanisms include epithelial barriers, phagocytes, NK cells, and plasma proteins, for example, of the complement system. The reaction of innate immunity is often manifested as inflammation. Innate immunity, unlike adaptive immunity, does not have fine antigen specificity or memory.
- The defense reactions of adaptive immunity develop slowly, but are more potent and specialized.
- Microbes and other foreign antigens are captured by dendritic cells and transported to lymph nodes, where the antigens are recognized by naïve lymphocytes. The lymphocytes are activated to proliferate and differentiate into effector and memory cells.
- Cell-mediated immunity is the reaction of T lymphocytes, designed to combat cell-associated microbes (e.g., phagocytosed microbes and microbes in the cytoplasm of infected cells). Humoral immunity is mediated by antibodies and is effective against extracellular microbes (in the circulation and mucosal lumens).
- CD4+ helper T cells help B cells to make antibodies, activate macrophages to destroy ingested microbes, stimulate recruitment of leukocytes, and regulate all immune responses to protein antigens. The functions of CD4+ T cells are mediated by secreted proteins called cytokines. CD8+ cytotoxic T lymphocytes kill cells that express antigens in the cytoplasm that are seen as foreign (e.g., virus-infected and tumor cells) and can also produce cytokines.
- Antibodies secreted by plasma cells neutralize microbes and block their infectivity, and promote the phagocytosis and destruction of pathogens. Antibodies also confer passive immunity to neonates.

The brief outline of basic immunology presented here provides a foundation for considering the diseases of the immune system. We first discuss the immune reactions that cause injury, called *hypersensitivity* reactions, and then disorders caused by the failure of tolerance to self antigens, called *autoimmune disorders*, and the rejection of transplants. This is followed by diseases caused by a defective immune system, called *immunodeficiency diseases*. We close with a consideration of *amyloidosis*, a disorder that is often associated with immune and inflammatory diseases.

Hypersensitivity: Immunologically Mediated Tissue Injury

Injurious immune reactions, called *hypersensitivity*, are the basis of the pathology associated with immunologic diseases. This term arose from the idea that individuals who have been previously exposed to an antigen manifest detectable reactions to that antigen and are therefore said to be *sensitized*. Hypersensitivity implies an excessive or harmful reaction to antigen. There are several important general features of hypersensitivity disorders.

- **Hypersensitivity reactions can be elicited by exogenous environmental antigens (microbial and nonmicrobial) or endogenous self antigens.** Humans live in an environment teeming with substances capable of eliciting immune responses. Exogenous antigens include those in dust, pollens, foods, drugs, microbes, and various chemicals. The immune responses against such exogenous antigens may take a variety of forms, ranging from annoying but trivial discomforts, such as itching of the skin, to potentially fatal diseases, such as bronchial asthma and anaphylaxis. Some of the most common reactions to environmental antigens cause the group of diseases known as *allergy*. Immune responses against self, or autologous, antigens, result in *autoimmune diseases*.
- **Hypersensitivity usually results from an imbalance between the effector mechanisms of immune responses and the control mechanisms that serve to normally limit such responses.** In fact, in many hypersensitivity diseases, it is suspected that the underlying cause is a failure of normal regulation. We will return to this concept when we consider autoimmunity.
- **The development of hypersensitivity diseases (both allergic and autoimmune) is often associated with the inheritance of particular susceptibility genes.** HLA genes and many non-HLA genes have been implicated in different diseases; specific examples will be described in the context of the diseases.
- **The mechanisms of tissue injury in hypersensitivity reactions are the same as the effector mechanisms of defense against infectious pathogens.** The problem in hypersensitivity is that these reactions are poorly controlled, excessive, or misdirected (e.g., against normally harmless environmental and self antigens).

Classification of Hypersensitivity Diseases

Hypersensitivity diseases can be classified on the basis of the immunologic mechanism that mediates the disease (Table 6-1). This classification is of value in distinguishing the manner in which the immune response causes tissue injury and disease, and the accompanying pathologic and clinical manifestations. However, it is now increasingly recognized that multiple mechanisms may be operative in any one hypersensitivity disease. The main types of hypersensitivity reactions are the following:

- **In immediate hypersensitivity (type I hypersensitivity), the injury is caused by T_H2 cells, IgE antibodies, and mast cells and other leukocytes.** Mast cells release mediators that act on vessels and smooth muscle and proinflammatory cytokines that recruit inflammatory cells.
- **In antibody-mediated disorders (type II hypersensitivity), secreted IgG and IgM antibodies injure cells by promoting their phagocytosis or lysis and injure tissues by inducing inflammation.** Antibodies may also

Table 6-1 Mechanisms of Hypersensitivity Reactions

Type	Immune Mechanisms	Histopathologic Lesions	Prototypical Disorders
Immediate (type I) hypersensitivity	Production of IgE antibody → immediate release of vasoactive amines and other mediators from mast cells; later recruitment of inflammatory cells	Vascular dilation, edema, smooth muscle contraction, mucus production, tissue injury, inflammation	Anaphylaxis; allergies; bronchial asthma (atopic forms)
Antibody-mediated (type II) hypersensitivity	Production of IgG, IgM → binds to antigen on target cell or tissue → phagocytosis or lysis of target cell by activated complement or Fc receptors; recruitment of leukocytes	Phagocytosis and lysis of cells; inflammation; in some diseases, functional derangements without cell or tissue injury	Autoimmune hemolytic anemia; Goodpasture syndrome
Immune complex–mediated (type III) hypersensitivity	Deposition of antigen-antibody complexes → complement activation → recruitment of leukocytes by complement products and Fc receptors → release of enzymes and other toxic molecules	Inflammation, necrotizing vasculitis (fibrinoid necrosis)	Systemic lupus erythematosus; some forms of glomerulonephritis; serum sickness; Arthus reaction
Cell-mediated (type IV) hypersensitivity	Activated T lymphocytes → (1) release of cytokines, inflammation and macrophage activation; (2) T cell–mediated cytotoxicity	Perivascular cellular infiltrates; edema; granuloma formation; cell destruction	Contact dermatitis; multiple sclerosis; type 1 diabetes; tuberculosis

Ig, immunoglobulin.

interfere with cellular functions and cause disease without tissue injury.

- **In immune complex–mediated disorders (type III hypersensitivity), IgG and IgM antibodies bind antigens usually in the circulation, and the antigen-antibody complexes deposit in tissues and induce inflammation.** The leukocytes that are recruited (neutrophils and monocytes) produce tissue damage by release of lysosomal enzymes and generation of toxic free radicals.
- **In cell-mediated immune disorders (type IV hypersensitivity), sensitized T lymphocytes (T_H1 and T_H17 cells and CTLs) are the cause of the tissue injury.** T_H2 cells induce lesions that are part of immediate hypersensitivity reactions and are not considered a form of type IV hypersensitivity.

Immediate (Type I) Hypersensitivity

Immediate, or type I, hypersensitivity is a rapid immunologic reaction occurring in a previously sensitized individual that is triggered by the binding of an antigen to IgE antibody on the surface of mast cells. These reactions are often called *allergy*, and the antigens that elicit them are *allergens*. Immediate hypersensitivity may occur as a systemic disorder or as a local reaction. The systemic reaction most often follows injection of an antigen into a sensitized individual (e.g., by a bee sting), but can also follow antigen ingestion (e.g., peanut allergens). Sometimes, within minutes the patient goes into a state of shock, which may be fatal. Local reactions are diverse and vary depending on the portal of entry of the allergen. They may take the form of localized cutaneous rash or blisters (skin allergy, hives), nasal and conjunctival discharge (allergic rhinitis and conjunctivitis), hay fever, bronchial asthma, or allergic gastroenteritis (food allergy).

Many local type I hypersensitivity reactions have two well-defined phases (Fig. 6-13). The *immediate reaction* is characterized by vasodilation, vascular leakage, and depending on the location, smooth muscle spasm or glandular secretions. These changes usually become evident within minutes after exposure to an allergen and tend to

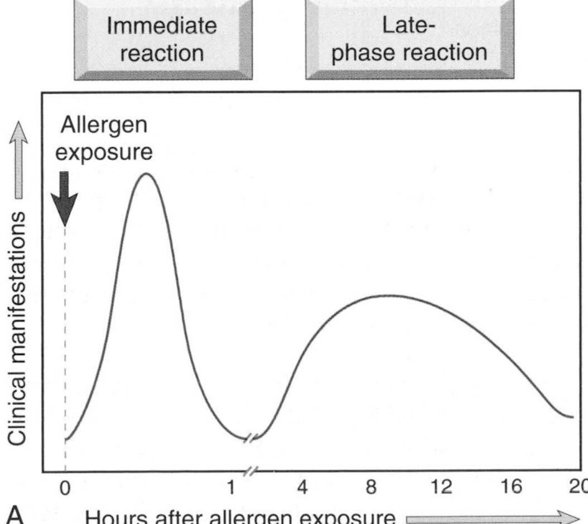

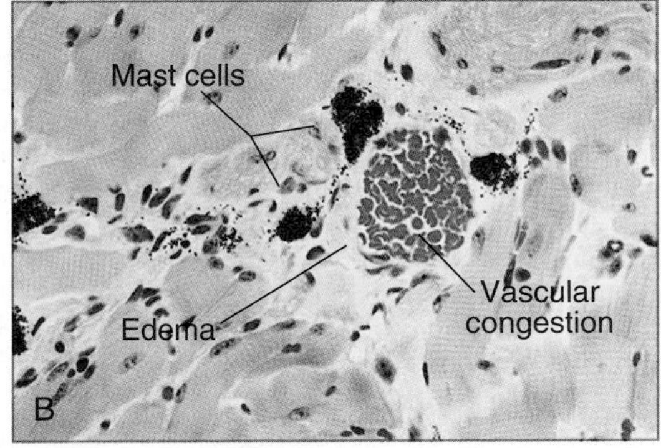

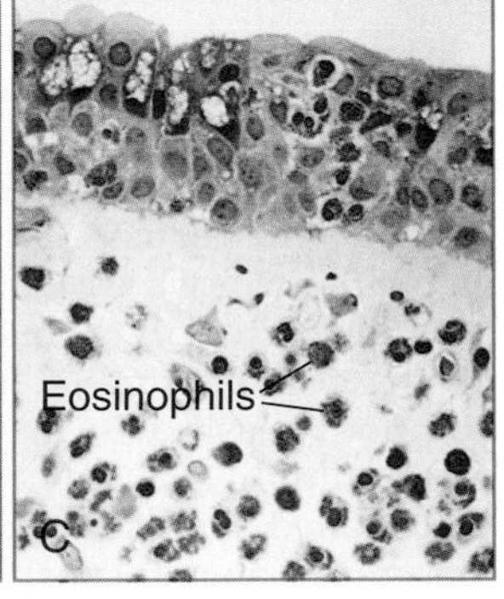

Figure 6-13 Phases of immediate hypersensitivity reactions. **A,** Kinetics of the immediate and late-phase reactions. The immediate vascular and smooth muscle reaction to allergen develops within minutes after challenge (allergen exposure in a previously sensitized individual), and the late-phase reaction develops 2 to 24 hours later. The immediate reaction **(B)** is characterized by vasodilation, congestion, and edema, and the late-phase reaction **(C)** is characterized by an inflammatory infiltrate rich in eosinophils, neutrophils, and T cells. (Courtesy Dr. Daniel Friend, Department of Pathology, Brigham and Women's Hospital, Boston, Mass.)

subside in a few hours. In many instances (e.g., allergic rhinitis and bronchial asthma), a second, *late-phase reaction* sets in 2 to 24 hours later without additional exposure to antigen and may last for several days. This late-phase reaction is characterized by infiltration of tissues with eosinophils, neutrophils, basophils, monocytes, and CD4+ T cells, as well as tissue destruction, typically in the form of mucosal epithelial cell damage.

Most immediate hypersensitivity disorders are caused by excessive T_H2 responses and these cells play a central role by stimulating IgE production and promoting inflammation. These T_H2-mediated disorders show a characteristic sequence of events (Fig. 6-14), described next.

Activation of T_H2 Cells and Production of IgE Antibody

The first step in the generation of T_H2 cells is the presentation of the antigen to naive CD4+ helper T cells, probably by dendritic cells that capture the antigen from its site of entry. For reasons that are still not understood, only some environmental antigens elicit strong T_H2 responses and thus serve as allergens. In response to antigen and other stimuli, including cytokines such as IL-4 produced at the local site, the T cells differentiate into T_H2 cells. The newly minted T_H2 cells produce a number of cytokines upon subsequent encounter with the antigen; as mentioned earlier, the signature cytokines of this subset are IL-4, IL-5, and IL-13. IL-4 acts on B cells to stimulate class switching to IgE and promotes the development of additional T_H2 cells. IL-5 is involved in the development and activation of eosinophils, which are important effectors of type I hypersensitivity (discussed later). IL-13 enhances IgE production and acts on epithelial cells to stimulate mucus secretion. In addition, T_H2 cells (as well as mast cells and epithelial cells) produce chemokines that attract more T_H2 cells, as well as other leukocytes, to the reaction site.

Sensitization and Activation of Mast Cells

Because mast cells are central to the development of immediate hypersensitivity, we first review some of their salient characteristics. *Mast cells* are bone marrow–derived cells that are widely distributed in the tissues. They are abundant near blood vessels and nerves and in subepithelial tissues, which explains why local immediate hypersensitivity reactions often occur at these sites. Mast cells have cytoplasmic membrane-bound granules that contain a variety of biologically active mediators, described later. The granules also contain acidic proteoglycans that bind basic dyes such as toluidine blue. (*Mast* in German refers to fattening of animals, and the name of these cells came from the erroneous belief that their granules fed the tissue where the cells were located.) As is detailed next, mast cells (and their circulating counterpart, basophils) are activated by the cross-linking of high-affinity IgE Fc receptors; in addition, mast cells may also be triggered by several other stimuli, such as complement components C5a and C3a (called *anaphylatoxins* because they elicit reactions that mimic anaphylaxis), both of which act by binding to receptors on the mast cell membrane. Other mast cell secretagogues include some chemokines (e.g., IL-8), drugs such as codeine and morphine, adenosine, melittin (present in bee venom), and physical stimuli (e.g., heat, cold, sunlight). Basophils are similar to mast cells in many respects, including the presence of cell surface IgE Fc receptors as well as cytoplasmic granules. In contrast to mast cells, however, basophils are not normally present in tissues but rather circulate in the blood in extremely small numbers. Similar to other granulocytes, basophils can be recruited to inflammatory sites.

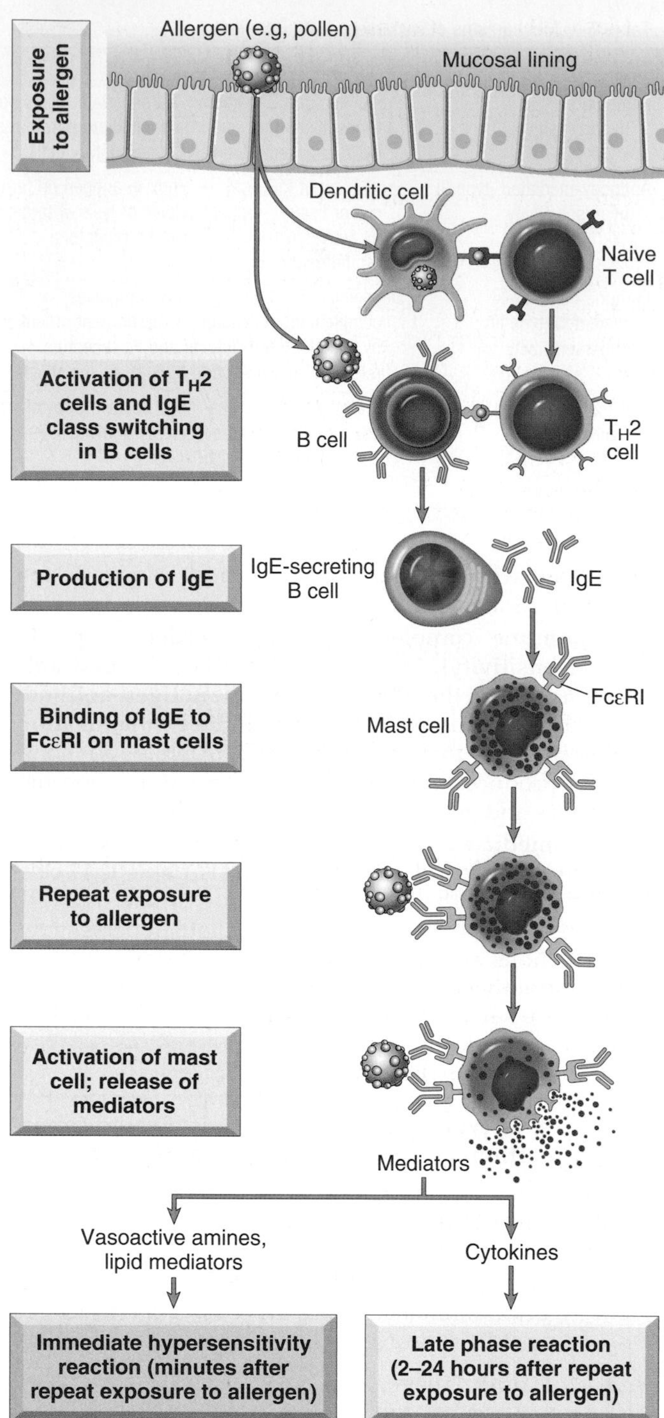

Figure 6-14 Sequence of events in immediate (type I) hypersensitivity. Immediate hypersensitivity reactions are initiated by the introduction of an allergen, which stimulates T_H2 responses and IgE production in genetically susceptible individuals. IgE binds to Fc receptors (FcεRI) on mast cells, and subsequent exposure to the allergen activates the mast cells to secrete the mediators that are responsible for the pathologic manifestations of immediate hypersensitivity. See text for abbreviations.

Mast cells and basophils express a high-affinity receptor, called FcεRI, which is specific for the Fc portion of IgE and therefore avidly binds IgE antibodies. IgE-coated mast cells are said to be *sensitized*, because they are sensitive to subsequent encounter with the specific antigen. **When a mast cell, armed with IgE antibodies previously produced in response to an antigen, is exposed to the same antigen, the cell is activated, leading eventually to the release of an arsenal of powerful mediators responsible for the clinical features of immediate hypersensitivity reactions.** In the first step in the sequence of mast cell activation, the antigen binds to the IgE antibodies previously attached to the mast cells. Multivalent antigens bind to and cross-link adjacent IgE antibodies. The underlying Fcε receptors are brought together, and this activates signal transduction pathways from the cytoplasmic portion of the receptors. These signals lead to the production of mediators that are responsible for the initial, sometimes explosive, symptoms of immediate hypersensitivity, and they also set into motion the events that lead to the late-phase reaction.

Mediators of Immediate Hypersensitivity

Mast cell activation leads to degranulation, with the discharge of preformed (primary) mediators that are stored in the granules, and de novo synthesis and release of secondary mediators, including lipid products and cytokines (Fig. 6-15).

Preformed Mediators. Mediators contained within mast cell granules are the first to be released and can be divided into three categories:

- *Vasoactive amines.* The most important mast cell-derived amine is *histamine* (Chapter 3). Histamine causes intense smooth muscle contraction, increased vascular permeability, and increased mucus secretion by nasal, bronchial, and gastric glands.
- *Enzymes.* These are contained in the granule matrix and include neutral proteases (chymase, tryptase) and several acid hydrolases. The enzymes cause tissue damage and lead to the generation of kinins and activated components of complement (e.g., C3a) by acting on their precursor proteins.
- *Proteoglycans.* These include heparin, a well-known anticoagulant, and chondroitin sulfate. The proteoglycans serve to package and store the amines in the granules.

Lipid Mediators. The major *lipid mediators* are arachidonic acid–derived products (Chapter 3). Reactions in the mast cell membranes lead to activation of phospholipase A_2, an enzyme that converts membrane phospholipids to *arachidonic acid.* This is the parent compound from which leukotrienes and prostaglandins are produced by the 5-lipoxygenase and cyclooxygenase pathways, respectively.

- *Leukotrienes.* Leukotrienes C_4 and D_4 are the most potent vasoactive and spasmogenic agents known. On a molar basis, they are several thousand times more active than histamine in increasing vascular permeability and causing bronchial smooth muscle contraction. Leukotriene B_4 is highly chemotactic for neutrophils, eosinophils, and monocytes.

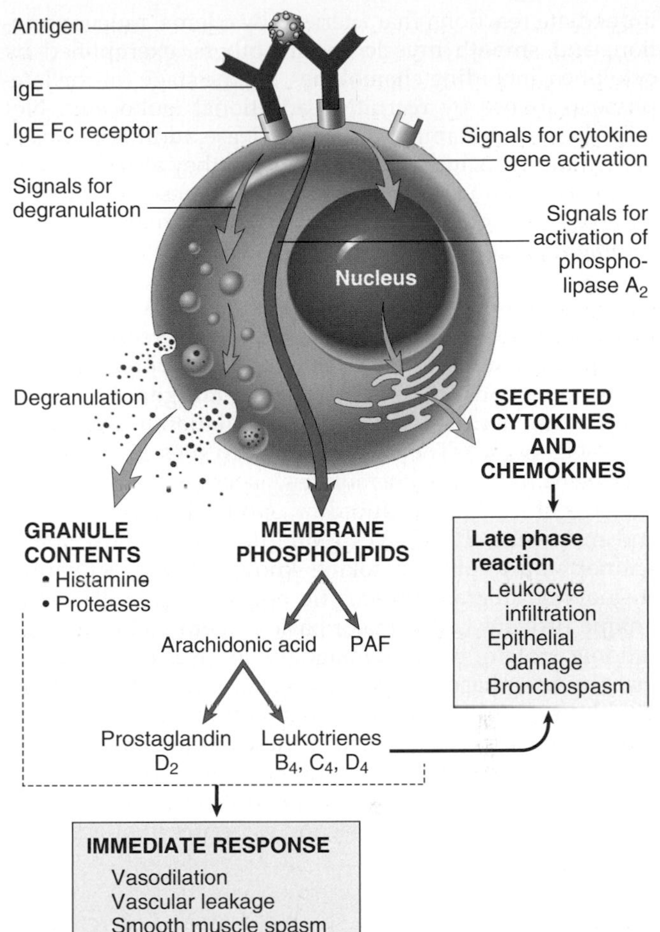

Figure 6-15 Mast cell mediators. Upon activation, mast cells release various classes of mediators that are responsible for the immediate and late-phase reactions. PAF, Platelet-activating factor.

- *Prostaglandin D_2.* This is the most abundant mediator produced in mast cells by the cyclooxygenase pathway. It causes intense bronchospasm as well as increased mucus secretion.
- *Platelet-activating factor (PAF).* PAF (Chapter 3) is a lipid mediator produced by some mast cell populations but it is not derived from arachidonic acid. It causes platelet aggregation, release of histamine, bronchospasm, increased vascular permeability, and vasodilation. Its role in immediate hypersensitivity reactions is not well established.

Cytokines. Mast cells are sources of many cytokines, which may play an important role at several stages of immediate hypersensitivity reactions. The cytokines include: TNF, IL-1, and chemokines, which promote leukocyte recruitment (typical of the late-phase reaction); IL-4, which amplifies the T_H2 response; and numerous others. The inflammatory cells that are recruited by mast cell-derived TNF and chemokines are additional sources of cytokines and of histamine-releasing factors that cause further mast cell degranulation.

These mediators are responsible for the manifestations of immediate hypersensitivity reactions. Some, such as histamine and leukotrienes, are released rapidly from sensitized mast cells and are responsible for the intense immediate reactions characterized by edema, mucus secretion, and smooth muscle spasm; others, exemplified by cytokines, including chemokines, set the stage for the late-phase response by recruiting additional leukocytes. Not only do these inflammatory cells release additional waves of mediators (including cytokines), but they also cause epithelial cell damage. Epithelial cells themselves are not passive bystanders in this reaction; they can also produce soluble mediators, such as chemokines.

Late-Phase Reaction

In the late-phase reaction, leukocytes are recruited that amplify and sustain the inflammatory response without additional exposure to the triggering antigen. *Eosinophils* are often an abundant leukocyte population in these reactions (Fig. 6-13C). They are recruited to sites of immediate hypersensitivity by chemokines, such as eotaxin, and others that may be produced by epithelial cells, T_H2 cells, and mast cells. The T_H2 cytokine IL-5 is the most potent eosinophil-activating cytokine known. Upon activation, eosinophils liberate proteolytic enzymes as well as two unique proteins called major basic protein and eosinophil cationic protein, which damage tissues. It is now believed that the late-phase reaction is a major cause of symptoms in some type I hypersensitivity disorders, such as allergic asthma. Therefore, treatment of these diseases requires the use of broad-spectrum antiinflammatory drugs, such as steroids, rather than anti-histamine drugs, which are of benefit in the immediate reaction as occurs in allergic rhinitis (hay fever).

Development of Allergies

Susceptibility to immediate hypersensitivity reactions is genetically determined. An increased propensity to develop immediate hypersensitivity reactions is called *atopy*. Atopic individuals tend to have higher serum IgE levels and more IL-4–producing T_H2 cells than does the general population. A positive family history of allergy is found in 50% of atopic individuals. The basis of familial predisposition is not clear, but studies in patients with asthma reveal linkage to polymorphisms in several genes. Some of these genes are located in the chromosome 5q31 region; these include genes encoding the cytokines IL-3, IL-4, IL-5, IL-9, IL-13, and GM-CSF. This locus has attracted great attention because of the known roles of many of these cytokines in the allergic reaction, but how the disease-associated polymorphisms influence the development of allergies is not known. Linkage has also been noted to 6p, close to the HLA complex, suggesting that the inheritance of certain HLA alleles permits reactivity to certain allergens.

Environmental factors are also important in the development of allergic diseases. Exposure to environmental pollutants, which is common in industrialized societies, is an important predisposing factor for allergy. In fact, it is known that dogs and cats diverged from humans about 95 million years ago and chimpanzees only about 4-5 million years ago, suggesting that chimps share more genes with us than do dogs and cats. Nevertheless, dogs and cats, who live in the same environment as humans, develop allergies and chimps do not. This simple observation suggests that environmental factors may be more important in the development of allergic disease than genetics. Viral infections of the airways are important triggers for bronchial asthma, an allergic disease affecting the lungs (Chapter 15). Bacterial skin infections are strongly associated with atopic dermatitis.

It is estimated that 20% to 30% of immediate hypersensitivity reactions are triggered by non-antigenic stimuli such as temperature extremes and exercise, and do not involve T_H2 cells or IgE; such reactions are sometimes called *nonatopic allergy*. It is believed that in these cases mast cells are abnormally sensitive to activation by various nonimmune stimuli.

The incidence of many allergic diseases is increasing in developed countries, and seems to be related to a decrease in infections during early life. These observations have led to an idea, sometimes called the *hygiene hypothesis*, that early childhood and even prenatal exposure to microbial antigens educates the immune system in such a way that subsequent pathologic responses against common environmental allergens are prevented. Thus, too much hygiene in childhood may increase allergies later in life. This hypothesis, however, is difficult to prove, and the underlying mechanisms are not defined.

With this consideration of the basic mechanisms of type I hypersensitivity, we turn to some clinically important examples of IgE-mediated disease. These reactions can lead to a wide spectrum of injury and clinical manifestations (Table 6-2).

Systemic Anaphylaxis

Systemic anaphylaxis is characterized by vascular shock, widespread edema, and difficulty in breathing. It may occur in sensitized individuals in hospital settings after administration of foreign proteins (e.g., antisera), hormones, enzymes, polysaccharides, and drugs (e.g., the antibiotic penicillin), or in the community setting following exposure to food allergens (e.g., peanuts, shellfish) or insect toxins (e.g., those in bee venom). Extremely small doses of antigen may trigger anaphylaxis, for example, the tiny amounts used in skin testing for various forms of allergies. Because of the risk of severe allergic reactions to minute quantities of peanuts, U.S. agencies are considering a ban on peanut snacks served in the confined quarters of commercial airplanes. Within minutes after exposure, itching, hives, and skin erythema appear, followed shortly thereafter by a striking contraction of respiratory bronchioles and respiratory distress. Laryngeal edema results in hoarseness and further compromises breathing. Vomiting, abdominal

Table 6-2 Examples of Disorders Caused by Immediate Hypersensitivity

Clinical Syndrome	Clinical and Pathologic Manifestations
Anaphylaxis (may be caused by drugs, bee sting, food)	Fall in blood pressure (shock) cause by vascular dilation; airway obstruction due to laryngeal edema
Bronchial asthma	Airway obstruction caused by bronchial smooth muscle hyperactivity; inflammation and tissue injury caused by late-phase reaction
Allergic rhinitis, sinusitis (hay fever)	Increased mucus secretion; inflammation of upper airways, sinuses
Food allergies	Increased peristalsis due to contraction of intestinal muscles

cramps, diarrhea, and laryngeal obstruction follow, and the patient may go into shock and even die within the hour. The risk of anaphylaxis must be borne in mind when certain therapeutic agents are administered. Although patients at risk can generally be identified by a previous history of some form of allergy, the absence of such a history does not preclude the possibility of an anaphylactic reaction.

Local Immediate Hypersensitivity Reactions

About 10% to 20% of the population suffers from allergies involving localized reactions to common environmental allergens, such as pollen, animal dander, house dust, foods, and the like. Specific diseases include urticaria, allergic rhinitis (hay fever), bronchial asthma, and food allergies; these are discussed elsewhere in this text.

KEY CONCEPTS

Immediate (Type I) Hypersensitivity

- These are also called allergic reactions, or allergies
- They are induced by environmental antigens (allergens) that stimulate strong T_H2 responses and IgE production in genetically susceptible individuals
- IgE coats mast cells by binding to Fcε receptors; reexposure to the allergen leads to cross-linking of the IgE and FcεRI, activation of mast cells, and release of mediators.
- The principal mediators are histamine, proteases, and other granule contents, prostaglandins and leukotrienes, and cytokines.
- The mediators are responsible for the immediate vascular and smooth muscle reactions and the late-phase reaction (inflammation).
- The clinical manifestations may be local or systemic, and range from mildly annoying rhinitis to fatal anaphylaxis.

Antibody-Mediated (Type II) Hypersensitivity

Antibodies that react with antigens present on cell surfaces or in the extracellular matrix cause disease by destroying these cells, triggering inflammation, or interfering with normal functions. The antibodies may be specific for normal cell or tissue antigens (*autoantibodies*) or for exogenous antigens, such as chemical or microbial proteins, that bind to a cell surface or tissue matrix. The antibody-dependent mechanisms that cause tissue injury and disease are illustrated in Figure 6-16 and described next. These reactions are the cause of several important diseases (Table 6-3).

Opsonization and Phagocytosis

Phagocytosis is largely responsible for depletion of cells coated with antibodies. Cells opsonized by IgG antibodies are recognized by phagocyte Fc receptors, which are specific for the Fc portions of some IgG subclasses. In addition, when IgM or IgG antibodies are deposited on the surfaces of cells, they may activate the complement system by the classical pathway. Complement activation generates by-products, mainly C3b and C4b, which are deposited on the surfaces of the cells and recognized by phagocytes that express receptors for these proteins. The net result is phagocytosis of the opsonized cells and their destruction (Fig. 6-16*A*). Complement activation on cells also leads to the formation of the membrane attack complex, which disrupts membrane integrity by "drilling holes" through the lipid bilayer, thereby causing osmotic lysis of the cells. This mechanism of killing is probably effective only with cells that have thin cell walls, such as *Neisseria* bacteria.

Antibody-mediated destruction of cells may occur by another process called *antibody-dependent cellular cytotoxicity (ADCC)*. Cells that are coated with IgG antibody are killed by a variety of effector cells, mainly NK cells and macrophages, which bind to the target by their receptors for the Fc fragment of IgG, and cell lysis proceeds without phagocytosis. The contribution of ADCC to common hypersensitivity diseases is uncertain.

Clinically, antibody-mediated cell destruction and phagocytosis occur in the following situations: (1) transfusion reactions, in which cells from an incompatible donor react with and are opsonized by preformed antibody in the host (Chapter 14); (2) hemolytic disease of the newborn (erythroblastosis fetalis), in which there is an antigenic difference between the mother and the fetus, and IgG antierythrocyte antibodies from the mother cross the placenta and cause destruction of fetal red cells (Chapter 10); (3) autoimmune hemolytic anemia, agranulocytosis, and thrombocytopenia, in which individuals produce antibodies to their own blood cells, which are then destroyed (Chapter 14); and (4) certain drug reactions, in which a drug acts as a "hapten" by attaching to plasma membrane proteins of red cells and antibodies are produced against the drug-protein complex.

Inflammation

When antibodies deposit in fixed tissues, such as basement membranes and extracellular matrix, the resultant injury is due to inflammation. The deposited antibodies activate complement, generating by-products, including chemotactic agents (mainly C5a), which direct the migration of polymorphonuclear leukocytes and monocytes, and anaphylatoxins (C3a and C5a), which increase vascular permeability (Fig. 6-16*B*). The leukocytes are activated by engagement of their C3b and Fc receptors. This results in the production of other substances that damage tissues, such as lysosomal enzymes, including proteases capable of digesting basement membrane, collagen, elastin, and cartilage, and reactive oxygen species.

Antibody-mediated inflammation is the mechanism responsible for tissue injury in some forms of *glomerulonephritis*, *vascular rejection* in organ grafts, and other disorders (Table 6-3).

Cellular Dysfunction

In some cases, antibodies directed against cell surface receptors impair or dysregulate function without causing cell injury or inflammation (Fig. 6-16C). For example, in *myasthenia gravis*, antibodies reactive with acetylcholine receptors in the motor end plates of skeletal muscles block neuromuscular transmission and therefore cause muscle weakness. The converse (i.e., antibody-mediated stimulation of cell function) is the basis of *Graves disease*. In this disorder, antibodies against the thyroid-stimulating hormone receptor on thyroid epithelial cells stimulate the cells, resulting in hyperthyroidism.

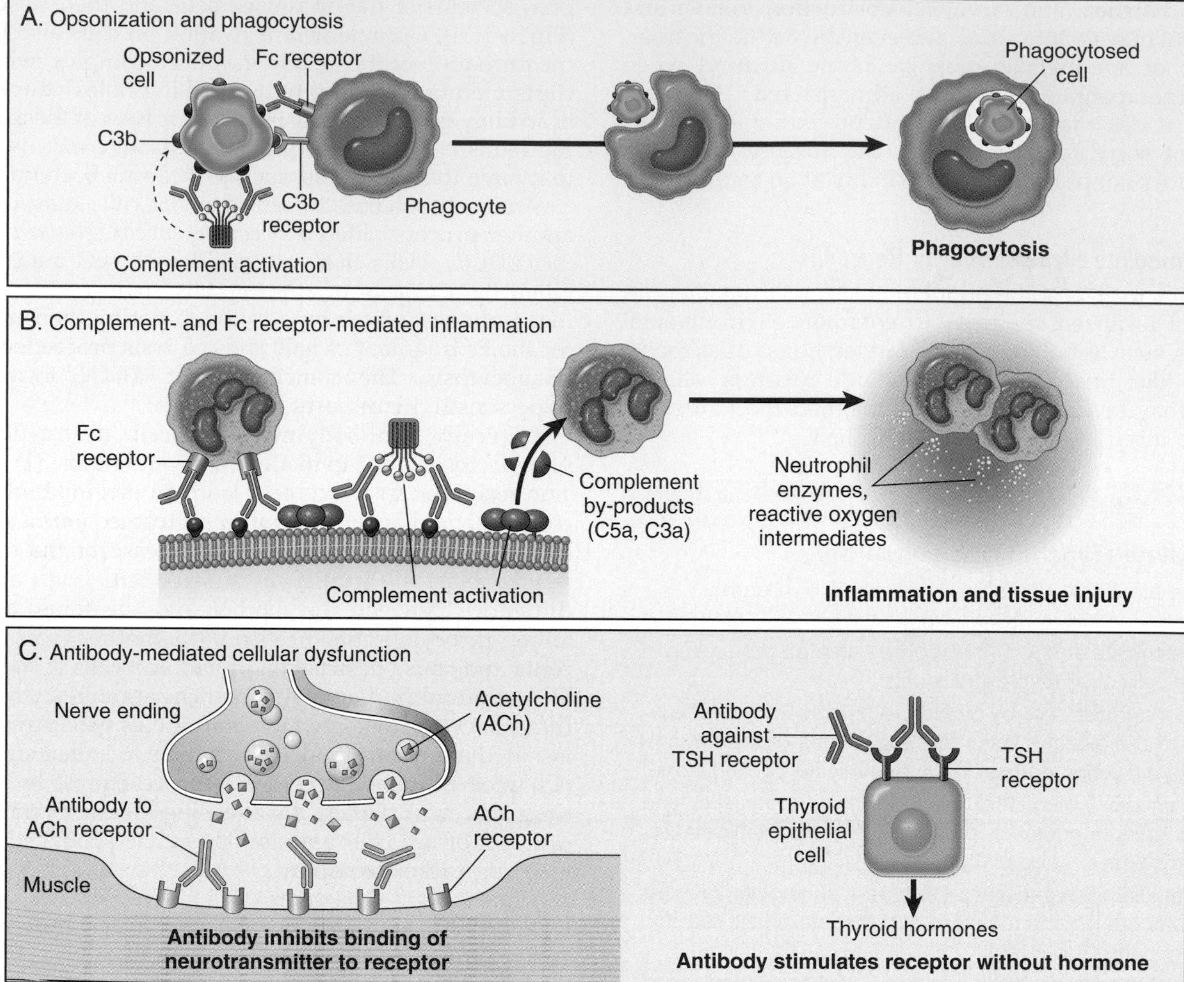

Figure 6-16 Mechanisms of antibody-mediated injury. **A,** Opsonization of cells by antibodies and complement components and ingestion by phagocytes. **B,** Inflammation induced by antibody binding to Fc receptors of leukocytes and by complement breakdown products. **C,** Antireceptor antibodies disturb the normal function of receptors. In these examples, antibodies to the acetylcholine (ACh) receptor impair neuromuscular transmission in myasthenia gravis, and antibodies against the thyroid-stimulating hormone (TSH) receptor activate thyroid cells in Graves disease.

Table 6-3 Examples of Antibody-Mediated Diseases (Type II Hypersensitivity)

Disease	Target Antigen	Mechanisms of Disease	Clinicopathologic Manifestations
Autoimmune hemolytic anemia	Red cell membrane proteins (Rh blood group antigens, I antigen)	Opsonization and phagocytosis of red cells	Hemolysis, anemia
Autoimmune thrombocytopenic purpura	Platelet membrane proteins (GpIIb : IIIa integrin)	Opsonization and phagocytosis of platelets	Bleeding
Pemphigus vulgaris	Proteins in intercellular junctions of epidermal cells (epidermal cadherin)	Antibody-mediated activation of proteases, disruption of intercellular adhesions	Skin vesicles (bullae)
Vasculitis caused by ANCA	Neutrophil granule proteins, presumably released from activated neutrophils	Neutrophil degranulation and inflammation	Vasculitis
Goodpasture syndrome	Noncollagenous protein in basement membranes of kidney glomeruli and lung alveoli	Complement- and Fc receptor–mediated inflammation	Nephritis, lung hemorrhage
Acute rheumatic fever	Streptococcal cell wall antigen; antibody cross-reacts with myocardial antigen	Inflammation, macrophage activation	Myocarditis, arthritis
Myasthenia gravis	Acetylcholine receptor	Antibody inhibits acetylcholine binding, down-modulates receptors	Muscle weakness, paralysis
Graves disease (hyperthyroidism)	TSH receptor	Antibody-mediated stimulation of TSH receptors	Hyperthyroidism
Insulin-resistant diabetes	Insulin receptor	Antibody inhibits binding of insulin	Hyperglycemia, ketoacidosis
Pernicious anemia	Intrinsic factor of gastric parietal cells	Neutralization of intrinsic factor, decreased absorption of vitamin B_{12}	Abnormal erythropoiesis, anemia

ANCA, Antineutrophil cytoplasmic antibodies; TSH, thyroid-stimulating hormone.

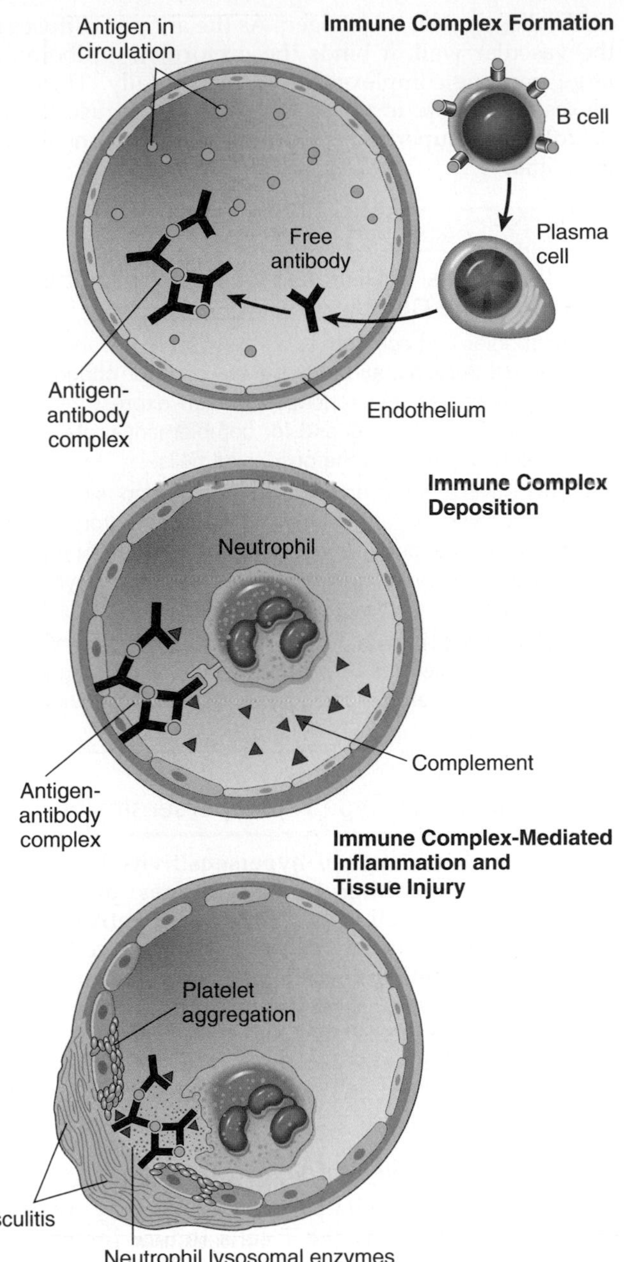

Figure 6-17 Immune complex disease. The sequential phases in the induction of systemic immune complex–mediated diseases (type III hypersensitivity).

Immune Complex–Mediated (Type III) Hypersensitivity

Antigen-antibody complexes produce tissue damage mainly by eliciting inflammation at the sites of deposition. The pathologic reaction is usually initiated when antigen combines with antibody in the circulation, creating immune complexes that typically deposit in vessel walls. Less frequently, the complexes may be formed at sites where antigen has been "planted" previously (called in situ immune complexes). The antigens that form immune complexes may be *exogenous*, such as a foreign protein that is injected or produced by an infectious microbe, or *endogenous*, if the individual produces antibody against self antigens (autoimmunity). Examples of immune complex disorders and the antigens involved are listed in Table 6-4. Immune complex–mediated diseases tend be *systemic*, but often preferentially involve the kidney (glomerulonephritis), joints (arthritis), and small blood vessels (vasculitis), all of which are common sites of immune complex deposition.

Systemic Immune Complex Disease

Acute serum sickness is the prototype of a systemic immune complex disease; it was once a frequent sequela to the administration of large amounts of foreign serum (e.g., serum from immunized horses used for protection against diphtheria). In modern times the disease is infrequent, and usually seen in individuals who receive antibodies from other individuals or species. Nevertheless, it is an informative model that has taught us a great deal about systemic immune complex disorders.

The pathogenesis of systemic immune complex disease can be divided into three phases (Fig. 6-17).

1. **Formation of immune complexes.** The introduction of a protein antigen triggers an immune response that results in the formation of antibodies, typically about a week after the injection of the protein. These antibodies are secreted into the blood, where they react with the antigen still present in the circulation and form antigen-antibody complexes.
2. **Deposition of immune complexes.** In the next phase the circulating antigen-antibody complexes are deposited in various tissues. The factors that determine whether immune complex formation will lead to tissue deposition and disease are not fully understood, but the major influences seem to be the characteristics of the complexes and local vascular alterations. In general, complexes that are of medium size, formed in slight antigen excess, are the most pathogenic. Organs where

Table 6-4 Examples of Immune Complex–Mediated Diseases

Disease	Antigen Involved	Clinicopathologic Manifestations
Systemic lupus erythematosus	Nuclear antigens (circulating or "planted" in kidney)	Nephritis, skin lesions, arthritis, others
Poststreptococcal glomerulonephritis	Streptococcal cell wall antigen(s); may be "planted" in glomerular basement membrane	Nephritis
Polyarteritis nodosa	Hepatitis B virus antigens in some cases	Systemic vasculitis
Reactive arthritis	Bacterial antigens (e.g., *Yersinia*)	Acute arthritis
Serum sickness	Various proteins, e.g., foreign serum protein (horse antithymocyte globulin)	Arthritis, vasculitis, nephritis
Arthus reaction (experimental)	Various foreign proteins	Cutaneous vasculitis

blood is filtered at high pressure to form other fluids, like urine and synovial fluid, are sites where immune complexes become concentrated and tend to deposit; hence, immune complex disease often affects glomeruli and joints.

3. **Inflammation and tissue injury.** Once immune complexes are deposited in the tissues, they initiate an acute inflammatory reaction. During this phase (approximately 10 days after antigen administration), clinical features such as fever, urticaria, joint pains (arthralgias), lymph node enlargement, and proteinuria appear. Wherever complexes deposit the tissue damage is similar. The mechanisms of inflammation and injury were discussed above, in the discussion of antibody-mediated injury. The resultant inflammatory lesion is termed *vasculitis* if it occurs in blood vessels, *glomerulonephritis* if it occurs in renal glomeruli, *arthritis* if it occurs in the joints, and so on.

It is clear that complement-fixing antibodies (i.e., IgG and IgM) and antibodies that bind to leukocyte Fc receptors (some subclasses of IgG) induce the pathologic lesions of immune complex disorders. The important role of complement in the pathogenesis of the tissue injury is supported by the observations that complement proteins can be detected at the site of injury and, during the active phase of the disease, consumption of complement leads to a decrease in serum levels of C3. In fact, serum C3 levels can, in some cases, be used to monitor disease activity.

MORPHOLOGY

The principal morphologic manifestation of immune complex injury is acute vasculitis, associated with necrosis of the vessel wall and intense neutrophilic infiltration. The necrotic tissue and deposits of immune complexes, complement, and plasma protein appear as a smudgy eosinophilic area of tissue destruction, an appearance termed **fibrinoid necrosis** (see Fig. 2-15). When deposited in the kidney, the complexes can be seen on immunofluorescence microscopy as granular lumpy deposits of immunoglobulin and complement and on electron microscopy as electron-dense deposits along the glomerular basement membrane (see Figs. 6-31 and 6-32).

If the disease results from a single large exposure to antigen, such as *acute serum sickness*, the lesions tend to resolve as a result of catabolism of the immune complexes. A form of *chronic serum sickness* results from repeated or prolonged exposure to an antigen. This occurs in several diseases, such as systemic lupus erythematosus (SLE), which is associated with persistent antibody responses to autoantigens. In many diseases, the morphologic changes and other findings suggest immune complex deposition but the inciting antigens are unknown. Included in this category are membranous glomerulonephritis and several vasculitides.

Local Immune Complex Disease (Arthus Reaction)

The *Arthus reaction* is a localized area of tissue necrosis resulting from acute immune complex vasculitis, usually elicited in the skin. The reaction can be produced experimentally by intracutaneous injection of antigen in a previously immunized animal that contains circulating antibodies against the antigen. As the antigen diffuses into the vascular wall, it binds the preformed antibody, and large immune complexes are formed locally. These complexes precipitate in the vessel walls and cause fibrinoid necrosis, and superimposed thrombosis worsens the ischemic injury.

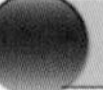

KEY CONCEPTS

Pathogenesis of Diseases Caused by Antibodies and Immune Complexes

- Antibodies can coat (opsonize) cells, with or without complement proteins, and target these cells for phagocytosis by phagocytes (macrophages), which express receptors for the Fc tails of IgG and for complement proteins. The result is depletion of the opsonized cells.
- Antibodies and immune complexes may deposit in tissues or blood vessels, and elicit an acute inflammatory reaction by activating complement, with release of breakdown products, or by engaging Fc receptors of leukocytes. The inflammatory reaction causes tissue injury.
- Antibodies can bind to cell surface receptors or other essential molecules and cause functional derangements (either inhibition or unregulated activation) without cell injury.

T Cell–Mediated (Type IV) Hypersensitivity

The cell-mediated type of hypersensitivity is caused by inflammation resulting from cytokines produced by CD4+ T cells and cell killing by CD8+ T cells (Fig. 6-18). CD4+ T cell–mediated hypersensitivity induced by environmental and self antigens is the cause of many chronic inflammatory diseases, including autoimmune diseases (Table 6-5). CD8+ cells may also be involved in some of these autoimmune diseases and may be the dominant effector cells in certain reactions, especially those that follow viral infections.

CD4+ T Cell–Mediated Inflammation

In CD4+ T cell–mediated hypersensitivity reactions, cytokines produced by the T cells induce inflammation that may be chronic and destructive. The prototype of T cell–mediated inflammation is *delayed-type hypersensitivity (DTH)*, a tissue reaction to antigens given to immune individuals. In this reaction, an antigen administered into the skin of a previously immunized individual results in a detectable cutaneous reaction within 24 to 48 hours (hence the term *delayed*, in contrast to immediate hypersensitivity). Both T_H1 and T_H17 cells contribute to organ-specific diseases in which inflammation is a prominent aspect of the pathology. The inflammatory reaction associated with T_H1 cells is dominated by activated macrophages, and that triggered by T_H17 cells has a greater neutrophil component.

The inflammatory reactions stimulated by CD4+ T cells can be divided into sequential stages.

Activation of CD4+ T Cells. As described earlier, naive CD4+ T cells recognize peptides displayed by dendritic cells and secrete IL-2, which functions as an autocrine growth factor to stimulate proliferation of the antigen-responsive T cells. The subsequent differentiation of

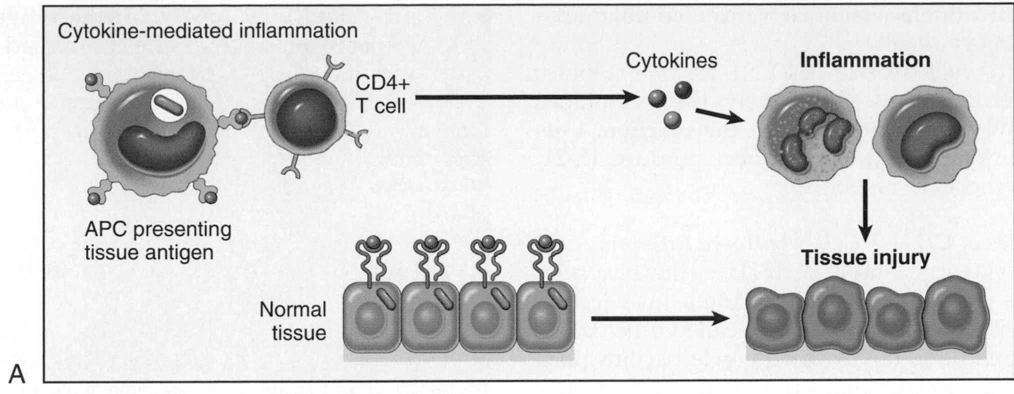

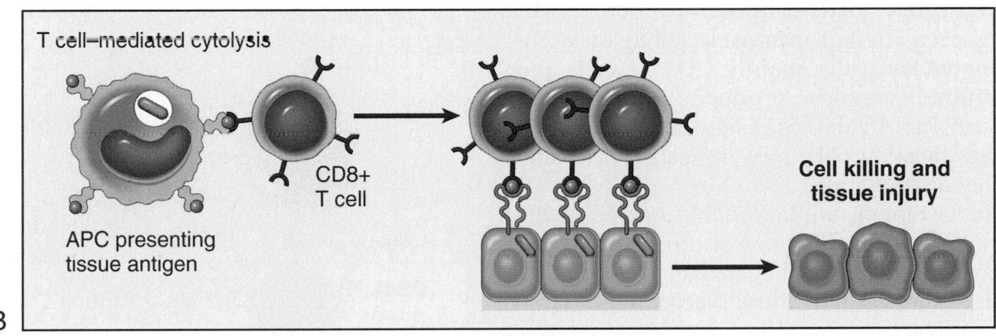

Figure 6-18 Mechanisms of T cell–mediated (type IV) hypersensitivity reactions. **A,** CD4+ T_H1 cells (and sometimes CD8+ T cells, not shown) respond to tissue antigens by secreting cytokines that stimulate inflammation and activate phagocytes, leading to tissue injury. CD4+ T_H17 cells contribute to inflammation by recruiting neutrophils (and, to a lesser extent, monocytes). **B,** In some diseases, CD8+ cytotoxic T lymphocytes (CTLs) directly kill tissue cells. APC, Antigen-presenting cell.

antigen-stimulated T cells to T_H1 or T_H17 cells is driven by the cytokines produced by APCs at the time of T-cell activation. In some situations the APCs (dendritic cells and macrophages) produce IL-12, which induces differentiation of CD4+ T cells to the T_H1 subset. IFN-γ produced by these effector cells promotes further T_H1 development, thus amplifying the reaction. If the APCs produce inflammatory cytokines such as IL-1, IL-6, and a close relative of IL-12 called *IL-23*, these stimulate differentiation of T cells to the T_H17 subset. Some of the differentiated effector cells enter the circulation and may remain in the memory pool of T cells for long periods, sometimes years.

Responses of Differentiated Effector T Cells. Upon repeat exposure to an antigen, T_H1 cells secrete cytokines, mainly IFN-γ, which are responsible for many of the manifestations of delayed-type hypersensitivity. IFN-γ-activated ("classically activated") macrophages are altered in several ways: their ability to phagocytose and kill microorganisms is markedly augmented; they express more class II MHC molecules on the surface, thus facilitating further antigen presentation; they secrete TNF, IL-1, and chemokines, which promote inflammation (Chapter 3); and they produce more IL-12, thereby amplifying the T_H1 response. Thus, activated macrophages serve to eliminate the offending

Table 6-5 T Cell–Mediated Diseases

Disease	Specificity of Pathogenic T Cells	Principal Mechanisms of Tissue Injury	Clinicopathologic Manifestations
Rheumatoid arthritis	Collagen? Citrullinated self proteins?	Inflammation mediated by T_H17 (and T_H1?) cytokines; role of antibodies and immune complexes?	Chronic arthritis with inflammation, destruction of articular cartilage
Multiple sclerosis	Protein antigens in myelin (e.g., myelin basic protein)	Inflammation mediated by T_H1 and T_H17 cytokines, myelin destruction by activated macrophages	Demyelination in CNS with perivascular inflammation; paralysis,
Type 1 diabetes mellitus	Antigens of pancreatic islet β cells (insulin, glutamic acid decarboxylase, others)	T cell–mediated inflammation, destruction of islet cells by CTLs	Insulitis (chronic inflammation in islets), destruction of β cells; diabetes
Inflammatory bowel disease	Enteric bacteria; self antigens?	Inflammation mediated by T_H1 and T_H17 cytokines	Chronic intestinal inflammation, obstruction
Psoriasis	Unknown	Inflammation mediated mainly by T_H17 cytokines	Destructive plaques in the skin
Contact sensitivity	Various environmental chemicals (e.g., urushiol from poison ivy or poison oak)	Inflammation mediated by T_H1 (and T_H17?) cytokines	Epidermal necrosis, dermal inflammation, causing skin rash and blisters

Examples of human T cell–mediated diseases are listed. In many cases, the specificity of the T cells and the mechanisms of tissue injury are inferred based on the similarity with experimental animal models of the diseases.

antigen; if the activation is sustained, continued inflammation and tissue injury result.

Activated T_H17 cells secrete IL-17, IL-22, chemokines, and several other cytokines. Collectively, these cytokines recruit neutrophils and monocytes to the reaction, thus promoting inflammation. T_H17 cells also produce IL-21, which amplifies the T_H17 response.

Clinical Examples of CD4+ T Cell–Mediated Inflammatory Reactions. The classic example of DTH is the *tuberculin reaction,* which is produced by the intracutaneous injection of purified protein derivative (PPD, also called tuberculin), a protein-containing antigen of the tubercle bacillus. In a previously sensitized individual, reddening and induration of the site appear in 8 to 12 hours, reach a peak in 24 to 72 hours, and thereafter slowly subside. Morphologically, delayed-type hypersensitivity is characterized by the accumulation of mononuclear cells, mainly CD4+ T cells and macrophages, around venules, producing perivascular "cuffing" (Fig. 6-19). In fully developed lesions, the venules show marked endothelial hypertrophy, reflecting cytokine-mediated endothelial activation.

With certain persistent or nondegradable antigens, such as tubercle bacilli colonizing the lungs or other tissues, the infiltrate is dominated by macrophages over a period of 2 or 3 weeks. With sustained activation, macrophages often undergo a morphologic transformation into *epithelioid cells,* large epithelium-like cells with abundant cytoplasm. A microscopic aggregation of epithelioid cells, usually surrounded by a collar of lymphocytes, is referred to as a *granuloma* (Fig. 6-20*A*). This pattern of inflammation, called *granulomatous inflammation* (Chapter 3), is typically associated with strong T_H1-cell activation and high-level production of cytokines such as IFN-γ (Fig. 6-20*B*). It can also be caused by indigestible foreign bodies, which activate macrophages without eliciting an adaptive immune response.

Contact dermatitis is a common example of tissue injury resulting from DTH reactions. It may be evoked by contact with urushiol, the antigenic component of poison ivy or poison oak, and presents as a vesicular dermatitis. It is thought that in these reactions, the environmental chemical binds to and structurally modifies some self proteins and peptides derived from these modified proteins are recognized by T cells and elicit the reaction. Chemicals may also modify HLA molecules, making them appear foreign to T cells. The same mechanism is responsible for most *drug reactions,* among the most common immunologic reactions

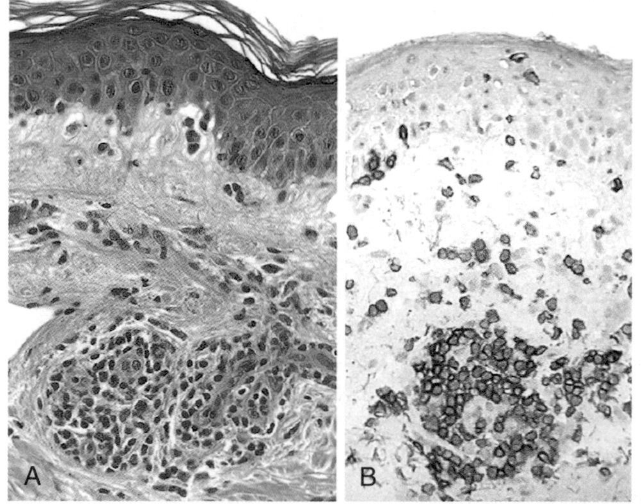

Figure 6-19 Delayed hypersensitivity reaction in the skin. **A,** Perivascular accumulation ("cuffing") of mononuclear inflammatory cells (lymphocytes and macrophages), with associated dermal edema and fibrin deposition. **B,** Immunoperoxidase staining reveals a predominantly perivascular cellular infiltrate that marks positively with anti-CD4 antibodies. (Courtesy Dr. Louis Picker, Department of Pathology, University of Texas Southwestern Medical School, Dallas, Texas.)

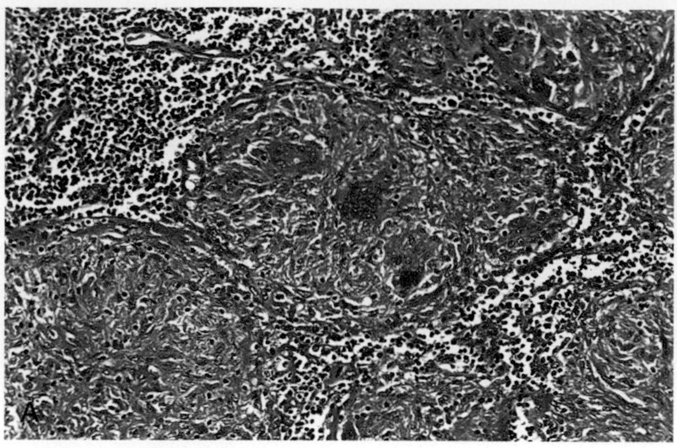

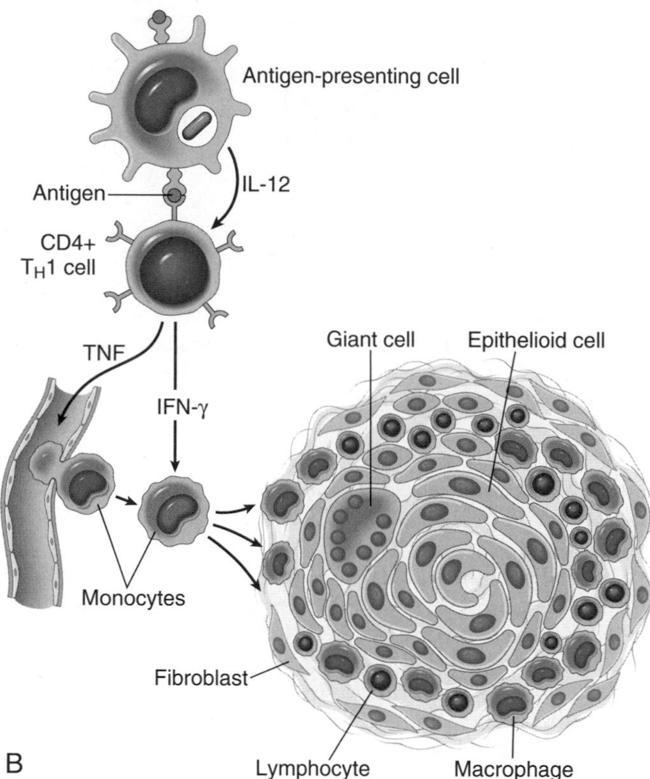

Figure 6-20 Granulomatous inflammation. **A,** A section of a lymph node shows several granulomas, each made up of an aggregate of epithelioid cells and surrounded by lymphocytes. The granuloma in the center shows several multinucleate giant cells. **B,** The events that give rise to the formation of granulomas in type IV hypersensitivity reactions, illustrating the role of T_H1 cytokines. In some granulomas (e.g., in schistosomiasis), T_H2 cells contribute to the lesions. The role of T_H17 cells in granuloma formation is not known. (**A,** Courtesy Dr. Trace Worrell, Department of Pathology, University of Texas Southwestern Medical School, Dallas, Texas.)

of humans. In these reactions, the drug (often a reactive chemical) alters self proteins, including MHC molecules, and the "neoantigens" are recognized as foreign by T cells, leading to cytokine production and inflammation. These often manifest as skin rashes.

CD4+ T cell–mediated inflammation is the basis of tissue injury in many organ-specific and systemic autoimmune diseases, such as rheumatoid arthritis and multiple sclerosis, as well as diseases probably caused by uncontrolled reactions to bacterial commensals, such as inflammatory bowel disease (Table 6-5).

CD8+ T Cell–Mediated Cytotoxicity

In this type of T cell–mediated reaction, CD8+ CTLs kill antigen-expressing target cells. Tissue destruction by CTLs may be an important component of some T cell–mediated diseases, such as type 1 diabetes. CTLs directed against cell surface histocompatibility antigens play an important role in graft rejection, to be discussed later. They also play a role in reactions against viruses. In a virus-infected cell, viral peptides are displayed by class I MHC molecules and the complex is recognized by the TCR of CD8+ T lymphocytes. The killing of infected cells leads to the elimination of the infection, but in some cases it is responsible for cell damage that accompanies the infection (e.g., in viral hepatitis). Tumor-associated antigens are also presented on the cell surface, and CTLs are involved in the host response to transformed cells (Chapter 7).

The principal mechanism of T cell–mediated killing of targets involves *perforins* and *granzymes*, preformed mediators contained in the lysosome-like granules of CTLs. CTLs that recognize the target cells secrete a complex consisting of perforin, granzymes, and other proteins which enters target cells by endocytosis. In the target cell cytoplasm, perforin facilitates the release of the granzymes from the complex. Granzymes are proteases that cleave and activate caspases, which induce apoptosis of the target cells (Chapter 2). Activated CTLs also express Fas ligand, a molecule with homology to TNF, which can bind to Fas expressed on target cells and trigger apoptosis.

CD8+ T cells also produce cytokines, notably IFN-γ, and are involved in inflammatory reactions resembling DTH, especially following virus infections and exposure to some contact sensitizing agents.

KEY CONCEPTS

Mechanisms of T Cell–Mediated Hypersensitivity Reactions

- Cytokine-mediated inflammation: CD4+ T cells are activated by exposure to a protein antigen and differentiate into T_H1 and T_H17 effector cells. Subsequent exposure to the antigen results in the secretion of cytokines. IFN-γ activates macrophages to produce substances that cause tissue damage and promote fibrosis, and IL-17 and other cytokines recruit leukocytes, thus promoting inflammation.
- The classical T cell–mediated inflammatory reaction is delayed type hypersensitivity.
- T cell–mediated cytotoxicity: CD8+ cytotoxic T lymphocytes (CTLs) specific for an antigen recognize cells expressing the target antigen and kill these cells. CD8+ T cells also secrete IFN-γ.

Now that we have described how the immune system can cause tissue damage, we turn to diseases in which normal control mechanisms fail. The prototypes of such diseases are autoimmune disorders, which are the result of failure of tolerance to self antigens.

Autoimmune Diseases

Immune reactions against self antigens—*autoimmunity*—are an important cause of certain diseases in humans, estimated to affect at least 1% to 2% of the US population. A growing number of diseases have been attributed to autoimmunity (Table 6-6). It should be noted, however, that the mere presence of autoantibodies does not indicate an autoimmune disease exists. Autoantibodies can be found in the serum of apparently normal individuals, particularly in older age groups. Furthermore, innocuous autoantibodies are sometimes produced after damage to tissues and may serve a physiologic role in the removal of tissue breakdown products. How, then, does one define *pathologic autoimmunity*? Ideally, at least three requirements should be met before a disorder is categorized as truly caused by autoimmunity: (1) the presence of an immune reaction specific for some self antigen or self tissue; (2) evidence that such a reaction is not secondary to tissue damage but is of primary pathogenic significance; and (3) the absence of another well-defined cause of the disease. Similarity with experimental models of proven autoimmunity is also often used to support this mechanism in human diseases. Disorders in which chronic inflammation is a prominent component are sometimes grouped under *immune-mediated inflammatory diseases*; these may be autoimmune, or the immune

Table 6-6 Autoimmune Diseases

Organ-Specific	Systemic
Diseases Mediated by Antibodies	
Autoimmune hemolytic anemia	Systemic lupus erythematosus
Autoimmune thrombocytopenia	
Autoimmune atrophic gastritis of pernicious anemia	
Myasthenia gravis	
Graves disease	
Goodpasture syndrome	
Diseases Mediated by T Cells*	
Type 1 diabetes mellitus	Rheumatoid arthritis
Multiple sclerosis	Systemic sclerosis (scleroderma)† Sjögren syndrome†
Diseases Postulated to Be Autoimmune	
Inflammatory bowel diseases (Crohn disease, ulcerative colitis)‡	
Primary biliary cirrhosis†	Polyarteritis nodosa†
Autoimmune (chronic active) hepatitis	Inflammatory myopathies†

*A role for T cells has been demonstrated in these disorders, but antibodies may also be involved in tissue injury.
†An autoimmune basis of these disorders is suspected but the supporting evidence is not strong.
‡These disorders may result from excessive immune responses to commensal enteric microbes, autoimmunity, or a combination of the two.

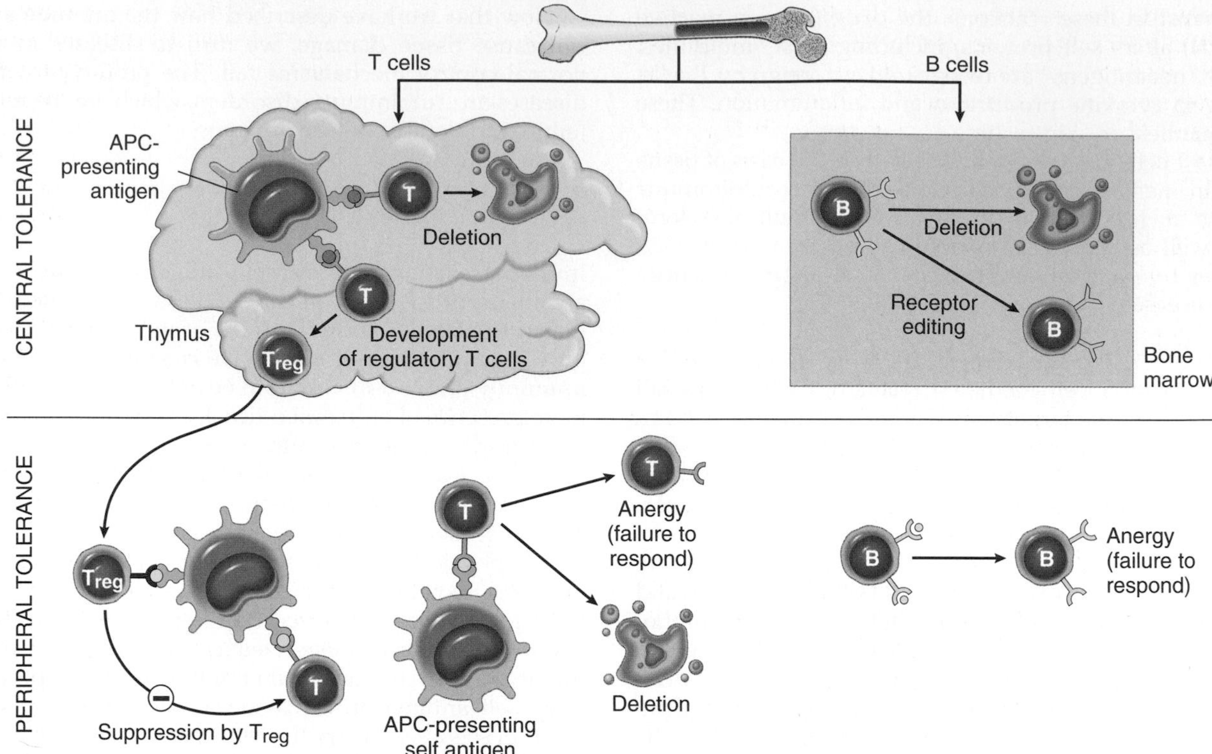

Figure 6-21 Mechanisms of immunologic tolerance to self antigens. The principal mechanisms of central and peripheral self-tolerance in T and B cells are illustrated. APC, Antigen-presenting cell.

response may be directed against normally harmless microbes such as gut commensal bacteria.

The clinical manifestations of autoimmune disorders are extremely varied. On one end are conditions in which the immune responses are directed against a single organ or tissue, resulting in *organ-specific disease*, and on the other end are diseases in which the autoimmune reactions are against widespread antigens, resulting in *systemic* or *generalized disease*. Examples of organ-specific autoimmune diseases are type 1 diabetes mellitus, in which the autoreactive T cells and antibodies are specific for β cells of the pancreatic islets, and multiple sclerosis, in which autoreactive T cells react against central nervous system myelin. The best example of systemic autoimmune disease is SLE, in which a diversity of antibodies directed against DNA, platelets, red cells, and protein-phospholipid complexes result in widespread lesions throughout the body. In the middle of the spectrum falls Goodpasture syndrome, in which antibodies to basement membranes of lung and kidney induce lesions in these organs.

It is obvious that autoimmunity results from the loss of self-tolerance, and the question arises as to how this happens. Before we look for answers to this question, we review the mechanisms of immunologic tolerance to self antigens.

Immunologic Tolerance

Immunologic tolerance is the phenomenon of unresponsiveness to an antigen induced by exposure of lymphocytes to that antigen. *Self-tolerance* refers to lack of responsiveness to an individual's own antigens, and it underlies our ability to live in harmony with our cells and tissues. Because the antigen receptors of lymphocytes are generated by somatic recombination of genes in a random fashion, lymphocytes with receptors capable of recognizing self antigens are generated constantly, and these cells have to be eliminated or inactivated as soon as they recognize self antigens, to prevent them from causing harm.

The mechanisms of self-tolerance can be broadly classified into two groups: central tolerance and peripheral tolerance (Fig. 6-21). Each of these is considered briefly.

Central Tolerance

In this process, immature self-reactive T and B lymphocyte clones that recognize self antigens during their maturation in the central (or generative) lymphoid organs (the thymus for T cells and the bone marrow for B cells) are killed or rendered harmless. The mechanisms of central tolerance in T and B cells show some similarities and differences.

- In developing T cells, random somatic gene rearrangements generate diverse TCRs. Such antigen-independent TCR generation produces many lymphocytes that express high-affinity receptors for self antigens. When immature lymphocytes encounter the antigens in the thymus, many of the cells die by apoptosis. This process, called *negative selection* or *deletion*, is responsible for eliminating self-reactive lymphocytes from the T-cell pool. A wide variety of autologous protein antigens, including antigens thought to be restricted to peripheral tissues, are processed and presented by thymic antigen-presenting cells in association with self MHC molecules and can, therefore, be recognized by potentially self-reactive T cells. A protein called AIRE (autoimmune regulator) stimulates expression of some "peripheral tissue-restricted" self antigens in the thymus and is thus critical for deletion of immature T cells specific for these antigens. Mutations in the *AIRE* gene are the cause of an autoimmune polyendocrinopathy (Chapter 24). In the CD4+ T-cell lineage, some of the cells that see self antigens in the thymus do not die but develop into regulatory T cells (described later).

- When developing B cells strongly recognize self antigens in the bone marrow, many of the cells reactivate the machinery of antigen receptor gene rearrangement and begin to express new antigen receptors, not specific for self antigens. This process is called *receptor editing;* it is estimated that a quarter to half of all B cells in the body may have undergone receptor editing during their maturation. If receptor editing does not occur, the self-reactive cells undergo apoptosis, thus purging potentially dangerous lymphocytes from the mature pool.

Central tolerance, however, is imperfect. Not all self antigens may be present in the thymus, and hence T cells bearing receptors for such autoantigens escape into the periphery. There is similar "slippage" in the B-cell system. Self-reactive lymphocytes that escape negative selection can inflict tissue injury unless they are deleted or muzzled in the peripheral tissues.

Peripheral Tolerance

Several mechanisms silence potentially autoreactive T and B cells in peripheral tissues; these are best defined for T cells. These mechanisms include the following:

- **Anergy. Lymphocytes that recognize self antigens may be rendered functionally unresponsive, a phenomenon called *anergy.*** We discussed earlier that activation of antigen-specific T cells requires two signals: recognition of peptide antigen in association with self MHC molecules on the surface of APCs and a set of costimulatory signals ("second signals") from APCs. These second signals are provided by certain T cell-associated molecules, such as CD28, that bind to their ligands (the costimulators B7-1 and B7-2) on APCs. If the antigen is presented to T cells without adequate levels of costimulators, the cells become anergic. Because costimulatory molecules are not expressed or are weakly expressed on resting dendritic cells in normal tissues, the encounter between autoreactive T cells and their specific self antigens displayed by these dendritic cells may lead to anergy. Several mechanisms of T-cell anergy have been demonstrated in various experimental systems. One of these, which has clinical implications, is that T cells that recognize self antigens receive an inhibitory signal from receptors that are structurally homologous to CD28 but serve the opposite functions. Two of these inhibitory receptors are CTLA-4, which (like CD28) binds to B7 molecules, and PD-1, which binds to two ligands that are expressed on a wide variety of cells. Because CTLA-4 has higher affinity for B7 molecules than does CD28, CTLA-4 may be preferentially engaged when the levels of B7 are low, as when APCs are presenting self antigens. Conversely, microbial products elicit innate immune reactions, during which B7 levels on APCs increase and the low-affinity receptor CD28 is engaged more. Thus, the affinities of the activating and inhibitory receptors and the level of expression of B7 may determine the outcome of T cell antigen recognition. The importance of these inhibitory mechanisms has been established by the finding that mice in which the gene encoding CTLA-4 or PD-1 is knocked out develop autoimmune diseases. Furthermore, polymorphisms in the *CTLA4* gene are associated with some autoimmune endocrine diseases in humans. Interestingly, some tumors and viruses may use the same pathways of immune regulation to evade immune attack. This realization has led to the development of antibodies that block CTLA-4 and PD-1 for tumor immunotherapy—by removing the brakes on the immune response, these antibodies promote responses against tumors.

  Anergy also affects mature B cells in peripheral tissues. It is believed that if B cells encounter self antigen in peripheral tissues, especially in the absence of specific helper T cells, the B cells become unable to respond to subsequent antigenic stimulation and may be excluded from lymphoid follicles, resulting in their death. B lymphocytes also express inhibitory receptors that may play a role in limiting their activation and preventing responses to self antigens.

- **Suppression by regulatory T cells. A population of T cells called *regulatory T cells* functions to prevent immune reactions against self antigens.** Regulatory T cells develop mainly in the thymus, as a result of recognition of self antigens (Fig. 6-21), but they may also be induced in peripheral lymphoid tissues. The best-defined regulatory T cells are CD4+ cells that express high levels of CD25, the α chain of the IL-2 receptor, and a transcription factor of the forkhead family, called FOXP3. Both IL-2 and FOXP3 are required for the development and maintenance of functional CD4+ regulatory T cells. Mutations in *FOXP3* result in severe autoimmunity in humans and mice; in humans these mutations are the cause of a systemic autoimmune disease called *IPEX* (an acronym for *i*mmune dysregulation, *p*olyendocrinopathy, *e*nteropathy, *X*-linked). In mice knockout of the gene encoding IL-2 or the IL-2 receptor α or β chain also results in severe multi-organ autoimmunity, because IL-2 is essential for the maintenance of regulatory T cells. Recent genome-wide association studies have revealed that polymorphisms in the *CD25* gene are associated with multiple sclerosis and other autoimmune diseases, raising the possibility of a regulatory T-cell defect contributing to these diseases. The mechanisms by which regulatory T cells suppress immune responses are not fully defined, but their inhibitory activity may be mediated in part by the secretion of immunosuppressive cytokines such as IL-10 and TGF-β, which inhibit lymphocyte activation and effector functions. Regulatory T cells also express CTLA-4, which may bind to B7 molecules on APCs and reduce their ability to activate T cells via CD28.

  Regulatory T cells may play a role in the acceptance of the fetus. Placental mammals face a unique challenge because the developing fetus expresses paternal antigens that are foreign to the mother yet have to be tolerated. There is emerging evidence that regulatory T cells prevent immune reactions against fetal antigens that are inherited from the father and therefore foreign to the mother. In line with this idea, during evolution, placentation appeared simultaneously with the ability to stably express the Foxp3 transcription factor. Experiments in mice have shown that fetal antigens induce long-lived Foxp3+ regulatory T cells, and depletion of these cells results in fetal loss. There is great interest in determining the contribution of regulatory T cells in human pregnancy and possible defects in these cells as the basis for recurrent spontaneous abortions.

- **Deletion by apoptosis. T cells that recognize self antigens may receive signals that promote their death by apoptosis.** Two mechanisms of deletion of mature T cells have been proposed, based mainly on studies in mice. It is postulated that if T cells recognize self antigens, they may express a pro-apoptotic member of the Bcl family, called Bim, without antiapoptotic members of the family like Bcl-2 and Bcl-x (whose induction requires the full set of signals for lymphocyte activation). Unopposed Bim triggers apoptosis by the mitochondrial pathway (Chapter 2). A second mechanism of activation-induced death of CD4+ T cells and B cells involves the Fas-Fas ligand system. Lymphocytes as well as many other cells express the death receptor Fas (CD95), a member of the TNF-receptor family. Fas ligand (FasL), a membrane protein that is structurally homologous to the cytokine TNF, is expressed mainly on activated T lymphocytes. The engagement of Fas by FasL induces apoptosis of activated T cells (Chapter 2). It is postulated that if self antigens engage antigen receptors of self-reactive T cells, Fas and FasL are co-expressed, leading to elimination of the cells via Fas-mediated apoptosis. Self-reactive B cells may also be deleted by FasL on T cells engaging Fas on the B cells. The importance of this mechanism in the peripheral deletion of autoreactive lymphocytes is highlighted by two mice that are natural mutants of Fas or FasL. These mice develop an autoimmune disease somewhat resembling human SLE, associated with generalized lymphoproliferation. In humans a similar disease is caused by mutations in the *FAS* gene; it is called the *autoimmune lymphoproliferative syndrome (ALPS).*

Some antigens are hidden (sequestered) from the immune system, because the tissues in which these antigens are located do not communicate with the blood and lymph. As a result, self antigens in these tissues fail to elicit immune responses and are essentially ignored by the immune system. This is believed to be the case for the testis, eye, and brain, all of which are called *immune-privileged sites* because it is difficult to induce immune responses to antigens introduced into these sites. If the antigens of these tissues are released, for example, as a consequence of trauma or infection, the result may be an immune response that leads to prolonged tissue inflammation and injury. This is the postulated mechanism for post-traumatic orchitis and uveitis.

Mechanisms of Autoimmunity: General Principles

The immune system normally exists in an equilibrium in which lymphocyte activation, which is required for defense against pathogens, is balanced by the mechanisms of tolerance, which prevent reactions against self antigens. The underlying cause of autoimmune diseases is the failure of tolerance, which allows responses to develop against self antigens. Understanding why tolerance fails in these diseases is an important goal of immunologists.

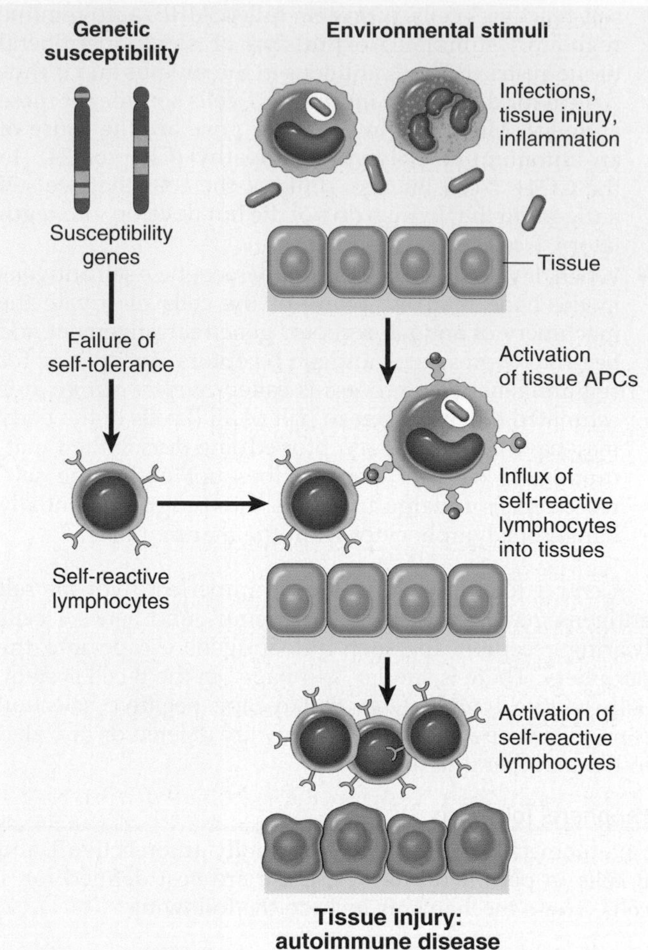

Figure 6-22 Pathogenesis of autoimmunity. Autoimmunity results from multiple factors, including susceptibility genes that may interfere with self-tolerance and environmental triggers (such as infections, tissue injury, and inflammation) that promote lymphocyte entry into tissues, activation of self-reactive lymphocytes, and tissue damage.

Autoimmunity arises from a combination of the inheritance of susceptibility genes, which may contribute to the breakdown of self-tolerance, and environmental triggers, such as infections and tissue damage, which promote the activation of self-reactive lymphocytes (Fig. 6-22). The genetics, as well as the gene-environment interactions, are complex and difficult to dissect, because of which much remains unknown about the enigma of autoimmunity. Nevertheless, some interesting clues have begun to emerge with the development of better technologies for defining genetic susceptibility and for studying patients.

It is thought that susceptibility genes and environmental triggers induce a number of changes that contribute to the development of autoimmunity:

- **Defective tolerance or regulation.** Fundamental to the development of autoimmune diseases is a failure of the mechanisms that maintain self-tolerance. As discussed later, some clues about how these mechanisms might be disrupted have come from the analysis of patients with rare inherited autoimmune disorders and from gene knockout mice that develop autoimmune lesions. However, despite the advances in understanding mechanisms of immune tolerance and regulation, it is not known why these may become defective in the majority of common autoimmune diseases.

- **Abnormal display of self antigens.** Abnormalities may include increased expression and persistence of self antigens that are normally cleared, or structural changes in these antigens resulting from enzymatic modifications or from cellular stress or injury. If these changes lead to the display of antigenic epitopes that are not expressed normally, the immune system may not be tolerant to these epitopes, thus allowing anti-self responses to develop.
- **Inflammation or an initial innate immune response.** As discussed earlier, the innate immune response is a strong stimulus for the subsequent activation of lymphocytes and the generation of adaptive immune responses. Microbes or cell injury may elicit local inflammatory reactions resembling innate immune responses, and these may be critical inducers of the autoimmune disease.

Although these are appealing hypotheses, which of these abnormalities actually play a role in a specific autoimmune disease in humans remains largely a matter of speculation.

Role of Susceptibility Genes

Most autoimmune diseases are complex multigenic disorders. It has been known for decades that autoimmunity has a genetic component. The incidence of many autoimmune diseases is greater in twins of affected individuals than in the general population, and greater in monozygotic than in dizygotic twins, proof that genetics contributes to the development of these disorders.

Association of HLA Alleles with Disease. **Among the genes known to be associated with autoimmunity, the greatest contribution is that of HLA genes** (Table 6-7). The most striking of these associations is between ankylosing spondylitis and *HLA-B27*; individuals who inherit this class I HLA allele have a 100-200 fold greater chance (odds ratio, or relative risk) of developing the disease compared with those who do not carry *HLA-B27*. Many autoimmune diseases are associated with different class II *HLA* alleles. Although it is reasonable to postulate that these associations reflect the ability of some HLA molecules to display self peptides, it has been difficult to show that disease-associated HLA molecules do so any better or worse than molecules that are not associated with autoimmunity. Thus, the mechanisms underlying these disease associations remain poorly understood. It is also important to understand that different HLA alleles may contribute to a disease but their presence is not, by itself, the cause of any disease. Thus, in the example of HLA-B27, the vast majority of individuals who inherit this allele never develop ankylosing spondylitis.

Table 6-7 Association of HLA Alleles and Inflammatory Diseases

Disease	HLA allele	Odds Ratio[†]
Rheumatoid arthritis (anti-CCP Ab positive)[‡]	DRB1, 1 SE allele[¶] DRB1, 2 SE alleles	4 12
Type 1 diabetes	DRB1*0301-DQA1*0501-DQB1*0201 haplotype DRB1*0401-DQA1*0301-DQB1*0302 haplotype DRB1*0301/0401 haplotype heterozygotes	4 8 35
Multiple sclerosis	DRB1*1501	3
Systemic lupus erythematosus	DRB1*0301 DRB1*1501	2 1.3
Ankylosing spondylitis	B*27 (mainly B*2705 and B*2702)	100-200
Celiac disease	DQA1*0501 DQB1*0201 haplotype	7

[†]The odds ratio reflects approximate values of increased risk of the disease associated with the inheritance of particular HLA alleles. The data are from European-derived populations.
[‡]Anti-CCP Ab = antibodies directed against cyclic citrullinated peptides. Data are from patients who test positive for these antibodies in the serum.
[¶]SE refers to shared epitope, so called because the susceptibility alleles map to one region of the DRB1 protein (positions 70-74).
Courtesy Dr. Michelle Fernando, Imperial College London.

In addition to autoimmune diseases, some inherited errors of metabolism, such as 21-hydroxylase deficiency and hereditary hemochromatosis, are also associated with particular HLA alleles (*HLA-BW47* and *HLA-A*, respectively). However, in these cases, the mutated genes causing 21-hydroxylase deficiency and hereditary hemochromatosis happen by chance to be located in the MHC locus, and the linked HLA alleles are innocent bystanders that are not culpable in either of these diseases.

Association of Non-MHC Genes with Autoimmune Diseases. Genome-wide association studies and family studies have shown that multiple non-MHC genes are associated with various autoimmune diseases (Table 6-8). Some of these genes are disease-specific, but many of the associations are seen in multiple disorders, suggesting that the products of these genes affect general mechanisms of immune regulation and self-tolerance. Three recently described genetic associations are especially interesting.

- Polymorphisms in a gene called *PTPN22*, which encodes a protein tyrosine phosphatase, are associated with rheumatoid arthritis, type 1 diabetes, and several other autoimmune diseases. Because these disorders have a fairly high prevalence (especially rheumatoid arthritis), *PTPN22* is said to be the gene that is most frequently implicated in autoimmunity. It is postulated that the disease-associated variants encode a phosphatase that is functionally defective and is thus unable to fully control the activity of tyrosine kinases, which are involved in many responses of lymphocytes and other cells. The net result is excessive lymphocyte activation.
- Polymorphisms in the gene for *NOD2* are associated with Crohn disease, a form of inflammatory bowel disease, especially in certain ethnic populations. NOD2, a member of the NOD-like receptor (NLR) family (discussed earlier), is a cytoplasmic sensor of microbes that is expressed in intestinal epithelial and other cells. According to one hypothesis, the disease-associated

Table 6-8 Selected Non–HLA Genes Associated with Autoimmune Diseases

Putative Gene Involved	Diseases	Postulated Function of Encoded Protein and Role of Mutation/Polymorphism in Disease
Genes involved in immune regulation:		
PTPN22	RA, T1D, IBD	Protein tyrosine phosphatase, may affect signaling in lymphocytes and may alter negative selection or activation of self-reactive T cells
IL23R	IBD, PS, AS	Receptor for the T_H17-inducing cytokine IL-23; may alter differentiation of CD4+ T cells into pathogenic $T_H17$effector cells
CTLA4	T1D, RA	Inhibits T cell responses by terminating activation and promoting activity of regulatory T cells; may interfere with self-tolerance
IL2RA	MS, T1D	α chain of the receptor for IL-2, which is a growth and survival factor for activated and regulatory T cells; may affect development of effector cells and/or regulation of immune responses
Genes involved in immune responses to microbes:		
NOD2	IBD	Cytoplasmic sensor of bacteria expressed in Paneth and other intestinal epithelial cells; may control resistance to gut commensal bacteria
ATG16	IBD	Involved in autophagy; possible role in defense against microbes and maintenance of epithelial barrier function
IRF5, IFIH1	SLE	Role in type I interferon production; type I IFN is involved in the pathogenesis of SLE (see text)

AS, Ankylosing spondylitis; IBD, inflammatory bowel disease; MS, multiple sclerosis; PS, psoriasis; RA, rheumatoid arthritis; SLE, systemic lupus erythematosus.
The probable linkage of these genes with various autoimmune diseases has been defined by genome-wide association studies (GWAS) and other methods for studying disease-associated polymorphisms.
Adapted from Zenewicz LA, Abraham C, Flavell RA, Cho JH: Unraveling the genetics of autoimmunity. Cell 2010;140:791.

variant is ineffective at sensing gut microbes, including commensal bacteria, resulting in entry of and chronic inflammatory responses against these normally well-tolerated organisms.

- Polymorphisms in the genes encoding the *IL-2 receptor (CD25)* and *IL-7 receptor* α chains are associated with multiple sclerosis and other autoimmune diseases. These cytokines may control the maintenance of regulatory T cells.

Many other polymorphisms have been described in particular autoimmune diseases, and we will mention some of these when we describe specific disorders. Although these genetic associations are beginning to reveal interesting clues about pathogenesis, the links between the genes, functions of their encoded proteins, and the diseases remain to be established.

We have previously mentioned that in mice and humans, gene knockouts and natural mutations affecting several individual genes result in autoimmunity. These genes include *AIRE, CTLA4, PD1, FAS, FASL,* and *IL2* and its receptor *CD25*. In addition, B cells express an Fc receptor that recognizes IgG antibodies bound to antigens and switches off further antibody production (a normal negative-feedback mechanism). Knockout of this receptor results in autoimmunity, presumably because the B cells can no longer be controlled. These examples provide valuable information about pathways of self-tolerance and immune regulation, but the diseases caused by these single gene mutations are rare and mutations in these genes are not the cause of most common autoimmune disorders.

Role of Infections

Autoimmune reactions may be triggered by infections. Two mechanisms have been postulated to explain the link between infections and autoimmunity (Fig. 6-23). First, infections may upregulate the expression of costimulators on APCs. If these cells are presenting self antigens, the result may be a breakdown of anergy and activation of T cells specific for the self antigens. Second, some microbes may express antigens that have the same amino acid sequences as self antigens. Immune responses against the microbial antigens may result in the activation of self-reactive lymphocytes. This phenomenon is called *molecular mimicry*. A clear example of such mimicry is rheumatic heart disease, in which antibodies against streptococcal proteins cross-react with myocardial proteins and cause myocarditis (Chapter 12). More subtle molecular mimicry may be involved in classic autoimmune diseases as well.

Microbes may induce other abnormalities that promote autoimmune reactions. Some viruses, such as Epstein-Barr virus (EBV) and HIV, cause polyclonal B-cell activation, which may result in production of autoantibodies. The tissue injury that is common in infections may release self antigens and structurally alter these antigens so that they are able to activate T cells that would not be tolerant to these new, modified antigens. Infections may induce the production of cytokines that recruit lymphocytes, including potentially self-reactive lymphocytes, to sites of self antigens.

Infections may protect against some autoimmune diseases. Although the role of infections in triggering autoimmunity has received a great deal of attention, recent epidemiologic studies suggest that the incidence of autoimmune diseases is increasing in developed countries as infections are better controlled. In some animal models (e.g., of type 1 diabetes) infections greatly reduce the incidence of disease. The underlying mechanisms are unclear; one possibility is that infections promote low-level IL-2 production, and this is essential for maintaining regulatory T cells.

Recently, there has been great interest in the idea that the normal gut and skin microbiome influences the development of autoimmunity. It is possible that different nonpathogenic microbes affect the relative proportions of effector and regulatory T cells, and shape the host response towards or away from aberrant activation. However, it is still not clear which microbes actually contribute to specific diseases in humans, or if the microbiome can be manipulated to prevent or treat these disorders.

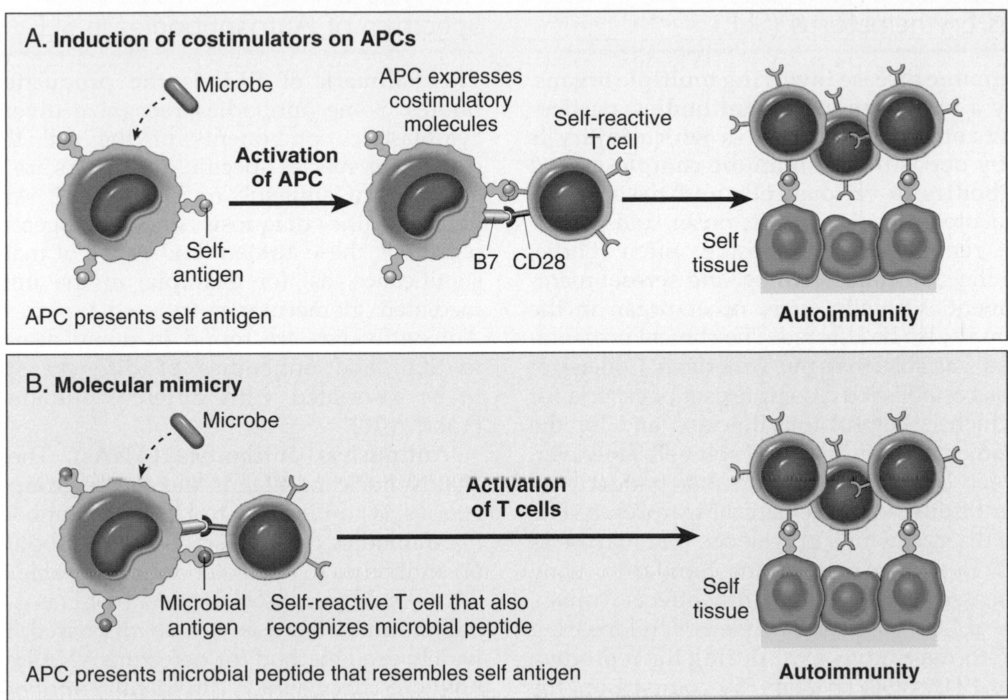

Figure 6-23 Postulated role of infections in autoimmunity. Infections may promote activation of self-reactive lymphocytes by inducing the expression of costimulators **(A),** or microbial antigens may mimic self antigens and activate self-reactive lymphocytes as a cross-reaction **(B).**

KEY CONCEPTS

Immunologic Tolerance and Autoimmunity

- Tolerance (unresponsiveness) to self antigens is a fundamental property of the immune system, and breakdown of tolerance is the basis of autoimmune diseases.
- Central tolerance: immature lymphocytes that recognize self antigens in the central (generative) lymphoid organs are killed by apoptosis; in the B-cell lineage, some of the self-reactive lymphocytes switch to new antigen receptors that are not self-reactive.
- Peripheral tolerance: mature lymphocytes that recognize self antigens in peripheral tissues become functionally inactive (anergic), or are suppressed by regulatory T lymphocytes, or die by apoptosis.
- The factors that lead to a failure of self-tolerance and the development of autoimmunity include (1) inheritance of susceptibility genes that may disrupt different tolerance pathways, and (2) infections and tissue injury that may expose self antigens and activate APCs and lymphocytes in the tissues.
- Autoimmune diseases are usually chronic and progressive, and the type of tissue injury is determined by the nature of the dominant immune response.

General Features of Autoimmune Diseases

Diseases caused by autoimmunity have some important general features.

- **Autoimmune diseases tend to be chronic, sometimes with relapses and remissions, and the damage is often progressive.** One reason for the chronicity is that the immune system contains many intrinsic amplification loops that allow small numbers of antigen-specific lymphocytes to accomplish their task of eradicating complex infections. When the response is inappropriately directed against self tissues, the same amplification mechanisms exacerbate and prolong the injury. Another reason for the persistence and progression of autoimmune disease is the phenomenon of *epitope spreading*, in which an immune response against one self antigen causes tissue damage, releasing other antigens, and resulting in the activation of lymphocytes by these newly encountered epitopes.
- **The clinical and pathologic manifestations of an autoimmune disease are determined by the nature of the underlying immune response.** Some of these diseases are caused by autoantibodies, whose formation may be associated with dysregulated germinal center reactions. Most chronic inflammatory diseases are caused by abnormal and excessive T_H1 and T_H17 responses; examples of these diseases include psoriasis, multiple sclerosis, and some types of inflammatory bowel disease. CD8+ CTLs contribute to killing of cells, such as islet β cells in type 1 diabetes. In some autoimmune diseases, such as rheumatoid arthritis, both antibodies and T cell–mediated inflammation may be involved.

With this background we can proceed to a discussion of specific autoimmune diseases. Table 6-6 lists both systemic and organ-specific autoimmune disorders. The systemic diseases tend to involve blood vessels and connective tissues, and therefore, they are often called *collagen vascular diseases* or *connective tissue diseases*. Our focus here is on selected systemic autoimmune diseases; organ-specific disorders are covered elsewhere in the book.

Systemic Lupus Erythematosus (SLE)

SLE is an autoimmune disease involving multiple organs, characterized by a vast array of autoantibodies, particularly antinuclear antibodies (ANAs), in which injury is caused mainly by deposition of immune complexes and binding of antibodies to various cells and tissues. The disease may be acute or insidious in its onset, and is typically a chronic, remitting and relapsing, often febrile, illness. Injury to the skin, joints, kidney, and serosal membranes is prominent. Virtually every other organ in the body, however, may also be affected. The clinical presentation of SLE is so variable that the American College of Rheumatology has established a complex set of criteria for this disorder, which is helpful for clinicians and for the design and assessment of clinical trials (Table 6-9). However, the disease is very heterogeneous, and any patient may present with any number of these clinical features. SLE is a fairly common disease, with a prevalence that may be as high as 1 in 2500 in certain populations. Similar to many autoimmune diseases, SLE predominantly affects women, with a frequency of 1 in 700 among women of childbearing age and a female-to-male ratio of 9:1 during the reproductive age group of 17 through 55 years. By comparison, the female-to-male ratio is only 2:1 for disease developing during childhood or after the age of 65. The prevalence of the disease is 2- to 3-fold higher in blacks and Hispanics than in whites. Although SLE often presents in the 20s and 30s, it may manifest at any age, even in early childhood.

Spectrum of Autoantibodies in SLE

The hallmark of SLE is the production of autoantibodies. Some antibodies recognize diverse nuclear and cytoplasmic components of the cell that are neither organ- nor species-specific, and others are directed against cell surface antigens of blood cells. Apart from their value in the diagnosis and management of patients with SLE, these autoantibodies are of major pathogenetic significance, as, for example, in the immune complex-mediated glomerulonephritis so typical of this disease. Autoantibodies are found in many diseases in addition to SLE, and antibodies of different specificities tend to be associated with different autoimmune disorders (Table 6-10).

Antinuclear antibodies (ANAs). These are directed against nuclear antigens and can be grouped into four categories: (1) antibodies to DNA, (2) antibodies to histones, (3) antibodies to nonhistone proteins bound to RNA, and (4) antibodies to nucleolar antigens. Table 6-10 lists several ANAs and their association with SLE as well as with other autoimmune diseases to be discussed later. The most widely used method for detecting ANAs is indirect immunofluorescence, which can identify antibodies that bind to a variety of nuclear antigens, including DNA, RNA, and proteins (collectively called *generic ANAs*). The pattern of nuclear fluorescence suggests the type of antibody present in the patient's serum. Four basic patterns are recognized (Fig. 6-24):

Table 6-9 1997 Revised Criteria for Classification of Systemic Lupus Erythematosus*

Criterion	Definition
1. Malar rash	Fixed erythema, flat or raised, over the malar eminences, tending to spare the nasolabial folds
2. Discoid rash	Erythematous raised patches with adherent keratotic scaling and follicular plugging; atrophic scarring may occur in older lesions
3. Photosensitivity	Rash as a result of unusual reaction to sunlight, by patient history or physician observation
4. Oral ulcers	Oral or nasopharyngeal ulceration, usually painless, observed by a physician
5. Arthritis	Nonerosive arthritis involving two or more peripheral joints, characterized by tenderness, swelling, or effusion
6. Serositis	Pleuritis—convincing history of pleuritic pain or rub heard by a physician or evidence of pleural effusion, or Pericarditis—documented by electrocardiogram or rub or evidence of pericardial effusion
7. Renal disorder	Persistent proteinuria >0.5 g/dL or >3 if quantitation not performed or Cellular casts—may be red blood cell, hemoglobin, granular, tubular, or mixed
8. Neurologic disorder	Seizures—in the absence of offending drugs or known metabolic derangements (e.g., uremia, ketoacidosis, or electrolyte imbalance), or Psychosis—in the absence of offending drugs or known metabolic derangements (e.g., uremia, ketoacidosis, or electrolyte imbalance)
9. Hematologic disorder	Hemolytic anemia—with reticulocytosis, or Leukopenia—$<4.0 \times 10^9$ cells/L (4000 cells/mm^3) total on two or more occasions, or Lymphopenia—$<1.5 \times 10^9$ cells/L (1500 cells/mm^3) on two or more occasions, or Thrombocytopenia—$<100 \times 10^9$ cells/L (100×10^3 cells/mm^3) in the absence of offending drugs
10. Immunologic disorder	Anti-DNA antibody to native DNA in abnormal titer, or Anti-Sm—presence of antibody to Sm nuclear antigen, or Positive finding of antiphospholipid antibodies based on (1) an abnormal serum level of IgG or IgM anticardiolipin antibodies, (2) a positive test for lupus anticoagulant using a standard test, or (3) a false-positive serologic test for syphilis known to be positive for at least 6 months and confirmed by negative *Treponema pallidum* immobilization or fluorescent treponemal antibody absorption test
11. Antinuclear antibody	An abnormal titer of antinuclear antibody by immunofluorescence or an equivalent assay at any point in time and in the absence of drugs known to be associated with drug-induced lupus syndrome

*This classification, based on 11 criteria, was proposed for the purpose of identifying patients in clinical studies. A person is said to have SLE if any four or more of the 11 criteria are present, serially or simultaneously, during any period of observation.

From Tan EM, et al: The revised criteria for the classification of systemic lupus erythematosus. Arthritis Rheum 1982;25:1271; and Hochberg MC: Updating the American College of Rheumatology revised criteria for the classification of systemic lupus erythematosus. Arthritis Rheum 1997;40:1725.

Table 6-10 Autoantibodies in Systemic Autoimmune Diseases

Disease	Specificity of Autoantibody	% Positive	Association with Specific Disease Features
Systemic lupus erythematosus (SLE)	Double-stranded DNA	40-60	Nephritis; specific for SLE
	U1-RNP	30-40	
	Smith (Sm) antigen (core protein of small RNP particles)	20-30	Specific for SLE
	Ro (SS-A)/La (SS-B) nucleoproteins	30-50	Congenital heart block; neonatal lupus
	Phospholipid-protein complexes (anti-PL)	30-40	Antiphospholipid syndrome (in ~10% of SLE patients)
	Multiple nuclear antigens ("generic ANAs")	95-100	Found in other autoimmune diseases, not specific.
Systemic sclerosis	DNA topoisomerase 1	30-70	Diffuse skin disease, lung disease; specific for systemic sclerosis
	Centromeric proteins (CENPs) A, B, C	20-40	Limited skin disease, ischemic digital loss, pulmonary hypertension
	RNA polymerase III	15-20	Acute onset, scleroderma renal crisis, cancer
Sjögren syndrome	Ro/SS-A La/SS-B	70-95	
Autoimmune myositis	Histidyl aminoacyl-tRNA synthetase, Jo1	25	Interstitial lung disease, Raynaud phenomenon
	Mi-2 nuclear antigen	5-10	Dermatomyositis, skin rash
	MDA5 (cytoplasmic receptor for viral RNA)	20-35 (Japanese)	Vascular skin lesions, interstitial lung disease
	TIF1γ nuclear protein	15-20	Dermatomyositis, cancer
Rheumatoid arthritis	CCP (cyclic citrullinated peptides); various citrullinated proteins	60-80	Specific for rheumatoid arthritis
	Rheumatoid factor (not specific)	60-70	

Listed autoantibodies are associated with high frequencies with particular diseases. "Generic" antinuclear antibodies (ANAs), which may react against many nuclear antigens, are positive in a large fraction of patients with SLE but are also positive in other autoimmune diseases. % positive refers to the approximate % of patients who test positive for each antibody.
The table was compiled with the help of Dr. Antony Rosen, Johns Hopkins University.

- *Homogeneous or diffuse nuclear staining* usually reflects antibodies to chromatin, histones, and, occasionally, double-stranded DNA.
- *Rim or peripheral staining* patterns are most often indicative of antibodies to double-stranded DNA and sometimes to nuclear envelope proteins.
- *Speckled pattern* refers to the presence of uniform or variable-sized speckles. This is one of the most commonly observed patterns of fluorescence and therefore the least specific. It reflects the presence of antibodies to non-DNA nuclear constituents such as Sm antigen, ribonucleoprotein, and SS-A and SS-B reactive antigens.
- *Nucleolar pattern* refers to the presence of a few discrete spots of fluorescence within the nucleus and represents antibodies to RNA. This pattern is reported most often in patients with systemic sclerosis.
- *Centromeric pattern.* Patients with systemic sclerosis often contain antibodies specific for centromeres, which give rise to this pattern.

The fluorescence patterns are not absolutely specific for the type of antibody, and because many autoantibodies may be present, combinations of patterns are frequent. Concerns have been raised about the sensitivity and subjective nature of this assay, and attempts are ongoing to replace it with ELISA for specific nuclear and other antigens. Nevertheless, the staining pattern is considered of diagnostic value, and the test remains in use. **Antibodies to double-stranded DNA and the so-called Smith (Sm) antigen are virtually diagnostic of SLE.**

Other Autoantibodies. In addition to ANAs, lupus patients have a host of other autoantibodies. Some are directed against blood cells, such as red cells, platelets, and lymphocytes; others react with proteins in complex with phospholipids. *Antiphospholipid antibodies* are present in 30% to 40% of lupus patients. They are actually directed against epitopes of plasma proteins that are revealed when the proteins are in complex with phospholipids. Included among these proteins are prothrombin, annexin V, β_2-glycoprotein I, protein S, and protein C. Antibodies against the phospholipid-β_2-glycoprotein complex also bind to cardiolipin antigen, used in syphilis serology, and therefore lupus patients may have a false-positive test result for syphilis. Some of these antibodies interfere with in vitro clotting tests, such as partial thromboplastin time. Therefore, these antibodies are sometimes referred to as *lupus anticoagulant*. Despite the observed clotting delays in vitro, however, patients with antiphospholipid antibodies have complications related to excessive clotting (a *hypercoagulable state*), such as thrombosis (Chapter 4).

Etiology and Pathogenesis of SLE

The fundamental defect in SLE is a failure of the mechanisms that maintain self-tolerance. Although what causes this failure of self-tolerance remains unknown, as is true of most autoimmune diseases, both genetic and environmental factors play a role.

Genetic Factors. SLE is a genetically complex disease with contributions from MHC and multiple non-MHC genes. Many lines of evidence support a genetic predisposition.

- Family members of patients have an increased risk of developing SLE. As many as 20% of clinically unaffected first-degree relatives of SLE patients reveal autoantibodies and other immunoregulatory abnormalities.
- There is a higher rate of concordance (>20%) in monozygotic twins when compared with dizygotic twins (1% to 3%).
- Studies of HLA associations support the concept that MHC genes regulate production of particular

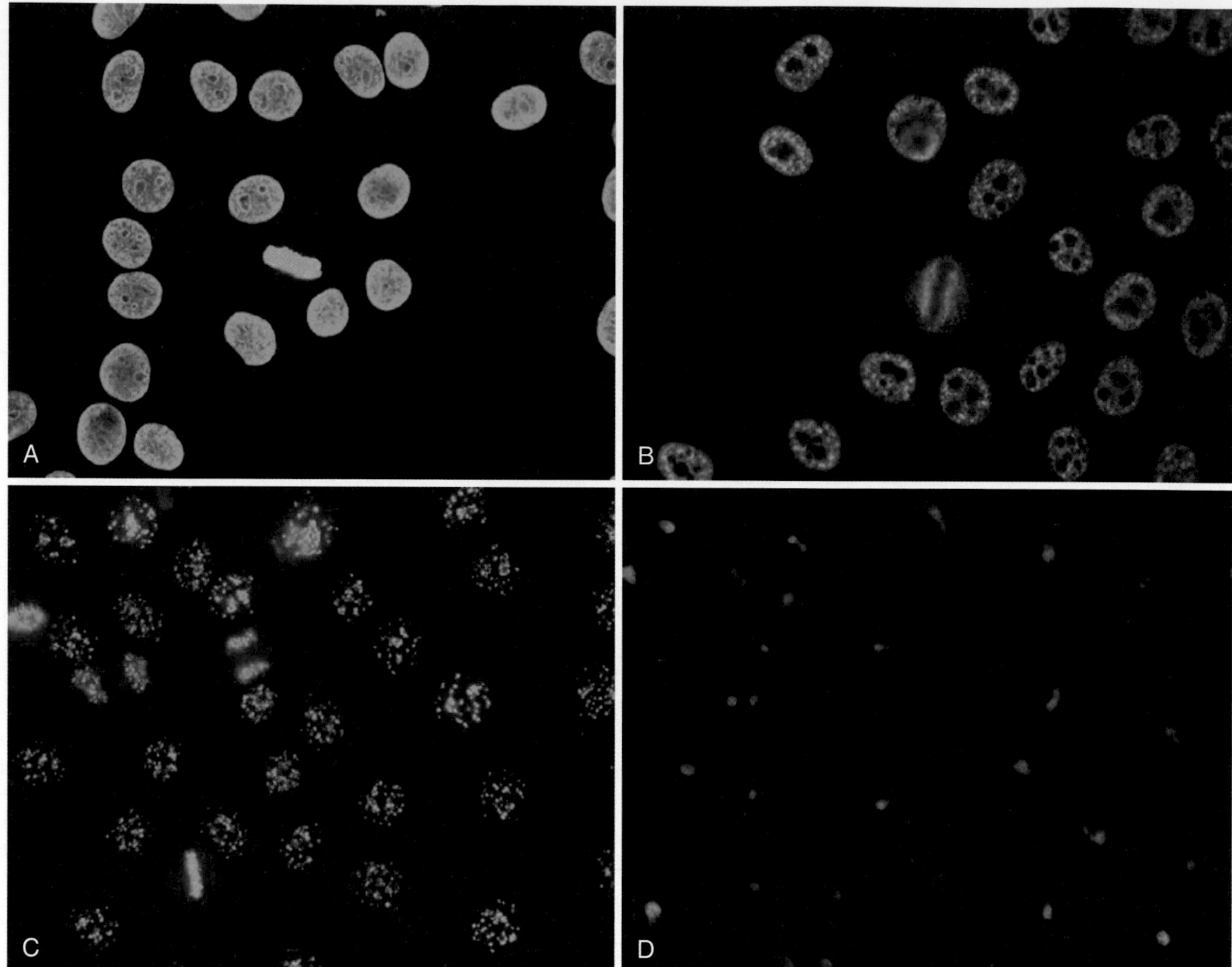

Figure 6-24 Staining patterns of antinuclear antibodies. **A,** Homogeneous or diffuse staining of nuclei is typical of antibodies reactive with dsDNA, nucleosomes and histones, and is common in SLE. **B,** Speckled pattern is seen with antibodies against various nuclear antigens, including Sm and RNPs. **C,** The pattern of staining of anti-centromere antibodies is seen in some cases of systemic sclerosis, Sjogren syndrome, and other diseases. **D,** Nucleolar pattern is typical of antibodies against nucleolar proteins. (Images reproduced from Wiik AS, et al, J. Autoimm. 35:276, 2010, with permission.)

autoantibodies. Specific alleles of the *HLA-DQ* locus have been linked to the production of anti–double-stranded DNA, anti-Sm, and antiphospholipid antibodies, although the relative risk is small.

- Some lupus patients have inherited deficiencies of early complement components, such as C2, C4, or C1q. Lack of complement may impair removal of circulating immune complexes by the mononuclear phagocyte system, thus favoring tissue deposition. Knockout mice lacking C4 or certain complement receptors are also prone to develop lupus-like autoimmunity. Various mechanisms have been invoked, including failure to clear immune complexes and loss of B-cell self-tolerance. It has also been proposed that deficiency of C1q results in defective phagocytic clearance of apoptotic cells. Many cells normally undergo apoptosis, and if they are not cleared their nuclear components may elicit immune responses.
- Genome-wide association studies have identified several genetic loci that may be associated with the disease. Many of these loci encode proteins involved in lymphocyte signaling and interferon responses, both of which may play a role in lupus pathogenesis, as discussed later. The relative risk for each locus is small, and even taken together these loci account for 20% or less of the genetic predisposition, suggesting an important role for environmental factors, discussed later.

Immunologic Factors. Recent studies in animal models and patients have revealed several immunologic aberrations that collectively may result in the persistence and uncontrolled activation of self-reactive lymphocytes.

- **Failure of self-tolerance in B cells** results from defective elimination of self-reactive B cells in the bone marrow or defects in peripheral tolerance mechanisms.
- **CD4+ helper T cells** specific for nucleosomal antigens also escape tolerance and contribute to the production of high-affinity pathogenic autoantibodies. The autoantibodies in SLE show characteristics of T cell-dependent antibodies produced in germinal centers, and increased

numbers of follicular helper T cells have been detected in the blood of SLE patients.

- **TLR engagement by nuclear DNA and RNA** contained in immune complexes may activate B lymphocytes. These TLRs function normally to sense microbial products, including nucleic acids. Thus, B cells specific for nuclear antigens may get second signals from TLRs and may be activated, resulting in increased production of antinuclear autoantibodies.
- **Type I interferons** play a role in lymphocyte activation in SLE. High levels of circulating type I interferons and a molecular signature in blood cells suggesting exposure to these cytokines has been reported in SLE patients and correlates with disease severity. Type I interferons are antiviral cytokines that are normally produced during innate immune responses to viruses. It may be that nucleic acids engage TLRs on dendritic cells and stimulate the production of interferons. In other words, self nucleic acids mimic their microbial counterparts. How interferons contribute to the development of SLE is unclear; these cytokines may activate dendritic cells and B cells and promote T_H1 responses, all of which may stimulate the production of pathogenic autoantibodies.
- Other cytokines that may play a role in unregulated B-cell activation include the TNF family member BAFF, which promotes survival of B cells. In some patients and animal models, increased production of BAFF has been reported, prompting attempts to block the cytokine or its receptor as therapy for SLE.

Environmental Factors. There are many indications that environmental factors must also be involved in the pathogenesis of SLE.

- **Exposure to ultraviolet (UV) light** exacerbates the disease in many individuals. UV irradiation may induce apoptosis in cells and may alter the DNA in such a way that it becomes immunogenic, perhaps because of enhanced recognition by TLRs. In addition, UV light may modulate the immune response, for example, by stimulating keratinocytes to produce IL-1, a cytokine known to promote inflammation.
- The **gender bias** of SLE is partly attributable to actions of sex hormones and partly related to genes on the X chromosome, independent of hormone effects.
- **Drugs** such as hydralazine, procainamide, and D-penicillamine can induce an SLE-like response in humans.

A Model for the Pathogenesis of SLE. It is clear from this discussion that the immunologic abnormalities in SLE—both documented and postulated—are varied and complex. Nevertheless, an attempt can be made to synthesize results from human studies and animal models into a hypothetical model of the pathogenesis of SLE (Fig. 6-25). UV irradiation and other environmental insults lead to the apoptosis of cells. Inadequate clearance of the nuclei of these cells results in a large burden of nuclear antigens. Underlying abnormalities in B and T lymphocytes are responsible for defective tolerance, because of which self-reactive lymphocytes survive and remain functional. These lymphocytes are stimulated by nuclear self antigens, and antibodies are produced against the antigens. Complexes of the antigens and antibodies bind to Fc receptors on B cells and dendritic cells, and may be internalized. The nucleic acid components engage TLRs and stimulate B cells to produce more autoantibodies. TLR stimuli also activate dendritic cells to produce interferons and other cytokines, which further enhance the immune response and cause more apoptosis. The net result is a cycle of antigen release and immune activation resulting in the production of high-affinity autoantibodies.

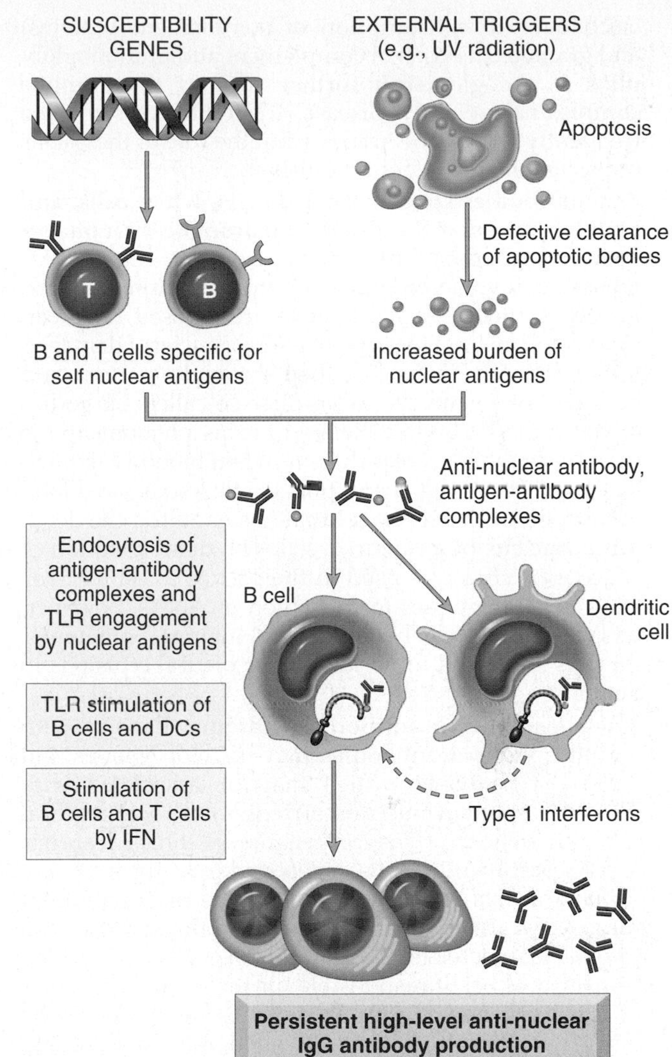

Figure 6-25 Model for the pathogenesis of systemic lupus erythematosus. In this hypothetical model, susceptibility genes interfere with the maintenance of self-tolerance and external triggers lead to persistence of nuclear antigens. The result is an antibody response against self nuclear antigens, which is amplified by the action of nucleic acids on dendritic cells (DCs) and B cells, and the production of type 1 interferons. TLRs, Toll-like receptors.

Mechanism of Tissue Injury. Different autoantibodies are the cause of most of the lesions of SLE.

- **Most of the systemic lesions are caused by immune complexes (type III hypersensitivity).** DNA-anti-DNA complexes can be detected in the glomeruli and small blood vessels. Low levels of serum complement (secondary to consumption of complement proteins) and granular deposits of complement and immunoglobulins in the glomeruli further support the immune complex nature of the disease. T cell infiltrates are also frequently seen in the kidneys, but the role of these cells in tissue damage is not established.

- **Autoantibodies specific for red cells, white cells, and platelets opsonize these cells and promote their phagocytosis and lysis.** There is no evidence that ANAs, which are involved in immune complex formation, can penetrate intact cells. If cell nuclei are exposed, however, the ANAs can bind to them. In tissues, nuclei of damaged cells react with ANAs, lose their chromatin pattern, and become homogeneous, to produce so-called LE bodies or hematoxylin bodies. Related to this phenomenon is the *LE cell*, which is readily seen when blood is agitated in vitro. The LE cell is any phagocytic leukocyte (blood neutrophil or macrophage) that has engulfed the denatured nucleus of an injured cell. The demonstration of LE cells in vitro was used in the past as a test for SLE. With new techniques for detection of ANAs, however, this test is now largely of historical interest. Sometimes, LE cells are found in pericardial or pleural effusions in patients.
- **Antiphospholipid antibody syndrome**. Patients with antiphospholipid antibodies may develop venous and arterial thromboses, which may be associated with recurrent spontaneous miscarriages and focal cerebral or ocular ischemia. This constellation of clinical features, in association with lupus, is referred to as the *secondary antiphospholipid antibody syndrome*. The mechanisms of thrombosis are not defined, and antibodies against clotting factors, platelets and endothelial cells have all been proposed as being responsible for thrombosis (Chapter 4). Some patients develop these autoantibodies and the clinical syndrome without associated SLE. They are said to have the *primary antiphospholipid antibody syndrome* (Chapter 4).
- The neuropsychiatric manifestations of SLE have been attributed to antibodies that react with neurons or receptors for various neurotransmitters and cross the blood brain barrier. However, this is not established and mechanisms involving other immune factors, such as cytokines, may also underlie the cognitive dysfunction and other CNS abnormalities that are associated with SLE.

Table 6-11 Clinical and Pathologic Manifestations of Systemic Lupus Erythematosus

Clinical Manifestation	Prevalence in Patients (%)*
Hematologic	100
Arthritis, arthralgia or myalgia	80-90
Skin	85
Fever	55-85
Fatigue	80-100
Weight loss	60
Renal	50-70
Neuropsychiatric	25-35
Pleuritis	45
Pericarditis	25
Gastrointestinal	20
Raynaud phenomenon	15-40
Ocular	5-15
Peripheral neuropathy	15

*Percentages are approximate and may vary with age, ethnicity, and other factors. Table compiled with the assistance of Dr. Meenakshi Jolly, Rush Medical Center, Chicago.

MORPHOLOGY

The morphologic changes in SLE are extremely variable. The frequency of individual organ involvement is shown in Table 6-11. The most characteristic lesions result from immune complex deposition in blood vessels, kidneys, connective tissue, and skin.

Blood Vessels. An acute necrotizing vasculitis involving capillaries, small arteries and arterioles may be present in any tissue. The arteritis is characterized by fibrinoid deposits in the vessel walls. In chronic stages, vessels undergo fibrous thickening with luminal narrowing.

Kidney. Up to 50% of SLE patients have clinically significant renal involvement. All of the glomerular lesions described later are the result of deposition of immune complexes that are regularly present in the mesangium or along the entire basement membrane and sometimes throughout the glomerulus. Both in situ formation and deposition of preformed circulating immune complexes may contribute to the injury, but the reason for the wide spectrum of histopathologic lesions (and clinical manifestations) in patients with lupus nephritis remains uncertain.

The kidney virtually always shows some evidence of renal abnormality if examined by electron microscopy and immunofluorescence. According to the currently accepted classification, six patterns of glomerular disease are seen in SLE. It should be noted that there is some overlap within these classes and over time lesions may evolve from one class to another. Thus, the exact percentage of patients with each of the six classes of lesions is difficult to determine. Suffice it to say that Class I is the least common and class IV is the most common pattern.

- **Minimal mesangial lupus nephritis** (class I) is very uncommon, and is characterized by immune complex deposition in the mesangium, identified by immunoflourescence and by electron microscopy, but without structural changes by light microscopy.
- **Mesangial proliferative lupus nephritis** (class II) is characterized by mesangial cell proliferation, often accompanied by accumulation of mesangial matrix, and granular mesangial deposits of immunoglobulin and complement without involvement of glomerular capillaries.
- **Focal lupus nephritis** (class III) is defined by involvement of fewer than 50% of all glomeruli. The lesions may be segmental (affecting only a portion of the glomerulus) or global (involving the entire glomerulus). Affected glomeruli may exhibit swelling and proliferation of endothelial and mesangial cells associated with leukocyte accumulation, capillary necrosis, and hyaline thrombi. There is also often extracapillary proliferation associated with focal necrosis and crescent formation (Fig. 6-26*A*). The clinical presentation ranges from mild hematuria and proteinuria to acute renal insufficiency. Red cell casts in the urine are common when the disease is active. Some patients progress to diffuse glomerulonephritis.

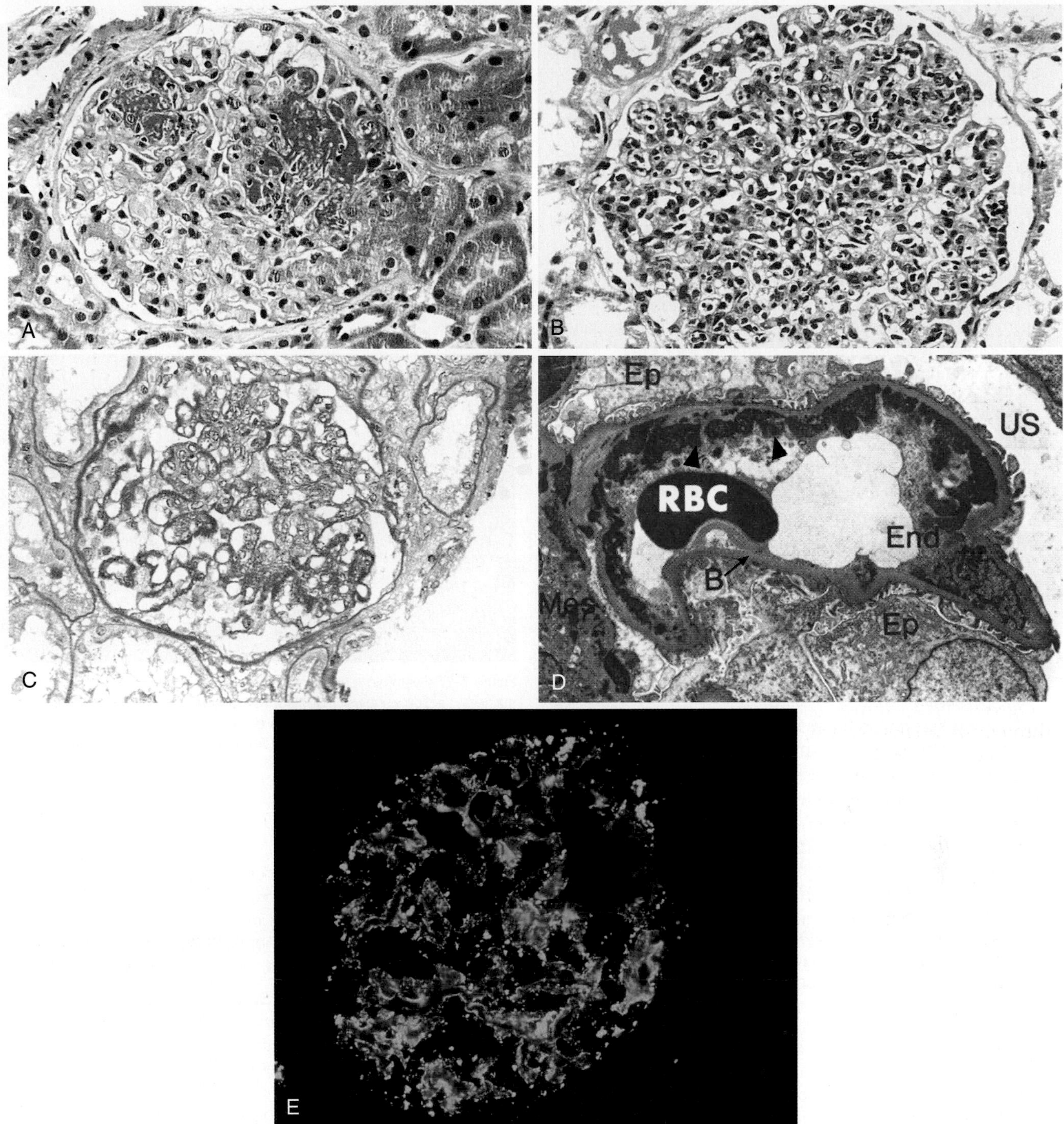

Figure 6-26 Lupus nephritis. **A,** Focal proliferative glomerulonephritis, with two focal necrotizing lesions at the 11 o'clock and 2 o'clock positions (H&E stain). Extracapillary proliferation is not prominent in this case. **B,** Diffuse proliferative glomerulonephritis. Note the marked increase in cellularity throughout the glomerulus (H&E stain). **C,** Lupus nephritis showing a glomerulus with several "wire loop" lesions representing extensive subendothelial deposits of immune complexes (periodic acid-Schiff stain). **D,** Electron micrograph of a renal glomerular capillary loop from a patient with SLE nephritis. Subendothelial dense deposits (*arrowheads*) correspond to "wire loops" seen by light microscopy. B *(with arrow)* refers to the basement membrane. **E,** Deposition of IgG antibody in a granular pattern, detected by immunofluorescence. B, Basement membrane; End, endothelium; Ep, epithelial cell with foot processes; Mes, mesangium; RBC, red blood cell in capillary lumen; US, urinary space. (**A-C,** Courtesy Dr. Helmut Rennke, Department of Pathology, Brigham and Women's Hospital, Boston, Mass. **D,** Courtesy Dr. Edwin Eigenbrodt, Department of Pathology, University of Texas, Southwestern Medical School, Dallas, Texas. **E,** Courtesy Dr. Jean Olson, Department of Pathology, University of California, San Francisco, Calif.)

The active (or proliferative) inflammatory lesions can heal completely or lead to chronic global or segmental glomerular scarring.

- **Diffuse lupus nephritis** (class IV) is the most common and severe form of lupus nephritis. The lesions are similar to those in class III, but differ in extent; typically, in class IV nephritis half or more of the glomeruli are affected. As in class III, the lesions may be segmental or global and on the basis of this, it can be subclassified as Class IV segmental (IV-S) or Class IV global (IV-G). Involved glomeruli show proliferation of endothelial, mesangial and epithelial cells (Fig. 6-26*B*), with the latter producing cellular crescents that fill Bowman's space (Chapter 20). Subendothelial immune complex deposits may create a circumferential thickening of the capillary wall, forming "wire loop" structures on light microscopy (Fig. 6-26*C*). Immune complexes can be readily detected by electron microscopy (Fig. 6-26*D*) and immunofluorescence (Fig. 6-26*E*). Lesions may progress to scarring of glomeruli. Patients with diffuse glomerulonephritis are usually symptomatic, showing hematuria as well as proteinuria. Hypertension and mild to severe renal insufficiency are also common.
- **Membranous lupus nephritis** (class V) is characterized by diffuse thickening of the capillary walls due to deposition of subepithelial immune complexes, similar to idiopathic membranous nephropathy, described in Chapter 20. The immune complexes are usually accompanied by increased production of basement membrane-like material. This lesion is usually accompanied by severe proteinuria or nephrotic syndrome, and may occur concurrently with focal or diffuse lupus nephritis.
- **Advanced sclerosing lupus nephritis** (class VI) is characterized by sclerosis of more than 90% of the glomeruli, and represents end-stage renal disease.
- Changes in the interstitium and tubules are frequently present in lupus nephritis patients. Rarely, **tubulointerstitial lesions** may be the dominant abnormality. Discrete immune complexes similar to those in glomeruli are present in the tubular or peritubular capillary basement membranes in many lupus nephritis patients, but the clinical significance of these extraglomerular deposits is not established. Often, there are well-organized B-cell follicles in the interstitium, with plasma cells that may be sources of autoantibodies.

Skin. Characteristic erythema affects the face along the bridge of the nose and cheeks (the "butterfly" rash) in approximately 50% of patients, but a similar rash may also be seen on the extremities and trunk. Urticaria, bullae, maculopapular lesions, and ulcerations also occur. Exposure to sunlight incites or accentuates the erythema. Histologically the involved areas show vacuolar degeneration of the basal layer of the epidermis (Fig. 6-27*A*). In the dermis, there is variable edema and perivascular inflammation. Vasculitis with fibrinoid necrosis may be prominent. Immunofluorescence microscopy shows deposition of immunoglobulin and complement along the dermoepidermal junction (Fig. 6-27*B*), which may also be present in uninvolved skin. This finding is not diagnostic of SLE and is sometimes seen in scleroderma or dermatomyositis.

Joints. Joint involvement is typically a nonerosive synovitis with little deformity, which contrasts with rheumatoid arthritis.

Central Nervous System. Neuropsychiatric symptoms of SLE have often been ascribed to acute vasculitis, but in histologic studies of the nervous system in such patients significant vasculitis is rarely present. Instead, noninflammatory occlusion of small vessels by intimal proliferation is sometimes noted, which may be due to endothelial damage by autoantibodies or immune complexes.

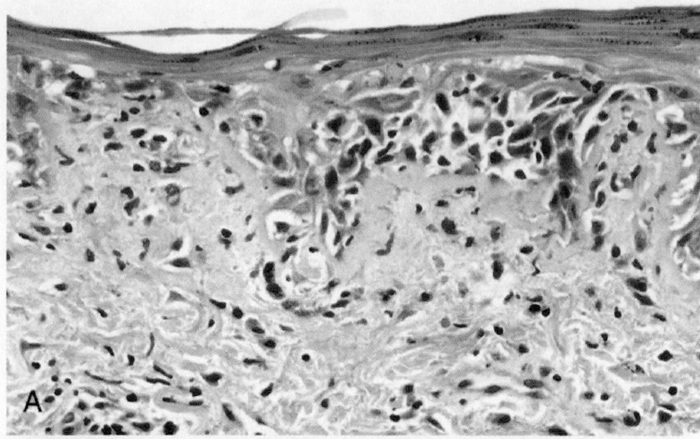

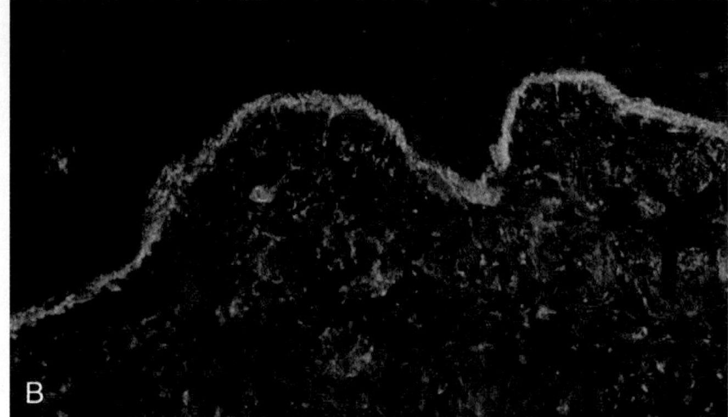

Figure 6-27 Systemic lupus erythematosus involving the skin. **A,** An H&E-stained section shows liquefactive degeneration of the basal layer of the epidermis and edema at the dermoepidermal junction. **B,** An immunofluorescence micrograph stained for IgG reveals deposits of Ig along the dermoepidermal junction. (A, Courtesy Dr. Jag Bhawan, Boston University School of Medicine, Boston, Mass. **B,** Courtesy Dr. Richard Sontheimer, Department of Dermatology, University of Texas Southwestern Medical School, Dallas, Texas.)

Pericarditis and Other Serosal Cavity Involvement. Inflammation of the serosal lining membranes may be acute, subacute, or chronic. During the acute phases, the mesothelial surfaces are sometimes covered with fibrinous exudate. Later they become thickened, opaque, and coated with a shaggy fibrous tissue that may lead to partial or total obliteration of the serosal cavity. Pleural and pericardial effusions may be present.

Cardiovascular system involvement may manifest as damage to any layer of the heart. Symptomatic or asymptomatic pericardial involvement is present in up to 50% of patients. Myocarditis, or mononuclear cell infiltration, is less common and may cause resting tachycardia and electrocardiographic abnormalities. Valvular abnormalities, primarily of the mitral and aortic valves, manifest as diffuse leaflet thickening that may be associated with dysfunction (stenosis and/or regurgitation). Valvular (or so-called Libman-Sacks) endocarditis was more common prior to the widespread use of steroids. This nonbacterial verrucous endocarditis takes the form of single or multiple 1- to 3-mm warty deposits on any heart valve, distinctively on either surface of the leaflets (Fig. 6-28). By comparison, the

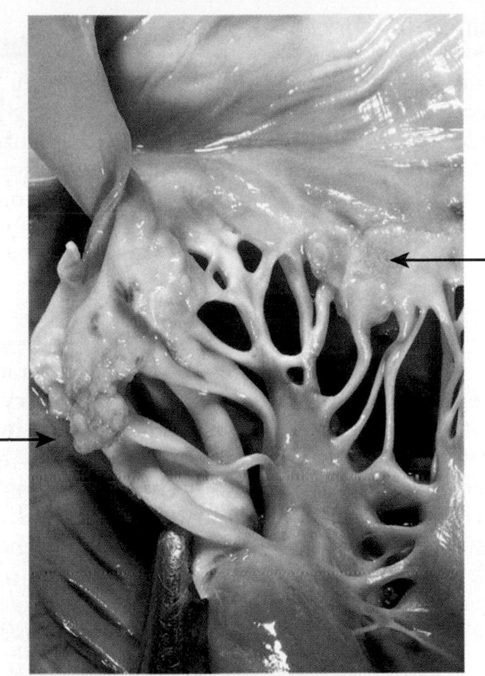

Figure 6-28 Libman-Sacks endocarditis of the mitral valve in lupus erythematosus. The vegetations attached to the margin of the thickened valve leaflet are indicated by *arrows*. (Courtesy Dr. Fred Schoen, Department of Pathology, Brigham and Women's Hospital, Boston, Mass.)

vegetations in infective endocarditis are considerably larger, and those in rheumatic heart disease (Chapter 12) are smaller and confined to the lines of closure of the valve leaflets.

An increasing number of patients have clinical evidence of coronary artery disease (angina, myocardial infarction) owing to coronary atherosclerosis. This complication is particularly notable in young patients with long-standing disease, and especially prevalent in those who have been treated with corticosteroids. The pathogenesis of accelerated coronary atherosclerosis is unclear but is probably multifactorial. Risk factors for atherosclerosis, including hypertension, obesity, and hyperlipidemia, are more commonly present in SLE patients than in the population at large. In addition, immune complexes and antiphospholipid antibodies may cause endothelial damage and promote atherosclerosis.

Spleen. Splenomegaly, capsular thickening, and follicular hyperplasia are common features. Central penicilliary arteries may show concentric intimal and smooth muscle cell hyperplasia, producing so-called onion-skin lesions.

Lungs. In addition to pleuritis and pleural effusions, which are present in almost 50% of patients, in some cases, there is chronic interstitial fibrosis and secondary pulmonary hypertension. None of these changes is specific for SLE.

Other Organs and Tissues. LE, or hematoxylin, bodies in the bone marrow or other organs are strongly indicative of SLE. Lymph nodes may be enlarged with hyperplastic follicles or even demonstrate necrotizing lymphadenitis.

Clinical Features. SLE is a multisystem disease that is highly variable in its clinical presentation, and its diagnosis relies on a constellation of clinical, serologic, and morphologic changes (Table 6-9). Typically, the patient is a young woman with some, but not necessarily all, of the following features: a butterfly rash over the face, fever, pain but no deformity in one or more peripheral joints (feet, ankles, knees, hips, fingers, wrists, elbows, shoulders), pleuritic chest pain, and photosensitivity. In many patients, however, the presentation of SLE is subtle and puzzling, taking forms such as a febrile illness of unknown origin, abnormal urinary findings, or joint disease masquerading as rheumatoid arthritis or rheumatic fever. "Generic" ANAs, detected by immunofluorescence assays, are found in virtually 100% of patients, but these are not specific for SLE. A variety of clinical findings may point toward renal involvement, including hematuria, red cell casts, proteinuria, and in some cases the classic nephrotic syndrome (Chapter 20). Laboratory evidence of some hematologic derangement is seen in virtually every case, but in some patients anemia or thrombocytopenia may be the presenting manifestation as well as the dominant clinical problem. In still others, mental aberrations, including psychosis or convulsions, or coronary artery disease may be prominent clinical problems. Patients with SLE are also prone to infections, presumably because of their underlying immune dysfunction and treatment with immunosuppressive drugs.

The course of the disease is variable and unpredictable. Rare acute cases result in death within weeks to months. More often, with appropriate therapy, the disease is characterized by flare-ups and remissions spanning a period of years or even decades. During acute flare-ups, increased formation of immune complexes results in complement activation, often leading to hypocomplementemia. Disease flares are usually treated with corticosteroids or other immunosuppressive drugs. Even without therapy, in some patients the disease may run an indolent course with relatively mild manifestations, such as skin changes and mild hematuria, for years. The outcome has improved significantly, and an approximately 90% 5-year and 80% 10-year survival can be expected. The most common causes of death are renal failure and intercurrent infections. Coronary artery disease is also becoming an important cause of death. Patients treated with steroids and immunosuppressive drugs incur the usual risks associated with such therapy.

As mentioned earlier, involvement of skin along with multisystem disease is fairly common in SLE. The following sections describe two syndromes in which the cutaneous involvement is the exclusive or most prominent feature.

Chronic Discoid Lupus Erythematosus. Chronic discoid lupus erythematosus is a disease in which the skin manifestations may mimic SLE, but systemic manifestations are rare. It is characterized by the presence of skin plaques showing varying degrees of edema, erythema, scaliness, follicular plugging, and skin atrophy surrounded by an elevated erythematous border. The face and scalp are usually affected, but widely disseminated lesions occasionally occur. The disease is usually confined to the skin, but 5% to 10% of patients with discoid lupus erythematosus develop multisystem manifestations after many years. Conversely, some patients with SLE may have prominent discoid lesions in the skin. Approximately 35% of patients show a positive test for generic ANAs, but antibodies to double-stranded DNA are rarely present. Immunofluorescence studies of skin biopsy specimens show deposition of immunoglobulin and C3 at the dermoepidermal junction similar to that in SLE.

Subacute Cutaneous Lupus Erythematosus. This condition also presents with predominant skin involvement and can be distinguished from chronic discoid lupus erythematosus by several criteria. The skin rash in this disease tends to be widespread, superficial, and nonscarring, although scarring lesions may occur in some patients. Most patients have mild systemic symptoms consistent with SLE. Furthermore, there is a strong association with antibodies to the SS-A antigen and with the *HLA-DR3* genotype. Thus, the term *subacute cutaneous lupus erythematosus* seems to define a group intermediate between SLE and lupus erythematosus localized only to skin.

Drug-Induced Lupus Erythematosus

A lupus erythematosus-like syndrome may develop in patients receiving a variety of drugs, including hydralazine, procainamide, isoniazid, and D-penicillamine, to name only a few. Somewhat surprisingly, anti-TNF therapy, which is effective in rheumatoid arthritis and other autoimmune diseases, can also cause drug-induced lupus. Many of these drugs are associated with the development of ANAs, but most patients do not have symptoms of lupus erythematosus. For example, 80% of patients receiving procainamide test positive for ANAs, but only one third of these manifest clinical symptoms, such as arthralgias, fever, and serositis. Although multiple organs are affected, renal and central nervous system involvement is distinctly uncommon. There are serologic and genetic differences from classic SLE, as well. Antibodies specific for double-stranded DNA are rare, but there is an extremely high frequency of antibodies specific for histones. Persons with the *HLA-DR4* allele are at a greater risk of developing a lupus erythematosus-like syndrome after administration of hydralazine, whereas those with *HLA-DR6* (but not *DR4*) are at high risk with procainamide. The disease remits after withdrawal of the offending drug.

KEY CONCEPTS

Systemic Lupus Erythematosus

- SLE is a systemic autoimmune disease caused by autoantibodies produced against numerous self antigens and the formation of immune complexes.
- The major autoantibodies, and the ones responsible for the formation of circulating immune complexes, are directed against nuclear antigens. Other autoantibodies react with erythrocytes, platelets, and various complexes of phospholipids with proteins.
- Disease manifestations include nephritis, skin lesions and arthritis (caused by the deposition of immune complexes), and hematologic and neurologic abnormalities.
- The underlying cause of the breakdown in self-tolerance in SLE is unknown; it may include excess or persistence of nuclear antigens, multiple inherited susceptibility genes, and environmental triggers (e.g., UV irradiation, which results in cellular apoptosis and release of nuclear proteins).

Rheumatoid Arthritis

Rheumatoid arthritis is a chronic inflammatory disease that affects primarily the joints but may involve extraarticular tissues such as the skin, blood vessels, lungs, and heart. Abundant evidence supports the autoimmune nature of the disease. Because the principal manifestations of the disease are in the joints, it is discussed in Chapter 26.

Sjögren Syndrome

Sjögren syndrome is a chronic disease characterized by dry eyes (*keratoconjunctivitis sicca*) and dry mouth (*xerostomia*) resulting from immunologically mediated destruction of the lacrimal and salivary glands. It occurs as an isolated disorder (primary form), also known as the sicca syndrome, or more often in association with another autoimmune disease (secondary form). Among the associated disorders, rheumatoid arthritis is the most common, but some patients have SLE, polymyositis, scleroderma, vasculitis, mixed connective tissue disease, or thyroiditis.

Etiology and Pathogenesis

The characteristic decrease in tears and saliva (*sicca syndrome*) is the result of lymphocytic infiltration and fibrosis of the lacrimal and salivary glands. The infiltrate contains predominantly activated CD4+ helper T cells and some B cells, including plasma cells. About 75% of patients have rheumatoid factor (an antibody reactive with self IgG) whether or not coexisting rheumatoid arthritis is present. ANAs are detected in 50% to 80% of patients by immunofluorescence assay. A host of other organ-specific and non-organ-specific antibodies have also been identified. Most important, however, are antibodies directed against two ribonucleoprotein antigens, SS-A (Ro) and SS-B (La) (Table 6-10), which can be detected in as many as 90% of patients by sensitive techniques. These antibodies are thus considered serologic markers of the disease. Patients with high titers of antibodies to SS-A are more likely to have early disease onset, longer disease duration, and extraglandular manifestations, such as cutaneous vasculitis and nephritis. These autoantibodies are also present in a smaller percentage of patients with SLE and hence are not diagnostic of Sjögren syndrome.

As with other autoimmune diseases, Sjögren syndrome shows some association, albeit weak, with certain HLA alleles. Studies of whites and blacks suggest linkage of the primary form with *HLA-B8*, *HLA-DR3*, and *DRW52* as well as *HLA-DQA1* and *HLA-DQB1* loci; in patients with anti-SS-A or anti-SS-B antibodies, specific alleles of *HLA-DQA1* and *HLA-DQB1* are frequent. This suggests that, as in SLE, inheritance of certain class II molecules predisposes to the development of particular autoantibodies.

Although the pathogenesis of Sjögren syndrome remains obscure, aberrant T-cell and B-cell activation are both implicated. The initiating trigger may be a viral infection of the salivary glands, which causes local cell death and release of tissue self antigens. In genetically susceptible individuals, CD4+ T cells and B cells specific for these self antigens may have escaped tolerance and are able to react. The result is inflammation, tissue damage, and, eventually, fibrosis. However, the role of particular cytokines or T cell subsets in the development of the lesions is not established. The nature of the autoantigens recognized by these lymphocytes is still mysterious. A cytoskeletal protein called α-fodrin is a candidate autoantigen, but its role in disease development has not been established yet. Sjögren syndrome-like disease is seen in some patients with human T-lymphotropic virus (HTLV), human immunodeficiency virus (HIV) or hepatitis C virus infections, but the link between these viruses and the autoimmune disorder is obscure.

MORPHOLOGY

As mentioned earlier, **lacrimal and salivary glands are the major targets of the disease,** although other exocrine glands, including those lining the respiratory and gastrointestinal tracts and the vagina, may also be involved. The earliest histologic finding in both the major and the minor salivary glands is periductal and perivascular lymphocytic infiltration. Eventually the lymphocytic infiltrate becomes extensive (Fig. 6-29), and in the larger salivary glands lymphoid follicles with germinal centers may be seen. The ductal lining epithelial cells may show hyperplasia, thus obstructing the ducts. Later there is atrophy of the acini, fibrosis, and hyalinization; still later in the course atrophy and replacement of parenchyma with fat are seen. In some cases the lymphoid infiltrate may be so intense as to give the appearance of a lymphoma. Indeed, these patients are at high risk for development of B-cell lymphomas, and molecular assessments of clonality may be necessary to distinguish intense reactive chronic inflammation from early involvement by lymphoma.

The lack of tears leads to drying of the corneal epithelium, which becomes inflamed, eroded, and ulcerated; the oral mucosa may atrophy, with inflammatory fissuring and ulceration; and dryness and crusting of the nose may lead to ulcerations and even perforation of the nasal septum.

Clinical Features. Sjögren syndrome occurs most commonly in women between the ages of 50 and 60. As might be expected, symptoms result from inflammatory destruction of the exocrine glands. The *keratoconjunctivitis* produces blurring of vision, burning, and itching, and thick secretions accumulate in the conjunctival sac. The *xerostomia* results in difficulty in swallowing solid foods, a decrease in the ability to taste, cracks and fissures in the mouth, and dryness of the buccal mucosa. Parotid gland enlargement is present in half the patients; dryness of the nasal mucosa, epistaxis, recurrent bronchitis, and pneumonitis are other symptoms. Manifestations of *extraglandular disease* are seen in one third of patients and include synovitis, diffuse pulmonary fibrosis, and peripheral neuropathy. These are more common in patients with high titers of antibodies specific for SS-A. In contrast to SLE, glomerular lesions are extremely rare in Sjögren syndrome. Defects of tubular function, however, including renal tubular acidosis, uricosuria, and phosphaturia, are often seen and are associated histologically with tubulointerstitial nephritis (Chapter 20). About 60% of patients have another accompanying autoimmune disorder, such as rheumatoid arthritis, and these patients also have the symptoms and signs of that disorder.

The combination of lacrimal and salivary gland inflammatory involvement was once called *Mikulicz disease.* The name has now been replaced by *Mikulicz syndrome*, broadened to include lacrimal and salivary gland enlargement from any cause, including sarcoidosis, lymphoma, and other tumors. *Biopsy of the lip (to examine minor salivary glands) is essential for the diagnosis of Sjögren syndrome.*

The lymph nodes of patients with Sjögren syndrome are often hyperplastic, but the most intense lymphocytic response is seen in the tissues that are the focal point of the autoimmune response, particularly the salivary and lacrimal glands. In early stages of the disease, this immune infiltrate consists of a mixture of polyclonal T and B cells. However, if the reaction continues unabated there is a strong tendency over time for individual clones within the population of B cells to gain a growth advantage, presumably because of the acquisition of somatic mutations. Emergence of a dominant B-cell clone is usually indicative of the development of a marginal zone lymphoma, a specific type of B-cell malignancy that often arises in the setting of chronic lymphocytic inflammation. About 5% of Sjögren patients develop lymphoma, an incidence that is 40-fold greater than normal. Certain other autoimmune disorders (e.g., Hashimoto thyroiditis) are also associated

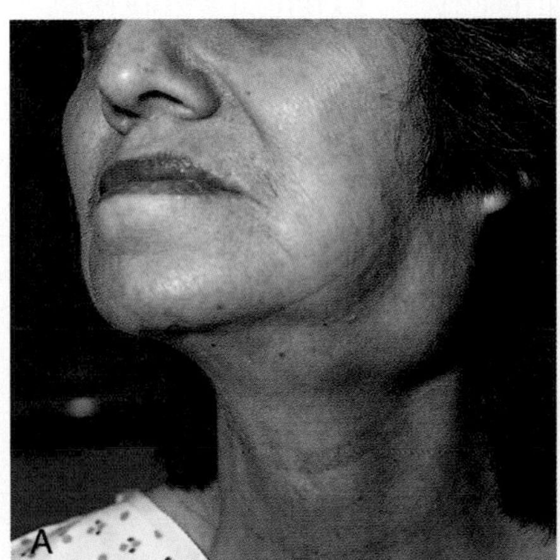

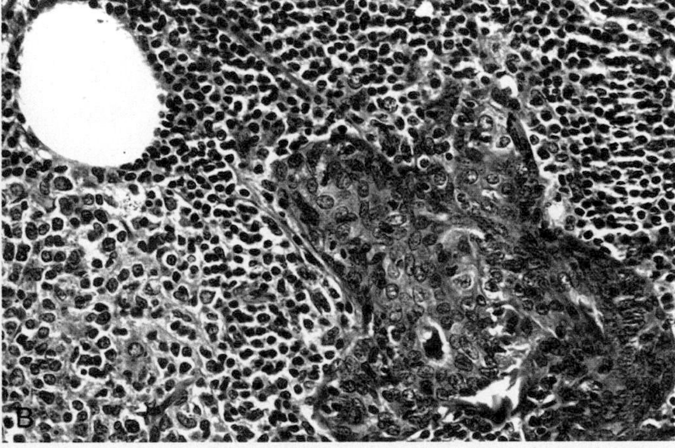

Figure 6-29 Sjögren syndrome. **A,** Enlargement of the salivary gland. **B,** Intense lymphocytic and plasma cell infiltration with ductal epithelial hyperplasia in a salivary gland. (**A,** Courtesy Dr. Richard Sontheimer, Department of Dermatology, University of Texas Southwestern Medical School, Dallas, Texas. **B,** Courtesy Dr. Dennis Burns, Department of Pathology, University of Texas Southwestern Medical School, Dallas, Texas.)

with a high risk of marginal zone lymphoma (Chapter 13), which typically arises within the organ or tissue that is the target of the autoimmune inflammation.

KEY CONCEPTS

Sjögren Syndrome

- Sjögren syndrome is an inflammatory disease that affects primarily the salivary and lacrimal glands, causing dryness of the mouth and eyes.
- The disease is believed to be caused by an autoimmune T-cell reaction against an unknown self antigen expressed in these glands, or immune reactions against the antigens of a virus that infects the tissues.

Systemic Sclerosis (Scleroderma)

Systemic sclerosis is characterized by: (1) chronic inflammation thought to be the result of autoimmunity, (2) widespread damage to small blood vessels, and (3) progressive interstitial and perivascular fibrosis in the skin and multiple organs. Although the term *scleroderma* is ingrained in clinical medicine, this disease is better named *systemic sclerosis* because it is characterized by excessive fibrosis throughout the body. The skin is most commonly affected, but the gastrointestinal tract, kidneys, heart, muscles, and lungs also are frequently involved. In some patients the disease seems to remain confined to the skin for many years, but in the majority it progresses to visceral involvement with death from renal failure, cardiac failure, pulmonary insufficiency, or intestinal malabsorption. The clinical heterogeneity of systemic sclerosis has been recognized by classifying the disease into two major categories: *diffuse scleroderma*, characterized by widespread skin involvement at onset, with rapid progression and early visceral involvement; and *limited scleroderma*, in which the skin involvement is often confined to fingers, forearms, and face. Visceral involvement occurs late; hence, the clinical course is relatively benign. Some patents with the limited disease also develop a combination of calcinosis, Raynaud phenomenon, esophageal dysmotility, sclerodactyly, and telangiectasia, called the *CREST syndrome*. Several other variants and related conditions, such as eosinophilic fasciitis, occur far less frequently and are not described here.

Etiology and Pathogenesis

The cause of systemic sclerosis is not known, but the **disease likely results from three interrelated processes—autoimmune responses, vascular damage, and collagen deposition** (Fig. 6-30).

- **Autoimmunity.** It is proposed that CD4+ T cells responding to an as yet unidentified antigen accumulate in the skin and release cytokines that activate inflammatory cells and fibroblasts. Although inflammatory infiltrates are typically sparse in the skin of patients with systemic sclerosis, activated CD4+ T cells can be found in many patients, and T_H2 cells have been isolated from the skin. Several cytokines produced by these T cells, including TGF-β and IL-13, can stimulate transcription of genes that encode collagen and other extracellular matrix proteins (e.g., fibronectin) in fibroblasts. Other cytokines recruit leukocytes and propagate the chronic inflammation.

  There is also evidence for inappropriate activation of humoral immunity, and the presence of various autoantibodies, notably ANAs, provides diagnostic and prognostic information. The role of these ANAs in the pathogenesis of the disease is unclear; it has been postulated that some of these antibodies may stimulate fibrosis, but the evidence in support of this idea is not convincing.
- **Vascular damage. Microvascular disease is consistently present early in the course of systemic sclerosis and may be the initial lesion.** Intimal proliferation is evident in the digital arteries of patients with systemic sclerosis. Capillary dilation with leaking, as well as destruction, is also common. Nailfold capillary loops are distorted early in the course of disease, and later they disappear. Telltale signs of endothelial activation and

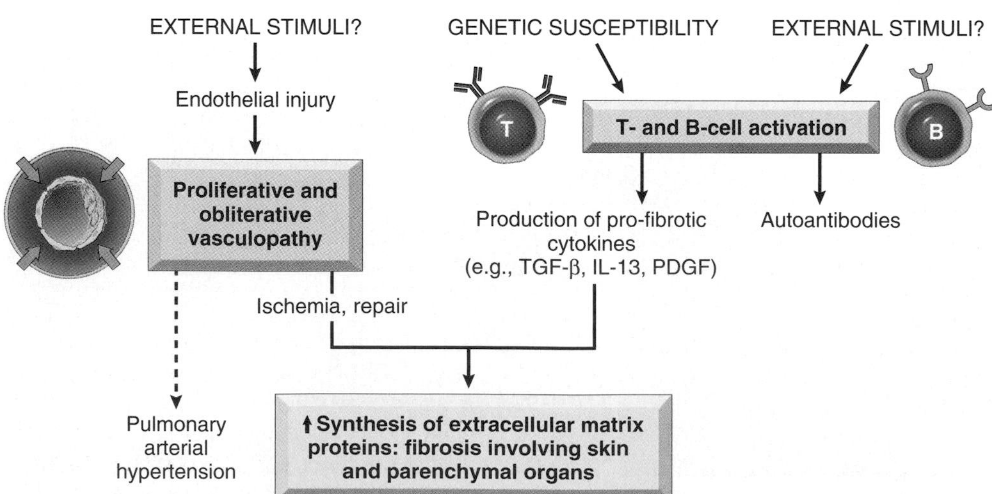

Figure 6-30 A model for the pathogenesis of systemic sclerosis. Unknown external stimuli cause vascular abnormalities and immune activation in genetically susceptible individuals, and both contribute to the excessive fibrosis.

injury (e.g., increased levels of von Willebrand factor) and increased platelet activation (increased percentage of circulating platelet aggregates) have also been noted. However, what causes the vascular injury is not known; it could be the initiating event or the result of chronic inflammation, with mediators released by inflammatory cells inflicting damage on microvascular endothelium. Repeated cycles of endothelial injury followed by platelet aggregation lead to release of platelet and endothelial factors (e.g., PDGF, TGF-β) that trigger perivascular fibrosis. Vascular smooth muscle cells also show abnormalities, such as increased expression of adrenergic receptors. Eventually, widespread narrowing of the microvasculature leads to ischemic injury and scarring.

- **Fibrosis.** The progressive fibrosis characteristic of the disease may be the culmination of multiple abnormalities, including the accumulation of alternatively activated macrophages, actions of fibrogenic cytokines produced by infiltrating leukocytes, hyperresponsiveness of fibroblasts to these cytokines, and scarring following upon ischemic damage caused by the vascular lesions. There is some evidence that fibroblasts from patients with systemic sclerosis have an intrinsic abnormality that causes them to produce excessive amounts of collagen, which is structurally normal. This idea is based on studies with cultured fibroblasts, and whether or how this abnormality relates to pathogenesis in vivo is unknown.

MORPHOLOGY

Virtually all organs can be involved in systemic sclerosis. Prominent changes occur in the skin, alimentary tract, musculoskeletal system, and kidney, but lesions also are often present in the blood vessels, heart, lungs, and peripheral nerves.

Skin. A great majority of patients have diffuse, sclerotic atrophy of the skin, which usually begins in the fingers and distal regions of the upper extremities and extends proximally to involve the upper arms, shoulders, neck, and face. Histologically, there are edema and perivascular infiltrates containing CD4+ T cells, together with swelling and degeneration of collagen fibers, which become eosinophilic. Capillaries and small arteries (150 to 500 μm in diameter) may show thickening of the basal lamina, endothelial cell damage, and partial occlusion. With progression of the disease, there is increasing fibrosis of the dermis, which becomes tightly bound to the subcutaneous structures. There is marked increase of compact collagen in the dermis, usually with thinning of the epidermis, loss of rete pegs, atrophy of the dermal appendages, and hyaline thickening of the walls of dermal arterioles and capillaries (Fig. 6-31*B*). Focal and sometimes diffuse subcutaneous calcifications may develop, especially in patients with the CREST syndrome. In advanced stages the fingers take on a tapered, clawlike appearance with limitation of motion in the joints, and the face becomes a drawn mask. Loss of blood supply may lead to cutaneous ulcerations and to atrophic changes in the terminal phalanges (Fig. 6-31*C*). Sometimes the tips of the fingers undergo autoamputation.

Alimentary Tract. The alimentary tract is affected in approximately 90% of patients. Progressive atrophy and collagenous fibrous replacement of the muscularis may develop at any level of the gut but are most severe in the esophagus. The lower two thirds of the esophagus often develops a rubber-hose–like inflexibility. The associated dysfunction of the lower esophageal sphincter gives rise to gastroesophageal reflux and its complications, including Barrett metaplasia (Chapter 17) and strictures. The mucosa is thinned and may be ulcerated, and there is excessive collagenization of the lamina propria and submucosa. Loss of villi and microvilli in the small bowel is the anatomic basis for the malabsorption syndrome sometimes encountered.

Musculoskeletal System. Inflammation of the synovium, associated with hypertrophy and hyperplasia of the synovial soft tissues, is common in the early stages; fibrosis later ensues. These changes are reminiscent of rheumatoid arthritis, but joint destruction is not common in systemic sclerosis. In a small subset of patients (approximately 10%), inflammatory myositis indistinguishable from polymyositis may develop.

Kidneys. Renal abnormalities occur in two-thirds of patients with systemic sclerosis. The most prominent are the vascular lesions. Interlobular arteries show intimal thickening as a result of deposition of mucinous or finely collagenous material, which stains histochemically for glycoprotein and acid mucopolysaccharides. There is also concentric proliferation of intimal cells. These changes may resemble those seen in malignant hypertension, but in scleroderma the alterations are restricted to vessels 150 to 500 μm in diameter and are not always associated with hypertension. Hypertension, however, does occur in 30% of patients with scleroderma, and in 20% it takes an ominously rapid, downhill course (malignant hypertension). In hypertensive patients, vascular alterations are more pronounced and are often associated with fibrinoid necrosis involving the arterioles together with thrombosis and infarction. Such patients often die of renal failure, which accounts for about 50% of deaths in persons with this disease. There are no specific glomerular changes.

Lungs. The lungs are involved in more than 50% of individuals with systemic sclerosis. This involvement may manifest as pulmonary hypertension and interstitial fibrosis. Pulmonary vasospasm, secondary to pulmonary vascular endothelial dysfunction, is considered important in the pathogenesis of pulmonary hypertension. Pulmonary fibrosis, when present, is indistinguishable from that seen in idiopathic pulmonary fibrosis (Chapter 15).

Heart. Pericarditis with effusion, myocardial fibrosis, and thickening of intramyocardial arterioles occur in one third of the patients. Clinical impairment by myocardial involvement, however, is less common.

Clinical Features. Systemic sclerosis has a female-to-male ratio of 3:1, with a peak incidence in the 50- to 60-year age group. Although systemic sclerosis shares many features with SLE, rheumatoid arthritis (Chapter 26), and polymyositis (Chapter 27), its distinctive features are the striking cutaneous changes, notably skin thickening. *Raynaud phenomenon,* manifested as episodic vasoconstriction of the arteries and arterioles of the extremities, is seen in virtually all patients and precedes other symptoms in 70% of cases. *Dysphagia* attributable to esophageal fibrosis and its resultant hypomotility are present in more than 50% of patients. Eventually, destruction of the esophageal wall leads to

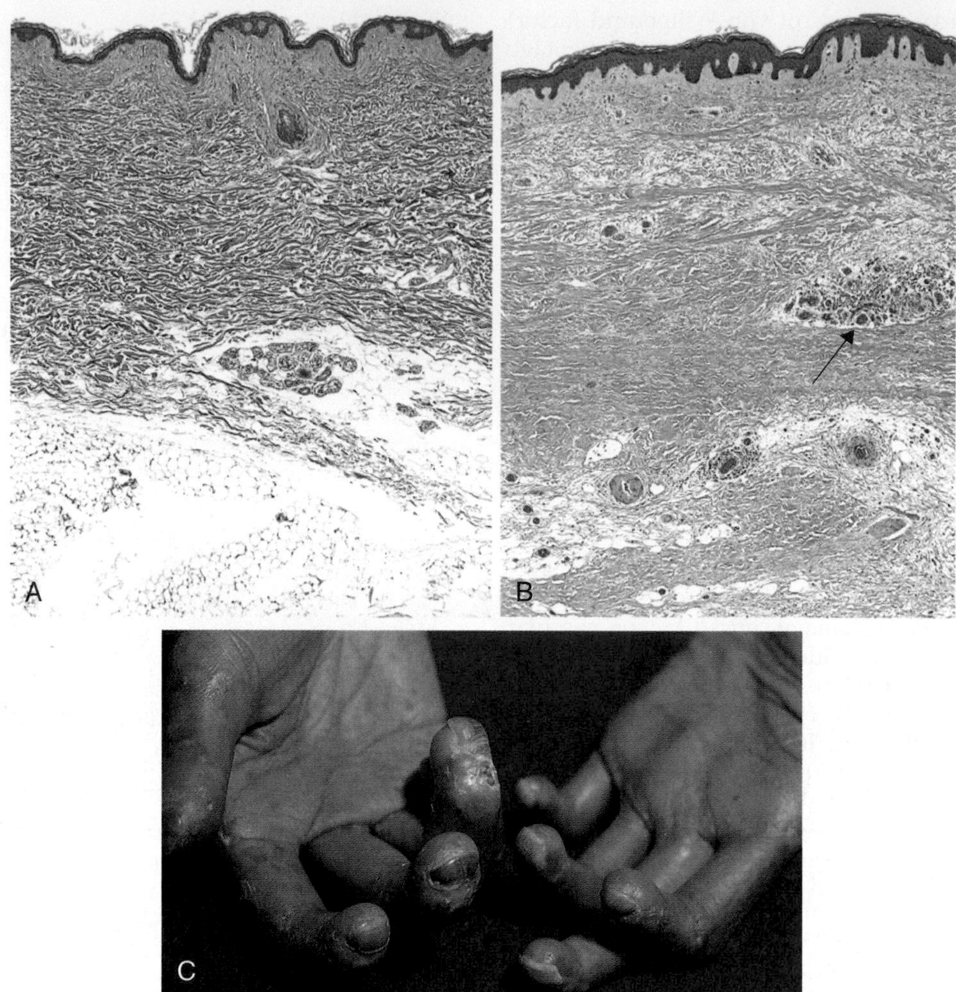

Figure 6-31 Systemic sclerosis. **A,** Normal skin. **B,** Skin biopsy from a patient with systemic sclerosis. Note the extensive deposition of dense collagen in the dermis with virtual absence of appendages (e.g., hair follicles) and foci of inflammation *(arrow)*. **C,** The extensive subcutaneous fibrosis has virtually immobilized the fingers, creating a clawlike flexion deformity. Loss of blood supply has led to cutaneous ulcerations. (**C,** Courtesy Dr. Richard Sontheimer, Department of Dermatology, University of Texas Southwestern Medical School, Dallas, Texas.)

atony and dilation, especially at its lower end. Abdominal pain, intestinal obstruction, or malabsorption syndrome with weight loss and anemia reflect involvement of the small intestine. Respiratory difficulties caused by the pulmonary fibrosis may result in right-sided cardiac dysfunction, and myocardial fibrosis may cause either arrhythmias or cardiac failure. Mild proteinuria occurs in as many as 30% of patients, but rarely is the proteinuria severe enough to cause a nephrotic syndrome. The most ominous manifestation is malignant hypertension (Chapter 11), with the subsequent development of fatal renal failure, but in its absence progression of the disease may be slow. The disease tends to be more severe in blacks, especially black women. As treatment of the renal crises has improved, pulmonary disease has become the major cause of death in systemic sclerosis.

Virtually all patients have ANAs that react with a variety of nuclear antigens. Two ANAs strongly associated with systemic sclerosis have been described. One of these, directed against *DNA topoisomerase* I (anti-Scl 70), is highly specific. Depending on the ethnic group and the assay, it is present in 10% to 20% of patients with diffuse systemic sclerosis. Patients who have this antibody are more likely to have pulmonary fibrosis and peripheral vascular disease. The other, an *anticentromere antibody*, is found in 20% to 30% of patients, who tend to have the CREST syndrome. Patients with this syndrome have relatively limited involvement of skin, often confined to fingers, forearms, and face, and calcification of the subcutaneous tissues. Involvement of the viscera, including esophageal lesions, pulmonary hypertension, and biliary cirrhosis, may not occur at all or occur late. In general these patients live longer than those with systemic sclerosis with diffuse visceral involvement at the outset.

KEY CONCEPTS

Systemic Sclerosis

- Systemic sclerosis (commonly called scleroderma) is characterized by progressive fibrosis involving the skin, gastrointestinal tract, and other tissues.

- Fibrosis may be the result of activation of fibroblasts by cytokines produced by T cells, but what triggers T-cell responses is unknown.
- Endothelial injury and microvascular disease are commonly present in the lesions of systemic sclerosis, perhaps causing chronic ischemia, but the pathogenesis of vascular injury is not known.

Inflammatory Myopathies

Inflammatory myopathies comprise an uncommon, heterogeneous group of disorders characterized by injury and inflammation of mainly the skeletal muscles, which are probably immunologically mediated. Three distinct disorders, *dermatomyositis*, *polymyositis*, and *inclusion-body myositis*, are included in this category. These may occur alone or with other immune-mediated diseases, particularly systemic sclerosis. These diseases are described in Chapter 27.

Mixed Connective Tissue Disease

The term *mixed connective tissue disease* is used to describe a disease with clinical features that are a mixture of the features of SLE, systemic sclerosis, and polymyositis. The disease is characterized serologically by high titers of antibodies to ribonucleoprotein particle-containing U1 ribonucleoprotein. Typically, mixed connective tissue disease presents with synovitis of the fingers, Raynaud phenomenon and mild myositis, but renal involvement is modest and there is a good response to corticosteroids, at least in the short term. Because the clinical features overlap with other diseases, it has been suggested that mixed connective tissue disease is not a distinct entity but that different patients represent subsets of SLE, systemic sclerosis, and polymyositis. The disease can, over time, evolve into classic SLE or systemic sclerosis. However, a subset of patients do not evolve into other diseases and the salutary response to steroids is not universal, suggesting that there may be an entity of mixed connective tissue disease distinct from other autoimmune diseases. Serious complications of mixed connective tissue disease include pulmonary hypertension, interstitial lung disease, and renal disease.

Polyarteritis Nodosa and Other Vasculitides

Polyarteritis nodosa belongs to a group of diseases characterized by necrotizing inflammation of the walls of blood vessels and showing strong evidence of an immunologic pathogenetic mechanism. The general term *noninfectious vasculitis* differentiates these conditions from those due to direct infection of the blood vessel wall (such as occurs in the wall of an abscess) and serves to emphasize that any type of vessel may be involved—arteries, arterioles, veins, or capillaries.

Noninfectious vasculitis is encountered in many clinical settings. A detailed classification and description of vasculitides is presented in Chapter 11, where the immunologic mechanisms are also discussed.

IgG4-Related Disease

IgG4-related disease (IgG4-RD) is a newly recognized constellation of disorders characterized by tissue infiltrates dominated by IgG4 antibody-producing plasma cells and lymphocytes, particularly T cells, storiform fibrosis, obliterative phlebitis, and usually increased serum IgG4. Although recognized only recently when extra-pancreatic manifestations were identified in patients with autoimmune pancreatitis, IgG4-related disease has now been described in virtually every organ system: the biliary tree, salivary glands, periorbital tissues, kidneys, lungs, lymph nodes, meninges, aorta, breast, prostate, thyroid, pericardium, and skin. Many medical conditions long viewed as confined to single organs are part of the IgG4-RD spectrum. These include Mikulicz syndrome (enlargement and fibrosis of salivary and lacrimal glands), Riedel thyroiditis, idiopathic retroperitoneal fibrosis, autoimmune pancreatitis, and inflammatory pseudotumors of the orbit, lungs, and kidneys, to name a few. The disease most often affects middle-aged and older men.

The pathogenesis of this condition is not understood, and although IgG4 production in lesions is a hallmark of the disease it is not known if this antibody type contributes to the pathology. The key role of B cells is supported by initial clinical trials in which depletion of B cells by anti–B cell reagents such as rituximab provided clinical benefit. It is unclear if the disease is truly autoimmune in nature, and no target autoantigens have been identified.

Rejection of Tissue Transplants

Transplant rejection is discussed here because it involves several of the immunologic reactions that underlie immune-mediated inflammatory diseases. A major barrier to transplantation is the process of *rejection*, in which the recipient's immune system recognizes the graft as being foreign and attacks it.

Mechanisms of Recognition and Rejection of Allografts

Rejection is a process in which T lymphocytes and antibodies produced against graft antigens react against and destroy tissue grafts. We next discuss how donor antigens from the graft are recognized by lymphocytes in the recipient and how the lymphocytes and their products destroy the graft.

Recognition of Graft Alloantigens by T and B Lymphocytes

The major antigenic differences between a donor and recipient that result in rejection of transplants are differences in HLA alleles. Grafts exchanged between individuals of the same species (the usual clinical situation) are called *allografts*, and grafts from one species to another (still an experimental procedure) are called *xenografts*. Because HLA genes are highly polymorphic, there are always some differences between individuals (except, of course, identical twins). Following transplantation, the recipient's T cells recognize donor antigens from the graft (the allogeneic

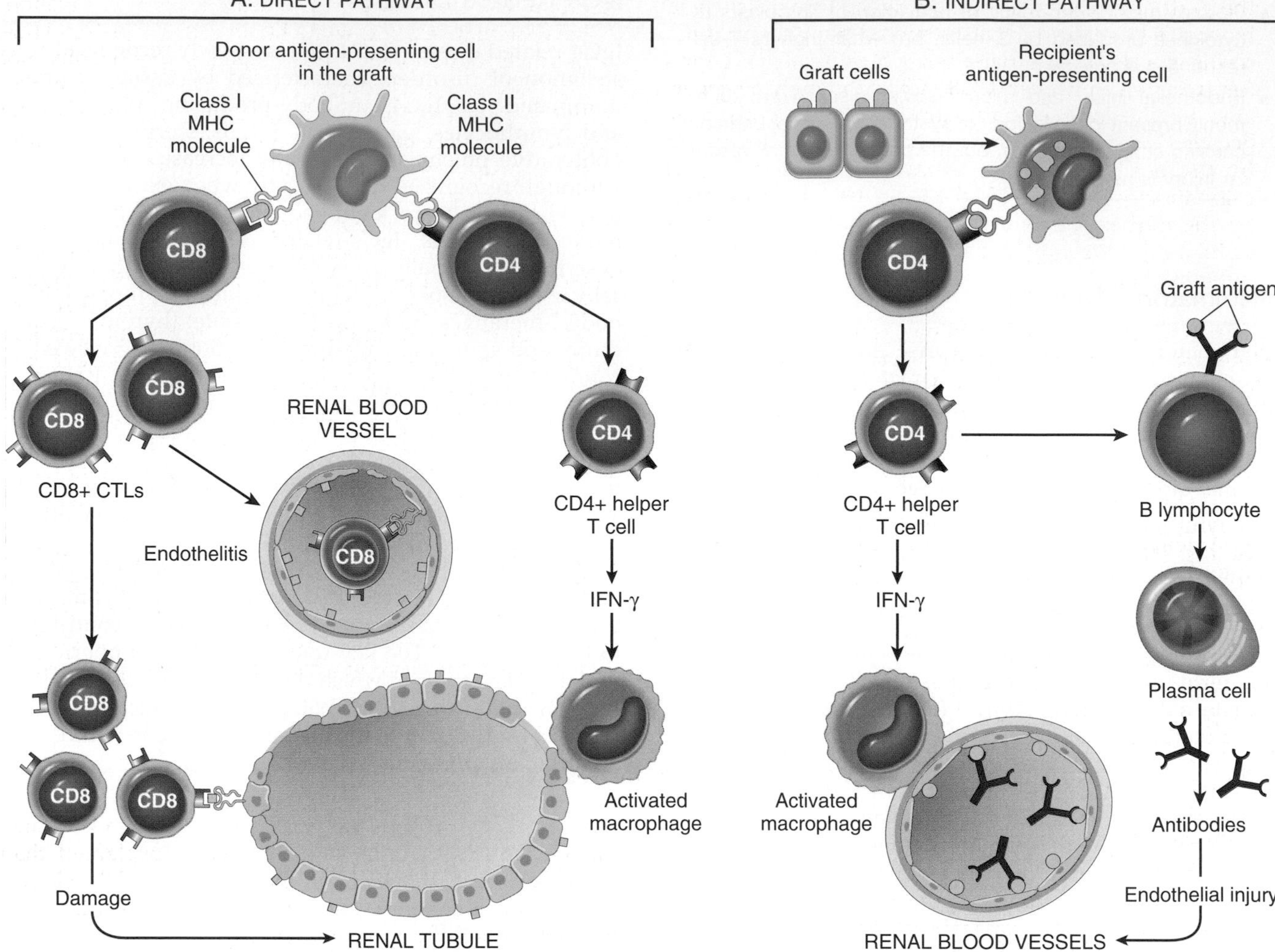

Figure 6-32 Recognition of alloantigens in organ grafts. **A,** In the direct pathway, donor class I and class II MHC antigens on antigen-presenting cells in the graft (along with costimulators, not shown) are recognized by host CD8+ cytotoxic T cells and CD4+ helper T cells, respectively. CD4+ cells proliferate and produce cytokines (e.g., IFN-γ), which induce tissue damage by a local inflammatory reaction. CD8+ T cells responding to graft antigens differentiate into CTLs that kill graft cells. **B,** In the indirect pathway graft antigens are picked up, processed, and displayed by host APCs and activate CD4+ T cells, which damage the graft by an inflammatory reaction and stimulate B lymphocytes to produce antibodies. An example of the reaction to kidney allografts is shown, but the same principles are applicable to all solid organ grafts.

antigens, or alloantigens) by two pathways, called *direct* and *indirect* (Fig. 6-32).

- **Direct pathway of allorecognition.** In the direct pathway, T cells of the transplant recipient recognize allogeneic (donor) MHC molecules on the surface of APCs in the graft. It is believed that dendritic cells carried in the donor organs are the most important APCs for initiating the antigraft response, because they not only express high levels of class I and II MHC molecules but also are endowed with costimulatory molecules (e.g., B7-1 and B7-2). The T cells of the host encounter the donor dendritic cells either within the grafted organ or after the dendritic cells migrate to the draining lymph nodes. CD8+ T cells recognize class I MHC molecules and differentiate into active CTLs. CD4+ helper T cells recognize allogeneic class II molecules and proliferate and differentiate into T_H1 (and possibly T_H17) effector cells. The direct recognition of allogeneic MHC molecules seems paradoxical to the rules of self MHC restriction: If T cells normally are restricted to recognizing foreign peptides displayed by self MHC molecules, why should these T cells recognize foreign MHC? The probable explanation is that allogeneic MHC molecules, with their bound peptides, resemble, or mimic, the self MHC–foreign peptide complexes that are recognized by self MHC–restricted T cells. In other words, recognition of allogeneic MHC molecules is a cross-reaction of T cells selected to recognize self MHC plus foreign peptides.
- **Indirect pathway of allorecognition.** In the indirect pathway, recipient T lymphocytes recognize MHC antigens of the graft donor after they are presented by the recipient's own APCs. This process involves the uptake and processing of MHC molecules from the grafted organ by host APCs. The peptides derived from the donor tissue are presented by the host's own MHC molecules, like any other foreign peptide. Thus, the indirect pathway is similar to the physiologic processing and presentation of other foreign (e.g., microbial) antigens. The indirect pathway generates CD4+ T cells that enter

the graft and recognize graft antigens being displayed by host APCs that have also entered the graft, and the result is a delayed hypersensitivity type of inflammatory reaction. However, CD8+ CTLs that may be generated by the indirect pathway cannot kill graft cells, because these CTLs recognize graft antigens presented by the host's APCs and cannot recognize the graft cells directly. Therefore, when T cells react to a graft by the indirect pathway, the principal mechanism of cellular rejection may be T-cell cytokine production and inflammation.

The frequency of T cells that can recognize the foreign antigens in a graft is much higher than the frequency of T cells specific for any microbe. For this reason, immune responses to allografts are stronger than responses to pathogens. Predictably, these strong reactions can destroy grafts rapidly, and their control requires powerful immunosuppressive agents.

B lymphocytes also recognize antigens in the graft, including HLA and other antigens that differ between donor and recipient. The activation of these B cells typically requires T cell help.

T Cell–Mediated Reactions

The critical role of T cells in transplant rejection has been documented in humans and in experimental animals. T cells can contribute to both acute and chronic rejection.

- **Acute cellular rejection,** also called *acute T cell–mediated rejection*, is most commonly seen within the initial months after transplantation and is heralded by clinical and biochemical signs of organ failure. It was thought that direct killing of graft cells by CD8+ CTLs is a major component of the reaction. However, more recent studies have established that an important component of this process is an inflammatory reaction in the graft triggered by cytokines secreted by activated CD4+ T cells. The inflammation results in increased vascular permeability and local accumulation of mononuclear cells (lymphocytes and macrophages), and graft injury is caused by the activated macrophages.
- T cells also contribute to **chronic rejection,** in which lymphocytes reacting against alloantigens in the vessel wall secrete cytokines that induce local inflammation and may stimulate the proliferation of vascular endothelial and smooth muscle cells.

Antibody-Mediated Reactions

Although T cells are pivotal in the rejection of organ transplants, antibodies produced against alloantigens in the graft are also important mediators of rejection. Antibody-mediated reactions can take three forms.

- **Hyperacute rejection occurs when preformed antidonor antibodies are present in the circulation of the recipient.** Such antibodies may be present in a recipient who has previously rejected a transplant. Multiparous women who develop antibodies against paternal HLA antigens shed from the fetus may have preformed antibodies that will react with grafts taken from their husbands or children, or even from unrelated individuals who share HLA alleles with the husbands. Prior blood transfusions can also lead to presensitization, because platelets and white blood cells are rich in HLA antigens and donors and recipients are usually not HLA-identical. Hyperacute rejection was a concern in the early days of kidney transplantation, but with the current practice of cross-matching, that is, testing recipient's serum for antibodies against donor's cells, it is no longer a significant clinical problem.
- **Acute antibody-mediated rejection** is caused by antidonor antibodies produced after transplantation. In recipients not previously sensitized to transplantation antigens, exposure to the class I and class II HLA antigens of the donor graft, as well as other antigens that differ between donor and recipient, may evoke antibodies. The antibodies formed by the recipient may cause injury by several mechanisms, including complement-dependent cytotoxicity, inflammation, and antibody-dependent cell-mediated cytotoxicity. The initial target of these antibodies in rejection seems to be the graft vasculature.
- **Chronic antibody-mediated rejection** usually develops insidiously, without preceding acute rejection, and primarily affects vascular components. Antibodies are detected in the circulation but are not readily identified within the graft. The mechanisms of the vascular lesions are not well understood.

Rejection of Kidney Grafts

Because kidneys were the first solid organs to be transplanted and more kidneys have been transplanted than any other organ, much of our understanding of the clinical and pathologic aspects of solid-organ transplantation is based on studies of renal allografts.

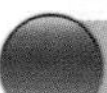

MORPHOLOGY

On the basis of the morphology and the underlying mechanism, rejection reactions are classified as hyperacute, acute, and chronic. The morphologic changes in these patterns are described later as they relate to renal transplants. Similar changes may occur in any other vascularized organ transplant and are discussed in relevant chapters.

Hyperacute Rejection

This form of rejection occurs within minutes or hours after transplantation. A hyperacutely rejecting kidney rapidly becomes cyanotic, mottled, and flaccid, and may excrete a mere few drops of bloody urine. Immunoglobulin and complement are deposited in the vessel wall, causing endothelial injury and fibrin-platelet thrombi (Fig. 6-33). Neutrophils rapidly accumulate within arterioles, glomeruli, and peritubular capillaries. As these changes become diffuse and intense, the glomeruli undergo thrombotic occlusion of the capillaries, and fibrinoid necrosis occurs in arterial walls. The kidney cortex then undergoes outright necrosis (infarction), and such nonfunctioning kidneys have to be removed.

Acute Rejection

This may occur within days of transplantation in the untreated recipient or may appear suddenly months or even years later, after immunosuppression is tapered or terminated. In any

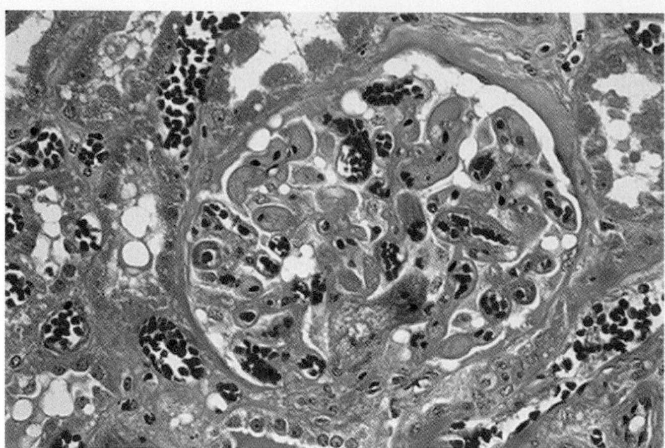

Figure 6-33 Hyperacute rejection. Hyperacute rejection of a kidney allograft showing platelet and fibrin thrombi, early neutrophil infiltration, and severe ischemic injury in a glomerulus.

one patient, cellular or humoral immune mechanisms may predominate.

- **Acute cellular (T cell-mediated) rejection.** Histologically, acute T cell–mediated rejection may be seen as two patterns.
  - In the **tubulointerstitial pattern** (sometimes called type I), there is extensive interstitial inflammation with infiltration of tubules, referred to as **tubulitis**, associated with focal tubular injury (Fig. 6-34*A*). As might be expected, immunohistochemical staining reveals both CD4+ and CD8+ T lymphocytes, which express markers of activated T cells, such as the α chain of the IL-2 receptor.
  - The **vascular pattern** shows inflammation of vessels (**endotheliitis**, type II) (Fig. 6-34*B*), sometimes with necrosis of vascular walls (type III). The affected vessels have swollen endothelial cells, and at places the lymphocytes can be seen between the endothelium and the vessel wall. The recognition of cellular rejection is important because, in the absence of an accompanying humoral rejection, patients respond well to immunosuppressive therapy.
- **Acute antibody-mediated rejection** is manifested mainly by damage to glomeruli and small blood vessels. Typically, the lesions consist of inflammation of glomeruli and peritubular capillaries, associated with deposition of the complement breakdown product C4d, which is produced during activation of the complement system by the antibody-dependent classical pathway (Fig. 6-35). Small vessels may also show focal thrombosis.

Cyclosporine, an immunosuppressive drug, is also nephrotoxic, and hence the histologic changes resulting from cyclosporine therapy (e.g., arteriolar hyaline deposits) may be superimposed.

Chronic Rejection

In recent years acute rejection has been largely controlled by immunosuppressive therapy, and chronic rejection has emerged as an increasingly frequent cause of graft failure. Patients with chronic rejection present clinically with progressive renal failure manifested by a rise in serum creatinine over a period of 4 to 6 months. Chronic rejection is dominated by vascular changes, which include (1) intimal thickening with inflammation, (2) glomerulopathy, with duplication of the basement membrane, likely secondary to chronic endothelial injury, and (3) peritubular capillaritis with multilayering of peritubular capillary basement membranes (Fig. 6-36). Interstitial fibrosis and tubular atrophy with loss of renal parenchyma may occur secondary to the vascular lesions. Chronically rejecting kidneys usually have interstitial mononuclear cell infiltrates, including NK cells and plasma cells.

Methods of Increasing Graft Survival

The value of HLA matching between donor and recipient varies in different solid-organ transplants. In kidney transplants, there is substantial benefit if all the polymorphic HLA alleles are matched (both inherited alleles of *HLA-A*, *-B*, and *DR*). However, HLA matching is usually not even done for transplants of liver, heart, and lungs, because other considerations, such as anatomic compatibility, severity of the underlying illness, and the need to minimize the time of organ storage, override the potential benefits of HLA matching.

Except for identical twins, who obviously express the same histocompatibility antigens, *immunosuppressive therapy* is a practical necessity in all other donor-recipient

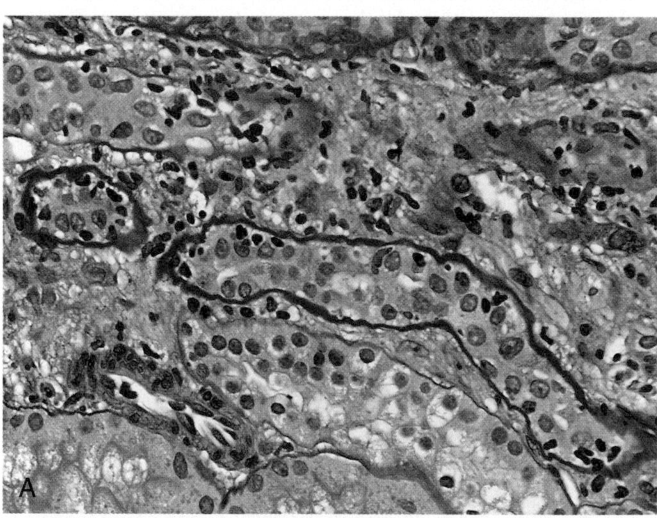

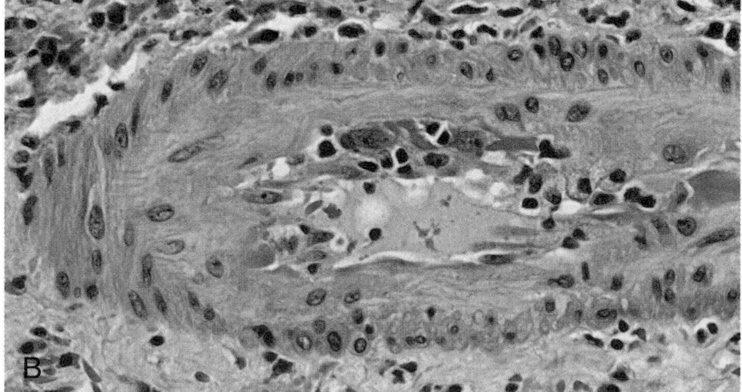

Figure 6-34 Acute T cell–mediated (cellular) rejection of a kidney allograft. **A,** Inflammatory cells in the interstitium and between epithelial cells of the tubules (tubulitis). **B,** Rejection vasculitis, with inflammatory cells attacking and undermining the endothelium (endotheliitis). (Courtesy Drs. Zoltan Laszik and Kuang-Yu Jen, Department of Pathology, University of California San Francisco.)

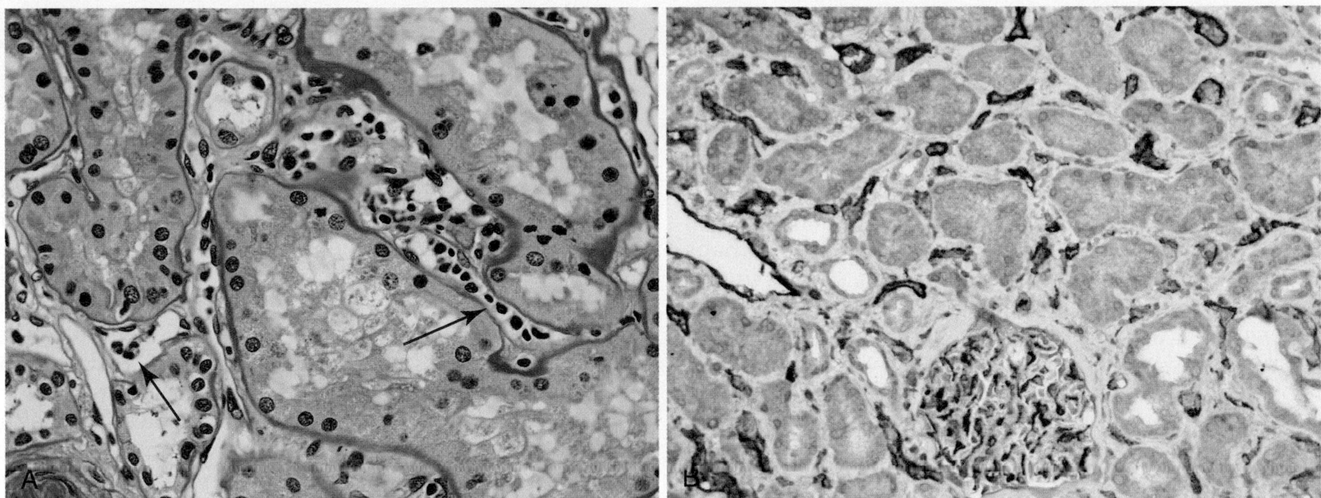

Figure 6-35 Acute antibody-mediated (humoral) rejection. **A,** Light micrograph showing inflammation (capillaritis) in peritubular capillaries (*arrows*). **B,** Immunoperoxidase stain shows C4d deposition in peritubular capillaries and a glomerulus. (Courtesy Dr. Zoltan Laszik, Department of Pathology, University of California San Francisco, Calif.)

combinations. Immunosuppressive drugs in current use include steroids (which reduce inflammation), mycophenolate mofetil (which inhibits lymphocyte proliferation), and tacrolimus (FK506). Tacrolimus, like its predecessor cyclosporine, is an inhibitor of the phosphatase calcineurin, which is required for activation of a transcription factor called nuclear factor of activated T cells (NFAT). NFAT stimulates transcription of cytokine genes, in particular, the gene that encodes IL-2. Thus, Tacrolimus inhibits T cell functions. Additional drugs that are used to treat rejection include T cell- and B cell-depleting antibodies, and pooled intravenous IgG (IVIG), which suppresses inflammation by unknown mechanisms. Plasmapheresis is used in cases of severe antibody-mediated rejection. Another, more recent, strategy for reducing antigraft immune responses is to prevent host T cells from receiving costimulatory signals from dendritic cells during the initial phase of sensitization. This can be accomplished by interrupting the interaction between the B7 molecules on the dendritic cells of the graft donor with the CD28 receptors on host T cells, for example, by administration of proteins that bind to B7 costimulators.

Although immunosuppression prolongs graft survival, it carries its own risks. The price paid in the form of increased susceptibility to opportunistic infections is not small. One of the most frequent infectious complications is reactivation of *polyoma virus*. The virus establishes latent infection of epithelial cells in the lower genitourinary tract of healthy individuals, and upon immunosuppression, it is reactivated, infects renal tubules, and may even cause graft

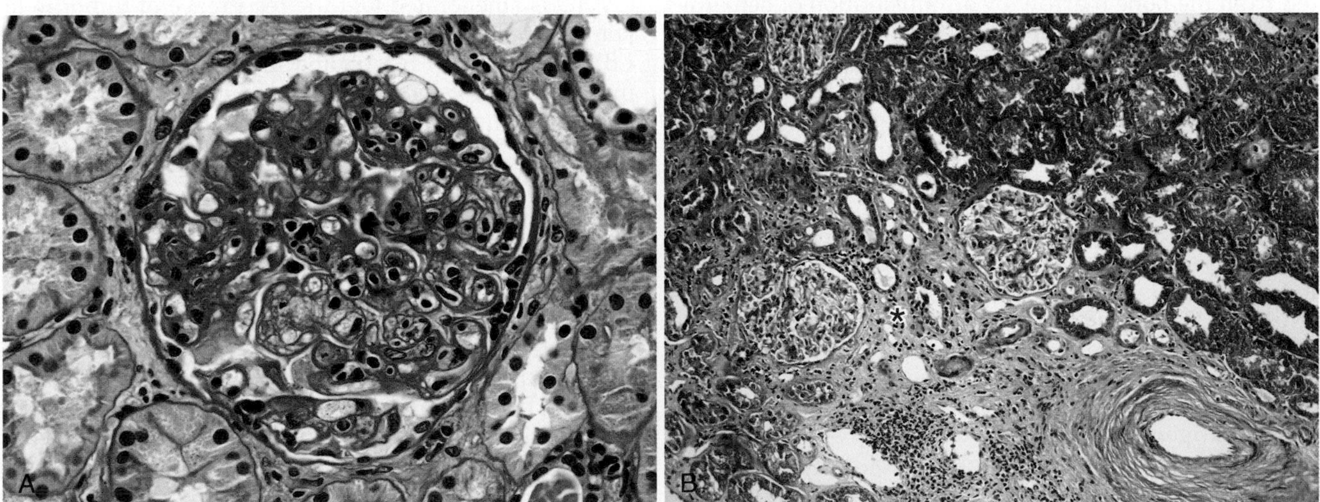

Figure 6-36 Chronic rejection of a kidney allograft. **A,** Transplant glomerulopathy, the characteristic manifestation of chronic antibody-mediated rejection. The glomerulus shows inflammatory cells within the capillary loops (glomerulitis), accumulation of mesangial matrix, and duplication of the capillary basement membrane. **B,** Interstitial fibrosis and tubular atrophy. In this trichrome stain, the blue area (*asterisk*) shows fibrosis, contrasted with the normal kidney on the top right. At the bottom right is an artery showing prominent arteriosclerosis. (Courtesy Dr. Zoltan Laszik, Department of Pathology, University of California San Francisco, Calif.)

failure. These patients are also at increased risk for developing EBV-induced lymphomas, human papillomavirus-induced squamous cell carcinomas, and Kaposi sarcoma (Chapter 11), all probably the result of reactivation of latent viral infections because of diminished host defenses. To circumvent the untoward effects of immunosuppression, much effort is being devoted to induce donor-specific tolerance in graft recipients. For instance, giving donor cells to graft recipients may prevent reactions to the graft, perhaps because the donor inoculum contains cells, such as immature dendritic cells, that induce tolerance to the donor alloantigens. This approach may result in long-term *mixed chimerism*, in which the recipient lives with the injected donor cells. Other strategies being tested include injecting regulatory T cells, and blocking the costimulatory signals that are required for lymphocyte activation, as mentioned above.

Transplantation of Other Solid Organs

In addition to the kidney, a variety of organs, such as the liver (Chapter 18), heart (Chapter 12), lungs, and pancreas, are also transplanted. The rejection reaction against liver transplants is not as vigorous as might be expected from the degree of HLA disparity. The molecular basis of this "privilege" is not understood.

Transplantation of Hematopoietic Stem Cells

Use of hematopoietic stem cell (HSC) transplants for hematologic malignancies, bone marrow failure syndromes (such as aplastic anemia), and disorders caused by inherited HSC defects (such as sickle cell anemia, thalassemia, and immunodeficiency states) is increasing in number each year. Transplantation of genetically "reengineered" hematopoietic stem cells obtained from affected patients may also be useful for somatic cell gene therapy, and is being evaluated in some immunodeficiencies. Historically, HSCs were obtained from the bone marrow, but now they usually are harvested from peripheral blood after they are mobilized from the bone marrow by administration of hematopoietic growth factors, or from the umbilical cord blood of newborn infants, a rich source of HSCs. In most of the conditions in which HSC transplantation is indicated, the recipient is irradiated or treated with high doses of chemotherapy to destroy the immune system (and sometimes, cancer cells) and to "open up" niches in the microenvironment of the marrow that nurture HSCs, thus allowing the transplanted HSCs to engraft. Several features distinguish HSC transplants from solid-organ transplants. Two problems that are unique to HSC transplantation are graft-versus-host disease (GVHD) and immunodeficiency.

GVHD occurs when immunologically competent cells or their precursors are transplanted into immunologically crippled recipients, and the transferred cells recognize alloantigens in the host and attack host tissues. It is seen most commonly in the setting of HSC transplantation but, rarely, may occur following transplantation of solid organs rich in lymphoid cells (e.g., the liver) or transfusion of unirradiated blood. When immune-compromised recipients receive HSC preparations from allogeneic donors, the immunocompetent T cells present in the donor inoculum recognize the recipient's HLA antigens as foreign and react against them. To try to minimize GVHD, HSC transplants are done between donor and recipient that are HLA-matched using precise DNA sequencing-based methods for molecular typing of HLA alleles.

- **Acute GVHD** occurs within days to weeks after allogeneic bone marrow transplantation. Although any organ may be affected, the major clinical manifestations result from involvement of the immune system and epithelia of the skin, liver, and intestines. Involvement of skin in GVHD is manifested by a generalized rash that may lead to desquamation in severe cases. Destruction of small bile ducts gives rise to jaundice, and mucosal ulceration of the gut results in bloody diarrhea. Although tissue injury may be severe, the affected tissues are usually not heavily infiltrated by lymphocytes. It is believed that in addition to direct cytotoxicity by CD8+ T cells, considerable damage is inflicted by cytokines released by the sensitized donor T cells.
- **Chronic GVHD** may follow the acute syndrome or may occur insidiously. These patients have extensive cutaneous injury, with destruction of skin appendages and fibrosis of the dermis. The changes may resemble systemic sclerosis (discussed earlier). Chronic liver disease manifested by cholestatic jaundice is also frequent. Damage to the gastrointestinal tract may cause esophageal strictures. The immune system is devastated, with involution of the thymus and depletion of lymphocytes in the lymph nodes. Not surprisingly, the patients experience recurrent and life-threatening infections. Some patients develop manifestations of autoimmunity, postulated to result from the grafted CD4+ helper T cells reacting with host B cells and stimulating these cells, some of which may be capable of producing autoantibodies.

Because GVHD is mediated by T lymphocytes contained in the transplanted donor cells, depletion of donor T cells before transfusion virtually eliminates the disease. This protocol, however, has proved to be a mixed blessing: GVHD is ameliorated, but the recurrence of tumor in leukemic patients as well as the incidence of graft failures and EBV-related B-cell lymphoma increase. It seems that the multifaceted T cells not only mediate GVHD but also are required for engraftment of the transplanted HSCs, suppression of EBV-infected B-cell clones, and control of leukemia cells. The latter *graft-versus-leukemia* effect can be quite dramatic. In fact, deliberate induction of graft-versus-leukemia effect by infusion of allogeneic T cells is used to treat chronic myelogenous leukemia that has relapsed after HSC transplantation.

Immunodeficiency is a frequent complication of HSC transplantation. The immunodeficiency may be a result of prior treatment, myeloablative preparation for the graft, a delay in repopulation of the recipient's immune system, and attack on the host's immune cells by grafted lymphocytes. Affected individuals are profoundly immunosuppressed and are easy prey to infections. Although many different types of organisms may infect patients, infection with cytomegalovirus is particularly important. This usually results from activation of previously silent infection. Cytomegalovirus-induced pneumonitis can be a fatal complication.

KEY CONCEPTS

Recognition and Rejection of Transplants (Allografts)

- The rejection response against solid organ transplants is initiated mainly by host T cells that recognize the foreign HLA antigens of the graft, either directly (on APCs in the graft) or indirectly (after uptake and presentation by host APCs).
- Types and mechanisms of rejection of solid organ grafts:
  - Hyperacute rejection. Preformed antidonor antibodies bind to graft endothelium immediately after transplantation, leading to thrombosis, ischemic damage, and rapid graft failure.
  - Acute cellular rejection. T cells destroy graft parenchyma (and vessels) by cytotoxicity and inflammatory reactions.
  - Acute humoral rejection. Antibodies damage graft vasculature.
  - Chronic rejection. Dominated by arteriosclerosis, this type is caused by T-cell activation and antibodies. The T-cells may secrete cytokines that induce proliferation of vascular smooth muscle cells, and the antibodies cause endothelial injury. The vascular lesions and T-cell reactions cause parenchymal fibrosis.
- Treatment of graft rejection relies on immunosuppressive drugs, which inhibit immune responses against the graft.
- Transplantation of hematopoietic stem cells (HSCs) requires careful matching of donor and recipient and is often complicated by graft-vs-host diseases (GVHD) and immune deficiency.

Immunodeficiency Syndromes

Immunodeficiencies can be divided into **primary** (or **congenital**) immunodeficiency disorders, which are genetically determined, and **secondary** (or **acquired**) immunodeficiencies, which may arise as complications of cancers, infections, malnutrition, or side effects of immunosuppression, irradiation, or chemotherapy for cancer and other diseases. Immunodeficiencies are manifested clinically by increased infections, which may be newly acquired or reactivation of latent infections. The primary immunodeficiency syndromes are accidents of nature that provide valuable insights into some of the critical molecules of the human immune system. Here we briefly discuss the more important and best-defined primary immunodeficiencies, to be followed by a more detailed description of acquired immunodeficiency syndrome (AIDS), the most devastating example of secondary immunodeficiency.

Primary Immunodeficiencies

Most primary immunodeficiency diseases are genetically determined and affect the defense mechanisms of innate immunity (phagocytes, NK cells, or complement) or the humoral and/or cellular arms of adaptive immunity (mediated by B and T lymphocytes, respectively). Although these disorders were once thought to be quite rare, some form of mild genetic immune deficiency is, in fact, present in many individuals. Most primary immunodeficiencies are detected in infancy, between 6 months and 2 years of life, the telltale signs being susceptibility to recurrent infections. Here we present selected examples of immunodeficiencies, beginning with defects in innate immunity and then defects in the maturation and activation of B and T lymphocytes. We conclude with immune defects associated with some systemic diseases.

Defects in Innate Immunity

Inherited defects in the early innate immune response typically affect leukocyte functions or the complement system, and all lead to increased vulnerability to infections (Table 6-12). Some of the defects whose molecular basis is defined are summarized next.

Defects in Leukocyte Function

- **Inherited defects in leukocyte adhesion**. Individuals with *leukocyte adhesion deficiency type 1* have a defect in the biosynthesis of the β_2 chain shared by the LFA-1 and Mac-1 integrins. *Leukocyte adhesion deficiency type 2* is caused by the absence of sialyl-Lewis X, the fucose-containing ligand for E- and P-selectins, as a result of a defect in a fucosyl transferase, the enzyme that attaches fucose moieties to protein backbones. The major clinical problem in both conditions is recurrent bacterial infections due to inadequate granulocyte function.

Table 6-12 Defects in Innate Immunity

Disease	Defect
Defects in Leukocyte Function	
Leukocyte adhesion deficiency 1	Defective leukocyte adhesion because of mutations in β chain of CD11/CD18 integrins
Leukocyte adhesion deficiency 2	Defective leukocyte adhesion because of mutations in fucosyl transferase required for synthesis of sialylated oligosaccharide (receptor for selectins)
Chédiak-Higashi syndrome	Decreased leukocyte functions because of mutations affecting protein involved in lysosomal membrane traffic
Chronic granulomatous disease	Decreased oxidative burst
X-linked	Phagocyte oxidase (membrane component)
Autosomal recessive	Phagocyte oxidase (cytoplasmic components)
Myeloperoxidase deficiency	Decreased microbial killing because of defective MPO-H_2O_2 system
Defects in the Complement System	
C2, C4 deficiency	Defective classical pathway activation, results in reduced resistance to infection and reduced clearance of immune complexes
C3 deficiency	Defects in all complement functions
Deficiency of complement regulatory proteins	Excessive complement activation; clinical syndromes include angioedema, paroxysmal hemoglobinuria, others

The table lists some of the more common inherited immune deficiencies affecting phagocytic leukocytes and the complement system.

Modified in part from Gallin JI: Disorders of phagocytic cells. In Gallin JI, et al (eds): Inflammation: Basic Principles and Clinical Correlates, 2nd ed. New York, Raven Press, 1992, pp 860, 861.

- **Inherited defects in phagolysosome function**. One such disorder is *Chédiak-Higashi syndrome,* an autosomal recessive condition characterized by defective fusion of phagosomes and lysosomes, resulting in defective phagocytes function and susceptibility to infections. The main leukocyte abnormalities are neutropenia (decreased numbers of neutrophils), defective degranulation, and delayed microbial killing. Leukocytes contain giant granules, which can be readily seen in peripheral blood smears and are thought to result from aberrant phagolysosome fusion. In addition, there are abnormalities in melanocytes (leading to albinism), cells of the nervous system (associated with nerve defects), and platelets (causing bleeding disorders). The gene associated with this disorder encodes a large cytosolic protein called LYST, which is believed to regulate lysosomal trafficking.
- **Inherited defects in microbicidal activity**. The importance of oxygen-dependent bactericidal mechanisms is shown by the existence of a group of congenital disorders called *chronic granulomatous disease*, which are characterized by defects in bacterial killing and render patients susceptible to recurrent bacterial infection. Chronic granulomatous disease results from inherited defects in the genes encoding components of *phagocyte oxidase*, the phagolysosomal enzyme that generates superoxide ($O_2^{\bar{\cdot}}$). The most common variants are an X-linked defect in one of the membrane-bound components (gp91phox) and autosomal recessive defects in the genes encoding two of the cytoplasmic components (p47phox and p67phox). The name of this disease comes from the macrophage-rich chronic inflammatory reaction that tries to control the infection when the initial neutrophil defense is inadequate. This often leads to collections of activated macrophages that wall off the microbes, forming granulomas.
- **Defects in TLR signaling**. Rare defects have been described in various TLRs. Defects in TLR3, a receptor for viral RNA, result in recurrent herpes simplex encephalitis, and defects in MyD88, the adaptor protein downstream of multiple TLRs, are associated with destructive bacterial pneumonias. It has been a surprise that these inherited abnormalities present with such restricted clinical phenotypes.

Deficiencies Affecting the Complement System

Hereditary deficiencies have been described for virtually all components of the complement system and several of the regulators. In addition, one disease, paroxysmal nocturnal hemoglobinuria, is marked by an acquired deficiency of complement regulatory factors.

- Deficiency of C2 is the most common complement protein deficiency. A deficiency of C2 or C4, early components of the classical pathway, is associated with increased bacterial or viral infections. However, many patients have no clinical manifestations, presumably because the alternative complement pathway is adequate for the control of most infections. Surprisingly, in some of these patients, as well as in patients with C1q deficiency, the dominant manifestation is SLE-like autoimmune disease, as discussed earlier.
- Deficiency of components of the alternative pathway (properdin and factor D) is rare. It is associated with recurrent pyogenic infections.
- The C3 component of complement is required for both the classical and alternative pathways, and hence a deficiency of this protein results in susceptibility to serious and recurrent pyogenic infections. There is also increased incidence of immune complex-mediated glomerulonephritis; in the absence of complement, immune complex-mediated inflammation is presumably caused by Fc receptor-dependent leukocyte activation.
- The terminal components of complement C5, 6, 7, 8, and 9 are required for the assembly of the membrane attack complex involved in the lysis of organisms. With a deficiency of these late-acting components, there is increased susceptibility to recurrent neisserial (gonococcal and meningococcal) infections; *Neisseria* bacteria have thin cell walls and are especially susceptible to the lytic actions of complement. Some patients inherit a defective form of mannose-binding lectin, the plasma protein that initiates the lectin pathway of complement. These individuals also show increased susceptibility to infections.
- A deficiency of C1 inhibitor (C1 INH) gives rise to *hereditary angioedema*. This autosomal dominant disorder is more common than complement deficiency states. The C1 inhibitor's targets are proteases, specifically C1r and C1s of the complement cascade, factor XII of the coagulation pathway, and the kallikrein system. With deficiency of C1 INH, unregulated activation of kallikrein may lead to increased production of vasoactive peptides such as bradykinin. Although the exact nature of the bioactive compound produced in hereditary angioedema is uncertain, these patients have episodes of edema affecting skin and mucosal surfaces such as the larynx and the gastrointestinal tract. This may result in life-threatening asphyxia or nausea, vomiting, and diarrhea after minor trauma or emotional stress. Acute attacks of hereditary angioedema can be treated with C1 inhibitor concentrates prepared from human plasma.
- Deficiencies of other complement regulatory proteins are the cause of paroxysmal nocturnal hemoglobinuria (Chapter 14) and some cases of hemolytic uremic syndrome (Chapter 20).

Defects in Adaptive Immunity

Defects in adaptive immunity are often subclassified on the basis of the primary component involved (i.e., B cells or T cells or both). However, these distinctions are not clear-cut; for instance, T-cell defects almost always lead to impaired antibody synthesis, and hence isolated deficiencies of T cells are often indistinguishable clinically from combined deficiencies of T and B cells. These immunodeficiencies result from abnormalities in lymphocyte maturation or activation. With advances in genetic analyses, the mutations responsible for many of these diseases have now been identified (Fig. 6-37).

Defects in Lymphocyte Maturation

Genetic deficiencies affecting the maturation of T or B lymphocytes present with abnormalities in cell-mediated or humoral immunity that are of varying severity.

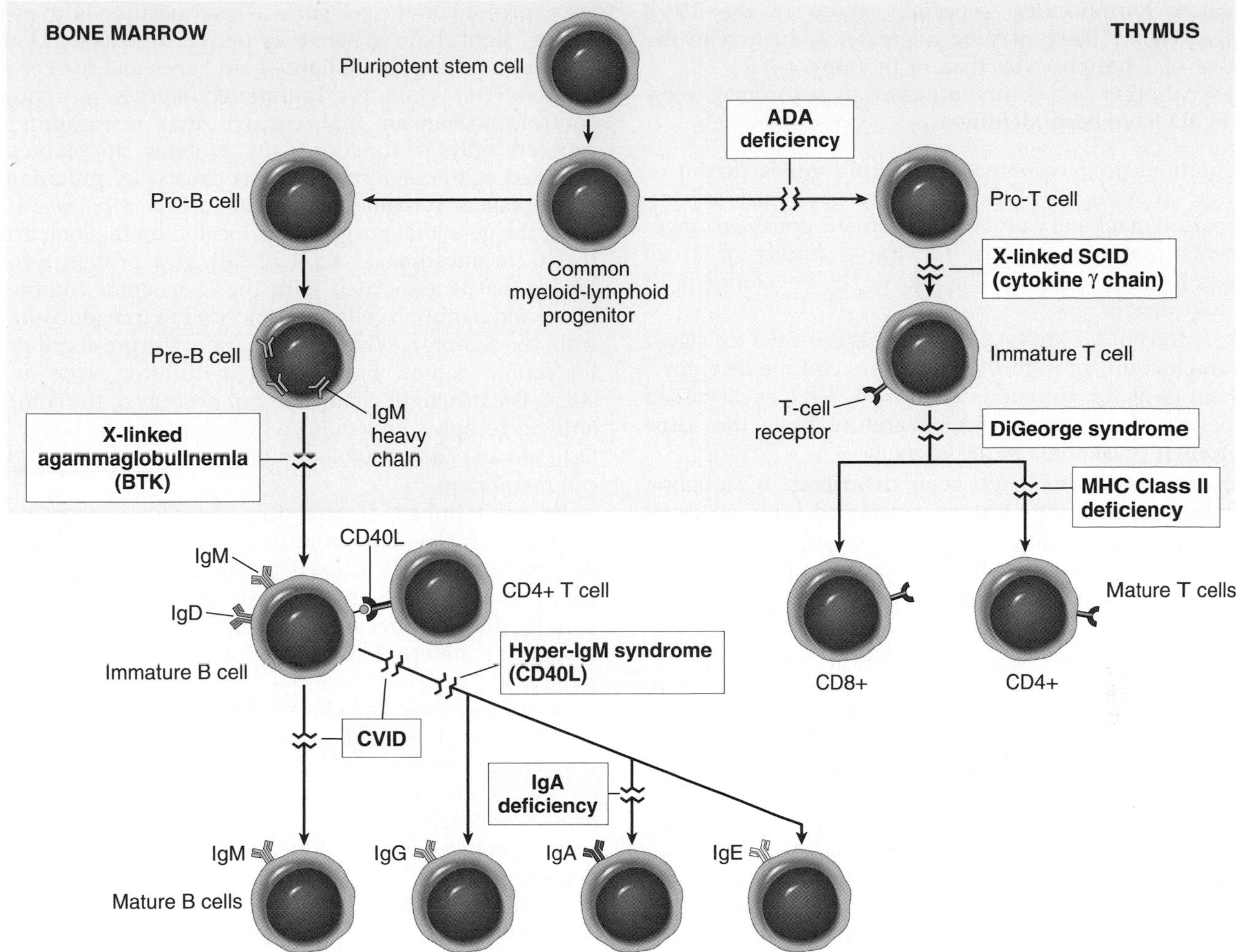

Figure 6-37 Primary immune deficiency diseases. Shown are the principal pathways of lymphocyte development and the blocks in these pathways in selected primary immune deficiency diseases. The affected genes are indicated in parentheses for some of the disorders. ADA, Adenosine deaminase; CD40L, CD40 ligand (also known as CD154); CVID, common variable immunodeficiency; SCID, severe combined immunodeficiency.

Severe Combined Immunodeficiency

Severe combined immunodeficiency (SCID) represents a constellation of genetically distinct syndromes, all having in common defects in both humoral and cell-mediated immune responses. Affected infants present with prominent thrush (oral candidiasis), extensive diaper rash, and failure to thrive. Some patients develop a morbilliform rash shortly after birth because maternal T cells are transferred across the placenta and attack the fetus, causing GVHD. Persons with SCID are extremely susceptible to recurrent, severe infections by a wide range of pathogens, including *Candida albicans*, *Pneumocystis jiroveci*, *Pseudomonas*, cytomegalovirus, varicella, and a whole host of bacteria. Without HSC transplantation, death occurs within the first year of life. Despite the common clinical manifestations, the underlying defects are quite varied in different forms of SCID, and in many cases the genetic lesion is not known. Often, the SCID defect resides in the T-cell compartment, with a secondary impairment of humoral immunity.

X-linked SCID. The most common form, accounting for 50% to 60% of cases, is X-linked, and hence SCID is more common in boys than in girls. The genetic defect in the X-linked form is a **mutation in the common γ-chain (γc) subunit of cytokine receptors**. This transmembrane protein is a signal-transducing component of the receptors for IL-2, IL-4, IL-7, IL-9, IL-11, IL-15, and IL-21. IL-7 is required for the survival and proliferation of lymphoid progenitors, particularly T-cell precursors. As a result of defective IL-7 receptor signaling, there is a profound defect in the earliest stages of lymphocyte development, especially T-cell development. T-cell numbers are greatly reduced, and although B cells may be normal in number, antibody synthesis is impaired because of lack of T-cell help. IL-15 is important for the maturation and proliferation of NK cells, and because the common γ chain is a component of the receptor for IL-15, these individuals often have a deficiency of NK cells as well.

Autosomal recessive SCID. The remaining forms of SCID are autosomal recessive disorders. The most common cause of autosomal recessive SCID is a **deficiency of the enzyme adenosine deaminase (ADA)**. Although the mechanisms by which ADA deficiency causes SCID are not entirely clear, it has been proposed that deficiency of ADA leads to accumulation of deoxyadenosine and its derivatives (e.g., deoxy-ATP), which are toxic to rapidly dividing immature lymphocytes, especially those of the T-cell lineage. Hence there may be a greater reduction in the number of T lymphocytes than of B lymphocytes.

Several other less common causes of autosomal recessive SCID have been identified:

- Mutations in recombinase-activating genes (RAG) or other components of the antigen receptor gene recombination machinery prevent the somatic gene rearrangements that are essential for the assembly of T-cell receptor and Ig genes. This blocks the development of T and B cells.
- An intracellular kinase called Jak3 is essential for signal transduction through the common cytokine receptor γ chain (which is mutated in X-linked SCID, as discussed above). Mutations of Jak3 therefore have the same effects as mutations in the γc chain.
- Several mutations have been described in signaling molecules, including kinases associated with the T-cell antigen receptor and components of calcium channels that are required for entry of calcium and activation of many signaling pathways.

The histologic findings in SCID depend on the underlying defect. In the two most common forms (γc mutation and ADA deficiency), the thymus is small and devoid of lymphoid cells. In X-linked SCID the thymus contains lobules of undifferentiated epithelial cells resembling fetal thymus, whereas in SCID caused by ADA deficiency, remnants of Hassall's corpuscles can be found. In both diseases, other lymphoid tissues are hypoplastic as well, with marked depletion of T-cell areas and in some cases both T-cell and B-cell zones.

Currently, HSC transplantation is the mainstay of treatment, but X-linked SCID is the first human disease in which gene therapy has been successful. For gene therapy a normal γc gene is expressed using a viral vector in HSCs taken from patients, and the cells are then transplanted back into the patients. The clinical experience is small, but some patients have shown reconstitution of their immune systems for over a year after therapy. Unfortunately, however, about 20% of these patients have developed T-cell lymphoblastic leukemia, highlighting the dangers of this particular approach to gene therapy. The uncontrolled T-cell proliferation may have been triggered by the activation of oncogenes by the integrated virus together with the growth advantage conferred by the introduced γc gene. Current trials are using new vectors with safety features built in. Patients with ADA deficiency have also been treated with HSC transplantation and, more recently, with administration of the enzyme or gene therapy involving the introduction of a normal *ADA* gene into T-cell precursors.

X-Linked Agammaglobulinemia (Bruton Agammaglobulinemia)

X-linked agammaglobulinemia is characterized by the failure of B-cell precursors (pro-B cells and pre-B cells) to develop into mature B cells. It is one of the more common forms of primary immunodeficiency. During normal B-cell maturation in the bone marrow, the Ig heavy-chain genes are rearranged first, in pre-B cells, and these are expressed on the cell surface in association with a "surrogate" light chain, where they deliver signals that induce rearrangement of the Ig light-chain genes and further maturation. This need for Ig-initiated signals is a quality control mechanism that ensures that maturation will proceed only if functional Ig proteins are expressed. X-linked agammaglobulinemia is caused by mutations in a cytoplasmic tyrosine kinase, called *Bruton tyrosine kinase (Btk)*; the gene that encodes it is located on the long arm of the X chromosome at Xq21.22. Btk is a protein tyrosine kinase that is associated with the Ig receptor complex of pre-B and mature B cells and is needed to transduce signals from the receptor. When it is mutated, the pre-B cell receptor cannot deliver signals, and maturation stops at this stage. Because light chains are not produced, the complete antigen receptor molecule (which contains Ig heavy and light chains) cannot be assembled and transported to the cell membrane.

As an X-linked disease, this disorder is seen almost entirely in males, but sporadic cases have been described in females, possibly caused by mutations in some other genes that function in the same pathway. **The disease usually does not become apparent until about 6 months of age, as maternal immunoglobulins are depleted.** In most cases, recurrent bacterial infections of the respiratory tract, such as acute and chronic pharyngitis, sinusitis, otitis media, bronchitis, and pneumonia, call attention to the underlying immune defect. Almost always the causative organisms are *Haemophilus influenzae, Streptococcus pneumoniae*, or *Staphylococcus aureus*. These organisms are normally opsonized by antibodies and cleared by phagocytosis. Because antibodies are important for neutralizing infectious viruses that are present in the bloodstream or mucosal secretions or being passed from cell to cell, individuals with this disease are also susceptible to certain viral infections, especially those caused by enteroviruses, such as echovirus, poliovirus, and coxsackievirus. These viruses infect the gastrointestinal tract, and from here they can disseminate to the nervous system via the blood. Thus, immunization with live poliovirus carries the risk of paralytic poliomyelitis, and echovirus can cause fatal encephalitis. For similar reasons, *Giardia lamblia*, an intestinal protozoan that is normally resisted by secreted IgA, causes persistent infections in persons with this disorder. In general, however, most intracellular viral, fungal, and protozoal infections are handled quite well by the intact T cell–mediated immunity.

The classic form of this disease has the following characteristics:

- B cells are absent or markedly decreased in the circulation, and the serum levels of all classes of immunoglobulins are depressed. Pre-B cells, which express the B-lineage marker CD19 but not membrane Ig, are found in normal numbers in the bone marrow.
- Germinal centers of lymph nodes, Peyer's patches, the appendix, and tonsils are underdeveloped.
- Plasma cells are absent throughout the body.
- T cell–mediated reactions are normal.

Autoimmune diseases, such as arthritis and dermatomyositis, occur in as many as 35% of individuals with this disease, which is paradoxical in association with an immune deficiency. It is likely that these autoimmune disorders are caused by a breakdown of self-tolerance resulting in autoimmunity, but chronic infections associated with the immune deficiency may play a role in inducing the inflammatory reactions. The treatment of X-linked agammaglobulinemia is replacement therapy with immunoglobulins. In the past, most patients succumbed to infection in infancy or early childhood. Prophylactic intravenous Ig therapy allows most individuals to reach adulthood.

DiGeorge Syndrome (Thymic Hypoplasia)

DiGeorge syndrome is a T-cell deficiency that results from failure of development of the third and fourth pharyngeal pouches. The latter give rise to the thymus, the parathyroids, some of the C cells of the thyroid, and the ultimobranchial body. Thus, individuals with this syndrome have a variable loss of T cell mediated immunity (resulting from hypoplasia or lack of the thymus), tetany (resulting from lack of the parathyroids), and congenital defects of the heart and great vessels. In addition, the appearance of the mouth, ears, and facies may be abnormal. Absence of cell-mediated immunity is caused by low numbers of T lymphocytes in the blood and lymphoid tissues and poor defense against certain fungal and viral infections. The T-cell zones of lymphoid organs—paracortical areas of the lymph nodes and the periarteriolar sheaths of the spleen—are depleted. Ig levels may be normal or reduced, depending on the severity of the T-cell deficiency.

In many cases, DiGeorge syndrome is not a familial disorder. It results from a deletion that maps to chromosome 22q11. This deletion is seen in more than 50% of patients, and DiGeorge syndrome is now considered a component of the *22q11 deletion syndrome*, discussed in Chapter 5. One gene in the deleted region is *TBX1*, which is required for development of the branchial arch and the great vessels. Notably, *TBX1* is involved by loss-of-function mutations in a few cases of DiGeorge syndrome that lack 22q11 deletions, strongly suggesting that its loss contributes to the observed phenotype.

Other Defects in Lymphocyte Maturation

Many other, rare causes of immunodeficiency resulting from defective lymphocyte maturation have been documented. One of these, the *bare lymphocyte syndrome*, is usually caused by mutations in transcription factors that are required for class II MHC gene expression. Lack of expression of class II MHC molecules prevents the development of CD4+ T cells. CD4+ T cells are involved in cellular immunity and provide help to B cells, and hence class II MHC deficiency results in combined immunodeficiency. Other defects are caused by mutations in antigen receptor chains or signaling molecules involved in T- or B-cell maturation.

Defects in Lymphocyte Activation and Function

With our improving understanding of the molecular pathways in lymphocyte activation and function, there has also been an increasing recognition of immune deficiencies caused by mutations affecting various components of these pathways. Some of the mutations cause well-defined syndromes, and others are rare but informative.

Hyper-IgM Syndrome

In this disorder the affected patients make IgM antibodies but are deficient in their ability to produce IgG, IgA, and IgE antibodies. It is now known that the defect in this disease affects the ability of helper T cells to deliver activating signals to B cells and macrophages. As discussed earlier in the chapter, many of the functions of CD4+ helper T cells require the engagement of CD40 on B cells, macrophages and dendritic cells by CD40L (also called CD154) expressed on antigen-activated T cells. This interaction triggers Ig class switching and affinity maturation in B cells, and stimulates the microbicidal functions of macrophages. Approximately 70% of individuals with hyper-IgM syndrome have the X-linked form of the disease, caused by mutations in the gene encoding CD40L located on Xq26. In the remaining patients the disease is inherited in an autosomal recessive pattern. Most of these patients have loss-of-function mutations involving either CD40 or the enzyme called activation-induced cytidine deaminase (AID), a DNA-editing enzyme that is required for Ig class switching and affinity maturation.

The serum of persons with this syndrome contains normal or elevated levels of IgM but no IgA or IgE and extremely low levels of IgG, although the number of B and T cells is normal. Clinically, patients present with recurrent pyogenic infections, because the level of opsonizing IgG antibodies is low. In addition, those with CD40L mutations are also susceptible to pneumonia caused by the intracellular organism *Pneumocystis jiroveci*, because CD40L-mediated macrophage activation, a key reaction of cell-mediated immunity, is also defective. Occasionally, the IgM antibodies react with blood cells, giving rise to autoimmune hemolytic anemia, thrombocytopenia, and neutropenia. In older patients there may be a proliferation of IgM-producing plasma cells that infiltrates the mucosa of the gastrointestinal tract.

Common Variable Immunodeficiency

This relatively frequent but poorly defined entity encompasses a heterogeneous group of disorders in which the common feature is hypogammaglobulinemia, generally affecting all the antibody classes but sometimes only IgG. The diagnosis of common variable immunodeficiency is based on exclusion of other well-defined causes of decreased antibody production.

Both sporadic and inherited forms of the disease occur. In familial forms there is no single pattern of inheritance. Relatives of such patients have a high incidence of selective IgA deficiency (see later). These studies suggest that at least in some cases, selective IgA deficiency and common variable immunodeficiency may represent different expressions of a common genetic defect in antibody synthesis. In contrast to X-linked agammaglobulinemia, most individuals with common variable immunodeficiency have normal or near-normal numbers of B cells in the blood and lymphoid tissues. These B cells, however, are not able to differentiate into plasma cells.

Both intrinsic B-cell defects and abnormalities in helper T cell–mediated activation of B cells may account for the antibody deficiency in this disease. Families have been reported in which the underlying abnormality is in a receptor for a cytokine called BAFF that promotes the survival and differentiation of B cells, or in a molecule called ICOS (inducible costimulator) that is homologous to CD28 and is involved in T-cell activation and in interactions between T and B cells. However, the known mutations account for a minority of cases.

The clinical manifestations of common variable immunodeficiency are caused by antibody deficiency, and hence they resemble those of X-linked agammaglobulinemia. The patients typically present with recurrent sinopulmonary pyogenic infections. In addition, about 20% of patients have recurrent herpesvirus infections. Serious enterovirus infections causing meningoencephalitis may also occur. Individuals with this disorder are also prone to the development of persistent diarrhea caused by *G. lamblia*. In contrast to X-linked agammaglobulinemia, common variable immunodeficiency affects both sexes equally, and the onset of symptoms is later, in childhood or adolescence. Histologically the B-cell areas of the lymphoid tissues (i.e., lymphoid follicles in nodes, spleen, and gut) are hyperplastic. The enlargement of B-cell areas may reflect incomplete activation, such that B cells can proliferate in response to antigen but do not produce antibodies.

As in X-linked agammaglobulinemia, these patients have a high frequency of autoimmune diseases (approximately 20%), including rheumatoid arthritis. The risk of lymphoid malignancy is also increased, and an increase in gastric cancer has been reported.

Isolated IgA Deficiency

Isolated IgA deficiency is a common immunodeficiency. In the United States it occurs in about 1 in 600 individuals of European descent. It is far less common in blacks and Asians. Affected individuals have extremely **low levels of both serum and secretory IgA**. It may be familial, or acquired in association with toxoplasmosis, measles, or some other viral infection. The association of IgA deficiency with common variable immunodeficiency was mentioned earlier. Most individuals with this disease are asymptomatic. Because IgA is the major antibody in external secretions, mucosal defenses are weakened, and infections occur in the respiratory, gastrointestinal, and urogenital tracts. Symptomatic patients commonly present with recurrent sinopulmonary infections and diarrhea. Some individuals with IgA deficiency are also deficient in the IgG2 and IgG4 subclasses of IgG. This group of patients is particularly prone to developing infections. In addition, IgA-deficient patients have a high frequency of respiratory tract allergy and a variety of autoimmune diseases, particularly SLE and rheumatoid arthritis. The basis of the increased frequency of autoimmune and allergic diseases is not known. When transfused with blood containing normal IgA, some of these patients develop severe, even fatal, anaphylactic reactions, because the IgA behaves like a foreign antigen (since the patients do not produce it and are not tolerant to it).

The defect in IgA deficiency is impaired differentiation of naive B lymphocytes to IgA-producing plasma cells. The molecular basis of this defect in most patients is unknown. Defects in a receptor for the B cell–activating cytokine, BAFF, have been described in some patients.

X-Linked Lymphoproliferative Syndrome

X-linked lymphoproliferative disease is characterized by an inability to eliminate Epstein-Barr virus (EBV), eventually leading to fulminant infectious mononucleosis and the development of B-cell tumors. In about 80% of cases, the disease is due to mutations in the gene encoding an adaptor molecule called *SLAM-associated protein (SAP)* that binds to a family of cell surface molecules involved in the activation of NK cells and T and B lymphocytes, including the signaling lymphocyte activation molecule (SLAM). Defects in SAP contribute to attenuated NK and T cell activation and result in increased susceptibility to viral infections. SAP is also required for the development of follicular helper T cells, and because of this defect XLP patients are unable to form germinal centers or produce high affinity antibodies, additional abnormalities that also likely contribute to susceptibility to viral infection. This immunodeficiency is most commonly manifested by severe EBV infection, including severe and sometimes fatal infectious mononucleosis (Chapter 8), but not other viral infections, for reasons that are not clear.

Other Defects in Lymphocyte Activation

Many rare cases of lymphocyte activation defects have been described, affecting antigen receptor signaling and various biochemical pathways. Defects in T_H1 responses are associated with atypical mycobacterial infections and defective T_H17 responses are the cause of chronic mucocutaneous candidiasis as well as bacterial infections of the skin (a disorder called *Job syndrome*).

Immunodeficiencies Associated with Systemic Diseases

In some inherited systemic disorders, immune deficiency is a prominent clinical problem. Two representative examples of such diseases are described next.

Wiskott-Aldrich Syndrome

Wiskott-Aldrich syndrome is an X-linked disease characterized by thrombocytopenia, eczema, and a marked vulnerability to recurrent infection, resulting in early death. The thymus is morphologically normal, at least early in the course of the disease, but there is progressive loss of T lymphocytes in the peripheral blood and in the T-cell zones (paracortical areas) of the lymph nodes, with variable defects in cellular immunity. Patients do not make antibodies to polysaccharide antigens, and the response to protein antigens is poor. IgM levels in the serum are low, but levels of IgG are usually normal. Paradoxically the levels of IgA and IgE are often elevated. Patients are also prone to developing B-cell lymphomas. The Wiskott-Aldrich syndrome is caused by mutations in the gene encoding *Wiskott-Aldrich syndrome protein (WASP)*, which is located at Xp11.23. WASP belongs to a family of proteins that are believed to link membrane receptors, such as antigen receptors, to cytoskeletal elements. The WASP protein may be involved in cytoskeleton-dependent responses, including cell migration and signal transduction, but the essential functions of this protein in lymphocytes and platelets are unclear. The only treatment is HSC transplantation.

Ataxia Telangiectasia

Ataxia telangiectasia is an autosomal-recessive disorder characterized by abnormal gait (ataxia), vascular malformations (telangiectases), neurologic deficits, increased

incidence of tumors, and immunodeficiency. The immunologic defects are of variable severity and may affect both B and T cells. The most prominent humoral immune abnormalities are defective production of isotype switched antibodies, mainly IgA and IgG2. The T cell defects, which are usually less pronounced, are associated with thymic hypoplasia. Patients experience upper and lower respiratory tract bacterial infections, multiple autoimmune phenomena, and increasingly frequent cancers with advancing age. The gene responsible for this disorder is located on chromosome 11 and encodes a protein called *ATM* (ataxia telangiectasia mutated) that is related structurally to phosphatidylinositol-3 (PI-3) kinase, but is a protein kinase. The ATM protein is a sensor of DNA damage (double-strand breaks) and it activates p53 by phosphorylation, which in turn can activate cell cycle checkpoints and apoptosis in cells with damaged DNA. ATM has also been shown to contribute to the stability of DNA double-strand break complexes during V(D)J recombination. Because of these abnormalities in DNA repair, the generation of antigen receptors may be abnormal. In addition, defective DNA repair may lead to abnormalities in the DNA recombination events that are involved in antibody isotype switching.

KEY CONCEPTS

Primary (Inherited) Immune Deficiency Diseases

- These diseases are caused by inherited mutations in genes involved in lymphocyte maturation or function, or in innate immunity.
- Deficiencies in innate immunity include defects of phagocyte function, complement, and innate immune receptors.
- Some of the common disorders affecting lymphocytes and the adaptive immune response are:
  - X-SCID: failure of T-cell and B-cell maturation; mutation in the common γ chain of a cytokine receptor, leading to failure of IL-7 signaling and defective lymphopoiesis
  - Autosomal recessive SCID: failure of T-cell development, secondary defect in antibody responses; approximately 50% of cases caused by mutation in the gene encoding ADA, leading to accumulation of toxic metabolites during lymphocyte maturation and proliferation
  - X-linked agammaglubulinemia (XLA): failure of B-cell maturation, absence of antibodies; caused by mutations in the *BTK* gene, which encodes B-cell tyrosine kinase, required for maturation signals from the pre-B cell and B-cell receptors
  - Common variable immunodeficiency: defects in antibody production; cause unknown in most cases
  - Selective IgA deficiency: failure of IgA production; cause unknown
  - X-linked hyper-IgM syndrome: failure to produce isotype-switched high-affinity antibodies (IgG, IgA, IgE); mutation in gene encoding CD40L
  - X-linked lymphoproliferative disease (XLP): defect in a signaling molecule causing defective responses against Epstein-Barr virus and lymphoproliferation
- These diseases present clinically with increased susceptibility to infections in early life.

Table 6-13 Causes of Secondary (Acquired) Immunodeficiencies

Cause	Mechanism
Human immunodeficiency virus infection	Depletion of CD4+ helper T cells
Irradiation and chemotherapy treatments for cancer	Decreased bone marrow precursors for all leukocytes
Involvement of bone marrow by cancers (metastases, leukemias)	Reduced site of leukocyte development
Protein-calorie malnutrition	Metabolic derangements inhibit lymphocyte maturation and function
Removal of spleen	Decreased phagocytosis of microbes

Secondary Immunodeficiencies

Secondary (acquired) immune deficiencies may be encountered in individuals with cancer, diabetes and other metabolic diseases, malnutrition, chronic infection, and in persons receiving chemotherapy or radiation therapy for cancer, or immunosuppressive drugs to prevent graft rejection or to treat autoimmune diseases (Table 6-13). As a group, the secondary immune deficiencies are more common than the disorders of primary genetic origin. Some of these secondary immunodeficiency states can be caused by defective lymphocyte maturation (when the bone marrow is damaged by radiation or chemotherapy or involved by tumors, such as leukemias and metastatic cancers), inadequate Ig synthesis (as in malnutrition), or lymphocyte depletion (from drugs or severe infections). The most common secondary immunodeficiency is AIDS, which is described in the next section.

Acquired Immunodeficiency Syndrome (AIDS)

AIDS is a disease caused by the retrovirus human immunodeficiency virus (HIV) and characterized by profound immunosuppression that leads to opportunistic infections, secondary neoplasms, and neurologic manifestations. The magnitude of this modern plague is truly staggering. By the end of 2009 (the last year for which complete US statistics are available), more than a million cases of AIDS had been reported in the United States, where AIDS is the second leading cause of death in men between ages 25 and 44, and the third leading cause of death in women in this age group. Although initially recognized in the United States, AIDS is a global problem. It has now been reported from more than 190 countries around the world, and the pool of HIV-infected persons in Africa and Asia is large and expanding. By the year 2011, HIV had infected 60 million people worldwide, and nearly 30 million adults and children have died of the disease. There are about 34 million people living with HIV, of whom 70% are in Africa and more than 20% in Asia; the prevalence rate of infection in adults in sub-Saharan Africa is more than 8%. It is estimated that 2.5 million people were newly infected with HIV in 2011 and 1.7 million deaths were caused by AIDS. In this dismal scenario, there may be some good news. Because of public health measures, the infection rate seems to be decreasing, and some authorities believe it may have peaked in the late 1990s. Furthermore, improved antiviral therapies have resulted in fewer people dying of the disease. However, these newer treatments are not readily available in many developing countries, and toxic side effects remain problems. The advent of these drugs raises its own tragic concern; because more people are living with HIV, the risk of spreading the infection will increase if vigilance is relaxed.

The enormous medical and social burden of AIDS has led to an explosion of research aimed at understanding HIV and its remarkable ability to cripple host defenses. The literature on HIV and AIDS is vast. Here we summarize the currently available data on the epidemiology, pathogenesis, and clinical features of HIV infection.

Epidemiology

Epidemiologic studies in the United States have identified five groups of adults at high risk for developing AIDS. The case distribution in these groups is as follows:

- **Homosexual or bisexual men** constitute the largest group, accounting for more than 50% of the reported cases. This includes about 5% who were intravenous drug abusers as well. Transmission of HIV in this category appears to be on the decline: in 2009 about 60% of new cases were attributed to male homosexual contacts.
- **Intravenous drug abusers** with no previous history of homosexuality are the next largest group, representing about 20% of infected individuals and 9% of new cases in 2009.
- **Hemophiliacs**, especially those who received large amounts of factor VIII or factor IX concentrates before 1985, make up about 0.5% of all cases.
- **Recipients of blood and blood components** who are not hemophiliacs but who received transfusions of HIV-infected whole blood or components (e.g., platelets, plasma) account for about 1% of patients. (Organs obtained from HIV-infected donors can also transmit the virus.)
- **Heterosexual contacts** of members of other high-risk groups (chiefly intravenous drug abusers) constitute about 20% of the patient population. About 30% of new cases in 2009 were attributable to heterosexual contact. Heterosexual transmission, although initially of less numerical importance in the United States, is globally the most common mode by which HIV is spread. In the past few years, even in the United States, the rate of increase of heterosexual transmission has outpaced transmission by other means. In sub-Saharan Africa, where the infection rate is estimated to be about 10,000 new cases every day, more than half the infected individuals are women. Spread of the virus is occurring most rapidly in female sex partners of male intravenous drug abusers. As a result, the number of women with AIDS is rising rapidly. In contrast to the experience in the United States, heterosexual transmission has always been the dominant mode of HIV infection in Asia and Africa.
- **HIV infection of the newborn**. The epidemiology of AIDS is quite different in children younger than 13 years. Close to 2% of all AIDS cases occur in this pediatric population, and worldwide more than 500,000 new cases and almost 400,000 deaths were reported in children in 2006. In this group, the vast majority acquired the infection by transmission of the virus from mother to child (discussed later).
- In approximately 5% of cases, the risk factors cannot be determined.

It should be apparent from the preceding discussion that transmission of HIV occurs under conditions that facilitate exchange of blood or body fluids containing the virus or virus-infected cells. **The three major routes of transmission are sexual contact, parenteral inoculation, and passage of the virus from infected mothers to their newborns.**

- **Sexual transmission** is clearly the dominant mode of infection worldwide, accounting for more than 75% of all cases of HIV transmission. Because the majority of infected people in the United States are men who have sex with men, most sexual transmission has occurred among homosexual men. The virus is carried in the semen, and it enters the recipient's body through abrasions in rectal or oral mucosa or by direct contact with mucosal lining cells. Viral transmission occurs in two ways: (1) direct inoculation into the blood vessels breached by trauma and (2) infection of dendritic cells or CD4+ cells within the mucosa. In addition to male-to-male and male-to-female transmission, there is evidence supporting female-to-male transmission.

  Sexual transmission of HIV is enhanced by coexisting sexually transmitted diseases, especially those associated with genital ulceration. In this regard, syphilis, chancroid, and herpes are particularly important. Other sexually transmitted diseases, including gonorrhea and chlamydia, are also cofactors for HIV transmission, perhaps because in these genital inflammatory states there is greater concentration of the virus and virus-containing cells in genital fluids, as a result of increased numbers of inflammatory cells in the semen.
- **Parenteral transmission** of HIV has occurred in three groups of individuals: intravenous drug abusers, hemophiliacs who received factor VIII and factor IX concentrates, and random recipients of blood transfusion. Of these three, intravenous drug users constitute by far the largest group. Transmission occurs by sharing of needles, syringes, and other paraphernalia contaminated with HIV-containing blood.

  Transmission of HIV by transfusion of blood or blood products, such as lyophilized factor VIII and factor IX concentrates, has been virtually eliminated. This fortunate outcome resulted from increasing use of recombinant clotting factors and from three public health measures: screening of donated blood and plasma for antibody to HIV, stringent purity criteria for factor VIII and factor IX preparations, and screening of donors on the basis of history. However, an extremely small risk of acquiring AIDS through transfusion of seronegative blood persists, because a recently infected individual may be antibody-negative. Currently, this risk is estimated to be 1 in more than 2 million units of blood transfused.
- As alluded to earlier, **mother-to-infant transmission** is the major cause of pediatric AIDS. Infected mothers can transmit the infection to their offspring by three routes: (1) in utero by transplacental spread, (2) during delivery through an infected birth canal, and (3) after birth by ingestion of breast milk. Of these, transmission during

birth (intrapartum) and in the immediate period thereafter (peripartum) is considered to be the most common mode in the United States. The reported transmission rates vary from 7% to 49% in different parts of the world. Higher risk of transmission is associated with high maternal viral load and low CD4+ T-cell counts as well as chorioamnionitis. Fortunately, antiretroviral therapy given to infected pregnant women in the United States has virtually eliminated mother-to-child transmission, but it remains a major source of infection in areas where these treatments are not readily available.

Much concern has arisen in the lay public and among health care workers about spread of HIV infection outside the high-risk groups. Extensive studies indicate that HIV infection cannot be transmitted by casual personal contact in the household, workplace, or school. Spread by insect bites is virtually impossible. Regarding transmission of HIV infection to health care workers, an extremely small but definite risk seems to be present. Seroconversion has been documented after accidental needle-stick injury or exposure of nonintact skin to infected blood in laboratory accidents. After needle-stick accidents, the risk of seroconversion is believed to be about 0.3%, and antiretroviral therapy given within 24 to 48 hours of a needle stick can reduce the risk of infection eightfold. By comparison, approximately 30% of those accidentally exposed to hepatitis B–infected blood become seropositive.

Etiology: The Properties of HIV

HIV is a nontransforming human retrovirus belonging to the lentivirus family. Included in this group are feline immunodeficiency virus, simian immunodeficiency virus, visna virus of sheep, bovine immunodeficiency virus, and the equine infectious anemia virus.

Two genetically different but related forms of HIV, called *HIV-1 and HIV-2*, have been isolated from patients with AIDS. HIV-1 is the most common type associated with AIDS in the United States, Europe, and Central Africa, whereas HIV-2 causes a similar disease principally in West Africa and India. Specific tests for HIV-2 are available, and blood collected for transfusion is routinely screened for both HIV-1 and HIV-2 seropositivity. The ensuing discussion relates primarily to HIV-1 and diseases caused by it, but the information is generally applicable to HIV-2 as well.

Structure of HIV

Similar to most retroviruses, the HIV-1 virion is spherical and contains an electron-dense, cone-shaped core surrounded by a lipid envelope derived from the host cell membrane (Fig. 6-38). **The virus core contains (1) the major capsid protein p24; (2) nucleocapsid protein p7/p9; (3) two copies of viral genomic RNA; and (4) the three viral enzymes (protease, reverse transcriptase, and integrase).** p24 is the most abundant viral antigen and is detected by an enzyme-linked immunoabsorbent assay that is widely used to diagnose HIV infection. The viral core is surrounded by a matrix protein called p17, which lies underneath the virion envelope. Studding the viral envelope are two viral glycoproteins, gp120 and gp41, which are critical for HIV infection of cells.

The HIV-1 RNA genome contains the *gag, pol,* and *env* genes, which are typical of retroviruses (Fig. 6-39). The

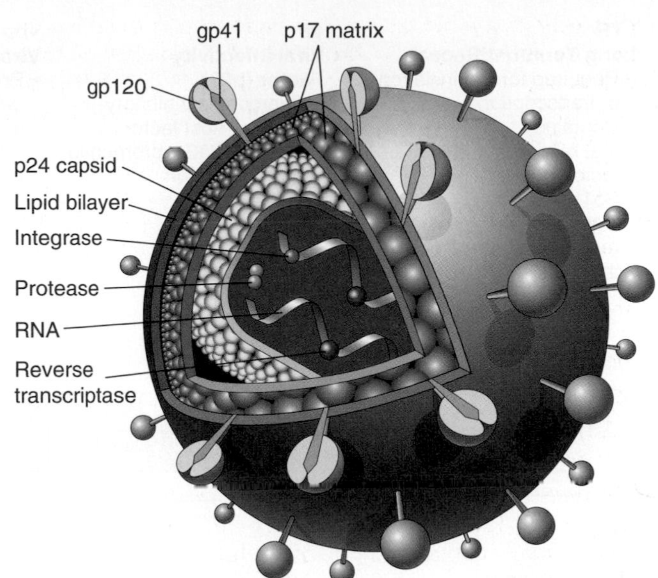

Figure 6-38 The structure of the human immune deficiency virus (HIV)-1 virion. The viral particle is covered by a lipid bilayer derived from the host cell and studded with viral glycoproteins gp41 and gp120.

products of the *gag* and *pol* genes are large precursor proteins that are cleaved by the viral protease to yield the mature proteins. In addition to these three standard retroviral genes, HIV contains several other accessory genes, including *tat, rev, vif, nef, vpr,* and *vpu*, which regulate the synthesis and assembly of infectious viral particles and the pathogenicity of the virus. For example, the product of the *tat* (transactivator) gene causes a 1000-fold increase in the transcription of viral genes and is critical for virus replication. The functions of other accessory proteins are indicated in Figure 6-39.

Molecular analysis of different HIV-1 isolates has revealed considerable variability in certain parts of the viral genome. Most variations are clustered in particular regions of the envelope glycoproteins. Because the humoral immune response against HIV-1 is targeted against its envelope, such variability poses problems for the development of a single antigen vaccine. On the basis of genetic analysis, HIV-1 can be divided into three subgroups, designated *M* (major), *O* (outlier), and *N* (neither *M* nor *O*). Group M viruses are the most common form worldwide, and they are further divided into several subtypes, or clades, designated A through K. Various subtypes differ in their geographic distribution; for example, subtype B is the most common form in western Europe and the United States, whereas subtype E is the most common clade in Thailand. Currently, clade C is the fastest spreading clade worldwide, being present in India, Ethiopia, and Southern Africa.

Pathogenesis of HIV Infection and AIDS

While HIV can infect many tissues, **the two major targets of HIV infection are the immune system and the central nervous system.** The effects of HIV infection on each of these two systems are discussed separately.

Profound immune deficiency, primarily affecting cell-mediated immunity, is the hallmark of AIDS. This results chiefly from infection and subsequent loss of CD4+ T cells

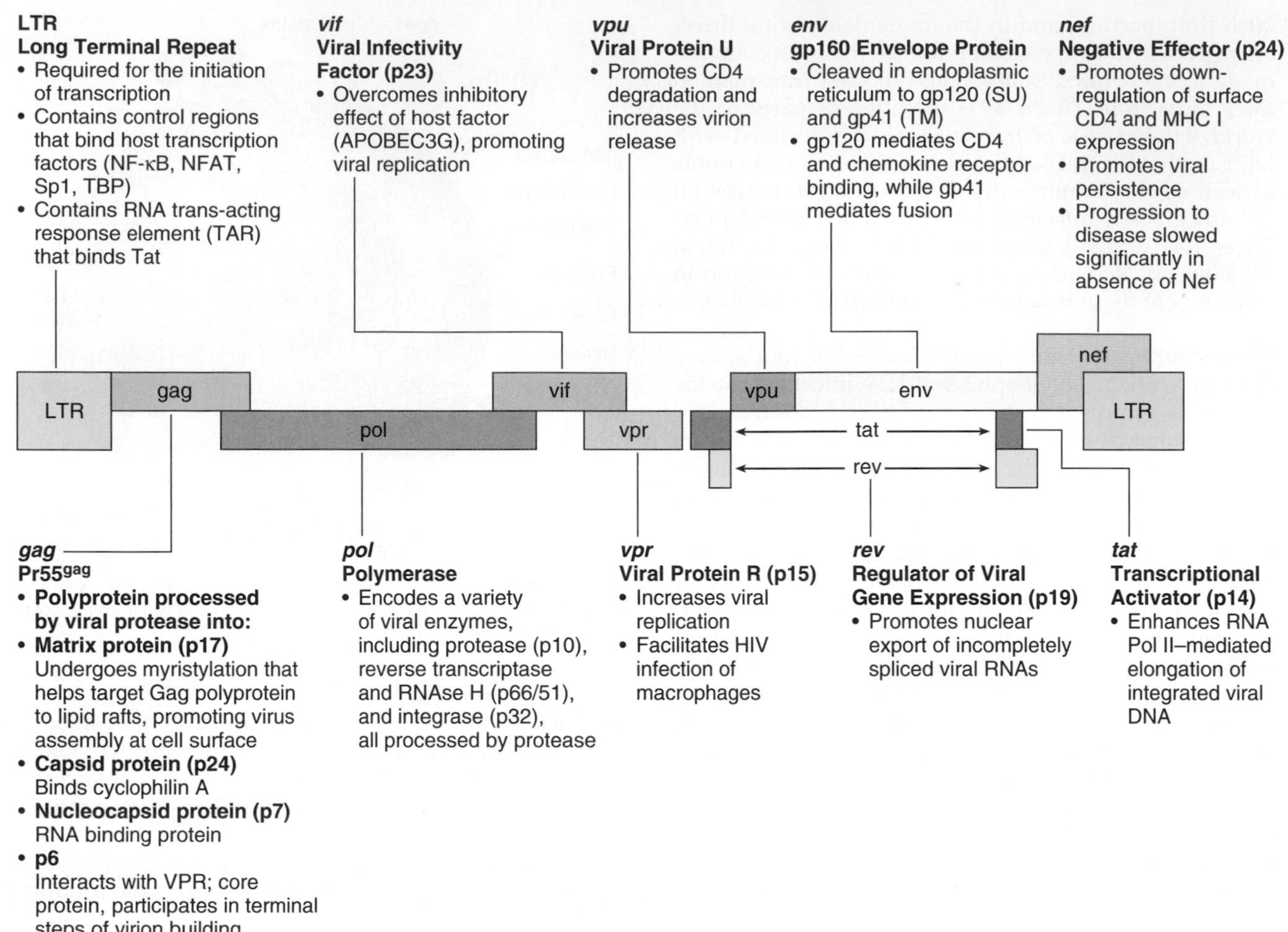

Figure 6-39 The HIV genome. Several viral genes and the functions of the encoded proteins are illustrated. The genes outlined in red are unique to HIV; others are shared by all retroviruses.

as well as impairment in the function of surviving helper T cells. As discussed later, macrophages and dendritic cells are also targets of HIV infection. HIV enters the body through mucosal tissues and blood and first infects T cells as well as dendritic cells and macrophages. The infection becomes established in lymphoid tissues, where the virus may remain latent for long periods. Active viral replication is associated with more infection of cells and progression to AIDS. We first describe the mechanisms involved in viral entry into T cells and macrophages and the replicative cycle of the virus within cells. This is followed by a more detailed review of the interaction between HIV and its cellular targets.

Life Cycle of HIV

The life cycle of HIV consists of infection of cells, integration of the provirus into the host cell genome, activation of viral replication, and production and release of infectious virus (Fig. 6-40). The molecules and mechanisms of each of these steps are understood in considerable detail.

Infection of Cells by HIV

HIV infects cells by using the CD4 molecule as receptor and various chemokine receptors as coreceptors (Fig. 6-40). The requirement for CD4 binding explains the selective tropism of the virus for CD4+ T cells and other CD4+ cells, particularly monocytes/macrophages and dendritic cells. Binding to CD4 is not sufficient for infection, however. HIV gp120 must also bind to other cell surface molecules (coreceptors) for entry into the cell. Chemokine receptors, particularly CCR5 and CXCR4, serve this role. HIV isolates can be distinguished by their use of these receptors: R5 strains use CCR5, X4 strains use CXCR4, and some strains (R5X4) are dual-tropic. R5 strains preferentially infect cells of the monocyte/macrophage lineage and are thus referred to as M-tropic, whereas X4 strains are T-tropic, preferentially infecting T cells. In approximately 90% of cases, the R5 (M-tropic) type of HIV is the dominant virus found in the blood of acutely infected individuals and early in the course of infection. Over the course of infection, however, T-tropic viruses gradually accumulate; these are especially virulent because T-tropic viruses are capable of infecting many T cells and even thymic T-cell precursors and cause greater T-cell depletion and impairment.

Molecular details of the deadly handshake between HIV glycoproteins and their cell surface receptors have been elucidated and are important to understand because they may provide the basis of anti-HIV therapy. The HIV envelope contains two glycoproteins, surface gp120 noncovalently attached to a transmembrane protein, gp41. **The initial step in infection is the binding of the gp120 envelope glycoprotein to CD4 molecules, which leads to**

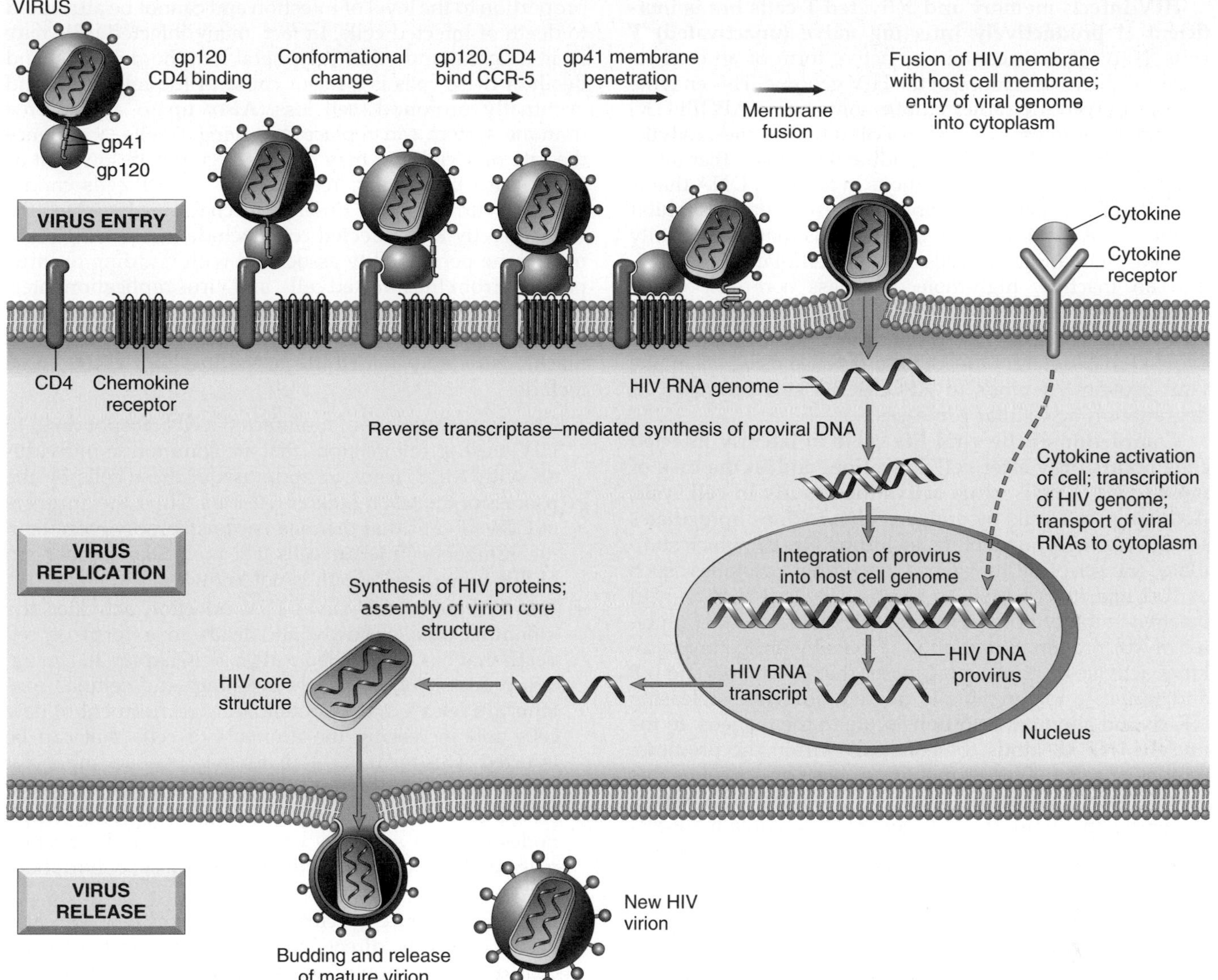

Figure 6-40 The life cycle of HIV showing the steps from viral entry to production of infectious virions. (Adapted with permission from Wain-Hobson S: HIV. One on one meets two. Nature 1996;384:117. Copyright 1996, Macmillan Magazines Limited.)

a conformational change that results in the formation of a new recognition site on gp120 for the coreceptors CCR5 or CXCR4. Binding to the coreceptors induces conformational changes in gp41 that result in the exposure of a hydrophobic region called the fusion peptide at the tip of gp41. This peptide inserts into the cell membrane of the target cells (e.g., T cells or macrophages), leading to fusion of the virus with the host cell. After fusion the virus core containing the HIV genome enters the cytoplasm of the cell. The requirement for HIV binding to coreceptors may have important implications for the pathogenesis of AIDS. Chemokines sterically hinder HIV infection of cells in culture by occupying their receptors, and therefore, the level of chemokines in the tissues may influence the efficiency of viral infection in vivo. Also, polymorphisms in the gene encoding CCR5 are associated with different susceptibility to HIV infection. About 1% of white Americans inherit two defective copies of the CCR5 gene and are resistant to infection and the development of AIDS associated with R5 HIV isolates. About 20% of individuals are heterozygous for this protective CCR5 allele; these persons are not protected from AIDS, but the onset of their disease after infection is somewhat delayed. Only rare homozygotes for the mutation have been found in African or East Asian populations.

Viral Replication

Once internalized, the RNA genome of the virus undergoes reverse transcription, leading to the synthesis of double-stranded complementary DNA (cDNA; proviral DNA) (Fig. 6-40). In quiescent T cells, HIV cDNA may remain in the cytoplasm in a linear episomal form. In dividing T cells, the cDNA circularizes, enters the nucleus, and is then integrated into the host genome. After this integration, the provirus may be silent for months or years, a form of latent infection. Alternatively, proviral DNA may be transcribed, with the formation of complete viral particles that bud from the cell membrane. Such productive infection, when associated with extensive viral budding, leads to death of infected cells.

HIV infects memory and activated T cells but is inefficient at productively infecting naive (unactivated) T cells. Naive T cells contain an active form of an enzyme that introduces mutations in the HIV genome. This enzyme has been given the rather cumbersome name APOBEC3G (for apolipoprotein B mRNA-editing, enzyme-catalytic, polypeptide-like 3G). It is a cytidine deaminase that introduces cytosine-to-uracil mutations in the viral DNA that is produced by reverse transcription. These mutations inhibit further DNA replication by mechanisms that are not fully defined. Activation of T cells converts cellular APOBEC3G into an inactive, high-molecular-mass complex, which explains why the virus can replicate in previously activated (e.g., memory) T cells and T-cell lines. HIV has also evolved to counteract this cellular defense mechanism; the viral protein Vif binds to APOBEC3G and promotes its degradation by cellular proteases.

Completion of the viral life cycle in latently infected cells occurs only after cell activation, and in the case of most CD4+ T cells virus activation results in cell lysis. Activation of T cells by antigens or cytokines upregulates several transcription factors, including NF-κB, which stimulate transcription of genes encoding cytokines such as IL-2 and its receptor. In resting T cells, NF-κB is held inactive in the cytoplasm in a complex with the IκB (inhibitor of κB) protein. Stimulation of cells by antigen or cytokines activates cytoplasmic kinases that phosphorylate IκB and target it for enzymatic degradation, thus releasing NF-κB and allowing it to translocate to the nucleus. In the nucleus, NF-κB binds to sequences within the promoter regions of several genes, including those of cytokines that are expressed in activated T cells. The long-terminal-repeat sequences that flank the HIV genome also contain NF-κB–binding sites that can be triggered by the same transcription factors. Imagine now a latently infected CD4+ cell that encounters an environmental antigen. Induction of NF-κB in such a cell (a physiologic response) activates the transcription of HIV proviral DNA (a pathologic outcome) and leads ultimately to the production of virions and to cell lysis. Furthermore, TNF and other cytokines produced by activated macrophages also stimulate NF-κB activity and thus lead to production of HIV RNA. Thus, it seems that HIV thrives when the host T cells and macrophages are physiologically activated, an act that can be best described as "subversion from within." Such activation in vivo may result from antigenic stimulation by HIV itself or by other infecting microorganisms. HIV-infected people are at increased risk for recurrent exposure to other infections, which lead to increased lymphocyte activation and production of proinflammatory cytokines. These, in turn, stimulate more HIV production, loss of additional CD4+ T cells, and more infection. Thus, it is easy to visualize how in individuals with AIDS a vicious cycle may be set up that culminates in inexorable destruction of the immune system.

Mechanism of T-Cell Depletion in HIV Infection

Loss of CD4+ T cells is mainly because of infection of the cells and the direct cytopathic effects of the replicating virus. In infected individuals, approximately 100 billion new viral particles are produced every day, and 1 to 2 billion CD4+ T cells die each day. Because the frequency of infected cells in the circulation is very low, for many years it was suspected that the immunodeficiency is out of proportion to the level of infection and cannot be attributed to death of infected cells. In fact, many infected cells may be in mucosal and other peripheral lymphoid organs, and death of these cells is a major cause of the relentless, and eventually profound, cell loss. Also, up to a point the immune system can replace the dying T cells, and hence the rate of T cell loss may appear deceptively low, but as the disease progresses, renewal of CD4+ T cells cannot keep up with their loss. Possible mechanisms by which the virus directly kills infected cells include increased plasma membrane permeability associated with budding of virus particles from the infected cells, and virus replication interfering with protein synthesis.

In addition to direct killing of cells by the virus, other mechanisms may contribute to the loss of T cells. These include:

- Chronic activation of uninfected cells, responding to HIV itself or to infections that are common in individuals with AIDS, leads to apoptosis of these cells by the process of *activation-induced cell death*. Thus, the numbers of CD4+ T cells that die may be considerably more than the numbers of infected cells. The molecular mechanism of this type of cell death is not known.
- Non-cytopathic (abortive) HIV infection activates the inflammasome pathway and leads to a form of cell death that has been called *pyroptosis* (Chapter 2). During this process, inflammatory cytokines and cellular contents are released, thus potentiating recruitment of new cells and increasing the numbers of cells that can be infected. This form of cell death may play an important role in spread of the infection.
- HIV infects cells in lymphoid organs (spleen, lymph nodes, tonsils) and may cause progressive destruction of the architecture and cellular composition of lymphoid tissues.
- Loss of immature precursors of CD4+ T cells can also occur, either by direct infection of thymic progenitor cells or by infection of accessory cells that secrete cytokines essential for CD4+ T-cell maturation.
- Fusion of infected and uninfected cells with formation of syncytia (giant cells) can occur. In tissue culture the gp120 expressed on productively infected cells binds to CD4 molecules on uninfected T cells, followed by cell fusion. Fused cells usually die within a few hours. This property of syncytia formation is generally confined to the T-tropic X4 type of HIV-1. For this reason, this type is often referred to as syncytia-inducing (SI) virus, in contrast to the R5 virus.
- Although marked reduction in CD4+ T cells, a hallmark of AIDS, can account for most of the immunodeficiency late in the course of HIV infection, there is evidence of qualitative defects in T cells even in asymptomatic HIV-infected persons. Reported defects include a reduction in antigen-induced T-cell proliferation, a decrease in T_H1-type responses relative to the T_H2 type, defects in intracellular signaling, and many more. The loss of T_H1 responses results in profound deficiency in cell-mediated immunity, leading to increased susceptibility to infections by viruses and other intracellular microbes. There is also a selective loss of the memory subset of CD4+ helper T cells early in the course of disease, which explains poor recall responses to previously encountered antigens.

Table 6-14 Major Abnormalities of Immune Function in AIDS

Lymphopenia
Predominantly caused by selective loss of the CD4+ helper T-cell subset
Decreased T-Cell Function In Vivo
Preferential loss of activated and memory T cells Decreased delayed-type hypersensitivity Susceptibility to opportunistic infections Susceptibility to neoplasms
Altered T-Cell Function In Vitro
Decreased proliferative response to mitogens, alloantigens, and soluble antigens Decreased cytotoxicity Decreased helper function for B-cell antibody production Decreased IL-2 and IFN-γ production
Polyclonal B-Cell Activation
Hypergammaglobulinemia and circulating immune complexes Inability to mount de novo antibody response to new antigens Poor responses to normal B-cell activation signals in vitro
Altered Monocyte or Macrophage Functions
Decreased chemotaxis and phagocytosis Decreased class II HLA expression Diminished capacity to present antigen to T cells

HLA, Human leukocyte antigen; IFN-γ, interferon-γ; IL-2, interleukin-2; TNF, tumor necrosis factor.

Low-level chronic or latent infection of T cells is an important feature of HIV infection. It is widely believed that integrated provirus, without viral gene expression (latent infection), can remain in the cells for months to years. Even with potent antiviral therapy, which practically sterilizes the peripheral blood, latent virus lurks within the CD4+ cells (both T cells and macrophages) in the lymph nodes. According to some estimates, 0.05% of CD4+ T cells in the lymph nodes are latently infected. Because most of these CD4+ T cells are memory cells, they are long-lived, with a life span of months to years, and thus provide a persistent reservoir of virus.

CD4+ T cells play a pivotal role in regulating both cellular and humoral immune responses. Therefore, loss of this "master regulator" has ripple effects on virtually every other component of the immune system, as summarized in Table 6-14.

HIV Infection of Non–T Cells

In addition to infection and loss of CD4+ T cells, **infection of macrophages and dendritic cells is also important in the pathogenesis of HIV infection**. Similar to T cells, the majority of the macrophages that are infected by HIV are found in the tissues and the number of blood monocytes infected by the virus may be low. In certain tissues, such as the lungs and brain, as many as 10% to 50% of macrophages are infected. Several aspects of HIV infection of macrophages should be emphasized:

- Although cell division is required for nuclear entry and replication of most retroviruses, HIV-1 can infect and multiply in terminally differentiated nondividing macrophages. This property of HIV-1 is dependent on the viral *vpr* gene. The Vpr protein allows nuclear targeting of the HIV preintegration complex through the nuclear pore.
- Infected macrophages bud relatively small amounts of virus from the cell surface, but these cells contain large numbers of virus particles often located in intracellular vacuoles. Even though macrophages allow viral replication, they are quite resistant to the cytopathic effects of HIV, in contrast to CD4+ T cells. Thus, macrophages may be reservoirs of infection whose output remains largely protected from host defenses. In late stages of HIV infection, when CD4+ T-cell numbers decline greatly, macrophages may be an important site of continued viral replication.
- Macrophages may act as portals of infection. Recall that in more than 90% of cases acute HIV infection is characterized by predominantly circulating M-tropic strains. This finding suggests that the initial infection of macrophages or dendritic cells may be important in the pathogenesis of HIV disease.
- Even uninfected monocytes are reported to have unexplained functional defects that may have important consequences for host defense. These defects include impaired microbicidal activity, decreased chemotaxis, decreased secretion of IL-1, inappropriate secretion of TNF, and poor capacity to present antigens to T cells. Also, even the low number of infected blood monocytes may be vehicles for HIV to be transported to various parts of the body, including the nervous system.

Studies have documented that, in addition to macrophages, two types of dendritic cells are also important targets for the initiation and maintenance of HIV infection: mucosal and follicular dendritic cells. It is thought that **mucosal dendritic cells are infected by the virus and may transport it to regional lymph nodes**, where the virus is transmitted to CD4+ T cells. Dendritic cells also express a lectin-like receptor that specifically binds HIV and displays it in an intact, infectious form to T cells, thus promoting infection of the T cells.

Follicular dendritic cells in the germinal centers of lymph nodes are potential reservoirs of HIV. Although some follicular dendritic cells may be susceptible to HIV infection, most virus particles are found on the surface of their dendritic processes. Follicular dendritic cells have receptors for the Fc portion of immunoglobulins, and hence they trap HIV virions coated with anti-HIV antibodies. The antibody-coated virions localized to follicular dendritic cells retain the ability to infect CD4+ T cells as they traverse the intricate meshwork formed by the dendritic processes of the follicular dendritic cells.

B Cell Function in HIV Infection. Although much attention has been focused on T cells, macrophages, and dendritic cells because they can be infected by HIV, individuals with AIDS also display profound abnormalities of B-cell function. Paradoxically, there is polyclonal activation of B cells, resulting in germinal center B-cell hyperplasia (particularly early in the disease course), bone marrow plasmacytosis, hypergammaglobulinemia, and formation of circulating immune complexes. This activation may result from multiple interacting factors: reactivation of or reinfection with cytomegalovirus and EBV, both of which are polyclonal B-cell activators, can occur; gp41 itself can promote B-cell growth and differentiation; and HIV-infected macrophages produce increased amounts of IL-6, which stimulates proliferation of B cells. Despite the presence of spontaneously activated B cells, patients with AIDS are unable to mount antibody responses to newly encountered antigens. This could be due, in part, to lack of T-cell help, but antibody responses against T-independent antigens are also suppressed, and hence there may be other intrinsic defects in B cells as well. Impaired humoral immunity renders these patients prey to disseminated infections caused by encapsulated bacteria, such as *S. pneumoniae* and *H. influenzae*, both of which require antibodies for effective opsonization and clearance.

Pathogenesis of Central Nervous System Involvement

The pathogenesis of neurologic manifestations deserves special mention because, in addition to the lymphoid system, the nervous system is a major target of HIV infection. Macrophages and microglia, cells in the central nervous system that belong to the macrophage lineage, are the predominant cell types in the brain that are infected with HIV. It is believed that HIV is carried into the brain by infected monocytes. In keeping with this, the HIV isolates from the brain are almost exclusively M-tropic. The mechanism of HIV-induced damage of the brain, however, remains obscure. Because neurons are not infected by HIV, and the extent of neuropathologic changes is often less than might be expected from the severity of neurologic symptoms, most workers believe that the neurologic deficit is caused indirectly by viral products and by soluble factors produced by infected microglia. Included among the soluble factors are the usual culprits, such as IL-1, TNF, and IL-6. In addition, nitric oxide induced in neuronal cells by gp41 has been implicated. Direct damage of neurons by soluble HIV gp120 has also been postulated.

Natural History of HIV Infection

Virus typically enters through mucosal epithelia. The subsequent pathologic and clinical manifestations of the infection can be divided into several phases: (1) an acute retroviral syndrome; (2) a middle, chronic phase, in which most individuals are asymptomatic; and (3) clinical AIDS (Figs. 6-41 and 6-42).

Primary Infection, Virus Dissemination, and the Acute Retroviral Syndrome

Acute (early) infection is characterized by infection of memory CD4+ T cells (which express CCR5) in mucosal lymphoid tissues, and death of many infected cells. Because the mucosal tissues are the largest reservoir of T cells in the body, and a major site of residence of memory T cells, this local loss results in considerable depletion of lymphocytes. Few infected cells are detectable in the blood and other tissues. Mucosal infection is often associated with damage to the epithelium, defects in mucosal barrier functions, and translocation of microbes across the epithelium.

Mucosal infection is followed by dissemination of the virus and the development of host immune responses. Dendritic cells in epithelia at sites of virus entry capture the virus and then migrate into the lymph nodes. Once in lymphoid tissues, dendritic cells may pass HIV on to CD4+ T cells through direct cell-cell contact. Within days after the first exposure to HIV, viral replication can be detected in

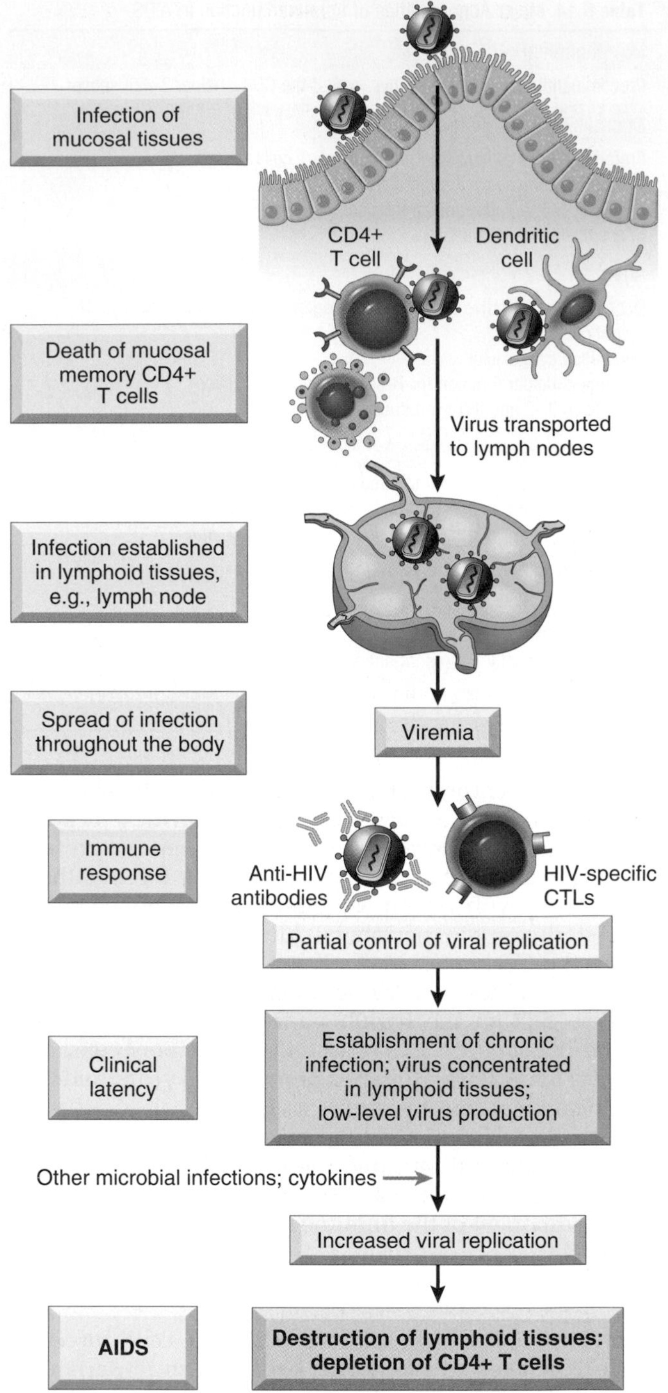

Figure 6-41 Pathogenesis of HIV-1 infection. The initial infection starts in mucosal tissues, involving mainly memory CD4+ T cells and dendritic cells, and spreads to lymph nodes. Viral replication leads to viremia and widespread seeding of lymphoid tissue. The viremia is controlled by the host immune response, and the patient then enters a phase of clinical latency. During this phase, viral replication in both T cells and macrophages continues unabated, but there is some immune containment of virus (not illustrated). There continues a gradual erosion of CD4+ cells and ultimately, CD4+ T-cell numbers decline, and the patient develops clinical symptoms of full-blown AIDS. CTL, Cytotoxic T lymphocyte.

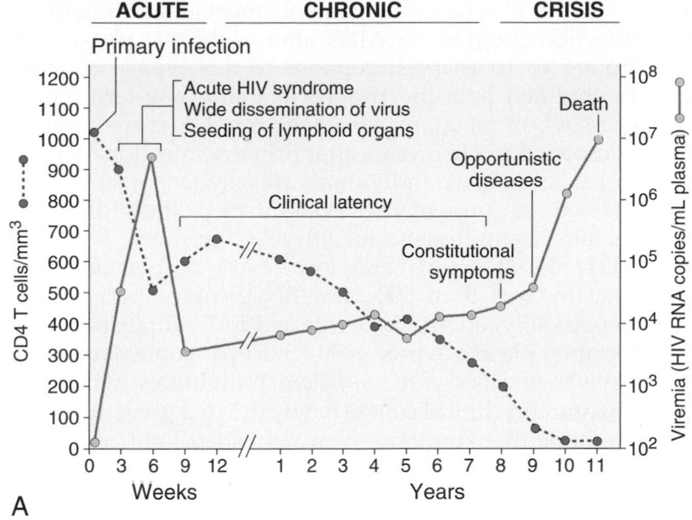

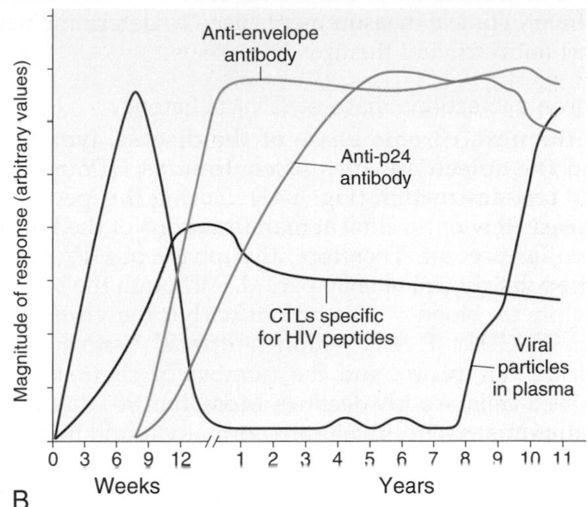

Figure 6-42 Clinical course of HIV infection. **A,** During the early period after primary infection there is dissemination of virus, development of an immune response to HIV, and often an acute viral syndrome. During the period of clinical latency, viral replication continues and the CD4+ T-cell count gradually decreases, until it reaches a critical level below which there is a substantial risk of AIDS-associated diseases. **B,** Immune response to HIV infection. A cytotoxic T lymphocyte (CTL) response to HIV is detectable by 2 to 3 weeks after the initial infection, and it peaks by 9 to 12 weeks. Marked expansion of virus-specific CD8+ T-cell clones occurs during this time, and up to 10% of a patient's CTLs may be HIV specific at 12 weeks. The humoral immune response to HIV peaks at about 12 weeks. (**A,** Redrawn from Fauci AS, Lane HC: Human immunodeficiency virus disease: AIDS and related conditions. In Fauci AS, et al (eds): Harrison's Principles of Internal Medicine, 14th ed. New York, McGraw-Hill, 1997, p 1791.)

the lymph nodes. This replication leads to viremia, during which high numbers of HIV particles are present in the patient's blood. The virus disseminates throughout the body and infects helper T cells, macrophages, and dendritic cells in peripheral lymphoid tissues.

As the HIV infection spreads, the individual mounts antiviral humoral and cell-mediated immune responses. These responses are evidenced by seroconversion (usually within 3 to 7 weeks of presumed exposure) and by the development of virus-specific CD8+ cytotoxic T cells. HIV-specific CD8+ T cells are detected in the blood at about the time viral titers begin to fall and are most likely responsible for the initial containment of HIV infection. These immune responses partially control the infection and viral production, and such control is reflected by a drop in viremia to low but detectable levels by about 12 weeks after the primary exposure.

The *acute retroviral syndrome* is the clinical presentation of the initial spread of the virus and the host response. It is estimated that 40% to 90% of individuals who acquire a primary infection develop this syndrome. This typically occurs 3 to 6 weeks after infection, and resolves spontaneously in 2 to 4 weeks. Clinically, this phase is associated with a self-limited acute illness with nonspecific symptoms, including sore throat, myalgias, fever, weight loss, and fatigue, resembling a flulike syndrome. Other clinical features, such as rash, cervical adenopathy, diarrhea, and vomiting, may also occur.

The extent of viremia, measured as HIV-1 RNA levels, in the blood is a useful surrogate marker of HIV disease progression and is of clinical value in the management of people with HIV infection. The viral load at the end of the acute phase reflects the equilibrium reached between the virus and the host response, and in a given patient it may remain fairly stable for several years. This level of steady-state viremia, called the *viral set point,* is a predictor of the rate of decline of CD4+ T cells, and, therefore, progression of HIV disease. In one study, only 8% of patients with a viral load of less than 4350 copies of viral mRNA per microliter of blood progressed to clinical AIDS in 5 years, whereas 62% of those with a viral load of greater than 36,270 copies developed AIDS in the same period.

Because the loss of immune containment is associated with declining CD4+ T-cell counts, the Centers for Disease Control (CDC) classification of HIV infection stratifies three categories on the basis of CD4+ cell counts: CD4+ cells greater than or equal to 500 cells/µL, 200 to 499 cells/µL, and fewer than 200 cells/µL (Table 6-15). For clinical management, blood CD4+ T-cell counts are perhaps the most reliable short-term indicator of disease progression.

Table 6-15 CDC Classification Categories of HIV Infection

Clinical Categories	CD4+ T-Cell Categories		
	1 ≥500 Cells/µL	2 200-499 Cells/µL	3 <200 Cells/µL
A. Asymptomatic, acute (primary) HIV, or persistent generalized lymphadenopathy	A1	A2	A3
B. Symptomatic, not A or C conditions	B1	B2	B3
C. AIDS indicator conditions: including constitutional disease, neurologic disease, or neoplasm			

Data from CDC. Centers for Disease Control and Prevention: 1993 revised classification system and expanded surveillance definition for AIDS among adolescents and adults. MMWR 1992;41(RR-17):1.

For this reason, CD4+ cell counts and not viral load are the primary clinical measurements used to determine when to start antiretroviral therapy.

Chronic Infection: Phase of Clinical Latency

In the next, chronic phase of the disease, lymph nodes and the spleen are sites of continuous HIV replication and cell destruction (Fig. 6-41). During this period of the disease, few or no clinical manifestations of the HIV infection are present. Therefore, this phase of HIV disease is called the clinical latency period. Although the majority of peripheral blood T cells do not harbor the virus, destruction of CD4+ T cells within lymphoid tissues continues during this phase, and the number of circulating blood CD4+ T cells steadily declines. More than 90% of the body's approximately 10^{12} T cells are normally found in lymphoid tissues, and it is estimated that HIV destroys up to 1×10^9 to 2×10^9 CD4+ T cells every day. Early in the course of the disease, the body may continue to make new CD4+ T cells, and therefore CD4+ T cells can be replaced almost as quickly as they are destroyed. At this stage, up to 10% of CD4+ T cells in lymphoid organs may be infected, but the frequency of circulating CD4+ T cells that are infected at any one time may be less than 0.1% of the total CD4+ T cells. Eventually, over a period of years, the continuous cycle of virus infection, T-cell death, and new infection leads to a steady decline in the number of CD4+ T cells in the lymphoid tissues and the circulation.

Concomitant with this loss of CD4+ T cells, host defenses begin to wane, and the proportion of the surviving CD4+ cells infected with HIV increases, as does the viral burden per CD4+ cell. Not unexpectedly, HIV RNA levels increase as the host begins to lose the battle with the virus. How HIV escapes immune control is not entirely clear, but several mechanisms have been proposed. These include destruction of the CD4+ T cells that are critical for effective immunity, antigenic variation, and down-modulation of class I MHC molecules on infected cells so that viral antigens are not recognized by CD8+ CTLs. During this period the virus may evolve and switch from relying solely on CCR5 to enter its target cells to relying on either CXCR4 or both CCR5 and CXCR4. This coreceptor switch is associated with more rapid decline in CD4+ T-cell counts, presumably because of greater infection of T cells.

In this chronic phase of infection, patients are either asymptomatic or develop minor opportunistic infections, such as oral candidiasis (thrush), vaginal candidiasis, herpes zoster, and perhaps mycobacterial tuberculosis (the latter being particularly common in resource-poor regions such as sub-Saharan Africa). Autoimmune thrombocytopenia may also be noted (Chapter 14).

AIDS

The final phase is progression to AIDS, characterized by a breakdown of host defense, a dramatic increase in plasma virus, and severe, life-threatening clinical disease. Typically the patient presents with long-lasting fever (>1 month), fatigue, weight loss, and diarrhea. After a variable period, serious opportunistic infections, secondary neoplasms, or clinical neurologic disease (grouped under the rubric *AIDS indicator diseases*, discussed later) emerge, and the patient is said to have developed AIDS.

In the absence of treatment, most patients with HIV infection progress to AIDS after a chronic phase lasting from 7 to 10 years. Exceptions to this typical course are exemplified by rapid progressors and long-term nonprogressors. In *rapid progressors* the middle, chronic phase is telescoped to 2 to 3 years after primary infection. About 5% to 15% of infected individuals are *long-term nonprogressors*, defined as untreated HIV-1–infected individuals who remain asymptomatic for 10 years or more, with stable CD4+ T-cell counts and low levels of plasma viremia (usually less than 500 viral RNA copies per milliliter). Remarkably, about 1% of infected individuals have undetectable plasma virus (<50-75 RNA copies/mL); these have been called *elite controllers*. Individuals with such an uncommon clinical course have attracted great attention in the hope that studying them may shed light on host and viral factors that influence disease progression. Studies thus far indicate that this group is heterogeneous with respect to the variables that influence the course of the disease. In most cases, the viral isolates do not show qualitative abnormalities, suggesting that the course of the disease cannot be attributed to a "wimpy" virus. In all cases there is evidence of a vigorous anti-HIV immune response, but the immune correlates of protection are still unknown. Some of these individuals have high levels of HIV-specific CD4+ and CD8+ T-cell responses, and these levels are maintained over the course of infection. The inheritance of particular HLA alleles seems to correlate with resistance to disease progression, perhaps reflecting the ability to mount antiviral T cell responses. Further studies, it is hoped, will provide the answers to this and other questions critical to understanding disease progression.

Clinical Features of AIDS

The clinical manifestations of HIV infection can be readily surmised from the foregoing discussion. They range from a mild acute illness to severe disease. Because the salient clinical features of the acute early and chronic middle phases of HIV infection were described earlier, here we summarize the clinical manifestations of the terminal phase, AIDS. At the outset it should be pointed out that the clinical manifestations and opportunistic infections associated with HIV infection may differ in different parts of the world. Also, the course of the disease has been greatly modified by new antiretroviral therapies, and many complications that were once devastating are now infrequent.

In the United States, the typical adult patient with AIDS presents with fever, weight loss, diarrhea, generalized lymphadenopathy, multiple opportunistic infections, neurologic disease, and, in many cases, secondary neoplasms. The infections and neoplasms listed in Table 6-16 are included in the surveillance definition of AIDS.

Opportunistic Infections. **Opportunistic infections account for the majority of deaths in untreated patients with AIDS.** Many of these infections represent reactivation of latent infections, which are normally kept in check by a robust immune system but are not completely eradicated because the infectious agents have evolved to coexist with their hosts. The actual frequency of infections varies in different regions of the world, and has been markedly reduced by the advent of highly active antiretroviral therapy (HAART), which relies on a combination of three

Table 6-16 AIDS-Defining Opportunistic Infections and Neoplasms Found in Patients with HIV Infection

Infections
Protozoal and Helminthic Infections
Cryptosporidiosis or isosporidiosis (enteritis)
Pneumocystosis (pneumonia or disseminated infection)
Toxoplasmosis (pneumonia or CNS infection)
Fungal Infections
Candidiasis (esophageal, tracheal, or pulmonary)
Cryptococcosis (CNS infection)
Coccidioidomycosis (disseminated)
Histoplasmosis (disseminated)
Bacterial Infections
Mycobacteriosis ("atypical," e.g., *Mycobacterium avium-intracellulare*, disseminated or extrapulmonary; *Mycobacterium tuberculosis*, pulmonary or extrapulmonary)
Nocardiosis (pneumonia, meningitis, disseminated)
Salmonella infections, disseminated
Viral Infections
Cytomegalovirus (pulmonary, intestinal, retinitis, or CNS infections)
Herpes simplex virus (localized or disseminated infection)
Varicella-zoster virus (localized or disseminated infection)
Progressive multifocal leukoencephalopathy
Neoplasms
Kaposi sarcoma
Primary lymphoma of brain
Invasive cancer of uterine cervix

CNS, Central nervous system.

or four drugs that block different steps of the HIV life cycle. A brief summary of selected opportunistic infections is provided here.

- Approximately 15% to 30% of untreated HIV-infected people develop pneumonia at some time during the course of the disease, caused by the fungus *Pneumocystis jiroveci* (reactivation of a prior latent infection). Before the advent of HAART, this infection was the presenting feature in about 20% of cases, but the incidence is much less in patients who respond to HAART.
- Many patients present with an opportunistic infection other than *P. jiroveci* pneumonia. Among the most common pathogens are *Candida*, cytomegalovirus, atypical and typical mycobacteria, *Cryptococcus neoformans*, *Toxoplasma gondii*, *Cryptosporidium*, herpes simplex virus, papovaviruses, and *Histoplasma capsulatum*.
- *Candidiasis* is the most common fungal infection in patients with AIDS, and infection of the oral cavity, vagina, and esophagus are its most common clinical manifestations. In asymptomatic HIV-infected individuals oral candidiasis is a sign of immunologic decompensation, and it often heralds the transition to AIDS. Invasive candidiasis is infrequent in patients with AIDS, and it usually occurs when there is drug-induced neutropenia or use of indwelling catheters.
- *Cytomegalovirus* may cause disseminated disease, although, more commonly, it affects the eye and gastrointestinal tract. Chorioretinitis was seen in approximately 25% of patients before the advent of HAART, but this has decreased dramatically after the initiation of HAART. Cytomegalovirus retinitis occurs almost exclusively in patients with CD4+ T cell counts less than 50 per microliter. Gastrointestinal disease, seen in 5% to 10% of cases, manifests as esophagitis and colitis, the latter associated with multiple mucosal ulcerations.
- Disseminated bacterial infection with *atypical mycobacteria* (mainly *Mycobacterium avium-intracellulare*) also occurs late, in the setting of severe immunosuppression. Coincident with the AIDS epidemic, the incidence of tuberculosis has risen dramatically. Worldwide, almost a third of all deaths in AIDS patients are attributable to tuberculosis, but this complication remains uncommon in the United States. Patients with AIDS have reactivation of latent pulmonary disease as well as outbreaks of primary infection. In contrast to infection with atypical mycobacteria, *M. tuberculosis* manifests itself early in the course of AIDS. As with tuberculosis in other settings, the infection may be confined to lungs or may involve multiple organs. The pattern of expression depends on the degree of immunosuppression; dissemination is more common in patients with very low CD4+ T-cell counts. Most worrisome are reports indicating that a growing number of isolates are resistant to multiple antimycobacterial drugs.
- *Cryptococcosis* occurs in about 10% of AIDS patients. As in other settings with immunosuppression, meningitis is the major clinical manifestation of cryptococcosis. *Toxoplasma gondii*, another frequent invader of the central nervous system in AIDS, causes encephalitis and is responsible for 50% of all mass lesions in the central nervous system.
- *JC virus*, a human papovavirus, is another important cause of central nervous system infections in HIV-infected patients. It causes progressive multifocal leukoencephalopathy (Chapter 28). *Herpes simplex virus infection* is manifested by mucocutaneous ulcerations involving the mouth, esophagus, external genitalia, and perianal region. *Persistent diarrhea*, which is common in untreated patients with advanced AIDS, is often caused by infections with protozoans such as *Cryptosporidium*, *Isospora belli*, or microsporidia. These patients have chronic, profuse, watery diarrhea with massive fluid loss. Diarrhea may also result from infection with enteric bacteria, such as *Salmonella* and *Shigella*, as well as *M. avium-intracellulare.*

Tumors. Patients with AIDS have a high incidence of certain tumors, especially *Kaposi sarcoma (KS)*, B-cell lymphoma, cervical cancer in women, and anal cancer in men. It is estimated that 25% to 40% of untreated HIV-infected individuals will eventually develop a malignancy. A common feature of these tumors is that they are caused by oncogenic DNA viruses, specifically Kaposi sarcoma herpesvirus (Kaposi sarcoma), EBV (B-cell lymphoma), and human papillomavirus (cervical and anal carcinoma). Even in healthy people, any of these viruses may establish latent infections that are kept in check by a competent immune system. The increased risk of malignancy in AIDS patients exists mainly because of failure to contain the infections and reactivation of the viruses, as well as decreased immunity against the tumors.

Kaposi Sarcoma. Kaposi sarcoma, a vascular tumor that is otherwise rare in the United States, is the most common neoplasm in patients with AIDS. The morphology of KS and its occurrence in patients not infected with HIV are discussed in Chapter 11. At the onset of the AIDS epidemic, up to 30% of infected homosexual or bisexual men had KS, but in recent years, with use of HAART there has been a dramatic decline in its incidence. In contrast, in areas of sub-Saharan Africa where HIV infection is both frequent and largely untreated, Kaposi sarcoma is one of the most common tumors.

The lesions of KS are characterized by the proliferation of spindle-shaped cells that express markers of both endothelial cells (vascular or lymphatic) and smooth muscle cells. There is also a profusion of slitlike vascular spaces, suggesting that the lesions may arise from primitive mesenchymal precursors of vascular channels. In addition, KS lesions display chronic inflammatory cell infiltrates. Many of the features of KS suggest that it is not a malignant tumor (despite its ominous name). For instance, spindle cells in many KS lesions are polyclonal or oligoclonal, although more advanced lesions occasionally show monoclonality. The current model of KS pathogenesis is that the spindle cells produce proinflammatory and angiogenic factors, which recruit the inflammatory and neovascular components of the lesion, and the latter components supply signals that aid in spindle cell survival and growth.

There is compelling evidence that KS is caused by the *KS herpesvirus* (KSHV), also called *human herpesvirus 8* (HHV8). Exactly how KSHV infection leads to KS is still unclear. Like other herpesviruses, KSHV establishes latent infection, during which several proteins are produced with potential roles in stimulating spindle cell proliferation and preventing apoptosis. These include a viral homologue of cyclin D and several inhibitors of p53. However, KSHV infection, while necessary for KS development, is not sufficient, and additional cofactors are needed. In the AIDS-related form, that cofactor is clearly HIV. (The relevant cofactors for HIV-negative KS remain unknown.) HIV-mediated immune suppression may aid in widespread dissemination of KSHV in the host.

KSHV infection is not restricted to endothelial cells. The virus is related phylogenetically to the lymphotropic subfamily of herpesviruses (γ-herpesvirus); in keeping with this, its genome is found in B cells of infected subjects. In fact, KSHV infection is also linked to rare B-cell lymphomas in AIDS patients (called *primary effusion lymphoma*) and to multicentric Castleman disease, a B-cell lymphoproliferative disorder.

Clinically, AIDS-associated KS is quite different from the sporadic form (Chapter 11). In HIV-infected individuals the tumor is usually widespread, affecting the skin, mucous membranes, gastrointestinal tract, lymph nodes, and lungs. These tumors also tend to be more aggressive than classic KS.

Lymphomas. Lymphoma occurs at a markedly increased rate in individuals with AIDS, making it one of several AIDS-defining conditions. Roughly 5% of AIDS patients present with lymphoma, and approximately another 5% develop lymphoma during their subsequent course. With the advent of effective antiretroviral therapy, the incidence of lymphoma has fallen substantially in some HIV-infected populations. However, even in the era of retroviral therapy, lymphoma continues to occur in HIV-infected people at an incidence that is at least 10-fold greater than the population average. These epidemiologic findings suggest that the association of lymphoma and HIV infection is only partially explained by T-cell immunodeficiency. Indeed, based on molecular characterization of HIV-associated lymphomas and the epidemiologic considerations above, at least two mechanisms appear to underlie the increased risk of B-cell tumors in HIV infected individuals (Fig. 6-43).

- **Unchecked proliferation of B cells infected with oncogenic herpesviruses in the setting of profound T cell depletion (AIDS).** T-cell immunity is required to restrain the proliferation of B cells infected with oncogenic viruses such as EBV and KSHV. With the appearance of severe T-cell depletion late in the course of HIV infection, this control is lost. As a result AIDS patients are at high risk of developing aggressive B cell lymphomas composed of tumor cells infected by oncogenic viruses, particularly EBV.

  By adulthood, most normal individuals are infected by EBV. Once immunity is established, EBV persists in such individuals as a latent infection in approximately 1 in 100,000 B cells, most of which have a memory B-cell

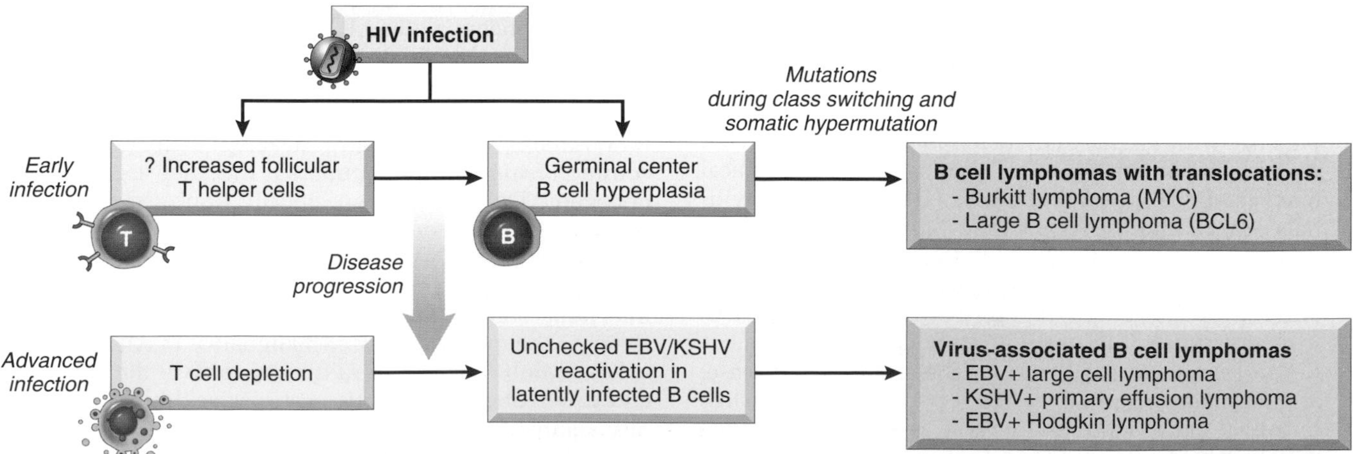

Figure 6-43 A model for the pathogenesis of B-cell lymphomas in HIV infection. HIV infection results in several changes that may cooperate to produce B-cell lymphomas.

phenotype. Activation of such cells, by antigen or by cytokines, reawakens an EBV-encoded program of gene expression that drives B-cell proliferation. Patients with AIDS have high levels of several cytokines, some of which, including IL-6, are growth factors for B cells. These patients are also chronically infected with pathogens that may lead to B-cell stimulation. In the absence of T-cell immunity, these activated, EBV infected clones proliferate and eventually acquire additional somatic mutations, leading to their outgrowth as full-blown EBV-positive B-cell lymphomas. The tumors often occur in extranodal sites, such as the central nervous system, but also the gut, the orbit, and the lungs, and elsewhere. AIDS patients are also prone to rare lymphomas that present as malignant effusions (so-called primary effusion lymphoma), which are remarkable in that the tumor cells are usually coinfected by both EBV and KSHV, a highly unusual example of cooperativity between two oncogenic viruses.

- **Germinal center B-cell hyperplasia in the setting of early HIV infection.** As mentioned, even in the face of effective antiretroviral therapy, the overall rate of lymphoma in the HIV-infected population remains elevated, even in those with normal CD4+ T-cell counts. As might be anticipated, the majority of the lymphomas that arise in patients with preserved CD4 T-cell counts are not associated with EBV or KSHV. What then explains the continued increased risk of lymphoma? The answer is not known, but it may be related to the profound germinal center B-cell hyperplasia that occurs early in HIV infection. Recall that in germinal centers, B cells diversify their immunoglobulin genes via lesions introduced into their DNA by the enzyme activation-induced deaminase (AID). This process is imperfect, and there is experimental evidence showing that AID can cause mutations in oncogenes implicated in B-cell lymphomagenesis. Of note, the aggressive B cell tumors that arise outside of the setting of full-blown AIDS in HIV-infected individuals, such as Burkitt lymphoma and diffuse large B-cell lymphoma, are often associated with mutations in oncogenes such as *MYC* and *BCL6* that bear the molecular hallmarks of "mistakes" made during attempted immunoglobulin class-switching and somatic hypermutations, two AID-dependent events that occur in germinal center B cells. Thus, the striking germinal center B-cell hyperplasia that occurs early in HIV infection may contribute to lymphomagenesis by simply increasing the number of B cells that are "at-risk" for acquiring potential lymphoma-initiating events.

Several other EBV-related proliferations also merit mention. Hodgkin lymphoma, an unusual B cell tumor associated with a pronounced tissue inflammatory response (Chapter 13), also occurs at increased frequency in HIV-infected individuals. In virtually all instances of HIV-associated Hodgkin lymphoma, the characteristic tumor cells (Reed-Sternberg cells) are infected with EBV. Many (but not all) HIV patients with Hodgkin lymphoma have low CD4 counts at the time of disease presentation. EBV infection also is responsible for oral hairy leukoplakia (white projections on the tongue), which results from EBV-driven squamous cell proliferation of the oral mucosa (Chapter 16).

Other Tumors. In addition to KS and lymphomas, patients with AIDS also have an increased occurrence of carcinoma of the uterine cervix and of anal cancer. This is most likely due to reactivation of latent human papillomavirus (HPV) infection in the setting of immunosuppression. This virus is intimately associated with squamous cell carcinoma of the cervix and its precursor lesions, cervical dysplasia and carcinoma in situ (Chapters 7 and 22). HPV-associated cervical dysplasia is 10 times more common in HIV-infected women as compared with uninfected women attending family planning clinics. Hence it is recommended that gynecologic examination be part of a routine work-up of HIV-infected women.

Central Nervous System Disease. Involvement of the central nervous system is a common and important manifestation of AIDS. Ninety percent of patients demonstrate some form of neurologic involvement at autopsy, and 40% to 60% have clinically apparent neurologic dysfunction. Importantly, in some patients, neurologic manifestations may be the sole or earliest presenting feature of HIV infection. In addition to opportunistic infections and neoplasms, several virally determined neuropathologic changes occur. These include a self-limited meningoencephalitis occurring at the time of seroconversion, aseptic meningitis, vacuolar myelopathy, peripheral neuropathies, and, most commonly, a progressive encephalopathy designated clinically as HIV-associated neurocognitive disorder (Chapter 28).

Effect of Antiretroviral Drug Therapy on the Clinical Course of HIV Infection. The advent of new antiretroviral drugs that target the viral reverse transcriptase, protease, and integrase has changed the clinical face of AIDS. These drugs are given in combination to reduce the emergence of mutants that develop resistance to any one; treatment regimens are commonly called *highly active antiretroviral therapy (HAART)* or *combination antiretroviral therapy.* Over 25 antiretroviral drugs from six distinct drug classes have been developed for the management of HIV infection. When a combination of at least three effective drugs is used in a motivated, compliant patient, HIV replication is reduced to below the level of detection (<50 copies RNA per milliliter) and remains there indefinitely (as long as the patient adheres to therapy). Even when a drug-resistant virus breaks through, there are several second- and third-line options to combat the virus. Once the virus is suppressed, the progressive loss of CD4+ T cells is halted. Over a period of several years the peripheral CD4+ T-cell count slowly increases and often returns to a normal level. With the use of these drugs, in the United States the annual death rate from AIDS has decreased from its peak of 16 to 18 per 100,000 people in 1995-1996 to less than 4 per 100,000. Many AIDS-associated disorders, such as opportunistic infections with *P. jiroveci* and Kaposi sarcoma, are very uncommon now. Effective antiretroviral therapy has reduced the transmission of the virus, especially from infected mothers to newborns. However, because of the reduced mortality, more people are living with HIV, and since they are not virus-free, there is a fear that the risk of spreading the infection may increase if vigilance is relaxed. Indeed, there is compelling evidence that even treated patients who remain asymptomatic, with virtually undetectable plasma virus for years, develop active infection if they stop the treatment.

Despite these dramatic improvements, several new complications associated with HIV infection and its treatment have emerged. Some patients with advanced disease who are given antiretroviral therapy develop a paradoxical clinical deterioration during the period of recovery of the immune system. This occurs despite increasing CD4+ T-cell counts and decreasing viral load. This disorder has been called the *immune reconstitution inflammatory syndrome*. Its basis is not understood but is postulated to be a poorly regulated host response to the high antigenic burden of persistent microbes. Perhaps a more important complication of long-term HAART pertains to adverse side-effects of the drugs. These include lipoatrophy (loss of facial fat), lipoaccumulation (excess fat deposition centrally), elevated lipids, insulin resistance, peripheral neuropathy, premature cardiovascular kidney and liver disease. Finally, non-AIDS morbidity is far more common than classic AIDS-related morbidity in long-term HAART-treated patients. Major causes of morbidity are cancer, and accelerated cardiovascular, kidney, and liver disease. The mechanism for these non-AIDS related complications is not known, but persistent inflammation and T-cell dysfunction may be playing a role.

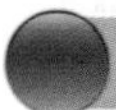

MORPHOLOGY

The anatomic changes in the tissues (with the exception of lesions in the brain) are neither specific nor diagnostic. Common pathologic features of AIDS include opportunistic infections, KS, and B cell lymphomas. Most of these lesions are discussed elsewhere, because they also occur in individuals who do not have HIV infection. Lesions in the central nervous system are described in Chapter 28.

Biopsy specimens from enlarged lymph nodes in the early stages of HIV infection reveal a marked hyperplasia of B cell follicles. The follicles are enlarged and often take on unusual, serpiginous shapes. The mantle zones that surround the follicles are attenuated, and the germinal centers impinge on interfollicular T cell areas. This hyperplasia of B cells is the morphologic reflection of the polyclonal B-cell activation and hypergammaglobulinemia seen in HIV-infected individuals.

With disease progression, the frenzy of B-cell proliferation subsides and gives way to a pattern of severe lymphoid involution. The lymph nodes are depleted of lymphocytes, and the organized network of follicular dendritic cells is disrupted. The germinal centers may even become hyalinized. During this advanced stage viral burden in the nodes is reduced, in part because of the disruption of the follicular dendritic cells. These "burnt-out" lymph nodes are atrophic and small and may harbor numerous opportunistic pathogens, often within macrophages. Because of profound immunosuppression, the inflammatory response to infections both in the lymph nodes and at extranodal sites may be sparse or atypical. For example, mycobacteria may not evoke granuloma formation because CD4+ cells are deficient. In the empty-looking lymph nodes and in other organs, the presence of infectious agents may not be readily apparent without special stains. As might be expected, lymphoid involution is not confined to the nodes; in later stages of AIDS, the spleen and thymus also are converted to "wastelands" that are virtually devoid of lymphocytes.

Despite spectacular advances in our understanding of HIV infection, the long-term prognosis of patients with AIDS remains dismal. Although with effective drug therapy the mortality rate has declined in the United States, the treated patients still carry viral DNA in their lymphoid tissues. Can there be a cure with persistent virus? Although a considerable effort has been mounted to develop a vaccine, many hurdles remain to be crossed before vaccine-based prophylaxis becomes a reality. Molecular analyses have revealed an alarming degree of variation in viral isolates from patients; this renders the task of producing a vaccine extremely difficult. Recent efforts have focused on producing antibodies against relatively invariant portions of HIV proteins. The task of developing an effective vaccine is complicated by the fact that the correlates of immune protection are not fully understood. At present, therefore, prevention, public health measures, and antiretroviral drugs remain the mainstays in the fight against AIDS.

KEY CONCEPTS

Pathogenesis and Course of HIV Infection and AIDS

- Virus entry into cells: requires CD4 and co-receptors, which are receptors for chemokines; involves binding of viral gp120 and fusion with the cell mediated by viral gp41 protein; main cellular targets are CD4+ helper T cells, macrophages, and DCs
- Viral replication: provirus genome integrates into host cell DNA; viral gene expression is triggered by stimuli that activate infected cells (e.g., infectious microbes, cytokines produced during normal immune responses)
- Progression of infection: acute infection of mucosal T cells and DCs; viremia with dissemination of virus; latent infection of cells in lymphoid tissue; continuing viral replication and progressive loss of CD4+ T cells
- Mechanisms of immune deficiency:
  - Loss of CD4+ T cells: T-cell death during viral replication and budding (similar to other cytopathic infections); apoptosis as a result of chronic stimulation; decreased thymic output; functional defects
  - Defective macrophage and DC functions
  - Destruction of architecture of lymphoid tissues (late)
- Clinical manifestations of AIDS include opportunistic infections, tumors such as B-cell lymphomas, and CNS abnormalities.

Amyloidosis

Amyloidosis is a condition associated with a number of inherited and inflammatory disorders in which extracellular deposits of fibrillar proteins are responsible for tissue damage and functional compromise. These abnormal fibrils are produced by the aggregation of misfolded proteins (which are soluble in their normal folded configuration). The fibrillar deposits bind a wide variety of proteoglycans and glycosaminoglycans, including heparan sulfate and dermatan sulfate, and plasma proteins, notably serum amyloid P component (SAP). The presence of abundant charged sugar groups in these adsorbed proteins give the deposits staining characteristics that were thought to resemble starch (amylose). Therefore, the deposits were called *amyloid*, a name that is firmly entrenched despite the realization that the deposits are unrelated to starch.

Amyloid is deposited in the extracellular space in various tissues and organs of the body in a variety of clinical settings. Because amyloid deposition appears insidiously and sometimes mysteriously, its clinical recognition ultimately depends on morphologic identification of this distinctive substance in appropriate biopsy specimens. With the light microscope and hematoxylin and eosin stains, amyloid appears as an amorphous, eosinophilic, hyaline, extracellular substance. *With progressive accumulation, it encroaches on and produces pressure atrophy of adjacent cells.* To differentiate amyloid from other hyaline materials (e.g., collagen, fibrin), a variety of histochemical techniques, described later, are used. Perhaps most widely used is the Congo red stain, which under ordinary light imparts a pink or red color to tissue deposits, but far more striking and specific is the green birefringence of the stained amyloid when observed by polarizing microscopy (see later).

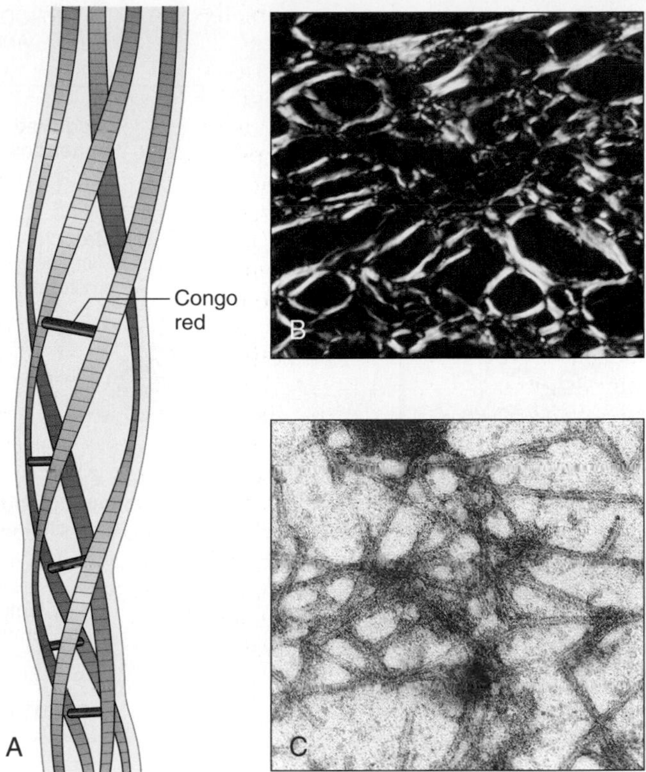

Figure 6-44 Structure of amyloid. **A,** A schematic diagram of an amyloid fiber showing four fibrils (there can be as many as six in each fiber) wound around one another with regularly spaced binding of the Congo red dye. **B,** Congo red staining shows apple-green birefringence under polarized light, a diagnostic feature of amyloid. **C,** Electron micrograph of 7.5- to 10-nm amyloid fibrils. (From Merlini G, Bellotti V: Molecular mechanisms of amyloidosis. N Engl J Med 2003;349:583-596, with permission of the Massachusetts Medical Society.)

Properties of Amyloid Proteins

Even though all amyloid deposits have a similar appearance and staining characteristics, amyloid is not a single chemical entity. In fact, more than 20 (at last count, 23) different proteins can aggregate and form fibrils with the appearance of amyloid. There are three major and several minor biochemical forms, which are deposited by different pathogenetic mechanisms. Therefore, amyloidosis should not be considered a single disease; rather it is a group of diseases having in common the deposition of similar-appearing proteins. At the heart of the morphologic similarity is the remarkably uniform physical organization of amyloid protein, which we consider first.

Physical Nature of Amyloid. By electron microscopy, all types of amyloid consist of continuous, nonbranching fibrils with a diameter of approximately 7.5 to 10 nm. X-ray crystallography and infrared spectroscopy demonstrate a characteristic cross-β-pleated sheet conformation (Fig. 6-44). This conformation is seen regardless of the clinical setting or chemical composition and is responsible for the distinctive Congo red staining and birefringence of amyloid.

Chemical Nature of Amyloid. Approximately 95% of the amyloid material consists of fibril proteins, the remaining 5% being the P component and other glycoproteins. The three most common forms of amyloid are the following:

- **The AL (amyloid light chain) protein is made up of complete immunoglobulin light chains, the amino-terminal fragments of light chains, or both.** Most of the AL proteins analyzed are composed of λ light chains or their fragments, but κ chains are present in some cases. The amyloid fibril protein of the AL type is produced from free Ig light chains secreted by a monoclonal population of plasma cells, and its deposition is associated with certain forms of plasma cell tumors (Chapter 13).
- **The AA (amyloid-associated) type of amyloid fibril protein is derived from a unique non-Ig protein made by the liver.** It has a molecular weight of 8500 and consists of 76 amino acid residues. AA fibrils are derived by proteolysis from a larger (12,000 daltons) precursor in the serum called SAA (serum amyloid-associated) protein that is synthesized in the liver and circulates bound to high density lipoproteins. The production of SAA protein is increased in inflammatory states as part of the acute phase response; therefore, this form of amyloidosis is associated with chronic inflammation, and is often called *secondary amyloidosis*.
- **β-amyloid protein (Aβ) constitutes the core of cerebral plaques found in Alzheimer disease** as well as the amyloid deposited in walls of cerebral blood vessels in individuals with this disease. The Aβ protein is a 4000-dalton peptide that is derived by proteolysis from a much larger transmembrane glycoprotein, called *amyloid precursor protein*. This form of amyloid is discussed in Chapter 28.

As mentioned, multiple other biochemically distinct proteins can also deposit as amyloid in a variety of clinical settings. Among these rarer causes of amyloidosis, the proteins most often involved are the following:

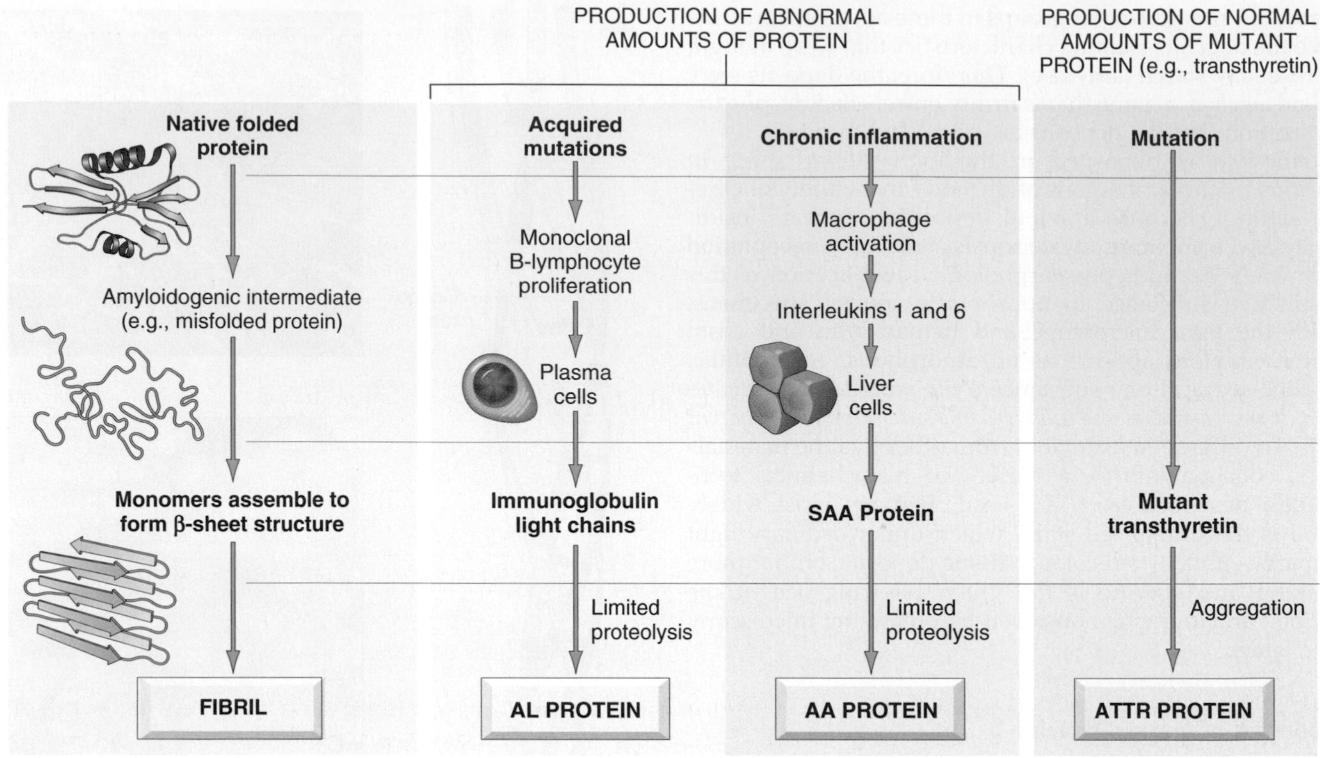

Figure 6-45 Pathogenesis of amyloidosis, showing the proposed mechanisms underlying deposition of the major forms of amyloid fibrils.

- *Transthyretin (TTR)* is a normal serum protein that binds and transports thyroxine and retinol. Several distinct mutant forms of TTR (and its fragments) are deposited in a group of genetically determined disorders referred to as familial amyloid polyneuropathies. Normal TTR is also deposited in the heart of aged individuals (senile systemic amyloidosis).
- *β_2-microglobulin*, a component of MHC class I molecules and a normal serum protein, has been identified as the amyloid fibril subunit ($A\beta_2m$) in amyloidosis that complicates the course of patients on long-term hemodialysis.
- In a minority of cases of prion disease in the central nervous system, the misfolded *prion proteins* aggregate in the extracellular space and acquire the structural and staining characteristics of amyloid protein.
- In addition, other minor components are always present in amyloid. These include serum amyloid P component, proteoglycans, and highly sulfated glycosaminoglycans. Serum amyloid P protein may contribute to amyloid deposition by stabilizing the fibrils and decreasing their clearance.

Pathogenesis and Classification of Amyloidosis

Amyloidosis results from abnormal folding of proteins, which become insoluble, aggregate, and deposit as fibrils in extracellular tissues. Normally, misfolded proteins are degraded intracellularly in proteasomes, or extracellularly by macrophages. It appears that in amyloidosis, these quality control mechanisms fail, leading to accumulation of a misfolded protein outside cells. The proteins that form amyloid fall into two general categories (Fig. 6-45): (1) normal proteins that have an inherent tendency to fold improperly, associate and form fibrils, and do so when they are produced in increased amounts; and (2) mutant proteins that are prone to misfolding and subsequent aggregation. The mechanisms of deposition of different types of amyloid are discussed below along with classification.

Because a given biochemical form of amyloid (e.g., AA) may be associated with amyloid deposition in diverse clinical settings, we follow a combined biochemical-clinical classification for our discussion (Table 6-17). Amyloid may be *systemic* (generalized), involving several organ systems, or it may be *localized*, when deposits are limited to a single organ, such as the heart.

On clinical grounds, the systemic, or generalized, pattern is subclassified into *primary amyloidosis*, when it is associated with some plasma cell disorder, or *secondary amyloidosis*, when it occurs as a complication of an underlying chronic inflammatory or tissue-destructive process. *Hereditary* or *familial amyloidosis* constitutes a separate, albeit heterogeneous group, with several distinctive patterns of organ involvement.

Primary Amyloidosis: Plasma Cell Disorders Associated with Amyloidosis. Amyloid in this category is usually systemic in distribution and is of the AL type. With approximately 2000 to 3000 new cases every year in the United States, this is the most common form of amyloidosis. In all cases, the disorder is caused by a clonal proliferation of plasma cells that synthesize an Ig that is prone to form amyloid due to its intrinsic physiochemical properties. Best defined is the occurrence of systemic amyloidosis in 5% to 15% of individuals with multiple myeloma, a plasma-cell

Table 6-17 Classification of Amyloidosis

Clinicopathologic Category	Associated Diseases	Major Fibril Protein	Chemically Related Precursor Protein
Systemic (Generalized) Amyloidosis			
Immunocyte dyscrasias with amyloidosis (primary amyloidosis)	Multiple myeloma and other monoclonal plasma cell proliferations	AL	Immunoglobulin light chains, chiefly λ type
Reactive systemic amyloidosis (secondary amyloidosis)	Chronic inflammatory conditions	AA	SAA
Hemodialysis-associated amyloidosis	Chronic renal failure	$A\beta_2m$	β_2-microglobulin
Hereditary Amyloidosis			
Familial Mediterranean fever		AA	SAA
Familial amyloidotic neuropathies (several types)		ATTR	Transthyretin
Systemic senile amyloidosis		ATTR	Transthyretin
Localized Amyloidosis			
Senile cerebral	Alzheimer disease	Aβ	APP
Endocrine	Type 2 diabetes		
Medullary carcinoma of thyroid		A Cal	Calcitonin
Islets of Langerhans		AIAPP	Islet amyloid peptide
Isolated atrial amyloidosis		AANF	Atrial natriuretic factor

tumor characterized by multiple osteolytic lesions throughout the skeletal system (Chapter 13). The malignant plasma cells synthesize abnormal amounts of a single Ig (monoclonal gammopathy), producing an M (myeloma) protein spike on serum electrophoresis. In addition to the synthesis of whole Ig molecules, the malignant plasma cells often secrete free, unpaired κ or λ light chains (referred to as *Bence-Jones protein*). These may be found in the serum, and due to their small molecular size, Bence-Jones proteins are excreted and concentrated in the urine. In primary amyloidosis, the free light chains are not only present in serum and urine but are also deposited in tissues as amyloid. It should be noted, however, that the great majority of myeloma patients who have free light chains in serum and urine do not develop amyloidosis. Clearly, not all free light chains are equally likely to produce amyloid, and it is believed that the *amyloidogenic potential* of any particular light chain is largely determined by its specific amino acid sequence.

Most persons with AL amyloid do not have classic multiple myeloma or any other overt B-cell neoplasm; such cases have been traditionally classified as primary amyloidosis, because their clinical features derive from the effects of amyloid deposition without any other associated disease. In virtually all such cases, however, monoclonal immunoglobulins or free light chains, or both, can be found in the serum or urine. Most of these patients also have a modest increase in the number of plasma cells in the bone marrow, which presumably secrete the precursors of AL protein. Thus, these patients have an underlying monoclonal proliferation of plasma cells (*monoclonal gammopathy*) in which production of an abnormal protein, rather than production of tumor masses, is the predominant manifestation.

Reactive Systemic Amyloidosis. The amyloid deposits in this pattern are systemic in distribution and are composed of AA protein. This category was previously referred to as *secondary amyloidosis* because it is secondary to an associated inflammatory condition. At one time, tuberculosis, bronchiectasis, and chronic osteomyelitis were the most important underlying conditions, but with the advent of effective antimicrobial chemotherapy the importance of these conditions has diminished. More commonly now, reactive systemic amyloidosis complicates rheumatoid arthritis, other connective tissue disorders such as ankylosing spondylitis, and inflammatory bowel disease, particularly Crohn disease and ulcerative colitis. Among these the most frequent associated condition is rheumatoid arthritis. Amyloidosis is reported to occur in approximately 3% of patients with rheumatoid arthritis and is clinically significant in one half of those affected. Heroin abusers who inject the drug subcutaneously also have a high occurrence rate of generalized AA amyloidosis. The chronic skin infections associated with "skin-popping" of narcotics seem to be responsible for the amyloidosis. Reactive systemic amyloidosis may also occur in association with solid tumors, the most common being renal cell carcinoma and Hodgkin lymphoma.

In this form of amyloidosis, SAA synthesis by liver cells is stimulated by cytokines such as IL-6 and IL-1 that are produced during inflammation; thus, long-standing inflammation leads to a sustained elevation of SAA levels. However, increased production of SAA by itself is not sufficient for the deposition of amyloid. There are two possible explanations for this. According to one view, SAA is normally degraded to soluble end products by the action of monocyte-derived enzymes. Conceivably, individuals who develop amyloidosis have an enzyme defect that results in incomplete breakdown of SAA, thus generating insoluble AA molecules. Alternatively, a genetically determined structural abnormality in the SAA molecule may render it resistant to degradation by macrophages.

Heredofamilial Amyloidosis. A variety of familial forms of amyloidosis have been described. Most of them are rare and occur in limited geographic areas. The most common and best studied is an autosomal recessive condition called *familial Mediterranean fever*. This is an "autoinflammatory" syndrome associated with excessive production of the cytokine IL-1 in response to inflammatory stimuli. It is characterized clinically by attacks of fever accompanied by inflammation of serosal surfaces, including peritoneum, pleura, and synovial membrane. The gene for familial Mediterranean fever encodes a protein called *pyrin* (for its relation to fever), which is one of a complex of proteins that regulate inflammatory reactions via the production of proinflammatory cytokines (Chapter 3). This disorder is encountered largely in individuals of Armenian, Sephardic Jewish, and Arabic origins. It is sometimes associated with widespread amyloidosis. The amyloid fibril proteins are made up of AA proteins, suggesting that this form of amyloidosis is related to the recurrent bouts of inflammation.

In contrast to familial Mediterranean fever, a group of autosomal dominant familial disorders is characterized by deposition of amyloid predominantly in peripheral and autonomic nerves. These familial amyloidotic polyneuropathies have been described in different parts of the world. As mentioned before, in all of these genetic disorders, the fibrils are made up of mutant TTRs. In these disorders, TTRs are deposited as amyloid fibrils because genetically determined alterations of structure appear to render the TTRs prone to misfolding and aggregation, and resistant to proteolysis.

Hemodialysis-Associated Amyloidosis. Patients on long-term hemodialysis for renal failure can develop amyloidosis as a result of deposition of β_2-microglobulin. This protein is present in high concentrations in the serum of persons with renal disease and in the past, it was retained in the circulation because it could not be filtered through dialysis membranes. Patients sometimes presented with carpal tunnel syndrome because of β_2-microglobulin deposition. With new dialysis filters, the incidence of this complication has decreased substantially.

Localized Amyloidosis. Sometimes, amyloid deposits are limited to a single organ or tissue without involvement of any other site in the body. The deposits may produce grossly detectable nodular masses or be evident only on microscopic examination. Nodular deposits of amyloid are most often encountered in the lung, larynx, skin, urinary bladder, tongue, and the region about the eye. Frequently, there are infiltrates of lymphocytes and plasma cells in the periphery of these amyloid masses. At least in some cases, the amyloid consists of AL protein and may therefore represent a localized form of plasma cell-derived amyloid.

Endocrine Amyloid. Microscopic deposits of localized amyloid may be found in certain endocrine tumors, such as medullary carcinoma of the thyroid gland, islet tumors of the pancreas, pheochromocytomas, and undifferentiated carcinomas of the stomach, and in the islets of Langerhans in individuals with type 2 diabetes mellitus. In these settings the amyloidogenic proteins seem to be derived either from polypeptide hormones (e.g., medullary carcinoma) or from unique proteins (e.g., islet amyloid polypeptide). In medullary carcinomas of the thyroid, the presence of amyloid is an essential diagnostic feature.

Amyloid of Aging. Several well-documented forms of amyloid deposition occur with aging. *Senile systemic amyloidosis* refers to the systemic deposition of amyloid in elderly patients (usually in their 70s and 80s). Because of the dominant involvement and related dysfunction of the heart, this form was previously called *senile cardiac amyloidosis*. Those who are symptomatic present with a restrictive cardiomyopathy and arrhythmias (Chapter 12). The amyloid in this form is derived from normal TTR. In addition to the sporadic senile systemic amyloidosis, another form, affecting predominantly the heart, that results from the deposition of a mutant form of TTR has also been recognized. Approximately 4% of the black population in the United States expresses this mutant form of TTR, and cardiomyopathy has been identified in both homozygous and heterozygous patients. The precise prevalence of patients with this mutation who develop clinically manifest cardiac disease is not known.

MORPHOLOGY

There are no consistent or distinctive patterns of organ or tissue distribution of amyloid deposits in any of the categories cited. Nonetheless, a few generalizations can be made. In amyloidosis secondary to chronic inflammatory disorders, kidneys, liver, spleen, lymph nodes, adrenals, and thyroid, as well as many other tissues, are typically affected. Although amyloidosis associated with plasma cell proliferations cannot reliably be distinguished from the secondary form by its organ distribution, it more often involves the heart, gastrointestinal tract, respiratory tract, peripheral nerves, skin, and tongue. The localization of amyloid deposits in the hereditary syndromes is varied. In familial Mediterranean fever the amyloidosis may be widespread, involving the kidneys, blood vessels, spleen, respiratory tract, and (rarely) liver. The localization of amyloid in the remaining hereditary syndromes can be inferred from the designation of these entities.

Whatever the clinical disorder, the amyloidosis may or may not be apparent on macroscopic examination. When amyloid accumulates in larger amounts, the organ is frequently enlarged and the tissue appears gray with a waxy, firm consistency. **Histologically, the amyloid deposition is always extracellular and begins between cells,** often closely adjacent to basement membranes (Fig. 6-46*A*). As the amyloid accumulates, it encroaches on the cells, in time surrounding and destroying them. In the form associated with plasma cell proliferation, perivascular and vascular deposits are common.

The histologic diagnosis of amyloid is based almost entirely on its staining characteristics. The most common staining technique uses the dye Congo red, which under ordinary light imparts a pink or red color to amyloid deposits. Under polarized light the Congo red-stained amyloid shows so-called apple-green birefringence (Fig. 6-46*B*). This reaction is shared by all forms of amyloid and is caused by the crossed β-pleated configuration of amyloid fibrils. Confirmation can be obtained by electron microscopy, which reveals amorphous nonoriented thin fibrils. AA, AL, and ATTR types of amyloid can also be distinguished by specific immunohistochemical staining.

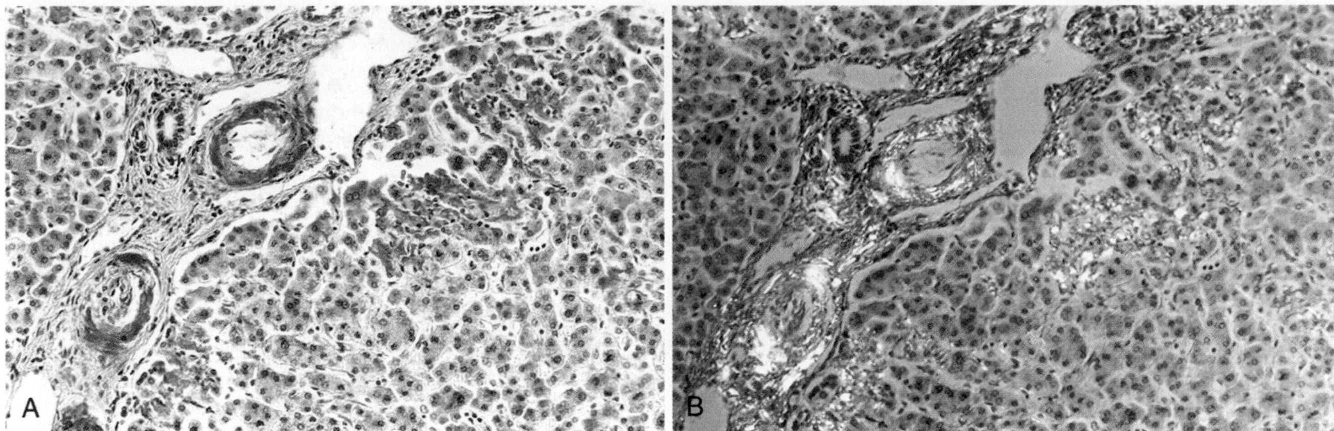

Figure 6-46 Amyloidosis. **A,** A section of the liver stained with Congo red reveals pink-red deposits of amyloid in the walls of blood vessels and along sinusoids. **B,** Note the yellow-green birefringence of the deposits when observed by polarizing microscope. (Courtesy Dr. Trace Worrell and Sandy Hinton, Department of Pathology, University of Texas Southwestern Medical School, Dallas, Texas.)

The pattern of organ involvement in different clinical forms of amyloidosis is variable.

Kidney. Amyloidosis of the kidney is the most common and potentially the most serious form of organ involvement. Grossly, the kidneys may be of normal size and color, or, in advanced cases, they may be shrunken because of ischemia caused by vascular narrowing induced by the deposition of amyloid within arterial and arteriolar walls.

Histologically, the amyloid is deposited primarily in the glomeruli, but the interstitial peritubular tissue, arteries, and arterioles are also affected. The glomerular deposits first appear as subtle thickenings of the mesangial matrix, accompanied usually by uneven widening of the basement membranes of the glomerular capillaries. In time the mesangial depositions and the deposits along the basement membranes cause capillary narrowing and distortion of the glomerular vascular tuft. With progression of the glomerular amyloidosis, the capillary lumens are obliterated, and the obsolescent glomerulus is flooded by confluent masses or interlacing broad ribbons of amyloid (Fig. 6-47).

Spleen. Amyloidosis of the spleen may be inapparent grossly or may cause moderate to marked splenomegaly (up to 800 g). For completely mysterious reasons, one of two patterns of deposition is seen. In one, the deposits are largely limited to the splenic follicles, producing tapioca-like granules on gross inspection, designated sago spleen. In the other pattern, the amyloid involves the walls of the splenic sinuses and connective tissue framework in the red pulp. Fusion of the early deposits gives rise to large, maplike areas of amyloidosis, creating what has been designated lardaceous spleen.

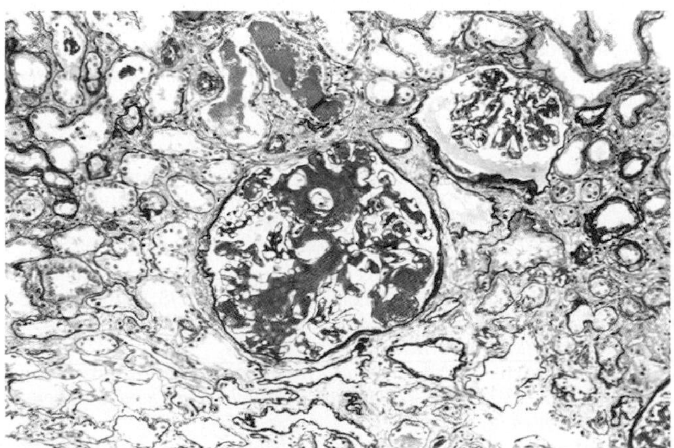

Figure 6-47 Amyloidosis of the kidney. The glomerular architecture is almost totally obliterated by the massive accumulation of amyloid.

Liver. The deposits may be inapparent grossly or may cause moderate to marked hepatomegaly. Amyloid appears first in the space of Disse and then progressively encroaches on adjacent hepatic parenchymal cells and sinusoids (Fig. 6-46). In time, deformity, pressure atrophy, and disappearance of hepatocytes occur, causing total replacement of large areas of liver parenchyma. Vascular involvement and deposits in Kupffer cells are frequent. Normal liver function is usually preserved despite sometimes quite severe involvement of the liver.

Heart. Amyloidosis of the heart (Chapter 12) may occur in any form of systemic amyloidosis. It is also the major organ involved in senile systemic amyloidosis. The heart may be enlarged and firm, but more often it shows no significant changes on gross inspection. Histologically the deposits begin as focal subendocardial accumulations and within the myocardium between the muscle fibers. Expansion of these myocardial deposits eventually causes pressure atrophy of myocardial fibers. When the amyloid deposits are subendocardial, the conduction system may be damaged, accounting for the electrocardiographic abnormalities noted in some patients.

Other Organs. Nodular depositions in the tongue may cause macroglossia, giving rise to the designation tumor-forming amyloid of the tongue. The respiratory tract may be involved focally or diffusely from the larynx down to the smallest bronchioles. As mentioned earlier, a distinct form of amyloid is found in the brains of patients with Alzheimer disease. It may be present in so-called plaques as well as blood vessels (Chapter 28). Amyloidosis of peripheral and autonomic nerves is a feature of several familial amyloidotic neuropathies. Depositions of amyloid in patients on long-term hemodialysis are most prominent in the carpal ligament of the wrist, resulting in compression of the median nerve (carpal tunnel syndrome). These patients may also have extensive amyloid deposition in the joints.

Clinical Features. Amyloidosis may be found as an unsuspected anatomic change, having produced no clinical manifestations, or it may cause serious clinical problems and even death. The symptoms depend on the magnitude of the deposits and on the sites or organs affected. Clinical manifestations at first are often entirely nonspecific, such as weakness, weight loss, light-headedness, or syncope. Somewhat more specific findings appear later and most often relate to renal, cardiac, and gastrointestinal involvement.

Renal involvement gives rise to proteinuria that may be severe enough to cause the nephrotic syndrome (Chapter 20). Progressive obliteration of glomeruli in advanced cases ultimately leads to renal failure and uremia. Renal failure is a common cause of death. *Cardiac amyloidosis* may present as an insidious congestive heart failure. The most serious aspects of cardiac amyloidosis are conduction disturbances and arrhythmias, which may prove fatal. Occasionally, cardiac amyloidosis produces a restrictive pattern of cardiomyopathy and masquerades as chronic constrictive pericarditis (Chapter 12). *Gastrointestinal amyloidosis* may be entirely asymptomatic, or it may present in a variety of ways. Amyloidosis of the tongue may cause sufficient enlargement and inelasticity to hamper speech and swallowing. Depositions in the stomach and intestine may lead to malabsorption, diarrhea, and disturbances in digestion. *Vascular amyloidosis* causes vascular fragility that may lead to bleeding, sometimes massive, that can occur spontaneously or following seemingly trivial trauma. Additionally, in some cases AL amyloid binds and inactivates factor X, a critical coagulation factor, leading to a life-threatening bleeding disorder.

The diagnosis of amyloidosis depends on the histologic demonstration of amyloid deposits in tissues. The most common sites biopsied are the kidney, when renal manifestations are present, or rectal or gingival tissues in patients suspected of having systemic amyloidosis. Examination of abdominal fat aspirates stained with Congo red can also be used for the diagnosis of systemic amyloidosis. The test is quite specific, but its sensitivity is low. In suspected cases of AL amyloidosis, serum and urine protein electrophoresis and immunoelectrophoresis should be performed. Bone marrow aspirates in such cases often show monoclonal plasmacytosis, even in the absence of overt multiple myeloma. Scintigraphy with radiolabeled serum amyloid P (SAP) component is a rapid and specific test, since SAP binds to the amyloid deposits and reveals their presence. It also gives a measure of the extent of amyloidosis and can be used to follow patients undergoing treatment.

The prognosis for individuals with generalized amyloidosis is poor. Those with AL amyloidosis (not including multiple myeloma) have a median survival of 2 years after diagnosis. Persons with myeloma-associated amyloidosis have an even poorer prognosis. The outlook for individuals with reactive systemic amyloidosis is somewhat better and depends to some extent on the control of the underlying condition. Resorption of amyloid after treatment of the associated condition has been reported, but this is a rare occurrence. New therapeutic strategies aimed at correcting protein misfolding and inhibiting fibrillogenesis are being developed.

KEY CONCEPTS

Amyloidosis

- Amyloidosis is a disorder characterized by the extracellular deposits of misfolded proteins that aggregate to form insoluble fibrils.
- The deposition of these proteins may result from: excessive production of proteins that are prone to misfolding and aggregation; mutations that produce proteins that cannot fold properly and tend to aggregate; defective or incomplete proteolytic degradation of extracellular proteins.
- Amyloidosis may be localized or systemic. It is seen in association with a variety of primary disorders, including monoclonal B-cell proliferations (in which the amyloid deposits consist of immunoglobulin light chains); chronic inflammatory diseases such as rheumatoid arthritis (deposits of amyloid A protein, derived from an acute-phase protein produced in inflammation); Alzheimer disease (amyloid b protein); familial conditions in which the amyloid deposits consist of mutants of normal proteins (e.g., transthyretin in familial amyloid polyneuropathies); amyloidosis associated with dialysis (deposits of β_2-microglobulin, whose clearance is defective).
- Amyloid deposits cause tissue injury and impair normal function by causing pressure on cells and tissues. They do not evoke an inflammatory response.

SUGGESTED READINGS

Innate Immunity

Goubau D, Deddouche S, Reis E, et al: Cytosolic sensing of viruses. *Immunity* 38:855–69, 2013. *[An excellent review on the numerous mechanisms used by cells to recognize viral DNA and RNA.]*

Kumar H, Kawai T, Akira S: Pathogen recognition by the innate immune system. *Int Rev Immunol* 30:16–34, 2011. *[A comprehensive review of the receptors used by the innate immune system to sense microbes.]*

Park H, Bourla AB, Kastner DL, et al: Lighting the fires within: the cell biology of autoinflammatory diseases. *Nat Rev Immunol* 12:570–80, 2012. *[A discussion of the inflammasome, and autoinflammatory diseases resulting from gain-of-function mutations in components of the inflammasome as well as other disorders involving abnormal inflammasome activity.]*

Schenten D, Medzhitov R: The control of adaptive immune responses by the innate immune system. *Adv Immunol* 109:87–124, 2011. *[A thoughtful discussion of how innate immune responses provide the danger signals that stimulate adaptive immunity.]*

Walker JA, Barlow JL, McKenzie AN: Innate lymphoid cells–how did we miss them? *Nat Rev Immunol* 13:75–87, 2013. *[A discussion of a recently appreciated family of cells of innate immunity, and their functions in host defense and immune regulation.]*

Cell-Mediated Immunity

Liao W, Lin JX, Leonard WJ: Interleukin-2 at the crossroads of effector responses, tolerance, and immunotherapy. *Immunity* 38:13–25, 2013. *[An excellent review of the established and newly discovered functions of a well-known cytokine, IL-2.]*

O'Shea JJ, Paul WE: Mechanisms underlying lineage commitment and plasticity of helper CD4+ T cells. *Science* 327:1098, 2010. *[An excellent review of the development and functions of helper T cell subsets, and the uncertainties in the field.]*

Pulendran B, Artis D: New paradigms in type 2 immunity. *Science* 337:431–5, 2012. *[A discussion of the mechanisms and functions of TH2 responses.]*

(Note: articles on TH17 cells are listed below, under "Other Hypersensitivity Reactions".)

Humoral Immunity

Craft JE: Follicular helper T cells in immunity and systemic autoimmunity. *Nat Rev Rheumatol* 8:337–47, 2012. *[A discussion of the properties and generation of follicular helper T cells and their roles in antibody production and autoimmunity.]*

Crotty S: Follicular helper CD4 T cells (TFH). *Annu Rev Immunol* 29:621–63, 2011. *[A comprehensive review of the development and functions of follicular helper T cells.]*

Goodnow CC, Vinuesa CG, Randall KL, et al: Control systems and decision making for antibody production. *Nat Immunol* 11:681–8, 2010. *[An excellent discussion of the major control points in the process of antibody production.]*

Victora GD, Nussenzweig MC: Germinal centers. *Annu Rev Immunol* 30:429–57, 2012. *[An excellent review of the properties and formation of germinal centers and their roles in antibody responses and autoimmune diseases.]*

Immune Regulation

Chaudhry A, Rudensky AY: Control of inflammation by integration of environmental cues by regulatory T cells. *J Clin Invest* 123: 939–44, 2013. *[A thoughtful discussion of how regulatory T cells control inflammatory responses and maintain homeostasis in the immune system.]*

Josefowicz SZ, Lu LF, Rudensky AY: Regulatory T cells: mechanisms of differentiation and function. *Annu Rev Immunol* 30:531–64, 2012. *[A detailed examination of the generation and functions of regulatory T cells.]*

Ohkura N, Kitagawa Y, Sakaguchi S: Development and maintenance of regulatory T cells. *Immunity* 38:414–23, 2013. *[An excellent review of the molecular mechanisms underlying the generation, maintenance, and stability of regulatory T cells.]*

Sakaguchi S, Miyara M, Costantino CM, et al: FOXP3+ regulatory T cells in the human immune system. *Nat Rev Immunol* 10:490, 2010. *[An excellent discussion of the properties and role of regulatory T cells in humans.]*

Immediate Hypersensitivity, Allergy

Galli SJ: The development of allergic inflammation. *Nature* 454:445, 2008. *[An excellent review of the mechanisms of inflammation in allergic diseases.]*

Galli SJ, Tsai M: IgE and mast cells in allergic disease. *Nat Med* 18: 693–704, 2012. *[An excellent review of the roles of IgE antibody and mast cells in chronic allergic diseases.]*

Gurish MF, Austen KF: Developmental origin and functional specialization of mast cell subsets. *Immunity* 37:25–33, 2012. *[A modern discussion of mast cell populations in different tissues, and their development and functions.]*

Holgate ST: Innate and adaptive immune responses in asthma. *Nat Med* 2012;18:673–83. *[A comprehensive discussion of the roles of TH2 cells, cytokines, and other cells of the immune system in the development and resolution of asthma.]*

Holloway JW, Yang IA, Holgate ST: Genetics of allergic disease. *J Allergy Clin Immunol* 125:S81–94, 2010. *[An update on susceptibility genes for allergic disease and what they tell us about pathophysiology.]*

Kauffmann F, Demenais F: Gene-environment interactions in asthma and allergic diseases: challenges and perspectives. *J Allergy Clin Immunol* 130:1229–40, 2012. *[A thoughtful discussion of the complex interactions between susceptibility genes and environmental influences that may underlie allergic diseases.]*

Other Hypersensitivity Reactions

Jancar S, Sanchez Crespo M: Immune complex–mediated tissue injury: a multistep paradigm. *Trends Immunol* 26:48, 2005. *[A summary of the mechanisms of immune complex–mediated tissue injury.]*

Maddur MS, Miossec P, Kaveri SV, et al: Th17 cells: biology, pathogenesis of autoimmune and inflammatory diseases, and therapeutic strategies. *Am J Pathol* 181:8–18, 2012. *[An excellent review of the development and lineage relationships of TH17 cells and their roles in autoimmune and other inflammatory diseases.]*

Sturfelt G, Truedsson L: Complement in the immunopathogenesis of rheumatic disease. *Nat Rev Rheumatol* 8:458–68, 2012. *[A review of complement deficiencies and the role of the complement system in autoimmune diseases.]*

Weaver CT, Elson CO, Fouser LA, et al: The Th17 pathway and inflammatory diseases of the intestines, lungs, and skin. *Annu Rev Pathol* 8:477–512, 2013. *[A detailed discussion of the biology of TH17 cells and their involvement in inflammatory diseases.]*

Immunological Tolerance

Basten A, Silveira PA: B-cell tolerance: mechanisms and implications. *Curr Opin Immunol* 22:566–74, 2010. *[A comprehensive review of the molecular mechanisms of central and peripheral tolerance in B cells, and how the choice between activation and tolerance is determined.]*

Kyewski B, Klein L: A central role for central tolerance. *Annu Rev Immunol* 24:571, 2006. *[A discussion of the mechanisms of central tolerance, with a focus on T cells.]*

Mueller DL: Mechanisms maintaining peripheral tolerance. *Nat Immunol* 11:21, 2010. *[A discussion of the mechanisms of peripheral tolerance, with an emphasis on T cells.]*

Odorizzi PM, Wherry EJ: Inhibitory receptors on lymphocytes: insights from infections. *J Immunol* 188:2957–65, 2012. *[An excellent review of the inhibitory receptors used by T lymphocytes to control their activation, the roles of these receptors in influencing the outcomes of infections, and the potential of targeting these receptors for the immunotherapy of cancer and chronic infections.]*

Schwartz RH: Historical overview of immunological tolerance. *Cold Spring Harb Perspect Biol* 4:a006908, 2012. *[A thoughtful summary of the mechanisms of tolerance, the experimental studies behind the elucidation of these mechanisms, and how they may be disrupted to give rise to autoimmunity.]*

Mechanisms of Autoimmunity: General

Cheng MH, Anderson MS: Monogenic autoimmunity. *Annu Rev Immunol* 30:393–427, 2012. *[An excellent review of autoimmune syndromes caused by single-gene mutations, and what they teach us about pathways of immunological tolerance.]*

Goodnow CC: Multistep pathogenesis of autoimmune disease. *Cell* 130:25, 2007. *[An excellent discussion of the checkpoints that prevent autoimmunity and why these might fail.]*

Mathis D, Benoist C: Microbiota and autoimmune disease: the hosted self. *Cell Host Microbe* 10:297–301, 2011. *[A review of the evidence that the microbiome influences immune activation and autoimmunity, and the relevance of these findings to human autoimmune diseases.]*

Palmer MT, Weaver CT: Autoimmunity: increasing suspects in the CD4+ T cell lineage. *Nat Immunol* 11:36, 2010. *[A thoughtful discussion of the central role of CD4+ T cells in the pathogenesis of autoimmune diseases.]*

Voight BF, Cotsapas C: Human genetics offers an emerging picture of common pathways and mechanisms in autoimmunity. *Curr Opin Immunol* 24:552–7, 2012. *[A discussion of the genetic associations with autoimmune diseases and the implications for understanding pathways of autoimmunity.]*

Wehrens EJ, Prakken BJ, van Wijk F: T cells out of control–impaired immune regulation in the inflamed joint. *Nat Rev Rheumatol* 9:34–42, 2013. *[A review of how abnormalities in immune regulation may contribute to inflammation and tissue injury in autoimmune diseases.]*

Zenewicz L, Abraham C, Flavell RA, et al: Unraveling the genetics of autoimmunity. *Cell* 140:791, 2010. *[An update on susceptibility genes for autoimmune diseases, how these are identified, and their significance.]*

Systemic Lupus Erythematosus

Banchereau J, Pascual V: Type I interferon in systemic lupus erythematosus and other autoimmune diseases. *Immunity* 25:383, 2006. *[A review of the recently discovered role of interferons in SLE and other autoimmune diseases, and the potential for targeting this family of cytokines for therapy.]*

Liu Z, Davidson A: Taming lupus-a new understanding of pathogenesis is leading to clinical advances. *Nat Med* 18:871–82, 2012. *[An excellent review of recent advances in understanding the genetics of lupus and the roles of innate and adaptive immune responses in the disease, and how these advances are shaping the development of novel therapies.]*

Tsokos GC: Systemic lupus erythematosus. *New Engl J Med* 365:2110, 2011. *[An excellent review of the clinical features and pathogenesis of lupus.]*

Sjogren Syndrome, Systemic Sclerosis, and Other Systemic Autoimmune Diseases

Giannakopoulos B, Krilis SA: The pathogenesis of the antiphospholipid syndrome. *New Engl J Med* 368:1033, 2013. *[An excellent review of the clinical features and pathogenesis of this enigmatic syndrome.]*

Jennette JC, Falk RJ, Hu P, et al: Pathogenesis of antineutrophil cytoplasmic autoantibody-associated small-vessel vasculitis. *Annu Rev Pathol* 8:139–60, 2013. *[A comprehensive review of the clinical and pathologic features and pathogenesis of small vessel vasculitis.]*

Katsumoto TR, Whitfield ML, Connolly MK: The pathogenesis of systemic sclerosis. *Annu Rev Pathol* 6:509, 2011. *[An excellent review of the pathogenesis of systemic sclerosis, and the many unanswered questions.]*

Mahajan VS, Mattoo H, Deshpande V, et al: IgG4-related disease. *Annu Rev Pathol* 9, in press, 2014. *[An excellent review of the clinical and pathologic features and likely autoimmune pathogenesis of a quite recently identified multisystem fibrotic disease.]*

Voulgarelis M, Tzioufas AG: Pathogenetic mechanisms in the initiation and perpetuation of Sjögren's syndrome. *Nat Rev Rheumatol* 6:529, 2010. *[A good discussion of what is known and not known about the pathogenesis of Sjögren syndrome.]*

Rejection of Transplants

Gras S, Kjer-Nielsen L, Chen Z, et al: The structural bases of direct T-cell allorecognition: implications for T-cell-mediated transplant rejection. *Immunol Cell Biol* 89:388–95, 2011. *[An excellent review of the molecular basis of T cell recognition of allogeneic MHC molecules.]*

Kinnear G, Jones ND, Wood KJ: Costimulation blockade: current perspectives and implications for therapy. *Transplantation* 95:527–35, 2013. *[An excellent update on the role of costimulators in T cell activation and the therapeutic targeting of costimulatory pathways to treat transplant rejection.]*

Mitchell RN: Graft vascular disease: immune response meets the vessel wall. *Annu Rev Pathol* 4:19, 2009. *[A review of the mechanisms that lead to vascular disease in chronic graft rejection.]*

Nagy ZA: Alloreactivity: an old puzzle revisited. *Scand J Immunol* 75:463–70, 2012. *[A thoughtful discussion of the evolution of ideas about allorecognition, and the current understanding of the phenomenon.]*

Nankivell BJ, Alexander SI: Rejection of the kidney allograft. *N Engl J Med* 363:1451, 2010. *[Good review of the mechanisms of recognition and rejection of allografts and the development of new strategies for treating rejection.]*

Tang Q, Bluestone JA, Kang SM: CD4(+)Foxp3(+) regulatory T cell therapy in transplantation. *J Mol Cell Biol* 4:11–21, 2012. *[An excellent review of the potential for Treg therapy of graft rejection and the challenges facing clinical application.]*

Wood KJ, Goto R: Mechanisms of rejection: current perspectives. *Transplantation* 93:1–10, 2012. *[An excellent review of the steps in the recognition of alloantigens and the activation of alloreactive lymphocytes, and the mechanisms of graft rejection.]*

Primary Immunodeficiency Diseases

Fischer A: Human primary immunodeficiency diseases. *Immunity* 28:835, 2008. *[An excellent summary of primary immunodeficiencies affecting the innate and adaptive immune systems.]*

Notarangelo LD: Functional T cell immunodeficiencies (with T cells present). *Annu Rev Immunol* 31:195–225, 2013. *[A detailed review of inherited defects in T cell survival and activation, independent of their maturation.]*

Parvaneh N, Casanova JL, Notarangelo LD, et al: Primary immunodeficiencies: a rapidly evolving story. *J Allergy Clin Immunol* 131:314–23, 2013. *[An excellent review of newly described primary immunodeficiency syndromes.]*

Pieper K, Grimbacher B, Eibel H: B-cell biology and development. *J Allergy Clin Immunol* 131:959–71, 2013. *[A review of the development of B cells and inherited defects causing developmental disorders with immunodeficiency.]*

HIV and Aids

Douek DC, Roederer M, Koup RA: Emerging concepts in the immunopathogenesis of AIDS. *Annu Rev Med* 60:471, 2009. *[A balanced discussion of the pathogenesis of AIDS, and the still unresolved issues.]*

Moir S, Chun TW, Fauci AS: Pathogenic mechanisms of HIV disease. *Annu Rev Pathol* 6:223, 2011. *[A discussion of current concepts of the mechanisms by which HIV causes immunodeficiency.]*

Walker B, McMichael A: The T-cell response to HIV. *Cold Spring Harb Perspect Med* 2:a007054, 2012. *[An excellent review of the development, control and functions of T cell responses to HIV infection, and how the virus evades these responses.]*

Amyloidosis

Buxbaum JN, Linke RP: A molecular history of the amyloidoses. *J Mol Biol* 421:142–59, 2012. *[A thoughtful review of how our understanding of amyloid proteins and their role in disease has evolved, and the molecular studies that have led to current concepts.]*

Obici L, Merlini G: AA amyloidosis: basic knowledge, unmet needs and future treatments. *Swiss Med Wkly* 142:w13580, 2012. *[A thorough review of the most common form of amyloid, including its formation and pathologic effects, and strategies for treating diseases caused by amyloid deposition.]*

Pepys MB: Amyloidosis. *Annu Rev Med* 57:223, 2006. *[An excellent review of the pathogenesis, clinical features and therapeutic approaches in amyloidosis.]*

See TARGETED THERAPY available online at www.studentconsult.com

CHAPTER 7

Neoplasia

CHAPTER CONTENTS

Cancer is the second leading cause of death in the United States; only cardiovascular diseases exact a higher toll. Even more agonizing than the mortality rate is the emotional and physical suffering inflicted by cancers. Patients and the public often ask, "When will there be a cure for this scourge?" The answer to this simple question is difficult, because cancer is not one disease but many disorders with widely different natural histories and responses to treatments. Some cancers, such as Hodgkin lymphoma, are curable, whereas others, such as pancreatic adenocarcinoma, are virtually always fatal. The only hope for controlling cancer lies in learning more about its causes and pathogenesis. Fortunately, great strides have been made in understanding its molecular basis and some good news has emerged: cancer mortality for both men and women in the United States declined during the last decade of the twentieth century and has continued its downward course in the twenty-first.

In this chapter, we describe the vocabulary of tumor biology and pathology and then review the morphologic characteristics that define neoplasia and allow benign and malignant tumors to be identified and distinguished. Also reviewed is the epidemiology of cancer, which provides a measure of the impact of cancer on human populations as well as clues to its environmental causes, insights that have led to effective prevention campaigns against certain cancers. Building on this foundation, we then discuss the biologic properties of tumors and the molecular basis of carcinogenesis, emphasizing the critical role that genetic alterations play in the development of neoplasia.

Finally, we turn to cancer diagnosis, focusing on new technologies that are helping to direct the use of cancer drugs that are targeted at particular molecular lesions. Throughout, we give examples of new analytic methods and therapies that are not only changing our approach to cancer treatment but also providing new insights into cancer pathophysiology.

Nomenclature

Neoplasia means "new growth," and a new growth is called a *neoplasm. Tumor* originally applied to the swelling caused by inflammation, but the nonneoplastic usage of tumor has almost vanished; thus, the term is now equated with neoplasm. *Oncology* (Greek *oncos* = tumor) is the study of tumors or neoplasms.

Although all physicians know what they mean when they use the term *neoplasm*, it has been surprisingly difficult to develop an accurate definition. In the premolecular era, the eminent British oncologist Willis came closest: "A neoplasm is an abnormal mass of tissue, the growth of which exceeds and is uncoordinated with that of the normal tissues and persists in the same excessive manner after cessation of the stimuli which evoked the change." In the modern era, a neoplasm can be defined as a disorder of cell growth that is triggered by a series of acquired mutations affecting a single cell and its clonal progeny. As discussed later, the causative mutations give the neoplastic cells a survival and growth advantage, resulting in excessive proliferation that is independent of physiologic growth signals (autonomous).

All tumors have two basic components: (1) neoplastic cells that constitute the tumor *parenchyma* and (2) *reactive stroma* made up of connective tissue, blood vessels, and variable numbers of cells of the adaptive and innate immune system. The classification of tumors and their biologic behavior are based primarily on the parenchymal component, but their growth and spread are critically dependent on their stroma. In some tumors, connective tissue is scant and so the neoplasm is soft and fleshy. In other cases, the parenchymal cells stimulate the formation of an abundant collagenous stroma, referred to as *desmoplasia.* Some demoplastic tumors—for example, some cancers of the female breast—are stony hard or *scirrhous.*

Benign Tumors. **A tumor is said to be *benign* when its gross and microscopic appearances are considered relatively innocent, implying that it will remain localized, will not spread to other sites, and is amenable to local surgical removal;** understandably, the patient generally survives. However, "benign" tumors may cause significant morbidity and are sometimes even fatal.

In general, benign tumors are designated by attaching the suffix *-oma* to the name of the cell type from which the tumor originates. Tumors of mesenchymal cells generally follow this rule. For example, a benign tumor arising in fibrous tissue is called a *fibroma,* whereas a benign cartilaginous tumor is a *chondroma.* In contrast, the nomenclature of benign epithelial tumors is more complex; some are classified based on their cells of origin, others on microscopic pattern, and still others on their macroscopic architecture.

Adenoma is applied to benign epithelial neoplasms derived from glands, although they may or may not form glandular structures. On this basis, a benign epithelial neoplasm that arises from renal tubular cells growing in the form of numerous tightly clustered small glands is termed an *adenoma,* as is a heterogeneous mass of adrenal cortical cells growing as a solid sheet. Benign epithelial neoplasms producing microscopically or macroscopically visible fingerlike or warty projections from epithelial surfaces are referred to as *papillomas.* Those that form large cystic masses, such as in the ovary, are referred to as *cystadenomas.* Some tumors produce papillary patterns that protrude into cystic spaces and are called papillary cystadenomas. When a neoplasm—benign or malignant—produces a macroscopically visible projection above a mucosal surface and projects, for example, into the gastric or colonic lumen, it is termed a *polyp.* If the polyp has glandular tissue, it is called an adenomatous polyp (Fig. 7-1).

Malignant Tumors. Malignant tumors are collectively referred to as *cancers,* derived from the Latin word for crab, because they tend to adhere to any part that they seize on in an obstinate manner. **Malignant tumors can invade and destroy adjacent structures and spread to distant sites (metastasize) to cause death.** Not all cancers pursue so deadly a course. Some are discovered early enough to be excised surgically or are treated successfully with chemotherapy or radiation, but the designation *malignant* always raises a red flag.

The nomenclature of malignant tumors essentially follows the same schema used for benign neoplasms, with certain additions. Malignant tumors arising in solid mesenchymal tissues are usually called *sarcomas* (Greek *sar* = fleshy; e.g., fibrosarcoma, chondrosarcoma, leiomyosarcoma, and rhabdomyosarcoma), whereas those arising from blood-forming cells are designated *leukemias* (literally, white blood) or *lymphomas* (tumors of lymphocytes or their precursors). Malignant neoplasms of epithelial cell origin, derived from any of the three germ layers, are called *carcinomas.* Thus, cancers arising in the ectodermally derived epidermis, the mesodermally derived renal tubules, and the endodermally derived lining of the gastrointestinal tract are all termed carcinomas. Carcinomas may be further qualified. *Squamous cell carcinoma* denotes a cancer in which the tumor cells resemble stratified squamous epithelium, and *adenocarcinoma* denotes a lesion in which the neoplastic epithelial cells grow in a glandular pattern. Sometimes the tissue or organ of origin can be identified and is added as a descriptor, as in renal cell adenocarcinoma or bronchogenic squamous cell carcinoma. Not infrequently, a cancer is composed of cells of unknown tissue origin, and must be designated merely as an undifferentiated malignant tumor.

Mixed Tumors. In most benign and malignant neoplasms, all of the parenchymal cells closely resemble one another. Infrequently, however, divergent differentiation of a single neoplastic clone creates a *mixed tumor,* such as the mixed tumor of salivary gland. These tumors contain epithelial components scattered within a myxoid stroma that may contain islands of cartilage or bone (Fig. 7-2). All of these elements arise from a single clone capable of capable of

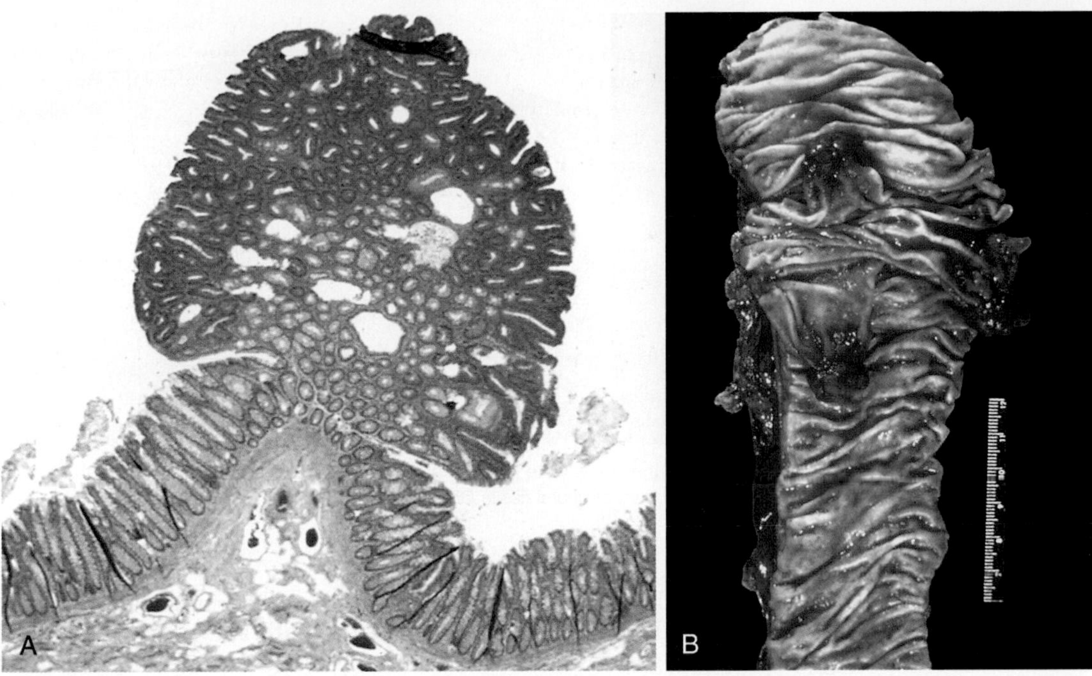

Figure 7-1 Colonic polyp. **A,** An aedonmatous (glandular) polyp is projecting into the colonic lumen and is attached to the mucosa by a distinct stalk. **B,** Gross appearance of several colonic polyps.

producing both epithelial and myoepithelial cells; thus, the preferred designation of this neoplasm is *pleomorphic adenoma*. The great majority of neoplasms, even mixed tumors, are composed of cells from a single germ layer. An exception is a tumor called a *teratoma*, which contains recognizable mature or immature cells or tissues belonging to more than one germ cell layer (and sometimes all three). Teratoma originates from totipotential germ cells that are normally present in the ovary and testis and sometimes also found in abnormal midline embryonic rests. Such cells can differentiate into any of the cell types found in the adult body and so, not surprisingly, may give rise to neoplasms that contain, in a helter-skelter fashion, bone, epithelium, muscle, fat, nerve, and other tissues. A particularly common pattern is seen in the *ovarian cystic teratoma (dermoid cyst)*, which differentiates principally along ectodermal lines to create a cystic tumor lined by skin replete with hair, sebaceous glands, and tooth structures (Fig. 7-3).

The nomenclature of the more common types of tumors is presented in Table 7-1. It is evident from this list that there are some inappropriate but deeply entrenched usages. For instance, benign-sounding designations such as lymphoma, melanoma, mesothelioma, and seminoma are used for certain malignant neoplasms. It is also important to recognize that ominous sounding terms are applied to some trivial lesions. *Hamartomas* are disorganized but benign masses composed of cells indigenous to the involved site. Once thought to be a developmental malformation unworthy of the -oma designation, many in fact have clonal chromosomal aberrations that are acquired through somatic mutations and on this basis are now considered neoplasms. *Choristoma* is the term applied to a heterotopic rest of cells. For example, a small nodule of well-developed and normally organized pancreatic tissue may be found in the submucosa of the stomach, duodenum, or small intestine. The term choristoma, suggesting a neoplasm, imparts a gravity to these lesions that is far beyond their actual significance.

Characteristics of Benign and Malignant Neoplasms

Nothing is more important to the individual with a tumor than being told "It is benign," and so the differentiation

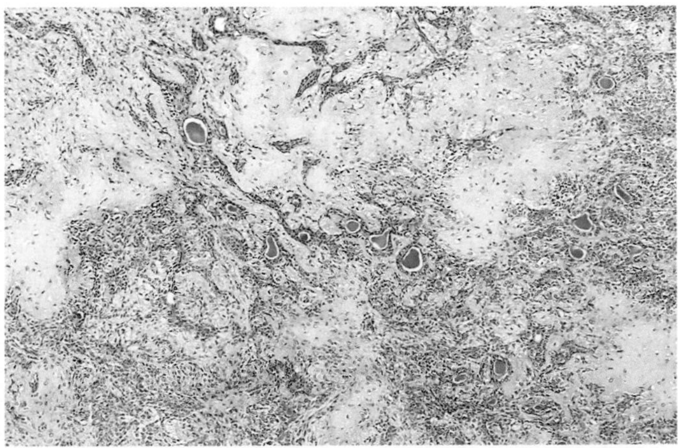

Figure 7-2 This mixed tumor of the parotid gland contains epithelial cells forming ducts and myxoid stroma that resemble cartilage. (Courtesy Dr. Trace Worrell, University of Texas Southwestern Medical School, Dallas, Texas.)

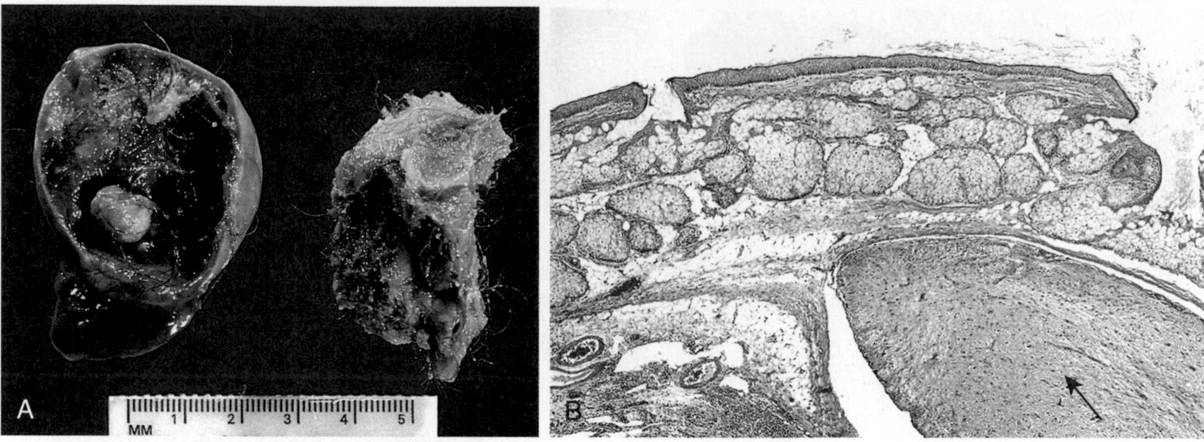

Figure 7-3 **A,** Gross appearance of an opened cystic teratoma of the ovary. Note the presence of hair, sebaceous material, and tooth. **B,** A microscopic view of a similar tumor shows skin, sebaceous glands, fat cells, and a tract of neural tissue *(arrow).*

between benign and malignant tumors is one of the most important distinctions a pathologist can make. Although an innocent face may mask an ugly nature, in general, benign and malignant tumors can be distinguished on the basis of a number of histologic and anatomic features, (described below). Malignant tumors also tend to grow more rapidly than benign tumors, but there are so many exceptions that growth rate is not a very useful discriminator between benignity and malignancy. In fact, even cancers exhibit remarkably varied growth rates, from slow-growing tumors associated with survival for years, often without treatment, to rapidly growing tumors that may be lethal within months or weeks.

Differentiation and Anaplasia

Differentiation refers to the extent to which neoplastic parenchymal cells resemble the corresponding normal

Table 7-1 Nomenclature of Tumors

Tissue of Origin	Benign	Malignant
Composed of one parenchymal cell type		
Tumors of Mesenchymal Origin		
Connective tissue and derivatives	Fibroma Lipoma Chondroma Osteoma	Fibrosarcoma Liposarcoma Chondrosarcoma Osteogenic sarcoma
Vessels and surface coverings		
Blood vessels	Hemangioma	Angiosarcoma
Lymph vessels	Lymphangioma	Lymphangiosarcoma
Mesothelium	Benign fibrous tumor	Mesothelioma
Brain coverings	Meningioma	Invasive meningioma
Blood Cells and Related Cells		
Hematopoietic cells		Leukemias
Lymphoid tissue		Lymphomas
Muscle		
Smooth	Leiomyoma	Leiomyosarcoma
Striated	Rhabdomyoma	Rhabdomyosarcoma
Tumors of Epithelial Origin		
Stratified squamous	Squamous cell papilloma	Squamous cell carcinoma
Basal cells of skin or adnexa		Basal cell carcinoma
Tumors of Epithelial Origin (cont'd)		
Epithelial lining of glands or ducts	Adenoma Papilloma Cystadenoma	Adenocarcinoma Papillary carcinomas Cystadenocarcinoma
Respiratory passages	Bronchial adenoma	Bronchogenic carcinoma
Renal epithelium	Renal tubular adenoma	Renal cell carcinoma
Liver cells	Hepatic adenoma	Hepatocellular carcinoma
Urinary tract epithelium (transitional)	Transitional cell papilloma	Transitional cell carcinoma
Placental epithelium	Hydatidiform mole	Choriocarcinoma
Testicular epithelium (germ cells)		Seminoma Embryonal carcinoma
Tumors of Melanocytes	Nevus	Malignant melanoma
More than one neoplastic cell type—mixed tumors, usually derived from one germ cell layer		
Salivary glands	Pleomorphic adenoma (mixed tumor of salivary origin)	Malignant mixed tumor of salivary gland origin
Renal anlage		Wilms tumor
More than one neoplastic cell type derived from more than one germ cell layer—teratogenous		
Totipotential cells in gonads or in embryonic rests	Mature teratoma, dermoid cyst	Immature teratoma, teratocarcinoma

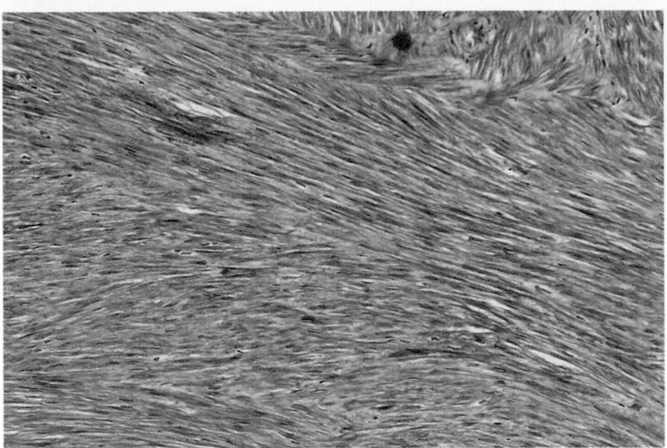

Figure 7-4 Leiomyoma of the uterus. This benign, well-differentiated tumor contains interlacing bundles of neoplastic smooth muscle cells that are virtually identical in appearance to normal smooth muscle cells in the myometrium.

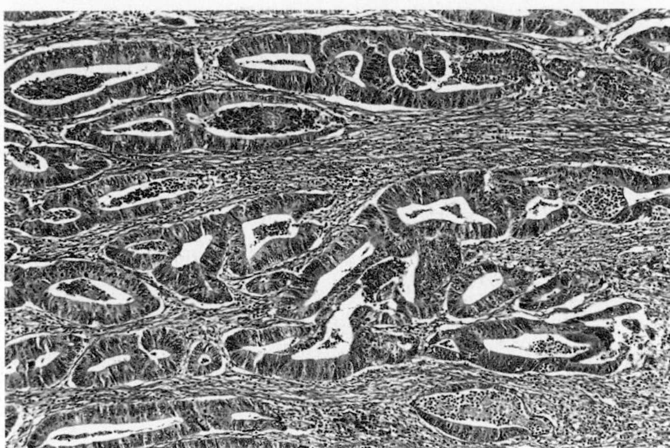

Figure 7-6 Malignant tumor (adenocarcinoma) of the colon. Note that compared with the well-formed and normal-looking glands characteristic of a benign tumor (Fig. 7-5), the cancerous glands are irregular in shape and size and do not resemble the normal colonic glands. This tumor is considered differentiated because gland formation is seen. The malignant glands have invaded the muscular layer of the colon. (Courtesy Dr. Trace Worrell, University of Texas Southwestern Medical School, Dallas, Texas.)

parenchymal cells, both morphologically and functionally; lack of differentiation is called *anaplasia*. In general, benign tumors are well differentiated (Figs. 7-4 and 7-5). The neoplastic cell in a tumor of benign adipocytes—a lipoma—so closely resembles normal adipocytes that it may be impossible to recognize the tumor by microscopic examination of individual cells. Only the growth of these cells into a discrete mass discloses the neoplastic nature of the lesion. One may get so close to the tree that one loses sight of the forest. In well-differentiated benign tumors, mitoses are usually rare and are of normal configuration.

In contrast, **while malignant neoplasms exhibit a wide range of parenchymal cell differentiation, most exhibit morphologic alterations that betray their malignant nature** (Fig. 7-6). There are exceptions, however. At one end of the spectrum, certain well-differentiated adenocarcinomas of the thyroid, for example, form normal-appearing follicles, and some squamous cell carcinomas contain cells that appear identical to normal squamous epithelial cells (Fig. 7-7). Thus, the morphologic distinction between well-differentiated malignant tumors and benign tumors may be quite subtle. At the other end of the spectrum lie tumors exhibiting little or no evidence of differentiation (Fig. 7-8). In between the two extremes lie tumors that are loosely referred to as moderately well differentiated.

Malignant neoplasms that are composed of poorly differentiated cells are said to be *anaplastic*. **Lack of differentiation, or anaplasia, is considered a hallmark of malignancy.** The term *anaplasia* means "to form backward," implying a reversal of differentiation to a more primitive level. Whether cancers in fact arise from "reverse

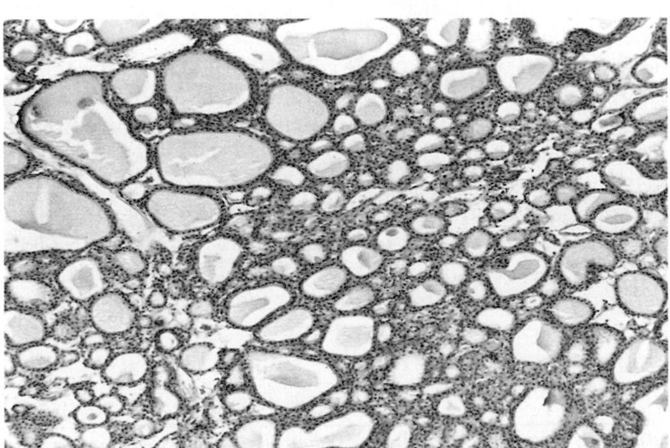

Figure 7-5 Benign tumor (adenoma) of the thyroid. Note the normal-looking (well-differentiated), colloid-filled thyroid follicles. (Courtesy Dr. Trace Worrell, University of Texas Southwestern Medical School, Dallas, Texas.)

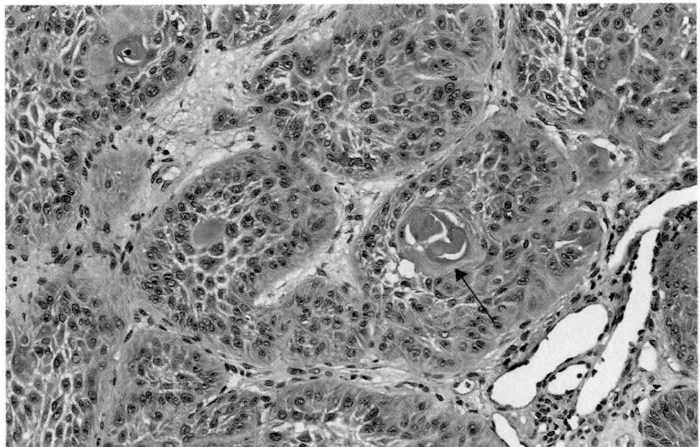

Figure 7-7 Well-differentiated squamous cell carcinoma of the skin. The tumor cells are strikingly similar to normal squamous epithelial cells, with intercellular bridges and nests of keratin pearls *(arrow)*. (Courtesy Dr. Trace Worrell, University of Texas Southwestern Medical School, Dallas, Texas.)

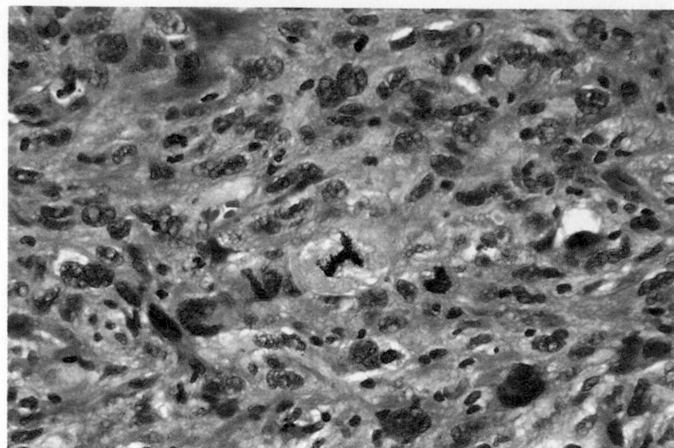

Figure 7-8 Anaplastic tumor showing cellular and nuclear variation in size and shape. The prominent cell in the center field has an abnormal tripolar spindle.

differentiation" of mature normal cells or instead from incomplete differentiation of less mature cells is an important fundamental issue that is discussed later.

Lack of differentiation, or anaplasia, is often associated with many other morphologic changes.

- **Pleomorphism**. Cancer cells often display pleomorphism—variation in size and shape (Fig. 7-9). Thus, cells within the same tumor are not uniform, but range from small cells with an undifferentiated appearance, to *tumor giant cells* many times larger than their neighbors. Some tumor giant cells possess only a single huge polymorphic nucleus, while others may have two or more large, hyperchromatic nuclei (Fig. 7-9). These giant cells are not to be confused with inflammatory Langhans or foreign body giant cells, which are derived from macrophages and contain many small, normal-appearing nuclei.
- **Abnormal nuclear morphology**. Characteristically, the nuclei are disproportionately large for the cell, with a nuclear-to-cytoplasm ratio that may approach 1:1 instead of the normal 1:4 or 1:6. The nuclear shape is variable and often irregular, and the chromatin is often coarsely clumped and distributed along the nuclear membrane, or more darkly stained than normal *(hyperchromatic)*. Abnormally large nucleoli are also commonly seen.
- **Mitoses**. Unlike in benign tumors and some well-differentiated malignant neoplasms, in undifferentiated tumors, many cells are in mitosis, reflecting the high proliferative activity of the parenchymal cells. The presence of mitoses, however, does not necessarily indicate that a tumor is malignant or that the tissue is neoplastic. Mitoses are indicative of rapid cell growth. Hence, cells in mitosis are often seen in normal tissues exhibiting rapid turnover, such as the epithelial lining of the gut and nonneoplastic proliferations such as hyperplasias. More important as a morphologic feature of malignancy are *atypical, bizarre mitotic figures*, sometimes with tripolar, quadripolar, or multipolar spindles (Fig. 7-8).
- **Loss of polarity**. In addition to the cytologic abnormalities, the orientation of anaplastic cells is markedly disturbed. Sheets or large masses of tumor cells grow in an anarchic, disorganized fashion.
- **Other changes**. Growing tumor cells obviously require a blood supply, but often the vascular stroma is insufficient, and as a result in many rapidly growing malignant tumors develop large central areas of ischemic necrosis.

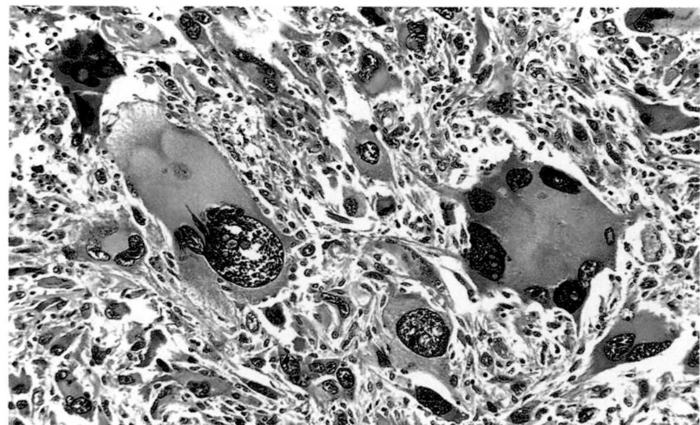

Figure 7-9 Pleomorphic tumor of the skeletal muscle (rhabdomyosarcoma). Note the marked cellular and nuclear pleomorphism, hyperchromatic nuclei, and tumor giant cells. (Courtesy Dr. Trace Worrell, University of Texas Southwestern Medical School, Dallas, Texas.)

As one might surmise, the better the differentiation of the transformed cell, the more completely it retains the functional capabilities of its normal counterpart. Thus, benign neoplasms and well-differentiated carcinomas of endocrine glands frequently secrete hormones characteristic of their origin. Increased levels of these hormones in the blood are used clinically to detect and follow such tumors. Well-differentiated squamous cell carcinomas of the epidermis synthesize keratin, and well-differentiated hepatocellular carcinomas elaborate bile. Highly anaplastic undifferentiated cells, whatever their tissue of origin, lose their resemblance to the normal cells from which they have arisen. In some instances, new and unanticipated functions emerge. Thus, some tumors express fetal proteins that are not produced by comparable cells in the adult, while others express proteins that are normally only found in other types of adult cells. For example, bronchogenic carcinomas may produce corticotropin, parathyroid-like hormone, insulin, glucagon, and other hormones, giving rise to paraneoplastic syndromes (described later). Despite such exceptions, rapidly growing anaplastic tumors are less likely to have specialized functional activity. The cells in benign tumors are almost always well differentiated and resemble their normal cells of origin; the cells in cancer are more or less differentiated, but some derangement of differentiation is always present.

Metaplasia and Dysplasia. *Metaplasia* is defined as the replacement of one type of cell with another type (Chapter 2). Metaplasia is nearly always found in association with tissue damage, repair, and regeneration. Often the replacing cell type is better suited to some alteration in

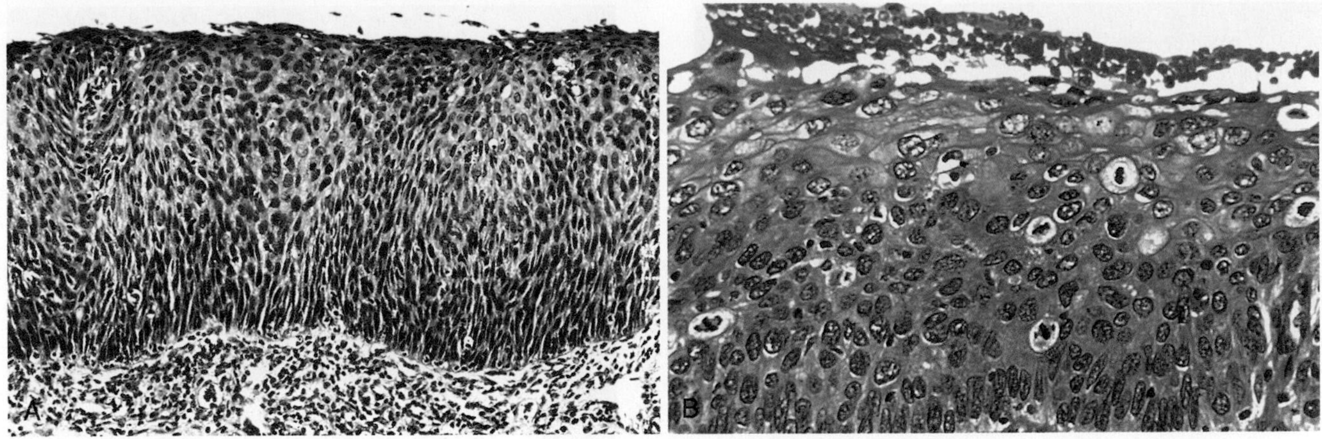

Figure 7-10 A, Carcinoma in situ. A low-power view shows that the epithelium is entirely replaced by atypical dysplastic cells. There is no orderly differentiation of squamous cells. The basement membrane is intact, and there is no tumor in the subepithelial stroma. **B,** A high-power view of another region shows failure of normal differentiation, marked nuclear and cellular pleomorphism, and numerous mitotic figures extending toward the surface.

the local environment. For example, gastroesophageal reflux damages the squamous epithelium of the esophagus, leading to its replacement by glandular (gastric or intestinal) epithelium more suited to an acidic environment.

Dysplasia is a term that literally means "disordered growth." It is encountered principally in epithelia and is characterized by a constellation of changes that include a loss in the uniformity of the individual cells as well as a loss in their architectural orientation. Dysplastic cells may exhibit considerable pleomorphism and often contain large hyperchromatic nuclei with a high nuclear-to-cytoplasmic ratio. The architecture of the tissue may be disorderly. For example, in dysplastic squamous epithelium the normal progressive maturation of tall cells in the basal layer to flattened squames on the surface may fail in part or entirely, leading to replacement of the epithelium by basal-appearing cells with hyperchromatic nuclei. In addition, mitotic figures are more abundant than in the normal tissue and rather than being confined to the basal layer may instead be seen at all levels, including surface cells.

When dysplastic changes are marked and involve the full thickness of the epithelium, but the lesion does not penetrate the basement membrane, it is considered a preinvasive neoplasm and is referred to as *carcinoma in situ* (Fig. 7-10**). Once the tumor cells breach the basement membrane, the tumor is said to be *invasive*.** Dysplastic changes are often found adjacent to foci of invasive carcinoma, and in some situations, such as in long-term cigarette smokers and persons with Barrett esophagus, severe epithelial dysplasia frequently antedates the appearance of cancer. Moreover, some mutations associated with full blown cancers (described later) may be present in even "mild" dysplasias. Thus, although **dysplasia may be a precursor to malignant transformation, it does not always progress to cancer**. With removal of the inciting causes, mild to moderate dysplasias that do not involve the entire thickness of epithelium may be completely reversible. Even carcinoma in situ may persist for years before it becomes invasive. Finally, while it should be noted that dysplasia often occurs in metaplastic epithelium, not all metaplastic epithelium is dysplastic.

Local Invasion

The growth of cancers is accompanied by progressive infiltration, invasion, and destruction of the surrounding tissue, whereas nearly all benign tumors grow as cohesive expansile masses that remain localized to their site of origin and lack the capacity to infiltrate, invade, or metastasize to distant sites. Because benign tumors grow and expand slowly, they usually develop a rim of compressed fibrous tissue called a *capsule* that separates them from the host tissue. This capsule consists largely of extracellular matrix deposited by stromal cells such as fibroblasts, which are activated by hypoxic damage resulting from the pressure of the expanding tumor. Such encapsulation does not prevent tumor growth, but it creates a tissue plane that makes the tumor discrete, readily palpable, moveable (non-fixed), and easily excisable by surgical enucleation (Figs. 7-11 and 7-12). There are a few exceptions to this rule, however. For example, hemangiomas (neoplasms composed of tangled blood vessels) are often unencapsulated and permeate the site in which they arise (e.g., the dermis of the skin and the liver); when such lesions are extensive, they may be unresectable.

In contrast, malignant tumors are, in general, poorly demarcated from the surrounding normal tissue, and a well-defined cleavage plane is lacking (Figs. 7-13 and 7-14). Slowly expanding malignant tumors, however, may develop an apparently enclosing fibrous capsule and may push along a broad front into adjacent normal structures. Histologic examination of such "pseudoencapsulated" masses almost always shows rows of cells penetrating the margin and infiltrating the adjacent structures, a crablike pattern of growth that constitutes the popular image of cancer.

Next to the development of metastases, invasiveness is the most reliable feature that differentiates cancers from benign tumors. Most malignant tumors do not recognize normal anatomic boundaries and can be expected to penetrate the wall of the colon or uterus, for example, or fungate through the surface of the skin. Such invasiveness makes their surgical resection difficult or impossible, and even if the tumor appears well circumscribed it is

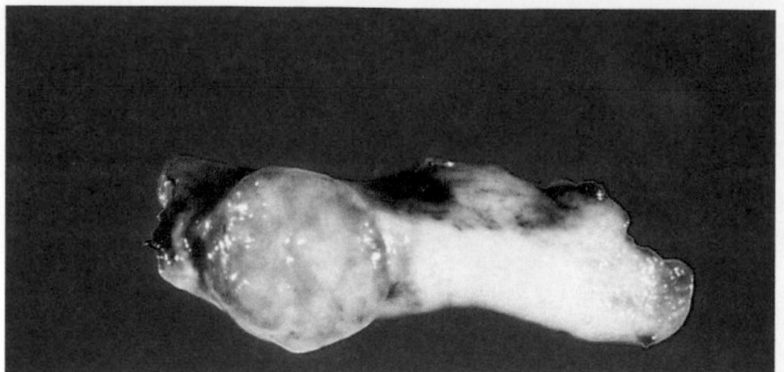

Figure 7-11 Fibroadenoma of the breast. The tan-colored, encapsulated small tumor is sharply demarcated from the whiter breast tissue.

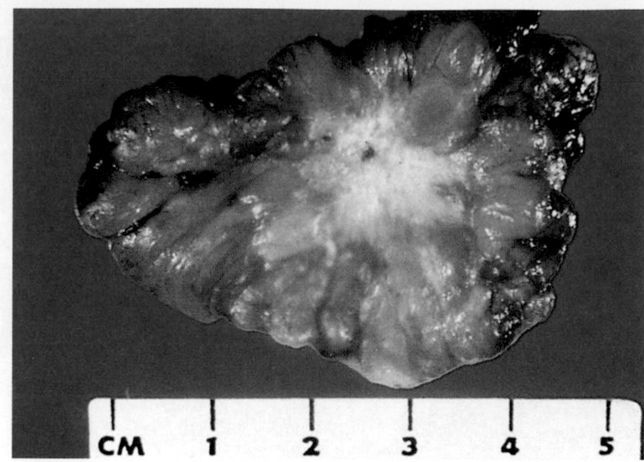

Figure 7-13 Cut section of an invasive ductal carcinoma of the breast. The lesion is retracted, infiltrating the surrounding breast substance, and would be stony hard on palpation. (Courtesy Dr. Trace Worrell, University of Texas Southwestern Medical School, Dallas, Texas.)

necessary to remove a considerable margin of apparently normal tissues adjacent to the infiltrative neoplasm in order to ensure complete local excision. As noted earlier, some cancers seem to evolve from a preinvasive stage referred to as *carcinoma in situ.* This commonly occurs in carcinomas of the skin, breast, and certain other sites and is best illustrated by carcinoma of the uterine cervix (Chapter 21). In situ epithelial cancers display the cytologic features of malignancy without invasion of the basement membrane. They may be considered one step removed from invasive cancer; with time, most penetrate the basement membrane and invade the subepithelial stroma.

Metastasis

Metastasis is defined by the spread of a tumor to sites that are physically discontinuous with the primary tumor, and unequivocally marks a tumor as malignant, as by definition benign neoplasms do not metastasize. The invasiveness of cancers permits them to penetrate into blood vessels, lymphatics, and body cavities, providing the opportunity for spread. All malignant tumors can metastasize, but some do so very infrequently. Examples include malignant neoplasms of the glial cells in the central nervous system, called *gliomas,* and basal cell carcinomas of the skin. Both of these cancers invade early in their course, but rarely metastasize. It is evident then that the properties of invasion and metastasis are separable.

In general, the likelihood of a primary tumor metastasizing correlates with lack of differentiation, aggressive local invasion, rapid growth, and large size. There are innumerable exceptions, however. Small, well-differentiated, slowly growing lesions sometimes metastasize widely; conversely, some rapidly growing, large lesions remain localized for years. Many factors relating to both invader and host are involved.

Approximately 30% of newly diagnosed solid tumors (excluding skin cancers other than melanomas) present with metastases. Metastatic spread strongly reduces the possibility of cure; hence, short of prevention of cancer, no achievement would be of greater benefit to patients than an effective means to block metastasis, with the important caveat that many tumors destined to kill the patient have already spread at the time of initial diagnosis. Blood cancers (the leukemias and lymphomas, sometimes called

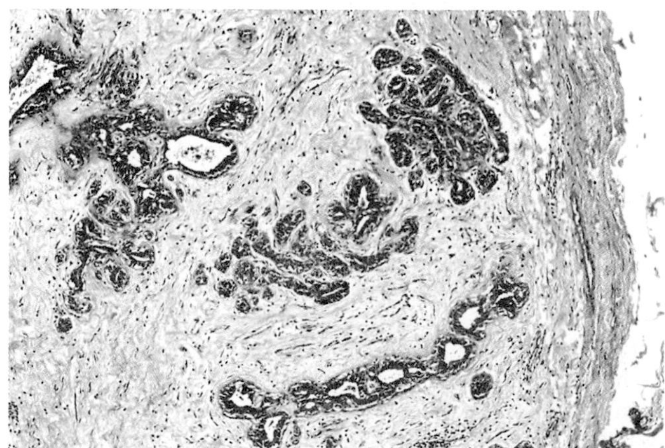

Figure 7-12 Microscopic view of fibroadenoma of the breast seen in Figure 7-11. The fibrous capsule *(right)* delimits the tumor from the surrounding tissue. (Courtesy Dr. Trace Worrell, University of Texas Southwestern Medical School, Dallas, Texas.)

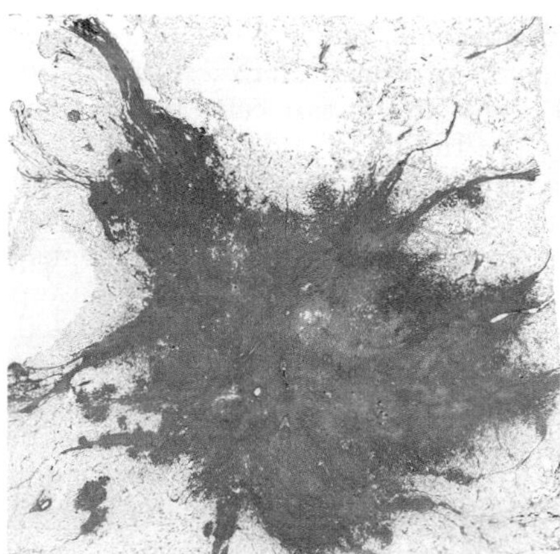

Figure 7-14 Low power microscopic view of invasive breast cancer. Note the irregular infiltrative borders without a well-defined capsule and intense stromal reaction. (Courtesy Dr. Susan Lester, Brigham and Women's Hospital, Boston, Mass.)

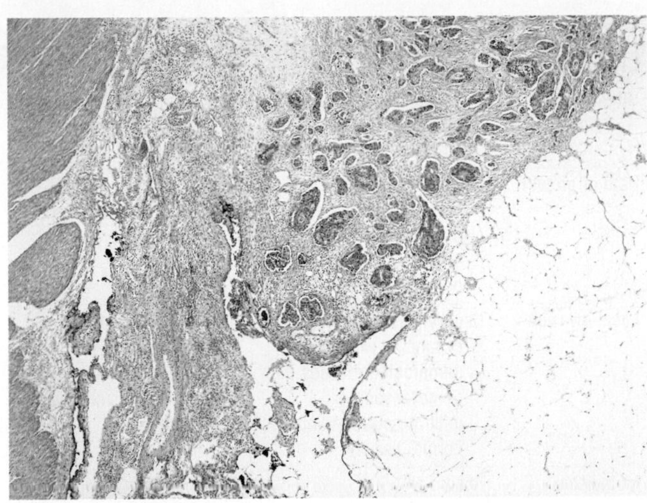

Figure 7-15 Colon carcinoma invading pericolonic adipose tissue. (Courtesy Dr. Shuji Ogino, Dana Farber Cancer Institute, Boston, Mass.)

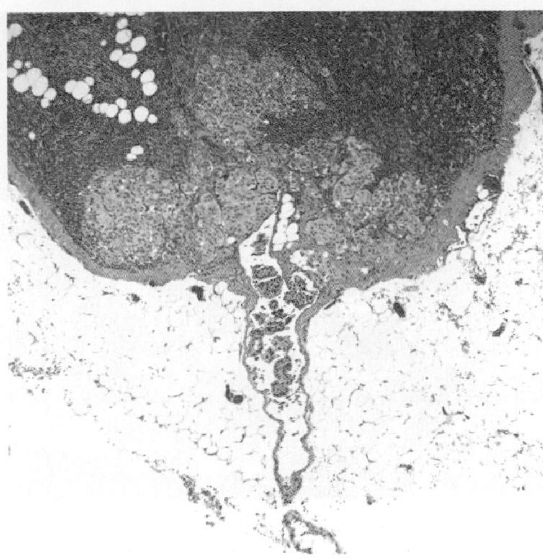

Figure 7-16 Axillary lymph node with metastatic breast carcinoma. Note the aggregates of tumor cells within the substance of the node and the dilated lymphatic channel. (Courtesy Dr. Susan Lester, Brigham and Women's Hospital, Boston, Mass.)

liquid tumors) are derived from blood-forming cells that normally have the capacity to enter the bloodstream and travel to distant sites; as a result, leukemias and lymphomas are often disseminated at diagnosis and are always taken to be malignant.

Pathways of Spread

Dissemination of cancers may occur through one of three pathways: (1) direct seeding of body cavities or surfaces, (2) lymphatic spread, and (3) hematogenous spread. Although iatrogenic spread of tumor cells on surgical instruments may occur—it is the reason, for example, why biopsies of testicular masses are never done—it is generally rare and not discussed further.

Seeding of Body Cavities and Surfaces. Seeding of body cavities and surfaces may occur whenever a malignant neoplasm penetrates into a natural "open field" lacking physical barriers. Most often involved is the peritoneal cavity (Fig. 7-15), but any other cavity—pleural, pericardial, subarachnoid, and joint spaces—may be affected. Such seeding is particularly characteristic of carcinomas arising in the ovaries, which, not infrequently, spread to peritoneal surfaces, which become coated with a heavy cancerous glaze. Remarkably, the tumor cells may remain confined to the surface of the abdominal viscera without penetrating into the substance. Sometimes mucus-secreting appendiceal carcinomas or ovarian carcinomas fill the peritoneal cavity with a gelatinous neoplastic mass referred to as *pseudomyxoma peritonei.*

Lymphatic Spread. **Transport through lymphatics is the most common pathway for the initial dissemination of carcinomas** (Fig. 7-16). Sarcomas may also use this route. Tumors do not contain functional lymphatics, but lymphatic vessels located at the tumor margins are apparently sufficient for the lymphatic spread of tumor cells. The emphasis on lymphatic spread for carcinomas and hematogenous spread for sarcomas is misleading, because ultimately there are numerous interconnections between the vascular and the lymphatic systems. The pattern of lymph node involvement follows the natural routes of lymphatic drainage. Because carcinomas of the breast usually arise in the upper outer quadrants, they generally disseminate first to the axillary lymph nodes. Cancers of the inner quadrants drain to the nodes along the internal mammary arteries. Thereafter, the infraclavicular and supraclavicular nodes may become involved. Carcinomas of the lung arising in the major respiratory passages metastasize first to the perihilar tracheobronchial and mediastinal nodes. Local lymph nodes, however, may be bypassed—so-called skip metastasis—because of venous-lymphatic anastomoses or because inflammation or radiation has obliterated lymphatic channels.

In breast cancer, determining the involvement of axillary lymph nodes is important for assessing the future course of the disease and for selecting suitable therapeutic strategies. To avoid the considerable surgical morbidity associated with a full axillary lymph node dissection, *biopsy of sentinel nodes* is often used to assess the presence or absence of metastatic lesions in the lymph nodes. **A sentinel lymph node is defined as "the first node in a regional lymphatic basin that receives lymph flow from the primary tumor."** Sentinel node mapping can be done by injection of radiolabeled tracers or colored dyes, and examination of frozen sections of the sentinel lymph node performed during surgery can guide the surgeon to the appropriate therapy. Sentinel node examination has also been used for detecting the spread of melanomas, colon cancers, and other tumors.

In many cases, the regional nodes serve as effective barriers to further dissemination of the tumor, at least for a while. Conceivably, after arrest within the node the cells may be destroyed by a tumor-specific immune response. Drainage of tumor cell debris or tumor antigens, or both, also induces reactive changes within nodes. Thus, enlargement of nodes may be caused by the spread and growth of cancer cells or reactive hyperplasia (Chapter 13). Therefore, nodal enlargement in proximity to a cancer, while it must arouse suspicion, does not necessarily equate with dissemination of the primary lesion.

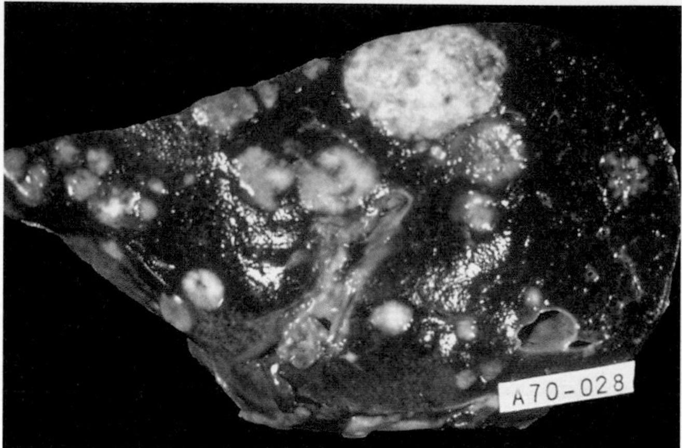

Figure 7-17 A liver studded with metastatic cancer.

Table 7-2 Comparisons Between Benign and Malignant Tumors

Characteristics	Benign	Malignant
Differentiation/ anaplasia	Well differentiated; structure sometimes typical of tissue of origin	Some lack of differentiation (anaplasia); structure often atypical
Rate of growth	Usually progressive and slow; may come to a standstill or regress; mitotic figures rare and normal	Erratic, may be slow to rapid; mitotic figures may be numerous and abnormal
Local invasion	Usually cohesive, expansile, well-demarcated masses that do not invade or infiltrate surrounding normal tissues	Locally invasive, infiltrating surrounding tissue; sometimes may be misleadingly cohesive and expansile
Metastasis	Absent	Frequent; more likely with large undifferentiated primary tumors

Hematogenous Spread. Hematogenous spread is typical of sarcomas but is also seen with carcinomas. Arteries, with their thicker walls, are less readily penetrated than are veins. Arterial spread may occur, however, when tumor cells pass through the pulmonary capillary beds or pulmonary arteriovenous shunts or when pulmonary metastases themselves give rise to additional tumor emboli. In such vascular spread, several factors influence the patterns of distribution of the metastases. With venous invasion, the bloodborne cells follow the venous flow draining the site of the neoplasm, and the tumor cells often come to rest in the first capillary bed they encounter. Understandably the liver (Fig. 7-17) and the lungs (Fig. 7-18) are most frequently involved in such hematogenous dissemination, because all portal area drainage flows to the liver and all caval blood flows to the lungs. Cancers arising in close proximity to the vertebral column often embolize through the paravertebral plexus, and this pathway is involved in the frequent vertebral metastases of carcinomas of the thyroid and prostate.

Certain cancers have a propensity for invasion of veins. Renal cell carcinoma often invades the branches of the renal vein and then the renal vein itself, from where it may grow in a snakelike fashion up the inferior vena cava, sometimes reaching the right side of the heart. Hepatocellular carcinomas often penetrate portal and hepatic radicles to grow within them into the main venous channels. Remarkably, such intravenous growth may not be accompanied by widespread dissemination. Histologic evidence of penetration of small vessels at the site of the primary neoplasm is obviously an ominous feature.

Many observations suggest that mere anatomic localization of the neoplasm and natural pathways of venous drainage do not wholly explain the systemic distributions of metastases. For example, breast carcinoma preferentially spreads to bone, bronchogenic carcinomas tend to involve the adrenals and the brain, and neuroblastomas spread to the liver and bones. Conversely, skeletal muscles and the spleen, despite receiving a high percentage of the cardiac output and having large vascular beds, are rarely the site of secondary deposits. The probable basis of such tissue-specific homing of tumor cells is discussed later.

The distinguishing features of benign and malignant tumors are summarized in Table 7-2 and Figure 7-19. Having completed our overview of the morphology and behavior of neoplasms, we now discuss the pathogenesis of neoplasia, starting with clues gleaned from studies of the epidemiology of cancer.

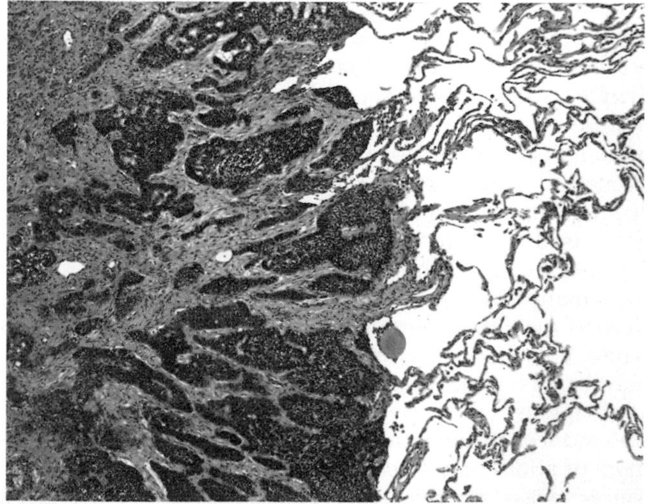

Figure 7-18 Microscopic view of lung metastasis. A colonic adenocarcinoma has formed a metastatic nodule in the lung. (Courtesy Dr. Shuji Ogino, Dana Farber Cancer Institute, Boston, Mass.)

KEY CONCEPTS

Characteristics of Benign and Malignant Neoplasms

- Benign and malignant tumors can be distinguished from one another based on the degree of differentiation, rate of growth, local invasiveness, and distant spread.
- Benign tumors resemble the tissue of origin and are well differentiated; malignant tumors are less well differentiated or completely undifferentiated (anaplastic).
- Benign tumors are more likely to retain functions of their cells of origin, whereas malignant tumors sometimes acquire unexpected functions due to derangements in differentiation.

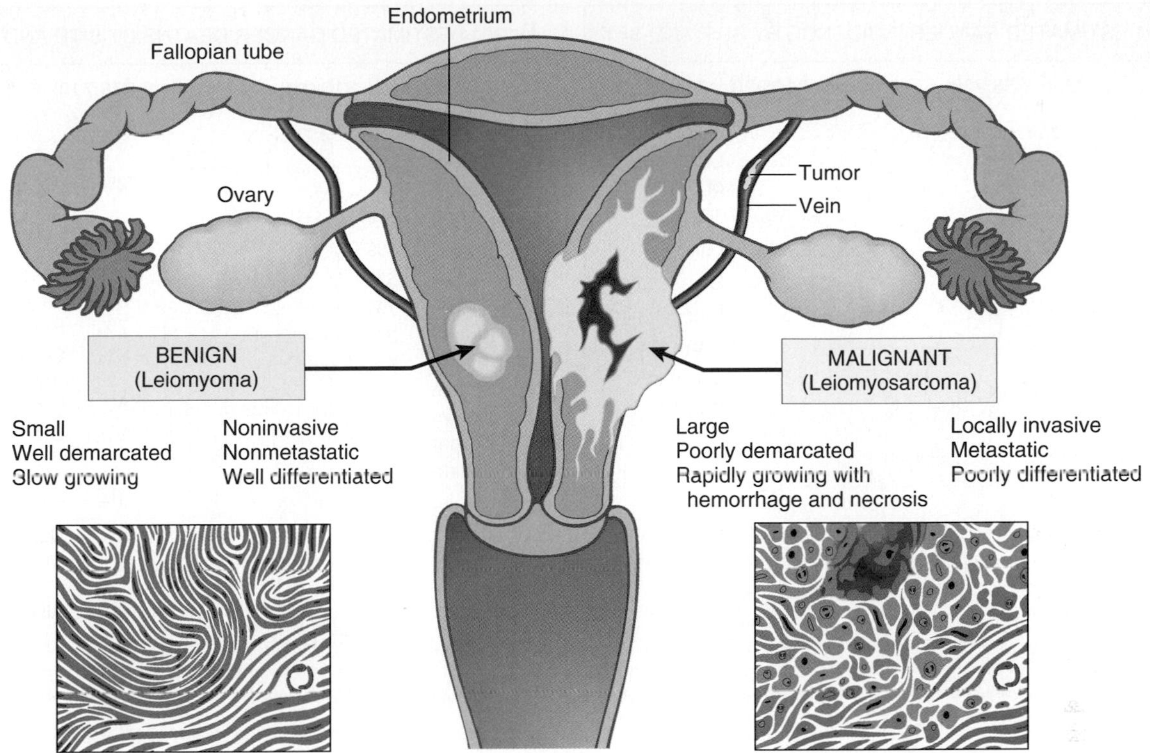

Figure 7-19 Comparison between a benign tumor of the myometrium (leiomyoma) and a malignant tumor of the same origin (leiomyosarcoma).

- Benign tumors are slow growing, while malignant tumors generally grow faster.
- Benign tumors are circumscribed and have a capsule; malignant tumors are poorly circumscribed and invade surrounding normal tissues.
- Benign tumors remain localized at the site of origin, whereas malignant tumors metastasize to distant sites.

Epidemiology of Cancer

Study of cancer patterns in populations has contributed substantially to knowledge about its origins. Epidemiologic studies have established the causative link between smoking and lung cancer, and comparison of diet and cancer rates in the Western world and the developing world has implicated high dietary fat and low fiber in the development of colon cancer. Major insights into the causes of cancer can be obtained by epidemiologic studies that relate particular environmental, racial (possibly hereditary), and cultural influences to the occurrence of specific neoplasms. Certain diseases associated with an increased risk of developing cancer also provide clues to the pathogenesis of cancer. In the following sections, we discuss the overall incidence of cancer and then review factors relating to the patient and the environment that influence the predisposition to cancer.

The Global Impact of Cancer

In 2008, it was estimated that there were about 12.7 million new cancer cases worldwide, leading to 7.6 million deaths (21,000 deaths per day). Due to increasing population size and age, by 2030 it is projected that the number of cancer cases and cancer-related deaths worldwide will increase to 21.4 million and 13.2 million, respectively. Cancer is ubiquitous in human populations; the only certain way to avoid cancer is to not be born, as to live is to incur risk. However, there is remarkable geographic variation in the incidence of specific cancers that is believed to stem mainly from differences in exposure to environmental carcinogens (discussed later), suggesting that many (and perhaps even most) cancers are preventable. The major organ sites affected and the estimated frequency of cancer deaths in the United States are shown in Figure 7-20. The most common tumors in men arise in the prostate, lung, and colon/rectum. In women, cancers of the breast, lung, and colon/rectum are the most frequent. Cancers of the lung, female breast, prostate, and colon/rectum constitute more than 50% of cancer diagnoses and cancer deaths in the United States. In contrast, in the developing world the most common cancers involve the lung, stomach, and liver in men and the breast, cervix, and lung in women.

Most longitudinal data pertaining to cancer incidence comes from developed countries. Age-adjusted death rates (deaths per 100,000 population) for many cancers have changed significantly over the years in the United States. In the last 50 years of the twentieth century, the overall age-adjusted cancer death rate increased significantly in both men and women. However, in men the cancer incidence rate has been stable since 1995 and the cancer death rate has decreased 18.4% since 1990. Similarly, in women the cancer incidence rate also stabilized in 1995 and the cancer death rate has decreased 10.4% since 1991. Among men, nearly 80% of the decrease is accounted for by lower

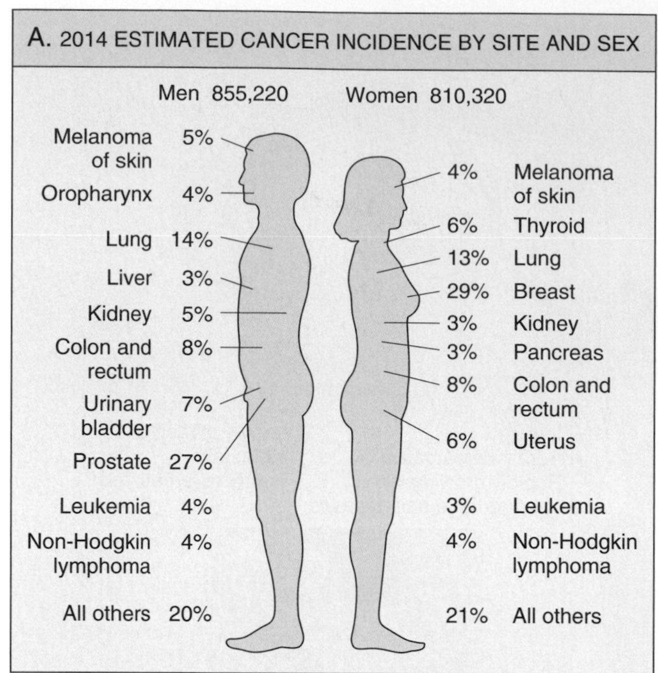

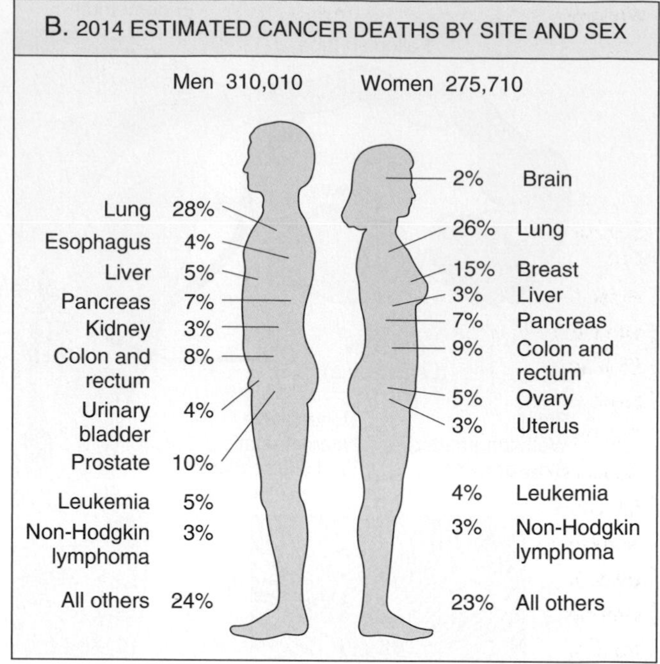

Figure 7-20 Cancer incidence **(A)** and mortality **(B)** by site and sex. Excludes basal cell and squamous cell skin cancers and in situ carcinomas, except urinary bladder. (Adapted from American Cancer Society. Cancer Statistics 2011.)

death rates from lung, prostate, and colorectal cancers; among women, nearly 60% of the decrease is due to reductions in death rates from breast and colorectal cancers. Decreased use of tobacco products is responsible for the reduction in lung cancer deaths, while improved detection and treatment are responsible for the decrease in death rates for colorectal, female breast, and prostate cancer.

The last half-century has also seen a sharp decline in the number of deaths caused by cervical cancer in the United States, which is attributable to the Papanicolaou (Pap) smear test, which enables detection of precursor lesions and early, curable cancers. A downward trend in deaths from stomach cancer in both sexes has been observed that is attributed to a reduction in unknown dietary carcinogens. However, between 1990-1991 and 2004, lung cancer death rates in women, and liver and intrahepatic bile duct cancer death rates in men, increased substantially, offsetting some of the improvement in survival from other cancers. Indeed, although carcinomas of the breast occur about 2.5 times more frequently than those of the lung in women, lung cancer now causes more deaths in women. Deaths due to primary liver cancers, which declined between 1930 and 1970, have approximately doubled over the past 40 years. This number is expected to increase further over the coming decades as a large number of individuals infected with the hepatitis C virus (HCV) begin to develop hepatocellular carcinoma.

Although race is not a clearly defined biological variable, it can define groups at risk for certain cancers. The disparity in cancer mortality rates between white and black Americans persists, but African Americans had the largest decline in cancer mortality during the past decade. Hispanics living in the United States have a lower frequency of the most common tumors seen in the white non-Hispanic population but a higher incidence of tumors of the stomach, liver, uterine cervix, and gallbladder, as well as certain leukemias.

Environmental Factors

Although both genetic and environmental factors contribute to the development of cancer, environmental influences appear to be the dominant risk factors for most cancers. Evidence supporting a central role for environmental factors can be found in the wide geographic variation that exists in the incidence of specific forms of cancer (Fig. 7-21). For example, the most common tumor of men in the United States and most of the developed world is prostate cancer, but in certain countries or regions (most located in the developing world), cancers of the liver, stomach, esophagus, bladder, lung, oropharynx, and the immune system rise to the top of the list. Similarly, the incidence of breast cancer is generally much higher in women in developed countries than in most parts of the developing world. Although racial predispositions cannot be ruled out, it is believed that environmental influences—some known, some not—underlie most of these differences in cancer incidence.

Among the best established environmental factors affecting cancer risk are the following:

- **Infectious agents**. About 15% of all cancers worldwide are believed to be caused directly or indirectly by infectious agents, with the burden of cancers linked to infections being roughly three times higher in the developing world than in the developed world. For example, *human papilloma virus* (HPV), an agent that is spread through sexual contact, is responsible for a large majority of cases of cervical carcinoma and an increasing fraction of head and neck cancers. Specific infectious agents and their associated cancers are discussed later in this chapter.
- **Smoking**. Cigarette smoking has been called the single most important environmental factor contributing to premature death in the United States. Smoking,

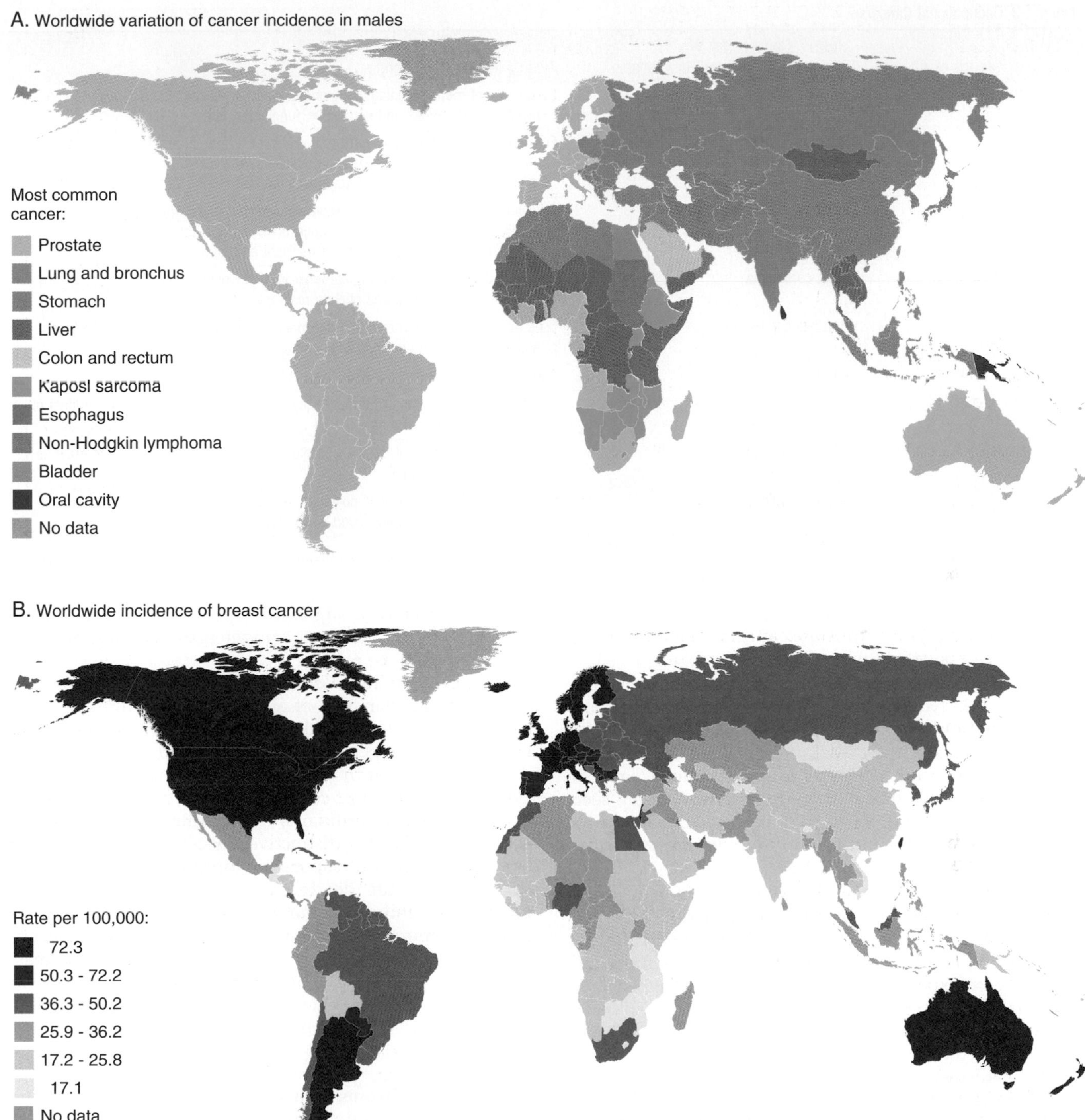

Figure 7-21 Geographic variation in cancer incidence. **A,** Most common cancers in males by country. **B,** Variation in breast cancer incidence in women by country. (Adapted from Global Cancer Facts & Figures, 2nd ed. Atlanta, American Cancer Society, 2011.)

particularly of cigarettes, has been implicated in cancer of the mouth, pharynx, larynx, esophagus, pancreas, bladder, and most significantly, about 90% of lung cancer deaths (Chapter 9).

- **Alcohol consumption**. Alcohol abuse alone increases the risk of carcinomas of the oropharynx (excluding lip), larynx, and esophagus and, by the development of alcoholic cirrhosis, hepatocellular carcinoma. Alcohol and tobacco together synergistically increase the risk of cancers in the upper airways and digestive tract.
- **Diet**. Although the precise dietary factors that affect cancer risk remain a matter of debate, wide geographic variation in the incidences of colorectal carcinoma, prostate carcinoma, and breast carcinoma has been ascribed to differences in diet.
- **Obesity**. Given that there is an obesity epidemic in the United States that is spreading to other parts of the world (Chapter 9), it is concerning that weight is strongly associated with cancer risk. Overall, the most overweight individuals in the U.S. population have 52% (men) to 62% (women) higher death rates from cancer

Table 7-3 Occupational Cancers

Agents or Groups of Agents	Human Cancers for Which Reasonable Evidence Is Available	Typical Use or Occurrence
Arsenic and arsenic compounds	Lung carcinoma, skin carcinoma	By-product of metal smelting; component of alloys, electrical and semiconductor devices, medications and herbicides, fungicides, and animal dips
Asbestos	Lung, esophageal, gastric, and colon carcinoma; mesothelioma	Formerly used for many applications because of fire, heat, and friction resistance; still found in existing construction as well as fire-resistant textiles, friction materials (i.e., brake linings), underlayment and roofing papers, and floor tiles
Benzene	Acute myeloid leukemia	Principal component of light oil; despite known risk, many applications exist in printing and lithography, paint, rubber, dry cleaning, adhesives and coatings, and detergents; formerly widely used as solvent and fumigant
Beryllium and beryllium compounds	Lung carcinoma	Missile fuel and space vehicles; hardener for lightweight metal alloys, particularly in aerospace applications and nuclear reactors
Cadmium and cadmium compounds	Prostate carcinoma	Uses include yellow pigments and phosphors; found in solders; used in batteries and as alloy and in metal platings and coatings
Chromium compounds	Lung carcinoma	Component of metal alloys, paints, pigments, and preservatives
Nickel compounds	Lung and oropharyngeal carcinoma	Nickel plating; component of ferrous alloys, ceramics, and batteries; by-product of stainless-steel arc welding
Radon and its decay products	Lung carcinoma	From decay of minerals containing uranium; potentially serious hazard in quarries and underground mines
Vinyl chloride	Hepatic angiosarcoma	Refrigerant; monomer for vinyl polymers; adhesive for plastics; formerly inert aerosol propellant in pressurized containers

Modified from Stellman JM, Stellman SD: Cancer and workplace. CA Cancer J Clin 1996;46:70.

than do their slimmer counterparts; it follows that approximately 14% of cancer deaths in men and 20% in women can be attributed to obesity.

- **Reproductive history**. There is strong evidence that lifelong cumulative exposure to estrogen stimulation, particularly if unopposed by progesterone, increases the risk of cancers of the breast and endometrium, tissues that are responsive to these hormones. Indeed, some of the differences in breast cancer incidence that are seen across the world are believed be related to cultural mores that affect the timing and number of pregnancies a woman has during her lifetime.
- **Environmental carcinogens**. There is no paucity of well-characterized environmental carcinogens: they lurk in the ambient environment, in the workplace (Table 7-3), in food, and in personal practices. Individuals may be exposed to carcinogenic factors when they go outside (e.g., ultraviolet [UV] rays, smog), drink well water (e.g., arsenic, particularly in Bangladesh), take certain medications (e.g., methotrexate), go to work (e.g., asbestos), or even while lounging at home (e.g., grilled meat, high-fat diet, alcohol).

It appears that almost everything one does to earn a livelihood or for pleasure is fattening, immoral, illegal, or, even worse, carcinogenic!

Age

Age has an important influence on the likelihood of being afflicted with cancer. Most carcinomas occur in the later years of life (>55 years). Cancer is the main cause of death among women aged 40 to 79 and among men aged 60 to 79; the decline in deaths after age 80 is due to the lower number of individuals who reach this age. The rising incidence of cancer with age is likely explained by the accumulation of somatic mutations associated with the emergence of malignant neoplasms (discussed later). The decline in immune competence that accompanies aging may also be a factor.

Tragically, children are not spared; cancer accounts for slightly more than 10% of all deaths in children younger than age 15 in the United States, second only to accidents. However, the types of cancers that predominate in children are significantly different from those seen in adults. Carcinomas, the most common general category of tumor in adults, are extraordinarily rare among children. Instead, acute leukemia and distinctive neoplasms of the central nervous system are responsible for approximately 60% of childhood cancer deaths. The common neoplasms of infancy and childhood include the so-called small round blue cell tumors such as neuroblastoma, Wilms tumor, retinoblastoma, acute leukemias, and rhabdomyosarcomas. These are discussed in Chapter 10 and elsewhere in the text.

Acquired Predisposing Conditions

Acquired conditions that predispose to cancer can be divided into chronic inflammations, precursor lesions, and immunodeficiency states. Chronic inflammatory disorders and precursor lesions span a diverse set of conditions that are all associated with increased cellular replication, which appears to create a "fertile" soil for the development of malignant tumors. Indeed, repeated rounds of cell division may be required for neoplastic transformation, in that proliferating cells are the most at risk for accumulating the genetic lesions that lead to carcinogenesis. Tumors arising in the context of chronic inflammation are mostly carcinomas, but also include mesothelioma and several kinds of lymphoma. Immunodeficiency states predispose to virus-induced cancers. Each of these acquired predisposing conditions is described next.

Table 7-4 Chronic Inflammatory States and Cancer

Pathologic Condition	Associated Neoplasm(s)	Etiologic Agent
Asbestosis, silicosis	Mesothelioma, lung carcinoma	Asbestos fibers, silica particles
Inflammatory bowel disease	Colorectal carcinoma	
Lichen sclerosis	Vulvar squamous cell carcinoma	
Pancreatitis	Pancreatic carcinoma	Alcoholism, germline mutations (e.g., in the trypsinogen gene)
Chronic cholecystitis	Gallbladder cancer	Bile acids, bacteria, gallbladder stones
Reflux esophagitis, Barrett esophagus	Esophageal carcinoma	Gastric acid
Sjögren syndrome, Hashimoto thyroiditis	MALT lymphoma	
Opisthorchis, cholangitis	Cholangiocarcinoma, colon carcinoma	Liver flukes (*Opisthorchis viverrini*)
Gastritis/ulcers	Gastric adenocarcinoma, MALT lymphoma	*Helicobacter pylori*
Hepatitis	Hepatocellular carcinoma	Hepatitis B and/or C virus
Osteomyelitis	Carcinoma in draining sinuses	Bacterial infection
Chronic cervicitis	Cervical carcinoma	Human papillomavirus
Chronic cystitis	Bladder carcinoma	Schistosomiasis

Adapted from Tlsty TD, Coussens LM: Tumor stroma and regulation of cancer development. Ann Rev Pathol Mech Dis 2006;1:119.

Precursor lesions can be defined as localized morphologic changes that are associated with a high risk of cancer. Virtually all precursor lesions arise in epithelial surfaces and are associated with an increased risk of various forms of carcinoma.

- ***Chronic inflammation and cancer.*** A cause-and-effect relationship between chronic inflammation and cancer was first proposed by Virchow in 1863, and it is now appreciated that cancer risk is increased in individuals affected by a variety of chronic inflammatory diseases, including those with infectious and noninfectious etiologies (Table 7-4). As with any cause of tissue injury, each of these disorders is accompanied by a compensatory proliferation of cells that serves to repair the damage. In some cases, chronic inflammation may increase the pool of tissue stem cells, which may be particularly susceptible to transformation. Additionally the activated immune cells produce reactive oxygen species that are directly genotoxic. as well as inflammatory mediators that may promote bystander cell survival, even in the face of genomic damage. Chronic epithelial injury often leads to metaplasia, the replacement of one cell type with a second that is better able to survive the ongoing insult. In the short term, these changes can be adaptive; the organism must survive, and the damaged cells can be repaired or eliminated later. However, over longer time periods (years to decades) such alterations may allow cells with potentially oncogenic mutations to survive, eventually leading to cancer. Whatever the precise mechanism, the link between chronic inflammation and cancer has practical implications. For instance, diagnosis and effective treatment of *Helicobacter pylori* gastritis with antibiotics can quell a chronic inflammatory condition that might otherwise lead to the development of a gastric cancer.
- ***Precursor lesions and cancer.*** As mentioned, the term *precursor lesion* encompasses several entities that are associated with increased cancer risk. Precursor lesions do not inevitably progress to cancer; nevertheless, they are important to recognize because some precursor lesions can be detected by screening procedures and treated, thereby reducing the risk of developing cancer.

  Many precursor lesions arise in the setting of chronic inflammation and can be recognized by the presence of metaplasia: examples include *Barrett esophagus* (gastric and colonic metaplasia of the esophageal mucosa in the setting of gastric reflux); *squamous metaplasia* of the bronchial mucosa (in response to smoking) and the bladder mucosa (in response to schistosomiasis infection); and *colonic metaplasia* of the stomach (in the setting of pernicious anemia and chronic atrophic gastritis). Other precursor lesions are noninflammatory hyperplasias. One of the most common precursor lesions of this type is *endometrial hyperplasia*, which is caused by sustained estrogenic stimulation of the endometrium. Another relatively frequent precursor lesion is *leukoplakia*, a thickening of squamous epithelium that may occur in the oral cavity or on the penis or vulva and give rise to squamous carcinoma.

  The final group of precursor lesions is benign neoplasms that are at risk for malignant transformation. The classic example of a neoplastic precursor lesion is the colonic *villous adenoma*, which if left untreated progresses to cancer in about 50% of cases. It should be emphasized, however, that most benign tumors transform rarely (e.g., uterine leiomyomas, pleomorphic adenoma) and others not at all (e.g., lipomas). Why many benign tumors have a negligible risk of malignant transformation is an unsettled question; one possibility is that benign tumors at high risk for malignant transformation possess the cancer-enabling property of genomic instability (discussed later), whereas truly benign tumors do not.
- ***Immunodeficiency states and cancer.*** Patients who are immunodeficient, and particularly those who have deficits in T-cell immunity, are at increased risk for cancers, especially those caused by oncogenic viruses. These virally associated tumors include mainly lymphomas, but also certain carcinomas and even some sarcomas and sarcoma-like proliferations. The complex relationship between infections, immunity, and cancer are discussed later in this chapter.

Genetic Predisposition and Interactions Between Environmental and Inherited Factors

In some families cancer is an inherited trait, usually due to germline mutations in a tumor suppressor gene (described later). What then can be said about the influence of heredity on sporadic malignant neoplasms, which constitute roughly 95% of cancers in the United States? While the evidence suggests that these cancers are largely attributable to environmental factors or acquired predisposing conditions, lack of family history does not preclude an inherited component. It is generally difficult to sort out the hereditary and nonhereditary contributions because these factors often interact. The interaction between genetic and nongenetic factors is particularly complex when tumor development depends on the action of multiple contributory genes. Even in tumors with a well-defined inherited component, the risk of developing the tumor can be greatly influenced by nongenetic factors. For instance, breast cancer risk in females who inherit mutated copies of the *BRCA1* or *BRCA2* tumor suppressor genes (discussed later) is almost threefold higher for women born after 1940 than for women born before that year, perhaps because of changes in reproductive history. Furthermore, genetic factors can significantly influence the likelihood of developing environmentally induced cancers. Inherited variations (polymorphisms) of enzymes that metabolize procarcinogens to their active carcinogenic forms can influence cancer susceptibility. Of interest in this regard are genes that encode the cytochrome P-450 enzymes. As discussed later, a polymorphism in one of the P-450 loci confers an inherited susceptibility to lung cancers in cigarette smokers. More associations of this type are likely to be found.

KEY CONCEPTS

Epidemiology of Cancer

- The incidence of cancer varies with geography, age, race, and genetic background. Cancers are most common in adults older than 60 years of age, but occurs in adults at all ages and in children and infants. The geographic variation is thought to mainly stem from different environmental exposures.
- Important environmental factors implicated in carcinogenesis include infectious agents, smoking, alcohol, diet, obesity, reproductive history, and exposure to environmental carcinogens.
- The risk of cancer is increased by reparative proliferations caused by chronic inflammation or tissue injury, certain forms of hyperplasia, and immunodeficiency.
- Interactions between environmental factors and genetic factors may be important determinants of cancer risk.

Molecular Basis of Cancer: Role of Genetic and Epigenetic Alterations

Evidence for the genetic origins of cancer have been building up for over several decades. However, a full accounting of the extent of these genetic aberrations is only now coming to light, made possible by technologic advances in DNA sequencing and other methods that permit genome-wide analysis of cancer cells. The complexity of these data is daunting and the messages hidden within them have yet to be fully decoded, but certain "genomic themes" have emerged that are likely relevant to every cancer.

- **Nonlethal genetic damage lies at the heart of carcinogenesis.** The initial damage (or mutation) may be caused by environmental exposures, may be inherited in the germline, or may be spontaneous and random, falling into the category of "bad luck." The term environmental, used in this context, refers to any acquired mutation caused by exogenous agents, such as viruses or environmental chemicals, or by endogenous products of cellular metabolism.
- **A tumor is formed by the clonal expansion of a single precursor cell that has incurred genetic damage (i.e., tumors are clonal).** Alterations in DNA are heritable, being passed to daughter cells, and thus all cells within an individual tumor share the same set of mutations that were present at the moment of transformation. Such tumor-specific mutations are most often identified by DNA sequencing (e.g., point mutations) or by chromosomal analyses (e.g., chromosomal translocations and copy number changes, discussed later).
- **Four classes of normal regulatory genes—the growth-promoting proto-oncogenes, the growth-inhibiting tumor suppressor genes, genes that regulate programmed cell death (apoptosis), and genes involved in DNA repair—are the principal targets of cancer-causing mutations.** Mutations that activate *proto-oncogenes* generally cause an excessive increase in one of more normal functions of the encoded gene product, or sometimes impart a completely new function on the affected gene product that is oncogenic. Because these mutations cause a "gain-of-function," they can transform cells despite the presence of a normal copy of the same gene. Thus, in genetic parlance, oncogenes are dominant over their normal counterparts. Mutations that affect *tumor suppressor genes* generally cause a "loss-of-function," and in most instances both alleles must be damaged before transformation can occur. Thus, mutated tumor suppressor genes usually behave in a recessive fashion. However, there are exceptions: sometimes loss of only a single tumor suppressor gene allele (a state termed *haploinsufficiency*) reduces the activity of the encoded protein enough to release the brakes on cell proliferation and survival. Such a finding indicates that two "doses" of the gene are essential for normal function. *Apoptosis-regulating genes* may acquire abnormalities that result in less death and, therefore, enhanced survival of the cells. These abnormalities include gain-of-function mutations in genes whose products suppress apoptosis and loss-of-function mutations in genes whose products promote cell death. Loss-of-function mutations affecting *DNA repair genes* contribute to carcinogenesis indirectly by impairing the ability of the cell to recognize and repair nonlethal genetic damage in other genes. As a result, affected cells acquire mutations at an accelerated rate, a state referred to as a *mutator phenotype* that is marked by *genomic instability.*
- **Carcinogenesis results from the accumulation of complementary mutations in a stepwise fashion over time** (Fig. 7-22).
  - **Malignant neoplasms have several phenotypic attributes referred to as *cancer hallmarks,*** such as excessive growth, local invasiveness, and the ability to form distant metastases, which stem from genomic

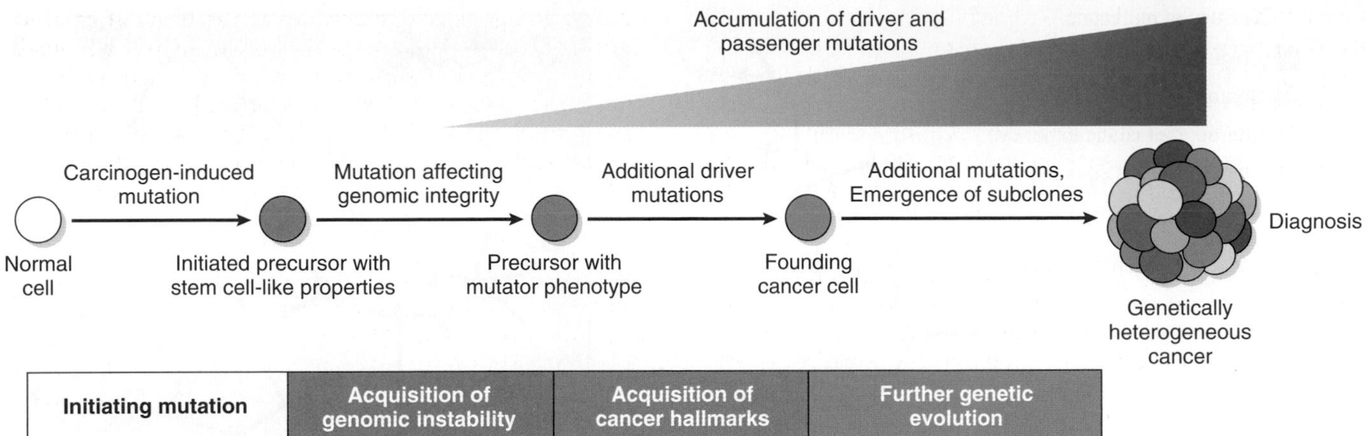

Figure 7-22 Development of a cancer through stepwise acquisition of complementary mutations. The order in which various driver mutations occur in initiated precursor cells is not known and may vary from tumor to tumor. See text for details.

alterations that change the expression and function of key genes and thereby impart a malignant phenotype.

- **Mutations that contribute to the development of the malignant phenotype are referred to as *driver mutations.*** The first driver mutation that starts a cell on the path to malignancy is the *initiating mutation,* which is typically maintained in all of the cells of the subsequent cancer. However, because no single mutation appears to be fully transforming, development of a cancer requires that the "initiated" cell acquire a number of additional driver mutations, each of which also contributes to the development of the cancer. The time over which this occurs is unknown in most cancers, but appears to be lengthy; even in aggressive cancers that clinically seem to appear "out of the blue," such as childhood acute lymphoblastic leukemia, cells bearing initiating mutations may be found in blood samples taken as long as a decade prior to diagnosis. The persistence of initiated cells during this long preclinical prodrome is consistent with the idea that cancers arise from cells with stem cell–like properties, so-called *cancer stem cells,* that have a capacity for self-renewal and long-term persistence.
- **Loss-of-function mutations in genes that maintain genomic integrity appear to be a common early step on the road to malignancy, particularly in solid tumors**. Mutations that lead to genomic instability not only increase the likelihood of acquiring driver mutations, but also greatly increase the frequency of mutations that have no phenotypic consequence, so-called *passenger mutations,* which are much more common than driver mutations. As a result, by the time a cell acquires all of the driver mutations that are needed for malignant behavior, it may bear hundreds or even thousands of acquired mutations.

Once established, tumors evolve genetically during their outgrowth and progression under the pressure of Darwinian selection (survival of the fittest). Early on, all of the cells in a tumor are genetically identical, being the progeny of a single founding transformed cell. However, by the time a tumor comes to clinical attention (generally when it attains a mass of about 1 gm, or about 10^9 cells), it has gone through a minimum of 30 cell doublings. This number is likely a substantial underestimation, because some fraction of cells in virtually all tumors die by apoptosis, and sometimes such cells are numerous. During this process, there is competition among tumor cells for access to nutrients and microenvironmental niches, and subclones with the capacity to overgrow their predecessors tend to "win" this Darwinian contest and dominate the tumor mass, only to be replaced by other, still malignant subclones. This pernicious tendency of tumors to become more aggressive over time is referred to as *tumor progression.* As a result, even though malignant tumors are clonal in origin, by the time they become clinically evident their constituent cells are often extremely heterogeneous genetically, particularly tumors with a mutator phenotype (Fig. 7-22).

A skeptical student might well ask, "How do we know that genetically distinct subclones really exist in any particular cancer?" Supportive data are now emerging from studies of solid cancers such as renal cell carcinoma, in which multiple regions of primary tumors and several different metastatic deposits have been subjected to extensive DNA sequencing (Fig. 7-23). As predicted, two types of mutations were identified in these studies: (1) mutations that were present in all tumor sites tested, which were presumably present in the founding cell at the moment of transformation, and (2) mutations that were unique to a subset of tumor sites, which were likely acquired after transformation during the outgrowth and spread of the tumor. This second type of mutation can be used to create tumor "family trees" showing the genetic relationships of various subclones. Remarkably, subclones within tumors appear to diverge genetically in a fashion that is very similar to the manner in which new species are thought to emerge in complex ecosystems; a cardinal example of the latter are the finches on the Galapagos Islands that inspired Darwin, in part, to propose evolution as the origin of the species. In the case of species, this genetic divergence occurs over a period of many millennia, whereas in tumors, subclones may arise and diverge on a timescale of years, months, or even weeks.

Selection of the fittest cells can explain not only the natural history of cancer, but also changes in tumor behavior following therapy. One of the most profound

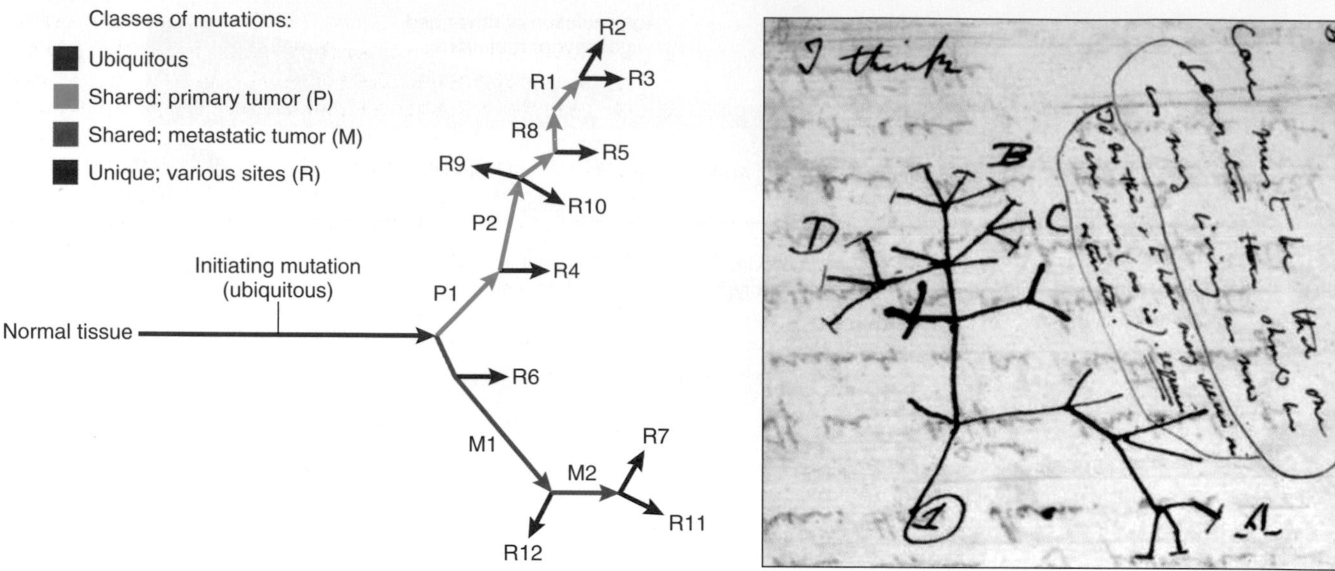

Figure 7-23 Tumor evolution. Evolution of a renal cell carcinoma *(left panel)* and Darwin's finches *(right panel)*. The renal cell carcinoma evolutionary tree is based on genetic comparisons drawn from sequencing of DNA obtained from different tumor sites; the finch evolutionary tree was surmised by Darwin based on morphologic comparisons of different species of finches on the Galapagos Islands. (*right panel*, from Notebook B: Transmutation of Species, Charles Darwin, 1837, p.26.)

selective pressures that cancer cells face is effective chemotherapy or radiotherapy given by treating physicians. Tumors that recur after therapy are almost always found to be resistant if the same treatment is given again, presumably because therapy selects for preexistent subclones that, by chance, have a genotype that allows them to survive.

It is increasingly apparent that **in addition to DNA mutations, epigenetic aberrations also contribute to the malignant properties of cancer cells.** Epigenetic modifications include DNA methylation, which tends to silence gene expression, and modifications of histones, the proteins that package DNA into chromatin, which depending on their nature may either enhance or dampen gene expression. Together, *DNA methylation* and *histone modifications* dictate which genes are expressed, which in turn determines the lineage commitment and differentiation state of both normal and neoplastic cells. Epigenetic modifications are usually passed on faithfully to daughter cells, but on occasion (just as with DNA mutations) alterations may occur that result in changes in gene expression. Aberrant DNA methylation in cancer cells is responsible for the silencing of some tumor suppressor genes, while tumor-specific changes in histone modifications may have far-ranging effects on gene expression in cancer cells (see later). The increasing awareness of the role of epigenetic alterations in cancer has revealed a new path forward for cancer treatment; unlike DNA mutations, epigenetic changes are potentially reversible by drugs that inhibit DNA- or histone-modifying factors. Thus, there is considerable interest in treating cancers with drugs that correct epigenetic abnormalities in cancer cells, with some encouraging early results.

We will return to these themes throughout the subsequent discussions, which turns to the cellular and molecular properties that underlie the malignant behavior of cancer cells.

Cellular and Molecular Hallmarks of Cancer

Over the past several decades, hundreds of genes that are mutated in cancer have been discovered. It is traditional to describe the functional consequences of these alterations one gene at a time. However, the blizzard of mutated genes emerging from the sequencing of cancer genomes has blanketed the landscape and revealed the limitations of trying to grasp the fundamental properties of cancer, gene by gene. For example, it is estimated that compilation of a reasonably complete catalog of the major genetic alterations in breast carcinoma will require whole genomic sequencing of thousands of tumors and will lead to the identification of dozens to hundreds of distinct driver mutations—and this is just one of hundreds of different kinds of cancer, some of which are substantially more genetically complex than breast carcinoma.

A much more tractable and conceptually satisfying way to think about the biology of cancer is to consider the common phenotypic properties that are imparted to cancer cells by their diverse genomic and epigenomic alterations. It appears that **all cancers display eight fundamental changes in cell physiology, which are considered the hallmarks of cancer**. These changes are illustrated in Figure 7-24 and consist of the following:

- **Self-sufficiency in growth signals**. Tumors have the capacity to proliferate without external stimuli, usually as a consequence of oncogene activation.
- **Insensitivity to growth-inhibitory signals**. Tumors may not respond to molecules that inhibit the proliferation of normal cells, usually because of inactivation of tumor suppressor genes that encode components of these growth inhibitory pathways.
- **Altered cellular metabolism**. Tumor cells undergo a metabolic switch to aerobic glycolysis (called the

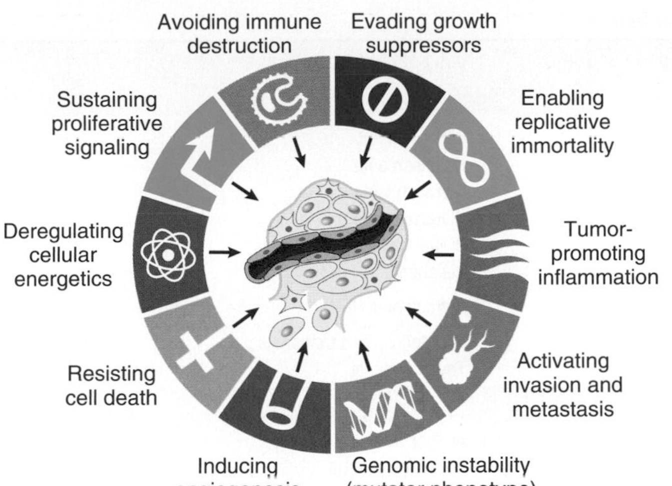

Figure 7-24 Hallmarks of cancer. (Adapted from Hanahan D, Weinberg RA. Hallmarks of cancer: the next generation. Cell 2011; 144:646.)

Warburg effect), which enables the synthesis of the macromolecules and organelles that are needed for rapid cell growth.

- **Evasion of apoptosis**. Tumors are resistant to programmed cell death.
- **Limitless replicative potential (immortality)**. Tumors have unrestricted proliferative capacity, a stem cell–like property that permits tumor cells to avoid cellular senescence and mitotic catastrophe.
- **Sustained angiogenesis**. Tumor cells, like normal cells, are not able to grow without a vascular supply to bring nutrients and oxygen and remove waste products. Hence, tumors must induce angiogenesis.
- **Ability to invade and metastasize**. Tumor metastases are the cause of the vast majority of cancer deaths and arise from the interplay of processes that are intrinsic to tumor cells and signals that are initiated by the tissue environment.
- **Ability to evade the host immune response**. You will recall that the cells of the innate and adaptive immune system can recognize and eliminate cells displaying abnormal antigens (e.g., a mutated oncoprotein). Cancer cells exhibit a number of alterations that allow them to evade the host immune response.

The acquisition of the genetic and epigenetic alterations that confer these hallmarks may be accelerated by **genomic instability** and by **cancer-promoting inflammation**. These are considered enabling characteristics because they promote cellular transformation and subsequent tumor progression.

In the following sections, each of the hallmarks and enabling characteristics of cancer cells is discussed, focusing on the most important contributing genes and cellular pathways. The discussion of cancer pathophysiology ends with a review of the roles that epigenetic changes and noncoding RNAs play in the disease.

Self-Sufficiency in Growth Signals: Oncogenes

Genes that promote autonomous cell growth in cancer cells are called *oncogenes*, and their unmutated cellular counterparts are called *proto-oncogenes*. **Oncogenes are created by mutations in proto-oncogenes and encode proteins called oncoproteins that have the ability to promote cell growth in the absence of normal growth-promoting signals**. *Oncoproteins* resemble the normal products of proto-oncogenes but bear mutations that are often inactivate internal regulatory elements; consequently, their activity in cells does not depend on external signals. Cells expressing oncoproteins are thus freed from the normal checkpoints and controls that limit growth, and as a result proliferate excessively.

To aid in the understanding of the nature and functions of oncoproteins and their role in cancer, it is necessary to briefly describe how normal cells respond to growth factors. Under physiologic conditions growth factor signaling pathways can be resolved into the following steps:

- The binding of a growth factor to its specific receptor
- Transient and limited activation of the growth factor receptor, which, in turn, activates several cytoplasmic signal-transducing proteins
- Transmission of the transduced signal to the nucleus via additional cytoplasmic effector proteins and second messengers or by a cascade of signal transduction molecules
- Induction and activation of nuclear regulatory factors that initiate DNA transcription
- Expression of factors that promote entry and progression of the cell into the cell cycle, ultimately resulting in cell division
- In parallel, changes in the expression of other genes that support cell survival and metabolic alterations that are needed for optimal growth

Aberrations in multiple signaling pathways have been identified in various tumors; many components of these pathways act as oncoproteins when mutated (Table 7-5). **Conversely, a number of tumor suppressors act by inhibiting one or more components of these pathways** (discussed later). In Chapter 1, the major signaling pathways that regulate cellular behavior are laid out, including the receptor tyrosine kinase pathway, the G protein–coupled receptor pathway, the JAK/STAT pathway, the WNT pathway, the Notch pathway, the Hedgehog pathway, the TGFβ/SMAD pathway, and the NF-κB pathway. Abnormalities in all these pathways are implicated in the development and progression of various cancers. This chapter focuses on the receptor tyrosine kinase pathway, because it appears to be the most frequently mutated oncogenic pathway in human neoplasms. Oncogenic mutations involving other signaling pathways are also mentioned, because many exemplify certain key concepts underlying cancer phenotypes and some are the targets of effective therapies.

Traditionally, oncoproteins have been likened to accelerators that speed the replication of cells and their DNA; by contrast, tumor suppressors have been viewed as brakes that slow or arrest this process. This view has merit and we will follow it in our initial description of the activities of oncogenes and tumor suppressors. However, the proliferation of cells not only requires the replication of DNA, but also sufficient biosynthesis of membrane, protein, and various macromolecules and organelles to enable a "mother" cell to divide and produce two complete

Table 7-5 Selected Oncogenes, Their Mode of Activation, and Associated Human Tumors

Category	Proto-Oncogene	Mode of Activation in Tumor	Associated Human Tumor
Growth Factors			
PDGF-β chain	*PDGFB*	Overexpression	Astrocytoma
Fibroblast growth factors	*HST1* *FGF3*	Overexpression Amplification	Osteosarcoma Stomach cancer Bladder cancer Breast cancer Melanoma
TGF-α	*TGFA*	Overexpression	Astrocytomas
HGF	*HGF*	Overexpression	Hepatocellular carcinomas Thyroid cancer
Growth Factor Receptors			
EGF-receptor family	*ERBB1 (EGFR)* *ERBB2 (HER)*	Mutation Amplification	Adenocarcinoma of lung Breast carcinoma
FMS-like tyrosine kinase 3	*FLT3*	Point mutation	Leukemia
Receptor for neurotrophic factors	*RET*	Point mutation	Multiple endocrine neoplasia 2A and B, familial medullary thyroid carcinomas
PDGF receptor	*PDGFRB*	Overexpression, translocation	Gliomas, leukemias
Receptor for KIT ligand	*KIT*	Point mutation	Gastrointestinal stromal tumors, seminomas, leukemias
ALK receptor	*ALK*	Translocation, fusion gene formation Point mutation	Adenocarcinoma of lung, certain lymphomas Neuroblastoma
Proteins Involved in Signal Transduction			
GTP-binding (G) proteins	*KRAS* *HRAS* *NRAS* *GNAQ* *GNAS*	Point mutation Point mutation Point mutation Point mutation Point mutation	Colon, lung, and pancreatic tumors Bladder and kidney tumors Melanomas, hematologic malignancies Uveal melanoma Pituitary adenoma, other endocrine tumors
Nonreceptor tyrosine kinase	*ABL*	Translocation Point mutation	Chronic myelogenous leukemia Acute lymphoblastic leukemia
RAS signal transduction	*BRAF*	Point mutation, Translocation	Melanomas, leukemias, colon carcinoma, others
Notch signal transduction	*NOTCH1*	Point mutation, Translocation Gene rearrangement	Leukemias, lymphomas, breast carcinoma
JAK/STAT signal transduction	*JAK2*	Translocation	Myeloproliferative disorders Acute lymphoblastic leukemia
Nuclear Regulatory Proteins			
Transcriptional activators	*MYC* *NMYC*	Translocation Amplification	Burkitt lymphoma Neuroblastoma
Cell Cycle Regulators			
Cyclins	*CCND1* (Cyclin D1)	Translocation Amplification	Mantle cell lymphoma, multiple myeloma Breast and esophageal cancers
Cyclin-dependent kinase	*CDK4*	Amplification or point mutation	Glioblastoma, melanoma, sarcoma

daughter cells. Cell growth pathways implicated in oncogenesis also initiate signals that promote and coordinate the biosynthesis of all of these cellular components (discussed later). This insight has led to the idea that it may be possible to target many aspects of oncogenic "pro-growth" signaling to therapeutic advantage, including the altered cellular metabolism that is characteristic of cancer cells.

Building on this framework, we next discuss the mechanisms by which cancer cells acquire self-sufficiency in growth signals.

Proto-oncogenes, Oncogenes, and Oncoproteins

Proto-oncogenes have multiple roles, but all participate at some level in signaling pathways that drive proliferation. Thus, pro-growth proto-oncogenes may encode growth factors, growth factor receptors, signal transducers, transcription factors, or cell cycle components. The corresponding oncogenes generally encode oncoproteins that serve functions similar to their normal counterparts, with the important difference that they are usually constitutively active. **As a result of this constitutive activity, pro-growth oncoproteins endow cells with self-sufficiency in growth.**

Two questions follow: (1) what are the functions of pro-growth oncoproteins and (2) how do the normally "civilized" proto-oncogenes turn into "enemies within?" The ensuing discussion uses receptor tyrosine kinases and downstream signaling components as examples. Receptor tyrosine kinase signaling is complex and has a number of major branchpoints and signaling nodes. Amongst these, Darwinian selection picks out the factors that have the

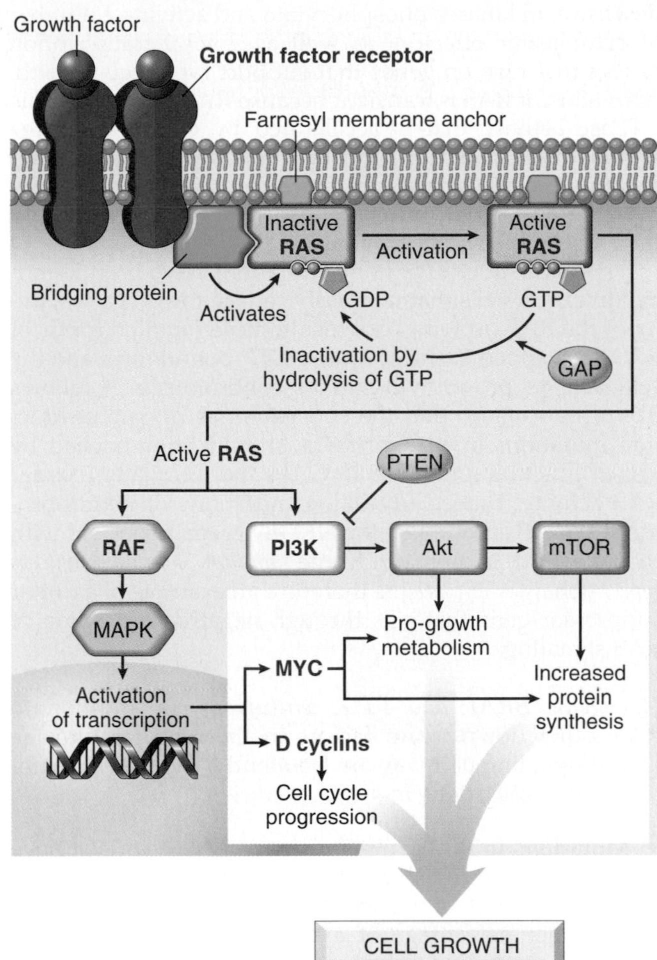

Figure 7-25 Growth factor signaling pathways in cancer. Growth factor receptors, RAS, PI3K, MYC, and D cyclins are oncoproteins that are activated by mutations in various cancers. GAPs apply brakes to RAS activation, and PTEN serves the same function for PI3K.

greatest impact on the malignant phenotype. Based on this logic, the signal transducer RAS, which operates immediately downstream from receptor tyrosine kinases, and two signaling "arms" that are downstream of RAS, the mitogen-activated protein kinase (MAPK) pathway and the phosphoinositidyl-3-kinase (PI3K)/AKT pathway, appear to be particularly important in promoting cancer cell growth (Fig. 7-25). Most (and possibly all) human cancers have molecular defects that affect one or more components of these pathways; examples are highlighted in Fig. 7-25 and are discussed in some detail below.

Growth Factors. Normal cells require stimulation by growth factors to proliferate. Most soluble growth factors are made by one cell type and act on a neighboring cell to stimulate proliferation (paracrine action). Some cancer cells, however, acquire the ability to synthesize the same growth factors to which they are responsive, creating an autocrine loop. For example, many brain tumors called *glioblastomas* express both platelet-derived growth factor (PDGF) and the PDGF receptor tyrosine kinases, and many sarcomas overexpress both transforming growth factor α (TGF-α) and its cognate receptor, epidermal growth factor receptor (EGFR), another member of the receptor tyrosine kinase family. In tumors in which an autocrine loop is an important pathogenic element, the growth factor gene itself is usually not altered or mutated. More commonly, signals transduced by other oncoproteins cause overexpression and increased secretion of growth factors , thereby initiating and amplifying the autocrine loop.

Growth Factor Receptors. A large number of oncogenes encode growth factor receptors, of which receptor tyrosine kinases are arguably the most important in cancer. Recall that receptor tyrosine kinases are transmembrane proteins with an extracellular ligand-binding domain and a cytoplasmic tyrosine kinase domain (Chapter 1). Normally, the receptor's kinase activity is activated transiently by binding of a specific growth factor to the extracellular domain, an event that induces a rapid change in receptor conformation to an active dimeric state. The activated receptor then autophosphorylates tyrosine residues in its own intracellular tail, and these modified residues serve as sites for recruitment of a number of signaling molecules, including RAS and PI3K, which have already been described as key players in receptor tyrosine kinase signaling. The oncogenic versions of these receptors are associated with mutations that lead to constitutive, growth factor–independent tyrosine kinase activity. Hence, the mutant receptors deliver continuous mitogenic signals to the cell, even in the absence of growth factor in the environment.

Receptor tyrosine kinases can be constitutively activated in tumors by multiple mechanisms, including point mutations, gene rearrangements, and gene amplifications. A few of the better characterized oncogenic mutations involving growth factor receptors are listed in Table 7-5; the following are salient examples of clinical importance:

- ***ERBB1*** encodes the epidermal growth factor receptor (EGFR), which is involved by point mutations in certain cancers. Of greatest clinical importance are several different *ERBB1* point mutations that are found in a subset of lung adenocarcinomas. These mutations result in constitutive activation of the EGFR tyrosine kinase.
- ***ERBB2*** encodes a different member of the receptor tyrosine kinase family, HER2. Rather than being activated by point mutations, the *ERBB2* gene is amplified in certain breast carcinomas, leading to overexpression of the HER2 receptor and constitutive tyrosine kinase activity.
- **Gene rearrangements** activate other receptor tyrosine kinases, such the tyrosine kinase ALK. For example, a deletion on chromosome 5 fuses part of the *ALK* gene with part of another gene called *EML4* in a subset of lung adenocarcinomas. The resulting *EML4-ALK* fusion gene encodes a chimeric EML4-ALK protein, again with constitutive tyrosine kinase activity.

The role of each of the mutations described earlier in promoting the growth and survival of tumor cells has been proven in no small part by the response of tumors bearing these mutations to therapeutic agents that specifically bind and inhibit these mutated receptor tyrosine kinases. For example, breast cancers with *ERBB2* amplification and overexpression of HER2 generally respond to treatment with antibodies or drugs that block HER2 activity. These inhibitors not only cause the cessation of tumor growth but also induce apoptosis and tumor regression, reflecting the ability of receptor tyrosine kinase signaling to augment cell survival as well as proliferation. Inhibitors of EGFR and ALK produce similar therapeutic responses in patients with lung adenocarcinomas harboring *ERBB1* mutations or *EML4-ALK* fusion genes, respectively.

Unfortunately, none of these targeted therapies cure advanced lung cancer. In treated patients tumors have often been found to have acquired activating mutations in some other signaling molecule, most often another tyrosine kinase, which sidesteps the effects of the drug, resulting in resistance to the targeted therapy. For example, lung cancers that develop resistance to EGFR inhibitors often have amplifications in a gene called *MET*, which encodes yet another receptor tyrosine kinase. This experience highlights one of the most daunting clinical problems in the treatment of advanced cancers—the presence of subclones within the genetically heterogeneous tumor cell population that are resistant to targeted therapies.

Downstream components of the receptor tyrosine kinase signaling pathway. As mentioned, receptor tyrosine kinase activation stimulates RAS and two major downstream signaling "arms," the MAPK cascade and the PI3K/AKT pathway. In line with the importance of these pathways in mediating cell growth, RAS, PI3K, and other components of these pathways are frequently involved by gain-of-function mutations in different types of cancer. Of interest, when *RAS* mutations are present in a tumor, activating mutations in receptor tyrosine kinases are almost always absent, at least within the dominant tumor clone, implying that in such tumors activated RAS can completely substitute for tyrosine kinase activity. Thus, lung adenocarcinomas fall into mutually exclusive molecular subtypes that are associated with mutations involving *RAS* or various tyrosine kinase genes, an insight that has important implications for targeted therapies in this type of cancer.

RAS Mutations. **Point mutations of *RAS* family genes constitute the most common type of abnormality involving proto-oncogenes in human tumors**. The *RAS* genes, of which there are three in humans (*HRAS, KRAS, NRAS*), were discovered initially in transforming retroviruses. Approximately 15% to 20% of all human tumors express mutated RAS proteins, but in some types of cancers the frequency of *RAS* mutations is much higher. For example, 90% of pancreatic adenocarcinomas and cholangiocarcinomas contain a *RAS* point mutation, as do about 50% of colon, endometrial, and thyroid cancers and about 30% of lung adenocarcinomas and myeloid leukemias. *RAS* mutations are not nearly as prevalent in other kinds of cancers, but are nevertheless detected at low frequencies in most.

Recall that RAS proteins are members of a family of membrane-associated small G proteins that bind guanosine nucleotides (guanosine triphosphate [GTP] and guanosine diphosphate [GDP]), similar to the larger trimolecular G proteins. They normally flip back and forth between an excited signal-transmitting state in which they are bound to GTP and a quiescent state in which they are bound to GDP. Stimulation of receptor tyrosine kinases by growth factors leads to exchange of GDP for GTP and subsequent conformational changes that generate active RAS, which in turn stimulates both the MAPK and PI3K/AKT arms of the receptor tyrosine kinase signaling pathway. These downstream kinases phosphorylate and activate a number of cytoplasmic effectors as well as several transcription factors that turn on genes that support rapid cell growth. Activation of RAS is transient because RAS has an intrinsic GTPase activity that is accelerated by *GTPase-activating proteins (GAPs)*, which bind to the active RAS and augment its GTPase activity by more than 1000-fold, thereby terminating signal transduction. Thus, GAPs prevent uncontrolled RAS activity.

Several distinct RAS point mutations have been identified in cancer cells that markedly reduce the GTPase activity of the RAS protein. As a result, these mutated forms of RAS are trapped in the activated GTP-bound form and the cell receives pro-growth signals continuously. It follows from this scenario that the consequences of gain-of-function mutations in RAS proteins should be mimicked by loss-of-function mutations in GAPs that normally restrain RAS activity. Indeed, disabling mutations of neurofibromin 1, a GAP encoded by the *NF1* gene, are associated with the inherited cancer syndrome *familial neurofibromatosis type 1* (Chapter 25). *NF1* is therefore an example of a tumor suppressor gene that acts through negative regulation of RAS signaling.

Oncogenic BRAF and PI3K Mutations. In addition to RAS, other downstream factors in the receptor tyrosine kinase signaling pathway are frequently involved by gain-of-function mutations in various cancers.

- **Mutations in *BRAF*,** a member of the *RAF* family, have been detected in close to 100% of hairy cell leukemias, more than 60% of melanomas, 80% of benign nevi, and a smaller percentage of a wide variety of other neoplasms, including colon carcinomas and dendritic cell tumors. BRAF is a serine/threonine protein kinase that sits at the top of a cascade of other serine/threonine kinases of the MAPK family. Like activating RAS mutations, activating mutations in BRAF stimulate each of these downstream kinases and ultimately activate transcription factors. Mutations in other MAPK family members downstream of BRAF are uncommon in cancer, suggesting only mutations affecting factors near the top of the RAS/MAPK cascade produce significant pro-growth signals in most cell types.
- **Mutations of the PI3K family of proteins** are also very common in certain cancers. PI3K is heterodimer comprised of a regulatory subunit and a catalytic subunit, of which several tissue-specific isoforms exist. Under normal circumstances, PI3K is recruited by receptor tyrosine kinase activation to plasma membrane-associated signaling protein complexes. Here, like BRAF, it activates a cascade of serine/threonine kinases, including AKT, which is a key signaling node. AKT has many substrates, several of which are particularly important. mTOR, a sensor of cellular nutrient status, is activated by AKT and in turn stimulates protein and lipid synthesis. BAD is a pro-apoptotic protein that inactivated by AKT, an effect that enhances cell survival. Similarly, FOXO transcription factors, which turn on genes that promote apoptosis, are also negatively regulated by AKT phosphorylation. Like RAS, PI3K is negatively regulated by an important "braking" factor called *PTEN*. Alterations in virtually all components of the

PI3K/AKT pathway have been found in various cancers, but as with the RAS/MAPK pathway, the factors at the top of the pathway, PI3K and its antagonist, PTEN, are most frequently mutated. PI3K mutations affect the catalytic subunits and generally result in an increase in enzyme activity. For example, about 30% of breast carcinomas have gain-of-function mutations involving the α-isoform of the PI3K catalytic subunit. As would be expected, *PTEN* is a tumor suppressor gene whose function is lost through mutation or epigenetic silencing in many cancers, particularly endometrial carcinomas (Chapter 21).

Because RAS proteins are so frequently mutated in human cancers, much effort has been spent to develop targeted therapy specific for these proteins. Unfortunately, none of the strategies designed to target RAS has so far been successful, in part because the vagaries of RAS protein structure and its mode of signaling make it a particularly difficult protein to inhibit with drugs. In contrast, treatment of patients with advanced melanomas harboring activating BRAF mutations with BRAF inhibitors have produced striking clinical responses. Such responses are strictly restricted to tumors with BRAF mutations, as morphologically identical melanomas without BRAF mutations never respond to BRAF inhibitors. This phenomenon, termed oncogene addiction (described below), highlights the need for molecular analysis to guide appropriate therapy. Multiple drugs that inhibit various PI3K isoforms have also been developed and are now being tested in the clinic.

Alterations in Nonreceptor Tyrosine Kinases. Mutations that confer oncogenic activity occur in several nonreceptor tyrosine kinases that normally localize to the cytoplasm or the nucleus. In many instances the mutations take the form of chromosomal translocations or rearrangements that create fusion genes encoding constitutively active tyrosine kinases. Despite their nonmembranous localization, most of these oncoproteins also activate the same signaling pathways as receptor tyrosine kinases. An important example of this oncogenic mechanism involves the ABL tyrosine kinase. In *chronic myelogenous leukemia* (CML) and some *acute lymphoblastic leukemias*, the *ABL* gene is translocated from its normal abode on chromosome 9 to chromosome 22 (Fig. 7-26), where it fuses with the *BCR* gene (see discussion of chromosomal translocations later in this chapter). The resultant chimeric gene encodes a constitutively active, oncogenic *BCR-ABL tyrosine kinase*. The most important contribution of the BCR moiety is that it promotes self-association of BCR-ABL, which appears to be sufficient to unleash tyrosine kinase activity of ABL. This is a recurrent mechanism in cancer, in that many different oncogenic tyrosine kinases consist of fusion proteins in which the non-tyrosine kinase partner drives self-association.

Treatment of CML has been revolutionized by the development of "designer" drugs with low toxicity and high therapeutic efficacy that inhibit the BCR-ABL kinase, another example of rational drug design emerging from an understanding of the molecular basis of cancer. The remarkable therapeutic response of CML to BCR-ABL inhibitors is one of the first and best examples of *oncogene addiction*, in which tumor cells are highly dependent on the activity of one or more oncogenes. Despite accumulation of mutations in other cancer-associated genes in CML cells, signaling through the BCR-ABL tyrosine kinase is required for most CML tumor cells to proliferate and survive, hence inhibition of its activity is a highly effective therapy. The presence of a *BCR-ABL* fusion gene defines CML and must be the initiating event in this disease; thus, additional mutations acquired by the founding clone are selected for their ability to complement the effects of constant signaling through BCR-ABL. BCR-ABL signaling can be seen as the central lodgepole around which a complex oncogenic structure is built. If the lodgepole is removed by inhibition of the BCR-ABL kinase, the entire structure collapses. Unfortunately, treatment of this "addiction" with BCR-ABL inhibitors does not lead to cure. Even though the proliferating component of the tumor is suppressed by BCR-ABL inhibitors and the patient seems completely well, rare CML "stem cells" harboring the *BCR-ABL* fusion gene persist, apparently because these cells do not require BCR-ABL signals for their survival. As a result, therapy with BCR-ABL inhibitors must be continued indefinitely;

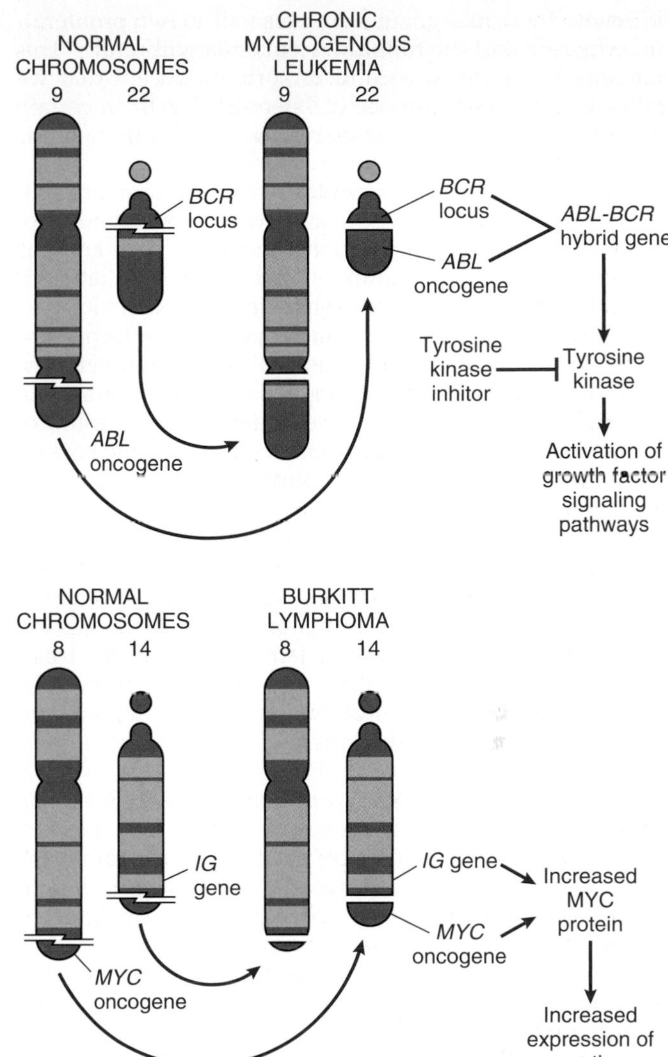

Figure 7-26 The chromosomal translocation and associated oncogenes in Burkitt lymphoma and chronic myelogenous leukemia.

otherwise these malignant stem cells will spawn proliferating offspring and the fullblown leukemia will return. This outcome highlights a second important concept that we will return to; the existence of "stem-like" cells in certain cancers that may be particularly resistant to therapeutic targeting.

In other instances, nonreceptor tyrosine kinases are activated by point mutations that abrogate the function of negative regulatory domains that normally hold enzyme activity in check. An example of this type of mutation is found in the nonreceptor tyrosine kinase JAK2. JAK2 participates in the JAK/STAT signaling pathway, which transduces mitogenic signals from growth factor and cytokine receptors that lack tyrosine kinase activity (as describe in Chapter 1). JAK/STAT activation alters the expression of target genes that bind STAT transcription factors. Several myeloproliferative disorders, particularly polycythemia vera, essential thrombocytosis, and primary myelofibrosis, are highly associated with activating point mutations in JAK2 that relieve the normal dependence of hematopoietic progenitors on growth factors such as erythropoietin (Chapter 13). Recognition of this molecular lesion has led to the clinical development of JAK2 inhibitors for treatment myeloproliferative disorders, and has stimulated searches for activating mutations in other nonreceptor tyrosine kinases in a wide variety of human cancers.

Transcription Factors. Just as all roads lead to Rome, all signal transduction pathways converge on the nucleus, where the expression of target genes that orchestrate the cell's orderly advance through the mitotic cycle is activated. Indeed, the ultimate consequence of deregulated mitogenic signaling pathways is inappropriate and continuous stimulation of nuclear transcription factors that drive growth-promoting genes. Thus, not surprisingly, growth autonomy may also occur as a consequence of mutations affecting the transcription factors that regulate the expression of pro-growth genes and cyclins. Transcription factors of this class include the products of the *MYC*, *MYB*, *JUN*, *FOS*, and *REL* proto-oncogenes. Of these, *MYC* is most commonly involved in human tumors, and hence a brief overview of its regulation and function follows.

MYC Oncogene. The *MYC* proto-oncogene is expressed in virtually all eukaryotic cells and belongs to the immediate early response genes, which are rapidly and transiently induced by RAS/MAPK signaling following growth factor stimulation of quiescent cells. Under normal circumstances, MYC protein concentrations are tightly controlled at the level of transcription, translation, and protein stability, and virtually all pathways that regulate growth impinge on MYC through one or more of these mechanisms. Several single nucleotide polymorphisms (SNPs) that are strongly linked to an elevated risk of cancers, such as prostate and ovarian carcinoma, fall within a large region devoid of recognizable genes that lies next to *MYC* on chromosome 8. Experimental data suggest that these genetic variants alter the function of enhancer elements that regulate *MYC* expression, and that increased cancer risk is associated with variants that bring about higher levels of *MYC* RNA expression in response to certain growth promoting signals.

How MYC promotes normal and neoplastic cell growth is incompletely understood, but a multitude of studies have shown that MYC has remarkably broad activities, several of which contribute not only to deregulated cell growth but also to several other hallmarks of cancer.

- **MYC activates the expression of many genes that are involved in cell growth.**
  - Some MYC target genes, like D cyclins, are directly involved in cell cycle progression.
  - MYC also upregulates the expression of rRNA genes and rRNA processing, thereby enhancing the assembly of ribosomes needed for protein synthesis.
  - MYC upregulates a program of gene expression that leads to metabolic reprogramming and the Warburg effect, another cancer hallmark (discussed later). Among the genes involved in metabolism that are upregulated by MYC are multiple glycolytic enzymes and factors involved in glutamine metabolism, both of which contribute to the generation of metabolic intermediates that are needed for synthesis of macromolecules such as DNA, proteins, and lipids.
  - Based on these protean effects, MYC can be considered a master transcriptional regulator of cell growth. Indeed, the fastest growing human tumors, such as Burkitt lymphoma, which virtually always bears a chromosomal translocation involving *MYC* (Fig. 7-26), are those with the highest levels of MYC.
- **In some contexts, MYC upregulates expression of telomerase**. As discussed later, telomerase is one of several factors that contribute to the endless replicative capacity (the immortalization) of cancer cells.
- **MYC is one of a handful of transcription factors that can act together to reprogram somatic cells into pluripotent stem cells** (Chapter 1). This capacity has led to suspicions that MYC may also contribute to cancer cell "stemness," another important aspect of the immortality of cancers.

Given the importance of MYC in regulation of cell growth, it should come as no surprise that it is deregulated in cancer through a variety of mechanisms. Sometimes deregulation involves genetic alterations of *MYC* itself. In addition to the *MYC* translocations in Burkitt lymphoma and a subset of other B and T cell tumors, *MYC* is amplified in some breast, colon, lung, and many other carcinomas. The functionally identical *NMYC* and *LMYC* genes are also amplified in neuroblastomas (Fig. 7-27) and small cell cancers of the lung, respectively. In many other instances, oncogenic mutations involving components of upstream signaling pathways elevate MYC protein levels by increasing *MYC* transcription, enhancing *MYC* mRNA translation, and/or stabilizing MYC protein. Thus, constitutive RAS/MAPK signaling (many cancers), Notch signaling (several hematologic cancers), Wnt signaling (colon carcinoma), and Hedgehog signaling (medulloblastoma) all transform cells in part through upregulation of *MYC*.

Cyclins and Cyclin-Dependent Kinases. As mentioned in Chapter 1, growth factors transduce signals that stimulate the orderly progression of cells through the various phases of the cell cycle, the process by which cells replicate their DNA in preparation for cell division. Progression of cells through the cell cycle is orchestrated by *cyclin-dependent kinases* (CDKs), which are activated by binding

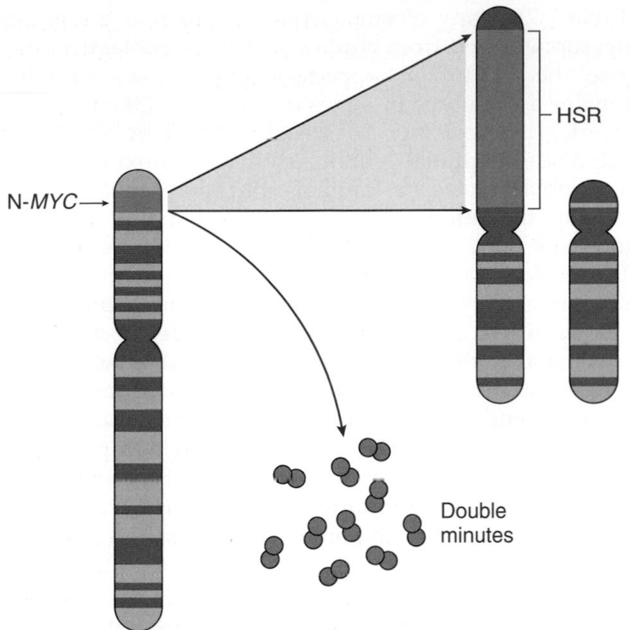

Figure 7-27 Amplification of the *NMYC* gene in human neuroblastomas. The *NMYC* gene, normally present on chromosome 2p, becomes amplified and is seen either as extra chromosomal double minutes or as a chromosomally integrated, homogeneous staining region (HSR). The integration involves other autosomes, such as 4, 9, or 13. (Modified from Brodeur GM: Molecular correlates of cytogenetic abnormalities in human cancer cells: implications for oncogene activation. In Brown EB (ed): Progress in Hematology, Vol 14. Orlando, FL, Grune & Stratton, 1986, p 229-256.)

Table 7-6 Cell Cycle Components and Inhibitors That Are Frequently Mutated in Cancer

Cell Cycle Component	Main Function
Cyclins and Cyclin-Dependent Kinases	
CDK4; D cyclins	Form a complex that phosphorylates RB, allowing the cell to progress through the G_1 restriction point
Cell Cycle Inhibitors	
CIP/KIP family: p21, p27 (CDKN1A-D)	Block the cell cycle by binding to cyclin-CDK complexes p21 is induced by the tumor suppressor p53 p27 responds to growth suppressors such as TGF-β
INK4/ARF family (CDKN2A-C)	p16/INK4a binds to cyclin D-CDK4 and promotes the inhibitory effects of RB p14/ARF increases p53 levels by inhibiting MDM2 activity
Cell Cycle Checkpoint Components	
RB	Tumor suppressive "pocket" protein that binds E2F transcription factors in its hypophosphorylated state, preventing G_1/S transition; also interacts with several transcription factors that regulate differentiation
p53	Tumor suppressor altered in the majority of cancers; causes cell cycle arrest and apoptosis. Acts mainly through p21 to cause cell cycle arrest. Causes apoptosis by inducing the transcription of pro-apoptotic genes such as *BAX*. Levels of p53 are negatively regulated by MDM2 through a feedback loop. p53 is required for the G_1/S checkpoint and is a main component of the G_2/M checkpoint.

to *cyclins*, so called because of the cyclic nature of their production and degradation. The CDK-cyclin complexes phosphorylate crucial target proteins that drive cells forward through the cell cycle. While cyclins arouse the CDKs, *CDK inhibitors* (CDKIs), of which there are many, silence the CDKs and exert negative control over the cell cycle (Table 7-6). Expression of these inhibitors is down-regulated by mitogenic signaling pathways, thus promoting the progression of the cell cycle.

There are two main cell cycle checkpoints one at the G_1/S transition and the other at the G_2/M transition, each of which is tightly regulated by a balance of growth promoting and growth suppressing factors, as well as by sensors of DNA damage (Chapter 1)**.** If activated, these DNA-damage sensors transmit signals that arrest cell cycle progression and, if cell damage cannot be repaired, initiate apoptosis. Understandably, defects in the G_1/S checkpoint are more important in cancer, in that these lead to dysregulated growth as well as a mutator phenotype, which (as mentioned) enables cancer development and progression. The major cancer-associated mutations that affect the G_1/S checkpoint can be broadly grouped into two classes:

- **Gain-of-function mutations in D cyclin genes and CDK4, oncogenes that promote G_1/S progression.** There are three D cyclin genes, D1, D2, and D3, which are functionally interchangeable and often dysregulated by acquired mutations in cancer, including chromosomal translocations in lymphoid tumors and gene amplification in a variety of solid tumors. Amplification of the *CDK4* gene also occurs in melanomas, sarcomas, and glioblastomas. Mutations affecting cyclin B and cyclin E and other CDKs also occur, but they are much less frequent, presumably because of the preeminent importance of the G_1/S transition in regulating tumor growth rates.
- **Loss-of-function mutations in tumor suppressor genes that inhibit G_1/S progression**. CDKIs that inhibit cyclin D/CDK complexes are frequently mutated or otherwise silenced in many human malignancies. For example, germline mutations of *p16* (*CDKN2A*) are present in 25% of melanoma-prone kindreds, and somatically acquired deletion or inactivation of *p16* is seen in 75% of pancreatic carcinomas, 40% to 70% of glioblastomas, 50% of esophageal cancers, 20% to 70% of acute lymphoblastic leukemias, and 20% of non–small-cell lung carcinomas, soft tissue sarcomas, and bladder cancers. Furthermore, the two most important tumor suppressor genes, *RB* and *TP53*, both encode proteins that inhibit G_1/S progression.

KEY CONCEPTS

Oncogenes, Oncoproteins, and Unregulated Cell Proliferation

Proto-oncogenes: normal cellular genes whose products promote cell proliferation

Oncogenes: mutated or overexpressed versions of proto-oncogenes that function autonomously, having lost dependence on normal growth promoting signals

Oncoprotein: a protein encoded by an oncogene that drives increased cell proliferation through one of several mechanisms

- Constitutive expression of growth factors and their cognate growth factor receptors, setting up an autocrine cell signaling loop
- Mutations in growth factor receptors, non-receptor tyrosine kinases, or downstream signaling molecules that lead to constitutive signaling, such as:
  - Activation of the EGF receptor tyrosine kinase by point mutations (lung cancer); activation of the HER2 receptor tyrosine kinase by gene amplification (breast cancer) ; activation of the JAK2 tyrosine kinase by point mutations (myeloproliferative disorders)
  - Activation of the ABL nonreceptor tyrosine kinase by chromosomal translocation and creation of a BCR-ABL fusion gene (chronic myelogenous leukemia, acute lymphoblastic leukemia)
  - Activation of RAS by point mutations (many cancers)
  - Activation of the PI3K and BRAF serine/threonine kinases by point mutations (many cancers)
- Increased expression of MYC, a master transcription factor that regulates genes needed for rapid cell growth by deregulation through chromosomal translocations (Burkitt lymphoma, other hematologic malignancies); gene amplication (neuroblastoma); increased activity of upstream signaling pathways (many cancers)
- Mutations that increase the activity of cyclin-dependent kinase 4 (CDK4)/D cyclin complexes, which promote cell cycle progression

Insensitivity to Growth Inhibition: Tumor Suppressor Genes

Whereas oncogenes drive the proliferation of cells, the products of most tumor suppressor genes apply brakes to cell proliferation, and abnormalities in these genes lead to failure of growth inhibition, another fundamental hallmark of carcinogenesis. Tumor suppressor proteins form a network of checkpoints that prevent uncontrolled growth. Many tumor suppressors, such as RB and p53, are part of a regulatory network that recognizes genotoxic stress from any source and responds by shutting down proliferation. Indeed, expression of an oncogene in normal cells with intact tumor suppressor genes leads to quiescence, or to permanent cell cycle arrest (oncogene-induced senescence, discussed later), rather than uncontrolled proliferation. Ultimately, the growth-inhibitory pathways may prod the cells into apoptosis. Another set of tumor suppressors seems to be involved in cell differentiation, causing cells to enter a postmitotic, differentiated pool without replicative potential. Similar to mitogenic signals, growth-inhibitory, pro-differentiation signals originate outside the cell and use receptors, signal transducers, and nuclear transcription regulators to accomplish their effects; tumor suppressors form a portion of these networks. Thus, the protein products of tumor suppressor genes may function as transcription factors, cell cycle inhibitors, signal transduction molecules, cell surface receptors, and regulators of cellular responses to DNA damage.

In this section, we describe tumor suppressor genes, their products, and possible mechanisms by which loss of their function contributes to unregulated cell growth (Table 7-7). Many of our current concepts of tumor suppressors evolved from studies of the retinoblastoma (*RB*) gene, the first tumor suppressor gene discovered, which remains a prototype of genes of this type. Like many discoveries in medicine, *RB* was identified by studying a rare disease, familial retinoblastoma. Approximately 40% of retinoblastomas are familial, with the predisposition to develop the tumor being transmitted as an autosomal dominant trait. Carriers of the retinoblastoma trait have a 10,000-fold increased risk of developing retinoblastoma (often in both eyes) as compared to the general population, and are also at greatly increased risk of developing osteosarcoma and other soft-tissue sarcomas. About 60% of retinoblastomas occur sporadically (virtually always in only one eye), and such patients are not at increased risk for other forms of cancer. To explain these two patterns of occurrence of retinoblastoma, Knudson proposed his now canonic **"two-hit" hypothesis of oncogenesis**. In molecular terms, Knudson's hypothesis can be stated as follows (Fig. 7-28):

- Two mutations (hits), involving both alleles of *RB* at chromosome locus 13q14, are required to produce retinoblastoma.
- In familial cases, children inherit one defective copy of the *RB* gene in the germline (the first hit), and the other copy is normal (Fig. 7-28). Retinoblastoma develops when the normal *RB* allele is mutated in retinoblasts as a result of a spontaneous somatic mutation (the second hit). Because such second hits seem to be virtually inevitable in a small fraction of retinoblasts, most individuals inheriting a germline defect in one *RB* allele develop unilateral or bilateral retinoblastoma, and the disease is inherited as an autosomal dominant trait.
- In sporadic cases both normal *RB* alleles must undergo somatic mutation in the same retinoblast (two hits). The probability of this event is low (explaining why retinoblastoma is an uncommon tumor in the general population), but the end result is the same: a retinal cell that has completely lost *RB* function and becomes cancerous.

Note that a child carrying an inherited mutant *RB* allele in all somatic cells is perfectly normal (except for the increased risk of developing cancer); it follows that one defective *RB* gene does not affect cell behavior. Thus, while the genetic trait (increased cancer risk) associated with germline mutations in *RB* is inherited in an autosomal dominant fashion, at the level of the individual cell, loss-of-function mutations in the *RB* gene behave in a recessive fashion.

Subsequent to the identification of *RB*, a large number of other tumor suppressor genes have been discovered, many through study of other types of familial cancers. In general, the major themes that were first appreciated through the study of familial retinoblastoma hold for these other famiial cancers: the risk of cancer is inherited as an autosomal dominant trait; tumors acquire a second hit in the sole normal tumor suppressor gene allele; and the same tumor suppressor gene is frequently mutated in sporadic tumors of the same type.

Some of the most important tumor suppressor genes, their associated familial syndromes, and their normal

Table 7-7 Selected Tumor Suppressor Genes and Associated Familial Syndromes and Cancers, Sorted by Cancer Hallmarks*

Gene	Protein	Function	Familial Syndromes	Sporadic Cancers
Inhibitors of Mitogenic Signaling Pathways				
APC	Adenomatous polyposis coli protein	Inhibitor of WNT signaling	Familial colonic polyps and carcinomas	Carcinomas of stomach, colon, pancreas; melanoma
NF1	Neurofibromin-1	Inhibitor of RAS/MAPK signaling	Neurofibromatosis type 1 (neurofibromas and malignant peripheral nerve sheath tumors)	Neuroblastoma, juvenile myeloid leukemia
NF2	Merlin	Cytoskeletal stability, Hippo pathway signaling	Neurofibromatosis type 2 (acoustic schwannoma and meningioma)	Schwannoma, meningioma
PTCH	Patched	Inhibitor of Hedgehog signaling	Gorlin syndrome (basal cell carcinoma, medulloblastoma, several benign tumors)	Basal cell carcinoma, medulloblastoma
PTEN	Phosphatase and tensin homologue	Inhibitor of PI3K/AKT signaling	Cowden syndrome (variety of benign skin, GI, and CNS growths; breast, endometrial, and thyroid carcinoma)	Diverse cancers, particularly carcinomas and lymphoid tumors
SMAD2, SMAD4	SMAD2, SMAD4	Component of the TGFβ signaling pathway, repressors of MYC and CDK4 expression, inducers of CDK inhibitor expression	Juvenile polyposis	Frequently mutated (along with other components of the TGFβ signaling pathway) in colonic and pancreatic carcinoma
Inhibitors of Cell Cycle Progression				
RB	Retinoblastoma (RB) protein	Inhibitor of G_1/S transition during cell cycle progression	Familial retinoblastoma syndrome (retinoblastoma, osteosarcoma, other sarcomas)	Retinoblastoma; osteosarcoma carcinomas of breast, colon, lung
CDKN2A	p16/INK4a and p14/ARF	p16: Negative regulator of cyclin-dependent kinases; p14, indirect activator of p53	Familial melanoma	Pancreatic, breast, and esophageal carcinoma, melanoma, certain leukemias
Inhibitors of "Pro-growth" Programs of Metabolism and Angiogenesis				
VHL	Von Hippel Lindau (VHL) protein	Inhibitor of hypoxia-induced transcription factors (e.g., HIF1α)	Von Hippel Lindau syndrome (cerebellar hemangioblastoma, retinal angioma, renal cell carcinoma)	Renal cell carcinoma
STK11	Liver kinase B1 (LKB1) or STK11	Activator of AMPK family of kinases; suppresses cell growth when cell nutrient and energy levels are low	Peutz-Jeghers syndrome (GI polyps, GI cancers, pancreatic carcinoma and other carcinomas)	Diverse carcinomas (5%-20% of cases, depending on type)
SDHB, SDHD	Succinate dehydrogenase complex subunits B and D	TCA cycle, oxidative phosphorylation	Familial paraganglioma, familial pheochromocytoma	Paraganglioma
Inhibitors of Invasion and Metastasis				
CDH1	E-cadherin	Cell adhesion, inhibition of cell motility	Familial gastric cancer	Gastric carcinoma, lobular breast carcinoma
Enablers of Genomic Stability				
TP53	p53 protein	Cell cycle arrest and apoptosis in response to DNA damage	Li-Fraumeni syndrome (diverse cancers)	Most human cancers
DNA Repair Factors				
BRCA1, BRCA2	Breast cancer-1 and breast cancer-2 (BRCA1 and BRCA2)	Repair of double-stranded breaks in DNA	Familial breast and ovarian carcinoma; carcinomas of male breast; chronic lymphocytic leukemia (BRCA2)	Rare
MSH2, MLH1, MSH6	MSH1, MLH1, MSH6	DNA mismatch repair	Hereditary nonpolyposis colon carcinoma	Colonic and endometrial carcinoma
Unknown Mechanisms				
WT1	Wilms tumor-1 (WT1)	Transcription factor	Familial Wilms tumor	Wilms tumor, certain leukemias
MEN1	Menin	Transcription factor	Multiple endocrine neoplasia-1 (MEN1; pituitary, parathyroid, and pancreatic endocrine tumors)	Pituitary, parathyroid, and pancreatic endocrine tumors

*Some tumor suppressors impact multiple cancer phenotypes (e.g., p53 affects cell cycle progression, genomic stability, susceptibility to cell death, and cellular metabolism); only a subset of major effects are given for each tumor suppressor gene listed. TCA, tricarboxylic acid.

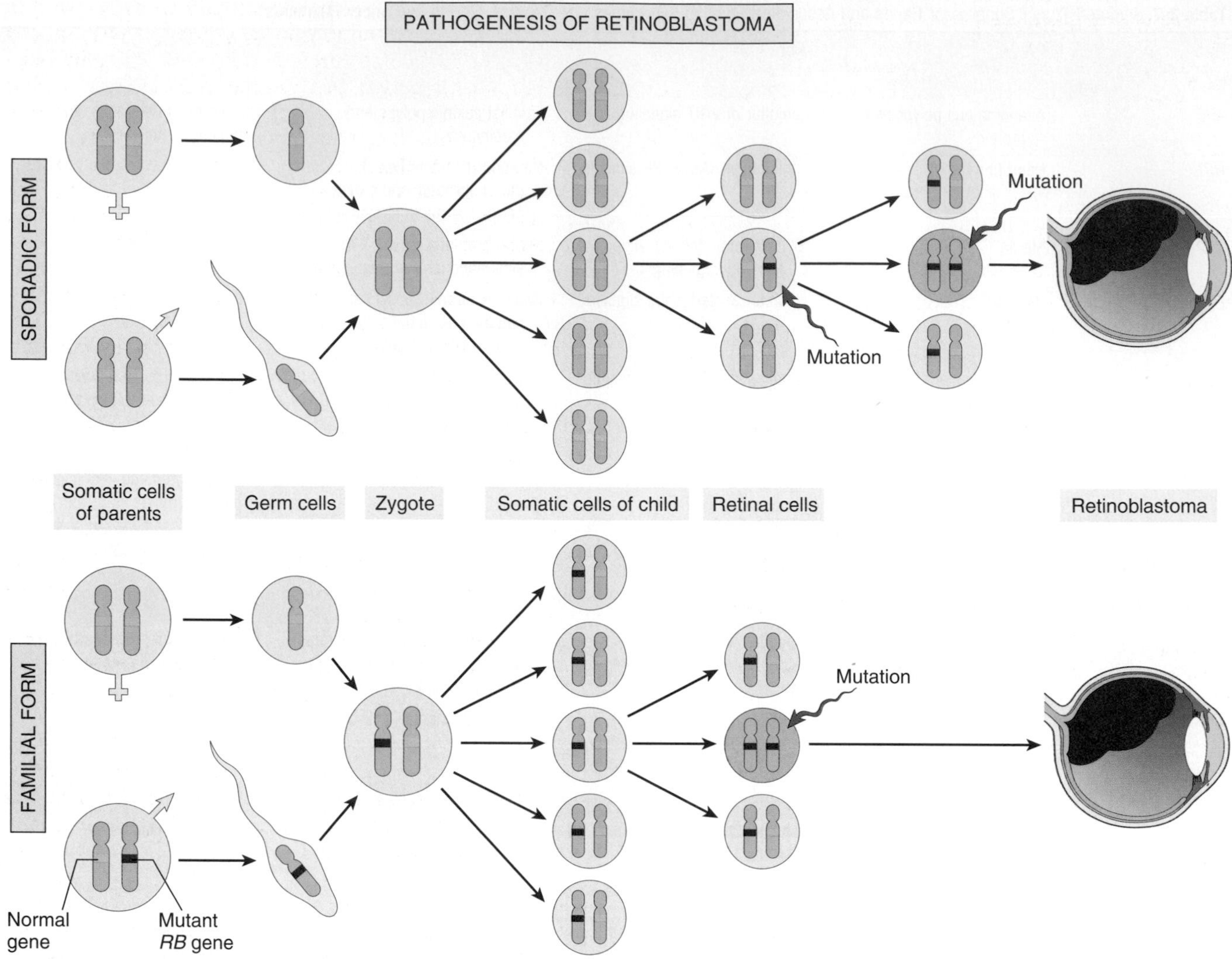

Figure 7-28 Pathogenesis of retinoblastoma. Two mutations of the *RB* locus on chromosome 13q14 lead to neoplastic proliferation of the retinal cells. In the sporadic form, both *RB* mutations in the tumor-founding retinal cell are acquired. In the familial form, all somatic cells inherit one mutated copy of *RB* gene from a carrier parent, and as a result only one additional *RB* mutation in a retinal cell is required for complete loss of RB function.

functions are listed in Table 7-7. Note that while tumor suppressors were initially thought of narrowly as proteins that put the brakes on cell cycle progression and DNA replication, it is now appreciated that some tumor suppressors prevent cellular transformation through other mechanisms, such as by altering cell metabolism (e.g., the serine-threonine kinase STK11, discussed later) or by ensuring genomic stability (e.g., the DNA repair factors BRCA1 and BRCA2). Thus, while most tumor suppressors have inhibitory effects on cell growth through one mechanism or another, a more inclusive definition of a tumor suppressor is simply a protein or gene that is associated with suppression of any of the various hallmarks of cancer.

We next consider consider how the major tumor suppressors function, focusing on those that are most frequently mutated in cancer or that highlight pathogenically important molecular mechanisms.

RB: Governor of Proliferation. **RB, a key negative regulator of the G_1/S cell cycle transition, is directly or indirectly inactivated in most human cancers.** RB also controls cellular differentiation. It exists in an active hypophosphorylated state in quiescent cells and an inactive hyperphosphorylated state in cells passing through the G_1/S cell cycle transition (Chapter 1). RB function may be compromised in two different ways:

- Loss-of-function mutations involving both *RB* alleles
- A shift from the active hypophosphorylated state to the inactive hyperphosphorylated state by gain-of-function mutations that upregulate CDK/cyclin D activity or by loss-of-function mutations that abrogate the activity of CDK inhibitors

As discussed previously, the decision of a cell to progress from G_1 into S is of great importance, since once a cell enters the S phase it is obligated to complete mitosis. High levels of CDK4/cyclin D, CDK6/cyclin D, and CDK2/cyclin E complexes lead to hyperphosphorylation and inhibition of RB, releasing E2F transcription factors that drive the expression of genes that are needed for progression to S phase (Fig. 7-29). Growth factor signaling pathways generally upregulate the activity of CDK/cyclin complexes

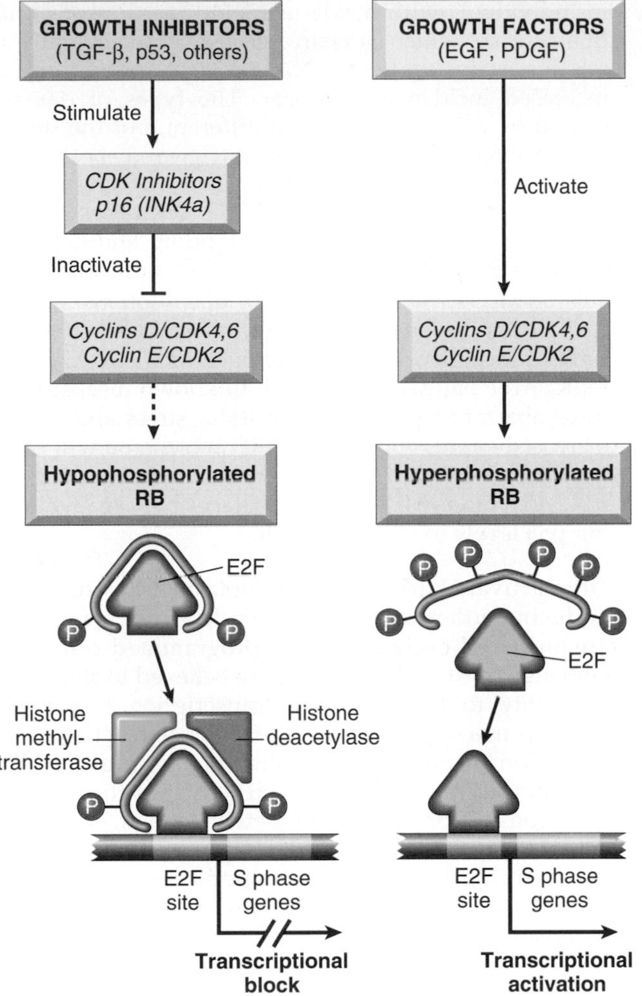

Figure 7-29 The role of RB in regulating the G_1-S checkpoint of the cell cycle. Hypophosphorylated RB in complex with the E2F transcription factors binds to DNA, recruits chromatin-remodeling factors (histone deacetylases and histone methyltransferases), and inhibits transcription of genes whose products are required for the S phase of the cell cycle. When RB is phosphorylated by the cyclin D-CDK4, cyclin D-CDK6, and cyclin E-CDK2 complexes, it releases E2F. The latter then activates transcription of S-phase genes. The phosphorylation of RB is inhibited by cyclin-dependent kinase inhibitors, because they inactivate cyclin-CDK complexes. Virtually all cancer cells show dysregulation of the G_1-S checkpoint as a result of mutation in one of four genes that regulate the phosphorylation of RB; these genes are *RB, CDK4*, the genes encoding cyclin D proteins, and *CDKN2A* (p16). TGF-β, transforming growth factor-β.

and drive cells through the G_1/S transition, whereas growth inhibitors tip the balance the other way by upregulating CDK inhibitors. RB is the point of integration of these opposing signals, making it a key player in regulation of cell cycle progression.

It was mentioned previously that germline and somatic loss-of-function mutations of the *RB* gene are associated with retinoblastoma and osteosarcoma, and analyses of cancer cell genomes have identified similar somatic *RB* mutations in a subset of glioblastomas, small-cell carcinomas of lung, breast cancers, and bladder carcinomas. However, given that RB is expressed in all cells, one may ask, why do patients with germline *RB* mutations preferentially develop only a few types of cancer? And, conversely, why aren't acquired mutations of *RB* found in all kinds of cancer? The reason why persons who inherit one defective allele of *RB* preferentially develop retinoblastoma is not understood, but a possible explanation is that other RB family members exist that may partially complement RB function in cell types other than retinoblasts.

With respect to the second question (i.e., why mutations of *RB* are not more widespread in human tumors), the answer is much simpler: mutations in other genes that control RB phosphorylation can mimic the effect of *RB* loss, and such genes are mutated in many cancers that have normal *RB* genes. Thus, for example, mutational activation of cyclin D or CDK4 and mutational inactivation of CDK inhibitors favors cell proliferation by facilitating the hyperphosphorylation and inactivation of RB. The current paradigm is that **loss of normal cell cycle control is central to malignant transformation and that at least one of four key regulators of the cell cycle (p16/INK4a, cyclin D, CDK4, RB) is dysregulated in the vast majority of human cancers**. In cells that harbor mutations in any one of these other genes, or in upstream factors that regulate their expression and function (e.g., receptor tyrosine kinases, RAS), RB may be functionally inactivated even if the *RB* gene itself is not mutated.

The transforming proteins of several oncogenic animal and human DNA viruses also act, in part, by neutralizing the growth-inhibitory activities of RB. In these cases, the RB protein is functionally inactivated by the binding of a viral protein and no longer acts as a cell cycle inhibitor. Simian virus 40 and polyomavirus large T antigens, adenovirus EIA protein, and HPV E7 protein all bind to the hypophosphorylated form of RB. The binding occurs in the same RB pocket that normally sequesters E2F transcription factors. Of note, in the case of HPV, viral types (such as HPV16) that confer a high risk for the development of cervical carcinoma express E7 protein variants with higher affinity for RB than do lower risk viral types. Thus, the RB protein, unable to bind the E2F transcription factors, is functionally inactivated by these viral oncoproteins, and the E2F factors are free to cause cell cycle progression.

KEY CONCEPTS

RB, Governor of the Cell Cycle

- When hypophosphorylated, RB exerts antiproliferative effects by binding and inhibiting E2F transcription factors that regulate genes required for cells to pass through the G1-S phase cell cycle checkpoint. Normal growth factor signaling leads to RB hyperphosphorylation and inactivation, thus promoting cell cycle progression.
- The antiproliferative effect of RB is abrogated in cancers through a variety of mechanisms, including:
  - Loss-of-function mutations affecting *RB*
  - Gene amplifications of CDK4 and cyclin D genes
  - Loss of cyclin-dependent kinase inhibitors (p16/INK4a)
  - Viral oncoproteins that bind and inhibit RB (E7 protein of HPV)

TP53*: *Guardian of the Genome. ***TP53*, a tumor suppressor gene that regulates cell cycle progression, DNA repair, cellular senescence, and apoptosis, is the most frequently mutated gene in human cancers.** Loss-of-function mutations in *TP53*, located on chromosome 17p13.1, are found in more than 50% of cancers. Moreover, *TP53* mutations occur with some frequency in virtually every type of cancer, including carcinomas of the lung, colon, and breast—the three leading causes of cancer death. In most cases, mutations are present in both *TP53* alleles and are acquired in somatic cells (not inherited in the germline). Less commonly, individuals inherit one mutated *TP53* allele. As in the case of the *RB* tumor suppressor and retinoblastoma, inheritance of a mutated copy of *TP53* predisposes individuals to malignant tumors because only one additional "hit" in the lone normal allele is needed to abrogate *TP53* function. Such individuals, said to have the *Li-Fraumeni syndrome*, have a 25-fold greater chance of developing a malignant tumor by age 50 than the general population. In contrast to individuals who inherit a mutant *RB* allele, the spectrum of tumors that develop in persons with the Li-Fraumeni syndrome is quite varied; the most common types of tumors are sarcomas, breast cancer, leukemias, brain tumors, and carcinomas of the adrenal cortex. People with the Li-Fraumeni syndrome often develop cancer at younger ages and are more likely to suffer from multiple primary tumors of varying types than are normal individuals.

These mutational data, while impressive, only begin to tell the tale of altered *TP53* function in cancer. *TP53* encodes the protein p53, which is tightly regulated at several levels. Analogous to RB, many tumors lacking *TP53* mutations have instead other mutations affecting proteins that regulate p53 function. For example, MDM2 and related proteins of the MDM2 family stimulate the degradation of p53; these proteins are frequently overexpressed in malignancies with normal *TP53* alleles. Indeed, the *MDM2* gene is amplified in 33% of human sarcomas, leading to a functional deficiency of p53 in these tumors. Also like RB, the transforming proteins of several DNA viruses bind p53 and promote its degradation. Best known of these viral oncoproteins is the E6 protein of high-risk human papilloma viruses, which have causative roles in cervical carcinoma and a subset of squamous cell carcinomas of the head and neck.

The frequent loss of p53 function in human tumors reflects its critical role in prevention of cancer development. p53 carries out this role by serving as the focal point of a large network of signals that sense cellular stress, primarily DNA damage, but also shortened telomeres, hypoxia, and stress caused by excessive pro-growth signaling, as may occur in cells bearing mutations in genes such as RAS and MYC. In nonstressed, healthy cells, p53 is held at bay through its aforementioned association with MDM2, an enzyme that ubiquitinylates p53, leading to its degradation by the proteasome. As a result, p53 is virtually undetectable in normal cells. In stressed cells, however, p53 is released from the inhibitory effects of MDM2 via two major mechanisms, which vary depending on the nature of the stress (Fig. 7-30).

- *DNA damage and hypoxia.* The key initiators of p53 activation following DNA damage or in cells exposed to hypoxia are two related protein kinases, ataxia-telangiectasia mutated (ATM) and ataxia-telangiectasia and Rad3 related (ATR). As the name implies, the *ATM* gene was originally identified as the germline mutation in individuals with ataxia-telangiectasia. Persons with this disease, which is characterized by an inability to repair certain kinds of DNA damage, suffer from an increased incidence of cancer. The types of damage sensed by ATM and ATR are different, but the downstream effects are similar. Once triggered, both ATM and ATR stimulate the phosphorylation of a number of proteins, including p53 and MDM2. These posttranslational modifications disrupt the binding and degradation of p53 by MDM2, allowing p53 to accumulate.
- *"Oncogenic" stress.* Activation of oncoproteins such as RAS leads to sustained, supraphysiologic signaling through pro-growth pathways such as the MAPK and PI3K/AKT pathways. Through unknown mechanisms, these aberrant signals create cellular stress and lead to increased expression of p14/ARF, which you will recall is encoded by the *CDKN2A* tumor suppressor gene. p14/ARF binds MDM2 and displaces p53, again allowing p53 levels to rise in the cell.

Once activated, p53 thwarts neoplastic transformation by inducing either transient cell cycle arrest, senescence (permanent cell cycle arrest), or programmed cell death (apoptosis). Most of these effects are believed to stem from p53's ability to function as a transcription factor. p53 binds DNA in a sequence-specific fashion and activates the transcription of hundreds of different target genes with p53-binding elements. The key target genes that execute the functions of p53 are not completely defined, but appear to fall into three major categories: (1) those that cause cell cycle arrest; (2) those that cause apoptosis; and (3) those that enhance catabolic metabolism or inhibit anabolic metabolism. The latter group of genes makes intuitive sense; there is no need for a cell that has stopped its cell cycle progression to continue to synthesize the large amounts of macromolecules (e.g., lipids and proteins) that are needed for cell growth and division. Also included in the list of p53 target genes are those encoding two kinds of regulatory RNAs, micro-RNA (mIRs) and long intervening noncoding (LINC) RNAs, which presumably help to coordinate the p53-dependent cellular response to stress.

Once p53 accumulates in a cell to levels that are sufficient to activate the transcription of target genes, several different outcomes are possible, each more serious than the last with respect to the ultimate fate of the affected cell:

- **Transient p53-induced cell cycle arrest.** Rapid onset, p53-mediated cell cycle arrest may be considered a primordial response to DNA damage. It occurs late in the G_1 phase and is caused in part by p53-dependent transcription of the *CDKN1A* gene, which encodes the CDK inhibitor p21. As discussed, p21 inhibits CDK4/D cyclin complexes, thereby maintaining RB in an active, hypophosphorylated state and blocking the progression of cells from G_1 phase to S phase. This pause in cell cycling is welcome, as it gives the cells "breathing time" to repair DNA damage. p53 also helps the process by inducing certain proteins, such as GADD45 (growth arrest and DNA damage), that enhance DNA repair. If DNA damage is repaired successfully, the signals responsible for p53 stabilization cease and p53 levels fall, releasing the cell cycle block. The cells may then revert to a normal state.

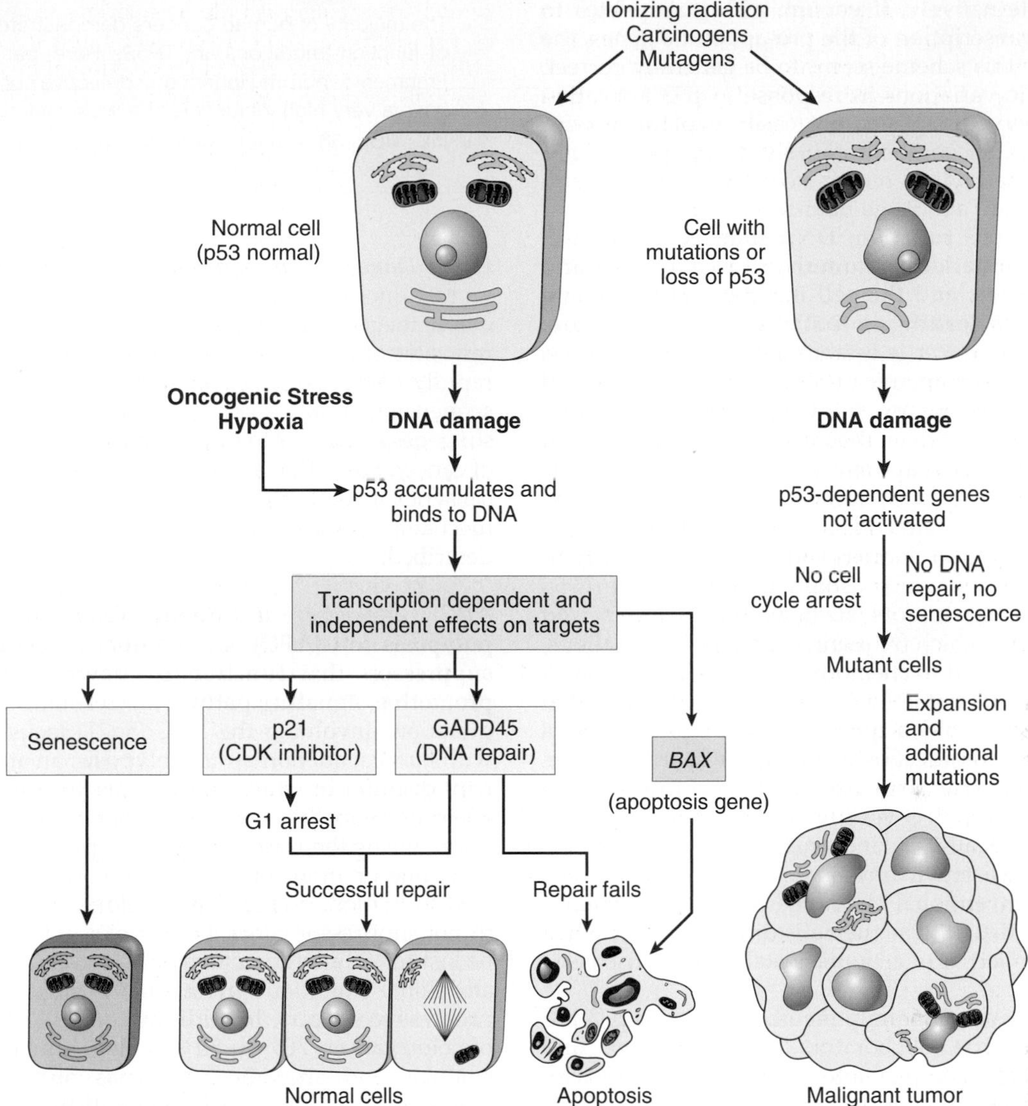

Figure 7-30 The role of p53 in maintaining the integrity of the genome. Activation of normal p53 by DNA-damaging agents or by hypoxia leads to cell cycle arrest in G_1 and induction of DNA repair by transcriptional upregulation of the cyclin-dependent kinase inhibitor *CDKN1A* (encoding the cyclin-dependent kinase inhibitor p21) and the *GADD45* genes. Successful repair of DNA allows cells to proceed with the cell cycle; if DNA repair fails, p53 triggers either apoptosis or senescence. In cells with loss or mutations of the p53 gene, DNA damage does not induce cell cycle arrest or DNA repair, and genetically damaged cells proliferate, giving rise eventually to malignant neoplasms.

- **p53-induced senescence.** Senescence is a state of permanent cell cycle arrest characterized by specific changes in morphology and gene expression that differentiate it from reversible cell cycle arrest. How cells become fixed in the senescence state is unclear. One plausible idea is that senescence is the product of epigenetic changes that result in the formation of heterochromatin at key loci, including genes that are required for progression of cells from the G_1 phase into S phase. Like other p53 responses, senescence may be stimulated in response to a variety of stresses, such as unopposed oncogene signaling, hypoxia, and shortened telomeres. The senescent cells, while not normal, are blocked from developing into tumors.
- **p53-induced apoptosis.** Apoptosis of cells with irreversible DNA damage is the ultimate protective mechanism against neoplastic transformation. p53 directs the transcription of several pro-apoptotic genes such as *BAX* and *PUMA* (described later), which are believed to tip the balance in favor of cell death via the intrinsic (mitochondrial) pathway.

What determines whether a cell repairs its DNA, becomes senescent, or undergoes apoptosis is uncertain, but both the duration and the level of p53 activation may be deciding factors. It appears that the affinity of p53 for its binding sites in the promoters and enhancers of DNA-repair genes is higher than its affinity for binding sites in pro-apoptotic genes. Thus, the DNA-repair pathway is stimulated first as p53 begins to accumulate. If p53 is sustained at this level due to ineffective DNA repair or other chronic stresses (e.g., that induced by a potentially oncogenic RAS mutation), epigenetic silencing of genes that are needed for cell cycle progression occurs, leading to senescence. Alternatively, if enough p53 accumulates to stimulate the transcription of the pro-apoptotic genes, the cell dies. While this scheme seems to be generally correct, cell-type-specific variations in response to p53 activation have been observed that are not easily explained, with some cell types succumbing rapidly to apoptosis, and others opting mainly for senescence. Thus, there is still much to be learned about the nuances of p53 function.

With loss of p53 function, DNA damage goes unrepaired, driver mutations accumulate in oncogenes and other cancer genes, and the cell marches blindly along a dangerous path leading to malignant transformation. Moreover, once a cancer is established, its p53 status has several important therapeutic implications. Irradiation and conventional chemotherapy, the two common modalities of cancer treatment, mediate their effects by inducing DNA damage and subsequent apoptosis. Tumors with wild type *TP53* alleles are more likely to be killed by such therapy than tumors with mutated *TP53* alleles. Such is the case with testicular teratocarcinomas and childhood acute lymphoblastic leukemias, which usually have wild type *TP53* alleles. In contrast, tumors such as lung cancers and colorectal cancers, which frequently carry *TP53* mutations, are relatively resistant to chemotherapy and irradiation. A second less obvious but even more nefarious result is that cells with defective p53 acquire a mutator phenotype, a tendency to acquire additional mutations at a high rate. Particularly in patients with advanced stage tumors with mutator phenotypes, it is very likely (and perhaps inevitable) that genetically distinct subclones will arise by chance that are resistant to any single therapy, whether this be radiation, conventional chemotherapy, or molecularly targeted cancer drugs. This theme is discussed later when the enabling properties of genomic instability are discussed more broadly.

The discovery of p53 family members p63 and p73 has revealed that p53 has collaborators. Indeed, p53, p63, and p73 are players in a complex interconnected network with significant crosstalk that is still being unraveled. p53 is ubiquitously expressed, while p63 and p73 show more tissue specificity. For example, p63 is essential for the differentiation of stratified squamous epithelia, while p73 has strong pro-apoptotic effects after DNA damage induced by chemotherapeutic agents.

KEY CONCEPTS

p53, Guardian of the Genome

- The p53 protein is the central monitor of stress in the cell and can be activated by anoxia, inappropriate signaling by mutated oncoproteins, or DNA damage. p53 controls the expression and activity of proteins involved in cell cycle arrest, DNA repair, cellular senescence, and apoptosis.
- DNA damage is sensed by complexes containing kinases of the ATM/ATR family; these kinases phosphorylate p53, liberating it from inhibitors such as MDM2. Active p53 then upregulates the expression of proteins such as the cyclin-dependent kinase inhibitor p21, thereby causing cell-cycle arrest at the G1-S checkpoint. This pause allows cells to repair DNA damage.
- If DNA damage cannot be repaired, p53 induces additional events that lead to cellular senescence or apoptosis.
- The majority of human cancers demonstrate biallelic loss-of-function mutations in *TP53*. Rare patients with Li-Fraumeni syndrome inherit one defective copy of *TP53* and have a very high incidence of a wide variety of cancers.
- Like RB, p53 is inactivated by viral oncoproteins, such as the E6 protein of HPV

Other Tumor Suppressor Genes. There is little doubt that more tumor suppressor genes remain to be discovered. Often, their location is suspected by the detection of recurrent sites of chromosomal deletions, which are now being rapidly identified and characterized by high throughput sequencing of cancer genomes. The known tumor suppressor genes all appear to impact one of more of the hallmarks of cancer. Some that are associated with well-defined clinical syndromes (Table 7-7) or that serve to highlight various mechanisms by which tumor suppressors function are described:

APC: Gatekeeper of Colonic Neoplasia. **Adenomatous polyposis coli (APC) is a member of the class of tumor suppressors that function by downregulating growth-promoting signaling pathways.** Germline loss-of-function mutations involving the *APC* (5q21) locus are associated with familial adenomatous polyposis, an autosomal dominant disorder in which individuals born with one mutant allele develop thousands of adenomatous polyps in the colon during their teens or 20s (Chapter 17). Almost invariably, one or more of these polyps undergoes malignant transformation, giving rise to colon cancer. As with other tumor suppressor genes, both copies of the *APC* gene must be lost for an adenoma to arise. As discussed later, several additional mutations must then occur for adenomas to progress to cancers. In addition to these hereditary forms of colon cancer, 70% to 80% of nonfamilial colorectal carcinomas and sporadic adenomas also show acquired defects involving both *APC* genes, firmly implicating *APC* loss of function in the pathogenesis of colonic tumors.

APC is a component of the WNT signaling pathway, which has a major role in controlling cell fate, adhesion, and cell polarity during embryonic development (Fig. 7-31). WNT signals through a family of cell surface receptors called frizzled (FRZ), and stimulates several pathways, the central one involving β-catenin and APC. A major function of the APC protein is to hold β-catenin activity in check. In the absence of WNT signaling, APC causes degradation of β-catenin, preventing its accumulation in the cytoplasm. APC does so by forming a macromolecular "destruction" complex that leads to the proteasomal degradation of β-catenin. Signaling by WNT blocks the formation of the destruction complex, stabilizing β-catenin and allowing it to translocate from the cytoplasm to the nucleus. Once in the nucleus β-catenin forms a transcription activation complex with the DNA-binding factor TCF. The β-catenin/TCF complex promotes the growth of colonic epithelial cells by increasing the transcription of *MYC*, *cyclin D1*, and other genes. Because inactivation of the *APC* gene disrupts the destruction complex, β-catenin survives and translocates to the nucleus, where it activates the transcription of pro-growth target genes in cooperation with TCF. Thus, cells that lose APC behave as if they are

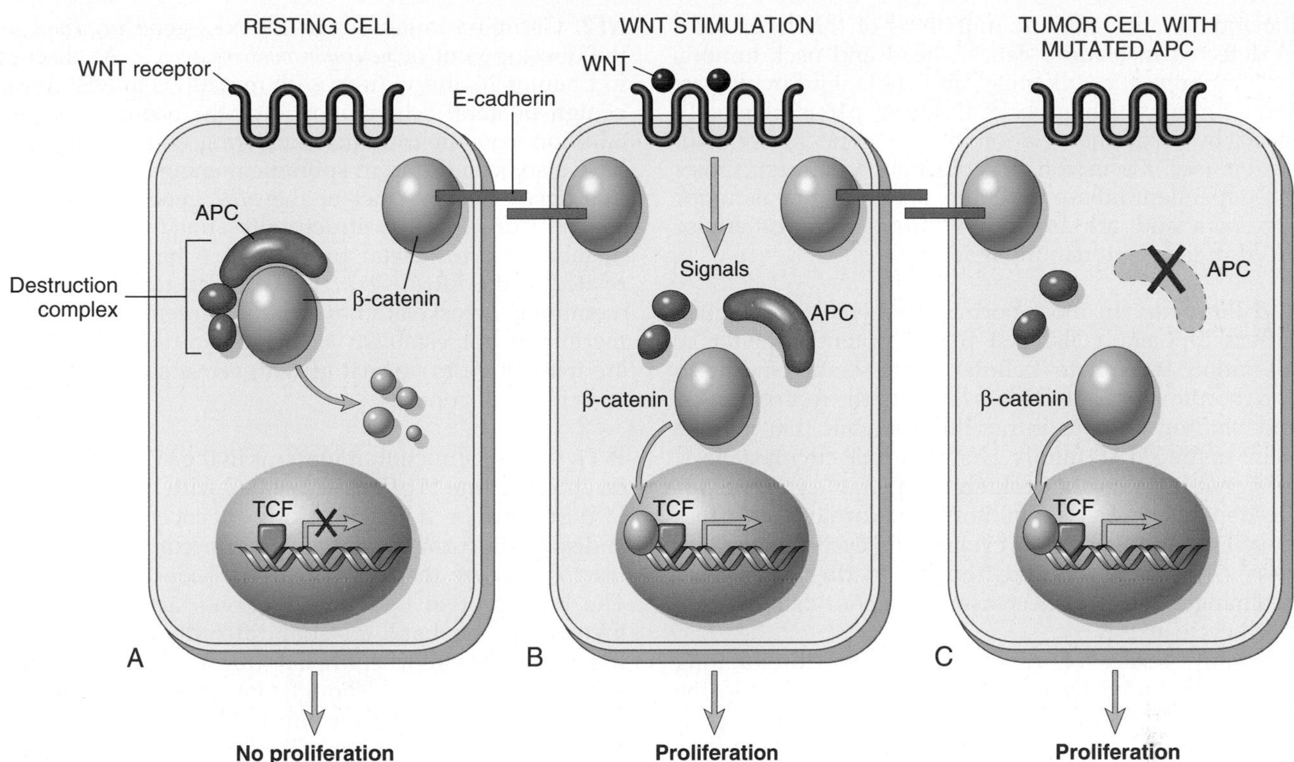

Figure 7-31 The role of APC in regulating the stability and function of β-catenin. APC and β-catenin are components of the WNT signaling pathway. **A,** In resting colonic epithelial cells (not exposed to WNT), β-catenin forms a macromolecular complex containing the APC protein. This complex leads to the destruction of β-catenin, and intracellular levels of β-catenin are low. **B,** When normal colonic epithelial cells are stimulated by WNT molecules, the *destruction complex* is deactivated, β-catenin degradation does not occur, and cytoplasmic levels increase. β-catenin translocates to the nucleus, where it binds to TCF, a transcription factor that activates genes involved in cell cycle progression. **C,** When *APC* is mutated or absent, as frequently occurs in colonic polyps and cancers, the destruction of β-catenin cannot occur. β-catenin translocates to the nucleus and coactivates genes that promote entry into the cell cycle, and cells behave as if they are under constant stimulation by the WNT pathway.

being continuously stimulated by WNT. The importance of the APC/β-catenin signaling pathway in tumorigenesis is attested to by the fact that many colon tumors with normal *APC* genes harbor mutations in β-catenin that prevent its APC-dependent destruction, allowing the mutant protein to accumulate in the nucleus and stimulate transcription. Thus, β-catenin, the target of APC, is itself a proto-oncoprotein. Dysregulation of the APC/β-catenin pathway is not restricted to colon cancers; for example, gain-of-function mutations in β-catenin are present in more than 50% of hepatoblastomas and in approximately 20% of hepatocellular carcinomas.

E-Cadherin. β-catenin binds to the cytoplasmic tail of E-cadherin, a cell surface protein that maintains intercellular adhesiveness. Loss of cell-cell contact, such as in a wound or injury to the epithelium, disrupts the interaction between E-cadherin and β-catenin, and also promotes increased translocation of β-catenin to the nucleus, where it stimulates genes that promote proliferation; this is an appropriate response to injury that can help repair the wound. Reestablishment of these E-cadherin contacts as the wound heals leads to β-catenin again being sequestered at the membrane and reduces in the proliferative signal; these cells are said to be "contact-inhibited." Loss-of-contact inhibition, by mutation of the E-cadherin/β-catenin axis, or by other changes, is a key characteristic of carcinomas. Furthermore, loss of E-cadherin can contribute to the malignant phenotype by allowing easy disaggregation of cells, which can then invade locally or metastasize. Reduced cell surface expression of E-cadherin has been noted in many carcinomas, including those that arise in the esophagus, colon, breast, ovary, and prostate. Germline loss-of-function mutations of the E-cadherin gene, known as *CDH1*, cause familial gastric carcinoma, and a variable proportion of sporadic gastric carcinomas are also associated with loss of E-cadherin expression. The molecular basis of reduced E-cadherin expression in sporadic cancers is varied. In a small proportion of cases, there are mutations in the E-cadherin gene (located on 16q); in other cancers, E-cadherin expression is reduced as a secondary effect of activating mutations in β-catenin genes. Additionally, E-cadherin may be downregulated by transcription repressors, such as SNAIL, that are implicated in epithelial-to-mesenchymal transition and metastasis (discussed later).

CDKN2A. The *CDKN2A* gene locus encodes two protein products: the p16/INK4a cyclin-dependent kinase inhibitor, which blocks CDK4/cyclin D-mediated phosphorylation of RB, thereby reinforcing the RB checkpoint; and p14/ARF, which activates the p53 pathway by inhibiting MDM2 and preventing destruction of p53. Thus, mutation or silencing of *CDKN2A* impacts both the RB and p53 tumor suppressor pathways. p16 also appears to be important in induction of cellular senescence (described later). Germline mutations in *CDKN2A* are associated with familial forms of melanoma, and sporadic mutations of this locus have been detected in bladder cancer, head and neck tumors, acute lymphoblastic leukemias, and cholangiocarcinomas. In some tumors, such as cervical cancer, p16 is frequently silenced by hypermethylation of the gene rather than mutation (see discussion of epigenetic changes). Other cyclin-dependent kinase inhibitors also function as tumor suppressors and are frequently mutated or otherwise silenced in many human malignancies.

TGF-β Pathway. In most normal epithelial, endothelial, and hematopoietic cells, TGF-β is a potent inhibitor of proliferation. It regulates cellular processes by binding to TGF-β receptors I and II. Dimerization of the receptor upon ligand binding initiates intracellular signals that involve proteins of the SMAD family. Under normal circumstances, these signals turn on antiproliferative genes (e.g., genes for cyclin-dependent kinase inhibitors) and turn off genes that drive cell growth (e.g., *MYC*, cyclins, and cyclin-dependent kinases). As can be inferred from our earlier discussion, these changes result in decreased phosphorylation of RB and cell cycle arrest.

In many forms of cancer these growth-inhibiting effects are impaired by loss-of-function mutations in the TGF-β signaling pathway. Mutations affecting the type II TGF-β receptor are common in cancers of the colon, stomach, and endometrium, while mutational inactivation of SMAD4 is common in pancreatic cancers. In many other cancers, loss of TGF-β-mediated growth inhibition occurs at the level of key target genes; examples include mutations that lead to loss of p21 function and/or persistent expression of *MYC*. In such cases other preserved elements of the TGF-β-induced program of gene expression may actually facilitate acquisition of cancer hallmarks, such as immune evasion or angiogenesis. Thus TGF-β signaling is a double-edged sword that can prevent or promote tumor growth, depending on the state of other genes in the cell.

PTEN. PTEN (*p*hosphatase and *ten*sin homologue) is a membrane-associated phosphatase encoded by a gene on chromosome 10q23 that is mutated in Cowden syndrome, an autosomal dominant disorder marked by frequent benign growths, such as skin appendage tumors, and an increased incidence of epithelial cancers, particularly of the breast (Chapter 21), endometrium, and thyroid. As already mentioned, PTEN acts as a tumor suppressor by serving as a brake on the PI3K/AKT arm of the receptor tyrosine kinase pathway. *PTEN* gene function is lost in many cancers through deletion, deleterious point mutations, or epigenetic silencing.

NF1. Individuals who inherit one mutant allele of the *NF1* gene develop numerous benign neurofibromas and optic nerve gliomas as a result of inactivation of the second copy of the gene. This condition is called *neurofibromatosis type 1* (Chapter 26). Some of the neurofibromas later develop into malignant peripheral nerve sheath tumors. As already discussed, *Neurofibromin*, the protein product of the *NF1* gene, contains a GTPase-activating domain that acts as a brake on RAS signaling. With loss of neurofibromin function, RAS tends to become trapped in an active, signal-emitting state.

NF2. Germline mutations in the *NF2* gene predispose to the development of *neurofibromatosis type 2*. As discussed in Chapter 26, individuals with mutations in *NF2* develop benign bilateral schwannomas of the acoustic nerve. In addition, somatic mutations affecting both alleles of *NF2* have also been found in sporadic meningiomas and ependymomas. The product of the *NF2* gene, called *neurofibromin 2* or *merlin*, is structurally similar to the red cell membrane cytoskeletal protein 4.1 (Chapter 13), and is related to the ERM (ezrin, radixin, and moesin) family of membrane cytoskeleton-associated proteins. Cells lacking merlin do not establish stable cell-to-cell junctions and are insensitive to normal growth arrest signals generated by cell-to-cell contact.

WT1. Loss-of-function mutations in the *WT1* gene, located on chromosome 11p13, is associated with the development of Wilms tumor, a pediatric kidney cancer. Both inherited and sporadic forms of Wilms tumor occur, and mutational inactivation of the *WT1* locus is seen in both forms. The WT1 protein is a transcriptional activator of genes involved in renal and gonadal differentiation. It regulates the mesenchymal-to-epithelial transition that occurs in kidney development. Though not precisely known, it is likely that the tumorigenic effect of WT1 deficiency is intimately connected with the role of the gene in the differentiation of genitourinary tissues.

Interestingly, although WT1 is a tumor suppressor in Wilms' tumor, a variety of adult cancers, including leukemias and breast carcinomas, overexpress WT1. Since these tissues do not normally express WT1 at all, *WT1* may function as an oncogene in these cancers. Thus, some genes that regulate development may act as a tumor suppressor in one epigenetic context (e.g., *WT1* in a renal progenitor cell) and an oncogene in a second (e.g., *WT1* in a hematopoietic stem cell), an example of "crosstalk" between genes and the epigenome that we discuss later.

PATCHED (PTCH). *PTCH1* is a tumor suppressor gene that encodes a cell membrane protein called PATCHED1. PATCHED proteins are negative regulators of the Hedgehog signaling pathway. Under normal circumstances, binding of soluble factors belonging to the Hedgehog family to PATCH receptors relieves this negative regulation and activates the pathway, which stimulates downstream transcription factors. In the absence of PATCHED proteins, there is unopposed Hedgehog signaling that increases the expression of a number of pro-growth genes, including *NMYC* and D cyclins. Germline loss-of-function mutations in *PTCH1* cause Gorlin syndrome, an inherited condition also known as nevoid basal cell carcinoma syndrome (Chapter 26) that is associated with greatly increased risks of basal cell carcinoma of the skin and of medulloblastoma, an aggressive cerebellar tumor that arises in children or adolescents. *PTCH1* mutations are also present in 20% to 50% of sporadic cases of basal cell carcinoma and 10% to 25% of sporadic cases of medulloblastoma. About one half of such mutations in basal cell carcinomas are of the type caused by UV exposure. Hedgehog pathway antagonists have been developed and are approved for treatment of advanced basal cell carcinoma, and are also being tested in medulloblastoma and other tumors associated with Hedgehog pathway activation.

VHL. **Germline loss-of-function mutations of the von Hippel-Lindau (*VHL*) gene on chromosome 3p are associated with hereditary renal cell cancers, pheochromocytomas, hemangioblastomas of the central nervous system, retinal angiomas, and renal cysts.** Mutations of the *VHL* gene have also been noted in sporadic renal cell cancers (Chapter 20). The VHL protein is a component of a ubiquitin ligase, a type of protein complex that covalently links ubiquitin chains to specific protein substrates, thereby promoting their degradation by the proteasome. A critical substrate for the VHL ubiquitin ligase is the transcription factor HIF1α (hypoxia-inducible transcription factor 1α). In the presence of oxygen, HIF1α is hydroxylated and binds to VHL, leading to its ubiquitination and degradation. In hypoxic environments the hydroxylation reaction does not occur, and HIF1α escapes recognition by VHL. As a result HIF1α accumulates in the nuclei of hypoxic cells and turns on many target genes, including genes encoding the growth/angiogenic factors vascular endothelial growth factor (VEGF) and PDGF, the glucose transporter GLUT1, and several glycolytic enzymes. Loss-of-function mutations in VHL also prevent the ubiquitination and degradation of HIF1α, even under normoxic conditions, and are accordingly associated with increased levels of angiogenic growth factors and alterations in cellular metabolism that favor growth.

STK11. **The *STK11* gene, also known as *LKB1*, encodes a serine/threonine kinase that is an important regulator of cellular metabolism.** Loss-of-function mutations of *STK11* give rise to Peutz-Jeghers syndrome, an autosomal dominant disorder associated with benign polyps of the gastrointestinal tract and an increased risk of multiple epithelial cancers, particularly gastrointestinal and pancreatic carcinomas. The function of *STK11* is still being elucidated, but it appears to have pleiotropic effects on multiple facets of cellular metabolism, including glucose uptake, gluconeogenesis, protein synthesis, mitochondrial biogenesis, and lipid metabolism. Sporadic mutations causing *STK11* loss-of-function are found in diverse carcinomas, a finding pointing to the important role of altered cellular metabolism in the establishment and maintenance of the transformed state (discussed later).

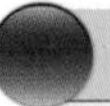

KEY CONCEPTS

Mechanism of Action of Major Tumor Suppressor Genes

APC: encodes a factor that negatively regulates the WNT pathway in colonic epithelium by promoting the formation of a complex that degrades β-catenin

- Mutated in familial adenomatous polyposis, autosomal dominant disorder associated with development of thousands of colonic polyps and early onset colon carcinoma; tumor development associated with loss of the single normal *APC* allele
- Mutated in about 70% of sporadic colon carcinomas; tumor development associated with acquired biallelic defects in *APC*

E-cadherin: cell adhesion molecule that plays an important role in contact-mediated growth inhibition of epithelial cells; also binds and sequesters β-catenin, a signaling protein that functions in the WNT pathway

- Germline loss-of-function mutations in the E-cadherin gene (*CDH1*) associated with autosomal dominant familial gastric carcinoma
- Loss of expression seen in many sporadic carcinomas; associated with loss of contact inhibition, loss of cohesiveness, increased invasiveness, and increased WNT signaling

CDKN2A: complex locus that encodes two tumor suppressive proteins, p16/INK4a, a cyclin-dependent kinase inhibitor that augments RB function, and ARF, which stabilizes p53

- Germline loss-of-function mutations are associated with autosomal dominant familial melanoma
- Biallelic loss-of-function seen in diverse cancers, including leukemias, melanomas, and carcinomas

TGF-β *pathway*: potent inhibitor of cellular proliferation in normal tissues

- Frequent loss-of-function mutations involving TGF-β receptors (colon, stomach, endometrium) or downstream signal transducers (SMADs, pancreas) in diverse carcinomas
- Complex role in carcinogenesis; may also have a pro-oncogenic role by enhancing the immune evasiveness of tumors

PTEN: encodes a lipid phosphatase that is an important negative regulator of PI3K/AKT signaling

- Germline loss-of-function mutations associated with Cowden syndrome, autosomal dominant disorder associated with a high risk of breast and endometrial carcinoma
- Biallelic loss-of-function common in diverse cancers

NF1: encodes neurofibromin 1, a GTPase that acts as a negative regulator of RAS

- Germline loss-of-function mutations cause neurofibromatosis type 1, autosomal dominant disorder associated with a high risk of neurofibromas and malignant peripheral nerve sheath tumors

NF2: encodes neurofibromin 2 (merlin), a cytoskeletal protein involved in contact inhibition

- Germline loss-of-function mutations cause neurofibromatosis type 2, autosomal dominant disorder associated with a high risk of bilateral schwannomas

WT1: encodes a transcription factor that is required for normal development of genitourinary tissues

- Germline loss-of-function mutations associated with Wilms tumor, a pediatric kidney cancer; similar *WT1* mutations also found in sporadic Wilms tumor

PTCH1: encodes membrane receptor that is a negative regulator of the Hedgehog signaling pathway

- Germline loss-of-function mutations cause Gorlin syndrome, autosomal dominant disorder associated with a high risk of basal cell carcinoma and medulloblastoma

- Acquired biallelic loss-of-function mutations of *PTCH1* are seen frequently in sporadic basal cell carcinomas and medulloblastomas

VHL: encodes a component of a ubiquitin ligase that is responsible for degradation of hypoxia-induced factors (HIFs), transcription factors that alter gene expression in response to hypoxia

- Germline loss-of-function mutations cause von Hippel-Lindau syndrome, autosomal dominant disorder associated with a high risk of renal cell carcinoma and pheochromocytoma
- Acquired biallelic loss-of mutations are common in sporadic renal cell carcinoma

Growth-Promoting Metabolic Alterations: The Warburg Effect

Even in the presence of ample oxygen, cancer cells demonstrate a distinctive form of cellular metabolism characterized by high levels of glucose uptake and increased conversion of glucose to lactose (fermentation) via the glycolytic pathway. This phenomenon, called the *Warburg effect* and also known as *aerobic glycolysis*, has been recognized for many years (indeed, Otto Warburg received the Nobel Prize in 1931 for discovery of the effect that bears his name). Clinically, the "glucose-hunger" of tumors is used to visualize tumors via positron emission tomography (PET) scanning, in which patients are injected with ^{18}F-fluorodeoxyglucose, a nonmetabolizable derivative of glucose that is preferentially taken up into tumor cells (as well as normal, actively dividing tissues such as the bone marrow). Most tumors are PET-positive, and rapidly growing ones are markedly so.

Warburg's discovery was largely neglected for many years, but over the past decade metabolism has become one of the most active areas of cancer research. Metabolic pathways (like signaling pathways) in normal and cancer cells are still being elucidated and the details are complex, but at the heart of the Warburg effect lies a simple question: why is it advantageous for a cancer cell to rely on seemingly inefficient glycolysis (which generates two molecules of ATP per molecule of glucose) instead of oxidative phosphorylation (which generates up to 36 molecules of ATP per molecule of glucose)? While pondering this question, it is important to recognize that rapidly growing normal cells, such as in embryonic tissues, also rely on aerobic fermentation. Thus, "Warburg metabolism" is not cancer specific, but instead is a general property of growing cells that becomes "fixed" in cancer cells.

The answer to this riddle is simple: **aerobic glycolysis provides rapidly dividing tumor cells with metabolic intermediates that are needed for the synthesis of cellular components, whereas mitochondrial oxidative phosphorylation does not.** The reason growing cells rely on aerobic glycolysis becomes readily apparent when one considers that a growing cell has a strict biosynthetic requirement; it must duplicate all of its cellular components—DNA, RNA, proteins, lipid, and organelles—before it can divide and produce two daughter cells. Recall that the net effect of oxidative phosphorylation is to take a single molecule of glucose, $C_6H_{12}O_6$, and combine it with six molecules of O_2 to produce six molecules of H_2O and six molecules of CO_2, which are lost through respiration. Thus, while "pure" oxidative phosphorylation yields abundant ATP, it fails to produce any carbon moieties that can be used to build cellular components that are needed for growth (proteins, lipids, and nucleic acids). Even cells that are not actively growing must shunt some metabolic intermediates away from oxidative phosphorylation in order to synthesize macromolecules that are needed for cellular maintenance.

By contrast, in actively growing cells only a small fraction of the cellular glucose is shunted through the oxidative phosphorylation pathway, such that on average each molecule of glucose that is metabolized produces approximately four molecules of ATP (instead of the two molecules that would be produced by "pure" glycolysis"). Presumably, this balance in glucose utilization (heavily biased toward aerobic fermentation, with a bit of oxidative phosphorylation) hits a metabolic "sweet spot" that is optimal for growth. It follows that growing cells do rely on mitochondrial metabolism. However, the main function of mitochondria in growing cells is not to generate ATP, but rather to carry out reactions that generate metabolic intermediates that can be shunted off and used as precursors in the synthesis of cellular building blocks. For example, lipid biosynthesis requires acetyl-CoA, and acetyl-CoA is largely synthesized in growing cells from intermediates such as citrate that are generated in mitochondria.

So how is this profound reprogramming of metabolism, the Warburg effect, triggered in growing normal and malignant cells? As might be guessed, **metabolic reprogramming is produced by signaling cascades downstream of growth factor receptors, the very same pathways that are deregulated by mutations in oncogenes and tumors suppressor genes in cancers.** Thus, whereas in rapidly growing normal cells aerobic glycolysis ceases when the tissue is no longer growing, in cancer cells this reprogramming persists due to the action of oncogenes and the loss of tumor suppressor gene function. Some of the important points of crosstalk between pro-growth signaling factors and cellular metabolism are shown in Fig. 7-32 and include the following:

- **PI3K/AKT signaling**. PI3K/AKT signaling upregulates the activity of glucose transporters and multiple glycolytic enzymes, thus increasing glycolysis; promotes shunting of mitochondrial intermediates to pathways leading to lipid biosynthesis; and stimulates factors that are required for protein synthesis.
- **Receptor tyrosine kinase activity**. In addition to transmitting growth signals to the nucleus, receptor tyrosine kinase signaling also influences metabolism. Rapidly dividing cells, both normal and malignant, express the M2 isoform of pyruvate kinase, which catalyzes the last step in the glycolytic pathway, the conversion of phosphoenolpyruvate to pyruvate. Receptor tyrosine kinases phosphorylate the M2 isoform of pyruvate kinase, a modification that attenuates its enzymatic activity. This creates a damming effect that leads to the build-up of upstream glycolytic intermediates, which are siphoned off for synthesis of DNA, RNA, and protein. Of note, in contrast to growing tissues and cancer cells, post-mitotic tissues with high demand for ATP such as the brain

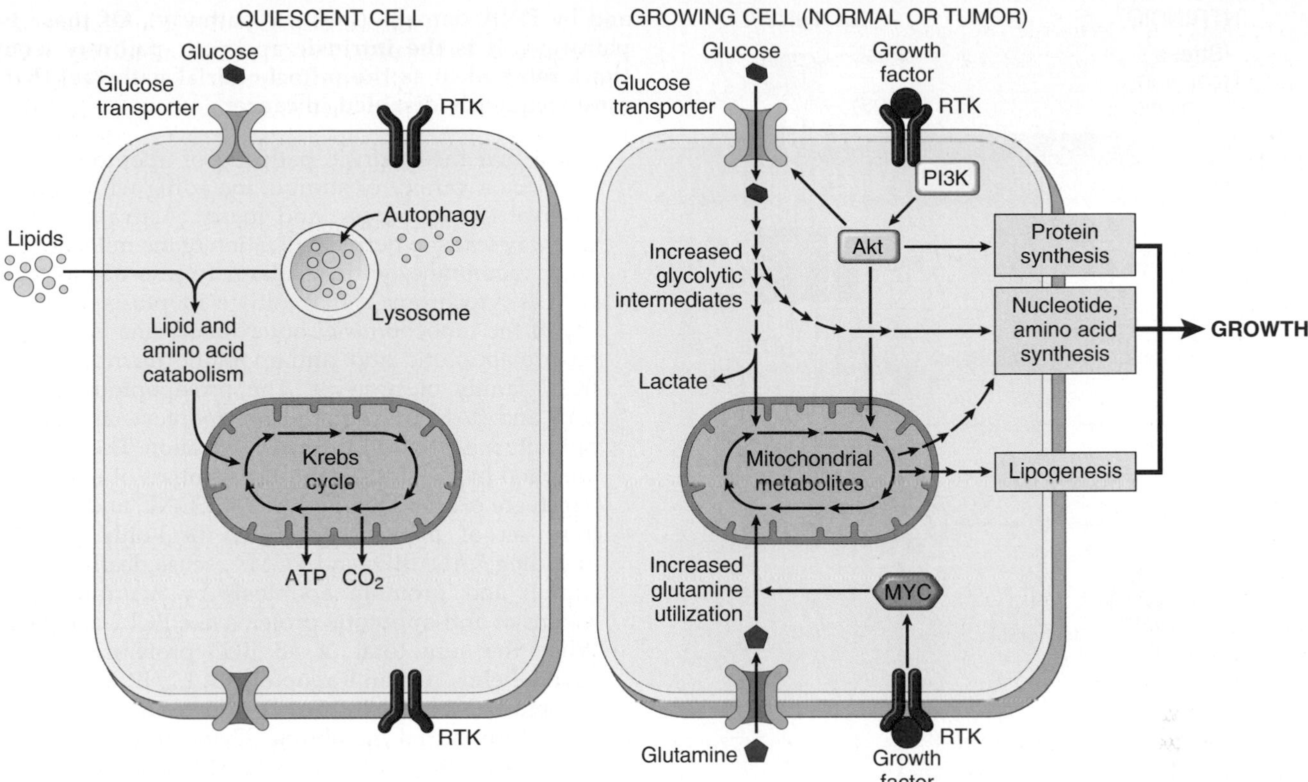

Figure 7-32 Metabolism and cell growth. Quiescent cells rely mainly on the Krebs cycle for ATP production; if starved, autophagy (self-eating) is induced to provide a source of fuel. When stimulated by growth factors, normal cells markedly upregulate glucose and glutamine uptake, which provide carbon sources for synthesis of nucleotides, proteins, and lipids. In cancers, oncogenic mutations involving growth factor signaling pathways and other key factors such as MYC deregulate these metabolic pathways, an alteration known as the *Warburg effect.*

express the M1 isoform of pyruvate kinase, which is insensitive to growth factor signaling pathways and efficiently funnels pyruvate, the last intermediate in the glycolytic pathway, into mitochondria where it is metabolized by oxidative phosphorylation to generate ATP, CO_2, and H_2O.

- **MYC**. As mentioned, pro-growth pathways upregulate expression of the transcription factor MYC, which drives changes in gene expression that support anabolic metabolism and cell growth. Among the most important metabolic factors that are upregulated by MYC are multiple glycolytic enzymes and glutaminase, which is required for mitochondrial utilization of glutamine.

The flipside of the coin is that tumor suppressors often inhibit metabolic pathways that support growth. We have already discussed the "braking" effect on PI3K/AKT signaling of PTEN, which opposes the Warburg effect, and how the STK11 tumor suppressor antagonizes metabolic changes that produce Warburg metabolism. Indeed, it may be that many (and perhaps all) tumor suppressors that induce growth arrest suppress the Warburg effect. For example, p53, arguably the most important tumor suppressor, upregulates target genes that collectively inhibit glucose uptake, glycolysis, lipogenesis, and the generation of NADPH (a key cofactor needed for the biosynthesis of macromolecules). Thus, it is increasingly clear that the functions of many oncoproteins and tumor suppressors are inextricably intertwined with cellular metabolism.

Autophagy. *Autophagy* is a state of severe nutrient deficiency in which cells not only arrest their growth, but also cannibalize their own organelles, proteins, and membranes as carbon sources for energy production (Chapter 2). If this adaptation fails, the cells die. Tumor cells often seem to be able to grow under marginal environmental conditions without triggering autophagy, suggesting that the pathways that induce autophagy are deranged. In keeping with this, several genes that promote autophagy are tumor suppressors. Whether autophagy is always bad from the vantage point of the tumor, however, remains a matter of active investigation and debate. For example, under conditions of severe nutrient deprivation tumor cells may use autophagy to become "dormant," a state of metabolic hibernation that allows cells to survive hard times for long periods. Such cells are believed to be resistant to therapies that kill actively dividing cells, and could therefore be responsible for therapeutic failures. Thus, autophagy may be a tumor's friend or foe depending on how the signaling pathways that regulate it are "wired" in a given tumor.

Evasion of Programmed Cell Death (Apoptosis)

Accumulation of neoplastic cells may result not only from activation of growth-promoting oncogenes or inactivation of growth-suppressing tumor suppressor genes, but also from mutations in the genes that regulate apoptosis. In the adult, cell death by apoptosis is a protective response to several pathologic conditions that might

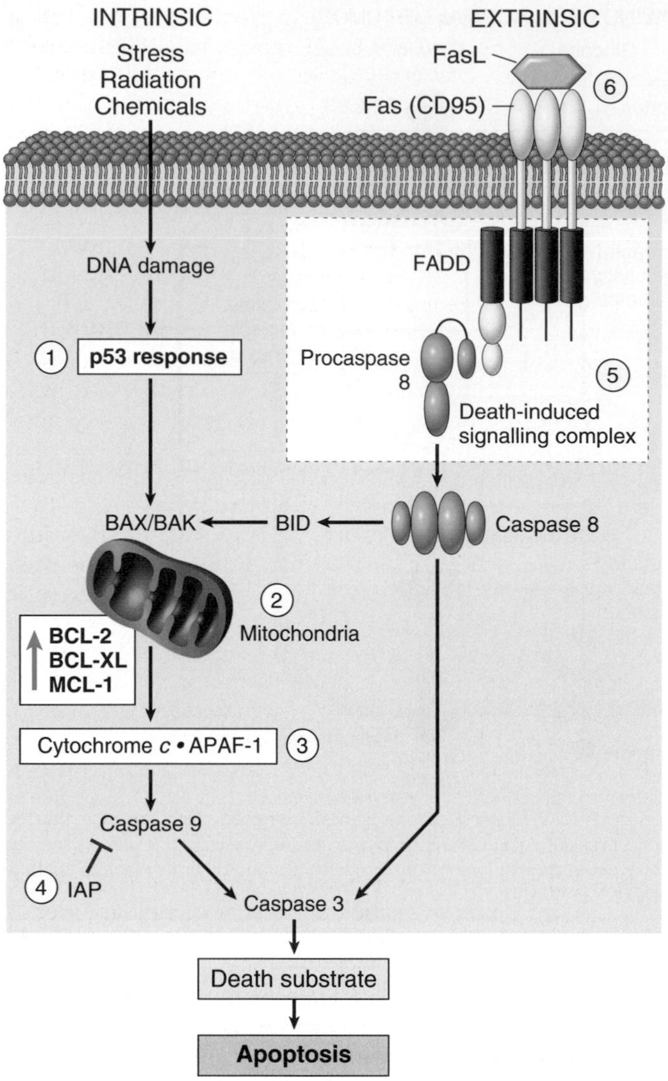

Figure 7-33 Intrinsic and extrinsic pathways of apoptosis and mechanisms used by tumor cells to evade cell death. (1) Loss of p53, leading to reduced function of pro-apoptotic factors such as BAX. (2) Reduced egress of cytochrome *c* from mitochondria as a result of upregulation of anti-apoptotic factors such as BCL2, BCL-XL, and MCL-1. (3) Loss of apoptotic peptidase activating factor 1 (APAF1). (4) Upregulation of inhibitors of apoptosis (IAP). (5) Reduced CD95 level. (6) Inactivation of death-induced signaling complex. FADD, Fas-associated via death domain.

contribute to malignancy if the cells remained viable. A cell with genomic injury can be induced to die, eliminating the chance that such a cell might go on to give rise to a neoplasm. A variety of signals, including DNA damage, deregulation of some of the most potent oncoproteins such as MYC, and loss of adhesion to the basement membrane (termed *anoikis*), can trigger apoptosis. Thus, apoptosis is a barrier that must be surmounted for cancer to develop and progress.

Biochemical Pathways That Lead To Programmed Cell Death. As discussed in Chapter 2, there are two distinct programs that activate apoptosis, the extrinsic and intrinsic pathways. Figure 7-33 shows, in simplified form, the sequence of events that lead to apoptosis by signaling through the death receptor CD95/Fas (extrinsic pathway) and by DNA damage (intrinsic pathway). **Of these two pathways, it is the intrinsic apoptotic pathway (sometimes referred to as the mitochondrial pathway) that is most frequently disabled in cancer.**

- Recall that the intrinsic pathway of apoptosis is triggered by a variety of stimuli, including withdrawal of survival factors, stress, and injury. Activation of this pathway leads to permeabilization of the mitochondrial outer membrane, with resultant release of molecules, such as cytochrome *c,* that initiate apoptosis. The integrity of the mitochondrial outer membrane is regulated by pro-apoptotic and anti-apoptotic members of the BCL2 family of proteins. The pro-apoptotic proteins BAX and BAK are required for apoptosis and directly promote mitochondrial permeabilization. Their action is inhibited by the anti-apoptotic members of this family, which are exemplified by BCL2, BCL-XL, and MCL1. A third set of proteins (so-called BH3-only proteins), including BAD, BID, and PUMA, sense death-inducing stimuli and promote apoptosis by neutralizing the actions of anti-apoptotic proteins like BCL2 and MCL1. When the sum total of all BH3 proteins expressed "overwhelms" the anti-apoptotic BCL2/BCL-XL/MCL1 barrier, BAX and BAK are activated and form pores in the mitochondrial membrane. Cytochrome *c* leaks into the cytosol, where it binds to APAF1, activating caspase 9. Caspase 9 then activates downstream caspases such as caspase 3, a typical *executioner caspase* that cleaves DNA and other substrates to cause cell death. Caspases are held in check in healthy cells by members of the *inhibitors of apoptosis protein* (IAP) family.
- The extrinsic pathway is initiated when CD95/Fas binds to its ligand, CD95L/FasL, leading to trimerization of the receptor and its cytoplasmic *death domains,* which attract the intracellular adaptor protein FADD. This protein recruits procaspase 8 to form the death-inducing signaling complex. Procaspase 8 is activated by cleavage into smaller subunits, generating caspase 8. Like caspase 9, caspase 8 then activates downstream executioner caspases. Additionally, caspase 8 can cleave and activate the BH3-only protein BID, activating the intrinsic pathway as well.

Within this framework it is possible to illustrate the multiple ways in which apoptosis is frustrated by cancer cells (Fig. 7-33). Of all these mechanisms, one of the best established is the role of BCL2 in protecting malignant lymphoid cells from apoptosis. As discussed later, approximately 85% of B-cell lymphomas of the follicular type (Chapter 13) carry a characteristic (14;18)(q32;q21) translocation. Recall that 14q32, the site where immunoglobulin heavy chain (IgH) genes are found, is also involved in the pathogenesis of Burkitt lymphoma. Juxtaposition of this transcriptionally active locus with *BCL2* (located at 18q21) causes overexpression of the BCL2 protein. This in turn protects lymphocytes from apoptosis and contributes to the survival of transformed B cells. Mice that are engineered to overexpress BCL2 in their B cells develop mainly lymphoid hyperplasia and autoimmune disorders and only infrequently get lymphoma; thus, overexpression of BCL2 must cooperate with other alterations (e.g., constitutive expression of MYC) to augment cancer development.

Nevertheless, most hematopoietic and solid tumors overexpress at least one member of the BCL2 family of anti-apoptotic proteins, suggesting that evasion of apoptosis is generally important in cancer development and progression. Furthermore, chemotherapy and radiation therapy kill cancer cells mainly by inducing apoptosis via the intrinsic pathway, and overexpression of BCL2 family members is believed to have an important role in the resistance of tumors to therapy. This appears to be particularly true for MCL-1, a BCL-2 family member that is normally subject to proteasomal degradation in the setting of DNA damage, but which is often found to be stabilized and overexpressed in drug-resistant cancers.

As mentioned earlier, p53 is an important pro-apoptotic protein that induces apoptosis in cells that are unable to repair DNA damage. The actions of p53 are mediated in part by transcriptional activation of BAX and PUMA, but there are also other connections between p53 and the apoptotic machinery. Thus, the apoptotic machinery in cancer may be thwarted by mutations affecting the component proteins directly, as well as by loss of sensors of genomic integrity such as p53.

The extrinsic pathway in less frequently altered in cancers, but nevertheless also has a role in some types, particularly certain lymphomas. Reduced levels of CD95/Fas may render the tumor cells less susceptible to apoptosis by CD95L/FasL. Other tumors have high levels of FLIP, a protein that can bind the death-induced signaling complex and prevent activation of caspase 8.

KEY CONCEPTS

Evasion of Apoptosis

- Apoptosis can be initiated through intrinsic or extrinsic pathways, both of which result in the activation of a proteolytic cascade of caspases that destroys the cell.
- Abnormalities of both pathways are found in cancer cells, but lesions that incapacitate the intrinsic (mitochondrial) pathway appear to be most common.
- In greater than 85% of follicular B-cell lymphomas, the anti-apoptotic gene *BCL2* is overexpressed due to a (14;18) translocation.
- Overexpression of other BCL2 family members such as MCL-1 is also linked to cancer cell survival and drug resistance.

Limitless Replicative Potential: The Stem Cell–Like Properties of Cancer Cells

All cancers contain cells that are immortal and have limitless replicative potential. Some cell lines established from cancers have now been proliferating ceaselessly in laboratories for more than 60 years, and it is reasonable to expect that they will continue to grow for as long as there are scientists to tend to them. How can it be that cancer cells have seemingly discovered the proverbial fountain of eternal youth? The answers are not completely known, but three interrelated factors appear critical to the immortality of cancer cells: (1) evasion of senescence; (2) evasion of mitotic crisis; (3) the capacity for self-renewal.

- **Evasion of senescence**. As was discussed in the section on cellular aging (Chapter 2), most normal human cells have the capacity to divide 60 to 70 times. After this, the cells become senescent, permanently leaving the cell cycle and never dividing again. The mechanisms that produce senescence are still not well understood, but the senescent state is associated with upregulation of tumor suppressors such as p53 and INK4a/p16 (perhaps in response to the accumulation of DNA damage over time). These tumor suppressors are believed to contribute to senescence in part by maintaining RB in a hypophosphorylated state, which favors cell cycle arrest. As already discussed, the RB-dependent G_1/S cell cycle checkpoint is disrupted in virtually all cancers by a wide variety of acquired genetic and epigenetic aberrations.
- **Evasion of mitotic crisis**. While cells that are resistant to senescence have increased replicative capacity, they are still not immortal; instead, they eventually enter into a phase referred to as *mitotic crisis* and die. This phenomenon has been ascribed to progressive shortening of *telomeres* at the ends of chromosomes. Telomeres are special DNA sequences at the ends of chromosomes that bind several types of protective protein complexes (Chapter 2). Most somatic cells do not express *telomerase*, the enzyme that is responsible for the maintenance of telomeres, and with each cell division their telomeres shorten. When the telomeric DNA is eroded, the exposed chromosome ends are "sensed" as double-stranded DNA breaks. If the affected cells have functional p53, the cell arrests its growth and may undergo apoptosis, but if p53 is dysfunctional, the nonhomologous end-joining pathway is activated and may join the "naked" ends of two chromosomes. This results in dicentric chromosomes that are pulled apart at anaphase, resulting in new double-stranded DNA breaks. The snowballing genomic damage caused by repeated "bridge-fusion-breakage" cycles eventually produces mitotic catastrophe and cell death (Fig. 7-34). Telomerase is expressed at very low levels in most somatic cells, and thus any cells that escape from senescence are very likely to die in mitotic crisis. However, if cells in crisis reactivate telomerase, the cells can restore their telomeres and survive; such cells may have suffered damage to oncogenes and tumor suppressor genes during crisis and are at high risk for malignant transformation. Alternatively, cancers may arise from stem cells (described later), which are normally long-lived in part because they continue to express telomerase. Whatever the mechanism, telomere maintenance is seen in virtually all types of cancers, and in 85% to 95% of cases this is due to upregulation of telomerase. The remaining tumors use another mechanism to maintain their telomeres termed *alternative lengthening of telomeres* that probably depends on DNA recombination.
- **Self-renewal**. Unlike most cells, tissue stem cells and germ cells express telomerase, making them resistant to mitotic crisis, and also somehow avoid the genetic and epigenetic alterations that trigger senescence. In addition, long-lived stem cells also possess another critical property, the capacity for self-renewal. In simple terms, self-renewal means that each time a stem cell divides at least one of the two daughter cells remains a stem cell.

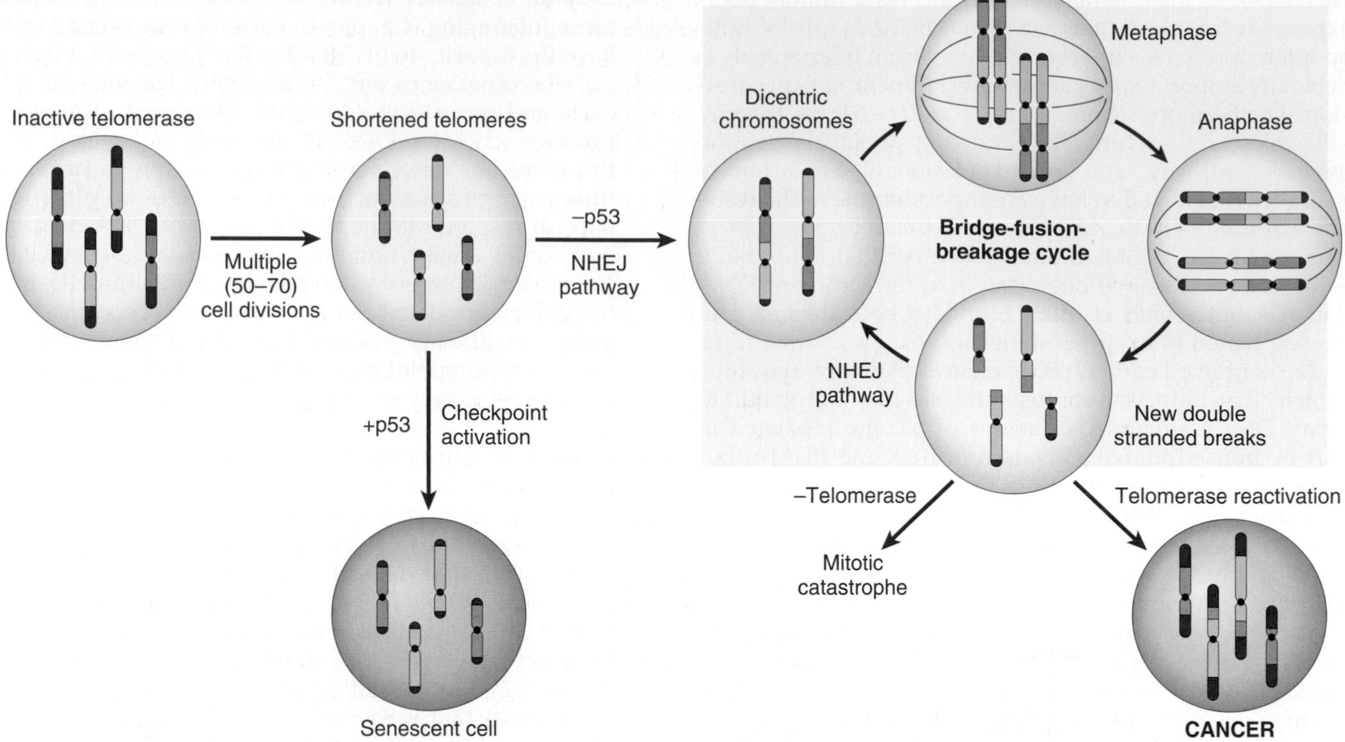

Figure 7-34 Escape of cells from senescence and mitotic catastrophe caused by telomere shortening. Replication of somatic cells, which do not express telomerase, leads to shortened telomeres. In the presence of competent checkpoints, cells undergo arrest and enter nonreplicative senescence. In the absence of checkpoints, DNA repair pathways, such as the nonhomologous end-joining (NHEJ) pathway are inappropriately activated, leading to the formation of dicentric chromosomes. At mitosis the dicentric chromosomes are pulled apart, generating random double-stranded breaks, which then activate DNA-repair pathways, leading to the random association of double-stranded ends and the formation, again, of dicentric chromosomes. Cells undergo numerous rounds of this bridge-fusion-breakage cycle, which generates massive chromosomal instability and numerous mutations. If cells fail to reexpress telomerase, they eventually undergo mitotic catastrophe and death. Reexpression of telomerase allows the cells to escape the bridge-fusion-breakage cycle, thus promoting their survival and tumorigenesis.

In a *symmetric division*, both daughter cells remain stem cells; such divisions may occur during embryogenesis, when stem cell pools are expanding, or during times of stress. In an *asymmetric division*, only one daughter cell remains a stem cell; in such circumstances, the non-stem cell daughter proceeds along some differentiation pathway, losing "stemness" but gaining one or more functions in the process. Such cells in "transit" to a differentiated state are often highly proliferative, but they eventually differentiate, stop dividing, and extinguish themselves.

The continued growth and maintenance of many tissues that contain short-lived cells, such as the formed elements of the bone marrow and blood and the epithelial cells of the gastrointestinal tract and skin, depends on a resident population of tissue stem cells that are capable of self-renewal. Following on this logic, because cancers are immortal and have limitless proliferative capacity, they too must contain cells that self-renew, so-called *cancer stem cells*. While the existence of cancer stem cells is accepted, there is ongoing debate about their identity and their numbers in particular cancers, due in large part to the difficulty in determining whether any particular cell is a cancer stem cell. Thus, the number of "stem cells" that are calculated to be present in a particular tumor can vary widely depending on methodology used to quantify stem cells, leading to uncertainty about whether cancer stem cells are rare or common in tumors.

Another open question is whether cancer stem cells arise from the transformation of tissue stem cells or from the conversion of conventional somatic cells to transformed cells with the acquired property of "stemness." The answer seems to be that both scenarios occur in different types of tumors (Fig. 7-35).

- In chronic myelogenous leukemia (CML), the *BCR-ABL* fusion gene that characterizes this tumor is present in a tumor cell subset that has all the properties of a normal hematopoietic stem cell. Thus, CML appears to originate from a transformed hematopoietic stem cell with an ingrained capacity for self-renewal. Similarly, certain epithelial tumors may arise from other adult stem cells, such as those that are present in colonic crypts.
- In contrast, studies of acute myeloid leukemia have shown that the cancer stem cells in this disease arise from more differentiated hematopoietic progenitors that acquire an abnormal capacity for self-renewal. How this occurs is unclear, but it is believed that certain mutated transcription factors, such as a PML-RARA fusion protein that is associated with acute promyelocytic leukemia (described later) may have important roles in acquisition of "stemness" (Fig. 7-35). Recall that expression of a small number of transcription factors can result in the epigenetic reprogramming of a

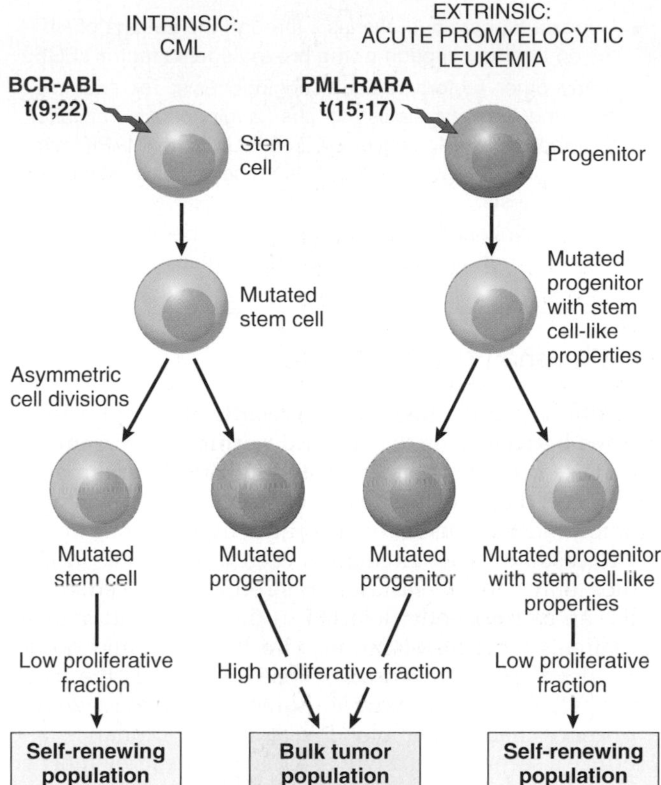

Figure 7-35 Origins of cells with self-renewing capacity in cancer. Cancer stem cells can arise from transformed tissue stem cells (e.g., hematopoietic stem cells in chronic myelogenous leukemia, CML) with intrinsic "stemness" or from proliferating cells that acquire a mutation that confers "stemness" (e.g., granulocyte progenitors in acute promyelocytic leukemia). In both instances, the cancer stem cells undergo asymmetric cell divisions that give rise to committed progenitors that proliferate more rapidly than the cancer stem cells; as a result, most of the malignant cells in both tumors lack self-renewing capacity.

differentiated somatic cell such as a fibroblast into a pluripotent stem cell. Thus, it is easy to imagine how mutations leading to misexpression of certain key transcription factors, such as MYC, might convert a somatic cell into a transformed cell with a capacity for self-renewal. A corollary of this idea is that, unlike normal stem cells and their more differentiated progeny, which have a fixed parent-offspring relationship, cancer cells within a tumor may be able to "de-differentiate" to a stem cell–like state. Indeed, there is evidence that cancers can repopulate their stem cell pools from non-stem cell populations, further complicating efforts to precisely define and selectively target cancer stem cells.

Despite these uncertainties, the concept of cancer stem cells has important implications for cancer therapy. Most notably, if cancer stem cells are essential for tumor persistence, it follows that these cells must be eliminated to eradicate the tumor. It is hypothesized that like normal stem cells, cancer stem cells have a high intrinsic resistance to conventional therapies due to a low rate of cell division and the expression of factors, such as multiple drug resistance-1 (MDR1), that counteract the effects of chemotherapeutic drugs. Thus, the limited success of current therapies may in part be explained by their failure to kill the malignant stem cells that lie at the root of cancer, an idea that is being actively tested in the laboratory.

KEY CONCEPTS

Limitless Replicative Potential

- A least some cells in all cancers must be stem cell–like; these cells are sometimes referred to as cancer stem cells. These may arise through transformation of a normal stem cell or through acquired genetic lesions that impart a stem-like state on a more mature cell.
- Cancer cells acquire lesions that inactivate senescence signals and reactivate telomerase, which act together to convey limitless replicative potential.

Angiogenesis

Even if a solid tumor possesses all of the genetic aberrations that are required for malignant transformation, it cannot enlarge beyond 1 to 2 mm in diameter unless it has the capacity to induce angiogenesis. Like normal tissues, tumors require delivery of oxygen and nutrients and removal of waste products; presumably the 1- to 2 mm zone represents the maximal distance across which oxygen, nutrients, and waste can diffuse from blood vessels. Growing cancers stimulate neoangiogenesis, during which vessels sprout from previously existing capillaries (Chapter 3). Neovascularization has a dual effect on tumor growth: perfusion supplies needed nutrients and oxygen, and newly formed endothelial cells stimulate the growth of adjacent tumor cells by secreting growth factors, such as insulin-like growth factors (IGFs) and PDGF. While the resulting tumor vasculature is effective at delivering nutrients and removing wastes, it is not entirely normal; the vessels are leaky and dilated, and have a haphazard pattern of connection, features that can be appreciated on angiograms. By permitting tumor cells access to these abnormal vessels, angiogenesis also contributes to metastasis. Angiogenesis is thus an essential facet of malignancy.

How do growing tumors develop a blood supply? The current paradigm is **that angiogenesis is controlled by a balance between angiogenesis promoters and inhibitors; in angiogenic tumors this balance is skewed in favor of promoters.** Early in their development, most human tumors do not induce angiogenesis. Starved of nutrients, these tumors remain small or in situ, possibly for years, until an *angiogenic switch* terminates this stage of vascular quiescence. The molecular basis of the angiogenic switch involves increased production of angiogenic factors and/or loss of angiogenic inhibitors. These factors may be produced by the tumor cells themselves or by inflammatory cells (e.g., macrophages) or other stromal cells associated with the tumors. Proteases, either elaborated by the tumor cells or by stromal cells in response to the tumor, are also involved in regulating the balance between angiogenic and antiangiogenic factors. Many proteases can release proangiogenic basic fibroblast growth factors (bFGF) that are stored in the ECM; conversely, the angiogenesis inhibitors angiostatin and endostatin are produced by proteolytic cleavage of plasminogen and collagen, respectively.

The local balance of angiogenic and antiangiogenic factors is influenced by several factors:

- Relative lack of oxygen due to hypoxia stabilizes HIF1α, an oxygen-sensitive transcription factor mentioned earlier, which then activates the transcription of the proangiogenic cytokines VEGF and bFGF. These factors create an angiogenic gradient that stimulates the proliferation of endothelial cells and guides the growth of new vessels toward the tumor. VEGF also increases the expression of ligands that activate the Notch signaling pathway, which regulates the branching and density of the new vessels (Chapter 3).
- Mutations involving tumor suppressors and oncogenes in cancers also tilt the balance in favor of angiogenesis. For example, p53 can stimulate expression of antiangiogenic molecules, such as thrombospondin-1, and repress expression of proangiogenic molecules such as VEGF. Thus, loss of p53 in tumor cells not only removes cell cycle checkpoints and alters tumor cell metabolism but also provides a more permissive environment for angiogenesis.
- The transcription of VEGF is also influenced by signals from the RAS-MAP kinase pathway, and gain-of-function mutations in *RAS* or *MYC* upregulate the production of VEGF. bFGF and VEGF are commonly expressed in a wide variety of tumor cells, and elevated levels can be detected in the serum and urine of a significant fraction of cancer patients.

The idea that angiogenesis is essential if solid tumors are to grow to clinically significant sizes has provided a powerful impetus for the development of therapeutic agents that block angiogenesis. These agents are now a part of the armamentarium that oncologists use against cancers; a cardinal example is bevacizumab, a monoclonal antibody that neutralizes VEGF activity and is approved for use in the treatment of multiple cancers. However, angiogenesis inhibitors have not been nearly as effective as was hoped based on preclinical studies conducted using mouse models of cancer; they can prolong life, but usually for only a few months and at very high financial cost. The mechanisms that underlie the persistence and ultimate progression of cancers in the face of therapy with angiogenesis inhibitors are not yet clear. Perhaps there is emergence of tumor subclones that by virtue of greater invasive and metastatic potential gain ready access to existing host vessels. The modest benefit of anti-angiogenic therapy highlights the pernicious nature of advanced cancers, which can even elude therapies directed at stromal support cells such as endothelium that are genomically stable and thus presumably "immune" to the Darwinian pressures that lead cancer cells to acquire more malignant phenotypes over time. Improvements are only possible with greater understanding of the "escape routes" through which tumor cells sidestep the effects of the angiogenesis inhibitors that are now in use.

KEY CONCEPTS

Angiogenesis

- Vascularization of tumors is essential for their growth and is controlled by the balance between angiogenic and anti-angiogenic factors that are produced by tumor and stromal cells.
- Hypoxia triggers angiogenesis through the actions of HIF-1α on the transcription of the proangiogenic factor VEGF.
- Many other factors regulate angiogenesis; for example, p53 induces synthesis of the angiogenesis inhibitor thombospondin-1, while RAS, MYC, and MAPK signaling all upregulate VEGF expression and stimulate angiogenesis.
- VEGF inhibitors are used to treat a number of advanced cancers and prolong the clinical course, but are not curative.

Invasion and Metastasis

Invasion and metastasis are the results of complex interactions between cancer cells and normal stroma and are the major causes of cancer-related morbidity and mortality. Hence, they are the subjects of intense scrutiny. Studies in mice and humans reveal that although millions of cells are released into the circulation each day from a primary tumor, only a few metastases are produced. Indeed, tumor cells can be frequently detected in the blood and marrow of patients with breast cancer who have not, and do not ever, develop overt metastatic disease. Why is the metastatic process so inefficient? For tumor cells to emerge from a primary mass, enter blood vessels or lymphatics, and produce a secondary growth at a distant site, they must go through a series of steps (summarized in Fig. 7-36), each of which is inefficient and subject to a multitude of controls; hence, at any point in the sequence, the breakaway cells may not survive. In this discussion, the metastatic cascade is divided into two phases: (1) invasion of the extracellular matrix (ECM) and (2) vascular dissemination, homing of tumor cells, and colonization. Subsequently, the molecular genetics of the metastatic cascade, as currently understood, are presented.

Invasion of Extracellular Matrix

The structural organization and function of normal tissues is to a great extent determined by interactions between cells and the ECM. As discussed in Chapter 1, tissues are organized into compartments separated from each other by two types of ECM: basement membrane and interstitial connective tissue. Although organized differently, each of these components of ECM is made up of collagens, glycoproteins, and proteoglycans. As shown in Figure 7-36, tumor cells must interact with the ECM at several stages in the metastatic cascade. A carcinoma must first breach the underlying basement membrane, then traverse the interstitial connective tissue, and ultimately gain access to the circulation by penetrating the vascular basement membrane. This process is repeated in reverse when tumor cell emboli extravasate at a distant site. Invasion of the ECM initiates the metastatic cascade and is an active process that can be resolved into several steps (Fig. 7-37):

- "Loosening up" of tumor cell–tumor cell interactions
- Degradation of ECM
- Attachment to novel ECM components
- Migration and invasion of tumor cells

Dissociation of cancer cells from one another is often the result of alterations in intercellular adhesion molecules and is the first step in the process of invasion.

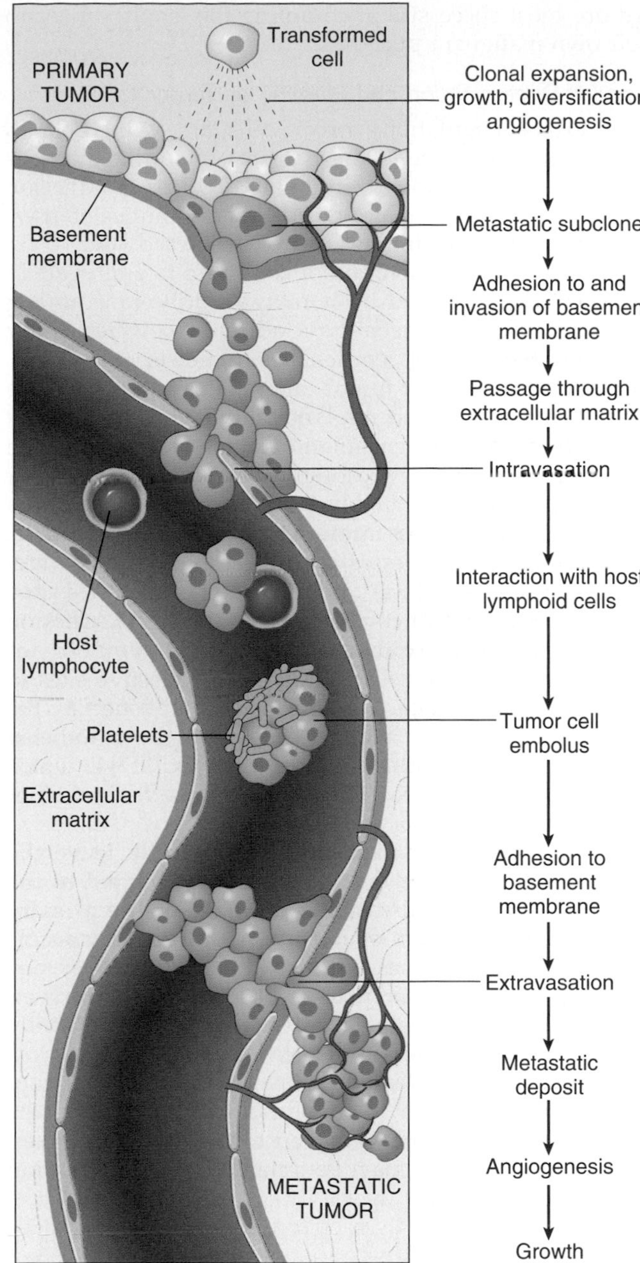

Figure 7-36 The metastatic cascade. Sequential steps involved in the hematogenous spread of a tumor.

Normal epithelial cells are tightly glued to each other and the ECM by a variety of adhesion molecules. Cell-cell interactions are mediated by the cadherin family of transmembrane glycoproteins. *E-cadherins* mediate the homotypic adhesion of epithelial cells, serving to both hold the cells together and to relay signals between the cells. In several epithelial tumors, including adenocarcinomas of the colon, stomach, and breast, E-cadherin function is lost. Presumably, this reduces the ability of cells to adhere to each other and facilitates their detachment from the primary tumor and their advance into the surrounding tissues.

Degradation of the basement membrane and interstitial connective tissue is the second step in invasion. Tumor cells may accomplish this by either secreting proteolytic enzymes themselves or by inducing stromal cells (e.g., fibroblasts and inflammatory cells) to elaborate proteases. Many different families of proteases, such as matrix metalloproteinases (MMPs), cathepsin D, and urokinase plasminogen activator, have been implicated in tumor cell invasion. MMPs regulate tumor invasion not only by remodeling insoluble components of the basement membrane and interstitial matrix but also by releasing

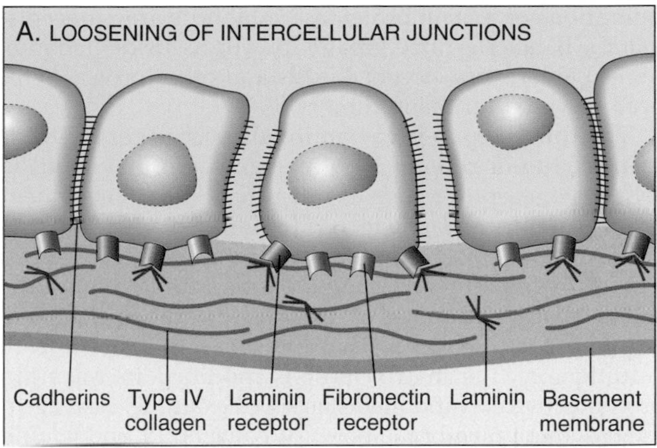

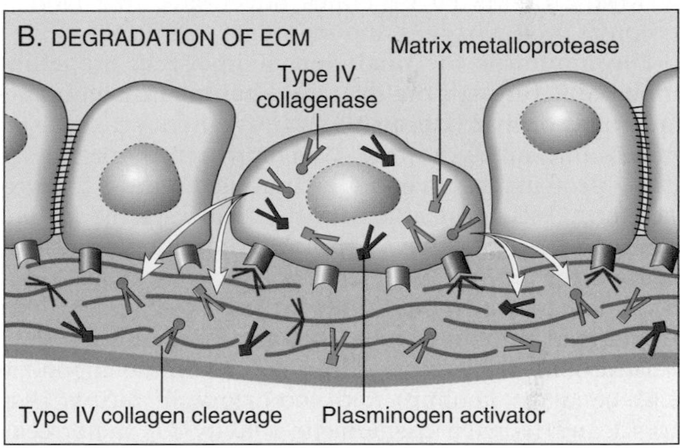

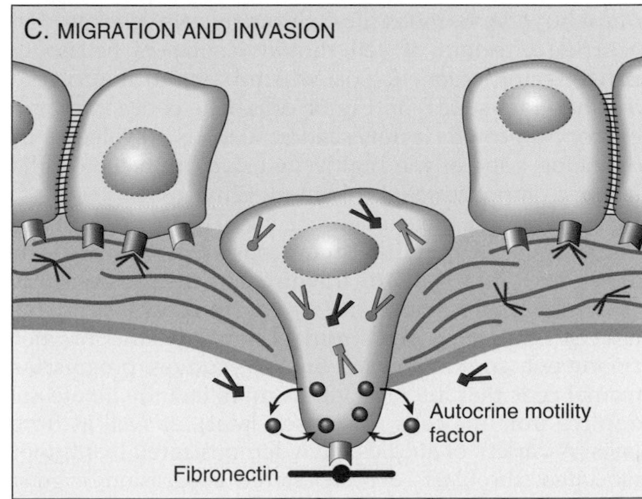

Figure 7-37 Sequence of events in the invasion of epithelial basement membranes by tumor cells. Tumor cells detach from each other because of reduced adhesiveness and attract inflammatory cells. Proteases secreted from tumor cells and inflammatory cells degrade the basement membrane. Binding of tumor cells to proteolytically generated binding sites and tumor cell migration follow.

ECM-sequestered growth factors. Indeed, cleavage products of collagen and proteoglycans also have chemotactic, angiogenic, and growth-promoting effects. For example, MMP9 is a gelatinase that cleaves type IV collagen of the epithelial and vascular basement membrane and also stimulates release of VEGF from ECM-sequestered pools. Benign tumors of the breast, colon, and stomach show little type IV collagenase activity, whereas their malignant counterparts overexpress this enzyme. Concurrently, the concentrations of metalloproteinase inhibitors are reduced so that the balance is tilted greatly toward tissue degradation. Indeed, overexpression of MMPs and other proteases has been reported for many tumors.

The third step in invasion involves changes in attachment of tumor cells to ECM proteins. Normal epithelial cells have receptors, such as integrins, for basement membrane laminin and collagens that are polarized at their basal surface; these receptors help to maintain the cells in a resting, differentiated state. Loss of adhesion in normal cells leads to induction of apoptosis, while, not surprisingly, tumor cells are resistant to this form of cell death. Additionally, the matrix itself is modified in ways that promote invasion and metastasis. For example, cleavage of the basement membrane proteins collagen IV and laminin by MMP2 or MMP9 generates novel sites that bind to receptors on tumor cells and stimulate migration.

Locomotion is the final step of invasion, propelling tumor cells through the degraded basement membranes and zones of matrix proteolysis. Migration is a multistep process that involves many families of receptors and signaling proteins that eventually impinge on the actin cytoskeleton. Cells must attach to the matrix at the leading edge, detach from the matrix at the trailing edge, and contract the actin cytoskeleton to ratchet forward. Such movement seems to be stimulated and directed by tumor cell-derived cytokines, such as autocrine motility factors. In addition, cleavage products of matrix components (e.g., collagen, laminin) and some growth factors (e.g., IGFs I and II) have chemotactic activity for tumor cells. Furthermore, proteolytic cleavage liberates growth factors bound to matrix molecules. Stromal cells also produce paracrine effectors of cell motility, such as hepatocyte growth factor/scatter factor, which binds to the receptor tyrosine kinase MET on tumor cells. The concentration of hepatocyte growth factor/scatter factor is elevated at the advancing edge of the highly invasive brain tumor glioblastoma, supporting its role in motility.

It has become clear in recent years that the ECM and stromal cells surrounding tumor cells are not a mere static barrier for tumor cells to traverse but instead constitute a varied environment in which reciprocal signaling between tumor cells and stromal cells may either promote or prevent tumorigenesis and/or tumor progression. Stromal cells that interact with tumors include innate and adaptive immune cells (discussed later), as well as fibroblasts. A variety of studies have demonstrated that tumor-associated fibroblasts exhibit altered expression of genes that encode ECM molecules, proteases, protease inhibitors, and various growth factors. Thus, tumor cells reside in a complex and ever-changing milieu composed of ECM, growth factors, fibroblasts, and immune cells, with significant cross-talk among all the components. It is easy to imagine that tumors come to be dominated by subclones that are most successful at co-opting this environment to their own malignant purposes.

Vascular Dissemination and Homing of Tumor Cells

Once in the circulation, tumor cells are vulnerable to destruction by a variety of mechanisms, including mechanical shear stress, apoptosis stimulated by loss of adhesion (termed *anoikis*), and innate and adaptive immune defenses. The details of tumor immunity are considered later.

Within the circulation, tumor cells tend to aggregate in clumps. This is favored by homotypic adhesions among tumor cells as well as heterotypic adhesion between tumor cells and blood cells, particularly platelets (Fig. 7-36). Formation of platelet-tumor aggregates may enhance tumor cell survival and implantability. Tumor cells may also bind and activate coagulation factors, resulting in the formation of emboli. Arrest and extravasation of tumor emboli at distant sites involves adhesion to the endothelium, followed by egress through the basement membrane. Involved in these processes are adhesion molecules (integrins, laminin receptors) and proteolytic enzymes, discussed earlier. Of particular interest is the CD44 adhesion molecule, which is expressed on normal T lymphocytes and is used by these cells to migrate to selective sites in lymphoid tissues. Such migration is accomplished by the binding of CD44 to hyaluronate on high endothelial venules. Solid tumors also often express CD44, which appears to enhance their spread to lymph nodes and other metastatic sites.

The site at which circulating tumor cells leave the capillaries to form secondary deposits is related to the anatomic location and vascular drainage of the primary tumor and the tropism of particular tumors for specific tissues. Most metastases occur in the first capillary bed available to the tumor. Many observations, however, suggest that natural pathways of drainage do not wholly explain the distribution of metastases. For example, prostatic carcinoma preferentially spreads to bone, bronchogenic carcinomas tend to involve the adrenals and the brain, and neuroblastomas spread to the liver and bones. Such organ tropism may be related to the following mechanisms:

- Tumor cells may have adhesion molecules whose ligands are expressed preferentially on the endothelial cells of the target organ.
- Chemokines have an important role in determining the target tissues for metastasis. For instance, some breast cancer cells express the chemokine receptors CXCR4 and CCR7.
- In some cases, the target tissue may be a nonpermissive environment—"unfavorable soil," so to speak, for the growth of tumor seedlings. For example, although well-vascularized, skeletal muscle and spleen are rarely sites of metastasis.

Alas, tumor cells do not read textbooks of pathology, and there is still much to be learned about the factors that govern their spread. Despite their "cleverness" in escaping their tissue of origin, circulating tumor cells are quite inefficient in colonizing distant organs. Moreover, even when metastases are established, they may grow to only small, clinically insignificant sizes. Indeed, the concept of *dormancy*, referring to the prolonged survival of micrometastases without progression, is well described in melanoma and in breast and prostate cancer. Although the molecular mechanisms of colonization are still being unraveled in mouse models, a consistent theme seems to be that tumor cells secrete cytokines, growth factors, and ECM molecules that act on the resident stromal cells, which in turn make the metastatic site habitable for the cancer cell. For example, breast cancer metastases to bone are osteolytic because of the activation of osteoclasts in the metastatic site. Breast cancer cells secrete parathyroid hormone-related protein (PTHRP), which stimulates osteoblasts to make RANK ligand (RANKL). RANKL then activates osteoclasts, which degrade the bone matrix and release growth factors embedded within it, like IGF and TGF-β. With a better molecular understanding of the mechanisms of metastasis our ability to target them therapeutically will be greatly enhanced.

Molecular Genetics of Metastasis Development

Why do only some tumors metastasize? What are the genetic and epigenetic changes that allow metastases? Why is the metastatic process so inefficient? Several competing theories have been proposed to explain how the metastatic phenotype arises.

- The *clonal evolution model* suggests that as mutations accumulate in genetically unstable cancer cells and the tumor become heterogeneous (Fig. 7-38*A*), a rare subset of tumor cell subclones acquires a pattern of gene expression that is permissive for all steps involved in metastasis.
- A subset of breast cancers has a metastatic gene expression signature similar to that found in metastases, although no clinical evidence for metastasis is apparent. It is hypothesized that in these tumors with a "*metastasis signature*" most if not all cells develop a predilection for metastatic spread during early stages of carcinogenesis (Fig. 7-38*B*).
- A third idea that combines the two above supposes that the metastatic signature is necessary but not sufficient for metastasis, and that additional mutations are needed for metastasis to occur (Fig. 7-38*C*).
- Finally, there is evidence the capacity for metastasis involves not only properties intrinsic to the cancer cells but also the characteristics of their microenvironment, such as the components of the stroma, the presence of infiltrating immune cells, and angiogenesis (Fig. 7-38*D*).

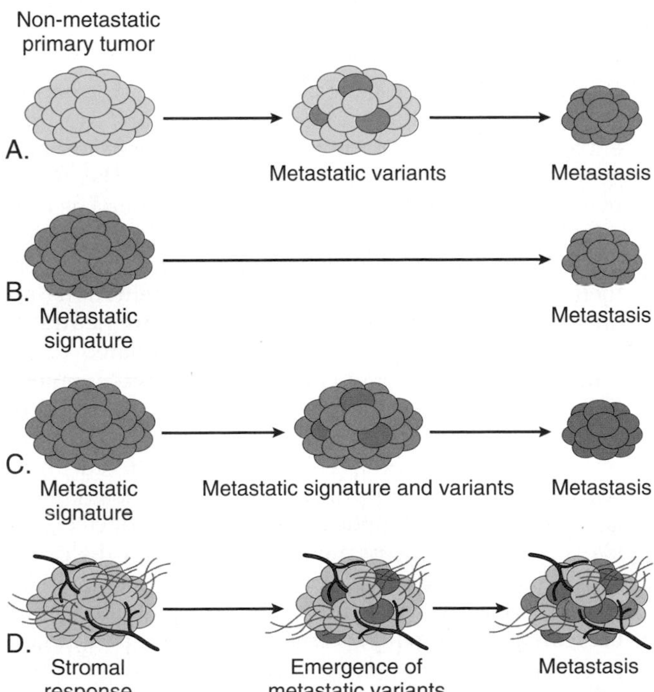

Figure 7-38 Mechanisms of metastasis development within a primary tumor. A nonmetastatic primary tumor is shown (light blue) on the left side of all diagrams. Four models are presented: **A,** Metastasis is caused by rare variant clones that develop in the primary tumor. **B,** Metastasis is caused by the gene expression pattern of most cells of the primary tumor, referred to as a metastatic signature. **C,** A combination of **A** and **B**, in which metastatic variants appear in a tumor with a metastatic gene signature. **D,** Metastasis development is greatly influenced by the tumor stroma, which may regulate angiogenesis, local invasiveness, and resistance to immune elimination, allowing cells of the primary tumor, as in **C**, to become metastatic.

One open question in the field is whether there are genes whose principal or sole contribution to tumorigenesis is to control metastasis. This question is of more than academic interest, because if altered forms of certain genes promote or suppress the metastatic phenotype, their detection in a primary tumor would have both prognostic and therapeutic implications. Because metastasis is a complex phenomenon involving a variety of steps and pathways, it is thought that "metastasis oncogenes" or "metastasis suppressor genes" are few in number. A metastasis suppressor gene is defined as a gene whose loss promotes the development of metastasis without an effect on the primary tumor. At least a dozen genes lost in metastatic lesions have been confirmed to function as "metastasis suppressors." Their molecular functions are varied and not completely clear; however, most appear to affect various signaling pathways.

Among candidates for metastasis oncogenes are *SNAIL* and *TWIST*, which encode transcription factors whose primary function is to promote epithelial-to-mesenchymal transition (EMT). In EMT, carcinoma cells downregulate certain epithelial markers (e.g., E-cadherin) and upregulate certain mesenchymal markers (e.g., vimentin and smooth muscle actin). These changes are believed to favor the development of a promigratory phenotype that is essential for metastasis. Loss of E-cadherin expression seems to be a key event in EMT, and SNAIL and TWIST are transcriptional repressors that downregulate E-cadherin expression. EMT has been documented mainly in breast cancers; whether it is a general phenomenon in other solid tumors remains to be established.

Role of Stromal Elements in Metastasis

In the preceding sections we have seen seen several examples of interaction between tumor cells and stromal elements. For example, macrophages in the stroma secrete matrix-degrading proteases, and cleavage of ECM proteins can release latent angiogenic factors and growth factors, such as TGFβ. Successful tumor cells must co-opt these and other interactions and use them to promote their growth and invasion, and it follows that these interactions, and the stromal cells themselves, are potential targets in cancer treatment. We have already discussed the use of angiogenesis inhibitors in cancer patients; of even greater potential benefit are therapies that overcome another hallmark of cancer cells—the ability to evade the host immune response (discussed next).

KEY CONCEPTS

Invasion and Metastasis

- Ability to invade tissues, a hallmark of malignancy, occurs in four steps: loosening of cell-cell contacts, degradation of ECM, attachment to novel ECM components, and migration of tumor cells.
- Cell-cell contacts are lost by the inactivation of E-cadherin through a variety of pathways.
- Basement membranes and interstitial matrix degradation is mediated by proteolytic enzymes secreted by tumor cells and stromal cells, such as matrix metalloproteases and cathepsins.
- Proteolytic enzymes also release growth factors sequestered in the ECM and generate chemotactic and angiogenic fragments from cleavage of ECM glycoproteins.
- The metastatic site of many tumors can be predicted by the location of the primary tumor. Many tumors arrest in the first capillary bed they encounter (lung and liver, most commonly).
- Some tumors show organ tropism, probably due to expression of adhesion or chemokine receptors whose ligands are expressed by endothelial cells the metastatic site.
- Genes that promote epithelial-mesenchymal transitions, like *TWIST* and *SNAIL*, may be important metastasis genes in epithelial tumors

Evasion of Host Defense

Long one of the "holy grails" of oncology, the promise of therapies that enable the host immune system to recognize and destroy cancer cells is finally coming to fruition, largely due to a clearer understanding of the ways by which cancer cells evade the host response. Paul Ehrlich first conceived the idea that tumor cells can be recognized as "foreign" and eliminated by the immune system. Subsequently, Lewis Thomas and Macfarlane Burnet formalized this concept by coining the term *immune surveillance,* which implies that a normal function of the immune system is to constantly "scan" the body for emerging malignant cells and destroy them. This idea has been supported by many observations—the presence of lymphocytic infiltrates around tumors and reactive changes in lymph nodes draining sites of cancer; experimental results, mostly with transplanted tumors; the increased incidence of some cancers in immunodeficient people and mice; the direct demonstration of tumor-specific T cells and antibodies in patients; and most recently and most directly, the response of advanced cancers to therapeutic agents that act by stimulating latent host T-cell responses (described later).

The fact that cancers occur in immunocompetent individuals indicates that immune surveillance is imperfect; however, that some tumors escape such policing does not preclude the possibility that many others were aborted. Assuming that the immune system is capable of recognizing and eliminating nascent cancers, it follows that the tumors that do grow out must be composed of cells that are either invisible to the host immune system or that release factors that actively suppress host immunity. The term *cancer immunoediting* has been used to describe the ability of the immune system to shape and mold the immunogenic properties of tumor cells in a fashion that ultimately leads to the darwinian selection of subclones that are best able to avoid immune elimination. In support of this idea, in the past several years it has become evident that tumors produce a number of factors that promote immune tolerance and immune suppression, and that therapeutic agents that neutralize these factors can lead to tumor regression, even in patients with advanced cancers. These encouraging clinical responses constitute strong evidence that evasion of host immunity is indeed a hallmark of many, if not all, human cancers.

The following section explores some of the important questions about tumor immunity: What is the nature of tumor antigens? What host effector systems recognize tumor cells? How do tumors evade these host mechanisms? And, how can immune reactions against tumors be exploited therapeutically?

Tumor Antigens

Antigens found in tumors that elicit an immune response have been demonstrated in many experimentally induced tumors and in some human cancers. Tumor antigens can be classified according to their molecular structure and source.

The main classes of tumor antigen are as follows (Fig. 7-39):

- **Products of mutated genes.** Neoplastic transformation, as discussed, results from genetic alterations in protooncogenes and tumor suppressor genes; these mutated genes encode variant proteins that have never been seen by the immune system and are thus recognized as nonself. Additionally, because of genetic instability, cancers often harbor a high burden of mutations throughout their genomes. Most of these acquired mutations are likely to be "passengers," mutations that are neutral in terms of cancer cell fitness and thus unrelated to the transformed phenotype. However, by chance, some of these passenger mutations may fall in the coding sequences of genes and give rise to protein variants that serve as tumor antigens. The products of altered protooncogenes, tumor suppressor genes, and "passenger" genes are translated in the cytoplasm of tumor cells, and like any cytoplasmic protein, they may enter the class I MHC antigen-processing pathway and be recognized by CD8+ T cells. In addition, these proteins may enter the class II antigen-processing pathway in antigen-presenting cells that have phagocytosed dead tumor cells, and thus be recognized by CD4+ T cells also. Some cancer patients have circulating CD4+ and CD8+ T cells that can respond to peptides derived from mutated oncoproteins such as RAS, p53, and BCR-ABL. In animals, immunization with mutated RAS or p53 proteins induces CTLs and rejection responses against tumors expressing these mutated proteins. However, the tumor-specific neoantigens that are recognized by CTLs in patients with cancer are for the most part currently unknown.

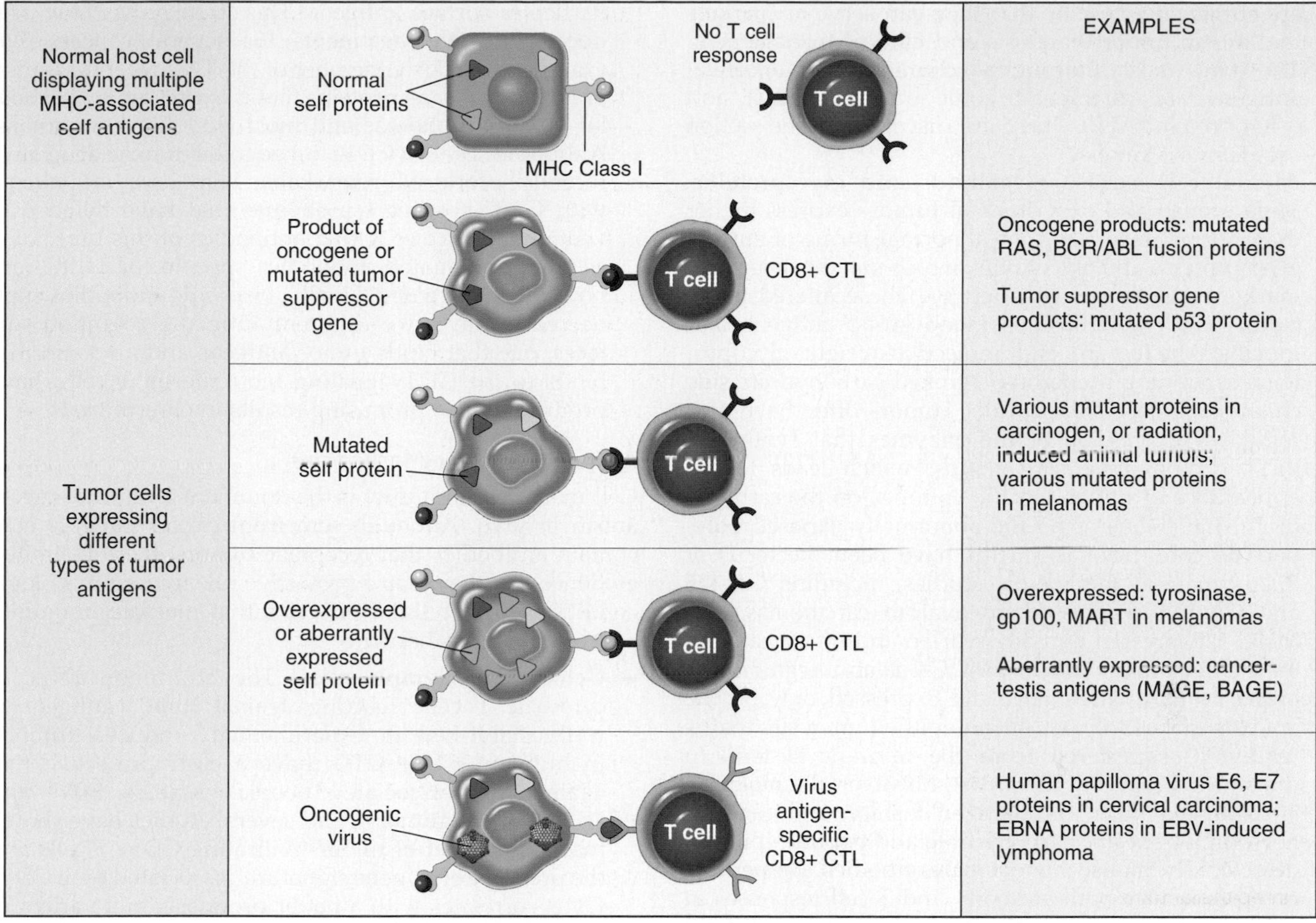

Figure 7-39 Tumor antigens recognized by CD8+ T cells. (Modified from Abbas AK, Lichtman AH: Cellular and Molecular Immunology, 5th ed. Philadelphia, WB Saunders, 2003.)

- **Overexpressed or aberrantly expressed cellular proteins.** Tumor antigens may also be normal cellular proteins that are abnormally expressed in tumor cells. One such antigen is tyrosinase, an enzyme involved in melanin biosynthesis that is expressed only in normal melanocytes and melanomas. It may be surprising that the immune system is able to respond to this normal self-antigen. The probable explanation is that tyrosinase is normally produced in such small amounts and in so few normal cells that it is not recognized by the immune system and fails to induce tolerance. Another group of tumor antigens, the *cancer-testis antigens*, are encoded by genes that are silent in all adult tissues except germ cells in the testis—hence their name. Although the protein is present in the testis it is not expressed on the cell surface in an antigenic form, because sperm do not express MHC class I antigens. Thus, for all practical purposes these antigens are tumor specific. Prototypic of this group is the melanoma antigen gene (MAGE) family. Although originally described in melanomas, MAGE antigens are expressed by a variety of tumor types. For example, MAGE-1 is expressed on 37% of melanomas and a variable number of lung, liver, stomach, and esophageal carcinomas. There are several other members of the MAGE family, variously called RAGE, GAGE, and other fanciful acronyms.
- **Tumor antigens produced by oncogenic viruses.** Several viruses are associated with cancers. Not surprisingly, these viruses produce proteins that are recognized as foreign by the immune system. The most potent of these antigens are proteins produced by latent DNA viruses; examples in humans include human papilloma virus (HPV) and Epstein-Barr virus (EBV). There is abundant evidence that CTLs recognize antigens of these viruses and that a competent immune system plays a role in surveillance against virus-induced tumors because of its ability to recognize and kill virus-infected cells. In fact, the concept of immune surveillance against tumors is best established for DNA virus-induced tumors.
- **Oncofetal antigens.** Oncofetal antigens are proteins that are expressed at high levels on cancer cells and in normal developing (fetal) tissues. Although originally believed to be completely specific for tumors and fetal tissues, as techniques for detecting these antigens have improved, it became clear that their expression in adults is not limited to tumors. Amounts of these proteins are increased in tissues and in the circulation in various inflammatory conditions, and they are even found in small quantities in normal tissues. There is no evidence that oncofetal antigens are important inducers or targets of antitumor immunity. However, oncofetal proteins

are sufficiently specific that they can serve as markers that aid in tumor diagnosis and clinical management. The two most thoroughly characterized oncofetal antigens are carcinoembryonic antigen (CEA) and α-fetoprotein (AFP). These are discussed in the section on "Tumor Markers."

- **Altered cell surface glycolipids and glycoproteins.** Most human and experimental tumors express higher than normal levels and/or abnormal forms of surface glycoproteins and glycolipids, which may be diagnostic markers and targets for therapy. These altered molecules include gangliosides, blood group antigens, and mucins. Mucins are high-molecular-weight glycoproteins containing numerous O-linked carbohydrate side chains on a core polypeptide. Tumors often have dysregulated expression of the enzymes that synthesize these carbohydrate side chains, which leads to the appearance of tumor-specific epitopes on the carbohydrate side chains or on the abnormally exposed polypeptide core. Several mucins have been the focus of diagnostic and therapeutic studies, including CA-125 and CA-19-9, expressed on ovarian carcinomas, and MUC-1, expressed on both ovarian and breast carcinomas. Unlike many mucins, MUC-1 is an integral membrane protein that is normally expressed only on the apical surface of breast ductal epithelium, a site that is relatively sequestered from the immune system. In ductal carcinomas of the breast, however, the molecule is expressed in an unpolarized fashion and contains new, tumor-specific carbohydrate and peptide epitopes detectable by mouse monoclonal antibodies. The peptide epitopes induce both antibody and T-cell responses in cancer patients and are therefore considered candidates for tumor vaccines in patients with breast cancer and possibly ovarian cancer as well.
- **Cell type–specific differentiation antigens.** Tumors express molecules that are normally present on the cells of origin. These antigens are called *differentiation antigens* because they are specific for particular lineages or differentiation stages of various cell types. Such differentiation antigens are typically normal self-antigens, and therefore they do not induce immune responses in tumor-bearing hosts. Their importance is as potential targets for immunotherapy and for identifying the tissue of origin of tumors. There are now several examples of monoclonal antibodies that recognize cell type specific antigens that are highly effective anti-tumor agents. Antibodies against CD20, a transmembrane protein that is expressed on the surface of all normal mature B cells, have broad cytocidal activity against mature B-cell lymphomas and leukemias and are widely used in the treatment of these tumors. These antibodies are believed to induce cell killing through several mechanisms, including opsonization and phagocytosis of tumor cells, antibody-dependent cell-mediated cytotoxicity and complement fixation. Anti-CD20 antibodies also kill normal B cells, but because hematopoietic stem cells are spared, normal B cells reemerge following treatment.

Monoclonal antibodies may also be covalently coupled to drugs, toxins, or radiochemicals; in this instance, the antibody serves as guided missile that delivers a therapeutic warhead to cancers expressing particular surface antigens. This strategy has now produced effective treatments for several cancers. For example, CD30 is a member of the TNF receptor family of transmembrane proteins that is expressed by particular T cell lymphomas and most Hodgkin lymphomas. Antibodies against CD30 linked to a cytotoxic drug have recently produced remarkable responses in patients with CD30-positive lymphomas that have failed conventional therapies. Other antibodies of this type, such as toxin-conjugated antibodies specific for HER2, are now being evaluated. Finally, bispecific antibodies engineered to have two different antigen recognition surfaces, one that binds tumor antigens and a second that binds to the CD3 signaling molecule on T cells, have produced some promising results in clinical trials.

Antitumor Effector Mechanisms

Cell-mediated immunity is the dominant antitumor mechanism in vivo. Although sera from cancer patients may contain antibodies that recognize tumors, there is limited evidence that they play a protective role under physiologic conditions. The cellular effectors that mediate immunity are described in Chapter 6.

- **Cytotoxic T lymphocytes**. The antitumor effect of cytotoxic T cells reacting against tumor antigens is well established in experimentally induced tumors. In humans, CD8+ CTLs have a clear protective role against virus-associated neoplasms (e.g., EBV- and HPV-induced tumors), and several studies have shown that the number of tumor-infiltrating CD8+ T cells and the presence of a "gene signature" associated with CD8+ CTLs correlates with a better prognosis in a variety of cancers, not only those caused by oncogenic viruses.
- **Natural killer cells.** NK cells are lymphocytes that are capable of destroying tumor cells without prior sensitization and thus may provide the first line of defense against tumor cells. After activation with IL-2 and IL-15, NK cells can lyse a wide range of human tumors, including many that seem to be nonimmunogenic for T cells. While the importance of NK cells in host response against spontenous tumors is still not well established, cytokines that activate NK cells are being used for immunotherapy.
- **Macrophages**. Activated macrophages exhibit cytotoxicity against tumor cells in vitro. T cells, NK cells, and macrophages may collaborate in antitumor reactivity, because interferon-γ, a cytokine secreted by T cells and NK cells, is a potent activator of macrophages. Activated macrophages may kill tumors by mechanisms similar to those used to kill microbes (e.g., production of reactive oxygen species; Chapter 2).

Immune Surveillance and Escape

Given the many potential antitumor mechanisms, is there any evidence that they operate in vivo to prevent emergence of neoplasms? One strong argument for the existence of immune surveillance is the increased frequency of cancers in the setting of immunodeficiency. Persons with congenital immunodeficiencies develop cancers at about 200 times the rate in immunocompetent individuals. Immunosuppressed transplant recipients and persons with AIDS also have an increased incidence of malignancies.

Most (but not all) of these neoplasms are aggressive lymphomas composed of mature B cells. Particularly illustrative is the rare X-linked recessive immunodeficiency disorder termed *XLP (X-linked lymphoproliferative syndrome)*, caused by mutations in the gene encoding an adapter protein, SAP, which participates in NK and T-cell signaling pathways. In affected boys, EBV infection does not take the usual self-limited form of infectious mononucleosis but instead evolves into a chronic or sometimes fatal form of infectious mononucleosis or, even worse, a lymphoma comprised of EBV-infected B cells.

Most cancers occur in persons who do not suffer from any overt immunodeficiency. It is evident, then, that tumor cells must develop mechanisms to escape or evade the immune system in immunocompetent hosts. Several such mechanisms may be operative (Fig. 7-40).

- **Selective outgrowth of antigen-negative variants.** During tumor progression, strongly immunogenic subclones may be eliminated, an example of immunoediting that has already been discussed.
- **Loss or reduced expression of MHC molecules.** Tumor cells may fail to express normal levels of HLA class I molecules, thereby escaping attack by cytotoxic T cells. Such cells, however, may trigger NK cells if the tumor cells express ligands for NK cell activating receptors.
- **Activation of immunoregulatory pathways.** An important emerging concept is that tumor cells actively inhibit tumor immunity by engaging normal pathways of immune regulation that serve as "checkpoints" in immune responses. Through a variety of mechanisms, tumor cells may downregulate the expression of costimulatory factors on antigen-presenting cells, such as dendritic cells; as a result, the antigen presenting cells fail to engage the stimulatory receptor CD28 and instead activate the inhibitory receptor CTLA-4 on effector T cells. This not only prevents sensitization but also may induce long-lived unresponsiveness in tumor-specific T cells. Tumor cells also may upregulate the expression of PD-L1 and PD-L2, cell surface proteins that activate the programmed death-1 (PD-1) receptor on effector T cells. PD-1, like CTLA-4, may inhibit T cell activation. Antibodies that block the inhibitory CTLA-4 or PD-1 receptors have produced promising results in clinical trials conducted in patients with advanced-stage solid tumors. Additional clinical trials are being planned using both PD-1 and CTLA-4 blocking antibodies in combination with each other and with conventional or targeted chemotherapy. The success of these agents has led to a new paradigm in cancer immunotherapy, sometimes called "checkpoint blockade". This is centered on the idea that treatments that remove the "brakes" imposed by tumors on host anti-tumor immune responses can be highly effective in treating cancer.
- **Secretion of immunosuppressive factors by cancer cells.** Tumors may secrete several products that inhibit the host immune response. TGF-β is secreted in large quantities by many tumors and is a potent immunosuppressant. Other tumors secrete galectins, sugar-rich lectin-like factors that skew T-cell responses so as to favor immunosuppression. Many other soluble factors produced by tumors are also suspected of inhibiting the host immune response, including interleukin-10, prostaglandin E2, certain metabolites derived from tryptophan, and VEGF, which can inhibit the diapedesis of T cells from the vasculature into the tumor bed.
- **Induction of regulatory T cells (Tregs).** Some studies suggest that tumors produce factors that favor the development of immunosuppressive regulatory T cells, which could also contribute to "immunoevasion."

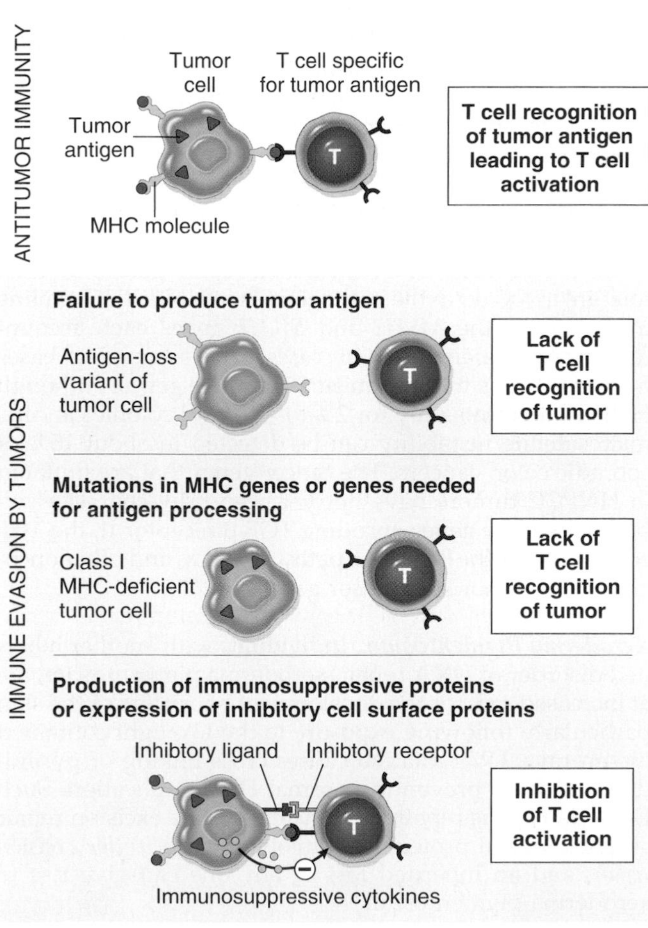

Figure 7-40 Mechanisms by which tumors evade the immune system. Tumors may evade immune responses by losing expression of antigens or major histocompatibility complex (MHC) molecules or by producing immunosuppressive cytokines or ligands such as PD-L1 for inhibitory receptors on T cells. (Reprinted from Abbas AK, Lichtman AH, Pillai S: Cellular and Molecular Immunology, 7th ed. Philadelphia, WB Saunders, 2012.)

Thus, it seems that there is no dearth of mechanisms by which tumor cells can outwit the host immune system. Nevertheless, the aforementioned response of tumors to immunomodulatory agents, such as antibodies that block CTLA-4 and PD-1, has generated tremendous excitement around the potential of modern cancer immunotherapy. The major challenges now are to determine which immune evasion mechanisms are most important in human cancers (preferably using sensitive and specific biomarker tests that can be performed on each individual patient's cancer) and to develop a broader set of therapies that overcome these mechanisms and induce effective host immunity.

KEY CONCEPTS

Evasion of Immune Surveillance

- Tumor cells can be recognized by the immune system as non-self and destroyed.
- Antitumor activity is mediated by predominantly cell-mediated mechanisms. Tumor antigens are presented on the cell surface by MHC class I molecules and are recognized by CD8+ CTLs.
- The different classes of tumor antigens include products of mutated proto-oncogenes, tumor suppressor genes, overexpressed or aberrantly expressed proteins, tumor antigens produced by oncogenic viruses, oncofetal antigens, altered glycolipids and glycoproteins, and cell type-specific differentiation antigens.
- Immunosuppressed patients have an increased risk for development of cancer, particularly types caused by oncogenic DNA viruses.
- In immunocompetent patients, tumors may avoid the immune system by several mechanisms, including selective outgrowth of antigen-negative variants, loss or reduced expression of histocompatibility antigens, and immunosuppression mediated by expression of certain factors (e.g., TGF-β, PD-1 ligand, galectins) by the tumor cells.
- Antibodies that overcome these mechanisms of immune evasion are showing promise in clinical trials conducted in patients with advanced cancer.

Genomic Instability

Genetic aberrations that increase mutation rates are very common in cancers and expedite the acquisition of driver mutations that are required for transformation and subsequent tumor progression. Although humans literally swim in environmental agents that are mutagenic (e.g., chemicals, radiation, sunlight), cancers are relatively rare outcomes of these encounters. This state of affairs results from the ability of normal cells to repair DNA damage, the death of cells with irreparable damage (see "Evasion of Apoptosis" earlier), and other mechanisms, such as oncogene-induced senescence and immune surveillance.

We have previously discussed is the role of the *TP53* tumor suppressor gene in protecting the genome from potentially oncogenic damage, both by arresting cell division to provide time for repair of DNA damage caused by environmental mutagens and by initiating apoptosis in irreparably damaged cells. The importance of DNA repair in maintaining the integrity of the genome is further highlighted by several inherited disorders in which genes that encode proteins involved in DNA repair are defective. Individuals born with such inherited defects in DNA-repair proteins are at a greatly increased risk of developing cancer. Moreover, defects in repair mechanisms are present in certain kinds of sporadic human cancers. Mutations in DNA-repair genes themselves are not oncogenic, but their abnormalities greatly enhance the occurrence of mutations in other genes during the process of normal cell division. Typically, genomic instability occurs when both copies of the DNA repair gene are lost; however, some work has suggested that haploinsufficiency of at least a subset of these genes may also promote cancer. As explained below, defects in three types of DNA-repair systems—mismatch repair, nucleotide excision repair, and recombination repair—contribute to different types of cancers.

Hereditary Nonpolyposis Colon Cancer Syndrome. Hereditary nonpolyposis colon cancer (HNPCC) syndrome is an autosomal dominant disorder characterized by familial carcinomas of the colon affecting predominantly the cecum and proximal colon (Chapter 17). It results from defects in a family of genes encoding a group of proteins that work together to carry out *DNA mismatch repair.* When a strand of DNA is being replicated, these proteins act as "spell checkers." For example, if there is an erroneous pairing of G with T rather than the normal A with T, the mismatch-repair factors correct the defect. Individuals with HNPCC syndrome inherit one abnormal copy of a mismatch repair gene. Trouble arises when cells acquire loss-of-function mutations, presumably at random, in their normal alleles. With "proofreading" function lost, errors gradually accumulate throughout the genome, and some of these errors may by chance activate proto-oncogenes or inactivate tumor suppressor genes. With time, a cancer may result. Thus, DNA-repair genes behave like tumor suppressor genes in their mode of inheritance, but in contrast to tumor suppressor genes (and oncogenes), they affect cell growth only indirectly—by allowing mutations in other genes during the process of normal cell division.

One of the hallmarks of patients with mismatch-repair defects is *microsatellite instability.* Microsatellites are tandem repeats of one to six nucleotides found throughout the genome. In normal people the length of these microsatellites remains constant. However, in people with HNPCC, these satellites are unstable and increase or decrease in length in tumor cells, creating alleles not found in normal cells of the same patient.

Of the various DNA mismatch-repair genes, at least four are involved in the pathogenesis of HNPCC. Germline mutations in the *MSH2* and *MLH1* genes each account for approximately 30% of cases. The remaining cases have mutations in other mismatch repair genes. Although HNPCC accounts only for 2% to 4% of all colonic cancers, microsatellite instability can be detected in about 15% of sporadic colon cancers. The cancer genes that are mutated in HNPCC tumors have not yet been fully characterized but include the genes encoding TGF-β receptor II, the TCF component of the β-catenin pathway, *BAX,* and other oncogenes and tumor suppressor genes.

Xeroderma Pigmentosum. Individuals with another inherited disorder of DNA repair, xeroderma pigmentosum, are at increased risk for the development of cancers of the skin particularly following exposure to the UV light contained in sun rays. UV radiation causes cross-linking of pyrimidine residues, preventing normal DNA replication. Such DNA damage is repaired by the nucleotide excision repair system. Several proteins are involved in *nucleotide excision repair,* and an inherited loss of any one can give rise to xeroderma pigmentosum.

Diseases with Defects in DNA Repair by Homologous Recombination. Several rare autosomal recessive cancer syndromes have been described that are characterized by hypersensitivity to certain kinds of DNA-damaging agents, such as ionizing radiation (*Bloom syndrome* and *ataxia-telangiectasia*), or DNA cross-linking agents, such as many chemotherapeutic drugs (*Fanconi anemia*). The phenotype of these diseases is complex and includes, in addition to predisposition to cancer, features such as neural symptoms (ataxia-telangiectasia), bone marrow aplasia (Fanconi anemia), and developmental defects (Bloom syndrome).

- As mentioned earlier, the gene mutated in ataxia-telangiectasia, *ATM*, is important in recognizing and responding to DNA damage caused by ionizing radiation. Persons with Bloom syndrome have a predisposition to a very broad spectrum of tumors. The defective gene encodes a helicase that participates in DNA repair by homologous recombination.
- There are 13 genes that make up the Fanconi anemia complex; mutation of any one of these genes can result in the phenotype. Interestingly, *BRCA2*, which is mutated in some individuals with familial breast cancer, is also mutated in a subset of persons with Fanconi anemia.
- Mutations in two genes, *BRCA1* and *BRCA2*, account for 25% of cases of familial breast cancer. In addition to breast cancer, women with *BRCA1* mutations have a substantially higher risk of epithelial ovarian cancers, and men have a slightly higher risk of prostate cancer. Likewise, mutations in the *BRCA2* gene increase the risk of breast cancer in both men and women as well as cancer of the ovary, prostate, pancreas, bile ducts, stomach, melanocytes, and B lymphocytes. Although their functions have not been elucidated fully, cells that lack these genes develop chromosomal breaks and severe aneuploidy. It appears that the Fanconi anemia proteins and the BRCA proteins form a DNA-damage response network whose purpose is to repair certain types of DNA damage using the homologous recombination repair pathway. Defects in this pathway leads to the activation of the salvage nonhomologous end joining pathway, formation of dicentric chromosomes, bridge-fusion-breakage cycles, and massive aneuploidy. Although linkage of *BRCA1* and *BRCA2* to familial breast cancers is established, these genes are rarely inactivated in sporadic cases of breast cancer. In this regard, *BRCA1* and *BRCA2* are different from other tumor suppressor genes, such as *APC* and *p53*, which are inactivated in both familial and sporadic cancers.

Cancers Resulting from Mutations Induced by Regulated Genomic Instability: Lymphoid Neoplasms. A special type of DNA damage plays a central role in the pathogenesis of tumors of B and T lymphocytes. As described in Chapter 6, adaptive immunity relies on the ability of B and T cells to diversify their antigen receptor genes. Early B and T cells both express a pair of gene products, RAG1 and RAG2, that carry out V(D)J segment recombination, permitting the asembly of functional antigen receptor genes. In addition, after encountering antigen mature B cells express a specialized enzyme called antigen-induced cytosine deaminase (AID), which catalyzes both immunoglobulin gene class switch recombination and somatic hypermutation. Errors during antigen receptor gene assembly and diversification are responsible for many of the mutations that cause lymphoid neoplasms (Chapter 13).

KEY CONCEPTS

Genomic Instability as Enabler of Malignancy

- Persons with inherited mutations of genes involved in DNA repair systems are at greatly increased risk for the development of cancer.
- Patients with HNPCC syndrome have defects in the mismatch repair system, leading to development of carcinomas of the colon. These patients' genomes show microsatellite instability, characterized by changes in length of short repeats throughout the genome.
- Patients with xeroderma pigmentosum have a defect in the nucleotide excision repair pathway and are at increased risk for the development of cancers of the skin exposed to UV light, because of an inability to repair pyrimidine dimers.
- Syndromes involving defects in the homologous recombination DNA repair system constitute a group of disorders—Bloom syndrome, ataxia-telangiectasia, and Fanconi anemia—that are characterized by hypersensitivity to DNA-damaging agents, such as ionizing radiation. *BRCA1* and *BRCA2*, which are mutated in familial breast cancers, are involved in DNA repair.
- Mutations incurred in lymphoid cells due to expression of gene products that induce genomic instability (RAG1, RAG2, AID) are important causes of lymphoid neoplasms.

Cancer-Enabling Inflammation

Infiltrating cancers provoke a chronic inflammatory reaction, leading some to liken them to "wounds that do not heal." In patients with advanced cancers, this inflammatory reaction can be so extensive as to cause systemic signs and symptoms, such as anemia (due to inflammation-induced sequestration of iron and downregulation of erythropoietin production, Chapter 14), fatigue, and cachexia (described later). However, studies carried out on cancers in animal models suggest that inflammatory cells also modify the local tumor microenvironment to enable many of the hallmarks of cancer. These effects may stem from direct interactions between inflammatory cells and tumor cells, or through indirect effects of inflammatory cells on other resident stromal cells, particularly cancer-associated fibroblasts and endothelial cells. Proposed cancer-enabling effects of inflammatory cells and resident stromal cells include the following:

- **Release of factors that promote proliferation**. Infiltrating leukocytes and activated stromal cells have been shown to secrete a wide variety of growth factors, such as EGF, and proteases that can liberate growth factors from the extracellular matrix (ECM).
- **Removal of growth suppressors**. As mentioned, the growth of epithelial cells is suppressed by cell-cell and cell-ECM interactions. Proteases released by inflammatory cells can degrade the adhesion molecules that mediate these interactions, removing a barrier to growth.
- **Enhanced resistance to cell death**. Recall that detachment of epithelial cells from basement membranes and from cell-cell interactions can lead to a particular form of cell death called *anoikis*. It is suspected that tumor-associated macrophages may prevent anoikis by

expressing adhesion molecules such as integrins that promote direct physical interactions with tumor cells. There is also substantial evidence that stromal cell–cancer cell interactions increase the resistance of cancer cells to chemotherapy, presumably by activating signaling pathways that promote cell survival in the face of stresses such as DNA damage.

- **Inducing angiogenesis**. Inflammatory cells release numerous factors, including VEGF, which can stimulate angiogenesis.
- **Activating invasion and metastasis**. Proteases released from macrophages foster tissue invasion by remodeling the ECM, while factors such as TNF and EGF may directly stimulate tumor cell motility. As mentioned, other factors released from stromal cells, such as TGF-β, may promote epithelial-mesenchymal transitions, which is considered to be a key event in the process of invasion and metastasis.
- **Evading immune destruction**. A variety of soluble factors released by macrophages and other stromal cells are believed to contribute to the immunosuppressive microenvironment of tumors, including TGF-β and a number of other factors that either favor the recruitment of immunosuppressive T regulatory cells or suppress the function of CD8+ cytotoxic T cells. Furthermore, there is abundant evidence in murine cancer models and emerging evidence in human disease that advanced cancers contain mainly alternatively activated (M2) macrophages (Chapter 3), cells induced by cytokines such as IL-4 and IL-13. These macrophages produce cytokines that promote angiogenesis, fibroblast proliferation, and collagen deposition, all of which are commonly observed in invasive cancers. In addition, they appear to suppress effective host immune responses to cancer cells through mechanisms that remain to be elucidated.

A thorough understanding of how cancers "manipulate" inflammatory cells to support their growth and survival remains elusive. However, the results from animal studies are intriguing and raise the possibility of therapies directed at tumor-induced inflammation and its downstream consequences. Of note in this regard, COX2 inhibitors have been shown to decrease the incidence of colonic adenomas and are now approved for treatment of patients with familial adenomatous polyposis.

Dysregulation of Cancer-Associated Genes

The genetic damage that activates oncogenes or inactivates tumor suppressor genes may be subtle (e.g., point mutations) or may involve segments of chromosomes large enough to be detected in a routine karyotype. Activation of oncogenes and loss of function of tumor suppressor genes by mutations were discussed earlier in this chapter. Here we first discuss chromosomal abnormalities and then end this section by discussing the epigenetic changes that contribute to carcinogenesis and the role of noncoding RNAs.

Chromosomal Changes

Certain chromosomal abnormalities are highly associated with particular neoplasms and inevitably lead to the dysregulation of genes with an integral role in the pathogenesis of that tumor type. Specific recurrent chromosomal abnormalities have been identified in most leukemias and lymphomas, many sarcomas, and an increasing number of carcinomas. In addition, whole chromosomes may be gained or lost. Although changes in chromosome number (aneuploidy) and structure are generally considered to be late phenomena in cancer progression, in some cases (e.g., in cells that have lost their telomeres, Figure 7-34), it can be an early event that initiates the transformation process.

Historically, chromosomal changes in cancer were identified through karyotyping, the morphologic identification of metaphase chromosomes prepared from clinical specimens. Today, however, cancer cell karyotypes are being reconstructed in research labs from deep sequencing of cancer cell genomes, and it is possible that conventional karyotyping will be supplanted by other methods even in clinical laboratories in the years to come. Whatever technology is used, the study of chromosomal changes in tumor cells is important. First, genes in the vicinity of recurrent chromosomal breakpoints or deletions are very likely to be either oncogenes (e.g., *MYC*, *BCL2*, *ABL*) or tumor suppressor genes (e.g., *APC*, *RB*). Second, certain karyotypic abnormalities have diagnostic value or important prognostic or therapeutic implications. For example, tests that detect and quantify *BCR-ABL* fusion genes or their mRNA products are essential for the diagnosis of CML and are used to monitor the response to BCR-ABL kinase inhibitors. Many additional chromosomal aberrations that are characteristic of specific tumor types are presented in later chapters.

Chromosomal Translocations. Any type of chromosomal rearrangement—translocations, inversions, amplifications, and even small deletions—can activate proto-oncogenes, but chromosomal translocation is the most common mechanism described to date. Notable examples of oncogenes activated by chromosomal translocations are listed in Table 7-8. Translocations can activate proto-oncogenes in two ways:

- By promoter or enhancer substitution, in which the translocation results in overexpression of a proto-oncogene by swapping its regulatory elements with those of another gene, typically one that is highly expressed.
- By formation of a fusion gene in which the coding sequences of two genes are fused in part or in whole, leading to the expression of a novel chimeric protein with oncogenic properties.

Overexpression of a proto-oncogene caused by translocation is exemplified by Burkitt lymphoma. Virtually all Burkitt lymphomas have a translocation involving chromosome 8q24, where the *MYC* gene resides, and one of the three chromosomes that carry an immunoglobulin gene. At its normal locus, *MYC* is tightly controlled, and is most highly expressed in actively dividing cells. In Burkitt lymphoma the most common translocation moves the *MYC*-containing segment of chromosome 8 to chromosome 14q32 (See Fig. 7-26), placing it close to the immunoglobulin heavy chain (*IGH*) gene. The genetic notation for the translocation is t(8:14)(q24;q32). The molecular

Table 7-8 Selected Examples of Oncogenes Created by Translocations

Malignancy	Translocation	Affected Genes*
Chronic myelogenous leukemia (CML)	(9;22)(q34;q11)	*ABL* 9q34 *BCR* 22q11
Acute myeloid leukemia (AML)	(8;21)(q22;q22) (15;17)(q22;q21)	*AML* 8q22 *ETO* 21q22 *PML* 15q22 *RARA* 17q21
Burkitt lymphoma	(8;14)(q24;q32)	*MYC* 8q24 *IGH* 14q32
Mantle cell lymphoma	(11;14)(q13;q32)	*CCND1* 11q13 *IGH* 14q32
Follicular lymphoma	(14;18)(q32;q21)	*IGH* 14q32 *BCL2* 18q21
Ewing sarcoma	(11;22)(q24;q12)	*FLI1* 11q24 *EWSR1* 22q12
Prostatic adenocarcinoma	(7:21)(p22;q22) (17:21)(p21;q22)	*TMPRSS2* (21q22.3) *ETV1* (7p21.2) *ETV4* (17q21)

*Genes in bold type are involved in multiple rearrangements.

mechanisms of the translocation-mediated overexpression of *MYC* are variable, as are the precise breakpoints within the *MYC* gene. In most cases the translocation removes regulatory sequences of the *MYC* gene and replaces them with the control regions of the *IGH* gene, which is highly expressed in B-cells. The *MYC* coding sequences remain intact and the MYC protein is constitutively expressed at high levels. The almost invariable presence of *MYC* translocations in Burkitt lymphomas attests to the importance of *MYC* overactivity in the pathogenesis of this tumor.

There are many other examples of translocations involving oncogenes and antigen receptor loci in lymphoid tumors. For these (or any other) translocations to occur, double-stranded DNA breaks must occur simultaneously in at least two places in the genome and the free DNA ends must then be joined to create two new derivative chromosomes. In lymphoid cells most of these molecular misadventures are believed to occur during attempts at normal antigen receptor gene recombination (which occurs in both B- and T-cell progenitors) or class-switch recombination (which is confined to antigen-stimulated mature B cells). Not unexpectedly, tumors with translocations involving immunoglobulin genes are always of B-cell origin, and tumors with translocations involving T cell receptor genes are always of T-cell origin. The affected genes are diverse, but as with translocations involving *MYC*, the net effect is overexpression of some protein with oncogenic activity.

The *Philadelphia chromosome*, characteristic of CML and a subset of B-cell acute lymphoblastic leukemias (Chapter 13), provides the prototypic example of a chromosomal rearrangement that creates a fusion gene encoding a chimeric oncoprotein. In this instance, the two chromosome breaks lie within the *ABL* gene on chromosome 9 and within the *BCR* (*b*reakpoint *c*luster *r*egion) gene on chromosome 22 (Fig. 7-26). Non-homologous end-joining then leads to a reciprocal translocation that creates an oncogenic *BCR-ABL* fusion gene on the derivative chromosome 22 (the so-called Philadelphia chromosome).

The *BCR-ABL* fusion gene encodes a chimeric BCR-ABL protein with constitutive tyrosine kinase activity. Although the translocations are cytogenetically identical in CML and B-cell acute lymphoblastic leukemias (B-ALL), the structure of the resulting *BCR-ABL* fusion genes and proteins they encode usually differ slightly in these two tumors. Since the discovery of *BCR-ABL* in CML, many other fusion oncogenes encoding constitutively active tyrosine kinases have been described in a broad array of human cancers. Like BCR-ABL, these fusion proteins drive oncogenic signaling pathways and have sometimes proven to be targets of effective therapies.

Other oncogenic fusion genes encode nuclear factors that regulate transcription or chromatin structure. In contrast to overactive tyrosine kinases, less is generally known about how nuclear oncoproteins function. An exception with important clinical consequences is found in a form of leukemia called *acute promyelocytic leukemia* (APML). APML is virtually always associated with a reciprocal translocation between chromosomes 15 and 17 that produces a *PML-RARA* fusion gene (Fig. 7-41). How this fusion gene functions is now reasonably well understood.

- The fusion gene encodes a chimeric protein consisting of part of a protein called PML and part of the retinoic acid receptor-α (RARα). Normal RARα binds to DNA and activates transcription in the presence of retinoids. Among the RARα responsive genes are a number that are needed for the differentiation of myeloid progenitors into neutrophils.
- The PML-RARα oncoprotein has diminished affinity for retinoids, such that at physiologic levels retinoids do not bind to PML-RARα to any significant degree. In this "unliganded" state, it retains the capacity to bind DNA, but instead of activating transcription, it inhibits transcription through recruitment of transcriptional repressors. This interferes with the expression of genes that are needed for differentiation, leading to a "pile-up" of proliferating myeloid progenitors that replace normal bone marrow elements.
- When given in pharmacologic doses, all-trans retinoic acid binds to PML-RARα and causes a conformational change that results in the displacement of repressor complexes and the recruitment of different complexes that activate transcription. This exchange overcomes the block in gene expression, causing the neoplastic myeloid progenitors to differentiate into neutrophils and die, clearing the marrow over several days and allowing for recovery of normal hematopoiesis.

This highly effective therapy is the first example of *differentiation therapy*, in which immortal tumor cells are induced to differentiate into their mature progeny, which have limited life spans. It has also spurred efforts to develop drugs that target other nuclear oncoproteins, despite the inherent difficulty of the problem.

Deletions. Chromosomal deletions are another very prevalent structural abnormality in tumor cells. Deletion of specific regions of chromosomes is associated with the loss of particular tumor suppressor genes.

As we discussed earlier, deletions involving chromosome 13q14, the site of the *RB* gene, are associated with retinoblastoma, and deletion of the *VHL* tumor suppressor gene on chromosome 3p is a very common event in renal cell carcinomas. Ongoing sequencing of cancer cell genomes will undoubtedly reveal many more examples of deletions

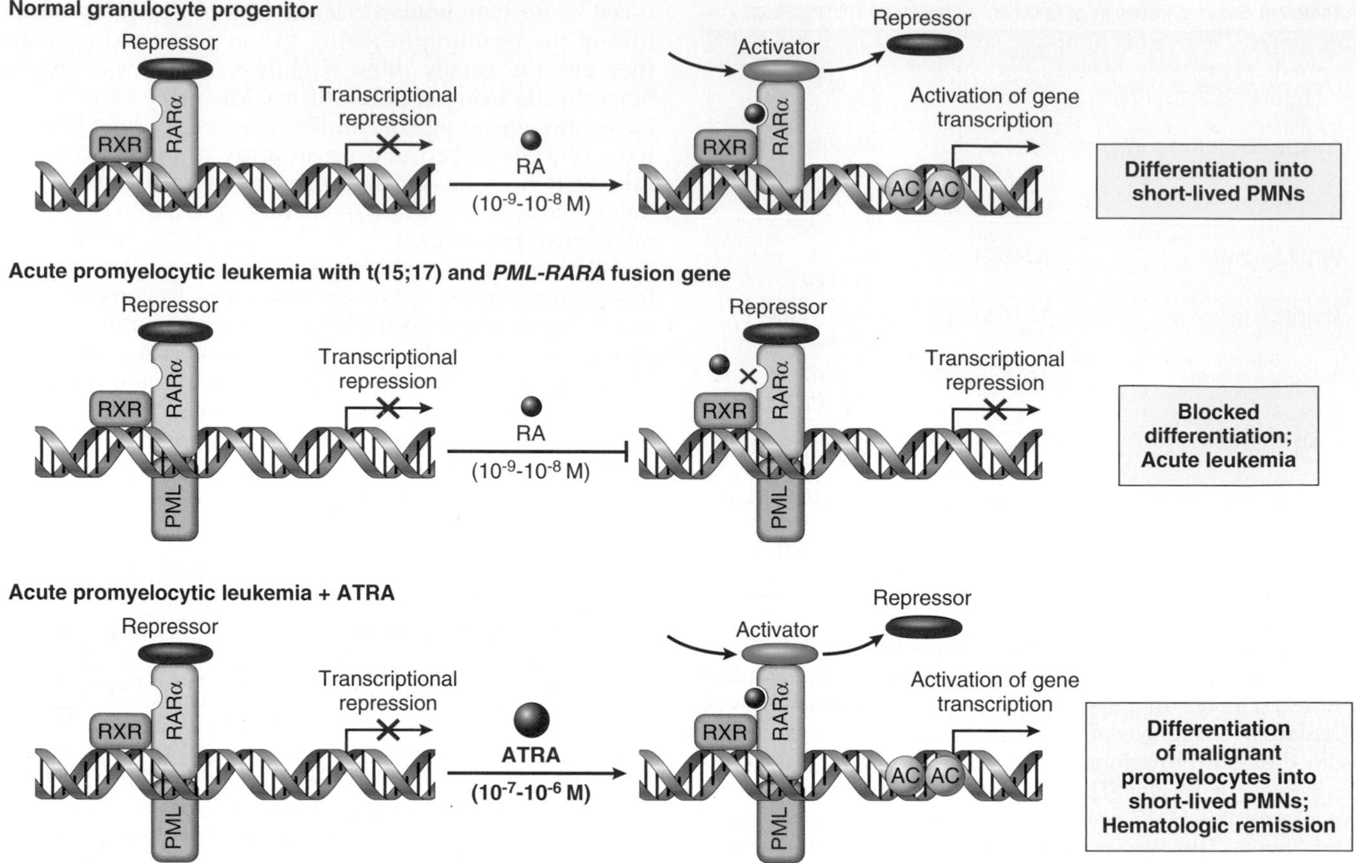

Figure 7-41 Molecular pathogenesis of acute promyelocytic leukemia and basis for response to all-trans retinoic acid. ATRA, all-trans retinoic acid; RA, retinoic acid; RXR, binding partner for normal RARa and PML-RARa fusion protein encoded by a chimeric gene created by the (15;17) translocation in acute promyelocytic leukemia.

involving tumor suppressor genes, as well as small insertions of DNA from one site into another. It should be noted that not all deletions lead to loss of gene function; a few activate oncogenes through the same mechanisms as chromosomal translocations. For example, about 25% of T-cell acute lymphoblastic leukemias have small deletions of chromosome 1 that juxtapose the *TAL1* proto-oncogene with a nearby active promoter, leading to overexpression of the TAL1 transcription factor. Similarly, deletions involving chromosome 5 in a subset of lung cancers produce an oncogenic *EML4-ALK* fusion gene encoding a constitutively active tyrosine kinase. It is likely that more "cryptic" deletions that activate oncogenes will be discovered through deep sequencing of cancer genomes.

Gene Amplification. Overexpression of oncogenes may also result from reduplication and amplification of their DNA sequences. Such amplification may produce up to several hundred copies of the oncogene in the tumor cell. In some cases the amplified genes produce chromosomal changes that can be identified microscopically. Two mutually exclusive patterns are seen: (1) multiple small extrachromosomal structures called *double minutes* and (2) *homogeneous staining regions.* The latter derive from the insertion of the amplified genes into new chromosomal locations, which may be distant from the normal location of the involved oncogene. The affected chromosomal regions lack a normal pattern of light and dark-staining bands, appearing homogeneous in karyotypes (Fig. 7-27). From a clinical perspective the most important amplifications are *NMYC* in neuroblastoma and *ERBB2* in breast cancers. *NMYC* is amplified in 25% to 30% of neuroblastomas, and its amplification is associated with poor prognosis. *ERBB2* amplification occurs in about 20% of breast cancers. As already mentioned, antibody therapy directed against the HER2 receptor encoded by *ERBB2* is an effective therapy for this molecular subset of breast cancers.

Chromothrypsis. The true extent of chromosome rearrangements in cancer is only now coming into view thanks to sequencing of entire cancer cell genomes, which allows for comprehensive "reconstruction" of chromosomes from DNA sequences. Genomic sequencing has revealed not only many simple rearrangements (e.g., small deletions, duplications, or inversions) that were not appreciated by prior methods, but also much more dramatic chromosome "catastrophes" termed *chromothrypsis* (literally, chromosome shattering). Chromothrypsis is observed in 1% to 2% of cancers as a whole, but is found in up to 25% of osteosarcomas and other bone cancers and at relatively high frequency in gliomas as well. It appears to result from a single event in which dozens to hundreds of chromosome breaks occur within part or across the entirety of a single chromosome or several chromosomes. The genesis of these breaks is unknown, but DNA repair mechanisms are activated in affected cells that stitch the pieces together in a haphazard way, creating many chromosome rearrangements and also resulting in the loss of some chromosome segments. It is hypothesized that such catastrophic events by chance simultaneously activate oncogenes and inactivate tumor suppressors, thereby expediting the process of carcinogenesis.

KEY CONCEPTS

Genetic Lesions in Cancer

- Tumor cells may acquire several types of oncogenic mutations, including point mutations and other nonrandom chromosomal abnormalities, such as translocations, deletions, and gene amplifications.
- Balanced translocations contribute to carcinogenesis by overexpression of oncogenes or generation of novel fusion proteins with altered signaling capacity. Deletions frequently cause loss of tumor suppressor gene function, and occasionally activate proto-oncogenes. Gene amplification generally increases the expression and function of oncogenes.
- Genomic sequencing has revealed numerous "cryptic" (subcytogenetic) rearrangements, mainly small deletions and insertions ("indels"), as well as chromothrypsis, in which a chromosome is "shattered" and then reassembled in a haphazard way.

Epigenetic Changes

Epigenetic changes have important roles in many aspects of the malignant phenotype, including the expression of cancer genes, the control of differentiation and self-renewal, and even drug sensitivity and drug resistance. As discussed in Chapter 1, "epigenetics" refers to factors other than the sequence of DNA that regulate gene expression (and, thereby, cellular phenotype). Recall that these factors include histones modifications catalyzed by enzymes associated with chromatin regulatory complexes; DNA methylation, a modification created by DNA methyltransferases; and other less well characterized proteins that regulate the higher order organization of DNA (e.g., looping of enhancer elements onto gene promoters).

It has been recognized for more than a hundred years that the nuclei of cancer cells display abnormal morphologies, which (as discussed earlier) may take the form of hyperchromasia, chromatin clumping, or chromatin clearing (so-called vesicular nuclear chromatin). These altered appearances stem from disturbances of chromatin organization, the basis of which has been obscure. One of the most notable findings emerging from the sequencing of cancer genomes has been the identification of numerous mutations involving genes that encode epigenetic regulatory proteins (Table 7-9). As a result, it is now suspected that the altered morphologic appearance of cancer cells reflects acquired genetic defects in factors that maintain the epigenome. Indeed, methods that allow genome-wide assessment of the cell's epigenome are now available and have begun to reveal widespread epigenetic alterations in cancers, which can be broadly divided into the following categories:

Table 7-9 Examples of Epigenomic Regulatory Genes that are Mutated in Cancer

Gene(s)	Function	Tumor (Approximate Frequency of Mutation)
DNMT3A	DNA methylation	Acute myeloid leukemia (20%)
MLL1	Histone methylation	Acute leukemia in infants (90%)
MLL2	Histone methylation	Follicular lymphoma (90%)
CREBBP/ EP300	Histone acetylation	Diffuse large B cell lymphoma (40%)
ARID1A	Nucleosome positioning/chromatin remodeling	Ovarian clear cell carcinoma (60%), endometrial carcinoma (30%-40%)
SNF5	Nucleosome positioning/chromatin remodeling	Malignant rhabdoid tumor (100%)
PBRM1	Nucleosome positioning/chromatin remodeling	Renal carcinoma (30%)

- **Silencing of tumor suppressor genes by local hypermethylation of DNA.** Some cancer cells exhibit selective hypermethylation of the promoters of tumor suppressor genes that results in their transcriptional silencing. Typically, hypermethylation occurs on only one allele and the function of the other copy of the affected tumor suppressor gene is lost through another mechanism, such as a disabling point mutation or a deletion. One of several examples of a tumor suppressor gene that is hypermethylated in several cancers is *CDKN2A*, which you will recall is a complex locus that encodes two tumor suppressors, p14/ARF and p16/INK4a, that enhance p53 and RB activity, respectively.
- **Global changes in DNA methylation.** In addition to local hypermethylation of tumor suppressor genes, many tumors exhibit abnormal patterns of DNA methylation throughout their genomes, sometimes in the form of hypermethylation and other times as hypomethylation. Tumors commonly exhibiting abnormal DNA methylation, such as acute myeloid leukemia, sometimes have mutations in genes encoding DNA methyltransferases or other factors that influence DNA methylation (Table 7-9), suggesting that the observed alterations have a genetic basis. The most obvious potential consequence of global changes in methylation is altered expression of multiple genes, which may be overexpressed or underexpressed compared to normal depending on the nature of local changes. In addition, however, mice engineered to have hypomethylated genomes also exhibit chromosomal instability; thus, altered DNA methylation may contribute to tumorigenesis in several ways.
- **Changes in histones.** Cancer cells often demonstrate changes in histones near genes that influence cellular behavior. As with changes in DNA methylation, in an increasing number of instances it appears that these alterations have a genetic basis, being attributable to mutations that affect the activities of protein complexes that "write", "read" and "erase" histone marks, or that position nucleosomes on DNA (Table 7-9). Details have yet to emerge, but it is virtually certain that these lesions somehow alter the expression of sets of genes that contribute to the malignant phenotype.

Much remains to be deciphered about the state of the "epigenome" in various cancers and its contribution to the malignant state, but several aspects of the relationship merit emphasis.

- The lineage-specificity of certain oncogenes and tumor suppressor genes has an epigenetic basis. You may have noticed that tumor suppressors and oncoproteins can be broadly divided into two classes, those that are mutated or otherwise dysregulated in many cancers (e.g., RAS, MYC, p53), and those that are mutated in a restricted subset of tumors (e.g., VHL in renal cell carcinomas, APC in colon carcinoma) and are thus lineage restricted. A cancer cell's lineage or differentiation state, like that of normal cells, is generated by epigenetic modifications that produce a pattern of gene expression that characterizes that particular cell type. It follows that lineage-restricted cancer genes only act within epigenetic contexts in which key oncogenic targets are controlled by these genes.
- The epigenome is an attractive therapeutic target. Because the epigenetic state of a cell depends on reversible modifications that are carried out by enzymes (which are generally good drug targets), there is intense interest in developing drugs that target epigenomic modifiers in cancer and other diseases. Inhibitors of histone deacetylases, chromatin erasers that remove acetyl groups from histones, are approved for use in certain lymphoid tumors, and DNA methylation inhibitors are now being used to treat myeloid tumors, based in part on the idea that these drugs may reactivate tumor suppressor genes. Other drugs that target specific chromatin writers and chromatin readers are also now being tested in clinical trials.
- Cancers may exhibit considerable epigenetic heterogeneity. Just as genomic instability gives rise to genetic heterogeneity in cancers, it is feared that cancers will also prove to have extensive epigenetic heterogeneity from cell to cell within individual tumors. One consequence of such heterogeneity may be drug resistance. For example, epigenetic alterations can lead to the resistance of lung cancer cells to inhibitors of EGF receptor signaling. When the inhibitors are removed, the lung cancer cells revert to their prior inhibitor-sensitive state. If widespread, such epigenetic plasticity may join genetic heterogeneity as yet another barrier to the development of curative cancer therapies.

Noncoding RNAs and Cancer

As discussed in Chapter 1, microRNAs (miRs) are small noncoding, single-stranded RNAs, approximately 22 nucleotides in length, that mediate sequence-specific inhibition of messenger RNA (mRNA) translation through the action of the RNA-induced silencing complex (RISC). Given that miRs control normal cell growth, differentiation, and cell survival, it is not surprising that they play a role in carcinogenesis. Altered miR expression, sometimes stemming from amplifications and deletions of miR loci, has been identified in many cancers. Decreased expression of certain miRs increases the translation of oncogenic mRNAs; such mIRs have tumor suppressive activity. Conversely, overexpression of other mIRs represss the expression of tumor suppressor genes; such mIRs promote tumor development and are often referred to as *onco-mIRs.* Specific examples of contributions of mIRs to cancer are numerous; the following are among the best established:

- **OncomiRs**. miR-200 has been shown to promote epithelial-mesenchymal transitions believed to be important in invasiveness and metastasis; and miR-155, originally identified at the site of retroviral insertions in avian lymphomas, is overexpressed in many human B cell lymphomas and indirectly upregulates a large number of genes that promote proliferation, including *MYC*.
- **Tumor suppressive miRs**. Deletions affecting certain tumor suppressive miRs, such as miR-15 and miR-16, are among the most frequent genetic lesions in chronic lymphocytic leukemia, a common tumor of older adults. In this context, it appears that their loss leads to upregulation of the anti-apoptotic protein BCL-2.
- **Tumor suppressive properties of mIR processing factors**. Study of families that are prone to the development of an unusual collection of neoplasms, including certain rare ovarian and testicular tumors, unexpectedly identified heterozygous germline defects in *DICER*, a gene that encodes an endonuclease that is required for the processing and production of functional mIRs. Thus, *DICER* is tumor suppressive in certain cellular contexts. Whether the tumor suppressive function of DICER stems from its involvement in processing of miRs remains to be established.

The involvement of miRs is likely the proverbial tip-of-the-iceberg with respect to the role of noncoding RNAs in cancer. Systematic genomic analyses have revealed that more than 60% of the genome is transcribed into RNAs, most of which are noncoding and believed to have regulatory functions (Chapter 1). These noncoding RNAs fall into several classes: piwi-interacting RNAs (piRNAs), the most common type of small noncoding RNA, which (like miRs) are believed to have a role in post-transcriptional gene silencing; snoRNAs, which are important in maturation of rRNA and the assembly of ribosomes; and long intervening noncoding RNAs (lincRNAs), some of which regulate the activity of chromatin "writers," the factors that modify histones and thereby control gene expression. Abnormalities in the expression of these regulatory RNAs have also been implicated in several human diseases, including cancer, and many more examples of cancer-associations are likely to be forthcoming.

Molecular Basis of Multistep Carcinogenesis

Given that malignant tumors must acquire multiple "hallmarks" of cancer, it follows that cancers result from the stepwise accumulation of multiple mutations that act in complementary ways to produce a fully malignant tumor. The notion that malignant tumors arise from a protracted sequence of events is supported by epidemiologic, experimental, and molecular studies, and the study of oncogenes and tumor suppressor genes has provided a firm molecular footing for the concept of multistep carcinogenesis. Genome-wide sequencing of cancers has revealed as few as ten or so mutations in certain leukemias

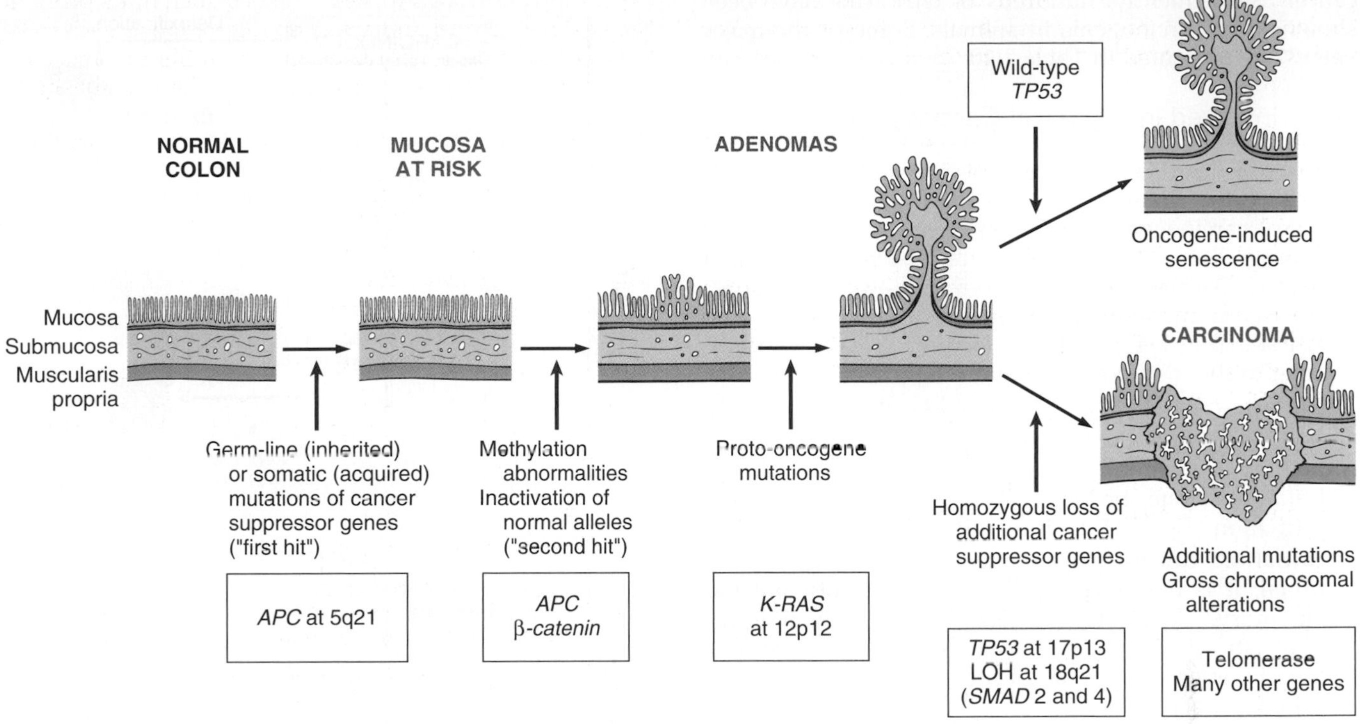

Figure 7-42 Molecular model for the evolution of colorectal cancers through the adenoma-carcinoma sequence. Although *APC* mutation is an early event and loss of *TP53* occurs late in the process of tumorigenesis, the timing for the other changes may be variable. Note also that individual tumors may not have all of the changes listed. *Top right*, cells that gain oncogene signaling without loss of *TP53* eventually enter oncogene-induced senescence. LOH, loss-of-heterozygosity.

to many thousands of mutations in tumors that arise following chronic exposure to carcinogens, such as lung cancers associated with cigarette smoking. Although the presence of multiple mutations is consistent with the idea that no single mutation will suffice to produce a cancer, as already mentioned it is often difficult to determine which mutations in a tumor drive oncogenesis and which are "passengers," mutations that provide no advantage to the tumor cell and are merely along for the ride.

A more direct answer to the question "how many mutations does it take to establish a fully malignant tumor?" comes from experimental attempts to transform normal human cells with combinations of oncogenes, some derived from transforming viruses (described later). For example, normal human epithelial cells can be transformed by the following combination of events: (1) activation of RAS; (2) inactivation of RB; (3) inactivation of p53; (4) inactivation of PP2A, a tumor suppressive phosphatase that is a negative regulator of many signaling pathways; and (5) constitutive expression of telomerase. Cells bearing all of these alterations are immortal and produce invasive, fully malignant growths when injected into immunodeficient mice.

Unlike in the laboratory, these events presumably never occur simultaneously during the natural development of a human cancer, but instead occur in a stepwise fashion. What is the evidence that this is so? A classic example of incremental acquisition of the malignant phenotype is found in colon carcinoma. Many of these cancers evolve through a series of morphologically identifiable stages: colon epithelial hyperplasia followed by formation of adenomas that progressively enlarge and ultimately undergo malignant transformation (Chapter 17). Molecular analyses of proliferations at each of these stages have indeed shown that precancerous lesions have fewer mutations than adenocarcinomas and suggest a tendency to acquire particular mutations in the sequence illustrated in Figure 7-42. According to this scheme, inactivation of the *APC* tumor suppressor gene occurs first, followed by activation of *RAS* and, ultimately, loss of a tumor suppressor gene on 18q and loss of *TP53*. While multiple mutations, including gain of oncogenes and loss of tumor suppressors, are required for carcinogenesis, the precise temporal sequence of mutations does not appear to be fixed and may be different in each organ and tumor type.

Similar evidence for stepwise progression also exists for other recognizable precursor lesions to epithelial cancers, such as dysplasias of the cervix, hyperplasias of the endometrium, and the evolution of oral cancers. These are described in subsequent chapters.

Carcinogenic Agents and Their Cellular Interactions

More than 200 years ago the London surgeon Sir Percival Pott correctly attributed scrotal skin cancer in chimney sweeps to chronic exposure to soot. Based on this observation, the Danish Chimney Sweeps Guild ruled that its members must bathe daily. No public health measure since that time has achieved so much in controlling a form of cancer! Subsequently, hundreds of chemicals have been shown to be carcinogenic in animals. Some of the major agents are presented in Table 7-10.

Steps Involved in Chemical Carcinogenesis

As discussed earlier, carcinogenesis is a multistep process. This is readily demonstrated in experimental models of chemical carcinogenesis, in which the stages of initiation and progression during cancer development were first described. The classic experiments that allowed the distinction between initiation and promotion were performed on mouse skin (Fig. 7-43), and revealed the following concepts relating to the initiation-promotion sequence:

- **Initiation** results from exposure of cells to a sufficient dose of a carcinogenic agent; an initiated cell is altered, making it potentially capable of giving rise to a tumor. Initiation alone, however, is not sufficient for tumor formation (Fig. 7-43, treatment group 1).
- **Initiation causes permanent DNA damage (mutations); it is therefore rapid and irreversible and has "memory."** Thus, tumors are produced even if the application of the promoting agent is delayed for several months after a single application of the initiator (Fig. 7-43, treatment group 3).
- **Promoters can induce tumors to arise from initiated cells, but they are nontumorigenic by themselves.** Furthermore, tumors do not result when the promoting agent is applied before, rather than after, the initiating agent (Fig. 7-43, treatment group 4). This indicates that, in contrast to the effects of initiators, the cellular changes resulting from the application of promoters do not affect DNA directly and are reversible. As discussed later, promoters enhance the proliferation of initiated cells, an effect that may contribute to the acquisition of additional mutations.

Although the concepts of initiation and promotion have been derived largely from experiments involving induction of skin cancer in mice, they are also useful concepts when considering the roles of certain factors that contribute to human cancers. With this brief overview, initiation and promotion can be examined in more detail (Fig. 7-44). All initiating chemical carcinogens are highly reactive electrophiles (have electron-deficient atoms) that can react with nucleophilic (electron-rich) sites in the cell. Their targets are DNA, RNA, and proteins, and in some cases these interactions cause cell death. Initiation, obviously, inflicts nonlethal damage to the DNA that cannot be repaired. The mutated cell then passes on the DNA lesions to its daughter cells. Chemicals that can cause initiation of carcinogenesis can be classified into two categories: direct acting and indirect acting.

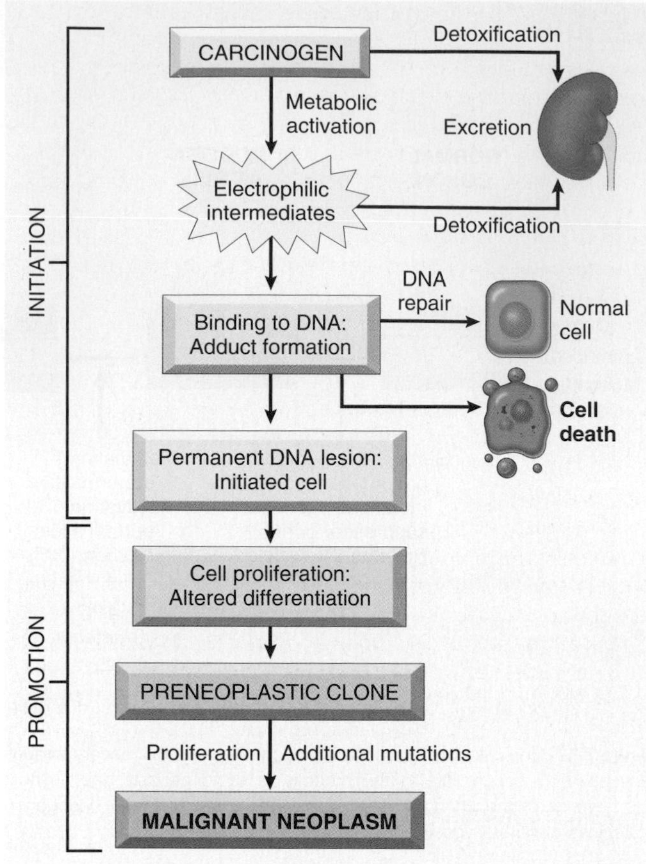

Figure 7-44 General schema of events in chemical carcinogenesis. Note that promoters cause clonal expansion of the initiated cell, thus producing a preneoplastic clone. Further proliferation induced by the promoter or other factors causes accumulation of additional mutations and emergence of a malignant tumor.

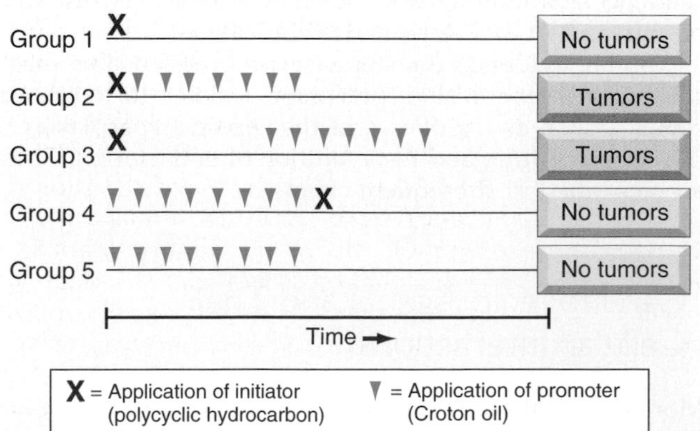

Figure 7-43 Experiments demonstrating the initiation and promotion phases of carcinogenesis in mice. Group 2: application of promoter repeated at twice-weekly intervals for several months. Group 3: application of promoter delayed for several months and then applied twice weekly.

Direct-Acting Carcinogens

Direct-acting carcinogens require no metabolic conversion to become carcinogenic. Most are weak carcinogens but some are important because they are cancer chemotherapeutic drugs (e.g., alkylating agents). Tragically, in some instances these agents have successfully cured, controlled, or delayed recurrence of certain types of cancer (e.g., leukemia, lymphoma, and ovarian carcinoma), only to evoke later a second form of cancer, usually acute myeloid leukemia. The risk of induced cancer is low, but its existence dictates judicious use of such agents.

Indirect-Acting Carcinogens

The designation indirect-acting carcinogen refers to chemicals that require metabolic conversion to become active carcinogens; the carcinogenic product of metabolism is called an *ultimate carcinogen*. Some of the most potent indirect chemical carcinogens—the polycyclic hydrocarbons—are present in fossil fuels. Others, for example, benzo[*a*] pyrene (the active component of soot, which Potts showed to be carcinogenic), are formed during the high-temperature combustion of tobacco in cigarettes and are implicated in the causation of lung cancer. Polycyclic hydrocarbons may also be produced from animal fats during the process of broiling or grilling meats and are present in smoked meats and fish. The principal active products in many hydrocarbons are epoxides, which form covalent adducts (addition products) with molecules in the cell, principally DNA, but also with RNA and proteins.

The aromatic amines and azo dyes are another class of indirect-acting carcinogens that were widely used in the past in the aniline dye and rubber industries. Many other occupational carcinogens are listed in Table 7-10.

Most chemical carcinogens require metabolic activation for conversion into ultimate carcinogens (Fig. 7-44). Certain metabolic pathways may inactivate (detoxify) the procarcinogen or its derivatives. Most of the known carcinogens are metabolized by *cytochrome P-450-dependent mono-oxygenases*. The genes that encode these enzymes are polymorphic, and the activity and inducibility of these enzymes vary significantly among individuals (described further in Chapter 9). Because these enzymes are essential for the activation of procarcinogens, the susceptibility to carcinogenesis is related in part to the particular polymorphic variants that an individual inherits. Thus, it may be possible to assess cancer risk in a given individual by genetic analysis of such enzyme polymorphisms.

Table 7-10 Major Chemical Carcinogens

Direct-Acting Carcinogens
Alkylating Agents
β-Propiolactone
Dimethyl sulfate
Diepoxybutane
Anticancer drugs (cyclophosphamide, chlorambucil, nitrosoureas, and others)
Acylating Agents
1-Acetyl-imidazole
Dimethylcarbamyl chloride
Procarcinogens That Require Metabolic Activation
Polycyclic and Heterocyclic Aromatic Hydrocarbons
Benz[*a*]anthracene
Benzo[*a*]pyrene
Dibenz[*a,h*]anthracene
3-Methylcholanthrene
7,12-Dimethylbenz[*a*]anthracene
Aromatic Amines, Amides, Azo Dyes
2-Naphthylamine (β-naphthylamine)
Benzidine
2-Acetylaminofluorene
Dimethylaminoazobenzene (butter yellow)
Natural Plant and Microbial Products
Aflatoxin B_1
Griseofulvin
Cycasin
Safrole
Betel nuts
Others
Nitrosamine and amides
Vinyl chloride, nickel, chromium
Insecticides, fungicides
Polychlorinated biphenyls

The metabolism of polycyclic aromatic hydrocarbons, such as benzo[*a*]pyrene by the product of the P-450 gene, *CYP1A1*, provides an instructive example. Approximately 10% of the white population has a highly inducible form of this enzyme that is associated with an increased risk of lung cancer in smokers. Light smokers with the susceptible *CYP1A1* genotype have a sevenfold higher risk of developing lung cancer compared with smokers without the permissive genotype. It should be appreciated, however, that not all variation in the activation or detoxification of carcinogens is genetically determined. Age, sex, and nutritional status also influence the internal dose of toxicants produced and hence the risk of cancer development in a particular individual.

Molecular Targets of Chemical Carcinogens. Because malignant transformation results from mutations, it comes as no surprise that most chemical initiating agents target DNA and are mutagenic. There is no single or unique alteration associated with cancer initiation. Nor is there any apparent predisposition for initiators to cause mutations in particular genes; presumably, mutations occur throughout the genome and cells that by chance suffer damage to the "usual suspects", oncogenes and tumor suppressors such as *RAS* and *TP53*, gain a potential selective advantage and are at risk for subsequent transformation.

This is not to say that mutations induced by carcinogens occur in an entirely random fashion. Because of their chemical structures, some carcinogens interact preferentially with particular DNA sequences or bases, and thus produce mutations that are clustered at "hotspots" or that are enriched for particular base substitutions. One illustrative example of a chemical carcinogen associated with a mutational "hotspot" is *aflatoxin* B_1, a naturally occurring agent produced by some strains of a mold called *Aspergillus*. *Aspergillus* grows on improperly stored grains and nuts, and there is a strong correlation between the dietary level of this food contaminant and the incidence of hepatocellular carcinoma in parts of Africa and the Far East. Interestingly, aflatoxin B_1-associated hepatocellular carcinomas tend to have a particular mutation in *TP53*, a G:C→T:A transversion in codon 249 that produces an arginine to serine substitution in the p53 protein. In contrast, *TP53* mutations are infrequent in liver tumors from areas where aflatoxin contamination of food does not occur, and few of these mutations involve codon 249. Similarly, lung cancers associated with smoking have a 10-fold higher mutational burden on average than lung cancers in nonsmokers, and these excess mutations are strongly skewed toward particular base substitutions known to be caused by carcinogens in cigarette smoke (the proverbial "smoking gun"). With sequencing of cancer genomes becoming routine, it is likely that other "carcinogen signatures" will be discovered; these associations may prove useful in epidemiologic studies of chemical carcinogenesis.

Additional potential carcinogens in the workplace and at home include vinyl chloride, arsenic, nickel, chromium, insecticides, fungicides, and polychlorinated biphenyls. Finally, nitrites used as food preservatives have caused concern, in that they cause nitrosylation of amines contained in the food. The nitrosoamines so formed are suspected to be carcinogenic.

Promotion of Chemical Carcinogenesis

Promoters are chemical agents that are not mutagenic, but which instead stimulate cellular proliferation. It is self-evident that in the absence of proliferation, tumors cannot arise. In tissues that are normally quiescent, such as the liver, the mitogenic stimulus may be provided by the initiating agent. This occurs if the carcinogenic initiator is toxic and kills a large number of cells, thereby stimulating regeneration of the surviving cells. In classic experimental systems, however, the carcinogenic potential of initiators is only revealed upon the subsequent administration of promoters (e.g., phorbol esters, hormones, phenols, and drugs), which by definition are nontumorigenic. Application of promoters leads to proliferation and clonal expansion of initiated (mutated) cells. Driven to proliferate, subclones of the initiated cells suffer various additional mutations, and eventually a cancerous clone with all the necessary hallmark characteristics may emerge. It is likely that many factors contributing to oncogenesis in humans also act by stimulating proliferation and thus can be thought of conceptually as tumor promoters; examples include unopposed estrogenic stimulation of the endometrium and breast, and chronic inflammatory processes associated with tissue repair (e.g., inflammatory bowel disease, chronic hepatitis, and Barrett esophagus).

KEY CONCEPTS

Chemical Carcinogenesis

- Chemical carcinogens have highly reactive electrophile groups that directly damage DNA, leading to mutations and eventually cancer.
- Direct-acting agents do not require metabolic conversion to become carcinogenic, while indirect-acting agents are not active until converted to an ultimate carcinogen by endogenous metabolic pathways. Hence, polymorphisms of endogenous enzymes such as cytochrome P-450 may influence carcinogenesis.
- After exposure of a cell to a mutagen or an initiator, tumorigenesis can be enhanced by exposure to promoters, which stimulate proliferation of the mutated cells.
- Examples of human carcinogens are direct-acting agents (e.g., alkylating agents used for chemotherapy), indirect acting agents (e.g., benzo[a]pyrene, azo dyes, aflatoxin), and promoters or agents that cause pathologic hyperplasias of the endometrium or regenerative activity in the liver.

Radiation Carcinogenesis

Radiant energy, in the form of the UV rays of sunlight or as ionizing electromagnetic and particulate radiation, is carcinogenic. UV light is clearly implicated in the causation of skin cancers, and ionizing radiation exposure from medical or occupational exposure, nuclear plant accidents, and atomic bomb detonations has produced a variety of cancers. Although the contribution of radiation to the total human burden of cancer is probably small, the well-known latency of damage caused by radiant energy and its cumulative effect require extremely long periods of observation and make it difficult to ascertain its full significance. An increased incidence of breast cancer has become apparent decades later among women exposed during childhood to atomic bomb tests. The incidence peaked during 1988-1992 and then declined. Moreover, possible additive or synergistic effects of radiation with other potentially carcinogenic factors add another dimension to the picture.

Ultraviolet Rays

Exposure to UV rays derived from the sun, particularly in fair-skinned individuals, is associated with an increased incidence of squamous cell carcinoma, basal cell carcinoma, and melanoma of the skin. The degree of risk depends on the type of UV rays, the intensity of exposure, and the quantity of the light-absorbing "protective mantle" of melanin in the skin. Persons of European origin who have fair skin that repeatedly becomes sunburned but stalwartly refuses to tan and who live in locales receiving a great deal of sunlight (e.g., Queensland, Australia, close to the equator) have among the highest incidence of skin cancers (melanomas, squamous cell carcinomas, and basal cell carcinomas) in the world. Nonmelanoma skin cancers are associated with total cumulative exposure to UV radiation, whereas melanomas are associated with intense intermittent exposure—as occurs with sunbathing. The UV portion of the solar spectrum can be divided into three wavelength ranges: UVA (320-400 nm), UVB (280-320 nm), and UVC (200-280 nm). Of these, UVB is believed to be responsible for the induction of cutaneous cancers. UVC, although a potent mutagen, is not considered significant because it is filtered out by the ozone layer surrounding the earth (hence the concern about ozone depletion).

The carcinogenicity of UVB light is due to formation of pyrimidine dimers in DNA. If the energy in a photon of UV light is absorbed by DNA, the result is a chemical reaction that leads to covalent crosslinking of pyrimidine bases, particularly adjacent thymidine residues in the same strand of DNA. This distorts the DNA helix and prevents proper pairing of the dimer with bases in the opposite DNA strand. Pyrimidine dimers are repaired by the nucleotide excision repair pathway. There are five steps in nucleotide excision repair, and in mammalian cells the process may involve 30 or more proteins. It is postulated that with excessive sun exposure, the capacity of the nucleotide excision repair pathway is overwhelmed, and error-prone nontemplated DNA-repair mechanisms become operative that provide for the survival of the cell at the cost of genomic mutations that, in some instances, lead to cancer. The importance of the nucleotide excision repair pathway of DNA repair is most graphically illustrated by the high frequency of cancers in individuals with the hereditary disorder *xeroderma pigmentosum* (discussed previously). The role of UV exposure in the etiology of melanoma has been somewhat controversial. However, recent sequencing of melanoma genomes has revealed a very large number of mutations that appear to stem from nontemplated error-prone repair of pyrimidine dimers, reinforcing the belief that sun exposure has an important causative role in this potentially lethal cancer.

Ionizing Radiation

Electromagnetic (x-rays, γ rays) and particulate (α particles, β particles, protons, neutrons) radiations are all carcinogenic. The evidence is so voluminous that a few examples suffice. Many individuals pioneering the use of x-rays developed skin cancers. Miners of radioactive elements in central Europe and the Rocky Mountain region of the United States have a tenfold increased incidence of lung cancers compared to the rest of the population. Most telling is the follow-up of survivors of the atomic bombs dropped on Hiroshima and Nagasaki. Initially there was a marked increase in the incidence of certain forms of leukemia after an average latent period of about 7 years. Subsequently the incidence of many solid tumors with longer latent periods (e.g., carcinomas of the breast, colon, thyroid, and lung) increased. Of great concern in the current era of widespread use of computerized tomography (CT scans) are studies that have shown that children who get two or three CT scans have a threefold higher risk of leukemia, and those that received five to 10 such scans have a threefold higher risk of brain tumors. The overall risk in children is very low (roughly one excess leukemia and one excess brain tumor over 10 years per 10,000 CT scans), but nevertheless emphasizes the need to minimize radiation exposure whenever possible.

In humans there is a hierarchy of vulnerability of different tissues to radiation-induced cancers. Most frequent are myeloid leukemias (tumors of granulocytes and their precursors; Chapter 13). Cancer of the thyroid follows closely but only in the young. In the intermediate category are cancers of the breast, lungs, and salivary glands. In contrast, skin, bone, and the gastrointestinal tract are relatively resistant to radiation-induced neoplasia, even though the gastrointestinal epithelial cells are vulnerable to the acute cell-killing effects of radiation, and the skin is "first in line" for all external radiation. Nonetheless, the physician must not forget: practically *any* cell can be transformed into a cancer cell by sufficient exposure to radiant energy.

KEY CONCEPTS

Radiation Carcinogenesis

- Ionizing radiation causes chromosome breakage, translocations, and, less frequently, point mutations, leading to genetic damage and carcinogenesis.
- UV rays induce the formation of pyrimidine dimers within DNA, leading to mutations. Therefore, UV rays can give rise to squamous cell carcinomas and melanomas of the skin. Individuals with defects in the repair of pyrimidine dimers suffer from Xeroderma pigmentosa and are at particularly high risk.
- Exposure to radiation during imaging procedures such as CT scans is linked to a very small, but measurable, increase in cancer risk in children.

Microbial Carcinogenesis

Many RNA and DNA viruses have proved to be oncogenic in animals as disparate as frogs and primates. Despite intense scrutiny, however, only a few viruses have been linked with human cancer. Our discussion focuses on human oncogenic viruses as well as the role of the bacterium *Helicobacter pylori* in gastric cancer.

Oncogenic RNA Viruses

Human T-Cell Leukemia Virus Type 1. Although the study of animal retroviruses has provided spectacular insights into the molecular basis of cancer, only one human retrovirus, human T-cell leukemia virus type 1 (HTLV-1), is firmly implicated in the pathogenesis of cancer in humans.

HTLV-1 causes *adult T-cell leukemia/lymphoma* (ATLL), a tumor that is endemic in certain parts of Japan, the Caribbean basin, South America, and Africa, and found sporadically elsewhere, including the United States. Worldwide, it is estimated that 15 to 20 million people are infected with HTLV-1. Similar to the human immunodeficiency virus, which causes AIDS, HTLV-1 has tropism for CD4+ T cells, and hence this subset of T cells is the major target for neoplastic transformation. Human infection requires transmission of infected T cells via sexual intercourse, blood products, or breastfeeding. Leukemia develops in only 3% to 5% of the infected individuals, typically after a long latent period of 40 to 60 years. A high fraction of the leukemias express the transcription factor FoxP3, a marker of regulatory T cells (Tregs) that act to suppress immune responses. It is hypothesized that the neoplastic expansion of Tregs in ATLL may underlie the susceptibility of affected patients to opportunistic infections, which are a frequent cause of death.

There is little doubt that HTLV-1 infection of T lymphocytes is necessary for leukemogenesis, but the molecular mechanisms of transformation are not certain. In contrast to several murine retroviruses, HTLV-1 does not contain an oncogene, and no consistent integration next to a proto-oncogene has been discovered. In leukemic cells, however, viral integration shows a clonal pattern. In other words, although the site of viral integration in host chromosomes is random (the viral DNA is found at different locations in different cancers), the site of integration is identical within all cells of a given cancer. This would not occur if HTLV-1 were merely a passenger that infects cells after transformation; rather, it means that HTLV-1 must have been present at the moment of transformation, placing it at the "scene of the crime."

The HTLV-1 genome contains the *gag*, *pol*, *env*, and long-terminal-repeat regions typical of all retroviruses, but, in contrast to other leukemia viruses, it contains another gene referred to as *tax*. **Several aspects of HTLV-1's transforming activity are attributable to Tax,** the protein product of this gene. Tax is essential for viral replication, because it stimulates transcription of viral RNA from the 5′ long terminal repeat. However, Tax also alters the transcription of several host cell genes and interacts with certain host cell signaling proteins. By doing so, Tax contributes to the acquisition of several cancer hallmarks, including the following:

- **Increased pro-growth signaling and cell survival.** Tax interacts with PI3K and thereby stimulates AKT; as discussed earlier, these kinases participate in the cascade that promotes both cell survival and metabolic alterations that enhance cell growth. Tax also directly upregulates the expression of cyclin D2 and represses the expression of multiple CDK inhibitors, changes that promote cell cycle progression. Finally, Tax can activate the transcription factor NF-κB, which promotes the survival of many cell types, including lymphocytes.

- **Increased genomic instability.** Tax may also cause genomic instability by interfering with DNA-repair functions and inhibiting cell cycle checkpoints activated by DNA damage. In line with these defects, HTLV-1-associated leukemias tend to be highly aneuploid.

The precise steps that lead to the development of adult T-cell leukemia/lymphoma are still not known, but a plausible scenario is as follows. Infection by HTLV-1 causes the expansion of a nonmalignant polyclonal cell population through stimulatory effects of Tax on cell proliferation. The proliferating T cells are at increased risk of mutations and genomic instability due to the effects of Tax, and possibly other viral factors as well. This instability allows the accumulation of mutations and chromosomal abnormalities, and eventually a monoclonal neoplastic T-cell population emerges.

Oncogenic DNA Viruses

As with RNA viruses, several oncogenic DNA viruses that cause tumors in animals have been identified. Of the various human DNA viruses, five—HPV, Epstein-Barr virus (EBV), hepatitis B virus (HBV), Merkel cell polyoma virus, and Kaposi sarcoma herpesvirus, also called human herpesvirus 8—have been implicated in the causation of human cancer. Merkel cell polyomavirus has been identified in Merkel cell carcinomas and is described in Chapter 25. Kaposi sarcoma herpesvirus is discussed in Chapters 6 and 11. Although not a DNA virus, hepatitis C virus (HCV) is also associated with cancer and is discussed here briefly.

Human Papillomavirus. At least 70 genetically distinct types of HPV have been identified. Some types (e.g., 1, 2, 4, and 7) cause benign squamous papillomas (warts) in humans. In contrast, high-risk HPVs (e.g., types 16 and 18) have been implicated in the genesis of squamous cell carcinomas of the cervix, anogenital region, and head and neck (particularly tumors arising in the tonsillar mucosa). These cancers are sexually transmitted diseases, caused by transmission of HPV. In contrast to cervical cancers, genital warts have low malignant potential and are associated with low-risk HPVs, predominantly HPV-6 and HPV-11. Interestingly, in benign warts, the HPV genome is maintained in a nonintegrated episomal form, while in cancers the HPV genome is integrated into the host genome, suggesting that integration of viral DNA is important for malignant transformation. As with HTLV-1, the site of viral integration in host chromosomes is random, but the pattern of integration is clonal. Cells in which the viral genome has integrated show significantly more genomic instability. Because the integration site is random, there is no consistent association with a host proto-oncogene. Rather, integration interrupts the viral DNA within the E1/E2 open reading frame, leading to loss of the E2 viral repressor and overexpression of the oncoproteins E6 and

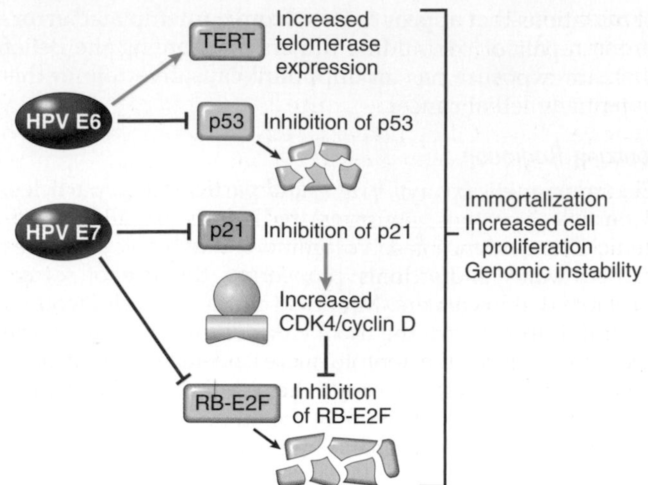

Figure 7-45 Transforming effects of HPV E6 and E7 proteins. The net effect of HPV E6 and E7 proteins is to immortalize cells and remove the restraints on cell proliferation (see Fig. 7-29). TERC, telomerase catalytic subunit. (Modified from Münger K, Howley PM: Human papillomavirus immortalization and transformation functions. Virus Res 2002;89:213-228.)

E7. Indeed, **the oncogenic potential of HPV can largely be explained by the activities of the two viral genes encoding E6 and E7** (Fig. 7-45).

- **Oncogenic activities of E6.** The E6 protein binds to and mediates the degradation of p53, and also stimulates the expression of TERT, the catalytic subunit of telomerase, which you will recall contributes to the immortalization of cells. E6 from high-risk HPV types has a higher affinity for p53 than E6 from low-risk HPV types. Interestingly the E6-p53 interaction may offer some clues regarding polymorphisms and risk factors for development of cervical cancer. Human *TP53* is polymorphic at codon 72, encoding either a proline or arginine residue at that position. The p53 Arg72 variant is much more susceptible to degradation by E6. Not surprisingly, infected individuals with the Arg72 polymorphism are more likely to develop cervical carcinomas.
- **Oncogenic activities of E7.** The E7 protein has effects that complement those of E6, all of which are centered on speeding cells through the G_1-S cell cycle checkpoint. It binds to the RB protein and displaces the E2F transcription factors that are normally sequestered by RB, promoting progression through the cell cycle. As with E6 proteins and p53, E7 proteins from high-risk HPV types have a higher affinity for RB than do E7 proteins from low-risk HPV types. E7 also inactivates the CDK inhibitors p21 and p27. Finally, E7 proteins from high-risk HPVs (types 16, 18, and 31) also bind and presumably activate cyclins E and A.

To summarize, **high-risk HPV types express oncogenic proteins that inactivate tumor suppressors, activate cyclins, inhibit apoptosis, and combat cellular senescence.** Thus, it is evident that HPV proteins promote many of the hallmarks of cancer. The primacy of HPV infection in the causation of cervical cancer is confirmed by the effectiveness of HPV vaccines in preventing cervical cancer. However, infection with HPV itself is not sufficient for carcinogenesis. For example, when human keratinocytes are transfected with DNA from HPV types 16, 18, or 31 in vitro, they are immortalized but do not form tumors in experimental animals. Co-transfection with a mutated *RAS* gene results in full malignant transformation. In addition to such genetic co-factors, HPV in all likelihood also acts in concert with environmental factors. These include cigarette smoking, coexisting microbial infections, dietary deficiencies, and hormonal changes, all of which have been implicated in the pathogenesis of cervical cancers. A high proportion of women infected with HPV clear the infection by immunologic mechanisms, but others do not, some for unknown reasons, some because of acquired immune abnormalities, such as those that result from HIV infection. As might be expected, women who are coinfected with high-risk HPV types and HIV have an elevated risk of cervical cancer.

Epstein-Barr Virus. EBV, a member of the herpesvirus family, has been implicated in the pathogenesis of several human tumors: the African form of Burkitt lymphoma; B-cell lymphomas in immunosuppressed individuals (particularly in those with HIV infection or undergoing immunosuppressive therapy after organ or bone marrow transplantation); a subset of Hodgkin lymphoma; nasopharyngeal and some gastric carcinomas; and rare forms of T-cell lymphoma and natural killer (NK) cell lymphoma. The most common EBV-associated tumors are those derived from B cells and nasopharyngeal carcinoma; other EBV-associated neoplasms are discussed elsewhere in this book.

EBV infects B lymphocytes and possibly epithelial cells of the oropharynx. The virus uses the complement receptor CD21 to attach to and infect B cells. The infection of B cells is latent; that is, there is no viral replication and the cells are not killed. However, B cells latently infected with EBV express viral proteins that result in the ability to propagate indefinitely in vitro (immortalization). The molecular basis of B-cell proliferation induced by EBV is complex, but as with other viruses it involves the "hijacking" of several normal signaling pathways. One EBV gene, latent membrane protein-1 (*LMP-1),* acts as an oncogene, in that its expression in transgenic mice induces B-cell lymphomas. LMP-1 behaves like a constitutively active CD40 receptor, a key recipient of helper T-cell signals that stimulate B-cell growth (Chapter 6). LMP-1 activates the NF-κB and JAK/STAT signaling pathways and promotes B-cell survival and proliferation, all of which occur autonomously (i.e., without T cells or other outside signals) in EBV-infected B cells. Concurrently, LMP-1 prevents apoptosis by activating BCL2. Thus, the virus "borrows" normal B-cell activation pathways to expand the pool of latently infected cells. Another EBV gene, *EBNA-2,* encodes a nuclear protein that mimics a constitutively active Notch receptor. EBNA-2 transactivates several host genes, including cyclin D and the *SRC* family of proto-oncogenes. In addition, the EBV genome contains a gene encoding a viral cytokine, vIL-10, that was "borrowed" from the host genome. This viral cytokine can prevent macrophages and monocytes from activating T cells and is required for EBV-dependent transformation of B cells. In immunologically normal individuals, EBV-driven polyclonal B-cell proliferation in vivo is readily controlled, and the individual either remains asymptomatic or develops a self-limited episode of infectious mononucleosis (Chapter 8). Evasion of the immune system seems to be a key step in EBV-related oncogenesis.

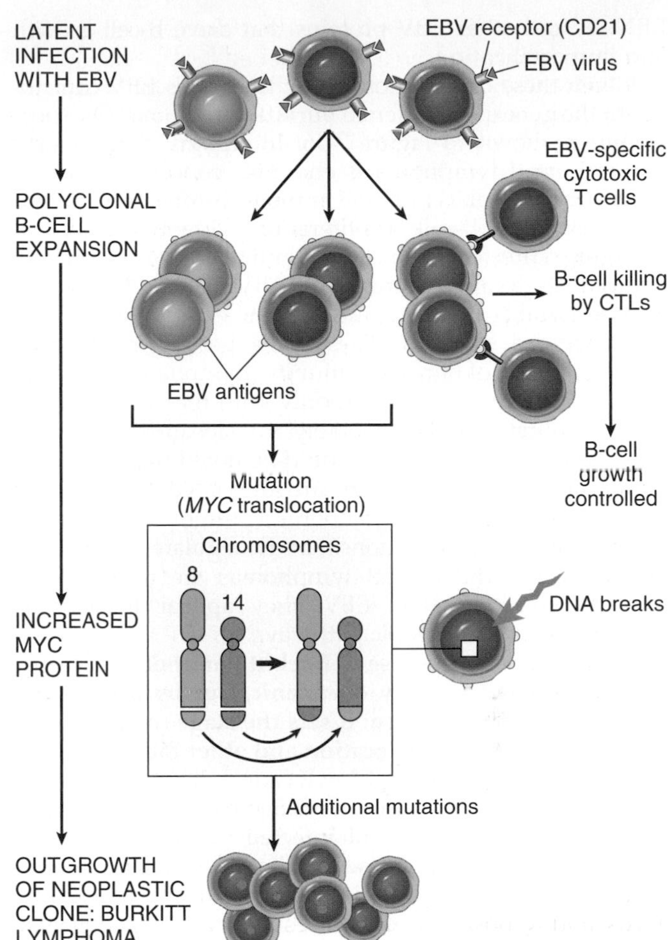

Figure 7-46 Possible evolution of EBV-induced Burkitt lymphoma.

Burkitt lymphoma is a neoplasm of B lymphocytes that is endemic in central Africa and New Guinea, areas where it is the most common childhood tumor. A morphologically identical lymphoma occurs sporadically throughout the world. The association between endemic Burkitt lymphoma and EBV is quite strong (Fig. 7-46):

- More than 90% of African tumors carry the EBV genome
- One hundred percent of the patients have elevated antibody titers against viral capsid antigens
- Serum antibody titers against viral capsid antigens are correlated with the risk of developing the tumor

Although EBV is intimately involved in the causation of Burkitt lymphoma, several observations suggest that additional factors are also involved. (1) EBV infection is not limited to the geographic locales where Burkitt lymphoma is found; in fact, it is a ubiquitous virus that infects almost all humans worldwide. (2) The EBV genome is found in only 15% to 20% of sufferers of Burkitt lymphoma outside Africa. (3) There are significant differences in the patterns of viral gene expression in EBV-transformed (but not tumorigenic) B-cell lines and Burkitt lymphoma cells. Most notably, Burkitt lymphoma cells do not express LMP-1,

EBNA2, and other EBV proteins that drive B-cell growth and immortalization.

Given these observations, how then does EBV contribute to the genesis of endemic Burkitt lymphoma? One possibility is shown in Figure 7-46. In regions of the world where Burkitt lymphoma is endemic, concomitant infections such as malaria impair immune competence, allowing sustained B-cell proliferation. Eventually, T-cell immunity directed against EBV antigens such as EBNA2 and LMP-1 eliminates most of the EBV-infected B cells, but a small number of cells downregulate expression of these immunogenic antigens. These cells persist indefinitely, even in the face of normal immunity. Lymphoma cells may emerge from this population only with the acquisition of specific mutations, most notably translocations that activate the *MYC* oncogene. It should be noted that in nonendemic areas 80% of tumors are unrelated to EBV, but virtually all endemic and sporadic tumors possess the t(8;14) or other translocations that dysregulate *MYC*. Thus, although sporadic Burkitt lymphomas are triggered by mechanisms other than EBV, they appear to develop through similar oncogenic pathways.

In summary, **in the case of Burkitt lymphoma, it seems that EBV is not directly oncogenic, but by acting as a polyclonal B-cell mitogen, it sets the stage for the acquisition of the (8;14) translocation and other mutations that ultimately produce a full-blown cancer.** In most individuals, EBV infection is readily controlled by effective immune responses, and virtually all infected individuals remain asymptomatic or develop self-limited infectious mononucleosis. In regions of Africa where Burkitt lymphoma is endemic, poorly understood cofactors (e.g., chronic malaria) may favor the acquisition of additional genetic events (e.g., the t(8;14)) that lead to transformation.

The role played by EBV is more direct in EBV-positive B-cell lymphomas in immunosuppressed patients. Some persons with AIDS or who receive immunosuppressive therapy for preventing allograft rejection develop EBV-positive B-cell tumors, often at multiple sites and within extranodal tissues such as the gut or the central nervous system. These proliferations are polyclonal at the outset but can evolve into monoclonal neoplasms. In contrast to Burkitt lymphoma, the tumors in immunosuppressed patients uniformly express LMP-1 and EBNA2, which are antigenic and can be recognized by cytotoxic T cells. Also, in contrast to Burkitt lymphoma, they usually lack *MYC* translocations. These potentially lethal proliferations can be subdued if the immunological status of the host improves, as may occur with withdrawal of immunosuppressive drugs in transplant recipients.

Nasopharyngeal carcinoma is also associated with EBV infection. This tumor is endemic in southern China, in some parts of Africa, and in the Inuit population of the Arctic. In contrast to Burkitt lymphoma, 100% of nasopharyngeal carcinomas obtained from all parts of the world contain EBV. The structure of the viral genome is identical (clonal) in all of the tumor cells within individual tumors, excluding the possibility that EBV infection occurred after tumor development. Antibody titers to viral capsid antigens are greatly elevated, and in endemic areas patients develop IgA antibodies before the appearance of the tumor. The uniform association of EBV with nasopharyngeal carcinoma suggests that EBV has a central role in the genesis of the tumor, but (as with Burkitt lymphoma) the restricted geographic distribution indicates that genetic or environmental cofactors, or both, also contribute to tumor development. Unlike Burkitt lymphoma, LMP-1 is expressed in nasopharyngeal carcinoma cells and, as in B cells, activates the NF-κB pathway. NF-κB in turn upregulates the expression of factors such as VEGF, FGF-2, MMP9, and COX2 that may contribute to oncogenesis.

The relationship of EBV to the pathogenesis of Hodgkin lymphoma, yet another EBV-associated tumor, is discussed in Chapter 13.

Hepatitis B and C Viruses. Epidemiologic studies strongly suggest a close association between hepatitis B and C virus infection and the occurrence of liver cancer (Chapter 18). It is estimated that 70% to 85% of hepatocellular carcinomas worldwide are caused by infection with hepatitis B virus (HBV) or hepatitis C virus (HCV). HBV is endemic in countries of the Far East and Africa; correspondingly, these areas have the highest incidence of hepatocellular carcinoma. Despite compelling epidemiologic and experimental evidence incriminating HBV and HCV, the mode of action of these viruses in liver tumorigenesis is not fully elucidated. The HBV and HCV genomes do not encode any viral oncoproteins, and although the HBV DNA is integrated within the human genome, there is no consistent pattern of integration in liver cells. Indeed, **while the oncogenic effects of HBV and HCV are multifactorial, the dominant effect seems to be immunologically mediated chronic inflammation and hepatocyte death leading to regeneration and, over time, genomic damage.** It is also suspected that in the setting of unresolved chronic inflammation, as occurs in viral hepatitis or chronic gastritis caused by *H. pylori* (see later), the immune response may become maladaptive, promoting rather than preventing tumorigenesis.

As with any cause of hepatocellular injury, chronic viral infection leads to the compensatory proliferation of hepatocytes. This regenerative process is aided and abetted by a plethora of growth factors, cytokines, chemokines, and other bioactive substances. These are produced by activated immune cells and promote cell survival, tissue remodeling, and angiogenesis (Chapter 3). The activated immune cells also produce other mediators, such as reactive oxygen species, that are genotoxic and mutagenic. One key molecular step seems to be activation of the NF-κB pathway in hepatocytes in response to mediators derived from the activated immune cells. Activation of the NF-κB pathway within hepatocytes blocks apoptosis, allowing the dividing hepatocytes to incur genotoxic stress and to accumulate mutations. Although this seems to be the dominant mechanism in the pathogenesis of virus-induced hepatocellular carcinoma, the HBV genome also contains genes that may directly promote the development of cancer. For example, an HBV gene known as *HBx* can activate a variety of transcription factors and several signal transduction pathways. In addition, viral integration can cause structural changes in chromosomes that dysregulate oncogenes and tumor suppressor genes.

Although not a DNA virus, HCV is also strongly linked to the pathogenesis of liver cancer. The molecular mechanisms used by HCV are less well defined than are those of HBV. In addition to chronic liver cell injury and compensatory regeneration, components of the HCV genome, such as the HCV core protein, may have a direct effect on tumorigenesis, possibly by activating a variety of growth-promoting signal transduction pathways.

Helicobacter pylori

First incriminated as a cause of peptic ulcers, *H. pylori* now has acquired the dubious distinction of being the first bacterium classified as a carcinogen. Indeed, *H. pylori* infection is implicated in the genesis of both gastric adenocarcinomas and gastric lymphomas.

The scenario for the development of gastric adenocarcinoma is similar to that of HBV- and HCV-induced liver cancer, as it involves increased epithelial cell proliferation in a background of chronic inflammation. As in viral hepatitis, the inflammatory milieu contains numerous genotoxic agents, such as reactive oxygen species. There is an initial development of chronic gastritis, followed by gastric atrophy, intestinal metaplasia of the lining cells, dysplasia, and cancer. This sequence takes decades to complete and occurs in only 3% of infected patients. Like HBV and HCV, the *H. pylori* genome also contains genes directly implicated in oncogenesis. Strains associated with gastric adenocarcinoma have been shown to contain a "pathogenicity island" that contains cytotoxin-associated A (*CagA*) gene. Although *H. pylori* is noninvasive, *CagA* penetrates into gastric epithelial cells, where it has a variety of effects, including the initiation of a signaling cascade that mimics unregulated growth factor stimulation.

As mentioned earlier, *H. pylori* is associated with an increased risk for the development of gastric lymphomas as well. The gastric lymphomas are of B-cell origin, and because the tumors recapitulate some of the features of normal Peyer's patches, they are often called lymphomas of mucosa-associated lymphoid tissue, or MALTomas (also discussed in Chapters 13 and 17). Their molecular pathogenesis is incompletely understood but seems to involve strain-specific *H. pylori* factors, as well as host genetic factors, such as polymorphisms in the promoters of inflammatory cytokines such as IL-1β and tumor necrosis factor (TNF). It is thought that *H. pylori* infection leads to the appearance of *H. pylori*-reactive T cells, which in turn stimulate a polyclonal B-cell proliferation. In chronic infections, currently unknown mutations may be acquired that give individual cells a growth advantage. These cells grow out into a monoclonal "MALToma" that nevertheless remains dependent on T-cell stimulation of B-cell pathways that activate the transcription factor NF-κB. At this stage, eradication of *H. pylori* by antibiotic therapy "cures" the lymphoma by removing the antigenic stimulus for T cells. At later stages, however, additional mutations may be acquired that cause constitutive NF-κB activation. At this point, the MALToma no longer requires the antigenic stimulus of the bacterium for growth and survival and develops the capacity to spread beyond the stomach to other tissues.

KEY CONCEPTS

Viral and Bacterial Oncogenesis

HTLV-1: a retrovirus that is endemic in Japan, the Caribbean, and parts of South America and Africa that causes adult T-cell leukemia/lymphoma

- HTLV-1 encodes the viral protein Tax, which turns on pro-growth and pro-survival signaling pathways (PI3K/AKT, NF-κB), leading to a polyclonal expansion of T cells.
- After a long latent period (decades), a small fraction of HTLV-1–infected individuals develop adult T-cell leukemia/lymphoma, a CD4+ tumor that arises from an HTLV-1 infected cell, presumably due to acquisition of additional mutations in the host cell genome.

HPV: an important cause of benign warts, cervical cancer, and oropharyngeal cancer

- Oncogenic types of HPV encode two viral oncoproteins, E6 and E7, that bind to Rb and p53, respectively, with high affinity and neutralize their function.
- Development of cancer is associated with integration of HPV into the host genome and additional mutations needed for acquisition of cancer hallmarks.
- HPV cancers can be prevented by vaccination against high-risk HPV types.

EBV: ubiquitous herpesvirus implicated in the pathogenesis of Burkitt lymphomas, B-cell lymphomas in patients with T-cell immunosuppression (HIV infection, transplant recipients), and several other cancers

- The EBV genome harbors several genes encoding proteins that trigger B cell signaling pathways; in concert, these signals are potent inducers of B cell growth and transformation.
- In the absence of T-cell immunity, EBV-infected B cells can rapidly "grow out" as aggressive B-cell tumors.
- In the presence of normal T-cell immunity, a small fraction of infected patients develop EBV-positive B-cell tumors (Burkitt lymphoma, Hodgkin lymphoma) or carcinomas (nasopharyngeal, gastric carcinoma)

Hepatitis B virus and hepatitis C virus: cause of between 70% and 85% of hepatocellular carcinomas worldwide

- Oncogenic effects are multifactorial; dominant effect seems to be immunologically mediated chronic inflammation, hepatocellular injury, and reparative hepatocyte proliferation.
- HBx protein of HBV and the HCV core protein can activate signal transduction pathways that also may contribute to carcinogenesis.

H. pylori: implicated in gastric adenocarcinoma and MALT lymphoma

- Pathogenesis of *H. pylori*-induced gastric cancers is multifactorial, including chronic inflammation and reparative gastric cell proliferation.
- *H. pylori* pathogenicity genes, such as *CagA,* also may contribute by stimulating growth factor pathways.
- Chronic *H. pylori* infection leads to polyclonal B-cell proliferations that may give rise to a monoclonal B-cell tumor (MALT lymphoma) of the stomach as a result of accumulation of mutations.

Clinical Aspects of Neoplasia

Ultimately the importance of neoplasms lies in their effects on patients. Although malignant tumors are of course more threatening than benign tumors, any tumor, even a benign one, may cause morbidity and mortality.

Local and Hormonal Effects

Location is a critical determinant of the clinical effects of both benign and malignant tumors. Tumors may impinge upon vital tissues and impair their functions, cause death of involved tissues, and provide a nidus for infection. A small (1 cm) pituitary adenoma, although benign and possibly nonfunctional, can compress and destroy the surrounding normal gland and thus lead to serious hypopituitarism. Cancers arising within or metastatic to an endocrine gland may cause an endocrine insufficiency by destroying the gland. Neoplasms in the gut, both benign and malignant, may cause obstruction as they enlarge. Infrequently, peristaltic movement telescopes the neoplasm and its affected segment into the downstream segment, producing an obstructing intussusception (Chapter 17). Symptoms produced by a cancer due to its position can (ironically) be lifesaving; for example, the few survivors of pancreatic cancer are those whose tumors "fortuitously" obstruct bile ducts early in their course, leading to the appearance of jaundice and other symptoms at a stage of the disease when surgical cure is still possible.

Benign and malignant neoplasms arising in endocrine glands can cause clinical problems by producing hormones. Such functional activity is more typical of benign than of malignant tumors, which may be so undifferentiated to have lost such capability. A benign beta-cell adenoma of the pancreatic islets less than 1 cm in diameter may produce sufficient insulin to cause fatal hypoglycemia. In addition, nonendocrine tumors may elaborate hormones or hormone-like products and give rise to paraneoplastic syndromes (discussed later). The erosive and destructive growth of cancers or the expansile pressure of a benign tumor on any natural surface, such as the skin or mucosa of the gut, may cause ulcerations, secondary infections, and bleeding. Melena (blood in the stool) and hematuria, for example, are characteristic of neoplasms of the gut and urinary tract. Neoplasms, benign as well as malignant, may cause problems in varied ways, but all are far less common than our next topic, the cachexia of malignancy.

Cancer Cachexia

Individuals with cancer commonly suffer progressive loss of body fat and lean body mass accompanied by profound weakness, anorexia, and anemia, referred to as *cachexia.* Cancer cachexia is associated with:

- Equal loss of both fat and lean muscle
- Elevated basal metabolic rate
- Evidence of systemic inflammation (e.g., an increase in acute phase reactants, Chapter 6)

The mechanisms that underlie cancer cachexia are not understood. Inflammation related to the interplay between cancer and the immune system is likely to have a role. TNFα (originally known as cachectin) is a leading suspect among several mediators released from immune cells that may contribute to cachexia. Humoral factors released from tumor cells such as proteolysis inducing factor have been implicated in the loss of muscle mass, which is discussed further in Chapter 9.

Paraneoplastic Syndromes

Some cancer-bearing individuals develop signs and symptoms that cannot readily be explained by the anatomic distribution of the tumor or by the elaboration of hormones indigenous to the tissue from which the tumor arose; these are known as paraneoplastic syndromes. These occur in about 10% of persons with cancer. Despite their relative infrequency, paraneoplastic syndromes are important to recognize, for several reasons:

- They may be the earliest manifestation of an occult neoplasm.
- In affected patients they can cause significant clinical problems and may even be lethal.
- They may mimic metastatic disease and therefore confound treatment.

A classification of paraneoplastic syndromes and their presumed origins is presented in Table 7-11. A few comments on some of the more common and interesting syndromes follow.

Endocrinopathies are frequently encountered paraneoplastic syndromes. The responsible cancers are not of endocrine origin and the secretory activity of such tumors is referred to as ectopic hormone production. *Cushing syndrome* is the most common endocrinopathy. Approximately 50% of individuals with this endocrinopathy have carcinoma of the lung, chiefly the small-cell type. It is caused by excessive production of corticotropin or corticotropin-like peptides. The precursor of corticotropin is a large molecule known as pro-opiomelanocortin. Lung cancer patients with Cushing syndrome have elevated serum levels of both pro-opiomelanocortin and corticotropin. The former is not found in serum of patients with excess corticotropin produced by the pituitary.

Hypercalcemia is probably the most common paraneoplastic syndrome; in fact, symptomatic hypercalcemia is more often related to some form of cancer than to hyperparathyroidism. Two general processes are involved in cancer-associated hypercalcemia: (1) *osteolysis* induced by cancer, whether primary in bone, such as multiple myeloma, or metastatic to bone from any primary lesion, and (2) the production of *calcemic humoral substances* by extraosseous neoplasms. Only the second mechanism is considered to be paraneoplastic; hypercalcemia due to primary or secondary involvement of the skeleton by tumor is <u>not</u> a paraneoplastic syndrome.

Several humoral factors have been associated with paraneoplastic hypercalcemia of malignancy. The most important, *parathyroid hormone-related protein* (PTHRP), is a molecule related to, but distinct from, parathyroid hormone (PTH). PTHRP resembles the native hormone only in its N terminus. It has some biologic actions similar to those of PTH, and both hormones share a G protein–coupled receptor, known as PTH/PTHRP receptor (often referred to as PTH-R or PTHRP-R). In contrast to PTH, PTHRP is produced in small amounts by many normal tissues, including keratinocytes, muscles, bone, and ovary. It regulates calcium transport in the lactating breast and across the placenta, and seems to modulate pulmonary development and remodeling. Tumors most often associated with paraneoplastic hypercalcemia are carcinomas of the breast, lung, kidney, and ovary. In breast cancers, hypercalcemia

Table 7-11 Paraneoplastic Syndromes

Clinical Syndromes	Major Forms of Underlying Cancer	Causal Mechanism
Endocrinopathies		
Cushing syndrome	Small-cell carcinoma of lung Pancreatic carcinoma Neural tumors	ACTH or ACTH-like substance
Syndrome of inappropriate antidiuretic hormone secretion	Small-cell carcinoma of lung Intracranial neoplasms	Antidiuretic hormone or atrial natriuretic hormones
Hypercalcemia	Squamous cell carcinoma of lung Breast carcinoma Renal carcinoma Adult T-cell leukemia/lymphoma	Parathyroid hormone-related protein (PTHRP), TGF-α, TNF, IL-1
Hypoglycemia	Ovarian carcinoma Fibrosarcoma Other mesenchymal sarcomas	Insulin or insulin-like substance
Polycythemia	Renal carcinoma Cerebellar hemangioma Hepatocellular carcinoma	Erythropoietin
Nerve and Muscle syndromes		
Myasthenia	Bronchogenic carcinoma Thymic neoplasms	Immunologic
Disorders of the central and peripheral nervous system	Breast carcinoma	
Dermatologic Disorders		
Acanthosis nigricans	Gastric carcinoma Lung carcinoma Uterine carcinoma	Immunologic; secretion of epidermal growth factor
Dermatomyositis	Bronchogenic carcinoma Breast carcinoma	Immunologic
Osseous, Articular, and Soft Tissue Changes		
Hypertrophic osteoarthropathy and clubbing of the fingers	Bronchogenic carcinoma Thymic neoplasms	Unknown
Vascular and Hematologic Changes		
Venous thrombosis (Trousseau phenomenon)	Pancreatic carcinoma Bronchogenic carcinoma Other cancers	Tumor products (mucins that activate clotting)
Disseminated intravascular coagulation	Acute promyelocytic leukemia Prostatic carcinoma	Tumor products that activate clotting
Nonbacterial thrombotic endocarditis	Advanced cancers	Hypercoagulability
Red cell aplasia	Thymic neoplasms	Unknown
Others		
Nephrotic syndrome	Various cancers	Tumor antigens, immune complexes

ACTH, Adrenocorticotropic hormone; IL, interleukin; TGF, transforming growth factor; TNF, tumor necrosis factor.

due to PTHRP production is often exacerbated by osteolytic bone metastases. The most common lung neoplasm associated with hypercalcemia is squamous cell carcinoma. In addition to PTHRP, several other factors, such as IL-1, TGF-α, TNF, and dihydroxyvitamin D, have also been causally implicated in the hypercalcemia of malignancy.

The *neuromyopathic paraneoplastic syndromes* take diverse forms, such as peripheral neuropathies, cortical cerebellar degeneration, a polymyopathy resembling polymyositis, and a myasthenic syndrome similar to *myasthenia gravis* (Chapter 27). The cause of these syndromes is poorly understood. In some cases, antibodies, presumably induced against tumor cell antigens (Chapter 28) that cross-react with neuronal cell antigens, have been detected. It is postulated that some visceral cancers ectopically express certain neural antigens. For some unknown reason, the immune system recognizes these antigens as foreign and mounts an immune response.

Acanthosis nigricans is a disorder characterized by gray-black patches of thickened, hyperkeratotic skin with a velvety appearance. It occurs rarely as a genetically determined disease in juveniles or adults (Chapter 25). In addition, in about 50% of the cases, particularly in those over age 40, the appearance of such lesions is associated with some form of cancer. Sometimes the skin changes appear before the cancer is discovered.

Hypertrophic osteoarthropathy is encountered in 1% to 10% of patients with lung carcinoma. Rarely, other forms of cancer are involved. This disorder is characterized by (1) periosteal new bone formation, primarily at the distal ends of long bones, metatarsals, metacarpals, and proximal phalanges; (2) arthritis of the adjacent joints; and (3) clubbing of the digits. Although the osteoarthropathy is seldom seen in noncancer patients, clubbing of the fingertips may be encountered in liver diseases, diffuse lung disease, congenital cyanotic heart disease, ulcerative colitis, and other disorders. The cause of hypertrophic osteoarthropathy is unknown.

Several vascular and hematologic manifestations may appear in association with a variety of forms of cancer. As mentioned in the discussion of thrombosis (Chapter 4), *migratory thrombophlebitis* (Trousseau syndrome) may be encountered in association with deep-seated cancers, most often carcinomas of the pancreas or lung. *Disseminated intravascular coagulation* may complicate a diversity of clinical disorders (Chapter 14); among cancers, it is most commonly associated with acute promyelocytic leukemia and prostatic adenocarcinoma. Bland, small, nonbacterial fibrinous vegetations sometimes form on the cardiac valve leaflets (more often on left-sided valves), particularly in individuals with advanced mucin-secreting adenocarcinomas. These lesions, called *nonbacterial thrombotic endocarditis*, are described further in Chapter 12. The vegetations are potential sources of emboli that can further complicate the course of the cancer.

Grading and Staging of Tumors

Methods to quantify the probable clinical aggressiveness of a given neoplasm and its apparent extent and spread in the individual patient are necessary for making an accurate prognosis and for comparing end results of various treatment protocols. For instance, the results of treating well-differentiated thyroid adenocarcinoma that is localized to the thyroid gland will be different from those obtained from treating highly anaplastic thyroid cancers that have invaded the neck organs. Systems have been developed to express, at least in semiquantitative terms, the level of differentiation, or grade, and extent of spread of a cancer within the patient, or stage, as parameters of the clinical gravity of the disease.

- **Grading.** Grading of a cancer is based on the degree of differentiation of the tumor cells and, in some cancers, the number of mitoses or architectural features. Grading schemes have evolved for each type of malignancy, and generally range from two categories (low grade and high grade) to four categories. Criteria for the individual grades vary in different types of tumors and so are not detailed here, but all attempt, in essence, to judge the extent to which the tumor cells resemble or fail to resemble their normal counterparts. Although histologic grading is useful, the correlation between histologic appearance and biologic behavior is less than perfect. In recognition of this problem and to avoid spurious quantification, it is common practice to characterize a particular neoplasm in descriptive terms, for example, well-differentiated, mucin-secreting adenocarcinoma of the stomach, or poorly differentiated pancreatic adenocarcinoma.
- **Staging.** The staging of solid cancers is based on the size of the primary lesion, its extent of spread to regional lymph nodes, and the presence or absence of blood-borne metastases. The major staging system currently in use is the American Joint Committee on Cancer Staging. This system uses a classification called the *TNM system—T* for primary tumor, *N* for regional lymph node involvement, and *M* for metastases. TNM staging varies for specific forms of cancer, but there are general principles. The primary lesion is characterized as T1 to T4 based on increasing size. T0 is used to indicate an in situ lesion. N0 would mean no nodal involvement, whereas N1 to N3 would denote involvement of an increasing number and range of nodes. M0 signifies no distant metastases, whereas M1 or sometimes M2 indicates the presence of metastases and some judgment as to their number.

KEY CONCEPTS

Clinical Aspects of Tumors

Cachexia: progressive loss of body fat and lean body mass, accompanied by profound weakness, anorexia, and anemia, that is caused by release of factors by the tumor or host immune cells

Paraneoplastic syndromes: symptom complexes in individuals with cancer that cannot be explained by tumor spread or release of hormones that are indigenous to the tumor "cell of origin." For example:

- Endocrinopathies (Cushing syndrome, hypercalcemia)
- Neuropathic syndromes (polymyopathy, peripheral neuropathies, neural degeneration, myasthenic syndromes)
- Skin disorders (acanthosis nigricans)
- Skeletal and joint abnormalities (hypertrophic osteoarthritis)
- Hypercoagulability (migratory thrombophlebitis, disseminated intravascular coagulation, nonbacterial thrombotic endocarditis)

Grading: determined by cytologic appearance; based on the idea that behavior and differentiation are related, with poorly differentiated tumors having more aggressive behavior

Staging: determined by surgical exploration or imaging, is based on size, local and regional lymph node spread, and distant metastases; of greater clinical value than grading

Laboratory Diagnosis of Cancer

Every year the approach to laboratory diagnosis of cancer becomes more complex, more sophisticated, and more specialized. For virtually every neoplasm mentioned in this text, the experts have characterized several subcategories; we must walk, however, before we can run. Each of the following sections attempts to present the state of the art, avoiding details of technologies.

Histologic and Cytologic Methods. The laboratory diagnosis of cancer is, in most instances, not difficult. The two ends of the benign-malignant spectrum pose no problem; however, in the middle lies a gray zone that novices dread and where experts tread cautiously. The focus here is on the roles of the clinician (often a surgeon) and the pathologist in facilitating the correct diagnosis.

Clinical data are invaluable for accurate pathologic diagnosis, but often clinicians underestimate its value. Radiation changes in the skin or mucosa can be similar to those associated with cancer. Sections taken from a healing fracture can mimic an osteosarcoma. Moreover, the laboratory evaluation of a lesion can be only as good as the specimen made available for examination. It must be adequate, representative, and properly preserved. Several sampling approaches are available: (1) excision or biopsy, (2) needle aspiration, and (3) cytologic smears. When excision of a small lesion is not possible, selection of an appropriate site for biopsy of a large mass requires awareness that the periphery may not be representative and the center largely necrotic. Appropriate preservation involves such actions as prompt immersion of at least a portion of the specimen in a fixative (usually a formalin solution) and (depending on the differential diagnosis) rapid allocation of tissue for other studies such as cytogenetics, flow cytometry, and molecular diagnostics (described later). Requesting "quick-frozen section" diagnosis is sometimes desirable, for example, in determining the nature of a mass lesion, in evaluating the margins of an excised cancer to ascertain that the entire neoplasm has been removed, or in making decisions about what additional studies beyond histology are needed. This method permits histologic evaluation within minutes. In experienced, competent hands, frozen-section diagnosis is highly accurate, but there are particular instances in which the better histologic detail provided by the more time-consuming routine methods is needed—for example, when extremely radical surgery, such as the amputation of an extremity, may be indicated. Better to wait a day or two, despite the delay, than to perform inadequate or unnecessary surgery.

Fine-needle aspiration of tumors is another approach that is widely used. The procedure involves aspirating cells and attendant fluid with a small-bore needle, followed by cytologic examination of the stained smear. This method is used most commonly for the assessment of readily palpable lesions in sites such as the breast, thyroid, and lymph nodes. Modern imaging techniques permit extension of the method to lesions in deep-seated structures, such as pelvic lymph nodes and pancreas. Fine-needle aspiration is less invasive and more rapidly performed than are needle biopsies. It obviates surgery and its attendant risks. Although it entails some difficulties, such as small sample size and sampling errors, in experienced hands it is reliable, rapid, and useful.

Cytologic smears provide yet another method for the detection of cancer (Chapter 22). This approach is widely used to screen for carcinoma of the cervix, often at an in situ stage, but it is also used to evaluate many other forms of suspected malignancy in which tumor cells are easily accessible or shed, such as endometrial carcinoma, lung carcinoma, bladder and prostatic tumors, and gastric carcinomas; for the identification of tumor cells in abdominal, pleural, joint, and cerebrospinal fluids; and, less commonly, with other forms of neoplasia.

As pointed out earlier, cancer cells have lowered cohesiveness and exhibit a range of morphologic changes encompassed by the term anaplasia. Thus, shed cells can be evaluated for the features of anaplasia indicative of their origin from a tumor (Figs. 7-47 and 7-48). In these cases, judgment must be rendered based on the features of individual cells or, at most, a clump of cells, without the supporting evidence of loss of orientation of one cell to another, and (most importantly) evidence of invasion. This

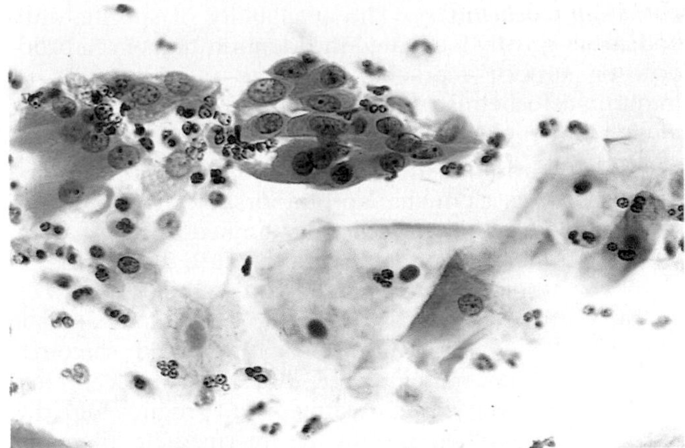

Figure 7-47 A normal cervicovaginal smear shows large, flattened squamous cells and groups of metaplastic cells; interspersed are neutrophils. There are no malignant cells. (Courtesy Dr. P. K. Gupta, University of Pennsylvania, Philadelphia, Pa.)

method permits differentiation among normal, dysplastic, and malignant cells and, in addition, permits the recognition of cellular changes characteristic of carcinoma in situ. The gratifying control of cervical cancer through screening with Pap smears is the best testament to the value of cytology.

Although histology and exfoliative cytology remain the foundation of cancer diagnosis, they have inherent limits; for example, it can be difficult to determine the nature of a poorly differentiated tumor of any type, and some specific tumor types are notoriously difficult to distinguish based on their morphologic appearance alone (e.g., various types of acute leukemias and lymphomas). These limitations have spurred the widespread application of immunohistochemistry and flow cytometry, which can be used to make these diagnostic distinctions. Another rapidly expanding modality is molecular diagnostics, which is being used increasingly to identify cancers that are amenable to treatment with so-called targeted therapies, drugs that are directed at mutated oncoproteins. Only some highlights of these diagnostic modalities are presented.

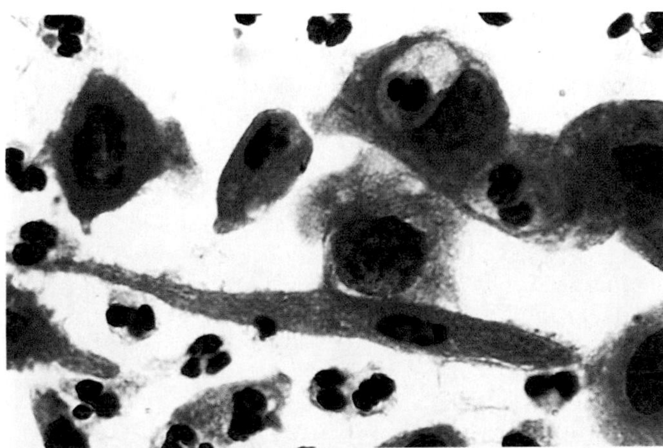

Figure 7-48 An abnormal cervicovaginal smear shows numerous malignant cells that have pleomorphic, hyperchromatic nuclei; interspersed are normal polymorphonuclear leukocytes. (Courtesy Dr. P. K. Gupta, University of Pennsylvania, Philadelphia, Pa.)

Immunohistochemistry. The availability of specific antibodies has greatly facilitated the identification of cell products or surface markers. Examples of the utility of immunohistochemistry in the diagnosis or management of malignant neoplasms follow.

- **Categorization of undifferentiated malignant tumors.** In many cases malignant tumors of diverse origin resemble each other because of limited differentiation. These tumors are often quite difficult to distinguish on the basis of routine hematoxylin and eosin (H&E)-stained tissue sections. For example, certain anaplastic carcinomas, lymphomas, melanomas, and sarcomas may look quite similar, but they must be accurately identified because their treatment and prognosis are different. Antibodies specific to intermediate filaments have proved to be of particular value in such cases, because solid tumor cells often contain intermediate filaments characteristic of their cell of origin. For example, the presence of cytokeratins, detected by immunohistochemistry, points to an epithelial origin (carcinoma) (Fig. 7-49), whereas desmin is specific for neoplasms of muscle cell origin. Other useful immunohistochemical markers include lineage-specific membrane proteins (e.g., CD20, a marker of B-cell tumors) and transcription factors.
- **Determination of site of origin of metastatic tumors.** Many cancer patients present with metastases. In some the primary site is obvious or readily detected on the basis of clinical or radiologic features. In cases in which the origin of the tumor is obscure, immunohistochemical detection of tissue-specific or organ-specific antigens in a biopsy specimen of the metastatic deposit can lead to the identification of the tumor source. For example, prostate-specific antigen (PSA) and thyroglobulin are markers of carcinomas of the prostate and thyroid, respectively.
- **Detection of molecules that have prognostic or therapeutic significance.** Immunohistochemical detection of hormone (estrogen/progesterone) receptors in breast cancer cells is of prognostic and therapeutic value because these cancers are susceptible to antiestrogen therapy (Chapter 23). In general, receptor-positive breast cancers have a better prognosis than receptor negative tumors. Protein products of oncogenes such as *ERBB2* in breast cancers can also be detected by immunostaining. Breast cancers with strong immunohistochemical staining for the protein product of the *ERBB2* gene product, HER2, generally have a poor prognosis, but are amenable to treatment with antibodies that block the activity of the HER2 receptor. Because high-level expression of HER2 is caused by amplification of *ERBB2*, fluorescent in situ hybridization (FISH) to confirm *ERBB2* gene amplification is sometimes used as an adjunct to immunohistochemical studies. Similarly, immunohistochemical stains for ALK protein can be used to identify lung cancers and lymphomas expressing constitutively active ALK fusion proteins.

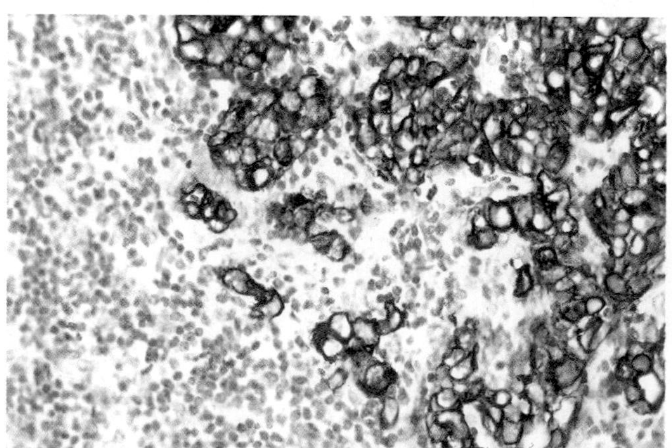

Figure 7-49 Anticytokeratin immunoperoxidase stain of a tumor of epithelial origin (carcinoma). (Courtesy Dr. Melissa Upton, University of Washington, Seattle, Wash.)

Flow Cytometry. Flow cytometry can rapidly and quantitatively measure several individual cell characteristics, but is mainly used to identify cellular antigens expressed by "liquid" tumors, those that arise from blood-forming tissues. These include B- and T-cell lymphomas and leukemias, as well as myeloid neoplasms. An advantage of flow cytometry over immunohistochemistry is that multiple antigens can be assessed simultaneously on individual cells using combinations of specific antibodies linked to different fluorescent dyes. Monoclonal antibodies directed against various lymphohematopoietic cells are listed in Chapter 13.

Circulating Tumor Cells. Instrumentation that permits detection, quantification, and characterization of rare solid tumors cells (e.g., carcinoma, melanoma) circulating in the blood is being explored as a diagnostic modality. Some of the latest devices rely on three-dimensional flow cells coated with antibodies specific for tumor cells of interest (e.g., carcinoma cells) that efficiently capture rare tumor cells present in the blood. Such methods currently fall in the realm of clinical research, but have the potential to permit earlier diagnosis, to gauge the risk of metastasis, and to provide a minimally invasive means of assessing the response of tumor cells to therapy.

Molecular and Cytogenetic Diagnostics. Several molecular or cytogenetic techniques—some established, others emerging—have been used for diagnosis and, in some cases, for predicting behavior of tumors.

- **Diagnosis of malignant neoplasms.** Although molecular methods are not the primary modality of cancer diagnosis, they are of considerable value in selected cases. T and B cell tumors are derived from single cells with unique antigen receptor gene rearrangements, whereas reactive lymphoid proliferations contain many different lymphocyte clones, each with a different set of rearrangements antigen receptor genes. For this reason, PCR-based evaluation of rearranged T-cell receptor or immunoglobulin genes allows distinction between monoclonal (neoplastic) and polyclonal (reactive) proliferations. Many hematopoietic neoplasms (leukemias and lymphomas) are associated with specific translocations that activate oncogenes. Detection of such translocations, usually by routine cytogenetic analysis or by FISH (Chapter 5), is often extremely helpful in diagnosis. Diagnosis of sarcomas (Chapter 26) with characteristic translocations is also aided by molecular techniques, in part because chromosome preparations are often difficult to obtain from solid tumors. For example, many sarcomas of childhood, so-called round blue cell tumors (Chapter 10), can be difficult to distinguish from each other on the basis of morphology. However, the presence of the characteristic (11;22)(q24;q12) translocation, established by PCR, in one of these tumors confirms the diagnosis of Ewing sarcoma. Another diagnostic platform that is finding increasing use is **DNA microarrays,** either tiling arrays, which cover the entire human genome, or single-nucleotide polymorphism arrays (SNP chips), which allow high-resolution mapping of copy number changes (either deletions or amplifications) genome-wide.

- **Prognosis of malignant neoplasms.** Certain genetic alterations are associated with poor prognosis, and hence their detection allows stratification of patients for therapy. For example, amplification of the *NMYC* gene and deletions of 1p bode poorly for patients with neuroblastoma, and oligodendrogliomas in which the only genomic abnormality is the loss of chromosomes 1p and 19q respond well to therapy and are associated with long-term survival when compared to tumors with intact 1p and 19q but with EGF receptor amplification.
- **Detection of minimal residual disease.** After treatment of patients with leukemia or lymphoma, the presence of minimal disease or the onset of relapse can be monitored by PCR-based amplification of nucleic acid sequences unique to the malignant clone. For example, detection of *BCR-ABL* transcripts by PCR gives a measure of the residual leukemia cells in treated patients with CML. The prognostic importance of minimal residual disease has been established in acute leukemia and is being evaluated in other neoplasms.
- **Diagnosis of hereditary predisposition to cancer.** As discussed earlier, germline mutations in several tumor suppressor genes, including *BRCA1*, *BRCA2*, and the *RET* proto-oncogene, are associated with a high risk of developing specific cancers. Thus, detection of these mutated alleles may allow the patient and physician to devise an aggressive screening program, consider the option of prophylactic surgery, and counsel relatives, who may also be at risk. Such analysis usually requires detection of a specific mutation (e.g., *RET* gene) or sequencing of the entire gene. The latter is necessitated when several different cancer-associated mutations are known to exist. Although the detection of mutations in such cases is relatively straightforward, the ethical issues surrounding presymptomatic diagnosis are complex.
- **Guiding therapy with oncoprotein-directed drugs.** An increasing number of chemotherapeutic agents target oncoproteins that are only present in a subset of cancers of a particular type. Thus, the molecular identification of genetic lesions that produce these oncoproteins is essential for optimal treatment of patients. Current examples of genetic lesions that guide therapy and are frequently tested for in molecular diagnostic laboratories include the *PML-RARA* fusion gene in acute promyelocytic leukemia; the *BCR-ABL* fusion gene in chronic myelogenous leukemia and acute lymphoblastic leukemia; *ERBB1* (EGFR) mutations and *ALK* gene rearrangements in lung cancer; and *BRAF* mutations in melanoma.

Molecular Profiles of Tumors: The Future of Cancer Diagnostics

Until recently, molecular studies of tumors involved the analysis of individual genes. However, the past few years have seen the introduction of revolutionary technologies that can rapidly sequence an entire genome; assess epigenetic modifications genome-wide (the epigenome); quantify all of the RNAs expressed in a cell population (the transcriptome); measure many proteins simultaneously (the proteome); and take a snapshot of all of the cell's metabolites (the metabolome). Thus, we have entered the age of "omics!"

The most common method for large-scale analysis of RNA expression in use today in research laboratories is based on DNA microarrays, but newer methods that involve RNA sequencing have appeared that offer a more comprehensive and quantitative assessment of RNA expression. However, RNA is prone to degradation and is a more difficult analyte to work with than DNA in clinical practice. Furthermore, DNA sequencing is technically simpler that RNA sequencing, permitting the development of methods that rely on massively parallel sequencing (so-called next generation [NextGen] sequencing). The increases in DNA sequencing capacity and speed that such methods have enabled over the past decade have been breath taking, and are matched by equally remarkable decreases in cost. The first reasonably complete draft of the sequence of the human genome, released in 2003, took 12 years of work and cost about $2,700,000,000. At present, using NextGen sequencing, certain cancer centers are completing the process of whole genome sequencing for individual tumors in 28 days, which includes the time required for the extraordinarily complex task of assembling and analyzing the sequencing data. The cost of whole genome sequencing has now fallen under $3,000, and is continuing to drop; there is no doubt that the long promised $1,000 genome is now in sight.

These advances have enabled the systematic sequencing and cataloging of genomic alterations in various human cancers, much of it within a large consortium sponsored by the National Cancer Institute called The Cancer Genome Atlas (TCGA). The complexity of the genetic aberrations identified in these genome-wide studies has inspired informaticians to create new ways of displaying the data, such as circos plots (Fig. 7-50), which provide a snapshot of all of the genetic alterations that exist in a particular tumor.

The main impact of cancer genome sequencing to date has been in the area of research: identification of new mutations that underlie various cancers; description of the full panoply of genetic lesions that are found in individual cancers; and a greater appreciation of the genetic heterogeneity that exists in individual cancers from area to area. As noted, a few centers are piloting the use of whole genome sequencing to manage patients, but most efforts in the clinical realm are focused on developing sequencing methods that permit identification of therapeutically "actionable" genetic lesions in a timely fashion at a reasonable cost. Such approaches seem particularly applicable to

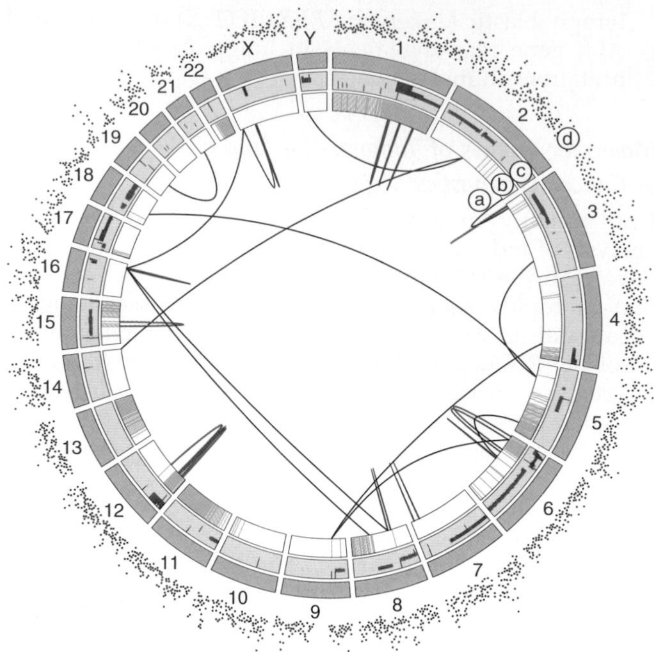

Figure 7-50 A circos plot showing genetic alterations in a single lung cancer in a male patient. Each of the 24 chromosomes in the cancer is displayed in a circle. The positions of various tumor-specific aberrations are mapped onto these chromosomes as follows: **a,** Structural rearrangements in chromosomes. The blue lines denote intrachromosomal rearrangements, while the red lines denote interchromosomal rearrangements. **b,** Regions of loss of heterozygosity and allelic imbalance (overrepresentation of one allele versus the second) are in green. **c,** Copy number profiles, showing copy number losses (in red), and copy gains (in blue). **d,** Point mutations, represented as red dots.

tumors such as lung carcinomas, which are genetically diverse and require a "personalized" approach if targeted therapy is to succeed. Thus, the current trend in molecular diagnostic laboratories is to develop methods that permit several hundred exons of key genes to be sequenced simultaneously at sufficient "depth" (fold coverage of the sequence in question) to reliably detect any mutations that might be present in as few as 5% of tumor cells. A second method that is moving rapidly into clinical practice involves the use of DNA arrays to identify changes in DNA copy number, such as amplifications and deletions. Arrays containing probes that span the entire genome at some standard spacing can detect all but the smallest copy number aberrations, providing information that is complementary to that obtained from DNA sequencing. Other "omics", such as proteomics and epigenomics, are currently being used mainly in the realm of clinical research, but with many drugs that target the cancer epigenome moving into the clinic, it can be anticipated that tests directed at assessing the state of the epigenome that predict response to such agents are soon to follow.

The excitement created by the development of new techniques for the global molecular analysis of tumors has led some scientists to predict that the end of histopathology is in sight. Indeed, with the advent of targeted therapies, it can be argued that we are in the midst of a paradigm shift in which the most important part of the work-up of a cancer sample is the identification of molecular targets, rather than histopathologic diagnosis (Fig. 7-51). For example, it is now appreciated that histopathologically distinct cancers all often harbor the same gain-of-function mutation in the serine/threonine kinase BRAF, a component of the RAS signaling pathway (Fig. 7-52). In principle, all of these diverse "BRAFomas" are candidates for treatment with BRAF inhibitors. However, early studies have shown that the effectiveness of BRAF inhibitors vary widely depending on histologic subtype: hairy cell leukemias with BRAF mutations appear to have sustained responses, melanomas respond transiently, and colon carcinomas respond little, if at all, for reasons that remain to be determined. In this specific case, one could argue that the lineage distinctions that seem to predict response to BRAF inhibitors could be made by expression profiling. However, histopathologic inspection of tumors also provides information about other important characteristics of cancers, such as anaplasia, invasiveness, and tumor heterogeneity. Histopathology coupled with in situ biomarker tests performed on tissue sections also remains the best way to assess tumor : stromal cell interactions, such angiogenesis and host immune responses; the latter may have an increasingly important role in guiding therapeutic interventions that are designed to counteract immune evasion by tumors. Thus, what lies ahead is not the replacement of one set of techniques by another. On the contrary, for the foreseeable future the most accurate diagnosis and assessment of prognosis in cancer patients will be arrived at by a combination of morphologic and molecular techniques.

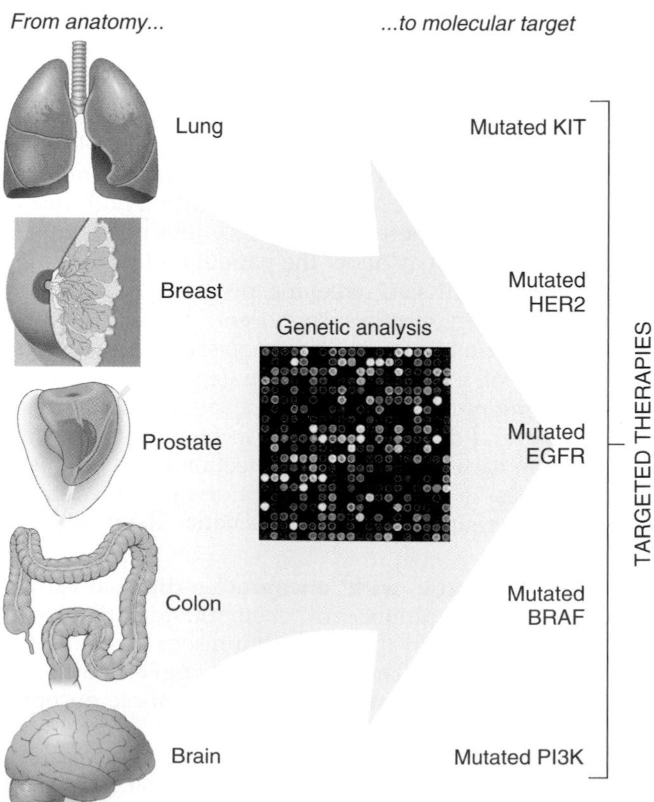

Figure 7-51 A paradigm shift: classification of cancer according to therapeutic targets rather than cell of origin and morphology. (Courtesy Dr. Levi Garraway, Dana Farber Cancer Institute.)

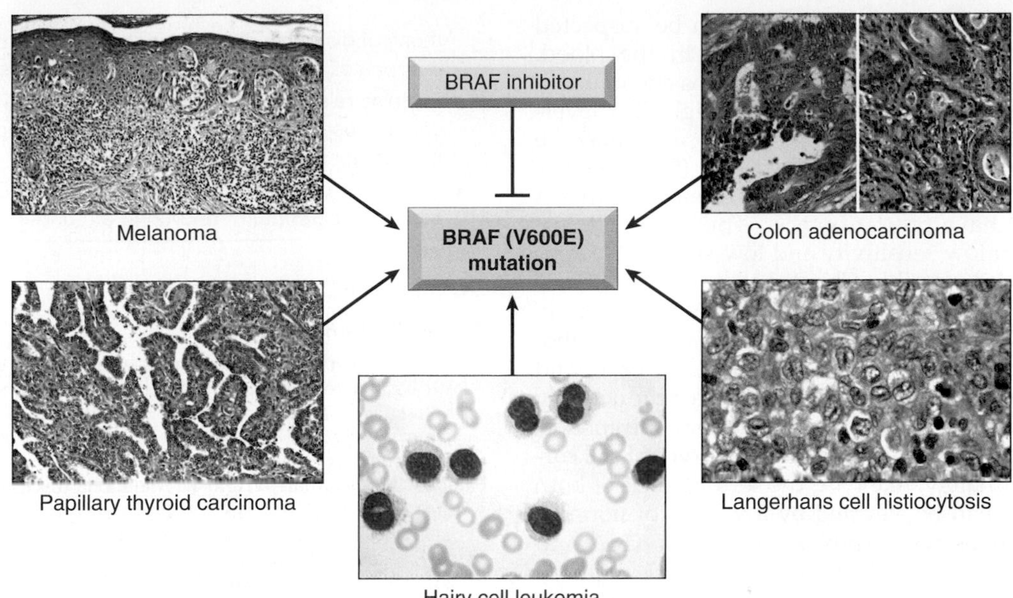

Figure 7-52 Diverse tumor types with a common molecular pathogenesis.

Tumor Markers

Biochemical assays for tumor-associated enzymes, hormones, and other tumor markers in the blood cannot be used for definitive diagnosis of cancer; however, they contribute to the detection of cancer and in some instances are useful in determining the effectiveness of therapy or the appearance of a recurrence.

A host of tumor markers have been described, and new candidates are identified every year. Only a few have stood the test of time and proved to have clinical usefulness.

The application of several markers, listed in Table 7-12, is considered in the discussion of specific forms of neoplasia in other chapters, so only a few widely used examples suffice here. Blood tests for *prostate specific antigen* (PSA), a marker for prostatic adenocarcinoma, are frequently used

Table 7-12 Selected Tumor Markers

Tumor Markers	Tumor Types
Hormones	
Human chorionic gonadotropin	Trophoblastic tumors, nonseminomatous testicular tumors
Calcitonin	Medullary carcinoma of thyroid
Catecholamine and metabolites	Pheochromocytoma and related tumors
Ectopic hormones	See Table 7-11
Oncofetal Antigens	
α-Fetoprotein	Liver cell cancer, nonseminomatous germ cell tumors of testis
Carcinoembryonic antigen	Carcinomas of the colon, pancreas, lung, stomach, and heart
Isoenzymes	
Prostatic acid phosphatase	Prostate cancer
Neuron-specific enolase	Small-cell cancer of lung, neuroblastoma
Specific Proteins	
Immunoglobulins	Multiple myeloma and other gammopathies
Prostate-specific antigen and prostate-specific membrane antigen	Prostate cancer
Mucins and Other Glycoproteins	
CA-125	Ovarian cancer
CA-19-9	Colon cancer, pancreatic cancer
CA-15-3	Breast cancer
Cell-Free DNA Markers	
TP53, APC, RAS mutants in stool and serum	Colon cancer
TP53, RAS mutants in stool and serum	Pancreatic cancer
TP53, RAS mutants in sputum and serum	Lung cancer
TP53 mutants in urine	Bladder cancer

in clinical practice. Prostatic carcinoma can be suspected when elevated levels of PSA are found in the blood. However, PSA screening highlights problems encountered with virtually every tumor marker. Although PSA levels are often elevated in cancer, PSA levels also may be elevated in benign prostatic hyperplasia (Chapter 18). Furthermore, there is no PSA level that ensures that a person does not have prostate cancer. Thus, the PSA test suffers from both low sensitivity and low specificity, limitations discussed in detail in Chapter 18.

Other tumor markers occasionally used in clinical practice include *carcinoembryonic antigen* (CEA), which is elaborated by carcinomas of the colon, pancreas, stomach, and breast, and *alpha-fetoprotein* (AFP), which is produced by hepatocellular carcinomas, yolk sac remnants in the gonads, and occasionally teratocarcinomas and embryonal cell carcinomas. Unfortunately, like PSA, the serum levels of both of these markers can be elevated by a variety of nonneoplastic conditions as well. Thus, as with PSA, CEA and AFP assays lack both specificity and sensitivity required for the early detection of cancers, but they are useful for detection of recurrences after excision. With successful resection of the tumor, these markers disappear from the serum; their persistence or reappearance almost always signifies tumor lurking within.

Other widely used markers include *human chorionic gonadotropin* (HCG) for testicular tumors, *CA-125* for ovarian tumors, and *immunoglobulin* in multiple myeloma and other secretory plasma cell tumors. The development of tests to detect cancer markers in blood and body fluids is an active area of research, and are focused in particular on the analysis of DNA that is shed from dying tumor cells. Some of the cell-free DNAs being evaluated as tumor markers include mutated *APC, TP53,* and *RAS* sequences in the stool of individuals with colorectal carcinomas; mutated *TP53* and hypermethylated genes in the sputum of persons with lung cancer and in the saliva of persons with head and neck cancers; and mutated *TP53* in the urine of patients with bladder cancer.

With all of the advances in genomic analyses and targeted therapies, one can safely predict that we are on the cusp of the golden age of tumor diagnosis and treatment. Those of you who are in medical school now can safely assume that the expectations for rapid advances in cancer diagnosis and therapy will be realized while you are still in practice. Get ready!

KEY CONCEPTS

Laboratory Diagnosis of Cancer

- Several sampling approaches exist for the diagnosis of tumors, including excision, biopsy, fine-needle aspiration, and cytologic smears.
- Immunohistochemistry and flow cytometry studies help in the diagnosis and classification of tumors, because distinct protein expression patterns define different entities.
- Molecular analyses are used to determine diagnosis, prognosis, the detection of minimal residual disease, and the diagnosis of hereditary predisposition to cancer.
- Molecular profiling of tumors by RNA expression profiling, DNA sequencing, and DNA copy number arrays are useful in molecular stratification of otherwise identical tumors or those of distinct histogenesis that share a mutation for the purpose of targeted treatment and prognostication.
- Proteins released by tumors into the serum, such as PSA, can be used to screen populations for cancer and to monitor for recurrence after treatment.
- Assays of circulating tumor cells and of DNA shed into blood, stool, sputum, and urine are under development.

SUGGESTED READINGS

Cancer Epidemiology

de Martel C, Ferlay J, Franceschi S, et al: Global burden of cancers attributable to infections in 2008: a review and synthetic analysis. *Lancet Oncol* 13:607–15, 2012. *[A recent analysis that estimates that approximately 16% of cancers (2 million cases per year) are attributable to infectious agents]*

Faulds MH, Dahlman-Wright K: Metabolic diseases and cancer risk. *Curr Opin Oncol* 24:58–61, 2012. *[A review focused on evidence linking metabolic disorders such obesity and diabetes to increased cancer risk]*

Liang J, Shang Y: Estrogen and Cancer. *Annu Rev Physiol* 75:225–40, 2013. *[A summary of epidemiologic evidence connecting hyperestrogenism to cancer and of current understanding of the oncogenic mechanisms of estrogen signaling]*

Roberts DL, Dive C, Renehan AG: Biological mechanisms linking obesity and cancer risk: new perspectives. *Annu Rev Med* 61:301–16, 2010. *[Discussion of possible biological processes that increase cancer risk in the obese]*

Cancer "Evolution"

Gerlinger M, Rowan AJ, Horswell S, et al: Intratumor heterogeneity and branched evolution revealed by multiregion sequencing. *N Engl J Med* 366:883–92, 2012. *[A paper highlighting the challenges that genomic instability and genomic evolution of cancers present to molecular diagnosticians and clinicians employing targeted therapies to treat cancer]*

Greaves M, Maley CC: Clonal evolution in cancer. *Nature* 481:306–13, 2012. *[A discussion of the iterative processes of clonal expansion, genetic diversification and clonal selection that promote cancer evolution and ultimately lead to therapeutic failure]*

Ma QC, Ennis CA, Aparicio S: Opening Pandora's Box–the new biology of driver mutations and clonal evolution in cancer as revealed by next generation sequencing. *Curr Opin Genet Dev* 22:3–9, 2012. *[A review summarizing driver mutations and their roles in directing clonal patterns of tumor evolution]*

Hallmarks of Cancer

Hanahan D, Weinberg RA: Hallmarks of cancer: the next generation. *Cell* 144:646–74, 2011. *[An update of a classic paper describing the key features common to all cancers]*

Oncogenes

Cilloni D, Saglio G: Molecular pathways: BCR-ABL. *Clin Cancer Res* 18:930–7, 2012. *[A discussion of the functional consequences and clinical significance of aberrant tyrosine kinase activity in chronic myeloid leukemia mediated by the constitutive enzyme activity of BCR-ABL]*

Dang CV: MYC on the path to cancer. *Cell* 149:22–35, 2012. *[A review of the widespread oncogenic role of the transcription factor MYC in cancer]*

Pao W, Chmielecki J: Rational, biologically based treatment of EGFR-mutant non-small-cell lung cancer. *Nat Rev Cancer* 10:760–74, 2010. *[A review summarizing recent work aimed at treating and ultimately curing lung cancers associated with activating mutations in the receptor tyrosine kinase EGFR]*

Pylayeva-Gupta Y, Grabocka E, Bar-Sagi D: RAS oncogenes: weaving a tumorigenic web. *Nat Rev Cancer* 11:761–74, 2011. *[A description of how RAS oncogenes activate multiple downstream signaling pathways to drive cellular transformation and oncogenesis]*

Tumor Suppressor Genes

Goh AM, Coffill CR, Lane DP: The role of mutant p53 in human cancer. *J Pathol* 223:116–26, 2011. *[Discussion of emerging oncogenic roles of mutant p53 proteins]*

Manning AL, Dyson NJ: RB: mitotic implications of a tumour suppressor. *Nat Rev Cancer* 12:220–6, 2012. *[In addition to the well established roles of RB in control of cell cycle progression and proliferation, this review describes other emerging tumor suppressive functions, such as maintenance of genomic stability]*

Roy R, Chun J, Powell SN: BRCA1 and BRCA2: different roles in a common pathway of genome protection. *Nat Rev Cancer* 12:68–78, 2012. *[A discussion of the concerted roles of the BRCA1 and BRCA2 tumor suppressor proteins in protecting the genome from double-strand DNA damage during DNA replication]*

Song MS, Salmena L, Pandolfi PP: The functions and regulation of the PTEN tumour suppressor. *Nat Rev Mol Cell Biol* 13:283–96, 2012. *[A detailed discussion of the tumor suppressive role of the the lipid phosphatase PTEN]*

Cancer Cell Metabolism

Ward PS, Thompson CB: Metabolic reprogramming: a cancer hallmark even warburg did not anticipate. *Cancer Cell* 21:297–308, 2012. *[A review making the case that altered cancer metabolism is a fundamental hallmark of cancer cells]*

Autophagy

Lozy F, Karantza V: Autophagy and cancer cell metabolism. *Semin Cell Dev Biol* 23:395–401, 2012. *[A discussion of how cellular metabolism and autophagy may contribute to the ability of cancer cells to adapt to environmental stressors and survive radiation and chemotherapy]*

Mah LY, Ryan KM: Autophagy and cancer. *Cold Spring Harb Perspect Biol* 4:a008821, 2012. *[A review of the possible interplay between autophagy and various aspects of tumor suppression, including cellular responses to nutrient and hypoxic stress, control of programmed cell death, and tumor-associated immune responses]*

Evasion of Apoptosis

Kilbride SM, Prehn JH: Central roles of apoptotic proteins in mitochondrial function. *Oncogene* 32:2703–11, 2013. *[A review focusing on the mechanistic roles of pro-apoptotic members of the BCL-2 family in controlling mitochondrial activity and the implications of these activities for cancer cell biology]*

Llambi F, Green DR: Apoptosis and oncogenesis: give and take in the BCL-2 family. *Curr Opin Genet Dev* 21:12–20, 2011. *[A discussion of the complex and sometimes paradoxical roles of BCL-2 family members in cancer]*

Cancer Stem Cells

Magee JA, Piskounova E, Morrison SJ: Cancer stem cells: impact, heterogeneity, and uncertainty. *Cancer Cell* 21:283–96, 2012. *[A critical review of the cancer stem cell model, with an eye towards its applicability to genetically and epigenetically heterogeneous human cancers]*

Martinez P, Blasco MA: Telomeric and extra-telomeric roles for telomerase and the telomere-binding proteins. *Nat Rev Cancer* 11:161–76, 2011. *[A review discussing the role of telomeric proteins in immortalization of cancer cells and other emerging non-telomeric functions that may also contribute to oncogenesis]*

Angiogenesis

Bottsford-Miller JN, Coleman RL, Sood AK: Resistance and Escape From Antiangiogenesis Therapy: Clinical Implications and Future Strategies. *J Clin Oncol* 30:4026–34, 2012. *[A discussion of how tumors escape from anti-angiogenic therapy and possible solutions to this limitation]*

Fokas E, McKenna WG, Muschel RJ: The impact of tumor microenvironment on cancer treatment and its modulation by direct and indirect antivascular strategies. *Cancer Metastasis Rev* 31:823–42, 2012. *[A discussion of the pro-oncogenic role of the tumor microenvironment in cancer and its implications for development of new therapies]*

Invasion and Metastasis

Spano D, Heck C, De Antonellis P, et al: Molecular networks that regulate cancer metastasis. *Semin Cancer Biol* 22:234–49, 2012. *[A review that addresses some of the genetic events and critical factors that contributes to acquisition of the metastatic phenotype during oncogenesis]*

Tiwari N, Gheldof A, Tatari M, et al: EMT as the ultimate survival mechanism of cancer cells. *Semin Cancer Biol* 22:194–207, 2012. *[A far-ranging discussion of the possible roles of epithelial-mesenchymal transition in metastasis and other cancer hallmarks]*

Evasion of Host Defense

Brahmer JR, Tykodi SS, Chow LQ, et al: Safety and activity of anti-PD-L1 antibody in patients with advanced cancer. *N Engl J Med* 366:2455–65, 2012. Also, Topalian SL, Hodi FS, Brahmer JR, et al: Safety, activity, and immune correlates of anti-PD-1 antibody in cancer. *N Engl J Med* 366:2443–54, 2012. *[Two back-to-back landmark papers describing the anti-cancer activity of antibodies that interfere with the activity of PD-1, a signaling receptor that inhibits T cell function]*

Cancer Enabling Inflammation

Coussens LM, Zitvogel L, Palucka AK: Neutralizing tumor-promoting chronic inflammation: a magic bullet? *Science* 339:286–91, 2013. *[A discussion of clinical and experimental studies describing protumorigenic roles for immune cells that elicit cancer-associated inflammation]*

De Palma M, Lewis CE: Macrophage regulation of tumor responses to anticancer therapies. *Cancer Cell* 23:277–86, 2013. *[A discussion of the pro and anti oncogenic effects of different subsets of tumor-associated macrophages]*

Hanahan D, Coussens LM: Accessories to the crime: functions of cells recruited to the tumor microenvironment. *Cancer Cell* 21:309–22, 2012. *[A detailed discussion of the possible roles of stromal cells in aiding and abetting cancer cells]*

Chromosomal Aberrations

Forment JV, Kaidi A, Jackson SP: Chromothripsis and cancer: causes and consequences of chromosome shattering. *Nat Rev Cancer* 12:663–70, 2012. *[A review describing how chromothripsis occurs and its potential diagnostic, prognostic and therapeutic implications in cancer]*

Gostissa M, Alt FW, Chiarle R: Mechanisms that promote and suppress chromosomal translocations in lymphocytes. *Annu Rev Immunol* 29:319–50, 2011. *[A discussion of pathogenic insights gleaned from experimental models of oncogenic chromosomal translocations in lymphocytes]*

Epigenetics and Cancer

Baylin SB, Jones PA: A decade of exploring the cancer epigenome - biological and translational implications. *Nat Rev Cancer* 11:726–34, 2011. *[A discussion of recent discoveries that link epigenetic abnormalities in cancer to mutations in genes that control DNA methylation, the packaging and the function of DNA in chromatin, and metabolism]*

Lindsley RC, Ebert BL: Molecular pathophysiology of myelodysplastic syndromes. *Annu Rev Pathol* 30:3376–82, 2012. *[A review of the pervasive role of epigenetic abnormalities in this group of myeloid malignancies]*

You JS, Jones PA: Cancer genetics and epigenetics: two sides of the same coin? *Cancer Cell* 22:9–20, 2012. *[A review discussing the origins and interplay of mutations and epignetic aberrations in cancer cells]*

Non-coding RNAs

Esteller M: Non-coding RNAs in human disease. *Nat Rev Genet* 12: 861–74, 2011. *[A review that discusses the roles of various classes of non-coding RNAs in human disease, including cancer]*

Lujambio A, Lowe SW: The microcosmos of cancer. *Nature* 482:347–55, 2012. *[A discussion of the roles of micro-RNAs in cancer]*

Environmental Carcinogens

Berger MF, Hodis E, Heffernan TP, et al: Melanoma genome sequencing reveals frequent PREX2 mutations. *Nature* 485:502–6, 2012. *[A study that describes and quantifies the mutational impact of sun-exposure on melanoma genomes]*

Pleasance ED, Stephens PJ, O'Meara S, et al: A small-cell lung cancer genome with complex signatures of tobacco exposure. *Nature* 463:184–90, 2010. *[A study that describes and quantifies the mutational impact of carcinogens in tobacco smoke on lung cancer genomes]*

Microbial Carcinogenesis

Cabibbo G, Maida M, Genco C, et al: Causes of and prevention strategies for hepatocellular carcinoma. *Semin Oncol* 39:374–83, 2012. *[A discussion of the various environmental factors implicated in hepatocellular carcinoma, including hepatitis viruses]*

Magrath I: Epidemiology: clues to the pathogenesis of Burkitt lymphoma. *Br J Haematol* 156:744–56, 2012. *[A discussion of the roles of Epstein-Barr virus and malaria in genesis of this aggressive B cell malignancy]*

Moody CA, Laimins LA: Human papillomavirus oncoproteins: pathways to transformation. *Nat Rev Cancer* 10:550–60, 2010. *[A review focused on the oncogenic activities of HPV E6 and E7 proteins]*

Peleteiro B, La Vecchia C, Lunet N: The role of Helicobacter pylori infection in the web of gastric cancer causation. *Eur J Cancer Prev* 21:118–25, 2012. *[A review that proposes a conceptual framework for understanding the role of H. pylori infection in gastric cancer]*

Cancer Cachexia and Paraneoplastic Syndromes

Azar L, Khasnis A: Paraneoplastic rheumatologic syndromes. *Curr Opin Rheumatol* 25:44–9, 2013. *[A review focused on paraneoplastic synovitis, bone disease, myositis, and vasculitis]*

Graus F, Dalmau J: Paraneoplastic neurological syndromes. *Curr Opin Neurol* ;25:795- 801, 2012. *[A review describing paraneoplastic neurological syndromes and the impact of antibodies against surface antigens in their management]*

Lucia S, Esposito M, Rossi Fanelli F, et al: Cancer Cachexia: From Molecular Mechanisms to Patient's Care. *Crit Rev Oncog* 17:315–21, 2012. *[A review of cancer cachexia mechanisms and their implications for development of effective therapies]*

Cancer Diagnostics

Alix-Panabieres C, Schwarzenbach H, Pantel K: Circulating tumor cells and circulating tumor DNA. *Annu Rev Med* 63:199–215, 2012. *[A review discussing the detection, characterization, and diagnostic implications of rare circulating tumor cells and free nucleic acids derived from tumors]*

Kohlmann A, Grossmann V, Haferlach T: Integration of next-generation sequencing into clinical practice: are we there yet? *Semin Oncol* 39:26–36, 2012. *[A discussion of how and when deep sequencing may impact cancer diagnosis, therapy selection, and monitoring of response to therapy]*

Pao W, Iafrate AJ, Su Z: Genetically informed lung cancer medicine. *J Pathol* 223:230–40, 2011. *[A review of the rapid adoption and application of genomic analysis to the diagnosis and treatment of lung cancer]*

See TARGETED THERAPY available online at www.studentconsult.com

CHAPTER 8

Infectious Diseases

Alexander J. McAdam • Danny A. Milner • Arlene H. Sharpe

CHAPTER CONTENTS

General Principles of Microbial Pathogenesis

Despite the availability of effective vaccines and antibiotics, infectious diseases remain an important health problem throughout the world. In the United States and other high-income countries, infectious diseases are particularly important causes of death among older adults and in people who are immunosuppressed or who suffer from debilitating chronic diseases. In the developing world, inadequate access to medical care and malnutrition contribute to a heavy burden of infectious diseases. In these areas, six of the ten leading causes of death are infectious diseases. Tragically, most of these deaths occur in children, with respiratory and diarrheal infections taking the greatest toll.

How Microorganisms Cause Disease

Over the past few years, it has become evident that humans and other animals harbor a complex ecosystem of microbial flora (the *microbiome*) that has important roles in health and disease. It is estimated that the normal human body harbors 10 times more microbial cells than human cells! Most of these commensal organisms coexist happily with their human hosts, occupying microenvironmental niches that might otherwise be filled by potential pathogens, and in doing so help to prevent infectious disease. However, under conditions where normal host defenses are breached or attenuated (described below), even "healthy" microbial flora may cause symptomatic infections and can even be fatal.

Most infectious diseases are caused by pathogenic, noncommensal organisms, which exhibit a wide range of virulence. Highly infectious microbes produce disease in a high fraction of healthy individuals, sometimes at "doses" of only a few organisms. Other microbes are minimally pathogenic, requiring large exposures and concomitant breaches of host defenses to cause disease. We will start our review of infectious disease at the beginning of the process, the establishment of a "beachhead" in the host, and then discuss dissemination and transmission of infection, before turning to specific infectious diseases.

Routes of Entry of Microbes

Microbes can enter the host by breaching epithelial surfaces, inhalation, ingestion, or sexual transmission (Table 8-1). In general, respiratory, gastrointestinal, and genitourinary tract infections in otherwise healthy persons are caused by virulent microorganisms with the ability to damage or penetrate the epidermis or mucosal epithelium. By contrast, skin infections in healthy persons are mainly caused by less virulent organisms that enter the skin through superficial injuries.

Skin

The intact keratinized epidermis protects against infection by serving as a strong mechanical barrier and by producing antimicrobial *fatty acids* and *defensins*, small peptides that are toxic to bacteria. These and other substances secreted by the skin create an environmental niche that is occupied by potential opportunistic organisms. Certain fungi (*dermatophytes*) can cause superficial infections of the intact stratum corneum, hair, and nails, but **most skin infections are initiated by mechanical injury of the epidermis**. The injury may range from minor trauma (superficial pricks and abrasions), to large wounds, burns, and pressure-related ulcers, particularly in diabetics. In the hospital setting, infections may stem from intravenous catheters in patients or needle sticks in healthcare workers. Some pathogens penetrate the skin via an insect or animal bite; vectors for such infections include a wide range of unpleasant characters, such as fleas, ticks, mosquitoes, mites, lice, and rabid animals. In general, microorganisms can not traverse the unbroken skin; exceptions include the larvae of *Schistosoma*, which release enzymes that dissolve the adhesive proteins that hold keratinocytes together.

Gastrointestinal Tract

Most gastrointestinal pathogens are transmitted by food or drink contaminated with fecal material. When hygiene fails, diarrheal disease becomes rampant. The gastrointestinal tract has several local defenses. Of these, *acidic gastric secretions* are particularly important since they are highly effective at killing certain organisms. Healthy volunteers do not become infected with *Vibrio cholerae* unless they are fed 10^{11} organisms, but neutralizing stomach acid reduces the necessary infectious dose by 10,000-fold. A *viscous layer of mucus* covers the gut throughout its length, protecting the surface epithelium. *Pancreatic enzymes* and

Table 8-1 Routes of Microbial Infecton

Site	Major Local Defense(s)	Basis for Failure of Local Defense	Pathogens (examples)
Skin	Epidermal barrier	Mechanical defects (punctures, burns, ulcers)	*S. aureus, Candida albicans, Pseudomonas aeuginosa*
		Needle sticks	HIV, hepatitis viruses
		Arthropod and animal bites	Yellow fever, plague, Lyme disease, malaria, rabies
		Direct penetration	Schistosoma
GI Tract	Epithelial barrier	Attachment and local proliferation of microbes	*Vibrio cholerae, Giardia*
		Attachment and local invasion of microbes	*Shigella, Salmonella, Campylobacter*
		Uptake through M cells	Poliovirus, certain pathogenic bacteria
	Acidic secretions	Acid-resistant cysts and eggs	Many protozoa and helminths
	Bile and pancreatic enzymes	Resistant microbial external coats	Hepatitis A, rotavirus, Norovirus
	Normal protective flora	Broad spectrum antibiotic use	*Clostridium difficile*
Respiratory Tract	Mucociliary clearance	Attachment and local proliferation of microbes	Influenza viruses
		Ciliary paralysis by toxins	*Haemophilus influenzae, M. pneumoniae, Bordtella pertusis*
	Resident alveolar macrophages	Resistance to killing by phagocytes	*M. tuberculosis*
Urogenital Tract	Urination	Obstruction, microbial attachment and local proliferation	*E. coli*
	Normal vaginal flora	Antibiotic use	*Candida albicans*
	Intact epidermal/epithelial barrier	Microbial attachment and local proliferation	*N. gonococcus*
		Direct infection/local invasion	Herpes viruses, syphilis
		Local trauma	Various sexually transmitted diseases, e.g., human papilloma virus

bile detergents can destroy organisms with envelopes, such as certain viruses. As in the skin, antimicrobial *defensins* are produce by gut epithelial cells. *IgA antibodies*, produced in mucosal lymphoid tissues such as Peyer patches and secreted into the gut lumen (Chapter 18), can neutralize potential pathogens. *Peristalsis* can clear organisms, preventing their local overgrowth. Finally, as already mentioned, the *normal gut flora* creates a microenvironment that discourages colonization by potential pathogens, such as *Clostridium difficile*.

Gastrointestinal tract infections may occur when local defenses are circumvented by a pathogen, or when they are so weakened that even normal flora produce disease. Many notorious gastrointestinal pathogens are intrinsically resistant to local defenses, particularly those that enter the host by ingestion. *Norovirus* (the scourge of the cruise ship industry) is a non-enveloped virus that is resistant to inactivation by acid, bile, and pancreatic enzymes and hence easily spread in places where people are crowded together. Similarly, intestinal protozoa and some intestinal helminths transmitted as cysts or eggs, respectively, have acid-resistant outer coats, and some bacteria, such as *Shigella*, are also resistant to acid; hence, as few as 100 organisms of each can cause illness.

Enteropathogenic pathogens may establish symptomatic gastrointestinal disease through several distinct mechanisms:

- *Adhesion and local proliferation*. Examples include *V. cholerae* and enterotoxigenic *Escherichia coli*, which bind to the intestinal epithelium and multiply in the overlying mucous layer. Here, these organisms elaborate potent exotoxins that are responsible for symptomatic disease.
- *Adhesion and mucosal invasion*. Pathogens such as *Shigella*, *Salmonella enterica*, *Campylobacter jejuni*, and *Entamoeba histolytica* invade the intestinal mucosa and lamina propria and cause ulceration, inflammation, and hemorrhage that manifest clinically as dysentery.
- *"Hijacking" of host pathways of antigen uptake*. You will recall that mucosal lymphoid tissues such as Peyer patches are covered by specialized epithelial cells called M cells, which are responsible for uptake and delivery of antigens to underlying lymphoid tissues. Ironically, multiple infectious agents, including poliovirus, are taken up into the host through this same pathway.

There are several caveats to the themes laid out above. Some organisms contaminating food can produce gastrointestinal disease without ever establishing an infection in the host. A cardinal example is *S. aureus*, which elaborates a powerful exotoxin during its growth in contaminated food that is responsible for acute food poisoning. Diminished local defenses due to loss of gastric acidity, broad-spectrum antibiotic treatment, ileus, or mechanical obstruction may exacerbate infections caused by virulent pathogens and allow organisms of low pathogenecity to establish disease. Other opportunistic organisms such as *Candida* only produce gastrointestinal disease when the immune system is weakened. In this setting, *Candida* has a particular predilection for establishing infections in squamous mucosae (e.g., oral thrush, esophagitis), but may also involve other sites.

Respiratory Tract

A plethora of microorganisms, including viruses, bacteria, and fungi, are inhaled daily, mainly in dust or aerosol particles. The distance these particles travel into the respiratory system is inversely proportional to their size. Large particles are trapped in the mucociliary blanket that lines the nose and the upper respiratory tract. Microorganisms trapped in the mucus layer are transported by ciliary action to the back of the throat, where they are swallowed and cleared. By contrast, particles smaller than 5 microns are carried into the alveoli, where they are phagocytosed by resident alveolar macrophages or by neutrophils recruited to the lung by cytokines.

The microorganisms that infect the healthy respiratory tract evade local defenses through several different mechanisms. Some pathogenic respiratory viruses attach to and enter epithelial cells in the lower respiratory tract and pharynx. For example, influenza viruses have envelope proteins called hemagglutinins that bind to sialic acid on the surface of epithelial cells. Attachment induces the host cell to endocytose the virus, leading to viral entry and replication. The resulting damage to the respiratory epithelium sets the stage for superinfection by *S. pneumoniae* and *S. aureus*, often leading to serious pneumonias. Certain bacterial respiratory pathogens, including *Haemophilus influenzae, M. pneumoniae,* and *Bordetella pertussis*, release toxins that enhance their ability to establish an infection by impairing ciliary activity. Another important mechanism of establishing respiratory infection is primary resistance to killing following phagocytosis. A classic example is *Mycobacterium tuberculosis*, which gains a foothold in alveoli by surviving within the phagolysosomes of macrophages.

Other organisms establish disease when local or systemic defenses are impaired. Chronic impairment of mucociliary defense mechanisms occurs in smokers and in people with cystic fibrosis, while acute injury occurs in patients undergoing mechanical ventilation and in those who aspirate gastric acid. Many other infectious agents cause respiratory infections primarily in the setting of systemic immunodeficiency. Examples include fungal infections by *P. jiroveci* in AIDS patients and by *Aspergillus* species in patients with neutropenia.

Urogenital Tract

Urine is sterile, and the urinary tract is protected from infection by regular emptying during micturition. Urinary tract pathogens (e.g., *E. coli*) almost always gain access via the urethra and must be able to adhere to urothelium to avoid being washed away. Anatomy plays an important role in dictating risk. Women have more than 10 times as many urinary tract infections as men because the distance between the urinary bladder and skin (i.e., the length of the urethra) is 5 cm in women versus 20 cm in men. Understandably, **obstruction of urinary flow or reflux of urine compromises normal defenses and increases susceptibility to urinary tract infections**.

From puberty until menopause the vagina is protected from pathogens by lactobacilli, which ferment glucose to lactic acid, producing a low pH environment that suppresses the growth of pathogens. Antibiotics can kill the lactobacilli and allow overgrowth of yeast, causing vaginal candidiasis. The uterine cervix is covered by squamous mucosa that is also resistant to infection. However, minor trauma may expose immature proliferating epithelial cells that are susceptible to infection by human papilloma viruses, an important sexually transmitted pathogen that is the cause of most cases of cervical carcinoma (Chapters 7 and 22).

Vertical Transmission

Vertical transmission of infectious agents from mother to fetus or newborn child is a common mode of transmission of certain pathogens, and may occur through several different routes.

- *Placental-fetal transmission.* This is most likely to occur when the mother is infected with a pathogen during pregnancy. Some of the resulting infections interfere with fetal development, and understandably the degree and type of damage depend on the age of the fetus at the time of infection. For example, rubella infection during the first trimester can lead to heart malformations, mental retardation, cataracts, or deafness, while rubella infection during the third trimester has little effect.
- *Transmission during birth.* This mode of transmission is caused by contact with infectious agents during passage through the birth canal. Examples include gonococcal and chlamydial conjunctivitis.
- *Postnatal transmission in maternal milk.* Agents transmitted in this fashion include cytomegalovirus (CMV), human immunodeficiency virus (HIV), and hepatitis B virus (HBV).

Spread and Dissemination of Microbes Within the Body

While some disease-causing microorganisms remain localized to the initial site of infection, others have the capacity to invade tissues and spread to distant sites via the lymphatics, the blood, or the nerves (Fig. 8-1). Pathogens can spread within the body in several ways. Some extracellular pathogens secrete enzymes that break down tissues, allowing the organisms to advance virtually unimpeded. For example, *S. aureus* secretes hyaluronidase, which degrades the extracellular matrix between host cells, allowing the microbes to follow tissue planes of least resistance. Eventually the organisms may travel through the lymphatics to regional lymph nodes and the blood, potentially leading to bacteremia and spread to distant organs, such as heart and bone. Certain viruses, such as rabies, poliovirus, and *Varicella*, spread to the central nervous system by infecting peripheral nerves and then traveling intracellularly along axons. However, the most common and efficient mode of microbial dissemination is through the bloodstream. Some blood-borne pathogens, such as certain viruses (e.g., poliovirus, hepatitis B virus), most bacteria and fungi, some protozoa (e.g., African trypanosomes), and helminths are transported free in plasma, while others are carried within leukocytes (e.g., herpesviruses, HIV, mycobacteria, and certain fungi and protozoa) or red cells (e.g., malarial parasites).

The consequences of blood-borne spread of pathogens vary widely depending on the virulence of the organism, the magnitude of the infection, the pattern of seeding, and host factors such as immune status. Sporadic

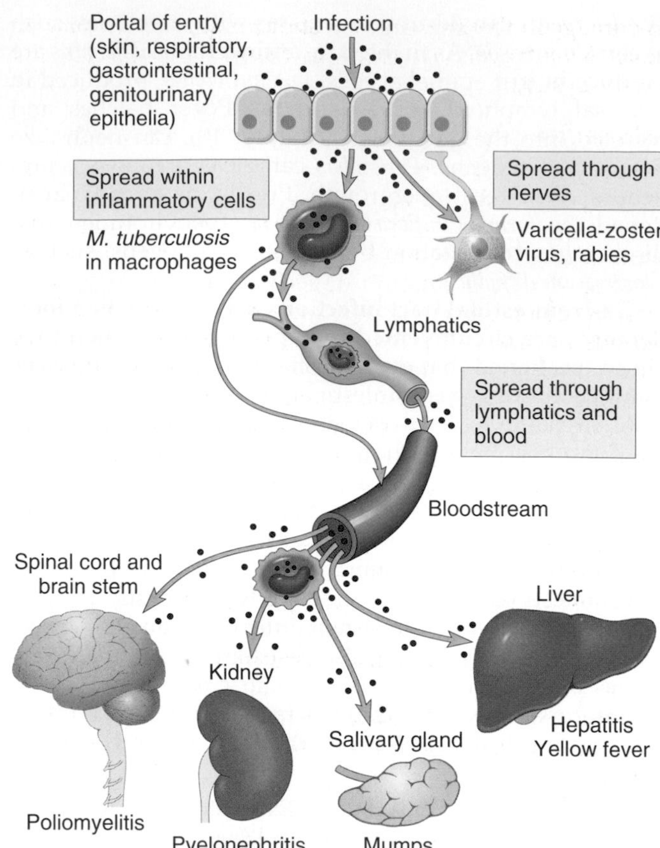

Figure 8-1 Routes of entry and dissemination of microbes. To enter the body, microbes penetrate the epithelial or mucosal barriers. Infection may remain localized at the site of entry or spread to other sites in the body. Most common microbes (selected examples are shown) spread through the lymphatics or bloodstream (either freely or within inflammatory cells). However, certain viruses and bacterial toxins may also travel through nerves. (Adapted from Mims CA: The Pathogenesis of Infectious Disease, 4th ed. San Diego, Academic Press, 1996.)

bloodstream invasion by low-virulence or nonvirulent microbes (e.g., during brushing of teeth) is common but is quickly controlled by normal host defenses. By contrast, disseminated viremia, bacteremia, fungemia, or parasitemia by virulent pathogens often produces severe illness and is a serious threat to life. As discussed in Chapter 4, such infections may produce a systemic inflammatory response syndrome that manifests as fever, low blood pressure, and coagulopathies that may progress to organ failure and death if unchecked, even in previously healthy individuals. In other instances, the major signs of spread of the infection are related to tissue seeding. These may take the form of a single large infectious nidus (an abscess or tuberculoma), multiple small sites of infection (e.g., miliary tuberculosis or *Candida* microabscesses), or infection of the heart and vessels (infectious endocarditis and mycotic aneurysm).

Other microbes cause characteristic patterns of disease because of tropism for specific tissues. These include already mentioned neurotropic viruses (rabies, poliovirus, varicella) and certain parasites. For example, after penetrating the skin, *Schistosoma mansoni* parasites localize to blood vessels of the portal system and mesentery, leading to damage in the liver and intestine. Similarly, *Schistosoma hematobium* travels to vessels in the urinary bladder and causes cystitis.

Release from the Body and Transmission of Microbes

Infectious microbes use a variety of "exit strategies" to ensure their transmission from one host to the next. Depending on the location of of infection, release may be accomplished by skin shedding, coughing, sneezing, voiding of urine or feces, during sexual contact, or through insect vectors. Some pathogens are released for only brief periods of time or periodically during disease flares, but others, such as the enteric pathogen *S. typhi*, may be shed for long periods by asymptomatic carrier hosts. Once released, pathogens also show wide variation in hardiness. Some survive for extended periods of time in dust, food, or water. Bacterial spores, protozoan cysts, and helminth eggs can remain viable in a cool and dry environment for months to years. By contrast, some fragile pathogens persist outside of the body for only short periods of time and must be passed quickly from person to person, often by direct contact.

Most pathogens are transmitted from person to person by respiratory, fecal-oral, or sexual routes. Viruses and bacteria spread by the respiratory route are infectious only when lesions are open to the airways. With coughing, the pathogens are aerosolized in droplets and released into the air. Some respiratory pathogens, including influenza viruses, are spread in large droplets that travel no more than 3 feet from the source, but others, including *M. tuberculosis* and varicella-zoster virus, spread in small droplets or within dust particles that can travel much longer distances.

Understandably, most enteric pathogens are spread by the fecal-oral route, that is, by ingestion of stool-contaminated water or food. Water-borne viruses involved in epidemic outbreaks that are spread in this fashion include hepatitis A and E viruses, poliovirus, and rotavirus. Other important pathogens spread by the fecal-oral route include *V. cholerae*, *Shigella*, *Campylobacter jejuni*, and *Salmonella*. Some parasitic helminthes (e.g., hookworms, schistosomes) shed eggs in stool that hatch as larvae that are capable of penetrating the skin of the next host. Sexual transmission often entails prolonged intimate or mucosal contact and is responsible for spread of a wide variety of pathogens, including viruses (e.g., *Herpes simplex*, HIV, human papilloma virus), bacteria (*T. pallidum*, *Gonococcus*), protozoa (*Candida*) and even arthropods (*Phthiris pubis*, or crab lice).

Besides these major routes of transmission, pathogens exist that exploit virtually every imaginable means for spreading to a new host. Saliva is responsible for transmitting viruses that replicate in the salivary gland or oropharynx, including Epstein-Barr virus and rabies virus, which may be spread by an amorous kiss or a frenzied bite, respectively. Protozoa and helminths have evolved particularly complex life cycles that often involve intermediate hosts bearing successive developmental stages of the pathogen. Some of the most important human pathogens are protozoa that are spread through blood meals taken by arthropod vectors (mosquitoes, ticks, mites). Finally, a few pathogens can be transmitted from animals to humans (termed *zoonotic infections*), either by direct contact, consumption of animal products, or via an invetebrate vector.

KEY CONCEPTS

Transmission and Dissemination of Microbes

- Transmission of infections can occur by contact (direct and indirect), respiratory route, fecal-oral route, sexual transmission, vertical transmission or insect/arthropod vectors.
- A pathogen can establish infection if it possesses virulence factors that overcome normal host defenses or if the host defenses are compromised.
- Host defenses against infection include:
  - Skin: tough keratinized barrier, low pH, fatty acids
  - Respiratory system: alveolar macrophages, mucociliary clearance by bronchial epithelium, IgA
  - GI system: acidic gastric pH, viscous mucus, pancreatic enzymes and bile, defensins, IgA, and normal flora
  - Urogenital tract: repeated flushing and acidic environment created by commensal flora
- Pathogens can proliferate locally, at the site of initial infection, or spread to other sites by direct extension (invasion) or by transport in the lymphatics, the blood, or nerves.

Host-Pathogen Interactions

Host Defenses against Infection

The outcome of infection is determined by the virulence of the microbe and the nature of the host immune response, which may either eliminate the infection or, in some cases, exacerbate or even be the principal cause of tissue damage. The host has a large and complex armamentarium of defenses against pathogens, including physical barriers and components of the innate and adaptive immune systems, which were discussed extensively in Chapter 6. The complexity of the immune system is a testimony to the remarkable selective pressures that infectious diseases place on humans and other animals; there is little doubt that the ability to survive in a world full of pathogenic microbes was (and remains) one of the most important forces shaping human evolution. Unfortunately, Darwinian forces also drive the continuing evolution of a remarkable array of highly diverse microbes, which are constantly threatening to get a step ahead of host defenses.

We will return to the issue of newly emerging infections later in this Chapter. In the next section, we discuss the various mechanisms by which pathogens evade the host and cause disease.

Immune Evasion by Microbes

Most pathogenic microbes have developed one or more strategies that allow them to evade host defenses (Fig. 8-2). The mechanisms of evasion are probably even more numerous than the mechanisms of effective host response, as any microbe that by chance acquires resistance to an effective host response is likely, over time, to rise in prevalence in the microbial population. Some salient examples of immune evasion by microbes are as follows:

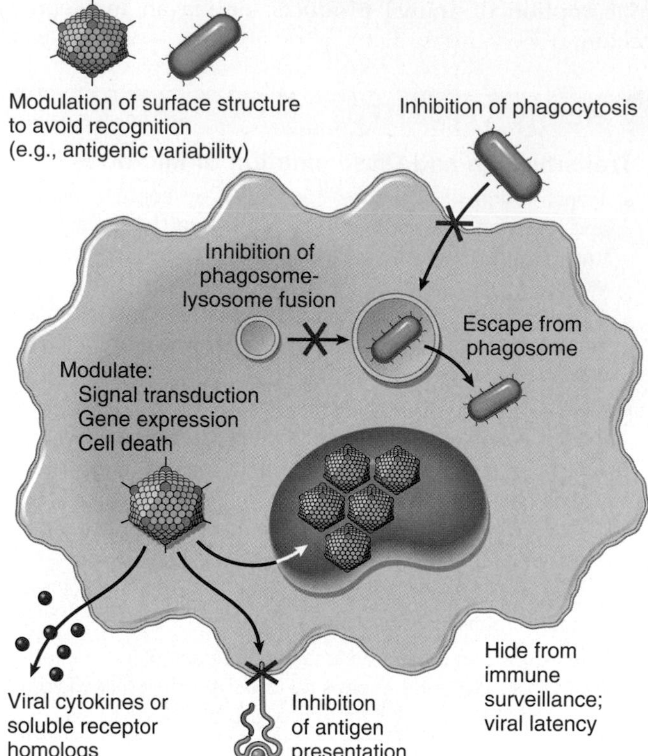

Figure 8-2 An overview of mechanisms used by viral and bacterial pathogens to evade innate and adaptive immunity. (Modified with permission from Finlay B, McFadden G: Anti-immunology: evasion of the host immune system by bacterial and viral pathogens. Cell 2006;124:767-782.)

- *Antigenic variation.* This is an important mechanism for escape from antibody-mediated host defenses. Antibodies against microbial antigens can block microbial adhesion and uptake into cells, act as opsinins to facilitate phagocytosis, and fix complement, and cytotoxic T cells recognize microbial antigens expressed in the context of MHC molecules on the surface of infected host cells. To escape recognition, microbes have many strategies that allow them to "change their coats" by expressing different surface antigens. Spirochetes belonging to *Borrelia* species and trypanosomes have sophisticated genetic mechanisms that allow them to periodically switch their major surface proteins. Influenza viruses have a complex RNA genome that allows for frequenct recombination events, permitting antigenic "drift" and "shifts". In a less elegant but nevertheless effective fashion, other microbes simply generate numerous genetic variants through mutation. For example, there are over 90 different serotypes of *S. pneumoniae*, each with different capsular polysaccharides. Similarly, the low fidelity of viral RNA polymerases of HIV and many respiratory viruses (including influenza virus) create viral antigenic variation (Table 8-2).
- *Resistance to antimicrobial peptides.* You will recall from Chapter 6 that epithelial cells and some leukocytes produce cationic antimicrobial peptides such as defensins and cathelicidins that are toxic to microbes, in part by forming pores in microbial membranes. These peptides can also augment anti-microbial immunity by inducing the production of pro-inflammatory chemokines and cytokines. Resistance to these peptides is a factor in the virulence of a number of pathogens, including *Shigella* ssp, *S. aureus,* and *Candida*. Microbial strategies to avoid killing by peptides include changes in net surface charge and membrane hydrophobicity that prevent antimicrobial peptide insertion and pore formation, secretion of proteins that inactivate or degrade the peptides, and pumps that export the peptides.
- *Resistance to killing by phagocytes.* Phagocytosis and killing of bacteria by neutrophils and macrophages are a critical host defense against extracellular bacteria; accordingly, pathogens have evolved a wealth of resistance mechanisms at virtually every level of the process. The carbohydrate capsule on the surface of many bacteria that cause pneumonia or meningitis (*S. pneumoniae, N. meningitidis, H. influenzae*) prevents phagocytosis of the organisms by neutrophils. *E. coli* that cause meningitis in newborns synthesize a special capsule containing sialic acid that will not bind C3b, which is critical for activation of the alternative complement pathway and opsonization-directed phagocytosis. *S. aureus* expresses protein A, which binds the Fc portion of antibodies and so inhibits phagocytosis. Other bacteria make proteins that variously kill phagocytes, prevent their migration, or diminish their oxidative burst. Finally, some pathogens are resistance to intracellular killing in phagocytes, including mycobacteria, *Listeria, Cryptococcus neoformans,* and certain protozoa (e.g., leishmania, trypanosomes, toxoplasmas).
- *Evasion of apoptosis and manipulation of host cell metabolism.* Some viruses produce proteins that interfere with apoptosis of the host cell, which may buy them the time necessary to replicate, enter latency, or even transform host cells. Microbes that replicate intracellularly (viruses, some bacteria, fungi and protozoa) also express factors that modulate autophagy, which appears to enhance their ability to evade degradation and to replicate.
- *Resistance to cytokine-, chemokine- and complement-mediated host defense.* Many virues express factors that interfere with the actions of cytokines, chemokines, or complement. For example, some viruses produce soluble homologues of IFN-α/β or IFN-γ receptors that function as "decoys" and sop up and inhibit the actions of secreted IFNs. Viruses also produce proteins that inhibit the JAK/STAT pathway, a key signaling cascade that

Table 8-2 Mechanisms of Antigenic Variation

Type	Example	Disease
High mutation rate	HIV Influenza virus	AIDS Influenza
Genetic reassortment	Influenza virus Rotavirus	Influenza Diarrhea
Genetic rearrangement (e.g., gene recombination, gene conversion, site-specific inversion)	*Borrelia burgdorferi* *Neisseria gonorrhoeae* *Trypanosoma* sp. *Plasmodium* sp.	Lyme disease Gonorrhea African sleeping sickness Malaria
Large diversity of serotypes	Rhinoviruses *Streptococcus pneumoniae*	Colds Pneumonia Meningitis

lies downstream of IFN receptors. Other viruses produce proteins that inactivate or inhibit double-stranded RNA–dependent protein kinase (PKR), an important mediator of the antiviral effects of IFN, or produce proteins that block complement activation.

- *Evasion of recognition by CD4+ helper T cells and CD8+ cytotoxic T cells.* This is also an important mode of immune evasion by viruses, which involves several different mechanisms. Several DNA viruses (e.g., HSV, CMV, and EBV) bind to or alter localization of major histocompatibility complex (MHC) class I proteins, impairing peptide presentation to CD8+ T cells. Downregulation of MHC class I molecules could lead to targeting by NK cells, but herpesviruses also express MHC class I homologues that inhibit NK cells by engaging NK cell inhibitory receptors (Chapter 6). Herpesviruses also can target MHC class II molecules for degradation, impairing antigen presentation to CD4+ T helper cells.
- Another strategy exploits *immunoregulatory mechanisms to downregulate anti-microbial T cell responses.* During chronic viral infections, antigen-specific T cells initially acquire effector functions but gradually lose their potency as infection progresses. This loss of function, termed T cell exhaustion, is a feature of chronic infections by HIV, hepatitis C virus, and hepatitis B virus. A major mechanism regulating T cell exhaustion is upregulation of immunoinhibitory T cell pathways. The PD-1 pathway, which normally functions to maintain T cell tolerance to self-antigens, is an important mediator of T cell exhaustion during chronic viral infection.
- The ultimate means of avoiding the immune system is to "lie low" by establishing a state of *latent infection* in which few if any viral genes are expressed. Examples include latent infections of neurons by *herpes simplex* and *Varicella* and of B lymphocytes by Epstein-Barr virus. These latent infections persist in an asymptomatic state throughout life, but may produce disease if the viruses are "awakened" from their latent state and enter a phase of viral replication. Other pathogens infect leukocytes, and in doing so interfere with their function, leading to persistent infection. A classic example is HIV, which infects CD4+ T cells and by doing so sets the stage for T cell dysfunction and persistent, progressive disease.

KEY CONCEPTS

Immune evasion by microbes

After bypassing host tissue barriers, infectious microorganisms must also evade host innate and adaptive immunity to successfully proliferate and be transmitted to the next host. Strategies include:

- Antigenic variation
- Inactivating antibodies or complement
- Resisting phagocytosis, e.g. by producing a capsule
- Suppressing the host adaptive immune response, e.g. by interfering with cytokines or inhibiting MHC expression and antigen presentation.
- Establishing latency, during which viruses survive in a silent state in infected cells.

Injurious Effects of Host Immunity

As mentioned earlier, while generally beneficial, the host immune response to microbes can sometimes be the major cause of tissue injury. The granulomatous inflammatory reaction to *M. tuberculosis* sequesters the bacilli and prevents their spread, but it also can produce tissue damage and fibrosis. Similarly, damage to hepatocytes following hepatitis B virus and hepatitis C virus infection is mainly due to the effects of the immune response on infected liver cells rather than cytopathic effects of the virus. Humoral immune responses to microbes also can have pathologic consequences. Following infection with *S. pyogenes,* antibodies produced against the streptococcal M protein can cross-react with cardiac proteins and damage the heart, leading to rheumatic heart disease. Similarly, poststreptococcal glomerulonephritis is caused by immune complexes formed between antistreptococcal antibodies and circulating streptococcal antigens; these complexes deposit in the renal glomeruli, producing inflammation in the kidney.

Inflammation elicited by microbes also underlies a wide variety of chronic inflammatory disorders as well as some forms of cancer. A cycle of inflammation and epithelial injury is involved in the pathogenesis of inflammatory bowel disease, with microbes playing at least a peripheral role (Chapter 17). Viruses (hepatitis B virus, hepatitis C virus) and bacteria (*H. pylori*) that are not known to carry or activate oncogenes are associated with cancers, presumably because these microbes trigger chronic inflammation, which provides fertile ground for the development of cancer (Chapter 7).

Infections in People with Immunodeficiencies

Inherited or acquired defects in innate and adaptive immunity (Chapter 6) often impair only part of the immune system, rendering the affected individual susceptible to specific types of infections. These rare disorders have served to illuminate important aspects of specific components of host defense, as well as the unique vulnerabilities of certain pathogens. The following are some specific examples:

- *Antibody deficiencies*, as seen in patients with X-linked agammaglobulinemia, lead to increased susceptibility to infections by extracellular bacteria, including *S. pneumoniae, H. influenzae,* and *S. aureus,* as well as a few viruses (rotavirus and enteroviruses).
- *Complement defects* in early components of the complement cascade lead to susceptibility to infections by encapsulated bacteria, such as *S. pneumoniae,* whereas deficiencies of the late membrane attack complex components (C5-C9) are associated with *Neisseria* infections.
- *Defects in neutrophil function* lead to increased susceptibility to infections with *S. aureus,* some gram-negative bacteria, and fungi.
- *Defects in Toll-like receptor (TLR) signaling pathways* have varied effects. Mutations in MyD88 or IRAK4, which are downstream of several TLRs, predispose to pyogenic bacterial infections, particularly invasive infections with *S. pneumoniae,* while impaired TLR3 responses are associated with childhood herpes simplex virus encephalitis.

- *T-cell defects* lead to susceptibility to intracellular pathogens, particularly viruses and some parasites. Inherited mutations that impair the generation of T_H1 cells (such as mutations in IL-12 or IFN-γ receptors, or the transcription factor STAT1) are associated with atypical mycobacterial infections. By contrast, defects that impair the generation of T_H17 cells (such as mutations in STAT3) are associated with chronic mucocutaneous candidiasis.

Even more common are acquired immunodeficiencies. Worldwide, the most common cause of immunodeficiency is infection with HIV, the cause of AIDS. While most organisms that infect people with AIDS were common pathogens before the era of HIV, others were uncommon (cryptococcus, pneumocystis), and one, Kaposi sarcoma herpesvirus (KSHV), also called human herpesvirus-8 (HHV-8), was discovered as a result of research in AIDS patients.

Other causes of acquired immunodeficiencies include infiltrative processes that suppress bone marrow function (such as leukemia), immunosuppressive drugs used to treat patients with autoimmune diseases and organ transplant recipients, as well as drugs used to treat cancer, and hematopoietic stem cell transplantation. Therapy to prevent rejection of organ transplants leads to severe immunosuppression, making transplant recipients very susceptible to infectious diseases. Patients receiving hematopoietic stem cell transplants have profound defects in innate and adaptive immunity during the time that it takes for the donated stem cells to engraft, and become susceptible to infection with almost any organism, including opportunistic organisms that seldom cause disease in healthy people (e.g., *Aspergillus* species and *Pseudomonas* species).

Decline of immune responses can result in reactivation of latent infection and severe pathologic manifestations. Such reactivation is seen in latent viral infections (e.g., herpesviruses) and some bacterial infections (e.g., tuberculosis). At least some of the increased incidence of certain infections in the elderly may be due to age-related declines in immune function.

Diseases of organ systems other than the immune system also can make patients susceptible to diseases due to specific microorganisms. People with cystic fibrosis commonly get respiratory infections with *P. aeruginosa*, *S. aureus*, and *Burkholdaria cepacia*. Lack of splenic function in people with sickle cell disease makes them susceptible to infection with encapsulated bacteria such as *S. pneumoniae*, which are normally opsonized and phagocytosed by splenic macrophages. Burns destroy skin, removing this barrier to microbes and allowing infection with pathogens such as *P. aeruginosa*. Finally, malnutrition can impair immune defenses.

Host Damage

Infectious agents establish infection and damage tissues by three mechanisms:

- They can contact or enter host cells and cause cell death directly, or cause changes in cellular metabolism and proliferation that can eventually lead to transformation.
- They may release toxins that kill cells at a distance, release enzymes that degrade tissue components, or damage blood vessels and cause ischemic necrosis.
- They can induce host immune responses that, though directed against the invader, cause additional tissue damage. As already mentioned, the defensive responses of the host constitute a double-edged sword: They are necessary to overcome the infection but at the same time may directly contribute to tissue damage.

Here we describe some of the mechanisms whereby viruses and bacteria damage host tissues.

Mechanisms of Viral Injury

Viruses can directly damage host cells by entering them and replicating at the host's expense. The predilection for viruses to infect certain cells and not others is called *tropism* and may be determined by physical factors, surface proteins that are required for viral entry, and other factors that are required for viral replication. Each is discussed below briefly.

A major determinant of tissue tropism is the presence of viral receptors on host cells. Viruses have surface proteins that bind to particular proteins found on the surface of host cells. Many of these host cell proteins normally function as receptors for host factors. For example, HIV glycoprotein gp120 binds to CD4 on T cells and to the chemokine receptors CXCR4 (mainly on T cells) and CCR5 (mainly on macrophages) (Chapter 6), while Epstein-Barr virus binds to complement receptor 2 (also known as CR2 or CD21) on B cells. Other tropisms are explained by different kinds of cell-lineage specific factors. For example, JC virus infection, which causes leukoencephalopathy (Chapter 28), is restricted to oligodendroglial cells in the CNS; this is because the expression of JC viral genes needed for a productive infection requires host transcription factors that are only expressed in glial cells, and not in neurons or endothelial cells.

Physical barriers also can contribute to tissue tropism. For example, enteroviruses replicate in the intestine in part because they can resist inactivation by acids, bile, and digestive enzymes. Rhinoviruses infect host cells only within the upper respiratory tract because they replicate optimally at the lower temperatures found in sites exposed to the ambient atmosphere.

Once viruses are inside host cells, they can damage or kill the cells by a number of mechanisms (Fig. 8-3):

- *Direct cytopathic effects.* Some viruses kill cells by preventing synthesis of critical host macromolecules (e.g., host cell DNA, RNA, or proteins), or by producing degradative enzymes and toxic proteins. For example, poliovirus inactivates cap-binding protein, which is essential for translation of host cell mRNAs but leaves translation of poliovirus mRNAs unaffected. Herpes simplex virus produces proteins that inhibit the synthesis of cellular DNA and mRNA, as well as other proteins that degrade host DNA. Viruses can induce cell death by a variety of means, including by activating so-called death receptors (members of the TNF receptor family) on the plasma membrane and by triggering the intracellular apoptotic machinery. During the course of productive viral infection, large amounts of viral proteins are synthesized in infected cells, including unfolded or

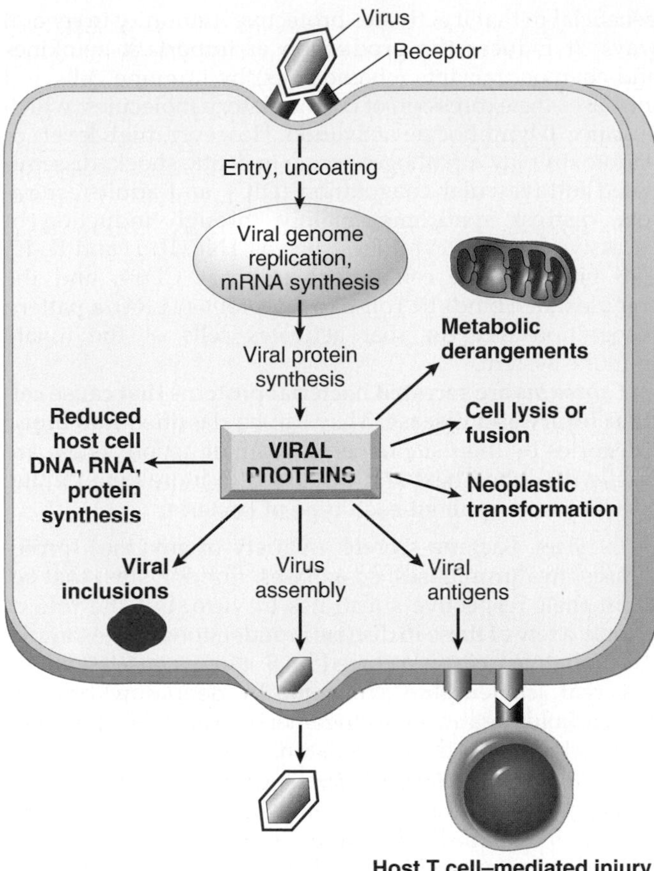

Figure 8-3 Mechanisms by which viruses cause injury to cells.

misfolded proteins that activate the ER stress response; this, too, activates pro-apoptotic pathways. Finally, some viruses encode proteins that are pro-apoptotic; the HIV vpr protein is one such example.

- *Anti-viral immune responses.* Host lymphocytes can recognize and destroy virus-infected cells. Cytotoxic T lymphocytes (CTLs) are important for defense against viral infections, but CTLs also can be responsible for tissue injury, as discussed previously.
- *Transformation of infected cells.* Oncogenic viruses can stimulate cell growth and survival by a variety of mechanisms, including expression of virus-encoded oncogenes, expression of viral proteins that inactivate key tumor suppressors, and insertional mutagenesis, in which expression of host genes is altered by the insertion of the viral genome into the genes or the flanking host genome. The mechanisms of viral transformation are numerous and are discussed in Chapter 7.

Mechanisms of Bacterial Injury

***Bacterial Virulence.* Bacterial damage to host tissues depends on the ability of the bacteria to adhere to host cells, to invade cells and tissues, or to deliver toxins.** Pathogenic bacteria have *virulence genes* that encode proteins that confer these properties. An example of the importance of such genes can be found in the various strains of *Salmonella*. All *Salmonella* strains that infect humans are closely related enough to form a single species, meaning that they share many "housekeeping" genes. Differences in a relatively small number of pathogenicity genes determine whether an isolate of *Salmonella* causes life-threatening typhoid fever or self-limited enteritis. Virulence genes are frequently found grouped together in clusters called *pathogenicity islands*.

***Mobile genetic elements* such as plasmids and bacteriophages can transmit functionally important genes to bacteria, including genes that influence pathogenicity and drug resistance.** Genes for toxins are sometimes found in plasmids but are more often found in the genomes of bacteriophages, including the genes that encode the toxins responsible for the pathogenesis of cholera, diphtheria and botulism. Genes for acquired antibiotic resistance traits are more frequently found on plasmids, which can spread not only within bacterial species but also between more distantly related organisms. For example, a plasmid with genes for vancomycin resistance can spread not only between species of *Enterococcus*, but also to more distantly related (and virulent) *S. aureus*.

Many bacteria coordinately regulate gene expression within a large population by a process called *quorum sensing*. For example, bacteria can induce expression of virulence factors as they grow to high concentration in tissue. This may allow bacteria growing in discrete host sites, such as an abscess or consolidated pneumonia, to overcome host defenses. *S. aureus* coordinately regulates virulence factors by secreting *autoinducer peptides*. As the bacteria increase in numbers, the level of the autoinducer peptide increases, stimulating toxin production. Within the population, some bacteria produce the autoinducer peptide and others respond to it by secreting toxins. Thus, because of quorum sensing, unicellular bacteria acquire some of the more complex properties of multicellular organisms, in which different cells perform different functions.

Communities of bacteria can also form *biofilms* in which the organisms live within a viscous layer of extracellular polysaccharides that adhere to host tissues or devices such as intravascular catheters and artificial joints. In addition to enhancing adherence to host tissues, biofilms increase the virulence of bacteria by protecting the microbes from immune effector mechanisms and increasing their resistance to antimicrobial drugs. Biofilm formation seems to be particularly important in the persistence and relapse of bacterial endocarditis, artificial joint infections, and respiratory infections in people with cystic fibrosis.

Bacterial Adherence to Host Cells. Adhesins are bacterial surface proteins that bind bacteria to host cells or extracellular matrix. Adhesins are limited in structural type but have a broad range of host cell specificity. *Streptococcus pyogenes* adheres to host tissues using the adhesins protein F and teichoic acid, which project from the bacterial cell wall and bind to fibronectin on the surface of host cells and in the extracellular matrix.

Pili are filamentous proteins on the surface of bacteria that act as adhesins. The stalks of pili are composed of conserved repeating subunits, while the variable subunits on the tips of the pili determine the tissue-binding specificity of the bacteria. For example, strains of *E. coli* that cause urinary tract infections specifically express a pilus which binds to a gal(α1-4)gal moiety expressed on uroepithelial cells. Pili can be targets of the host antibody response and, in turn, some bacteria such as N. gonorrhoeae, vary their pili to escape from the host immune system.

Virulence of Intracellular Bacteria. Bacteria have evolved a variety of mechanisms for entering host cells. Some bacteria use the host immune response to gain entry into macrophages. Opsonization of bacteria with antibodies or the complement protein C3b promotes phagocytosis of bacteria by macrophages. Like many bacteria, *M. tuberculosis* activates the alternative complement pathway, resulting in opsonization with C3b. Once coated with C3b, *M. tuberculosis* binds to the CR3 complement receptor on macrophages, enters the macrophages, and replicates within phagosomes. Gram-negative bacteria use a complex secretion system to enter epithelial cells. This type III secretion system consists of needle-like structures projecting from the bacterial surface that bind to host cells. These proteins then form pores in the host cell membrane and inject bacterial proteins that mediate the rearrangement of the host cell cytoskeleton in a fashion that facilitates bacterial entry. Once inside the host cell, other bacteria such as *Listeria monocytogenes* modify the actin cytoskeleton to promote the direct spreading of the organism to neighboring cells, allowing the bacteria to evade immune effector mechanisms.

After bacteria enter the host cell, their fate (and that of the infected cell) varies greatly depending on the organism. *Shigella* and *E. coli* inhibit host protein synthesis, replicate rapidly, and lyse the host cell within hours. Most bacteria are killed within macrophages when the phagosome fuses with an acidic lysosome to form a phagolysosome, but certain bacteria elude this host defense. For example, *M. tuberculosis* blocks fusion of the lysosome with the phagosome, allowing it to proliferate unchecked within the macrophage. Other bacteria avoid destruction in macrophages by leaving the phagosome and entering the cytoplasm. *L. monocytogenes* produces a pore-forming protein called listeriolysin O and two phospholipases that degrade the phagosome membrane, allowing the bacterium to escape into the cytoplasm.

Facultative intracellular bacteria infect epithelial cells (*Shigella* and enteroinvasive *E. coli*), macrophages (*M. tuberculosis, M. leprae*), or both (*S. typhi*). The growth of bacteria in cells can allow them to escape from certain effector mechanisms of the immune response (e.g., antibodies and complement), and can also facilitate the spread of the bacteria. An example of the latter is the migration of infected macrophages carrying *M. tuberculosis* from the lung to draining lymph nodes and other more distant sites.

Bacterial Toxins. Any bacterial substance that contributes to illness can be considered a toxin. Toxins are classified as *endotoxins*, which are components of the bacterial cell, and *exotoxins*, which are proteins that are secreted by the bacterium.

***Bacterial endotoxin* is a lipopolysaccharide (LPS) in the outer membrane of Gram-negative bacteria that both stimulates host immune responses and injures the host.** Lipid A, which anchors LPS in the host cell membrane through long-chain fatty acids, has the endotoxin activity of LPS. Lipid A is connected to a conserved core carbohydrate chain, which is attached to a variable carbohydrate chain called the O antigen. The response to lipid A is beneficial in that it activates protective immunity in several ways. It induces the production of important cytokines and chemoattractants (chemokines) by immune cells and increases the expression of costimulatory molecules, which enhance T-lymphocyte activation. However, high levels of endotoxin play a pathogenic role in septic shock, disseminated intravascular coagulation (DIC), and adult respiratory distress syndrome, mainly through induction of excessive levels of cytokines such as TNF, IL-1, and IL-12. LPS binds to the cell-surface receptor CD14, and the complex then binds to Toll-like receptor 4 (TLR4), a pattern recognition receptor that activates cells of the innate immune system.

***Exotoxins* are secreted bacterial proteins that cause cellular injury and disease.** They can be classified into broad categories by their site or mechanism of action. These are briefly described next and discussed in more detail in the specific sections about each type of bacteria.

- *Enzymes.* Bacteria secrete a variety of enzymes (proteases, hyaluronidases, coagulases, fibrinolysins) that act on their respective substrates in vitro, but the role of only a few of these in disease is understood. For example, exfoliative toxins produced by *S. aureus* cause staphylococcal scalded skin syndrome by degrading proteins that hold keratinocytes together, causing the epidermis to detach from the deeper skin.
- *Toxins that alter intracellular signaling or regulatory pathways.* Most of these toxins have an active (A) subunit with enzymatic activity and a binding (B) subunit that binds to receptors on the cell surface and delivers the A subunit into the cell cytoplasm. The effects of these toxins are diverse and depend on the binding specificity of the B domain and the cellular pathways affected by the A domain. A-B toxins are made by many bacteria including *Bacillus anthracis, V. cholerae*, and some strains of *E. coli*.
- *Neurotoxins* produced by *Clostridium botulinum* and *Clostridium tetani* inhibit release of neurotransmitters, resulting in paralysis. These toxins do not kill neurons; instead, the A domains interact specifically with proteins involved in secretion of neurotransmitters at the synaptic junction. Both tetanus and botulism can result in death from respiratory failure due to paralysis of the chest and diaphragm muscles.
- *Superantigens* are bacterial toxins that stimulate very large number of T lymphocytes by binding to conserved portions of the T-cell receptor, leading to massive T-lymphocyte proliferation and cytokine release. The high levels of cytokines can lead to capillary leak and shock. Superantigens made by *S. aureus* and *S. pyogenes* cause toxic shock syndrome (TSS).

KEY CONCEPTS

How Microorganisms Cause Disease

- Diseases caused by microbes involve interplay between microbial virulence factors and host responses.
- Infectious agents cause death or dysfunction by directly interacting with the cell.

- Injury may be due to local or systemic release of microbial products including endotoxin (LPS), exotoxins or superantigens.
- Pathogens can induce immune responses that cause tissue damage. Absence of an immune response may reduce damage induced by some infections; conversely, immune compromise can allow uncontrolled expansion of opportunistic agents or of microorganisms that can directly cause injury.

Sexually Transmitted Infections

A variety of organisms can be transmitted through sexual contact (Table 8-3). Groups at greater risk for sexually transmitted infections (STIs) include adolescents, men who have sex with men, and people who use illegal drugs parenterally. While the increased risk among these groups is partially due to unsafe sexual practices, limited access to health care is often a contributing factor. The presence of an STI in children, unless acquired during birth, strongly suggests sexual abuse.

Some pathogens, such as *C. trachomatis* and *N. gonorrhoeae,* are almost always spread by sexual intercourse, whereas others, such as *Shigella* species and *E. histolytica,* are typically spread by other means, but are also occasionally spread by oral-anal sex. To reduce the spread of STIs, it is expected that these infections be reported to public health authorities so that people who have had intimate contact with the person may be tested and treated.

Although the various pathogens that cause STIs differ in many ways, some general features should be noted.

- *STIs may become established and spread from the urethra, vagina, cervix, rectum, or oral pharynx.* Organisms that cause STIs depend on direct contact for person-to-person spread because these pathogens do not survive in the environment. Transmission of STIs often occurs from asymptomatic people who do not realize that they have an infection.
- *Infection with one STI-associated organism increases the risk for additional STIs.* This is mainly because the risk factors are the same for all STIs. In addition, the epithelial injury caused by *N. gonorrhoeae* or *C. trachomatis* can increase the chance of co-infection with the other, as well as the risk of HIV infection if there is concomitant exposure.
- *The microbes that cause STIs can be spread from a pregnant woman to the fetus and cause severe damage to the fetus or child.* Perinatally acquired *C. trachomatis* causes conjunctivitis, and neonatal HSV infection is much more likely to cause visceral and CNS disease than is infection acquired later in life. Syphilis frequently causes miscarriage. HIV infection may be fatal to children infected with the virus prenatally or perinatally. Diagnosis of STIs in pregnant women is critical, because intrauterine or neonatal transmission of STIs can often be prevented by treatment of the mother or newborn. Antiretroviral treatment of pregnant women with HIV infection and their newborn infants can reduce the transmission of HIV to offspring from 25% to less than 2%.

Syphilis is discussed later in this chapter, and other STIs are described in Chapters 21 and 22.

Spectrum of Inflammatory Responses to Infection

In contrast to the vast molecular diversity of microbes, the morphologic patterns of tissue responses to microbes are limited, as are the mechanisms directing these responses.

Table 8-3 Classification of Important Sexually Transmitted Diseases

Pathogens	Disease or Syndrome and Population Principally Affected		
	Males	Females	Both
Viruses			
Herpes simplex virus			Primary and recurrent herpes, neonatal herpes
Hepatitis B virus			Hepatitis
Human papillomavirus	Cancer of penis (some cases)	Cervical dysplasia and cancer, vulvar cancer	Condyloma acuminatum
Human immunodeficiency virus			Acquired immunodeficiency syndrome
Chlamydiae			
Chlamydia trachomatis	Urethritis, epididymitis, proctitis	Urethral syndrome, cervicitis, bartholinitis, salpingitis and sequelae	Lymphogranuloma venereum
Mycoplasmas			
Ureaplasma urealyticum	Urethritis		
Bacteria			
Neisseria gonorrhoeae	Epididymitis, prostatitis, urethral stricture	Cervicitis, endometritis, bartholinitis, salpingitis, and sequelae (infertility, ectopic pregnancy, recurrent salpingitis)	Urethritis, proctitis, pharyngitis, disseminated gonococcal infection
Treponema pallidum			Syphilis
Haemophilus ducreyi			Chancroid
Klebsiella granulomatis			Granuloma inguinale (donovanosis)
Protozoa			
Trichomonas vaginalis	Urethritis, balanitis	Vaginitis	

Table 8-4 Spectrum of Inflammatory Responses to Infection

Type of Response	Pathogenesis	Examples
Suppurative (Purulent) Infection	Increased vascular permeability Leukocyte infiltration (neutrophils) Chemoattractants from bacteria Formation of "pus"	Staphylococcal pneumonia Tissue abscesses
Mononuclear and granulomatous inflammation	Mononuclear cell infiltrates (monocytes, macrophages, plasma cells, lymphocytes) Cell-mediated immune response to pathogens ("persistent antigen") Formation of granulomata	Syphilis Tuberculosis
Cytopathic-cytoproliferative reactions	Viral transformation of cells Necrosis or proliferation (including multinucleation) Linked to neoplasia	Human Papilloma Virus Herpesvirus
Tissue necrosis	Toxin or lysis mediated destruction Lack of inflammatory cells Rapidly progressive processes	*Clostridium perfringens* Hepatitis B
Chronic inflammation/ scarring	Repetitive injury leads to fibrosis Loss of normal parenchyma	Chronic hepatitis (cirrhosis)
No reaction	Severe immune compromise	*Mycobacterium avium* in untreated AIDS (T-cell deficiency) Mucormycosis in bone marrow transplant patients (neutropenia)

Therefore, many pathogens produce similar reaction patterns, and few features are unique or pathognomonic for a particular microorganism. Moreover, sometimes the nature of the interaction between the microorganism and the host determines the histologic features of the inflammatory response. Thus, pyogenic bacteria, which normally evoke vigorous leukocyte responses, may cause rapid tissue necrosis with little leukocyte exudation in a profoundly neutropenic host. Similarly, in a normal patient, *M. tuberculosis* causes well-formed granulomas with few mycobacteria present, whereas in an AIDS patient the same mycobacteria multiply profusely in macrophages, which fail to coalesce into granulomas, which are summarized in Table 8-4 and described below.

There are five major histologic patterns of tissue reaction in infections.

Suppurative (Purulent) Inflammation

This pattern is characterized by increased vascular permeability and leukocytic infiltration, predominantly of neutrophils (Fig. 8-4). The neutrophils are attracted to the site of infection by release of chemoattractants from the "pyogenic" (pus-forming) bacteria that evoke this response, mostly extracellular gram-positive cocci and gram-negative rods. Masses of dying and dead neutrophils and liquefactive necrosis of the tissue form pus. The sizes of purulent lesions range from tiny microabscesses formed in multiple organs during bacterial sepsis secondary to a colonized heart valve, to diffuse involvement of entire lobes of the lung in pneumonia. How destructive the lesions are depends on their location and the organism involved. For example, pneumococci usually spare alveolar walls and cause lobar pneumonia that resolves completely, whereas staphylococci and *Klebsiella* species destroy alveolar walls and form abscesses that heal with scar formation. Bacterial pharyngitis resolves without sequelae, whereas untreated acute bacterial inflammation of a joint can destroy the joint in a few days.

Mononuclear and Granulomatous Inflammation

Diffuse, predominantly mononuclear, interstitial infiltrates are a common feature of all chronic inflammatory processes, but when they develop acutely, they often are a response to viruses, intracellular bacteria, or intracellular parasites. In addition, spirochetes and helminths provoke chronic inflammatory responses. Which mononuclear cell predominates within the inflammatory lesion depends on the host immune response to the organism. For example, plasma cells are abundant in the primary and secondary lesions of syphilis (Fig. 8-5), whereas lymphocytes predominate in HBV infection or viral infections of the brain. The presence of these lymphocytes reflects cell-mediated immune responses against the pathogen or pathogen-infected cells. At the other extreme, macrophages may become filled with organisms, as occurs in *M. avium-intracellulare* infections in AIDS patients, who cannot mount an effective immune response to the organisms. *Granulomatous inflammation* is a distinctive form of

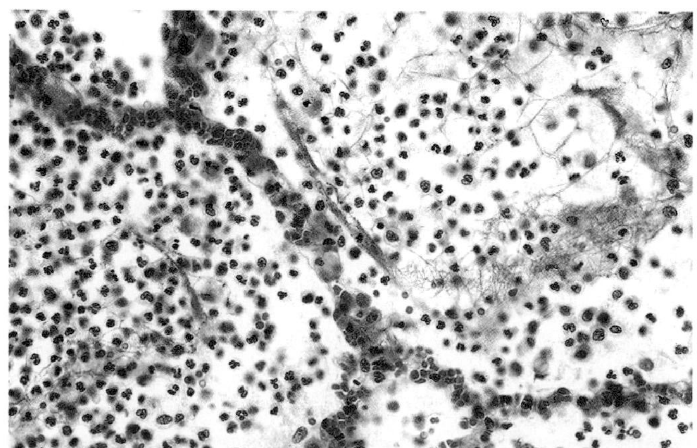

Figure 8-4 Suppurative (purulent) infection. Pneumococcal pneumonia with extensive neutrophilic infiltrate.

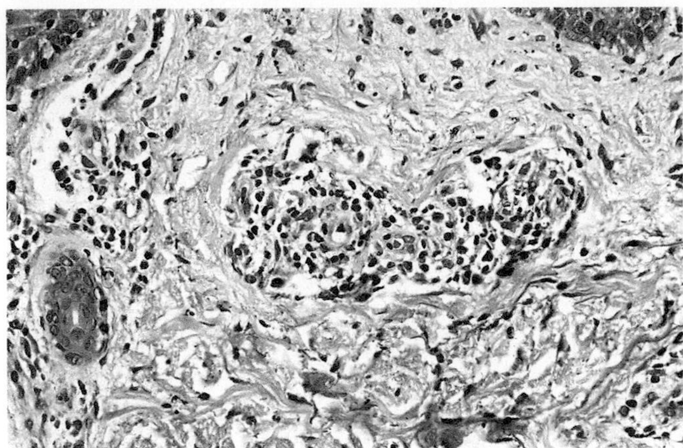

Figure 8-5 Secondary syphilis in the dermis with perivascular lymphoplasmacytic infiltrate and endothelial proliferation.

mononuclear inflammation usually evoked by infectious agents that resist eradication and are capable of stimulating strong T cell–mediated immunity (e.g., *M. tuberculosis, Histoplasma capsulatum,* schistosome eggs). Granulomatous inflammation is characterized by accumulation and aggregation of activated macrophages called "epithelioid" cells, some of which may fuse to form giant cells. Granulomas may contain a central area of caseous necrosis (see Chapter 3 and "Tuberculosis" in this chapter).

Cytopathic-Cytoproliferative Reaction

These reactions are usually produced by viruses. The lesions are characterized by cell necrosis or cellular proliferation, usually with sparse inflammatory cells. Some viruses replicate within cells and make viral aggregates that are visible as inclusion bodies (e.g., herpesviruses or adenovirus) or induce cells to fuse and form multinucleated cells called polykaryons (e.g., measles virus or herpesviruses). Focal cell damage in the skin may cause epithelial cells to become detached, forming blisters (Fig. 8-6). Some viruses can cause epithelial cells to proliferate (e.g., venereal warts caused by HPV or the umbilicated papules of molluscum contagiosum caused by poxviruses). Finally, viruses can contribute to the development of malignant neoplasms (Chapter 7).

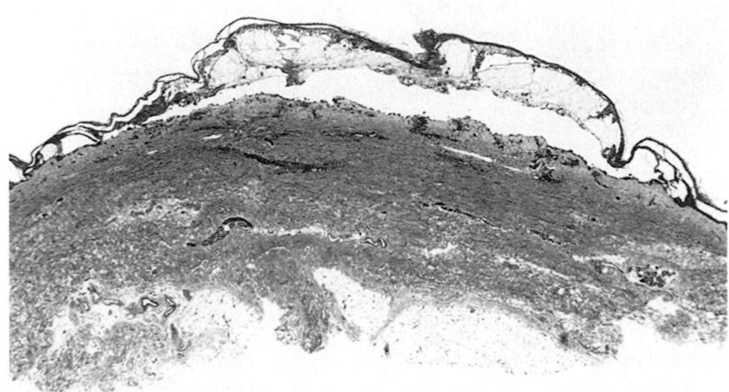

Figure 8-6 Herpesvirus blister in mucosa. See Figure 8-9 for viral inclusions.

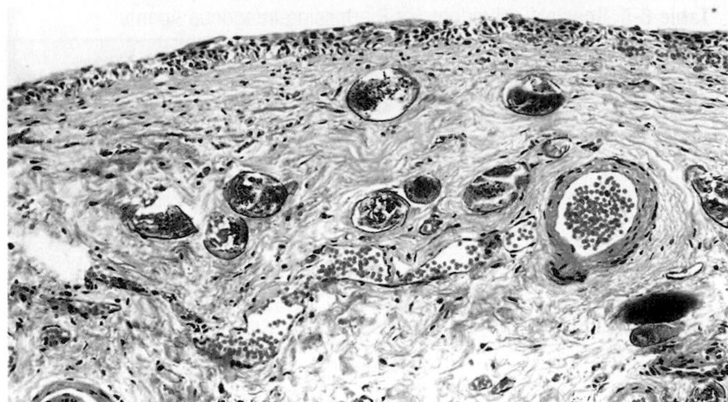

Figure 8-7 *Schistosoma haematobium* infection of the bladder with numerous calcified eggs and extensive scarring.

Tissue Necrosis

Clostridium perfringens and other organisms such as *C. diphtheriae* that secrete powerful toxins cause such rapid and severe necrosis (gangrenous necrosis) that tissue damage is the dominant feature. The parasite *E. histolytica* causes colonic ulcers and liver abscesses characterized by extensive tissue destruction with liquefactive necrosis and little inflammatory infiltrate. Some viruses can cause widespread and severe necrosis of host cells associated with inflammation, as exemplified by total destruction of the temporal lobes of the brain by herpesvirus or the liver by HBV.

Chronic Inflammation and Scarring

Many infections elicit chronic inflammation, which can lead either to complete healing or to extensive scarring. For example, chronic HBV infection may cause cirrhosis of the liver, in which dense fibrous septae surround nodules of regenerating hepatocytes with complete loss of normal liver architecture and consequent changes in blood flow.. Sometimes the exuberant scarring response is the major cause of dysfunction (e.g., the "pipestem" fibrosis of the liver or fibrosis of the bladder wall caused by schistosomal eggs [Fig. 8-7] or the constrictive fibrous pericarditis in tuberculosis).

These patterns of tissue reaction are useful guidelines for analyzing microscopic features of infectious processes, but they rarely appear in pure form because different types of host reactions often occur at the same time. For example, the lung of an AIDS patient may be infected with CMV, which causes cytolytic changes, and at the same time by *Pneumocystis,* which causes interstitial inflammation. Similar patterns of inflammation also can be seen in tissue responses to physical or chemical agents and in inflammatory diseases of unknown cause (Chapter 3).

Special Techniques for Diagnosing Infectious Agents

The gold standards for diagnosis of infections are culture, biochemical or serologic identification, and, in some cases, molecular diagnosis, depending on the organism in question. Some infectious agents or their products can be directly observed in hematoxylin and eosin–stained

Table 8-5 Special Techniques for Diagnosing Infectious Agents

Techniques	Infectious Agents
Gram stain	Most bacteria
Acid-fast stain	Mycobacteria, nocardiae (modified)
Silver stains	Fungi, legionellae, *Pneumocystis*
Periodic acid-Schiff	Fungi, amebae
Mucicarmine	Cryptococci
Giemsa	*Campylobacter*, leishmaniae, malaria parasites
Antibody stains	All classes
Culture	All classes
DNA probes	All classes

sections (e.g., the inclusion bodies formed by CMV and herpes simplex virus [HSV]; bacterial clumps, which usually stain blue; *Candida* and *Mucor* among the fungi; most protozoans; and all helminths). Many infectious agents, however, are best visualized by special stains that identify organisms on the basis of particular characteristics of their cell wall or coat—Gram, acid-fast, silver, mucicarmine, and Giemsa stains—or by staining with specific antibodies (Table 8-5). Regardless of the staining technique, organisms are typically easiest to identify at the advancing edge of a lesion rather than at its center, particularly if there is necrosis. Acute infections can be diagnosed serologically by detecting pathogen-specific antibodies in the serum. The presence of specific IgM antibody shortly after the onset of symptoms is often diagnostic. Alternatively, specific antibody titers can be measured during the early, acute infection and again 4-6 weeks later during the convalescent period; a four-fold rise in titer is usually considered diagnostic.

Nucleic acid amplification tests, such as polymerase chain reaction (PCR) and transcription-mediated amplification, are increasingly being used for rapid identification of microbes. These molecular diagnostic assays have become routine for diagnosis of gonorrhea, chlamydial infection, tuberculosis, and herpes encephalitis. In some cases, molecular assays are much more sensitive than conventional testing. PCR testing of cerebrospinal fluid (CSF) for HSV encephalitis has a sensitivity of about 80%, while viral culture of CSF has a sensitivity of less than 10%. Similarly, nucleic acid testing for genital *Chlamydia* detects 10% to 30% more infections than does conventional *Chlamydia* culture. In other cases, such as gonorrhea, the sensitivity of nucleic acid testing is similar to that of culture. In people infected with HIV, quantification of HIV RNA is an important guide to management of antiretroviral therapy. The management of HBV and HCV infections is similarly guided by nucleic acid–based viral quantification or typing to predict resistance to antiviral drugs. Mass spectroscopy is another technique that identifies specific components of an infectious agent by size and charge distribution and can allow for the rapid identification of cultured bacteria.

This concludes our discussion of the general principles of the pathogenesis and pathology of infectious disease. We now turn to specific infections caused by viruses, bacteria, fungi, and parasites, and focuses on their *pathogenic mechanisms* and *pathologic changes* rather than details of clinical features, which are available in clinical textbooks. Infections that typically involve a specific organ are discussed in other chapters.

Viral Infections

Viruses are the cause of many clinically important acute and chronic infections, which may affect virtually every organ system (Table 8-6).

Acute (Transient) Infections

The viruses that cause transient infections are structurally heterogeneous, but all elicit effective immune responses that eliminate the pathogens, limiting the durations of the infections. However, specific viruses exhibit widely differing degrees of genetic diversity, a variable that has an important impact on the susceptibility of the host to re-infection by viruses of the same type. The mumps virus, for example, has only one genetic subtype and infects people only once, whereas other viruses, such as influenza viruses, can repeatedly infect the same individual because

Table 8-6 Selected Human Viruses and Viral Diseases

Organ System	Species	Disease
Respiratory	Adenovirus	Upper and lower respiratory tract infections, conjunctivitis, diarrhea
	Rhinovirus	Upper respiratory tract infection
	Influenza viruses A, B	Influenza
	Respiratory syncytial virus	Bronchiolitis, pneumonia
Digestive	Mumps virus	Mumps, pancreatitis, orchitis
	Rotavirus	Childhood gastroenteritis
	Norovirus	Gastroenteritis
	Hepatitis A virus	Acute viral hepatitis
	Hepatitis B virus	Acute or chronic hepatitis
	Hepatitis D virus	With HBV, acute or chronic hepatitis
	Hepatitis C virus	Acute or chronic hepatitis
	Hepatitis E virus	Enterically transmitted hepatitis
Systemic with skin eruptions	Measles virus	Measles (rubeola)
	Rubella virus	German measles (rubella)
	Varicella-zoster virus	Chickenpox, shingles
	Herpes simplex virus 1	Oral herpes ("cold sore")
	Herpes simplex virus 2	Genital herpes
Systemic with hematopoietic disorders	Cytomegalovirus	Cytomegalic inclusion disease
	Epstein-Barr virus	Infectious mononucleosis
	HIV-1 and HIV-2	AIDS
Arboviral and hemorrhagic fevers	Dengue virus 1-4	Dengue hemorrhagic fever
	Yellow fever virus	Yellow fever
Skin/genital warts	Papillomavirus	Condyloma; cervical carcinoma
Central nervous system	Poliovirus	Poliomyelitis
	JC virus	Progressive multifocal leukoencephalopathy (opportunistic)

new genetic variants arise periodically in nature. Immunity to some viruses wanes with time, and this too may allow the same virus to infect the host repeatedly (e.g., respiratory syncytial virus).

Measles

Measles is an acute viral infection that affects multiple organs and causes a wide range of disease, from mild, self-limited infections to severe systemic manifestations. Measles (rubeola) virus is a leading cause of vaccine-preventable death and illness worldwide. More than 20 million people acquire measles each year. In 2010, measles accounted for an estimated 139,000 deaths globally, the majority in children in developing countries. Because of poor nutrition and lack of access to medical care, children in developing countries are 10 to 1000 times more likely to die of measles than are children in developed countries. Measles can produce severe disease in people with defects in cellular immunity (e.g., people infected with HIV or people with a hematologic malignancy). Epidemics of measles occur among unvaccinated individuals. In the United States, the incidence of measles has decreased dramatically since 1963, when a measles vaccine was licensed, and endemic transmission was eliminated in 2000. The diagnosis may be made clinically, by serology, or by detection of viral antigen in nasal exudates or urinary sediments.

Pathogenesis. Measles virus is a single-stranded RNA virus of the paramyxovirus family, which includes mumps, respiratory syncytial virus, parainfluenza virus (a cause of croup), and human metapneumovirus. There is only one serotype of measles virus. Measles virus is transmitted by respiratory droplets. Three cell-surface receptors have been identified for the virus: CD46 (a complement-regulatory protein that inactivates C3 convertases), signaling lymphocytic activation molecule (SLAM, a molecule involved in T-cell activation), and nectin 4 (adherens junction protein). CD46 is expressed on all nucleated cells, while SLAM is expressed on cells of the immune system, and nectin 4 is expressed on epithelial cells. All of these receptors bind the viral hemagglutinin protein.

Measles can replicate in a variety of cell types, including epithelial cells and leukocytes. The virus initially multiplies within the respiratory tract and then spreads to local lymphoid tissues. Replication of the virus in lymphatic tissue is followed by viremia and systemic dissemination to many tissues, including the conjunctiva, skin, respiratory tract, urinary tract, small blood vessels, lymphatic system, and CNS. Most children develop T-cell–mediated immunity to measles virus that helps control the viral infection and produces the measles rash. Hence, the rash is less frequent in people with deficiencies in cell-mediated immunity. In addition, in malnourished children with poor medical care, measles virus may cause croup, pneumonia, diarrhea and protein-losing enteropathy, keratitis leading to scarring and blindness, encephalitis, and hemorrhagic rashes ("black measles").

Antibody-mediated immunity to measles virus protects against reinfection. Measles also can cause transient but profound immunosuppression, resulting in secondary bacterial and viral infections, which are responsible for much of measles-related morbidity and mortality. Alterations of both innate and adaptive immune responses occur following measles infection, including defects in dendritic cell and lymphocyte function. Subacute sclerosing panencephalitis (Chapter 28) and measles inclusion body encephalitis (in immunocompromised individuals) are rare late complications of measles. The pathogenesis of subacute sclerosing panencephalitis is not well understood, but a replication-defective variant of measles may be involved in this persistent viral infection.

MORPHOLOGY

The blotchy, reddish brown rash of measles virus infection on the face, trunk, and proximal extremities is produced by dilated skin vessels, edema, and a mononuclear perivascular infiltrate. Ulcerated mucosal lesions in the oral cavity near the opening of the Stensen ducts (the pathognomonic **Koplik spots**) are marked by necrosis, neutrophilic exudate, and neovascularization. The lymphoid organs typically have marked follicular hyperplasia, large germinal centers, and randomly distributed multinucleate giant cells, called **Warthin-Finkeldey cells**, which have eosinophilic nuclear and cytoplasmic inclusion bodies. These are pathognomonic of measles and are also found in the lung and sputum (Fig. 8-8). The milder forms of measles pneumonia show the same peribronchial and interstitial mononuclear cell infiltration that is seen in other nonlethal viral infections.

Mumps

Mumps is an acute systemic viral infection usually associated with pain and swelling of the salivary glands. Like measles virus, mumps virus is a member of the paramyxovirus family. Mumps virus has two types of surface glycoproteins, one with hemagglutinin and neuraminidase activities and the other with cell fusion and cytolytic activities. Mumps viruses enter the upper respiratory tract through inhalation of respiratory droplets, spread to draining lymph nodes where they replicate in lymphocytes (preferentially in activated T cells), and then spread through the blood to the salivary and other glands. Mumps virus infects salivary gland ductal epithelial cells, resulting in desquamation of involved cells, edema, and inflammation that leads to the classic salivary gland pain and swelling.

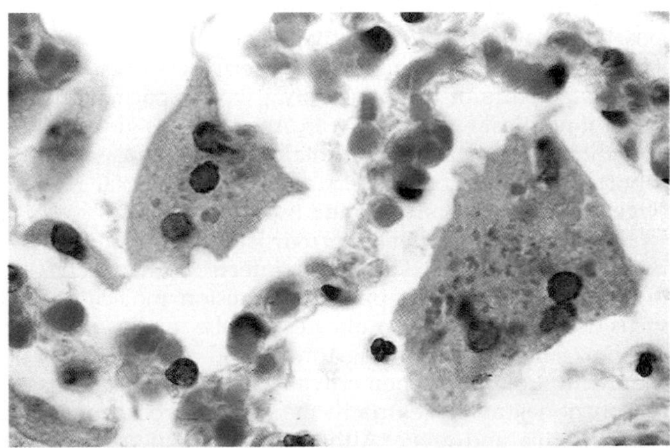

Figure 8-8 Measles giant cells in the lung. Note the glassy eosinophilic intranuclear inclusions.

Mumps virus also can spread to other sites, including the CNS, testis, ovary, and pancreas. Aseptic meningitis is the most common extrasalivary gland complication of mumps infection, occurring in up to 15% of cases. The mumps vaccine has reduced the incidence of mumps by 99% in the United States. The diagnosis is usually made clinically, but serology, viral culture, or PCR assays can be used for definitive diagnosis.

MORPHOLOGY

Mumps parotitis is bilateral in 70% of cases. The affected glands are enlarged, have a doughy consistency, and are moist, glistening, and reddish-brown on cross-section. On microscopic examination the gland interstitium is edematous and diffusely infiltrated by macrophages, lymphocytes, and plasma cells, which compress acini and ducts. Neutrophils and necrotic debris may fill the duct lumen and cause focal damage to the lining epithelium.

In **mumps orchitis** testicular swelling may be marked, caused by edema, mononuclear cell infiltration, and focal hemorrhages. Because the testis is tightly contained within the tunica albuginea, parenchymal swelling may compromise the blood supply and cause areas of infarction. The testicular damage can lead to scarring, atrophy, and, if severe, sterility.

Infection and damage of acinar cells in the **pancreas** may release digestive enyzmes, causing parenchymal and fat necrosis and neutrophil-rich inflammation. **Mumps encephalitis** causes perivenous demyelination and perivascular mononuclear cuffing.

Poliovirus Infection

Poliovirus causes an acute systemic viral infection, leading to a wide range of manifestations, from mild, self-limited infections to paralysis of limb muscles and respiratory muscles. Poliovirus is a spherical, unencapsulated RNA virus of the enterovirus genus. Other enteroviruses cause childhood diarrhea as well as rashes (coxsackievirus A), conjunctivitis (enterovirus 70), viral meningitis (coxsackieviruses and echovirus), and myopericarditis (coxsackievirus B). There are three serotypes of poliovirus, each of which is included in the Salk formalin-fixed (killed) vaccine and the Sabin oral, attenuated (live) vaccine. These vaccines have nearly eradicated polio, because the poliovirus infects only humans, shows limited genetic variation, and is effectively neutralized by antibodies generated by immunization. Nevertheless, this scourge persists in parts of the developing world, particularly in areas of political unrest and war. According to global polio surveillance data, in 2013, a total of 328 polio cases were reported from Afghanistan, Cameroon, Ethiopia, Kenya, Nigeria, Pakistan, Somalia, and Syria.

Poliovirus, like other enteroviruses, is transmitted by the fecal-oral route. The virus infects human cells by binding to CD155, an epithelial adhesion molecule. The virus is ingested and replicates in the mucosa of the pharynx and gut, including tonsils and Peyer patches in the ileum. Poliovirus then spreads through lymphatics to lymph nodes and eventually the blood, producing transient viremia and fever. Although most poliovirus infections are asymptomatic, in about 1 of 100 infected persons poliovirus invades the CNS and replicates in motor neurons of the spinal cord (spinal poliomyelitis) or brain stem (bulbar poliomyelitis). Antiviral antibodies control the disease in most cases; it is not known why they fail to contain the virus in some individuals. Viral spread to the nervous system may be through the blood or by retrograde transport of the virus along axons of motor neurons. Rare cases of poliomyelitis that occur after vaccination are caused by mutations of the attenuated viruses to wild-type forms. The diagnosis can be made by viral culture or PCR of throat secretions or stool, or by serology. The neurologic features and neuropathology of poliovirus infection are described in Chapter 28.

West Nile Virus

West Nile Virus is an acute systemic viral infection that causes a mild, self-limited infection or neuroinvasive disease associated with long-term neurologic sequelae. West Nile virus is an arthropod-borne virus (arbovirus) of the flavivirus group, which also includes viruses that cause dengue fever and yellow fever. West Nile virus has a broad geographic distribution in the Old World, including Africa, the Middle East, Europe, Southeast Asia, and Australia. It was first detected in the United States in 1999 during an outbreak in New York City, and has since spread across the United States; in the year 2013, a least one case was reported in 44 states. West Nile virus is transmitted by mosquitoes to birds and to mammals. Infected birds develop prolonged viremia and are the major reservoir for the virus. Humans are incidental hosts. Most affected patients acquire the infection from a mosquito bite; less commonly, human-to-human transmission occurs by blood transfusion, organ transplantation, breast-feeding, or transplacental spread.

After inoculation by a mosquito, West Nile virus replicates in skin dendritic cells, which then migrate to lymph nodes. Here, the virus replicates further, enters the bloodstream, and, in some individuals, crosses the blood-brain barrier. In the CNS, the virus infects neurons. Chemokines have critical roles in recruiting leukocytes to the CNS, where they assist in viral clearance. The chemokine receptor CCR5 contributes to resistance to neuroinvasive infection, hence mutations in both copies of the CCR5 gene that lead to loss of function are associated with an increased rate of symptomatic infection. Recall that in HIV infection the role of this receptor is the opposite—CCR5 loss-of-function is protective because HIV uses the receptor to infect host T cells (Chapter 6).

West Nile virus infection is usually asymptomatic, but in 20% of infected individuals it gives rise to a fever, headache, myalgia, fatigue, anorexia, and nausea. A maculopapular rash is seen in approximately half the cases. CNS complications (meningitis, encephalitis, meningoencephalitis) occur in about 1 in 150 clinically apparent infections. Meningoencephalitis has a mortality of about 10% and results in long-term cognitive and neurologic impairment in many survivors. Perivascular and leptomeningeal chronic inflammation, microglial nodules (Chapter 28), and neuronophagia predominantly involving the temporal lobes and brain stem have been observed in patients who died of West Nile virus infection. Immunosuppressed persons and older adults appear to be at the greatest risk for severe disease. Rare complications include hepatitis, myocarditis, and pancreatitis. The diagnosis is usually made by serology, but viral culture and PCR-based tests are also used.

Viral Hemorrhagic Fever

Viral hemorrhagic fever (VHF) is a severe life-threatening multisystem syndrome in which there is vascular dysregulation and damage, leading to shock. VHF is caused by enveloped RNA viruses belonging to four different genera: Arenaviridae, Filoviridae, Bunyaviridae, and Flaviviridae. These viruses can produce a spectrum of illnesses, ranging from a mild acute disease characterized by fever, headache, myalgia, rash, neutropenia, and thrombocytopenia to severe, life-threatening disease in which there is sudden hemodynamic deterioration and shock. All these viruses pass through an animal or insect host during their life cycles and therefore their ranges are restricted to areas in which their hosts reside. Humans are incidental hosts who are infected when they come into contact with infected hosts (typically rodents) or insect vectors (mosquitoes and ticks). Some viruses that cause hemorrhagic fever (Ebola, Marburg, Lassa) also can spread from person to person.

The pathogenesis of the infection and its complications vary among the different viruses but there are some common features. Damage to blood vessels is often prominent. It may be caused by direct infection of and damage to endothelial cells, or infection of macrophages and dendritic cells leading to production of inflammatory cytokines. There may be hemorrhagic manifestations, including petechiae, caused by a combination of thrombocytopenia or platelet dysfunction, endothelial injury, cytokine-induced disseminated intravascular coagulation, and deficiency of clotting factors because of hepatic injury. Hemorrhages may be prominent in some infections (e.g. Congo-Crimean fever) but are rarely life-threatening. Necrosis of tissues secondary to the vascular lesions and hemorrhages may be seen and varies from mild and focal to massive, but the attendant inflammatory response is usually minimal.

Latent Infections (Herpesvirus Infections)

Latency is defined as the persistence of viral genomes in cells that do not produce infectious virus. Dissemination of the infection and tissue injury stem from reactivation of the latent virus. The viruses that most frequently establish latent infections in humans are *herpesviruses*. These are large encapsulated viruses with double-stranded DNA genomes that encode approximately 70 proteins. Herpesviruses cause acute infection followed by latent infection in which the viruses persist in a noninfectious form with periodic reactivation and shedding of infectious virus.

There are eight types of human herpesviruses, belonging to three subgroups that are defined by the type of cell most frequently infected and the site of latency: α-group viruses, including HSV-1, HSV-2, and VZV, which infect epithelial cells and produce latent infection in neurons; lymphotropic β-group viruses, including CMV, human herpesvirus-6 (which causes exanthem subitum, also known as roseola infantum and sixth disease, a benign rash of infants), and human herpesvirus-7 (a virus without a known disease association), which infect and produce latent infection in a variety of cell types; and the γ-group viruses EBV and KSHV/HHV-8, the cause of Kaposi sarcoma, which produce latent infection mainly in lymphoid cells. In addition, herpesvirus simiae (monkey B virus) is an Old World monkey virus that resembles HSV-1 and can cause fatal neurologic disease in animal handlers, usually resulting from an animal bite.

Herpes Simplex Viruses

HSV-1 and HSV-2 differ serologically but are closely related genetically and cause a similar set of primary and recurrent infections. Both viruses replicate in the skin and the mucous membranes at the site of entry of the virus (usually oropharynx or genitals), where they produce infectious virions and cause vesicular lesions of the epidermis. The viruses spread to sensory neurons that innervate these primary sites of replication. Viral nucleocapsids are transported along axons to the neuronal cell bodies, where the viruses establish latent infection. In immunocompetent hosts, primary HSV infection resolves in a few weeks, although the virus remains latent in nerve cells. During latency the viral DNA remains within the nucleus of the neuron, and only latency-associated viral RNA transcripts (LATs) are synthesized. No viral proteins appear to be produced during latency. LATs may contribute to latency by conferring resistance to apoptosis, silencing lytic gene expression through heterochromatin formation, and serving as precursors for microRNAs that downregulate expression of critical HSV lytic genes. Reactivation of HSV-1 and HSV-2 may occur repeatedly with or without symptoms, and results in the spread of virus from the neurons to the skin or to mucous membranes. Reactivation can occur in the presence of host immunity, because HSVs have developed ways to avoid immune recognition. For example, HSVs can evade antiviral CTLs by inhibiting the MHC class I recognition pathway, and elude humoral immune defenses by producing receptors for the Fc domain of immunoglobulin and inhibitors of complement.

In addition to causing cutaneous lesions, HSV-1 is the major infectious cause of corneal blindness in the United States. Corneal epithelial disease is thought to be due to direct viral damage, while corneal stromal disease appears to be immune-mediated. HSV-1 is also the major cause of fatal sporadic encephalitis in the United States. When the infection spreads to the brain, it usually involves the temporal lobes and orbital gyri of the frontal lobes. Inherited mutations in TLR3 or components of its signaling pathway increase the risk of HSV encephalitis. In addition, neonates and individuals with compromised cellular immunity (e.g., secondary to HIV infection or chemotherapy) may suffer disseminated herpesvirus infections. HSV-2 infection increases the risk of HIV transmission by four-fold and increases the risk of HIV acquisition by two- to three-fold.

MORPHOLOGY

HSV-infected cells contain large, pink to purple **intranuclear inclusions** (Cowdry type A) that consist of viral replication proteins and virions at various stage of assembly that push the host cell chromatin out to the edges of the nucleus (Fig. 8-9). Due to cell fusion, HSVs also produces inclusion-bearing multinucleated syncytia.

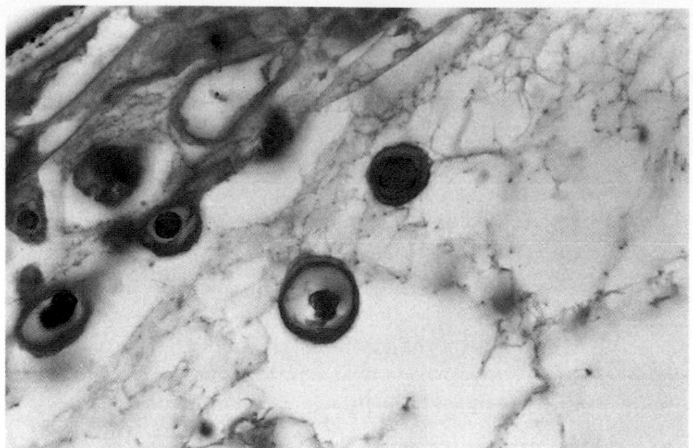

Figure 8-9 A herpesvirus blister showing glassy intranuclear viral inclusion bodies.

HSV-1 and HSV-2 cause lesions ranging from self-limited cold sores and gingivostomatitis to life-threatening disseminated visceral infections and encephalitis. **Fever blisters or cold sores** favor the facial skin around mucosal orifices (lips, nose), where their distribution is frequently bilateral and independent of skin dermatomes. Intraepithelial vesicles (blisters), which are formed by intracellular edema and ballooning degeneration of epidermal cells, frequently burst and crust over, but some may result in superficial ulcerations.

Gingivostomatitis, which is usually encountered in children, is caused by HSV-1. It is a vesicular eruption extending from the tongue to the retropharynx and causing cervical lymphadenopathy. Swollen, erythematous HSV lesions of the fingers or palm (herpetic whitlow) occur in infants and, occasionally, in health care workers.

Genital herpes is more often caused by HSV-2 than by HSV-1. It is characterized by vesicles on the genital mucous membranes as well as on the external genitalia that are rapidly converted into superficial ulcerations, rimmed by an inflammatory infiltrate (Chapter 22). Herpesvirus (usually HSV-2) can be transmitted to neonates during passage through the birth canal of infected mothers. Although HSV-2 infection in the neonate may be mild, more commonly it is fulminating with generalized lymphadenopathy, splenomegaly, and necrotic foci throughout the lungs, liver, adrenals, and CNS.

Two forms of **corneal lesions** are caused by HSV (Chapter 29). **Herpes epithelial keratitis** shows typical virus-induced cytolysis of the superficial epithelium. In contrast, **herpes stromal keratitis** is characterized by infiltrates of mononuclear cells around keratinocytes and endothelial cells, leading to neovascularization, scarring, opacification of the cornea, and eventual blindness. Here, the damage is caused by an immunologic reaction to the HSV infection, rather than the cytopathic effects of the virus itself.

Herpes simplex encephalitis is described in Chapter 28.

Disseminated skin and visceral herpes infections are usually encountered in hospitalized patients with some form of underlying cancer or immunosuppression. **Herpes esophagitis** is frequently complicated by superinfection with bacteria or fungi. **Herpes bronchopneumonia**, sometimes stemming from intubation of a patient with active oral lesions, is often necrotizing, and **herpes hepatitis** may cause liver failure.

Varicella-Zoster Virus (VZV)

Acute infection with VZV causes chickenpox and reactivation of latent VZV causes shingles (also called *herpes zoster*). Chickenpox is mild in children but more severe in adults and in immunocompromised people. Shingles is a source of morbidity in older and immunosuppressed persons. Like HSV, VZV infects mucous membranes, skin, and neurons and causes a self-limited primary infection in immunocompetent individuals. Also like HSV, VZV evades immune responses and establishes a latent infection in sensory ganglia. In contrast to HSV, VZV is transmitted in epidemic fashion by respiratory aerosols, disseminates hematogenously, and causes widespread vesicular skin lesions. Latent VZV infection is seen in neurons and/or satellite cells around neurons in the dorsal root ganglia. Reactivation and clinical recurrences causing shingles are uncommon but may occur many years after the primary infection. Localized recurrence of VZV is most frequent and painful in dermatomes innervated by the trigeminal ganglia, where the virus is most likely to be latent. VZV rarely recurs in immunocompetent individuals (in only 1-4% of infected individuals), but immunosuppressed or older persons can have multiple recurrences of VZV. For this reason, vaccination to prevent shingles is now recommended in all patients over age 60 years, and in younger adults with chronic disorders that may impair immunity. VZV infection is diagnosed by viral culture or detection of viral antigens in cells scraped from superficial lesions.

MORPHOLOGY

The **chickenpox** rash occurs approximately 2 weeks after respiratory infection. Lesions appear in multiple waves centrifugally from the torso to the head and extremities. Each lesion progresses rapidly from a macule to a vesicle, which resembles a dewdrop on a rose petal. On histologic examination, chickenpox lesions show intraepithelial vesicles (Fig. 8-10) with intranuclear inclusions in epithelial cells at the base of the vesicles. After a few days most chickenpox vesicles rupture, crust over, and heal by regeneration, leaving no scars. However, bacterial superinfection of vesicles that are ruptured by trauma may lead to destruction of the basal epidermal layer and residual scarring.

Shingles occurs when VZV that has long remained latent in the dorsal root ganglia after a previous chickenpox infection is reactivated and infects sensory nerves that carry it to one or

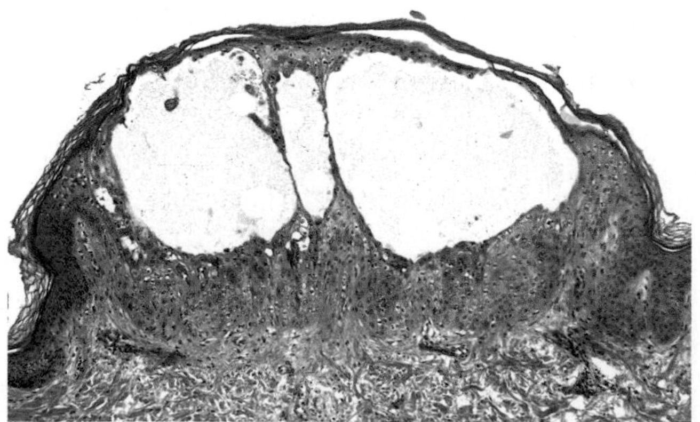

Figure 8-10 Skin lesion of chickenpox (varicella-zoster virus) with intraepithelial vesicle.

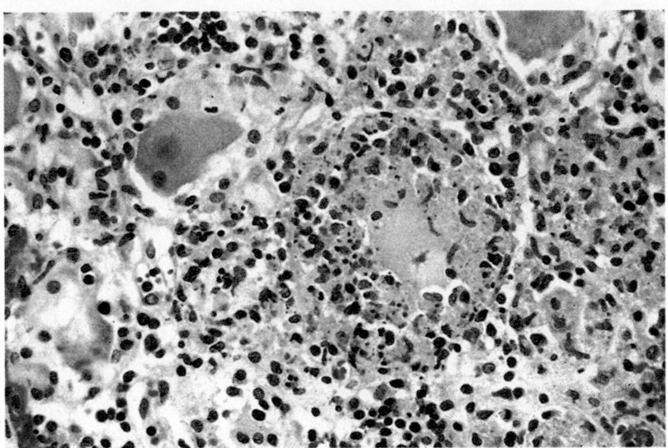

Figure 8-11 Dorsal root ganglion with varicella-zoster virus infection. Note the ganglion cell necrosis and associated inflammation. (Courtesy Dr. James Morris, Radcliffe Infirmary, Oxford, England.)

more dermatomes. There, the virus infects keratinocytes and causes vesicular lesions, which, unlike chickenpox, are often associated with intense itching, burning, or sharp pain because of concomitant radiculoneuritis. This pain is especially severe when the trigeminal nerves are involved; rarely, the geniculate nucleus is involved, causing facial paralysis (Ramsay Hunt syndrome). The sensory ganglia contain a dense, predominantly mononuclear infiltrate, with herpetic intranuclear inclusions within neurons and their supporting cells (Fig. 8-11). VZV can also cause interstitial pneumonia, encephalitis, transverse myelitis, and necrotizing visceral lesions, particularly in immunosuppressed people.

Cytomegalovirus

Cytomegalovirus (CMV), a β-group herpesvirus, can produce a variety of disease manifestations, depending on the age of the host, and, more importantly, on the host's immune status. CMV latently infects monocytes and their bone marrow progenitors and can be reactivated when cellular immunity is depressed. CMV causes an asymptomatic or mononucleosis-like infection in healthy individuals but devastating systemic infections in neonates and in immunocompromised people, in whom the virus may infect many different cell types and tissues. As its name implies, CMV-infected cells exhibit gigantism of both the entire cell and its nucleus, which typically contains a large inclusion surrounded by a clear halo ("owl's eye").

Transmission of CMV can occur by several mechanisms, depending on the age group affected. These include the following:

- *Transplacental transmission,* from a newly acquired or primary infection in a mother who does not have protective antibodies (congenital CMV).
- *Neonatal transmission,* through cervical or vaginal secretions at birth, or later through breast milk from a mother who has active infection (perinatal CMV).
- *Transmission through saliva* during preschool years, especially in day care centers. Toddlers so infected readily transmit the virus to their parents.
- *Transmission by the genital route* is the dominant mode after about 15 years of age. Spread may also occur via respiratory secretions and the fecal-oral route.
- *Iatrogenic transmission,* at any age through organ transplants or blood transfusions.

Acute CMV infection induces transient but severe immunosuppression. CMV can infect dendritic cells and impair antigen processing and the ability of dendritic cells to stimulate T lymphocytes. Similar to other herpesviruses, CMV can evade immune defenses by downmodulating MHC class I and II molecules and by producing homologues of TNF receptor, IL-10, and MHC class I molecules. Interestingly, CMV can evade NK cells by producing ligands that block activating receptors and class I–like proteins that engage inhibitory receptors. Thus, CMV both hides from and actively suppresses immune responses.

MORPHOLOGY

Infected cells are strikingly enlarged, often to a diameter of 40 μm, and show cellular and nuclear pleomorphism. Prominent **intranuclear basophilic inclusions** spanning half the nuclear diameter are usually set off from the nuclear membrane by a clear halo (Fig. 8-12). Within the cytoplasm of infected cells, smaller basophilic inclusions can also be seen. In the glandular organs, the parenchymal epithelial cells are infected; in the brain, the neurons; in the lungs, the alveolar macrophages and epithelial and endothelial cells; and in the kidneys, the tubular epithelial and glomerular endothelial cells. Disseminated CMV causes focal necrosis with minimal inflammation in virtually any organ.

Congenital Infections. Infection acquired in utero may take many forms. In approximately 95% of cases it is asymptomatic. However, sometimes when the virus is acquired from a mother with primary infection (who does not have protective antibodies), classic *cytomegalic inclusion disease* develops. Cytomegalic inclusion disease resembles erythroblastosis fetalis. Affected infants may suffer intrauterine growth retardation, and present with jaundice, hepatosplenomegaly, anemia, bleeding due to thrombocytopenia, and encephalitis. In fatal cases the brain is often smaller than normal (microcephaly) and may show foci of calcification. Diagnosis of neonatal CMV is made by viral culture or PCR amplification of viral DNA in urine or saliva.

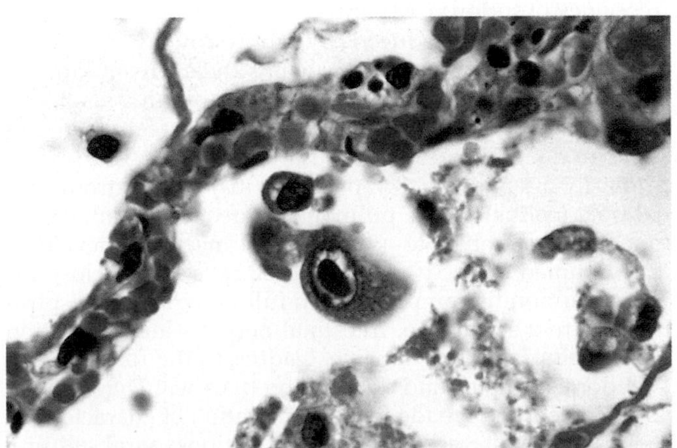

Figure 8-12 Cytomegalovirus: distinct nuclear and ill-defined cytoplasmic inclusions in the lung.

The infants who survive usually have permanent deficits, including intellectual disability, hearing loss, and other neurologic impairments. The congenital infection is not always devastating, however, and may take the form of interstitial pneumonitis, hepatitis, or a hematologic disorder. Most infants with this milder form of cytomegalic inclusion disease recover, although a few develop intellectual disability later. Uncommonly, a totally asymptomatic infection may be followed months to years later by neurologic sequelae, including delayed-onset intellectual disability and deafness.

Perinatal Infections. Infection acquired during passage through the birth canal or from breast milk is usually asymptomatic due to protective maternal anti-CMV antibodies, which are transmitted to the fetus across the placenta. Despite the lack of symptoms, many of these infants continue to excrete CMV in their urine or saliva for months to years. Subtle effects on hearing and intelligence later in life have been reported in some studies. Much less commonly, infected infants develop interstitial pneumonitis, failure to thrive, rash, or hepatitis.

Cytomegalovirus Mononucleosis. In healthy young children and adults the disease is nearly always asymptomatic. In surveys around the world, 50% to 100% of adults have antibodies to CMV, indicating previous exposure. **The most common clinical manifestation of CMV infection in immunocompetent hosts beyond the neonatal period is an infectious mononucleosis-like illness, with fever, atypical lymphocytosis, lymphadenopathy, and hepatitis, marked by hepatomegaly and abnormal liver function tests.** The diagnosis is made by serology. Most people recover without any sequelae, but the virus may continue to be excreted in body fluids for months to years. Irrespective of the presence or absence of symptoms, infected individuals remain seropositive for life and the virus is never cleared, persisting in latently infected leukocytes.

CMV in Immunosuppressed Individuals. **Immunocompromised individuals (e.g., transplant recipients, HIV-infected individuals) are susceptible to severe CMV infection;** these may be either primary infections or reactivation of latent CMV. In the past, CMV was the most common opportunistic viral pathogen in AIDS , but the frequency of serious CMV infection in HIV-positive people has been greatly reduced by antiretroviral treatment. Recipients of solid-organ transplants (heart, liver, kidney) also may contract CMV from the donor organ.

In all these settings, serious, even life-threatening, disseminated CMV infections in immunosuppressed people primarily affect the lungs (pneumonitis) and gastrointestinal tract (colitis). In the pulmonary infection an interstitial mononuclear infiltrate with foci of necrosis develops, accompanied by the typical enlarged cells with inclusions. The pneumonitis can progress to full-blown acute respiratory distress syndrome. Intestinal necrosis and ulceration can develop and be extensive, leading to the formation of pseudomembranes and debilitating diarrhea. Diagnosis of CMV infections is made by demonstration of characteristic morphologic alterations in tissue sections, viral culture, rising antiviral antibody titer, detection of CMV antigens, and PCR-based detection of CMV DNA. The antigen-detection and PCR-based assays have revolutionized the approach to monitoring CMV infection in people after transplantation.

Chronic Productive Infections

In some infections the immune system is unable to eliminate the virus, and continued viral replication leads to persistent viremia. The high mutation rate of viruses such as HIV and HBV may contribute to their escape from control by the immune system. HIV and HBV infection are described in Chapters 6 and 18, respectively.

Transforming Viral Infections

Some viruses can transform infected cells into benign or malignant tumor cells. Oncogenic viruses can stimulate cell growth and survival by a variety of mechanisms, as discussed in Chapter 7. Several viruses have been implicated in the causation of human cancer, including EBV, HPV, HBV, and HTLV-1. EBV is discussed here; others are discussed in later chapters.

Epstein-Barr Virus (EBV)

EBV causes infectious mononucleosis, a benign, self-limited lymphoproliferative disorder, and is associated with the pathogenesis of several human tumors, most commonly certain lymphomas and nasopharyngeal carcinoma. Infectious mononucleosis is discussed here and EBV-associated neoplasms are discussed in Chapter 7.

Infectious mononucleosis is characterized by fever, sore throat, generalized lymphadenopathy, splenomegaly, and the appearance in the blood of atypical activated T lymphocytes (mononucleosis cells). Some people develop hepatitis, meningoencephalitis, and pneumonitis. Infectious mononucleosis occurs principally in late adolescents or young adults among upper socioeconomic classes in developed nations. In the rest of the world, primary infection with EBV occurs in childhood and is usually asymptomatic.

Pathogenesis. EBV is transmitted by close human contact, frequently through the saliva during kissing. EBV infects B cells and possibly epithelial cells of the oropharynx. It has been hypothesized that EBV initially infects oropharyngeal epithelial cells and then spreads to underlying lymphoid tissue (tonsils and adenoids), where mature B cells are infected (Fig. 8-13). Of note, people with X-linked agammaglobulinemia, who lack B cells, do not become latently infected with EBV or shed virus, suggesting that B cells are the main reservoir of infection. An EBV envelope glycoprotein binds CD21 (CR2), the receptor for the C3d component of complement (Chapter 3), which is present on B cells. Infection of B cells may take one of two forms. In a minority of B cells, infection is lytic, leading to viral replication and eventual cell lysis accompanied by release of virions, which may infect other B cells. In most B cells, however, EBV establishes latent infection, during which the virus persists as an extrachromosomal episome.

A small number of EBV-encoded proteins are believed to be particularly important in the establishment of latency, as follows:

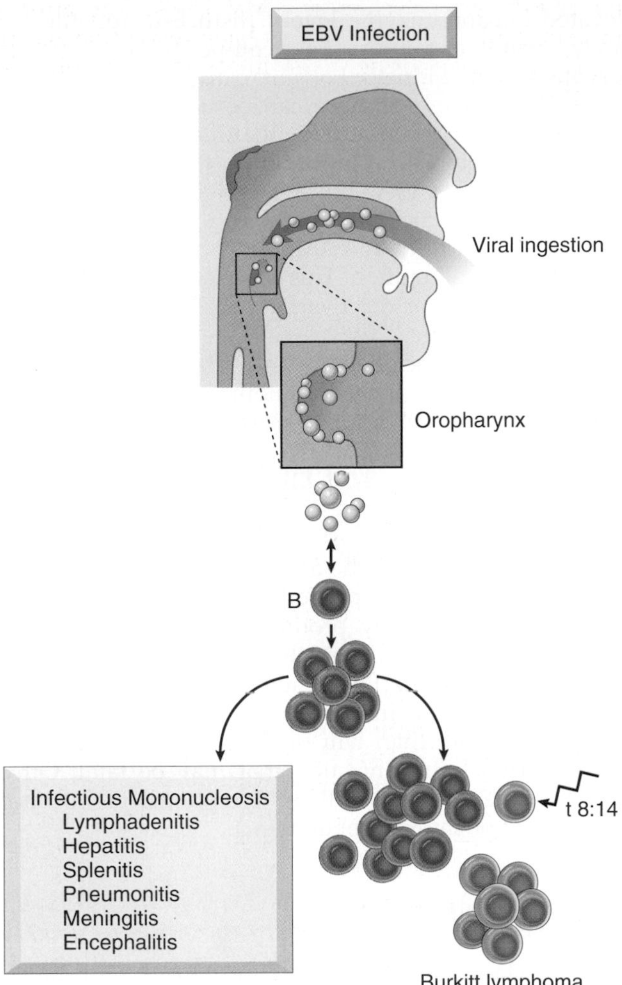

Figure 8-13 Outcomes of Epstein-Barr virus (EBV) infection. In an individual with normal immune function, infection is usually either asymptomatic or leads to mononucleosis. In the setting of cellular immunodeficiency, the proliferation of infected B cells may be uncontrolled, leading to the development of B-cell neoplasms. In other instances, persons without overt evidence of immunodeficiency develop EBV-positive tumors, which are usually (but not always) also derived from B cells. One secondary genetic event that collaborates with EBV to cause B-cell transformation is a balanced 8;14 chromosomal translocation, which is seen in Burkitt lymphoma. EBV is also implicated in the pathogenesis of nasopharyngeal carcinoma, Hodgkin lymphoma, and certain other rare non-Hodgkin lymphomas.

- *Epstein-Barr nuclear antigen 1 (EBNA1)* binds the EBV genome to host cell chromosomes during mitosis, thereby ensuring that viral episomes are partitioned evenly to daughter cells when infected cells divide.
- *Latent membrane protein 1 (LMP1)* drives B-cell activation and proliferation. LMP1 does so by mimicking a constitutively active form of CD40, a B cell surface receptor. Like activated CD40, LMP1 binds to TNF receptor–associated factors (TRAFs), adaptor molecules that trigger downstream events that activate NF-κB and the JAK/STAT signaling pathway. In addition, LMP1 prevents apoptosis by activating Bcl-2.
- *EBNA2* also promotes B-cell activation and replication. It turns on the transcription of several host cell genes, including genes that encode proteins that drive cell cycle entry, such as cyclin D.
- EBV produces a *homologue of IL-10* (vIL-10), which inhibits macrophages and dendritic cells and suppresses antiviral T cell responses.

As a result of the actions of these EBV proteins, B cells that are latently infected with EBV are activated and begin to proliferate and to disseminate. This uncontrolled, expanding polyclonal population of EBV-infected B cells secretes antibodies with many specificities, including antibodies that recognize sheep or horse red cells. These so-called heterophile antibodies are detected in diagnostic tests for mononucleosis. EBV-infected B cells may also produce autoantibodies, for example against platelets, leading to transient immune mediated thrombocytopenia in a small subset of patients with mononucleosis.

EBV is shed in the saliva. It is not known whether the source of the virus is B cells, oropharyngeal epithelial cells, or both.

The symptoms of infectious mononucleosis appear upon initiation of the host immune response. Cellular immunity mediated by CD8+ cytotoxic T cells and NK cells is the most important component of this response. The *atypical lymphocytes* seen in the blood, characteristic of this disease, are mainly EBV-specific CD8+ cytotoxic T cells, but also include CD16+ NK cells. The reactive proliferation of T cells is largely centered in lymphoid tissues, which accounts for the lymphadenopathy and splenomegaly. Early in the course of the infection, IgM antibodies are formed against viral capsid antigens; later, IgG antibodies are formed that persist for life. In otherwise healthy persons, the fully developed humoral and cellular responses to EBV act as brakes on viral shedding, resulting in the elimination of B cells expressing the full complement of EBV latency-associated genes. In hosts with acquired defects in cellular immunity (e.g., AIDS, organ transplantation), reactivation of EBV can lead to B-cell proliferation, which can progress through a multistep process to EBV-associated B-cell lymphomas. EBV also contributes to the development of some cases of Burkitt lymphoma (Chapter 13), in which a chromosomal translocation (most commonly an 8:14 translocation) involving the *MYC* oncogene is the critical oncogenic event (Fig. 8-13).

MORPHOLOGY

The major alterations involve the blood, lymph nodes, spleen, liver, CNS, and, occasionally, other organs. The **peripheral blood** shows absolute lymphocytosis; more than 60% of white blood cells are lymphocytes. Between 5% and 80% of these are large, **atypical lymphocytes**, 12 to 16 µm in diameter, characterized by an abundant cytoplasm containing multiple clear vacuolations, an oval, indented, or folded nucleus, and scattered cytoplasmic azurophilic granules (Fig. 8-14). These atypical lymphocytes, most of which express CD8, are sufficiently distinctive to strongly suggest the diagnosis.

The **lymph nodes** are typically discrete and enlarged throughout the body, particularly in the posterior cervical, axillary, and inguinal regions. On histologic examination the most striking feature is the expansion of paracortical areas due to activation of T cells (immunoblasts). A minor population of EBV-infected B cells expressing *EBNA2*, *LMP1*, and other

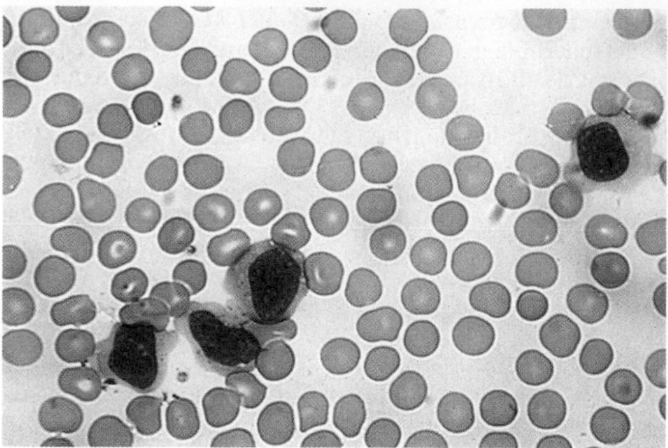

Figure 8-14 Atypical lymphocytes in infectious mononucleosis.

latency-specific genes can also be detected in the paracortex using specific antibodies. EBV-infected B cells resembling Reed-Sternberg cells (the malignant cells of Hodgkin lymphoma, Chapter 13) may be found. B-cell areas (follicles) may also show mild hyperplasia. The T-cell proliferation is sometimes so exuberant that it is difficult to distinguish the nodal morphology from that seen in malignant lymphomas. Similar changes commonly occur in the tonsils and lymphoid tissue of the oropharynx.

The **spleen** is enlarged in most cases, weighing between 300 and 500 gm. It is usually soft and fleshy, with a hyperemic cut surface. The histologic changes are analogous to those of the lymph nodes, showing an expansion of white pulp follicles and red pulp sinusoids due to the presence of numerous activated T cells. These spleens are especially vulnerable to rupture, possibly in part because the rapid increase in size produces a tense, fragile splenic capsule.

The **liver** is usually involved to some degree, although hepatomegaly is at most moderate. On histologic examination, atypical lymphocytes are seen in the portal areas and sinusoids, and scattered, isolated cells or foci of parenchymal necrosis may be present. This histologic picture is similar to that of other forms of viral hepatitis.

Clinical Features. EBV in young children classically presents with fever, sore throat, lymphadenitis, and the other features mentioned earlier. However, malaise, fatigue, and lymphadenopathy are the common presentation in young adults with infectious mononucleosis and can raise the specter of leukemia or lymphoma; EBV also can present as a fever of unknown origin without significant lymphadenopathy or other localized findings, hepatitis resembling one of the hepatotropic viral syndromes, or a febrile rash resembling rubella. **The diagnosis depends on the following findings (in increasing order of specificity): (1) lymphocytosis with the characteristic atypical lymphocytes in the peripheral blood, (2) a positive heterophile antibody reaction (Monospot test), and (3) a rising titer of specific antibodies for EBV antigens (viral capsid antigens, early antigens, or Epstein-Barr nuclear antigen).** In most patients, infectious mononucleosis resolves within 4 to 6 weeks, but sometimes the fatigue lasts longer. One or more complications occasionally supervene. Perhaps most common is marked hepatic dysfunction with jaundice, elevated hepatic enzyme levels, disturbed appetite, and rarely, even liver failure. Other complications involve the nervous system, kidneys, bone marrow, lungs, eyes, heart, and spleen. Splenic rupture can occur even with minor trauma, leading to hemorrhage that may be fatal.

A more serious complication in those lacking T-cell immunity, such as HIV-infected individuals, or individuals receiving immunosuppressive therapy (e.g., bone marrow or solid-organ transplant recipients), is unimpeded B-cell proliferation. This process can be initiated by an acute infection or reactivation of latent B cell infection and usually begins as polyclonal B-cell proliferation that transforms to monoclonal B-cell lymphoma. As detailed in Chapter 13, EBV also causes another distinctive form of lymphoma, called *Burkitt lymphoma*, particularly in certain geographic locales.

Serious consequences of EBV infection occur in individuals suffering from the X-linked lymphoproliferation syndrome (also known as *Duncan disease*), a disorder caused by mutations in the *SH2D1A* gene, which encodes a signaling protein that participates in T-cell and NK-cell activation and antibody production. This rare inherited immunodeficiency is characterized by an ineffective immune response to EBV. Patients are usually normal until they are acutely infected with EBV, often during adolescence. In more than half of the cases, EBV causes an acute overwhelming infection that may be fatal. Others succumb to EBV-positive B-cell lymphoma or infections related to hypogammaglobulinemia.

Bacterial Infections

Different classes of bacteria are responsible for diverse infections (Table 8-7).

Gram-Positive Bacterial Infections

Common gram-positive pathogens include *Staphylococcus*, *Streptococcus*, and *Enterococcus*, each of which causes many types of infections. Diphtheria, listeriosis, anthrax, and nocardiosis are less common infections also caused by gram-positive rods and discussed here. *Clostridia* are discussed with the anaerobes.

Staphylococcal Infections

***S. aureus* causes a myriad of skin lesions (boils, carbuncles, impetigo, and scalded-skin syndrome) as well as abscesses, sepsis, osteomyelitis, pneumonia, endocarditis, food poisoning, and toxic shock syndrome** (Fig. 8-15). *S. aureus* are pyogenic gram-positive cocci that form clusters resembling bunches of grapes. The general characteristics of *S. aureus* infection are reviewed here. Specific organ infections are described in other chapters. Coagulase-negative staphylococci, such as *S. epidermidis*, cause opportunistic infections in catheterized patients, patients with prosthetic cardiac valves, and drug addicts. *S. saprophyticus* is a common cause of urinary tract infections in young women.

Pathogenesis. *S. aureus* produces a multitude of virulence factors, which include surface proteins involved in adherence and evasion of the host immune response, secreted

Table 8-7 Selected Human Bacterial Pathogens and Associated Diseases

Organ System	Species	Frequent Disease Presentations
Respiratory	*Streptococcus pyogenes*	Pharyngitis
	Corynebacterium diphtheria	Diphtheria
	Bordetella pertussis	Pertussis
	Streptococcus pneumonia	Lobar pneumonia
	Mycobacterium tuberculosis	Tuberculosis
	Legionella pneumophila	Legionnaire disease
Gastrointestinal	*Helicobacter pylori*	Peptic ulcers
	Vibrio cholerae, enterotoxigenic *E. coli*	Noninflammatory gastroenteritis
	Shigella species, *Salmonella* species, *Campylobacter jejuni*, enterohemorrhagic *E. coli*	Inflammatory gastroenteritis
	Salmonolla typhi	Entcric (typhoid) fever
	Clostridium difficile	Pseudomembranous colitis
Nervous system	*Neisseria meningitidis*, *Streptococcus pneumonia*, *Haemophilus influenza*, *Listeria monocytogenes*	Acute meningitis
	Clostridium tetani, *Clostridium botulinum*	Paralytic intoxications, tetanus and botulism
Urogenital	*Escherichia coli*, *Pseudomonas aeruginosa*, *Enterococcus* species	Urinary tract infections
	Neisseria gonorrhoeae	Gonorrhea
	Chlamydia trachomatis	Chlamydia
	Treponema pallidum	Syphilis
Skin and adjacent soft tissue	*Staphylococcus aureus*	Abscess, cellulitis
	Streptococcus pyogenes	Impetigo, erysipelas, necrotizing fasciitis
	Clostridium perfringens	Gas gangrene
	Bacillus anthracis	Cutaneous anthrax
	Pseudomonas aeruginosa	Burn infections
	Mycobacterium leprae	Leprosy
Disseminated infections	*Yersinia pestis*	Plague
	Borrelia burgdorferi	Lyme disease
	Brucella species	Brucellosis (undulant fever)
Disseminated neonatal infection	*Streptococcus agalactiae*, *Listeria monocytogenes*	Neonatal bacteremia, meningitis
	Treponema pallidum	Congenital syphilis

enzymes that degrade host structures, secreted toxins that damage host cells, and proteins that cause antibiotic resistance. *S. aureus* expresses surface receptors for fibrinogen (called *clumping factor*), fibronectin, and vitronectin, and uses these molecules to bind to host endothelial cells. Staphylococci infecting prosthetic valves and catheters have a polysaccharide capsule that allows them to attach to artificial materials and resist host cell phagocytosis. Staphylococci also have on their surface protein A, which binds the Fc portion of immunoglobulins, allowing the organism to escape antibody-mediated killing.

Bacterial Toxins. *S. aureus* produces multiple *membrane-damaging (hemolytic) toxins*. These include α-toxin, a protein that intercalates into the plasma membrane of host cells, forming pores that allow toxic levels of calcium to leak into cells; β-toxin, a sphingomyelinase; and δ-toxin, which is a detergent-like peptide. Staphylococcal γ-toxin and leukocidin lyse red cells and phagocytes, respectively.

The *exfoliative A and B toxins* produced by *S. aureus* are serine proteases that cleave the desmosomal protein desmoglein 1, which holds epidermal cells tightly together. This causes keratinocytes to detach from one another and from the underlying basement membrane, resulting in a loss of barrier function that often leads to secondary skin infections. Exfoliation may occur locally at the site of infection (bullous impetigo) or may result in widespread loss of the superficial epidermis (staphylococcal scalded-skin syndrome).

Superantigens produced by *S. aureus* cause food poisoning and toxic shock syndrome. Toxic shock syndrome came to public attention because of its association with the use of hyperabsorbent tampons, which became colonized with *S. aureus* during use. It is now clear that toxic shock syndrome can be caused by growth of *S. aureus* at many sites, most commonly the vagina and infected surgical sites. This syndrome is characterized by hypotension (shock), renal failure, coagulopathy, liver disease, respiratory distress, a generalized erythematous rash, and soft tissue necrosis at the site of infection. If not promptly treated, it can be fatal. Toxic shock syndrome can also be caused by *Streptococcus pyogenes.* Bacterial superantigens cause polyclonal T cell proliferation by binding to conserved portions of MHC molecules and to relatively conserved portions of T-cell receptor β chains. In this manner superantigens may stimulate up to 20% of T lymphocytes, leading to release of cytokines such as TNF and IL-1, in such large amounts that they may trigger the systemic inflammatory response syndrome (Chapter 4). Superantigens produced by *S. aureus* also cause vomiting, presumably by affecting the CNS or the enteric nervous system.

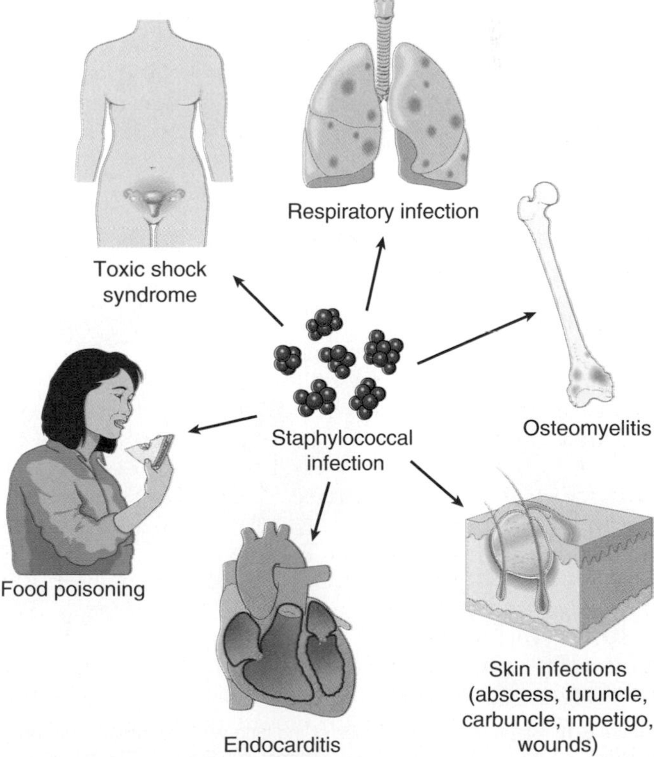

Figure 8-15 The many consequences of staphylococcal infection.

Antibiotic resistance is a growing problem in treatment of *S. aureus* infections. Methicillin-resistant *S. aureus* (MRSA) are resistant to nearly all penicillin and cephalosporin antibiotics. Until recently, MRSA was mainly found in healthcare facilities, but community-acquired MRSA infections are now common in many areas. As a result, empirical treatment of staphylococcal infections with penicillin and cephalosporin antibiotics is less likely to be effective.

MORPHOLOGY

Whether the lesion is located in the skin, lungs, bones, or heart valves, *S. aureus* causes pyogenic inflammation that is distinctive for its local destruction of host tissue. Excluding impetigo, which is restricted to the superficial epidermis, staphylococcal skin infections are centered around the hair follicles where they begin. A **furuncle**, or **boil**, is a focal suppurative inflammation of the skin and subcutaneous tissue. They may be solitary or multiple or recur in successive crops. Furuncles are most frequent in moist, hairy areas, such as the face, axillae, groin, legs, and submammary folds. Beginning in a single hair follicle, a boil develops into a growing and deepening abscess that eventually "comes to a head" by thinning and rupturing the overlying skin. A **carbuncle** is a deeper suppurative infection that spreads laterally beneath the deep subcutaneous fascia and then burrows superficially to erupt in multiple adjacent skin sinuses. Carbuncles typically appear beneath the skin of the upper back and posterior neck, where fascial planes favor their spread. **Hidradenitis** is chronic suppurative infection of apocrine glands, most often in the axilla. Infections of the nail bed (**paronychia**) or on the palmar side of the fingertips (**felons**) are exquisitely painful. They may follow trauma or embedded splinters and, if deep enough, destroy the bone of the terminal phalanx or detach the fingernail.

S. aureus lung infections (Fig. 8-16) have a polymorphonuclear infiltrate similar to that of *S. pneumoniae* infections (Fig. 8-4), but cause much more tissue destruction. Lung infections usually arise from a hematogenous source, such as an infected thrombus, or in the setting of a predisposing condition such as influenza.

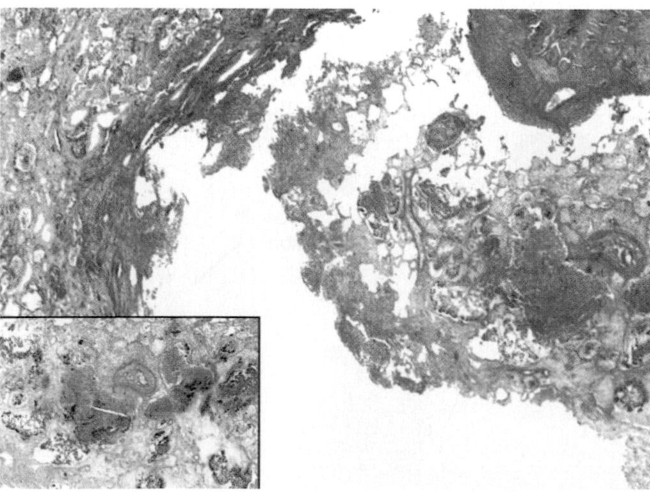

Figure 8-16 Staphylococcal abscess of the lung with extensive neutrophilic infiltrate and destruction of the alveoli (contrast with Fig. 8-4). The inset shows the same area on Gram stain highlighting clusters of bacteria.

Staphylococcal scalded-skin syndrome, also called Ritter disease, most frequently occurs in children with *S. aureus* infection of the nasopharynx or skin. There is a sunburn-like rash that spreads over the entire body and evolves into fragile bullae that lead to partial or total skin loss. The desquamation of the epidermis in staphylococcal scalded-skin syndrome occurs at the level of the granulosa layer, distinguishing it from toxic epidermal necrolysis, or Lyell disease, which is secondary to drug hypersensitivity and causes desquamation at the level of the epidermal-dermal junction (Chapter 25).

Streptococcal and Enterococcal Infections

Streptococci cause suppurative infections of the skin, oropharynx, lungs, and heart valves. They are also responsible for a number of postinfectious syndromes, including rheumatic fever (Chapter 12), immune complex glomerulonephritis (Chapter 20), and erythema nodosum (Chapter 25). These bacteria are gram-positive cocci that grow in pairs or chains. β-hemolytic streptococci are typed according to their surface carbohydrate (Lancefield) antigens. *S. pyogenes* (group A) causes pharyngitis, scarlet fever, erysipelas, impetigo, rheumatic fever, toxic shock syndrome, and glomerulonephritis. *S. agalactiae* (group B) colonizes the female genital tract and causes sepsis and meningitis in neonates and chorioamnionitis in pregnancy. *S. pneumoniae*, the most important α-hemolytic streptococcus, is a common cause of community-acquired pneumonia in older adults and meningitis in children and adults. The viridans-group streptococci include α-hemolytic and nonhemolytic streptococci found in normal oral flora that are a common cause of endocarditis. *S. mutans* is the major cause of dental caries. Streptococcal infections are diagnosed by culture, and, in those with pharyngitis, by the rapid streptococcal antigen test.

Enterococci are gram-positive cocci that grow in chains. They are often resistant to commonly used antibiotics and are a significant cause of endocarditis and urinary tract infections.

Pathogenesis. The different species of streptococci produce many virulence factors and toxins. *S. pyogenes, S. agalactiae,* and *S. pneumoniae* have capsules that resist phagocytosis. *S. pyogenes* also expresses M protein, a surface protein that prevents bacteria from being phagocytosed, and a complement C5a peptidase that degrades this chemotactic peptide. *S. pyogenes* secretes a phage-encoded pyrogenic exotoxin that causes fever and rash in scarlet fever. Poststreptococcal acute rheumatic fever is probably caused by antistreptococcal M protein antibodies and T cells that cross-react with cardiac proteins. Virulent *S. pyogenes* have been referred to as flesh-eating bacteria because they cause a rapidly progressive necrotizing fasciitis. Although the antiphagocytic capsule is the most important virulence factor of *S. pneumoniae,* it also produces pneumolysin, a toxin that inserts into host cell membranes and lyses cells, greatly increasing tissue damage. *S. mutans* produces caries by metabolizing sucrose to lactic acid (which causes demineralization of tooth enamel) and by secreting high-molecular-weight glucans that promote aggregation of bacteria and plaque formation.

Enterococci are low-virulence bacteria, although they do have an antiphagocytic capsule and produce enzymes that

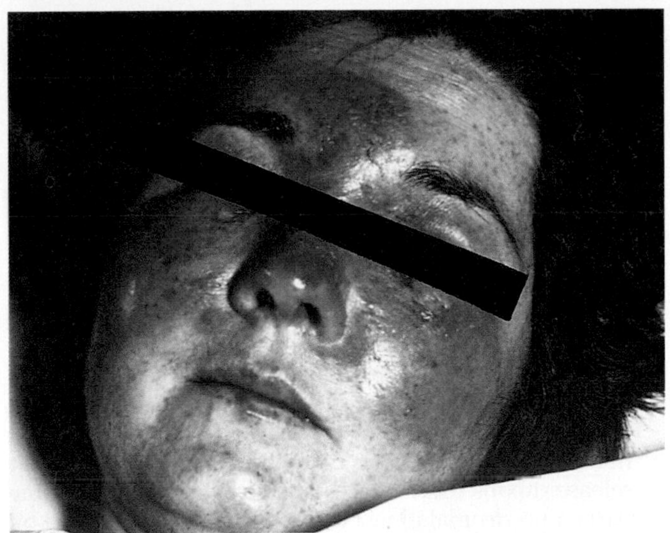

Figure 8-17 Streptococcal erysipelas.

injure host tissues. The emergence of enterococci as pathogens is primarily due to their resistance to antibiotics.

MORPHOLOGY

Streptococcal infections are characterized by diffuse interstitial neutrophilic infiltrates with minimal destruction of host tissues. The skin lesions caused by streptococci (furuncles, carbuncles, and impetigo) resemble those of staphylococci.

Erysipelas is caused by exotoxins from superficial infection with *S. pyogenes*. It is characterized by rapidly spreading erythematous cutaneous swelling that may begin on the face or, less frequently, on the body or an extremity. The rash has a sharp, well-demarcated, serpiginous border and may form a "butterfly" distribution on the face (Fig. 8-17). On histologic examination there is a diffuse, edematous, neutrophilic inflammatory reaction in the dermis and epidermis extending into the subcutaneous tissues. Microabscesses may be formed, but tissue necrosis is usually minor.

Streptococcal pharyngitis, which is the major antecedent of poststreptococcal glomerulonephritis (Chapter 20), is marked by edema, epiglottic swelling, and punctate abscesses of the tonsillar crypts, sometimes accompanied by cervical lymphadenopathy. Swelling associated with severe pharyngeal infection may encroach on the airways, especially if there is peritonsillar or retropharyngeal abscess formation.

Scarlet fever, associated with pharyngitis caused by *S. pyogenes*, is most common between the ages of 3 and 15 years. It is manifested by a punctate erythematous rash that is most prominent over the trunk and inner aspects of the arms and legs. The face is also involved, but usually a small area about the mouth remains relatively unaffected, producing circumoral pallor. The skin usually becomes hyperkeratotic and scaly during defervescence.

S. pneumoniae is an important cause of lobar pneumonia (described in Chapter 15 and pictured in Fig. 8-4).

Diphtheria

Diphtheria is caused by *Corynebacterium diphtheriae*, a slender gram-positive rod with clubbed ends that spreads from person to person in respiratory droplets or skin exudate. Respiratory diphtheria causes pharyngeal or, less often, nasal or laryngeal infection. There is toxin-mediated formation of a gray pharyngeal membrane, and damage to the heart, nerves, and other organs. Cutaneous diphtheria causes chronic ulcers with a dirty gray membrane, but does not cause systemic damage. *C. diphtheriae* produces a phage-encoded A-B toxin that blocks host cell protein synthesis. The A fragment does this by catalyzing the covalent transfer of adenosine diphosphate (ADP)-ribose to elongation factor-2 (EF-2). This inhibits EF-2 function, which is required for the translation of mRNA into protein. A single molecule of diphtheria toxin can kill a cell by ADP-ribosylating, and thereby inactivating, more than a million EF-2 molecules. Immunization with diphtheria toxoid (formalin-fixed toxin) stimulates production of toxin-neutralizing antibodies that protect people from the lethal effects of the toxin.

MORPHOLOGY

Inhaled *C. diphtheriae* carried in respiratory droplets proliferate at the site of attachment on the mucosa of the nasopharynx, oropharynx, larynx, or trachea. The bacteria also form satellite lesions in the esophagus or lower airways. Release of exotoxin causes necrosis of the epithelium, accompanied by an outpouring of a dense fibrinosuppurative exudate. The coagulation of this exudate on the ulcerated necrotic surface creates a tough, dirty gray to black, superficial membrane, sometimes called **pseudo-membrane** because it is not formed by viable tissue (Fig. 8-18). There is an intense neutrophilic infiltration in the underlying tissues with marked vascular congestion, interstitial edema, and fibrin exudation. When the membrane sloughs off its inflamed and vascularized bed, bleeding and asphyxiation may occur. With control of the infection, the membrane is coughed up or removed by enzymatic digestion, and the inflammatory reaction subsides.

Although the bacterial invasion remains localized, with entry of exotoxin into the blood and its systemic distribution, there may be fatty change in the myocardium with isolated myofiber necrosis, polyneuritis with degeneration of the myelin sheaths and axis cylinders, and (less commonly) fatty change and focal necroses of parenchymal cells in the liver, kidneys, and adrenals.

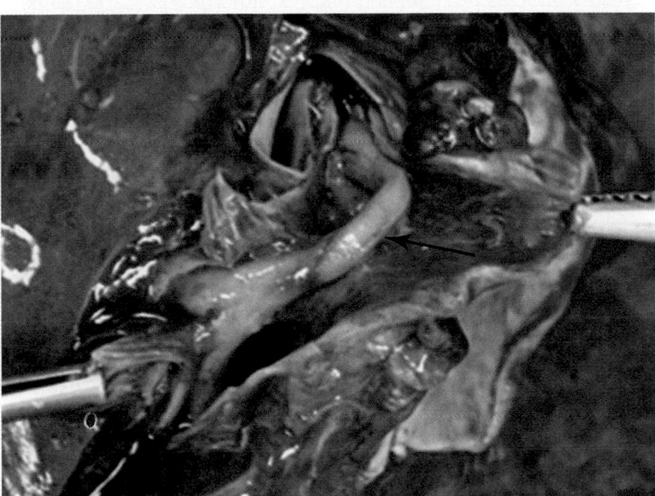

Figure 8-18 Membrane of diphtheria *(arrow)* lying within a transverse bronchus. (Courtesy Dr. Robin A. Cooke, Department of Anatomical Pathology, Princess Alexandria Hospital, Brisbane, Australia.)

Listeriosis

Listeria monocytogenes is a gram-positive bacillus that causes severe food-borne infections in vulnerable hosts. Outbreaks of *L. monocytogenes* infection have been linked to contaminated dairy products, chicken, and hot dogs. Pregnant women, neonates, older adults, and immunosuppressed persons are particularly susceptible to severe *L. monocytogenes* infection. In pregnant women, *L. monocytogenes* causes an amnionitis that may result in abortion, stillbirth, or neonatal sepsis. In neonates and immunosuppressed adults, it can cause disseminated disease (granulomatosis infantiseptica of the newborn) and an exudative meningitis.

L. monocytogenes is a facultative intracellular pathogen, and therefore, T cells play a particularly important role in the host immune response. The bacteria bind to receptors on host epithelial cells and macrophages and are phagocytosed. The bacteria escape from the phagolysosome using a pore-forming protein, listeriolysin O, and two phospholipases. In the host cell cytoplasm, Act A, a bacterial surface protein, binds to host cell cytoskeletal proteins and induces actin polymerization. This in turn generates sufficient force to propel the bacteria into adjacent, uninfected host cells. Resting macrophages fail to kill the intracellular bacteria, whereas macrophages that are activated by IFN-γ can. Accordingly, an effective host response to *L. monocytogenes* depends on IFN-γ produced by NK cells early in the course of the infection and T cells in chronic infection. Patients with defects in cell-mediated immunity, such as those with reduced levels of CD4+ lymphocytes, are at increased risk for listeriosis.

MORPHOLOGY

In acute infections, *L. monocytogenes* evokes an exudative pattern of inflammation with numerous neutrophils. The meningitis it causes is macroscopically and microscopically indistinguishable from that resulting from infection with other pyogenic bacteria (Chapter 28). **The finding of gram-positive, mostly intracellular bacilli in the CSF is virtually diagnostic.** More varied lesions may be encountered in neonates and immunosuppressed adults. Focal abscesses alternating with grayish or yellow nodules representing necrotic amorphous tissue debris can occur in any organ, including the lung, liver, spleen, and lymph nodes. In infections of longer duration, macrophages appear in large numbers, but granulomas are rare. Infants born with *L. monocytogenes* sepsis often have a papular red rash over the extremities, and listerial abscesses can be seen in the placenta. A smear of the meconium will disclose the gram-positive bacilli.

Anthrax

Anthrax is characterized by necrotizing inflammatory lesions in the skin or gastrointestinal tract or systemically. It is caused by *Bacillus anthracis*, a large, spore-forming gram-positive rod-shaped bacterium found in environmental sources. Livestock become infected by spores in their environment or feed. Humans usually become infected by eating or handling meat or products (e.g., wool or hides) from infected animals. There are a small number of cases of anthrax each year, most of which occur in the developing world. Anthrax spores can be made into a fine powder, creating a potent biologic weapon that is a potential bioterrorism threat. In 1979, accidental release of *B. anthracis* spores at a military research institute in Russia killed 66 people. In 2001, 22 people in the United States were infected with *B. anthracis*, mostly through spores delivered in the mail.

There are three major forms of anthrax.

- *Cutaneous anthrax*, which makes up 95% of naturally occurring infections, begins as a painless, pruritic papule that develops into a vesicle within 2 days. As the vesicle enlarges, striking edema may occur around it, with development of regional lymphadenopathy. After the vesicle ruptures, the remaining ulcer becomes covered with a characteristic black eschar, which dries and falls off as the person recovers. Bacteremia is rare.
- *Inhalational anthrax* occurs when airborne spores are inhaled. The spores are carried by phagocytes to lymph nodes where they germinate, producing bacilli that release toxins that cause hemorrhagic mediastinitis. After a prodromal illness of 1 to 6 days characterized by fever, cough, and chest or abdominal pain, there is abrupt onset of increased fever, hypoxia, and sweating. Frequently, meningitis develops from bacteremia. Inhalational anthrax rapidly leads to shock and frequently death within 1 to 2 days.
- *Gastrointestinal anthrax* is usually contracted by eating undercooked meat contaminated with *B. anthracis*. Initially, the person has nausea, abdominal pain, and vomiting, followed by severe, bloody diarrhea and, sometimes, bacteremia. Mortality is approximately 40%.

Pathogenesis. *B. anthracis* produces potent toxins and an antiphagocytic polyglutamyl capsule. The mechanisms of action of anthrax toxins are well understood (Fig. 8-19). They have A and B subunits. The B subunit is also called the *protective antigen*, because antibodies against it protect against the toxins. Following infection the B subunit is released into the circulation and binds to a cell surface

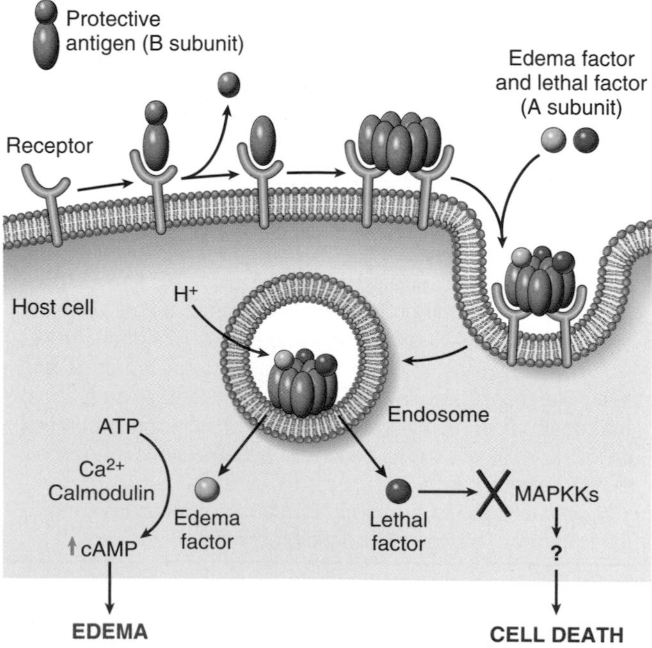

Figure 8-19 Mechanism of action of anthrax toxins. Note that each B subunit binds either EF or LF but not both (as shown for simplicity). (Adapted from Mourez M, Lacy DB, Cunningham K, et al: 2001: A year of major advances in anthrax toxin research. Trends Microbiol 2002;10:287.)

receptor that is highly expressed on endothelial cells. Then a host protease removes a fragment of the B subunit, and the remaining fragment self-associates to form a heptamer. The B unit is not toxic, but serves to deliver the toxic A units into cells. Anthrax toxin has two alternate A subunits: *edema factor* (EF) and *lethal factor* (LF), each named for the effect of the toxin in experimental animals. One to three molecules of the EF or LF bind to a B subunit heptamer, and this complex is endocytosed into the host cell. Each B heptamer binds either EF or LF. The low pH of the endosome causes a conformational change in the B heptamer, which then forms a channel in the endosome membrane through which the EF or LF moves into the cytoplasm. In the cytoplasm, EF binds to calcium and calmodulin to form an adenylate cyclase. The active enzyme converts ATP to intracellular cyclic adenosine monophosphate (cAMP), altering cell function. LF has a different mechanism of action. LF is a protease that destroys mitogen-activated protein kinase kinases (MAPKKs). These kinases regulate the activity of MAPKs, which are important regulators of cell growth and differentiation (Chapter 1). The mechanism of cell death caused by dysregulation of MAPKs is not understood.

MORPHOLOGY

Anthrax lesions at any site are typified by necrosis and exudative inflammation rich in neutrophils and macrophages. The presence of large, boxcar-shaped gram-positive extracellular bacteria in chains, seen histopathologically or grown in culture, suggests the diagnosis.

Inhalational anthrax causes numerous foci of hemorrhage in the mediastinum and hemorrhagic lymphadenitis of hilar and peribronchial lymph nodes. The lungs typically show a perihilar interstitial pneumonia with infiltration of macrophages and neutrophils and pulmonary vasculitis. Hemorrhagic lung lesions associated with vasculitis are also present in about half of cases. Mediastinal lymph nodes are expanded by edema and by macrophages containing phagocytosed apoptotic lymphocytes. *B. anthracis* is most likely to be seen in the alveolar capillaries and venules and, to a lesser degree, within the alveolar space and draining hilar lymph nodes (Fig. 8-20). In fatal cases, however, the organism may be found in multiple organs (spleen, liver, intestines, kidneys, adrenal glands, and meninges).

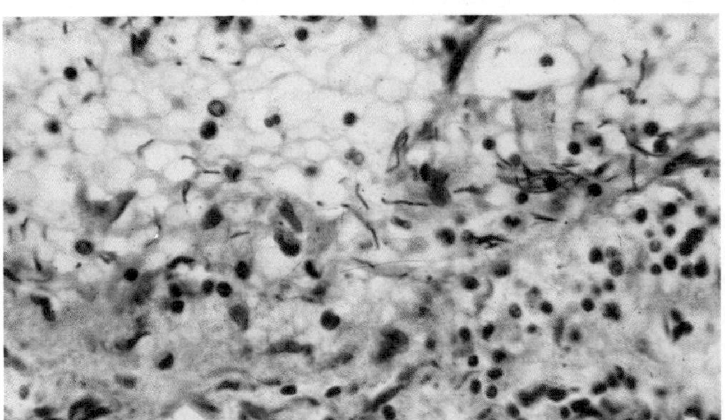

Figure 8-20 *Bacillus anthracis* in the subcapsular sinus of a hilar lymph node of a patient who died of inhalational anthrax. (Courtesy Dr. Lev Grinberg, Department of Pathology, Hospital 40, Ekaterinburg, Russia, and Dr. David Walker, UTMB Center for Biodefense and Emerging Infectious Diseases, Galveston, Texas.)

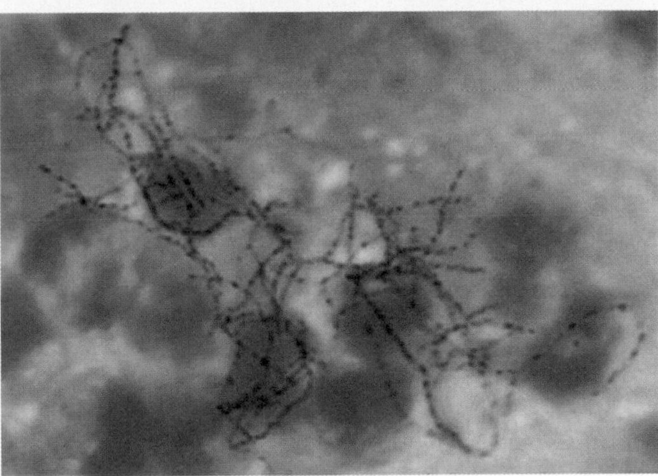

Figure 8-21 *Nocardia asteroides* in a Gram-stained sputum sample. Note the beaded, branched gram-positive organisms and leukocytes. (Courtesy Dr. Ellen Jo Baron, Stanford University Medical Center, Stanford, Calif.)

Nocardia

***Nocardia* are aerobic gram-positive bacteria found in soil that cause opportunistic infections.** The organism grows in distinctive branched chains. In culture, *Nocardia* form thin aerial filaments resembling hyphae. Despite this morphologic similarity to molds, *Nocardia* are true bacteria.

Nocardia asteroides causes respiratory infections, most often in patients with defects in immunity due to prolonged steroid use, HIV infection, or diabetes mellitus. Respiratory infection with *N. asteroides* causes an indolent illness with fever, weight loss, and cough, which may be mistaken for tuberculosis or malignancy. In some cases *N. asteroides* infections disseminate from the lungs to the CNS. Infections of the CNS are also indolent and cause varying neurologic deficits depending on the site of the lesions. *Nocardia brasiliensis* causes skin infections following injuries contaminated with soil. Manifestations include cellulitis, lymphocutaneous disease, and actinomycetoma with formation of nodules that progress to form chronic draining fistulae.

MORPHOLOGY

Nocardia appear in tissue as slender gram-positive organisms arranged in branching filaments (Fig. 8-21). Irregular staining gives the filaments a beaded appearance. *Nocardia* stain with modified acid-fast stains (Fite-Faraco stain), unlike *Actinomyces*, which may appear similar on Gram stain of tissue. *Nocardia* elicit a suppurative response with central liquefaction and surrounding granulation and fibrosis. Granulomas do not form.

Gram-Negative Bacterial Infections

Only a few gram-negative bacteria are discussed in this section. A number of important gram-negative pathogens are discussed in the appropriate chapters of organ systems, including bacterial causes of gastrointestinal infections and urinary tract infections. Anaerobic gram-negative organisms are considered later in this chapter. Gram-negative bacterial infections are usually diagnosed by culture.

Neisserial Infections

Neisseria are gram-negative diplococci that are flattened on the adjoining sides, giving the pair the shape of a coffee bean. These aerobic bacteria have stringent nutritional requirements and grow best on enriched media such as lysed sheep's blood agar. The two clinically significant *Neisseria* are *N. meningitidis* and *N. gonorrhoeae*.

***N. meningitidis* is a significant cause of bacterial meningitis, particularly among adolescents and young adults.** The organism is a common colonizer of the oropharynx and is spread by the respiratory route. An immune response leads to elimination of the colonizing organism in most people, and this response is protective against subsequent infection with the same serotype of bacteria. There are several capsular serotypes of *N. meningitidis*, however five of them cause most cases of disease. Invasive disease mainly occurs when people encounter new strains to which they are not immune, as may happen to young children or to young adults living in crowded quarters such as military barracks or college dormitories. *N. meningitidis* is endemic in the United States, but epidemics occur periodically in sub-Saharan Africa and cause thousands of deaths. Conjugate vaccines for *N. meningitidis* composed of capsular polysaccharides conjugated to antigenic proteins are available and are highly effective at preventing disease.

Even in the absence of preexisting immunity, only a small fraction of people infected with *N. meningitidis* develop meningitis. The bacteria must invade respiratory epithelial cells and travel to their basolateral side to enter the blood. In the blood, the bacterial capsule inhibits opsonization and destruction of the bacteria by complement proteins. The importance of complement as a first-line defense against *N. meningitidis* is shown by the increased rates of serious infection among people who have inherited defects in the complement proteins (C5 to C9) that form the membrane attack complex, or patients with paroxysmal nocturnal hemoglobinuria (Chapter 14) who are being treated with an antibody inhibitor of the membrane attack complex. If *N. meningitidis* escapes the host response, the consequences can be severe. Although antibiotic treatment greatly reduces the mortality of *N. meningitidis* infection, about 10% of infected patients still die The pathology of pyogenic meningitis is discussed in Chapter 28.

***N. gonorrhoeae* is an important cause of sexually transmitted disease (STD)**, with more than 300,000 cases reported each year in the United States. It is second only to *C. trachomatis* among bacterial STDs. Infection in men causes urethritis. In women, *N. gonorrhoeae* infection is often asymptomatic and so may go unnoticed. Untreated gonorrhea may lead to pelvic inflammatory disease, which can cause infertility or ectopic pregnancy (Chapter 22). Infection is diagnosed by culture and PCR tests.

Although *N. gonorrhoeae* infection usually manifests locally in the genital or cervical mucosa, pharynx, or anorectum, disseminated infections may occur. Like *N. meningitidis*, *N. gonorrhoeae* is much more likely to become disseminated in people who lack the complement proteins that form the membrane attack complex. Disseminated infection of adults and adolescents usually causes septic arthritis accompanied by a rash of hemorrhagic papules and pustules. Neonatal *N. gonorrhoeae* infection causes conjunctivitis that may lead to blindness and, rarely, sepsis. The eye infection, which is preventable by instillation of silver nitrate or antibiotics in the newborn's eyes, remains an important cause of blindness in some developing nations.

Pathogenesis. *Neisseria* organisms adhere to and invade nonciliated epithelial cells at the site of entry (nasopharynx, urethra, or cervix). Adherence of *N. gonorrhoeae* to epithelial cells is initially mediated by long pili, which bind to CD46, a protein expressed on all human nucleated cells. OPA proteins (so named because they make bacterial colonies opaque), located in the outer membrane of the bacteria, increase binding of *Neisseria* organisms to epithelial cells and promote entry of bacteria into cells.

Neisseria use antigenic variation as a strategy to escape the immune response. The existence of multiple capsular serotypes of *N. meningitidis* results in meningitis in some people on exposure to a new strain, as discussed above. In addition, *Neisseria* species also can generate new antigens by special genetic mechanisms, which permit a single bacterial clone to change its expressed antigens and escape immune defenses. Such mechanisms involve both pili and OPA proteins:

- Recombination of genes encoding pili proteins. The pili are composed of polypeptides encoded by the pilin gene, which consists of a promoter and coding sequences for 10 to 15 pili protein variants. At any point in time, only one of these coding sequences is adjacent to the promoter, allowing it to be expressed. Periodically, homologous recombination shuttles one of the other pilin coding sequences next to the promoter, resulting in expression of a different pili variant.
- Expression of different OPA proteins. Each *OPA* gene has several repeats of a five-nucleotide sequence, which are frequently deleted or duplicated. These changes shift the reading frame of the gene so that it encodes new sequences. Stop codons are also introduced by the additions and deletions, which determine whether each *OPA* gene is expressed or silent. Thus, *Neisseria* can express one, none, or multiple OPA proteins at any time.

Pertussis

Pertussis, or whooping cough, caused by the gram-negative coccobacillus *Bordetella pertussis*, is an acute, highly communicable illness characterized by paroxysms of violent coughing followed by a loud inspiratory "whoop." In the United States, the incidence of pertussis has risen dramatically, with large epidemics occurring in 2005, 2010, and 2012. Although the reasons for this increase are not clear, the acellular pertussis vaccine currently in use is less effective than the vaccine used before 1997, and this may be a factor in the changing epidemiology of this disease. In areas of the developing world where vaccination is not widely practiced, pertussis kills hundreds of thousands of children each year. The diagnosis is best made by PCR, because culture is less sensitive.

Pathogenesis. *B. pertussis* colonizes the brush border of the bronchial epithelium and also invades macrophages. It contains a filamentous hemagglutinin that binds to carbohydrates on the surface of respiratory epithelial cells, as well as to CR3 (Mac-1) integrins on macrophages. Pertussis

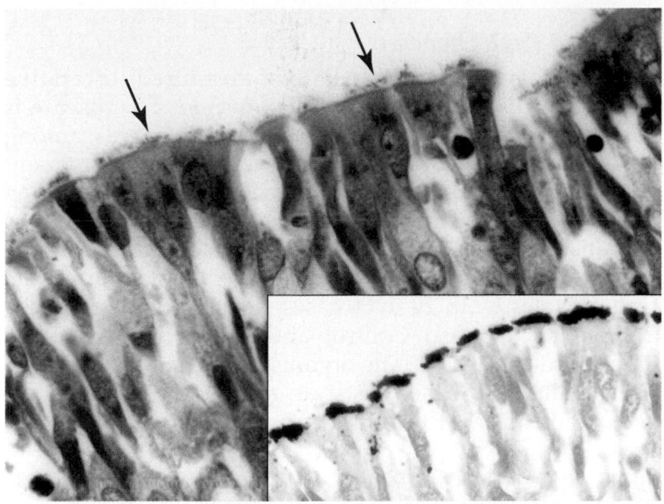

Figure 8-22 Whooping cough showing a haze of bacilli *(arrows)* entangled with the cilia of bronchial epithelial cells. The inset highlights the haze of bacilli by immunohistochemistry using a monoclonal antibody reactive to the lipooligosaccharide A of *Bordetella pertussis*. (Images courtesy Dr. Christopher Paddock of the Centers for Disease Control, Atlanta, Ga.)

toxin is a typical A-B toxin that is composed of five subunits. The A unit, like cholera toxin, ADP-ribosylates and inactivates guanine nucleotide-binding proteins, so these G proteins can no longer transduce signals. The B component contains four subunits that bind to extracellular molecules and allow the A subunit to enter cells. The B subunit can also bind to cell surface molecules such as TLR-4 and through these it can initiate signaling events in cells. Collectively, pertussis toxin subunits impair host defenses by inhibiting neutrophils and macrophages and paralyzing cilia, among other effects.

B. pertussis also produces a toxic adenylate cyclase that enters host cells and converts ATP to cAMP. The rise in cAMP inhibits phagocytosis and the oxidative burst in neutrophils, and can cause apoptosis of macrophages. In addition, pertussis toxin inhibits neutrophil recruitment into the airways and has inhibitory effects on macrophages; the mechanisms underlying these effects are not understood.

MORPHOLOGY

Bordetella bacteria cause a laryngotracheobronchitis that in severe cases features bronchial mucosal erosion, hyperemia, and copious mucopurulent exudate (Fig. 8-22). Unless superinfected, the lung alveoli remain open and intact. In parallel with a striking peripheral lymphocytosis (up to 90%), there is hypercellularity and enlargement of the mucosal lymph follicles and peribronchial lymph nodes.

Pseudomonas *Infection*

***Pseudomonas aeruginosa* is an opportunistic aerobic gram-negative bacillus that is a frequent, deadly pathogen of people with cystic fibrosis, severe burns, or neutropenia.** Many people with cystic fibrosis die of pulmonary failure secondary to chronic infection with *P. aeruginosa. P. aeruginosa* can be very resistant to antibiotics, making these infections difficult to treat. It often infects extensive skin burns, which can lead to sepsis. *P. aeruginosa* is a common cause of hospital-acquired infections; it has been cultured from washbasins, respirator tubing, nursery cribs, and even antiseptic-containing bottles. It also causes corneal keratitis in wearers of contact lenses, endocarditis and osteomyelitis in intravenous drug abusers, external otitis (swimmer's ear) in healthy individuals, and severe external otitis in people with diabetes.

Pathogenesis. *P. aeruginosa* produces several toxins that contribute to local tissue damage. The organism secretes an A-B exotoxin called *exotoxin* A that, like diphtheria toxin, inhibits protein synthesis by ADP-ribosylating the ribosomal protein EF-2, leading to the death of host cells. *P. aeruginosa* also secretes damaging enzymes that destroy extracellular matrix (elastase), kill leukocytes (leukocidin), and destroy cell membranes (hemolysins). In the lungs of people with cystic fibrosis, *P. aeruginosa* secretes a mucoid exopolysaccharide called *alginate*, which forms a biofilm that protects bacteria from antibodies, complement, phagocytes, and antibiotics. The organism rapidly develops antibiotic resistance through other mechanisms as well, making treatment difficult.

MORPHOLOGY

Pseudomonas causes a **necrotizing pneumonia** that is distributed through the terminal airways in a fleur-de-lis pattern, with striking pale necrotic centers and red, hemorrhagic peripheral areas. On microscopic examination, masses of organisms are seen that tend to be most concentrated in the walls of blood vessels, where host cells undergo coagulative necrosis (Fig. 8-23). This picture of gram-negative **bacterial vasculitis** accompanied by thrombosis and hemorrhage, although not pathognomonic, is highly suggestive of *P. aeruginosa* infection.

Bronchial obstruction caused by mucus plugging and subsequent *P. aeruginosa* infection are frequent complications of cystic fibrosis. Despite antibiotic treatment and the host immune response, chronic *P. aeruginosa* infection may result in bronchiectasis and pulmonary fibrosis (Chapter 15).

In skin burns, *P. aeruginosa* proliferates widely, penetrating deeply into the veins and spreading hematogenously.

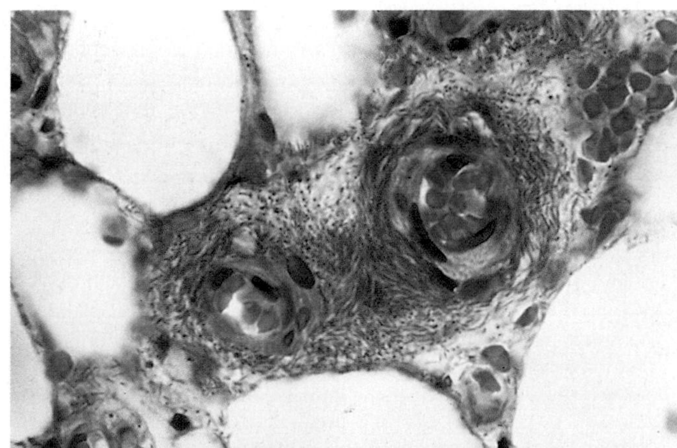

Figure 8-23 *Pseudomonas* vasculitis in which masses of organisms form a perivascular blue haze.

Well-demarcated necrotic and hemorrhagic oval skin lesions, called **ecthyma gangrenosum**, often appear. Disseminated intravascular coagulation is a frequent complication of *P. aeruginosa* bacteremia.

Plague

***Yersinia pestis* is a gram-negative facultative intracellular bacterium that causes an invasive, frequently fatal, infection called *plague*.** It is transmitted from rodents to humans by fleabites or, less often, from one human to another by aerosols. Plague, also named *Black Death,* caused three great pandemics that killed an estimated 100 million people in Egypt and Byzantium in the sixth century; one quarter of Europe's population in the fourteenth and fifteenth centuries; and tens of millions in India, Myanmar, and China at the beginning of the twentieth century. Most cases now occur in Africa, but the organism is endemic in many parts of the world, including nations in the former Soviet Union, the Americas, and Asia. Wild rodents in the rural western United States are infected with *Y. pestis*, and are the source of 10 to 15 human cases every year. *Y. enterocolitica* and *Y. pseudotuberculosis* are genetically similar to *Y. pestis;* these bacteria cause fecal-orally transmitted ileitis and mesenteric lymphadenitis.

Y. pestis ensures its own spread by forming a biofilm that obstructs the gut of the infected flea. The starving flea bites and regurgitates before it feeds, and thus infects the rodent or human that it is biting. The bacteria spread from the site of inoculation to lymphoid tissues, where they proliferate and inhibit the host from mounting an effective response. *Y. pestis* has a plasmid-borne complex of genes, the Yop virulon, which encodes a type III secretion system, a hollow syringe-like structure that projects from the bacterial surface, binds to host cells, and injects bacterial proteins, called *Yops* (*Yersinia* outercoat proteins), into the cell. YopE, YopH, and YopT block phagocytosis by inactivating molecules that regulate actin polymerization. YopJ inhibits the signaling pathways that are activated by LPS, blocking the production of inflammatory cytokines.

MORPHOLOGY

Yersinia pestis causes lymph node enlargement (buboes), pneumonia, or sepsis with a striking neutrophilia. The distinctive histologic features include (1) massive proliferation of the organisms, (2) early appearance of protein-rich and polysaccharide-rich effusions with few inflammatory cells, (3) necrosis of tissues and blood vessels with hemorrhage, thrombosis, and marked tissue swelling, and (4) neutrophilic infiltrates that accumulate adjacent to necrotic areas as healing begins.

In **bubonic plague** the infected fleabite is usually on the legs, where it forms a small pustule or ulcer. The draining lymph nodes enlarge dramatically within a few days and become soft, pulpy, and plum colored, and may infarct or rupture through the skin. In **pneumonic plague** there is a severe, confluent, hemorrhagic and necrotizing bronchopneumonia, often with fibrinous pleuritis. In **septicemic plague** lymph nodes throughout the body as well as organs rich in mononuclear phagocytes develop foci of necrosis. Fulminant bacteremia also induces disseminated intravascular coagulation with widespread hemorrhages and thrombi.

Chancroid (Soft Chancre)

Chancroid is an acute, sexually transmitted, ulcerative infection caused by *Haemophilus ducreyi*. The disease is most common in tropical and subtropical areas among lower socioeconomic groups and men who have frequent sex with prostitutes. Chancroid is one of the most common causes of genital ulcers in Africa and Southeast Asia, where it probably serves as an important cofactor in the transmission of HIV infection. Chancroid is uncommon in the United States, with 20 to 50 cases per year reported to the Centers for Disease Control and Prevention (CDC) in the past several years. The organism is difficult to grow in culture and PCR-based tests are not widely available, so chancroid is likely to be underdiagnosed.

MORPHOLOGY

Four to 7 days after inoculation, a tender erythematous papule involving the external genitalia develops. In males, the primary lesion is usually on the penis; in females, most lesions occur in the vagina or the periurethral area. Over several days, the surface of the primary lesion erodes to produce an irregular, painful ulcer. In contrast to the primary chancre of syphilis, the ulcer of chancroid is not indurated, and multiple lesions may be present. The base of the ulcer is covered by shaggy, yellow-gray exudate. The regional lymph nodes become enlarged and tender in about 50% of cases within 1 to 2 weeks after primary infection. If the infection is not treated, the enlarged nodes (buboes) may erode the overlying skin to produce chronic, draining ulcers.

Microscopically, the ulcer of chancroid contains a superficial zone of neutrophilic debris and fibrin, and an underlying zone of granulation tissue containing areas of necrosis and thrombosed vessels. A dense, lymphoplasmacytic inflammatory infiltrate is present beneath the layer of granulation tissue. Coccobacilli are sometimes demonstrable in Gram or silver stains, but they are often obscured by other bacteria that colonize the ulcer base.

Granuloma Inguinale

Granuloma inguinale, or donovanosis, is a sexually transmitted chronic inflammatory disease caused by *Klebsiella granulomatis* (formerly called *Calymmatobacterium donovani*), a minute, encapsulated, coccobacillus. Granuloma inguinale is uncommon in the United States and Western Europe but is endemic in rural areas in some developing countries. Untreated cases are characterized by the development of extensive scarring, often associated with lymphatic obstruction and lymphedema (elephantiasis) of the external genitalia. Culture of the organism is difficult, and PCR assays are not widely available, so the diagnosis is made by microscopic examination of smears or biopsy samples of the ulcer.

MORPHOLOGY

Granuloma inguinale begins as a raised papular lesion on the moist stratified squamous epithelium of the genitalia or, rarely, the oral mucosa or pharynx. The lesion eventually ulcerates and develops abundant granulation tissue, which manifests grossly as a protuberant, soft, painless mass. As the lesion enlarges, its borders become raised and indurated. Disfiguring scars may develop in untreated cases and are sometimes associated with urethral, vulvar, or anal **strictures**. Regional lymph nodes typically are spared or show only nonspecific reactive changes, in contrast to chancroid.

Microscopic examination of active lesions reveals marked epithelial hyperplasia at the borders of the ulcer, sometimes mimicking carcinoma (pseudoepitheliomatous hyperplasia). A mixture of neutrophils and mononuclear inflammatory cells is present at the base of the ulcer and beneath the surrounding epithelium. The organisms are demonstrable in Giemsa-stained smears of the exudate as minute, encapsulated coccobacilli (Donovan bodies) in macrophages. Silver stains (e.g., the Warthin-Starry stain) may also demonstrate the organism.

Mycobacteria

Bacteria in the genus *Mycobacterium* are slender, aerobic rods that grow in straight or branching chains. Mycobacteria have a unique waxy cell wall composed of unusual glycolipids and lipids including mycolic acid, which makes them acid-fast, meaning they will retain stains even on treatment with a mixture of acid and alcohol. They are weakly gram positive.

Tuberculosis

Tuberculosis is a serious chronic pulmonary and systemic disease caused most often by *M. tuberculosis*. The source of transmission is humans with active tuberculosis who release mycobacteria present in sputum. Oropharyngeal and intestinal tuberculosis contracted by drinking milk contaminated with *M. bovis* is rare in countries where milk is routinely pasteurized, but it is still seen in countries that have tuberculous dairy cows and unpasteurized milk.

Epidemiology. According to the World Health Organization (WHO), tuberculosis is estimated to affect more than a billion individuals worldwide, with 8.7 million new cases and 1.4 million deaths each year. But there is significant progress toward WHO targets for reduction in cases of tuberculosis. Globally, between 2010 and 2011, new cases of tuberculosis fell at a rate of 2.2%, and mortality has decreased by 41% since 1990. Infection with HIV makes people susceptible to rapidly progressive tuberculosis; 13% of the people who developed tuberculosis in 2011 were HIV-positive. In 2011 there were 10,528 new cases of tuberculosis in the United States, 62% of which occurred in foreign-born people.

Tuberculosis flourishes wherever there is poverty, crowding, and chronic debilitating illness. In the United States, tuberculosis is mainly a disease of older adults, immigrants from high-burden countries, racial and ethnic minorities, and people with AIDS. Certain disease states also increase the risk: diabetes mellitus, Hodgkin lymphoma, chronic lung disease (particularly silicosis), chronic renal failure, malnutrition, alcoholism, and immunosuppression.

It is important that infection with *M. tuberculosis* be differentiated from active disease. Most infections are acquired by person-to-person transmission of airborne organisms from an active case to a susceptible host. In most healthy people primary tuberculosis is asymptomatic, although it may cause fever and pleural effusion. Generally, the only evidence of infection, if any remains, is a tiny, fibrocalcific pulmonary nodule at the site of the infection. Viable organisms may remain dormant in such lesions for decades. If immune defenses are lowered, the infection may be reactivated, producing communicable and potentially life-threatening disease.

Infection typically leads to the development of delayed hypersensitivity to *M. tuberculosis* antigens, which can be detected by the tuberculin (PPD, or Mantoux) skin test. About 2 to 4 weeks after infection, intracutaneous injection of purified protein derivative of *M. tuberculosis* induces a visible and palpable induration that peaks in 48 to 72 hours. *A positive tuberculin test signifies T-cell–mediated immunity to mycobacterial antigens* but does not differentiate between infection and active disease. False-negative reactions may occur in the setting of certain viral infections, sarcoidosis, malnutrition, Hodgkin lymphoma, immunosuppression, and (notably) overwhelming active tuberculous disease. False-positive reactions may result from infection by atypical mycobacteria or prior vaccination with BCG *(Bacillus Calmette-Guerin)*, an attenuated strain of *M. bovis* that is used as a vaccine in some countries.

Pathogenesis. **The outcome of infection in a previously unexposed, immunocompetent person depends on the development of anti-mycobacterial T-cell–mediated immunity.** These T cells control the host response to the bacteria and also result in development of pathologic lesions, such as caseating granulomas and cavitation.

Infection by *M. tuberculosis* proceeds in steps, from initial infection of macrophages to a subsequent T_H1 response that both contains the bacteria and causes tissue damage (Fig. 8-24). Early in infection, *M. tuberculosis* replicates essentially unchecked within macrophages, while later in infection, the cell response stimulates macrophages to contain the proliferation of the bacteria. The steps in infection are the following.

- *Entry into macrophages. M. tuberculosis* enters macrophages by phagocytosis mediated by several receptors expressed on the phagocyte, including mannose binding lectin and CR3.
- *Replication in macrophages. M. tuberculosis* inhibits maturation of the phagosome and blocks formation of the phagolysosome, allowing the bacterium to replicate unchecked within the vesicle, protected from the microbicidal mechanisms of lysosomes. The bacterium blocks phagolysosome formation by inhibiting Ca^{2+} signals and the recruitment and assembly of the proteins that mediate phagosome-lysosome fusion. Thus, during the earliest stage of primary tuberculosis (<3 weeks) in the nonsensitized individual, bacteria proliferate in the pulmonary alveolar macrophages and air spaces, resulting in bacteremia and seeding of multiple sites. Despite the bacteremia, most people at this stage are asymptomatic or have a mild flu-like illness.
- Multiple pathogen associated molecular patterns (Chapter 6) of *M. tuberculosis*, including lipoproteins and glycolipids, are recognized by innate immune receptors, including Toll-like receptors such as TLR2.

A. INFECTION BEFORE ACTIVATION OF CELL MEDIATED IMMUNITY

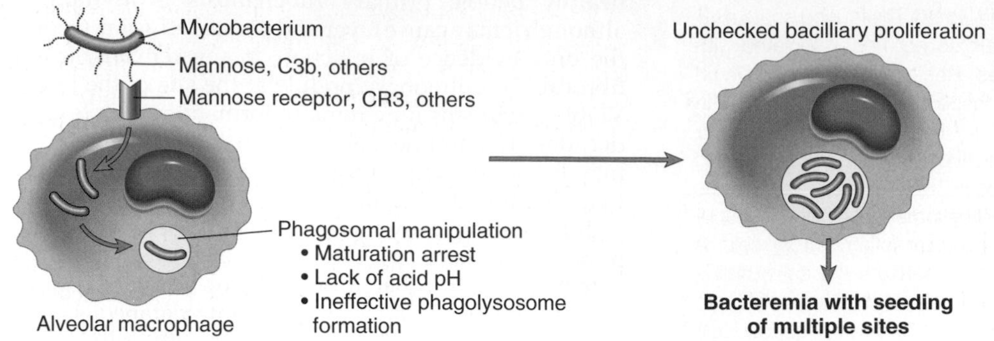

B. INITIATION AND CONSEQUENCES OF CELL MEDIATED IMMUNITY

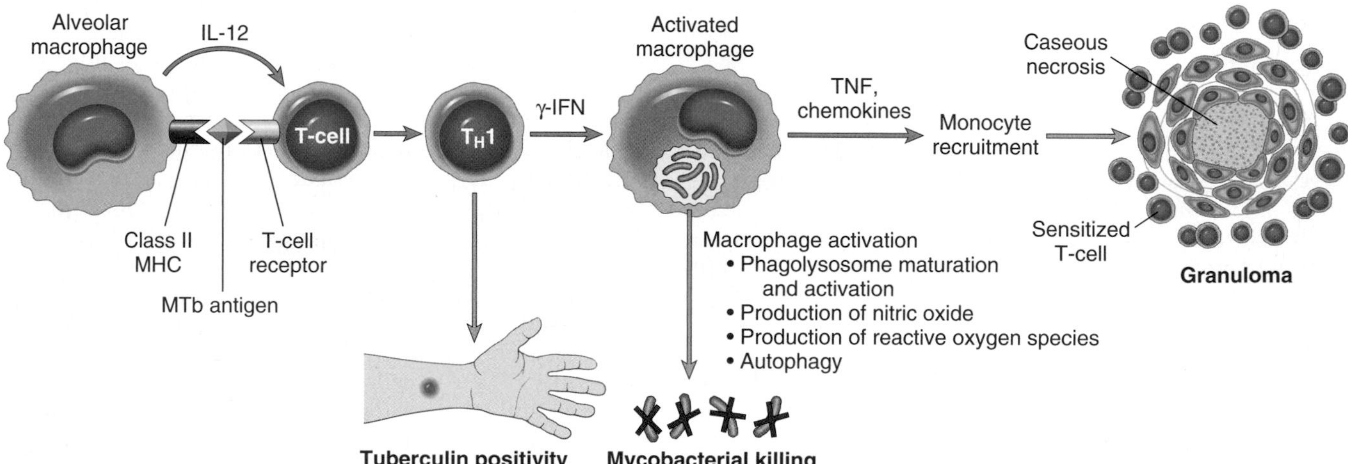

Figure 8-24 The sequence of events in primary pulmonary tuberculosis, commencing with inhalation of virulent *Mycobacterium tuberculosis* organisms and culminating with the development of cell-mediated immunity to the organism. **A,** Events occurring during early infection, before activation of T-cell–mediated immunity. **B,** The initiation and consequences of T-cell–mediated immunity. The development of resistance to the organism is accompanied by the appearance of a positive tuberculin test. γ-IFN, interferon-γ; MHC, major histocompatibility complex; MTB, *M. tuberculosis*; TNF, tumor necrosis factor.

This initiates and enhances the innate and adaptive immune responses to *M. tuberculosis,* as described below.

- *The T_H1 response.* About 3 weeks after infection, a T-helper 1 (T_H1) response is mounted that activates macrophages, enabling them to become bactericidal. The response is initiated by mycobacterial antigens that enter draining lymph nodes and are displayed to T cells. Differentiation of T_H1 cells depends on IL-12, which is produced by antigen-presenting cells that have encountered the mycobacteria. Stimulation of TLR2 by mycobacterial ligands promotes production of IL-12 by dendritic cells.
- *T_H1-mediated macrophage activation and killing of bacteria.* T_H1 cells, both in lymph nodes and in the lung, produce IFN-γ. **IFN-γ is the critical mediator that enables macrophages to contain the *M. tuberculosis* infection.** First, IFN-γ stimulates maturation of the phagolysosome in infected macrophages, exposing the bacteria to a lethal acidic, oxidizing environment. Second, IFN-γ stimulates expression of inducible nitric oxide synthase, which produces nitric oxide (NO). NO combines with other oxidants to create reactive nitrogen intermediates, which appear to be particularly important for killing of mycobacterium. Third, IFN-γ mobilizes antimicrobial peptides (defensins) against the bacteria. Finally, IFN-γ stimulates autophagy, a process that sequesters and then destroys damaged organelles and intracellular bacteria such as *M. tuberculosis.*
- *Granulomatous inflammation and tissue damage.* **In addition to stimulating macrophages to kill mycobacteria, the T_H1 response orchestrates the formation of granulomas and caseous necrosis.** Macrophages activated by IFN-γ differentiate into the "epithelioid histiocytes" that aggregate to form granulomas; some epithelioid cells may fuse to form giant cells. In many people this response halts the infection before significant tissue destruction or illness occur. In other people the infection progresses due to advanced age or immunosuppression, and the ongoing immune response results in caseation necrosis. Activated macrophages also secrete TNF and chemokines, which promote recruitment of more monocytes. The importance of TNF is underscored by the fact that patients with rheumatoid arthritis who are treated with a TNF antagonist have an increased risk of tuberculosis reactivation.

- *Role of other immune cells.* In addition to the T_H1 response, NKT cells that recognize mycobacterial lipid antigens bound to CD1 on antigen-presenting cells, or T cells that express a $\gamma\delta$ T-cell receptor, also make IFN-γ. However, it is clear that T_H1 cells have a central role in this process, since defects in any of the steps in generating a T_H1 response result in absence of resistance and disease progression.
- *Host susceptibility to disease.* People with genetic deficiencies in the IL-12 pathway and the IFN-γ pathway, including STAT1 a signal transducer for IFN-γ, are vulnerable to severe mycobacterial infections. Polymorphisms in a large number of genes, including HLA, IFN-γ, IFN-γ receptor, and TLR2 have been found to be associated with susceptibility to tuberculosis, but the contribution of these associations to disease development is still under investigation.
- *Immunological state in active tuberculosis.* It is not entirely clear why some people progress from latent to active tuberculosis. Recent studies demonstrate that neutrophils in the blood of people with active tuberculosis express a group of genes that are upregulated by type I and type II interferons. The expression levels of these interferon-responsive genes correspond to the extent of lung disease as assessed by radiographic analysis. Furthermore, the expression levels of these genes fall in response to treatment for tuberculosis. This type of analysis suggests that an early interferon response is a harbinger of development of active disease, and has potential utility for diagnosis of active tuberculosis or for monitoring the extent of or response to treatment of active disease. A caveat is that while most patients with latent tuberculosis do not have this pattern of gene expression, 10 to 20% of them do.

In summary, immunity to *M. tuberculosis* is primarily mediated by T_H1 cells, which stimulate macrophages to kill the bacteria. This immune response, while largely effective, comes at the cost of accompanying tissue destruction. Reactivation of the infection or re-exposure to the bacilli in a previously sensitized host results in rapid mobilization of a defensive reaction but also increased tissue necrosis. Just as T-cell immunity and resistance are correlated, so, too, the loss of T-cell immunity (indicated by tuberculin negativity in a previously tuberculin-positive individual) may be an ominous sign that resistance to the organism has faded.

Clinical Features. Clinical tuberculosis is separated into two important pathophysiologic types: "primary" tuberculosis, which occurs in the nonimmune host, and "secondary" tuberculosis, which occurs in the host who is immune to *M. tuberculosis.* The many clinical-pathologic patterns of tuberculosis are shown in Figure 8-25.

Primary tuberculosis is the form of disease that develops in a previously unexposed and therefore unsensitized, person. Clinically significant disease develops in about 5% of newly infected people. With primary tuberculosis the source of the organism is exogenous. In most people, the primary infection is contained, but in others, primary tuberculosis is progressive. The diagnosis of progressive primary tuberculosis in adults can be difficult. In contrast to secondary tuberculosis (apical disease with cavitation; see later), progressive primary tuberculosis more often resembles an acute bacterial pneumonia with consolidation of the lobe, hilar adenopathy, and pleural effusion. Lymphohematogenous dissemination following primary infection may result in the development of tuberculous meningitis and miliary tuberculosis (discussed later).

Secondary tuberculosis is the pattern of disease that arises in a previously sensitized host. It may follow shortly after primary tuberculosis, but more commonly it appears many years after the initial infection, usually when host resistance is weakened. It most commonly stems from reactivation of a latent infection, but may also result from exogenous reinfection in the face of waning host immunity or when a large inoculum of virulent bacilli overwhelms the host immune system. Reactivation is more common in low-prevalence areas, while reinfection plays an important role in regions of high contagion.

Secondary pulmonary tuberculosis classically involves the apex of the upper lobes of one or both lungs. Because of the preexistence of hypersensitivity, the bacilli elicit a prompt and marked tissue response that tends to wall off the focus of infection. As a result, the regional lymph nodes are less prominently involved early in secondary disease than they are in primary tuberculosis. On the other hand, cavitation occurs readily in the secondary form. Indeed, cavitation is almost inevitable in neglected secondary tuberculosis, and erosion of the cavities into an airway is an important source of infection because the person now coughs sputum that contains bacteria.

Localized secondary tuberculosis may be asymptomatic. When manifestations appear, they are usually insidious in onset. Systemic symptoms, probably related to cytokines released by activated macrophages (e.g., TNF and IL-1), often appear early in the course and include malaise, anorexia, weight loss, and fever. Commonly, the fever is low grade and remittent (appearing late each afternoon and then subsiding), and night sweats occur. With progressive pulmonary involvement, increasing amounts of sputum, at first mucoid and later purulent, appear. Some degree of hemoptysis is present in about half of all cases of pulmonary tuberculosis. Pleuritic pain may result from extension of the infection to the pleural surfaces. Extrapulmonary manifestations of tuberculosis are legion and depend on the organ system involved.

The diagnosis of pulmonary disease is based in part on the history and on physical and radiographic findings of consolidation or cavitation in the apices of the lungs. Ultimately, however, tubercle bacilli must be identified. Acid-fast smears and cultures of the sputum of patients suspected of having tuberculosis should be performed. Culture on solid agar media show growth at 3 to 6 weeks, but culture in liquid media can provide an answer within 2 weeks. PCR amplification of *M. tuberculosis* DNA allows for even more rapid diagnosis. A PCR test has recently come into use that both identifies the presence of *M. tuberculosis* and, if the organism is detected, whether it is resistant to rifampin. This PCR assay is as sensitive as culture in acid-fast smear-positive samples, but it is slightly less sensitive in smear-negative tuberculosis, and substantially less sensitive in children. Thus, culture remains the gold standard because it also allows testing of drug susceptibility. Multidrug resistance is now seen more commonly than

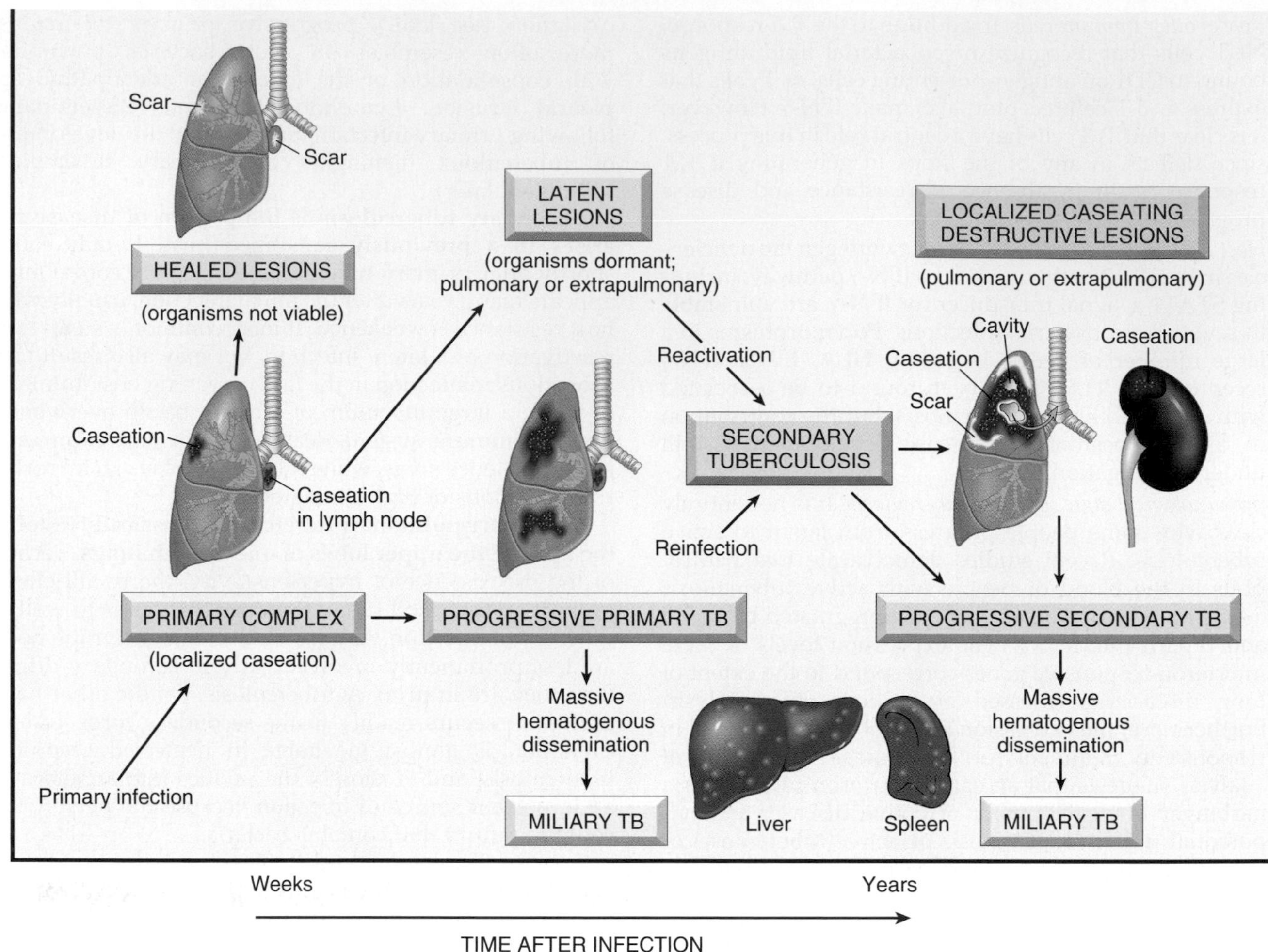

Figure 8-25 The natural history and spectrum of tuberculosis. (Adapted from a sketch provided by Professor R.K. Kumar, The University of New South Wales, School of Pathology, Sydney, Australia.)

it was in past years; hence, all newly diagnosed cases in the United States are treated with at least four drugs, unless the susceptibility of the bacterium from the source case is known. The prognosis is generally good if infections are localized to the lungs, except when they are caused by drug-resistant strains or occur in aged, debilitated, or immunosuppressed individuals, who are at high risk for developing extrapulmonary tuberculosis as well as progression of pulmonary disease.

All stages of HIV infection are associated with an increased risk of tuberculosis. The use of HAART reduces the risk of tuberculosis in people with HIV infection, but even with HAART, people infected with HIV are more likely to develop symptomatic tuberculosis. A low CD4 count before starting HAART is an important risk factor for development of tuberculosis, which underscores the role of the immune response in keeping reactivation of *M. tuberculosis* in check. Pulmonary manifestations of tuberculosis in HIV-infected individuals are extremely variable, ranging from focal lesions to multifocal infiltrates to localized apical disease with cavitation. The extent of immunodeficiency also determines the frequency of extrapulmonary involvement, rising from 10% to 15% in mildly immunosuppressed people to greater than 50% in those with severe immune deficiency. Other atypical features of tuberculosis in HIV-positive people include an increased frequency of false-negative sputum smears and tuberculin tests (the latter sometimes referred to as "anergy"), and the absence of characteristic granulomas in tissues, particularly in the late stages of HIV. The increased frequency of sputum smear-negativity is paradoxical because these immunosuppressed patients typically have higher bacterial loads. The likely explanation is that cavitation and bronchial damage are more severe in immunocompetent individuals, resulting in more bacilli in expelled sputum. In contrast, the absence of bronchial wall destruction due to reduced T-cell–mediated hypersensitivity results in the excretion of fewer bacilli in the sputum.

MORPHOLOGY

Primary Tuberculosis. In countries where consumption of infected milk has been eliminated, primary tuberculosis almost always begins in the lungs. Typically, the inhaled bacilli implant in the distal airspaces of the lower part of the upper lobe or the upper part of the lower lobe, usually close to the pleura. As sensitization develops, a 1- to 1.5-cm area of gray-white inflammation with consolidation emerges, known as the Ghon focus. In most cases, the center of this focus undergoes caseous necrosis. Tubercle bacilli, either free or within phagocytes, drain to the regional nodes, which also often caseate. **This combination of parenchymal lung lesion and nodal involvement is referred to as the Ghon complex** (Fig. 8-26). During the first few weeks there is also lymphatic and hematogenous dissemination to other parts of the body. In approximately 95% of cases, development of cell-mediated immunity controls the infection. Hence, the Ghon complex undergoes progressive fibrosis, often followed by radiologically detectable calcification (Ranke complex), and despite seeding of other organs, no lesions develop.

Histologically, sites of active involvement are marked by a characteristic granulomatous inflammatory reaction that forms both caseating and noncaseating tubercles (Fig. 8-27*A* to *C*). Individual tubercles are microscopic; it is only when multiple granulomas coalesce that they become macroscopically visible. The granulomas are usually enclosed within a fibroblastic rim punctuated by lymphocytes. Multinucleated giant cells are present in the granulomas. Immunocompromised people do not form the characteristic granulomas and their macrophages contain many bacilli (Fig. 8-27*D*).

Secondary Tuberculosis. The initial lesion is usually a small focus of consolidation, less than 2 cm in diameter, within 1 to 2 cm of the apical pleura. Such foci are sharply circumscribed,

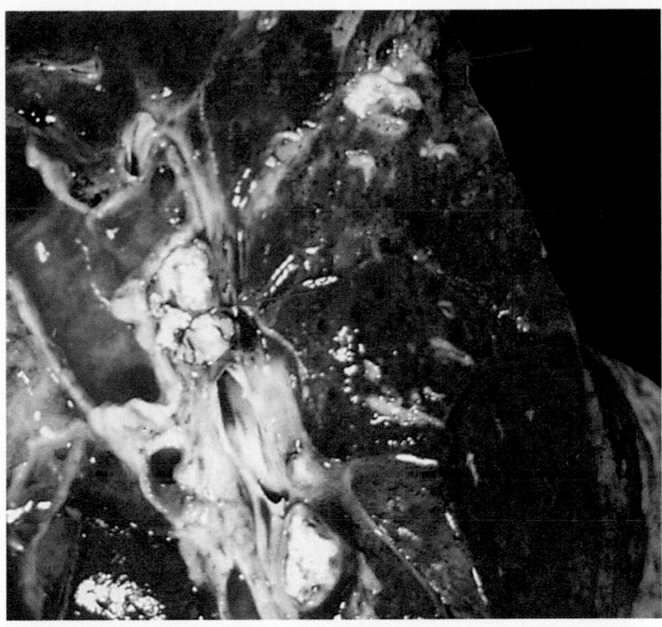

Figure 8-26 Primary pulmonary tuberculosis, Ghon complex. The gray-white parenchymal focus is under the pleura in the lower part of the upper lobe *(red arrow)*. Hilar lymph nodes with caseation are seen on the left *(blue arrow)*.

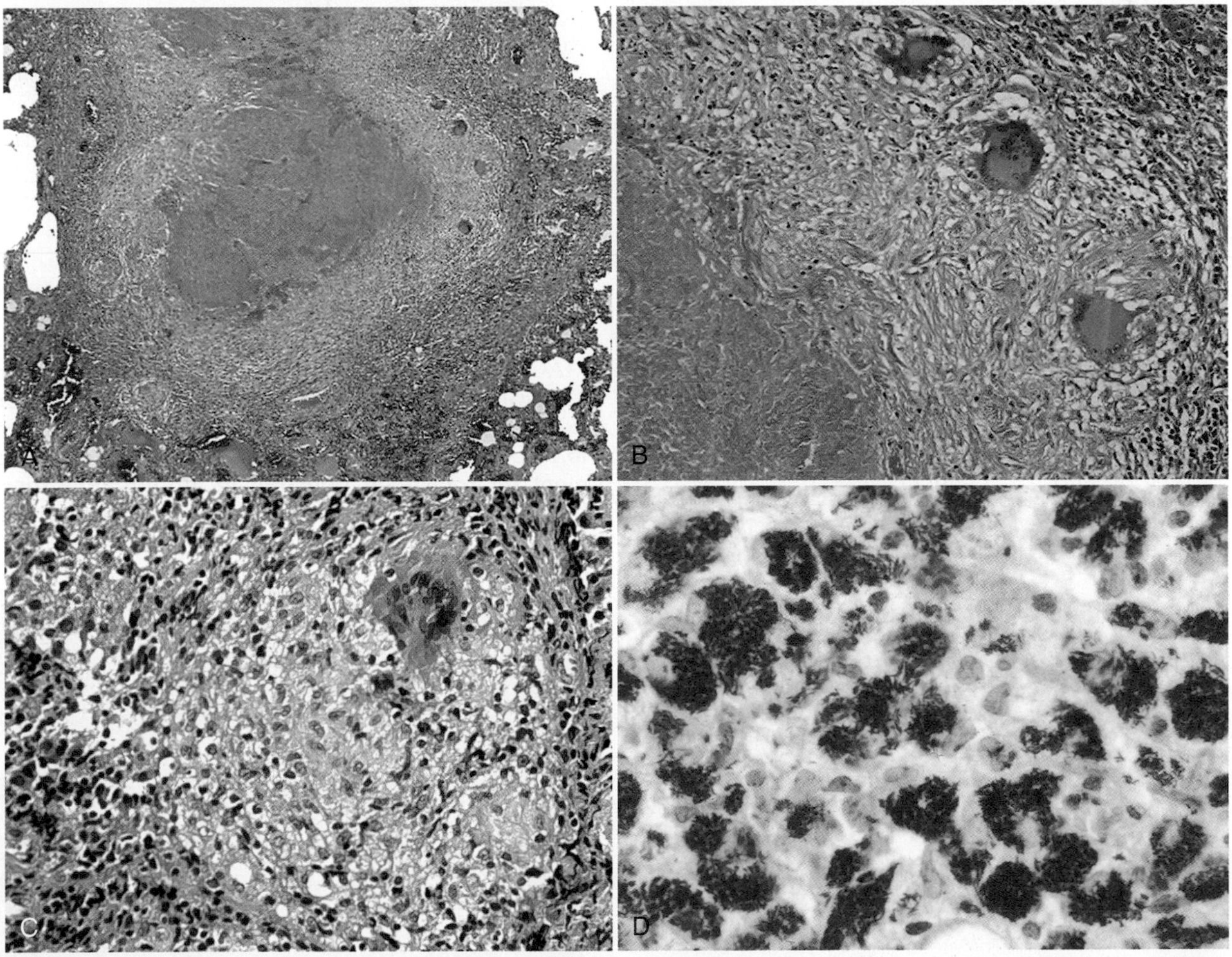

Figure 8-27 The morphologic spectrum of tuberculosis. Characteristic tubercle at low magnification **(A)** and high magnification **(B)** shows central granular caseation surrounded by epithelioid and multinucleate giant cells. This is the usual response in people who have developed cell-mediated immunity to the organism. *Inset:* Acid-fast stain shows rare positive (red) organisms. **C,** Occasionally, even in immunocompetent patients, tubercular granulomas may not show central caseation; hence regardless of the presence or absence of caseous necrosis, use of special stain for acid-fast organisms is indicated when granulomas are present. **D,** In this specimen from an immunocompromised patient, sheets of foamy macrophages packed with mycobacteria are seen (acid-fast stain).

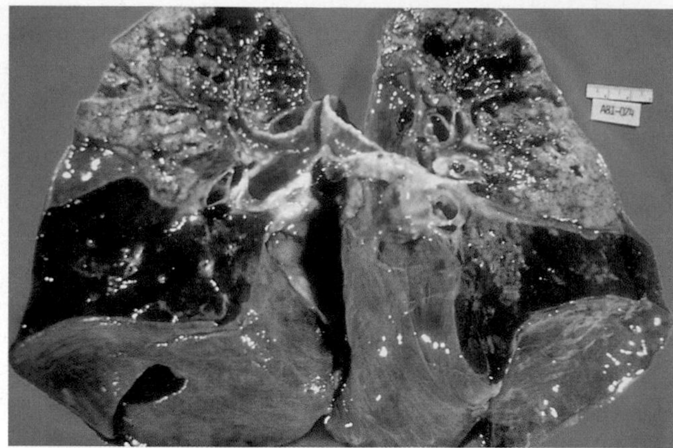

Figure 8-28 Secondary pulmonary tuberculosis. The upper parts of both lungs are riddled with gray-white areas of caseation and multiple areas of softening and cavitation.

firm and gray-white to yellow in color and have variable degrees of central caseation and peripheral fibrosis (Fig. 8-28). In immunocompetent individuals, the initial parenchymal focus undergoes progressive fibrous encapsulation, leaving only fibrocalcific scars. Histologically, the active lesions show characteristic coalescent tubercles with central caseation. Tubercle bacilli can often be identified with acid-fast stains in early exudative and caseous phases of granuloma formation but are usually too few to be found in the late, fibrocalcific stages. Localized, apical, secondary pulmonary tuberculosis may heal with fibrosis either spontaneously or after therapy, or the disease may progress and extend along several different pathways.

Progressive pulmonary tuberculosis may ensue in older adults and immunosuppressed people. The apical lesion expands into adjacent lung and eventually erodes into bronchi and vessels. This evacuates the caseous center, creating a ragged, irregular cavity that is poorly walled off by fibrous tissue. Erosion of blood vessels results in hemoptysis. With adequate treatment the process may be arrested, although healing by fibrosis often distorts the pulmonary architecture. The cavities, now free of inflammation, may persist or become fibrotic. If the treatment is inadequate or if host defenses are impaired, the infection may spread via airways, lymphatic channels, or the vascular system. **Miliary pulmonary disease** occurs when organisms draining through lymphatics enter the venous blood and circulate back to the lung. Individual lesions are either microscopic or small, visible (2-mm) foci of yellow-white consolidation scattered through the lung parenchyma (the adjective "miliary" is derived from the resemblance of these foci to millet seeds). Miliary lesions may expand and coalesce, resulting in consolidation of large regions or even whole lobes of the lung. With progressive pulmonary tuberculosis, the pleural cavity is invariably involved, and serous **pleural effusions**, **tuberculous empyema**, or **obliterative fibrous pleuritis** may develop. Progressive primary tuberculosis that occurs in immunosuppressed individuals spreads in a similar manner.

Endobronchial, **endotracheal**, and **laryngeal tuberculosis** may develop by spread through lymphatic channels or from expectorated infectious material. The mucosal lining may be studded with minute granulomatous lesions that may only be apparent microscopically.

Systemic miliary tuberculosis occurs when bacteria disseminate through the systemic arterial system. Miliary tuberculosis is most prominent in the liver, bone marrow, spleen, adrenals, meninges, kidneys, fallopian tubes, and epididymis, but could involve any organ (Fig. 8-29).

Isolated tuberculosis may appear in any of the organs or tissues seeded hematogenously and may be the presenting manifestation. Organs that are commonly involved include the meninges (tuberculous meningitis), kidneys (renal tuberculosis), adrenals (formerly an important cause of Addison disease), bones (osteomyelitis), and fallopian tubes (salpingitis). When the vertebrae are affected, the disease is referred to as **Pott disease**. Paraspinal "cold" abscesses in these patients may track along tissue planes and present as an abdominal or pelvic mass.

Lymphadenitis is the most frequent presentation of extrapulmonary tuberculosis, usually occurring in the cervical region ("scrofula"). In HIV-negative individuals, lymphadenitis tends to be unifocal and localized. HIV-positive people, on the other hand, almost always have multifocal disease, systemic symptoms, and either pulmonary or other organ involvement by active tuberculosis.

As previously mentioned, **intestinal tuberculosis** contracted by the drinking of contaminated milk is common in countries where bovine tuberculosis is present and milk is not pasteurized. In countries where milk is pasteurized, intestinal tuberculosis is more often caused by the swallowing of coughed-up infective material in patients with advanced pulmonary disease. Typically the organisms are seeded to mucosal lymphoid aggregates of the small and large bowel, which then undergo granulomatous inflammation that can lead to ulceration of the overlying mucosa, particularly in the ileum. Healing creates strictures.

Mycobacterium avium *Complex*

Mycobacterium avium and *M. intracellulare* are separate species, but the infections they cause are so similar that they are simply referred to as *M. avium* complex, or MAC. MAC is common in soil, water, dust, and domestic animals. **Clinically significant infection with MAC is uncommon except among people with T-cell immunodeficiency due to AIDS, and immunosuppression resulting from treatment for transplant rejection or autoimmune diseases.** In patients with marked T-cell immunodeficiency, MAC

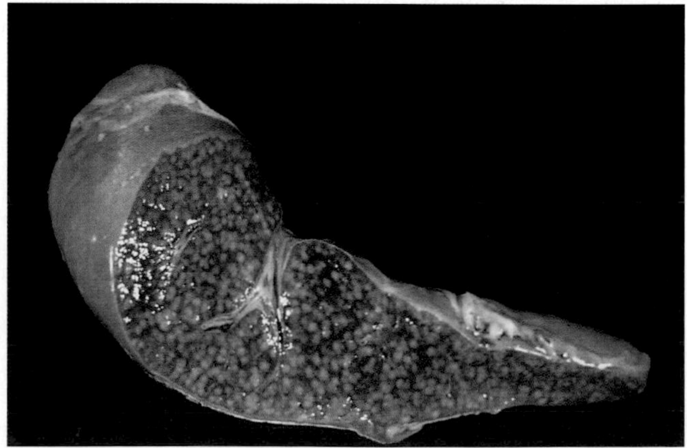

Figure 8-29 Miliary tuberculosis of the spleen. The cut surface shows numerous gray-white tubercles.

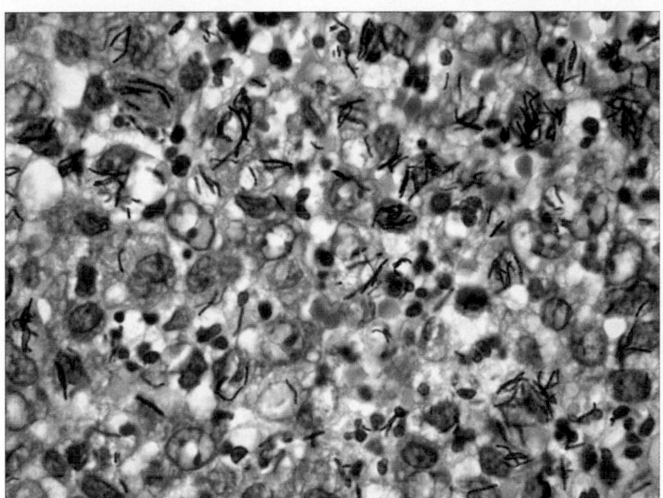

Figure 8-30 *Mycobacterium avium* infection in a patient with AIDS, showing massive infection with acid-fast organisms. This pattern is more common in patients with acquired immunodeficiencies.

causes widely disseminated infections, and organisms proliferate abundantly in many organs, including the lungs and gastrointestinal system. Patients are feverish, with drenching night sweats and weight loss. In the rare case of MAC in a person without HIV, the organisms primarily infect the lung, causing a productive cough and sometimes fever and weight loss.

MORPHOLOGY

The hallmark of MAC infections in patients with HIV is abundant acid-fast bacilli within macrophages (Fig. 8-30). Depending on the severity of immune deficiency, MAC infections can be widely disseminated throughout the mononuclear phagocyte system, causing enlargement of involved lymph nodes, liver, and spleen, or localized to the lungs. There may be a yellowish pigmentation to these organs secondary to the large number of organisms present in swollen macrophages. Granulomas, lymphocytes, and tissue destruction are rare.

Leprosy

Leprosy, or *Hansen disease,* is a slowly progressive infection caused by *M. leprae* that mainly affects the skin and peripheral nerves. Despite its low communicability, leprosy remains endemic among people living in several developing tropical nations.

Pathogenesis. The source of infection and route of transmission are not known, however human respiratory secretions or soil are likely origins. *M. leprae* is taken up by macrophages and disseminates in the blood, but it replicates primarily in relatively cool tissues of the skin and extremities. It proliferates best at 32° to 34°C, the temperature of the human skin. Like *M. tuberculosis, M. leprae* secretes no toxins, and its virulence is based on properties of its cell wall, which is similar enough to that of *M. tuberculosis* that immunization with BCG confers some protection against *M. leprae* infection. Cell-mediated immunity is manifested by delayed-type hypersensitivity reactions to dermal injections of a bacterial extract called *lepromin.*

***M. leprae* causes two strikingly different patterns of disease, called tuberculoid and lepromatous. The helper T-lymphocyte response to *M. leprae* determines whether an individual has tuberculoid or lepromatous leprosy.** People with the less severe *tuberculoid leprosy* have dry, scaly skin lesions that lack sensation. They often have asymmetric involvement of large peripheral nerves. The more severe form, *lepromatous leprosy,* includes symmetric skin thickening and nodules. In lepromatous leprosy, widespread invasion of the mycobacteria into Schwann cells and into endoneural and perineural macrophages damages the peripheral nervous system. In advanced cases of lepromatous leprosy, *M. leprae* is present in sputum and blood. People can also have intermediate forms of disease, called *borderline leprosy.*

As mentioned earlier, tuberculoid and lepromatous leprosy are associated with different T cell responses. People with tuberculoid leprosy have a T_H1 response associated with production of IL-2 and IFN-γ. As with *M. tuberculosis,* IFN-γ functions to mobilize an effective host macrophage response and hence the microbial burden is low. Lepromatous leprosy is associated with a weak T_H1 response and, in some cases, a relative increase in the T_H2 response. The net result is weak cell-mediated immunity and an inability to control the bacteria, which can be readily visualized in tissue sections. Occasionally, most often in the lepromatous form, antibodies are produced against *M. leprae* antigens. Paradoxically, these antibodies are usually not protective, but they may form immune complexes with free antigens that can lead to erythema nodosum, vasculitis, and glomerulonephritis.

MORPHOLOGY

Tuberculoid leprosy begins with localized flat, red skin lesions that enlarge and develop irregular shapes with indurated, elevated, hyperpigmented margins and depressed pale centers (central healing). Neuronal involvement dominates tuberculoid leprosy. Nerves become enclosed within granulomatous inflammatory reactions and, if small (e.g., the peripheral twigs), are destroyed (Fig. 8-31). Nerve degeneration causes skin anesthesias and skin and muscle atrophy that render the person liable to trauma of the affected parts, leading to the development of chronic skin ulcers. Contractures, paralyses, and autoamputation of fingers or toes may ensue. Facial nerve involvement can lead to paralysis of the eyelids, with keratitis and corneal ulcerations. On microscopic examination, all sites of involvement have granulomatous lesions closely resembling those found in tuberculosis. Because of the strong host defense, bacilli are almost never found, hence the name **paucibacillary** leprosy. The presence of granulomas and absence of bacteria reflect strong T-cell immunity. Because leprosy pursues an extremely slow course, spanning decades, most patients die with leprosy rather than of it.

Lepromatous leprosy involves the skin, peripheral nerves, anterior eye chamber, upper airways (down to the larynx), testes, hands, and feet. The vital organs and CNS are rarely affected, presumably because the core temperature is too high for growth of *M. leprae*. Lepromatous lesions contain large aggregates of lipid-laden macrophages (lepra cells), often filled with masses ("globi") of acid-fast bacilli (Fig. 8-32). Because of the abundant bacteria, lepromatous leprosy is referred to as

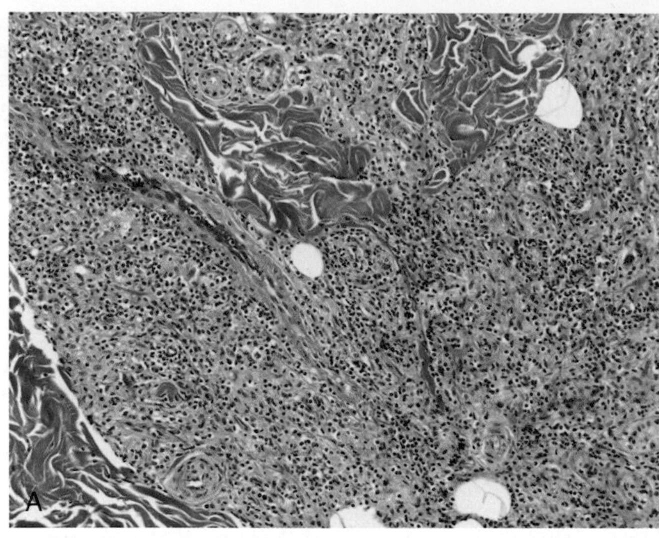

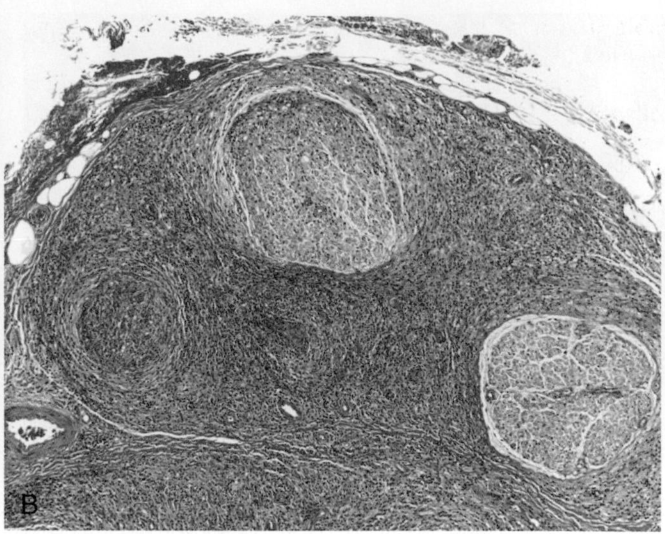

Figure 8-31 Two types of inflammatory infiltrates common in leprosy are: **A**, dense dermal macrophage infiltration surrounding adnexa, vessels, and nerves (resulting in subcutaneous nodules) and **B,** dense chronic lymphocytic and histiocytic infiltration into large nerve bundles (resulting in mononeuropathy).

multibacillary. Macular, papular, or nodular lesions form on the face, ears, wrists, elbows, and knees. With progression, the nodular lesions coalesce to yield a distinctive leonine facies. Most skin lesions are hypoesthetic or anesthetic. Lesions in the nose may cause persistent inflammation and bacilli-laden discharge. The peripheral nerves, particularly the ulnar and peroneal nerves where they approach the skin surface, are symmetrically invaded with mycobacteria, with minimal inflammation. Loss of sensation and trophic changes in the hands and feet follow the nerve lesions. Lymph nodes contain aggregates of bacteria-filled foamy macrophages in the paracortical (T cell) areas and reactive germinal centers. In advanced disease, aggregates of macrophages are also present in the splenic red pulp and the liver. The testes are usually extensively involved, leading to destruction of the seminiferous tubules and consequent sterility.

Spirochetes

Spirochetes are gram-negative, slender corkscrew-shaped bacteria with axial periplasmic flagella wound around a helical protoplasm. The bacteria are covered in a membrane called an outer sheath, which may mask bacterial antigens from the host immune response. *Treponema pallidum* subsp. *pallidum* is the microaerophilic spirochete that causes syphilis, a chronic venereal disease with multiple clinical presentations. Other closely related treponemes cause yaws *(Treponema pallidum* subsp. *pertenue)* and pinta *(Treponema pallidum* subsp. *carateum)*.

Syphilis

Syphilis is a chronic sexually transmitted disease with varied clinical and pathologic manifestations. The causative spirochete, *T. pallidum* subsp. *pallidum,* hereafter referred to simply as *T. pallidum,* is too slender to be seen in Gram stain, but it can be visualized by silver stains and immunofluorescence techniques (Fig. 8-33). Transplacental transmission of *T. pallidum* occurs readily, and active disease during pregnancy results in congenital syphilis. *T. pallidum* cannot be grown in culture. Public health programs and penicillin treatment reduced the number of cases of syphilis in the United States from the late 1940s until the 1970s. The number of cases has been relatively

Figure 8-32 Lepromatous leprosy. Acid-fast bacilli ("red snappers") within macrophages.

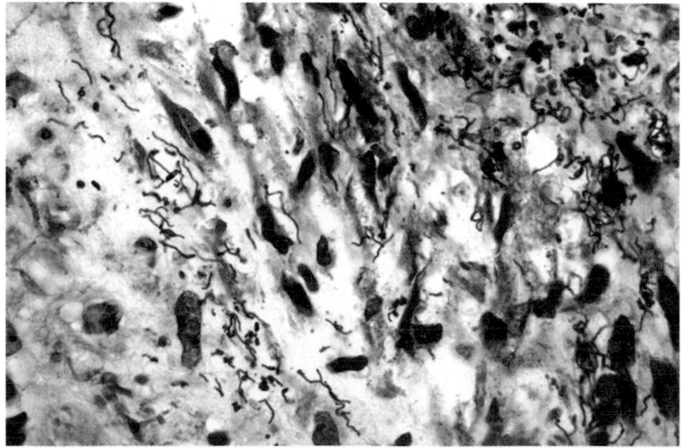

Figure 8-33 *Treponema pallidum* (Steiner silver stain) showing several spirochetes in histologic sections of placental syphilis.

stable in recent years, with approximately 14,000 being reported in 2010.

Pathogenesis. Proliferative endarteritis affecting small vessels with a surrounding plasma cell-rich infiltrate is characteristic of all stages of syphilis. Much of the pathology of syphilis can be ascribed to the ischemia produced by the vascular lesions. The pathogenesis of endarteritis is unknown.

The immune response to *T. pallidum* reduces the burden of bacteria and can lead to resolution of local lesions but does not reliably eliminate the systemic infection. Superficial sites of infection (chancres and rashes) have an intense inflammatory infiltrate that includes T cells, plasma cells and macrophages that surround the bacteria. The infiltrating CD4+ T cells are $T_{H}1$ cells that may activate macrophages to kill the bacteria. Treponeme-specific antibodies are detectable and these activate complement in the lesion and opsonize the bacteria for phagocytosis by macrophages. In many patients, the organism persists despite these host responses. A protein in the outer membrane of *T. pallidum*, TprK, accumulates structural diversity during the course of infection through gene conversion (recombination) between silent donor sites and the *tprK* gene and this might contribute to antigenic diversity that allows the organism to persist.

Syphilis is divided into three stages, with distinct clinical and pathologic manifestations (Fig. 8-34).

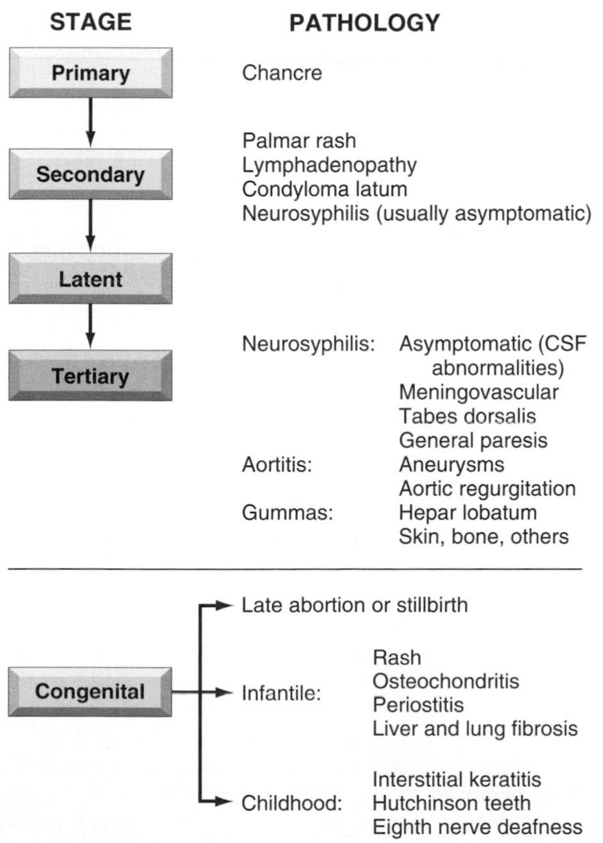

STAGE	PATHOLOGY	
Primary	Chancre	
Secondary	Palmar rash Lymphadenopathy Condyloma latum Neurosyphilis (usually asymptomatic)	
Latent		
Tertiary	Neurosyphilis:	Asymptomatic (CSF abnormalities) Meningovascular Tabes dorsalis General paresis
	Aortitis:	Aneurysms Aortic regurgitation
	Gummas:	Hepar lobatum Skin, bone, others
Congenital	Late abortion or stillbirth	
	Infantile:	Rash Osteochondritis Periostitis Liver and lung fibrosis
	Childhood:	Interstitial keratitis Hutchinson teeth Eighth nerve deafness

Figure 8-34 Protean manifestations of syphilis.

Primary Syphilis. This stage, occurring approximately 3 weeks after infection, features a single firm, nontender, raised, red lesion (chancre) located at the site of treponemal invasion on the penis, cervix, vaginal wall, or anus. The chancre heals with or without therapy. Spirochetes are plentiful within the chancre and spread from there throughout the body by hematologic and lymphatic dissemination.

Secondary Syphilis. This stage is marked by painless, superficial lesions of the skin and mucosal surfaces. It occurs 2 to 10 weeks after the primary chancre in approximately 75% of untreated people. Skin lesions frequently occur on the palms or soles of the feet, may be maculopapular, scaly, or pustular. Moist areas of the skin, such as the anogenital region, inner thighs, and axillae, may have *condylomata lata*, which are broad-based, elevated plaques. Silvery-gray superficial erosions may form on the oral, pharyngeal and genital mucous membranes. Lymphadenopathy, mild fever, malaise, and weight loss are also common in secondary syphilis. Asymptomatic neurosyphilis (discussed below) occurs in 8-40% of patients and symptomatic neurosyphilis, with meningitis, visual changes or hearing changes, occurs in 1-2%. Secondary syphilis lasts several weeks and then the person enters the latent stage of the disease.

Tertiary Syphilis. Tertiary syphilis has three main manifestations: cardiovascular syphilis, neurosyphilis, and so-called *benign tertiary syphilis*. These may occur alone or in combination. Tertiary syphilis occurs in one third of untreated patients, usually after a latent period of 5 years or more.

- *Cardiovascular syphilis*, in the form of syphilitic aortitis, accounts for more than 80% of cases of tertiary disease. The pathogenesis of this vascular lesion is not known, but the scarcity of treponemes and the intense inflammatory infiltrate suggest that the immune response plays a role. The aortitis leads to slowly progressive dilation of the aortic root and arch, which causes aortic valve insufficiency and aneurysms of the proximal aorta (Chapter 11).
- *Neurosyphilis* may be symptomatic or asymptomatic. Symptomatic neurosyphilis is discussed in Chapter 28. Asymptomatic neurosyphilis, which accounts for about one third of neurosyphilis cases, is initially suspected on detection of CSF abnormalities such as pleocytosis (increased numbers of inflammatory cells), elevated protein levels, or decreased glucose, and is confirmed by detection of antibodies stimulated by the spirochetes (discussed later) in the CSF. Antibiotics are given for a longer time if the spirochetes have spread to the CNS, so patients with tertiary syphilis should be tested for neurosyphilis even if they do not have neurologic symptoms.
- *Benign tertiary syphilis* is characterized by the formation of *gummas* in bone, skin, and the mucous membranes of the upper airway and mouth. Gummas are nodular lesions probably related to the development of delayed hypersensitivity to the bacteria. Skeletal involvement characteristically causes pain, tenderness, swelling, and pathologic fractures. Gummas in the skin and mucous membranes may produce nodular lesions or, rarely,

destructive, ulcerative lesions. Gummas are rare because of the use of effective antibiotics.

Congenital Syphilis. Congenital syphilis occurs most frequently during maternal primary or secondary syphilis, when the spirochetes are most numerous. Intrauterine death and perinatal death each occurs in approximately 25% of cases of untreated congenital syphilis.

Manifestations of congenital syphilis are divided into those that occur in the first 2 years of life (infantile syphilis) and those that occur later (tardive syphilis). Infantile syphilis is often manifested by nasal discharge and congestion (snuffles) in the first few months of life. A desquamating or bullous rash can lead to sloughing of the skin, particularly of the hands and feet and around the mouth and anus. Hepatomegaly and skeletal abnormalities are common. Late manifestations develop in nearly half of untreated children with neonatal syphilis.

Serologic Tests for Syphilis. Serology remains the mainstay of diagnosis of syphilis. Serologic tests include nontreponemal antibody tests and antitreponemal antibody tests. Nontreponemal tests measure antibody to cardiolipin, a phospholipid present in both host tissues and *T. pallidum*. These antibodies are detected in the rapid plasma reagin (RPR) and Venereal Disease Research Laboratory (VDRL) tests. Treponemal antibody tests measure antibodies that specifically react with *T. pallidum*. These include the fluorescent treponemal antibody absorption test and the *T. pallidum* enzyme immunoassay test.

The use of these tests is complex because of differences in the antibody responses they measure and imperfections in the tests.

- Both treponemal and nontreponemal tests are only moderately sensitive (~70%-85%) for primary syphilis.
- Both types of tests are very sensitive (>95%) for secondary syphilis.
- Treponemal tests are very sensitive for tertiary and latent syphilis. In contrast, nontreponemal antibody titers fall with time and so nontreponemal tests are somewhat less sensitive for tertiary or latent syphilis.
- Nontreponemal antibody levels fall with successful treatment of syphilis, and so changes in the titers detected in these tests can be used to monitor therapy.
- Treponemal tests, which are nonquantitative, remain positive even after successful therapy.
- Both nontreponemal and treponemal tests can be used to screen for syphilis, but positive results should be confirmed using a test of the other type (e.g., confirm nontreponemal positive test results with a treponemal test). Confirmatory testing is needed because false-positive results can occur in both nontreponemal and treponemal tests. Causes of false-positive results in these tests include pregnancy, autoimmune diseases, and infections other than syphilis.

MORPHOLOGY

In primary syphilis a chancre occurs on the penis or scrotum of 70% of men and on the vulva or cervix of 50% of women. The chancre is a slightly elevated, firm, reddened papule, up to several centimeters in diameter, that erodes to create a clean-based shallow ulcer. The contiguous induration creates a button-like mass directly adjacent to the eroded skin, providing the basis for the designation hard chancre (Fig. 8-35). On histologic examination, the chancre contains an intense infiltrate of plasma cells, with scattered macrophages and lymphocytes and a proliferative endarteritis. The endarteritis starts with endothelial cell activation and proliferation and progresses to intimal fibrosis (Fig. 8-5). The regional nodes are usually enlarged due to nonspecific acute or chronic lymphadenitis, plasma cell–rich infiltrates, or granulomas.

In secondary syphilis widespread mucocutaneous lesions involve the oral cavity, palms of the hands, and soles of the feet. The rash frequently consists of discrete red-brown macules less than 5 mm in diameter, but it may be follicular, pustular, annular, or scaling. Red lesions in the mouth or vagina contain the most organisms and are the most infectious. Histologically, the mucocutaneous lesions of secondary syphilis show the same plasma cell infiltrate and obliterative endarteritis as the primary chancre, although the inflammation is often less intense.

Tertiary syphilis most frequently involves the aorta; the CNS; and the liver, bones, and testes. The aortitis is caused by endarteritis of the vasa vasorum of the proximal aorta. Occlusion of the vasa vasorum results in scarring of the media of the proximal aortic wall, causing a loss of elasticity. There may be narrowing of the coronary artery ostia caused by subintimal scarring with resulting myocardial ischemia. The morphologic and clinical features of syphilitic aortitis are discussed in greater detail with diseases of the blood vessels (Chapter 11).

Neurosyphilis takes one of several forms, designated meningovascular syphilis, tabes dorsalis, and general paresis (Chapter 28).

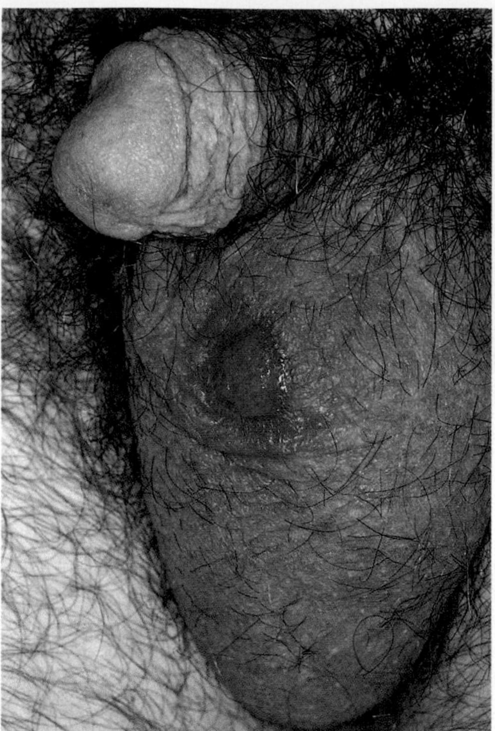

Figure 8-35 Syphilitic chancre in the scrotum (see Fig. 8-35 for the histopathology of syphilis). (Courtesy Dr. Richard Johnson, Beth Israel-Deaconess Hospital, Boston, Mass.)

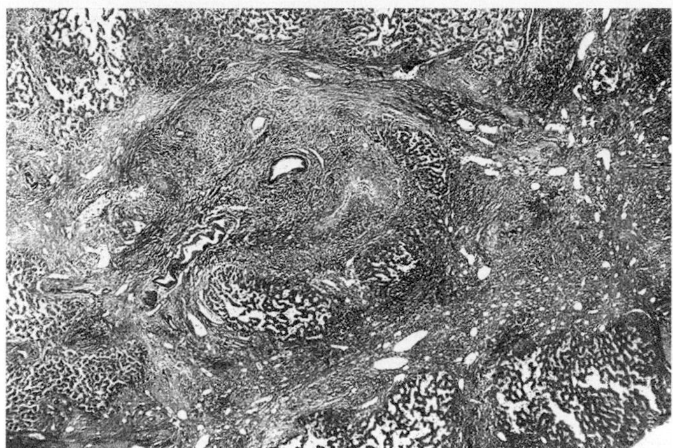

Figure 8-36 Trichrome stain of liver shows a gumma (scar), stained blue, caused by tertiary syphilis (the hepatic lesion is also known as hepar lobatum).

Syphilitic gummas are white-gray and rubbery, occur singly or multiply, and vary in size from microscopic lesions resembling tubercles to large tumor-like masses. They occur in most organs but particularly in skin, subcutaneous tissue, bone, and joints. In the liver, scarring as a result of gummas may cause a distinctive hepatic lesion known as hepar lobatum (Fig. 8-36). On histologic examination, the gummas have centers of coagulated, necrotic material and margins composed of plump, palisading macrophages and fibroblasts surrounded by large numbers of mononuclear leukocytes, chiefly plasma cells. Treponemes are scant in gummas and are difficult to demonstrate.

The rash of **congenital syphilis** is more severe than that of adult secondary syphilis. It is a bullous eruption of the palms and soles of the feet associated with epidermal sloughing. **Syphilitic osteochondritis and periostitis** affect all bones, but lesions of the nose and lower legs are most distinctive. Destruction of the vomer causes collapse of the bridge of the nose and, later on, the characteristic saddle nose deformity. Periostitis of the tibia leads to excessive new bone growth on the anterior surfaces and anterior bowing, or saber shin. There is also widespread disturbance in endochondral bone formation. The epiphyses become widened as the cartilage overgrows, and cartilage is found in displaced islands within the metaphysis.

The **liver** is often severely affected in congenital syphilis. Diffuse fibrosis permeates lobules to isolate hepatic cells into small nests, accompanied by the characteristic lymphoplasmacytic infiltrate and vascular changes. Gummas are occasionally found in the liver, even in early cases. The **lungs** may be affected by a diffuse interstitial fibrosis. In the syphilitic stillborn, the lungs appear pale and airless (pneumonia alba). The generalized spirochetemia may lead to diffuse interstitial inflammatory reactions in virtually any other organ (e.g., the pancreas, kidneys, heart, spleen, thymus, endocrine organs, and CNS).

The late manifestations of congenital syphilis include a distinctive **triad of interstitial keratitis, Hutchinson teeth, and eighth-nerve deafness**. In addition to interstitial keratitis, the ocular changes include choroiditis and abnormal retinal pigmentation. Hutchinson teeth are small incisors shaped like a screwdriver or a peg, often with notches in the enamel. Eighth-nerve deafness and optic nerve atrophy develop secondary to meningovascular syphilis.

Lyme Disease

Lyme disease is a common arthropod-borne illness caused by the spirochete, *Borrelia burgdorferi*, which can be localized or disseminated with a tendency to cause persistent chronic arthritis. It is named for the Connecticut town where there was an epidemic of arthritis associated with skin erythema in the mid-1970s. It is caused by several subspecies of the spirochete *Borrelia burgdorferi,* which is transmitted from rodents to people by *Ixodes* deer ticks. Lyme disease is endemic in the United States, Europe, and Japan. In the United States there were approximately 33,000 confirmed and probable cases reported in 2011. Most cases occur in the northeastern states and the upper Midwest. In endemic areas, *B. burgdorferi* infects up to 50% of ticks, which may also be infected with *Ehrlichia* and *Babesia*. Serology is the main method of diagnosis, but PCR can be done on infected tissue.

Lyme disease involves multiple organ systems and is divided into three stages (Fig. 8-37).

- In *stage 1 (localized infection)* spirochetes multiply and spread in the dermis at the site of a tick bite, causing an expanding area of redness, often with a pale center. This lesion, called *erythema migrans,* may be accompanied by fever and lymphadenopathy. The rash spontaneously disappears in 4 to 12 weeks.
- In *stage 2 (disseminated infection)* spirochetes spread hematogenously throughout the body and cause secondary skin lesions, lymphadenopathy, migratory joint and muscle pain, cardiac arrhythmias, and meningitis often associated with cranial nerve involvement.
- *Stage 3 (persistent infection)* manifests many months after the tick bite. *B. burgdorferi* usually causes a chronic arthritis sometimes with severe damage to large joints. Less often, patients will have polyneuropathy and encephalitis that vary from mild to debilitating.

Pathogenesis. *B. burgdorferi* does not produce LPS or exotoxins that damage the host. **Much of the pathology associated with *B. burgdorferi* is thought to be secondary to the immune response against the bacteria and the inflammation that accompanies it.** The initial immune response is stimulated by binding of bacterial lipoproteins to TLR2

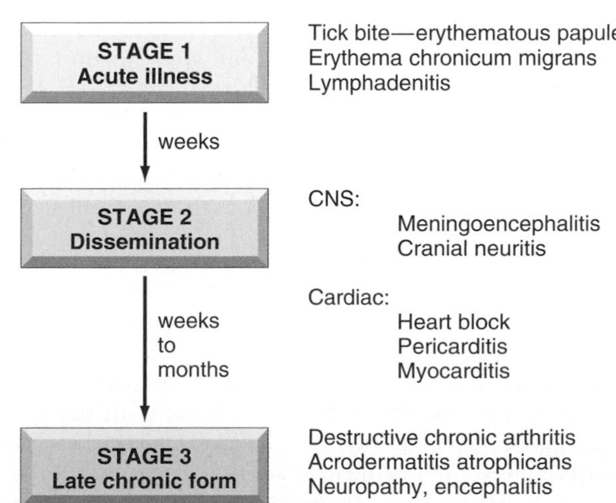

Figure 8-37 Clinical stages of Lyme disease.

on macrophages. In response, these cells release proinflammatory cytokines (IL-6 and TNF) and generate bactericidal reactive nitrogen intermediates, reducing but usually not eliminating the infection.

The inflammatory lesions are likely triggered by T cells and cytokines. *Borrelia*-specific antibodies, made 2 to 4 weeks after infection, direct complement-mediated phagocytosis and killing of the bacteria; however, *B. burgdorferi* escapes the antibody response through antigenic variation. Similar to *Borrelia hermsii*, a cause of endemic relapsing fever, *B. burgdorferi* has a plasmid with a single promoter sequence and multiple coding sequences for an antigenic surface protein, VlsE, each of which can shuttle into position next to the promoter and be expressed. Thus, as the antibody response to one VlsE protein is mounted, bacteria expressing an alternate VlsE protein can escape immune recognition. Chronic manifestations of Lyme disease, such as the late arthritis, are probably caused by the immune response against persistent bacteria.

MORPHOLOGY

Skin lesions caused by *B. burgdorferi* are characterized by edema and a lymphocytic-plasma cell infiltrate. In early Lyme arthritis, the synovium resembles early rheumatoid arthritis, with villous hypertrophy, lining-cell hyperplasia, and abundant lymphocytes and plasma cells in the subsynovium. A distinctive feature of Lyme arthritis is an arteritis, which produces onionskin-like lesions resembling those seen in lupus (Chapter 6). In late Lyme disease there may be extensive erosion of the cartilage in large joints. In Lyme meningitis the CSF is hypercellular, due to a marked lymphoplasmacytic infiltrate, and contains antispirochete IgGs.

Anaerobic Bacteria

Many anaerobic bacteria are normal flora in sites of the body that have low oxygen levels. The anaerobic flora cause disease (abscesses or peritonitis) when they are introduced into normally sterile sites or when the balance of organisms is upset and pathogenic anaerobes overgrow (e.g., *Clostridium difficile* colitis with antibiotic treatment). Environmental anaerobes also cause disease (tetanus, botulism, and gas gangrene).

Abscesses Caused by Anaerobes

Commensal bacteria from adjacent sites (oropharynx, intestine, and female genital tract) are the usual cause of abscesses, so the species found in an abscess often reflect the normal flora in that site. Abscesses are usually caused by mixed anaerobic and facultative aerobic bacterial infections. Because most anaerobes that cause abscesses are part of the normal flora, it is not surprising that these organisms do not produce significant toxins.

The bacteria found in head and neck abscesses reflect oral and pharyngeal flora. Common anaerobes at this site include the gram-negative bacilli *Prevotella* and *Porphyromonas* species, often mixed with the facultative *S. aureus* and *S. pyogenes*. *Fusobacterium necrophorum*, an oral commensal, causes Lemierre syndrome, characterized by infection of the lateral pharyngeal space and septic jugular vein thrombosis. Abdominal abscesses are caused by the anaerobes of the gastrointestinal tract, including gram-positive *Peptostreptococcus* and *Clostridium* species, as well as gram-negative *Bacteroides fragilis* and *E. coli*. Genital tract infections in women (e.g., Bartholin cyst abscesses and tubo-ovarian abscesses) are caused by anaerobic gram-negative bacilli, such as *Prevotella* species, often mixed with *E. coli* or *Streptococcus agalactiae*.

MORPHOLOGY

Abscesses caused by anaerobes contain discolored and foul-smelling pus that is often poorly walled off. Otherwise, these lesions pathologically resemble those of the common pyogenic infections. Gram stain reveals mixed infection with gram-positive and gram-negative rods and gram-positive cocci mixed with neutrophils.

Clostridial Infections

Clostridium species are gram-positive bacilli that grow under anaerobic conditions and produce spores that are present in the soil. Four types of disease are caused by *Clostridium*:

- *C. perfringens, C. septicum*, and other species cause cellulitis and myonecrosis of traumatic and surgical wounds (*gas gangrene*), uterine myonecrosis often associated with illegal abortions, mild food poisoning, and infection of the small bowel associated with ischemia or neutropenia that often leads to severe sepsis.
- *C. tetani*, the cause of *tetanus*, proliferates in puncture wounds and in the umbilical stump of newborn infants and releases a potent neurotoxin that causes increased muscle tone and generalized spasms of skeletal muscles (lockjaw). Tetanus toxoid (formalin-fixed tetanus toxin) is part of the DPT (diphtheria, pertussis, and tetanus) immunization, and this has greatly decreased the incidence of tetanus worldwide.
- *C. botulinum*, the cause of *botulism*, grows in inadequately cooked foods and releases a potent neurotoxin that blocks synaptic release of acetylcholine and causes flaccid paralysis of respiratory and skeletal muscles.
- *C. difficile* overgrows other intestinal flora in antibiotic-treated people, releases toxins, and causes *pseudomembranous colitis* (Chapter 17).

Clostridial infections can be diagnosed by culture (cellulitis, myonecrosis), toxin assays (pseudomembranous colitis), or both (botulism).

Pathogenesis. *Clostridium perfringens* does not grow in the presence of oxygen, so tissue death is essential for growth of the bacteria in the host. **These bacteria release collagenase and hyaluronidase that degrade extracellular matrix proteins and contribute to bacterial invasiveness, but their most powerful virulence factors are the many toxins they produce.** *C. perfringens* secretes 14 toxins, the most important of which is α-toxin. This toxin has multiple actions. It is a phospholipase C that degrades lecithin, a major component of cell membranes, and so destroys red cells, platelets, and muscle cells, causing myonecrosis. It also has a sphingomyelinase activity that contributes to nerve sheath damage.

Ingestion of food contaminated with *C. perfringens* causes a brief diarrhea. Spores, usually in contaminated meat, survive cooking, and the organism proliferates in cooling food. *C. perfringens* enterotoxin forms pores in the epithelial cell membranes, lysing the cells and disrupting tight junctions between epithelial cells.

The neurotoxins produced by *C. botulinum* and *C. tetani* both inhibit release of neurotransmitters, resulting in paralysis. Botulism toxin, eaten in contaminated foods or absorbed from wounds infected with *C. botulinum*, binds gangliosides on motor neurons and is transported into the cell. In the cytoplasm, the A fragment of botulism toxin cleaves a protein, called synaptobrevin, that mediates fusion of neurotransmitter-containing vesicles with the neuron membrane. By blocking vesicle fusion, botulism toxin prevents the release of acetylcholine at the neuromuscular junction, resulting in flaccid paralysis. If the respiratory muscles are affected, botulism can lead to death. The widespread use of botulism toxin (Botox) in cosmetic surgery is based on its ability to cause paralysis of strategically chosen muscles on the face. Tetanus toxin causes a violent spastic paralysis by blocking release of γ-aminobutyric acid, a neurotransmitter that inhibits motor neurons.

C. difficile produces toxin A, an enterotoxin that stimulates chemokine production and thus attracts leukocytes, and toxin B, a cytotoxin, which causes distinctive cytopathic effects in cultured cells. Both toxins are glucosyl transferases and are part of a pathogenicity island that is absent from the chromosomes of nonpathogenic strains of *C. difficile*.

MORPHOLOGY

The most significant lesions are caused by *C. perfringens*; these are described next. **Clostridial cellulitis**, which originates in wounds, can be differentiated from infection caused by pyogenic cocci by its foul odor, its thin, discolored exudate, and the relatively quick and wide tissue destruction. On microscopic examination, the amount of tissue necrosis is disproportionate to the number of neutrophils and gram-positive bacteria present (Fig. 8-38). Clostridial cellulitis, which often has granulation tissue at its borders, is treatable by debridement and antibiotics.

In contrast, **clostridial gas gangrene** is life-threatening and is characterized by marked edema and enzymatic necrosis of involved muscle cells 1 to 3 days after injury. An extensive fluid exudate, which is lacking in inflammatory cells, causes swelling of the affected region and the overlying skin, which develops large bullous vesicles that rupture. Gas bubbles caused by bacterial fermentation appear within the gangrenous tissues. As the infection progresses, the inflamed muscles become soft, blue-black, friable, and semifluid as a result of the massive proteolytic action of the released bacterial enzymes. On microscopic examination there is severe **myonecrosis**, extensive hemolysis, and marked vascular injury, with thrombosis. *C. perfringens* is also associated with dusk-colored, wedge-shaped infarcts in the small bowel, particularly in neutropenic people. Regardless of the site of entry, when *C. perfringens* disseminates hematogenously there is widespread formation of gas bubbles.

Despite the severe neurologic damage caused by botulinum and tetanus toxins, the neuropathologic changes are subtle and nonspecific.

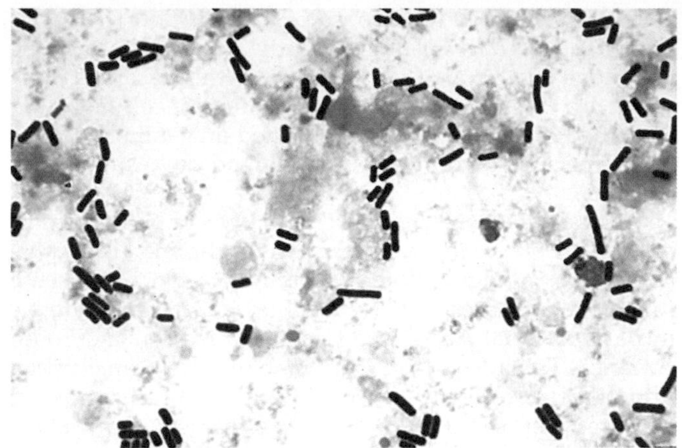

Figure 8-38 Boxcar-shaped gram-positive *Clostridium perfringens* intermingled with necrotic debris in gangrenous tissue.

Obligate Intracellular Bacteria

Obligate intracellular bacteria proliferate only within host cells, although some may survive outside of cells. These organisms are well adapted to the intracellular environment, with membrane pumps to capture amino acids and ATP for energy. Some are unable to synthesize ATP at all (e.g., *Chlamydia*), while others synthesize at least some of their own ATP (e.g., the rickettsiae).

Chlamydial Infections

C. trachomatis is a small gram-negative bacterium that is an obligate intracellular parasite. *C. trachomatis* exists in two forms during its unique life cycle. The infectious form, called the *elementary body,* is a metabolically inactive, spore-like structure. Host cells take up the elementary body by receptor-mediated endocytosis. The bacteria prevent fusion of the endosome and lysosome by an unknown mechanism. Inside the endosome the elementary body differentiates into a metabolically active form, called the *reticulate body*. The reticulate body uses ATP and amino acids from the host cell to replicate and forms new infectious elementary bodies.

The various diseases caused by *C. trachomatis* infection are associated with different serotypes of the bacteria: urogenital infections and inclusion conjunctivitis (serotypes D through K), lymphogranuloma venereum (serotypes L1, L2, and L3), and an ocular infection of children, trachoma (serotypes A, B, and C). The venereal infections caused by *C. trachomatis* are discussed here.

Genital infection by *C. trachomatis* is the most common sexually transmitted bacterial disease in the world. In 2010, approximately 1.3 million cases of genital chlamydia were reported to the CDC. Before the identification of *C. trachomatis,* people infected with this organism were diagnosed with nongonococcal urethritis.

Genital *C. trachomatis* infections (other than lymphogranuloma venereum, discussed later) are associated with clinical features that are similar to those caused by *N. gonorrhoeae.* Patients may develop epididymitis, prostatitis, pelvic inflammatory disease, pharyngitis, conjunctivitis, perihepatic inflammation, and proctitis. Unlike *N. gonorrhoeae* urethritis, *C. trachomatis* urethritis in men may be asymptomatic and so may go untreated. Both *N. gonorrhoeae* and *C. trachomatis* frequently cause asymptomatic infections in women. *C. trachomatis* urethritis can be diagnosed by culture of the bacteria in human cell lines, but amplified nucleic acid tests performed on genital swabs or urine specimens are more sensitive and have supplanted cultures.

Genital infection with the L serotypes of *C. trachomatis* causes *lymphogranuloma venereum*, a chronic, ulcerative disease. Lymphogranuloma venereum is a sporadic disease in the United States and Western Europe, but it is endemic in parts of Asia, Africa, the Caribbean region, and South America. The infection initially manifests as a small, often unnoticed, papule on the genital mucosa or nearby skin. Two to 6 weeks later, growth of the organism and the host response in draining lymph nodes produce swollen, tender lymph nodes, which may coalesce and rupture. If not treated, the infection can subsequently cause fibrosis and strictures in the anogenital tract. Rectal strictures are particularly common in women.

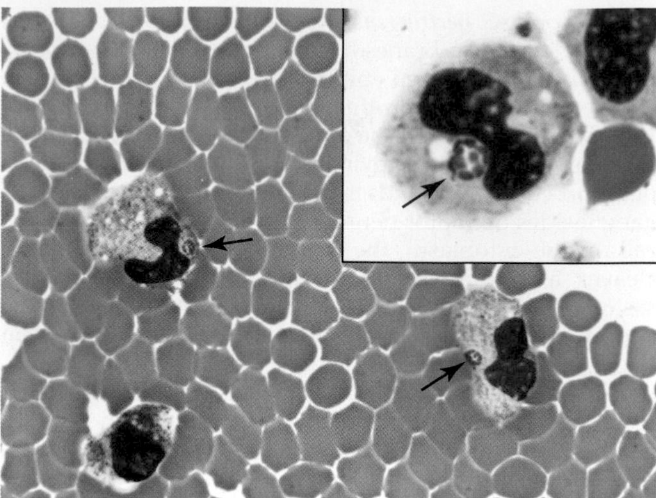

Figure 8-39 Peripheral blood granulocytes (band neutrophils) containing *Anaplasma* inclusions *(arrows)*. (Courtesy Dr. Tad Weiczorek, Faulkner Hospital, Boston, Mass.)

MORPHOLOGY

The features of *C. trachomatis* **urethritis** are virtually identical to those of gonorrhea. The primary infection is characterized by a mucopurulent discharge containing a predominance of neutrophils. Organisms are not visible in Gram-stained smears or sections.

The lesions of **lymphogranuloma venereum** contain a mixed granulomatous and neutrophilic inflammatory response. Variable numbers of chlamydial inclusions are seen in the cytoplasm of epithelial cells or inflammatory cells. Regional lymphadenopathy is common, usually occurring within 30 days of infection. Lymph node involvement is characterized by a granulomatous inflammatory reaction associated with irregularly shaped foci of necrosis containing neutrophils (stellate abscesses). With time, the inflammatory reaction is dominated by nonspecific chronic inflammatory infiltrates and extensive fibrosis. The latter, in turn, may cause local lymphatic obstruction, lymphedema, and strictures. In active lesions, the diagnosis of lymphogranuloma venereum may be made by demonstration of the organism in biopsy sections or smears of exudate. In more chronic cases, the diagnosis rests with the demonstration of antibodies to the appropriate chlamydial serotypes in the patient's serum.

Rickettsial Infections

Members of the *Rickettsiales* are vector-borne obligate intracellular bacteria that cause epidemic and scrub typhus, spotted fevers (*Rickettsia rickettsii* and others), ehrlichiosis, and anaplasmosis. These organisms have the structure of gram-negative, rod-shaped bacteria, although they stain poorly with Gram stain.

- *Epidemic typhus* (caused by *Rickettsia prowazekii*) is transmitted from person to person by body lice. It is associated with wars and poverty, when individuals live in close contact with poor hygiene. Manifestations include a rash that is initially macular, progressing to a petechial, maculopapular rash on the entire body except the face, palms, and soles.
- *Scrub typhus* (caused by *Orienta tsutsugamushi*) is transmitted by chiggers. It is endemic in areas of Asia, Australia, and some islands in the western Pacific and Indian oceans. Fever, headache, myalgia and cough are usual symptoms, sometimes accompanied by a characteristic eschar and associated lymphadenopathy from the chigger bite.
- *Rocky Mountain spotted fever* (caused by *Rickettsia rickettsia*) is transmitted to humans by dog ticks. It is most common in the southeastern and south-central United States. It begins as a nonspecific severe illness with fever, myalgias, and gastrointestinal distress, and progresses to a widespread macular then petechial rash that can involve the palms and soles.
- *Ehrlichiosis* (caused by *Ehrlichia chaffeensis*) and *anaplasmosis* (*Anaplasma phagocytophilum*) are tick-transmitted diseases. The bacteria predominantly infect monocytes (*Ehrlichia chaffeensis*) or neutrophils (*Anaplasma phagocytophilum*). Characteristic cytoplasmic inclusions (morulae), composed of masses of bacteria that occasionally take the shape of a mulberry, are present in leukocytes (Fig. 8-39). Ehrlichiosis and anaplasmosis are characterized by abrupt onset of fever, headache, and malaise, and may progress to respiratory insufficiency, renal failure, and shock. Rash occurs in approximately 40% of people with *E. chaffeensis* infections.

Rickettsial diseases are usually diagnosed clinically and confirmed by serology or immunostaining of the organisms.

Pathogenesis. **The severe manifestations of rickettsial infections are primarily due to infection of endothelial cells and the consequent endothelial dysfunction and injury.** The rickettsiae that cause typhus and spotted fevers predominantly infect vascular endothelial cells, especially those in the lungs and brain. The bacteria enter the endothelial cells by endocytosis, but they escape from the endosome into the cytoplasm. The organisms proliferate in the endothelial cell cytoplasm and then either lyse the cell (typhus group) or spread from cell to cell (spotted fever group). The widespread endothelial dysfunction can cause shock, peripheral and pulmonary edema, and disseminated intravascular coagulation, as well as renal failure and a variety of CNS manifestations that can include coma.

The innate immune response to rickettsial infection is mounted by NK cells, which produce IFN-γ, reducing bacterial proliferation. Subsequent cytotoxic T lymphocyte responses are critical for elimination of rickettsial infections. IFN-γ and TNF produced by activated NK cells and T cells stimulate the production of bactericidal nitric oxide derivatives. Cytotoxic T cells lyse infected cells, reducing bacterial proliferation.

MORPHOLOGY

Typhus Fever. In mild cases the gross changes are limited to a rash and small hemorrhages due to the vascular lesions. In more severe cases, there may be areas of necrosis of the skin and gangrene of the tips of the fingers, nose, earlobes, scrotum, penis, and vulva. In such cases, irregular ecchymotic hemorrhages may be found internally, principally in the brain, heart muscle, testes, serosal membrane, lungs, and kidneys.

The most prominent microscopic changes are small vessel lesions and focal areas of hemorrhage and inflammation in various organs and tissues. Endothelial swelling in the capillaries, arterioles, and venules may narrow the lumens of these vessels. A cuff of mononuclear inflammatory cells usually surrounds the affected vessel. The vascular lumens are sometimes thrombosed. Necrosis of the vessel wall is unusual in typhus (compared with Rocky Mountain spotted fever). Vascular thromboses lead to gangrenous necrosis of the skin and other structures in a minority of cases. In the brain, characteristic typhus nodules are composed of focal microglial proliferations with an infiltrate of mixed T lymphocytes and macrophages (Fig. 8-40).

Scrub typhus, or mite-borne infection, is usually a milder version of typhus fever. The rash is usually transitory or might not appear. Vascular necrosis or thrombosis is rare, but there may be a prominent inflammatory lymphadenopathy.

Rocky Mountain Spotted Fever. A hemorrhagic rash that extends over the entire body, including the palms of the hands and soles of the feet, is the hallmark of Rocky Mountain spotted fever. An eschar at the site of the tick bite is uncommon with Rocky Mountain spotted fever but is often seen with *R. akari*, *R. africae*, and *R. conorii* infection. The vascular lesions that underlie the rash often lead to acute necrosis, fibrin extravasation, and occasionally thrombosis of the small blood vessels, including arterioles (Fig. 8-41). In severe Rocky Mountain spotted fever, foci of necrotic skin appear, particularly on the fingers, toes, elbows, ears, and scrotum. The perivascular inflammatory response, similar to that of typhus, is seen in the brain, skeletal muscle, lungs, kidneys, testes, and heart muscle. The vascular lesions in the brain may involve larger vessels and produce microinfarcts. A noncardiogenic pulmonary edema causing adult respiratory distress syndrome is the major cause of death in patients with Rocky Mountain spotted fever.

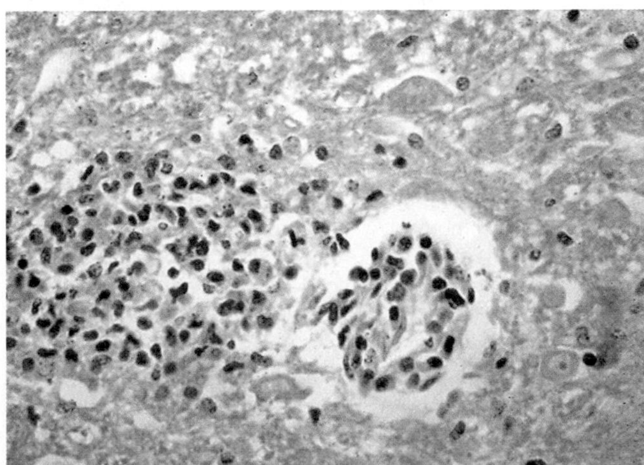

Figure 8-40 Typhus nodule in the brain.

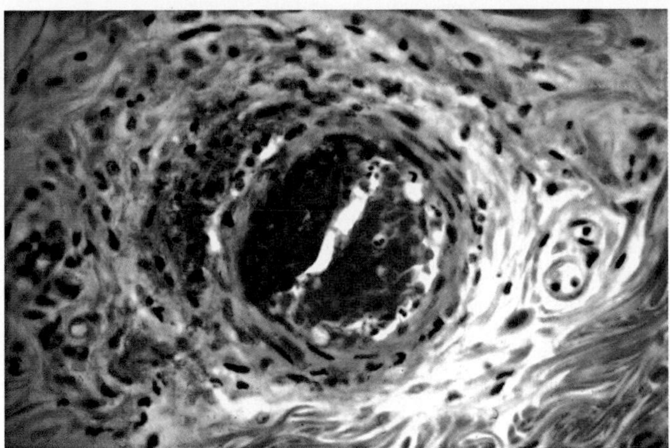

Figure 8-41 Rocky Mountain spotted fever with a thrombosed vessel and vasculitis.

Fungal Infections

Fungi are eukaryotes with cell walls that grow as multicellular filaments (mold) or individual cells alone or in chains (yeast). Cell walls give fungi their shape. Yeasts are round to oval and mainly reproduce by budding. Some yeasts, such as *Candida albicans*, can produce buds that fail to detach and become elongated, producing a chain of elongated yeast cells called *pseudohyphae*. Molds consist of threadlike filaments (hyphae) that grow and divide at their tips. They can produce round cells, called *conidia,* that easily become airborne, disseminating the fungus. Many medically important fungi are dimorphic, existing as yeast or molds, depending on environmental conditions (yeast form at human body temperature and a mold form at room temperature). Fungal infections can be diagnosed by histologic examination, although definitive identification of some species requires culture.

Fungal infections, also called *mycoses*, are of four major types:

- *Superficial and cutaneous mycoses* are common and limited to the very superficial or keratinized layers of skin, hair, and nails.
- *Subcutaneous mycoses* involve the skin, subcutaneous tissues, and lymphatics and rarely disseminate systemically.

- *Endemic mycoses* are caused by dimorphic fungi that can produce serious systemic illness in healthy individuals.
- *Opportunistic mycoses* can cause life-threatening systemic diseases in individuals who are immunosuppressed or who carry implanted prosthetic devices or vascular catheters. Some of the fungi that cause opportunistic mycoses are discussed below; those involving specific organs are discussed in other chapters.

Yeast

Candidiasis

Most *Candida* infections originate when the normal commensal flora breach the skin or mucosal barriers. Residing normally in the skin, mouth, gastrointestinal tract, and vagina, *Candida* species usually live as benign commensals and seldom produce disease in healthy people. *Candida* species, usually *C. albicans*, are the most frequent cause of human fungal infections. These infections may be confined to the skin or mucous membranes or may disseminate widely. In otherwise healthy people *Candida* cause vaginitis and diaper rash. Individuals with diabetes and burn patients are particularly susceptible to superficial candidiasis. In individuals with indwelling intravenous lines or catheters, or undergoing peritoneal dialysis, *Candida* can spread into the bloodstream. Severe disseminated candidiasis most commonly occurs in patients who are neutropenic due to leukemia, chemotherapy, or hematopoietic stem cell transplantation, and may cause shock and disseminated intravascular coagulation.

Pathogenesis. A single strain of *Candida* can be successful as a commensal or a pathogen. *Candida* can shift between different phenotypes. Phenotypic switching involves coordinated regulation of phase-specific genes and provides a way for *Candida* to adapt to changes in the host environment (produced by antibiotic therapy, the immune response, or altered host physiology). These variants can exhibit altered colony morphology, cell shape, antigenicity, and virulence.

Candida produce a large number of functionally distinct adhesins that mediate adherence to host cells and contribute to virulence. These adhesins include (1) an integrin-like protein, which binds to fibrinogen, fibronectin, and laminin; (2) a protein that binds to epithelial cells; and (3) several agglutinins that bind to endothelial cells or fibronectin. Adhesion is an important determinant of virulence, since strains with reduced adherence to cells in vitro are avirulent in experimental models in vivo. Differential expression of adhesins by yeast and filamentous forms leads to recognition of distinct receptors on host cells.

Candida produce a number of enzymes that contribute to invasiveness, including at least nine secreted aspartyl proteinases, which may promote tissue invasion by degrading extracellular matrix proteins, and catalases, which may enable the organism to resist oxidative killing by phagocytic cells.

The ability of *C. albicans* to grow as biofilms also contributes to its capacity to cause disease. *Candida* biofilms are microbial communities consisting of mixtures of yeast, filamentous forms, and fungal-derived extracellular matrix. *C. albicans* can form biofilms on implanted medical devices that reduce the organism's susceptibility to immune responses and antifungal drug therapy.

Neutrophils, macrophages and T_H17 cells are important for protection against *Candida* infection.

- Neutrophils and macrophages phagocytose *Candida*, and oxidative killing by these phagocytes is a first line of host defense. The important role of neutrophils and macrophages is illustrated by the increased risk of *Candida* infections in individuals with neutropenia or defects in NADPH oxidase or myeloperoxidase. Filamentous forms, but not yeast, can escape from phagosomes and enter the cytoplasm and proliferate.
- *Candida* yeast activate dendritic cells through multiple pathways, more so than do the filamentous forms of the fungi. For example, β-1,3-glucan expressed by the yeast engages dectin on dendritic cells and induces IL-6 and IL-23 production, which promotes T_H17 responses. The T_H17 responses elicited by *Candida* are responsible for recruiting neutrophils and monocytes (Chapter 6). These responses are critical for protection against *Candida* infection, as shown by recurrent mucocutaneous candidiasis in individuals with either low T-cell counts due to HIV infection or inherent defects in T_H17 cell development.

MORPHOLOGY

In tissue sections, *C. albicans* can appear as yeast, pseudohyphae, and, less commonly, true hyphae, defined by the presence of septae (Fig. 8-42). Pseudohyphae, an important diagnostic clue, are a chain of budding yeast cells joined end to end at constrictions. All forms may be present together in the same tissue. The organisms may be seen in routine hematoxylin and eosin stains, but a variety of special fungal stains (Gomori methenamine-silver, periodic acid-Schiff) are commonly used to better visualize them.

Most commonly candidiasis takes the form of a superficial infection on mucosal surfaces of the oral cavity **(thrush)**. Florid proliferation of the fungi creates gray-white, dirty-looking pseudomembranes composed of matted organisms and inflammatory debris. Deep to the surface, there is mucosal hyperemia and inflammation. This form of candidiasis is seen in newborns, debilitated people, children receiving oral steroids for asthma, and following a course of broad-spectrum antibiotics that destroy competing normal bacterial flora. The other major risk group includes HIV-positive patients; people with oral thrush for no obvious reason should be evaluated for HIV infection.

Candida esophagitis is commonly seen in AIDS patients and in those with hematolymphoid malignancies. These patients present with dysphagia (painful swallowing) and retrosternal pain; endoscopy demonstrates white plaques and pseudomembranes resembling oral thrush on the esophageal mucosa (Fig. 8-42).

Candida vaginitis is common, especially in women who are diabetic, pregnant, or on oral contraceptive pills. It is usually associated with intense itching and a thick, curdlike discharge.

Cutaneous candidiasis can present in many different forms, including infection of the nail proper (onychomycosis), nail folds (paronychia), hair follicles (folliculitis), moist, intertriginous skin, such as armpits or webs of the fingers and toes (intertrigo), and penile skin (balanitis). Diaper rash is a cutaneous

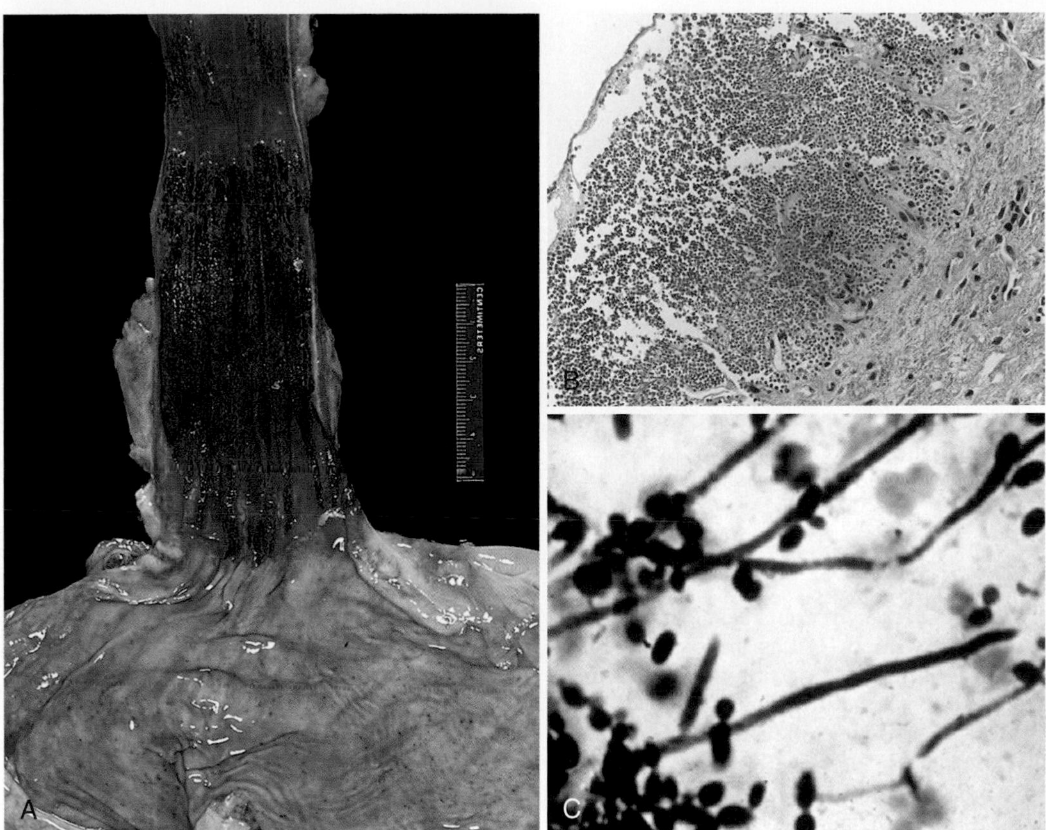

Figure 8-42 The morphology of *Candida* infections. **A,** Severe candidiasis of the distal esophagus. **B,** Hematoxylin and eosin stain of esophageal candidiasis reveals the dense mat of *Candida*. **C,** Characteristic pseudohyphae and budding yeast of *Candida*. (**C**. Courtesy Dr. Dominick Cuvuoti, Department of Pathology, University of Texas Southwestern Medical School, Dallas, Texas).

candidal infection seen in the perineum of infants, the region in contact with wet diapers.

Invasive candidiasis is caused by bloodborne dissemination of organisms to various tissues or organs. Common patterns include (1) renal abscesses, (2) myocardial abscesses and endocarditis, (3) brain microabscesses and meningitis, (4) endophthalmitis (virtually any eye structure can be involved), and (5) hepatic abscesses. In any of these locations, depending on the immune status of the infected person, the fungus may evoke little inflammation cause the usual suppurative response, or occasionally produce granulomas. People with acute leukemias who are profoundly neutropenic after chemotherapy are particularly prone to developing systemic disease. *Candida* endocarditis is the most common fungal endocarditis, usually occurring in the setting of prosthetic heart valves or in intravenous drug abusers. In the latter group the tricuspid valve is involved.

Cryptococcosis

Two species of cryptococcus are known to cause disease in humans, *C. neoformans* and *C. gattii*, both of which grow as encapsulated yeasts. It has long been recognized that while *C. neoformans* may cause meningoencephalitis in otherwise healthy individuals, it more frequently presents as an opportunistic infection in people with AIDS, leukemia, lymphoma, systemic lupus erythematosus, or sarcoidosis, as well as in immunosuppressed transplant recipients. Many of these patients receive high-dose corticosteroids, a major risk factor for *C. neoformans* infection. *Cryptococcus neoformans* is present in the soil and in bird (particularly pigeon) droppings and infects people when it is inhaled.

C. gattii was an obscure infectious agent until 1999, when it was identified as the cause of an outbreak of cryptococcal disease in the American Pacific Northwest and contiguous areas of British Columbia. It has subsequently been linked to cryptococcal infections worldwide. Because most current tests used to diagnose cryptococcal infections (discussed later) do not distinguish between *C. gatti* and *C. neoformans*, the true incidence of infections caused by these two agents is currently uncertain. Based on findings from areas where *C. gattii* is now specifically tested for, it appears that *C. gattii* is more likely than *C. neoformans* to cause disease in immunologically normal individuals and to present with large lesions that produce mass effects or that mimic the radiologic appearance of a neoplasm. *C. gattii* is associated with certain species of trees, is found in soil, and like *C. neoformans* is acquired by inhalation.

Pathogenesis. **Cryptococcus has several virulence factors that enable it to evade host defenses**, as follows:

- *Polysaccharide capsule*. Glucuronoxylomannan inhibits phagocytosis by alveolar macrophages, leukocyte migration, and recruitment of inflammatory cells. *C. neoformans* can undergo phenotypic switching, which leads to changes in the structure and size of the capsular polysaccharide, providing a means to evade immune responses.

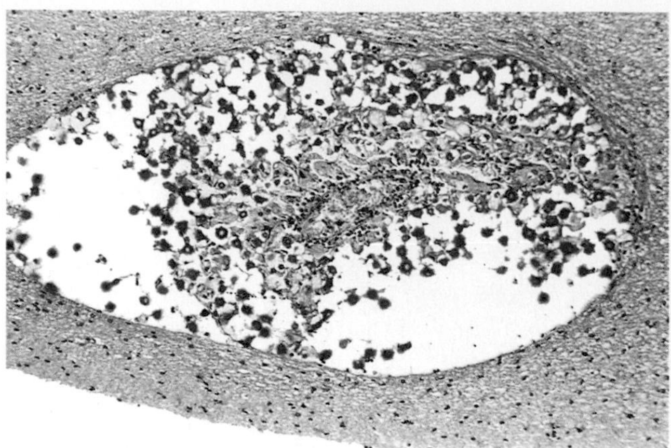

Figure 8-43 Mucicarmine stain of cryptococci (staining red) in a Virchow-Robin perivascular space of the brain (soap-bubble lesion).

- *Melanin production*. Laccase in the yeast catalyzes the formation of melanin which (1) has antioxidant properties, (2) decreases antibody-mediated phagocytosis, (3) counteracts the effects of antifungal agents, (4) binds iron, (5) and provides cell wall integrity.
- *Enzymes*. Serine proteinase cleaves fibronectin and other basement membrane proteins, which may aid tissue invasion. Mannitol dehydrogenase produces mannitol, which leads to osmotic edema and inhibits killing of the yeast by neutrophils and reactive oxygen species.

MORPHOLOGY

Cryptococcus has yeast but not pseudohyphal or hyphal forms. **The 5- to 10-μm cryptococcal yeast has a highly characteristic thick gelatinous capsule containing a polysaccharide that stains intense red with periodic acid-Schiff and mucicarmine in tissues** (Fig. 8-43) and can be detected with antibody-coated beads in an agglutination assay. India ink preparations create a negative image, visualizing the thick capsule as a clear halo within a dark background. Although the lung is the primary site of infection, pulmonary involvement is usually mild and asymptomatic, even while the fungus is spreading to the CNS. *C. gattii* appears to be particularly likely to form a solitary pulmonary granuloma similar to the circumscribed (coin) lesions caused by *Histoplasma*.

The major lesions caused by cryptococcus are in the CNS, involving the meninges, cortical gray matter, and basal nuclei. The host response to cryptococci is extremely variable. In immunosuppressed people, organisms may evoke virtually no inflammatory reaction, so gelatinous masses of fungi grow in the meninges or expand the perivascular Virchow-Robin spaces within the gray matter, producing the so-called soap-bubble lesions (Fig. 8-43). In severely immunosuppressed persons, *C. neoformans* may disseminate widely to the skin, liver, spleen, adrenals, and bones. In nonimmunosuppressed people or in those with protracted disease, the fungi induce a chronic granulomatous reaction composed of macrophages, lymphocytes, and foreign body-type giant cells. Suppuration also may occur, as well as a rare granulomatous arteritis of the circle of Willis.

Molds

Aspergillosis

***Aspergillus* is a ubiquitous mold that causes allergies (allergic bronchopulmonary aspergillosis) in otherwise healthy people and serious sinusitis, pneumonia, and invasive disease in immunocompromised individuals.** The major conditions that predispose to *Aspergillus* infection are neutropenia and use of corticosteroids. *Aspergillus fumigatus* is the most common pathogenic species of the fungus.

Pathogenesis. *Aspergillus* species are transmitted as airborne conidia, and the lung is the major portal of entry. The small size of *A. fumigatus* spores, approximately 2 to 3 μm, enables them to reach alveoli. Alveolar macrophages recognize *Aspergillus* through TLR2 and the lectin dectin-1, which recognizes β-1,3-glucan when it is exposed on the swollen conidia. Both receptors activate phagocytes to ingest and kill the conidia. In immunosuppressed states, conidia can germinate into hyphae, which then invade tissues. TLRs can recognize products of the fungal hyphae and trigger the release of pro-inflammatory mediators, including TNF-α, IL-β, and chemokines. Neutrophils produce reactive oxygen intermediates that kill hyphae. Invasive aspergillosis is highly associated with neutropenia and impaired neutrophil defenses.

***Aspergillus* produces several virulence factors, including adhesins, antioxidants, enzymes, and toxins.** Conidia, whose cell walls are built of β-1, 3-glucan and galactomannan (both molecules can be measured in serum as markers of invasiveness), can bind to fibrinogen, laminin, complement, fibronectin, collagen, albumin, and surfactant proteins, but receptor-ligand interactions are not well defined. *Aspergillus* produces several antioxidant defenses, including melanin pigment, mannitol, catalases, and superoxide dismutases. This fungus also produces phospholipases, proteases, and toxins, but their roles in pathogenicity are not clear. The carcinogen aflatoxin is made by *Aspergillus* species growing on the surface of peanuts and may contribute to liver cancer in Africa. Sensitization to *Aspergillus* spores produces an allergic alveolitis (Chapter 15). Allergic bronchopulmonary aspergillosis, associated with hypersensitivity arising from superficial colonization of the bronchial mucosa, often occurs in asthmatic people.

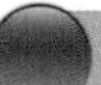

MORPHOLOGY

Colonizing aspergillosis (aspergilloma) refers to growth of the fungus in pulmonary cavities and minimal or no invasion of the tissues (the nose also is often colonized). The cavities are usually the result of prior tuberculosis, bronchiectasis, old infarcts, or abscesses. Proliferating masses of hyphae form brownish "fungus balls" lying free within the cavities. The surrounding inflammatory reaction may be sparse, or there may be chronic inflammation and fibrosis. People with aspergillomas usually have recurrent hemoptysis.

Invasive aspergillosis is an opportunistic infection that is confined to immunosuppressed hosts. The primary lesions are usually in the lung, but widespread hematogenous dissemination with involvement of the heart valves and brain is common.

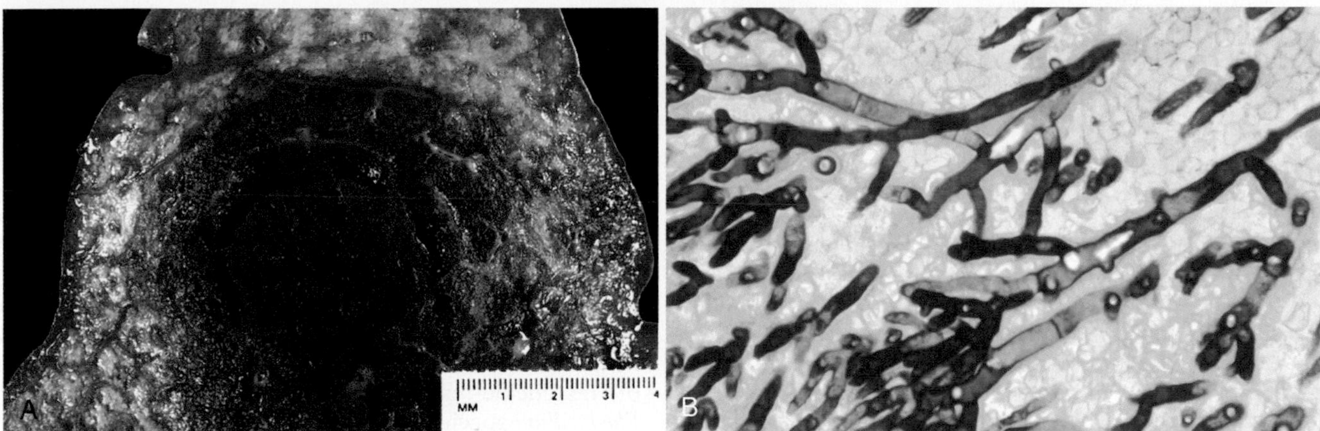

Figure 8-44 *Aspergillus* infection. **A,** Invasive aspergillosis of the lung in a bone marrow transplant patient. **B,** Gomori methenamine-silver (GMS) stain shows septate hyphae with acute-angle branching, consistent with *Aspergillus*.

The pulmonary lesions take the form of necrotizing pneumonia with sharply delineated, rounded, gray foci and hemorrhagic borders; they are often referred to as target lesions (Fig. 8-44*A*). ***Aspergillus* forms fruiting bodies (usually in lung cavities) and septate filaments, 5 to 10 μm thick, branching at acute angles (40 degrees)** (Fig. 8-44*B*). *Aspergillus* hyphae cannot be distinguished from *Pseudallescheria boydii* and *Fusarium* species by morphology alone. *Aspergillus* has a tendency to invade blood vessels, therefore areas of hemorrhage and infarction are usually superimposed on the necrotizing, inflammatory tissue reactions. Rhinocerebral *Aspergillus* infection in immunosuppressed individuals resembles that caused by Mucormycoses (e.g., *Mucor*, *Rhizopus*).

Zygomycosis (Mucormycosis)

Mucormycotina are widely distributed in nature and cause no harm to immunocompetent individuals, but they infect immunosuppressed people, causing mucormycosis. Mucormycosis (formerly zygomycosis) is an opportunistic infection caused by bread mold fungi, including *Mucor, Rhizopus, Lichtheimia (formerly Absidia),* and *Cunninghamella*, which belong to the family Mucormycetes. Major predisposing factors are neutropenia, corticosteroid use, diabetes mellitus, iron overload, and breakdown of the cutaneous barrier (e.g., as a result of burns, surgical wounds, or trauma).

Pathogenesis. Immune responses to Mucormycotina differ from other fungi and the organisms have variable natural resistance. As with *Aspergillus*, Mucormycotina are transmitted by airborne asexual spores. Inhaled spores commonly produce infection in the sinuses and the lungs, but percutaneous exposure or ingestion can also lead to infection. Macrophages provide the initial defense by phagocytosis and non-oxidative killing of germinating sporangiospores. Mucormycotina hyphal components are recognized by TLR2, which results in a pro-inflammatory cascade of cytokines including IL-6 and TNF-α. Neutrophils have a key role in killing hyphae after germination by directly damaging hyphae walls. If the macrophages or neutrophils are compromised in numbers or function, the probability of an established and then invasive infection is greatly increased. There is natural variation in resistance to both phagocytosis of spores and neutrophil damage to hyphae depending on the species of Mucormycotina causing infection; thus, some infections can appear more aggressive than others despite a similar host milieu. Lastly, the availability of free iron (a promoter of Mucormycotina growth) increases probability of infection, as seen in people with diabetes (increased free iron due to ketoacidosis and/or glycosylation-induced poor iron affinity) and patients on chronic iron chelation treatment (where deferoxamine acts as a siderophore within the fungi).

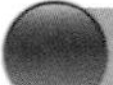

MORPHOLOGY

Mucormycetes form nonseptate hyphae of variable width (6-50 μm) with frequent right angle branching, distinct from *Aspergillus* hyphae, that are readily demonstrated by hematoxylin and eosin or special fungal stains (Fig. 8-45). The three primary sites of invasion are the nasal sinuses, lungs, and gastrointestinal tract, depending on whether the spores (which are widespread in dust and air) are inhaled or ingested. Most commonly in individuals with diabetes, the fungus may spread from nasal sinuses to the orbit and brain, giving rise to **rhinocerebral mucormycosis**. The Mucormycotina cause local tissue necrosis, invade arterial walls, and penetrate the periorbital tissues and cranial vault. Meningoencephalitis follows,

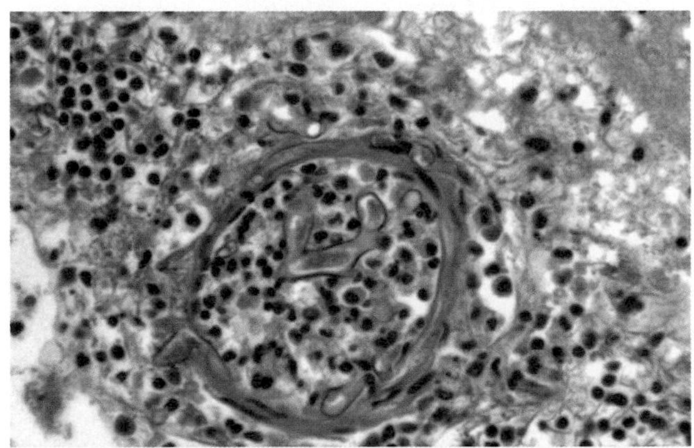

Figure 8-45 Meningeal blood vessels with angioinvasive *Mucor* species. Note the irregular width and near right-angle branching of the hyphae. Compare with Aspergillus, Fig. 8-44.

sometimes complicated by cerebral infarctions when fungi invade arteries and induce thrombosis.

Lung involvement with Mucormycotina may be secondary to rhinocerebral disease, or it may be primary in people with severe immunodeficiency. The lung lesions combine areas of hemorrhagic pneumonia with vascular thrombi and distal infarctions.

Dimorphic Fungi

The medically important dimorphic fungi are discussed in Chapter 15 and include blastomyces, histoplasma, and coccidioidomyces. Suffice it to say that **they grow as yeast in human tissue but as a hyaline mold under some laboratory culture conditions, typically at room temperature.** On histological examination, the organisms have characteristic yeast appearances but can be somewhat difficult to speciate if organisms are rare. The immune response can range from suppurative to granulomatous depending on the organism and stage of disease. If concurrent cultures from a sample begin to demonstrate hyaline mold, this indicates that the organism is dimorphic and specific treatment can be started.

Parasitic Infections

Protozoa

Protozoa are unicellular eukaryotic organisms. The parasitic protozoa are transmitted by insects or by the fecal-oral route and, in humans, mainly reside in the blood or intestine (Table 8-8). Most protozoal infections are diagnosed by microscopic examination of blood smears or lesions.

Malaria

Malaria, caused by the intracellular parasite *Plasmodium,* affects more than 160 million people worldwide and kills more than 500,000 people each year. According to the WHO, 90% of deaths from malaria occur in sub-Saharan Africa, where malaria is a leading cause of death in children younger than 5 years old. *Plasmodium falciparum* (the cause of severe cerebral malaria) and the four other malaria parasites that infect humans (*P. vivax, P. ovale, P. knowlesi,* and *P. malariae*) are all transmitted by female Anopheles mosquitoes, which are widely distributed throughout Africa, Asia, and Latin America. Nearly all of the approximately 1500 new cases of malaria each year in the United States occur in travelers or immigrants. Mass spraying to eliminate the mosquito vectors was successful initially but ultimately failed when DDT was removed from the market due to environmental concerns. Worldwide public health efforts to control malaria today face the challenges of insecticide-resistant mosquitoes and drug-resistant *Plasmodium* species. Currently, a combination of mosquito control and anti-malarial drugs is viewed as the means to decrease the incidence.

Table 8-8 Selected Human Protozoal Diseases

Location	Species	Disease
Luminal or epithelial	*Entamoeba histolytica*	Amebic dysentery; liver abscess
	Balantidium coli	Colitis
	Giardia lamblia	Diarrheal disease, malabsorption
	Isospora belli, Cryptosporidium sp.	Chronic enterocolitis or malabsorption or both
	Trichomonas vaginalis	Urethritis, vaginitis
Central nervous system	*Naegleria fowleri*	Meningoencephalitis
	Acanthamoeba sp.	Meningoencephalitis or ophthalmitis
Bloodstream	*Plasmodium* sp.	Malaria
	Babesia microti, B. bovis	Babesiosis
	Trypanosoma sp.	African sleeping sickness
Intracellular	*Trypanosoma cruzi*	Chagas disease
	Leishmania donovani	Kala-azar
	Leishmania sp.	Cutaneous and mucocutaneous leishmaniasis
	Toxoplasma gondii	Toxoplasmosis

Life Cycle and Pathogenesis. The life cycles of the *Plasmodium* species are similar, although *P. falciparum* differs in ways that contribute to its greater virulence. *P. vivax, P. ovale, P. knowlesi,* and *P. malariae* cause low levels of parasitemia, mild anemia, and, in very rare instances, splenic rupture and nephrotic syndrome. ***P. falciparum* infection is associated with high levels of parasitemia, that may lead to severe anemia, cerebral symptoms, renal failure, pulmonary edema, and death, depending on the susceptibility of the host.**

The life cycle of *Plasmodium* species is simple, as it involves only humans and mosquitoes, but the development of the parasite is complex, as it passes through several morphologically distinct forms. The infectious stage of *Plasmodium,* the *sporozoite,* is found in the salivary glands of female mosquitoes. When the mosquito takes a blood meal, sporozoites are released into the human's blood and, within minutes, attach to and invade liver cells by binding to the hepatocyte receptor for the serum proteins thrombospondin and properdin (Fig. 8-46). Within liver cells, malaria parasites multiply, releasing as many as 30,000 *merozoites* (asexual, haploid forms) when each infected hepatocyte ruptures. During *P. falciparum* infection, rupture usually occurs within 8 to 12 weeks. In contrast, *P. vivax* and *P. ovale* form latent *hypnozoites* in hepatocytes, which cause relapses of malaria weeks to months after initial infection. The infection of the liver and development of merozoites is called the *exoerythrocytic* stage. This stage is asymptomatic. Once released from the liver, *Plasmodium* merozoites use a lectin-like molecule to bind to sialic acid residues on glycophorin molecules on the surface of red cells and invade by active membrane penetration. Within the red cells (*erythrocytic* stage) the parasites grow in a membrane-bound digestive vacuole, hydrolyzing hemoglobin through secreted enzymes. The *trophozoite* is the first stage of the parasite in the red cell and is defined by the presence of a single chromatin mass. The next stage, the *schizont,* has multiple chromatin masses, each of which develops into a merozoite. Upon lysis of the red cell, the new merozoites infect additional red cells. Paroxysmal fever, chills, and rigors characteristic of malaria occur when the merozoites are released into the blood. As discussed later, release of merozoites induces the host cells to produce cytokines such as TNF that cause fever. The periodicity of such paroxysms (every 48-72 hours) varies with

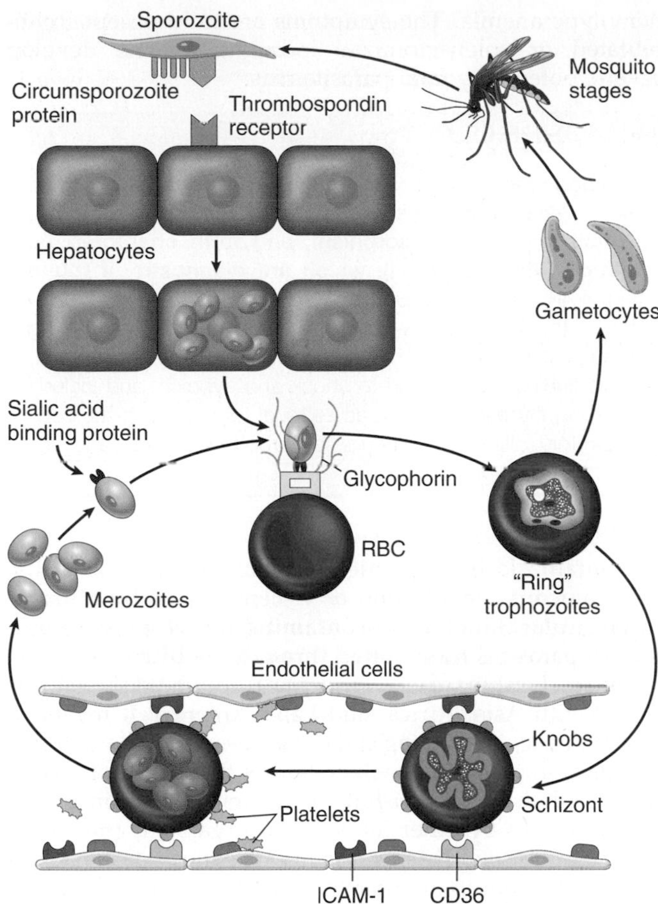

Figure 8-46 Life cycle of *Plasmodium falciparum*. Both exoerythocytic and erythrocytic stages are depicted. ICAM-1, Intercellular adhesion molecule 1; RBC, red blood cell. (Drawn by Dr. Jeffrey Joseph, Beth Israel-Deaconess Hospital, Boston, MA.)

the species of the malarial parasite. Although most malaria parasites within the red cells develop into merozoites, some parasites develop, under specific conditions, into sexual forms called *gametocytes* that infect the mosquito when it takes its blood meal.

Plasmodium falciparum causes more severe disease than the other *Plasmodium* species do. Several features of *P. falciparum* account for its greater pathogenicity:

- *P. falciparum* is able to infect red blood cells of any age, whereas other species infect only young or old red cells, which are a smaller fraction of the red cell pool.
- *P. falciparum* causes infected red cells to clump together (rosette) and to stick to endothelial cells lining small blood vessels (sequestration), which blocks blood flow. Several proteins, including *P. falciparum* erythrocyte membrane protein 1 (PfEMP1), associate and form knobs on the surface of red cells (Fig. 8-46). PfEMP1 binds to ligands on endothelial cells, including CD36, thrombospondin, VCAM-1, ICAM-1, and E-selectin. Red cell sequestration decreases tissue perfusion and leads to ischemia, which is responsible for the manifestations of cerebral malaria, the major cause of death in children with malaria.
- In *P. falciparum* infection, GPI-linked proteins, including merozoite surface antigens, are released from infected red cells and induce cytokine production by host cells. These cytokines, including TNF, IFN-γ, and IL-1, suppress production of red blood cells, increase fever, stimulate the production of reactive nitrogen species (leading to tissue damage), and induce expression of endothelial receptors for PfEMP1 (increasing sequestration).

Host resistance to *Plasmodium* can be intrinsic or acquired. Intrinsic resistance stems from inherited alterations that reduce the susceptibility of red cells to productive *Plasmodium* infections. Resistance may also be acquired following repeated or prolonged exposure to *Plasmodium* species, which stimulates a partially protective immune response.

Several types of mutations affecting red cells are highly prevalent in parts of the world where malaria is endemic and are absent in other parts of the world. Most of these mutations are deleterious in homozygous form, suggesting that they are maintained in populations due to a selective advantage for heterozygous carriers against malaria. The mutations fall into four broad classes.

- Point mutations in globin genes—sickle cell disease (HbS), HbC disease (hemoglobinopathies)
- Mutations leading to globin deficiencies—α- and β-thalassemia
- Mutations affecting red cell enzymes—glucose-6-phosphate dehydrogenase (G6PD) deficiency
- Mutations causing red cell membrane defects—absence of DARC (Duffy surface blood group), band 3, spectrin

P. vivax enters red cells by binding to the Duffy blood group antigen, and most of the population of West Africa is not susceptible to infection by *P. vivax* because they do not have the Duffy antigen. The mechanisms of the protective effects of the other three types of mutations are less well understood, but likely involve a favorable shift in the balance between the growth of intraerythrocytic parasites and their clearance by host phagocytes.

Individuals living where *Plasmodium* is endemic often gain partial immune-mediated resistance to malaria, evidenced by reduced illness despite infection. Antibodies and T lymphocytes specific for *Plasmodium* reduce disease manifestations, although the parasite has developed strategies to evade the host immune response. *P. falciparum* uses antigenic variation to escape from antibody responses to PfEMP1. Each haploid *P. falciparum* genome has about 50 *var* genes, each encoding a variant of PfEMP1. The mechanism of *var* regulation is not known, but at least 2% of the parasites switch PfEMP1 genes each generation. Cytotoxic T cells may also be important in resistance to *P. falciparum*. Current vaccine trials have demonstrated decreases in severe disease but only modest efficacy against clinical infection.

MORPHOLOGY

The diagnostic test for malaria infection is examination of a Giemsa-stained peripheral blood smear, which permits the asexual stages of the parasite to be identified within infected red cells. Insertion of parasite proteins into the red cell membrane leads to recognition by macrophages,

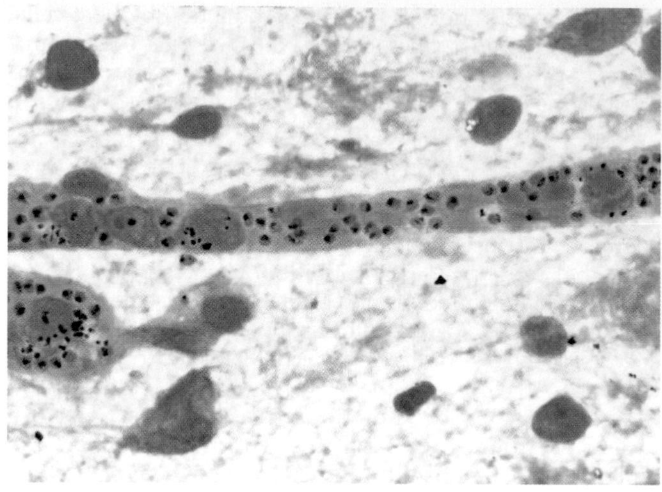

Figure 8-47 Field's stain of *Plasmodium falciparum*-infected red cells marginating within a capillary in cerebral malaria.

particularly in the spleen. Plasmodium falciparum infection leads to **splenomegaly**, due to both congestion and hyperplasia of the red pulp, and the spleen may eventually exceed 1000 gm in weight. In chronic infections, the spleen becomes increasingly fibrotic and brittle, with a thick capsule and fibrous trabeculae. The parenchyma is gray or black because the phagocytes contain granular, brown-black, faintly birefringent hemozoin pigment. Macrophages with engulfed parasitized red cells are also numerous.

With progression of malaria, the liver becomes enlarged and pigmented. Kupffer cells are heavily laden with malarial pigment, parasites, and cellular debris, while some pigment is also present in the parenchymal cells. Pigmented phagocytic cells may be found dispersed throughout the bone marrow, lymph nodes, subcutaneous tissues, and lungs. The kidneys are often enlarged and congested with a dusting of pigment in the glomeruli and hemoglobin casts in the tubules.

In **cerebral malaria** caused by *P. falciparum*, brain vessels are plugged with parasitized red cells (Fig. 8-47). Around the vessels there are ring hemorrhages that are probably related to local hypoxia incident to the vascular stasis and small focal inflammatory reactions (called **malarial** or **Dürck granulomata**). With more severe hypoxia, there is degeneration of neurons, focal ischemic softening, and occasionally scant inflammatory infiltrates in the meninges.

Nonspecific focal hypoxic lesions in the heart may be induced by the progressive anemia and circulatory stasis in chronically infected people. In some, the myocardium shows focal interstitial infiltrates. Finally, in the nonimmune patient, pulmonary edema or shock with disseminated intravascular coagulation may cause death, sometimes in the absence of other characteristic lesions.

Babesiosis

Babesia microti and *Babesia divergens* are malaria-like protozoans transmitted by the same deer ticks that carry Lyme disease and granulocytic ehrlichiosis. The white-footed mouse is the reservoir for *B. microti*, and in some areas, nearly all mice have a persistent low-level parasitemia. *B. microti* survives well in refrigerated blood, and several cases of transfusion-acquired babesiosis have been reported. *Babesia* parasitize red cells and cause fever and hemolytic anemia. The symptoms are mild except in debilitated or splenectomized individuals, who develop severe, potentially fatal parasitemias.

MORPHOLOGY

In blood smears, *Babesia* organisms superficially resemble *P. falciparum* ring stages, but lack hemozoin pigment, exhibit greater pleomorphism, and form characteristic tetrads (Maltese cross), which are diagnostic, if found (Fig. 8-48). The level of *B. microti* parasitemia is a good indication of the severity of infection (about 1% in mild cases and up to 30% in splenectomized persons). In fatal cases the anatomic findings are related to shock and hypoxia, and include jaundice, hepatic necrosis, acute renal tubular necrosis, adult respiratory distress syndrome, erythrophagocytosis, and visceral hemorrhages.

Leishmaniasis

Leishmaniasis is a chronic inflammatory disease of the skin, mucous membranes, or viscera caused by obligate intracellular, kinetoplast-containing (kinetoplastid) protozoan parasites transmitted through the bite of infected sandflies. Leishmaniasis is endemic throughout the Middle East, South Asia, Africa, and Latin America. It may also be epidemic, as is tragically the case in Sudan, India, Bangladesh, and Brazil, where tens of thousands of people have died of visceral leishmaniasis. Leishmanial infection, like infections by other intracellular organisms (mycobacteria, *Histoplasma, Toxoplasma,* and trypanosomes), is exacerbated by conditions that interfere with T-cell function, such as AIDS. Culture or histologic examination is used to diagnose the infection.

***Pathogenesis.* The life cycle of *Leishmania* involves two forms: the promastigote, which develops and lives extracellularly in the sandfly vector, and the amastigote, which multiplies intracellularly in host macrophages.** Mammals, including rodents, dogs, and foxes, are reservoirs of *Leishmania*. When sandflies bite infected humans or animals, macrophages harboring amastigotes are ingested. The amastigotes differentiate into promastigotes, multiply within the digestive tract of the sandfly and migrate to the salivary gland, where they are poised for transmission by the fly bite. When the infected fly bites a person, the slender, flagellated infectious promastigotes

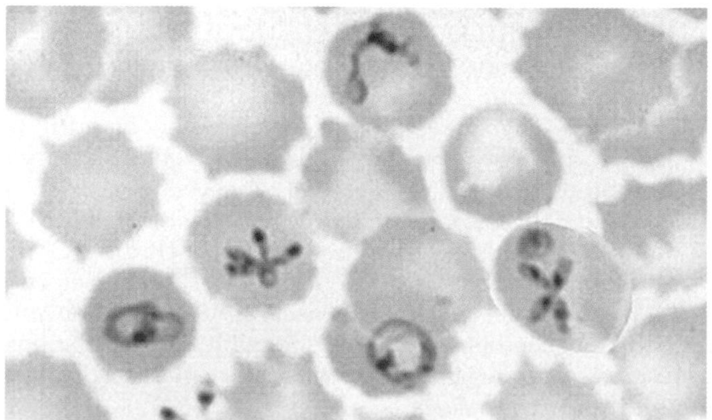

Figure 8-48 Erythrocytes with *Babesia*, including the distinctive Maltese cross form. (Courtesy Lynne Garcia, LSG and Associates, Santa Monica, Calif.)

are released into the host dermis along with the sandfly saliva, which potentiates parasite infectivity. The promastigotes are phagocytosed by macrophages, and the acidity within the phagolysosome induces them to transform into round amastigotes that lack flagella but contain a single mitochondrion with its DNA massed into a unique suborganelle, the kinetoplast. Amastigotes proliferate within macrophages, and dying macrophages release progeny amastigotes that can infect additional macrophages.

How far the amastigotes spread throughout the body depends on the *Leishmania* species and host, and determines the extent of disease. There are several forms of disease and that are caused by different species of *Leishmania*.

- Cutaneous disease
  - Old World—*Leishmania major* and *Leishmania tropica*
  - New World—*Leishmania mexicana* and *Leishmania braziliensis*
- Mucocutaneous disease (also called *espundia*)
  - New World—*L. braziliensis*
- Visceral disease involving the liver, spleen, and bone marrow
  - Old World—*Leishmania donovani* and *Leishmania infantum*
  - New World—*Leishmania chagasi*

Tropism of *Leishmania* species seems to be linked in part to the optimal temperature for their growth. Parasites that cause visceral disease grow best at 37°C, whereas parasites that cause mucocutaneous disease grow better at lower temperatures. However, cutaneous *Leishmania* species often are viscerotropic in HIV patients.

Leishmania manipulate innate host defenses to facilitate their entry and survival in macrophages. Promastigotes produce two abundant surface glycoconjugates that contribute to their virulence.

- Lipophosphoglycan forms a dense glycocalyx that both activates complement (leading to C3b deposition on the parasite surface) and inhibits complement action (by preventing membrane attack complex insertion into the parasite membrane). Thus, the parasite becomes coated with C3b but avoids destruction by the membrane attack complex. Instead, the C3b on the surface of the parasite binds to Mac-1 and CR1 on macrophages, targeting the promastigote for phagocytosis.
- Gp63 is a zinc-dependent proteinase that cleaves complement and some lysosomal antimicrobial enzymes. Gp63 also binds to fibronectin receptors on macrophages and promotes promastigote adhesion to macrophages.

Leishmania amastigotes also produce molecules that facilitate their survival and replication within macrophages. Amastigotes reproduce in macrophage phagolysosomes, which normally have a pH of 4.5. However, the amastigotes protect themselves from this hostile environment by expressing a proton-transporting ATPase, which maintains the phagolysosome pH at 6.5.

The primary mechanisms of resistance and susceptibility to *Leishmania* are mediated through T_H1 and T_H2 responses. Parasite-specific CD4+ T_H1 cells are needed to control *Leishmania* in mice and humans. *Leishmania* evade host immunity by impairing the development of the T_H1 response. In animal models, mice that are resistant to *Leishmania* infection produce high levels of T_H1-derived IFN-γ, which activates macrophages to kill the parasites through reactive oxygen species. By contrast, mouse strains that are susceptible to leishmaniasis mount a dominant T_H2 response. T_H2 cytokines such as IL-4, IL-13, and IL-10 prevent effective killing of *Leishmania* by inhibiting the microbicidal activity of macrophages.

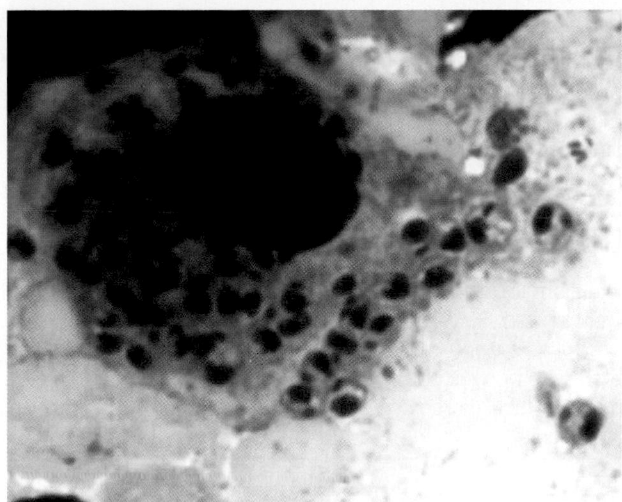

Figure 8-49 Giemsa stain of a tissue macrophage with *Leishmania donovani* parasites.

MORPHOLOGY

Leishmania species produce four different types of lesions in humans: visceral, cutaneous, mucocutaneous, and diffuse cutaneous. In **visceral leishmaniasis**, parasites invade macrophages throughout the mononuclear phagocyte system (Fig. 8-49), and cause severe systemic disease marked by hepatosplenomegaly, lymphadenopathy, pancytopenia, fever, and weight loss. The spleen may weigh as much as 3 kg. Phagocytic cells are enlarged and filled with *Leishmania*, many plasma cells are present, and the normal architecture of the spleen is obscured. In the late stages, the liver becomes increasingly fibrotic. Phagocytic cells crowd the bone marrow and also may be found in the lungs, gastrointestinal tract, kidneys, pancreas, and testes. Often there is hyperpigmentation of the skin in individuals of South Asian ancestry, which is why the disease is called *kala-azar* (*black fever* in Hindi). In the kidneys there may be an immune complex-mediated mesangioproliferative glomerulonephritis, and in advanced cases there may be amyloid deposition. People with advanced leishmaniasis can develop life-threatening secondary bacterial infections, such as pneumonia, sepsis or tuberculosis. Hemorrhages related to thrombocytopenia may also be fatal.

Cutaneous leishmaniasis is a relatively mild, localized disease consisting of ulcers on exposed skin. The lesion begins as a papule surrounded by induration, changes into a shallow and slowly expanding ulcer, often with heaped-up borders, and usually heals by involution within 6 to 18 months without treatment. On microscopic examination, the lesion shows granulomatous inflammation, usually with many giant cells and few parasites.

Mucocutaneous leishmaniasis is found only in the New World. Moist, ulcerating, or nonulcerating lesions develop in the nasopharyngeal areas and, with progression, may be highly destructive and disfiguring. Microscopic examination reveals a mixed inflammatory infiltrate composed of parasite-containing macrophages with lymphocytes and plasma cells. Later, the tissue inflammatory response becomes granulomatous, and the number of parasites declines. Eventually, the lesions remit and scar, although reactivation may occur after long intervals by mechanisms that are not currently understood.

Diffuse cutaneous leishmaniasis is a rare form of dermal infection found in Ethiopia and adjacent East Africa and in Central and South America. Diffuse cutaneous leishmaniasis begins as a single skin nodule, which continues spreading until the entire body is covered by nodular lesions. Microscopically, they contain aggregates of foamy macrophages stuffed with leishmania.

African Trypanosomiasis

African trypanosomes are kinetoplastid parasites that proliferate as extracellular forms in the blood and cause sustained or intermittent fevers, lymphadenopathy, splenomegaly, progressive brain dysfunction (sleeping sickness), cachexia, and death. *Trypanosoma brucei rhodesiense* infection, which occurs in East Africa and is often acute and virulent, is a zoonotic infection that is best combated by reducing infected fly populations. *Trypanosoma brucei gambiense* infection occurring in West Africa tends to spread from human to human via fly bites and requires active case detection and treatment. Tsetse flies (genus *Glossina*) transmit African *Trypanosoma* to humans either from the reservoir of parasites found in wild and domestic animals *(T. brucei rhodesiense)* or from other humans *(T. brucei gambiense)*. Within the fly, the parasites multiply in the stomach and then in the salivary glands before developing into nondividing trypomastigotes, which are transmitted to humans and animals with the next blood meal.

Pathogenesis. African trypanosomes are covered by a single, abundant, glycolipid-anchored protein called the *variant surface glycoprotein (VSG)*. As parasites proliferate in the bloodstream, the host produces antibodies to the VSG, which, in association with phagocytes, kill most of the organisms, causing a spike of fever. A small number of parasites, however, undergo a genetic rearrangement and produce a different VSG on their surface and so escape the host immune response. These successor trypanosomes multiply until the host mounts a new anti-VSG response and kills most of them, but then another clone with a distinct VSG takes over. In this way, African trypanosomes cause waves of fever before they finally invade the CNS. Trypanosomes have many VSG genes, only one of which is expressed at a time. The parasite uses an elegant mechanism to turn VSG genes on and off. Although VSG genes are scattered throughout the trypanosome genome, only VSG genes found within *bloodstream expression sites* near the ends of chromosomes (the telomeres) are transcribed. New VSG genes are periodically moved into the bloodstream expression sites, mainly by homologous recombination. A specialized RNA polymerase that transcribes VSG genes associates with only a single bloodstream expression site, limiting expression to one VSG gene at a time.

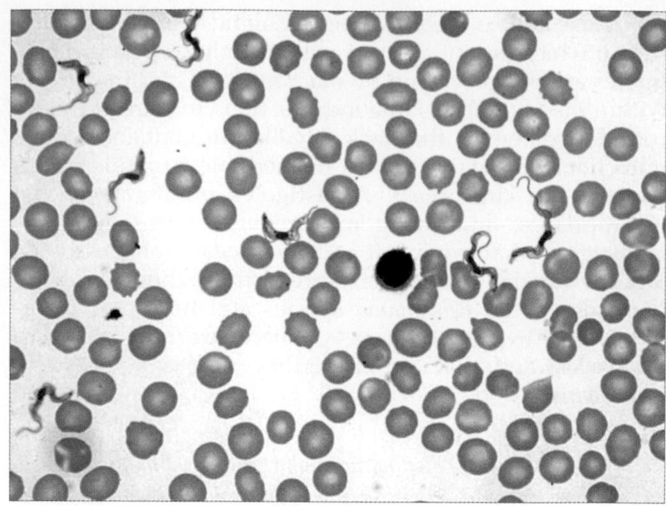

Figure 8-50 Slender bloodstream parasites of African trypanosomiasis.

MORPHOLOGY

A large, red, rubbery chancre forms at the site of the insect bite and contains numerous parasites surrounded by a dense, predominantly mononuclear, inflammatory infiltrate. With chronicity, the lymph nodes and spleen enlarge due to infiltration by lymphocytes, plasma cells, and macrophages, which are filled with dead parasites. Trypanosomes, which are small and difficult to visualize (Fig. 8-50), concentrate in capillary loops, such as the choroid plexus and glomeruli. When parasites breach the blood-brain barrier and invade the CNS, a leptomeningitis develops that extends into the perivascular Virchow-Robin spaces, and eventually a demyelinating panencephalitis occurs. Plasma cells containing cytoplasmic globules filled with immunoglobulins are frequent and are referred to as **Mott cells**. Chronic disease leads to progressive cachexia; patients, devoid of energy and normal mentation, literally waste away.

Chagas Disease

***Trypanosoma cruzi* is a kinetoplastid, intracellular protozoan parasite that causes American trypanosomiasis (Chagas disease).** Chagas disease occurs rarely in the United States and Mexico but is more common in South America, particularly Brazil. *T. cruzi* parasites infect many animals, including cats, dogs, and rodents. The parasites are transmitted between animals and to humans by triatomine bugs (also known as kissing bugs or reduviids), which hide in the cracks of loosely constructed houses, feed on the sleeping inhabitants, and pass the parasites in the feces; the infectious parasites enter the host through damaged skin or through mucous membranes. At the site of skin entry there may be a transient, erythematous nodule. Another important route of infection is oral ingestion of the parasites due to contamination of food products with triatomine bugs and/or their feces. Once in the host, *T. cruzi* invades human cells through interaction with a variety of molecules including TLRs, kinins, and receptors for TGF, EGF, tyrosine kinases, and LDL.

Pathogenesis. While most intracellular pathogens avoid the toxic contents of lysosomes, *T. cruzi* actually requires brief exposure to the acidic phagolysosome for development of amastigotes, the intracellular stage of the parasite.

To ensure exposure to lysosomes, *T. cruzi* trypomastigotes elevate the concentration of cytoplasmic calcium in host cells, which promotes fusion of the phagosome and lysosome. In addition to enhancing amastigote development, the low pH of the lysosome activates pore-forming proteins that disrupt the lysosomal membrane, releasing the parasite into the cell cytoplasm. Parasites reproduce as rounded amastigotes in the cytoplasm of host cells and then develop flagella, lyse host cells, enter the bloodstream, and penetrate smooth, skeletal, and heart muscles.

Chagas disease primarily affects the heart and in endemic areas, it is a major cause of sudden death due to cardiac arrhythmia. In acute Chagas disease, which is mild in most individuals, cardiac damage results from direct invasion of myocardial cells by the organisms and the subsequent inflammation. Rarely, acute Chagas disease presents with high parasitemia, fever, or progressive cardiac dilation and failure, often with generalized lymphadenopathy or splenomegaly. In chronic Chagas disease, which occurs in 20% of people 5 to 15 years after initial infection, the mechanism of cardiac damage has two components.

- The presence of persistent *T. cruzi* parasites leads to a continued immune response with a striking inflammatory infiltration of the myocardium, even though only scant organisms may be present.
- The parasite also may induce autoimmune responses, such that antibodies and T cells that recognize parasite proteins cross-react with host myocardial cells, nerve cells, and extracellular proteins such as laminin. For example, cross-reactive antibodies may induce electrophysiologic dysfunction of the heart.

Damage to myocardial cells and to conductance pathways causes a dilated cardiomyopathy and cardiac arrhythmias. In addition, damage to the myenteric plexus causes dilation of the colon (megacolon) and esophagus. This is particularly common in Brazilian endemic areas where as many as 50% of the patients with lethal carditis have colonic and esophageal disease.

MORPHOLOGY

In lethal **acute myocarditis**, the changes are diffusely distributed throughout the heart. Clusters of amastigotes cause swelling of individual myocardial fibers and create intracellular pseudocysts. There is focal myocardial cell necrosis accompanied by extensive, dense, acute interstitial inflammatory infiltration throughout the myocardium, often associated with four-chamber cardiac dilation (Chapter 12).

In **chronic Chagas disease** the heart is typically dilated, rounded, and increased in size and weight. Often, there are mural thrombi that, in about half of autopsy cases, have given rise to pulmonary or systemic emboli or infarctions. On histologic examination, there are interstitial and perivascular inflammatory infiltrates composed of lymphocytes, plasma cells, and monocytes. There are scattered foci of myocardial cell necrosis and interstitial fibrosis, especially toward the apex of the left ventricle, which may undergo aneurysmal dilation and thinning. Even with dilation of the esophagus and colon, parasites cannot be found within ganglia of myenteric plexus. Chronic Chagas cardiomyopathy is often treated by cardiac transplantation.

Metazoa

Metazoa are multicellular, eukaryotic organisms. The parasitic metazoa are contracted by consuming the parasite, often in undercooked meat, or by direct invasion of the host through the skin or via insect bites. Metazoa dwell in many sites of the body, including the intestine, skin, lung, liver, muscle, blood vessels, and lymphatics. The infections are diagnosed by microscopic identification of larvae or ova in excretions or tissues, and by serology.

Strongyloidiasis

Strongyloides stercoralis infects tens of million people worldwide and is endemic in the southeastern United States, South America, sub-Saharan Africa, and Southeast Asia. **The worms live in the soil and infect humans when larvae penetrate the skin, travel in the circulation to the lungs, and then travel up the trachea to be swallowed.** Female worms reside in the mucosa of the small intestine, where they produce eggs by asexual reproduction (parthenogenesis). Most of the larvae are passed in the stool and then may contaminate soil to continue the cycle of infection.

In immunocompetent hosts, *S. stercoralis* may cause diarrhea, bloating, and occasionally malabsorption. Unlike other parasitic worms, *S. stercoralis* larvae hatched in the gut can invade the colon mucosa and reinitiate infection (autoinfection). Immunocompromised hosts, particularly people on prolonged corticosteroid therapy, can have very high worm burdens (hyperinfection) due to uncontrolled autoinfection, leading to fatal disease. Corticosteroids inhibit the functions of eosinophils that accumulate in tissues in response to infection, induce apoptosis in immune cells, and stimulate female *Strongyloides* directly to increase infective larvae production. In addition, other disease states which perturb immune control mechanisms (e.g., organ transplantation, lymphoma, HIV/AIDS, HTLV-1) have increased risks. Hyperinfection can be complicated by sepsis caused by intestinal bacteria, which enter the blood following damage to the intestinal wall by the invading larvae.

MORPHOLOGY

In mild strongyloidiasis, worms, mainly larvae, are present in the duodenal crypts but are not seen in the underlying tissue. There is an eosinophil-rich infiltrate in the lamina propria with mucosal edema. Hyperinfection with *S. stercoralis* results in invasion of larvae into the colonic submucosa, lymphatics, and blood vessels, with an associated mononuclear infiltrate. There are many adult worms, larvae, and eggs in the crypts of the duodenum and ileum (Fig. 8-51). Worms of all stages may be found in other organs, including skin and lungs, and may even be found in large numbers in sputum.

Tapeworms (Cestodes): Cysticercosis and Hydatid Disease

Taenia solium and *Echinococcus granulosus* are cestode parasites (tapeworms) that cause cysticercosis and hydatid infections, respectively. Both diseases are caused by larvae that develop after ingestion of tapeworm eggs. These tapeworms have a complex life cycle requiring two mammalian hosts: a definitive host, in which the worm reaches sexual

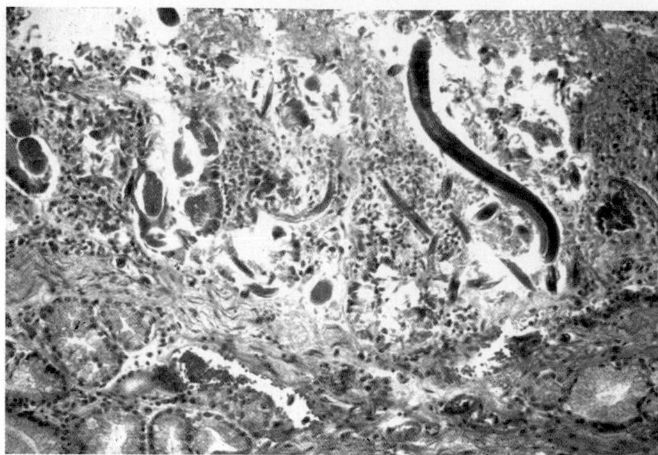

Figure 8-51 *Strongyloides* hyperinfection in a patient treated with high-dose cortisone. A female, her eggs, and rhabditoid larvae are in the duodenal crypts; filariform larvae are entering the blood vessels and muscularis mucosa. (Courtesy Dr. Franz C. Von Lichtenberg, Brigham and Women's Hospital, Boston, Mass.)

maturity, and an intermediate host, in which the worm does not reach sexual maturity.

Taenia solium tapeworms consist of a head (scolex) that has suckers and hooklets that attach to the intestinal wall, a neck, and many flat segments called *proglottids* that contain both male and female reproductive organs. New proglottids develop behind the scolex. The most distal proglottids are mature and contain many eggs, and they can detach and be shed in the feces. *T. solium* can be transmitted to humans in two ways, ingestion of larval cysts or eggs, with distinct outcomes.

- Larval cysts, called cysticerci, are ingested in undercooked pork and attach to the intestinal wall, where they develop into mature adult tapeworms. These can grow to many meters in length and produce mild abdominal symptoms. The parasite life cycle is completed with this mode of infection and cysticercosis does not develop.
- When intermediate hosts (pigs or humans) ingest eggs in food or water contaminated with human feces, the larvae hatch, penetrate the gut wall, disseminate hematogenously, and encyst in many organs, giving rise to clinical symptoms of cysticercosis. The most serious manifestations result from encystment in the brain (neurocysticercosis). Convulsions, increased intracranial pressure, and other neurologic disturbances may occur. Adult tapeworms are not produced with this mode of infection since larval cysts lodged in various tissues cannot develop into mature worms. Viable *T. solium* cysts often do not produce symptoms and can evade host immune defenses by producing taeniaestatin and paramyosin, which seem to inhibit complement activation. When the cysticerci die and degenerate, an inflammatory response develops.

Taenia saginata, the beef tapeworm, and *Diphyllobothrium latum*, the fish tapeworm, are acquired by eating undercooked meat or fish. In humans these parasites live only in the gut, and do not form cysticerci.

Hydatid disease is caused by ingestion of eggs of echinococcal species. For *Echinococcus granulosus* the definitive host is the dog and the usual intermediate hosts are sheep. For *Echinococcus multilocularis* the fox is the most important definitive host, and rodents are intermediate hosts. Humans are accidental intermediate hosts, infected by ingestion of food contaminated with eggs shed by dogs or foxes. Eggs hatch in the duodenum and invade the liver, lungs, or bones.

MORPHOLOGY

Cysticerci may be found in any organ, but the more common locations include the brain, muscles, skin, and heart. Cerebral symptoms depend on the precise location of the cysts, which may be intraparenchymal, attached to the arachnoid, or freely floating in the ventricular system. The cysts are ovoid and white to opalescent, often grape-sized, and contain an invaginated scolex with hooklets that are bathed in clear cyst fluid (Fig. 8-52). The cyst wall is more than 100 μm thick, is rich in glycoproteins, and evokes little host inflammatory response when it is intact. When cysts degenerate, however, there is inflammation, followed by focal scarring, and calcifications, which may be visible by radiography.

About two thirds of human *E. granulosus* cysts are found in the liver, 5% to 15% in the lung, and the rest in bones and brain or other organs. In the various organs the larvae lodge within the capillaries and first incite an inflammatory reaction composed principally of mononuclear leukocytes and eosinophils. Many such larvae are destroyed, but others encyst. The cysts begin at microscopic levels and progressively increase in size, so that in 5 years or more they may have achieved dimensions of more than 10 cm in diameter. Enclosing an opalescent fluid is an inner, nucleated, germinative layer and an outer, opaque, non-nucleated layer. The outer non-nucleated layer is distinctive and has innumerable delicate laminations. Outside this opaque layer, there is a host inflammatory reaction that produces a zone of fibroblasts, giant cells, and mononuclear and eosinophilic cells. In time a dense fibrous capsule forms. Daughter cysts often develop within the large mother cyst. These appear first as minute projections of the germinative layer that develop central vesicles and thus form tiny brood capsules. Degenerating scolices of the worm produce a fine, sandlike sediment within the hydatid fluid (hydatid sand).

Trichinosis

Trichinella is a species of nematode parasite that is acquired by ingestion of larvae in undercooked meat from infected

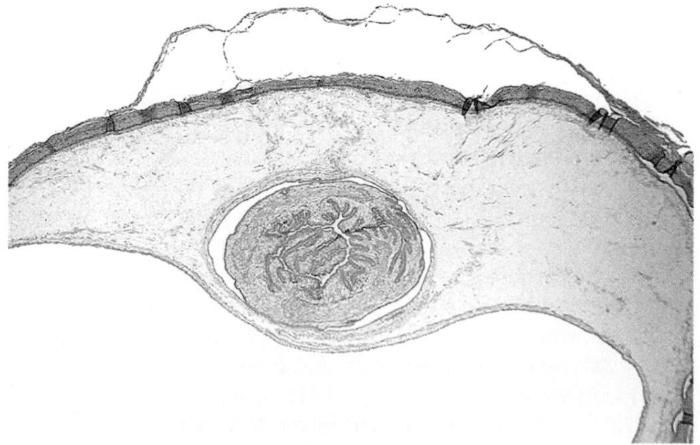

Figure 8-52 Portion of a cysticercus cyst in the skin.

animals (usually pigs, boars, or horses) that have themselves been infected by eating rats or meat products containing *T. spiralis, T. nativa,* or *T. britovi*. In the United States the number of *T. spiralis*–infected pigs has been greatly reduced by laws requiring proper cooking of food fed to hogs; the number of reported human infections in the United States is now less than 20 cases each year. Still, trichinosis remains widespread in other parts of the world, where undercooked meat, including noncommercial livestock and game (e.g., bear), is commonly eaten.

The life cycle of *T. spiralis* begins in the human intestine but ends within muscle as humans are dead-end hosts. In the human gut, *T. spiralis* larvae develop into adults that mate and release new larvae, which penetrate into the tissues. Larvae disseminate hematogenously and penetrate muscle cells, causing fever, myalgias, marked eosinophilia, and periorbital edema. Less commonly, the larvae lodge in the heart, lungs, and brain, and patients can develop dyspnea, encephalitis, and cardiac failure. In striated skeletal muscle, *T. spiralis* larvae become intracellular parasites, increase dramatically in size, and modify the host muscle cell (referred to as the *nurse cell*) so that it loses its striations, gains a collagenous capsule, and develops a plexus of new blood vessels around itself. The nurse cell-parasite complex is largely asymptomatic, and the worm may persist for years before it dies and calcifies. Antibodies to larval antigens, which include an immunodominant carbohydrate epitope called *tyvelose*, may reduce reinfection and are useful for serodiagnosis of the disease.

***Trichinella spiralis* and other invasive nematodes stimulate a T_H2 response,** with production of IL-4, IL-5, IL-10, and IL-13. The cytokines produced by T_H2 cells activate eosinophils and mast cells, both of which are associated with the inflammatory response to these parasites. In animal models of *T. spiralis* infection, the T_H2 response is associated with increased contractility of the intestine, which expels adult worms from the gut and subsequently reduces the number of larvae in the muscles. While the T_H2 response indirectly reduces the number of larvae in muscle by eliminating adults from the intestine, it is not clear whether the intramuscular inflammatory response, which is composed of mononuclear cells and eosinophils, is effective against the larvae.

MORPHOLOGY

During the invasive phase of trichinosis, cell destruction can be widespread with heavy infections and may be lethal. In the heart there is a patchy interstitial myocarditis characterized by many eosinophils and scattered giant cells. The myocarditis can lead to scarring. Larvae in the heart do not encyst and are difficult to identify, because they die and disappear. In the lungs, trapped larvae cause focal edema and hemorrhages, sometimes with an allergic eosinophilic infiltrate. In the CNS, larvae cause a diffuse lymphocytic and eosinophilic infiltrate, with focal gliosis in and about small capillaries of the brain.

Trichinella spiralis preferentially encysts in striated skeletal muscles with the richest blood supply, including the diaphragm and the extraocular, laryngeal, deltoid, gastrocnemius, and intercostal muscles (Fig. 8-53). Coiled larvae are approximately 1 mm long and are surrounded by membrane-bound vacuoles within nurse cells, which in turn are surrounded by new blood vessels and an eosinophil-rich mononuclear cell infiltrate. This infiltrate is greatest around dying parasites, which eventually calcify and leave behind scars that are sufficiently characteristic to suggest the diagnosis of trichinosis.

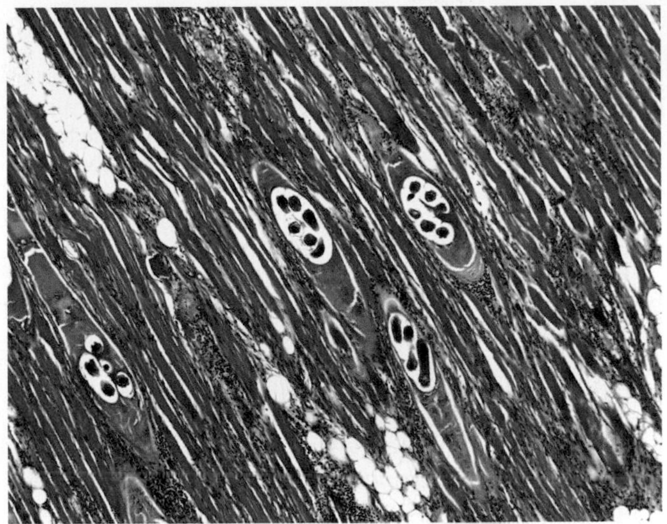

Figure 8-53 Multiple coiled *Trichinella spiralis* larvae within skeletal muscle cells.

Schistosomiasis

Schistosomiasis infects approximately 230 million persons and kills more than 200,000 individuals annually. The affected organs and hence the site of major disease vary with the species. *Shistosoma* mansoni and *S. japonicum* affect the liver and the gut predominantly. Most deaths are due to hepatic cirrhosis, which is caused by *S. mansoni* in Latin America, Africa, and the Middle East and by *S. japonicum* and *S. mekongi* in East Asia. By contrast, *S. haematobium*, found in Africa, causes chronic granulomatous bladder inflammation that may lead to hematuria, obstructive uropathy, and carcinoma. *Schistosoma* flukes, like all trematodes, require passage through freshwater snails that live in the slow-moving water of tropical rivers, lakes, and irrigation ditches, ironically linking agricultural development with spread of the disease. Acute schistosomiasis in humans can be a severe febrile illness that peaks about 2 months after infection. Severe hepatic fibrosis is a serious manifestation of chronic schistosomiasis (see later).

Pathogenesis. **Much of the pathology of schistosomiasis is caused by host inflammatory reactions to different stages of the parasite.** The life cycle of *Schistosoma* involves stepwise infection of several human tissues, each associated with host inflammatory responses. After release from snails, ciliated miracidium larvae mature into infectious schistosome larvae (cercariae) that swim through fresh water and penetrate human skin with the aid of powerful proteolytic enzymes that degrade the keratinized layer. There is minimal skin reaction. Schistosomes migrate through the skin into the peripheral vasculature and lymphatics, travel to the lungs and heart, from where they are disseminated widely, including the mesenteric, splanchnic and portal circulation, ultimately reaching the hepatic vessels where they mature (*S. mansoni* and *S. japonicum*).

Mature male-female worm pairs then migrate once again and settle in the venous system (commonly the portal or pelvic veins). Females produce hundreds to thousands of eggs per day which secrete proteases and elicit localized inflammatory reactions. This inflammatory response to egg migration is necessary for passive transfer across the intestine and, in the case of *S. haemtobium*, bladder walls, allowing the eggs to be shed in stool or urine, respectively. Infection of freshwater snails completes the life cycle.

Eggs that are carried by the portal circulation into the hepatic parenchyma can cause severe chronic inflammation in the liver. This immune response to *S. mansoni* and *S. japonicum* eggs is responsible for the most serious complication of schistosomiasis , liver fibrosis. The helper T-cell response in the early stage is dominated by T_H1 cells that produce IFN-γ, which stimulates macrophages to secrete high levels of the cytokines TNF, IL-1, and IL-6 that cause fever. Chronic schistosomiasis is associated with a dominant T_H2 response, associated with the presence of alternatively activated macrophages. Both types of helper T cells contribute to the formation of granulomas surrounding eggs in the liver. Hepatic fibrosis is a serious manifestation of chronic schistosomiasis in which T_H2 cells and alternatively activated macrophages may play the major role.

MORPHOLOGY

In early *S. mansoni* or *S. japonicum* infections, white, pinhead-sized granulomas are scattered throughout the gut and liver. At the center of the granuloma is the schistosome egg, which contains a miracidium; this degenerates over time and calcifies. The granulomas are composed of macrophages, lymphocytes, neutrophils, and eosinophils, which are distinctive for helminth infections (Fig. 8-54). The liver is darkened by regurgitated heme-derived pigments from the schistosome gut, which, like malaria pigments, are iron-free and accumulate in Kupffer cells and splenic macrophages.

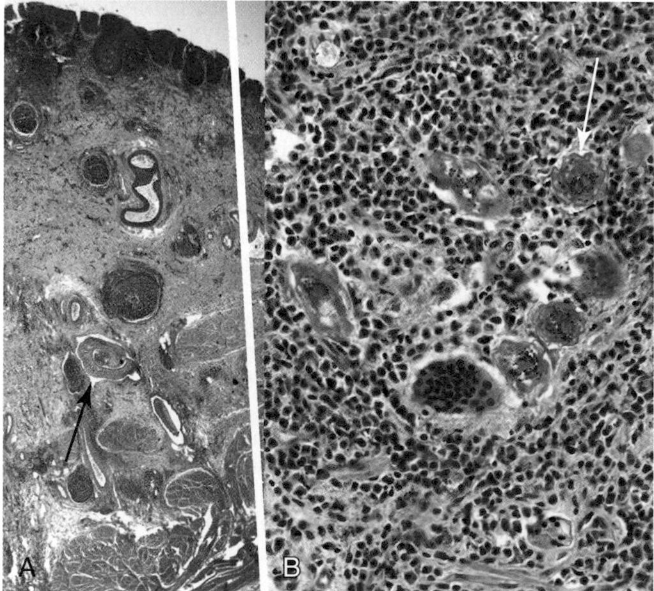

Figure 8-54 *Schistosoma hematobium* infection of the bladder (left) showing dense fibrosis, scattered granulomas, and a cross section of adult worms in a vessel *(arrow)*. High magnification (right) demonstrates miracidium-containing eggs *(arrow)*, prominent eosinophils, histiocytes, and giant cells.

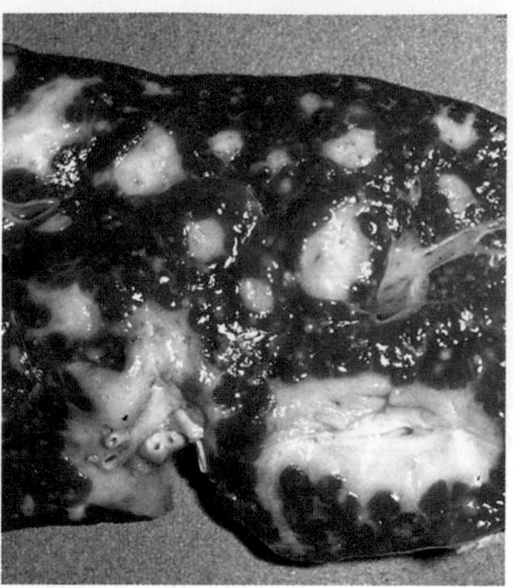

Figure 8-55 Pipe-stem fibrosis of the liver due to chronic *Schistosoma japonicum* infection.

In late *S. mansoni* or *S. japonicum* infections, inflammatory patches or pseudopolyps may form in the colon. The surface of the liver is bumpy, and cut surfaces reveal granulomas and widespread fibrosis and portal enlargement without intervening regenerative nodules. Because these fibrous triads resemble the stem of a clay pipe, the lesion is named **pipestem fibrosis** (Fig. 8-55). The fibrosis often obliterates the portal veins, leading to portal hypertension, severe congestive splenomegaly, esophageal varices, and ascites. Schistosome eggs, diverted to the lung through portal collaterals, may produce granulomatous pulmonary arteritis with intimal hyperplasia, progressive arterial obstruction, and ultimately heart failure (cor pulmonale). On histologic examination, arteries in the lungs show disruption of the elastic layer by granulomas and scars, luminal organizing thrombi, and angiomatoid lesions similar to those of idiopathic pulmonary hypertension (Chapter 15). Patients with hepatosplenic schistosomiasis also have an increased frequency of mesangioproliferative or membranous glomerulopathy (Chapter 20), in which glomeruli contain deposits of immunoglobulin and complement but rarely schistosome antigen.

In *S. haematobium* infection, inflammatory cystitis due to massive egg deposition and granulomas appears early, leading to mucosal erosions and hematuria. Later, the granulomas calcify and develop a sandy appearance, which, if severe, may line the wall of the bladder and cause a dense concentric rim (calcified bladder) on radiographic films. The most frequent complication of *S. haematobium* infection is inflammation and fibrosis of the ureteral walls, leading to obstruction, hydronephrosis, and chronic pyelonephritis. There is also an association between urinary schistosomiasis and squamous cell carcinoma of the bladder (Chapter 21).

Lymphatic Filariasis

Lymphatic filariasis is transmitted by mosquitoes and is caused by closely related nematodes, *Wuchereria bancrofti* and *Brugia* species (*B. malayi* or *B. timori*), which are responsible for 90% and 10%, respectively, of the 90 million infections worldwide. In endemic areas, which include parts of Latin America, sub-Saharan Africa, and Southeast Asia, filariasis causes a spectrum of diseases.

- Asymptomatic microfilaremia
- Recurrent lymphadenitis
- Chronic lymphadenitis with swelling of the dependent limb or scrotum (elephantiasis)
- Tropical pulmonary eosinophilia.

As is the case with leprosy and leishmanial infections, some of the different disease manifestations caused by lymphatic filariae are likely related to variations in host T-cell responses to the parasites.

Pathogenesis. Infective larvae released by mosquitoes into the tissues during a blood meal develop within lymphatic channels into adult males and females, which mate and release microfilariae that enter into the bloodstream. When they bite infected individuals the mosquitoes can take up the microfilariae and transmit the disease. The filarial genome project has led to the identification of a number of filarial molecules that enable the organism to evade or inhibit immune defenses. *Brugia malayi* produces:

- Several surface glycoproteins with antioxidant function, which may protect from superoxide and free oxygen radicals
- Homologs of cystatins, cysteine protease inhibitors, which can impair the MHC class II antigen-processing pathway
- Serpins, serine protease inhibitors, which can inhibit neutrophil proteases, critical inflammatory mediators
- Homologs of TGF-β, which can bind to mammalian TGF-β receptors and downregulate inflammatory responses.

In addition, symbiotic *Wolbachia* bacteria infect filarial nematodes and contribute to pathogenesis of disease. *Wolbachia* are required for nematode development and reproduction, and antibiotics that eradicate *Wolbachia* impair nematode survival and fertility. It has been hypothesized that LPS from *Wolbachia* also stimulates inflammatory responses.

Immunologic responses to the filarial worms produce damage to the human host. In chronic lymphatic filariasis, damage to the lymphatics is caused directly by the adult parasites and by a T_H1-mediated immune response, which stimulates the formation of granulomas around the adult parasites. There may be an *IgE-mediated hypersensitivity* response to microfilariae in *tropical pulmonary eosinophilia.* IgE and eosinophils may be stimulated by IL-4 and IL-5, respectively, secreted by filaria-specific T_H2 helper T cells. Tropical pulmonary eosinophilia is seen most commonly in either individuals of Southern Asian or northern Latin American descent, suggesting that host factors contribute to this disorder (Chapter 15).

MORPHOLOGY

Chronic filariasis is characterized by **persistent lymphedema** of the extremities, scrotum, penis, or vulva (Fig. 8-56). Frequently there is hydrocele and lymph node enlargement. In severe and long-lasting infections, chylous weeping of the enlarged scrotum may ensue, or a chronically swollen leg may develop tough subcutaneous fibrosis and epithelial hyperkeratosis, termed **elephantiasis**. Elephantoid skin shows dilation of the dermal lymphatics, widespread lymphocytic infiltrates and focal cholesterol deposits; the epidermis is thickened and hyperkeratotic. Adult filarial worms—live, dead, or calcified—are present in the draining lymphatics or nodes, surrounded by (1) mild or no inflammation, (2) an intense eosinophilia with hemorrhage and fibrin (recurrent filarial funiculoepididymitis), or (3) granulomas. Over time, the dilated lymphatics develop polypoid infoldings. In the testis, hydrocele fluid, which often contains cholesterol crystals, red cells, and hemosiderin, induces thickening and calcification of the tunica vaginalis.

Lung involvement by microfilariae is marked by eosinophilia caused by T_H2 responses and cytokine production (tropical eosinophilia) or by dead microfilariae surrounded by stellate, hyaline, eosinophilic precipitates embedded in small epithelioid granulomas (Meyers-Kouwenaar bodies). Typically, these patients lack other manifestations of filarial disease.

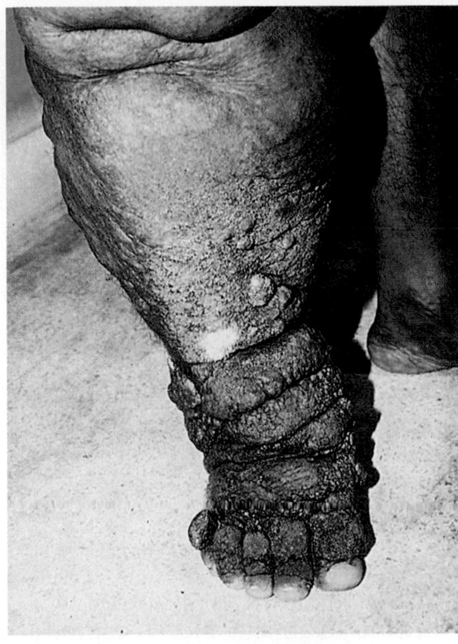

Figure 8-56 Massive edema and elephantiasis caused by filariasis of the leg. (Courtesy Dr. Willy Piessens, Harvard School of Public Health, Boston, Mass.)

Onchocerciasis

Onchocerca volvulus is a filarial nematode **that is the leading cause of preventable blindness in sub-Saharan Africa**. It is transmitted by black flies and affects 18 million people in Africa, South America, and Yemen. An aggressive campaign of ivermectin treatment has dramatically reduced the incidence of *Onchocerca* infection in West Africa. Since vector's preferred habitat is near fast moving water there is higher incidence of human disease near rivers, accounting for the name *river blindness* given to this disease. It is estimated that there are 270,000 people who are blind due to onchocerciasis.

The disease attributable to onchocerciasis is primarily due to inflammation induced by microfilaria. Adult *O. volvulus* parasites mate in the dermis, where they are surrounded by a mixed infiltrate of host cells that produces a characteristic subcutaneous nodule *(onchocercoma)*. Inseminated females produce microfilariae, which accumulate in the skin and disseminate to the eye chambers.

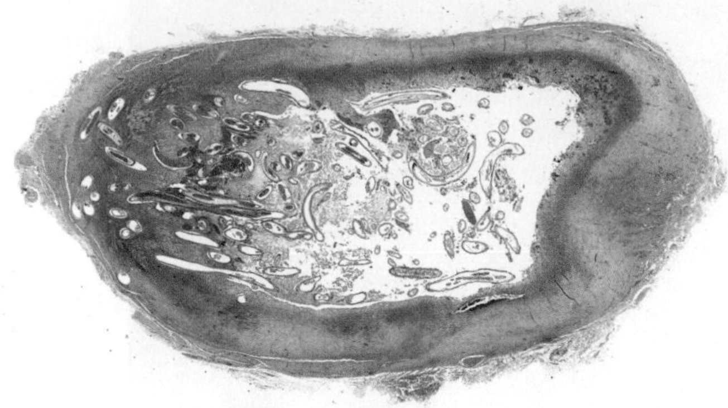

Figure 8-57 Microfilaria-laden gravid female of *Onchocerca volvulus* in a subcutaneous fibrous nodule.

Ivermectin kills only immature worms, not adult worms, so parasites repopulate the host a few months after treatment. Doxycycline treatment blocks reproduction of *O. volvus* for up to 24 months by killing *Wolbachia*, already mentioned as symbiotic bacteria that are required for the fertility of the filarial species.

MORPHOLOGY

Onchocerca volvulus causes chronic, itchy dermatitis with focal darkening or loss of pigment and scaling, referred to as *leopard, lizard, or elephant skin*. Foci of epidermal atrophy and elastic fiber breakdown may alternate with areas of hyperkeratosis, hyperpigmentation with pigment incontinence, dermal atrophy, and fibrosis. The subcutaneous onchocercoma is composed of a fibrous capsule surrounding adult worms and a mixed chronic inflammatory infiltrate that includes fibrin, neutrophils, eosinophils, lymphocytes, and giant cells (Fig. 8-57). The progressive eye lesions begin with punctate keratitis along with small, fluffy opacities of the cornea caused by degenerating microfilariae, which evoke an eosinophilic infiltrate. This is followed by a sclerosing keratitis that opacifies the cornea, beginning at the scleral limbus. Keratitis is sometimes accentuated by treatment with antifilarial drugs (Mazzotti reaction). Microfilariae in the anterior chamber cause iridocyclitis and glaucoma, whereas involvement of the choroid and retina results in atrophy and loss of vision.

Emerging Infectious Diseases

The rapidly expanding human population juxtaposed with environmental infractions allow the emergence of new pathogens and the re-emergence of old infectious agents. Although infectious diseases such as leprosy have been known since biblical times, and parasitic schistosomes and mycobacteria have been demonstrated in Egyptian mummies, a surprising number of new infectious agents continue to be discovered (Table 8-9). The infectious causes of some diseases with significant morbidity and mortality were previously unrecognized, because some of the infectious agents are difficult to culture; examples include *Helicobacter pylori* gastritis, HBV and HCV, and *Legionella pneumophila*. Some infectious agents are genuinely new to humans, e.g., HIV, which causes AIDS, and *B. burgdorferi*, which causes Lyme disease. Other infections have become much more common because of immunosuppression caused by AIDS or therapy for transplant rejection and some cancers (e.g., CMV, Kaposi sarcoma herpesvirus, *Mycobacterium avium-intracellulare, Pneumocystis jiroveci*, and *Cryptosporidium parvum*). Finally, infectious diseases that are common in one area may be introduced into a new area. For example, West Nile virus has been common in Europe, Asia, and Africa for years but was first described in the United States in 1999.

Human demographics and behavior are important contributors to the emergence of infectious diseases. AIDS was first recognized in the United States as predominantly a disease of homosexuals and injection drug users, but heterosexual transmission is now common. In sub-Saharan Africa, the area of the world with the highest number of AIDS cases, it is predominantly a heterosexual disease. Changes in the environment occasionally drive rates of infectious diseases. Reforestation of the eastern United States has led to massive increases in the populations of deer and mice, which carry the ticks that transmit Lyme disease, babesiosis, and ehrlichiosis. Failure of DDT to control the mosquitoes that transmit malaria and the development of drug-resistant parasites have dramatically increased the morbidity and mortality of *Plasmodium falciparum* infection in Asia, Africa, and Latin America. Microbial adaptation to widespread antibiotic use contributed to the emergence of drug resistance in many species of bacteria, including *M. tuberculosis, N. gonorrhoeae, S. aureus*, and *E. faecium*. Infections with antibiotic-resistant

Table 8-9 Some Recently Recognized Infectious Agents and Manifestations

Date Recognized	Infectious Agent	Manifestations
1977	Ebola virus	Epidemic Ebola hemorrhagic fever
	Hantaan virus	Hemorrhagic fever with renal syndrome
	Legionella pneumophila	Legionnaire disease
	Campylobacter jejuni	Enteritis
1980	HTLV-I	T-cell lymphoma or leukemia, HTLV-associated myelopathy
1981	*Staphylococcus aureus*	Toxic shock syndrome
1982	*Escherichia coli* 0157:H7	Hemorrhagic colitis, hemolytic-uremic syndrome
	Borrelia burgdorferi	Lyme disease
1983	HIV	AIDS
	Helicobacter pylori	Gastric ulcers
1988	Hepatitis E	Enterically transmitted hepatitis
1989	Hepatitis C	Hepatitis C
1992	*Vibrio cholerae* 0139	New epidemic cholera strain
	Bartonella henselae	Cat-scratch disease
1995	KSHV (HHV-8)	Kaposi sarcoma in AIDS
1999	West Nile virus	West Nile fever, neuroinvasive disease
2003	SARS coronavirus	Severe acute respiratory syndrome

bacteria are a continuing problem due to widespread use of antibiotics (e.g., MRSA and vancomycin-resistant *Enterococcus*). Human commercial use of dense populations of domestic animals (e.g., pigs, chickens) juxtaposed to habitat destruction of other disease reservoirs (e.g., bats and wild birds) can lead to acquisition of either unique traits in common pathogens such as influenza or emergence of unique viruses such as severe acute respiratory syndrome (SARS) virus and West Nile Virus. Because these pathogens are novel, humans lack immunity and so these infections can quickly spread through the population as pandemics, as was seen with influenza A H1N1 in 2009.

Agents of Bioterrorism. Sadly, the anthrax attacks in the United States in 2001 transformed the theoretical threat of bioterrorism into reality. The CDC has evaluated the microorganisms that pose the greatest danger as weapons on the basis of the efficiency with which disease can be transmitted, how difficult the microorganisms are to produce and distribute, what can be done to defend against them, and the extent to which they are likely to alarm the public and produce widespread fear.

- Category A agents pose the highest risk and can be readily disseminated or transmitted from person to person, can cause high mortality with potential for major public health impact, might cause public panic and social disruption, and might require special action for public health preparedness. For example, smallpox is a category A agent because of its high transmissibility in any climate or season, case mortality rate of 30% or greater, and lack of effective antiviral therapy. This agent can be easily disseminated because of the stability of the virus in aerosol form and the very small dose needed for infection. Smallpox naturally spreads from person to person mainly by direct contact with virus in skin lesions or contaminated clothing or bedding. Symptoms appear after 7 to 17 days. Initially there is high fever, headache, and backache, followed by the appearance of the rash, which first appears on the mucosa of the mouth and pharynx, face, and forearms and later spreads to the trunk and legs and becomes vesicular and later pustular. Because people can be contagious during the incubation period, this virus has the potential to continue to spread throughout an unprotected population. Since vaccination ended in the United States in 1972 and vaccination immunity has waned, the population is highly susceptible to smallpox. Recent concern that smallpox could be used for bioterrorism has led to a return of vaccination for selected groups in the United States and Israel.
- Category B agents are relatively easy to disseminate, produce moderate morbidity but low mortality, and require specific diagnostic and disease surveillance. Many of these agents are foodborne or waterborne. Examples include *Brucella* sp., *Vibrio cholerae*, and ricin toxin from castor beans.
- Category C agents include emerging pathogens that could be engineered for mass dissemination because of availability, ease of production and dissemination, potential for high morbidity and mortality, and great impact on health. Examples include Hantavirus and Nipahvirus.

SUGGESTED READINGS

General Principles of Microbial Pathogenesis

Casanova JL, Abel L, Quintana-Murci L: Human TLRs and IL-1Rs in host defense: natural insights from evolutionary, epidemiological, and clinical genetics. *Annu Rev Immunol* 29:447–91, 2011.

Honda K, Littman DR: The microbiome in infectious disease and inflammation. *Annu Rev Immunol* 30:759–95, 2012.

Mims C, Nash A, Stephen J: *Mims' Pathogenesis of Infectious Disease*, ed 5, London; San Diego, 2000, Academic Press.

Noriega V, Redmann V, Gardner T, et al: Diverse immune evasion strategies by human cytomegalovirus. *Immunol Res* 54:140–51, 2012.

Relman DA: Microbial genomics and infectious diseases. *N Engl J Med* 365:347–57, 2011.

Virology

Balfour HH Jr, Odumade OA, Schmeling DO, et al: Behavioral, Virologic, and Immunologic Factors Associated With Acquisition and Severity of Primary Epstein Barr Virus Infection in University Students. *J Infect Dis* 2012.

Griffin DE, Lin WH, Pan CH: Measles virus, immune control, and persistence. *FEMS Microbiol Rev* 36:649–62, 2012.

Kew O: Reaching the last one per cent: progress and challenges in global polio eradication. *Curr Opin Virol* 2:188–98, 2012.

Koelle DM, Corey L: Herpes simplex: insights on pathogenesis and possible vaccines. *Annu Rev Med* 59:381–95, 2008.

Lim JK, McDermott DH, Lisco A, et al: CCR5 deficiency is a risk factor for early clinical manifestations of West Nile virus infection but not for viral transmission. *J Infect Dis* 201:178–85, 2010.

Mulholland EK, Griffiths UK, Biellik R: Measles in the 21st century. *N Engl J Med* 366:1755–7, 2012.

Paessler S, Walker DH: Pathogenesis of the Viral Hemorrhagic Fevers. *Annu Rev Pathol* 2012.

Rickinson AB, Fox CP: Epstein-Barr Virus and Infectious Mononucleosis: What Students Can Teach Us. *J Infect Dis* 2012.

Schmidt AC: Response to dengue fever—the good, the bad, and the ugly? *N Engl J Med* 363:484–7, 2010.

Simmons CP, Farrar JJ, Nguyen v V, et al: Dengue. *N Engl J Med* 366:1423–32, 2012.

Speck SH, Ganem D: Viral latency and its regulation: lessons from the gamma-herpesviruses. *Cell Host Microbe* 8:100–15, 2010.

Bacteriology

Barrios-Payan J, Saqui-Salces M, Jeyanathan M, et al: Extrapulmonary locations of mycobacterium tuberculosis DNA during latent infection, *J Infect Dis* 206:1194–205, 2012.

Botelho-Nevers E, Raoult D: Host, pathogen and treatment-related prognostic factors in rickettsioses. *Eur J Clin Microbiol Infect Dis* 30:1139–50, 2011.

Cherry JD: Epidemic pertussis in 2012—the resurgence of a vaccine-preventable disease. *N Engl J Med* 367:785–7, 2012.

Ho EL, Lukehart SA: Syphilis: using modern approaches to understand an old disease. *J Clin Invest* 121:4584–92, 2011.

Mann EE, Wozniak DJ: Pseudomonas biofilm matrix composition and niche biology. *FEMS Microbiol Rev* 36:893–916, 2012.

Mediavilla JR, Chen L, Mathema B, et al: Global epidemiology of community-associated methicillin resistant Staphylococcus aureus (CA-MRSA). *Curr Opin Microbiol* 15:588–95, 2012.

Melican K, Dumenil G: Vascular colonization by Neisseria meningitidis. *Curr Opin Microbiol* 15:50–6, 2012.

Singh B, Fleury C, Jalalvand F, et al: Human pathogens utilize host extracellular matrix proteins laminin and collagen for adhesion and invasion of the host. *FEMS Microbiol Rev* 36:1122–80, 2012.

Wessels MR: Clinical practice. Streptococcal pharyngitis. *N Engl J Med* 364:648–55, 2011.

Zumla A, Raviglione M, Hafner R, et al: Tuberculosis. *N Engl J Med* 368:745–55, 2013.

Fungi

Dagenais TR, Keller NP: Pathogenesis of Aspergillus fumigatus in Invasive Aspergillosis. *Clin Microbiol Rev* 22:447–65, 2009.

Gamaletsou MN, Sipsas NV, Roilides E, et al: Rhino-orbital-cerebral mucormycosis. *Curr Infect Dis Rep* 14:423–34, 2012.

Karkowska-Kuleta J, Rapala-Kozik M, Kozik A: Fungi pathogenic to humans: molecular bases of virulence of Candida albicans, Cryptococcus neoformans and Aspergillus fumigatus. *Acta Biochim Pol* 56:211–24, 2009.

Netea MG, Marodi L: Innate immune mechanisms for recognition and uptake of Candida species. *Trends Immunol* 31:346–53, 2010.

Puel A, Cypowyj S, Marodi L, et al: Inborn errors of human IL-17 immunity underlie chronic mucocutaneous candidiasis. *Curr Opin Allergy Clin Immunol* 12:616–22, 2012.

Wuthrich M, Deepe GS Jr, Klein B: Adaptive immunity to fungi. *Annu Rev Immunol* 30:115–48, 2012.

Parasitology

Barron L, Wynn TA: Macrophage activation governs schistosomiasis-induced inflammation and fibrosis. *Eur J Immunol* 41:2509–14, 2011.

Duffield JS, Lupher M, Thannickal VJ, et al: Host responses in tissue repair and fibrosis. *Annu Rev Pathol* 8:241–76, 2013.

Larkin BM, Smith PM, Ponichtera HE, et al: Induction and regulation of pathogenic Th17 cell responses in schistosomiasis. *Semin Immunopathol* 34:873–88, 2012.

Lescure FX, Le Loup G, Freilij H, et al: Chagas disease: changes in knowledge and management. *Lancet Infect Dis* 10:556–70, 2010.

Machado FS, Dutra WO, Esper L, et al: Current understanding of immunity to Trypanosoma cruzi infection and pathogenesis of Chagas disease. *Semin Immunopathol* 34:753–70, 2012.

Marcos LA, Terashima A, Dupont HL, et al: Strongyloides hyperinfection syndrome: an emerging global infectious disease. *Trans R Soc Trop Med Hyg* 102:314–8, 2008.

Teixeirs AR, Hecht MM, Guimaro MC, et al: Pathogenesis of Chagas disease: parasite persistence and autoimmunity. *Clin Microbiol Rev* 24:592–630, 2011.

See TARGETED THERAPY available online at www.studentconsult.com

CHAPTER 9

Environmental and Nutritional Diseases

CHAPTER CONTENTS

Many diseases are caused or influenced by environmental factors. Broadly defined, the term *environment* encompasses the various indoor, outdoor, and occupational settings in which human beings live and work. In each of these settings, the air people breathe, the food and water they consume, and the toxic agents they are exposed to are major determinants of health. The environmental factors that influence our health pertain to individual behavior ("personal environment") and include tobacco use, alcohol ingestion, recreational drug consumption, diet, and the like, or the external (ambient and workplace) environment. In general, in developed countries personal behavior has a larger effect on health than the ambient environment, but new threats related to global warming (described later) may change this equation.

The term *environmental disease* refers to conditions caused by exposure to chemical or physical agents in the ambient, workplace, and personal environment, including diseases of nutritional origin. Disease related to environmental exposures mostly comes to the public's attention after dramatic events, such as the methyl mercury contamination of Minamata Bay in Japan in the 1960s, the exposure to dioxin in Seveso, Italy, in 1976, the leakage of methyl isocyanate gas in Bhopal, India, in 1984, the intentional contamination of Tokyo subways by the organophosphate pesticide sarin in 1995, and the Fukushima nuclear meltdown following the tsunami in 2011. Fortunately, these types of disasters are rare, but more subtle forms of environmental disease caused by chronic exposure to relatively low levels of contaminants, occupational injuries, and nutritional deficiencies are extremely common. The International Labor Organization has estimated that work-related injuries and illnesses kill approximately 2 million people per year globally (more deaths than are caused by road accidents and wars combined). In the United States in 2012, there were nearly 3 million occupational injuries and illnesses. Disease related to malnutrition is even more pervasive. In 2010, it was estimated that 925 million people were malnourished—one in every seven persons worldwide. Children are disproportionately affected by undernutrition, which accounts for more than 50% of childhood mortality worldwide. Estimating the burden of disease in the general population caused by nonoccupational exposures to toxic agents is complicated by the diversity of agents and difficulties in determining the extent and duration of exposures. But whatever the precise numbers, it is clear that environmental diseases are major causes of disability and suffering, and constitute a heavy financial burden, particularly in developing countries.

In this chapter, we first consider two key issues in global health: the global burden of disease, and the emerging problem of the health effects of climate change. We then discuss the mechanisms of toxicity of chemical and physical agents, and address specific environmental disorders, including those of nutritional origin.

Environmental Effects on Global Disease Burden

Since 1990 a World Health Organization project entitled "The Global Burden of Disease" (GBD) has set the standard for reporting global health information. The GBD estimates the burden imposed by environmental disease, including those caused by communicable and nutritional diseases. It does so in part by applying a metric called *DALY* (disability-adjusted life year), which is defined as the sum of years of life lost due to premature mortality and years of life lost to disability in a population. DALY reporting provides a high degree of uniformity for health information gathered about acute and chronic diseases in different parts of the world and at multiple locations in a single country. A comparison of causes of morbidity and mortality from 1990 to 2010 generated by the GBD project has revealed the following trends:

- **On a worldwide basis, there were dramatic increases in mortality due to HIV/AIDS and associated infections**, which peaked in 2006. Other changes included an 11.2% decrease in aggregate deaths from infectious disease, maternal, neonatal, and nutritional disorders; a 39.2% increase in deaths from noncommunicable diseases (e.g., cancer, cardiovascular diseases, and diabetes); and a 9.2% increase in deaths from injuries (Fig. 9-1). All are attributable in part to aging of the world's population from a mean age of 26.1 years to a mean age of 29.5 years. As a consequence of these shifts, the global healthy life expectancy at birth, an estimate of expected years of life free of disability, rose for men from 54.4 years to 58.3 years and for women from 57.8 years to 61.8 years.
- **Undernutrition is the single leading global cause of health loss (defined as morbidity and premature death).** It is estimated that about one third of the disease burden in developing countries is, directly or indirectly,

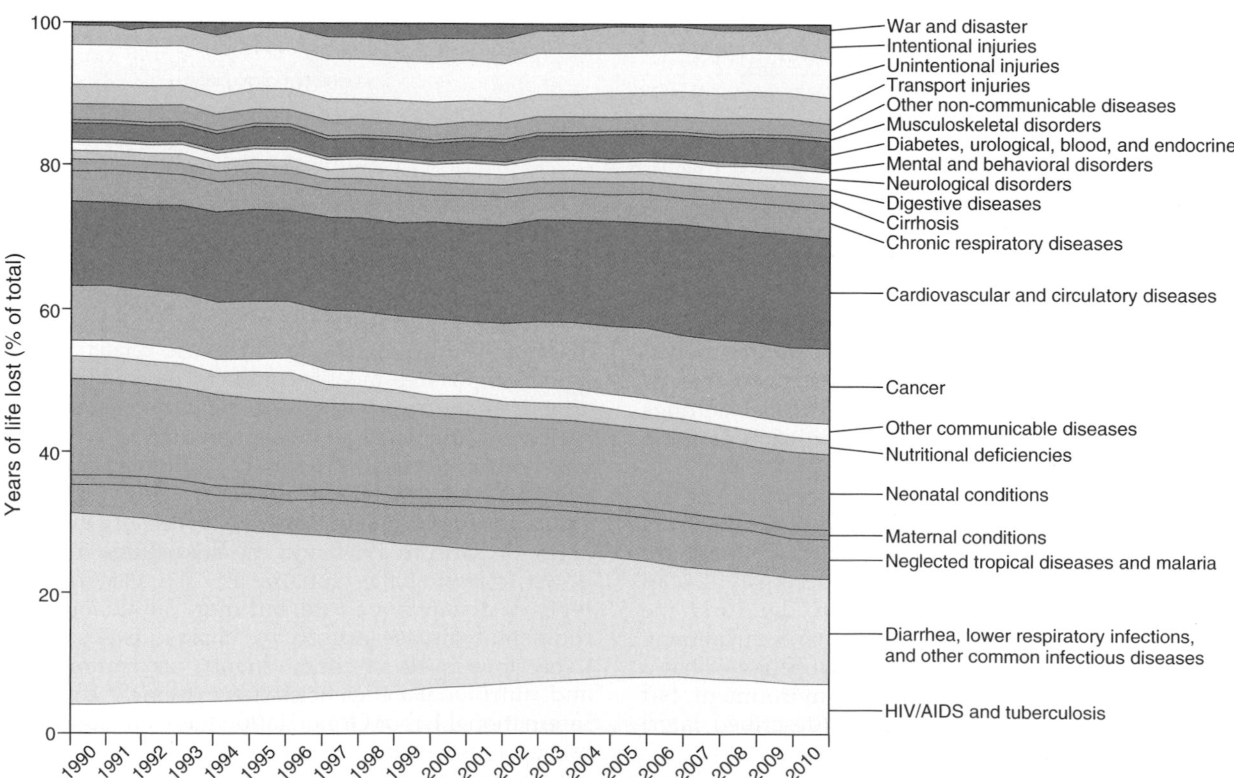

Figure 9-1 The changing global burden of disease, 1990-2010. Estimated percentage of years of life lost to diseases, accidents, war, and disaster is shown for this 20-year period.

due to poor general nutrition or deficiencies in specific nutrients that increase the risk of infections.

- **Ischemic heart disease and cerebrovascular disease remain the leading causes of death in developed countries.** In these countries the main risk factors associated with loss of healthy life are smoking, high blood pressure, obesity, high cholesterol, and alcohol abuse.
- **In developing countries, five of the 10 leading causes of death are infectious diseases:** respiratory infections, human immunodeficiency virus/acquired immunodeficiency syndrome (HIV/AIDS), diarrheal diseases, tuberculosis, and malaria. In 2010, HIV/AIDS and related infections such as tuberculosis were responsible for about 45% of years of life lost in Southern sub-Saharan Africa and about 10% in Southeast Asia.
- **In the postnatal period, about 50% of all deaths in children younger than 5 years of age are attributed to only three conditions, all preventable: pneumonia, diarrheal diseases, and malaria.** Nevertheless, thanks largely to public health measures, some progress has been made on this front; worldwide, deaths in children younger than 5 years of age declined from approximately 11.5 million in 1990 to approximately 7 million in 2010, even though the number of live births increased steadily during this time.

Emerging infectious diseases also constitute an important component of the global burden of disease. Emerging infections are defined as infectious disorders whose incidence has recently increased or could reasonably be expected to increase in the near future. Their emergence may occur by chance, but often finds its basis in some change in environmental and socioeconomic conditions. Categories of emerging infectious diseases include: (1) *diseases caused by newly evolved strains or organisms*, such as multidrug-resistant tuberculosis, chloroquine-resistant malaria, and methicillin-resistant *Staphylococcus aureus*; (2) *diseases caused by pathogens endemic in other species that recently "jumped" to human populations*, such as HIV; and (3) *diseases caused by pathogens that have been present in human populations but show a recent increase in incidence.* An example of the latter is dengue fever, which due to warming climate appears poised to spread into the southern United States.

Health Effects of Climate Change

Without immediate action, climate change stands to become the preeminent global cause of environmental disease in the twenty-first century and beyond. Temperature measurements show that the earth has warmed at an accelerating rate over the past 50 years, perhaps at a rate greater than in any period during the preceding 1000 years. Since 1960 the global average temperature has increased by approximately 0.6°C, with the greatest increases seen over land areas between 40 degrees north and 70 degrees north. Notably, nine of the 10 hottest years in the meteorologic record have occurred in the twenty-first century. These increases in global temperature have been accompanied by the rapid loss of glacial and sea ice, leading to predictions that the iconic glaciers of Glacier National Park in Montana and Mt. Kilimanjaro in Tanzania may disappear by the year 2025, and that the Arctic Ocean will be completely ice-free in summer by no later than the year 2040.

Although politicians quibble, among scientists there is a general acceptance that climate change is, at least in part, man-made. The principal culprit is the rising atmospheric level of greenhouse gases, particularly carbon dioxide (CO_2) released through the burning of fossil fuels (Fig. 9-2*A*), as well as ozone (an important air pollutant, discussed later) and methane. These gases, along with water vapor, produce the so-called greenhouse effect by absorbing and re-emitting infrared energy radiated from the Earth's surface that otherwise would be lost into space. The annual average level of atmospheric CO_2 in late 2012 (about 391 ppm) was higher than at any point in approximately 650,000 years and, without changes in human behavior, is expected to increase to between 500 to 1200 ppm by the end of this century—levels not experienced for tens of millions of years. This increase stems not only from increased CO_2 production but also from deforestation and the attendant decrease in carbon fixation by plants.

Depending on which computer model is used, increased levels of greenhouse gases are projected to cause the global temperature to rise by 2°C to 5°C by the year 2100 (Fig. 9-2*B*). Part of the uncertainty about the extent of the

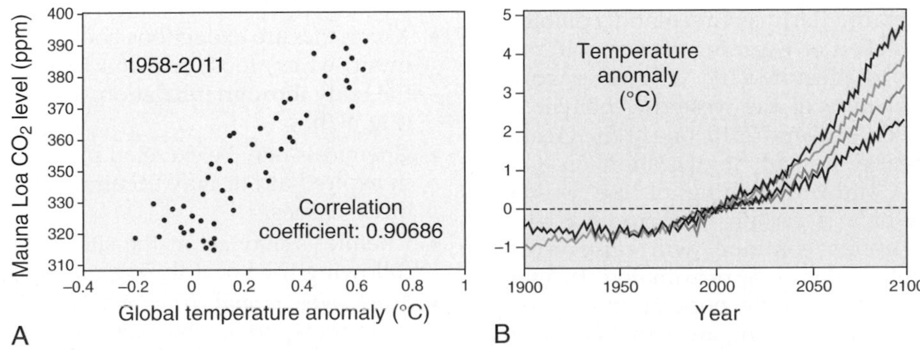

Figure 9-2 Climate change, past and future. **A,** Correlation of CO_2 levels measured at the Mauna Loa Observatory in Hawaii with average global temperature trends over the past 50 years. "Global temperature" in any given year was deduced at the Hadley Center (United Kingdom) from measurements taken at more than 3000 weather stations located around the globe. **B,** Predicted temperature increases during the twenty-first century. Different computer models plot anticipated rises in global temperatures of 2°C to 5°C by the year 2100. (**A,** Courtesy Dr. Richard Aster, Department of Geophysics, Colorado State University, Fort Collins, Colo.)

temperature increase stems from questions about the degree to which positive-feedback loops will exacerbate factors driving the process. Examples of such self-reinforcing loops are increases in surface heat absorption due to loss of reflective ice and snow; increases in water vapor due to greater evaporation from warming rivers, lakes, and oceans; large releases of CO_2 and methane from organic matter in thawing Arctic "permafrost" and submarine methane hydrates; and decreased sequestration of CO_2 in oceans due to reduced growth of organisms, such as diatoms, that serve as carbon sinks. Increased heat energy in the oceans and atmosphere is also projected to increase the variability and severity of weather events, such as floods, droughts, and storms. An additional worrisome effect of increased atmospheric CO_2 concentrations is increasing acidity of the oceans, which may disrupt marine ecosystems and fisheries.

The health impacts of climate change will depend on its extent and rapidity, the nature and severity of the ensuing consequences, and humankind's ability to mitigate the damage. Even in the best case scenario, however, climate change is expected to have a serious negative impact on human health by increasing the incidence of a number of diseases, including the following:

- *Cardiovascular, cerebrovascular, and respiratory diseases,* all of which will be worsened by heat waves and air pollution
- *Gastroenteritis, cholera, and other foodborne and waterborne infectious diseases,* caused by contamination as a consequence of floods and disruption of clean water supplies and sewage treatment, after heavy rains and other environmental disasters
- *Vector-borne infectious diseases, such as malaria and dengue fever,* due to changes in vector number and geographic distribution related to increased temperatures, crop failures, and more extreme weather variation (e.g., more frequent and severe El Niño events)
- *Malnutrition,* caused by changes in local climate that disrupt crop production. Such changes are anticipated to be most severe in tropical locations, in which average temperatures may already be near or above crop tolerance levels; it is estimated that by 2080, agricultural productivity may decline by 10% to 25% in some developing countries as a consequence of climate change.

Beyond these disease-specific effects, it is estimated that melting of glacial ice, particularly in Greenland, combined with the thermal expansion of warming oceans, will raise sea levels by at least 1 to 2 feet by 2100. Of greater worry, temperatures in the vicinity of the western Antarctic ice sheet rose 2.4°C between 1958 and 2010, one of the greatest increases in temperature seen at any location on earth during this period. Complete melting of the western Antarctic ice shelf, which is certain to occur in coming centuries if current trends continue, will raise oceans levels by an additional 5 meters—approximately 16.5 feet. Approximately 10% of the world's population—roughly 600 million people—live in low-lying areas that are at risk for flooding even if the rise in ocean levels is at the low end of these estimates. The resulting displacement of people will disrupt lives and commerce, creating conditions ripe for political unrest, war, and poverty, the "vectors" of malnutrition, sickness, and death.

Both developed and developing countries will suffer the consequences of climate change, but the burden will be greatest in developing countries, which to date have been least culpable for increases in greenhouse gases to date. This equation is changing rapidly, however, owing to the growth of the economies of India and China, which has recently surpassed the United States to become the largest producer of CO_2 in the world. The urgent challenge is to develop new renewable energy resources that stem the production of greenhouse gases.

Toxicity of Chemical and Physical Agents

***Toxicology* is defined as the science of poisons. It studies the distribution, effects, and mechanisms of action of toxic agents.** More broadly, it also includes the study of the effects of physical agents such as radiation and heat. Approximately 4 billion pounds of toxic chemicals, including 72 million pounds of recognized carcinogens, are released per year in the United States. Of about 100,000 chemicals in commercial use in the United States, only a very small proportion has been tested experimentally for health effects. Several agencies in the United States set permissible levels of exposure to known environmental hazards (e.g., the maximum level of carbon monoxide in air that is noninjurious or the tolerable levels of radiation that are harmless or "safe"). Factors such as the complex interaction between various pollutants, and the age, genetic predisposition, and the different tissue sensitivities of exposed persons, create wide variations in individual sensitivity to toxic agents, limiting the value of establishing rigid "safe levels" for entire populations. Nevertheless, such cut-offs are useful for comparative studies of the effects of harmful agents between specific populations, and for estimating risk of disease in heavily exposed individuals.

We now consider some basic principles relevant to the effects of toxic chemicals and drugs.

- The *definition of a poison* is not straightforward. It is basically a quantitative concept strictly dependent on *dosage*. The quote from Paracelsus in the sixteenth century that "all substances are poisons; the right dosage differentiates a poison from a remedy" is even more valid today, given the proliferation of pharmaceutical drugs with potentially harmful effects.
- *Xenobiotics* are exogenous chemicals in the environment in air, water, food, and soil that may be absorbed into the body through inhalation, ingestion, and skin contact (Fig. 9-3).
- Chemicals may be excreted in urine or feces; eliminated in expired air; or may accumulate in bone, fat, brain, or other tissues.
- Chemicals may act at the site of entry or at other sites following transport through the blood.
- *Most solvents and drugs are lipophilic,* which facilitates their transport in the blood by lipoproteins and their penetration through the plasma membrane into cells.
- Most solvents, drugs, and xenobiotics are metabolized to form inactive water-soluble products *(detoxification),* or are *activated to form toxic metabolites.* The reactions that metabolize xenobiotics into nontoxic products, or

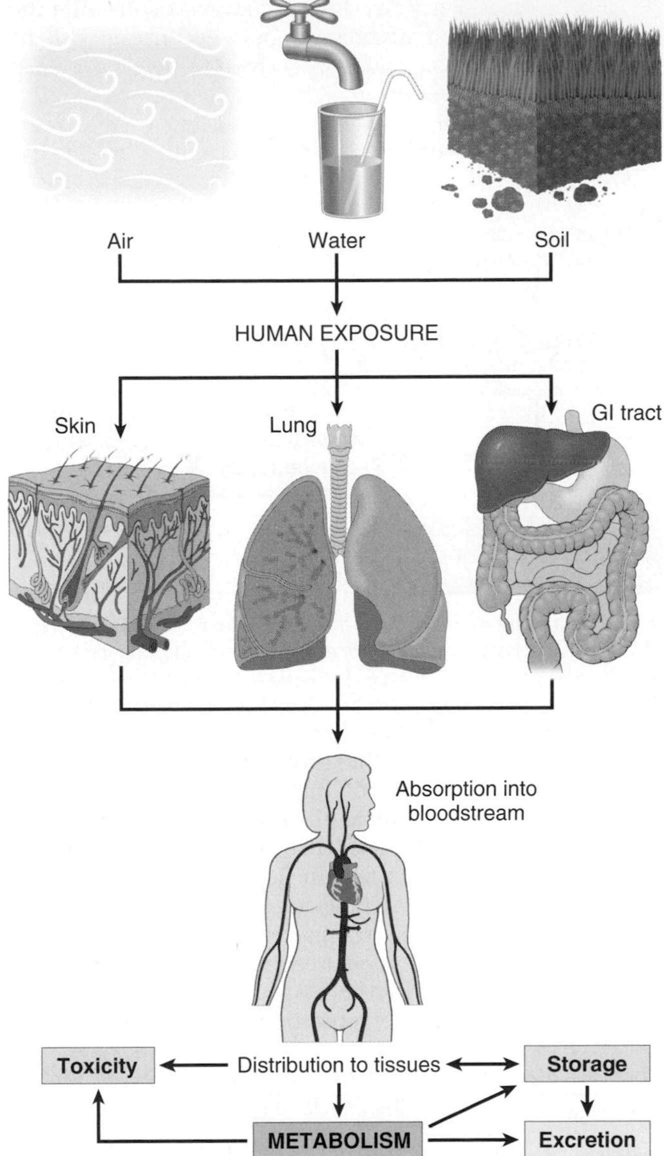

Figure 9-3 Human exposure to pollutants. Pollutants in the air, water, and soil are absorbed through the lungs, gastrointestinal tract, and skin. In the body they may act at the site of absorption but are generally transported through the bloodstream to various organs where they may be stored or metabolized. Xenobiotics may be metabolized to water-soluble compounds that are excreted, or to toxic metabolites, a process referred to as activation.

that activate xenobiotics to generate toxic compounds (Figs. 9-3 and 9-4), occur in two phases. In *phase I* reactions, chemicals undergo hydrolysis, oxidation, or reduction. Products of phase I reactions are often metabolized into water-soluble compounds through *phase II* reactions, which include glucuronidation, sulfation, methylation, and conjugation with glutathione. Water-soluble compounds are readily excreted. Enzymes that catalyze the biotransformation of xenobiotics and drugs are known as *drug-metabolizing enzymes.*

- The most important catalyst of phase I reactions is the *cytochrome P-450 enzyme system* (*abbreviated as CYP*) located primarily in the endoplasmic reticulum of the liver but also present in skin, lungs, and gastrointestinal mucosa, and other organs. CYPs are a large family of heme-containing enzymes, each with preferred substrate specificities. **The P-450 system catalyzes reactions that either detoxify xenobiotics or, less commonly, convert xenobiotics into active compounds that cause cellular injury.** Both types of reactions may produce, as a byproduct, *reactive oxygen species (ROS)*, which can cause cellular damage (Chapter 2). Examples of metabolic activation of chemicals through CYPs are the production of the toxic trichloromethyl free radical from carbon tetrachloride in the liver, and the generation of a DNA-binding metabolite from benzo[*a*]pyrene, a carcinogen present in cigarette smoke. CYPs participate in the metabolism of a large number of common therapeutic drugs such as acetaminophen, barbiturates, warfarin, and anticonvulsants, and also in alcohol metabolism (discussed later).

There is great variation in the activity of CYPs among individuals. The variation may be a consequence of genetic polymorphisms in specific CYPs, but more commonly it is due to exposure to drugs or chemicals that induce or diminish CYP activity. Known CYP inducers include environmental chemicals, drugs, smoking, alcohol, and hormones. In contrast, fasting or starvation can decrease CYP activity.

Inducers of CYP do so by binding to nuclear receptors, which then heterodimerize with the retinoic X receptor (RXR) to form a transcriptional activation complex that associates with promoter elements located in the 5′-flanking region of CYP genes. Nuclear receptors participating in CYP induction responses include the aryl hydrocarbon receptor, the peroxisome proliferator-activated receptors *(PPAR)*, and two orphan nuclear receptors, constitutive androstane receptor (CAR), and pregnane X receptor (PXR).

This brief overview of the general mechanisms of toxicity provides the background for the discussion of environmental diseases presented in this chapter.

Environmental Pollution

Air Pollution

Air pollution is a significant cause of morbidity and mortality worldwide, particularly among at-risk individuals with preexisting pulmonary or cardiac disease. Air is precious to life, but can also carry many potential causes of disease. Airborne microorganisms have long been major causes of morbidity and mortality, especially in developing countries. More widespread are airborne chemical and particulate pollutants, especially in industrialized nations. Here, we consider these hazards in outdoor and indoor air.

Outdoor Air Pollution

The ambient air in industrialized nations is contaminated with an unsavory mixture of gaseous and particulate pollutants, more heavily in cities and in proximity to heavy industry. In the United States, the Environmental Protection Agency monitors and sets allowable upper limits for six pollutants: sulfur dioxide, carbon monoxide, ozone, nitrogen dioxide, lead, and particulate matter. Collectively, these agents produce the well-known *smog* (smoke and fog) that sometimes stifles large cities such as Beijing, Los

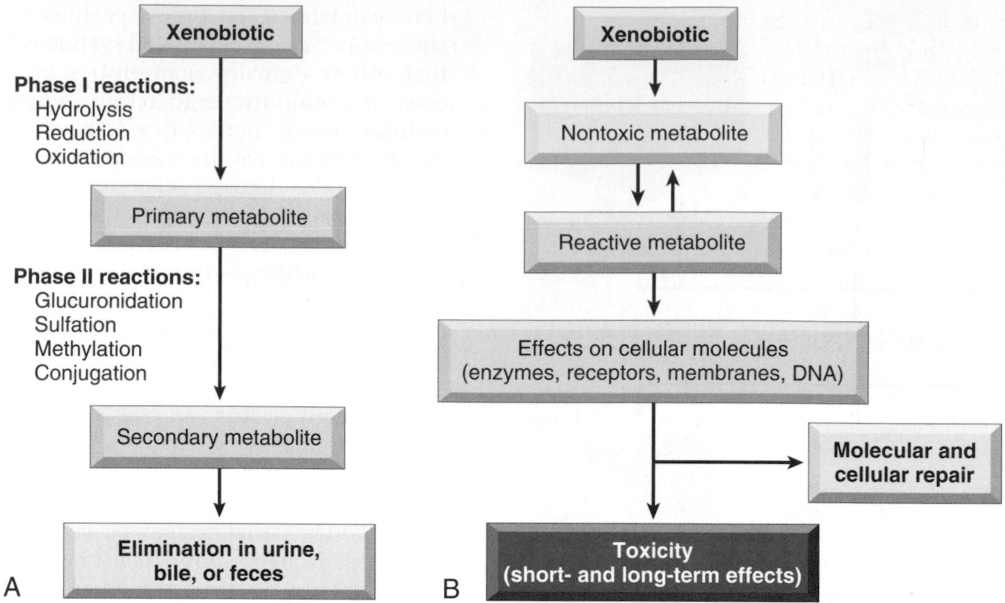

Figure 9-4 Xenobiotic metabolism. **A,** Xenobiotics can be metabolized to nontoxic metabolites and eliminated from the body (detoxification). **B,** Xenobiotic metabolism may also result in the formation of a reactive metabolite that is toxic to cellular components. If repair is not effective, short- and long-term effects develop. (Based on Hodgson E: A Textbook of Modern Toxicology, 3rd ed. Hoboken, NJ, Wiley, 2004.)

Angeles, Houston, Cairo, New Delhi, Mexico City, and São Paulo. It may seem that air pollution is a modern phenomenon, but this is hardly the case. John Evelyn wrote in 1661 that inhabitants of London suffered from "Catharrs, Phthisicks and Consumptions" (bronchitis, pneumonia, and tuberculosis) and breathed "nothing but an impure and thick mist, accompanied by a fuliginous and filthy vapour, which renders them obnoxious to a thousand inconveniences, corrupting the lungs, and disordering the entire habit of their bodies." The first environmental control law, proclaimed by Edward I in 1306, was straightforward in its simplicity: "whoever should be found guilty of burning coal shall suffer the loss of his head." What has changed in modern times is the nature and sources of air pollutants, and the types of regulations that control their emission.

Although the lungs bear the brunt of the adverse consequences, air pollutants can affect many organ systems. Except for some comments on smoking, pollutant-caused lung diseases are discussed in Chapter 15. Major health effects of outdoor pollutants are summarized in Table 9-1. Ozone, sulfur dioxide, particulates, and carbon monoxide are discussed here.

Ozone (O_3) is produced by interaction of ultraviolet (UV) radiation and oxygen (O_2) in the stratosphere and naturally accumulates in the so-called ozone layer 10 to 30 miles above the earth's surface. This layer protects life on earth by absorbing the most dangerous UV radiation emitted by the sun. During the past 35 years, the stratospheric ozone layer decreased in both thickness and extent due to the widespread use of chlorofluorocarbon gases in air conditioners and refrigerators and as aerosol propellents. When released into the atmosphere, these gases drift up into the stratosphere and participate in chemical reactions that destroy ozone. Due to prevailing stratospheric air currents, the resulting depletion has been most profound in polar regions, particularly over Antarctica during the winter months. Recognition of the problem led in 1987 to the Montreal Protocol, a series of international agreements that currently calls for a complete phase-out of chlorofluorocarbon use by 2020. Decreased use of chlorofluorocarbons over the past 25 years has reduced the size of the yearly ozone "hole" over Antarctica, suggesting that this global environmental challenge is being met successfully.

In contrast to the "good" ozone in the stratosphere, ozone that accumulates in the lower atmosphere *(ground-level ozone)* is one of the most pernicious air pollutants.

Table 9-1 Health Effects of Outdoor Air Pollutants

Pollutant	Populations at Risk	Effects
Ozone	Healthy adults and children	Decreased lung function Increased airway reactivity Lung inflammation
	Athletes, outdoor workers Asthmatics	Decreased exercise capacity Increased hospitalizations
Nitrogen dioxide	Healthy adults Asthmatics Children	Increased airway reactivity Decreased lung function Increased respiratory infections
Sulfur dioxide	Healthy adults Individuals with chronic lung disease	Increased respiratory symptoms Increased mortality
	Asthmatics	Increased hospitalization Decreased lung function
Acid aerosols	Healthy adults Children Asthmatics	Altered mucociliary clearance Increased respiratory infections Decreased lung function Increased hospitalizations
Particulates	Children Individuals with chronic lung or heart disease	Increased respiratory infections Decreased lung function
	Asthmatics	Excess mortality Increased attacks

Data from Bascom R, et al: Health effects of outdoor air pollution. Am J Respir Crit Care Med 153:477, 1996.

Ground-level ozone is a gas formed by the reaction of nitrogen oxides and volatile organic compounds in the presence of sunlight. These chemicals are released by industrial emissions and motor vehicle exhaust. Ozone toxicity is in large part mediated by the production of free radicals, which injure epithelial cells along the respiratory tract and type I alveolar cells, and cause the release of inflammatory mediators. Healthy individuals exposed to ozone experience upper respiratory tract inflammation and mild symptoms (decreased lung function and chest discomfort), but exposure is much more dangerous for people with asthma or emphysema.

Even low levels of ozone may be detrimental to the lung function of normal individuals when mixed with other air pollutants. Unfortunately, air pollutants often combine to create a veritable "witches' brew" of ozone and other agents such as *sulfur dioxide* and particulates. Sulfur dioxide is produced by power plants burning coal and oil, from copper smelting, and as a byproduct of paper mills. Released into the air, it may be converted into sulfuric acid and sulfuric trioxide, which cause a burning sensation in the nose and throat, difficulty in breathing, and asthma attacks in susceptible individuals.

Particulate matter (known as "soot") is a particularly important cause of morbidity and mortality related to pulmonary inflammation and secondary cardiovascular effects. Based on studies of large cities in the United States, it is estimated that there is a 0.5% increase in overall daily mortality for every 10 mg/m^3 increase in 10 μm particles in outdoor air, mainly due to exacerbations of pulmonary and cardiac disease. Particulates are emitted by coal- and oil-fired power plants, by industrial processes burning these fuels, and by diesel exhaust. Although the particles have not been well characterized chemically or physically, *fine or ultrafine particles less than 10 μm in diameter* are the most harmful. They are readily inhaled into the alveoli, where they are phagocytosed by macrophages and neutrophils, which respond by releasing a number of inflammatory mediators. In contrast, particles that are greater than 10 μm in diameter are of lesser consequence, because they are generally removed in the nose, or trapped by the mucociliary epithelium of the airways.

Carbon monoxide is a systemic asphyxiant that is an important cause of accidental and suicidal death. Carbon monoxide (CO) is a nonirritating, colorless, tasteless, odorless gas that is produced during any process that results in the incomplete oxidation of hydrocarbons. From the standpoint of human health, the most important environmental source of CO is the burning of carbonaceous materials, as occurs in automotive engines, furnaces, and cigarettes. CO is short-lived in the atmosphere, being rapidly oxidized to carbon dioxide (CO_2); thus, elevated levels in ambient air are transient and occur only in close proximity to sources of CO. Chronic poisoning may occur in individuals working in environments such as tunnels, underground garages, and in highway toll booths with high exposures to automobile fumes. Of greater concern is acute toxicity. In a small, closed garage, the average running car can produce sufficient CO to induce coma or death within 5 minutes, and CO concentrations can also rapidly rise to toxic levels with improper use of gasoline-powered generators (e.g., during power outages) or following mine fires. CO kills in part by inducing central nervous system (CNS) depression, which appears so insidiously that victims are often unaware of their plight. Hemoglobin has 200-fold greater affinity for CO than for oxygen, and the resultant carboxyhemoglobin cannot carry O_2. Systemic hypoxia develops when the hemoglobin is 20% to 30% saturated with CO; unconsciousness and death are likely with 60% to 70% saturation.

MORPHOLOGY

Chronic poisoning by CO develops because carboxyhemoglobin, once formed, is remarkably stable. Even with low-level, but persistent, exposure to CO, carboxyhemoglobin may rise to life-threatening levels in the blood. The slowly developing hypoxia can insidiously evoke widespread ischemic changes in the central nervous system; these are particularly marked in the basal ganglia and lenticular nuclei. With cessation of exposure to CO, the patient usually recovers, but there may be permanent neurologic sequelae, such as impairment of memory, vision, hearing, and speech. The diagnosis is made by measuring carboxyhemoglobin levels in the blood.

Acute poisoning by CO is generally a consequence of accidental exposure or suicide attempt. In light-skinned individuals, **acute poisoning is marked by a characteristic generalized cherry-red color of the skin and mucous membranes,** which result from high levels of carboxyhemoglobin. This effect of CO on coloration may result in a failure to recognize the oxygen-starved state of the victim (and parenthetically is used by the meat industry in the United States to keep meat appearing fresh—caveat emptor!). If death occurs rapidly, morphologic changes may not be present; with longer survival the brain may be slightly edematous, with punctate hemorrhages and hypoxia-induced neuronal changes. The morphologic changes are not specific and stem from systemic hypoxia.

Indoor Air Pollution

As we increasingly "button up" our homes to exclude the environment, the potential for pollution of the indoor air increases. The most common pollutant is *tobacco smoke* (discussed later), but additional offenders are CO, nitrogen dioxide (both already mentioned as outdoor pollutants), and asbestos (Chapter 15). Volatile substances containing polycyclic aromatic hydrocarbons generated by cooking oils and coal burning are important indoor pollutants in some regions of China. Only a few comments about other agents are made here.

- *Wood smoke*, containing various oxides of nitrogen and carbon particulates, is an irritant that may predispose to lung infections and may contain polycyclic hydrocarbons, important carcinogens.
- *Bioaerosols* range from microbiologic agents capable of causing infectious diseases such as Legionnaires disease, viral pneumonia, and the common cold, to less threatening but nonetheless distressing allergens derived from pet dander, dust mites, and fungi and molds responsible for rhinitis, eye irritation, and asthma.
- *Radon*, a radioactive gas derived from uranium widely present in soil and in homes, can cause lung cancer in uranium miners. However, it does not seem that low-level chronic exposures in the home increase lung cancer risk, at least for nonsmokers.

- Exposure to *formaldehyde*, used in the manufacture of building materials (e.g., cabinetry, furniture, adhesives) may be a health problem in refugees from environmental disasters living in poorly ventilated trailers. At concentrations of 0.1 ppm or higher, it causes breathing difficulties and a burning sensation in the eyes and throat, and can trigger asthma attacks. Formaldehyde is classified as a carcinogen for humans and animals.
- The so-called *sick building syndrome* remains an elusive problem; it may be a consequence of exposure to one or more indoor pollutants, possibly due to poor ventilation.

KEY CONCEPTS

Environmental Diseases and Environmental Pollution

- Environmental diseases are conditions caused by exposure to chemical or physical agents in the ambient, workplace, and personal environments.
- Exogenous chemicals known as *xenobiotics* enter the body through inhalation, ingestion, and skin contact, and can either be eliminated or accumulate in fat, bone, brain, and other tissues.
- Xenobiotics can be converted into nontoxic products, or activated to generate toxic compounds, through a two-phase reaction process that involves the cytochrome P-450 system.
- The most common and important air pollutants are ozone (which in combination with oxides and particulate matter forms smog), sulfur dioxide, acid aerosols, and particles less than 10 μm in diameter.
- Carbon monoxide poisoning an important cause of death from accidents and suicide; it binds hemoglobin with high affinity, leading to systemic asphyxiation associated with CNS depression.
- A variety of pollutants, including smokes, bioaerosols, radon, and formaldehyde, may accumulate in indoor air and cause disease.

Metals as Environmental Pollutants

Lead, mercury, arsenic, and cadmium are the heavy metals most commonly associated with harmful effects in humans.

Lead

Lead is a readily absorbed metal that binds to sulfhydryl groups in proteins and interferes with calcium metabolism, effects that lead to hematologic, skeletal, neurologic, gastrointestinal, and renal toxicities. Lead exposure may occur through contaminated air, food and water. For most of the twentieth century the major sources of lead in the environment were lead-containing house paints and gasoline. Although limits have been set for the amounts of lead contained in residential paints and use of leaded gasoline in road vehicles was banned in the United States in 1996, lead contamination remains an important health hazard, particularly for children. The large-scale recall of toys containing lead in 2007 alerted the general public to the dangers of lead exposures. There are many sources of lead in the environment, such as from mining, foundries, batteries, and spray painting, which constitute occupational hazards. However, *flaking lead paint* in older houses and soil contamination pose major hazards to youngsters. During the past 30 years, the median blood level of lead in preschool children in the United States decreased from 15 μg/dL to the present level of less than 2 μg/dL due to public health measures. Nevertheless, blood levels of lead in children living in older homes containing lead-based paint or lead-contaminated dust often exceed 5 μg/dL, the level at which the Centers for Disease Control and Prevention (CDC) recommends that measures be taken to limit further exposure. While treatment for lead poisoning in children is currently mandated only when blood lead levels are ≥45 μg/dL, it is believed that *subclinical lead poisoning* may occur in children with blood lead levels considerably below this mark. The results of low-level lead poisoning include subtle deficits in intellectual capacity, behavioral problems such as hyperactivity, and poor organizational skills. Lead poisoning, although less common in adults, occurs mainly as an occupational hazard in those involved in the manufacturing of batteries, pigments, car radiators, and tin cans. The main clinical features of lead poisoning in children and adults are shown in Figures 9-5 and 9-6.

Most of the absorbed lead (80% to 85%) is incorporated into bone and developing teeth, where it competes with calcium; its half-life in bone is 20 to 30 years. High levels of lead cause *CNS disturbances* in adults and children, but *peripheral neuropathies* predominate in adults. Children absorb more than 50% of ingested lead (compared with

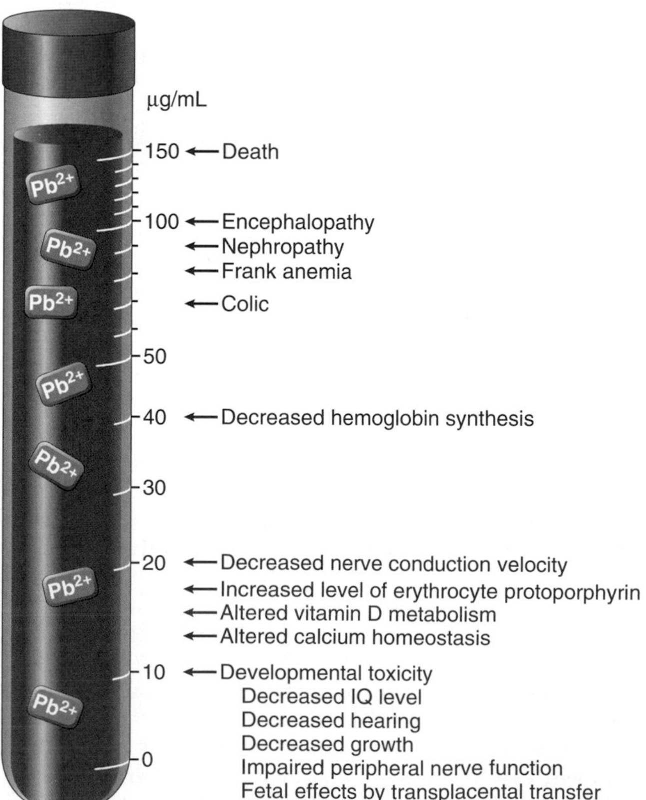

Figure 9-5 Effects of lead poisoning in children related to blood levels. (Modified from Bellinger DC, Bellinger AM: Childhood lead poisoning: the tortuous path from science to policy. J Clin Invest 116:853; 2006.)

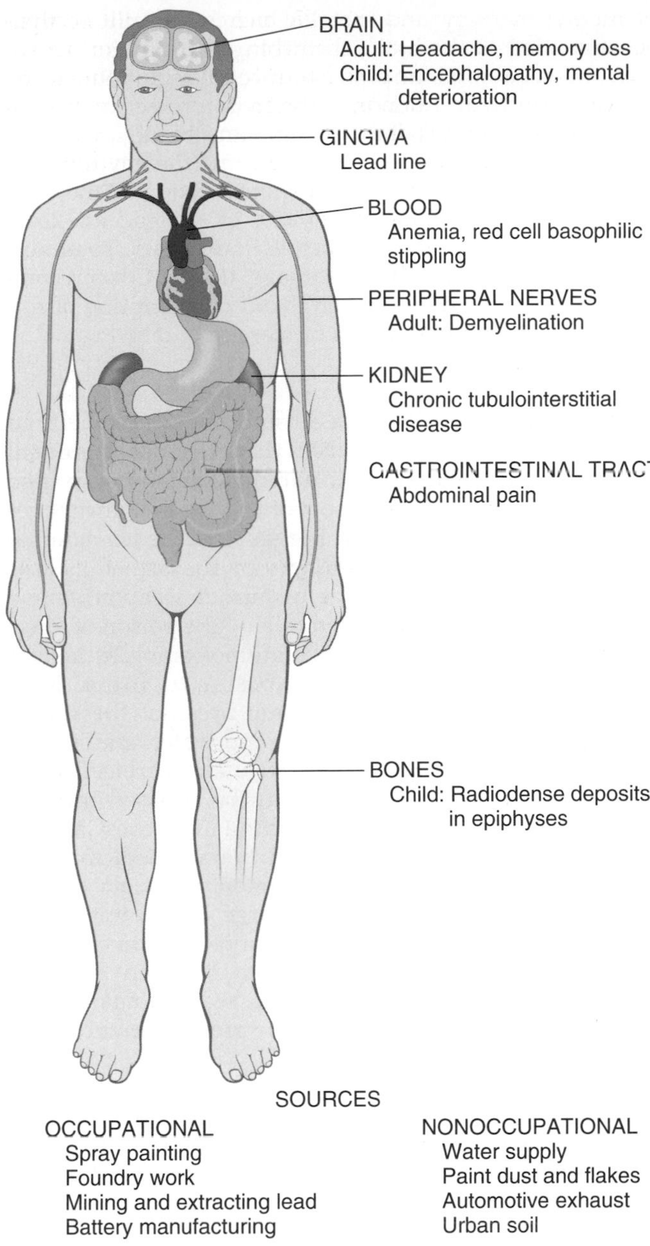

Figure 9-6 Pathologic features of lead poisoning in adults.

≤15% in adults); the higher intestinal absorption and the more permeable blood-brain barrier of children create a high susceptibility to brain damage. The neurotoxic effects of lead are attributed to the inhibition of neurotransmitters caused by the disruption of calcium homeostasis. Other effects of lead exposure include the following:

- Lead interferes with the normal remodeling of cartilage and primary bone trabeculae in the epiphyses in children. This causes increased bone density detected as radiodense "lead lines" (Fig. 9-7; another type of lead line appears in the gums as a result of hyperpigmentation).
- Lead inhibits the healing of fractures by increasing chondrogenesis and delaying cartilage mineralization.
- Lead inhibits the activity of two enzymes involved in heme synthesis, δ-aminolevulinic acid dehydratase and ferrochelatase. Ferrochelatase catalyzes the incorporation of iron into protoporphyrin, and its inhibition causes a rise in protoporphyrin levels. The resulting heme deficiency causes various abnormalities, but the most obvious is a *microcytic hypochromic anemia* stemming from the suppression of hemoglobin synthesis.

The diagnosis of lead poisoning requires constant awareness of its prevalence. In children it may be suspected on the basis of neurologic and behavioral changes, or by unexplained microcytic anemia. Definitive diagnosis requires the detection of elevated blood levels of lead and free (or zinc-bound) red cell protoporphyrin.

MORPHOLOGY

The major anatomic targets of lead toxicity are the bone marrow and blood, nervous system, gastrointestinal tract, and kidneys (Fig. 9-6).

Blood and marrow changes occur fairly rapidly and are characteristic. The inhibition of ferrochelatase by lead may result in the appearance of a few **ring sideroblasts**, red cell precursors with iron-laden mitochondria that are detected with a Prussian blue stain. In the peripheral blood the defect in hemoglobin synthesis appears as a **microcytic, hypochromic anemia** that is often accompanied by mild **hemolysis**. Even more distinctive is a **punctate basophilic stippling of the red cells.**

Brain damage is prone to occur in children. It can be very subtle, producing mild dysfunction, or it can be massive and lethal. In young children, sensory, motor, intellectual, and psychologic impairments have been described, including reduced IQ, learning disabilities, retarded psychomotor development, blindness, and, in more severe cases, psychoses,

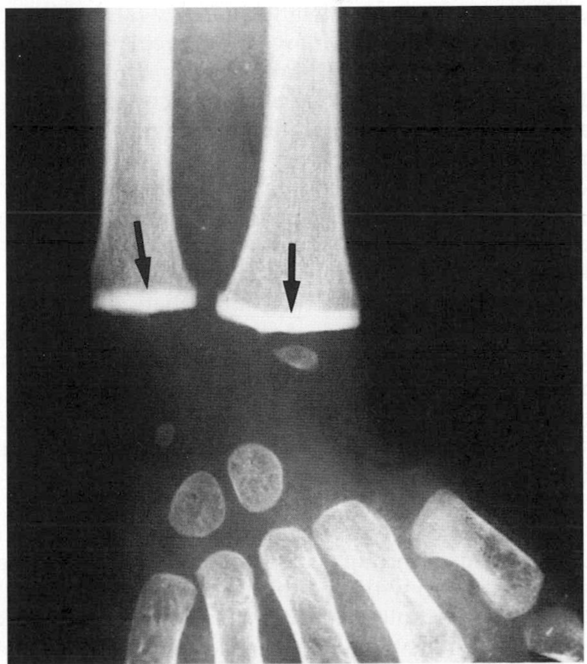

Figure 9-7 Lead poisoning. Impaired remodeling of calcified cartilage in the epiphyses *(arrows)* of the wrist has caused a marked increase in their radiodensity, so that they are as radiopaque as the cortical bone. (Courtesy Dr. G. W. Dietz, Department of Radiology, University of Texas Southwestern Medical School, Dallas, Texas.)

seizures, and coma (Fig. 9-5). Lead toxicity in the mother may impair brain development in the prenatal infant. The anatomic changes underlying the more subtle functional deficits are ill-defined, but there is concern that some of the defects may be permanent. At the more severe end of the spectrum lies marked brain edema, demyelination of the cerebral and cerebellar white matter, and necrosis of cortical neurons accompanied by diffuse astrocytic proliferation. In adults the CNS is less often affected, but frequently **a peripheral demyelinating neuropathy** appears, typically involving the motor nerves of the most commonly used muscles. Thus, the extensor muscles of the wrist and fingers are often the first to be affected (causing wrist-drop), followed by paralysis of the peroneal muscles (causing foot-drop).

The **gastrointestinal tract** is also a major source of clinical manifestations. Lead "colic" is characterized by extremely severe, poorly localized abdominal pain.

Kidneys may develop proximal tubular damage associated with intranuclear inclusions consisting of protein aggregates. Chronic renal damage leads eventually to interstitial fibrosis and possibly renal failure. Decreases in uric acid excretion can lead to gout ("saturnine gout").

Mercury

Like lead, mercury binds to sulfhydryl groups in certain proteins with high affinity, leading to damage in the CNS and the kidney. Mercury has had many uses throughout history, for example, as a pigment in cave paintings, a cosmetic, a remedy for syphilis, and a component of diuretics. Alchemists tried (without much success) to produce gold from mercury. Poisoning from inhalation of mercury vapors has long been recognized and is associated with tremor, gingivitis, and bizarre behavior, such as that displayed by the Mad Hatter in *Alice in Wonderland*. There are three forms of mercury: metallic mercury (also referred to as elemental mercury), inorganic mercury compounds (mostly mercuric chloride), and organic mercury (mostly methyl mercury). Today, the main sources of exposure to mercury are contaminated fish (methyl mercury) and mercury vapors released from metallic mercury in dental amalgams, a possible occupational hazard for dental workers. In some areas of the world, mercury used in gold mining has contaminated rivers and streams.

Inorganic mercury from the natural degassing of the earth's crust or from industrial contamination is converted to organic compounds such as methyl mercury by bacteria. Methyl mercury enters the food chain, and in carnivorous fish such as swordfish, shark, and bluefish, may be concentrated to levels a million-fold higher than in the surrounding water. Disasters caused by the consumption of fish contaminated by the release of methyl mercury from industrial sources in Minamata Bay and the Agano River in Japan caused widespread mortality and morbidity. Acute exposure through consumption of bread made from grain treated with a methyl mercury-based fungicide in Iraq in 1971 resulted in hundreds of deaths and thousands of hospitalizations. The medical disorders associated with the Minamata episode became known as *Minamata disease* and include cerebral palsy, deafness, blindness, mental retardation, and major CNS defects in children exposed in utero. For unclear reasons, *the developing brain is extremely sensitive to methyl mercury*. The lipid solubility of methyl mercury and metallic mercury facilitate their accumulation in the brain, disturbing neuromotor, cognitive, and behavioral functions. Intracellular glutathione, by acting as sulfhydryl donor, is the main protective mechanism against mercury-induced CNS and kidney damage.

Mercury continues to be released into the environment by power plants and other industrial sources, and there are serious concerns about the effects of chronic low-level exposure to methyl mercury in the food supply. To protect against potential fetal brain damage, the CDC has recommended that pregnant women avoid consumption of fish known to contain high levels of mercury.

Arsenic

Arsenic salts interfere with several aspects of cellular metabolism, leading to toxicities that are most prominent in the gastrointestinal tract, nervous system, skin, and heart. Arsenic was the poison of choice in Renaissance Italy, with members of the Borgia and Medici families being highly skilled practitioners of the art of its use. Because of its favored use as a murder weapon among royal families, arsenic has been called "the poison of kings and the king of poisons." Deliberate poisoning by arsenic is exceedingly rare today, but exposure to arsenic is an important health problem in many areas of the world. Arsenic is found naturally in soils and water, and is used in products such as wood preservers and herbicides and other agricultural products. It may be released into the environment from mines and smelting industries. Arsenic is present in Chinese and Indian herbal medicine, and arsenic trioxide is a frontline treatment for acute promyelocytic leukemia (Chapter 7). Large concentrations of inorganic arsenic are present in ground water in countries such as Bangladesh, Chile, and China. Between 35 and 77 million people in Bangladesh drink water contaminated with arsenic, constituting one of the greatest environmental cancer risks yet uncovered.

The most toxic forms of arsenic are the trivalent compounds arsenic trioxide, sodium arsenite, and arsenic trichloride. If ingested in large quantities, arsenic causes *acute gastrointestinal, cardiovascular, and CNS toxicities* that are often fatal. These effects may be attributed in part to interference with mitochondrial oxidative phosphorylation, since trivalent arsenic can replace the phosphates in adenosine triphosphate. However, arsenic also has pleiotropic effects on the activity of a number of other enzymes and ion channels, and these too may contribute to certain toxicities.

- *Neurologic effects* usually occur 2 to 8 weeks after exposure and consist of a sensorimotor neuropathy that causes paresthesias, numbness, and pain.
- Chronic exposure to arsenic causes *skin changes* consisting of hyperpigmentation and hyperkeratosis
- The most serious consequence of chronic exposure is the *increased risk for the development of cancers*, particularly of the lungs, bladder and skin. Arsenic-induced skin tumors differ from those induced by sunlight; they are often multiple and usually appear on the palms and soles. The mechanisms of arsenic carcinogenesis in skin and lung have not been elucidated but may involve defects in nucleotide excision repair mechanisms that protect against DNA damage.

- Finally, there is also evidence that chronic exposure to arsenic in drinking water can cause non-malignant respiratory disease.

Cadmium

Cadmium is preferentially toxic to the kidneys and the lungs through uncertain mechanisms that may involve increased production of reactive oxygen species. In contrast to the other metals discussed in this section, cadmium toxicity is a relatively modern problem. It is an occupational and environmental pollutant generated by mining, electroplating, and production of nickel-cadmium batteries, which are usually disposed of as household waste. Cadmium can contaminate the soil and plants directly or through fertilizers and irrigation water. Food is the most important source of cadmium exposure for the general population. Its toxic effects require its uptake into cells via transporters such as ZIP8, which normally serves as a transporter for zinc.

The principal toxic effects of excess cadmium take the form of *obstructive lung disease* caused by necrosis of alveolar epithelial cells, and *renal tubular damage* that may progress to *end-stage renal disease*. A survey completed in 2008 showed that 5% of the U.S. population age 20 years and older have urinary cadmium levels that may produce subtle kidney injury and calcium loss. Cadmium exposure can also cause skeletal abnormalities associated with calcium loss. Cadmium-containing water used to irrigate rice fields in Japan caused a disease in postmenopausal women known as "Itai-Itai" (ouch-ouch), a combination of osteoporosis and osteomalacia associated with renal disease. Finally, cadmium exposure is also associated with an elevated risk of lung cancer, which has been demonstrated in workers exposed occupationally and in populations living near zinc smelters. Cadmium is not directly genotoxic and most likely produces DNA damage through the generation of reactive oxygen species (Chapter 2).

KEY CONCEPTS

Toxic Effects of Heavy Metals

- Lead, mercury, arsenic, and cadmium are the heavy metals most commonly associated with toxic effects in humans.
- Children absorb more ingested lead than adults; the main source of exposure for children is lead-containing paint in older housing.
- Excess lead causes CNS defects in children and peripheral neuropathy in adults. It also interferes with the remodeling of cartilage and causes anemia by interfering with hemoglobin synthesis.
- The major source of exposure to mercury is contaminated fish. The developing brain is highly sensitive to methyl mercury, which accumulates in the CNS.
- Exposure of the fetus to high levels of mercury in utero may lead to Minamata disease, characterized by cerebral palsy, deafness, and blindness.
- Arsenic is naturally found in soil and water and is a component of some wood preservatives and herbicides. Excess arsenic interferes with mitochondrial oxidative phosphorylation and the function of a variety of proteins. It causes toxic effects in the gastrointestinal tract, CNS, and cardiovascular system; long-term exposure causes skin lesions and carcinomas.
- Cadmium from nickel-cadmium batteries and chemical fertilizers can contaminate soil. Excess cadmium causes obstructive lung disease and kidney damage.

Occupational Health Risks: Industrial and Agricultural Exposures

More than 10 million occupational injuries occur annually in the United States and approximately 65,000 people die as a consequence of work-related accidents and illnesses. Work-related accidents are the biggest occupational health problem in developing countries, while work-related diseases are more frequent in industrialized countries. Industrial exposures to toxic agents are as varied as the industries themselves. They range from mere irritation of the respiratory mucosa by formaldehyde or ammonia fumes; to lung cancer induced by exposure to asbestos, arsenic, or uranium mining; to leukemia caused by chronic exposure to benzene. Human diseases associated with occupational exposures are listed in Table 9-2. Following are examples of important agents that contribute to occupational diseases. Toxicity caused by metals is discussed earlier in this chapter.

- *Organic solvents* are widely used in huge quantities worldwide. Some, such as *chloroform* and *carbon tetrachloride*, are found in degreasing and dry cleaning agents and paint removers. Acute exposure to high levels of vapors from these agents can cause dizziness and confusion, leading to CNS depression and even coma. Lower levels are toxic for the liver and kidneys. Occupational exposure of rubber workers to *benzene* and *1,3-butadiene* increases the risk of leukemia. Benzene is oxidized by hepatic CYP2E1 to toxic metabolites that disrupt the differentiation of hematopoietic cells in the bone marrow, leading to dose-dependent marrow aplasia and an increased risk of acute myeloid leukemia.
- *Polycyclic hydrocarbons* may be released during the combustion of fossil fuels, particularly when coal and gas are burned at high temperatures (e.g., in steel foundries), and are present in tar and soot (Pott identified soot as the cause of scrotal cancers in chimney sweeps in 1775; Chapter 7). Polycyclic hydrocarbons are among the most potent carcinogens, and industrial exposures have been implicated in the development of lung and bladder cancer.
- *Organochlorines* (and halogenated organic compounds in general) are synthetic lipophilic products that resist degradation. Important organochlorines used as pesticides include *DDT (dichlorodiphenyltrichloroethane)*, lindane, aldrin, and dieldrin. Nonpesticide organochlorines include *polychlorinated biphenyls (PCBs)* and *dioxin* (TCDD; 2,3,7,8-tetrachlorodibenzo-*p*-dioxin). DDT was banned in the United States in 1973, but *p*, *p*′-DDE, a long-lasting DDT metabolite, is still detectable in the blood of a sizable minority of U.S. inhabitants. DDT is

Table 9-2 Human Diseases Associated with Occupational Exposures

Organ/System	Effect	Toxicant
Cardiovascular system	Heart disease	Carbon monoxide, lead, solvents, cobalt, cadmium
Respiratory system	Nasal cancer	Isopropyl alcohol, wood dust
	Lung cancer	Radon, asbestos, silica, bis(chloromethyl)ether, nickel, arsenic, chromium, mustard gas, uranium
	Chronic obstructive lung disease	Grain dust, coal dust, cadmium
	Hypersensitivity	Beryllium, isocyanates
	Irritation	Ammonia, sulfur oxides, formaldehyde
	Fibrosis	Silica, asbestos, cobalt
Nervous system	Peripheral neuropathies	Solvents, acrylamide, methyl chloride, mercury, lead, arsenic, DDT
	Ataxic gait	Chlordane, toluene, acrylamide, mercury
	Central nervous system depression	Alcohols, ketones, aldehydes, solvents
	Cataracts	Ultraviolet radiation
Urinary system	Renal toxicity	Mercury, lead, glycol ethers, solvents
	Bladder cancer	Naphthylamines, 4-aminobiphenyl, benzidine, rubber products
Reproductive system	Male infertility	Lead, phthalate plasticizers, cadmium
	Female infertility/stillbirths	Lead, mercury
	Teratogenesis	Mercury, polychlorinated biphenyls
Hematopoietic system	Leukemia	Benzene
Skin	Folliculitis and acneiform dermatosis	Polychlorinated biphenyls, dioxins, herbicides
	Cancer	Ultraviolet radiation
Gastrointestinal tract	Liver angiosarcoma	Vinyl chloride

Data from Leigh JP, et al: Occupational injury and illness in the United States. Estimates of costs, morbidity, and mortality, Arch Intern Med 157:1557, 1997; Mitchell FL: Hazardous waste. In Rom WN (ed): Environmental and Occupational Medicine, 2nd ed. Boston, Little, Brown, 1992, p 1275; and Levi PE: Classes of toxic chemicals. In Hodgson E, Levi PE (eds): A Textbook of Modern Toxicology. Stamford, CT, Appleton & Lange, 1997, p 229.

on the list of recommended insecticides for indoor uses in areas in which malaria is endemic. PCB (another banned substance), dioxin, and PBDEs (polybrominated diphenyl ethers used as flame retardants) are also detectable in a large proportion of the U.S. population. Most organochlorines disrupt hormonal balance because of antiestrogenic or antiandrogenic activity.

- *Dioxins* and *PCBs* can cause skin disorders such as folliculitis and a dermatosis known as *chloracne* that is characterized by acne, cyst formation, hyperpigmentation, and hyperkeratosis, generally around the face and behind the ears. These toxins can also cause abnormalities in the liver and CNS. Because PCBs induce CYPs, workers exposed to these substances may show abnormal drug metabolism. Environmental disasters in Japan and China in the late 1960s caused by the consumption of rice oil contaminated by PCBs during its production poisoned about 2000 people in each episode. The primary manifestation of the disease (Yusho in Japan; Yu-Cheng in China) was chloracne and hyperpigmentation of the skin and nails. Aficionados of political intrigues may recall that Viktor Yushenko, a former President of Ukraine, was poisoned by dioxins and suffered severe disfigurement as a result.
- Inhalation of mineral dusts causes chronic, nonneoplastic lung diseases known as *pneumoconioses.* This term also includes diseases induced by organic and inorganic particulates, and chemical fume- and vapor-induced nonneoplastic lung diseases. The most common pneumoconioses are caused by exposures to *coal dust* (e.g., mining of hard coal), *silica* (e.g., sandblasting, stone cutting), *asbestos* (e.g., mining, fabrication, insulation work), and *beryllium* (e.g, mining, fabrication). Exposure to these agents nearly always occurs in the workplace. However, the increased risk of cancer as a result of asbestos exposure extends to the family members of asbestos workers and to other individuals exposed outside the workplace. Pneumoconioses and their pathogenesis are discussed in Chapter 15.
- Exposure to *vinyl chloride* used in the synthesis of polyvinyl resins leads to the development of angiosarcoma of the liver, an uncommon type of hepatic tumor.
- *Bisphenol A* (BPA) is used in the synthesis of polycarbonate food and water containers and of epoxy resins that line almost all food bottles and cans; as a result, exposure to BPA is virtually ubiquitous in humans. BPA has long been known as a potential endocrine disruptor. Several large retrospective studies have linked elevated urinary BPA levels to heart disease in adult populations. In addition, infants who drink from BPA-containing containers may be particularly susceptible to its endocrine effects. In 2010, Canada was the first country to list BPA as a toxic substance, and the largest makers of baby bottles and "sippy" cups have stopped using BPA in the manufacturing process. The extent of the human health risks associated with BPA remains uncertain, however, and requires further study.

Effects of Tobacco

Smoking is the most readily preventable cause of death in humans. The main culprit is cigarette smoking, but smokeless tobacco (e.g., snuff, chewing tobacco) is also harmful to health and an important cause of oral cancer. The use of tobacco products not only creates personal risks, but passive tobacco inhalation from the environment *("second-hand smoke")* can cause lung cancer in nonsmokers. Two thirds of smokers live in 10 countries, led by China, which accounts for nearly 30%, and India with about 10%, followed by Indonesia, Russia, the United States, Japan, Brazil, Bangladesh, Germany, and Turkey. In the United States alone, tobacco is responsible for more than 400,000 deaths annually, one third of these attributable to lung cancer. Indeed, tobacco is the leading exogenous cause of human cancers, including 90% of lung cancers.

From 1998 to 2007 in the United States, the incidence of smoking declined modestly, but this trend failed to continue, and approximately 20% of adults remain smokers. More disturbing, the world's most populous country, China, has become the world's largest producer and consumer of cigarettes. China has approximately 350 million smokers who in aggregate consume about 33% of all cigarettes smoked worldwide. It is estimated that more than 1 million people in China die each year of smoking-related diseases; this rate is projected to rise to 8 million deaths each year by 2050. Worldwide, cigarette smoking causes more than 4 million deaths annually, mostly from cardiovascular disease, various types of cancers, and chronic respiratory problems. These figures are expected to rise to 8 million tobacco-related deaths by 2020, the major increase occurring in developing countries. Of people alive today, an estimated 500 million will die of tobacco-related illnesses.

Tobacco reduces overall survival through dose-dependent effects that are often expressed as pack-years, the average number of cigarette packs smoked each day multiplied by the number of years of smoking. The cumulative effects of smoking over time are striking. For instance, while about 75% of nonsmokers are alive at age 70, only about 50% of smokers survive to that age (Fig. 9-8). The only good news is that cessation of smoking greatly reduces, within 5 years, overall mortality and the risk of death from cardiovascular diseases. Lung cancer mortality decreases by 21% within 5 years, but the excess risk persists for 30 years.

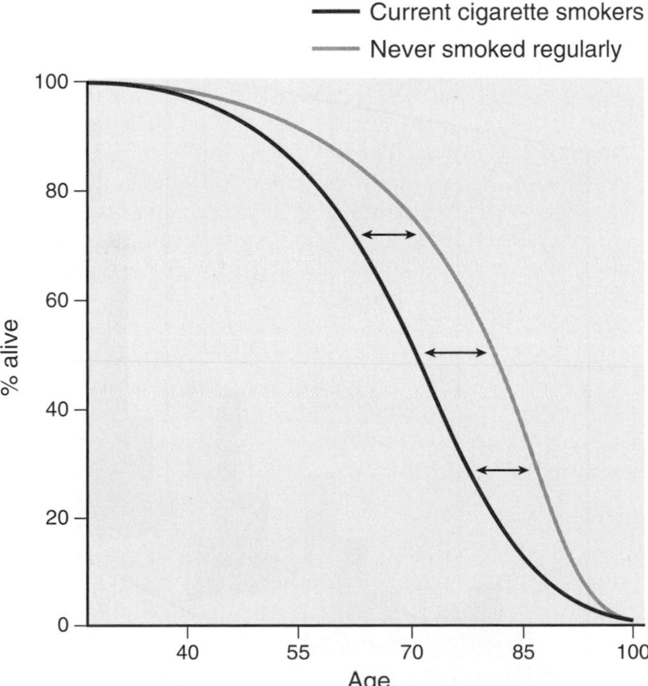

Figure 9-8 The effects of smoking on survival. The study compared age-specific death rates for current cigarette smokers with that of individuals who never smoked regularly (British Doctors Study). Measured at age 75, the difference in survival between smokers and nonsmokers is 7.5 years. (Modified from Stewart BW, Kleihues P (eds): World Cancer Report. Lyon, IARC Press, 2003.)

Table 9-3 Effects of Selected Tobacco Smoke Constituents

Substance	Effect
Tar	Carcinogenesis
Polycyclic aromatic hydrocarbons	Carcinogenesis
Nicotine	Ganglionic stimulation and depression; tumor promotion
Phenol	Tumor promotion; mucosal irritation
Benzo[a]pyrene	Carcinogenesis
Carbon monoxide	Impaired oxygen transport and utilization
Formaldehyde	Toxicity to cilia; mucosal irritation
Nitrogen oxides	Toxicity to cilia; mucosal irritation
Nitrosamine	Carcinogenesis

The number of potentially noxious chemicals in tobacco smoke is extraordinary. Tobacco contains between 2000 and 4000 substances, more than 60 of which have been identified as carcinogens. Table 9-3 provides only a partial list and includes various types of injuries produced by these agents. *Nicotine*, an alkaloid present in tobacco leaves, is not a direct cause of tobacco-related diseases, but is strongly addictive. Without it, it would be easy for smokers to stop the habit. Nicotine binds to nicotinic acetylcholine receptors in the brain, and stimulates the release of catecholamines from sympathetic neurons. This activity is responsible for the acute effects of smoking, such as the increase in heart rate and blood pressure, and the elevation in cardiac contractility and output.

Smoking and Lung Cancer. Agents in smoke have a direct irritant effect on the tracheobronchial mucosa, producing *inflammation* and *increased mucus production (bronchitis).* Cigarette smoke also causes the recruitment of leukocytes to the lung, with increased local elastase production and subsequent injury to lung tissue, leading to *emphysema.* Components of cigarette smoke, particularly *polycyclic hydrocarbons and nitrosamines* (Table 9-4), are potent carcinogens in animals and are directly involved in the development of lung cancer in humans (Chapter 15). CYPs (cytochrome P-450 phase I enzymes) and phase II enzymes increase the water solubility of the carcinogens, facilitating their excretion. However, some intermediates produced by CYPs are electrophilic and form DNA adducts. If such

Table 9-4 Suspected Organ-Specific Carcinogens in Tobacco Smoke

Organ	Carcinogen
Lung, larynx	Polycyclic aromatic hydrocarbons 4-(Methylnitrosoamino)-1-(3-pyridyl)-1-butanone (NNK) Polonium 210
Esophagus	*N*'-Nitrosonornicotine (NNN)
Pancreas	NNK
Bladder	4-Aminobiphenyl, 2-naphthylamine
Oral cavity (smoking)	Polycyclic aromatic hydrocarbons, NNK, NNN
Oral cavity (snuff)	NNK, NNN, polonium 210

Data from Szczesny LB, Holbrook JH: Cigarette smoking. In Rom WH (ed): Environmental and Occupational Medicine, 2nd ed. Boston, Little, Brown, 1992, p 1211.

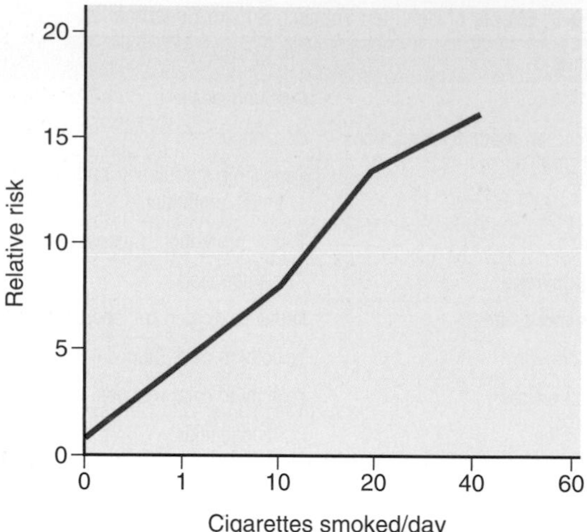

Figure 9-9 The risk of lung cancer is determined by the number of cigarettes smoked. (Modified from Stewart BW, Kleihues P (eds): World Cancer Report. Lyon, IARC Press, 2003.)

adducts persist, they can cause mutations in oncogenes and tumor suppressors (Chapter 7). Most tellingly, deep sequencing of the genomes of lung cancers that occur in smokers has revealed the presence of thousands of mutations of a type that is produced by carcinogens in tobacco smoke in experimental settings. The risk of developing lung cancer is related to the number of pack years or cigarettes smoked per day (Fig. 9-9). Moreover, smoking increases the risk of other carcinogenic influences. Witness the ten-fold higher incidence of lung carcinomas in asbestos workers and uranium miners who smoke over those who do not smoke, and the interaction between tobacco consumption and alcohol in the development of oral cancers (Fig. 9-10).

Smoking and Other Diseases. In addition to lung cancer, smoking is linked to many other malignant and nonmalignant disorders that affect numerous organ systems (Fig. 9-11).

- Cigarette smoking is associated with *cancers of the esophagus, pancreas, bladder, kidney, cervix,* and *bone marrow.*
- The toll taken by nonmalignant conditions associated with smoking is even more terrible. The most common diseases caused by cigarette smoking involve the lung and include *emphysema, chronic bronchitis,* and *chronic obstructive pulmonary disease,* conditions that are discussed in Chapter 15.
- Cigarette smoking is also strongly linked to the development of *atherosclerosis* and its major complication, *myocardial infarction.* The causal mechanisms probably relate to several factors, including increased platelet aggregation, decreased myocardial oxygen supply (because of significant lung disease coupled with the hypoxia related to the CO content of cigarette smoke) accompanied by an increased oxygen demand, and a decreased threshold for ventricular fibrillation. Smoking has a multiplicative effect on the incidence of myocardial infarction when combined with hypertension and hypercholesterolemia.
- In addition to having deleterious effects on the smoker, smoking also harms the developing fetus. Maternal smoking increases the risk of *spontaneous abortions* and *preterm births* and results in *intrauterine growth retardation* (Chapter 10). Birth weights of infants born to mothers who stopped smoking before pregnancy are, however, normal.
- Exposure to *environmental tobacco smoke (passive smoke inhalation)* is associated with some of the same detrimental effects that result from active smoking. It is estimated that the relative risk of lung cancer in nonsmokers exposed to environmental smoke is about 1.3 times higher than that of nonsmokers who are not exposed to smoke. In the United States, approximately 3000 lung cancer deaths in nonsmokers older than 35 years can be attributed each year to environmental tobacco smoke. Even more striking is the increased risk of coronary atherosclerosis and fatal myocardial infarction. Studies report that every year 30,000 to 60,000 cardiac deaths in the United States are associated with exposure to passive smoke. Passive smoke inhalation in nonsmokers can be estimated by measuring the blood levels of *cotinine*, a metabolite of nicotine. During the period of 1999 to 2008, the prevalence of elevated cotinine levels in nonsmokers in the United States fell from 52% to 40% thanks to bans on smoking in public places, but exposure to environmental tobacco smoke in the home remains a major public health concern, particularly for children who may develop respiratory illnesses and asthma.

It is clear that the transient pleasure of smoking comes with a heavy long-term price. A new part of the picture is electronic cigarettes, devices that simulate cigarette

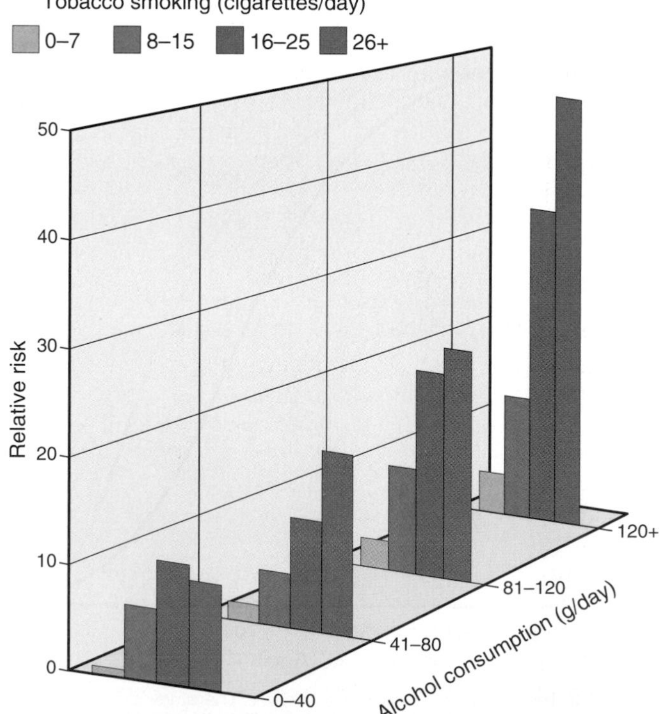

Figure 9-10 Multiplicative increase in the risk of laryngeal cancer from the interaction between cigarette smoking and alcohol consumption. (Modified from Stewart BW, Kleihues P (eds): World Cancer Report. Lyon, IARC Press, 2003.)

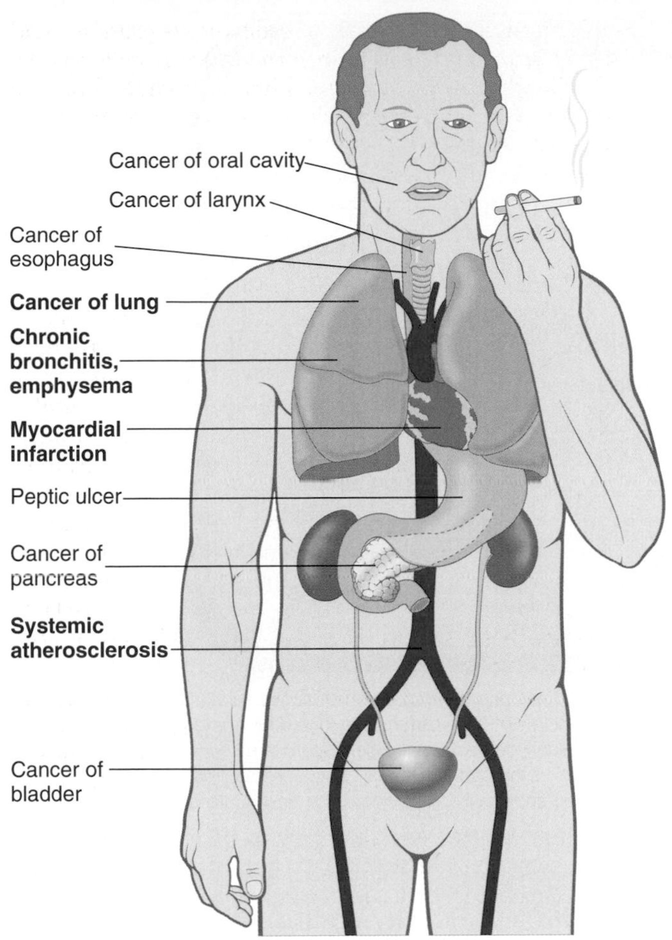

Figure 9-11 Summary of the adverse effects of smoking: those that are more common are in boldface.

smoking by delivering vaporized nicotine and flavorings, which are rising in popularity. As of 2013, however, the WHO has not indicated if these devices are effective in helping smokers to quit or if they have adverse health effects of their own.

KEY CONCEPTS

Health Effects of Tobacco

- Smoking is the most prevalent preventable cause of human death.
- Tobacco smoke contains more than 2000 compounds. Among these are nicotine, which is responsible for tobacco addiction, and potent carcinogens—mainly, polycyclic aromatic hydrocarbons, nitrosamines, and aromatic amines.
- Approximately 90% of lung cancers occur in smokers. Smoking is also associated with an increased risk of cancers of the oral cavity, larynx, esophagus, stomach, bladder, and kidney, as well as some forms of leukemia. Cessation of smoking reduces the risk of lung cancer.
- Smokeless tobacco use is an important cause of oral cancers. Tobacco consumption interacts with alcohol in multiplying the risk of oral, laryngeal, and esophageal cancer and increases the risk of lung cancers from occupational exposures to asbestos, uranium, and other agents.
- Tobacco use is an important risk factor for development of atherosclerosis and myocardial infarction, peripheral vascular disease, and cerebrovascular disease. In the lungs, in addition to cancer, it predisposes to emphysema, chronic bronchitis, and chronic obstructive disease.
- Maternal smoking increases the risk of abortion, premature birth, and intrauterine growth retardation.

Effects of Alcohol

Ethanol consumption in moderate amounts is generally not injurious (and may even protect against some disorders), but in excessive amounts alcohol causes serious physical and psychological damage. In this section we describe the steps of alcohol metabolism and the major health consequences associated with alcohol abuse.

Despite all the attention given to illicit drugs such as cocaine and heroin, alcohol abuse is a far more widespread hazard and claims many more lives. Fifty percent of adults in the Western world drink alcohol, and about 5% to 10% have chronic alcoholism. It is estimated that there are more than 10 million chronic alcoholics in the United States and that alcohol consumption is responsible for more than 100,000 deaths annually. More than 50% of these deaths result from accidents caused by drunken driving and alcohol-related homicides and suicides, and about 15,000 annual deaths are a consequence of cirrhosis of the liver. Worldwide, alcohol accounts for approximately 1.8 million deaths per year (3.2% of all deaths).

After consumption, ethanol is absorbed unaltered in the stomach and small intestine. It is then distributed to all the tissues and fluids of the body in direct proportion to the blood level. Less than 10% is excreted unchanged in the urine, sweat, and breath. The amount exhaled is proportional to the blood level and forms the basis of the breath test used by law enforcement agencies. A concentration of 80 mg/dL in the blood constitutes the legal definition of drunk driving in the United States. For an average individual, this alcohol concentration may be reached after consumption of three standard drinks, about three (12 ounce) bottles of beer, 15 ounces of wine, or 4 to 5 ounces of 80 proof distilled spirits. Drowsiness occurs at 200 mg/dL, stupor at 300 mg/dL, and coma, with possible respiratory arrest, at higher levels. The rate of metabolism affects the blood alcohol level. Chronic alcoholics can tolerate levels of up to 700 mg/dL, a situation that is partially explained by accelerated ethanol metabolism caused by a fivefold to 10-fold induction of liver CYPs (discussed later). The effects of alcohol also vary by age, sex, and body fat.

Most of the alcohol in the blood is oxidized to *acetaldehyde* in the liver by three enzyme systems consisting of alcohol dehydrogenase, the microsomal ethanol-oxidizing system, and catalase (Fig. 9-12). The main enzyme system involved in alcohol metabolism is alcohol dehydrogenase, located in the cytosol of hepatocytes. At high blood alcohol levels, the microsomal ethanol-oxidizing system participates in its metabolism. Catalase, which uses hydrogen peroxide as its substrate, is of minor importance, metabolizing no more than 5% of ethanol in the liver. Acetaldehyde

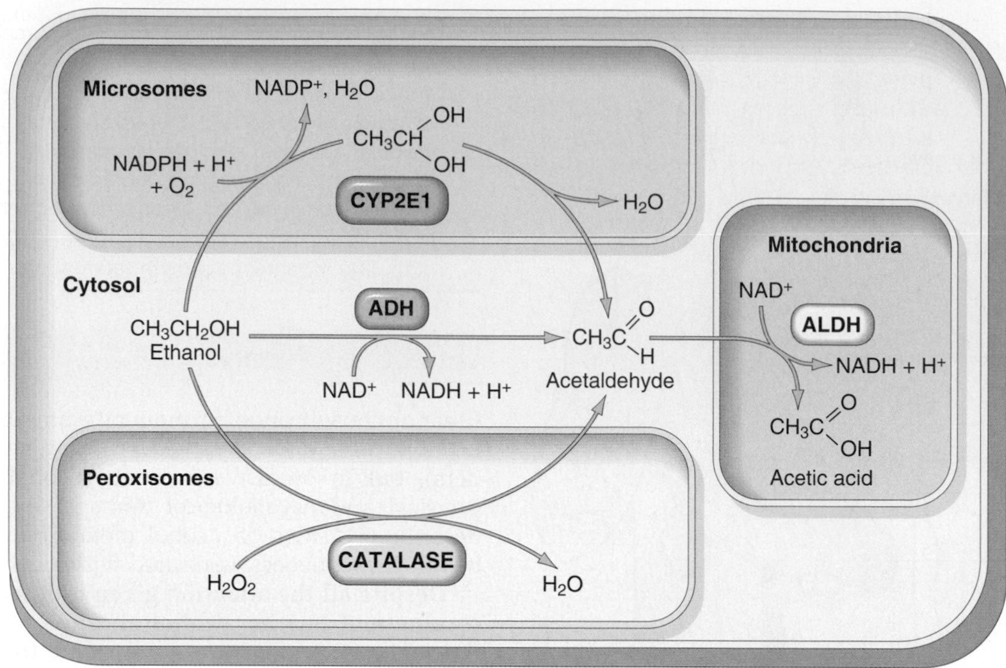

Figure 9-12 Metabolism of ethanol: oxidation of ethanol to acetaldehyde by three different routes and the generation of acetic acid. Note that oxidation by ADH (alcohol dehydrogenase) takes place in the cytosol; the cytochrome P-450 system and its CYP2E1 isoform are located in the endoplasmic reticulum (microsomes), and catalase is located in peroxisomes. Oxidation of acetaldehyde by ALDH (aldehyde dehydrogenase) occurs in mitochondria. ADH oxidation is the most important route; catalase is involved in only 5% of ethanol metabolism. Oxidation through CYPs may also generate reactive oxygen species (not shown). (From Parkinson A: Biotransformation of xenobiotics. In Klassen CD [ed]: Casarett and Doull's Toxicology: The Basic Science of Poisons, 6th ed. New York, McGraw-Hill, 2001, p 133.)

produced by alcohol metabolism is converted to *acetate* by acetaldehyde dehydrogenase, which is then utilized in the mitochondrial respiratory chain.

The microsomal oxidation system involves CYPs, particularly CYP2E1 located in the smooth endoplasmic reticulum. Induction of CYPs by alcohol explains the increased susceptibility of alcoholics to other compounds metabolized by the same enzyme system, which include drugs, anesthetics, carcinogens, and industrial solvents. Note, however, that when alcohol is present in the blood at high concentrations, it competes with other CYP2E1 substrates and delays drug catabolism, potentiating the depressant effects of narcotic, sedative, and psychoactive drugs in the CNS.

The oxidation of ethanol produces toxic metabolites and disrupts certain metabolic pathways, the most important of which include the following:

- *Acetaldehyde*, the direct product of alcohol oxidation, has many toxic effects and is responsible for some of the acute effects of alcohol and for the development of oral cancers. The efficiency of alcohol metabolism varies between populations, depending on the expression levels of alcohol dehydrogenase and acetaldehyde dehydrogenase isozymes, and the presence of genetic variants that alter enzyme activity. About 50% of Asians have very low alcohol dehydrogenase activity, due to the substitution of lysine for glutamine at residue 487 (the normal allele is termed ALDH2*1 and the inactive variant is designated as ALDH2*2). The ALDH2*2 protein has dominant-negative activity, such that even one copy of the ALDH2*2 allele reduces acetaldehyde dehydrogenase activity significantly. Individuals homozygous for the ALDH2*2 allele are completely unable to oxidize acetaldehyde and cannot tolerate alcohol, experiencing nausea, flushing, tachycardia, and hyperventilation after its ingestion.
- Alcohol oxidation by alcohol dehydrogenase causes the reduction of nicotinamide adenine dinucleotide (NAD) to NADH, with a consequent decrease in NAD and increase in NADH. NAD is required for fatty acid oxidation in the liver and for the conversion of lactate into pyruvate. Its deficiency is a main cause of the accumulation of fat in the liver of alcoholics. The increase in the NADH/NAD ratio in alcoholics also causes lactic acidosis.
- Metabolism of ethanol in the liver by CYP2E1 produces reactive oxygen species, which cause lipid peroxidation of hepatocyte cell membranes. Alcohol also causes the release of endotoxin (lipopolysaccharide) from gram-negative bacteria in the intestinal flora, which stimulates the production of TNF (tumor necrosis factor) and other cytokines from macrophages and Kupffer cells, leading to hepatic injury. However, it must be said that the mechanisms by which alcohol causes liver injury remain to be completely defined.

The adverse effects of ethanol can be classified as acute or chronic.

Acute alcoholism exerts its effects mainly on the CNS, but it may induce hepatic and gastric changes that are reversible if alcohol consumption is discontinued. Even with moderate intake of alcohol, multiple fat droplets accumulate in the cytoplasm of hepatocytes *(fatty change* or *hepatic steatosis).* The gastric changes are *acute gastritis* and *ulceration.* In the CNS, alcohol is a depressant, first affecting subcortical structures (probably the high brain stem reticular formation) that modulate cerebral cortical activity. Consequently, there is stimulation and disordered cortical, motor, and intellectual behavior. At progressively higher blood levels, cortical neurons and then lower medullary centers are depressed, including those that regulate respiration. Respiratory arrest may follow.

Chronic alcoholism affects not only the liver and stomach, but virtually all other organs and tissues as well. Chronic alcoholics suffer significant morbidity and have a shortened life span, related principally to damage to the liver, gastrointestinal tract, CNS, cardiovascular system, and pancreas.

- The *liver* is the main site of chronic injury. In addition to fatty change mentioned above, chronic alcoholism causes alcoholic hepatitis and cirrhosis, as described in Chapter 18. Cirrhosis is associated with portal hypertension and an increased risk for the development of hepatocellular carcinoma.
- In the *gastrointestinal tract,* chronic alcoholism can cause massive bleeding from gastritis, gastric ulcer, or esophageal varices (associated with cirrhosis), which may be fatal.
- *Thiamine (vitamin B_1) deficiency* is common in chronic alcoholics. The principal lesions resulting from this deficiency are *peripheral neuropathies* and the *Wernicke-Korsakoff syndrome* (see Table 9-9 in this chapter and Chapter 28); cerebral atrophy, cerebellar degeneration, and optic neuropathy may also occur.
- Alcohol has diverse effects on the cardiovascular system. Injury to the myocardium may produce dilated congestive cardiomyopathy (*alcoholic cardiomyopathy,* discussed in Chapter 12). Chronic alcoholism is also associated with an increased incidence of hypertension, and heavy alcohol consumption, with attendant liver injury, results in decreased levels of HDL, increasing the likelihood of coronary heart disease.
- Excessive alcohol intake increases the risk of *acute and chronic pancreatitis* (Chapter 19).
- The use of ethanol during pregnancy can cause *fetal alcohol syndrome,* which is marked by microcephaly, growth retardation, and facial abnormalities in the newborn, and reduction in mental functions as the child grows older. It is difficult to establish the minimal amount of alcohol consumption that can cause fetal alcohol syndrome, but consumption during the first trimester of pregnancy is particularly harmful. It has been estimated that the prevalence of frequent and binge drinking among pregnant women is approximately 6% and that fetal alcohol syndrome affects 1 to 4.8 per 1000 children born in the United States.
- Chronic alcohol consumption is associated with an *increased incidence of cancer* of the oral cavity, esophagus, liver, and, in women, possibly the breast. Acetaldehyde is considered to be the main agent associated with alcohol-induced laryngeal and esophageal cancer, in that acetaldehyde-DNA adducts have been detected in some tumors from these tissues. Individuals with one copy of the ALDH2*2 allele who drink are at a higher risk for developing cancer of the esophagus. As mentioned earlier, alcohol and cigarette smoke synergize in the causation of various cancers.
- Ethanol is a substantial source of energy (empty calories). Chronic alcoholism leads to malnutrition and nutritional deficiencies, particularly of the B vitamins.

Not all is gloom and doom, however. Moderate amounts of alcohol (about 20-30 gm/day, corresponding to approximately 250 mL of wine) have been reported to increase high-density lipoprotein (HDL) levels, inhibit platelet aggregation, and lower fibrinogen levels, providing a possible basis for protective effects against coronary heart disease. More broadly, epidemiologic studies have linked light to moderate alcohol consumption with increased overall survival as compared to teetotalers and heavy drinkers. Although it remains uncertain whether these survival benefits are due to alcohol consumption *per se* or to other covariates (e.g., having a lifestyle that permits one to enjoy a good glass of wine on a daily basis), it seems that the old saying is true, at least with respect to alcohol—all things in moderation!

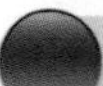

KEY CONCEPTS

Alcohol—Metabolism and Health Effects

- Acute alcohol abuse causes drowsiness at blood levels of approximately 200 mg/dL. Stupor and coma develop at higher levels.
- Alcohol is oxidized to acetaldehyde in the liver by alcohol dehydrogenase, by the cytochrome P-450 system, and by catalase, which is of minor importance. Acetaldehyde is converted to acetate in mitochondria and utilized in the respiratory chain.
- Alcohol oxidation by alcohol dehydrogenase depletes NAD, leading to accumulation of fat in the liver and metabolic acidosis.
- The main effects of chronic alcoholism are fatty liver, alcoholic hepatitis, and cirrhosis, which leads to portal hypertension and increases the risk for development of hepatocellular carcinoma.
- Chronic alcoholism can cause bleeding from gastritis and gastric ulcers, peripheral neuropathy associated with thiamine deficiency, alcoholic cardiomyopathy, and acute and chronic pancreatitis.
- Chronic alcoholism is a major risk factor for cancers of the oral cavity, larynx, and esophagus. The risk is greatly increased by concurrent smoking or use of smokeless tobacco.

Injury by Therapeutic Drugs and Drugs of Abuse

Injury by Therapeutic Drugs (Adverse Drug Reactions)

Adverse drug reactions refer to untoward effects of drugs that are given in conventional therapeutic settings. These reactions are extremely common in the practice of medicine; an exotic, but easily seen example is discoloration of the skin caused by the antibiotic minocycline (Fig. 9-13).

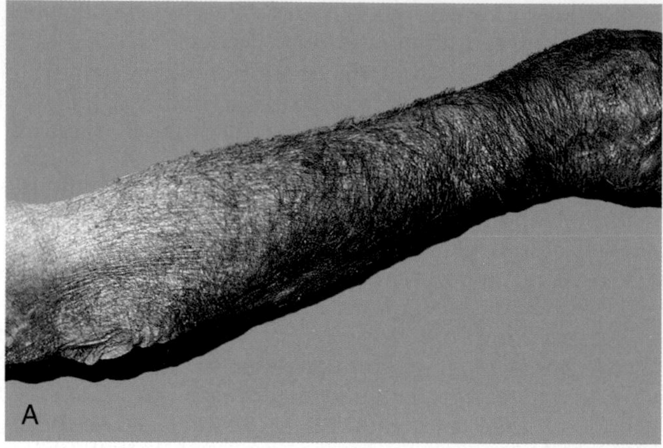

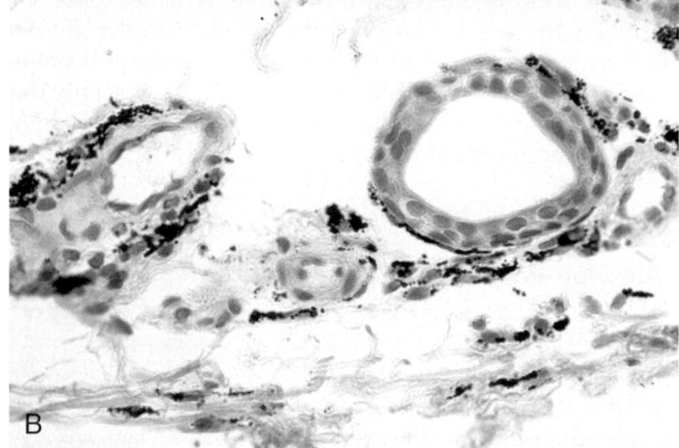

Figure 9-13 Adverse drug reaction. Skin pigmentation caused by minocycline, a long-acting tetracycline derivative. **A,** Diffuse blue-gray pigmentation of the forearm; **B,** Deposition of drug metabolite/iron/melanin pigment particles in the dermis. (Courtesy Dr. Zsolt Argenyi, Department of Pathology, University of Washington, Seattle, Wash.)

Much more common are drug reactions that are due to direct actions of the drug or to immunologically based hypersensitivity reactions. Drug-induced hypersensitivity reactions most commonly present as skin rashes, but they may also mimic autoimmune disorders such as systemic lupus erythematosus (Chapter 6), hemolytic anemia, and immune thrombocytopenia (Chapter 13). Adverse drug reactions affect almost 10% of patients admitted to a hospital.

The number of fatal adverse drug reactions is debated, but by some accounts may be as high as 140,000 deaths per year. Table 9-5 lists common pathologic findings in adverse drug reactions and the drugs most frequently involved. Many of the drugs that produce adverse reactions, such as antineoplastic agents, are highly potent, and the adverse reactions are accepted risks of the treatment. In this section, adverse reactions to commonly used drugs are examined, first discussing the unwelcome effects of anticoagulants, menopausal hormone therapy (MHT), oral contraceptives (OCs), and anabolic steroids and then discussing the effects of acetaminophen and aspirin, because all are commonly used.

Anticoagulants

In 2011, the two drugs that most frequently caused adverse reactions reported to the Food and Drug Administration were the oral anticoagulants warfarin and dabigatran. Warfarin is an antagonist of vitamin K, and dabigatran is a direct inhibitor of thrombin. The principal complications associated with both of these medications are bleeding, which can be fatal, and thrombotic complications such as embolic stroke stemming from undertreatment. Warfarin is inexpensive and its effects are easy to monitor, but many drugs and foods rich in vitamin K either interfere with its metabolism or abrogate its function. As a result, maintaining anticoagulation in a relatively safe therapeutic range can be problematic. Pharmacologic interactions of drugs with dabigatran metabolism have not been described, but many bleeding complications nevertheless occur. It is primarily used to prevent thromboembolism in patients

Table 9-5 Common Adverse Drug Reactions and Their Agents

Reaction	Major Offenders
Bone Marrow And Blood Cells*	
Granulocytopenia, aplastic anemia, pancytopenia	Antineoplastic agents, immunosuppressives, chloramphenicol
Hemolytic anemia, thrombocytopenia	Penicillin, methyldopa, quinidine, heparin
Cutaneous	
Urticaria, macules, papules, vesicles, petechiae, exfoliative dermatitis, fixed drug eruptions, abnormal pigmentation	Antineoplastic agents, sulfonamides, hydantoins, some antibiotics, and many other agents
Cardiac	
Arrhythmias	Theophylline, hydantoins, digoxin
Cardiomyopathy	Doxorubicin, daunorubicin
Renal	
Glomerulonephritis	Penicillamine
Acute tubular necrosis	Aminoglycoside antibiotics, cyclosporin, amphotericin B
Tubulointerstitial disease with papillary necrosis	Phenacetin, salicylates
Pulmonary	
Asthma	Salicylates
Acute pneumonitis	Nitrofurantoin
Interstitial fibrosis	Busulfan, nitrofurantoin, bleomycin
Hepatic	
Fatty change	Tetracycline
Diffuse hepatocellular damage	Halothane, isoniazid, acetaminophen
Cholestasis	Chlorpromazine, estrogens, contraceptive agents
Systemic	
Anaphylaxis	Penicillin
Lupus erythematosus syndrome (drug-induced lupus)	Hydralazine, procainamide
Bleeding	Warfarin, dabigatran
Central Nervous System	
Tinnitus and dizziness	Salicylates
Acute dystonic reactions and parkinsonian syndrome	Phenothiazine antipsychotics
Respiratory depression	Sedatives

*Affected in almost half of all drug-related deaths.

with atrial fibrillation who are at high risk for thrombotic stroke.

Menopausal Hormone Therapy (MHT)

The most common type of MHT (previously referred to as hormone replacement therapy, or HRT) consists of the administration of estrogens together with a progestogen. Because of the risk of uterine cancer, estrogen therapy alone is used only in hysterectomized women. Initially used to counteract "hot flashes" and other symptoms of menopause, early clinical studies suggested that MHT use in postmenopausal women could prevent or slow the progression of osteoporosis (Chapter 26) and reduce the likelihood of myocardial infarction. However, subsequent randomized clinical trials have produced decidedly mixed results. In 2002, the Women's Health Initiative stunned the medical community by reporting that a large prospective placebo controlled trial failed to find support for some of the presumed beneficial effects of the therapy. This study involved approximately 17,000 women who were taking a combination of estrogen (conjugated equine estrogens) and a synthetic progestin (medroxyprogesterone acetate). Although MHT did reduce the number of fractures in women on treatment, researchers also reported that after 5 years of treatment, combination MHT increased the risk of breast cancer (Chapter 23), stroke, and venous thromboembolism and had no effect on the incidence of coronary heart disease. The shockwaves produced by these findings led to a drastic decrease in the use of MHT, from 16 million prescriptions in 2001 to 6 million in 2006, which was accompanied by an apparent drop in the incidence of newly diagnosed breast cancers. But during the past few years there has been a reappraisal of the risks and benefits of MHT. These newer analyses showed that MHT effects depend on the type of hormone therapy regimen used (combination estrogen-progestin versus estrogen alone), the age and risk factor status of the woman at the start of treatment, the duration of the treatment, and possibly the hormone dose, formulation, and route of administration. The current risk:benefit consensus can be summarized as follows:

- Combination estrogen-progestin increases the risk of breast cancer after a median time of 5 to 6 years. In contrast, estrogen alone in women with hysterectomy is associated with a borderline reduction in risk of breast cancer.
- MHT may have a protective effect on the development of atherosclerosis and coronary disease in women younger than age 60 years, but there is no protection in women who started MHT at an older age. These data support the notion that there may be a critical therapeutic window for MHT effects on the cardiovascular system. Protective effects in younger women depend in part on the response of estrogen receptors and healthy vascular endothelium. However, MHT should not be used for prevention of cardiovascular disease or other chronic diseases.
- MHT increases the risk of stroke and venous thromboembolism (VTE), including deep vein thrombosis and pulmonary embolism. The increase in VTE is more pronounced during the first 2 years of treatment and in women who have other risk factors such as immobilization and hypercoagulable states caused by prothrombin or factor V Leiden mutations (Chapter 4). Whether risks of VTE and stroke are lower with transdermal than oral routes of estrogen administration warrants further study.

As can be appreciated from these associations, assessment of risks and benefits when considering the use of MHT in women is complex. The current feeling is that these agents have a role in the management of menopausal symptoms in early menopause but should not be used long term for chronic disease prevention.

Oral Contraceptives (OCs)

Worldwide, more than 100 million women use hormonal contraception. OCs nearly always contain a synthetic estradiol and a variable amount of a progestin, but some preparations contain only progestins. They act by inhibiting ovulation or preventing implantation. Currently prescribed OCs contain a much smaller amount of estrogens (as little as 20 μg of ethinyl estradiol) than the earliest formulations, and are associated with fewer side effects. Transdermal and implantable formulations have also become available. Hence, the results of epidemiologic studies should be interpreted in the context of the dosage and the delivery system. Nevertheless, there is good evidence to support the following conclusions:

- *Breast carcinoma*: The prevailing opinion is that OCs *do not* increase breast cancer risk.
- *Endometrial cancer and ovarian cancers*: OCs have a protective effect against these tumors.
- *Cervical cancer*: OCs may increase risk of cervical carcinomas in women infected with human papillomavirus, although it is unclear whether the increased risk merely reflects greater sexual activity in women on OCs.
- *Thromboembolism*: Most studies indicate that OCs, including the newer low-dose (less than 50 μg of estrogen) preparations, are associated with a threefold to sixfold increased risk of venous thrombosis and pulmonary thromboembolism due to a hypercoagulable state induced by elevated hepatic synthesis of coagulation factors. This risk may be even higher with newer "third-generation" OCs that contain synthetic progestins, particularly in women who are carriers of the factor V Leiden mutation. To put this complication into context, however, the risk of thromboembolism associated with OC use is two to six times lower than the risk of thromboembolism associated with pregnancy.
- *Cardiovascular disease*: There is considerable uncertainty about the risk of atherosclerosis and myocardial infarction in users of OCs. It seems that OCs do not increase the risk of coronary artery disease in women younger than 30 years or in older women who are nonsmokers, but the risk does approximately double in women older than 35 years who smoke.
- *Hepatic adenoma*: There is a well-defined association between the use of OCs and this rare benign hepatic tumor, especially in older women who have used OCs for prolonged periods. The tumor appears as a large, solitary, and well-encapsulated mass.

Ultimately, the pros and cons of OCs must be viewed in the context of their wide applicability and acceptance as a form of contraception that protects against unwanted pregnancies.

Anabolic Steroids

The use of steroids to increase performance by baseball players, track-and-field athletes, and wrestlers has received wide publicity during the past decade. Anabolic steroids are synthetic versions of testosterone, and for performance enhancement they are used at doses that are about 10 to 100 times higher than therapeutic indications. The high concentration of testosterone and its derivatives inhibits production and release of luteinizing hormone and follicle-stimulating hormone by a feedback mechanism, and increases the amount of estrogens, which are produced from anabolic steroids. Anabolic steroids have multiple adverse effects including stunted growth in adolescents, acne, gynecomastia, and testicular atrophy in males, and growth of facial hair and menstrual changes in women. Other effects include psychiatric disturbances and an increased risk of myocardial infarction. Hepatic cholestasis may develop in individuals receiving orally administered anabolic steroids.

Acetaminophen

Acetaminophen is the most commonly used analgesic in the United States. It is present in more than 300 products, alone or in combination with other agents. Hence, acetaminophen toxicity is common, being responsible for more than 50,000 emergency room visits per year. In the United States, it is the cause of about 50% of cases of acute liver failure, with 30% mortality. Intentional overdose (attempted suicide) is the most common cause of acetaminophen toxicity in Great Britain, but unintentional overdose is the most frequent cause in the United States, representing almost 50% of the total intoxication cases.

At therapeutic doses, about 95% of acetaminophen undergoes detoxification in the liver by phase II enzymes and is excreted in the urine as glucuronate or sulfate conjugates (Fig. 9-14). About 5% or less is metabolized through the activity of CYPs (primarily CYP2E) to NAPQI (*N*-acetyl-*p*-benzoquinoneimine), a highly reactive metabolite. NAPQI is normally conjugated with glutathione (GSH), but when acetaminophen is taken in large doses unconjugated *NAPQI* accumulates and causes hepatocellular injury, leading to *centrilobular necrosis* that may progress to *liver failure*. The injury produced by NAPQI involves two mechanisms: (1) covalent binding to hepatic proteins, which causes damage to cellular membranes and mitochondrial dysfunction, and (2) depletion of GSH, making hepatocytes more susceptible to reactive oxygen species-induced injury. Because alcohol induces CYP2E in the liver, toxicity can occur at lower doses in chronic alcoholics.

The window between the usual dose (0.5 gm) and the toxic dose (15 to 25 gm) is large, and the drug is ordinarily very safe. Toxicity begins with nausea, vomiting, diarrhea, and sometimes shock, followed in a few days by evidence of jaundice. Overdoses of acetaminophen can be treated at its early stages (within 12 hours) by administration of *N-acetylcysteine,* which restores GSH levels. In serious overdose liver failure ensues, starting with centrilobular necrosis that may extend to entire lobules; in such circumstances liver transplantation is the only hope for survival. Some patients also show evidence of concurrent renal damage.

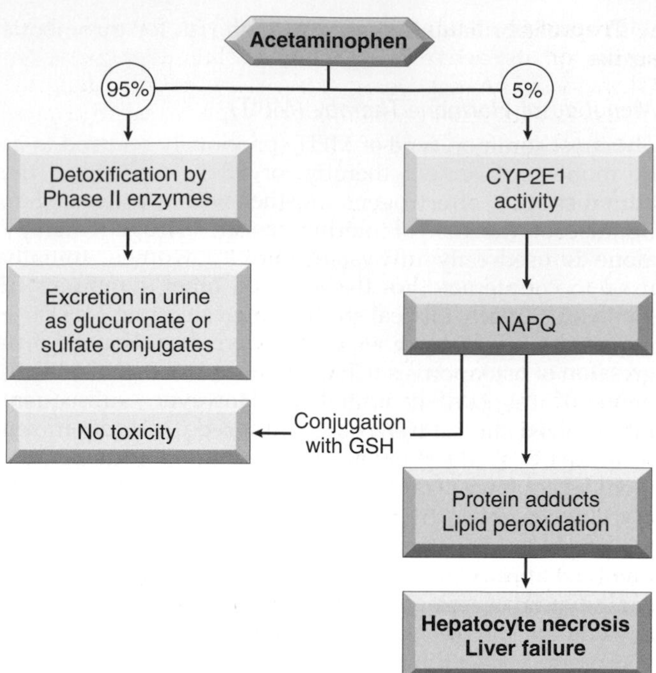

Figure 9-14 Acetaminophen metabolism and toxicity. (See text for details.) (Courtesy Dr. Xavier Vaquero, Department of Pathology, University of Washington, Seattle, Wash.)

Aspirin (Acetylsalicylic Acid)

Aspirin overdose may result from accidental ingestion of a large number of tablets by young children; in adults overdose is frequently suicidal. Much less commonly, salicylate poisoning is caused by the excessive use of ointments containing oil of wintergreen (methyl salicylate). Acute salicylate overdose causes alkalosis as a consequence of the stimulation of the respiratory center in the medulla. This is followed by metabolic acidosis and accumulation of pyruvate and lactate, caused by uncoupling of oxidative phosphorylation and inhibition of the Krebs cycle. Metabolic acidosis enhances the formation of non-ionized forms of salicylates, which diffuse into the brain and produce effects from nausea to coma. Ingestion of 2 to 4 gm by children or 10 to 30 gm by adults may be fatal, but survival has been reported after ingestion of doses five times larger.

Chronic aspirin toxicity (salicylism) may develop in persons who take 3 gm or more daily for long periods of time for treatment of chronic pain or inflammatory conditions. Chronic salicylism is manifested by headaches, dizziness, ringing in the ears (tinnitus), hearing impairment, mental confusion, drowsiness, nausea, vomiting, and diarrhea. The CNS changes may progress to convulsions and coma. The morphologic consequences of chronic salicylism are varied. Most often there is an acute erosive gastritis (Chapter 17), which may produce overt or covert gastrointestinal bleeding and lead to gastric ulceration. A bleeding tendency may appear concurrently with chronic toxicity, because aspirin acetylates platelet cyclooxygenase and irreversibly blocks the production of thromboxane A_2, an activator of platelet aggregation. Petechial hemorrhages may appear in the skin and internal viscera, and bleeding from gastric ulcerations may be exaggerated. With the recognition of gastric ulceration and bleeding as an important complication of ingestion of large doses of aspirin, chronic toxicity is now quite uncommon.

Proprietary analgesic mixtures of aspirin and phenacetin or its active metabolite, acetaminophen, when taken over several years, can cause tubulointerstitial nephritis with renal papillary necrosis, referred to as *analgesic nephropathy* (Chapter 20).

Injury by Nontherapeutic Agents (Drug Abuse)

According to the United Nations Office on Drugs and Crime, it is estimated in the year 2010 approximately 153 million to 300 million people between 15 and 64 years of age used an illicit substance at least once. In most instances, occasional users of illicit "recreational" drugs suffer no apparent long-term health effects, but (depending on the drug) acute effects may take a significant toll in the form of accidents, violence, or even fatal drug-related complications. Drug abuse generally involves the repeated or chronic use of mind-altering substances, beyond therapeutic or social norms, and may lead to drug addiction and overdose, both serious public health problems. Common drugs of abuse are listed in Table 9-6. Considered here are cocaine, heroin, amphetamines, and marijuana, among others.

Cocaine

Globally, cocaine use is greatest in North America, Western and Central Europe, Australia, and New Zealand; in each of these countries, it is estimated from 1% to 2% of adults younger than age 65 years used cocaine in 2010. According to national surveys, the numbers of users in the United States has decline substantially in recent years, from approximately 2.4 million in 2006 to approximately 1.5 million in 2010.

Cocaine is extracted from the leaves of the coca plant, and is usually prepared as a water-soluble powder, cocaine hydrochloride. Sold on the street, it is liberally diluted with talcum powder, lactose, or other look-alikes. Cocaine can be snorted or dissolved in water and injected subcutaneously or intravenously. Crystallization of the pure alkaloid yields nuggets of *crack*, so called because of the cracking or popping sound it makes when heated to produce vapors that are inhaled. The pharmacologic actions of cocaine and crack are identical, but crack is far more potent.

Table 9-6 Common Drugs of Abuse

Class	Molecular Target	Example
Opioid narcotics	Mu opioid receptor (agonist)	Heroin, Hydromorphone (Dilaudid) Oxycodone (OxyContin) Methadone (Dolophine) Meperidine (Demerol)
Sedative-hypnotics	$GABA_A$ receptor (agonist)	Barbiturates Ethanol Methaqualone (Quaalude) Glutethimide (Doriden) Ethchlorvynol (Placidyl)
Psychomotor stimulants	Dopamine transporter (antagonist)	Cocaine
	Serotonin receptors (toxicity)	Amphetamines 3,4-methylenedioxymethamphetamine (MDMA, ecstasy)
Phencyclidine-like drugs	NMDA glutamate receptor channel (antagonist)	Phencyclidine (PCP, angel dust) Ketamine
Cannabinoids	CBI cannabinoid receptors (agonist)	Marijuana Hashish
Hallucinogens	Serotonin 5-HT_2 receptors (agonist)	Lysergic acid diethylamide (LSD) Mescaline Psilocybin

GABA, γ-aminobutyric acid; 5-HT_2, 5-hydroxytryptamine; NMDA, *N*-methyl D-aspartate.
From Hyman SE: A 28-year-old man addicted to cocaine. JAMA 286:2586, 2001.

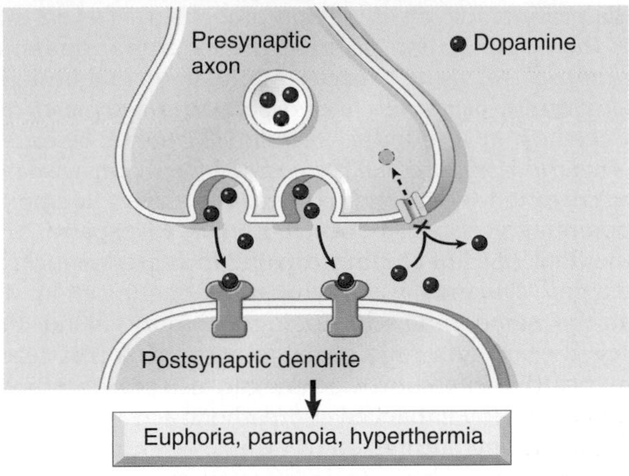

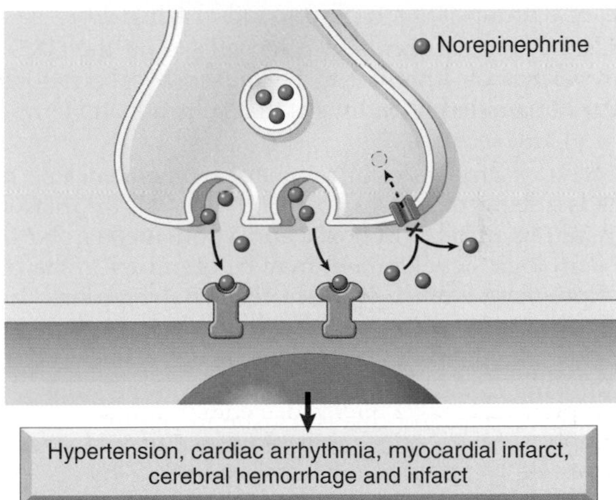

Figure 9-15 The effect of cocaine on neurotransmission. The drug inhibits reuptake of the neurotransmitters dopamine and norepinephrine in the central and peripheral nervous systems.

Cocaine produces an intense euphoria and stimulation, making it one of the most addictive drugs. Experimental animals will press a lever more than 1000 times and forgo food and drink to obtain it. In the cocaine user, although physical dependence generally does not occur, the psychologic withdrawal is profound and can be extremely difficult to treat. Intense cravings are particularly severe in the first several months after abstinence and can recur for years.

The acute and chronic effects of cocaine on various organ systems are as follows:

- *Cardiovascular effects*. The most serious physical effects of cocaine relate to its acute action on the cardiovascular system, where it behaves as a sympathomimetic (Fig. 9-15). It facilitates neurotransmission both in the CNS, where it blocks the reuptake of dopamine, and at adrenergic nerve endings, where it blocks the reuptake of both epinephrine and norepinephrine while stimulating the presynaptic release of norepinephrine. The net effect is the accumulation of these two neurotransmitters in synapses, resulting in excess stimulation, manifested by *tachycardia, hypertension,* and *peripheral vasoconstriction.* Cocaine may also induce *myocardial ischemia* by causing *coronary artery vasoconstriction* and by enhancing platelet aggregation and thrombus formation. Cigarette smoking potentiates cocaine-induced coronary vasospasm. Thus, the dual effect of cocaine, causing increased myocardial oxygen demand by its sympathomimetic action, and, at the same time, decreasing coronary blood flow, sets the stage for myocardial ischemia that may lead to myocardial infarction. Cocaine can also precipitate *lethal arrhythmias* by enhanced sympathetic activity as well as by disrupting normal ion (K^+, Ca^{2+}, Na^+) transport in the myocardium. These toxic effects are not necessarily dose related, and a fatal event may occur in a first time user with what is a typical mood-altering dose.

- *CNS.* The most common acute effects on the CNS are hyperpyrexia (thought to be caused by aberrations of the dopaminergic pathways that control body temperature) and seizures.
- *Effects on pregnancy.* In pregnant women, cocaine may cause acute decreases in blood flow to the placenta, resulting in fetal hypoxia and spontaneous abortion. Neurologic development may be impaired in the fetus of pregnant women who are chronic drug users.
- *Other effects.* Chronic cocaine use may cause (1) perforation of the nasal septum in snorters, (2) decreased lung diffusing capacity in those who inhale the smoke, and (3) development of dilated cardiomyopathy.

Opiates

In 2010, there were an estimated 13 to 21 million users of opiates worldwide, with the highest levels of use being in North America (an estimated 4% of people between 15 and 64 years of age). Opiate drugs of abuse include synthetic prescription opiates such as oxycodone (OxyContin) and "street drugs," most notably heroin. Heroin is an addictive opioid derived from the poppy plant that is closely related to morphine. Its use is even more harmful than that of cocaine. As sold on the street, it is cut (diluted) with an agent (often talc or quinine); thus, the size of the dose is not only variable but also usually unknown to the buyer. Heroin, along with any contaminating substances, is usually self-administered intravenously or subcutaneously. The effects on the CNS are varied and include euphoria, hallucinations, somnolence, and sedation. Heroin has a wide range of other adverse physical effects related to (1) the pharmacologic action of the agent, (2) reactions to the cutting agents or contaminants, (3) hypersensitivity reactions to the drug or its adulterants (quinine itself has neurologic, renal, and auditory toxicity), and (4) diseases contracted incident to the use of contaminated needles. Some of the most important adverse effects of heroin follow:

- *Sudden death.* Sudden death, usually related to overdose, is an ever-present risk, because drug purity is generally unknown (ranging from 2% to 90%). The yearly mortality among heroin users in the United States is estimated to be between 1% and 3%. Sudden death can also occur if heroin is taken after tolerance for the drug, built up over time, is lost (as during a period of incarceration). The mechanisms of death include profound respiratory depression, arrhythmia and cardiac arrest, and severe pulmonary edema.
- *Pulmonary injury.* Pulmonary complications include moderate to severe edema, septic embolism from endocarditis, lung abscess, opportunistic infections, and foreign-body granulomas from talc and other adulterants. Although granulomas occur principally in the lung, they are sometimes found in the mononuclear phagocyte system, particularly in the spleen, liver, and lymph nodes that drain the upper extremities. Examination under polarized light often highlights trapped talc crystals, sometimes enclosed within foreign-body giant cells.
- *Infections.* Infectious complications are common. The four sites most commonly affected are the skin and subcutaneous tissue, heart valves, liver, and lungs. In a series of addicted patients admitted to the hospital, more than 10% had endocarditis, which often takes a distinctive form involving right-sided heart valves, particularly the tricuspid. Most cases are caused by *S. aureus*, but fungi and a multitude of other organisms have also been implicated. Viral hepatitis is the most common infection among addicted persons and is acquired by the sharing of dirty needles. In the United States, this practice has also led to a very high incidence of HIV infection in intravenous drug abusers.
- *Skin.* Cutaneous lesions are probably the most frequent telltale sign of heroin addiction. Acute changes include abscesses, cellulitis, and ulcerations due to subcutaneous injections. Scarring at injection sites, hyperpigmentation over commonly used veins, and thrombosed veins are the usual sequelae of repeated intravenous inoculations.
- *Kidneys.* Kidney disease is a relatively common hazard. The two forms most frequently encountered are amyloidosis (generally secondary to skin infections) and focal and segmental glomerulosclerosis; both induce proteinuria and the nephrotic syndrome.

Abuse of oxycodone, an oral opiate available by prescription for treatment of pain, has increased sharply in recent years in the United States. According to the National Institute of Drug Abuse, approximately 5% of high school seniors took oxycodone in the year 2010, sometimes with tragic results due to the potent respiratory suppressant effect of the drug. The overall number of yearly fatalities attributed to abuse of prescription opiates in the United States rose from approximately 3000 in 1999 to approximately 12,000 deaths in 2008. Most of this increase is attributable to abuse of oxycodone, which has surpassed heroin as the leading cause of opiate-related death in the United States.

Amphetamines and Related Drugs

Methamphetamine. This addictive drug, known as *"speed"* or *"meth,"* is closely related to amphetamine but has stronger effects in the CNS. Methamphetamine use rose rapidly in the United States in the early 2000s, peaking in the year 2005, but has fallen steadily since that time. According to national surveys, use of methamphetamine fell to approximately 350,000 users in 2010, a decrease of more than 50% since 2006. Methamphetamine acts by releasing dopamine in the brain, which inhibits presynaptic neurotransmission at corticostriatal synapses, slowing glutamate release. Methamphetamine produces a feeling of euphoria, which is followed by a "crash." Long-term use leads to violent behaviors, confusion, and psychotic features that include paranoia and hallucinations.

MDMA. MDMA (3,4 methylenedioxymethamphetamine) is popularly known as *ecstasy*. MDMA is used mainly by young people between the ages of 14 and 34 years in North America, Europe, and Australia. It is generally taken orally. Its effects, which include euphoria and hallucinogen-like feelings that last 4 to 6 hours, are partly attributable to an increase in serotonin release in the CNS. As the drug wears off, this increased release coupled with its ability to interfere with serotonin synthesis causes a subsequent a post-use drop in serotonin that is only slowly replenished. MDMA use also reduces the number of serotonergic axon terminals in the striatum and the cortex, and it may increase the peripheral effects of dopamine and adrenergic agents. MDMA tablets may be spiked with other drugs, including methamphetamine and cocaine, which greatly enhance the effects on the CNS.

Marijuana

It is estimated that between 2.6% to 5% of adults worldwide (119 million to 224 million people) used marijuana (or "pot") in 2010, making it far and away the most widely used illicit drug globally. Several states in the United States have legalized the "recreational" use of marijuana in 2013, and more appear poised to follow; thus, its status as an illicit drug is undergoing reevaluation.

Marijuana is made from the leaves of the *Cannabis sativa* plant, which contain the psychoactive substance Δ^9-tetrahydrocannabinol (THC). About 5% to 10% of THC is absorbed when it is smoked in a hand-rolled cigarette ("joint"). Despite numerous studies, the central question of whether the drug has persistent adverse physical and functional effects remains unresolved. Some of the untoward anecdotal effects may be allergic or idiosyncratic reactions or possibly related to contaminants in the preparations rather than to the pharmacologic effects of marijuana. Among the beneficial effects of marijuana is its potential use to treat nausea secondary to cancer chemotherapy and as an agent capable of decreasing pain in some chronic conditions that are otherwise difficult to treat. The functional and organic CNS consequences of marijuana smoking have received most scrutiny. Its use distorts sensory perception and impairs motor coordination, but these acute effects generally clear in 4 to 5 hours. With continued use these changes may progress to cognitive and psychomotor impairments, such as inability to judge time, speed, and distance, a potential cause of automobile accidents. Marijuana increases the heart rate and sometimes blood pressure, and it may cause angina in a person with coronary artery disease.

The respiratory system is also affected by chronic marijuana smoking; laryngitis, pharyngitis, bronchitis, cough and hoarseness, and asthma-like symptoms have all been described, along with mild but significant airway obstruction. Marijuana cigarettes contain a large number of carcinogens that are also present in tobacco. Smoking a marijuana cigarette, compared with a tobacco cigarette, is associated with a threefold increase in the amount of tar inhaled and retained in the lungs, presumably because of the larger puff volume, deeper inhalation, and longer breath holding.

In addition to the use of THC as a recreational drug, a large number of studies have characterized the *endogenous cannabinoid system*, which consists of the *cannabinoid receptors CB1 and CB2*, and the endogenous lipid ligands known as *endocannabinoids*. This system participates in the regulation of the hypothalamic-pituitary-adrenal axis, and modulates the control of appetite, food intake, and energy balance, as well as fertility and sexual behavior.

Other Drugs

The variety of drugs that have been tried by those seeking "new experiences" (e.g., "highs," "lows," "out-of-body experiences") defies belief. These drugs include various stimulants, depressants, analgesics, and hallucinogens (Table 9-6). Among these are PCP (phencyclidine, an anesthetic agent), analgesics such as Vicodin, and ketamine, an anesthetic agent used in animal surgery. Most drugs of abuse are used by males more often than by females. The exception is prescription tranquilizers, which are abused by women about twice as often as by men and which often lead to chronic dependencies.

Chronic inhalation of vapors of spray paints, paint thinners, and some glues that contain toluene ("glue sniffing" or "huffing") can cause cognitive abnormalities and magnetic resonance imaging–detectable brain damage that ranges from mild to severe dementia. Because inhalants are used haphazardly and in various combinations, not much is known about the long-time deleterious effects of most of these agents. However, their acute effects are clear: they cause bizarre and often aggressive behavior that leads to violence or depressed mood and suicidal ideation.

New drugs of abuse emerge yearly. An example is so-called *bath salts*, intentionally misnamed substances that appeared in 2010 and have nothing to do with bathing. Bath salts usually contain 4-methyl-meth-cathinone and methylenedioxypyrovalerone, chemicals that have amphetamine-like effects when snorted or eaten. Bath salts have been associated with agitation, psychosis, myocardial infarction, and suicide. They will no doubt be declared illegal, only to be replaced by the next generation of illicit "designer" drugs.

KEY CONCEPTS

Drug Injury

- Drug injury may be caused by therapeutic drugs (adverse drug reactions) or nontherapeutic agents (drug abuse).
- Antineoplastic agents, anticoagulants, MHT preparations and oral contraceptives, acetaminophen, and aspirin are among the therapeutic drugs involved most frequently.
- MHT increases the risk of endometrial and breast cancers and thromboembolism and does not appear to protect against ischemic heart disease. Oral contraceptives have a protective effect against endometrial and ovarian cancers

but increase the risk of thromboembolism and hepatic adenomas.

- Overdose of acetaminophen may cause centrilobular liver necrosis, leading to liver failure. Early treatment with agents that restore GSH levels may limit toxicity. Aspirin blocks the production of thromboxane A_2, which may produce gastric ulceration and bleeding.
- The common drugs of abuse include sedative-hypnotics (barbiturates, ethanol), psychomotor stimulants (cocaine, methamphetamine, ecstasy), opioid narcotics (heroin, oxycodone), hallucinogens, and cannabinoids (marijuana)

Injury by Physical Agents

Injury induced by physical agents is divided into the following categories: mechanical trauma, thermal injury, electrical injury, and injury produced by ionizing radiation. Each type is considered separately.

Mechanical Trauma

Mechanical forces may inflict a variety of forms of damage. The type of injury depends on the shape of the colliding object, the amount of energy discharged at impact, and the tissues or organs that bear the impact. Bone and head injuries result in unique damage and are discussed elsewhere (Chapters 26 and 28). All soft tissues react similarly to mechanical forces, and the patterns of injury can be divided into abrasions, contusions, lacerations, incised wounds, and puncture wounds. This is just a small sampling of the various forms of trauma encountered by forensic pathologists, who deal with wounds produced by shooting, stabbing, blunt force, traffic accidents, and other causes. In addition to morphologic analyses, forensic pathology now includes molecular methods for identity testing and sophisticated methods to detect the presence of foreign substances. Details about the practice of forensic pathology can be found in specialized textbooks.

Thermal Injury

Both excessive heat and excessive cold are important causes of injury. Burns are the most common cause of thermal injury and are discussed first; a brief discussion of hyperthermia and hypothermia follows.

Thermal Burns

In the United States, approximately 450,000 persons per year receive medical treatment for burn injuries. Eighty percent of burns are caused by fire or by scalding, the latter being a major cause of injury in children. It is estimated that approximately 3500 persons die each year as a consequence of injuries caused by fire and smoke inhalation, mostly originating in homes. Since the 1970s, marked decreases have been seen in both mortality rates and the length of hospitalizations of burn patients. In recent years there were approximately 45,000 hospitalizations per year for burns; among those treated in specialized burn centers (about 55% of those hospitalized), the survival rate was more than 95%, a remarkable testimony to improvements in the care of patients with severe burns. These improvements have been achieved by a better understanding of the systemic effects of massive burns, the prevention of wound infection, and the use of treatments that promote the healing of skin surfaces.

The clinical significance of a burn injury depends on the following factors:

- Depth of the burns
- Percentage of body surface involved
- Internal injuries caused by the inhalation of hot and toxic fumes
- Promptness and efficacy of therapy, especially fluid and electrolyte management and prevention or control of wound infections

Burns used to be classified as first degree to fourth degree, according to the depth of the injury (first-degree burns being the most superficial), but are now classified as superficial, partial thickness, and full-thickness burns.

- *Superficial burns* (formerly known as *first-degree burns*) are confined to the epidermis.
- *Partial thickness burns* (formerly known as *second-degree burns*) involve injury to the dermis.
- *Full-thickness burns* (formerly known as *third-degree burns*) extend to the subcutaneous tissue. Full-thickness burns may also involve damage to muscle tissue underneath the subcutaneous tissue (these were known formerly as fourth-degree burns).

Shock, sepsis, and *respiratory insufficiency* are the greatest threats to life in burn patients. Particularly in burns of more than 20% of the body surface, there is a rapid (within hours) shift of body fluids into the interstitial compartments, both at the burn site and systemically, due to the *systemic inflammatory response syndrome*, leading to shock (Chapter 4). Because of widespread vascular leakiness, generalized edema, including pulmonary edema, can be severe. An important pathophysiologic effect of burns is the development of a *hypermetabolic state* associated with excess heat loss and an increased need for nutritional support. It is estimated that when more than 40% of the body surface is burned, the resting metabolic rate may double.

The burn site is ideal for the growth of microorganisms; the serum and debris provide nutrients, and the burn injury compromises blood flow, blocking effective inflammatory responses. As a result, virtually all burns become colonized with bacteria. Infections are defined by the presence of greater than 10^5 bacteria per gram of tissue, and invasive local infection is defined by the presence of greater than 10^5 bacteria per gram in unburned tissue adjacent to the burn. The most common offender is the opportunist *Pseudomonas aeruginosa,* but antibiotic-resistant strains of other common hospital-acquired bacteria, such as methicillin-resistant *S. aureus,* and fungi, particularly *Candida* species, may also be involved. Furthermore, cellular and humoral defenses against infections are compromised, and both lymphocyte and phagocyte functions are impaired. Direct bacteremic spread and release of toxic substances such as endotoxin from the local site have dire consequences. Pneumonia or septic shock with renal failure and/or the acute respiratory distress syndrome (Chapter 15) are the most common serious sequelae.

Organ system failure resulting from burn sepsis has greatly diminished during the past 30 years, because of the introduction of techniques for early excision and grafting of the burn wound. Removal of the burn wound decreases infection and reduces the need for reconstructive surgery. Grafting is done with split-thickness skin grafts; dermal substitutes, which serve as a bed for cell repopulation, may be used in large full-thickness burns.

Injury to the airways and lungs may develop within 24 to 48 hours after the burn and may result from the direct effect of heat on the mouth, nose, and upper airways or from the inhalation of heated air and noxious gases in the smoke. Water-soluble gases, such as chlorine, sulfur oxides, and ammonia, may react with water to form acids or alkalis, particularly in the upper airways, producing inflammation and swelling, which may lead to partial or complete airway obstruction. Lipid-soluble gases, such as nitrous oxide and products of burning plastics, are more likely to reach deeper airways, producing pneumonitis.

In burn survivors the development of hypertrophic scars, both at the site of the original burn and at donor graft sites, and itching may become long-term, difficult-to-treat problems. Hypertrophic scarring is a common complication of burn injury marked by excessive deposition of collagen in the healing wound bed; its etiology is not well understood.

MORPHOLOGY

Grossly, full-thickness burns are white or charred, dry, and painless (because of destruction of nerve endings), whereas, depending on the depth, partial-thickness burns are pink or mottled with blisters and painful. Histologically, devitalized tissue reveals coagulative necrosis, adjacent to vital tissue that quickly accumulates inflammatory cells and marked exudation.

Hyperthermia

Prolonged exposure to elevated ambient temperatures can result in heat cramps, heat exhaustion, and heat stroke.

- *Heat cramps* result from loss of electrolytes via sweating. Cramping of voluntary muscles, usually in association with vigorous exercise, is the hallmark. Heat-dissipating mechanisms are able to maintain normal core body temperature.
- *Heat exhaustion* is probably the most common hyperthermic syndrome. Its onset is sudden, with prostration and collapse, and it results from a failure of the cardiovascular system to compensate for hypovolemia caused by dehydration. After a period of collapse, which is usually brief, equilibrium is spontaneously re-established if the victim is able to rehydrate.
- *Heat stroke* is associated with high ambient temperatures, high humidity, and exertion. Older adults, individuals undergoing intense physical stress (including young athletes and military recruits), and persons with cardiovascular disease are at particularly high risk for heat stroke. Thermoregulatory mechanisms fail, sweating ceases, and the core body temperature rises to more than 40°C, leading to multiorgan dysfunction that can be rapidly fatal. The hyperthermia is accompanied by marked generalized vasodilation, with peripheral pooling of blood and a decreased effective circulating blood volume. Hyperkalemia, tachycardia, arrhythmias, and other systemic effects are common. Particularly important, however, are sustained contractions of skeletal muscle that can exacerbate the hyperthermia and lead to muscle necrosis (rhabdomyolysis). These phenomena appear to stem from nitrosylation of ryanodine receptor 1 (RYR1), which is located in the sarcoplasmic reticulum of skeletal muscle. RYR1 regulates the release of calcium from the sarcoplasm. Heat stroke deranges RYR1 function and allows calcium to leak into the cytoplasm, where it stimulates muscle contraction and heat production. Inherited mutations in *RYR1* occur in the condition called *malignant hyperthermia*, characterized by a "heat-stroke–like" rise in core body temperature and muscle contractures following exposure to common anesthetics. *RYR1* mutations may also increase the susceptibility to heat stroke in humans and produce heat intolerance in mice. Of interest, mice with *RYR1* mutations are protected from heat stroke by drugs that inhibit calcium leakage from the sarcoplasm, suggesting that it may be possible to develop specific therapies for those who develop or are at high risk for heat stroke and malignant hyperthermia.

Hypothermia

Prolonged exposure to low ambient temperature leads to hypothermia, a condition seen all too frequently in homeless persons. High humidity, wet clothing, and dilation of superficial blood vessels resulting from the ingestion of alcohol hasten the lowering of body temperature. At a body temperature of about 90°F, loss of consciousness occurs, followed by bradycardia and atrial fibrillation at lower core temperatures.

Hypothermia causes injury by two mechanisms:

- *Direct effects* are probably mediated by physical disruptions within cells by high salt concentrations caused by the crystallization of intra- and extracellular water.
- *Indirect effects* result from circulatory changes, which vary depending on the rate and duration of the temperature drop. Slow chilling may induce vasoconstriction and increase vascular permeability, leading to edema and hypoxia. Such changes are typical of "trench foot." This condition developed in soldiers who spent long periods of time in waterlogged trenches during the First World War (1914-1918), frequently causing gangrene that necessitated amputation. With sudden, persistent chilling, the vasoconstriction and increased viscosity of the blood in the local area may cause ischemic injury and degenerative changes in peripheral nerves. In this situation, vascular injury and edema become evident only after the temperature begins to return to normal. However, during the period of ischemia, hypoxic changes and infarction of the affected tissues (e.g., gangrene of toes or feet) may develop.

Electrical Injury

Electrical injuries, which are often fatal, can arise from contact with low-voltage currents (i.e., in the home and workplace) or high-voltage currents carried by high-power lines or produced by lightning. Injuries are of two types: (1) burns and (2) ventricular fibrillation or cardiac and respiratory center failure, resulting from disruption of normal electrical impulses. The type of injury and the severity and extent of burns depend on the strength (amperage), duration, and path of the electric current within the body.

Voltage in the household and workplace (120 or 220 V) is high enough that with low resistance at the site of contact (as when the skin is wet), sufficient current can pass through the body to cause serious injury, including *ventricular fibrillation*. If the current flow is sustained, it may generate enough heat to produce burns at the site of entry and exit as well as in internal organs. An important characteristic of alternating current, the type supplied to most homes, is that it induces tetanic muscle spasm, so that when a live wire or switch is grasped, irreversible clutching is likely to occur, prolonging the period of current flow. This results in a greater likelihood of developing extensive electrical burns and, in some cases, spasm of the chest wall muscles, producing death from asphyxia. Currents generated from high-voltage sources cause similar damage; however, because of the large current flows generated, these are more likely to produce paralysis of medullary centers and extensive burns. Lightning is a classic cause of high-voltage electrical injury. Magnetic fields and microwave radiation, when sufficiently intense, may also produce burns, usually of the skin and subjacent connective tissue, and may also interfere with cardiac pacemakers.

Injury Produced by Ionizing Radiation

Radiation is energy that travels in the form of waves or high-speed particles. Radiation has a wide range of energies that span the electromagnetic spectrum; it can be divided into nonionizing and ionizing radiation. The energy of nonionizing radiation such as UV and infrared light, microwave, and sound waves, can move atoms in a molecule or cause them to vibrate, but is not sufficient to displace bound electrons from atoms. By contrast, *ionizing radiation* has sufficient energy to remove tightly bound electrons. Collision of electrons with other molecules releases electrons in a reaction cascade, referred to as ionization. The main sources of ionizing radiation are *x-rays* and *gamma rays* (electromagnetic waves of very high frequencies), *high-energy neutrons*, *alpha particles* (composed of two protons and two neutrons), and *beta particles*, which are essentially electrons. At equivalent amounts of energy, alpha particles induce heavy damage in a restricted area, whereas x-rays and gamma rays dissipate energy over a longer, deeper course, and produce considerably less damage per unit of tissue. About 50% of the total dose of ionizing radiation received by the U.S. population is human-made, mostly originating from medical devices and radioisotopes. In fact, the exposure of patients to ionizing radiation during radiologic imaging tests roughly doubled between the early 1980s and 2006, mainly because of much more widespread use of CT scans.

Ionizing radiation is a double-edged sword. It is indispensable in medical practice, being used in the treatment of cancer, in diagnostic imaging, and in therapeutic or diagnostic radioisotopes, but it also produces adverse short- and long-term effects such as *fibrosis*, *mutagenesis*, *carcinogenesis*, and *teratogenesis*.

Radiation Units. Several somewhat confusing terms are used to describe radiation dose, which can be quantified according to the amount of radiation emitted by a source, the amount of radiation that is absorbed by a person, and the biologic effect of the radiation. Commonly used terms are as follows:

- *Curie* (Ci) represents the disintegrations per second of a radionuclide (radioisotope). One Ci is equal to 3.7×10^{10} disintegrations per second. This is an expression of the amount of radiation emitted by a source.
- *Gray* (Gy) is a unit that expresses the energy absorbed by the target tissue per unit mass. One Gray corresponds to absorption of 10^4 erg/gm of tissue. A Centigray (cGy), which is the absorption of 100 erg/gm of tissue, is equivalent to 100 Rad (radiation absorbed dose), abbreviated as R. The cGy terminology has now replaced the Rad in medical practice.
- *Sievert* (Sv) is a unit of equivalent dose that depends on the biologic rather than the physical effects of radiation (it replaced a unit called "Rem"). For the same absorbed dose, various types of radiation produce different amounts of damage. The equivalent dose controls for this variation and thereby provides a uniform measure of biologic dose. The equivalent dose (expressed in *Sieverts*) corresponds to the absorbed dose (expressed in Grays) multiplied by the relative biologic effectiveness of the radiation. The relative biologic effectiveness depends on the type of radiation, the type and volume of the exposed tissue, the duration of the exposure, and some other biologic factors (discussed below). The effective dose of x-rays in radiographs and computed tomography is commonly expressed in milliSieverts (mSv). For x-radiation, 1 mSv = 1 mGy.

Main Determinants of the Biologic Effects of Ionizing Radiation. In addition to the physical properties of the radiation, its biologic effects depend heavily on the following factors.

- *Rate of delivery* significantly modifies the biologic effect. Although the effect of radiant energy is cumulative, divided doses may allow cells to repair some of the damage between exposures. Thus, fractionated doses of radiant energy have a cumulative effect only to the extent that repair during the "recovery" intervals is incomplete. Radiation therapy of tumors exploits the general capability of normal cells to repair themselves and recover more rapidly than tumor cells, and thus not sustain as much cumulative radiation damage.
- *Field size* has a great influence on the consequences of irradiation. The body can sustain relatively high doses of radiation when delivered to small, carefully shielded fields, whereas smaller doses delivered to larger fields may be lethal.
- *Cell proliferation.* Because ionizing radiation damages DNA, rapidly dividing cells are more vulnerable to injury than are quiescent cells (Fig. 9-16). Except at extremely high doses that impair DNA transcription,

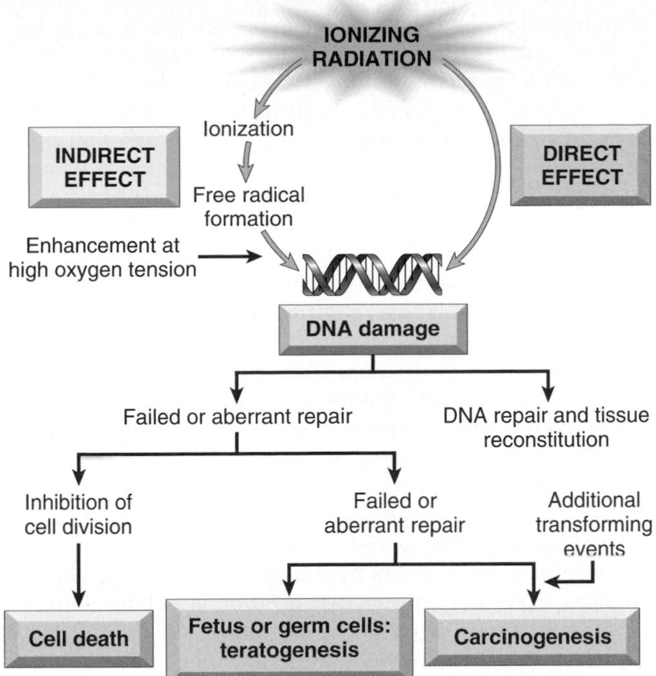

Figure 9-16 Effects of ionizing radiation on DNA and its consequences. The effects on DNA can be direct, or most importantly, indirect, through free radical formation.

irradiation does not kill nondividing cells, such as neurons and muscle cells. However, as discussed in Chapter 7, in dividing cells DNA damage is detected by sensors that produce signals leading to the upregulation of p53, the "guardian of the genome". p53 in turn upregulates the expression of genes that initially lead to cell cycle arrest and, if the DNA damage is too great to be repair, genes that cause cell death through apoptosis. Understandably, therefore, tissues with a high rate of cell division, such as *gonads, bone marrow, lymphoid tissue,* and the *mucosa of the gastrointestinal tract*, are extremely vulnerable to radiation, and the injury is manifested early after exposure.

- *Oxygen effects and hypoxia*. The production of reactive oxygen species from reactions with free radicals generated by radiolysis of water is the major mechanism by which DNA is damaged by ionizing radiation. Poorly vascularized tissues with low oxygenation, such as the center of rapidly growing tumors, are generally less sensitive to radiation therapy than nonhypoxic tissues.
- *Vascular damage*. Damage to endothelial cells, which are moderately sensitive to radiation, may cause narrowing or occlusion of blood vessels leading to impaired healing, fibrosis, and chronic ischemic atrophy. These changes may appear months or years after exposure (Fig. 9-17). Late effects in tissues with a low rate of cell proliferation, such as the brain, kidney, liver, muscle, and subcutaneous tissue, may include cell death, atrophy, and fibrosis. These effects are associated with vascular damage and the release of proinflammatory mediators in irradiated areas.

Figure 9-18 shows the overall consequences of radiation exposure. These consequences vary according to the dose of radiation and the type of exposure. Table 9-7 lists the estimated threshold doses for acute effects of radiation aimed at specific organs; Table 9-8 lists the syndromes caused by exposure to various doses of total-body radiation.

MORPHOLOGY

Cells surviving radiant energy damage show a wide range of structural **changes in chromosomes** that are related to double-stranded DNA breaks, including deletions, translocations, and fragmentation. The mitotic spindle often becomes disorderly, and polyploidy and aneuploidy may be encountered. **Nuclear swelling** and condensation and clumping of chromatin may appear; disruption of the nuclear membrane may also be noted. Apoptosis may occur. Several **abnormal nuclear morphologies** may be seen. Giant cells with pleomorphic nuclei or more than one nucleus may appear and persist for years after exposure. At extremely high doses of radiant energy, markers of cell death, such as nuclear pyknosis and lysis, appear quickly.

In addition to affecting DNA and nuclei, radiant energy may induce a variety of **cytoplasmic changes**, including cytoplasmic swelling, mitochondrial distortion, and degeneration of the endoplasmic reticulum. Plasma membrane breaks and focal defects may be seen. The histologic constellation of cellular pleomorphism, giant-cell formation, conformational changes in nuclei, and abnormal mitotic figures creates a more than passing similarity between radiation-injured cells and cancer cells, a problem that plagues the pathologist when evaluating irradiated tissues for the possible persistence of tumor cells.

Vascular changes and interstitial fibrosis are also prominent in irradiated tissues (Fig. 9-19). During the immediate postirradiation period, vessels may show only dilation. With time, or with higher doses, a variety of degenerative changes appear, including endothelial cell swelling and vacuolation, or even necrosis and dissolution of the walls of small vessels such as capillaries and venules. Affected vessels may rupture or thrombose. Still later, endothelial cell proliferation and collagenous hyalinization and thickening of the intima are seen in irradiated vessels, resulting in marked narrowing or even obliteration of the vascular lumens. At this time, an increase in interstitial collagen in the irradiated field usually becomes evident, leading to scarring and contractions.

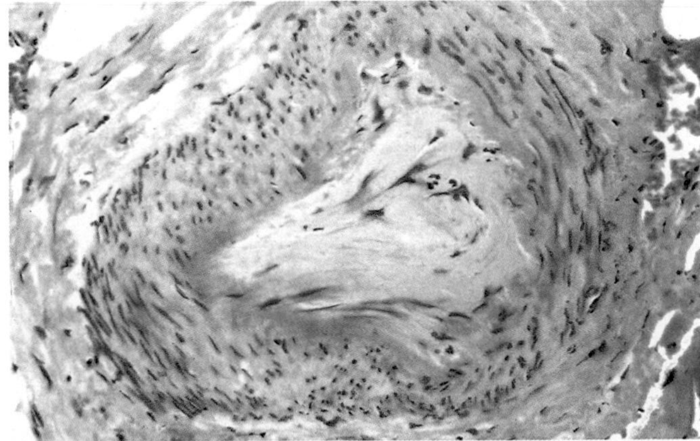

Figure 9-17 Radiation-induced chronic vascular injury with subintimal fibrosis occluding the lumen. (American Registry of Pathology © 1990.)

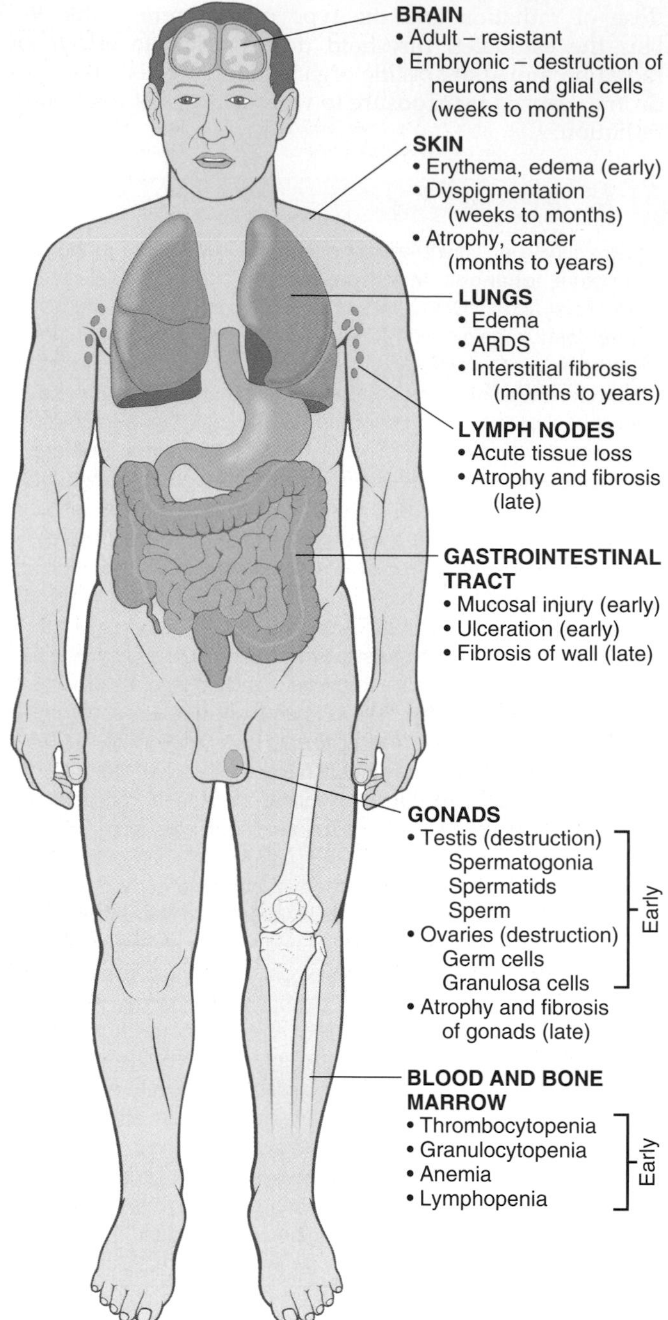

Figure 9-18 Overview of the major morphologic consequences of radiation injury. Early changes occur in hours to weeks; late changes occur in months to years. ARDS, Acute respiratory distress syndrome.

Total-Body Irradiation. Exposure of large areas of the body to even very small doses of radiation may have devastating effects. Doses below 1 Sv produce minimal symptoms, if any. However, higher levels of exposure cause health effects known as *acute radiation syndromes*, which at progressively higher doses involve the hematopoietic, gastrointestinal, and central nervous systems. The syndromes associated with total-body exposure to ionizing radiation are presented in Table 9-8.

Acute Effects on Hematopoietic and Lymphoid Systems. The hematopoietic and lymphoid systems are extremely susceptible to radiation injury and deserve special mention. With high dose levels and large exposure fields, *severe lymphopenia* may appear within hours of irradiation, along with shrinkage of the lymph nodes and spleen. Radiation kills lymphocytes directly, both in the circulation and in tissues (nodes, spleen, thymus, gut). With sublethal doses of radiation, regeneration from viable precursors is prompt, leading to restoration of a normal blood lymphocyte count within weeks to months. Hematopoietic precursors in the bone marrow are also quite sensitive to radiant energy, which produces a dose-dependent *marrow aplasia*. The acute effects of marrow irradiation on peripheral blood counts reflects the kinetics of turnover of the formed elements—the granulocytes, platelets, and red cells, which have half-lives of less than a day, 10 days, and 120 days, respectively. After a brief rise in the circulating neutrophil count, *neutropenia* appears within several days. Neutrophil counts reach their nadir, often at counts near zero, during the second week. If the patient survives, recovery of the normal granulocyte count may require 2 to 3 months. *Thrombocytopenia* appears by the end of the first week, with the platelet count nadir occurring somewhat later than that of granulocytes; recovery is similarly delayed. *Anemia* appears after 2 to 3 weeks and may persist for months. Understandably, higher doses of radiation produce more severe cytopenias and more prolonged periods of recovery. Very high doses kill marrow stem cells and induce permanent aplasia (*aplastic anemia*) marked by a failure of blood count recovery, whereas with lower doses the aplasia is transient.

Fibrosis. A common consequence of radiation therapy for cancer is the development of fibrosis in the tissues included in the irradiated field (Fig. 9-19). Fibrosis may occur weeks or months after irradiation as a consequence of the replacement of dead parenchymal cells by connective tissue, leading to the formation of scars and adhesions. Vascular damage, the death of tissue stem cells, and the release of cytokines and chemokines that promote inflammation and fibroblast activation are the main contributors to the development of radiation-induced fibrosis (Figs. 9-20 and 9-21). Common sites of fibrosis after radiation treatment are the lungs, the salivary glands after radiation therapy for head and neck cancers, and colorectal and pelvic areas after treatment for cancer of the prostate, rectum, or cervix.

DNA Damage and Carcinogenesis. Ionizing radiation can cause multiple types of DNA damage, including single-base damage, single- and double-stranded breaks, and

Table 9-7 Estimated Threshold Doses for Acute Radiation Effects on Specific Organs

Health Effect	Organ	Dose (Sv)
Temporary sterility	Testes	0.15
Depression of hematopoiesis	Bone marrow	0.50
Reversible skin effects (e.g., erythema)	Skin	1-2
Permanent sterility	Ovaries	2.5-6
Temporary hair loss	Skin	3-5
Permanent sterility	Testis	3.5
Cataract	Lens of eye	5

Table 9-8 Effects of Total-Body Ionizing Radiation

	0-1 Sv	1-2 Sv	2-10 Sv	10-20 Sv	>50 Sv
Main site of injury	None	Lymphocytes	Bone marrow	Small bowel	Brain
Main signs and symptoms	None	Moderate granulocytopenia Lymphopenia	Leukopenia, hemorrhage, hair loss, vomiting	Diarrhea, fever, electrolyte imbalance, vomiting	Ataxia, coma, convulsions, vomiting
Time of development	–	1 day to 1 week	2-6 weeks	5-14 days	1-4 hours
Lethality	None	None	Variable (0% to 80%)	100%	100%

DNA-protein cross-links. In surviving cells, simple defects may be repaired by various enzyme systems present in most mammalian cells. The most serious damage to DNA consists of *double-stranded breaks (DSBs).* Two types of mechanisms can repair DSBs in mammalian cells: *homologous recombination* and *nonhomologous end joining (NHEJ),* with NHEJ being the most common repair pathway. DNA repair through NHEJ often produces mutations, including short deletions or duplications, or gross chromosomal aberrations such as translocations and inversions. If the replication of cells containing DSBs is not stopped by cell cycle checkpoint controls (Chapter 1), cells with chromosomal damage persist and may initiate carcinogenesis many years later. More recently it has been recognized that these abnormal cells also produce a "bystander effect," that is, they alter the behavior of nonirradiated surrounding cells through the production of growth factors and cytokines. Bystander effects are referred to as non-target effects of radiation.

Cancer Risks from Exposures to Radiation. Any cell capable of division that has sustained a mutation has the potential to become cancerous. Thus, an increased incidence of neoplasms may occur in any organ after exposure to ionizing radiation. The level of radiation required to increase the risk of cancer development is difficult to determine, but there is little doubt that acute or prolonged exposures that result in doses of greater than 100 mSv cause serious consequences, including cancer. Proof of this risk is found in the increased incidence of leukemias and solid tumors in several organs (e.g., thyroid, breast, and lungs) in survivors of the atomic bombings of Hiroshima and Nagasaki; the high number of thyroid cancers in survivors of the Chernobyl accident; the high incidence of thyroid tumors, and the elevated frequency of leukemias and birth defects, in inhabitants of the Marshall Islands exposed to nuclear fallout; and the development of "second cancers," such as acute myeloid leukemia, myelodysplastic syndrome, and solid tumors, in individuals who received radiation therapy for cancers such as Hodgkin lymphoma. The long-term cancer risks caused by radiation exposures in the range of 5 to 100 mSv are much more difficult to establish, because accurate measurements of risks require large population groups ranging from 50,000 to 5 million people. Nevertheless, for x-rays and gamma rays there is good evidence for a statistically significant increase in the risk of cancer at acute doses of greater than 50 mSv and "reasonable" evidence for acute doses of greater than 5 mSv; as a point of reference, a single posteroanterior chest radiograph, a lateral chest film chest radiograph, and a computed tomography of the chest deliver effective doses to the lungs of 0.01, 0.15, and 10 mSv, respectively. It is believed that the risk of secondary cancers following irradiation is greatest in children. This is based in part on

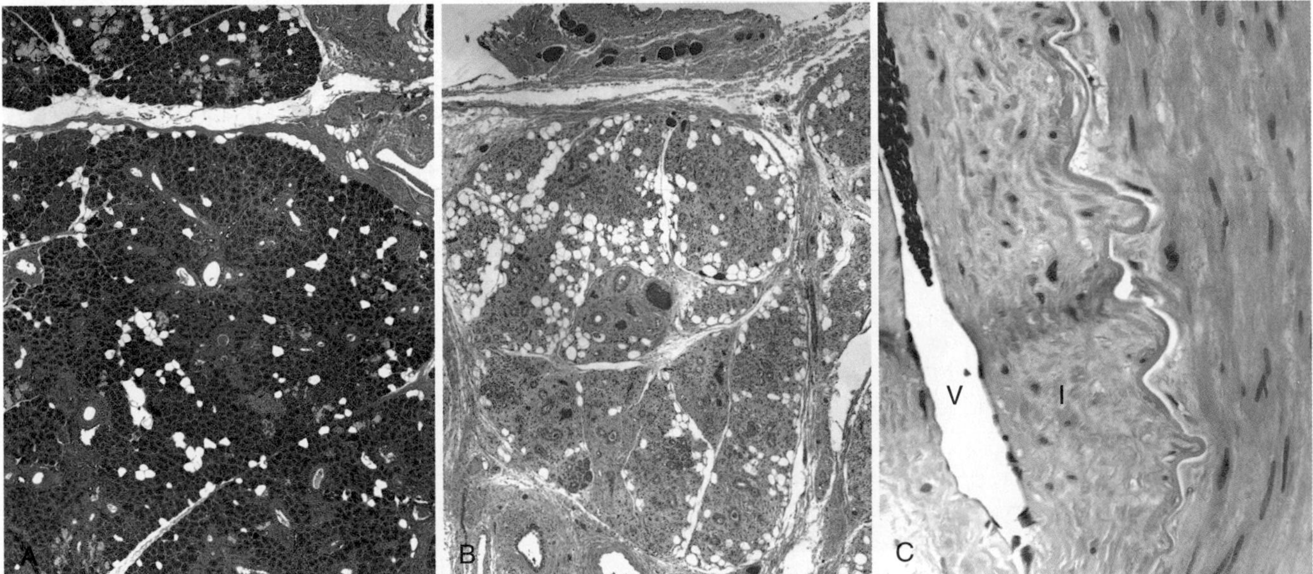

Figure 9-19 Fibrosis and vascular changes in salivary glands produced by radiation therapy of the neck region. **A,** Normal salivary gland; **B,** fibrosis caused by radiation; **C,** fibrosis and vascular changes consisting of fibrointimal thickening and arteriolar sclerosis. V, vessel lumen; I, thickened intima. (Courtesy Dr. Melissa Upton, Department of Pathology, University of Washington, Seattle, Wash.)

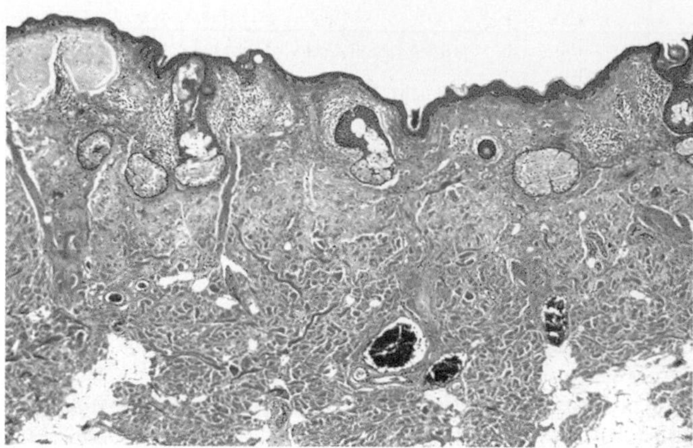

Figure 9-20 Chronic radiation dermatitis with atrophy of epidermis, dermal fibrosis, and telangiectasia of the subcutaneous blood vessels. (American Registry of Pathology © 1990.)

a recent large-scale epidemiologic study showing that children who receive at least two CT scans have very small but measurable increased risks for leukemia and malignant brain tumors, and on older studies showing that radiation therapy to the chest is particularly likely to produce breast cancers when administered to adolescent females.

Increased risk of cancer development may also be associated with occupational exposures. *Radon* gas is a ubiquitous product of the spontaneous decay of uranium. Its carcinogenic effects are largely attributable to two decay products, *polonium 214* and *polonium 218* (or "radon daughters"), which emit alpha particles. Polonium 214 and 218 produced from inhaled radon tend to deposit in the lung, and chronic exposure in uranium miners may give rise to lung carcinomas. Risks are also present in homes in which the levels of radon are very high, comparable to those found in mines. However, there is little evidence to suggest that radon contributes to the risk of lung cancer in the average household. For historical reasons, we also mention here the development of osteogenic sarcomas after radium exposure in radium dial painters, chemists, radiologists, and patients exposed to radium as a treatment for various ailments during the first part of the twentieth century.

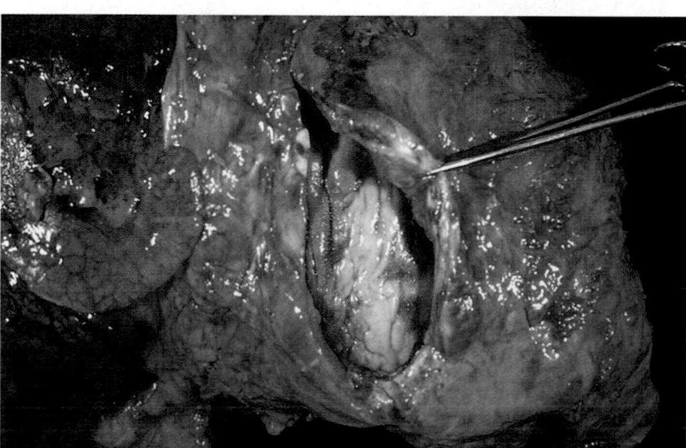

Figure 9-21 Extensive mediastinal fibrosis after radiotherapy for carcinoma of the lung. Note the markedly thickened peri cardium. (From the teaching collection of the Department Pathology, Southwestern Medical School, Dallas, TX.)

KEY CONCEPTS

Radiation Injury

- Ionizing radiation may injure cells directly or indirectly by generating free radicals from water or molecular oxygen
- Ionizing radiation damages DNA; therefore, rapidly dividing cells such as germ cells, and those in the bone marrow and gastrointestinal tract are very sensitive to radiation injury
- DNA damage that is not adequately repaired may result in mutations that predispose affected cells to neoplastic transformation
- Ionizing radiation may cause vascular damage and sclerosis, resulting in ischemic necrosis of parenchymal cells and their replacement by fibrous tissue

Nutritional Diseases

Malnutrition, also referred to as *protein energy malnutrition or PEM*, is a consequence of inadequate intake of proteins and calories, or deficiencies in the digestion or absorption of proteins, resulting in the loss of fat and muscle tissue, weight loss, lethargy, and generalized weakness. Millions of people in developing nations are malnourished and starving, or living on the cruel edge of starvation. In the industrial world and, more recently, also in developing countries, *obesity* has become a major public health problem due to its association with the development of diseases such as diabetes, atherosclerosis, and cancer.

The sections that follow barely skim the surface of nutritional disorders. Particular attention is devoted to PEM, anorexia nervosa and bulimia, deficiencies of vitamins and trace minerals, obesity, and a brief overview of the relationships of diet to atherosclerosis and cancer. Other nutrients and nutritional issues are discussed in the context of specific diseases.

Dietary Insufficiency

An appropriate diet should provide (1) sufficient energy, in the form of carbohydrates, fats, and proteins, for the body's daily metabolic needs; (2) amino acids and fatty acids to be used as building blocks for synthesis of proteins and lipids; and (3) vitamins and minerals, which function as coenzymes or hormones in vital metabolic pathways or, as in the case of calcium and phosphate, as important structural components. In *primary malnutrition*, one or all of these components are missing from the diet. By contrast, in *secondary malnutrition*, malnutrition results from malabsorption, impaired utilization or storage, excess loss, or increased need for nutrients.

There are several conditions that may lead to primary or secondary malnutrition.

- *Poverty*. Homeless persons, aged individuals, and children of the poor often suffer from PEM as well as trace nutrient deficiencies. In poor countries, poverty, crop failures, livestock deaths, and drought, often in times of war and political upheaval, create the setting for the malnourishment of children and adults.

- *Infections.* PEM increases susceptibility to many common infectious diseases. Conversely, infections have a negative effect on nutrition, thus establishing a vicious cycle.
- *Acute and chronic illnesses.* The basal metabolic rate becomes accelerated in many illnesses resulting in increased daily requirements for all nutrients. Failure to recognize these nutritional needs may delay recovery. PEM is often present in patients with wasting diseases, such as *advanced cancers* and *AIDS* (discussed later).
- *Chronic alcoholism.* Alcoholic persons may sometimes suffer PEM but more frequently have deficiencies of vitamins, especially thiamine, pyridoxine, folate, and vitamin A, as a result of poor diet, defective gastrointestinal absorption, abnormal nutrient utilization and storage, increased metabolic needs, and an increased rate of loss. A failure to recognize the likelihood of thiamine deficiency in persons with chronic alcoholism may result in irreversible brain damage (e.g., *Wernicke encephalopathy* and *Korsakoff psychosis*, discussed in Chapter 28).
- *Ignorance and failure of diet supplementation.* Even the affluent may fail to recognize that infants, adolescents, and pregnant women have increased nutritional needs. Ignorance about the nutritional content of various foods is also a contributing factor. Some examples are: iron deficiency in infants fed exclusively artificial milk diets; polished rice used as the mainstay of a diet may lack adequate amounts of thiamine; lack of iodine from food and water in regions removed from the oceans, unless supplementation is provided.
- *Self-imposed dietary restriction. Anorexia nervosa, bulimia,* and less overt eating disorders affect many individuals who are concerned about body image and are obsessed with body weight (anorexia and bulimia are discussed later).
- *Other causes.* Additional causes of malnutrition include gastrointestinal diseases and malabsorption syndromes, genetic diseases, specific drug therapies (which block uptake or utilization of particular nutrients), and inadequate total parenteral nutrition.

Protein-Energy Malnutrition

Severe PEM is a serious, often lethal disease that preferentially affects children. It is common in low-income countries, where it affects up to 30% of children and is a major factor in high death rates among children younger than 5 years of age. It is estimated that malnutrition is responsible for approximately 50% of deaths in infancy and childhood each year in developing countries. In developed countries, PEM often occurs in older and debilitated patients in nursing homes and hospitals, but also occurs with disturbing frequency in children living in poverty, even in the United States.

Malnutrition is determined according to the *body mass index* (BMI, weight in kilograms divided by height in meters squared). A BMI less than 16 kg/m^2 is considered malnutrition (normal range 18.5 to 25 kg/m^2). In more practical ways, a child whose weight falls to less than 80% of normal (provided in standard tables) is considered malnourished. However, loss of weight may be masked by generalized edema, as discussed later. Other helpful parameters are the evaluation of fat stores (thickness of skin folds), muscle mass (reduced circumference of mid-arm), and serum proteins (albumin and transferrin levels provide a measure of the adequacy of the visceral protein compartment).

Marasmus and Kwashiorkor. In malnourished children, PEM presents as a range of clinical syndromes, all characterized by a dietary intake of protein and calories inadequate to meet the body's needs. The two ends of the spectrum of PEM syndromes are known as *marasmus* and *kwashiorkor*. From a functional standpoint, there are two differentially regulated protein compartments in the body: the somatic compartment, represented by proteins in skeletal muscles, and the visceral compartment, represented by protein stores in the visceral organs, primarily the liver. As we shall see, the somatic compartment is affected more severely in marasmus, and the visceral compartment is depleted more severely in kwashiorkor.

A child is considered to have *marasmus* when weight falls to 60% of normal for sex, height, and age. A marasmic child suffers growth retardation and loss of muscle, the latter resulting from catabolism and depletion of the somatic protein compartment. This seems to be an adaptive response that provides the body with amino acids as a source of energy. The visceral protein compartment, which is presumably more precious and critical for survival, is only marginally depleted, and hence serum albumin levels are either normal or only slightly reduced. In addition to muscle proteins, subcutaneous fat is also mobilized and used as fuel. The production of leptin (discussed later) is low, which may stimulate the hypothalamic-pituitary-adrenal axis to produce high levels of cortisol that contribute to lipolysis. With such losses of muscle and subcutaneous fat, the *extremities are emaciated;* by comparison, the head appears too large for the body (Fig. 9-22*A*). Anemia and manifestations of multiple vitamin deficiencies are present, and there is evidence of *immune deficiency*, particularly T-cell-mediated immunity. Hence, concurrent infections are usually present, which impose additional nutritional demands. Unfortunately, images of children dead or near death with marasmus, have become commonplace in television and newspaper reports of famine and disasters in various areas of the world.

Kwashiorkor occurs when protein deprivation is relatively more severe than the deficit in total calories (Fig. 9-22*B*). This is the most common form of PEM seen in African children who have been weaned too early and subsequently fed, almost exclusively, a carbohydrate diet (kwashiorkor, from the Ga language in Ghana, describes a disease in an young child that occurs following the arrival or another baby). The prevalence of kwashiorkor is also high in impoverished countries of Southeast Asia. Less severe forms may occur worldwide in persons with chronic diarrheal states in which protein is not absorbed or in those with chronic protein loss due to conditions such as protein-losing enteropathies, the nephrotic syndrome, or after extensive burns. Cases of kwashiorkor resulting from fad diets or replacement of milk by rice-based beverages have been reported in the United States.

In kwashiorkor, marked protein deprivation is associated with severe depletion of the visceral protein compartment, and the resultant hypoalbuminemia gives rise to

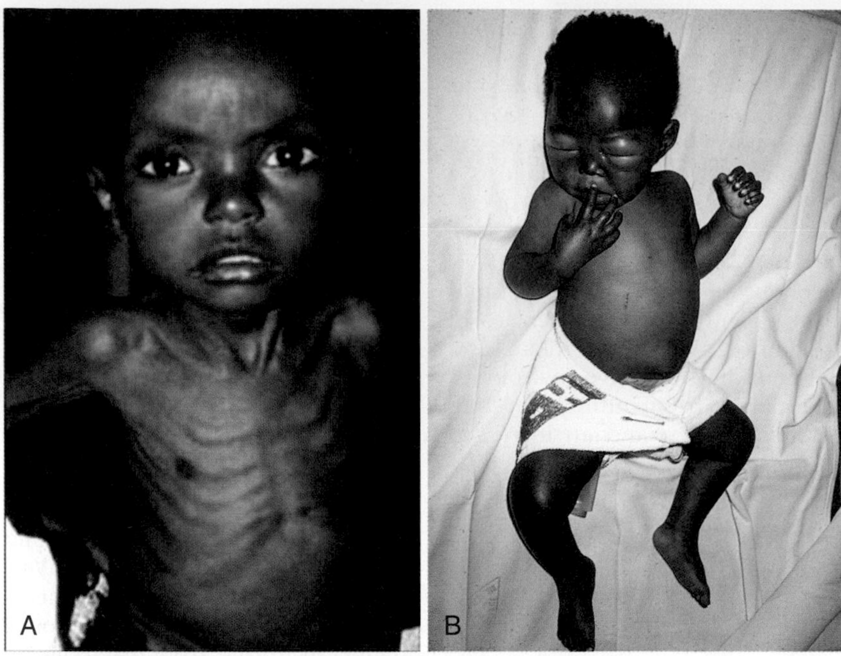

Figure 9-22 Childhood malnutrition. **A,** Marasmus. Note the loss of muscle mass and subcutaneous fat; the head appears to be too large for the emaciated body. **B,** Kwashiorkor. The infant shows generalized edema, seen as ascites and puffiness of the face, hands, and legs. (**A,** From Clinic Barak, Reisebericht Kenya.)

generalized or *dependent edema* (Fig. 9-22*B*). The loss of weight in these patients is masked by the increased fluid retention. In further contrast to marasmus, there is relative sparing of subcutaneous fat and muscle mass. Children with kwashiorkor have characteristic *skin lesions,* with alternating zones of hyperpigmentation, areas of desquamation, and hypopigmentation, giving a "flaky paint" appearance. *Hair changes* include overall loss of color or alternating bands of pale and darker hair. Other features that differentiate kwashiorkor from marasmus include an enlarged, *fatty liver* (resulting from reduced synthesis of the carrier protein component of lipoproteins), and the development of apathy, listlessness, and loss of appetite. Vitamin deficiencies are likely to be present, as are *defects in immunity* and *secondary infections.* As already stated, marasmus and kwashiorkor are two ends of a spectrum, and considerable overlap exists between these conditions.

PEM in the developed world. In the United States, secondary PEM often develops in chronically ill, older, and bedridden patients. An 18-item questionnaire known as the *Mininutritional Assessment* (MNA) is often used to measure the nutritional status of older persons. It is estimated that more than 50% of older residents in nursing homes in the United States are malnourished. Weight loss of more than 5% associated with PEM increases the risk of mortality in nursing home patients by almost five-fold. The most obvious signs of secondary PEM include: (1) depletion of subcutaneous fat in the arms, chest wall, shoulders, or metacarpal regions; (2) wasting of the quadriceps and deltoid muscles; and (3) ankle or sacral edema. Bedridden or hospitalized malnourished patients have an increased risk of infection, sepsis, impaired wound healing, and death after surgery.

MORPHOLOGY

The main anatomic changes in PEM are (1) growth failure, (2) peripheral edema in kwashiorkor, and (3) loss of body fat and atrophy of muscle, more marked in marasmus.

The **liver** in kwashiorkor, but not in marasmus, is enlarged and fatty; superimposed cirrhosis is rare. In kwashiorkor (rarely in marasmus) the **small bowel** shows a decrease in the mitotic index in the crypts of the glands, associated with mucosal atrophy and loss of villi and microvilli. In such cases concurrent loss of small intestinal enzymes occurs, most often manifested as disaccharidase deficiency. Hence, infants with kwashiorkor initially may not respond well to full-strength, milk-based diets. With treatment, the mucosal changes are reversible.

The **bone marrow** in both kwashiorkor and marasmus may be hypoplastic, mainly as a result of decreased numbers of red cell precursors. The peripheral blood commonly reveals mild to moderate anemia, which is often multifactorial in origin; nutritional deficiencies of iron, folate, and protein, as well as the suppressive effects of infection (anemia of chronic disease) may all contribute. Depending on the predominant factor, the red cells may be microcytic, normocytic, or macrocytic.

The **brain** in infants who are born to malnourished mothers and who suffer PEM during the first 1 or 2 years of life has been reported by some to show cerebral atrophy, a reduced number of neurons, and impaired myelinization of white matter.

Many other changes may be present, including (1) thymic and lymphoid atrophy (more marked in kwashiorkor than in marasmus), (2) anatomic alterations induced by intercurrent infections, particularly with all manner of endemic worms and other parasites, and (3) deficiencies of other required nutrients such as iodine and vitamins.

Cachexia. PEM is a common complication in patients with AIDS or advanced cancers, and in these settings it is known as *cachexia*. Cachexia occurs in about 50% of cancer patients, most commonly in individuals with gastrointestinal, pancreatic, and lung cancers, and is responsible for about 30% of cancer deaths. It is a highly debilitating condition characterized by extreme weight loss, fatigue, muscle atrophy, anemia, anorexia, and edema. Mortality is generally the consequence of atrophy of the diaphragm and other respiratory muscles.

The precise causes of cachexia are not known, but it is clear that mediators secreted by tumors and during chronic inflammatory reactions contribute to its development:

- *Proteolysis-inducing factor*, which is a glycosylated polypeptide excreted in the urine of weight-losing patients with pancreatic, breast, colon, and other cancers
- *Lipid-mobilizing factor*, which increases fatty acid oxidation, and proinflammatory cytokines, such as TNF (originally known as *cachectin*), and IL-6.

Proteolysis-inducing factor and proinflammatory cytokines cause skeletal muscle breakdown through the NF-κB-induced activation of the ubiquitin proteasome pathway, which promotes the degradation of skeletal muscle structural proteins such as myosin heavy chain by upregulating the expression of several muscle-specific ubiquitin ligases. Other data implicate acquired abnormalities of the myofibril dystrophin-glycoprotein complex (Fig. 9-23), the same membrane complex that is defective in several forms of muscular dystrophy (Chapter 27).

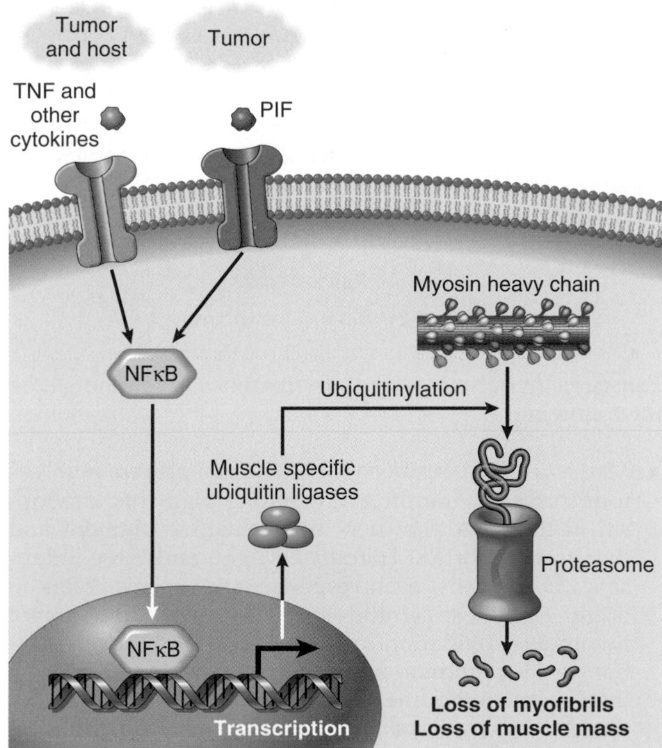

Figure 9-23 Mechanisms of cancer cachexia. Proteolysis-inducing factor (PIF) produced by tumors and TNF and other cytokines produced by host immune cells activate NF-κB and initiate the transcription of the muscle-specific ubiquitin ligases. These ligases in turn ubiquitinate structural components of myofibrils such as myosin heavy chain, leading to their degradation by the proteasome.

Anorexia Nervosa and Bulimia

Anorexia nervosa is self-induced starvation, resulting in marked weight loss; *bulimia* is a condition in which the patient binges on food and then induces vomiting. Anorexia nervosa has the highest death rate of any psychiatric disorder. Bulimia is more common than anorexia nervosa, and generally has a better prognosis; it is estimated to occur in 1% to 2% of women and 0.1% of men, with an average onset at 20 years of age. These eating disorders occur primarily in previously healthy young women who have developed an obsession with body image and thinness. The neurobiologic underpinnings of these diseases are unknown, but it has been suggested that altered serotonin metabolism may be an important component.

The clinical findings in anorexia nervosa are generally similar to those in severe PEM. In addition, effects on the endocrine system are prominent. *Amenorrhea*, resulting from decreased secretion of gonadotropin-releasing hormone, and subsequent decreased secretion of luteinizing hormone and follicle-stimulating hormone, is so common that its presence is consider a diagnostic feature. Other common findings related to *decreased thyroid hormone release* include cold intolerance, bradycardia, constipation, and changes in the skin and hair. In addition, dehydration and electrolyte abnormalities are frequently present. The skin becomes dry and scaly. *Bone density is decreased*, most likely because of low estrogen levels, mimicking the postmenopausal acceleration of osteoporosis. Anemia, lymphopenia, and hypoalbuminemia may be present. A major complication of anorexia nervosa (and also bulimia) is an increased susceptibility to *cardiac arrhythmia* and *sudden death*, resulting from hypokalemia.

In bulimia, *binge eating* is the norm. Large amounts of food, principally carbohydrates, are ingested, only to be followed by induced vomiting. Although menstrual irregularities are common, amenorrhea occurs in less than 50% of bulimic patients because weight and gonadotropin levels remain near normal. The major medical complications relate to frequent vomiting and the chronic use of laxatives and diuretics. They include (1) *electrolyte imbalances* (hypokalemia), which predispose the patient to cardiac arrhythmias; (2) *pulmonary aspiration* of gastric contents; and (3) *esophageal and gastric rupture*. Nevertheless, there are no specific signs or symptoms; thus, the diagnosis of bulimia relies on a comprehensive psychologic assessment of the person.

Vitamin Deficiencies

Thirteen vitamins are necessary for health; vitamins A, D, E, and K are *fat-soluble*, and all others are *water-soluble*. The distinction between fat- and water-soluble vitamins is important. Fat-soluble vitamins are more readily stored in the body, but they may be poorly absorbed in fat malabsorption disorders, caused by disturbances of digestive functions (Chapter 17). Certain vitamins can be synthesized endogenously—vitamin D from precursor steroids, vitamin K and biotin by the intestinal microflora, and niacin from tryptophan, an essential amino acid.

Notwithstanding this endogenous synthesis, a dietary supply of all vitamins is essential for health.

A deficiency of vitamins may be primary (dietary in origin) or secondary to disturbances in intestinal absorption, transport in the blood, tissue storage, or metabolic conversion. In the following sections, vitamins A, D, and C are presented in some detail because of their wide-ranging activities and the morphologic changes of deficient states. This is followed by presentation in tabular form of the main consequences of deficiencies of the remaining vitamins (E, K, and the B complex) and some essential minerals. However, it should be emphasized that deficiency of a single vitamin is uncommon, and that single or multiple vitamin deficiencies may be associated with PEM.

Vitamin A

The major functions of vitamin A are maintenance of normal vision, regulation of cell growth and differentiation, and regulation of lipid metabolism. Vitamin A is the name given to a group of related compounds that include *retinol* (vitamin A alcohol), *retinal* (vitamin A aldehyde), *and retinoic acid* (vitamin A acid), which have similar biologic activities.

Retinol is the chemical name given to vitamin A. It is the transport form and, as retinol ester, also the storage form. The generic term *retinoids* encompasses vitamin A in its various forms and both natural and synthetic chemicals that are structurally related to vitamin A, but may not necessarily have vitamin A–like biologic activity. Animal-derived foods such as liver, fish, eggs, milk, and butter are important dietary sources of preformed vitamin A. Yellow and leafy green vegetables such as carrots, squash, and spinach supply large amounts of carotenoids, provitamins that can be metabolized to active vitamin A in the body. Carotenoids contribute approximately 30% of the vitamin A in human diets; the most important of these is β-carotene, which is efficiently converted to vitamin A. The Recommended Dietary Allowance for vitamin A is expressed in retinol equivalents, to take into account both preformed vitamin A and β-carotene.

Vitamin A is a fat-soluble vitamin, and its absorption requires bile, pancreatic enzymes, and some level of antioxidant activity in the food. Retinol (generally ingested as retinol ester) and β-carotene are absorbed in the intestine, where β-carotene is also converted to retinol (Fig. 9-24). Retinol is then transported in chylomicrons to the liver for esterification and storage. Uptake in liver cells takes place through the apolipoprotein E receptor. More than 90% of the body's vitamin A reserves are stored in the liver, predominantly in the perisinusoidal stellate (Ito) cells. In healthy persons who consume an adequate diet, these reserves are sufficient to meet the body's demands for at least 6 months. Retinol esters stored in the liver can be mobilized; before release, retinol binds to a specific retinol-binding protein (RBP), synthesized in the liver. The uptake of retinol/RBP in peripheral tissues is dependent on cell surface receptors specific for RBP. After uptake, retinol binds to a cellular RBP, and the RBP is released back into the blood. Retinol may also be stored in peripheral tissues as retinol ester or may be oxidized to form retinoic acid, which has important effects on epithelial differentiation and growth.

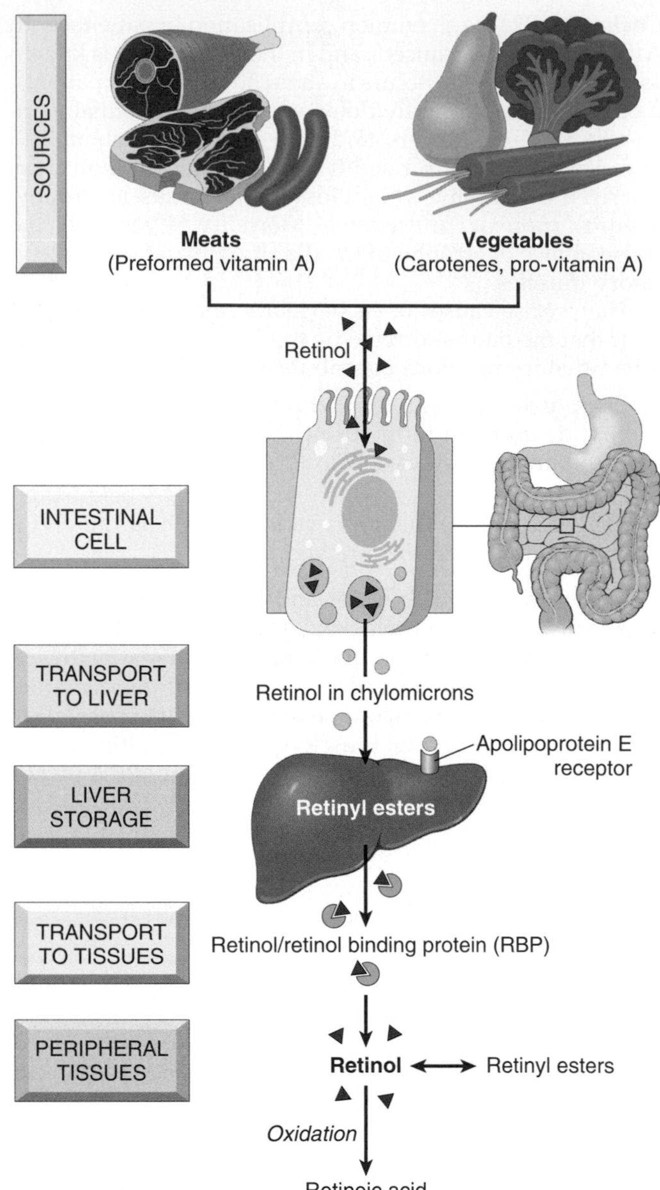

Figure 9-24 Vitamin A metabolism.

Function. In humans, the main functions of vitamin A are the following:

- *Maintenance of normal vision.* The visual process involves four forms of vitamin A–containing pigments: rhodopsin in the rods, the most light-sensitive pigment and therefore important in reduced light, and three iodopsins in cone cells, each responsive to specific colors in bright light. The synthesis of rhodopsin from retinol involves (1) oxidation to all-*trans*-retinal, (2) isomerization to 11-*cis*-retinal, and (3) covalent association with the 7-transmembrane rod protein opsin to form rhodopsin. A photon of light causes the isomerization of 11-*cis*-retinal to all-*trans*-retinal, which dissociates from rhodopsin. This induces a conformational change in opsin, triggering a series of downstream events that generate a nerve impulse, which is transmitted via neurons from the retina to the brain. During dark adaptation, some of the all-*trans*-retinal is reconverted to

11-*cis*-retinal, but most is reduced to retinol and lost to the retina, dictating the need for continuous supply.

- *Cell growth and differentiation.* Vitamin A and retinoids play an important role in the orderly differentiation of mucus-secreting epithelium; when a deficiency state exists, the epithelium undergoes *squamous metaplasia,* differentiating into a keratinizing epithelium. Activation of retinoic acid receptors (RARs) by their ligands causes the release of corepressors and the obligatory formation of heterodimers with another retinoid receptor, known as the *retinoic X receptor* (RXR). Both RAR and RXR have three isoforms, α, β, and γ. The RAR/RXR heterodimers bind to retinoic acid response elements located in the regulatory regions of genes that encode receptors for growth factors, tumor suppressor genes, and secreted proteins. Through these effects, retinoids regulate cell growth and differentiation, cell cycle control, and other biologic responses. *All-trans-retinoic acid*, a potent acid derivative of vitamin A, has the highest affinity for RARs compared with other retinoids.
- *Metabolic effects of retinoids.* The retinoic X receptor (RXR), believed to be activated by 9-*cis* retinoic acid, can form heterodimers with other nuclear receptors, such as (as we have seen) nuclear receptors involved in drug metabolism, the peroxisome proliferator-activated receptors (PPARs), and vitamin D receptors. PPARs are key regulators of fatty acid metabolism, including fatty acid oxidation in fat tissue and muscle, adipogenesis, and lipoprotein metabolism. The association between RXR and PPARγ provides an explanation for the metabolic effects of retinoids on adipogenesis.
- *Host resistance to infections.* Vitamin A supplementation can reduce morbidity and mortality from some forms of diarrhea, and in preschool children with measles, supplementation can improve the clinical outcome. The beneficial effect of vitamin A in diarrheal diseases may be related to the maintenance and restoration of the integrity of the epithelium of the gut. The effects of vitamin A on infections also derive in part from its ability to stimulate the immune system, although the mechanisms are not entirely clear. Infections may reduce the bioavailability of vitamin A by inhibiting retinol binding protein synthesis in the liver through the acute-phase response associated with many infections. The drop in hepatic retinol binding protein causes a decrease in circulating retinol, which reduces the tissue availability of vitamin A.

In addition, retinoids, β-carotene, and some related carotenoids function as photoprotective and antioxidant agents.

Retinoids are used clinically for the treatment of skin disorders such as severe acne and certain forms of psoriasis, and also in the treatment of acute promyelocytic leukemia. As discussed in Chapter 7, all-*trans*-retinoic acid induces the differentiation and subsequent apoptosis of acute promyelocytic leukemia cells through its ability to bind to a PML-RARα fusion protein that characterizes this form of cancer. A different isomer, 13-*cis* retinoic acid, has been used with some success in the treatment of childhood neuroblastoma.

Vitamin A Deficiency. Vitamin A deficiency occurs worldwide either as a consequence of general undernutrition or as a secondary deficiency in individuals with conditions that cause malabsorption of fats. In children, stores of vitamin A are depleted by infections, and the absorption of the vitamin is poor in newborn infants. Adult patients with malabsorption syndromes, such as celiac disease, Crohn disease, and colitis, may develop vitamin A deficiency, in conjunction with depletion of other fat-soluble vitamins. Bariatric surgery and, in older persons, continuous use of mineral oil as a laxative may lead to deficiency. The pathologic effects of vitamin A deficiency are summarized in Figure 9-25.

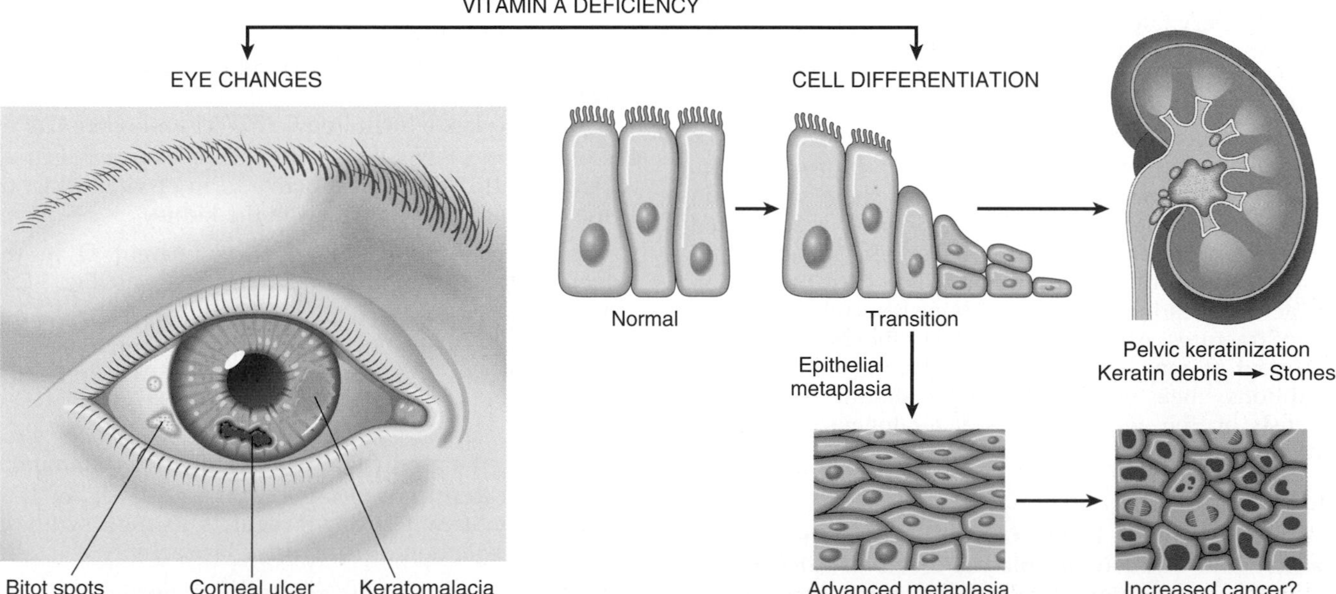

Figure 9-25 Vitamin A deficiency, its major consequences in the eye and in the production of keratinizing metaplasia of specialized epithelial surfaces, and its possible role in epithelial metaplasia. Not depicted are night blindness and immune deficiency.

As already discussed, vitamin A is a component of rhodopsin and other visual pigments. Not surprisingly, one of the earliest manifestations of vitamin A deficiency is impaired vision, particularly in reduced light *(night blindness)*. Other effects of deficiency are related to the role of vitamin A in maintaining the differentiation of epithelial cells. Persistent deficiency gives rise to *epithelial metaplasia* and *keratinization*. The most devastating changes occur in the eyes and are referred to as *xerophthalmia* (dry eye). First, there is dryness of the conjunctiva (xerosis conjunctivae) as the normal lacrimal and mucus-secreting epithelium is replaced by keratinized epithelium. This is followed by a buildup of keratin debris in small opaque plaques *(Bitot spots)* that progresses to erosion of the roughened corneal surface, softening and destruction of the cornea *(keratomalacia)*, and blindness.

In addition to the ocular epithelium, the epithelium lining the upper respiratory passage and urinary tract also undergoes *squamous metaplasia*. Loss of the mucociliary epithelium of the airways predisposes to secondary pulmonary infections, and desquamation of keratin debris in the urinary tract predisposes to renal and urinary bladder stones. Hyperplasia and *hyperkeratinization of the epidermis* with plugging of the ducts of the adnexal glands may produce follicular or papular dermatosis. Another very serious consequence is immune deficiency, which is responsible for higher mortality rates from common infections such as measles, pneumonia, and infectious diarrhea. In parts of the world where deficiency of vitamin A is prevalent, dietary supplements reduce mortality by 20% to 30%.

Vitamin A Toxicity. Both short- and long-term excesses of vitamin A may produce toxic manifestations, a point of concern because of the megadoses touted by certain sellers of supplements. The consequences of acute hypervitaminosis A were first described by Gerrit de Veer in 1597, a ship's carpenter stranded in the Arctic, who recounted in his diary the serious symptoms that he and other members of the crew developed after eating polar bear liver. With this cautionary tale in mind, the adventurous eater should be aware that acute vitamin A toxicity has also been described in individuals who ingested the livers of whales, sharks, and even tuna.

The symptoms of acute vitamin A toxicity include headache, dizziness, vomiting, stupor, and blurred vision, symptoms that may be confused with those of a brain tumor (*pseudotumor cerebri*). Chronic toxicity is associated with weight loss, anorexia, nausea, vomiting, and bone and joint pain. Retinoic acid stimulates osteoclast production and activity, leading to increased bone resorption and high risk of fractures. Although synthetic retinoids used for the treatment of acne are not associated with these types of conditions, their use in pregnancy should be avoided because of the well-established teratogenic effects of retinoids.

Vitamin D

The major function of the fat-soluble vitamin D is the maintenance of adequate plasma levels of calcium and phosphorus to support metabolic functions, bone mineralization, and neuromuscular transmission. Vitamin D is required for the prevention of bone diseases known as *rickets* (in children whose epiphyses have not already closed), *osteomalacia* (in adults), and *hypocalcemic tetany*. This latter condition is a convulsive state caused by an insufficient extracellular concentration of ionized calcium, which is required for normal neural excitation and the relaxation of muscles. Rickets was nearly endemic in large European cities and poor areas of New York and Boston at the end of the nineteenth century. Although cod liver oil was recognized for its anti-rachitic properties in the early part of that century, it took almost 100 years for it to be accepted by the medical profession as an effective preventive agent (it did not help that cod liver oil consumed in fishing villages in Northern Europe, Scandinavia, and Iceland was a dark, foul-smelling liquid). In addition to its effects on calcium and phosphorus homeostasis, vitamin D has effects in nonskeletal tissues.

Metabolism of Vitamin D. **The major source of vitamin D for humans is its endogenous synthesis from a precursor, 7-dehydrocholesterol, in a photochemical reaction that requires solar or artificial UV light in the range of 290 to 315 nm (UVB radiation).** This reaction results in the synthesis of *cholecalciferol*, known as *vitamin D_3*. Herein, the term *vitamin D* is used to refer to this compound. Under usual conditions of sun exposure, about 90% of the required vitamin D is endogenously synthesized the skin. However, individuals with dark skin generally have a lower level of vitamin D production because of melanin pigmentation. Dietary sources, such as deep-sea fish, plants, and grains, contribute the remaining required vitamin D and depend on adequate intestinal fat absorption. In plants, vitamin D is present in a precursor form (ergosterol), which is converted to vitamin D in the body.

The main steps of vitamin D metabolism are summarized as follows):

1. Photochemical synthesis of vitamin D from 7-dehydrocholesterol in the skin and absorption of vitamin D from foods and supplements in the gut
2. Binding of vitamin D from both of these sources to plasma α_1-globulin *(D-binding protein or DBP)* and transport into the liver
3. Conversion of vitamin D into 25-hydroxycholecalciferol (25-OH-D) in the liver, through the action of 25-hydroxylases, including CYP27A1 and other CYPs
4. Conversion of 25-OH-D into *1,25-dihydroxyvitamin D*, [1α,25$(OH)_2D_3$], the most active form of vitamin D, by the enzyme 1α-hydroxylase in the kidney

The production of 1,25-dihydroxyvitamin D in the kidney is regulated by three main mechanisms (Fig. 9-26):

- *Hypocalcemia stimulates secretion of parathyroid hormone (PTH),* which in turn augments the conversion of 25-OH-D into 1,25-dihydroxyvitamin D by activating 1α-hydroxylase
- *Hypophosphatemia directly activates 1α-hydroxylase,* increasing the production of 1,25-dihydroxyvitamin D
- *Through a feedback mechanism,* increased levels of 1,25-dihydroxyvitamin D down-regulate its own synthesis through inhibition of 1α-hydroxylase activity

Functions. Like retinoids and steroid hormones, 1,25-dihydroxyvitamin D acts by binding to a high-affinity nuclear receptor (*vitamin D receptor)*, which associates with

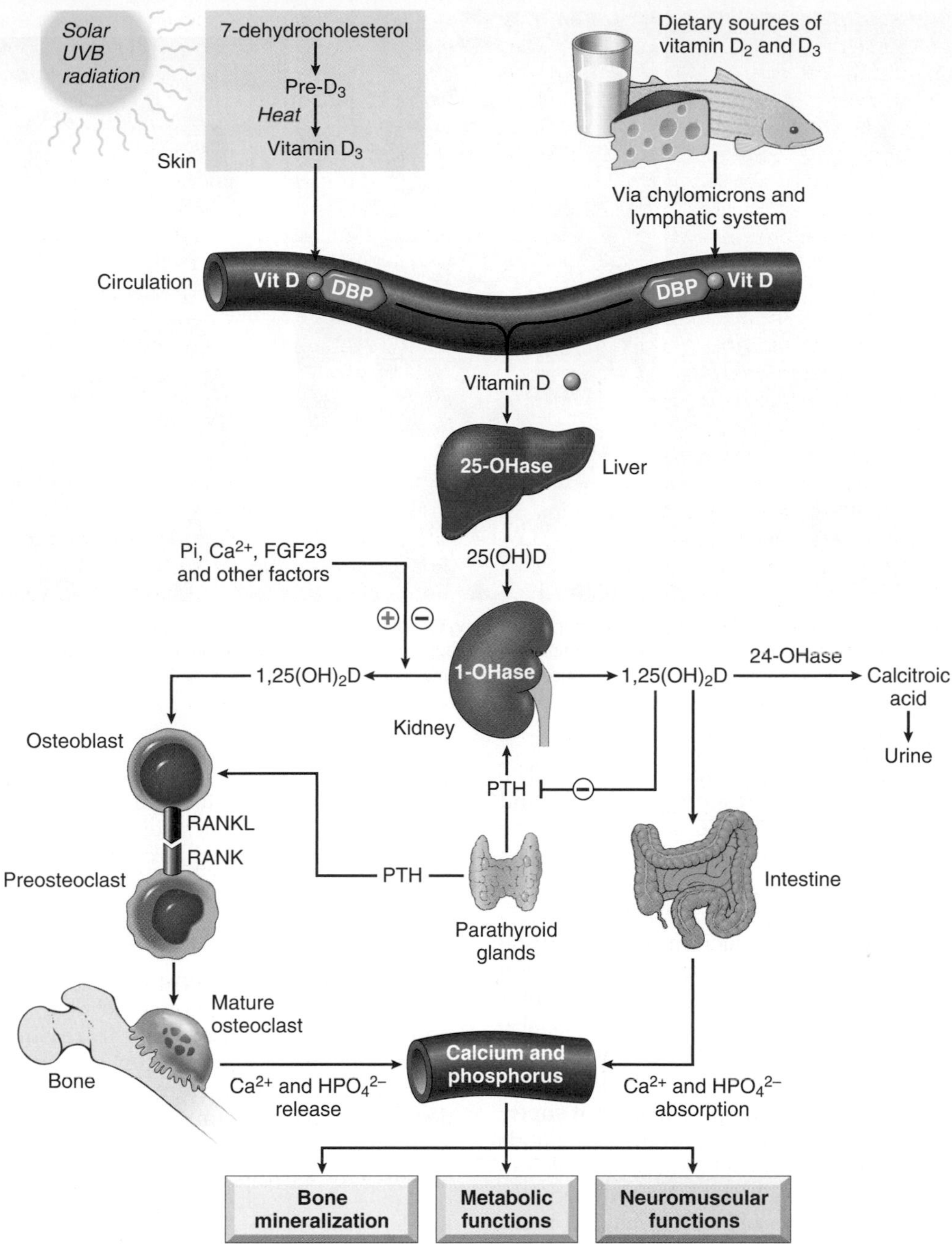

Figure 9-26 Vitamin D metabolism. Vitamin D is produced from 7-dehydrocholesterol in the skin or is ingested in the diet. It is converted in the liver into 25(OH) D, and in kidney into 1,25(OH)$_2$D (1,25-dihydroxyvitamin D), the active form of the vitamin. 1,25(OH)$_2$D stimulates the expression of RANKL, an important regulator of osteoclast maturation and function, on osteoblasts, and enhances the intestinal absorption of calcium and phosphorus in the intestine. DBP, Vitamin D–binding protein (α_1-globulin); FGF23, fibroblast growth factor 23.

the already mentioned RXR. This heterodimeric complex binds to vitamin D response elements located in the regulatory sequences of vitamin D target genes. The receptors for 1,25-dihydroxyvitamin D are present in most cells of the body. In the small intestine, bones, and kidneys, signals transduced via these receptors regulate plasma levels of calcium and phosphorus. Beyond its role on skeletal homeostasis, vitamin D has immunomodulatory and antiproliferative effects. 1,25-dihydroxyvitamin D also appears to act through mechanisms that do not require the transcription of target genes. These alternative mechanisms involve the binding of 1,25-dihydroxyvitamin D to a membrane-associated vitamin D receptor (mVDR), leading to the activation of protein kinase C and opening of calcium channels.

Effects of Vitamin D on Calcium and Phosphorus Homeostasis. The main functions of 1,25-dihydroxyvitamin D on calcium and phosphorus homeostasis are the following:

- *Stimulation of intestinal calcium absorption.* 1,25-dihydroxyvitamin D stimulates intestinal absorption of calcium in the duodenum through the interaction of 1,25-dihydroxyvitamin D with nuclear vitamin D

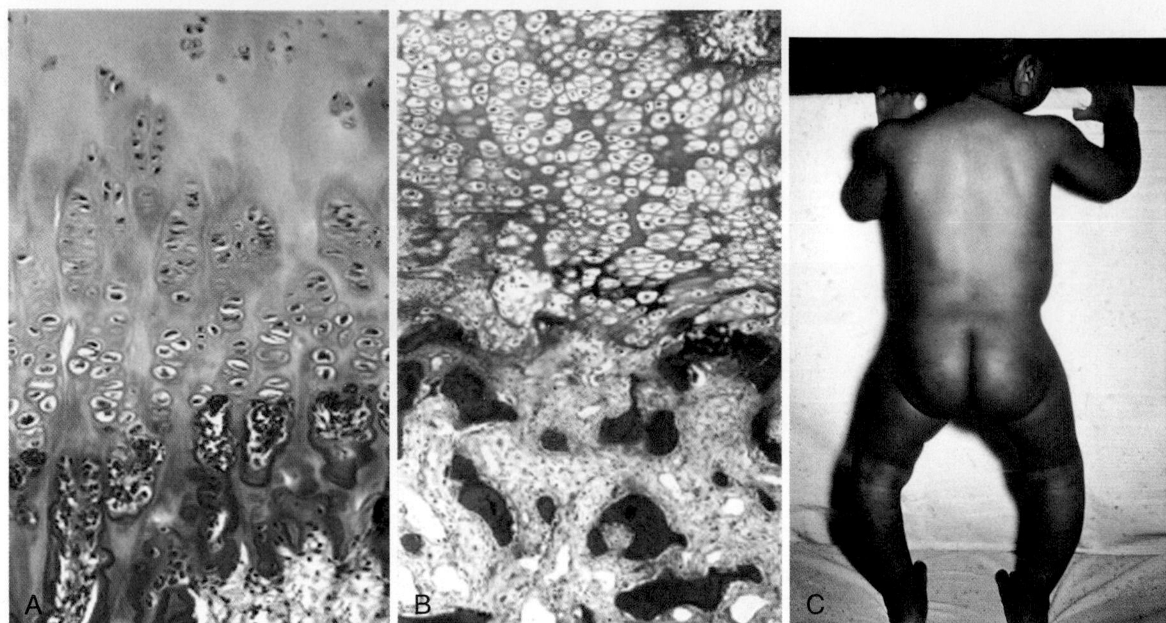

Figure 9-27 Rickets. **A,** Normal costochondral junction of a young child illustrating formation of cartilage palisades and orderly transition from cartilage to new bone. **B,** Detail of a rachitic costochondral junction in which the palisades of cartilage is lost. Darker trabeculae are well-formed bone; paler trabeculae consist of uncalcified osteoid. **C,** Rickets: note bowing of legs due to formation of poorly mineralized bones. (**B,** Courtesy Dr. Andrew E. Rosenberg, Massachusetts General Hospital, Boston, Mass.)

receptor and the formation of a complex with RXR. The complex binds to vitamin D response elements and activates the transcription of TRPV6 (a member of the transient receptor potential vanilloid family), which encodes a critical calcium transport channel.

- *Stimulation of calcium reabsorption in the kidney.* 1,25-dihydroxyvitamin D increases calcium influx in distal tubules of the kidney through the increased expression of TRPV5, another member of the transient receptor potential vanilloid family. TRPV5 expression is also regulated by PTH in response to hypocalcemia.
- *Interaction with PTH in the regulation of blood calcium.* Vitamin D maintains calcium and phosphorus at supersaturated levels in the plasma. The parathyroid glands have a key role in the regulation of extracellular calcium concentrations. These glands have a calcium receptor that senses even small changes in blood calcium concentrations. In addition to their effects on calcium absorption in the intestine and kidneys already described, both 1,25-dihydroxyvitamin D and PTH enhance the expression of RANKL (receptor activator of NF-κB ligand) on osteoblasts. RANKL binds to its receptor (RANK) located in preosteoclasts, thereby inducing the differentiation of these cells into mature osteoclasts (Chapter 26). Through the secretion of hydrochloric acid and activation of proteases such as cathepsin K, osteoclasts dissolve bone and release calcium and phosphorus into the circulation.
- *Mineralization of bone.* Vitamin D contributes to the mineralization of osteoid matrix and epiphyseal cartilage in both flat and long bones. It stimulates osteoblasts to synthesize the calcium-binding protein osteocalcin, involved in the deposition of calcium during bone development. Flat bones develop by intramembranous bone formation, in which mesenchymal cells differentiate directly into osteoblasts, which synthesize the collagenous osteoid matrix on which calcium is deposited. Long bones develop by endochondral ossification, through which growing cartilage at the epiphyseal plates is provisionally mineralized and then progressively resorbed and replaced by osteoid matrix that is mineralized to create bone (Fig. 9-27*A*).

When *hypocalcemia* occurs due to vitamin D deficiency (Fig. 9-28), PTH production is elevated, causing: (1) activation of renal 1α-hydroxylase, increasing the amount of active vitamin D and calcium absorption; (2) increased resorption of calcium from bone by osteoclasts; (3) decreased renal calcium excretion; and (4) increased renal excretion of phosphate. The latter is explained by increased synthesis in bone of fibroblast growth factor 23 (FGF-23), one of a group of agents known as *phosphatonins* that block phosphate absorption in the intestine and phosphate reabsorption in the kidney. Although a normal serum level of calcium may be restored, hypophosphatemia persists, impairing the mineralization of bone. Increased production of FGF-23 may be responsible for tumor-induced osteomalacia and some forms of hypophosphatemic rickets.

Deficiency States. The normal reference range for circulating 25-(OH)-D is 20 to 100 ng/mL; concentrations of less than 20 ng/mL constitute vitamin D deficiency.

Rickets in growing children and osteomalacia in adults are skeletal diseases with worldwide distributions. They may result from diets deficient in calcium and vitamin D, but an equally important cause of vitamin D deficiency is limited exposure to sunlight. This most often affects inhabitants of northern latitudes, but can even be a problem in tropical countries, in heavily veiled women, and in children born to mothers who have frequent pregnancies

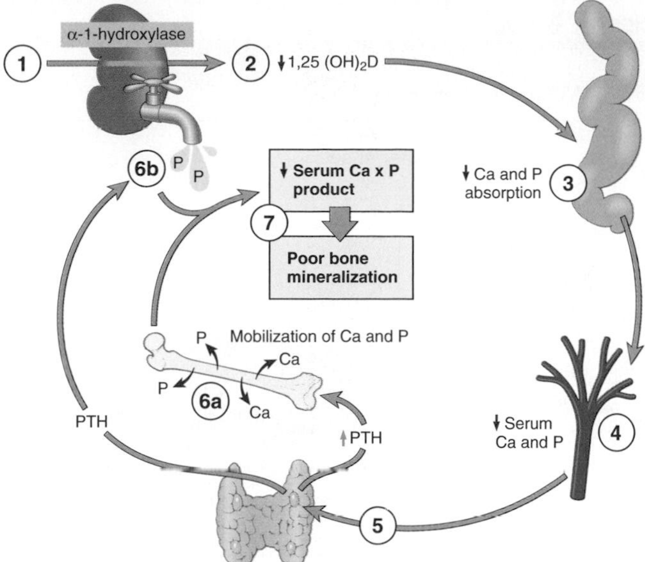

Figure 9-28 Vitamin D deficiency. There is inadequate substrate for the renal 1α-hydroxylase (1), yielding a deficiency of $1,25(OH)_2D$ (2), and deficient absorption of calcium and phosphorus from the gut (3), with consequently depressed serum levels of both (4). The hypocalcemia activates the parathyroid glands (5), causing mobilization of calcium and phosphorus from bone (6a). Simultaneously, the parathyroid hormone (PTH) induces wasting of phosphate in the urine (6b) and calcium retention. As a result, the serum levels of calcium are normal or nearly normal, but phosphate levels are low; hence, mineralization is impaired (7).

followed by lactation. In all of these situations, vitamin D deficiency can be prevented by a diet high in fish oils. Other, less common causes of rickets and osteomalacia include renal disorders causing decreased synthesis of 1,25-dihydroxyvitamin D, phosphate depletion, malabsorption disorders, and some rare inherited disorders. Although rickets and osteomalacia rarely occur outside high-risk groups, milder forms of vitamin D deficiency (also called *vitamin D insufficiency*), leading to an increased risk of bone loss and hip fractures, are quite common in older adults in the United States and Europe. Some genetically determined variants of the vitamin D receptors are also associated with an accelerated loss of bone minerals with aging and certain familial forms of osteoporosis (Chapter 26).

MORPHOLOGY

Vitamin D deficiency in both rickets and osteomalacia results in an **excess of unmineralized matrix**. The following sequence ensues in rickets:

- Overgrowth of epiphyseal cartilage due to inadequate provisional calcification and failure of the cartilage cells to mature and disintegrate
- Persistence of distorted, irregular masses of cartilage, which project into the marrow cavity
- Deposition of osteoid matrix on inadequately mineralized cartilaginous remnants
- Disruption of the orderly replacement of cartilage by osteoid matrix, with enlargement and lateral expansion of the osteochondral junction (Fig. 9-27*B*)
- Abnormal overgrowth of capillaries and fibroblasts in the disorganized zone resulting from microfractures and stresses on the inadequately mineralized, weak, poorly formed bone
- Deformation of the skeleton due to the loss of structural rigidity of the developing bones

The gross skeletal changes in rickets depend on the severity and duration of the process and, in particular, the stresses to which individual bones are subjected. During the nonambulatory stage of infancy, the head and chest sustain the greatest stresses. The softened occipital bones may become flattened, and the parietal bones can be buckled inward by pressure; with the release of the pressure, elastic recoil snaps the bones back into their original positions **(craniotabes)**. An excess of osteoid produces **frontal bossing** and a **squared appearance to the head**. Deformation of the chest results from overgrowth of cartilage or osteoid tissue at the costochondral junction, producing the **"rachitic rosary."** The weakened metaphyseal areas of the ribs are subject to the pull of the respiratory muscles and thus bend inward, creating anterior protrusion of the sternum **(pigeon breast deformity)**. When an ambulating child develops rickets, deformities are likely to affect the spine, pelvis, and tibia, causing **lumbar lordosis** and **bowing of the legs** (Fig. 9-27*C*).

In adults with **osteomalacia**, the lack of vitamin D deranges the normal bone remodeling that occurs throughout life. The newly formed osteoid matrix laid down by osteoblasts is inadequately mineralized, thus producing the excess of persistent osteoid that is characteristic of osteomalacia. Although the contours of the bone are not affected, the bone is weak and vulnerable to gross fractures or microfractures, which are most likely to affect vertebral bodies and femoral necks. The unmineralized osteoid appears as a thickened layer of matrix (which stains pink in hematoxylin and eosin preparations) arranged about the more basophilic, normally mineralized trabeculae.

Nonskeletal Effects of Vitamin D. As mentioned earlier, the vitamin D receptor is present in various cells and tissues that do not participate in calcium and phosphorus homeostasis. In addition, macrophages, keratinocytes, and tissues such as breast, prostate, and colon can produce 1,25-dihydroxyvitamin D. Within macrophages, synthesis of 1,25-dihydroxyvitamin D occurs through the activity of CYP27B located in the mitochondria. It appears that pathogen-induced activation of Toll-like receptors in macrophages causes increased expression of vitamin D receptor and CYP27B, leading to local synthesis of 1,25-dihydroxyvitamin D and activation of vitamin-D-dependent gene expression in macrophages and other neighboring immune cells. The net effect of this altered gene expression on the immune response remains to be determined. One recent clinical trial in patients with tuberculosis showed that vitamin D supplements increased lymphocyte counts, altered circulating levels of multiple cytokines and chemokines, and enhanced clearance of *Mycobacterium tuberculosis* from sputum, suggesting the vitamin D has complex effects that may, on the whole, be beneficial in this setting. Other regulatory effects of vitamin D in the innate and adaptive immune system have been reported, but the data are often contradictory. It has also been reported that low levels of 1,25-dihydroxyvitamin D (<20 ng/mL) are associated with a 30% to 50% increase in

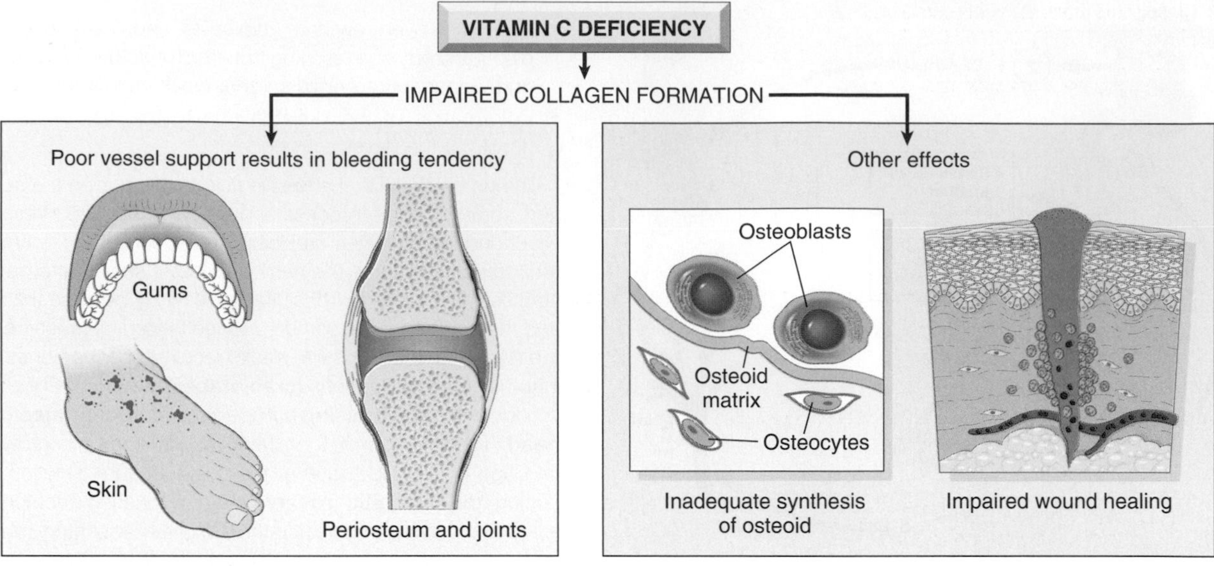

Figure 9-29 Major consequences of vitamin C deficiency caused by impaired formation of collagen.

the incidence of colon, prostate, and breast cancers, but whether vitamin D supplementation can reduce cancer risk has not been firmly established.

Vitamin D Toxicity. Prolonged exposure to normal sunlight does not produce an excess of vitamin D, but megadoses of orally administered vitamin can lead to hypervitaminosis. In children, hypervitaminosis D may take the form of metastatic calcifications of soft tissues such as the kidney; in adults it causes bone pain and hypercalcemia. The toxic potential of this vitamin is so great that in sufficiently large doses it is a potent rodenticide.

Vitamin C (Ascorbic Acid)

A deficiency of water-soluble vitamin C leads to the development of *scurvy*, characterized principally by bone

Table 9-9 Vitamins: Major Functions and Deficiency Syndromes

Vitamin	Functions	Deficiency Syndromes
Fat-soluble		
Vitamin A	A component of visual pigment Maintenance of specialized epithelia Maintenance of resistance to infection	Night blindness, xerophthalmia, blindness Squamous metaplasia Vulnerability to infection, particularly measles
Vitamin D	Facilitates intestinal absorption of calcium and phosphorus and mineralization of bone	Rickets in children Osteomalacia in adults
Vitamin E	Major antioxidant; scavenges free radicals	Spinocerebellar degeneration
Vitamin K	Cofactor in hepatic carboxylation of procoagulants—factors II (prothrombin), VII, IX, and X; and protein C and protein S	Bleeding diathesis (Chapter 14)
Water-soluble		
Vitamin B_1 (thiamine)	As pyrophosphate, is coenzyme in decarboxylation reactions	Dry and wet beriberi, Wernicke syndrome, Korsakoff syndrome (Chapter 28)
Vitamin B_2 (riboflavin)	Converted to coenzymes flavin mononucleotide and flavin adenine dinucleotide, cofactors for many enzymes in intermediary metabolism	Ariboflavinosis, cheilosis, stomatitis, glossitis, dermatitis, corneal vascularization
Niacin	Incorporated into nicotinamide adenine dinucleotide (NAD) and NAD phosphate, involved in a variety of redox reactions	Pellagra—"three Ds": dementia, dermatitis, diarrhea
Vitamin B_6 (pyridoxine)	Derivatives serve as coenzymes in many intermediary reactions	Cheilosis, glossitis, dermatitis, peripheral neuropathy (Chapter 28) Maintenance of myelinization of spinal cord tracts
Vitamin B_{12}	Required for normal folate metabolism and DNA synthesis	Megaloblastic pernicious anemia and degeneration of posterolateral spinal cord tracts (Chapter 14)
Vitamin C	Serves in many oxidation-reduction (redox) reactions and hydroxylation of collagen	Scurvy
Folate	Essential for transfer and use of one-carbon units in DNA synthesis	Megaloblastic anemia, neural tube defects (Chapter 14)
Pantothenic acid	Incorporated in coenzyme A	No nonexperimental syndrome recognized
Biotin	Cofactor in carboxylation reactions	No clearly defined clinical syndrome

Table 9-10 Selected Trace Elements and Deficiency Syndromes

Element	Function	Basis of Deficiency	Clinical Features
Zinc	Component of enzymes, principally oxidases	Inadequate supplementation in artificial diets Interference with absorption by other dietary constituents Inborn error of metabolism	Rash around eyes, mouth, nose, and anus called acrodermatitis enteropathica Anorexia and diarrhea Growth retardation in children Depressed mental function Depressed wound healing and immune response Impaired night vision Infertility
Iron	Essential component of hemoglobin as well as several iron-containing metalloenzymes	Inadequate diet Chronic blood loss	Hypochromic microcytic anemia (Chapter 14)
Iodine	Component of thyroid hormone	Inadequate supply in food and water	Goiter and hypothyroidism (Chapter 24)
Copper	Component of cytochrome *c* oxidase, dopamine β-hydroxylase, tyrosinase, lysyl oxidase, and unknown enzymes involved in cross-linking collagen	Inadequate supplementation in artificial diet Interference with absorption	Muscle weakness Neurologic defects Abnormal collagen cross-linking
Fluoride	Mechanism unknown	Inadequate supply in soil and water Inadequate supplementation	Dental caries (Chapter 16)
Selenium	Component of glutathione peroxidase Antioxidant with vitamin E	Inadequate amounts in soil and water	Myopathy Cardiomyopathy (Keshan disease)

disease in growing children and by hemorrhages and healing defects in both children and adults. Sailors of the British Royal Navy were nicknamed "limeys," because at the end of the eighteenth century the Navy began to provide lime and lemon juice (rich sources of vitamin C) to sailors to prevent scurvy during their long sojourn at sea. It was not until 1932 that ascorbic acid was identified and synthesized. Ascorbic acid is not synthesized endogenously in humans; therefore, we are entirely dependent on the diet for this nutrient. Vitamin C is present in milk and some animal products (liver, fish) and is abundant in a variety of fruits and vegetables. All but the most restricted diets provide adequate amounts of vitamin C.

Function. Ascorbic acid functions in a variety of biosynthetic pathways by accelerating hydroxylation and amidation reactions. The best established function of vitamin C is the *activation of prolyl and lysyl hydroxylases* from inactive precursors, providing for *hydroxylation of procollagen.* Inadequately hydroxylated procollagen cannot acquire a stable helical configuration, so it is poorly secreted from the fibroblast. Those molecules that are secreted are adequately cross-linked, lack tensile strength, and are more soluble and vulnerable to enzymatic degradation. Collagen, which normally has the highest content of hydroxyproline of any polypeptide, is most affected, particularly in blood vessels, accounting for the predisposition to hemorrhages in scurvy. In addition, a deficiency of vitamin C suppresses the rate of synthesis of procollagen, independent of effects on proline hydroxylation.

Vitamin C also has *antioxidant properties.* Vitamin C can scavenge free radicals directly and can act indirectly by regenerating the antioxidant form of vitamin E.

Deficiency States. Consequences of vitamin C deficiency (scurvy) are illustrated in Figure 9-29. Because of the abundance of ascorbic acid in many foods, scurvy has ceased to be a global problem. It is sometimes encountered even in affluent populations as a secondary deficiency, particularly among older individuals, persons who live alone, and chronic alcoholics, groups that often have erratic and inadequate eating patterns. Occasionally, scurvy occurs in patients undergoing peritoneal dialysis and hemodialysis and among food faddists. The condition also sometimes appears in infants who are maintained on formulas of evaporated milk without supplementation of vitamin C.

Vitamin C Excess. The popular notion that megadoses of vitamin C protect against the common cold, or at least allay the symptoms, has not been borne out by controlled clinical studies. Such slight relief as may be experienced is probably due to the mild antihistamine action of ascorbic acid. Similarly, there is no evidence that large doses of vitamin C protect against cancer development. The physiologic availability of excess vitamin C is limited due to its inherent instability, poor intestinal absorption, and rapid urinary excretion. Fortunately, toxicities related to high doses of vitamin C are rare, consisting of possible iron overload (due to increase absorption), hemolytic anemia in those with glucose-6-phosphate dehydrogenase (G6PD) deficiency (Chapter 14), and calcium oxalate kidney stones.

Other vitamins and some essential minerals are listed and briefly described in Tables 9-9 and 9-10 and are discussed in other chapters.

KEY CONCEPTS

Nutritional Diseases

- Primary PEM is a common cause of childhood deaths in poor countries. The two main primary PEM syndromes are marasmus and kwashiorkor. Secondary PEM occurs in the chronically ill and in patients with advanced cancer (as a result of cachexia).
- Kwashiorkor is characterized by hypoalbuminemia, generalized edema, fatty liver, skin changes, and defects in immunity. It is caused by diets low in protein but normal in calories.
- Marasmus is characterized by emaciation resulting from loss of muscle mass and fat with relative preservation of

serum albumin. It is caused by diets severely lacking in calories—both protein and nonprotein.
- Anorexia nervosa is self-induced starvation; it is characterized by amenorrhea and multiple manifestations of low thyroid hormone levels. Bulimia is a condition in which food binges alternate with induced vomiting.
- Vitamins A and D are fat-soluble vitamins with a wide range of activities. Vitamin A is required for vision, epithelial differentiation, and immune function. Vitamin D is a key regulator of calcium and phosphate homeostasis.
- Vitamin C and members of the vitamin B family are water-soluble. Vitamin C is needed for collagen synthesis and collagen cross-linking and tensile strength. B vitamins have diverse roles in cellular metabolism.

Obesity

Excess adiposity (obesity) and excess body weight are associated with increased incidence of several of the most important diseases of humans, including type 2 diabetes, dyslipidemias, cardiovascular disease, hypertension, and cancer. Obesity is defined as an accumulation of adipose tissue that is of sufficient magnitude to impair health. As with weight loss, excess weight is best assessed by *the body mass index,* or BMI. For practical reasons, *body weight*, which generally correlates well with BMI, is often used as a surrogate for BMI measurements. The normal BMI range is 18.5 to 25 kg/m^2, although the range may differ for different countries. Individuals with BMI greater than 30 kg/m^2 are classified as obese; those with BMI between 25 kg/m^2 and 30 kg/m^2 are considered overweight. Unless otherwise noted, the term *obesity* herein applies to both the truly obese and the overweight.

Not only the total body weight but also the distribution of the stored fat is of importance in obesity. *Central, or visceral, obesity,* in which fat accumulates in the trunk and in the abdominal cavity (in the mesentery and around viscera), is associated with a much higher risk for several diseases than is excess accumulation of fat diffusely in subcutaneous tissue.

Obesity is a major public health problem in developed countries and an emerging health problem in developing nations, such as India. Globally, the World Health Organization estimates that by 2015, 700 million adults will be obese. In certain countries, obesity coexists with malnutrition in individual families. In the United States obesity has reached epidemic proportions. The prevalence of obesity increased from 13% to 32% between 1960 and 2004, and by 2010, 35.7% of adult in the United States were obese, as were 16.9% of children. Indeed, in 2009, it was estimated that the health care cost of obesity and related diseases had risen to $147 billion annually in the United States, a price tag that appears bound to rise further as the nation's collective waistline expands. The increase in obesity in the United States has been associated with the higher caloric content of the diet, mostly caused by increased consumption of refined sugars, sweetened beverages, and vegetable oils.

At its simplest level, obesity is a disease of caloric imbalance that results from an excess intake of calories that exceeds their consumption by the body. However, the pathogenesis of obesity is complex and incompletely understood. Ongoing research has identified intricate humoral and neural mechanisms that control appetite and satiety. These neurohumoral mechanisms respond to genetic, nutritional, environmental, and psychologic signals, and trigger a metabolic response through the stimulation of centers located in the hypothalamus. There is little doubt that genetic influences play an important role in weight control, but obesity is a disease that depends on the interaction between multiple factors. After all, regardless of genetic makeup, obesity would not occur without intake of food.

In a simplified way the neurohumoral mechanisms that regulate energy balance can be subdivided into three components (Figs. 9-30 and 9-31):

- The *peripheral or afferent system* generates signals from various sites. Its main components are *leptin* and *adiponectin* produced by fat cells, *ghrelin* from the stomach, *peptide YY (PYY)* from the ileum and colon, and *insulin* from the pancreas.
- The *arcuate nucleus in the hypothalamus* processes and integrates neurohumoral peripheral signals and generates efferent signals. It contains two subsets of first-order neurons: (1) *POMC* (pro-opiomelanocortin) and *CART* (cocaine and amphetamine-regulated transcripts) neurons, and (2) neurons containing *NPY* (neuropeptide Y) and *AgRP* (agouti-related peptide). These first-order neurons communicate with second-order neurons in the hypothalmus.
- The *efferent system* is organized along two pathways, anabolic and catabolic, that control food intake and energy expenditure, respectively. The hypothalamic system also communicates with forebrain and midbrain centers that control the autonomic nervous system.
- POMC/CART neurons enhance energy expenditure and weight loss through the production of the anorexigenic α-melanocyte-stimulating hormone (MSH), and the activation of the melanocortin receptors 3 and 4 (MC3/4R) in second-order neurons. These second order neurons are in turn responsible for producing factors such as thyroid releasing hormone (TSH) and corticotropin releasing hormone (CRH) that increase the basal metabolic rate and anabolic metabolism, thus favoring weight loss. By contrast, the NPY/AgRP neurons promote food intake (orexigenic effect) and weight gain, through the activation of Y1/5 receptors in secondary neurons. These secondary neurons then release factors such as melanin-concentrating hormone (MCH) and orexin, which stimulate appetite.

Three important components of the afferent system, which regulates appetite and satiety, are leptin, adiponectin, and gut hormones.

Leptin. The name *leptin* is derived from the Greek term *leptos*, meaning "thin." Leptin, a 16-kD hormone synthesized by fat cells, is the product of the *ob* gene. The leptin receptor (OB-R) belongs to the type I cytokine receptor superfamily, which includes the gp130, granulocyte-colony-stimulating factor, IL-2, and IL-6 receptors. Mice genetically deficient in leptin (*ob/ob mice*) or leptin receptors (*db/db mice*) fail to sense the adequacy of fat stores, overeat, and gain weight, behaving as if they are undernourished. Thus, the obesity of these animals is a consequence of the

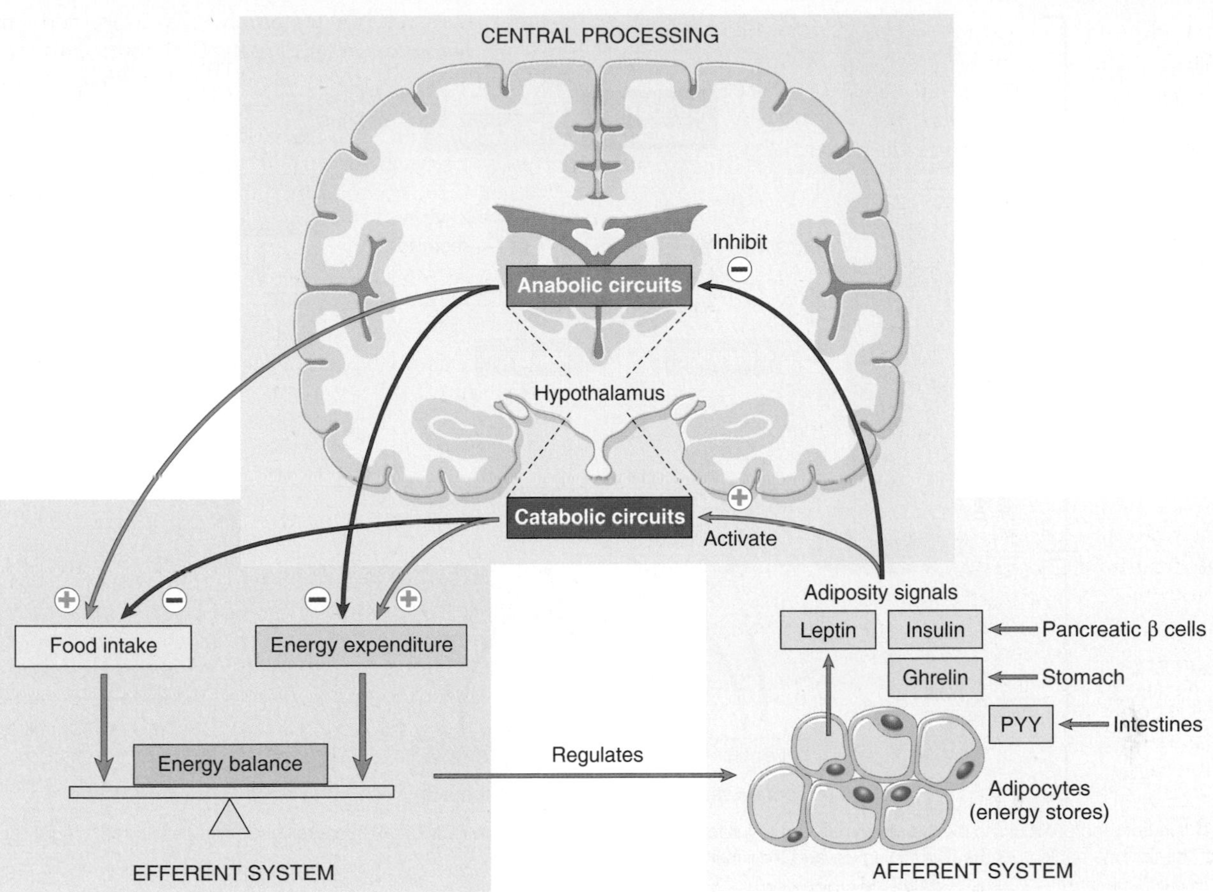

Figure 9-30 Regulation of energy balance. Adipose tissues generate afferent signals that influence the activity of the hypothalamus, which is the central regulator of appetite and satiety. These signals decrease food intake by inhibiting anabolic circuits, and enhance energy expenditure through the activation of catabolic circuits. PYY, Peptide YY. See text for details.

lack of the signal for energy sufficiency that is normally provided by leptin.

While the precise mechanisms that regulate the output of leptin from adipose tissue have not been completely defined, it has been established that leptin secretion is stimulated when fat stores are abundant. It is believed that insulin-stimulated glucose metabolism is an important factor in the regulation of leptin levels. Leptin levels are also regulated by multiple additional posttranscriptional mechanisms that affect its synthesis, secretion, and turnover. In the hypothalamus, leptin stimulates POMC/CART neurons that produce anorexigenic neuropeptides (primarily melanocyte-stimulating hormone) and inhibits NPY/AgRP neurons that produce feeding-inducing (orexigenic) neuropeptides (Figs. 9-30 and 9-31). In individuals with stable weight, the activities of the opposing POMC/CART and NPY/AgRP pathways are properly balanced. However, when there are inadequate stores of body fat, leptin secretion is diminished and food intake is increased.

Humans with loss-of-function mutations in the leptin system develop early-onset severe obesity, but this is a rare condition. Mutations of melanocortin receptor 4 (MC4R) and its downstream pathways are more frequent, being responsible for about 5% of massive obesity. In these individuals, sensing of satiety (anorexigenic signal) is not generated, and hence they behave as if they are undernourished. Haploinsufficiency of brain-derived neurotrophic factor (BDNF), an important component of signaling downstream of MC4R in the hypothalamus, is associated with obesity in patients with the WAGR syndrome (a very rare condition that includes Wilms tumor, aniridia, genitourinary defects, and mental retardation in addition to obesity, Chapter 10). Although the defects in leptin and MC4R detected so far are uncommon, they underscore the importance of these systems in the control of energy balance and body weight. Perhaps other genetic or acquired defects in these pathways may have pathogenic effects in more common forms of obesity. For instance, it has been proposed that leptin resistance is prevalent in humans; it has also been noted that obese children have lower circulating levels of BDNF.

Leptin regulates not only food intake but also energy expenditure, through a distinct set of pathways. Thus, an abundance of leptin stimulates physical activity, heat production, and energy expenditure. The neurohumoral mediators of leptin-induced energy expenditure are less well defined. *Thermogenesis*, an important catabolic effect mediated by leptin, is controlled in part by hypothalamic signals that increase the release of norepinephrine from sympathetic nerve endings in adipose tissue. In addition to these effects, leptin can function as a proinflammatory cytokine and participates in the regulation of hematopoiesis and lymphopoiesis. The OB-R receptor is similar structurally to the IL-6 receptor and activates the JAK/STAT pathway.

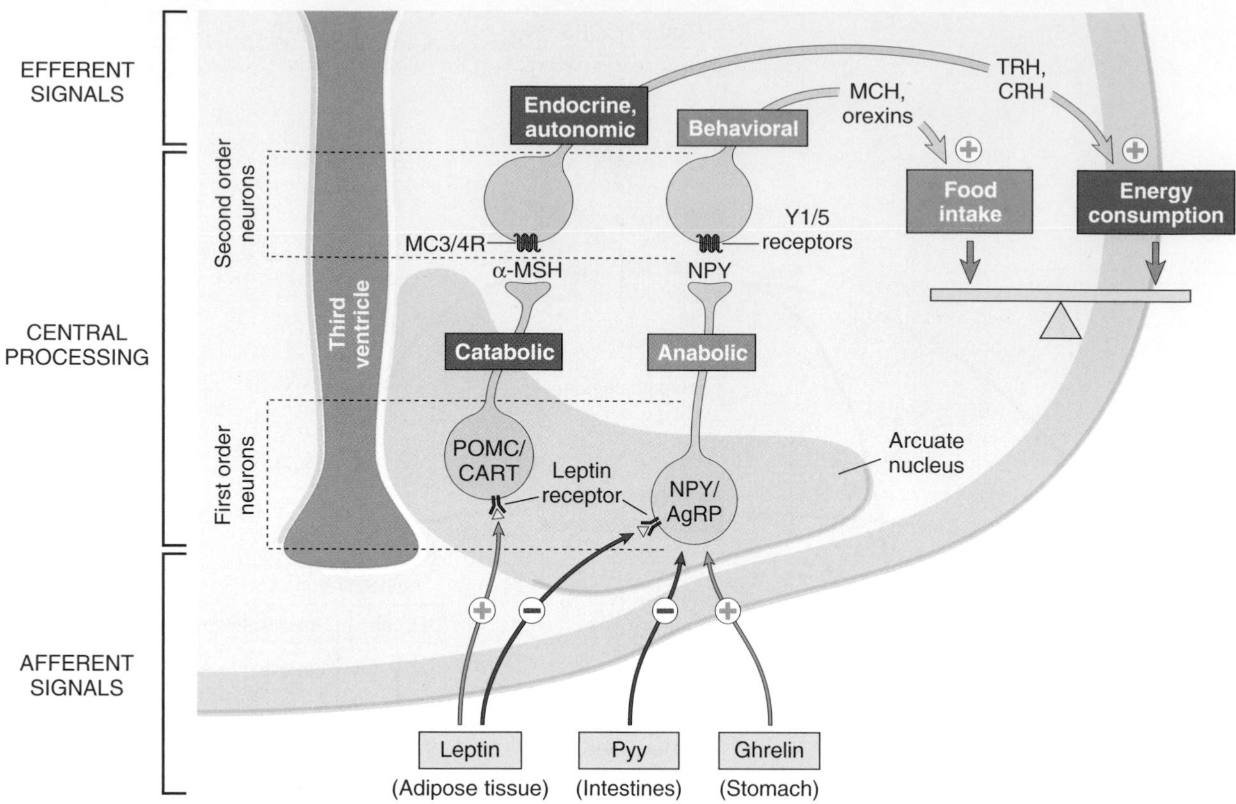

Figure 9-31 Neurohumoral circuits in the hypothalamus that regulate energy balance. Shown are POMC/CART anorexigenic neurons and NPY/AgRP orexigenic neurons in the arcuate nucleus of the hypothalamus, and their pathways. See text for details.

Adiponectin. Injections of adiponectin in mice stimulate fatty acid oxidation in muscle, causing a decrease in fat mass. This hormone is produced mainly by adipocytes. Its levels in the blood are very high, about 1000 times higher than those of other polypeptide hormones, and are lower in obese than in lean individuals. Adiponectin, which has been called a "fat-burning molecule" and the "guardian angel against obesity," directs fatty acids to muscle for their oxidation. It decreases the influx of fatty acids to the liver and the total hepatic triglyceride content, and also decreases the glucose production in the liver, causing an increase in insulin sensitivity and protecting against the metabolic syndrome (described later). Adiponectin circulates as a complex of three, six, or even more aggregates of the monomeric form, and binds to two receptors, AdipoR1 and AdipoR2. These receptors are found in many tissues, including the brain, but AdipoR1 and AdipoR2 are most highly expressed in skeletal muscle and liver, respectively. Binding of adiponectin to its receptors triggers signals that activate cAMP-dependent protein kinase (protein kinase A), which in turn phosphorylates and inactivates acetyl coenzyme A carboxylase, a key enzyme required for fatty acid synthesis.

Gut Hormones. Gut peptides act as short-term meal initiators and terminators. They include ghrelin, PYY, pancreatic polypeptide, insulin, and amylin among others. *Ghrelin* is produced in the stomach and in the arcuate nucleus of the hypothalamus. It is the only known gut hormone that increases food intake (orexigenic effect). Its injection in rodents elicits voracious feeding, even after repeated administration. Long-term injections cause weight gain, by increasing caloric intake and reducing energy utilization. Ghrelin acts by binding the growth hormone secretagogue receptor, which is abundant in the hypothalamus and the pituitary. Although the precise mechanisms of ghrelin action have not been identified, it most likely stimulates NPY/AgRP neurons to increase food intake. Ghrelin levels rise before meals and fall between 1 and 2 hours after eating. In obese individuals the postprandial suppression of ghrelin is attenuated and may contribute to overeating.

PYY is secreted from endocrine cells in the ileum and colon. Plasma levels of PYY are low during fasting and increase shortly after food intake. Intravenous administration of PYY reduces energy intake, and its levels generally increase after gastric bypass surgery. By contrast, levels of PYY generally decrease in individuals with the *Prader-Willi syndrome* (caused by loss of imprinted genes on chromosome 15q11-q13), a disorder marked by hyperphagia and obesity. These observations have led to ongoing work to produce PYYs for the treatment of obesity. *Amylin*, a peptide secreted with insulin from pancreatic β-cells that reduces food intake and weight gain, is also being evaluated for the treatment of obesity and diabetes. Both PYY and amylin act centrally by stimulating POMC/CART neurons in the hypothalamus, causing a decrease in food intake.

Actions of Adipocytes. In addition to leptin and adiponectin, adipose tissue produces cytokines such as TNF, IL-6, IL-1, and IL-18, chemokines, and steroid hormones. The

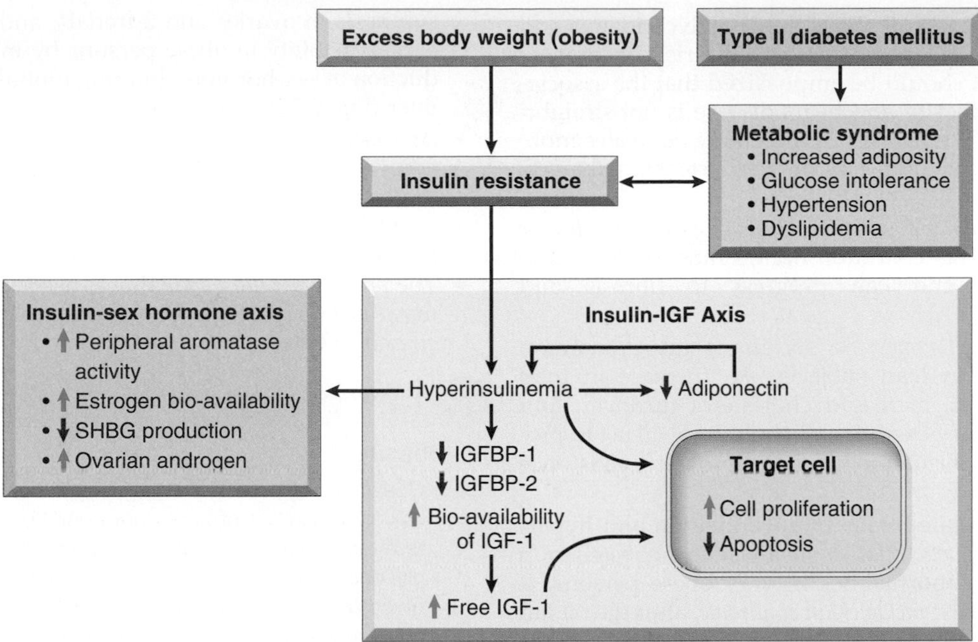

Figure 9-32 Obesity, metabolic syndrome, and cancer. Obesity and excessive weight are precursors of the metabolic syndrome, which is associated with insulin resistance, type 2 diabetes, and hormonal changes. Increases in insulin and IGF-1 (insulin-like growth factor-1) stimulate cell proliferation and inhibit apoptosis and may contribute to tumor development. IGF, Insulin-like growth factor; IGFBP, insulin-like growth factor-binding protein; SHBG, sex hormone-binding globulin. (Modified from Renehan AG, et al: Obesity and cancer risk: the role of the insulin-IGF axis. Trends Endocrinol Metab 17:328, 2006.)

increased production of cytokines and chemokines by adipose tissue in obese patients creates a chronic proinflammatory state marked by high levels of circulating C-reactive protein. This relationship may be more than a one-way street, as emerging evidence suggests that immune cells, particularly tissue macrophages, have important roles in regulating adipocyte function. Through this panoply of mediators, adipose tissue participates in the control of energy balance and energy metabolism, functioning as a link between lipid metabolism, nutrition, and inflammatory responses. Thus, the adipocyte, which was relegated to an obscure and passive role as the "Cinderella of cells of metabolism," is now "the Belle of the Ball" at the forefront of metabolic research.

Regulation of adipocyte numbers. The total number of adipocytes is established during childhood and adolescence (yet another reason to be concerned about childhood obesity), and is higher in obese than in lean individuals. In adults, it is estimated that approximately 10% of adipocytes are renewed annually, regardless of the level of the individual's body mass, but the number of adipocytes remains constant. Thus, adipocyte numbers are tightly controlled, and loss of fat mass in an adult person occurs through shrinkage of existing adipocytes. The well-known difficulty in maintaining weight losses from dieting is not well understood but appears to be related to homeostatic mechanisms that keep body fat constant over time. Thus, unless lowered caloric intake and/or increase energy expenditure is sustained, body weight inexorably returns to prediet levels. In a sense, therefore, the number of adipocytes create a set point for body weight.

Other emerging factors associated with obesity: role of the gut microbiome. A surprising and potentially important new explanation for the development of obesity has focused on alterations in the gut microbiome. Diet has marked effects on the bacterial makeup of the colon, and the bacterial flora in turn can have large effects on the ability of the host to break down certain dietary constituents (e.g., fiber) and absorb nutrients, as well as on epithelial integrity and inflammation. In response to these changes, expression of gut factors such as PYY that feedback on central appetite centers may also be altered. The data showing that gut flora can influence obesity are strong in certain mouse models, but the relevance of these models to human obesity, although tantalizing, remain to be proven.

General Consequences of Obesity

Obesity, particularly *central obesity,* increases the risk for a number of conditions, including type 2 diabetes and cardiovascular disease (Fig. 9-32). Obesity is the main driver of a cluster of alterations known as the *metabolic syndrome* characterized by visceral or intra-abdominal adiposity, insulin resistance, hyperinsulinemia, glucose intolerance, hypertension, hypertriglyceridemia, and low HDL cholesterol (Chapter 11).

- Obesity is associated with *insulin resistance* and *hyperinsulinemia,* important features of type 2 diabetes (Chapter 24), and weight loss is associated with improvements in these abnormalities. Excess insulin, in turn, may play a role in the retention of sodium, expansion of blood volume, production of excess norepinephrine, and smooth muscle proliferation that are the hallmarks of hypertension. Regardless of the nature of the pathogenic mechanisms, the risk of developing *hypertension* among previously normotensive persons increases proportionately with weight.

- Obese persons generally have hypertriglyceridemia and low HDL, both of which increase the risk of *coronary artery disease*. It should be emphasized that the association between obesity and heart disease is not straightforward, and such linkage as there may be relates more to the associated diabetes and hypertension than to weight.
- Obesity is associated with *nonalcoholic fatty liver disease* (Chapter 18). This condition occurs most often in diabetic patients and can progress to fibrosis and cirrhosis.
- *Cholelithiasis (gallstones)* is six times more common in obese than in lean subjects. An increase in total body cholesterol, increased cholesterol turnover, and augmented biliary excretion of cholesterol all act to predispose to the formation of cholesterol-rich gallstones (Chapter 18).
- Obesity is associated with hypoventilation and hypersomnolence. *Hypoventilation syndrome* is a constellation of respiratory abnormalities in very obese persons. It has been called the *pickwickian syndrome*, after the fat lad who was constantly falling asleep in Charles Dickens' Pickwick Papers. *Hypersomnolence*, both at night and during the day, is often associated with apneic pauses during sleep (sleep apnea), polycythemia, and eventual right-sided heart failure (*cor pulmonale*).
- Marked adiposity predisposes to the development of degenerative joint disease *(osteoarthritis)*. This form of arthritis, which typically appears in older persons, is attributed in large part to the cumulative effects of increased load on weight-bearing joints.

Obesity and Cancer

In 2007, the National Cancer Institute estimated that 4% of cancers in men and 7% of cancers in women were attributable to obesity, numbers that can be expected to rise as obesity increases. The clearest associations with increased risk were for cancers of the esophagus, pancreas, colon and rectum, breast, endometrium, kidney, thyroid, and gallbladder. The mechanisms by which obesity promotes cancer development are unknown, but several non-mutually exclusive possibilities have been proposed:

- *Elevated insulin levels*. Insulin resistance leads to hyperinsulinemia (Fig. 9-32), which has multiple effects that may directly or indirectly contribute to cancer. For example, hyperinsulinemia inhibits the production of the IGF-binding proteins IGFBP-1 and IGFBP-2, thereby causing a rise in levels of free insulin-like growth factor-1 (IGF-1). IGF-1 is a mitogen, and its receptor, IGFR-1, is highly expressed in many human cancers. It binds with high affinity to the IGFR-1 receptor, and with low affinity to the insulin receptor, which are also expressed on many cancers. Upon stimulation by IGF-1, IGFR-1 activates the RAS and PI3K/AKT pathways, which promote the growth of both normal and neoplastic cells (Chapter 7).
- Obesity has effects on *steroid hormones* that regulate cell growth and differentiation in the breast, uterus, and other tissues. Specifically, obesity increases the synthesis of estrogen from androgen precursors through an effect of adipose tissue aromatases, increases androgen synthesis in ovaries and adrenals, and enhances estrogen availability in obese persons by inhibiting the production of sex-hormone-binding globulin (SHBG) in the liver (Fig. 9-32).
- As discussed earlier, *adiponectin*, secreted mostly from adipose tissue, is an abundant hormone that is inversely correlated with obesity and acts as an insulin-sensitizing agent. Thus, the decreased levels of adiponectin in obese persons contribute to hyperinsulinemia.
- The *proinflammatory state* that is associated with obesity may itself be carcinogenic, through mechanisms discussed in Chapter 7.

KEY CONCEPTS

Obesity

- Obesity is a disorder of energy regulation. It increases the risk for a number of important conditions such as insulin resistance, type 2 diabetes, hypertension, and hypertriglyceridemia, which are associated with the development of coronary artery disease, as well as certain cancers, nonalcoholic fatty liver disease, and gallstones.
- The regulation of energy balance is complex. It has three main components: (1) afferent signals, provided mostly by insulin, leptin, ghrelin, and peptide YY; (2) the central hypothalamic system, which integrates afferent signals and triggers the efferent signals; and (3) efferent signals, which control energy balance.
- Leptin plays a key role in energy balance. Its output from adipose tissues is regulated by the abundance of fat stores. Leptin binding to its receptors in the hypothalamus increases energy consumption by stimulating POMC/CART neurons and inhibiting NPY/AgRP neurons.

Diet, Cancer, and Atherosclerosis

Diet and Cancer

As you will recall from Chapter 7, the incidence of specific cancers varies as much as 100-fold in different geographic areas. It is well known that differences in incidence of various cancers are not fixed and can be modified by environmental factors, including changes in diet. For instance, the incidence of colon cancer in Japanese men and women 55 to 60 years of age was negligible about 50 years ago, but it is now higher than that in men of the same age in the United Kingdom. Studies have also shown a progressive increase in colon cancers in Japanese populations as they moved from Japan to Hawaii and from there to the continental United States. Nevertheless, despite extensive experimental and epidemiologic research, relatively few mechanisms that link diets and specific types of cancer have been established.

With respect to carcinogenesis, three aspects of the diet are of major concern: (1) the content of exogenous carcinogens, (2) the endogenous synthesis of carcinogens from dietary components, and (3) the lack of protective factors.

- Regarding *exogenous* substances, *aflatoxin* is involved in the development of hepatocellular carcinomas in parts of Asia and Africa, generally in cooperation with hepatitis B virus. Exposure to aflatoxin causes a specific mutation in codon 249 of the *TP53* gene; when found in hepatocellular carcinomas, this mutation serves as a molecular signature for aflatoxin exposure. Debate continues about the carcinogenicity of food additives, artificial sweeteners, and contaminating pesticides.

- The concern about *endogenous* synthesis of carcinogens or enhancers of carcinogenicity from components of the diet relates principally to gastric carcinomas. *Nitrosamines and nitrosamides* are implicated in the generation of these tumors, as they have been clearly shown to induce gastric cancer in animals. These compounds can be formed in the body from nitrites and amines or amides derived from digested proteins. Sources of nitrites include sodium nitrite added to foods as a preservative, and nitrates, present in common vegetables, which are reduced in the gut by bacterial flora. There is, then, the potential for endogenous production of carcinogenic agents from dietary components, which might well have an effect on the stomach.
- *High animal fat intake combined with low fiber intake has been implicated in the causation of colon cancer.* It has been estimated that doubling the average level of total fiber consumption to about 40 gm/day per person in most populations decreases the risk of colon cancer by 50%. The most plausible explanation for this association is that high fat intake increases the level of bile acids in the gut, which in turn modifies intestinal flora, favoring the growth of microaerophilic bacteria. Bile acid metabolites produced by these bacteria may function as carcinogens. The *protective effect of a high-fiber diet* might relate to (1) increased stool bulk and decreased transit time, which decreases the exposure of mucosa to putative offenders, and (2) the capacity of certain fibers to bind carcinogens and thereby protect the mucosa. However, attempts to document these theories in clinical and experimental studies have not generated consistent results.
- Although epidemiologic data show a strong positive correlation between total dietary fat intake and breast cancer, it is still unclear whether increased fat consumption has a causal relationship to breast cancer development.
- Vitamins C and E, β-carotenes, and selenium have been assumed to have anticarcinogenic effects because of their antioxidant properties. However, thus far there is no convincing evidence that these antioxidants act as chemopreventive agents. As discussed earlier in this chapter, retinoids are effective agents in the therapy of acute promyelocytic leukemia, and associations between low levels of vitamin D and cancer of the colon, prostate, and breast have been reported.

Thus, despite many tantalizing trends and proclamations by "diet gurus," thus far there is no definitive proof that a particular diet can cause or prevent cancer. On the other hand, given the relationships between obesity and cancer development, prevention of obesity through the consumption of a healthy diet is a commonsense measure that goes a long way in preserving good health. Concern persists that carcinogens lurk in things as pleasurable as a juicy steak, a rich ice cream, and in nuts contaminated with aflatoxin.

Diet and Atherosclerosis

The contribution of diet to atherogenesis is an important and controversial issue. The central question is "can dietary modification—specifically, reduction in the consumption of cholesterol and saturated animal fats (e.g., eggs, butter, beef)—reduce serum cholesterol levels and prevent or retard the development of atherosclerosis (most importantly, coronary heart disease)?" The average adult in the United States consumes a large amount of fat and cholesterol daily, with a ratio of saturated fatty acids to polyunsaturated fatty acids of about 3:1. Lowering this ratio to 1:1 causes a 10% to 15% reduction in the serum cholesterol level within a few weeks. Given the strong association of hypercholesterolemia with risk of atherosclerosis (Chapter 11), it is plausible that a low-fat diet might lower risk. A corollary of this idea is that supplementation of diet with "good" fats, for example, fish oil fatty acids belonging to the omega-3 family, might protect against atherosclerosis. However, recent studies have shown that omega-3 fatty acid supplements do not lower the risk of cardiovascular disease. Still, there remains much interest in the role that caloric restriction and special diets may play in the control of body weight and prevention of cardiovascular disease.

Caloric restriction has been convincingly demonstrated to decrease the incidence of some diseases and to increase life span in experimental animals. The basis of this striking observation is not entirely clear but seems to depend on activation of sirtuins and on lowering of insulin and IGF-1 levels (Chapter 2). In calorie-restricted animals there is also less age-related decline in immunologic functions, less oxidative damage, and greater resistance to carcinogenesis.

Not surprisingly, there are a large number of commercial diets that are reported by proponents to decrease the risk of heart disease. Among those are the low-carbohydrate diets (e.g., the Atkins Diet, the Zone, Sugar Busters, Protein Power) and others such as The Miami Diet/Hollywood 48-Hour Miracle Diet, and the South Beach Diet. The effect of these diets on heart disease, if any, is highly controversial.

Most diets dictate what you cannot eat (of course, your favorite foods!). A better strategy is to simply focus on eating an enjoyable and healthy diet rich in fish, vegetables, whole grains, fruits, olive and peanut oils (to replace saturated and *trans* fats), complex carbohydrates (instead of simple carbohydrates contained in sweets and soft drinks), and low in salt (to control hypertension).

Even lowly garlic has been touted to protect against heart disease (and also against, devils, werewolves, vampires, and, alas, kisses), although research has yet to prove this effect unequivocally. Of these, the effect on kisses is the best established!

SUGGESTED READINGS

Climate Change and Global Health

Global Burden of Disease Study 2010, *Lancet*, epublished December 13, 2012. *[An entire issue of this journal devoted to a detailed summary of the latest global disease data from the GBD project]*

Jones KE, et al: Global trends in emerging infectious diseases. *Nature* 451:990, 2008. *[A discussion of the risk of emergence of new infectious diseases.]*

McMichael AJ, Woodruff RE, Hales S. Climate change and human health: present and future risks. *Lancet* 367:859, 2006. *[A slightly older but still relevant assessment of the likely impact of climate change on human health.]*

Environmental Chemicals

Casals-Casas C, Desvergne B: Endocrine disruptors: from endocrine to metabolic disruption. *Annu Rev Phys* 73:135, 2011. *[An update discussing the scope and possible consequences of human exposure to this class of chemical.]*

Centers for Disease Control and Prevention: Third National Report on Human Exposure to Environmental Chemicals, 2005. *[A survey of environmental chemicals, with comments on exposure and health risk trends.]*

Air Pollution

McCreanor J, et al: Respiratory effects of exposure to diesel traffic in persons with asthma. *N Engl J Med* 357:2348, 2007. *[A paper discussing the danger of particulates in diesel exhaust to patients with asthma.]*

Mills NL, et al: Ischemic and thrombotic effects of dilute diesel-exhaust inhalation in men with coronary heart disease. *N Engl J Med* 357:1075, 2007. *[A paper discussing the interaction of exhaust particulates and atherosclerotic heart disease.]*

Pope CA, Ezzati M, Dockery DW: Fine-particulate air pollution and life expectancy in the United States. *N Engl J Med* 360:376, 2009. *[A paper correlating increases in life expectancy in major U.S. cities with decreases in fine-particulate air pollution.]*

Toxic Metals

Bellinger DC: Lead. *Pediatrics* 113:1016, 2004. *[A comprehensive overview of lead toxicity.]*

Clarkson TW, Magos L, Myers GJ: The toxicology of mercury—current exposures and clinical manifestations. *N Engl J Med* 349:1731, 2003. *[An older but still relevant overview of the subject.]*

Tobacco and Alcohol

Boffetta P, Hecht S, Gray N, et al: Smokeless tobacco and cancer. *Lancet Oncol* 9:667, 2009. *[A review of cancer risks associated with smokeless tobacco worldwide.]*

Seitz HK, Stickel F: Molecular mechanisms of alcohol-mediated carcinogenesis. *Nat Rev Cancer* 7:599, 2007. *[A review of the multifactorial effects of alcohol that may contribute to cancer development.]*

Radiation

Brenner DJ, Hall EJ: Computed tomography—an increasing source of radiation exposure. *N Engl J Med* 357:2277, 2007. *[A paper highlighting the increasing exposure of patients to imaging-related radiation.]*

Matthew JD, et al: Cancer risk in 680,000 people exposed to computed tomography scans in childhood or adolescence: data linkage study of 11 million Australians. *BMJ* 346:f2360, 2013. *[A recent paper showing that children who have undergone CT scans have a 24% increased risk of cancer, adding to accruing evidence that CT scans increase the risk of secondary cancers in children and adolescents.]*

Stone HB, et al: Effects of radiation on normal tissue: consequences and mechanisms. *Lancet Oncol* 4:529, 2003. *[A discussion of the deleterious effects of radiation on tissues and cells.]*

Estrogens and Progestins

Manson JE, Hsia J, Johnson KC, et al: Estrogen plus progestin and the risk of coronary heart disease. *N Engl J Med* 349:523, 2003. *[A landmark study from the Women's Health Initiative.]*

Ravdin PM, Cronin KA, Howlader N, et al: The decrease in breast cancer incidence in 2003 in the United States. *N Engl J Med* 356:1670, 2007. *[An paper documenting the decrease in breast cancer that followed its linkage to MHT.]*

Hormones and Nutritional Disorders

Hollick MF: Vitamin D deficiency. *N Engl J Med* 357:266, 2007. *[A comprehensive review of vitamin D deficiency.]*

Tang X-H, Gudas LJ: Retinoids, retinoic acid receptors, and cancer. *Annu Rev Pathol* 6:345, 2011. *[A review of the role of retinoids in cancer, with a focus on solid tumors.]*

Obesity and Metabolic Syndrome

Froguel P, Blakemore AIF: The power of the extreme in elucidating obesity. *N Engl J Med* 359:891, 2008. *[A discussion of the implications of rare obesity genes for understanding typical sporadic obesity.]*

Gregor MF, Hotamisligil GS: Inflammatory mechanisms in obesity. *Annu Rev Immunol* 29:445, 2011. *[A concise discussion of current views of the pro-inflammatory state associated with obesity.]*

Jornayvaz FR, Samuel VT, Shulman GI: The role of muscle insulin resistance in the pathogenesis of atherogenic dyslipidemia and nonalcoholic fatty liver disease associated with the metabolic syndrome. *Annu Rev Nutr* 30:273, 2010. *[A discussion of the metabolic syndrome from the perspective of the role of insulin resistance in skeletal muscle.]*

Roberts DL, Dive C, Renehan AG: Biological mechanisms linking obesity and cancer risk: new perspectives. *Annu Rev Med* 61:301, 2010. *[A discussion of the possible interactions between obesity and cancer.]*

Suzuki K, Simpson KA, Minnion JS, et al: The role of gut hormones and the hypothalamus in appetite regulation. *Endocr J* 57:359, 2010. *[A review of the interplay between the gut and the hypothalamus in regulating food consumption.]*

Tilg H, Kaser A. Gut microbiome, obesity, and metabolic dysfunction. *J Clin Invest* 121:2126, 2011. *[A review discussing the evidence, for and against, of a role for the gut microbiome in the metabolic syndrome.]*

See TARGETED THERAPY available online at www.studentconsult.com 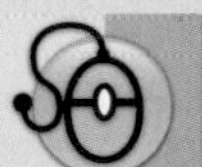

CHAPTER 10

Diseases of Infancy and Childhood

Anirban Maitra

CHAPTER CONTENTS

Children are not merely little adults, and their diseases are not merely variants of adult diseases. Many childhood conditions are unique to, or at least take distinctive forms in, this stage of life and so are discussed separately in this chapter. Diseases originating in the perinatal period are important in that they account for significant morbidity and mortality. As would be expected, the chances for survival of live-born infants improve with each passing week. This progress represents, at least in part, a triumph of improved medical care. Better prenatal care, more effective methods of monitoring the condition of the fetus, and judicious resort to cesarean section before term when there is evidence of fetal distress, have all contributed toward bringing into this world live-born infants who in past years might have been stillborn. This has resulted in an increased number of *high-risk infants* in the population. Nonetheless, the infant mortality rate in the United States has shown a decline from a level of 20 deaths per 1000 live births in 1970 to about 6.1 deaths in 2010, the latest year for which complete data are available. Although the death rate has continued to decline for all infants, African Americans continue to have an infant mortality rate more than twice (12.4 deaths per 1000 live births) that of American whites (5.3 deaths). Worldwide, infant mortality rates vary widely, from as low as 1.8 deaths per 1000 live births in Luxembourg, to as high as 180 deaths in the African subcontinent. Rather dismayingly, the United States ranks thirty-first in infant mortality rates among developed nations in the Western hemisphere.

Each stage of development of the infant and child is prey to a somewhat different group of disorders. The data available permit a survey of four time spans: (1) the neonatal period (the first 4 weeks of life), (2) infancy (the first year of life), (3) age 1 to 4 years, and (4) age 5 to 14 years.

The major causes of death in infancy and childhood are listed in Table 10-1. Congenital anomalies, disorders relating to short gestation (prematurity) and low birth weight, and sudden infant death syndrome (SIDS) represent the leading causes of death in the first 12 months of life. Once the infant survives the first year of life, the outlook brightens measurably. In the next two age groups—1 to 4 years and 5 to 9 years—unintentional injuries resulting from accidents have become the leading cause of death. Among the natural diseases, in order of importance, congenital anomalies and malignant neoplasms assume major significance. It would appear then that, in a sense, life is an obstacle course. Thankfully for the great majority, the obstacles are comfortably overcome.

The following discussion looks at specific conditions encountered during the various stages of infant and child development.

Table 10-1 Cause of Death Related with Age

Causes*	Rate†
Younger than 1 year	**660.6**
Congenital malformations, deformations, and chromosomal anomalies	
Disorders related to short gestation and low birth weight	
Sudden infant death syndrome (SIDS)	
Newborn affected by maternal complications of pregnancy	
Accidents (unintentional injuries)	
Newborn affected by complications of placenta, cord, and membranes	
Bacterial sepsis of newborn	
Respiratory distress of newborn	
Diseases of the circulatory system	
Neonatal hemorrhage	
1-4 Years	**28.3**
Accidents (unintentional injuries)	
Congenital malformations, deformations, and chromosomal abnormalities	
Assault (homicide)	
Malignant neoplasms	
Diseases of the heart‡	
5-9 Years	**12.5**
Accidents (unintentional injuries)	
Malignant neoplasms	
Congenital malformations, deformations, and chromosomal abnormalities	
Assault (homicide)	
Influenza and pneumonia	
10-14 Years	**15.7**
Accidents (unintentional injuries)	
Malignant neoplasms	
Intentional self-harm (suicide)	
Assault (homicide)	
Congenital malformations, deformations, and chromosomal anomalies	

*Causes are listed in decreasing order of frequency. All causes and rates are based on 2008 (final) and 2009 (preliminary) data.
†Rates are expressed per 100,000 population from all causes within each age group.
‡Excludes congenital heart disease.
Data source: Centers for Disease Control and Prevention/NCHS, National Vital Statistics System: mortality, 2009 and 2008 (www.cdc.gov/nchs/nvss/mortality_tables.htm).

Congenital Anomalies

Congenital anomalies are anatomic defects that are present at birth, but some, such as cardiac defects and renal anomalies, may not become clinically apparent until years later. The term *congenital* means "born with," but it does not imply or exclude a genetic basis for the birth defect. It is estimated that about 120,000 (1 in 33) babies are born with a birth defect each year in the United States. They are the most common cause of mortality in the first year and contribute significantly to morbidity and mortality throughout the early years of life. In a sense, anomalies found in live-born infants represent the less serious developmental failures in embryogenesis that are compatible with live birth. Perhaps 20% of fertilized ova are so anomalous that they are blighted from the outset. Others may be compatible with early fetal development, only to lead to spontaneous abortion. Less severe anomalies allow more prolonged intrauterine survival, with some disorders terminating in stillbirth and those still less significant permitting live birth despite the handicaps imposed.

Definitions

The process of morphogenesis (organ and tissue development) can be impaired by a variety of different errors.

- *Malformations* represent primary errors of morphogenesis, in which there is an *intrinsically abnormal developmental process* (Fig. 10-1). Malformations can be the result of a single gene or chromosomal defect, but are more commonly multifactorial in origin. Malformations may present in several patterns. Some, such as congenital heart defects and anencephaly (absence of the brain), involve single body systems, whereas in other cases multiple malformations involving many organs may coexist.
- *Disruptions* result from secondary destruction of an organ or body region that was previously normal in development; thus, in contrast to malformations, disruptions arise from an *extrinsic disturbance in morphogenesis. Amniotic bands,* denoting rupture of amnion with resultant formation of "bands" that encircle, compress, or attach to parts of the developing fetus, are the classic example of a disruption (Fig. 10-2). A variety of environmental agents may cause disruptions (see later). Understandably, disruptions are not heritable and hence are not associated with risk of recurrence in subsequent pregnancies.
- *Deformations,* like disruptions, also represent an *extrinsic disturbance of development* rather than an intrinsic error of morphogenesis. Deformations are common problems, affecting approximately 2% of newborn infants to varying degrees. Fundamental to the pathogenesis of deformations is localized or generalized compression of the growing fetus by *abnormal biomechanical forces,* leading eventually to a variety of structural abnormalities. The most common underlying factor responsible for deformations is *uterine constraint.* Between the thirty-fifth and thirty-eighth weeks of gestation, rapid increase in the size of the fetus outpaces the growth of the uterus, and the relative amount of amniotic fluid (which normally acts as a cushion) also decreases. Thus, even the normal fetus is subjected to some form of uterine constraint. Several factors increase the likelihood of excessive compression of the fetus resulting in deformations. *Maternal factors* include first pregnancy, small uterus, malformed (bicornuate) uterus, and leiomyomas. *Fetal or placental factors* include oligohydramnios, multiple fetuses, and abnormal fetal presentation. An example of a deformation is clubfeet, often a component of Potter sequence, described later.
- A *sequence* is a cascade of anomalies triggered by one initiating aberration. Approximately half the time, congenital anomalies occur singly; in the remaining cases, multiple congenital anomalies are recognized. In some instances the constellation of anomalies may be explained by a single, localized aberration in organogenesis (malformation, disruption, or deformation) that

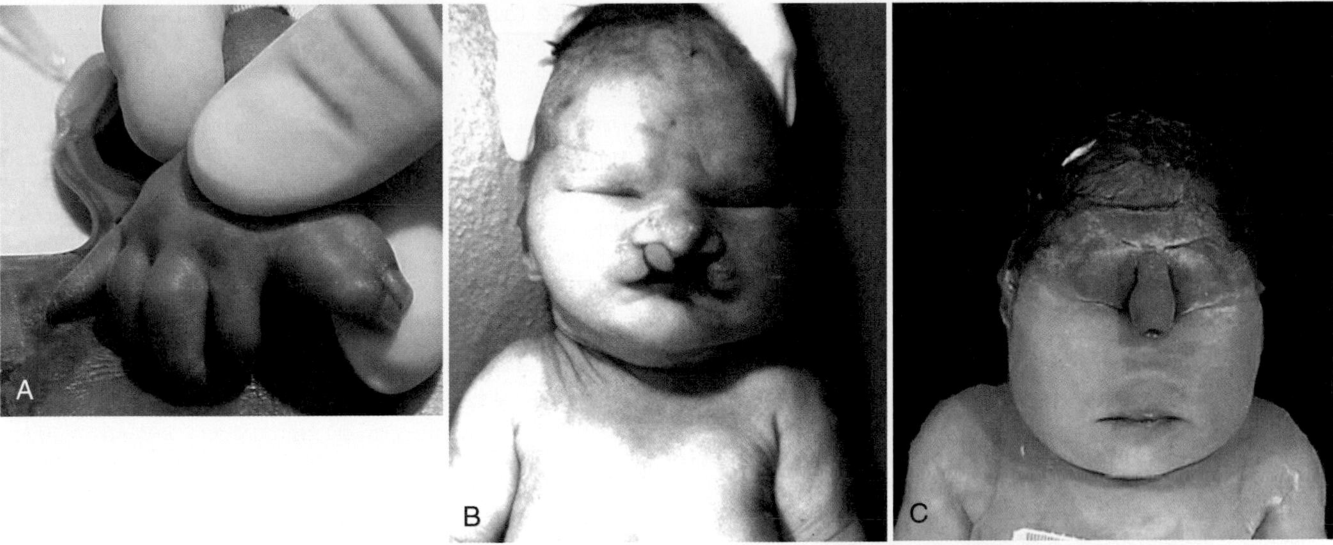

Figure 10-1 Examples of malformations. *Polydactyly* (one or more extra digits) and *syndactyly* (fusion of digits), both of which are illustrated in **A**, have little functional consequence when they occur in isolation. Similarly, *cleft lip* (**B**), with or without associated *cleft palate*, is compatible with life when it occurs as an isolated anomaly; in the present case, however, this neonate had an underlying *malformation syndrome* (trisomy 13) and died of severe cardiac defects. **C,** The stillbirth illustrated represents a severe and essentially lethal malformation, wherein the midface structures are fused or ill-formed; in almost all cases, this degree of external dysmorphogenesis is associated with severe internal anomalies such as maldevelopment of the brain and cardiac defects. (**A** and **C**, Courtesy Dr. Reade Quinton; **B**, Courtesy Dr. Beverly Rogers, Department of Pathology, University of Texas Southwestern Medical Center, Dallas, Texas.)

sets into motion secondary effects in other organs. A good example is the *oligohydramnios* (or *Potter*) *sequence* (Fig. 10-3). Oligohydramnios (decreased amniotic fluid) may be caused by a variety of unrelated maternal, placental, or fetal abnormalities. Causes of oligohydramnios include chronic leakage of amniotic fluid because of rupture of the amnion, uteroplacental insufficiency resulting from maternal hypertension or severe toxemia, and renal agenesis in the fetus (because fetal urine is a major constituent of amniotic fluid). The fetal compression associated with significant oligohydramnios, in turn, results in a classic phenotype in the newborn infant, including flattened facies and positional abnormalities of the hands and feet (Fig. 10-4). The hips may be dislocated. Growth of the chest wall and the contained lungs is also compromised so that the lungs are frequently hypoplastic, occasionally to the degree that they are the cause of fetal demise. Nodules in the amnion *(amnion nodosum)* are frequently present.

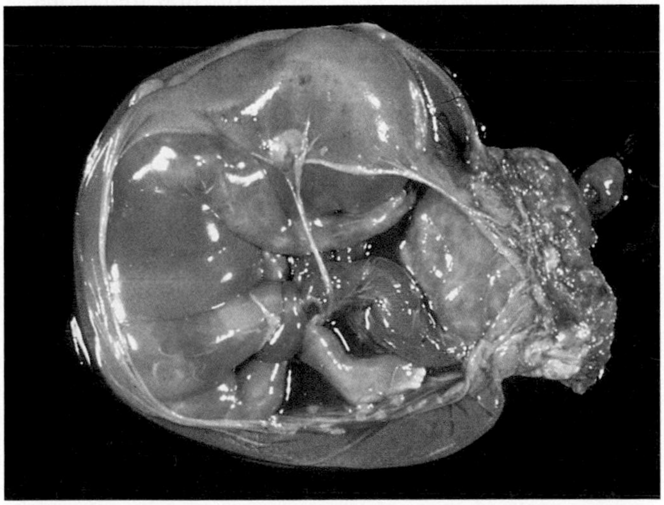

Figure 10-2 Disruption of morphogenesis by an amniotic band. Note the placenta at the right of the diagram and the band of amnion extending from the top portion of the amniotic sac to encircle the leg of the fetus. (Courtesy Dr. Theonia Boyd, Children's Hospital of Boston, Boston, Mass.)

- A *malformation syndrome* is a constellation of congenital anomalies, believed to be pathologically related, that, in contrast to a sequence, cannot be explained on the basis of a single, localized, initiating defect. Syndromes are most often caused by a single etiologic agent, such as a viral infection or specific chromosomal abnormality, which simultaneously affects several tissues.

In addition to the aforementioned general definitions, a few organ-specific terms should be defined. Agenesis

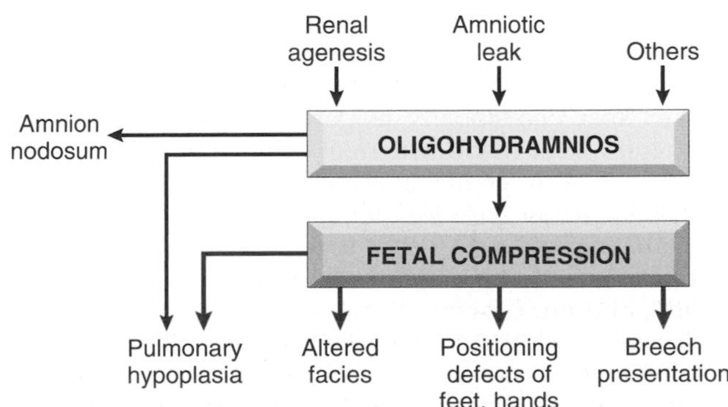

Figure 10-3 Schematic diagram of the pathogenesis of the oligohydramnios sequence.

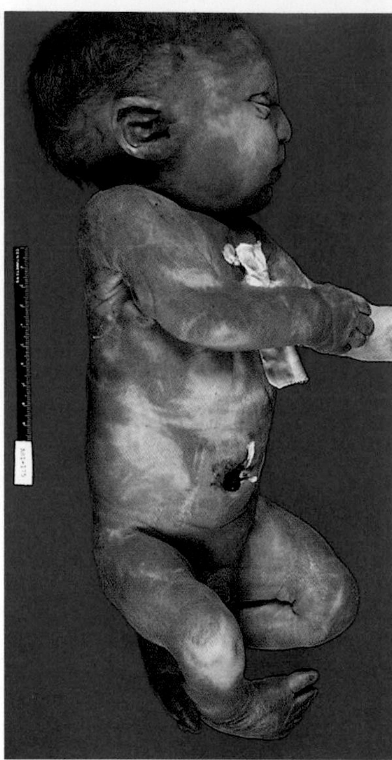

Figure 10-4 Infant with oligohydramnios sequence. Note the flattened facial features and deformed right foot (talipes equinovarus).

Table 10-2 Causes of Congenital Anomalies in Humans

Cause	Frequency (%)
Genetic	
Chromosomal aberrations	10-15
Mendelian inheritance	2-10
Environmental	
Maternal/placental infections Rubella Toxoplasmosis Syphilis Cytomegalovirus Human immunodeficiency virus	2-3
Maternal disease states Diabetes Phenylketonuria Endocrinopathies	6-8
Drugs and chemicals Alcohol Folic acid antagonists Androgens Phenytoin Thalidomide Warfarin 13-*cis*-retinoic acid Others	1
Irradiations	1
Multifactorial	20-25
Unknown	40-60

Adapted from Stevenson RE, et al (eds): Human Malformations and related Anomalies. New York, Oxford University Press, 1993, p 115.

refers to the complete absence of an organ and its associated primordium. A closely related term, aplasia, also refers to the absence of an organ but one that occurs due to failure of growth of the existing primordium. *Atresia* describes the absence of an opening, usually of a hollow visceral organ, such as the trachea and intestine. *Hypoplasia* refers to incomplete development or decreased size of an organ with decreased numbers of cells, whereas *hyperplasia* refers to the converse, that is, the enlargement of an organ due to increased numbers of cells. An abnormality in an organ or a tissue as a result of an increase or a decrease in the size (rather than the number) of individual cells defines *hypertrophy* or *hypotrophy*, respectively. Finally, *dysplasia*, in the context of malformations (versus *neoplasia*) describes an abnormal organization of cells.

Causes of Anomalies

At one time, it was believed that the presence of a visible, external anomaly was divine punishment for wickedness, a belief that occasionally jeopardized the mother's life. Although we are learning a great deal about the molecular bases of some congenital anomalies, *the exact cause remains unknown in at least one half to three fourths of the cases.* **The common known causes of congenital anomalies can be grouped into three major categories: genetic, environmental, and multifactorial** (Table 10-2).

Genetic causes of malformations include all of the previously discussed mechanisms of genetic disease (Chapter 5). Virtually all chromosomal syndromes are associated with congenital malformations. Examples include Down syndrome and other trisomies, Turner syndrome, and Klinefelter syndrome. Most chromosomal disorders arise during gametogenesis and hence are not familial. Single-gene mutations, characterized by mendelian inheritance, may underlie major malformations. For example, holoprosencephaly is the most common developmental defect of the forebrain and midface in humans; the Hedgehog signaling pathway plays a critical role in the morphogenesis of these structures, and loss-of-function mutations of individual components within this pathway are reported in families with a history of recurrent holoprosencephaly.

Environmental influences, such as viral infections, drugs, and irradiation to which the mother was exposed during pregnancy, may cause fetal anomalies. Among the viral infections listed in Table 10-2, rubella was a major scourge of the nineteenth and early twentieth centuries. Fortunately, maternal rubella and the resultant *rubella embryopathy* have been virtually eliminated in developed countries as a result of maternal rubella vaccination. A variety of drugs and chemicals have been suspected to be teratogenic, but perhaps less than 1% of congenital malformations are caused by these agents. The list includes thalidomide, alcohol, anticonvulsants, warfarin (oral anticoagulant), and 13-*cis*-retinoic acid, which is used in the treatment of severe acne. For example, *thalidomide,* once used as a tranquilizer in Europe, causes an extremely high incidence (50% to 80%) of limb malformations. *Alcohol,* when consumed even in modest amounts during pregnancy, is an important environmental teratogen. Affected infants show prenatal and postnatal growth retardation, facial anomalies (microcephaly, short palpebral fissures, maxillary

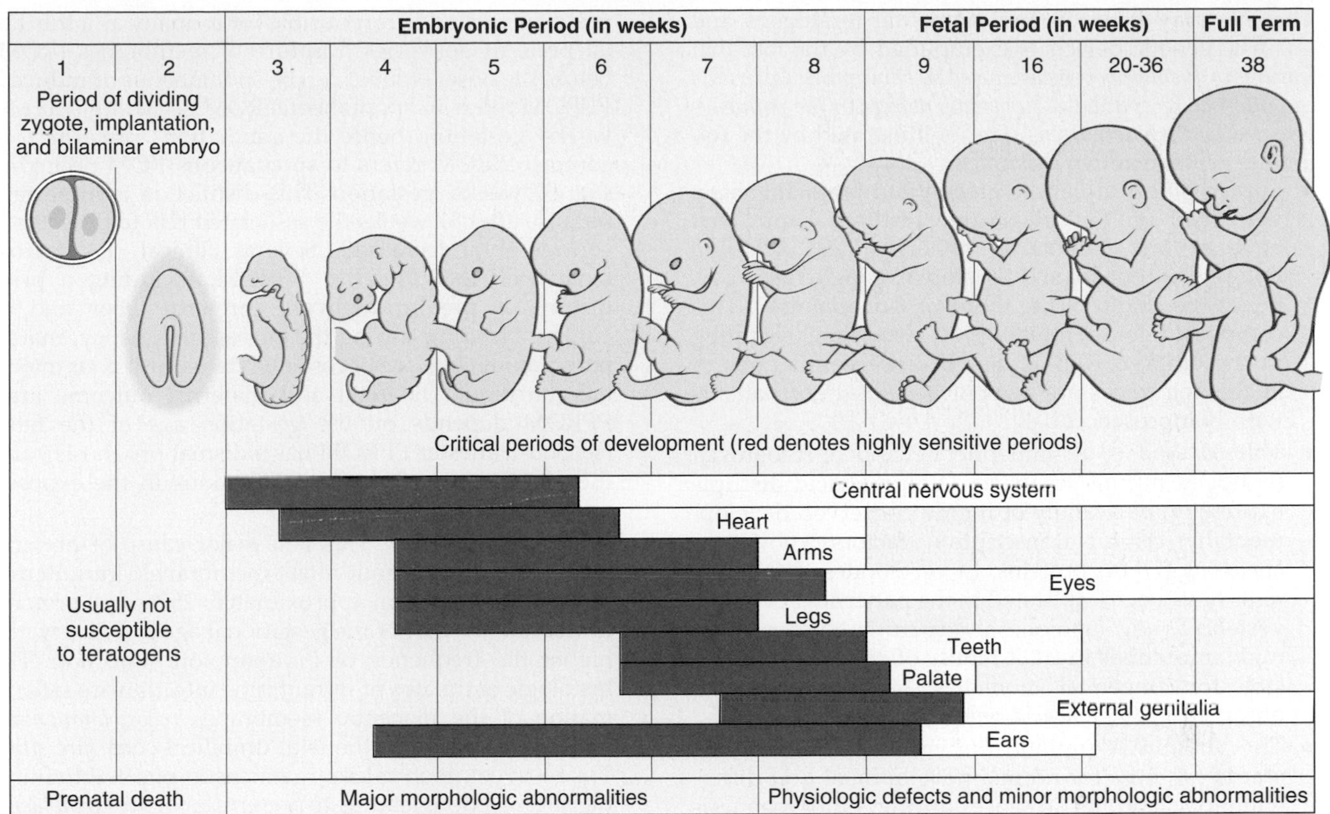

Figure 10-5 Critical periods of development for various organ systems and the resultant malformations. (Modified and redrawn from Moore KL: The Developing Human, 5th ed. Philadelphia, WB Saunders, 1993, p 156.)

hypoplasia), and psychomotor disturbances. These in combination are labeled the *fetal alcohol syndrome* (also discussed in Chapter 9). While cigarette smoke-derived nicotine has not been convincingly demonstrated to be a teratogen, there is a high incidence of spontaneous abortions, premature labor, and placental abnormalities in pregnant smokers; babies born to mothers who smoke often have a low birth weight and may be prone to the SIDS. *In light of these findings, it is best to avoid nicotine exposure altogether during pregnancy.* Among maternal conditions listed in Table 10-2, *diabetes mellitus* is a common entity, and despite advances in antenatal obstetric monitoring and glucose control, the incidence of major malformations in infants of diabetic mothers stands between 6% and 10% in most series. Maternal hyperglycemia-induced fetal hyperinsulinemia results in fetal macrosomia (organomegaly and increased body fat and muscle mass); cardiac anomalies, neural tube defects, and other central nervous system (CNS) malformations are some of the major anomalies seen in *diabetic embryopathy.*

Multifactorial inheritance, which implies the interaction of environmental influences with two or more genes of small effect, is the most common genetic cause of congenital malformations. Included in this category are some relatively common malformations such as cleft lip, cleft palate and neural tube defects. The importance of environmental contributions to multifactorial inheritance is underscored by the dramatic reduction of the incidence of neural tube defects by periconceptional intake of folic acid in the diet.

Pathogenesis. The pathogenesis of congenital anomalies is complex and still poorly understood, but two general principles of developmental pathology are relevant regardless of the etiologic agent.

1. *The timing of the prenatal teratogenic insult has an important impact on the occurrence and the type of anomaly produced* (Fig. 10-5). The intrauterine development of humans can be divided into two phases: (1) the embryonic period occupying the first 9 weeks of pregnancy and (2) the fetal period terminating at birth.
   - In the *early embryonic period* (first 3 weeks after fertilization), an injurious agent damages either enough cells to cause death and abortion or only a few cells, presumably allowing the embryo to recover without developing defects. *Between the third and the ninth weeks, the embryo is extremely susceptible to teratogenesis,* and the peak sensitivity during this period occurs between the fourth and the fifth weeks. During this period organs are being crafted out of the germ cell layers.
   - The *fetal period* that follows organogenesis is marked chiefly by the further growth and maturation of the organs, with greatly reduced susceptibility to teratogenic agents. Instead, the fetus is susceptible to growth retardation or injury to already formed organs. It is therefore possible for a given agent to produce different anomalies if exposure occurs at different times of gestation.

2. The interplay between environmental teratogens and intrinsic genetic defects is exemplified by the fact that *features of dysmorphogenesis caused by environmental insults can often be recapitulated by genetic defects in the pathways targeted by these teratogens.* This is illustrated by the following representative examples.
   - *Cyclopamine* is a plant teratogen and pregnant sheep who feed on this plant give birth to lambs that have severe craniofacial abnormalities including holoprosencephaly and "cyclopia" (single fused eye, hence the origin of the moniker cyclopamine). This compound is an inhibitor of Hedgehog signaling in the embryo, and as stated earlier, mutations of Hedgehog genes are present in subsets of patients with holoprosencephaly.
   - *Valproic acid* is an antiepileptic and a recognized teratogen during pregnancy. Valproic acid disrupts expression of a family of highly conserved developmentally critical transcription factors known as *homeobox* (HOX) proteins. In vertebrates, HOX proteins have been implicated in the patterning of limbs, vertebrae, and craniofacial structures. Not surprisingly, mutations in *HOX* family of genes are responsible for congenital anomalies that mimic features observed in *valproic acid embryopathy*.
   - The vitamin A (retinol) derivative *all-trans-retinoic acid* is essential for normal development and differentiation, and its absence during embryogenesis results in a constellation of malformations affecting multiple organ systems, including the eyes, genitourinary system, cardiovascular system, diaphragm, and lungs (see Chapter 9 for effects of for vitamin A deficiency in the postnatal period). Conversely, *excessive exposure to retinoic acid is also teratogenic.* Infants born to mothers treated with retinoic acid for severe acne have a predictable phenotype *(retinoic acid embryopathy)*, including CNS, cardiac, and craniofacial defects, such as *cleft lip and cleft palate*. The latter may stem from retinoic acid–mediated deregulation of components of the transforming growth factor-β (TGF-β) signaling pathway, which is involved in palatogenesis. Mice with knockout of the *Tgfb3* gene uniformly develop cleft palate, once again illustrating the functional relationship between teratogenic exposure and signaling pathways in the causation of congenital anomalies.

Prematurity and Fetal Growth Restriction

Prematurity, defined by a gestational age less than 37 weeks, is the second most common cause of neonatal mortality, behind only congenital anomalies (Table 10-1). The American College of Obstetrics and Gynecology estimates that 12% of all births in the United States are preterm deliveries, and despite extensive research into this area, this rate has increased over the last two decades. The major risk factors for prematurity include:

- *Preterm premature rupture of placental membranes* (PPROM): PPROM complicates about 3% of all pregnancies and is responsible for as many as a third of all preterm deliveries. Rupture of membranes (ROM) before the onset of labor can be spontaneous or induced. PPROM refers to spontaneous ROM occurring *before* 37 weeks' gestation (hence the annotation "preterm"). In contrast, PROM refers to spontaneous ROM occurring *after* 37 weeks' gestation. This distinction is important because after 37 weeks the associated risk to the fetus is considerably decreased. Several clinical risk factors have been identified for PPROM, including a prior history of preterm delivery, preterm labor and/or vaginal bleeding during the current pregnancy, maternal smoking, low socioeconomic status, and poor maternal nutrition. The fetal and maternal outcome after PPROM depends on the gestation age of the fetus (second-trimester PPROM has a dismal prognosis), and the effective prophylaxis of infections in the exposed amniotic cavity.
- *Intrauterine infection:* This is a major cause of preterm labor with and without intact membranes. Intrauterine infection is present in approximately 25% of all preterm births, and the earlier the gestational age at delivery, the higher the frequency of intra-amniotic infection. The histologic correlates of intrauterine infection are inflammation of the placental membranes *(chorioamnionitis)* and inflammation of the fetal umbilical cord *(funisitis)*. The most common microorganisms implicated in intrauterine infections leading to preterm labor are *Ureaplasma urealyticum*, *Mycoplasma hominis*, *Gardnerella vaginalis* (the dominant organism found in "bacterial vaginosis," a polymicrobial infection), *Trichomonas*, gonorrhea, and *Chlamydia*. In developing countries, malaria and HIV are significant contributors to the burden of preterm labor and prematurity. Recent studies have begun to elucidate the molecular mechanisms of inflammation-induced preterm labor. Endogenous Toll-like receptors (TLRs), which bind bacterial components as natural ligands (Chapter 6), have emerged as key players in this process. It is postulated that signals produced by TLR engagement deregulate prostaglandin expression, which in turn induces uterine smooth muscle contractions.
- *Uterine, cervical, and placental structural abnormalities:* Uterine distortion (e.g., uterine fibroids), compromised structural support of the cervix ("cervical incompetence"), *placenta previa*, and *abruptio placentae* (Chapter 22) are associated with an increased risk of prematurity.
- *Multiple gestation* (twin pregnancy).

The hazards of prematurity are manifold for the newborn and may give rise to one or more of the following:

- Neonatal respiratory distress syndrome, also known as hyaline membrane disease
- Necrotizing enterocolitis
- Sepsis
- Intraventricular and germinal matrix hemorrhage

Fetal Growth Restriction

Although preterm infants have low birth weights, it is usually appropriate once adjusted for their gestational age. In contrast, as many as one third of infants who weigh less than 2500 gm are born at term and are therefore undergrown rather than immature. These small-for-gestational-age (SGA) infants suffer from *fetal growth restriction*. Fetal growth restriction (FGR) may result from fetal, maternal, or placental abnormalities, although in many cases the specific cause is unknown.

Fetal Abnormalities. Fetal influences are those that intrinsically reduce growth potential of the fetus despite an adequate supply of nutrients from the mother. Prominent among such fetal conditions are *chromosomal disorders, congenital anomalies, and congenital infections*. Chromosomal abnormalities may be detected in up to 17% of fetuses sampled for FGR and in up to 66% of fetuses with documented ultrasonographic malformations. Among the first group, the abnormalities include triploidy (7%), trisomy 18 (6%), trisomy 21 (1%), trisomy 13 (1%), and a variety of deletions and translocations (2%). *Fetal infection* should be considered in all infants with FGR. Those most commonly responsible for FGR are the TORCH group of infections (toxoplasmosis, rubella, cytomegalovirus, herpesvirus, and other viruses and bacteria, such as syphilis). Infants who are SGA because of fetal factors usually have symmetric growth restriction (also referred to as *proportionate FGR*), meaning that all organ systems are similarly affected.

Placental Abnormalities. During the third trimester of pregnancy, vigorous fetal growth places particularly heavy demands on the uteroplacental blood supply. Therefore, the adequacy of placental growth in the preceding midtrimester is extremely important, and *uteroplacental insufficiency is an important cause of growth restriction*. This insufficiency may result from *umbilical-placental vascular anomalies* (such as single umbilical artery, abnormal cord insertion, placental hemangioma), *placental abruption, placenta previa, placental thrombosis and infarction, placental infection*, or *multiple gestations* (Chapter 22). In some cases the placenta may be small without any detectable underlying cause. Placental causes of FGR tend to result in *asymmetric* (or disproportionate) growth retardation of the fetus with relative sparing of the brain. Physiologically, this general type of FGR is viewed as a down-regulation of growth in the latter half of gestation because of limited availability of nutrients or oxygen.

Maternal Abnormalities. By far the most common factors associated with SGA infants are maternal conditions that result in decreased placental blood flow. Vascular diseases, such as *preeclampsia (toxemia of pregnancy)* and *chronic hypertension*, are often the underlying cause. Another class of maternal diseases increasingly being recognized in the setting of FGR are *thrombophilias*, such as the acquired antiphospholipid antibody syndrome (Chapter 6). Inherited diseases of hypercoagulability are also associated with recurrent early pregnancy losses. The list of other maternal conditions associated with SGA infants is long, but some of the avoidable factors worth mentioning are maternal *narcotic abuse, alcohol intake*, and *heavy cigarette smoking. Drugs* causing FGR include both classic teratogens, such as chemotherapeutic agents, and some commonly administered therapeutic agents, such as phenytoin (Dilantin). *Maternal malnutrition* (in particular, prolonged hypoglycemia) may also affect fetal growth, but the association between SGA infants and the nutritional status of the mother is complex.

The SGA infant faces a difficult course, not only during the struggle for survival in the perinatal period, but also in childhood and adult life. Depending on the underlying cause of FGR and, to a lesser extent, the degree of prematurity, there is a significant risk of morbidity in the form of a major handicap, cerebral dysfunction, learning disability, or hearing and visual impairment.

Neonatal Respiratory Distress Syndrome

There are many causes of respiratory distress in the newborn. The most common cause is respiratory distress syndrome (RDS), also known as *hyaline membrane disease* because of the deposition of a layer of hyaline proteinaceous material in the peripheral airspaces of infants who succumb to this condition. Others include excessive sedation of the mother, fetal head injury during delivery, aspiration of blood or amniotic fluid, and intrauterine hypoxia brought about by coiling of the umbilical cord about the neck. An estimated 24,000 cases of RDS are reported annually in the United States. Thankfully, improvements in management of this condition have sharply decreased deaths due to respiratory insufficiency from as many as 5000 per year a decade earlier to less than 900 cases per year currently.

In untreated infants (not receiving surfactant), RDS generally presents in a stereotypical fashion, with characteristic clinical findings. The infant is almost always preterm but has weight appropriate for gestational age, and there are strong, but not invariable, associations with *male gender, maternal diabetes*, and delivery by *cesarean section*. Resuscitation may be necessary at birth, but usually within a few minutes rhythmic breathing and normal color are reestablished. Soon afterward, often within 30 minutes, breathing becomes more difficult, and within a few hours cyanosis becomes evident. Fine rales can now be heard over both lung fields. A chest x-ray film at this time usually reveals uniform minute reticulogranular densities, producing a so-called *ground-glass picture*. In the full-blown condition the respiratory distress persists, cyanosis increases, and even the administration of 80% oxygen by a variety of ventilatory methods fails to improve the situation. If therapy staves off death for the first 3 or 4 days, however, the infant has an excellent chance of recovery.

Pathogenesis. **Immaturity of the lungs is the most important substrate on which RDS develops.** It may be encountered in full-term infants but is much more frequent in those "born before their time into this breathing world." The incidence of RDS is inversely proportional to gestational age. It occurs in about 60% of infants born at less than 28 weeks of gestation, 30% of those born between 28 to 34 weeks' gestation, and less than 5% of those born after 34 weeks' gestation.

The fundamental defect in RDS is a deficiency of pulmonary surfactant. As described in Chapter 15, surfactant consists predominantly of dipalmitoyl phosphatidylcholine (lecithin), smaller amounts of phosphatidylglycerol, and two groups of surfactant-associated proteins. The first group is composed of hydrophilic glycoproteins SP-A and SP-D, which play a role in pulmonary host defense (innate immunity). The second group consists of hydrophobic surfactant proteins SP-B and SP-C, which, in concert with the surfactant lipids, are involved in the reduction of surface tension at the air-liquid barrier in the alveoli of the lung. With reduced surface tension in the alveoli, less pressure is required to keep them patent and hence aerated. The importance of surfactant proteins in normal lung function can be gauged by the occurrence of severe respiratory failure in neonates with congenital deficiency of surfactant caused by mutations in the *SFTPB* or *SFTBC* genes.

Surfactant production by type II alveolar cells is accelerated after the thirty-fifth week of gestation in the fetus. At birth, the first breath of life requires high inspiratory pressures to expand the lungs. With normal levels of surfactant, the lungs retain up to 40% of the residual air volume after the first breath; thus, subsequent breaths require far lower inspiratory pressures. With a deficiency of surfactant, the lungs collapse with each successive breath, and so infants must work as hard with each successive breath as they did with the first. The problem of *stiff* atelectatic lungs is compounded by the *soft* thoracic wall that is pulled in as the diaphragm descends. Progressive atelectasis and reduced lung compliance then lead to a train of events as depicted in Figure 10-6, resulting in protein-rich, fibrin-rich exudation into the alveolar spaces with the formation of hyaline membranes. The fibrin-hyaline membranes are barriers to gas exchange, leading to carbon dioxide retention and hypoxemia. The hypoxemia itself further impairs surfactant synthesis, and a vicious cycle ensues.

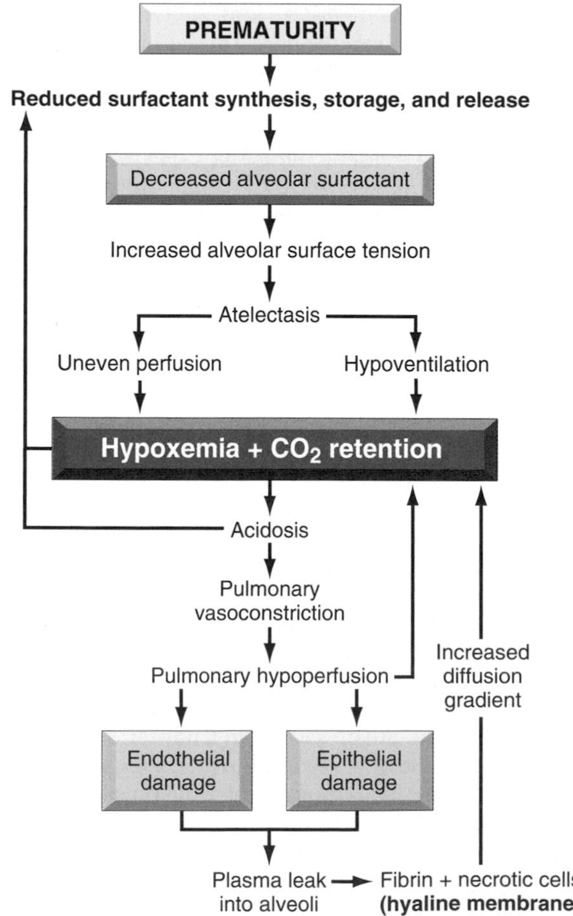

Figure 10-6 Schematic outline of the pathophysiology of respiratory distress syndrome (see text).

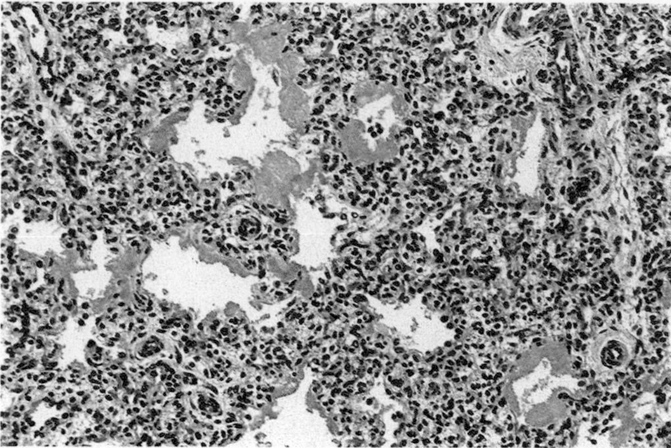

Figure 10-7 Hyaline membrane disease. There is alternating atelectasis and dilation of the alveoli. Note the eosinophilic thick hyaline membranes lining the dilated alveoli.

Surfactant synthesis is modulated by a variety of hormones and growth factors, including cortisol, insulin, prolactin, thyroxine, and TGF-β. *The role of glucocorticoids is particularly important.* Conditions associated with intrauterine stress and FGR that increase corticosteroid release lower the risk of developing RDS. Surfactant synthesis can be suppressed by the compensatory high blood levels of insulin in infants of diabetic mothers, which counteracts the effects of steroids. This may explain, in part, why infants of diabetic mothers have a higher risk of developing RDS. Labor is known to increase surfactant synthesis; hence, cesarean section before the onset of labor may increase the risk of RDS.

MORPHOLOGY

The lungs are distinctive on gross examination. Though of normal size, they are solid, airless, and reddish purple, similar to the color of the liver, and they usually sink in water. Microscopically, alveoli are poorly developed, and those that are present are collapsed (Fig. 10-7). When the infant dies early in the course of the disease, necrotic cellular debris can be seen in the terminal bronchioles and alveolar ducts. The necrotic material becomes incorporated within **eosinophilic hyaline membranes** lining the respiratory bronchioles, alveolar ducts, and alveoli. The membranes are largely made up of fibrin admixed with cell debris derived chiefly from necrotic type II pneumocytes. The sequence of events that leads to the formation of hyaline membranes is depicted in Figure 10-6. There is a remarkable paucity of neutrophilic inflammatory reaction associated with these membranes. The lesions of hyaline membrane disease are never seen in stillborn infants.

In infants who survive more than 48 hours, reparative changes occur in the lungs. The alveolar epithelium proliferates under the surface of the membrane, and may detach into the airspace where it undergoes partial digestion or phagocytosis by macrophages.

Clinical Features. The classic clinical presentation before the era of treatment with exogenous surfactant was described earlier. Currently, the actual clinical course and prognosis for neonatal RDS vary, depending on the maturity and birth weight of the infant and the promptness of institution of therapy. *A major thrust in the control of RDS focuses on prevention, either by delaying labor until the fetal lung reaches maturity or by inducing maturation of the lung in the fetus at risk.* Critical to these objectives is the ability to assess fetal lung maturity accurately. Because pulmonary secretions are discharged into the amniotic fluid, analysis of amniotic fluid phospholipids provides a good estimate of the level of surfactant in the alveolar lining. Prophylactic administration of exogenous surfactant at birth to extremely premature infants (gestational age < 28 weeks) has been shown to be very beneficial, such that it is now uncommon for infants to die of acute RDS.

In uncomplicated cases, recovery begins to occur within 3 or 4 days. In affected neonates, oxygen is required. However, high concentration of ventilator-administered oxygen for prolonged periods is associated with two well-known complications: *retrolental fibroplasia* (also called *retinopathy of prematurity*) in the eyes, and *bronchopulmonary dysplasia.* Fortunately, both complications are now infrequent as a result of gentler ventilation techniques, antenatal glucocorticoid therapy, and prophylactic surfactant treatments.

- Retinopathy of prematurity has a two-phase pathogenesis. During the *hyperoxic* phase of RDS therapy (phase I), expression of the proangiogenic vascular endothelial growth factor (VEGF) is markedly decreased, causing endothelial cell apoptosis; VEGF levels rebound after return to relatively hypoxic room air ventilation (phase II), inducing retinal vessel proliferation (*neovascularization*) characteristic of the lesions in the retina.
- *The major abnormality in bronchopulmonary dysplasia is* striking decrease in alveolar septation (manifested as large, simplified alveolar structures) and a dysmorphic capillary configuration. Thus, the current view is that bronchopulmonary dysplasia is caused by a potentially reversible impairment in the development of alveolar septation at the so-called "saccular" stage. Multiple factors—hyperoxemia, hyperventilation, prematurity, inflammatory cytokines, and vascular maldevelopment—contribute to bronchopulmonary dysplasia and probably act additively or synergistically to promote injury. The levels of a variety of proinflammatory cytokines (TNF, interleukin-1β [IL-1β], IL-6, and IL-8) are increased in the alveoli of infants who develop bronchopulmonary dysplasia, suggesting a role for these cytokines in arresting pulmonary development.

Infants who recover from RDS are also at increased risk for developing a variety of other complications associated with preterm birth; most important among these are *patent ductus arteriosus, intraventricular hemorrhage,* and *necrotizing enterocolitis.* Thus, although technologic advances help save the lives of many infants with RDS, it also brings to the surface the exquisite fragility of the immature neonate.

Necrotizing Enterocolitis

Necrotizing enterocolitis is most common in premature infants, with the incidence of the disease being inversely proportional to the gestational age. It occurs in approximately 1 out of 10 very low birth weight infants (<1500 gm). Approximately 2500 cases occur annually in the United States.

The pathogenesis of necrotizing enterocolitis is uncertain, but is in all likelihood multifactorial. In addition to prematurity, most cases are associated with enteral feeding, suggesting that some postnatal insult (such as introduction of bacteria) sets in motion the cascade culminating in tissue destruction. While infectious agents likely play a role in the pathogenesis of necrotizing enterocolitis, no single bacterial pathogen has been linked to the disease. A large number of inflammatory mediators have been associated with necrotizing enterocolitis, and their discussion is beyond the scope of this book. One particular mediator, platelet activating factor (PAF), has been implicated in increasing mucosal permeability by promoting enterocyte apoptosis and compromising intercellular tight junctions, thus adding "fuel to the fire." Stool and serum samples of infants with necrotizing enterocolitis demonstrate higher PAF levels than age-matched controls. Ultimately, breakdown of mucosal barrier functions permits transluminal migration of gut bacteria, leading to a vicious cycle of inflammation, mucosal necrosis, and further bacterial entry, eventually culminating in sepsis and shock (Chapter 4).

The clinical course is fairly typical, with the onset of bloody stools, abdominal distention, and development of circulatory collapse. Abdominal radiographs often demonstrate gas within the intestinal wall *(pneumatosis intestinalis).*

MORPHOLOGY

Necrotizing enterocolitis typically involves the terminal ileum, cecum, and right colon, although any part of the small or large intestines may be involved. The involved segment is distended, friable, and congested, or it can be frankly gangrenous; intestinal perforation with accompanying peritonitis may be seen. Microscopically, mucosal or transmural coagulative necrosis, ulceration, bacterial colonization, and submucosal gas bubbles may be seen (Fig. 10-8). Reparative changes, such as the formation of granulation tissue and fibrosis, may begin shortly after the acute episode. When detected early on, necrotizing enterocolitis can be often managed conservatively, but many cases (20% to 60%) require resection of the necrotic segments of bowel. Necrotizing enterocolitis is associated with high perinatal mortality; those who survive often develop post-necrotizing enterocolitis strictures from fibrosis caused by the healing process.

Perinatal Infections

In general, fetal and perinatal infections are acquired through one of two primary routes—transcervically (also referred to as ascending) or transplacentally (hematologic). Occasionally, infections occur by a combination of the two routes in that an ascending microorganism infects the endometrium and then invades the fetal bloodstream via the chorionic villi.

Transcervical (Ascending) Infections

Most bacterial and a few viral (e.g., herpes simplex II) infections are acquired by the cervicovaginal route. Such infections may be acquired in utero or around the time of

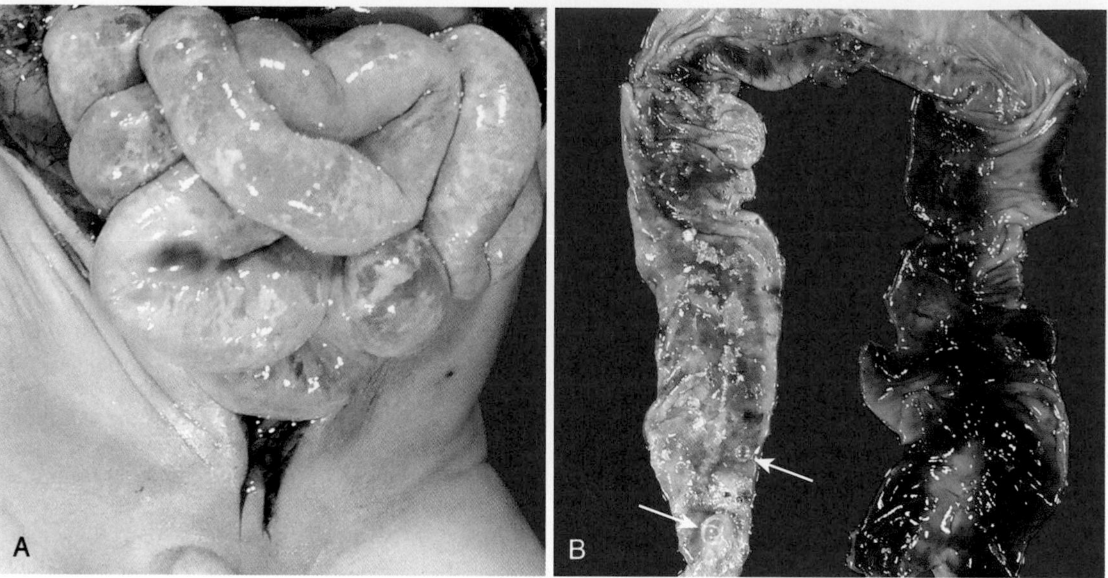

Figure 10-8 Necrotizing enterocolitis (NEC). **A,** Postmortem examination in a severe case of NEC shows the entire small bowel is markedly distended with a perilously thin wall (usually this implies impending perforation). **B,** The congested portion of the ileum corresponds to areas of hemorrhagic infarction and transmural necrosis microscopically. Submucosal gas bubbles *(pneumatosis intestinalis)* can be seen in several areas *(arrows).*

birth. In general the fetus acquires the infection either by inhaling infected amniotic fluid into the lungs shortly before birth or by passing through an infected birth canal during delivery. As stated before, preterm birth is a common and unfortunate consequence of infection. Preterm birth due to infection may be related either to damage and rupture of the amniotic sac as a direct consequence of the inflammation or to the induction of labor by prostaglandins released from infiltrating neutrophils. Inflammation of the placental membranes and cord are usually seen, but the presence or absence and severity of chorioamnionitis do not necessarily correlate with the severity of the fetal infection. In the fetus infected by inhalation of amniotic fluid, pneumonia, sepsis, and meningitis are the most common sequelae.

Transplacental (Hematologic) Infections

Most parasitic (e.g., toxoplasma, malaria) and viral infections and a few bacterial infections (i.e., *Listeria, Treponema*) gain access to the fetal bloodstream transplacentally via the chorionic villi. This hematogenous transmission may occur at any time during gestation or occasionally, as may be the case with hepatitis B and HIV, at the time of delivery via maternal-to-fetal transfusion. The clinical manifestations of these infections are highly variable, depending largely on the gestational timing and microorganism involved.

Parvovirus B19, which causes erythema infectiosum or "fifth disease of childhood" in immunocompetent older children, can infect 1% to 5% of seronegative (non-immune) pregnant women, and the vast majority have a normal pregnancy outcome. Adverse pregnancy outcomes in a minority of intrauterine infections include spontaneous abortion (particularly in the second trimester), stillbirth, hydrops fetalis (see later), and congenital anemia. Parvovirus B19 has a particular tropism for erythroid cells, and diagnostic viral inclusions can be seen in early erythroid progenitors in infected infants (Fig. 10-9).

The *TORCH group of infections* (see earlier) are grouped together because they may evoke similar clinical and pathologic manifestations, including *fever, encephalitis, chorioretinitis, hepatosplenomegaly, pneumonitis, myocarditis, hemolytic anemia, and vesicular or hemorrhagic skin lesions.* Such infections occurring early in gestation may also cause chronic sequelae in the child, including growth and mental retardation, cataracts, congenital cardiac anomalies, and bone defects.

Sepsis

Perinatal sepsis can be grouped clinically based on early onset (within the first 7 days of life) versus late onset (from 7 days to 3 months). Most cases of early-onset sepsis are acquired at or shortly before birth and tend to result in clinical signs and symptoms of pneumonia, sepsis, and occasionally meningitis within 4 or 5 days of life. Group B

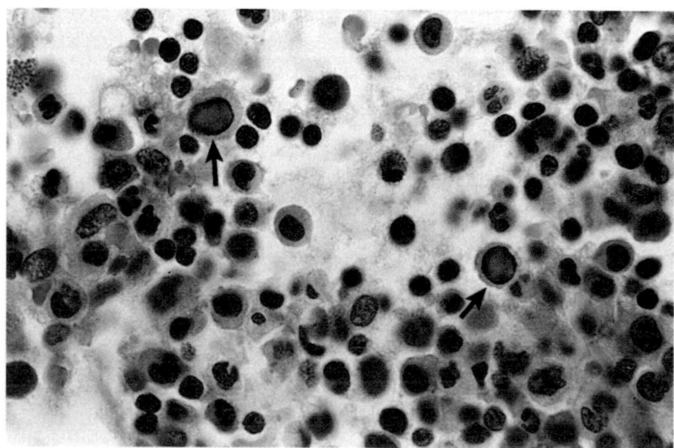

Figure 10-9 Bone marrow from an infant infected with parvovirus B19. The *arrows* indicate two erythroid precursors with large homogeneous intranuclear inclusions and a surrounding peripheral rim of residual chromatin.

streptococcus is the most common cause of early-onset sepsis as well as early-onset bacterial meningitis. Infections with *Listeria* and *Candida* have longer latent periods between the time of microorganism inoculation and the appearance of clinical symptoms and present as late-onset sepsis.

Fetal Hydrops

Fetal hydrops refers to the accumulation of edema fluid in the fetus during intrauterine growth. Until recently, hemolytic anemia caused by Rh blood group incompatibility between mother and fetus *(immune hydrops)* was the most common cause, but with the successful prophylaxis of this disorder during pregnancy, causes of *nonimmune hydrops* have emerged as the principal culprits (Table 10-3). The intrauterine fluid accumulation can be quite variable, from progressive, generalized edema of the fetus *(hydrops fetalis)*, a usually lethal condition, to more localized degrees of edema, such as isolated pleural and peritoneal effusions, or postnuchal fluid accumulation (*cystic hygroma*, see later) that are compatible with life.

Immune Hydrops

Immune hydrops is a hemolytic disease caused by blood group antigen incompatibility between mother and fetus. When the fetus inherits red cell antigenic determinants from the father that are foreign to the mother, a maternal immune reaction may occur. *The major antigens known to induce clinically significant immunologic reactions are certain of the Rh antigens and the ABO blood groups.* The reaction occurs in second and subsequent pregnancies in an Rh-negative mother with an Rh-positive father.

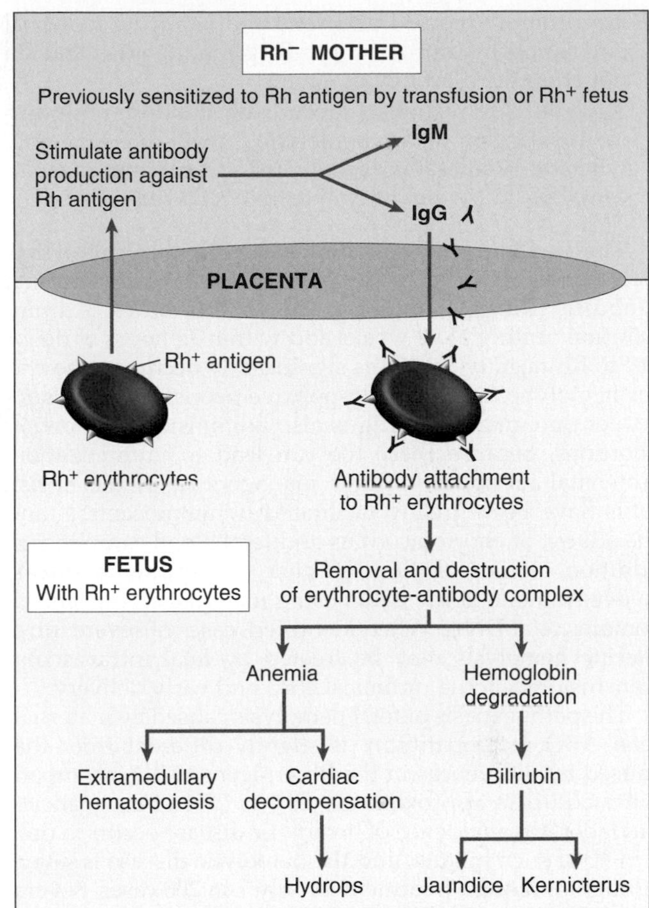

Figure 10-10 Pathogenesis of immune hydrops fetalis (see text).

Table 10-3 Selected Causes of Nonimmune Fetal Hydrops

Cardiovascular
Malformations Tachyarrhythmia High-output failure
Chromosomal
Turner syndrome Trisomy 21, trisomy 18
Thoracic Causes
Cystic adenomatoid malformation Diaphragmatic hernia
Fetal Anemia
Homozygous α-thalassemia Parvovirus B19 Immune hydrops (Rh and ABO)
Twin Gestation
Twin-to-twin transfusion
Infection (excluding parvovirus)
Cytomegalovirus Syphilis Toxoplasmosis
Genitourinary Tract Malformations
Tumors
Genetic/Metabolic Disorders

The cause of fetal hydrops may be undetermined ("idiopathic") in up to 20% of cases.
Data from Machin GA: Hydrops, cystic hygroma, hydrothorax, pericardial effusions, and fetal ascites. In Gilbert-Barness E, et al (eds): Potter's Pathology of the Fetus, Infant, and Child. St. Louis, Mosby, 2007, p 33.

Etiology and Pathogenesis. The underlying basis of immune hydrops is the immunization of the mother by blood group antigens on fetal red cells and the free passage of antibodies from the mother through the placenta to the fetus (Fig. 10-10). Fetal red cells may reach the maternal circulation during the last trimester of pregnancy, when the cytotrophoblast is no longer present as a barrier, or during childbirth itself. The mother thus becomes sensitized to the foreign antigen. The initial exposure to Rh antigen evokes the formation of IgM antibodies,that unlike IgG antibodies, do not cross the placenta. Thus, Rh disease is uncommon with the first pregnancy. Exposure during a subsequent pregnancy generally leads to a brisk IgG antibody response and the risk of immune hydrops.

Of the numerous antigens included in the Rh system, only the D antigen is a major cause of Rh incompatibility. Several factors influence the immune response to Rh-positive fetal red cells that reach the maternal circulation.

- Concurrent ABO incompatibility protects the mother against Rh immunization, because the fetal red cells

are promptly coated and removed from the maternal circulation by anti-A or anti-B IgM antibodies that do not cross the placenta.
- The antibody response depends on the dose of immunizing antigen; hence, hemolytic disease develops only when the mother has experienced a significant transplacental bleed (>1 mL of Rh-positive fetal red cells).

The incidence of maternal Rh isoimmunization has decreased significantly since the use of Rhesus immune globulin (RhIg) containing anti-D antibodies. Administration of RhIg at 28 weeks and within 72 hours of delivery to Rh-negative mothers significantly decreases the risk for hemolytic disease in Rh-positive neonates and in subsequent pregnancies; RhIg is also administered following abortions, because these too can lead to immunization. Antenatal identification and management of the at-risk fetus have been greatly facilitated by amniocentesis and the advent of chorionic villus and fetal blood sampling. In addition, cloning of the *RHD* gene has resulted in efforts to determine fetal Rh status using maternal serum since it contains fetal DNA. When identified, cases of severe intrauterine hemolysis may be treated by fetal intravascular transfusions via the umbilical cord and early delivery.

The pathogenesis of fetal hemolysis caused by maternal-fetal ABO incompatibility is slightly different from that caused by differences in the Rh antigens. ABO incompatibility occurs in approximately 20% to 25% of pregnancies, but laboratory evidence of hemolytic disease occurs in only 1 in 10 of such infants, and the hemolytic disease is severe enough to require treatment in only 1 in 200 cases. Several factors account for this. First, as mentioned, most anti-A and anti-B antibodies are of the IgM type and hence do not cross the placenta. Second, neonatal red cells express blood group antigens A and B poorly. Third, many cells other than red cells express A and B antigens and thus absorb some of the transferred antibody. ABO hemolytic disease occurs almost exclusively in infants of group A or B who are born of group O mothers. For reasons unknown, certain group O women possess IgG antibodies directed against group A or B antigens (or both) even without prior sensitization. Therefore, the firstborn may be affected. Fortunately, even with transplacentally acquired antibodies, lysis of the infant's red cells is minimal. There is no effective protection against ABO reactions.

There are two consequences of excessive destruction of red cells in the neonate (Fig. 10-10). The severity of these changes varies considerably, depending on the degree of hemolysis and the maturity of the infant.

- *Anemia* is a direct result of red cell loss. If hemolysis is mild, increased red cell production may suffice to maintain near normal levels of red cells. However, with more severe hemolysis, progressive anemia develops and may result in hypoxic injury to the heart and liver. Because of liver injury, plasma protein synthesis decreases, and levels of these proteins may drop to as low as 2 to 2.5 mg/dL. Cardiac hypoxia may lead to cardiac decompensation and failure. The combination of reduced plasma oncotic pressure and increased hydrostatic pressure in the circulation (secondary to cardiac failure) results in generalized edema and anasarca, culminating in hydrops fetalis.
- *Jaundice* develops because hemolysis produces unconjugated bilirubin (Chapter 18). Bilirubin also passes through the infant's poorly developed blood-brain barrier. Being water insoluble, bilirubin blinds to lipids in the brain, and can damage the CNS, causing *kernicterus* (see Fig. 10-13).

Nonimmune Hydrops

The three major causes of nonimmune hydrops include cardiovascular defects, chromosomal anomalies, and fetal anemia (Table 10-3). Both structural and functional cardiovascular defects, such as congenital malformations and arrhythmias, may result in intrauterine cardiac failure and hydrops. Among the chromosomal anomalies, 45,X karyotype (Turner syndrome) and the trisomies 21 and 18 are associated with fetal hydrops because of the accompanying structural cardiac anomalies. In Turner syndrome, abnormalities of lymphatic drainage from the neck may lead to postnuchal fluid accumulation *(cystic hygromas)* as well. Fetal anemia, not caused by Rh- or ABO-associated antibodies, can also result in hydrops. In fact, in some parts of the world (e.g., Southeast Asia), severe fetal anemia due to homozygous α-thalassemia, resulting from deletion of all four α-globin genes, is probably the most common cause of nonimmune hydrops (Chapter 14). Transplacental infection by parvovirus B19 is rapidly emerging as an important cause of hydrops (see earlier). The virus gains preferential entry into erythroid precursors (normoblasts), where it replicates, leading to apoptosis of red cell progenitors and isolated red cell aplasia. Parvoviral intranuclear inclusions can be seen within circulating and marrow erythroid precursors (Fig. 10-9). Approximately 10% of cases of nonimmune hydrops are related to monozygous twin pregnancies and twin-to-twin transfusion occurring through anastomoses between the two circulations.

MORPHOLOGY

The anatomic findings in fetuses with intrauterine fluid accumulation vary with both the severity of the disease and the underlying etiology. As previously noted, hydrops fetalis represents the most severe and generalized manifestation (Fig. 10-11), and lesser degrees of edema such as isolated pleural, peritoneal, or postnuchal fluid collections can occur. Accordingly, infants may be stillborn, die within the first few days, or recover completely. The presence of dysmorphic features suggests a chromosomal abnormality; postmortem examination may reveal an underlying cardiac anomaly.

In hydrops associated with fetal anemia, both fetus and placenta are characteristically pale; in most cases the liver and spleen are enlarged from cardiac failure and congestion. Additionally, the bone marrow demonstrates compensatory hyperplasia of erythroid precursors (parvovirus-associated red cell aplasia being a notable exception), and extramedullary hematopoiesis is present in the liver, spleen, and lymph nodes, and possibly other tissues such as the kidneys, lungs, and even the heart. The increased hematopoietic activity accounts for the presence in the peripheral circulation of large numbers of immature red cells, including reticulocytes, normoblasts, and erythroblasts **(erythroblastosis fetalis)** (Fig. 10-12).

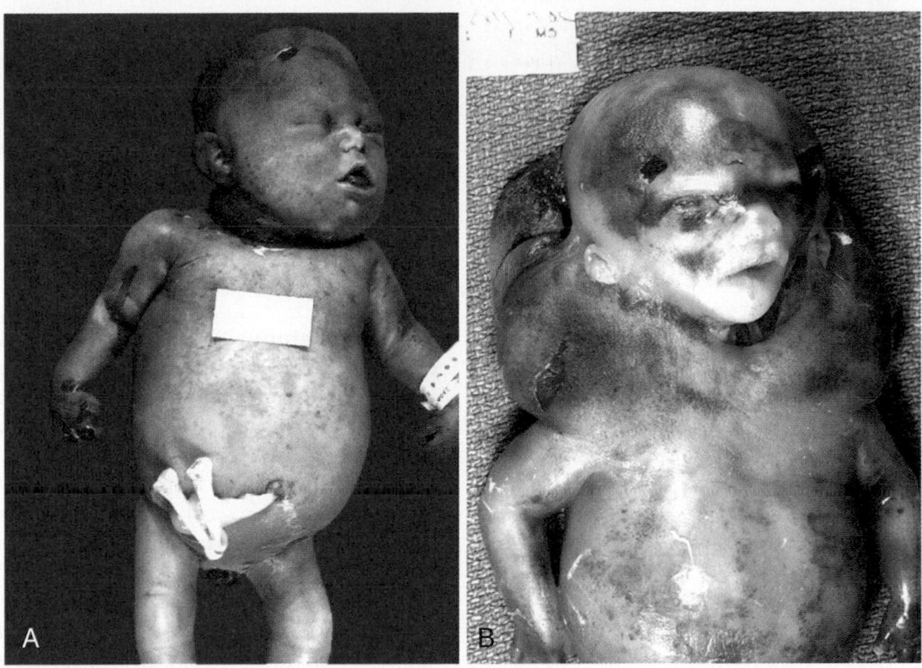

Figure 10-11 Hydrops fetalis. **A,** There is generalized accumulation of fluid in the fetus. **B,** Fluid accumulation is particularly prominent in the soft tissues of the neck, and this condition has been termed *cystic hygroma.* Cystic hygromas are characteristically seen, but not limited to, constitutional chromosomal anomalies such as 45,X karyotypes. (Courtesy Dr. Beverly Rogers, Department of Pathology, University of Texas Southwestern Medical Center, Dallas, Texas.)

The most serious threat in fetal hydrops is CNS damage, known as **kernicterus** (Fig. 10-13). The affected brain is enlarged and edematous and, when sectioned, has a bright yellow color, particularly the basal ganglia, thalamus, cerebellum, cerebral gray matter, and spinal cord. The precise level of bilirubin that induces kernicterus is unpredictable, but neural damage usually requires a blood bilirubin level greater than 20 mg/dL in term infants; in premature infants this threshold may be considerably lower.

Clinical Features. The clinical manifestations of fetal hydrops vary with the severity of the disease and can be inferred from the preceding discussion. Minimally affected infants display pallor, possibly accompanied by hepatosplenomegaly (to which may be added jaundice with more severe hemolytic reactions), whereas the most gravely ill neonates present with intense jaundice, generalized edema, and signs of neurologic injury. These infants may be supported by a variety of measures, including phototherapy (visual light oxidizes toxic unconjugated bilirubin to harmless, readily excreted, water-soluble dipyrroles) and, in severe cases, total exchange transfusion of the infant.

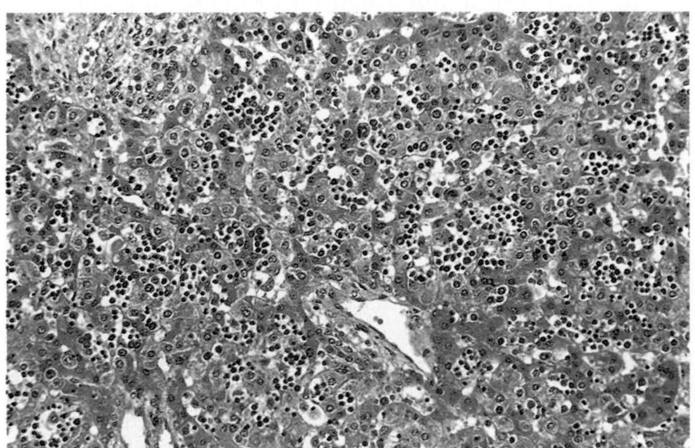

Figure 10-12 Numerous islands of extramedullary hematopoiesis (small blue cells) are scattered among mature hepatocytes in the liver of this infant with nonimmune hydrops fetalis.

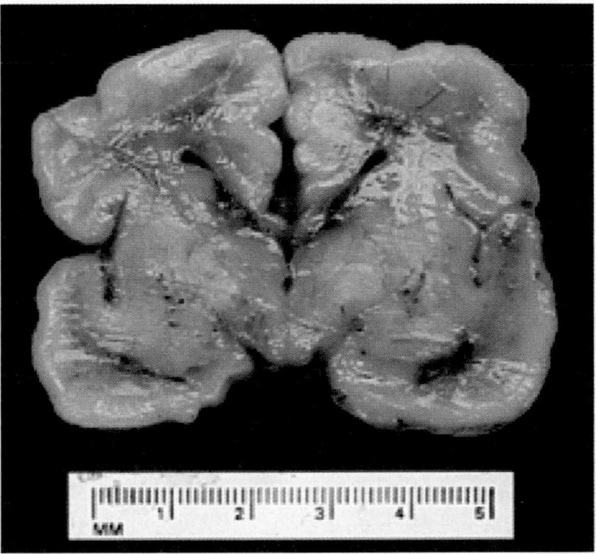

Figure 10-13 Kernicterus. Note the yellow discoloration of the brain parenchyma due to bilirubin accumulation, which is most prominent in the basal ganglia deep to the ventricles.

Inborn Errors of Metabolism and Other Genetic Disorders

Inborn errors of metabolism are well-characterized genetic abnormalities that give rise to metabolic disorders. Since Sir Archibald Garrod coined the term in 1908, the number of such diseases that have been recognized has increased exponentially and a comprehensive discussion of these diseases is beyond the scope of this chapter. *Most inborn errors of metabolism are rare diseases that are generally inherited as autosomal recessive or X-linked traits* (Chapter 5). Mitochondrial disorders (Chapter 5) form a distinct entity by themselves. Some of the clinical features that suggest an underlying metabolic disorder in a neonate are listed in Table 10-4. Three genetic disorders of metabolism, phenylketonuria (PKU), galactosemia, and cystic fibrosis, are selected for discussion here. PKU and galactosemia are reviewed because their early diagnosis (via neonatal screening programs) is particularly important and with appropriate dietary regimens early death or mental retardation can be prevented. Cystic fibrosis is included because it is one of the most common, potentially lethal diseases occurring in individuals of Caucasian descent.

Phenylketonuria

There are several variants of this inborn error of metabolism, which affects 1 in 10,000 live-born Caucasian infants. The most common form, referred to as *classic phenylketonuria*, is quite common in persons of Scandinavian descent and is distinctly uncommon in African American and Jewish populations.

Table 10-4 Abnormalities Suggesting Inborn Errors of Metabolism

General
Dysmorphic features Deafness Self-mutilation Abnormal hair Abnormal body or urine odor ("sweaty feet"; "mousy or musty"; "maple syrup") Hepatosplenomegaly; cardiomegaly Hydrops
Neurologic
Hypotonia or hypertonia Coma Persistent lethargy Seizures
Gastrointestinal
Poor feeding Recurrent vomiting Jaundice
Eyes
Cataract Cherry red macula Dislocated lens Glaucoma
Muscle, Joints
Myopathy Abnormal mobility

Adapted from Barness LA, Gilbert-Barness E: Metabolic diseases. In Gilbert-Barness E, et al (eds): Potter's Pathology of the Fetus, Infant, and Child. St. Louis, Mosby, 2007.

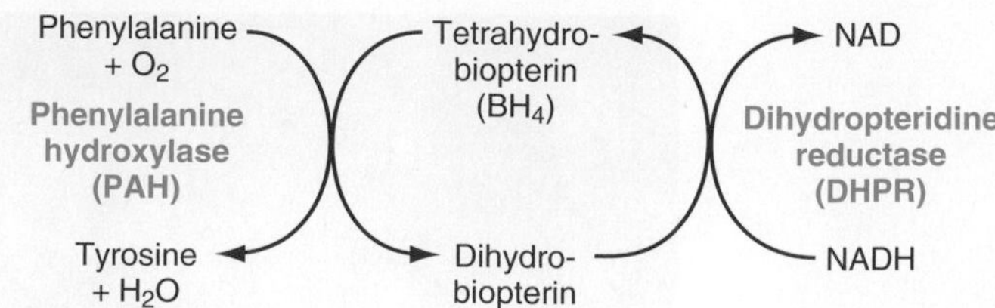

Figure 10-14 The phenylalanine hydroxylase system. Deficiency of PAH and DHPR can give rise to phenylketonuria.

Phenylketonuria (PKU) is an autosomal recessive disorder caused by a severe deficiency of the enzyme phenylalanine hydroxylase (PAH) and the resultant hyperphenylalaninemia. Affected infants are normal at birth but within a few weeks develop a rising plasma phenylalanine level, which impairs brain development. Usually by 6 months of life *severe mental retardation* becomes evident; fewer than 4% of untreated phenylketonuric children have IQs greater than 50 or 60. About one third of these children are never able to walk, and two thirds cannot talk. *Seizures,* other neurologic abnormalities, *decreased pigmentation of hair and skin,* and *eczema* often accompany the *mental retardation* in untreated children. Hyperphenylalaninemia and the resultant mental retardation can be avoided by restricting phenylalanine intake early in life. Hence, several screening procedures are routinely performed to detect PKU in the immediate postnatal period.

Many female PKU patients, if treated with dietary restriction early in life, reach childbearing age and are clinically asymptomatic. Most of them have marked hyperphenylalaninemia, because dietary treatment is discontinued after they reach adulthood. Between 75% and 90% of children born to such women are mentally retarded and microcephalic, and 15% have congenital heart disease, even though the infants themselves are heterozygotes. This syndrome, termed *maternal PKU,* results from the teratogenic effects of phenylalanine or its metabolites that cross the placenta and affect specific fetal organs during development. The presence and severity of the fetal anomalies directly correlate with the maternal phenylalanine level, so *it is imperative that maternal dietary restriction of phenylalanine be initiated before conception and continued throughout pregnancy.*

The biochemical abnormality in PKU is an inability to convert phenylalanine into tyrosine. In normal children, less than 50% of the dietary intake of phenylalanine is necessary for protein synthesis. The remainder is converted to tyrosine by the phenylalanine hydroxylase system (Fig. 10-14). When phenylalanine metabolism is blocked because of a lack of PAH enzyme, minor shunt pathways come into play, yielding several intermediates that are excreted in large amounts in the urine and in the sweat. These impart a *strong musty or mousy odor* to affected infants. It is believed that excess phenylalanine or its metabolites contribute to the brain damage in PKU. Concomitant lack of tyrosine (Fig. 10-14), a precursor of melanin, is responsible for the light color of hair and skin.

At the molecular level, approximately 500 mutant alleles of the *PAH* gene have been identified, only some of which cause a severe deficiency of the enzyme and thus result in classic PKU. Infants with mutations resulting in a complete lack of PAH activity present with the classic features of PKU, while those with up to 6% residual activity present

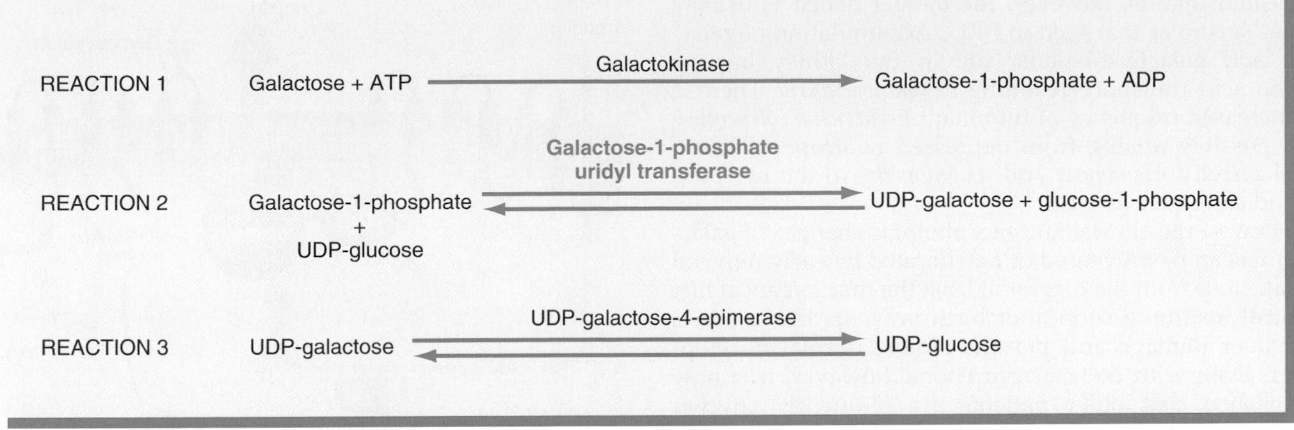

Figure 10-15 Pathways of galactose metabolism. ADP, Adenosine diphosphate; ATP, adenosine triphosphate; UDP, uridine diphosphate.

with milder disease. Moreover, some mutations result in only modest elevations of blood phenylalanine levels without associated neurologic damage. This latter condition, referred to as *benign hyperphenylalaninemia*, is important to recognize, because these individuals may well have positive screening tests but do not develop the stigmata of classic PKU. Because of the numerous disease-causing alleles of the phenylalanine hydroxylase gene, molecular diagnosis is not feasible, and measurement of serum phenylalanine levels is necessary to differentiate benign hyperphenylalaninemia from PKU; the levels in the latter are typically five-fold or more above normal. Once a biochemical diagnosis is established, the specific mutation causing PKU can be determined. With the identification of the mutation, carrier testing of at-risk family members can be performed.

While 98% of PKU is attributable to mutations in PAH, approximately 2% occur due to abnormalities in synthesis or recycling of the cofactor *tetrahydrobiopterin* BH_4 (Fig. 10-14). *It is clinically important to recognize these variant forms of PKU, because they cannot be treated by dietary restriction of phenylalanine.*

Galactosemia

Galactosemia is an autosomal recessive disorder of galactose metabolism resulting from accumulation of galactose-1-phosphate in tissues. Normally, lactose, the major carbohydrate of mammalian milk, is split into glucose and galactose in the intestinal microvilli by lactase. Galactose is then converted to glucose in three steps (Fig. 10-15). *Two variants of galactosemia have been identified. In the more common variant there is a total lack of galactose-1-phosphate uridyl transferase* (also known as *GALT*) *involved in reaction 2. The rare variant arises from a deficiency of galactokinase, involved in reaction 1.* Because galactokinase deficiency leads to a milder form of the disease not associated with mental retardation, it is not considered in this discussion. As a result of the transferase deficiency, *galactose-1-phosphate* accumulates in many locations, including the liver, spleen, lens of the eye, kidneys, heart muscle, cerebral cortex, and erythrocytes. Alternative metabolic pathways are activated, leading to the production of *galactitol* (a polyol metabolite of galactose) and *galactonate*, an oxidized by-product of excess galactose, both of which also accumulate in the tissues. Long-term toxicity in galactosemia has been variously imputed to these metabolic intermediates. Heterozygotes may have a mild enzyme deficiency but are spared the clinical and pathologic consequences of the homozygous state.

The clinical picture is variable, probably reflecting the heterogeneity of mutations in the galactose-1-phosphate uridyl transferase gene. The liver, eyes, and brain bear the brunt of the damage. The early-to-develop *hepatomegaly* is due largely to fatty change, but in time widespread scarring that closely resembles the cirrhosis of alcohol abuse may supervene (Fig. 10-16). *Opacification of the lens (cataract)* develops, probably because the lens absorbs water and swells as galactitol, produced by alternative metabolic pathways, accumulates and increases osmotic pressure. Nonspecific alterations appear in the CNS, including *loss of nerve cells, gliosis, and edema, particularly in the dentate nuclei of the cerebellum and the olivary nuclei of the medulla.* Similar changes may occur in the cerebral cortex and white matter.

These infants *fail to thrive* almost from birth. *Vomiting* and *diarrhea* appear within a few days of milk ingestion. *Jaundice* and *hepatomegaly* usually become evident during the first week of life and may seem to be a continuation of the physiologic jaundice of the newborn. The *cataracts* develop within a few weeks, and within the first 6 to 12 months of life *mental retardation* may be detected. Even in

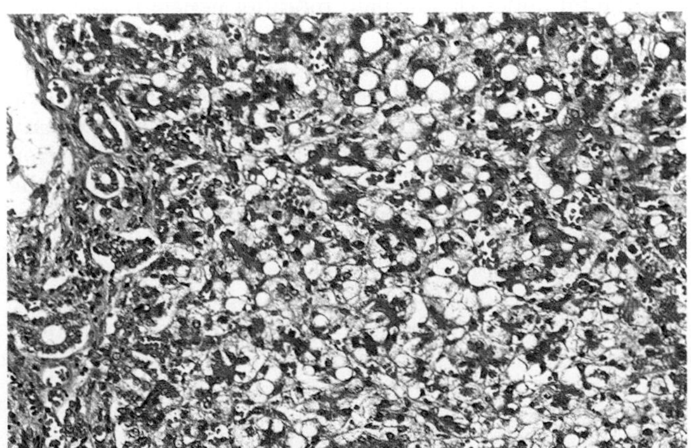

Figure 10-16 Galactosemia. The liver shows extensive fatty change and a delicate fibrosis. (Courtesy Dr. Wesley Tyson, The Children's Hospital, Denver, Colo.)

untreated infants, however, the mental deficit is usually not as severe as that seen in PKU. Accumulation of galactose and galactose-1-phosphate in the kidney impairs amino acid transport, resulting in *aminoaciduria.* There is an increased frequency of fulminant *Escherichia coli septicemia,* possibly arising from depressed neutrophil bactericidal activity. *Hemolysis* and *coagulopathy* in the newborn period can occur as well.

Many of the clinical and morphologic changes of galactosemia can be prevented or ameliorated by early removal of galactose from the diet for at least the first 2 years of life. Control instituted soon after birth prevents the cataracts and liver damage and permits almost normal development. Even with dietary restrictions, however, it is now established that older patients are frequently affected by a speech disorder and gonadal failure (especially premature ovarian failure) and, less commonly, ataxia.

Cystic Fibrosis (Mucoviscidosis)

Cystic fibrosis is an inherited disorder of ion transport that affects fluid secretion in exocrine glands and in the epithelial lining of the respiratory, gastrointestinal, and reproductive tracts. In many individuals this disorder leads to abnormally viscous secretions that obstruct organ passages, resulting in most of the clinical features of this disorder, such as *chronic lung disease secondary to recurrent infections, pancreatic insufficiency, steatorrhea, malnutrition, hepatic cirrhosis, intestinal obstruction, and male infertility.* These manifestations may appear at any point in life from before birth to much later in childhood or even in adolescence.

With an incidence of 1 in 2500 live births, *cystic fibrosis is the most common lethal genetic disease that affects Caucasian populations.* The carrier frequency in the United States is 1 in 20 among Caucasians but significantly lower in African Americans, Asians, and Hispanics. Although cystic fibrosis follows an *autosomal recessive* transmission pattern, recent data suggest that *even heterozygote carriers have a higher incidence of respiratory and pancreatic diseases* as compared with the general population. In addition, despite the classification of cystic fibrosis as a "mendelian" disorder, there is a wide degree of phenotypic variation that results from diverse mutations in the gene associated with cystic fibrosis, the tissue-specific effects of the encoded gene product, and the influence of so-called modifier genes.

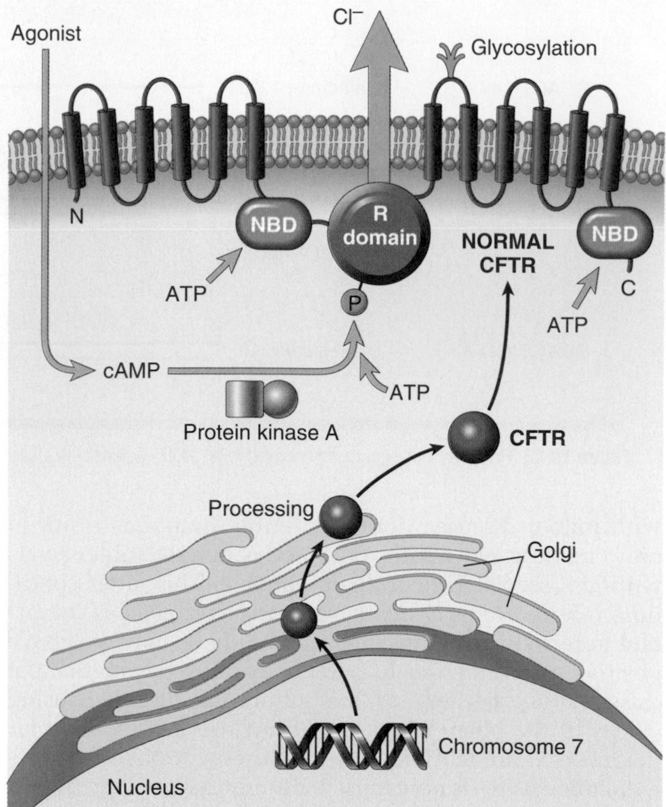

Figure 10-17 *Top*, Normal cystic fibrosis transmembrane conductance regulator (CFTR) structure and activation. CFTR consists of two transmembrane domains, two nucleotide-binding domains (NBDs), and a regulatory R domain. Agonists (e.g., acetylcholine) bind to epithelial cells and increase cyclic adenosine monophosphate (cAMP), which activates protein kinase A, the latter phosphorylating the CFTR at the R domain using ATP. This results in opening of the chloride channel. *Bottom*, CFTR from gene to protein. The most common mutation in the *CFTR* gene results in defective protein folding in the Golgi/endoplasmic reticulum and degradation of CFTR before it reaches the cell surface. Other mutations affect synthesis of CFTR, NBDs, and R domains, as well as membrane-spanning domains. (See text for details.)

Cystic Fibrosis Gene: Normal Structure and Function. In normal duct epithelia, chloride is transported by plasma membrane channels (chloride channels). **The primary defect in cystic fibrosis results from abnormal function of an epithelial chloride channel protein encoded by the cystic fibrosis transmembrane conductance regulator (CFTR) gene on chromosome 7q31.2.** The 1480-amino acid polypeptide encoded by CFTR has two transmembrane domains (each containing six α-helices), two cytoplasmic nucleotide-binding domains (NBDs), and a regulatory domain (R domain) that contains protein kinase A and C phosphorylation sites (Fig. 10-17). The two transmembrane domains form a channel through which chloride passes. Activation of the CFTR channel is mediated by agonist-induced increases in cyclic adenosine monophosphate (cAMP), followed by activation of a protein kinase A that phosphorylates the R domain. Adenosine triphosphate (ATP) binding and hydrolysis occurs at the NBD and is essential for the opening and closing of the channel pore in response to cAMP-mediated signaling. Several important facets of CFTR function have emerged in recent years:

- *CFTR regulates multiple additional ion channels and cellular processes.* Although initially characterized as a chloride-conductance channel, it is now recognized that CFTR can regulate multiple ion channels and cellular processes, primarily through interactions involving its NBDs. These include so-called outwardly rectified chloride channels, inwardly rectified potassium channels (Kir6.1), the epithelial sodium channel (ENaC), gap junction channels, and cellular processes involved in ATP transport and mucus secretion. Of these, the interaction of CFTR with the ENaC has possibly the most pathophysiologic relevance in cystic fibrosis. The ENaC is situated on the apical surface of exocrine epithelial cells and is responsible for sodium uptake from the

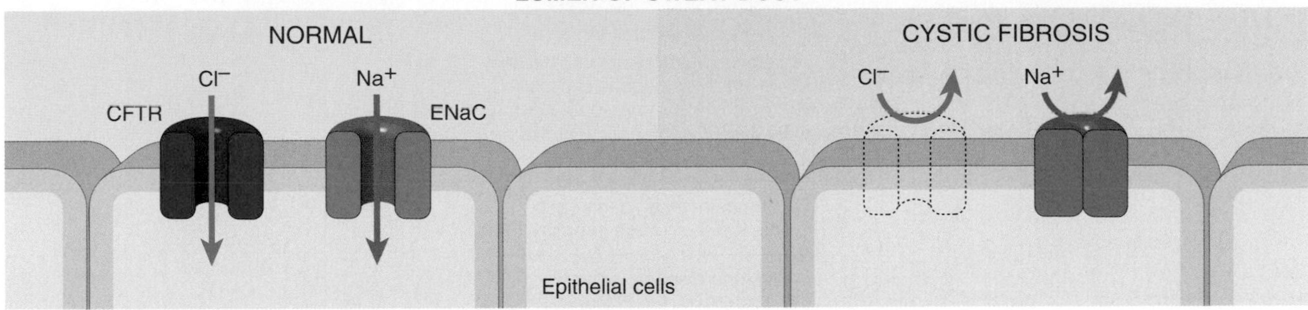

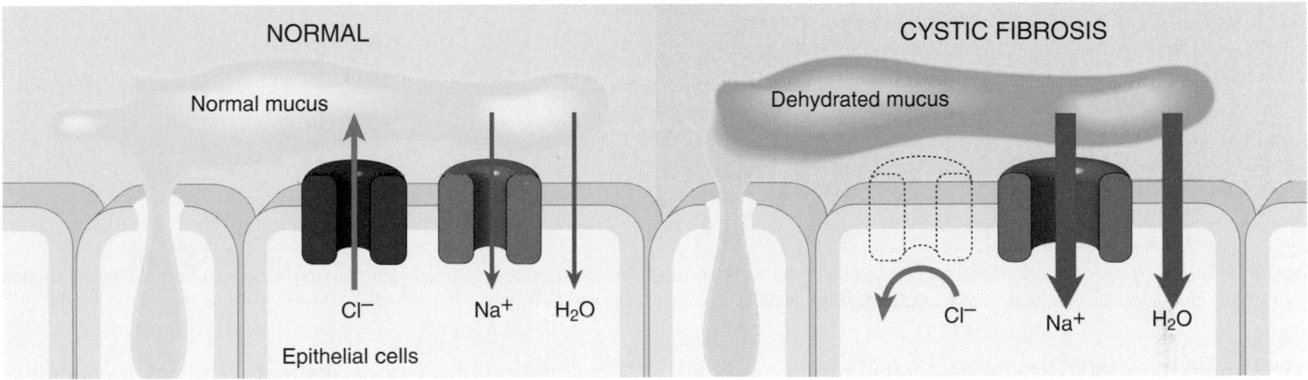

Figure 10-18 Chloride channel defect in the sweat duct *(top)* causes increased chloride and sodium concentration in sweat. In the airway *(bottom)*, patients with cystic fibrosis have decreased chloride secretion and increased sodium and water reabsorption leading to dehydration of the mucus layer coating epithelial cells, defective mucociliary action, and mucus plugging of airways. CFTR, Cystic fibrosis transmembrane conductance regulator; ENaC, epithelial sodium channel.

luminal fluid, rendering it (the luminal fluid) hypotonic. The ENaC is *inhibited* by normally functioning CFTR; hence, *in cystic fibrosis, ENaC activity increases, markedly augmenting sodium uptake across the apical membrane.* The importance of this phenomenon is discussed later in the context of pulmonary and gastrointestinal pathology in cystic fibrosis. The one exception to this rule happens to be the human sweat ducts, where ENaC activity *decreases* as a result of *CFTR* mutations; therefore, a hypertonic luminal fluid containing high sweat sodium chloride (the *sine qua non* of classic cystic fibrosis) is formed. This is the basis for the "salty" sweat that mothers can often detect in their affected infants.

- *The functions of* CFTR *are tissue-specific; therefore, the impact of a mutation in* CFTR *is also tissue-specific.* The major function of CFTR in the *sweat gland ducts* is to reabsorb luminal chloride ions and augment sodium reabsorption via the ENaC (see earlier). Therefore, in the sweat ducts, loss of CFTR function leads to decreased reabsorption of sodium chloride and production of hypertonic sweat (Fig. 10-18). However, in the *respiratory and intestinal epithelium,* the CFTR is one of the most important avenues for *active luminal secretion of chloride.* At these sites, *CFTR* mutations result in loss or reduction of chloride secretion into the lumen (Fig. 10-18). Active luminal sodium absorption is increased (due to loss of inhibition of ENaC activity), and both of these ion changes increase passive water reabsorption from the lumen, *lowering the water content of the surface fluid layer coating mucosal cells.* Thus, unlike the sweat ducts, there is no difference in the salt concentration of the surface fluid layer coating the respiratory and intestinal mucosal cells in normal individuals versus those with cystic fibrosis. Instead, *the pathogenesis of respiratory and intestinal complications in cystic fibrosis seems to stem from an isotonic but low-volume surface fluid layer.* In the lungs, this dehydration leads to defective mucociliary action and the accumulation of hyperconcentrated, viscid secretions that obstruct the air passages and predispose to recurrent pulmonary infections.
- CFTR *regulates transport of bicarbonate ions.* The bicarbonate transport function of CFTR is mediated by reciprocal interactions with a family of anion exchangers called SLC26, which are co-expressed on the apical surface with CFTR. In some *CFTR* mutants chloride transport is completely or substantially preserved, while *bicarbonate transport is markedly abnormal.* Alkaline fluids are secreted by normal tissues, in contrast fluids that are acidic (due to absence of bicarbonate ions) are secreted by epithelia harboring these mutant *CFTR* alleles. The acidity of secretions results in decreased luminal pH that can lead to a variety of adverse effects such as increased mucin precipitation and plugging of ducts, and increased binding of bacteria to plugged mucins. *Pancreatic insufficiency, a feature of classic cystic fibrosis, is virtually always present when there are CFTR mutations with abnormal bicarbonate conductance.*

Cystic Fibrosis Gene: Mutational Spectra and Genotype-Phenotype Correlation. Since the *CFTR* gene was cloned

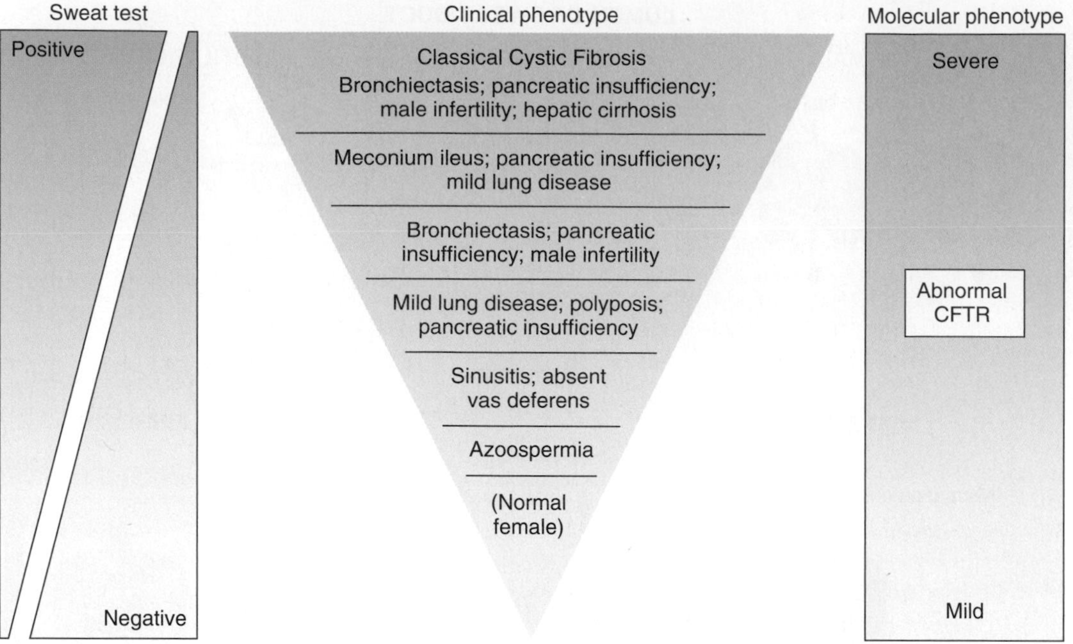

Figure 10-19 The many clinical manifestations of mutations in the cystic fibrosis gene, from most severe to asymptomatic. (Redrawn from Wallis C: Diagnosing cystic fibrosis: blood, sweat, and tears. Arch Dis Child 76:85, 1997.)

in 1989, more than 1800 disease-associated mutations have been identified. The mutations can be grouped into six classes based on their effect on the CFTR protein:

- Class I: *Defective protein synthesis.* These mutations are associated with complete lack of CFTR protein at the apical surface of epithelial cells.
- Class II: *Abnormal protein folding, processing, and trafficking.* These mutations result in defective processing of the protein from the endoplasmic reticulum to the Golgi apparatus; the protein does not become fully folded and glycosylated and is instead degraded before it reaches the cell surface. The most common class II mutation is a deletion of three nucleotides coding for phenylalanine at amino acid position 508 (ΔF508). Worldwide, this mutation can be found in approximately 70% of cystic fibrosis patients. Class II mutations are also associated with complete lack of CFTR protein at the apical surface of epithelial cells.
- Class III: *Defective regulation.* Mutations in this class prevent activation of CFTR by abrogating ATP binding and hydrolysis, an essential prerequisite for ion transport (see earlier). Thus, there is a normal amount of CFTR on the apical surface, but it is nonfunctional.
- Class IV: *Decreased conductance.* These mutations typically occur in the transmembrane domain of *CFTR*, which forms the ionic pore for chloride transport. There is a normal amount of CFTR at the apical membrane, but with reduced function. This class is usually associated with a milder phenotype.
- Class V: *Reduced abundance.* These mutations typically affect intronic splice sites or the *CFTR* promoter, such that there is a reduced amount of normal protein. As discussed subsequently, class V mutations are also associated with a milder phenotype.
- Class VI: *Altered function in regulation of ion channels.* As previously described, CFTR is involved in the regulation of multiple distinct cellular ion channels, of which its role in regulating bicarbonate secretion through relevant apical channels is required for maintaining luminal pH balance. Mutations in this class affect the regulatory role of CFTR. In some cases, a given mutation affects the conductance by CFTR as well as regulation of other ion channels. For example, the ΔF508 mutation is both a class II and class VI mutation.

Because cystic fibrosis is an autosomal recessive disease, affected individuals harbor mutations on both alleles. However, the nature of mutations on each of the two alleles can have a remarkable effect on the overall phenotype, as well as on organ-specific manifestations (Fig. 10-19). Thus, two "severe" mutations (for example, a combination of Class I, II or III mutations in any permutation) that produce virtual absence of membrane CFTR function are associated with the classic cystic fibrosis phenotype (pancreatic insufficiency, sinopulmonary infections, and gastrointestinal symptoms), while the presence of a "mild" (class IV or V) mutation on one or both alleles results in a less severe phenotype. This general dictum of genotype-phenotype correlation is most consistent for pancreatic disease, wherein the presence of one allele with a mild mutation associated with some CFTR activity can prevent the pancreatic insufficiency that is virtually always seen with homozygosity for "severe" mutations. By contrast, genotype-phenotype correlations are far less consistent in pulmonary disease, due to the effect of secondary modifiers (see later). As genetic testing for *CFTR* mutations has expanded, *it has become evident that some patients who present with clinical features apparently unrelated to cystic fibrosis may also harbor* CFTR *mutations.* These include individuals with *idiopathic chronic pancreatitis, late-onset chronic pulmonary disease, idiopathic bronchiectasis,* and *obstructive azoospermia* caused by bilateral absence of the vas deferens (see detailed discussion of individual phenotypes later). Most of these patients do not demonstrate other features of cystic fibrosis, despite the presence of bi-allelic *CFTR* mutations; these patients are classified as having *nonclassic* or *atypical cystic fibrosis.* Identifying these individuals is important not only for subsequent management, but also for genetic counseling.

Genetic and Environmental Modifiers. **Although cystic fibrosis remains one of the best-known examples of the "one gene, one disease" axiom, there is now considerable evidence that genes other than CFTR modify the frequency and severity of certain organ-specific manifestations, especially pulmonary manifestations and neonatal meconium ileus.** Not surprisingly, polymorphisms in genes whose products modulate neutrophil function in response to bacterial infections act as modifier loci for the severity of pulmonary disease in cystic fibrosis. Examples of such modifier genes include *mannose binding lectin 2 (MBL2), transforming growth factor β1 (TGFB1)* and *interferon related developmental regulator 1 (IFRD1).* It is postulated that polymorphisms in these genes regulate the resistance of the lungs to exogenous infections with virulent microbes (see later), thus modifying the natural history of cystic fibrosis. Similarly, several other genetic modifiers appear to influence the incidence of meconium ileus in cystic fibrosis, although the degree of association is less stringent than that observed for pulmonary manifestations.

Environmental modifiers may also explain the significant phenotypic differences between individuals who share the same *CFTR* genotype. This is best exemplified in pulmonary disease, where *CFTR* genotype and phenotype correlations can be perplexing. As stated earlier, defective mucociliary action because of deficient hydration of the mucus results in an inability to clear bacteria from the airways. *Pseudomonas aeruginosa* species, in particular, colonize the lower respiratory tract, first intermittently and then chronically. Concurrent viral infections predispose to such colonization. The static mucus creates a hypoxic microenvironment in the airway surface fluid, which in turn favors the production of *alginate,* a mucoid polysaccharide capsule, by the colonizing bacteria. Alginate production permits the formation of a biofilm that protects the bacteria from antibodies and antibiotics, allowing them to evade host defenses, and produce a chronic destructive lung disease. Antibody- and cell-mediated immune reactions induced by the organisms result in further pulmonary destruction, but are ineffective against the organism. It is evident, therefore, that in addition to genetic factors (e.g., class of mutation), a plethora of environmental modifiers (e.g., virulence of organisms, efficacy of therapy, intercurrent and concurrent infections by other organisms, exposure to tobacco and allergens) can influence the severity and progression of lung disease in cystic fibrosis.

MORPHOLOGY

The anatomic changes are highly variable in distribution and severity. In individuals with nonclassic cystic fibrosis, the disease is quite mild and does not seriously disturb their growth and development. In others, the pancreatic involvement is severe and impairs intestinal absorption because of the pancreatic insufficiency (Chapter 19), and so malabsorption stunts development and post-natal growth. In others, the mucus secretion defect leads to defective mucociliary action, obstruction of bronchi and bronchioles, and crippling fatal pulmonary infections. In all variants, the **sweat glands are morphologically unaffected.**

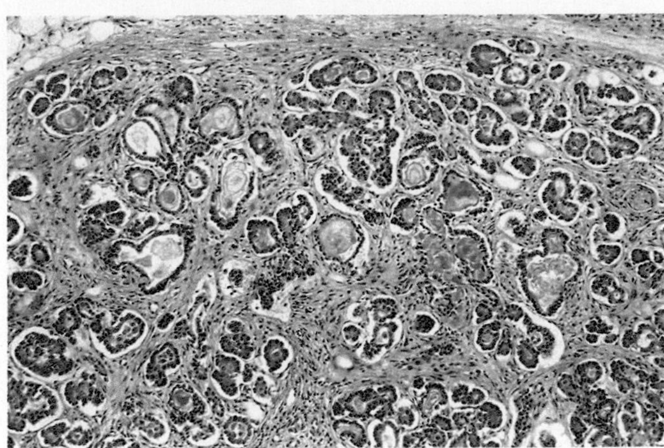

Figure 10-20 Pancreas in cystic fibrosis. The ducts are dilated and plugged with eosinophilic mucin, and the parenchymal glands are atrophic and replaced by fibrous tissue.

Pancreatic abnormalities are present in approximately 85% to 90% of patients with cystic fibrosis. In the milder cases, there may be only accumulations of mucus in the small ducts with some dilation of the exocrine glands. In more severe cases, usually seen in older children or adolescents, the ducts are completely plugged, causing atrophy of the exocrine glands and progressive fibrosis (Fig. 10-20). Atrophy of the exocrine portion of the pancreas may occur, leaving only the islets within a fibrofatty stroma. The loss of pancreatic exocrine secretion impairs fat absorption, and the associated avitaminosis A may contribute to squamous metaplasia of the lining epithelium of the ducts in the pancreas, which are already injured by the inspissated mucus secretions. Thick viscid plugs of mucus may also be found in the small intestine of infants. Sometimes these cause small-bowel obstruction, known as **meconium ileus**.

The **liver involvement** follows the same basic pattern. Bile canaliculi are plugged by mucus material, accompanied by ductular proliferation and portal inflammation. Hepatic **steatosis** is not an uncommon finding in liver biopsies. Over time, **focal biliary cirrhosis** develops in approximately a third of patients (Chapter 18), which can eventually involve the entire liver, resulting in diffuse hepatic nodularity. Such severe hepatic involvement is encountered in less than 10% of patients.

The **salivary glands** frequently show histologic changes similar to those described in the pancreas: progressive dilation of ducts, squamous metaplasia of the lining epithelium, and glandular atrophy followed by fibrosis.

The **pulmonary changes** are the most serious complications of this disease (Fig. 10-21). These stem from the viscous mucus secretions of the submucosal glands of the respiratory tree leading to secondary obstruction and infection of the air passages. The bronchioles are often distended with thick mucus associated with marked hyperplasia and hypertrophy of

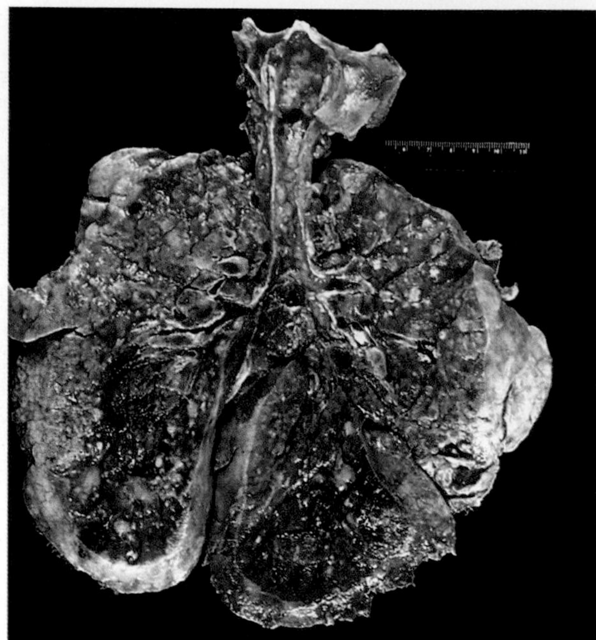

Figure 10-21 Lungs of a patient dying of cystic fibrosis. There is extensive mucus plugging and dilation of the tracheobronchial tree. The pulmonary parenchyma is consolidated by a combination of both secretions and pneumonia—the green color associated with *Pseudomonas* infections. (Courtesy Dr. Eduardo Yunis, Children's Hospital of Pittsburgh, Pittsburgh, Pa.)

the mucus-secreting cells. Superimposed infections give rise to severe chronic bronchitis and bronchiectasis (Chapter 15). In many instances, lung abscesses develop. *Staphylococcus aureus*, *Haemophilus influenzae*, and *Pseudomonas aeruginosa* are the three most common organisms responsible for lung infections. As mentioned earlier, a mucoid form of *P. aeruginosa* (alginate-producing) is particularly frequent and causes chronic inflammation. Even more sinister is the increasing frequency of infection with another group of pseudomonads, the *Burkholderia cepacia* complex, which includes at least nine different species; of these, infections with *B. cenocepacia* are the most common in cystic fibrosis patients. This opportunistic bacterium is particularly hardy, and infection with this organism has been associated with fulminant illness ("cepacia syndrome"), longer hospital stays, and increased mortality. Other opportunistic bacterial pathogens include *Stenotrophomonas maltophilia* and *nontuberculous mycobacteria*; *allergic bronchopulmonary aspergillosis* also occurs with increased frequency in cystic fibrosis.

Azoospermia and infertility are found in 95% of the males who survive to adulthood; **congenital bilateral absence of the vas deferens** is a frequent finding in these patients. In some males, bilateral absence of the vas deferens may be the only feature suggestive of an underlying *CFTR* mutation.

Clinical Features. Few childhood diseases are as protean as cystic fibrosis in clinical manifestations (Table 10-5). The symptoms are extremely varied and may appear at birth to years later, and involve one organ system or many. Approximately 5% to 10% of the cases come to clinical attention at birth or soon after because of *meconium ileus.* Distal intestinal obstruction can also occur in older individuals, manifesting as recurrent episodes of right lower quadrant pain sometimes associated with a palpable mass of meconium, with or without associated intussusception, in the right iliac fossa.

Exocrine pancreatic insufficiency occurs in the majority (85% to 90%) of patients with cystic fibrosis and is associated with "severe" *CFTR* mutations on *both* alleles (e.g., *ΔF508/ΔF508*), whereas 10% to 15% of patients with one "severe" and one "mild" *CFTR* mutation *(ΔF508/R117H)* or two "mild" *CFTR* mutations retain enough pancreatic exocrine function so as not to require enzyme supplementation (*pancreas-sufficient* phenotype). Pancreatic insufficiency is associated with protein and fat malabsorption and increased fecal loss. Manifestations of malabsorption (e.g., large, foul-smelling stools, abdominal distention, and poor weight gain) may appear during the first year of life. The faulty fat absorption may induce deficiency of the fat-soluble vitamins, resulting in manifestations of avitaminosis A, D, or K. Hypoproteinemia may be severe enough to cause generalized edema. Persistent diarrhea may result in rectal prolapse in up to 10% of children with this disease. The *pancreas-sufficient* phenotype is usually not associated with other gastrointestinal complications, and in general, these individuals demonstrate excellent growth and development. A subset of patients with pancreas-sufficient cystic fibrosis have recurrent bouts of pancreatitis associated with acute abdominal pain and

Table 10-5 Clinical Features and Diagnostic Criteria for Cystic Fibrosis

Clinical Features of Cystic Fibrosis

1. *Chronic sinopulmonary disease manifested by*
   a. Persistent colonization/infection with typical cystic fibrosis pathogens, including *Staphylococcus aureus*, nontypeable *Haemophilus influenzae*, mucoid and nonmucoid *Pseudomonas aeruginosa, Burkholderia cepacia*
   b. Chronic cough and sputum production
   c. Persistent chest radiograph abnormalities (e.g., bronchiectasis, atelectasis, infiltrates, hyperinflation)
   d. Airway obstruction manifested by wheezing and air trapping
   e. Nasal polyps; radiographic or computed tomographic abnormalities of paranasal sinuses
   f. Digital clubbing
2. *Gastrointestinal and nutritional abnormalities, including*
   a. Intestinal: meconium ileus, distal intestinal obstruction syndrome, rectal prolapse
   b. Pancreatic: pancreatic insufficiency, recurrent acute pancreatitis, chronic pancreatitis
   c. Hepatic: chronic hepatic disease manifested by clinical or histologic evidence of focal biliary cirrhosis, or multilobular cirrhosis, prolonged neonatal jaundice
   d. Nutritional: failure to thrive (protein-calorie malnutrition), hypoproteinemia, edema, complications secondary to fat-soluble vitamin deficiency
3. *Salt-loss syndromes: acute salt depletion, chronic metabolic alkalosis*
4. *Male urogenital abnormalities resulting in obstructive azoospermia (congenital bilateral absence of vas deferens)*

Criteria for Diagnosis of Cystic Fibrosis

One or more characteristic phenotypic features,
OR a history of cystic fibrosis in a sibling,
OR a positive newborn screening test result
AND
An increased sweat chloride concentration on two or more occasions
OR identification of two cystic fibrosis mutations,
OR demonstration of abnormal epithelial nasal ion transport

Adapted with permission from Rosenstein BJ, Cutting GR: The diagnosis of cystic fibrosis: a consensus statement. J Pediatr 132:589, 1998.

occasionally, life-threatening complications. These patients have other features of classic cystic fibrosis, such as pulmonary disease. By contrast, *"idiopathic" chronic pancreatitis* can also occur as an isolated late-onset finding in the absence of other stigmata of cystic fibrosis (Chapter 19); bi-allelic *CFTR* mutations (usually one "mild," one "severe") are demonstrable in the majority of these individuals who have *nonclassic or atypical cystic fibrosis. Endocrine pancreatic insufficiency* (i.e., diabetes) is uncommon in cystic fibrosis and is caused by severe destruction of pancreatic parenchyma including the islets.

Cardiorespiratory complications, such as persistent lung infections, obstructive pulmonary disease, and *cor pulmonale*, are the most common cause of death (~80%) in patients in the United States. By age 18, 80% of patients with classic cystic fibrosis harbor *P. aeruginosa*, and 3.5% harbor *B. cepacia*. With the indiscriminate use of antibiotic prophylaxis against *Staphylococcus*, there has been an unfortunate resurgence of resistant strains of *Pseudomonas* in many patients. Individuals who carry one "severe" and one "mild" *CFTR* mutation may develop late-onset mild pulmonary disease, another example of nonclassic or atypical cystic fibrosis. Patients with mild pulmonary disease usually have little or no pancreatic disease. Adult-onset *"idiopathic" bronchiectasis*, has been linked to *CFTR* mutations in a subset of cases. *Recurrent sinonasal polyps* can occur in 10% to 25% of individuals with cystic fibrosis; hence, children who present with this finding should be tested for cystic fibrosis.

Significant *liver disease* occurs late in the natural history of cystic fibrosis and is gaining in clinical importance as life expectancies increase. In fact, after cardiopulmonary and transplantation-related complications, liver disease is the most common cause of death in cystic fibrosis. Most studies suggest that symptomatic or biochemical liver disease has its onset at or around puberty, with a prevalence of approximately 13% to 17%. However, *asymptomatic hepatomegaly* may be present in up to a third of individuals. Obstruction of the common bile duct may occur due to stones or sludge; it presents with abdominal pain and the acute onset of jaundice. As previously noted, *diffuse biliary cirrhosis* develops in less than 10% of individuals with cystic fibrosis.

Approximately 95% of males with cystic fibrosis are *infertile*, as a result of obstructive azoospermia. As mentioned earlier, this is most commonly due to congenital bilateral absence of the vas deferens, which is caused in 80% of cases by bi-allelic *CFTR* mutations.

In most cases, the diagnosis of cystic fibrosis is based on persistently elevated sweat electrolyte concentrations (often the mother makes the diagnosis by recognizing her infant's abnormally salty sweat), characteristic clinical findings (sinopulmonary disease and gastrointestinal manifestations), an abnormal newborn screening test, or a family history. A minority of patients with cystic fibrosis, especially those with at least one "mild" *CFTR* mutation, may have a normal or near-normal sweat test (<60 mM/L). Measurement of nasal transepithelial potential difference in vivo can be a useful adjunct under these circumstances; individuals with cystic fibrosis demonstrate a significantly more negative baseline nasal potential difference than controls. Sequencing the *CFTR* gene is the gold standard for diagnosis of cystic fibrosis. Therefore, in patients with suggestive clinical findings or family history (or both), genetic analysis may be warranted.

There have been major improvements in the management of acute and chronic complications for cystic fibrosis, including more potent antimicrobial therapies, pancreatic enzyme replacement, and bilateral lung transplantation. New treatment modalities for restoring mutant CFTR function are being tested in clinical trials. For example, the first-in-class of a group of agents known as CFTR "potentiators" has been recently approved for use in a minority (~3%-5%) of cystic fibrosis patients that harbor a G155D mutation in the *CFTR* gene. This particular mutation is a class IV alteration, in which functionally defective CFTR is present in otherwise normal amounts at the cell membrane; the orally bioavailable CFTR "potentiator" partially restores the critical ion transport functions to the defective channel. Overall, improvements in the management of cystic fibrosis has extended the median life expectancy to close to 40 years and increasingly, a lethal disease of childhood is changing into a chronic disease of adults.

Sudden Infant Death Syndrome (SIDS)

According to the National Institute of Child Health and Human Development, **SIDS is defined as "the sudden death of an infant under 1 year of age which remains unexplained after a thorough case investigation, including performance of a complete autopsy, examination of the death scene, and review of the clinical history."** It is important to emphasize that many cases of sudden death in infancy may have an unexpected anatomic or biochemical basis discernible at autopsy (Table 10-6), and these should not be labeled as SIDS, but rather as *sudden unexpected infant death (SUID)*. The Centers for Disease Control and Prevention estimates that SIDS accounts for approximately half of the cases of SUID in the United States. An aspect of SIDS that is not stressed in the definition is that the infant usually dies while asleep, mostly in the prone or side position, hence the pseudonyms of *crib death* or *cot death*.

Epidemiology. As infantile deaths due to nutritional problems and infections have come under control in developed countries, SIDS has assumed greater importance, including in the United States. SIDS is the leading cause of death between age 1 month and 1 year in this country and the third leading cause of death overall in infancy, after congenital anomalies and diseases of prematurity and low birth weight. Mostly because of nationwide SIDS awareness campaigns by organizations such as the American Academy of Pediatrics, there has been a significant drop in SIDS-related mortality in the past decade, from an estimated 120 deaths per 100,000 live births in 1992 to 54 per 100,000 in 2005. This number translates to about 2000 deaths due to SIDS in the US. Worldwide, in countries where unexpected infant deaths are diagnosed as SIDS only after postmortem examination, the death rates from SIDS range from 10 per 100,000 live births in the Netherlands to 80 per 100,000 in New Zealand.

Approximately 90% of all SIDS deaths occur during the first 6 months of life, most between ages 2 and 4 months. This narrow window of peak susceptibility is a unique characteristic that is independent of other risk factors (to

Table 10-6 Risk Factors and Postmortem Findings Associated with Sudden Infant Death Syndrome

Parental
Young maternal age (age younger than 20 years)
Maternal smoking during pregnancy
Drug abuse in *either* parent, specifically paternal marijuana and maternal opiate, cocaine use
Short intergestational intervals
Late or no prenatal care
Low socioeconomic group
African-American and American Indian ethnicity (? socioeconomic factors)
Infant
Brain stem abnormalities, associated with delayed development of arousal and cardiorespiratory control
Prematurity and/or low birth weight
Male sex
Product of a multiple birth
SIDS in a prior sibling
Antecedent respiratory infections
Germline polymorphisms in autonomic nervous system genes
Environment
Prone or side sleep position
Sleeping on a soft surface
Hyperthermia
Co-sleeping in first 3 months of life
Postmortem Abnormalities Detected in Cases of Sudden Unexpected Infant Death (SUID)*
Infections
Viral myocarditis
Bronchopneumonia
Unsuspected congenital anomaly
Congenital aortic stenosis
Anomalous origin of the left coronary artery from the pulmonary artery
Traumatic child abuse
Intentional suffocation (filicide)
Genetic and metabolic defects
Long QT syndrome (*SCN5A* and *KCNQ1* mutations)
Fatty acid oxidation disorders (*MCAD, LCHAD, SCHAD* mutations)
Histiocytoid cardiomyopathy (*MTCYB* mutations)
Abnormal inflammatory responsiveness (partial deletions in *C4a* and *C4b*)

*SIDS is not the only cause of SUIDs, but rather is a *diagnosis of exclusion*. Therefore, performance of an autopsy may often reveal findings that would explain the cause of an SUID. These cases should *not*, strictly speaking, be labeled as "SIDS." SCN5A, sodium channel, voltage-gated, type V, alpha polypeptide; KCNQ1, potassium voltage-gated channel, KQT-like subfamily, member 1; MCAD, medium-chain acyl coenzyme A dehydrogenase; LCHAD, long-chain 3-hydroxyacyl coenzyme A dehydrogenase; SCHAD, short-chain 3-hydroxyacyl coenzyme A dehydrogenase; MTCYB, mitochondrial cytochrome *b*; C4, complement component 4.

be described) and the geographic locale. Most infants who die of SIDS die at home, usually during the night after a period of sleep. For many years, prolonged apnea was considered to be a risk factor for SIDS. Infants who developed a so-called *"apparent life-threatening event"* (ALTE), characterized by some combination of apnea, marked change in color or muscle tone, choking or gagging, were considered at risk for subsequent SIDS. However, epidemiologic studies have demonstrated that these "life-threatening events" and SIDS have different risk factors and ages of onset, and are probably unrelated entities. Children experiencing ALTEs are often premature or have a mechanical basis for respiratory compromise. This distinction might explain why home apnea monitors, which have proliferated among American families for "SIDS prevention," have had minimal impact on reducing the risk of SIDS.

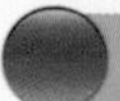

MORPHOLOGY

In infants who have died of suspected SIDS, a variety of findings have been reported at postmortem examination. They are usually subtle and of uncertain significance and are not present in all cases. Multiple petechiae are the most common finding (~80% of cases); these are usually present on the thymus, visceral and parietal pleura, and epicardium. Grossly, the lungs are usually congested, and vascular engorgement with or without pulmonary edema is demonstrable microscopically in the majority of cases. These changes possibly represent agonal events, because they are found with comparable frequencies in *explained* sudden deaths in infancy. Within the upper respiratory system (larynx and trachea), there may be some histologic evidence of recent infection (correlating with the clinical symptoms), although the changes are not sufficiently severe to account for death and should not detract from the diagnosis of SIDS. The CNS demonstrates astrogliosis of the brain stem and cerebellum. Sophisticated morphometric studies have revealed quantitative brain-stem abnormalities such as hypoplasia of the arcuate nucleus or a decrease in brain-stem neuronal populations in several cases; these observations are not uniform, however. Nonspecific findings include frequent persistence of hepatic extramedullary hematopoiesis and periadrenal brown fat; it is tempting to speculate that these latter findings relate to chronic hypoxemia, retardation of normal development, and chronic stress. Thus, autopsy usually fails to provide a clear cause of death, and this may well be related to the etiologic heterogeneity of SIDS. The importance of a postmortem examination rests in identifying other causes of SUID, such as unsuspected infection, congenital anomaly, or a genetic disorder (Table 10-6), the presence of any of which would *exclude* a diagnosis of SIDS; and in ruling out the unfortunate possibility of traumatic child abuse.

Pathogenesis. The circumstances surrounding SIDS have been explored in great detail, and it is generally accepted that it is a *multifactorial condition,* with a variable mixture of contributing factors. **A "triple-risk" model of SIDS has been proposed, which postulates the intersection of three overlapping factors: (1) a vulnerable infant, (2) a critical developmental period in homeostatic control, and (3) an exogenous stressor.** According to this model, several factors make the infant vulnerable to sudden death during the critical developmental period (i.e., the first 6 months of life). These vulnerability factors may relate to the parents or the infant, while the exogenous stressor(s) are environmental (Table 10-6).

While numerous factors have been proposed to account for a vulnerable infant, *the most compelling hypothesis is that SIDS reflects a delayed development of "arousal" and cardiorespiratory control.* The brain stem, and in particular the medulla oblongata, plays a critical role in the body's "arousal" response to noxious stimuli such as episodic hypercarbia, hypoxia, and thermal stress encountered during sleep. The serotonergic (5-HT) system of the medulla is implicated in these "arousal" responses, as well as regulation of other critical homeostatic functions such as respiratory drive, blood pressure, and upper airway reflexes. Abnormalities in serotonin-dependent signaling in the brain stem may be the underlying basis for SIDS in some infants.

Epidemiologic and genetic studies have identified additional vulnerability factors for SIDS in the "triple-risk" model. Infants who are born before term or who are low birth weight are at increased risk, and risk increases with decreasing gestational age or birth weight. As stated, male sex is associated with a slightly greater incidence of SIDS. SIDS in a prior sibling is associated with a fivefold relative risk of recurrence, highlighting the importance of a genetic predisposition; *traumatic child abuse must be carefully excluded under these circumstances.* Most SIDS babies have an immediate prior history of a mild respiratory tract infection, but no single causative organism has been isolated. These infections may predispose an already vulnerable infant to even greater impairment of cardiorespiratory control and delayed arousal. In this context, *laryngeal chemoreceptors* have emerged as a putative "missing link" between upper respiratory tract infections, the prone position, and SIDS. When stimulated, these laryngeal chemoreceptors typically elicit an inhibitory cardiorespiratory reflex. Stimulation of the chemoreceptors is augmented by respiratory tract infections, which increase the volume of secretions, and by the prone position, which impairs swallowing and clearing of the airways even in healthy infants. In a previously vulnerable infant with impaired arousal, the resulting inhibitory cardiorespiratory reflex may prove fatal. Genetic vulnerability factors in the infant include polymorphisms of genes related to serotonergic signaling and autonomic innervation, pointing to the importance of these processes in the pathophysiology of SIDS.

In addition to infant vulnerability factors, several maternal risk factors have also been identified. *Maternal smoking during pregnancy* has consistently emerged as a risk factor in epidemiologic studies of SIDS, with children exposed to in utero nicotine having more than double the risk of SIDS as compared with children born to nonsmokers. Young maternal age, frequent childbirths, and inadequate prenatal care are all risk factors associated with increased incidence of SIDS in the offspring.

Among the potential "environmental stressors," prone or side sleeping positions, sleeping with parents in the first 3 months, sleeping on soft surfaces, and thermal stress are probably the most important modifiable risk factors for SIDS. The prone or side positions predispose an infant to one or more recognized noxious stimuli (hypoxia, hypercarbia, and thermal stress) during sleep. The side position was considered a reliable alternative to the prone sleeping position, but *the American Academy of Pediatrics now recognizes the supine sleeping position as the only safe position that reduces the risk of SIDS.* This "Back to Sleep" campaign has resulted in substantial reductions in SIDS-related deaths since its inception in 1994.

As has been stated, SIDS is far from the only cause of SUIDs. **In fact, SIDS is a diagnosis of exclusion, requiring careful examination of the death scene and a complete postmortem examination.** The latter can reveal an unsuspected cause of sudden death in as many as 20% or more of "SIDS" babies. Infections (e.g., viral myocarditis or bronchopneumonia) are the most common causes of sudden "unexpected" death, followed by unsuspected congenital anomalies. In part as a result of advancements in molecular diagnostics and knowledge of the human genome, several genetic causes of sudden "unexpected" infant death have emerged. For example, fatty acid oxidation disorders, characterized by defects in mitochondrial fatty acid oxidative enzymes, may be responsible for as many as 5% of SUIDs. Other newly emerging genetic causes of sudden death are listed in Table 10-6.

Tumors and Tumor-like Lesions of Infancy and Childhood

Only 2% of all malignant tumors occur in infancy and childhood; nonetheless, cancer (including leukemia) accounts for about 9% of deaths in the United States in children older than age 4 and up to age 14 years, and only accidents cause significantly more deaths. Benign tumors are even more common than cancers. Most benign tumors are of little concern, but on occasion they cause serious complications by virtue of their location or rapid increase in size.

It is sometimes difficult to separate, on morphologic grounds, true tumors or neoplasms from tumor-like lesions in the infant and child. In this context, two special categories of tumor-like lesions should be distinguished from true tumors.

- The term *heterotopia* (or *choristoma*) is applied to microscopically normal cells or tissues that are present in abnormal locations. Examples of heterotopias include a rest of pancreatic tissue found in the wall of the stomach or small intestine, or a small mass of adrenal cells found in the kidney, lungs, ovaries, or elsewhere. These heterotopic rests are usually of little significance, but they can be confused clinically with neoplasms. Rarely, they are sites of origin of true neoplasms, producing paradoxes such as an adrenal carcinoma arising in the ovary.
- The term *hamartoma* refers to an excessive, focal overgrowth of cells and tissues native to the organ in which it occurs. Although the cellular elements are mature and identical to those found in the remainder of the organ, they do not reproduce the normal architecture of the surrounding tissue. The line of demarcation between a hamartoma and a benign neoplasm is often unclear, since both lesions can be clonal. Hemangiomas, lymphangiomas, rhabdomyomas of the heart, adenomas of the liver, and developmental cysts within the kidneys, lungs, or pancreas are interpreted by some as hamartomas and by others as true neoplasms. Their unequivocally benign histology, however, does not preclude bothersome and rarely life-threatening clinical problems in some cases.

Benign Tumors and Tumor-Like Lesions

Virtually any tumor may be encountered in children, but within this wide array hemangiomas, lymphangiomas, fibrous lesions, and teratomas deserve special mention. You will notice that the most common neoplasms of childhood are so-called soft-tissue tumors of mesenchymal derivation. This contrasts with adults, in whom the most common tumors, benign or malignant, have an epithelial origin. Benign tumors of various tissues are described in

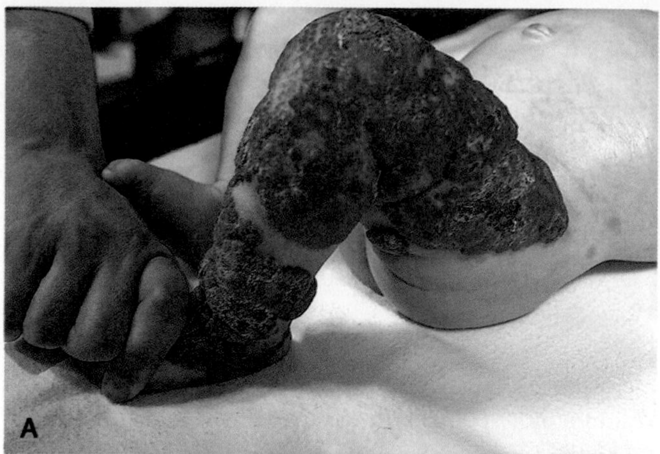

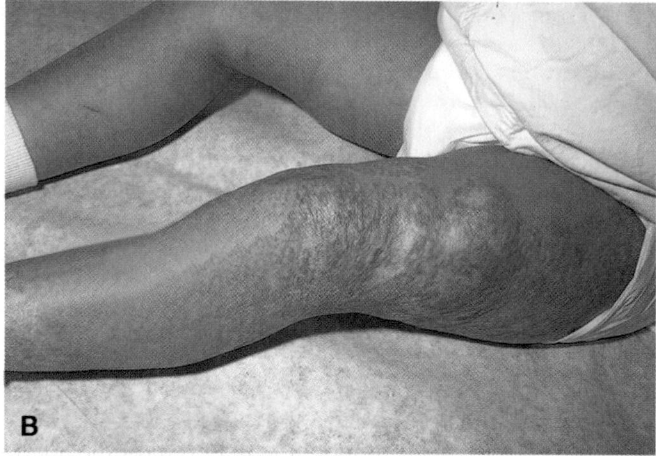

Figure 10-22 Congenital capillary hemangioma at birth (**A**) and at age 2 years (**B**) after spontaneous regression. (Courtesy Dr. Eduardo Yunis, Children's Hospital of Pittsburgh, Pittsburgh, Pa.)

greater detail in appropriate chapters; here a few comments are made about their special features in childhood.

Hemangioma. *Hemangiomas are the most common tumors of infancy* (Chapter 11). Architecturally, they do not differ from those occurring in adults. Both cavernous and capillary hemangiomas may be encountered, although the latter are often more cellular than in adults, a feature that is deceptively worrisome. In children, most are located in the skin, particularly on the face and scalp, where they produce flat to elevated, irregular, red-blue masses; some of the flat, larger lesions (considered by some to represent vascular ectasias) are referred to as *port-wine stains.* Hemangiomas may enlarge along with the growth of the child, but in many instances they spontaneously regress (Fig. 10-22). In addition to their cosmetic significance, they can represent one facet of the hereditary disorder von Hippel-Lindau disease (Chapter 28). A subset of CNS cavernous hemangiomas can occur in the familial setting; these families harbor mutations in one of three *cerebral cavernous malformation* (CCM) genes.

Lymphatic Tumors. A wide variety of lesions are of lymphatic origin. Some of them—*lymphangiomas*—are hamartomatous or neoplastic, whereas others seem to represent abnormal dilations of preexisting lymph channels known as *lymphangiectasis.* The *lymphangiomas* are usually characterized by cystic and cavernous spaces. Lesions of this nature may occur in the skin but are more often encountered in the deeper regions of the neck, axilla, mediastinum, retroperitoneal tissue, and elsewhere. Although histologically benign, they tend to increase in size after birth, owing to the accumulation of fluid and the budding of preexisting spaces. In this manner they may encroach on vital structures, such as those in the mediastinum or nerve trunks in the axilla, and give rise to clinical problems. *Lymphangiectasis,* in contrast, usually presents as a diffuse swelling of part or all of an extremity; considerable distortion and deformation may occur as a consequence of the spongy, dilated subcutaneous and deeper lymphatics. The lesion is not progressive, however, and does not extend beyond its original location. Nonetheless, it creates cosmetic problems that are often difficult to correct surgically.

Fibrous Tumors. Fibrous tumors occurring in infants and children range from sparsely cellular proliferations of spindle-shaped cells (designated as *fibromatosis*) to richly cellular lesions indistinguishable from fibrosarcomas occurring in adults (designated as *congenital-infantile fibrosarcomas*). Biologic behavior cannot be predicted based on histology alone, however, in that despite their histologic similarities with adult fibrosarcomas, the congenital-infantile variants have an excellent prognosis. *A characteristic chromosomal translocation, t(12;15)(p13;q25), has been described in congenital-infantile fibrosarcomas, which results in generation of an ETV6-NTRK3 fusion transcript.* The normal *ETV6* gene product is a transcription factor, while the *NTRK3* gene product (also known as TRKC) is a tyrosine kinase. Like other tyrosine kinase fusion proteins found in human neoplasms, ETV6-TRKC is constitutively active and stimulates signaling through the oncogenic RAS and PI-3K/AKT pathways (Chapter 7). Among soft-tissue tumors, the ETV6-NTRK3 fusion transcript is unique to infantile fibrosarcomas, making it a useful diagnostic marker.

Teratomas. Teratomas illustrate the relationship of histologic maturity to biologic behavior. Teratomas may occur as benign, well-differentiated cystic lesions (mature teratomas), as lesions of indeterminate potential (immature teratomas), or as unequivocally malignant teratomas (usually admixed with another germ cell tumor component such as endodermal sinus tumor) (Chapter 21). They exhibit two peaks in incidence: the first at approximately 2 years of age and the second in late adolescence or early adulthood. The first peak is congenital neoplasms; the later occurring lesions may also be of prenatal origin but are more slowly growing. *Sacrococcygeal teratomas* are the most common teratomas of childhood, accounting for 40% or more of cases (Fig. 10-23). They occur with a frequency of 1 in 20,000 to 40,000 live births, and are four times more common in girls than boys. In view of the overlap in the mechanisms underlying teratogenesis and oncogenesis, it is interesting that approximately 10% of sacrococcygeal teratomas are associated with congenital anomalies, primarily defects of the hindgut and cloacal region and other midline defects (e.g., meningocele, spina bifida) not believed to result from local effects of the tumor.

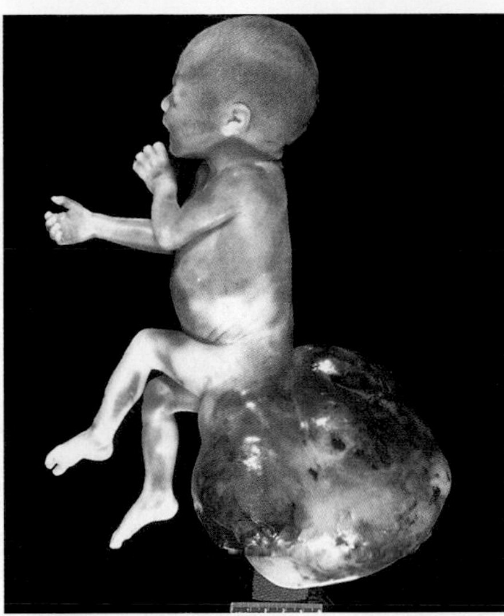

Figure 10-23 Sacrococcygeal teratoma. Note the size of the lesion compared with that of the stillbirth.

Approximately 75% of these tumors are mature teratomas, and about 12% are unequivocally malignant and lethal. The remainder is immature teratomas; their malignant potential correlates with the amount of immature tissue, usually immature neuroepithelial elements, that are present. Most of the benign teratomas are encountered in younger infants (<4 months), whereas children with malignant lesions tend to be somewhat older. Other sites for teratomas in childhood include the testis (Chapter 21), ovaries (Chapter 22), and various midline locations, such as the mediastinum, retroperitoneum, and head and neck.

Malignant Tumors

Cancers of infancy and childhood differ biologically and histologically from their counterparts occurring later in life. The main differences, some of which have already been alluded to, include the following:

- Incidence and type of tumor
- Relatively frequent demonstration of a close relationship between abnormal development (teratogenesis) and tumor induction (oncogenesis)
- Prevalence of underlying familial or genetic aberrations spontaneously
- Tendency of fetal and neonatal malignancies to regress or differentiate spontaneously
- Improved survival or cure of many childhood tumors, so that more attention is now being devoted to minimizing the adverse delayed effects of chemotherapy and radiation therapy in survivors, including the development of second malignancies

Incidence and Types. The most frequent childhood cancers arise in the hematopoietic system, nervous tissue (including the central and sympathetic nervous system, adrenal medulla, and retina), soft tissues, bone, and kidney. This is in sharp contrast to adults, in whom the skin, lung, breast, prostate, and colon are the most common sites of tumors.

Neoplasms that exhibit sharp peaks in incidence in children younger than age 10 years include (1) leukemia (principally acute lymphoblastic leukemia), (2) neuroblastoma, (3) Wilms tumor, (4) hepatoblastoma, (5) retinoblastoma, (6) rhabdomyosarcoma, (7) teratoma, (8) Ewing sarcoma, and posterior fossa neoplasms—principally (9) juvenile astrocytoma, (10) medulloblastoma, and (11) ependymoma. Other forms of cancer are also common in childhood but do not have the same striking early peak. The approximate age distribution of these cancers is indicated in Table 10-7. Within this large array, leukemia alone accounts for more deaths in children younger than age 15 years than all of the other tumors combined.

Histologically, many of the malignant non-hematopoietic pediatric neoplasms are unique. In general, they tend to have a more primitive *(embryonal)* undifferentiated appearance, are often characterized by sheets of cells with small, round nuclei, and frequently show features of organogenesis specific to the site of tumor origin. Because of this latter characteristic, these tumors are frequently designated by the suffix *-blastoma,* for example, nephroblastoma (Wilms tumor), hepatoblastoma, and neuroblastoma. Because of their primitive histologic appearance, many childhood tumors have been collectively referred to as *small round blue cell tumors.* The differential diagnosis of such tumors includes neuroblastoma, Wilms tumor, lymphoma (Chapter 13), rhabdomyosarcoma (Chapter 27), Ewing sarcoma/primitive neuroectodermal tumor (Chapter 26), medulloblastoma (Chapter 28), and retinoblastoma (Chapter 29). If the anatomic site of origin is known, diagnosis is usually possible on histologic grounds alone. Occasionally, a combination of chromosome analysis, immunoperoxidase stains, or electron microscopy is required. Two of these tumors are particularly illustrative and are discussed here: the neuroblastic tumors, specifically neuroblastoma, and Wilms tumor. The remaining tumors are discussed in their respective organ-specific chapters.

Neuroblastic Tumors

The term neuroblastic tumor includes tumors of the sympathetic ganglia and adrenal medulla that are derived from primordial neural crest cells populating these sites. As a family, neuroblastic tumors demonstrate certain characteristic features including *spontaneous or therapy-induced*

Table 10-7 Common Malignant Neoplasms of Infancy and Childhood

0 to 4 Years	5 to 9 Years	10 to 14 Years
Leukemia	Leukemia	
Retinoblastoma	Retinoblastoma	
Neuroblastoma	Neuroblastoma	
Wilms tumor		
Hepatoblastoma	Hepatocellular carcinoma	Hepatocellular carcinoma
Soft tissue sarcoma (especially rhabdomyosarcoma)	Soft tissue sarcoma	Soft-tissue sarcoma
Teratomas		
Central nervous system tumors	Central nervous system tumors	Osteogenic sarcoma
	Ewing sarcoma	Thyroid carcinoma
	Lymphoma	Hodgkin disease

differentiation of primitive neuroblasts into mature elements, spontaneous tumor regression, and a *wide range of clinical behavior and prognosis,* which often mirror the extent of histologic differentiation. Neuroblastoma is the most important member of this family. It is the most common extracranial solid tumor of childhood, and the most frequently diagnosed tumor of infancy. The prevalence is about one case in 7000 live births, and there are approximately 700 cases diagnosed each year in the United States. The median age at diagnosis is 18 months; approximately 40% of cases are diagnosed in infancy. Most neuroblastomas occur sporadically, but 1% to 2% are familial, and in such cases the neoplasms may involve both of the adrenals or multiple primary autonomic sites. Germline mutations in the *anaplastic lymphoma kinase (ALK)* gene (Chapter 13) have recently been identified as a major cause of familial predisposition to neuroblastoma. Somatic gain-of-function *ALK* mutations are also observed in less than 10% of sporadic neuroblastomas. Tumors harboring *ALK* mutations in either the germline or somatic setting may be amenable to treatment using small molecule inhibitors that target the activity of this kinase.

Despite the remarkable progress made in the therapy of this disease, long-term prognosis for the high-risk subsets remains modest, with a 5-year survival in the range of 40%. As will be evident later, age and stage have a remarkable effect on prognosis, and, in general, children younger than 18 months of age tend to have a significantly better prognosis than older individuals at comparable disease burdens.

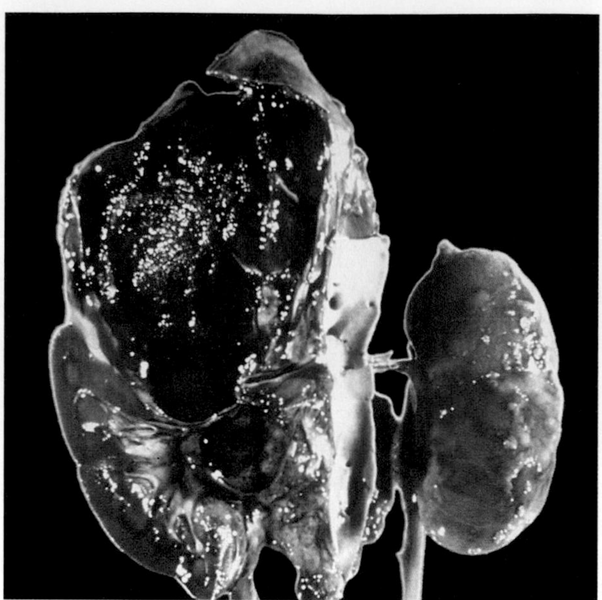

Figure 10-24 Adrenal neuroblastoma in a 6-month-old child. The hemorrhagic, partially encapsulated tumor has displaced the opened left kidney and is impinging on the aorta and left renal artery. (Courtesy Dr. Arthur Weinberg, University of Texas Southwestern Medical School, Dallas, Texas.)

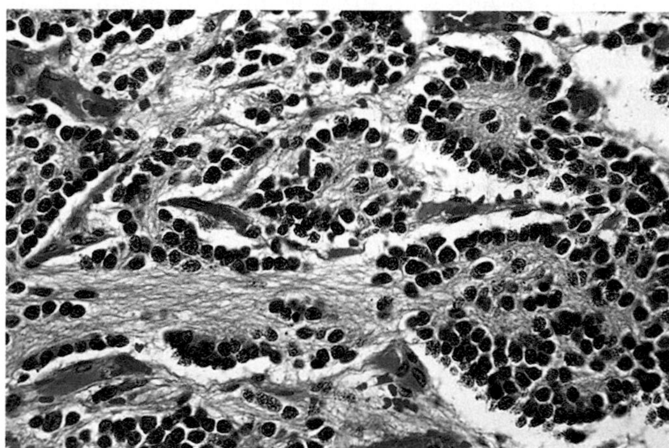

Figure 10-25 Adrenal neuroblastoma. This tumor is composed of small cells embedded in a finely fibrillar matrix.

MORPHOLOGY

In childhood about 40% of neuroblastomas arise in the adrenal medulla. The remainder occur anywhere along the sympathetic chain, with the most common locations being the paravertebral region of the abdomen (25%) and posterior mediastinum (15%). Tumors may arise in numerous other sites, including the pelvis, the neck, and within the brain (cerebral neuroblastomas).

Neuroblastomas range in size from minute nodules (so-called **in situ lesions**) to large masses more than 1 kg in weight (Fig. 10-24). In situ neuroblastomas are reported to occur 40 times more frequently than clinically overt tumors. The great majority of these silent lesions spontaneously regress, leaving only a focus of fibrosis or calcification in the adult; this has led some to question the neoplastic connotation for the in situ lesions, arguing instead in favor of labeling them as developmental anomalies ("rests").

Some neuroblastomas are often sharply demarcated by a fibrous pseudo-capsule, but others are far more infiltrative and invade surrounding structures, including the kidneys, renal vein, and vena cava, and envelop the aorta. On transection, they are composed of soft, gray-tan, tissue. Larger tumors have areas of necrosis, cystic softening, and hemorrhage. Occasionally, foci of punctate intra-tumoral calcification can be palpated.

Histologically, classic neuroblastomas are composed of small, primitive-appearing cells with dark nuclei, scant cytoplasm, and poorly defined cell borders growing in solid sheets. Such tumors may be difficult to differentiate morphologically from other small round blue cell tumors. Mitotic activity, nuclear breakdown ("karyorrhexis"), and pleomorphism may be prominent. The background often demonstrates a faintly eosinophilic fibrillary material (**neuropil**) that corresponds to neuritic processes of the primitive neuroblasts. Typically, rosettes (**Homer-Wright pseudorosettes**) can be found in which the tumor cells are concentrically arranged about a central space filled with neuropil (Fig. 10-25). Other helpful features include positive immunohistochemical reactions for neuron-specific enolase and ultrastructural demonstration of small, membrane-bound, cytoplasmic catecholamine-containing secretory granules; the latter contain characteristic central dense cores surrounded by a peripheral halo (dense core granules). Some neoplasms show signs of maturation that can be spontaneous or therapy-induced. Larger cells having more abundant cytoplasm, large vesicular nuclei, and a prominent nucleolus, representing *ganglion cells* in various stages of maturation, may be found in tumors admixed with primitive neuroblasts (**ganglioneuroblastoma**). Even better differentiated lesions contain many more

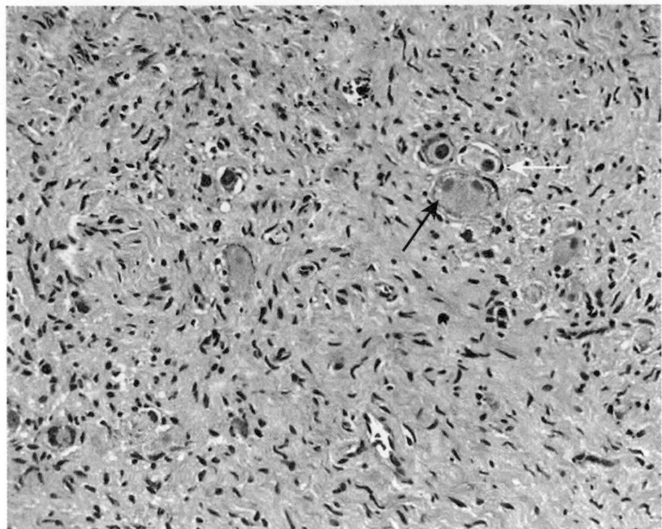

Figure 10-26 Ganglioneuromas, arising from spontaneous or therapy-induced maturation of neuroblastomas, are characterized by clusters of large cells with vesicular nuclei and abundant eosinophilic cytoplasm, representing neoplastic ganglion cells *(arrow)*. Spindle-shaped Schwann cells are present in the background stroma.

large cells resembling mature ganglion cells with few if any residual neuroblasts; such neoplasms merit the designation **ganglioneuroma** (Fig. 10-26). Maturation of neuroblasts into ganglion cells is usually accompanied by the appearance of **Schwann cells**. In fact, the presence of a so-called schwannian stroma composed of organized fascicles of neuritic processes, mature Schwann cells, and fibroblasts is a histologic prerequisite for the designation of ganglioneuroblastoma and ganglioneuroma; ganglion cells in and of themselves do not fulfill the criteria for maturation. The origin of Schwann cells in neuroblastoma remains an issue of contention; some investigators believe they represent a reactive population recruited by the tumor cells. However, studies using microdissection techniques have demonstrated that the Schwann cells harbor at least a subset of the same genetic alterations found in neuroblasts, and therefore are a component of the malignant clone. Irrespective of histogenesis, documenting the presence of schwannian stroma is essential, because its presence is associated with a **favorable outcome** (Table 10-8).

Metastases, when they develop, appear early and widely. In addition to local infiltration and lymph node spread, there is a pronounced tendency to spread through the bloodstream to the liver, lungs, bone marrow, and bones.

Staging. The International Neuroblastoma Staging System, which is the most widely used staging scheme worldwide, is detailed here:

- **Stage 1:** Localized tumor with complete gross excision, with or without microscopic residual disease; representative ipsilateral nonadherent lymph nodes negative for tumor (nodes adherent to the primary tumor may be positive for tumor).
- **Stage 2A:** Localized tumor with incomplete gross resection; representative ipsilateral nonadherent lymph nodes negative for tumor microscopically.
- **Stage 2B:** Localized tumor with or without complete gross excision; ipsilateral nonadherent lymph nodes positive for tumor; enlarged contralateral lymph nodes, which are negative for tumor microscopically.
- **Stage 3:** Unresectable unilateral tumor infiltrating across the midline with or without regional lymph node involvement; or localized unilateral tumor with contralateral regional lymph node involvement.
- **Stage 4:** Any primary tumor with dissemination to distant lymph nodes, bone, bone marrow, liver, skin, and/or other organs *(except as defined for stage 4S)*.
- **Stage 4S** ("S" = special): Localized primary tumor (as defined for stages 1, 2A, or 2B) with dissemination limited to skin, liver, and/or bone marrow; *stage 4S is limited to infants younger than 1 year.*

Unfortunately, most (60% to 80%) children present with stage 3 or 4 tumors, and only 20% to 40% present with stage 1, 2A, 2B, or 4S neuroblastomas. The staging system is of paramount importance in determining prognosis.

Clinical Course and Prognostic Features. In young children, under age 2 years, neuroblastomas generally present with large abdominal masses, fever, and possibly weight loss. In older children, they may not come to attention until metastases produce manifestations, such as bone pain, respiratory symptoms, or gastrointestinal complaints. Neuroblastomas may metastasize widely through the hematogenous and lymphatic systems, particularly to liver, lungs, bones, and bone marrow. Proptosis and ecchymosis may also be present, due to spread to the periorbital region, a common metastatic site. Bladder and bowel dysfunction may be caused by paraspinal neuroblastomas that impinge on nerves. In neonates, disseminated neuroblastomas may present with multiple cutaneous metastases

Table 10-8 Prognostic Factors in Neuroblastomas

Variable	Favorable	Unfavorable
Stage*	Stage 1, 2A, 2B, 4S	Stage 3, 4
Age*	<18 months	>18 months
Histology*		
Evidence of schwannian stroma and gangliocytic differentiation†	Present	Absent
Mitosis-karyorrhexis index‡	<200/5000 cells	>200/5000 cells
DNA ploidy*	Hyperdiploid (whole chromosomal gains)	Near-diploid (Segmental chromosomal losses; chromothripsis)
*MYCN**	Not amplified	Amplified
Chromosome 1p loss	Absent	Present
Chromosome 11q loss	Absent	Present
TRKA expression	Present	Absent
TRKB expression	Absent	Present
Mutations of neuritogenesis genes	Absent	Present

*Corresponds to the most commonly used parameters in clinical practice for assessment of prognosis and risk stratification.

†It is not only the presence but also the amount of schwannian stroma that confers the designation of a favorable histology. At least *50% or more schwannian stroma* is required before a neoplasm can be classified as ganglioneuroblastoma or ganglioneuroma.

‡Mitotic karyorrhexis index (MKI) is defined as the number of mitotic or karyorrhectic cells per 5000 tumor cells in random foci.

that cause deep blue discoloration of the skin (earning the unfortunate designation of "*blueberry muffin baby*"). *About 90% of neuroblastomas, regardless of location, produce catecholamines* (similar to the catecholamines associated with pheochromocytomas), which are an important diagnostic feature (i.e., elevated blood levels of catecholamines and elevated urine levels of the metabolites vanillylmandelic acid [VMA] and homovanillic acid [HVA]). Despite the elaboration of catecholamines, hypertension is much less frequent with these neoplasms than with pheochromocytomas (Chapter 24). Ganglioneuromas, unlike their malignant counterparts, tend to produce either asymptomatic mass lesions or symptoms related to compression.

The course of neuroblastomas is extremely variable. Several clinical, histopathologic, molecular, and biochemical factors have been identified that have a bearing on prognosis (Table 10-8); based on the collection of prognostic factors present in a given patient, they are classified either as "low," "intermediate," or "high" risk. With improvements in therapy, long-term survival exceeds 90% of patients in the first two groups, while less than 50% of patients in the high-risk category are long-term survivors. The most pertinent prognostic factors include the following:

- *Age and stage are the most important determinants of outcome.* Neuroblastomas at stages 1, 2A, or 2B tend to have an excellent prognosis, irrespective of age ("low" or "intermediate" risk); the one notable exception to this rule are tumors exhibiting amplification of the *MYCN* oncogene. Infants with localized primary tumors and widespread metastases to the liver, bone marrow, and skin (stage 4S) represent a special subtype, wherein it is not uncommon for the disease to regress spontaneously. The biologic basis of this welcome behavior is not clear. *The age of 18 months has emerged as a critical point of dichotomy in terms of prognosis.* Children younger than 18 months of age, and especially those in the first year of life, have an excellent prognosis regardless of the stage of the neoplasm. Children older than 18 months fall into at least the "intermediate" risk category, while those with higher stage tumors or with confounding unfavorable prognostic variables like *MYCN* amplification in the neoplastic cells are considered "high" risk.
- *Morphology is an independent prognostic variable in neuroblastic tumors.* An age-linked morphologic classification of neuroblastic tumors has recently been proposed that divides them into *favorable* and *unfavorable* histologic subtypes. The specific morphologic features that bear on prognosis are listed in Table 10-8.
- *Amplification of the MYCN oncogene in neuroblastomas is a molecular event that has possibly the most profound impact on prognosis,* particularly when it occurs in tumors that would otherwise portend a good outcome. The presence of *MYCN* amplification "bumps" the tumor into a "high"-risk category, irrespective of age, stage, or histology. *MYCN* is located on the distal short arm of chromosome 2 (2p23-p24). Amplification of *MYCN* does not karyotypically manifest at the resident 2p23-p24 site, but rather as extrachromosomal double minute chromosomes or homogeneously staining regions on other chromosomes (Fig. 10-27). *MYCN* amplification is present in about 20% to 30% of primary tumors, most presenting as advanced-stage disease, and the degree of amplification correlates with worse prognosis. *MYCN* amplification is currently the most important genetic abnormality used in risk stratification of neuroblastic tumors (see later).
- *Ploidy* of the tumor cells correlates with outcome in children less than 2 years of age but loses its independent prognostic significance in older children. Broadly, neuroblastomas can be divided into two categories: *near-diploid* and *hyper-diploid* (*whole chromosome gains*), with the latter being associated with a better prognosis. It is postulated that neuroblastomas with hyperdiploidy have an underlying defect in the mitotic machinery, leading to nondisjunction and whole chromosome gains, but otherwise relatively banal karyotypes. On the contrary, the more aggressive near-diploid tumors

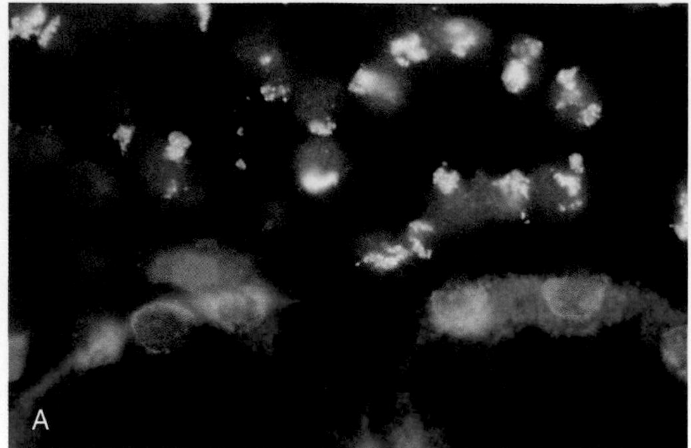

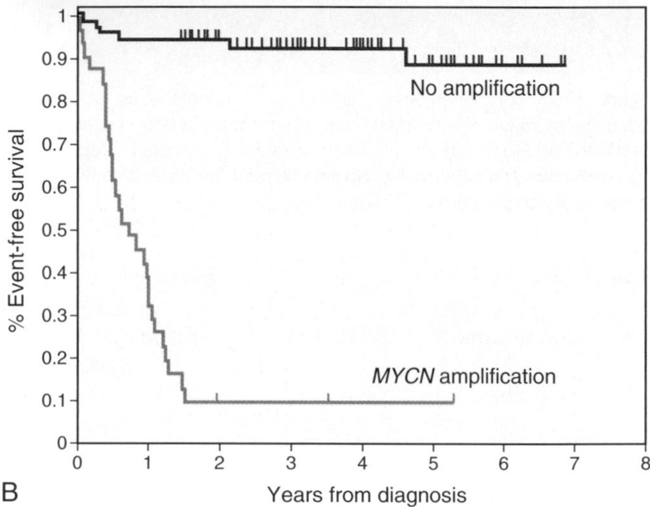

Figure 10-27 **A**, Fluorescence in situ hybridization using a fluorescein-labeled cosmid probe for *N-myc* on a tissue section. Note the neuroblastoma cells on the upper half of the photo with large areas of staining (*yellow-green*); this corresponds to amplified *N-MYC* in the form of homogeneously staining regions. Renal tubular epithelial cells in the lower half of the photograph show no nuclear staining and background (*green*) cytoplasmic staining. **B**, A Kaplan-Meier survival curve of infants younger than 1 year of age with metastatic neuroblastoma. The 3-year event-free survival of infants whose tumors lacked *MYCN* amplification was 93%, whereas those with tumors that had *MYCN* amplification had only a 10% event free survival. (**A,** Courtesy Dr. Timothy Triche, Children's Hospital, Los Angeles, Calif.; **B,** Reproduced with permission from Brodeur GM: Neuroblastoma: biological insights into a clinical enigma. Nat Rev Cancer 3:203-216; 2003.)

harbor generalized genomic instability, with multiple segmental chromosomal aberrations that result in a complex karyotype with adverse prognostic implications. One peculiar form of segmental aberration described recently in aggressive neuroblastomas is called *chromothripsis* (Chapter 7), which involves localized fragmentation of a chromosome segment followed by random assembly of the fragments. In a subset of neuroblastomas, chromothripsis can result in amplification of *MYCN* or other oncogenes, or losses in tumor suppressor loci.

While *age, stage, histology,, MYCN status,* and *DNA ploidy* are currently the "core" criteria used for the purposes of formal risk stratification and therapeutic decision, several emerging molecular variables have been described with prognostic implications. The most pertinent ones include the following:

- *Hemizygous deletion of the distal short arm of chromosome 1* in the region of band p36 has been demonstrated in 25% to 35% of primary tumors. Loss of 1p36 in neuroblastomas has a strong correlation with *MYCN* amplification, as well as advanced disease stage, and is associated with an increased risk of disease relapse in localized tumors. *Hemizygous loss of chromosome 11q* genetic material is another adverse prognostic factor, and may be the most common deletion event in neuroblastomas.
- *The expression of specific neurotrophin receptors* is also a prognostic marker for neuroblastoma. The neurotrophin receptors are a family of tyrosine kinase receptors, notably TrkA, TrkB, and TrkC (also known as NTRK3, see earlier), that regulate the growth, survival, and differentiation of neural cells. High TrkA expression is a favorable prognostic factor in neuroblastomas, generally associated with low-stage tumors lacking *MYCN* amplification that occur in younger patients. In contrast, elevated TrkB expression is associated with unfavorable biological characteristics, including *MYCN* amplification and a higher disease stage.
- Lastly, the application of next generation sequencing techniques to unravel the neuroblastoma genome has identified recurrent mutations in genes whose products are involved in *neuritogenesis* (a process in neuronal differentiation which includes the sprouting of neurites that will subsequently lead to the formation of axons). Selected examples of mutated genes within this functional class include *alpha thalassemia / mental retardation, X-linked* (*ATRX*) and *protein tyrosine phosphatase, receptor type D* (*PTPRD*). Mutations of neuritogenesis associated genes were generally present in more aggressive, higher-stage neuroblastomas (including those arising in the absence of *MYCN* amplification), and these alterations are postulated to lead to defects in neuronal differentiation within the neoplastic cells, likely underlying their poorly differentiated histology.

Although discussion of the treatment modalities for neuroblastoma is beyond the scope of this book, we mention in passing two promising experimental approaches. The first involves the use of retinoids as an adjunct therapy for inducing the differentiation of neuroblastoma. Recall that the retinoic acid pathway plays a critical role in cellular differentiation during embryogenesis. The second is focused on tumors harboring activating *ALK* mutations because they are potentially susceptible to targeted inhibitors of the encoded kinase, and such agents are currently undergoing evaluation in clinical trials.

Finally, we should mention the current status of screening programs for neuroblastoma. Because the vast majority of neuroblastomas release catecholamines into the circulation, detection of catecholamine metabolites (VMA and HVA) in urine could, in principle, form the basis for screening for asymptomatic tumors in children. However, two large studies in Europe and North America have failed to demonstrate improved mortality rates with population screening, because most tumors detected had favorable biologic characteristics. Therefore, community-based screening programs for neuroblastomas are not currently advocated.

Wilms Tumor

Wilms tumor afflicts approximately 1 in every 10,000 children in the United States, making it the most common primary renal tumor of childhood and the fourth most common pediatric malignancy in the United States. The peak incidence for Wilms tumor is between 2 and 5 years of age, and 95% of tumors occur before the age of 10 years. Approximately 5% to 10% of Wilms tumors involve both kidneys, either simultaneously *(synchronous)* or one after the other *(metachronous)*. Bilateral Wilms tumors have a median age of onset approximately 10 months earlier than tumors restricted to one kidney, and these patients are presumed to harbor a germline mutation in one of the Wilms tumor-predisposing genes (see later). The biology of this tumor illustrates several important aspects of childhood neoplasms, such as the relationship between *malformations* and *neoplasia*, the histologic similarities between *organogenesis* and *oncogenesis*, the *two-hit theory* of recessive tumor suppressor genes (Chapter 7), the role of *premalignant lesions*, and perhaps most importantly, the potential for *judicious treatment modalities* to dramatically affect prognosis and outcome. Improvements in the cure rates for Wilms tumor (from as low as 30% a few decades ago, to approximately 90% currently) represent one of the greatest successes of pediatric oncology.

Pathogenesis and Genetics. *The risk of Wilms tumor is increased with at least three recognizable groups of congenital malformations associated with distinct chromosomal loci.* Although Wilms tumors arising in this setting account for no more than 10% of cases, these *syndromic tumors* have provided important insight into the biology of this neoplasm.

- The first group of patients has the *WAGR syndrome*, characterized by *W*ilms tumor, *a*niridia, *g*enital anomalies, and mental *r*etardation. Their lifetime risk of developing Wilms tumor is approximately 33%. Individuals with WAGR syndrome carry constitutional (germline) deletions of 11p13. Studies on these patients led to the identification of the first Wilms tumor-associated gene, *WT1*, and a contiguously deleted autosomal dominant gene for aniridia, *PAX6*, both located on chromosome 11p13. Patients with deletions restricted to *PAX6*, with normal *WT1* function, develop sporadic aniridia, but they are not at increased risk for Wilms tumors. The presence of germline *WT1* deletions in WAGR syndrome represents the "first hit"; the development of Wilms tumor in these patients frequently correlates with the occurrence of a nonsense or frameshift mutation in the second *WT1* allele ("second hit").

- A second group of patients at much higher risk for Wilms tumor (~90%) have the *Denys-Drash syndrome*, which is characterized by *gonadal dysgenesis* (male pseudohermaphroditism) and *early-onset nephropathy* leading to renal failure. The characteristic glomerular lesion in these patients is a *diffuse mesangial sclerosis* (Chapter 20). As in patients with WAGR, these patients also demonstrate germline abnormalities in *WT1*. In patients with the Denys-Drash syndrome, however, the genetic abnormality is a *dominant-negative missense mutation* in the zinc-finger region of the WT1 protein that affects its DNA-binding properties. This mutation interferes with the function of the remaining wild-type allele, yet strangely, it is sufficient only in causing genitourinary abnormalities, but not tumorigenesis; Wilms tumors arising in Denys-Drash syndrome demonstrate bi-allelic inactivation of *WT1*. In addition to Wilms tumors, these individuals are also at increased risk for developing germ cell tumors called *gonadoblastomas* (Chapter 21), almost certainly a consequence of disruption in normal gonadal development.

  WT1 encodes a DNA-binding transcription factor that is expressed within several tissues, including the kidney and gonads, during embryogenesis. The WT1 protein is critical for normal renal and gonadal development. WT1 has multiple binding partners, and the choice of this partner can affect whether WT1 functions as a transcriptional activator or repressor in a given cellular context. Numerous transcriptional targets of WT1 have been identified, including genes encoding glomerular podocyte-specific proteins and proteins involved in induction of renal differentiation. Despite the importance of *WT1* in nephrogenesis and its unequivocal role as a tumor suppressor gene, only about 10% of patients with sporadic (nonsyndromic) Wilms tumors demonstrate *WT1* mutations, suggesting that the majority of these tumors are caused by mutations in other genes.

- A third group, that is clinically distinct from these previous two groups of patients but also with an increased risk of developing Wilms tumor are children with *Beckwith-Wiedemann syndrome* (BWS), characterized by enlargement of body organs (organomegaly), macroglossia, hemihypertrophy, omphalocele, and abnormal large cells in the adrenal cortex (adrenal cytomegaly). BWS has served as a model for a nonclassical mechanism of tumorigenesis in humans—*genomic imprinting* (Chapter 5). The chromosomal region implicated in BWS has been localized to band 11p15.5 ("WT2"), distal to the *WT1* locus. This region contains multiple genes that are normally expressed from only one of the two parental alleles, with transcriptional silencing (i.e., imprinting) of the other parental homologue by methylation of the promoter region. Unlike WAGR or Denys-Drash syndromes, the genetic basis for BWS is considerably more heterogeneous in that no single 11p15.5 gene is involved in all cases. Moreover, the phenotype of BWS, including the predisposition to tumorigenesis, is influenced by the specific "WT2" imprinting abnormalities present. One of the genes in this region—insulin-like growth factor-2 (*IGF2*) —is normally expressed solely from the *paternal allele*, while the maternal allele is silenced by imprinting. In some Wilms tumors, *loss of imprinting* (i.e., re-expression of the maternal *IGF2* allele) can be demonstrated, leading to overexpression of the IGF-2 protein. In other instances there is a selective deletion of the imprinted maternal allele, combined with duplication of the transcriptionally active paternal allele in the tumor *(uniparental paternal disomy)*, which has an identical functional effect in terms of overexpression of IGF-2. Because the IGF-2 protein is an embryonal growth factor, it could conceivably explain the features of overgrowth associated with BWS, as well as the increased risk for Wilms tumors in these patients. Of all the "WT2" genes, imprinting abnormalities of *IGF2* have the strongest relationship to tumor predisposition in BWS. A subset of patients with BWS harbor mutations of the cell cycle regulator *CDKN1C* (also known as *p57* or *KIP2*); however, these patients have a significantly lower risk for developing Wilms tumors. In addition to Wilms tumors, patients with BWS are also at increased risk for developing hepatoblastoma, pancreatoblastoma, adrenocortical tumors, and rhabdomyosarcomas.

Recent genetic studies have also elucidated the role of β-catenin in Wilms tumor. It will be recalled (Chapter 7) that β-catenin belongs to the developmentally important *WNT (wingless)* signaling pathway. Gain-of-function mutations of the gene encoding β-catenin have been demonstrated in approximately 10% of sporadic Wilms tumors; there is a significant overlap between the presence of *WT1* and β-catenin mutations, suggesting a synergistic role for these events in the genesis of Wilms tumors.

Nephrogenic rests are putative precursor lesions of Wilms tumors and are seen in the renal parenchyma adjacent to approximately 25% to 40% of unilateral tumors; this frequency rises to nearly 100% in cases of bilateral Wilms tumors. In many instances the nephrogenic rests share genetic alterations with the adjacent Wilms tumor, pointing to their preneoplastic status. The appearance of nephrogenic rests varies from expansile masses that resemble Wilms tumors (hyperplastic rests) to sclerotic rests consisting predominantly of fibrous tissue and occasional admixed immature tubules or glomeruli. It is important to document the presence of nephrogenic rests in the resected specimen, because these patients are at an increased risk of developing Wilms tumors in the contralateral kidney and require frequent and regular surveillance for many years.

MORPHOLOGY

Grossly, Wilms tumor tends to present as a large, solitary, well-circumscribed mass, although 10% are either bilateral or multicentric at the time of diagnosis. On cut section, the tumor is soft, homogeneous, and tan to gray with occasional foci of hemorrhage, cyst formation, and necrosis (Fig. 10-28).

Microscopically, Wilms tumors are characterized by recognizable attempts to recapitulate different stages of nephrogenesis. **The classic triphasic combination of blastemal, stromal, and epithelial cell types is observed in the vast majority**

of lesions, although the percentage of each component is variable (Fig. 10-29*A*). Sheets of small blue cells with few distinctive features characterize the blastemal component. Epithelial differentiation is usually in the form of abortive tubules or glomeruli. Stromal cells are usually fibrocytic or myxoid in nature, although skeletal muscle differentiation is not uncommon. Rarely, other heterologous elements are identified, including squamous or mucinous epithelium, smooth muscle, adipose tissue, cartilage, and osteoid and neurogenic tissue. Approximately 5% of tumors reveal **anaplasia**, defined as the presence of cells with large, hyperchromatic, pleomorphic nuclei and abnormal mitoses (Fig. 10-29*B*). The presence of anaplasia correlates with the presence of *TP53* mutations and the emergence of resistance to chemotherapy. Recall that p53 elicits pro-apoptotic signals in response to DNA damage (Chapter 7). The loss of p53 function might explain the relative unresponsiveness of anaplastic cells to cytotoxic chemotherapy.

Clinical Features. Most children with Wilms tumors present with a large abdominal mass that may be unilateral or, when very large, may extend across the midline and down into the pelvis. Hematuria, pain in the abdomen after some traumatic incident, intestinal obstruction, and appearance of hypertension are other patterns of presentation. In a considerable number of these patients, pulmonary metastases are present at the time of primary diagnosis.

As stated, most patients with Wilms tumor can expect to be cured of their malignancy. Anaplastic histology remains a critical determinant of adverse prognosis. Even anaplasia restricted to the kidney (i.e., without extra-renal spread) confers an increased risk of recurrence and death, emphasizing the need for accurate identification of this histologic feature. Molecular parameters that correlate with adverse prognosis include loss of genetic material on chromosomes 11q and 16q, and gain of chromosome 1q in the tumor cells. Along with the increased survival of individuals with Wilms tumor have come reports of an increased risk of developing second primary tumors, including bone and soft-tissue sarcomas, leukemia and lymphomas, and breast cancers. While some of these neoplasms result from the presence of a germline mutation in a cancer predisposition gene, others are a consequence of therapy, most commonly radiation administered to the cancer field. This tragic, albeit uncommon, outcome has mandated that radiation therapy be used judiciously in the treatment of this and other childhood cancers.

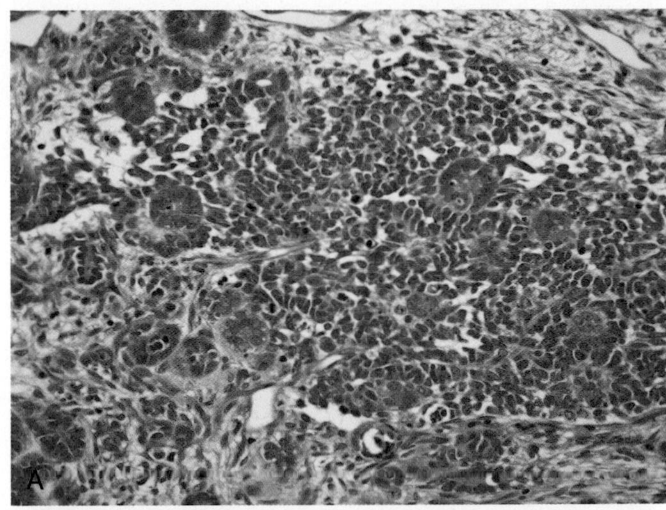

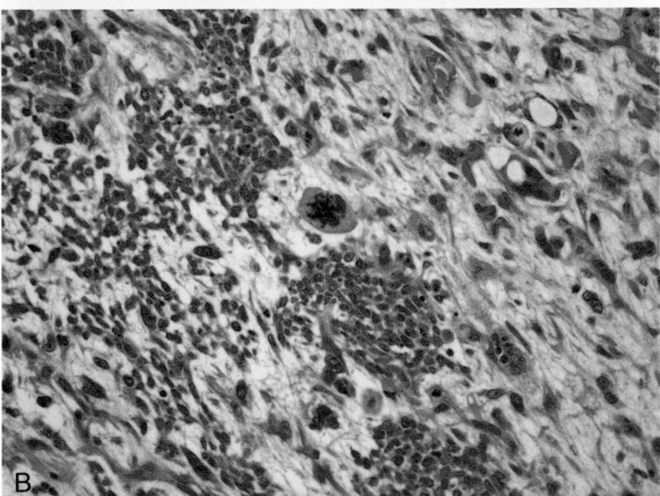

Figure 10-29 A, Wilms tumor with tightly packed blue cells consistent with the blastemal component and interspersed primitive tubules, representing the epithelial component. Although multiple mitotic figures are seen, none are atypical in this field. **B,** Focal anaplasia was present in this Wilms tumor in other areas, characterized by cells with hyperchromatic, pleomorphic nuclei, and abnormal mitoses.

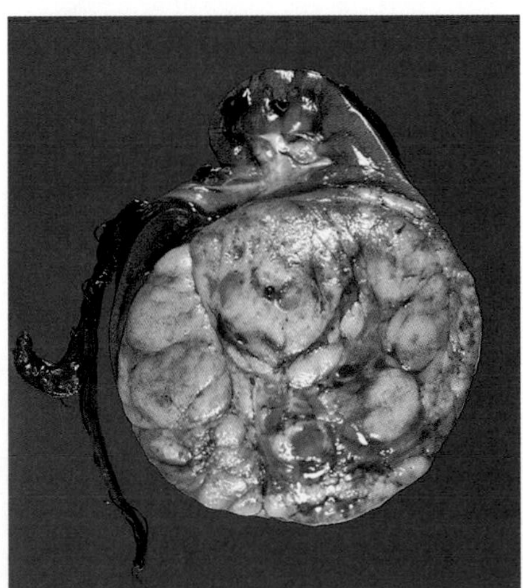

Figure 10-28 Wilms tumor in the lower pole of the kidney with the characteristic tan-to-gray color and well-circumscribed margins.

SUGGESTED READINGS

Congenital Anomalies

Bellini C, Hennekam RC: Non-immune hydrops fetalis: a short review of etiology and pathophysiology. *Am J Med Genet A* 158A:597-605, 2012. [*A well written review on non-immune hydrops, which accounts for the overhwelming majority of fetal hydrops in the Western world.*]

de Jong EP, Walther FJ, Kroes AC, et al: Parvovirus B19 infection in pregnancy: new insights and management. *Prenat Diagn* 31:419-25, 2011. [*A comprehesive review that discusses the epidemiology, natural history, and complications of intrauterine Parvovirus B19 infection, along with diagnostic and treatment guidelines.*]

Kochanek KD, Kirmeyer SE, Martin JA, et al: Annual summary of vital statistics: 2009. *Pediatrics* 129:338-48, 2012. [*A periodically updated release from the United States Centers for Disease Control, summarizing statistical data related to birth and death rates, congenital anomalies, causes of death, etc.*]

Cytsic Fibrosis and Inborn Errors of Metabolism

Cutting GR: Modifier genes in Mendelian disorders: the example of cystic fibrosis. *Ann N Y Acad Sci* 1214:57-69. 2010. [*An outstanding review on modifier genes in so-called monogenic disorders, using cystic fibrosis as a template.*]

Farrell PM, Rosenstein BJ, White TB, et al: Guidelines for diagnosis of cystic fibrosis in newborns through older adults: Cystic Fibrosis Foundation consensus report. *J Pediatr* 153:S4-S14, 2008. [A *somewhat dated, but gold standard consensus report on diagnostic criteria for cytsic fibrosis, including variant forms.*]

Mitchell JJ, Trakadis YJ, Scriver CR: Phenylalanine hydroxylase deficiency. *Genet Med* 13:697-707, 2011. [*A straightforward review on this prototype Mendelian disorder; useful if reader is seeking additional information beyond current chapter.*]

Ramsey BW, Davies J, McElvaney NG, et al: A CFTR potentiator in patients with cystic fibrosis and the G551D mutation. *N Engl J Med* 365:1663-72, 2011. [*An original research article describing one of the first therapeutic strategies in cystic fibrosis that works through potentiating the function of CFTR protein.*]

Ratjen F, McColley SA: Update in cystic fibrosis 2011. *Am J Respir Crit Care Med* 185:933-6, 2012. [*A clinically oriented review on cystic fibrosis that discusses many of the longer term sequela contributing to morbidity and mortality.*]

Diseases of Prematurity and SIDS

Casteels I, Cassiman C, Van Calster J, et al: Educational paper: Retinopathy of prematurity. *Eur J Pediatr* 171:887-93, 2012. [*A well rounded review on retinopathy of prematurity, which includes a discussion of how our understanding of the pathophysiology of this entity has evolved over time.*]

Gien J, Kinsella JP: Pathogenesis and treatment of bronchopulmonary dysplasia. *Curr Opin Pediatr* 23:305-13, 2011. [A*n outstanding review on bronchopulmonary dysplasia, which like the preceding reference, discusses how enhancements in understanding the pathophysiology of BPD have impacted prevention and treatment strategies.*]

Gower WA, Nogee LM: Surfactant dysfunction. *Paediatr Respir Rev* 12:223-9, 2011. [*A review discussing the genetic defects associated with surfactant dysfunction, and associated acute or chronic pulmonary disorders.*]

Kinney HC, Thach BT: The sudden infant death syndrome. *N Engl J Med* 361:795-805, 2009. [*A highly relevant review on SIDS, from one of the pioneering researchers elucidating the neuropathology of this condition.*]

Neu J, Walker WA: Necrotizing enterocolitis. *N Engl J Med* 364:255-64, 2011. [*An outstanding review on this condition from one of the leading physician scientists in this field; particularly exemplary photomicrographs and illustrations.*]

Tumors of Infancy and Childhood

Chau YY, Hastie ND: The role of Wt1 in regulating mesenchyme in cancer, development, and tissue homeostasis. *Trends Genet* 28:515-24, 2012. [*A comprehensive treatise on role of the Wt1 protein in development and in cancer.*]

Hamilton TE, Shamberger RC: Wilms tumor: recent advances in clinical care and biology. *Semin Pediatr Surg* 21:15-20, 2012. [*A review on Wilms tumor that discusses underlying genetic susceptibility, natural history, and treatment options.*]

Maris JM: Recent advances in neuroblastoma. *N Engl J Med* 362:2202-11, 2010. [*A well rounded review on neuroblastomas.*]

Molenaar JJ, Koster J, Zwijnenburg DA, et al: Sequencing of neuroblastoma identifies chromothripsis and defects in neuritogenesis genes. *Nature* 483:589-93, 2012. [*An original research article describing two new classes of recurrent genetic alterations in neuroblastomas.*]

Weksberg R, Shuman C, Beckwith JB: Beckwith-Wiedemann syndrome. *Eur J Hum Genet* 18:8-14, 2010. [*A review by Dr. Beckwith on the eponymously named syndrome that predisposes to several pediatric neoplasms, including Wilms tumor.*]

See TARGETED THERAPY available online at www.studentconsult.com 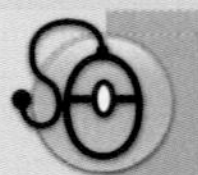

CHAPTER 11

Blood Vessels

Richard N. Mitchell

CHAPTER CONTENTS

Vascular pathology is responsible for more morbidity and mortality than any other category of human disease. Although the most clinically significant lesions involve arteries, venous disorders are not inconsequential. Two principal mechanisms underlie vascular disease:

- *Narrowing (stenosis)* or *complete obstruction* of vessel lumina, either progressively (e.g., by atherosclerosis) or precipitously (e.g., by thrombosis or embolism)
- *Weakening* of vessel walls, leading to dilation or rupture

To better appreciate the pathogenesis of vascular disorders, it is important to first understand normal blood vessels.

Vascular Structure and Function

The general architecture and cellular composition of blood vessels are similar throughout the cardiovascular system. However, structural specializations that reflect distinct functional roles characterize specific kinds of vessels (Fig. 11-1). For example, arterial walls are thicker than corresponding veins at the same level of branching to accommodate pulsatile flow and higher blood pressures. Arterial wall thickness gradually diminishes as the vessels become smaller, but the ratio of wall thickness to lumen diameter increases, allowing these muscular vessels to exert control over blood flow and pressure. Many disorders of the vasculature only affect particular types of vessels and thus have characteristic anatomic distributions. Thus, atherosclerosis affects mainly elastic and muscular arteries, hypertension affects small muscular arteries and arterioles, and different varieties of vasculitis characteristically involve only vessels of a certain caliber.

The basic constituents of the walls of blood vessels are endothelial cells and smooth muscle cells, admixed with a variety of extracellular matrix, including elastin, collagen, and glycosaminoglycans. The relative amount and configuration of the basic constituents differ along the vasculature owing to local adaptations to mechanical or metabolic needs. In arteries and veins, these constituents are organized into three concentric layers, the *intima, media,* and

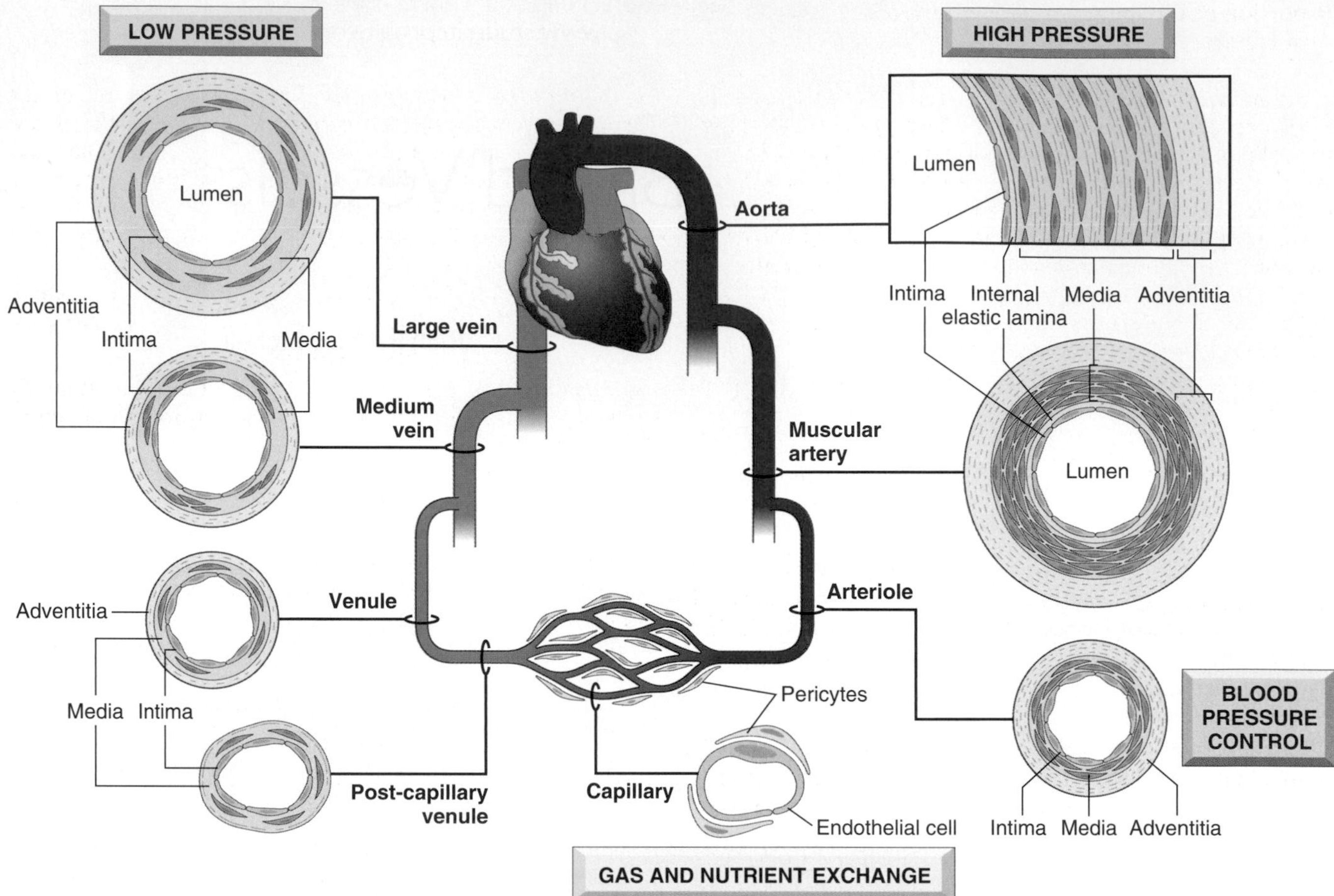

Figure 11-1 Regional specializations of the vasculature. Although the basic organization of the vasculature is constant, the thickness and composition of the various layers differ according to hemodynamic forces and tissue requirements. The aorta has substantial elastic tissue to accommodate high pulsatile forces, with the capacity to recoil and transmit energy into forward blood flow. The muscular arteries and arterioles have concentric rings of medial smooth muscle cells whose contractile state regulates vessel caliber and, thereby, blood flow and blood pressure. The venous system has relatively poorly developed medial layers that permit greater capacitance. The capillary wall permits ready diffusion of oxygen and nutrients because it is comprised only of an endothelial cell and sparse encircling pericytes. The differing structural and functional attributes leave the various parts of the vascular tree vulnerable to particular disorders. Thus, loss of aortic elastic tissue in a large artery may result in aneurysm, while stasis in a dilated venous bed may produce a thrombus.

adventitia, which are most anatomically distinct in the arteries.

- The *intima* normally consists of a single layer of endothelial cells sitting on a basement membrane underlaid by a thin layer of extracellular matrix; the intima is demarcated from the media by the *internal elastic lamina.*
- The *media* of vessels on the arterial side of the circulation varies in structure according to functional demands.
  - Arteries have several well-organized concentric layers of smooth muscle cells, while the smooth muscle cells of veins are arranged in a more haphazard fashion.
  - The media of elastic arteries (e.g., the aorta) has a high elastin content, allowing these vessels to expand during systole and recoil during diastole, a property that serves to propel the blood towards the tissues. With aging and the loss of elasticity, the aorta and larger arteries become less compliant, an alteration that tends to raise the systolic blood pressure. In addition, the arteries of older individuals often become progressively tortuous and dilated *(ectatic).*
  - In *muscular arteries,* the media is composed predominantly of circumferentially oriented smooth muscle cells. Arteriolar smooth muscle cell contraction *(vasoconstriction)* or relaxation *(vasodilation)* are regulated by inputs from the autonomic nervous system, and local metabolic factors. These responses change the size of the lumen and thus regulate regional blood flow and blood pressure.
  - *Arterioles are the principal points of physiologic resistance to blood flow.* Since the resistance to fluid flow is inversely proportional to the fourth power of the diameter (i.e., halving the diameter increases resistance 16-fold), small decreases in the lumen size of arterioles caused by structural changes or vasoconstriction can have profound effects on blood pressure.
- The *adventitia* lies external to the media and in many arteries is separated from the media by a well-defined *external elastic lamina.* The adventitia consists of loose connective tissue containing nerve fibers and the vasa vasorum (literally "vessels of the vessels"), small arterioles that are responsible for supplying the outer

portion of the media of large arteries with oxygen and nutrients.

As already alluded to, arteries are divided into three types based on their size and structural features: (1) large or *elastic arteries*, including the aorta, the major branches of the aorta (the innominate, subclavian, common carotid, and iliac arteries), and the pulmonary arteries; (2) medium-sized or *muscular arteries*, comprising smaller branches of the aorta (e.g., the coronary and renal arteries); and (3) small arteries (≤2 mm in diameter) and *arterioles* (20 to 100 μm in diameter), within tissues and organs.

Capillaries are approximately the diameter of a red cell (7 to 8 μm); they have an endothelial cell lining but no media, although variable numbers of *pericytes*, cells that resemble smooth muscle cells, typically lie just deep to the the endothelium. Collectively, capillaries have a huge cross-sectional area, and also have a relative low flow rate. The combination of thin walls and slow flow make capillaries ideally suited for the exchange of diffusible substances between blood and tissues. Because functionally useful oxygen diffusion in tissues is limited to a distance of only approximately 100 μm, the capillary network of most tissues is very rich. Tissues with high metabolic rates, such as myocardium and brain, have the highest density of capillaries.

Blood from capillary beds flows into postcapillary venules and then sequentially through collecting venules and small, medium, and large veins. In most inflammatory reactions, vascular leakage and leukocyte exudation occur preferentially from postcapillary venules (Chapter 3).

Relative to arteries at the same level of branching, veins have larger diameters, larger lumens, and thinner and less organized walls (Fig. 11-1). These structural features augment the capacity of the venous side of the circulation, which on average contains about two-thirds of total blood volume. Less rigid walls means that *veins are subject to dilation and compression, as well as infiltration by tumors and inflammatory processes*. Reverse flow (due to gravity) is prevented in the extremities by venous valves.

Lymphatics are thin-walled channels lined by specialized endothelium; they provide conduits to return interstitial tissue fluid and inflammatory cells to the bloodstream. *Lymphatics can also transport microbes and tumor cells, thus constituting an important potential pathway for disease dissemination.*

KEY CONCEPTS

Vascular Structure and Function

- All vessels except capillaries share a three-layered architecture consisting of an endothelium lined intima, a surrounding smooth muscle media, and supportive adventitia, admixed with extracellular matrix.
- The smooth muscle cell and matrix content of arteries, veins, and capillaries vary according to hemodynamic demands (e.g., pressure, pulsatility) and functional requirements.
- The specific composition of the vessel wall at any given site within the vascular tree influences the nature and consequences of pathologic injuries.

Vascular Anomalies

Although rarely symptomatic, anatomic variants of the usual vascular supply are important for treating physicians to recognize, as the failure to do so may lead to surgical complications and impede attempted therapeutic interventions (e.g., placement of coronary artery stents). Among congenital vascular anomalies, three are of particular medical significance:

- *Developmental* or *berry aneurysms* occur in cerebral vessels; when ruptured, these can be causes of fatal intracerebral hemorrhage (Chapter 28).
- *Arteriovenous fistulas* are direct connections (usually small) between arteries and veins that bypass the intervening capillary bed. They occur most commonly as developmental defects but can also result from rupture of an arterial aneurysm into the adjacent vein, from penetrating injuries that pierce arteries and veins, or from inflammatory necrosis of adjacent vessels; surgically generated arteriovenous fistulas provide vascular access for chronic hemodialysis. Like berry aneurysms, arteriovenous fistulas may rupture, leading to intracerebral hemorrhage. Large or multiple arteriovenous fistulas can produce clinically significant effects by shunting blood from the arterial to the venous circulations, forcing the heart to pump additional volume and leading to high-output cardiac failure.
- *Fibromuscular dysplasia* is a focal irregular thickening in medium and large muscular arteries, including renal, carotid, splanchnic, and vertebral vessels. The cause is unknown, but is probably developmental; first-degree relatives of affected individuals have an increased incidence. Segments of the vessel wall are focally thickened by a combination of medial and intimal hyperplasia and fibrosis, resulting in luminal stenosis; in the renal arteries, this can be a cause of renovascular hypertension (Chapter 20). Immediately adjacent vessel segments can have markedly attenuated media (on angiography, the vessels are said to have a "string of beads" appearance), leading to vascular outpouchings (*aneurysms*) that can rupture. Fibromuscular dysplasia can manifest at any age; although it is seen most frequently in young women, there is no association with oral contraceptives or increased estrogen expression.

Vascular Wall Response to Injury

The integrated functioning of endothelial cells and smooth muscle cells impacts vessel development as well as the physiologic and pathophysiologic responses to hemodynamic and biochemical stimuli. Their function (and dysfunction) are described briefly, followed by discussion of specific vascular disorders.

Endothelial cells form a specialized lining for blood vessels. Although endothelial cells throughout the vascular tree share many attributes, populations that line different portions of the vascular tree (large vessels vs. capillaries, arteries vs. veins) have distinct gene expression profiles, behaviors, and morphologic appearances. Thus, endothelial cells in liver sinusoids or in renal glomeruli are fenestrated (they have *holes*, presumably to facilitate filtration), while central nervous system endothelial cells (along with the associated perivascular cells) create an impermeable blood-brain barrier.

Endothelial cells are versatile multifunctional cells with a wealth of synthetic and metabolic properties. In the normal state they have several constitutive activities that are critical for vessel homeostasis and circulatory function. Endothelial cells have a nonthrombogenic surface that maintains blood in a fluid state (Chapter 4). They also modulate medial smooth muscle cell tone (thereby influencing vascular resistance), metabolize hormones such as angiotensin, regulate inflammation, and affect the growth of other cell types, particularly smooth muscle cells. Although interendothelial junctions are largely impermeable in normal vessels, vasoactive agents (e.g., histamine) allow the rapid egress of fluids, electrolytes and protein; in inflammation, even leukocytes can slip between adjacent endothelial cells (Chapter 3).

Endothelial cells can respond to various stimuli by adjusting their steady-state (constitutive) functions and by expressing newly acquired (inducible) properties—a process termed *endothelial activation* (Fig. 11-2). Inducers of endothelial activation include cytokines and bacterial products, which elicit inflammation and, in severe cases, septic shock (Chapter 4); hemodynamic stresses and lipid products, critical to the pathogenesis of atherosclerosis (see later); advanced glycation end-products (important in the pathologic sequelae of diabetes, Chapter 24); as well as viruses, complement components, and hypoxia. Activated endothelial cells, in turn, express adhesion molecules (Chapter 3) and produce cytokines and chemokines, growth factors, vasoactive molecules that result either in vasoconstriction or in vasodilation, major histocompatibility complex molecules, procoagulant and anticoagulant factors, and a variety of other biologically active products.

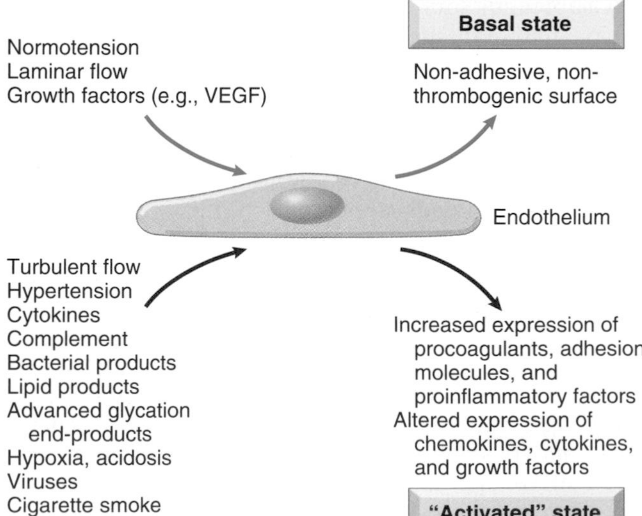

Figure 11-2 Basal and activated endothelial cell states. Normal blood pressure, laminar flow, and low growth factor levels promote a basal endothelial cell state that maintains a nonthrombotic, nonadhesive surface with appropriate vascular wall smooth muscle tone. Injury or exposure to certain mediators results in endothelial activation, a state where endothelial cells develop a procoagulant surface that can be adhesive for inflammatory cells, and also express factors that cause smooth muscle contraction and/or proliferation and matrix synthesis. VEGF, vascular endothelial growth factor.

Endothelial cells influence the vasoreactivity of the underlying smooth muscle cells through the production of both relaxing factors (e.g., nitric oxide [NO]) and contracting factors (e.g., endothelin). Normal endothelial cell function is characterized by a balance of these responses.

Endothelial dysfunction refers to an alteration in endothelial phenotype seen in many different conditions that is often both proinflammatory and prothrombogenic. It is responsible, at least in part, for the initiation of thrombus formation, atherosclerosis, and the vascular lesions of hypertension and other disorders. Certain forms of endothelial dysfunction are rapid in onset (within minutes), reversible, and independent of new protein synthesis (e.g., endothelial cell contraction induced by histamine and other vasoactive mediators that causes gaps in venular endothelium, Chapter 3). Other changes such as upregulation of adhesion molecules involve alterations in gene expression and protein synthesis and may require hours or even days to develop.

Vascular smooth muscle cells are the predominant cellular element of the vascular media, playing important roles in normal vascular repair and pathologic processes such as atherosclerosis. Smooth muscle cells have the capacity to proliferate when appropriately stimulated; they can also synthesize collagen, elastin, and proteoglycans and elaborate growth factors and cytokines. Smooth muscle cells are also responsible for the vasoconstriction or dilation that occurs in response to physiologic or pharmacologic stimuli.

Intimal Thickening: A Stereotyped Response to Vascular Injury

Vascular injury—associated with endothelial cell dysfunction or loss—stimulates smooth muscle cell recruitment and proliferation and associated matrix synthesis; the result is intimal thickening. Healing of injured vessels is analogous to the healing process that occurs in other damaged tissues (Chapter 3). Endothelial cells involved in repair may migrate from adjacent uninjured areas into denuded areas or may also be derived from circulating precursors. Medial smooth muscle cells or smooth muscle precursor cells also migrate into the intima, proliferate, and synthesize extracellular matrix in much the same way that fibroblasts fill in a wound (Fig. 11-3). The resulting neointima is typically completely covered by endothelial cells. This neointimal response occurs with any form of vascular damage or dysfunction, regardless of cause. *Thus, intimal thickening is the stereotypical response of the vessel wall to any insult.*

Neointimal smooth muscle cells have a phenotype that is distinct from that of medial smooth muscle cells. Specifically, rather than primarily functioning as contractile cells, neointimal smooth muscle cells are motile, undergo cell division, and acquire new biosynthetic capabilities. The function of neointimal smooth muscle cells is regulated by cytokines and growth factors derived from platelets, endothelial cells, and macrophages, as well as thrombin and activated complement factors. With time and restoration and/or normalization of the endothelial layer, intimal smooth muscle cells can return to a nonproliferative state. However, the healing response results in intimal thickening that may impede vascular flow.

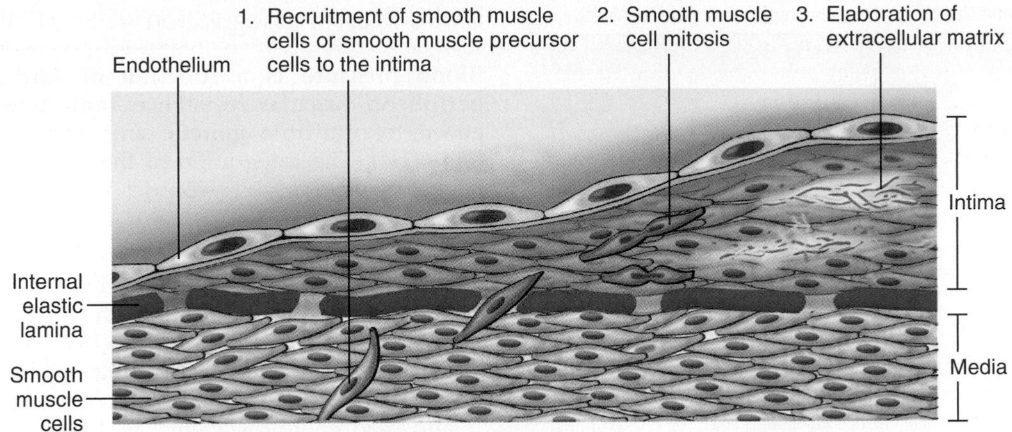

Figure 11-3 Stereotypical response to vascular injury. Schematic diagram of intimal thickening, emphasizing intimal smooth muscle cell migration and proliferation associated with extracellular matrix synthesis. The new intimal cells are shown in a different color to emphasize that they have a proliferative, synthetic, and noncontractile phenotype distinct from medial smooth muscle cells.

KEY CONCEPTS

Response of Vascular Wall Cells to Injury

- All vessels are lined by endothelium; although all endothelial cells share certain homeostatic properties, endothelial cells in specific vascular beds have special features that allow for tissue-specific functions (e.g., fenestrated endothelial cells in renal glomeruli).
- Endothelial cell function is tightly regulated in both the basal and activated states. Various physiologic and pathophysiologic stimuli induce endothelial activation and dysfunction that alter the endothelial cell phenotype (e.g., procoagulative vs. anticoagulative, proinflammatory vs. antiinflammatory, and nonadhesive vs. adhesive).
- Injury (of almost any type) to the vessel wall results in a stereotyped healing response involving smooth muscle cell proliferation, extracellular matrice deposition, and intimal expansion.
- The recruitment and activation of the smooth muscle cell involves signals from cells (e.g., endothelial cells, platelets, and macrophages), as well as mediators derived from coagulation and complement cascades.
- Excessive thickening of the intima may result in luminal stenosis and vascular obstruction.

Hypertensive Vascular Disease

Systemic and local tissue blood pressures must be maintained within a narrow range to prevent untoward consequences. Low blood pressure *(hypotension)* results in inadequate organ perfusion and can lead to tissue dysfunction or death. Conversely, high blood pressure *(hypertension)* can cause end-organ damage and is one of the major risk factors for atherosclerosis (see later).

Like height and weight, blood pressure is a continuously distributed variable, and detrimental effects of elevated blood pressure increase continuously as blood pressure rises—no rigidly defined threshold level of blood pressure identifies those who are at risk for cardiovascular disease. Both the systolic and diastolic blood pressure are important in determining risk; specifically, sustained diastolic pressures above 89 mm Hg or sustained systolic pressure above 139 mm Hg are associated with increased risk of atherosclerotic disease, and are thus considered clinically significant. Approximately 29% of individuals in the general population are hypertensive based on these criteria. However, such cutoffs do not reliably assess risk in all patients; for example, when other risk factors such as diabetes are present, lower thresholds are applicable.

Table 11-1 lists the major causes of hypertension. A small number of patients (approximately 5%) are said to have *secondary hypertension* resulting from an underlying renal or adrenal disease (e.g., primary aldosteronism, Cushing syndrome, or pheochromocytoma), renal artery stenosis, or other identifiable cause. *However, approximately 90% to 95% of hypertension is idiopathic—so-called essential hypertension.* Although the molecular pathways that regulate normal blood pressure are reasonably well understood, the causes of hypertension in most individuals remain unknown. It seems likely that hypertension is a multifactorial disorder, resulting from the cumulative effects of multiple genetic polymorphisms and interacting environmental factors.

The prevalence and vulnerability to complications of hypertension increase with age and are higher among African Americans. Besides increasing atherosclerotic risk, hypertension can cause cardiac hypertrophy and heart failure (*hypertensive heart disease*, Chapter 12), multi-infarct dementia (Chapter 28), aortic dissection (discussed later in this chapter), and renal failure (Chapter 20). Unfortunately, hypertension typically remains asymptomatic until late in its course and even severely elevated pressures can be clinically silent for years. Left untreated, roughly half of hypertensive patients die of ischemic heart disease (IHD) or congestive heart failure, and another third die of stroke. Treatment with blood pressure lowering drugs dramatically reduces the incidence and death rates attributable to all forms of hypertension-related pathology.

A small percentage of hypertensive persons (as much as 5%) show a rapidly rising blood pressure that, if untreated, leads to death within 1 to 2 years. This form of hypetension, called *malignant hypertension,* is characterized by severe hypertension (i.e., systolic pressure more than 200 mm Hg, diastolic pressure more than 120 mm Hg),

Table 11-1 Types and Causes of Hypertension (Systolic and Diastolic)

Essential hypertension
Accounts for 90% to 95% of all cases
Secondary hypertension
Renal
Acute glomerulonephritis Chronic renal disease Polycystic disease Renal artery stenosis Renal vasculitis Renin-producing tumors
Endocrine
Adrenocortical hyperfunction (Cushing syndrome, primary aldosteronism, congenital adrenal hyperplasia, licorice ingestion) Exogenous hormones (glucocorticoids, estrogen [including pregnancy-induced and oral contraceptives], sympathomimetics and tyramine-containing foods, monoamine oxidase inhibitors) Pheochromocytoma Acromegaly Hypothyroidism (myxedema) Hyperthyroidism (thyrotoxicosis) Pregnancy-induced
Cardiovascular
Coarctation of aorta Polyarteritis nodosa Increased intravascular volume Increased cardiac output Rigidity of the aorta
Neurologic
Psychogenic Increased intracranial pressure Sleep apnea Acute stress, including surgery

renal failure, and retinal hemorrhages and exudates, with or without papilledema. It can develop in previously normotensive persons but more often is superimposed on pre-existing "benign" hypertension.

This section briefly outlines normal blood pressure homeostasis, followed by a discussion of pathogenic mechanisms that underlie hypertension and a description of hypertension-associated pathologic changes in vessels.

Blood Pressure Regulation

Blood pressure is a function of cardiac output and peripheral vascular resistance, both of which are influenced by multiple genetic and environmental factors (Fig. 11-4). The integration of the various inputs ensures adequate systemic perfusion, despite differences in regional demand.

- *Cardiac output* is a function of stroke volume and heart rate. The most important determinant of stroke volume is the filling pressure, which is regulated through sodium homeostasis and its effect on blood volume. Heart rate and myocardial contractility (a second factor affecting stroke volume) are both regulated by the α- and β-adrenergic systems, which also have important effects on vascular tone.
- *Peripheral resistance* is regulated predominantly at the level of the arterioles by neural and hormonal inputs. Vascular tone reflects a balance between vasoconstrictors (including angiotensin II, catecholamines, and endothelin) and vasodilators (including kinins, prostaglandins, and nitric oxide). Resistance vessels also exhibit *autoregulation*, whereby increased blood flow induces vasoconstriction to protect tissues against hyperperfusion. Finally, blood pressure is fine-tuned by tissue pH and hypoxia to accommodate local metabolic demands.

Factors released from the kidneys, adrenals, and myocardium interact to influence vascular tone and to regulate blood volume by adjusting sodium balance (Fig. 11-5). The kidneys filter 170 L of plasma containing 23 moles of salt daily. Thus, with a typical daily diet containing 100 mEq of sodium, 99.5% of the filtered salt must be reabsorbed to maintain total body sodium levels. About 98% of the filtered sodium is reabsorbed by constitutively active sodium transporters. The small amount of remaining sodium is subject to resorption by the epithelial sodium channel (ENaC), which is tightly regulated by the renin-angiotensin system; it is this pathway that determines net sodium balance.

The kidneys and heart contain cells that sense changes in blood pressure or volume. In response, these cells

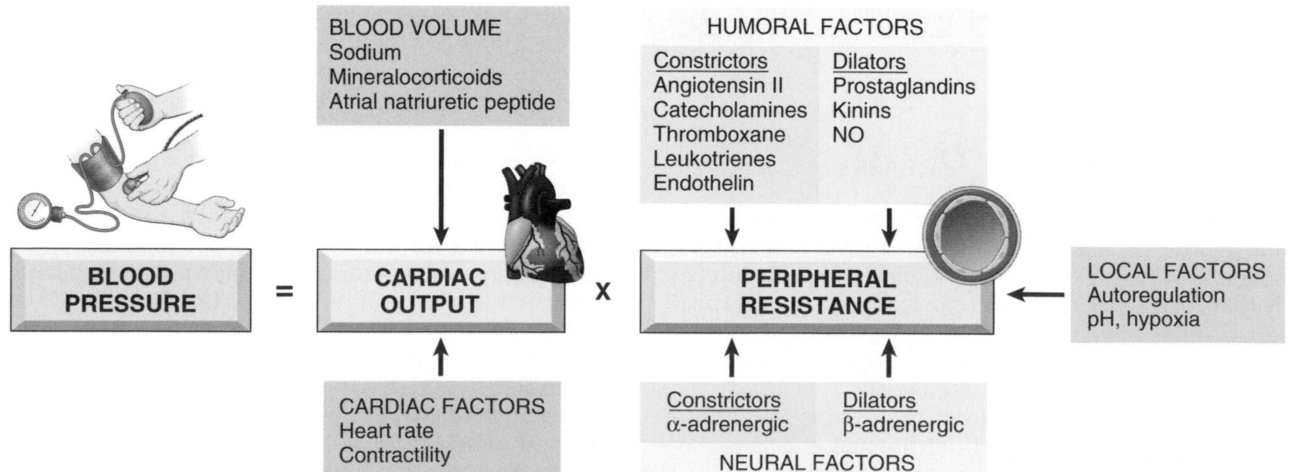

Figure 11-4 Blood pressure regulation. Diverse influences on cardiac output (e.g., blood volume and myocardial contractility) and peripheral resistance (neural, humoral, and local effectors) impact the output blood pressure.

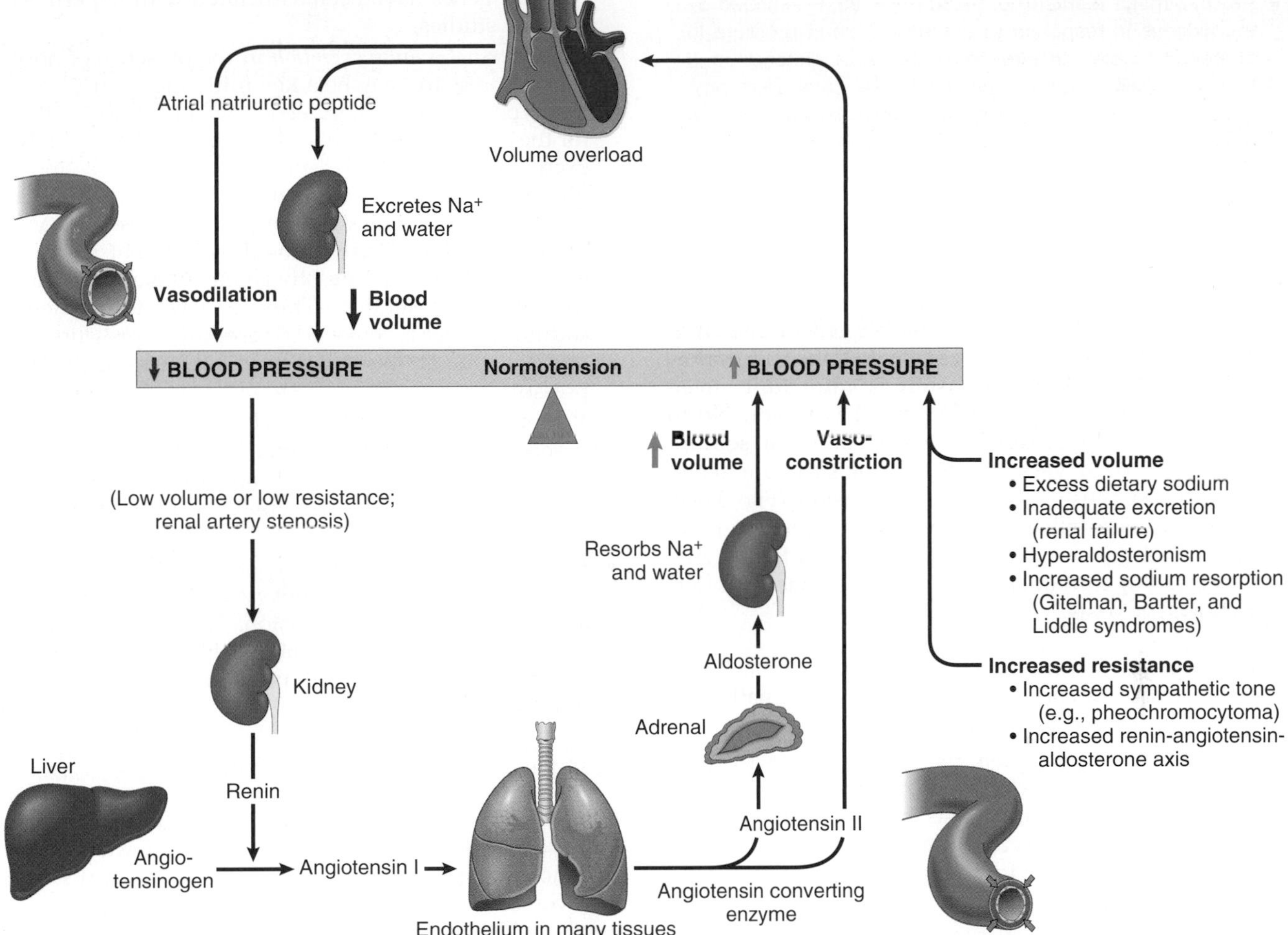

Figure 11-5 Interplay of renin-angiotensin-aldosterone and atrial natriuretic peptide in maintaining blood pressure homeostasis.

release circulating effectors that act in concert to maintain normal blood pressure. Kidneys influence peripheral resistance and sodium excretion/retention primarily through the renin-angiotensin system.

- *Renin* is a proteolytic enzyme produced by renal juxtaglomerular cells, myoepithelial cells that surround the glomerular afferent arterioles. Renin is released in response to low blood pressure in afferent arterioles, elevated levels of circulating catecholamines, or low sodium levels in the distal convoluted renal tubules. The latter occurs when the *glomerular filtration rate* falls (e.g., when the cardiac output is low), leading to increased sodium resorption by the proximal tubules.
- Renin cleaves *plasma angiotensinogen* to *angiotensin I*, which in turn is converted to *angiotensin II* by angiotensin-converting enzyme (ACE), mainly a product of vascular endothelium. Angiotensin II raises blood pressure by (1) inducing vascular contraction, (2) stimulating aldosterone secretion by the adrenal gland, and (3) increasing tubular sodium resorption. *Adrenal aldosterone* increases blood pressure by increasing sodium resorption (and thus water) in the distal convoluted tubule, which increases blood volume.
- The kidney also produces a variety of vascular relaxing substances (including prostaglandins and NO) that presumably counterbalance the vasopressor effects of angiotensin.

Myocardial natriuretic peptides are released from atrial and ventricular myocardium in response to volume expansion; these inhibit sodium resorption in the distal renal tubules, thus leading to sodium excretion and diuresis. They also induce systemic vasodilation.

KEY CONCEPTS

Blood Pressure Regulation

- Blood pressure is determined by vascular resistance and cardiac output.
- Vascular resistance is regulated at the level of the arterioles, influenced by neural and hormonal inputs.
- Cardiac output is determined by heart rate and stroke volume, which is strongly influenced by blood volume. Blood volume in turn is regulated mainly by renal sodium excretion or resorption.

- Renin, a major regulator of blood pressure, is secreted by the kidneys in response to decreased blood pressure in afferent arterioles. In turn, renin cleaves angiotensinogen to angiotensin I; subsequent peripheral catabolism produces angiotensin II, which regulates blood pressure by increasing vascular smooth muscle cell tone and by increasing adrenal aldosterone secretion and thereby renal sodium resorption.

Pathogenesis of Hypertension

Hypertension is a disorder with multiple genetic and environmental contributions. As already noted, **the vast majority (90% to 95%) of hypertension is idiopathic**. Even without knowing the specific lesions, it is reasonable to suppose that multiple small changes in renal sodium homeostasis and/or vessel wall tone or structure act in combination to cause essential hypertension (Fig. 11-5). Most other causes fall under the general rubric of renal disease, including renovascular hypertension (due to renal artery occlusion). Infrequently, hypertension has an underlying endocrine basis.

Pathogenesis of Secondary Hypertension. In many secondary forms of hypertension, the underlying pathways are reasonably well understood:

- In *renovascular hypertension*, renal artery stenosis causes decreased glomerular flow and pressure in the afferent arteriole of the glomerulus. This induces renin secretion, which, as already discussed, increases vascular tone and blood volume via the angiotensin-aldosterone pathway (Fig. 11-5).
- *Single-gene disorders* cause severe but rare forms of hypertension:
  - *Gene defects affecting enzymes involved in aldosterone metabolism (e.g., aldosterone synthase, 11β-hydroxylase, 17α-hydroxylase)*. These lead to an increase in secretion of aldosterone, increased salt and water resorption, plasma volume expansion and, ultimately, hypertension. *Primary hyperaldosteronism* is one of the most common causes of secondary hypertension (Chapter 24).
  - *Mutations affecting proteins that influence sodium reabsorption.* For example, the moderately severe form of salt-sensitive hypertension, called *Liddle syndrome*, is caused by gain-of-function mutations in an epithelial Na^+ channel protein that increase distal tubular reabsorption of sodium in response to aldosterone.

Mechanisms of Essential Hypertension

- *Genetic factors* influence blood pressure regulation, as shown by comparisons of monozygotic and dizygotic twins, and genetically related versus adopted children. Moreover, as noted earlier, several single-gene disorders cause relatively rare forms of hypertension (and hypotension) by altering net sodium reabsorption in the kidney. It is also suspected (but not yet proven) that variations in blood pressure may result from the cumulative effects of polymorphisms in several genes that affect blood pressure; for example, sequence variants in both the angiotensinogen and the angiotensin receptor genes have been associated with hypertension in some studies.
- *Reduced renal sodium excretion* in the presence of normal arterial pressure may be a key initiating event in essential hypertension and, indeed, a final common pathway for the pathogenesis of hypertension. Decreased sodium excretion may lead sequentially to an increase in fluid volume, increased cardiac output, and peripheral vasoconstriction, thereby elevating blood pressure. At the higher blood pressure, enough additional sodium is excreted by the kidneys to equal intake and prevent further fluid retention. Thus, a new steady state of sodium balance is achieved ("resetting of pressure natriuresis"), but at the expense of an increase in blood pressure.
- *Vasoconstrictive influences*, such as factors that induce vasoconstriction or stimuli that cause structural changes in the vessel wall, can lead to an increase in peripheral resistance and may also play a role in essential hypertension.
- *Environmental factors*, such as stress, obesity, smoking, physical inactivity, and heavy salt consumption are all implicated in hypertension. Indeed, the evidence linking dietary sodium intake with the prevalence of hypertension in different populations is particularly impressive.

Vascular Pathology in Hypertension

Hypertension not only accelerates atherogenesis (see later) but also causes degenerative changes in the walls of large and medium arteries that can lead to both aortic dissection and cerebrovascular hemorrhage. Hypertension is also associated with two forms of small blood vessel disease: hyaline arteriolosclerosis and hyperplastic arteriolosclerosis (Fig. 11-6).

MORPHOLOGY

Hyaline arteriolosclerosis. Arterioles show homogeneous, pink hyaline thickening with associated luminal narrowing (Fig. 11-6*A*). These changes reflect both plasma protein leakage across injured endothelial cells, as well as increased smooth muscle cell matrix synthesis in response to the chronic hemodynamic stresses of hypertension. Although the vessels of older patients (either normotensive or hypertensive) also frequently exhibit hyaline arteriosclerosis, it is more generalized and severe in patients with hypertension. The same lesions are also a common feature of diabetic microangiography; in that case, the underlying etiology is hyperglycemia-induced endothelial cell dysfunction (Chapter 24). In **nephrosclerosis** due to chronic hypertension, the arteriolar narrowing of hyaline arteriosclerosis causes diffuse impairment of renal blood supply and glomerular scarring (Chapter 20).

Hyperplastic Arteriolosclerosis. This lesion occurs in severe hypertension; vessels exhibit concentric, **laminated ("onion-skin")** thickening of the walls with luminal narrowing (Fig. 11-6*B*). The laminations consist of smooth muscle cells with thickened, reduplicated basement membrane; in malignant hypertension, they are accompanied by fibrinoid deposits and vessel wall necrosis **(necrotizing arteriolitis)**, particularly in the kidney (Chapter 20).

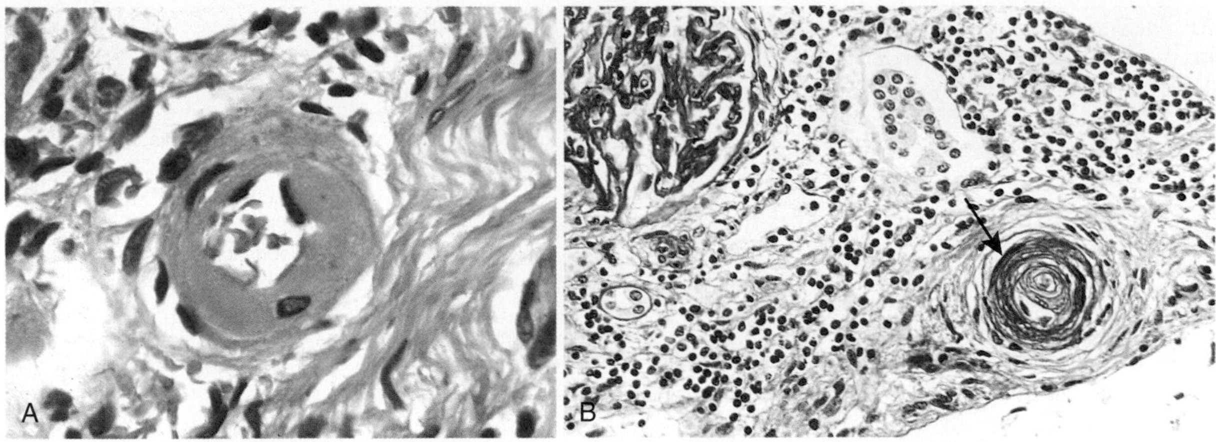

Figure 11-6 Vascular pathology in hypertension. **A,** Hyaline arteriolosclerosis. The arteriolar wall is thickened with increased protein deposition (hyalinized), and the lumen is markedly narrowed. **B,** Hyperplastic arteriolosclerosis (onion-skinning) causing luminal obliteration (periodic acid–Schiff [PAS] stain). (Courtesy Helmut Rennke, MD, Brigham and Women's Hospital, Boston, Mass.)

KEY CONCEPTS

Hypertension

- Hypertension is a common disorder , affecting roughly 30% of adults in the U.S.; it is a major risk factor for atherosclerosis, congestive heart failure, and renal failure.
- Essential hypertension represents 90% to 95% of cases and is a complex, multifactorial disorder, involving both environmental influences and genetic polymorphisms that influence sodium resorption and the renin-angiotensin-aldosterone system.
- Hypertension is occasionally caused by single gene disorders or is secondary to diseases of the kidney, adrenal, or other endocrine organs.
- Sustained hypertension requires participation of the kidney, which normally responds to hypertension by eliminating salt and water. In established hypertension, both increased blood volume and increased peripheral resistance contribute to the increased blood pressure.
- Histologically, hypertension is associated with thickening of arterial walls caused by hyaline deposits and, in severe cases, by proliferation of smooth muscle cells and reduplication of basement membranes.

Arteriosclerosis

Arteriosclerosis literally means "hardening of the arteries"; it is a generic term for arterial wall thickening and loss of elasticity. There are three general patterns, with different clinical and pathologic consequences:

- *Arteriolosclerosis* affects small arteries and arterioles, and may cause downstream ischemic injury. The two anatomic variants, hyaline and hyperplastic, are discussed earlier in relation to hypertension.
- *Mönckeberg medial sclerosis* is characterized by calcification of the walls of muscular arteries, typically involving the internal elastic membrane. Persons older than age 50 are most commonly affected. The calcifications do not encroach on the vessel lumen and are usually not clinically significant.
- *Atherosclerosis*, from Greek root words for "gruel" and "hardening," is the most frequent and clinically important pattern and is discussed here.

Atherosclerosis

Atherosclerosis underlies the pathogenesis of coronary, cerebral and peripheral vascular disease, and causes more morbidity and mortality (roughly half of all deaths) in the Western world than any other disorder. Because coronary artery disease is an important manifestation of the disease, epidemiologic data related to atherosclerosis mortality typically reflect deaths caused by ischemic heart disease (Chapter 12); indeed, myocardial infarction is responsible for almost a quarter of all deaths in the United States. Significant morbidity and mortality are also caused by aortic and carotid atherosclerotic disease and stroke.

The likelihood of atherosclerosis is determined by the combination of acquired (e.g., cholesterol levels, smoking, hypertension) and inherited (e.g., LDL receptor gene mutations) risk factors. Acting in concert they cause initimal lesions called *atheromas* (also called *atheromatous or atherosclerotic plaques*) that protrude into vessel lumens. An atheromatous plaque consists of a raised lesion with a soft grumous core of lipid (mainly cholesterol and cholesterol esters) covered by a fibrous cap (Fig. 11-7). Besides mechanically obstructing blood flow, atherosclerotic plaques can rupture leading to catastrophic obstructive vascular thrombosis. Atherosclerotic plaque can also increase the diffusion distance from the lumen to the media, leading to ischemic injury and weakening of the vessel wall, changes that may result in aneurysm formation.

Epidemiology. Although atherosclerosis-associated ischemic heart disease is ubiquitous among most developed nations, risk reduction and improved therapies have combined to moderate the associated mortality. At the same time, reduced mortality from infectious diseases and the adoption of Western lifestyles has led to increased

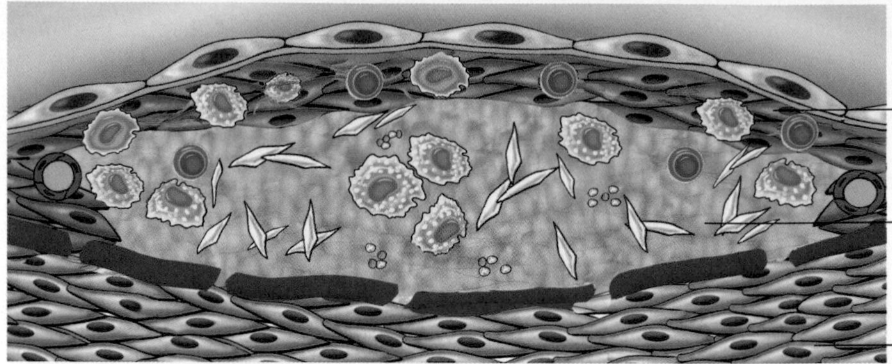

Figure 11-7 Basic structure of an atherosclerotic plaque. Note that atherosclerosis is an intimal-based process.

prevalence of ischemic heart disease in developing nations. As a result, the death rate for coronary artery disease in the United States now lags behind the death rates in most of Africa, India, and Southeast Asia. The countries of the former Soviet Union hold the dubious distinction of having the highest ischemic heart disease-associated mortality rates, three to five times higher than the United States, and seven to 12 times greater than Japan.

The prevalence and severity of atherosclerosis and ischemic heart disease among individuals and groups are related to a number of risk factors. Some of these factors are constitutional (and therefore less controllable), but others are acquired or related to specific behaviors and potentially amenable to intervention (Table 11-2). Risk factors have been identified through a number of prospective analyses (e.g., the Framingham Heart Study). *These risk factors have roughly multiplicative effect*. Thus, two factors increase risk approximately four-fold, and three (i.e., hyperlipidemia, hypertension, and smoking), increase risk by a factor of seven (Fig. 11-8).

Constitutional Risk Factors

- *Genetics*. Family history is the most important independent risk factor for atherosclerosis. Certain Mendelian disorders are strongly associated with atherosclerosis (e.g., familial hypercholesterolemia; Chapter 5), but these account for only a small percentage of cases. The well-established familial predisposition to atherosclerosis and ischemic heart disease is usually polygenic, relating to familial clustering of other established risk factors, such as hypertension or diabetes, or to inherited variants that influence other pathophysiologic processes, such as inflammation.

Table 11-2 Major Risk Factors for Atherosclerosis

Nonmodifiable (Constitutional)
Genetic abnormalities
Family history
Increasing age
Male gender
Modifiable
Hyperlipidemia
Hypertension
Cigarette smoking
Diabetes
Inflammation

- *Age* is a dominant influence. Although the development of atherosclerotic plaque is typically a progressive process, it does not usually become clinically manifest until lesions reach a critical threshold in middle age or later (see later). Thus, between ages 40 and 60, the incidence of myocardial infarction increases five-fold. Death rates from ischemic heart disease rise with each decade even into advanced age.
- *Gender*. Other factors being equal, premenopausal women are relatively protected against atherosclerosis and its consequences compared to age-matched men. Thus, myocardial infarction and other complications of atherosclerosis are uncommon in premenopausal women unless they are otherwise predisposed by diabetes, hyperlipidemia, or severe hypertension. After menopause, however, the incidence of atherosclerosis-related diseases increases in women and at older ages actually exceeds that of men. Although a favorable influence of estrogen has long been proposed to explain this effect, clinical trials of estrogen replacement have not been shown to protect against vascular disease; indeed, in some studies, post-menopausal estrogen replacement actually *increased* cardiovascular risk. The atheroprotective effect of estrogens may be related to the age at which the therapy is initiated; in younger postmenopausal women, coronary atherosclerosis is diminished by estrogen therapy, while older women appear not to benefit.

Modifiable Major Risk Factors

- ***Hyperlipidemia*—and more specifically hypercholesterolemia—is a major risk factor for atherosclerosis; even in the absence of other risk factors, hypercholesterolemia is sufficient to initiate lesion development.** The major component of serum cholesterol associated with increased risk is low-density lipoprotein (LDL) cholesterol ("bad cholesterol"). LDL is the complex that delivers cholesterol to peripheral tissues; in contrast, high-density lipoprotein (HDL) is the complex that mobilizes cholesterol from the periphery (including atheromas) and transports it to the liver for excretion in the bile. Consequently, higher levels of HDL ("good cholesterol") correlate with reduced risk.

  Understandably, dietary and pharmacologic approaches that lower LDL or total serum cholesterol, or raise serum HDL, are of considerable interest. High

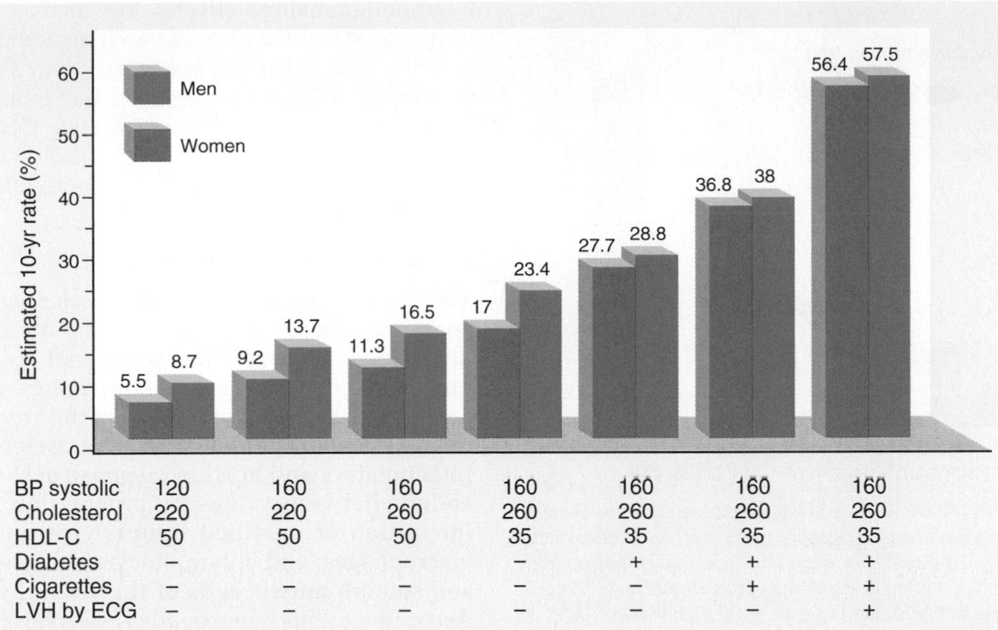

Figure 11-8 Estimated 10-year rate of coronary artery disease in 55-year old men and women as a function of established risk factors (hyperlipidemia, hypertension, smoking, and diabetes). BP, Blood pressure; ECG, electrocardiogram; HDL-C, high-density lipoprotein cholesterol; LVH, left ventricular hypertrophy. (From O'Donnell CJ, Kannel WB: Cardiovascular risks of hypertension: Lessons from observational studies. J Hypertension 16 (Suppl. 6):3, 1998.)

dietary intake of cholesterol and saturated fats (present in egg yolks, animal fats, and butter, for example) raises plasma cholesterol levels. Conversely, diets low in cholesterol and/or high in polyunsaturated fats lower plasma cholesterol levels. Omega-3 fatty acids (abundant in fish oils) are beneficial, whereas (trans)-unsaturated fats produced by artificial hydrogenation of polyunsaturated oils (used in baked goods and margarine) adversely affect cholesterol profiles. Exercise and moderate consumption of ethanol raise HDL levels whereas obesity and smoking lower it. *Statins* are a class of drugs that lower circulating cholesterol levels by inhibiting hydroxymethylglutaryl coenzyme A (HMG CoA) reductase, the rate-limiting enzyme in hepatic cholesterol biosynthesis (Chapter 5). In the past two decades, statins have been used widely to lower serum cholesterol levels, arguably one of the most significant success stories of translational research.

- *Hypertension* (see earlier) is another major risk factor for atherosclerosis; both systolic and diastolic levels are important. On its own, hypertension can increase the risk of ischemic heart disease by approximately 60% versus normotensive populations (Fig. 11-8). Chronic hypertension is the most common cause of left ventricular hypertrophy, and hence the latter is also a surrogate marker for cardiovascular risk.
- *Cigarette smoking* is a well-established risk factor in men and likely accounts for the increasing incidence and severity of atherosclerosis in women. Prolonged (years) smoking of one pack of cigarettes or more daily doubles the death rate from ischemic heart disease. Smoking cessation reduces that risk substantially.
- *Diabetes mellitus* induces hypercholesterolemia (Chapter 24) and markedly increases the risk of atherosclerosis. Other factors being equal, the incidence of myocardial infarction is twice as high in patients with diabetes than in those without. There is also an increased risk of stroke and a 100-fold increased risk of atherosclerosis-induced gangrene of the lower extremities.

Additional Risk Factors

As many as 20% of all cardiovascular events occur in the absence of overt risk factors (e.g., hypertension, hyperlipidemia, smoking, or diabetes). Indeed, more than 75% of cardiovascular events in previously healthy women occur with LDL cholesterol levels below 160 mg/dL (levels generally considered to connote low risk). Clearly, other factors also contribute to risk; among those that are proven or suspected are the following:

- *Inflammation.* Inflammation is present during all stages of atherogenesis and is intimately linked with atherosclerotic plaque formation and rupture (see later). With the increasing recognition that inflammation plays a significant causal role in ischemic heart disease, assessment of systemic inflammation has become important in overall risk stratification. While a number of circulating markers of inflammation correlate with ischemic heart disease risk, *C-reactive protein (CRP)* has emerged as one of the simplest to measure and one of the most sensitive.

  CRP is an acute phase reactant synthesized primarily by the liver. Its expression is increased by a number of inflammatory mediators, particularly IL-6, and it augments the innate immune response by binding to bacteria and activating the classical complement cascade. Whether CRP has any causal role in atherosclerosis is controversial. However, it is well established that plasma CRP is a strong, independent marker of risk for myocardial infarction, stroke, peripheral arterial disease,

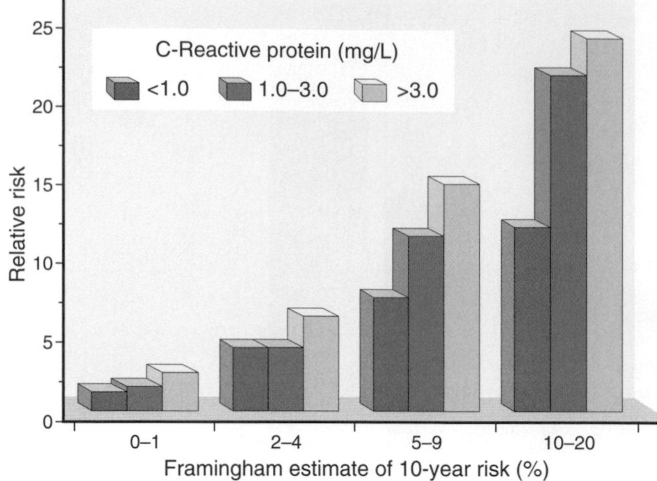

Figure 11-9 C reactive protein (CRP) predicts cardiovascular risk. Relative risk (y-axis) refers to the risk of a cardiovascular event (e.g., myocardial infarction). The x-axis is the 10-year risk of a cardiovascular event derived from established risk factors identified in the Framingham Heart Study. In each risk group, CRP values further stratify patients. (Data from Ridker PM, et al: Comparison of C-reactive protein and low-density lipoprotein cholesterol levels in the prediction of first cardiovascular events. N Engl J Med 347:1557, 2002.)

and sudden cardiac death, even among apparently healthy individuals (Fig. 11-9). Accordingly, CRP levels have been incorporated into risk stratification algorithms. CRP is also a useful marker for gauging the effects of risk reduction measures, such as smoking cessation, weight loss, exercise, and statins; each one of these reduce CRP levels.

- *Hyperhomocystinemia.* Serum homocysteine levels correlate with coronary atherosclerosis, peripheral vascular disease, stroke, and venous thrombosis. *Homocystinuria,* due to rare inborn errors of metabolism, results in elevated circulating homocysteine (>100 μmol/L) and is associated with premature vascular disease. Although low folate and vitamin B_{12} levels can increase homocysteine, supplemental vitamin ingestion does not affect the incidence of cardiovascular disease.
- *Metabolic syndrome.* Associated with central obesity (Chapter 9), this entity is characterized by insulin resistance, hypertension, dyslipidemia (elevated LDL and depressed HDL), hypercoagulability, and a proinflammatory state. The dyslipidemia, hyperglycemia, and hypertension are all cardiac risk factors, while the systemic hypercoagulable and proinflammatory state may contribute to endothelial dysfunction and/or thrombosis.
- *Lipoprotein a [Lp(a)]* is an altered form of LDL that contains the apolipoprotein B-100 portion of LDL linked to apolipoprotein A (apo A); Lp(a) levels are associated with coronary and cerebrovascular disease risk, independent of total cholesterol or LDL levels.
- *Factors affecting hemostasis.* Several markers of hemostatic and/or fibrinolytic function (e.g., elevated plasminogen activator inhibitor 1) are potent predictors of risk for major atherosclerotic events, including myocardial infarction and stroke. Platelet-derived factors, as well as thrombin—through both its procoagulant and proinflammatory effects—are increasingly recognized as major contributors to vascular pathology.
- *Other factors.* Factors associated with a less pronounced and/or difficult-to-quantitate risk include lack of exercise; competitive, stressful life style ("type A" personality); and obesity (the latter also being complicated by hypertension, diabetes, hypertriglyceridemia, and decreased HDL).

Pathogenesis of Atherosclerosis

The clinical importance of atherosclerosis has stimulated enormous interest in understanding the mechanisms that underlie its evolution and complications. The contemporary view of atherogenesis integrates the risk factors previously discussed and is called the "response to injury" hypothesis. **This model views atherosclerosis as a chronic inflammatory and healing response of the arterial wall to endothelial injury. Lesion progression occurs through interaction of modified lipoproteins, monocyte-derived macrophages, and T lymphocytes with endothelial cells and smooth muscle cells of the arterial wall** (Fig. 11-10). According to this schema, atherosclerosis progresses in the following sequence:

- *Endothelial injury and dysfunction,* causing (among other things) increased vascular permeability, leukocyte adhesion, and thrombosis
- *Accumulation of lipoproteins* (mainly LDL and its oxidized forms) in the vessel wall
- *Monocyte adhesion to the endothelium,* followed by migration into the intima and transformation into *macrophages* and *foam cells*
- *Platelet adhesion*
- *Factor release* from activated platelets, macrophages, and vascular wall cells, inducing *smooth muscle cell recruitment,* either from the media or from circulating precursors
- *Smooth muscle cell proliferation, extracellular matrix production,* and *recruitment of T cells.*
- *Lipid accumulation* both extracellularly and within cells (macrophages and smooth muscle cell)

Endothelial Injury. Endothelial cell injury is the cornerstone of the response-to-injury hypothesis. Endothelial loss due to *any* kind of injury—induced experimentally by mechanical denudation, hemodynamic forces, immune complex deposition, irradiation, or chemicals—results in intimal thickening. However, *early human lesions begin at sites of morphologically intact endothelium.* Thus, nondenuding *endothelial dysfunction* underlies most human atherosclerosis; the intact but dysfunctional endothelial cells exhibit increased endothelial permeability, enhanced leukocyte adhesion, and altered gene expression.

The specific pathways of and factors contributing to endothelial cell dysfunction in early atherosclerosis are not completely understood: etiologic culprits include toxins from cigarette smoke, homocysteine, and even infectious agents, according to some (blame the bugs!). Inflammatory cytokines (e.g., tumor necrosis factor [TNF]) can also stimulate pro-atherogenic endothelial gene expression. However, **the two most important causes of endothelial dysfunction are hemodynamic disturbances and hypercholesterolemia.**

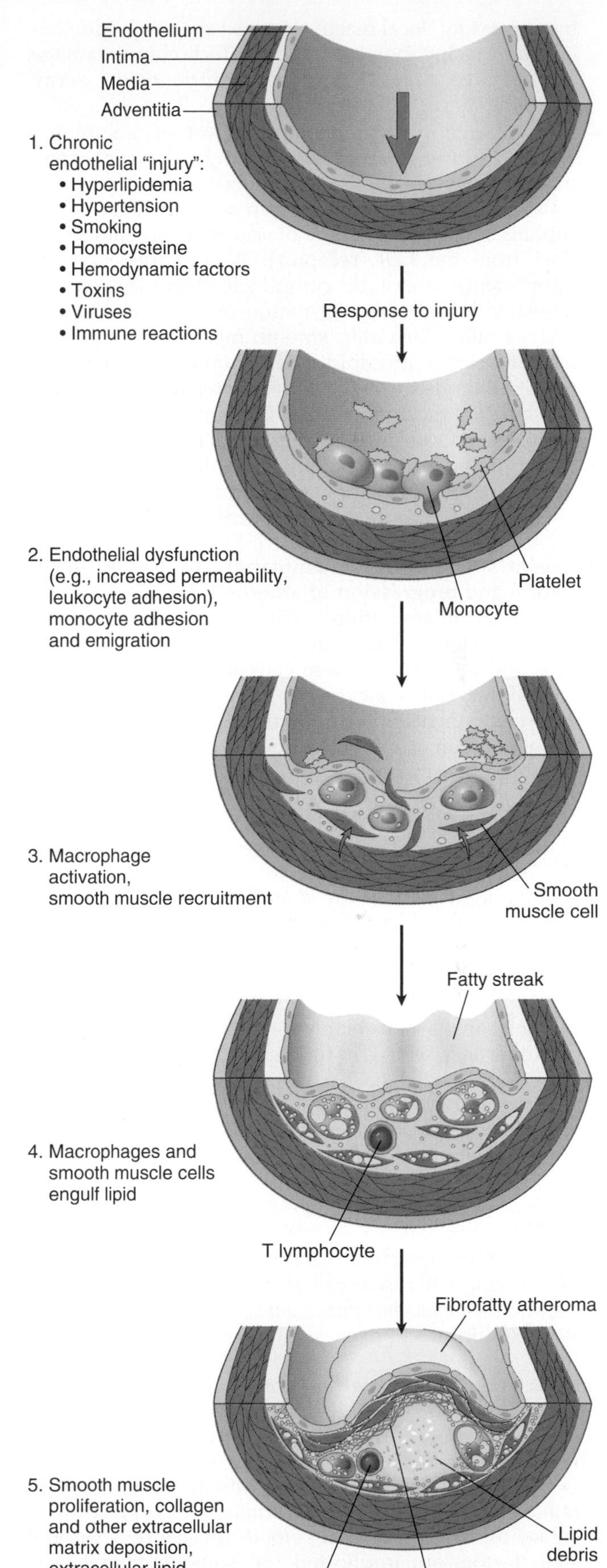

Figure 11-10 Evolution of arterial wall changes in the response to injury hypothesis. *1,* Normal. *2,* Endothelial injury with monocyte and platelet adhesion. *3,* Monocyte and smooth muscle cell migration into the intima, with macrophage activation. *4,* Macrophage and smooth muscle cell uptake of modified lipids, with further activation and recruitment of T cells. *5,* Intimal smooth muscle cell proliferation with extracellular matrix production, forming a well-developed plaque.

Hemodynamic Disturbances. The importance of hemodynamic turbulence in atherogenesis is illustrated by the observation that plaques tend to occur at ostia of exiting vessels, branch points, and along the posterior wall of the abdominal aorta, where there are disturbed flow patterns. In vitro studies have demonstrated that nonturbulent laminar flow leads to the induction of endothelial genes whose products (e.g., the antioxidant superoxide dismutase) actually *protect* against atherosclerosis. Such "atheroprotective" genes could explain the nonrandom localization of early atherosclerotic lesions.

Lipids. Lipids are transported in the bloodstream bound to specific apoproteins (forming lipoprotein complexes). *Dyslipoproteinemias* are lipoprotein abnormalities that may be present in the general population (and indeed, are found in many myocardial infarction survivors) include (1) increased LDL cholesterol levels, (2) decreased HDL cholesterol levels, and (3) increased levels of the abnormal lipoprotein (a). These may result from mutations that lead to defects in apoproteins or lipoprotein receptors, or arise from other underlying disorders that affect circulating lipid levels, such as nephrotic syndrome, alcoholism, hypothyroidism, or diabetes mellitus. All of these abnormalities are associated with an increased risk of atherosclerosis.

The evidence implicating hypercholesterolemia in atherogenesis includes:

- The dominant lipids in atheromatous plaques are cholesterol and cholesterol esters.
- Genetic defects in lipoprotein uptake and metabolism that cause hyperlipoproteinemia are associated with accelerated atherosclerosis. For example, familial hypercholesterolemia, caused by defective LDL receptors and inadequate hepatic LDL uptake (Chapter 5), can precipitate myocardial infarctions before age 20. Similarly, accelerated atherosclerosis occurs in animal models with engineered deficiencies in apolipoproteins or LDL receptors.
- Other genetic or acquired disorders (e.g., diabetes mellitus, hypothyroidism) that cause hypercholesterolemia lead to premature atherosclerosis.
- Epidemiologic analyses demonstrate a significant correlation between the severity of atherosclerosis and the levels of total plasma cholesterol or LDL.
- Lowering serum cholesterol by diet or drugs slows the rate of progression of atherosclerosis, causes regression of some plaques, and reduces the risk of cardiovascular events.

The mechanisms by which hyperlipidemia contributes to atherogenesis include the following:

- Chronic hyperlipidemia, particularly hypercholesterolemia, can directly impair endothelial cell function by increasing local reactive oxygen species production; besides causing membrane and mitochondrial damage, oxygen free radicals accelerate nitric oxide decay, damping its vasodilator activity.

- With chronic hyperlipidemia, lipoproteins accumulate within the intima, where they may aggregate or become oxidized by free radicals produced by inflammatory cells. Such modified LDL is then accumulated by macrophages through a variety of scavenger receptors (distinct from the LDL receptor). Because the modified lipoproteins cannot be completely degraded, chronic ingestion leads to the formation of lipid-filled macrophages called *foam cells;* smooth muscle cells can similarly transform into lipid-laden foam cells by ingesting modified lipids through LDL-receptor related proteins. Not only are the modified lipoproteins toxic to endothelial cells, smooth muscle cells, and macrophages, but their binding and uptake also stimulates the release of growth factors, cytokines, and chemokines that create a vicious cycle of monocyte recruitment and activation.

Inflammation. **Chronic inflammation contributes to the initiation and progression of atherosclerotic lesions.** It is believed that inflammation is triggered by the accumulation of cholesterol crystals and free fatty acids in macrophages and other cells. These cells sense the presence of abnormal materials via cytosolic innate immune receptors that are components of the inflammasome (Chapter 6). The resulting inflammasome activation leads to the production of the pro-inflammatory cytokine IL-1, which serves to recruit leukocytes, including monocytes. T lymphocytes are also activated, but what these T cells recognize and why these substances are detected as foreign "invaders" is not known. The net result of macrophage and T cell activation is the local production of cytokines and chemokines that recruit and activate more inflammatory cells. Activated macrophages produce reactive oxygen species that enhance LDL oxidation, and elaborate growth factors that drive smooth muscle cell proliferation. Activated T cells in the growing intimal lesions elaborate inflammatory cytokines, e.g., interferon-γ, which, in turn, can activate macrophages as well as endothelial cells and smooth muscle cells. These leukocytes and vascular wall cells release growth factors that promote smooth muscle cell proliferation and synthesis of extracellular matrix proteins. Thus, many of the lesions of atherosclerosis are attributable to the chronic inflammatory reaction in the vessel wall.

Infection. Although circumstantial evidence has been presented linking atherosclerosis to herpesvirus, cytomegalovirus, and *Chlamydophila pneumoniae*, there is no established causal role for infection.

Smooth Muscle Proliferation and Matrix Synthesis. Intimal smooth muscle cell proliferation and extracellular matrix deposition convert a fatty streak into a mature atheroma and contribute to the progressive growth of atherosclerotic lesions (Fig. 11-10). Intimal smooth muscle cells have a proliferative and synthetic phenotype distinct from the underlying medial smooth muscle cells. Several growth factors are implicated in smooth muscle cell proliferation, including platelet-derived growth factor (PDGF, released by locally adherent platelets, as well as macrophages, endothelial cells, and smooth muscle cells), fibroblast growth factor, and transforming growth factor-α (Chapter 1). These factors also stimulate smooth muscle cells to synthesize extracellular matrix (notably collagen), which stabilizes atherosclerotic plaques. In constrast, activated inflammatory cells in atheromas may increase the breakdown of extracellular matrix components, resulting in unstable plaques (see later).

Overview. Figure 11-11 summarizes the major pathogenic pathways in atherogenesis, emphasizing the multifactorial nature of the disease. This schematic highlights the concept of atherosclerosis as a chronic inflammatory response—and ultimately an attempt at vascular "healing"—driven by a variety of insults, including endothelial cell injury, lipid oxidation and accumulation, and inflammation. Atheromas are dynamic lesions consisting of dysfunctional endothelial cells, proliferating smooth muscle cells, and admixed T lymphocytes and macrophages. All four cell types are capable of liberating mediators that can influence atherogenesis. Thus, at early stages, intimal plaques are little more than aggregates of smooth muscle cells, macrophages, and foam cells; death of these cells releases lipids and necrotic debris. With progression, the atheroma is modified by extracellular matrix synthesized by smooth muscle cells; connective tissue is particularly prominent on the intimal aspect forming a fibrous cap, although lesions also typically retain a central core of lipid-laden cells and fatty debris that can become calcified. The intimal plaque may progressively encroach on the vessel lumen, or may compress the underlying media, leading to its degeneration; this in turn may expose thrombogenic factors such as tissue factor, resulting in thrombus formation and acute vascular occlusion.

MORPHOLOGY

Fatty streaks. Fatty streaks are composed of lipid-filled foamy macrophages. Beginning as multiple minute flat yellow spots, they eventually coalesce into elongated streaks 1 cm long or longer. These lesions are not sufficiently raised to cause any significant flow disturbances (Fig. 11-12). Although fatty streaks can evolve into plaques, not all are destined to become advanced lesions. Aortas of infants can exhibit fatty streaks, and such lesions are present in virtually all adolescents, even those without known risk factors. The observation that coronary fatty streaks begin to form in adolescence, at the same anatomic sites that later tend to develop plaques, suggests a temporal evolution of these lesions.

Atherosclerotic Plaque. The key processes in atherosclerosis are intimal thickening and lipid accumulation, which together form plaques (Figs. 11-7, 11-10, and 11-11). Atheromatous plaques are white-yellow and encroach on the lumen of the artery; superimposed thrombus over ulcerated plaques is red-brown. Plaques vary in size but can coalesce to form larger masses (Fig. 11-13).

Atherosclerotic lesions are patchy, usually involving only a portion of any given arterial wall and are rarely circumferential; on cross-section, the lesions therefore appear "eccentric" (see Fig. 11-14*A*). The focality of atherosclerotic lesions—despite the uniform exposure of vessel walls to such factors as cigarette

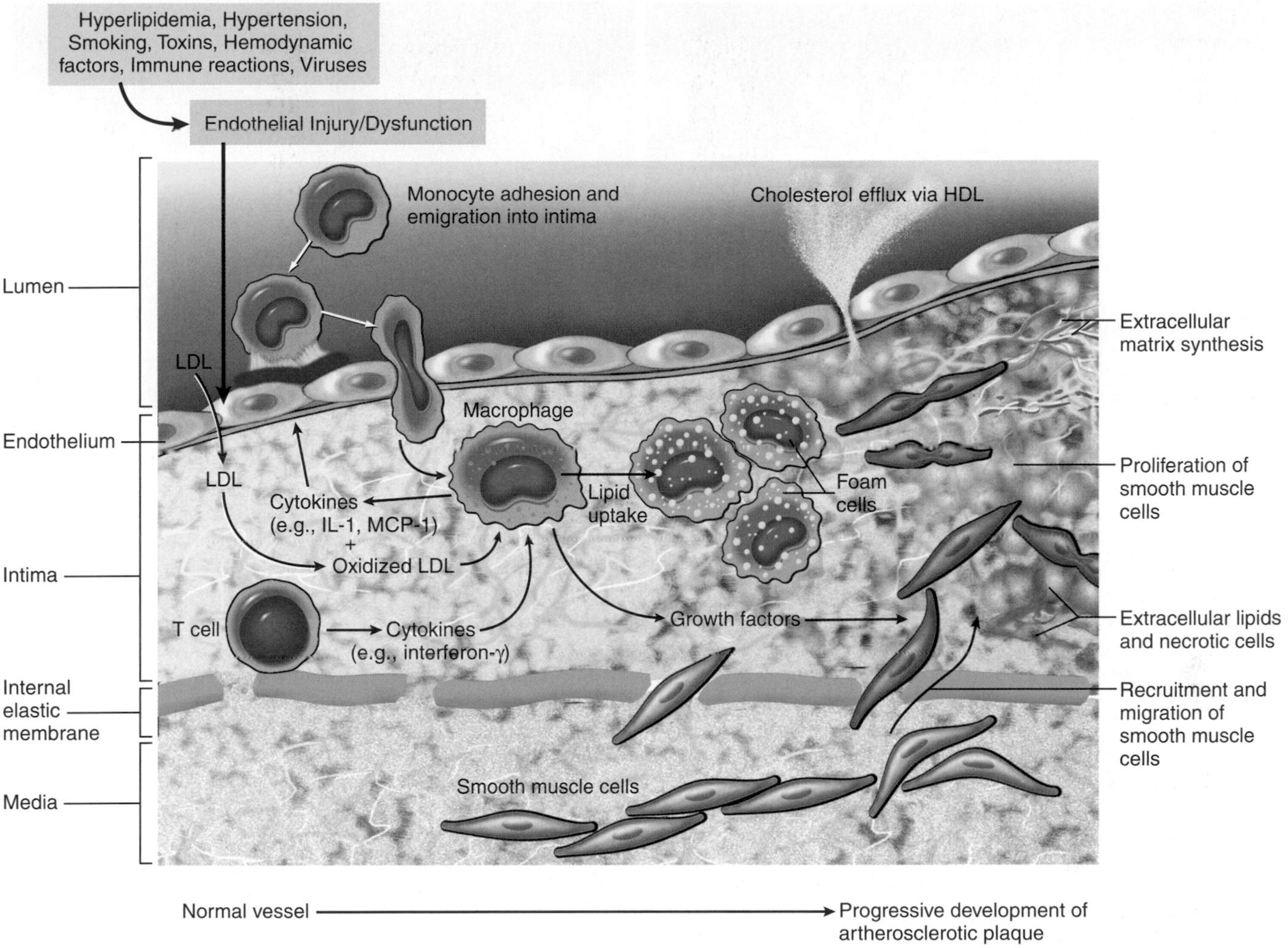

Figure 11-11 Sequence of cellular interactions in atherosclerosis. Hyperlipidemia, hyperglycemia, hypertension, and other influences cause endothelial dysfunction. This results in platelet adhesion and recruitment of circulating monocytes and T cells, with subsequent cytokine and growth factor release from inflammatory cells leading to smooth muscle cell migration and proliferation as well as further macrophage activation. Foam cells in atheromatous plaques derive from macrophages and smooth muscle cells that have accumulated modified lipids (e.g., oxidized and aggregated low density lipoprotein [LDL]) via scavenger and LDL-receptor-related proteins. Extracellular lipid is derived from insudation from the vessel lumen, particularly in the presence of hypercholesterolemia, as well as from degenerating foam cells. Cholesterol accumulation in the plaque reflects an imbalance between influx and efflux; high-density lipoprotein (HDL) likely helps clear cholesterol from these accumulations. In response to the elaborated cytokines and chemokines, smooth muscle cells migrate to the intima, proliferate, and produce extracellular matrix, including collagen and proteoglycans. IL-1, interleukin-1; MCP-1, monocyte chemoattractant protein-1.

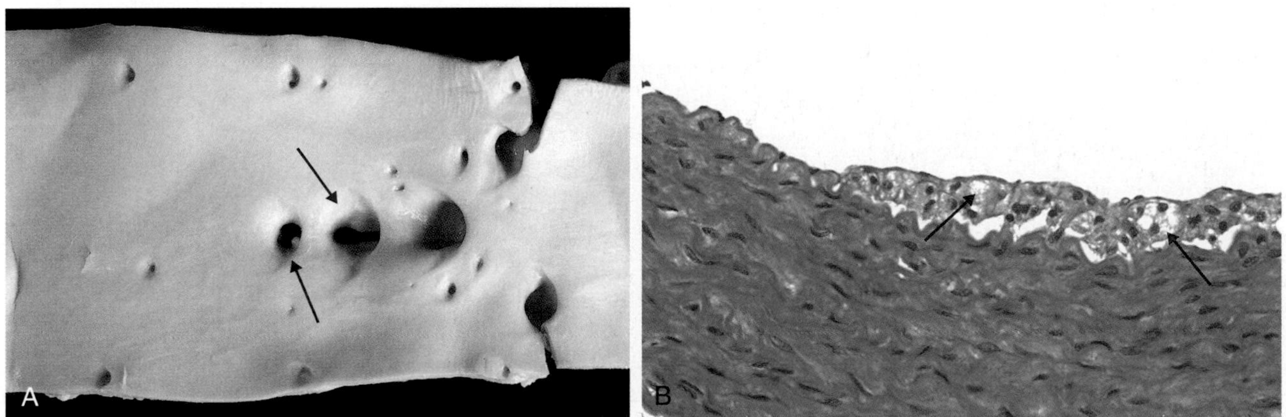

Figure 11-12 Fatty streak, a collection of foamy macrophages in the intima. **A,** Aorta with fatty streaks *(arrows),* associated largely with the ostia of branch vessels. **B,** Photomicrograph of fatty streak in an experimental hypercholesterolemic rabbit, demonstrating intimal, macrophage-derived foam cells *(arrows).* (**B**, Courtesy Myron I. Cybulsky, MD, University of Toronto, Canada.)

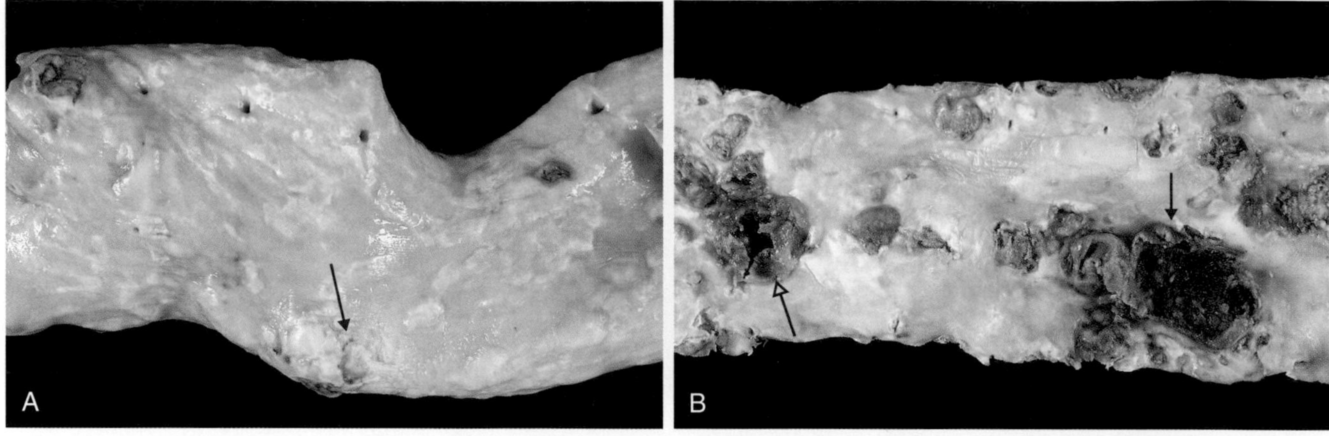

Figure 11-13 Gross views of atherosclerosis in the aorta. **A,** Mild atherosclerosis composed of fibrous plaques, one of which is denoted by the arrow. **B,** Severe disease with diffuse and complicated lesions including an ulcerated plaque *(open arrow),* and a lesion with overlying thrombus *(closed arrow).*

smoke toxins, elevated LDL, and hyperglycemia—is attributable to the vagaries of vascular hemodynamics. Local flow disturbances, such as turbulence at branch points, make certain portions of a vessel wall more susceptible to plaque formation. Although focal and sparsely distributed at first, with time atherosclerotic lesions can become larger, more numerous, and more broadly distributed. Moreover, in any given vessel, lesions at various stages often coexist.

In descending order, **the most extensively involved vessels are the lower abdominal aorta, the coronary arteries, the popliteal arteries, the internal carotid arteries, and the vessels of the circle of Willis.** In humans, the abdominal aorta is typically involved to a much greater degree than the thoracic aorta. Vessels of the upper extremities are usually spared, as are the mesenteric and renal arteries, except at their ostia. Although most individuals tend to have a consistent degree of atherosclerotic burden in the affected vasculature, severity of disease in one arterial distribution does not always predict its severity in another.

Atherosclerotic plaques have three principal components: (1) smooth muscle cells, macrophages, and T cells; (2) extracellular matrix, including collagen, elastic fibers, and proteoglycans; and (3) intracellular and extracellular lipid (Fig. 11-14). These components occur in varying proportions and configurations in different lesions. Typically, there is a superficial fibrous cap composed of smooth muscle cells and relatively dense collagen. Beneath and to the side of the cap (the "shoulder") is a more cellular area containing macrophages, T cells, and smooth muscle cells. Deep to the fibrous cap is a necrotic core, containing lipid (primarily cholesterol and cholesterol esters), debris from dead cells, foam cells (lipid-laden macrophages and smooth muscle cells), fibrin, variably organized thrombus, and other plasma proteins; the cholesterol content is frequently present as crystalline aggregates that are washed out during routine tissue processing and leave behind only empty "clefts." The periphery of the lesions demonstrate **neovascularization** (proliferating small blood vessels; Fig. 11-14C). Most atheromas contain abundant lipid, but some

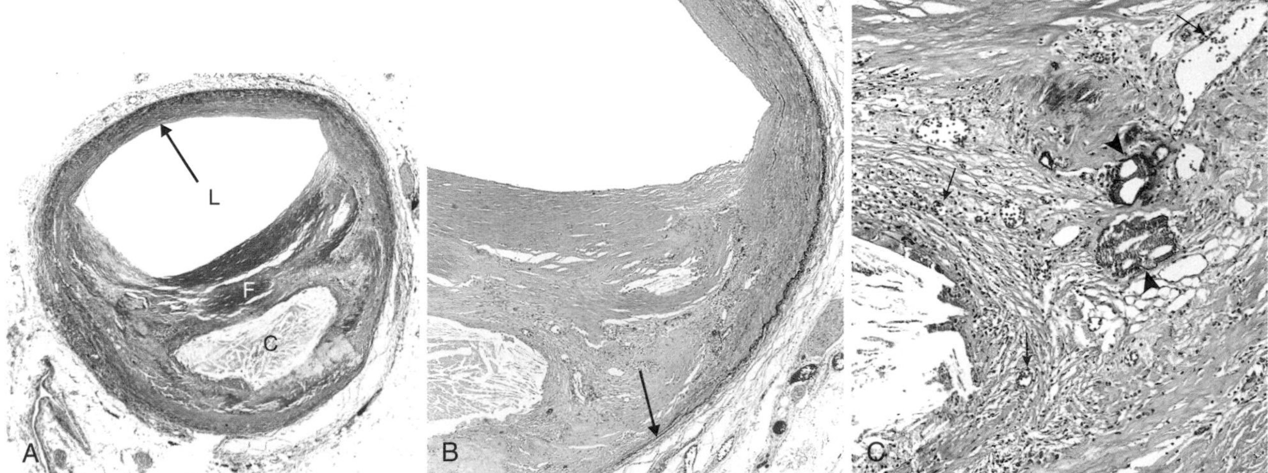

Figure 11-14 Histologic features of atheromatous plaque in the coronary artery. **A,** Overall architecture demonstrating fibrous cap (F) and a central necrotic core (C) containing cholesterol and other lipids. The lumen (L) has been moderately compromised. Note that a segment of the wall is plaque free *(arrow)*; the lesion is therefore "eccentric." In this section, collagen has been stained blue (Masson trichrome stain). **B,** Higher-power photograph of a section of the plaque shown in **A,** stained for elastin (black), demonstrating that the internal and external elastic laminae are attenuated and the media of the artery is thinned under the most advanced plaque *(arrow).* **C,** Higher magnification photomicrograph at the junction of the fibrous cap and core, showing scattered inflammatory cells, calcification *(arrowhead),* and neovascularization *(small arrows).*

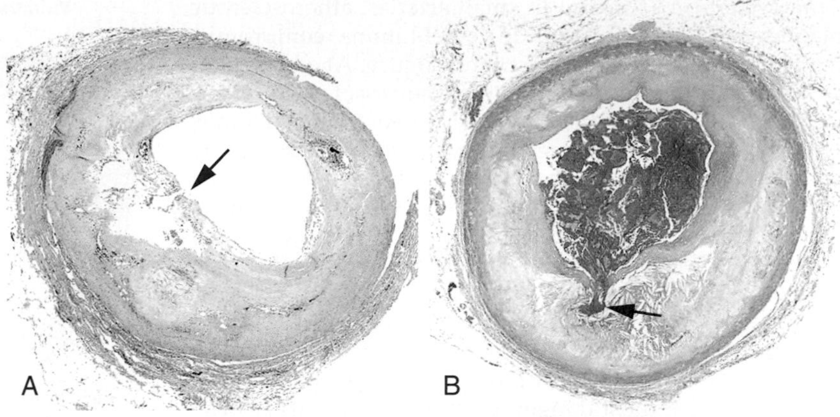

Figure 11-15 Atherosclerotic plaque rupture. **A,** Plaque rupture without superimposed thrombus, in a patient who died suddenly. **B,** Acute coronary thrombosis superimposed on an atherosclerotic plaque with focal disruption of the fibrous cap, triggering fatal myocardial infarction. In both **A** and **B,** an *arrow* points to the site of plaque rupture. (**B,** Reproduced from Schoen FJ: Interventional and Surgical Cardiovascular Patherosclerosisology: Clinical Correlations and Basic Principles. Philadelphia, WB Saunders, 1989, p 61.)

plaques ("fibrous plaques") are composed almost exclusively of smooth muscle cells and fibrous tissue.

Plaques generally continue to change and progressively enlarge through cell death and degeneration, synthesis and degradation (remodeling) of extracellular matrice, and organization of any superimposed thrombus. Moreover, atheromas often undergo calcification (Fig. 11-14*C*). Patients with advanced coronary calcification have increased risk for coronary events.

Atherosclerotic plaques are susceptible to the following clinically important pathologic changes:

- **Rupture, ulceration, or erosion** of the surface of atheromatous plaques exposes highly thrombogenic substances and leads to **thrombosis**, which may partially or completely occlude the vessel lumen (Fig. 11-15). If the patient survives, the clot may become organized and incorporated into the growing plaque.
- **Hemorrhage into a plaque.** Rupture of the overlying fibrous cap, or of the thin-walled vessels in the areas of neovascularization, can cause intraplaque hemorrhage; a contained hematoma may expand the plaque or induce plaque rupture.
- **Atheroembolism.** Plaque rupture can discharge atherosclerotic debris into the bloodstream, producing microemboli.
- **Aneurysm formation.** Atherosclerosis-induced pressure or ischemic atrophy of the underlying media, with loss of elastic tissue, causes weakness and potential rupture.

Consequences of Atherosclerotic Disease

Large elastic arteries (e.g., aorta, carotid, and iliac arteries) and large and medium-sized muscular arteries (e.g., coronary and popliteal arteries) are the major targets of atherosclerosis. Symptomatic atherosclerotic disease most often involves the arteries supplying the heart, brain, kidneys, and lower extremities. **Myocardial infarction (heart attack), cerebral infarction (stroke), aortic aneurysms, and peripheral vascular disease (gangrene of the legs) are the major consequences of atherosclerosis.** The natural history, principal morphologic features, and main pathogenic events are schematized in Figure 11-16.

We next describe the features of atherosclerotic lesions that are typically responsible for the clinicopathologic manifestations.

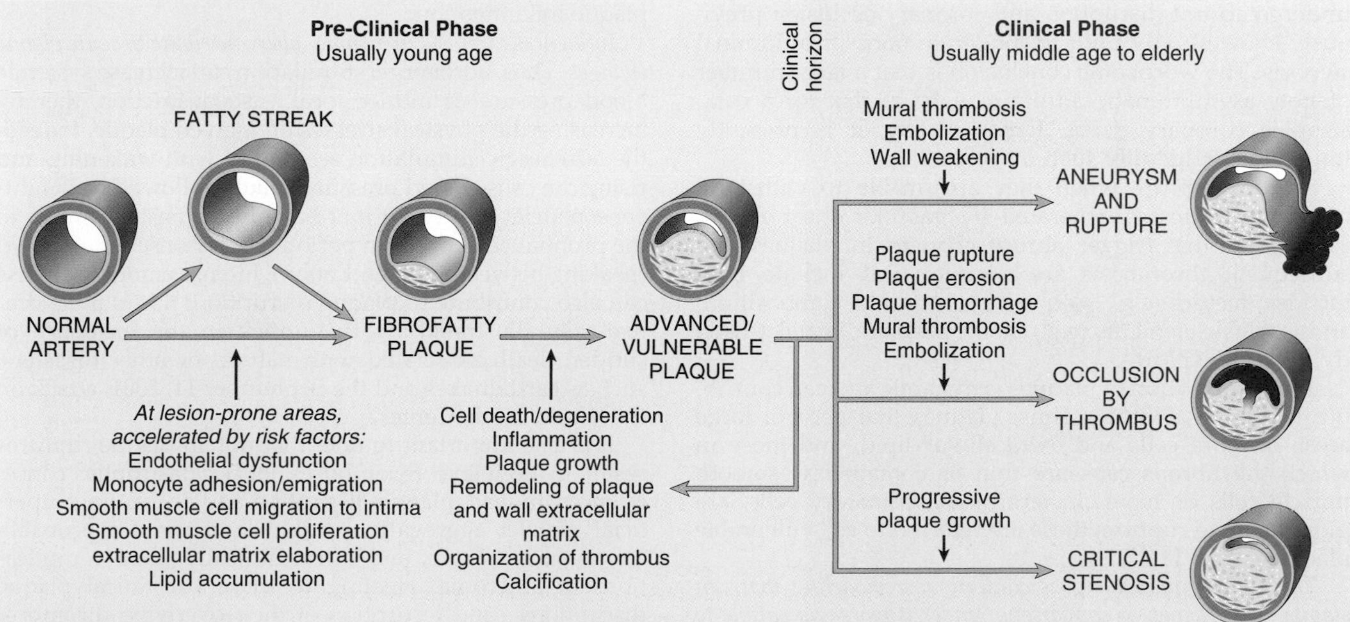

Figure 11-16 The natural history, morphologic features, main pathogenic events, and clinical complications of atherosclerosis.

Atherosclerotic Stenosis. In small arteries, atherosclerotic plaques can gradually occlude vessel lumina, compromising blood flow and causing ischemic injury. At early stages of stenosis, outward remodeling of the vessel media tends to preserve the size of the lumen. However, there are limits on the extent of remodeling, and eventually the expanding atheroma impinges on the lumen to such a degree that blood flow is compromised. *Critical stenosis* is the stage at which the occlusion is sufficiently severe to produce tissue ischemia. In the coronary (and other) circulations, this typically occurs at when the occlusion produces a 70% decrease in luminal cross-sectional area; with this degree of stenosis, chest pain may develop with exertion (so-called *stable angina*; see Chapter 12). Although acute plaque rupture (see later) is the most dangerous consequence, atherosclerosis also takes a toll through chronically diminished arterial perfusion: *mesenteric occlusion and bowel ischemia, sudden cardiac death, chronic ischemic heart disease, ischemic encephalopathy,* and *intermittent claudication* (diminished perfusion of the extremities) are all consequences of flow-limiting stenoses. The effects of vascular occlusion ultimately depend on arterial supply and the metabolic demand of the affected tissue.

Acute Plaque Change. Plaque erosion or rupture is typically promptly followed by partial or complete vascular thrombosis (Fig. 11-15), resulting in acute tissue infarction (e.g., myocardial or cerebral infarction) (Fig. 11-16). Plaque changes fall into three general categories:

- *Rupture/fissuring,* exposing highly thrombogenic plaque constituents
- *Erosion/ulceration,* exposing the thrombogenic subendothelial basement membrane to blood
- *Hemorrhage into the atheroma,* expanding its volume

It is now recognized that plaques that are responsible for myocardial infarction and other acute coronary syndromes are often asymptomatic before the acute change. Thus, pathologic and clinical studies show that the majority of plaques that undergo abrupt disruption and coronary occlusion previously showed only mild to moderate noncritical luminal stenosis. The worrisome conclusion is that a large number of now asymptomatic adults may be at risk for a catastrophic coronary event. Unfortunately, it is presently impossible to identify such individuals.

Plaques rupture when they are unable to withstand mechanical stresses generated by vascular shear forces. The events that trigger abrupt changes in plaques and subsequent thrombosis are complex and include both intrinsic factors (e.g., plaque structure and composition) and extrinsic elements (e.g., blood pressure, platelet reactivity, vessel spasm).

The composition of plaques is dynamic and can contribute to risk of rupture. Thus, plaques that contain large areas of foam cells and extracellular lipid, and those in which the fibrous caps are thin or contain few smooth muscle cells or have clusters of inflammatory cells, are more likely to rupture; these are referred to as "vulnerable plaques" (Fig. 11-17).

The fibrous cap undergoes continuous remodeling that can stabilize the plaque, or conversely, render it more susceptible to rupture. Collagen is the major structural component of the fibrous cap, and accounts for its mechanical strength and stability. Thus, the balance of collagen synthesis versus degradation affects cap integrity. Collagen in atherosclerotic plaque is produced primarily by smooth muscle cells so that loss of these cells results in a less sturdy cap. Moreover, collagen turnover is controlled by metalloproteinases (MMPs), enzymes elaborated largely by macrophages and smooth muscle cells within the atheromatous plaque; conversely, tissue inhibitors of metalloproteinases (TIMPs) produced by endothelial cells, smooth muscle cells, and macrophages modulate MMP activity. In general, plaque inflammation results in a net increase in collagen degradation and reduced collagen synthesis, thereby destabilizing the mechanical integrity of the fibrous cap (see later). The inflammatiion induced by cholesterol deposits themselves may contribute to plaque destabilization. Conversely, statins may have a beneficial therapeutic effect not only by reducing circulating cholesterol levels, but also by stabilizing plaques through a reduction in plaque inflammation.

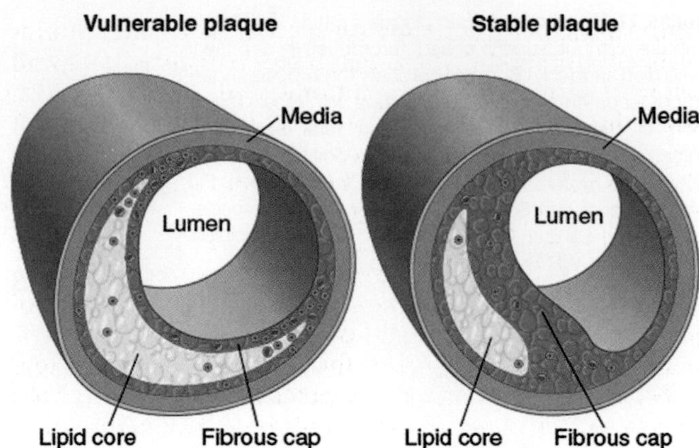

Figure 11-17 Vulnerable and stable atherosclerotic plaque. *Vulnerable plaques* have thin fibrous caps, large lipid cores, and greater inflammation. Stable plaques have thickened and densely collagenous fibrous caps with minimal inflammation and underlying atheromatous core. (Adapted from Libby P: Circulation 91:2844, 1995.)

Influences extrinsic to plaques also contribute to acute plaque changes. Thus, adrenergic stimulation can increase systemic blood pressure or induce local vasoconstriction, thereby increasing the physical stresses on a given plaque. Indeed, the adrenergic stimulation associated with wakening and rising can cause blood pressure spikes (followed by heightened platelet reactivity) that have been causally linked to the pronounced circadian periodicity for onset of acute MI (peaking between 6 AM and noon). Intense emotional stress can also contribute to plaque disruption; this is most dramatically illustrated by the uptick in the incidence of sudden death associated with natural or other disasters, such as earthquakes and the September 11, 2001, attack on the World Trade Center.

It is also important to note that not all plaque ruptures result in occlusive thromboses with catastrophic consequences. Indeed, plaque disruption and an ensuing superficial platelet aggregation and thrombosis are probably common, repetitive, and often clinically silent complications of atheroma. Healing of these subclinical plaque disruptions—and resorption of their overlying thrombi—is an important mechanism in the growth of atherosclerotic lesions.

Thrombosis. As mentioned earlier, partial or total thrombosis superimposed on a disrupted plaque is a central factor in acute coronary syndromes. In its most serious form, thrombosis leads to total occlusion of the affected vessel. In contrast, in other coronary syndromes (Chapter 12), luminal obstruction by the thrombus is incomplete, and may even wax and wane with time.

Mural thrombi in a coronary artery can also embolize. Indeed, small embolic fragments of thrombus can often be found in the distal intramyocardial circulation or in association with microinfarcts in patients with atherosclerosis who die suddenly. Finally, thrombin and other factors associated with thrombosis are potent activators of smooth muscle cells and can thereby contribute to the growth of atherosclerotic lesions.

Vasoconstriction. Vasoconstriction compromises lumen size, and, by increasing the local mechanical forces, can potentiate plaque disruption. Vasoconstriction at sites of atheroma may be stimulated by (1) circulating adrenergic agonists, (2) locally released platelet contents, (3) endothelial cell dysfunction with impaired secretion of endothelial-derived relaxing factors (nitric oxide) relative to contracting factors (endothelin), and (4) mediators released from perivascular inflammatory cells.

KEY CONCEPTS

Atherosclerosis

- Atherosclerosis is an intimal-based lesion composed of a fibrous cap and an atheromatous core; the constituents of the plaque include smooth muscle cells, extracellular matrices, inflammatory cells, lipids, and necrotic debris.
- Atherogenesis is driven by an interplay of vessel wall injury and inflammation. The multiple risk factors for atherosclerosis all cause endothelial cell dysfunction and influence inflammatory cell and smooth muscle cell recruitment and stimulation.
- Atherosclerotic plaques develop and grow slowly over decades. Stable plaques can produce symptoms related to chronic ischemia by narrowing vessel lumens, whereas unstable plaques can cause dramatic and potentially fatal ischemic complications related to acute plaque rupture, thrombosis, or embolization.
- Stable plaques tend to have a dense fibrous cap, minimal lipid accumulation and little inflammation, whereas "vulnerable" unstable plaques have thin caps, large lipid cores, and relatively dense inflammatory infiltrates.

Aneurysms and Dissection

An aneurysm is a localized abnormal dilation of a blood vessel or the heart that may be congenital or acquired (Fig. 11-18). When an aneurysm involves an attenuated but intact arterial wall or thinned ventricular wall of the heart, it is called a "true" aneurysm. Atherosclerotic, syphilitic, and congenital vascular aneurysms, as well as ventricular aneurysms that follow transmural myocardial infarctions are of this type. In contrast, a *false aneurysm* (also called *pseudo-aneurysm*) is a defect in the vascular wall leading to an extravascular hematoma that freely communicates with the intravascular space ("pulsating hematoma"). Examples include a ventricular rupture after myocardial infarction that is contained by a pericardial adhesion, or a leak at the sutured junction of a vascular graft with a natural artery. An arterial *dissection* arises when blood enters a defect in the arterial wall and tunnels between its layers. Dissections are often but not always aneurysmal (see later). Both true and false aneurysms as well as dissections can rupture, often with catastrophic consequences.

Descriptively, aneurysms are classified by macroscopic shape and size (Fig. 11-18). *Saccular aneurysms* are spherical outpouchings involving only a portion of the vessel wall; they vary from 5 to 20 cm in diameter and often contain thrombus. *Fusiform aneurysms* are diffuse, circumferential dilations of a long vascular segment; they vary in diameter (up to 20 cm) and in length and can involve extensive portions of the aortic arch, abdominal aorta, or even the iliacs. These types are not specific for any disease or clinical manifestations.

Pathogenesis of Aneurysms. To maintain their structural and functional integrity, arterial walls constantly remodel

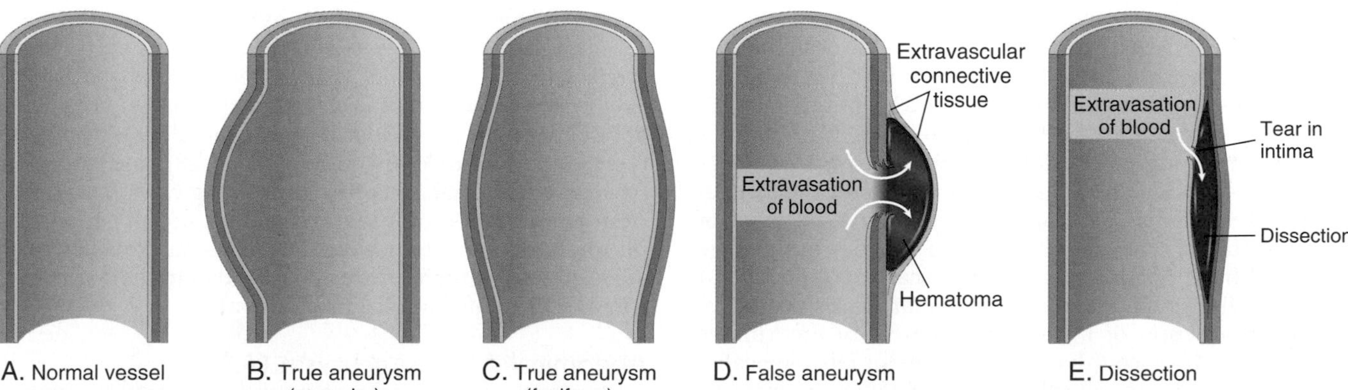

Figure 11-18 Aneurysms. **A,** Normal vessel. **B,** True aneurysm, saccular type. The wall focally bulges outward and may be attenuated but is otherwise intact. **C,** True aneurysm, fusiform type. There is circumferential dilation of the vessel, without rupture. **D,** False aneurysm. The wall is ruptured, and there is a collection of blood (hematoma) that is bounded externally by adherent extravascular tissues. **E,** Dissection. Blood has entered (dissected) the wall of the vessel and separated the layers. Although this is shown as occurring through a tear in the lumen, dissections can also occur by rupture of the vessels of the vasa vasorum within the media.

by synthesizing, degrading, and repairing damage to their extracellular matrix constituents. Aneurysms can occur when the structure or function of the connective tissue within the vascular wall is compromised. Although we cite here examples of inherited defects in connective tissues, weakening of vessel walls is important in the more common, sporadic forms of aneurysms as well.

- *The intrinsic quality of the vascular wall connective tissue is poor.* In *Marfan syndrome*, for example (Chapter 5), defective synthesis of the scaffolding protein *fibrillin* leads to aberrant TGF-β activity and weakening of elastic tissue; in the aorta, this may result in progressive dilation. *Loeys-Dietz syndrome* is another cause of aneurysms; in this disorder, mutations in TGF-β receptors lead to defective synthesis of elastin and collagens I and III. Aneurysms in such individuals can rupture fairly easily (even at small size) and are thus considered to follow an "aggressive" course. Weak vessel walls due to defective type III collagen synthesis are also a hallmark of the vascular forms of *Ehlers-Danlos syndrome* (Chapter 5), and altered collagen cross-linking associated with vitamin C deficiency (scurvy) is an example of a nutritional basis for aneurysm formation, that is thankfully rare these days.
- *The balance of collagen degradation and synthesis is altered by inflammation and associated proteases.* In particular, increased matrix metalloprotease (MMP) expression, especially by macrophages in atherosclerotic plaque or in vasculitis, likely contributes to aneurysm development; these enzymes have the capacity to degrade virtually all components of the extracellular matrix in the arterial wall (collagens, elastin, proteoglycans, laminin, fibronectin). Decreased expression of tissue inhibitors of metalloproteases (TIMPs) can also contribute to the extracellular matrix degradation. The risk of aneurysm formation in the setting of inflammatory lesions (e.g., atherosclerosis) may be associated with MMP and/or TIMP polymorphisms, or altered by the nature of the local inflammatory response. For example, abdominal aortic aneurysms (AAA; see later) are associated with local production of cytokines (such as IL-4 and IL-10) that stimulate release of elastolytic MMP from macrophages.
- *The vascular wall is weakened through loss of smooth muscle cells or the synthesis of noncollagenous or nonelastic extracellular matrix.* Ischemia of the inner media occurs when there is atherosclerotic thickening of the intima, which increases the distance that oxygen and nutrients must diffuse. Systemic hypertension can also cause significant narrowing of arterioles of the vasa vasorum (e.g., in the aorta), which causes outer medial ischemia. Medial ischemia may lead to "degenerative changes" of the aorta, whereby smooth muscle cell loss—or change in synthetic phenotype—leads to scarring (and loss of elastic fibers), inadequate extracellular matrix synthesis, and production of increasing amounts of amorphous ground substance (glycosaminoglycan). Histologically, these changes are collectively recognized as *cystic medial degeneration* (Fig. 11-19), which can be seen in a variety of settings, including Marfan syndrome and scurvy.

Tertiary syphilis is another rare cause of aortic aneurysms. The obliterative endarteritis characteristic of late-stage syphilis shows a predilection for small vessels, including those of the vasa vasorum of the thoracic aorta. This leads to ischemic injury of the aortic media and aneurysmal dilation, which sometimes involves the aortic valve annulus.

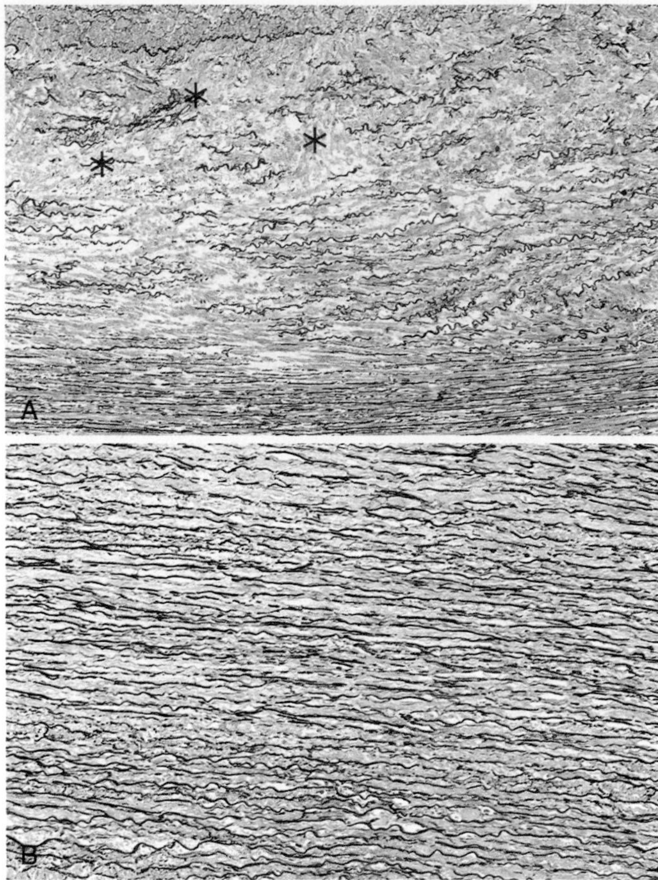

Figure 11-19 Cystic medial degeneration. **A,** Cross-section of aortic media from a patient with Marfan syndrome, showing elastin fragmentation and areas devoid of elastin that resemble cystic spaces but are actually filled with proteoglycans *(asterisks).* **B,** Normal media for comparison, showing the regular layered pattern of elastic tissue. In both **A** and **B**, elastin is stained black.

The two most important causes of aortic aneurysms are atherosclerosis and hypertension; atherosclerosis is a greater factor in AAAs, while hypertension is the most common etiology associated with ascending aortic aneurysms. Other factors that weaken vessel walls and lead to aneurysms include trauma, vasculitis (see later), congenital defects (e.g., fibromuscular dysplasia and *berry aneurysms* typically in the circle of Willis; Chapter 28), and infections *(mycotic aneurysms).* Mycotic aneurysms can originate (1) from embolization of a septic embolus, usually as a complication of infective endocarditis; (2) as an extension of an adjacent suppurative process; or (3) by circulating organisms directly infecting the arterial wall.

Abdominal Aortic Aneurysm (AAA)

Aneurysms occurring as a consequence of atherosclerosis form most commonly in the abdominal aorta and common iliac arteries. A variety of factors discussed earlier collaborate to weaken the media and predispose to aneurysm formation.

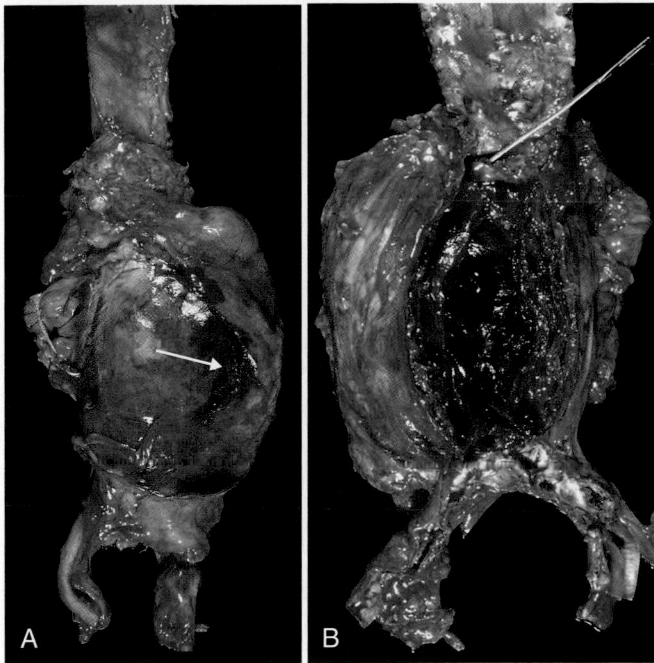

Figure 11-20 Abdominal aortic aneurysm. **A,** External view, gross photograph of a large aortic aneurysm that ruptured (rupture site is indicated by the *arrow*). **B,** Opened view, with the location of the rupture tract indicated by a probe. The wall of the aneurysm is exceedingly thin, and the lumen is filled by a large quantity of layered but largely unorganized thrombus.

AAAs occur more frequently in men and in smokers, rarely developing before age 50. Atherosclerosis is a major cause of AAA, but other factors clearly contribute since the incidence is less than 5% in men older than age 60 years, despite the almost universal presence of abdominal aortic atherosclerosis in this population.

MORPHOLOGY

Usually positioned below the renal arteries and above the bifurcation of the aorta, AAA can be saccular or fusiform, up to 15 cm in diameter, and up to 25 cm in length (Fig. 11-20). There is severe complicated atherosclerosis with destruction and thinning of the underlying aortic media; the aneurysm frequently contains a bland, laminated, poorly organized mural thrombus. AAA can occasionally affect the renal and superior or inferior mesenteric arteries, either by direct extension or by occluding vessel ostia with mural thrombi. Not infrequently, AAA is accompanied by smaller aneurysms of the iliac arteries.

Even though they are less common than the usual atherosclerotic aneurysm, three AAA variants merit special mention because of their unusual features:

- **Inflammatory AAA** account for 5% to 10% of all AAA; these typically occur in younger patients, who often present with back pain and elevated inflammatory markers (e.g., elevation of C-reactive protein). Inflammatory aneurysms are characterized by abundant lymphoplasmacytic inflammation with many macrophages (and even giant cells) associated with dense periaortic scarring that can extend into the anterior retroperitoneum. The cause is a presumed localized immune response to the abdominal aortic wall; remarkably, most cases are not associated with inflammation of other arteries.
- A subset of inflammatory AAA may be a vascular manifestation of a recently recognized entity called **immunoglobulin G4 (IgG4)-related disease**. This is a disorder marked by (in most cases) high plasma levels of IgG4 and tissue fibrosis associated with frequent infiltrating IgG4-expressing plasma cells. It may affect a variety of tissues, including pancreas, biliary system, and salivary gland. The affected individuals have aortitis and periaortitis that weaken the wall sufficiently in some cases to give rise to aneurysms. Recognition of this entity is important since it responds well to steroid therapy.
- **Mycotic AAA** are lesions that have become infected by the lodging of circulating microorganisms in the wall. In such cases, suppuration further destroys the media, potentiating rapid dilation and rupture.

Clinical Features. Most cases of AAA are asymptomatic and are discovered incidentally on physical exam as an abdominal mass (often palpably pulsating) that may mimic a tumor. The other clinical manifestations of AAA include:

- Rupture into the peritoneal cavity or retroperitoneal tissues with massive, potentially fatal hemorrhage
- Obstruction of a vessel branching off from the aorta, resulting in ischemic injury to the supplied tissue; for example, iliac (leg), renal (kidney), mesenteric (gastrointestinal tract), or vertebral arteries (spinal cord)
- Embolism from atheroma or mural thrombus
- Impingement on an adjacent structure, for example, compression of a ureter or erosion of vertebrae

The risk of rupture is directly related to the size of the aneurysm, varying from nil for AAA 4 cm or less in diameter, to 1% per year for AAA between 4 and 5 cm, 11% per year for AAA between 5 and 6 cm, and 25% per year for aneurysms larger than 6 cm. Most aneurysms expand at a rate of 0.2 to 0.3 cm/year, but 20% expand more rapidly. In general, aneurysms 5 cm or larger are managed aggressively, usually by surgical bypass with prosthetic grafts, although treatment via endoluminal approaches using stent grafts (expandable wire frames covered by a cloth sleeve) rather than surgery is now available for selected patients. Timely surgery is critical; operative mortality for unruptured aneurysms is approximately 5%, whereas emergency surgery after rupture carries a mortality rate of more than 50%. It is worth reiterating that because atherosclerosis is a systemic disease, a patient with AAA is also very likely to have atherosclerosis in other vascular beds and is at a significantly increased risk of IHD and stroke.

Thoracic Aortic Aneurysm

Thoracic aortic aneurysms are most commonly associated with hypertension, although other causes such as Marfan syndrome and Loeys-Dietz syndrome are increasingly recognized. These can present with signs and symptoms referable to (1) respiratory difficulties due to encroachment on the lungs and airways, (2) difficulty in swallowing due to compression of the esophagus, (3) persistent cough due to compression of the recurrent laryngeal nerves, (4) pain caused by erosion of bone (i.e., ribs and vertebral bodies), (5) cardiac disease as the aortic aneurysm leads to aortic valve dilation with valvular insufficiency or narrowing of

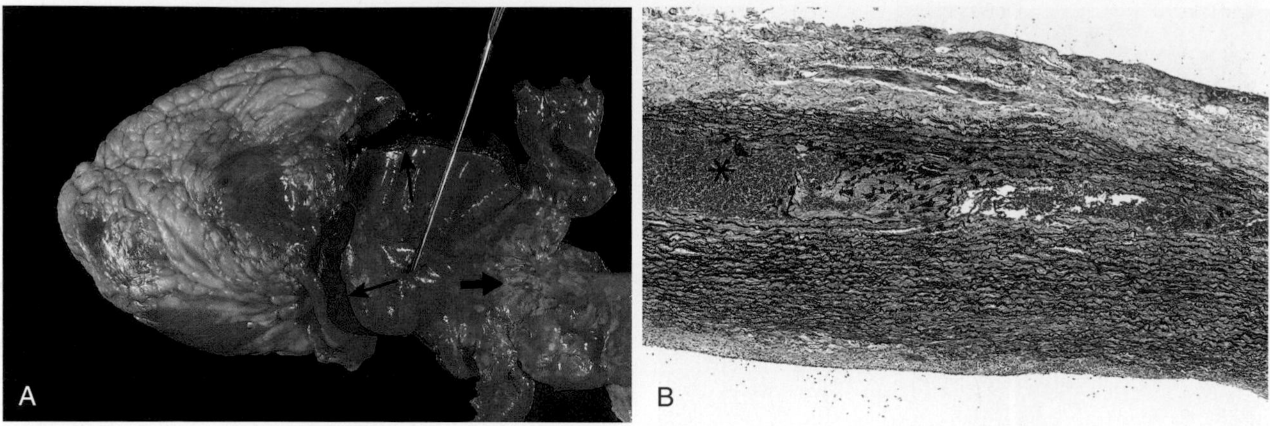

Figure 11-21 Aortic dissection. **A,** Gross photograph of an opened aorta with proximal dissection originating from a small, oblique intimal tear (probe), allowing blood to enter the media and creating a retrograde intramural hematoma *(narrow arrows).* Note that the intimal tear has occurred in a region largely free of atherosclerotic plaque and that propagation of the intramural hematoma distally is arrested where atherosclerosis begins *(broad arrow).* **B,** Histologic view of the dissection demonstrating an aortic intramural hematoma *(asterisk).* Aortic elastic layers are black and blood is red (Movat stain).

the coronary ostia causing myocardial ischemia, and (6) rupture. Most patients with syphilitic aneurysms die of heart failure secondary to aortic valvular incompetence.

Aortic Dissection

Aortic dissection occurs when blood separates the laminar planes of the media to form a blood-filled channel within the aortic wall (Fig. 11-21); this can be catastrophic if the dissection then ruptures through the adventitia and hemorrhages into adjacent spaces. Aortic dissection may or may not be associated with radiologically detectable aortic dilation.

Aortic dissection occurs principally in two groups of patients: (1) men aged 40 to 60 years with antecedent hypertension (more than 90% of cases) and (2) younger adults with systemic or localized abnormalities of connective tissue affecting the aorta (e.g., Marfan syndrome). Dissections can be iatrogenic, for example, following arterial cannulations during coronary catheterization procedures or cardiopulmonary bypass. Rarely, pregnancy is associated with aortic (or other vessel) dissection (roughly 10 to 20 cases per million births). This typically occurs during or after the third trimester, and may be related to hormone-induced vascular remodeling and the hemodynamic stresses of the perinatal period. Dissection is unusual in the presence of substantial atherosclerosis or other cause of medial scarring such as syphilis, presumably because the medial fibrosis inhibits propagation of the dissecting hematoma.

Pathogenesis. **Hypertension is the major risk factor for aortic dissection.** Aortas of hypertensive patients have medial hypertrophy of vasa vasorum associated with degenerative changes such as loss of medial smooth muscle cells and disorganized extracellular matrix, suggesting that ischemic injury (due to diminished flow through the vasa vasorum, possibly exacerbated by high wall pressures) is contributory. Other dissections occur in the setting of inherited or acquired connective tissue disorders with defective vascular extracellular matrix (e.g., Marfan syndrome, Ehlers-Danlos syndrome, defects in copper metabolism). However, recognizable medial damage appears to be neither a prerequisite for dissection nor a reliable predictor of its occurrence. Regardless of the underlying etiology, the trigger for the intimal tear and initial intramural aortic hemorrhage is not known in most cases. Once a tear has occurred, blood flow under systemic pressure dissects through the media, leading to progression of the hematoma. Accordingly, aggressive pressure-reducing therapy may be effective in limiting an evolving dissection. In some cases, disruption of penetrating vessels of the vasa vasorum can give rise to an intramural hematoma *without* an intimal tear.

MORPHOLOGY

In most cases, no specific underlying causal pathology is identified in the aortic wall. The most frequent preexisting histologically detectable lesion is **cystic medial degeneration** (Fig. 11-19), and inflammation is characteristically absent. However, since dissections can occur in the setting of rather trivial medial degeneration, and marked degenerative changes are frequently seen at autopsies of patients who are completely free from dissection, the relationship of the structural changes to the pathogenesis of dissection is uncertain.

An aortic dissection usually initiates with an intimal tear. In the vast majority of spontaneous dissections, the tear occurs in the ascending aorta, usually within 10 cm of the aortic valve (Fig. 11-21*A*). Such tears are typically transverse with sharp, jagged edges up to 1 to 5 cm in length. The dissection can extend retrograde toward the heart as well as distally, sometimes into the iliac and femoral arteries. The dissecting hematoma spreads characteristically along the laminar planes of the aorta, usually between the middle and outer thirds (Fig. 11-21*B*). It can rupture through the adventitia causing massive hemorrhage (e.g., into the thoracic or abdominal cavities) or cardiac tamponade (hemorrhage into the pericardial sac). In some (lucky) instances, the dissecting hematoma reenters the lumen of the aorta through a second distal intimal tear, creating a new false vascular channel ("double-barreled aorta"). This averts a fatal extraaortic hemorrhage, and over time, such false channels can be endothelialized to become recognizable **chronic dissections**.

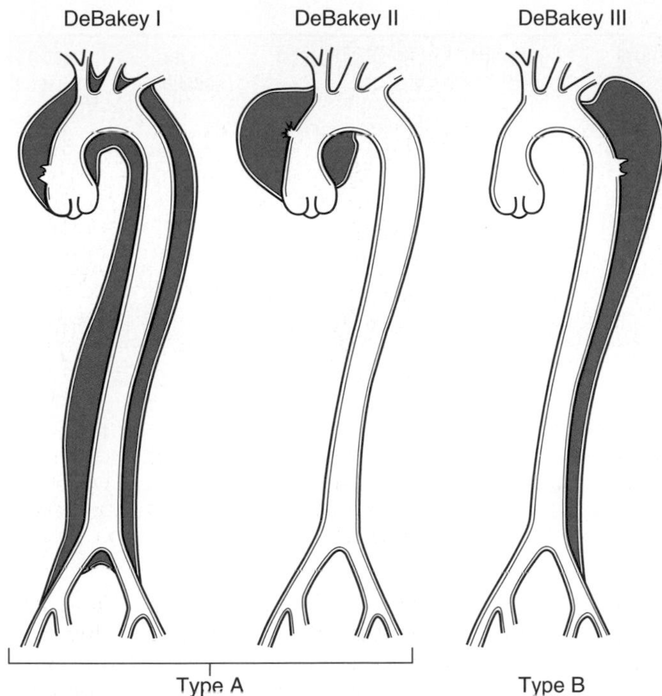

Figure 11-22 Classification of dissections. Type A (proximal) involves the ascending aorta, either as part of a more extensive dissection (DeBakey I) or in isolation (DeBakey II). Type B (distal or DeBakey III) dissections arise after the take-off of the great vessels. Type A dissections typically have the most serious complications and greatest associated mortality.

Clinical Features. The morbidity and mortality associated with dissections depend on which part of the aorta is involved; the most serious complications occur with dissections between the aortic valve and the distal arch. Accordingly, aortic dissections are generally classified into two types (Fig. 11-22).

- The more common (and dangerous) *proximal* lesions (called *type A dissections*), involving either both the ascending and descending aorta or just the ascending aorta only (types I and II of the DeBakey classification)
- *Distal lesions not involving the ascending part* and usually beginning distal to the subclavian artery (called *type B dissections* or DeBakey type III)

The classic clinical symptoms of aortic dissection are the sudden onset of excruciating pain, usually beginning in the anterior chest, radiating to the back between the scapulae, and moving downward as the dissection progresses; the pain can be confused with that of myocardial infarction.

The most common cause of death is rupture of the dissection into the pericardial, pleural, or peritoneal cavities. Retrograde dissection into the aortic root can also disrupt the aortic valve annulus. Common clinical manifestations include cardiac tamponade and aortic insufficiency. Dissections can also extend into the great arteries of the neck, or into the coronary, renal, mesenteric, or iliac arteries, causing vascular obstruction and ischemic consequences such as myocardial infarction; involvement of spinal arteries can cause transverse myelitis.

In type A dissections, rapid diagnosis and institution of intensive antihypertensive therapy coupled with surgical plication of the aortic intimal tear can save 65% to 85% of patients. However, mortality approaches 70% in those who present with hemorrhage or symptoms related to distal ischemia, and the overall 10-year survival is only 40% to 60%. Most type B dissections can be managed conservatively; patients have a 75% survival rate whether they are treated with surgery or antihypertensive medication only.

KEY CONCEPTS

Aneurysms and Dissections

- Aneurysms are congenital or acquired dilations of the heart or blood vessels that involve the entire thickness of the wall. Complications are related to rupture, thrombosis, and embolization.
- Dissections occur when blood enters the wall of a vessel and separates the various layers. Complications arise due to rupture or obstruction of vessels branching off the aorta.
- Aneurysms and dissections result from structural weakness of the vessel wall caused by loss of smooth muscle cells or insufficient extracellular matrix, which can result from ischemia, genetic defects, or defective matrix remodeling.

Vasculitis

Vasculitis is a general term for vessel wall inflammation. The clinical features of the various vasculitides are protean and largely depend on the vascular bed affected (e.g., CNS vs. heart vs. small bowel). Besides the findings referable to the specific tissues involved, the clinical manifestations typically include constitutional signs and symptoms such as fever, myalgias, arthralgias, and malaise.

Vessels of any type in virtually any organ can be affected, but most vasculitides affect small vessels ranging in size from arterioles to capillaries to venules. There are exceptions, however, and, several of the vasculitides tend to affect only vessels of a particular size or location. Thus, there are entities that primarily affect the aorta and medium-sized arteries, while others principally affect only smaller arterioles. Some 20 primary forms of vasculitis are recognized, and classification schemes attempt (with variable success) to group them according to vessel diameter, role of immune complexes, presence of specific autoantibodies, granuloma formation, organ specificity, and even population demographics (Table 11-3 and Fig. 11-23). As we will see, there is considerable clinical and pathologic overlap among these entities.

The two common pathogenic mechanisms of vasculitis are immune-mediated inflammation and direct invasion of vascular walls by infectious pathogens. *Infections can also indirectly induce a noninfectious vasculitis,* for example, by generating immune complexes or triggering a cross-reactive immune response. In any given patient, it is critical to distinguish between infectious and immunologic mechanisms, because immunosuppressive therapy is appropriate for immune-mediated vasculitis but could very well be counter-productive for infectious vasculitides. Physical and chemical injury, such as from irradiation, mechanical trauma, and toxins, can also cause vasculitis.

Table 11-3 Primary Forms of Vasculitis

	Giant Cell Arteritis	Granulomatosis with Polyangiitis	Churg-Strauss Syndrome	Polyarteritis Nodosa	Leukocytoclastic Vasculitis	Buerger Disease	Behçet Disease
Sites of Involvement							
Aorta	+	–	–	–	–	–	–
Medium-sized arteries	+	+	+	+	–	+	+
Small-sized arteries	–	+	+	+	+	+	+
Capillaries	–	–	–	–	+	–	+
Veins	–	–	–	–	+	+	+
Inflammatory Cells Present							
Lymphocytes	+	+	+	±	±	±	±
Macrophages	+	+	+	±	±	±	±
Neutrophils	Rare	+	+	±	±	±	Required
Eosinophils	Very rare	±	Required	±	±	±	±
Other Features							
Granulomas	± *	Required *	±	–	–	–	–
Giant cells	Often; not required	±	–	–	–	–	–
Thrombosis	±	±	±	±	±	Required	±
Serum ANCA positivity	–	+	+	±	–	–	–
Clinical history	>40 y years old, ± polymyalgia rheumatica	Any	Asthma, atopy	Any	Any	Young male smoker	Orogenital ulcers

*The granulomas of giant cell arteritis are found within the vessel wall as part of the inflammation comprising the vasculitis, but need not be present to render the diagnosis. The granulomas of granulomatosis with polyangiitis are larger, spanning between vessels, and associated with areas of tissue necrosis.
From Seidman MA, Mitchell RN: Surgical pathology of small-and medium-sized vessels. In Current Concepts in Cardiovascular Pathology, Philadelphia, Saunders, 2012.

Noninfectious Vasculitis

The major cause of noninfectious vasculitis is a local or systemic immune response. Immunologic injury in noninfectious vasculitis may be caused by:

- Immune complex deposition
- Antineutrophil cytoplasmic antibodies
- Antiendothelial cell antibodies
- Autoreactive T cells

Immune Complex-Associated Vasculitis

This form of vasculitis can be seen in systemic immunologic disorders such as systemic lupus erythematosus (Chapter 6) that are associated with autoantibody

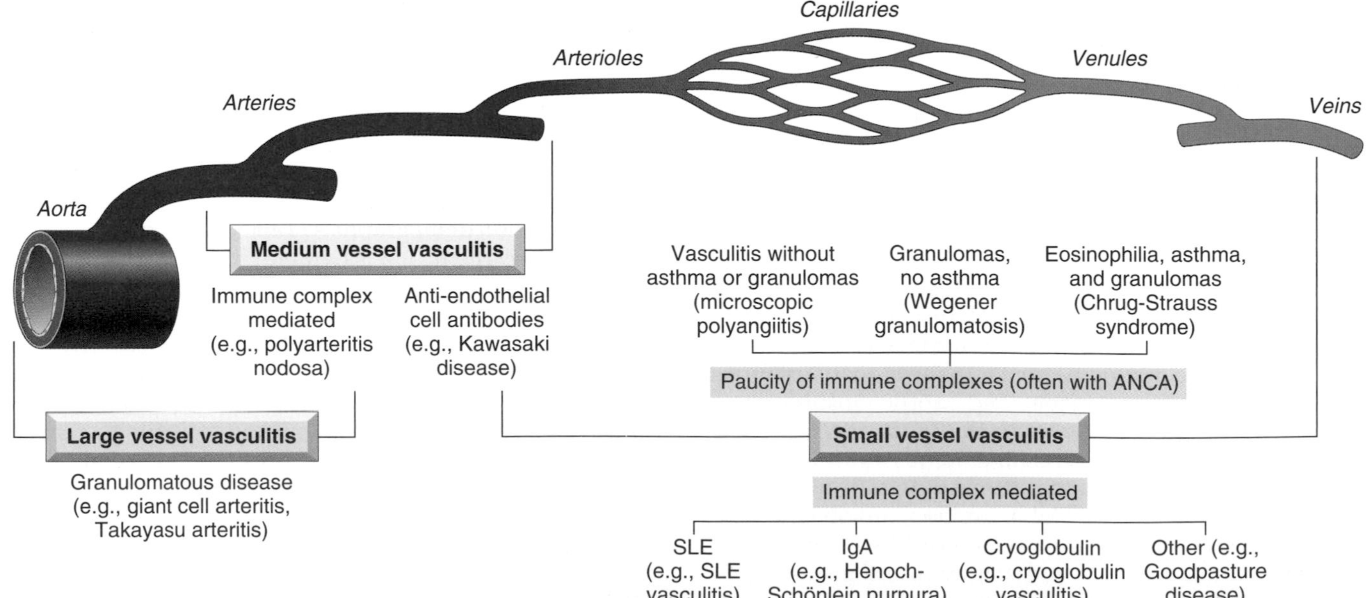

Figure 11-23 Vascular sites typically involved with the more common forms of vasculitis, as well as their presumptive etiologies. Note that there is a substantial overlap in distributions. ANCA, Antineutrophil cytoplasmic antibody; SLE, systemic lupus erythematosus.

production and formation of immune complexes that deposit in vessels. The vascular lesions resemble those found in experimental immune complex–mediated disorders, such as the Arthus phenomenon and serum sickness, and in many cases contain readily identifiable antibody and complement. Often, however, this type of vasculitis presents a number of diagnostic challenges. Only rarely is the specific antigen responsible for immune complex formation identified. Also, in most cases it is not clear whether the pathogenic antigen-antibody complexes are deposited from the circulation or form in situ. Indeed, the sensitivity and specificity of circulating immune complex assays in such diseases are extremely low. In many suspected cases, even the antigen-antibody deposits are scarce. In such instances, the immune complexes may have been degraded by the time of biopsy; alternatively, other mechanisms may underlie such "pauci-immune" vasculitides.

Immune complex deposition is also implicated in the following vasculitides:

- *Drug hypersensitivity vasculitis.* In some cases (e.g., penicillin), drugs act as haptens by binding to serum proteins or vessel wall constituents; other agents are themselves foreign proteins (e.g., streptokinase). Regardless, antibodies directed against the drug-modified proteins or foreign molecules result in immune complex formation. The clinical manifestations can be mild and self-limiting, or severe and even fatal; skin lesions are most common. It is always important to consider drug hypersensitivity as a cause of vasculitis since discontinuation of the offending agent usually leads to resolution.
- *Vasculitis secondary to infections.* Antibodies to microbial constituents can form immune complexes that circulate and deposit in vascular lesions. In up to 30% of patients with polyarteritis nodosa (see later), the vasculitis is attributable to immune complexes composed of hepatitis B surface antigens (HBsAg) and anti-HBsAg antibody.

Antineutrophil Cytoplasmic Antibodies

Many patients with vasculitis have circulating antibodies that react with neutrophil cytoplasmic antigens, so-called *antineutrophil cytoplasmic antibodies (ANCAs)*. ANCAs are a heterogeneous group of autoantibodies directed against constituents (mainly enzymes) of neutrophil primary granules, monocyte lysosomes, and endothelial cells. ANCAs are very useful diagnostic markers; their titers generally mirror clinical severity, and a rise in titers after periods of quiescence is predictive of disease recurrence. Although a number of ANCAs have been described, two are most important. These were previously grouped according to the intracellular distribution of the target antigens (cytoplasmic [c-ANCA] or perinuclear [p-ANCA]), but are now classified according to their antigen specificity:

- *Anti-proteinase-3 (PR3-ANCA, previously c-ANCA).* PR3 is a neutrophil azurophilic granule constituent that shares homology with numerous microbial peptides, raising the possibility that the generation of PR3-ANCAs is triggered by certain infections. PR3-ANCAs are associated with polyangiitis (see later).
- *Anti-myeloperoxidase (MPO-ANCA, previously p-ANCA).* MPO is a lysosomal granule constituent involved in oxygen free radical generation (Chapter 3). MPO-ANCAs are induced by several therapeutic agents, particularly propylthiouracil. MPO-ANCAs are associated with microscopic polyangiitis and Churg-Strauss syndrome (see later).

The close association between ANCA titers and disease activity suggests a pathogenic role for these antibodies. Of note, ANCAs can directly activate neutrophils, stimulating the release of reactive oxygen species and proteolytic enzymes; in vascular beds, such activation also leads to destructive interactions between inflammatory cells and endothelial cells. While the antigenic targets of ANCA are primarily intracellular (and therefore not usually accessible to circulating antibodies), it is now clear that ANCA antigens (especially PR3) are either constitutively expressed at low levels on the plasma membrane or are translocated to the cell surface in activated and apoptotic leukocytes.

A plausible mechanism for ANCA vasculitis is the following:

- Drugs or cross-reactive microbial antigens induce ANCA formation; alternatively, leukocyte surface expression or release of PR3 and MPO (in the setting of infections) incites ANCA development in a susceptible host.
- Subsequent infection, endotoxin exposure, or inflammatory stimulus elicits cytokines such as TNF that upregulate the surface expression of PR3 and MPO on neutrophils and other cell types.
- ANCAs react with these cytokine-activated cells, causing either direct injury (e.g., to endothelial cells) or further activation (e.g., of neutrophils).
- ANCA-activated neutrophils cause tissue injury by releasing granule contents and reactive oxygen species.

Since ANCA autoantibodies are directed against cellular constituents and do not form circulating immune complexes, the vascular lesions do not typically contain demonstrable antibody and complement. Thus, ANCA-associated vasculitides are often described as "pauci-immune." Interestingly, ANCA directed against proteins other than PR3 and MPO are often seen in patients with nonvasculitic inflammatory disorders, such as inflammatory bowel disease, sclerosing cholangitis, and rheumatoid arthritis.

Antiendothelial Cell Antibodies

Antibodies to endothelial cells, perhaps induced by defects in immune regulation, may predispose to certain vasculitides, for example, Kawasaki disease (see later).

The following discussion presents several of the best characterized and generally recognized vasculitides; there is substantial overlap among the different entities. Moreover, it should be kept in mind that some patients with vasculitis do not have a classic constellation of findings that allows them to be neatly pigeon-holed into one specific diagnosis.

Giant Cell (Temporal) Arteritis

Giant cell (temporal) arteritis is the most common form of vasculitis among older individuals in the United States and Europe. **It is a chronic inflammatory disorder of large to small-sized arteries that principally affects arteries in the head**—especially the temporal arteries—but also the vertebral and ophthalmic arteries. Ophthalmic arterial involvement can lead abruptly to permanent blindness; consequently, giant cell arteritis is a medical emergency requiring prompt recognition and treatment. Lesions also occur in other arteries, including the aorta (giant cell aortitis).

Pathogenesis. Most evidence suggests that giant cell arteritis stems from a T-cell–mediated immune response against one of handful of vessel wall antigens that drives subsequent proinflammatory cytokine production (particularly TNF). Anti-endothelial cell and anti-smooth muscle cell antibodies can also be demonstrated in roughly two thirds of patients, although it is unclear whether these are causal or a consequence of other immune injury. A cellular immune etiology is supported by the characteristic granulomatous response, a correlation with certain MHC class II haplotypes, and a prompt therapeutic response to steroids. The extraordinary predilection for a single vascular site (temporal artery) remains unexplained.

MORPHOLOGY

Involved arterial segments develop **intimal thickening** (with occasional thromboses) **that reduces the luminal diameter**. Classic lesions exhibit medial **granulomatous inflammation** centered on the internal elastic lamina that produce **elastic lamina fragmentation**; there is an infiltrate of T cells (CD4+ > CD8+) and macrophages. Although multinucleated giant cells are seen in approximately 75% of adequately biopsied specimens (Fig. 11-24), granulomas and giant cells can be rare or absent. Inflammatory lesions are only focally distributed along the vessel and long segments of relatively normal artery may be interposed. The healed stage is marked by medial attenuation and scarring with intimal thickening, typically with residual elastic tissue fragmentation and adventitial fibrosis.

Clinical Features. Giant cell arteritis is rare before age 50. Symptoms may be only vague and constitutional—fever, fatigue, weight loss—or there may be facial pain or headache, most intense along the course of the superficial temporal artery, which can be painful to palpation. Ocular symptoms (associated with involvement of the ophthalmic artery) appear abruptly in about 50% of patients; these range from diplopia to complete vision loss. Diagnosis depends on biopsy and histologic confirmation. However, because giant cell arteritis can be extremely focal within an artery, adequate biopsy requires at least a 1-cm segment; even then, a negative biopsy result does not exclude the diagnosis. Corticosteroids or anti-TNF therapies are typically effective.

Takayasu Arteritis

This is a granulomatous vasculitis of medium and larger arteries characterized principally by ocular disturbances and marked weakening of the pulses in the upper extremities (hence the name *pulseless disease*). Takayasu arteritis manifests with transmural fibrous thickening of the aorta—particularly the aortic arch and great vessels—with severe luminal narrowing of the major branch vessels (Fig. 11-25). Takayasu aortitis shares many attributes with giant cell aortitis, including clinical features and histology. Indeed, the distinction is typically made based on the age of the patient: in patients older than 50, the diagnosis is giant cell aortitis, while in those younger than 50, it is Takayasu

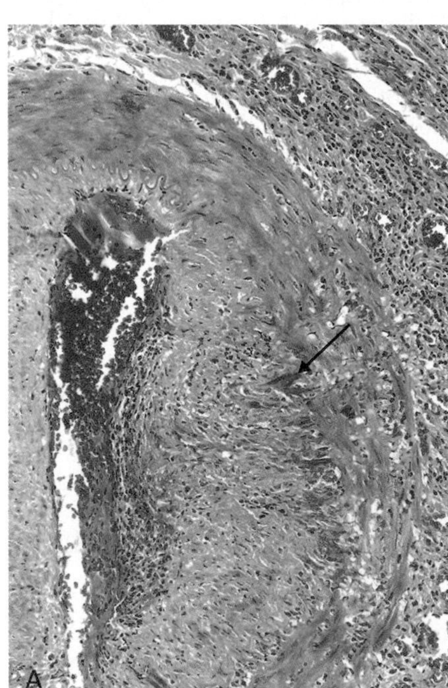

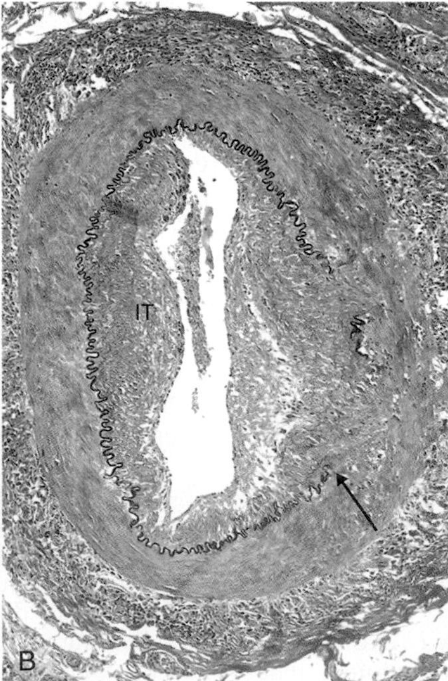

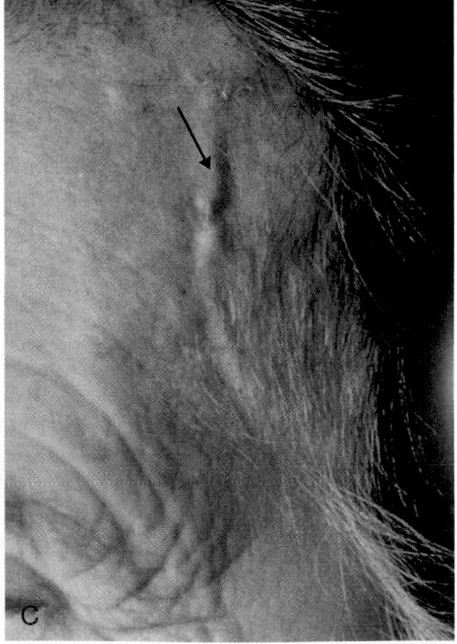

Figure 11-24 Giant cell (temporal) arteritis. **A,** Hematoxylin and eosin stain of section of temporal artery showing giant cells at the degenerated internal elastic lamina in active arteritis *(arrow)*. **B,** Elastic tissue stain demonstrating focal destruction of internal elastic lamina *(arrow)* and intimal thickening (IT) characteristic of long-standing or healed arteritis. **C,** The temporal artery of a patient with classic giant cell arteritis shows a thickened, nodular, and tender segment of a vessel on the surface of head *(arrow)*. (**C,** From Salvarani C, et al. Polymyalgia rheumatica and giant-cell arteritis. N Engl J Med 347:261, 2002.)

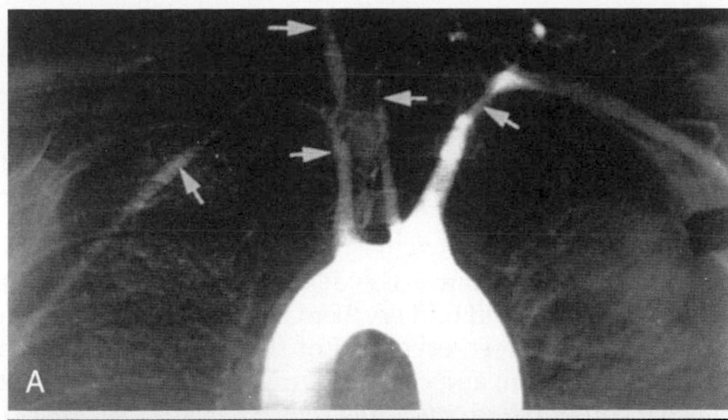

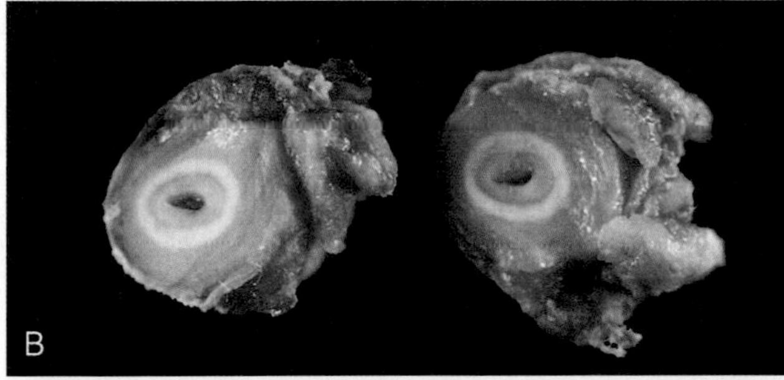

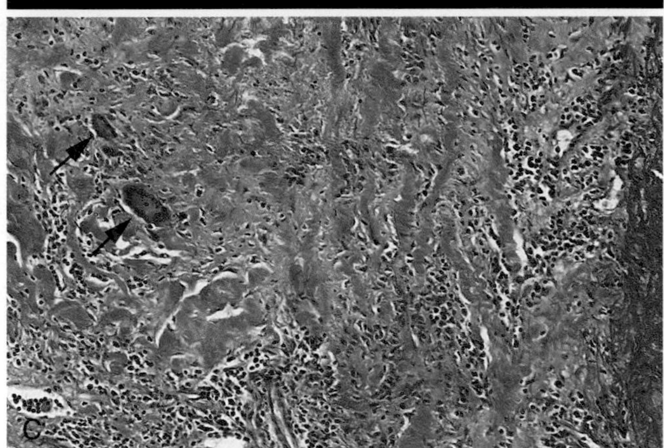

Figure 11-25 Takayasu arteritis. **A,** Aortic arch angiogram showing narrowing of brachiocephalic, carotid, and subclavian arteries *(arrows)*. **B,** Gross photograph of two cross-sections of the right carotid artery taken at autopsy of the patient shown in **A,** demonstrating marked intimal thickening and adventitial fibrosis with minimal residual lumen. **C,** Histologic appearance in active Takayasu aortitis, illustrating destruction and fibrosis of the arterial media associated with mononuclear infiltrates and inflammatory giant cells *(arrows)*.

aortitis. Although historically associated with the Japanese population and a subset of HLA haplotypes, Takayasu aortitis has a global distribution. An autoimmune etiology is likely.

MORPHOLOGY

Takayasu arteritis classically involves the aortic arch. In a third of patients, it also affects the remainder of the aorta and its branches, with **pulmonary artery** involvement in half the cases; **coronary and renal arteries** may be similarly affected. There is irregular thickening of the vessel wall with intimal hyperplasia; when the aortic arch is involved, the great vessel lumina can be markedly narrowed or even obliterated (Fig. 11-25*A* and *B*). Histologically, the changes range from adventitial mononuclear infiltrates with perivascular cuffing of the vasa vasorum, to intense mononuclear inflammation in the media, to granulomatous inflammation, replete with giant cells and patchy medial necrosis. The histology (Fig. 11-25*C*) is indistinguishable from giant cell (temporal) arteritis. As the disease progresses, collagenous scarring, with admixed chronic inflammatory infiltrates, occurs in all three layers of the vessel wall. Occasionally, aortic root involvement causes dilation and aortic valve insufficiency.

Clinical Features. Initial symptoms are usually nonspecific, including fatigue, weight loss, and fever. With progression, vascular symptoms appear and dominate the clinical picture, including reduced blood pressure and weak pulses in the carotids and the upper extremities; ocular disturbances, including visual defects, retinal hemorrhages, and total blindness; and neurologic deficits. Involvement of the more distal aorta may lead to claudication of the legs; pulmonary artery involvement can cause pulmonary hypertension. Narrowing of the coronary ostia may lead to myocardial infarction, and involvement of the renal arteries leads to systemic hypertension in roughly half of patients. The course of the disease is variable. In some there is rapid progression, while others enter a quiescent stage after 1 to 2 years, permitting long-term survival, albeit with visual or neurologic deficits.

Polyarteritis Nodosa

Polyarteritis nodosa (PAN) is a systemic vasculitis of small- or medium-sized muscular arteries, typically involving renal and visceral vessels but sparing the pulmonary circulation. There is no association with ANCA, but about 30% of patients with PAN have chronic hepatitis B and deposits containing HBsAg-HBsAb complexes in affected vessels, indicating an immune complex–mediated etiology in that subset. The cause remains unknown in the remaining cases; there may be etiologic and clinical distinctions between classic idiopathic PAN, the cutaneous forms of PAN, and the PAN associated with chronic hepatitis.

MORPHOLOGY

Classic polyarteritis nodosa is characterized by **segmental transmural necrotizing inflammation of small- to medium-sized arteries**. Vessels of the kidneys, heart, liver, and gastrointestinal tract are involved in descending order of frequency. Lesions usually involve only part of the vessel circumference with a predilection for branch points. The inflammatory process weakens the arterial wall and can lead to aneurysms or even rupture. Impaired perfusion with ulcerations, infarcts, ischemic atrophy, or hemorrhages may be the first sign of disease.

During the acute phase, there is transmural inflammation of the arterial wall with a mixed infiltrate of neutrophils, eosinophils, and mononuclear cells, frequently accompanied by **fibrinoid necrosis** (Fig. 11-26). Luminal thrombosis can occur. Later, the acute inflammatory infiltrate is replaced by fibrous (occasionally nodular) thickening of the vessel wall that can extend into the adventitia. Characteristically, all stages of activity (from early to late) may coexist in different vessels or even within the same vessel, suggesting ongoing and recurrent insults.

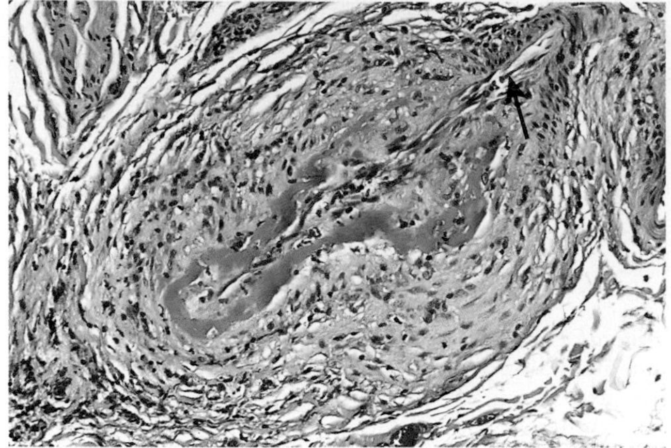

Figure 11-26 Polyarteritis nodosa. There is segmental fibrinoid necrosis and thrombotic occlusion of the lumen of this small artery. Note that part of the vessel wall at the upper right *(arrow)* is uninvolved. (Courtesy Sidney Murphree, MD, Department of Pathology, University of Texas Southwestern Medical School, Dallas, Texas.)

Clinical Features. Although typically a disease of young adults, PAN can also occur in pediatric and geriatric populations. Clinical manifestations result from ischemia and infarction of affected tissues and organs. The course is frequently remitting and episodic, with long symptom-free intervals. Because the vascular involvement is widely scattered, the clinical signs and symptoms of PAN can be quite variable. A "classic" presentation can involve some combination of rapidly accelerating hypertension due to renal artery involvement; abdominal pain and bloody stools caused by vascular gastrointestinal lesions; diffuse myalgias; and peripheral neuritis, predominantly affecting motor nerves. Renal involvement is often prominent and a major cause of mortality. Untreated, PAN is typically fatal; however, immunosuppression can yield remissions or cures in 90% of cases.

Kawasaki Disease

***Kawasaki disease* is an acute febrile, usually self-limited illness of infancy and childhood (80% of patients are 4 years old or younger); it is associated with an arteritis affecting large to medium-sized, and even small vessels.** Its clinical significance stems primarily from a predilection for coronary artery involvement that can cause aneurysms that rupture or thrombose, resulting in acute myocardial infarctions. Originally described in Japan, the disease has a worldwide distribution and is the leading cause of acquired heart disease in children.

The pathogenesis of Kawasaki disease is unknown. A variety of infectious agents (mostly viral) have been implicated in triggering the disease in genetically susceptible individuals. The vascular damage is primarily mediated by activated T cells and monocytes/macrophages.

MORPHOLOGY

The vasculitis resembles that seen in polyarteritis nodosa. There is a dense transmural inflammatory infiltrate, although the fibrinoid necrosis is usually less prominent than in PAN. The acute vasculitis typically subsides spontaneously or in response to treatment, but aneurysm formation due to wall damage can supervene. As with other arteritides, healed lesions can also exhibit obstructive intimal thickening. Pathologic changes outside the cardiovascular system are rarely significant.

Clinical Features. Kawasaki disease typically presents with conjunctival and oral erythema and blistering, edema of the hands and feet, erythema of the palms and soles, a desquamative rash, and cervical lymph node enlargement (hence its other name, *mucocutaneous lymph node syndrome*). Approximately 20% of untreated patients develop cardiovascular sequelae, ranging from asymptomatic coronary arteritis, to coronary artery ectasia, to giant coronary artery aneurysms (7 to 8 mm) leading to rupture or thrombosis, myocardial infarction, and sudden death. If the disease is recognized early in its course, treatment with intravenous immunoglobulin and aspirin sharply reduce the risk of symptomatic coronary artery disease.

Microscopic Polyangiitis

Microscopic polyangiitis is a *necrotizing vasculitis that generally affects capillaries, as well as small arterioles and venules.* It is also called hypersensitivity vasculitis or leukocytoclastic vasculitis. Unlike polyarteritis nodosa, *all lesions of microscopic polyangiitis tend to be of the same age in any given patient and are distributed more widely.* The skin, mucous membranes, lungs, brain, heart, gastrointestinal tract, kidneys, and muscle can all be involved; *necrotizing glomerulonephritis* (90% of patients) and pulmonary capillaritis are particularly common. Microscopic angiitis can be a feature of a number of immune disorders, such as Henoch-Schönlein purpura, essential mixed cryoglobulinemia, and vasculitis associated with connective tissue disorders.

Pathogenesis. In some cases, antibody responses to antigens such as drugs (e.g., penicillin), microorganisms (e.g., streptococci), heterologous proteins, or tumor proteins have been implicated. These can either lead to immune complex deposition or trigger secondary immune responses (e.g., the development of ANCAs) that are pathogenic. Indeed, most cases are associated with MPO-ANCA. Recruitment and activation of neutrophils within affected vascular beds is likely responsible for the disease manifestations.

MORPHOLOGY

Microscopic polyangiitis is characterized by segmental fibrinoid necrosis of the media and focal transmural necrotizing lesions; granulomatous inflammation is absent. These lesions morphologically resemble PAN but typically spare medium-sized and larger arteries; consequently, infarcts are uncommon. In some areas (typically postcapillary venules), only infiltrating neutrophils, many undergoing apoptosis, are seen, giving rise to the term **leukocytoclastic vasculitis** (Fig. 11-27*A*). Although immunoglobulins and complement components can be demonstrated in early skin lesions, little or no immunoglobulin are found in most lesions (so-called "pauci-immune injury").

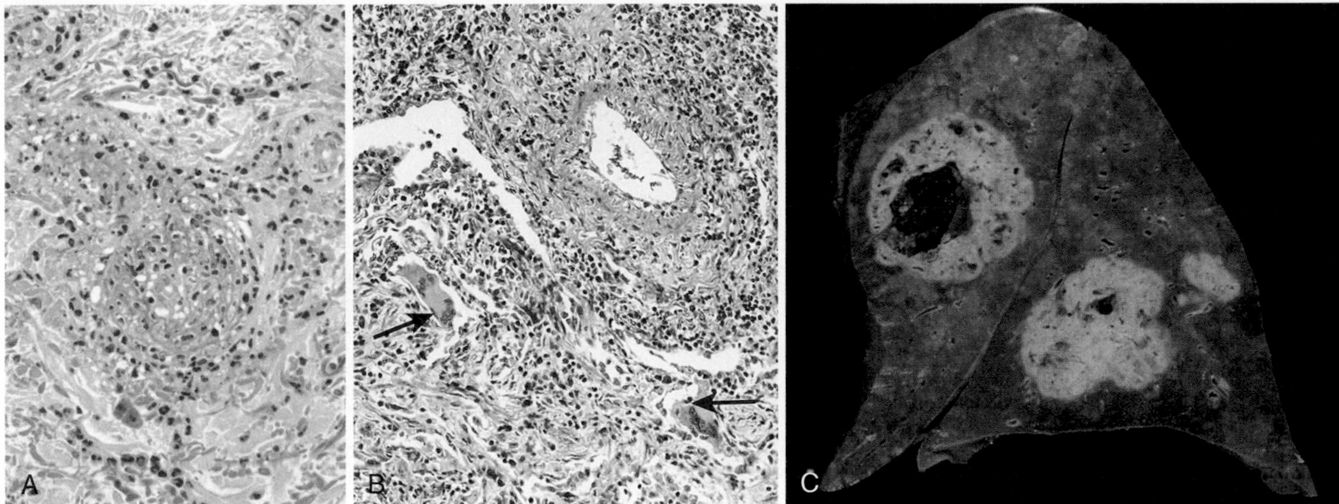

Figure 11-27 Small vessel vasculitis. **A,** Leukocytoclastic vasculitis (microscopic polyangiitis) with fragmentation of neutrophils in and around blood vessel walls. **B** and **C**, Granulomatosis with polyangiitis. **B,** Vasculitis of a small artery with adjacent granulomatous inflammation including epithelioid cells and giant cells *(arrows)*. **C,** Gross photo from the lung of a patient with fatal granulomatosis with polyangiitis, demonstrating large nodular centrally cavitating lesions. (**A,** Courtesy Scott Granter, MD, Brigham and Women's Hospital, Boston, Mass.; **C,** Courtesy Sidney Murphree, MD, Department of Pathology, University of Texas Southwestern Medical School, Dallas, Texas.)

Clinical Features. Depending on the vascular bed involved, major clinical features include hemoptysis, hematuria and proteinuria, bowel pain or bleeding, muscle pain or weakness, and palpable cutaneous purpura. Except in those in whom widespread renal or brain involvement develop, immunosuppression induces remission and markedly improves long-term survival.

Churg-Strauss Syndrome

Churg-Strauss syndrome is a small-vessel necrotizing vasculitis classically associated with asthma, allergic rhinitis, lung infiltrates, peripheral hypereosinophilia, and extravascular necrotizing granulomata. Also called allergic granulomatosis and angiitis, it is a relatively rare disease (roughly one in a million people). Vascular lesions can be histologically similar to polyarteritis nodosa or microscopic polyangiitis, but are also characteristically accompanied by granulomas and eosinophils. ANCAs (mostly MPO-ANCAs) are present in less than half the cases, and suggest that there are distinct subsets of patients with the syndrome. Nevertheless, when present, the ANCAs are likely involved in the pathogenesis of the vascular lesions.

Churg- Strauss syndrome is a multisystem diseases with cutaneous involvement (palpable purpura), gastrointestinal tract bleeding, and renal disease (primarily as focal and segmental glomerulosclerosis). Myocardial involvement may give rise to cardiomyopathy; the heart is involved in 60% of patients and accounts for almost half of the deaths in the syndrome. Involvement of the heart is associated with the presence of eosinophilic infiltrates. The syndrome may be a consequence of hyperresponsiveness to an allergic stimulus; in patients with asthma, leukotriene receptor antagonists have been reported to be a trigger.

Behçet Disease

Behçet disease is a small- to medium-vessel neutrophilic vasculitis that classically presents as a clinical triad of recurrent oral aphthous ulcers, genital ulcers, and uveitis. There can also be gastrointestinal and pulmonary manifestations, with disease mortality related to severe neurologic involvement or rupture of vascular aneurysms. There is an association with certain HLA haplotypes (HLA-B51, in particular) and a cross-reactive immune response to certain microorganisms is implicated. T_H17 cells (Chapter 6) play a significant role by contributing to the recruitment of neutrophils, which are seen infiltrating vessels walls. However, the findings are nonspecific and the diagnosis requires an appropriate clinical story. Immunosuppression with steroids or TNF-antagonist therapies are generally effective.

Granulomatosis with Polyangiitis

Previously called Wegener granulomatosis, granulomatosis with polyangiitis is a necrotizing vasculitis characterized by a triad of:

- *Necrotizing granulomas* of the upper respiratory tract (ear, nose, sinuses, throat) or the lower respiratory tract (lung) or both.
- *Necrotizing or granulomatous vasculitis* affecting small- to medium-sized vessels (e.g., capillaries, venules, arterioles, and arteries), most prominent in the lungs and upper airways but involving other sites as well.
- *Focal necrotizing, often crescentic, glomerulonephritis.*

"Limited" forms of this disease may be restricted to the respiratory tract. Conversely, a widespread form of the disease can affect eyes, skin, and other organs, notably the heart; clinically, this resembles PAN except that there is also respiratory involvement.

Pathogenesis. Granulomatosis with polyangiitis likely represents a form of T-cell–mediated hypersensitivity response to normally "innocuous" inhaled microbial or other environmental agents; such a pathogenesis is supported by the presence of granulomas and a dramatic response to immunosuppressive therapy. PR3-ANCAs are also present in up to 95% of cases; they are a useful marker of disease activity and may participate in disease

pathogenesis. Following immunosuppression, a rising PR3-ANCA titer is often a harbinger of relapse; most patients in remission have a negative test or falling titers.

MORPHOLOGY

Upper respiratory tract lesions range from inflammatory sinusitis with mucosal granulomas to ulcerative lesions of the nose, palate, or pharynx, rimmed by **granulomas with geographic patterns of central necrosis and accompanying vasculitis** (Fig. 11-27*B*). The necrotizing granulomas are surrounded by a zone of proliferating fibroblasts associated with giant cells and leukocytic infiltrate, reminiscent of mycobacterial or fungal infections. Multiple granulomas can coalesce to produce radiographically visible nodules that can also cavitate; late stage disease may be marked by extensive necrotizing granulomatous involvement of the parenchyma (Fig. 11-27*C*), and alveolar hemorrhage may be prominent. Lesions may ultimately undergo progressive fibrosis and organization.

A spectrum of renal lesions can be seen (Chapter 20). In early stages, glomeruli exhibit only focal necrosis with isolated capillary loop thrombosis (**focal and segmental necrotizing glomerulonephritis**); there is minimal parietal cell proliferation in the Bowman capsule. More advanced glomerular lesions are characterized by diffuse necrosis with exuberant parietal cell proliferation resulting in crescent formation (**crescentic glomerulonephritis**).

Clinical Features. Males are affected more often than females, at an average age of about 40 years. Classic features include persistent pneumonitis with bilateral nodular and cavitary infiltrates (95%), chronic sinusitis (90%), mucosal ulcerations of the nasopharynx (75%), and evidence of renal disease (80%). Other features include rashes, myalgias, articular involvement, neural inflammation, and fever. Left untreated, the disease is usually rapidly fatal, with 80% mortality within 1 year. Treatment with steroids, cyclophosphamide, and more recently TNF antagonists have turned this formerly fatal condition into a chronic relapsing and remitting disease.

Thromboangiitis Obliterans (Buerger Disease)

***Thromboangiitis obliterans (Buerger disease)* is characterized by segmental, thrombosing, acute and chronic inflammation of medium-sized and small arteries, principally the tibial and radial arteries, with occasional secondary extension into the veins and nerves of the extremities.** It is a distinctive disease that often leads to vascular insufficiency, typically of the extremities. It occurs almost exclusively in heavy cigarette smokers, usually before age 35.

Pathogenesis. The strong relationship with cigarette smoking may stem from either a direct idiosyncratic endothelial cell toxicity caused by some component of tobacco, or an immune response to components of tobacco smoke that modify host vascular wall proteins. Most patients have hypersensitivity to intradermally injected tobacco extracts, and their vessels exhibit impaired endothelium-dependent vasodilation when challenged with acetylcholine. There is an increased prevalence in certain ethnic groups (Israeli, Indian subcontinent, Japanese) and an association with particular HLA haplotypes.

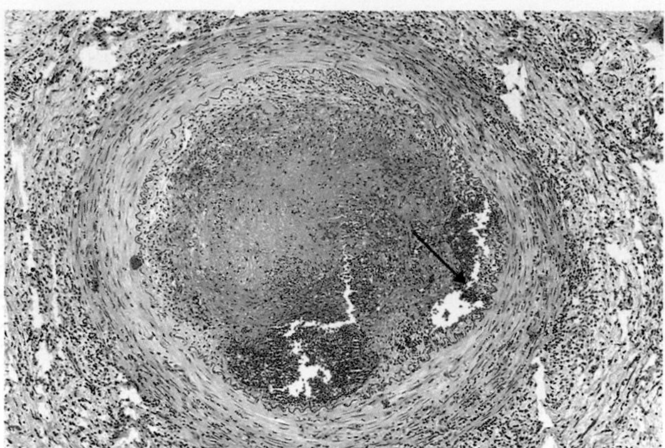

Figure 11-28 Thromboangiitis obliterans (Buerger disease). The lumen is occluded by a thrombus containing abscesses *(arrow)*, and the vessel wall is infiltrated with leukocytes.

MORPHOLOGY

Thromboangiitis obliterans is characterized by a **focal acute and chronic vasculitis of small- and medium-sized arteries,** predominantly of the extremities. On histology, there is acute and chronic inflammation, accompanied by luminal thrombosis. The thrombus can contain small **microabscesses** composed of neutrophils surrounded by granulomatous inflammation (Fig. 11-28); the thrombus may eventually organize and recanalize. The inflammatory process extends into contiguous veins and nerves (rare with other forms of vasculitis), and with time all three structures can be encased in fibrous tissue.

Clinical Features. Early manifestations include cold-induced Raynaud phenomenon (see later), leg pain induced by exercise that is relieved on rest (*intermittent claudication*), instep foot pain induced by exercise (*instep claudication*), and a superficial nodular phlebitis (venous inflammation). The vascular insufficiency of Buerger disease tends to be accompanied by severe pain—even at rest—undoubtedly due to the neural involvement. Chronic extremity ulcerations develop, progressing over time (occasionally precipitously) to frank gangrene. Smoking abstinence in the early stages of the disease can often ameliorate further attacks; however, once established, the vascular lesions typically do not respond to smoking abstinence.

Vasculitis Associated with Other Noninfectious Disorders

Vasculitis resembling hypersensitivity angiitis or classic polyarteritis nodosa can sometimes be associated with other disorders, such as rheumatoid arthritis, systemic lupus erythematosus, malignancy, or systemic illnesses such as mixed cryoglobulinemia, antiphospholipid antibody syndrome (Chapter 4), and Henoch-Schönlein purpura. *Rheumatoid vasculitis* occurs predominantly in the setting of long-standing, severe rheumatoid arthritis and usually affects small- and medium-sized arteries, leading to visceral infarction; it may also cause a clinically significant aortitis. Identifying the underlying pathology has therapeutic significance. For example, although *lupus vasculitis* and antiphospholipid antibody syndrome can be morphologically and clinically similar, immunosuppressive therapy is required in the former, and anticoagulant therapy is indicated in the latter.

Infectious Vasculitis

Arteritis can be caused by the direct invasion of infectious agents, usually bacteria (*Pseudomonas* being the classic example) or fungi, in particular *Aspergillus* and *Mucor* species. Vascular invasion can be part of a localized tissue infection (e.g., bacterial pneumonia or adjacent to abscesses), or—less commonly—can arise from hematogenous spread of microorganisms during septicemia or embolization from infective endocarditis.

Vascular infections can weaken arterial walls and culminate in *mycotic aneurysms* (see earlier), or can induce thrombosis and infarction. Thus, inflammation-induced thrombosis of meningeal vessels in bacterial meningitis can eventually cause infarction of the underlying brain.

> **KEY CONCEPTS**
>
> **Vasculitis**
>
> - Vasculitis is defined as inflammation of vessel walls; it is frequently associated with systemic manifestations (including fever, malaise, myalgias, and arthralgias) and organ dysfunction that depends on the pattern of vascular involvement.
> - Vasculitis can result from infections, but more commonly has an immunologic basis, including immune complex deposition, formation of anti-neutrophil antibodies (ANCA), or T cell responses to vascular wall antigens.
> - Different forms of vasculitis tend to specifically affect vessels of a particular caliber and location, and the clinical manifestations depend on the pattern of vessel involvement.

Disorders of Blood Vessel Hyperreactivity

Several disorders are characterized by inappropriate or exaggerated vasoconstriction of blood vessels.

Raynaud Phenomenon

Raynaud phenomenon results from exaggerated vasoconstriction of arteries and arterioles in the extremities, particularly the fingers and toes, but also occasionally the nose, earlobes, or lips. The restricted blood flow induces paroxysmal pallor, and even cyanosis in severe cases; involved digits classically show "red, white, and blue" color changes from most proximal to most distal, correlating with proximal vasodilation, central vasoconstriction, and more distal cyanosis (Fig. 11-29). Raynaud phenomenon can be a primary entity or secondary to other disorders.

Primary Raynaud phenomenon (previously called Raynaud disease) is caused by exaggerated central and local vasomotor responses to cold or emotion; it affects 3% to 5% of the general population and has a predilection for young women. It tends to symmetrically affect the extremities, and the severity and extent of involvement typically remains static over time. Structural changes in the arterial walls are absent except in long-standing disease, when intimal thickening can develop. The course is usually benign, but chronicity can lead to atrophy of the skin, subcutaneous tissues, and muscles. Ulceration and ischemic gangrene are rare.

Secondary Raynaud phenomenon refers to vascular insufficiency due to arterial disease caused by other entities including SLE, scleroderma, Buerger disease, or even atherosclerosis. Clinically, secondary Raynaud phenomenon tends to have asymmetric involvement of the extremities and progressively worsens in extent and severity over time.

Since Raynaud phenomenon may be the first manifestation of immune-mediated vasculitides, any patient with

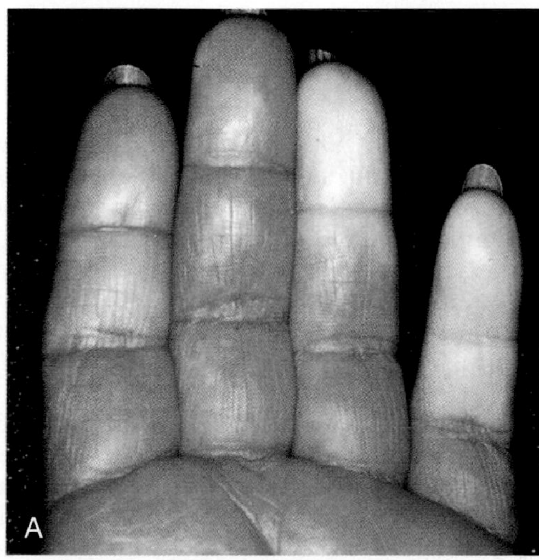

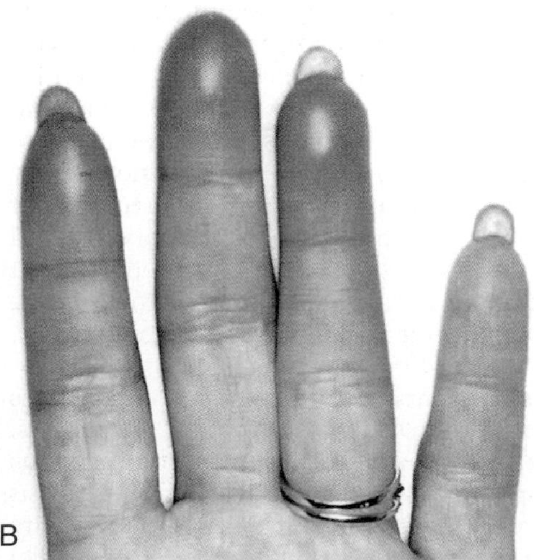

Figure 11-29 Raynaud phenomenon. **A,** Sharply demarcated pallor of the distal fingers resulting from spasm of the digital arteries. **B,** Cyanosis of the fingertips. (Reproduced from Salvarani C, et al: Polymyalgia rheumatica and giant-cell arteritis. N Engl J Med 347:261, 2002.)

new symptoms should be evaluated. Of these, some 10% will eventually manifest an underlying disorder.

Myocardial Vessel Vasospasm

Excessive constriction of coronary arteries or myocardial arterioles may cause ischemia, and persistent vasospasm can even cause myocardial infarction. In addition to intrinsic hyper-reactivity of medial smooth muscle cells, as described earlier for primary Raynaud disease, high levels of vasoactive mediators can precipitate prolonged myocardial vessel contraction. Such agents can be endogenous (e.g., epinephrine released by pheochromocytomas) or exogenous (cocaine or phenylephrine). Elevated thyroid hormone causes a similar effect by increasing the sensitivity of vessels to circulating catecholamines, while autoantibodies and T cells in scleroderma (Chapter 6) can cause vascular instability and vasospasm. In some individuals, extreme psychological stress and the attendant release of catecholamines can lead to pathologic vasospasm.

When vasospasm of cardiac arterial or arteriolar beds (so-called *cardiac Raynaud*) is of sufficient duration (20 to 30 minutes), myocardial infarction occurs. Elevated levels of catechols also increase heart rate and myocardial contractility, exacerbating ischemia caused by the vasospasm. The outcome may be sudden cardiac death (likely caused by a fatal arrhythmia) or an ischemic dilated cardiomyopathy, so-called *Takotsubo cardiomyopathy* (also called "broken heart syndrome" because of the association with emotional duress; Chapter 12). Histologically, acute cases may show microscopic areas of necrosis characterized by myocyte hypercontraction (*contraction band necrosis*); subacute and chronic cases may exhibit microscopic foci of granulation tissue and/or scar.

Veins and Lymphatics

Varicose veins and phlebothrombosis/thrombophlebitis together account for at least 90% of clinical venous disease.

Varicose Veins

Varicose veins are abnormally dilated, tortuous veins produced by prolonged, increased intraluminal pressure leading to vessel dilation and incompetence of the venous valves. The *superficial veins* of the upper and lower leg are commonly involved because venous pressures in these sites can be markedly elevated (up to 10 times normal) by prolonged dependent posture. Roughly 10% to 30% of adults develop lower extremity varicosities; obesity and pregnancy increase risk by creating mass effects that impede venous drainage. A familial predilection to varicose veins reflects defective venous wall development.

Clinical Features. Incompetence of the venous valves leads to stasis, congestion, edema, pain, and thrombosis. Secondary tissue ischemia results from chronic venous congestion and poor vessel drainage leading to *stasis dermatitis* (also called "brawny induration"; the brawny color comes from the hemolysis of extravasated red cells) and ulcerations; poor wound healing and superimposed infections are common additional complications. *Notably, embolism from these superficial veins is very rare, in contrast to the relatively frequent thromboembolism that arises from thrombosed deep veins* (see later and Chapter 4).

Varicosities in two other sites also deserve mention:

- *Esophageal varices.* Liver cirrhosis (less frequently, portal vein obstruction or hepatic vein thrombosis) causes portal vein hypertension (Chapter 18). Portal hypertension leads to the opening of portosystemic shunts that increase blood flow into veins at the gastroesophageal junction (forming *esophageal varices*), the rectum (forming *hemorrhoids*), and periumbilical veins of the abdominal wall (forming a *caput medusa*). Esophageal varices are the most important since their rupture can lead to massive (even fatal) upper gastrointestinal hemorrhage.
- *Hemorrhoids* can also result from primary varicose dilation of the venous plexus at the anorectal junction (e.g., through prolonged pelvic vascular congestion due to pregnancy or straining to defecate). Hemorrhoids are uncomfortable and may be a source of bleeding; they can also thrombose and are prone to painful ulceration.

Thrombophlebitis and Phlebothrombosis

Thrombophlebitis and phlebothrombosis are largely interchangeable designations for venous thrombosis and inflammation; involvement of deep leg veins accounts for more than 90% of cases. The periprostatic venous plexus in males and the pelvic venous plexus in females are additional sites, as are the large veins in the skull and the dural sinuses (especially in the setting of infection or inflammation). Portal vein thrombosis may occur with peritoneal infections (peritonitis, appendicitis, salpingitis, and pelvic abscesses), as well as certain thrombophilic conditions associated with platelet hyperactivity (e.g., polycythemia vera, Chapter 13).

Prolonged immobilization resulting in venous stasis is the most important risk factor for deep venous thrombosis (DVT) in the lower extremities. This can occur with extended bedrest or even sitting during lengthy trips in an airplane or automobile; postoperative patients are also at risk, in part, due to immobilization. Clearly, DVT can develop in the setting of any other mechanical factor that slows venous return; these include congestive heart failure, pregnancy, and obesity.

Systemic hypercoagulability, including genetic hypercoagulability syndromes (Chapter 4), *often also plays a role in potentiating thrombophlebitis.* In patients with cancer, particularly adenocarcinomas, hypercoagulability occurs as a paraneoplastic syndrome related to elaboration of procoagulant factors by tumor cells (Chapter 7). In this setting, venous thromboses classically appear in one location, disappear, and then occur in another site, so-called *migratory thrombophlebitis (Trousseau sign).*

Thrombi in the legs tend to produce few, if any, reliable signs or symptoms. Indeed, local manifestations, including vein dilation, edema, cyanosis, heat, erythema, or pain may be entirely absent, especially in bedridden patients. In some cases, pain can be elicited by pressure over affected veins, squeezing the calf muscles, or forced dorsiflexion of the foot (*Homan sign*). However, these findings are notoriously unreliable; hence their absence does not exclude a diagnosis of DVT.

Pulmonary embolism is the most common serious clinical complication of DVT, and is often the first manifestation of thrombophlebitis (Chapter 4). It results from fragmentation or detachment of the venous thrombus. Depending on the size and number of emboli, the outcome can range from no symptoms to death.

Superior and Inferior Vena Cava Syndromes

The *superior vena cava syndrome* is usually caused by neoplasms that compress or invade the superior vena cava, such as bronchogenic carcinoma or mediastinal lymphoma. Less commonly, other space occupying lesions in the mediastinum such as aortic aneurysms can be the cause of compression. The resulting obstruction produces a characteristic clinical complex including marked dilation of the veins of the head, neck, and arms with cyanosis. Pulmonary vessels can also be compressed, inducing respiratory distress.

The *inferior vena cava syndrome* can be caused by neoplasms that compress or invade the inferior vena cava (IVC) or by thrombosis of the hepatic, renal, or lower extremity veins that propagates cephalad. Certain neoplasms—particularly hepatocellular carcinoma and renal cell carcinoma—show a striking tendency to grow within veins, and these can ultimately occlude the IVC. IVC obstruction induces marked lower extremity edema, distention of the superficial collateral veins of the lower abdomen, and—with renal vein involvement—massive proteinuria.

Lymphangitis and Lymphedema

Although primary disorders of lymphatic vessels are extremely uncommon, secondary processes frequently develop in association with inflammation or malignancies.

Lymphangitis represents acute inflammation elicited by the spread of bacterial infections into lymphatics; group A β-hemolytic streptococci are the most common agent, although any microbe can be causal. Affected lymphatics are dilated and filled with an exudate of neutrophils and monocytes; the infiltrates can extend through the vessel wall, and in severe cases, can produce cellulitis or focal abscesses. Lymphangitis is manifested by red, painful subcutaneous streaks (the inflamed lymphatics), and painful enlargement of the draining lymph nodes *(lymphadenitis)*. If bacteria are not successfully contained within the lymph nodes, subsequent escape into the venous circulation can result in bacteremia or sepsis.

Primary lymphedema can occur as an isolated congenital defect (simple congenital lymphedema) or as the familial *Milroy disease (heredofamilial congenital lymphedema)*, which results in lymphatic agenesis or hypoplasia. *Secondary* or *obstructive lymphedema* stems from blockage of a previously normal lymphatic; examples include:

- Malignant tumors obstructing lymphatic channels or the regional lymph nodes
- Surgical procedures that remove regional groups of lymph nodes (e.g., axillary lymph nodes in radical mastectomy)
- Postirradiation fibrosis
- Filariasis
- Postinflammatory thrombosis and scarring

Regardless of the cause, lymphedema increases the hydrostatic pressure in the lymphatics distal to the obstruction and causes increased interstitial fluid accumulation. Persistent edema and subsequent deposition of interstitial connective tissue leads to a *peau d'orange* (orange peel) appearance of the overlying skin, seen typically in skin overlying breast cancers after the draining lymphatics are clogged with tumor cells; ulcers may develop due to inadequate tissue perfusion. Rupture of dilated lymphatics (e.g., secondary to obstruction from a tumor) leads to milky accumulations of lymph designated as *chylous ascites* (abdomen), *chylothorax*, and *chylopericardium*.

Vascular Tumors

Tumors of blood vessels and lymphatics constitute a spectrum from benign hemangiomas to intermediate lesions that are locally aggressive but infrequently metastasize, to rare, highly malignant angiosarcomas (Table 11-4). Congenital or developmental malformations and nonneoplastic reactive vascular proliferations (e.g., *bacillary angiomatosis*) can also present as tumor-like lesions. Because the growth of vascular neoplasms appears to depend on the same signaling pathways that regulate angiogenesis, treatment with inhibitors of blood vessel formation (antiangiogenic therapy) is a rational therapy that is being explored.

Vascular neoplasms can be endothelial-derived (e.g., hemangioma, lymphangioma, angiosarcoma) or can arise from cells that support or surround blood vessels (e.g., glomus tumor, hemangiopericytoma). Primary tumors of large vessels (aorta, pulmonary artery, and vena cava) are mostly connective tissue sarcomas. Although a benign well-differentiated hemangioma can usually be readily discriminated from an anaplastic high-grade angiosarcoma, the distinction between benign and malignant can

Table 11-4 Classification of Vascular Tumors and Tumor-Like Conditions

Benign Neoplasms, Developmental and Acquired Conditions
Hemangioma
Capillary hemangioma
Cavernous hemangioma
Pyogenic granuloma
Lymphangioma
Simple (capillary) lymphangioma
Cavernous lymphangioma (cystic hygroma)
Glomus tumor
Vascular ectasias
Nevus flammeus
Spider telangiectasia (arterial spider)
Hereditary hemorrhagic telangiectasis (Osler-Weber-Rendu disease)
Reactive vascular proliferations
Bacillary angiomatosis
Intermediate-Grade Neoplasms
Kaposi sarcoma
Hemangioendothelioma
Malignant Neoplasm
Angiosarcoma
Hemangiopericytoma

occasionally be difficult. Two general rules of thumb are helpful:

- Benign tumors usually produce obvious vascular channels filled with blood cells (e.g. capillaries filled with red cells) lined by a monolayer of normal-appearing endothelial cells.
- Malignant tumors are more cellular and more proliferative, and exhibit cytologic atypia; they usually do not form well-organized vessels. The endothelial derivation of neoplastic proliferations that do not form distinct vascular lumina can usually be confirmed by immunohistochemical demonstration of endothelial cell-specific markers such as CD31 or von Willebrand factor.

Benign Tumors and Tumor-Like Conditions

Vascular Ectasias. *Ectasia* is a generic term for any local dilation of a structure, while *telangiectasia* is used to describe a permanent dilation of preexisting small vessels (capillaries, venules, and arterioles) that form a discrete red lesion—usually in the skin or mucous membranes. These can be congenital or acquired and *are not true neoplasms;* some of them are malformations and others are hamartomas:

- *Nevus flammeus* (a "birthmark"), the most common form of vascular ectasia, is a light pink to deep purple flat lesion on the head or neck composed of dilated vessels. Most ultimately regress spontaneously.
- The so-called *port wine stain* is a special form of nevus flammeus. These lesions tend to grow during childhood, thicken the skin surface, and do not fade with time. Such lesions in the distribution of the trigeminal nerve are associated with the *Sturge-Weber syndrome* (also called *encephalotrigeminal angiomatosis*). This uncommon congenital disorder is associated with facial port wine nevi, ipsilateral venous angiomas in the cortical leptomeninges, mental retardation, seizures, hemiplegia, and skull radio-opacities. Thus, a large facial telangiectasia in a child with mental deficiency may indicate the presence of additional vascular malformations.
- *Spider telangiectasias* are nonneoplastic vascular lesions grossly resembling a spider. These manifest as radial, often pulsatile arrays of dilated subcutaneous arteries or arterioles (resembling spider legs) about a central core (resembling a spider's body) that blanch with pressure. These commonly occur on the face, neck, or upper chest and are most frequently associated with hyperestrogenic states, such as pregnancy or liver cirrhosis.
- *Hereditary hemorrhagic telangiectasia (Osler-Weber-Rendu disease)* is an autosomal dominant disorder caused by mutations in genes that encode components of the TGF-β signaling pathway. The telangiectasias are malformations composed of dilated capillaries and veins that are present at birth. They are widely distributed over the skin and oral mucous membranes, as well as in the respiratory, gastrointestinal, and urinary tracts. The lesions can spontaneously rupture, causing serious epistaxis (nosebleed), gastrointestinal bleeding, or hematuria.

Hemangioma. Hemangiomas are very common tumors characterized by increased numbers of normal or abnormal vessels filled with blood (Fig. 11-30). These lesions constitute 7% of all benign tumors of infancy and childhood; most are present from birth and initially increase in size, but many eventually regress spontaneously. While hemangiomas typically are localized lesions confined to the head and neck, they can occasionally be more extensive (*angiomatosis*) and can occur internally. Nearly one third of these internal lesions are found in the liver. Malignant transformation is rare. Several histologic and clinical variants have been described:

- *Capillary hemangiomas* are the most common type; these occur in the skin, subcutaneous tissues, and mucous membranes of the oral cavities and lips, as well as in the liver, spleen, and kidneys (Fig. 11-30*A*). Histologically, they are composed of thin-walled capillaries with scant stroma (Fig. 11-30*B*).
- *Juvenile hemangiomas* (so-called "strawberry type" hemangiomas) of the newborn are extremely common (1 in 200 births) and can be multiple. These arise in the skin and grow rapidly for a few months, but then fade by 1 to 3 years of age and completely regress by age 7 in the vast majority of cases.
- *Cavernous hemangiomas* are composed of large, dilated vascular channels. As compared to capillary hemangiomas, *cavernous hemangiomas* are more infiltrative, frequently involve deep structures, and do not spontaneously regress. On histologic examination, the mass is unencapsulated, has infiltrative borders, and is composed of *large, cavernous blood-filled vascular* spaces separated by connective tissue stroma (Fig. 11-30*C*). Intravascular thrombosis and associated dystrophic calcification are common. They can be locally destructive, and as a result some may require surgery. More often the tumors are of little clinical significance, but they can be cosmetically troublesome and are vulnerable to traumatic ulceration and bleeding. Moreover, cavernous hemangiomas detected by imaging studies may be difficult to distinguish from their malignant counterparts. Brain hemangiomas are also problematic, as they can cause symptoms related to compression of adjacent tissue or rupture. Cavernous hemangiomas are one component of *von Hippel-Lindau disease* (Chapter 28), in which vascular lesions are commonly found in the cerebellum, brain stem, retina, pancreas, and liver.
- *Pyogenic granulomas* are capillary hemangiomas that present as rapidly growing red pedunculated lesions on the skin, gingival, or oral mucosa. They bleed easily and are often ulcerated (Fig. 11-30*D*). Roughly a quarter of lesions develop after trauma, reaching a size of 1 to 2 cm within a few weeks. Curettage and cautery is usually curative. *Pregnancy tumor* (granuloma gravidarum) is a pyogenic granuloma that occurs infrequently (1% of patients) in the gingiva of pregnant women. These lesions may spontaneously regress (especially after pregnancy), or undergo fibrosis, but occasionally require surgical excision.

Lymphangiomas. Lymphangiomas are the benign lymphatic counterparts of hemangiomas.

- *Simple (capillary) lymphangiomas* are slightly elevated or sometimes pedunculated lesions up to 1 to 2 cm in diameter that occur predominantly in the head,

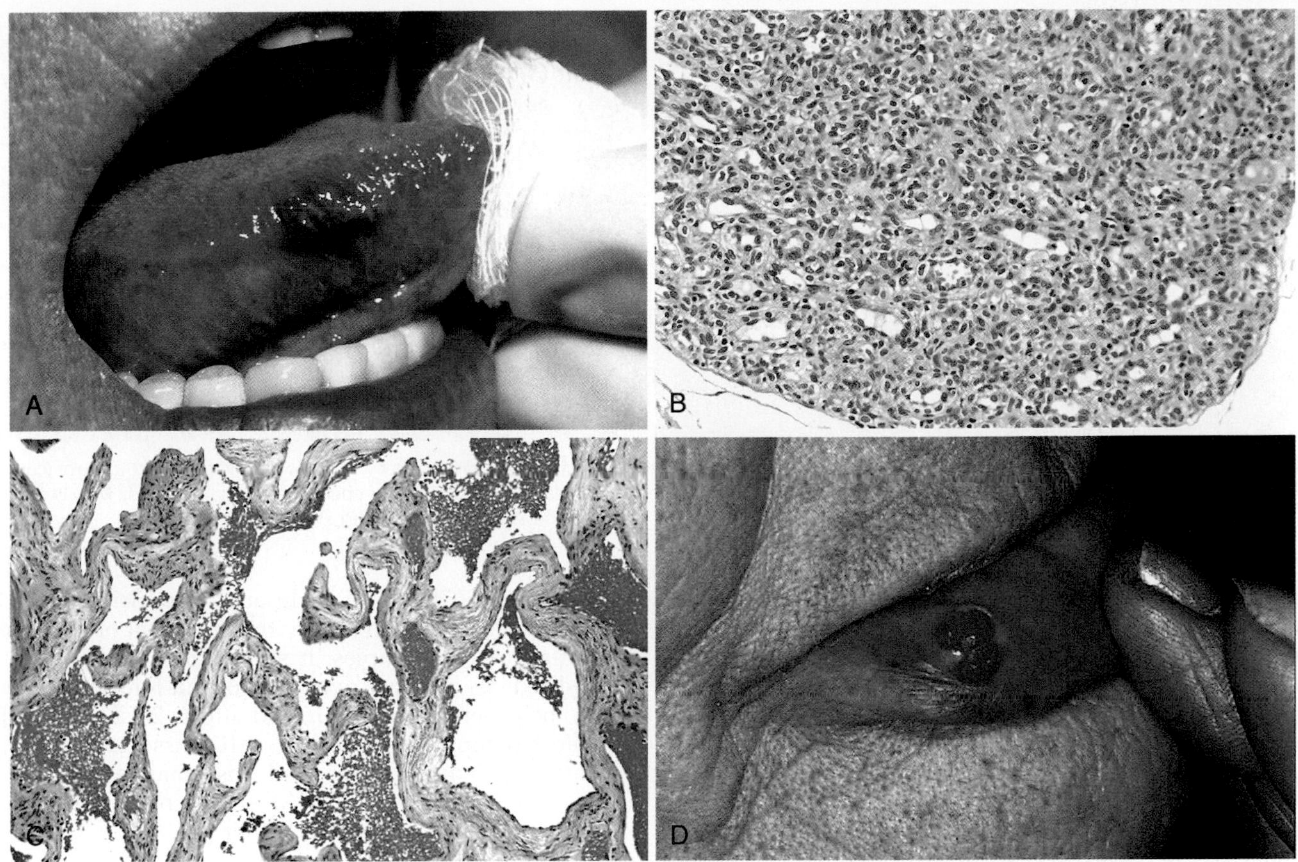

Figure 11-30 Hemangiomas. **A,** Hemangioma of the tongue. **B,** Histology of juvenile capillary hemangioma. **C,** Histology of cavernous hemangioma. **D,** Pyogenic granuloma of the lip. (**A** and **D,** Courtesy John Sexton, MD, Beth Israel Hospital, Boston, Mass.; **B,** courtesy Christopher DM Fletcher, MD, Brigham and Women's Hospital, Boston, Mass.; **C,** courtesy Thomas Rogers, MD, University of Texas Southwestern Medical School, Dallas, Texas.)

neck, and axillary subcutaneous tissues. Histologically, lymphangiomas exhibit networks of endothelium-lined spaces that can be *distinguished from capillary channels only by the absence of red cells.*

- *Cavernous lymphangiomas (cystic hygromas)* are typically found in the neck or axilla of children, and more rarely in the retroperitoneum. Cavernous lymphangiomas can occasionally be enormous (up to 15 cm in diameter) and may fill the axilla or produce gross deformities about the neck. Of note, cavernous lymphangiomas of the neck are common in Turner syndrome. These lesions are composed of massively dilated lymphatic spaces lined by endothelial cells and separated by intervening connective tissue stroma containing lymphoid aggregates. The tumor margins are indistinct and unencapsulated, making definitive resection difficult.

Glomus Tumor (Glomangioma). Glomus tumors are benign but exquisitely painful tumors *arising from modified smooth muscle cells of the glomus bodies,* arteriovenous structures involved in thermoregulation. Although they may superficially resemble hemangiomas, glomangiomas arise from smooth muscle cells rather than endothelial cells. They are most commonly found in the distal portion of the digits, especially under the fingernails. Excision is curative.

Bacillary Angiomatosis. *Bacillary angiomatosis* is a vascular proliferation in immunocompromised hosts (e.g., patients with AIDS) caused by opportunistic gram-negative bacilli of the *Bartonella* family. Lesions can involve the skin, bone, brain, and other organs. Two species are implicated:

- *Bartonella henselae,* whose principal reservoir is the domestic cat; this organism causes *cat-scratch disease* (a necrotizing granulomatous disorder of lymph nodes) in immunocompetent hosts.
- *Bartonella quintana,* which is transmitted by human body lice; this microbe was the cause of "trench fever" in World War I.

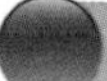

MORPHOLOGY

Skin lesions are red papules and nodules, or rounded subcutaneous masses; histologically, there is capillary proliferation with prominent epithelioid endothelial cells exhibiting nuclear atypia and mitoses (Fig. 11-31). Lesions contain stromal neutrophils, nuclear dust, and the causal bacteria.

Although difficult to cultivate in the laboratory, the *Bartonella* culprits can be unequivocally demonstrated using molecular methods such as polymerase chain reaction with species-specific primers. All the species are able to adhere to endothelial cells and are internalized in vacuoles. With *B. henselae* infection, the vascular proliferation results from induction of host hypoxia-inducible factor-1 (HIF-1) by the bacteria, which in turn drives

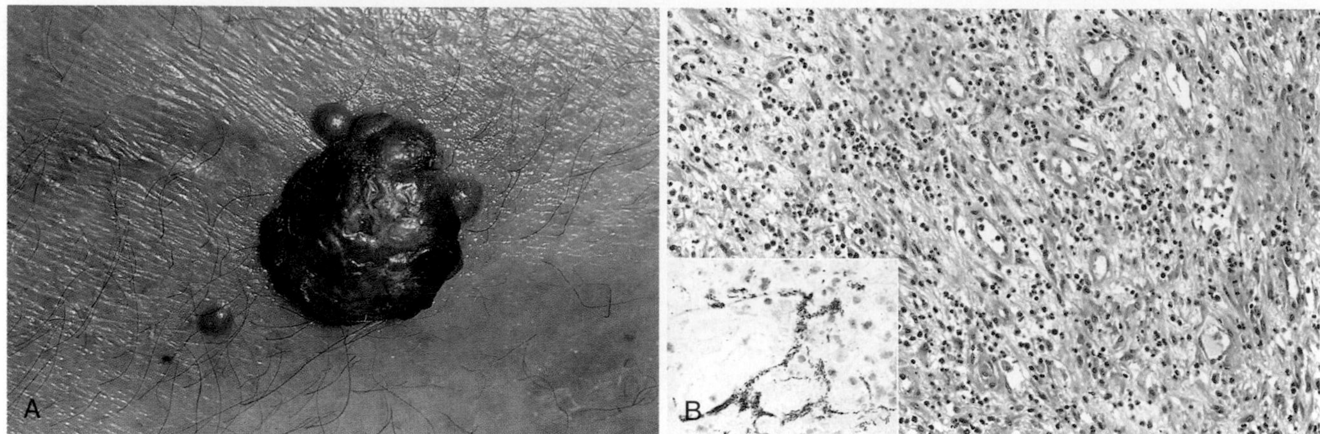

Figure 11-31 Bacillary angiomatosis. **A,** Characteristic cutaneous lesion. **B,** Histologic appearance with acute neutrophilic inflammation and vascular (capillary) proliferation. Inset, modified silver (Warthin-Starry) stain demonstrates clusters of tangled bacilli (black). (**A,** courtesy Richard Johnson, MD, Beth Israel Deaconess Medical Center, Boston; **B** and *inset,* courtesy Scott Granter, MD, Brigham and Women's Hospital, Boston, Mass.)

vascular endothelial growth factor (VEGF) production. The infections (and lesions) are cleared by macrolide antibiotics (including erythromycin).

Intermediate-Grade (Borderline) Tumors

Kaposi Sarcoma. **Kaposi sarcoma (KS) is vascular neoplasm caused by human herpesvirus 8 (HHV8) that is highly associated with acquired immunodeficiency syndrome (AIDS).** It also occurs much less commonly in other settings. Four forms of KS are recognized, based on population demographics and risks:

- *Classic KS* is a disorder of older men of Mediterranean, Middle Eastern, or Eastern European descent (especially Ashkenazic Jews); it is uncommon in the United States. It can be associated with malignancy or altered immunity, but is not associated with HIV infection. Classic KS manifests as multiple red-purple skin plaques or nodules, usually in the distal lower extremities; these progressively increase in size and number and spread proximally. Although persistent, the tumors are typically asymptomatic and remain localized to the skin and subcutaneous tissue.
- *Endemic African KS* typically occurs in HIV-seronegative individuals younger than age 40 and can follow an indolent or aggressive course; it involves lymph nodes much more frequently than the classic variant. In combination with AIDS-associated KS (see later), KS is now the most common tumor in central Africa. A particularly severe form, with prominent lymph node and visceral involvement, occurs in prepubertal children; the prognosis is poor, with an almost 100% mortality within 3 years.
- *Transplant-associated KS* occurs in solid organ transplant recipients in the setting of T-cell immunosuppression. The risk of KS is increased 100-fold in transplant recipients, pursuing an aggressive course that characteristically involves lymph nodes, mucosa, and viscera; cutaneous lesions may be absent. Lesions often regress with attenuation of immunosuppression, but at the risk of organ rejection.
- *AIDS-associated (epidemic) KS* is an AIDS-defining illness, and *worldwide, it represents the most common HIV-related malignancy* (Chapter 6). Although the incidence of KS has fallen more than 80% with the advent of aggressive antiretroviral therapies, it still occurs in HIV-infected individuals at a rate over a thousand-fold greater than in the general population, and affects 2-3% of the HIV-infected population in the US. AIDS-associated KS often involves lymph nodes and disseminates widely to viscera early in its course. Most patients eventually die of opportunistic infections rather KS.

Pathogenesis. Virtually all KS lesions are infected by *human herpesvirus 8 (HHV8),* also known as Kaposi sarcoma herpesvirus. Like Epstein-Barr virus, HHV8 is a γ-herpesvirus. It is transmitted sexually and by poorly understood nonsexual routes potentially including oral secretions and cutaneous exposures (of note, the prevalence of endemic African KS is inversely related to the wearing of shoes). HHV8 and altered T-cell immunity are likely required for KS development; in older adults, diminished T-cell immunity may be related to aging. Because the development and progression of KS are tightly linked to immune function, its molecular pathogenesis is discussed in detail in Chapter 6.

MORPHOLOGY

In **classic KS** (and sometimes in other variants), the cutaneous lesions progress through three stages:

- **Patches** are red-purple macules typically confined to the distal lower extremities (Fig. 11-32*A*). Histology shows only dilated irregular endothelial cell–lined vascular spaces with interspersed lymphocytes, plasma cells, and macrophages (sometimes containing hemosiderin). The lesions can be difficult to distinguish from granulation tissue.
- With time, lesions spread proximally and become larger, violaceous, **raised plaques** (Fig. 11-32*A*) composed of dermal accumulations of dilated, jagged vascular channels lined and surrounded by plump spindle cells. Scattered between the vascular channels are extravasated erythrocytes, hemosiderin-laden macrophages, and other mononuclear inflammatory cells.

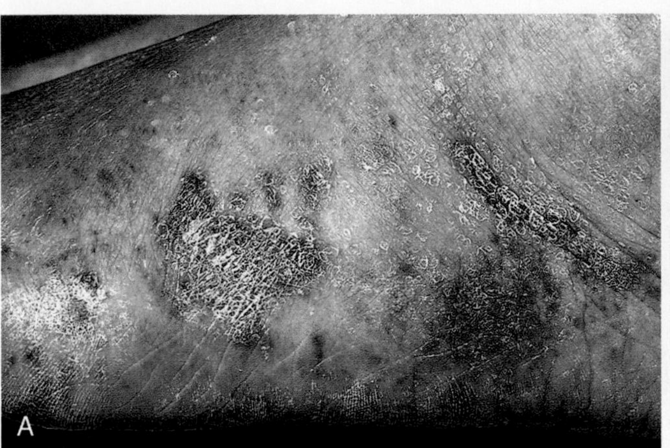

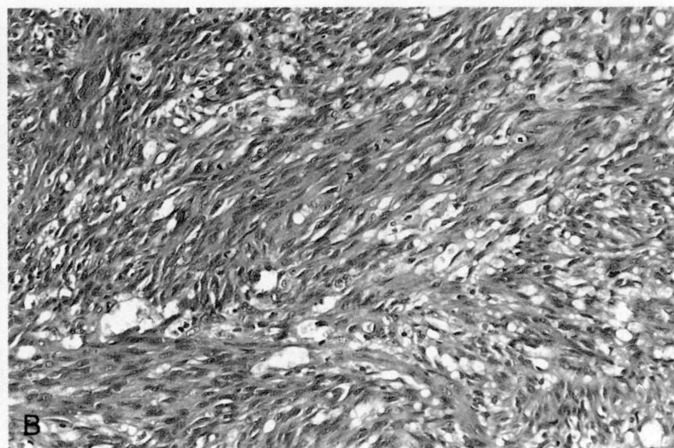

Figure 11-32 Kaposi sarcoma. **A,** Gross photograph, illustrating coalescent red-purple macules and plaques of the skin. **B,** Histologic appearance of the nodular stage of KS, demonstrating sheets of plump, proliferating spindle cells. (**B,** Courtesy Christopher DM Fletcher, MD, Brigham and Women's Hospital, Boston, Mass.)

- Eventually, lesions become **nodular** and more distinctly neoplastic. These lesions are composed of sheets of plump, proliferating spindle cells, mostly in the dermis or subcutaneous tissues (Fig. 11-32*B*), encompassing small vessels and slitlike spaces containing red cells. Marked hemorrhage, hemosiderin pigment, and mononuclear inflammation are present; mitotic figures are common, as are round, pink, cytoplasmic globules representing degenerating red cells within phagolysosomes. The nodular stage often heralds nodal and visceral involvement, particularly in the African and AIDS-associated variants.

Clinical Features. The course of KS varies widely and is significantly influenced by the clinical setting. Most primary KSHV infections are asymptomatic. Classic KS is—at least initially— largely restricted to the surface of the body, and surgical resection is usually adequate for an excellent prognosis. Radiation can be used for multiple lesions in a restricted area and chemotherapy yields satisfactory results for more disseminated disease, including nodal involvement. In immunosuppression-associated KS, withdrawal of immunosuppression (perhaps with adjunct chemotherapy or radiotherapy) is often effective. Antiretroviral therapy treatment has greatly decreased that frequency of KS in HIV infected patients, emphasizing the central role that T cell immunodeficiency has in the disease. Interferon-α and angiogenesis inhibitors are variably effective, while newer strategies aimed at specific kinases that lie downtream of VEGF receptors show promise.

Hemangioendothelioma. *Hemangioendotheliomas* encompass a spectrum of vascular neoplasms with clinical behaviors *intermediate between benign, well-differentiated hemangiomas and frankly anaplastic angiosarcomas,* described later.

Epithelioid hemangioendothelioma is an example; it is a vascular tumor of adults occurring around medium- and large-sized veins. Well-defined vascular channels are inconspicuous, and neoplastic cells are plump and often cuboidal (resembling epithelial cells). The clinical behavior is extremely variable; most are cured by excision, but up to 40% recur, 20% to 30% eventually metastasize, and perhaps 15% of patients die of their tumor.

Malignant Tumors

Angiosarcoma. *Angiosarcoma* is a malignant endothelial neoplasm that primarily affects older adults. There is equal gender predilection, and the tumor may occur at any site, but most often involves skin, soft tissue, breast, and liver.

Hepatic angiosarcoma is associated with carcinogenic exposures, including arsenic (e.g., in pesticides), Thorotrast (a radioactive contrast agent formerly used for radiologic imaging), and polyvinyl chloride (a widely used plastic). All of these agents have long latencies between initial exposure and eventual tumor development. The increased frequency of angiosarcoma among polyvinyl chloride workers is one of the well-documented instances of human chemical carcinogenesis.

Angiosarcoma can also arise in the setting of lymphedema, classically in the ipsilateral upper extremity several years after radical mastectomy (i.e., with lymph node resection) for breast cancer; the tumor presumably arises from lymphatic vessels *(lymphangiosarcoma).* Angiosarcoma has also been induced by radiation and are rarely associated with foreign material introduced into the body either iatrogenically or accidentally.

Angiosarcomas are locally invasive and can readily metastasize; 5-year survival rates approach 30%.

MORPHOLOGY

Cutaneous angiosarcoma can begin as multiple deceptively small and asymptomatic red papules or nodules; these eventually become large, fleshy masses of red-tan to gray-white tissue with margins blurring imperceptibly into surrounding structures (Fig. 11-33*A*). Central areas of necrosis and hemorrhage are frequent.

Microscopically, **all degrees of differentiation can be seen,** from plump, atypical endothelial cells forming vascular channels (Fig. 11-33*B*) to wildly undifferentiated tumors with a solid spindled appearance and no discernible blood vessels that may be difficult to distinguish from carcinomas and melanomas. The endothelial origin of these tumors can be demonstrated by immunohistochemical staining for CD31 or von Willebrand factor (Fig. 11-33*C*).

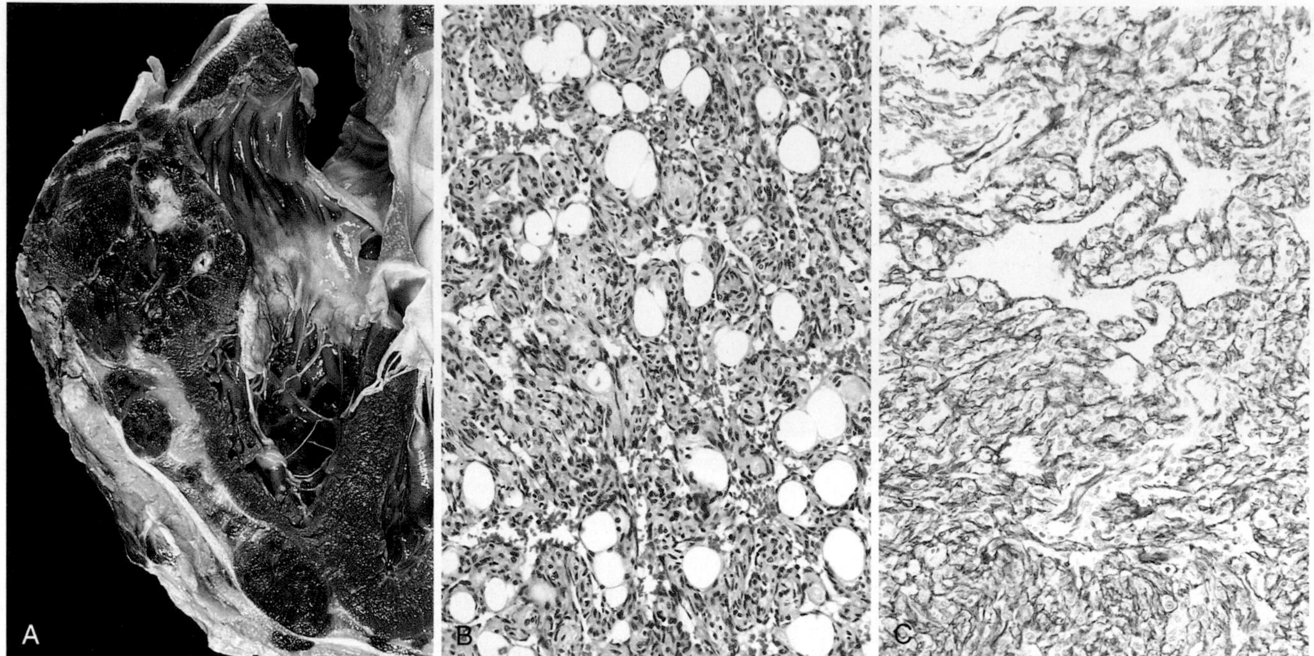

Figure 11-33 Angiosarcoma. **A,** Angiosarcoma involving the right ventricle. **B,** Moderately differentiated angiosarcoma with dense clumps of atypical cells lining distinct vascular lumens. **C,** Immunohistochemical staining for the endothelial cell marker CD31, demonstrating the endothelial nature of the tumor cells.

Hemangiopericytoma. Hemangiopericytomas have been considered tumors that arise from pericytes, the myofibroblast-like cells associated with capillaries and venules. Recent studies suggest that tumors of pericytes are very rare and the vast majority of those previously assigned to this group are derived from other cells such as fibroblasts and are classified as such. One example is the solitary fibrous tumor that arises on the pleura.

KEY CONCEPTS

Vascular Tumors

- Vascular ectasias are not neoplasms, but rather dilations of existing vessels.
- Vessel neoplasms can derive from either blood vessels or lymphatics, and can be composed of endothelial cells (hemangioma, lymphangioma, angiosarcoma) or other components of vascular wall cells
- Most vascular tumors are benign (e.g., hemangiomas), some have an intermediate, locally aggressive behavior (e.g., Kaposi sarcoma), and others are highly malignant (e.g., angiosarcoma).
- Benign tumors typically form obvious vascular channels lined by normal-appearing endothelial cells. Malignant tumors are more often solid and cellular, exhibit cytologic atypia, and lack well-defined vessels.

Pathology of Vascular Intervention

The morphologic changes that occur in vessels following therapeutic intervention (e.g., stenting or bypass surgery) largely recapitulate the changes that occur in the setting of any vascular insult. Local trauma or thrombosis (e.g., due to a stent), or abnormal mechanical forces (e.g., a saphenous vein inserted into the arterial circulation as a coronary artery bypass graft), all induce the same stereotypical healing responses. Analogous to the various insults that drive atherosclerosis, any therapeutic intervention that injures the endothelium also tends to induce intimal thickening by recruiting smooth muscle cells and promoting extracellular matrice deposition.

Endovascular Stenting

Arterial stenoses (especially those in coronary arteries) can be dilated by transiently inflating a balloon catheter to pressures sufficient to rupture the occluding plaque (*balloon angioplasty*); in doing so, a (hopefully) limited *arterial dissection* is also induced. Although most patients improve symptomatically following angioplasty alone, *abrupt reclosure* can occur as a result of compression of the lumen by an extensive circumferential or longitudinal dissection, by vessel wall spasm, or by thrombosis. Thus, more than 90% of endovascular coronary procedures now involve both angioplasty and concurrent *coronary stent* placement.

Coronary stents are expandable tubes of metallic mesh. They provide a larger and more regular lumen, "tack down" the intimal flaps and dissections that occur during angioplasty, and mechanically limit vascular spasm. Nevertheless, due to endothelial injury, *thrombosis* is an important immediate post-stenting complication, and patients must receive potent antithrombotic agents (primarily platelet antagonists) to prevent acute catastrophic thrombotic occlusions. The *long-term* success of angioplasty is limited by the development of *proliferative in-stent restenosis*. This intimal thickening is due to smooth muscle cell ingrowth, proliferation, and matrix synthesis, all driven by the initial vascular wall injury; it causes clinically

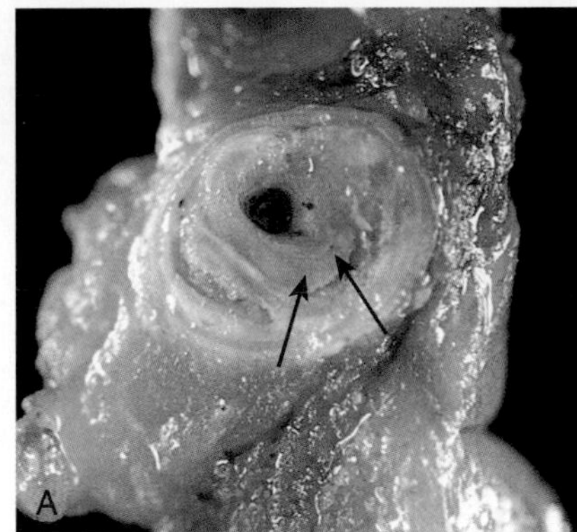

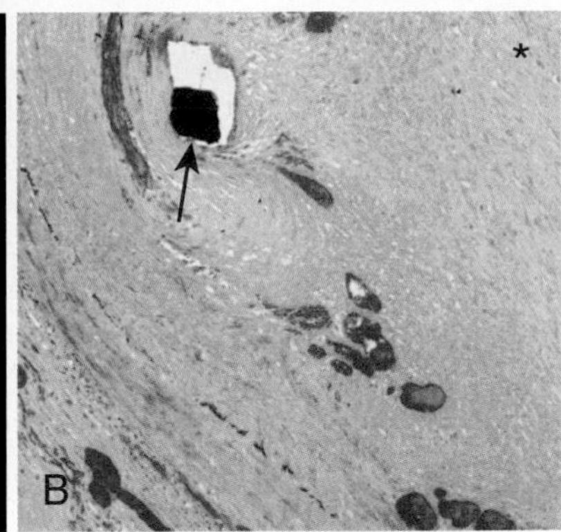

Figure 11-34 Restenosis after angioplasty and stenting. **A,** Gross view demonstrating residual yellow atherosclerotic plaque *(arrows)* and a new, tan-white concentric intimal lesion inside of that plaque. **B,** Histologic view shows a thickened neointima separating and overlying the stent wires (the black diamond indicated by the *arrow*), which encroaches on the lumen (indicated by the *asterisk*); Movat stain with matrix staining gray-green. (***B,*** Reproduced from Schoen FJ, Edwards WD. Pathology of cardiovascular interventions, including endovascular therapies, revascularization, vascular replacement, cardiac assist/replacement, arrhythmia control, and repaired congenital heart disease. In Silver MD, Gotlieb AI, Schoen FJ (eds): Cardiovascular Pathology, 3rd ed. Philadelphia, Churchill Livingstone, 2001.)

significant luminal occlusion in up to a third of patients within 6 to 12 months of stenting (Fig. 11-34).

The newest generation of *drug-eluting stents* is designed to avoid this complication by leaching antiproliferative drugs (e.g., paclitaxel or sirolimus) into the adjacent vessel wall to block smooth muscle cell activation. Although the duration of drug elution is short (days to weeks), these drug-eluting stents nevertheless reduce the incidence of restenosis at 1 year by 50% to 80%. However, because of the antiproliferative effect of the drug-eluting stents, the time to reendothelialization is prolonged and patients require extended courses of anticoagulation to prevent stent thrombosis.

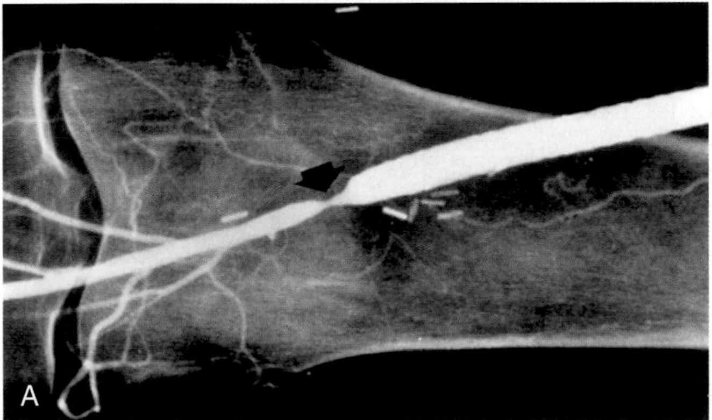

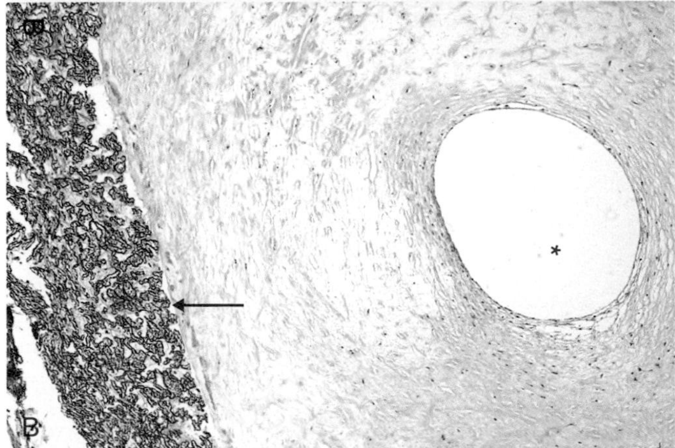

Figure 11-35 Intimal hyperplasia at the distal anastomosis of a synthetic femoral-popliteal graft. **A,** Angiogram demonstrating constriction *(arrow)*. **B,** Photomicrograph demonstrating Gore-Tex graft *(arrow)* with prominent intimal proliferation and very small residual lumen *(asterisk)*. (**A,** Courtesy Anthony D. Whittemore, MD, Brigham and Women's Hospital, Boston, Mass.)

Vascular Replacement

Synthetic or autologous vascular grafts are increasingly used to replace damaged vessels or bypass diseased arteries. Large-bore (12- to 18-mm) synthetic conduits function well in high-flow locations such as the aorta; unfortunately, small-diameter artificial grafts (≤8 mm in diameter) generally fail as a result of early thrombosis or late intimal hyperplasia, the latter at the junction of the graft with the native vasculature (Fig. 11-35).

Consequently, when small-bore vessel replacement is required (e.g., in coronary bypass surgeries), the grafts are fashioned from saphenous veins (taken from the patient's own leg) or left internal mammary arteries. The long-term patency of saphenous vein grafts is only 50% at 10 years; grafts occlude due to thrombosis (typically early), intimal thickening (months to years postoperatively), and vein graft atherosclerosis—sometimes with superimposed plaque rupture, thrombi, or aneurysms (usually more than 2 to 3 years). By contrast, 90% or more of internal mammary artery grafts are patent at 10 years. With the advent of stenting (and better control of risk factors such as hyperlipidemia), the frequency of coronary arterial bypass surgery has decreased in recent years.

SUGGESTED READINGS

Vascular Structure and Function

Monahan-Earley R, Dvorak AM, Aird WC: Evolutionary origins of the blood vascular system and endothelium. *J Thromb Haemost* 11(Suppl 1):46, 2013. *[Interesting discussion of the evolutionary basis for vascular development, including cogent explanations for endothelial heterogeneity.]*

Semenza G: Vasculogenesis, angiogenesis, and arteriogenesis: mechanisms of blood vessel formation and remodeling. *J Cell Biochem* 102:840, 2007. *[Good overview of physiologic and developmental blood vessel formation and remodeling.]*

Vascular Wall Response to Injury

Gimbrone MA Jr, Garcia-Cardeña G: Vascular endothelium, hemodynamics, and the pathobiology of atherosclerosis. *Cardiovasc Pathol* 22:9, 2013. *[Well-written review on endothelial responses to mechanical forces from one of the leading groups in the field.]*

Pober JS, Min W, Bradley JR: Mechanisms of endothelial dysfunction, injury, and death. *Annu Rev Pathol Mech Dis* 4:71, 2009. *[Well-written and scholarly review of the etiology and outcomes of endothelial injury.]*

Hypertensive Vascular Disease

Coffman TM: Under pressure: the search for the essential mechanisms of hypertension. *Nature Med* 17:1402, 2011. *[Current and well-written review of the current state of the field including recent translational advances.]*

Lifton RP, et al: Molecular mechanisms of human hypertension. *Cell* 104:545, 2001. *[A well-written overview of the genetics and molecular pathways that underlie hypertension; although older, it still provides a good framework for understanding the multiple intersecting mechanisms of essential hypertension]*

Singh M, Mensah GA, Bakris G: Pathogenesis and clinical physiology of hypertension. *Cardiol Clin* 28:545, 2010. *[Excellent and up-to-date overview of normal blood pressure regulation and the interaction of genetics and environment in the pathophysiology of hypertension.]*

Atherosclerosis

Finn AV, et al: Concept of vulnerable/unstable plaque. *Arterioscler Thromb Vasc Biol* 30:1282, 2010. *[Good overview of the evolving concepts regarding plaque stability.]*

Grebe A, Latz E: Cholesterol crystals and inflammation. *Curr Rheumatol Rep* 15:313, 2013. *[A review of the activation of the inflammasome by cholesterol crystals, and its role in atherosclerosis.]*

Libby P, et al: Inflammation in atherosclerosis: from pathophysiology to practice. *J Am Coll Cardiol* 54:2129, 2009. *[Excellent overview of the role of inflammation in atherosclerotic disease.]*

Ridker P: C-reactive protein and the prediction of cardiovascular events among those at intermediate risk: moving an inflammatory hypothesis towards consensus. *J Am Coll Cardiol* 49:2129, 2007. *[A solid opinion piece pulling regarding the utility of inflammatory markers in providing additional independent information for predicting for cardiovascular events.]*

Rocha VZ, Libby P: Obesity, inflammation, and atherosclerosis. *Nat Rev Cardiol* 6:399, 2009. *[Good review of the interaction of risk factors, including the potential role of the metabolic syndrome in atherosclerotic disease.]*

Ross R: Atherosclerosis-an inflammatory disease. *N Engl J Med* 340:115, 1999. *[The key paper that eloquently laid out the response-to-injury hypothesis for atherosclerosis.]*

Witztum JL, Lichtman AH: The influence of innate and adaptive immune responses on atherosclerosis. *Annu Rev Pathol Mech Dis* 9:73, 2014. *[A recent update on the involvement of different components of the inflammatory response in atherosclerosis.]*

Aneurysms and Dissection

Gillis E, Van Laer L, Loeys BL: Genetics of Thoracic Aortic Aneurysm: At the Crossroad of Transforming Growth Factor-β Signaling and Vascular Smooth Muscle Cell Contractility. *Circ Res* 113:327, 2013. *[Up-to-date discussion of the molecular and cellular basis for thoracic aneurysms and dissections.]*

Michel JB, et al: Novel aspects of the pathogenesis of aneurysms of the abdominal aorta in humans. *Cardiovasc Res* 90:18, 2011. *[Good discussion of the molecular pathways underlying human abdominal aortic aneurysm formation.]*

Vasculitis

Jennette J, et al: Pathogenesis of antineutrophil cytoplasmic autoantibody-associated small vessel vasculitis. *Annu Rev Pathol Mech Dis* 8:139, 2013. *[Excellent recent review of discussing how ANCAs activate neutrophils and other inflammatory cells.]*

Kallenberg CG: Pathophysiology of ANCA-associated small vessel vasculitis. *Curr Rheumatol Rep* 12:399, 2010. *[Recent overview of the pathogenesis of the ANCA-associated vasculitides.]*

Veins and Lymphatics

Goldhaber SZ: Venous thromboembolism: epidemiology and magnitude of the problem. *Best Pract Res Clin Haematol* 25:235, 2012. *[Thorough clinically-oriented overview of deep venous thrombosis and pulmonary embolism, including epidemiology, mechanism of disease, and therapy.]*

Vascular Tumors

Ganem D: KSHV infection and pathogenesis of Kaposi's sarcoma. *Annu Rev Pathol* 1:273, 2006. *[Excellent, scholarly review of the pathologic mechanisms underlying Kaposi sarcoma.]*

Penel N, et al: Angiosarcoma: State of the art and perspectives. *Crit Rev Oncol Hematol* 2010. *[Extensive clinical summary of this aggressively malignant vascular tumor.]*

Pathology of Vascular Intervention

Inoue T, et al: Vascular inflammation and repair: implications for re-endothelialization, restenosis, and stent thrombosis. *JACC Cardiovasc Interv* 4:1057, 2011. *[Excellent overview of the inflammatory pathways that influence the outcomes of percutaneous vessel interventions.]*

Kim FY, et al: Saphenous vein graft disease: review of pathophysiology, prevention, and treatment. *Cardiol Rev* 21:101, 2013. *[Good overview of the pathogenesis and clinical issues relating to venous bypass grafting, germane to all graft stenosis.]*

See TARGETED THERAPY available online at www.studentconsult.com

CHAPTER 12

The Heart

Frederick J. Schoen • Richard N. Mitchell

CHAPTER CONTENTS

The human heart is a remarkably efficient, durable, and reliable pump, distributing more than 6000 liters of blood through the body each day, and beating 30 to 40 million times a year—providing tissues with vital nutrients and facilitating waste excretion. Consequently, cardiac dysfunction can have devastating physiologic consequences. Cardiovascular disease (including coronary artery disease, stroke, and peripheral vascular disease) is the number one cause of worldwide mortality, with about 80% of the burden occurring in developing countries. In the United States alone, cardiovascular disease accounts for roughly a third of all deaths, totaling about 800,000 individuals—or nearly 1.5 times the number of deaths caused by all forms of cancer combined.

Disruption of *any* element of the heart—myocardium, valves, conduction system, and coronary vasculature—can adversely affect pumping efficiency, thus leading to morbidity and mortality. The major categories of cardiac disease described in this chapter include congenital heart abnormalities, ischemic heart disease, hypertensive heart disease, diseases of the cardiac valves, and primary myocardial disorders. A few comments about pericardial diseases and cardiac neoplasms, as well as cardiac transplantation, are also presented. This chapter begins with a brief review of the normal heart since most cardiac diseases manifest as structural and/or functional changes in one or more cardiac components. General principles underlying cardiac hypertrophy and failure—common end points of several of the different forms of heart disease—are also discussed.

Cardiac Structure and Specializations

Heart weight varies with body habitus, averaging approximately 0.4% to 0.5% of body weight (250 to 320 gm in females and 300 to 360 gm in males); the right ventricle wall thickness is usually 0.3 to 0.5 cm, while the left ventricle wall is 1.3 to 1.5 cm thick. Increases in heart weight or ventricular thickness above these normal limits indicates *hypertrophy*, and an enlarged chamber size implies *dilation*; both can represent compensatory changes in response to heart disease and to volume and/or pressure overloads (see later). Increased cardiac weight or size (or both)—resulting from hypertrophy and/or dilation—is called *cardiomegaly*.

Myocardium

The pumping function of the heart is accomplished via the coordinated contraction (during *systole*) and relaxation (during *diastole*) of the cardiac myocytes that comprise the *myocardium*. Left ventricular myocytes are arranged circumferentially in a spiral orientation that helps to generate a coordinated wave of contraction that spreads from the apex to the base of the heart. In contrast, right ventricular myocytes have a somewhat less structured organization. The contractile apparatus within myocytes is organized into a series of subunits called *sarcomeres*, composed of highly ordered networks of thick filaments (primarily *myosin* in the center of the sarcomere) interlaced with thin filaments (largely *actin*, attached to the end of the sarcomere) and regulatory proteins such as troponin and tropomyosin. The actin and myosin filaments partially overlap with each other, giving rise to the striated appearance of cardiac myocytes (overlapping areas of actin and myosin are dark while the intervening areas are light).

Contraction results as myosin filaments ratchet adjacent actin filaments toward the center—shortening individual sarcomeres, and collectively leading to myocyte shortening. The amount of force generated is determined by the distance each sarcomere contracts. Thus, moderate ventricular dilation during diastole creates a greater distance over which the sarcomere can subsequently shorten and augment the force of systolic contraction. This compensatory mechanism serves to accommodate differing volume and pressure demands. Unfortunately, there is an upper limit to the benefit of increased stretching during diastole. With excessive dilation, the overlap of the actin and myosin filaments is reduced and the force of contraction decreases sharply, leading to heart failure.

Atrial myocytes are relatively haphazardly arranged, and thus generate weaker contractile forces than the ventricles. Some atrial cells have distinctive cytoplasmic electron-dense storage granules that contain *atrial natriuretic peptide*; this is a peptide hormone that promotes arterial vasodilation and stimulates renal salt and water elimination (*natriuresis* and *diuresis*), actions that are beneficial in the setting of hypertension and congestive heart failure.

The coordinated beating of cardiac myocytes depends on *intercalated discs*—specialized intercellular junctions that facilitate cell-to-cell mechanical and electrical (ionic) coupling. Within the intercalated discs (and at the lateral borders of adjacent myocytes), *gap junctions* facilitate synchronized waves of myocyte contraction by permitting rapid movement of ions (e.g., sodium, potassium, calcium) between adjoining cells. Abnormalities in the spatial distribution of gap junctions in a variety of heart diseases can cause electromechanical dysfunction (*arrhythmia*) and/or heart failure.

Valves

The four cardiac valves—tricuspid, pulmonary, mitral, and aortic—maintain unidirectional blood flow. Valve function depends on the mobility, pliability, and structural integrity of the *leaflets* of the *atrioventricular* valves (tricuspid and mitral) or *cusps* of the *semilunar valves* (aortic and pulmonary). Cardiac valves are lined by endothelium and share a similar, tri-layered architecture:

- A dense collagenous core (*fibrosa*) at the outflow surface and connected to the valvular supporting structures
- A central core of loose connective tissue (*spongiosa*)
- A layer rich in elastin (*ventricularis* or *atrialis* depending on which chamber it faces) on the inflow surface

The collagen of the ventricularis is largely responsible for the mechanical integrity of a valve, while the elastic tissue of the atrialis/ventricularis imparts a rapid recoil to achieve prompt valve closure. The proteoglycan-rich spongiosa facilitates the interactions of the collagenous (relatively stiff) and elastic layers during the cardiac cycle. Crucial to function are the valvular interstitial cells, the most abundant cell type in the heart valves, and distributed throughout all of its layers. Valvular interstitial cells synthesize extracellular matrix (ECM) and express matrix degrading enzymes (including matrix metalloproteinases [MMPs], along with inhibitors that remodel collagen and other matrix components. Valvular interstitial cells comprise a diverse and dynamic population of resident cells that can alter their phenotypes and functions in response to changing hemodynamic stresses.

The function of the semilunar valves depends on the integrity and coordinated movements of the cuspal attachments. Thus, dilation of the aortic root can hinder coaptation of the aortic valve cusps during closure and result in valvular regurgitation. In contrast, the competence of the atrioventricular valves depends on the proper function not only the leaflets but also the tendinous cords and the attached papillary muscles of the ventricular wall. Left ventricular dilation, a ruptured tendinous cord, or papillary muscle dysfunction can all interfere with valve closure, causing valvular insufficiency.

Because they are thin enough to be nourished by diffusion from the blood, normal leaflets and cusps have only scant blood vessels limited to the proximal portion. **Pathologic changes of valves are largely of three types: damage to collagen that weakens the leaflets, exemplified by mitral valve prolapse; nodular calcification beginning in interstitial cells, as in calcific aortic stenosis; and fibrotic thickening, the key feature in rheumatic heart disease** (see later).

Conduction System

Coordinated contraction of the cardiac muscle depends on propagation of electrical impulses—accomplished through specialized excitatory and conducting myocytes within the cardiac conduction system that regulate heart rate and rhythm. The frequency of electrical impulses that course through the conduction system is sensitive to neural inputs (e.g., vagal stimulation), extrinsic adrenergic agents (e.g., adrenaline), hypoxia, and potassium concentration (i.e., hyperkalemia can block signal transmission altogether). Inputs from the autonomic nervous system can increase the heart rate to twice normal within seconds, and are important for physiologic responses to exercise or other states associated with increased oxygen demand.

The components of the conduction system include:

- *Sinoatrial (SA) node* pacemaker (at the junction of the right atrial appendage and superior vena cava)
- *Atrioventricular (AV) node* (located in the right atrium along the atrial septum)
- *Bundle of His*, connecting the right atrium to the ventricular septum
- Subsequent divisions into the right and left bundle branches that stimulate their respective ventricles via further arborization into the *Purkinje network*

The cells of the cardiac conduction system depolarize spontaneously, enabling them to function as cardiac pacemakers. Because the normal rate of spontaneous depolarization in the SA node (60 to 100 beats/minute) is faster than the other components, it normally sets the pace. The AV node has a gatekeeper function; by delaying the transmission of signals from the atria to the ventricles, it ensures that atrial contraction precedes ventricular systole.

Blood Supply

Cardiac myocytes rely almost exclusively on oxidative phosphorylation for their energy needs. Besides a high density of mitochondria (20% to 30% of myocyte volume), myocardial energy generation also requires a constant supply of oxygenated blood—rendering myocardium extremely vulnerable to ischemia. Nutrients and oxygen are delivered via the *coronary arteries*, with takeoffs immediately distal to the aortic valve. These initially course along the external surface of the heart *(epicardial coronary arteries)* and then penetrate the myocardium *(intramural arteries)*, subsequently branching into arterioles, and eventually forming a rich arborizing vascular network so that each myocyte contacts roughly three capillaries.

There are three major epicardial coronary arteries (so-called because they form a crown or *corona* at the base of the heart):

- Left anterior descending (LAD) and left circumflex (LCX) arteries arise from the left (main) coronary artery
- Right coronary artery

The divisions of the LAD are called *diagonal* branches, and those of the LCX are *marginal branches.* The right and left coronary arteries function as end arteries, although anatomically most hearts have numerous intercoronary anastomoses (connections called collateral circulation). Blood flow to the myocardium occurs during ventricular diastole, following closure of the aortic valve, and when the microcirculation is not compressed by cardiac contraction. At rest, diastole comprises approximately two thirds of the cardiac cycle; with tachycardia (increased heart rate), the relative duration of diastole also shortens, thus potentially compromising cardiac perfusion.

Cardiac Stem Cells

Although cardiac regeneration in metazoans (e.g., newts and zebrafish) is well described, the myocardium of higher order animals is classically depicted as a permanent cell population without replicative potential. However, increasing evidence points to the presence of bone marrow–derived precursors—as well as a small population of stem cells within the myocardium—that are capable of repopulating the mammalian heart. Besides self-renewal, these cardiac stem cells generate all cell lineages seen within the myocardium. They constitute up to 5% to 10% of normal atrial cellularity, but represent only roughly 1 in 100,000 cells in a normal ventricle.

Cardiac stem cells have a very slow rate of proliferation, which is greatest in neonates, and decreases with age. The human adult heart replaces roughly 1% of its total population each year, so that by the age of 50 years, almost 45% of the total cardiomyocytes have been renewed. While stem cell numbers and progeny increase after myocardial injury or hypertrophy, albeit to a limited extent, hearts that suffer myocardial cell loss (e.g., due to infarction) do not recover any significant function in the necrotic zone (one of several features that distinguish humans from fish and newts). Nevertheless, the potential for stimulating proliferation and differentiation of these cells in vivo is tantalizing since it could facilitate recovery of myocardial function following irreversible myocardial damage. Similarly, ex vivo expansion and subsequent administration of stem cells is another strategy being explored in the unfulfilled quest to heal a broken heart. Until then a trip to the local jewelry store will have to suffice!

Effects of Aging on the Heart

The prevalence of most forms of heart disease increases with each advancing decade. Consequently, as the average population in developed countries ages, changes in the cardiovascular system that accrue with aging become increasingly significant (Table 12-1).

Epicardial fat increases, while the detritus of years of intracellular catabolism and oxidant stress accumulate in the form of intracellular lipofuscin. *Basophilic degeneration*, a gray-blue byproduct of glycogen metabolism within cardiac myocytes, is also increased. The size of the left ventricular cavity, particularly in the base-to-apex dimension, is reduced; this volume change is exacerbated by systemic hypertension and bulging of the basal ventricular septum into the left ventricular outflow tract (termed *sigmoid septum*).

Valvular aging changes include calcification of the mitral annulus and aortic valve, the latter frequently leading to aortic stenosis. In addition, the valves can develop fibrous thickening, and the mitral leaflets tend to buckle back toward the left atrium during ventricular systole, simulating a prolapsing (myxomatous) mitral valve. As this happens, increasing volume and pressure overloads lead to left atrial dilation, and with it, an increased incidence of atrial arrhythmias (e.g., fibrillation). With time, small filiform processes *(Lambl excrescences)* form on the closure lines of aortic and mitral valves, probably resulting from the organization of small thrombi.

The aorta becomes progressively stiffer, owing to the fragmentation and loss of elastic tissue and increased collagen deposition, along with the accumulation of atherosclerotic plaque. The result is less elasticity, and increased

Table 12-1 Changes in the Aging Heart

Chambers
Increased left atrial cavity size Decreased left ventricular cavity size Sigmoid-shaped ventricular septum
Valves
Aortic valve calcific deposits Mitral valve annular calcific deposits Fibrous thickening of leaflets Buckling of mitral leaflets toward the left atrium Lambl excrescences
Epicardial Coronary Arteries
Tortuosity Diminished compliance Calcific deposits Atherosclerotic plaque
Myocardium
Decreased mass Increased subepicardial fat Brown atrophy Lipofuscin deposition Basophilic degeneration Amyloid deposits
Aorta
Dilated ascending aorta with rightward shift Elongated (tortuous) thoracic aorta Sinotubular junction calcific deposits Elastic fragmentation and collagen accumulation Atherosclerotic plaque

pressure spikes with each cardiac contraction that are transmitted to distal organs.

Compared with younger myocardium, "elderly" myocardium has fewer myocytes, increased collagenized connective tissue and, often the deposition of extracellular amyloid (most commonly due to poorly catabolized transthyretin; see Chapter 6).

Most importantly, the progressive atherosclerosis (Chapter 11)—over a period of 50 to 60 years—finally ends up causing significant stenosis, or weakens the wall sufficiently to give rise to catastrophic dissection of the aortic wall (see later).

Overview of Cardiac Pathophysiology

Cardiovascular dysfunction can be attributed to one (or more) of six principal mechanisms:

- *Pump failure.* In some conditions, the myocardium contracts weakly during systole and there is inadequate cardiac output. Conversely, myocardium may relax insufficiently during diastole to permit adequate ventricular filling.
- *Flow obstruction.* Lesions can obstruct blood flow through a vessel (e.g., atherosclerotic plaque) or prevent valve opening or otherwise cause increased ventricular chamber pressure (e.g., aortic valvular stenosis, systemic hypertension, or aortic coarctation). In the case of a valvular blockage, the increased pressure overloads the chamber that pumps against the obstruction.
- *Regurgitant flow.* A portion of the output from each contraction flows backward through an incompetent valve, adding a volume overload to the affected atria or ventricles (e.g., left ventricle in aortic regurgitation; left atrium and left ventricle in mitral regurgitation).
- *Shunted flow.* Blood can be diverted from one part of the heart to another (e.g., from the left ventricle to the right ventricle), through defects that can be congenital or acquired (e.g., following myocardial infarction). Shunted flow can also occur between blood vessels, as in patent ductus arteriosus (PDA).
- *Disorders of cardiac conduction.* Conduction defects or arrhythmias due to uncoordinated generation or transmission of impulses (e.g., atrial or ventricular fibrillation) lead to nonuniform and inefficient myocardial contractions, and may in fact be lethal.
- *Rupture of the heart or a major vessel.* In such circumstances (e.g., gunshot to the left ventricle, or aortic dissection and rupture), there is cataclysmic exsanguination, either into body cavities or externally.

Most cardiovascular disease results from a complex interplay of genetics and environmental factors; these may disrupt signaling pathways that control morphogenesis, impact myocyte survival after injury, or affect contractility or electrical conduction in the face of biomechanical stressors. Indeed, the pathogenesis of many congenital heart defects involves an underlying genetic abnormality whose expression is modified by environmental or maternal factors (see later). Moreover, genes that control the development of the heart may also regulate the response to various forms of injury including aging. Subtle polymorphisms can significantly impact the risk of many forms of heart disease, and, as discussed later, a number of adult-onset heart disorders have a fundamentally genetic basis. Thus, cardiovascular genetics provides an important window on the pathogenesis of heart disease and increasingly molecular diagnoses are becoming a critical part of its classification.

Heart Failure

Heart failure, often called *congestive heart failure (CHF),* is a common, usually progressive condition with a poor prognosis. Each year in the United States, CHF affects more than 5 million individuals (approximately 2% of the population), necessitating more than a million hospitalizations, and contributing to the death of nearly 300,000 people.

CHF occurs when the heart is unable to pump blood at a rate sufficient to meet the metabolic demands of the tissues or can do so only at an elevated filling pressure. It is the common end stage of many forms of chronic heart disease, often developing insidiously from the cumulative effects of chronic work overload (e.g., in valve disease or hypertension) or ischemic heart disease (e.g., following myocardial infarction with heart damage). However, acute hemodynamic stresses, such as fluid overload, abrupt valvular dysfunction, or myocardial infarction, can all precipitate sudden CHF.

When cardiac workload increases or cardiac function is compromised, several physiologic mechanisms maintain arterial pressure and organ perfusion:

- *Frank-Starling mechanism,* in which increased filling volumes dilate the heart and thereby increase subsequent actin-myosin cross-bridge formation, enhancing contractility and stroke volume
- *Myocardial adaptations, including hypertrophy with or without cardiac chamber dilation.* In many pathologic states, heart failure is preceded by cardiac hypertrophy, the compensatory response of the myocardium to increased mechanical work. The collective molecular, cellular, and structural changes that occur as a response to injury or changes in loading conditions are called *ventricular remodeling.*
- *Activation of neurohumoral* systems to augment heart function and/or regulate filling volumes and pressures
  - Release of norepinephrine by adrenergic cardiac nerves of the autonomic nervous system (which increases heart rate and augments myocardial contractility and vascular resistance)
  - Activation of the renin-angiotensin-aldosterone system
  - Release of atrial natriuretic peptide. The latter two factors act to adjust filling volumes and pressures.

These adaptive mechanisms may be adequate to maintain normal cardiac output in the face of acute perturbations, but their capacity to do so may ultimately be overwhelmed. Moreover, superimposed pathologic changes, such as myocyte apoptosis, intracellular cytoskeletal alterations, and extracellular matrix deposition, may cause further structural and functional disturbances. Heart failure can result from progressive deterioration of myocardial contractile function *(systolic dysfunction)*—reflected as a decrease in ejection fraction (EF, the percentage of blood volume ejected from the ventricle during systole; normal is approximately 45% to 65%). Reduction in EF can occur with ischemic injury, inadequate adaptation to pressure or volume overload due to hypertension or valvular disease, or ventricular dilation. Increasingly, heart failure is recognized as resulting from an inability of the heart chamber to expand and fill sufficiently during diastole *(diastolic dysfunction),* for example, due to left ventricular hypertrophy, myocardial fibrosis, constrictive pericarditis, or amyloid deposition.

Cardiac Hypertrophy: Pathophysiology and Progression to Heart Failure

Sustained increase in mechanical work due to pressure or volume overload (e.g., systemic hypertension or aortic stenosis) or trophic signals (e.g., those mediated through the activation of β-adrenergic receptors) cause myocytes to increase in size *(hypertrophy)*; cumulatively, this increases the size and weight of the heart (Fig. 12-1). Hypertrophy requires increased protein synthesis, thus enabling the assembly of additional sarcomeres, as well as increasing the numbers of mitochondria. Hypertrophic myocytes also have enlarged nuclei, attributable to increased DNA ploidy resulting from DNA replication in the absence of cell division. The pattern of hypertrophy reflects the nature of the stimulus. In *pressure-overload hypertrophy* (e.g., due to hypertension or aortic stenosis), new sarcomeres are predominantly assembled in parallel to the long axes of cells, expanding the cross-sectional area of myocytes in ventricles and causing a concentric increase in wall thickness. In contrast, *volume-overload hypertrophy* is characterized by new sarcomeres being assembled in series within existing sarcomeres, leading primarily to ventricular dilation. As a result, in dilation due to volume overload, or dilation that accompanies failure of a previously pressure overloaded heart, the wall thickness may be increased, normal, or less than normal. Consequently, heart weight, rather than wall thickness, is the best measure of hypertrophy in dilated hearts.

Cardiac hypertrophy can be substantial in clinical heart disease. Heart weights of two to three times normal are common in patients with systemic hypertension, ischemic heart disease, aortic stenosis, mitral regurgitation, or dilated cardiomyopathy, and heart weights can be three- to four-fold greater than normal in those with aortic regurgitation or hypertrophic cardiomyopathy.

Important changes at the tissue and cell level occur with cardiac hypertrophy. Importantly, myocyte hypertrophy is not accompanied by a proportional increase in capillary numbers. As a result, the supply of oxygen and nutrients to the hypertrophied heart, particularly one undergoing pressure overload hypertrophy, is more tenuous than in the normal heart. At the same time, oxygen consumption by the hypertrophied heart is elevated due to the increased workload that drives the process. Hypertrophy is also often accompanied by deposition of fibrous tissue (interstitial fibrosis). Molecular changes include the expression of immediate-early genes (e.g., *FOS, JUN, MYC,* and *EGR1*) (Chapter 2). With prolonged hemodynamic overload, there may be a shift to a gene expression pattern resembling that seen during fetal cardiac development (including selective expression of embryonic/fetal forms of β-myosin heavy chain, natriuretic peptides, and collagen).

At a functional level, cardiac hypertrophy is associated with heightened metabolic demands due to increases in mass, heart rate, and contractility (inotropic state, or force of contraction), all of which increase cardiac oxygen consumption. *As a result of these changes, the hypertrophied heart is vulnerable to ischemia-related decompensation,* which can evolve to cardiac failure and eventually lead to death.

The proposed sequence of initially beneficial—and later harmful—events in response to increased cardiac work is summarized in Figure 12-2. *The molecular and cellular changes in hypertrophied hearts that initially mediate enhanced function may themselves contribute to the development of heart failure.* This can occur through:

- Abnormal myocardial metabolism
- Alterations of intracellular handling of calcium ions
- Myocyte apoptosis
- Reprogramming of gene expression, which may occur in part through changes in expression of miRNAs, small noncoding RNAs that inhibit gene expression (Chapter 1).

The degree of structural abnormality of the heart in CHF does not always reflect the severity of dysfunction, and the structural, biochemical, and molecular basis for myocardial contractile failure can be obscure.

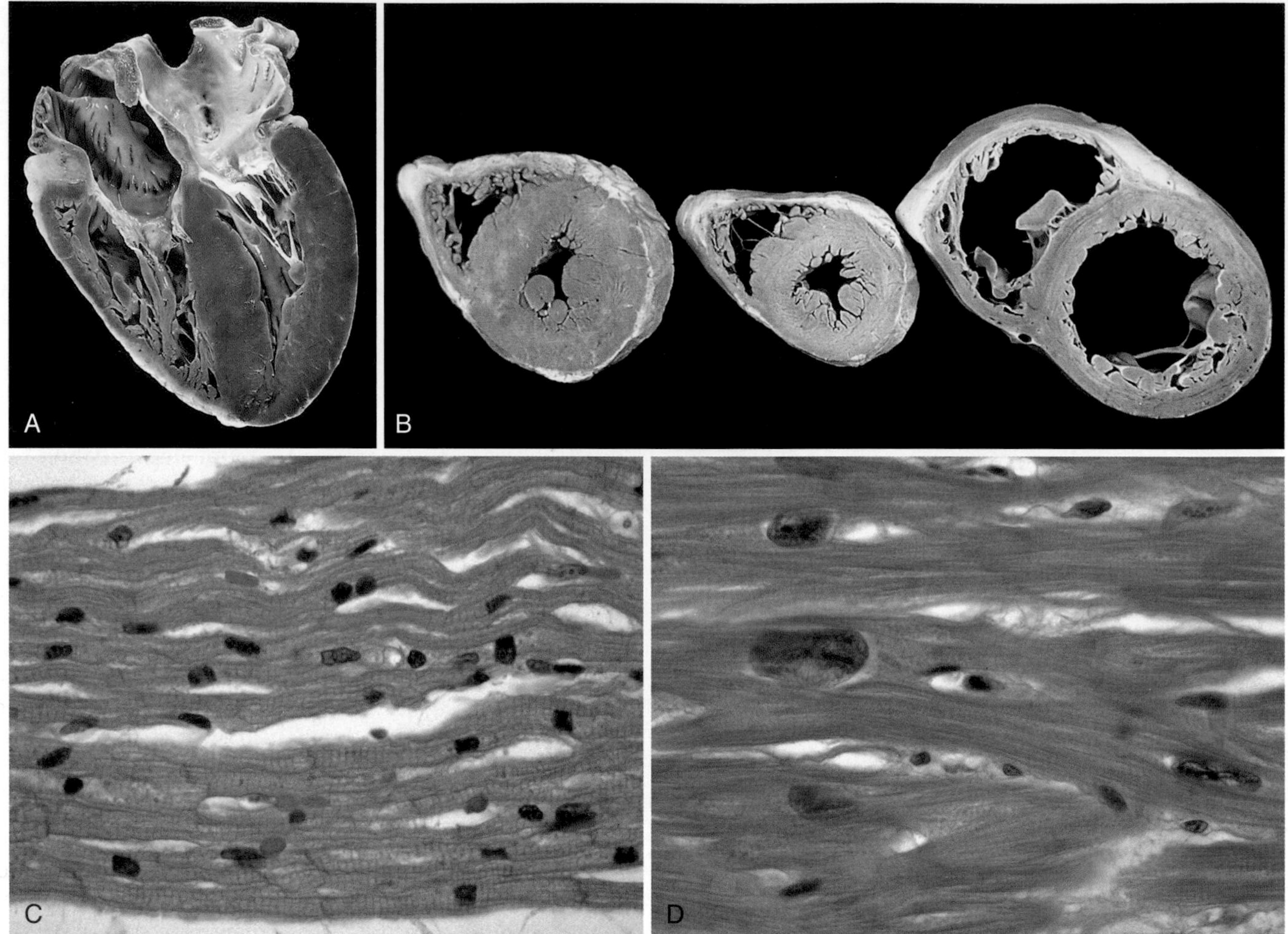

Figure 12-1 Left ventricular hypertrophy. **A,** Pressure hypertrophy due to left ventricular outflow obstruction. The left ventricle is on the lower right in this apical four-chamber view of the heart. **B,** Left ventricular hypertrophy with and without dilation, viewed in transverse heart sections. Compared with a normal heart *(center)*, the pressure-hypertrophied hearts (*left* and in **A**) have increased mass and a thick left ventricular wall, while the hypertrophied, dilated heart *(right)* has increased mass and a normal wall thickness. **C,** Normal myocardium. **D,** Hypertrophied myocardium (panels **C** and **D** are photomicrographs at the same magnification). Note the increases in both cell size and nuclear size in the hypertrophied myocytes. (**A,B,** Reproduced with permission from Edwards WD: Cardiac anatomy and examination of cardiac specimens. In Emmanouilides GC, et al [eds]: Moss and Adams Heart Disease in Infants, Children, and Adolescents: Including the Fetus and Young Adults, 5th ed. Philadelphia, Williams & Wilkins, 1995, p 86.)

At autopsy, the hearts of patients with CHF are generally heavy and dilated, and may be relatively thin-walled; they exhibit microscopic evidence of hypertrophy, but the extent of these changes is extremely variable. In hearts that have suffered myocardial infarction, loss of pumping capacity due to myocyte death leads to work-related hypertrophy of the surrounding viable myocardium. In valvular heart disease, the increased pressure or volume overloads the myocardium globally. Increased heart mass owing to disease is correlated with excess cardiac mortality and morbidity; indeed, cardiomegaly is an independent risk factor for sudden death.

In contrast to pathologic hypertrophy (which is often associated with contractile impairment), hypertrophy induced by regular strenuous exercise has varied effects on the heart depending on the type of exercise. Aerobic exercise (e.g., long distance running) tends to be associated with volume-load hypertrophy that may be accompanied by increases in capillary density (unlike other forms of hypertrophy) and decreases in resting heart rate and blood pressure—effects that are all beneficial. These changes are sometimes referred to as *physiologic hypertrophy*. Static exercise (e.g., weight lifting) is associated with pressure hypertrophy and appears more likely to be associated with deleterious changes.

Whatever its basis, CHF is characterized by variable degrees of decreased cardiac output and tissue perfusion (sometimes called forward failure), as well as pooling of blood in the venous capacitance system (backward failure); the latter may cause pulmonary edema, peripheral edema, or both. As a result, many of the significant clinical features and morphologic changes noted in CHF are actually secondary to injuries induced by hypoxia and congestion in tissues away from the heart.

The cardiovascular system is a closed circuit. Thus, although left-sided and right-sided failure can occur independently, failure of one side (particularly the left) often produces excessive strain on the other, terminating in global heart failure. Despite this interdependence, it is easiest to understand the pathology of heart failure by considering right- and left-sided heart failure separately.

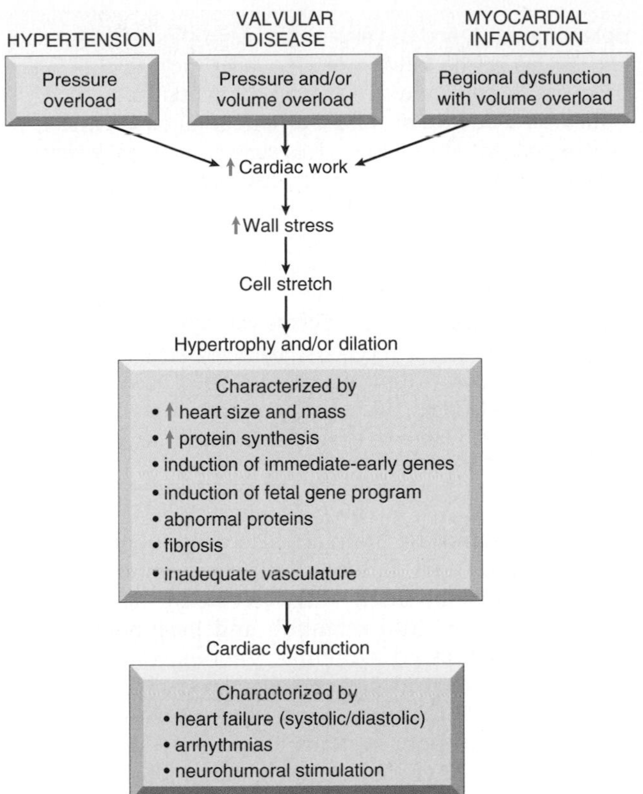

Figure 12-2 Schematic representation of the causes and consequences of cardiac hypertrophy.

Left-Sided Heart Failure

Left-sided heart failure is most often caused by:

- Ischemic heart disease
- Hypertension
- Aortic and mitral valvular diseases
- Primary myocardial diseases

The clinical and morphologic effects of left-sided CHF are a consequence of passive congestion (blood backing up in the pulmonary circulation), stasis of blood in the left-sided chambers, and inadequate perfusion of downstream tissues leading to organ dysfunction.

MORPHOLOGY

Heart. The heart findings depend on the disease process, ranging from myocardial infarcts, to stenotic or regurgitant valves, to intrinsic myocardial pathology. Except for failure caused by mitral valve stenosis or unusual restrictive cardiomyopathies (described later), the left ventricle is usually hypertrophied and often dilated, sometimes massively. The microscopic changes are nonspecific: primarily myocyte hypertrophy and variable degrees of interstitial fibrosis. Impaired left ventricular function usually causes secondary dilation of the left atrium, which increases the risk of atrial fibrillation. This in turn results in stasis of blood, particularly in the atrial appendage, which is a common site of thrombus formation.

Lungs. Pulmonary congestion and **edema** produce heavy, wet lungs, as described elsewhere (Chapters 4 and 15). Pulmonary changes—from mildest to most severe—include (1) perivascular and interstitial edema, particularly in the interlobular septa, responsible for the characteristic Kerley B and C lines noted on chest X-ray study in CHF, (2) progressive edematous widening of alveolar septa, and (3) accumulation of edema fluid in the alveolar spaces. Some red cells and plasma proteins extravasate into the edema fluid within the alveolar spaces, where they are phagocytosed and digested by macrophages, which store the iron recovered from hemoglobin in the form of hemosiderin. These *hemosiderin-laden macrophages* (also known as **heart failure cells**) are telltale signs of previous episodes of pulmonary edema. Pleural effusions arise from elevated pleural capillary pressure and the resultant transudation of fluid into the pleural cavities.

Early left-sided heart failure symptoms are related to pulmonary congestion and edema and may be subtle. Initially, cough and *dyspnea* (breathlessness) may occur only with exertion. As CHF progresses, worsening pulmonary edema may cause *orthopnea* (dyspnea when supine, relieved by sitting or standing) or *paroxysmal nocturnal dyspnea* (dyspnea usually occurring at night that is so severe that it induces a feeling of suffocation). Dyspnea at rest may follow. *Atrial fibrillation*, an uncoordinated, chaotic contraction of the atrium, exacerbates CHF owing to the loss of the atrial "kick" and its 10% to 15% contribution to ventricular filling.

A reduced ejection fraction leads to diminished renal perfusion, causing activation of the renin-angiotensin-aldosterone system as a compensatory mechanism to correct the "perceived" hypotension. This leads to salt and water retention, with expansion of the interstitial and intravascular fluid volumes (Chapters 4 and 11) that then exacerbate the ongoing pulmonary edema. If the hypoperfusion of the kidney becomes sufficiently severe, impaired excretion of nitrogenous products may cause azotemia (called *prerenal azotemia* because of its vascular origin; Chapter 20). In far-advanced CHF, cerebral hypoperfusion can give rise to *hypoxic encephalopathy* (Chapter 28), with irritability, loss of attention span, and restlessness that can progress to stupor and coma with ischemic cerebral injury.

Left-sided heart failure can be divided into systolic and diastolic failure:

- *Systolic failure* is defined by insufficient ejection fraction (pump failure), and can be caused by any of the many disorders that damage or derange the contractile function of the left ventricle.
- In *diastolic failure*, the left ventricle is abnormally stiff and cannot relax during diastole. Thus, although cardiac function is relatively preserved at rest, the heart is unable to increase its output in response to increases in the metabolic demands of peripheral tissues (e.g., during exercise). Moreover, because the left ventricle cannot expand normally, any increase in filling pressure is immediately transferred back into the pulmonary circulation, producing rapid onset pulmonary edema (*flash pulmonary edema*). Diastolic failure predominantly occurs in patients older than age 65 years and for unclear reasons is more common in women. Hypertension is the most common underlying etiology; diabetes mellitus, obesity, and bilateral renal artery stenosis may also

contribute to risk. Reduced left ventricular relaxation may stem from myocardial fibrosis (e.g., in cardiomyopathies and ischemic heart disease), and infiltrative disorders associated with restrictive cardiomyopathies (e.g., cardiac amyloidosis). Diastolic failure may appear in older patients without any known predisposing factors, possibly as an exaggeration of the normal stiffening of the heart with age. Constrictive pericarditis (discussed later) can also limit myocardial relaxation and therefore mimics primary diastolic dysfunction.

Right-Sided Heart Failure

Right-sided heart failure is most commonly caused by left-sided heart failure, as any increase in pressure in the pulmonary circulation from left-sided failure inevitably burdens the right side of the heart. Consequently, the causes of right-sided heart failure include all of those that induce left-sided heart failure. Isolated right-sided heart failure is infrequent and typically occurs in patients with one of a variety of disorders affecting the lungs; hence it is often referred to as *cor pulmonale.* Besides parenchymal lung diseases, cor pulmonale can also arise secondary to disorders that affect the pulmonary vasculature, for example, primary pulmonary hypertension (Chapter 15), recurrent pulmonary thromboembolism (Chapter 4), or conditions that cause pulmonary vasoconstriction (obstructive sleep apnea, altitude sickness). *The common feature of these disorders is pulmonary hypertension* (discussed later), which results in hypertrophy and dilation of the right side of the heart. In extreme cases, leftward bulging of the interventricular septum can even cause left ventricular dysfunction. The major morphologic and clinical effects of primary right-sided heart failure differ from those of left-sided heart failure in that pulmonary congestion is minimal while engorgement of the systemic and portal venous systems is pronounced.

MORPHOLOGY

Heart. As in left-heart failure, the cardiac morphology varies with cause. Rarely, structural defects such as tricuspid or pulmonary valvular abnormalities or endocardial fibrosis (as in carcinoid heart disease) may be present. However, since isolated right heart failure is most often caused by lung disease, most cases exhibit only hypertrophy and dilation of the right atrium and ventricle.

Liver and Portal System. Congestion of the hepatic and portal vessels may produce pathologic changes in the liver, the spleen, and the GI tract. The liver is usually increased in size and weight **(congestive hepatomegaly)** due to prominent **passive congestion**, greatest around the central veins (Chapter 4). Grossly, this is reflected as congested red-brown pericentral zones, with relatively normal-colored tan periportal regions, producing the characteristic "nutmeg liver" appearance (Chapter 4). In some instances, especially when left-sided heart failure with hypoperfusion is also present, severe centrilobular hypoxia produces **centrilobular necrosis**. With longstanding severe right-sided heart failure, the central areas can become fibrotic, eventually culminating in **cardiac cirrhosis** (Chapter 18). Portal venous hypertension also causes enlargement of the spleen with platelet sequestration **(congestive splenomegaly)**, and can also contribute to chronic congestion and edema of the bowel wall. The latter may be sufficiently severe as to interfere with nutrient (and/or drug) absorption.

Pleural, Pericardial, and Peritoneal Spaces. Systemic venous congestion can lead to fluid accumulation in the pleural, pericardial, or peritoneal spaces (**effusions**; peritoneal effusions are also called **ascites**). Large pleural effusions can impact lung inflation, causing atelectasis, and substantial ascites can also limit diaphragmatic excursion, causing dyspnea on a purely mechanical basis.

Subcutaneous Tissues. Edema of the peripheral and dependent portions of the body, especially ankle (pedal) and pretibial edema, is a hallmark of right-sided heart failure. In chronically bedridden patients presacral edema may predominate. Generalized massive edema (**anasarca**) may also occur.

The kidney and the brain are also prominently affected in right-sided heart failure. Renal congestion is more marked with right-sided than left-sided heart failure, leading to greater fluid retention and peripheral edema, and more pronounced azotemia. Venous congestion and hypoxia of the central nervous system can also produce deficits of mental function akin to those seen in left-sided heart failure with poor systemic perfusion.

Although we have discussed right and left heart failure separately, it is again worth emphasizing that in many cases of chronic cardiac decompensation, patients present in biventricular CHF with symptoms reflecting both right-sided and left-sided heart failure.

Standard therapy for CHF is mainly pharmacologic. Drugs that relieve fluid overload (e.g., diuretics), that block the renin-angiotensin-aldosterone axis (e.g., angiotensin converting enzyme inhibitors), and that lower adrenergic tone (e.g., beta-1 adrenergic blockers) are all particularly beneficial. The efficacy of the latter two classes of drugs supports the concept that neurohumoral changes in CHF (e.g., renin and norepinephrine elevations) are maladaptive contributions to heart failure.

Newer approaches to improving cardiac function include mechanical assist devices, and resynchronization of electrical impulses to maximize cardiac efficiency. Interestingly, some patients treated by mechanical assist can recover sufficient function to be weaned from the device. There is also considerable enthusiasm for novel therapies, including cell-based approaches, although several hurdles remain in their implementation.

KEY CONCEPTS

Heart Failure

- CHF occurs when the heart is unable to provide adequate perfusion to meet the metabolic requirements of peripheral tissues; inadequate cardiac output is usually accompanied by increased congestion of the venous circulation.
- Left-sided heart failure is most commonly due to ischemic heart disease, systemic hypertension, mitral or aortic valve disease, and primary diseases of the myocardium; symptoms are mainly a consequence of pulmonary congestion and edema, although systemic hypoperfusion can cause secondary renal and cerebral dysfunction.

- Right heart failure is most often due to left heart failure, and less commonly to primary pulmonary disorders; symptoms are chiefly related to peripheral edema and visceral congestion.

Congenital Heart Disease

Congenital heart disease (CHD) is a general term designating abnormalities of the heart or great vessels that are present at birth. Most congenital heart disease arises from faulty embryogenesis during gestational weeks 3 through 8, when major cardiovascular structures form and begin to function. The most severe anomalies are incompatible with intrauterine survival and significant heart malformations are common among premature infant and stillborns. On the other hand, defects that affect individual chambers or discrete regions of the heart are often compatible with embryologic maturation and eventual live birth. In this category are septation defects, unilateral obstructions, and outflow tract anomalies. Septal defects, or "holes in the heart", include atrial septal defects (ASDs) or ventricular septal defects (VSDs). Stenotic lesion can be at the level of the cardiac valve or entire cardiac chamber, as in hypoplastic left heart syndrome. Outflow tract anomalies include inappropriate routing of the great vessels from the ventricular mass. These forms of congenital heart disease usually produce clinically important manifestations only after birth—unveiled by the transition from fetal to perinatal circulation.

Incidence. With an incidence of up to 5%, congenital cardiovascular malformations are among the most prevalent birth defects and are the most common type of pediatric heart disease. Approximately 1% of individuals have significant forms of congenital heart disease that are diagnosed in the first year of life. However, milder forms of congenital heart disease such as bicuspid semilunar valves, with an incidence itself of 1-2%, may not become evident until adulthood. Twelve disorders account for about 85% of cases; their frequencies are listed in Table 12-2.

Table 12-2 Frequencies of Congenital Cardiac Malformations*

Malformation	Incidence per Million Live Births	%
Ventricular septal defect	4482	42
Atrial septal defect	1043	10
Pulmonary stenosis	836	8
Patent ductus arteriosus	781	7
Tetralogy of Fallot	577	5
Coarctation of the aorta	492	5
Atrioventricular septal defect	396	4
Aortic stenosis	388	4
Transposition of the great arteries	388	4
Truncus arteriosus	136	1
Total anomalous pulmonary venous connection	120	1
Tricuspid atresia	118	1
Total	9757	

*Presented as upper quartile of 44 published studies. Percentages do not add up to 100% because of rounding.

Source: Hoffman JIE, Kaplan S: The incidence of congenital heart disease. J Am Coll Cardiol 39:1890, 2002.

The number of individuals who survive into adulthood with congenital heart disease is increasing rapidly and is estimated at nearly 1 million individuals in the United States. Many have benefited from advances in early postnatal (and even intrauterine) surgical repair of their structural defects. In some cases, however, surgical repairs fail to restore complete normalcy; patients may have already sustained pulmonary or myocardial changes that are no longer reversible, or may suffer from arrhythmias due to surgical scarring. Other factors that impact the long-term outcome include risks associated with the use of prosthetic materials and devices (e.g., substitute valves or myocardial patches), and the cardiovascular stressors associated with childbearing that may tip a repaired heart into failure.

Cardiac Development. The diverse malformations seen in congenital heart disease are caused by errors that occur during cardiac morphogenesis (Fig. 12-3). The earliest cardiac precursors originate in lateral mesoderm and move to the midline in two migratory waves to create a crescent of cells consisting of the first and second heart fields by about day 15 of development. Both fields contain multipotent progenitor cells that can produce all of the major cell types of the heart: endocardium, myocardium, and smooth muscle cells. However, each heart field is differentially marked by the expression of distinct gene sets. Thus, the first heart field expresses the transcription factor Hand1, whereas the second heart field expresses the transcription factor Hand2 and the secreted protein fibroblast growth factor-10.

Even at this very early stage of development, each heart field is destined to give rise to particular portions of the heart. Thus, the left ventricle largely derives from cells originating in the first heart field, whereas cells from the second heart field become the outflow tract, right ventricle, and most of the atria. By day 20, the initial cell crescent develops into a beating tube, which loops to the right and begins to form the basic heart chambers roughly 8 days later. At the same time, two other critical events occur: (1) neural crest–derived cells migrate into the outflow tract, where they participate in the septation of the outflow tract and the formation of the aortic arches, and (2) interstitial connective tissue that will become the future atrioventricular canal and outflow tract enlarges to produce swellings known as endocardial cushions. By day 50, further septation of the ventricles, atria, and atrioventricular valves produces a four-chambered heart.

Proper orchestration of these remarkable transformations depends on a network of transcription factors that are regulated by a number of signaling pathways, particularly the Wnt, hedgehog, vascular endothelial growth factor (VEGF), bone morphogenetic factor, TGFβ, fibroblast growth factor, and Notch pathways (Chapter 1). In addition, specific micro-RNAs play critical roles in cardiac development by coordinating patterns and levels of transcription factor expression. The heart is a mechanical organ that generates pulsatile blood from its earliest stages of development. It is therefore likely that hemodynamic forces play an important role in cardiac development, just as they influence adaptations in the adult heart such as hypertrophy and dilation.

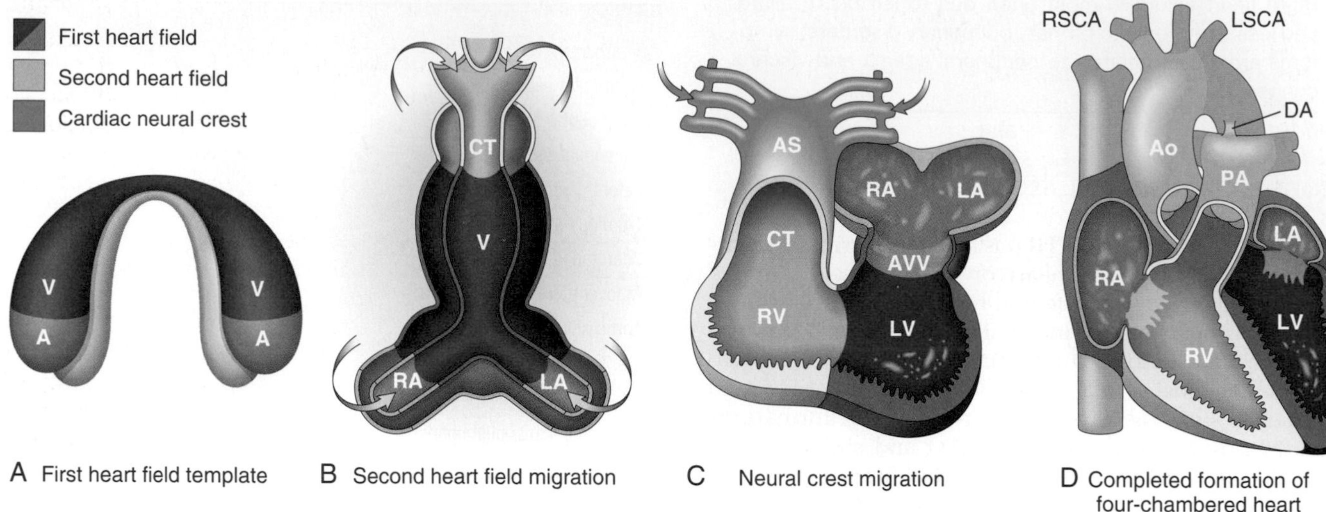

Figure 12-3 Human cardiac development, emphasizing three main sources of cells. **A,** Day 15. First heart field (FHF) cells (shown in red) form a crescent shape in the anterior embryo with second heart field (SHF) cells (shown in yellow) near the FHF. **B,** Day 21. SHF cells lie dorsal to the straight heart tube and begin to migrate *(arrows)* into the anterior and posterior ends of the tube to form the right ventricle, conotruncus (CT), and part of the atria (A). **C,** Day 28. Following rightward looping of the heart tube, cardiac neural crest cells (shown in blue) also migrate *(arrow)* into the outflow tract from the neural folds to septate the outflow tract and pattern the bilaterally symmetric aortic arch arteries. **D,** Day 50. Septation of the ventricles, atria, and atrioventricular valves (AVV) results in the appropriately configured four-chambered heart. Ao, Aorta; AS, aortic sac; DA, ductus arteriosus; LA, left atrium; LCA, left carotid artery; LSCA, left subclavian artery; LV, left ventricle; PA, pulmonary artery; RA, right atrium; RCA, right carotid artery; RSCA, right subclavian artery; V, ventricle. (Modified with permission from Srivastava D: Making or breaking the heart: from lineage determination to morphogenesis. Cell 126:1037, 2006.)

Many of the inherited defects that affect heart development involve genes that encode transcription factors; these typically cause partial loss of function and are autosomal dominant (discussed later). Even relatively minor decrements in activity can result in significant defects. Moreover, transient environmental stresses during the first trimester of pregnancy that alter the activity of these same genes could conceivably lead to acquired defects that mimic those produced by heritable mutations.

Etiology and Pathogenesis. **Sporadic genetic abnormalities are the major known causes of congenital heart disease.** They can take the form of single gene mutations, small chromosomal losses, and additions or deletions of whole chromosomes (trisomies and monosomies). In the case of single gene mutations, the affected genes encode proteins belonging to several different functional classes (Table 12-3); as noted earlier, many of these involve transcription factors. Since affected patients are heterozygous for such mutations, it follows that a 50% reduction in the activity of these factors (or even less) may be sufficient to derange cardiac development.

Moreover, many of the transcription factors interact in large protein complexes, providing a rationale for why mutations in any one of several genes can produce similar defects. Thus, GATA4, TBX5, and NKX2-5, three transcription factors that are mutated in some patients with atrial and ventricular septal defects, all bind to one another and co-regulate the expression of target genes required for proper cardiac development. Of further interest, GATA4 and TBX20 are also mutated in rare forms of adult-onset cardiomyopathy (discussed later), indicating important roles not only in development but also in maintaining normal function of the postnatal heart.

Table 12-3 Selected Examples of Gene Defects Associated with Congenital Heart Disease*

Disorder	Gene(s)	Gene Product Function
Nonsyndromic		
ASD or conduction defects	*NKX2.5*	Transcription factor
ASD or VSD	*GATA4*	Transcription factor
Tetralogy of Fallot	*ZFPM2* or *NKX2.5*	Transcription factors
Syndromic†		
Alagille syndrome—pulmonary artery stenosis or tetralogy of Fallot	*JAG1* or *NOTCH2*	Signaling proteins or receptors
Char syndrome—PDA	*TFAP2B*	Transcription factor
CHARGE syndrome—ASD, VSD, PDA, or hypoplastic right side of the heart	*CHD7*	Helicase-binding protein
DiGeorge syndrome—ASD, VSD, or outflow tract obstruction	*TBX1*	Transcription factor
Holt-Oram syndrome—ASD, VSD, or conduction defect	*TBX5*	Transcription factor
Noonan syndrome—pulmonary valve stenosis, VSD, or hypertrophic cardiomyopathy	*PTPN11, KRAS, SOS1*	Signaling proteins

ASD, Atrial septal defect; CHARGE, posterior *c*oloboma, *h*eart defect, choanal *a*tresia, *r*etardation, *g*enital and *e*ar anomalies; PDA, patent ductus arteriosus; VSD, ventricular septal defect.
*Different mutations can cause the same phenotype, and mutations in some genes can cause multiple phenotypes (e.g., *NKX2.5*). Many of these congenital lesions also can occur sporadically, without specific genetic mutation.
†Only the cardiac manifestations of the syndrome are listed; the other skeletal, facial, neurologic, and visceral changes are not.

Other single gene mutations associated with congenital heart disease can alter structural proteins or affect signaling pathway molecules. Thus, mutations in genes encoding various components of the Notch pathway (Chapter 1) are associated with a variety of congenital heart defects, including bicuspid aortic valve (*NOTCH1*, discussed later) and tetralogy of Fallot (*JAG1* and *NOTCH2*). As described in Chapter 11, fibrillin mutations underlie Marfan syndrome—associated with valvular defects and aortic aneurysms. Although fibrillin is an important structural protein in the ECM, it is also an important negative regulator of TGF-β signaling, and hyperactive TGF-β signaling contributes to the cardiovascular abnormalities in Marfan syndrome and Loeys-Dietz syndrome.

A notable example of a small chromosomal lesion causing congenital heart disease is deletion of chromosome 22q11.2, occurring in up to 50% of patients with DiGeorge syndrome. In this syndrome, the fourth branchial arch and the derivatives of the third and fourth pharyngeal pouches (which contribute to the formation of the thymus, parathyroids, and heart) develop abnormally. The syndrome is therefore associated with multiple deficits (memorable through the mnemonic CATCH-22: *c*ardiac abnormality, *a*bnormal facies, *t*hymic aplasia, *c*left palate, and *h*ypocalcemia, all on chromosome 22). Of the 30 or so genes present on this chromosome segment, deletion specifically of the *TBX1* transcription factor gene is probably the culprit lesion. TBX1 regulates neural crest migration, as well as the expansion of cardiac progenitors in the second heart field. Interestingly, deletions in this region are also associated with mental illness, including schizophrenia.

Other important genetic causes of congenital heart disease include chromosomal aneuploidies, particularly Turner syndrome (monosomy X) and trisomies 13, 18, and 21. Indeed, *the most common genetic cause of congenital heart disease is trisomy 21 (Down syndrome)*; roughly 40% of patients with Down syndrome have one or more heart defects, most often affecting structures derived from the second heart field (e.g., the atrioventricular septae). The mechanisms by which aneuploidy causes congenital heart disease likely involve the dysregulated expression of multiple genes.

Despite these genetic advances, our understanding of the mechanisms underlying congenital heart disease remains rudimentary. Most affected patients have no identifiable genetic risk, and even in those that do, the nature and severity of the defect are highly variable. Thus, *environmental factors*, alone or in combination with genetic factors, are also increasingly implicated in congenital heart disease. Examples include congenital rubella infection, gestational diabetes, and teratogen exposure (including some therapeutic drugs). Nutritional factors may also influence risk. For instance, folate supplementation during early pregnancy may reduce congenital heart disease risk.

Clinical Features. Most of the various structural anomalies in congenital heart disease can be organized into three major categories:

- Malformations causing a *left-to-right shunt*
- Malformations causing a *right-to-left shunt*
- Malformations causing an *obstruction*

A *shunt* is an abnormal communication between chambers or blood vessels. Abnormal channels permit blood flow down pressure gradients from the left (systemic) side to the right (pulmonary) side of the circulation or vice versa. When blood from the right side of the circulation flows directly into the left side *(right-to-left shunt)*, hypoxemia and *cyanosis* (a dusky blueness of the skin and mucous membranes) result because the pulmonary circulation is bypassed and poorly oxygenated venous blood shunts directly into the systemic arterial supply. In addition, right-to-left shunts can allow emboli from the peripheral veins to bypass the lungs and directly enter the systemic circulation *(paradoxical embolism)*. Severe, long-standing cyanosis also causes a peculiar distal blunting and enlargement ("clubbing") of the tips of the fingers and toes (called *hypertrophic osteoarthropathy*), as well as *polycythemia*. The most important causes of right-to-left shunts are Tetralogy of Fallot, transposition of the great arteries, persistent truncus arteriosus, tricuspid atresia, and total anomalous pulmonary venous connection.

In contrast, *left-to-right shunts* (e.g., ASD, VSD, and patent ductus arteriosus [PDA]) increase pulmonary blood flow, but are not *initially* associated with cyanosis. However, left-to-right shunts chronically elevate both volume and pressure in the normally low-pressure, low-resistance pulmonary circulation. To maintain relatively normal distal pulmonary capillary and venous pressures, the muscular pulmonary arteries (<1 mm in diameter) initially respond by undergoing medial hypertrophy and vasoconstriction. However, prolonged pulmonary arterial vasoconstriction stimulates the development of irreversible obstructive intimal lesions analogous to the arteriolar changes seen in systemic hypertension; pulmonary arteries can even develop frank atherosclerotic lesions (Chapter 11). The right ventricle also responds to the pulmonary vascular changes by undergoing progressive right ventricular hypertrophy. Eventually, pulmonary vascular resistance approaches systemic levels, and the original left-to-right shunt becomes a right-to-left shunt that introduces poorly oxygenated blood into the systemic circulation *(Eisenmenger syndrome)*.

Once irreversible pulmonary hypertension develops, the structural defects of congenital heart disease are considered irreparable; subsequent right heart failure can lead to the patient's death. This provides the rationale for early intervention to close significant left-to-right shunts.

Obstructive congenital heart disease occurs when there is abnormal narrowing of chambers, valves, or blood vessels; these include coarctation of the aorta, aortic valvular stenosis, and pulmonary valvular stenosis. A complete obstruction is called an *atresia*. In some disorders (e.g., Tetralogy of Fallot [TOF]), an obstruction (pulmonary stenosis) and a shunt (right-to-left through a VSD) are both present.

The altered hemodynamics of congenital heart disease usually cause cardiac dilation or hypertrophy (or both). However, some defects induce a decrease in the volume and muscle mass of a cardiac chamber; this is called *hypoplasia* if it occurs before birth and *atrophy* if it develops postnatally.

Left-to-Right Shunts

Left-to-right shunts are the most common congenital heart disease; these include ASD, VSD, and PDA as shown in

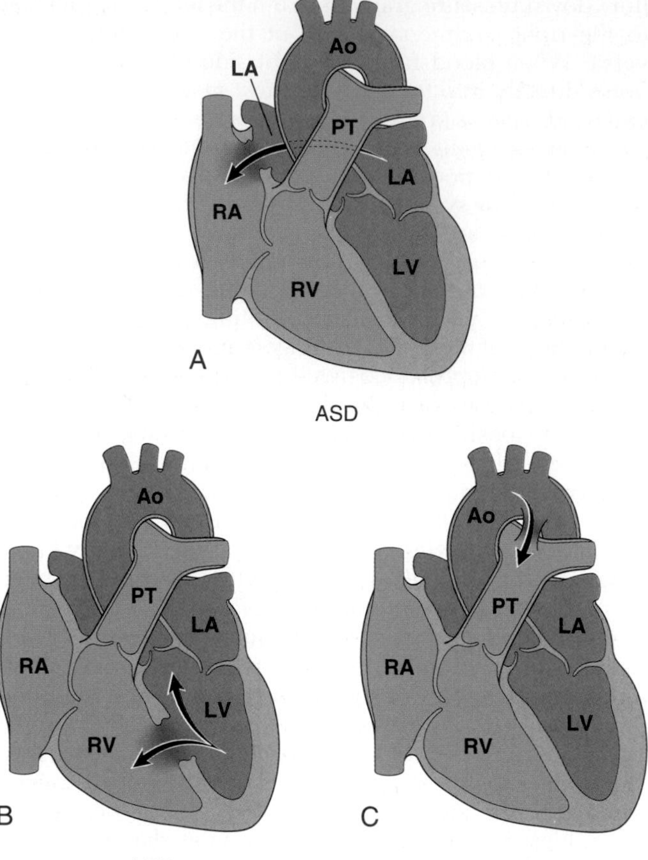

Figure 12-4 Common congenital left-to-right shunts (*arrows* indicate the direction of blood flow). **A,** Atrial septal defect (ASD). **B,** Ventricular septal defect (VSD). With VSD the shunt is left-to-right, and the pressures are the same in both ventricles. Pressure hypertrophy of the right ventricle and volume hypertrophy of the left ventricle are generally present. **C,** Patent ductus arteriosus (PDA). Ao, Aorta; LA, left atrium; LV, left ventricle; PT, pulmonary trunk; RA, right atrium; RV, right ventricle.

Figure 12-4. ASD typically increases only right ventricular and pulmonary outflow volumes, while VSD and PDA cause both increased pulmonary blood flow and pressure. Depending on their size and location, manifestations of these shunts range in severity from no symptoms at all to fulminant heart failure.

Atrial Septal Defect

ASDs are abnormal, fixed openings in the atrial septum caused by incomplete tissue formation that allows communication of blood between the left and right atria; ASDs are usually asymptomatic until adulthood (Table 12-2 and Fig. 12-4*A*). ASD should not be confused with *patent foramen ovale* (*PFO*; see later), which represents the failure to close a foramen (hole) that is part of normal development. Both ASD and PFO result from defects in the formation of the interatrial septum; a brief summary of the developmental stages of this structure follows:

- The *septum primum* is a crescent-shaped membranous ingrowth that sits posteriorly between the right and left atria and partially separates them; the remaining anterior opening, called the *ostium primum,* allows movement of blood from the right to left atrium during fetal development.
- Before the growing septum primum completely obliterates the ostium primum, it develops a second posterior opening called the *ostium secundum*.
- The *septum secundum* is a subsequent membranous ingrowth located to the right and anterior of the septum primum.
- As the septum secundum grows, it also leaves a small opening called the *foramen ovale* that is continuous with the ostium secundum—the foramen ovale/ostium secundum permits continued right-to-left shunting of blood during intrauterine development.
- The septum secundum continues to enlarge until it forms a flap of tissue that covers the foramen ovale on its left side.

This flap of tissue opens and closes in response to pressure gradients between the left and right atria; the valve opens only when the pressure is greater in the right atrium. In fetal life, the lungs are nonfunctional, and the pressure in the *pulmonary circulation* is greater than that of the *systemic circulation*; thus, the right atrium is under higher pressures than the left atrium, and the valve of the foramen ovale is normally open. At birth, with lung expansion, the pulmonary vascular pressures drop, and the right atrial pressures fall below those in the left atrium. As a result, the valve of the foramen ovale closes—and usually permanently seals (see later).

MORPHOLOGY

ASDs are classified according to their location. **Secundum ASD** (90% of all ASD) result from a deficient septum secundum formation near the center of the atrial septum. These are usually not associated with other anomalies, may be of any size, and can be multiple or fenestrated. **Primum anomalies** (5% of ASD) occur adjacent to the AV valves and are often associated with AV valve abnormalities and/or a VSD. **Sinus venosus defects** (5%) are located near the entrance of the superior vena cava and can be associated with anomalous pulmonary venous return to the right atrium.

Clinical Features. ASDs result in a left-to-right shunt, largely because pulmonary vascular resistance is considerably less than systemic vascular resistance and because the compliance (distensibility) of the right ventricle is much greater than that of the left. Pulmonary blood flow may be two to eight times normal. A murmur is often present as a result of excessive flow through the pulmonary valve and/or through the ASD. Despite the right-sided volume overload, ASDs are generally well tolerated and usually do not become symptomatic before age 30; irreversible pulmonary hypertension is unusual. ASD closure (surgical or catheter-based) reverses the hemodynamic abnormalities and prevents the complications, including heart failure, paradoxical embolization, and irreversible pulmonary vascular disease. Mortality is low, and long-term survival is comparable to that of the normal population.

Patent Foramen Ovale. The foramen ovale closes permanently in approximately 80% of people by 2 years of age. However, in the remaining 20%, the unsealed flap can open if right-sided pressures become elevated. Thus, sustained pulmonary hypertension or even transient increases in right-sided pressures, for example, during a bowel movement, coughing, or sneezing, can produce brief periods of right-to-left shunting, with the possibility of paradoxical embolism.

Ventricular Septal Defect

VSDs are incomplete closures of the ventricular septum, allowing free communication of blood between the left to right ventricles; they are the most common form of congenital heart disease (Table 12-2 and Fig. 12-4*B*).

MORPHOLOGY

VSDs are classified according to their size and location. Most are about the size of the aortic valve orifice, and about 90% occur in the region of the membranous interventricular septum (**membranous VSD**; Fig. 12-5). The remainder occur below the pulmonary valve **(infundibular VSD)** or within the muscular septum. Although most VSDs are single, those in the muscular septum may be multiple.

Clinical Features. Most VSDs that clinically manifest in the pediatric age group are associated with other congenital cardiac anomalies such as Tetralogy of Fallot; only 20% to 30% are isolated. Conversely, if a VSD is first detected only in an adult, it is usually an isolated defect. The functional consequences of a VSD depend on the size of the defect and whether there are associated right-sided malformations. Thus, large VSDs cause difficulties virtually from birth; smaller lesions are generally well tolerated for years and may not be recognized until much later in life. Moreover, approximately 50% of small muscular VSDs close spontaneously. Large defects are usually membranous or infundibular, and they generally cause significant left-to-right shunting, leading to early right ventricular hypertrophy and pulmonary hypertension. Over time, large unclosed VSDs almost universally lead to irreversible pulmonary vascular disease, ultimately resulting in shunt reversal, cyanosis, and death. Surgical or catheter-based closure of asymptomatic VSD is generally delayed beyond infancy, in hope of spontaneous closure. Early correction, however, must be performed for large defects to prevent the development of irreversible obstructive pulmonary vascular disease.

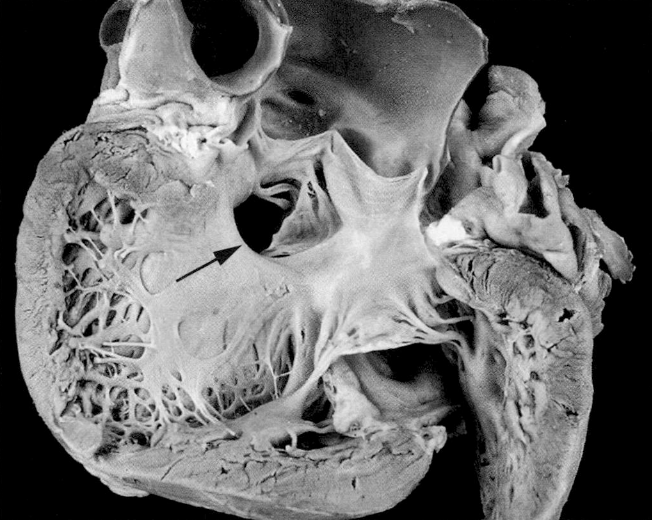

Figure 12-5 A ventricular septal defect (membranous type), denoted by the arrow. (Courtesy William D. Edwards, MD, Mayo Clinic, Rochester, Minn.)

Patent Ductus Arteriosus

The *ductus arteriosus* arises from the pulmonary artery and joins the aorta just distal to the origin of the left subclavian artery. During intrauterine life, it permits blood flow from the pulmonary artery to the aorta, thereby bypassing the unoxygenated lungs. Shortly after birth in healthy term infants, the ductus constricts and is functionally closed after 1 to 2 days; this occurs in response to increased arterial oxygenation, decreased pulmonary vascular resistance, and declining local levels of prostaglandin E_2. Complete structural obliteration occurs within the first few months of extrauterine life to form the *ligamentum arteriosum.* Ductal closure is often delayed (or even absent) in infants with hypoxia (due to respiratory distress or heart disease), or when PDA occurs in association with other congenital defects, particularly VSDs that increase pulmonary vascular pressures. PDAs account for about 7% of cases of congenital heart disease (Table 12-2 and Fig. 12-4C), and 90% of these are isolated defects.

PDA produces a characteristic continuous harsh "machinery-like" murmur. The clinical impact of a PDA depends on its diameter and the cardiovascular status of the individual. PDA is usually asymptomatic at birth, and a narrow PDA may have no effect on the child's growth and development. Because the shunt is initially left-to-right, there is no cyanosis. However, with large shunts, the additional volume and pressure overloads eventually produce obstructive changes in small pulmonary arteries, leading to reversal of flow and its associated consequences. In general, isolated PDA should be closed as early in life as is feasible. Conversely, preservation of ductal patency (by administering prostaglandin E) may be life saving for infants with various congenital malformations that obstruct the pulmonary or systemic outflow tracts. In aortic valve atresia, for example, a PDA may provide the entire systemic blood flow.

Right-to-Left Shunts

The diseases in this group cause cyanosis early in postnatal life (*cyanotic* congenital heart disease). Tetralogy of Fallot, the most common in this group, and transposition of the great arteries are illustrated schematically in Figure 12-6. The others include persistent truncus arteriosus, tricuspid atresia, and total anomalous pulmonary venous connection.

Tetralogy of Fallot

The four cardinal features of TOF are (1) VSD, (2) obstruction of the right ventricular outflow tract (subpulmonary stenosis), (3) an aorta that overrides the VSD, and (4) right ventricular hypertrophy (Fig. 12-6*A*). All of these features result embryologically from anterosuperior displacement of the infundibular septum.

MORPHOLOGY

The heart is typically enlarged and is classically "boot-shaped" due to marked right ventricular hypertrophy. The VSD is usually large with the aortic valve at the superior border, thereby

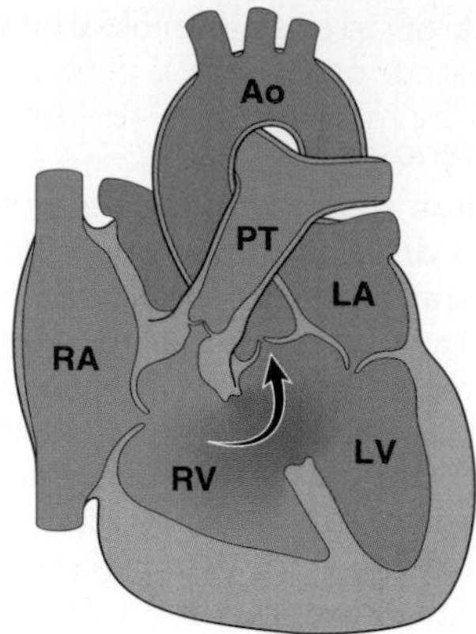

A Classic tetralogy of Fallot

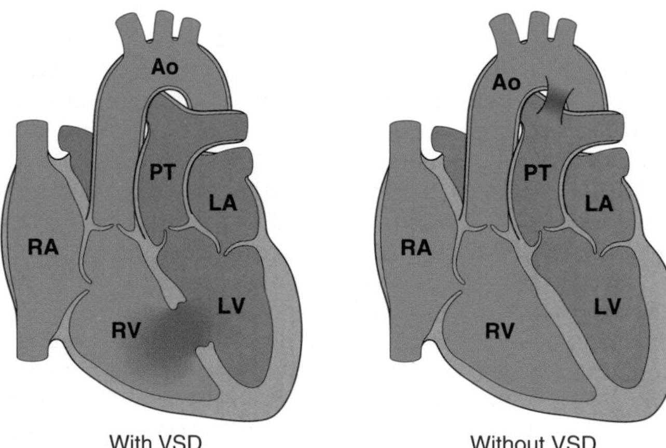

B Complete transposition

Figure 12-6 Common congenital right-to-left shunts *(cyanotic congenital heart disease).* **A,** Tetralogy of Fallot. The direction of shunting across the ventricular septal defect (VSD) depends on the degree of the subpulmonary stenosis; when severe, a right-to-left shunt results (*arrow*). **B,** Transposition of the great arteries with and without VSD. Ao, Aorta; LA, left atrium; LV, left ventricle; PT, pulmonary trunk; RA, right atrium; RV, right ventricle.

overriding the defect and both ventricular chambers. The obstruction to right ventricular outflow is most often due to narrowing of the infundibulum (subpulmonic stenosis) but can be accompanied by pulmonary valvular stenosis. Sometimes there is complete atresia of the pulmonary valve and variable portions of the pulmonary arteries, such that blood flow through a PDA, dilated bronchial arteries, or both, is necessary for survival. Aortic valve insufficiency or an ASD may also be present; a right aortic arch is present in about 25% of cases.

Clinical Features. Even untreated, patients with TOF can survive into adult life; 10% of untreated patients are alive at 20 years and 3% survive for 40 years. The clinical consequences depend primarily on the severity of the subpulmonary stenosis, since this determines the direction of blood flow. If the subpulmonary stenosis is mild, the abnormality resembles an isolated VSD, and the shunt may be left-to-right, without cyanosis (so-called "pink tetralogy"). *With more severe right ventricular outflow obstruction, right-sided pressures approach or exceed left-sided pressures, and right-to-left shunting develops, producing cyanosis (classic TOF).* Most infants with TOF are cyanotic from birth or soon thereafter. The more severe the subpulmonic stenosis, the more hypoplastic are the pulmonary arteries (i.e., smaller and thinner-walled), and the larger is the overriding aorta. As the child grows and the heart increases in size, the pulmonic orifice does not expand proportionally, making the obstruction progressively worse. The subpulmonary stenosis, however, protects the pulmonary vasculature from pressure overload, and right ventricular failure is rare because the right ventricle is decompressed by the shunting of blood into the left ventricle and aorta. Complete surgical repair is possible but becomes complicated for individuals with pulmonary atresia and dilated bronchial arteries.

Transposition of the Great Arteries

TGA produces ventriculoarterial discordance. Thus, the aorta lies anterior and arises from the right ventricle, while the pulmonary artery is relatively posterior and emanates from the left ventricle (Fig. 12-7; see also Fig. 12-6*B*). The atrium-to-ventricle connections are normal (concordant), with the right atrium joining the right ventricle and the left atrium emptying into the left ventricle. The embryologic defect in complete TGA stems from abnormal formation of the truncal and aortopulmonary septa. The result is separation of the systemic and pulmonary circulations, a condition incompatible with postnatal life unless a shunt exists for adequate mixing of blood.

The outlook for infants with TGA depends on the degree of blood "mixing," the magnitude of tissue hypoxia, and the ability of the right ventricle to maintain the systemic circulation. Patients with TGA and a VSD (approximately 35%) often have a stable shunt. However, dependence on a patent foramen ovale or ductus arteriosus for blood mixing (approximately 65%) is problematic. These systemic-to-pulmonary connections tend to close early and thus require intervention to create a new shunt within the first few days of life (e.g., balloon atrial septostomy). With

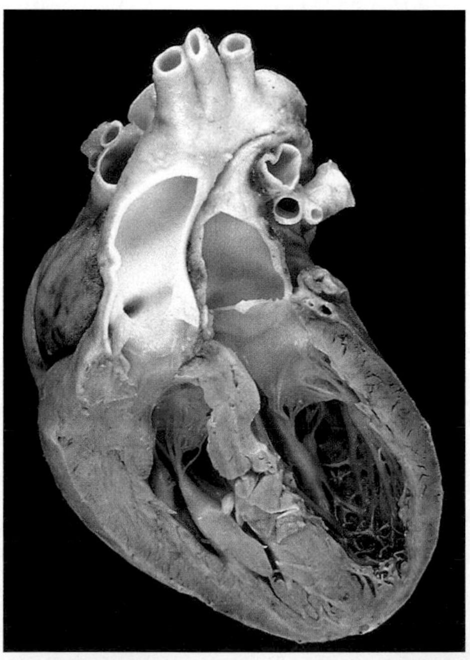

Figure 12-7 Transposition of the great arteries. (Courtesy William D. Edwards, MD, Mayo Clinic, Rochester, Minn.)

time, right ventricular hypertrophy becomes prominent, because this chamber functions as the systemic ventricle. Concurrently, the left ventricle becomes thin-walled (atrophic) as it supports the low-resistance pulmonary circulation. Without surgery, most patients die within months. However, improving surgical interventions allow many patients with TGA to survive into adulthood.

Tricuspid Atresia

Tricuspid atresia represents complete occlusion of the tricuspid valve orifice. It results embryologically from unequal division of the AV canal; thus, the mitral valve is larger than normal, and there is right ventricular underdevelopment (hypoplasia). The circulation can be maintained by right-to-left shunting through an interatrial communication (ASD or patent foramen ovale), in addition to a VSD that affords communication between the left ventricle and the pulmonary artery arising from the hypoplastic right ventricle. Cyanosis is present virtually from birth, and there is a high early mortality.

Obstructive Lesions

Congenital obstruction to blood flow can occur at the level of the heart valves or within a great vessel. Common examples include aortic or pulmonary valve stenosis or atresia, and coarctation of the aorta. Obstruction can also occur within a chamber, as with subpulmonary stenosis in TOF.

Coarctation of the Aorta

Coarctation (narrowing, constriction) of the aorta ranks high in frequency among the common structural anomalies. It is twice as common in males as in females; interestingly, females with Turner syndrome are also frequently affected (Chapter 5). There are two classic forms: (1) an "infantile" form—often symptomatic in early childhood—with tubular hypoplasia of the aortic arch proximal to a PDA, and (2) an "adult" form with a discrete ridgelike infolding of the aorta just opposite the closed ductus arteriosus *(ligamentum arteriosum)* distal to the arch vessels (Fig. 12-8). Encroachment on the aortic lumen is variable, sometimes leaving only a small channel and at other times producing only minimal narrowing. Although coarctation of the aorta may occur as a solitary defect, in 50% of cases it is accompanied by a bicuspid aortic valve and may also be associated with congenital aortic stenosis, ASD, VSD, mitral regurgitation, or berry aneurysms of the circle of Willis.

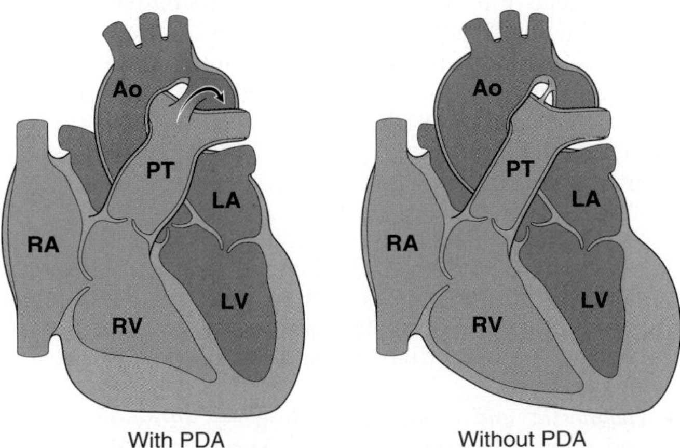

Figure 12-8 Schematic of aortic coarctation with and without patent ductus arteriosus (PDA). Ao, Aorta; LA, left atrium; LV, left ventricle; PT, pulmonary trunk; RA, right atrium; RV, right ventricle; PDA, patent ductus arteriosus. (Courtesy William D. Edwards, MD, Mayo Clinic, Rochester, Minn.)

Clinical manifestations depend on the severity of the narrowing and the patency of the ductus arteriosus. *Coarctation of the aorta with a PDA* usually manifests early in life; indeed, it may cause signs and symptoms immediately after birth. In such cases, the delivery of unsaturated blood through the PDA produces cyanosis localized to the lower half of the body. Many such infants do not survive the neonatal period without surgical or catheter-based intervention to occlude the PDA.

The outlook is different with *coarctation of the aorta without a PDA*, unless the aortic constriction is severe. Most children are asymptomatic, and the disease may go unrecognized until well into adult life. Typically there is hypertension in the upper extremities with weak pulses and hypotension in the lower extremities, associated with manifestations of arterial insufficiency (i.e., claudication and coldness). Particularly characteristic is the development of collateral circulation between the pre-coarctation and post-coarctation arteries through enlarged intercostal and internal mammary arteries, often producing radiographically visible erosions ("notching") of the undersurfaces of the ribs.

With significant coarctations, murmurs are present throughout systole; sometimes a vibratory "thrill" is also present. The long-standing pressure overload leads to concentric left ventricular hypertrophy. With uncomplicated coarctation of the aorta, surgical resection and end-to-end anastomosis or replacement of the affected aortic segment by a prosthetic graft yields excellent results.

Pulmonary Stenosis and Atresia

Pulmonary stenosis or atresia is a relatively frequent malformation leading to obstruction at the level of the pulmonary valve. This can be mild to severe; the lesion can also be isolated or part of a more complex anomaly—either TOF or TGA. Right ventricular hypertrophy typically develops, and there is sometimes poststenotic dilation of the pulmonary artery due to injury of the wall by "jetting" blood. With coexistent subpulmonary stenosis (as in TOF), the pulmonary trunk is not dilated and may in fact be hypoplastic. When the valve is entirely atretic, there is no communication between the right ventricle and lungs. In such cases the anomaly is associated with a hypoplastic right ventricle and an ASD; blood reaches the lungs through a PDA. Mild stenosis may be asymptomatic and compatible with long life, whereas symptomatic cases require surgical correction.

Aortic Stenosis and Atresia

Congenital narrowing and obstruction of the aortic valve can occur at three locations: valvular, subvalvular, and supravalvular. Congenital aortic stenosis is an isolated lesion in 80% of cases. With *valvular aortic stenosis* the cusps may be hypoplastic (small), dysplastic (thickened, nodular), or abnormal in number (usually acommissural or unicommissural). In severe congenital aortic stenosis or atresia, obstruction of the left ventricular outflow tract leads to hypoplasia of the left ventricle and ascending aorta, sometimes accompanied by dense, porcelain-like left ventricular endocardial fibroelastosis. The ductus must be open to allow blood flow to the aorta and coronary arteries, and the constellation of findings is called the *hypoplastic left heart syndrome*. Unless a palliative procedure is done to preserve PDA patency, duct closure in the first week of life is generally lethal. However, less severe congenital aortic stenosis can be compatible with long survival.

Subaortic stenosis is caused by a thickened ring or collar of dense endocardial fibrous tissue below the level of the cusps. *Supravalvular aortic stenosis* is a congenital aortic dysplasia with thickening of ascending aortic wall and consequent luminal constriction. In some cases it is a component of a multiorgan developmental disorder resulting from deletions on chromosome 7 that include the gene for elastin. Other features of the syndrome include hypercalcemia, cognitive abnormalities, and characteristic facial anomalies (*Williams-Beuren syndrome*). Elastin gene mutations may cause supravalvular stenosis by disrupting elastin–smooth muscle cell interactions during aortic morphogenesis.

Subaortic stenosis is usually associated with a prominent systolic murmur and sometimes a thrill. Pressure hypertrophy of the left ventricle develops as a consequence of the obstruction to blood flow, but congenital stenoses are well tolerated unless very severe. Although mild stenoses can often be managed conservatively with antibiotic prophylaxis (to prevent endocarditis) and avoidance of strenuous activity, the resulting left ventricular hypertrophy still carries a risk of sudden death with exertion.

KEY CONCEPTS

Congenital Heart Disease

- Congenital heart disease represents defects of cardiac chambers or the great vessels; these either result in shunting of blood between the right and left circulation or cause outflow obstructions. Lesions range from relatively asymptomatic to rapidly fatal. Environmental (toxic or infectious) and genetic causes both contribute, and the manifestations depend on the timing of the environmental insult or which step in cardiac development is affected.
- Left-to-right shunts are most common and are typically associated with ASDs, VSDs, or a PDA. These lesions result in chronic right-sided pressure and volume overloads that eventually cause pulmonary hypertension with reversal of flow and right-to-left shunts with cyanosis (*Eisenmenger syndrome*).
- Right-to-left shunts are most commonly caused by TOF or TGA. These are cyanotic lesions from the outset and are associated with polycythemia, hypertrophic osteoarthropathy, and paradoxical emboli.
- Obstructive lesions include aortic coarctation; the clinical severity of the lesion depends on the degree of stenosis and the patency of the ductus arteriosus.

Ischemic Heart Disease

Ischemic heart disease (IHD) represents a group of pathophysiologically related syndromes resulting from ***myocardial ischemia*** **— an imbalance between myocardial supply (perfusion) and cardiac demand for oxygenated blood.** Ischemia not only limits tissue oxygenation (and thus ATP generation), but also reduces the availability of nutrients and the removal of metabolic wastes (Chapter 2). Thus, cardiac ischemia is generally less well tolerated than hypoxia *per se*, such as may occur with severe anemia, cyanotic heart disease, or advanced lung disease.

In more than 90% of cases, myocardial ischemia results from reduced blood flow due to obstructive atherosclerotic lesions in the epicardial coronary arteries; consequently, IHD is frequently referred to as coronary artery disease (CAD). In most cases there is a long period (up to decades) of silent, slow progression of coronary lesions before the sudden onset of symptoms. Thus, IHD is often the late manifestation of coronary atherosclerosis that began during childhood or adolescence (Chapter 11).

IHD can present as one or more of the following clinical syndromes:

- *Myocardial infarction (MI)*, where ischemia causes frank cardiac necrosis
- *Angina pectoris* (literally "chest pain"), where ischemia is not severe enough to cause infarction, but the symptoms nevertheless portend infarction risk
- *Chronic IHD with heart failure*
- *Sudden cardiac death (SCD).*

In addition to coronary atherosclerosis, myocardial ischemia can be caused by coronary emboli, myocardial vessel inflammation, or vascular spasm. Moreover, otherwise modest vascular occlusions may become consequential in the setting of increased cardiac energy demand (e.g., myocardial hypertrophy or increased heart rate), hypoxemia, or systemic hypotension (e.g., shock). Some conditions can have multiple deleterious effects. Thus, tachycardia increases oxygen demand (because of more contractions per unit time) while decreasing functional supply (by decreasing the relative time spent in diastole, when cardiac perfusion occurs).

Epidemiology. IHD is the leading cause of death in the United States (one of every six deaths in 2008; more than 400,000 individuals) and other developed nations (approximately 7 million total per year). As high as these numbers are, they represent a substantial improvement relative to just one to two generations ago. Since peaking in 1963, the overall death rate from IHD has fallen in the United States by approximately 50%. This remarkable improvement can be attributed to:

- *Prevention*, achieved by modifying important risk factors, such as smoking, blood cholesterol, and hypertension. Additional risk reduction and prevention may potentially be achieved by maintenance of normal blood glucose levels in diabetic patients, control of obesity, and exercise.
- *Diagnostic and therapeutic advances*, allowing earlier and more effective treatments. The latter include new medications, including the use of cholesterol lowering drugs such as statins, coronary care units, thrombolysis for MI, percutaneous transluminal coronary angioplasty, endovascular stents, coronary artery bypass graft (CABG) surgery, and improved control of heart

failure and arrhythmias via left ventricular assist devices, implantable defibrillators, and cardiac resynchronization with pacemakers. Even a simple daily prophylactic aspirin can have therapeutic benefit.

Continuing this encouraging trend will be challenging, particularly in view of the increased longevity of "baby boomers" (which will lead to a doubling of individuals older than age 65 by 2050), the "obesity epidemic," and other factors. Increasingly, new therapeutic advances will depend on understanding the genetic determinants of coronary atherosclerosis and IHD. For example, the observation that MIs occur in only a fraction of individuals with coronary disease suggests that simple control of atherosclerotic risk factors is only part of the story. For example, MI risk—but not coronary atherosclerosis—is associated with genetic variants that modify leukotriene B4 metabolism.

Pathogenesis. **The dominant cause of IHD syndromes is insufficient coronary perfusion relative to myocardial demand; in the vast majority of cases, this is due to chronic, progressive atherosclerotic narrowing of the epicardial coronary arteries, and variable degrees of superimposed acute plaque change, thrombosis, and vasospasm.** The individual elements and their interactions are discussed next.

Chronic Vascular Occlusion. More than 90% of patients with IHD have atherosclerosis involving one or more of the epicardial coronary arteries (Chapter 11). The clinical manifestations of coronary atherosclerosis are generally due to progressive narrowing of the lumen leading to stenosis ("fixed" obstructions), or to acute plaque erosion or rupture with thrombosis, all of which compromise blood flow. A fixed lesion obstructing greater than 75% of vascular cross-sectional area defines significant coronary artery disease; this is generally the threshold for symptomatic ischemia precipitated by exercise (typically manifesting as angina). With this degree of obstruction, compensatory coronary arterial vasodilation is no longer sufficient to meet even moderate increases in myocardial demand. Obstruction of 90% of the cross-sectional area of the lumen can lead to inadequate coronary blood flow even at rest. Progressive myocardial ischemia induced by slowly developing occlusions may stimulate the formation of collateral vessels over time, which can often protect against myocardial ischemia and infarction and mitigate the effects of high-grade stenoses.

Although only a single major coronary epicardial vessel may be affected, two or all three—the LAD, LCX, and RCA—are often involved by obstructive atherosclerosis. Clinically significant plaques can be located anywhere along the course of the vessels, particularly the RCA, although they tend to predominate within the first several centimeters of the LAD and LCX. Sometimes the major epicardial branches are also involved (i.e., LAD diagonal branches, LCX obtuse marginal branches, or posterior descending branch of the RCA), but atherosclerosis of the intramural (penetrating) branches is rare.

Acute Plaque Change. The risk of an individual developing clinically important IHD depends in part on the number, distribution, structure, and degree of obstruction of atheromatous plaques. However, the varied clinical manifestations of IHD cannot be explained by the anatomic disease burden alone. This is particularly true for the so-called acute coronary syndromes, namely unstable angina, acute MI, and sudden death. These acute coronary syndromes are typically initiated by an unpredictable and abrupt conversion of a stable atherosclerotic plaque to an unstable and potentially life-threatening atherothrombotic lesion through rupture, superficial erosion, ulceration, fissuring, or deep hemorrhage (Chapter 11). In most instances, plaque changes—typically associated with intralesional inflammation—precipitate the formation of a superimposed thrombus that partially or completely occludes the artery.

Consequences of Myocardial Ischemia. The common feature of the acute coronary syndromes is downstream myocardial ischemia.

- *Stable angina* results from increases in myocardial oxygen demand that outstrip the ability of stenosed coronary arteries to increase oxygen delivery; it is usually not associated with plaque disruption.
- *Unstable angina* is caused by plaque disruption that results in thrombosis and vasoconstriction, and leads to severe but transient reductions in coronary blood flow. In some cases, microinfarcts can occur distal to disrupted plaques due to thromboemboli.
- *Myocardial infarction (MI)* is often the result of acute plaque change that induces an abrupt thrombotic occlusion, resulting in myocardial necrosis.
- *Sudden cardiac death* may be caused by regional myocardial ischemia that induces a fatal ventricular arrhythmia.

Each of these important syndromes is discussed in detail next, followed by an examination of the important myocardial consequences.

Angina Pectoris

Angina pectoris is characterized by paroxysmal and usually recurrent attacks of substernal or precordial chest discomfort caused by transient (15 seconds to 15 minutes) myocardial ischemia that is insufficient to induce myocyte necrosis. The pain itself is likely a consequence of the ischemia-induced release of adenosine, bradykinin, and other molecules that stimulate sympathetic and vagal afferent nerves. There are three overlapping patterns of angina pectoris caused by varying combinations of decreased perfusion, increased demand, and coronary arterial pathology. Importantly, not all ischemic events are perceived by patients; silent ischemia is particularly common in the geriatric population and in the setting of diabetic neuropathy.

- *Stable (typical) angina* is the most common form of angina; it is *caused by an imbalance in coronary perfusion (due to chronic stenosing coronary atherosclerosis) relative to myocardial demand*, such as that produced by physical activity, emotional excitement or psychological stress. Typical angina pectoris is variously described as a deep, poorly localized pressure, squeezing, or burning sensation (like indigestion), but unusually as pain, and is usually relieved by rest (decreasing demand) or administering vasodilators, such as nitroglycerin and calcium channel blockers (increasing perfusion).

- *Prinzmetal variant angina is an uncommon form of episodic myocardial ischemia; it is caused by coronary artery spasm.* Although individuals with Prinzmetal variant angina may well have significant coronary atherosclerosis, the anginal attacks are unrelated to physical activity, heart rate, or blood pressure. Prinzmetal angina generally responds promptly to vasodilators.
- *Unstable or crescendo angina* refers to *a pattern of increasingly frequent, prolonged (>20 min), or severe angina or chest discomfort that is described as frank pain, precipitated by progressively lower levels of physical activity or even occurring at rest.* In most patients, unstable angina is caused by the disruption of an atherosclerotic plaque with superimposed partial thrombosis and possibly embolization or vasospasm (or both). Approximately one-half of patients with unstable angina have evidence of myocardial necrosis; for others, acute MI may be imminent.

Myocardial Infarction

Myocardial infarction, also commonly referred to as "heart attack," is the death of cardiac muscle due to prolonged severe ischemia. Roughly 1.5 million individuals in the United States suffer an MI annually.

Incidence and Risk Factors. MI can occur at virtually any age; nearly 10% of myocardial infarcts occur in people younger than age 40, and 45% occur in people younger than age 65. Nevertheless, MI frequency rises progressively with increasing age. The incidence of MI also strongly correlates with genetic and behavioral predispositions to atherosclerosis. Blacks and whites are equally affected. Through middle age, male gender increases the relative risk of MI; indeed, women are generally protected against MI during their reproductive years. However, postmenopausal decline in estrogen production is usually associated with accelerated CAD, and IHD is the most common cause of death in older women. Unfortunately, postmenopausal hormonal replacement therapy has not been shown to be protective, and in fact, in some cases, may be detrimental.

Pathogenesis

Coronary Arterial Occlusion. The following sequence of events likely underlies most MIs (see Chapter 11 for additional details):

- A coronary artery atheromatous plaque undergoes an acute change consisting of intraplaque hemorrhage, erosion or ulceration, or rupture or fissuring.
- When exposed to subendothelial collagen and necrotic plaque contents, platelets adhere, become activated, release their granule contents, and aggregate to form microthrombi.
- Vasospasm is stimulated by mediators released from platelets.
- Tissue factor activates the coagulation pathway, adding to the bulk of the thrombus.
- Within minutes, the thrombus can expand to completely occlude the vessel lumen.

Compelling evidence for this sequence derives from (1) autopsy studies of patients dying of acute MI; (2) angiographic studies demonstrating a high frequency of thrombotic occlusion early after MI; (3) the high success rate of coronary revascularization following MI (i.e., thrombolysis, angioplasty, stent placement, and surgery); and (4) the demonstration of residual disrupted atherosclerotic lesions by angiography after thrombolysis. Coronary angiography performed within 4 hours of MI onset shows coronary thrombosis in almost 90% of cases. However, angiography after 12 to 24 hours reveals thrombosis only about 60% of the time, suggesting resolution due to fibrinolysis, relaxation of spasm, or both.

In approximately 10% of cases, transmural MI occurs in the absence of the typical coronary atherothrombosis. In such situations, other mechanisms may be responsible for the reduced coronary blood flow, including:

- *Vasospasm* with or without coronary atherosclerosis, perhaps in association with platelet aggregation or due to drug ingestion (e.g., cocaine or ephedrine)
- *Emboli* from the left atrium in association with atrial fibrillation, a left-sided mural thrombus, vegetations of infective endocarditis, intracardiac prosthetic material; or *paradoxical emboli* from the right side of the heart or the peripheral veins, traversing a patent foramen ovale and into the coronary arteries
- *Ischemia without detectable or significant coronary atherosclerosis and thrombosis* may be caused by disorders of small intramural coronary vessels (e.g., vasculitis), hematologic abnormalities (e.g., sickle cell disease), amyloid deposition in vascular walls, vascular dissection, marked hypertrophy (e.g., aortic stenosis), lowered systemic blood pressure (e.g., shock), or inadequate myocardial "protection" during cardiac surgery.

Myocardial Response. **Coronary arterial obstruction diminishes blood flow to a region of myocardium (Fig. 12-9), causing ischemia, rapid myocardial dysfunction, and eventually—with prolonged vascular compromise—myocyte death.** The anatomic region supplied by that artery is referred to as the *area at risk.* The outcome depends predominantly on the severity and duration of flow deprivation (Fig. 12-10).

The early biochemical consequence of myocardial ischemia is the cessation of aerobic metabolism within seconds, leading to inadequate production of high-energy phosphates (e.g., creatine phosphate and adenosine triphosphate) and accumulation of potentially noxious metabolites (e.g., lactic acid) (Fig. 12-10*A*). Because of the exquisite dependence of myocardial function on oxygen and nutrients, myocardial contractility ceases within a minute or so of the onset of severe ischemia. Such loss of function actually precipitates heart failure long before myocyte death occurs.

As detailed in Chapter 2, ultrastructural changes (including myofibrillar relaxation, glycogen depletion, cell and mitochondrial swelling) also develop within a few minutes of the onset of ischemia. Nevertheless, these early manifestations of ischemic injury are potentially reversible. Indeed, experimental and clinical evidence shows that only severe ischemia (blood flow 10% or less of normal) lasting 20 to 30 minutes or longer leads to irreversible damage (necrosis) of cardiac myocytes. This delay in the onset of

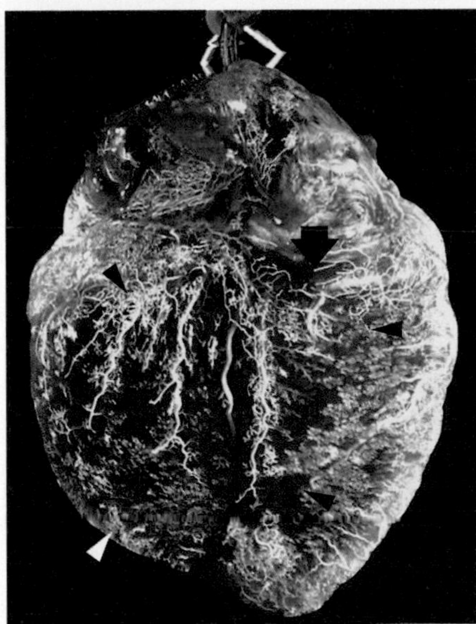

Figure 12-9 Postmortem angiogram showing the posterior aspect of the heart of a patient who died during the evolution of acute myocardial infarction, demonstrating total occlusion of the distal right coronary artery by an acute thrombus *(arrow)* and a large zone of myocardial hypoperfusion involving the posterior left and right ventricles, as indicated by *arrowheads*, and having almost absent filling of capillaries. The heart has been fixed by coronary arterial perfusion with glutaraldehyde and cleared with methyl salicylate, followed by intracoronary injection of silicone polymer (yellow). (Photograph courtesy Lewis L. Lainey. Reproduced with permission from Schoen FJ: Interventional and Surgical Cardiovascular Pathology: Clinical Correlations and Basic Principles. Philadelphia, WB Saunders, 1989, p. 60.)

permanent myocardial injury provides the rationale for rapid diagnosis in acute MI—to permit early coronary intervention to establish reperfusion and salvage as much "at risk" myocardium as possible.

The earliest detectable feature of myocyte necrosis is the disruption of the integrity of the sarcolemmal membrane, allowing intracellular macromolecules to leak out of necrotic cells into the cardiac interstitium and ultimately into the microvasculature and lymphatics. This escape of intracellular myocardial proteins into the circulation forms the basis for blood tests that can sensitively detect irreversible myocyte damage, and are important for managing MI (see later). With prolonged severe ischemia, injury to the microvasculature follows injury to the cardiac myocytes. The temporal progression of these events is summarized in Table 12-4.

Table 12-4 Approximate Time of Onset of Key Events in Ischemic Cardiac Myocytes

Feature	Time
Onset of ATP depletion	Seconds
Loss of contractility	<2 min
ATP reduced	
to 50% of normal	10 min
to 10% of normal	40 min
Irreversible cell injury	20-40 min
Microvascular injury	>1 hr

ATP, Adenosine triphosphate.

The progression of ischemic necrosis in the myocardium is summarized in Figure 12-11. Due to the myocardial perfusion pattern from epicardium to endocardium, ischemia is most pronounced in the subendocardium; thus, irreversible injury of ischemic myocytes occurs first in the subendocardial zone. With more extended ischemia, a *wavefront* of cell death moves through the myocardium to encompass progressively more of the transmural thickness and breadth of the ischemic zone. The precise location, size, and specific morphologic features of an acute MI depend on:

- The location, severity, and rate of development of coronary obstructions due to atherosclerosis and thromboses
- The size of the vascular bed perfused by the obstructed vessels
- The duration of the occlusion
- The metabolic and oxygen needs of the myocardium at risk

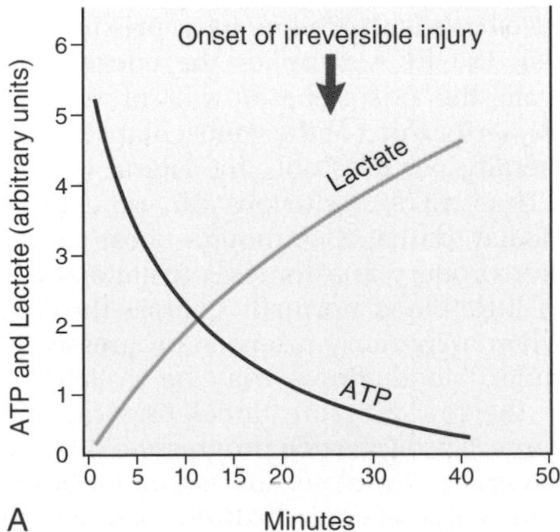

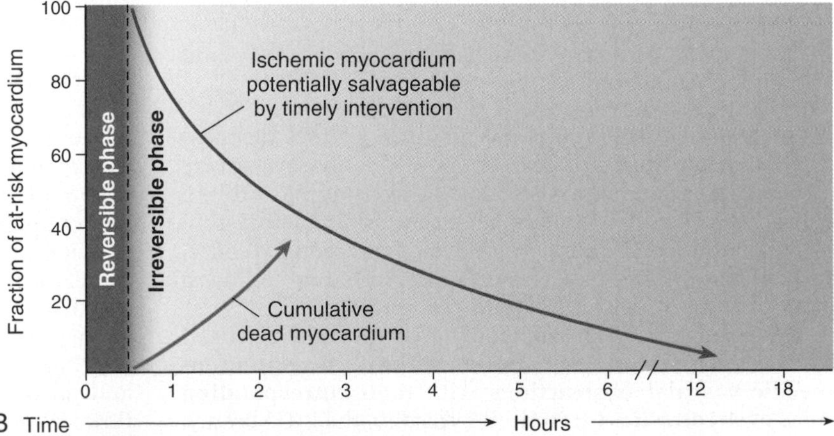

Figure 12-10 Temporal sequence of early biochemical findings and progression of necrosis after onset of severe myocardial ischemia. **A,** Early changes include loss of adenosine triphosphate (ATP) and accumulation of lactate. **B,** For approximately 30 minutes after the onset of even the most severe ischemia, myocardial injury is potentially reversible. Thereafter, progressive loss of viability occurs that is complete by 6 to 12 hours. The benefits of reperfusion are greatest when it is achieved early, and are progressively lost when reperfusion is delayed. (Modified with permission from Antman E: Acute myocardial infarction. In Braunwald E, et al [eds]: Heart Disease: A Textbook of Cardiovascular Medicine, 6th ed. Philadelphia, WB Saunders, 2001, pp 1114 1231.)

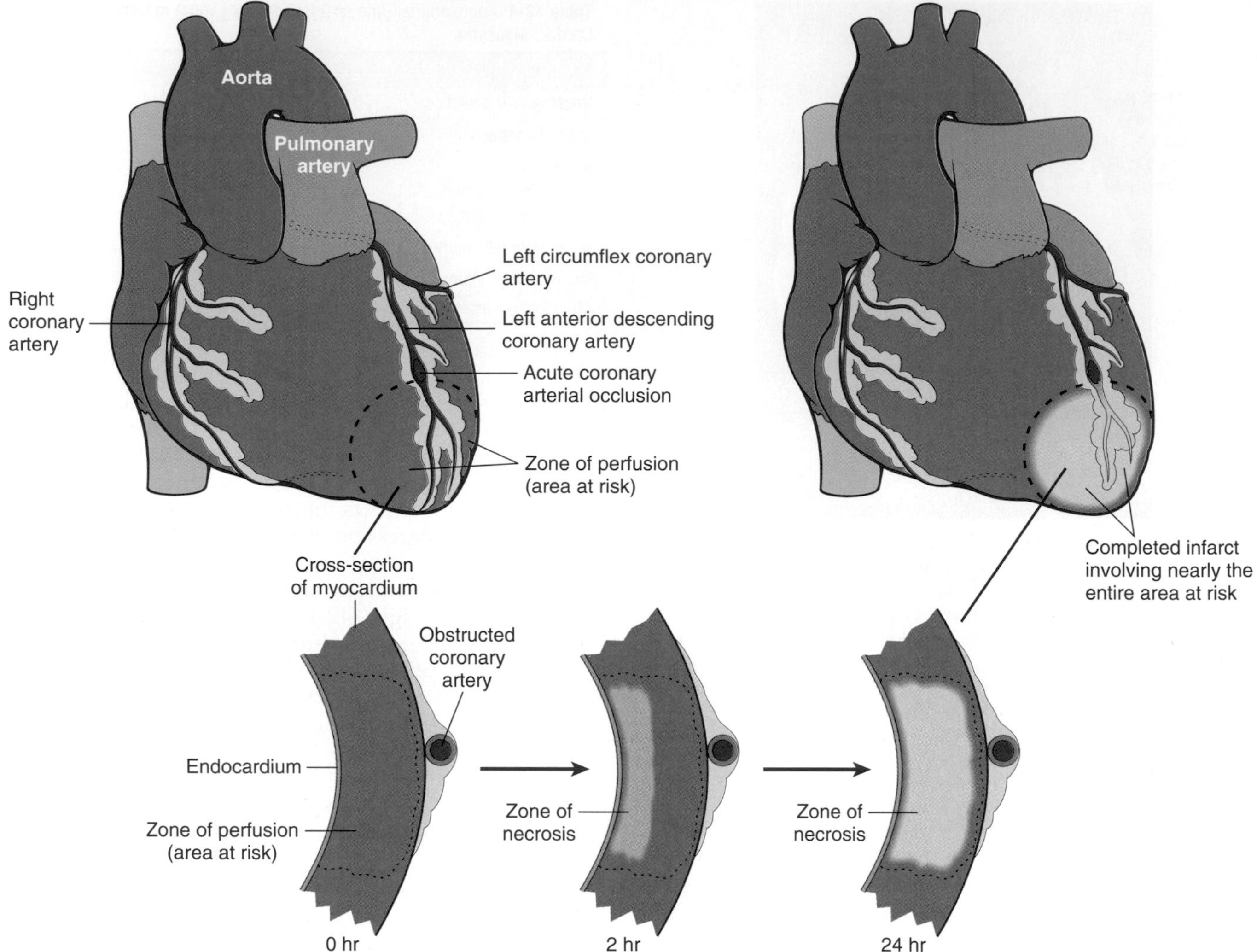

Figure 12-11 Progression of myocardial necrosis after coronary artery occlusion. Necrosis begins in a small zone of the myocardium beneath the endocardial surface in the center of the ischemic zone. The area that depends on the occluded vessel for perfusion is the "at risk" myocardium (*shaded*). Note that a very narrow zone of myocardium immediately beneath the endocardium is spared from necrosis because it can be oxygenated by diffusion from the ventricle.

- The extent of collateral blood vessels
- The presence, site, and severity of coronary arterial spasm
- Other factors, such as heart rate, cardiac rhythm, and blood oxygenation

Necrosis involves approximately half of the thickness of the myocardium in 2 to 3 hours of the onset of severe myocardial ischemia, and is usually transmural within 6 hours. However, in instances where chronic sublethal ischemia has induced a more well-developed coronary collateral circulation, the progression of necrosis may follow a more protracted course (12 hours or longer).

Knowledge of the areas of myocardium perfused by the major coronary arteries allows correlation of specific vascular obstructions with their corresponding areas of myocardial infarction. Typically, the LAD branch of the left coronary artery supplies most of the apex of the heart, the anterior wall of the left ventricle, and the anterior two thirds of the ventricular septum. By convention, the coronary artery—either RCA or LCX—that perfuses the posterior third of the septum is called "dominant" (even though the LAD and LCX collectively perfuse the majority of the left ventricular myocardium). In a *right dominant circulation* (present in approximately 80% of individuals), the RCA supplies the entire right ventricular free wall, the posterobasal wall of the left ventricle, and the posterior third of the ventricular septum, while the LCX generally perfuses only the lateral wall of the left ventricle. Thus, RCA occlusions can potentially lead to left ventricular damage. Although most hearts have numerous intercoronary anastomoses (collateral circulation), relatively little blood normally courses through these. However, when a coronary artery is progressively narrowed over time, blood flows via the collaterals from the high- to the low-pressure circulating causing the channels to enlarge. Through such progressive dilation and growth of collaterals, stimulated by ischemia, blood flow is provided to areas of myocardium that would otherwise be deprived of adequate perfusion. Indeed, in the setting of extensive collateralization, the normal epicardial perfusion territories may be so expanded that subsequent occlusion leads to infarction in paradoxical distributions.

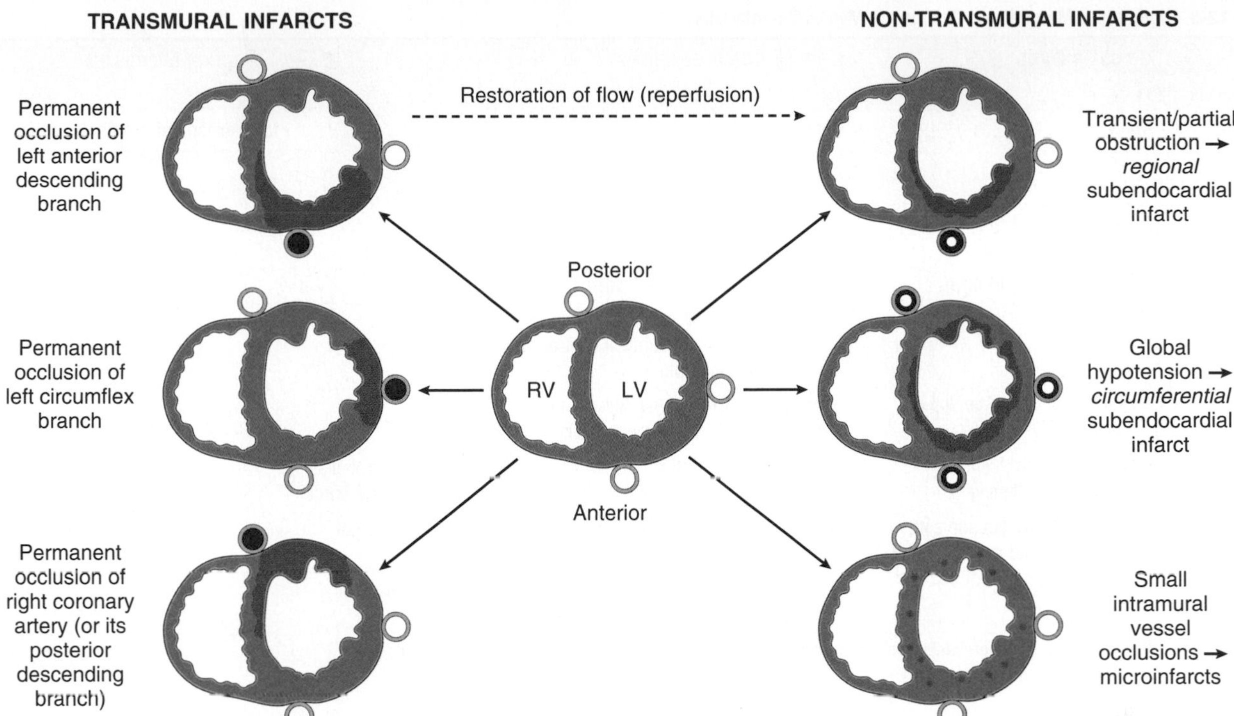

Figure 12-12 Distribution of myocardial ischemic necrosis correlates with the location and nature of decreased perfusion. *Left,* The positions of transmural acute infarcts resulting from occlusions of the major coronary arteries; *top to bottom,* left anterior descending, left circumflex, and right coronary arteries. *Right,* The types of infarcts that result from a partial or transient occlusion, global hypotension, or intramural small vessel occlusions.

Patterns of Infarction. The distribution of myocardial necrosis correlates with the location and cause of the decreased perfusion (Fig. 12-12).

- *Transmural infarction.* Myocardial infarcts caused by occlusion of an epicardial vessel (in the absence of any therapeutic intervention) are typically transmural—the necrosis involves virtually the full thickness of the ventricular wall in the distribution of the affected coronary. This pattern of infarction is usually associated with a combination of chronic coronary atherosclerosis, acute plaque change, and superimposed thrombosis (discussed earlier).
- *Subendocardial (nontransmural) infarction.* As the subendocardial zone is normally the least perfused region of myocardium, this area is most vulnerable to any reduction in coronary flow. A subendocardial infarct—typically involving roughly the inner third of the ventricular wall—can occur as a result of a plaque disruption followed by a coronary thrombus that becomes lysed (therapeutically or spontaneously) before myocardial necrosis extends across the full thickness of the wall. Subendocardial infarcts can also result from prolonged, severe reduction in systemic blood pressure, as in shock superimposed on chronic, otherwise noncritical, coronary stenoses. In the subendocardial infarcts that occur as a result of global hypotension, myocardial damage is usually circumferential, rather than being limited to the distribution of a single major coronary artery.
- *Multifocal microinfarction.* This pattern is seen when there is pathology involving only smaller intramural vessels. This may occur in the setting of microembolization, vasculitis, or vascular spasm, for example, due to endogenous catechols (epinephrine) or drugs (cocaine or ephedrine). Elevated levels of catechols also increase heart rate and myocardial contractility, exacerbating ischemia caused by the vasospasm. The outcome of such vasospasm can be sudden cardiac death (usually caused by a fatal arrhythmia) or an ischemic dilated cardiomyopathy, so-called *takotsubo cardiomyopathy* (also called "broken heart syndrome" because of the association with emotional duress).

Owing to the characteristic electrocardiographic changes resulting from myocardial ischemia or necrosis in various distributions, a transmural infarct is sometimes referred to as an "ST elevation myocardial infarct" (STEMI) and a subendocardial infarct as a "non–ST elevation infarct" (NSTEMI). Depending on the extent and location of the vascular involvement, microinfarctions show nonspecific changes or can even be electrocardiographically silent.

MORPHOLOGY

The temporal evolution of the morphologic changes in acute MI and subsequent healing are summarized in Table 12-5.

Nearly all transmural infarcts involve at least a portion of the left ventricle (comprising the free wall and ventricular septum) and encompass nearly the entire perfusion zone of the occluded coronary artery save for a narrow rim (approximately 0.1 mm) of preserved subendocardial myocardium that is preserved by diffusion of oxygen and nutrients from the ventricular lumen.

Of MIs caused by a right coronary obstruction, 15% to 30% extend from the posterior free wall of the septal portion of the left ventricle into the adjacent right ventricular wall. Isolated

Table 12-5 Evolution of Morphologic Changes in Myocardial Infarction

Time	Gross Features	Light Microscope	Electron Microscope
Reversible Injury			
0-½ hr	None	None	Relaxation of myofibrils; glycogen loss; mitochondrial swelling
Irreversible Injury			
½-4 hr	None	Usually none; variable waviness of fibers at border	Sarcolemmal disruption; mitochondrial amorphous densities
4-12 hr	Dark mottling (occasional)	Early coagulation necrosis; edema; hemorrhage	
12-24 hr	Dark mottling	Ongoing coagulation necrosis; pyknosis of nuclei; myocyte hypereosinophilia; marginal contraction band necrosis; early neutrophilic infiltrate	
1-3 days	Mottling with yellow-tan infarct center	Coagulation necrosis, with loss of nuclei and striations; brisk interstitial infiltrate of neutrophils	
3-7 days	Hyperemic border; central yellow-tan softening	Beginning disintegration of dead myofibers, with dying neutrophils; early phagocytosis of dead cells by macrophages at infarct border	
7-10 days	Maximally yellow-tan and soft, with depressed red-tan margins	Well-developed phagocytosis of dead cells; granulation tissue at margins	
10-14 days	Red-gray depressed infarct borders	Well-established granulation tissue with new blood vessels and collagen deposition	
2-8 wk	Gray-white scar, progressive from border toward core of infarct	Increased collagen deposition, with decreased cellularity	
>2 mo	Scarring complete	Dense collagenous scar	

infarction of the right ventricle is unusual (only 1% to 3% of cases), as is infarction of the atria.

The frequencies of involvement of each of the three main arterial trunks and the corresponding sites of myocardial lesions resulting in infarction (in the typical right dominant heart) are as follows (Fig. 12-12*A*):

- Left anterior descending coronary artery (40% to 50%): infarcts involving the anterior wall of left ventricle near the apex; the anterior portion of ventricular septum; and the apex circumferentially
- Right coronary artery (30% to 40%): infarcts involving the inferior/posterior wall of left ventricle; posterior portion of ventricular septum; and the inferior/posterior right ventricular free wall in some cases
- Left circumflex coronary artery (15% to 20%): infarcts involving the lateral wall of left ventricle except at the apex

Other locations of critical coronary arterial lesions causing infarcts are sometimes encountered, such as the left main coronary artery, the secondary (diagonal) branches of the left anterior descending coronary artery, or the marginal branches of the left circumflex coronary artery.

The gross and microscopic appearance of an infarct depends on the duration of survival of the patient following the MI. Areas of damage undergo a progressive sequence of morphologic changes involving typical ischemic coagulative necrosis (the predominant mechanism of cell death in MI, although apoptosis may also occur), followed by inflammation and repair that closely parallels responses to injury in other tissues.

Early morphologic recognition of acute MI can be difficult, particularly when death occurs within a few hours of the onset of symptoms. MIs less than 12 hours old are usually not apparent on gross examination. However, if the infarct preceded death by 2 to 3 hours, it is possible to highlight the area of necrosis by immersion of tissue slices in a solution of **triphenyltetrazolium chloride**. This gross histochemical stain imparts a brick-red color to intact, noninfarcted myocardium where lactate dehydrogenase activity is preserved. Because dehydrogenases leak out through the damaged membranes of dead cells, an infarct appears as an unstained pale zone (Fig. 12-13). By 12 to 24 hours after infarction, an MI can usually be identified grossly as a reddish-blue area of discoloration caused by stagnated, trapped blood. Thereafter, the infarct becomes

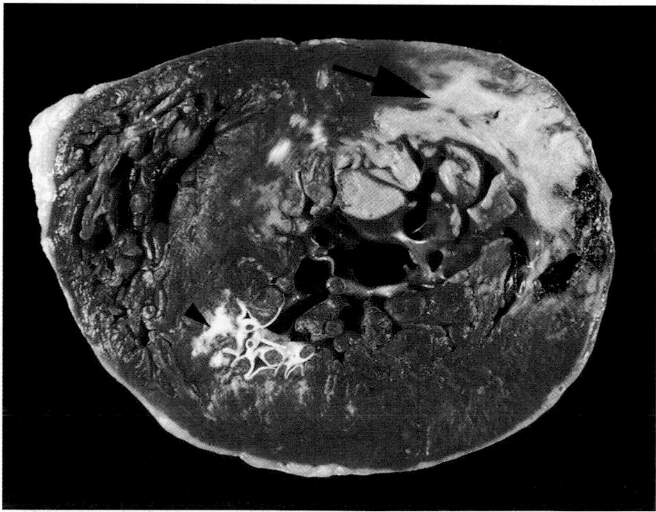

Figure 12-13 Acute myocardial infarct, predominantly of the posterolateral left ventricle, demonstrated histochemically by a lack of staining by triphenyltetrazolium chloride in areas of necrosis *(arrow)*. The staining defect is due to the lactate dehydrogenase leakage that follows cell death. Note the myocardial hemorrhage at one edge of the infarct that was associated with cardiac rupture, and the anterior scar *(arrowhead)*, indicative of old infarct. Specimen is oriented with the posterior wall at the top.

progressively more sharply defined, yellow-tan, and soft. By 10 days to 2 weeks, it is rimmed by a hyperemic zone of highly vascularized granulation tissue. Over the succeeding weeks, the injured region evolves to a fibrous scar.

The histopathologic changes also proceed in a fairly predictable sequence (Fig. 12-14). The typical changes of coagulative necrosis become detectable in the first 6 to 12 hours. "Wavy fibers" may be present at the periphery of the infarct; these changes probably result from the forceful systolic tugs of the viable fibers on immediately adjacent, noncontractile dead fibers, causing stretching and folding. An additional sublethal ischemic change may be seen in the margins of infarcts: so-called myocyte vacuolization or **myocytolysis**, which reflects intracellular accumulations of salt and water within the sarcoplasmic reticulum. The necrotic muscle elicits acute inflammation (most prominent between 1 and 3 days). Thereafter, macrophages remove the necrotic myocytes (most noticeable by 3 to 7 days), and the damaged zone is progressively replaced by the ingrowth of highly vascularized granulation tissue (most prominent at 1 to 2 weeks); as healing progresses, this is replaced by fibrous tissue. In most instances, scarring is well advanced by the end of the sixth week, but the efficiency of repair depends on the size of the original lesion, as well as the relative metabolic and inflammatory state of the host.

Since healing requires the participation of inflammatory cells, immune suppression (e.g., due to steroids) can impair the vigor of the healing response. Moreover, delivering inflammatory cells to the site of necrosis requires intact vasculature; since blood vessels often survive only at the edges of an infarct, MIs typically heal from the margins toward the center. Consequently, a large infarct may not heal as quickly or as completely as a small one. A healing infarct can also appear nonuniform, with the most advanced healing at the periphery. Once a lesion is completely healed, it is impossible to determine its age (i.e., the dense fibrous scar of 8-week-old and 10-year-old infarcts looks virtually identical).

The following discussion considers the changes that result from interventions that can limit infarct size by salvaging myocardium that is not yet necrotic.

Infarct Modification by Reperfusion. **Reperfusion is the restoration of blood flow to ischemic myocardium threatened by infarction; the goal is to salvage cardiac muscle at risk and limit infarct size.** The cardiology adage that *"time is myocardium"* succinctly captures the impetus to intervene promptly once ongoing infarction is diagnosed; patient outcome materially worsens with progressively larger infarcts. Not only does reperfusion improve short- and long-term survival, but it also impacts short- and long-term myocardial function. Thus, prompt reperfusion is the preeminent objective for treatment of patients with MI. This can be accomplished by a host of coronary interventions, that is, thrombolysis, angioplasty, stent placement, or coronary artery bypass graft [CABG] surgery. The goal is to dissolve, mechanically alter, or bypass the lesion that precipitated the acute infarction. The benefits of reperfusion correlate with (1) the rapidity of reestablishing

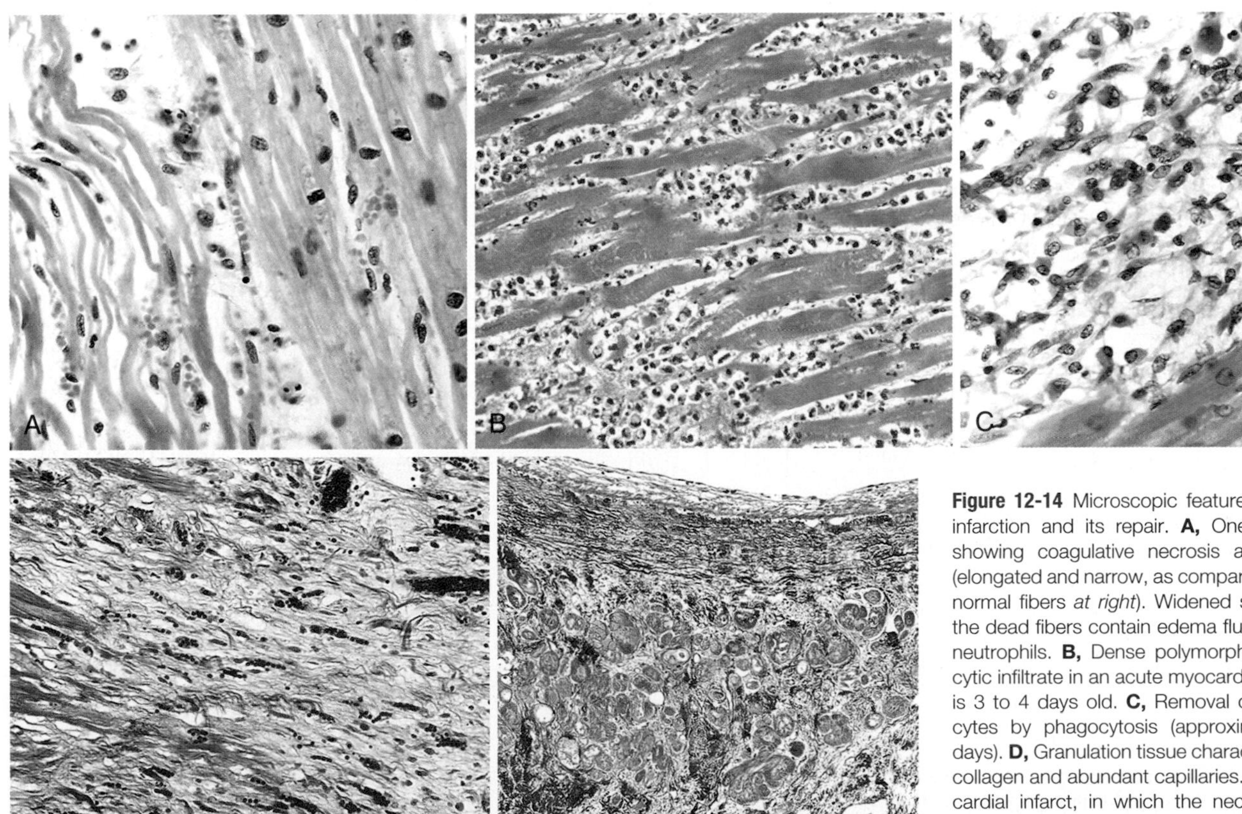

Figure 12-14 Microscopic features of myocardial infarction and its repair. **A,** One-day-old infarct showing coagulative necrosis and wavy fibers (elongated and narrow, as compared with adjacent normal fibers *at right*). Widened spaces between the dead fibers contain edema fluid and scattered neutrophils. **B,** Dense polymorphonuclear leukocytic infiltrate in an acute myocardial infarction that is 3 to 4 days old. **C,** Removal of necrotic myocytes by phagocytosis (approximately 7 to 10 days). **D,** Granulation tissue characterized by loose collagen and abundant capillaries. **E,** Healed myocardial infarct, in which the necrotic tissue has been replaced by a dense collagenous scar. The residual cardiac muscle cells show evidence of compensatory hypertrophy.

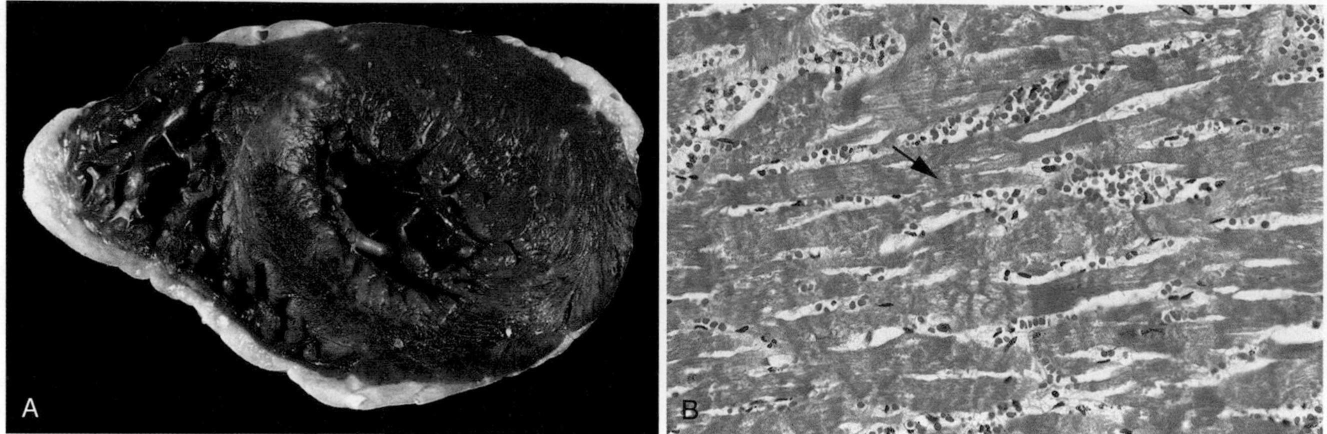

Figure 12-15 Consequences of myocardial ischemia followed by reperfusion. Gross **(A)** and microscopic **(B)** appearance of myocardium modified by reperfusion. **A,** Large, densely hemorrhagic, anterior wall acute myocardial infarction in a patient with left anterior descending artery thrombus treated with streptokinase, a fibrinolytic agent (triphenyl tetrazolium chloride-stained heart slice). Specimen oriented with posterior wall at top. **B,** Myocardial necrosis with hemorrhage and contraction bands, visible as dark bands spanning some myofibers *(arrow).*

coronary blood flow (the first 3 to 4 hours following obstruction are critical) and (2) the extent of restoration of blood flow and correction of the underlying causal lesion. Indeed, thrombolysis can remove a thrombus occluding a coronary artery, but does not alter the underlying atherosclerotic plaque that initiated it. In contrast, percutaneous transluminal coronary angioplasty (PTCA) with stent placement not only eliminates a thrombotic occlusion but also relieves some of the original obstruction and instability caused by the underlying disrupted plaque. CABG provides a new conduit for flow bypassing the area of vessel blockage.

The typical appearance of reperfused myocardium is illustrated in Figure 12-15. Reperfused infarcts are usually hemorrhagic because the vasculature is injured during ischemia and there is bleeding after flow is restored. Microscopic examination reveals that irreversibly injured myocytes exhibit *contraction bands,* intensely eosinophilic intracellular "stripes" composed of closely packed sarcomeres. These result from the exaggerated contraction of sarcomeres when perfusion is reestablished, at which time the interior of cells with damaged membranes is exposed to a high concentration of calcium ions from the plasma. Thus, *reperfusion not only salvages reversibly injured cells but also alters the morphology of lethally injured cells.*

The effects of reperfusion on myocardial viability and function are discussed later and summarized in Figure 12-16. Although clearly beneficial, reperfusion can trigger deleterious complications, including arrhythmias as well as damage superimposed on the original ischemia, so-called *reperfusion injury.* This term encompasses various forms of damage that can occur after restoration of flow to "vulnerable" myocardium that is ischemic but not yet irreversibly damaged (Fig. 12-16*B*). As discussed in Chapter 2, reperfusion injury may be mediated by oxidative stress, calcium overload, and inflammatory cells recruited after tissue reperfusion. Reperfusion-induced microvascular injury not only results in hemorrhage but can also cause

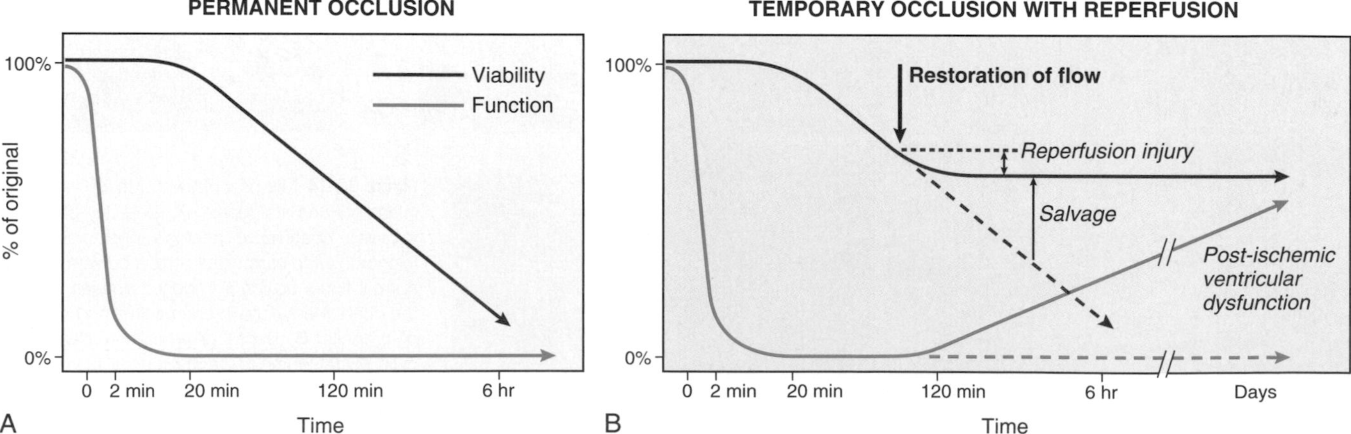

Figure 12-16 Effects of reperfusion on myocardial viability and function. Following coronary occlusion, contractile function is lost within 2 minutes and viability begins to diminish after approximately 20 minutes. If perfusion is not restored (**A**), then nearly all myocardium in the affected region suffers death. **B,** If flow is restored, then some necrosis is prevented, myocardium is salvaged, and at least some function can return. The earlier reperfusion occurs, the greater the degree of salvage. However, the process of reperfusion itself may induce some damage *(reperfusion injury)*, and return of function of salvaged myocardium may be delayed for hours to days *(postischemic ventricular dysfunction* or *stunning).*

endothelial swelling that occludes capillaries and may limit the reperfusion of critically injured myocardium (called *no-reflow*). Although the clinical significance of myocardial reperfusion injury is debated, it has been estimated that up to 50% (or more) of the ultimate infarct size can be attributed to its effects.

Biochemical abnormalities (and their functional consequences) may also persist for days to weeks in reperfused myocytes. Such changes are thought to underlie a phenomenon referred to as *stunned myocardium,* a state of prolonged cardiac failure induced by short-term ischemia that usually recovers after several days. Myocardium that is subjected to chronic, sublethal ischemia may also enter into a state of lowered metabolism and function called *hibernation*. Subsequent revascularization (e.g., by CABG surgery, angioplasty, or stenting) often restores normal function to such hibernating myocardium.

Clinical Features. **MI is diagnosed by clinical symptoms, laboratory tests for the presence of myocardial proteins in the plasma, and characteristic electrocardiographic changes.** Patients with MI classically present with prolonged (more than 30 minutes) chest pain described as crushing, stabbing, or squeezing, associated with a rapid, weak pulse; profuse sweating (diaphoresis), and nausea and vomiting are common, and can suggest involvement of the posterior-inferior ventricle with secondary vagal stimulation. Dyspnea due to impaired contractility of the ischemic myocardium and the resultant pulmonary congestion and edema is a frequent symptom. However, in as many as 25% of patients the onset is entirely asymptomatic (e.g., in the setting of diabetic neuropathy) and the disease is discovered only by electrocardiographic changes or laboratory tests that show evidence of myocardial damage (see later).

The laboratory evaluation of MI is based on measuring the blood levels of proteins that leak out of irreversibly damaged myocytes; the most useful of these molecules are cardiac-specific troponins T and I (cTnT and cTnI), and the MB fraction of creatine kinase (CK-MB) (Fig. 12-17). The diagnosis of myocardial injury is established when blood levels of these cardiac biomarkers are elevated. The rate of appearance of these markers in the peripheral circulation depends on several factors, including their intracellular location and molecular weight, the blood flow and lymphatic drainage in the area of the infarct, and the rate of elimination of the marker from the blood.

The most sensitive and specific biomarkers of myocardial damage are cardiac-specific proteins, particularly cTnT and cTnI (proteins that regulate calcium-mediated contraction of cardiac and skeletal muscle). *Troponins I* and *T* are not normally detectable in the circulation. Following an MI, levels of both begin to rise at 3-12 hours; cTnT levels peak somewhere between 12-48 hours while cTnI levels are maximal at 24 hours. *Creatine kinase* is an enzyme expressed in brain, myocardium, and skeletal muscle; it is a dimer composed of two isoforms designated "M" and "B." While MM homodimers are found predominantly in cardiac and skeletal muscle, and BB homodimers in brain, lung, and many other tissues, MB heterodimers are principally localized to cardiac muscle (with considerably lesser amounts found in skeletal muscle). Thus, the MB form of creatine kinase (CK-MB) is sensitive but not specific, since it can also be elevated after skeletal muscle injury. CK-MB begins to rise within 3 to 12 hours of the onset of MI, peaks at about 24 hours, and returns to normal within approximately 48 to 72 hours.

To summarize:

- Time to elevation of CKMB, cTnT and cTnI is 3 to 12 hrs
- CK-MB and cTnI peak at 24 hours
- CK-MB returns to normal in 48-72 hrs, cTnI in 5-10 days, and cTnT in 5 to 14 days

Consequences and Complications of Myocardial Infarction. Extraordinary progress has been made in the treatment of patients with acute MI. Concurrent with the decrease in the overall mortality of IHD since the 1960s,

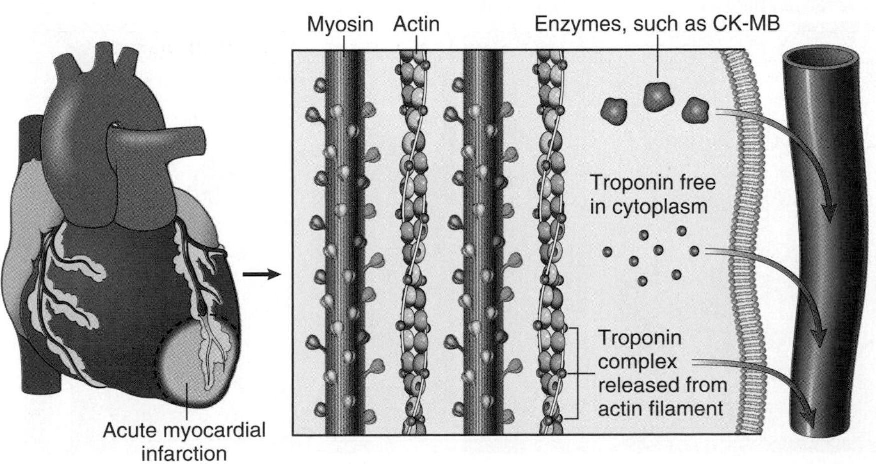

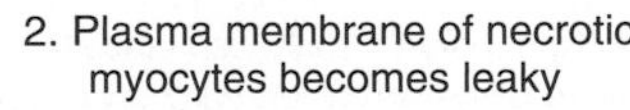

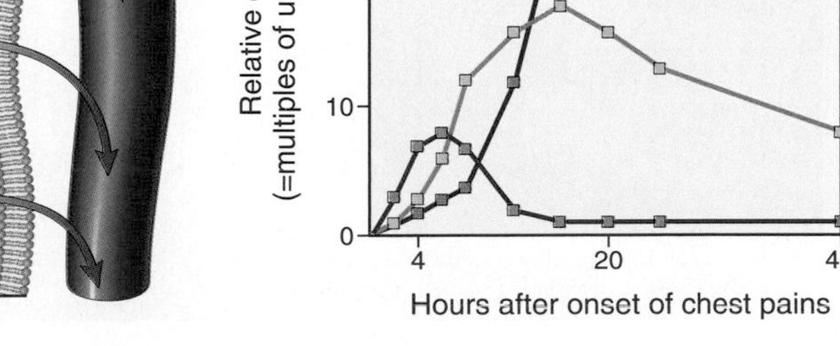

Figure 12-17 Release of myocyte proteins in myocardial infarction. Some of these proteins, for example, troponin I or troponin T, and creatine kinase, MB fraction (CK-MB) are routinely used as diagnostic biomarkers.

the in-hospital death rate has declined from around 30% to approximately 5% in patients receiving timely therapy. Factors associated with a poorer prognosis include advanced age, female gender, diabetes mellitus, and—due to the cumulative loss of functional myocardium—previous MI. Half of the deaths associated with acute MI occur within 1 hour of onset, most commonly due to a fatal arrhythmia; most of these individuals never reach the hospital. MI therapeutic interventions include:

- Morphine to relieve pain and improve dyspneic symptoms
- Prompt reperfusion to salvage myocardium
- Antiplatelet agents such as aspirin, P2Y12 receptor inhibitors, and GPIIb/IIIa inhibitors
- Anticoagulant therapy with unfractionated heparin, low-molecular-weight heparin, direct thrombin inhibitors, and/or factor Xa inhibitors to prevent coronary artery clot propagation
- Nitrates to induce vasodilation and reverse vasospasm
- Beta blockers to decrease myocardial oxygen demand and to reduce risk of arrhythmias
- Antiarrhythmics to manage arrhythmias
- Angiotensin-converting enzyme (ACE) inhibitors to limit ventricular dilation
- Oxygen supplementation to improve blood oxygen saturation

Despite these interventions, many patients have one or more complications following acute MI (Fig. 12-18):

- *Contractile dysfunction.* Myocardial infarcts produce abnormalities in left ventricular function roughly proportional to their size. There is usually some degree of left ventricular failure with hypotension, pulmonary vascular congestion, and interstitial pulmonary transudates, which can progress to pulmonary edema and respiratory impairment. Severe "pump failure" *(cardiogenic shock)* occurs in 10% to 15% of patients following acute MI, generally with large infarcts involving more than 40% of the left ventricle. Cardiogenic shock has a nearly 70% mortality rate; it accounts for two thirds of in-hospital deaths in those patients admitted for MI.

  Right ventricular infarcts can cause right-sided heart failure associated with pooling of blood in the venous circulation and systemic hypotension.

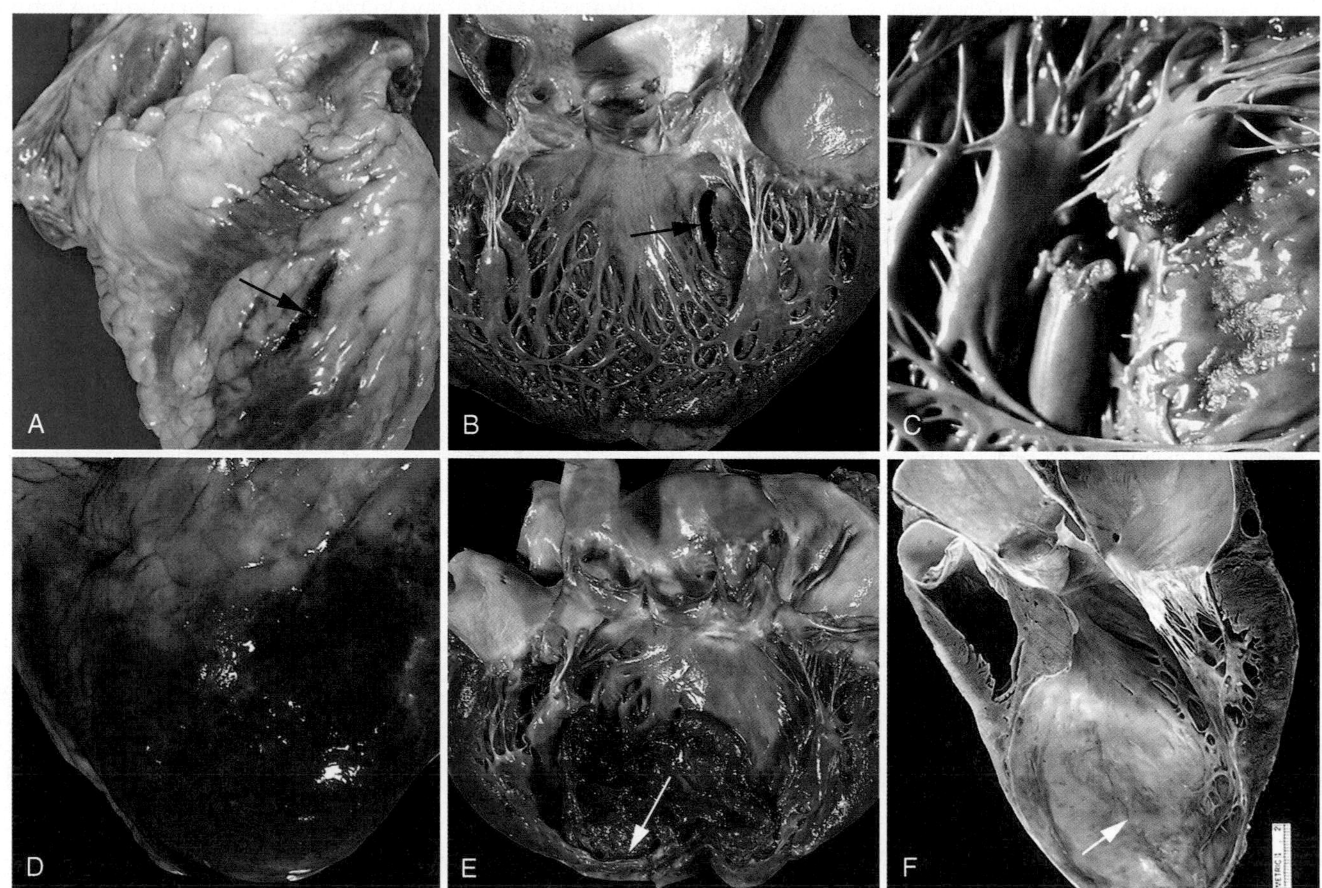

Figure 12-18 Complications of myocardial infarction. **A,** Anterior myocardial rupture in an acute infarct *(arrow).* **B,** Rupture of the ventricular septum *(arrow).* **C,** Complete rupture of a necrotic papillary muscle. **D,** Fibrinous pericarditis, showing a dark, roughened epicardial surface overlying an acute infarct. **E,** Early expansion of anteroapical infarct with wall thinning *(arrow)* and mural thrombus. **F,** Large apical left ventricular aneurysm. The left ventricle is on the right in this apical four-chamber view of the heart. (**A-E,** Reproduced with permission from Schoen FJ: Interventional and Surgical Cardiovascular Pathology: Clinical Correlations and Basic Principles. Philadelphia, WB Saunders, 1989; **F,** Courtesy William D. Edwards, MD, Mayo Clinic, Rochester, Minn.)

- *Arrhythmias.* Many patients have *myocardial irritability* and/or conduction disturbances following MI that lead to potentially fatal arrhythmias. MI-associated arrhythmias include sinus bradycardia, atrial fibrillation, heart block, tachycardia, ventricular premature contractions, ventricular tachycardia, and ventricular fibrillation. Because of the location of portions of the atrioventricular conduction system (bundle of His) in the inferoseptal myocardium, infarcts involving this site can also be associated with heart block (see also the discussion concerning arrhythmias).
- *Myocardial rupture.* The various forms of cardiac rupture typically occur when there is transmural necrosis of a ventricle. These include:
  - Rupture of the ventricular free wall (most common), with hemopericardium and cardiac tamponade (Fig. 12-18*A*)
  - Rupture of the ventricular septum (less common), leading to an *acute VSD* and left-to-right shunting (Fig. 12-18*B*)
  - Papillary muscle rupture (least common), resulting in the acute onset of severe mitral regurgitation (Fig. 12-18*C*)

  Free-wall rupture occurs most frequently 2 to 4 days after MI, when coagulative necrosis, neutrophilic infiltration, and lysis of the myocardial connective tissue have appreciably weakened the infarcted myocardium; the anterolateral wall at the mid-ventricular level is the most common site. Risk factors for free-wall rupture include age older than 60, first MI, large, transmural and anterior MI, absence of left ventricular hypertrophy, and preexisting hypertension. Ventricular rupture occurs less frequently in patients with prior MI because associated fibrotic scarring tends to inhibit myocardial tearing. While acute free-wall ruptures are usually rapidly fatal, a fortuitously located pericardial adhesion can abort a rupture and result in a *false aneurysm* (localized hematoma communicating with the ventricular cavity). The wall of a false aneurysm consists only of epicardium and adherent parietal pericardium and thus many still ultimately rupture.
- *Ventricular aneurysm.* In contrast to the *false aneurysms* mentioned earlier, *true aneurysms* of the ventricular wall are bounded by myocardium that has become scarred. Aneurysms of the ventricular wall are a late complication of large transmural infarcts that experience early expansion. The thin scar tissue wall of an aneurysm paradoxically bulges during systole (Fig. 12-18*F*). Complications of ventricular aneurysms include mural thrombus, arrhythmias, and heart failure; rupture of the tough fibrotic wall does not usually occur.
- *Pericarditis.* A fibrinous or fibrinohemorrhagic pericarditis usually develops about the second or third day following a transmural infarct as a result of underlying myocardial inflammation (*Dressler syndrome*; Fig. 12-18*D*).
- Infarct *expansion.* As a result of the weakening of necrotic muscle, there may be disproportionate stretching, thinning, and dilation of the infarct region (especially with anteroseptal infarcts), which is often associated with mural thrombus (Fig. 12-18*E*).
- *Mural thrombus.* With any infarct, the combination of a local abnormality in contractility (causing stasis) and endocardial damage (creating a thrombogenic surface) can foster *mural thrombosis* and potentially *thromboembolism.*
- *Papillary muscle dysfunction.* Although papillary muscle rupture after an MI may certainly result in precipitous onset of mitral (or tricuspid) valve incompetence, most post-infarct regurgitation results from ischemic dysfunction of a papillary muscle (and underlying myocardium), or later from ventricular dilation or from papillary muscle fibrosis and shortening.
- *Progressive late heart failure* (chronic IHD) is discussed later.

The risk of postinfarct complications and the prognosis of the patient depend primarily on the infarct size, location, and fraction of the wall thickness involved (subendocardial or transmural). Thus, large transmural infarcts yield a higher probability of cardiogenic shock, arrhythmias, and late CHF. Patients with anterior transmural infarcts are at greatest risk for free-wall rupture, expansion, mural thrombi, and aneurysm. In contrast, posterior transmural infarcts are more likely to be complicated by conduction blocks, right ventricular involvement, or both; when acute VSDs occur in this area they are more difficult to manage. Moreover, female gender, age older than 70 years, diabetes mellitus and previous MI are poor prognostic factors in patients with ST elevation myocardial infarcts. With subendocardial infarcts, only rarely do pericarditis, rupture, and aneurysms occur.

In addition to the sequence of repair in the infarcted tissues described earlier, the noninfarcted segments of the ventricle undergo hypertrophy and dilation; collectively, these changes are termed *ventricular remodeling.* The compensatory hypertrophy of noninfarcted myocardium is initially hemodynamically beneficial. However, this adaptive effect may be overwhelmed by ventricular dilation (with or without ventricular aneurysm) and increased oxygen demand, which can exacerbate ischemia and depress cardiac function. There may also be changes in ventricular shape and stiffening of the ventricle due to scar formation and hypertrophy that further diminish cardiac output. Some of these deleterious effects appear to be reduced by ACE inhibitors, which lessen the ventricular remodeling that can occurs after infarction.

Long-term prognosis after MI depends on many factors, the most important of which are the residual left ventricular function and the extent of any vascular obstructions in vessels that perfuse the remaining viable myocardium. The overall total mortality within the first year can be as high as 30%; thereafter, each passing year is associated with an additional 3% to 4% mortality among survivors. Infarct prevention (through control of risk factors) in individuals who have never experienced MI *(primary prevention)* and prevention of reinfarction in MI survivors *(secondary prevention)* are important strategies that have received much attention and achieved considerable success.

The relationship of the causes, pathophysiology, and consequences of MI are summarized in Figure 12-19, including the possible outcomes of chronic IHD and sudden death, discussed below.

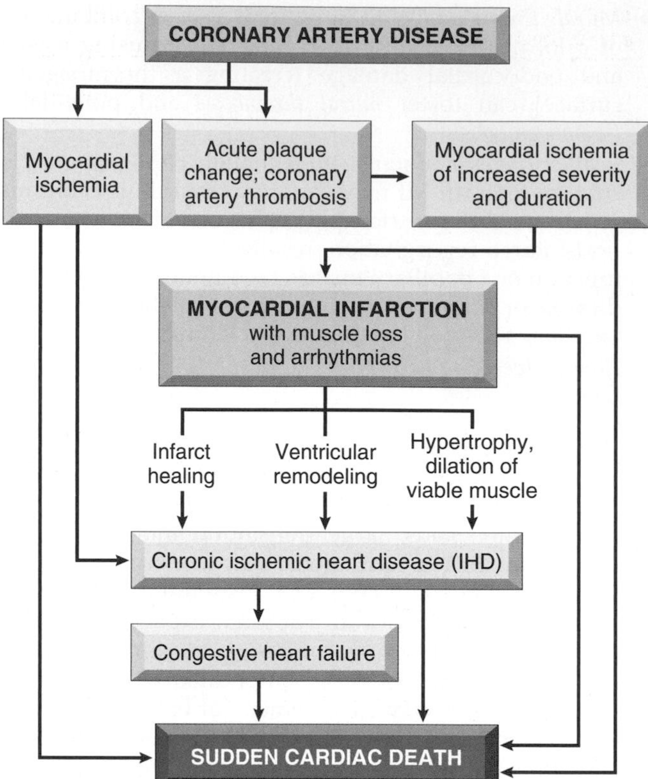

Figure 12-19 Schematic for the causes and outcomes of ischemic heart disease (IHD), showing the interrelationships among coronary artery disease, acute plaque change, myocardial ischemia, myocardial infarction, chronic IHD, congestive heart failure, and sudden cardiac death.

Chronic Ischemic Heart Disease

The designation chronic IHD (often called *ischemic cardiomyopathy* by clinicians) is used here to describe progressive congestive heart failure as a consequence of accumulated ischemic myocardial damage and/or inadequate compensatory responses. In most instances there has been prior MI and sometimes previous coronary arterial interventions and/or bypass surgery. Chronic IHD usually appears postinfarction due to the functional decompensation of hypertrophied noninfarcted myocardium (see earlier discussion of cardiac hypertrophy). However, in other cases severe obstructive coronary artery disease may present as chronic congestive heart failure in the absence of prior infarction. Patients with chronic IHD account for almost 50% of cardiac transplant recipients.

MORPHOLOGY

Hearts from patients with chronic IHD have cardiomegaly, with left ventricular hypertrophy and dilation. Invariably there is some degree of stenotic coronary atherosclerosis. Discrete scars representing healed infarcts are usually present. The mural endocardium often has patchy fibrous thickenings (due to abnormal wall shear forces), and mural thrombi may be present. Microscopic findings include myocardial hypertrophy, diffuse subendocardial vacuolization, and fibrosis.

KEY CONCEPTS

Ischemic Heart Disease

- The vast majority of ischemic heart disease is due to coronary artery atherosclerosis; vasospasm, vasculitis, or embolism are less common causes.
- Cardiac ischemia results from a mismatch in coronary supply and myocardial demand, and presents as different, albeit overlapping syndromes:
  - *Angina pectoris* is chest pain due to inadequate perfusion, and is typically due to atherosclerotic disease with greater than 70% fixed stenosis (so-called critical stenosis).
  - *Unstable angina* results from a small fissure or rupture of atherosclerotic plaque triggering platelet aggregation, vasoconstriction, and formation of a mural thrombus that need not necessarily be occlusive.
  - *Acute myocardial infarction* typically results from acute thromboses after plaque disruption; most occur in plaques that did not previously exhibit critical stenosis.
  - *Sudden cardiac death* usually results from a fatal arrhythmia, typically without significant acute myocardial damage.
  - *Chronic ischemic heart disease* is progressive heart failure due to ischemic injury, either from prior infarctions or chronic low-grade ischemia.
- Myocardial ischemia leads to loss of function within 1 to 2 minutes, but causes necrosis only after 20 to 40 minutes. Myocardial infarction is diagnosed based on symptoms, electrocardiographic changes, and measurement of serum CK-MB and troponins. Gross and histologic changes of infarction require hours to days to develop.
- Infarction can be modified by therapeutic intervention (e.g., thrombolysis or stenting), which salvages myocardium at risk, but potentially induces reperfusion-related injury.
- Complications of infarction include: ventricular rupture, papillary muscle rupture, aneurysm formation, mural thrombus, arrhythmia, pericarditis, and CHF.

Arrhythmias

Abnormalities in myocardial conduction can be sustained or sporadic *(paroxysmal)*. Aberrant rhythms can be initiated anywhere in the conduction system, from SA node down to the level of an individual myocyte; they are typically designated as originating from the atrium *(supraventricular)* or within the ventricular myocardium. Arrhythmias can manifest as *tachycardia* (fast heart rate), *bradycardia* (slow heart rate), an irregular rhythm with normal ventricular contraction, chaotic depolarization without functional ventricular contraction (*ventricular fibrillation*), or no electrical activity at all *(asystole)*. Patients may be unaware of a rhythm disorder, or may note a "racing heart" or *palpitations* (irregular rhythm); loss of adequate cardiac output due to sustained arrhythmia can produce light-headedness (near syncope), loss of consciousness *(syncope),* or *sudden cardiac death* (see later)

Ischemic injury is the most common cause of rhythm disorders, either through direct damage, or through the dilation of heart chambers that alters conduction system firing.

- If the SA node is damaged (e.g., *sick sinus syndrome*), other fibers or even the AV node can take over pacemaker function, albeit at a much slower intrinsic rate (causing bradycardia).
- If the atrial myocytes become "irritable" and depolarize independently and sporadically (as occurs with atrial dilation), the signals are variably transmitted through the AV node leading to the random "irregularly irregular" heart rate of *atrial fibrillation*.
- If the AV node is dysfunctional, varying degrees of *heart block* occur, ranging from simple prolongation of the P-R interval on the electrocardiogram (ECG; *first degree heart block*), to intermittent transmission of the signal *(second degree heart block)*, to complete failure *(third degree heart block)*.

As already discussed, coordinated cardiac contraction depends on the orderly transmission of electrical currents from myocyte to myocyte via gap junctions. Thus, abnormalities in the structure or spatial distribution of gap junctions, which are seen in a variety of disorders (e.g., IHD and dilated cardiomyopathies), can cause arrhythmias. Ischemia, myocyte hypertrophy, and inflammation (e.g., myocarditis or sarcoidosis) also promote increased "irritability" that leads to spontaneous aberrant myocyte depolarization; because of the electrical interconnection of myocytes, such random events can cause inappropriate firing of adjacent cells and create abnormal electrical circuits (so-called reentry circuits) that lead to *ventricular tachycardia*, which may progress to fatal ventricular fibrillation. Likewise, deposition of nonconducting material (e.g., amyloid), and even small areas of fibrosis, can disrupt myocyte-to-myocyte signaling, again sowing the seeds for development of reentry circuits that can give rise to potentially fatal arrythmias.

Heritable conditions associated with arrhythmias are important to recognize, since they may alert physicians to the need for intervention to prevent sudden cardiac death (discussed later) in the proband and their family members. Some of these disorders are associated with recognizable anatomic abnormalities (e.g., congenital anomalies, hypertrophic cardiomyopathy, mitral valve prolapse). However, other heritable disorders precipitate arrythmias and sudden death in the absence of structural cardiac pathology (so-called primary electrical disorders). These syndromes can only be diagnosed by genetic testing, which is performed in those with a positive family history or an unexplained nonlethal arrhythmia.

The primary electrical abnormalities of the heart that predispose to arrhythmias are listed in Table 12-6. The most important of these are the so-called *channelopathies*, which are caused by mutations in genes that are required for normal ion channel function. These disorders (mostly with autosomal dominant inheritance) either involve genes that encode the structural components of ion channels (including Na^+, K^+, and Ca^+ channels), or accessory proteins that are essential for normal channel function. Ion channels are responsible for conducting the electrical currents that mediate contraction of the heart, and it is thus not surprising that defects in these channels may provoke arrythmias. The prototype is the *long QT syndrome*, characterized by prolongation of the QT segment in ECGs and susceptibility to malignant ventricular arrhythmias. Ion channels are needed for the normal function of many tissues, and certain channelopathies are also associated with skeletal muscle disorders and diabetes. Nevertheless, the most common channelopathies are isolated disorders of the heart, and their most feared consequence is sudden cardiac death (discussed below).

Table 12-6 Selected Examples of Causal Genes in Inherited Arrhythmogenic Diseases*

Disorder	Gene	Function
Long QT syndrome†	*KCNQ1*	K^+ channel (LOF)
	KCNH2	K^+ channel (LOF)
	SCN5A	Na^+ channel (GOF)
	CAV3	Caveolin, Na^+ current (GOF)
Short QT syndrome†	*KCNQ1*	K^+ channel (GOF)
	KCNH2	K^+ channel (GOF)
Brugada syndrome†	*SCN5A*	Na^+ channel (LOF)
	CACNB2b	Ca^{++} channel (LOF)
	SCN1b	Na^+ channel (LOF)*
CPVT syndrome†	*RYR2*	Diastolic Ca^{++} release (GOF)
	CASQ2	Diastolic Ca^{++} release (LOF)

*Different mutations can cause the same general syndrome and mutations in some genes can cause multiple different phenotypes; thus, loss of function (LOF) mutations may cause long QT intervals, whereas gain of function (GOF) mutations result in short repolarization intervals.

†**Long QT syndrome** manifests as arrhythmias associated with excessive prolongation of the cardiac repolarization; patients often present with stress-induced syncope or sudden cardiac death (SCD), and some forms are associated with swimming. **Short QT syndrome** patients have arrhythmias associated with abbreviated repolarization intervals; they can present with palpitations, syncope, and SCD. **Brugada syndrome** manifests as ECG abnormalities (ST segment elevations and right bundle branch block) in the absence of structural heart disease; patients classically present with syncope or SCD during rest or sleep, or after large meals. **CPVT** does not have characteristic ECG changes; patients often present in childhood with life-threatening arrhythmias due to adrenergic stimulation (stress-related).

LOF, Loss of function mutations; GOF, gain of function mutations; CPVT, catecholaminergic polymorphic ventricular tachycardia.

Modified from Cerrone M , Priori SG: Genetics of sudden death: focus on inherited channelopathies. Eur Heart J, 2011:32, 2109-2118.

Sudden Cardiac Death (SCD)

SCD is most commonly defined as unexpected death from cardiac causes either without symptoms, or within 1 to 24 hours of symptom onset (different authors use different criteria); this happens in some 300,000 to 400,000 individuals each year in the United States alone. Coronary artery disease is the leading cause of SCD, responsible for 80% to 90% of cases; unfortunately, SCD is often the first manifestation of IHD. Interestingly, there is typically only chronic severe atherosclerotic disease; acute plaque disruption is found in only 10% to 20% of cases. Healed remote MIs are present in about 40%.

With younger victims, other nonatherosclerotic causes are more common etiologies for SCD:

- Hereditary or acquired abnormalities of the cardiac conduction system
- Congenital coronary arterial abnormalities
- Mitral valve prolapse
- Myocarditis or sarcoidosis
- Dilated or hypertrophic cardiomyopathy
- Pulmonary hypertension
- Myocardial hypertrophy. Increased cardiac mass is an independent risk factor for SCD; thus, some young individuals who die suddenly—including athletes—have

hypertensive hypertrophy or unexplained increased cardiac mass as the only finding.

- Other miscellaneous causes, such as pericardial tamponade, pulmonary embolism, systemic metabolic and hemodynamic alterations, catecholamines, and drugs of abuse, particularly cocaine and methamphetamine.

The mechanism of SCD is most often a lethal arrhythmia (e.g., asystole or ventricular fibrillation). Notably, infarction need not occur; 80% to 90% of patients who suffer SCD but are successfully resuscitated do not show any enzymatic or ECG evidence of myocardial necrosis—even when the original cause was ischemic heart disease. Although ischemic injury (and other pathologies) can directly affect the major components of the conduction system, most cases of fatal arrhythmia are triggered by electrical irritability of myocardium distant from the major elements of the conduction system.

The prognosis of patients vulnerable to SCD is markedly improved by pharmaceutical intervention, and particularly by implantation of automatic cardioverter defibrillators that can sense and electrically counteract episodes of ventricular fibrillation.

MORPHOLOGY

Marked coronary atherosclerosis with a critical (>75% cross-sectional area) stenosis involving one or more of the three major vessels is present in 80% to 90% of SCD victims; only 10% to 20% of cases are of nonatherosclerotic origin. Usually there are high-grade stenoses (>90% of area); in approximately one half, acute plaque disruption is observed, and in approximately 25% diagnostic changes of acute MI are seen. This suggests that many patients who die suddenly are suffering an MI, but the short interval from onset to death precludes the development of diagnostic myocardial changes. However, in one study of those who had been successfully resuscitated from a sudden cardiac arrest, a new MI occurred in only 39% of the patients. Thus, most SCD is not associated with acute MI; most of these deaths are thought to result from myocardial ischemia-induced irritability that initiates malignant ventricular arrhythmias. Scars of previous infarcts and subendocardial myocyte vacuolization indicative of severe chronic ischemia are common in such patients.

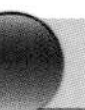

KEY CONCEPTS

Arrhythmias

- Arrhythmias can be caused by ischemic or structural changes in the conduction system or by intrinsic myocyte electrical instability. In structurally normal hearts, arrhythmias are more often due to mutations in ion channels that cause aberrant repolarization or depolarization.
- SCD typically results from ventricular fibrillation, and is most frequently a consequence of coronary artery disease. Myocardial irritability typically results from nonlethal ischemia or from preexisting fibrosis from previous myocardial injury. SCD is less often due to acute plaque rupture with thrombosis that induces a rapidly fatal arrhythmia.

Hypertensive Heart Disease

Hypertensive heart disease (HHD) is a consequence of the increased demands placed on the heart by hypertension, causing pressure overload and ventricular hypertrophy. Although most commonly seen in the left heart as the result of systemic hypertension, pulmonary hypertension can cause right-sided HHD, or *cor pulmonale.*

Systemic (Left-Sided) Hypertensive Heart Disease

Hypertrophy of the heart is an adaptive response to the pressure overload of chronic hypertension. However, such compensatory changes may be ultimately maladaptive and can lead to myocardial dysfunction, cardiac dilation, CHF, and in some cases sudden death. *The minimal pathologic criteria for the diagnosis of systemic HHD are the following: (1) left ventricular hypertrophy (usually concentric) in the absence of other cardiovascular pathology and (2) a clinical history or pathologic evidence of hypertension in other organs (e.g., kidney).* The Framingham Study established unequivocally that even mild hypertension (levels only slightly above 140/90 mm Hg)—if sufficiently prolonged—induces left ventricular hypertrophy. Approximately 30% of the population of the United States suffers from hypertension of at least this degree. The pathogenesis of hypertension is discussed in Chapter 11.

MORPHOLOGY

Hypertension induces left ventricular pressure overload hypertrophy, initially without ventricular dilation. As a result, the left ventricular wall thickening increases the weight of the heart disproportionately to the increase in overall cardiac size (Fig. 12-20*A*). The thickness of the left ventricular wall may exceed 2.0 cm, and the heart weight may exceed 500 gm. In time the increased thickness of the left ventricular wall, often associated with increased interstitial connective tissue, imparts a stiffness that impairs diastolic filling, frequently with consequent left atrial enlargement.

Microscopically, the earliest change of systemic HHD is an increase in the transverse diameter of myocytes, which may be difficult to appreciate on routine microscopy. At a more advanced stage variable degrees of cellular and nuclear enlargement become apparent, often accompanied by interstitial fibrosis.

Compensated systemic HHD may be asymptomatic, producing only electrocardiographic or echocardiographic evidence of left ventricular enlargement. In many patients, systemic HHD comes to attention due to new atrial fibrillation induced by left atrial enlargement, or by progressive CHF. Depending on the severity, duration, and underlying basis of the hypertension, and on the adequacy of therapeutic control, the patient may (1) enjoy normal longevity and die of unrelated causes, (2) develop IHD due to both the potentiating effects of hypertension on coronary atherosclerosis and the ischemia induced by increased oxygen demand from the hypertrophic muscle, (3) suffer renal damage or cerebrovascular stroke as direct effects of

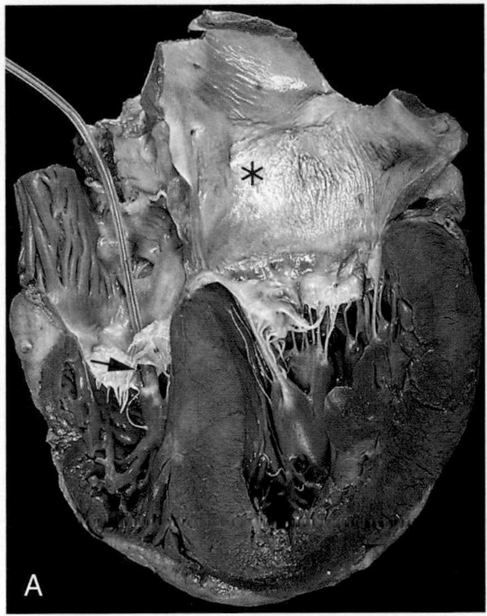

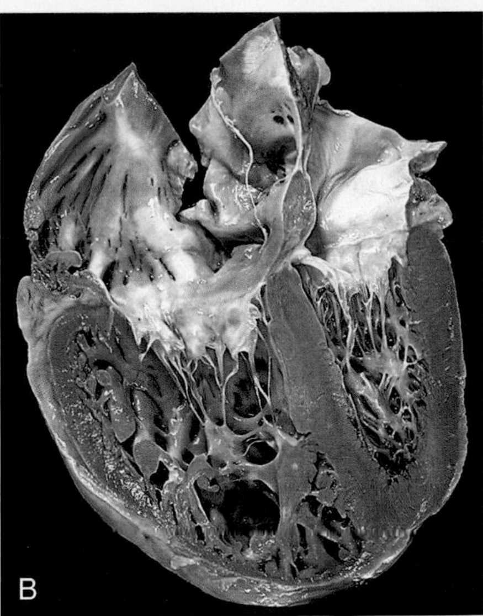

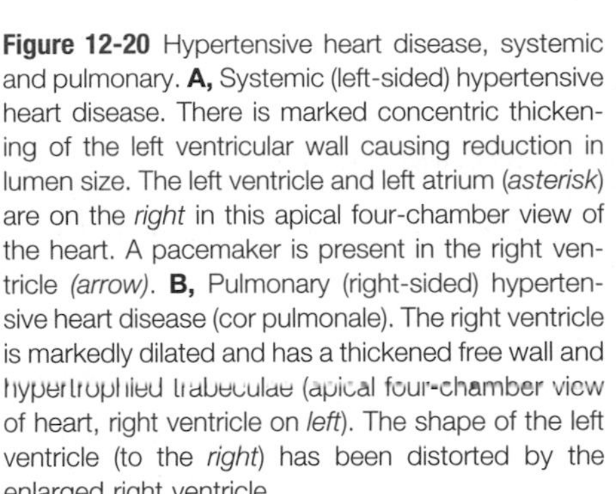
Figure 12-20 Hypertensive heart disease, systemic and pulmonary. **A,** Systemic (left-sided) hypertensive heart disease. There is marked concentric thickening of the left ventricular wall causing reduction in lumen size. The left ventricle and left atrium (*asterisk*) are on the *right* in this apical four-chamber view of the heart. A pacemaker is present in the right ventricle *(arrow)*. **B,** Pulmonary (right-sided) hypertensive heart disease (cor pulmonale). The right ventricle is markedly dilated and has a thickened free wall and hypertrophied trabeculae (apical four-chamber view of heart, right ventricle on *left*). The shape of the left ventricle (to the *right*) has been distorted by the enlarged right ventricle.

hypertension, or (4) experience progressive heart failure or SCD. Effective control of hypertension can prevent cardiac hypertrophy, or can lead to its regression; with normalization of the blood pressure, the associated risks of HHD are diminished.

Pulmonary (Right-Sided) Hypertensive Heart Disease (Cor Pulmonale)

Normally, because the pulmonary vasculature is the low pressure side of the circulation, the right ventricle has a thinner and more compliant wall than the left ventricle. Isolated pulmonary HHD, or *cor pulmonale,* stems from right ventricular pressure overload. Chronic cor pulmonale is characterized by right ventricular hypertrophy, dilation, and potentially right-sided failure. Typical causes of *chronic* cor pulmonale are disorders of the lungs, especially chronic parenchymal diseases such as emphysema, and primary pulmonary hypertension (Table 12-7; see also Chapter 15). *Acute* cor pulmonale can follow massive pulmonary embolism. Nevertheless, it should also be remembered that pulmonary hypertension *most commonly occurs as a complication of left-sided heart disease.*

MORPHOLOGY

In acute cor pulmonale there is marked dilation of the right ventricle without hypertrophy. On cross-section the normal crescent shape of the right ventricle is transformed to a dilated ovoid. In chronic cor pulmonale the right ventricular wall thickens, sometimes up to 1.0 cm or more (Fig. 12-20*B*). More subtle right ventricular hypertrophy may take the form of thickening of the muscle bundles in the outflow tract, immediately below the pulmonary valve, or thickening of the moderator band, the muscle bundle that connects the ventricular septum to the anterior right ventricular papillary muscle. Sometimes, the hypertrophied right ventricle compresses the left ventricular chamber, or leads to regurgitation and fibrous thickening of the tricuspid valve.

Table 12-7 Disorders Predisposing to Cor Pulmonale

Diseases of the Pulmonary Parenchyma
Chronic obstructive pulmonary disease
Diffuse pulmonary interstitial fibrosis
Pneumoconioses
Cystic fibrosis
Bronchiectasis
Diseases of the Pulmonary Vessels
Recurrent pulmonary thromboembolism
Primary pulmonary hypertension
Extensive pulmonary arteritis (e.g., granulomatosis with polyangiitis)
Drug-, toxin-, or radiation-induced vascular obstruction
Extensive pulmonary tumor microembolism
Disorders Affecting Chest Movement
Kyphoscoliosis
Marked obesity (sleep apnea, pickwickian syndrome)
Neuromuscular diseases
Disorders Inducing Pulmonary Arterial Constriction
Metabolic acidosis
Hypoxemia
Chronic altitude sickness
Obstruction of major airways
Idiopathic alveolar hypoventilation

KEY CONCEPTS

Hypertensive Heart Disease

- Hypertensive heart disease can affect either the left ventricle or the right ventricle; the latter is called *cor pulmonale*. Elevated pressures induce myocyte hypertrophy and interstitial fibrosis that increases wall thickness and myocardial stiffness.
- The chronic pressure overload of systemic hypertension causes left ventricular concentric hypertrophy, often associated with left atrial dilation due to impaired diastolic filling of the ventricle. Persistently elevated pressure overload can cause ventricular failure with dilation.
- Cor pulmonale results from pulmonary hypertension due to primary lung parenchymal or vascular disorders. There is commonly right ventricular and right atrial hypertrophy; right ventricular and atrial dilation can occur.

Valvular Heart Disease

Valvular disease can come to clinical attention due to stenosis, insufficiency (synonyms: regurgitation or incompetence), or both. *Stenosis is the failure of a valve to open completely, which impedes forward flow. Insufficiency results from failure of a valve to close completely, thereby allowing reversed flow.* These abnormalities can be present alone or coexist, and may involve only a single valve, or more than one valve. *Functional regurgitation* is used to describe the incompetence of a valve stemming from an abnormality in one of its support structures, as opposed to a primary valve defect. For example, dilation of the right or left ventricle can pull the ventricular papillary muscles down and outward, thereby preventing proper closure of otherwise normal mitral or tricuspid leaflets. Functional mitral valve regurgitation is particularly common and clinically important in IHD, as well as in dilated cardiomyopathy.

The clinical consequences of valve dysfunction vary depending on the valve involved, the degree of impairment, the tempo of disease onset, and the rate and quality of compensatory mechanisms. For example, sudden destruction of an aortic valve cusp by infection (infective endocarditis; see later) can cause acute, massive, and rapidly fatal regurgitation. In contrast, rheumatic mitral stenosis typically develops indolently over years, and its clinical effects can be well tolerated for extended periods. Certain conditions can complicate valvular heart disease by increasing the demands on the heart; for example, the increased output demands of pregnancy can exacerbate valve disease and lead to unfavorable maternal or fetal outcomes. Valvular stenosis or insufficiency often produces secondary changes, both proximal and distal to the affected valve, particularly in the myocardium. Generally, valvular stenosis leads to pressure overload cardiac hypertrophy, whereas mitral or aortic valvular insufficiency leads to volume overload; both situations can culminate in heart failure. In addition, the ejection of blood through narrowed stenotic valves can produce high speed "jets" of blood that injure the endocardium where they impact.

Valvular abnormalities can be congenital (discussed earlier) or acquired. *Acquired valvular stenosis* has relatively few causes; it is almost always a consequence of a remote or chronic injury of the valve cusps that declares itself clinically only after many years. In contrast, *acquired valvular insufficiency* can result from intrinsic disease of the valve cusps or damage to or distortion of the supporting structures (e.g., the aorta, mitral annulus, tendinous cords, papillary muscles, ventricular free wall). Thus, valvular insufficiency has many causes and may appear acutely, as with rupture of the cords, or chronically in disorders associated with leaflet scarring and retraction.

The causes of acquired heart valve diseases are summarized in Table 12-8. The most frequent causes of the major functional valvular lesions are:

- *Aortic stenosis:* calcification and sclerosis of anatomically normal or congenitally bicuspid aortic valves
- *Aortic insufficiency:* dilation of the ascending aorta, often secondary to hypertension and/or aging
- *Mitral stenosis:* rheumatic heart disease
- *Mitral insufficiency:* myxomatous degeneration (*mitral valve prolapse*)

Table 12-8 Major Etiologies of Acquired Heart Valve Disease

Mitral Valve Disease	Aortic Valve Disease
Mitral Stenosis	**Aortic Stenosis**
Postinflammatory scarring (rheumatic heart disease)	Postinflammatory scarring (rheumatic heart disease) Senile calcific aortic stenosis Calcification of congenitally deformed valve
Mitral Regurgitation	**Aortic Regurgitation**
Abnormalities of Leaflets and Commissures Postinflammatory scarring Infective endocarditis Mitral valve prolapse Drugs (e.g., fen-phen)	Postinflammatory scarring (rheumatic heart disease)
Abnormalities of Tensor Apparatus Rupture of papillary muscle Papillary muscle dysfunction (fibrosis) Rupture of chordae tendineae	Degenerative aortic dilatation Syphilitic aortitis Ankylosing spondylitis Rheumatoid arthritis Marfan syndrome
Abnormalities of Left Ventricle and/or Annulus LV enlargement (myocarditis, dilated cardiomyopathy) Calcification of mitral ring	

LV, Left ventricular.

Modified from Schoen FJ: Surgical pathology of removed natural and prosthetic valves. Hum Pathol 18:558, 1987.

Calcific Valvular Degeneration

Heart valves are subjected to high levels of repetitive mechanical stress, particularly at the hinge points of the cusps and leaflets; this is a consequence of (1) 30 to 40 million or more cardiac contractions per year, (2) substantial tissue deformations during each contraction, and (3) transvalvular pressure gradients in the closed phase of each contraction of approximately 120 mm Hg for the mitral and 80 mm Hg for the aortic valve. It is therefore not surprising that these delicate structures can suffer cumulative damage and calcification that lead to clinically important dysfunction.

Calcific Aortic Stenosis

The most common of all valvular abnormalities, calcific aortic stenosis is usually the consequence of age-associated "wear and tear" of either anatomically normal valves or congenitally bicuspid valves (in approximately 1% of the population). The prevalence of aortic stenosis is estimated at 2% and is increasing as the general population ages. Aortic stenosis of previously normal valves (termed senile calcific aortic stenosis) usually comes to clinical attention in the seventh to ninth decades of life, whereas stenotic bicuspid valves tend to become clinically significant 1 to 2 decades earlier.

Aortic valve calcification is likely a consequence of recurrent chronic injury due to hyperlipidemia, hypertension, inflammation, and other factors similar to those implicated in atherosclerosis. Bicuspid valves incur greater mechanical stress than normal tricuspid valves, which may explain their accelerated stenosis. The chronic progressive injury leads to valvular degeneration and incites the deposition of hydroxyapatite (the same calcium salt found in bone). Although this model provides a good starting point for understanding calcific degeneration, it is increasingly clear that the valve injury of calcific aortic stenosis differs in some important respects from atherosclerosis. Most notably, the abnormal valves contain cells resembling osteoblasts that synthesize bone matrix proteins and promote the deposition of calcium salts. Moreover, interventions that improve atherosclerotic risk (e.g., statins), do not appear to significantly impact valvular calcific degeneration.

MORPHOLOGY

The gross morphologic hallmark of nonrheumatic, calcific aortic stenosis (involving either tricuspid or bicuspid valves) is mounded calcified masses within the aortic cusps that ultimately protrude through the outflow surfaces into the sinuses of Valsalva, and prevent cuspal opening. The free edges of the cusps are usually not involved (Fig. 12-21*A*). Microscopically, the layered architecture of the valve is largely preserved. The calcific process begins in the valvular fibrosa on the outflow surface of the valve, at the points of maximal cusp flexion (near the margins of attachment). Inflammation is variable, and metaplastic bone (and even bone marrow) may be seen. In aortic stenosis, the functional valve area is decreased by large nodular calcific deposits that can eventually cause measurable outflow obstruction; this subjects the left ventricular myocardium to progressively increasing pressure overload.

In contrast to rheumatic (and congenital) aortic stenosis (see Fig. 12-23*E*), commissural fusion is not usually seen. The mitral valve is generally normal, although some patients may have direct extension of aortic valve calcific deposits onto the anterior mitral leaflet. In contrast, virtually all patients with rheumatic aortic stenosis also have concomitant and characteristic structural abnormalities of the mitral valve (see later discussion).

Clinical Features. In calcific aortic stenosis (superimposed on a previously normal or bicuspid aortic valve), the obstruction to left ventricular outflow leads to gradual narrowing of the valve orifice (valve area approximately 0.5 to 1 cm^2 in severe aortic stenosis; normal approximately 4 cm^2) and an increasing pressure gradient across the calcified valve, reaching 75 to 100 mm Hg in severe cases. Left ventricular pressures rise to 200 mm Hg or more in such instances, producing concentric left ventricular (pressure overload) hypertrophy. The hypertrophied myocardium tends to be ischemic (as a result of diminished microcirculatory perfusion, often complicated by coronary atherosclerosis), and angina pectoris may occur. Both systolic and diastolic myocardial function may be impaired; eventually, cardiac decompensation and CHF can ensue. The onset of symptoms (angina, CHF, or syncope) in aortic stenosis heralds cardiac decompensation and carries an extremely poor prognosis. If untreated, most patients with aortic stenosis will die within 5 years of developing angina, within 3 years of developing syncope, and within 2 years of CHF onset. Treatment requires surgical valve replacement, as medical therapy is ineffective in severe symptomatic aortic stenosis.

Calcific Stenosis of Congenitally Bicuspid Aortic Valve

Bicuspid aortic valve (BAV) is a developmental abnormality with prevalence in the population of approximately 1%. Some cases of BAV show familial clustering, often with associated aorta or left ventricular outflow tract malformations. While the heritability of BAV is well-established, and three loci on chromosomes 18q, 5q, and 13q have been identified in kindred studies, the specific genes that are responsible for the disorder remain largely unknown. Thus far, only loss-of-function mutations in *NOTCH1* (mapping to chromosome 9q34.3) have been specifically associated with BAV in a few families; tantalizingly, modulation of Notch activity in animal models also impacts valvular calcification.

In a congenitally bicuspid aortic valve, there are only two functional cusps, usually of unequal size, with the larger cusp having a midline *raphe*, resulting from incomplete commissural separation during development; less frequently the cusps are of equal size and the raphe is absent. The raphe is frequently a major site of calcific deposits. Once stenosis is present, the clinical course is similar to that described earlier for calcific aortic stenosis. Valves that become bicuspid because of an acquired deformity (e.g., rheumatic valve disease) have a

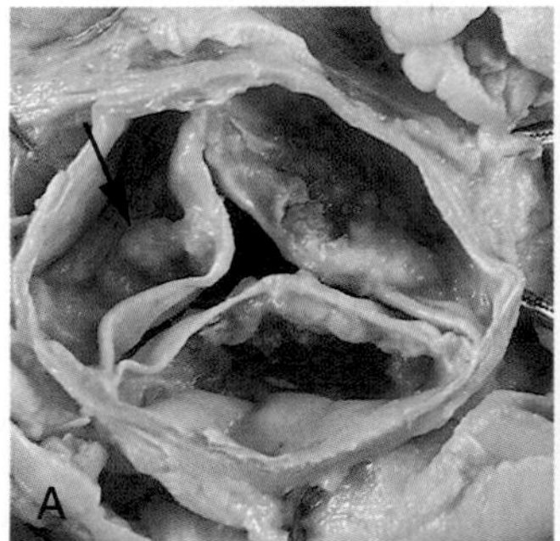

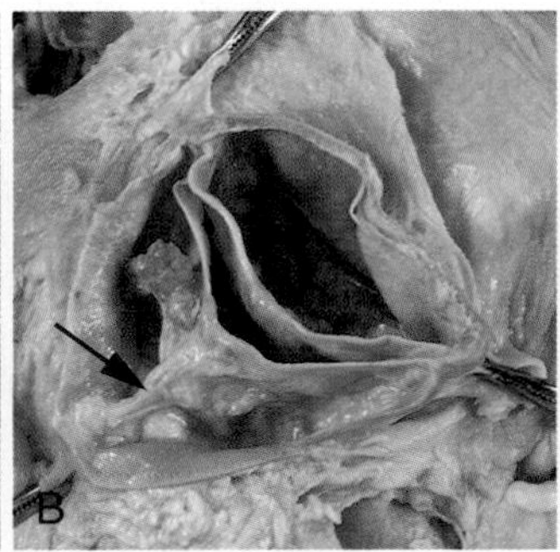

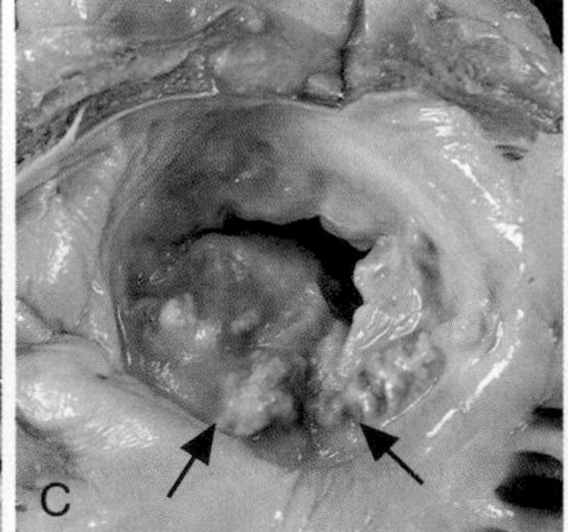

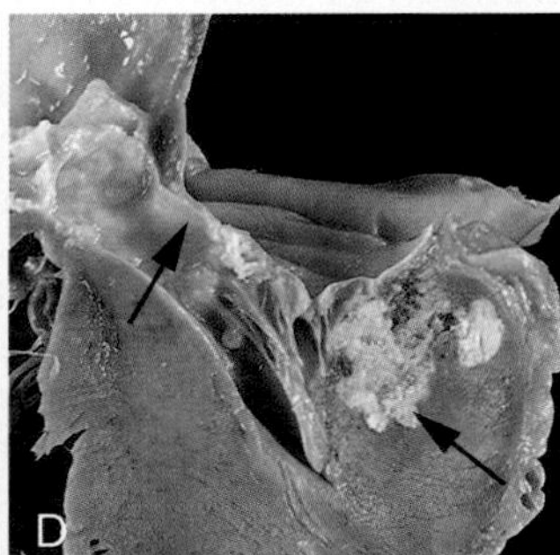

Figure 12-21 Calcific valvular degeneration. **A,** Calcific aortic stenosis of a previously normal valve (viewed from aortic aspect). Nodular masses of calcium are heaped up within the sinuses of Valsalva *(arrow)*. Note that the commissures are not fused, as occurs with postrheumatic aortic valve stenosis (see Fig. 12-23*E*). **B,** Calcific aortic stenosis of a congenitally bicuspid valve. One cusp has a partial fusion at its center, called a *raphe (arrow)*. **C** and **D,** Mitral annular calcification, with calcific nodules at the base (attachment margin) of the anterior mitral leaflet *(arrows)*. **C,** Left atrial view. **D,** Cut section of myocardium showing the lateral wall with dense calcification that extends into the underlying myocardium (*arrow*).

fused commissure that produces a conjoined cusp that is generally twice the size of the nonconjoined cusp. BAVs may also become incompetent as a result of aortic dilation, cusp prolapse, or infective endocarditis. The mitral valve is generally normal in patients with a congenitally bicuspid aortic valve.

Although BAV is usually asymptomatic early in life, late complications include aortic stenosis or regurgitation, infective endocarditis, and aortic dilation and/or dissection. In particular, BAVs are predisposed to progressive calcification, similar to that occurring in aortic valves with initially normal anatomy (Fig. 12-21*B*); calcified BAV comprise approximately 50% of cases of aortic stenosis in adults. Structural abnormalities of the aortic wall also commonly accompany BAV, even when the valve is hemodynamically normal, and this may potentiate aortic dilation or aortic dissection (see later).

Mitral Annular Calcification

As opposed to the predominantly cuspal involvement in aortic valve calcification, degenerative calcific deposits in the mitral valve typically develop in the fibrous annulus. Grossly, these appear as irregular, stony hard, occasionally ulcerated nodules (2 to 5 mm in thickness) at the base of the leaflets (Fig. 12-21*C*, *D*). Mitral annular calcification usually does not affect valvular function. However, in exceptional cases it can lead to:

- Regurgitation by interfering with physiologic contraction of the valve ring
- Stenosis by impairing opening of the mitral leaflets
- Arrhythmias and occasionally sudden death by penetration of calcium deposits to a depth sufficient to impinge on the atrioventricular conduction system.

Because calcific nodules may also provide a site for thrombus formation, patients with mitral annular calcification have an increased risk of embolic stroke, and the calcific nodules can become a nidus for infective endocarditis. Heavy calcific deposits are sometimes visualized on echocardiography or seen as distinctive, ringlike opacities on chest radiographs. Mitral annular calcification is most common in women older than age 60 and individuals with mitral valve prolapse (see later).

Mitral Valve Prolapse (Myxomatous Degeneration of the Mitral Valve)

In mitral valve prolapse (MVP), one or both mitral valve leaflets are "floppy" and *prolapse*, or balloon back, into the left atrium during systole. MVP affects approximately 2-3% of adults in the United States with an approximate 7:1 female-to-male ratio; it is most often an incidental finding on physical examination, but in a small minority of affected individuals may lead to serious complications.

Pathogenesis. The etiologic basis for the changes that weaken the valve leaflets and associated structures is unknown in most cases. Uncommonly, MVP is associated with heritable disorders of connective tissue including Marfan syndrome, caused by fibrillin-1 (*FBN-1*) mutations (Chapter 5). Fibrillin-1 defects alter cell-matrix interactions and dysregulate TGF-β signaling. Interestingly, mice with mutated *FBN-1* develop a form of mitral valve prolapse that is prevented by TGF-β inhibitors, indicating that excess TGF-β activity can cause the characteristic structural laxity and myxomatous changes. Whether similar mechanisms contribute to sporadic MVP is unknown. Genetic linkage analyses have also mapped inherited forms of MVP to loci involved in the remodeling of valvular extracellular matrix and cell:cell adhesion.

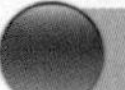

MORPHOLOGY

The characteristic anatomic change in MVP is interchordal ballooning (hooding) of the mitral leaflets or portions thereof (Fig. 12-22*A-C*). The affected leaflets are often enlarged, redundant, thick, and rubbery. The associated tendinous cords may be elongated, thinned, or even ruptured, and the annulus may be dilated. The tricuspid, aortic, or pulmonary valves may also be affected. The key histologic change in the tissue is marked thickening of the spongiosa layer with deposition of mucoid (myxomatous) material, called **myxomatous degeneration**; there is also attenuation of the collagenous fibrosa layer of the valve, on which the structural integrity of the leaflet depends (Fig. 12-22*E*). Secondary changes reflect the stresses and tissue injury incident to the billowing leaflets: (1) fibrous thickening of the valve leaflets, particularly where they rub against each other; (2) linear fibrous thickening of the left ventricular endocardial surface where the abnormally long cords snap or rub against it; (3) thickening of the mural endocardium of the left ventricle or atrium as a consequence of friction-induced injury induced by the prolapsing, hypermobile leaflets; (4) thrombi on the atrial surfaces of the leaflets or the atrial walls (Fig. 12-22*B*); and (5) focal calcifications at the base of the posterior mitral leaflet (Fig. 12-22*C*). Notably, mitral valve myxomatous degeneration can also occur as a secondary consequence of regurgitation of other etiologies (e.g., ischemic dysfunction).

Clinical Features. Most individuals diagnosed with MVP are asymptomatic; in such cases, the condition is discovered incidentally by auscultation of mid-systolic clicks, sometimes followed by a mid to late systolic murmur. The diagnosis is confirmed by echocardiography. A minority of patients have chest pain mimicking angina (although not exertional in nature), and a subset has dyspnea, presumably related to valvular insufficiency. Although the great majority of persons with MVP have no untoward effects, approximately 3% develop one of four serious complications: (1) infective endocarditis; (2) mitral insufficiency, sometimes with chordal rupture; (3) stroke or other systemic infarct, resulting from embolism of leaflet thrombi; or (4) arrhythmias, both ventricular and atrial. Rarely, MVP is the only finding in sudden cardiac death.

The risk of serious complications is very low in MVP discovered incidentally in young asymptomatic patients; the risk is higher for men, older patients, and those with arrhythmias or mitral regurgitation. Valve repair or replacement surgery can be done for symptomatic patients or those with increased risk for significant complications; indeed, in the United States, MVP is the most common cause for mitral valve surgery.

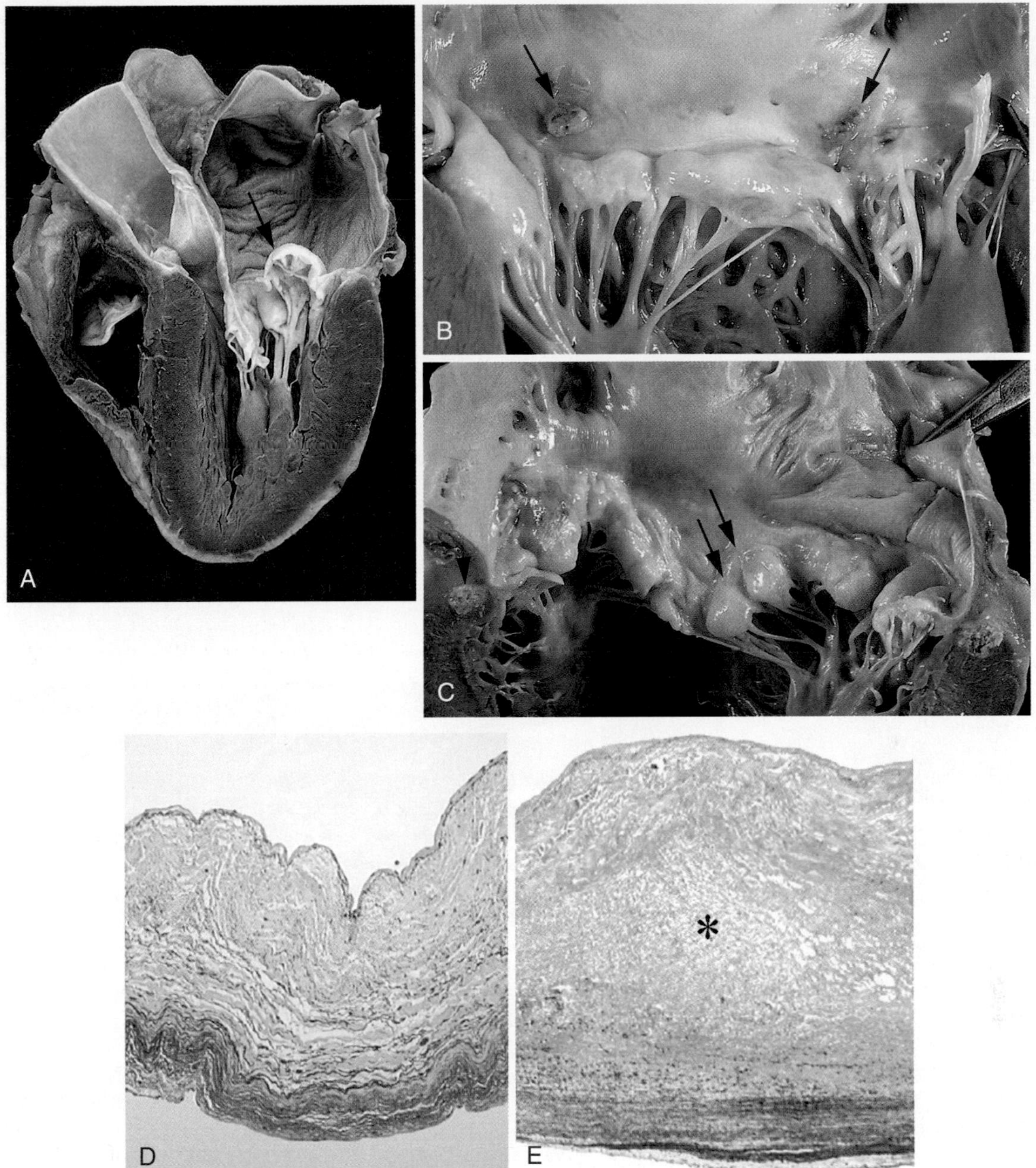

Figure 12-22 Myxomatous degeneration of the mitral valve. **A,** Long axis view (left ventricle is on the *right*) demonstrating hooding with prolapse of the posterior mitral leaflet into the left atrium *(arrow)*. **B,** Opened valve, showing pronounced hooding of the posterior mitral leaflet with thrombotic plaques at sites of leaflet-left atrium contact *(arrows)*. **C,** Opened valve with pronounced hooding *(double arrows)* in a patient who died suddenly. Note also mitral annular calcification *(arrowhead)*. Normal heart valve **(D)** and myxomatous mitral valve **(E)**. In myxomatous valves, collagen in the fibrosa is loose and disorganized, proteoglycan deposition *(asterisk)* in the spongiosa is markedly expanded, and elastin in the atrialis is disorganized. (**A,** Courtesy William D. Edwards, MD, Mayo Clinic, Rochester, Minn; **D, E,** Movat pentachrome stain, in which collagen is yellow, elastin is black, and proteoglycans are blue). From Rabkin E, et al: Activated interstitial myofibroblasts express catabolic enzymes and mediate matrix remodeling in myxomatous heart valves. Circulation 104:2525-2532, 2001.)

Rheumatic Fever and Rheumatic Heart Disease

Rheumatic fever (RF) is an acute, immunologically mediated, multisystem inflammatory disease classically occurring a few weeks after an episode of group A streptococcal pharyngitis; occasionally, RF can follow streptococcal infections at other sites, such as the skin. Acute rheumatic carditis is a common manifestation of active RF and may progress over time to chronic rheumatic heart disease (RHD), mainly manifesting as valvular abnormalities.

RHD is characterized principally by deforming fibrotic valvular disease, particularly involving the mitral valve; *indeed, RHD is virtually the only cause of mitral stenosis*. The incidence and mortality rate of RF and RHD have declined remarkably in many parts of the world over the past century, as a result of improved sanitation, and rapid diagnosis and treatment of streptococcal pharyngitis. Nevertheless, in developing countries, and in many crowded, economically depressed urban areas, RHD remains an important public health problem, affecting an estimated 15 million people.

Pathogenesis. **Acute rheumatic fever results from host immune responses to group A streptococcal antigens that cross-react with host proteins.** In particular, antibodies and CD4+ T cells directed against streptococcal M proteins can also in some cases recognize cardiac self-antigens. Antibody binding can activate complement, as well as recruit Fc-receptor bearing cells (neutrophils and macrophages); cytokine production by the stimulated T cells leads to macrophage activation (e.g., within Aschoff bodies). Damage to heart tissue may thus be caused by a combination of antibody- and T cell–mediated reactions (Chapter 6).

MORPHOLOGY

Key pathologic features of acute RF and chronic RHD are shown in Figure 12-23. During acute RF, focal inflammatory lesions are found in various tissues. Distinctive lesions occur in the heart, called **Aschoff bodies**, consisting of foci of T lymphocytes, occasional plasma cells, and plump activated macrophages called **Anitschkow cells** (pathognomonic for RF). These macrophages have abundant cytoplasm and central round-to-ovoid nuclei (occasionally binucleate) in which the chromatin condenses into a central, slender, wavy ribbon (hence the designation "caterpillar cells").

During acute RF, diffuse inflammation and Aschoff bodies may be found in any of the three layers of the heart, resulting in pericarditis, myocarditis, or endocarditis (**pancarditis**).

Inflammation of the endocardium and the left-sided valves typically results in fibrinoid necrosis within the cusps or tendinous cords. Overlying these necrotic foci and along the lines of closure are small (1 to 2 mm) vegetations, called **verrucae**. Thus, RHD is one of the forms of vegetative valve disease, each of which exhibit their own characteristic morphologic features (Fig. 12-24). Subendocardial lesions, perhaps exacerbated by regurgitant jets, can induce irregular thickenings called **MacCallum plaques**, usually in the left atrium.

The cardinal anatomic changes of the mitral valve in chronic RHD are **leaflet thickening, commissural fusion and shortening, and thickening and fusion of the tendinous cords** (Fig. 12-23*D*). In chronic disease the mitral valve is virtually always involved. The mitral valve is affected in isolation in roughly two thirds of RHD, and along with the aortic valve in another 25% of cases. Tricuspid valve involvement is

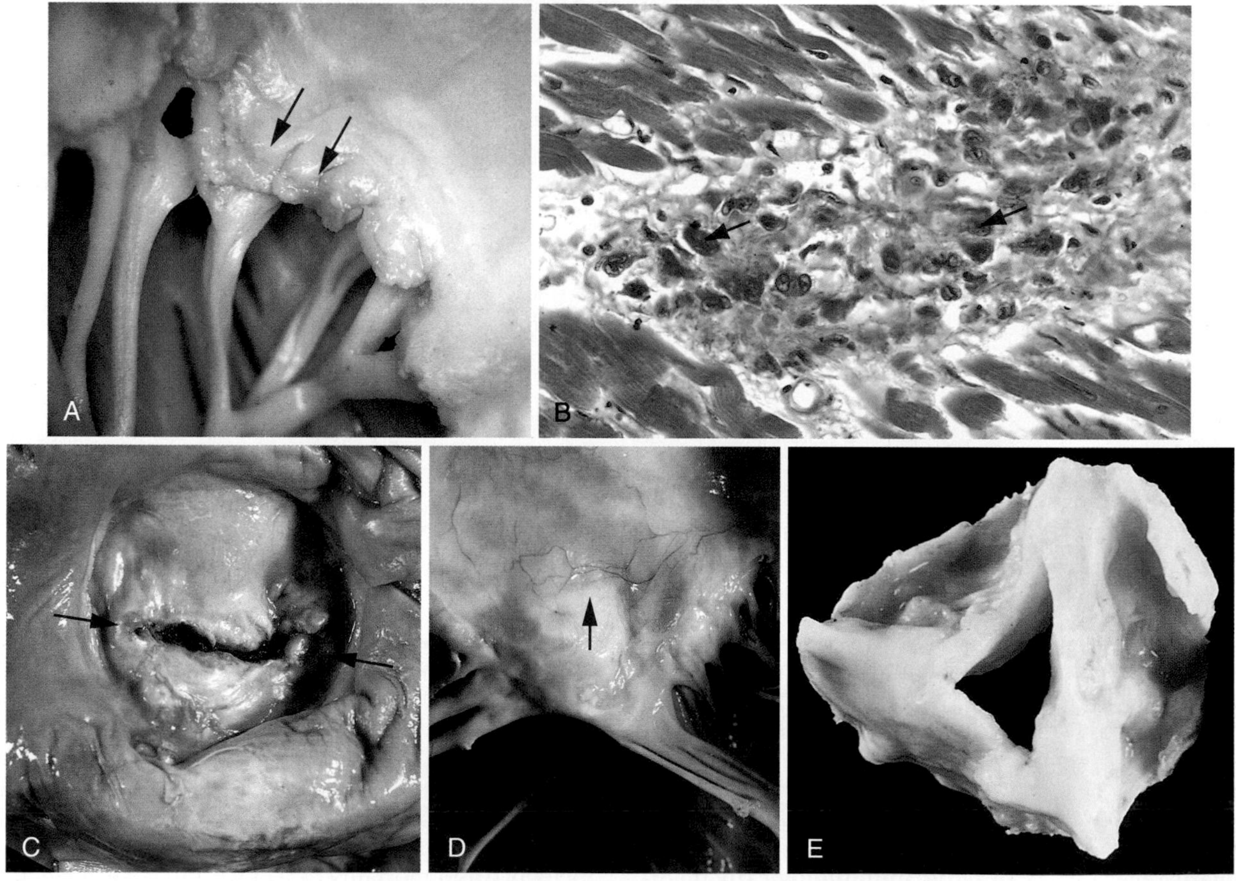

Figure 12-23 Acute and chronic rheumatic heart disease. **A,** Acute rheumatic mitral valvulitis superimposed on chronic rheumatic heart disease. Small vegetations (verrucae) are visible along the line of closure of the mitral valve leaflet *(arrows)*. Previous episodes of rheumatic valvulitis have caused fibrous thickening and fusion of the chordae tendineae. **B,** Microscopic appearance of an *Aschoff body* in a patient with acute rheumatic carditis. The myocardium exhibits a circumscribed nodule of mixed mononuclear inflammatory cells with associated necrosis; within the inflammation, large activated macrophages show prominent nucleoli, as well as chromatin condensed into long, wavy ribbons (caterpillar cells; *arrows*). **C** and **D,** Mitral stenosis with diffuse fibrous thickening and distortion of the valve leaflets and commissural fusion (*arrows*, **C**), and thickening of the chordae tendineae (**D**). Note neovascularization of anterior mitral leaflet (*arrow*, **D**). **E,** Surgically resected specimen of rheumatic aortic stenosis, demonstrating thickening and distortion of the cusps with commissural fusion. (**E,** Reproduced from Schoen FJ, St. John-Sutton M: Contemporary issues in the pathology of valvular heart disease. Hum Pathol 18:568, 1967.)

infrequent, and the pulmonary valve is only rarely affected. Because of the increase in calcific aortic stenosis (see earlier) and the reduced frequency of RHD, rheumatic aortic stenosis now accounts for a small fraction of cases of acquired aortic stenosis.

In rheumatic mitral stenosis, calcification and fibrous bridging across the valvular commissures create "fish mouth" or "buttonhole" stenoses. With tight mitral stenosis, the left atrium progressively dilates and may harbor mural thrombi that can embolize. Long-standing congestive changes in the lungs may induce pulmonary vascular and parenchymal changes; over time, these can lead to right ventricular hypertrophy. The left ventricle is largely unaffected by isolated pure mitral stenosis. Microscopically, valves show organization of the acute inflammation, with post-inflammatory neovascularization and transmural fibrosis that obliterate the leaflet architecture. Aschoff bodies are rarely seen in surgical specimens or autopsy tissue from patients with chronic RHD, as a result of the long intervals between the initial insult and the development of the chronic deformity.

Clinical Features. RF is characterized by a constellation of findings: (1) migratory polyarthritis of the large joints, (2) pancarditis, (3) subcutaneous nodules, (4) erythema marginatum of the skin, and (5) Sydenham chorea, a neurologic disorder with involuntary rapid, purposeless movements. The diagnosis is established by the so-called Jones criteria: evidence of a preceding group A streptococcal infection, with the presence of two of the major manifestations listed earlier or one major and two minor manifestations (nonspecific signs and symptoms that include fever, arthralgia, or elevated blood levels of acute-phase reactants).

Acute RF typically appears 10 days to 6 weeks after a group A streptococcal infection in about 3% of patients. It occurs most often in children between ages 5 and 15, but first attacks can occur in middle to later life. Although pharyngeal cultures for streptococci are negative by the time the illness begins, antibodies to one or more streptococcal enzymes, such as streptolysin O and DNase B, can be detected in the sera of most patients with RF. The predominant clinical manifestations are carditis and arthritis, the latter more common in adults than in children. Arthritis typically begins with migratory polyarthritis (accompanied by fever) in which one large joint after another becomes painful and swollen for a period of days and then subsides spontaneously, leaving no residual disability. Clinical features related to *acute carditis* include pericardial friction rubs, tachycardia, and arrhythmias. Myocarditis can cause cardiac dilation that may culminate in functional mitral valve insufficiency or even heart failure. Approximately 1% of affected individuals die of fulminant RF involvement of the heart.

After an initial attack there is increased vulnerability to reactivation of the disease with subsequent pharyngeal infections, and the same manifestations are likely to appear with each recurrent attack. Damage to the valves is cumulative. Turbulence induced by ongoing valvular deformities leads to additional fibrosis. Clinical manifestations appear years or even decades after the initial episode of RF and depend on which cardiac valves are involved. In addition to various cardiac murmurs, cardiac hypertrophy and dilation, and heart failure, individuals with chronic RHD may suffer from arrhythmias (particularly atrial fibrillation in the setting of mitral stenosis), thromboembolic complications, and infective endocarditis (see later). The long-term prognosis is highly variable. Surgical repair or prosthetic replacement of diseased valves has greatly improved the outlook for persons with RHD.

Infective Endocarditis

Infective endocarditis (IE) is a microbial infection of the heart valves or the mural endocardium that leads to the formation of *vegetations* composed of thrombotic debris and organisms, often associated with destruction of the underlying cardiac tissues. The aorta, aneurysms, other blood vessels, and prosthetic devices can also become infected. Although fungi and other classes of microorganisms can be responsible, most infections are bacterial *(bacterial endocarditis)*. Prompt diagnosis, identification of the offending agent, and effective treatment of IE is important in limiting morbidity and mortality.

Traditionally, IE has been classified on clinical grounds into acute and subacute forms. This subdivision reflects the range of the disease severity and tempo, which are determined in large part by the virulence of the infecting microorganism and whether underlying cardiac disease is present. *Acute infective endocarditis* is typically caused by infection of a previously normal heart valve by a highly virulent organism (e.g., *Staphylococcus aureus*) that rapidly produces necrotizing and destructive lesions. These infections may be difficult to cure with antibiotics alone, and usually require surgery. Despite appropriate treatment, death can ensue within days to weeks. In contrast, *subacute IE* is characterized by organisms with lower virulence (e.g., viridans streptococci) that cause insidious infections of deformed valves with overall less destruction. In such cases the disease may pursue a protracted course of weeks to months, and cures can be achieved with antibiotics.

Pathogenesis. Although highly virulent organisms can infect previously normal valves, a variety of cardiac and vascular abnormalities increase the risk of developing IE. Rheumatic heart disease with valvular scarring has historically been the major antecedent disorder; as RHD becomes less common, it has been supplanted by mitral valve prolapse, degenerative calcific valvular stenosis, bicuspid aortic valve (whether calcified or not), artificial (prosthetic) valves, and unrepaired and repaired congenital defects.

The causal organisms differ among the major high-risk groups. Endocarditis of native but previously damaged or otherwise abnormal valves is caused most commonly (50% to 60% of cases) by *Streptococcus viridans*, a normal component of the oral cavity flora. In contrast, more virulent *S. aureus* organisms commonly found on the skin can infect either healthy or deformed valves and are responsible for 20% to 30% of cases overall; notably, *S. aureus* is the major offender in IE among intravenous drug abusers. Other bacterial causes include enterococci and the so-called HACEK group (*Haemophilus, Actinobacillus, Cardiobacterium, Eikenella*, and *Kingella*), all commensals in the oral cavity. Prosthetic valve endocarditis is caused most commonly by coagulase-negative staphylococci (e.g., *S. epidermidis*). Other agents causing endocarditis include gram-negative

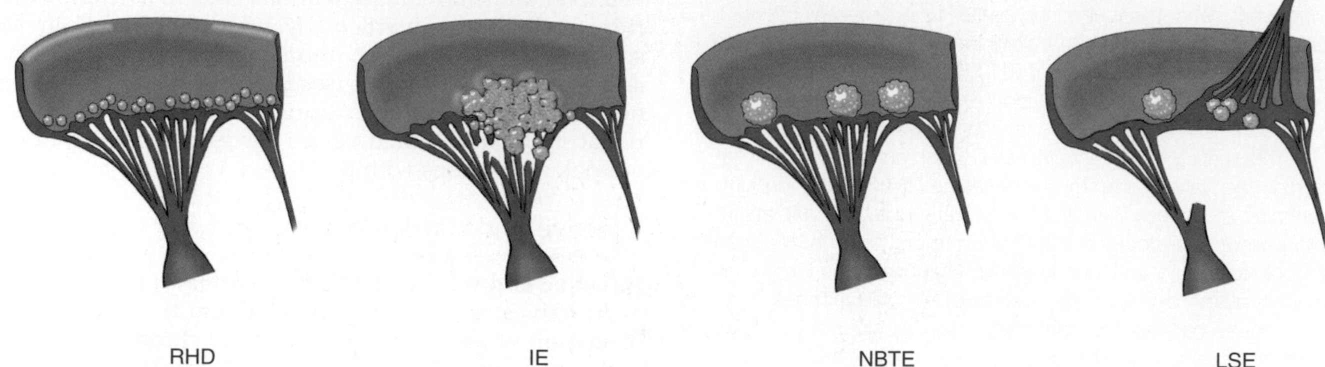

Figure 12-24 Comparison of the four major forms of vegetative endocarditis. The rheumatic fever phase of rheumatic heart disease (RHD) is marked by small, warty vegetations along the lines of closure of the valve leaflets. Infective endocarditis (IE) is characterized by large, irregular masses on the valve cusps that can extend onto the chordae (see Fig. 12-25*A*). Nonbacterial thrombotic endocarditis (NBTE) typically exhibits small, bland vegetations, usually attached at the line of closure. One or many may be present (see Figure 12-26). Libman-Sacks endocarditis (LSE) has small or medium-sized vegetations on either or both sides of the valve leaflets.

bacilli and fungi. In about 10% of all cases of endocarditis, no organism can be isolated from the blood ("culture-negative" endocarditis); reasons include prior antibiotic therapy, difficulties in isolating the offending agent, or because deeply embedded organisms within the enlarging vegetation are not released into the blood.

Foremost among the factors predisposing to endocarditis are those that cause microorganism seeding into the blood stream (bacteremia or fungemia). The source may be an obvious infection elsewhere, a dental or surgical procedure, a contaminated needle shared by intravenous drug users, or seemingly trivial breaks in the epithelial barriers of the gut, oral cavity, or skin. In patients with valve abnormalities, or with known bacteremia, IE risk can be lowered by antibiotic prophylaxis.

MORPHOLOGY

Vegetations on heart valves are the classic hallmark of IE; these are friable, bulky, potentially destructive lesions containing fibrin, inflammatory cells, and bacteria or other organisms (Figs. 12-24 and 12-25). The aortic and mitral valves are the most common sites of infection, although the valves of the right heart may also be involved, particularly in intravenous drug abusers. Vegetations can be single or multiple and may involve more than one valve; they can occasionally erode into the underlying myocardium and produce an abscess (ring abscess; Fig. 12-25*B*). Vegetations are prone to embolization; because the embolic fragments often contain virulent organisms, abscesses frequently develop where they lodge, leading to sequelae such as septic infarcts or mycotic aneurysms.

The vegetations of subacute endocarditis are associated with less valvular destruction than those of acute endocarditis, although the distinction can be subtle. Microscopically, the vegetations of subacute IE typically exhibit granulation tissue at their bases indicative of healing. With time, fibrosis, calcification, and a chronic inflammatory infiltrate can develop.

Clinical Features. Acute endocarditis has a stormy onset with rapidly developing fever, chills, weakness, and lassitude. Although fever is the most consistent sign of IE, it can be slight or absent, particularly in older adults, and the only manifestations may be nonspecific fatigue, loss of

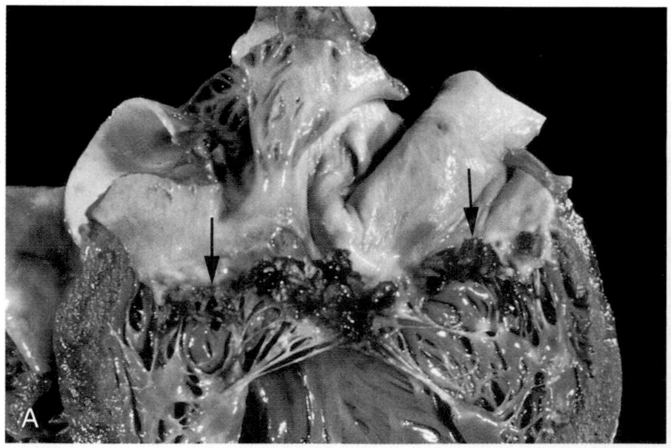

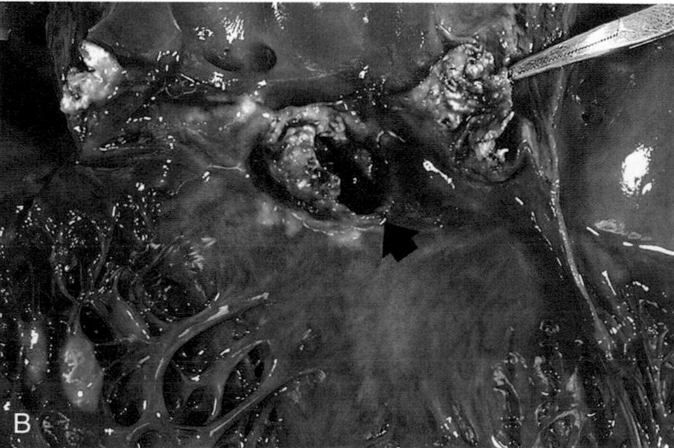

Figure 12-25 Infective (bacterial) endocarditis. **A,** Endocarditis of mitral valve (subacute, caused by *Streptococcus viridans*). The large, friable vegetations are denoted by *arrows*. **B,** Acute endocarditis of congenitally bicuspid aortic valve (caused by *Staphylococcus aureus)* with extensive cuspal destruction and ring abscess *(arrow)*.

Table 12-9 Diagnostic Criteria for Infective Endocarditis*

Pathologic Criteria
Microorganisms, demonstrated by culture or histologic examination, in a vegetation, embolus from a vegetation, or intracardiac abscess
Histologic confirmation of active endocarditis in vegetation or intracardiac abscess
Clinical Criteria
Major
Blood culture(s) positive for a characteristic organism or persistently positive for an unusual organism
Echocardiographic identification of a valve-related or implant-related mass or abscess, or partial separation of artificial valve
New valvular regurgitation
Minor
Predisposing heart lesion or intravenous drug use
Fever
Vascular lesions, including arterial petechiae, subungual/splinter hemorrhages, emboli, septic infarcts, mycotic aneurysm, intracranial hemorrhage, Janeway lesions†
Immunological phenomena, including glomerulonephritis, Osler nodes,† Roth spots,§ rheumatoid factor
Microbiologic evidence, including a single culture positive for an unusual organism
Echocardiographic findings consistent with but not diagnostic of endocarditis, including worsening or changing of a preexistent murmur

*Diagnosis by these guidelines, often called the Duke Criteria, requires either pathologic or clinical criteria; if clinical criteria are used, 2 major, 1 major + 3 minor, or 5 minor criteria are required for diagnosis.

†Janeway lesions are small erythematous or hemorrhagic, macular, nontender lesions on the palms and soles and are the consequence of septic embolic events.

‡Osler nodes are small, tender subcutaneous nodules that develop in the pulp of the digits or occasionally more proximally in the fingers and persist for hours to several days.

§Roth spots are oval retinal hemorrhages with pale centers.

Modified from Durack DT, et al: New criteria for diagnosis of infective endocarditis: utilization of specific echocardiographic findings. Am J Med, 96:200, 1994, and Karchmer AW: Infective Endocarditis. In Braunwald E, Zipes DP, Libby P (eds): Heart Disease. A Textbook of Cardiovascular Medicine, 6th ed. Philadelphia, WB Saunders, 2001, p 1723.

weight, and a flulike syndrome. Murmurs are present in 90% of patients with left-sided IE, either from a new valvular defect or from a preexisting abnormality. The so-called modified Duke criteria (Table 12-9) facilitate evaluation of individuals with suspected IE that takes into account predisposing factors, physical findings, blood culture results, echocardiographic findings, and laboratory information.

Complications of IE generally begin within the first few weeks of onset, and can include glomerular antigen-antibody complex deposition causing glomerulonephritis (Chapter 20). Earlier diagnosis and effective treatment has nearly eliminated some previously common clinical manifestations of long-standing IE—for example, microthromboemboli (manifest as splinter or subungual hemorrhages), erythematous or hemorrhagic nontender lesions on the palms or soles (Janeway lesions), subcutaneous nodules in the pulp of the digits (Osler nodes), and retinal hemorrhages in the eyes (Roth spots).

Noninfected Vegetations

Noninfected (sterile) vegetations occur in nonbacterial thrombotic endocarditis and the endocarditis of systemic lupus erythematosus (SLE), called Libman-Sacks endocarditis (see later).

Nonbacterial Thrombotic Endocarditis

Nonbacterial thrombotic endocarditis (NBTE) is characterized by the deposition of small sterile thrombi on the leaflets of the cardiac valves (Figs. 12-24 and 12-26). The lesions are 1 to 5 mm in size, and occur as single or multiple vegetations along the line of closure of the leaflets or cusps. Histologically, they comprise bland thrombi that are loosely attached to the underlying valve; the vegetations are not invasive and do not elicit any inflammatory reaction. Thus, although the local effect of the vegetations is usually trivial, they can be the source of systemic emboli that produce significant infarcts in the brain, heart, or elsewhere.

NBTE is often encountered in debilitated patients, such as those with cancer or sepsis—hence the previous term *marantic endocarditis* (root word *marasmus*, relating to malnutrition). It frequently occurs concomitantly with deep venous thromboses, pulmonary emboli, or other findings suggesting an underlying systemic hypercoagulable state (Chapter 4). Indeed, there is a striking association with mucinous adenocarcinomas, potentially relating to the procoagulant effects of tumor-derived mucin or tissue

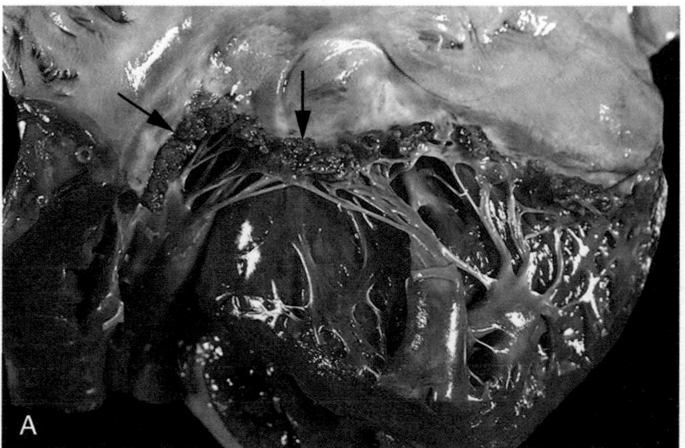

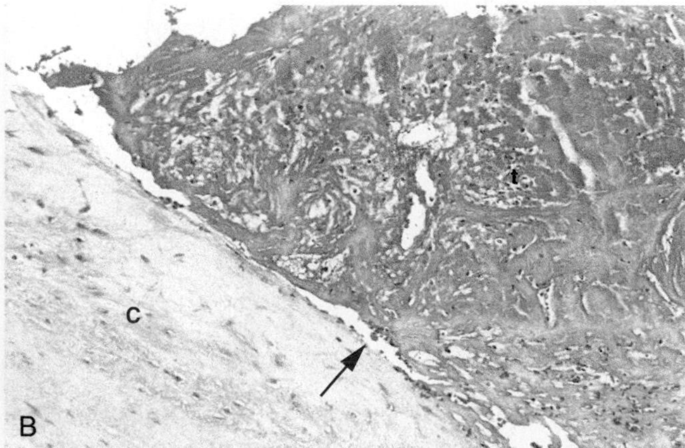

Figure 12-26 Nonbacterial thrombotic endocarditis (NBTE). **A,** Nearly complete row of thrombotic vegetations along the line of closure of the mitral valve leaflets *(arrows)*. **B,** Photomicrograph of NBTE, showing bland thrombus, with virtually no inflammation in the valve cusp (c) or the thrombotic deposit (t). The thrombus is only loosely attached to the cusp *(arrow)*.

factor that can also cause migratory thrombophlebitis (Trousseau syndrome, Chapter 4). Endocardial trauma, as from an indwelling catheter, is another well-recognized predisposing condition, and right-sided valvular and endocardial thrombotic lesions frequently track along the course of pulmonary artery catheters.

Endocarditis of Systemic Lupus Erythematosus (Libman-Sacks Disease)

Mitral and tricuspid valvulitis with small, sterile vegetations, called *Libman-Sacks endocarditis,* is occasionally encountered in systemic lupus erythematosus. Due to the use of steriods, the incidence of this complication has been greatly reduced. The lesions are small (1 to 4 mm in diameter), single or multiple, sterile, pink vegetations with a warty (verrucous) appearance. They may be located on the undersurfaces of the atrioventricular valves, on the valvular endocardium, on the chords, or on the mural endocardium of atria or ventricles. Histologically the vegetations consist of a finely granular, fibrinous eosinophilic material containing cellular debris including nuclear remnants. Vegetations are often associated with an intense valvulitis, characterized by fibrinoid necrosis of the valve substance and reflecting the activation of complement and recruitment of Fc-receptor-bearing cells.

Thrombotic heart valve lesions with sterile vegetations or rarely fibrous thickening can occur in the setting of the antiphospholipid syndrome, which can also induce a hypercoagulable state (Chapter 4). The mitral valve is more frequently involved than the aortic valve, and regurgitation is the usual functional abnormality.

Carcinoid Heart Disease

The *carcinoid syndrome* **refers to a systemic disorder marked by flushing, diarrhea, dermatitis, and bronchoconstriction that is caused by bioactive compounds such as serotonin released by *carcinoid tumors*** (Chapter 17). *Carcinoid heart disease* refers to the cardiac manifestations caused by the bioactive compounds and occurs in roughly half of the patients in whom the systemic syndrome develops. Cardiac lesions do not typically occur until there is a massive hepatic metastatic burden, since the liver normally catabolizes circulating mediators before they can affect the heart. Classically, endocardium and valves of the right heart are primarily affected since they are the first cardiac tissues bathed by the mediators released by gastrointestinal carcinoid tumors. The left side of the heart is afforded some measure of protection because the pulmonary vascular bed degrades the mediators. However, left heart carcinoid lesions can occur in the setting of atrial or septal defects and right-to-left flow, or can be elicited by primary pulmonary carcinoid tumors.

Pathogenesis. The mediators elaborated by carcinoid tumors include serotonin (5-hydroxytryptamine), kallikrein, bradykinin, histamine, prostaglandins, and tachykinins. Although it is not clear which of these is causal, plasma levels of serotonin and urinary excretion of the serotonin metabolite 5-hydroxyindoleacetic acid correlate with the severity of the cardiac lesions. The valvular plaques in carcinoid syndrome are also similar to lesions that occur in patients taking fenfluramine (an appetite suppressant) or ergot alkaloids (for migraine headaches); interestingly, these agents affect systemic serotonin metabolism. Similarly, left-sided plaques have been reported following methysergide or ergotamine therapy for migraines; notably, these drugs are metabolized to serotonin as they pass through the pulmonary vasculature. Despite this tantalizing evidence, however, it is not known how serotonin might induce the observed cardiac changes, nor has it been proven that treatment with serotonin inhibitors has any effect on the development or progression of heart lesions.

MORPHOLOGY

The cardiovascular lesions associated with the carcinoid syndrome are distinctive, glistening white intimal plaquelike thickenings of the endocardial surfaces of the cardiac chambers and valve leaflets (Fig. 12-27). The lesions are composed of smooth muscle cells and sparse collagen fibers embedded in an acid mucopolysaccharide-rich matrix material. Underlying structures are intact. With right-sided involvement, typical findings are tricuspid insufficiency and pulmonary stenosis.

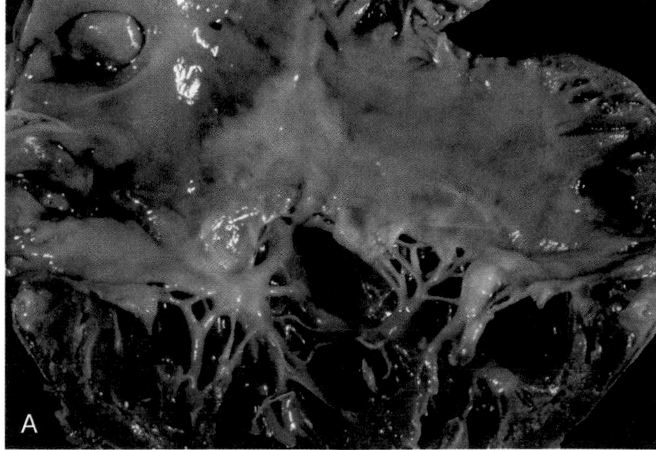

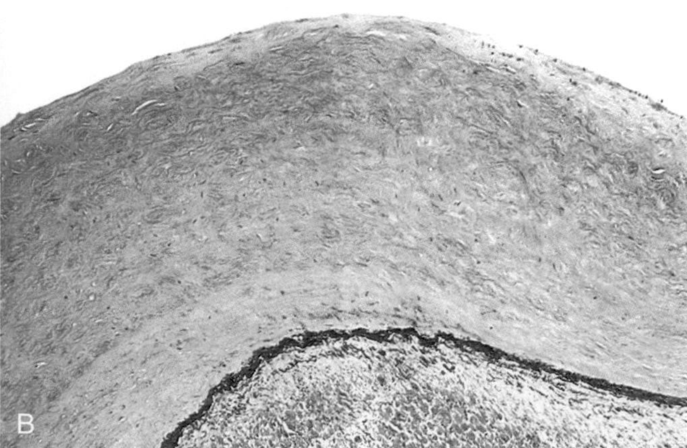

Figure 12-27 Carcinoid heart disease. **A,** Characteristic endocardial fibrotic lesion involving the right ventricle and tricuspid valve. **B,** Microscopic appearance of carcinoid heart disease with intimal thickening. Movat stain shows myocardial elastic tissue (black) underlying the acid mucopolysaccharide-rich lesion (blue-green). The underlying myocardium is unaffected.

Complications of Prosthetic Valves

Replacement of damaged cardiac valves with prostheses is a common and often lifesaving mode of therapy. There are two types of valvular prostheses:

- *Mechanical valves*. These consist of different configurations of rigid nonphysiologic material, such as caged balls, tilting disks, or hinged semicircular flaps (bi-leaflet tilting disk valves).
- *Tissue valves* (*bioprostheses*). Porcine aortic valves or bovine pericardium are preserved in a dilute glutaraldehyde solution and then mounted on a prosthetic frame. Alternatively, frozen human valves from deceased donors (called cryopreserved "homografts") can also be used. Tissue valves are flexible and function similarly to natural semilunar valves. However, the chemical treatment of the animal valves cross-links the valvular proteins, especially collagen, and renders the tissue nonviable. Similarly, the freezing and thawing of human homografts may also render them largely nonviable.

Approximately 60% of substitute valve recipients develop a serious prosthesis-related problem within 10 years after the surgery. The complications that occur depend on which type of valve has been implanted (Table 12-10 and Fig. 12-28).

- *Thromboembolism* is the major consideration with mechanical valves (Fig. 12-28*A*); this may take the form of either thrombotic occlusion of the prosthesis or emboli released from thrombi formed on the valve. Because blood flow in all mechanical devices is nonlaminar, foci of turbulence and stasis are produced by prostheses that predispose to thrombus formation. The risk of such complications necessitates long-term anticoagulation in all individuals with mechanical valves, with the attendant risk of hemorrhagic stroke or other forms of serious bleeding.
- *Structural deterioration* rarely causes failure of mechanical valves in current use. However, virtually all bioprostheses eventually become incompetent due to calcification and/or tearing (Fig. 12-28*B*).
- *Infective endocarditis* is a potentially serious complication of any valve replacement. The vegetations of prosthetic valve endocarditis are usually located at the prosthesis-tissue interface, and often cause the formation of a ring abscess, which can eventually lead to a paravalvular regurgitant blood leak. In addition, vegetations may directly involve the tissue of bioprosthetic valvular cusps. The major organisms causing such infections are staphylococcal skin contaminants (e.g., *S. epidermidis*), *S. aureus*, streptococci, and fungi.
- Other complications include paravalvular leak due to inadequate healing, obstruction due to overgrowth of fibrous tissue during healing, valve-orifice disproportion (where the effective valve area is too small for the needs of the patient, leading to a relative stenosis), intravascular hemolysis due to high shear forces, or excessive noise owing to hard contacts of moving rigid parts.

Table 12-10 Complications of Cardiac Valve Prostheses

Thrombosis/thromboembolism
Anticoagulant-related hemorrhage
Prosthetic valve endocarditis
Structural deterioration (intrinsic)
Wear, fracture, poppet failure in ball valves, cuspal tear, calcification
Other forms of dysfunction
Inadequate healing (paravalvular leak), exuberant healing (obstruction), hemolysis

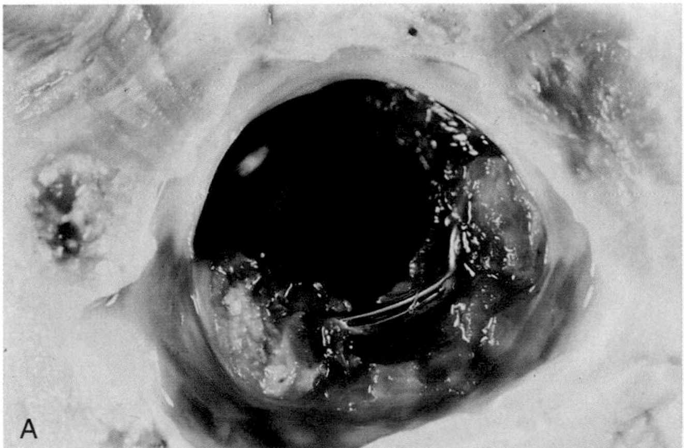

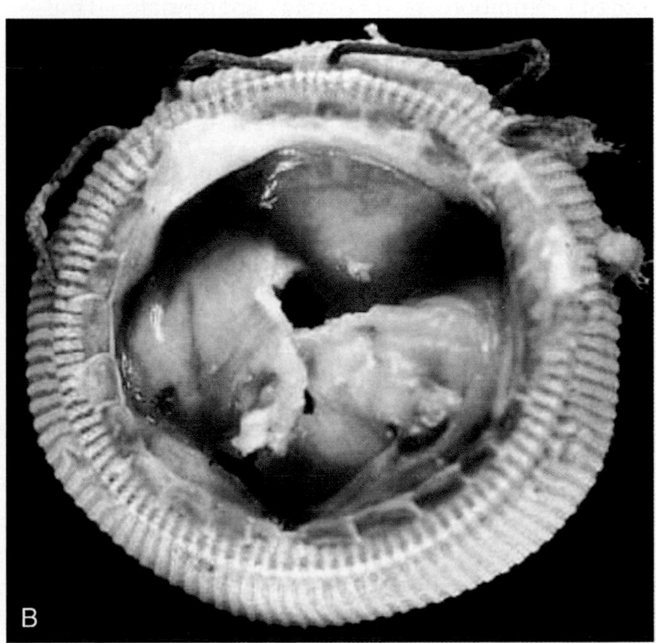

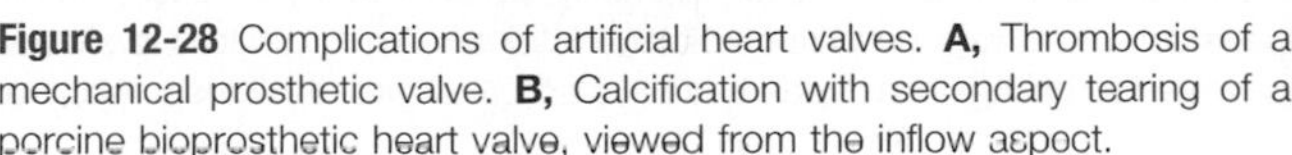

Figure 12-28 Complications of artificial heart valves. **A,** Thrombosis of a mechanical prosthetic valve. **B,** Calcification with secondary tearing of a porcine bioprosthetic heart valve, viewed from the inflow aspect.

KEY CONCEPTS

Valvular Heart Disease

- Valve pathology can lead to occlusion (*stenosis*) and/or to regurgitation (*insufficiency*); acquired aortic and mitral valves stenoses account for approximately two thirds of all valve disease.
- Valve calcification is a degenerative process that typically results in stenosis; abnormal matrix synthesis and turnover result in myxomatous degeneration and insufficiency.
- Inflammatory valve diseases lead to post-inflammatory neovascularization and scarring. Rheumatic heart disease results from anti-streptococcal antibodies that cross-react with cardiac tissues; it most commonly affects the mitral valve and is responsible for 99% of acquired mitral stenoses.
- Infective endocarditis can be aggressive and rapidly destroy normal valves (acute IE), or can be indolent and minimally destructive of previously abnormal valves (subacute IE). Systemic embolization can produce septic infarcts.
- Nonbacterial thrombotic endocarditis occurs on previously normal valves due to hypercoagulable states; embolization is an important complication.
- Mechanical prosthetic valves have thrombotic or hemorrhagic complications related to the nonlaminar flow of blood and the need for chronic anti-coagulation. Bioprosthetic valves are nonviable and are therefore susceptible to long-term calcification and/or degeneration with tearing. Both types of valves have an increased risk of developing endocarditis relative to native valves.

Cardiomyopathies

Although the term *cardiomyopathy* (literally, heart muscle disease) has been historically applied to any cardiac dysfunction resulting from a myocardial abnormality, a more nuanced definition is probably appropriate. Thus—stimulated by the recognition of new phenotypes and the advent of more sophisticated molecular characterization—an expert panel has suggested: "*[C]ardiomyopathies are a heterogeneous group of diseases of the myocardium associated with mechanical and/or electrical dysfunction that usually (but not invariably) exhibit inappropriate ventricular hypertrophy or dilatation and are due to a variety of causes that frequently are genetic. Cardiomyopathies either are confined to the heart or are part of generalized systemic disorders, often leading to cardiovascular death or progressive heart failure-related disability.*"

Thus, cardiomyopathies manifest as failure of myocardial performance; this can be mechanical (e.g., diastolic or systolic dysfunction) leading to CHF, or can culminate in life-threatening arrhythmias. *Primary* cardiomyopathies can be genetic or acquired diseases of myocardium, whereas *secondary* cardiomyopathies have myocardial involvement as a component of a systemic or multiorgan disorder. A major advance in our understanding of cardiomyopathies stems from the frequent identification of underlying genetic causes, including mutations in myocardial proteins involved in contraction, cell-cell contacts, and the cytoskeleton. These, in turn, lead to abnormal contraction or relaxation, or to dysregulated ion transport across cell membranes. Although chronic myocardial dysfunction secondary to ischemia, valvular abnormalities, or hypertension can cause significant ventricular dysfunction (as described previously), these conditions should not be denoted as cardiomyopathies.

Cardiomyopathies can be classified according to a variety of criteria, including the underlying genetic basis of dysfunction; indeed, we have already discussed a number of the arrhythmia-inducing channelopathies, which may be included in cardiomyopathies. However, we will confine our list of cardiomyopathies to disorders that produce anatomic abnormalities in the heart. These fall into three pathologic patterns (Fig. 12-29 and Table 12-11):

- Dilated cardiomyopathy (including arrhythmogenic right ventricular cardiomyopathy)
- Hypertrophic cardiomyopathy
- Restrictive cardiomyopathy

Among the three major patterns, dilated cardiomyopathy is most common (90% of cases), and restrictive cardiomyopathy is the least frequent. Within each pattern, there is a spectrum of clinical severity, and in some cases clinical features overlap among the groups. In addition, each of these patterns can be caused by a specific identifiable cause, or can be idiopathic (Tables 12-11 and 12-12).

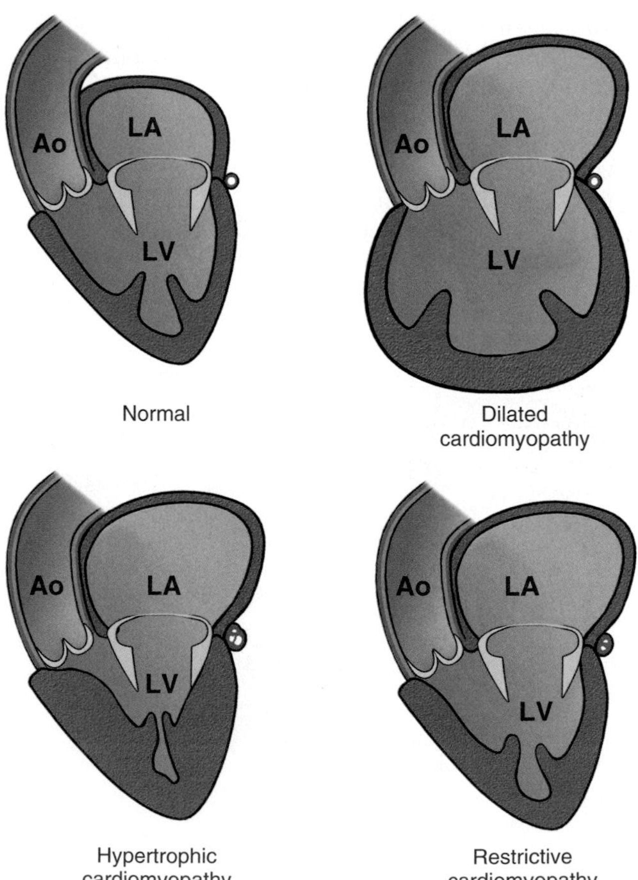

Figure 12-29 The three major morphologic patterns of cardiomyopathy. Dilated cardiomyopathy leads primarily to systolic dysfunction, whereas restrictive and hypertrophic cardiomyopathies result in diastolic dysfunction. Note the changes in atrial and/or ventricular wall thickness. Ao, Aorta; LA, left atrium; LV, left ventricle.

Table 12-11 Cardiomyopathy and Indirect Myocardial Dysfunction: Functional Patterns and Causes

Functional Pattern	Left Ventricular Ejection Fraction*	Mechanisms of Heart Failure	Causes of Phenotype	Indirect Myocardial Dysfunction (Mimicking Cardiomyopathy)
Dilated	<40%	Impairment of contractility (systolic dysfunction)	Genetic; alcohol; peripartum; myocarditis; hemochromatosis; chronic anemia; doxorubicin (Adriamycin) toxicity; sarcoidosis; idiopathic	Ischemic heart disease; valvular heart disease; hypertensive heart disease; congenital heart disease
Hypertrophic	50% to 80%	Impairment of compliance (diastolic dysfunction)	Genetic; Friedreich ataxia; storage diseases; infants of diabetic mother	Hypertensive heart disease; aortic stenosis
Restrictive	45% to 90%	Impairment of compliance (diastolic dysfunction)	Amyloidosis; radiation-induced fibrosis; idiopathic	Pericardial constriction

*Normal, approximately 50% to 65%.

Dilated Cardiomyopathy

Dilated cardiomyopathy (DCM) is characterized morphologically and functionally by progressive cardiac dilation and contractile (systolic) dysfunction, usually with concomitant hypertrophy. Many cases are familial, but the DCM phenotype can result from diverse causes, both primary and secondary.

Table 12-12 Conditions Associated with Heart Muscle Diseases

Cardiac Infections
Viruses Chlamydia Rickettsia Bacteria Fungi Protozoa
Toxins
Alcohol Cobalt Catecholamines Carbon monoxide Lithium Hydrocarbons Arsenic Cyclophosphamide Doxorubicin (Adriamycin) and daunorubicin
Metabolic
Hyperthyroidism Hypothyroidism Hyperkalemia Hypokalemia Nutritional deficiency (protein, thiamine, other avitaminoses) Hemochromatosis
Neuromuscular Disease
Friedreich ataxia Muscular dystrophy Congenital atrophies
Storage Disorders and Other Depositions
Hunter-Hurler syndrome Glycogen storage disease Fabry disease Amyloidosis
Infiltrative
Leukemia Carcinomatosis Sarcoidosis Radiation-induced fibrosis
Immunologic
Myocarditis (several forms) Posttransplant rejection

Pathogenesis. By the time of diagnosis, DCM has typically progressed to end-stage disease; the heart is dilated and poorly contractile. Unfortunately, at that point, even an exhaustive evaluation frequently fails to suggest a specific etiology. Increasingly, familial (genetic) forms of DCM are recognized, but the final pathology can also result from various acquired myocardial insults; as this implies, several different pathways can lead to DCM (Fig. 12-31).

- *Genetic Influences.* DCM is familial in at least 30% to 50% of cases, in which it is caused by mutations in a diverse group of more than 20 genes encoding proteins involved in the cytoskeleton, sarcolemma, and nuclear envelope (laminin A/C). In particular, mutations in *TTN*, a gene that encodes titin (so-called because it is the largest protein expressed in humans), may account for approximately 20% of all cases of DCM (Fig. 12-30).

  In the genetic forms of DCM, autosomal dominant inheritance is the predominant pattern; X-linked, autosomal recessive, and mitochondrial inheritance are less common. In some families there are deletions in mitochondrial genes that result in defects in oxidative phosphorylation; in others there are mutations in genes encoding enzymes involved in β-oxidation of fatty acids. Mitochondrial defects typically manifest in the pediatric population, while X-linked DCM typically presents after puberty and into early adulthood. X-linked cardiomyopathy can also be associated with mutations affecting the membrane-associated dystrophin protein that couples cytoskeleton to the extracellular matrix; recall that dystrophin is mutated in the most common skeletal myopathies (i.e., Duchenne and Becker muscular dystrophies; Chapter 27). Some patients and families with dystrophin gene mutations have DCM as the primary clinical feature. Interestingly, and probably resulting from the common developmental origin of contractile myocytes and conduction elements, congenital abnormalities of conduction may also be associated with DCM.
- *Myocarditis.* Sequential endomyocardial biopsies have documented progression from myocarditis to DCM. In other studies, the detection of the genetic fingerprints of coxsackie B and other viruses within myocardium of patients with DCM suggests that viral myocarditis can be causal (see later discussion).
- *Alcohol and other toxins. Alcohol abuse* is strongly associated with the development of DCM, raising the

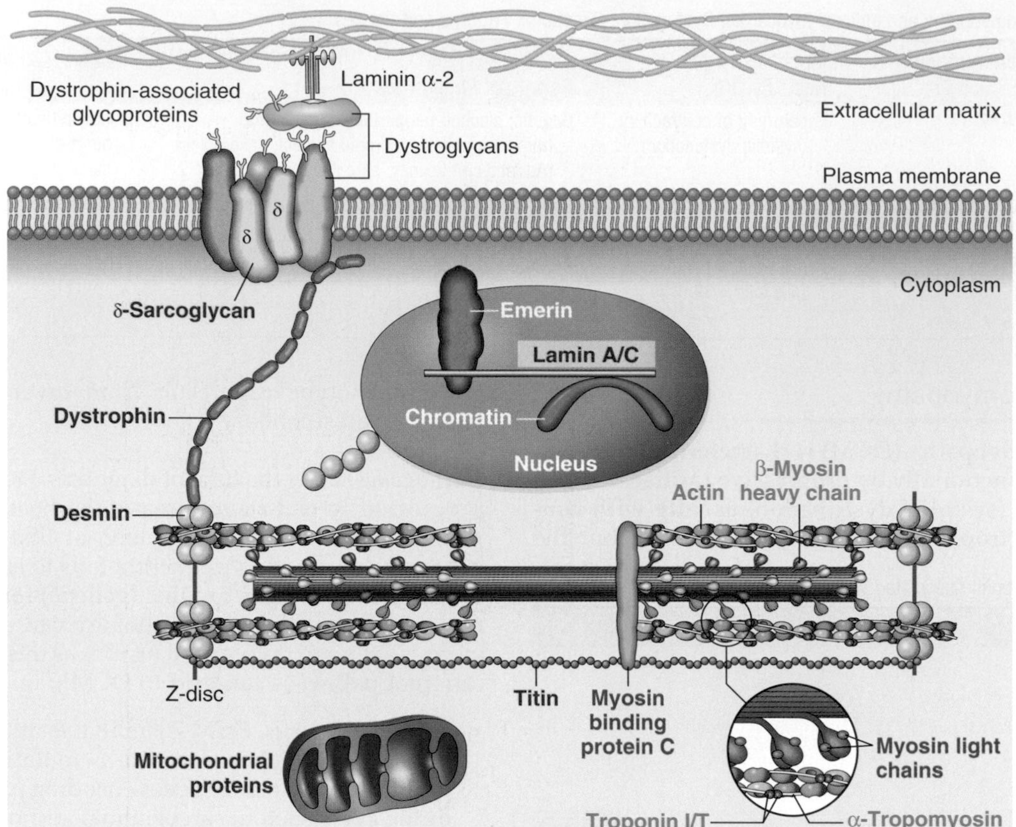

Figure 12-30 Schematic of a myocyte, showing key proteins mutated in dilated cardiomyopathy (red labels), hypertrophic cardiomyopathy (blue labels), or both (green labels). Mutations in titin (the largest known human protein at approximately 30,000 amino acids) account for approximately 20% of all dilated cardiomyopathy. Titin spans the sarcomere and connects the Z and M bands thereby limiting the passive range of motion of the sarcomere as it is stretched. Titin also functions like a molecular spring, with domains that unfold when the protein is stretched and refold when the tension is removed, thereby impacting the passive elasticity of striated muscle.

possibility that ethanol toxicity (Chapter 9) or a secondary nutritional disturbance can underlie myocardial injury. Alcohol or its metabolites (especially acetaldehyde) have a direct toxic effect on the myocardium. Moreover, chronic alcoholism may be associated with thiamine deficiency, which can lead to beriberi heart disease (also indistinguishable from DCM). Nevertheless, no morphologic features serve to distinguish *alcoholic cardiomyopathy* from DCM of other causes.

In other cases, some other toxic insult can progress to eventual myocardial failure. Particularly important is myocardial injury caused by certain chemotherapeutic agents, including doxorubicin (Adriamycin), and even targeted cancer therapeutics (e.g., tyrosine kinase inhibitors). Cobalt is an example of a heavy metal with cardiotoxicity and has caused DCM in the setting of inadvertent tainting (e.g., in beer production).

- *Childbirth.* A special form of DCM, termed *peripartum cardiomyopathy*, can occur late in pregnancy or up to months postpartum. The mechanism underlying this entity is poorly understood but is probably multifactorial. Pregnancy-associated hypertension, volume overload, nutritional deficiency, other metabolic derangements, or an as yet poorly characterized immunological reaction have been proposed as causes. Recent work suggests that the primary defect is a microvascular angiogenic imbalance within the myocardium leading to functional ischemic injury. Thus, peripartum cardiomyopathy can be elicited in mouse models by increased levels of circulating antiangiogenic mediators including vascular endothelial growth factor inhibitors (e.g., sFLT1, as occurs with preeclampsia) or antiangiogenic cleavage products of the hormone prolactin (which rises late in pregnancy). Proangiogenic approaches, including the blockade of prolactin secretion by bromocriptine, represent new therapeutic strategies for treating this disease.
- *Iron overload* in the heart can result from either hereditary hemochromatosis (Chapter 18) or from multiple transfusions. DCM is the most common manifestation of such iron excess, and may be caused by interference with metal-dependent enzyme systems or to injury from iron-mediated production of reactive oxygen species.
- *Supraphysiologic stress* can also result in DCM. This can happen with persistent tachycardia, hyperthyroidism, or even during development, as in the fetuses of insulin-dependent diabetic mothers. *Excess catecholamines*, in particular, may result in multifocal myocardial contraction band necrosis that can eventually progress to DCM. This can happen in individuals with *pheochromocytomas*, tumors that elaborate epinephrine (Chapter 24); use of cocaine or vasopressor agents such as dopamine can have similar consequences. Such "catecholamine effect" also occurs in the setting of intense autonomic stimulation, for example, secondary to intracranial

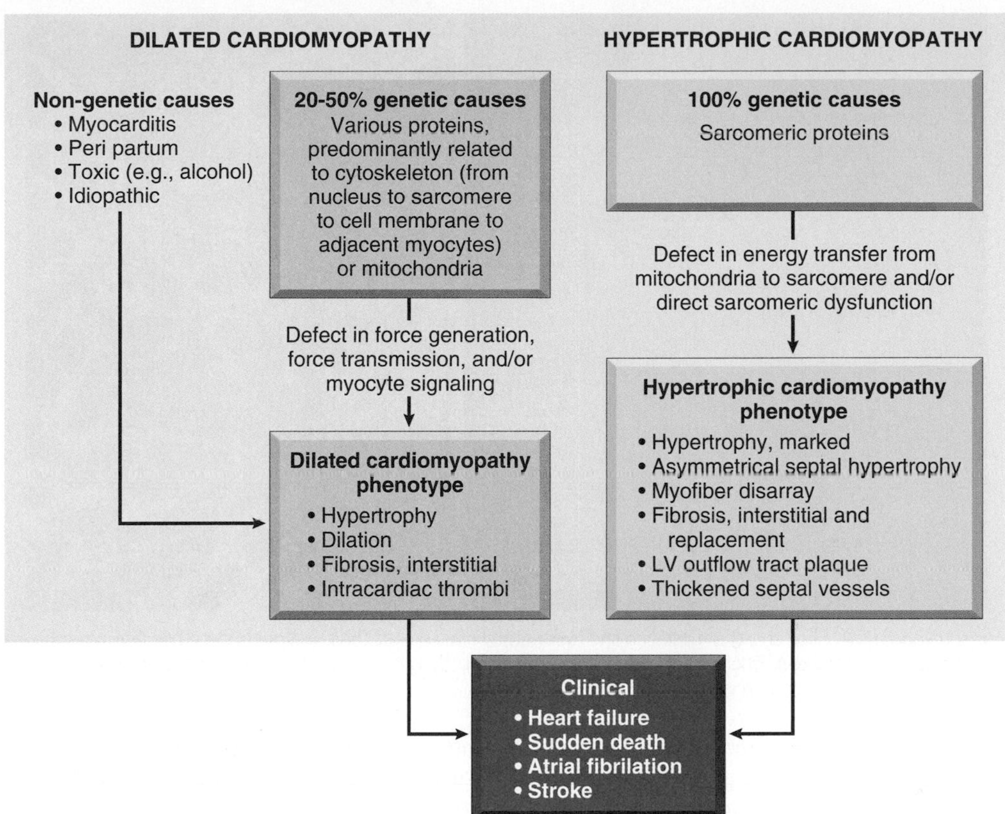

Figure 12-31 Causes and consequences of dilated and hypertrophic cardiomyopathy. Some dilated cardiomyopathies and virtually all hypertrophic cardiomyopathies are genetic in origin. The genetic causes of dilated cardiomyopathy involve mutations in any of a wide range of genes. They encode proteins predominantly of the cytoskeleton, but also the sarcomere, mitochondria, and nuclear envelope. In contrast, all of the mutated genes that cause hypertrophic cardiomyopathy encode proteins of the sarcomere. Although these two forms of cardiomyopathy differ greatly in subcellular basis and morphologic phenotypes, they share a common set of clinical complications. LV, left ventricle.

lesions or emotional duress. Thus, *takotsubo cardiomyopathy* is an entity characterized by left ventricular contractile dysfunction following extreme psychological stress; affected myocardium may be stunned or show multifocal contraction band necrosis. For unclear reasons, the left ventricular apex is most often affected leading to "apical ballooning" that resembles a "takotsubo," Japanese for "fishing pot for trapping octopus" (hence, the name).

The mechanism of catecholamine cardiotoxicity is uncertain, but likely relates either to direct myocyte toxicity due to calcium overload or to focal vasoconstriction in the coronary arterial macro- or microcirculation in the face of an increased heart rate. Similar changes may be encountered in individuals who have recovered from hypotensive episodes or have been resuscitated from a cardiac arrest; in such cases, the damage is a result of ischemia-reperfusion (see earlier) with subsequent inflammation.

MORPHOLOGY

In DCM the heart is usually enlarged, heavy (often weighing two to three times normal), and flabby, due to dilation of all chambers (Fig. 12-32). Mural thrombi are common and may be a source of thromboemboli. There are no primary valvular alterations; if mitral (or tricuspid) regurgitation is present, it results from left (or right) ventricular chamber dilation (*functional regurgitation*). Either the coronary arteries are free of significant narrowing or the obstructions present are insufficient to explain the degree of cardiac dysfunction.

The histologic abnormalities in DCM are nonspecific and usually do not point to a specific etiology. Most muscle cells are hypertrophied with enlarged nuclei, but some are attenuated, stretched, and irregular. Interstitial and endocardial fibrosis of variable degree is present, and small subendocardial scars may replace individual cells or groups of cells, probably reflecting healing of previous ischemic necrosis of myocytes caused by hypertrophy-induced imbalance between perfusion and demand. Moreover, the severity of morphologic changes may not reflect either the degree of dysfunction or the patient's prognosis.

Clinical Features. DCM can occur at any age, including in childhood, but it most commonly affects individuals between the ages of 20 and 50. **It presents with slowly progressive signs and symptoms of CHF including dyspnea, easy fatigability, and poor exertional capacity. At the end stage, ejection fractions are typically less than 25%** (normal = 50% to 65%). Secondary mitral regurgitation and abnormal cardiac rhythms are common, and embolism from intracardiac thrombi can occur. Death usually results from progressive cardiac failure or arrhythmia, and can occur suddenly. Although the annual mortality is high (10% to 50%), some severely affected patients respond well to pharmacologic therapy. Cardiac transplantation is also

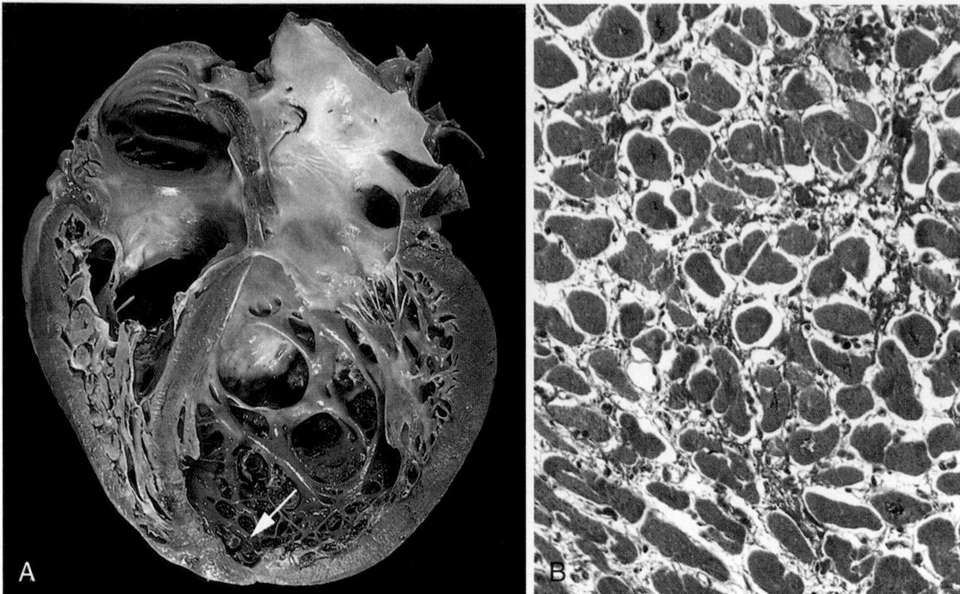

Figure 12-32 Dilated cardiomyopathy. **A,** Four-chamber dilatation and hypertrophy are evident. There is a mural thrombus (*arrow*) at the apex of the left ventricle (on the *right* in this apical four-chamber view). The coronary arteries were patent. **B,** Histologic section demonstrating variable myocyte hypertrophy and interstitial fibrosis (collagen is highlighted as blue in this Masson trichrome stain).

increasingly performed, and long-term ventricular assist can be beneficial. Interestingly, in some patients, relatively short-term mechanical cardiac support can induce durable improvement of cardiac function.

Arrhythmogenic Right Ventricular Cardiomyopathy

Arrhythmogenic right ventricular cardiomyopathy (ARVC) is an inherited disease of myocardium causing right ventricular failure and rhythm disturbances (particularly ventricular tachycardia or fibrillation) with sudden death. Left-sided involvement with left-sided heart failure may also occur. Morphologically, the right ventricular wall is severely thinned due to loss of myocytes, accompanied by extensive fatty infiltration and fibrosis (Fig. 12-33). Although myocardial inflammation may be present, ARVC is not considered an inflammatory cardiomyopathy. Classical ARVC has autosomal dominant inheritance with a variable penetrance. The disease has been attributed to defective cell adhesion proteins in the desmosomes that link adjacent cardiac myocytes. *Naxos syndrome* is a disorder characterized by arrhythmogenic right ventricular cardiomyopathy and hyperkeratosis of plantar palmar skin surfaces specifically associated with mutations in the gene encoding the desmosome-associated protein plakoglobin.

Hypertrophic Cardiomyopathy

Hypertrophic cardiomyopathy (HCM) is a common (incidence, 1 in 500), clinically heterogeneous, genetic

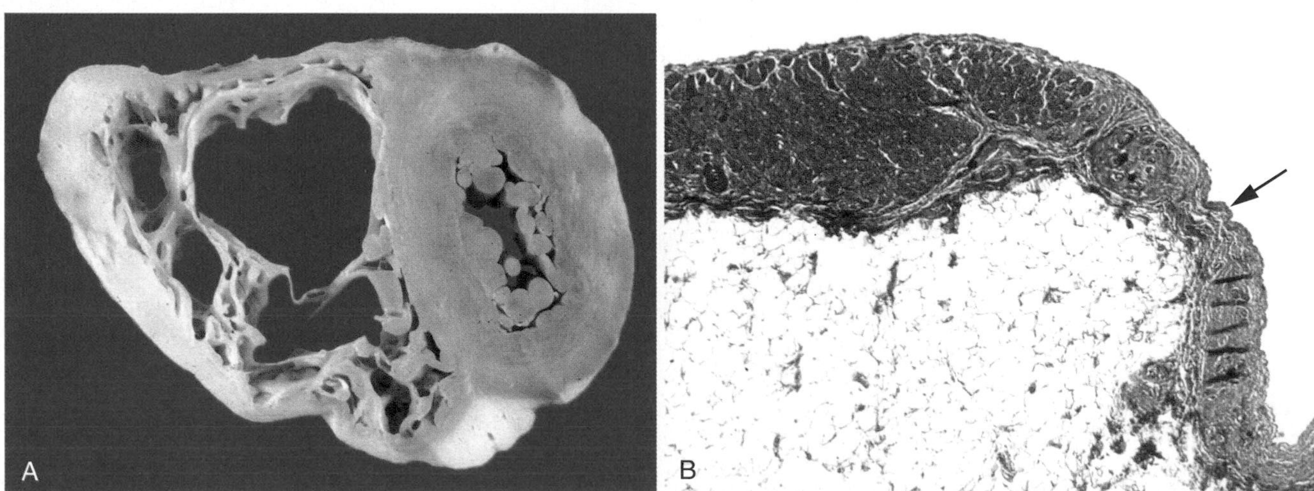

Figure 12-33 Arrhythmogenic right ventricular cardiomyopathy. **A,** Gross photograph, showing dilation of the right ventricle and near-transmural replacement of the right ventricular free-wall by fat and fibrosis. The left ventricle has a virtually normal configuration in this case, but can also be involved by the disease process. **B,** Histologic section of the right ventricular free wall, demonstrating replacement of myocardium (red) by fibrosis (blue, *arrow*) and fat (Masson trichrome stain).

disorder characterized by myocardial hypertrophy, poorly compliant left ventricular myocardium leading to abnormal diastolic filling, and (in about one third of cases) intermittent ventricular outflow obstruction. It is the leading cause of left ventricular hypertrophy unexplained by other clinical or pathologic causes. The heart is thick-walled, heavy, and *hyper*contracting, in striking contrast to the flabby, *hypo*contracting heart of DCM. HCM causes primarily diastolic dysfunction; systolic function is usually preserved. The two most common diseases that must be distinguished clinically from HCM are deposition diseases (e.g., amyloidosis, Fabry disease) and hypertensive heart disease coupled with age-related subaortic septal hypertrophy (see earlier discussion under Hypertensive Heart Disease). Occasionally, valvular or congenital subvalvular aortic stenosis can also mimic HCM.

Pathogenesis. In most cases, the pattern of transmission is autosomal dominant with variable penetrance. HCM is caused by mutations in any one of several genes that encode sarcomeric proteins; there are more than 400 different known mutations in nine different genes, most being missense mutations. Mutations causing HCM are found most commonly in the gene encoding β-myosin heavy chain (β-MHC), followed by the genes coding for cardiac TnT, α-tropomyosin, and myosin-binding protein C (MYBP-C); overall, these account for 70% to 80% of all cases. Different affected families may have distinct mutations involving the same protein. For example, approximately 50 different mutations of β-MHC are known to cause HCM. The prognosis of HCM varies widely and correlates strongly with specific mutations. Although it is clear that these genetic defects are critical to the etiology of HCM, the sequence of events leading from mutations to disease is still poorly understood.

As discussed above, HCM is a disease caused by mutations in proteins of the sarcomere. Although such sarcomeric alterations have been thought to be pathologic on the basis of abnormal cardiac contraction causing a secondary compensatory hypertrophy, newer evidence suggests that HCM may instead arise from defective energy transfer from its source of generation (mitochondria) to its site of use (sarcomeres). In addition, the interstitial fibrosis in HCM probably occurs secondary to exaggerated responses of the myocardial fibroblasts to the primary myocardial dysfunction. In contrast, DCM is mostly associated with abnormalities of cytoskeletal proteins (Fig. 12-30), and can be conceptualized as a disease of abnormal force generation, force transmission, or myocyte signaling. To complicate matters, mutations in certain genes, depicted in Figure 12-30, can give rise to either HCM or DCM, depending on the site and nature of the mutation.

MORPHOLOGY

The essential feature of HCM is **massive myocardial hypertrophy, usually without ventricular dilation** (Fig. 12-34). The classic pattern involves disproportionate thickening of the ventricular septum relative to the left ventricle free wall (with a ratio of septum to free wall greater than 3:1), termed **asymmetric septal hypertrophy**. In about 10% of cases, the hypertrophy is concentric and symmetrical. On longitudinal sectioning, the normally round-to-ovoid left ventricular cavity may be compressed into a "banana-like" configuration by bulging of the ventricular septum into the lumen (Fig. 12-34*A*). Although marked hypertrophy can involve the entire septum, it is usually most prominent in the subaortic region. The left ventricular outflow tract often exhibits a fibrous endocardial plaque associated with thickening of the anterior mitral leaflet. Both findings result from contact of the anterior mitral leaflet with the septum during ventricular systole; they correlate with the echocardiographic "systolic anterior motion" of the anterior leaflet, with functional left ventricular outflow tract obstruction during mid-systole.

The most important histologic features of HCM myocardium are (1) massive myocyte hypertrophy, with transverse myocyte diameters frequently greater than 40 μm (normal, approximately 15 μm); (2) haphazard disarray of bundles of myocytes, individual myocytes, and contractile elements in sarcomeres within cells (termed **myofiber disarray**); and (3) interstitial and replacement fibrosis (Fig. 12-34*B*).

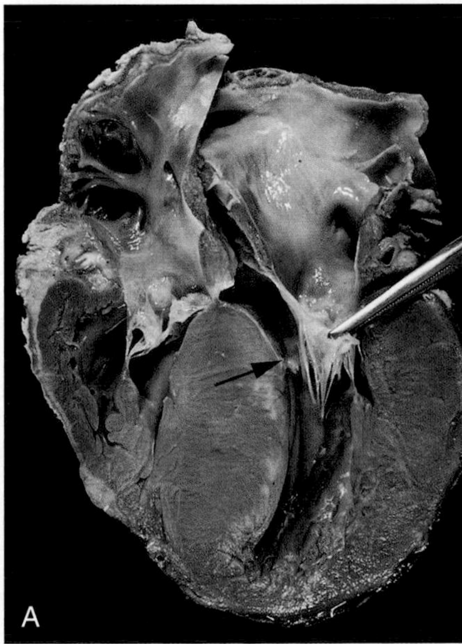

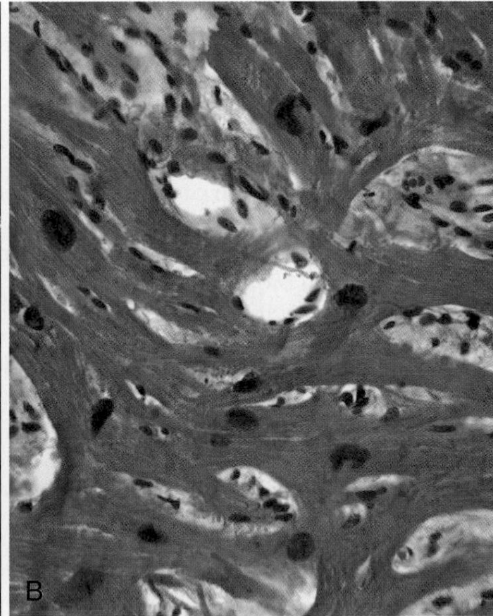

Figure 12-34 Hypertrophic cardiomyopathy with asymmetric septal hypertrophy. **A,** The septal muscle bulges into the left ventricular outflow tract, and the left atrium is enlarged. The anterior mitral leaflet has been reflected away from the septum to reveal a fibrous endocardial plaque *(arrow)* (see text). **B,** Histologic appearance demonstrating myocyte disarray, extreme hypertrophy, and exaggerated myocyte branching, as well as the characteristic interstitial fibrosis (collagen is blue in this Masson trichrome stain).

Clinical Features. **The central abnormality in HCM is reduced stroke volume due to impaired diastolic filling.** This is a consequence of a reduced chamber size, as well as the reduced compliance of the massively hypertrophied left ventricle. In addition, approximately 25% of patients with HCM have dynamic obstruction to the left ventricular outflow. The compromised cardiac output in conjunction with a secondary increase in pulmonary venous pressure explains the exertional dyspnea seen in these patients. Auscultation discloses a harsh systolic ejection murmur, caused by the ventricular outflow obstruction as the anterior mitral leaflet moves toward the ventricular septum during systole. Because of the massive hypertrophy, high left ventricular chamber pressure, and frequently thick-walled intramural arteries, focal myocardial ischemia commonly results, even in the absence of concomitant coronary artery disease. Major clinical problems in HCM are atrial fibrillation, mural thrombus formation leading to embolization and possible stroke, intractable cardiac failure, ventricular arrhythmias, and, not infrequently, sudden death, especially with certain specific mutations. Indeed, HCM is one of the most common causes of sudden, otherwise unexplained death in young athletes.

The natural history of HCM is highly variable. Most patients can be helped by pharmacologic intervention (e.g., β-adrenergic blockade) to decrease heart rate and contractility. Some benefit can also be gained by reducing the septal myocardial mass, thus relieving the outflow tract obstruction. This can be achieved either by surgical excision of muscle or by carefully controlled septal infarction through a catheter-based infusion of alcohol.

Restrictive Cardiomyopathy

Restrictive cardiomyopathy is characterized by a primary decrease in ventricular compliance, resulting in impaired ventricular filling during diastole. Because the contractile (systolic) function of the left ventricle is usually unaffected, the functional abnormality can be confused with that of constrictive pericarditis or HCM. Restrictive cardiomyopathy can be idiopathic or associated with distinct diseases or processes that affect the myocardium, principally radiation fibrosis, amyloidosis, sarcoidosis, metastatic tumors, or the deposition of metabolites that accumulate due to inborn errors of metabolism.

The morphologic features are not distinctive. The ventricles are of approximately normal size or slightly enlarged, the cavities are not dilated, and the myocardium is firm and noncompliant. Biatrial dilation is commonly observed. Microscopically, there may be only patchy or diffuse interstitial fibrosis, which can vary from minimal to extensive. Endomyocardial biopsy can often reveal a specific etiology. An important specific subgroup is amyloidosis (described later).

Several other restrictive conditions merit brief mention.

- *Endomyocardial fibrosis* is principally a disease of children and young adults in Africa and other tropical areas, characterized by fibrosis of the ventricular endocardium and subendocardium that extends from the apex upward, often involving the tricuspid and mitral valves. The fibrous tissue markedly diminishes the volume and compliance of affected chambers and so causes a restrictive functional defect. Ventricular mural thrombi sometimes develop, and indeed the endocardial fibrosis may result from thrombus organization. The etiology is unknown.
- *Loeffler endomyocarditis* also results in endomyocardial fibrosis, typically with large mural thrombi, with an overall morphology similar to the tropical disease. However, in addition to the cardiac changes, there is often a peripheral eosinophilia and eosinophilic infiltrates in multiple organs, including the heart. The release of toxic products of eosinophils, especially major basic protein, is postulated to initiate endomyocardial necrosis, followed by scarring of the necrotic area, layering of the endocardium by thrombus, and finally organization of the thrombus. Many patients with Loeffler endomyocarditis have a myeloproliferative disorder associated with chromosomal rearrangements involving either the platelet-derived growth factor receptor (PDGFR)-α or -β genes (Chapter 13). These rearrangements produce fusion genes that encode constitutively active PDGFR tyrosine kinases. Treatment of such patients with the tyrosine kinase inhibitor imatinib has resulted in hematologic remissions associated with reversal of the endomyocarditis, which is otherwise often rapidly fatal.
- *Endocardial fibroelastosis* is an uncommon heart disease characterized by fibroelastic thickening that typically involves the left ventricular endocardium. It is most common in the first 2 years of life; in a third of cases, it is accompanied by aortic valve obstruction or other congenital cardiac anomalies. Endocardial fibroelastosis may actually represent a common morphologic endpoint of several different insults including viral infections (e.g., intrauterine exposure to mumps) or mutations in the gene for tafazzin, which affects mitochondrial inner membrane integrity. Diffuse involvement may be responsible for rapid and progressive cardiac decompensation and death.

Myocarditis

Myocarditis is a diverse group of pathologic entities in which infectious microorganisms and/or a primary inflammatory process cause myocardial injury. Myocarditis should be distinguished from conditions such as ischemic heart disease, where myocardial inflammation is secondary to other causes.

Pathogenesis. In the United States, *viral infections* are the most common cause of myocarditis. *Coxsackie viruses A* and *B* and other enteroviruses probably account for most of the cases. Other less common etiologic agents include cytomegalovirus, HIV, and influenza (Table 12-13). In some (but not all) cases, the responsible virus can be ascertained by serologic studies or by identifying viral nucleic acid sequences in myocardial biopsies. Depending on the pathogen and the host, viruses can potentially cause myocardial injury either as a direct cytopathic effect, or by eliciting a destructive immune response. Inflammatory cytokines produced in response to myocardial injury can also cause *myocardial dysfunction* that is out of proportion to the degree of actual myocyte damage.

Table 12-13 Major Causes of Myocarditis

Infections
Viruses (e.g., coxsackievirus, ECHO, influenza, HIV, cytomegalovirus)
Chlamydiae (e.g., *Chlamydophyla psittaci*)
Rickettsiae (e.g., *Rickettsia typhi*, typhus fever)
Bacteria (e.g., *Corynebacterium diphtheriae, Neisseria meningococcus, Borrelia* (Lyme disease)
Fungi (e.g., *Candida*)
Protozoa (e.g., *Trypanosoma cruzi* [Chagas disease], toxoplasmosis)
Helminths (e.g., trichinosis)
Immune-Mediated Reactions
Postviral
Poststreptococcal (rheumatic fever)
Systemic lupus erythematosus
Drug hypersensitivity (e.g., methyldopa, sulfonamides)
Transplant rejection
Unknown
Sarcoidosis
Giant cell myocarditis

HIV, Human immunodeficiency virus.

Nonviral agents are also important causes of infectious myocarditis, particularly the protozoan *Trypanosoma cruzi*, the agent of Chagas disease. Chagas disease is endemic in some regions of South America, with myocardial involvement in most infected individuals. About 10% of patients die during an acute attack; others develop a chronic immune-mediated myocarditis that may progress to cardiac insufficiency in 10 to 20 years. Trichinosis (*Trichinella spiralis*) is the most common helminthic disease associated with myocarditis. Parasitic diseases, including toxoplasmosis, and bacterial infections such as Lyme disease and diphtheria, can also cause myocarditis. In the case of diphtheritic myocarditis, the myocardial injury is a consequence of diphtheria toxin release by the causal organism, *Corynebacterium diphtheriae* (Chapter 8). Myocarditis occurs in approximately 5% of patients with Lyme disease, a systemic illness caused by the bacterial spirochete *Borrelia burgdorferi* (Chapter 8); it manifests primarily as a self-limited conduction system disorder that may require a temporary pacemaker. AIDS-associated myocarditis may reflect inflammation and myocyte damage without a clear etiologic agent, or a myocarditis attributable directly to HIV or to an opportunistic pathogen.

There are also noninfectious causes of myocarditis. Broadly speaking they are either immunologically mediated (*hypersensitivity myocarditis*) or idiopathic conditions with distinctive morphology (*giant cell myocarditis*) suspected to be of immunologic origin (Table 12-13).

MORPHOLOGY

Grossly, the heart in myocarditis may appear normal or dilated; some hypertrophy may be present depending on disease duration. In advanced stages the ventricular myocardium is flabby and often mottled by either pale foci or minute hemorrhagic lesions. Mural thrombi may be present.

Active myocarditis is characterized by an interstitial inflammatory infiltrate associated with focal myocyte necrosis (Fig. 12-35). A diffuse, mononuclear, predominantly lymphocytic infiltrate is most common (Fig. 12-35*A*). Although endomyocardial biopsies are diagnostic in some cases, they can be spuriously negative because inflammatory involvement of the myocardium may be focal or patchy. If the patient survives the acute phase of myocarditis, the inflammatory lesions either resolve, leaving no residual changes, or heal by progressive fibrosis.

Hypersensitivity myocarditis has interstitial infiltrates, principally perivascular, composed of lymphocytes, macrophages, and a high proportion of eosinophils (Fig. 12-35*B*). A morphologically distinctive form of myocarditis, called **giant-cell myocarditis**, is characterized by a widespread inflammatory cellular infiltrate containing multinucleate giant cells (fused macrophages) interspersed with lymphocytes, eosinophils, plasma cells, and macrophages. Focal to frequently extensive necrosis is present (Fig. 12-35*C*). This variant likely represents the fulminant end of the myocarditis spectrum and carries a poor prognosis.

The myocarditis of **Chagas disease** is distinctive by virtue of the parasitization of scattered myofibers by trypanosomes accompanied by a mixed inflammatory infiltrate of neutrophils, lymphocytes, macrophages, and occasional eosinophils (Fig. 12-35*D*).

Clinical Features. The clinical spectrum of myocarditis is broad. At one end, the disease is entirely asymptomatic, and patients can expect a complete recovery without sequelae; at the other extreme is the precipitous onset of heart failure or arrhythmias, occasionally with sudden death. Between these extremes are the many levels of involvement associated with symptoms such as fatigue, dyspnea, palpitations, precordial discomfort, and fever. The clinical features of myocarditis can mimic those of acute MI. As noted previously, patients can develop dilated cardiomyopathy as a late complication of myocarditis.

Other Causes of Myocardial Disease

Cardiotoxic Drugs. Cardiac complications of cancer therapy are an important clinical problem; cardiotoxicity has been associated with conventional chemotherapeutic agents, tyrosine kinase inhibitors, and certain forms of immunotherapy. The anthracyclines doxorubicin and daunorubicin are the chemotherapeutic agents most often associated with toxic myocardial injury; they cause dilated cardiomyopathy with heart failure attributed primarily to peroxidation of lipids in myocyte membranes. Anthra cycline toxicity is dose-dependent, with the cardiotoxicity risk increasing when cumulative life-time doses exceed 500 mg/m^2.

Many other therapeutic agents, including lithium, phenothiazines, and chloroquine can idiosyncratically induce myocardial injury and sometimes sudden death. Common findings in affected myocardium include myofiber swelling, cytoplasmic vacuolization, and fatty change. Discontinuing the offending agent often leads to prompt resolution, without apparent sequelae. Occasionally, however, more extensive damage produces myocyte necrosis that can evolve to a dilated cardiomyopathy.

Amyloidosis. Amyloidosis results from the extracellular accumulation of protein fibrils that are prone to forming insoluble β-pleated sheets (Chapter 6). Cardiac

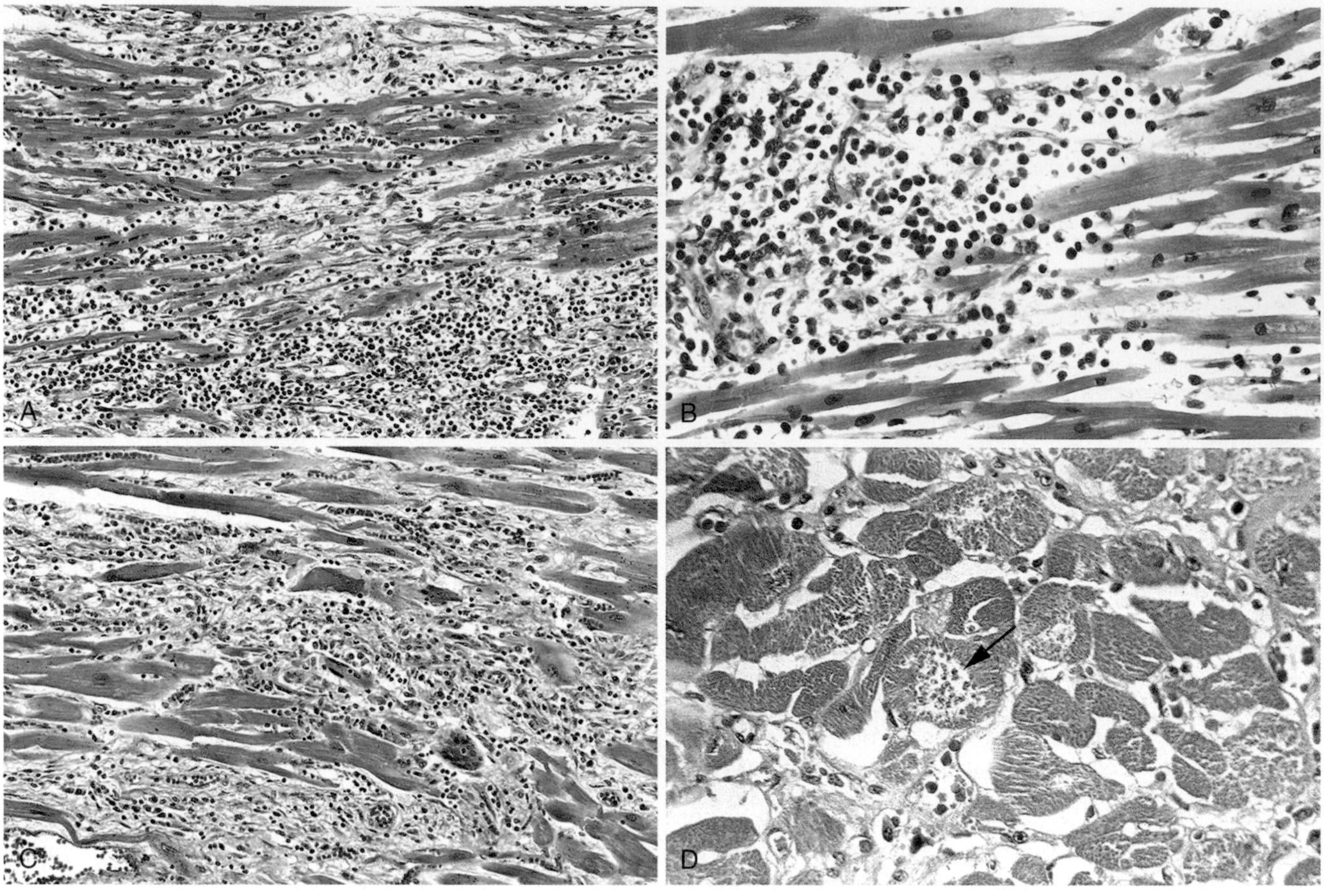

Figure 12-35 Myocarditis. **A,** Lymphocytic myocarditis, associated with myocyte injury. **B,** Hypersensitivity myocarditis, characterized by interstitial inflammatory infiltrate composed largely of eosinophils and mononuclear inflammatory cells, predominantly localized to perivascular and expanded interstitial spaces. **C,** Giant-cell myocarditis, with mononuclear inflammatory infiltrate containing lymphocytes and macrophages, extensive loss of muscle, and multinucleated giant cells (fused macrophages). **D,** The myocarditis of Chagas disease. A myofiber distended with trypanosomes *(arrow)* is present along with individual myofiber necrosis, and modest amounts of inflammation.

amyloidosis can appear as a consequence of systemic amyloidosis (e.g., due to myeloma or inflammation-associated amyloid) or can be restricted to the heart, particularly in the aged (*senile cardiac amyloidosis*). Senile cardiac amyloidosis characteristically occurs in individuals 70 years and older, and has a far better prognosis than systemic amyloidosis. Senile cardiac amyloid deposits are largely composed of *transthyretin,* a normal serum protein synthesized in the liver that *trans*ports *thy*roxine and *retin*ol-binding protein. Mutant forms of transthyretin can accelerate the cardiac (and associated systemic) amyloid deposition; 4% of African-Americans have a transthyretin mutation substituting isoleucine for valine at position 122 that produces a particularly amyloidogenic protein, responsible for autosomal dominant familial transthyretin amyloidosis. Isolated atrial amyloidosis can also occur secondary to deposition of atrial natriuretic peptide, but its clinical significance is uncertain.

Cardiac amyloidosis most frequently produces a restrictive cardiomyopathy, but it can also be asymptomatic, manifest as dilation or arrhythmias, or mimic ischemic or valvular disease. The varied presentations depend on the predominant location of the deposits, for example, interstitium, conduction system, vasculature, or valves.

MORPHOLOGY

In cardiac amyloidosis the heart varies in consistency from normal to firm and rubbery. The chambers are usually of normal size, but can be dilated and have thickened walls. Small, semitranslucent nodules resembling drips of wax may be seen on the atrial endocardial surface, particularly on the left. Histologically, hyaline eosinophilic deposits of amyloid may be found in the interstitium, conduction tissue, valves, endocardium, pericardium, and small intramural coronary arteries (Fig. 12-36); they can be distinguished from other deposits by special stains such as Congo red, which produces classic apple-green birefringence when viewed under polarized light (Fig. 12-36*B*). Intramural arteries and arterioles may have sufficient amyloid in their walls to compress and occlude their lumens, inducing myocardial ischemia ("small-vessel disease").

KEY CONCEPTS

Cardiomyopathy

- Cardiomyopathy is intrinsic cardiac muscle disease; there may be specific causes, or it can be idiopathic.

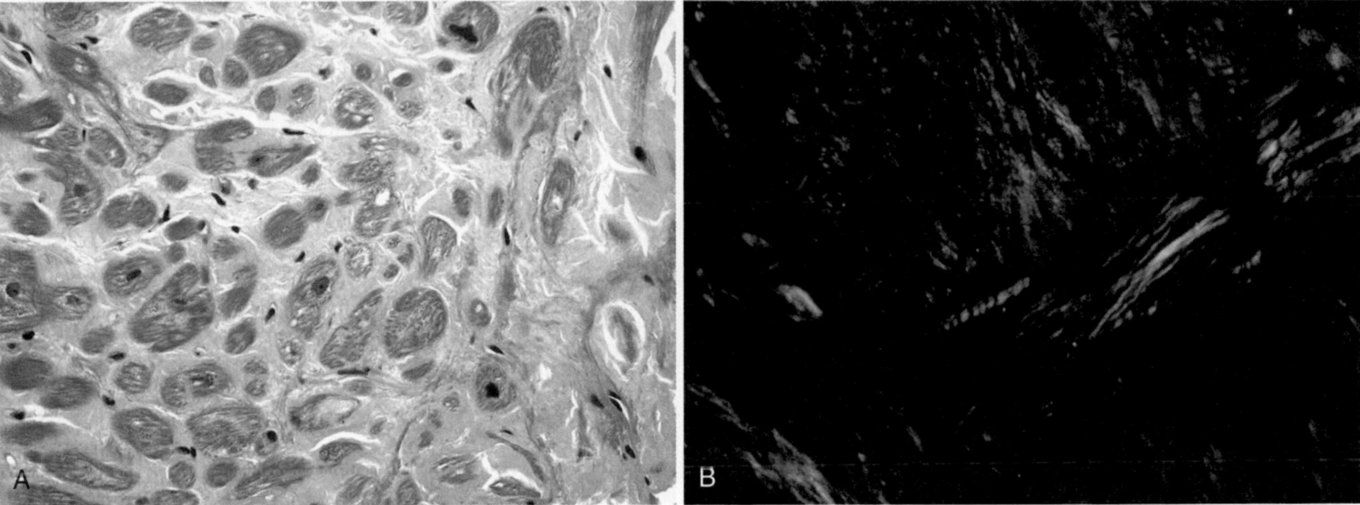

Figure 12-36 Cardiac amyloidosis. **A,** Hematoxylin and eosin stain, showing amyloid appearing as amorphous pink material around myocytes. **B,** Congo red stain viewed under polarized light, in which amyloid shows characteristic apple-green birefringence (compared with collagen, which appears white).

- There are three general pathophysiologic categories of cardiomyopathy: dilated (90%), hypertrophic, and restrictive (least common).
- Dilated cardiomyopathy results in systolic (contractile) dysfunction. Causes include myocarditis, toxic exposures (e.g., alcohol), and pregnancy. In 20% to 50% of cases, genetic cytoskeletal protein defects are causal, with titin mutations representing up to 20% of cases of dilated cardiomyopathy.
- Hypertrophic cardiomyopathy results in diastolic (relaxation) dysfunction. Virtually all cases are due to autosomal dominant mutations in the proteins comprising the contractile apparatus, in particular β-myosin heavy chain.
- Restrictive cardiomyopathy results in a stiff, noncompliant myocardium and can be due to deposition (e.g., amyloid), increased interstitial fibrosis (e.g., due to radiation), or endomyocardial scarring.
- Myocarditis is myocardial damage caused by inflammatory infiltrates secondary to infections or immune reactions. Coxsackie A and B viruses are the most common causes in the United States. Clinically, myocarditis can be asymptomatic, give rise to acute heart failure, or evolve into dilated cardiomyopathy.

Pericardial Disease

The most important pericardial disorders cause fluid accumulation, inflammation, fibrous constriction, or some combination of these processes, usually in association with other cardiac pathology or a systemic disease; isolated pericardial disease is unusual.

Pericardial Effusion and Hemopericardium

Normally, the pericardial sac contains less than 50 mL of thin, clear, straw-colored fluid. Under various circumstances the parietal pericardium may be distended by serous fluid *(pericardial effusion)*, blood (*hemopericardium*), or pus (*purulent pericarditis*). With long-standing cardiac enlargement or with slowly accumulating fluid, the pericardium has time to dilate. This permits a slowly accumulating pericardial effusion to become quite large without interfering with cardiac function. Thus, with chronic effusions of less than 500 mL in volume, the only clinical significance is a characteristic globular enlargement of the heart shadow on chest radiographs. In contrast, rapidly developing fluid collections of as little as 200 to 300 mL—e.g., due to hemopericardium caused by a ruptured MI or aortic dissection—can produce clinically devastating compression of the thin-walled atria and venae cavae, or the ventricles themselves; cardiac filling is thereby restricted, producing potentially fatal *cardiac tamponade.*

Pericarditis

Pericardial inflammation can occur secondary to a variety of cardiac, thoracic, or systemic disorders, metastases from remote neoplasms, or cardiac surgical procedures. Primary pericarditis is unusual and almost always of viral origin. The major causes of pericarditis are listed in Table 12-14. Most evoke an acute pericarditis, but a few, such as tuberculosis and fungi, produce chronic reactions.

Acute Pericarditis

Serous pericarditis is characteristically produced by noninfectious inflammatory diseases, including rheumatic fever, SLE, and scleroderma, as well as tumors and uremia. An infection in the tissues contiguous to the pericardium—for example, a bacterial pleuritis—may incite sufficient irritation of the parietal pericardial serosa to cause a sterile serous effusion that can progress to serofibrinous pericarditis and ultimately to a frank suppurative reaction. In some instances a well-defined viral infection elsewhere—upper respiratory tract infection, pneumonia, parotitis—antedates the pericarditis and serves as the primary focus of infection. Infrequently, usually in young adults, a viral pericarditis occurs as an apparent primary infection that may be accompanied by myocarditis *(myopericarditis).* Tumors can cause a serous pericarditis by lymphatic

Table 12-14 Causes of Pericarditis

Infectious Agents
Viruses
Pyogenic bacteria
Tuberculosis
Fungi
Other parasites
Presumably Immunologically Mediated
Rheumatic fever
Systemic lupus erythematosus
Scleroderma
Postcardiotomy
Postmyocardial infarction (Dressler) syndrome
Drug hypersensitivity reaction
Miscellaneous
Myocardial infarction
Uremia
Following cardiac surgery
Neoplasia
Trauma
Radiation

invasion or direct contiguous extension into the pericardium. Histologically, serous pericarditis elicits a mild inflammatory infiltrate in the epipericardial fat consisting predominantly of lymphocytes; tumor-associated pericarditis may also exhibit neoplastic cells. Organization into fibrous adhesions rarely occurs.

Fibrinous and serofibrinous pericarditis are *the most frequent types of pericarditis*; these are composed of serous fluid variably admixed with a fibrinous exudate. Common causes include acute MI (Fig. 12-18*D*), postinfarction (Dressler) syndrome (an autoimmune response appearing days-weeks after an MI), uremia, chest radiation, rheumatic fever, SLE, and trauma. A fibrinous reaction also follows routine cardiac surgery.

MORPHOLOGY

In fibrinous pericarditis the surface is dry, with a fine granular roughening. In serofibrinous pericarditis a more intense inflammatory process induces the accumulation of larger amounts of yellow to brown turbid fluid, containing leukocytes, erythrocytes, and fibrin. As with all inflammatory exudates, fibrin may be lysed with resolution of the exudate, or can become organized (Chapter 3).

Symptoms of fibrinous pericarditis characteristically include pain (sharp, pleuritic, and position dependent) and fever; congestive failure may also be present. *A loud pericardial friction rub is the most striking clinical finding.* However, the collection of serous fluid can actually prevent rubbing by separating the two layers of the pericardium.

Purulent or suppurative pericarditis reflects an active infection caused by microbial invasion of the pericardial space; this can occur through:

- Direct extension from neighboring infections, such as an empyema of the pleural cavity, lobar pneumonia, mediastinal infections, or extension of a ring abscess through the myocardium or aortic root
- Seeding from the blood
- Lymphatic extension
- Direct introduction during cardiotomy

The exudate ranges from a thin cloudy fluid to frank pus up to 400 to 500 mL in volume. The serosal surfaces are reddened, granular, and coated with the exudate (Fig. 12-37). Microscopically there is an acute inflammatory reaction, which sometimes extends into surrounding structures to induce *mediastinopericarditis*. Complete resolution is infrequent, and organization by scarring is the usual outcome. The intense inflammatory response and the subsequent scarring frequently produce *constrictive pericarditis*, a serious consequence (see later). Clinical findings in the active phase resemble those seen in fibrinous pericarditis, although the frank infection leads to more marked systemic symptoms including spiking fevers and rigors.

Hemorrhagic pericarditis has an exudate composed of blood mixed with a fibrinous or suppurative effusion; it is most commonly caused by the spread of a malignant neoplasm to the pericardial space. In such cases, cytologic examination of fluid removed through a pericardial tap often reveals neoplastic cells. Hemorrhagic pericarditis can also be found in bacterial infections, in persons with an underlying bleeding diathesis, and in tuberculosis. Hemorrhagic pericarditis often follows cardiac surgery and is occasionally responsible for significant blood loss or even tamponade, requiring re-operation. The clinical significance is similar to that of fibrinous or suppurative pericarditis.

Caseous pericarditis is, until proved otherwise, tuberculous in origin; infrequently, fungal infections evoke a similar reaction. Pericardial involvement occurs by direct spread from tuberculous foci within the tracheobronchial nodes. Caseous pericarditis is a common antecedent of disabling, fibrocalcific, chronic constrictive pericarditis.

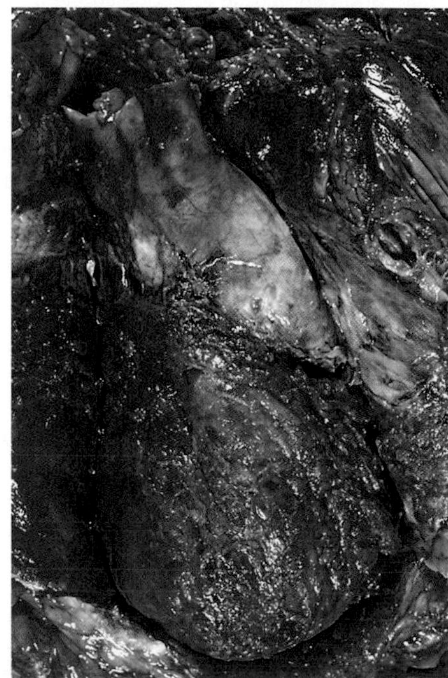

Figure 12-37 Acute suppurative pericarditis arising from direct extension of an adjacent pneumonia. Extensive purulent exudate is evident.

Chronic or Healed Pericarditis. In some cases organization merely produces plaque-like fibrous thickenings of the serosal membranes ("soldier's plaque") or thin, delicate adhesions that rarely cause impairment of cardiac function. In other cases, fibrosis in the form of mesh-like stringy adhesions completely obliterates the pericardial sac. In most instances, this *adhesive pericarditis* has no effect on cardiac function.

Adhesive mediastinopericarditis may follow infectious pericarditis, previous cardiac surgery, or mediastinal irradiation. The pericardial sac is obliterated, and adherence of the external aspect of the parietal layer to surrounding structures strains cardiac function. With each systolic contraction, the heart pulls not only against the parietal pericardium but also against the attached surrounding structures. Systolic retraction of the rib cage and diaphragm, pulsus paradoxus, and a variety of other characteristic clinical findings may be observed. The increased workload causes occasionally severe cardiac hypertrophy and dilation.

In *constrictive pericarditis* the heart is encased in a dense, fibrous or fibrocalcific scar that limits diastolic expansion and cardiac output, features that mimic a restrictive cardiomyopathy. A prior history of pericarditis may or may not be present. The fibrous scar can be up to a centimeter in thickness, obliterating the pericardial space and sometimes calcifying; in extreme cases it can resemble a plaster mold *(concretio cordis)*. Because of the dense enclosing scar, cardiac hypertrophy and dilation cannot occur. Cardiac output may be reduced at rest, but more importantly the heart has little if any capacity to increase its output in response to increased systemic demands. Signs of constrictive pericarditis include distant or muffled heart sounds, elevated jugular venous pressure, and peripheral edema. Treatment consists of surgical resection of the shell of constricting fibrous tissue (pericardiectomy).

Heart Disease Associated with Rheumatologic Disorders

The heart (vessels, myocardium, valves, or pericardium) can be significantly impacted by chronic rheumatologic diseases (e.g., rheumatoid arthritis, SLE, systemic sclerosis, ankylosing spondylitis, and psoriatic arthritis). Indeed, as improved therapies lead to longer life expectancies, the cardiovascular manifestations of such systemic inflammation are increasingly recognized. In addition, ischemic heart disease can be accelerated in the setting of systemic inflammation.

Although rheumatoid arthritis is primarily a joint disorder, it also has several extra-articular manifestations, including subcutaneous rheumatoid nodules, vasculitis, and neutropenia (Chapter 26). The heart is also involved in 20-40% of severe cases. The most common finding is a *fibrinous pericarditis* that may progress to fibrous thickening of the visceral and parietal pericardium and dense adhesions. Granulomatous rheumatoid nodules resembling the subcutaneous nodules may also occur in the myocardium, endocardium, valves, and aortic root. *Rheumatoid valvulitis* can lead to marked fibrous thickening and secondary calcification of the aortic valve cusps, producing changes resembling those of chronic rheumatic valvular disease. The Libman-Sacks valvular lesions associated with SLE were discussed previously.

Tumors of the Heart

Primary tumors of the heart are rare; in contrast, metastatic tumors to the heart occur in about 5% of persons dying of cancer. The most common primary cardiac tumors, in descending order of frequency (overall, including adults and children) are myxomas, fibromas, lipomas, papillary fibroelastomas, rhabdomyomas, and angiosarcomas. The five most common tumors are all benign and collectively account for 80% to 90% of primary tumors of the heart.

Primary Cardiac Tumors

Myxomas are the most common primary tumor of the adult heart (Fig. 12-38). These are benign neoplasms thought to arise from primitive multipotent mesenchymal cells. Although sporadic myxomas do not show consistent genetic alterations, familial syndromes associated with myxomas have activating mutations in the *GNAS1* gene, encoding a subunit of G protein (Gsα) (in association with McCune-Albright syndrome) or null mutations in *PRKAR1A*, encoding a regulatory subunit of a cyclic-AMP-dependent protein kinase (*Carney complex*). About 90% of myxomas arise in the atria, with a left-to-right ratio of approximately 4:1.

MORPHOLOGY

The tumors are usually single, but can rarely be multiple. The region of the fossa ovalis in the atrial septum is the favored site of origin. Myxomas range from small (<1 cm) to large (≥10 cm), and can be sessile or pedunculated lesions (Fig. 12-38*A*). They vary from globular hard masses mottled with hemorrhage to soft, translucent, papillary, or villous lesions having a gelatinous appearance. The pedunculated form is often sufficiently mobile to move during systole into the atrioventricular valve

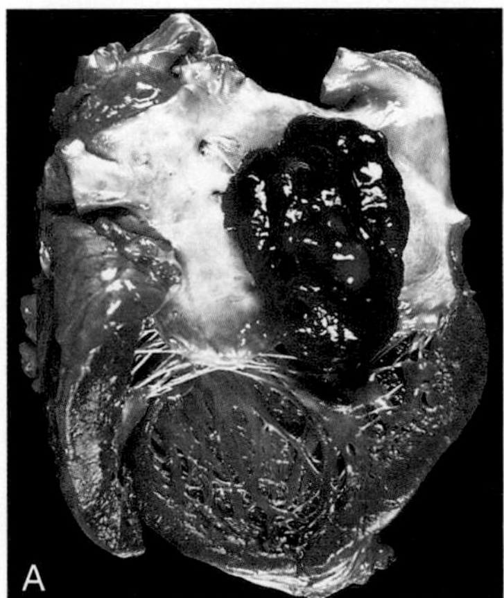

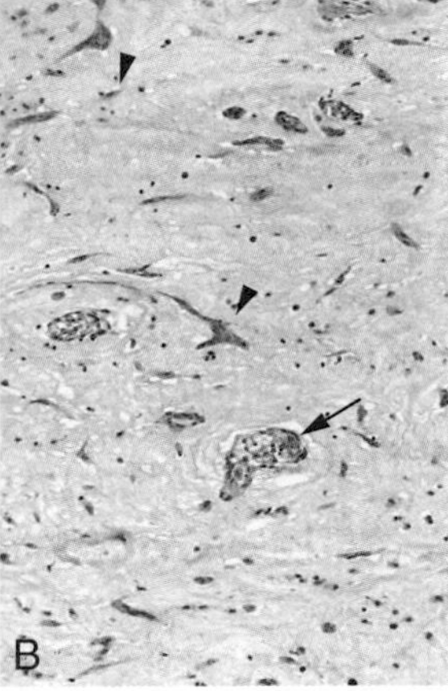

Figure 12-38 Atrial myxoma. **A,** A large pedunculated lesion arises from the region of the fossa ovalis and extends into the mitral valve orifice. **B,** Abundant amorphous extracellular matrix contains scattered multinucleate myxoma cells (*arrowheads*) in various groupings, including abnormal vessel-like formations *(arrow)*.

opening, causing intermittent obstruction that may be position-dependent. Sometimes mobile tumors exert a "wrecking-ball" effect, causing damage to the valve leaflets.

Histologically, myxomas are composed of stellate or globular myxoma cells embedded within an abundant acid mucopolysaccharide ground substance (Fig. 12-38*B*). Peculiar vessel-like or gland-like structures are characteristic. Hemorrhage and mononuclear inflammation are usually present.

The major clinical manifestations are due to valvular "ball-valve" obstruction, embolization, or a syndrome of constitutional symptoms, such as fever and malaise. Sometimes fragmentation and systemic embolization calls attention to these lesions. Constitutional symptoms are probably due to the elaboration by some myxomas of the cytokine interleukin-6, a major mediator of the acute-phase response. Echocardiography provides the opportunity to identify these masses noninvasively. Surgical removal is usually curative; rarely, presumably with incomplete excision, the neoplasm can recurs months to years later.

Lipoma. Lipomas are localized, well-circumscribed, benign tumors composed of mature fat cells that can occur in the subendocardium, subepicardium, or myocardium. They may be asymptomatic, or produce ball-valve obstructions or arrhythmias. Lipomas are most often located in the left ventricle, right atrium, or atrial septum. In the atrial septum, nonneoplastic depositions of fat sometimes occur that are called "lipomatous hypertrophy." These lesions include white and brown adipose tissue, as well as small interspersed areas of myocardium.

Papillary Fibroelastoma. *Papillary fibroelastomas* are curious, usually incidental, sea-anemone-like lesions, most often identified at autopsy. They may embolize and thereby become clinically important. Clonal cytogenetic abnormalities have been reported, suggesting that fibroelastomas are unusual benign neoplasms. They resemble the much smaller, usually trivial, *Lambl excrescences* that may represent remotely organized thrombus on the aortic valves of older individuals.

MORPHOLOGY

Papillary fibroelastomas are usually (>80%) located on valves, particularly the ventricular surfaces of semilunar valves and the atrial surfaces of atrioventricular valves. Each lesion, typically 1 to 2 cm in diameter, consists of a distinctive cluster of hairlike projections up to 1 cm in length. Histologically, the projections are covered by a surface endothelium surrounding a core of myxoid connective tissue with abundant mucopolysaccharide matrix and elastic fibers.

Rhabdomyoma. *Rhabdomyomas* are the most frequent primary tumor of the pediatric heart, and are commonly discovered in the first years of life because of obstruction of a valvular orifice or cardiac chamber. Approximately half of cardiac rhabdomyomas are due to sporadic mutations; the other 50% of cases are associated with tuberous sclerosis (Chapter 28), with mutations in the *TSC1* or *TSC2* tumor suppressor gene. The *TSC1* and *TSC2* proteins (hamartin and tuberin, respectively) function in a complex that inhibits the activity of the mammalian target of rapamycin (mTOR), a kinase that stimulates cell growth and regulates cell size. *TSC1* or *TSC2* expression is often absent in tuberous sclerosis-associated rhabdomyomas, providing a mechanism for myocyte overgrowth. Because rhabdomyomas often regress spontaneously, they may be considered as hamartomas rather than true neoplasms.

MORPHOLOGY

Rhabdomyomas are gray-white myocardial masses that can be small or up to several centimeters in diameter. They are usually multiple and involve the ventricles preferentially, protruding into the lumen. Microscopically, they are composed of bizarre, markedly enlarged myocytes. Routine histologic processing often artifactually reduces the abundant cytoplasm to thin strands that stretch from the nucleus to the surface membrane, an appearance referred to as "spider" cells.

Sarcoma. Cardiac *angiosarcomas* and other sarcomas are not clinically or morphologically distinctive from their counterparts in other locations, and so require no further comment here.

Cardiac Effects of Noncardiac Neoplasms

With enhanced patient survival due to diagnostic and therapeutic advances, significant cardiovascular effects of noncardiac neoplasms and their therapy are increasingly encountered (Table 12-15). The pathologic consequences include direct tumor infiltration, effects of circulating mediators, and therapeutic complications.

The most frequent metastatic tumors involving the heart are carcinomas of the lung and breast, melanomas, leukemias, and lymphomas. Metastases can reach the heart and pericardium by retrograde lymphatic extension (most carcinomas), by hematogenous seeding (many tumors), by direct contiguous extension (primary carcinoma of the lung, breast, or esophagus), or by venous extension (tumors of the kidney or liver). Clinical symptoms are most often associated with pericardial spread, which can cause

Table 12-15 Cardiovascular Effects of Noncardiac Neoplasms

Direct Consequences of Tumor
Pericardial and myocardial metastases
Large vessel obstruction
Pulmonary tumor emboli
Indirect Consequences of Tumor (Complications of Circulating Mediators)
Nonbacterial thrombotic endocarditis
Carcinoid heart disease
Pheochromocytoma-associated heart disease
Myeloma-associated amyloidosis
Effects of Tumor Therapy
Chemotherapy
Radiation therapy

Modified from Schoen FJ, et al: Cardiac effects of non-cardiac neoplasms. Cardiol Clin 2:657, 1984.

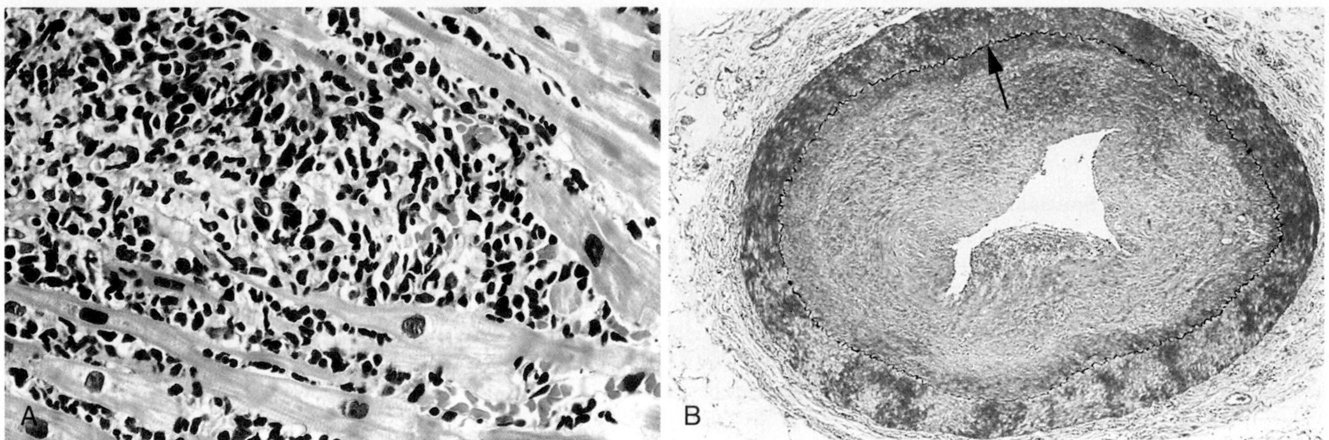

Figure 12-39 Complications of heart transplantation. **A,** Cardiac allograft rejection typified by lymphocytic infiltrate associated with cardiac myocyte damage. **B,** Allograft arteriopathy, with severe diffuse concentric intimal thickening producing critical stenosis. The internal elastic lamina *(arrow)* and media are intact (Movat pentachrome stain, elastin black). (**B,** Reproduced with permission from Salomon RN, et al: Human coronary transplantation-associated arteriosclerosis. Evidence for chronic immune reaction to activated graft endothelial cells. Am J Pathol 138:791, 1991.)

symptomatic pericardial effusions or a mass-effect that is sufficient to restrict cardiac filling. Myocardial metastases are usually clinically silent or have nonspecific features, such as a generalized defect in ventricular contractility or compliance. Bronchogenic carcinoma or malignant lymphoma may infiltrate the mediastinum extensively, causing encasement, compression, or invasion of the superior vena cava with resultant obstruction to blood coming from the head and upper extremities *(superior vena cava syndrome)*. Renal cell carcinoma often invades the renal vein, and may grow as a continuous column of tumor up the inferior vena cava and into the right atrium, blocking venous return to the heart.

Noncardiac tumors may also affect cardiac function indirectly, sometimes via circulating tumor-derived substances. The consequences include nonbacterial thrombotic endocarditis, carcinoid heart disease, pheochromocytoma-associated myocardial damage and myeloma-associated AL-type amyloidosis.

Complications of chemotherapy were discussed earlier in this chapter. Radiation used to treat breast, lung, or mediastinal neoplasms can cause pericarditis, pericardial effusion, myocardial fibrosis, and chronic pericardial disorders. Other cardiac effects of radiation therapy include accelerated coronary artery disease and mural and valvular endocardial fibrosis.

Cardiac Transplantation

Transplantation of cardiac allografts is now frequently performed (approximately 3000 per year worldwide) for severe, intractable heart failure of diverse causes—most commonly DCM and IHD. Three major factors have contributed to the improved outcome of cardiac transplantation since the first human to human transplant in 1967: (1) more effective immunosuppressive therapy (including the use of cyclosporin A, glucocorticoids, and other agents), (2) careful selection of candidates, and (3) early histopathologic diagnosis of acute allograft rejection by endomyocardial biopsy.

Of the major complications, allograft rejection is the primary problem requiring surveillance; routine endomyocardial biopsy is the only reliable means of diagnosing acute cardiac rejection before substantial myocardial damage has occurred and at a stage that is reversible in the majority of instances. Classic *cellular rejection* is characterized by interstitial lymphocytic inflammation with associated myocyte damage; the histology resembles myocarditis (Fig. 12-39*A*). There may also be interstitial edema due to vascular injury, and local cytokine elaboration can impact myocardial contractility without necessarily eliciting myocyte damage. Increasingly, *antibody-mediated rejection* is also recognized as a pathologic mechanism of injury; donor-specific antibodies directed against major histocompatibility complex proteins lead to complement activation and the recruitment of Fc-receptor-bearing cells. Mild rejection may resolve spontaneously, while prompt recognition of more severe episodes allows successful treatment by augmenting baseline levels of immunosuppression; occasionally aggressive anti-T cell or anti-B cell immunotherapy, with or without plasmapheresis may be necessary.

Allograft arteriopathy is the single most important long-term limitation for cardiac transplantation. It is a late, progressive, diffusely stenosing intimal proliferation in the coronary arteries (Fig. 12-39*B*), leading to ischemic injury. Within 5 years of transplantation, 50% of patients develop significant allograft arteriopathy, and virtually all patients have lesions within 10 years. The pathogenesis of allograft arteriopathy involves immunologic responses that induce local production of growth factors that promote intimal smooth muscle cell recruitment and proliferation with ECM synthesis. Allograft arteriopathy is a particularly vexing problem because it can lead to silent MI (transplant patients have denervated hearts and do not experience angina), progressive CHF, or sudden cardiac death.

Other postoperative problems include infection and malignancies, particularly Epstein-Barr virus-associated B-cell lymphomas that arise in the setting of chronic T-cell immunosuppression. Despite these problems, the overall outlook is good; the 1-year survival is 90% and 5-year survival is greater than 60%.

SUGGESTED READINGS

General

Zipe DP, et al, editors: *Braunwald's Heart Disease: A Textbook of Cardiovascular Medicine*, ed 9, Philadelphia, 2011, Elsevier Saunders. [*An outstanding and authoritative text, with excellent sections on heart failure and atherosclerotic cardiovascular disease.*]

Cardiac Structure and Specializations

Rasmussen TL, Raveendran G, Zhang J, et al: Getting to the heart of myocardial stem cells and cell therapy. *Circulation* 123:1771, 2011. [*A well-written overview of the challenges and current state of the art regarding stem cell therapies in heart disease.*]

Heart Failure

Ashrafian H, Frenneaux MP, Opie LH, et al: Metabolic mechanisms in heart failure. *Circulation* 116:434, 2007. [*Good review of the molecular pathways underlying myocardial decompensation.*]

Neubauer S: The failing heart—an engine out of fuel. *N Engl J Med* 356:1140, 2007. [*Well-written overview of the mechanisms and therapeutic approaches in congestive failure.*]

Congenital Heart Disease

Bruneau BG: The developmental genetics of congenital heart disease. *Nature* 451:943, 2008. [*Succinct overview of the relationships between cardiac development and congenital heart disease.*]

Dinardo JA: Heart failure associated with adult congenital heart disease. *Semin Cardiothorac Vasc Anesth* 17:44, 2013. [*Well-written summary of the consequences of congenital heart disorders seen in the adult population.*]

Huang JB, Liu YL, Sun PW, et al: Molecular mechanisms of congenital heart disease. *Cardiovasc Pathol* 19:e183, 2010. [*Comprehensive review of the genes and pathways underlying congenital heart disease.*]

MacGrogan D, Nus M, de la Pompa JL: Notch signaling in cardiac development and disease. *Curr Top Dev Biol* 92:333, 2010. [*A scholarly review of the role of Notch in cardiac development.*]

Ischemic Heart Disease

Hausenloy DJ, Yellon DM: Myocardial ischemia-reperfusion injury: a neglected therapeutic target. *J Clin Invest* 123:92, 2013. [*Nice discussion of the mechanisms and possible therapeutic approaches in ischemia-reperfusion injury.*]

Libby P, Theroux P: Pathophysiology of coronary artery disease. *Circulation* 111:3481, 2005. [*A well-written review of the pathways, as well as the diagnostic and therapeutic implications of atherosclerotic coronary disease.*]

Nabel EG, Braunwald E: A tale of coronary artery disease and myocardial infarction. *N Engl J Med* 366:54, 2012. [*A terrific overview of the history of our understanding of the pathophysiology of coronary artery disease, and the successes of informed therapeutic interventions.*]

Ovize M, Baxter GF, Di Lisa F, et al: Postconditioning and protection from reperfusion injury: where do we stand? Position paper from the Working Group of Cellular Biology of the Heart of the European Society of Cardiology. *Cardiovasc Res* 87:406, 2010. [*A good overview of the mechanisms and potential therapeutic interventions for ischemia-reperfusion injury and for ischemic pre-conditioning in limiting infarct size.*]

Yellon DM, Hausenloy DJ: Myocardial reperfusion injury. *N Engl J Med* 357:1121, 2007. [*Great review of the mechanisms and potential therapeutic approaches to limiting reperfusion injury after MI.*]

Arrhythmias

Cerrone M, Priori SG: Genetics of sudden death: focus on inherited channelopathies. *Eur Heart J* 32:2109, 2011. [*Up-to-date, well-organized description of the known ion channel disorders that cause sudden cardiac death.*]

Hypertensive Heart Disease

Farber HW, Loscalzo J: Pulmonary arterial hypertension. *N Engl J Med* 351:1655, 2004. [*Although a little older, this remains an excellent review of right-sided hypertension-associated pathology.*]

Valvular Heart Disease

Bhattacharyya S, Davar J, Dreyfus G, et al: Carcinoid heart disease. *Circulation* 116:2860, 2007. [*Good review of the current thinking on pathophysiology, diagnosis, and treatment of this entity.*]

Guilherme L, Köhler KF, Kalil J: Rheumatic heart disease: mediation by complex immune events. *Adv Clin Chem* 53:31, 2011. [*A well-written and scholarly discussion of the pathogenic mechanisms regarding rheumatic heart disease.*]

Hill EE, Herijgers P, Herregods MC, et al: Evolving trends in infective endocarditis. *Clin Microbiol Infect* 12:5, 2006. [*Good, clinically-oriented overview of the developments in microorganisms, diagnosis, and therapies for infective endocarditis.*]

Li C, Xu S, Gotlieb AI, et al: The response to valve injury. A paradigm to understand the pathogenesis of heart valve disease. *Cardiovasc Pathol* 20:183, 2011. [*Nice overview of pathologic concepts in valvular disease.*]

New SE, Aikawa E: Molecular imaging insights into early inflammatory stages of arterial and aortic valve calcification. *Circ Res* 108:1381, 2011. [*A good overview of the mechanisms leading to degenerative calcification on valves and vessels.*]

Schoen FJ: Cardiac valves and valvular pathology. Update on function, disease, repair, and replacement. *Cardiovasc Pathol* 14:189, 2005. [*Excellent review on mechanisms of valve disease and therapeutic approaches.*]

Cardiomyopathies

Azaouagh A, Churzidse S, Konorza T, et al: Arrhythmogenic right ventricular cardiomyopathy/dysplasia: a review and update. *Clin Res Cardiol* 100:383, 2011. [*Excellent up-to-date look at this entity and its genetic causes.*]

Cooper LT Jr: Myocarditis. *N Engl J Med* 360:1526, 2009. [*A nice review of etiology, pathogenesis, and clinical features.*]

Herman DS, Lam L, Taylor MR, et al: Truncations of titin causing dilated cardiomyopathy. *N Engl J Med* 366:619, 2012. [*Elucidation of the common association of titin mutations with dilated cardiomyopathy.*]

Maron BJ, Towbin JA, Thiene G, et al: Contemporary definitions and classification of the cardiomyopathies: an American Heart Association Scientific Statement from the Council on Clinical Cardiology, Heart Failure and Transplantation Committee; Quality of Care and Outcomes Research and Functional Genomics and Translational Biology Interdisciplinary Working Groups; and Council on Epidemiology and Prevention. *Circulation* 113:1807, 2006. [*Consensus document regarding an updated classification of cardiomyopathies, heavily weighted to genetic etiologies rather than pathophysiologic manifestations.*]

Patten IS, Rana S, Shahul S, et al: Cardiac angiogenic imbalance leads to peripartum cardiomyopathy. *Nature* 485:333, 2012. [*New perspective on the mechanisms underlying pregnancy-associated cardiomyopathy.*]

Seidman CE, Seidman JG: Identifying sarcomere gene mutations in hypertrophic cardiomyopathy: a personal history. *Circ Res* 108:743, 2011. [*A well-written and authoritative overview of the genetics and pathophysiology of hypertrophic cardiomyopathy from one of the leading groups in the world.*]

Tumors of the Heart

Cheng H, Force T: Molecular mechanisms of cardiovascular toxicity of targeted cancer therapeutics. *Circ Res* 106:21, 2010. [*Excellent and thoughtful review of the common pathways involved in tumorigenesis and cardiac development and homeostasis.*]

Sawyer DB: Anthracyclines and heart failure. *New Engl J Med* 38:1154, 2013. [*Succinct overview of chemotherapeutic cardiotoxicity.*]

Cardiac Transplantation

Kittleson MM, Kobashigawa JA: Antibody-mediated rejection. *Curr Opin Organ Transplant* 17:551, 2012. [*Good succinct review of the mechanisms, diagnosis, and therapeutic interventions in antibody-mediated rejection.*]

Mitchell RN: Graft vascular disease: immune response meets the vessel wall. *Annu Rev Pathol* 4:19, 2009. [*Comprehensive overview of allograft arteriopathy, including animal models, pathogenic mechanisms, clinical diagnosis, and therapy.*]

See TARGETED THERAPY available online at www.studentconsult.com

CHAPTER 13

Diseases of White Blood Cells, Lymph Nodes, Spleen, and Thymus

CHAPTER CONTENTS

The components of the hematopoietic system have been traditionally divided into the *myeloid tissues,* which include the bone marrow and the cells derived from it (e.g., red cells, platelets, granulocytes, and monocytes), and the *lymphoid tissues,* consisting of the thymus, lymph nodes, and spleen. It is important to recognize, however, that this subdivision is artificial with respect to both the normal physiology of hematopoietic cells and the diseases affecting them. For example, although bone marrow contains relatively few lymphocytes, it is the source of all lymphoid progenitors, and the home of long-lived plasma cells and memory lymphocytes. Similarly, neoplastic disorders of myeloid progenitor cells (myeloid leukemias) originate in the bone marrow but secondarily involve the spleen and (to a lesser degree) the lymph nodes. Some red cell disorders (e.g., immunohemolytic anemia, discussed in Chapter 14) result from the formation of autoantibodies, indicating a primary disorder of lymphocytes. Thus, it is not possible to draw neat lines between diseases involving the myeloid and lymphoid tissues.

Recognizing this difficulty, we somewhat arbitrarily divide diseases of the hematopoietic tissues into two chapters. In this chapter we discuss white cell diseases and disorders affecting the spleen and thymus. In Chapter 14 we consider diseases of red cells and those affecting hemostasis. Before delving into specific diseases, we will briefly discuss the origins of hematopoietic cells, since many disorders of white cells and red cells involve disturbances of their normal development and maturation.

Development and Maintenance of Hematopoietic Tissues

Blood cell progenitors first appear during the third week of embryonic development in the yolk sac. Cells derived from the yolk sac are the source of long-lived tissue macrophages, such as microglial cells in the brain and Kupffer cells in the liver (Chapter 3), but the contribution of the yolk sac to blood formation, mainly in the form of embryonic red blood cells, is only transient. Definitive *hematopoietic stem cells* (HSCs) arise several weeks later in the mesoderm of the intraembryonic aorta/gonad/mesonephros region. During the third month of embryogenesis, HSCs migrate to the liver, which becomes the chief site of blood cell formation until shortly before birth. HSCs also take up residence in the fetal placenta; this pool of HSCs is of uncertain physiologic relevance, but has taken on

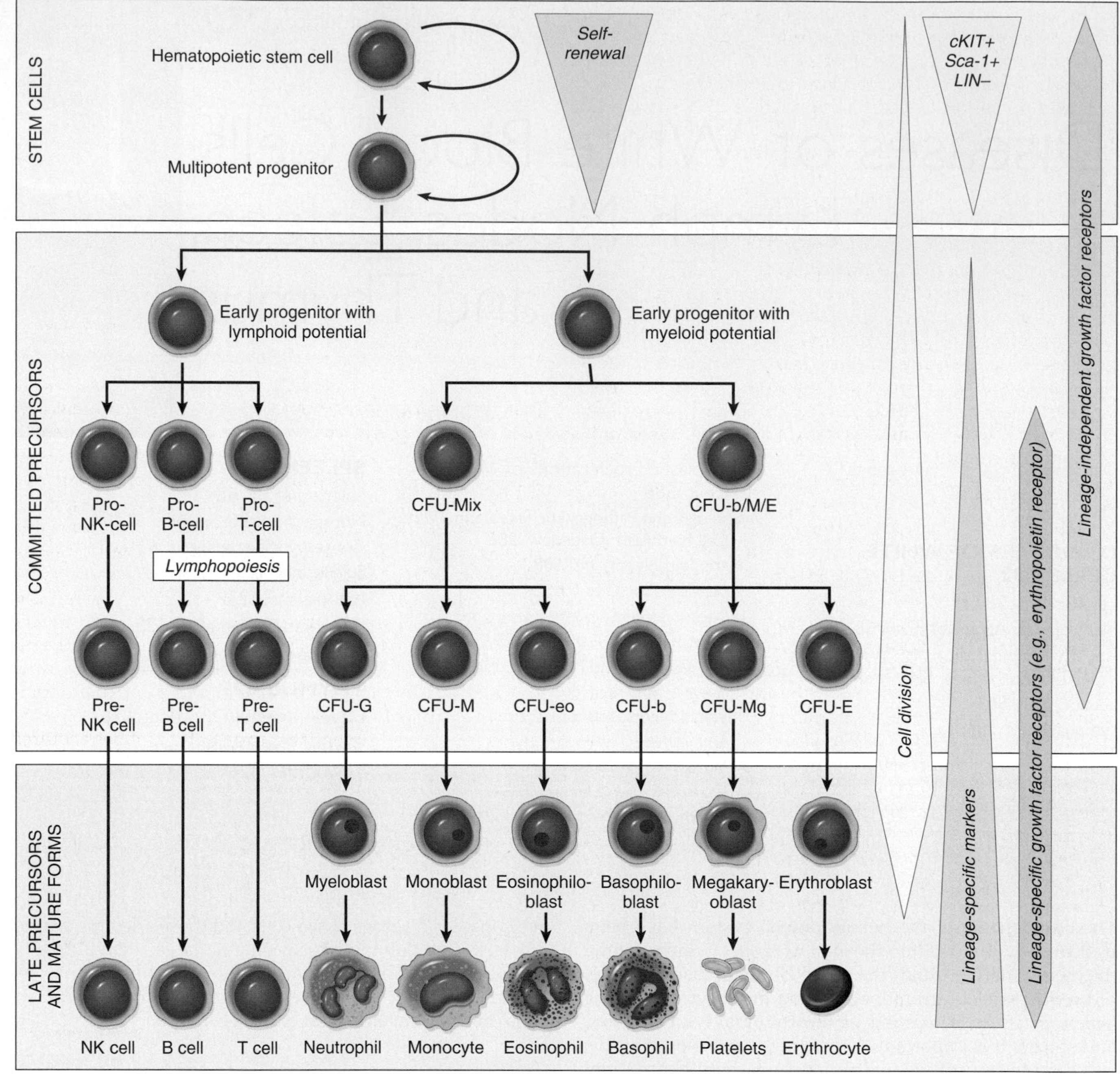

Figure 13-1 Differentiation of blood cells. CFU, Colony forming unit; LIN–, negative for lineage-specific markers.

substantial clinical importance, as HSCs harvested at birth from umbilical cord blood are being used increasingly in therapeutic hematopoietic stem cell transplantation. By the fourth month of development, HSCs shift in location yet again, taking up residence in the bone marrow. By birth, marrow throughout the skeleton is hematopoietically active and hepatic hematopoiesis dwindles to a trickle, persisting only in widely scattered foci that become inactive soon after birth. Until puberty, hematopoietically active marrow is found throughout the skeleton, but soon thereafter it becomes restricted to the axial skeleton. Thus, in normal adults, only about half of the marrow space is hematopoietically active.

The formed elements of blood—red cells, granulocytes, monocytes, platelets, and lymphocytes—have a common origin from HSCs, pluripotent cells that sit at the apex of a hierarchy of bone marrow progenitors (Fig. 13-1). Most evidence supporting this scheme comes from studies in mice, but human hematopoiesis is believed to proceed in a similar way. HSCs give rise to several kinds of early progenitor cells with a restricted differentiation potential, such that they ultimately produce mainly myeloid cells or lymphoid cells. The origins of lymphoid cells are revisited when tumors derived from these cells are discussed. These early progenitors in turn give "birth" to progenitors that are further constrained to differentiation along particular lineages. Some of these cells are referred to as *colony-forming units* (CFUs) (Fig. 13-1), because they produce colonies composed of specific kinds of mature cells when grown in culture. From the various committed progenitors are derived the morphologically recognizable precursors, such as myeloblasts, proerythroblasts, and megakaryoblasts, which are the immediate progenitors of mature granulocytes, red cells, and platelets.

HSCs have two essential properties that are required for the maintenance of hematopoiesis: pluripotency and the capacity for self-renewal. Pluripotency refers to the ability of a single HSC to generate all mature blood cells. When an HSC divides, at least one daughter cell must self-renew to avoid stem cell depletion. Self-renewing divisions occur within a specialized marrow niche, in which stromal cells and secreted factors nurture and protect the HSCs. As one might surmise from their ability to migrate during embryonic development, HSCs are not sessile. Particularly under conditions of marked stress, such as severe anemia or acute inflammation, HSCs are mobilized from the bone marrow and appear in the peripheral blood. In fact, HSCs used in transplantation are now mainly collected from the peripheral blood of donors treated with granulocyte colony stimulating factor (G-CSF), one of the factors that can mobilize a fraction of marrow HSCs from their stem cell niches.

The marrow response to short-term physiologic needs is regulated by hematopoietic growth factors through effects on the committed progenitors. Because mature blood elements are terminally differentiated cells with finite life spans, their numbers must be constantly replenished. In current models of hematopoiesis, some divisions of HSCs give rise to cells referred to as *multipotent progenitors*, which are more proliferative than HSCs but have a lesser capacity for self-renewal (Fig. 13-1). Division of multipotent progenitors gives rise to at least one daughter cell that leaves the stem cell pool and begins to differentiate. Once past this threshold, these newly committed cells lose the capacity for self-renewal and commence an inexorable journey down a road that leads to terminal differentiation and death. However, as these progenitors differentiate, they also begin to proliferate more rapidly in response to growth factors, expanding their numbers. Some growth factors, such as stem cell factor (also called *KIT ligand*) and FLT3-ligand, act through receptors that are expressed on very early committed progenitors. Others, such as erythropoietin, granulocyte-macrophage colony-stimulating factor (GM-CSF), G-CSF, and thrombopoietin, act through receptors that are only expressed on committed progenitors with more restricted differentiation potentials. Feedback loops involving these lineage-specific growth factors tune the marrow output, allowing the numbers of formed blood elements (red cells, white cells, and platelets) to be maintained within appropriate ranges (Table 13-1).

Many diseases alter the production of blood cells. The marrow is the ultimate source of most cells of the innate and adaptive immune system and responds to infectious or inflammatory challenges by increasing its output of granulocytes under the direction of specific growth factors and cytokines. By contrast, many other disorders are associated with defects in hematopoiesis that lead to deficiencies of one or more types of blood cells. Primary tumors of hematopoietic cells are among the most important diseases that interfere with marrow function, but certain genetic diseases, infections, toxins, and nutritional deficiencies, as well as chronic inflammation from any cause, can also decrease the production of blood cells by the marrow.

Tumors of hematopoietic origin are often associated with mutations that block progenitor cell maturation or abrogate their growth factor dependence. The net effect of such derangements is an unregulated clonal expansion of hematopoietic elements, which replace normal marrow progenitors and often spread to other hematopoietic tissues. In some instances, these tumors originate from transformed HSCs that retain the ability to differentiate along multiple lineages, whereas in other instances the origin is a more differentiated progenitor that has acquired an abnormal capacity for self-renewal (Chapter 7).

Table 13-1 Adult Reference Ranges for Blood Cells*

Cell Type	
White cells ($\times 10^3/\mu L$)	4.8-10.8
Granulocytes (%)	40-70
Neutrophils ($\times 10^3/\mu L$)	1.4-6.5
Lymphocytes ($\times 10^3/\mu L$)	1.2-3.4
Monocytes ($\times 10^3/\mu L$)	0.1-0.6
Eosinophils ($\times 10^3/\mu L$)	0-0.5
Basophils ($\times 10^3/\mu L$)	0-0.2
Red cells ($\times 10^3/\mu L$)	4.3-5, men; 3.5-5, women
Platelets ($\times 10^3/\mu L$)	150-450

*Reference ranges vary among laboratories. The reference ranges for the laboratory providing the result should always be used.

MORPHOLOGY

The bone marrow is a unique microenvironment that supports the orderly proliferation, differentiation, and release of blood cells. It is filled with a network of thin-walled sinusoids lined by a single layer of endothelial cells, which are underlaid by a discontinuous basement membrane and adventitial cells. Within the interstitium lie clusters of hematopoietic cells and fat cells. Differentiated blood cells enter the circulation by transcellular migration through the endothelial cells.

The normal marrow is organized in subtle, but important, ways. For example, normal **megakaryocytes** lie next to sinusoids and extend cytoplasmic processes that bud off into the bloodstream to produce platelets, while red cell precursors often surround macrophages (so-called *nurse cells*) that provide some of the iron needed for the synthesis of hemoglobin. Processes that distort the marrow architecture, such as deposits of metastatic cancer or granulomatous disorders, can cause the abnormal release of immature precursors into the peripheral blood, a finding that is referred to as **leukoerythroblastosis**.

Marrow aspirate smears provide the best assessment of the morphology of hematopoietic cells. The most mature marrow precursors can be identified based on their morphology alone. Immature precursors ("blast" forms) of different types are morphologically similar and must be identified definitively using lineage-specific antibodies and histochemical markers (described later under white cell neoplasms). Biopsies are a good means for estimating marrow activity. In normal adults, the ratio of fat cells to hematopoietic elements is about 1 : 1. In hypoplastic states (e.g., aplastic anemia) the proportion of fat cells is greatly increased; conversely, fat cells often disappear when the marrow is involved by hematopoietic tumors and in diseases characterized by compensatory hyperplasias (e.g., hemolytic anemias), and neoplastic proliferations such as leukemias. Other disorders (e.g., metastatic cancers and granulomatous diseases) induce local marrow fibrosis. Such lesions are usually inaspirable and best seen in biopsies.

DISORDERS OF WHITE CELLS

Disorders of white blood cells can be classified into two broad categories: *proliferative disorders*, in which there is an expansion of leukocytes, and *leukopenias*, which are defined as a deficiency of leukocytes. Proliferations of white cells can be *reactive* or *neoplastic*. Reactive proliferations in the setting of infections or inflammatory processes, when leukocytes are needed for an effective host response, are fairly common. Neoplastic disorders, though less frequent, are much more important clinically. In the following discussion we will first describe the leukopenic states and summarize the common reactive disorders, and then consider in some detail the malignant proliferations of white cells.

Leukopenia

The number of circulating white cells may be markedly decreased in a variety of disorders. An abnormally low white cell count *(leukopenia)* usually results from reduced numbers of neutrophils *(neutropenia, granulocytopenia)*. *Lymphopenia* is less common; in addition to congenital immunodeficiency diseases (Chapter 6), it is most commonly observed in advanced human immunodeficiency virus (HIV) infection, following therapy with glucocorticoids or cytotoxic drugs, autoimmune disorders, malnutrition, and certain acute viral infections. In the latter setting lymphopenia actually stems from lymphocyte redistribution rather than a decrease in the number of lymphocytes in the body. Acute viral infections induce production of type I interferons, which activate T lymphocytes and change the expression of surface proteins that regulate T cell migration. These changes result in the sequestration of activated T cells in lymph nodes and increased adherence to endothelial cells, both of which contribute to lymphopenia. Granulocytopenia is more common and is often associated with diminished granulocyte function, and thus merits further discussion.

Neutropenia, Agranulocytosis

Neutropenia, a reduction in the number of neutrophils in the blood, occurs in a wide variety of circumstances. *Agranulocytosis,* a clinically significant reduction in neutrophils, has the serious consequence of making individuals susceptible to bacterial and fungal infections.

Pathogenesis. **Neutropenia can be caused by (1) inadequate or ineffective granulopoiesis, or (2) increased destruction or sequestration of neutrophils in the periphery.** Inadequate or ineffective granulopoiesis is observed in the setting of:

- *Suppression of hematopoietic stem cells,* as occurs in aplastic anemia (Chapter 14) and a variety of infiltrative marrow disorders (e.g., tumors, granulomatous disease); in these conditions granulocytopenia is accompanied by anemia and thrombocytopenia
- *Suppression of committed granulocytic precursors* by exposure to certain drugs (discussed later)
- Disease states associated with *ineffective hematopoiesis,* such as megaloblastic anemias (Chapter 14) and myelodysplastic syndromes, in which defective precursors die in the marrow
- Rare *congenital conditions* (e.g., Kostmann syndrome) in which inherited defects in specific genes impair granulocytic differentiation

Accelerated destruction or sequestration of neutrophils occurs with

- *Immunologically mediated injury* to neutrophils, which can be idiopathic, associated with a well-defined immunologic disorder (e.g., systemic lupus erythematosus), or caused by exposure to drugs
- *Splenomegaly,* in which splenic enlargement leads to sequestration of neutrophils and modest neutropenia, sometimes associated with anemia and often with thrombocytopenia
- *Increased peripheral utilization,* which can occur in overwhelming bacterial, fungal, or rickettsial infections

The most common cause of agranulocytosis is *drug toxicity*. Certain drugs, such as alkylating agents and antimetabolites used in cancer treatment, produce agranulocytosis in a predictable, dose-related fashion. Because such drugs cause a generalized suppression of hematopoiesis, production of red cells and platelets is also affected. Agranulocytosis can also occur as an idiosyncratic reaction to a large variety of agents. The roster of implicated drugs includes aminopyrine, chloramphenicol, sulfonamides, chlorpromazine, thiouracil, and phenylbutazone. The neutropenia induced by chlorpromazine and related phenothiazines results from a toxic effect on granulocytic precursors in the bone marrow. In contrast, agranulocytosis following administration of other drugs, such as sulfonamides, probably stems from antibody-mediated destruction of mature neutrophils through mechanisms similar to those involved in drug-induced immunohemolytic anemias (Chapter 14).

In some patients with acquired idiopathic neutropenia, autoantibodies directed against neutrophil-specific antigens are detected. Severe neutropenia can also occur in association with monoclonal proliferations of large granular lymphocytes (so-called *LGL leukemia*). The mechanism of this neutropenia is not clear; suppression of granulocytic progenitors by products of the neoplastic cell (usually a CD8+ cytotoxic T cell) is considered most likely.

MORPHOLOGY

The alterations in the **bone marrow** vary with cause. With excessive destruction of neutrophils in the periphery, the marrow is usually hypercellular due to a compensatory increase in granulocytic precursors. Hypercellularity is also the rule with neutropenias caused by ineffective granulopoiesis, as occurs in megaloblastic anemias and myelodysplastic syndromes. Agranulocytosis caused by agents that suppress or destroy granulocytic precursors is understandably associated with marrow hypocellularity.

Infections are a common consequence of agranulocytosis. Ulcerating necrotizing lesions of the gingiva, floor of the mouth, buccal mucosa, pharynx, or elsewhere in the oral cavity (agranulocytic angina) are quite characteristic. These are typically deep, undermined, and covered by gray to green-black necrotic membranes from which numerous bacteria or fungi can be isolated. Less frequently, similar ulcerative lesions occur in the skin, vagina, anus, or gastrointestinal tract. Severe life-threatening invasive bacterial or fungal infections may occur in the lungs, urinary tract, and kidneys. The neutropenic patient is at particularly high risk for deep fungal infections caused by *Candida* and *Aspergillus*. Sites of infection often show a massive growth of organisms with little leukocytic response. In the most dramatic instances, bacteria grow in colonies (botryomycosis) resembling those seen on agar plates.

Clinical Features. The symptoms and signs of neutropenia are related to infection, and include malaise, chills, and fever, often followed by marked weakness and fatigability. With agranulocytosis, infections are often overwhelming and may cause death within hours to days.

Serious infections are most likely when the neutrophil count falls below 500 per mm^3. Because infections are often fulminant, broad-spectrum antibiotics must be given expeditiously whenever signs or symptoms appear. In some instances, such as following myelosuppressive chemotherapy, neutropenia is treated with G-CSF, a growth factor that stimulates the production of granulocytes from marrow precursors.

Reactive Proliferations of White Cells and Lymph Nodes

Leukocytosis

Leukocytosis refers to an increase in the number of white cells in the blood. It is a common reaction to a variety of inflammatory states.

Pathogenesis. The peripheral blood leukocyte count is influenced by several factors, including:

- The size of the myeloid and lymphoid precursor and storage cell pools in the bone marrow, thymus, circulation, and peripheral tissues
- The rate of release of cells from the storage pools into the circulation
- The proportion of cells that are adherent to blood vessel walls at any time (the marginal pool)
- The rate of extravasation of cells from the blood into tissues

Table 13-2 Mechanisms and Causes of Leukocytosis

Increased Production in the Marrow
Chronic infection or inflammation (growth factor-dependent) Paraneoplastic (e.g., Hodgkin lymphoma; growth factor-dependent) Myeloproliferative disorders (e.g., chronic myeloid leukemia; growth factor-independent)
Increased Release from Marrow Stores
Endotoxemia Infection Hypoxia
Decreased Margination
Exercise Catecholamines
Decreased Extravasation into Tissues
Glucocorticoids

As discussed in Chapter 3, leukocyte homeostasis is maintained by cytokines, growth factors, and adhesion molecules through their effects on the commitment, proliferation, differentiation, and extravasation of leukocytes and their progenitors. Table 13-2 summarizes the major mechanisms of neutrophilic leukocytosis and its causes, the most important of which is infection. In acute infection there is a rapid increase in the egress of mature granulocytes from the bone marrow pool, an alteration that may be mediated through the effects of tumor necrosis factor (TNF) and interleukin-1 (IL-1). If the infection or an inflammatory process is prolonged, IL-1, TNF, and other inflammatory mediators stimulate macrophages, bone marrow stromal cells and T cells to produce increased amounts of hematopoietic growth factors. These factors enhance the proliferation and differentiation of committed granulocytic progenitors and, over several days, cause a sustained increase in neutrophil production.

Some growth factors preferentially stimulate the production of a single type of leukocyte. For example, IL-5 mainly stimulates eosinophil production, while G-CSF induces neutrophilia. Such factors are differentially produced in response to various pathogenic stimuli and, as a result, the five principal types of leukocytosis (neutrophilia, eosinophilia, basophilia, monocytosis, and lymphocytosis) tend to be observed in different clinical settings (Table 13-3).

In sepsis or severe inflammatory disorders (e.g., Kawasaki disease), leukocytosis is often accompanied by morphologic changes in the neutrophils, such as toxic granulations, Döhle bodies, and cytoplasmic vacuoles (Fig. 13-2). *Toxic granules*, which are coarser and darker than the normal neutrophilic granules, represent abnormal azurophilic (primary) granules. *Döhle bodies* are patches of dilated endoplasmic reticulum that appear as sky-blue cytoplasmic "puddles."

In most instances it is not difficult to distinguish reactive and neoplastic leukocytoses, but uncertainties may arise in two settings. Acute viral infections, particularly in

Table 13-3 Causes of Leukocytosis

Type of Leukocytosis	Causes
Neutrophilic leukocytosis	Acute bacterial infections, especially those caused by pyogenic organisms; sterile inflammation caused by, for example, tissue necrosis (myocardial infarction, burns)
Eosinophilic leukocytosis (eosinophilia)	Allergic disorders such as asthma, hay fever, parasitic infestations; drug reactions; certain malignancies (e.g., Hodgkin and some non-Hodgkin lymphomas); automimmune disorders (e.g., pemphigus, dermatitis herpetiformis) and some vasculitides; atheroembolic disease (transient)
Basophilic leukocytosis (basophilia)	Rare, often indicative of a myeloproliferative disease (e.g., chronic myelogenous leukemia)
Monocytosis	Chronic infections (e.g., tuberculosis), bacterial endocarditis, rickettsiosis, and malaria; autoimmune disorders (e.g., systemic lupus erythematosus); inflammatory bowel diseases (e.g., ulcerative colitis)
Lymphocytosis	Accompanies monocytosis in many disorders associated with chronic immunologic stimulation (e.g., tuberculosis, brucellosis); viral infections (e.g., hepatitis A, cytomegalovirus, Epstein-Barr virus); *Bordetella pertussis* infection

children, can cause the appearance of large numbers of activated lymphocytes that resemble neoplastic lymphoid cells. At other times, particularly in severe infections, many immature granulocytes appear in the blood, mimicking a myeloid leukemia *(leukemoid reaction)*. Special laboratory studies (discussed later) are helpful in distinguishing reactive and neoplastic leukocytoses.

Lymphadenitis

Following their initial development from precursors in the central (also called primary) lymphoid organs,—the bone marrow for B cells and the thymus for T cells—, lymphocytes circulate through the blood and, under the influence of specific cytokines and chemokines, home to lymph nodes, spleen, tonsils, adenoids, and Peyer's patches, which constitute the peripheral (secondary) lymphoid tissues. Lymph nodes, the most widely distributed and easily accessible lymphoid tissue, are frequently examined for diagnostic purposes. They are discrete encapsulated structures that contain well-organized B-cell and T-cell zones, which are richly invested with phagocytes and antigen-presenting cells (see Fig. 6-8, Chapter 6).

The activation of resident immune cells leads to morphologic changes in lymph nodes. Within several days of antigenic stimulation, the primary follicles enlarge and develop pale-staining *germinal centers*, highly dynamic structures in which B cells acquire the capacity to make high-affinity antibodies against specific antigens. Paracortical T-cell zones may also undergo hyperplasia. The degree and pattern of the morphologic changes are dependent on the inciting stimulus and the intensity of the response. Trivial injuries and infections induce subtle changes, while more significant infections inevitably produce nodal enlargement and sometimes leave residual scarring. For this reason, lymph nodes in adults are almost never "normal" or "resting," and it is often necessary to distinguish morphologic changes secondary to past experience from those related to present disease. Infections and inflammatory stimuli often elicit regional or systemic immune reactions within lymph nodes. Some that produce distinctive morphologic patterns are described in other chapters. Most, however, cause stereotypical patterns of lymph node reaction designated acute and chronic nonspecific lymphadenitis.

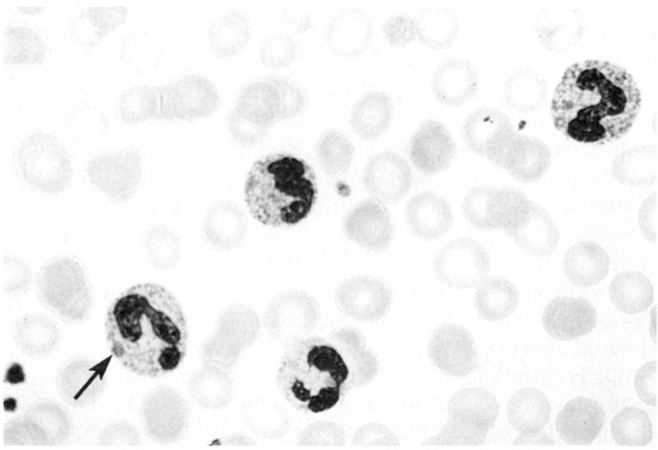

Figure 13-2 Reactive changes in neutrophils. Neutrophils containing coarse purple cytoplasmic granules (toxic granulations) and blue cytoplasmic patches of dilated endoplasmic reticulum (Döhle bodies, *arrow*) are observed in this peripheral blood smear prepared from a patient with bacterial sepsis.

Acute Nonspecific Lymphadenitis

Acute lymphadenitis in the cervical region is most often due to drainage of microbes or microbial products from infections of the teeth or tonsils, while in the axillary or inguinal regions it is most often caused by infections in the extremities. Acute lymphadenitis also occurs in mesenteric lymph nodes draining acute appendicitis. Other self-limited infections may also cause acute mesenteric adenitis and induce symptoms mimicking acute appendicitis, a differential diagnosis that plagues the surgeon. Systemic viral infections (particularly in children) and bacteremia often produce acute generalized lymphadenopathy.

MORPHOLOGY

The nodes are swollen, gray-red, and engorged. Microscopically, there is prominence of large reactive germinal centers containing numerous mitotic figures. Macrophages often contain particulate debris derived from dead bacteria or necrotic cells. When pyogenic organisms are the cause, neutrophils are prominent and the centers of the follicles may undergo necrosis; sometimes the entire node is converted to a bag of pus. With less severe reactions, scattered neutrophils infiltrate about the follicles and accumulate within the lymphoid sinuses. The endothelial cells lining the sinuses undergo hyperplasia.

Nodes involved by acute lymphadenitis are enlarged and painful. When abscess formation is extensive the nodes become fluctuant. The overlying skin is red. Sometimes, suppurative infections penetrate through the capsule of the node and track to the skin to produce draining sinuses. Healing of such lesions is associated with scarring.

Chronic Nonspecific Lymphadenitis

Chronic immunologic stimuli produce several different patterns of lymph node reaction, as described later.

MORPHOLOGY

Follicular hyperplasia is caused by stimuli that activate humoral immune responses. It is defined by the presence of large oblong germinal centers (secondary follicles), which are surrounded by a collar of small resting naive B cells (the mantle zone) (Fig. 13-3). Germinal centers are normally polarized, consisting of two distinct regions: (1) a dark zone containing proliferating blastlike B cells (centroblasts) and (2) a light zone composed of B cells with irregular or cleaved nuclear contours (centrocytes). Interspersed between the germinal B centers is an inconspicuous network of antigen-presenting follicular dendritic cells and macrophages (often referred to as **tingible-body macrophages**) containing the nuclear debris of B cells, which undergo apoptosis if they fail to produce an antibody with a high affinity for antigen.

Causes of follicular hyperplasia include rheumatoid arthritis, toxoplasmosis, and early stages of infection with HIV. This form of hyperplasia is morphologically similar to follicular lymphoma (discussed later). Features favoring a reactive (nonneoplastic) hyperplasia include (1) preservation of the lymph node architecture, including the interfollicular T-cell zones and the sinusoids; (2) marked variation in the shape and size of the follicles; and (3) the presence of frequent mitotic figures, phagocytic macrophages, and recognizable light and dark zones, all of which tend to be absent from neoplastic follicles.

Paracortical hyperplasia is caused by stimuli that trigger T-cell–mediated immune responses, such as acute viral infections (e.g., infectious mononucleosis). The T-cell regions typically contain immunoblasts, activated T cells three to four times the size of resting lymphocytes that have round nuclei, open chromatin, several prominent nucleoli, and moderate amounts of pale cytoplasm. The expanded T-cell zones encroach on and, in particularly exuberant reactions, efface the B-cell follicles. In such cases immunoblasts may be so numerous that special studies are needed to exclude a lymphoid neoplasm. In addition, there is often a hypertrophy of sinusoidal and vascular endothelial cells, sometimes accompanied by infiltrating macrophages and eosinophils.

Sinus histiocytosis (also called *reticular hyperplasia*) refers to an increase in the number and size of the cells that line lymphatic sinusoids. Although nonspecific, this form of hyperplasia may be particularly prominent in lymph nodes draining cancers such as carcinoma of the breast. The lining lymphatic endothelial cells are markedly hypertrophied and macrophages are greatly increased in numbers, resulting in the expansion and distension of the sinuses.

Characteristically, lymph nodes in chronic reactions are nontender, as nodal enlargement occurs slowly over time and acute inflammation with associated tissue damage is absent. Chronic lymphadenitis is particularly common in inguinal and axillary nodes, which drain relatively large areas of the body and are frequently stimulated by immune reactions to trivial injuries and infections of the extremities.

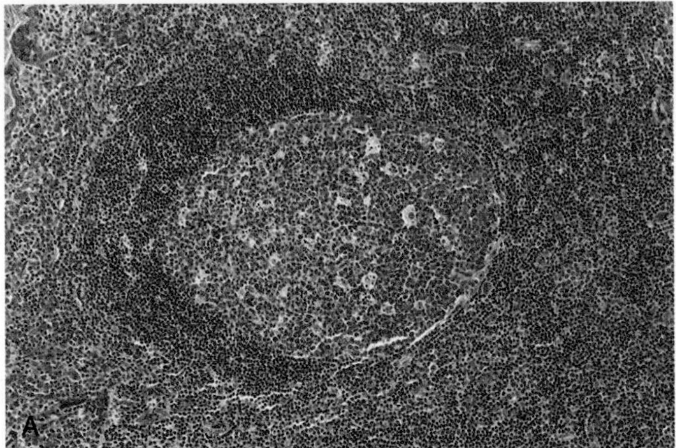

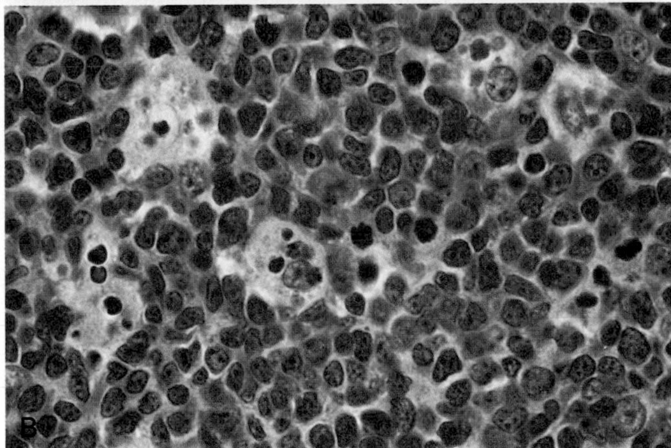

Figure 13-3 Follicular hyperplasia. **A,** Low-power view showing a reactive follicle and surrounding mantle zone. The dark-staining mantle zone is more prominent adjacent to the germinal-center light zone in the left half of the follicle. The right half of the follicle consists of the dark zone. **B,** High-power view of the dark zone shows several mitotic figures and numerous macrophages containing phagocytosed apoptotic cells (tingible bodies).

Furthermore, chronic immune reactions can promote the appearance of organized collections of immune cells in nonlymphoid tissues. These collections are sometimes called tertiary lymphoid organs. A classic example is that of chronic gastritis caused by *Helicobacter pylori,* in which aggregates of mucosal lymphocytes are seen that simulate the appearance of Peyer patches. A similar phenomenon occurs in rheumatoid arthritis, in which B-cell follicles often appear in the inflamed synovium. Lymphotoxin, a cytokine required for the formation of normal Peyer patches, is probably involved in the establishment of these "extranodal" inflammation-induced collections of lymphoid cells.

Hemophagocytic Lymphohistiocytosis

Hemophagocytic lymphohistiocytosis (HLH) is a reactive condition marked by cytopenias and signs and symptoms of systemic inflammation related to macrophage activation. For this reason, it is also sometimes referred to as *macrophage activation syndrome.* Some forms are familial and may appear early in life, even in infants, while other forms are sporadic and may affect people of any age.

Pathogenesis. **The common feature of all forms of HLH is systemic activation of macrophages and CD8+ cytotoxic**

T cells. The activated macrophages phagocytose blood cell progenitors in the marrow and formed elements in the peripheral tissues, while the "stew" of mediators released from macrophages and lymphocytes suppress hematopoiesis and produce symptoms of systemic inflammation. These effects lead to cytopenias and a shock-like picture, sometimes referred to as "cytokine storm" or the systemic inflammatory response syndrome (Chapter 4).

Familial forms of HLH are associated with several different mutations, all of which impact the ability of cytotoxic T cells and NK to properly form or deploy cytotoxic granules. How these defects lead to HLH is not known. One idea with some experimental support is based on the premise that cytotoxic T cells keep immune responses in check by lysing antigen-bearing dendritic cells or activated macrophages; if this regulatory mechanism fails, hyperactivation of the immune system and the clinical syndrome of HLH ensue. Unbridled HLH is associated with extremely high levels of inflammatory mediators such as interferon-γ, TNFα, IL-6, and IL-12, as well as soluble IL-2 receptor. Some "sporadic" cases in adults also prove to have mutations in the same set of genes, while in other adult-onset patients the cause is unknown. The most common trigger for HLH is infection, particularly with Epstein-Barr virus (EBV).

Clinical Features. Most patients present with an acute febrile illness associated with splenomegaly and hepatomegaly. Hemophagocytosis is usually seen on bone marrow examination, but is neither sufficient nor required to make the diagnosis. Laboratory studies typically reveal anemia, thrombocytopenia, and very high levels of plasma ferritin and soluble IL-2 receptor, both indicative of severe inflammation, as well as elevated liver function tests and triglyceride levels, both related to hepatitis. Coagulation studies may show evidence of disseminated intravascular coagulation. If untreated, this picture can progress rapidly to multiorgan failure, shock, and death.

Treatment involves the use of immunosuppressive drugs and "mild" chemotherapy. Patients with germline mutations that cause HLH or who have persistent/resistant disease are candidates for hematopoietic stem cell transplantation. Without treatment, the prognosis is grim, particularly in those with familial forms of the disease, who typically survive for less than 2 months. With prompt treatment, with or without subsequent hematopoietic stem cell transplantation, roughly half of patients survive, though many do so with significant sequelae, such as renal damage in adults and growth and mental retardation in children.

Neoplastic Proliferations of White Cells

Malignancies are clinically the most important disorders of white cells. These diseases fall into several broad categories:

- *Lymphoid neoplasms* include a diverse group of tumors of B-cell, T-cell, and NK-cell origin. In many instances the phenotype of the neoplastic cell closely resembles that of a particular stage of normal lymphocyte maturation, a feature that is used in the diagnosis and classification of these disorders.
- *Myeloid neoplasms* arise from early hematopoietic progenitors. Three categories of myeloid neoplasia are recognized: *acute myeloid leukemias,* in which immature progenitor cells accumulate in the bone marrow; *myelodysplastic syndromes,* which are associated with ineffective hematopoiesis and resultant peripheral blood cytopenias; and *chronic myeloproliferative disorders,* in which increased production of one or more terminally differentiated myeloid elements (e.g., granulocytes) usually leads to elevated peripheral blood counts.
- The *histiocytoses* are uncommon proliferative lesions of macrophages and dendritic cells. Although "histiocyte" (literally, "tissue cell") is an archaic morphologic term, it is still often used. A special type of immature dendritic cell, the Langerhans cell, gives rise to a spectrum of neoplastic disorders referred to as the *Langerhans cell histiocytoses.*

Etiologic and Pathogenetic Factors in White Cell Neoplasia: Overview

As discussed see in the following sections, the neoplastic disorders of white cells are extremely varied. Before we delve into this complexity, it is worth considering a few themes of general relevance to their etiology and pathogenesis.

Chromosomal Translocations and Other Acquired Mutations. **Nonrandom chromosomal abnormalities, most commonly translocations, are present in the majority of white cell neoplasms.** Many specific rearrangements are associated with particular neoplasms, suggesting a critical role in their genesis (Chapter 7).

- **The genes that are mutated or otherwise altered often play crucial roles in the development, growth, or survival of the normal counterpart of the malignant cell.** As a consequence, certain mutations are strongly associated with specific tumor types, so much so that is some instances they are required for particular diagnoses. In some instances, the mutation produces a "dominant-negative" protein that interferes with a normal function (a loss of function); in others the result is an inappropriate increase in some normal activity (a gain of function).
- **Oncoproteins created by genomic aberrations often block normal maturation, turn on pro-growth signaling pathways, or protect cells from apoptotic cell death.** Figure 13-4 highlights some of the more common or better characterized oncogenic events that serve as oncogenic driver mutations in particular kinds of white cell malignancies.
  - Many oncoproteins cause an arrest in differentiation, often at a stage when cells are proliferating rapidly. The importance of this block in maturation is most evident in the acute leukemias, in which dominant-negative oncogenic mutations involving transcription factors are often present that interfere with early stages of lymphoid or myeloid cell differentiation.
  - Other mutations in transcriptional regulators seem to directly enhance the self-renewal of tumors cells,

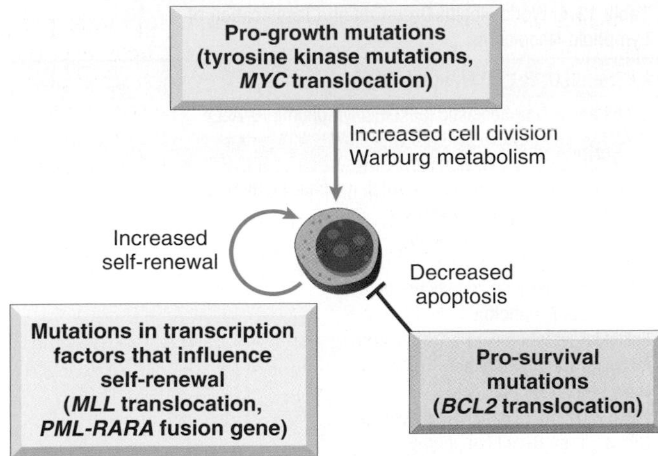

Figure 13-4 Pathogenesis of white cell malignancies. Various tumors harbor mutations that principally effect maturation or enhance self-renewal, drive growth, or prevent apoptosis. Exemplary examples of each type of mutation are listed; details are provided later under specific tumor types.

giving such cells stem-cell–like properties. These types of mutations often collaborate with mutations that produce a constitutively active tyrosine kinase; oncogenic tyrosine kinases activate RAS and its two downstream signaling arms, the PI3K/AKT and MAPK pathways (Chapter 7), and thereby drive cell growth and Warburg metabolism.

- Finally, mutations that inhibit apoptosis are prevalent in certain hematologic malignancies.

- **Proto-oncogenes are often activated in lymphoid cells by errors that occur during antigen receptor gene rearrangement and diversification.** Among lymphoid cells, potentially oncogenic mutations occur most frequently in germinal center B cells during attempted antibody diversification. After antigen stimulation, B cells enter germinal centers and upregulate the expression of activation-induced cytosine deaminase (AID), a specialized DNA-modifying enzyme that is essential for two types of immunoglobulin (Ig) gene modifications: *class switching*, an intragenic recombination event in which the IgM heavy-chain constant gene segment is replaced with a different constant segment (e.g., IgG_3), leading to a switch in the class (isotype) of antibody produced; and *somatic hypermutation*, which creates point mutations within Ig genes that may increase antibody affinity for antigen (Chapter 6). Certain proto-oncogenes, such as *MYC*, are activated in germinal center B-cell lymphomas by translocations to the transcriptionally active Ig locus. Remarkably, AID expression is sufficient to induce *MYC/Ig* translocations in normal germinal center B cells, apparently because AID creates lesions in DNA that lead to chromosomal breaks. Other proto-oncogenes, such as *BCL6*, a transcription factor that has an important role in many B cell malignancies, are frequently activated in germinal center B-cell lymphomas by point mutations that also seem to stem from "mistargeted" DNA breaks induced by AID. A different type of regulated genomic instability is unique to precursor B and T cells, which express a V(D)J recombinase that cuts DNA at specific sites within the Ig and T-cell receptor loci, respectively. This process is essential for the assembly of productive antigen receptor genes, but sometimes goes awry, leading to the joining of portions of other genes to antigen receptor gene regulatory elements. Particularly in tumors of precursor T cells, proto-oncogenes are often deregulated by their involvement in such aberrant recombination events.

Inherited Genetic Factors. As discussed in Chapter 7, individuals with genetic diseases that promote genomic instability, such as Bloom syndrome, Fanconi anemia, and ataxia telangiectasia, are at increased risk of acute leukemia. In addition, both Down syndrome (trisomy 21) and type I neurofibromatosis are associated with an increased incidence of childhood leukemia.

Viruses. Three lymphotropic viruses—human T-cell leukemia virus-1 (HTLV-1), Epstein-Barr virus (EBV), and Kaposi sarcoma herpesvirus/human herpesvirus-8 (KSHV/HHV-8)—have been implicated as causative agents in particular lymphomas. The possible mechanisms of transformation by viruses are discussed in Chapter 7. HTLV-1 is associated with adult T-cell leukemia/lymphoma. EBV is found in a subset of Burkitt lymphoma, 30% to 40% of Hodgkin lymphoma (HL), many B-cell lymphomas arising in the setting of T-cell immunodeficiency, and rare NK-cell lymphomas. In addition to Kaposi sarcoma (Chapter 11), KSHV is associated with an unusual B-cell lymphoma that presents as a malignant effusion, often in the pleural cavity.

Chronic Inflammation. Several agents that cause localized chronic inflammation predispose to lymphoid neoplasia, which almost always arises within the inflamed tissue. Examples include the associations between *H. pylori* infection and gastric B-cell lymphomas (Chapter 17), gluten-sensitive enteropathy and intestinal T-cell lymphomas, and even breast implants, which are associated with an unusual subtype of T cell lymphoma. This can be contrasted with HIV infection, which is associated with an increased risk of B-cell lymphomas that may arise within virtually any organ. Early in the course, T-cell dysregulation by HIV infection causes a systemic hyperplasia of germinal center B cells that is associated with an increased incidence of germinal center B-cell lymphomas. In advanced infection (acquired immunodeficiency syndrome), severe T-cell immunodeficiency further elevates the risk for B-cell lymphomas, particularly those associated with EBV and KSHV/HHV-8. These relationships are discussed in more detail in Chapter 6.

Iatrogenic Factors. Ironically, radiation therapy and certain forms of chemotherapy used to treat cancer increase the risk of subsequent myeloid and lymphoid neoplasms. This association stems from the mutagenic effects of ionizing radiation and chemotherapeutic drugs on hematolymphoid progenitor cells.

Smoking. The incidence of acute myeloid leukemia is increased 1.3- to 2-fold in smokers, presumably because of exposure to carcinogens, such as benzene, in tobacco smoke.

Lymphoid Neoplasms

Definitions and Classifications

One confusing aspect of the lymphoid neoplasms concerns the use of the terms *lymphocytic leukemia* and *lymphoma. Leukemia* is used for neoplasms that present with widespread involvement of the bone marrow and (usually, but not always) the peripheral blood. *Lymphoma* is used for proliferations that arise as discrete tissue masses. Originally these terms were attached to what were considered distinct entities, but with time and increased understanding these divisions have blurred. Many entities called "lymphoma" occasionally have leukemic presentations, and evolution to "leukemia" is not unusual during the progression of incurable "lymphomas." Conversely, tumors identical to "leukemias" sometimes arise as soft-tissue masses without detectable bone marrow disease. Hence, when applied to particular neoplasms, the terms *leukemia* and *lymphoma* merely reflect the usual tissue distribution of each disease at presentation.

Within the large group of lymphomas, *Hodgkin lymphoma* is segregated from all other forms, which constitute the *non-Hodgkin lymphomas (NHLs).* Hodgkin lymphoma has distinctive pathologic features and is treated in a unique fashion. Another special group of B cell tumors, which differs from most lymphomas, is the *plasma cell neoplasms.* These most often arise in the bone marrow and only infrequently involve lymph nodes or the peripheral blood. Taken together, the diverse lymphoid neoplasms constitute a complex, clinically important group of cancers, with about 100,000 new cases being diagnosed each year in the United States.

The clinical presentation of the various lymphoid neoplasms is most often determined by the anatomic distribution of disease. Two thirds of NHLs and virtually all Hodgkin lymphomas present as enlarged nontender lymph nodes (often > 2 cm). The remaining one third of NHLs present with symptoms related to the involvement of extranodal sites (e.g., skin, stomach, or brain). The lymphocytic leukemias most often come to attention because of signs and symptoms related to the suppression of normal hematopoiesis by tumor cells in the bone marrow. Finally, the most common plasma cell neoplasm, multiple myeloma, causes bony destruction of the skeleton and often presents with pain due to pathologic fractures. Other symptoms related to lymphoid tumors are frequently caused by proteins secreted from the tumor cells or from immune cells that are responding to the tumor. Specific examples include the plasma cell tumors, in which much of the pathophysiology is related to the secretion of whole antibodies or Ig fragments; Hodgkin lymphoma, which is often associated with fever related to the release of cytokines from inflammatory cells responding to the tumor cells; and peripheral T-cell lymphomas, tumors of functional T cells that often release a number of inflammatory cytokines and chemokines.

Historically, few areas of pathology evoked as much controversy as the classification of lymphoid neoplasms, but consensus has been reached through use of objective molecular diagnostic tools. The current World Health Organization (WHO) classification scheme (Table 13-4) uses morphologic, immunophenotypic, genotypic, and clinical features to sort the lymphoid neoplasms into five broad categories, which are separated according to the cell of origin:

1. Precursor B-cell neoplasms (neoplasms of immature B cells)
2. Peripheral B-cell neoplasms (neoplasms of mature B cells)
3. Precursor T-cell neoplasms (neoplasms of immature T cells)
4. Peripheral T-cell and NK-cell neoplasms (neoplasms of mature T cells and NK cells)
5. Hodgkin lymphoma (neoplasms of Reed-Sternberg cells and variants)

Before discussing the specific entities of the WHO classification, some important principles relevant to the lymphoid neoplasms should be emphasized.

- Lymphoid neoplasia can be suspected from the clinical features, but histologic examination of lymph nodes or other involved tissues is required for diagnosis.

Table 13-4 World Health Organization Classification of Lymphoid Neoplasms

I. Precursor B-Cell Neoplasms
B-cell acute lymphoblastic leukemia/lymphoma (B-ALL)
II. Peripheral B-Cell Neoplasms
Chronic lymphocytic leukemia/small lymphocytic lymphoma
B-cell prolymphocytic leukemia
Lymphoplasmacytic lymphoma
Splenic and nodal marginal zone lymphomas
Extranodal marginal zone lymphoma
Mantle cell lymphoma
Follicular lymphoma
Marginal zone lymphoma
Hairy cell leukemia
Plasmacytoma/plasma cell myeloma
Diffuse large B-cell lymphoma
Burkitt lymphoma
III. Precursor T-Cell Neoplasms
T-cell acute lymphoblastic leukemia/lymphoma (T-ALL)
IV. Peripheral T-Cell and NK-Cell Neoplasms
T-cell prolymphocytic leukemia
Large granular lymphocytic leukemia
Mycosis fungoides/Sézary syndrome
Peripheral T-cell lymphoma, unspecified
Anaplastic large-cell lymphoma
Angioimmunoblastic T-cell lymphoma
Enteropathy-associated T-cell lymphoma
Panniculitis-like T-cell lymphoma
Hepatosplenic γδT-cell lymphoma
Adult T-cell leukemia/lymphoma
Extranodal NK/T-cell lymphoma
NK-cell leukemia
V. Hodgkin Lymphoma
Classical subtypes
Nodular sclerosis
Mixed cellularity
Lymphocyte-rich
Lymphocyte depletion
Lymphocyte predominance

NK, Natural killer.

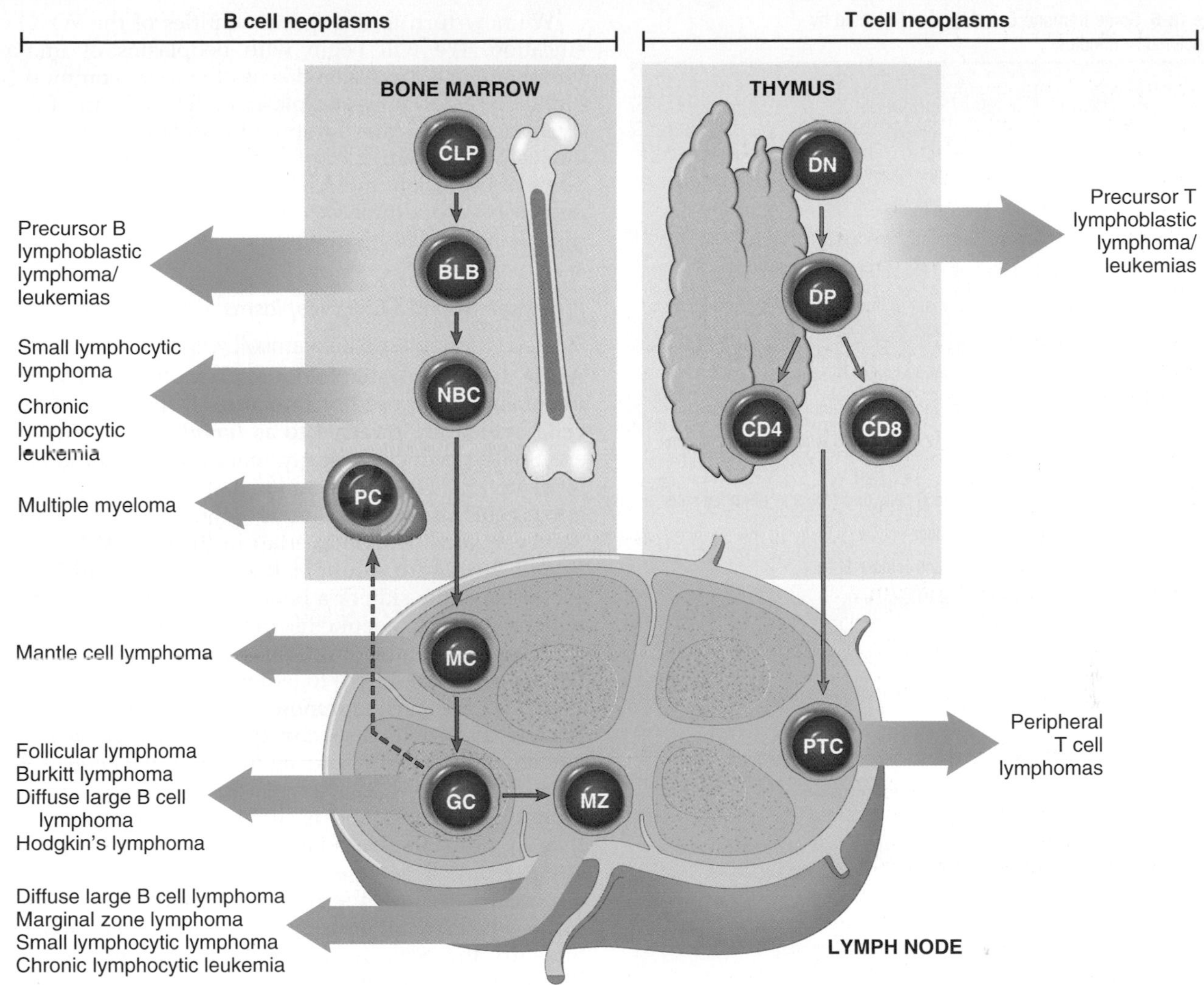

Figure 13-5 Origin of lymphoid neoplasms. Stages of B- and T-cell differentiation from which specific lymphoid tumors emerge are shown. CLP, Common lymphoid precursor; BLB, pre-B lymphoblast; DN, CD4/CD8 double-negative pro-T cell; DP, CD4/CD8 double-positive pre-T cell; GC, germinal-center B cell; MC, mantle B cell; MZ, marginal zone B cell; NBC, naive B cell; PTC, peripheral T cell.

- **Antigen receptor gene rearrangement generally precedes transformation of lymphoid cells; hence, all daughter cells derived from the malignant progenitor share the same antigen receptor gene configuration and sequence, and synthesize identical antigen receptor proteins (either Igs or T-cell receptors)**. In contrast, normal immune responses are comprised of polyclonal populations of lymphocytes that express many different antigen receptors. Thus, analyses of antigen receptor genes and their protein products can be used to distinguish reactive (polyclonal) and malignant (monoclonal) lymphoid proliferations. In addition, each antigen receptor gene rearrangement produces a unique DNA sequence that constitutes a highly specific clonal marker, which can be used to detect small numbers of residual malignant lymphoid cells after therapy.
- **Most lymphoid neoplasms resemble some recognizable stage of B- or T-cell differentiation** (Fig. 13-5), a feature that is used in their classification. The vast majority (85% to 90%) of lymphoid neoplasms are of B-cell origin, with most of the remainder being T-cell tumors; only rarely are tumors of NK cell origin encountered. Markers recognized by antibodies that are helpful in the characterization of lymphomas and leukemias are listed in Table 13-5.
- **Lymphoid neoplasms are often associated with immune abnormalities.** Both a loss of protective immunity (susceptibility to infection) and a breakdown of tolerance (autoimmunity) can be seen, sometimes in the same patient. In a further ironic twist, individuals with inherited or acquired immunodeficiency are themselves at high risk of developing certain lymphoid neoplasms, particularly those caused by oncogenic viruses (e.g., EBV).
- **Neoplastic B and T cells tend to recapitulate the behavior of their normal counterparts.** Like normal lymphocytes, neoplastic B and T cells home to certain tissue sites, leading to characteristic patterns of involvement. For example, follicular lymphomas home to germinal centers in lymph nodes, whereas cutaneous T-cell lymphomas home to the skin. Like their normal counterparts, particular adhesion molecules and chemokine receptors govern the homing of the neoplastic lymphoid cells. Variable numbers of neoplastic B and T

Table 13-5 Some Immune Cell Antigens Detected by Monoclonal Antibodies

Antigen Designation	Normal Cellular Distribution
Primarily T-Cell Associated	
CD1	Thymocytes and Langerhans cells
CD3	Thymocytes, mature T cells
CD4	Helper T cells, subset of thymocytes
CD5	T cells and a small subset of B cells
CD8	Cytotoxic T cells, subset of thymocytes, and some NK cells
Primarily B-Cell Associated	
CD10	Pre-B cells and germinal-center B cells
CD19	Pre-B cells and mature B cells but not plasma cells
CD20	Pre-B cells after CD19 and mature B cells but not plasma cells
CD21	EBV receptor; mature B cells and follicular dendritic cells
CD23	Activated mature B cells
CD79a	Marrow pre-B cells and mature B cells
Primarily Monocyte or Macrophage Associated	
CD11c	Granulocytes, monocytes, and macrophages; also expressed by hairy cell leukemias
CD13	Immature and mature monocytes and granulocytes
CD14	Monocytes
CD15	Granulocytes; Reed-Sternberg cells and variants
CD33	Myeloid progenitors and monocytes
CD64	Mature myeloid cells
Primarily NK-Cell Associated	
CD16	NK cells and granulocytes
CD56	NK cells and a subset of T cells
Primarily Stem Cell and Progenitor Cell Associated	
CD34	Pluripotent hematopoietic stem cells and progenitor cells of many lineages
Activation Markers	
CD30	Activated B cells, T cells, and monocytes; Reed-Sternberg cells and variants
Present on All Leukocytes	
CD45	All leukocytes; also known as leukocyte common antigen (LCA)

CD, Cluster designation; EBV, Epstein-Barr virus; NK, natural killer.

lymphoid cells also recirculate through the lymphatics and peripheral blood to distant sites; as a result most lymphoid tumors are widely disseminated at the time of diagnosis. Notable exceptions to this rule include Hodgkin lymphomas, which are sometimes restricted to one group of lymph nodes, and marginal zone B-cell lymphomas, which are often restricted to sites of chronic inflammation.

- **Hodgkin lymphoma spreads in an orderly fashion, whereas most forms of NHL spread widely early in their course in a less predictable fashion.** Hence, while lymphoma staging provides generally useful prognostic information, it is of most utility in guiding therapy in Hodgkin lymphoma.

We now turn to the specific entities of the WHO classification. We will begin with neoplasms of immature lymphoid cells, and then discuss the more common Non-Hodgkin lymphomas and plasma cell neoplasms, followed by a selection of rarer lymphoid neoplams that are pathogenically informative or of particular clinical importance. Some of the salient molecular and clinical features of these neoplasms are summarized in Table 13-6. We will finish by discussing the Hodgkin lymphomas.

Precursor B- and T-Cell Neoplasms

Acute Lymphoblastic Leukemia/Lymphoma

Acute lymphoblastic leukemia/lymphomas (ALLs) are neoplasms composed of immature B (pre-B) or T (pre-T) cells, which are referred to as *lymphoblasts.* About 85% are B-ALLs, which typically manifest as childhood acute "leukemias." The less common T-ALLs tend to present in adolescent males as thymic "lymphomas." There is, however, considerable overlap in the clinical behavior of B- and T-ALL; for example, B-ALL uncommonly presents as a mass in the skin or a bone, and many T-ALLs present with or evolve to a leukemic picture. Because of their morphologic and clinical similarities, the various forms of ALL will be considered here together.

ALL is the most common cancer of children. Approximately 2500 new cases are diagnosed each year in the United States, most occurring in individuals younger than 15 years of age. ALL is almost three times as common in whites as in blacks and is slightly more frequent in boys than in girls. Hispanics have the highest incidence of any ethnic group. B-ALL peaks in incidence at about the age of 3, perhaps because the number of normal bone marrow pre-B cells (the cell of origin) is greatest very early in life. Similarly the peak incidence of T-ALL is in adolescence, the age when the thymus reaches maximum size. B- and T-ALL also occur less frequently in adults of all ages.

Pathogenesis. **Many of the chromosomal aberrations seen in ALL dysregulate the expression and function of transcription factors required for normal B- and T-cell development.** Up to 70% of T-ALLs have gain-of-function mutations in *NOTCH1*, a gene that is essential for T-cell development. On the other hand, a high fraction of B-ALLs have loss-of-function mutations in genes that are required for B-cell development, such as *PAX5*, *E2A*, and *EBF*, or a balanced t(12;21) involving the genes *ETV6* and *RUNX1*, two genes that are needed in very early hematopoietic precursors. All of these varied mutations disturb the differentiation of lymphoid precursors and promote maturation arrest, and in doing they induce increased self-renewal, a stem cell–like phenotype. Similar themes are relevant in the genesis of AML (discussed later).

In keeping with the multistep origin of cancer (Chapter 7), single mutations are not sufficient to produce ALL. The identity of these complementary mutations is incomplete, but aberrations that drive cell growth, such as mutations that increase tyrosine kinase activity and RAS signaling, are commonly present. Emerging data from deep sequencing of ALL genomes is rapidly filling in the remaining gaps. Early returns suggest that fewer than 10 mutations are sufficient to produce full-blown ALL; hence, compared to solid tumors, ALL is a genetically simple tumor.

Table 13-6 Summary of Major Types of Lymphoid Leukemias and Non-Hodgkin Lymphomas

Diagnosis	Cell of Origin	Genotype	Salient Clinical Features
Neoplasms of Immature B and T Cells			
B-cell acute lymphoblastic leukemia/lymphoma*	Bone marrow precursor B cell	Diverse chromosomal translocations; t(12;21) involving *RUNX1* and *ETV6* present in 25%	Predominantly children; symptoms relating to marrow replacement and pancytopenia; aggressive
T-cell acute lymphoblastic leukemia/lymphoma	Precursor T cell (often of thymic origin)	Diverse chromosomal translocations, *NOTCH1* mutations (50%-70%)	Predominantly adolescent males; thymic masses and variable bone marrow involvement; aggressive
Neoplasms of Mature B Cells			
Burkitt lymphoma*	Germinal-center B cell	Translocations involving *MYC* and Ig loci, usually t(8;14); subset EBV-associated	Adolescents or young adults with extranodal masses; uncommonly presents as "leukemia"; aggressive
Diffuse large B-cell lymphoma†	Germinal-center or postgerminal center B cell	Diverse chromosomal rearrangements, most often of *BCL6* (30%), *BCL2* (10%), or *MYC* (5%)	All ages, but most common in older adults; often appears as a rapidly growing mass; 30% extranodal; aggressive
Extranodal marginal zone lymphoma	Memory B cell	t(11;18), t(1;14), and t(14;18) creating *MALT1-IAP2*, *BCL10-IgH*, and *MALT1-IgH* fusion genes, respectively	Arises at extranodal sites in adults with chronic inflammatory diseases; may remain localized; indolent
Follicular lymphoma†	Germinal-center B cell	t(14;18) creating *BCL2-IgH* fusion gene	Older adults with generalized lymphadenopathy and marrow involvement; indolent
Hairy cell leukemia	Memory B cell	Activating *BRAF* mutations	Older males with pancytopenia and splenomegaly; indolent
Mantle cell lymphoma	Naive B cell	t(11;14) creating *CyclinD1-IgH* fusion gene	Older males with disseminated disease; moderately aggressive
Multiple myeloma/solitary plasmacytoma†	Post-germinal-center bone marrow homing plasma cell	Diverse rearrangements involving *IgH*; 13q deletions	Myeloma: older adults with lytic bone lesions, pathologic fractures, hypercalcemia, and renal failure; moderately aggressive Plasmacytoma: isolated plasma cell masses in bone or soft tissue; indolent
Small lymphocytic lymphoma/chronic lymphocytic leukemia	Naive B cell or memory B cell	Trisomy 12, deletions of 11q, 13q, and 17p	Older adults with bone marrow, lymph node, spleen, and liver disease; autoimmune hemolysis and thrombocytopenia in a minority; indolent
Neoplasms of Mature T Cells or NK Cells			
Adult T-cell leukemia/lymphoma	Helper T cell	HTLV-1 provirus present in tumor cells	Adults with cutaneous lesions, marrow involvement, and hypercalcemia; occurs mainly in Japan, West Africa, and the Caribbean; aggressive
Peripheral T-cell lymphoma, unspecified	Helper or cytotoxic T cell	No specific chromosomal abnormality	Mainly older adults; usually presents with lymphadenopathy; aggressive
Anaplastic large-cell lymphoma	Cytotoxic T cell	Rearrangements of *ALK* (anaplastic large cell lymphoma kinase) in a subset	Children and young adults, usually with lymph node and soft-tissue disease; aggressive
Extranodal NK/T-cell lymphoma	NK-cell (common) or cytotoxic T cell (rare)	EBV-associated; no specific chromosomal abnormality	Adults with destructive extranodal masses, most commonly sinonasal; aggressive
Mycosis fungoides/Sézary syndrome	Helper T cell	No specific chromosomal abnormality	Adult patients with cutaneous patches, plaques, nodules, or generalized erythema; indolent
Large granular lymphocytic leukemia	Two types: cytotoxic T cell and NK cell	Point mutations in *STAT3*	Adult patients with splenomegaly, neutropenia, and anemia, sometimes, accompanied by autoimmune disease

*Most common tumors in children
†Most common tumors in adults.
EBV, Epstein-Barr virus; *HIV*, human immunodeficiency virus; *Ig*, immunoglobulin; *NK*, natural killer.

Approximately 90% of ALLs have numerical or structural chromosomal changes. Most common is hyperploidy (>50 chromosomes), but hypoploidy and a variety of balanced chromosomal translocations are also seen. Changes in chromosome numbers are of uncertain pathogenic significance, but are important because they frequently correlate with immunophenotype and sometimes prognosis. For example, hyperdiploidy and hypodiploidy are seen only in B-ALL. In addition, B- and T-ALL are associated with completely different sets of translocations, indicating that they are pathogenetically distinct.

MORPHOLOGY

In leukemic presentations, **the marrow is hypercellular and packed with lymphoblasts,** which replace the normal marrow elements. Mediastinal thymic masses occur in 50% to 70% of T-ALLs, which are also more likely to be associated with lymphadenopathy and splenomegaly. In both B- and T-ALL, the tumor cells have scant basophilic cytoplasm and nuclei somewhat larger than those of small lymphocytes (Fig. 13-6*A*). The nuclear chromatin is delicate and finely stippled, and nucleoli are usually small and often demarcated by a rim of condensed chromatin. In many cases the nuclear membrane is deeply subdivided, imparting a convoluted appearance. In keeping with the aggressive clinical behavior, the mitotic rate is high. As with other rapidly growing lymphoid tumors, interspersed macrophages ingesting apoptotic tumor cells may impart a "starry sky" appearance (shown in Fig. 13-15).

Because of their different responses to chemotherapy, ALL must be distinguished from acute myeloid leukemia (AML), a neoplasm of immature myeloid cells that can cause identical signs and symptoms. **Compared with myeloblasts, lymphoblasts have more condensed chromatin, less conspicuous nucleoli, and smaller amounts of cytoplasm that usually lacks granules.** However, these morphologic distinctions are not absolute and definitive diagnosis relies on stains performed with antibodies specific for B- and T-cell antigens (Fig. 13-6*B* and *C*). Histochemical stains are also helpful, in that (in contrast to myeloblasts) lymphoblasts are myeloperoxidase-negative and often contain periodic acid-Schiff–positive cytoplasmic material.

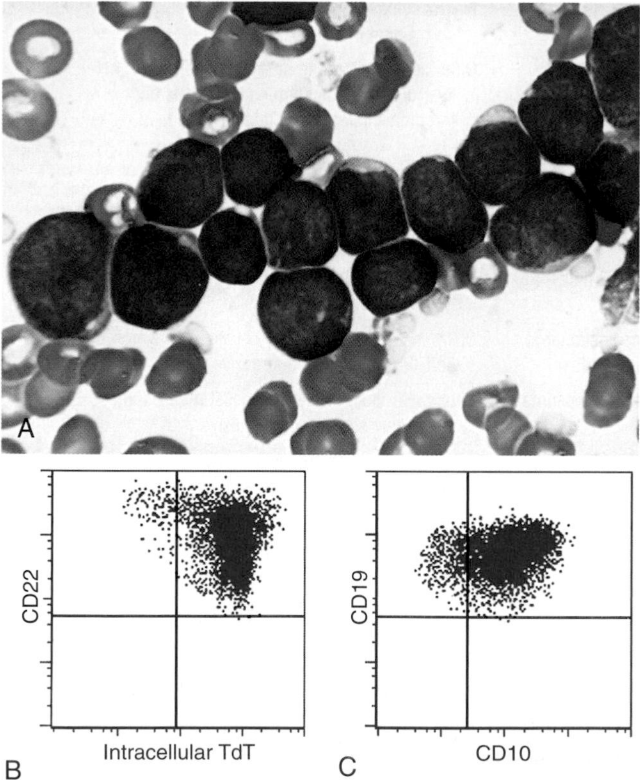

Figure 13-6 **A,** Acute lymphoblastic leukemia/lymphoma. Lymphoblasts with condensed nuclear chromatin, small nucleoli, and scant agranular cytoplasm. **B** and **C** represent the phenotype of the ALL shown in **A,** analyzed by flow cytometry. **B,** Note that the lymphoblasts represented by the red dots express terminal deoxynucleotidyl-transferase (TdT) and the B-cell marker CD22. **C,** The same cells are positive for two other markers, CD10 and CD19, commonly expressed on pre-B lymphoblasts. Thus, this is a B-ALL. (**A,** Courtesy Dr. Robert W. McKenna, Department of Pathology, University of Texas Southwestern Medical School, Dallas, Texas; **B** and **C,** courtesy Dr. Louis Picker, Oregon Health Science Center, Portland, Ore.)

Immunophenotype. Immunostaining for terminal deoxynucleotidyl transferase (TdT), a specialized DNA polymerase that is expressed only in pre-B and pre-T lymphoblasts, is positive in more than 95% of cases (Fig. 13-6*B*). B- and T-ALLs are distinguished with stains for B- and T-cell–specific markers (summarized later).

B-ALLs are arrested at various stages of pre–B-cell development. The lymphoblasts usually express the pan B-cell marker CD19 and the transcription factor PAX5, as well as CD10. In very immature B-ALLs, CD10 is negative. Alternatively, more mature "late pre-B" ALLs express CD10, CD19, CD20, and cytoplasmic IgM heavy chain (μ chain).

Similarly, T-ALLs are arrested at various stages of pre–T-cell development. In most cases the cells are positive for CD1, CD2, CD5, and CD7. The more immature tumors are usually negative for surface CD3, CD4, and CD8, whereas "late" pre–T-cell tumors are positive for these markers.

Clinical Features. Although ALL and AML are genetically and immunophenotypically distinct, they are clinically very similar. In both, the accumulation of neoplastic "blasts" in the bone marrow suppresses normal hematopoiesis by physical crowding, competition for growth factors, and other poorly understood mechanisms. The common features and those more characteristic of ALL are the following:

- *Abrupt stormy onset* within days to a few weeks of the first symptoms
- *Symptoms related to depression of marrow function,* including fatigue due to anemia; fever, reflecting infections secondary to neutropenia; and bleeding due to thrombocytopenia
- *Mass effects caused by neoplastic infiltration* (which are more common in ALL), including bone pain resulting from marrow expansion and infiltration of the subperiosteum; generalized lymphadenopathy, splenomegaly, and hepatomegaly; testicular enlargement; and in T-ALL, complications related to compression of large vessels and airways in the mediastinum
- *Central nervous system manifestations* such as headache, vomiting, and nerve palsies resulting from meningeal spread, all of which are also more common in ALL

Prognosis. Pediatric ALL is one of the great success stories of oncology. With aggressive chemotherapy about 95% of children with ALL obtain a complete remission, and 75% to 85% are cured. Despite these achievements, however, ALL remains the leading cause of cancer deaths in children, and only 35% to 40% of adults are cured. Several factors are associated with a worse prognosis: (1) age younger than 2 years, largely because of the strong association of infantile ALL with translocations involving the *MLL* gene; (2) presentation in adolescence or adulthood; and (3) peripheral blood blast counts greater than 100,000, which probably reflects a high tumor burden. Favorable prognostic markers include (1) age between 2 and 10 years, (2) a low white cell count, (3) hyperdiploidy, (4) trisomy of chromosomes 4, 7, and 10, and (5) the presence of a t(12;21). Notably, the molecular detection of residual disease after therapy is predictive of a worse outcome in both B- and T-ALL and is being used to guide new clinical trials.

Although most chromosomal aberrations in ALL alter the function of transcription factors, the t(9;22) instead creates a fusion gene that encodes a constitutively active BCR-ABL tyrosine kinase (described in more detail under chronic myelogenous leukemia). In B-ALL, the BCR-ABL protein is usually 190 kDa in size and has stronger tyrosine kinase activity than the form of BCR-ABL that is found in chronic myelogenous leukemia, in which a BCR-ABL protein of 210 kDa in size is usually seen. Treatment of t(9;22)-positive ALLs with BCR-ABL kinase inhibitors in combination with conventional chemotherapy is highly effective and has greatly improved the outcome for this molecular subtype of B-ALL in children. The outlook for adults with ALL remains more guarded, in part because of differences in the molecular pathogenesis of adult and childhood ALL, but also because older adults cannot tolerate the very intensive chemotherapy regimens that are curative in children.

Peripheral B-Cell Neoplasms

Chronic Lymphocytic Leukemia, Small Lymphocytic Lymphoma

Chronic lymphocytic leukemia (CLL) and small lymphocytic lymphoma (SLL) differ only in the degree of peripheral blood lymphocytosis. Most affected patients have sufficient lymphocytosis to fulfill the diagnostic requirement for CLL (absolute lymphocyte count > 5000 per mm^3). **CLL is the most common leukemia of adults in the Western world.** There are about 15,000 new cases of CLL each year in the United States. The median age at diagnosis is 60 years, and there is a 2:1 male predominance. In contrast, SLL constitutes only 4% of NHLs. CLL/SLL is much less common in Japan and other Asian countries than in the West.

Pathogenesis. Unlike most other lymphoid malignancies, chromosomal translocations are rare in CLL/SLL. **The most common genetic anomalies are deletions of 13q14.3, 11q, and 17p, and trisomy 12q.** Molecular characterization of the region deleted on chromosome 13 has implicated two microRNAs, miR-15a and miR-16-1, as possible tumor suppressor genes. DNA sequencing has revealed that the Ig genes of some CLL/SLL are somatically hypermutated, whereas others are not, suggesting that the cell of origin may be either a postgerminal center memory B cell or a naive B cell. For unclear reasons, tumors with unmutated Ig segments (those putatively of naive B-cell origin) pursue a more aggressive course. Deep sequencing of CLL genomes has also revealed gain-of-function mutations involving the NOTCH1 receptor in 10% to 18% of tumors, as well as frequent mutations in genes that regulate RNA splicing.

The growth of CLL/SLL cells is largely confined to proliferation centers (described below), where tumor cells receive critical cues from the microenvironment. Stromal cells in proliferation centers seem to express a variety of factors that stimulate the activity of the transcription factor NF-κB, which promotes cell growth and survival. In addition, experimental models of CLL suggest that tumor cells rely on signals generated by the B-cell receptor (membrane bound immunoglobulin) for growth and survival. These signals are transduced by a cascade of kinases that include the Bruton tyrosine kinase (BTK), which is defective in patients with congenital X-linked agammaglobulinemia (Chapter 6). Of note, BTK inhibitors now being tested in clinical trials have produced sustained responses in a high fraction of CLL patients, indicating that human CLL cells are also dependent on this signaling pathway.

MORPHOLOGY

Lymph nodes are diffusely effaced by an infiltrate of predominantly small lymphocytes 6 to 12 μm in diameter with round to slightly irregular nuclei, condensed chromatin, and scant cytoplasm (Fig. 13-7). Admixed are variable numbers of larger activated lymphocytes that often gather in loose aggregates referred to as **proliferation centers**, which contain mitotically active cells. When present, **proliferation centers are pathognomonic for CLL/SLL**. The blood contains large numbers of small round lymphocytes with scant cytoplasm (Fig. 13-8). Some of these cells are usually disrupted in the process of making smears, producing so-called **smudge cells**. The bone marrow is almost always involved by interstitial infiltrates or aggregates of tumor cells. Infiltrates are also virtually always seen in the splenic white and red pulp and the hepatic portal tracts (Fig. 13-9).

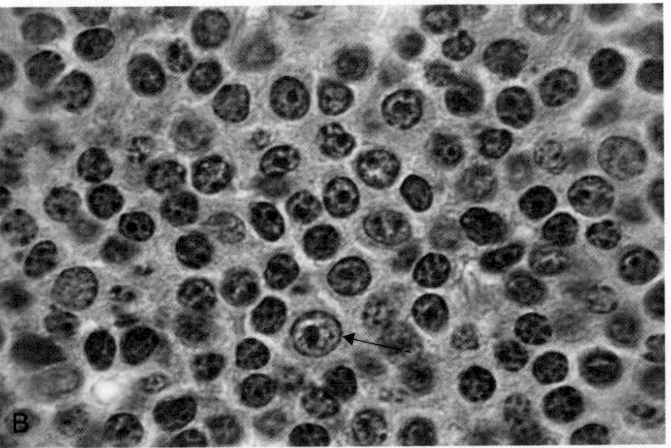

Figure 13-7 Small lymphocytic lymphoma/chronic lymphocytic leukemia (lymph node). **A,** Low-power view shows diffuse effacement of nodal architecture. **B,** At high power the majority of the tumor cells are small round lymphocytes. A "prolymphocyte," a larger cell with a centrally placed nucleolus, is also present in this field *(arrow)*. (**A,** Courtesy Dr. José Hernandez, Department of Pathology, University of Texas Southwestern Medical School, Dallas, Texas.)

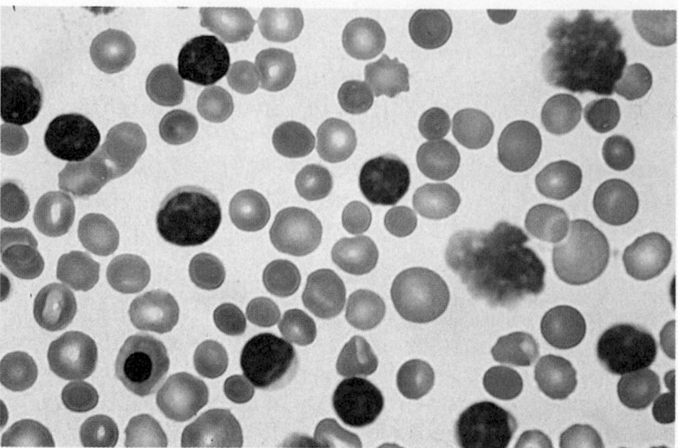

Figure 13-8 Chronic lymphocytic leukemia. This peripheral blood smear is flooded with small lymphocytes with condensed chromatin and scant cytoplasm. A characteristic finding is the presence of disrupted tumor cells (smudge cells), two of which are present in this smear. A coexistent autoimmune hemolytic anemia (Chapter 14) explains the presence of spherocytes (hyperchromatic, round erythrocytes). A nucleated erythroid cell is present in the lower left-hand corner of the field. In this setting, circulating nucleated red cells could stem from premature release of progenitors in the face of severe anemia, marrow infiltration by tumor (leukoerythroblastosis), or both.

Immunophenotype. CLL/SLL has a distinctive immunophenotype. The tumor cells express the pan B-cell markers CD19 and CD20, as well as CD23 and CD5, the latter a marker that is found on a small subset of normal B cells. Low-level expression of surface Ig (usually IgM or IgM and IgD) is also typical.

Clinical Features. Patients are often asymptomatic at diagnosis. When symptoms appear, they are nonspecific and include easy fatigability, weight loss, and anorexia. Generalized lymphadenopathy and hepatosplenomegaly are present in 50% to 60% of symptomatic patients. The leukocyte count is highly variable; leukopenia can be seen in individuals with SLL and marrow involvement, while counts in excess of 200,000/mm^3 are sometimes seen in CLL patients with heavy tumor burdens. A small monoclonal Ig "spike" is present in the blood of some patients.

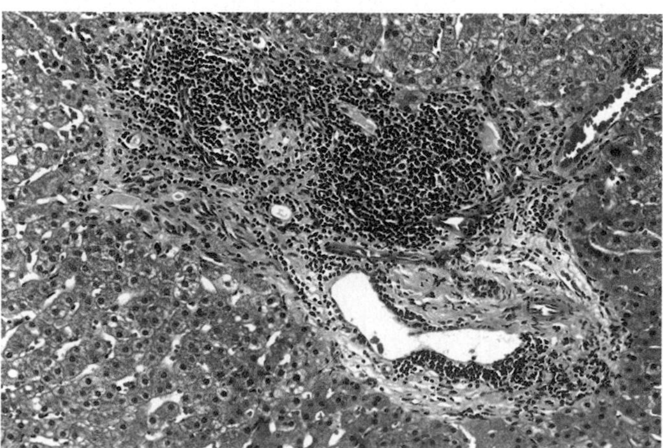

Figure 13-9 Small lymphocytic lymphoma/chronic lymphocytic leukemia involving the liver. Low-power view of a typical periportal lymphocytic infiltrate. (Courtesy Dr. Mark Fleming, Department of Pathology, Children's Hospital, Boston, Mass.)

At the other end of the spectrum are asymptomatic patients with monoclonal B cells in their peripheral blood but in numbers that are too few to merit the diagnosis of CLL. These abnormal B cells often have some of the same genetic aberrations that are seen in CLL, such as 13q deletions and trisomy 12, yet only about 1% of such patients progress to symptomatic CLL per year, presumably due to acquisition of additional genetic lesions.

CLL/SLL disrupts normal immune function through uncertain mechanisms. Hypogammaglobulinemia is common and contributes to an increased susceptibility to infections, particularly those caused by bacteria. Conversely, 10% to 15% of patients develop hemolytic anemia or thrombocytopenia due to autoantibodies made by non-neoplastic B cells.

The course and prognosis are extremely variable and depend primarily on the clinical stage. Overall median survival is 4 to 6 years, but is more than 10 years in individuals with minimal tumor burdens at diagnosis. Other variables that correlate with a worse outcome include (1) the presence of deletions of 11q and 17p, (2) a lack of somatic hypermutation, (3) the expression of ZAP-70, a protein that augments signals produced by the Ig receptor, and (4) the presence of *NOTCH1* mutations. Symptomatic patients are generally treated with "gentle" chemotherapy and immunotherapy with antibodies against proteins found on the surface of CLL/SLL cells, particularly CD20. Hematopoietic stem cell transplantation is being offered to the relatively young. The most promising new therapy is BTK inhibitors, described earlier.

Another factor that impacts patient survival is the tendency of CLL/SLL to transform to a more aggressive tumor. Most commonly this takes the form of a transformation to diffuse large B-cell lymphoma, so-called *Richter syndrome* (approximately 5% to 10% of patients). Transformation to diffuse large B-cell lymphoma is often heralded by the development of a rapidly enlarging mass within a lymph node or the spleen. Transformation probably stems from the acquisition of additional, still mutations that increase growth. Large-cell transformation is an ominous event, with most patients surviving less than 1 year.

Follicular Lymphoma

Follicular lymphoma is the most common form of indolent NHL in the United States, affecting 15,000 to 20,000 individuals per year. It usually presents in middle age and afflicts males and females equally. It is less common in Europe and rare in Asian populations.

Pathogenesis. **Follicular lymphoma likely arises from germinal center B cells and is strongly associated with chromosomal translocations involving *BCL2*.** Its hallmark is a (14;18) translocation that juxtaposes the *IGH* locus on chromosome 14 and the *BCL2* locus on chromosome 18. The t(14;18) is seen in up to 90% of follicular lymphomas, and leads to overexpression of BCL2 (see Fig. 13-12). BCL2 antagonizes apoptosis (Chapter 7) and promotes the survival of follicular lymphoma cells. Notably, while normal germinal centers contain numerous B cells undergoing apoptosis, follicular lymphoma is characteristically devoid of apoptotic cells. Deep sequencing of follicular lymphoma genomes have identified mutations in the *MLL2* gene in about 90% of cases as well. *MLL2* encodes a histone

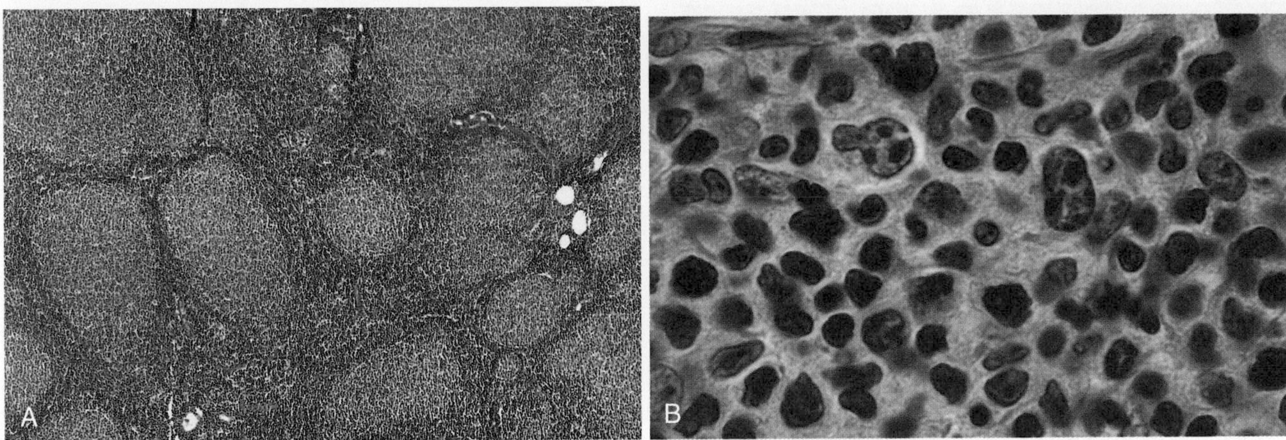

Figure 13-10 Follicular lymphoma (lymph node). **A,** Nodular aggregates of lymphoma cells are present throughout lymph node. **B,** At high magnification, small lymphoid cells with condensed chromatin and irregular or cleaved nuclear outlines (centrocytes) are mixed with a population of larger cells with nucleoli (centroblasts). (**A,** Courtesy Dr. Robert W. McKenna, Department of Pathology, University of Texas Southwestern Medical School, Dallas, Texas.)

methyltransferase that regulates gene expression, suggesting that epigenetic abnormalities have an important role in this neoplasm; however, the functional significance of *MLL2* mutations has yet to be deciphered.

Particularly early in the disease, follicular lymphoma cells growing in lymph nodes are found within a network of reactive follicular dendritic cells admixed with macrophages and T cells. Expression profiling studies have shown that differences in the genes expressed by these reactive cells are predictive of outcome, implying that the response of follicular lymphoma cells to therapy is influenced by the surrounding microenvironment.

MORPHOLOGY

In most cases, a predominantly nodular or nodular and diffuse growth pattern is observed in involved lymph nodes (Fig. 13-10*A*). Two principal cell types are present in varying proportions: (1) small cells with irregular or cleaved nuclear contours and scant cytoplasm, referred to as **centrocytes** (small cleaved cells); and (2) larger cells with open nuclear chromatin, several nucleoli, and modest amounts of cytoplasm, referred to as **centroblasts** (Fig. 13-10*B*). In most follicular lymphomas, small cleaved cells are in the majority. Peripheral blood involvement sufficient to produce lymphocytosis (usually less than 20,000 cells/mm^3) is seen in about 10% of cases. Bone marrow involvement occurs in 85% of cases and characteristically takes the form of paratrabecular lymphoid aggregates. The splenic white pulp (Fig. 13-11) and hepatic portal triads are also frequently involved.

Immunophenotype. The neoplastic cells closely resemble normal germinal center B cells, expressing CD19, CD20, CD10, surface Ig, and BCL6. Unlike CLL/SLL and mantle cell lymphoma, CD5 is not expressed. BCL2 is expressed in more than 90% of cases, in distinction to normal follicular center B cells, which are BCL2-negative (Fig. 13-12).

Clinical Features. Follicular lymphoma tends to present with painless, generalized lymphadenopathy. Involvement of extranodal sites, such as the gastrointestinal tract, central nervous system, or testis, is relatively uncommon. Although incurable, it usually follows an indolent waxing and waning course. Survival (median, 7 to 9 years) is not improved by aggressive therapy; hence, the usual approach is to palliate patients with low-dose chemotherapy or immunotherapy (e.g., anti-CD20 antibody) when they become symptomatic.

Histologic transformation occurs in 30% to 50% of follicular lymphomas, most commonly to diffuse large B-cell lymphoma. Less commonly, tumors resembling Burkitt lymphoma emerge that are associated with chromosomal translocations involving *MYC*. Like normal germinal center B cells, follicular lymphomas have ongoing somatic hypermutation, which may promote transformation by causing point mutations or chromosomal aberrations. The median survival is less than 1 year after transformation.

Diffuse Large B-Cell Lymphoma

Diffuse large B-cell lymphoma (DLBCL) is the most common form of NHL. Each year in the United States there are about 25,000 new cases. There is a slight male

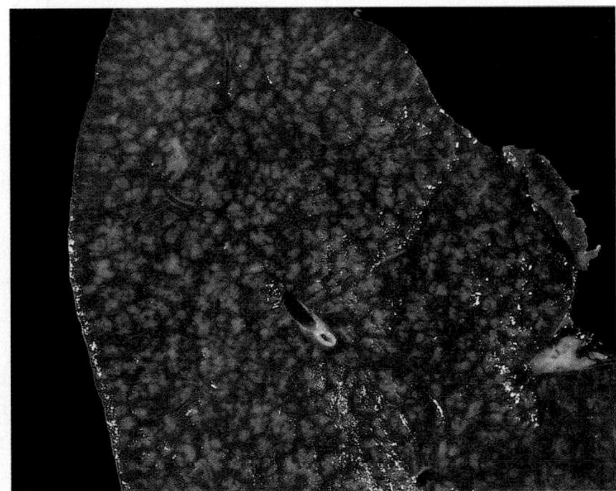

Figure 13-11 Follicular lymphoma (spleen). Prominent nodules represent white pulp follicles expanded by follicular lymphoma cells. Other indolent B-cell lymphomas (small lymphocytic lymphoma, mantle cell lymphoma, marginal zone lymphoma) can produce an identical pattern of involvement. (Courtesy Dr. Jeffrey Jorgenson, Department of Hematopathology, MD Anderson Cancer Center, Houston, Texas.)

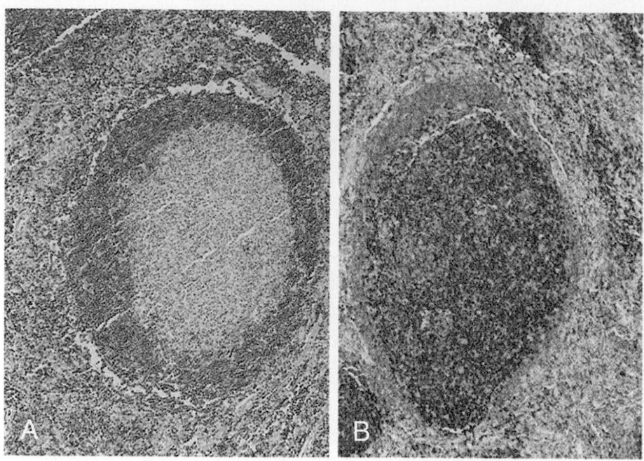

Figure 13-12 BCL2 expression in reactive and neoplastic follicles. BCL2 protein was detected by using an immunohistochemical technique that produces a brown stain. In reactive follicles **(A),** BCL2 is present in mantle zone cells but not follicular-center B cells, whereas follicular lymphoma cells **(B)** show strong BCL2 staining. (Courtesy Dr. Jeffrey Jorgenson, Department of Hematopathology, MD Anderson Cancer Center, Houston, Texas.)

predominance. The median patient age is about 60 years, but DLBCL also occurs in young adults and children.

Pathogenesis. Genetic, gene expression profiling, and immunohistochemical studies indicate that DLBCL is molecularly heterogeneous. One frequent pathogenic event is dysregulation of BCL6, a DNA-binding zinc-finger transcriptional repressor that is required for the formation of normal germinal centers. About 30% of DLBCLs contain various translocations that have in common a breakpoint in *BCL6* at chromosome 3q27. Acquired mutations in *BCL6* promoter sequences that abrogate *BCL6* autoregulation (an important negative-regulatory mechanism) are seen even more frequently. It is hypothesized that both types of lesions are inadvertent byproducts of somatic hypermutation that result in overexpression of *BCL6*, which has several important consequences. BCL6 represses the expression of factors that normally serve to promote germinal center B-cell differentiation, growth arrest, and apoptosis, and each of these effects is believed to contribute to the development of DLBCL. Mutations similar to those found in *BCL6* are also seen in multiple other oncogenes, including *MYC*, suggesting that somatic hypermutation in DLBCL cells is "mistargeted" to a wide variety of loci.

Another 10% to 20% of tumors are associated with the t(14;18) (discussed earlier under Follicular Lymphoma), which leads to the overexpression of the antiapoptotic protein BCL2. Tumors with *BCL2* rearrangements usually lack *BCL6* rearrangements, suggesting that these rearrangements define two distinct molecular classes of DLBCL. Some tumors with *BCL2* rearrangements may arise from unrecognized underlying follicular lymphomas, which frequently transform to DLBCL. Roughly 5% of DLBCLs are associated with translocations involving *MYC;* these tumors may have a distinctive biology and are discussed further under Burkitt Lymphoma (later). Finally, deep sequencing of DLBCL genomes has identified frequent mutations in genes encoding histone acetyltransferases such as p300 and CREBP, proteins that regulate gene expression by modifying histones and altering chromatin structure. This association has sparked interest in using drugs that target the epigenome as therapies for DLBCL.

MORPHOLOGY

The common features are a relatively **large cell size** (usually four to five times the diameter of a small lymphocyte) and a **diffuse pattern of growth** (Fig. 13-13). In other respects, substantial morphologic variation is seen. Most commonly, the tumor cells have a round or oval nucleus that appears vesicular due to margination of chromatin to the nuclear membrane, but large multilobated or cleaved nuclei are prominent in some cases. Nucleoli may be two to three in number and located adjacent to the nuclear membrane, or single and centrally placed. The cytoplasm is usually moderately abundant and may be pale or basophilic. More anaplastic tumors may even contain multinucleated cells with large inclusion-like nucleoli that resemble Reed-Sternberg cells (the malignant cell of Hodgkin lymphoma).

Immunophenotype. These mature B-cell tumors express CD19 and CD20 and show variable expression of germinal center B-cell markers such as CD10 and BCL6. Most have surface Ig.

Special Subtypes. Several subtypes of DLBCL are sufficiently distinctive to merit brief discussion.

- *Immunodeficiency-associated large B-cell lymphoma* occurs in the setting of severe T-cell immunodeficiency (e.g., advanced HIV infection and allogeneic bone marrow transplantation). The neoplastic B cells are usually infected with EBV, which plays a critical pathogenic role. Restoration of T-cell immunity may lead to regression of these proliferations.
- *Primary effusion lymphoma* presents as a malignant pleural or ascitic effusion, mostly in patients with advanced HIV infection or older adults. The tumor cells are often anaplastic in appearance and typically fail to express surface B- or T-cell markers, but have clonal IgH gene rearrangements. In all cases the tumor cells are infected with KSHV/HHV-8, which appears to have a causal role.

Clinical Features. DLBCL typically presents as a rapidly enlarging mass at a nodal or extranodal site. It can arise

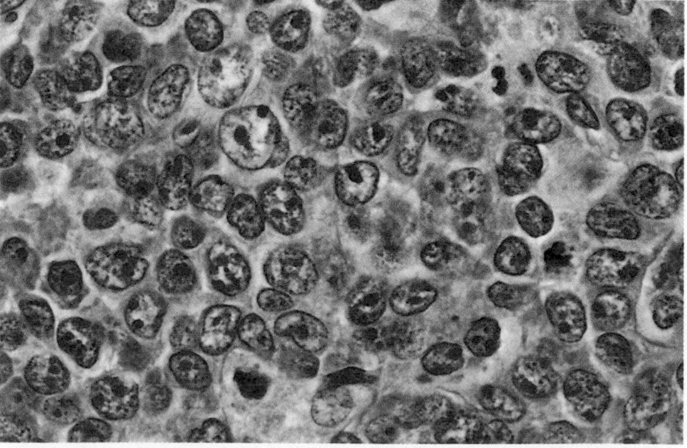

Figure 13-13 Diffuse large B-cell lymphoma. Tumor cells have large nuclei, open chromatin, and prominent nucleoli. (Courtesy Dr. Robert W. McKenna, Department of Pathology, University of Texas Southwestern Medical School, Dallas, Texas.)

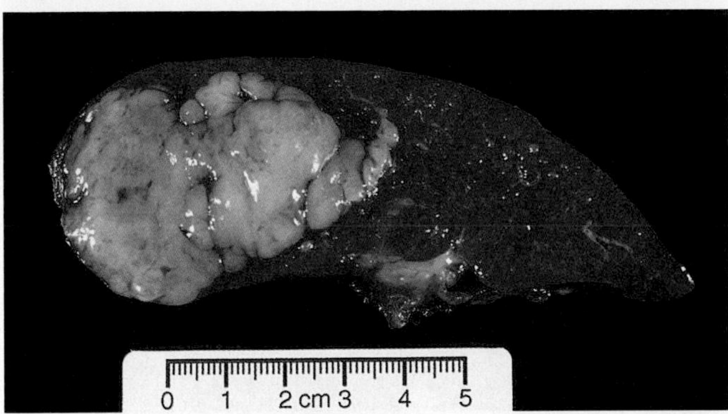

Figure 13-14 Diffuse large B-cell lymphoma involving the spleen. The isolated large mass is typical. In contrast, indolent B-cell lymphomas usually produce multifocal expansion of white pulp (see Fig. 13-11). (Courtesy Dr. Mark Fleming, Department of Pathology, Children's Hospital, Boston, Mass.)

virtually anywhere in the body. Waldeyer ring, the oropharyngeal lymphoid tissue that includes the tonsils and adenoids, is involved commonly. Primary or secondary involvement of the liver and spleen may take the form of large destructive masses (Fig. 13-14). Extranodal sites include the gastrointestinal tract, skin, bone, brain, and other tissues. Bone marrow involvement is relatively uncommon and usually occurs late in the course. Rarely, a leukemic picture emerges.

DLBCLs are aggressive tumors that are rapidly fatal without treatment. With intensive combination chemotherapy, 60% to 80% of patients achieve a complete remission, and 40% to 50% are cured. Adjuvant therapy with anti-CD20 antibody improves both the initial response and the overall outcome. Individuals with limited disease fare better than those with widespread disease or bulky tumor masses. Expression profiling has identified distinct molecular subtypes with differing clinical outcomes and has provided the rationale for new therapies directed at inhibiting the NF-κB and B cell receptor signaling pathways. Of note, about 5% of DLBCLs have *MYC* translocations, and these cases of DLBCL may be difficult to distinguish from Burkitt lymphoma (described later) by conventional diagnostic tests. In fact, recent data suggest that DLBCLs with *MYC* translocations have a worse prognosis than those without and may be better treated with chemotherapy regimens that are now standard for Burkitt lymphoma.

Burkitt Lymphoma

Within the category of Burkitt Lymphoma fall (1) African (endemic) Burkitt lymphoma, (2) sporadic (nonendemic) Burkitt lymphoma, and (3) a subset of aggressive lymphomas occurring in individuals infected with HIV. Burkitt lymphomas occurring in each of these settings are histologically identical but differ in some clinical, genotypic, and virologic characteristics.

Pathogenesis. **All forms of Burkitt lymphoma are highly associated with translocations of the *MYC* gene on chromosome 8 that lead to increased MYC protein levels.** MYC is a master transcriptional regulator that increases the expression of genes that are required for aerobic glycolysis, the so-called Warburg effect (Chapter 7). When nutrients such as glucose and glutamine are available, Warburg metabolism allow cells to biosynthesize all of the building blocks—nucleotides, lipids, proteins—that are needed for growth and cell division. Consequently, Burkitt lymphoma is believed to be the fastest growing human tumor. The translocation partner for *MYC* is usually the IgH locus [t(8;14)] but may also be the Ig κ [t(2;8)] or λ [t(8;22)] light chain loci. The breakpoints in the IgH locus in sporadic Burkitt lymphoma are usually found in the class switch regions, whereas the breakpoints in endemic Burkitt lymphoma tend to lie within more 5′ V(D)J sequences. The basis for this subtle molecular distinction is not known, but both types of translocations can be induced in germinal center B cells by AID, a specialized DNA-modifying enzyme required for both Ig class switching and somatic hypermutation (see earlier). The net effect of these translocations is similar; the *MYC* coding sequence is repositioned adjacent to strong Ig promoter and enhancer elements, which drive increased *MYC* expression. In addition, the translocated *MYC* allele often harbors point mutations that further increase its activity.

Essentially all endemic Burkitt lymphomas are latently infected with EBV, which is also present in about 25% of HIV-associated tumors and 15% to 20% of sporadic cases. The configuration of the EBV DNA is identical in all tumor cells within individual cases, indicating that infection precedes transformation. Although this places EBV at the "scene of the crime," its precise role in the genesis of Burkitt lymphoma remains poorly understood.

MORPHOLOGY

Involved tissues are effaced by a diffuse infiltrate of intermediate-sized lymphoid cells 10 to 25 μm in diameter with round or oval nuclei, coarse chromatin, several nucleoli, and a moderate amount of cytoplasm (Fig. 13-15). **The tumor exhibits a high mitotic index and contains numerous apoptotic cells**, the nuclear remnants of which are phagocytosed by interspersed benign macrophages. These phagocytes have abundant clear cytoplasm, creating a characteristic **"starry sky" pattern**. When the bone marrow is involved, aspirates reveal tumor cells with slightly clumped nuclear chromatin, two to five distinct nucleoli, and **royal blue cytoplasm containing clear cytoplasmic vacuoles**.

Immunophenotype. These are tumors of mature B cells that express surface IgM, CD19, CD20, CD10, and BCL6, a phenotype consistent with a germinal center B-cell origin. Unlike other tumors of germinal center origin, Burkitt lymphoma almost always fails to express the antiapoptotic protein BCL2.

Clinical Features. Both endemic and sporadic Burkitt lymphomas are found mainly in children or young adults; overall, it accounts for about 30% of childhood NHLs in the United States. Most tumors manifest at extranodal sites. Endemic Burkitt lymphoma often presents as a mass involving the mandible and shows an unusual predilection for involvement of abdominal viscera, particularly the kidneys, ovaries, and adrenal glands. In contrast, sporadic Burkitt lymphoma most often appears as a mass involving the ileocecum and peritoneum. Involvement of the bone marrow and peripheral blood is uncommon, especially in endemic cases.

Burkitt lymphoma is very aggressive but responds well to intensive chemotherapy. Most children and young adults can be cured. The outcome is more guarded in older adults.

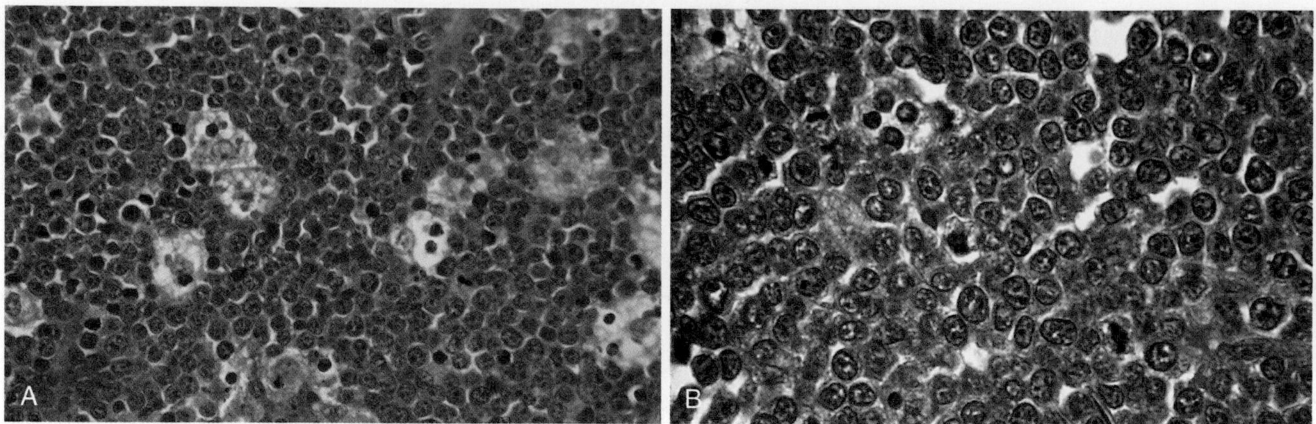

Figure 13-15 Burkitt lymphoma. **A,** At low power, numerous pale tingible body macrophages are evident, producing a "starry sky" appearance. **B,** At high power, tumor cells have multiple small nucleoli and high mitotic index. The lack of significant variation in nuclear shape and size lends a monotonous appearance. (**B,** Courtesy Dr. José Hernandez, Department of Pathology, University of Texas Southwestern Medical School, Dallas, Tex.)

KEY CONCEPTS

Common Forms of Lymphoid Leukemia and Lymphoma

Acute Lymphoblastic Leukemia/Lymphoblastic Lymphoma

- Most common type of cancer in children, may be derived from either precursor B of T cells
- Highly aggressive tumors manifest with signs and symptoms of bone marrow failure, or as rapidly growing masses.
- Tumor cells contain genetic lesions that block differentiation, leading to the accumulation of immature, nonfunctional blasts.

Small Lymphocytic Lymphoma/Chronic Lymphocytic Leukemia

- Most common leukemia of adults
- Tumor of mature B cells that usually manifests with bone marrow and lymph node involvement
- Indolent course, commonly associated with immune abnormalities, including an increased susceptibility to infection and autoimmune disorders

Follicular Lymphoma

- Most common indolent lymphoma of adults
- Tumor cells recapitulate the growth pattern of normal germinal center B cells; most cases are associated with a (14;18) translocation that results in the overexpression of BCL2.

Diffuse Large B-Cell Lymphoma

- Most common lymphoma of adults
- Heterogeneous group of mature B-cell tumors that shares a large cell morphology and aggressive clinical behavior
- Rearrangements or mutations of *BCL6* gene are recognized associations; one third carry a (14;18) translocation involving *BCL2* and may arise from follicular lymphomas.

Burkitt Lymphoma

- Very aggressive tumor of mature B cells that usually arises at extranodal sites.
- Strongly associated with translocations involving the *MYC* proto-oncogene
- Tumor cells often are latently infected by EBV.

Plasma Cell Neoplasms and Related Disorders

These B-cell proliferations contain neoplastic plasma cells that virtually always secrete a monoclonal Ig or Ig fragment, which serve as tumor markers and often have pathologic consequences. Collectively, the plasma cell neoplasms (often referred to as *dyscrasias*) account for about 15% of the deaths caused by lymphoid neoplasms. The most common and deadly of these neoplasms is multiple myeloma, of which there are about 15,000 new cases per year in the United States.

A monoclonal Ig identified in the blood is referred to as an *M component*, in reference to myeloma. Because complete M components have molecular weights of 160,000 or higher, they are restricted to the plasma and extracellular fluid and excluded from the urine in the absence of glomerular damage. However, **neoplastic plasma cells often synthesize excess light chains along with complete Igs**. Occasionally only light chains are produced, and rare tumors secrete only heavy chains. Highly sensitive tests for free light chains in the blood are now available. In patients with plasma cell tumors, the level of free light chains is usually elevated and is markedly skewed toward one light chain (e.g., kappa) at the expense of the second (e.g., lambda). Because free light chains are small in size, they are also excreted in the urine, where they are referred to as *Bence-Jones proteins*.

Terms used to describe the abnormal Igs associated with plasma cell neoplasms include *monoclonal gammopathy, dysproteinemia,* and *paraproteinemia*. These abnormal proteins are associated with the following clinicopathologic entities:

- *Multiple myeloma (plasma cell myeloma)*, the most important plasma cell neoplasm, usually presents as tumorous masses scattered throughout the skeletal system. *Solitary myeloma* (*plasmacytoma*) is an infrequent variant that presents as a single mass in bone or soft tissue. *Smoldering myeloma* refers to another uncommon variant defined by a lack of symptoms and a high plasma M component.
- *Waldenström macroglobulinemia* is a syndrome in which high levels of IgM lead to symptoms related to hyperviscosity of the blood. It occurs in older adults, most commonly in association with lymphoplasmacytic lymphoma (described later).

- *Heavy-chain disease* is a rare monoclonal gammopathy that is seen in association with a diverse group of disorders, including lymphoplasmacytic lymphoma and an unusual small bowel marginal zone lymphoma that occurs in malnourished populations (so-called *Mediterranean lymphoma*). The common feature is the synthesis and secretion of free heavy-chain fragments.
- *Primary or immunocyte-associated amyloidosis* results from a monoclonal proliferation of plasma cells secreting light chains (usually of λ isotype) that are deposited as amyloid. Some patients have overt multiple myeloma, but others have only a minor clonal population of plasma cells in the marrow.
- *Monoclonal gammopathy of undetermined significance (MGUS)* is applied to patients without signs or symptoms who have small to moderately large M components in their blood. MGUS is very common in older adults and has a low but constant rate of transformation to symptomatic monoclonal gammopathies, most often multiple myeloma.

With this background, we now turn to some of the specific clinicopathologic entities. Primary amyloidosis was discussed along with other disorders of the immune system in Chapter 6.

Multiple Myeloma. **Multiple myeloma is a plasma cell neoplasm commonly associated with lytic bone lesions, hypercalcemia, renal failure, and acquired immune abnormalities.** Although bony disease dominates, it can spread late in its course to lymph nodes and extranodal sites. Multiple myeloma causes 1% of all cancer deaths in Western countries. Its incidence is higher in men and people of African descent. It is chiefly a disease of older adults, with a peak age of incidence of 65 to 70 years.

Pathogenesis. Multiple myeloma is associated with frequent rearrangements involving the IgH locus and various proto-oncogenes. Included among the loci that are recurrently involved in translocations with the Ig heavy-chain gene on chromosome 14q32 are the cell cycle-regulatory genes cyclin D1 on chromosome 11q13 and cyclin D3 on chromosome 6p21. Deletions of chromosome 17p that involve the *TP53* tumor suppressor locus also occur and are associated with a poor outcome. Late-stage, highly aggressive forms of the disease such as plasma cell leukemia are associated with acquisition of rearrangements involving *MYC*. More recent deep sequencing of myeloma genomes has identified frequent mutations involving components of the NF-κB pathway, which supports B-cell survival. Based on these studies, it is evident that myeloma molecularly heterogeneous.

The proliferation and survival of myeloma cells are dependent on several cytokines, most notably IL-6. IL-6 is an important growth factor for plasma cells. It is produced by the tumor cells themselves and by resident marrow stromal cells. High serum levels of IL-6 are seen in patients with active disease and are associated with a poor prognosis. Myeloma cell growth and survival are also augmented by direct physical interactions with bone marrow stromal cells, which is a focus of new therapeutic approaches.

Factors produced by neoplastic plasma cells mediate bone destruction, the major pathologic feature of multiple myeloma. Of particular importance, myeloma-derived MIP1α up-regulates the expression of the receptor activator of NF-κB ligand (RANKL) by bone marrow stromal cells, which in turn activates osteoclasts. Other factors released from tumor cells, such as modulators of the Wnt pathway, are potent inhibitors of osteoblast function. The net effect is a marked increase in bone resorption, which leads to hypercalcemia and pathologic fractures.

MORPHOLOGY

Multiple myeloma usually presents as destructive plasma cell tumors (plasmacytomas) involving the axial skeleton. The bones most commonly affected (in descending order of frequency) are the vertebral column, ribs, skull, pelvis, femur, clavicle, and scapula. Lesions begin in the medullary cavity, erode cancellous bone, and progressively destroy the bony cortex, often leading to pathologic fractures; these are most common in the vertebral column, but may occur in any affected bone. **The bone lesions appear radiographically as punched-out defects, usually 1 to 4 cm in diameter** (Fig. 13-16), and consist of soft, gelatinous, red tumor masses. Less commonly, widespread myelomatous bone disease produces diffuse demineralization (osteopenia) rather than focal defects.

Even away from overt tumor masses, the marrow contains an increased number of plasma cells, which usually constitute more than 30% of the cellularity. The plasma cells may infiltrate the interstitium or be present in sheets that completely replace normal elements. Like their benign counterparts, malignant plasma cells have a perinuclear clearing due to a prominent Golgi apparatus and an eccentrically placed nucleus (Fig. 13-17). Relatively normal-appearing plasma cells, **plasmablasts** with vesicular nuclear chromatin and a prominent single nucleolus, or **bizarre, multinucleated cells** may predominate. Other cytologic variants stem from the dysregulated synthesis and secretion of Ig, which often leads to intracellular accumulation of intact or partially degraded protein. Such variants include **flame cells** with fiery red cytoplasm, **Mott cells** with multiple grapelike cytoplasmic droplets, and cells containing a variety of other inclusions, including **fibrils, crystalline rods, and globules**. The globular inclusions are referred to as **Russell bodies** (if cytoplasmic) or **Dutcher bodies** (if nuclear). In advanced disease, plasma cell infiltrates may be present in the spleen, liver, kidneys, lungs, lymph nodes, and other soft tissues.

Commonly, the high level of M proteins causes red cells in peripheral blood smears to stick to one another in linear arrays, a finding referred to as **rouleaux formation**. Rouleaux formation is characteristic but not specific, as it may be seen in other conditions in which Ig levels are elevated, such as lupus erythematosus and early HIV infection. Rarely, tumor cells flood the peripheral blood, giving rise to **plasma cell leukemia**.

Bence Jones proteins are excreted in the kidney and contribute to a form of renal disease called **myeloma kidney**. This important complication is discussed in detail in Chapter 20.

Immunophenotype. Plasma cell tumors are positive for CD138, an adhesion molecule also known as syndecan-1, and often express CD56, a feature that can be helpful in identifying small populations of neoplastic cells.

Clinical Features. The clinical features of multiple myeloma stem from (1) the effects of plasma cell growth in

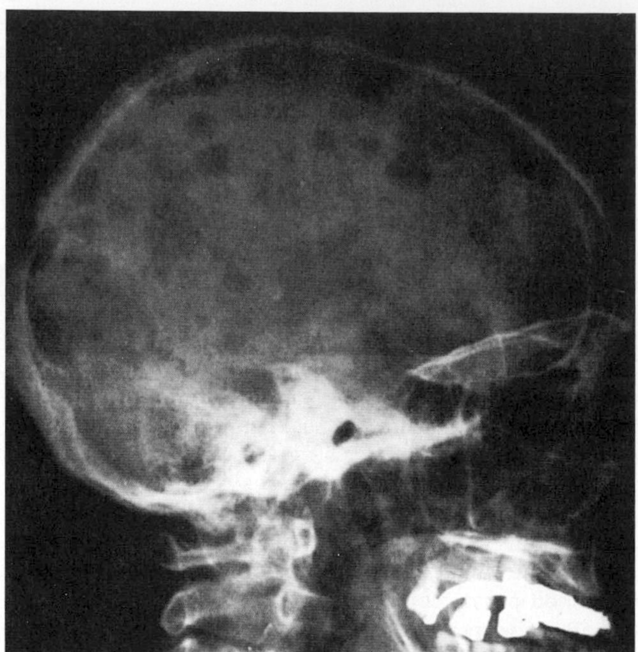

Figure 13-16 Multiple myeloma of the skull (radiograph, lateral view). The sharply punched-out bone lesions are most obvious in the calvarium.

tissues, particularly the bones; (2) the production of excessive Igs, which often have abnormal physicochemical properties; and (3) the suppression of normal humoral immunity.

Bone resorption often leads to *pathologic fractures* and *chronic pain*. The attendant *hypercalcemia* can give rise to neurologic manifestations, such as confusion, weakness, lethargy, constipation, and polyuria, and contributes to renal dysfunction. Decreased production of normal Igs sets the stage for *recurrent bacterial infections*. Cellular immunity is relatively unaffected. Of great significance is *renal insufficiency*, which trails only infections as a cause of death. The pathogenesis of renal failure (Chapter 20), which occurs in up to 50% of patients, is multifactorial. However, the single most important factor seems to be *Bence-Jones proteinuria*, as the excreted light chains are toxic to renal tubular epithelial cells. Certain light chains (particularly those of the λ6 and λ3 families) are prone to cause *amyloidosis* of the AL type (Chapter 6), which can exacerbate renal dysfunction and deposit in other tissues as well.

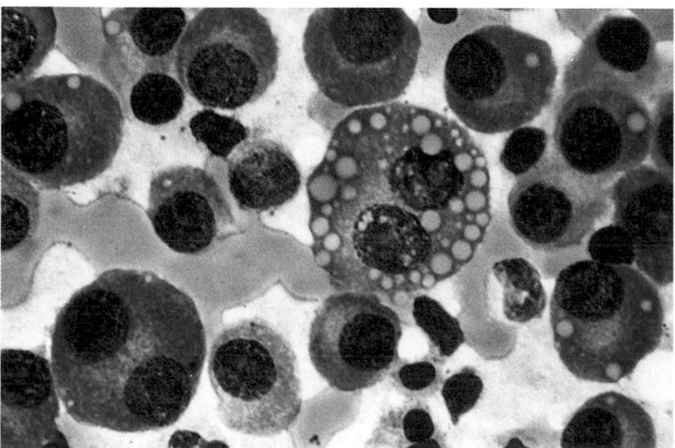

Figure 13-17 Multiple myeloma (bone marrow aspirate). Normal marrow cells are largely replaced by plasma cells, including forms with multiple nuclei, prominent nucleoli, and cytoplasmic droplets containing Ig.

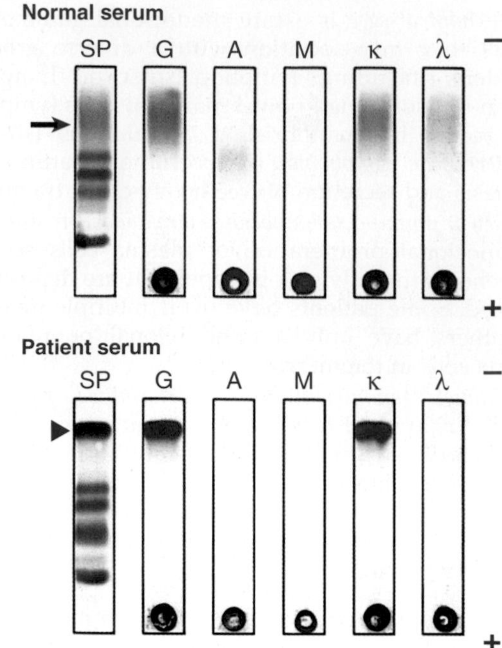

Figure 13-18 M protein detection in multiple myeloma. Serum protein electrophoresis (SP) is used to screen for a monoclonal immunoglobulin (M protein). Polyclonal IgG in normal serum (*arrow*) appears as a broad band; in contrast, serum from a patient with multiple myeloma contains a single sharp protein band (*arrowhead*) in this region of the electropherogram. The suspected monoclonal Ig is confirmed and characterized by immunofixation. In this procedure, proteins separated by electrophoresis within a gel are reacted with specific antisera. After extensive washing, proteins that are cross-linked by antisera are retained and detected with a protein stain. Note the sharp band in the patient serum is cross-linked by antisera specific for IgG heavy chain (G) and kappa light chain (κ), indicating the presence of an IgGκ M protein. Levels of polyclonal IgG, IgA (A), and lambda light chain (λ) are also decreased in the patient serum relative to normal, a finding typical of multiple myeloma. (Courtesy Dr. David Sacks, Department of Pathology, Brigham and Women's Hospital, Boston, Mass.)

In 99% of patients, laboratory analyses reveal increased levels of Igs in the blood and/or light chains (Bence-Jones proteins) in the urine. The monoclonal Igs are usually first detected as abnormal protein "spikes" in serum or urine electrophoresis and then further characterized by immunofixation (Fig. 13-18). Most myelomas are associated with more than 3 gm/dL of serum Ig and/or more than 6 mg/dL of urine Bence-Jones protein. The most common monoclonal Ig ("M protein") is IgG (approximately 55% of patients), followed by IgA (approximately 25% of cases). Myelomas expressing IgM, IgD, or IgE occur but are rare. Excessive production and aggregation of M proteins, usually of the IgA and or IgG_3 subtype, leads to symptoms related to hyperviscosity (described under lymphoplasmacytic lymphoma) in about 7% of patients. Both free light chains and a serum M protein are observed together in 60% to 70% of patients. However, in about 20% of patients only free light chains are present. Around 1% of myelomas are nonsecretory; hence, the absence of detectable M proteins does not completely exclude the diagnosis.

The clinicopathologic diagnosis of multiple myeloma rests on radiographic and laboratory findings. It can be strongly suspected when the distinctive radiographic changes are present, but definitive diagnosis requires a bone marrow examination. Marrow involvement often gives rise to a normocytic normochromic anemia, sometimes accompanied by moderate leukopenia and thrombocytopenia.

The prognosis is variable, but has improved in recent years with new therapeutic approaches. The median survival is 4 to 7 years, and cures have yet to be achieved. Patients with multiple bony lesions, if untreated, rarely survive for more than 6 to 12 months, whereas patients with "smoldering myeloma" may be asymptomatic for many years. Translocations involving cyclin D1 are associated with a good outcome, whereas deletions of 13q, deletions of 17p, and the t(4;14) all portend a more aggressive course.

New therapies are bringing hope. Myeloma cells are sensitive to inhibitors of the proteasome, a cellular organelle that degrades unwanted and misfolded proteins. As discussed in Chapter 2, misfolded proteins activate apoptotic pathways. Myeloma cells are prone to the accumulation of misfolded, unpaired Ig chains. Proteasome inhibitors may induce cell death by exacerbating this inherent tendency, and also seem to retard bone resorption through effects on stromal cells. Thalidomide and related compounds such as lenalidomide also have activity against myeloma. Interestingly, this may also involve changes in protein degradation, as lenalidamide appears to activate ubiquitin ligases, thereby targeting proteins for proteolysis that are required for myeloma growth. Biphosphonates, drugs that inhibit bone resorption, reduce pathologic fractures and limit the hypercalcemia. Hematopoietic stem cell transplantation prolongs life but has not yet proven to be curative.

Solitary Myeloma (Plasmacytoma). About 3% to 5% of plasma cell neoplasms present as a solitary lesion of bone or soft tissue. The bone lesions tend to occur in the same locations as in multiple myeloma. Extraosseous lesions are often located in the lungs, oronasopharynx, or nasal sinuses. Modest elevations of M proteins in the blood or urine may be found in some patients. Solitary osseous plasmacytoma almost inevitably progresses to multiple myeloma, but this can take 10 to 20 years or longer. In contrast, extraosseous plasmacytomas, particularly those involving the upper respiratory tract, are frequently cured by local resection.

Smoldering Myeloma. This entity defines a middle ground between multiple myeloma and monoclonal gammopathy of uncertain significance. Plasma cells make up 10% to 30% of the marrow cellularity, and the serum M protein level is greater than 3 gm/dL, but patients are asymptomatic. About 75% of patients progress to multiple myeloma over a 15-year period.

Monoclonal Gammopathy of Uncertain Significance. MGUS is the most common plasma cell dyscrasia, occurring in about 3% of persons older than 50 years of age and in about 5% of individuals older than 70 years of age. By definition, patients are asymptomatic and the serum M protein level is less than 3 gm/dL. **Approximately 1% of patients with MGUS develop a symptomatic plasma cell neoplasm, usually multiple myeloma, per year**, a rate of conversion that remains roughly constant over time. The clonal plasma cells in MGUS contain many of the same chromosomal translocations and deletions that are found in full-blown multiple myeloma, indicating that MGUS is an early stage of myeloma development. As in patients with smoldering myeloma, progression to multiple myeloma is unpredictable; hence, periodic assessment of serum M component levels and Bence Jones proteinuria is warranted.

Lymphoplasmacytic Lymphoma. Lymphoplasmacytic lymphoma is a B-cell neoplasm of older adults that usually presents in the sixth or seventh decade of life. Although bearing a superficial resemblance to CLL/SLL, it differs in that a substantial fraction of the tumor cells undergo terminal differentiation to plasma cells. Most commonly, the plasma cell component secretes monoclonal IgM, often in amounts sufficient to cause a hyperviscosity syndrome known as *Waldenström macroglobulinemia*. Unlike multiple myeloma, complications stemming from the secretion of free light chains (e.g., renal failure and amyloidosis) are relatively rare and bone destruction does not occur.

Pathogenesis. Recent deep sequencing studies have shown that virtually all cases of lymphoplasmacytic lymphoma are associated with acquired mutations in *MYD88*. The *MYD88* gene encodes an adaptor protein that participates in signaling events that activate NF-κB and also augment signals downstream of the B-cell receptor (Ig) complex, both of which may promote the growth and survival of the tumor cells.

MORPHOLOGY

Typically, the marrow contains an infiltrate of lymphocytes, plasma cells, and plasmacytoid lymphocytes in varying proportions, often accompanied by mast cell hyperplasia (Fig. 13-19). Some tumors also contain a population of larger lymphoid cells with more vesicular nuclear chromatin and prominent nucleoli. Periodic acid-Schiff-positive inclusions containing Ig are frequently seen in the cytoplasm (**Russell bodies**) or the nucleus (**Dutcher bodies**) of some of the plasma cells. At diagnosis the tumor has usually disseminated to the lymph nodes, spleen, and liver. Infiltration of the nerve roots, meninges, and more rarely the brain can also occur with disease progression.

Immunophenotype. The lymphoid component expresses B-cell markers such as CD20 and surface Ig, whereas the plasma cell component secretes the same Ig that is expressed on the surface of the lymphoid cells. This is usually IgM but can also be IgG or IgA.

Clinical Features. The dominant presenting complaints are nonspecific and include weakness, fatigue, and weight loss. Approximately half the patients have *lymphadenopathy, hepatomegaly, and splenomegaly.* Anemia caused by marrow infiltration is common. About 10% of patients have *autoimmune hemolysis* caused by *cold agglutinins*, IgM antibodies that bind to red cells at temperatures of less than 37°C (Chapter 14).

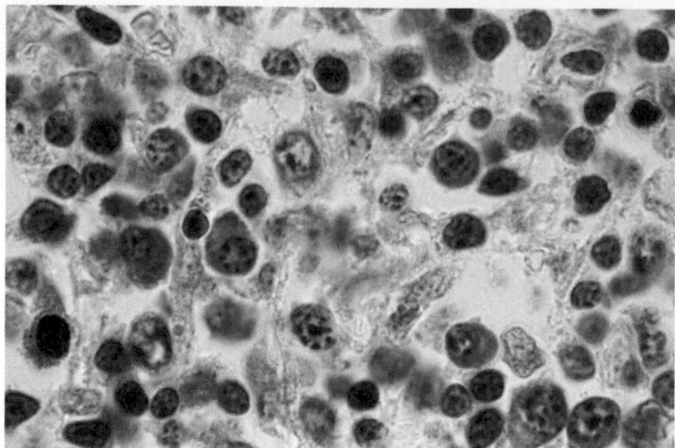

Figure 13-19 Lymphoplasmacytic lymphoma. Bone marrow biopsy shows a characteristic mixture of small lymphoid cells exhibiting various degrees of plasma cell differentiation. In addition, a mast cell with purplish red cytoplasmic granules is present at the left-hand side of the field.

Patients with IgM-secreting tumors have additional signs and symptoms stemming from the physicochemical properties of IgM. Because of its large size, at high concentrations IgM greatly increases the viscosity of the blood, giving rise to a *hyperviscosity syndrome* characterized by the following:

- *Visual impairment* associated with venous congestion, which is reflected by striking tortuosity and distention of retinal veins; retinal hemorrhages and exudates can also contribute to the visual problems
- *Neurologic problems* such as headaches, dizziness, deafness, and stupor, all stemming from sluggish blood flow and sludging
- *Bleeding* related to the formation of complexes between macroglobulins and clotting factors as well as interference with platelet functions
- *Cryoglobulinemia* resulting from the precipitation of macroglobulins at low temperatures, which produces symptoms such as Raynaud phenomenon and cold urticaria

Lymphoplasmacytic lymphoma is an incurable progressive disease. Because most IgM is intravascular, symptoms caused by the high IgM levels (e.g., hyperviscosity and hemolysis) can be alleviated by plasmapheresis. Tumor growth can be controlled for a time with low doses of chemotherapeutic drugs and immunotherapy with anti-CD20 antibody. Transformation to large-cell lymphoma occurs but is uncommon. Median survival is about 4 years.

KEY CONCEPTS

Plasma Cell Neoplasms

Multiple Myeloma

- Plasma cell tumor that manifests with multiple lytic bone lesions associated with pathologic fractures and hypercalcemia
- Neoplastic plasma cells suppress normal humoral immunity and secrete partial immunoglobulins that are nephrotoxic
- Associated with diverse translocations involving the IgH locus; frequent dysregulation and overexpression of D cyclins
- May be associated with AL amyloidosis (as may other neoplasms later)

Other Plasma Cell Neoplasms

- MGUS (monoclonal gammopathy of unknown significance): common in older adults, progresses to myeloma at a rate of 1% per year
- Smoldering myeloma: disseminated disease that pursues an unusually indolent course
- Solitary osseous plasmacytoma: solitary bone lesion identical to disseminated myeloma; most progress to myeloma within 7 to 10 years
- Extramedullary plasmacytoma: solitary mass, usually in the upper aerodigestive tract; rarely progresses to systemic disease
- Lymphoplasmacytic lymphoma: B cell lymphoma that exhibits plasmacytic differentiation; clinical symptoms dominated by hyperviscosity related to high levels of tumor-derived IgM; highly associated with mutations in the *MYD88* gene

Mantle Cell Lymphoma

Mantle cell lymphoma is an uncommon lymphoid neoplasm that makes up about 2.5% of NHL in the United States and 7% to 9% of NHL in Europe. It usually presents in the fifth to sixth decades of life and shows a male predominance. As the name implies, the tumor cells closely resemble the normal mantle zone B cells that surround germinal centers.

Pathogenesis. **Virtually all mantle cell lymphomas have an (11;14) translocation involving the IgH locus on chromosome 14 and the cyclin D1 locus on chromosome 11 that leads to overexpression of cyclin D1.** This translocation is detected in about 70% of cases by standard karyotyping and in virtually all tumors by fluorescence in situ hybridization. The resulting up-regulation of cyclin D1 promotes G1- to S-phase progression during the cell cycle, as was described in Chapter 7.

MORPHOLOGY

At diagnosis the majority of patients have generalized lymphadenopathy, and 20% to 40% have peripheral blood involvement. Frequent sites of extranodal involvement include the bone marrow, spleen, liver, and gut. Occasionally, mucosal involvement of the small bowel or colon produces polyp-like lesions (lymphomatoid polyposis); of all forms of NHL, mantle cell lymphoma is most likely to spread in this fashion.

Nodal tumor cells may surround reactive germinal centers to produce a nodular appearance at low power, or diffusely efface the node. **Typically, the proliferation consists of a homogeneous population of small lymphocytes with irregular to occasionally deeply clefted (cleaved) nuclear contours** (Fig. 13-20). Large cells resembling centroblasts and proliferation centers are absent, distinguishing mantle cell lymphoma from follicular lymphoma and CLL/SLL, respectively. In most cases the nuclear chromatin is condensed, nucleoli are inconspicuous, and the cytoplasm is scant. Occasionally, tumors composed of intermediate-sized cells with more open chromatin and a brisk mitotic rate are observed; immunophenotyping is necessary to distinguish these "blastoid" variants from ALL.

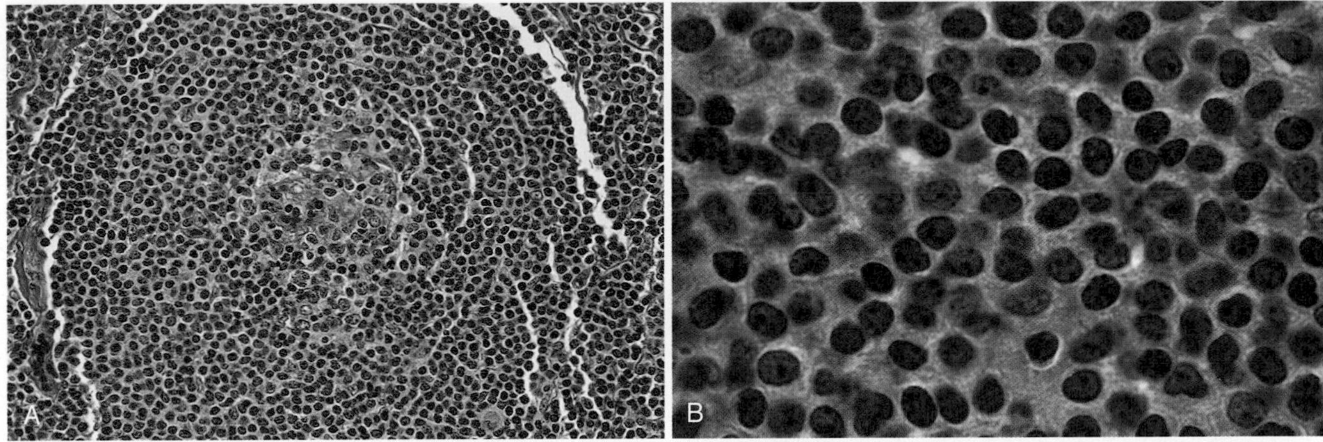

Figure 13-20 Mantle cell lymphoma. **A,** At low power, neoplastic lymphoid cells surround a small, atrophic germinal center, producing a mantle zone pattern of growth. **B,** High-power view shows a homogeneous population of small lymphoid cells with somewhat irregular nuclear outlines, condensed chromatin, and scant cytoplasm. Large cells resembling prolymphocytes (seen in chronic lymphocytic leukemia) and centroblasts (seen in follicular lymphoma) are absent.

Immunophenotype. Mantle cell lymphomas express high levels of cyclin D1. Most tumors are also express CD19, CD20, and moderately high levels of surface Ig (usually IgM and IgD with κ or λ light chain). It is usually CD5+ and CD23–, which help to distinguish it from CLL/SLL. The IgH genes lack somatic hypermutation, supporting an origin from a naive B cell.

Clinical Features. The most common presentation is painless lymphadenopathy. Symptoms related to involvement of the spleen (present in ~50% of cases) and gut are also common. The prognosis is poor; the median survival is only 3 to 4 years. This lymphoma is not curable with conventional chemotherapy, and most patients eventually succumb to organ dysfunction caused by tumor infiltration. The blastoid variant and a "proliferative" expression profiling signature are associated with even shorter survivals. Hematopoietic stem cell transplantation and proteasome inhibitors are newer therapeutic approaches that show some promise.

Marginal Zone Lymphomas

The category of marginal zone lymphoma encompasses a heterogeneous group of B-cell tumors that arise within lymph nodes, spleen, or extranodal tissues. The extranodal tumors were initially recognized at mucosal sites and are often referred to as mucosa-associated lymphoid tumors (or "MALTomas"). In most cases, the tumor cells show evidence of somatic hypermutation and are considered to be of memory B-cell origin.

Although all marginal zone lymphomas share certain features, those occurring at extranodal sites deserve special attention because of their unusual pathogenesis and three exceptional characteristics.

- They often arise within tissues involved by chronic inflammatory disorders of autoimmune or infectious etiology; examples include the salivary gland in Sjögren disease, the thyroid gland in Hashimoto thyroiditis, and the stomach in *Helicobacter* gastritis.
- They remain localized for prolonged periods, spreading systemically only late in their course.
- They may regress if the inciting agent (e.g., *Helicobacter pylori)* is eradicated.

These characteristics suggest that **extranodal marginal zone lymphomas arising in chronically inflamed tissues lie on a continuum between reactive lymphoid hyperplasia and full-blown lymphoma.** The disease begins as a polyclonal immune reaction. With the acquisition of still-unknown initiating mutations, a B-cell clone emerges that still depends on antigen-stimulated T-helper cells for signals that drive growth and survival. At this stage, withdrawal of the responsible antigen causes tumor involution. A clinically relevant example is found in gastric "MALToma," in which antibiotic therapy directed against *H. pylori* often leads to tumor regression (Chapter 17). With time, however, tumors may acquire additional mutations that render their growth and survival antigen-independent, such as the (11;18), (14;18), or (1;14) chromosomal translocations, which are relatively specific for extranodal marginal zone lymphomas. All of these translocations up-regulate the expression and function of BCL10 or MALT1, protein components of a signaling complex that activates NF-κB and promotes the growth and survival of B cells. With further clonal evolution, spread to distant sites and transformation to diffuse large B-cell lymphoma may occur. This theme of polyclonal to monoclonal transition during lymphomagenesis is also applicable to the pathogenesis of EBV-induced lymphoma and is discussed more fully in Chapter 7.

Hairy Cell Leukemia

This rare but distinctive B-cell neoplasm constitutes about 2% of all leukemias. It is predominantly a disease of middle-aged white males, with a median age of 55 and a male-to-female ratio of 5:1.

Pathogenesis. **Hairy cell leukemias are associated in more than 90% of cases with activating point mutations in the serine/threonine kinase BRAF,** which is positioned immediately downstream of RAS in the MAPK signaling cascade (Chapter 7). The specific mutation, a valine to glutamate substitution at residue 600, is also found in diverse other neoplasms, including many melanomas and Langerhans cell histiocytosis (discussed later).

MORPHOLOGY

Hairy cell leukemia derives its picturesque name from the appearance of the leukemic cells, which have **fine hairlike projections** that are best recognized under the phase-contrast microscope (Fig. 13-21). On routine peripheral blood smears, hairy cells have round, oblong, or reniform nuclei and moderate amounts of pale blue cytoplasm with threadlike or bleblike extensions. The number of circulating cells is highly variable. The marrow is involved by a diffuse interstitial infiltrate of cells with oblong or reniform nuclei, condensed chromatin, and pale cytoplasm. Because these cells are enmeshed in an extracellular matrix composed of reticulin fibrils, they usually cannot be aspirated (a clinical difficulty referred to as a "dry tap") and are only seen in marrow biopsies. The splenic red pulp is usually heavily infiltrated, leading to obliteration of white pulp and a beefy red gross appearance. Hepatic portal triads are also involved frequently.

Immunophenotype. Hairy cell leukemias typically express the pan-B-cell markers CD19 and CD20, surface Ig (usually IgG), and certain relatively distinctive markers, such as CD11c, CD25, CD103, and annexin A1.

Clinical Features. Clinical manifestations result largely from infiltration of the bone marrow, liver, and spleen. *Splenomegaly*, often massive, is the most common and sometimes the only abnormal physical finding. *Hepatomegaly* is less common and not as marked; lymphadenopathy is rare. *Pancytopenia* resulting from marrow involvement and splenic sequestration is seen in more than half the cases. About one third of those affected present with *infections*. There is an increased incidence of atypical mycobacterial infections, possibly related to frequent unexplained monocytopenia.

Hairy cell leukemia follows an indolent course. For unclear reasons, this tumor is exceptionally sensitive to "gentle" chemotherapeutic regimens, which produce long-lasting remissions. Tumors often relapse after 5 or more years, yet generally respond well when retreated with the same agents, a feature that is highly unusual among human cancers. BRAF inhibitors appear to produce excellent responses in tumors that have failed conventional chemotherapy. The overall prognosis is excellent.

Peripheral T-Cell and NK-Cell Neoplasms

These categories include a heterogeneous group of neoplasms having phenotypes resembling mature T cells or NK cells. Peripheral T-cell tumors make up about 5% to 10% of NHLs in the United States and Europe, while NK cell tumors are rare. By contrast, for unknown reasons both T cell and NK cell tumors are relatively more common in the Far East. Only the most common diagnoses and those of particular pathogenetic interest will be discussed.

Peripheral T-Cell Lymphoma, Unspecified

Although the WHO classification includes a number of distinct peripheral T-cell neoplasms, many of these lymphomas are not easily categorized and are lumped into a "wastebasket" diagnosis, *peripheral T-cell lymphoma, unspecified*. As might be expected, no morphologic feature is pathognomonic, but certain findings are characteristic. These tumors efface lymph nodes diffusely and are typically composed of a pleomorphic mixture of variably sized malignant T cells (Fig. 13-22). There is often a prominent infiltrate of reactive cells, such as eosinophils and macrophages, probably attracted by tumor-derived cytokines. Brisk neoangiogenesis may also be seen.

By definition, all peripheral T-cell lymphomas are derived from mature T cells. They usually express CD2, CD3, CD5, and either αβ or γδ T-cell receptors. Some also express CD4 or CD8; such tumors are taken to be of helper or cytotoxic T-cell origin, respectively. However, many tumors have phenotypes that do not resemble any known normal T cell. In difficult cases where the differential diagnosis lies between lymphoma and a florid reactive process, DNA analysis is used to confirm the presence of clonal T-cell receptor rearrangements.

Most patients present with generalized lymphadenopathy, sometimes accompanied by eosinophilia, pruritus, fever, and weight loss. Although cures of peripheral T-cell lymphoma have been reported, these tumors have a significantly worse prognosis than comparably aggressive mature B-cell neoplasms (e.g., diffuse large B-cell lymphoma).

Anaplastic Large-Cell Lymphoma (ALK Positive)

This uncommon entity is defined by the presence of rearrangements in the *ALK* gene on chromosome 2p23. These

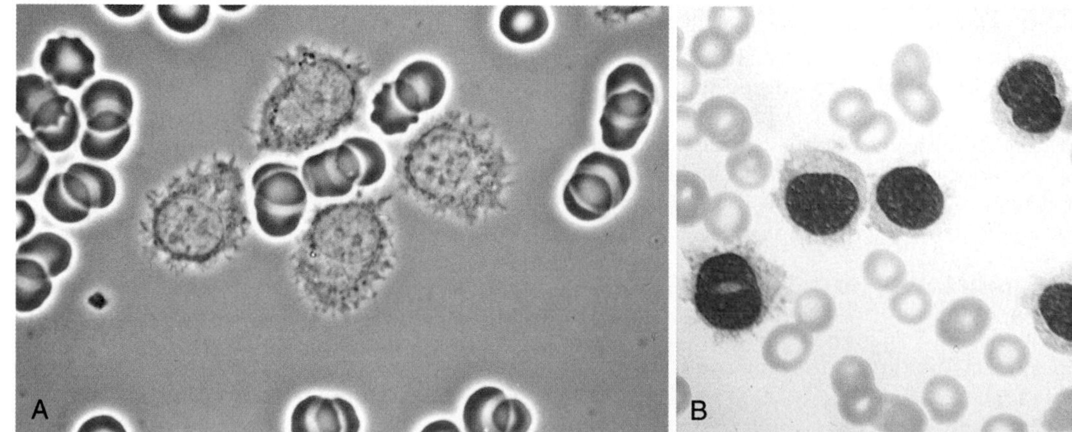

Figure 13-21 Hairy cell leukemia (peripheral blood smear). **A,** Phase-contrast microscopy shows tumor cells with fine hairlike cytoplasmic projections. **B,** In stained smears, these cells have round or folded nuclei and modest amounts of pale blue, agranular cytoplasm.

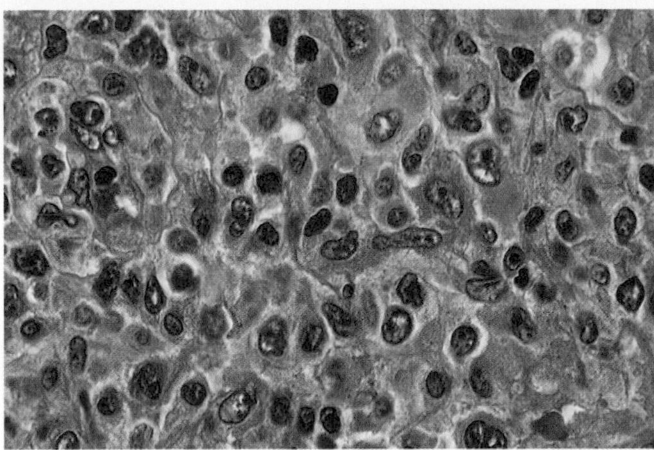

Figure 13-22 Peripheral T cell lymphoma, unspecified (lymph node). A spectrum of small, intermediate, and large lymphoid cells, many with irregular nuclear contours, is visible.

rearrangements break the *ALK* locus and lead to the formation of chimeric genes encoding ALK fusion proteins, constitutively active tyrosine kinases that trigger the RAS and JAK/STAT signaling pathways.

As the name implies, this tumor is typically composed of large anaplastic cells, some containing horseshoe-shaped nuclei and voluminous cytoplasm (so-called *hallmark cells*) (Fig. 13-23*A*). The tumor cells often cluster about venules and infiltrate lymphoid sinuses, mimicking the appearance of metastatic carcinoma. ALK is not expressed in normal lymphocytes; thus, the detection of ALK protein in tumor cells (Fig. 13-23*B*) is a reliable indicator of an *ALK* gene rearrangement.

T-cell lymphomas with *ALK* rearrangements tend to occur in children or young adults, frequently involve soft tissues, and carry a very good prognosis (unlike other aggressive peripheral T-cell neoplasms). The cure rate with chemotherapy is 75% to 80%. Inhibitors of ALK have been developed and are being evaluated as a form of selective, targeted therapy. Morphologically similar tumors lacking *ALK* rearrangements occur in older adults and have a substantially worse prognosis. Both the ALK+ and ALK- tumors usually express CD30, a member of the TNF receptor family; of note, recombinant antibodies that bind and kill CD30-expressing cells have produced promising responses in patients with anaplastic large cell lymphoma and Hodgkin lymphoma, another CD30+ tumor (described later).

Adult T-Cell Leukemia/Lymphoma

This neoplasm of CD4+ T cells is only observed in adults infected by human T-cell leukemia retrovirus type 1 (HTLV-1), which was discussed in Chapter 7. It occurs mainly in regions where HTLV-1 is endemic, namely southern Japan, West Africa, and the Caribbean basin. Common findings include skin lesions, generalized lymphadenopathy, hepatosplenomegaly, peripheral blood lymphocytosis, and hypercalcemia. The appearance of the tumor cells varies, but cells with multilobated nuclei ("cloverleaf" or "flower" cells) are frequently observed. The tumor cells contain clonal HTLV-1 provirus, which is believed to play a critical pathogenic role. Notably, HTLV-1 encodes a protein called Tax that is a potent activator of NF-κB, which, as previously discussed, enhances lymphocyte growth and survival.

Most patients present with rapidly progressive disease that is fatal within months to 1 year despite aggressive chemotherapy. Less commonly, the tumor involves only the skin and follows a much more indolent course, like that of mycosis fungoides (described below). It should be noted that in addition to adult T-cell leukemia/lymphoma, HTLV-1 infection sometimes gives rise to a progressive demyelinating disease of the central nervous system and spinal cord (Chapter 28).

Mycosis Fungoides/Sézary Syndrome

Mycosis fungoides and Sézary syndrome are different manifestations of a tumor of CD4+ helper T cells that home to the skin. Clinically, the cutaneous lesions of *mycosis fungoides* typically progress through three somewhat distinct stages, an inflammatory *premycotic phase*, a *plaque phase*, and a *tumor phase* (Chapter 25). Histologically,

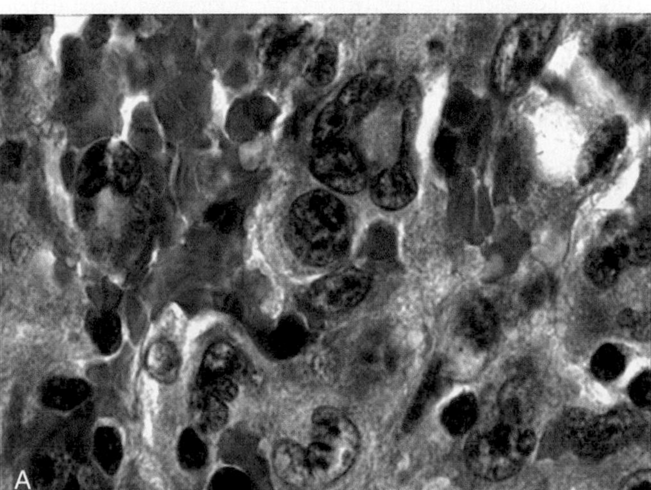

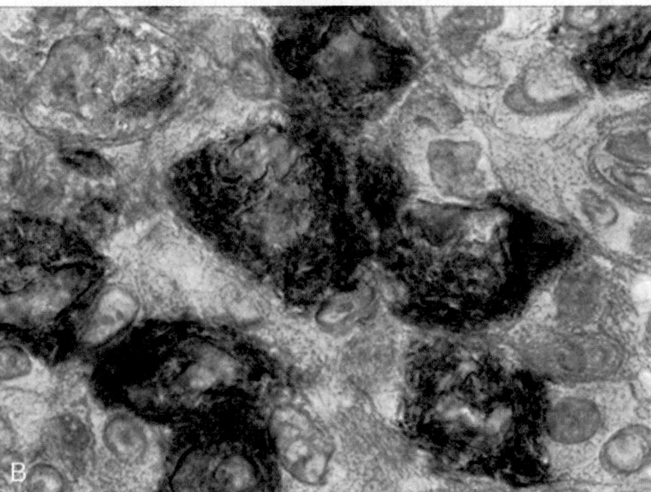

Figure 13-23 Anaplastic large-cell lymphoma. **A,** Several "hallmark" cells with horseshoe-like or "embryoid" nuclei and abundant cytoplasm lie near the center of the field. **B,** Immunohistochemical stain demonstrating the presence of ALK fusion protein. (Courtesy Dr. Jeffrey Kutok, Department of Pathology, Brigham and Women's Hospital, Boston, Mass.)

the epidermis and upper dermis are infiltrated by neoplastic T cells, which often have a cerebriform appearance due to marked infolding of the nuclear membrane. Late disease progression is characterized by extracutaneous spread, most commonly to lymph nodes and bone marrow.

Sézary syndrome is a variant in which skin involvement is manifested as a *generalized exfoliative erythroderma*. In contrast to mycosis fungoides, the skin lesions rarely proceed to tumefaction, and there is an associated leukemia of "Sézary" cells with characteristic cerebriform nuclei.

The tumor cells express the adhesion molecule cutaneous leukocyte antigen (CLA) and the chemokine receptors CCR4 and CCR10, all of which contribute to the homing of normal CD4+ T cells to the skin. Although cutaneous disease dominates the clinical picture, sensitive molecular analyses have shown that the tumor cells circulate through the blood, marrow, and lymph nodes even early in the course. Nevertheless, these are indolent tumors, with a median survival of 8 to 9 years. Transformation to aggressive T-cell lymphoma occurs occasionally as a terminal event.

Large Granular Lymphocytic Leukemia

T-cell and NK-cell variants of this rare neoplasm are recognized, both of which occur mainly in adults. Individuals with T-cell disease usually present with mild to moderate lymphocytosis and splenomegaly. Lymphadenopathy and hepatomegaly are usually absent. NK-cell disease often presents in an even more subtle fashion, with little or no lymphocytosis or splenomegaly.

Recent work has shown that 30% to 40% of large granular lymphocytic leukemias have acquired mutations in the transcription factor STAT3, which functions downstream of cytokine receptors. These mutations occur in both T-cell and NK-cell forms of the disease and appear to result in cytokine-independent activation of STAT3, which is now postulated to have a major role in the pathogenesis of these heretofore mysterious proliferations.

The tumor cells are large lymphocytes with abundant blue cytoplasm and a few coarse azurophilic granules, best seen in peripheral blood smears. The marrow usually contains sparse interstitial lymphocytic infiltrates, which can be difficult to appreciate without immunohistochemical stains. Infiltrates are also usually present in the spleen and liver. As might be expected, T-cell variants are CD3+, whereas NK-cell large granular lymphocytic leukemias are CD3–, CD56+.

Despite the relative paucity of marrow infiltration, ***neutropenia* and *anemia* dominate the clinical picture**. Neutropenia is often accompanied by a striking decrease in late myeloid forms in the marrow. Rarely, *pure red cell aplasia* is seen. There is also an increased incidence of rheumatologic disorders. Some patients with *Felty syndrome*, a triad of rheumatoid arthritis, splenomegaly, and neutropenia, have this disorder as an underlying cause. The basis for these varied clinical abnormalities is unknown, but autoimmunity, provoked in some way by the tumor, seems likely.

The course is variable, being largely dependent on the severity of the cytopenias and their responsiveness to low-dose chemotherapy or steroids. In general, tumors of T-cell origin pursue an indolent course, whereas NK-cell tumors behave more aggressively.

Extranodal NK/T-Cell Lymphoma

This neoplasm is rare in the United States and Europe, but constitutes as many as 3% of NHLs in Asia. It presents most commonly as a destructive nasopharyngeal mass; less common sites of presentation include the testis and the skin. The tumor cell infiltrate typically surrounds and invades small vessels, leading to extensive *ischemic necrosis*. In touch preparations, *large azurophilic granules* are seen in the cytoplasm of the tumor cells that resemble those found in normal NK cells.

Extranodal NK/T-cell lymphoma is highly associated with EBV. Within individual patients, all of the tumor cells contain identical EBV episomes, indicating that the tumor originates from a single EBV-infected cell. How EBV gains entry is uncertain, since the tumor cells do not express CD21, the surface protein that serves as the B-cell EBV receptor. Most tumors are CD3– and lack T-cell receptor rearrangements and express NK-cell markers, supporting an NK-cell origin. No consistent chromosome aberration has been described.

Most extranodal NK/T-cell lymphomas are highly aggressive neoplasms that respond well to radiation therapy but are resistant to chemotherapy. Thus, the prognosis is poor in patients with advanced disease.

KEY CONCEPTS

Uncommon Lymphoid Neoplasms

Mantle cell lymphoma: Tumor of naive B cells that pursues a moderately aggressive course and is highly associated with translocations involving the cyclin D1 gene

Marginal zone lymphoma: Indolent tumors of antigen-primed B cells that arise at sites of chronic immune stimulation and often remain localized for long periods of time

Hairy cell leukemia: Morphologically distinct, very indolent tumor of mature B cells that is highly associated with mutations in the BRAF serine/threonine kinase

Peripheral NK/T cell lymphomas and leukemias

- Anaplastic large cell lymphoma: Aggressive T cell tumor, associated in a subset with activating mutations in the ALK tyrosine kinase
- Adult T cell leukemia/lymphoma: Aggressive tumor of CD4+ T cells that is uniformly associated with HTLV-1 infection
- Large granular lymphocytic leukemia: Indolent tumor of cytotoxic T cells or NK cells that is associated with mutations in the transcription factor STAT3 and with autoimmune phenomena and cytopenias
- Extranodal NK/T cell lymphoma: Aggressive tumor, usually derived from NK cells, that is strongly associated with EBV infection

Hodgkin Lymphoma

Hodgkin lymphoma (HL) encompasses a group of lymphoid neoplasms that differ from NHL in several respects (Table 13-7). While NHLs frequently occur at extranodal sites and spread in an unpredictable fashion, **HL arises in a single node or chain of nodes and spreads first to**

Table 13-7 Differences between Hodgkin and Non-Hodgkin Lymphomas

Hodgkin Lymphoma	Non-Hodgkin Lymphoma
More often localized to a single axial group of nodes (cervical, mediastinal, para-aortic)	More frequent involvement of multiple peripheral nodes
Orderly spread by contiguity	Noncontiguous spread
Mesenteric nodes and Waldeyer ring rarely involved	Waldeyer ring and mesenteric nodes commonly involved
Extranodal presentation rare	Extranodal presentation common

anatomically contiguous lymphoid tissues. HL also has distinctive morphologic features. It is characterized by the presence of neoplastic giant cells called *Reed-Sternberg cells.* These cells release factors that induce the accumulation of reactive lymphocytes, macrophages, and granulocytes, which typically make up greater than 90% of the tumor cellularity. In the vast majority of HLs, the neoplastic Reed-Sternberg cells are derived from germinal center or postgerminal center B cells.

Hodgkin lymphoma accounts for 0.7% of all new cancers in the United States; there are about 8000 new cases each year. The average age at diagnosis is 32 years. It is one of the most common cancers of young adults and adolescents, but also occurs in the aged. It was the first human cancer to be successfully treated with radiation therapy and chemotherapy, and is curable in most cases.

Classification. The WHO classification recognizes five subtypes of HL:

1. Nodular sclerosis
2. Mixed cellularity
3. Lymphocyte-rich
4. Lymphocyte depletion
5. Lymphocyte predominance

In the first four subtypes—nodular sclerosis, mixed cellularity, lymphocyte-rich, and lymphocyte depletion—the Reed-Sternberg cells have a similar immunophenotype. These subtypes are often lumped together as *classical* forms of HL. In the remaining subtype, lymphocyte predominance, the Reed-Sternberg cells have a distinctive B-cell immunophenotype that differs from that of the "classical" types.

Pathogenesis. The origin of the neoplastic Reed-Sternberg cells of classical HL has been explained through elegant studies relying on molecular analysis of single isolated Reed-Sternberg cells and variants. In the vast majority of cases, the Ig genes of Reed-Sternberg cells have undergone both V(D)J recombination and somatic hypermutation, establishing an origin from a germinal center or postgerminal center B cell. Despite having the genetic signature of a B cell, the Reed-Sternberg cells of classical HL fail to express most B-cell–specific genes, including the Ig genes. The cause of this wholesale reprogramming of gene expression has yet to be fully explained, but presumably is the result of widespread epigenetic changes of uncertain etiology.

Activation of the transcription factor NF-κB is a common event in classical HL. This can occur by several mechanisms:

- NF-κB may be activated either by EBV infection or by some other mechanism and turns on genes that promote lymphocyte survival and proliferation.
- EBV^+ tumor cells express latent membrane protein-1 (LMP-1), a protein encoded by the EBV genome that transmits signals that up-regulate NF-κB.
- Activation of NF-κB may occur in EBV-tumors as a result of acquired loss-of-function mutations in IκB or A20 (also known as *TNF alpha-induced protein 3, or TNFAIP3*), which are both negative regulators of NF-κB.
- It is hypothesized that activation of NF-κB by EBV or other mechanisms rescues "crippled" germinal center B cells that cannot express Igs from apoptosis, setting the stage for the acquisition of other unknown mutations that collaborate to produce Reed-Sternberg cells.

Little is known about the basis for the morphology of Reed-Sternberg cells and variants, but it is intriguing that EBV-infected B cells resembling Reed-Sternberg cells are found in the lymph nodes of individuals with infectious mononucleosis, strongly suggesting that EBV-encoded proteins play a part in the remarkable metamorphosis of B cells into Reed-Sternberg cells.

The florid accumulation of reactive cells in tissues involved by classical HL occurs in response to a wide variety of cytokines (e.g., IL-5, IL-10, and M-CSF) chemokines (e.g.,eotaxin), and other factors (e.g., immunomodulatory factor galectin-1) that are secreted by Reed-Sternberg cells. Once attracted, the reactive cells produce factors that support the growth and survival of the tumor cells and further modify the reactive cell response. For example, eosinophils and T cells express ligands that activate the CD30 and CD40 receptors found on Reed-Sternberg cells, producing signals that up-regulate NF-κB. Other examples of "cross-talk" between Reed-Sternberg cells and surrounding reactive cells are provided in Figure 13-28. Some of the factors produced by RS cells give rise to a state of immunodeficiency by impairment of T helper and cytotoxic cells and enhancing the generation of regulatory T cells (as discussed later).

Reed-Sternberg cells are aneuploid and possess diverse clonal chromosomal aberrations. Copy number gains in the *REL* proto-oncogene on chromosome 2p are particularly common and may also contribute to increases in NF-κB activity.

MORPHOLOGY

Identification of Reed-Sternberg cells and their variants is essential for the diagnosis. **Diagnostic Reed-Sternberg cells are large cells (45 μm in diameter) with multiple nuclei or a single nucleus with multiple nuclear lobes, each with a large inclusion-like nucleolus about the size of a small lymphocyte (5 to 7 μm in diameter)** (Fig. 13-24*A*). The cytoplasm is abundant. Several Reed-Sternberg cell variants are also recognized. **Mononuclear variants** contain a single nucleus with a large inclusion-like nucleolus (Fig. 13-24*B*). **Lacunar cells** (seen in the nodular sclerosis subtype) have more delicate, folded, or multilobate nuclei and abundant pale cytoplasm that is often disrupted during the cutting of sections, leaving the nucleus sitting in an empty hole (a lacuna) (Fig.

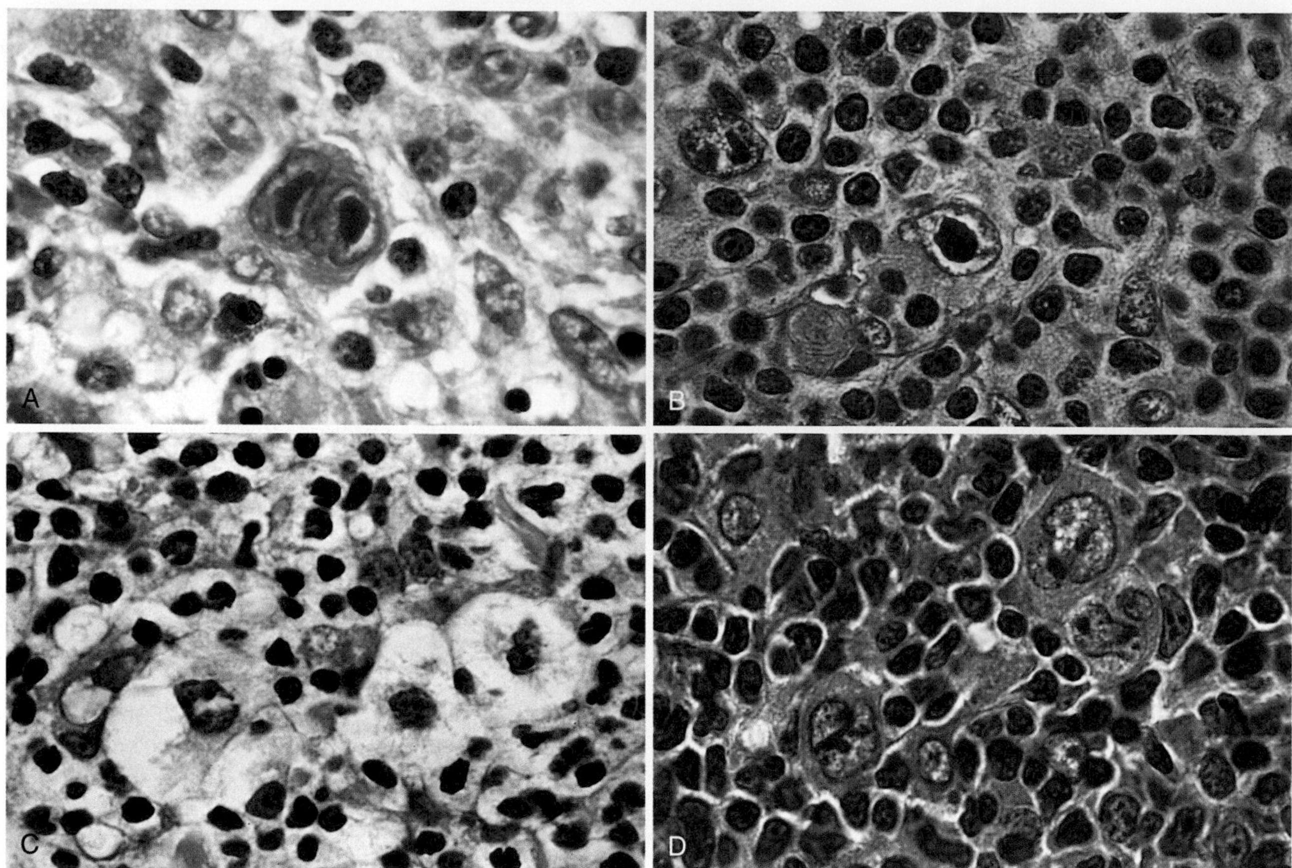

Figure 13-24 Reed-Sternberg cells and variants. **A,** Diagnostic Reed-Sternberg cell, with two nuclear lobes, large inclusion-like nucleoli, and abundant cytoplasm, surrounded by lymphocytes, macrophages, and an eosinophil. **B,** Reed-Sternberg cell, mononuclear variant. **C,** Reed-Sternberg cell, lacunar variant. This variant has a folded or multilobated nucleus and lies within a open space, which is an artifact created by disruption of the cytoplasm during tissue sectioning. **D,** Reed-Sternberg cell, lymphohistiocytic variant. Several such variants with multiply infolded nuclear membranes, small nucleoli, fine chromatin, and abundant pale cytoplasm are present. (**A,** Courtesy Dr. Robert W. McKenna, Department of Pathology, University of Texas Southwestern Medical School, Dallas, Tex.)

13-24*C*). In classical forms of HL, Reed-Sternberg cells undergo a peculiar form of cell death in which the cells shrink and become pyknotic, a process described as "mummification." **Lymphohistiocytic variants** (L&H cells) with polypoid nuclei, inconspicuous nucleoli, and moderately abundant cytoplasm are characteristic of the lymphocyte predominance subtype (Fig. 13-24*D*).

HL must be distinguished from other conditions in which cells resembling Reed-Sternberg cells can be seen, such as infectious mononucleosis, solid tissue cancers, and large-cell NHLs. The diagnosis of HL depends on the identification of Reed-Sternberg cells in a background of non-neoplastic inflammatory cells. The Reed-Sternberg cells of HL also have a characteristic immunohistochemical profile.

With this as background, we turn to the subclasses of HL, pointing out some of the salient morphologic and immunophenotypic features of each (Table 13-8). The clinical manifestations common to all are presented later.

Nodular Sclerosis Type. This is the most common form of HL, constituting 65% to 70% of cases. It is characterized by the presence of lacunar variant Reed-Sternberg cells and the **deposition of collagen in bands that divide involved lymph nodes into circumscribed nodules** (Fig. 13-25). The fibrosis may be scant or abundant. The Reed-Sternberg cells are found in a polymorphous background of T cells, eosinophils, plasma cells, and macrophages. Diagnostic Reed-Sternberg cells are often uncommon. The Reed-Sternberg cells in this and other "classical" HL subtypes have a characteristic immunophenotype; they are positive for PAX5 (a B-cell transcription factor), CD15, and CD30, and negative for other B-cell markers, T-cell markers, and CD45 (leukocyte common antigen). As in other forms of HL, involvement of the spleen, liver, bone marrow, and other organs and tissues can appear in due course in the form of irregular tumor nodules resembling those seen in lymph nodes. This subtype is uncommonly associated with EBV.

The nodular sclerosis type occurs with equal frequency in males and females. It has a propensity to involve the lower cervical, supraclavicular, and mediastinal lymph nodes of adolescents or young adults. The prognosis is excellent.

Mixed-Cellularity Type. This form of HL constitutes about 20% to 25% of cases. Involved lymph nodes are diffusely effaced by a heterogeneous cellular infiltrate, which includes T cells, eosinophils, plasma cells, and benign macrophages admixed with Reed-Sternberg cells (Fig. 13-26). **Diagnostic Reed-Sternberg cells and mononuclear variants are usually plentiful. The Reed-Sternberg cells are infected with EBV in about 70% of cases.** The immunophenotype is identical to that observed in the nodular sclerosis type.

Mixed-cellularity HL is more common in males. Compared with the lymphocyte predominance and nodular sclerosis subtypes, it is more likely to be associated with older age, systemic symptoms such as night sweats and weight loss, and

Table 13-8 Subtypes of Hodgkin Lymphoma

Subtype	Morphology and Immunophenotype	Typical Clinical Features
Nodular sclerosis	Frequent lacunar cells and occasional diagnostic RS cells; background infiltrate composed of T lymphocytes, eosinophils, macrophages, and plasma cells; fibrous bands dividing cellular areas into nodules. RS cells CD15+, CD30+; usually EBV–	Most common subtype; usually stage I or II disease; frequent mediastinal involvement; equal occurrence in males and females (F = M), most patients young adults
Mixed cellularity	Frequent mononuclear and diagnostic RS cells; background infiltrate rich in T lymphocytes, eosinophils, macrophages, plasma cells; RS cells CD15+, CD30+; 70% EBV+	More than 50% present as stage III or IV disease; M greater than F; biphasic incidence, peaking in young adults and again in adults older than 55
Lymphocyte rich	Frequent mononuclear and diagnostic RS cells; background infiltrate rich in T lymphocytes; RS cells CD15+, CD30+; 40% EBV–	Uncommon; M greater than F; tends to be seen in older adults
Lymphocyte depletion	Reticular variant: Frequent diagnostic RS cells and variants and a paucity of background reactive cells; RS cells CD15+, CD30+; most EBV+	Uncommon; more common in older males, HIV-infected individuals, and in developing countries; often presents with advanced disease
Lymphocyte predominance	Frequent L&H (popcorn cell) variants in a background of follicular dendritic cells and reactive B cells; RS cells CD20+, CD15–, C30–; EB–	Uncommon; young males with cervical or axillary lymphadenopathy; mediastinal

L&H, lymphohistiocytic; RS cell, Reed-Sternberg cell.

advanced tumor stage. Nonetheless, the overall prognosis is very good.

Lymphocyte-Rich Type. This is an uncommon form of classical HL in which **reactive lymphocytes make up the vast majority of the cellular infiltrate**. In most cases, involved lymph nodes are diffusely effaced, but vague nodularity due to the presence of residual B-cell follicles is sometimes seen. This entity is distinguished from the lymphocyte predominance type by the presence of frequent mononuclear variants and diagnostic Reed-Sternberg cells with a "classical" immunophenotypic profile. It is associated with EBV in about 40% of cases and has a very good to excellent prognosis.

Lymphocyte Depletion Type. This is the least common form of HL, amounting to less than 5% of cases. It is characterized by a paucity of lymphocytes and a relative abundance of Reed-Sternberg cells or their pleomorphic variants. The immunophenotype of the Reed-Sternberg cells is identical to that seen in other classical types of HL. Immunophenotyping is essential, since most tumors suspected of being lymphocyte depletion HL actually prove to be large-cell NHLs. **The Reed-Sternberg cells are infected with EBV in over 90% of cases.**

Lymphocyte depletion HL occurs predominantly in older adults, in HIV+ individuals of any age, and in nonindustrialized countries. Advanced stage and systemic symptoms are frequent, and the overall outcome is somewhat less favorable than in the other subtypes.

Lymphocyte Predominance Type. This uncommon "nonclassical" variant of HL accounts for about 5% of cases. Involved nodes are effaced by a nodular infiltrate of small lymphocytes admixed with variable numbers of macrophages (Fig. 13-27). "Classical" Reed-Sternberg cells are usually difficult to find. Instead, this tumor contains so-called L&H (lymphocytic and histiocytic) variants, which have a multilobed nucleus resembling a popcorn kernel ("popcorn cell"). Eosinophils and plasma cells are usually scant or absent.

In contrast to the Reed-Sternberg cells found in classical forms of HL, **L&H variants express B-cell markers typical of germinal-center B cells**, such as CD20 and BCL6, and are usually negative for CD15 and CD30. The typical nodular pattern of growth is due to the presence of expanded B-cell follicles, which are populated with L&H variants, numerous reactive B cells, and follicular dendritic cells. The IgH genes of

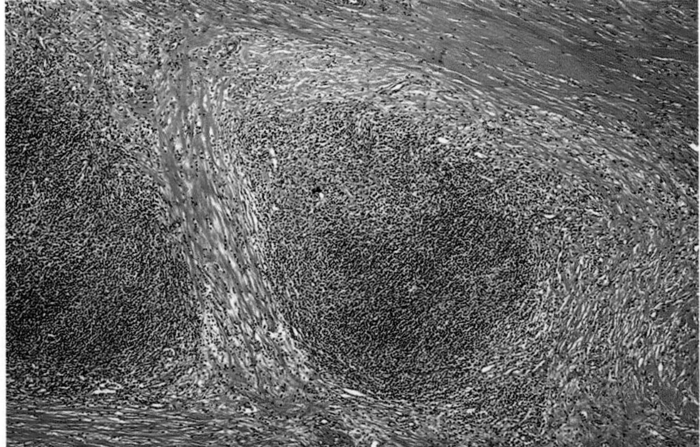

Figure 13-25 Hodgkin lymphoma, nodular sclerosis type. A low-power view shows well-defined bands of pink, acellular collagen that subdivide the tumor into nodules. (Courtesy Dr. Robert W. McKenna, Department of Pathology, University of Texas Southwestern Medical School, Dallas, Tex.)

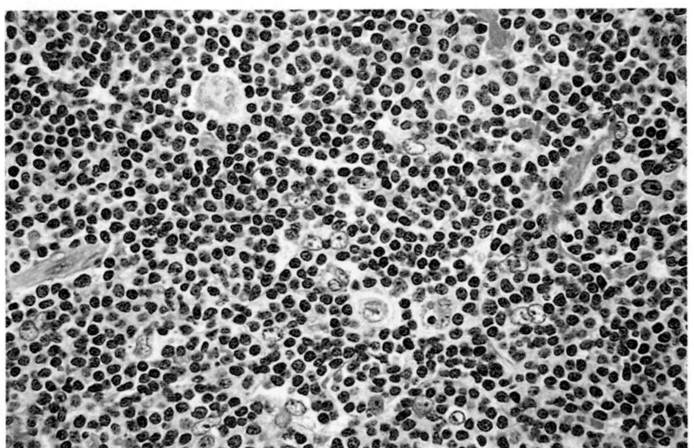

Figure 13-26 Hodgkin lymphoma, mixed-cellularity type. A diagnostic, binucleate Reed-Sternberg cell is surrounded by reactive cells, including eosinophils (bright red cytoplasm), lymphocytes, and histiocytes. (Courtesy Dr. Robert W. McKenna, Department of Pathology, University of Texas Southwestern Medical School, Dallas, Tex.)

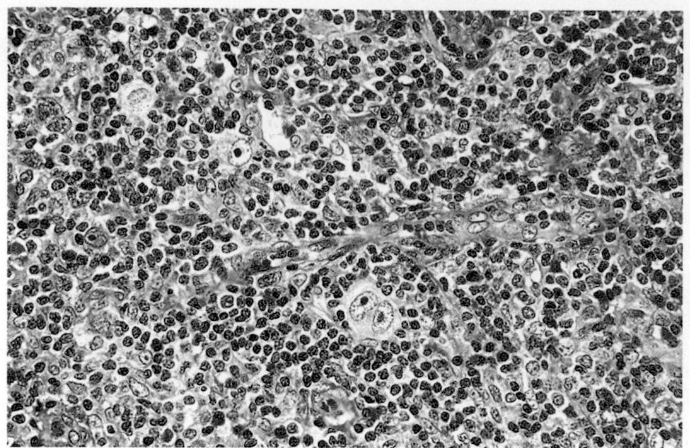

Figure 13-27 Hodgkin lymphoma, lymphocyte predominance type. Numerous mature-looking lymphocytes surround scattered, large, pale-staining lymphohistiocytic variants ("popcorn" cells). (Courtesy Dr. Robert W. McKenna, Department of Pathology, University of Texas Southwestern Medical School, Dallas, Tex.)

the L&H variants show evidence of ongoing somatic hypermutation, a modification that occurs only in germinal center B cells. In 3% to 5% of cases, this type transforms into a tumor resembling diffuse large B-cell lymphoma. EBV is not associated with this subtype.

A majority of patients are males, usually younger than 35 years of age, who typically present with cervical or axillary lymphadenopathy. Mediastinal and bone marrow involvement is rare. In some series, this form of HL is more likely to recur than the classical subtypes, but the prognosis is excellent.

Clinical Features. HL most commonly present as painless lymphadenopathy. Patients with the nodular sclerosis or lymphocyte predominance types tend to have stage I-II disease and are usually free of systemic manifestations. Patients with disseminated disease (stages III-IV) or the mixed-cellularity or lymphocyte depletion subtypes are more likely to have constitutional symptoms, such as fever, night sweats, and weight loss. Cutaneous immune unresponsiveness (also called anergy) resulting from depressed cell-mediated immunity is seen in most cases. The mix of factors released from Reed-Sternberg cells (Fig. 13-28) suppress T_H1 immune responses and may contribute to immune dysregulation.

The spread of HL is remarkably stereotyped: nodal disease first, then splenic disease, hepatic disease, and finally involvement of the marrow and other tissues. Staging involves physical examination, radiologic imaging of the abdomen, pelvis, and chest, and biopsy of the bone marrow (Table 13-9). With current treatment protocols, tumor stage rather than histologic type is the most important prognostic variable. The cure rate of patients with stages I and IIA is close to 90%. Even with advanced disease (stages IVA and IVB), disease-free survival at 5 years is 60% to 70%.

Low-stage localized HL can be cured with involved field radiotherapy, and indeed cure of such patients was one of the early success stories in oncology. However, it was subsequently recognized that long-term survivors treated with radiotherapy had a much higher incidence of certain malignancies, including lung cancer, melanoma, and breast cancer. Patients treated with early chemotherapy regimens containing alkylating agents also had a high

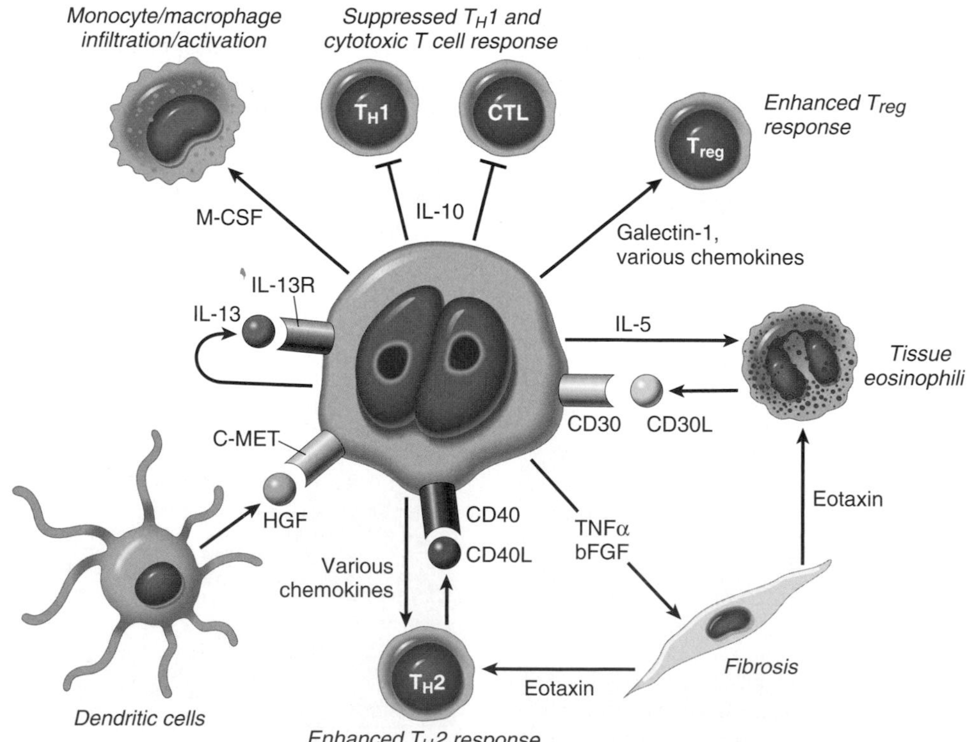

Figure 13-28 Proposed signals mediating "cross-talk" between Reed-Sternberg cells and surrounding normal cells in classical forms of Hodgkin lymphoma. *CD30L,* CD30 ligand; *bFGF,* basic fibroblast growth factor; *M-CSF,* monocyte colony-stimulating factor; *HGF,* hepatocyte growth factor (binds to the c-MET receptor); *TGFβ,* transforming growth factor β; *TNFα,* tumor necrosis factor α; *CTL,* CD8+ cytotoxic T cell; *T_H1* and *T_H2,* CD4+ T helper cell subsets; *Treg,* regulatory T cell.

Table 13-9 Clinical Staging of Hodgkin and Non-Hodgkin Lymphomas (Ann Arbor Classification)

Stage	Distribution of Disease
I	Involvement of a single lymph node region (I) or a single extralymphatic organ or site (IE)
II	Involvement of two or more lymph node regions on the same side of the diaphragm alone (II) or localized involvement of an extralymphatic organ or site (IIE)
III	Involvement of lymph node regions on both sides of the diaphragm without (III) or with (IIIE) localized involvement of an extralymphatic organ or site
IV	Diffuse involvement of one or more extralymphatic organs or sites with or without lymphatic involvement
All stages are further divided on the basis of the absence (A) or presence (B) of the following symptoms: unexplained fever, drenching night sweats, and/or unexplained weight loss of greater than 10% of normal body weight.	

Data from Carbone PT, et al: Symposium (Ann Arbor): Staging in Hodgkin's disease. *Cancer Res* 31:1707, 1971.

incidence of secondary tumors, particularly acute myeloid leukemia. These sobering results spurred the development of current treatment regimens, which minimize the use of radiotherapy and employ less genotoxic chemotherapeutic agents; as a result, the incidence of secondary tumors appears to have been reduced markedly, without any loss of therapeutic efficacy. Anti-CD30 antibodies have produced excellent responses in patients with disease that has failed conventional treatments and represent a promising targeted therapy.

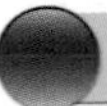

KEY CONCEPTS

Hodgkin Lymphoma

- Unusual tumor consisting mostly of reactive lymphocytes, macrophages, eosinophils, plasma cells and stromal cells mixed with rare tumor giant cells called Reed-Sternberg cells and variants
- Two broad types, classical (which has several subtypes) and lymphocyte predominant, which are distinguished based on morphologic and immunophenotypic grounds
- Reed-Sternberg cells of classical types make multiple cytokines and chemokines that influence the host response, and the host response in turn makes factors that support the growth of the tumor cells
- Classical forms are frequently associated with acquired mutations that activate the transcription factor NF-κB and with EBV infection
- Lymphocyte predominance type expresses B cell markers and is not associated with EBV

Myeloid Neoplasms

The common feature of this heterogeneous group of neoplasms is an origin from hematopoietic progenitor cells. These diseases primarily involve the marrow and to a lesser degree the secondary hematopoietic organs (the spleen, liver, and lymph nodes), and usually present with symptoms related to altered hematopoiesis. Three broad categories of myeloid neoplasia exist:

- *Acute myeloid leukemias,* in which an accumulation of immature myeloid forms (blasts) in the bone marrow suppresses normal hematopoiesis
- *Myelodysplastic syndromes,* in which defective maturation of myeloid progenitors gives rise to ineffective hematopoiesis, leading to cytopenias
- *Myeloproliferative disorders,* in which there is usually increased production of one or more types of blood cells

The pathogenesis of myeloid neoplasms is best understood in the context of normal hematopoiesis, which involves a hierarchy of hematopoietic stem cells, committed progenitors, and more differentiated elements (Fig. 13-1). Normal hematopoiesis is finely tuned by homeostatic feedback mechanisms involving cytokines and growth factors that modulate the production of red cells, white cells, and platelets in the marrow. These mechanisms are deranged in marrows involved by myeloid neoplasms, which "escape" from normal homeostatic controls and suppress the function of residual normal stem cells. The specific manifestations of the different myeloid neoplasms are influenced by

- *The position of the transformed cell within the hierarchy of progenitors* (i.e., a pluripotent hematopoietic stem cell versus a more committed progenitor)
- *The effect of the transforming events on differentiation,* which may be inhibited, skewed, or deranged by particular oncogenic mutations

Given that all myeloid neoplasms originate from transformed hematopoietic progenitors, it is not surprising that divisions between these neoplasms are sometimes blurred. Myeloid neoplasms, like other malignancies, tend to evolve over time to more aggressive forms of disease. In particular, both myelodysplastic syndromes and myeloproliferative disorders often "transform" to AML. In one of the most important myeloproliferative disorders, chronic myelogenous leukemia (CML), transformation to acute lymphoblastic leukemia is also seen, indicating that it originates from a transformed pluripotent hematopoietic stem cell.

Acute Myeloid Leukemia

Acute myeloid leukemia (AML) is a tumor of hematopoietic progenitors caused by acquired oncogenic mutations that impede differentiation, leading to the accumulation of immature myeloid blasts in the marrow. The replacement of the marrow with blasts produces marrow failure and complications related to anemia, thrombocytopenia, and neutropenia. AML occurs at all ages, but the incidence rises throughout life, peaking after 60 years of age. There are about 13,000 new cases each year in the United States.

Classification. AML is quite heterogeneous, reflecting the complexities of myeloid cell differentiation. The current WHO classification subdivides AML into four categories (Table 13-10). The first includes forms of AML that are associated with particular genetic aberrations, which are important because they correlate with prognosis and guide therapy. Also included are categories of AML arising after a myelodysplastic disorder (MDS) or with MDS-like features, and therapy-related AML. AMLs in these two categories have distinct genetic features and respond poorly to

Table 13-10 Major Subtypes of AML in the WHO Classification

Class	Prognosis	Morphology/Comments
I. AML with Genetic Aberrations		
AML with t(8;21)(q22;q22); *RUNX1/ETO* fusion gene	Favorable	Full range of myelocytic maturation; Auer rods easily found; abnormal cytoplasmic granules
AML with inv(16)(p13;q22); *CBFB/MYH*11 fusion gene	Favorable	Myelocytic and monocytic differentiation; abnormal eosinophilic precursors with abnormal basophilic granules
AML with t(15;17)(q22;11-12); *RARA/PML* fusion gene	Intermediate	Numerous Auer rods, often in bundles within individual progranulocytes; primary granules usually very prominent, but inconspicuous in microgranular variant; high incidence of DIC
AML with t(11q23;v); diverse *MLL* fusion genes	Poor	Usually some degree of monocytic differentiation
AML with normal cytogenetics and mutated *NPM*	Favorable	Detected by immunohistochemical staining for NPM
II. AML with MDS-like Features		
With prior MDS	Poor	Diagnosis based on clinical history
AML with multilineage dysplasia	Poor	Maturing cells with dysplastic features typical of MDS
AML with MDS-like cytogenetic aberrations	Poor	Associated with 5q-, 7q-, 20q-aberrations
III. AML, therapy-related	Very poor	If following alkylator therapy or radiation therapy, 2- to 8-year latency period, MDS-like cytogenetic aberrations (e.g., 5q-, 7q-); if following topoisomerase II inhibitor (e.g., etoposide) therapy, 1- to 3-year latency, translocations involving *MLL* (11q23)
IV. AML, Not Otherwise Specified		
AML, minimally differentiated	Intermediate	Negative for myeloperoxidase; myeloid antigens detected on blasts by flow cytometry
AML without maturation	Intermediate	>3% of blasts positive for myeloperoxidase
AML with myelocytic maturation	Intermediate	Full range of myelocytic maturation
AML with myelomonocytic maturation	Intermediate	Myelocytic and monocytic differentiation
AML with monocytic maturation	Intermediate	Nonspecific esterase-positive monoblasts and pro-monocytes predominate in marrow; may see monoblasts or mature monocytes in the blood
AML with erythroid maturation	Intermediate	Erythroid/myeloid subtype defined by >50% dysplastic maturing erythroid precursors and >20% myeloblasts; pure erythroid subtype defined by >80% erythroid precursors without myeloblasts
AML with megakaryocytic maturation	Intermediate	Blasts of megakaryocytic lineage predominate; detected with antibodies against megakaryocyte-specific markers (GPIIb/IIIa or vWF); often associated with marrow fibrosis; most common AML in Down syndrome

AML, Acute myeloid leukemia; DIC, disseminated intravascular coagulation; MDS, myelodysplasia; NPM, nucleophosmin; vWF, von Willebrand factor.

therapy. A fourth "wastebasket" category includes AMLs lacking any of these features. These are classified based on the degree of differentiation and the lineage of the leukemic blasts. Given the increasing role of cytogenetic and molecular features in directing therapy, a further shift toward genetic classification of AML is both inevitable and desirable.

Pathogenesis. **Many of the recurrent genetic aberrations seen in AML disrupt genes encoding transcription factors that are required for normal myeloid differentiation.** For example, the two most common chromosomal rearrangements, t(8;21) and inv(16), disrupt the *RUNX1* and *CBFB* genes, respectively. These two genes encode polypeptides that bind one another to form a RUNX1/CBF1β transcription factor that is required for normal hematopoiesis. The t(8;21) and the inv(16) create chimeric genes encoding fusion proteins that interfere with the function of RUNX1/CBF1β and block the maturation of myeloid cells. However, experiments in mouse models indicate that genetic lesions that merely block the maturation of myeloid progenitors are not sufficient to cause AML. Thus other genetic changes (discussed next) are also essential.

There is increasing evidence that mutations that lead to activation of growth factor signaling pathways collaborate with transcription factor aberrations to produce AML. One example is found in AML with the t(15;17), acute promyelocytic leukemia. The t(15;17) creates yet another fusion gene encoding a chimeric protein consisting of the retinoic acid receptor-α (RARα) fused to a portion of a protein called PML (after the tumor). As discussed in Chapter 7, this fusion protein interferes with the terminal differentiation of granulocytes, an effect that can be overcome by treatment with either all-trans retinoic acid or arsenic trioxide. However, expression of the PML-RARa fusion protein in the bone marrow cells of mice produces disease only in aged mice, suggesting that PML-RARα is not sufficient. Indeed, AMLs with the t(15;17) (a subtype referred to as acute promyelocytic leukemia) also have frequent activating mutations in FLT3, a receptor tyrosine kinase that transmits signals that mimic normal growth factor signaling, thereby increasing cellular proliferation and survival. As might be predicted, the combination of PML-RARα and activated FLT3 is a potent inducer of AML in mice. Other similar observations in human AML and in mouse models indicate that aberrant activation of growth factor signaling pathways is a common feature of AML.

Deep sequencing of AML genomes has also revealed unexpectedly frequent mutations affecting factors that impact the state of the "epigenome," suggesting the epigenetic alterations have a central role in AML.

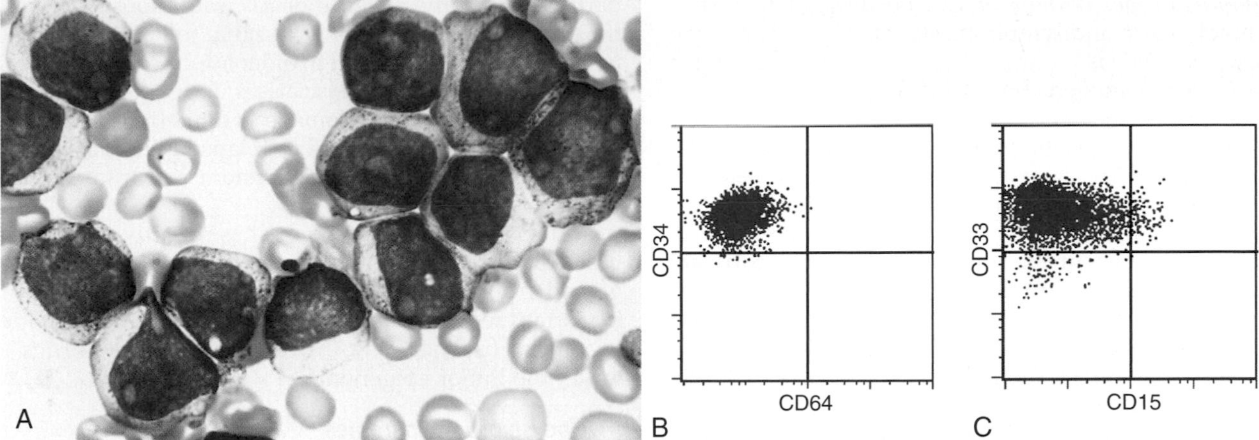

Figure 13-29 **A,** Acute myeloid leukemia without maturation (FAB M1 subtype). Myeloblasts have delicate nuclear chromatin, prominent nucleoli, and fine azurophilic granules in the cytoplasm. **B,** In the flow cytometric analysis shown, the myeloid blasts, represented by the red dots, express CD34, a marker of multipotent stem cells, but do not express CD64, a marker of mature myeloid cells. **C,** The same myeloid blasts express CD33, a marker of immature myeloid cells, and a subset express CD15, a marker of more mature myeloid cells. Thus, these blasts are myeloid cells showing limited maturation. (**A,** Courtesy Dr. Robert W. McKenna Department of Pathology, University of Texas Southwestern Medical School, Dallas, Tex; **B** and **C,** courtesy Dr. Louis Picker, Oregon Health Science Center, Portland, Ore.)

Gene expression is regulated by two types of epigenetic modifications, DNA methylation and posttranslational modifications of histones (e.g., acetylation, methylation, phosphorylation). Some of the most commonly mutated genes in AML encode factors that influence DNA methylation or histone modifications. Another 15% of tumors have mutations involving genes encoding components of the cohesin complex, proteins that regulate the three-dimensional structure of chromatin. The precise mechanism by which these mutations contribute to the development of AML remains to be determined and is a "hot" area of current research.

MORPHOLOGY

The diagnosis of AML is based on the presence of at least 20% myeloid blasts in the bone marrow. Several types of myeloid blasts are recognized, and individual tumors may have more than one type of blast or blasts with hybrid features. **Myeloblasts** have delicate nuclear chromatin, two to four nucleoli, and more voluminous cytoplasm than lymphoblasts (Fig. 13-29A). The cytoplasm often contains fine, peroxidase-positive azurophilic granules. **Auer rods**, distinctive needle-like azurophilic granules, are present in many cases; they are particularly numerous in AML with the t(15;17) (acute promyelocytic leukemia) (Fig. 13-30*A*). **Monoblasts** (Fig. 13-30*B*) have folded or lobulated nuclei, lack Auer rods, and are nonspecific esterase-positive. In some AMLs, blasts show megakaryocytic differentiation, which is often accompanied by marrow fibrosis caused by the release of fibrogenic cytokines. Rarely, the blasts of AML show erythroid differentiation.

The number of leukemic cells in the blood is highly variable. Blasts may be more than 100,000/mm^3, but are under 10,000/mm^3 in about 50% of patients. **Occasionally, blasts are entirely absent from the blood (aleukemic leukemia).** For this reason, a bone marrow examination is essential to exclude acute leukemia in pancytopenic patients.

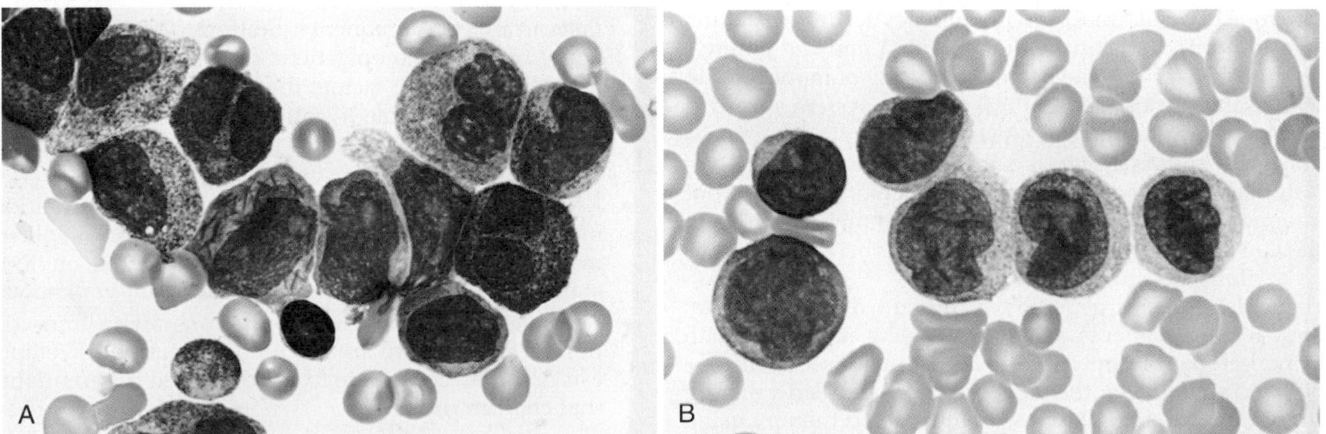

Figure 13-30 Acute myeloid leukemia subtypes. **A,** Acute promyelocytic leukemia with the t(15;17) (FAB M3 subtype). Bone marrow aspirate shows neoplastic promyelocytes with abnormally coarse and numerous azurophilic granules. Other characteristic findings include the presence of several cells with bilobed nuclei and a cell in the center of the field that contains multiple needle-like Auer rods. **B,** Acute myeloid leukemia with monocytic differentiation (FAB M5b subtype). Peripheral smear shows one monoblast and five promonocytes with folded nuclear membranes. (Courtesy Dr. Robert W. McKenna, Department of Pathology, University of Texas Southwestern Medical School, Dallas, Tex.)

Immunophenotype. Because it can be difficult to distinguish myeloblasts and lymphoblasts morphologically, the diagnosis of AML is confirmed by performing stains for myeloid-specific antigens (Fig. 13-29*B,C*).

Cytogenetics. Cytogenetic analysis has a central role in the classification of AML. Karyotypic aberrations are detected in 50% to 70% of cases with standard techniques and in approximately 90% of cases using special high-resolution banding. Particular chromosomal abnormalities correlate with certain clinical features. AMLs arising de novo in younger adults are commonly associated with balanced chromosomal translocations, particularly t(8;21), inv(16), and t(15;17). In contrast, AMLs following myelodysplastic syndromes or exposure to DNA-damaging agents (such as chemotherapy or radiation therapy) often have deletions or monosomies involving chromosomes 5 and 7 and usually lack chromosomal translocations. The exception to this rule is AML occurring after treatment with topoisomerase II inhibitors, which is strongly associated with translocations involving the *MLL* gene on chromosome 11q23. AML in older adults is also more likely to be associated with "bad" aberrations, such as deletions of chromosomes 5q and 7q.

Clinical Features. Most patients present within weeks or a few months of the onset of symptoms with complaints related to *anemia, neutropenia, and thrombocytopenia,* most notably fatigue, fever, and spontaneous mucosal and cutaneous bleeding. You will remember that these findings are very similar to those produced by ALL. Thrombocytopenia results in a bleeding diathesis, which is often prominent. Cutaneous petechiae and ecchymoses, serosal hemorrhages into the linings of the body cavities and viscera, and mucosal hemorrhages into the gingivae and urinary tract are common. Procoagulants and fibrinolytic factors released by leukemic cells, especially in AML with the t(15;17), exacerbate the bleeding tendency. Infections are frequent, particularly in the oral cavity, skin, lungs, kidneys, urinary bladder, and colon, and are often caused by opportunists such as fungi, *Pseudomonas,* and commensals.

Signs and symptoms related to involvement of tissues other than the marrow are usually less striking in AML than in ALL, but tumors with monocytic differentiation often infiltrate the skin (leukemia cutis) and the gingiva; this probably reflects the normal tendency of monocytes to extravasate into tissues. Central nervous system spread is less common than in ALL. AML occasionally presents as a localized soft-tissue mass known variously as a myeloblastoma, granulocytic sarcoma, or chloroma. Without systemic treatment, such tumors inevitably progress to full-blown AML over time.

Prognosis. AML is generally a difficult disease to treat; about 60% of patients achieve complete remission with chemotherapy, but only 15% to 30% remain free of disease for 5 years. However, the outcome varies markedly among different molecular subtypes. With targeted therapy using all-trans retinoic acid and arsenic salts (described in Chapter 7), AMLs with the t(15;17) now have the best prognosis of any type, being curable in more than 80% of patients. AMLs with t(8;21) or inv(16) have a relatively good prognosis with conventional chemotherapy, particularly in the absence of *KIT* mutations. In contrast, the prognosis is dismal for AMLs that follow MDS or genotoxic therapy, or that occur in older adults, possibly because in these contexts the disease arises out of a background of hematopoietic stem cell damage or depletion. These "high-risk" forms of AML (as well as relapsed AML of all types) are treated with hematopoietic stem cell transplantation when possible.

Sequencing of AML genomes has recently revealed new molecular predictors of outcome. It is certain that insights gained from DNA sequencing will have an increasingly important role in selecting therapy and stratifying patients in clinical trials of new therapeutics, such as drugs that target the tumor epigenome.

Myelodysplastic Syndromes

The term "myelodysplastic syndrome" (MDS) refers to a group of clonal stem cell disorders characterized by maturation defects that are associated with ineffective hematopoiesis and a high risk of transformation to AML. In MDS the bone marrow is partly or wholly replaced by the clonal progeny of a neoplastic multipotent stem cell that retains the capacity to differentiate but does so in an ineffective and disordered fashion. These abnormal cells stay within the bone marrow and hence the patients have peripheral blood cytopenias.

MDS may be either primary (idiopathic) or secondary to previous genotoxic drug or radiation therapy (t-MDS). t-MDS usually appears from 2 to 8 years after the genotoxic exposure. All forms of MDS can transform to AML, but transformation occurs with highest frequency and most rapidly in t-MDS. Although characteristic morphologic changes are typically seen in the marrow and the peripheral blood, the diagnosis frequently requires correlation with other laboratory tests. Cytogenetic analysis is particularly helpful, since certain chromosomal aberrations (discussed later) are often observed.

Pathogenesis. The pathogenesis of MDS is poorly understood, but important new insights have come from recent deep sequencing of MDS genomes, which has identified a number of recurrently mutated genes. These genes can be lumped into three major functional categories, as follows:

- *Epigenetic factors.* Frequent mutations are seen involving many of the same epigenetic factors that are mutated in AML, including factors that regulate DNA methylation and histone modifications; thus, like AML, dysregulation of the epigenome appears to be important in the genesis of MDS.
- *RNA splicing factors.* A subset of tumors has mutations involving components of the 3′ end of the RNA splicing machinery. The impact of these mutations on RNA splicing and other nuclear functions is not yet known.
- *Transcription factors.* These mutations affect transcription factors that are are required for normal myelopoiesis and may contribute to the deranged differentiation that characterizes MDS.

In addition, roughly 10% of MDS cases have loss-of-function mutations in the tumor suppressor gene *TP53,* which correlate with the presence of a complex karyotype and particularly poor clinical outcomes. Both primary MDS and t-MDS are associated with similar recurrent

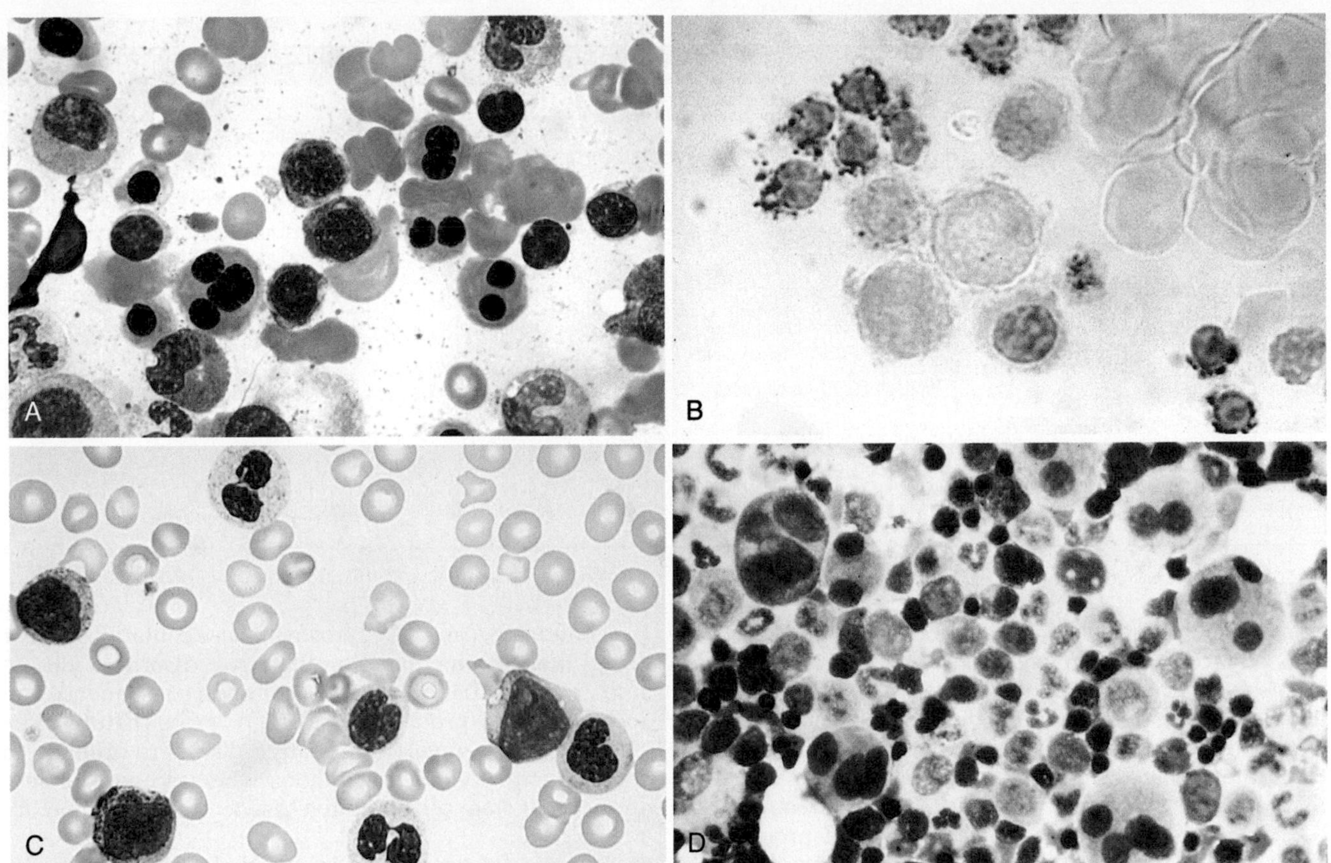

Figure 13-31 Myelodysplasia. Characteristic forms of dysplasia are shown. **A,** Nucleated red cell progenitors with multilobated or multiple nuclei. **B,** Ringed sideroblasts, erythroid progenitors with iron-laden mitochondria seen as blue perinuclear granules (Prussian blue stain). **C,** Pseudo-Pelger-Hüet cells, neutrophils with only two nuclear lobes instead of the normal three to four, are observed at the top and bottom of this field. **D,** Megakaryocytes with multiple nuclei instead of the normal single multilobated nucleus. (**A, B, D,** Marrow aspirates; **C,** peripheral blood smear.)

chromosomal abnormalities, including monosomies 5 and 7, deletions of 5q, 7q, and 20q, and trisomy 8.

As with aneuploidy in other cancers, it is not known how these aberrations contribute to MDS. One idea with some experimental support is that the gain or loss of single copies of key genes is sufficient to give cells a growth advantage, and that aneuploidy is one way to achieve this result. For example, subtle increases in the notorious oncoprotein MYC is sufficient to stimulate cell growth. Notably, the *MYC* gene is located on chromosome 8, and trisomy 8 is one of the most common forms of aneuploidy in a wide range of myeloid tumors. Similarly, the region that is commonly lost on chromosome 5q contains a gene encoding the ribosomal protein RPS14. In experimental systems, loss of one copy of RPS14 produces ineffective erythropoiesis, one of the hallmarks of MDS.

MORPHOLOGY

Although the marrow is usually hypercellular at diagnosis, it is sometimes normocellular or, less commonly, hypocellular. The most characteristic finding is disordered (dysplastic) differentiation affecting the erythroid, granulocytic, monocytic, and megakaryocytic lineages to varying degrees (Fig. 13-31). Within the erythroid series, common abnormalities include **ring sideroblasts**, erythroblasts with iron-laden mitochondria visible as perinuclear granules in Prussian blue-stained aspirates or biopsies; **megaloblastoid maturation**, resembling that seen in vitamin B_{12} and folate deficiency (Chapter 14); and **nuclear budding abnormalities**, recognized as nuclei with misshapen, often polyploid, outlines. Neutrophils frequently contain decreased numbers of secondary granules, toxic granulations, and/or Döhle bodies. **Pseudo-Pelger-Hüet cells**, neutrophils with only two nuclear lobes, are commonly observed, and neutrophils are seen occasionally that completely lack nuclear segmentation. Megakaryocytes with single nuclear lobes or multiple separate nuclei (**pawn ball megakaryocytes**) are also characteristic. **Myeloid blasts** may be increased but make up less than 20% of the overall marrow cellularity. The blood often contains pseudo-Pelger-Hüet cells, giant platelets, macrocytes, and poikilocytes, accompanied by a relative or absolute monocytosis. Myeloid blasts usually make up less than 10% of the leukocytes in the blood.

Clinical Features. Primary MDS is predominantly a disease of older adults; the mean age of onset is 70 years. In up to half of the cases, it is discovered incidentally on routine blood testing. When symptomatic, it presents with weakness, infections, and hemorrhages, all due to pancytopenia.

Primary MDS is divided into eight categories based on morphologic and cytogenetic features in the WHO

Table 13-11 Tyrosine Kinase Mutations in Myeloproliferative Disorders

Disorder	Mutation	Frequency*	Consequences†
Chronic myelogenous leukemia	*BCR-ABL* fusion gene	100%	Constitutive ABL kinase activation‡
Polycythemia vera	*JAK2* point mutations	>95%	Constitutive JAK2 kinase activation
Essential thrombocythemia	*JAK2* point mutations *MPL* point mutations	50% to 60% 5% to 10%	Constitutive JAK2 kinase activation Constitutive MPL kinase activation
Primary myelofibrosis	*JAK2* point mutations *MPL* point mutations	50% to 60% 5% to 10%	Constitutive JAK2 kinase activation Constitutive MPL kinase activation
Systemic mastocytosis	*KIT* point mutations	>90%	Constitutive KIT kinase activation
Chronic eosinophilic leukemia§	*FIP1L1-PDGFRA* fusion gene *PDE4DIP-PDGFRB* fusion gene	Common Rare	Constitutive PDGFRα kinase activation Constitutive PDGFRβ kinase activation‡
Stem cell leukemia‖	Various *FGFR1* fusion genes	100%	Constitutive FGFR1 kinase activation¶

*Refers to frequency within a diagnostic category.
†All stimulate ligand-independent pro-growth and survival signals.
‡Responds to imatinib therapy.
§Associated with Loeffler endocarditis (Chapter 12).
‖Rare disorder originating in pluripotent hematopoietic stem cells that presents with concomitant myeloproliferative disorder and lymphoblastic leukemia/lymphoma.
¶Responds to PKC412 therapy.

classification, details of which are beyond our scope. A prognostic scoring system has been developed that groups patients into 5 major prognostic groups. In brief, worse outcomes are (understandably) predicted by higher blast counts and more severe cytopenias, as well as the presence of multiple clonal chromosomal abnormalities.

The median survival in primary MDS varies from 9 to 29 months, but some individuals in good prognostic groups may live for 5 years or more. Overall, progression to AML occurs in 10% to 40% of individuals and is usually accompanied by the appearance of additional cytogenetic abnormalities. Patients often succumb to the complications of thrombocytopenia (bleeding) and neutropenia (infection). The outlook is even grimmer in t-MDS, which has a median survival of only 4 to 8 months. In t-MDS, cytopenias tend to be more severe and progression to AML is often rapid.

Treatment options are fairly limited. In younger patients, allogeneic hematopoietic stem cell transplantation offers hope for reconstitution of normal hematopoiesis and possible cure. Older patients with MDS are treated supportively with antibiotics and blood product transfusions. Thalidomide-like drugs (see prior discussion in myeloma) and DNA methylation inhibitors improve the effectiveness of hematopoiesis and the peripheral blood counts in a subset of patients. The presence of isolated 5q- is correlated with a hematologic response to thalidomide-like drugs, but as yet response to DNA methylation inhibitors is unpredictable.

Myeloproliferative Disorders

The common pathogenic feature of the myeloproliferative disorders is the presence of mutated, constitutively activated tyrosine kinases or other acquired aberrations in signaling pathways that lead to growth factor independence. Hematopoietic growth factors act on normal progenitors by binding to surface receptors and activating tyrosine kinases, which turn on pathways that promote growth and survival (Chapter 7). The mutated tyrosine kinases found in the myeloproliferative disorders circumvent normal controls and lead to the growth factor-independent proliferation and survival of marrow progenitors. Because the tyrosine kinase mutations underlying the various myeloproliferative disorders do not impair differentiation, the most common consequence is an increase in the production of one or more mature blood elements. Most myeloproliferative disorders originate in multipotent myeloid progenitors, whereas others arise in pluripotent stem cells that give rise to both lymphoid and myeloid cells.

There is a considerable degree of clinical and morphologic overlap among the myeloproliferative disorders. The common features include:

- *Increased proliferative drive* in the bone marrow
- Homing of the neoplastic stem cells to secondary hematopoietic organs, producing *extramedullary hematopoiesis*
- Variable transformation to a spent phase characterized by *marrow fibrosis* and peripheral blood *cytopenias*
- Variable transformation to *acute leukemia*

Certain myeloproliferative disorders are strongly associated with activating mutations in specific tyrosine kinases. This insight and the availability of kinase inhibitors have increased the importance of molecular tests for tyrosine kinase mutations, both for purposes of diagnosis and the selection of therapy. This discussion is confined to the more common myeloproliferative disorders, which are classified based on clinical, laboratory, and molecular criteria. Systemic mastocytosis, a distinctive myeloproliferative disorder that is associated with mutations in the KIT tyrosine kinase, is discussed under disorders of the skin (Chapter 25). The association of various myeloproliferative disorders with specific tyrosine kinase mutations (including rare disorders not discussed here) is summarized in Table 13-11.

Chronic Myelogenous Leukemia

Chronic myelogenous leukemia (CML) is distinguished from other myeloproliferative disorders by the presence of a chimeric *BCR-ABL* gene derived from portions of the *BCR* gene on chromosome 22 and the *ABL* gene on chromosome 9. *BCR-ABL* directs the synthesis of a constitutively active BCR-ABL tyrosine kinase (Fig. 13-32), which

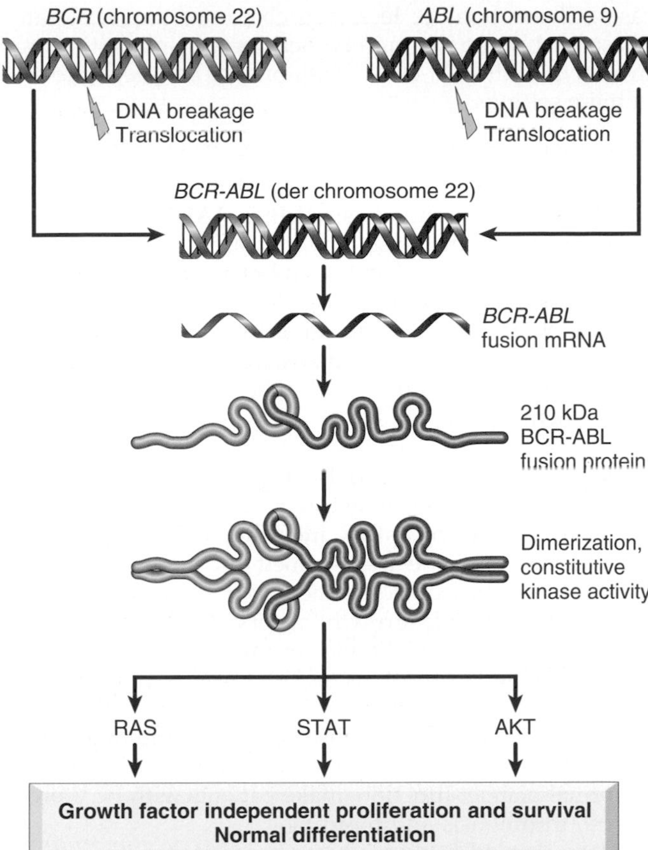

Figure 13-32 Pathogenesis of chronic myeloid leukemia. Breakage and joining of *BCR* and *ABL* creates a chimeric *BCR-ABL* fusion gene that encodes a constitutively active BCR-ABL tyrosine kinase. BCR-ABL activates multiple downstream pathways, which drive growth factor-independent proliferation and survival of bone marrow progenitors. Because BCR-ABL does not interfere with differentiation, the net result is an increase in mature elements in the peripheral blood, particularly granulocytes and platelets.

in CML is usually 210 kDa in size. In more than 90% of cases, *BCR-ABL* is created by a reciprocal (9;22)(q34;q11) translocation (the so-called *Philadelphia chromosome* [Ph]). In the remaining cases the *BCR-ABL* fusion gene is formed by cytogenetically complex or cryptic rearrangements and must be detected by other methods, such as fluorescence in situ hybridization or polymerase chain reaction (PCR)-based tests. The cell of origin is a pluripotent hematopoietic stem cell.

Pathogenesis. Tyrosine kinases are normally regulated by ligand-mediated dimerization and autophosphorylation, which creates an activated kinase capable of phosphorylating other protein substrates (Chapters 3 and 7). The BCR moiety of BCR-ABL contains a dimerization domain that self-associates, leading to the activation of the ABL tyrosine kinase moiety. The ABL kinase in turn phosphorylates proteins that induce signaling through the same pro-growth and pro-survival pathways that are turned on by hematopoietic growth factors, including the RAS and JAK/STAT pathways. For unknown reasons, BCR-ABL preferentially drives the proliferation of granulocytic and megakaryocytic progenitors, and also causes the abnormal release of immature granulocytic forms from the marrow into the blood.

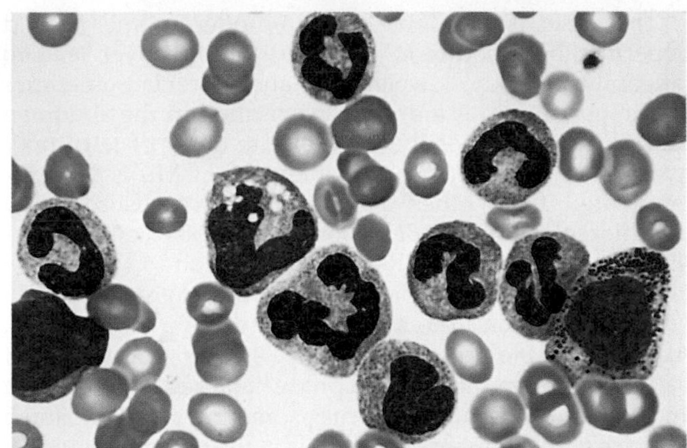

Figure 13-33 Chronic myelogenous leukemia. Peripheral blood smear shows many mature neutrophils, some metamyelocytes, and a myelocyte. (Courtesy Dr. Robert W. McKenna, Department of Pathology, University of Texas Southwestern Medical School, Dallas, Tex.)

MORPHOLOGY

The marrow is markedly **hypercellular** because of massively increased numbers of maturing granulocytic precursors, which usually include an elevated proportion of eosinophils and basophils. Megakaryocytes are also increased and usually include small, dysplastic forms. Erythroid progenitors are present in normal or mildly decreased numbers. A characteristic finding is the presence of scattered macrophages with abundant wrinkled, green-blue cytoplasm so-called sea-blue histiocytes. Increased deposition of reticulin is typical, but overt marrow fibrosis is rare early in the course. The blood reveals a **leukocytosis, often exceeding 100,000 cells/mm^3** (Fig. 13-33), which consists predominantly of neutrophils, band forms, metamyelocytes, myelocytes, eosinophils, and basophils. Blasts usually make up less than 10% of the circulating cells. Platelets are also usually increased, sometimes markedly. The spleen is often greatly enlarged as a result of extensive extramedullary hematopoiesis (Fig. 13-34) and often contains infarcts of varying age. Extramedullary hematopoiesis can also produce mild hepatomegaly and lymphadenopathy.

Clinical Features. CML is primarily a disease of adults but also occurs in children and adolescents. The peak incidence is in the fifth to sixth decades of life. There are about 4500 new cases per year in the United States.

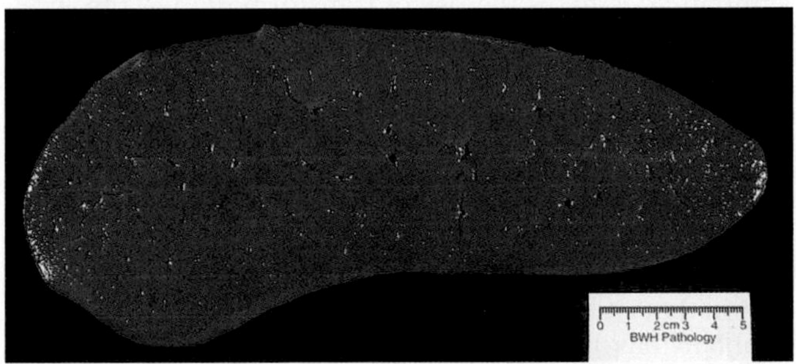

Figure 13-34 Chronic myeloid leukemia (spleen). Enlarged spleen (2630 gm; normal: 150 to 200 gm) with greatly expanded red pulp stemming from neoplastic hematopoiesis. (Courtesy Dr. Daniel Jones, Department of Pathology, MD Anderson Cancer Center, Houston, Tex.)

The onset is insidious. Mild-to-moderate anemia and hypermetabolism due to increased cell turnover lead to fatigability, weakness, weight loss, and anorexia. Sometimes the first symptom is a dragging sensation in the abdomen caused by splenomegaly, or the acute onset of left upper quadrant pain due to splenic infarction. CML is best differentiated from other myeloproliferative disorders by detection of the *BCR-ABL* fusion gene through either chromosomal analysis or PCR-based tests.

The natural history is one of slow progression; even without treatment, the median survival is about 3 years. After a variable period averaging 3 years, about 50% of patients enter an "accelerated phase" marked by increasing anemia and thrombocytopenia, sometimes accompanied by a rise in the number of basophils in the blood. Additional clonal cytogenetic abnormalities, such as trisomy 8, isochromosome 17q, or duplication of the Ph chromosome, often appear. Within 6 to 12 months, the accelerated phase terminates in a picture resembling acute leukemia (*blast crisis*). In the other 50% of patients, blast crises occur abruptly without an accelerated phase. In 70% of crises, the blasts are of myeloid origin (myeloid blast crisis), whereas in most of the remainder the blasts are of pre–B cell origin (lymphoid blast crisis). This is taken as evidence that CML originates from a pluripotent stem cell with both myeloid and lymphoid potential.

Given that we have seen that acute leukemias often stem from complementary mutations involving a transcription factor and a tyosine kinase, it might be predicted that blast crisis would be caused by an acquired mutation in a key transcriptional regulator. This prediction has been realized in lymphoid blast crisis, in which 85% of cases are associated with mutations that interfere with the activity of Ikaros, a transcription factor that regulates the differentiation of hematopoietic progenitors. The same types of Ikaros mutations are also seen in BCR-ABL-positive B-ALL, suggesting that these two varieties of aggressive leukemia have a similar pathogenic basis.

Understanding of the pathogenesis of CML has led to the use of drugs that target BCR-ABL. Treatment with BCR-ABL inhibitors results in sustained hematologic remissions in greater than 90% of patients, with generally tolerable side effects. These inhibitors markedly decrease the number of BCR-ABL-positive cells in the marrow and elsewhere, but do not extinguish the CML "stem cell," which persists at low levels. As a result, it is not clear if BCR-ABL inhibitors are ever truly curative. However, this form of targeted therapy controls blood counts and substantially decreases the risk of transformation to the accelerated phase and blast crisis, which is the greatest threat to the patient. It may be that by lowering the proliferative drive of the BCR-ABL-positive progenitors, BCR-ABL inhibitors decrease the rate at which these cells acquire mutations that lead to disease progression.

The other major threat to the patient is the emergence of resistance to first generation BCR-ABL inhibitors, which in about 50% of cases stems from mutations in BCR-ABL and in the remaining cases mutations in other kinases. This problem has been overcome in part by development of second and third generation kinase inhibitors that are active against mutated forms of BCR-ABL. For relatively young patients, hematopoietic stem cell transplantation performed in the stable phase is curative in about 75% of cases. The outlook is less favorable once the accelerated phase or blast crisis supervenes, as transplantation and treatment with BCR-ABL inhibitors are both less effective in these settings.

Polycythemia Vera

Polycythemia vera is strongly associated with activating point mutations in the tyrosine kinase JAK2. Polycythemia vera (PCV) is characterized by increased marrow production of red cells, granulocytes, and platelets (panmyelosis), but it is the increase in red cells (polycythemia) that is responsible for most of the clinical symptoms. PCV must be differentiated from relative polycythemia resulting from hemoconcentration and other causes of absolute polycythemia (Chapter 14).

Pathogenesis. **JAK2 participates in the JAK/ STAT pathway, which lies downstream of multiple hematopoietic growth factor receptors, including the erythropoietin receptor.** In PCV the transformed progenitor cells have markedly decreased requirements for erythropoietin and other hematopoietic growth factors due to constitutive JAK2 signaling. Accordingly, serum erythropoietin levels in PCV are low, whereas secondary forms of polycythemia have high erythropoietin levels. The elevated hematocrit leads to increased blood viscosity and sludging. These hemodynamic factors, together with thrombocytosis and abnormal platelet function, make patients with PCV prone to both thrombosis and bleeding.

More than 97% of cases are associated with a mutation in *JAK2* that results in a valine-to-phenylalanine substitution at residue 617; other *JAK2* mutations are found in most (and perhaps all) of the remaining cases. The mutated forms of JAK2 found in PCV render hematopoietic cell lines growth factor-independent, and when expressed in murine bone marrow progenitors cause a PCV-like syndrome that is associated with marrow fibrosis. In 25% to 30% of cases the tumor cells contain two mutated copies of *JAK2*, a genotype that is associated with higher white cell counts, more significant splenomegaly, symptomatic pruritus, and a greater rate of progression to the spent phase.

The proliferative drive in PCV (and other myeloproliferative disorders associated with JAK2 mutations) is less than in CML, which is associated with more pronounced marrow hypercellularity, leukocytosis, and splenomegaly. Presumably, JAK2 signals are quantitatively weaker or qualitatively different from those produced by BCR-ABL (Fig. 13-32).

MORPHOLOGY

The marrow is hypercellular, but some residual fat is usually present. **The increase in red cell progenitors is subtle and usually accompanied by an increase in granulocytic precursors and megakaryocytes as well.** At diagnosis, a moderate to marked increase in reticulin fibers is seen in about 10% of marrows. Mild organomegaly is common, being caused early in the course largely by congestion; at this stage extramedullary hematopoiesis is minimal. The peripheral blood often contains increased numbers of basophils and abnormally large platelets.

Late in the course, PCV often progresses to a **spent phase** characterized by extensive marrow fibrosis that displaces hematopoietic cells. This is accompanied by increased extramedullary hematopoiesis in the spleen and liver, often leading to prominent organomegaly (Fig. 13-35). Transformation to AML, with its typical features, occurs in about 1% of patients.

Clinical Features. PCV is uncommon, having an incidence of 1 to 3 per 100,000 per year. It appears insidiously, usually in adults of late middle age. Most symptoms are related to the increased red cell mass and hematocrit. Usually, there is also an increased total blood volume. Together, these factors cause abnormal blood flow, particularly on the low-pressure venous side of the circulation, which becomes greatly distended. Patients are plethoric and cyanotic due to stagnation and deoxygenation of blood in peripheral vessels. Headache, dizziness, hypertension, and gastrointestinal symptoms are common. Intense pruritus and peptic ulceration may occur, both possibly resulting from the release of histamine from basophils. High cell turnover gives rise to hyperuricemia; symptomatic gout is seen in 5% to 10% of cases.

More ominously, the abnormal blood flow and platelet function lead to an increased risk of both major bleeding and thrombotic episodes. About 25% of patients first come to attention due to deep venous thrombosis, myocardial infarction, or stroke. Thromboses sometimes also occur in the hepatic veins (producing Budd-Chiari syndrome) and the portal and mesenteric veins (leading to bowel infarction). It should be remembered that thrombotic complications sometimes precede the appearance of the typical hematologic findings. Minor hemorrhages (epistaxis, bleeding gums) are common, and life-threatening hemorrhages occur in 5% to 10% of cases.

The hemoglobin concentration ranges from 14 to 28 gm/dL, and the hematocrit is usually 60% or more. Sometimes chronic bleeding leads to iron deficiency, which can suppress erythropoiesis sufficiently to lower the hematocrit into the normal range, an example of two defects counteracting one another to "correct" a laboratory abnormality. The white cell count ranges from 12,000 to 50,000 cells/mm^3, and the platelet count is often greater than 500,000 platelets/mm^3. The platelets usually exhibit morphologic abnormalities such as giant forms and are often defective in functional aggregation studies.

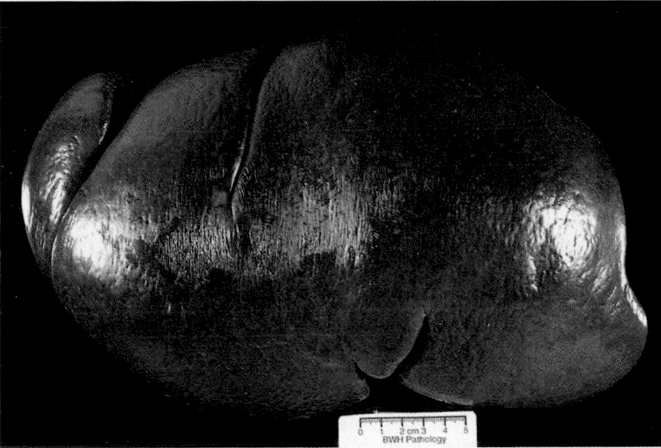

Figure 13-35 Polycythemia vera, spent phase. Massive splenomegaly (3020 gm; normal: 150 to 200 gm) largely due to extramedullary hematopoiesis occurring in the setting of advanced marrow myelofibrosis. (Courtesy Dr. Mark Fleming, Department of Pathology, Children's Hospital, Boston, Mass.)

Without treatment, death from bleeding or thrombosis occurs within months of diagnosis. However, simply maintaining the red cell mass at nearly normal levels by phlebotomy extends the median survival to about 10 years. JAK2 inhibitors are in preclinical development and represent a promising form of targeted therapy.

Extended survival with treatment has revealed that PCV tends to evolve to a "spent phase," during which clinical and anatomic features of primary myelofibrosis develop. The disease undergoes this transition in about 15% to 20% of patients after an average period of 10 years. It is marked by the appearance of obliterative fibrosis in the bone marrow (myelofibrosis) and extensive extramedullary hematopoiesis, principally in the spleen, which enlarges greatly. The mechanisms underlying the progression to the spent phase are not known.

In about 2% of patients, PCV transforms to AML. Surprisingly, the AML clone often lacks *JAK2* mutations, suggesting that the causative *JAK2* mutations occur in an abnormal stem cell that already harbors potentially oncogenic mutations, and therefore is "at risk" for giving rise to several different myeloid tumors. Unlike CML, transformation to ALL is rarely observed, consistent with the cell of origin being a progenitor committed to myeloid differentiation.

Essential Thrombocytosis

Essential thrombocytosis (ET) is often associated with activating point mutations in JAK2 (50% of cases) or MPL (5% to 10% of cases), a receptor tyrosine kinase that is normally activated by thrombopoietin. In addition, recent DNA sequencing studies have revealed that most of the remaining cases have mutations in calreticulin, a protein with several described functions in the endoplasmic reticulum and the cytoplasm. Since JAK2 and calreticulin mutations are mutually exclusive, it is hypothesized that the calreticulin mutations also increase JAK-STAT signaling through currently unknown mechanisms.

ET manifests clinically with elevated platelet counts and is separated from PCV and primary myelofibrosis based on the absence of polycythemia and marrow fibrosis, respectively. In those cases without tyrosine kinase mutations, causes of reactive thrombocytosis, such as inflammatory disorders and iron deficiency, must be excluded before the diagnosis can be established.

Constitutive JAK2 or MPL signaling renders the progenitors thrombopoietin-independent and leads to hyperproliferation. The *JAK2* mutation is the same as that found in almost all cases of PCV. Why some patients with *JAK2* mutations present with PCV and others with ET is not understood. Some cases of "ET" may in fact be PCV disguised by iron deficiency (which is more common in individuals diagnosed with ET), but this is probably true of only a small fraction of patients. As mentioned, most cases without JAK2 or MPL mutations have calreticulin mutations instead.

Bone marrow cellularity is usually only mildly increased, but megakaryocytes are often markedly increased in

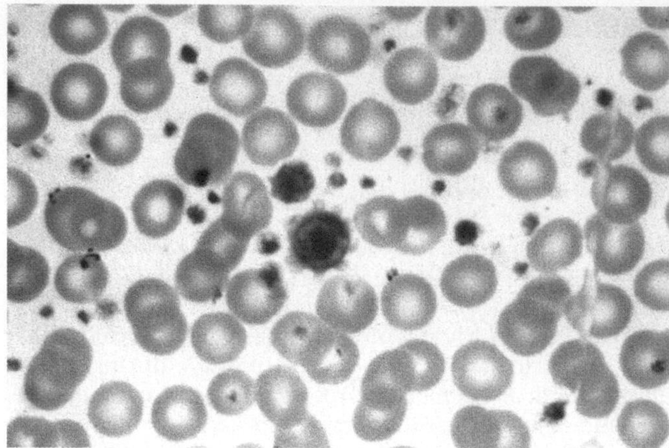

Figure 13-36 Essential thrombocytosis. Peripheral blood smear shows marked thrombocytosis, including giant platelets approximating the size of surrounding red cells.

number and include abnormally large forms. Delicate reticulin fibrils are often seen, but the overt fibrosis of primary myelofibrosis (see later) is absent. Peripheral smears usually reveal abnormally large platelets (Fig. 13-36), often accompanied by mild leukocytosis. Modest degrees of extramedullary hematopoiesis may occur, producing mild organomegaly in about 50% of patients. Uncommonly, a spent phase of marrow fibrosis or transformation to AML supervenes.

The incidence of ET is 1 to 3 per 100,000 per year. It usually occurs past the age of 60 but may also be seen in young adults. Dysfunctions of platelets derived from the neoplastic clone can lead to thrombosis and hemorrhage, the major clinical manifestations. Platelets are not only increased in numbers but also frequently demonstrate qualitative abnormalities in functional tests. The types of thrombotic events resemble those observed in PCV; they include deep venous thrombosis, portal and hepatic vein thrombosis, and myocardial infarction. One characteristic symptom is *erythromelalgia*, a throbbing and burning of hands and feet caused by occlusion of small arterioles by platelet aggregates, which may also be seen in PCV.

ET is an indolent disorder with long asymptomatic periods punctuated by occasional thrombotic or hemorrhagic crises. Median survival times are 12 to 15 years. Thrombotic complications are most likely in patients with very high platelet counts and homozygous *JAK2* mutations. Therapy consists of "gentle" chemotherapeutic agents that suppress thrombopoiesis.

Primary Myelofibrosis

The hallmark of primary myelofibrosis is the development of obliterative marrow fibrosis. The replacement of the marrow by fibrous tissue reduces bone marrow hematopoiesis, leading to cytopenias and extensive extramedullary hematopoiesis. Histologically, the appearance is identical to the spent phase that occurs occasionally late in the course of other myeloproliferative disorders. This similarity also extends to the underlying pathogenesis.

Activating JAK2 mutations are present in 50% to 60% of cases and activating MPL mutations in an additional 1% to 5% of cases of primary myelofibrosis. As with ET, most of the remaining cases have been recently observed to have mutations in calreticulin that are hypothesized to give rise to increased JAK-STAT signaling.

The chief pathologic feature is the extensive deposition of collagen in the marrow by non-neoplastic fibroblasts. The fibrosis inexorably displaces hematopoietic elements, including stem cells, from the marrow and eventually leads to marrow failure. It is probably caused by the inappropriate release of fibrogenic factors from neoplastic megakaryocytes. Two factors synthesized by megakaryocytes have been implicated: *platelet-derived growth factor* and *TGF-β*. As you recall, platelet-derived growth factor and TGF-β are fibroblast mitogens. In addition, TGF-β promotes collagen deposition and causes angiogenesis, both of which are observed in myelofibrosis.

As marrow fibrosis progresses, circulating hematopoietic stem cells take up residence in niches in secondary hematopoietic organs, such as the spleen, the liver, and the lymph nodes, leading to the appearance of extramedullary hematopoiesis. For incompletely understood reasons, red cell production at extramedullary sites is disordered. This factor and the concomitant suppression of marrow function result in moderate to severe anemia. It is not clear whether primary myelofibrosis is truly distinct from PCV and ET, or merely reflects unusually rapid progression to the spent phase.

MORPHOLOGY

Early in the course, the marrow is often hypercellular due to increases in maturing cells of all lineages, a feature reminiscent of PCV. Morphologically, the erythroid and granulocytic precursors appear normal, but megakaryocytes are large, dysplastic, and abnormally clustered. At this stage fibrosis is minimal, and the blood may show leukocytosis and thrombocytosis. **With progression, the marrow becomes more hypocellular and diffusely fibrotic.** Clusters of atypical megakaryocytes with unusual nuclear shapes (described as "cloud-like") are seen, and hematopoietic elements are often found within dilated sinusoids, which is a manifestation of severe architectural distortion cause by the fibrosis. Very late in the course, the fibrotic marrow space may be converted into bone, a change called "osteosclerosis." These features are identical to those seen in the spent phase of other myeloproliferative disorders.

Fibrotic obliteration of the marrow space leads to extensive extramedullary hematopoiesis, principally in the spleen, which is usually markedly enlarged, sometimes up to 4000 gm. Grossly, such spleens are firm and diffusely red to gray. As in CML, subcapsular infarcts are common (see Fig. 13-40). Initially, extramedullary hematopoiesis is confined to the sinusoids, but later it expands into the cords. The liver may be enlarged moderately by sinusoidal foci of extramedullary hematopoiesis. Hematopoiesis can also appear within lymph nodes, but significant lymphadenopathy is uncommon.

The marrow fibrosis is reflected in several characteristic blood findings (Fig. 13-37). Marrow distortion leads to the premature release of nucleated erythroid and early granulocyte progenitors (**leukoerythroblastosis**), and immature cells also enter the circulation from sites of extramedullary hematopoiesis. **Teardrop-shaped red cells** (dacryocytes), cells that were probably damaged during the birthing process in the fibrotic marrow, are also often seen. Although characteristic of primary

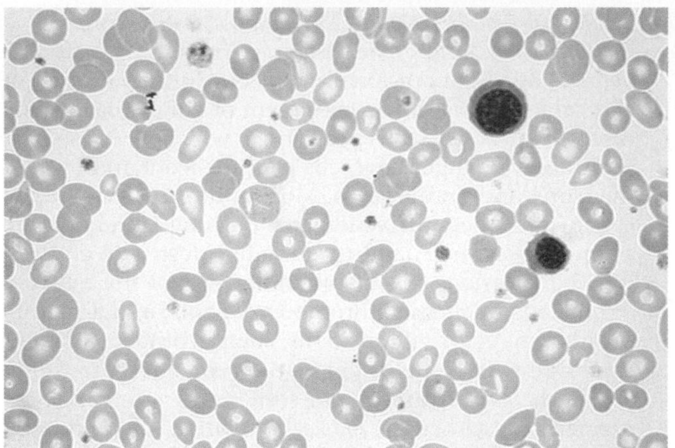

Figure 13-37 Primary myelofibrosis (peripheral blood smear). Two nucleated erythroid precursors and several teardrop-shaped red cells (dacryocytes) are evident. Immature myeloid cells were present in other fields. An identical picture can be seen in other diseases producing marrow distortion and fibrosis.

myelofibrosis, leukoerythroblastosis and teardrop red cells are seen in many infiltrative disorders of the marrow, including granulomatous diseases and metastatic tumors. Other common, albeit nonspecific, blood findings include abnormally large platelets and basophilia.

Clinical Features. Primary myelofibrosis is less common than PCV and ET and usually occurs in individuals older than 60 years of age. Except when preceded by another myeloproliferative disorder, it comes to attention because of progressive anemia and splenomegaly, which produces a sensation of fullness in the left upper quadrant. Nonspecific symptoms such as fatigue, weight loss, and night sweats result from an increase in metabolism associated with the expanding mass of hematopoietic cells. Hyperuricemia and secondary gout due to a high rate of cell turnover can complicate the picture.

Laboratory studies typically show a moderate to severe normochromic normocytic anemia accompanied by leukoerythroblastosis. The white cell count is usually normal or mildly reduced, but can be markedly elevated (80,000 to 100,000 cells/mm^3) early in the course. The platelet count is usually normal or elevated at the time of diagnosis, but thrombocytopenia may supervene as the disease progresses. These blood findings are not specific; bone marrow biopsy is essential for diagnosis.

Primary myelofibrosis is a much more difficult disease to treat than PCV or ET. The course is variable, but the median survival is in the range of 3 to 5 years. Threats to life include intercurrent infections, thrombotic episodes, bleeding related to platelet abnormalities, and transformation to AML, which occurs in 5% to 20% of cases. When myelofibrosis is extensive, AML sometimes arises at extramedullary sites, including lymph nodes and soft tissues. JAK2 inhibitors have recently been approved to treat this disease and are effective at decreasing the splenomegaly and constitutional symptoms. Hematopoietic stem cell transplantation offers some hope for cure in those young and fit enough to withstand the procedure.

KEY CONCEPTS

Myeloid Neoplasms

Myeloid tumors occur mainly in adults and fall into three major groups:

Acute myeloid leukemias (AMLs)

- Aggressive tumors comprised of immature myeloid lineage blasts, which replace the marrow and suppress normal hematopoiesis
- Associated with diverse acquired mutations that lead to expression of abnormal transcription factors, which interfere with myeloid differentiation
- Often also associated with mutations in genes encoding growth factor receptor signaling pathway components or regulators of the epigenome

Myeloproliferative disorders

- Myeloid tumors in which production of formed myeloid elements is initially increased, leading to high blood counts and extramedullary hematopoiesis
- Commonly associated with acquired mutations that lead to constitutive activation of tyrosine kinases, which mimic signals from normal growth factors. The most common pathogenic kinases are BCR-ABL (associated with CML) and mutated JAK2 (associated with polycythemia vera and primary myelofibrosis).
- All can transform to acute leukemia and to a spent phase of marrow fibrosis associated with anemia, thrombocytopenia, and splenomegaly.

Myelodysplastic Syndromes

- Poorly understood myeloid tumors characterized by disordered and ineffective hematopoiesis and dysmaturation
- Recently shown to frequently harbor mutations in splicing factors and epigenetic regulators
- Manifest with one or more cytopenias and progress in 10% to 40% of cases to AML

Langerhans Cell Histiocytosis

The term *histiocytosis* is an "umbrella" designation for a variety of proliferative disorders of dendritic cells or macrophages. Some, such as rare "histiocytic" lymphomas, are clearly malignant, whereas others, such as reactive proliferations of macrophages in lymph nodes, are clearly benign. Lying between these two extremes are the Langerhans cell histiocytoses, a spectrum of proliferations of a special type of immature dendritic cell called the Langerhans cell (Chapter 6).

The origin and nature of the proliferating cells in Langerhans cell histiocytosis has been controversial, leading to discussion of whether it is better considered a neoplasm or a reactive process. Recent sequencing has largely settled this score, as the majority of cases have mutations that are known to be oncogenic in other contexts. The most common mutation is an activating valine-to-glutamate substitution at residue 600 in BRAF, already discussed for its role in hairy cell leukemia, which is present in 55% to 60% of cases. Less common mutations have also been detected in TP53, RAS, and the tyrosine kinase MET. Thus, there seems no doubt that many of these proliferations are neoplastic in origin.

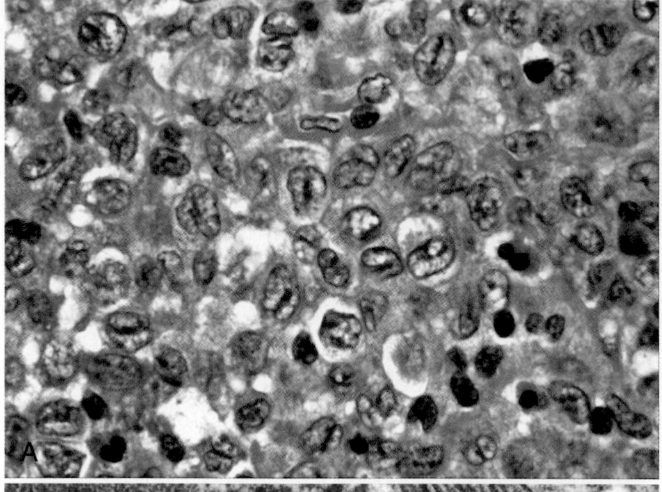

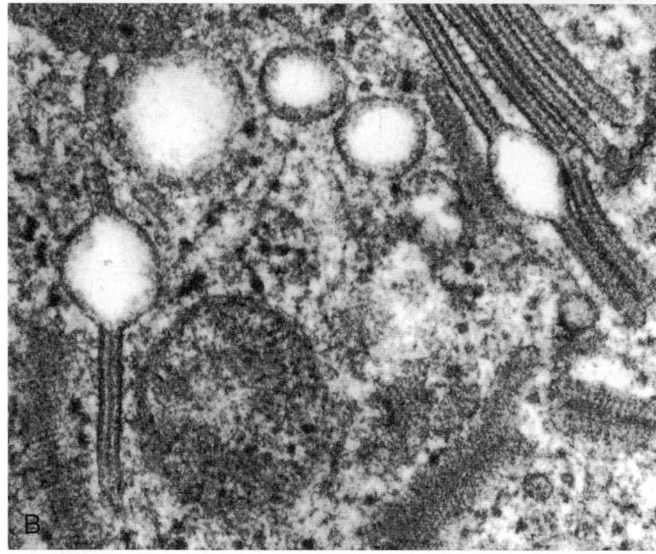

Figure 13-38 Langerhans cell histiocytosis. **A,** Langerhans cells with folded or grooved nuclei and moderately abundant pale cytoplasm are mixed with a few eosinophils. **B,** An electron micrograph shows rodlike Birbeck granules with characteristic periodicity and dilated terminal end. (**B,** Courtesy Dr. George Murphy, Department of Pathology, Brigham and Women's Hospital, Boston, Mass.)

Regardless of the clinical picture, the proliferating Langerhans cells have abundant, often vacuolated cytoplasm and vesicular nuclei containing linear grooves or folds (Fig. 13-38*A*). The presence of *Birbeck granules* in the cytoplasm is characteristic. Birbeck granules are pentalaminar tubules, often with a dilated terminal end producing a tennis racket-like appearance (Fig. 13-38*B*), which contain the protein langerin. In addition, the tumor cells also typically express HLA-DR, S-100, and CD1a.

Langerhans cell histiocytosis presents as several clinicopathologic entities:

- *Multifocal multisystem Langerhans cell histiocytosis (Letterer-Siwe disease)* occurs most frequently before 2 years of age but occasionally affects adults. A dominant clinical feature is the development of cutaneous lesions resembling a seborrheic eruption, which is caused by infiltrates of Langerhans cells over the front and back of the trunk and on the scalp. Most of those affected have concurrent hepatosplenomegaly, lymphadenopathy, pulmonary lesions, and (eventually) destructive osteolytic bone lesions. Extensive infiltration of the marrow often leads to anemia, thrombocytopenia, and a predisposition to recurrent infections, such as otitis media and mastoiditis. In some instances the tumor cells are quite anaplastic; such tumors are sometimes referred to as Langerhans cell sarcoma. The course of untreated disease is rapidly fatal. With intensive chemotherapy, 50% of patients survive 5 years.
- *Unifocal and multifocal unisystem Langerhans cell histiocytosis (eosinophilic granuloma)* is characterized by proliferations of Langerhans cells admixed with variable numbers of eosinophils, lymphocytes, plasma cells, and neutrophils. Eosinophils are usually, but not always, a prominent component of the infiltrate. It typically arises within the medullary cavities of bones, most commonly the calvarium, ribs, and femur. Less commonly, unisystem lesions of identical histology arise in the skin, lungs, or stomach. *Unifocal lesions* most commonly affect the skeletal system in older children or adults. Bone lesions can be asymptomatic or cause pain, tenderness, and, in some instances, pathologic fractures. Unifocal disease is indolent and may heal spontaneously or be cured by local excision or irradiation. *Multifocal unisystem disease* usually affects young children, who present with multiple erosive bony masses that sometimes expand into adjacent soft tissue. Involvement of the posterior pituitary stalk of the hypothalamus leads to diabetes insipidus in about 50% of patients. The combination of calvarial bone defects, diabetes insipidus, and exophthalmos is referred to as the *Hand-Schüller-Christian* triad. Many patients experience spontaneous regression; others can be treated successfully with chemotherapy.
- *Pulmonary Langerhans cell histiocytosis* represents a special category of disease, most often seen in adult smokers, which may regress spontaneously upon cessation of smoking. These lesions have been described as reactive proliferations of Langerhans cells, but fully 40% are associated with BRAF mutations, suggesting that in many instances, they too are neoplastic in origin.

One factor that contributes to the homing of neoplastic Langerhans cells is the aberrant expression of chemokine receptors. For example, while normal epidermal Langerhans cells express CCR6, their neoplastic counterparts express both CCR6 and CCR7. This allows the neoplastic cells to migrate into tissues that express the relevant chemokines—CCL20 (a ligand for CCR6) in skin and bone, and CCL19 and 21 (ligands for CCR7) in lymphoid organs.

SPLEEN

The spleen is an ingeniously designed filter for the blood and a site of immune responses to blood-borne antigens. Normally in the adult it weighs about 150 gm and is enclosed within a thin, glistening, slate-gray connective tissue capsule. Its cut surface reveals extensive red pulp dotted with gray specks, which are the white pulp follicles. These consist of an artery with an eccentric collar of T lymphocytes, the so-called periarteriolar lymphatic sheath. At intervals this sheath expands to form lymphoid nodules composed mainly of B lymphocytes, which are capable of developing into germinal centers identical to those seen in lymph nodes in response to antigenic stimulation (Fig. 13-39).

The red pulp of the spleen is traversed by numerous thin-walled vascular sinusoids, separated by the splenic cords or "cords of Billroth." The endothelial lining of the sinusoid is discontinuous, providing a passage for blood cells between the sinusoids and cords. The cords contain a labyrinth of macrophages loosely connected through long dendritic processes to create both a physical and a functional filter. As it traverses the red pulp, the blood takes two routes to reach the splenic veins. Some flows through capillaries into the cords, from which blood cells squeeze through gaps in the discontinuous basement of the endothelial lining to reach the sinusoids; this is the so-called open circulation or slow compartment. In the other "closed circuit," blood passes rapidly and directly from the capillaries to the splenic veins. Although only a small fraction of the blood pursues the "open" route, during the course of a day the entire blood volume passes through the cords, where it is closely examined by macrophages.

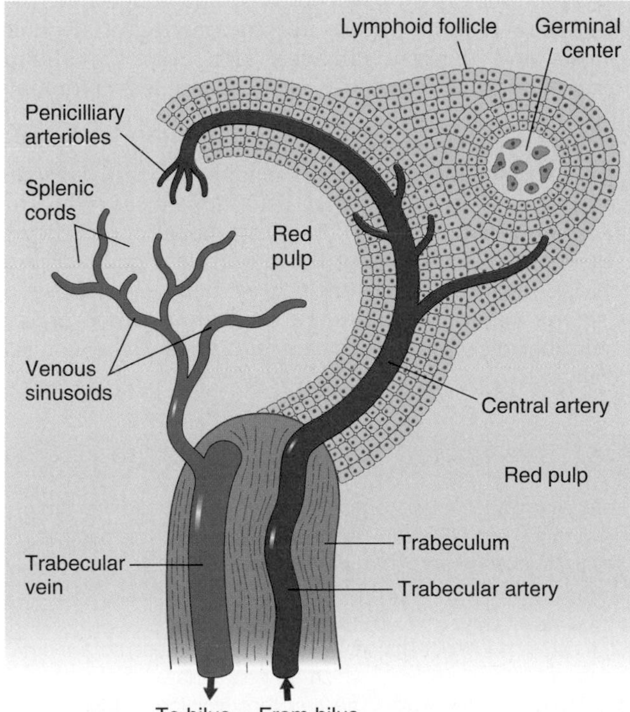

Figure 13-39 Normal splenic architecture. (Modified from Faller DV: Diseases of the spleen. In Wyngaarden JB, Smith LH (eds): *Cecil Textbook of Medicine*, 18th ed. Philadelphia, WB Saunders, 1988, p 1036.)

The spleen has four functions that impact disease states:

1. *Phagocytosis of blood cells and particulate matter.* As is discussed under the hemolytic anemias (Chapter 14), red cells undergo extreme deformation during passage from the cords into the sinusoids. In conditions in which red cell deformability is decreased, red cells become trapped in the cords and are more readily phagocytosed by macrophages. Splenic macrophages are also responsible for "pitting" of red cells, the process by which inclusions such as *Heinz bodies* and *Howell-Jolly bodies* are excised, and for the removal of particles, such as bacteria, from the blood.
2. *Antibody production.* Dendritic cells in the periarterial lymphatic sheath trap antigens and present them to T lymphocytes. T- and B-cell interaction at the edges of white pulp follicles leads to the generation of antibody-secreting plasma cells, which are found mainly within the sinuses of the red pulp. The spleen seems to be an important site of production of antibodies against microbial polysaccharides, as well as autoantibodies against a variety of self antigens.
3. *Hematopoiesis.* During fetal development, the spleen may be a minor site of hematopoiesis, but this normally disappears by birth. However, the spleen can become a major site of compensatory extramedullary hematopoiesis in the setting of severe chronic anemia (e.g., in patients with thalassemia, described in Chapter 14) and in patients with myeloproliferative disorders, such as chronic myelogenous leukemia and primary myelofibrosis.
4. *Sequestration of formed blood elements.* The normal spleen contains only about 30 to 40 mL of red cells, but this volume increases greatly with splenomegaly. The normal spleen also harbors approximately 30% to 40% of the total platelet mass in the body. With splenomegaly up to 80% to 90% of the total platelet mass can be sequestered in the interstices of the red pulp, producing thrombocytopenia. Similarly, the enlarged spleen can trap white cells and thereby induce leukopenia.

As the largest unit of the mononuclear phagocyte system, the spleen is involved in all systemic inflammations, generalized hematopoietic disorders, and many metabolic disturbances. In each, the spleen undergoes enlargement *(splenomegaly)*, which is the major manifestation of disorders of this organ. It is rarely the primary site of disease. Splenic insufficiency due to splenectomy or autoinfarction (as in sickle-cell disease) has one major clinical manifestation, an increased susceptibility to sepsis cause by encapsulated bacteria such as pneumococci, meningococci, and *Haemophilus influenzae*. The decrease in phagocytic capacity and antibody production that result from asplenia both contribute to the increased risk of sepsis, which may be fatal. All asplenic individuals should be vaccinated against these agents to reduce the risk of this tragic complication.

Splenomegaly

When sufficiently enlarged, the spleen causes a dragging sensation in the left upper quadrant and, through pressure on the stomach, discomfort after eating. In addition, enlargement can cause a syndrome known as *hypersplenism*, which is characterized by anemia, leukopenia, thrombocytopenia, alone or in combination. The probable cause of the cytopenias is increased sequestration of formed elements and the consequent enhanced phagocytosis by the splenic macrophages.

Table 13-12 lists major disorders associated with splenomegaly. Splenomegaly in virtually all the conditions mentioned has been discussed elsewhere. A few disorders are left to consider.

Nonspecific Acute Splenitis

Enlargement of the spleen occurs in any blood-borne infection. The nonspecific splenic reaction in these infections is caused both by the microbiologic agents themselves and by cytokines that are released as part of the immune response.

Table 13-12 Disorders Associated with Splenomegaly

I. Infections
Nonspecific splenitis of various blood-borne infections (particularly infectious endocarditis)
Infectious mononucleosis
Tuberculosis
Typhoid fever
Brucellosis
Cytomegalovirus
Syphilis
Malaria
Histoplasmosis
Toxoplasmosis
Kala-azar
Trypanosomiasis
Schistosomiasis
Leishmaniasis
Echinococcosis
II. Congestive States Related to Portal Hypertension
Cirrhosis of the liver
Portal or splenic vein thrombosis
Cardiac failure
III. Lymphohematogenous Disorders
Hodgkin lymphoma
Non-Hodgkin lymphomas and lymphocytic leukemias
Multiple myeloma
Myeloproliferative disorders
Hemolytic anemias
IV. Immunologic-Inflammatory Conditions
Rheumatoid arthritis
Systemic lupus erythematosus
V. Storage Diseases
Gaucher disease
Niemann-Pick disease
Mucopolysaccharidoses
VI. Miscellaneous Disorders
Amyloidosis
Primary neoplasms and cysts
Secondary neoplasms

MORPHOLOGY

The spleen is enlarged (200 to 400 gm) and soft. Microscopically, the major feature is acute congestion of the red pulp, which may encroach on and virtually efface the lymphoid follicles. Neutrophils, plasma cells, and occasionally eosinophils are usually present throughout the white and red pulp. At times the white pulp follicles may undergo necrosis, particularly when the causative agent is a hemolytic streptococcus. Rarely, abscess formation occurs.

Congestive Splenomegaly

Chronic venous outflow obstruction causes a form of splenic enlargement referred to as *congestive splenomegaly*. Venous obstruction may be caused by intrahepatic disorders that retard portal venous drainage, or arise from extrahepatic disorders that directly impinge upon the portal or splenic veins. All of these disorders ultimately lead to portal or splenic vein hypertension. *Systemic, or central, venous congestion* is encountered in cardiac decompensation involving the right side of the heart, as can occur in tricuspid or pulmonic valvular disease, chronic cor pulmonale, or following left-sided heart failure. Systemic congestion is associated with only moderately enlarged spleens that rarely exceed 500 gm in weight.

Cirrhosis of the liver is the main cause of massive congestive splenomegaly. The "pipe-stem" hepatic fibrosis of schistosomiasis causes particularly severe congestive splenomegaly, while the diffuse fibrous scarring of alcoholic cirrhosis and pigment cirrhosis also evokes profound enlargements. Other forms of cirrhosis are less commonly implicated.

Congestive splenomegaly is also caused by obstruction of the extrahepatic portal vein or splenic vein. This can stem from *spontaneous portal vein thrombosis*, which is usually associated with some intrahepatic obstructive disease, or inflammation of the portal vein *(pylephlebitis)*, such as follows intraperitoneal infections. Thrombosis of the splenic vein can be caused by infiltrating tumors arising in neighboring organs, such as carcinomas of the stomach or pancreas.

MORPHOLOGY

Long-standing splenic congestion produces marked enlargement (1000 to 5000 gm). The organ is firm, and the capsule is usually thickened and fibrous. Microscopically, the red pulp is congested early in the course but becomes increasingly fibrotic and cellular with time. The elevated portal venous pressure stimulates the deposition of collagen in the basement membrane of the sinusoids, which appear dilated because of the rigidity of their walls. The resultant slowing of blood flow from the cords to the sinusoids prolongs the exposure of the blood cells to macrophages, resulting in excessive destruction (hypersplenism).

Splenic Infarcts

Splenic infarcts are common lesions caused by the occlusion of the major splenic artery or any of its branches. The lack of extensive collateral blood supply predisposes to infarction following vascular occlusion. The spleen, along with kidneys and brain, ranks as one of the most frequent sites where emboli lodge. In normal-sized spleens, infarcts are most often caused by emboli that arise from the heart. The infarcts can be small or large, single or multiple, or even involve the entire organ. They are usually bland, except in individuals with infectious endocarditis of the mitral or aortic valves, in whom septic infarcts are common. Infarcts are also common in markedly enlarged spleens, regardless of cause, presumably because the blood supply is tenuous and easily compromised.

MORPHOLOGY

Bland infarcts are characteristically pale, wedge-shaped, and subcapsular in location. The overlying capsule is often covered with fibrin (Fig. 13-40). In septic infarcts this appearance is modified by the development of suppurative necrosis. In the course of healing, large depressed scars often develop.

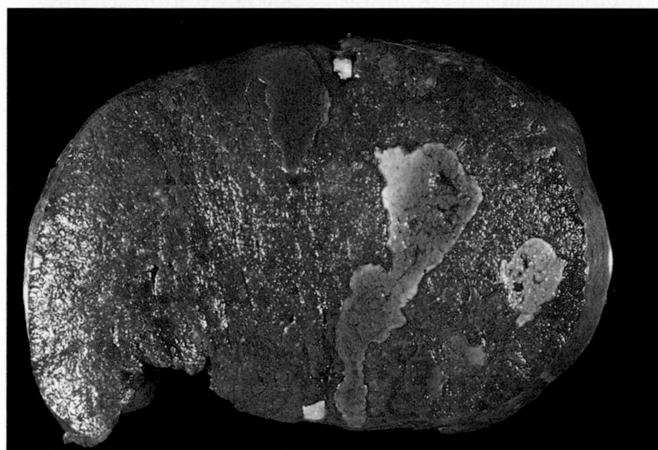

Figure 13-40 Splenic infarcts. Multiple well-circumscribed infarcts are present in this spleen, which is massively enlarged (2820 gm; normal: 150 to 200 gm) by extramedullary hematopoiesis secondary to a myeloproliferative disorder (myelofibrosis). Recent infarcts are hemorrhagic, whereas older, more fibrotic infarcts are a pale yellow-gray color.

Neoplasms

Neoplastic involvement of the spleen is rare except in myeloid and lymphoid tumors, which often cause splenomegaly (discussed earlier). Benign fibromas, osteomas, chondromas, lymphangiomas, and hemangiomas may arise in the spleen. Of these, lymphangiomas and hemangiomas are most common and often cavernous in type.

Congenital Anomalies

Complete absence of the spleen is rare and is usually associated with other congenital abnormalities, such as situs inversus and cardiac malformations. *Hypoplasia* is a more common finding.

Accessory spleens (spleniculi) are common, being present singly or multiply in 20% to 35% of postmortem examinations. They are small, spherical structures that are histologically and functionally identical to the normal spleen. They can be found at any place within the abdominal cavity. Accessory spleens are of great clinical importance in some hematologic disorders, such as hereditary spherocytosis and immune thrombocytopenia purpura, where splenectomy is used as a treatment. If an accessory spleen is overlooked, the therapeutic benefit of removal of the definitive spleen may be reduced or lost entirely.

Rupture

Splenic rupture is usually precipitated by blunt trauma. Much less often, it occurs in the apparent absence of a physical blow. Such "spontaneous ruptures" never involve truly normal spleens but rather stem from some minor physical insult to a spleen made fragile by an underlying condition. The most common predisposing conditions are infectious mononucleosis, malaria, typhoid fever, and lymphoid neoplasms, which may cause the spleen to enlarge rapidly, producing a thin, tense capsule that is susceptible to rupture. This dramatic event often precipitates intraperitoneal hemorrhage, which must be treated by prompt splenectomy to prevent death from blood loss. Chronically enlarged spleens are unlikely to rupture because of the toughening effect of extensive reactive fibrosis.

THYMUS

Once an organ buried in obscurity, the thymus now has a starring role in cell-mediated immunity (Chapter 6). Here, our interest centers on the disorders of the gland itself.

The thymus is embryologically derived from the third and, inconstantly, the fourth pair of pharyngeal pouches. At birth it weighs 10 to 35 gm. It grows until puberty, when it achieves a maximum weight of 20 to 50 gm, and thereafter undergoes progressive involution to little more than 5 to 15 gm in older adults. The thymus can also involute in children and young adults in response to severe illness and HIV infection.

The fully developed thymus is composed of two fused, well-encapsulated lobes. Fibrous extensions of the capsule divide each lobe into numerous lobules, each with an outer cortical layer enclosing the central medulla. Diverse types of cells populate the thymus, but thymic epithelial cells and immature T lymphocytes, also called thymocytes, predominate. The cortical, peripheral, epithelial cells are polygonal in shape and have an abundant cytoplasm with dendritic extensions that contact adjacent cells. In contrast, the epithelial cells in the medulla are densely packed, often spindle-shaped, and have scant cytoplasm devoid of interconnecting processes. Whorls of medullary epithelial cells create *Hassall corpuscles,* with their characteristic keratinized cores.

As you know from the earlier consideration of the thymus in relation to immunity, progenitor cells migrate from the marrow to the thymus and mature into T cells, which are exported to the periphery, but only after they have been educated in the "thymic university" to distinguish between self and non-self antigens. During adulthood the thymic production of T cells slowly declines as the organ atrophies.

Macrophages, dendritic cells, a minor population of B lymphocytes, rare neutrophils and eosinophils, and scattered myoid (muscle-like) cells are also found within the thymus. The myoid cells are of particular interest because of the suspicion that they play some role in the development of myasthenia gravis, a musculoskeletal disorder of immune origin.

Pathologic changes within the thymus are limited and will be described here. The changes associated with myasthenia gravis are considered in Chapter 27.

Developmental Disorders

Thymic hypoplasia or *aplasia* is seen in DiGeorge syndrome, which is marked by severe defects in cell-mediated immunity and variable abnormalities of parathyroid development associated with hypoparathyroidism. As discussed in Chapter 5, DiGeorge syndrome is often associated with other developmental defects as part of the 22q11 deletion syndrome.

Isolated *thymic cysts* are uncommon lesions that are usually discovered incidentally postmortem or during surgery. They rarely exceed 4 cm in diameter, can be spherical or arborizing, and are lined by stratified to columnar epithelium. The fluid contents can be serous or mucinous and are often modified by hemorrhage.

While isolated cysts are not clinically significant, neoplastic thymic masses (whatever their origin) compress and distort adjacent normal thymus and sometimes cause cysts to form. Therefore, the presence of a cystic thymic lesion in a symptomatic patient should provoke a thorough search for a neoplasm, particularly a lymphoma or a thymoma.

Thymic Hyperplasia

The term *thymic hyperplasia* is a bit misleading, since it usually applies to the appearance of B-cell germinal centers within the thymus, a finding that is referred to as *thymic follicular hyperplasia.* Such B-cell follicles are present in only small numbers in the normal thymus. Although follicular hyperplasia can occur in a number of chronic inflammatory and immunologic states, it is most frequently encountered in myasthenia gravis, in which it is found in 65% to 75% of cases (Chapter 27). Similar thymic changes are sometimes encountered in Graves disease, systemic lupus erythematosus, scleroderma, rheumatoid arthritis, and other autoimmune disorders.

In other instances, a morphologically normal thymus is simply large for the age of the patient. As mentioned, the size of the thymus varies widely, and whether this constitutes a true hyperplasia or is merely a variant of normal is unclear. The main significance of this form of thymic "hyperplasia" is that it may be mistaken radiologically for a thymoma, leading to unnecessary surgical procedures.

Thymomas

A diversity of neoplasms may arise in the thymus—germ cell tumors, lymphomas, carcinoids, and others—but **the designation "thymoma" is restricted to tumors of thymic epithelial cells.** Such tumors typically also contain benign immature T cells (thymocytes).

The WHO has created a classification system based on histology for thymomas, but its clinical utility remains uncertain. We will instead use a classification that relies on the most important prognostic features, the surgical stage and the presence or absence of overt cytologic features of

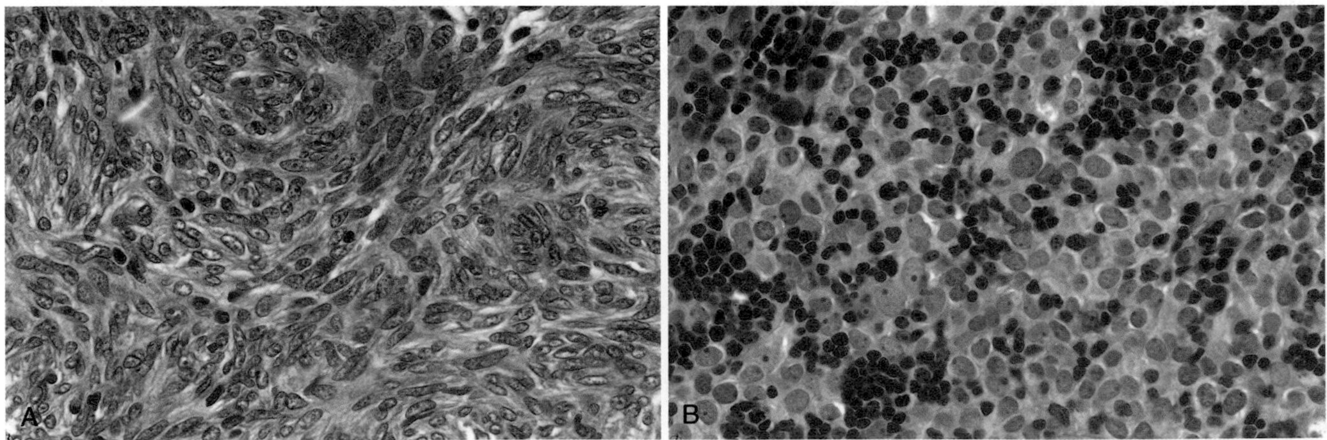

Figure 13-41 Thymoma. **A,** Benign thymoma (medullary type). The neoplastic epithelial cells are arranged in a swirling pattern and have bland, oval to elongated nuclei with inconspicuous nucleoli. Only a few small, reactive lymphoid cells are interspersed. **B,** Malignant thymoma, type I. The neoplastic epithelial cells are polygonal and have round to oval, bland nuclei with inconspicuous nucleoli. Numerous small, reactive lymphoid cells are interspersed. The morphologic appearance of this tumor is identical to that of benign thymomas of the cortical type. In this case, however, the tumor was locally aggressive, invading adjacent lung and pericardium.

malignancy. In this simple system there are only three histologic subtypes:

- Tumors that are cytologically benign and noninvasive
- Tumors that are cytologically benign but invasive or metastatic
- Tumors that are cytologically malignant (thymic carcinoma)

In all categories, the tumors usually occur in adults older than 40 years of age; thymomas are rare in children. Males and females are affected equally. Most arise in the anterior superior mediastinum, but sometimes they occur in the neck, thyroid, pulmonary hilus, or elsewhere. They are uncommon in the posterior mediastinum. Thymomas account for 20% to 30% of tumors in the anterosuperior mediastinum, which is also a common location for certain lymphomas.

MORPHOLOGY

Macroscopically, thymomas are lobulated, firm, gray-white masses of up to 15 to 20 cm in size. They sometimes have areas of cystic necrosis and calcification. Most are encapsulated, but 20% to 25% of the tumors penetrate the capsule and infiltrate perithymic tissues and structures.

Noninvasive thymomas are most often composed of medullary-type epithelial cells or a mixture of medullary and cortical type epithelial cells. The medullary type epithelial cells are elongated or spindle-shaped (Fig. 13-41*A*). There is usually a sparse infiltrate of thymocytes, which often recapitulate the phenotype of medullary thymocytes. In mixed thymomas there is an admixture of polygonal cortical type epithelial cells and a denser infiltrate of thymocytes. The medullary and mixed patterns together account for about 50% of all thymomas. Tumors that have a substantial proportion of medullary-type epithelial cells are usually noninvasive.

Invasive thymoma refers to a tumor that is cytologically benign but locally invasive. These tumors are much more likely to metastasize. The epithelial cells are most commonly of the cortical variety, with abundant cytoplasm and rounded vesicular nuclei (Fig. 13-41*B*), and are usually mixed with numerous thymocytes. In some cases, the neoplastic cells show cytologic atypia, a feature that correlates with a propensity for more aggressive behavior. These tumors account for about 20% to 25% of all thymomas. **By definition, invasive thymomas penetrate through the capsule into surrounding structures.** The extent of invasion has been subdivided into various stages, which are beyond our scope. With minimal invasion, complete excision yields a 5-year survival rate of greater than 90%, whereas extensive invasion is associated with a 5-year survival rate of less than 50%.

Thymic carcinoma represents about 5% of thymomas. Macroscopically, they are usually fleshy, obviously invasive masses, sometimes accompanied by metastases to sites such as the lungs. Microscopically, most are **squamous cell carcinomas**. The next most common variant is **lymphoepithelioma-like carcinoma**, a tumor composed of sheets of cells with indistinct borders that bears a close histologic resemblance to nasopharyngeal carcinoma. About 50% of lymphoepithelioma-like carcinomas contain monoclonal EBV genomes, consistent with a role for EBV in their pathogenesis. A variety of other less common histologic patterns of thymic carcinoma have been described; all exhibit cytologic atypia seen in other carcinomas.

Clinical Features. About 40% of thymomas present with symptoms stemming from impingement on mediastinal structures. Another 30% to 45% are detected in the course of evaluating patients with myasthenia gravis. The rest are discovered incidentally during imaging studies or cardiothoracic surgery. In addition to myasthenia gravis, other associated autoimmune disorders include hypogammaglobulinemia, pure red cell aplasia, Graves disease, pernicious anemia, dermatomyositis-polymyositis, and Cushing syndrome. The basis for these associations is still obscure, but the thymocytes that arise within thymomas give rise to long-lived CD4+ and CD8+ T cells, and cortical thymomas rich in thymocytes are more likely to be associated with autoimmune disease. Hence, it seems likely that abnormalities in the selection or "education" of T cells maturing within the environment of the neoplasm contribute to the development of diverse autoimmune disorders.

SUGGESTED READINGS

Hematopoietic Stem Cells

Rossi L, Lin KK, Boles NC, et al: Less is more: unveiling the functional core of hematopoietic stem cells through knockout mice. *Cell Stem Cell* 11:302, 2012. *[A summary of insights gained into genes that regulate HSC function through use of knockout mice.]*

Wang LD, Wagers AJ: Dynamic niches in the origination and differentiation of haematopoietic stem cells. *Nat Rev Mol Cell Biol* 12:643, 2011. *[A discussion of the nature and biology of the marrow stem cell niche.]*

White Cell Neoplasms

Badalian-Very G, Vergilio J-A, Fleming M, et al: Pathogenesis of Langerhans cell histiocytosis. *Annu Rev Pathol* epublished 8/6/2012. *[A comprehensive review of controversies and new insights into the pathogenesis of unusual tumor.]*

Jaffe ES, Harris NL, Stein H, et al: Classification of lymphoid neoplasms: the microscope as a tool for disease discovery. *Blood* 112:4384, 2008. *[An overview of the origins and utility of the most recent WHO classification of lymphoid neoplasms.]*

Kridel R, Sehn LH, Gascoyne RD: Pathogenesis of follicular lymphoma. *J Clin Invest* 122:3424, 2012. *[Discussion of new insights into the pathogenesis of this disease that have emerged from deep sequencing and expression profiling.]*

Lenz G, Staudt LM: Aggressive lymphomas. *N Engl J Med* 362:1417, 2010. *[An excellent brief review of the molecular origins of aggressive B cell lymphomas.]*

Lindsley RC, Ebert BL: Molecular pathophysiology of myelodysplastic syndromes. *Annu Rev Pathol* epublished 9/1/12. *[Update on the rapidly moving field of the molecular genetics of MDS.]*

Molyneux EM, Rochford R, Griffin B, et al: Burkitt's lymphoma. *Lancet* 379:1234, 2012. *[A review of the pathogenesis and treatment of Burkitt's lymphoma.]*

Palumbo A, Anderson KC: Multiple myeloma. *N Engl J Med* 364:1046, 2011. *[A review of the pathogenesis and treatment of multiple myeloma.]*

Patel JP, Gonen M, Figueroa ME, et al: Prognostic relevance of integrated genetic profiling in acute myeloid leukemia. *N Engl J Med* 366:1079, 2012. *[Landmark paper showing that focused deep sequencing of AML genomes can be used to predict outcome in patients treated with conventional chemotherapy.]*

Pui CH, Mullighan CG, Evans WE, et al: Pediatric acute lymphoblastic leukemia: where are we going and how do we get there. *Blood* 120:1165, 2012. *[A review of the pathogenesis, diagnosis, and treatment of ALL.]*

Schmitz R, Stanelle J, Hansmann ML, et al: Pathogenesis of classical and lymphocyte-predominant Hodgkin lymphoma. *Annu Rev Pathol* 4:151, 2009. *[A concise review of Hodgkin lymphoma pathogenesis.]*

Shih AH, Abdel-Wahab O, Patel JP, et al: The role of epigenetic regulators in myeloid malignancies. *Nat Rev Cancer* 12:599, 2012. *[Update on the rapidly emerging data suggesting that epigenetic aberrations have broadly important roles in myeloid neoplasms.]*

Vardiman JW, Thiele J, Arber DA, et al: The 2008 revision of the World Health Organization (WHO) classification of myeloid neoplasms and acute leukemia. *Blood* 114:937, 2008. *[A report providing the rationale for the WHO classification of myeloid neoplasms.]*

The Cancer Genome Atlas Research Network: Genomic and Epigenomic Landscapes of Adult De Novo Acute Myeloid Leukemia. *N Eng J Med* epublished May 1, 2013. *[A landmark paper that using next generation sequencing and other genomic approaches to systematically describe the scope of genetic aberrations in acute myeloid leukemia.]*

Disorders That Affect the Spleen and Thymus

Choi SS, Kim KD, Chung KY: Prognostic and clinical relevance of the World Health Organization schema for the classification of thymic epithelial tumors: a clinicopathologic study of 108 patients and literature review. *Chest* 127:755, 2005. *[A large clinicopathologic series that shows that stage is the best predictor of outcome in thymoma.]*

See TARGETED THERAPY available online at www.studentconsult.com

CHAPTER 14

Red Blood Cell and Bleeding Disorders

CHAPTER CONTENTS

In this chapter we will first consider diseases of red cells. By far, the most common and important are the anemias, red cell deficiency states that usually have a nonneoplastic basis. We will then complete our review of blood diseases by discussing the major bleeding disorders and complications of blood transfusion.

Anemias

Anemia is defined as a reduction of the total circulating red cell mass below normal limits. Anemia reduces the oxygen-carrying capacity of the blood, leading to tissue hypoxia. In practice, the measurement of red cell mass is not easy, and anemia is usually diagnosed based on a reduction in the *hematocrit* (the ratio of packed red cells to total blood volume) and the *hemoglobin concentration* of the blood to levels that are below the normal range. These values correlate with the red cell mass except when there are changes in plasma volume caused by fluid retention or dehydration.

There are many classifications of anemia. We will follow one based on underlying mechanisms that is presented in Table 14-1. A second clinically useful approach classifies anemia according to alterations in red cell morphology, which often point to particular causes. Morphologic characteristics providing etiologic clues include red cell size (normocytic, microcytic, or macrocytic); degree of hemoglobinization, reflected in the color of red cells (normochromic or hypochromic); and shape. In general, microcytic hypochromic anemias are caused by disorders of hemoglobin synthesis (most often iron deficiency), while macrocytic anemias often stem from abnormalities that impair the maturation of erythroid precursors in the bone marrow. Normochromic, normocytic anemias have diverse etiologies; in some of these anemias, specific abnormalities of red cell shape (best appreciated through visual inspection of peripheral smears) provide an important clue as to the cause. The other indices can also be assessed qualitatively in smears, but precise measurement is carried out in clinical laboratories with special instrumentation. The most useful red cell indices are as follows:

Table 14-1 Classification of Anemia According to Underlying Mechanism

Mechanism	Specific Examples
Blood Loss	
Acute blood loss	Trauma
Chronic blood loss	Gastrointestinal tract lesions, gynecologic disturbances*
Increased Red Cell Destruction (Hemolysis)	
Inherited genetic defects	
Red cell membrane disorders	Hereditary spherocytosis, hereditary elliptocytosis
Enzyme deficiencies	
Hexose monophosphate shunt enzyme deficiencies	G6PD deficiency, glutathione synthetase deficiency
Glycolytic enzyme deficiencies	Pyruvate kinase deficiency, hexokinase deficiency
Hemoglobin abnormalities	
Deficient globin synthesis	Thalassemia syndromes
Structurally abnormal globins (hemoglobinopathies)	Sickle cell disease, unstable hemoglobins
Acquired genetic defects	
Deficiency of phosphatidylinositol-linked glycoproteins	Paroxysmal nocturnal hemoglobinuria
Antibody-mediated destruction	Hemolytic disease of the newborn (Rh disease), transfusion reactions, drug-induced, autoimmune disorders
Mechanical trauma	
Microangiopathic hemolytic anemias	Hemolytic uremic syndrome, disseminated intravascular coagulation, thrombotic thrombocytopenia purpura
Cardiac traumatic hemolysis	Defective cardiac valves
Repetitive physical trauma	Bongo drumming, marathon running, karate chopping
Infections of red cells	Malaria, babesiosis
Toxic or chemical injury	Clostridial sepsis, snake venom, lead poisoning
Membrane lipid abnormalities	Abetalipoproteinemia, severe hepatocellular liver disease
Sequestration	Hypersplenism
Decreased Red Cell Production	
Inherited genetic defects	
Defects leading to stem cell depletion	Fanconi anemia, telomerase defects
Defects affecting erythroblast maturation	Thalassemia syndromes
Nutritional deficiencies	
Deficiencies affecting DNA synthesis	B_{12} and folate deficiencies
Deficiencies affecting hemoglobin synthesis	Iron deficiency anemia
Erythropoietin deficiency	Renal failure, anemia of chronic disease
Immune-mediated injury of progenitors	Aplastic anemia, pure red cell aplasia
Inflammation-mediated iron sequestration	Anemia of chronic disease
Primary hematopoietic neoplasms	Acute leukemia, myelodysplasia, myeloproliferative disorders (Chapter 13)
Space-occupying marrow lesions	Metastatic neoplasms, granulomatous disease
Infections of red cell progenitors	Parvovirus B19 infection
Unknown mechanisms	Endocrine disorders, hepatocellular liver disease

G6PD, Glucose-6-phosphate dehydrogenase.
*Most often cause of anemia is iron deficiency, not bleeding per se.

- *Mean cell volume*: the average volume of a red cell expressed in femtoliters (fL)
- *Mean cell hemoglobin*: the average content (mass) of hemoglobin per red cell, expressed in picograms
- *Mean cell hemoglobin concentration*: the average concentration of hemoglobin in a given volume of packed red cells, expressed in grams per deciliter
- *Red cell distribution width*: the coefficient of variation of red cell volume

Adult reference ranges for red cell indices are shown in Table 14-2.

Whatever its cause, when sufficiently severe anemia leads to certain clinical findings. Patients appear pale. Weakness, malaise, and easy fatigability are common complaints. The lowered oxygen content of the circulating blood leads to dyspnea on mild exertion. Hypoxia can cause fatty change in the liver, myocardium, and kidney. If fatty changes in the myocardium are sufficiently severe, cardiac failure can develop and compound the tissue hypoxia caused by the deficiency of O_2 in the blood. On occasion, the myocardial hypoxia manifests as angina pectoris, particularly when complicated by pre-existing coronary artery disease. With acute blood loss and shock,

Table 14-2 Adult Reference Ranges for Red Cells*

Measurement (units)	Men	Women
Hemoglobin (gm/dL)	13.6-17.2	12.0-15.0
Hematocrit (%)	39-49	33-43
Red cell count ($\times 10^6/\mu L$)	4.3-5.9	3.5-5.0
Reticulocyte count (%)	0.5-1.5	
Mean cell volume (fL)	82-96	
Mean cell hemoglobin (pg)	27-33	
Mean cell hemoglobin concentration (gm/dL)	33-37	
Red cell distribution width	11.5-14.5	

*Reference ranges vary among laboratories. The reference ranges for the laboratory providing the result should always be used in interpreting test results.

oliguria and anuria can develop as a result of renal hypoperfusion. Central nervous system hypoxia can cause headache, dimness of vision, and faintness.

Anemias of Blood Loss

Acute Blood Loss

The effects of acute blood loss are mainly due to the loss of intravascular volume, which if massive can lead to cardiovascular collapse, shock, and death. The clinical features depend on the rate of hemorrhage and whether the bleeding is external or internal. If the patient survives, the blood volume is rapidly restored by the intravascular shift of water from the interstitial fluid compartment. This fluid shift results in hemodilution and a lowering of the hematocrit. The reduction in oxygenation triggers increased secretion of erythropoietin from the kidney, which stimulates the proliferation of committed erythroid progenitors (CFU-E) in the marrow (see Fig. 13-1). It takes about 5 days for the progeny of these CFU-Es to mature and appear as newly released red cells (reticulocytes) in the peripheral blood. The iron in hemoglobin is recaptured if red cells extravasate into tissues, whereas bleeding into the gut or out of the body leads to iron loss and possible iron deficiency, which can hamper the restoration of normal red cell counts.

Significant bleeding results in predictable changes in the blood involving not only red cells, but also white cells and platelets. If the bleeding is sufficiently massive to cause a decrease in blood pressure, the compensatory release of adrenergic hormones mobilizes granulocytes from the intravascular marginal pool and results in *leukocytosis* (see Fig. 13-2). Initially, red cells appear normal in size and color (normocytic, normochromic). However, as marrow production increases there is a striking increase in the reticulocyte count (*reticulocytosis*), which reaches 10% to 15% after 7 days. Reticulocytes are larger in size than normal red cells (macrocytes) and have a blue-red polychromatophilic cytoplasm. Early recovery from blood loss is also often accompanied by *thrombocytosis*, which results from an increase in platelet production.

Chronic Blood Loss

Chronic blood loss induces anemia only when the rate of loss exceeds the regenerative capacity of the marrow or when iron reserves are depleted and iron deficiency anemia appears (see later).

Hemolytic Anemias

Hemolytic anemias share the following features:

- A shortened red cell life span below the normal 120 days
- Elevated erythropoietin levels and a compensatory increase in erythropoiesis
- Accumulation of hemoglobin degradation products that are created as part of the process of red cell hemolysis

The physiologic destruction of senescent red cells takes place within macrophages, which are abundant in the spleen, liver, and bone marrow. This process appears to be triggered by age-dependent changes in red cell surface proteins, which lead to their recognition and phagocytosis. In the great majority of hemolytic anemias the premature destruction of red cells also occurs within phagocytes, an event that is referred to as *extravascular hemolysis.* If persistent, extravascular hemolysis leads to a hyperplasia of phagocytes manifested by varying degrees of *splenomegaly.*

Extravascular hemolysis is generally caused by alterations that render the red cell less deformable. Extreme changes in shape are required for red cells to navigate the splenic sinusoids successfully. Reduced deformability makes this passage difficult, leading to red cell sequestration and phagocytosis by macrophages located within the splenic cords. Regardless of the cause, the principal clinical features of extravascular hemolysis are *anemia, splenomegaly, and jaundice.* Some hemoglobin inevitably escapes from phagocytes, which leads to variable decreases in plasma *haptoglobin*, an α_2-globulin that binds free hemoglobin and prevents its excretion in the urine. Because much of the pathologic destruction of red cells occurs in the spleen, individuals with extravascular hemolysis often benefit from splenectomy.

Less commonly, *intravascular hemolysis* predominates. Intravascular hemolysis of red cells may be caused by mechanical injury, complement fixation, intracellular parasites (e.g., falciparum malaria, Chapter 8), or exogenous toxic factors. Causes of mechanical injury include trauma caused by cardiac valves, thrombotic narrowing of the microcirculation, or repetitive physical trauma (e.g., marathon running and bongo drum beating). Complement fixation occurs in a variety of situations in which antibodies recognize and bind red cell antigens. Toxic injury is exemplified by clostridial sepsis, which results in the release of enzymes that digest the red cell membrane.

Whatever the mechanism, intravascular hemolysis is manifested by *anemia, hemoglobinemia, hemoglobinuria, hemosiderinuria, and jaundice.* The large amounts of free hemoglobin released from lysed red cells are promptly bound by haptoglobin, producing a complex that is rapidly cleared by mononuclear phagocytes. As serum haptoglobin is depleted, free hemoglobin oxidizes to *methemoglobin,* which is brown in color. The renal proximal tubular cells reabsorb and catabolize much of the filtered hemoglobin and methemoglobin, but some passes out in the urine, imparting a red-brown color. Iron released from hemoglobin can accumulate within tubular cells, giving rise to *renal hemosiderosis.* Concomitantly, heme groups derived from hemoglobin-haptoglobin complexes are catabolized to bilirubin within mononuclear phagocytes, leading to jaundice. Unlike in extravascular hemolysis, splenomegaly is not seen.

In all types of uncomplicated hemolytic anemias, the excess serum bilirubin is unconjugated. The level of hyperbilirubinemia depends on the functional capacity of the liver and the rate of hemolysis. When the liver is normal, jaundice is rarely severe. Excessive bilirubin excreted by the liver into the gastrointestinal tract leads to increased formation and fecal excretion of urobilin (Chapter 18), and often leads to the formation of gallstones derived from heme pigments.

MORPHOLOGY

Certain changes are seen in hemolytic anemias regardless of cause or type. Anemia and lowered tissue oxygen tension trigger the production of erythropoietin, which stimulates erythroid differentiation and leads to the appearance of **increased numbers of erythroid precursors (normoblasts)** in the marrow (Fig. 14-1). Compensatory increases in erythropoiesis result in a **prominent reticulocytosis** in the peripheral blood. The phagocytosis of red cells leads to the accumulation of the iron containing pigment **hemosiderin**, particularly in the spleen, liver, and bone marrow. Such iron accumulation is referred to as **hemosiderosis**. If the anemia is severe, **extramedullary hematopoiesis** can appear in the liver, spleen, and lymph nodes. With chronic hemolysis, elevated biliary excretion of bilirubin promotes the formation of **pigment gallstones** (cholelithiasis).

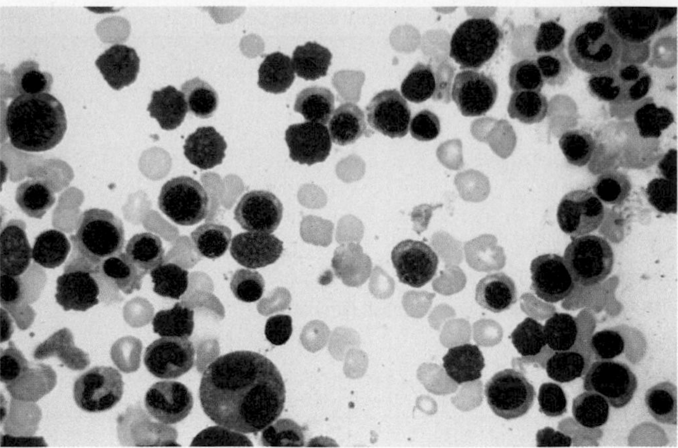

Figure 14-1 Marrow smear from a patient with hemolytic anemia. The marrow reveals increased numbers of maturing erythroid progenitors (normoblasts). (Courtesy Dr. Steven Kroft, Department of Pathology, University of Texas Southwestern Medical School, Dallas, Texas.)

The hemolytic anemias can be classified in a variety of ways; here, we rely on the underlying mechanisms (Table 14-1). We begin by discussing the major inherited forms of hemolytic anemia, and then move on to the acquired forms that are most common or of particular pathophysiologic interest.

Hereditary Spherocytosis

Hereditary spherocytosis (HS) is an inherited disorder caused by intrinsic defects in the red cell membrane skeleton that render red cells spheroid, less deformable, and vulnerable to splenic sequestration and destruction. The prevalence of HS is highest in northern Europe, where rates of 1 in 5000 are reported. An autosomal dominant inheritance pattern is seen in about 75% of cases. The remaining patients have a more severe form of the disease that is usually caused by the inheritance of two different defects (a state known as compound heterozygosity).

Pathogenesis. The remarkable deformability and durability of the normal red cell are attributable to the physicochemical properties of its specialized membrane skeleton (Fig. 14-2), which lies closely apposed to the internal surface of the plasma membrane. Its chief protein component, spectrin, consists of two polypeptide chains, α and β, which form intertwined (helical) flexible heterodimers. The "head" regions of spectrin dimers self-associate to form tetramers, while the "tails" associate with actin oligomers. Each actin oligomer can bind multiple spectrin tetramers, thus creating a two-dimensional spectrin-actin skeleton that is connected to the cell membrane by two distinct interactions. The first, involving the proteins ankyrin and band 4.2, binds spectrin to the transmembrane ion transporter, band 3. The second, involving protein 4.1, binds the "tail" of spectrin to another transmembrane protein, glycophorin A.

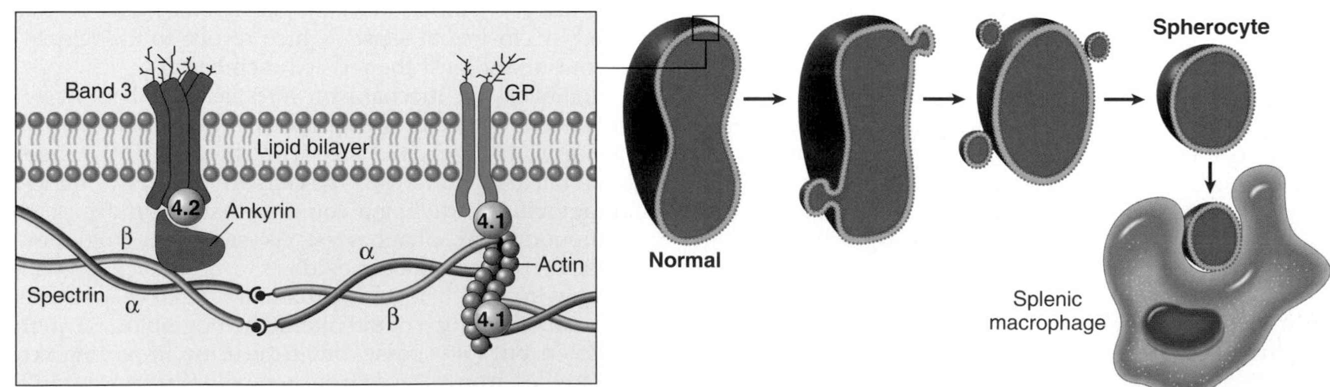

Figure 14-2 Role of the red cell membrane skeleton in hereditary spherocytosis. The left panel shows the normal organization of the major red cell membrane skeletal proteins. Various mutations involving α-spectrin, β-spectrin, ankyrin, band 4.2, or band 3 that weaken the interactions between these proteins cause red cells to lose membrane fragments. To accommodate the resultant change in the ratio of surface area to volume these cells adopt a spherical shape. Spherocytic cells are less deformable than normal ones and therefore become trapped in the splenic cords, where they are phagocytosed by macrophages. GP, Glycophorin.

HS is caused by diverse mutations that lead to an insufficiency of membrane skeletal components. As a result of these alterations, the life span of the affected red cells is decreased on average to 10 to 20 days from the normal 120 days. The pathogenic mutations most commonly affect ankyrin, band 3, spectrin, or band 4.2, the proteins involved in one of the two tethering interactions, presumably because this complex is particularly important in stabilizing the lipid bilayer. Most mutations cause frameshifts or introduce premature stop codons, such that the mutated allele fails to produce any protein. The resulting deficiency of the affected protein reduces the assembly of the skeleton as a whole, destabilizing the overlying plasma membrane. Young HS red cells are normal in shape, but the destabilized lipid bilayer sheds membrane fragments as red cells age in the circulation. The loss of membrane relative to cytoplasm "forces" the cells to assume the smallest possible diameter for a given volume, namely, a sphere. Compound heterozygosity for two defective alleles understandably results in a more severe membrane skeleton deficiency.

The invariably beneficial effects of splenectomy prove that the spleen has a cardinal role in the premature demise of spherocytes. The travails of spherocytic red cells are fairly well defined. In the life of the portly inflexible spherocyte, the spleen is the villain. Normal red cells must undergo extreme deformation to leave the cords of Billroth and enter the sinusoids. Because of their spheroidal shape and reduced deformability, the hapless spherocytes are trapped in the splenic cords, where they are easy prey for macrophages. The splenic environment also somehow exacerbates the tendency of HS red cells to lose membrane along with K^+ ions and H_2O; prolonged splenic exposure (erythrostasis), depletion of red cell glucose, and diminished red cell pH have all been suggested to contribute to these abnormalities (Fig. 14-3). After splenectomy the spherocytes persist, but the anemia is corrected.

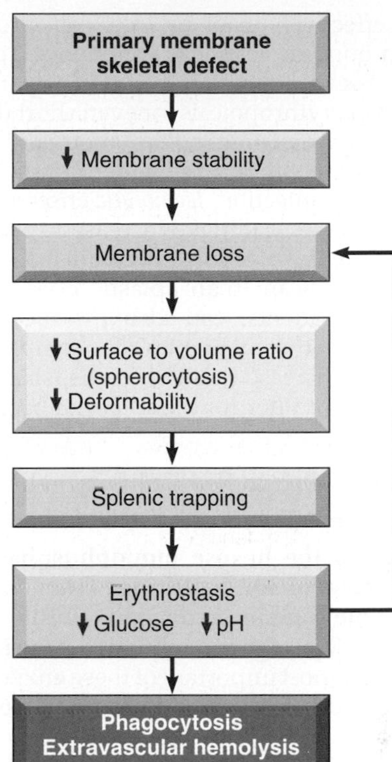

Figure 14-3 Pathophysiology of hereditary spherocytosis.

MORPHOLOGY

The most specific morphologic finding is **spherocytosis**, apparent on smears as small, dark-staining (hyperchromic) red cells lacking the central zone of pallor (Fig. 14-4). Spherocytosis is distinctive but not pathognomonic, as spherocytes are also seen in other disorders associated with membrane loss, such as in autoimmune hemolytic anemia. Other features are common to all hemolytic anemias. These include reticulocytosis, marrow erythroid hyperplasia, hemosiderosis, and mild jaundice. **Cholelithiasis** (pigment stones) occurs in 40% to 50% of affected adults. Moderate **splenomegaly** is characteristic (500-1000 gm); in few other hemolytic anemias is the spleen enlarged as much or as consistently. Splenomegaly results from congestion of the cords of Billroth and increased numbers of phagocytes.

Clinical Features. The diagnosis is based on family history, hematologic findings, and laboratory evidence. In two thirds of the patients the red cells are abnormally sensitive to *osmotic lysis* when incubated in hypotonic salt solutions, which causes the influx of water into spherocytes with little margin for expansion. HS red cells also have an *increased mean cell hemoglobin concentration*, due to dehydration caused by the loss of K^+ and H_2O.

The characteristic clinical features are *anemia, splenomegaly, and jaundice*. The severity varies greatly. In a small minority (mainly compound heterozygotes) HS presents at birth with marked jaundice and requires exchange transfusions. In 20% to 30% of patients the disease is so mild as to be virtually asymptomatic; here the decreased red cell survival is readily compensated for by increased erythropoiesis. In most, however, the compensatory changes are outpaced, producing a chronic hemolytic anemia of mild to moderate severity.

The generally stable clinical course is sometimes punctuated by *aplastic crises,* usually triggered by an acute parvovirus infection. Parvovirus infects and kills red cell

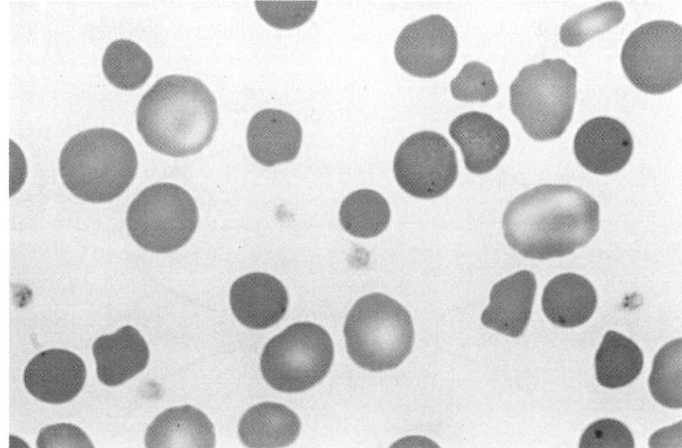

Figure 14-4 Hereditary spherocytosis (peripheral smear). Note the anisocytosis and several dark-appearing spherocytes with no central pallor. Howell-Jolly bodies (small dark nuclear remnants) are also present in red cells of this asplenic patient. (Courtesy Dr. Robert W. McKenna, Department of Pathology, University of Texas Southwestern Medical School, Dallas, Texas.)

progenitors, effectively causing red cell production to cease until an immune response commences, generally in 1 to 2 weeks. Because of the reduced life span of HS red cells, cessation of erythropoiesis for even short time periods leads to sudden worsening of the anemia. Transfusions may be necessary to support the patient until the immune response clears the infection. *Hemolytic crises* are produced by intercurrent events leading to increased splenic destruction of red cells (e.g., infectious mononucleosis); these are clinically less significant than aplastic crises. Gallstones, found in many patients, can also produce symptoms. Splenectomy treats the anemia and its complications, but brings with it an increased risk of sepsis, since the spleen acts as an important filter for blood borne bacteria.

Hemolytic Disease Due to Red Cell Enzyme Defects: Glucose-6-Phosphate Dehydrogenase Deficiency

Abnormalities in the hexose monophosphate shunt or glutathione metabolism resulting from deficient or impaired enzyme function reduce the ability of red cells to protect themselves against oxidative injuries and lead to hemolysis. The most important of these enzyme derangements is the hereditary deficiency of glucose-6-phosphate dehydrogenase (G6PD) activity. G6PD reduces nicotinamide adenine dinucleotide phosphate (NADP) to NADPH while oxidizing glucose-6-phosphate (Fig. 14-5). NADPH then provides reducing equivalents needed for conversion of oxidized glutathione to reduced glutathione, which protects against oxidant injury by participating as a cofactor in reactions that neutralize compounds such as H_2O_2 (Fig. 14-5).

G6PD deficiency is a recessive X-linked trait, placing males at higher risk for symptomatic disease. Several hundred G6PD genetic variants are known, but most are harmless. Two variants, designated G6PD$^-$ and G6PD Mediterranean, cause most of the clinically significant hemolytic anemias. G6PD$^-$ is present in about 10% of American blacks; G6PD Mediterranean, as the name implies, is prevalent in the Middle East. The high frequency of these variants in each population is believed to stem from a protective effect against *Plasmodium falciparum* malaria (discussed later). G6PD variants associated with hemolysis result in misfolding of the protein, making it more susceptible to proteolytic degradation. Compared with the most common normal variant, G6PD B, the half-life of G6PD$^-$ is moderately reduced, whereas that of G6PD Mediterranean is more markedly abnormal. Because mature red cells do not synthesize new proteins, G6PD$^-$ or G6PD Mediterranean enzyme activities fall quickly to levels inadequate to protect against oxidant stress as red cells age. Thus, older red cells are much more prone to hemolysis than younger ones.

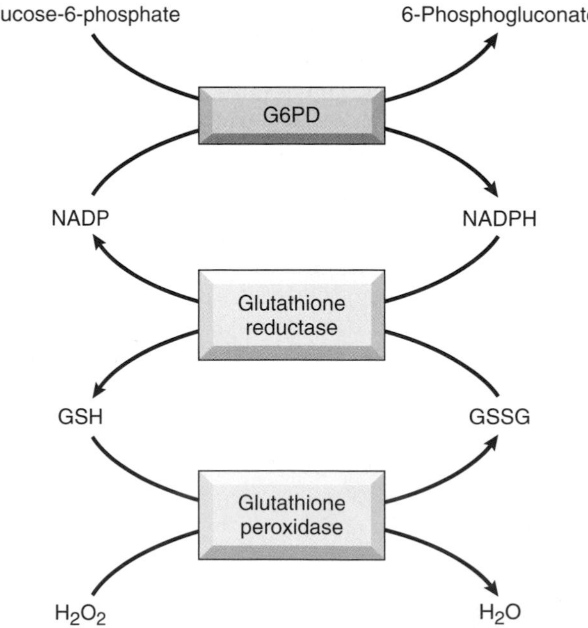

Figure 14-5 Role of glucose-6-phosphate dehydrogenase (G6PD) in defense against oxidant injury. The disposal of H_2O_2, a potential oxidant, is dependent on the adequacy of reduced glutathione (GSH), which is generated by the action of the reduced form of nicotinamide adenine dinucleotide (NADPH). The synthesis of NADPH is dependent on the activity of G6PD. GSSG, Oxidized glutathione.

The episodic hemolysis that is characteristic of G6PD deficiency is caused by exposures that generate oxidant stress. The most common triggers are *infections,* in which oxygen-derived free radicals are produced by activated leukocytes. Many infections can trigger hemolysis; viral hepatitis, pneumonia, and typhoid fever are among those most likely to do so. The other important initiators are *drugs* and certain *foods.* The oxidant drugs implicated are numerous, including antimalarials (e.g., primaquine and chloroquine), sulfonamides, nitrofurantoins, and others. Some drugs cause hemolysis only in individuals with the more severe Mediterranean variant. The most frequently cited food is the *fava bean,* which generates oxidants when metabolized. "Favism" is endemic in the Mediterranean, Middle East, and parts of Africa where consumption is prevalent. Uncommonly, G6PD deficiency presents as neonatal jaundice or a chronic low-grade hemolytic anemia in the absence of infection or known environmental triggers.

Oxidants cause both *intravascular and extravascular hemolysis* in G6PD-deficient individuals. Exposure of G6PD-deficient red cells to high levels of oxidants causes the cross-linking of reactive sulfhydryl groups on globin chains, which become denatured and form membrane-bound precipitates known as *Heinz bodies.* These are seen as dark inclusions within red cells stained with crystal violet (Fig. 14-6). Heinz bodies can damage the membrane sufficiently to cause intravascular hemolysis. Less severe membrane damage results in decreased red cell deformability. As inclusion-bearing red cells pass through the splenic cords, macrophages pluck out the Heinz bodies. As a result of membrane damage, some of these partially devoured cells retain an abnormal shape, appearing to have a bite taken out of them (Fig. 14-6). Other less severely damaged cells become spherocytes due to loss of membrane surface area. Both bite cells and spherocytes are trapped in splenic cords and removed rapidly by phagocytes.

Acute intravascular hemolysis, marked by anemia, hemoglobinemia, and hemoglobinuria, usually begins 2 to 3 days following exposure of G6PD-deficient individuals to oxidants. The hemolysis is greater in individuals with the highly unstable G6PD Mediterranean variant. Because only older red cells are at risk for lysis, the episode is self-limited, as hemolysis ceases when only younger G6PD-replete red cells remain (even if the patient

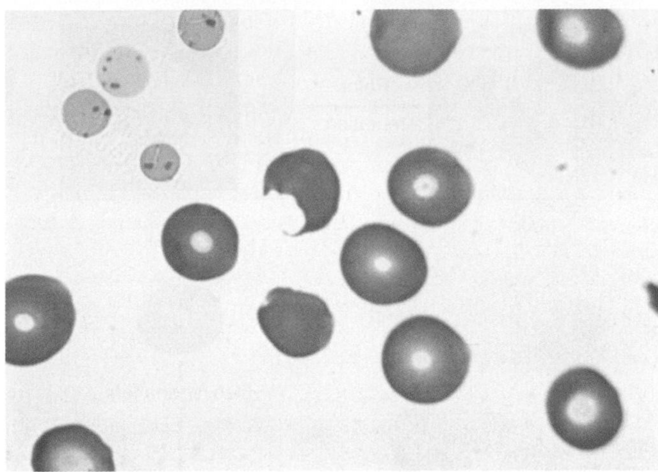

Figure 14-6 Glucose-6-phosphate dehydrogenase deficiency: effects of oxidant drug exposure (peripheral blood smear). *Inset,* Red cells with precipitates of denatured globin (Heinz bodies) revealed by supravital staining. As the splenic macrophages pluck out these inclusions, "bite cells" like the one in this smear are produced. (Courtesy Dr. Robert W. McKenna, Department of Pathology, University of Texas Southwestern Medical School, Dallas, Texas.)

continues to take the offending drug). The recovery phase is heralded by reticulocytosis. Because hemolytic episodes related to G6PD deficiency occur intermittently, features related to chronic hemolysis (e.g., splenomegaly, cholelithiasis) are absent.

Sickle Cell Disease

Sickle cell disease is a common hereditary hemoglobinopathy caused by a point mutation in β-globin that promotes the polymerization of deoxygenated hemoglobin, leading to red cell distortion, hemolytic anemia, microvascular obstruction, and ischemic tissue damage. Several hundred different hemoglobinopathies caused by mutations in globin genes are known, but only those associated with sickle cell disease are prevalent enough in the United States to merit discussion. Hemoglobin is a tetrameric protein composed of two pairs of globin chains, each with its own heme group. Normal adult red cells contain mainly HbA ($\alpha_2\beta_2$), along with small amounts of HbA$_2$ ($\alpha_2\delta_2$) and fetal hemoglobin (HbF; $\alpha_2\gamma_2$). Sickle cell disease is caused by a point mutation in the sixth codon of β-globin that leads to the replacement of a glutamate residue with a valine residue. The abnormal physiochemical properties of the resulting sickle hemoglobin (HbS) are responsible for the disease.

About 8% to 10% of African Americans, or roughly 2 million individuals, are heterozygous for HbS, a largely asymptomatic condition known as sickle cell trait. The offspring of two heterozygotes has a 1 in 4 chance of being homozygous for the sickle mutation, a state that produces symptomatic sickle cell disease. In such individuals, almost all the hemoglobin in the red cell is HbS ($\alpha_2\beta^S{}_2$). There are about 70,000 individuals with sickle cell disease in the United States. In certain populations in Africa the prevalence of heterozygosity is as high as 30%.

This high frequency stems from protection afforded by HbS against falciparum malaria. Population studies have shown that the sickle hemoglobin mutation has arisen independently at least six times in areas in which falciparum malaria is endemic, providing clear evidence of strong Darwinian selection for this trait. Parasite densities are lower in infected AS children than in AA children, and AS children are significantly less likely to have severe disease or to die from malaria. While mechanistic details are lacking two scenarios to explain these observations are favored:

- Metabolically active intracellular parasites consume O2 and decrease intracellular pH, both of which promote hemoglobin sickling in AS red cells. These distorted and stiffened cells may be cleared more rapidly by phagocytes in the spleen and liver, helping to keep parasite loads down.
- Another effect of sickling is that it impairs the formation of membrane knobs containing a protein made by the parasite called PfEMP-1. These membrane knobs are implicated in adhesion of infected red cells to endothelium, which is believed to have an important pathogenic role in the most severe form of the disease, cerebral malaria.

It has been suggested that G6PD deficiency and thalassemias also protect against malaria by increasing the clearance and decreasing the adherence of infected red cells, possibly by raised levels of oxidant stress and causing membrane damage in the parasite-bearing cells.

Pathogenesis. The major pathologic manifestations—chronic hemolysis, microvascular occlusions, and tissue damage—all stem from the tendency of HbS molecules to stack into polymers when deoxygenated. Initially, this process converts the red cell cytosol from a freely flowing liquid into a viscous gel. With continued deoxygenation HbS molecules assemble into long needle-like fibers within red cells, producing a distorted sickle or holly-leaf shape.

Several variables affect the rate and degree of sickling:

- *Interaction of HbS with the other types of hemoglobin in the cell.* In heterozygotes with sickle cell trait, about 40% of the hemoglobin is HbS and the rest is HbA, which interferes with HbS polymerization. As a result, red cells in heterozygous individuals do not sickle except under conditions of profound hypoxia. HbF inhibits the polymerization of HbS even more than HbA; hence, infants do not become symptomatic until they reach 5 or 6 months of age, when the level of HbF normally falls. However, in some individuals HbF expression remains at relatively high levels, a condition known as hereditary persistence of HbF; in these individuals, sickle cell disease is much less severe. Another variant hemoglobin is HbC, in which lysine is substituted for glutamate in the sixth amino acid residue of β-globin. HbC is also common in regions where HbS is found; overall, about 2% to 3% of American blacks are HbC heterozygotes and about 1 in 1250 are compound HbS/HbC heterozygotes. In HbSC red cells the percentage of HbS is 50%, as compared with only 40% in HbAS cells. Moreover, HbSC cells tend to lose salt and water and become dehydrated, which increases the intracellular concentration of HbS. Both of these factors increase the tendency for HbS to polymerize. As a result, individuals who are compound heterozygotes for HbS and HbC have a symptomatic sickling disorder (termed *HbSC disease*), but it is milder than sickle cell disease.

- *Mean cell hemoglobin concentration* (MCHC). Higher HbS concentrations increase the probability that aggregation and polymerization will occur during any given period of deoxygenation. Thus, intracellular dehydration, which increases the MCHC, facilitates sickling. Conversely, conditions that decrease the MCHC reduce the disease severity. This occurs when the individual is homozygous for HbS but also has coexistent α-thalassemia, which reduces Hb synthesis and leads to milder disease.
- *Intracellular pH.* A decrease in pH reduces the oxygen affinity of hemoglobin, thereby increasing the fraction of deoxygenated HbS at any given oxygen tension and augmenting the tendency for sickling.
- *Transit time of red cells through microvascular beds.* As will be discussed, much of the pathology of sickle cell disease is related to vascular occlusion caused by sickling within microvascular beds. Transit times in most normal microvascular beds are too short for significant aggregation of deoxygenated HbS to occur, and as a result sickling is confined to microvascular beds with slow transit times. Blood flow is sluggish in the normal spleen and bone marrow, which are prominently affected in sickle cell disease, and also in vascular beds that are inflamed. The movement of blood through inflamed tissues is slowed because of the adhesion of leukocytes to activated endothelial cells and the transudation of fluid through leaky vessels. As a result, inflamed vascular beds are prone to sickling and occlusion.

Sickling causes cumulative damage to red cells through several mechanisms. As HbS polymers grow, they herniate through the membrane skeleton and project from the cell ensheathed by only the lipid bilayer. This severe derangement in membrane structure causes the influx of Ca^{2+} ions, which induce the cross-linking of membrane proteins and activate an ion channel that permits the efflux of K^+ and H_2O. With repeated episodes of sickling, red cells become increasingly dehydrated, dense, and rigid (Fig. 14-7). Eventually, the most severely damaged cells are converted to end-stage, nondeformable, irreversibly sickled cells, which retain a sickle shape even when fully oxygenated. The severity of the hemolysis correlates with the percentage of irreversibly sickled cells, which are rapidly sequestered and removed by mononuclear phagocytes (extravascular hemolysis). Sickled red cells are also mechanically fragile, leading to some intravascular hemolysis as well.

The pathogenesis of the *microvascular occlusions*, which are responsible for the most serious clinical features, is far less certain. Microvascular occlusions are not related to the number of irreversibly sickled cells in the blood, but instead may be dependent upon more subtle red cell membrane damage and local factors, such as inflammation or vasoconstriction, that tend to slow or arrest the movement of red cells through microvascular beds (Fig. 14-7). As mentioned above, sickle red cells express higher than normal levels of adhesion molecules and are sticky. Mediators released from granulocytes during inflammatory reactions up-regulate the expression of adhesion molecules on endothelial cells (Chapter 3) and further enhance the tendency for sickle red cells to get arrested during transit through the microvasculature. The stagnation of red cells within

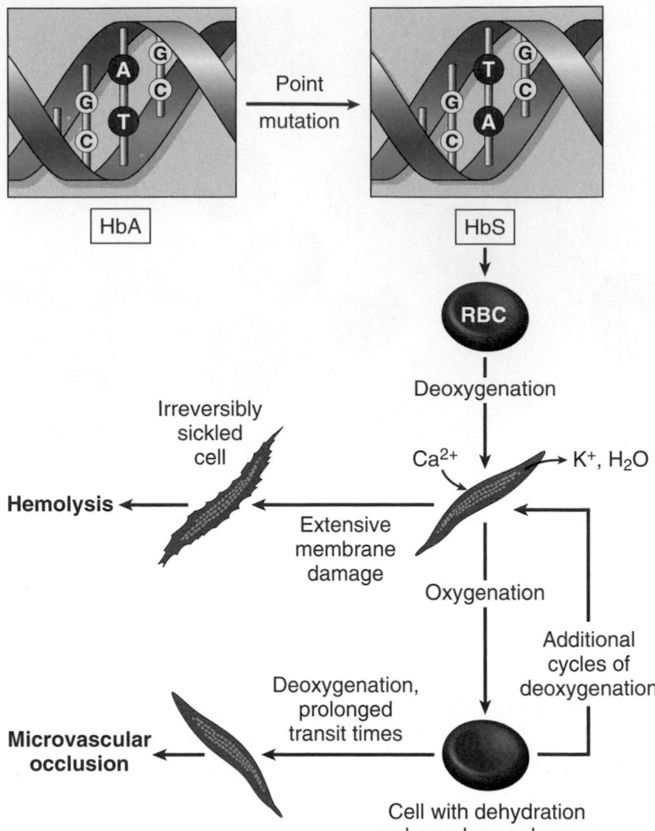

Figure 14-7 Pathophysiology of sickle cell disease.

inflamed vascular beds results in extended exposure to low oxygen tension, sickling, and vascular obstruction. Once started, it is easy to envision how a vicious cycle of sickling, obstruction, hypoxia, and more sickling ensues. Depletion of nitric oxide (NO) may also play a part in the vascular occlusions. Free hemoglobin released from lysed sickle red cells can bind and inactivate NO, which is a potent vasodilator and inhibitor of platelet aggregation. The reduction in active NO leads to increased vascular tone (narrowing vessels) and enhances platelet aggregation, both of which may contribute to red cell stasis, sickling, and (in some instances) thrombosis.

MORPHOLOGY

In sickle cell anemia, the peripheral blood demonstrates variable numbers of **irreversibly sickled cells**, reticulocytosis, and target cells, which result from red cell dehydration (Fig. 14-8). **Howell-Jolly bodies** (small nuclear remnants) are also present in some red cells due to the asplenia (see later). The bone marrow is hyperplastic as a result of a compensatory erythroid hyperplasia. Expansion of the marrow leads to bone resorption and secondary new bone formation, resulting in prominent cheekbones and changes in the skull that resemble a "crewcut" on x-ray studies. Extramedullary hematopoiesis can also appear. The increased breakdown of hemoglobin can cause pigment gallstones and hyperbilirubinemia.

In early childhood, the spleen is enlarged up to 500 gm by red pulp congestion, which is caused by the trapping of sickled red cells in the cords and sinuses (Fig. 14-9). With time, however, the chronic erythrostasis leads to splenic infarction,

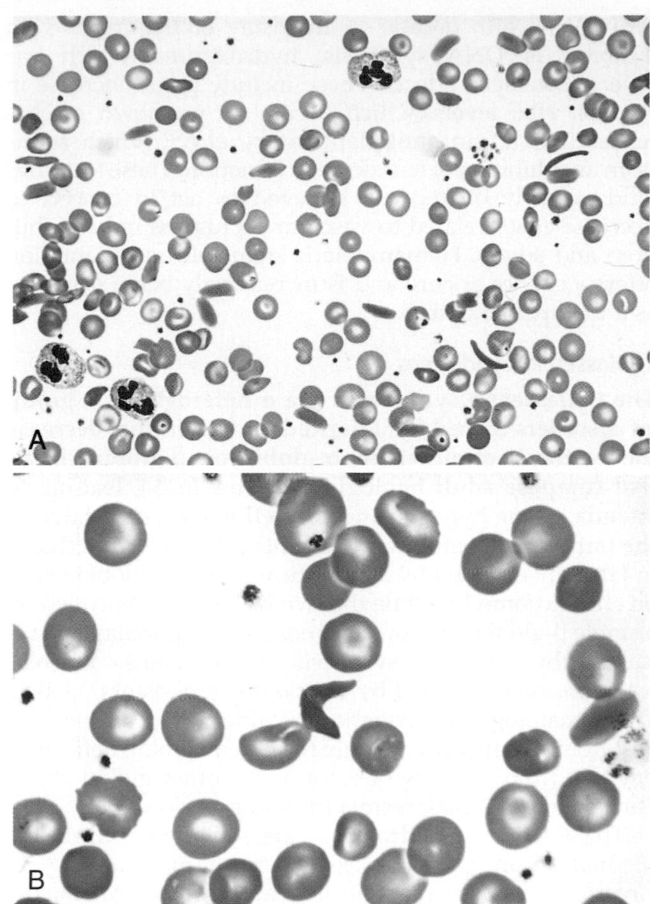

Figure 14-8 Sickle cell disease (peripheral blood smear). **A,** Low magnification shows sickle cells, anisocytosis, and poikilocytosis. **B,** Higher magnification shows an irreversibly sickled cell in the center. (Courtesy Dr. Robert W. McKenna, Department of Pathology, University of Texas Southwestern Medical School, Dallas, Texas.)

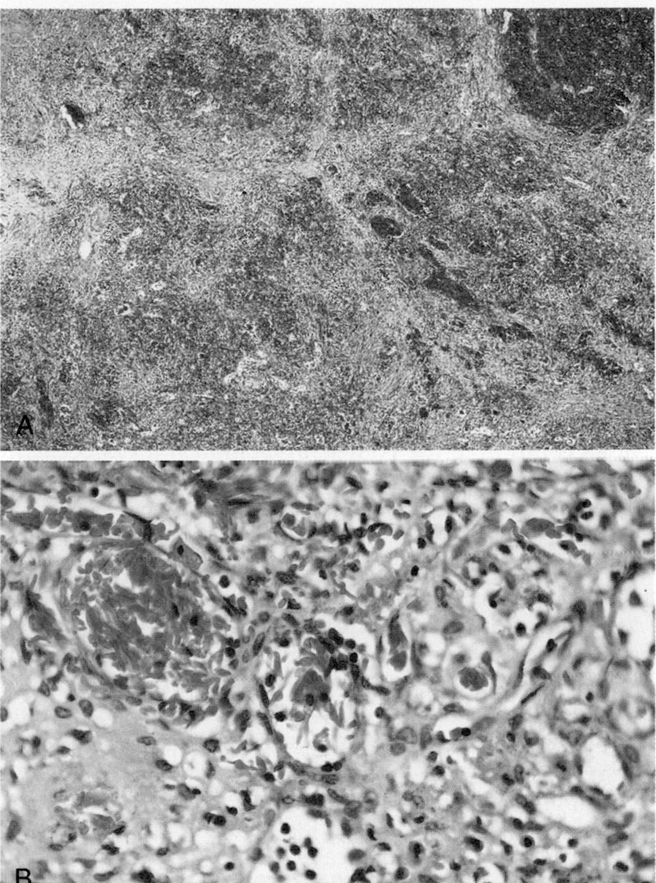

Figure 14-9 **A,** Spleen in sickle cell disease (low power). Red pulp cords and sinusoids are markedly congested; between the congested areas, pale areas of fibrosis resulting from ischemic damage are evident. **B,** Under high power, splenic sinusoids are dilated and filled with sickled red cells. (Courtesy Dr. Darren Wirthwein, Department of Pathology, University of Texas Southwestern Medical School, Dallas, Texas.)

fibrosis, and progressive shrinkage, so that by adolescence or early adulthood only a small nubbin of fibrous splenic tissue is left; this process is called **autosplenectomy** (Fig. 14-10). Infarctions caused by vascular occlusions can occur in many other tissues as well, including the bones, brain, kidney, liver, retina, and pulmonary vessels, the latter sometimes producing cor pulmonale. In adult patients, vascular stagnation in subcutaneous tissues often leads to leg ulcers; this complication is rare in children.

Clinical Features

Sickle cell disease causes a moderately severe hemolytic anemia (hematocrit 18% to 30%) that is associated with reticulocytosis, hyperbilirubinemia, and the presence of irreversibly sickled cells. Its course is punctuated by a variety of "crises." *Vaso-occlusive crises,* also called *pain crises,* are episodes of hypoxic injury and infarction that cause severe pain in the affected region. Although infection, dehydration, and acidosis (all of which favor sickling) can act as triggers, in most instances no predisposing cause is identified. The most commonly involved sites are the bones, lungs, liver, brain, spleen, and penis. In children, painful bone crises are extremely common and often difficult to distinguish from acute osteomyelitis. These frequently manifest as the *hand-foot syndrome* or dactylitis of the bones of the hands or feet, or both. *Acute chest syndrome* is a particularly dangerous type of vaso-occlusive crisis involving the lungs, which typically presents with fever, cough, chest pain, and pulmonary infiltrates. Pulmonary inflammation (such as may be induced by a

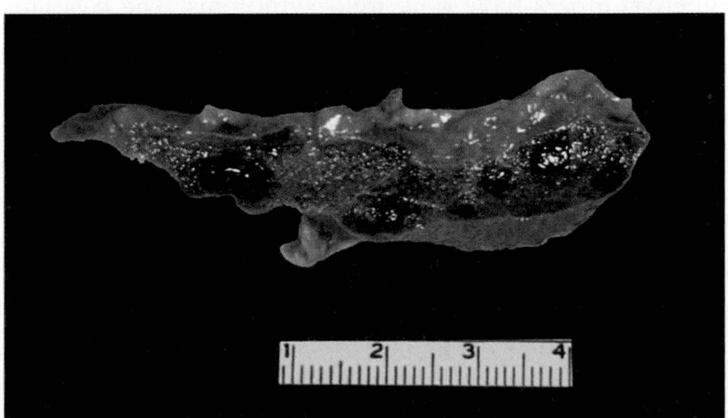

Figure 14-10 "Autoinfarcted" splenic remnant in sickle cell disease. (Courtesy Drs. Dennis Burns and Darren Wirthwein, Department of Pathology, University of Texas Southwestern Medical School, Dallas, Texas.)

simple infection) may cause blood flow to become sluggish and "spleenlike," leading to sickling and vaso-occlusion. This compromises pulmonary function, creating a potentially fatal cycle of worsening pulmonary and systemic hypoxemia, sickling, and vaso-occlusion. *Priapism* affects up to 45% of males after puberty and may lead to hypoxic damage and erectile dysfunction. Other disorders related to vascular obstruction, particularly *stroke* and retinopathy leading to *loss of visual acuity* and even blindness, can take a devastating toll. Factors proposed to contribute to stroke include the adhesion of sickle red cells to arterial vascular endothelium and vasoconstriction caused by the depletion of NO by free hemoglobin.

Although occlusive crises are the most common cause of patient morbidity and mortality, several other acute events complicate the course. *Sequestration crises* occur in children with intact spleens. Massive entrapment of sickle red cells leads to rapid splenic enlargement, hypovolemia, and sometimes shock. Both sequestration crises and the acute chest syndrome may be fatal and sometimes require prompt treatment with exchange transfusions. *Aplastic crises* stem from the infection of red cell progenitors by parvovirus B19, which causes a transient cessation of erythropoiesis and a sudden worsening of the anemia.

In addition to these dramatic crises, chronic tissue hypoxia takes a subtle but important toll. Chronic hypoxia is responsible for a generalized impairment of growth and development, as well as organ damage affecting the spleen, heart, kidneys, and lungs. Sickling provoked by hypertonicity in the renal medulla causes damage that eventually leads to hyposthenuria (the inability to concentrate urine), which increases the propensity for dehydration and its attendant risks.

Increased susceptibility to infection with encapsulated organisms is another threat. This is due in large part to altered splenic function, which is severely impaired in children by congestion and poor blood flow, and completely absent in adults because of splenic infarction. Defects of uncertain etiology in the alternative complement pathway also impair the opsonization of bacteria. *Pneumococcus pneumoniae* and *Haemophilus influenzae* septicemia and meningitis are common, particularly in children, but can be reduced by vaccination and prophylactic antibiotics.

It must be emphasized that there is great variation in the clinical manifestations of sickle cell disease. Some individuals are crippled by repeated vaso-occlusive crises, whereas others have only mild symptoms. The basis for this wide range in disease expression is not understood; both modifying genes and environmental factors are suspected.

The diagnosis is suggested by the clinical findings and the presence of irreversibly sickled red cells and is confirmed by various tests for sickle hemoglobin. In general, these involve mixing a blood sample with an oxygen-consuming reagent, such as metabisulfite, which induces sickling of red cells if HbS is present. Hemoglobin electrophoresis is also used to demonstrate the presence of HbS and exclude other sickle syndromes, such as HbSC disease. Prenatal diagnosis is possible by analysis of fetal DNA obtained by amniocentesis or chorionic biopsy.

The outlook for patients with sickle cell disease has improved considerably over the past 10 to 20 years. About 90% of patients survive to age 20, and close to 50% survive beyond the fifth decade. A mainstay of treatment is an inhibitor of DNA synthesis, hydroxyurea, which has several beneficial effects. These include (1) an increase in red cell HbF levels, which occurs by unknown mechanisms; and (2) an antiinflammatory effect, which stems from an inhibition of leukocyte production. These activities (and possibly others) are believed to act in concert to decrease crises related to vascular occlusions in both children and adults. Hematopoietic stem cell transplantation offers a chance at cure and is increasingly being explored as a therapeutic option.

Thalassemia Syndromes

The thalassemia syndromes are a heterogeneous group of disorders caused by inherited mutations that decrease the synthesis of either the α-globin or β-globin chains that compose adult hemoglobin, HbA ($\alpha_2\beta_2$), leading to anemia, tissue hypoxia, and red cell hemolysis related to the imbalance in globin chain synthesis. The two α chains in HbA are encoded by an identical pair of α-globin genes on chromosome 16, while the two β chains are encoded by a single β-globin gene on chromosome 11. β-thalassemia is caused by deficient synthesis of β chains, whereas α-thalassemia is caused by deficient synthesis of α chains. The hematologic consequences of diminished synthesis of one globin chain stem not only from hemoglobin deficiency but also from a relative excess of the other globin chain, particularly in β-thalassemia (described below).

Thalassemia syndromes are endemic in the Mediterranean basin (indeed, *thalassa* means "sea" in Greek), as well as the Middle East, tropical Africa, the Indian subcontinent, and Asia, and in aggregate are among the most common inherited disorders of humans. As with sickle cell disease and other common inherited red cell disorders, their prevalence seems to be explained by the protection they afford heterozygous carriers against malaria. Although we discuss the thalassemia syndromes with other inherited forms of anemia associated with hemolysis, it is important to recognize that the defects in globin synthesis that underlie these disorders cause anemia through two mechanisms: decreased red cell production, and decreased red cell lifespan.

β-Thalassemias

The β-thalassemias are caused by mutations that diminish the synthesis of β-globin chains. The clinical severity varies widely due to heterogeneity in the causative mutations. We will begin our discussion with the molecular lesions in β-thalassemia and then relate the clinical variants to specific underlying molecular defects.

Molecular Pathogenesis. The causative mutations fall into two categories: (1) β^0 *mutations*, associated with absent β-globin synthesis, and (2) β^+ *mutations*, characterized by reduced (but detectable) β-globin synthesis. Sequencing of β-thalassemia genes has revealed more than 100 different causative mutations, mostly consisting of point mutations. Details of these mutations and their effects are found in specialized texts. Figure 14-11 gives a few illustrative examples.

- *Splicing mutations.* These are the most common cause of β^+-thalassemia. Most of these mutations lie within

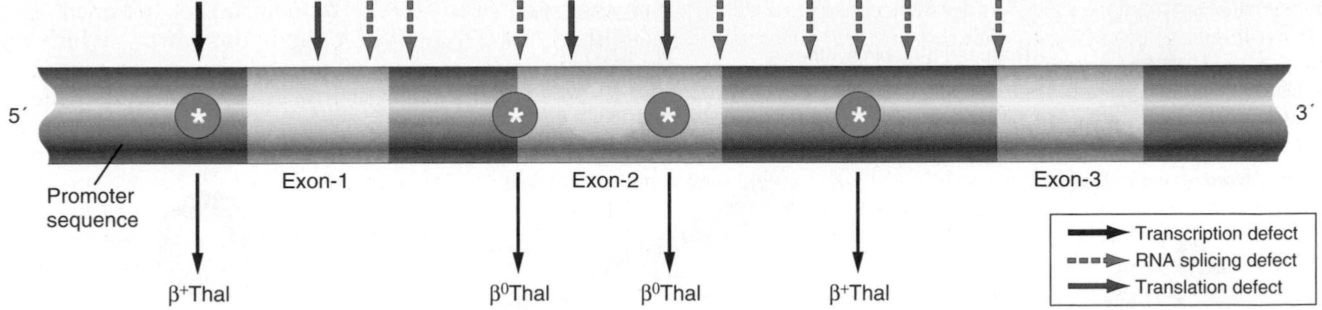

Figure 14-11 Distribution of β-globin gene mutations associated with β-thalassemia. Arrows denote sites where point mutations giving rise to $β^0$ or $β^+$ thalassemia have been identified.

introns, while a few are located within exons. Some of these mutations destroy the normal RNA splice junctions and completely prevent the production of normal β-globin mRNA, resulting in $β^0$-thalassemia. Others create an "ectopic" splice site within an intron. Because the flanking normal splice sites remain, both normal and abnormal splicing occurs and some normal β-globin mRNA is made, resulting in $β^+$ thalassemia.

- *Promoter region mutations.* These mutations reduce transcription by 75% to 80%. Some normal β-globin is synthesized; thus, these mutations are associated with $β^+$-thalassemia.
- *Chain terminator mutations.* These are the most common cause of $β^0$-thalassemia. Two subtypes of mutations fall into this category. The most common type creates a new stop codon within an exon; the other introduces small insertions or deletions that shift the mRNA reading frames (frameshift mutations; see Chapter 5). Both block translation and prevent the synthesis of any functional β-globin.

Impaired β-globin synthesis results in anemia by two mechanisms (Fig. 14-12). The deficit in HbA synthesis produces "underhemoglobinized" hypochromic, microcytic red cells with subnormal oxygen transport capacity. Even more important is the diminished survival of red cells and their precursors, which results from the imbalance in α- and β-globin synthesis. Unpaired α chains precipitate within red cell precursors, forming insoluble inclusions. These inclusions cause a variety of untoward effects, but membrane damage is the proximal cause of most red cell pathology. Many red cell precursors succumb to membrane damage and undergo apoptosis. In severe β-thalassemia, it is estimated that 70% to 85% of red cell precursors suffer this fate, which leads to *ineffective erythropoiesis*. Those red cells that are released from the marrow also contain inclusions and have membrane damage, leaving theme prone to splenic sequestration and *extravascular hemolysis*.

In severe β-thalassemia, ineffective erythropoiesis creates several additional problems. Erythropoietic drive in the setting of severe uncompensated anemia leads to massive erythroid hyperplasia in the marrow and extensive extramedullary hematopoiesis. The expanding mass of red cell precursors erodes the bony cortex, impairs bone growth, and produces skeletal abnormalities (described later). Extramedullary hematopoiesis involves the liver, spleen, and lymph nodes, and in extreme cases produces extraosseous masses in the thorax, abdomen, and pelvis. The metabolically active erythroid progenitors steal nutrients from other tissues that are already oxygen-starved, causing severe cachexia in untreated patients.

Another serious complication of ineffective erythropoiesis is excessive absorption of dietary iron. Ineffective erythropoiesis suppresses hepcidin, a critical negative regulator of iron absorption (see Iron Deficiency Anemia). Increased absorption of iron from the gut due to low hepcidin levels and the iron load of repeated blood transfusions inevitably lead to severe iron accumulation unless preventive steps are taken. Secondary injury to parenchymal organs, particularly the liver, often follows and sometimes induces *secondary hemochromatosis* (Chapter 18).

Clinical Syndromes. The relationships of clinical phenotypes to underlying genotypes are summarized in Table 14-3. Clinical classification of β-thalassemia is based on the severity of the anemia, which in turn depends on the genetic defect ($β^+$ or $β^0$) and the gene dosage (homozygous or heterozygous). In general, individuals with two β-thalassemia alleles ($β^+/β^+$,$β^+/β^0$, or $β^0/β^0$) have a severe, transfusion-dependent anemia called β-*thalassemia major.* Heterozygotes with one β-thalassemia gene and one normal gene ($β^{+}/β$ or $β^0/β$) usually have a mild asymptomatic microcytic anemia. This condition is referred to as *β-thalassemia minor* or *β-thalassemia trait.* A third genetically heterogeneous variant of moderate severity is called β-*thalassemia intermedia.* This category includes milder variants of $β^+/β^+$ or $β^+/β^0$-thalassemia and unusual forms of heterozygous β-thalassemia. Some patients with β-thalassemia intermedia have two defective β-globin genes and an α-thalassemia gene defect, which improves the effectiveness of erythropoiesis and red cell survival by lessening the imbalance in α- and β-chain synthesis. In other rare but informative cases, individuals have a single β-globin defect and one or two extra copies of normal α-globin genes (stemming from a gene duplication event), which worsens the chain imbalance. These unusual forms of the disease serve to emphasize the cardinal role of unpaired α-globin chains in the pathology. The clinical and morphologic features of β-thalassemia intermedia are not described separately but can be surmised from the following discussions of β-thalassemia major and β-thalassemia minor.

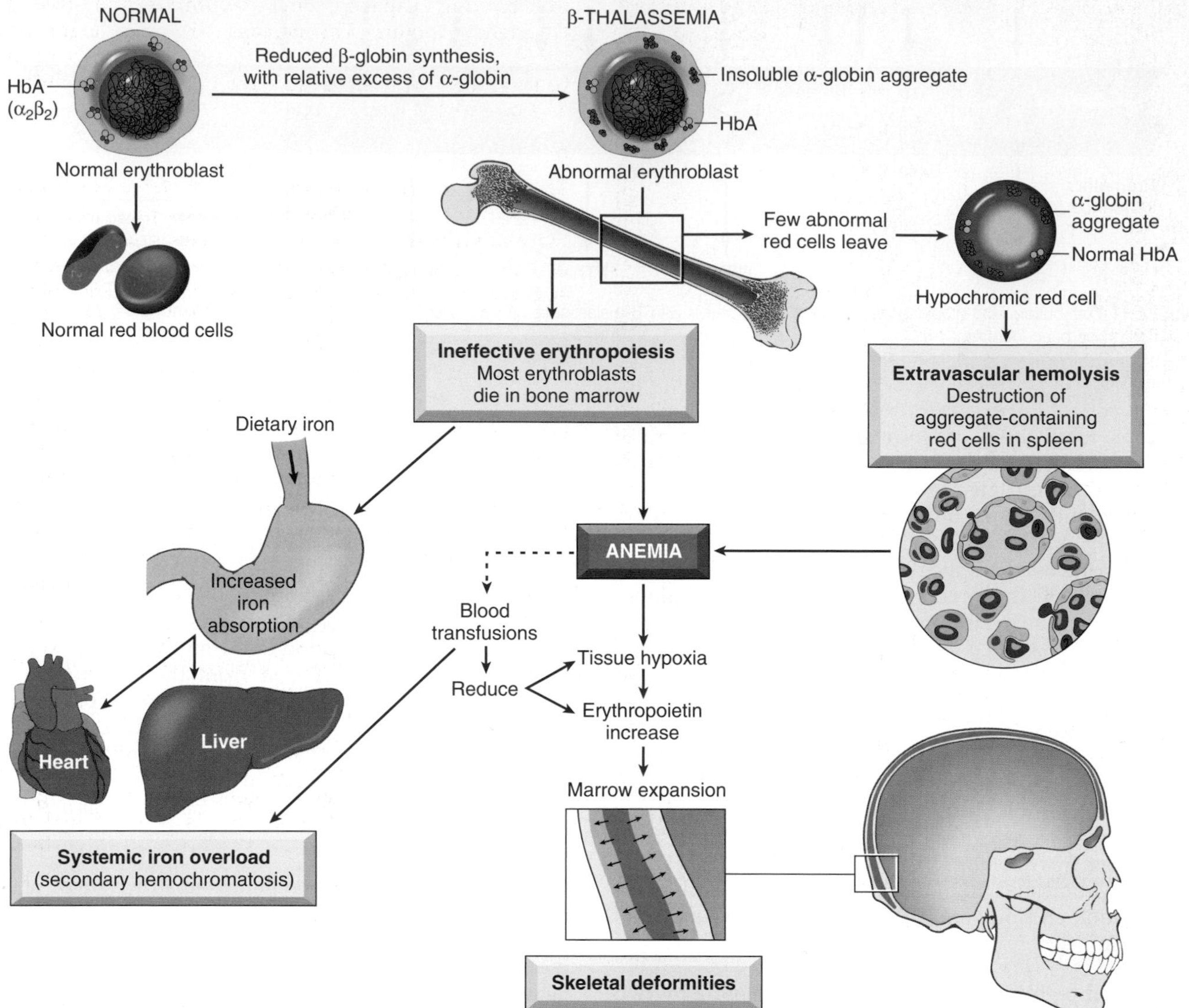

Figure 14-12 Pathogenesis of β-thalassemia major. Note that the aggregates of unpaired α-globin chains, a hallmark of the disease, are not visible in routinely stained blood smears. Blood transfusions are a double-edged sword, diminishing the anemia and its attendant complications, but also adding to the systemic iron overload.

β-Thalassemia Major. β-Thalassemia major is most common in Mediterranean countries, parts of Africa, and Southeast Asia. In the United States the incidence is highest in immigrants from these areas. The anemia manifests 6 to 9 months after birth as hemoglobin synthesis switches from HbF to HbA. In untransfused patients, hemoglobin levels are 3 to 6 gm/dL. The red cells may completely lack HbA (β^0/β^0 genotype) or contain small amounts (β^+/β^+ or β^0/β^+ genotypes). The major red cell hemoglobin is HbF, which is markedly elevated. HbA_2 levels are sometimes high but more often are normal or low.

MORPHOLOGY

Blood smears show severe red cell abnormalities, including marked variation in size (**anisocytosis**) and shape (**poikilocytosis**), **microcytosis**, and **hypochromia**. Target cells (so called because hemoglobin collects in the center of the cell), basophilic stippling, and fragmented red cells are also common. Inclusions of aggregated α chains are efficiently removed by the spleen and not easily seen. The reticulocyte count is elevated, but it is lower than expected for the severity of anemia because of the ineffective erythropoiesis. Variable numbers of poorly hemoglobinized nucleated red cell precursors (normoblasts) are seen in the peripheral blood as a result of "stress" erythropoiesis and abnormal release from sites of extramedullary hematopoiesis.

Other major alterations involve the bone marrow and spleen. In the untransfused patient there is a striking expansion of hematopoietically active marrow. In the bones of the face and skull the burgeoning marrow erodes existing cortical bone and induces new bone formation, giving rise to a "crewcut" appearance on x-ray studies (Fig. 14-13). Both phagocyte hyperplasia and extramedullary hematopoiesis contribute to enlargement of the spleen, which can weigh as much as 1500 gm. The liver and the lymph nodes can also be enlarged by extramedullary hematopoiesis.

Hemosiderosis and secondary hemochromatosis, the two manifestations of iron overload (Chapter 18), occur in almost all patients. The deposited iron often damages organs, most notably the heart, liver, and pancreas.

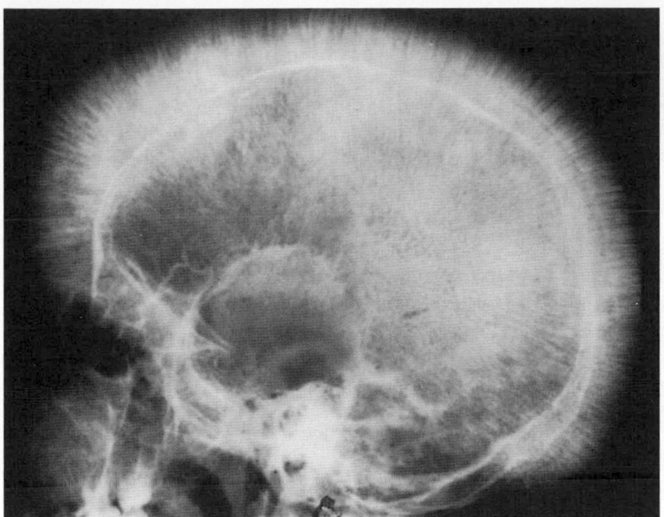

Figure 14-13 Thalassemia. X-ray film of the skull showing new bone formation on the outer table, producing perpendicular radiations resembling a crewcut. (Courtesy Dr. Jack Reynolds, Department of Radiology, University of Texas Southwestern Medical School, Dallas, Texas.)

The clinical course of β-thalassemia major is brief unless blood transfusions are given. Untreated children suffer from growth retardation and die at an early age from the effects of anemia. In those who survive long enough, the cheekbones and other bony prominences are enlarged and distorted. Hepatosplenomegaly due to extramedullary hematopoiesis is usually present. Although blood transfusions improve the anemia and suppress complications related to excessive erythropoiesis, they lead to complications of their own. Cardiac disease resulting from progressive iron overload and secondary hemochromatosis (Chapter 18) is an important cause of death, particularly in heavily transfused patients, who must be treated with iron chelators to prevent or reduce this complication. With transfusions and iron chelation, survival into the third decade is possible, but the overall outlook remains guarded. Hematopoietic stem cell transplantation is the only therapy offering a cure and is being used increasingly. Prenatal diagnosis is possible by molecular analysis of DNA.

β-Thalassemia Minor. β-Thalassemia minor is much more common than β-thalassemia major and understandably affects the same ethnic groups. Most patients are heterozygous carriers of a β^+ or β^0 allele. These patients are usually asymptomatic. Anemia, if present, is mild. The peripheral blood smear typically shows some red cell abnormalities, including hypochromia, microcytosis, basophilic stippling, and target cells. Mild erythroid hyperplasia is seen in the bone marrow. Hemoglobin electrophoresis usually reveals an increase in HbA_2 ($\alpha_2\delta_2$) to 4% to 8% of the total hemoglobin (normal, 2.5% ± 0.3%), which is a reflection of an elevated ratio of δ-chain to β-chain synthesis. HbF levels are generally normal or occasionally slightly increased.

Recognition of β-thalassemia trait is important for two reasons: (1) it superficially resembles the hypochromic microcytic anemia of iron deficiency, and (2) it has implications for genetic counseling. Iron deficiency can usually be excluded through measurement of serum iron, total iron-binding capacity, and serum ferritin (see Iron Deficiency Anemia). The increase in HbA_2 is diagnostically useful, particularly in individuals (such as women of child-bearing age) who are at risk for both β-thalassemia trait and iron deficiency.

α-Thalassemias

The α-thalassemias are caused by inherited deletions that result in reduced or absent synthesis of α-globin chains. Normally, there are four α-globin genes, and the severity of α-thalassemia depends on how many α-globin genes are affected. As in β-thalassemias, the anemia stems both from a lack of adequate hemoglobin and the presence of excess unpaired globin chains (β, γ, and δ), which vary in type at different ages. In newborns with α-thalassemia, excess unpaired γ-globin chains form γ_4 tetramers known as *hemoglobin Barts,* whereas in older children and adults excess β-globin chains form β_4 tetramers known as *HbH*. Because free β and γ chains are more soluble than free α chains and form fairly stable homotetramers, hemolysis and ineffective erythropoiesis are less severe than in β-thalassemias. A variety of molecular lesions give rise to α-thalassemia, but gene deletion is the most common cause of reduced α-chain synthesis.

Clinical Syndromes. The clinical syndromes are determined and classified by the number of α-globin genes that are deleted. Each of the four α-globin genes normally contributes 25% of the total α-globin chains. α-Thalassemia syndromes stem from combinations of deletions that remove one to four α-globin genes. Not surprisingly, the severity of the clinical syndrome is proportional to the number of α-globin genes that are deleted. The different types of α-thalassemia and their salient clinical features are listed in Table 14-3.

Silent Carrier State. Silent carrier state is associated with the deletion of a single α-globin gene, which causes a barely detectable reduction in α-globin chain synthesis. These individuals are completely asymptomatic but have slight microcytosis.

α-Thalassemia Trait. α-Thalassemia trait is caused by the deletion of two α-globin genes from a single chromosome (α/α −/−) or the deletion of one α-globin gene from each of the two chromosomes (α/− α/−) (Table 14-3). The former genotype is more common in Asian populations, the latter in regions of Africa. Both genotypes produce similar quantitative deficiencies of α-globin and are clinically identical, but have different implications for the children of affected individuals, who are at risk of clinically significant α-thalassemia (HbH disease or hydrops fetalis) only when at least one parent has the −/− haplotype. As a result, symptomatic α-thalassemia is relatively common in Asian populations and rare in black African populations. The clinical picture in α-thalassemia trait is identical to that described for β-thalassemia minor, that is, small red cells (microcytosis), minimal or no anemia, and no abnormal physical signs. HbA_2 levels are normal or low.

Hemoglobin H Disease. HbH disease is caused by deletion of three α-globin genes. As discussed, HbH disease is most common in Asian populations. With only one normal

Table 14-3 Clinical and Genetic Classification of Thalassemias

Clinical Syndromes	Genotype	Clinical Features	Molecular Genetics
β-Thalassemias			
β-Thalassemia major	Homozygous β-thalassemia (β^0/β^0, β^+/β^+, β^0/β^+)	Severe; requires blood transfusions	Mainly point mutations that lead to defects in the transcription, splicing, or translation of β-globin mRNA
β-Thalassemia intermedia	Variable (β^0/β^+, β^+/β^+, β^0/β, β^+/β)	Severe but does not require regular blood transfusions	
β-Thalassemia minor	Heterozygous β-thalassemia (β^0/β, β^+/β)	Asymptomatic with mild or absent anemia; red cell abnormalities seen	
α-Thalassemias			
Silent carrier	–/α α/α	Asymptomatic; no red cell abnormality	Mainly gene deletions
α-Thalassemia trait	–/– α/α (Asian) –/α –/α (black African, Asian)	Asymptomatic, like β-thalassemia minor	
HbH disease	–/– –/α	Severe; resembles β-thalassemia intermedia	
Hydrops fetalis	–/– –/–	Lethal in utero without transfusions	

α-globin gene, the synthesis of α chains is markedly reduced, and tetramers of β-globin, called HbH, form. HbH has an extremely high affinity for oxygen and therefore is not useful for oxygen delivery, leading to tissue hypoxia disproportionate to the level of hemoglobin. Additionally, HbH is prone to oxidation, which causes it to precipitate and form intracellular inclusions that promote red cell sequestration and phagocytosis in the spleen. The result is a moderately severe anemia resembling β-thalassemia intermedia.

Hydrops Fetalis. Hydrops fetalis is the most severe form of α-thalassemia and is caused by deletion of all four α-globin genes. In the fetus, excess γ-globin chains form tetramers (hemoglobin Barts) that have such a high affinity for oxygen that they deliver little to tissues. Survival in early development is due to the expression of ζ chains, an embryonic globin that pairs with γ chains to form a functional $\zeta_2\gamma_2$ Hb tetramer. Signs of fetal distress usually become evident by the third trimester of pregnancy. In the past, severe tissue anoxia led to death in utero or shortly after birth; with intrauterine transfusion many such infants are now saved. The fetus shows severe pallor, generalized edema, and massive hepatosplenomegaly similar to that seen in hemolytic disease of the newborn (Chapter 10). There is a lifelong dependence on blood transfusions for survival, with the associated risk of iron overload. Hematopoietic stem cell transplantation can be curative.

Paroxysmal Nocturnal Hemoglobinuria

Paroxysmal nocturnal hemoglobinuria (PNH) is a disease that results from acquired mutations in the phosphatidylinositol glycan complementation group A gene (*PIGA*), an enzyme that is essential for the synthesis of certain membrane-associated complement regulatory proteins. PNH has an incidence of 2 to 5 per million in the United States. Despite its rarity, it has fascinated hematologists because it is the only hemolytic anemia caused by an acquired genetic defect. Recall that proteins are anchored into the lipid bilayer in two ways. Most have a hydrophobic region that spans the cell membrane; these are called transmembrane proteins. The others are attached to the cell membrane through a covalent linkage to a specialized phospholipid called glycosylphosphatidylinositol (GPI). In PNH, these GPI-linked proteins are deficient because of somatic mutations that inactivate PIGA. *PIGA* is X-linked and subject to lyonization (random inactivation of one X chromosome in cells of females; Chapter 5). As a result, a single acquired mutation in the active *PIGA* gene of any given cell is sufficient to produce a deficiency state. Because the causative mutations occur in a hematopoietic stem cell, all of its clonal progeny (red cells, white cells, and platelets) are deficient in GPI-linked proteins. Typically the mutant clone coexists with the progeny of normal stem cells that are not PIGA deficient.

Remarkably, most normal individuals harbor small numbers of bone marrow cells with *PIGA* mutations identical to those that cause PNH. It is hypothesized that these cells increase in numbers (thus producing clinically evident PNH) only in rare instances where they have a selective advantage, such as in the setting of autoimmune reactions against GPI-linked antigens. Such a scenario might explain the frequent association of PNH and aplastic anemia, a marrow failure syndrome (discussed later) that has an autoimmune basis in many individuals.

PNH blood cells are deficient in three GPI-linked proteins that regulate complement activity: (1) decay-accelerating factor, or CD55; (2) membrane inhibitor of reactive lysis, or CD59; and (3) C8 binding protein. Of these factors, the most important is CD59, a potent inhibitor of C3 convertase that prevents the spontaneous activation of the alternative complement pathway.

Red cells deficient in these GPI-linked factors are abnormally susceptible to lysis or injury by complement. This manifests as *intravascular hemolysis*, which is caused by the C5b-C9 membrane attack complex. The hemolysis is paroxysmal and nocturnal in only 25% of cases; chronic hemolysis without dramatic hemoglobinuria is more typical. The tendency for red cells to lyse at night is explained by a slight decrease in blood pH during sleep, which increases the activity of complement. The anemia is variable but usually mild to moderate in severity. The loss of heme iron in the urine (hemosiderinuria) eventually leads to iron deficiency, which can exacerbate the anemia if untreated.

Thrombosis is the leading cause of disease-related death in individuals with PNH. About 40% of patients suffer

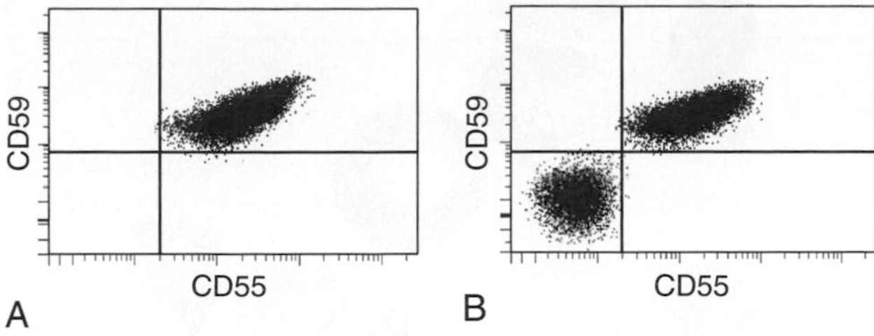

Figure 14-14 Paroxysmal nocturnal hemoglobinuria (PNH). **A,** Flow cytogram of blood from a normal individual shows that the red cells express two phosphatidylinositol glycan (PIG)-linked membrane proteins, CD55 and CD59, on their surfaces. **B,** Flow cytogram of blood from a patient with PNH shows a population of red cells that is deficient in both CD55 and CD59. As is typical of PNH, a second population of CD55+/CD59+ red cells that is derived from residual normal hematopoietic stem cells is also present. (Courtesy Dr. Scott Rodig, Department of Pathology, Brigham and Women's Hospital, Boston, Mass.)

from venous thrombosis, often involving the hepatic, portal, or cerebral veins. About 5% to 10% of patients eventually develop acute myeloid leukemia or a myelodysplastic syndrome, possibly because hematopoietic stem cells have suffered some type of genetic damage.

PNH is diagnosed by flow cytometry, which provides a sensitive means for detecting red cells that are deficient in GPI-linked proteins such as CD59 (Fig. 14-14). The cardinal role of complement activation in PNH pathogenesis has been proven by therapeutic use of a monoclonal antibody called Eculizumab that prevents the conversion of C5 to C5a. This inhibitor not only reduces the hemolysis and attendant transfusion requirements, but also lowers the risk of thrombosis by up to 90%. How complement activation leads to thrombosis in patients with PNH is not clear; the absorption of NO by free hemoglobin (discussed under sickle cell disease) may be one contributing factor. The drawbacks to C5 inhibitor therapy are its high cost and an increased risk of serious or fatal meningococcal infections (as is true in individuals with inherited complement defects). Immunosuppressive drugs are sometimes beneficial for those with evidence of marrow aplasia. The only cure is hematopoietic stem cell transplantation.

Immunohemolytic Anemias

Hemolytic anemias in this category are caused by antibodies that bind to red cells, leading to their premature destruction. Although these disorders are commonly referred to as *autoimmune hemolytic anemias*, the designation immunohemolytic anemia is preferred because in some instances the immune reaction is initiated by an ingested drug. Immunohemolytic anemia can be classified based on the characteristics of the responsible antibody (Table 14-4).

The diagnosis of immunohemolytic anemia requires the detection of antibodies and/or complement on red cells from the patient. This is done using the *direct Coombs antiglobulin test*, in which the patient's red cells are mixed with sera containing antibodies that are specific for human immunoglobulin or complement. If either immunoglobulin or complement is present on the surface of the red cells, the antibodies cause agglutination, which is easily appreciated visually as clumping. In the *indirect Coombs antiglobulin test*, the patient's serum is tested for its ability to agglutinate commercially available red cells bearing particular defined antigens. This test is used to characterize the antigen target and temperature dependence of the responsible antibody. Quantitative immunologic tests to measure such antibodies directly are also available.

Table 14-4 Classification of Immunohemolytic Anemias

Warm Antibody Type (IgG Antibodies Active at 37°C)
Primary (idiopathic)
Secondary
Autoimmune disorders (particularly systemic lupus erythematosus)
Drugs
Lymphoid neoplasms
Cold Agglutinin Type (IgM Antibodies Active Below 37°C)
Acute (mycoplasmal infection, infectious mononucleosis)
Chronic
Idiopathic
Lymphoid neoplasms
Cold Hemolysin Type (IgG Antibodies Active Below 37°C)
Rare; occurs mainly in children following viral infections

Warm Antibody Type. Warm antibody type is the most common form of immunohemolytic anemia. About 50% of cases are idiopathic (primary); the others are related to a predisposing condition (Table 14-4) or exposure to a drug. Most causative antibodies are of the IgG class; less commonly, IgA antibodies are the culprits. The red cell hemolysis is mostly extravascular. IgG-coated red cells bind to Fc receptors on phagocytes, which remove red cell membrane during "partial" phagocytosis. As in hereditary spherocytosis, the loss of membrane converts the red cells to spherocytes, which are sequestered and destroyed in the spleen. Moderate splenomegaly due to hyperplasia of splenic phagocytes is usually seen.

As with other autoimmune disorders, the cause of primary immunohemolytic anemia is unknown. In many cases, the antibodies are directed against the Rh blood group antigens. The mechanisms of drug-induced immunohemolytic anemia are better understood. Two different mechanisms have been described.

- *Antigenic drugs.* In this setting hemolysis usually follows large, intravenous doses of the offending drug and occurs 1 to 2 weeks after therapy is initiated. These drugs, exemplified by penicillin and cephalosporins, bind to the red cell membrane and are recognized by antidrug antibodies. Sometimes the antibodies bind only to the drug, as in penicillin-induced hemolysis. In other cases, such as in quinidine-induced hemolysis, the antibodies recognize a complex of the drug and a membrane protein. The responsible antibodies sometimes fix complement and cause intravascular hemolysis, but more often they act as opsonins that promote extravascular hemolysis within phagocytes.
- *Tolerance-breaking drugs.* These drugs, of which the antihypertensive agent α-methyldopa is the prototype, induce in some unknown manner the production of antibodies against red cell antigens, particularly the Rh blood group antigens. About 10% of patients taking α-methyldopa develop autoantibodies, as assessed by the direct Coombs test, and roughly 1% develop clinically significant hemolysis.

Cold Agglutinin Type. Cold agglutinin type of immunohemolytic anemia is caused by IgM antibodies that bind red cells avidly at low temperatures (0°C to 4°C). It is less common than warm antibody immunohemolytic anemia, accounting for 15% to 30% of cases. Cold agglutinin antibodies sometimes appear transiently following certain infections, such as with *Mycoplasma pneumoniae*, Epstein-Barr virus, cytomegalovirus, influenza virus, and human immunodeficiency virus (HIV). In these settings the disorder is self-limited and the antibodies rarely induce clinically important hemolysis. Chronic cold agglutinin immunohemolytic anemia occurs in association with certain B-cell neoplasms or as an idiopathic condition.

Clinical symptoms result from binding of IgM to red cells in vascular beds where the temperature may fall below 30°C, such as in exposed fingers, toes, and ears. IgM binding agglutinates red cells and fixes complement rapidly. As the blood recirculates and warms, IgM is released, usually before complement-mediated hemolysis can occur. However, the transient interaction with IgM is sufficient to deposit sublytic quantities of C3b, an excellent opsonin, which leads to the removal of affected red cells by phagocytes in the spleen, liver, and bone marrow. The hemolysis is of variable severity. Vascular obstruction caused by agglutinated red cells results in pallor, cyanosis, and Raynaud phenomenon (Chapter 11) in body parts exposed to cold temperature.

Cold Hemolysin Type. Cold hemolysins are autoantibodies responsible for an unusual entity known as *paroxysmal cold hemoglobinuria*. This rare disorder causes substantial, sometimes fatal, intravascular hemolysis and hemoglobinuria. The autoantibodies are IgGs that bind to the P blood group antigen on the red cell surface in cool, peripheral regions of the body. Complement-mediated lysis occurs when the cells recirculate to warm central regions, because the complement cascade functions more efficiently at 37°C. Most cases are seen in children following viral infections; in this setting the disorder is transient, and most of those affected recover within 1 month.

Treatment of warm antibody immunohemolytic anemia centers on the removal of initiating factors (i.e., drugs); when this is not feasible, immunosuppressive drugs and splenectomy are the mainstays. Chronic cold agglutinin immunohemolytic anemia caused by IgM antibodies is more difficult to treat.

Hemolytic Anemia Resulting from Trauma to Red Cells

The most significant hemolysis caused by trauma to red cells is seen in individuals with cardiac valve prostheses and microangiopathic disorders. Artificial mechanical cardiac valves are more frequently implicated than are bioprosthetic porcine or bovine valves. The hemolysis stems from shear forces produced by turbulent blood flow and pressure gradients across damaged valves. *Microangiopathic hemolytic anemia* is most commonly seen with disseminated intravascular coagulation, but it also occurs in thrombotic thrombocytopenic purpura (TTP), hemolytic-uremic syndrome (HUS), malignant hypertension, systemic lupus erythematosus, and disseminated cancer. The common pathogenic feature in these disorders is a microvascular lesion that results in luminal narrowing, often due to the deposition of fibrin and platelets. These vascular changes produce shear stresses that mechanically injure passing red cells. Regardless of the cause, traumatic damage leads to the appearance of red cell fragments (*schistocytes*), "burr cells," "helmet cells," and "triangle cells" in blood smears (Fig. 14-15).

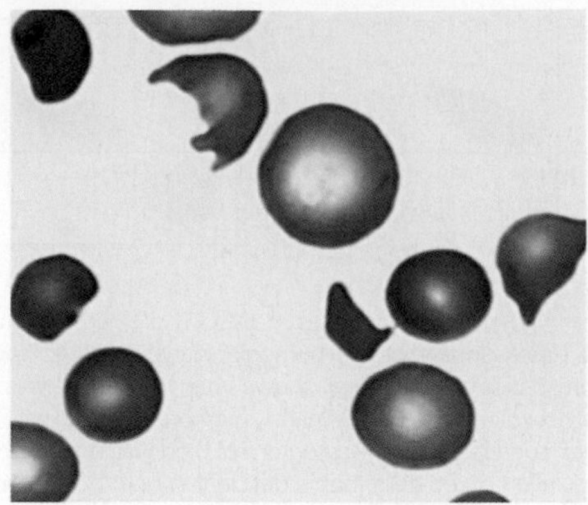

Figure 14-15 Microangiopathic hemolytic anemia. A peripheral blood smear from a person with hemolytic-uremic syndrome shows several fragmented red cells. (Courtesy Dr. Robert W. McKenna, Department of Pathology, University of Texas Southwestern Medical School, Dallas, Texas.)

KEY CONCEPTS

Hereditary Spherocytosis

- Autosomal dominant disorder caused by mutations that affect the red cell membrane skeleton, leading to loss of membrane and eventual conversion of red cells to spherocytes, which are phagocytosed and removed in the spleen
- Manifested by anemia, splenomegaly

Thalassemias

- Autosomal codominant disorders caused by mutations in α- or β-globin that reduce hemoglobin synthesis, resulting in a microcytic, hypochromic anemia.
- In β-thalassemia, unpaired α-globin chains form aggregates that damage red cell precursors and further impair erythropoiesis.

Sickle Cell Anemia

- Autosomal recessive disorder resulting from a mutation in β-globin that causes deoxygenated hemoglobin to self-associate into long polymers that distort (sickle) the red cell
- Blockage of vessels by sickled cells causes pain crises and tissue infarction, particularly of the marrow and spleen
- Red cell membrane damage caused by repeated bouts of sickling results in a moderate to severe hemolytic anemia

Glucose-6-Phosphate Dehydrogenase Deficiency

- X-linked disorder caused by mutations that destabilize G6PD, making red cells susceptible to oxidant damage

Immunohemolytic Anemias

- Caused by antibodies against either normal red cell constituents or antigens modified by haptens (e.g., drugs)
- Antibody binding results in either red cell opsonization and extravascular hemolysis or (uncommonly) complement fixation and intravascular hemolysis

Anemias of Diminished Erythropoiesis

Although the anemias that stem from the inadequate production of red cells are heterogeneous, they can be classified into several major categories based on pathophysiology (Table 14-1). The most common and important anemias associated with red cell underproduction are those caused by nutritional deficiencies, followed by those that arise secondary to renal failure and chronic inflammation. Also included are less common disorders that lead to generalized bone marrow failure, such as aplastic anemia, primary hematopoietic neoplasms (Chapter 13), and infiltrative disorders that lead to marrow replacement (e.g., metastatic cancer and disseminated granulomatous disease). We first discuss the extrinsic causes of diminished erythropoiesis, which are more common and clinically important, and then nonneoplastic intrinsic causes.

Megaloblastic Anemias

The common theme among the various causes of megaloblastic anemia is an impairment of DNA synthesis that leads to ineffective hematopoiesis and distinctive morphologic changes, including abnormally large erythroid precursors and red cells. The causes of megaloblastic anemias are given in Table 14-5. The following discussion first describes the common features and then turns to the two principal types: pernicious anemia (the major form of vitamin B_{12} deficiency anemia) and folate deficiency anemia.

Some of the metabolic roles of vitamin B_{12} and folate are considered later. For now it suffices that vitamin B_{12} and folic acid are coenzymes required for the synthesis of thymidine, one of the four bases found in DNA. A deficiency of these vitamins or impairment in their metabolism results in defective nuclear maturation due to deranged or inadequate DNA synthesis, with an attendant delay or block in cell division.

Table 14-5 Causes of Megaloblastic Anemia

Vitamin B_{12} Deficiency
Decreased Intake
Inadequate diet, vegetarianism
Impaired Absorption
Intrinsic factor deficiency
Pernicious anemia
Gastrectomy
Malabsorption states
Diffuse intestinal disease (e.g., lymphoma, systemic sclerosis)
Ileal resection, ileitis
Competitive parasitic uptake
Fish tapeworm infestation
Bacterial overgrowth in blind loops and diverticula of bowel
Folic Acid Deficiency
Decreased Intake
Inadequate diet, alcoholism, infancy
Impaired Absorption
Malabsorption states
Intrinsic intestinal disease
Anticonvulsants, oral contraceptives
Increased Loss
Hemodialysis
Increased Requirement
Pregnancy, infancy, disseminated cancer, markedly increased hematopoiesis
Impaired Utilization
Folic acid antagonists
Unresponsive to Vitamin B_{12} or Folic Acid Therapy
Metabolic Inhibitors of DNA Synthesis and/or Folate Metabolism (e.g., Methotrexate)

Modified from Beck WS: Megaloblastic anemias. In Wyngaarden JB, Smith LH (eds): Cecil Textbook of Medicine, 18th ed. Philadelphia, WB Saunders, 1988, p. 900.

MORPHOLOGY

Certain peripheral blood findings are shared by all megaloblastic anemias. The presence of red cells that are macrocytic and oval **(macro-ovalocytes)** is highly characteristic. Because they are larger than normal and contain ample hemoglobin, most macrocytes lack the central pallor of normal red cells and even appear "hyperchromic," but the MCHC is not elevated. There is marked variation in the size (anisocytosis) and shape (poikilocytosis) of red cells. The reticulocyte count is low. Nucleated red cell progenitors occasionally appear in the circulating blood when anemia is severe. Neutrophils are also larger than normal (macropolymorphonuclear) and show **nuclear hypersegmentation**, having five or more nuclear lobules instead of the normal three to four (Fig. 14-16).

The marrow is usually markedly hypercellular as a result of increased hematopoietic precursors, which often completely replace the fatty marrow. **Megaloblastic changes** are detected at all stages of erythroid development. The most primitive cells (promegaloblasts) are large, with a deeply basophilic cytoplasm, prominent nucleoli, and a distinctive, fine nuclear chromatin pattern (Fig. 14-17). As these cells differentiate and begin to accumulate hemoglobin, the nucleus retains its finely distributed chromatin and fails to develop the clumped pyknotic chromatin typical of normoblasts. While nuclear maturation is delayed, cytoplasmic maturation and hemoglobin accumulation proceed at a normal pace, leading to nuclear-to-cytoplasmic asynchrony. Because DNA synthesis is impaired in all proliferating cells, granulocytic precursors also display dysmaturation in the form of **giant metamyelocytes and band forms**. Megakaryocytes, too, can be abnormally large and have bizarre, multilobate nuclei.

The marrow hyperplasia is a response to increased levels of growth factors, such as erythropoietin. However, the derangement in DNA synthesis causes most precursors to undergo apoptosis in the marrow (an example of ineffective hematopoiesis) and leads to pancytopenia. The anemia is further exacerbated by a mild degree of red cell hemolysis of uncertain etiology.

Anemias of Vitamin B_{12} Deficiency: Pernicious Anemia

Pernicious anemia is a specific form of megaloblastic anemia caused by an autoimmune gastritis that impairs the production of intrinsic factor, which is required for vitamin B_{12} uptake from the gut.

Normal Vitamin B_{12} Metabolism. Vitamin B_{12} is a complex organometallic compound also known as cobalamin. Under normal circumstances humans are totally dependent on dietary vitamin B_{12}. Microorganisms are the source of cobalamin in the food chain. Plants and vegetables contain little cobalamin, save that contributed by microbial

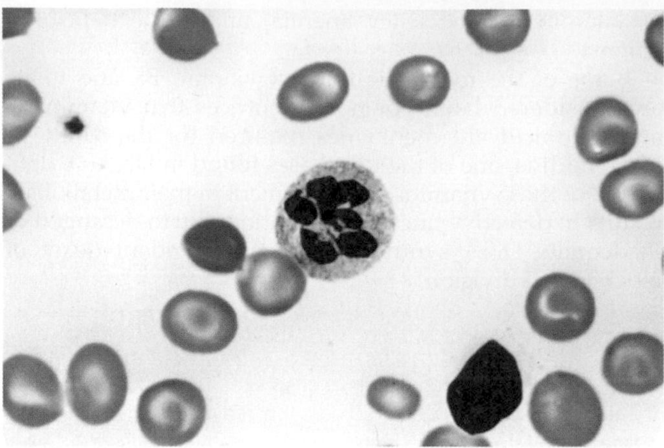

Figure 14-16 Megaloblastic anemia. A peripheral blood smear shows a hypersegmented neutrophil with a six-lobed nucleus. (Courtesy Dr. Robert W. McKenna, Department of Pathology, University of Texas Southwestern Medical School, Dallas, Texas.)

contamination, and strictly vegetarian or macrobiotic diets do not provide adequate amounts of this essential nutrient. The daily requirement is 2 to 3 μg. A diet that includes animal products contains significantly larger amounts and normally results in the accumulation of intrahepatic stores of vitamin B_{12} that are sufficient to last for several years.

Absorption of vitamin B_{12} requires intrinsic factor, which is secreted by the parietal cells of the fundic mucosa (Fig. 14-18). Vitamin B_{12} is freed from binding proteins in food through the action of pepsin in the stomach and binds to a salivary protein called *haptocorrin*. In the duodenum, bound vitamin B_{12} is released from haptocorrin by the action of pancreatic proteases and it associates with intrinsic factor. This complex is transported to the ileum, where it is endocytosed by ileal enterocytes that express a receptor for intrinsic factor called *cubilin* on their surfaces. Within ileal cells, vitamin B_{12} associates with a major carrier

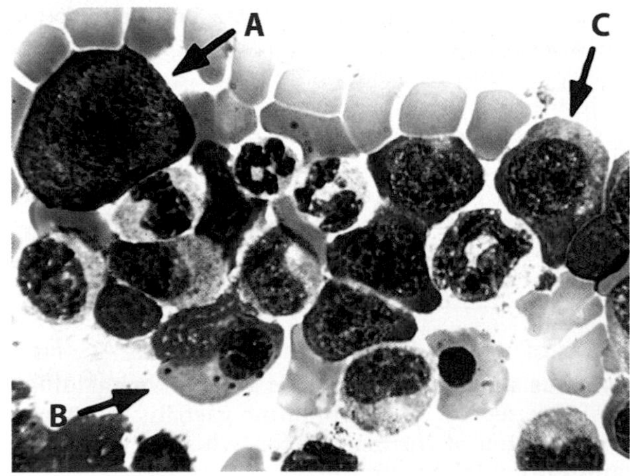

Figure 14-17 Megaloblastic anemia (bone marrow aspirate). **A** to **C**, Megaloblasts in various stages of differentiation. Note that the orthochromatic megaloblast (**B**) is hemoglobinized (as revealed by cytoplasmic color), but in contrast to normal orthochromatic normoblasts, the nucleus is not pyknotic. The early erythroid precursors (**A** and **C**) and the granulocytic precursors are also large and have abnormally immature chromatin. (Courtesy Dr. Jose Hernandez, Department of Pathology, University of Texas Southwestern Medical School, Dallas, Texas.)

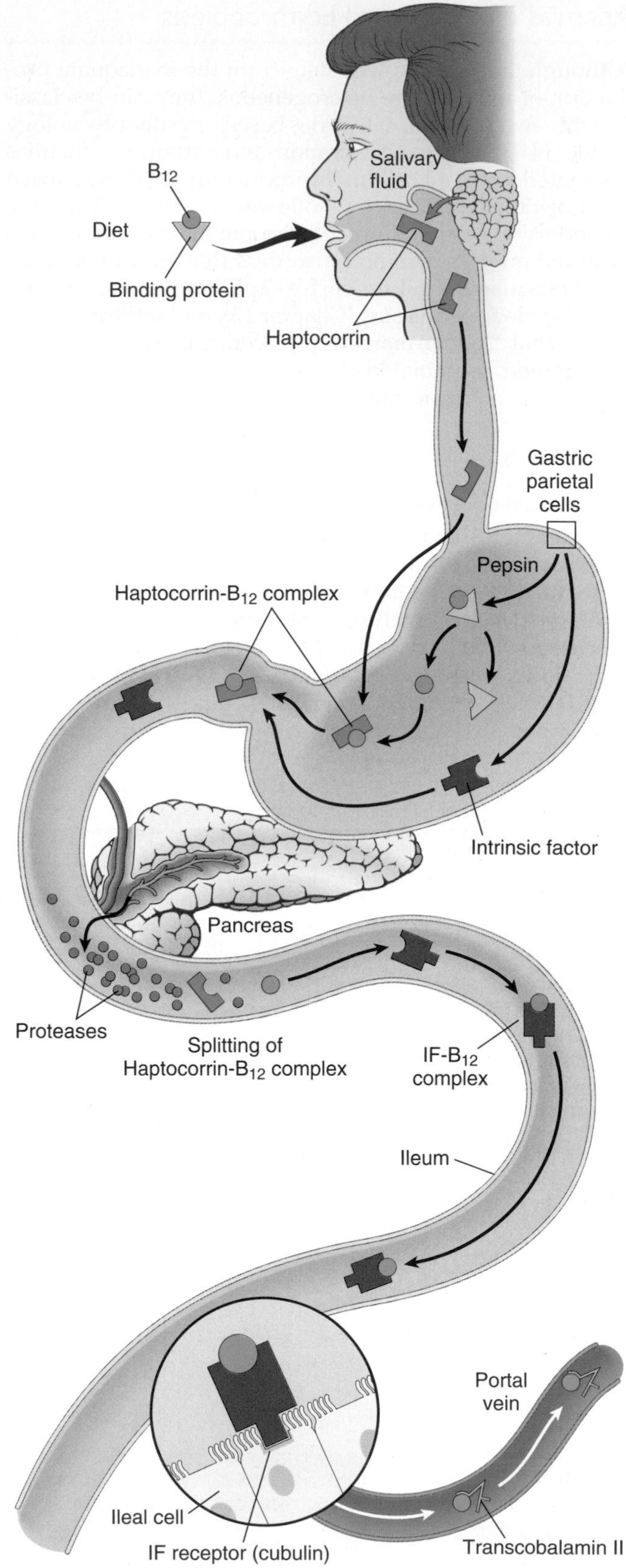

Figure 14-18 Schematic illustration of vitamin B_{12} absorption. IF, Intrinsic factor; haptocorrin, cubilin, see text.

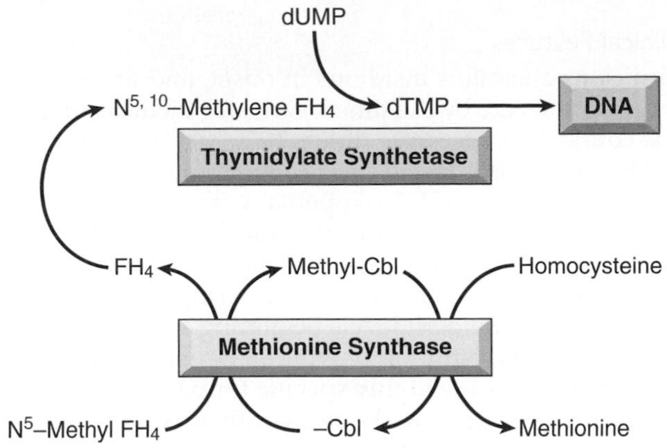

Figure 14-19 Relationship of N^5-methyl FH_4, methionine synthase, and thymidylate synthetase. In cobalamin (Cbl) deficiency, folate is sequestered as N^5-methyl FH_4. This ultimately deprives thymidylate synthetase of its folate coenzyme ($N^{5,10}$-methylene FH_4), thereby impairing DNA synthesis. FH_4, Tetrahydrofolic acid.

protein, transcobalamin II, and is secreted into the plasma. Transcobalamin II delivers vitamin B_{12} to the liver and other cells of the body, including rapidly proliferating cells in the bone marrow and the gastrointestinal tract. In addition to this major pathway, there is also a poorly understood alternative uptake mechanism that is not dependent on intrinsic factor or an intact terminal ileum. Up to 1% of a large oral dose can be absorbed by this pathway, making it feasible to treat pernicious anemia with high doses of oral vitamin B_{12}.

Biochemical Functions of Vitamin B_{12}. Only two reactions in humans are known to require vitamin B_{12}. In one, methylcobalamin serves as an essential cofactor in the conversion of homocysteine to methionine by methionine synthase (Fig. 14-19). In the process, methylcobalamin yields a methyl group that is recovered from N^5-methyltetrahydrofolic acid (N^5-methyl FH_4), the principal form of folic acid in plasma. In the same reaction, N^5-methyl FH_4 is converted to tetrahydrofolic acid (FH_4). FH_4 is crucial, because it is required (through its derivative $N^{5,10}$-methylene FH_4) for the conversion of deoxyuridine monophosphate (dUMP) to deoxythymidine monophosphate (dTMP), a building block for DNA. It is postulated that the fundamental cause of the impaired DNA synthesis in vitamin B_{12} deficiency is the reduced availability of FH_4, most of which is "trapped" as N^5-methyl FH_4. The FH_4 deficit may be further exacerbated by an "internal" folate deficiency caused by a failure to synthesize metabolically active polyglutamylated forms. This stems from the requirement for vitamin B_{12} in the synthesis of methionine, which contributes a carbon group needed in the metabolic reactions that create folate polyglutamates (Fig. 14-20). Whatever the mechanism, lack of folate is the proximate cause of anemia in vitamin B_{12} deficiency, because the anemia improves with administration of folic acid.

The neurologic complications associated with vitamin B_{12} deficiency are more enigmatic, because they are not improved (and may actually be worsened) by folate administration. The other known reaction that depends on vitamin B_{12} is the isomerization of methylmalonyl coenzyme A to succinyl coenzyme A, which requires adenosylcobalamin as a prosthetic group on the enzyme methylmalonyl-coenzyme A mutase. A deficiency of vitamin B_{12} thus leads to increased plasma and urine levels of methylmalonic acid. Interruption of this reaction and the consequent buildup of methylmalonate and propionate (a precursor) could lead to the formation and incorporation of abnormal fatty acids into neuronal lipids. It has been suggested that this biochemical abnormality predisposes to myelin breakdown and thereby produces the neurologic complications of vitamin B_{12} deficiency (Chapter 28). However, rare individuals with hereditary deficiencies of methylmalonyl-coenzyme A mutase do not suffer from the neurologic abnormalities seen in vitamin B_{12} deficiency, casting doubt on this explanation.

Pernicious Anemia

Incidence. Although somewhat more prevalent in Scandinavian and other Caucasian populations, pernicious anemia occurs in all racial groups, including blacks and Hispanics. It is a disease of older adults; the median age at diagnosis is 60 years, and it is rare in people younger than 30. A genetic predisposition is strongly suspected, but no definable genetic pattern of transmission has been discerned. As described later, many affected individuals have a tendency to form antibodies against multiple self-antigens.

Pathogenesis. Pernicious anemia is believed to result from an autoimmune attack on the gastric mucosa. Histologically, there is a *chronic atrophic gastritis* marked by a loss of parietal cells, a prominent infiltrate of lymphocytes and plasma cells, and megaloblastic changes in mucosal cells similar to those found in erythroid precursors. Three types of autoantibodies are present in many, but not all, patients. About 75% of patients have a *type I antibody* that blocks the binding of vitamin B_{12} to intrinsic factor. Type I antibodies are found in both plasma and gastric juice. *Type II antibodies* prevent binding of the intrinsic factor-vitamin B_{12} complex to its ileal receptor. These antibodies are also found in a large proportion of patients with pernicious anemia. *Type III antibodies* are present in 85% to 90% of patients and recognize the α and β subunits of the gastric proton pump, which is normally localized to the microvilli of the canalicular system of the gastric parietal cell. Type III

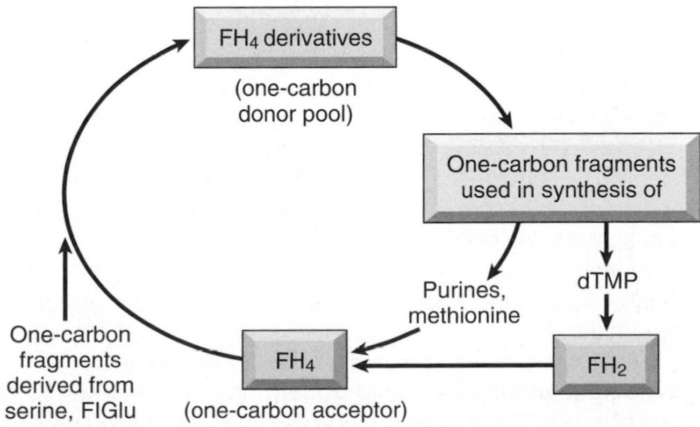

Figure 14-20 Role of folate derivatives in the transfer of one-carbon fragments for synthesis of biologic macromolecules. FH_4, Tetrahydrofolic acid; FH_2, dihydrofolic acid; FIGlu, formiminoglutamate; dTMP, deoxythymidine monophosphate.

antibodies are not specific, in that they are found in as many as 50% of older adults with idiopathic chronic gastritis not associated with pernicious anemia.

Autoantibodies are of diagnostic utility, but they are not thought to be the primary cause of the gastric pathology; rather, it seems that an autoreactive T-cell response initiates gastric mucosal injury and triggers the formation of autoantibodies. When the mass of intrinsic factor-secreting cells falls below a threshold (and reserves of stored vitamin B_{12} are depleted), anemia develops. The common association of pernicious anemia with other autoimmune disorders, particularly autoimmune thyroiditis and adrenalitis, is also consistent with an underlying immune basis. The tendency to develop pernicious anemia (as well as other autoimmune disorders) is linked to genetic variants involving the inflammasome, suggesting that altered innate immunity may also play some role.

Vitamin B_{12} deficiency is associated with disorders other than pernicious anemia. Most of these impair absorption of the vitamin at one of the steps outlined earlier (Table 14-5). With achlorhydria and loss of pepsin secretion (which occurs in some older adults), vitamin B_{12} is not readily released from proteins in food. With gastrectomy, intrinsic factor is not available for uptake in the ileum. With loss of exocrine pancreatic function, vitamin B_{12} cannot be released from haptocorrin-vitamin B_{12} complexes. Ileal resection or diffuse ileal disease can remove or damage the site of intrinsic factor-vitamin B_{12} complex absorption. Certain tapeworms (particularly those acquired by eating raw fish) compete with the host for B_{12} and can induce a deficiency state. In some settings, such as pregnancy, hyperthyroidism, disseminated cancer, and chronic infection, an increased demand for vitamin B_{12} can produce a relative deficiency, even with normal absorption.

MORPHOLOGY

The findings in the bone marrow and blood in pernicious anemia are similar to those described earlier for all megaloblastic anemias. The stomach typically shows diffuse chronic gastritis (Chapter 17). The most characteristic alteration is **fundic gland atrophy**, affecting both chief cells and parietal cells, the latter being virtually absent. The glandular epithelium is replaced by mucus-secreting goblet cells that resemble those lining the large intestine, a form of metaplasia referred to as **intestinalization**. Some of the cells as well as their nuclei may increase to double the normal size, a "megaloblastic" change analogous to that seen in the marrow. With time, the tongue may become shiny, glazed, and "beefy" **(atrophic glossitis)**. The gastric atrophy and metaplastic changes are due to autoimmunity and not vitamin B_{12} deficiency; hence, parenteral administration of vitamin B_{12} corrects the megaloblastic changes in the marrow and the epithelial cells of the alimentary tract, but gastric atrophy and achlorhydria persist.

Central nervous system lesions are found in about three fourths of all cases of florid pernicious anemia but can also be seen in the absence of overt hematologic findings. The principal alterations involve the cord, where there is **demyelination of the dorsal and lateral spinal tracts,** sometimes followed by loss of axons. These changes give rise to spastic paraparesis, sensory ataxia, and severe paresthesias in the lower limbs. Less frequently, degenerative changes occur in the ganglia of the posterior roots and in peripheral nerves (Chapter 28).

Clinical Features

Pernicious anemia is insidious in onset, and the anemia is often quite severe by the time it comes to medical attention. The course is progressive unless halted by therapy.

The diagnosis is based on (1) a moderate to severe megaloblastic anemia, (2) leukopenia with hypersegmented granulocytes, (3) low serum vitamin B_{12}, and (4) elevated serum levels of homocysteine and methylmalonic acid. The diagnosis is confirmed by an outpouring of reticulocytes and a rise in hematocrit levels beginning about 5 days after parenteral administration of vitamin B_{12}. Serum antibodies to intrinsic factor are highly specific for pernicious anemia. Their presence attests to the cause rather than the presence or absence of vitamin B_{12} deficiency.

Persons with atrophy and metaplasia of the gastric mucosa associated with pernicious anemia have an increased risk of gastric carcinoma (Chapter 17). Elevated homocysteine levels are a risk factor for atherosclerosis and thrombosis, and it is suspected that vitamin B_{12} deficiency may increase the incidence of vascular disease on this basis. With parenteral or high-dose oral vitamin B_{12}, the anemia is cured and the progression of the peripheral neurologic disease can be reversed or at least halted, but the changes in the gastric mucosa and the risk of carcinoma are unaffected.

Anemia of Folate Deficiency

A deficiency of folic acid (more properly, pteroylmonoglutamic acid) results in a megaloblastic anemia having the same pathologic features as that caused by vitamin B_{12} deficiency. FH_4 derivatives act as intermediates in the transfer of one-carbon units such as formyl and methyl groups to various compounds (Fig. 14-20). FH_4 serves as an acceptor of one-carbon fragments from compounds such as serine and formiminoglutamic acid. The FH_4 derivatives so generated in turn donate the acquired one-carbon fragments in reactions synthesizing various metabolites. FH_4, then, can be viewed as the biologic "middleman" in a series of swaps involving one-carbon moieties. The most important metabolic processes depending on such transfers are (1) purine synthesis; (2) the conversion of homocysteine to methionine, a reaction also requiring vitamin B_{12}; and (3) deoxythymidylate monophosphate (dTMP) synthesis. In the first two reactions, tetrahydrofolate (FH_4) is regenerated from its one-carbon carrier derivatives and is available to accept another one-carbon moiety and reenter the donor pool. In the synthesis of dTMP, a dihydrofolate (FH_2) is produced that must be reduced by dihydrofolate reductase for reentry into the FH_4 pool. The reductase step is significant, because this enzyme is susceptible to inhibition by various drugs. Among the molecules whose synthesis is dependent on folates, dTMP is perhaps the most important biologically, because it is required for DNA synthesis. It should be apparent from this discussion that **suppressed synthesis of DNA, the common denominator of folic acid and vitamin B_{12} deficiency, is the immediate cause of megaloblastosis**.

Etiology. The three major causes of folic acid deficiency are (1) decreased intake, (2) increased requirements, and (3) impaired utilization (Table 14-5). Humans are entirely dependent on dietary sources for their folic acid requirement, which is 50 to 200 μg daily. Most normal diets contain ample amounts. The richest sources are green vegetables such as lettuce, spinach, asparagus, and broccoli. Certain fruits (e.g., lemons, bananas, melons) and animal sources (e.g., liver) contain lesser amounts. The folic acid in these foods is largely in the form of folylpolyglutamates. Despite their abundance in raw foods, polyglutamates are sensitive to heat; boiling, steaming, or frying of foods for 5 to 10 minutes destroys up to 95% of the folate content. Intestinal conjugases split the polyglutamates into monoglutamates that are readily absorbed in the proximal jejunum. During intestinal absorption they are modified to 5-methyltetrahydrofolate, the normal transport form of folate. The body's reserves of folate are relatively modest, and a deficiency can arise within weeks to months if intake is inadequate.

Decreased intake can result from either a nutritionally inadequate diet or impairment of intestinal absorption. A normal diet contains folate in excess of the minimal daily adult requirement. Inadequate dietary intakes are almost invariably associated with grossly deficient diets. Such dietary inadequacies are most frequently encountered in chronic alcoholics, the indigent, and the very old. In alcoholics with cirrhosis, other mechanisms of folate deficiency such as trapping of folate within the liver, excessive urinary loss, and disordered folate metabolism have also been implicated. Under these circumstances, the megaloblastic anemia is often accompanied by general malnutrition and manifestations of other avitaminoses, including cheilosis, glossitis, and dermatitis. Malabsorption syndromes, such as sprue, can lead to inadequate absorption of this nutrient, as can diffuse infiltrative diseases of the small intestine (e.g., lymphoma). In addition, certain drugs, particularly the anticonvulsant phenytoin and oral contraceptives, interfere with absorption.

Despite normal intake of folic acid, a *relative deficiency* can be encountered when requirements are increased. Conditions in which this is seen include pregnancy, infancy, derangements associated with hyperactive hematopoiesis (hemolytic anemias), and disseminated cancer. In all these circumstances the demands of increased DNA synthesis render normal intake inadequate.

Folic acid antagonists, such as methotrexate, inhibit dihydrofolate reductase and lead to a deficiency of FH_4. With inhibition of folate metabolism, all rapidly growing cells are affected, but particularly the cells of the bone marrow and the gastrointestinal tract. Many chemotherapeutic drugs used in the treatment of cancer damage DNA or inhibit DNA synthesis through other mechanisms; these can also cause megaloblastic changes in rapidly dividing cells.

As mentioned at the outset, the megaloblastic anemia that results from a deficiency of folic acid is identical to that encountered in vitamin B_{12} deficiency. Thus, the diagnosis of folate deficiency can be made only by demonstration of decreased folate levels in the serum or red cells. As in vitamin B_{12} deficiency, serum homocysteine levels are increased, but methylmalonate concentrations are normal. Importantly, neurologic changes do not occur.

Although prompt hematologic response heralded by reticulocytosis follows the administration of folic acid, it should be remembered that the hematologic symptoms of vitamin B_{12} deficiency anemia also respond to folate therapy. As already mentioned, folate does not prevent (and may even exacerbate) the neurologic deficits seen in vitamin B_{12} deficiency states. It is thus essential to exclude vitamin B_{12} deficiency in megaloblastic anemia before initiating therapy with folate.

Iron Deficiency Anemia

Deficiency of iron is the most common nutritional disorder in the world and results in a clinical signs and symptoms that are mostly related to inadequate hemoglobin synthesis. Although the prevalence of iron deficiency anemia is higher in developing countries, this form of anemia is common in the United States, particularly in toddlers, adolescent girls, and women of childbearing age. The factors underlying the iron deficiency differ somewhat in various population groups and can be best considered in the context of normal iron metabolism.

Iron Metabolism. The normal daily Western diet contains about 10 to 20 mg of iron, most in the form of heme contained in animal products, with the remainder being inorganic iron in vegetables. About 20% of heme iron (in contrast to 1% to 2% of nonheme iron) is absorbable, so the average Western diet contains sufficient iron to balance fixed daily losses. The total body iron content is normally about 2.5 gm in women and as high as 6 gm in men, and can be divided into functional and storage compartments (Table 14-6). About 80% of the functional iron is found in hemoglobin; myoglobin and iron-containing enzymes such as catalase and the cytochromes contain the rest. The storage pool represented by hemosiderin and ferritin contains about 15% to 20% of total body iron. The major sites of iron storage are the liver and mononuclear phagocytes. Healthy young females have smaller stores of iron than do males, primarily because of blood loss during menstruation, and often develop iron deficiency due to excessive losses or increased demands associated with menstruation and pregnancy, respectively.

Iron in the body is recycled between the functional and storage pools (Fig. 14-21). It is transported in plasma by an iron-binding glycoprotein called *transferrin*, which is synthesized in the liver. In normal individuals, transferrin is about one third saturated with iron, yielding serum iron levels that average 120 μg/dL in men and 100 μg/dL in women. The major function of plasma transferrin is to deliver iron to cells, including erythroid precursors, which require iron to synthesize hemoglobin. Erythroid precursors possess high-affinity receptors for transferrin that mediate iron import through receptor-mediated endocytosis.

Table 14-6 Iron Distribution in Healthy Young Adults (mg)

Pool	Men	Women
Total	3450	2450
Functional	2100	1750
Hemoglobin	300	250
Myoglobin	50	50
Enzymes		
Storage	1000	400
Ferritin, hemosiderin		

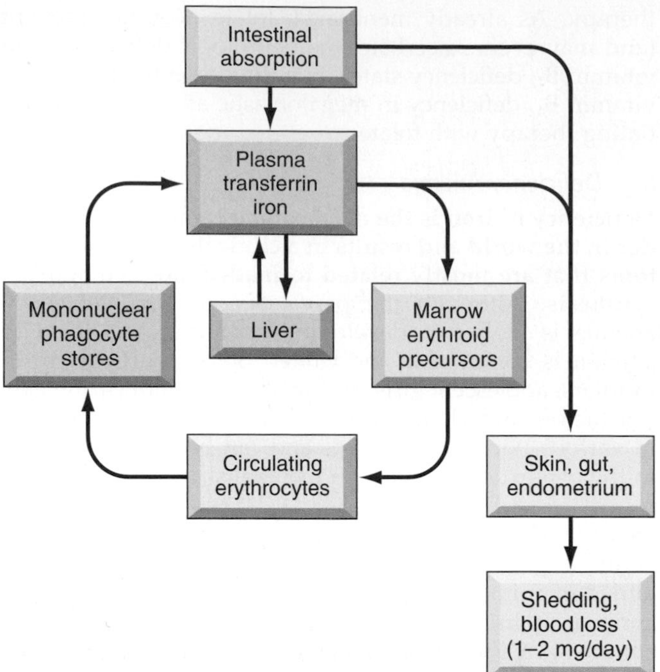

Figure 14-21 Iron metabolism. Iron absorbed from the gut is bound to plasma transferrin and transported to the marrow, where it is delivered to developing red cells and incorporated into hemoglobin. Mature red cells are released into the circulation and, after 120 days, are ingested by macrophages, primarily in the spleen, liver, and bone marrow. Here iron is extracted from hemoglobin and recycled to plasma transferrin. At equilibrium, iron absorbed from the gut is balanced by losses in shed keratinocytes, enterocytes, and (in women) endometrium.

Free iron is highly toxic (Chapter 18), and it is therefore important that storage iron be sequestered. This is achieved by binding of iron in the storage pool to either ferritin or hemosiderin. *Ferritin* is a ubiquitous protein-iron complex that is found at highest levels in the liver, spleen, bone marrow, and skeletal muscles. In the liver, most ferritin is stored within the parenchymal cells; in other tissues, such as the spleen and the bone marrow, it is found mainly in macrophages. Hepatocyte iron is derived from plasma transferrin, whereas storage iron in macrophages is derived from the breakdown of red cells. Intracellular ferritin is located in the cytosol and in lysosomes, in which partially degraded protein shells of ferritin aggregate into *hemosiderin* granules. Iron in hemosiderin is chemically reactive and turns blue-black when exposed to potassium ferrocyanide, which is the basis for the *Prussian blue stain*. With normal iron stores, only trace amounts of hemosiderin are found in the body, principally in macrophages in the bone marrow, spleen, and liver, most being stored as ferritin. In iron-overloaded cells, most iron is stored in hemosiderin.

Because plasma ferritin is derived largely from the storage pool of body iron, its levels correlate well with body iron stores. In iron deficiency, serum ferritin is below 12 μg/L, whereas in iron overload values approaching 5000 μg/L may be seen. Of physiologic importance, the storage iron pool can be readily mobilized if iron requirements increase, as may occur after loss of blood.

Iron is both essential for cellular metabolism and highly toxic in excess, and total body iron stores must therefore be regulated meticulously. Iron balance is maintained by regulating the absorption of dietary iron in the proximal duodenum. There is no regulated pathway for iron excretion, which is limited to the 1 to 2 mg lost each day through the shedding of mucosal and skin epithelial cells. In contrast, as body iron stores increase, absorption falls, and vice versa.

The pathways responsible for the absorption of iron are now understood in reasonable detail (Fig. 14-22), and differ partially for nonheme and heme iron. Luminal nonheme iron is mostly in the Fe^{3+} (ferric) state and must first be reduced to Fe^{2+} (ferrous) iron by ferrireductases, such as b cytochromes and STEAP3. Fe^{2+} iron is then transported across the apical membrane by divalent metal transporter 1 (DMT1). The absorption of nonheme iron is variable and often inefficient, being inhibited by substances in the diet that bind and stabilize Fe^{3+} iron and enhanced by substances that stabilize Fe^{2+} iron (described later). Frequently, less than 5% of dietary nonheme iron is absorbed. In contrast, about 25% of the heme iron derived from hemoglobin, myoglobin, and other animal proteins is absorbed. Heme iron is moved across the apical membrane into the cytoplasm through transporters that are incompletely characterized. Here, it is metabolized to release Fe^{2+} iron, which enters a common pool with nonheme Fe^{2+} iron.

Iron that enters the duodenal cells can follow one of two pathways: transport to the blood or storage as mucosal iron. This distribution is influenced by body iron stores. Fe^{2+} iron destined for the circulation is transported from the cytoplasm across the basolateral enterocyte membrane by ferroportin. This process is coupled to the oxidation of Fe^{2+} iron to Fe^{3+} iron, which is carried out by the iron oxidases hephaestin and ceruloplasmin. Newly absorbed Fe^{3+} iron binds rapidly to the plasma protein transferrin, which delivers iron to red cell progenitors in the marrow (Fig. 14-21). Both DMT1 and ferroportin are widely distributed in the body and are involved in iron transport in other tissues as well. For example, DMT1 also mediates the uptake of "functional" iron (derived from endocytosed transferrin) across lysosomal membranes into the cytosol of red cell precursors in the bone marrow, and ferroportin plays an important role in the release of storage iron from macrophages.

Iron absorption is regulated by *hepcidin*, a small circulating peptide that is synthesized and released from the liver in response to increases in intrahepatic iron levels. Hepcidin inhibits iron transfer from the enterocyte to plasma by binding to ferroportin and causing it to be endocytosed and degraded. As a result, as hepcidin levels rise, iron becomes trapped within duodenal cells in the form of mucosal ferritin and is lost as these cells are sloughed. Thus, when the body is replete with iron, high hepcidin levels inhibit its absorption into the blood. Conversely, with low body stores of iron, hepcidin synthesis falls and this in turn facilitates iron absorption. By inhibiting ferroportin, hepcidin not only reduces iron uptake from enterocytes but also suppresses iron release from macrophages, which are an important source of the iron that is used by erythroid precursors to make hemoglobin. This, as we shall see, is important in the pathogenesis of anemia of chronic diseases.

Alterations in hepcidin have a central role in diseases involving disturbances of iron metabolism. This is illustrated by the following examples.

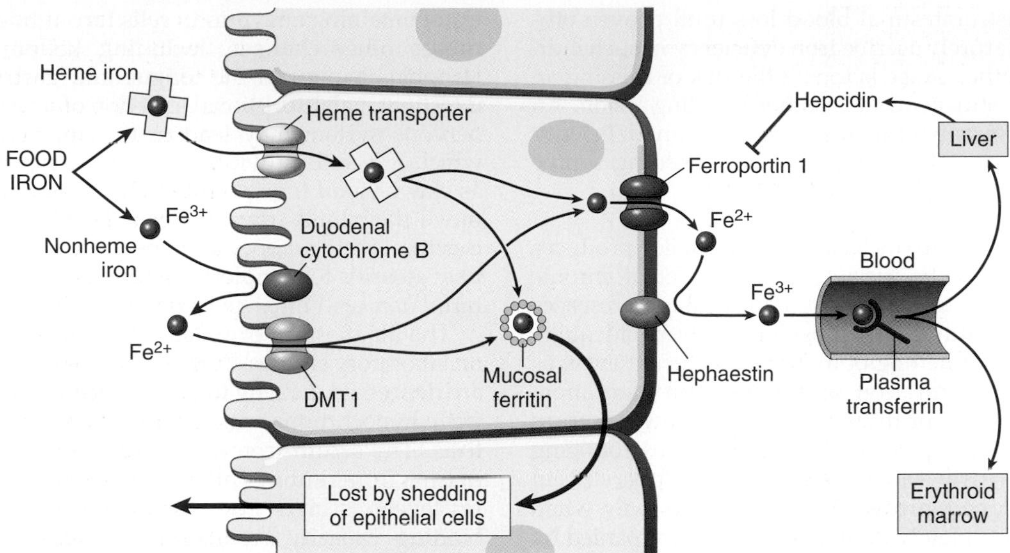

Figure 14-22 Regulation of iron absorption. Duodenal epithelial cell uptake of heme and nonheme iron is depicted. When the storage sites of the body are replete with iron and erythropoietic activity is normal, plasma hepcidin levels are high. This leads to down-regulation of ferroportin and trapping of most of the absorbed iron, which is lost when duodenal epithelial cells are shed into the gut. Conversely, when body iron stores decrease or when erythropoiesis is stimulated, hepcidin levels fall and ferroportin activity increases, allowing a greater fraction of the absorbed iron to be transferred to plasma transferrin. *DMT1*, Divalent metal transporter 1.

- As will be described subsequently, the *anemia of chronic disease* (perhaps more accurately referred to as the anemia of chronic inflammation) is caused in part by inflammatory mediators that increase hepatic hepcidin production.
- A rare form of microcytic anemia is caused by mutations that disable TMPRSS6, a hepatic transmembrane serine protease that normally suppresses hepcidin production when iron stores are low. Affected patients have high hepcidin levels, resulting in reduced iron absorption and failure to respond to iron therapy.
- Conversely, hepcidin activity is inappropriately low in both primary and secondary *hemochromatosis*, a syndrome caused by systemic iron overload.
- Secondary hemochromatosis can occur in diseases associated with *ineffective erythropoiesis*, such as β-thalassemia major and myelodysplastic syndromes (Chapter 13). Through incompletely understood mechanisms, ineffective erythropoiesis suppresses hepatic hepcidin production, even when iron stores are high. As discussed in Chapter 18, the various inherited forms of primary hemochromatosis are associated with mutations in hepcidin or the genes that regulate hepcidin expression.

Etiology. **Iron deficiency can result from (1) dietary lack, (2) impaired absorption, (3) increased requirement, or (4) chronic blood loss.** To maintain a normal iron balance, about 1 mg of iron must be absorbed from the diet every day. Because only 10% to 15% of ingested iron is absorbed, the daily iron requirement is 7 to 10 mg for adult men and 7 to 20 mg for adult women. Because the average daily dietary intake of iron in the Western world is about 15 to 20 mg, most men ingest more than adequate iron, whereas many women consume marginally adequate amounts of iron. The bioavailability of dietary iron is as important as the overall content. Heme iron is much more absorbable than inorganic iron, the absorption of which is influenced by other dietary contents. Absorption of inorganic iron is enhanced by ascorbic acid, citric acid, amino acids, and sugars in the diet, and inhibited by tannates (found in tea), carbonates, oxalates, and phosphates.

Dietary lack is rare in developed countries, where on average about two thirds of the dietary iron is in the readily absorbed heme form provided by meat. The situation is different in developing countries, where food is less abundant and most iron in the diet is found in plants in the poorly absorbable inorganic form. Dietary iron inadequacy occurs in even privileged societies in the following groups:

- *Infants,* who are at high risk due to the very small amounts of iron in milk. Human breast milk provides only about 0.3 mg/L of iron. Cow's milk contains about twice as much iron, but its bioavailability is poor.
- *The impoverished,* who can have suboptimal diets for socioeconomic reasons at any age
- *Older adults,* who often have restricted diets with little meat because of limited income or poor dentition
- *Teenagers* who subsist on "junk" food

Impaired absorption is found in sprue, other causes of fat malabsorption (steatorrhea), and chronic diarrhea. Gastrectomy impairs iron absorption by decreasing the acidity of the proximal duodenum (which enhances uptake), and also by increasing the speed with which gut contents pass through the duodenum. Specific items in the diet, as is evident from the preceding discussion, can also affect absorption.

Increased requirement is an important cause of iron deficiency in growing infants, children, and adolescents, as well as premenopausal women, particularly during pregnancy. Economically deprived women having multiple, closely spaced pregnancies are at exceptionally high risk.

Chronic blood loss is the most common cause of iron deficiency in the Western world. External hemorrhage or bleeding into the gastrointestinal, urinary, or genital tracts depletes iron reserves. Iron deficiency in adult men and postmenopausal women in the Western world must be attributed to gastrointestinal blood loss until proven otherwise. To prematurely ascribe iron deficiency in such individuals to any other cause is to run the risk of missing an occult gastrointestinal cancer or other bleeding lesion. An alert clinician investigating unexplained iron deficiency anemia occasionally discovers an occult bleeding source such as a cancer and thereby saves a life.

Pathogenesis. Whatever its basis, iron deficiency produces a *hypochromic microcytic anemia.* At the outset of chronic blood loss or other states of negative iron balance, reserves in the form of ferritin and hemosiderin may be adequate to maintain normal hemoglobin and hematocrit levels as well as normal serum iron and transferrin saturation. Progressive depletion of these reserves first lowers serum iron and transferrin saturation levels without producing anemia. In this early stage there is increased erythroid activity in the bone marrow. Anemia appears only when iron stores are completely depleted and is accompanied by lower than normal serum iron, ferritin, and transferrin saturation levels.

MORPHOLOGY

The bone marrow reveals a mild to moderate increase in erythroid progenitors. A diagnostically significant finding is the **disappearance of stainable iron from macrophages in the bone marrow**, which is best assessed by performing Prussian blue stains on smears of aspirated marrow. In peripheral blood smears, the red cells are small **(microcytic)** and pale **(hypochromic)**. Normal red cells with sufficient hemoglobin have a zone of central pallor measuring about one third of the cell diameter. In established iron deficiency the zone of pallor is enlarged; hemoglobin may be seen only in a narrow peripheral rim (Fig. 14-23). Poikilocytosis in the form of small, elongated red cells (pencil cells) is also characteristically seen.

Clinical Features

The clinical manifestations of the anemia are nonspecific and were detailed earlier. The dominating signs and symptoms frequently relate to the underlying cause of the anemia, for example, gastrointestinal or gynecologic disease, malnutrition, pregnancy, and malabsorption. In severe and long-standing iron deficiency, depletion of iron-containing enzymes in cells throughout the body also causes other changes, including koilonychia, alopecia, atrophic changes in the tongue and gastric mucosa, and intestinal malabsorption. Depletion of iron from the central nervous system may lead to the appearance of pica, in which affected individuals consume non-foodstuffs such as clay or food ingredients such as flour, and periodically move their limbs during sleep. Esophageal webs appear together with microcytic hypochromic anemia and atrophic glossitis to complete the triad of major findings in the rare *Plummer-Vinson syndrome* (Chapter 17).

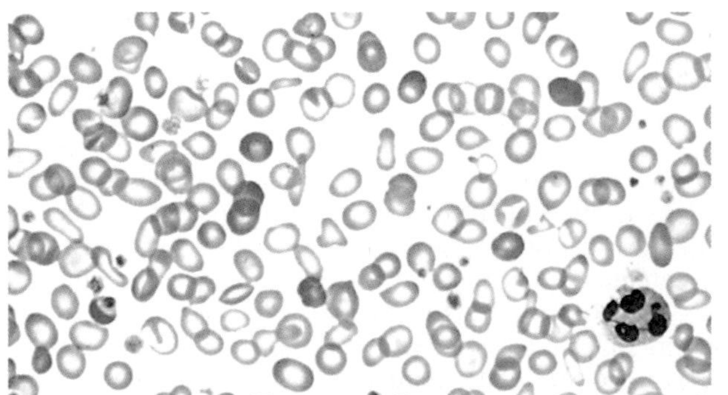

Figure 14-23 Hypochromic microcytic anemia of iron deficiency (peripheral blood smear). Note the small red cells containing a narrow rim of peripheral hemoglobin. Scattered fully hemoglobinized cells, present due to recent blood transfusion, stand in contrast. (Courtesy Dr. Robert W. McKenna, Department of Pathology, University of Texas Southwestern Medical School, Dallas, Texas.)

The diagnosis of iron deficiency anemia ultimately rests on laboratory studies. Both the hemoglobin and hematocrit are depressed, usually to a moderate degree, in association with hypochromia, microcytosis, and modest poikilocytosis. The serum iron and ferritin are low, and the total plasma iron-binding capacity (reflecting elevated transferrin levels) is high. Low serum iron with increased iron-binding capacity results in a reduction of transferrin saturation to below 15%. Reduced iron stores inhibit hepcidin synthesis, and its serum levels fall. In uncomplicated iron deficiency, oral iron supplementation produces an increase in reticulocytes in about 5 to 7 days that is followed by a steady increase in blood counts and the normalization of red cell indices.

Anemia of Chronic Disease

Impaired red cell production associated with chronic diseases that produce systemic inflammation is perhaps the most common cause of anemia among hospitalized patients in the United States. This form of anemia stems from a reduction in the proliferation of erythroid progenitors and impaired iron utilization. The chronic illnesses associated with this form of anemia can be grouped into three categories:

1. Chronic microbial infections, such as osteomyelitis, bacterial endocarditis, and lung abscess
2. Chronic immune disorders, such as rheumatoid arthritis and regional enteritis
3. Neoplasms, such as carcinomas of the lung and breast, and Hodgkin lymphoma

The anemia of chronic disease occurs in the setting of persistent systemic inflammation and is associated with low serum iron, reduced total iron-binding capacity, and abundant stored iron in tissue macrophages. Several effects of inflammation contribute to the observed abnormalities. Most notably, certain inflammatory mediators, particularly interleukin-6 (IL-6), stimulate an increase in the hepatic production of hepcidin. As was discussed under the anemia of iron deficiency, hepcidin inhibits ferroportin function in macrophages and reduces the transfer of iron from the storage pool to developing erythroid precursors in the bone marrow. As a result, the erythroid precursors are starved for iron in the midst of plenty. In addition, these progenitors do not proliferate adequately because erythropoietin levels are inappropriately low for the degree of anemia. The precise mechanism underlying this reduction in erythropoietin is uncertain, but transgenic mice expressing high levels of hepcidin develop a microcytic anemia associated with low erythropoietin levels, suggesting that hepcidin directly or indirectly suppresses erythropoietin production.

What might be the reason for iron sequestration in the setting of inflammation? The best guess is that it enhances the body's ability to fend off certain types of infection, particularly those caused by bacteria (e.g., *H. influenzae*) that require iron for pathogenicity. In this regard it is interesting to consider that hepcidin is structurally related to defensins, a family of peptides that have intrinsic antibacterial activity. This connection further highlights the poorly understood but intriguing relationship between inflammation, innate immunity, and iron metabolism.

The anemia is usually mild, and the dominant symptoms are those of the underlying disease. The red cells can be normocytic and normochromic, or hypochromic and microcytic, as in anemia of iron deficiency. The presence of increased storage iron in marrow macrophages, a high serum ferritin level, and a reduced total iron-binding capacity readily rule out iron deficiency as the cause of anemia. Only successful treatment of the underlying condition reliably corrects the anemia. However, some patients, particularly those with cancer, benefit from administration of erythropoietin.

Aplastic Anemia

Aplastic anemia refers to a syndrome of chronic primary hematopoietic failure and attendant *pancytopenia* (anemia, neutropenia, and thrombocytopenia). In the majority of patients autoimmune mechanisms are suspected, but inherited or acquired abnormalities of hematopoietic stem cells also seem to contribute in at least a subset of patients.

Table 14-7 Major Causes of Aplastic Anemia

Acquired
Idiopathic
Acquired stem cell defects
Immune mediated
Chemical Agents
Dose related
Alkylating agents
Antimetabolites
Benzene
Chloramphenicol
Inorganic arsenicals
Idiosyncratic
Chloramphenicol
Phenylbutazone
Organic arsenicals
Methylphenylethylhydantoin
Carbamazepine
Penicillamine
Gold salts
Physical Agents
Whole-body irradiation
Viral Infections
Hepatitis (unknown virus)
Cytomegalovirus infections
Epstein-Barr virus infections
Herpes zoster (varicella zoster)
Inherited
Fanconi anemia
Telomerase defects

Etiology. The most common circumstances associated with aplastic anemia are listed in Table 14-7. Most cases of "known" etiology follow exposure to chemicals and drugs. Certain drugs and agents (including many cancer chemotherapy drugs and the organic solvent benzene) cause marrow suppression that is dose related and reversible. In other instances, aplastic anemia arises in an unpredictable, idiosyncratic fashion following exposure to drugs that normally cause little or no marrow suppression. The implicated drugs include chloramphenicol and gold salts.

Persistent marrow aplasia can also appear after a variety of *viral infections,* most commonly viral hepatitis of the non-A, non-B, non-C, non-G type, which is associated with 5% to 10% of cases. Why aplastic anemia develops in certain individuals is not understood.

Whole-body *irradiation* can destroy hematopoietic stem cells in a dose-dependent fashion. Persons who receive therapeutic irradiation or are exposed to radiation in nuclear accidents (e.g., Chernobyl) are at risk for marrow aplasia.

Specific abnormalities underlie some cases of aplastic aplasia.

- *Fanconi anemia* is a rare autosomal recessive disorder caused by defects in a multiprotein complex that is required for DNA repair (Chapter 7). Marrow hypofunction becomes evident early in life and is often accompanied by multiple congenital anomalies, such as hypoplasia of the kidney and spleen and bone anomalies, which most commonly involve the thumbs or radii.
- Inherited defects in *telomerase* are found in 5% to 10% of adult onset aplastic anemia. Telomerase is required for cellular immortality and limitless replication (Chapters 1 and 7). It might be anticipated, therefore, that partial deficits in telomerase activity could result in premature hematopoietic stem cell exhaustion and marrow aplasia.
- Even more common than telomerase mutations are abnormally short telomeres, which are found in the marrow cells of as many as half of those affected with aplastic anemia. It is unknown whether this shortening is due to other unappreciated telomerase defects or is a consequence of excessive stem cell replication.

In most instances, however, no initiating factor can be identified; about 65% of cases fall into this *idiopathic* category.

Pathogenesis. The pathogenesis of aplastic anemia is not fully understood. Indeed, it is unlikely that a single mechanism underlies all cases. However, **two major etiologies have been invoked: an extrinsic, immune-mediated suppression of marrow progenitors, and an intrinsic abnormality of stem cells** (Fig. 14-24).

Experimental studies have focused on a model in which activated T cells suppress hematopoietic stem cells. Stem cells may first be antigenically altered by exposure to drugs, infectious agents, or other unidentified environmental insults. This provokes a cellular immune response, during which activated T_H1 cells produce cytokines such as interferon-γ (IFN-γ) and TNF that suppress and kill hematopoietic progenitors. This scenario is supported by several observations.

- Analysis of the few remaining marrow stem cells from aplastic anemia marrows has revealed that genes

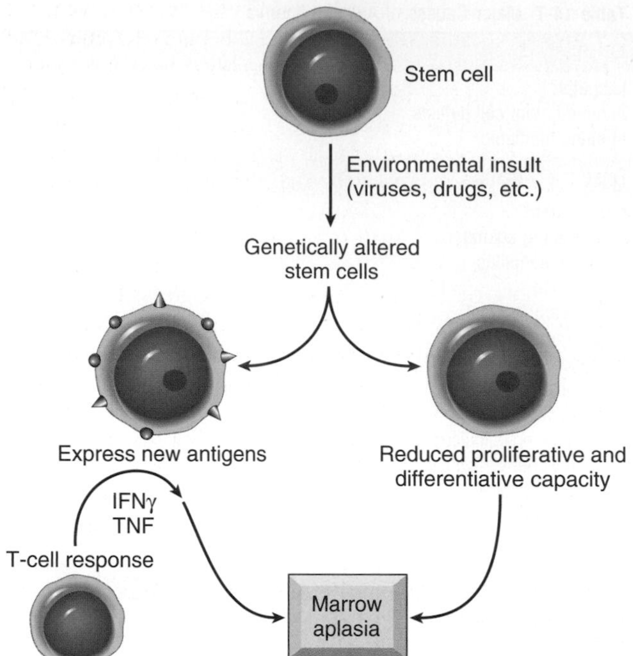

Figure 14-24 Pathophysiology of aplastic anemia. Damaged stem cells can produce progeny expressing neoantigens that evoke an autoimmune reaction, or give rise to a clonal population with reduced proliferative capacity. Either pathway could lead to marrow aplasia. See text for abbreviations.

involved in apoptosis and death pathways are up-regulated; of note, the same genes are up-regulated in normal stem cells exposed to interferon-γ.

- Even more compelling (and clinically relevant) evidence comes from experience with immunosuppressive therapy. Antithymocyte globulin and other immunosuppressive drugs such as cyclosporine produce responses in 60% to 70% of patients. It is proposed that these therapies work by suppressing or killing autoreactive T-cell clones. The antigens recognized by the autoreactive T cells are not well defined. In some instances GPI-linked proteins may be the targets, possibly explaining the previously noted association of aplastic anemia and PNH.

Alternatively, the notion that aplastic anemia results from a fundamental stem cell abnormality is supported by the presence of karyotypic aberrations in many cases; the occasional transformation of aplasias into myeloid neoplasms, typically myelodysplasia or acute myeloid leukemia; and the association with abnormally short telomeres. Some marrow insult (or a predisposition to DNA damage) presumably results in sufficient injury to limit the proliferative and differentiation capacity of stem cells. If the damage is extensive enough, aplastic anemia results. These two mechanisms are not mutually exclusive, because genetically altered stem cells might also express "neoantigens" that could serve as targets for a T-cell attack.

MORPHOLOGY

The markedly hypocellular bone marrow is largely devoid of hematopoietic cells; often only fat cells, fibrous stroma, and scattered lymphocytes and plasma cells remain. Marrow aspirates often yield little material (a "dry tap"); hence, aplasia is best appreciated in marrow biopsies (Fig. 14-25). Other nonspecific pathologic changes are related to granulocytopenia and thrombocytopenia, such as mucocutaneous bacterial infections and abnormal bleeding, respectively. If the anemia necessitates multiple transfusions, systemic hemosiderosis can appear.

Clinical Features

Aplastic anemia can occur at any age and in either sex. The onset is usually insidious. Initial manifestations vary somewhat, depending on which cell line is predominantly affected, but pancytopenia ultimately appears, with the expected consequences. Anemia can cause progressive weakness, pallor, and dyspnea; thrombocytopenia is heralded by petechiae and ecchymoses; and neutropenia manifests as frequent and persistent minor infections or the sudden onset of chills, fever, and prostration. Splenomegaly is characteristically absent; if it is present, the diagnosis of aplastic anemia should be seriously questioned. The red cells are usually slightly macrocytic and normochromic. Reticulocytopenia is the rule.

The diagnosis rests on examination of a bone marrow biopsy. It is important to distinguish aplastic anemia from other causes of pancytopenia, such as "aleukemic"

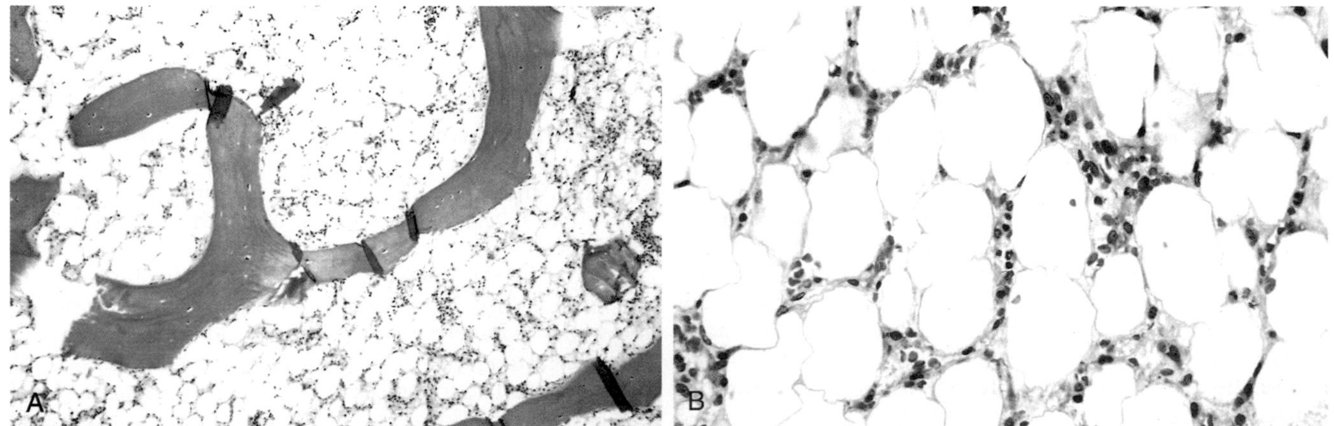

Figure 14-25 Aplastic anemia (bone marrow biopsy). Markedly hypocellular marrow contains mainly fat cells. **A,** Low power. **B,** High power. (Courtesy Dr. Steven Kroft, Department of Pathology, University of Texas Southwestern Medical School, Dallas, Texas.)

leukemia and myelodysplastic syndromes (Chapter 13), which can have identical clinical manifestations. In aplastic anemia, the marrow is hypocellular (and usually markedly so), whereas myeloid neoplasms are associated with hypercellular marrows filled with neoplastic progenitors.

The prognosis is variable. Bone marrow transplantation is the treatment of choice in those with a suitable donor and provides a 5-year survival of more than 75%. Older patients or those without suitable donors often respond well to immunosuppressive therapy.

Pure Red Cell Aplasia

Pure red cell aplasia is a primary marrow disorder in which only erythroid progenitors are suppressed. In severe cases, red cell progenitors are completely absent from the marrow. It may occur in association with neoplasms, particularly thymoma and large granular lymphocytic leukemia (Chapter 13), drug exposures, autoimmune disorders, and parvovirus infection (see later). With the exception of those with parvovirus infection, it is likely that most cases have an autoimmune basis. When a thymoma is present, resection leads to hematologic improvement in about half of the patients. In patients without thymoma, immunosuppressive therapy is often beneficial. Plasmapheresis may also be helpful in unusual patients with pathogenic autoantibodies, such as neutralizing antibodies to erythropoietin that appear de novo or following the administration of recombinant erythropoietin.

A special form of red cell aplasia occurs in individuals infected with parvovirus B19, which preferentially infects and destroys red cell progenitors. Normal individuals clear parvovirus infections within 1 to 2 weeks; as a result, the aplasia is transient and clinically unimportant. However, in persons with moderate to severe hemolytic anemias, even a brief cessation of erythropoiesis results in rapid worsening of the anemia, producing an aplastic crisis. In those who are severely immunosuppressed (e.g., persons with advanced HIV infection), an ineffective immune response sometimes permits the infection to persist, leading to chronic red cell aplasia and a moderate to severe anemia.

Other Forms of Marrow Failure

***Myelophthisic anemia* describes a form of marrow failure in which space-occupying lesions replace normal marrow elements.** The commonest cause is metastatic cancer, most often carcinomas arising in the breast, lung, and prostate. However, any infiltrative process (e.g., granulomatous disease) involving the marrow can produce identical findings. Myelophthisic anemia is also a feature of the spent phase of myeloproliferative disorders (Chapter 13). All of the responsible diseases cause marrow distortion and fibrosis, which act to displace normal marrow elements and disturb mechanisms that regulate the egress of red cells and granulocytes from the marrow. The latter effect causes the abnormal release of nucleated erythroid precursors and immature granulocytic forms *(leukoerythroblastosis)* into peripheral smears, and the appearance of *teardrop-shaped red cells,* which are believed to be deformed during their tortuous escape from the fibrotic marrow.

***Chronic renal failure,* whatever its cause, is almost invariably associated with an anemia that tends to be roughly proportional to the severity of the uremia.** The basis of anemia in renal failure is multifactorial, but the dominant cause is the diminished synthesis of erythropoietin by the damaged kidneys, which leads to inadequate red cell production. Other contributors are an extracorpuscular defect that reduces red cell life span, and iron deficiency due to platelet dysfunction and increased bleeding, which is often encountered in uremia. Administration of recombinant erythropoietin results in a significant improvement of the anemia, although an optimal response may require concomitant iron replacement therapy.

Hepatocellular liver disease, whether toxic, infectious, or cirrhotic, is associated with anemia attributed to decreased marrow function. Folate and iron deficiencies caused by poor nutrition and excessive bleeding often exacerbate anemia in this setting. Erythroid progenitors are preferentially affected; depression of the white cell count and platelets is less common but also occurs. The anemia is often slightly macrocytic due to lipid abnormalities associated with liver failure, which cause red cell membranes to acquire phospholipid and cholesterol as they circulate in the peripheral blood.

Endocrine disorders, particularly hypothyroidism, may also be associated with a mild normochromic, normocytic anemia.

KEY CONCEPTS

Megaloblastic Anemia

- Caused by deficiencies of folate or vitamin B_{12} that lead to inadequate synthesis of thymidine and defective DNA replication
- Results in enlarged abnormal hematopoietic precursors (megaloblasts), ineffective hematopoiesis, macrocytic anemia, and (in most cases) pancytopenia
- B_{12} deficiency also associated with neurologic damage, particularly in the posterior and lateral tracts of the spinal cord

Iron Deficiency Anemia

- Caused by chronic bleeding or inadequate iron intake; results in insufficient hemoglobin synthesis and hypochromic, microcytic red cells

Anemia of Chronic Disease

- Caused by inflammatory cytokines, which increase hepcidin levels and thereby sequester iron in macrophages, and also suppress erythropoietin production

Aplastic Anemia

- Caused by bone marrow failure (hypocellularity) due to diverse causes, including exposures to toxins and radiation, idiosyncratic reactions to drugs and viruses, and inherited defects in telomerase and DNA repair

Pure Red Cell Aplasia

- Acute: Parvovirus B19 infection (may persist in immunosuppressed patients)
- Chronic: Associated with thymoma, large granular lymphocytic leukemia, presence of neutralizing antibodies against erythropoietin, and other autoimmune phenomenon

Other Causes of Underproduction Anemias

- Marrow replacement (tumors, granulomatous disease; so-called myelophthisic anemias), renal failure, endocrine disorders, liver failure

Polycythemia

Polycythemia denotes an abnormally high red cell count, usually with a corresponding increase in the hemoglobin level. It may be relative when there is hemoconcentration due to decreased plasma volume, or absolute when there is an increase in the total red cell mass. *Relative polycythemia* results from dehydration, such as occurs with deprivation of water, prolonged vomiting or diarrhea, or excessive use of diuretics. It is also associated with an obscure condition of unknown etiology called stress polycythemia, or Gaisböck syndrome. Affected individuals are usually hypertensive, obese, and anxious ("stressed"). *Absolute polycythemia* is *primary* when it results from an intrinsic abnormality of hematopoietic precursors and *secondary* when the red cell progenitors are responding to increased levels of erythropoietin. A pathophysiologic classification of polycythemia divided along these lines is given in Table 14-8.

The most common cause of primary polycythemia is *polycythemia vera,* a myeloproliferative disorder associated with mutations that lead to erythropoietin-independent growth of red cell progenitors (Chapter 13). Much less commonly, primary polycythemia results from familial mutations in the erythropoietin receptor that induce erythropoietin-independent receptor activation. One such individual won Olympic gold medals in cross-country skiing, having benefited from this natural form of blood doping! Secondary polycythemia may be caused by compensatory or pathologic increases in erythropoietin secretion. Causes of the latter include erythropoietin-secreting tumors and rare, but illustrative, inherited defects that lead to the stabilization of HIF-1α, a hypoxia-induced factor that stimulates the transcription of the erythropoietin gene.

Bleeding Disorders: Hemorrhagic Diatheses

Excessive bleeding can result from (1) increased fragility of vessels, (2) platelet deficiency or dysfunction, and (3) derangement of coagulation, alone or in combination. Before discussing specific bleeding disorders, it is helpful to review the common laboratory tests used in the evaluation of a bleeding diathesis. The normal hemostatic response involves the blood vessel wall, the platelets, and the clotting cascade (Chapter 4). Tests used to evaluate different aspects of hemostasis are the following:

Table 14-8 Pathophysiologic Classification of Polycythemia

Relative
Reduced plasma volume (hemoconcentration)
Absolute
Primary (Low Erythropoietin)
Polycythemia vera
Inherited erythropoietin receptor mutations (rare)
Secondary (High Erythropoietin)
Compensatory
Lung disease
High-altitude living
Cyanotic heart disease
Paraneoplastic
Erythropoietin-secreting tumors (e.g., renal cell carcinoma, hepatocellular carcinoma, cerebellar hemangioblastoma)
Hemoglobin mutants with high O_2 affinity
Inherited defects that stabilize HIF-1α
Chuvash polycythemia (homozygous *VHL* mutations)
Prolyl hydroxylase mutations

HIF-1α, Hypoxia-induced factor 1α.

- *Prothrombin time (PT).* This test assesses the extrinsic and common coagulation pathways. The clotting of plasma after addition of an exogenous source of tissue thromboplastin (e.g., brain extract) and Ca^{2+} ions is measured in seconds. A prolonged PT can result from deficiency or dysfunction of factor V, factor VII, factor X, prothrombin, or fibrinogen.
- *Partial thromboplastin time (PTT).* This test assesses the intrinsic and common clotting pathways. The clotting of plasma after addition of kaolin, cephalin, and Ca^{2+} ions is measured in seconds. Kaolin activates the contact-dependent factor XII, and cephalin substitutes for platelet phospholipids. Prolongation of the PTT can be due to deficiency or dysfunction of factors V, VIII, IX, X, XI, or XII, prothrombin, or fibrinogen, or to interfering antibodies to phospholipid (Chapter 4).
- *Platelet counts.* These are obtained on anticoagulated blood using an electronic particle counter. The reference range is 150×10^3 to 300×10^3 platelets/μL. Abnormal platelet counts are best confirmed by inspection of a peripheral blood smear, in that clumping of platelets can cause spurious "thrombocytopenia" during automated counting, and high counts may be indicative of a myeloproliferative disorder, such as essential thrombocythemia (Chapter 13).
- *Tests of platelet function.* At present, no single test provides an adequate assessment of the complex functions of platelets. Specialized tests that can be useful in particular clinical settings include tests of platelet aggregation, which measure the ability of platelets to aggregate in response to agonists like thrombin; and quantitative and qualitative tests of von Willebrand factor, which plays an important role in platelet adhesion to the extracellular matrix (Chapter 4). An older test, the bleeding time, has some value but is time-consuming and difficult to standardize and is therefore performed infrequently. Newer instrument-based assays that provide quantitative measures of platelet function show promise but remain imperfect at predicting bleeding risk, presumably because of difficulties in simulating in vivo clotting in the laboratory.

More specialized tests are available to measure the levels of specific clotting factors, fibrinogen, fibrin split products, and the presence of circulating anticoagulants.

Bleeding Disorders Caused by Vessel Wall Abnormalities

Disorders within this category are relatively common, but do not usually cause serious bleeding problems. Most often, they present with small hemorrhages (petechiae and purpura) in the skin or mucous membranes, particularly the gingivae. On occasion, however, more significant hemorrhages occur into joints, muscles, and subperiosteal locations, or take the form of menorrhagia, nosebleeds, gastrointestinal bleeding, or hematuria. The platelet count and tests of coagulation (PT, PTT) are usually normal, pointing by exclusion to the underlying problem.

The varied clinical conditions in which abnormalities in the vessel wall cause bleeding include the following:

- *Infections* often induce petechial and purpuric hemorrhages, particularly meningococcemia, other forms of septicemia, infective endocarditis, and several of the rickettsioses. The involved mechanisms include microbial damage to the microvasculature (vasculitis) and disseminated intravascular coagulation. Failure to recognize meningococcemia as a cause of petechiae and purpura can be catastrophic for the patient.
- *Drug reactions* sometimes induce cutaneous petechiae and purpura without causing thrombocytopenia. In many instances the vascular injury is mediated by the deposition of drug-induced immune complexes in vessel walls, which leads to hypersensitivity (*leukocytoclastic*) vasculitis (Chapter 11).
- *Scurvy* and the *Ehlers-Danlos syndrome* are associated with microvascular bleeding that results from collagen defects that weaken vessel walls. The same mechanism may account for the spontaneous purpura that are commonly seen in older adults and the skin hemorrhages that are seen with *Cushing syndrome,* in which the protein-wasting effects of excessive corticosteroid production cause loss of perivascular supporting tissue.
- *Henoch-Schönlein purpura* is a systemic immune disorder of unknown cause that is characterized by a purpuric rash, colicky abdominal pain, polyarthralgia, and acute glomerulonephritis (Chapter 20). All these changes result from the deposition of circulating immune complexes within vessels throughout the body and within the glomerular mesangial regions.
- *Hereditary hemorrhagic telangiectasia* (also known as *Weber-Osler-Rendu syndrome*) is an autosomal dominant disorder that can be caused by mutations in at least five different genes, most of which modulate TGF-β signaling. It is characterized by dilated, tortuous blood vessels with thin walls that bleed readily. Bleeding can occur anywhere, but it is most common under the mucous membranes of the nose (epistaxis), tongue, mouth, and eyes, and throughout the gastrointestinal tract.
- *Perivascular amyloidosis* can weaken blood vessel walls and cause bleeding. This complication is most common with amyloid light-chain (AL) amyloidosis (Chapter 6) and often manifests as mucocutaneous petechiae.

Among these conditions, serious bleeding is most often associated with hereditary hemorrhagic telangiectasia. The bleeding in each is nonspecific, and the diagnosis of these entities is based on the recognition of other more specific associated findings.

Bleeding Related to Reduced Platelet Number: Thrombocytopenia

Reduction in platelet number (*thrombocytopenia*) constitutes an important cause of generalized bleeding. A count less than 100,000 platelets/μL is generally considered to constitute thrombocytopenia. Platelet counts in the range of 20,000 to 50,000 platelets/μL can aggravate posttraumatic bleeding, while platelet counts less than 20,000 platelets/μL may be associated with spontaneous (nontraumatic) bleeding. Bleeding resulting from thrombocytopenia is associated with a normal PT and PTT.

Platelets are critical for hemostasis, in that they form temporary plugs that stop bleeding and promote key reactions in the coagulation cascade (Chapter 4). Spontaneous bleeding associated with thrombocytopenia most often involves small vessels. Common sites for such hemorrhages are the skin and the mucous membranes of the gastrointestinal and genitourinary tracts. Most feared, however, is *intracranial bleeding,* which is a threat to any patient with a markedly depressed platelet count.

The causes of thrombocytopenia fall into four major categories (Table 14-9).

Table 14-9 Causes of Thrombocytopenia

Decreased Production of Platelets
Selective impairment of platelet production
Drug-induced: alcohol, thiazides, cytotoxic drugs
Infections: measles, human immunodeficiency virus (HIV)
Nutritional deficiencies
B_{12}, folate deficiency (megaloblastic leukemia)
Bone marrow failure
Aplastic anemia (see Table 14-7)
Bone marrow replacement
Leukemia, disseminated cancer, granulomatous disease
Ineffective hematopoiesis
Myelodysplastic syndromes (Chapter 13)
Decreased Platelet Survival
Immunologic destruction
Primary autoimmune
Chromic immune thrombocytopenic purpura
Acute immune thrombocytopenic purpura
Secondary autoimmune
Systemic lupus erythematosus, B-cell lymphoid neoplasms
Alloimmune: posttransfusion and neonatal
Drug-associated: quinidine, heparin, sulfa compounds
Infections: HIV, infectious mononucleosis (transient, mild), dengue fever
Nonimmunologic destruction
Disseminated intravascular coagulation
Thrombotic microangiopathies
Giant hemangiomas
Sequestration
Hypersplenism
Dilution
Transfusions

- *Decreased platelet production.* This can result from conditions that depress marrow output generally (such as aplastic anemia and leukemia) or affect megakaryocytes somewhat selectively. Examples of the latter include certain drugs and alcohol, which may suppress platelet production through uncertain mechanisms when taken in large amounts; HIV, which may infect megakaryocytes and inhibit platelet production; and myelodysplastic syndromes (Chapter 13), which may occasionally present with isolated thrombocytopenia.

- *Decreased platelet survival.* This important mechanism of thrombocytopenia can have an immunological or nonimmunologic basis. In *immune thrombocytopenia,* destruction is caused by the deposition of antibodies or immune complexes on platelets. Antibodies to platelets can recognize self-antigens (autoantibodies) or non-self antigens (alloantibodies). Autoimmune thrombocytopenia is discussed in the following section. *Alloantibodies* can arise when platelets are transfused or cross the placenta from the fetus into the pregnant mother. In the latter case, IgG antibodies made in the mother can cause clinically significant thrombocytopenia in the fetus. This is reminiscent of hemolytic disease of the newborn, in which red cells are the target (Chapter 10). The most important nonimmunologic causes are *disseminated intravascular coagulation* and the *thrombotic microangiopathies,* in which unbridled, often systemic, platelet activation reduces platelet life span. Nonimmunologic destruction of platelets may also be caused by *mechanical injury,* such as in individuals with prosthetic heart valves.
- *Sequestration.* The spleen normally sequesters 30% to 35% of the body's platelets, but this can rise to 80% to 90% when the spleen is enlarged, producing moderate degrees of thrombocytopenia.
- *Dilution.* Massive transfusions can produce a dilutional thrombocytopenia. With prolonged blood storage the number of viable platelets decreases; thus, plasma volume and red cell mass are reconstituted by transfusion, but the number of circulating platelets is relatively reduced.

Chronic Immune Thrombocytopenic Purpura (ITP)

Chronic ITP is caused by autoantibody mediated destruction of platelets. It can occur in the setting of a variety of predisposing conditions and exposures (secondary) or in the absence of any known risk factors (primary or idiopathic). The contexts in which chronic ITP occurs secondarily are numerous and include individuals with systemic lupus erythematosus (Chapter 6), HIV infection, and B-cell neoplasms such as chronic lymphocytic leukemia (Chapter 13). The diagnosis of primary chronic ITP is made only after secondary causes are excluded.

Pathogenesis. The autoantibodies, most often directed against platelet membrane glycoproteins IIb-IIIa or Ib-IX, can be demonstrated in the plasma and bound to the platelet surface in about 80% of patients. In the overwhelming majority of cases, the antiplatelet antibodies are of the IgG class.

As in autoimmune hemolytic anemias, antiplatelet antibodies act as opsonins that are recognized by IgG Fc receptors expressed on phagocytes (Chapter 6), leading to increased platelet destruction. The thrombocytopenia is usually markedly improved by splenectomy, indicating that the spleen is the major site of removal of opsonized platelets. The splenic red pulp is also rich in plasma cells, and part of the benefit of splenectomy (a frequent treatment for chronic ITP) may stem from the removal of a source of autoantibodies. In some instances the autoantibodies may also bind to and damage megakaryocytes, leading to decreases in platelet production that further exacerbate the thrombocytopenia.

MORPHOLOGY

The principal changes of thrombocytopenic purpura are found in the spleen, bone marrow, and blood, but they are not specific. Secondary changes related to the bleeding diathesis may be found in any tissue or structure in the body.

The spleen is of normal size. Typically, there is congestion of the sinusoids and enlargement of the splenic follicles, often associated with prominent reactive germinal centers. In many instances scattered megakaryocytes are found within the sinuses, possibly representing a mild form of extramedullary hematopoiesis driven by elevated levels of thrombopoietin. **The marrow reveals a modestly increased number of megakaryocytes**. Some are apparently immature, with large, nonlobulated, single nuclei. These findings are not specific but merely reflect accelerated thrombopoiesis, being found in most forms of thrombocytopenia resulting from increased platelet destruction. The importance of bone marrow examination is to rule out thrombocytopenias resulting from bone marrow failure or other primary bone marrow disorders. The secondary changes relate to the hemorrhages that are dispersed throughout the body. The **peripheral blood often reveals abnormally large platelets** (megathrombocytes), which are a sign of accelerated thrombopoiesis.

Clinical Features

Chronic ITP occurs most commonly in adult women younger than 40 years of age. The female-to-male ratio is 3:1. It is often insidious in onset and is characterized by bleeding into the skin and mucosal surfaces. Cutaneous bleeding is seen in the form of pinpoint hemorrhages (*petechiae*), which are especially prominent in the dependent areas where the capillary pressure is higher. Petechiae can become confluent, giving rise to *ecchymoses.* Often there is a history of easy bruising, nosebleeds, bleeding from the gums, and hemorrhages into soft tissues from relatively minor trauma. The disease may manifest first with melena, hematuria, or excessive menstrual flow. Subarachnoid hemorrhage and intracerebral hemorrhage are serious and sometimes fatal complications, but fortunately they are rare in treated patients. Splenomegaly and lymphadenopathy are uncommon in primary disease, and their presence should lead one to consider other diagnoses, such as ITP secondary to a B-cell neoplasm.

The clinical signs and symptoms are not specific but rather reflective of the thrombocytopenia. The findings of a low platelet count, normal or increased megakaryocytes in the bone marrow, and large platelets in the peripheral blood are taken as presumptive evidence of accelerated platelet destruction. The PT and PTT are normal. Tests for platelet autoantibodies are not widely available. Therefore, the diagnosis is one of exclusion and can be made only after other causes of thrombocytopenia (such as those listed in Table 14-9) have been ruled out.

Almost all patients respond to glucocorticoids (which inhibit phagocyte function), but many eventually relapse. Those with moderately severe thrombocytopenia (platelet counts > 30,000/mL) can be followed carefully, and some of these individuals may have spontaneous remissions over a period of a year or more. In individuals with severe thrombocytopenia, splenectomy normalizes the platelet count in about two thirds of patients, but with the attendant increased risk of bacterial sepsis. Immunomodulatory agents such as intravenous immunoglobulin or anti-CD20 antibody (rituximab) are often effective in patients who relapse after splenectomy or for whom splenectomy is contraindicated. Peptides that mimic the effects of thrombopoietin (so-called *TPO-mimetics*) are also effective in stimulating platelet production and improving platelet counts.

Acute Immune Thrombocytopenic Purpura

Like chronic ITP, this condition is caused by autoantibodies to platelets, but its clinical features and course are distinct. Acute ITP is mainly a disease of childhood occurring with equal frequency in both sexes. Symptoms appear abruptly, often 1 to 2 weeks after a self-limited viral illness, which appears to trigger the development of autoantibodies through uncertain mechanisms. Unlike chronic ITP, acute ITP is self-limited, usually resolving spontaneously within 6 months. Glucocorticoids are given only if the thrombocytopenia is severe. In about 20% of children, usually those without a viral prodrome, thrombocytopenia persists; these less fortunate children have a childhood form of chronic ITP that follows a course similar to the adult disease.

Drug-Induced Thrombocytopenia

Drugs can induce thrombocytopenia through direct effects on platelets and secondary to immunologically mediated platelet destruction. The drugs most commonly implicated are quinine, quinidine, and vancomycin, all of which bind platelet glycoproteins and in one way or another create antigenic determinants that are recognized by antibodies. Much more rarely, drugs induce true autoantibodies through unknown mechanisms. Thrombocytopenia, which may be severe, is also a common consequence of platelet inhibitory drugs that bind glycoprotein IIb/IIIa; it is hypothesized that these drugs induce conformational changes in glycoprotein IIb/IIIa and create an immunogenic epitope.

Heparin-induced thrombocytopenia (HIT) has a distinctive pathogenesis and is of particular importance because of its potential for severe clinical consequences. Thrombocytopenia occurs in about 5% of persons receiving heparin and is of two types:

- Type I thrombocytopenia occurs rapidly after the onset of therapy and is of little clinical importance, sometimes resolving despite the continuation of therapy. It most likely results from a direct platelet-aggregating effect of heparin.
- Type II thrombocytopenia is less common but of much greater clinical significance. It occurs 5 to 14 days after therapy begins (or sooner if the person has been sensitized to heparin) and, paradoxically, often leads to life-threatening venous and arterial thrombosis. This severe form of HIT is caused by antibodies that recognize complexes of heparin and platelet factor 4, which is a normal component of platelet granules. Binding of antibody to these complexes activates platelets and promotes thrombosis, even in the setting of thrombocytopenia. Unless therapy is immediately discontinued and an alternative nonheparin anticoagulant instituted, clots within large arteries may lead to vascular insufficiency and limb loss, and emboli from deep venous thrombosis can cause fatal pulmonary thromboembolism. The risk of severe HIT is lowered, but not completely eliminated, by the use of low-molecular-weight heparin preparations. Unfortunately, once severe HIT develops even low-molecular-weight heparins exacerbate the thrombotic tendency and must be avoided.

HIV-Associated Thrombocytopenia

Thrombocytopenia is one of the most common hematologic manifestations of HIV infection. Both impaired platelet production and increased destruction contribute. CD4 and CXCR4, the receptor and coreceptor, respectively, for HIV, are found on megakaryocytes, allowing these cells to be infected. HIV-infected megakaryocytes are prone to apoptosis and their ability to produce platelets is impaired. HIV infection also causes B-cell hyperplasia and dysregulation, which predisposes to the development of autoantibodies. In some instances the antibodies are directed against platelet membrane glycoprotein IIb-III complexes. As in other immune cytopenias, the autoantibodies opsonize platelets, promoting their destruction by mononuclear phagocytes in the spleen and elsewhere. The deposition of immune complexes on platelets may also contribute to the accelerated loss of platelets in some patients who are HIV infected.

Thrombotic Microangiopathies: Thrombotic Thrombocytopenic Purpura (TTP) and Hemolytic-Uremic Syndrome (HUS)

The term *thrombotic microangiopathy* encompasses a spectrum of clinical syndromes that includes TTP and HUS. They are caused by insults that lead to excessive activation of platelets, which deposit as thrombi in small blood vessels.

According to its original description, TTP was defined as the pentad of fever, thrombocytopenia, microangiopathic hemolytic anemia, transient neurologic deficits, and renal failure. HUS is also associated with microangiopathic hemolytic anemia and thrombocytopenia but is distinguished by the absence of neurologic symptoms, the prominence of acute renal failure, and its frequent occurrence in children. With time, experience, and increased mechanistic insight, however, these distinctions have blurred. Many adult patients with "TTP" lack one or more of the five criteria, and some patients with "HUS" have fever and neurologic dysfunction.

In both conditions, intravascular thrombi cause a *microangiopathic hemolytic anemia* and widespread *organ dysfunction*, and the attendant consumption of platelets leads to thrombocytopenia. It is believed that the varied clinical manifestations of TTP and HUS are related to differing proclivities for thrombus formation in tissues. While disseminated intravascular coagulation (discussed later) and thrombotic microangiopathies share features such as microvascular occlusion and microangiopathic hemolytic anemia, they are pathogenically distinct. In TTP and HUS (unlike in disseminated intravascular coagulation), activation of the coagulation cascade is not of primary importance, and hence laboratory tests of coagulation, such as the PT and PTT, are usually normal.

Table 14-10 Thrombotic Microangiopathies: Causes and Associations

Thrombotic Thrombocytopenic Purpura
Deficiency of ADAMTS13
Inherited Acquired (autoantibodies)
Hemolytic Uremic Syndrome
Typical: *Escherichia coli* strain 0157:H7 infection
Endothelial damage by Shiga-like toxin
Atypical: alternative complement pathway inhibitor deficiencies
(complement factor H, membrane cofactor protein (CD46), or factor I) Inherited Acquired (autoantibodies)
Miscellaneous associations
Drugs (cyclosporine, chemotherapeutic agents) Radiation, bone marrow transplantation Other infections (HIV, pneumococcal sepsis) Conditions associated with autoimmunity (systemic lupus erythematosus, HIV infection, lymphoid neoplasms)

HIV, Human immunodeficiency virus.

Although certain features of the various thrombotic microangiopathies overlap, the triggers for the pathogenic platelet activation are distinctive and provide a more satisfying and clinically relevant way of thinking about these disorders; these are summarized in Table 14-10. **TTP is usually associated with a deficiency in a plasma enzyme called *ADAMTS13*,** also designated "vWF metalloprotease." ADAMTS13 normally degrades very high-molecular-weight multimers of von Willebrand factor (vWF). In its absence, these multimers accumulate in plasma and tend to promote platelet activation and aggregation. Superimposition of endothelial cell injury (caused by some other condition) may further promote the formation of platelet microaggregates, thus initiating or exacerbating clinically evident TTP.

The deficiency of ADAMTS13 can be inherited or acquired. In the acquired form, an autoantibody that inhibits the metalloprotease activity of ADAMTS13 is present. Less commonly, patients inherit an inactivating mutation in *ADAMTS13*. In those with hereditary ADAMTS13 deficiency, the onset is often delayed until adolescence and the symptoms are episodic. Thus, factors other than ADAMTS13 (e.g., some superimposed vascular injury or prothrombotic state) must be involved in triggering full-blown TTP.

TTP is an important diagnosis to consider in any patient presenting with thrombocytopenia and microangiopathic hemolytic anemia, because delays in diagnosis can be fatal. With plasma exchange, which removes autoantibodies and provides functional ADAMTS13, TTP (which once was uniformly fatal) can be treated successfully in more than 80% of patients.

In contrast, HUS is associated with normal levels of ADAMTS13 and is initiated by several other distinct defects. "Typical" HUS is strongly associated with infectious gastroenteritis caused by *Escherichia coli* strain O157:H7, which elaborates a Shiga-like toxin. This toxin is absorbed from the inflamed gastrointestinal mucosa into the circulation, where it alters endothelial cell function in some manner that results in platelet activation and aggregation. Children and older adults are at highest risk. Those affected present with bloody diarrhea, and a few days later HUS makes its appearance. With appropriate supportive care complete recovery is possible, but irreversible renal damage and death can occur in more severe cases.

"Atypical" HUS is often associated with defects in complement factor H, membrane cofactor protein (CD46), or factor I, three proteins that normally act to prevent excessive activation of the alternative complement pathway. Deficiencies of these proteins can be caused by inherited defects or acquired inhibitory autoantibodies and are associated with a remitting, relapsing course. Unlike TTP, the basis for the platelet activation in typical and atypical HUS is unclear. Therapeutic antibodies that inhibit the activation of the complement factor C5 are effective in preventing thrombosis in patients with inherited deficiencies of complement regulatory proteins, proving that excessive complement activation underlies the pathogenesis of this form of HUS. Similarly, immunosuppression can be beneficial to patients with inhibitory antibodies against complement regulatory factors. Typical HUS is treated supportively. Patients who survive the acute insult usually recover, but some have permanent renal damage and eventually require dialysis or renal transplantation. The impact of HUS and TTP on the kidneys is discussed further in Chapter 20.

Thrombotic microangiopathies resembling HUS can also be seen following exposures to other agents that damage endothelial cells (e.g., certain drugs and radiation therapy). The prognosis in these settings is guarded, because the HUS is often complicated by chronic, life-threatening conditions.

Bleeding Disorders Related to Defective Platelet Functions

Qualitative defects of platelet function can be inherited or acquired. Several inherited disorders characterized by abnormal platelet function and normal platelet count have been described. A brief discussion of these rare diseases is warranted because they provide excellent models for investigating the molecular mechanisms of platelet function.

Inherited disorders of platelet function can be classified into three pathogenically distinct groups: (1) defects of adhesion, (2) defects of aggregation, and (3) disorders of platelet secretion (release reaction).

- *Bernard-Soulier syndrome* illustrates the consequences of defective adhesion of platelets to subendothelial matrix. Bernard-Soulier syndrome is caused by an inherited deficiency of the platelet membrane glycoprotein complex Ib-IX. This glycoprotein is a receptor for vWF and is essential for normal platelet adhesion to the subendothelial extracellular matrix (Chapter 4). Affected patients have a variable, often severe, bleeding tendency.
- Bleeding due to *defective platelet aggregation* is exemplified by *Glanzmann thrombasthenia,* which is also transmitted as an autosomal recessive trait. Thrombasthenic platelets fail to aggregate in response to adenosine diphosphate (ADP), collagen, epinephrine, or thrombin because of deficiency or dysfunction of glycoprotein IIb-IIIa, an integrin that participates in "bridge formation" between platelets by binding fibrinogen. The associated bleeding tendency is often severe.

- *Disorders of platelet secretion* are characterized by the defective release of certain mediators of platelet activation, such as thromboxanes and granule-bound ADP. The biochemical defects underlying these so-called *storage pool disorders* are varied, complex, and beyond the scope of our discussion.

Among the *acquired defects* of platelet function, two are clinically significant. The first is caused by ingestion of *aspirin and other nonsteroidal anti-inflammatory drugs*. Aspirin is a potent, irreversible inhibitor of the enzyme cyclooxygenase, which is required for the synthesis of thromboxane A_2 and prostaglandins (Chapter 3). These mediators play important roles in platelet aggregation and subsequent release reactions (Chapter 4). The antiplatelet effects of aspirin form the basis for its use in the prophylaxis of coronary thrombosis (Chapter 12). *Uremia* (Chapter 20) is the second condition exemplifying an acquired defect in platelet function. The pathogenesis of platelet dysfunction in uremia is complex and involves defects in adhesion, granule secretion, and aggregation.

Hemorrhagic Diatheses Related to Abnormalities in Clotting Factors

Inherited or acquired deficiencies of virtually every coagulation factor have been reported as causes of bleeding diatheses. Bleeding due to isolated coagulation factor deficiencies most commonly manifests as *large posttraumatic ecchymoses or hematomas*, or *prolonged bleeding* after a laceration or any form of surgical procedure. Unlike bleeding seen with thrombocytopenia, bleeding due to coagulation factor deficiencies often occurs into the gastrointestinal and urinary tracts and into weight-bearing joints (hemarthrosis). Typical stories include the patient who oozes blood for days after a tooth extraction or who develops a hemarthrosis after minor stress on a knee joint.

Hereditary deficiencies typically affect a single clotting factor. The most common and important inherited deficiencies of coagulation factors affect factor VIII (hemophilia A), and factor IX (hemophilia B). Deficiencies of vWF (von Willebrand disease) are also discussed here, as this factor influences both coagulation and platelet function. Rare inherited deficiencies of each of the other coagulation factors have also been described.

Acquired deficiencies usually involve multiple coagulation factors and can be based on decreased protein synthesis or a shortened half-life. Vitamin K deficiency (Chapter 9) results in the impaired synthesis of factors II, VII, IX, X and protein C. Many of these factors are made in the liver and are therefore deficient in severe parenchymal liver disease. Alternatively, in disseminated intravascular coagulation, multiple coagulation factors are consumed and are therefore deficient. Acquired deficiencies of single factors occur, but they are rare. These are usually caused by inhibitory autoantibodies.

The Factor VIII-vWF Complex

The two most common inherited disorders of bleeding, hemophilia A and von Willebrand disease, are caused by qualitative or quantitative defects involving factor VIII and vWF, respectively. Before we discuss these disorders it will be helpful to review the structure and function of these two proteins, which exist together in the plasma as part of a single large complex.

Factor VIII and vWF are encoded by separate genes and are synthesized in different cells. Factor VIII is an essential cofactor of factor IX, which converts factor X to factor Xa (Fig. 14-26; Chapter 4). It is made in several tissues; sinusoidal endothelial cells and Kupffer cells in the liver seem to be major sources. Once factor VIII reaches the

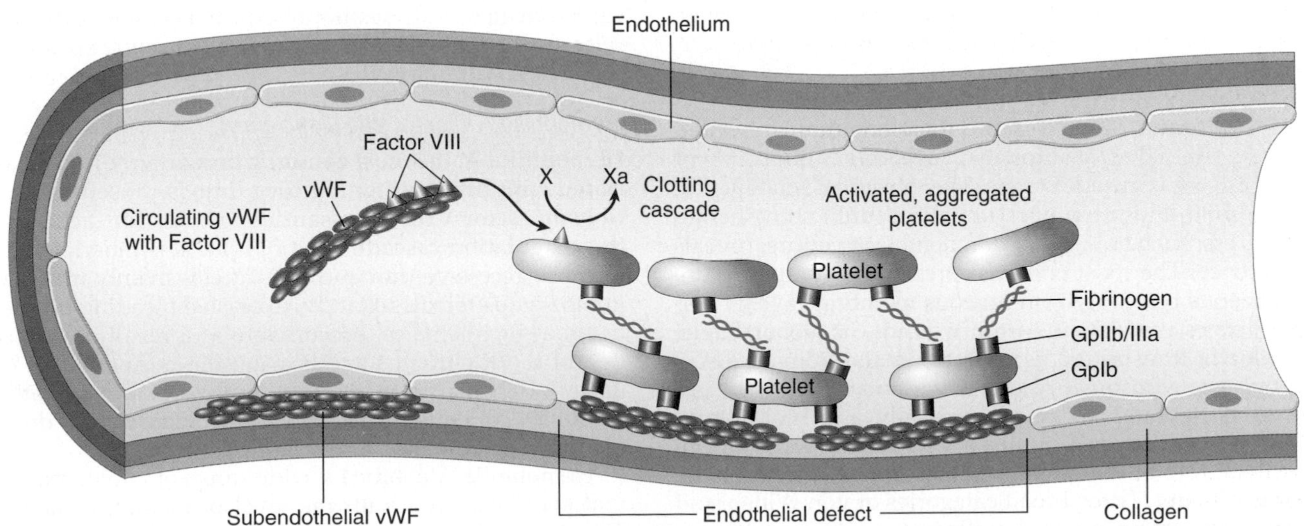

Figure 14-26 Structure and function of factor VIII-von Willebrand factor (vWF) complex. Factor VIII is synthesized in the liver and kidney, and vWF is made in endothelial cells and megakaryocytes. The two associate to form a complex in the circulation. vWF is also present in the subendothelial matrix of normal blood vessels and the α-granules of platelets. Following endothelial injury, exposure of subendothelial vWF causes adhesion of platelets, primarily via the glycoprotein Ib (GpIb) platelet receptor. Circulating vWF and vWF released from the α-granules of activated platelets can bind exposed subendothelial matrix, further contributing to platelet adhesion and activation. Activated platelets form hemostatic aggregates; fibrinogen participates in aggregation through bridging interactions with the glycoprotein IIb/IIIa (GpIIb/IIIa) platelet receptor. Factor VIII takes part in the coagulation cascade as a cofactor in the activation of factor X on the surface of activated platelets.

circulation, it binds to vWF, which is produced by endothelial cells and, to a lesser degree, by megakaryocytes, which are the source of the vWF that is found in platelet α-granules. vWF stabilizes factor VIII, which has a half-life of about 2.4 hours when free and 12 hours when bound to vWF in the circulation.

Circulating vWF exists as multimers containing as many as 100 subunits that can exceed 20×10^6 daltons in molecular mass. In addition to factor VIII, these multimers interact with several other proteins involved in hemostasis, including collagen, heparin, and possibly platelet membrane glycoproteins. The most important function of vWF is to promote the adhesion of platelets to the subendothelial matrix. This occurs through bridging interactions between platelet glycoprotein Ib-IX, vWF, and matrix components such as collagen. Some vWF is secreted from endothelial cells directly into the subendothelial matrix, where it lies ready to promote platelet adhesion if the endothelial lining is disrupted (Fig. 14-26). Endothelial cells and platelets also release vWF into the circulation. Upon vascular injury, this second pool of vWF binds collagen in the subendothelial matrix to further augment platelet adhesion. vWF multimers may also promote platelet aggregation by binding to activated GpIIb/IIIa integrins; this activity may be of particular importance under conditions of high shear stress (such as occurs in small vessels).

Factor VIII and vWF protein levels are measured by immunological techniques. Factor VIII function is measured specifically by performing coagulation assays with mixtures of patient plasma and factor VIII-deficient plasma. vWF function is assessed using the ristocetin agglutination test. This assay is performed by mixing the patient's plasma with formalin-fixed platelets and ristocetin, a small molecule that binds and "activates" vWF. Ristocetin induces multivalent vWF multimers to bind platelet glycoprotein Ib-IX and form interplatelet "bridges." The resulting clumping (agglutination) of platelets is measured in a device called an aggregometer. Thus, the degree to which patient plasma promotes ristocetin-dependent platelet agglutination reflects the vWF activity of the sample.

Von Willebrand Disease

Von Willebrand disease is the most common inherited bleeding disorder of humans, affecting about 1% of adults in the United States. The bleeding tendency is usually mild and often goes unnoticed until some hemostatic stress, such as surgery or a dental procedure, reveals its presence. The most common presenting symptoms are spontaneous bleeding from mucous membranes (e.g., epistaxis), excessive bleeding from wounds, or menorrhagia. It is usually transmitted as an autosomal dominant disorder, but rare autosomal recessive variants also exist.

Von Willebrand disease is clinically and molecularly heterogeneous; several hundred vWF variants have been described, few of which have been formally proven to be disease-causing. Three broad categories of von Willebrand disease are recognized, each with a range of phenotypes:

- **Type 1 and type 3 von Willebrand disease are associated with *quantitative defects* in vWF. Type 1, an autosomal dominant disorder characterized by a mild to moderate vWF deficiency**, accounts for about 70% of all cases. Incomplete penetrance and variable expressivity are commonly observed, but it generally is associated with mild disease. **Type 3 (an autosomal recessive disorder) is associated with very low levels of vWF and correspondingly severe clinical manifestations.** Because a severe deficiency of vWF has a marked effect on the stability of factor VIII, some of the bleeding characteristics resemble those seen in hemophilia. Type 1 disease is associated with a spectrum of mutations, including point substitutions that interfere with maturation of the vWF protein or that result in rapid clearance from the plasma. Type 3 disease is usually caused by deletions or frameshift mutations involving both alleles.
- **Type 2 von Willebrand disease is characterized by qualitative defects in vWF**; there are several subtypes, of which type 2A is the most common. It is inherited as an autosomal dominant disorder. vWF is expressed in normal amounts, but missense mutations are present that lead to defective multimer assembly. Large and intermediate multimers, representing the most active forms of vWF, are missing from plasma. Type 2 von Willebrand disease accounts for 25% of all cases and is associated with mild to moderate bleeding.

Patients with von Willebrand disease have defects in platelet function despite a normal platelet count. The plasma level of active vWF, measured as the ristocetin cofactor activity, is reduced. Because vWF stabilizes factor VIII, a deficiency of vWF gives rise to a secondary decrease in factor VIII levels. This may be reflected by a prolongation of the PTT in von Willebrand disease types 1 and 3. However, except in rare type 3 patients, adverse complications typical of severe factor VIII deficiency, such as bleeding into the joints, are not seen.

Even within families in which a single defective vWF allele is segregating, wide variability in clinical expression is common. This is due in part to modifying genes that influence circulating levels of vWF, which show a wide range in normal populations. Persons with von Willebrand disease facing hemostatic challenges (dental work, surgery) can be treated with desmopressin, which stimulates vWF release, or with infusions of plasma concentrates containing factor VIII and vWF.

Hemophilia A (Factor VIII Deficiency)

Hemophilia A, the most common hereditary disease associated with life-threatening bleeding, is caused by mutations in factor VIII, an essential cofactor for factor IX in the coagulation cascade. Hemophilia A is inherited as an X-linked recessive trait and thus affects mainly males and homozygous females. Rarely, excessive bleeding occurs in heterozygous females, presumably as a result of inactivation of the X chromosome bearing the normal factor VIII allele by chance in most cells (unfavorable lyonization). About 30% of patients have no family history; their disease is caused by new mutations.

Hemophilia A exhibits a wide range of clinical severity that correlates well with the level of factor VIII activity. Those with less than 1% of normal levels have severe disease; those with 2% to 5% of normal levels have moderately severe disease; and those with 6% to 50% of normal levels have mild disease. The varying degrees of factor VIII deficiency are largely explained by heterogeneity in the causative mutations. As with β-thalassemia, the genetic lesions include deletions, nonsense mutations that create stop codons, and mutations that cause errors in mRNA splicing. The most severe deficiencies result from an inversion involving the X chromosome that completely abolishes the synthesis of factor VIII. Less commonly, severe hemophilia A is associated with point mutations in factor VIII that impair the function of the protein. In such cases factor VIII protein levels may be normal by immunoassay. Mutations permitting some active factor VIII to be synthesized are associated with mild to moderate disease. The disease in such patients may be modified by other genetic factors that influence factor VIII expression levels, which vary widely in normal individuals.

In all symptomatic cases there is a tendency toward easy bruising and massive hemorrhage after trauma or operative procedures. In addition, "spontaneous" hemorrhages frequently occur in regions of the body that are susceptible to trauma, particularly the joints, where they are known as *hemarthroses*. Recurrent bleeding into the joints leads to progressive deformities that can be crippling. Petechiae are characteristically absent.

Patients with hemophilia A have a prolonged PTT and a normal PT, results that point to an abnormality of the intrinsic coagulation pathway. Factor VIII-specific assays are required for diagnosis. As explained in Chapter 4, the bleeding diathesis reflects the pre-eminent role of the factor VIIIa/factor IXa complex in activation of factor X in vivo. The precise explanation for the tendency of hemophiliacs to bleed at particular sites (joints, muscles, and the central nervous system) remains uncertain.

Hemophilia A is treated with infusions of recombinant factor VIII. About 15% of patients with severe hemophilia A develop antibodies that bind and inhibit factor VIII, probably because the protein is perceived as foreign, having never been "seen" by the immune system. These antibody inhibitors can be a very difficult therapeutic challenge. Before the development of recombinant factor VIII therapy, thousands of hemophiliacs received plasma-derived factor VIII concentrates containing HIV, and many developed AIDS (Chapter 6). The risk of HIV transmission has been eliminated but tragically too late for an entire generation of hemophiliacs. Efforts to develop somatic gene therapy for hemophilia are ongoing.

Hemophilia B (Christmas Disease, Factor IX Deficiency)

Severe factor IX deficiency produces a disorder clinically indistinguishable from factor VIII deficiency (hemophilia A). This should not be surprising, given that factors VIII and IX function together to activate factor X. A wide spectrum of mutations involving the gene that encodes factor IX is found in hemophilia B. Like hemophilia A, it is inherited as an X-linked recessive trait and shows variable clinical severity. In about 15% of these patients, factor IX protein is present but is nonfunctional. As with hemophilia A, the PTT is prolonged and the PT is normal. Diagnosis of Christmas disease (named after the first patient identified with this condition, and not the holiday) is possible only by assay of the factor levels. The disease is treated with infusions of recombinant factor IX.

Disseminated Intravascular Coagulation (DIC)

DIC is an acute, subacute, or chronic thrombohemorrhagic disorder characterized by the excessive activation of coagulation and the formation of thrombi in the microvasculature of the body. It occurs as a secondary complication of many different disorders. Sometimes the coagulopathy is localized to a specific organ or tissue. As a consequence of the thrombotic diathesis there is consumption of platelets, fibrin, and coagulation factors and, secondarily, activation of fibrinolysis. DIC can present with signs and symptoms relating to the tissue hypoxia and infarction caused by the myriad microthrombi; with hemorrhage caused by the depletion of factors required for hemostasis and the activation of fibrinolytic mechanisms; or both.

Etiology and Pathogenesis. At the outset, it must be emphasized that DIC is not a primary disease. It is a coagulopathy that occurs in the course of a variety of clinical conditions. In discussing the general mechanisms underlying DIC, it is useful to briefly review the normal process of blood coagulation and clot removal (Chapter 4).

Clotting in vivo is thought to be initiated by exposure of tissue factor, which combines with factor VII to activate both factor X directly and to activate factor IX. Activation of factor X leads to the generation of *thrombin*, the central player in clotting. At sites where the endothelium is disrupted, thrombin converts fibrinogen to fibrin, feeds back to activate factors IX, VIII, and V, stimulates fibrin cross-linking, inhibits fibrinolysis, and activates platelets, all of which augment the formation of a stable clot. To prevent runaway clotting, this process must be sharply limited to the site of tissue injury. Remarkably, as thrombin is swept away in the bloodstream and encounters uninjured vessels, it is converted to an anticoagulant through binding to *thrombomodulin*, a protein found on the surface of endothelial cells. The thrombin-thrombomodulin complex activates protein C, which is an important inhibitor of factor V and factor VIII. Other activated coagulation factors are removed from the circulation by the liver, and as you will recall, the blood also contains several potent fibrinolytic factors, such as plasmin. These and additional checks and balances normally ensure that just enough clotting occurs at the right place and time.

From this brief review it should be clear that DIC could result from pathologic activation of coagulation or the impairment of clot-inhibiting mechanisms. Because the latter rarely constitute primary mechanisms of DIC, we will focus on the abnormal initiation of clotting.

Two major mechanisms trigger DIC: (1) release of tissue factor or other, poorly characterized procoaagulants, into the circulation, and (2) widespread injury to the endothelial cells. Procoagulants such as tissue factor can be derived from a variety of sources, such as the placenta in obstetric complications or tissues injured by trauma or burns. Mucus released from certain adenocarcinomas may also act as procoagulants by directly activate factor X.

Endothelial injury can initiate DIC in several ways. Injuries that cause endothelial cell necrosis expose the subendothelial matrix, leading to the activation of platelets and the coagulation pathway. However, even subtle endothelial injuries can unleash procoagulant activity. One mediator of endothelial injury is TNF, which is implicated in DIC occurring with sepsis. TNF induces endothelial cells to express tissue factor on their cell surfaces and to decrease the expression of thrombomodulin, shifting the checks and balances that govern hemostasis towards coagulation. In addition, TNF up-regulates the expression of adhesion molecules on endothelial cells, thereby promoting the adhesion of leukocytes, which can damage endothelial cells by releasing reactive oxygen species and preformed proteases. Widespread endothelial injury may also be produced by deposition of antigen-antibody complexes (e.g., systemic lupus erythematosus), temperature extremes (e.g., heat stroke, burns), or microorganisms (e.g., meningococci, rickettsiae). Even subtle endothelial injury can unleash procoagulant activity by enhancing membrane expression of tissue factor.

DIC is most likely to be associated with obstetric complications, malignant neoplasms, sepsis, and major trauma. The triggers in these conditions are often multiple and interrelated. For example, in bacterial infections *endotoxins* can inhibit the endothelial expression of thrombomodulin directly or indirectly by stimulating immune cells to make TNF, and can also activate factor XII. *Antigen-antibody complexes* formed in response to the infection can activate the classical complement pathway, giving rise to complement fragments that secondarily activate both platelets and granulocytes. In *massive trauma, extensive surgery,* and *severe burns,* the major trigger is the release of procoagulants such as tissue factor. In *obstetric conditions,* procoagulants derived from the placenta, dead retained fetus, or amniotic fluid may enter the circulation. *Hypoxia, acidosis, and shock,* which often coexist in very ill patients, can also cause widespread endothelial injury, and supervening infections can complicate the problems further. *Among cancers, acute promyelocytic leukemia and adenocarcinomas* of the lung, pancreas, colon, and stomach are most frequently associated with DIC.

The possible consequences of DIC are twofold (Fig. 14-27).

- *Widespread deposition of fibrin* within the microcirculation. This leads to *ischemia* of the more severely affected or more vulnerable organs and a *microangiopathic hemolytic anemia,* which results from the fragmentation of red cells as they squeeze through the narrowed microvasculature.
- Consumption of platelets and clotting factors and the activation of plasminogen, leading to a *hemorrhagic diathesis.* Plasmin not only cleaves fibrin, but it also digests factors V and VIII, thereby reducing their concentration further. In addition, fibrin degradation products resulting from fibrinolysis inhibit platelet aggregation, fibrin polymerization, and thrombin.

MORPHOLOGY

Thrombi are most often found in the brain, heart, lungs, kidneys, adrenals, spleen, and liver, in decreasing order of frequency, but any tissue can be affected. Affected kidneys may have small thrombi in the glomeruli that evoke only reactive swelling of endothelial cells or, in severe cases, microinfarcts or even **bilateral renal cortical necrosis**. Numerous fibrin thrombi may be found in alveolar capillaries, sometimes associated with pulmonary edema and fibrin exudation, creating "hyaline membranes" reminiscent of acute respiratory distress syndrome (Chapter 15). In the central nervous system, fibrin thrombi can cause microinfarcts, occasionally complicated by simultaneous hemorrhage, which can sometimes lead to variable neurologic signs and symptoms. The manifestations in the endocrine glands are of considerable interest. In meningococcemia, fibrin thrombi within the microcirculation of the adrenal cortex are the probable basis for the massive adrenal hemorrhages seen in **Waterhouse-Friderichsen syndrome** (Chapter 24). An unusual form of DIC occurs in association with giant hemangiomas (**Kasabach-Merritt syndrome**), in which thrombi form within the neoplasm because of stasis and recurrent trauma to fragile blood vessels.

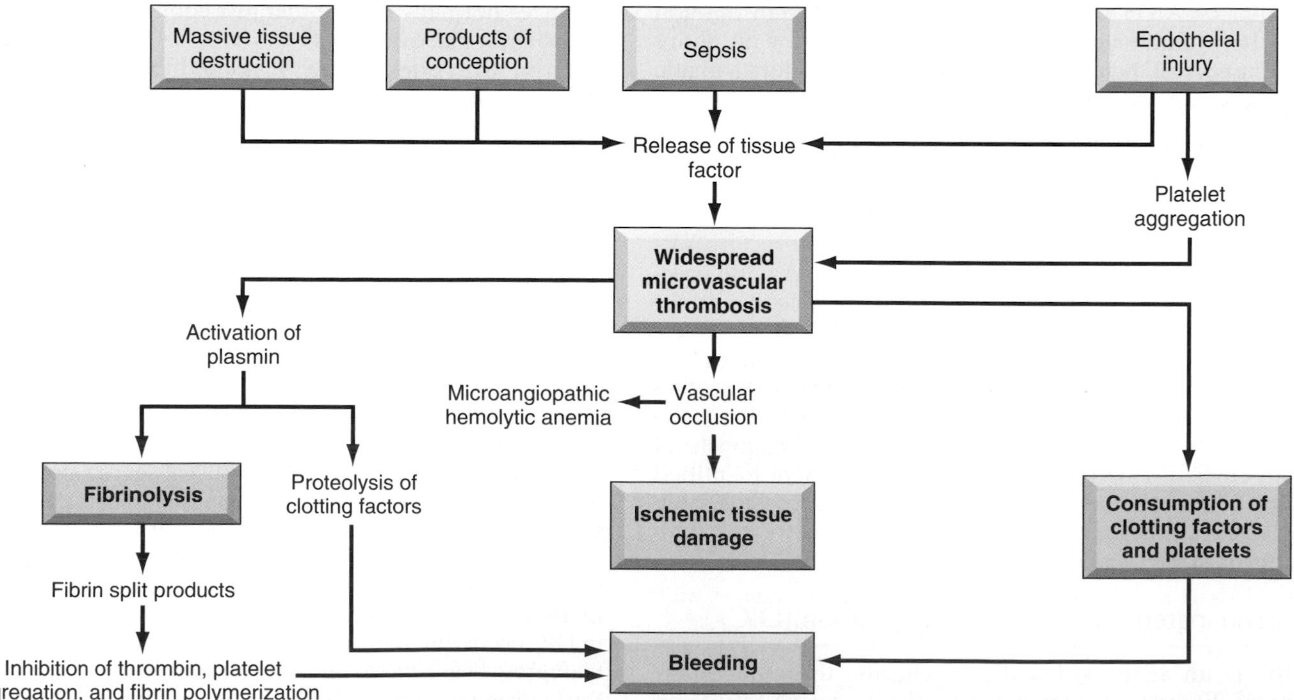

Figure 14-27 Pathophysiology of disseminated intravascular coagulation.

Clinical Features. The onset can be fulminant, as in endotoxic shock or amniotic fluid embolism, or insidious and chronic, as in cases of carcinomatosis or retention of a dead fetus. Overall, about 50% of the affected are obstetric patients having complications of pregnancy. In this setting the disorder tends to be reversible with delivery of the fetus. About 33% of the affected patients have carcinomatosis. The remaining cases are associated with the various entities previously listed.

It is almost impossible to detail all the potential clinical presentations, but a few common patterns are worthy of description. These include *microangiopathic hemolytic anemia*; dyspnea, cyanosis, and respiratory failure; convulsions and coma; oliguria and acute renal failure; and sudden or progressive circulatory failure and shock. In general, acute DIC, associated with obstetric complications or major trauma, for example, is dominated by a bleeding diathesis, whereas chronic DIC, such as occurs in cancer patients, tends to present with thrombotic complications. The diagnosis is based on clinical observation and laboratory studies, including measurement of fibrinogen levels, platelets, the PT and PTT, and fibrin degradation products.

The prognosis is highly variable and largely depends on the underlying disorder. The only definitive treatment is to remove or treat the inciting cause. The management requires meticulous maneuvering between the Scylla of thrombosis and the Charybdis of bleeding diathesis. Administration of anticoagulants or procoagulants has been advocated in specific settings, but not without controversy.

KEY CONCEPTS

Immune Thrombocytopenic Purpura

- Caused by autoantibodies against platelet antigens
- May be triggered by drugs, infections, or lymphomas, or may be idiopathic

Thrombotic Thrombocytopenic Purpura and Hemolytic Uremic Syndrome

- Both manifest with thrombocytopenia, microangiopathic hemolytic anemia, and renal failure; fever and CNS involvement are more typical of TTP.
- *TTP*: Caused by acquired or inherited deficiencies of ADAMTS 13, a plasma metalloprotease that cleaves very-high-molecular-weight multimers of von Willebrand factor (vWF). Deficiency of ADAMTS 13 results in abnormally large vWF multimers that activate platelets.
- *Hemolytic uremic syndrome*: caused by deficiencies of complement regulatory proteins or agents that damage endothelial cells, such as a Shiga-like toxin elaborated by *E. coli* strain O157:H7. The abnormalities initiate platelet activation, platelet aggregation, and microvascular thrombosis.

Von Willebrand Disease

- Autosomal dominant disorder caused by mutations in vWF, a large protein that promotes the adhesion of platelets to subendothelial collagen
- Typically causes a mild to moderate bleeding disorder resembling that associated with thrombocytopenia

Hemophilia

- *Hemophilia A*: X-linked disorder caused by mutations in factor VIII. Affected males typically present with severe bleeding into soft tissues and joints and have a PTT.
- *Hemophilia B*: X-linked disorder caused by mutations in coagulation factor IX. It is clinically identical to hemophilia A.

Disseminated Intravascular Coagulation

- Syndrome in which systemic activation of the coagulation leads to consumption of coagulation factors and platelets
- Can produce bleeding, vascular occlusion and tissue hypoxemia, or both
- Common triggers: sepsis, major trauma, certain cancers, obstetric complications

Complications of Transfusion

Blood products are often rightly called the gift of life, permitting people to survive traumatic injuries and procedures such as hematopoietic stem cell transplantation and complex surgical procedures that would otherwise prove fatal. Over 5 million red cell transfusions are given in US hospitals each year. Thanks to improved screening of donors, blood products (packed red blood cells, platelets, and fresh-frozen plasma) are safer than ever before.

Nevertheless, complications still occur. Most are minor and transient. The most common is referred to as a *febrile nonhemolytic reaction*, which takes the form of fever and chills, sometimes with mild dyspnea, within 6 hours of a transfusion of red cells or platelets. These reactions are thought to be caused by inflammatory mediators derived from donor leukocytes. The frequency of these reactions increases with the storage age of the product and is decreased by measures that limit donor leukocyte contamination. Symptoms respond to antipyretics and are short-lived.

Other transfusion reactions are uncommon or rare, but can have severe and sometimes fatal consequences, and therefore merit discussion.

Allergic Reactions

Severe, potentially fatal allergic reactions may occur when blood products containing certain antigens are given to previously sensitized recipients. These are most likely to occur in patients with IgA deficiency, which has a frequency of 1:300 to 1:500 people. In this instance, the reaction is triggered by IgG antibodies that recognize IgA in the infused blood product. Fortunately, most patients with IgA deficiency do not develop such antibodies, and these severe reactions are rare, occurring in 1 in 20,000 to 1 in 50,000 transfusions. *Urticarial allergic reactions* may be triggered by the presence an allergen in the donated blood product that is recognized by IgE antibodies in the recipient. These are considerably more common, occurring in 1% to 3% of transfusions, but are generally mild. In most instances symptoms respond to antihistamines and do not require discontinuation of the transfusion.

Hemolytic Reactions

***Acute hemolytic reactions* are usually caused by preformed IgM antibodies against donor red cells that fix**

complement. They most commonly stem from an error in patient identification or tube labeling that allows a patient to receive an ABO incompatible unit of blood. Pre-existing high affinity "natural" IgM antibodies, usually against polysaccharide blood group antigens A or B, bind to red cells and rapidly induce complement mediated lysis, intravascular hemolysis, and hemoglobinuria. Fever, shaking chills, and flank pain appear rapidly. The direct Coombs test is typically positive, unless all of the donor red cells have lysed. The signs and symptoms are due to complement activation rather than intravascular hemolysis *per se*, as osmotic lysis of red cells (e.g., by mistakenly infusing red cells and 5% dextrose in water simultaneously) produces hemoglobinuria without any of the other symptoms of a hemolytic reaction. In severe cases the process may rapidly progress to DIC, shock, acute renal failure, and occasionally death.

Delayed hemolytic reactions **are caused by antibodies that recognize red cell antigens that the recipient was sensitized to previously, for example, through a prior blood transfusion.** These are typically caused by IgG antibodies to foreign protein antigens and are associated with a positive direct Coombs test and laboratory features of hemolysis (e.g., low haptoglobin and elevated LDH). Antibodies to antigens such as Rh, Kell, and Kidd often induce sufficient complement activation to cause severe and potentially fatal reactions identical to those resulting from ABO mismatches. Other antibodies that do not fix complement typically result in red cell opsonization, extravascular hemolysis, and spherocytosis, and are associated with relatively minor signs and symptoms.

Transfusion-Related Acute Lung Injury

TRALI is a severe, frequently fatal complication in which factors in a transfused blood product trigger the activation of neutrophils in the lung microvasculature. The incidence of TRALI is low, probably less than 1 per 10,000 transfusions, but it may occur more frequently in patients with preexisting lung disease. Though its pathogenesis is incompletely understood, current models favor a "two hit" hypothesis. The first is a priming event that leads to increased sequestration and sensitization of neutrophils in the microvasculature of the lung. It is postulated that this event may involve endothelial activation, for example by inflammatory mediators. The primed neutrophils are then activated by a factor present in the transfused blood product, which constitutes the second hit.

A variety of factors have been implicated as "second hits", but the leading candidates are antibodies in the transfused blood product that recognize antigens expressed on neutrophils. By far the most common antibodies associated with TRALI are those that bind major histocompatibility complex (MHC) antigens, particularly MHC class I antigens. These antibodies are often found in multiparous women, who generate such antibodies in response to foreign MHC antigens expressed by the fetus. Rarely, donor antibodies to neutrophil-specific antigens trigger TRALI. Although TRALI has been associated with virtually all plasma-containing blood products, it is more likely to occur following transfusion of products containing high levels of donor antibodies, such as fresh frozen plasma and platelets. The presentation is dramatic, sudden onset respiratory failure, during or soon after a transfusion. Diffuse bilateral pulmonary infiltrates that do not respond to diuretics are seen on chest imaging. Other associated findings include fever, hypotension and hypoxemia. The treatment is largely supportive and the outcome is guarded; mortality is 5% in uncomplicated cases and up to 67% in those who were severely ill. TRALI is important to recognize, because donor products that induce the complication in one patient are much more likely to do so in a second. Indeed, recent measures to exclude multiparous women from plasma donation have resulted in the incidence of TRALI being cut in half.

Infectious Complications

Virtually any infectious agent can be transmitted through blood products, but bacterial and viral infections are most likely to be so. Most *bacterial infections* are caused by skin flora, indicating that the contamination occurred at the time that the product is taken from the donor. Significant bacterial contamination (sufficient to produce symptoms) is much more common in platelet preparations than red cell preparations, due in large part to the fact that platelets (unlike red cells) must be stored at room temperature, conditions that are favorable for bacterial growth. Rates of bacterial infection secondary to platelet transfusion can be as high as 1 in 5000, with infections secondary to red cell transfusions being several orders of magnitude less frequent. Many of the symptoms (fever, chills, hypotension) resemble those of hemolytic and non-hemolytic transfusion reactions, and it may be necessary to start broad-spectrum antibiotics prospectively in symptomatic patients while awaiting laboratory results.

Advances in donor selection, donor screening, and infectious disease testing have dramatically decreased the incidence of viral transmission by blood products. However on rare occasions when the donor is acutely infected but the virus is not yet detectable with current nucleic acid testing technology, there can be transfusion-related transmission of viruses such as HIV, hepatitis C, and hepatitis B. Rates of transmission of HIV, hepatitis C, and hepatitis B are estimated to be 1 in 2 million, 1 in 1 million, and 1 in 500,000, respectively. There also remains a low risk of "exotic" infectious agents such as West Nile virus, trypanosomiasis, and babesiosis.

SUGGESTED READINGS

Red Cell Disorders

An X, Mohandas N: Disorders of the red cell membrane. *Br J Haematol* 141:367, 2008. *[An excellent overview of inherited red cell membrane defects.]*

Ganz T, Nemeth E: Hepcidin and disorders of iron metabolism. *Annu Rev Med* 62:347, 2011. *[A review focused on disorders of iron metabolism that are mediated by altered hepcidin levels, including the anemia of chronic inflammation.]*

Higgs DR, Engel JD, Stamatoyannopoulos G: Thalassemia. *Lancet* 379:373, 2012. *[A review of the molecular pathogenesis of thalassemia syndromes and current approaches to therapy.]*

Kassim AA, Debaun MR: Sickle cell disease, vasculopathy, and therapeutics. *Annu Rev Med* epublished 11/30/2012. *[A thorough discussion of the role of vasculopathy in tissue damage in sickle cell disease.]*

Parker CJ: Paroxysmal nocturnal hemoglobinuria. *Curr Opin Hematol* 19:141, 2012. *[Discussion of the natural history of PNH and the therapeutic impact of antibodies that inhibit the C5b–C9 membrane attack complex.]*

Platt OS: Hydroxyurea for the treatment of sickle cell disease. *N Engl J Med* 358:1362, 2008. *[A review focused on the beneficial effects of hydroxyurea in sickle cell disease.]*

Young NS, Bacigalupo A, Marsh JC: Aplastic anemia: pathophysiology and treatment. *Biol Blood Marrow Transplant* 16:S119, 2010. *[A discussion of the role of the immune system and telomerase mutations in aplastic anemia.]*

Bleeding Disorders

Arepally GM, Ortel TL: Heparin-induced thrombocytopenia. *Annu Rev Med* 61:77, 2010. *[A discussion of pathogenesis, clinical features, diagnostic criteria, and therapeutic approaches in HIT.]*

De Meyer SF, Deckmyn H, Vanhoorelbeke K: von Willebrand factor to the rescue. *Blood* 113:5049, 2009. *[An update on the molecular pathogenesis and treatment of vWD.]*

Noris M, Remuzzi G: Atypical hemolytic uremic syndrome. *N Engl J Med* 361:1676, 2009. *[An article focused on the role of excessive activation of the alternative complement pathway in some forms of HUS.]*

Pawlinski R, Mackman N: Cellular sources of tissue factor in endotoxemia and sepsis. *Thromb Res* 125(S1):S70, 2010. *[An overview of the role of cellular procoagulants in DIC associated with bacterial infection.]*

Stasi R: Immune thrombocytopenia: pathophysiologic and clinical update. *Semin Thromb Hemost* 38:454, 2012. *[Discussion of the role of T cells in immune thrombocytopenia and treatment with immunomodulatory agents and growth factors.]*

Zhou Z, Nguyen TC, Guchhait P, et al: Von Willebrand factor, ADAMTS-13, and thrombotic thrombocytopenia purpura. *Semin Thromb Hemost* 36:71, 2010. *[A review focused on the role of vWF deregulation and ADAMTS 13 deficiency in TTP.]*

See TARGETED THERAPY available online at
www.studentconsult.com 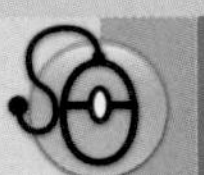

CHAPTER 15

The Lung

Aliya N. Husain

CHAPTER CONTENTS

The lungs are ingeniously constructed to carry out their cardinal function, the exchange of gases between inspired air and blood. Developmentally, the respiratory system is an outgrowth from the ventral wall of the foregut. The midline trachea develops two lateral outpocketings, the lung buds. The lung buds eventually divide into branches called lobar bronchi, three on the right and two on the left, thus giving rise to three lobes on the right and two on the left.

The lobar bronchi allow passage of air from the outside into the lung. They have firm cartilaginous walls that provide mechanical support, and are lined with columnar ciliated epithelium with abundant subepithelial glands that produce mucus, which impedes the entry of microbes. The mainstem bronchus is more vertical and directly in line with the trachea. Consequently, aspirated foreign materials, such as vomitus, blood, and foreign bodies, tend to enter the right lung more often than the left. The right and left lobar bronchi branch dichotomously, giving rise to progressively smaller airways. Accompanying the branching airways is the double arterial supply to the lungs, derived from the pulmonary and bronchial arteries.

Progressive branching of the bronchi forms *bronchioles,* which are distinguished from bronchi by the lack of cartilage and submucosal glands within their walls. Further branching of bronchioles leads to the *terminal bronchioles,* which are less than 2 mm in diameter. The part of the lung distal to the terminal bronchiole is called the *acinus;* it is roughly spherical, with a diameter of about 7 mm. An acinus is composed of *respiratory bronchioles* (each of which gives off several alveoli from its sides), *alveolar ducts,* and *alveolar sacs,* the blind ends of the respiratory passages, whose walls are formed entirely of alveoli, which are the site of gas exchange (see Fig. 15-6). A cluster of three to five terminal bronchioles, each with its appended acinus, is referred to as the pulmonary *lobule.*

Except for the vocal cords, which are covered by stratified squamous epithelium, the entire respiratory tree, including the larynx, trachea, and bronchioles, is lined by pseudostratified, tall, columnar, ciliated epithelial cells. The bronchial mucosa also contains a population of neuroendocrine cells that have neurosecretory-type granules and can release a variety of factors, including serotonin, calcitonin, and gastrin-releasing peptide (bombesin). Numerous mucus-secreting goblet cells and submucosal glands are dispersed throughout the walls of the trachea and bronchi (but not the bronchioles).

The microscopic structure of the alveolar walls (or alveolar septa) consists of the following (Fig. 15-1):

- An intertwining network of *anastomosing capillaries* lined with endothelial cells
- *Basement membrane and surrounding interstitial tissue,* which separate the endothelial cells from the alveolar lining epithelial cells. In thin portions of the alveolar septum, the basement membranes of epithelium and endothelium are fused, whereas in thicker portions they are separated by an interstitial space *(pulmonary interstitium)* containing fine elastic fibers, small bundles of collagen, a few fibroblast-like interstitial cells, smooth muscle cells, mast cells, and rare lymphocytes and monocytes.
- *Alveolar epithelium,* a continuous layer of two cell types: flattened, platelike *type I pneumocytes,* covering 95% of the alveolar surface, and rounded *type II pneumocytes.* Type II cells synthesize *surfactant* (which forms a very thin layer over the alveolar cell membranes) and are involved in the repair of alveolar epithelium through their ability to give rise to type I cells.
- *Alveolar macrophages,* loosely attached to the epithelial cells or lying free within the alveolar spaces

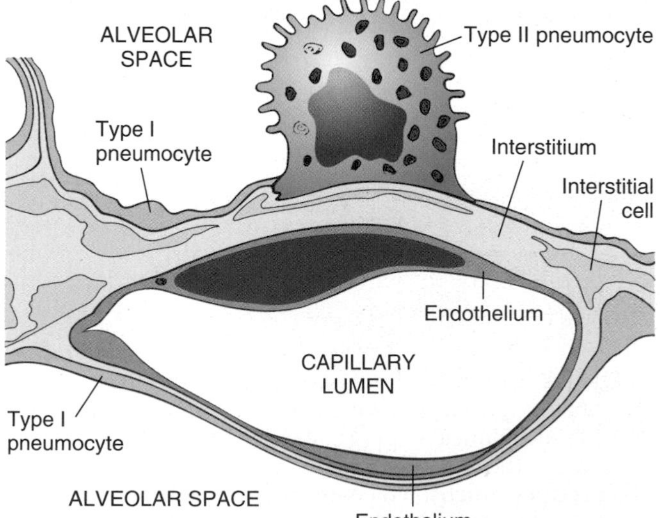

Figure 15-1 Microscopic structure of the alveolar wall. Note that the basement membrane *(yellow)* is thin on one side and widened where it is continuous with the interstitial space. Portions of interstitial cells are shown.

The alveolar walls are perforated by numerous *pores of Kohn,* which permit the passage of bacteria and exudate between adjacent alveoli (see Fig. 15-34*B*).

Congenital Anomalies

Developmental anomalies of the lung are rare; the more common of these include the following:

- *Pulmonary hypoplasia* is the defective development of both lungs (one may be more affected than the other) resulting in decreased weight, volume, and acini for body weight and gestational age. It is caused by abnormalities that compress the lung or impede normal lung expansion in utero, such as congenital diaphragmatic hernia and oligohydramnios. Severe hypoplasia is fatal in the early neonatal period.
- *Foregut cysts* arise from abnormal detachments of primitive foregut and are most often located in the hilum or middle mediastinum. Depending on the wall structure, these cysts are classified as bronchogenic (most common), esophageal, or enteric. A bronchogenic cyst is rarely connected to the tracheobronchial tree. Microscopically, the cyst is lined by ciliated pseudostratified columnar epithelium. The wall contains bronchial glands, cartilage, and smooth muscle. They usually present due to compression of nearby structures or are found incidentally.
- *Pulmonary sequestration* refers to a discrete area of lung tissue that (1) lacks any connection to the airway system and (2) has a abnormal blood supply arising from the aorta or its branches. *Extralobar sequestrations* are external to the lung and most commonly come to attention in infants as mass lesions. They may be associated with other congenital anomalies. *Intralobar sequestrations* occur within the lung. They usually present in older children, often due to recurrent localized infection or bronchiectasis.

Other less common congenital abnormalities include tracheal and bronchial anomalies (atresia, stenosis, tracheoesophageal fistula), vascular anomalies, congenital pulmonary airway malformation and congenital lobar overinflation (emphysema).

Atelectasis (Collapse)

Atelectasis refers either to incomplete expansion of the lungs (neonatal atelectasis) or to the collapse of previously

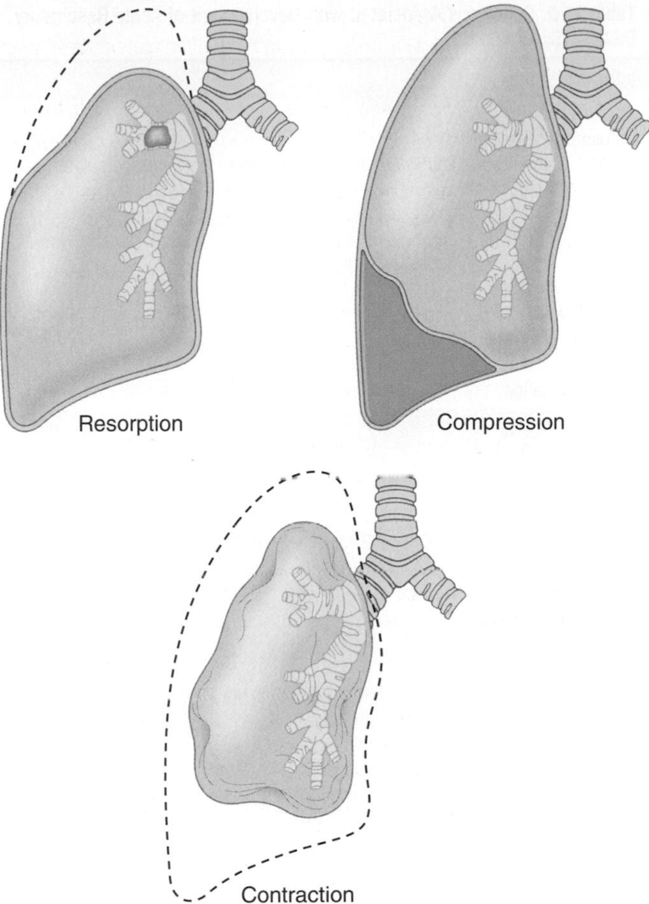

Figure 15-2 Various forms of acquired atelectasis. Dashed lines indicate normal lung volume.

inflated lung, producing areas of relatively airless pulmonary parenchyma. The main types of acquired atelectasis, which is encountered principally in adults, are the following (Fig. 15-2).

- *Resorption atelectasis* stems from complete obstruction of an airway. Over time, air is resorbed from the dependent alveoli, which collapse. Since lung volume is diminished, the mediastinum shifts *toward* the atelectatic lung. Airway obstruction is most often caused by excessive secretions (e.g., mucus plugs) or exudates within smaller bronchi, as may occur in bronchial asthma, chronic bronchitis, bronchiectasis, and postoperative states. Aspiration of foreign bodies and, rarely, fragments of bronchial tumors may also lead to airway obstruction and atelectasis.
- *Compression atelectasis* results whenever significant volumes of fluid (transudate, exudate or blood), tumor, or air (*pneumothorax*) accumulate within the pleural cavity. With compression atelectasis, the mediastinum shifts *away* from the affected lung.
- *Contraction atelectasis* occurs when focal or generalized pulmonary or pleural fibrosis prevents full lung expansion.

Significant atelectasis reduces oxygenation and predisposes to infection. Except in cases caused by contraction, atelectasis is a reversible disorder.

Pulmonary Edema

Pulmonary edema (leakage of excessive interstitial fluid which accumulates in alveolar spaces) can result from hemodynamic disturbances (hemodynamic or cardiogenic pulmonary edema) or from direct increases in capillary permeability, as a result of microvascular injury (Table 15-1). A general consideration of edema is given in Chapter 3, and pulmonary congestion and edema are described briefly in the context of congestive heart failure (Chapter 11). Whatever the clinical setting, pulmonary congestion and edema produce heavy, wet lungs. Therapy and outcome depend on the underlying etiology.

Hemodynamic Pulmonary Edema

Hemodynamic pulmonary edema is due to *increased hydrostatic pressure,* as occurs most commonly in left-sided congestive heart failure. Fluid accumulates initially in the basal regions of the lower lobes because hydrostatic pressure is greatest in these sites (dependent edema). Histologically, the alveolar capillaries are engorged, and an intra-alveolar transudate appears as finely granular pale pink material. Alveolar microhemorrhages and *hemosiderin-laden macrophages ("heart failure" cells)* may be present. In long-standing pulmonary congestion (e.g., as seen in mitral stenosis), hemosiderin-laden macrophages are abundant, and fibrosis and thickening of the alveolar walls cause the soggy lungs to become firm and brown *(brown induration).* These changes not only impair normal respiratory function but also predispose to infection.

Table 15-1 Classification and Causes of Pulmonary Edema

Hemodynamic Edema
Increased hydrostatic pressure (increased pulmonary venous pressure)
Left-sided heart failure (common) Volume overload Pulmonary vein obstruction
Decreased oncotic pressure (less common)
Hypoalbuminemia Nephrotic syndrome Liver disease Protein-losing enteropathies
Lymphatic obstruction (rare)
Edema Due to Alveolar Wall Injury (Microvascular or Epithelial Injury)
Direct Injury
Infections: bacterial pneumonia Inhaled gases: high concentration oxygen, smoke Liquid aspiration: gastric contents, near-drowning Radiation
Indirect Injury
Septicemia Blood transfusion related Burns Drugs and chemicals: chemotherapeutic agents (bleomycin), other medications (methadone, amphotericin B), heroin, cocaine, kerosene, paraquat Shock, trauma
Edema of Undetermined Origin
High altitude Neurogenic (central nervous system trauma)

Edema Caused by Microvascular (Alveolar) Injury

Noncardiogenic pulmonary edema is due to injury to the alveolar septa. Primary injury to the vascular endothelium or damage to alveolar epithelial cells (with secondary microvascular injury) produces an inflammatory exudate that leaks into the interstitial space and, in more severe cases, into the alveoli. In most forms of pneumonia the edema remains localized and is overshadowed by the manifestations of infection. When diffuse, however, alveolar edema is an important contributor to a serious and often fatal condition, *acute respiratory distress syndrome* (discussed below).

Acute Lung Injury and Acute Respiratory Distress Syndrome (Diffuse Alveolar Damage)

Acute lung injury (ALI) (also called noncardiogenic pulmonary edema) is characterized by the abrupt onset of significant hypoxemia and bilateral pulmonary infiltrates in the absence of cardiac failure. Acute respiratory distress syndrome (ARDS) is a manifestation of severe ALI. Both ARDS and ALI are associated with inflammation-associated increases in pulmonary vascular permeability, edema and epithelial cell death. The histologic manifestation of these diseases is *diffuse alveolar damage* (DAD).

ALI is a well-recognized complication of diverse conditions, including both direct injuries to the lungs and systemic disorders (Table 15-2). In many cases, a combination of predisposing conditions is responsible (e.g., shock, oxygen therapy, and sepsis). Nonpulmonary organ dysfunction may also be present in severe cases.

Table 15-2 Conditions Associated with Development of Acute Respiratory Distress Syndrome

Infection
Sepsis*
Diffuse pulmonary infections*
Viral, *Mycoplasma*, and *Pneumocystis* pneumonia; miliary tuberculosis
Gastric aspiration*
Physical/Injury
Mechanical trauma, including head injuries*
Pulmonary contusions
Near-drowning
Fractures with fat embolism
Burns
Ionizing radiation
Inhaled Irritants
Oxygen toxicity
Smoke
Irritant gases and chemicals
Chemical Injury
Heroin or methadone overdose
Acetylsalicylic acid
Barbiturate overdose
Paraquat
Hematologic Conditions
Transfusion associated lung injury (TRALI)
Disseminated intravascular coagulation
Pancreatitis
Uremia
Cardiopulmonary Bypass
Hypersensitivity Reactions
Organic solvents
Drugs

*More than 50% of cases of acute respiratory distress syndrome are associated with these four conditions.

Pathogenesis. ALI/ARDS is initiated by injury of pneumocytes and pulmonary endothelium, setting in motion a viscous cycle of increasing inflammation and pulmonary damage (Fig. 15-3).

- *Endothelial activation* is an important early event. In some instances, endothelial activation is secondary to pneumocyte injury, which is sensed by resident alveolar macrophages. In response, these immune sentinels secrete mediators such as TNF that act on the neighboring endothelium. Alternatively, circulating inflammatory mediators may activate pulmonary endothelium directly in the setting of severe tissue injury or sepsis. Some of these mediators injure endothelial cells, while others (notably cytokines) activate endothelial cells to express increased levels of adhesion molecules, procoagulant proteins and chemokines.
- *Adhesion and extravasation of neutrophils.* Neutrophils adhere to the activated endothelium and migrate into the interstitium and the alveoli, where they degranulate and release inflammatory mediators, including proteases, reactive oxygen species, and cytokines. Macrophage migration inhibitory factor (MIF) released into the local milieu also helps to sustain the ongoing proinflammatory response. The result is increased recruitment and adhesion of leukocytes, causing more endothelial injury, and local thrombosis. This cycle of inflammation and endothelial damage lies at the heart of ALI/ARDS.
- *Accumulation of intraalveolar fluid and formation of hyaline membranes.* Endothelial activation and injury make pulmonary capillaries leaky, allowing interstitial and intraalveolar edema fluid to form. Damage and necrosis of type II alveolar pneumocytes leads to surfactant abnormalities, further compromising alveolar gas exchange. Ultimately, the inspissated protein-rich edema fluid and debris from dead alveolar epithelial cells organize into hyaline membranes, a characteristic feature of ALI/ARDS.
- *Resolution of injury* is impeded in ALI/ARDS due to epithelial necrosis and inflammatory damage that impairs the ability of remaining cells to assist with edema resorption. Eventually, however, if the inflammatory stimulus lessens, macrophages remove intraalveolar debris and release fibrogenic cytokines such as transforming growth factor β (TGF-β) and platelet-derived growth factor (PDGF). These factors stimulate fibroblast growth and collagen deposition, leading to fibrosis of alveolar walls. Bronchiolar stem cells proliferate to replace pneumocytes. Endothelial restoration occurs through proliferation of uninjured capillary endothelium.

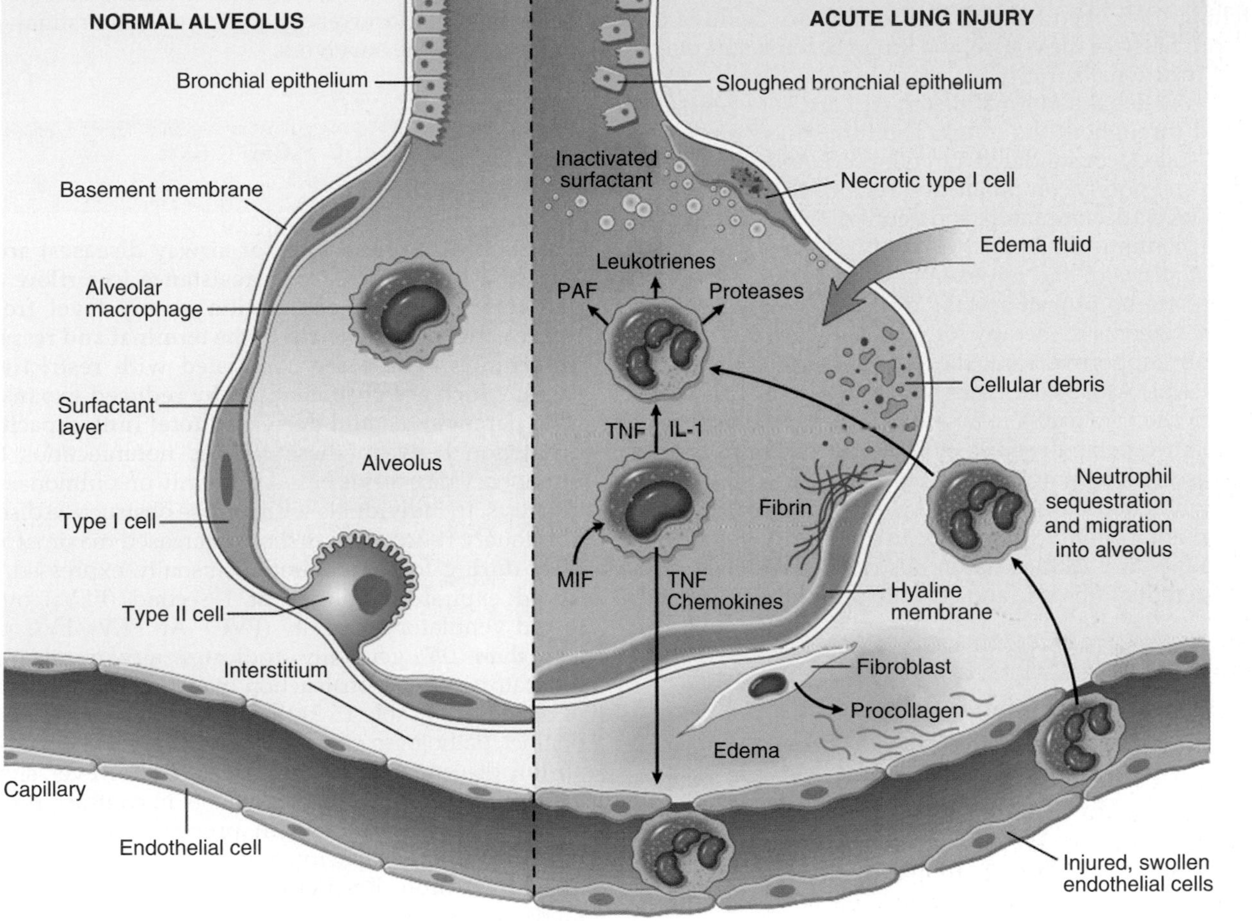

Figure 15-3 The normal alveolus *(left side)* compared with the injured alveolus in the early phase of acute lung injury and acute respiratory distress syndrome. (Modified with permission from Matthay MA, Ware LB, Zimmerman GA: The acute respiratory distress syndrome. J Clin Invest 122:2731, 2012.) *IL-1,* interleukin-1; *MIF,* migration inhibitory factor; *PAF,* platelet activating factor; *TNF,* tumor necrosis factor.

Epidemiologic studies have shown that ALI/ARDS is more common and associated with a worse prognosis in chronic alcoholics and in smokers. Genetic studies have identified a number of genes that increase the risk of ARDS, including variants that map to genes linked to inflammation and coagulation.

MORPHOLOGY

In the acute stage, the lungs are heavy, firm, red, and boggy. They exhibit congestion, interstitial and intra-alveolar edema, inflammation, fibrin deposition, and **diffuse alveolar damage**. The alveolar walls become lined with waxy **hyaline membranes** (Fig. 15-4) that are morphologically similar to those seen in hyaline membrane disease of neonates (Chapter 10). Alveolar hyaline membranes consist of fibrin-rich edema fluid mixed with the cytoplasmic and lipid remnants of necrotic epithelial cells. In the organizing stage, type II pneumocytes proliferate, and granulation tissue forms in the alveolar walls and spaces. In most cases the granulation tissue resolves, leaving minimal functional impairment. Sometimes, however, fibrotic thickening (scarring) of the alveolar septa ensues. Fatal cases often have superimposed bronchopneumonia.

Clinical Course. Individuals who develop ALI are usually hospitalized for one of the predisposing conditions listed earlier. Profound *dyspnea and tachypnea* herald ALI, followed by increasing *cyanosis and hypoxemia, respiratory failure,* and the appearance of *diffuse bilateral infiltrates* on radiographic examination. Hypoxemia may be refractory

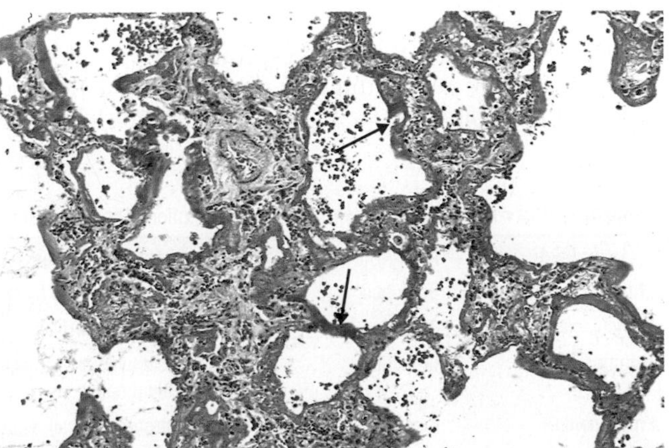

Figure 15-4 Diffuse alveolar damage (acute respiratory distress syndrome). Some of the alveoli are collapsed, while others are distended. Many are lined by hyaline membranes *(arrows)*.

to oxygen therapy due to ventilation perfusion mismatching (described below), and respiratory acidosis can develop. Early in the course, the lungs become stiff due to loss of functional surfactant.

The functional abnormalities in ALI are not evenly distributed throughout the lungs. The lungs have areas that are infiltrated, consolidated, or collapsed (and thus poorly aerated and poorly compliant) and regions that have nearly normal levels of compliance and ventilation. Poorly aerated regions continue to be perfused, producing *ventilation-perfusion mismatch* and hypoxemia.

There are no proven specific treatments; however, due to improvements in therapy for sepsis, mechanical ventilation, and supportive care, the mortality rate among the 200,000 ALI/ARDS cases seen yearly in the United States has decreased from 60% to about 40%, with the majority of deaths attributable to sepsis or multiorgan failure and, in some cases, direct lung injury. Most survivors recover pulmonary function but many have persistent impairment in physical and cognitive functions. In a minority of patients, the exudate and diffuse tissue destruction result in scarring, interstitial fibrosis, and chronic pulmonary disease.

KEY CONCEPTS

Acute Respiratory Distress Syndrome

- ARDS is a clinical syndrome of progressive respiratory insufficiency caused by diffuse alveolar damage in the setting of sepsis, severe trauma, or diffuse pulmonary infection.
- Damage to endothelial and alveolar epithelial cells, with inflammation, are the key initiating events and the basis of lung damage.
- The characteristic histologic picture is that of hyaline membranes lining alveolar walls. Edema, scattered neutrophils and macrophages, and epithelial necrosis are also present.

Acute Interstitial Pneumonia

Acute interstitial pneumonia is a term that is used to describe widespread ALI of unknown etiology associated with a rapidly progressive clinical course. It is sometimes referred to as idiopathic ALI-DAD. It is an uncommon disorder that occurs at a mean age of 59 years and has no sex predilection. Patients present with acute respiratory failure often following an illness of less than 3 weeks' duration that resembles an upper respiratory tract infection. The radiographic and pathologic features are identical to those of the organizing stage of ALI. The mortality rate varies from 33% to 74%, with most deaths occurring within 1 to 2 months. Recurrences and chronic interstitial disease may occur in the survivors.

Obstructive and Restrictive Lung Diseases

Obstructive lung diseases (or airway diseases) are characterized by an increase in resistance to airflow due to partial or complete obstruction at any level from the trachea and larger bronchi to the terminal and respiratory bronchioles. These are contrasted with restrictive diseases, which are characterized by reduced expansion of lung parenchyma and decreased total lung capacity. The distinction between these chronic noninfectious diffuse pulmonary diseases is based primarily on pulmonary function tests. In individuals with diffuse obstructive disorders, pulmonary function tests show decreased maximal airflow rates during forced expiration, usually expressed as the forced expiratory volume at 1 second (FEV_1) over the forced ventilatory capacity (FVC). An FEV_1/FVC ratio of less than 0.7 generally indicates airway obstruction. Expiratory airflow obstruction may be caused by a variety of conditions (Table 15-3) that are ideally distinguished by distinct pathologic changes and different mechanisms of airflow obstruction. As discussed later, however, such neat distinctions are not always possible. In contrast, restrictive diseases are associated with proportionate decreases in both total lung capacity and FEV_1, leading to normal FEV_1/FVC ratio. Restrictive defects occur in two broad kinds of conditions: (1) *chest wall disorders* (e.g., severe obesity, pleural diseases, kyphoscoliosis, and neuromuscular diseases such as poliomyelitis) and (2) *chronic interstitial and infiltrative diseases*, such as pneumoconioses and interstitial fibrosis.

Obstructive Lung Diseases

Common obstructive lung diseases include emphysema, chronic bronchitis, asthma, and bronchiectasis, each of which has distinct pathologic features and clinical characteristics (Table 15-3). Emphysema and chronic bronchitis are often clinically grouped together and referred to as *chronic obstructive pulmonary disease* (COPD), since the majority of patients have features of both, almost certainly because they share a major trigger—cigarette

Table 15-3 Disorders Associated with Airflow Obstruction: The Spectrum of Chronic Obstructive Pulmonary Disease

Clinical Term	Anatomic Site	Major Pathologic Changes	Etiology	Signs/Symptoms
Chronic bronchitis	Bronchus	Mucous gland hyperplasia, hypersecretion	Tobacco smoke, air pollutants	Cough, sputum production
Bronchiectasis	Bronchus	Airway dilation and scarring	Persistent or severe infections	Cough, purulent sputum, fever
Asthma	Bronchus	Smooth muscle hyperplasia, excess mucus, inflammation	Immunologic or undefined causes	Episodic wheezing, cough, dyspnea
Emphysema	Acinus	Airspace enlargement; wall destruction	Tobacco smoke	Dyspnea
Small-airway disease, bronchiolitis*	Bronchiole	Inflammatory scarring/obliteration	Tobacco smoke, air pollutants, miscellaneous	Cough, dyspnea

*Can be seen with any form of obstructive lung disease or as an isolated finding.

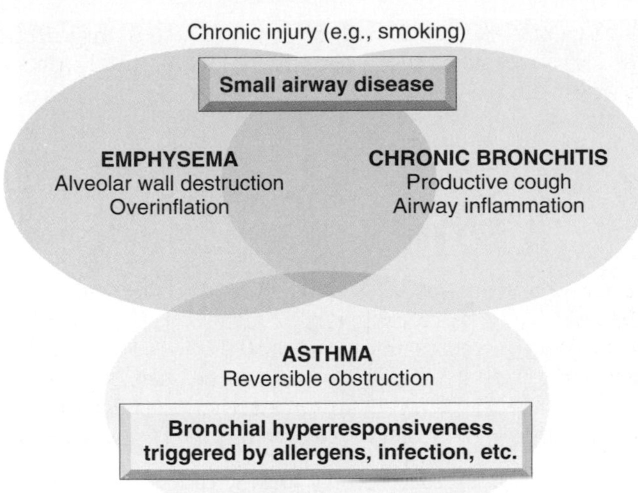

Figure 15-5 Schematic representation of overlap between chronic obstructive lung diseases.

smoking. In addition, small-airway disease, a variant of chronic bronchiolitis, is now known to contribute to obstruction both in emphysema and chronic bronchitis. While asthma is distinguished from chronic bronchitis and emphysema by the presence of reversible bronchospasm, some patients with otherwise typical asthma also develop an irreversible component (Fig. 15-5). Conversely, some patients with otherwise typical COPD have a reversible component. It is clinically common to label such patients as having COPD/asthma.

COPD is a major public health problem. It is the fourth leading cause of morbidity and mortality in the United States and is projected to rank fifth by 2020 as a worldwide burden of disease. There is a clear-cut association between heavy cigarette smoking and emphysema, and women and African Americans are more susceptible than other groups. About 35-50% of heavy smokers develop COPD; conversely 80% of COPD is due to smoking. Other risk factors include environmental and occupational pollutants, airway hyperresponsiveness and genetic polymorphisms.

Recognizing that there is overlap between various forms of COPD, it is still useful to discuss each individually in order to highlight the pathophysiologic basis of different causes of airflow obstruction.

Emphysema

Emphysema is characterized by irreversible enlargement of the airspaces distal to the terminal bronchiole, accompanied by destruction of their walls without obvious fibrosis. Small airway fibrosis (distinct from chronic bronchitis) has recently been to shown to be present in patients with emphysema; it is a significant contributor to airflow obstruction. Emphysema is classified according to its anatomic distribution within the lobule. Recall that the lobule is a cluster of acini, the terminal respiratory units. Based on the segments of the respiratory units that are involved, emphysema is classified into four major types: (1) *centriacinar*, (2) *panacinar*, (3) *paraseptal*, and (4) *irregular*. Of these, only the first two cause clinically significant airflow obstruction (Fig. 15-6). Centriacinar emphysema is the most common form, constituting more than 95% of clinically significant cases.

- ***Centriacinar (centrilobular) emphysema.*** In this type of emphysema the central or proximal parts of the acini, formed by respiratory bronchioles, are affected, whereas distal alveoli are spared (Figs. 15-6*B* and 15-7*A*). Thus, both emphysematous and normal airspaces exist within the same acinus and lobule. The lesions are more common and usually more severe in the upper lobes, particularly in the apical segments. Inflammation around bronchi and bronchioles is common. In severe centriacinar emphysema, the distal acinus may also be involved, making differentiation from panacinar emphysema difficult. Centriacinar emphysema occurs predominantly in heavy smokers, often in association with chronic bronchitis (COPD).
- ***Panacinar (panlobular) emphysema.*** In this type, the acini are uniformly enlarged from the level of the respiratory bronchiole to the terminal blind alveoli (Figs. 15-6*C* and 15-7*B*). The prefix "pan" refers to the entire acinus, not the entire lung. In contrast to centriacinar emphysema, panacinar emphysema tends to occur more commonly in the lower zones and in the anterior margins of the lung, and it is usually most severe at the bases. This type of emphysema is associated with *α_1-antitrypsin deficiency* (Chapter 17).
- ***Distal acinar (paraseptal) emphysema.*** In this type, the proximal portion of the acinus is normal, and the distal part is predominantly involved. The emphysema is more striking adjacent to the pleura, along the lobular

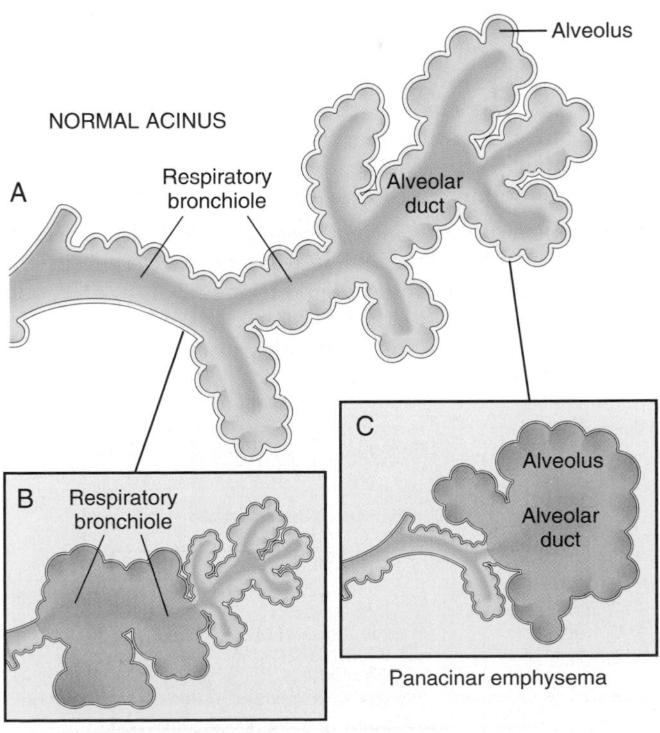

Figure 15-6 Clinically signficant patterns of emphysema. **A,** Structure of the normal acinus. **B,** Centriacinar emphysema with dilation that initially affects the respiratory bronchioles. **C,** Panacinar emphysema with initial distention of the alveolus and alveolar duct.

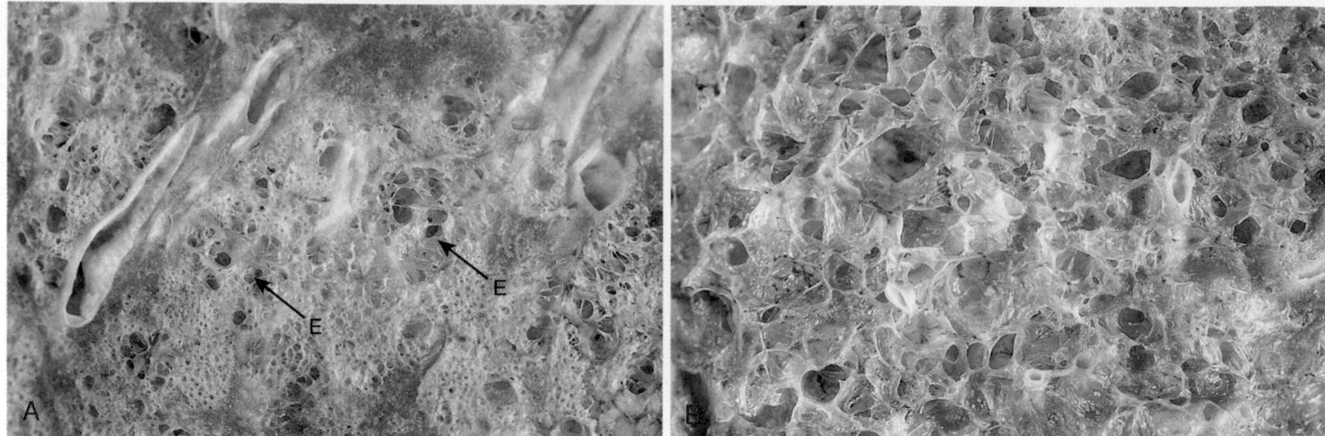

Figure 15-7 A, Centriacinar emphysema. Central areas show marked emphysematous damage (E), surrounded by relatively spared alveolar spaces. **B,** Panacinar emphysema involving the entire pulmonary lobule.

connective tissue septa, and at the margins of the lobules. It occurs adjacent to areas of fibrosis, scarring, or atelectasis and is usually more severe in the upper half of the lungs. The characteristic findings are of multiple, continuous, enlarged airspaces from less than 0.5 cm to more than 2.0 cm in diameter, sometimes forming cystlike structures. This type of emphysema probably underlies many cases of spontaneous pneumothorax in young adults.

- ***Airspace enlargement with fibrosis (irregular emphysema).*** Irregular emphysema, so named because the acinus is irregularly involved, is almost invariably associated with scarring. In most instances it occurs in small foci and is clinically insignificant.

Pathogenesis. Inhaled cigarette smoke and other noxious particles cause lung damage and inflammation, which results in parenchymal destruction (emphysema) and airway disease (bronchiolitis and chronic bronchitis). Factors that influence the development of emphysema include the following (Fig. 15-8):

- *Inflammatory mediators and leukocytes.* A wide variety of mediators have been shown to be increased in the affected parts (including leukotriene B_4, IL-8, TNF, and others) These mediators are released by resident epithelial cells and macrophages, and attract inflammatory cells from the circulation (chemotactic factors), amplify the inflammatory process (proinflammatory cytokines) and induce structural changes (growth factors).
- *Protease-antiprotease imbalance.* Several proteases are released from the inflammatory cells and epithelial cells that break down connective tissue components. In patients who develop emphysema, there is a relative deficiency of protective antiproteases, which in some instances has a genetic basis (further discussed later).
- *Oxidative stress.* Substances in tobacco smoke, alveolar damage, and inflammatory cells all produce oxidants, which may beget more tissue damage and inflammation. The role of oxidants is supported by mouse models in which the *NRF2* gene is inactivated. *NRF2* encodes a transcription factor that serves as a sensor for oxidants in alveolar epithelial cells and many other cells types. Intracellular oxidants activate *NRF2*, which upregulates the expression of multiple genes that protect cells from oxidant damage. Mice without *NRF2* are significantly more sensitive to tobacco smoke than normal mice, and genetic variants in *NRF2*, *NRF2* regulators, and *NRF2* target genes are all associated with smoking-related lung disease in humans.
- *Infection.* Although infection is not thought to play a role in the initiation of tissue destruction, bacterial and/or viral infections may exacerbate the associated inflammation and chronic bronchitis.

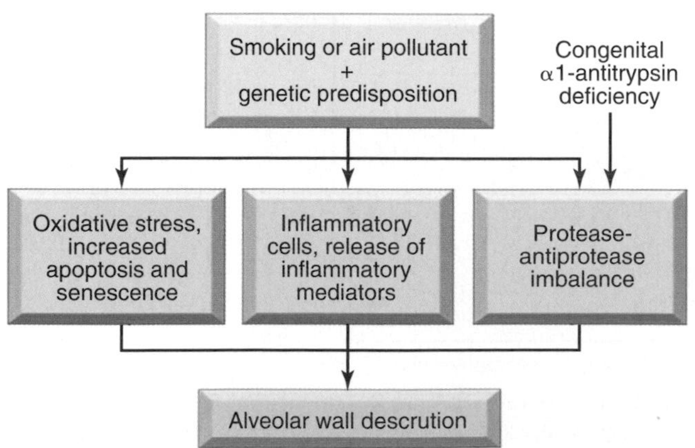

Figure 15-8 Pathogenesis of emphysema. See text for details.

The idea that proteases are important is based in part on the observation that patients with a genetic deficiency of the antiprotease α_1-antitrypsin have a markedly enhanced tendency to develop pulmonary emphysema, which is compounded by smoking. About 1% of all patients with emphysema have this defect. α_1-antitrypsin, normally present in serum, tissue fluids, and macrophages, is a major inhibitor of proteases (particularly elastase) secreted by neutrophils during inflammation. α_1-antitrypsin is encoded by the proteinase inhibitor *(Pi)* locus on chromosome 14. The *Pi* locus is polymorphic, and approximately 0.012% of the US population is homozygous for the *Z* allele, a genotype that is associated with markedly decreased serum levels of α_1-antitrypsin. More than 80% of these individuals develop symptomatic panacinar emphysema, which occurs at an earlier age and is of greater severity if the individual smokes. It is postulated that any injury (e.g., that induced by smoking) that increases the activation and influx of neutrophils into the lung leads to local release of proteases, which in the absence of α_1-antitrypsin activity result in excessive digestion of elastic tissue and emphysema.

Several other genetic variants have been linked to risk of emphysema. Among these are variants associated with the nicotinic acetylcholine receptor, which are hypothesized to influence the addictiveness of tobacco smoke and thus the behavior of smokers. Not surprisingly, the same variants are also linked to lung cancer risk, emphasizing the importance of smoking in both of these diseases.

A number of factors contribute to airway obstruction in emphysema. Small airways are normally held open by the elastic recoil of the lung parenchyma, and the loss of elastic tissue in the walls of alveoli that surround respiratory bronchioles reduces radial traction and thus causes the respiratory bronchioles to collapse during expiration. This leads to functional airflow obstruction despite the absence of mechanical obstruction. In addition, even young smokers often have small airway inflammation associated with the following changes:

- Goblet cell hyperplasia, with mucus plugging of the lumen
- Inflammatory infiltrates in bronchial walls consisting of neutrophils, macrophages, B cells (sometimes forming follicles), and T cells
- Thickening of the bronchiolar wall due to smooth muscle hypertrophy and peribronchial fibrosis

Together these changes narrow the bronchiolar lumen and contribute to airway obstruction.

MORPHOLOGY

Advanced emphysema produces voluminous lungs, often overlapping the heart and hiding it when the anterior chest wall is removed. Generally, the upper two thirds of the lungs are more severely affected. Large apical blebs or bullae are more characteristic of irregular emphysema secondary to scarring and of distal acinar emphysema. Large alveoli can easily be seen on the cut surface of fixed lungs (Fig. 15-7).

Microscopically, abnormally large alveoli are separated by thin septa with only focal centriacinar fibrosis. There is loss of attachments of the alveoli to the outer wall of small airways. The pores of Kohn are so large that septa appear to be floating or protrude blindly into alveolar spaces with a club-shaped end. Prolonged vasoconstriction leads to changes of pulmonary arterial hypertension. As alveolar walls are destroyed, there is a decrease in the capillary bed area. With advanced disease, there are even larger abnormal airspaces and possibly blebs or bullae, which often deform and compress the respiratory bronchioles and vasculature of the lung. Inflammatory changes in small airways were described earlier.

Clinical Course. Symptoms do not appear until at least one third of the functioning pulmonary parenchyma is damaged. *Dyspnea* usually appears first, beginning insidiously but progressing steadily. In some patients, cough or wheezing is the chief complaint, easily confused with asthma. Cough and expectoration are extremely variable and depend on the extent of the associated bronchitis.

Table 15-4 Emphysema and Chronic Bronchitis

	Predominant Bronchitis	Predominant Emphysema
Age (yr)	40-45	50-75
Dyspnea	Mild; late	Severe; early
Cough	Early; copious sputum	Late; scanty sputum
Infections	Common	Occasional
Respiratory insufficiency	Repeated	Terminal
Cor pulmonale	Common	Rare; terminal
Airway resistance	Increased	Normal or slightly increased
Elastic recoil	Normal	Low
Chest radiograph	Prominent vessels; large heart	Hyperinflation; small heart
Appearance	Blue bloater	Pink puffer

Weight loss is common and can be so severe as to suggest an occult cancer. Classically, the patient with severe emphysema is barrel-chested and dyspneic, with obviously prolonged expiration, sits forward in a hunched-over position, and breathes through pursed lips. *Impaired expiratory airflow,* best measured through spirometry, is the key to diagnosis.

In individuals with severe emphysema, cough is often slight, overdistention is severe, diffusion capacity is low, and blood gas values are relatively normal at rest. Such patients may overventilate and remain well oxygenated, and therefore are somewhat ingloriously designated *pink puffers* (Table 15-4). Development of cor pulmonale and eventually congestive heart failure, related to secondary pulmonary hypertension, is associated with a poor prognosis. Death in most patients with emphysema is due to (1) coronary artery disease, (2) respiratory failure, (3) right-sided heart failure, or (4) massive collapse of the lungs secondary to pneumothorax. Treatment options include smoking cessation, oxygen therapy, long-acting bronchodilators with inhaled corticosteroids, physical therapy, bullectomy, and, in selected patients, lung volume reduction surgery and lung transplantation. α_1-AT replacement therapy is being evaluated.

KEY CONCEPTS

Emphysema

- Emphysema is a chronic obstructive airway disease characterized by permanent enlargement of air spaces distal to terminal bronchioles. It is a component of COPD (chronic obstructive pulmonary disease) along with chronic bronchitis.
- Subtypes include centriacinar (most common, smoking related), panacinar (seen in α_1-antitrypsin deficiency), distal acinar and irregular.
- Smoking and inhaled pollutants cause ongoing accumulations of inflammatory cells, releasing elastases and oxidants, which destroy the alveolar walls.
- Most patients with emphysema also have some degree of chronic bronchitis, which is to be expected since cigarette smoking is an underlying risk factor for both.

Other Forms of Emphysema

The following are conditions to which the term emphysema is applied because they are associated with lung overinflation or focal emphysematous change

- ***Compensatory hyperinflation.*** This term is sometimes used to designate dilation of alveoli in response to loss of lung substance elsewhere. It is best exemplified by the hyperexpansion of residual lung parenchyma following surgical removal of a diseased lung or lobe.
- ***Obstructive overinflation.*** In this condition the lung expands because air is trapped within it. A common cause is subtotal obstruction of the airways by a tumor or foreign object. Another example is *congenital lobar overinflation* in infants, probably resulting from hypoplasia of bronchial cartilage and sometimes associated with other congenital cardiac and lung abnormalities. Overinflation in obstructive lesions occurs either (1) because the obstructive agent acts as ball valve, allowing air to enter on inspiration while preventing its exodus on expiration, or (2) because *collaterals* bring in air behind the obstruction. These collaterals consist of the *pores of Kohn* and other direct accessory bronchioloalveolar connections (the *canals of Lambert*). Obstructive overinflation can be a life-threatening emergency, because the affected portion distends sufficiently to compress the remaining lung.
- ***Bullous emphysema.*** This is a descriptive term for large subpleural blebs or bullae (spaces greater than 1 cm in diameter in the distended state) that can occur in any form of emphysema (Fig. 15-9). These localized accentuations of emphysema occur near the apex, sometimes near old tuberculous scarring. On occasion, rupture of the bullae may give rise to pneumothorax.
- ***Interstitial emphysema***. Entrance of air into the connective tissue stroma of the lung, mediastinum, or subcutaneous tissue produces *interstitial emphysema.* In most instances, alveolar tears in pulmonary emphysema provide the avenue of entrance of air into the stroma of the lung, but rarely, chest wounds that allow entry of air or fractured ribs that puncture the lung substance underlie this disorder. Alveolar tears are usually caused by rapid increases in pressure within alveolar sacs, such as occurs when there is a combination of coughing and bronchiolar obstruction. Premature children on positive pressure ventilation adults who are being artificially ventilated are most at risk.

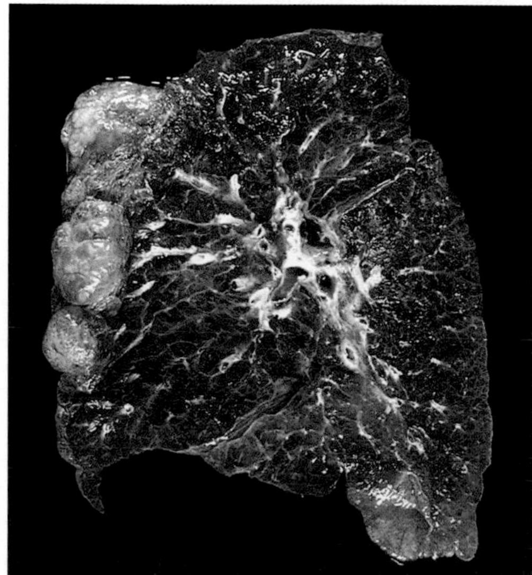

Figure 15-9 Bullous emphysema. Note the large subpleural bullae *(upper left)*.

Chronic Bronchitis

Chronic bronchitis is defined clinically as persistent cough with sputum production for at least 3 months in at least 2 consecutive years, in the absence of any other identifiable cause. Common in habitual smokers and inhabitants of smog-laden cities, chronic bronchitis is one end of the spectrum of COPD, with emphysema being the other. Most patients lie somewhere in between, having features of both. When chronic bronchitis persists for years, it may accelerate decline in lung function, lead to cor pulmonale and heart failure, or cause atypical metaplasia and dysplasia of the respiratory epithelium, providing a rich soil for cancerous transformation.

Pathogenesis. The primary or initiating factor in the genesis of chronic bronchitis is exposure to noxious or irritating inhaled substances such as tobacco smoke (90% of patients are smokers) and dust from grain, cotton, and silica.

- *Mucus hypersecretion.* The earliest feature of chronic bronchitis is hypersecretion of mucus in the large airways, associated with hypertrophy of the submucosal glands in the trachea and bronchi. The basis for mucus hypersecretion is incompletely understood, but it appears to involve inflammatory mediators such as histamine and IL-13. With time, there is also a marked increase in goblet cells in small airways—small bronchi and bronchioles—leading to excessive mucus production that contributes to airway obstruction. It is thought that both the submucosal gland hypertrophy and the increase in goblet cells are protective reactions against tobacco smoke or other pollutants (e.g., sulfur dioxide and nitrogen dioxide).
- *Inflammation.* Inhalants that induce chronic bronchitis cause cellular damage, eliciting both acute and chronic inflammatory responses involving neutrophils, lymphocytes, and macrophages. Long-standing inflammation and accompanying fibrosis involving small airways (small bronchi and bronchioles, less than 2 to 3 mm in diameter) can also lead to chronic airway obstruction. This feature is similar to that described earlier in emphysema and is a common denominator in COPD.
- *Infection.* Infection does not initiate chronic bronchitis, but is probably significant in maintaining it and may be critical in producing acute exacerbations.

It should be recognized that cigarette smoke predisposes to chronic bronchitis in several ways. Not only does it damage airway lining cells, leading to chronic inflammation, but it also interferes with the ciliary action of the respiratory epithelium, preventing the clearance of mucus and increasing the risk of infection.

MORPHOLOGY

Grossly, there is hyperemia, swelling, and edema of the mucous membranes, frequently accompanied by excessive mucinous or mucopurulent secretions. Sometimes, heavy casts of secretions and pus fill the bronchi and bronchioles. The characteristic features are mild chronic inflammation of the airways (predominantly lymphocytes) and enlargement of the mucus-secreting glands of the trachea and bronchi. Although the numbers of goblet cells increase slightly, the **major change is in the size of mucous glands (hyperplasia)**. This increase can be assessed by the ratio of the thickness of the mucous gland layer to the thickness of the wall between the epithelium and the cartilage (**Reid index**). The Reid index (normally 0.4) is increased in chronic bronchitis, usually in proportion to the severity and duration of the disease. The bronchial epithelium may exhibit squamous metaplasia and dysplasia. There is marked narrowing of bronchioles caused by mucus plugging, inflammation, and fibrosis. In the most severe cases, there may be obliteration of lumen due to fibrosis (**bronchiolitis obliterans**).

Clinical Features. The cardinal symptom of chronic bronchitis is a persistent cough productive of sparse sputum. For many years no other respiratory functional impairment is present, but eventually dyspnea on exertion develops. With the passage of time, and usually with continued smoking, other elements of COPD may appear, including hypercapnia, hypoxemia, and mild cyanosis (*"blue bloaters"*). Differentiation of pure chronic bronchitis from that associated with emphysema can be made in the classic case (Table 15-4), but, as has been mentioned, many patients with COPD have both conditions. Long-standing severe chronic bronchitis commonly leads to cor pulmonale and cardiac failure. Death may also result from further impairment of respiratory function due to superimposed acute infections.

KEY CONCEPTS

Chronic Bronchitis

- Chronic bronchitis is defined as persistent productive cough for at least 3 consecutive months in at least 2 consecutive years.
- Cigarette smoking is the most important risk factor; air pollutants also contribute.
- The dominant pathologic features are mucus hypersecretion and persistent inflammation.
- Histologic examination demonstrates enlargement of mucous-secreting glands, goblet cell hyperplasia, chronic inflammation, and bronchiolar wall fibrosis.

Asthma

Asthma is a chronic disorder of the conducting airways, usually caused by an immunological reaction, which is marked by episodic bronchoconstriction due to increased airway sensitivity to a variety of stimuli; inflammation of the bronchial walls; and increased mucus secretion. The disease is manifested by recurrent episodes of wheezing, breathlessness, chest tightness, and cough, particularly at night and/or in the early morning. These symptoms are usually associated with widespread but variable bronchoconstriction and airflow limitation that is at least partly reversible, either spontaneously or with treatment. Some of the stimuli that trigger attacks in patients would have little or no effect in subjects with normal airways. Rarely, a state of unremitting attacks, called acute severe asthma (formerly known as *status asthmaticus*), may prove fatal; usually, such patients have had a long history of asthma. Between the attacks, patients may be virtually asymptomatic. Of note, there has been a significant increase in the incidence of asthma in the Western world over the past 40 to 50 years, which may be reaching a plateau now. More recently, although treatment for asthma has improved substantially, the prevalence of asthma continues to increase in low and middle income countries and in some ethnic groups in which prevalence was previously low.

Asthma may be categorized as *atopic* (evidence of allergen sensitization and immune activation, often in a patient with allergic rhinitis or eczema) or *non-atopic* (no evidence of allergen sensitization). In either type, episodes of bronchospasm can have diverse triggers, such as respiratory infections (especially viral infections), exposure to irritants (e.g., smoke, fumes), cold air, stress, and exercise. There is some evidence that sub-classifying asthma according to its clinical features and underlying biology is clinically useful. One example is early-onset allergic asthma associated with T_H2 helper T cell inflammation, a feature seen in about half of the patients. This form of asthma responds well to corticosteroids. However, there is no current consensus as to definitions and diagnostic criteria. Asthma may also be classified according to the agents or events that trigger bronchoconstriction. These include seasonal, exercise-induced, drug-induced (e.g., aspirin), and occupational asthma, and asthmatic bronchitis in smokers.

Atopic Asthma. This most common type of asthma is a **classic example of IgE-mediated (type I) hypersensitivity reaction**, discussed in detail in Chapter 6. The disease usually begins in childhood and is triggered by environmental allergens, such as dusts, pollens, cockroach or animal dander, and foods, which most frequently act in synergy with other proinflammatory environmental cofactors, most notable respiratory viral infections. A positive family history of asthma is common, and a skin test with the offending antigen in these patients results in an immediate wheal-and-flare reaction. Atopic asthma may also be diagnosed based on high total serum IgE levels or evidence of allergen sensitization by serum radioallergosorbent tests (called RAST), which can detect the presence of IgE antibodies that are specific for individual allergens.

Non-Atopic Asthma. Individuals with non-atopic asthma do not have evidence of allergen sensitization and skin test results are usually negative. A positive family history of asthma is less common in these patients. Respiratory infections due to viruses (e.g., rhinovirus, parainfluenza virus and respiratory syncytial virus) are common triggers in non-atopic asthma. Inhaled air pollutants, such as smoking, sulfur dioxide, ozone, and nitrogen dioxide, may also contribute to the chronic airway inflammation and hyperreactivity in some cases. As already mentioned, in some instances attacks may be triggered by seemingly innocuous events, such as exposure to cold and even exercise.

Drug-Induced Asthma. Several pharmacologic agents provoke asthma. *Aspirin-sensitive asthma* is an uncommon type, occurring in individuals with recurrent rhinitis and nasal polyps. These individuals are exquisitely sensitive to small doses of aspirin as well as other nonsteroidal anti-inflammatory medications, and they experience not only asthmatic attacks but also urticaria. Aspirin (and other non-steroidal anti-inflammatory drugs) triggers asthma in these patients by inhibiting the cyclooxygenase pathway of arachidonic acid metabolism, leading to a rapid decrease in prostaglandin E_2. Normally prostaglandin E_2 inhibits enzymes that generate proinflammatory mediators such as leukotrienes B_4, C_4, D_4 and E_4, which are believed to have central roles in aspirin-induced asthma.

Occupational Asthma. This form of asthma may be triggered by fumes (epoxy resins, plastics), organic and chemical dusts (wood, cotton, platinum), gases (toluene), or other chemicals (formaldehyde, penicillin products). Only minute quantities of chemicals are required to induce the attack, which usually occurs after repeated exposure. The underlying mechanisms vary according to stimulus and include type I reactions, direct liberation of bronchoconstrictor substances, and hypersensitivity responses of unknown origin.

Pathogenesis. **Atopic asthma is caused by a T_H2 and IgE response to environmental allergens in genetically predisposed individuals.** Airway inflammation is central to disease pathophysiology and causes airway dysfunction partly through the release of potent inflammatory mediators and partly through remodeling of the airway wall. As the disease becomes more severe, there is increased local secretion of growth factors, which induce mucus gland hypertrophy, smooth muscle proliferation, angiogenesis, fibrosis and nerve proliferation. Varying combinations of these processes help explain the different asthma subtypes, their response to treatment and their natural history over a person's lifetime.

The contributions of the immune response, genetics and environment are discussed separately below, although they are closely intertwined.

T_H2 Responses, IgE and Inflammation. **A fundamental abnormality in asthma is an exaggerated T_H2 response to normally harmless environmental antigens** (Fig 15-10). T_H2 cells secrete cytokines that promote inflammation and stimulate B cells to produce IgE and other antibodies. These cytokines include IL-4, which stimulates the production of IgE; IL-5, which activates locally recruited eosinophils; and IL-13, which stimulates mucus secretion from bronchial submucosal glands and also promotes IgE production by B cells. The T cells and epithelial cells secrete chemokines that recruit more T cells and eosinophils, thus exacerbating the reaction. As in other allergic reactions (Chapter 6), IgE binds to the Fc receptors on submucosal mast cells, and repeat exposure to the allergen triggers the mast cells to release granule contents and produce cytokines and other mediators, which collectively induce the *early-phase (immediate hypersensitivity) reaction* and the *late-phase reaction*.

The early reaction is dominated by bronchoconstriction, increased mucus production, variable degrees of vasodilation, and increased vascular permeability. Bronchoconstriction is triggered by direct stimulation of subepithelial vagal (parasympathetic) receptors through both central and local reflexes triggered by mediators produced by mast cells and other cells in the reaction. The late-phase reaction is dominated by recruitment of leukocytes, notably eosinophils, neutrophils, and more T cells. Although T_H2 cells are the dominant T cell type involved in the disease, other T cells that contribute to the inflammation include T_H17 (IL-17 producing) cells, which recruit neutrophils.

Many mediators produced by leukocytes and epithelial cells have been implicated in the asthmatic response. The long list of "suspects" in acute asthma can be ranked based on the clinical efficacy of pharmacologic intervention with antagonists of specific mediators.

- Mediators whose role in bronchospasm is clearly supported by efficacy of pharmacologic intervention are: (1) *leukotrienes C_4, D_4*, and *E_4*, which cause prolonged bronchoconstriction as well as increased vascular permeability and increased mucus secretion, and (2) *acetylcholine*, released from intrapulmonary parasympathetic nerves, which can cause airway smooth muscle constriction by directly stimulating muscarinic receptors.
- A second group includes agents present at the "scene of the crime" but whose actual role in acute allergic asthma seems relatively minor on the basis of lack of efficacy of potent antagonists or synthesis inhibitors: (1) *histamine*, a potent bronchoconstrictor; (2) *prostaglandin D_2*, which elicits bronchoconstriction and vasodilatation; and (3) *platelet-activating factor*, which causes aggregation of platelets and release of serotonin from their granules. These mediators might yet prove important in certain types of chronic or nonallergic asthma.
- Finally, a large third group comprises the "suspects" for whom specific antagonists or inhibitors are not available or have been insufficiently studied as yet. Several promising focused therapies for asthma that target the IL-13/IL-4 signal transduction pathways are in development, including anti-IL-13 monoclonal antibodies and IL-4 receptor antagonists. Other targets include IL-1, TNF, IL-6, chemokines (e.g., eotaxin, also known as CCL11), neuropeptides, nitric oxide, bradykinin, and endothelins.

It is thus clear that multiple mediators contribute to the acute asthmatic response. Moreover, the composition of this "mediator soup" might vary among individuals or different types of asthma. The appreciation of the importance of inflammatory cells and mediators in asthma has led to greater emphasis on anti-inflammatory drugs, such as corticosteroids, in its treatment.

Genetic Susceptibility. **Susceptibility to atopic asthma is multigenic and often associated with increased incidence of other allergic disorders, such as allergic rhinitis (hay fever) and eczema.** The genetic polymorphisms linked to asthma and other allergic disorders were described in Chapter 6. Suffice it to say here that many of these are likely to influence immune responses and the subsequent inflammatory reaction. Some of the stronger or more interesting associations include the following:

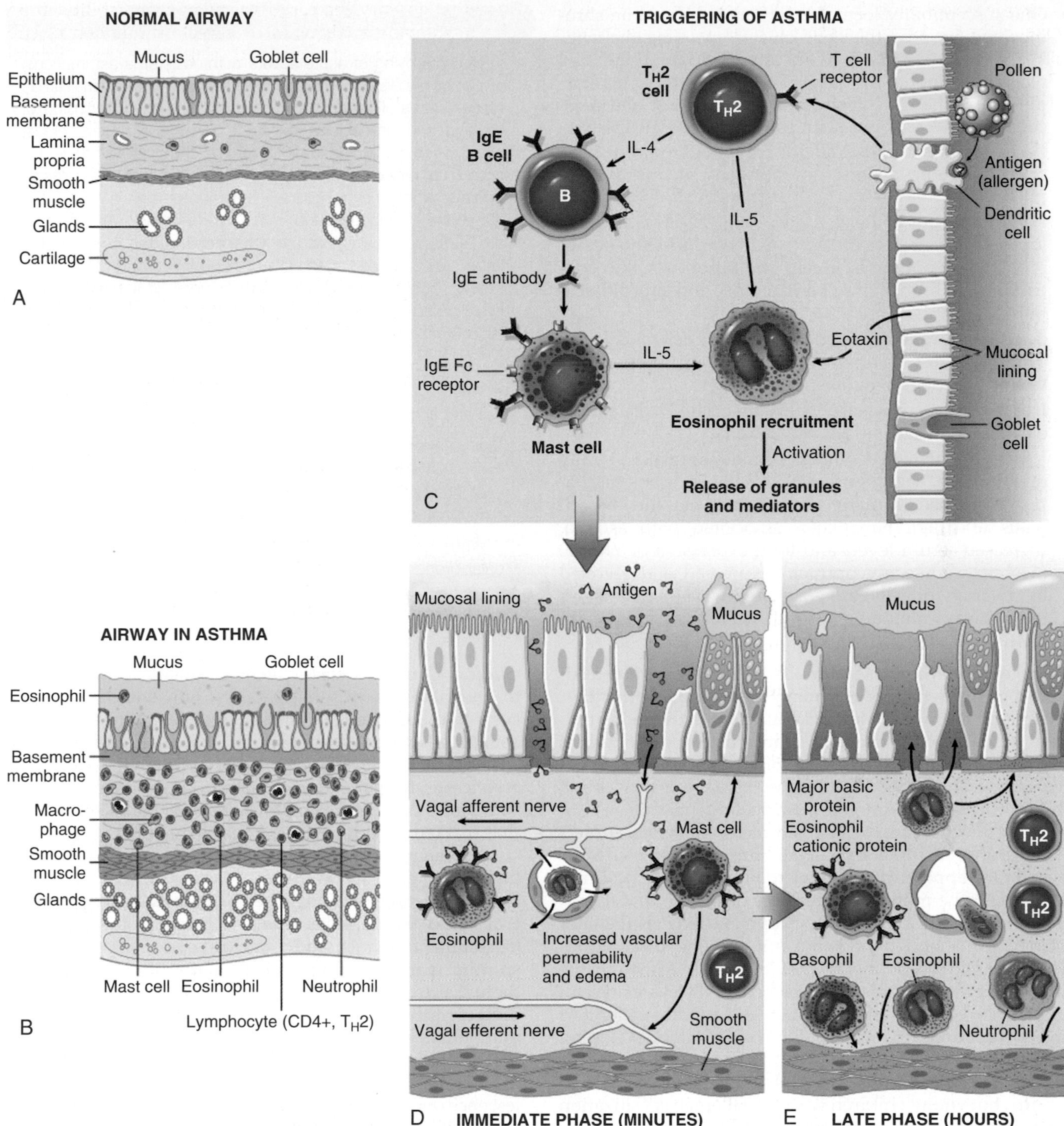

Figure 15-10 A and **B,** Comparison of a normal airway and an airway involved by asthma. The asthmatic airway is marked by accumulation of mucus in the bronchial lumen secondary to an increase in the number of mucus-secreting goblet cells in the mucosa and hypertrophy of submucosal glands; intense chronic inflammation due to recruitment of eosinophils, macrophages, and other inflammatory cells; thickened basement membrane; and hypertrophy and hyperplasia of smooth muscle cells. **C,** Inhaled allergens (antigen) elicit a T_H2-dominated response favoring IgE production and eosinophil recruitment. **D,** On re-exposure to antigen (Ag), the immediate reaction is triggered by Ag-induced cross-linking of IgE bound to Fc receptors on mast cells. These cells release preformed mediators that directly and via neuronal reflexes induce bronchospasm, increased vascular permeability, mucus production, and recruitment of leukocytes. **E,** Leukocytes recruited to the site of reaction (neutrophils, eosinophils, and basophils; lymphocytes and monocytes) release additional mediators that initiate the late phase of asthma. Several factors released from eosinophils (e.g., major basic protein, eosinophil cationic protein) also cause damage to the epithelium.

- One susceptibility locus for asthma is located on chromosome 5q, near the gene cluster encoding the cytokines IL-3, IL-4, IL-5, IL-9, and IL-13 and the IL-4 receptor. Among the genes in this cluster, polymorphisms in the *IL13* gene have the strongest and most consistent associations with asthma or allergic disease.
- Particular class II HLA alleles are linked to production of IgE antibodies against some antigens, such as ragweed pollen.
- Polymorphisms in the gene encoding ADAM33, a metalloproteinase, may be linked to increased proliferation of bronchial smooth muscle cells and fibroblasts, thus contributing to bronchial hyperreactivity and subepithelial fibrosis.
- β_2-adrenergic receptor gene variants are associated with differential in vivo airway hyper-responsiveness and in vitro response to β-agonist stimulation.
- IL-4 receptor gene variants are associated with atopy, elevated total serum IgE, and asthma.
- Variants in several members of the mammalian family of chitinases, enzymes that cleave chitin, a polysaccharide contained in many human parasites and the cell walls of fungi, have been associated with asthma. Increased serum levels and lung expression of YKL-40 (a chitinase-like glycoprotein expressed and secreted by a variety of cells) are correlated with disease severity, airway remodeling, and decreased pulmonary function.

Environmental Factors. **Asthma is a disease of industrialized societies where the majority of people live in cities.** This likely has two main explanations. Firstly, industrialized environments contain many airborne pollutants that can serve as allergens to initiate the T_H2 response. Secondly, city life tends to limit the exposure of very young children to certain antigens, particularly microbial antigens, and exposure to such antigens seems to protect children from asthma and atopy. This protective effect is even more apparent if the microbial exposure occurred throughout the mother's pregnancy. The idea that microbial exposure during early development reduces the later incidence of allergic (and some autoimmune) diseases has been popularized as the *hygiene hypothesis.* Although the underlying mechanisms of this protective effect are unclear, it has spurred trials of probiotics and putative allergens given to children to decrease their risk of later developing allergies.

Infections themselves are not a cause or trigger for asthma, but young children with aeroallergen sensitization who develop lower respiratory tract viral infections (rhinovirus type C, respiratory syncytial virus) have a 10- to 30-fold increased risk of developing persistent and/or severe asthma. Both viral and bacterial infections (identified by cultures and non-culture tools) are associated with acute exacerbations of the disease.

Over time, repeated bouts of allergen exposure and immune reactions result in structural changes in the bronchial wall, referred to as "*airway remodeling*." These changes, described later in greater detail, include hypertrophy and hyperplasia of bronchial smooth muscle, epithelial injury, increased airway vascularity, increased subepithelial mucus gland hypertrophy, and deposition of subepithelial collagen.

MORPHOLOGY

In patients dying of acute severe asthma (status asthmaticus) the lungs are distended by overinflation and contain small areas of atelectasis. The most striking gross finding is occlusion of bronchi and bronchioles by thick, tenacious mucus plugs, which often contain shed epithelium. A characteristic finding in sputum or bronchoalveolar lavage specimens is **Curschmann spirals**, which may result from extrusion of mucus plugs from subepithelial mucous gland ducts or bronchioles. Also present are numerous eosinophils and **Charcot-Leyden crystals**; the latter are composed of an eosinophil protein called galectin-10. The other characteristic histologic findings of asthma, collectively called **"airway remodeling"** (Fig. 15-10*B*, and 15-11), include:

- Thickening of airway wall
- Subbasement membrane fibrosis (due to deposition of type I and III collagen)
- Increased vascularity
- An increase in the size of the submucosal glands and number of airway goblet cells
- Hypertrophy and/or hyperplasia of the bronchial wall muscle

While acute airflow obstruction is primarily attributed to muscular bronchoconstriction, acute edema, and mucus plugging, airway remodeling may also contribute to chronic irreversible airway obstruction as well.

Clinical Course. A classic acute asthmatic attack lasts up to several hours. In some patients, however, the cardinal symptoms of chest tightness, dyspnea, wheezing, and coughing (with or without sputum production) are present at a low level constantly. In its most severe form, *status asthmaticus,* the paroxysm persists for days and even weeks, sometimes causing airflow obstruction that is so extreme that marked cyanosis or even death ensues.

The diagnosis is based on demonstration of an increase in airflow obstruction (from baseline levels), difficulty with exhalation (prolonged expiration, wheeze), peripheral blood eosinophilia, and the finding of eosinophils, Curschmann spirals, and Charcot-Leyden crystals in the sputum (particularly in patients with atopic asthma). In the usual case with intervals of freedom from respiratory difficulty, the disease is more discouraging and disabling than lethal, and most individuals with asthma are able to maintain a productive life. Therapy is based on severity of the disease. Up to 50% of childhood asthma remits in adolescence only to return in adulthood in a significant number of patients. In other cases there is a variable decline in baseline lung function.

KEY CONCEPTS

Asthma

- Asthma is characterized by reversible bronchoconstriction caused by airway hyperresponsiveness to a variety of stimuli.
- Atopic asthma is caused by a T_H2 and IgE-mediated immunologic reaction to environmental allergens and is characterized by acute-phase (immediate) and late-phase

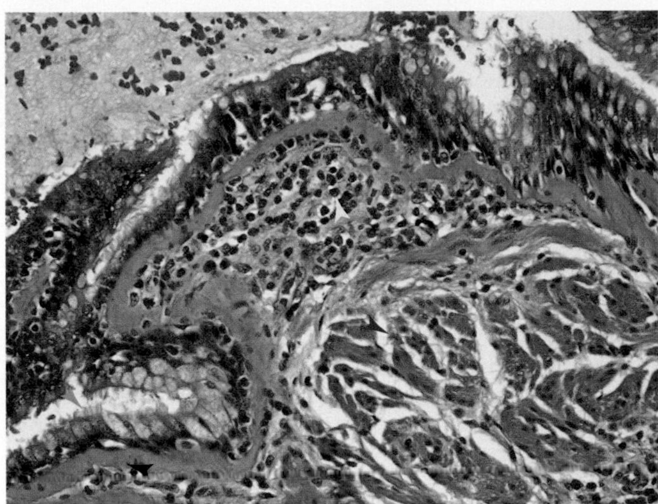

Figure 15-11 Bronchus from an asthmatic patient showing goblet cell hyperplasia *(green arrowhead)*, subbasement membrane fibrosis *(black arrowhead)*, eosinophilic inflammation *(yellow arrowhead)*, and muscle hypertrophy *(blue arrowhead)*.

reactions. The T_H2 cytokines IL 4, IL-5, and IL13 are important mediators. IL17 and IL9 are also being shown to be important in some asthmatics.

- Triggers for nonatopic asthma are less clear but include viral infections and inhaled air pollutants, which can also trigger atopic asthma.
- Eosinophils are key inflammatory cells found in almost all subtypes of asthma; other inflammatory cells include mast cells, neutrophils and T lymphocytes.
- Airway remodeling (sub-basement membrane fibrosis, hypertrophy of bronchial glands, and smooth muscle hyperplasia) adds an irreversible component to the obstructive disease.

Bronchiectasis

Bronchiectasis is a disorder in which destruction of smooth muscle and elastic tissue by chronic necrotizing infections leads to permanent dilation of bronchi and bronchioles. Because of better control of lung infections, bronchiectasis is now uncommon. It may still develop in association with a variety of conditions, including the following:

- *Congenital or hereditary conditions*, including cystic fibrosis, intralobar sequestration of the lung, immunodeficiency states, and primary ciliary dyskinesia and Kartagener syndromes
- *Infections*, including necrotizing pneumonia caused by bacteria, viruses, or fungi; this may be a single severe episode or recurrent infections
- *Bronchial obstruction*, due to tumor, foreign bodies, or mucus impaction; in each instance the bronchiectasis is localized to the obstructed lung segment
- Other conditions, including rheumatoid arthritis, systemic lupus erythematosus, inflammatory bowel disease, COPD, and posttransplantation (chronic lung rejection, and chronic graft-versus-host disease after bone marrow transplantation)
- One fourth to one half of cases are *idiopathic*, lacking the aforementioned associations.

Pathogenesis. Obstruction and infection are the major conditions associated with bronchiectasis, and it is likely that both are necessary for the development of full-fledged lesions. After bronchial obstruction, normal clearing mechanisms are impaired, resulting in pooling of secretions distal to the obstruction and secondary infection and inflammation. Conversely, severe infections of the bronchi lead to inflammation, often with necrosis, fibrosis, and eventually dilation of airways.

Both mechanisms are readily apparent in a severe form of bronchiectasis that is associated with cystic fibrosis (Chapter 10). In cystic fibrosis the primary defect in ion transport leads to defective mucociliary action and airway obstruction by thick viscous secretions. This sets the stage for chronic bacterial infections, which cause widespread damage to airway walls. With destruction of supporting smooth muscle and elastic tissue, the bronchi become markedly dilated, while smaller bronchioles are progressively obliterated as a result of fibrosis (bronchiolitis obliterans).

In *primary ciliary dyskinesia*, an autosomal recessive syndrome with a frequency of 1 in 15,000 to 40,000 births, ciliary dysfunction due to defects in ciliary motor proteins (e.g., mutations involving dynein) contributes to the retention of secretions and recurrent infections that in turn lead to bronchiectasis. Ciliary function is necessary during development to ensure proper rotation of the developing organs in the chest and abdomen; it is absence, their location becomes a matter of chance. As a result, approximately half of the patients with primary ciliary dyskinesia have *Kartagener syndrome*, marked by situs inversus or a partial lateralizing abnormality associated with bronchiectasis and sinusitis. The lack of ciliary activity interferes with bacterial clearance, predisposes the sinuses and bronchi to infection, and affects cell motility during embryogenesis, resulting in the situs inversus. Males with this condition tend to be infertile, as a result of sperm dysmotility.

Allergic bronchopulmonary aspergillosis occurs in patients with asthma and cystic fibrosis who develop periods of exacerbation and remission that may lead to proximal bronchiectasis and fibrotic lung disease. It is a condition that results from a hypersensitivity reaction to the fungus *Aspergillus fumigatus*. Sensitization to *Aspergillus* in the allergic host leads to activation of T_H2 helper T cells, which play a key role in recruiting eosinophils and other leukocytes. Characteristically, there are high serum IgE levels, serum antibodies to *Aspergillus*, intense airway inflammation with eosinophils, and the formation of mucus plugs, which play a primary role in its pathogenesis.

MORPHOLOGY

Bronchiectasis usually affects the lower lobes bilaterally, particularly air passages that are vertical, and is most severe in the more distal bronchi and bronchioles. When tumors or aspiration of foreign bodies lead to bronchiectasis, the involvement may be localized to a single lung segment. **The airways are dilated, sometimes up to four times normal size.** Characteristically, the bronchi and bronchioles are so dilated that they can be

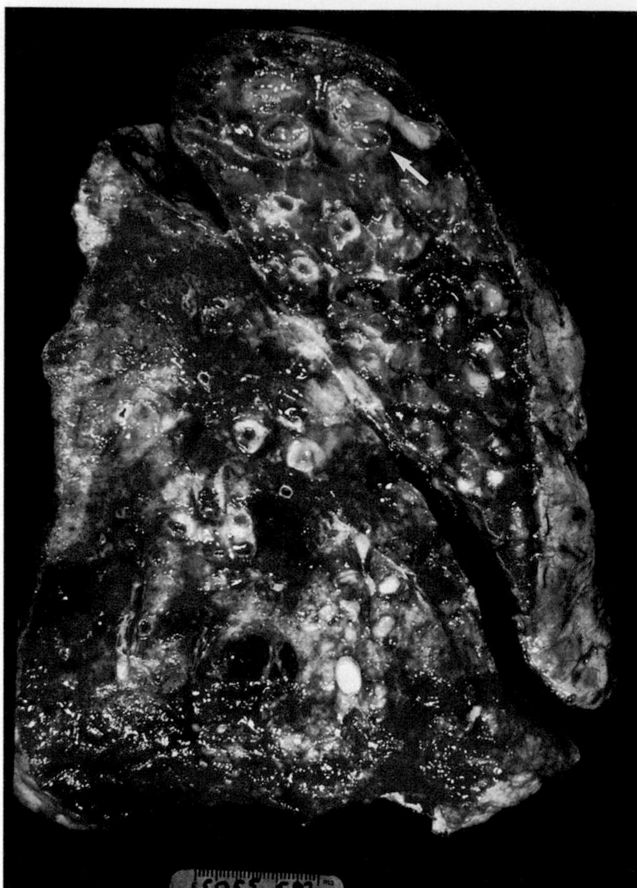

Figure 15-12 Bronchiectasis in a patient with cystic fibrosis, who underwent lung transplantation. Cut surface of lung shows markedly distended peripheral bronchi filled with mucopurulent secretions.

followed almost to the pleural surfaces. By contrast, in the normal lung, the bronchioles cannot be followed by eye beyond a point 2 to 3 cm from the pleural surfaces. On the cut surface of the lung, the dilated bronchi appear cystic and are filled with mucopurulent secretions (Fig. 15-12).

The histologic findings vary with the activity and chronicity of the disease. In the full-blown, active case there is an intense acute and chronic inflammatory exudation within the walls of the bronchi and bronchioles, associated with desquamation of the lining epithelium and extensive areas of ulceration. There may be pseudostratification of the columnar cells or squamous metaplasia of the remaining epithelium. In some instances necrosis destroys the bronchial or bronchiolar walls and forms a lung abscess. Fibrosis of the bronchial and bronchiolar walls and peribronchiolar fibrosis develop in the more chronic cases, leading to varying degrees of subtotal or total obliteration of bronchiolar lumens.

A large variety of bacteria can be found in the usual case of bronchiectasis. These include staphylococci, streptococci, pneumococci, enteric organisms, anaerobic and microaerophilic bacteria, and (particularly in children) *Haemophilus influenzae* and *Pseudomonas aeruginosa*. In allergic bronchopulmonary aspergillosis, a few fungal hyphae can be seen on special stains within the mucoinflammatory contents of the dilated segmental bronchi. In late stages the fungus may infiltrate the bronchial wall.

Clinical Course. Bronchiectasis causes severe, persistent cough; expectoration of foul smelling, sometimes bloody sputum; dyspnea and orthopnea in severe cases; and, on occasion, hemoptysis, which may be massive. Symptoms are often episodic and are precipitated by upper respiratory tract infections or the introduction of new pathogenic agents. Paroxysms of cough are particularly frequent when the patient rises in the morning, as the change in position causes collections of pus and secretions to drain into the bronchi. Obstructive respiratory insufficiency can lead to marked dyspnea and cyanosis. However, due to current treatment with better antibiotics and physical therapy, outcome has improved considerably and life expectancy has almost doubled. Hence cor pulmonale, brain abscesses, and amyloidosis are less frequent complications of bronchiectasis currently than in the past.

Chronic Diffuse Interstitial (Restrictive) Diseases

Restrictive lung disorders occur in two general conditions: (1) *chronic interstitial and infiltrative diseases*, such as pneumoconioses and interstitial fibrosis of unknown etiology; and (2) *chest wall disorders* (e.g., neuromuscular diseases such as poliomyelitis, severe obesity, pleural diseases, and kyphoscoliosis), which are not discussed here.

Chronic interstitial pulmonary diseases are a heterogeneous group of disorders characterized predominantly by inflammation and fibrosis of the pulmonary interstitium. Many of the entities are of unknown cause and pathogenesis, and some have an intra-alveolar as well as an interstitial component. There is frequent overlap in histologic features among the different conditions. These disorders account for about 15% of noninfectious diseases seen by pulmonary physicians.

In general, the clinical and pulmonary functional changes are those of *restrictive lung disease*. Patients have dyspnea, tachypnea, end-inspiratory crackles, and eventual cyanosis, without wheezing or other evidence of airway obstruction. The classic functional abnormalities are reductions in diffusion capacity, lung volume, and lung compliance. Chest radiographs show bilateral lesions that take the form of small nodules, irregular lines, or *ground-glass shadows*, all corresponding to areas of interstitial fibrosis. Eventually, secondary pulmonary hypertension and right-sided heart failure associated with cor pulmonale may result. Although the entities can often be distinguished in the early stages, the advanced forms are hard to differentiate because all result in scarring and gross destruction of the lung, often referred to as *end-stage lung* or *honeycomb lung*. Diffuse restrictive diseases are categorized based on histology and clinical features (Table 15-5).

Fibrosing Diseases

Idiopathic Pulmonary Fibrosis

Idiopathic pulmonary fibrosis (IPF) refers to a clinicopathologic syndrome marked by progressive interstitial pulmonary fibrosis and respiratory failure. In Europe the term *cryptogenic fibrosing alveolitis* is more popular. IPF has

Table 15-5 Major Categories of Chronic Interstitial Lung Disease

Fibrosing
Usual interstitial pneumonia (idiopathic pulmonary fibrosis) Nonspecific interstitial pneumonia Cryptogenic organizing pneumonia Connective tissue disease-associated Pneumoconiosis Drug reactions Radiation pneumonitis
Granulomatous
Sarcoidosis Hypersensitivity pneumonitis
Eosinophilic
Smoking Related
Desquamative interstitial pneumonia Respiratory bronchiolitis associated interstitial lung disease
Other
Langerhans cell histiocytosis Pulmonary alveolar proteinosis Lymphoid interstitial pneumonia

characteristic radiologic, pathologic, and clinical features. The histologic pattern of fibrosis is referred to as usual interstitial pneumonia (UIP), which can often be diagnosed based on its characteristic appearance in CT scans. The UIP pattern can also be seen in other diseases, notably connective tissue diseases, chronic hypersensitivity pneumonia, and asbestosis; these must be distinguished from IPF based on other clinical, laboratory, and histological features.

Pathogenesis. While the cause of IPF remains unknown, it appears that the fibrosis arises in genetically predisposed individuals who are prone to aberrant repair of recurrent alveolar epithelial cell injuries caused by environmental exposures (Fig. 15-13). The implicated factors are as follows:

- *Environmental factors.* Most important among these is cigarette smoking, which increases the risk of IPF several fold. IPF incidence is also increased in individuals who are exposed to metal fumes and wood dust, or who work in certain occupations, including farming, hairdressing, and stone-polishing. It is hypothesized that exposure to environmental irritants or toxins in each of these contexts causes recurrent alveolar epithelial cell damage. Gastric reflux has also been recently implicated.
- *Genetic factors.* The vast majority of individuals who smoke or who have other environmental exposures linked to IPF do not develop the disorder, indicating that additional factors are required for its development. Chief among the suspects are inherited genetic variants. One group of genetic lesions of particular interest is germline loss-of-function mutations in the *TERT* and *TERC* genes, which encode components of telomerase. You will recall that telomerase is an enzyme that maintains the ends of chromosomes (the telomeres) and thereby prevents cellular senescence. Up to 15% of familial IPF is associated with telomerase gene defects, and up to 25% of sporadic IPF cases are associated with abnormal telomerase shortening in peripheral blood lymphocytes; the cause of this shortening is currently unknown, and it is not yet known whether such individuals also have telomere shortening in their alveolar epithelial cells. Other, rare familial forms of IPF are associated with mutations in genes encoding components of surfactant; these mutations create folding defects in the affected proteins, leading to activation of the unfolded protein response in type II pneumocytes. This in turn appears to make pneumocytes more sensitive to environmental insults, enhancing the consequent cellular dysfunction and injury. Finally, roughly one-third of IPF cases are associated with a common genetic variant that greatly increases the secretion of MUC5B, a mucin that may make alveolar epithelial cells susceptible to injury or exaggerate downstream events that lead to fibrosis.
- *Age.* IPF is a disease of older individuals, rarely appearing before the age of 50 years. Whether this association stems from aging-related telomere shortening or from other acquired changes associated with aging is unknown.

It is easy to imagine how some of the factors cited herein might combine to exacerbate alveolar epithelial cell damage and senescence, which seems to be the initiating event

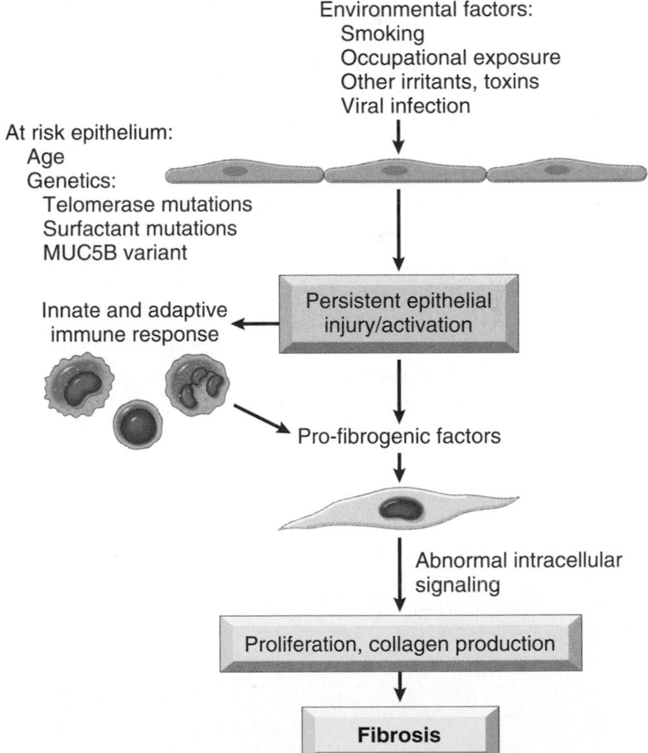

Figure 15-13 Proposed pathogenic mechanisms in idiopathic pulmonary fibrosis. Environmental factors that are potentially injurious to alveolar epithelium interact with genetic or aging-related factors that place epithelium at risk to create a persistent epithelial injury. Factors secreted from injured/activated epithelium, possibly augmented by factors released from innate and adaptive immune cells responding to "danger" signals produced by damaged epithelium, activate interstitial fibroblasts. There is some evidence that these activated fibroblasts exhibit signaling abnormalities that lead to increased signaling through the PI3K/AKT pathway. The activated fibroblasts synthesize and deposit collagen, leading to interstitial fibrosis and eventual respiratory failure.

in IPF, but it must be admitted that the pathogenesis of IPF is complex and poorly understood. For example, it is unknown precisely how alveolar epithelial cell damage translates into interstitial fibrosis. One model holds that the injured epithelial cells are the source of profibrogenic factors such as TGF-β, whereas a second, nonmutually exclusive model proposes that innate and adaptive immune cells produce such factors as part of the host response to epithelial cell damage. Other work has described abnormalities in the fibroblasts themselves that involve changes in intracellular signaling and features reminiscent of epithelial mesenchymal transition (Chapter 7), but a causal link to fibrosis has not been established.

MORPHOLOGY

Grossly, the pleural surfaces of the lung are cobblestoned as a result of the retraction of scars along the interlobular septa. The cut surface shows firm, rubbery white areas of fibrosis, which occurs preferentially in the lower lobes, the **subpleural regions**, and along the **interlobular septa**. Microscopically, the hallmark is **patchy interstitial fibrosis**, which varies in intensity (Fig. 15-14) and age. The earliest lesions contain exuberant fibroblastic proliferation **(fibroblastic foci)**. With time these areas become more collagenous and less cellular. Quite typical is the coexistence of both early and late lesions (Fig. 15-15). The dense fibrosis causes the destruction of alveolar architecture and formation of cystic spaces lined by hyperplastic type II pneumocytes or bronchiolar epithelium (**honeycomb fibrosis**). With adequate sampling, these diagnostic histologic changes (i.e., areas of dense collagenous fibrosis with relatively normal lung and fibroblastic foci) can be identified even in advanced IPF. There is mild to moderate inflammation within the fibrotic areas, consisting of mostly lymphocytes admixed with a few plasma cells, neutrophils, eosinophils, and mast cells. Foci of squamous metaplasia and smooth muscle hyperplasia may be present, along with pulmonary arterial hypertensive changes (intimal fibrosis and medial thickening). In acute exacerbations diffuse alveolar damage may be superimposed on these chronic changes.

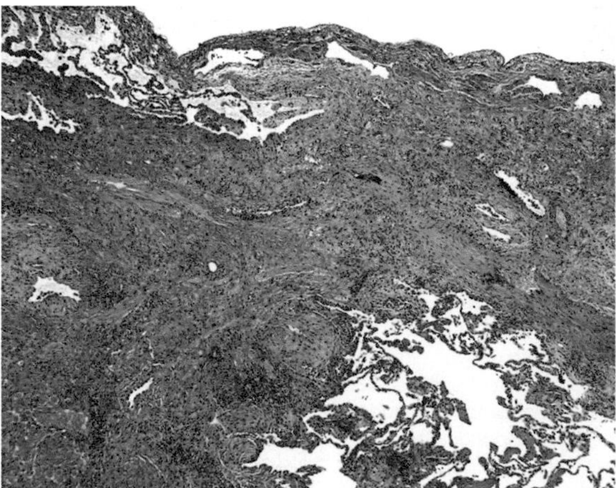

Figure 15-14 Usual interstitial pneumonia. The fibrosis is more pronounced in the subpleural region. (Courtesy Dr. Nicole Cipriani, Department of Pathology, University of Chicago, Chicago, Ill.)

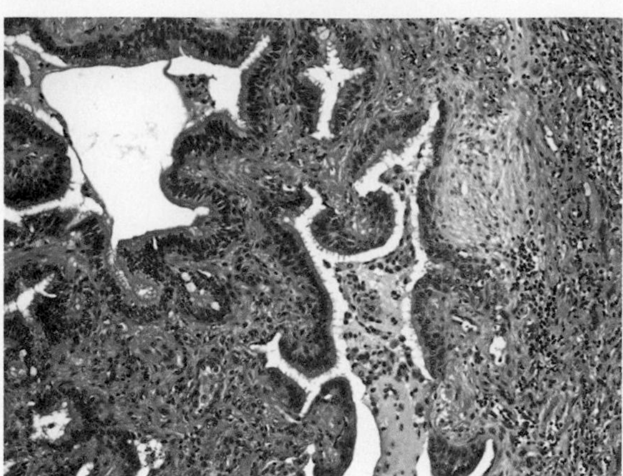

Figure 15-15 Usual interstitial pneumonia. Fibroblastic focus with fibers running parallel to surface and bluish myxoid extracellular matrix. Honeycombing is present on the left.

Clinical Course. IPF begins insidiously with gradually increasing *dyspnea on exertion* and dry cough. Most patients are 55 to 75 years old at presentation. Hypoxemia, *cyanosis*, and clubbing occur late in the course. The progression in an individual patient is unpredictable. Usually there is a gradual deterioration in pulmonary status despite medical treatment with immunosuppressive drugs such as steroids, cyclophosphamide, or azathioprine. Other IPF patients have acute exacerbations of the underlying disease and follow a rapid downhill clinical course. The median survival is about 3 years after diagnosis. Lung transplantation is the only definitive therapy.

Nonspecific Interstitial Pneumonia

The concept of nonspecific interstitial pneumonia emerged when it was realized that there is a group of patients with diffuse interstitial lung disease whose lung biopsies lack the diagnostic features of any of the other well-characterized interstitial diseases. Despite its "nonspecific" name, this entity is important to recognize, since these patients have a much better prognosis than do those with usual interstitial pneumonia. Nonspecific interstitial pneumonia may be idiopathic or associated with connective tissue disease.

MORPHOLOGY

On the basis of its histology, nonspecific interstitial pneumonia is divided into cellular and fibrosing patterns. The cellular pattern consists primarily of mild to moderate chronic interstitial inflammation, containing lymphocytes and a few plasma cells, in a uniform or patchy distribution. The fibrosing pattern consists of diffuse or patchy interstitial fibrotic lesions of roughly the same stage of development, an important distinction from usual interstitial pneumonia. Fibroblastic foci, honeycombing, hyaline membranes and granulomas are absent.

Clinical Course. Patients present with dyspnea and cough of several months' duration. They are more likely to be female nonsmokers in their sixth decade of life. Key features on high-resolution computed tomography are bilateral, symmetric, predominantly lower lobe reticular opacities. Those having the cellular pattern are somewhat younger than those with the fibrosing pattern and have a better prognosis.

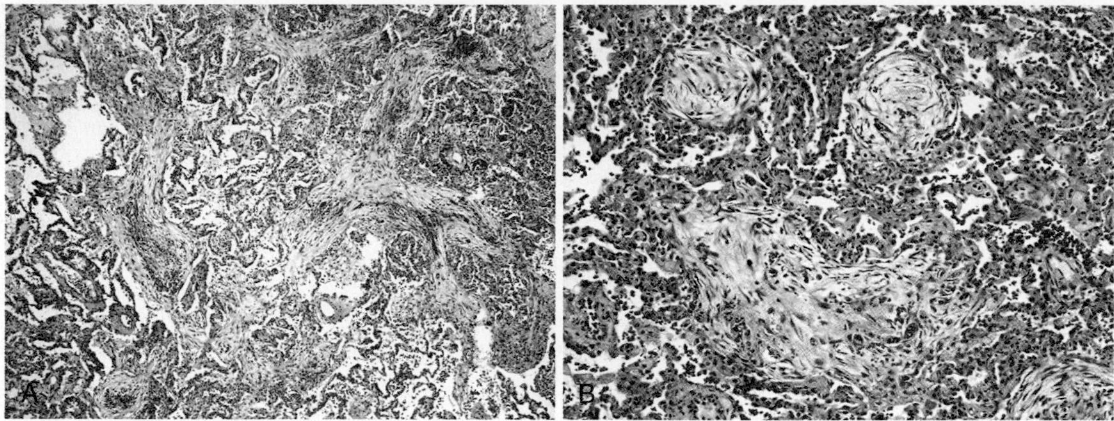

Figure 15-16 Cryptogenic organizing pneumonia. Some alveolar spaces are filled with balls of fibroblasts (Masson bodies), while the alveolar walls are relatively normal. **A,** Low power. **B,** High power.

Cryptogenic Organizing Pneumonia

Cryptogenic organizing pneumonia is synonymous with the popular term *bronchiolitis obliterans organizing pneumonia*; however, the former is now preferred, since it conveys the essential features of a clinicopathologic syndrome of unknown etiology and avoids confusion with airway diseases such as bronchiolitis obliterans. Patients present with cough and dyspnea and have patchy subpleural or peribronchial areas of airspace consolidation radiographically. Histologically, cryptogenic organizing pneumonia is characterized by the presence of polypoid plugs of loose organizing connective tissue (Masson bodies) within alveolar ducts, alveoli, and often bronchioles (Fig. 15-16). The connective tissue is all of the same age, and the underlying lung architecture is normal. There is no interstitial fibrosis or honeycomb lung. Some patients recover spontaneously, but most need treatment with oral steroids for 6 months or longer for complete recovery.

It is important to recognize that organizing pneumonia with intra-alveolar fibrosis is most often seen as a response to infections or inflammatory injury of the lungs. These include viral and bacterial pneumonia, inhaled toxins, drugs, connective tissue disease, and graft-versus-host disease in bone marrow transplant recipients. The prognosis for these patients is dependent on the underlying disorder.

Pulmonary Involvement in Autoimmune Diseases

Many autoimmune diseases (also referred to a connective tissue diseases because of their frequent association with arthritis), most notably systemic lupus erythematosus, rheumatoid arthritis, progressive systemic sclerosis (scleroderma), and dermatomyositis-polymyositis, can involve the lung at some point in their course. Pulmonary involvement can take different histologic patterns; nonspecific interstitial pneumonia, usual interstitial pneumonia, vascular sclerosis, organizing pneumonia, and bronchiolitis are the most common.

- *Rheumatoid arthritis*: pulmonary involvement may occur in 30% to 40% of patients as (1) chronic pleuritis, with or without effusion; (2) diffuse interstitial pneumonitis and fibrosis; (3) intrapulmonary rheumatoid nodules; (4) follicular bronchiolitis; or (5) pulmonary hypertension
- *Systemic sclerosis* (scleroderma): diffuse interstitial fibrosis (nonspecific interstitial pattern more common than usual interstitial pattern) and pleural involvement
- *Lupus erythematosus*: patchy, transient parenchymal infiltrates, or occasionally severe lupus pneumonitis, as well as pleurisy and pleural effusions.

Pulmonary involvement in these diseases has a variable prognosis that is determined by the extent and histologic pattern of involvement.

KEY CONCEPTS

Chronic Interstitial Lung Diseases

- Diffuse interstitial fibrosis of the lung gives rise to restrictive lung diseases characterized by reduced lung compliance and reduced forced vital capacity (FVC). The ratio of FEV_1 to FVC is normal.
- Idiopathic pulmonary fibrosis is prototypic of restrictive lung diseases. It is characterized by patchy interstitial fibrosis fibroblastic foci and formation of cystic spaces (honeycomb lung). This histologic pattern is known as usual interstitial pneumonia.
- The cause of idiopathic pulmonary fibrosis is unknown, but genetic analyses point to roles for senescence of alveolar epithelium (due to telomere shortening), cell stress related to protein misfolding, abnormal signaling in alveolar fibroblasts, and altered mucin production. The resulting injury to alveolar epithelial cells set in motion event that lead to increase local production of fibrogenic cytokines such as TGF-β
- The other diseases that cause diffuse interstitial fibrosis are heterogeneous poorly understood, but most have better prognoses that idiopathic pulmonary fibrosis.

Pneumoconioses

The term *pneumoconiosis,* originally coined to describe the nonneoplastic lung reaction to inhalation of mineral dusts encountered in the workplace, now also includes diseases induced by organic as well as inorganic particulates and chemical fumes and vapors. A simplified

Table 15-6 Lung Diseases Caused by Air Pollutants

Agent	Disease	Exposure
Mineral Dusts		
Coal dust	Anthracosis Macules Progressive massive fibrosis Caplan syndrome	Coal mining (particularly hard coal)
Silica	Silicosis Caplan syndrome	Metal casting work, sandblasting, hard rock mining, stone cutting, others
Asbestos	Asbestosis Pleural plaques Caplan syndrome Mesothelioma Carcinoma of the lung, larynx, stomach, colon	Mining, milling, manufacturing, and installation and removal of insulation
Beryllium	Acute berylliosis Beryllium granulomatosis Lung carcinoma (?)	Mining, manufacturing
Iron oxide	Siderosis	Welding
Barium sulfate	Baritosis	Mining
Tin oxide	Stannosis	Mining
Organic Dusts That Induce Hypersensitivity Pneumonitis		
Moldy hay Bagasse Bird droppings	Farmer's lung Bagassosis Bird-breeder's lung	Farming Manufacturing wallboard, paper Bird handling
Organic Dusts That Induce Asthma		
Cotton, flax, hemp	Byssinosis	Textile manufacturing
Red cedar dust	Asthma	Lumbering, carpentry
Chemical Fumes and Vapors		
Nitrous oxide, sulfur dioxide, ammonia, benzene, insecticides	Bronchitis, asthma Pulmonary edema ARDS Mucosal injury Fulminant poisoning	Occupational and accidental exposure

ARDS, Acute respiratory distress syndrome.

classification is presented in Table 15-6. Where implemented, regulations limiting worker exposure have resulted in a marked decrease in dust-associated diseases.

Although the pneumoconioses result from well-defined occupational exposure to specific airborne agents, ambient air pollution also has deleterious effects on the general population, especially in urban areas (Chapter 9), and can have serious, sometimes fatal effects on those with COPD or heart disease. Pollution increases the risk of asthma, especially in children. Efforts to reduce air pollution have been effective in the west, but industrialization in other parts of the world, particularly China, has produced dangerous levels of air pollution. Even in the U.S. improvements are possible, as some data suggest that even low levels of air pollution can have deleterious effects on health.

Pathogenesis. The development of a pneumoconiosis depends on (1) the amount of dust retained in the lung and airways; (2) the size, shape, and buoyancy of the particles; (3) particle solubility and physiochemical reactivity; and (4) the possible additional effects of other irritants (e.g., concomitant tobacco smoking). In most cases, these particles stimulate resident innate immune cells in the lung, leading to the diseases discussed later. The following general principles apply to pneumoconioses:

- The amount of dust retained in the lungs is determined by the dust concentration in ambient air, the duration of exposure, and the effectiveness of clearance mechanisms. Any influence, such as cigarette smoking, that impairs mucociliary clearance significantly increases the accumulation of dust in the lungs.
- The most dangerous particles are from 1 to 5 μm in diameter, because particles of this size may reach the terminal small airways and air sacs and settle in their linings.
- The solubility and cytotoxicity of particles, which are influenced to a considerable extent by their size, modify the pulmonary response. In general, small particles composed of injurious substances of high solubility may produce rapid-onset lung damage. Such particles are more likely to cause acute lung injury. Larger particles are more likely to resist dissolution and may persist within the lung parenchyma for years. These tend to evoke fibrosing collagenous pneumoconioses, such as is characteristic of *silicosis*.
- Other particles may be taken up by epithelial cells or may cross the epithelial cell lining and interact directly with fibroblasts and interstitial macrophages. Some may reach the lymphatics by direct drainage or within

migrating macrophages and thereby initiate an immune response to components of the particulates or to self-proteins modified by the particles or both.

- Finally, certain types of particles activate the inflammasome (Chapter 3) when phagocytosed by macrophages. These innate and adaptive immune responses amplify the intensity and the duration of the local reaction.
- Tobacco smoking worsens the effects of all inhaled mineral dusts, but particularly those caused by asbestos. The effects of inhaled particles are not confined to the lung alone, since solutes from particles can enter the blood and lung inflammation invokes systemic responses.

In general, only a small percentage of exposed people develop occupational respiratory diseases, implying a genetic predisposition to their development. Many of the diseases listed in Table 15-6 are quite uncommon. Hence only a selected few that cause fibrosis of the lung are presented next.

Coal Workers' Pneumoconiosis

Coal workers' pneumoconiosis is lung disease caused by inhalation of coal particles and other admixed forms of dust. Dust reduction measures in coal mines around the globe have drastically reduced its incidence. The spectrum of lung findings in coal workers is wide, varying from asymptomatic anthracosis, to simple coal workers' pneumoconiosis with little to no pulmonary dysfunction, to complicated coal workers' pneumoconiosis, or *progressive massive fibrosis,* in which lung function is compromised. Contaminating silica in the coal dust can favor progressive disease. In most cases, carbon dust itself is the major culprit, and studies have shown that complicated lesions contain much more dust than simple lesions. Coal workers may also develop emphysema and chronic bronchitis independent of smoking.

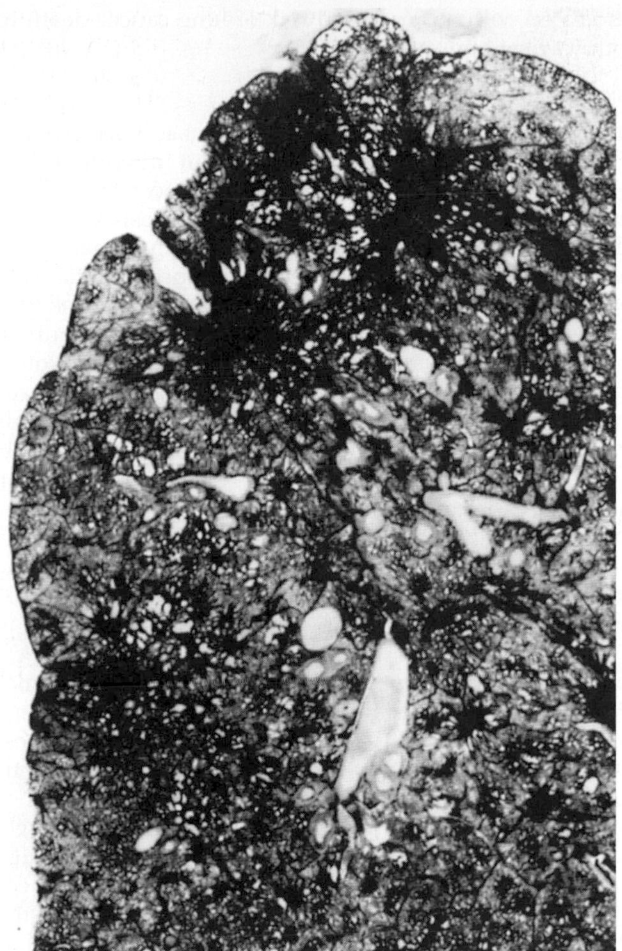

Figure 15-17 Progressive massive fibrosis superimposed on coal workers' pneumoconiosis. The large, blackened scars are located principally in the upper lobe. Note the extensions of scars into surrounding parenchyma and retraction of adjacent pleura. (Courtesy Drs. Werner Laquer and Jerome Kleinerman, the National Institute of Occupational Safety and Health, Morgantown, W.Va.)

MORPHOLOGY

Anthracosis is the most innocuous coal-induced pulmonary lesion in coal miners and is also seen to some degree in urban dwellers and tobacco smokers. Inhaled carbon pigment is engulfed by alveolar or interstitial macrophages, which then accumulate in the connective tissue along the lymphatics, including the pleural lymphatics, or in organized lymphoid tissue along the bronchi or in the lung hilus.

Simple coal workers' pneumoconiosis is characterized by **coal macules** (1 to 2 mm in diameter) and somewhat larger **coal nodules**. Coal macules consist of carbon-laden macrophages; nodules also contain a delicate network of collagen fibers. Although these lesions are scattered throughout the lung, the upper lobes and upper zones of the lower lobes are more heavily involved. They are located primarily adjacent to respiratory bronchioles, the site of initial dust accumulation. In due course dilation of adjacent alveoli occurs, sometimes giving rise to **centrilobular emphysema**.

Complicated coal workers' pneumoconiosis (progressive massive fibrosis) occurs on a background of simple disease and generally requires many years to develop. It is characterized by intensely blackened scars 1 cm or larger, sometimes up to 10 cm in greatest diameter. They are usually multiple (Fig. 15-17). Microscopically the lesions consist of dense collagen and pigment. The center of the lesion is often necrotic, most likely due to local ischemia.

Clinical Course. Coal workers' pneumoconiosis is usually benign, causing little decrement in lung function. Even mild forms of complicated coal workers' pneumoconiosis do not to affect lung function significantly. In a minority of cases (fewer than 10%), progressive massive fibrosis develops, leading to increasing pulmonary dysfunction, pulmonary hypertension, and cor pulmonale. Once progressive massive fibrosis develops, it may continue to worsen even if further exposure to dust is prevented. Unlike silicosis (discussed below), there is no convincing evidence that coal dust increases susceptibility to tuberculosis. There is also no compelling evidence that coal workers' pneumoconiosis in the absence of smoking predisposes to cancer. Domestic indoor use of "smoky coal" (bituminous) for cooking and heating is, however, associated with an increased risk of lung cancer death for both women and men.

Silicosis

Silicosis is a common lung disease caused by inhalation of proinflammatory crystalline silicon dioxide (silica) that usually presents after decades of exposure as slowly progressing, nodular, fibrosing pneumoconiosis. Currently, silicosis is the most prevalent chronic occupational disease in the world. Both dose and race are important in developing silicosis (African Americans are at higher risk than whites). As shown in Table 15-6, workers in a large number of occupations are at risk, including individuals involved with the repair, rehabilitation or demolition of concrete structures such as buildings and roads. Less commonly, the disease occurs in workers producing stressed denim by sandblasting, stone carvers, and jewelers using chalk molds. Occasionally, heavy exposure over months to a few years can result in acute silicosis, a disorder characterized by the accumulation of abundant lipoproteinaceous material within alveoli (identical morphologically to alveolar proteinosis, discussed later).

Pathogenesis. Silica occurs in both crystalline and amorphous forms, but crystalline forms (including quartz, cristobalite, and tridymite) are much more fibrogenic. Of these, quartz is most commonly implicated. After inhalation, the particles are phagocytosed by macrophages. The phagocytosed silica crystals activate the inflammasome, leading to the release of inflammatory mediators, particularly IL-1 and IL-18. The relatively benign response to silica in coal and hematite miners is thought to be due to coating of silica with other minerals, especially clay components, which render the silica less toxic. Although amorphous silicates are biologically less active than crystalline silica, heavy lung burdens of these minerals may also produce lesions.

MORPHOLOGY

Silicosis is characterized grossly in its early stages by tiny, barely palpable, discrete pale to blackened (if coal dust is also present) nodules in the hilar lymph nodes and upper zones of the lungs. As the disease progresses, these nodules coalesce into **hard, collagenous scars** (Fig. 15-18). Some nodules may undergo central softening and cavitation due to superimposed tuberculosis or to ischemia. Fibrotic lesions may also occur in the hilar lymph nodes and pleura. Sometimes, thin sheets of calcification occur in the lymph nodes and are seen radiographically as **eggshell calcification** (i.e., calcium surrounding a zone lacking calcification). If the disease continues to progress, expansion and coalescence of lesions may produce progressive massive fibrosis. Histologic examination reveals the hallmark lesion characterized by a central area of whorled collagen fibers with a more peripheral zone of dust-laden macrophages (Fig. 15-19). Examination of the nodules by polarized microscopy reveals the birefringent silicate particles (silica is weakly birefringent).

Clinical Course. Chest radiographs typically show a fine nodularity in the upper zones of the lung. Pulmonary functions are either normal or only moderately affected early in the course, and most patients do not develop shortness of breath until progressive massive fibrosis supervenes.

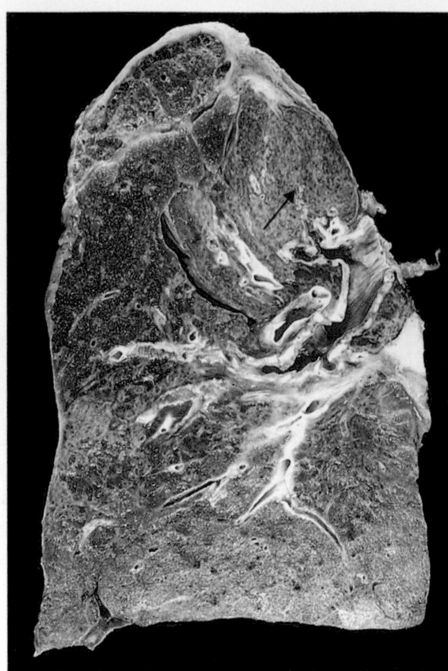

Figure 15-18 Advanced silicosis. Scarring has contracted the upper lobe into a small dark mass *(arrow)*. Note the dense pleural thickening. (Courtesy Dr. John Godleski, Brigham and Women's Hospital, Boston, Mass.)

The disease may continue to worsen even if the patient is no longer exposed. Silicosis is slow to kill, but impaired pulmonary function may severely limit activity. It is associated with an increased susceptibility to *tuberculosis*. This may be because crystalline silica inhibits the ability of pulmonary macrophages to kill phagocytosed mycobacteria. The onset of silicosis may be slow and insidious (10 to 30 years after exposure; most common), accelerated (within 10 years of exposure) or rapid (in weeks or months after intense exposure to fine dust high in silica; rare). Patients with silicosis have double the risk for developing lung cancer.

Asbestos-Related Diseases

Asbestos is a family of proinflammatory crystalline hydrated silicates that are associated with pulmonary

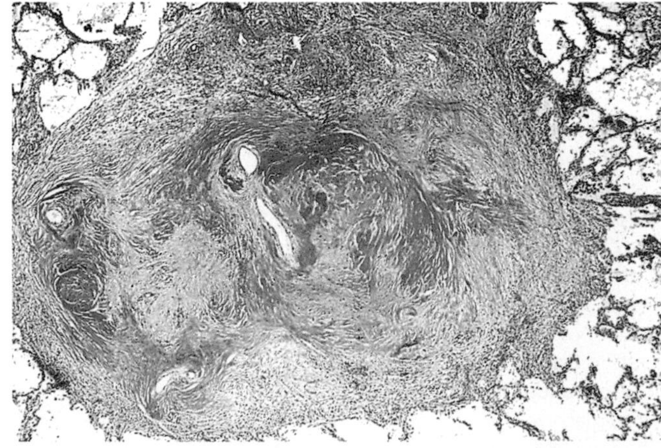

Figure 15-19 Several coalescent collagenous silicotic nodules. (Courtesy Dr. John Godleski, Brigham and Women's Hospital, Boston, Mass.)

fibrosis, carcinoma, mesothelioma, and other cancers. Use of asbestos is tightly restricted in many developed countries; however, there is little, if any, control in less developed parts of the world. Asbestos-related diseases include:

- Localized fibrous plaques or, rarely, diffuse pleural fibrosis
- Pleural effusions, recurrent
- Parenchymal interstitial fibrosis *(asbestosis)*
- Lung carcinoma
- Mesotheliomas
- Laryngeal, ovarian and perhaps other extrapulmonary neoplasms, including colon carcinomas; increased risk for systemic autoimmune diseases and cardiovascular disease has been proposed

An increased incidence of asbestos-related cancer in family members of asbestos workers has alerted the general public to the potential hazards of even low-level exposure to asbestos. However, the necessity of expensive asbestos abatement programs for environments such as schools with low, but measurable, airborne asbestos fiber counts remains a matter of contention.

Pathogenesis. **The disease-causing capabilities of the different forms of asbestos depend on concentration, size, shape, and solubility.** Asbestos occurs in two distinct geometric forms, *serpentine* and *amphibole*. The serpentine chrysotile form accounts for 90% of the asbestos used in industry. Amphiboles, even though less prevalent, are more pathogenic than chrysotiles, particularly with respect to induction of mesothelioma, a malignant tumor derived from the lining cells of pleural surfaces.

The greater pathogenicity of amphiboles is apparently related to their aerodynamic properties and solubility. Chrysotiles, with their more flexible, curled structure, are likely to become impacted in the upper respiratory passages and removed by the mucociliary elevator. Furthermore, once trapped in the lungs, chrysotiles are gradually leached from the tissues because they are more soluble than amphiboles. In contrast, the straight, stiff amphiboles may align themselves in the airstream and thus be delivered deeper into the lungs, where they can penetrate epithelial cells and reach the interstitium. Both amphiboles and serpentines are fibrogenic, and increasing doses are associated with a higher incidence of asbestos-related diseases.

In contrast to other inorganic dusts, asbestos can also act as a tumor initiator and promoter. Some of its oncogenic effects are mediated by reactive free radicals generated by asbestos fibers, which preferentially localize in the distal lung, close to the mesothelial layers. Toxic chemicals adsorbed onto the asbestos fibers also likely contribute to the oncogenicity of the fibers. For example, the adsorption of carcinogens in tobacco smoke onto asbestos fibers may be the basis for the remarkable synergy between tobacco smoking and the development of lung carcinoma in asbestos workers. Smoking also enhances the effect of asbestos by interfering with the mucociliary clearance of fibers. One study of asbestos workers found a fivefold increase of lung carcinoma with asbestos exposure alone, while asbestos exposure and smoking together led to a 55-fold increase in the risk.

As with silica crystals, **once phagocytosed by macrophages asbestos fibers activate the inflammasome and stimulate the release of proinflammatory factors and fibrogenic mediators.** The initial injury occurs at bifurcations of small airways and ducts, where asbestos fibers land, penetrate and are directly toxic to pulmonary parenchymal cells. Macrophages, both alveolar and interstitial, attempt to ingest and clear the fibers. Long-term deposition of fibers and persistent release of mediators (e.g., reactive oxygen species, proteases, cytokines, and growth factors) eventually lead to generalized interstitial pulmonary inflammation and interstitial fibrosis.

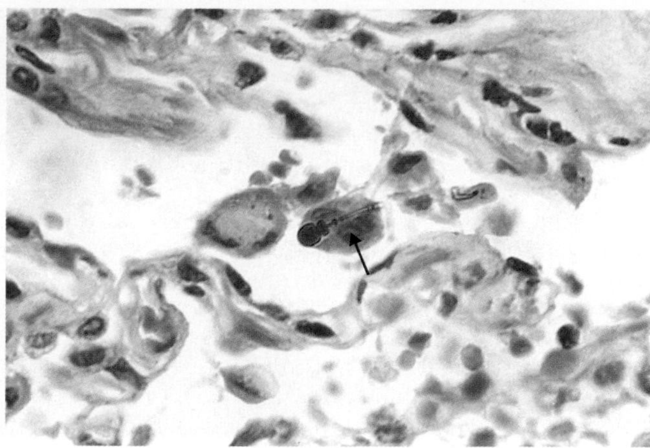

Figure 15-20 High-power detail of an asbestos body, revealing the typical beading and knobbed ends *(arrow)*.

MORPHOLOGY

Asbestosis is marked by **diffuse pulmonary interstitial fibrosis**, which is indistinguishable from diffuse interstitial fibrosis resulting from other causes, except for the presence of multiple **asbestos bodies**. Asbestos bodies are **golden brown, fusiform or beaded rods with a translucent center and consist of asbestos fibers coated with an iron-containing proteinaceous material** (Fig. 15-20). They arise when macrophages phagocytose asbestos fibers; the iron is presumably derived from phagocyte ferritin. Other inorganic particulates may become coated with similar iron-protein complexes and are called **ferruginous bodies**. Rare single asbestos bodies can be found in the lungs of normal people.

Asbestosis begins as fibrosis around respiratory bronchioles and alveolar ducts and extends to involve adjacent alveolar sacs and alveoli. The fibrous tissue distorts the architecture, creating enlarged airspaces enclosed within thick fibrous walls; eventually the affected regions become honeycombed. The pattern of fibrosis is similar to that seen in usual interstitial fibrosis, with fibroblastic foci and varying degrees of fibrosis, the only difference being the presence of numerous asbestos bodies. In contrast to coal workers' pneumoconiosis and silicosis, asbestosis begins in the lower lobes and subpleurally. The middle and upper lobes of the lungs become affected as fibrosis progresses. The scarring may trap and narrow pulmonary arteries and arterioles, causing pulmonary hypertension and cor pulmonale.

Pleural plaques, the most common manifestation of asbestos exposure, are well-circumscribed plaques of dense collagen (Fig. 15-21) that are often calcified. They develop most frequently on the anterior and posterolateral aspects of the **parietal pleura** and over the domes of the diaphragm. The size

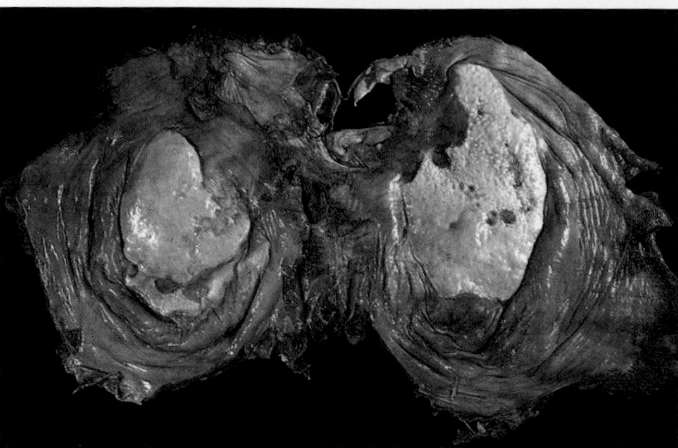

Figure 15-21 Asbestos-related pleural plaques. Large, discrete fibrocalcific plaques are seen on the pleural surface of the diaphragm. (Courtesy Dr. John Godleski, Brigham and Women's Hospital, Boston, Mass.)

and number of pleural plaques do not correlate with the level of exposure to asbestos or the time since exposure. They do not contain asbestos bodies; however, only rarely do they occur in individuals who have no history or evidence of asbestos exposure. Uncommonly, asbestos exposure induces pleural effusions, which are usually serous but may be bloody. Rarely, diffuse visceral pleural fibrosis may occur and, in advanced cases, bind the lung to the thoracic wall.

Both lung carcinomas and mesotheliomas (pleural and peritoneal) develop in workers exposed to asbestos (see sections on lung cancer and pleural tumors).

Clinical Course. The clinical findings in asbestosis are very similar to those caused by other diffuse interstitial lung diseases (discussed earlier). These rarely appear fewer than 10 years after first exposure and are more common after 20 to 30 years. Dyspnea is usually the first manifestation; at first, it is provoked by exertion, but later it is present even at rest. Cough associated with production of sputum, when present, is likely to be due to smoking rather than asbestosis. Chest x-ray studies reveal irregular linear densities, particularly in both lower lobes. With advancement of the pneumoconiosis, a honeycomb pattern develops. The disease may remain static or progress to respiratory failure, cor pulmonale, and death. Pleural plaques are usually asymptomatic and are detected on radiographs as circumscribed densities. Asbestosis complicated by lung or pleural cancer is associated with a particularly grim prognosis.

KEY CONCEPTS

Pneumoconioses

- Pneumoconioses encompass a group of chronic fibrosing diseases of the lung resulting from exposure to organic and inorganic particulates, most commonly mineral dust.
- Pulmonary alveolar macrophages play a central role in the pathogenesis of lung injury by promoting inflammation and producing reactive oxygen species and fibrogenic cytokines.
- Coal dust-induced disease varies from asymptomatic anthracosis to simple coal workers' pneumoconiosis (coal macules or nodules, and centrilobular emphysema), to progressive massive fibrosis (PMF), manifested by increasing pulmonary dysfunction, pulmonary hypertension, and cor pulmonale.
- Silicosis is the most common pneumoconiosis in the world, and crystalline silica (e.g., quartz) is the usual culprit. The lung disease is progressive even after exposure stops.
- The manifestations of silicosis can range from asymptomatic silicotic nodules to large areas of dense fibrosis; persons with silicosis also have an increased susceptibility to tuberculosis. There is two-fold increased risk of lung cancer.
- Asbestos fibers come in two forms; the stiff amphiboles have a greater fibrogenic and carcinogenic potential than the serpentine chrysotiles.
- Asbestos exposure is linked with six disease processes: (1) parenchymal interstitial fibrosis (asbestosis); (2) localized pleural plaques (asymptomatic) or rarely diffuse pleural fibrosis; (3) recurrent pleural effusions; (4) lung cancer; (5) malignant pleural and peritoneal mesotheliomas; and (6) laryngeal cancer.
- Cigarette smoking increases the risk of lung cancer in the setting of asbestos exposure; even family members of workers exposed to asbestos are at increased risk for cancer and mesothelioma.

Complications of Therapies

Drug-Induced Lung Diseases. An increasing number of prescription drugs have been found to cause a variety of both acute and chronic alterations in lung structure and function, interstitial fibrosis, bronchiolitis obliterans, and eosinophilic pneumonia. For example, cytotoxic drugs used in cancer therapy (e.g., bleomycin) cause pulmonary damage and fibrosis as a result of direct toxicity and by stimulating the influx of inflammatory cells into the alveoli. Amiodarone, a drug used to treat cardiac arrhythmias, is preferentially concentrated in the lung and causes significant pneumonitis in 5% to 15% of patients receiving it. Cough induced by ace inhibitors is very common.

Illicit intravenous drug abuse most often causes lung infections. In addition, particulate matter is introduced into the lung microvasculature where granulomas and fibrosis occur.

Radiation-Induced Lung Diseases. Radiation pneumonitis is a well-known complication of therapeutic radiation of thoracic tumors (lung, esophageal, breast, mediastinal). It most often involves the lung within the radiation port and occurs in both acute and chronic forms. *Acute radiation pneumonitis* (lymphocytic alveolitis or hypersensitivity pneumonitis) occurs 1 to 6 months after irradiation in 3% to 44% of patients, depending on dose and age. It is manifest by fever, dyspnea out of proportion to the volume of lung irradiated, pleural effusion, and infiltrates that usually correspond to an area of previous irradiation. With steroid therapy, these symptoms may resolve completely in some patients, while in others there is progression to *chronic radiation pneumonitis* (pulmonary fibrosis). The latter is a consequence of the repair of injured endothelial and epithelial cells. It may also occur without antecedent pulmonary symptoms. Morphologic changes are those of diffuse alveolar damage, including severe atypia of hyperplastic type II cells and fibroblasts. Epithelial cell atypia and foam cells within vessel walls are also characteristic of radiation damage.

Granulomatous Diseases

Sarcoidosis

Sarcoidosis is a systemic granulomatous disease of unknown cause that may involve many different tissues and organs. Sarcoidosis presents in many clinical patterns, but bilateral hilar lymphadenopathy or lung involvement is most common, occuring 90% of cases. Eye and skin lesions are next in frequency. Since other diseases, including mycobacterial and fungal infections and beryIliosis, can also produce noncaseating granulomas, the diagnosis is one of exclusion.

Sarcoidosis usually occurs in adults younger than 40 years of age, but can affect any age group. The prevalence is higher in women but varies widely in different countries and populations. In the United States the rates are highest in the Southeast and are 10 times higher in blacks than in whites. In contrast, the disease is rare among Chinese and Southeast Asians. Patterns of organ involvement also vary with race.

Pathogenesis. Although the etiology of sarcoidosis remains unknown, several lines of evidence suggest that it is a disease of disordered immune regulation in genetically predisposed individuals. It is not clear whether exposure to any environmental or infectious agent has a role in its pathogenesis.

Immunologic Factors. There are several immunologic abnormalities in the local milieu of sarcoid granulomas that suggest the involvement of a cell-mediated immune response to an unidentified antigen. These abnormalities include:

- Intra-alveolar and interstitial accumulation of CD4+ T cells, resulting in CD4/CD8 T-cell ratios ranging from 5:1 to 15:1, suggesting pathogenic involvement of CD4+ helper T cells. There is oligoclonal expansion of T-cell subsets as determined by analysis of T-cell receptor rearrangement, consistent with an antigen-driven proliferation.
- Increased levels of T cell-derived T_H1 cytokines such as IL-2 and IFN-γ, which may be responsible for T-cell expansion and macrophage activation, respectively.
- Increased levels of several cytokines in the local environment (IL-8, TNF, macrophage inflammatory protein 1α) that favor recruitment of additional T cells and monocytes and contribute to the formation of granulomas. TNF in particular is released at high levels by activated alveolar macrophages, and the TNF concentration in the bronchoalveolar fluid is a marker of disease activity.
- Impaired dendritic cell function.

Additionally, there are systemic immunologic abnormalities in individuals with sarcoidosis:

- Anergy to common skin test antigens such as *Candida* or tuberculosis purified protein derivative (PPD)

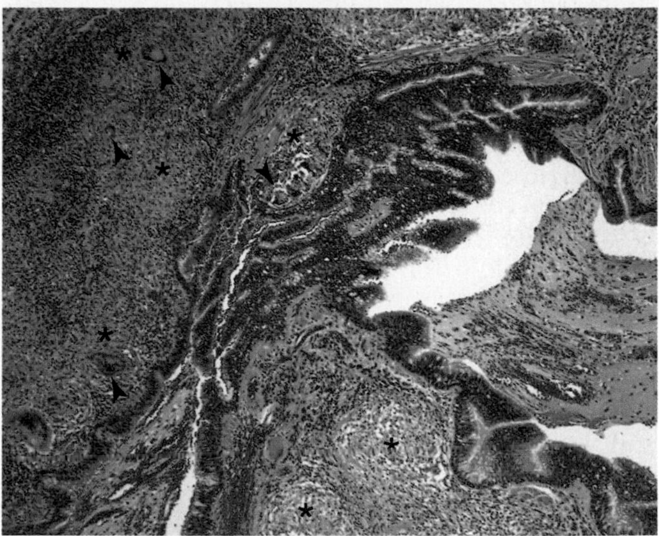

Figure 15-22 Bronchus with characteristic noncaseating sarcoidal granulomas (*asterisks*), with many multinucleated giant cells *(arrowheads)*. Note subepithelial location of granulomas.

- Polyclonal hypergammaglobulinemia, another manifestation of helper T-cell dysregulation

Genetic Factors. Evidence of genetic influences include familial and racial clustering of cases and the association with certain HLA genotypes (e.g., HLA-A1 and HLA-B8).

MORPHOLOGY

Virtually every organ in the body has been described as being affected by sarcoidosis, at least on rare occasions. Regardless of the tissue, involved tissues contain well-formed **nonnecrotizing granulomas** (Fig. 15-22) composed of aggregates of tightly clustered epithelioid macrophages, often with giant cells. Central necrosis is unusual. With chronicity the granulomas may become enclosed within fibrous rims or may eventually be replaced by hyaline fibrous scars. Laminated concretions composed of calcium and proteins known as **Schaumann bodies** and stellate inclusions known as **asteroid bodies** are found within giant cells in approximately 60% of the granulomas. Though characteristic, these microscopic features are not pathognomonic of sarcoidosis, because asteroid and Schaumann bodies may be encountered in other granulomatous diseases (e.g., tuberculosis).

The **lungs** are common sites of involvement. Macroscopically there is usually no demonstrable alteration, although in advanced cases the coalescence of granulomas produces small nodules that are palpable or visible as 1 to 2 cm, noncaseating, noncavitated consolidations. The lesions are distributed primarily along the lymphatics around bronchi and blood vessels, although alveolar lesions and pleural involvement are also seen. The relatively high frequency of granulomas in the bronchial submucosa accounts for the high diagnostic yield of bronchoscopic biopsies. There seems to be a strong tendency for lesions to heal in the lungs, so varying stages of fibrosis and hyalinization are often found. **Lymph nodes** are involved in almost all cases, particularly the hilar and mediastinal nodes, but any other node in the body may be involved. Nodes are characteristically enlarged, discrete, and sometimes calcified. The tonsils are affected in about one fourth to one third of cases.

The **spleen** is affected in about three fourths of cases, but it is enlarged in only one fifth. On occasion, granulomas may coalesce to form small nodules that are visible macroscopically. The **liver** is affected slightly less often than the spleen. It may be moderately enlarged and typically contains scattered granulomas, more in portal triads than in the lobular parenchyma. Needle biopsy can be diagnostic.

The **bone marrow** is involved in about one fifth of cases. Radiologically visible bone lesions have a particular tendency to involve phalangeal bones of the hands and feet, creating small circumscribed areas of bone resorption within the marrow cavity and a diffuse reticulated pattern throughout the cavity, with widening of the bony shafts or new bone formation on the outer surfaces.

Skin lesions, encountered in one fourth of cases, assume a variety of appearances, including discrete subcutaneous nodules; focal, slightly elevated, erythematous plaques; or flat lesions that are slightly reddened and scaling, resembling those of systemic lupus erythematosus. Lesions may also appear on the mucous membranes of the oral cavity, larynx, and upper respiratory tract. **Ocular involvement**, seen in one fourth of cases, takes the form of iritis or iridocyclitis, either bilaterally or unilaterally. Consequently, corneal opacities, glaucoma, and total loss of vision may occur. These ocular lesions are frequently accompanied by inflammation of the lacrimal glands and suppression of lacrimation. Bilateral sarcoidosis of the parotid, submaxillary, and sublingual glands constitutes the combined uveoparotid involvement designated as Mikulicz syndrome (Chapter 16). **Muscle** involvement is underdiagnosed, since it may be asymptomatic. Muscle weakness, aches, tenderness, and fatigue should prompt consideration of occult sarcoid myositis. which can be diagnosed by muscle biopsy. Sarcoid granulomas occasionally occur in the heart, kidneys, central nervous system (neurosarcoidosis, seen in 5% to15%), and endocrine glands, particularly in the pituitary, as well as in other body tissues.

Clinical Course. Because of its varying severity and inconstant tissue distribution, sarcoidosis may present with diverse features. It may be discovered unexpectedly on routine chest films as bilateral hilar adenopathy or may present with peripheral lymphadenopathy, cutaneous lesions, eye involvement, splenomegaly, or hepatomegaly. In the great majority of cases, however, individuals seek medical attention because of the insidious onset of respiratory abnormalities (shortness of breath, cough, chest pain, hemoptysis) or of constitutional signs and symptoms (fever, fatigue, weight loss, anorexia, night sweats).

Sarcoidosis follows an unpredictable course. It may be inexorably progressive, or marked by periods of activity interspersed with remissions, sometimes permanent, that may be spontaneous or induced by steroid therapy. Overall, 65% to 70% of affected patients recover with minimal or no residual manifestations. Twenty percent have permanent loss of some lung function or some permanent visual impairment. Of the remaining 10% to 15%, some die of cardiac or central nervous system damage, but most succumb to progressive pulmonary fibrosis and cor pulmonale.

KEY CONCEPTS

Sarcoidosis

- Sarcoidosis is a multisystem disease of unknown etiology; the diagnostic histopathologic feature is the presence of noncaseating granulomas in various tissues.
- Immunologic abnormalities include high levels of CD4+ T cells in the lung that secrete T_H1-dependent cytokines such as IFN-γ and IL-2 locally.
- Clinical manifestations include lymph node enlargement, eye involvement (sicca syndrome [dry eyes], iritis, or iridocyclitis), skin lesions (erythema nodosum, painless subcutaneous nodules), and visceral (liver, skin, marrow) involvement. Lung involvement occurs in 90% of cases, with formation of granulomas and interstitial fibrosis.

Hypersensitivity Pneumonitis

The term *hypersensitivity pneumonitis* describes a spectrum of immunologically mediated, predominantly interstitial, lung disorders caused by intense, often prolonged exposure to inhaled organic antigens. Affected individuals have an abnormal sensitivity or heightened reactivity to the causative antigen, which, in contrast to asthma, leads to pathologic changes that primarily involve the alveolar walls (thus the synonym "*extrinsic allergic alveolitis*"). It is important to recognize these diseases early in their course because progression to serious chronic fibrotic lung disease can be prevented by removal of the environmental agent.

Most commonly, hypersensitivity results from the inhalation of organic dust containing antigens made up of the spores of thermophilic bacteria, fungi, animal proteins, or bacterial products. Numerous syndromes are described, depending on the occupation or exposure of the individual. *Farmer's lung* results from exposure to dusts generated from humid, warm, newly harvested hay that permits the rapid proliferation of the spores of thermophilic actinomycetes. *Pigeon breeder's lung* (bird fancier's disease) is provoked by proteins from serum, excreta, or feathers of birds. *Humidifier* or *air-conditioner lung* is caused by thermophilic bacteria in heated water reservoirs. Pet birds and moldy basements are easily missed unless asked about specifically.

Several lines of evidence suggest that hypersensitivity pneumonitis is an immunologically mediated disease:

- Bronchoalveolar lavage specimens from the acute phase show increased levels of proinflammatory chemokines such as macrophage inflammatory protein 1α and IL-8.
- Bronchoalveolar lavage specimens also consistently demonstrate increased numbers of both CD4+ and CD8+ T lymphocytes.
- Most patients have specific antibodies against the causative antigen in their serum.
- Complement and immunoglobulins have been demonstrated within vessel walls by immunofluorescence.
- The presence of noncaseating granulomas in two thirds of the patients suggests that T-cell–mediated (type IV) hypersensitivity reactions against the implicated antigens are also common and have a pathogenic role.

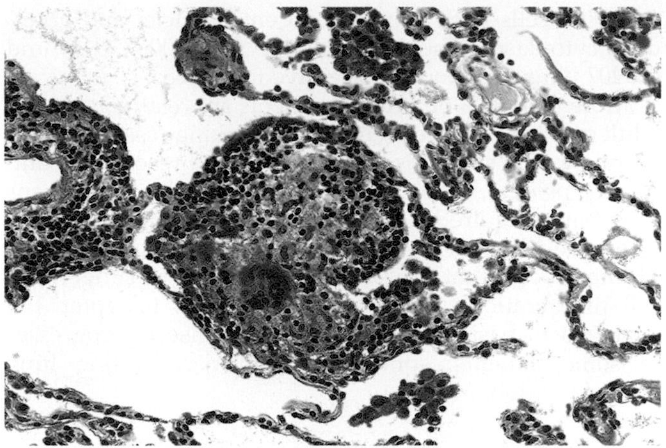

Figure 15-23 Hypersensitivity pneumonitis. Loosely formed interstitial granulomas and chronic inflammation are characteristic.

MORPHOLOGY

Histologic changes are characteristically centered on bronchioles. They include (1) interstitial pneumonitis, consisting primarily of lymphocytes, plasma cells, and macrophages (eosinophils are rare); (2) noncaseating granulomas in two thirds of patients (Fig. 15-23); and (3) interstitial fibrosis with fibroblastic foci, honeycombing, and obliterative bronchiolitis (in late stages). In more than half of patients, there is also evidence of an intra-alveolar infiltrate.

Clinical Features. The clinical manifestations are varied. Acute attacks, which follow inhalation of antigenic dust in sensitized patients, consist of recurring episodes of fever, dyspnea, cough, and leukocytosis. Micronodular interstitial infiltrates may appear in the chest radiograph, and pulmonary function tests show an acute restrictive disorder. Symptoms usually appear 4 to 6 hours after exposure and may last for 12 hours to several days. They recur with reexposure. If exposure is continuous and protracted, a chronic form of the disease supervenes, leading to progressive respiratory failure, dyspnea, and cyanosis and a decrease in total lung capacity and compliance—a picture similar to other forms of chronic interstitial disease.

Pulmonary Eosinophilia

Although relatively rare, there are several clinical and pathologic pulmonary entities that are characterized by an infiltration of eosinophils, recruited in part by elevated alveolar levels of eosinophil attractants such as IL-5.

Pulmonary eosinophilia is divided into the following categories:

- *Acute eosinophilic pneumonia with respiratory failure.* This is an acute illness of unknown cause. It has a rapid onset with fever, dyspnea, and hypoxemic respiratory failure. The chest radiograph shows diffuse infiltrates, and bronchoalveolar lavage fluid contains more than 25% eosinophils. Histology shows diffuse alveolar damage and many eosinophils. There is a prompt response to corticosteroids.
- *Secondary eosinophilia,* which occurs in a number of parasitic, fungal, and bacterial infections; in hypersensitivity pneumonitis; in drug allergies; and in association with asthma, allergic bronchopulmonary aspergillosis, or vasculitis (Churg-Strauss syndrome)
- *Idiopathic chronic eosinophilic pneumonia,* characterized by focal areas of cellular consolidation of the lung substance distributed chiefly in the periphery of the lung fields. Prominent in these lesions are heavy aggregates of lymphocytes and eosinophils within both the septal walls and the alveolar spaces. Interstitial fibrosis and organizing pneumonia are often present. These patients have cough, fever, night sweats, dyspnea, and weight loss, all of which respond to corticosteroid therapy. Chronic eosinophilic pneumonia is diagnosed when other causes of chronic pulmonary eosinophilia are excluded.

Smoking-Related Interstitial Diseases

Smoking-related diseases can be grouped into obstructive diseases (emphysema and chronic bronchitis, already discussed) and restrictive or interstitial diseases. A majority of individuals with idiopathic pulmonary fibrosis are smokers; however, the role of cigarette smoking in its pathogenesis has not been clarified yet. Desquamative interstitial pneumonia and respiratory bronchiolitis-associated interstitial lung disease are also smoking-associated interstitial lung diseases.

Desquamative Interstitial Pneumonia

Desquamative interstitial pneumonia is characterized by large collections of macrophages in the airspaces in a current or former smoker. The macrophages were originally thought to be desquamated pneumocytes, thus the misnomer "desquamative interstitial pneumonia."

MORPHOLOGY

The most striking finding is the accumulation of a large number of macrophages with abundant cytoplasm containing dusty brown pigment **(smokers' macrophages)** in the airspaces (Fig. 15-24). Finely granular iron may be seen in the macrophage cytoplasm. Some of the macrophages contain lamellar

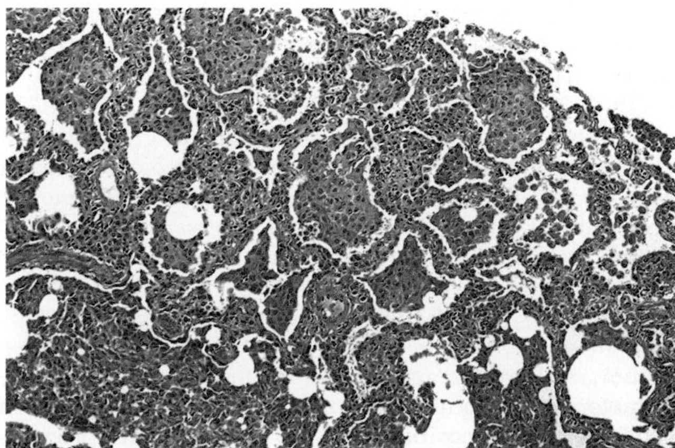

Figure 15-24 Desquamative interstitial pneumonia. Medium-power detail of lung demonstrates the accumulation of large numbers of macrophages within the alveolar spaces and only mild fibrous thickening of the alveolar walls.

bodies (composed of surfactant) within phagocytic vacuoles, presumably derived from necrotic type II pneumocytes. The alveolar septa are thickened by a sparse inflammatory infiltrate of lymphocytes, plasma cells, and occasional eosinophils. The septa are lined by plump, cuboidal pneumocytes. Interstitial fibrosis, when present, is mild. Emphysema is often present.

Desquamative interstitial pneumonia usually presents in the fourth or fifth decade of life, and is now equally common in men and women. Virtually all patients are cigarette smokers. Presenting symptoms include an insidious onset of dyspnea and dry cough over weeks or months, often associated with clubbing of digits. Pulmonary function tests usually show a mild restrictive abnormality with a moderate reduction of the diffusing capacity of carbon dioxide. Patients with desquamative interstitial pneumonia typically have an excellent response to steroid therapy and cessation of smoking but occasional patients may progress to interstitial fibrosis.

Respiratory Bronchiolitis-Associated Interstitial Lung Disease

Respiratory bronchiolitis-associated interstitial lung disease is marked by chronic inflammation and peribronchiolar fibrosis. It is a common histologic lesion in cigarette smokers. It is characterized by the presence of pigmented intraluminal macrophages within first- and second-order respiratory bronchioles. In its mildest form, it is most often an incidental finding in the lungs of smokers or ex-smokers. The term *respiratory bronchiolitis-associated interstitial lung disease* is used for patients who develop significant pulmonary symptoms, abnormal pulmonary function, and imaging abnormalities.

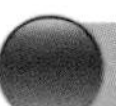

MORPHOLOGY

The changes are patchy at low magnification and have a bronchiolocentric distribution. Respiratory bronchioles, alveolar ducts, and peribronchiolar spaces contain aggregates of dusty brown macrophages **(smokers' macrophages)** similar to those seen in desquamative interstitial pneumonia. There is a patchy submucosal and peribronchiolar infiltrate of lymphocytes and histiocytes. Mild peribronchiolar fibrosis is also seen, which expands contiguous alveolar septa. Centrilobular emphysema is common but not severe. Desquamative interstitial pneumonia is often found in different parts of the same lung.

Symptoms are usually mild, consisting of gradual onset of dyspnea and cough in patients who are typically current smokers in the fourth or fifth decade of life with average exposures of over 30 pack-years of cigarette smoking. Cessation of smoking usually results in improvement.

Pulmonary Langerhans Cell Histiocytosis

Pulmonary Langerhans cell histiocytosis is a rare disease characterized by focal collections of Langerhans cells (often accompanied by eosinophils). As these lesions progress scarring occurs, leading to airway destruction and alveolar damage that result in the appearance of irregular cystic spaces. Imaging of the chest shows characteristic cystic and nodular abnormalities. Langerhans cells are immature dendritic cells with grooved, indented nuclei and abundant cytoplasm. They are positive for S100, CD1a, and CD207 (langerin) and are negative for CD68.

More than 95% of affected patients are relatively young adult smokers who get better after smoking cessation, suggesting that in some cases the lesions are a reactive inflammatory process. However, in other cases the Langerhans cells have acquired activating mutations in the serine/threonine kinase BRAF, a feature consistent with a neoplastic process that is also commonly seen in Langerhans cell proliferations involving other tissues (Chapter 13). A neoplastic basis may explain why the disease progresses in some patients, sometimes even necessitating lung transplantation.

Pulmonary Alveolar Proteinosis

Pulmonary alveolar proteinosis (PAP) is a rare disease caused by defects related to granulocyte-macrophage colony-stimulating factor (GM-CSF) or pulmonary macrophage dysfunction that results in the accumulation of surfactant in the intra-alveolar and bronchiolar spaces. PAP is characterized radiologically by bilateral patchy asymmetric pulmonary opacifications. There are three distinct classes of disease—autoimmune (formerly called acquired), secondary, and congenital—each with a similar spectrum of histologic changes.

- *Autoimmune PAP* is caused by circulating neutralizing antibodies specific for GM-CSF. It occurs primarily in adults, represents 90% of all cases of PAP, and lacks any familial predisposition. Knockout of the GM-CSF gene in mice induces PAP, and these mice are "cured" by treatment with GM-CSF. Loss of GM-CSF signaling blocks the terminal differentiation of alveolar macrophages impairing their ability to catabolize surfactant.
- *Secondary PAP* is uncommon and is associated with diverse diseases, including hematopoietic disorders, malignancies, immunodeficiency disorders, lysinuric protein intolerance (an inborn error of amino acid metabolism), and acute silicosis and other inhalational syndromes. It is speculated that these diseases somehow impair macrophage maturation or function, again leading to inadequate clearance of surfactant from alveolar spaces.
- *Hereditary PAP* is extremely rare, occurs in neonates and is caused by mutations that disrupt genes involved in GM-CSF signaling (GM-CSF and GM-CSF receptor gene mutations).

MORPHOLOGY

The disease is characterized by a peculiar homogeneous, granular precipitate containing surfactant proteins within the alveoli, causing focal-to-confluent consolidation of large areas of the lungs with minimal inflammatory reaction (Fig. 15-25). As a consequence there is a marked increase in the size and weight of the lung. The alveolar precipitate is periodic acid-Schiff positive, and contains cholesterol clefts and surfactant proteins (which can be demonstrated by immunohistochemical stains). Ultrastructurally, the surfactant lamellae in type II pneumocytes are normal.

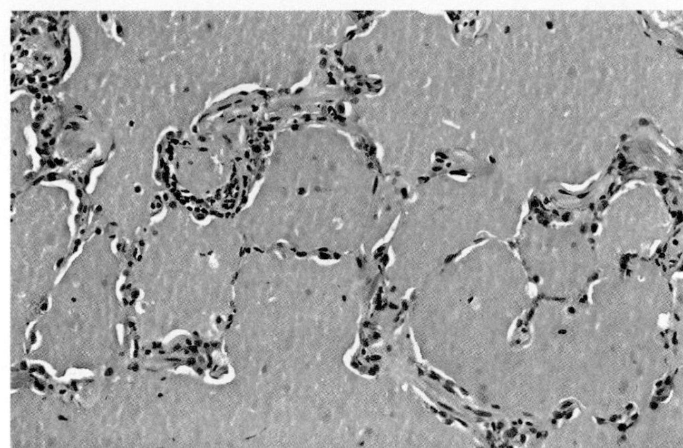

Figure 15-25 Pulmonary alveolar proteinosis. The alveoli are filled with a dense, amorphous, protein-lipid granular precipitate, while the alveolar walls are normal.

Adult patients, for the most part, present with cough and abundant sputum that often contains chunks of gelatinous material. Some have symptoms lasting for years, often with febrile illnesses. These patients are at risk for developing secondary infections with a variety of organisms. Progressive dyspnea, cyanosis, and respiratory insufficiency may occur, but other patients follow a benign course, with eventual resolution of the lesions. Whole-lung lavage is the standard of care and provides benefit regardless of the underlying defect. GM-CSF therapy is safe and effective in more than half of the patients with autoimmune PAP while therapy directed at the underlying disorder may be helpful in secondary PAP.

Surfactant Dysfunction Disorders

Surfactant dysfunction disorders are diseases caused by mutations in genes encoding proteins involved in surfactant trafficking or secretion. The mutated genes include the following:

- *ATP-binding cassette protein member 3* (*ABCA3*) is the most frequently mutated gene in sufactant dysfunction disorders. It is an autosomal recessive disorder and usually presents in the first few months of life with rapidly progressive respiratory failure followed by death. Less commonly it comes to attention in older children and in adults with chronic interstitial lung disease.
- *Surfactant protein C* is the second most commonly mutated gene in sufactant dysfunction disorders. It is autosomal dominant with variable penetrance and severity in 45% and sporadic in 55%. It has a highly variable course.
- *Surfactant protein B* is the least commonly mutated gene and is associated with an autosomal recessive form of sufactant dysfunction disorder. Typically, the infant is full term and rapidly develops progressive respiratory distress shortly after birth. Death ensues between 3 and 6 months of age.

MORPHOLOGY

There is variable amount of intra-alveolar pink granular material, type II pneumocyte hyperplasia, interstitial fibrosis and alveolar simplification. Immunohistochemical stains show the lack of surfactant proteins C and B in their respective deficiencies. Ultrastructurally, abnormalities in lamellar bodies in type II pneumocytes can be seen in all three; small lamellar bodies with electron dense cores are diagnostic for *ABCA3* mutation (Fig 15-26).

Diseases of Vascular Origin

Pulmonary Embolism and Infarction

Pulmonary embolism is an important cause of morbidity and mortality, particularly in patients who are bedridden, but also in a wide range of conditions that are associated with hypercoagulability. Blood clots that occlude the large pulmonary arteries are almost always embolic in origin. The usual source—thrombi in the deep veins of the leg (>95% of cases)—and the magnitude of the clinical problem were discussed in Chapter 4. Pulmonary embolism causes more than 50,000 deaths in the United States each year. Its incidence at autopsy has varied from 1% in the general population of hospital patients to 30% in patients dying after severe burns, trauma, or fractures. It is the sole or a major contributing cause of death in about 10% of adults who die acutely in hospitals. By contrast, large-vessel pulmonary thromboses are rare and develop only in the presence of pulmonary hypertension, pulmonary atherosclerosis, and heart failure.

Pathogenesis. **Pulmonary embolism usually occurs in patients with a predisposing condition that produces an increased tendency to clot (thrombophilia).** Patients often have cardiac disease or cancer, or have been immobilized for several days or weeks prior to the appearance of a

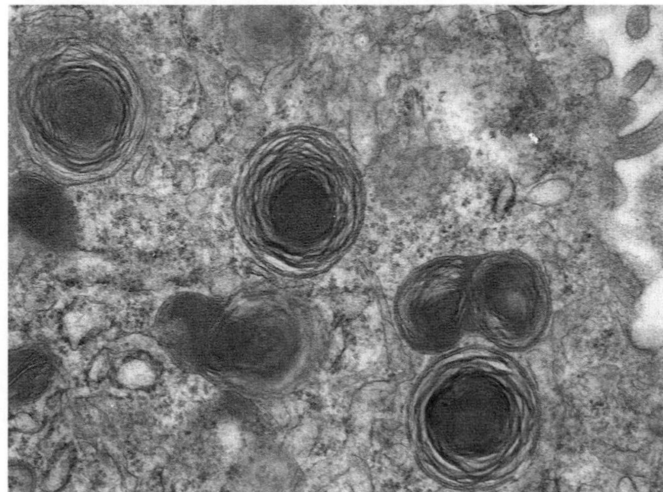

Figure 15-26 Pulmonary alveolar proteinosis associated with mutation of the *ABC3* gene. An electron micrograph shows type 2 pneumocytes containing small surfactant lamellae with electron dense cores, an appearance that is characteristic of cases associated with *ABCA3* mutations.

symptomatic embolism. Those with hip fractures are at particularly high risk. Hypercoagulable states, either primary (e.g., factor V Leiden, prothrombin mutations, and antiphospholipid syndrome) or secondary (e.g., obesity, recent surgery, cancer, oral contraceptive use, pregnancy), are important risk factors. Indwelling central venous lines can be a nidus for formation of right atrial thrombi, which can embolize to the lungs. Rarely pulmonary embolism may consist of fat, air, or tumor. Small bone marrow emboli are often seen in patients who die after chest compressions performed during resuscitative efforts.

The pathophysiologic response and clinical significance of pulmonary embolism depend on the extent to which pulmonary artery blood flow is obstructed, the size of the occluded vessels, the number of emboli, and the cardiovascular health of the patient. Emboli have two deleterious pathophysiologic consequences: *respiratory compromise* due to the nonperfused, although ventilated, segment; and *hemodynamic compromise* due to increased resistance to pulmonary blood flow caused by the embolic obstruction. Sudden death often ensues, largely as a result of the blockage of blood flow through the lungs. Death may also be caused by acute right-sided heart failure (*acute cor pulmonale*).

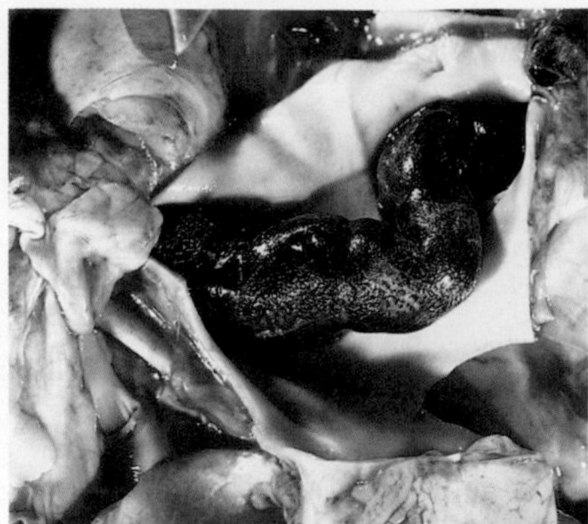

Figure 15-27 Large saddle embolus from the femoral vein lying astride the main left and right pulmonary arteries. (From the teaching collection of the Department of Pathology, University of Texas Southwestern Medical School, Dallas, Tex.)

MORPHOLOGY

Large emboli lodge in the main pulmonary artery or its major branches or at the bifurcation as a saddle embolus (Fig. 15-27). Smaller emboli travel out into the more peripheral vessels, where they may cause hemorrhage or infarction. In patients with adequate cardiovascular function, the bronchial arterial supply sustains the lung parenchyma; in this instance, hemorrhage may occur, but there is no infarction. In those in whom the cardiovascular function is already compromised, such as patients with heart or lung disease, infarction may occur. Overall, about 10% of emboli cause infarction. About three fourths of infarcts affect the lower lobes, and in more than half, multiple lesions occur. They vary in size from barely visible to massive lesions involving large parts of a lobe. Typically, they extend to the periphery of the lung as a wedge with the apex pointing toward the hilus of the lung. In many cases, an occluded vessel is identified near the apex of the infarct. Pulmonary embolus can be distinguished from a postmortem clot by the presence of the lines of Zahn in the thrombus (Chapter 4).

The pulmonary infarct is classically hemorrhagic and appears as a raised, red-blue area in the early stages (Fig. 15-28). Often, the apposed pleural surface is covered by a fibrinous exudate. The red cells begin to lyse within 48 hours, and the infarct becomes paler and eventually red-brown as hemosiderin is produced. With the passage of time, fibrous replacement begins at the margins as a gray-white peripheral zone and eventually converts the infarct into a contracted scar. Histologically, the hemorrhagic area shows ischemic necrosis of the alveolar walls, bronchioles, and vessels. If the infarct is caused by an infected embolus, the neutrophilic inflammatory reaction can be intense. Such lesions are referred to as **septic infarcts**, some which turn into abscesses.

Clinical Course. **A large pulmonary embolus is one of the few causes of virtually instantaneous death.** During cardiopulmonary resuscitation in such instances, the patient frequently is said to have *electromechanical dissociation,* in which the electrocardiogram has a rhythm but no pulses are palpated because no blood is entering the pulmonary arterial circulation. If the patient survives after a sizable pulmonary embolus, however, the clinical syndrome may mimic myocardial infarction, with severe chest pain, dyspnea, and shock. *Small emboli* are silent or induce only transient chest pain and cough. Pulmonary infarcts manifest as dyspnea, tachypnea, fever, chest pain, cough, and hemoptysis. An overlying fibrinous pleuritis may produce a pleural friction rub.

Findings on *chest radiograph* are variable and can be normal or disclose a pulmonary infarct, usually 12 to 36 hours after it has occurred, as a *wedge-shaped infiltrate*. The diagnosis of pulmonary embolism is usually made with spiral computed tomographic angiography. Rarely, other diagnostic methods, such as ventilation perfusion scanning or pulmonary angiography are required. Deep vein thrombosis can be diagnosed with duplex ultrasonography. After the initial acute insult, emboli often resolve via contraction and fibrinolysis, particularly in the relatively young. If unresolved, over the course of time multiple small emboli may lead to pulmonary hypertension and chronic cor

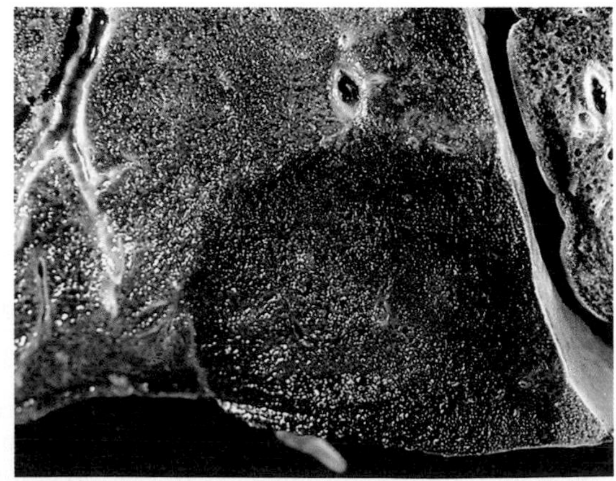

Figure 15-28 Acute hemorrhagic pulmonary infarct.

pulmonale. Perhaps most important is that a small embolus may presage a larger one. In the presence of an underlying predisposing condition, patients with a pulmonary embolus have a 30% chance of suffering a second embolus.

Prevention of pulmonary embolism is a major clinical challenge for which there is no easy solution. Prophylactic therapy includes early ambulation in postoperative and postpartum patients, elastic stockings and graduated compression stockings for bedridden patients, and anticoagulation in high-risk individuals. Treatment of pulmonary embolism includes anticoagulation and supportive measures; thrombolysis may have some benefit in those with severe complications (e.g., shock), but carries a high risk of bleeding. Those at risk of recurrent pulmonary embolism in whom anticoagulation is contraindicated may be fitted with an inferior vena cava filter (an "umbrella") that catches clots before they reach the lungs.

KEY CONCEPTS

Pulmonary Embolism

- Almost all large pulmonary artery thrombi are embolic in origin, usually arising from the deep veins of the lower leg.
- Risk factors include prolonged bed rest, leg surgery, severe trauma, CHF, use of oral contraceptives (especially those with high estrogen content), disseminated cancer, and genetic diseases of hypercoagulability.
- The vast majority (60% to 80%) of emboli are clinically silent, a minority (5%) cause acute cor pulmonale, shock, or death (typically from large "saddle emboli"), and the remaining cause pulmonary infarction.
- Risk of recurrence is high.

Pulmonary Hypertension

Pulmonary hypertension is defined as a mean pulmonary artery pressure greater than or equal to 25 mm Hg at rest. Based on underlying mechanisms, the World Health Organization has classified pulmonary hypertension into five groups. These groups are: (1) pulmonary arterial hypertension, a diverse collection of disorders that all primarily impact small pulmonary muscular arteries; (2) pulmonary hypertension secondary to left-heart failure; (3) pulmonary hypertension stemming from lung parenchymal disease or hypoxemia; (4) chronic thromboembolic pulmonary hypertension; and (5) pulmonary hypertension of multifactorial basis.

Pathogenesis. As can be gathered from the classification above, pulmonary hypertension has diverse causes. It is most frequently associated with structural cardiopulmonary conditions that increase pulmonary blood flow, pulmonary vascular resistance, or left heart resistance to blood flow. Some of the more common causes are the following:

- *Chronic obstructive or interstitial lung diseases* (group 3). These diseases obliterate alveolar capillaries, increasing pulmonary resistance to blood flow and, secondarily, pulmonary blood pressure.
- *Antecedent congenital or acquired heart disease* (group 2). Mitral stenosis, for example, causes an increase in left atrial pressure and pulmonary venous pressure that is eventually transmitted to the arterial side of the pulmonary vasculature, leading to hypertension.
- *Recurrent thromboemboli* (group 4). Recurrent pulmonary emboli may cause pulmonary hypertension by reducing the functional cross-sectional area of the pulmonary vascular bed, which in turn leads to an increase in pulmonary vascular resistance.
- *Autoimmune diseases* (group 1). Several of these diseases (most notably systemic sclerosis) involve the pulmonary vasculature and/or the interstitium, leading to increased vascular resistance and pulmonary hypertension.
- *Obstructive sleep apnea* (also group 3) is a common disorder that is associated with obesity and hypoxemia. It is now recognized to be a significant contributor to the development of pulmonary hypertension and cor pulmonale.

Uncommonly, pulmonary hypertension is encountered in patients in whom all known causes are excluded; this is referred to as *idiopathic pulmonary arterial hypertension*. However, this is a bit of a misnomer, as up to 80% of "idiopathic" pulmonary hypertension (sometimes referred to as primary pulmonary hypertension) has a genetic basis, sometimes being inherited in familes as an autosomal dominant trait. Within these families, there is incomplete penetrance, and only 10% to 20% of the family members actually develop overt disease.

As is often the case, much has been learned about the pathogenesis of pulmonary hypertension by investigating the molecular basis of the uncommon familial form of the disease. The first mutation to be discovered in familial pulmonary arterial hypertension was in the bone morphogenetic protein receptor type 2 (BMPR2). Inactivating germline mutations in the BMPR2 gene are found in 75% of the familial cases of pulmonary hypertension, and 25% of sporadic cases. Subsequently other mutations have been discovered that also converge on the BMPR2 pathway and affect intracellular signaling. It has also been demonstrated that BMPR2 is down-regulated in lungs from some idiopathic pulmonary arterial hypertension patients without mutation in its gene.

BMPR2 is a cell surface protein belonging to the TGF-β receptor superfamily, which binds a variety of cytokines, including TGF-β, bone morphogenetic protein (BMP), activin, and inhibin. Although originally described in the context of bone growth, BMP-BMPR2 signaling is now known to be important for embryogenesis, apoptosis, and cell proliferation and differentiation. Details remain to be worked out, but it appears that haploinsufficiency for BMPR2 leads to dysfunction and proliferation of endothelial cells and vascular smooth muscle cells. Because only 10% to 20% of individuals with *BMPR2* mutations develop disease, it is likely that modifier genes and/or environmental triggers also contribute to the pathogenesis of the disorder. A two-hit model has been proposed whereby a genetically susceptible individual with a *BMPR2* mutation requires additional genetic or environmental insults to develop the disease (Fig. 15-29).

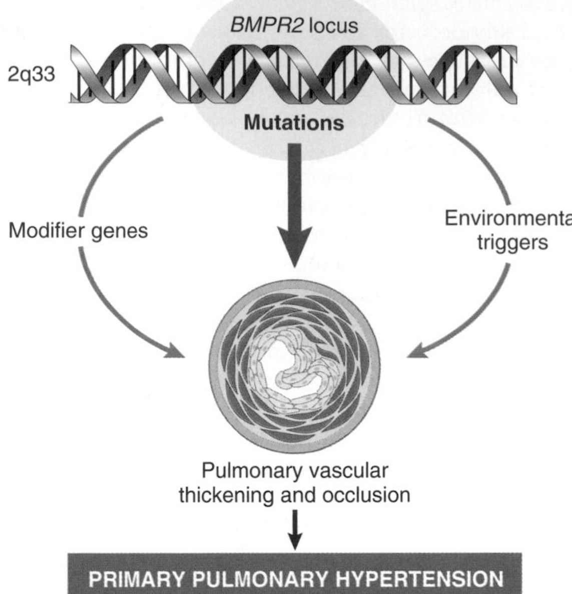

Figure 15-29 Pathogenesis of primary (idiopathic) pulmonary hypertension. See text for details.

MORPHOLOGY

Regardless of their etiology, all forms of pulmonary hypertension are associated with **medial hypertrophy of the pulmonary muscular and elastic arteries, pulmonary arterial atherosclerosis, and right ventricular hypertrophy**. The presence of many organizing or recanalized thrombi favors recurrent pulmonary emboli as the cause, and the coexistence of diffuse pulmonary fibrosis, or severe emphysema and chronic bronchitis, points to chronic hypoxia as the initiating event. The vessel changes can involve the entire arterial tree, from the main pulmonary arteries down to the arterioles (Fig. 15-30). In the most severe cases, atheromatous deposits form in the pulmonary artery and its major branches, resembling (but lesser in degree than) systemic atherosclerosis. The arterioles and small arteries (40 to 300 μm in diameter) are most prominently affected by striking medial hypertrophy and intimal fibrosis, sometimes narrowing the lumens to pinpoint channels. One extreme in the spectrum of pathologic changes is the plexiform lesion, so called because a tuft of capillary formations is present, producing a network, or web, that spans the lumens of dilated thin-walled, small arteries and may extend outside the vessel. Plexiform lesions are most prominent in idiopathic and familial pulmonary hypertension (group 1), unrepaired congenital heart disease with left-to-right shunts (group 2), and pulmonary hypertension associated with human immunodeficiency virus (HIV) infection and drugs (also group 1).

Clinical Course. Idiopathic pulmonary hypertension is most common in women who are 20 to 40 years of age and is also seen occasionally in young children. Clinical signs and symptoms in all forms of pulmonary hypertension become evident only in advanced disease. In cases of idiopathic disease, the presenting features are usually dyspnea and fatigue, but some patients have chest pain of the anginal type. Over time, severe respiratory distress, cyanosis, and right ventricular hypertrophy occur, and death from decompensated cor pulmonale, often with superimposed thromboembolism and pneumonia, usually ensues within 2 to 5 years in 80% of patients.

Treatment choices depend on the underlying cause. For those with secondary disease, therapy is directed at the trigger (e.g, thromboembolic disease or hypoxemia). A variety of vasodilators have been used with varying success in those with group 1 or refractory disease belonging to other groups. Lung transplantation provides definitive treatment for selected patients.

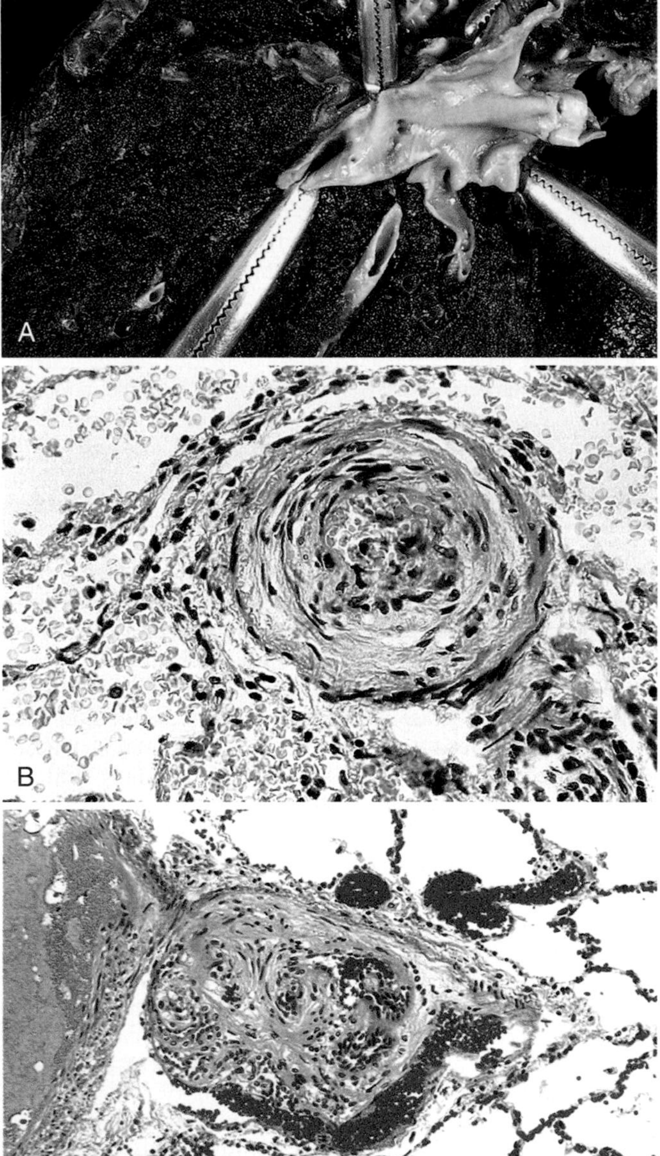

Figure 15-30 Vascular changes in pulmonary arterial hypertension. **A,** Atheroma formation, a finding usually limited to large vessels. **B,** Marked medial hypertrophy. **C,** Plexiform lesion of small arteries that is characteristic of advanced pulmonary hypertension.

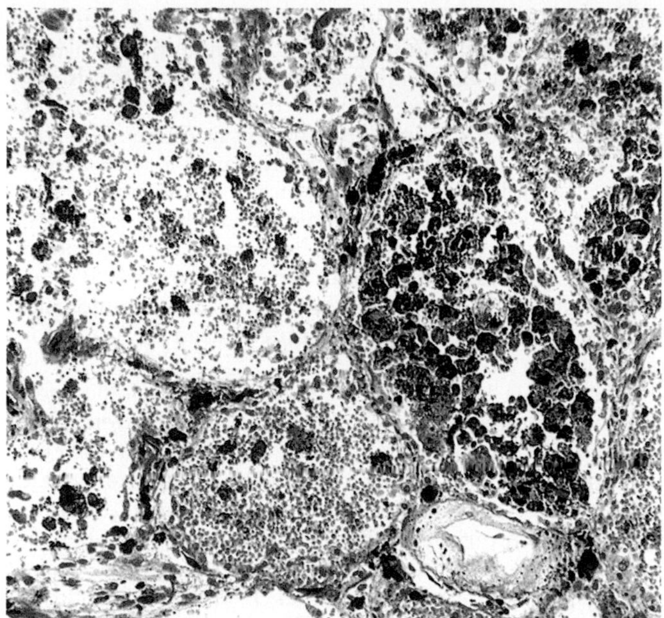

Figure 15-31 Diffuse pulmonary hemorrhage syndrome. There is acute intra-alveolar hemorrhage and hemosiderin-laden macrophages, reflecting previous hemorrhage (Prussian blue iron stain).

Diffuse Pulmonary Hemorrhage Syndromes

Pulmonary hemorrhage is a dramatic complication of some interstitial lung disorders. Among these so-called *pulmonary hemorrhage syndromes* (Fig. 15-31) are (1) Goodpasture syndrome, (2) idiopathic pulmonary hemosiderosis, and (3) vasculitis-associated hemorrhage, which is found in conditions such as hypersensitivity angiitis, Wegener granulomatosis, and systemic lupus erythematosus (Chapter 11).

Goodpasture Syndrome

Goodpasture syndrome is an uncommon autoimmune disease in which kidney and lung injury are caused by circulating autoantibodies against the noncollagenous domain of the α3 chain of collagen IV. When only renal disease is caused by this antibody, it is called anti-glomerular basement membrane disease. The term *Goodpasture syndrome* designates the 40% to 60% of patients who develop pulmonary hemorrhage in addition to renal disease. The antibodies initiate inflammatory destruction of the basement membrane in renal glomeruli and pulmonary alveoli, giving rise to *rapidly progressive glomerulonephritis* and a *necrotizing hemorrhagic interstitial pneumonitis.* Although any age can be affected, most cases occur in the teens or 20s, and in contrast to many other autoimmune diseases, there is a male preponderance. The majority of patients are active smokers.

Pathogenesis. The immunopathogenesis of the syndrome and the nature of the Goodpasture antigens are described in Chapter 20. The trigger that initiates the production of anti-basement membrane antibodies is still unknown. Because the epitopes that evoke anticollagen antibodies are normally hidden within the molecule, it is presumed that some environmental insult such as viral infection, exposure to hydrocarbon solvents (used in the dry cleaning industry), or smoking is required to unmask the cryptic epitopes. As in other autoimmune disorders, a genetic predisposition is indicated by association with certain HLA subtypes (e.g., HLA-DRB1*1501 and *1502).

MORPHOLOGY

In the classic case, the lungs are heavy, with areas of red-brown consolidation. Histologically, there is focal necrosis of alveolar walls associated with intra-alveolar hemorrhages. Often the alveoli contain hemosiderin-laden macrophages (Fig. 15-31). In later stages there may be fibrous thickening of the septae, hypertrophy of type II pneumocytes, and organization of blood in alveolar spaces. In many cases immunofluorescence studies reveal linear deposits of immunoglobulins along the basement membranes of the septal walls. The kidneys have the characteristic findings of focal proliferative glomerulonephritis in early cases or crescentic glomerulonephritis in patients with rapidly progressive glomerulonephritis. Diagnostic linear deposits of immunoglobulins and complement are seen by immunofluorescence studies along the glomerular basement membranes even in the few patients without renal disease.

Clinical Features. Most cases begin clinically with respiratory symptoms, principally hemoptysis, and radiographic evidence of focal pulmonary consolidations. Soon, manifestations of glomerulonephritis appear, leading to rapidly progressive renal failure. The most common cause of death is uremia. The once dismal prognosis for this disease has been markedly improved by intensive *plasmapheresis*. This procedure is thought to be beneficial by removing circulating antibasement membrane antibodies as well as chemical mediators of immunologic injury. Simultaneous immunosuppressive therapy inhibits further antibody production, ameliorating both lung hemorrhage and glomerulonephritis.

Idiopathic Pulmonary Hemosiderosis

Idiopathic pulmonary hemosiderosis is a rare disorder characterized by intermittent, diffuse alveolar hemorrhage. Most cases occur in young children, although the disease has been reported in adults as well. It usually presents with an insidious onset of productive cough, hemoptysis, and anemia associated with diffuse pulmonary infiltrations similar to Goodpasture syndrome.

The cause and pathogenesis are unknown, and no anti-basement membrane antibodies are detectable in serum or tissues. However, favorable response to long-term immunosuppression with prednisone and/or azathioprine indicates that an immunologic mechanism could be involved in the pulmonary capillary damage underlying alveolar bleeding. In addition, long-term follow-up of patients shows that some of them develop other immune disorders.

Polyangiitis With Granulomatosis

Previously called Wegener granulomatosis, this autoimmune disease most often involves the upper respiratory tract and/or the lungs, with hemoptysis being the common presenting symptom. Its features are discussed in Chapter

11. Here, it is enough to emphasize that a transbronchial lung biopsy might provide the only tissue available for diagnosis. Since the amount of tissue is small, necrosis and granulomatous vasculitis might not be present. Rather, the diagnostically important features are capillaritis and scattered, poorly formed granulomas (unlike those of sarcoidosis, which are rounded and well-defined).

Pulmonary Infections

Respiratory tract infections are more frequent than infections of any other organ and account for the largest number of workdays lost in the general population. The vast majority are upper respiratory tract infections caused by viruses (common cold, pharyngitis), but bacterial, viral, mycoplasmal, and fungal infections of the lung (pneumonia) still account for an enormous amount of morbidity and are the eighth leading cause of death (responsible for 2.3% of all deaths) in the United States. Pneumonia can be very broadly defined as any infection of the lung parenchyma.

Pulmonary anti-microbial defense mechanisms are described in Chapter 8. Pneumonia can result whenever these local defense mechanisms are impaired or the systemic resistance of the host is lowered. Factors that affect resistance in general include chronic diseases, immunologic deficiency, treatment with immunosuppressive agents, and leukopenia. The local defense mechanisms of the lung can be compromised by many factors, including:

- *Loss or suppression of the cough reflex* as a result of coma, anesthesia, neuromuscular disorders, drugs, or chest pain (may lead to *aspiration* of gastric contents)
- *Injury to the mucociliary apparatus* by either impairment of ciliary function or destruction of ciliated epithelium, due to cigarette smoke, inhalation of hot or corrosive gases, viral diseases, or genetic defects of ciliary function (e.g., the immotile cilia syndrome)
- *Accumulation of secretions* in conditions such as cystic fibrosis and bronchial obstruction
- *Interference with the phagocytic* or bactericidal action of alveolar macrophages by alcohol, tobacco smoke, anoxia, or oxygen intoxication
- *Pulmonary congestion and edema*

Defects in innate immunity (including neutrophil and complement defects) and humoral immunodeficiency typically lead to an increased incidence of infections with pyogenic bacteria. Germline mutations in MyD88 (an adaptor for several TLRs that is important for activation of the transcription factor NFκB) are also associated with destructive bacterial (pneumococcal) pneumonias. On the other hand, cell-mediated immune defects (congenital and acquired) lead to increased infections with intracellular microbes such as mycobacteria and herpesviruses as well as with microorganisms of very low virulence, such as *Pneumocystis jiroveci*.

Several other points should be emphasized. First, to paraphrase the French physician Louis Cruveilhier in 1919 (during the Spanish flu epidemic), "flu condemns, and additional infection executes". This is particularly true in debilitated patients. For example, the most common cause of death in viral influenza epidemics is superimposed bacterial pneumonia. Second, although the portal of entry for most bacterial pneumonias is the respiratory tract, hematogenous seeding of the lungs from another organ may occur and may be difficult to distinguish from primary pneumonia. Finally, many patients with chronic diseases acquire terminal pneumonia while hospitalized *(nosocomial infection)*. Bacteria common to the hospital environment may have acquired resistance to antibiotics; opportunities for spread are increased; invasive procedures, such as intubations and injections, are common; and bacteria may contaminate equipment used in respiratory care units.

Pneumonia is classified by the specific etiologic agent, which determines the treatment, or, if no pathogen can be isolated (which occurs in about 50% of cases), by the clinical setting in which the infection occurs. The latter considerably narrows the list of suspected pathogens, providing a guide for empirical antimicrobial therapy. As Table 15-7 indicates, pneumonia can arise in seven distinct clinical settings ("pneumonia syndromes"), and the implicated pathogens are reasonably specific to each category.

Community-Acquired Bacterial Pneumonias

Community-acquired acute pneumonia refers to lung infection in otherwise healthy individuals that is acquired from the normal environment (in contrast to hospital acquired pneumonia). It may be bacterial or viral. Clinical and radiologic features are usually insensitive in differentiating between them. Several newer biomarkers have been developed to identify patients with bacterial infection and to define their prognosis. Of these, C-reactive protein and procalcitonin, both acute-phase reactants produced primarily in the liver, are significantly elevated in bacterial more than in viral infections.

Often, the bacterial infection follows an upper respiratory tract viral infection. Bacterial invasion of the lung parenchyma causes the alveoli to be filled with an inflammatory exudate, thus causing consolidation ("solidification") of the pulmonary tissue. Many variables, such as the specific etiologic agent, the host reaction, and the extent of involvement, determine the precise form of pneumonia. Predisposing conditions include extremes of age, chronic diseases (congestive heart failure, COPD, and diabetes), congenital or acquired immune deficiencies, and decreased or absent splenic function (sickle cell disease or postsplenectomy, which puts the patient at risk for infection with encapsulated bacteria such as pneumococcus).

Streptococcus pneumoniae

***Streptococcus pneumoniae*, or *pneumococcus*, is the most common cause of community-acquired acute pneumonia.** Examination of Gram-stained sputum is an important step in the diagnosis of acute pneumonia. The presence of numerous neutrophils containing the typical gram-positive, lancet-shaped diplococci supports the diagnosis of pneumococcal pneumonia, but it must be remembered that *S. pneumoniae* is a part of the endogenous flora in 20% of adults, and therefore false-positive results may be obtained. Isolation of pneumococci from blood cultures is more specific but less sensitive (in the early phase of illness, only 20% to 30% of patients have positive blood cultures).

Table 15-7 Pneumonia Syndromes

Community-Acquired Acute Pneumonia
Streptococcus pneumoniae *Haemophilus influenzae* *Moraxella catarrhalis* *Staphylococcus aureus* *Legionella pneumophila* *Enterobacteriaceae (Klebsiella pneumoniae)* and *Pseudomonas* spp. *Mycoplasma pneumoniae* *Chlamydia* spp. *(C. pneumoniae, C. psittaci, C. trachomatis)* *Coxiella burnetii* (Q fever) Viruses: respiratory syncytial virus, parainfluenza virus and human metapneumovirus (children); influenza A and B (adults); adenovirus (military recruits);
Health Care-Associated Pneumonia
Staphylococcus aureus, methicillin-sensitive *Staphylococcus aureus*, methicillin-resistant *Pseudomonas aeruginosa* *Streptococcus pneumoniae*
Hospital-Acquired Pneumonia
Gram-negative rods, Enterobacteriaceae (*Klebsiella* spp., *Serratia marcescens, Escherichia coli*) and *Pseudomonas* spp. *Staphylococcus aureus* (usually methicillin-resistant)
Aspiration Pneumonia
Anaerobic oral flora (*Bacteroides, Prevotella, Fusobacterium, Peptostreptococcus*), admixed with aerobic bacteria (*Streptococcus pneumoniae, Staphylococcus aureus, Haemophilus influenzae, Pseudomonas aeruginosa*)
Chronic Pneumonia
Nocardia *Actinomyces* Granulomatous: *Mycobacterium* tuberculosis and atypical mycobacteria, *Histoplasma capsulatum, Coccidioides immitis, Blastomyces dermatitidis*
Necrotizing Pneumonia and Lung Abscess
Anaerobic bacteria (extremely common), with or without mixed aerobic infection *Staphylococcus aureus, Klebsiella pneumoniae, Streptococcus pyogenes*, and type 3 pneumococcus (uncommon)
Pneumonia in the Immunocompromised Host
Cytomegalovirus *Pneumocystis jiroveci* *Mycobacterium avium-intracellulare* Invasive aspergillosis Invasive candidiasis "Usual" bacterial, viral, and fungal organisms (listed herein)

Pneumococcal vaccines containing capsular polysaccharides from the common serotypes are used in individuals at high risk for pneumococcal sepsis.

Haemophilus influenzae

Haemophilus influenzae is a pleomorphic, gram-negative organism that occurs in encapsulated and nonencapsulated forms. There are six serotypes of the encapsulated form (types a to f), of which type b is the most virulent. Antibodies against the capsule protect the host from *H. influenzae* infection; hence the capsular polysaccharide b is incorporated in the widely used vaccine against *H. influenzae*. With routine use of *H. influenzae* conjugate vaccines, the incidence of disease caused by the b serotype has declined significantly. By contrast, infections with nonencapsulated forms, also called *nontypeable forms*, are increasing. They are less virulent, spread along the surface of the upper respiratory tract, and produce otitis media (infection of the middle ear), sinusitis, and bronchopneumonia. Neonates and children with comorbidities such as prematurity, malignancy, and immunodeficiency are at high risk for development of invasive infection.

H. influenzae pneumonia, which may follow a viral respiratory infection, is a pediatric emergency and has a high mortality rate. Descending laryngotracheobronchitis results in airway obstruction as the smaller bronchi are plugged by dense, fibrin-rich exudates containing neutrophils, similar to that seen in pneumococcal pneumonias. Pulmonary consolidation is usually lobular and patchy but may be confluent and involve the entire lung lobe. Before a vaccine became widely available, *H. influenzae* was a common cause of suppurative meningitis in children up to 5 years of age. *H. influenzae* also causes an acute, purulent conjunctivitis (pink eye) in children and, in predisposed older patients, may cause septicemia, endocarditis, pyelonephritis, cholecystitis, and suppurative arthritis. *H. influenzae* is the most common bacterial cause of acute exacerbation of COPD.

Moraxella catarrhalis

Moraxella catarrhalis is being increasingly recognized as a cause of bacterial pneumonia, especially in the elderly. It is the second most common bacterial cause of acute exacerbation of COPD. Along with *S. pneumoniae* and *H. influenzae*, *M. catarrhalis* constitutes one of the three most common causes of otitis media in children.

Staphylococcus aureus

Staphylococcus aureus is an important cause of secondary bacterial pneumonia in children and healthy adults following viral respiratory illnesses (e.g., measles in children and influenza in both children and adults). Staphylococcal pneumonia is associated with a high incidence of complications, such as lung abscess and empyema. *Intravenous drug users* are at high risk for development of staphylococcal pneumonia in association with endocarditis. It is also an important cause of hospital-acquired pneumonia.

Klebsiella pneumoniae

Klebsiella pneumoniae is the most frequent cause of gram-negative bacterial pneumonia. It commonly afflicts debilitated and malnourished people, particularly *chronic alcoholics*. Thick, mucoid, (often blood-tinged) sputum is characteristic, because the organism produces an abundant viscid capsular polysaccharide, which the patient may have difficulty expectorating.

Pseudomonas aeruginosa

Although *Pseudomonas aeruginosa* most commonly causes hospital-acquired infections, it is mentioned here because of its occurrence in cystic fibrosis and immunocompromised patients. It is common in patients who are neutropenic and it has a propensity to invade blood vessels with consequent extrapulmonary spread. *Pseudomonas* septicemia is a very fulminant disease.

Legionella pneumophila

Legionella pneumophila is the agent of Legionnaires' disease, an eponym for the epidemic and sporadic forms

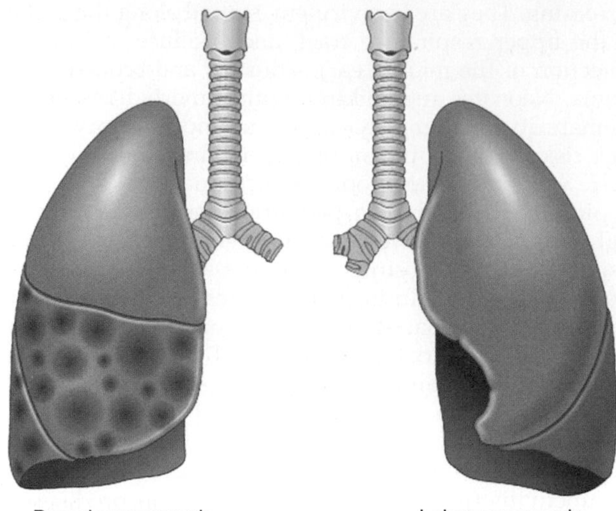

Figure 15-32 Comparison of bronchopneumonia and lobar pneumonia.

of pneumonia caused by this organism. It also causes Pontiac fever, a related self-limited upper respiratory tract infection. This organism flourishes in artificial aquatic environments, such as water-cooling towers and the tubing systems of domestic (potable) water supplies. The mode of transmission is either inhalation of aerosolized organisms or aspiration of contaminated drinking water. *Legionella* pneumonia is common in individuals with predisposing conditions such as cardiac, renal, immunologic, or hematologic disease. Organ transplant recipients are particularly susceptible. It can be quite severe, frequently requiring hospitalization, and immunosuppressed patients may have fatality rates of up to 50%. Rapid diagnosis is facilitated by demonstration of *Legionella* antigens in the urine or by a positive fluorescent antibody test on sputum samples; culture remains the diagnostic gold standard.

Mycoplasma pneumoniae

Mycoplasma infections are particularly common among children and young adults. They occur sporadically or as local epidemics in closed communities (schools, military camps, and prisons).

MORPHOLOGY

Bacterial pneumonia has two patterns of anatomic distribution: lobular bronchopneumonia and lobar pneumonia (Fig. 15-32). Patchy consolidation of the lung is the dominant characteristic of **bronchopneumonia** (Fig. 15-33), while consolidation of a large portion of a lobe or of an entire lobe defines **lobar pneumonia** (Fig. 15-34). These anatomic categorizations may be difficult to apply in individual cases because patterns overlap. The patchy involvement may become confluent, producing virtually total lobar consolidation; however, effective antibiotic therapy may limit involvement to a subtotal consolidation. Moreover, the same organisms may produce either pattern depending on patient susceptibility. **Most important from the clinical standpoint are identification of the causative agent and determination of the extent of disease.**

In **lobar pneumonia**, four stages of the inflammatory response have classically been described: congestion, red hepatization, gray hepatization, and resolution. In the first stage of **congestion** the lung is heavy, boggy, and red. It is characterized by vascular engorgement, intra-alveolar fluid with few neutrophils, and often the presence of numerous bacteria. The stage of **red hepatization** that follows is characterized by massive confluent exudation, as neutrophils, red cells, and fibrin fill the alveolar spaces (Fig. 15-35*A*). On gross examination, the lobe is red, firm, and airless, with a liver-like consistency, hence the term hepatization. The stage of **gray hepatization** that follows is marked by progressive disintegration of red cells and the persistence of a fibrinosuppurative exudate (Fig. 15-35*B*),

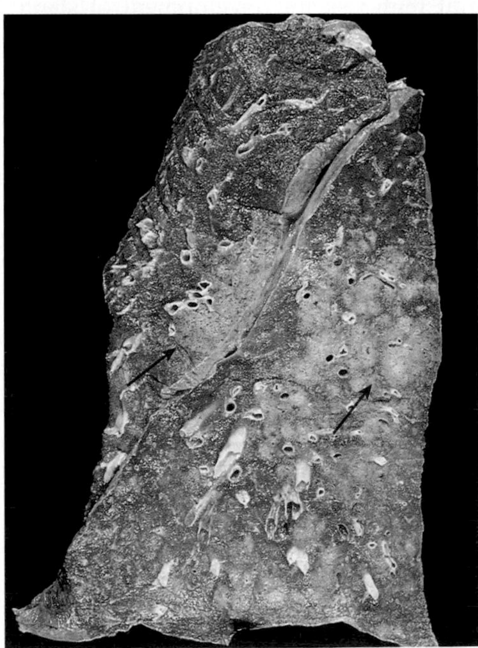

Figure 15-33 Bronchopneumonia. Section of lung showing patches of consolidation *(arrows)*.

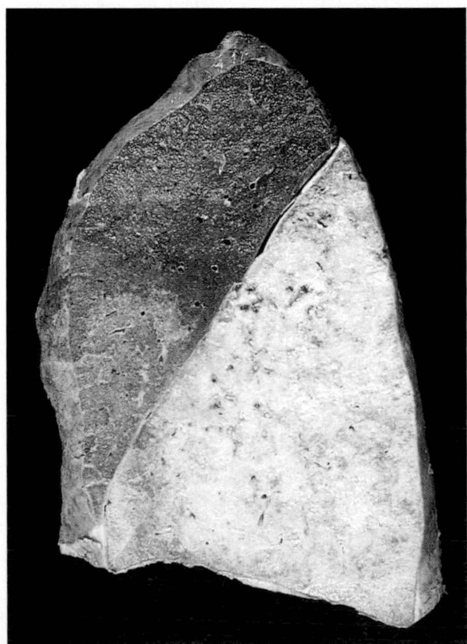

Figure 15-34 Lobar pneumonia—gray hepatization. The lower lobe is uniformly consolidated.

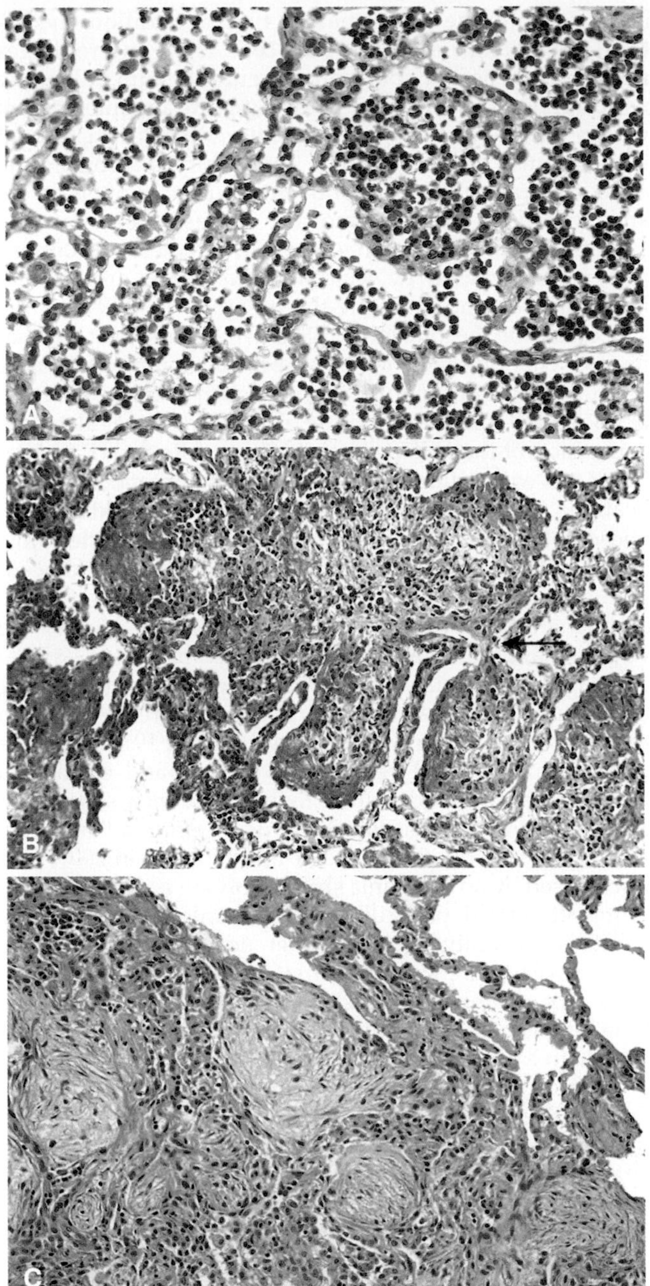

Figure 15-35 Stages of bacterial pneumonia. **A,** Acute pneumonia. The congested septal capillaries and numerous intra-alveolar neutrophils are characteristic of early red hepatization. Fibrin nets have not yet formed. **B,** Early organization of intra-alveolar exudate, seen focally to be streaming through the pores of Kohn *(arrow)*. **C,** Advanced organizing pneumonia. The exudates have been converted to fibromyxoid masses rich in macrophages and fibroblasts.

resulting in a color change to grayish-brown. In the final stage of **resolution** the exudate within the alveolar spaces is broken down by enzymatic digestion to produce granular, semifluid debris that is resorbed, ingested by macrophages, expectorated, or organized by fibroblasts growing into it (Fig. 15-35*C*). Pleural fibrinous reaction to the underlying inflammation, often present in the early stages if the consolidation extends to the surface **(pleuritis)**, may similarly resolve. More often it undergoes organization, leaving fibrous thickening or permanent adhesions.

Foci of **bronchopneumonia** are consolidated areas of acute suppurative inflammation. The consolidation may be confined to one lobe but is more often multilobar and frequently bilateral and basal because of the tendency of secretions to gravitate to the lower lobes. Well-developed lesions are slightly elevated, dry, granular, gray-red to yellow, and poorly delimited at their margins (Fig. 15-33). Histologically, the reaction usually elicits a neutrophil-rich exudate that fills the bronchi, bronchioles, and adjacent alveolar spaces (Fig. 15-35*A*).

Complications of pneumonia include (1) tissue destruction and necrosis, causing **abscess formation** (particularly common with type 3 pneumococci or *Klebsiella* infections); (2) spread of infection to the pleural cavity, causing the intrapleural fibrinosuppurative reaction known as **empyema**; and (3) **bacteremic dissemination** to the heart valves, pericardium, brain, kidneys, spleen, or joints, causing metastatic abscesses, endocarditis, meningitis, or suppurative arthritis.

Clinical Course. The major symptoms of community-acquired acute bacterial pneumonia are abrupt onset of high fever, shaking chills, and cough producting mucopurulent sputum; occasional patients may have hemoptysis. When pleuritis is present it is accompanied by pleuritic pain and pleural friction rub. The whole lobe is radiopaque in lobar pneumonia, whereas there are focal opacities in bronchopneumonia.

The clinical picture is markedly modified by the administration of antibiotics. Treated patients may be relatively afebrile with few clinical signs 48 to 72 hours after the initiation of antibiotics. The identification of the organism and the determination of its antibiotic sensitivity are the keystones to appropriate therapy. Fewer than 10% of patients with pneumonia severe enough to merit hospitalization now succumb, and in most such instances death results from a complication, such as empyema, meningitis, endocarditis, or pericarditis, or to some predisposing influence, such as debility or chronic alcoholism.

Community-Acquired Viral Pneumonia

Common viral infections include influenza virus types A and B, the respiratory syncytial viruses, human metapneumovirus, adenovirus, rhinoviruses, rubeola, and varicella viruses. Any of these agents can cause merely an upper respiratory tract infection, recognized as the common cold, or a more severe lower respiratory tract infection. Factors that favor such extension of the infection include extremes of age, malnutrition, alcoholism, and underlying debilitating illnesses.

Although the molecular details vary, all of the viruses that cause pneuomia produce disease through similar general mechanisms. These viruses have tropisms that allow them to attach to and enter respiratory lining cells. Viral replication and gene expression leads to cytopathic changes, inducing cell death and secondary inflammation. The resulting damage and impairment of local pulmonary defenses, such as mucociliary clearance, may predisopose to bacterial superinfections, which are often more serious than the viral infection itself.

Influenza Infections

Influenza viruses of type A infect humans, pigs, horses, and birds and are the major cause of pandemic and epidemic influenza infections. The influenza genome encodes a number of proteins, but the most important from the vantage point of viral virulence are the hemagglutin and neuramindase proteins. Hemagglutinin has three major subtypes (H1-H3), while neuraminidase has two (N1, N2). Both proteins are components of the influenza virus envelope, which consists of a lipid bilayer. Hemagglutinin is particularly important, as it serves to attach the virus to its cellular target via sialic acid residues on surface polysaccharides. Following uptake of the virus into endosomal vesicles, acidification of the endosome triggers a conformation change in hemagglutinin that allows the viral envelope to fuse with the host cell membrane, releasing the viral genomic RNAs into the cytoplasm of the cell. Neuraminidase in turn facilitates the release of newly formed virions that are budding from infected cells by cleaving sialic acid residues. Neutralizing host antibodies against viral hemagglutinin and neuraminidase prevent and ameliorate, respectively, infection with the influenza virus by interfering with these functions.

The viral genome is composed of eight single-stranded RNAs, each encoding one or more proteins. The RNAs are packaged into helices by nucleoproteins that determine the influenza virus type (A, B, or C). A single subtype of influenza virus A predominates throughout the world at a given time. Epidemics of influenza are caused by spontaneous mutations that alter antigenic epitopes on the viral hemagglutinin and neuraminidase proteins. These antigenic changes (*antigenic drift*) result in new viral strains that are sufficiently different to elude, at least in part, anti-influenza antibodies produced in members of the population in response to prior exposures to other flu strains. Usually, however, these new strains bear sufficient resemblance to prior strains that some members of the population are at least partially resistant to infection. By contrast, pandemics, which are longer and more widespread than epidemics, occur when both the hemagglutinin and the neuraminidase genes are replaced through recombination with animal influenza viruses *(antigenic shift)*. In this instance, essentially all individuals are susceptible to the new influenza virus. Viral assembly involves packaging of each of the 8 viral RNAs into single virions, and it is easy to see how infection of an animal by two different flu types could lead to swapping of genetic material within co-infected cells, creating a completely new viral strain. Thus, the unusual genome of influenza virus ensures that antigenic shifts leading to pandemics are inevitable.

If the host lacks protective antibodies, the virus infects pneumocytes and elicits several cytopathic changes. Shortly after entry into pneumocytes, the viral infection inhibits sodium channels, producing electrolyte and water shifts that lead to fluid accumulation in the alveolar lumen. This is followed by the death of the infected cells through several mechanisms, including inhibition of host cell mRNA translation and activation of caspases leading to apoptosis. The death of epithelial cells exacerbates the fluid accumulation and releases "danger signals" that activate resident macrophages. In addition, prior to their death, infected epithelial cells release a variety of inflammatory mediators, including several chemokines and cytokines, adding fuel to the inflammatory fire. In addition, mediators released from epithelial cells and macrophages activate the nearby pulmonary endothelium, allowing neutrophils to attach and extravasate into the interstitium within the first day or two of infection. In some cases viral infection may cause sufficient lung injury to produce the acute respiratory distress syndrome, but more often severe and sometimes fatal pulmonary disease stems from a superimposed bacterial pneumonia. Of these, secondary pneumonias caused by *Staphylococcus aureus* are particularly common and often life-threatening.

Control of the infection relies on several host mechanisms. The presence of viral products induces innate immune responses in infected cells, such as the production of α- and β-interferon. These mediators upregulate the expression of the *MX1* gene, which encodes a GTPase that interferes with influenza gene transcription and viral replication. As with other viral infections, natural killer cells and cytotoxic T cells can recognize and kill infected host cells, limiting viral replication and viral spread to adjacent pneumocytes. The cellular immune response is eventually augmented by development of antibody responses to the viral hemagglutinin and neuraminidase proteins.

Insight into future pandemics has come from studying those past. DNA analysis of viral genomes retrieved from the lungs of a soldier who died in the great 1918 influenza pandemic that killed between 20 million and 40 million people worldwide identified swine influenza sequences, consistent with this virus having its origin in a "antigenic shift". The first flu pandemic of this century, in 2009, was also caused by an antigenic shift involving a virus of swine origin. It caused particularly severe infections in young adults, apparently because older adults had antibodies against past influenza strains that conveyed at least partial protection. Comorbidities such as diabetes, heart disease, lung disease, and immunosuppression were also associated with a higher risk of severe infection.

What then might be the source of the next great pandemic? There is no certainty, but one concern is centered on avian influenza, which normally infects birds. One such strain, type H5N1, has spread throughout the world in wild and domestic birds. As of June 2011, a total of 562 H5N1 influenza virus infections and 325 deaths in humans (from 15 countries) have been reported to the World Health Organization (WHO). Nearly all cases have been acquired by close contact with domestic birds; most deaths resulted from pneumonia. Fortunately, the transmission of the current H5N1 avian virus is inefficient. However, if H5N1 influenza recombines with an influenza that is highly infectious for humans, a strain might result that is capable of sustained human-to-human transmission (and, thus, of causing the next great pandemic).

Human Metapneumovirus

Human metapneumovirus (MPV), a paramyxovirus discovered in 2001, is found worldwide and is associated with upper and lower respiratory tract infections. It can infect any age group but is most commonly seen in young children, elderly subjects, and immunocompromised patients. Human MPV can cause severe infections such as bronchiolitis and pneumonia and is responsible for 5% to 10% of hospitalizations and 12% to 20% of outpatient visits of children suffering from acute respiratory tract infections. Such infections are clinically indistinguishable from those caused by human respiratory syncytial virus and are often mistaken for influenza. The first human MPV infection occurs during early childhood, but reinfections are common throughout life, especially in older subjects. Diagnostic methods include PCR tests for viral RNA and direct immunofluorescence. Ribavirin is the only antiviral treatment that is currently available for human MPV infections; it is used mostly in immunocompromised patients with severe disease. Although work is ongoing, a clinically effective and safe vaccine has yet to be developed.

Severe Acute Respiratory Syndrome

Severe acute respiratory syndrome (SARS) first appeared in November 2002 in the Guangdong Province of China and subsequently spread to Hong Kong, Taiwan, Singapore, Vietnam, and Toronto, where large outbreaks also occurred. The ease of travel between continents clearly contributed to this initial rapid spread. The epidemic went no further, however, perhaps in part because of public health measures, and the last cases of SARS were laboratory-associated infections reported in April 2004. The cause of SARS was a new coronavirus. Many upper respiratory infections are caused by coronaviruses, but the SARS virus differed from other coronaviruses in that it infected the lower respiratory tract and spread throughout the body. SARS is a cardinal example of sudden emergence of a new infectious agent (Chapter 8), but since 2004 the virus has completely disappeared as mysteriously as its original debut. It is unknown if or when it will appear again.

MORPHOLOGY

All viral infections produce similar morphologic changes. Upper respiratory infections are marked by mucosal hyperemia and swelling, lymphomonocytic and plasmacytic infiltration of the submucosa, and overproduction of mucus secretions. The swollen mucosa and viscous exudate may plug the nasal channels, sinuses or the Eustachian tubes, leading to suppurative secondary bacterial infection. Virus-induced tonsillitis causing hyperplasia of the lymphoid tissue within the Waldeyer ring is frequent in children.

In viral **laryngotracheobronchitis** and **bronchiolitis** there is vocal cord swelling and abundant mucus production. Impairment of bronchociliary function invites bacterial superinfection with more marked suppuration. Plugging of small airways may give rise to focal lung atelectasis. With more severe bronchiolar involvement, widespread plugging of secondary and terminal airways by cell debris, fibrin, and inflammatory exudate may, if prolonged, lead to organization and fibrosis, resulting in obliterative bronchiolitis and permanent lung damage.

Lung involvement may be quite patchy or may involve whole lobes bilaterally or unilaterally. The affected areas are red-blue and congested. Pleuritis or pleural effusions are infrequent. The histologic pattern depends on the severity of the disease. **Predominant is an interstitial inflammatory reaction involving the walls of the alveoli.** The alveolar septa are widened and edematous and usually have a mononuclear inflammatory infiltrate of lymphocytes, macrophages, and occasionally plasma cells. In acute cases neutrophils may also be present. The alveoli may be free of exudate, but in many patients there is intra-alveolar proteinaceous material and a cellular exudate. When complicated by ARDS, pink hyaline membranes line the alveolar walls (Fig. 15-4). Eradication of the infection is followed by reconstitution of the normal lung architecture.

Superimposed bacterial infection modifies this picture by causing ulcerative bronchitis, bronchiolitis, and bacterial pneumonia. Some viruses, such as herpes simplex, varicella, and adenovirus, may be associated with necrosis of bronchial and alveolar epithelium and acute inflammation. Characteristic viral cytopathic changes are described in Chapter 8.

Clinical Course. The clinical course of viral infections is extremely varied. Many cases masquerade as severe upper respiratory tract infections or as *chest colds.* Even individuals with well-developed atypical pneumonia have few localizing symptoms. Cough may be absent, and the major manifestations may consist only of fever, headache, muscle aches, and pains in the legs. The edema and exudation are both strategically located to cause mismatching of ventilation and blood flow and thus evoke symptoms out of proportion to the scanty physical findings.

Viral infectons are usually mild and resolve spontaneously without any lasting sequelae. However, interstitial viral pneumonias may assume epidemic proportions, and in such instances even a low rate of complications can lead to significant morbidity and mortality, as is typically true of influenza epidemics.

Health Care-Associated Pneumonia

Health-care associated pneumonia was recently described as a distinct clinical entity associated with significant risk factors. These are: hospitalization of at least 2 days within the recent past; presentation from a nursing home or long-term care facility; attending a hospital or hemodialysis clinic; and recent intravenous antibiotic therapy, chemotherapy or wound care. The most common organisms isolated are methicillin-resistant *Staphylococcus aureus* and *P. aeruginosa.* These patients have a higher mortality than those with community-acquired pneumonia.

Hospital-Acquired Pneumonia

Hospital-acquired pneumonias are defined as pulmonary infections acquired in the course of a hospital stay. They are common in patients with severe underlying disease, immunosuppression, prolonged antibiotic therapy, or invasive access devices such as intravascular catheters. Patients on mechanical ventilation are at particularly high risk. Superimposed on an underlying disease (that caused hospitalization), hospital-acquired infections are serious and often life-threatening complications. Gram-positive cocci (mainly *S. aureus* and *S. pneumonia)* and gram-negative rods (Enterobacteriaceae and *Pseudomonas* species) are the most common isolates. There are similar organisms isolated in ventilator associated pneumonia but gram-negative bacilli are more common.

KEY CONCEPTS

Acute Pneumonia

- *S. pneumoniae* (the pneumococcus) is the most common cause of community-acquired acute pneumonia; the distribution of inflammation is usually lobar.

- Lobar pneumonias evolve through four stages: congestion, red hepatization, gray hepatization, and resolution.
- Other common causes of acute pneumonias in the community include *H. influenzae* and *M. catarrhalis* (both associated with acute exacerbations of COPD), *S. aureus* (usually secondary to viral respiratory infections), *K. pneumoniae* (observed in patients who are chronic alcoholics), *P. aeruginosa* (seen in persons with cystic fibrosis, in burn victims, and in patients with neutropenia), and *L. pneumophila*, seen particularly in organ transplant recipients.
- The term *atypical organisms* is used for *Mycoplasma pneumoniae, Chlamydophila pneumoniae, Coxiella burnetii*, and viruses (influenza viruses types A and B, human metapneumovirus) since they are not detectable on Gram stain nor do they grow on the standard bacteriologic culture media.
- Bacterial pneumonias are characterized by predominantly intra-alveolar neutrophilic inflammation while viral pneumonia shows interstitial lymphocytic inflammation. Characteristic viral inclusions may be seen.
- Lung abscess is often caused by anaerobic organisms or by mixed infections and frequently occur in debilitated individuals following aspiration of oral flora.

Aspiration Pneumonia

Aspiration pneumonia occurs in markedly debilitated patients or those who aspirate gastric contents either while unconscious (e.g., after a stroke) or during repeated vomiting. These patients have abnormal gag and swallowing reflexes that predispose to aspiration. The resultant pneumonia is partly chemical due to the irritating effects of gastric acid, and partly bacterial (from the oral flora). Typically, more than one organism is recovered on culture, aerobes being more common than anaerobes. This type of pneumonia is often necrotizing, pursues a fulminant clinical course, and is a frequent cause of death. In those who survive, lung abscess is a common complication.

Microaspiration, in contrast, occurs frequently in almost all people, especially those with gastroesophageal reflux disease. It usually results in small, poorly formed nonnecrotizing granulomas with multinucleated foreign body giant cell reaction. It is usually inconsequential, but may exacerbate other preexisting lung diseases such as asthma, interstitial fibrosis, and lung rejection.

Lung Abscess

The term *pulmonary abscess* describes a local suppurative process that produces necrosis of lung tissue. Oropharyngeal surgical or dental procedures, sinobronchial infections, and bronchiectasis play important roles in their development.

Etiology and Pathogenesis. Although under appropriate circumstances any pathogen can produce an abscess, the commonly isolated organisms include aerobic and anaerobic streptococci, *S. aureus*, and a host of gram-negative organisms. Mixed infections often occur because of the important causal role played by inhalation of foreign material. *Anaerobic organisms* normally found in the oral cavity, including members of the *Bacteroides, Fusobacterium*, and *Peptococcus* species, are the exclusive isolates in about 60% of cases. The causative organisms are introduced by the following mechanisms:

- *Aspiration of infective material* (the most frequent cause). This is particularly common in acute alcoholism, coma, anesthesia, sinusitis, gingivodental sepsis, and debilitation in which the cough reflexes are depressed. Aspiration first causes pneumonia which progresses to tissue necrosis and formation of lung abscess.
- *Antecedent primary lung infection.* Postpneumonic abscess formations are usually associated with *S. aureus*, *K. pneumoniae*, and type 3 pneumococcus. Posttransplant or otherwise immunosuppressed individuals are at special risk.
- *Septic embolism.* Infected emboli from thrombophlebitis in any portion of the systemic venous circulation or from the vegetations of infective bacterial endocarditis on the right side of the heart are trapped in the lung.
- *Neoplasia.* Secondary infection is particularly common in the bronchopulmonary segment obstructed by a primary or secondary malignancy *(postobstructive pneumonia)*.
- *Miscellaneous.* Direct traumatic penetrations of the lungs; spread of infections from a neighboring organ, such as suppuration in the esophagus, spine, subphrenic space, or pleural cavity; and hematogenous seeding of the lung by pyogenic organisms all may lead to lung abscess formation.

When all these causes are excluded, there are still cases in which no discernible basis for the abscess formation can be identified. These are referred to as *primary cryptogenic lung abscesses*.

MORPHOLOGY

Abscesses vary in diameter from a few millimeters to large cavities of 5 to 6 cm (Fig. 15-36). They may affect any part of the lung and may be single or multiple. Pulmonary abscesses due to aspiration are more common on the right (because of the

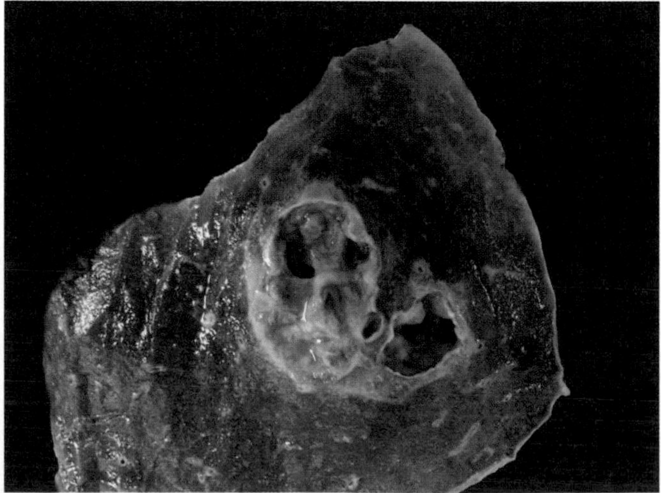

Figure 15-36 Cut surface of lung showing two abscesses. (Courtesy Dr. M. Kamran Mirza, University of Chicago, Chicago, Ill.)

more vertical right main bronchus) and are most often single. Abscesses that develop in the course of pneumonia or bronchiectasis are usually multiple, basal, and diffusely scattered. Septic emboli and pyemic abscesses are multiple and may affect any region of the lungs.

The **cardinal histologic change in all abscesses is suppurative destruction of the lung parenchyma within the central area of cavitation.** The abscess cavity may be filled with suppurative debris or, if there is communication with an air passage, may be partially drained to create an air-containing cavity. Superimposed saprophytic infections are prone to develop within the necrotic debris. Continued infection leads to large, poorly demarcated, fetid, green-black, multilocular cavities designated gangrene of the lung. In chronic cases considerable fibroblastic proliferation produces a fibrous wall.

Clinical Course. The manifestations of pulmonary abscesses are much like those of bronchiectasis and are characterized principally by cough, fever, and copious amounts of foul-smelling purulent or sanguineous sputum. Fever, chest pain, and weight loss are common. Clubbing of the fingers and toes may appear within a few weeks after the onset of an abscess. The diagnosis can be only suspected from the clinical findings and must be confirmed radiologically. Whenever an abscess is discovered in older individuals, it is important to rule out an underlying carcinoma, which is present in 10% to 15% of cases.

The course of abscesses is variable. With antimicrobial therapy, most resolve leaving behind a scar. Complications include extension of the infection into the pleural cavity, hemorrhage, the development of *brain abscesses* or *meningitis* from septic emboli, and (rarely) secondary amyloidosis (type AA).

Chronic Pneumonia

Chronic pneumonia is most often a localized lesion in the immunocompetent patient, with or without regional lymph node involvement. Typically, the inflammatory reaction is granulomatous, and is caused by bacteria (e.g., *M. tuberculosis*) or fungi (e.g., *Histoplasma capsulatum*). Tuberculosis of the lung and other organs was described in Chapter 8. Chronic pneumonias caused by fungi are discussed here.

Histoplasmosis

Histoplasma capsulatum infection is acquired by inhalation of dust particles from soil contaminated with bird or bat droppings that contain small spores (microconidia), the infectious form of the fungus. It is endemic along the Ohio and Mississippi rivers and the Caribbean. It is also found in Mexico, Central and South America, parts of eastern and southern Europe, Africa, eastern Asia and Australia. Like *M. tuberculosis, H. capsulatum* is an intracellular pathogen that is found mainly in phagocytes. The clinical presentations and morphologic lesions of histoplasmosis also strikingly resemble those of tuberculosis, including (1) a self-limited and often latent primary pulmonary involvement, which may result in coin lesions on chest radiography; (2) chronic, progressive, secondary lung disease, which is localized to the lung apices and causes cough, fever, and night sweats; (3) spread to extrapulmonary sites, including mediastinum, adrenals, liver, or meninges; and (4) widely disseminated disease in immunocompromised patients. Histoplasmosis can occur in immunocompetent individuals but as expected it is more severe in those with depressed cell mediated immunity.

The pathogenesis of histoplasmosis is incompletely understood. It is known that macrophages are the major target of infection. *H. capsulatum* may be internalized into macrophages after opsonization with antibody. *Histoplasma* yeasts can multiply within the phagosome, and lyse the host cells. *Histoplasma* infections are controlled by helper T cells that recognize fungal cell wall antigens and heat-shock proteins and subsequently secrete IFN-γ, which activates macrophages to kill intracellular yeasts. In addition, *Histoplasma* induces macrophages to secrete TNF, which recruits and stimulates other macrophages to kill *Histoplasma*.

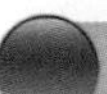

MORPHOLOGY

In the lungs of otherwise healthy adults, *Histoplasma* infections produce **granulomas**, which usually undergo caseation necrosis and coalesce to produce large areas of consolidation, but may also liquefy to form cavities (particularly in patients with COPD). With spontaneous resolution or effective treatment, these lesions undergo fibrosis and concentric calcification (tree-bark appearance) (Fig. 15-37*A*). Histologic differentiation from tuberculosis, sarcoidosis, and coccidioidomycosis requires identification of the 3- to 5-μm thin-walled yeast forms, which may persist in tissues for years.

In **fulminant disseminated histoplasmosis**, which occurs in immunosuppressed individuals, granulomas do not form; instead, there are focal accumulations of mononuclear phagocytes filled with fungal yeasts throughout the body (Fig. 15-37*B*).

The diagnosis of histoplasmosis is established by culture or identification of the fungus in tissue lesions. In addition, serologic tests for antibodies and antigen are also available. Antigen detection in body fluids is most useful in the early stages, because antibodies are formed 2 to 6 weeks after infection.

Blastomycosis

Blastomyces dermatitidis is a soil-inhabiting dimorphic fungus. It causes disease in the central and southeastern United States; infection also occurs in Canada, Mexico, the Middle East, Africa, and India. There are three clinical forms: *pulmonary blastomycosis, disseminated blastomycosis,* and a rare *primary cutaneous form* that results from direct inoculation of organisms into the skin. Pulmonary blastomycosis most often presents as an abrupt illness with productive cough, headache, chest pain, weight loss, fever, abdominal pain, night sweats, chills, and anorexia. Chest radiographs reveal lobar consolidation, multilobar infiltrates, perihilar infiltrates, multiple nodules, or miliary infiltrates. The upper lobes are most frequently involved. The pneumonia most often resolves spontaneously, but it may persist, or progress to a chronic lesion.

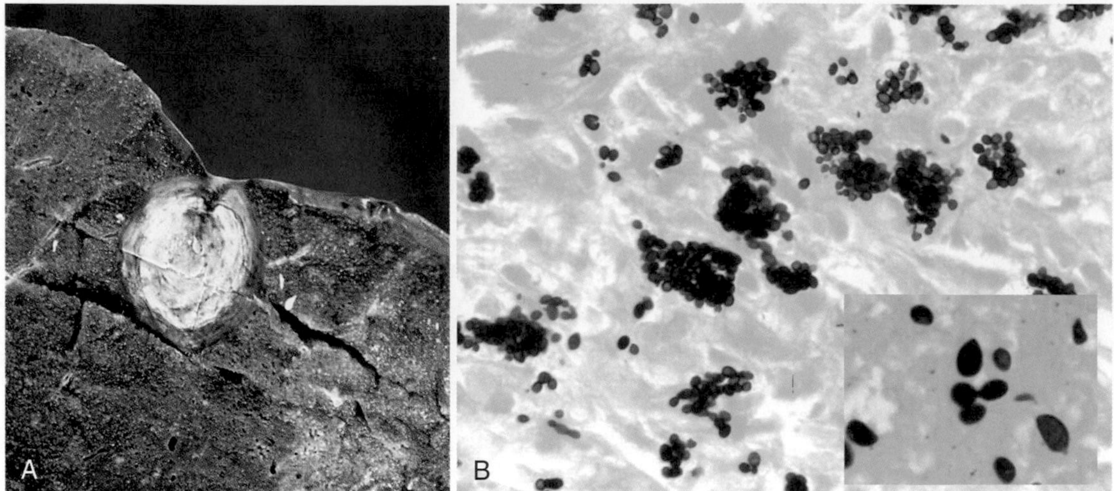

Figure 15-37 Histoplasmosis. **A,** Laminated *Histoplasma* granuloma of the lung. **B,** *Histoplasma capsulatum* yeast forms fill phagocytes in the lung of a patient with disseminated histoplasmosis, inset shows high power of pear-shaped thin-based budding yeasts (silver stain).

MORPHOLOGY

In the normal host, the lung lesions of blastomycosis are suppurative granulomas. Macrophages have a limited ability to ingest and kill *B. dermatitidis*, and the persistence of the yeast cells leads to continued recruitment of neutrophils. In tissue, *B. dermatitidis* is a round, 5- to 15-μm yeast cell that divides by broad-based budding. It has a thick, double-contoured cell wall, and visible nuclei (Fig. 15-38). Involvement of the skin and larynx is associated with marked epithelial hyperplasia, which may be mistaken for squamous cell carcinoma.

Coccidioidomycosis

Almost everyone who inhales the spores of *Coccidioides immitis* becomes infected and develops a delayed-type hypersensitivity reaction to the fungus. Indeed, more than 80% of people in endemic areas of the southwestern and western United States and in Mexico have a positive skin test reaction. One reason for the infectivity of *C. immitis* is that infective arthroconidia, when ingested by alveolar macrophages, block fusion of the phagosome and lysosome and so resist intracellular killing. As is the case with *Histoplasma*, most primary infections with *C. immitis* are asymptomatic, but 10% of infected people develop lung lesions, fever, cough, and pleuritic pains, accompanied by erythema nodosum or erythema multiforme (the San Joaquin Valley fever complex). Less than 1% of people develop disseminated *C. immitis* infection, which frequently involves the skin and meninges. Certain ethnic groups (e.g., Filipinos and African Americans) and the immunosuppressed are at particularly high risk for disseminated disease.

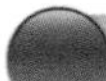

MORPHOLOGY

The primary and secondary lung lesions of *C. immitis* are similar to the granulomatous lesions of *Histoplasma*. Within macrophages or giant cells, *C. immitis* is present as thick-walled, nonbudding spherules 20 to 60 μm in diameter, often filled with small endospores. A pyogenic reaction is superimposed when the spherules rupture to release the endospores (Fig. 15-39). Rare progressive *C. immitis* disease involves the lungs, meninges, skin, bones, adrenals, lymph nodes, spleen, or liver. At all these sites, the inflammatory response may be purely granulomatous, pyogenic, or mixed. Purulent lesions dominate in patients with diminished resistance and with widespread dissemination.

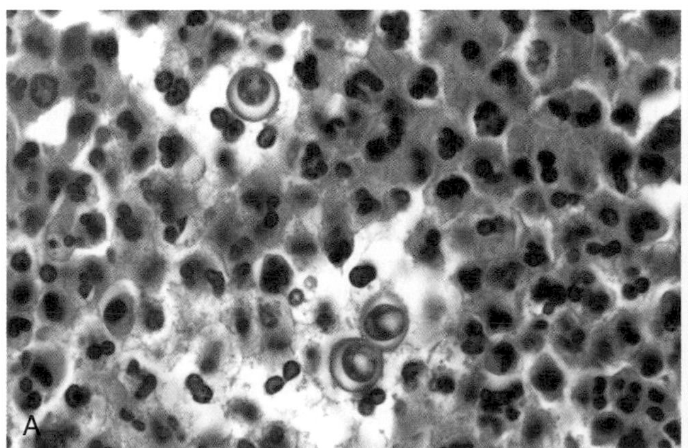

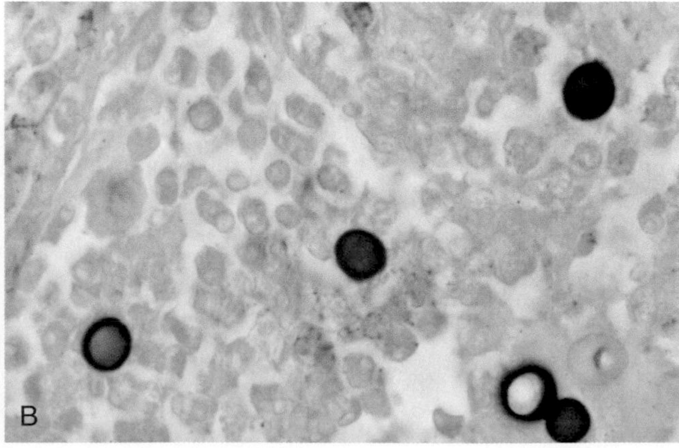

Figure 15-38 Blastomycosis. **A,** Rounded budding yeasts, larger than neutrophils, are present. Note the characteristic thick wall and nuclei (not seen in other fungi). **B,** Silver stain.

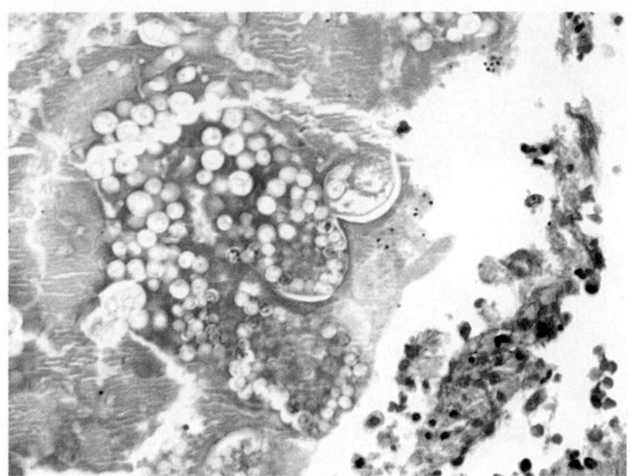

Figure 15-39 Coccidioidomycosis. Intact and ruptured spherules are seen.

Pneumonia in the Immunocompromised Host

The appearance of a pulmonary infiltrate, with or without signs of infection (e.g., fever), is one of the most common and serious complications in patients whose immune defenses are suppressed by disease, immunosuppressive therapy for organ or hematopoietic stem cell transplants, chemotherapy for tumors, or irradiation. A wide variety of so-called opportunistic infectious agents, many of which rarely cause infection in normal hosts, can cause these pneumonias, and often more than one agent is involved. Mortality from these opportunistic infections is high. Table 15-8 lists some of the opportunistic agents according to their prevalence and whether they cause local or diffuse pulmonary infiltrates. The differential diagnosis of such infiltrates includes drug reactions and involvement of the lung by tumor. The specific infections are discussed in Chapter 8. Of these, the ones that commonly involve the lung can be classified according to the etiologic agent: (1) bacteria (*P. aeruginosa, Mycobacterium* species, *L. pneumophila,* and *Listeria monocytogenes*), (2) viruses (cytomegalovirus [CMV] and herpesvirus), and (3) fungi (*P. jiroveci, Candida* species, *Aspergillus* species, the Phycomycetes, and *Cryptococcus neoformans*).

Table 15-8 Causes of Pulmonary Infiltrates in Immunocompromised Hosts

Diffuse Infiltrates	Focal Infiltrates
Common	
Cytomegalovirus	Gram-negative bacterial infections
Pneumocystis jiroveci	*Staphylococcus aureus*
Drug reaction	*Aspergillus*
	Candida
	Malignancy
Uncommon	
Bacterial pneumonia	*Cryptococcus*
Aspergillus	*Mucor*
Cryptococcus	*Pneumocystis jiroveci*
Malignancy	*Legionella pneumophila*

Pulmonary Disease in Human Immunodeficiency Virus Infection

Pulmonary disease accounts for 30% to 40% of hospitalizations in HIV-infected individuals. Although the use of potent antiretroviral agents and effective chemoprophylaxis has markedly altered the incidence and outcome of pulmonary disease in HIV-infected persons, the plethora of infectious agents and other pulmonary lesions make diagnosis and treatment a distinct challenge. Some of the individual microbial agents afflicting HIV-infected individuals have already been discussed; this section focuses only on the general principles of HIV-associated pulmonary disease.

- Despite the emphasis on opportunistic infections, it must be remembered that bacterial lower respiratory tract infections caused by the "usual" pathogens is one are among the most serious pulmonary disorders in HIV infection. The implicated organisms include *S. pneumoniae, S. aureus, H. influenzae,* and gram-negative rods. Bacterial pneumonias in HIV-infected persons are more common, more severe, and more often associated with bacteremia than in those without HIV infection.
- Not all pulmonary infiltrates in HIV-infected individuals are infectious in etiology. A host of noninfectious diseases, including Kaposi sarcoma (Chapters 6 and 11), non-Hodgkin lymphoma (Chapter 13), and lung cancer, occur with increased frequency and must be excluded.
- The CD4+ T-cell count determines the risk of infection with specific organisms. As a rule of thumb, bacterial and tubercular infections are more likely at higher CD4+ counts (>200 cells/mm^3). *Pneumocystis* pneumonia usually strikes at CD4+ counts less than 200 cells/mm^3, while cytomegalovirus, fungal, and *Mycobacterium avium* complex infections are uncommon until the very late stages of immunosuppression (CD4+ counts less than 50 cells/mm^3).

Finally, pulmonary disease in HIV-infected persons may result from more than one cause, and even common pathogens may present with atypical manifestations. Therefore, the diagnostic work-up of these patients may be more extensive (and expensive) than would be necessary in an immunocompetent individual.

Lung Transplantation

Indications for transplantation may include almost all non-neoplastic terminal lung diseases, provided that the patient does not have any other serious disease, which would preclude lifelong immunosuppressive therapy. The most common indications are end-stage emphysema, idiopathic pulmonary fibrosis, cystic fibrosis, and idiopathic/familial pulmonary arterial hypertension. While bilateral lung and heart-lung transplants are possible, in many cases a single-lung transplant is performed, offering sufficient improvement in pulmonary function for two recipients from a single (and all too scarce) donor. When bilateral chronic infection is present (e.g., cystic fibrosis, bronchiectasis), both lungs of the recipient must be replaced to remove the reservoir of infection.

With improving surgical and organ preservation techniques, postoperative complications (e.g., anastomotic dehiscence, vascular thrombosis, primary graft dysfunction) are fortunately becoming rare. The transplanted lung is subject to two major complications: infection and rejection.

- **Pulmonary infections** in lung transplant patients are essentially those of any immunocompromised host, discussed earlier. In the early posttransplant period (the first few weeks), bacterial infections are most common. With ganciclovir prophylaxis and matching of donor-recipient CMV status, CMV pneumonia occurs less frequently and is less severe, although some resistant strains are emerging. Most infections occur in the third to twelfth month after transplantation. *Pneumocystis jiroveci* pneumonia is rare, since almost all patients receive adequate prophylaxis, usually with Bactrim (trimethoprim-sulfamethoxazole). Fungal infections are mostly due to *Aspergillus* and *Candida* species, and they involve the bronchial anastomotic site and/or the lung.
- **Acute rejection** of the lung occurs to some degree in all patients despite routine immunosuppression. It most often appears several weeks to months after surgery but also may present years later or whenever immunosuppression is decreased. Patients present with fever, dyspnea, cough, and radiologic infiltrates. Since these are similar to the picture of infections, diagnosis often relies on transbronchial biopsy.
- **Chronic rejection** is a significant problem in at least half of all patients by 3 to 5 years posttransplant. It is manifested by cough, dyspnea, and an irreversible decrease in lung function tests due to pulmonary fibrosis.

MORPHOLOGY

The morphologic features of acute rejection are primarily those of inflammatory infiltrates (lymphocytes, plasma cells, and few neutrophils and eosinophils), either around small vessels, in the submucosa of airways, or both. The major morphologic correlate of chronic rejection is **bronchiolitis obliterans**, the partial or complete occlusion of small airways by fibrosis, with or without active inflammation (Fig. 15-40). Bronchiolitis obliterans is patchy and therefore difficult to diagnose via transbronchial biopsy. Bronchiectasis and pulmonary fibrosis may develop in long-standing cases.

Acute cellular airway rejection (the presumed forerunner of later, fibrous obliteration of these airways) is generally responsive to therapy, but the treatment of established bronchiolitis obliterans has been disappointing. Its progress may be slowed or even halted for some time, but it cannot be reversed. Infrequent complications of lung transplantation include accelerated pulmonary arteriosclerosis in the graft and EBV-associated B cell lymphoma. With continuing improvement in surgical, immunosuppressive, and antimicrobial therapies, the short-term outcome of lung transplantation has improved considerably, although it is still not as good as that for renal or cardiac transplantation. One-, five-, and ten-year survival rates are 79%, 53%, and 30%, respectively.

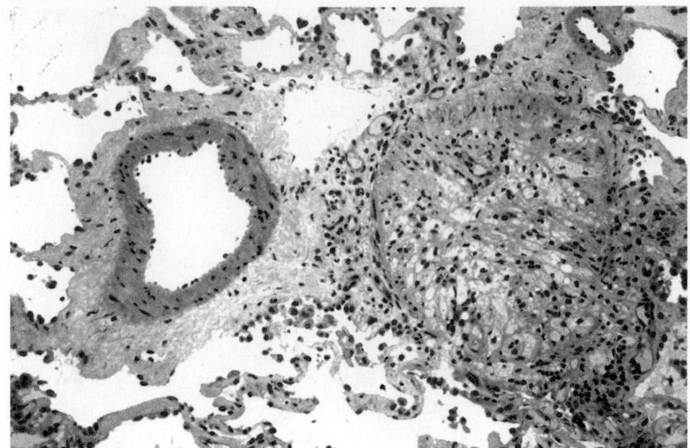

Figure 15-40 Chronic rejection of lung allograft associated with bronchiole (bronchiolitis obliterans). An adjacent pulmonary artery is normal. (Courtesy of Dr. Thomas Krausz, Department of Pathology, The University of Chicago, Pritzker School of Medicine, Chicago, IL.)

Tumors

A variety of benign and malignant tumors may arise in the lung, but 90% to 95% are carcinomas, about 5% are bronchial carcinoids, and 2% to 5% are mesenchymal and other miscellaneous neoplasms.

Carcinomas

Lung cancer is currently the most frequently diagnosed major cancer in the world (estimated 1.6 million new cases in 2008) **and the most common cause of cancer mortality worldwide** (1,380,000 deaths in 2008). This is largely due to the carcinogenic effects of cigarette smoke. Over the coming decades, changes in smoking habits will greatly influence lung cancer incidence and mortality as well as the prevalence of various histologic types of lung cancer.

The number of new cases of lung cancer occurring in 2012 in the United States was estimated to be 226,160 (note that in 1950 it was 18,000), accounting for about 14% of cancer diagnoses and 160,340 deaths, roughly 28% of all cancer-related deaths. As can be gathered from the sobering fact that the yearly mortality almost matches the yearly incidence, the overall outlook for affected patients remains bleak. Since the early 1990s, lung cancer incidence and mortality rates have been decreasing in men, due to the decreased smoking rates over the past 35 years. However, decreases in smoking patterns among women lag behind those of men. Since 1987 more women have died each year of lung cancer than of breast cancer, which for more than 40 years had been the major cause of cancer death in women. Cancer of the lung occurs most often between ages 40 and 70 years, with a peak incidence in the 50s or 60s. Only 2% of all cases appear before the age of 40.

Etiology and Pathogenesis. Most (but not all) lung cancers are associated with a well-known carcinogen—cigarette smoke. In addition there are other genetic and environmental factors which we will discuss after the role of tobacco smoking. The molecular changes to vary among the histologic subtypes, which will be described later. Suffice it to say that lung cancers can be broadly classified into small cell and non-small cell types and the latter group is made up of squamous cell and adenocarcinomas.

Tobacco Smoking. **About 80% of lung cancers occur in active smokers or those who stopped recently.** There is a nearly linear correlation between the frequency of lung cancer and pack-years of cigarette smoking. The increased risk becomes 60 times greater among habitual heavy smokers (two packs a day for 20 years) compared with nonsmokers. However, since lung cancer develops in only 11% of heavy smokers, there are other factors that predispose individuals to this deadly disease. For reasons not entirely clear, women have a higher susceptibility to carcinogens in tobacco than men. Although cessation of smoking decreases the risk for lung cancer over time, it may never return to baseline levels. In fact, genetic changes that predate lung cancer can persist for many years in the bronchial epithelium of former smokers. Passive smoking (proximity to cigarette smokers) increases the risk for lung cancer development to approximately twice that of nonsmokers. The smoking of pipes and cigars also increases the risk, but only modestly.

Although the duration and intensity of smoking are well correlated with cancer risk, not all persons exposed to tobacco smoke develop cancer. Some of this may be a matter of chance, but it is also likely that the mutagenic effect of carcinogens in smoke is modified by genetic variants. Recall that many chemicals (procarcinogens) are converted into carcinogens via activation by the highly polymorphic P-450 monooxygenase enzyme system (Chapter 9). Specific P-450 polymorphisms have an increased capacity to activate procarcinogens in cigarette smoke, and smokers with these genetic variants appear to incur a greater risk of lung cancer. Similarly, individuals whose peripheral blood lymphocytes show more numerous chromosomal breakages after exposure to tobacco-related carcinogens (mutagen sensitivity genotype) have a greater than 10-fold higher risk of developing lung cancer as compared with controls, presumably because of genetic variation in genes involved in DNA repair.

The histologic changes that correlate with steps along the path to neoplastic transformation are best documented for squamous cell carcinomas and are described in more detail later. There is a linear correlation between the intensity of exposure to cigarette smoke and the appearance of ever more worrisome epithelial changes. These begin with rather innocuous-appearing basal cell hyperplasia and squamous metaplasia and progress to squamous dysplasia and carcinoma in situ, the last stage before progression to invasive cancer.

Unfortunately, the carcinogenic effects of tobacco smoke extend to those who live and work with smokers. *Secondhand smoke*, or environmental tobacco smoke, contains numerous human carcinogens for which there is no safe level of exposure. It is estimated that each year about 3000 nonsmoking adults die of lung cancer as a result of breathing secondhand smoke. Cigar and pipe smoking also increase risk, although much less than smoking cigarettes. Smokeless tobacco is not a safe substitute for smoking cigarettes or cigars, as these products spare the lung but cause oral cancers and can lead to nicotine addiction.

Industrial Hazards. Certain industrial exposures, such as asbestos, arsenic, chromium, uranium, nickel, vinyl chloride and mustard gas, increase the risk of developing lung cancer. High-dose ionizing *radiation* is carcinogenic. There was an increased incidence of lung cancer among survivors of the Hiroshima and Nagasaki atomic bomb blasts, as well as in workers heavily involved in clean-up after the Chernobyl disaster. *Uranium* is weakly radioactive, but lung cancer rates among nonsmoking uranium miners are four times higher than those in the general population, and among smoking miners they are about 10 times higher. *Asbestos* exposure also increases the risk for lung cancer development. The latent period before the development of lung cancer is 10 to 30 years. Lung cancer is the most frequent malignancy in individuals exposed to asbestos, particularly when coupled with smoking. Asbestos workers who do not smoke have a five-fold greater risk of developing lung cancer than do nonsmoking control subjects, and those who smoke have a 55-fold greater risk.

Air Pollution. It is uncertain whether air pollution, by itself, increases the risk of lung cancer, but it likely adds to the risk in those who smoke or are exposed to secondhand smoke. It may do so through several different mechanisms. Chronic exposure to air particulates in smog may cause lung irritation, inflammation and repair, and you will recall that chronic inflammation and repair increases the risk of a variety of cancers (Chapter 7). A specific form of air pollution that may contribute to an increased risk of lung cancer is radon gas. Radon is a ubiquitous radioactive gas that has been linked epidemiologically to increased lung cancer in uranium miners, particularly those who smoke. This has generated concern that low-level exposure (e.g., in well-insulated homes in areas with naturally high levels of radon in soil) may also increase the incidence of lung cancers, but this point remains unsettled.

Molecular Genetics. As with other cancers (Chapter 7), smoking-related carcinomas of the lung arise by a stepwise accumulation of oncogenic "driver" mutations that result in the neoplastic transformation of pulmonary epithelial cells. Some of the genetic changes associated with cancers can be found in the "benign" bronchial epithelium of smokers without lung cancers, suggesting that large areas of the respiratory mucosa are mutagenized by exposure to carcinogens in tobacco smoke ("field effect"). On this fertile soil, those few cells that accumulate a sufficient panoply of complementary driver mutations to acquire all of the hallmarks of cancer (Chapter 7) develop into invasive carcinomas.

Lung carcinomas fall into several major histologic subgroups (described later), each with distinctive molecular features, as follows:

- *Squamous cell carcinoma* is highly associated with exposure to tobacco smoke and harbors diverse genetic aberrations, many of which are chromosome deletions involving tumor suppressor loci. These losses, especially those involving 3p, 9p (site of the *CDKN2A* gene), and 17p (site of the *TP53* gene) are early events in tumor evolution, being detected at an appreciable frequency in the histologically normal respiratory mucosal cells of smokers. Squamous cell carcinomas show the highest frequency of *TP53* mutations of all histologic types of lung carcinoma. p53 protein overexpression (as seen by immunohistochemical staining), a marker of *TP53* mutations, is also an early event, being reported in 10% to 50% of squamous dysplasias and 60% to 90% of squamous cell carcinoma in situ. Loss of expression of the retinoblastoma (RB) tumor suppressor is identified by immunohistochemistry in 15% of squamous cell carcinomas. The cyclin-dependent kinase inhibitor gene *CDKN2A* is inactivated and its protein product, p16, is lost in 65% of tumors. It has recently been recognized that many squamous cell carcinomas have amplification of *FGFR1*, a gene encoding the fibroblast growth factor receptor tyrosine kinase.

- *Small cell carcinoma* shows the strongest association with smoking and despite its divergent histologic features shares many molecular features with squamous cell carcinoma. This includes frequent loss-of-function aberrations involving *TP53* (75% to 90% of tumors), *RB* (close to 100% of tumors), and chromosome 3p deletions. Also common is amplification of genes of the *MYC* family.
- *Adenocarcinoma* is marked by oncogenic gain-of-function mutations involving components of growth factor receptor signaling pathways. All are found in a minority of tumors, but together they make up a substantial fraction of tumors as a whole. These include gain-of-function mutations in multiple genes encoding receptor tyrosine kinases, including *EGFR, ALK, ROS, MET,* and *RET,* which are all also mutated in other forms of cancer. Tumors without tyrosine kinase gene mutations often have mutations in the *KRAS* gene, which you will remember lies downstream of receptor tyrosine kinases in growth factor signaling pathways.

Lung Cancer in Never Smokers. The WHO estimates that 25% of lung cancer worldwide occurs in never smokers. This percentage is probably closer to 10% to 15% in Western countries. These cancers occur more commonly in women and most are adenocarcinomas. Cancers in nonsmokers are more likely to have *EGFR* mutations, and almost never have *KRAS* mutations; *TP53* mutations are not uncommon, but occur less frequently than in smoking-related cancers.

Table 15-9 Histologic Classification of Malignant Epithelial Lung Tumors

Tumor Classification
Squamous cell carcinoma
Papillary, clear cell, small cell, basaloid
Small-cell carcinoma
Combined small-cell carcinoma
Adenocarcinoma
Minimally invasive adenocarcinoma (nonmucinous, mucinous)
Lepidic, acinar; papillary, solid (according to predominant pattern)
Mucinous adenocarcinoma
Large-cell carcinoma
Large-cell neuroendocrine carcinoma
Adenosquamous carcinoma
Carcinomas with pleomorphic, sarcomatoid, or sarcomatous elements
Carcinoid tumor
Typical, atypical
Carcinomas of salivary gland type

Precursor (Preinvasive) Lesions. Four types of morphologic precursor epithelial lesions are recognized: (1) squamous dysplasia and carcinoma in situ, (2) atypical adenomatous hyperplasia, (3) adenocarcinoma in situ, and (4) diffuse idiopathic pulmonary neuroendocrine cell hyperplasia. It should be remembered that the term *precursor* does not imply that progression to cancer is inevitable. Currently it is not possible to distinguish between precursor lesions that progress and those that remain localized or regress.

Classification. Tumor classification is important for consistency in patient treatment and because it provides a basis for epidemiologic and biologic studies. The most recent classification is given in Table 15-9. Several histologic variants of each type of lung cancer are described; however, their clinical significance is still undetermined, except as mentioned herein. The relative proportions of the major categories are:

Figure 15-41 Atypical adenomatous hyperplasia. The epithelium is cuboidal and there is mild interstitial fibrosis.

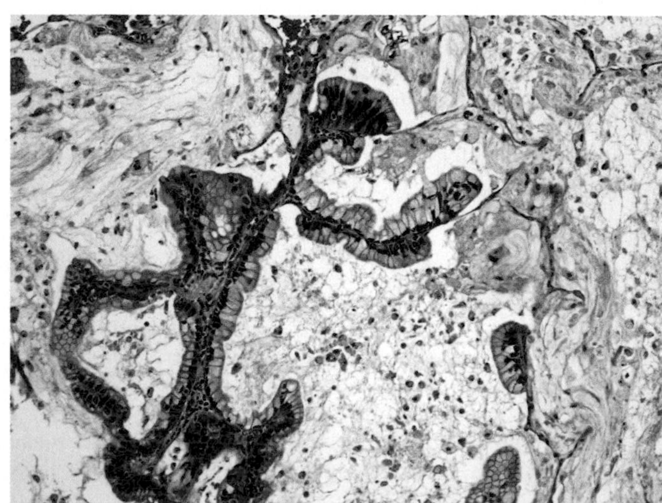

Figure 15-42 Adenocarcinoma in situ, mucinous subtype. Characteristic growth along pre-existing alveolar septa is evident, without invasion.

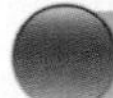

- Adenocarcinoma (38%)
- Squamous cell carcinoma (20%)
- Small cell carcinoma (14%)
- Large cell carcinoma (3%)
- Other (25%)

There may be mixtures of histologic patterns, even in the same cancer. Thus, combinations of squamous cell carcinoma and adenocarcinoma or small-cell and squamous cell carcinoma occur in about 10% of patients.

The incidence of adenocarcinoma has increased significantly in the last 2 decades. Adenocarcinoma is now the most common form of lung cancer in women and, in many studies, men as well. The basis for this change is unclear. A possible factor is the increase in women smokers, but this only highlights our lack of knowledge about why women tend to develop more adenocarcinomas. One possibility is that changes in cigarette type (filter tips, lower tar and nicotine) have caused smokers to inhale more deeply and thereby expose more peripheral airways and cells (with a predilection to adenocarcinoma) to carcinogens.

MORPHOLOGY

Lung carcinomas may arise in the peripheral lung (more often adenocarcinomas) or in the central/hilar region (more often squamous cell carcinomas), sometimes in association with recognizable precursor lesions.

Atypical adenomatous hyperplasia is a small lesion (≤5 mm) characterized by dysplastic pneumocytes lining alveolar walls that are mildly fibrotic (Fig. 15-41). It can be single or multiple and can be in the lung adjacent to invasive tumor or away from it.

Adenocarcinoma in situ (formerly called bronchioloalveolar carcinoma) is a lesion that is less than 3 cm and is composed entirely of dysplastic cells growing along preexisting alveolar septae. The cells have more dysplasia than atypical adenomatous hyperplasia and may or may not have intracellular mucin (mucinous and nonmucinous, respectively) (Fig. 15-42).

Adenocarcinoma is an invasive malignant epithelial tumor with glandular differentiation or mucin production by the tumor cells. Adenocarcinomas grow in various patterns, including acinar, lepidic, papillary, micropapillary, and solid with mucin formation. Compared with squamous cell cancers, the lesions are usually more peripherally located and tend to be smaller. They vary histologically from well-differentiated tumors with obvious glandular elements (Fig. 15-43*A*) to papillary lesions

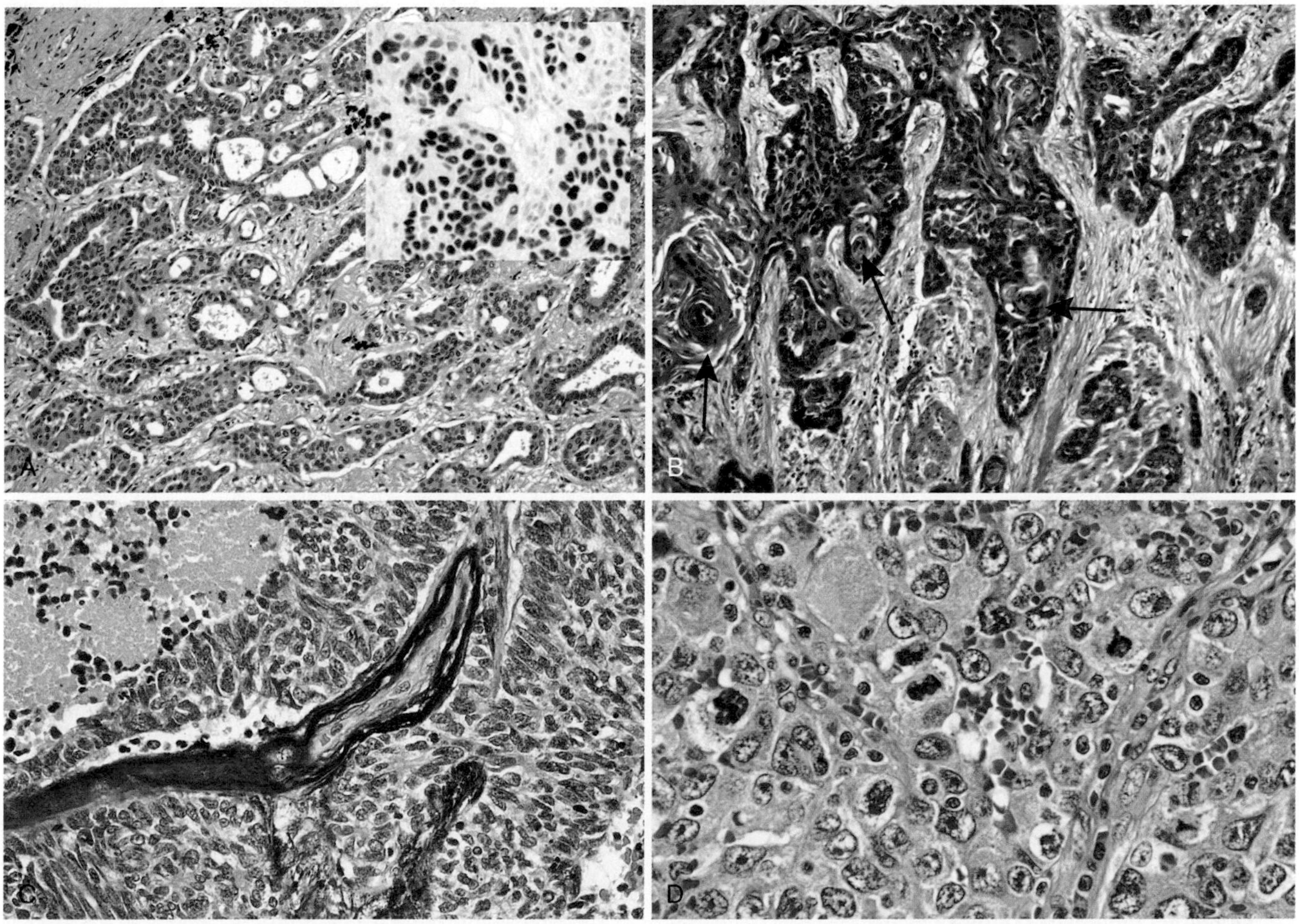

Figure 15-43 Histologic variants of lung carcinoma. **A,** Gland-forming adenocarcinoma; *inset* shows thyroid transcription factor 1 (TTF-1) expression, as detected by immunohistochemistry. **B,** Well-differentiated squamous cell carcinoma showing keratinization *(arrow)*. **C,** Small cell carcinoma. There are islands of small deeply basophilic cells and areas of necrosis. **D,** Large cell carcinoma. The tumor cells are pleomorphic and show no evidence of squamous or glandular differentiation.

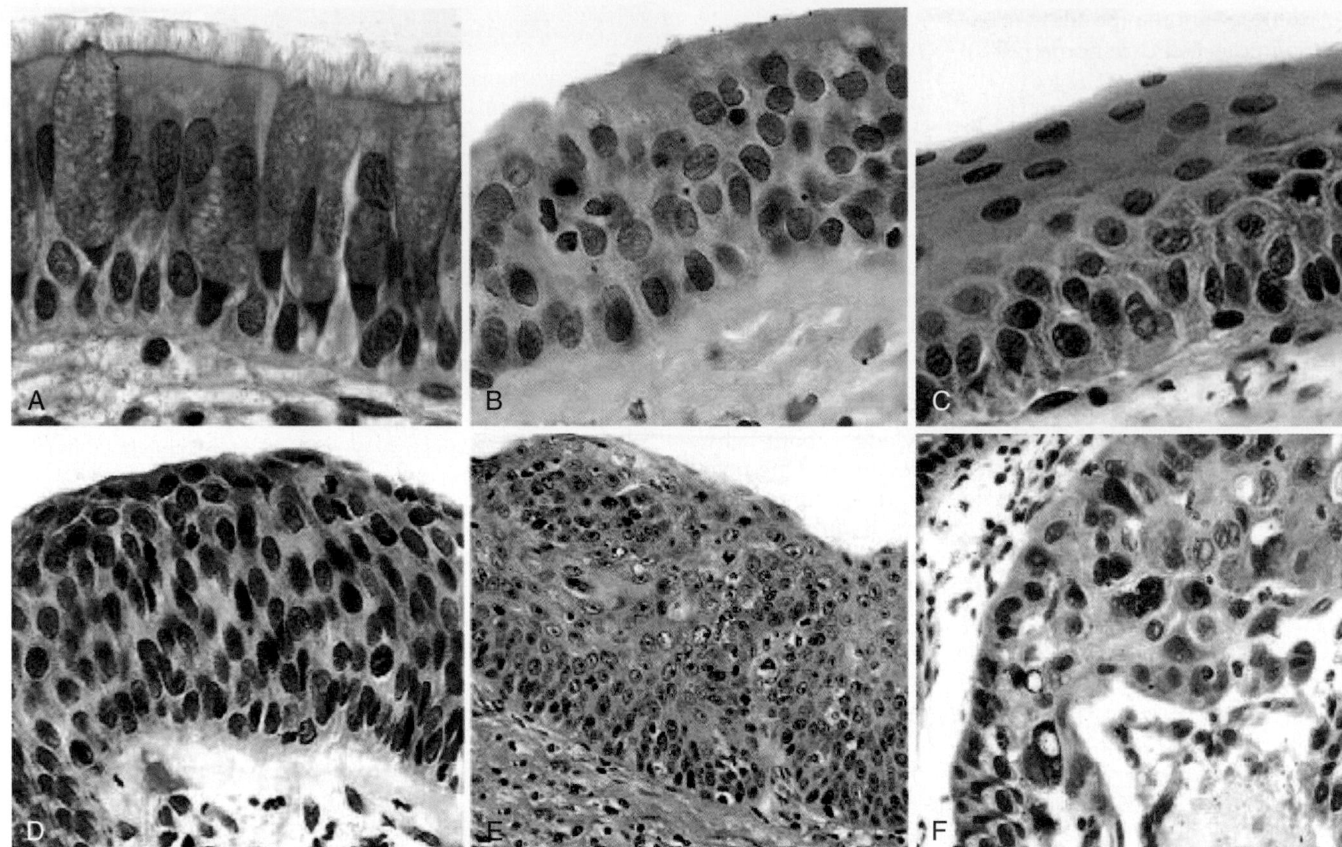

Figure 15-44 Precursor lesions of squamous cell carcinomas. Some of the earliest ("mild") changes in smoking-damaged respiratory epithelium include goblet cell hyperplasia **(A),** basal cell (or reserve cell) hyperplasia **(B),** and squamous metaplasia **(C).** More ominous changes include the appearance of squamous dysplasia **(D),** characterized by the presence of disordered squamous epithelium, with loss of nuclear polarity, nuclear hyperchromasia, pleomorphism, and mitotic figures. Squamous dysplasia may progress through the stages of mild, moderate, and severe dysplasia. Carcinoma-in-situ (CIS) **(E)**, the stage immediately preceding invasive squamous carcinoma **(F)**, by definition has not penetrated the basement membrane and has cytologic features similar to those in frank carcinoma. (**A-E,** Courtesy Dr. Adi Gazdar, Department of Pathology, University of Texas, Southwestern Medical School, Dallas. **F,** Reproduced with permission from Travis WD, et al [eds]: World Health Organization Histological Typing of Lung and Pleural Tumors. Heidelberg, Springer, 1999.)

resembling other papillary carcinomas to solid masses with only occasional mucin-producing glands and cells. The majority express thyroid transcription factor-1 (Fig 15-43*A* inset); first identified in the thyroid, this factor is required for normal lung development. At the periphery of the tumor there is often a lepidic pattern of spread, in which the tumor cells "crawl" along normal-appearing alveolar septae. Tumors (≤3 cm) with a small invasive component (≤5 mm) associated with scarring and a peripheral lepidic growth pattern are called **microinvasive adenocarcinoma**. These have a far better outcome than invasive carcinomas of the same size. **Mucinous adenocarcinomas** tend to spread aerogenously, forming satellite tumors. These may present as a solitary nodule or as multiple nodules, or an entire lobe may be consolidated by tumor, resembling lobar pneumonia and thus are less likely to be cured by surgery.

Squamous cell carcinoma is most commonly found in men and is **s**trongly associated with smoking. Precursors lesions that give rise to invasive squamous cell carcinoma are well characterized. Squamous cell carcinomas are often antedated by **squamous metaplasia** or **dysplasia** in the bronchial epithelium, which then transforms to **carcinoma in situ,** a phase that may last for several years (Fig. 15-44). By this time, atypical cells may be identified in cytologic smears of sputum or in bronchial lavage fluids or brushings (Fig. 15-45), although the lesion is asymptomatic and undetectable on radiographs. Eventually, an invasive squamous cell carcinoma appears. The tumor may then follow a variety of paths. It may grow exophytically into the bronchial lumen, producing an intraluminal mass. With further enlargement the bronchus becomes obstructed, leading to distal atelectasis and infection. The tumor may also penetrate the wall of the bronchus and infiltrate along the peribronchial tissue (Fig. 15-46) into the adjacent carina or mediastinum. In other instances, the tumor grows along a broad front to produce a cauliflower-like intraparenchymal mass that pushes lung substance ahead of it. As in almost all types of lung cancer, the neoplastic tissue is gray-white and firm to hard. Especially when the tumors are bulky, focal areas of hemorrhage or necrosis may appear to produce red or yellow-white mottling and softening. Sometimes these necrotic foci cavitate.

Histologically, squamous cell carcinoma is characterized by the presence of keratinization and/or intercellular bridges. Keratinization may take the form of squamous pearls or individual cells with markedly eosinophilic dense cytoplasm (Fig. 15-43*B*). These features are prominent in well-differentiated tumors, are easily seen but not extensive in moderately

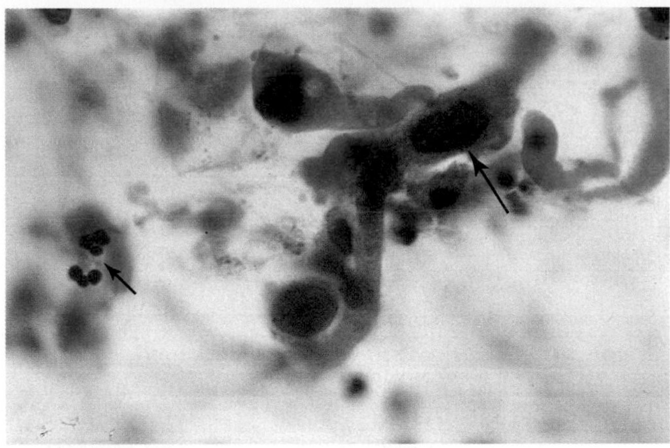

Figure 15-45 Cytologic diagnosis of lung cancer. A sputum specimen shows an orange-staining, keratinized squamous carcinoma cell with a prominent hyperchromatic nucleus *(large arrow)*. Note the size of the tumor cells compared with normal neutrophils (*small arrow*).

differentiated tumors, and are focally seen in poorly differentiated tumors. Mitotic activity is higher in poorly differentiated tumors. In the past, most squamous cell carcinomas were seen to arise centrally from the segmental or subsegmental bronchi. However, the incidence of squamous cell carcinoma of the peripheral lung is increasing. Squamous metaplasia, epithelial dysplasia, and foci of frank carcinoma in situ may be seen in bronchial epithelium adjacent to the tumor mass (Fig. 15-44).

Small cell carcinoma is a highly malignant tumor with a strong relationship to cigarette smoking; only about 1% occurs in nonsmokers. They may arise in major bronchi or in the periphery of the lung. There is no known preinvasive phase. They are the most aggressive of lung tumors, metastasizing widely and virtually always proving to be fatal.

Small cell carcinoma is comprised of relatively small cells with scant cytoplasm, ill-defined cell borders, finely granular nuclear chromatin (salt and pepper pattern), and absent or inconspicuous nucleoli (Fig. 15-43*C*). The cells are round, oval, or spindle-shaped, and nuclear molding is prominent. There is no absolute size for the tumor cells, but in general they are smaller than three times the diameter of a small resting lymphocyte (a size of about 25 microns). The mitotic count is high. The cells grow in clusters that exhibit neither glandular nor squamous organization. Necrosis is common and often extensive. Basophilic staining of vascular walls due to encrustation by DNA from necrotic tumor cells (Azzopardi effect) is frequently present. All small cell carcinomas are high grade. Combined small cell carcinoma is a variant in which typical small cell carcinoma is mixed with non-small cell histologies, such as large cell neuroendocrine carcinoma and even spindled cell morphologies resembling sarcoma.

Electron microscopy shows dense-core neurosecretory granules, about 100 nm in diameter, in two thirds of cases. The occurrence of neurosecretory granules, the expression of neuroendocrine markers such as chromogranin, synaptophysin, and CD57, and the ability of some of these tumors to secrete hormones (e.g., parathormone-related protein, a cause of paraneoplastic hypercalcemia) suggest that this tumor originates from neuroendocrine progenitor cells, which are present in the lining bronchial epithelium. Among the various types of lung cancer, small cell carcinoma is the one that is most commonly associated with ectopic hormone production (discussed later). Immunohistochemistry demonstrates high levels of the anti-apoptotic protein BCL2 in 90% of tumors.

Large cell carcinoma is an undifferentiated malignant epithelial tumor that lacks the cytologic features of other forms of lung cancer. The cells typically have large nuclei, prominent nucleoli, and a moderate amount of cytoplasm (Fig. 15-43*D*). Large cell carcinoma is a diagnosis of exclusion since is expresses none of the markers associated with adenocarcinoma (TTF-1, napsin A) and squamous cell carcinoma (p63, p40) (Fig 15-43*A* inset). One histologic variant is large cell neuroendocrine carcinoma, which has molecular features similar to those that characterize small cell carcinoma, but is comprised of tumor cells of larger size.

Any type of lung carcinoma may extend on to the pleural surface and then within the pleural cavity or into the pericardium. Metastases to the bronchial, tracheal, and mediastinal nodes can be found in most cases. The frequency of nodal involvement varies slightly with the histologic pattern but averages greater than 50%.

Distant spread of lung carcinoma occurs through both lymphatic and hematogenous pathways. These tumors often spread early throughout the body except for squamous cell carcinoma, which metastasizes outside the thorax late. Metastasis may be the first manifestation of an underlying occult pulmonary lesion. No organ or tissue is spared in the spread of these lesions, but the adrenals, for obscure reasons, are involved in more than half the cases. The liver (30% to 50%), brain (20%), and bone (20%) are additional favored sites of metastases.

Combined Carcinoma. Approximately 10% of all lung carcinomas have a combined histology, including two or more of the aforementioned types.

Secondary Pathology. Lung carcinomas have local effects that may cause several pathologic changes in the lung distal to the point of bronchial involvement. Partial obstruction may cause marked **focal emphysema;** total obstruction may lead to **atelectasis.** The impaired drainage of the airways is a common cause for **severe suppurative or ulcerative bronchitis** or **bronchiectasis. Pulmonary abscesses** sometimes call attention to an otherwise silent carcinoma. Compression or invasion of the superior vena cava can cause venous

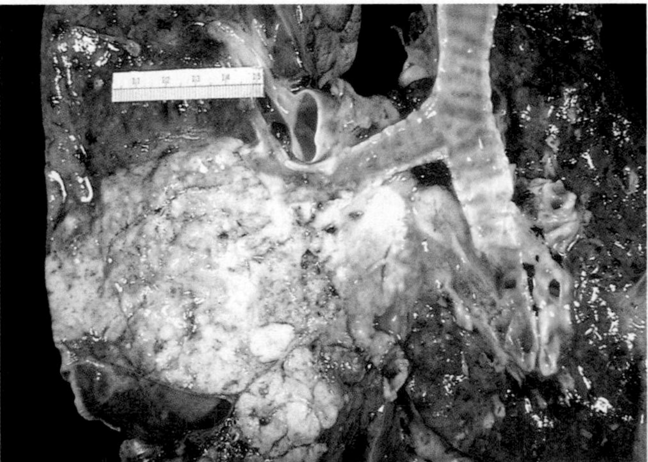

Figure 15-46 Lung carcinoma. The gray-white tumor infiltrates the lung parenchyma. Histologic sections identified this tumor as a squamous cell carcinoma.

congestion and edema of the head and arm, and, ultimately, circulatory compromise—the **superior vena cava syndrome.** Extension to the pericardial or pleural sacs may cause **pericarditis** (Chapter 11) or **pleuritis** with significant effusions.

Staging. A uniform TNM system for staging cancer according to its anatomic extent at the time of diagnosis is useful, particularly for comparing treatment results from different centers (Table 15-10).

Clinical Course. Lung cancer is one of the most insidious and aggressive neoplasms in the realm of oncology. In the usual case it is discovered in patients in their 50s or older whose symptoms are of several months' duration. The major presenting complaints are cough (75%), weight loss (40%), chest pain (40%), and dyspnea (20%). Some of the more common local manifestations of lung cancer and their pathologic bases are listed in Table 15-11. Not infrequently the tumor is discovered by its secondary spread during the course of investigation of an apparent primary or metastatic neoplasm elsewhere. Symptoms of metastases depend on the site, for example, back pain in bone metastases, headache, hemiparesis, cranial nerve damage, and seizures in brain metastases.

Table 15-10 International Staging System for Lung Cancer

TNM Staging			
Tis	Carcinoma in Situ		
T1	Tumor ≤ 3 cm without pleural or mainstem bronchus involvement (T1a, <2 cm; T1b, 2-3 cm)		
T2	Tumor 3-7 cm or involvement of mainstem bronchus 2 cm from carina, visceral pleural involvement, or lobar atelectasis (T2a, 3-5 cm; T2b, 5-7 cm)		
T3	Tumor >7 cm or one with involvement of parietal pleura, chest wall (including superior sulcus tumors), diaphragm, phrenic nerve, mediastinal pleura, parietal pericardium, mainstem bronchus < 2 cm from carina but without involvement of carina, or entire lung atelectasis, or separate tumor nodules in the same lobe		
T4	Any tumor with invasion of mediastinum, heart, great vessels, trachea, recurrent laryngeal nerve, esophagus, vertebral body, or carina or separate tumor nodules in a different ipsilateral lobe		
N0	No metastasis to regional lymph nodes		
N1	Ipsilateral hilar or peribronchial nodal involvement		
N2	Metastasis to ipsilateral mediastinal or subcarinal lymph nodes		
N3	Metastasis to contralateral mediastinal or hilar lymph nodes, ipsilateral or contralateral scalene, or supraclavicular lymph nodes		
M0	No distant metastasis		
M1	Distant metastasis (M1a, separate tumor nodule in contralateral lobe or pleural nodules or malignant pleural effusion; M1b, distant metastasis)		
Stage Grouping			
Stage IA	T1a, T1b	N0	M0
Stage IB	T2a	N0	M0
Stage IIA	T2b T1a, T1b, T2a	N0 N1	M0 M0
Stage IIB	T2b T3	N1 N0	M0 M0
Stage IIIA	T1, T2 T3 T4	N2 N1, N2 N0, N1	M0 M0 M0
Stage IIIB	Any T T4	N3 N2, N3	M0 M0
Stage IV	Any T	Any N	M1a, M1b

Table 15-11 Local Effects of Lung Tumor Spread

Clinical Feature	Pathologic Basis
Cough (50%-75%)	Involvement of central airways
Hemoptysis (25%-50%)	Hemorrhage from tumor in airway
Chest pain (20%)	Extension of tumor into mediastinum, pleura or chest wall
Pneumonia, abscess, lobar collapse	Airway obstruction by tumor
Lipoid pneumonia	Tumor obstruction; accumulation of cellular lipid in foamy macrophages
Pleural effusion	Tumor spread into pleura
Hoarseness	Recurrent laryngeal nerve invasion
Dysphagia	Esophageal invasion
Diaphragm paralysis	Phrenic nerve invasion
Rib destruction	Chest wall invasion
SVC syndrome	SVC compression by tumor
Horner syndrome	Sympathetic ganglia invasion
Pericarditis, tamponade	Pericardial involvement

SVC, Superior vena cava.

Despite some earlier studies that did not show any benefit, the first large-scale early detection trial produced a 20% reduction in lung cancer-related mortality by screening high-risk individuals with low-dose computed tomography. However, the outlook is still poor for most patients with lung carcinoma. Even with many incremental improvements in thoracic surgery, radiation therapy, and chemotherapy, the overall 5-year survival rate is only 16%. The 5-year survival rate is 52% for cases detected when the disease is still localized, 22% when there is regional metastasis and only 4% with distant metastases. In general, adenocarcinoma and squamous cell carcinoma tend to remain localized longer and have a slightly better prognosis than do the undifferentiated cancers, which are usually advanced by the time they are discovered.

Targeted treatment of patients with adenocarcinoma and activating mutations in EGFR (present in about 15% of all patients) or in other tyrosine kinases with specific inhibitors of the mutated kinases prolongs survival. Many tumors that recur carry new mutations that generate resistance to these inhibitors, proving that these drugs are "hitting" their target. In contrast, activating KRAS mutations (present in 30%) appear to be associated with a worse prognosis, regardless of treatment, in an already grim disease. New therapeutic targets are clearly needed.

Untreated, the survival time for patients with small-cell carcinoma is 6 to 17 weeks. This cancer is particularly sensitive to radiation therapy and chemotherapy, and cure rates of 15% to 25% for limited disease have been reported in some centers. However, most patients with small cell carcinoma have distant metastases at diagnosis. Thus, even with treatment, the mean survival after diagnosis is only about 1 year.

Paraneoplastic Syndromes. Lung carcinoma can be associated with several paraneoplastic syndromes (Chapter 7), some of which may antedate the development of a detectable pulmonary lesion. The hormones or hormone-like factors elaborated include:

- *Antidiuretic hormone* (ADH), inducing hyponatremia due to inappropriate ADH secretion
- *Adrenocorticotropic hormone* (ACTH), producing Cushing syndrome
- *Parathormone, parathyroid hormone-related peptide, prostaglandin E, and some cytokines,* all implicated in the hypercalcemia often seen with lung cancer
- *Calcitonin,* causing hypocalcemia
- *Gonadotropins,* causing gynecomastia
- *Serotonin and bradykinin,* associated with the carcinoid syndrome

The incidence of clinically significant syndromes related to these factors in lung cancer patients ranges from 1% to 10%, although a much higher proportion of patients show elevated serum levels of these (and other) peptide hormones. Any histologic type of tumor may occasionally produce any one of the hormones, but tumors that produce ACTH and ADH are predominantly small cell carcinomas, whereas those that produce hypercalcemia are mostly squamous cell carcinomas.

Other systemic manifestations of lung carcinoma include the *Lambert-Eaton myasthenic syndrome* (Chapter 26), in which muscle weakness is caused by auto-antibodies (possibly elicited by tumor ionic channels) directed to the neuronal calcium channel; *peripheral neuropathy,* usually purely sensory; dermatologic abnormalities, including *acanthosis nigricans* (Chapter 25); hematologic abnormalities, such as *leukemoid reactions,* hypercoagulable states such as *Trousseau syndrome* (deep vein thrombosis and thromboembolism); and finally, a peculiar abnormality of connective tissue called *hypertrophic pulmonary osteoarthropathy,* associated with clubbing of the fingers.

Apical lung cancers in the superior pulmonary sulcus tend to invade the neural structures around the trachea, including the cervical sympathetic plexus, and produce a group of clinical findings that includes severe pain in the distribution of the ulnar nerve and *Horner syndrome* (enophthalmos, ptosis, miosis, and anhidrosis) on the same side as the lesion. Such tumors are also referred to as *Pancoast tumors.*

KEY CONCEPTS

Carcinomas of the Lung

- The four major histologic subtypes are adenocarcinomas (most common), squamous cell carcinoma, large cell carcinoma, and small cell carcinoma.
- Each of these is clinically and genetically distinct. Small cell lung carcinomas are best treated by chemotherapy, because almost all are metastatic at presentation. The other carcinomas may be curable by surgery if limited to the lung. Combination chemotherapy also is available along with tyrosine kinase inhibitors for those with EGFR, ALK, ROS, and c-MET mutations.
- Smoking is the most important risk factor for lung cancer; in women and nonsmokers, adenocarcinomas are the most common cancers.
- Precursor lesions include squamous dysplasia for squamous cancer and atypical adenomatous hyperplasia and adenocarcinoma in situ (formerly bronchioloalveolar carcinoma) for adenocarcinomas.
- Tumors 3 cm or less in diameter characterized by pure growth along preexisting structures (lepidic pattern) without stromal invasion are now called *adenocarcinoma in situ.*
- Lung cancers, particularly small cell lung carcinomas, can cause paraneoplastic syndromes.

Neuroendocrine Proliferations and Tumors

The normal lung contains neuroendocrine cells within the epithelium as single cells or as clusters, the neuroepithelial bodies. While virtually all pulmonary neuroendocrine cell hyperplasias are secondary to airway fibrosis and/or inflammation, a rare disorder called *diffuse idiopathic pulmonary neuroendocrine cell hyperplasia* seems to be a precursor to the development of multiple tumorlets and typical or atypical carcinoids.

Neoplasms of neuroendocrine cells in the lung include benign *tumorlets,* small, inconsequential, hyperplastic nests of neuroendocrine cells seen in areas of scarring or chronic inflammation; *carcinoids;* and the (already discussed) highly aggressive small cell carcinoma and large cell neuroendocrine carcinoma of the lung. Carcinoid tumors are classified separately, since they differ significantly from carcinomas with evidence of neuroendocrine differentiation in terms of incidence and clinical, epidemiologic, histologic, and molecular characteristics. For example, in contrast to small cell and large cell neuroendocrine carcinomas, carcinoids may occur in patients with multiple endocrine neoplasia type 1.

Carcinoid Tumors

Carcinoid tumors represent 1% to 5% of all lung tumors. Most patients with these tumors are younger than 40 years of age, and the incidence is equal for both sexes. Approximately 20% to 40% of patients are nonsmokers. Carcinoid tumors are low-grade malignant epithelial neoplasms that are subclassified into *typical* and *atypical carcinoids.*

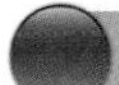

MORPHOLOGY

Carcinoids may arise centrally or may be peripheral. On gross examination, the central tumors grow as fingerlike or spherical polypoid masses that commonly project into the lumen of the bronchus and are usually covered by an intact mucosa (Fig. 15-47*A*). They rarely exceed 3 to 4 cm in diameter. Most are confined to the mainstem bronchi. Others, however, penetrate the bronchial wall to fan out in the peribronchial tissue, producing the so-called **collar-button lesion**. Peripheral tumors are solid and nodular.

Histologically, the tumor is composed of organoid, trabecular, palisading, ribbon, or rosette-like arrangements of cells separated by a delicate fibrovascular stroma. In common with the lesions of the gastrointestinal tract, the individual cells are quite regular and have uniform round nuclei and a moderate

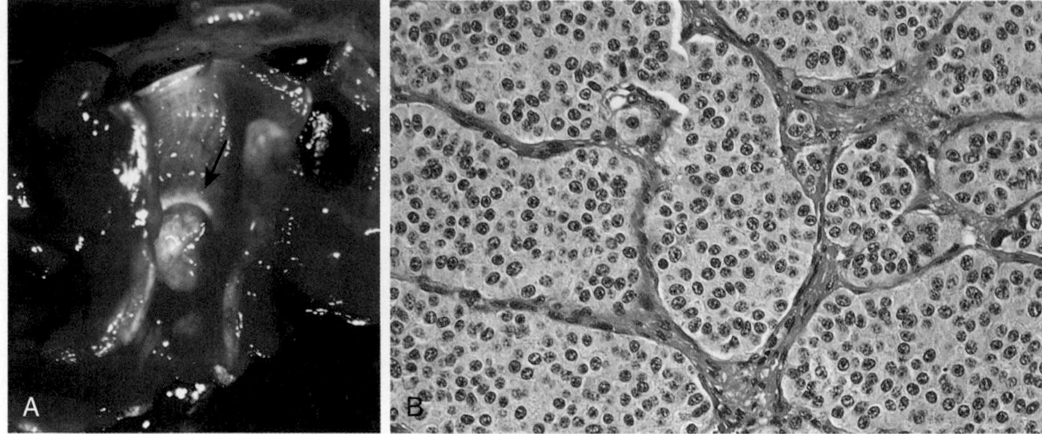

Figure 15-47 Bronchial carcinoid. **A,** Carcinoid growing as a spherical mass *(arrow)* protruding into the lumen of the bronchus. **B,** The tumor cells have small, rounded, uniform nuclei and moderate amounts of cytoplasm. (Courtesy Dr. Thomas Krausz, Department of Pathology, The University of Chicago, Pritzker School of Medicine, Chicago, Ill.)

amount of eosinophilic cytoplasm (Fig. 15-47*B*). Typical carcinoids have fewer than two mitoses per 10 high-power fields and lack necrosis, while atypical carcinoids have between two and 10 mitoses per 10 high-power fields and/or foci of necrosis. Atypical carcinoids also show increased pleomorphism, have more prominent nucleoli, and are more likely to grow in a disorganized fashion and invade lymphatics. On electron microscopy the cells exhibit the dense-core granules characteristic of other neuroendocrine tumors and, by immunohistochemistry, are found to contain serotonin, neuron-specific enolase, bombesin, calcitonin, or other peptides.

Clinical Features. The clinical manifestations of bronchial carcinoids emanate from their intraluminal growth, their capacity to metastasize, and the ability of some of the lesions to elaborate vasoactive amines. Persistent cough, hemoptysis, impairment of drainage of respiratory passages with secondary infections, bronchiectasis, emphysema, and atelectasis are all by-products of the intraluminal growth of these lesions.

Most interesting are functioning lesions capable of producing the classic *carcinoid syndrome*, characterized by intermittent attacks of diarrhea, flushing, and cyanosis. Approximately, 10 % of bronchial carcinoids give rise to this syndrome. Overall, most bronchial carcinoids do not have secretory activity and do not metastasize to distant sites but follow a relatively benign course for long periods and are therefore amenable to resection. The reported 5-year survival rates are 95% for typical carcinoids, 70% for atypical carcinoids, 30% for large cell neuroendocrine carcinoma, and 5% for small cell carcinoma, respectively.

Miscellaneous Tumors

Lesions of the complex category of benign and malignant mesenchymal tumors, such as inflammatory myofibroblastic tumor, fibroma, fibrosarcoma, lymphangioleiomyomatosis, leiomyoma, leiomyosarcoma, lipoma, hemangioma, and chondroma, may occur but are rare. Benign and malignant hematopoietic tumors, similar to those described in other organs, may also affect the lung, either as isolated lesions or, more commonly, as part of a generalized disorder. These include Langerhans cell histiocytosis, non-Hodgkin and Hodgkin lymphomas, lymphomatoid granulomatosis, an unusual EBV-positive B cell lymphoma, and low-grade extranodal marginal zone B-cell lymphoma (Chapter 13).

A lung *hamartoma* is a relatively common lesion that is usually discovered as an incidental, rounded radio-opacity *(coin lesion)* on a routine chest film. Most are, solitary, less than 3 to 4 cm in diameter, and well circumscribed. Pulmonary hamartoma consists of nodules of connective tissue intersected by epithelial clefts. Cartilage is the most common connective tissue, but there may also be cellular fibrous tissue and fat. The epithelial clefts are lined by ciliated columnar epithelium or nonciliated epithelium and probably represent entrapment of respiratory epithelium (Fig. 15-48). The traditional term *hamartoma* is retained for this lesion, but it is in fact a clonal neoplasm associated with chromosomal aberrations involving either 6p21 or 12q14-q15.

Lymphangioleiomyomatosis is a pulmonary disorder that primarily affects young woman of childbearing age. It is

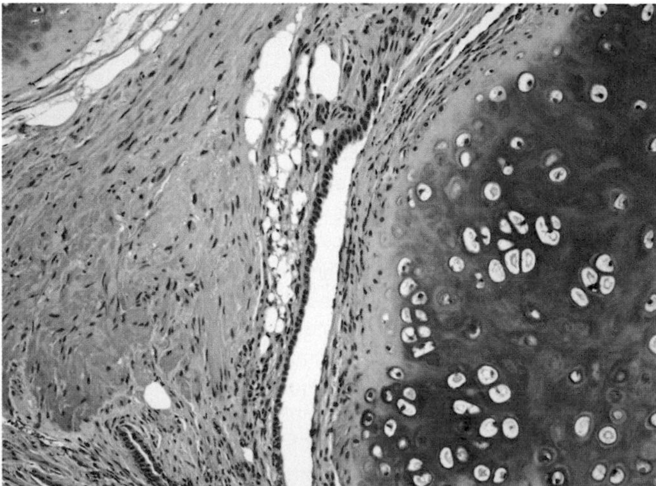

Figure 15-48 Pulmonary hamartoma. There are islands of cartilage, fat, smooth muscle, and entrapped respiratory epithelium.

characterized by a proliferation of perivascular epithelioid cells that express markers of both melanocytes and smooth muscle cells. The proliferation distorts the involved lung, leading to cystic, emphysema-like dilation of terminal airspaces, thickening of the interstitium, and obstruction of lymphatic vessels. The lesional epithelioid cells appear to frequently harbor loss of function mutations in the tumor suppressor *TSC2*, one of the loci linked to tuberous sclerosis (Chapter 28). You will recall that the protein encoded by *TSC2*, tuberin, is a negative regulator of mTOR, a key regulator of cellular metabolism. While *TSC2* mutations points to increased mTOR activity as a contributing factor, the disorder remains poorly understood. The strong tendency to affect young women suggests that estrogen contributes to the proliferation of perivascular epithelioid cells, which often express estrogen receptors. Patients most commonly present with dyspnea or spontaneous pneumothorax, the latter related to the emphysematous changes. The disease tends to be slowly progressive over a period of several decades. mTOR inhibitors are being tested in clinical trials, but lung transplantation is the only definitive treatment available currently.

Inflammatory myofibroblastic tumor, though rare, is more common in children, with an equal male-to-female ratio. Presenting symptoms include fever, cough, chest pain, and hemoptysis. It may also be asymptomatic. Imaging studies show a single (rarely multiple) round, well-defined, usually peripheral mass with calcium deposits in about a quarter of cases. Grossly, the lesion is firm, 3 to 10 cm in diameter, and grayish white. Microscopically, there is proliferation of spindle-shaped fibroblasts and myofibroblasts, lymphocytes, plasma cells, and peripheral fibrosis. Some of these tumors have activating rearrangements of the anaplastic lymphoma kinase (*ALK*) gene, located on 2p23, and treatment with ALK kinase inhibitors have produced sustained responses in such cases.

Tumors in the mediastinum either may arise in mediastinal structures or may be metastatic from the lung or other organs. They may also invade or compress the lungs. Table 15-12 lists the most common tumors in the various compartments of the mediastinum. Specific tumor types are discussed in appropriate sections of this book.

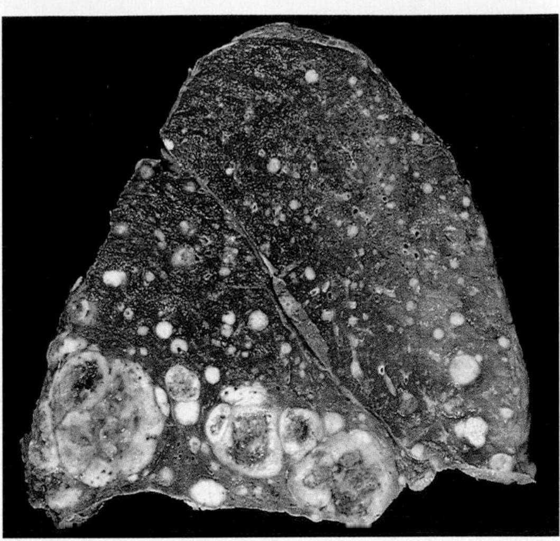

Figure 15-49 Numerous metastases to lung from a renal cell carcinoma. (Courtesy Dr. Michelle Mantel, Brigham and Women's Hospital, Boston, Mass.)

Metastatic Tumors

The lung is the most common site of metastatic neoplasms. Both carcinomas and sarcomas arising anywhere in the body may spread to the lungs via the blood or lymphatics or by direct continuity. Growth of contiguous tumors into the lungs occurs most often with esophageal carcinomas and mediastinal lymphomas.

MORPHOLOGY

The pattern of metastatic growth within the lungs is quite variable. In the usual case, multiple discrete nodules (cannonball lesions) are scattered throughout all lobes, more being at the periphery (Fig. 15-49). Other patterns include solitary nodule, endobronchial, pleural, pneumonic consolidation, and combinations of these. Foci of lepidic growth similar to adenocarcinoma in situ are seen occasionally with metastatic carcinomas and may be associated with any of the listed patterns.

Table 15-12 Mediastinal Tumors and Other Masses

Anterior Mediastinum
Thymoma
Teratoma
Lymphoma
Thyroid lesions
Parathyroid tumors
Metastatic carcinoma
Posterior Mediastinum
Neurogenic tumors (schwannoma, neurofibroma)
Lymphoma
Metastatic tumor (most are from the lung)
Bronchogenic cyst
Gastroenteric hernia
Middle Mediastinum
Bronchogenic cyst
Pericardial cyst
Lymphoma

Pleura

Pathologic involvement of the pleura is, most often, a secondary complication of some underlying disease. Secondary infections and pleural adhesions are particularly common findings at autopsy. Important primary disorders include (1) primary intrapleural bacterial infections that imply seeding of this space as an isolated focus in the course of a transient bacteremia and (2) a primary neoplasm of the pleura: mesothelioma (discussed later).

Pleural Effusion

Pleural effusion is a common manifestation of both primary and secondary pleural diseases, which may be inflammatory or noninflammatory. Normally, no more than 15 mL of serous, relatively acellular, clear fluid lubricates the pleural surface. Accumulation of pleural fluid occurs in the following settings:

- Increased hydrostatic pressure, as in congestive heart failure
- Increased vascular permeability, as in pneumonia
- Decreased osmotic pressure, as in nephrotic syndrome
- Increased intrapleural negative pressure, as in atelectasis
- Decreased lymphatic drainage, as in mediastinal carcinomatosis

Inflammatory Pleural Effusions

Serous, serofibrinous, and fibrinous pleuritis all have an inflammatory basis, differing only in the intensity and duration of the process. The most common causes of pleuritis are disorders associated with inflammation of the underlying lung, such as tuberculosis, pneumonia, lung infarcts, lung abscess, and bronchiectasis. Rheumatoid arthritis, systemic lupus erythematosus, uremia, diffuse systemic infections, other systemic disorders, and metastatic involvement of the pleura can also cause serous or serofibrinous pleuritis. Radiation used in therapy for tumors in the lung or mediastinum often causes a serofibrinous pleuritis. In most of these disorders, the serofibrinous reaction is only minimal, and the fluid exudate is resorbed with either resolution or organization of the fibrinous component. However, large amounts of fluid sometimes accumulate and compress the lung, causing respiratory distress.

A purulent pleural exudate *(empyema)* usually results from bacterial or mycotic seeding of the pleural space. Most commonly, this seeding occurs by contiguous spread of organisms from intrapulmonary infection, but occasionally, it occurs through lymphatic or hematogenous dissemination from a more distant source. Rarely, infections below the diaphragm, such as the subdiaphragmatic or liver abscess, may extend by continuity through the diaphragm into the pleural spaces, more often on the right side.

Empyema is characterized by loculated, yellow-green, creamy pus composed of masses of neutrophils admixed with other leukocytes. Although empyema may accumulate in large volumes (up to 500 to 1000 mL), usually the volume is small, and the pus becomes localized. Empyema may resolve, but more often the exudate organizes into dense, tough fibrous adhesions that frequently obliterate the pleural space or envelop the lungs; either can seriously restrict pulmonary expansion.

Hemorrhagic pleuritis manifested by sanguineous inflammatory exudates is infrequent and is found in hemorrhagic diatheses, rickettsial diseases, and neoplastic involvement of the pleural cavity. The sanguineous exudate must be differentiated from hemothorax (discussed later). When hemorrhagic pleuritis is encountered, careful search should be made for the presence of exfoliated tumor cells.

Noninflammatory Pleural Effusions

Noninflammatory collections of serous fluid within the pleural cavities are called *hydrothorax*. The fluid is clear and straw colored. Hydrothorax may be unilateral or bilateral, depending on the underlying cause. The most common cause of hydrothorax is cardiac failure, and for this reason it is usually accompanied by pulmonary congestion and edema. Transudates may also collect in any other systemic disease associated with generalized edema and are therefore found in renal failure and cirrhosis of the liver.

The escape of blood into the pleural cavity is known as *hemothorax*. It is almost invariably a fatal complication of a ruptured aortic aneurysm or vascular trauma or it may occur postoperatively.

Chylothorax is an accumulation of milky fluid, usually of lymphatic origin, in the pleural cavity. Chyle is milky white because it contains finely emulsified fats. Chylothorax is most often caused by thoracic duct trauma or obstruction that secondarily causes rupture of major lymphatic ducts. This disorder is typically caused by malignancies that obstruct the major lymphatic ducts. Usually such cancers arise within the thoracic cavity and invade the lymphatics locally, but occasionally more distant cancers metastasize via the lymphatics and grow within the right lymphatic or thoracic duct, producing obstruction.

Pneumothorax

Pneumothorax refers to air or gas in the pleural cavities and is most commonly associated with emphysema, asthma, and tuberculosis. It may be spontaneous, traumatic, or therapeutic. Spontaneous pneumothorax may complicate any form of pulmonary disease that causes rupture of an alveolus. An abscess cavity that communicates either directly with the pleural space or with the lung interstitial tissue may also lead to the escape of air. In the latter circumstance the air may dissect through the lung substance or back through the mediastinum (interstitial emphysema), eventually entering the pleural cavity. Traumatic pneumothorax is usually caused by some perforating injury to the chest wall, but sometimes the trauma pierces the lung and thus provides two avenues for the accumulation of air within the pleural spaces. Resorption of the air in the pleural space occurs in spontaneous and traumatic pneumothorax, provided that the original communication seals itself.

Of the various forms of pneumothorax, the one that attracts greatest clinical attention is so-called *spontaneous idiopathic pneumothorax*. This entity is encountered in relatively young people, seems to be due to rupture of small, peripheral, usually apical subpleural blebs, and usually subsides spontaneously as the air is resorbed. Recurrent attacks are common and can be quite disabling.

Pneumothorax may have as much clinical significance as a fluid collection in the lungs because it also causes compression, collapse, and atelectasis of the lung and may be responsible for marked respiratory distress. When the defect acts as a flap valve and permits the entrance of air during inspiration but fails to permit its escape during expiration, it effectively acts as a pump that creates the progressively increasing pressures of *tension pneumothorax*, which may be sufficient to compress vital mediastinal structures and the contralateral lung.

Pleural Tumors

The pleura may be involved by primary or secondary tumors. Secondary metastatic involvement is far more common than are primary tumors. The most frequent metastatic malignancies arise from primary neoplasms of the lung and breast. In addition to these cancers, malignancy

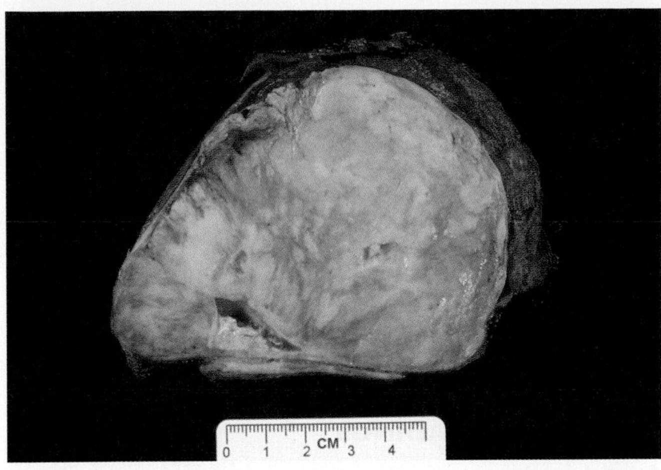

Figure 15-50 Solitary fibrous tumor. Cut surface is solid with a whorled appearance. (Courtesy Dr. Justine A. Barletta, Department of Pathology, Brigham and Women's Hospital, Boston, Mass.)

from any organ of the body may spread to the pleural spaces. Ovarian carcinomas, for example, tend to cause widespread implants in both the abdominal and thoracic cavities. In most metastatic involvements, a serous or serosanguineous effusion follows that often contains neoplastic cells. For this reason, careful cytologic examination of the sediment is of considerable diagnostic value.

Solitary Fibrous Tumor

Solitary fibrous tumor is a soft-tissue tumor with a propensity to occur in the pleura and, less commonly, in the lung, as well as other sites. The tumor is often attached to the pleural surface by a pedicle. It may be small (1 to 2 cm in diameter) or may reach an enormous size, but it tends to remain confined to the surface of the lung (Fig. 15-50).

MORPHOLOGY

Grossly, solitary fibrous tumor consists of dense fibrous tissue with occasional cysts filled with viscid fluid; microscopically, the tumor shows whorls of reticulin and collagen fibers among which are interspersed spindle cells resembling fibroblasts. Rarely, this tumor may be malignant, with pleomorphism, mitotic activity, necrosis, and large size (>10 cm). The tumor cells are CD34+ and keratin-negative by immunostaining, features that are helpful in distinguishing these lesions from malignant mesotheliomas (which show the opposite phenotype). The solitary fibrous tumor has no relationship to asbestos exposure.

It has recently been shown to be highly associated with a cryptic inversion of chromosome 12 involving the genes *NAB2* and *STAT6*. This rearrangement creates a *NAB2-STAT6* fusion gene that appears to be virtually unique to solitary fibrous tumor. It encodes a chimeric transcription factor that is hypothesized to be a key driver of tumor development.

Malignant Mesothelioma

Malignant mesotheliomas, although rare, have assumed great importance in the past few decades because of their increased incidence among people with heavy exposure to asbestos (see Pneumoconioses). Thoracic mesothelioma arises from either the visceral or the parietal pleura. In coastal areas with shipping industries in the United States and Great Britain, and in Canadian, Australian, and South African mining areas, as many as 90% of mesotheliomas are asbestos-related. The lifetime risk of developing mesothelioma in heavily exposed individuals is as high as 7% to 10%. There is a long latent period of 25 to 45 years for the development of asbestos-related mesothelioma, and there seems to be no increased risk of mesothelioma in asbestos workers who smoke. This is in contrast to the risk of asbestos-related lung carcinoma, already high, which is markedly magnified by smoking. Thus, for asbestos workers (particularly those who are also smokers), the risk of dying of lung carcinoma far exceeds that of developing mesothelioma.

Asbestos bodies (see Fig. 15-20) are found in increased numbers in the lungs of patients with mesothelioma. Another marker of asbestos exposure, the *asbestos plaque*, has been previously discussed (see Fig. 15-21).

Although several cytogenetic abnormalities have been detected, the most common is homozygous deletion of the tumor suppressor gene *CDKN2A/INK4a*, which occurs in about 80% of mesotheliomas. Demonstration of this deletion (usually by FISH) invovling chromosome 9p can be very helpful in distinguishing mesothelioma from reactive mesothelial proliferations. Deep sequencing of mesothelioma genomes is ongoing and may produce new insights.

MORPHOLOGY

Malignant mesothelioma is a diffuse lesion arising either from the visceral or parietal pleura, that spreads widely in the pleural space and is usually associated with extensive pleural effusion and direct invasion of thoracic structures. The affected lung becomes ensheathed by a thick layer of soft, gelatinous, grayish pink tumor tissue (Fig. 15-51).

Microscopically, malignant mesotheliomas may be epithelioid (60%), sarcomatoid (20%), or mixed (20%). This is in keeping

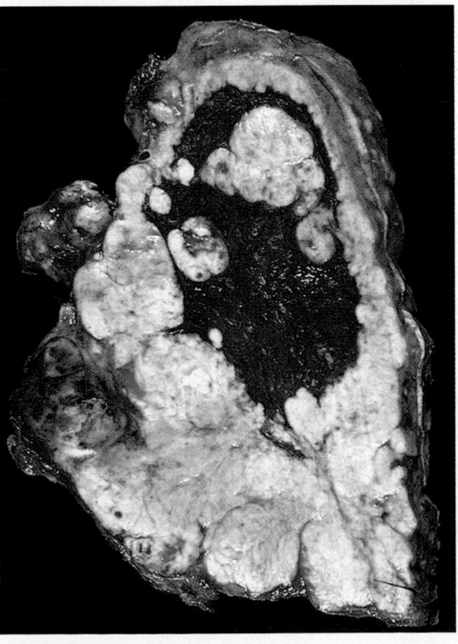

Figure 15-51 Malignant mesothelioma. Note the thick, firm, white pleural tumor tissue that ensheathes the lung.

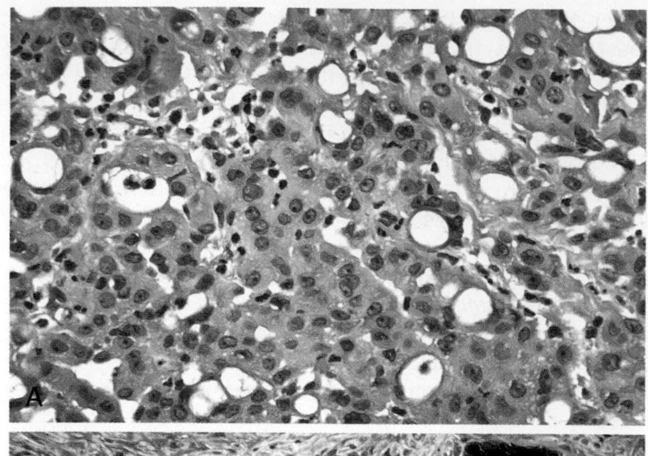

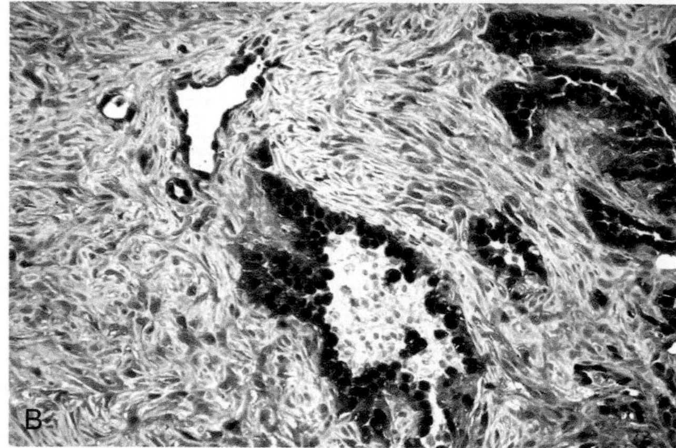

Figure 15-52 Histologic variants of malignant mesothelioma. **A,** Epithelioid type. **B,** Mixed type, stained for calretinin (immunoperoxidase method). The epithelial component is strongly positive (dark brown), while the sarcomatoid component is less so. (Courtesy Dr. Thomas Krausz, Department of Pathology, The University of Chicago, Pritzker School of Medicine, Chicago, Ill.)

with the fact that mesothelial cells have the potential to develop as epithelium-like cells or mesenchymal stromal cells.

The **epithelioid type** of mesothelioma consists of cuboidal, columnar, or flattened cells forming tubular or papillary structures resembling adenocarcinoma (Fig. 15-52*A*). Immunohistochemical stains are very helpful in differentiating it from pulmonary adenocarcinoma. Most mesotheliomas show strong positivity for keratin proteins, calretinin (Fig. 15-52*B*), Wilms tumor 1 (WT-1), cytokeratin 5/6, and D2-40. This panel of antibodies is diagnostic in a majority of cases when interpreted in the context of morphology and clinical presentation. The mesenchymal type of mesothelioma **(sarcomatoid type)** appears as a spindle cell sarcoma, resembling fibrosarcoma. Sarcomatoid mesotheliomas tend to have lower expression of many of the markers described previously and some may be positive only for keratin. The **mixed (biphasic) type** of mesothelioma contains both epithelioid and sarcomatoid patterns (Fig. 15-52*B*).

Clinical Course. The presenting complaints are chest pain, dyspnea, and, as noted, recurrent pleural effusions. Concurrent pulmonary asbestosis (fibrosis) is present in only 20% of individuals with pleural mesothelioma. The lung is invaded directly, and there is often metastatic spread to the hilar lymph nodes and, eventually, to the liver and other distant organs. Fifty percent of patients die within 12 months of diagnosis, and few survive longer than 2 years. Aggressive therapy (extrapleural pneumonectomy, chemotherapy, radiation therapy) seems to improve this poor prognosis in some patients.

Mesotheliomas also arise in the peritoneum, pericardium, tunica vaginalis, and genital tract (benign adenomatoid tumor; see Chapter 21). *Peritoneal mesotheliomas* are related to heavy asbestos exposure in 60% of male patients (the number is much lower in females). Although in about half cases the disease remains confined to the abdominal cavity, intestinal involvement frequently leads to death from intestinal obstruction or inanition.

SUGGESTED READINGS

Acute Lung Injury

Dushianthan A, et al: Acute respiratory distress syndrome and acute lung injury. *Postgrad Med J* 87:612, 2011. *[Succinct review of definitions, etiology, diagnosis and treatment of acute respiratory distress syndrome and acute lung injury.]*

Matthay MA, Zemans RL: The acute respiratory distress syndrome: Pathogenesis and treatment. *Annu Rev Pathol* 16:147, 2011. *[Updated view of the pathogenesis of acute respiratory distress syndrome]*

Obstructive Pulmonary Diseases

Hogg JC: A pathologist's view of airway obstruction in chronic obstructive pulmonary disease. *Am J Respir Crit Care Med* 186:v, 2012. *[A succinct editorial reviewing current knowledge about small airway involvement in COPD.]*

Mitzner W: Emphysema–a disease of small airways or lung parenchyma? *N Engl J Med* 365:1637, 2011. *[An editorial on the alveolar and small airway changes in emphysema.]*

Emphysema

Agusti A, Vestbo J: Current controversies and future perspectives in chronic obstructive pulmonary disease. *Am J Respir Crit Care Med* 184:507, 2011. *[Review of advances over the last decade in understanding COPD and remaining areas of uncertainties.]*

Huang YJ, et al: From microbe to microbiota: Considering microbial community composition in infections and airway diseases. *Am J Respir Crit Care Med* 185:691, 2012. *[Discussion of the role of the lung microbiome in health and in asthma, COPD and cystic fibrosis.]*

Tuder RM, et al: Lung disease associated with alpha1-antitrypsin deficiency. *Proc Am Thorac Soc* 7:381, 2010. *[Review of the broad range of activities of alpha1-antitrypsin and how its deficiency causes emphysema.]*

Tuder RM, Petrache I: Pathogenesis of chronic obstructive pulmonary disease. *J Clin Invest* 122:2749, 2012. *[Review article with emphasis on the pathogenesis of emphysema and how it is similar to aging.]*

Chronic Bronchitis

Kim V, Criner GJ: Chronic bronchitis and COPD. *Am J Respir Crit Care Med* (ePub ahead of print) 2012. *[Concise review of epidemiology, pathogenesis, clinical sequelae of mucous hyperplasia, and therapy of chronic bronchitis.]*

Asthma

Corren J, et al: Lebrikizumab treatment in adults with asthma. *N Engl J Med* 365:1088, 2011. *[Data from this study provide proof of the concept that anti–interleukin-13 therapy can be targeted to susceptible patients – a step forward in personalized therapy for asthma.]*

Fahy JV, Locksley RM: The airway epithelium as a regulator of Th2 responses in asthma. *Am J Respir Crit Care Med* 184:390, 2011. *[Summarizes and explains how epithelial cells regulate both innate and adaptive immune responses in the airway.]*

Galli SJ, Tsai M: IgE and mast cells in allergic disease. *Nat Med* 18:693, 2012. *[This review discusses the roles IgE and mast cells in immune responses that manifest clinically as asthma and other allergic disorders.]*

Holt PG, Sly PD: Viral infections and atopy in asthma pathogenesis: New rationales for asthma prevention and treatment. *Nat Med*

18:726, 2012. *[A detailed review of the role of viral infections and inflammatory responses in asthma exacerbations.]*

Holgate ST: Innate and adaptive immune responses in asthma. *Nat Med* 18:673, 2012. *[This review focuses on innate pathways that are important in asthma.]*

Wenzel SE: Asthma phenotypes: The evolution from clinical to molecular approaches. *Nat Med* 18:716, 2012. *[Review of the different asthma phenotypes and how this knowledge is used to guide therapy and further research.]*

Bronchiectasis

Bush A, Hogg C: Primary ciliary dyskinesia: Recent advances in epidemiology, diagnosis, management and relationship with the expanding spectrum of ciliopathy. *Expert Rev Respir Med* 6:663, 2012. *[Discussion of advances in primary ciliary dyskinesia genetics and other ciliopathies.]*

King PT: Pathogenesis of bronchiectasis. *Paediatr Respir Rev*, 12:104, 2011. *[This review describes the pathophysiology of noncystic fibrosis bronchiectasis.]*

Patterson K, Strek ME: Allergic bronchopulmonary aspergillosis. *Proc Am Thorac Soc* 7:237, 2010. *[Clear and succinct review of clinical features, diagnosis, treatment and outcomes of allergic bronchopulmonary aspergillosis.]*

Idiopathic pulmonary fibrosis

King TE Jr, et al: Idiopathic pulmonary fibrosis. *Lancet* 378:1949, 2011. *[A review of the clinical course, therapeutic options, and underlying mechanisms of idiopathic pulmonary fibrosis.]*

Steele MP, Schwartz DA: Molecular mechanisms in progressive idiopathic pulmonary fibrosis. *Annual Rev Med* 64:265, 2013. *[Discussion of genetic factors that increase the risk of IPF.]*

Nonspecific Interstitial Pneumonia

Travis WD, et al: Idiopathic nonspecific interstitial pneumonia: Report of an American thoracic society project. *Am J Respir Crit Care Med* 177:1338, 2008. *[Establishes idiopathic NSIP as a distinct clinical entity and describes its clinical, radiological and pathological features.]*

Organizing Pneumonia

Roberton BJ, Hansell DM: Organizing pneumonia: A kaleidoscope of concepts and morphologies. *Eur Radiol* 21:2244, 2011. *[Review of the pathology of organizing pneumonia, its clinical associations and radiologic findings.]*

Pneumoconiosis

Leung CC, et al: Silicosis. *Lancet* 379:2008, 2012. *[Review of pathogenesis, clinical features and complications of silicosis.]*

Park EK, et al: Elimination of asbestos use and asbestos-related diseases: An unfinished story. *Cancer Sci* 103:1751, 2012. *[Review commenting of increase in asbestos related diseases due to use in industrializing countries.]*

Sava F, Carlsten C: Respiratory health effects of ambient air pollution: An update. *Clin Chest Med* 33:759, 2011. *[Review discussing deleterious effects of co-exposures to air pollution, particularly in genetically predisposed individuals.]*

Radiation Pneumonitis

Krasin MJ, et al: Radiation-related treatment effects across the age spectrum: Differences and similarities or what the old and young can learn from each other. *Semin Radiat Oncol* 20:21, 2010. *[This study compares radiation related effects, including pneumonitis, pulmonary fibrosis, osteonecrosis, and fracture, across the age spectrum.]*

Sarcoidosis

O'Regan A, Berman JS: Sarcoidosis. *Ann Intern Med* 156:ITC5-1, 2012. *[Comprehensive review of pathogenesis, clinical manifestations, diagnosis, and prognosis of sarcoidosis.]*

Hypersensitivity Pneumonia

Selman M, et al: Hypersensitivity pneumonitis: Insights in diagnosis and pathobiology. *Am J Respir Crit Care Med* 186:314, 2012. *[Review of clinical forms, immunopathology, radiology, pathology and treatment of hypersensitivity pneumonitis.]*

Eosinophilic Lung Diseases

Fernandez Perez ER, Olson AL, Frankel SK: Eosinophilic lung diseases. *Med Clin North Am* 95:1163, 2011. *[Review of the clinical features, general diagnostic workup, and management of the eosinophilic lung diseases.]*

Smoking-related Interstitial Diseases

Tazelaar HD, et al: Desquamative interstitial pneumonia. *Histopathology* 58:509, 2011. *[Review of smoking-related DIP and its relationship to other interstitial lung diseases.]*

Pulmonary alveolar proteinosis

Borie R, et al: Pulmonary alveolar proteinosis. *Eur Respir Rev* 20:98, 2011. *[Review of the classification, pathogenesis and treatment of PAP.]*

Surfactant Dysfunction Disorders

Gower WA, Nogee LM: Surfactant dysfunction. *Paediatr Respir Rev* 12:223, 2011. *[Review of the clinical features, epidemiology, pathogenesis, molecular genetics, pathology and natural history of these rare disorders.]*

Pulmonary Hypertension

Paulin R, et al: From oncoproteins/tumor suppressors to microRNAs, the newest therapeutic targets for pulmonary arterial hypertension. *J Mol Med (Berl)* 89:1089, 2011. *[Review of discoveries in molecular pathogenesis of PAH and possible therapeutic implications.]*

Toshner M, Tajsic T, Morrell NW: Pulmonary hypertension: Advances in pathogenesis and treatment. *Br Med Bull* 94:21, 2010. *[Review of recent understanding of pathogenesis, pathology and treatment of PH.]*

Pulmonary hemorrhage Syndromes

Gibelin A, et al: Epidemiology and etiology of Wegener granulomatosis, microscopic polyangiitis, Churg-Strauss syndrome and Goodpasture syndrome: Vasculitides with frequent lung involvement. *Semin Respir Crit Care Med* 32:264, 2011. *[Review of the most common inflammatory conditions involving pulmonary vessels.]*

Pneumonia

Kimmel SR: The course and management of the 2009 H1N1 pandemic influenza. *Prim Care* 38:693, viii, 2011. *[Review of epidemiology, risk factors, treatment and vaccination for H1N1 influenza.]*

Mandell LA, et al: Infectious diseases society of America/American thoracic society consensus guidelines on the management of community-acquired pneumonia in adults. *Clin Infect Dis* 44(Suppl 2):S27, 2007. *[Provides the definitive standard for diagnosis and treatment of CAP.]*

Edwards KM, et al: Burden of human metapneumovirus infection in young children. *N Engl J Med* 368:633, 2013. *[Paper documenting the high frequency of metapneumovirus infection and its health impact in children under age 5.]*

Lung Transplantation

Christie JD, et al: The registry of the international society for heart and lung transplantation: 29th adult lung and heart-lung transplant report-2012. *J Heart Lung Transplant* 31:1073, 2012. *[Annual report of registry data including numbers of transplants, indications, and outcomes.]*

Lung Cancer

Cheng L, et al: Molecular pathology of lung cancer: Key to personalized medicine. *Mod Pathol* 25:347, 2012. *[Review summarizing molecular mechanisms and markers associated with primary and acquired resistance to EGFR-targeted therapy in lung adenocarcinomas.]*

Couraud S, et al: Lung cancer in never smokers–a review. *Eur J Cancer* 48:1299, 2012. *[Review focused on risk factors for lung cancer in non-smokers.]*

de Groot P, Munden RF: Lung cancer epidemiology, risk factors, and prevention. *Radiol Clin North Am* 50:863, 2012. *[Concise review of lung cancer, including genetics, molecular pathogenesis, pathology and mortality.]*

Hubaux R, et al: Arsenic, asbestos and radon: Emerging players in lung tumorigenesis. *Environ Health* 11:89, 2012. *[Comprehensive review of arsenic, asbestos, and radon associated molecular mechanisms responsible for lung cancer.]*

Perez-Moreno P, et al: Squamous cell carcinoma of the lung: Molecular subtypes and therapeutic opportunities. *Clin Cancer Res* 18:2443, 2012. *[Review focused on potentially "targetable" molecular defects in SCC of the lung.]*

Travis WD: Pathology of lung cancer. *Clin Chest Med* 32:669, 2011. *[Review of pathologic classification and microscopic features of lung cancer.]*

Pleura

Cardillo G, et al: Solitary fibrous tumors of the pleura. *Curr Opin Pulm Med* 18:339, 2012. *[Review of this rare entity with particular attention paid to clinical and pathologic characteristics that define long-term outcome.]*

Husain AN, et al: Guidelines for pathologic diagnosis of malignant mesothelioma: 2012 update of the consensus statement from the international mesothelioma interest group. *Arch Pathol Lab Med* (ePub ahead of print) 2012. [A practical guide for pathologic diagnosis of mesothelioma.]

See TARGETED THERAPY available online at www.studentconsult.com

CHAPTER 16

Head and Neck

Mark W. Lingen

CHAPTER CONTENTS

Diseases of the head and neck range from the common cold to uncommon neoplasms of the ear and nose. Those selected for discussion are assigned, sometimes arbitrarily, to one of the following anatomic sites: (1) oral cavity; (2) upper airways, including the nose, pharynx, larynx, and nasal sinuses; (3) ears; (4) neck; and (5) salivary glands.

ORAL CAVITY

Diseases of Teeth and Supporting Structures

Caries (Tooth Decay)

Dental caries is caused by focal demineralization of tooth structure (enamel and dentin) by acidic metabolites of fermenting sugars that are produced by bacteria. Caries is one of the most common diseases worldwide and is the main cause of tooth loss before age 35. Traditionally, the prevalence of caries has been higher in industrialized countries, where there is ready access to processed and refined foods containing large amounts of carbohydrates. However, global trends have changed the demographics. First, the rate of caries has markedly dropped in countries such as the United States, where improved oral hygiene has improved and fluoridation of the drinking water is widespread. Fluoride is incorporated into the crystalline structure of enamel, forming fluoroapatite, which contributes to the resistance to degradation by bacterial acids. Second, with the globalization of the world's economy, processed foods are being increasingly consumed in developing nations. With these trends, one can expect the rate of caries to increase dramatically in these regions of the world.

Gingivitis

Gingivitis is inflammation of the oral mucosa surrounding the teeth. It is the result of a poor oral hygiene and leads to the accumulation of dental plaque and calculus.

Dental plaque is a sticky, colorless, biofilm that collects between and on the surface of the teeth. It contains a mixture of bacteria, salivary proteins, and desquamated epithelial cells. If plaque is not removed, it becomes mineralized to form *calculus* (tartar). Plaque build-up beneath the gumline can lead to gingivitis, which is characterized by gingival erythema, edema, bleeding, changes in contour, and loss of soft tissue adaptation to the teeth. Gingivitis occurs at any age but is most prevalent and severe in adolescence (ranging from 40% to 60%). In addition, the bacteria in the plaque release acids from sugar-rich foods, thereby eroding the enamel surface and contributing to the development of caries. Gingivitis is a reversible disease; therapy is primarily aimed at reducing the accumulation of plaque and calculus via regular brushing, flossing, and dental visits.

Periodontitis

Periodontitis is an inflammatory process that affects the supporting structures of the teeth (periodontal ligaments) alveolar bone, and cementum. Periodontitis can lead to serious sequelae, including complete destruction of the periodontal ligament, which is responsible for the attachment of the teeth to the alveolar bone, leading to loosening and eventual loss of teeth. Periodontal disease is associated with a marked shift in the types and proportions of bacteria along the gingiva. Poor oral hygiene, with resultant change in oral flora, are believed to be important in the pathogenesis of periodontitis. For the most part, facultative gram-positive organisms colonize healthy gingival sites, while plaque within areas of active periodontitis contains anaerobic and microaerophilic gram-negative flora. Although 300 types of bacteria reside in the oral cavity, adult periodontitis is associated primarily with *Aggregatibacter (Actinobacillus) actinomycetemcomitans, Porphyromonas gingivalis,* and *Prevotella intermedia.*

While it typically presents without any associated disorders, periodontal disease can be a component of systemic disease, including acquired immunodeficiency syndrome (AIDS), leukemia, Crohn disease, diabetes mellitus, Down syndrome, sarcoidosis, and syndromes associated with defects in neutrophils (Chédiak-Higashi syndrome, agranulocytosis, and cyclic neutropenia). In addition, periodontal infections can be the origin of important systemic diseases, including infective endocarditis, and pulmonary and brain abscesses.

Inflammatory/Reactive Lesions

Aphthous Ulcers (Canker Sores)

Aphthous ulcers are common, often recurrent, exceedingly painful, superficial oral mucosal ulcerations of unknown etiology. They affect up to 40% of the population, and are most common in the first 2 decades of life. Aphthous ulcers tend to be prevalent within certain families and may also be associated with immunologic disorders including celiac disease, inflammatory bowel disease, and Behçet disease. The lesions appear as single or multiple, shallow, hyperemic ulcerations covered by a thin exudate and rimmed by a narrow zone of erythema (Fig. 16-1). The underlying inflammatory infiltrate is at first largely mononuclear, but secondary bacterial infection may result in a neutrophilic infiltrate. The lesions typically resolve spontaneously in 7 to 10 days, but may sometimes persist stubbornly for weeks, particularly in immunocompromised patients.

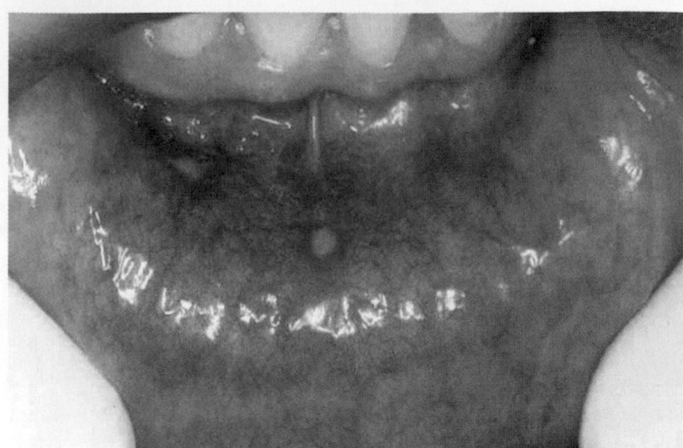

Figure 16-1 Aphthous ulcer. Single ulceration with an erythematous halo surrounding a yellowish fibrinopurulent membrane.

Fibrous Proliferative Lesions

The *irritation fibroma,* also called traumatic fibroma and focal fibrous hyperplasia, is a submucosal nodular mass of fibrous connective tissue stroma that occurs primarily on the buccal mucosa along the bite line or the gingiva (Fig. 16-2). It is believed to be a reactive proliferation caused by repetitive trauma. Treatment is complete surgical excision.

The ***pyogenic granuloma*** (Fig. 16-3) **is an inflammatory lesion typically found on the gingiva of children, young adults, and pregnant women (pregnancy tumor).** The surface of the lesion is often ulcerated and red to purple in color. In some cases, growth is alarmingly rapid, raising the fear of malignancy. Histologically these lesions demonstrate a highly vascular proliferation of organizing granulation tissue. Pyogenic granulomas can regress, mature into dense fibrous masses, or develop into a peripheral

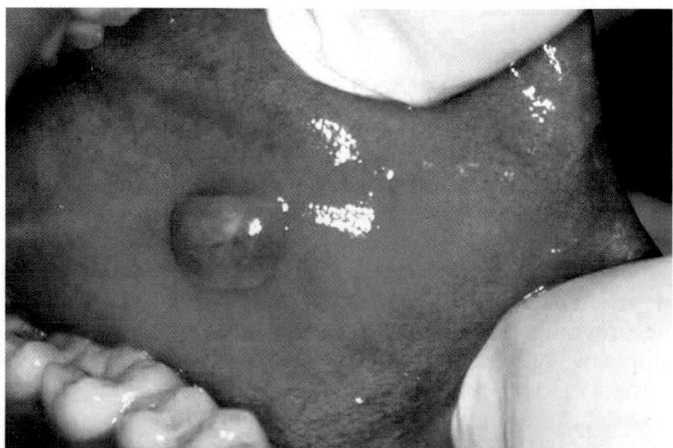

Figure 16-2 Fibroma. Smooth pink exophytic nodule on the buccal mucosa.

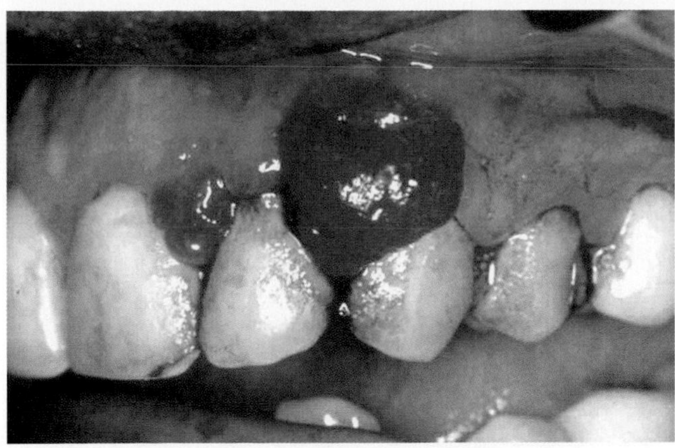

Figure 16-3 Pyogenic granuloma. Erythematous, hemorrhagic, and exophytic mass arising from the gingival mucosa.

ossifying fibroma. Complete surgical excision is the definitive treatment for these lesions.

The *peripheral ossifying fibroma* is a common gingival growth that is most likely reactive in nature rather than neoplastic. As mentioned, some may arise from a longstanding pyogenic granuloma, while others develop *de novo* from cells of the periodontal ligament. Peripheral ossifying fibromas appear as red, ulcerated, and nodular lesions of the gingiva. The peak incidence is in young and teenage females. Since the lesions have a recurrence rate of 15% to 20%, complete surgical excision down to the periosteum is the treatment of choice.

The *peripheral giant cell granuloma* is an uncommon lesion of the oral cavity, particularly the gingiva. Like the peripheral ossifying fibroma, peripheral giant cell granuloma most likely represents a reactive/inflammatory, rather than neoplastic, process. It is generally covered by intact gingival mucosa, but it may be ulcerated. Histologically, these lesions contain a striking aggregation of multinucleate, foreign body–like giant cells separated by a fibroangiomatous stroma. Although not encapsulated, these lesions are usually well delimited and easily excised. They should be differentiated from central giant-cell tumors found within the jaws and from the histologically similar but frequently multiple "brown tumors" seen in hyperparathyroidism (Chapter 24).

Infections

Herpes Simplex Virus Infections

Most orofacial herpetic infections are caused by herpes simplex virus type 1 (HSV-1) but oral HSV-2 (genital herpes) infections do occur. Primary infections typically occur in children between 2 and 4 years of age, are often asymptomatic, and do not cause significant morbidity. However, in 10% to 20% of cases, primary infections can present as *acute herpetic gingivostomatitis*, with abrupt onset of vesicles and ulcerations of the oral mucosa, particularly the gingiva. These lesions are also accompanied by lymphadenopathy, fever, anorexia, and irritability.

MORPHOLOGY

The vesicles range from lesions of a few millimeters to large bullae and are at first filled with a clear, serous fluid, but rapidly rupture to yield painful, red-rimmed, shallow ulcerations. On microscopic examination, there is intracellular and intercellular edema (acantholysis), creating clefts that may become transformed into macroscopic vesicles. Individual epidermal cells in the margins of the vesicle or lying free within the fluid sometimes develop eosinophilic **intranuclear viral inclusions,** or several cells may fuse to produce giant cells **(multinucleate polykaryons),** changes that are demonstrated by the diagnostic **Tzanck test**, based on microscopic examination of the vesicle fluid. The vesicles and shallow ulcers usually spontaneously clear within 3 to 4 weeks, but the virus treks along the regional nerves and eventually becomes dormant in the local ganglia (e.g., the trigeminal ganglion).

Infection is common and most adults harbor latent HSV-1. In some individuals, viral reactivation (recurrent herpetic stomatitis) occurs. The mechanisms of reactivation are poorly understood. It has been associated with trauma, allergies, exposure to ultraviolet light, upper respiratory tract infection, pregnancy, menstruation, immunosuppression, and exposure to temperature extremes. *Recurrent herpetic stomatitis* (in contrast to acute herpetic gingivostomatitis) occurs at the site of primary inoculation or in adjacent mucosa associated with the same ganglion. The lesions appear as groups of small (1 to 3 mm) vesicles on the lips (*Herpes labialis*), nasal orifices, buccal mucosa, gingiva, and hard palate. Although these lesions typically resolve in 7 to 10 days, they can persist in immunocompromised patients and may require systemic antiviral therapy.

Other viral infections that can involve the oral cavity as well as the head and neck region include herpes zoster, Epstein-Barr virus (EBV; mononucleosis, nasopharyngeal carcinoma, lymphoma), cytomegalovirus, enterovirus (herpangina, hand-foot-and-mouth disease, acute lymphonodular pharyngitis), and rubeola (measles).

Oral Candidiasis (Thrush)

***Candida albicans* is a normal component of the oral flora in approximately 50% of the population and is the most common fungal infection of the oral cavity.** Several factors seem to influence the likelihood of a clinical infection. These include the immune status of the individual, the strain of *C. albicans* present, and the composition of an individual's oral flora. There are three major clinical forms of oral candidiasis: *pseudomembranous, erythematous,* and *hyperplastic.* The pseudomembranous form is the most common and is also known as *thrush.* It is characterized by a superficial, gray to white inflammatory membrane composed of matted organisms enmeshed in a fibrinosuppurative exudate that can be readily scraped off to reveal an underlying erythematous inflammatory base. The infection typically remains superficial except in the setting of immunosuppression, such as in individuals with organ or bone marrow transplants, neutropenia, chemotherapy-induced immunosuppression, AIDS, and diabetes mellitus. In addition, broad-spectrum

Table 16-1 Oral Manifestations of Some Systemic Diseases

Systemic Disease	Associated Oral Changes
Infectious Diseases	
Scarlet fever	Fiery red tongue with prominent papillae (raspberry tongue); white-coated tongue through which hyperemic papillae project (strawberry tongue)
Measles	Spotty enanthema in the oral cavity often precedes the skin rash; ulcerations on the buccal mucosa about Stensen duct produce Koplik spots
Infectious mononucleosis	Acute pharyngitis and tonsillitis that may cause coating with a gray-white exudative membrane; enlargement of lymph nodes in the neck, palatal petechiae
Diphtheria	Characteristic dirty white, fibrinosuppurative, tough, inflammatory membrane over the tonsils and retropharynx
Human immunodeficiency virus	Predisposition to opportunistic oral infections, particularly herpes virus, *Candida*, and other fungi; oral lesions of Kaposi sarcoma and hairy leukoplakia (described in text)
Dermatologic Conditions*	
Lichen planus	Reticulate, lacelike, white keratotic lesions that sometimes ulcerate and rarely form bullae; seen in more than 50% of patients with cutaneous lichen planus; rarely, is the sole manifestation
Pemphigus	Vesicles and bullae prone to rupture, leaving hyperemic erosions covered with exudates
Bullous pemphigoid	Oral lesions (mucus membrane pemphigoid) resemble those of pemphigus but can be differentiated histologically
Erythema multiforme	Maculopapular, vesiculobullous eruption that sometimes follows an infection elsewhere, ingestion of drugs, development of cancer, or a collagen vascular disease; when there is widespread mucosal and skin involvement, it is referred to as *Stevens-Johnson syndrome*
Hematologic Disorders	
Pancytopenia (agranulocytosis, aplastic anemia)	Severe oral infections in the form of gingivitis, pharyngitis, tonsillitis; may extend to produce cellulitis of the neck (*Ludwig angina*)
Leukemia	With depletion of functioning neutrophils, oral lesions may appear like those in pancytopenia
Monocytic leukemia	Leukemic infiltration and enlargement of the gingivae, often with accompanying periodontitis
Miscellaneous	
Melanotic pigmentation	May appear in Addison disease, hemochromatosis, fibrous dysplasia of bone (Albright syndrome), and Peutz-Jeghers syndrome (gastrointestinal polyposis)
Phenytoin (Dilantin) ingestion	Striking fibrous enlargement of the gingivae
Pregnancy	A friable, red, pyogenic granuloma protruding from the gingiva ("pregnancy tumor")
Rendu-Osler-Weber syndrome	Autosomal dominant disorder with multiple congenital aneurysmal telangiectasias beneath mucosal surfaces of the oral cavity and lips

*See Chapter 25.

antibiotics that eliminate or alter the normal bacterial flora of the mouth can result in the development of oral candidiasis.

Deep Fungal Infections

In addition to their usual sites of infection, certain deep fungal infections have a predilection for the oral cavity and the head and neck region. Such fungi include histoplasmosis, blastomycosis, coccidioidomycosis, cryptococcosis, zygomycosis, and aspergillosis. With an increasing number of patients who are immunocompromised due to diseases such as AIDS or therapies for cancer and organ transplantation, the prevalence of fungal infections of the oral cavity has increased in recent years.

Oral Manifestations of Systemic Disease

The mouth is not merely a gateway for delicacies; it is also the site of oral lesions in many systemic diseases. In fact, *it is not uncommon for oral lesions to be the first sign of some underlying systemic condition.* Some of the more common disease associations and their oral changes are cited in Table 16-1. Only hairy leukoplakia is characterized in more detail here.

Hairy Leukoplakia

Hairy leukoplakia is a distinctive oral lesion on the lateral border of the tongue that is usually seen in immunocompromised patients and is caused by Epstein-Barr virus (EBV). It can be observed in patients infected with the human immunodeficiency virus (HIV) and may portend the development of AIDS. However, the lesions can also be found in patients who are immunocompromised for other reasons including cancer therapy, transplant associated immunosuppression, and advancing age. Hairy leukoplakia takes the form of *white, confluent patches of fluffy ("hairy"), hyperkeratotic thickenings, almost always situated on the lateral border of the tongue.* Unlike thrush, the lesion cannot be scraped off. The distinctive microscopic appearance consists of *hyperparakeratosis* and *acanthosis with "balloon cells" in the upper spinous layer.* Special stains can be used to demonstrate the presence of EBV RNA transcripts and proteins within the lesional cells. Sometimes there is superimposed candidal infection on the surface of the lesions, adding to the "hairiness."

Precancerous and Cancerous Lesions

Many epithelial and connective tissue tumors of the head and neck region (e.g., papillomas, hemangiomas, lymphomas) occur elsewhere in the body and are described adequately in other chapters. This discussion considers only squamous cell carcinoma and its associated precancerous lesions.

Leukoplakia and Erythroplakia

Leukoplakia is defined by the World Health Organization as "a white patch or plaque that cannot be scraped off and cannot be characterized clinically or pathologically as any other disease." This clinical term is reserved for lesions that are present in the oral cavity for no apparent reason. As such, white patches caused by obvious irritation or entities such as lichen planus and candidiasis are not considered to be leukoplakias. Approximately 3% of the world's population have leukoplakic lesions; 5% to 25% of these lesions are premalignant. **Thus, until proven otherwise by means of histologic evaluation, all leukoplakias must be considered precancerous.**

Related to leukoplakia, but much less common and much more ominous, is *erythroplakia,* which is a red, velvety, possibly eroded area within the oral cavity that usually remains level with or may be slightly depressed in relation to the surrounding mucosa (Fig. 16-4). The epithelium in such lesions tends to be markedly atypical, and the risk of malignant transformation is much higher than is leukoplakia. Intermediate forms are occasionally encountered that have the characteristics of both leukoplakia and erythroplakia, termed *speckled leukoerythroplakia.*

Both leukoplakia and erythroplakia may be seen in adults at any age, but they are usually found in persons aged 40 to 70, with a 2:1 male preponderance. Although these lesions have multifactorial origins, the use of tobacco (cigarettes, pipes, cigars, and certain forms of smokeless tobacco) is a common antecedent.

MORPHOLOGY

Leukoplakias may occur anywhere in the oral cavity (favored locations are buccal mucosa, floor of the mouth, ventral surface of the tongue, palate, and gingiva). They appear as solitary or multiple white patches or plaques, often with sharply demarcated borders. They may be slightly thickened and smooth or wrinkled and fissured, or they may appear as raised, sometimes corrugated, verrucous plaques (Fig. 16-5*A*). On histologic examination they present a spectrum of epithelial changes ranging from hyperkeratosis overlying a thickened, acanthotic but orderly mucosal epithelium to lesions with markedly dysplastic changes sometimes merging into carcinoma in situ (Fig. 16-5*B*).

The histologic changes in **erythroplakia** only rarely demonstrate orderly epidermal maturation; virtually all (approximately 90%) disclose severe dysplasia, carcinoma in situ, or minimally invasive carcinoma. Often, an intense subepithelial inflammatory reaction with vascular dilation is seen that likely contributes to the reddish clinical appearance.

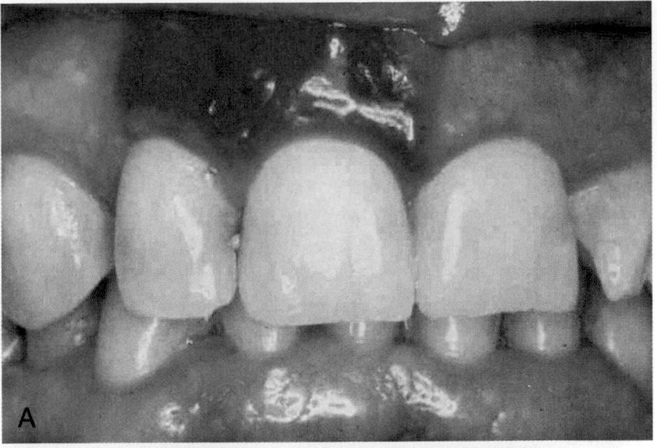

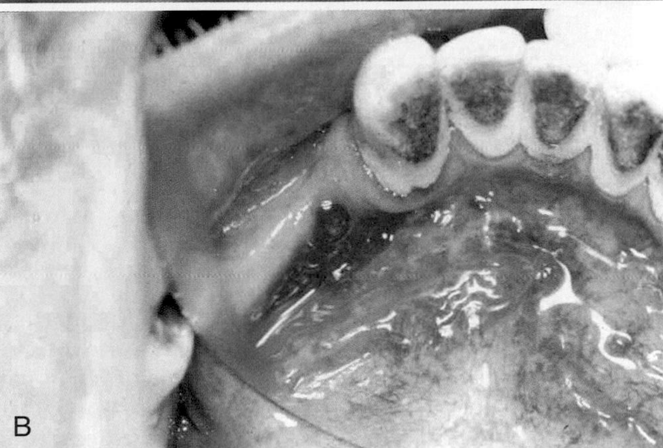

Figure 16-4 Erythroplakia. *A,* Lesion of the maxillary gingiva. *B,* Red lesion of the mandibular alveolar ridge. Biopsy of both lesions revealed carcinoma in situ.

Squamous Cell Carcinoma

Approximately 95% of cancers of the head and neck are squamous cell carcinomas (SCCs), with the remainder largely consisting of adenocarcinomas of salivary gland origin. Head and neck squamous cell carcinoma is the sixth most common neoplasm in the world. At current rates, approximately 45,000 cases in the United States and more than 650,000 cases worldwide will be diagnosed each year.

The pathogenesis of squamous cell carcinoma is multifactorial.

- Within North America and Europe, oral cavity SCC has classically been a disease of middle-aged individuals who have been chronic abusers of *smoked tobacco* and *alcohol*.
- In India and Asia, the chewing of betel quid and paan is a major regional predisposing influence. This concoction, considered a delicacy by some, contains ingredients such as areca nut, slaked lime, and tobacco, wrapped in a betel leaf; many of the ingredients of paan could give rise to potential carcinogens.
- *Actinic radiation* (sunlight) and, particularly, pipe smoking are known predisposing influences for cancer of the lower lip.
- The incidence of oral cavity SCC (particularly the tongue) in individuals younger than age 40, who have no known risk factors, has been on the rise.

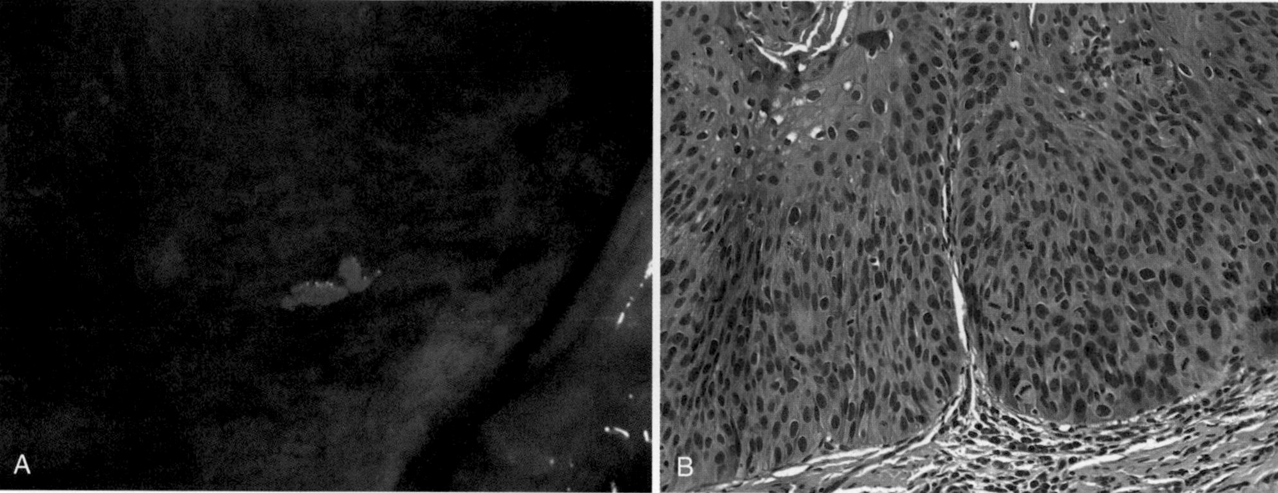

Figure 16-5 Leukoplakia. **A,** Clinical appearance of leukoplakias is highly variable. In this example, the lesion is relatively smooth and thin with well-demarcated borders. **B,** The histologic appearance of a leukoplakia showing severe dysplasia that is characterized by nuclear and cellular pleomorphism, numerous mitotic figures, and a loss of normal maturation.

The pathogenesis in this group of patients, who are nonsmokers and not infected with human papillomavirus (HPV), is unknown.

In the oropharynx, as many as 70% of SCCs, particularly those involving the tonsils, the base of the tongue, and the pharynx, harbor oncogenic variants of HPV, particularly HPV-16. HPV-associated SCC of the oropharynx has increased more than 2 -fold over the last 2 decades. It is predicted that by the year 2020, the incidence of HPV-associated head and neck SCC will surpass that of cervical cancer, in part because the anatomic sites of origin (tonsillar crypts, base of tongue, and oropharynx) are not readily accessible or amenable to cytologic screening (unlike the cervix) for premalignant lesions. Conversely, it should be noted that, unlike the oropharynx, HPV-associated SCC of the oral cavity is relatively uncommon.

Survival is dependent on a number of factors including the specific etiology of SCC. The 5-year survival rate of "classic" (smoking and alcohol related) early-stage SCC is approximately 80%, while survival drops to 20% for late-stage disease. Patients with HPV-positive SCC have greater long-term survival than those with HPV-negative tumors. The dismal outlook for the classic SCC is due to several factors, including the fact that the tumors are often diagnosed when the disease has already reached an advanced stage. Furthermore, the frequent development of multiple primary tumors markedly decreases survival. The rate of second primary tumors in these patients has been reported to be 3% to 7% per year, which is higher than for any other malignancy. This observation has led to the concept of "field cancerization," which postulates that multiple individual primary tumors develop independently in the upper aerodigestive tract as a result of years of chronic exposure of the mucosa to carcinogens. Because of such field cancerization, an individual who is fortunate to live 5 years after the detection of the initial primary tumor has an almost 35% chance of developing at least one new primary tumor within that period of time. An alternative hypotheses to explain multiple "primary" tumors is that they are actually intraepithelial metastases. The occurrence of new tumors can be particularly devastating for individuals whose initial lesions were small. The 5-year survival rate for the first primary tumor is considerably better than 50%, but in such individuals, second primary tumors are the most common cause of death. Therefore, the early detection of all premalignant lesions is critical for the long-term survival of these patients. Finally, the HPV vaccine, which is protective against cervical cancer, offers hope to stem the tide of HPV-associated head and neck SCC. Although clinical trails are ongoing, the vaccine has not yet been approved for this use.

Molecular Biology of Squamous Cell Carcinoma. As with other cancers, **the development of SCC is driven by the accumulation of mutations and epigenetic changes that alter the expression and function of oncogenes and tumor suppressor genes, leading to acquisition of cancer hallmarks (Chapter 7), such as resistance to cell death, increased proliferation, induction of angiogenesis, and the ability to invade and metastasize.** Deep sequencing of the classic SCC subset has revealed a large number of genetic alterations that bear a molecular signature consistent with tobacco carcinogen induced cancers (Fig. 16-6). These mutations frequently involve the p53 pathway as well as proteins responsible for the regulation of squamous differentiation, such as p63 and NOTCH 1. Conversely, HPV-associated SCCs contain far fewer and different genetic alterations and typically overexpress p16, a cyclin-dependent kinase inhibitor. In addition, owing to the expression of the HPV oncoproteins E6 and E7, there is inactivation of the p53 and RB pathways in much the same way as has been observed in cervical cancer (Chapter 22).

While the model outlined in Figure 16-6 is an acceptable working draft of the clinical, histologic, and molecular changes involved in development of carcinogen-induced SCC, it does not reflect the natural history of the disease for all lesions. Data regarding the incidence and timing of these changes in oral premalignancy are limited. Furthermore, it is not clear whether any of the genotypic changes, used individually or in a panel, can consistently predict which dysplastic lesions will progress to oral SCC. To complicate the matter further, SCC progression does not always occur in a linear fashion over a uniform period of time. Rather, there are subsets of lesions with histologic evidence of dysplasia that may or may not progress to

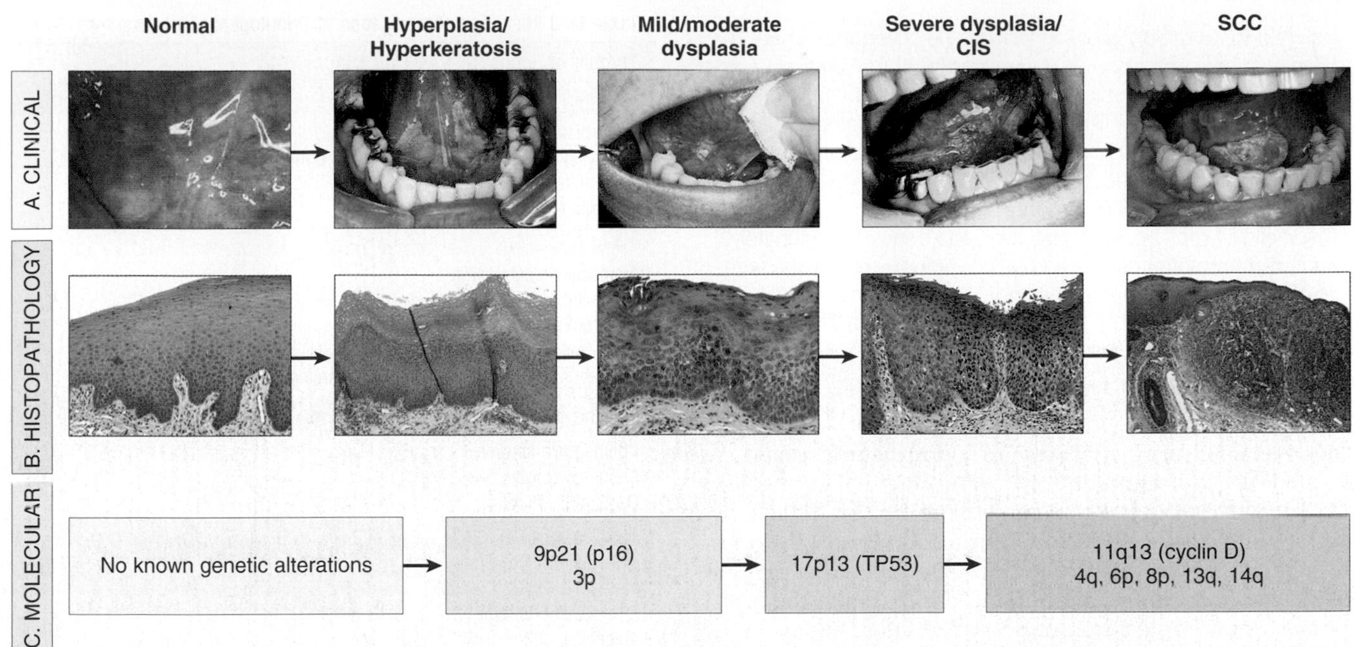

Figure 16-6 Clinical, histologic, and molecular progression of oral cancer. A, An idealized representation of the clinical progression of oral cancer. **B,** The histologic progression of squamous epithelium from normal, to hyperkeratosis, to mild/moderate dysplasia, to severe dysplasia, to cancer. **C,** The sites of the most common genetic alterations identified as important for cancer development. CIS, Carcinoma in situ; SCC, squamous cell carcinoma. (Clinical photographs courtesy of Sol Silverman, MD, from Silverman S: Oral Cancer. Hamilton, Ontario, Canada, BD Dekker, 2003.)

SCC. Similarly, histologically "normal" appearing mucosal lesions may truly be benign or they may represent molecularly premalignant lesions that have not yet developed morphologic changes consistent with dysplasia. Therefore, conventional histologic findings can only indicate that a given lesion may have malignant potential.

MORPHOLOGY

Squamous cell carcinoma may arise anywhere in the head and neck region that is lined by stratified squamous epithelium. For the "classic" oral cavity SCC, the favored locations are the ventral surface of the tongue, floor of the mouth, lower lip, soft palate, and gingiva (Fig. 16-7*A*). The "classic" malignancies are typically preceded by the presence of premalignant lesions that can be very heterogeneous in presentation (see earlier).

In the early stages, cancers of the oral cavity appear either as raised, firm, pearly plaques or as irregular, roughened, or verrucous areas of mucosal thickening, possibly mistaken for leukoplakia. Either pattern may be superimposed on a background of apparent leukoplakia or erythroplakia. As these lesions enlarge, they typically create ulcerated and protruding masses that have irregular and indurated (rolled) borders.

On histologic examination, these cancers begin as dysplastic lesions, which may or may not progress to full-thickness dysplasia (carcinoma in situ) before invading the underlying connective tissue stroma (Fig. 16-7*B*). This difference in progression should be contrasted with cervical cancer (Chapter 22), in which, typically, full-thickness dysplasia, representing carcinoma in situ, develops before invasion. Squamous cell carcinomas range from well-differentiated keratinizing neoplasms to anaplastic, sometimes sarcomatoid, tumors, and

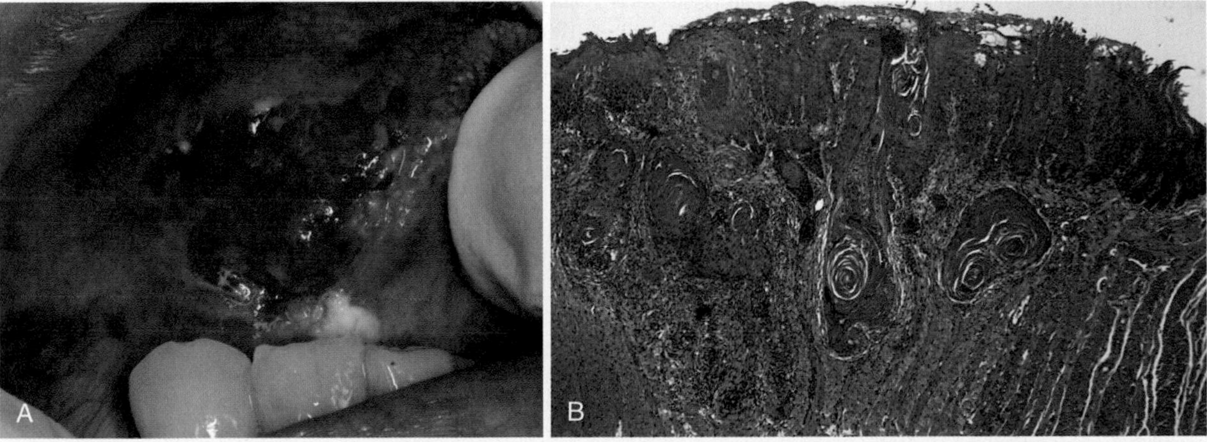

Figure 16-7 Squamous cell carcinoma. **A,** Clinical appearance demonstrating ulceration and induration of the oral mucosa. **B,** Histologic appearance demonstrating numerous nests and islands of malignant keratinocytes invading the underlying connective tissue stroma and skeletal muscle.

from slowly to rapidly growing lesions. However, the degree of histologic differentiation, as determined by the relative degree of keratinization, is not correlated with behavior. As a group these tumors tend to infiltrate locally before they metastasize to other sites. The routes of extension depend on the primary site. The favored sites of local metastasis are the cervical lymph nodes, while the most common sites of distant metastasis are mediastinal lymph nodes, lungs, liver, and bones. Unfortunately, such distant metastases are often already present at the time of discovery of the primary lesion.

Odontogenic Cysts and Tumors

The overwhelming majority of odontogenic cysts are derived from remnants of odontogenic epithelium present within the jaws. In contrast to the rest of the skeleton, epithelial-lined cysts are quite common in the jaws. In general, these cysts are subclassified as either inflammatory or developmental (Table 16-2). Only the most common of these lesions are described later.

The *dentigerous cyst* is defined as a cyst that originates around the crown of an unerupted tooth and is thought to be the result of fluid accumulation between the developing tooth and the dental follicle. Radiographically, these are unilocular lesions most often associated with impacted third molar (wisdom) teeth. Histologically, they are lined by a thin layer of stratified squamous epithelium. Often, there is a dense chronic inflammatory cell infiltrate in the connective tissue stroma. Complete removal of the lesion is curative.

The *odontogenic keratocyst (OKC)*, now called *keratocystic odontogenic tumor*, is an important lesion that must be differentiated from other odontogenic cysts because of its aggressive behavior. OKCs can be seen at any age but are most often diagnosed in patients between ages 10 and 40. They occur most commonly in males within the posterior mandible. Radiographically, OKCs present as well-defined unilocular or multilocular radiolucencies. Histologically, the cyst lining consists of a thin layer of keratinized stratified squamous epithelium with a prominent basal cell layer and a corrugated epithelial surface. Treatment requires complete removal of the lesion, because OKCs are locally aggressive and recurrence rates for inadequately removed lesions can reach 60%. About 80% of the lesions are solitary, but multiple OKCs occur in roughly 20% of patients, who should be evaluated for nevoid basal cell carcinoma syndrome (Gorlin syndrome), which is associated with mutations in the tumor suppressor gene *PTCH* (Patched) located on chromosome 9q22 (Chapter 25).

The *periapical cyst,* in contrast to the developmental cysts described earlier, is inflammatory in origin. These are common lesions found at the apex of teeth. They develop as a result of long-standing inflammation of the tooth (pulpitis), which may be caused by advanced carious lesions or by trauma to the tooth in question. The inflammatory process may result in necrosis of the pulpal tissue, which can traverse the length of the root and exit at the apex of the tooth into the surrounding alveolar bone. Over time, like any chronic inflammatory process, a lesion with granulation tissue may develop, and subsequent epithelialization may lead to the formation of a radicular cyst. While the term *periapical granuloma* is not the most appropriate terminology (the lesion does not show true granulomatous inflammation), this older name is still used. Periapical inflammatory lesions persist as a result of the continued presence of bacteria or other irritating agents in the area. Successful treatment, therefore, necessitates the complete removal of offending material and appropriate restoration of the tooth or extraction.

Odontogenic tumors are a group of lesions with diverse histologic appearances and clinical behavior. Some are true neoplasms (both benign and malignant), while others are more likely hamartomas. Odontogenic tumors are derived from odontogenic epithelium, ectomesenchyme, or both (Table 16-3). The two most common and clinically significant tumors are the following:

Table 16-2 Histologic Classification of Odontogenic Cysts

Inflammatory
Periapical cyst
Residual cyst
Paradental cyst
Developmental
Dentigerous cyst
Odontogenic keratocyst
Gingival cyst of newborn
Gingival cyst of adult
Eruption cyst
Lateral periodontal cyst
Glandular odontogenic cyst
Calcifying epithelial odontogenic cyst (Gorlin cyst)

Table 16-3 Histologic Classification of Odontogenic Tumors

Tumors of odontogenic epithelium
Benign
Ameloblastoma
Calcifying epithelial odontogenic tumor (Pindborg tumor)
Squamous odontogenic tumor
Adenomatoid odontogenic tumor
Malignant
Ameloblastic carcinoma
Malignant ameloblastoma
Clear-cell odontogenic carcinoma
Ghost cell odontogenic carcinoma
Primary intraosseous squamous cell carcinoma
Tumors of odontogenic ectomesenchyme
Odontogenic fibroma
Odontogenic myxoma
Cementoblastoma
Tumors of odontogenic epithelium and ectomesenchyme
Benign
Ameloblastic fibroma
Ameloblastic fibro-odontoma
Adenomatoid odontogenic tumor
Odontoameloblastoma
Complex odontoma
Compound odontoma
Calcifying cystic odontogenic tumor (calcifying odontogenic cyst)
Dentinogenic ghost cell tumor
Malignant
Ameloblastic fibrosarcoma

- *Ameloblastoma* arises from odontogenic epithelium and shows *no* ectomesenchymal differentiation. It is commonly cystic, slow growing, and locally invasive but has an indolent course in most cases. Treatment typically requires wide surgical resection to prevent recurrences.
- *Odontoma,* the most common type of odontogenic tumor, arises from epithelium but shows extensive depositions of enamel and dentin. Odontomas are probably hamartomas rather than true neoplasms and are cured by local excision.

KEY CONCEPTS

Oral Cavity

- **Caries** is the most common cause of tooth loss in persons younger than age 35 years. The primary cause is destruction of tooth structure by acid end-products of bacterial sugar fermentation.
- **Gingivitis** is a common and reversible inflammation of the mucosa surrounding the teeth.
- **Periodontitis** is a chronic inflammatory condition that results in the destruction of the supporting structures of the teeth with eventual loss of teeth. It is associated with poor oral hygiene and altered oral microbiota.
- **Aphthous ulcers** are painful superficial ulcers of unknown etiology.
- **Fibromas** and **pyogenic granulomas** are common reactive lesions of the oral mucosa.
- **Leukoplakias and erythroplakias** are oral mucosal lesions that may undergo malignant transformation.
- The majority of oral cavity and oropharyngeal cancers are **squamous cell carcinomas.** Oral cavity squamous cell carcinomas are classically linked to tobacco and alcohol use, but the incidence of HPV-associated lesions has risen dramatically in the oropharynx and base of the tongue.

UPPER AIRWAYS

The term *upper airways* is used here to include the nose, pharynx, and larynx and their related parts. Disorders of these structures are among the most common afflictions of humans, but fortunately the overwhelming majority of these disorders are more nuisance than threat.

Nose

Inflammatory diseases, mostly in the form of the common cold, are the most common disorders of the nose and accessory air sinuses. Most of these inflammatory conditions are viral in origin, but can be complicated by superimposed bacterial infections. Much less common are a few destructive inflammatory nasal diseases and primary tumors of the nasal cavity or maxillary sinus.

Inflammations

Infectious Rhinitis. Infectious rhinitis, commonly referred to as "common cold," is in most instances caused by one or more viruses. Major offenders are adenoviruses, echoviruses, and rhinoviruses. They evoke a profuse catarrhal discharge that is familiar to all and the bane of the kindergarten teacher. During the initial acute stages, the nasal mucosa is thickened, edematous, and red; the nasal cavities are narrowed; and the turbinates are enlarged. These changes may extend, to produce pharyngotonsillitis. Secondary bacterial infection enhances the inflammatory reaction and produces a mucopurulent or sometimes frankly suppurative exudate. But as all have learned from experience, these infections soon clear up—as the saying goes, in a week if treated but in 7 days if ignored.

Allergic Rhinitis. Allergic rhinitis (hay fever) is initiated by hypersensitivity reactions to one of a large group of allergens, most commonly the plant pollens, fungi, animal allergens, and dust mites. It affects 20% of the U.S. population. As is the case with asthma, allergic rhinitis is an IgE-mediated immune reaction with an early- and late-phase response (see "Immediate [Type I] Hypersensitivity" in Chapter 6). The allergic reaction is characterized by marked mucosal edema, redness, and mucus secretion, accompanied by a leukocytic infiltration in which eosinophils are prominent.

Nasal Polyps. Recurrent attacks of rhinitis may eventually lead to focal protrusions of the mucosa, producing so-called *nasal polyps*, which may reach 3 to 4 cm in length. On histologic examination these polyps consist of edematous mucosa having a loose stroma, often harboring hyperplastic or cystic mucous glands, infiltrated with a variety of inflammatory cells, including neutrophils, eosinophils, and plasma cells with occasional clusters of lymphocytes (Fig. 16-8). In the absence of bacterial infection, the mucosal covering of these polyps is intact, but with chronicity it may become ulcerated or infected. When multiple or large, the polyps may encroach on the airway and impair sinus drainage. Although the features of nasal polyps point to an allergic etiology, most people with nasal polyps are not atopic, and only 0.5% of atopic patients develop polyps.

Chronic Rhinitis. Chronic rhinitis is a sequel to repeated attacks of acute rhinitis, either microbial or allergic in origin, with the eventual development of superimposed bacterial infection. A deviated nasal septum or nasal polyps with impaired drainage of secretions contribute to the likelihood of microbial invasion. Frequently, there is superficial desquamation or ulceration of the mucosal epithelium and a variable inflammatory infiltrate of neutrophils, lymphocytes, and plasma cells subjacent to the epithelium. These suppurative infections sometimes extend into the air sinuses.

Sinusitis. Acute sinusitis is most commonly preceded by acute or chronic rhinitis, but maxillary sinusitis occasionally arises by extension of a periapical infection through the bony floor of the sinus. The offending agents are usually

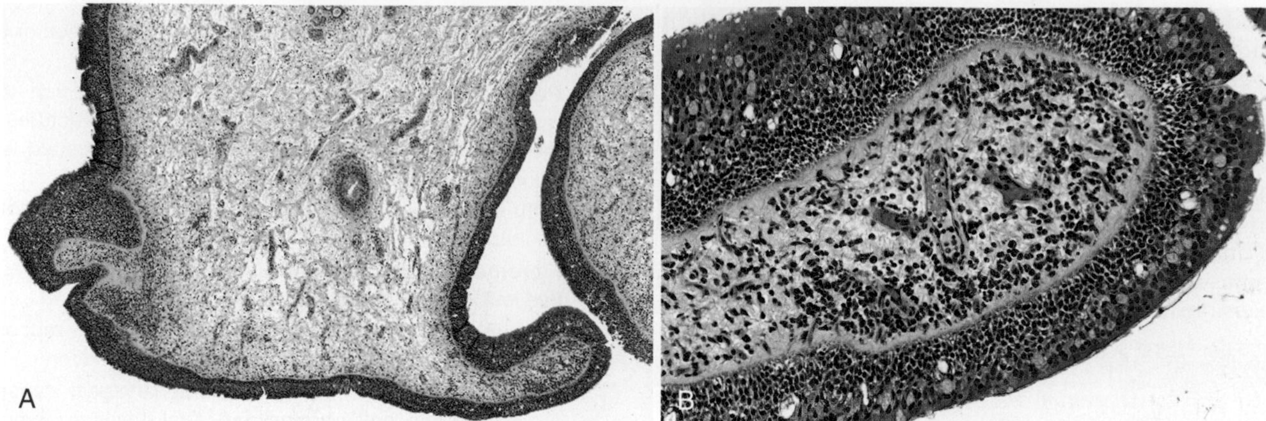

Figure 16-8 **A,** Nasal polyps. Low-power magnification showing edematous masses lined by epithelium. **B,** High-power view showing edema and eosinophil-rich inflammatory infiltrate.

inhabitants of the oral cavity, and the inflammatory reaction is entirely nonspecific. Impairment of drainage of the sinus by inflammatory edema of the mucosa is an important contributor to the process and, when complete, may impound the suppurative exudate, producing *empyema* of the sinus. Obstruction of the outflow, most often from the frontal and less commonly from the anterior ethmoid sinuses, occasionally leads to an accumulation of mucous secretions, producing a so-called *mucocele*.

Acute sinusitis may, in time, give rise to *chronic sinusitis*, particularly when there is interference with drainage. There is usually a mixed microbial flora, largely of normal inhabitants of the oral cavity. Particularly severe forms of chronic sinusitis are caused by fungi (e.g., mucormycosis), especially in patients with diabetes. Uncommonly, sinusitis is a component of *Kartagener syndrome*, which also includes bronchiectasis and situs inversus (Chapter 15). All these features are secondary to defective ciliary action. Although most instances of chronic sinusitis are more uncomfortable than disabling or serious, the infections have the potential of spreading into the orbit or of penetrating into the surrounding bone to give rise to osteomyelitis or spreading into the cranial vault, causing septic thrombophlebitis of a dural venous sinus.

Necrotizing Lesions of the Nose and Upper Airways

Necrotizing ulcerating lesions of the nose and upper respiratory tract may be produced by the following:

- Acute fungal infections (including mucormycosis; Chapter 8), particularly in patients with diabetes and immunosuppressed patients
- Granulomatosis with polyangiitis, previously called Wegener granulomatosis (Chapter 11)
- Extranodal NK/T-cell lymphoma, nasal type, is a lymphoma in which the tumor cells harbor EBV (Chapter 13). These neoplasms are typically seen in males who are in the fifth or sixth decade of life and most commonly occur in individuals of Asian and Latin American descent. Ulceration and superimposed bacterial infection frequently complicate the process. At one time these lesions were almost always rapidly fatal as a result of uncontrolled spread of the lymphoma and penetration into the cranial vault, or secondary bacterial infection and blood-borne dissemination of the infection. Currently, localized cases can often be controlled with radiotherapy, but relapse and recurrences remain common and are associated with poor outcomes.

Nasopharynx

Although the nasopharyngeal mucosa, related lymphoid structures, and glands may be involved in a wide variety of specific infections (e.g., diphtheria, infectious mononucleosis) and by neoplasms, the only disorders we describe here are nonspecific inflammations; tumors are discussed separately.

Inflammations

Pharyngitis and *tonsillitis* are frequent features of viral upper respiratory infections. Most commonly implicated are the rhinoviruses, echoviruses, and adenoviruses, and, less frequently, respiratory syncytial viruses and the various strains of influenza virus. In the usual case, there is reddening and edema of the nasopharyngeal mucosa, with reactive enlargement of nearby tonsils and lymph nodes. Bacterial infections may be superimposed on these viral infections, or may be primary invaders. The most common offenders are the β-hemolytic streptococci, but sometimes *Staphylococcus aureus* or other pathogens may be implicated. The inflamed nasopharyngeal mucosa may be covered by an exudative membrane (pseudomembrane), and the nasopalatine and palatine tonsils may be enlarged and covered by exudate. A typical appearance is of enlarged, reddened tonsils (due to reactive lymphoid hyperplasia) dotted by pinpoints of exudate emanating from the tonsillar crypts, so-called *follicular tonsillitis*.

The major importance of streptococcal "sore throats" lies in the possible development of late sequelae, such as rheumatic fever (Chapter 12) and glomerulonephritis (Chapter 20). Whether recurrent episodes of acute tonsillitis favor the development of chronic tonsillar enlargement is open to debate, but regardless of cause the enlargement of the lymphoid tissue invites the tender mercies of the ENT surgeon.

Tumors of the Nose, Sinuses, and Nasopharynx

Tumors in the nose, sinuses, and nasopharynx are infrequent but include the wide spectrum of mesenchymal and epithelial neoplasms. Distinctive types are described here.

Nasopharyngeal Angiofibroma. **Nasopharyngeal angiofibroma is a benign, highly vascular tumor that occurs almost exclusively in adolescent males who are often fair-skinned and red headed.** There is also an association with familial adenomatous polyps. It is believed to arise within the fibrovascular stroma of the posterolateral wall of the roof of the nasal cavity. Surgical removal is the treatment of choice. However, because of its locally aggressive nature and intracranial extension, recurrence rates can be as high as 20%. In about 9% of cases it is fatal, with death being caused by hemorrhage and intracranial extension.

Sinonasal (Schneiderian) Papilloma. **Sinonasal papilloma is a benign neoplasm arising from the respiratory or schneiderian mucosa lining the nasal cavity and paranasal sinuses.** These lesions occur in three forms: *exophytic* (most common), endophytic (*inverted*; most important biologically), and *cylindrical*. HPV DNA, often types 6 and 11, has been identified in the exophytic and endophytic lesions, but not the cylindrical type. Sinonasal papillomas are observed most commonly in adult males between the ages of 30 and 60. Because of its uniquely aggressive biologic behavior, only the endophytic form is discussed here. Endophytic sinonasal papillomas are benign but locally aggressive neoplasms occurring in both the nose and the paranasal sinuses. As the name implies, the papillomatous proliferation of squamous epithelium, instead of producing an exophytic growth, invaginates into the underlying stroma (Fig. 16-9). It has a high rate of recurrence if not adequately excised, with the potentially serious complication of invasion of the orbit or cranial vault. Furthermore, malignant transformation is observed in approximately 10% of cases.

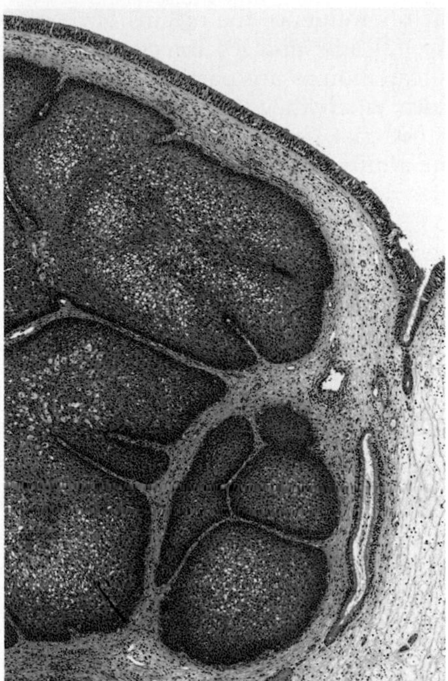

Figure 16-9 Inverted papilloma. The masses of squamous epithelium are growing inward; hence, the term *inverted*.

Olfactory Neuroblastoma (Esthesioneuroblastoma). **Olfactory neuroblastomas arise from the neuroectodermal olfactory cells present within the mucosa, particularly in the superior aspect of the nasal cavity.** There is a bimodal age distribution with peaks at 15 and 50 years of age. The patients typically present with nasal obstruction and/or epistaxis. Histologically, olfactory neuroblastomas are one of the small, blue, round cell neoplasms that include lymphoma, small cell carcinoma, Ewing sarcoma/peripheral neuroectodermal tumor, rhabdomyosarcoma, melanoma, and sinonasal undifferentiated carcinoma. Typically, olfactory neuroblastomas are composed of nests and lobules of well-circumscribed cells that are separated by a fibrovascular stroma. Many of the tumors also contain a fibrillary matrix that ultrastructurally corresponds to tangles of neuronal cell processes. Because these neoplasms are of neuroendocrine origin, the tumor cells contain membrane-bound secretory granules on electron microscopy and express neuron-specific enolase, synaptophysin, CD56, and chromogranin by immunohistochemistry. Depending on the stage and grade of a particular neoplasm, combinations of surgery, radiation therapy, and chemotherapy yield 5-year survival rates of 40% to 90%.

NUT Midline Carcinoma. This is an uncommon tumor that may occur in the nasopharynx, the salivary gland, or in other midline structures in the thorax or abdomen. It can occur at any age, from infancy to late adulthood. Its true incidence is not known, as it easily mistaken for squamous cell carcinoma, which it resembles morphologically. It is extremely aggressive and resistant to conventional therapy; as a result, most patients survive for less than a year following diagnosis.

Although rare, NUT midline carcinoma is pathogenically interesting. It is uniformly associated with translocations that create fusion genes encoding chimeric proteins comprised of most of NUT, a chromatin regulator, and a portion of a "chromatin reader" protein, usually BRD4. Drugs that displace BRD4-NUT from chromatin induce NUT midline carcinoma cells to terminally differentiate, a mechanism of oncogenesis that is common in acute leukemias but unusual for epithelial cancers. Targeted therapy with BRD4-NUT inhibitors is now being tested in the clinic and offers hope for those with this lethal form of cancer.

Nasopharyngeal Carcinoma. **Nasopharyngeal carcinoma is characterized by a distinctive geographic distribution, a close anatomic relationship to lymphoid tissue, and an association with EBV infection.** The nomenclature for nasopharyngeal carcinomas is in constant flux. However, at present the disease is thought to take one of three patterns: (1) keratinizing squamous cell carcinomas, (2) nonkeratinizing squamous cell carcinomas, and (3) undifferentiated/basaloid carcinomas that have an abundant non-neoplastic, lymphocytic infiltrate. The last pattern has often been called *lymphoepithelioma.* While widely used in clinical practice, this descriptive term should be avoided.

Three factors influence the origins of these neoplasms: (1) heredity, (2) age, and (3) infection with EBV. Nasopharyngeal carcinomas are particularly common in some parts of Africa, where they are the most frequent childhood cancer. In contrast, in southern China, they are very common in adults but rarely occur in children. In the United States they are rare in both adults and children. In addition to EBV infection, diets high in nitrosamines, such as fermented foods and salted fish, as well as other environmental insults such as smoking and chemical fumes, have been linked to the disease. In the nonkeratinizing form, most patients have anti-EBV antibodies against early antigens or viral capsid antigens.

MORPHOLOGY

On histologic examination, the keratinizing and nonkeratinizing squamous cell lesions resemble usual well-differentiated and poorly differentiated squamous cell carcinomas arising in other locations. The undifferentiated/basaloid variant is composed of large epithelial cells with oval or round vesicular nuclei, prominent nucleoli, and indistinct cell borders disposed in a syncytium-like array (Fig. 16-10*B*). Admixed with the epithelial cells are abundant, mature, normal-appearing lymphocytes, which are predominantly T cells. In addition, EBV genomes can be detected in the serum by PCR, or EBV encoded RNAs such as EBER-1 or proteins such as LMP-1 can be identified in the malignant epithelial cells by in situ hybridization (Fig. 16-10*B*) or immunohistochemistry, respectively.

Primary nasopharyngeal carcinomas are often clinically occult for long periods, and present with nasal obstruction, epistaxis, and often metastases to the cervical lymph nodes in as many as 70% of the patients. Radiotherapy is the standard treatment. For all types, there is an overall 5-year survival of approximately 60%. Depending on stage, the 5-year survival for the nonkeratinizing type is 70% to 98%, while the 5-year survival for the keratinizing form is approximately 20%. These differences in survival have been attributed to the fact that the undifferentiated carcinoma is the most radiosensitive, while the keratinizing squamous cell carcinoma is the least radiosensitive.

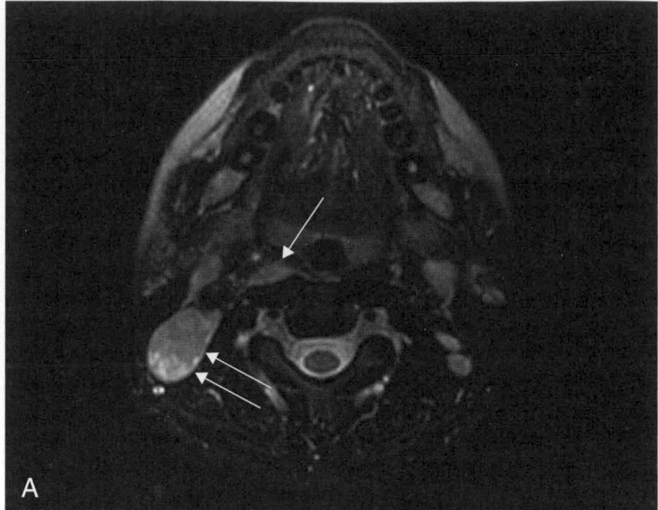

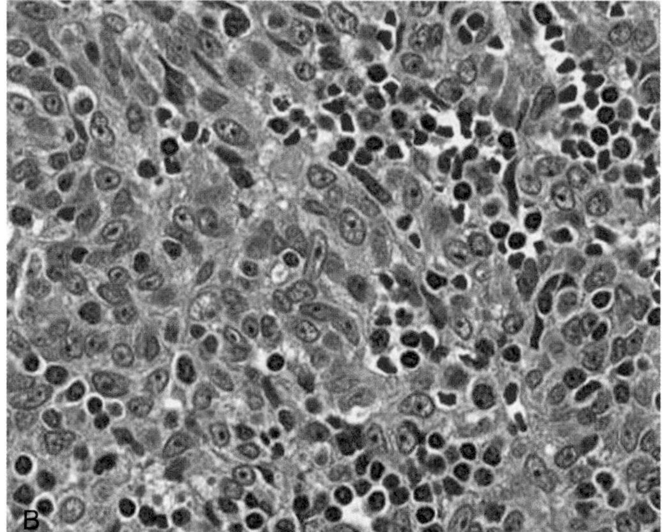

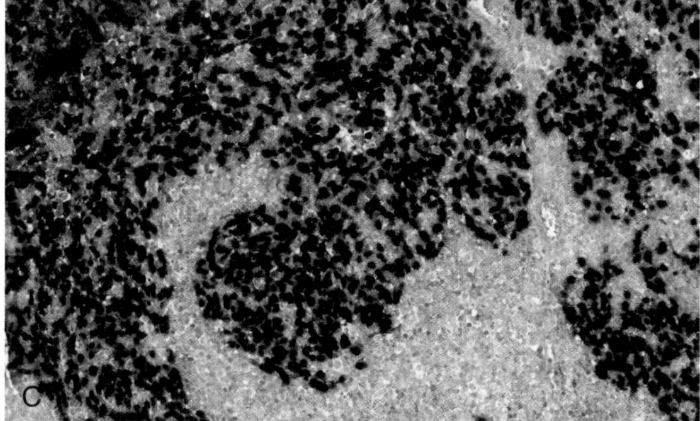

Figure 16-10 Nasopharyngeal carcinoma, undifferentiated type. **A,** Computed tomography study demonstrating thickening of the nasopharyngeal region (arrow) and an enlarged cervical lymph node (double arrow). **B,** The syncytium-like clusters of epithelium are surrounded by lymphocytes. **C,** In situ hybridization for EBER-1, a small nuclear RNA encoded by EBV.

Larynx

The most common disorders of the larynx are inflammatory. Tumors are uncommon but are amenable to resection, though often at the price of loss of natural voice.

Inflammations

Laryngitis may occur as the sole manifestation of allergic, viral, bacterial, or chemical insult, but it is more commonly part of a generalized upper respiratory tract infection or the result of heavy exposure to environmental toxins such as tobacco smoke. It may also occur in association with gastroesophageal reflux due to the irritating effect of gastric contents. The larynx may also be affected in systemic infections, such as tuberculosis and diphtheria. Although most infections are self-limited, they may at times be serious, especially in infancy or childhood, when mucosal congestion, exudation, or edema may cause laryngeal obstruction. In particular, in infants and young children with their small airways, laryngoepiglottitis, caused by respiratory syncytial virus, *Haemophilus influenzae*, or β-hemolytic streptococci may induce such sudden swelling of the epiglottis and vocal cords as to constitute a medical emergency. This form of disease is uncommon

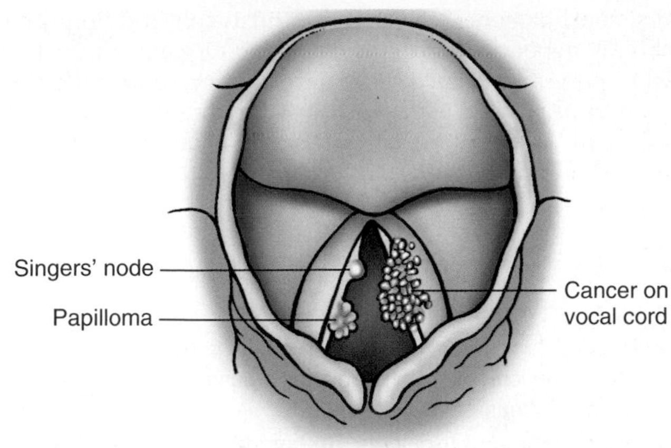

Figure 16-11 Diagrammatic comparison of a singer's nodule, a benign papilloma and an exophytic carcinoma of the larynx to highlight the difference in their clinical appearance.

in adults because of the larger size of the larynx and the stronger accessory muscles of respiration. *Croup* is the name given to laryngotracheobronchitis in children, in which the inflammatory narrowing of the airway produces the inspiratory stridor so frightening to parents. The most common form of laryngitis, encountered in heavy smokers, predisposes to squamous epithelial metaplasia and sometimes overt carcinoma.

Reactive Nodules (Vocal Cord Nodules and Polyps)

Reactive nodules, also called polyps, sometimes develop on the vocal cords, most often in heavy smokers or in individuals who impose great strain on their vocal cords *(singer's nodules)* (Fig. 16-11). By convention, singers' nodules are bilateral lesions and polyps are unilateral. Adults are most often affected. These nodules are smooth, rounded, sessile or pedunculated excrescences, generally only a few millimeters in the greatest dimension, located usually on the true vocal cords. They are typically covered by squamous epithelium that may become keratotic, hyperplastic, or even slightly dysplastic. The core of the nodule is a loose myxoid connective tissue that may be variably fibrotic or punctuated by numerous vascular channels. When nodules on opposing vocal cords impinge on each other, the mucosa may undergo ulceration. Because of their strategic location and accompanying inflammation, they characteristically change the character of the voice and often cause progressive hoarseness. They virtually never give rise to cancers.

Squamous Papilloma and Papillomatosis

Laryngeal squamous papillomas are benign neoplasms, usually located on the true vocal cords, that form soft, raspberry-like proliferations rarely more than 1 cm in diameter (Fig. 16-11). On histologic examination, the papillomas are made up of multiple slender, finger-like projections supported by central fibrovascular cores and covered by an orderly stratified squamous epithelium. When the papillomas are on the free edge of the vocal cord, trauma may lead to ulceration that can be accompanied by hemoptysis.

Papillomas are usually single in adults but are often multiple in children, in whom they are referred to as *juvenile laryngeal papillomatosis.* However, multiple recurring papillomas also occur in adults. *The lesions are caused by HPV types 6 and 11.* They do not become malignant, but frequently recur. They often spontaneously regress at puberty, but some affected patients endure numerous surgeries before this occurs.

Carcinoma of the Larynx

Carcinoma of the larynx is typically a squamous cell carcinoma seen in male chronic smokers.

Sequence of Hyperplasia-Dysplasia-Carcinoma. A spectrum of epithelial alterations is seen in the larynx. They range from *hyperplasia, atypical hyperplasia, dysplasia,* and *carcinoma in situ* to *invasive carcinoma.* Grossly, the epithelial changes vary from smooth, white or reddened focal thickenings, sometimes roughened by keratosis, to irregular verrucous or ulcerated white-pink lesions (Fig. 16-12).

There are all gradations of epithelial hyperplasia of the true vocal cords, and the likelihood of the development of an overt carcinoma is directly proportional to the grade of dysplasia when the lesion is first seen. Orderly hyperplasias have almost no potential for malignant transformation, but the risk rises to 1% to 2% during the span of 5 to 10 years with mild dysplasia and 5% to 10% with severe dysplasia. Only histologic evaluation can determine the gravity of the changes.

The epithelial alterations described above are most often related to tobacco smoke, the risk being proportional to the level of exposure. Indeed, up to the point of cancer, the changes often regress after cessation of smoking. Together

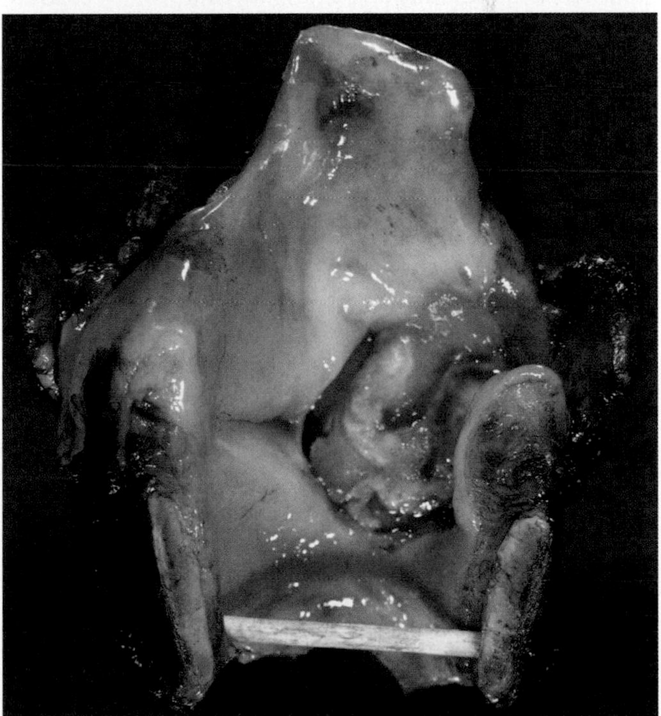

Figure 16-12 Laryngeal carcinoma. Note the large, ulcerated, fungating lesion involving the vocal cord and pyriform sinus.

smoking and alcohol increase the risk substantially. Other factors that may contribute to increased risk include nutritional factors, exposure to asbestos, irradiation, and infection with HPV.

MORPHOLOGY

About 95% of laryngeal carcinomas are typical squamous cell tumors. The tumor usually develops on the vocal cords, but it may also arise above or below the cords, on the epiglottis or aryepiglottic folds, or in the pyriform sinuses. Those confined within the larynx proper are termed **intrinsic**, whereas those that arise or extend outside the larynx are called **extrinsic**. Squamous cell carcinomas of the larynx follow the growth pattern of other squamous cell carcinomas. They begin as in situ lesions that later appear as pearly gray, wrinkled plaques on the mucosal surface, ultimately ulcerating and fungating (Fig. 16-12). The degree of anaplasia of the laryngeal tumors is highly variable. Sometimes massive tumor giant cells and multiple bizarre mitotic figures are seen. As expected with lesions arising from recurrent exposure to environmental carcinogens, adjacent mucosa may demonstrate squamous cell hyperplasia with foci of dysplasia or even carcinoma in situ.

Carcinoma of the larynx is most commonly seen in men in the sixth decade of life and often manifests clinically as persistent hoarseness, dysphagia, and dysphonia. Prognosis is highly dependent on clinical staging. Organ preservation techniques (laser surgery, microsurgery, and radiation therapy) are being used with greater frequency, particularly with early disease. Combined chemotherapy and radiation therapy, with or without salvage laryngectomy, may be required for more advanced or recurrent disease.

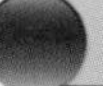

KEY CONCEPTS

Upper Airways

- **Rhinitis** can be infectious or allergic in nature. When recurrent it can lead to chronic rhinitis, sinusitis, and the development of nasal polyps.
- **Pharyngitis** and **tonsillitis** are common upper respiratory track viral infections typically caused by rhinoviruses, echoviruses, and adenoviruses.
- **Nasopharyngeal carcinoma** is most often caused by the EBV and is common among children in Africa and Asian adults.
- **Laryngitis** can be caused by a host of etiologies, including allergic, viral, bacterial, and chemical insults.
- **Vocal cord nodules** and **polyps** are reactive lesions seen in smokers or individuals who strain their vocal cords.
- **Laryngeal squamous cell carcinoma** is a disease of older males, related to smoking and alcohol use.

EARS

Although disorders of the ear rarely shorten life, many impair its quality. The most common aural disorders, in descending order of frequency, are (1) acute and chronic otitis (most often involving the middle ear and mastoid), sometimes leading to a cholesteatoma; (2) symptomatic otosclerosis; (3) aural polyps; (4) labyrinthitis; (5) carcinomas, largely of the external ear; and (6) paragangliomas, found mostly in the middle ear. Only those conditions that have distinctive morphologic features (save for labyrinthitis) are described. Paragangliomas are discussed later.

Inflammatory Lesions

Inflammations of the ear—*otitis media, acute or chronic*—occur mostly in infants and children. These lesions are typically viral in nature and produce a serous exudate but may become suppurative with superimposed bacterial infection. The most common bacteria in the acute infection are *Streptococcus pneumoniae,* non-typeable *H. influenzae,* and *Moraxella catarrhalis.*

Repeated bouts of acute otitis media with failure of resolution lead to chronic disease. The causative agents of chronic disease are usually *Pseudomonas aeruginosa, Staphylococcus aureus,* or a fungus; sometimes a mixed flora is the cause. Chronic infection has the potential to perforate the eardrum, encroach on the ossicles or labyrinth, spread into the mastoid spaces, and even penetrate into the cranial vault to produce a temporal cerebritis or abscess. Otitis media in the diabetic person, when caused by *P. aeruginosa,* is especially aggressive and spreads widely, causing destructive necrotizing otitis media.

Cholesteatomas, associated with chronic otitis media, are non-neoplastic, cystic lesions 1 to 4 cm in diameter, lined by keratinizing squamous epithelium or metaplastic mucus-secreting epithelium, and filled with amorphous debris (derived largely from desquamated epithelium). Sometimes they contain spicules of cholesterol. Their pathogenesis is not clear, but it is proposed that chronic inflammation and perforation of the eardrum with ingrowth of the squamous epithelium or metaplasia of the secretory epithelial lining of the middle ear are responsible for the formation of a squamous cell nest that becomes cystic. A chronic inflammatory reaction surrounds the keratinous cyst. Sometimes, the cyst ruptures, increasing the inflammatory reaction and inducing the formation of giant cells that enclose partially necrotic squames and other particulate debris. These lesions, by progressive enlargement, can erode into the ossicles, the labyrinth, the adjacent bone, or the surrounding soft tissue and sometimes produce visible neck masses.

Otosclerosis

As the name implies, **otosclerosis refers to abnormal bone deposition in the middle ear about the rim of the oval window into which the footplate of the stapes fits**. Both ears are usually affected. At first there is fibrous ankylosis of the footplate, followed in time by bony overgrowth anchoring it into the oval window. The degree of immobilization governs the severity of the hearing loss. This condition usually begins in the early decades of life; minimal degrees of this derangement are exceedingly common in the United States in young to middle-aged adults, but fortunately more severe symptomatic otosclerosis is relatively uncommon. In most instances it is familial, following an autosomal dominant transmission with variable penetrance. The basis for the osseous overgrowth is completely obscure, but it appears to represent uncoupling of normal bone resorption and bone formation. Thus, it begins with bone resorption, followed by fibrosis and vascularization of the temporal bone in the immediate vicinity of the oval window, in time replaced by dense new bone anchoring the footplate of the stapes. In most instances the process is slowly progressive over the span of decades, leading eventually to marked hearing loss.

Tumors

Epithelial and mesenchymal tumors that arise in the ear—external, middle, internal—all are rare save for basal cell or squamous cell carcinomas of the pinna (external ear). These carcinomas tend to occur in elderly men and are associated with sun exposure. By contrast, squamous cell carcinomas of the canal occur most often in middle-aged to elderly women and are not associated with sun exposure. Wherever they arise they morphologically resemble their counterparts in other skin locations, beginning as papules that extend and eventually erode and invade locally. Basal cell and squamous cell lesions of the pinna are locally invasive but they rarely spread. Squamous cell carcinomas arising in the external canal may invade the cranial cavity or metastasize to regional nodes, accounting for a 5-year mortality of about 50%.

KEY CONCEPTS

Ears

- **Infections** of the ear are common in children and typically viral in etiology. Chronic infections can be complicated by bacterial infections, which can lead to secondary complications including perforated eardrum as well as spreading to the ossicles or mastoid spaces.
- **Otosclerosis,** with its associated hearing loss, is caused by the abnormal deposition of bone in the middle ear.

NECK

Most of the conditions that involve the neck are described elsewhere (e.g., squamous cell and basal cell carcinomas of the skin, melanomas, lymphomas), or they are a component of a systemic disorder (e.g., generalized rashes, the lymphadenopathy of infectious mononucleosis or tonsillitis). What remains to be considered here are a few uncommon lesions unique to the neck.

Branchial Cyst (Cervical Lymphoepithelial Cyst)

The vast majority of these cysts are thought to arise from remnants of the second branchial arch and are most commonly observed in young adults between the ages of 20 and 40. These benign cysts usually appear on the upper lateral aspect of the neck along the sternocleidomastoid muscle. Clinically, the cysts are well circumscribed, 2 to 5 cm in diameter, with fibrous walls usually lined by stratified squamous or pseudostratified columnar epithelium. The cyst wall typically contains lymphoid tissue with prominent germinal centers. The contents of the cysts may be clear and watery or mucinous and may contain desquamated, granular cellular debris. The cysts enlarge slowly, are rarely the site of malignant transformation, and generally are readily excised. Similar lesions sometimes appear in the parotid gland or in the oral cavity beneath the tongue.

Thyroglossal Duct Cyst

Embryologically, the thyroid anlage begins in the region of the foramen cecum at the base of the tongue; as the gland develops it descends to its definitive midline location in the anterior neck. Remnants of this developmental tract may persist, producing cysts, 1 to 4 cm in diameter, which may be lined by stratified squamous epithelium, when located near the base of the tongue, or by pseudostratified columnar epithelium in lower locations. Transitional patterns are also encountered. The connective tissue wall of the cyst may harbor lymphoid aggregates or remnants of recognizable thyroid tissue. The treatment is excision. Malignant transformation within the lining epithelium has been reported but is rare.

Paraganglioma (Carotid Body Tumor)

Paraganglia are clusters of neuroendocrine cells associated with the sympathetic and parasympathetic nervous systems. As a result, these neoplasms can be seen in various regions of the body. While the most common location of these tumors is within the adrenal medulla, where they give rise to pheochromocytomas (Chapter 24), approximately 70% of extra-adrenal paragangliomas occur in the head and neck region. The pathogenesis of paragangliomas is not fully understood. However, loss of function mutations in genes encoding succinate dehydrogenase subunits or cofactors, proteins that participate in mitochondrial oxidative phosphorylation, occur frequently in both hereditary and spontaneous paragangliomas. How these mutations contribute to tumor development is not yet clear, but it is suspected that they do so by altering cellular metabolism, which you will recall is one of the hallmarks of neoplasia (Chapter 7). Interestingly, the incidence of these tumors is greater in people living at high altitudes.

Paragangliomas typically develop in two locations:

- Paravertebral paraganglia (e.g., organs of Zuckerkandl and, rarely, bladder). Such tumors have sympathetic connections and are chromaffin-positive, a stain that detects catecholamines.

- Paraganglia related to the great vessels of the head and neck, the so-called aorticopulmonary chain, including the *carotid bodies* (most common); aortic bodies; jugulotympanic ganglia; ganglion nodosum of the vagus nerve; and clusters located about the oral cavity, nose, nasopharynx, larynx, and orbit. These are innervated by the parasympathetic nervous system and infrequently release catecholamines.

MORPHOLOGY

The **carotid body tumor** is a prototype of a parasympathetic paraganglioma. It rarely exceeds 6 cm in diameter and arises close to or envelops the bifurcation of the common carotid artery. The tumor tissue is red-pink to brown. The microscopic features of all paragangliomas, wherever they arise, are remarkably uniform. They are chiefly composed of nests **(zellballen)** of round to oval chief cells (neuroectodermal in origin) that are surrounded by delicate vascular septae (Fig. 16-13). The tumor cells contain abundant, clear or granular, eosinophilic cytoplasm and uniform, round to ovoid, sometimes vesicular, nuclei. In most tumors there is little cellular pleomorphism, and mitoses are scant. The chief cells stain strongly for neuroendocrine markers such as chromogranin, synaptophysin, neuron-specific enolase, CD56, and CD57. In addition, there is a supporting network of spindle-shaped stromal cells, collectively called sustentacular cells, which are positive for S-100 protein. Electron microscopy often discloses well-demarcated neuroendocrine granules in paravertebral tumors, but their number can be highly variable and they tend to be scant in nonfunctioning tumors.

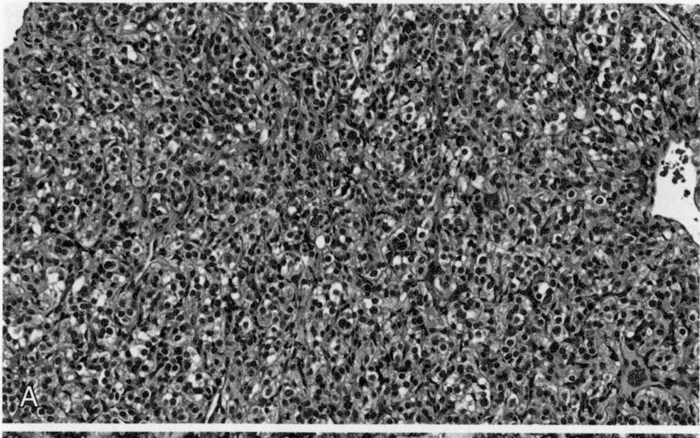

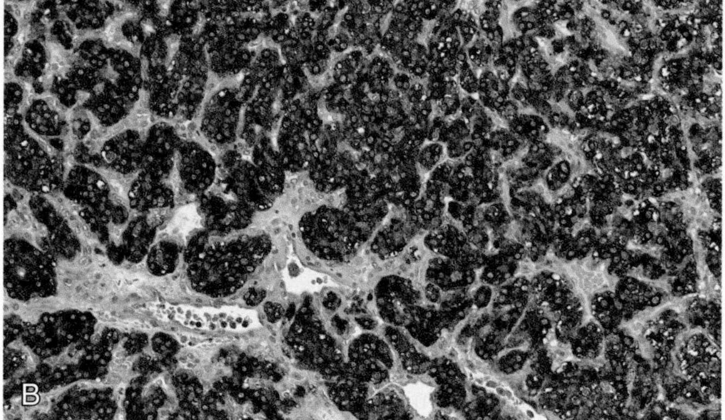

Figure 16-13 Carotid body tumor. **A,** Low-power view showing tumor clusters separated by septa (Zellballen). The septae are marked by bright red capillaries. **B,** Immunohistochemistry demonstrating positivity for chromogranin in the tumor cells.

Carotid body tumors (and paragangliomas in general) are rare. They are slow-growing and painless masses that usually arise in the fifth and sixth decades of life. They commonly occur singly and sporadically but may be familial, with autosomal dominant transmission in the multiple endocrine neoplasia 2 syndrome (Chapter 24); in this setting they are often multiple and sometimes bilateral. Carotid body tumors frequently recur after incomplete resection and, despite their benign appearance, may metastasize to regional lymph nodes and distant sites. About 50% ultimately prove fatal, largely because of infiltrative growth. Unfortunately, it is almost impossible to predict the clinical course of a carotid body tumor—mitoses, pleomorphism, and even vascular invasion are not reliable indicators.

KEY CONCEPTS

Neck

- **Branchial cysts** arise from the region of the second branchial pouch and are typically seen in young adults.
- **Thyroglossal duct cysts** arise as a result of incomplete descent of the thyroid analog from the foramen cecum in the base of the tongue.
- Seventy percent of **paragangliomas** are observed in the head and neck region that often develop in the fifth decade of life. While often sporadic in appearance, they may be associated with multiple endocrine neoplasia 2 syndrome.

SALIVARY GLANDS

There are three major salivary glands—parotid, submandibular, and sublingual—as well as innumerable minor salivary glands distributed throughout the mucosa of the oral cavity. Inflammatory or neoplastic disease may develop within any of these.

Xerostomia

Xerostomia is defined as a *dry mouth* resulting from a decrease in the production of saliva. Its incidence among various populations has been reported to be as high as 20% in individuals over the age of 70. It is a major feature of the autoimmune disorder Sjögren syndrome (Chapter 6), in which it is usually accompanied by dry eyes. A lack of salivary secretions is also a major complication of radiation therapy. However, xerostomia is most frequently a side-effect of many commonly prescribed classes of medications, including anticholinergic, antidepressant/antipsychotic, diuretic, antihypertensive, sedative, muscle relaxant, analgesic, and antihistamine drugs. Xerostomia may present as dry mucosa and/or atrophy of the papillae of the tongue, with fissuring and ulcerations. In conditions such as Sjögren syndrome, concomitant inflammatory enlargement of the salivary glands may also be observed. Complications of xerostomia include increased rates of dental caries, candidiasis, as well as difficulty in swallowing and speaking.

Inflammation (Sialadenitis)

Sialadenitis may be induced by trauma, viral or bacterial infection, or autoimmune disease. Mucoceles are the most common type of inflammatory salivary gland lesion. The most common form of viral sialadenitis is mumps, in which the major salivary glands, particularly the parotids, are affected (Chapter 8). Other glands (e.g., the pancreas and testes) may also be involved. As already discussed, autoimmunity underlies Sjögren syndrome, in which widespread inflammation of the salivary glands and the mucus-secreting glands of the mucosa induces xerostomia. Concomitant involvement of the lacrimal glands in Sjögren syndrome may also produce dry eyes—*keratoconjunctivitis sicca.*

Mucocele. This is the most common lesion of the salivary glands. It results from either blockage or rupture of a salivary gland duct, with consequent leakage of saliva into the surrounding connective tissue stroma. Mucoceles are most often found on the lower lip and are the result of trauma (Fig. 16-14*A*). They occur at all ages but are most common in toddlers, young adults, and the elderly, who are more prone to falling. Clinically, they present as fluctuant swellings of the lower lip that have a blue translucent hue. Patients may report a history of changes in the size of the lesion, particularly in association with meals. Histologically, mucoceles are pseudocysts with cyst-like spaces lined by inflammatory granulation tissue or by fibrous connective tissue. The cystic spaces are filled with mucin and inflammatory cells, particularly macrophages (Fig. 16-14*B*). Complete excision of the cyst and its accompanying minor salivary gland lobule is required, as incomplete excision may lead to recurrence.

Ranula is a term reserved for epithelial-lined cysts that arise when the duct of the sublingual gland has been damaged. A ranula may become so large that it develops into a "plunging ranula", a colorful description of a cyst that has dissected through the connective tissue stroma connecting the two bellies of the mylohyoid muscle.

Sialolithiasis and Nonspecific Sialadenitis. Nonspecific bacterial sialadenitis, most often involving the major salivary glands, particularly the submandibular glands, is a common condition, usually secondary to ductal obstruction produced by stones *(sialolithiasis).* The common offenders are *S. aureus* and *Streptococcus viridans.* The stone formation is sometimes related to obstruction of the orifices of the salivary glands by impacted food debris or by edema about the orifice after some injury. Frequently, no underlying cause can be detected. Decreased secretory function may also predispose to secondary bacterial invasion, as sometimes occurs in patients receiving long-term phenothiazines that suppress salivary secretion. Decreased salivary secretions caused by dehydration may lead to the development of bacterial suppurative parotitis in elderly patients with a recent history of major thoracic or abdominal surgery.

Whatever the origin, the obstructive process and bacterial invasion lead to a nonspecific inflammation of the affected glands that may be largely interstitial or, when induced by staphylococcal or other pyogens, may be associated with overt suppurative necrosis and abscess formation. Unilateral involvement of a single gland is the rule. The inflammatory involvement causes painful enlargement and sometimes a purulent ductal discharge.

Neoplasms

Despite their relatively simple morphology, the salivary glands give rise to no fewer than 30 histologically distinct tumors. A classification and the relative incidence of

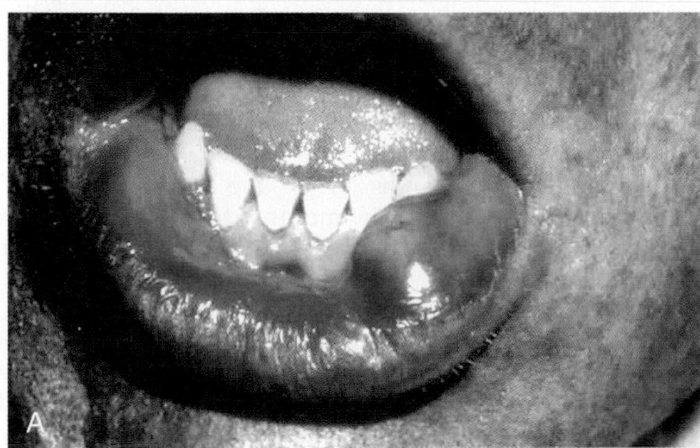

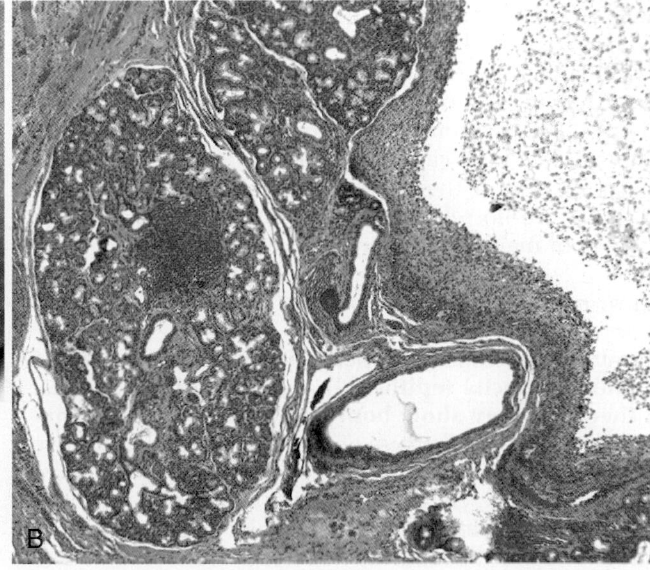

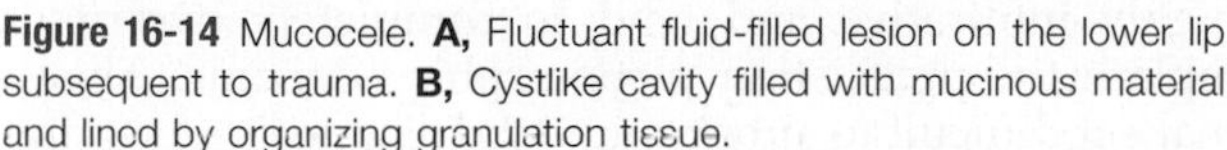

Figure 16-14 Mucocele. **A,** Fluctuant fluid-filled lesion on the lower lip subsequent to trauma. **B,** Cystlike cavity filled with mucinous material and lined by organizing granulation tissue.

Table 16-4 Histologic Classification and Incidence of the Most Common Benign and Malignant Tumors of the Salivary Glands

Benign	Malignant
Pleomorphic adenoma (50%) (mixed tumor)	Mucoepidermoid carcinoma (15%)
Warthin tumor (5%-10%)	Adenocarcinoma (NOS) (10%)
Oncocytoma (1%)	Acinic cell carcinoma (5%)
Other adenomas (5%-10%) Basal cell adenoma Canalicular adenoma	Adenoid cystic carcinoma (5%) Malignant mixed tumor (3%-5%) Squamous cell carcinoma (1%)
Ductal papillomas	Other carcinomas (2%)

NOS, Not otherwise specified.
Data from Ellis GL, Auclair PL: Tumors of the Salivary Glands. Atlas of Tumor Pathology, Fourth Series. Washington, DC, Armed Forces Institute of Pathology, 2008.

benign and malignant tumors is listed in Table 16-4; not included are the rare benign and malignant mesenchymal neoplasms.

As indicated in Table 16-4, a small number of neoplasms makes up more than 90% of salivary gland tumors, and so our discussion is restricted to these. Overall, these neoplasms are relatively uncommon and represent less than 2% of all tumors in humans. About 65% to 80% arise within the parotid, 10% in the submandibular gland, and the remainder in the minor salivary glands, including the sublingual glands. Approximately 15% to 30% of tumors in the parotid glands are malignant. In contrast, approximately 40% of submandibular, 50% of minor salivary gland, and 70% to 90% of sublingual tumors are cancerous. Thus, **the likelihood of a salivary gland tumor being malignant is more or less inversely proportional to the size of the gland.**

These tumors usually occur in adults, with a slight female predominance, but about 5% occur in children younger than age 16 years. Warthin tumors occur much more often in males than in females, perhaps reflecting the historically higher prevalence of smoking, a predisposing factor, among men. The benign tumors most often appear in the fifth to seventh decades of life. The malignant ones tend to appear somewhat later. Whatever the histologic pattern, neoplasms in the parotid glands produce distinctive swellings in front of and below the ear. In general, when they are first diagnosed, both benign and malignant lesions range from 4 to 6 cm in diameter and are mobile on palpation except in the case of neglected malignant tumors. Although benign tumors are known to have been present usually for many months to several years before coming to clinical attention, cancers are generally detected more quickly because of their rapid growth. Ultimately, however, there are no reliable clinical criteria to differentiate benign from malignant lesions.

Pleomorphic Adenoma

Pleomorphic adenomas are benign tumors that consist of a mixture of ductal (epithelial) and myoepithelial cells, and therefore they show both epithelial and mesenchymal differentiation. Because of their remarkable histologic diversity, these neoplasms have also been called *mixed tumors.* They represent about 60% of tumors in the parotid, are less common in the submandibular glands, and are relatively rare in the minor salivary glands. They reveal epithelial elements dispersed throughout the matrix along with varying degrees of myxoid, hyaline, chondroid (cartilaginous), and even osseous tissue. In some tumors the epithelial elements predominate; in others they are present only in widely dispersed foci.

Little is known about the origins of these neoplasms, except that radiation exposure increases the risk. Equally uncertain is the histogenesis of the various components. A currently popular view is that all neoplastic elements, including those that appear mesenchymal, are of either myoepithelial or ductal reserve cell origin (hence the designation *pleomorphic adenoma*). A high fraction of cases are associated with chromosomal rearrangements involving *PLAG1,* a gene encoding a transcription factor that is overexpressed as a result of these rearrangements. PLAG1 overexpression appears to upregulate expression of a number of genes that increase cell growth, such as components of growth factor receptor signaling pathways.

MORPHOLOGY

Most pleomorphic adenomas present as rounded, well-demarcated masses rarely exceeding 6 cm in the greatest dimension (Fig. 16-15). Although they are encapsulated, in some locations (particularly the palate) the capsule is not fully developed, and expansile growth produces protrusions into the surrounding gland, which may lead to recurrences if the tumor is merely enucleated. The cut surface is gray-white with myxoid and blue translucent areas of chondroid (cartilage-like).

The dominant histologic feature is the great heterogeneity mentioned. The epithelial elements resembling ductal cells or myoepithelial cells are arranged in duct formations, acini, irregular tubules, strands, or sheets of cells. These elements are typically dispersed within a mesenchyme-like background of loose myxoid tissue containing islands of cartilage and, rarely, foci of bone (Fig. 16-16). Sometimes the epithelial cells form well-developed ducts lined by cuboidal to columnar cells with an underlying layer of deeply chromatic, small myoepithelial cells. In other instances there may be strands or sheets of myoepithelial cells. Islands of well-differentiated squamous epithelium may also be present. In most cases there is no epithelial dysplasia or evident mitotic activity. There is no difference in biologic behavior between the tumors composed largely of epithelial elements and those composed largely of seemingly mesenchymal elements.

Clinical Features. These tumors present as painless, slow-growing, mobile, discrete masses within the parotid or submandibular areas or in the buccal cavity. The recurrence rate (perhaps months to years later) with parotidectomy is about 4% but, with simple enucleation approaches 25%.

A carcinoma arising in a pleomorphic adenoma is referred to variously as a *carcinoma ex pleomorphic adenoma* or a *malignant mixed tumor.* The incidence of malignant transformation increases with time, being about 2% for tumors present less than 5 years and almost 10% for those present for more than 15 years. The cancer usually takes the form of an adenocarcinoma or undifferentiated carcinoma. Like cancers elsewhere, these malignancies are highly infiltrative and tend to completely overrun and replace the preexisting pleomorphic adenoma. This may make it difficult to substantiate the diagnosis of carcinoma

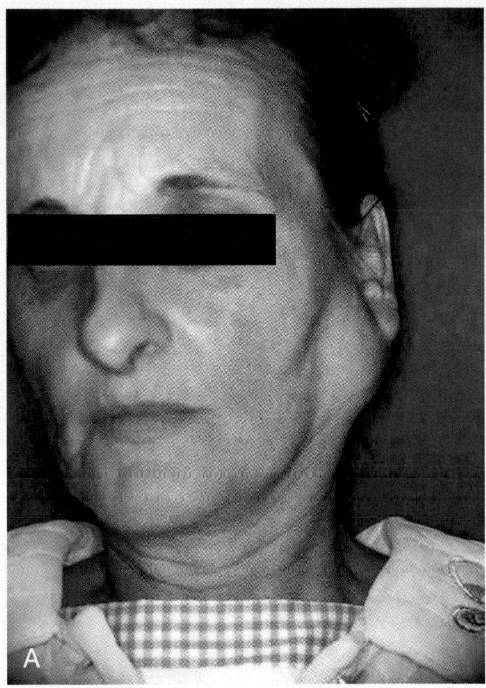

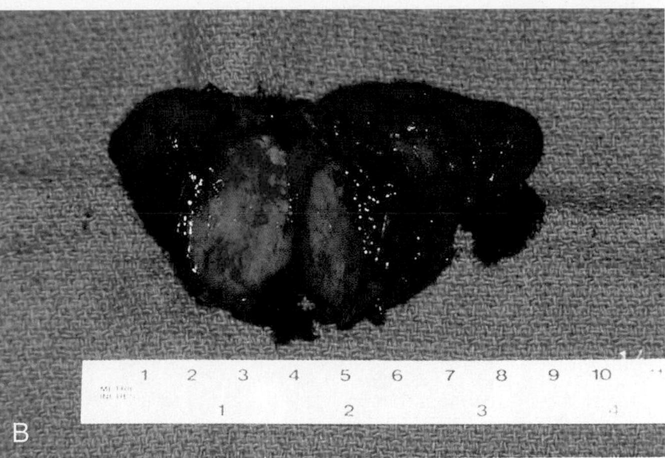

Figure 16-15 Pleomorphic adenoma. **A,** Slowly enlarging neoplasm in the parotid gland of many years duration. **B,** The bisected, sharply circumscribed, yellow-white tumor can be seen surrounded by normal salivary gland tissue.

ex pleomorphic adenoma, which requires that recognizable traces of pleomorphic adenoma be found. Regrettably, these cancers, when they appear, are among the most aggressive of all salivary gland malignant neoplasms, producing mortality rates of 30% to 50% at 5 years.

Warthin Tumor (Papillary Cystadenoma Lymphomatosum)

This curious benign neoplasm with its intimidating histologic name is the second most common salivary gland neoplasm. It arises almost *exclusively in the parotid gland* (the only tumor virtually restricted to the parotid) and occurs more commonly in males than in females, usually in the fifth to seventh decades of life. About 10% are multifocal and 10% bilateral. Smokers have eight times the risk of nonsmokers for developing these tumors.

MORPHOLOGY

Most Warthin tumors are round to oval encapsulated masses, 2 to 5 cm in diameter, usually arising in the superficial parotid gland, where they are readily palpable. Transection reveals a pale gray surface punctuated by narrow cystic or cleftlike spaces filled with mucinous or serous secretions. On microscopic examination these spaces are lined by a double layer of neoplastic epithelial cells resting on a dense lymphoid stroma sometimes bearing germinal centers (Fig. 16-17). The spaces are frequently narrowed by polypoid projections of the lymphoepithelial elements. The double layer of lining cells is distinctive; the upper layer consists of palisading columnar cells with abundant, finely granular, eosinophilic cytoplasm, while the lower layer is comprised of cuboidal to polygonal cells. The granular appearance of the cytoplasm of the upper layer of cells is due to the presence of numerous mitochondria, a feature referred to as "oncocytic". Secretory cells are dispersed in the columnar cell layer, accounting for the secretions within the dilated lumens. On occasion, there are foci of squamous metaplasia.

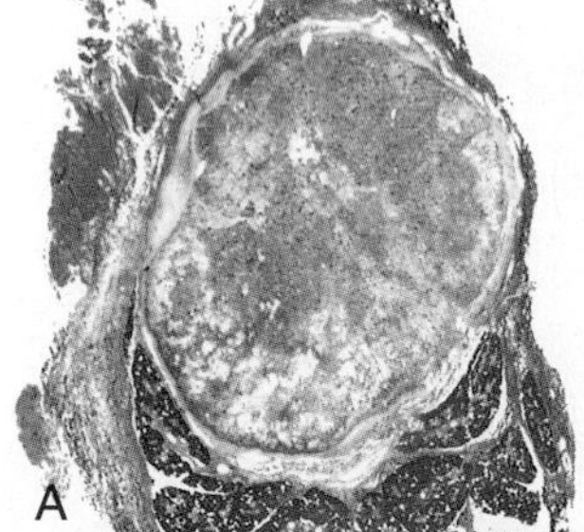

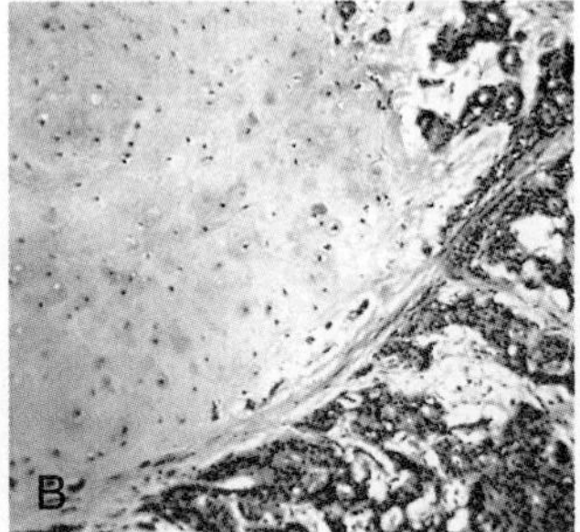

Figure 16-16 Pleomorphic adenoma. **A,** Low-power view showing a well-demarcated tumor with adjacent normal salivary gland parenchyma. **B,** High-power view showing epithelial cells and myoepithelial cells within a chondroid matrix material.

The histogenesis of these tumors has long been debated. The epithelial component of the tumor appears to be neoplastic, and presumably these cells make factors that serve as attractants for the lymphoid cells, which are believed to be reactive. Rarely, Warthin tumors have arisen within cervical lymph nodes, a finding that should not be mistaken for metastases. These neoplasms are benign, with recurrence rates of only 2% after resection.

Mucoepidermoid Carcinoma

These neoplasms are composed of variable mixtures of squamous cells, mucus-secreting cells, and intermediate

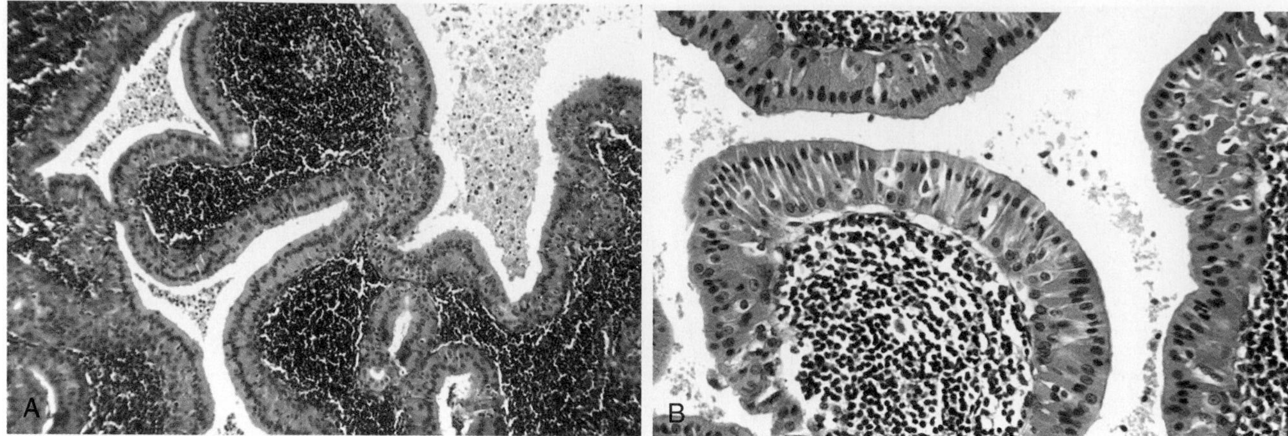

Figure 16-17 Warthin tumor. **A,** Low-power view showing epithelial and lymphoid elements. Note the follicular germinal center beneath the epithelium. **B,** Cystic spaces separate lobules of neoplastic epithelium consisting of a double layer of eosinophilic epithelial cells based on a reactive lymphoid stroma.

cells. They represent about 15% of all salivary gland tumors, and while they occur mainly (60% to 70%) in the parotids, they account for a large fraction of salivary gland neoplasms in the other glands, particularly the minor salivary glands. In more than half the cases, this tumor is associated with a balanced (11;19) (q21;p13) chromosomal translocation that creates a fusion gene composed of portions of the *MECT1* and *MAML2* genes. The *MECT1-MAML2* fusion gene is believed to play a key role in the genesis of this tumor, possibly by perturbing the Notch and cAMP-dependent signaling pathways. Overall, they are the most common form of primary malignant tumor of the salivary glands.

MORPHOLOGY

Mucoepidermoid carcinomas can grow as large as 8 cm in diameter and although they are apparently circumscribed, they lack well-defined capsules and are often infiltrative at the margins. Pale and gray-white on transection, they frequently contain small, mucin-containing cysts. The basic histologic pattern is that of cords, sheets, or cystic configurations of squamous, mucous, or intermediate cells (Fig. 16-18*A*). The hybrid cell types often have squamous features, with small to large mucus-filled vacuoles, best seen when highlighted with mucin stains (Fig. 16-18*B*). The tumor cells may be regular and benign appearing or, alternatively, highly anaplastic and unmistakably malignant. Accordingly, mucoepidermoid carcinomas are subclassified into low, intermediate, or high grade types.

The clinical course and prognosis depend on the grade of the neoplasm. Low-grade tumors may invade locally and recur in about 15% of cases, but only rarely do they metastasize and so yield a 5-year survival rate of more than 90%. By contrast, high-grade neoplasms and, to a lesser extent, intermediate-grade tumors are invasive and difficult to excise and so recur in about 25% to 30% of cases and, in 30% of cases, metastasize to distant sites. The 5-year survival rate in patients with these tumors is only 50%.

Other Salivary Gland Tumors

Two less common neoplasms merit brief description: adenoid cystic carcinoma and acinic cell carcinoma.

Adenoid cystic carcinoma is a relatively uncommon tumor, which in approximately 50% of cases is found in the minor salivary glands (in particular the palatine glands). Among the major salivary glands, the parotid and submandibular glands are the most common locations. Similar neoplasms

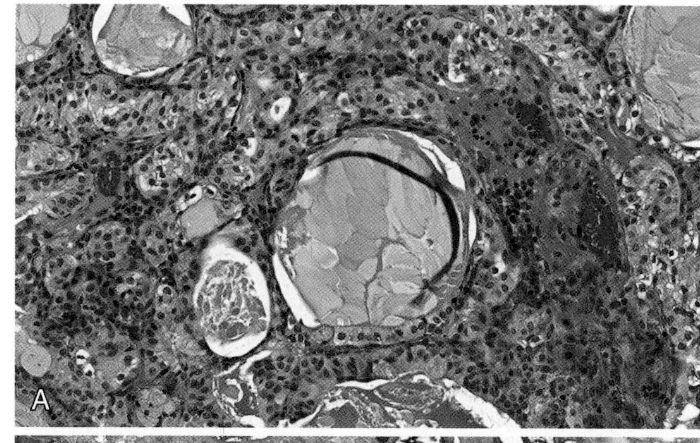

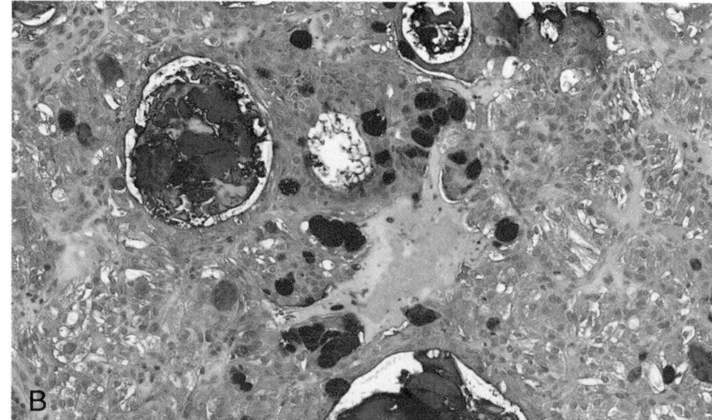

Figure 16-18 A, Mucoepidermoid carcinoma growing in nests composed of squamous cells as well as clear vacuolated cells containing mucin. **B,** Mucicarmine stains the mucin reddish pink.

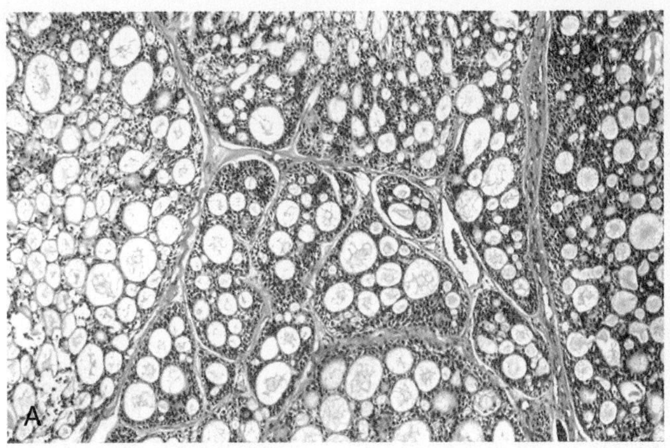
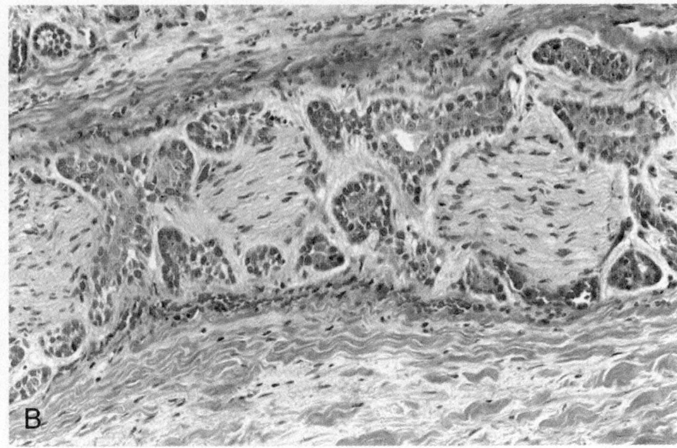

Figure 16-19 Adenoid cystic carcinoma in a salivary gland. **A,** Low-power view. The tumor cells have created a cribriform pattern enclosing secretions. **B,** Perineural invasion by tumor cells.

have been reported in the nose, sinuses, upper airways, breast, and elsewhere.

MORPHOLOGY

In gross appearance, they are generally small, poorly encapsulated, infiltrative, gray-pink lesions. On histologic evaluation, they are composed of small cells having dark, compact nuclei and scant cytoplasm. These cells tend to be disposed in tubular, solid, or cribriform patterns reminiscent of cylindromas arising in the adnexa of the skin (Chapter 25). The spaces between the tumor cells are often filled with a hyaline material thought to represent excess basement membrane (Fig. 16-19*A*). Other less common histologic patterns have been designated as tubular and solid variants.

Although slow growing, adenoid cystic carcinomas are unpredictable tumors with a tendency to invade perineural spaces (Fig. 16-19*B*), and they are stubbornly recurrent. Eventually, 50% or more disseminate widely to distant sites such as bone, liver, and brain, sometimes decades after attempted removal. Thus, although the 5-year survival rate is about 60% to 70%, it drops to about 30% at 10 years and 15% at 15 years. Neoplasms arising in the minor salivary glands have, on average, a poorer prognosis than those that arise in the parotid glands.

Acinic cell carcinoma is composed of cells resembling the normal serous acinar cells of salivary glands. It is relatively uncommon, representing only 2% to 3% of salivary gland tumors. Most arise in the parotids; the remainder arise in the submandibular glands. It rarely involves the minor glands, which normally have only a scant number of serous cells. Like Warthin tumor, it is sometimes bilateral or multicentric. The tumors are generally small, discrete lesions that may appear encapsulated. On histologic examination, they reveal a variable architecture and cell morphology. Most characteristically, the cells have clear cytoplasm but the cells are sometimes solid and at other times vacuolated. The tumor cells are disposed in sheets or microcystic, glandular, follicular, or papillary patterns. There is usually little anaplasia and few mitoses, but some tumors are occasionally slightly more pleomorphic.

The clinical course of these neoplasms is somewhat dependent on the level of pleomorphism. Overall, recurrence after resection is uncommon, but about 10% to 15% of these neoplasms metastasize to lymph nodes. The survival rate is in the range of 90% at 5 years and 60% at 20 years.

KEY CONCEPTS

Diseases of Salivary Glands

- **Sialadenitis** (inflammation of the salivary glands) can be caused by trauma, infection, or an autoimmune reaction.
- **Mucoceles** are caused by trauma to or blockage of a salivary gland duct, with consequent leakage of saliva into the surrounding connective tissue stroma.
- **Pleomorphic adenoma** is a benign, slow-growing neoplasm composed of a heterogenous mixture of epithelial and mesenchymal cells.
- **Mucoepidermoid carcinoma** is a malignant neoplasm of variable biological aggressiveness that is composed of a mixture of squamous and mucous cells.

SUGGESTED READINGS

Barnes L, Eveson JW, Reichart P, et al: *Pathology and genetics of head and neck tumors*, 2005, WHO, IARC, Chapter 6, Odontogenic Tumors, pp 284–327. [This chapter represents the most recent consensus regarding epidemiology, etiology, clinical features, and classification of odontogenic tumors.]

Dardick I: *Color Atlas/Text of Salivary Gland Pathology*, New York, 1996, Igaku-Shoin. [*Color atlas that discusses both normal salivary gland morphology and pathology. It also proposes hypotheses regarding the role of differentiation in the development as well as the histopathology of salivary gland neoplasia.*]

Ellis GL, Auclair PL: *Tumors of the salivary glands. AFIP atlas of tumor pathology*, Third series, Fascicle 9. Silver Spring MD, 2008, ARP Press. [*Comprehensive textbook on salivary gland pathology that is considered to be the gold standard.*]

Gillison ML, Broutian T, Pickard RK, et al: Human papilloma virus and rising oropharyngeal cancer incidence in the United States. *J Clin Oncol* 29:4294, 2011. [*A study using the Surveillance, Epidemiology, and End Results (SEER) Residual Tissue Repositories Program which demonstrated Increases in the population-level incidence and survival of oropharyngeal cancers in the United States since 1984 are caused by HPV infection.*]

Leemans CR, Braakhuis BJ, Brakenhoff RH: The molecular biology of head and neck cancer. *Nature Reviews Cancer* 11:9, 2011. [*An up to date discussion of the molecular biology of head and neck cancer.*]

Lingen MW, Xiao W, Schmitt A, et al: Low etiologic fraction for high-risk human papillomavirus in oral cavity squamous cell carcinomas. *Oral Oncol* 49:1, 2013. [*Manuscript estimated the etiologic fraction for HPV among consecutive, incident oral cavity squamous cell carcinomas at four North American hospitals and determined the etiologic fraction of HPV-positive cases was significantly lower than the oropharynx.*]

Phillipsen HP, Reichart PA: A revision of the 1992-edition of the WHO histological typing of odontogenic tumors. *J Oral Pathol Med* 31:253, 2002. [*A review article that outlines suggests revisions and updating to the nomenclature of odontogenic tumors.*]

Regezi JA, Sciubba JJ, Jordan RCK: *Oral Pathology: Clinical Pathologic Correlations*. 6th edition, 2011, Elsevier. [*A combined clinical and pathologic approach in an atlas-style text describing the major diseases of the oral cavity.*]

See TARGETED THERAPY available online at www.studentconsult.com 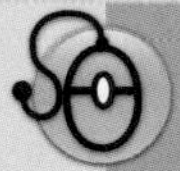

CHAPTER

17 The Gastrointestinal Tract

Jerrold R. Turner

CHAPTER CONTENTS

The gastrointestinal (GI) tract is a hollow tube extending from the oral cavity to the anus that consists of anatomically distinct segments, including the esophagus, stomach, small intestine, colon, rectum, and anus. Each of these segments has unique, complementary, and highly integrated functions, which together serve to regulate the intake, processing, and absorption of ingested nutrients and the disposal of waste products. The regional variations in structure and function are reflected in diseases of the GI tract, which often affect one or another segment preferentially. Accordingly, following consideration of several important congenital abnormalities, the discussion is organized anatomically. Disorders affecting more than one segment of the GI tract, such as Crohn disease, are discussed with the region that is involved most frequently.

CONGENITAL ABNORMALITIES

Depending on both the nature and timing of the insult during gestation, a variety of developmental anomalies can affect the GI tract. Importantly, because many organs develop simultaneously during embryogenesis, the presence of congenital GI disorders should prompt evaluation of other organs. Some defects are commonly associated with GI lesions.

Atresia, Fistulae, and Duplications

Atresia, fistulae, and duplications may occur in any part of the GI tract. When present within the esophagus they are discovered shortly after birth, usually due to regurgitation during feeding. Without prompt surgical repair, these lesions are incompatible with life. Absence, or *agenesis*, of the esophagus is extremely rare, but *atresia*, in which development is incomplete, is more common. In esophageal atresia a thin, noncanalized cord replaces a segment of esophagus, causing a mechanical obstruction (Fig. 17-1*A*). Atresia occurs most commonly at or near the tracheal bifurcation and is usually associated with a *fistula* connecting the upper or lower esophageal pouches to a bronchus or the trachea (17-1*B*). In other cases, a fistula can be present without atresia (Fig. 17-1*B, C*). Either form of fistula can lead to aspiration, suffocation, pneumonia, and severe fluid and electrolyte imbalances. Developmental abnormalities of the esophagus are associated with congenital heart defects, genitourinary malformations, and neurologic disease. Intestinal atresia is less common than esophageal atresia but frequently involves the duodenum. *Imperforate anus*, the most common form of congenital intestinal atresia, is due to a failure of the cloacal diaphragm to involute.

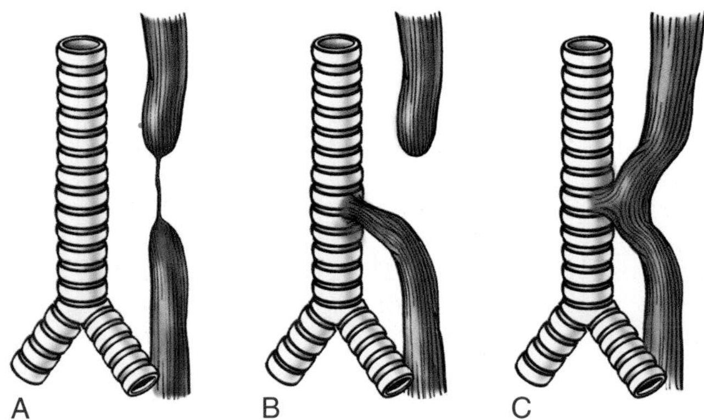

Figure 17-1 Esophageal atresia and tracheoesophageal fistula. **A,** Blind upper and lower esophagus with thin cord of connective tissue linking the two segments. **B,** Blind upper segment with fistula between lower segment and trachea. **C,** Fistula (without atresia) between patent esophagus and trachea. The developmental anomaly shown in **B** is the most common. (Adapted from Morson BC, Dawson IMP, eds: Gastrointestinal Pathology. Oxford, Blackwell Scientific Publications, 1972, p 8.)

Stenosis is an incomplete form of atresia in which the lumen is markedly reduced in caliber as a result of fibrous thickening of the wall. This results in either partial or complete obstruction. In addition to congenital forms, stenosis can be acquired as a consequence of inflammatory scarring, such as that caused by chronic gastroesophageal reflux, irradiation, systemic sclerosis, or caustic injury. Stenosis can involve any part of the GI tract, but the esophagus and small intestine are affected most often.

Diaphragmatic Hernia, Omphalocele, and Gastroschisis

Diaphragmatic hernia occurs when incomplete formation of the diaphragm allows the abdominal viscera to herniate into the thoracic cavity. When severe, the space-filling effect of the displaced viscera can cause pulmonary hypoplasia that is incompatible with life. *Omphalocele* occurs when closure of the abdominal musculature is incomplete and the abdominal viscera herniate into a ventral membranous sac: This may be repaired surgically, but as many as 40% of infants with an omphalocele have other birth defects. *Gastroschisis* is similar to omphalocele except that it involves all of the layers of the abdominal wall, from the peritoneum to the skin.

Ectopia

Ectopic tissues (developmental rests) are common in the GI tract. The most frequent site of *ectopic gastric mucosa* is the upper third of the esophagus, where it is referred to as an *inlet patch*. While generally asymptomatic, acid released by gastric mucosa within the esophagus can result in dysphagia, esophagitis, Barrett esophagus, or, rarely, adenocarcinoma. *Ectopic pancreatic tissue* occurs less frequently and can be found in the esophagus or stomach. Like inlet patches, these nodules are most often asymptomatic but they produce damage and local inflammation in some cases. When ectopic pancreatic tissue is present in the pylorus, inflammation and scarring may lead to obstruction. Because the rests may be present within any layer of the gastric wall, they can mimic invasive cancer. *Gastric heterotopia,* small patches of ectopic gastric mucosa in the small bowel or colon, may present with occult blood loss due to peptic ulceration of adjacent mucosa.

Meckel Diverticulum

A true diverticulum is a blind outpouching of the alimentary tract that communicates with the lumen and includes all three layers of the bowel wall. *The most common true diverticulum is the Meckel diverticulum, which occurs in the ileum.*

Meckel diverticulum occurs as a result of failed involution of the vitelline duct, which connects the lumen of the developing gut to the yolk sac. This solitary diverticulum extends from the antimesenteric side of the bowel (Fig. 17-2). The "rule of 2s" is often used to help remember characteristics of Meckel diverticula, which

- Occur in approximately 2% of the population
- Are generally present within 2 feet (60 cm) of the ileocecal valve
- Are approximately 2 inches (5 cm) long
- Are twice as common in males
- Are most often symptomatic by age 2 (only approximately 4% are ever symptomatic).

The mucosal lining of Meckel diverticula may resemble that of normal small intestine, but ectopic pancreatic or gastric tissue may also be present. The latter may secrete acid, cause peptic ulceration of adjacent small intestinal mucosa, and present with occult bleeding or abdominal pain resembling acute appendicitis or obstruction.

Less commonly, congenital diverticula occur in other parts of the small intestine and ascending colon. Virtually all other diverticula are acquired and either lack muscularis entirely or have an attenuated muscularis propria. The most common site of acquired diverticula is the sigmoid colon (discussed later).

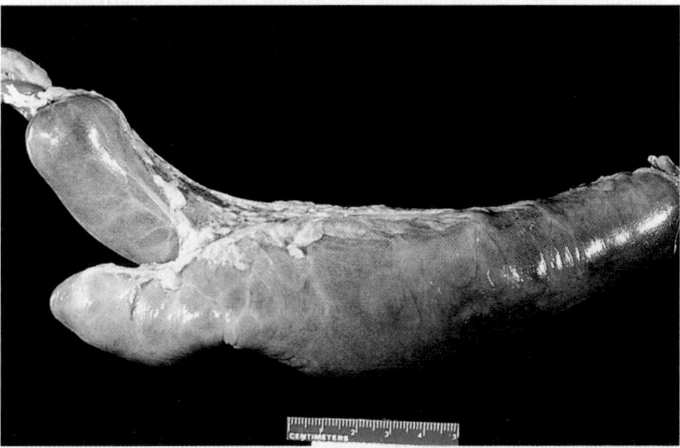

Figure 17-2 Meckel diverticulum. The blind pouch is located on the antimesenteric side of the small bowel.

Pyloric Stenosis

Congenital hypertrophic pyloric stenosis is three to five times more common in males and occurs once in 300 to 900 live births. Monozygotic twins have a high rate of concordance, with a 200-fold increased risk if one twin is affected. Incidence of congenital hypertrophic pyloric stenosis is also increased in dizygotic twins and siblings of affected individuals, although here the risk is only increased by 20-fold, reflecting a complex multifactorial pattern of inheritance. Consistent with a genetic basis, Turner syndrome and trisomy 18 also confer an increased risk of congenital hypertrophic pyloric stenosis. While the underlying mechanisms are not understood, erythromycin or azithromycin exposure, either orally or via mother's milk, in the first 2 weeks of life has been linked to increased disease incidence.

Congenital hypertrophic pyloric stenosis generally presents between the third and sixth weeks of life as new-onset regurgitation, projectile, nonbilious vomiting after feeding, and frequent demands for re-feeding. Physical examination reveals a firm, ovoid, 1 to 2 cm abdominal mass. In some cases abnormal left to right hyperperistalsis is evident during feeding and immediately before vomiting. This constellation of findings stems from hyperplasia of the pyloric muscularis propria, which obstructs the gastric outflow tract. Edema and inflammatory changes in the mucosa and submucosa may aggravate the narrowing. Surgical splitting of the muscularis (myotomy) is curative. Acquired pyloric stenosis occurs in adults as a consequence of antral gastritis or peptic ulcers close to the pylorus. Carcinomas of the distal stomach and pancreas may also narrow the pyloric channel due to fibrosis or malignant infiltration.

Hirschsprung Disease

Hirschsprung disease occurs in approximately 1 of 5000 live births. It may be isolated or occur in combination with other developmental abnormalities; 10% of all cases occur in children with Down syndrome and serious neurologic abnormalities are present in another 5%.

Pathogenesis. The enteric neuronal plexus develops from neural crest cells that migrate into the bowel wall during embryogenesis. Hirschsprung disease, also known as congenital aganglionic megacolon, results when the normal migration of neural crest cells from cecum to rectum is arrested prematurely or when the ganglion cells undergo premature death. This produces a distal intestinal segment that lacks both the Meissner submucosal and the Auerbach myenteric plexus ("aganglionosis"). Coordinated peristaltic contractions are absent and functional obstruction occurs, resulting in dilation proximal to the affected segment.

The mechanisms underlying defective neural crest cell migration in Hirschsprung disease are unknown, but a genetic component is present in nearly all cases, and 4% of patients' siblings are affected. Heterozygous loss-of-function mutations in the receptor tyrosine kinase *RET* account for the majority of familial cases and approximately 15% of sporadic cases. Mutations in at least seven other genes encoding proteins involved in enteric neurodevelopment, including the RET ligand glial-derived neurotrophic factor, endothelin, and the endothelin receptor, have also been described. However, these account for fewer than 30% of patients, suggesting that many other defects remain to be discovered. Because penetrance is incomplete, modifying genes or environmental factors must also be important. In addition, it is clear that sex-linked factors exist, since the disease is more common in males, but, when present in females, tends to involve longer aganglionic segments.

MORPHOLOGY

Diagnosis of Hirschsprung disease requires documenting the absence of ganglion cells within the affected segment. In addition to their characteristic morphology in hematoxylin and eosin–stained sections, ganglion cells can be identified using immunohistochemical stains for acetylcholinesterase.

The rectum is always affected, but the length of the additional involved segments varies widely, from the rectum and sigmoid colon in most cases to the entire colon in severe cases. The aganglionic region may have a grossly normal or contracted appearance. In contrast, the normally innervated proximal colon may undergo progressive dilation (Fig. 17-3) and, in time become massively distended **(megacolon)**, reaching diameters of as much as 20 cm. This may stretch and thin the colonic wall to the point of rupture, which occurs most frequently near the cecum. Mucosal inflammation or shallow ulcers may also be present in normally innervated segments, making gross identification of the extent of aganglionosis difficult. Hence, intraoperative frozen-section analysis is commonly used to confirm the presence of ganglion cells at the anastomotic margin.

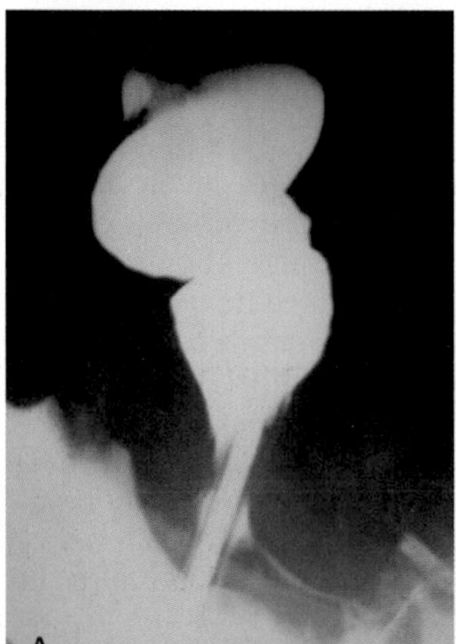

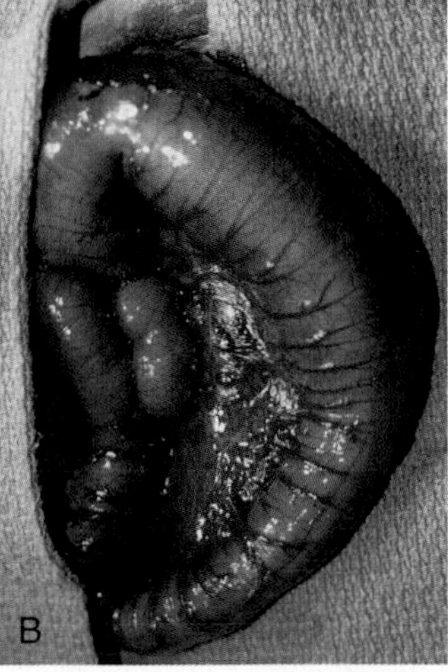

Figure 17-3 Hirschsprung disease. **A,** Preoperative barium enema study showing constricted rectum (bottom of the image) and dilated sigmoid colon. **B,** Corresponding intraoperative photograph showing constricted rectum and dilation of the sigmoid colon. (Courtesy Dr. Aliya Husain, The University of Chicago, Chicago, Ill.)

Clinical Features. Hirschsprung disease typically presents with a failure to pass meconium in the immediate postnatal period. Obstruction or constipation follows, often with visible, ineffective peristalsis, and may progress to abdominal distention and bilious vomiting. When only a few centimeters of rectum are involved occasional passage of stool may occur and obscure the diagnosis. The major threats to life are enterocolitis, fluid and electrolyte disturbances, perforation, and peritonitis. The primary mode of treatment is surgical resection of the aganglionic segment followed by anastomosis of the normal proximal colon to the rectum. Even after successful surgery, it may take years to attain normal bowel function and continence.

In contrast to the congenital megacolon of Hirschsprung disease, acquired megacolon may occur at any age as a result of Chagas disease, obstruction by a neoplasm or inflammatory stricture, toxic megacolon complicating ulcerative colitis, visceral myopathy, or in association with functional psychosomatic disorders. Of these, only Chagas disease (discussed later) is associated with loss of ganglion cells.

KEY CONCEPTS

Congenital malformations of the GI tract

- The GI tract is a common site of developmental abnormalities. In these cases, defects of other organs that develop in the same embryonic period should be sought.
- **Atresia, and fistulae,** are structural developmental anomalies that disrupt normal gastrointestinal transit and typically present early in life. **Imperforate anus** is the most common form of congenital intestinal atresia, while the esophagus is the most common site of fistulization.
- **Stenosis** may be developmental or acquired. Both forms are characterized by a thickened wall and partial or complete luminal obstruction. Acquired forms are often due to inflammatory scarring.
- **Diaphragmatic hernia** is characterized by incomplete diaphragm development and herniation of abdominal organs into the thorax. This often results in pulmonary hypoplasia. **Omphalocele** and **gastroschisis** refer to ventral herniation of abdominal organs.
- **Ectopia** refers to the presence of normally formed tissues in an abnormal site. This is common in the gastrointestinal tract, with **ectopic gastric mucosa** in the upper third of the esophagus being the most common form.
- The **Meckel diverticulum** is a true diverticulum, defined by the presence of all three layers of the bowel wall, that reflects failed involution of the vitelline duct. It is common and is a frequent site of gastric ectopia, which may result in occult bleeding.
- **Congenital hypertrophic pyloric stenosis** is a form of obstruction that presents between the third and sixth weeks of life. There is an ill-defined genetic component to this disease, which is most common in males.
- **Hirschsprung disease** is caused by the absence of neural crest derived ganglion cells within the colon. It causes functional obstruction of the affected bowel and proximal dilation. The defect always begins at the rectum, but extends proximally for variable lengths.

ESOPHAGUS

The esophagus develops from the cranial portion of the foregut and is recognizable by the third week of gestation. It is a hollow, highly distensible muscular tube that extends from the epiglottis in the pharynx to the gastroesophageal junction. Acquired diseases of the esophagus run the gamut from highly lethal cancers to the persistent "heartburn" of gastroesophageal reflux that may be chronic and incapacitating or merely an occasional annoyance.

Esophageal Obstruction

The esophagus is, essentially, a tube that delivers ingested solid food and fluids to the stomach. This can be impeded by structural, i.e. (mechanical) obstruction or functional obstruction. The latter results from disruption of the coordinated waves of peristaltic contractions that follow swallowing. Esophageal manometry allows separation of esophageal dysmotility into three principal forms, termed nutcracker esophagus, diffuse esophageal spasm, and hypertensive lower esophageal sphincter.

- *Nutcracker esophagus* describes patients with high-amplitude contractions of the distal esophagus that are, in part, due to loss of the normal coordination of inner circular layer and outer longitudinal layer smooth muscle contractions.
- *Diffuse esophageal spasm* is characterized by repetitive, simultaneous contractions of the distal esophageal smooth muscle.
- Lower esophageal sphincter dysfunction, such as high resting pressure or incomplete relaxation, are present in many patients with nutcracker esophagus or diffuse esophageal spasm. In the absence altered patterns of esophageal contraction, these sphincter abnormalities are termed *hypertensive lower esophageal sphincter*. As discussed below, these can be distinguished from achalasia in that the latter includes reduced esophageal peristaltic contractions.

Because wall stress is increased, esophageal dysmotility may result in development of small diverticulae, primarily the epiphrenic diverticulum located immediately above the lower esophageal sphincter. Similarly, impaired relaxation and spasm of the cricopharyngeus muscle after swallowing can result in increased pressure within the distal pharynx and development of a Zenker diverticulum (pharyngoesophageal diverticulum), which is located immediately above the upper esophageal sphincter. Zenker diverticulae are uncommon, but typically develop after age 50 and may reach several centimeters in size. When small they may be asymptomatic, but larger Zenker diverticulae may accumulate significant amounts of food, producing a mass and symptoms that include regurgitation and halitosis.

In contrast to functional obstruction, mechanical obstruction, which can be caused by strictures or cancer, presents as progressive dysphagia that begins with inability to swallow solids. With progression ingestion of liquids is also affected. Because obstruction develops slowly, patients may subconsciously modify their diet to favor soft foods and liquids and be unaware of their condition until the obstruction is nearly complete.

Benign *esophageal stenosis*, or narrowing of the lumen, is generally caused by fibrous thickening of the submucosa and is associated with atrophy of the muscularis propria as well as secondary epithelial damage. Although occasionally congenital, stenosis is most often due to inflammation and scarring that may be caused by chronic gastroesophageal reflux, irradiation, or caustic injury. In general, patients with functional obstruction or benign strictures maintain their appetite and weight, while, as discussed later, malignant strictures are often associated with weight loss.

Esophageal mucosal webs are idiopathic ledge-like protrusions of mucosa that may cause obstruction. These uncommon lesions typically occur in women older than age 40 and can be associated with gastroesophageal reflux, chronic graft-versus-host disease, or blistering skin diseases. In the upper esophagus, webs may be accompanied by iron-deficiency anemia, glossitis, and cheilosis as part of the *Paterson-Brown-Kelly* or *Plummer-Vinson syndrome*. In general, esophageal webs are semi-circumferential lesions that protrude less than 5 mm, have a thickness of 2 to 4 mm, and are composed of a fibrovascular connective tissue and overlying epithelium. The main symptom of webs is nonprogressive dysphagia associated with incompletely chewed food.

Esophageal rings, or *Schatzki rings*, are similar to webs, but are circumferential, thicker, and include mucosa, submucosa, and, occasionally, hypertrophic muscularis propria. When present in the distal esophagus, above the gastroesophageal junction, they are termed *A rings* and are covered by squamous mucosa; in contrast, those located at the squamocolumnar junction of the lower esophagus are designated *B rings* and may have gastric cardia-type mucosa on their undersurface.

Achalasia

Increased tone of the lower esophageal sphincter (LES), as a result of impaired smooth muscle relaxation, is an important cause of esophageal obstruction. Normally, release of nitric oxide and vasoactive intestinal polypeptide from inhibitory neurons, along with interruption of normal cholinergic signaling, allows the LES to relax during swallowing. *Achalasia is characterized by the triad of incomplete LES relaxation, increased LES tone, and aperistalsis of the esophagus.* Symptoms include dysphagia for solids and liquids, difficulty in belching, and chest pain. Although there is some increased risk for esophageal cancer, it is not considered great enough to warrant surveillance endoscopy.

Primary achalasia is the result of distal esophageal inhibitory neuronal, that is, ganglion cell, degeneration. This leads to increased tone, an inability to relax of the lower esophageal sphincter, and esophageal aperistalsis. Degenerative changes in the extraesophageal vagus nerve or the dorsal motor nucleus of the vagus may also occur. The cause is unknown; rare familial cases have been described.

Secondary achalasia may arise in Chagas disease, in which Trypanosoma cruzi infection causes destruction of the myenteric plexus, failure of peristalsis, and esophageal dilatation. Duodenal, colonic, and ureteric myenteric plexuses can also be affected in Chagas disease. Achalasia-like disease may be caused by diabetic autonomic neuropathy; infiltrative disorders such as malignancy, amyloidosis, or sarcoidosis; lesions of dorsal motor nuclei, particularly polio or surgical ablation; in association with Down syndrome; or as part of Allgrove (triple A) syndrome, an autosomal recessive disorder characterized by achalasia, alacrima, and adrenocorticotrophic hormone-resistant adrenal insufficiency. The association of some achalasia cases with remote herpes simplex virus 1 (HSV1) infection, linkage of immunoregulatory gene polymorphisms to achalasia, and occasional coexistence of Sjögren syndrome or autoimmune thyroid disease suggest that achalasia may also be driven by immune-mediated destruction of inhibitory esophageal neurons. Treatment modalities for both primary and secondary achalasia aim to overcome the mechanical obstruction, and include laparoscopic myotomy and pneumatic balloon dilatation. Botulinum neurotoxin (Botox) injection, to inhibit LES cholinergic neurons, can also be effective.

Esophagitis

Lacerations

Longitudinal mucosal tears near the gastroesophageal junction are termed *Mallory-Weiss tears,* and are most often associated with severe retching or vomiting secondary to acute alcohol intoxication. Normally, a reflex relaxation of the gastroesophageal musculature precedes the antiperistaltic contractile wave associated with vomiting. It is speculated that this relaxation fails during prolonged vomiting, with the result that refluxing gastric contents overwhelm the gastric inlet and cause the esophageal wall to stretch and tear. The roughly linear lacerations of Mallory-Weiss syndrome are longitudinally oriented and range in length from millimeters to several centimeters. These tears usually cross the gastroesophageal junction and may also be located in the proximal gastric mucosa. Up to 10% of upper GI bleeding, which often presents as hematemesis (Table 17-1), is due to superficial esophageal lacerations such as those associated with Mallory-Weiss syndrome. These do not generally require surgical intervention, and healing tends to be rapid and complete. In contrast, Boerhaave syndrome is a much less common but more serious disorder characterized by transmural tearing and rupture of the distal esophagus. This catastrophic event produces severe mediastinitis and generally requires surgical intervention. Because patients can present with severe chest pain, tachypnea, and shock, the initial differential diagnosis can include myocardial infarction.

Table 17-1 Esophageal Causes of Hematemesis

Lacerations (Mallory-Weiss syndrome)
Esophageal perforation (cancer or Boerhaave syndrome)
Varices (cirrhosis)
Esophageal-aortic fistula (usually with cancer)
Chemical and pill esophagitis
Infectious esophagitis (*Candida*, herpes)
Benign strictures
Vasculitis (autoimmune, cytomegalovirus)
Reflux esophagitis (erosive)
Eosinophilic esophagitis
Esophageal ulcers (many etiologies)
Barrett esophagus
Adenocarcinoma
Squamous cell carcinoma
Hiatal hernia

Chemical and Infectious Esophagitis

The stratified squamous mucosa of the esophagus may be damaged by a variety of irritants including alcohol, corrosive acids or alkalis, excessively hot fluids, and heavy smoking. Symptoms range from self-limited pain, particularly on swallowing, that is, *odynophagia,* to hemorrhage, stricture, or perforation in severe cases.

In children esophageal chemical injury is often secondary to accidental ingestion of household cleaning products; severe damage may follow attempted suicide in adults. Less severe chemical injury to the esophageal mucosa can occur when medicinal pills lodge and dissolve in the esophagus rather than passing into the stomach intact, a condition termed *pill-induced esophagitis.* Iatrogenic esophageal injury may be caused by cytotoxic chemotherapy, radiation therapy, or graft-versus-host disease. The esophagus may also be involved by the desquamative skin diseases bullous pemphigoid, epidermolysis bullosa and, rarely, Crohn disease.

Esophageal infections in otherwise healthy individuals are uncommon and most often due to herpes simplex virus. Infections in patients who are debilitated or immunosuppressed, as a result of disease or therapy, is more common and can be caused by herpes simplex virus, cytomegalovirus (CMV), or fungal organisms. Among fungi, candidiasis is most common, although mucormycosis and aspergillosis are also seen.

MORPHOLOGY

The morphology of chemical and infectious esophagitis varies with etiology. Dense infiltrates of neutrophils are present in most cases but may be absent following injury induced by chemicals (lye, acids, or detergent), which can lead to outright necrosis of the esophageal wall. Pill-induced esophagitis frequently occurs at the site of strictures that impede passage of luminal contents. When present, ulceration is accompanied by superficial necrosis with granulation tissue and eventual fibrosis.

Esophageal irradiation causes damage similar to that seen in other tissues and includes intimal proliferation and luminal narrowing of submucosal and mural blood vessels. The mucosal damage is, in part, secondary to this radiation-induced vascular injury as discussed in Chapter 9.

Infection by fungi or bacteria can either cause injury or complicate a preexisting ulcer. Nonpathogenic oral bacteria are frequently found in ulcer beds, while pathogenic organisms, which account for about 10% of infectious esophagitis, may invade the lamina propria and cause necrosis of overlying mucosa. Candidiasis, in its most advanced form, is characterized by adherent, gray-white **pseudomembranes** composed

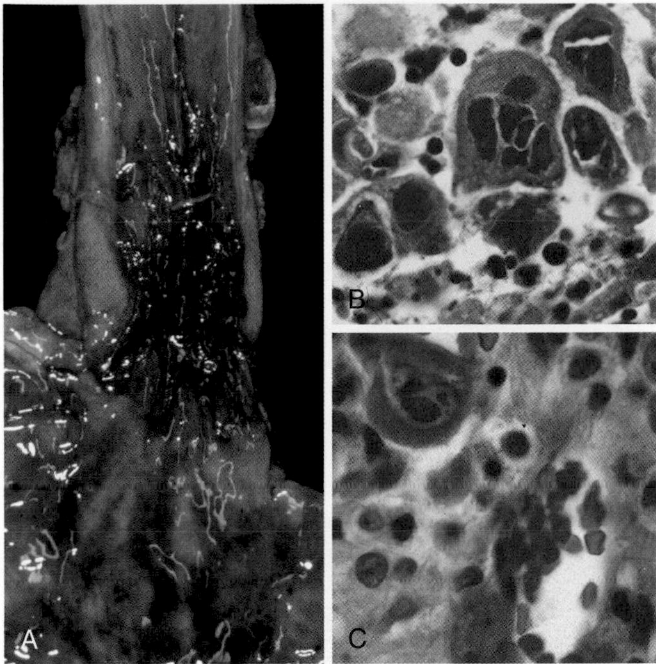

Figure 17-4 Viral esophagitis. **A,** Postmortem specimen with multiple, overlapping herpetic ulcers in the distal esophagus. **B,** Multinucleate squamous cells containing herpesvirus nuclear inclusions. **C,** Cytomegalovirus-infected endothelial cells with nuclear and cytoplasmic inclusions.

of densely matted fungal hyphae and inflammatory cells covering the esophageal mucosa.

The endoscopic appearance often provides a clue as to the infectious agent in viral esophagitis. Herpes viruses typically cause punched-out ulcers (Fig. 17-4*A*). Biopsy specimens demonstrate nuclear viral inclusions within a rim of degenerating epithelial cells at the margin of the ulcer (Fig. 17-4*B*). In contrast, CMV causes shallower ulcerations and characteristic nuclear and cytoplasmic inclusions within capillary endothelium and stromal cells (Fig. 17-4*C*). Although the histologic appearance is characteristic, immunohistochemical stains for virus-specific antigens are sensitive and specific ancillary diagnostic tools.

Histologic features of esophageal **graft-versus-host disease** are similar to those in the skin and include basal epithelial cell apoptosis, mucosal atrophy, and submucosal fibrosis without significant acute inflammatory infiltrates. The microscopic appearances of esophageal involvement in bullous pemphigoid, epidermolysis bullosa, and Crohn disease are also similar to those in the skin (Chapter 25).

Reflux Esophagitis

The stratified squamous epithelium of the esophagus is resistant to abrasion from foods but is sensitive to acid. Submucosal glands, which are most abundant in the proximal and distal esophagus, contribute to mucosal protection by secreting mucin and bicarbonate. More importantly, the tone of the lower esophageal sphincter prevents reflux of acidic gastric contents, which are under positive pressure and would otherwise enter the esophagus. Reflux of gastric contents into the lower esophagus is the most frequent cause of esophagitis and the most common outpatient GI diagnosis in the United States. The associated clinical condition is termed *gastroesophageal reflux disease (GERD).*

Pathogenesis. The most common cause of gastroesophageal reflux is transient lower esophageal sphincter relaxation. This is thought to be mediated via vagal pathways, and can be triggered by gastric distention, by gas or food, mild pharyngeal stimulation that does not trigger swallowing, and stress. Gastroesophageal reflux can also occur following swallow-induced lower esophageal sphincter relaxations or due to forceful opening of a relatively hypotensive lower esophageal sphincter by an abrupt increase in intraabdominal pressure, such as that due to coughing, straining, or bending. Other conditions that decrease lower esophageal sphincter tone or increase abdominal pressure and contribute to GERD include alcohol and tobacco use, obesity, central nervous system depressants, pregnancy, hiatal hernia (discussed later), delayed gastric emptying, and increased gastric volume. In many cases, no definitive cause is identified. Reflux of gastric juices is central to the development of mucosal injury in GERD. In severe cases, reflux of bile from the duodenum may exacerbate the damage.

MORPHOLOGY

Simple hyperemia, evident to the endoscopist as redness, may be the only alteration. In mild GERD the mucosal histology is often unremarkable. With more significant disease, eosinophils are recruited into the squamous mucosa followed by neutrophils, which are usually associated with more severe injury (Fig. 17-5*A*). Basal zone hyperplasia exceeding 20% of the total epithelial thickness and elongation of lamina propria papillae, such that they extend into the upper third of the epithelium, may also be present.

Clinical Features. GERD is most common in individuals older than age 40 but also occurs in infants and children. The most frequent clinical symptoms are heartburn, dysphagia, and regurgitation of sour-tasting gastric contents.

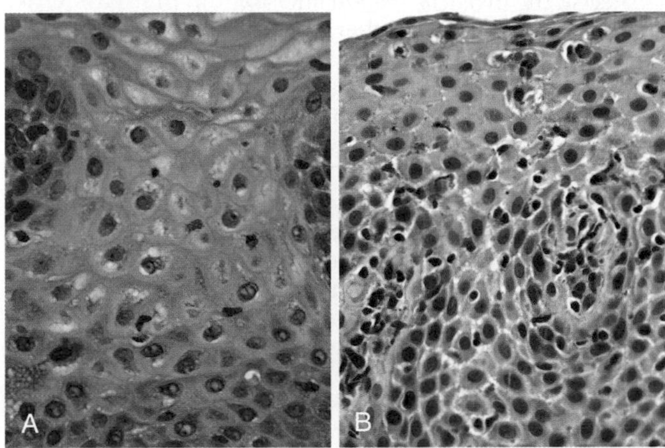

Figure 17-5 Esophagitis. **A,** Reflux esophagitis with scattered intraepithelial eosinophils and mild basal zone expansion. **B,** Eosinophilic esophagitis is characterized by numerous intraepithelial eosinophils. Abnormal squamous maturation is also apparent.

Rarely, chronic GERD is punctuated by attacks of severe chest pain that may be mistaken for heart disease. Treatment with proton pump inhibitors, which have replaced H_2 histamine receptor antagonists, to reduce gastric acidity typically provides symptomatic relief. While the severity of symptoms is not closely related to the degree of histologic damage, the latter tends to increase with disease duration. Complications of reflux esophagitis include ulceration, hematemesis, melena, stricture development, and Barrett esophagus.

Hiatal hernia can give rise to symptoms, such as heartburn and regurgitation of gastric juices, that are similar to those of GERD. It is characterized by separation of the diaphragmatic crura and protrusion of the stomach into the thorax through the resulting gap. Congenital hiatal hernias are recognized in infants and children, but many are acquired in later life. Hiatal hernia is symptomatic in fewer than 10% of adults, but can be a cause of lower esophageal sphincter incompetence.

Eosinophilic Esophagitis

The incidence of eosinophilic esophagitis is increasing markedly. Symptoms include food impaction and dysphagia in adults and feeding intolerance or GERD-like symptoms in children. The cardinal histologic feature is large numbers of intraepithelial eosinophils, particularly superficially (Fig. 17-5*B*). Their abundance can help to differentiate eosinophilic esophagitis from GERD, Crohn disease, and other causes of esophagitis. In addition, unlike patients with GERD, acid reflux is not prominent and high doses of proton pump inhibitors usually do not provide relief. *The majority of individuals with eosinophilic esophagitis are atopic* and many have atopic dermatitis, allergic rhinitis, asthma, or modest peripheral eosinophilia. Treatments include dietary restrictions to prevent exposure to food allergens, such as cow's milk and soy products, and topical or systemic corticosteroids.

Esophageal Varices

Venous blood from the GI tract passes through the liver, via the portal vein, before returning to the heart. This circulatory pattern is responsible for the first-pass effect in which drugs and other materials absorbed in the intestines are processed by the liver before entering the systemic circulation. Diseases that impede this flow cause portal hypertension and can lead to the development of esophageal varices, an important cause of esophageal bleeding.

Pathogenesis. **Portal hypertension results in the development of collateral channels at sites where the portal and caval systems communicate.** These collateral veins allow some drainage to occur, but at the same time they lead to development of congested subepithelial and submucosal venous plexi within the distal esophagus and proximal stomach. These vessels, termed *varices*, develop in the vast majority of cirrhotic patients, most commonly in association with alcoholic liver disease. Worldwide, hepatic schistosomiasis is the second most common cause of varices. A more detailed consideration of portal hypertension is given in Chapter 18.

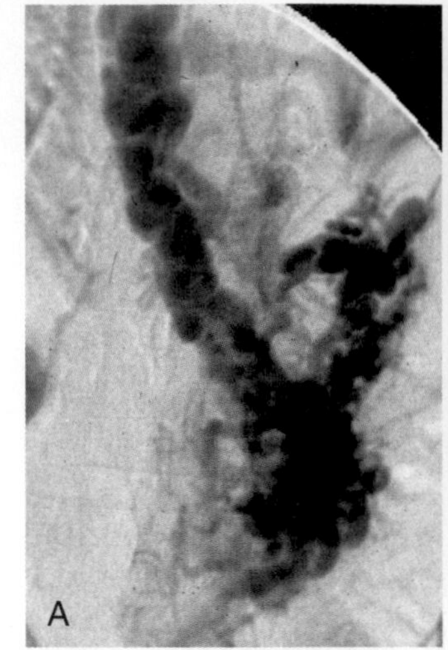

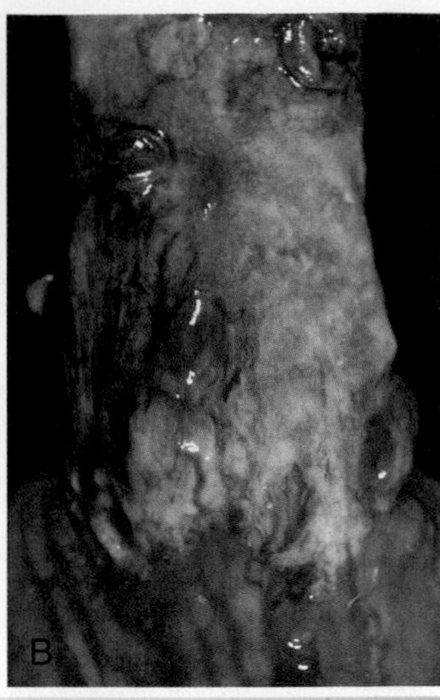

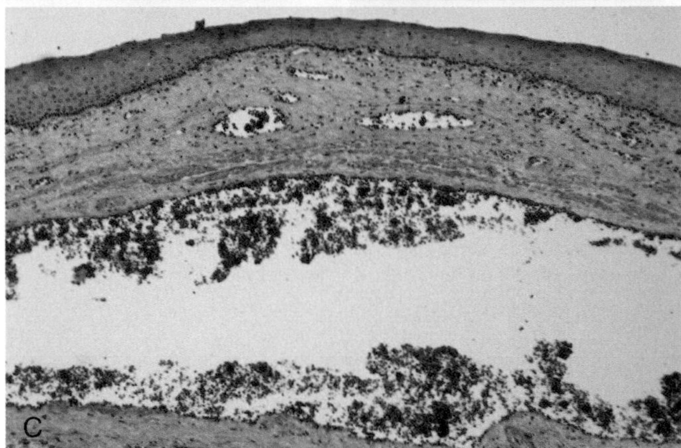

Figure 17-6 Esophageal varices. **A,** Although no longer used as a diagnostic approach, this angiogram demonstrates several tortuous esophageal varices. **B,** Collapsed varices are present in this postmortem specimen corresponding to the angiogram in **A**. The polypoid areas represent previous sites of variceal hemorrhage that have been ligated with bands. **C,** Dilated varices beneath intact squamous mucosa.

MORPHOLOGY

Varices are tortuous dilated veins lying primarily within the submucosa of the distal esophagus and proximal stomach (Fig. 17-6*A*). Venous channels directly beneath the esophageal epithelium may also become massively dilated. Varices may not be grossly obvious in surgical or postmortem specimens, because they collapse in the absence of blood flow (Fig. 17-6*B*) and are obscured by the overlying mucosa (Fig. 17-6*C*). Variceal rupture results in hemorrhage into the lumen or the esophageal wall, in which case the overlying mucosa appears ulcerated and necrotic. If rupture has occurred in the past, venous thrombosis, inflammation, and evidence of prior therapy may also be present.

Clinical Features. Gastroesophageal varices are present in nearly half of the patients with cirrhosis, and 25-40% of patients with cirrhosis develop variceal bleeding. Approximately 12% of previously asymptomatic varices bleed each year. Variceal hemorrhage is an emergency that can be treated medically by inducing splanchnic vasoconstriction or endoscopically by sclerotherapy (injection of thrombotic agents), balloon tamponade, or variceal ligation. Despite these interventions, 30% or more of patients with variceal hemorrhage die as a direct consequence of hemorrhage such as hypovolemic shock, hepatic coma, or other complications. Furthermore, more than 50% of patients who survive a first variceal bleed have recurrent hemorrhage within 1 year, and this carries a mortality rate similar to that of the first episode. Thus, patients with risk factors for hemorrhage, including large varices, elevated hepatic venous pressure gradient, previous bleeding, and advanced liver disease may be treated prophylactically with beta-blockers to reduce portal blood flow and with endoscopic variceal ligation. Despite the frequency and risks of variceal hemorrhage, it is important to recognize that cirrhosis patients with small varices that have never bled are at relatively low risk for bleeding and death, and that, even when varices are present, they are only one of several causes of hematemesis.

Barrett Esophagus

Barrett esophagus is a complication of chronic GERD that is characterized by intestinal metaplasia within the esophageal squamous mucosa. The incidence of Barrett esophagus is rising, and it is estimated to occur in as many as 10% of individuals with symptomatic GERD. Barrett esophagus is most common in white males and typically presents between 40 and 60 years of age. *The greatest concern in Barrett esophagus is that it confers an increased risk of esophageal adenocarcinoma.* Genomic sequencing of biopsies involved by Barrett esophagus has revealed the presence of mutations that are shared with esophageal adenocarcinoma, in keeping with the idea that Barrett esophagus is a precursor lesion to cancer. Potentially oncogenic mutations are more numerous when biopsies demonstrate dysplasia, which is detected in 0.2% to 2% of persons with Barrett esophagus each year. The presence of dysplasia, a preinvasive change, is associated with prolonged symptoms, longer segment length, increased patient age, and Caucasian race. Although the vast majority of esophageal adenocarcinomas are associated with Barrett esophagus, it is important to remember that most individuals with Barrett esophagus do not develop esophageal tumors.

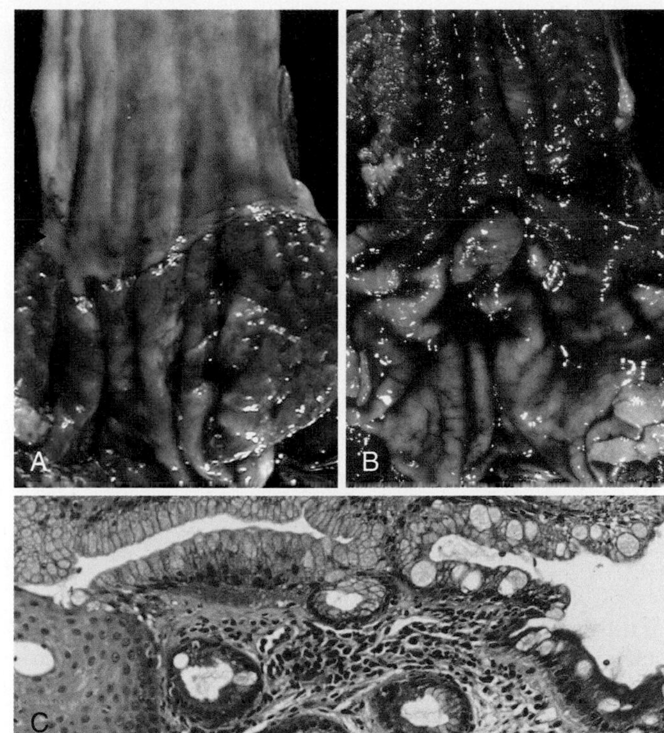

Figure 17-7 Barrett esophagus. **A,** Normal gastroesophageal junction. **B,** Barrett esophagus. Note the small islands of residual pale squamous mucosa within the Barrett mucosa. **C,** Histologic appearance of the gastroesophageal junction in Barrett esophagus. Note the transition between esophageal squamous mucosa (left) and Barrett metaplasia, with abundant metaplastic goblet cells (right).

MORPHOLOGY

Barrett esophagus can be recognized as one or several tongues or patches of red, velvety mucosa extending upward from the gastroesophageal junction. This metaplastic mucosa alternates with residual smooth, pale squamous (esophageal) mucosa and interfaces with light-brown columnar (gastric) mucosa distally (Fig. 17-7*A*, *B*). High-resolution endoscopes have increased the sensitivity of Barrett esophagus detection. This has led to subclassification of Barrett esophagus as long segment, which involves 3 cm or more, or short segment, in which less than 3 cm is involved. Available data suggest that the risk of dysplasia correlates with length of esophagus affected.

Diagnosis of Barrett esophagus requires endoscopic evidence of metaplastic columnar mucosa above the gastroesophageal junction. Microscopically, intestinal-type metaplasia is seen as replacement of the squamous esophageal epithelium with goblet cells. These are diagnostic of Barrett esophagus, and have distinct mucous vacuoles that stain pale blue by hematoxylin and eosin and impart the shape of a wine goblet to the remaining cytoplasm (Fig. 17-7*C*). Non-goblet columnar cells, such as gastric type foveolar cells, may also be present. However, whether the latter are sufficient for diagnosis is controversial.

When **dysplasia** is present, it is classified as low grade or high grade. Atypical mitoses, nuclear hyperchromasia, irregularly clumped chromatin, increased nuclear-to-cytoplasmic ratio, and a failure of epithelial cells to mature as they migrate to the esophageal surface are present in both grades of dysplasia (Fig. 17-8*A*). Gland architecture is frequently abnormal and is characterized by budding, irregular shapes, and cellular crowding. High-grade dysplasia (Fig. 17-8*B*) exhibits more severe cytologic and architectural changes. With progression, epithelial cells may invade the lamina propria, a feature that defines intramucosal carcinoma.

Clinical Features. **Barrett esophagus can only be identified thorough endoscopy and biopsy, which are usually prompted by GERD symptoms.** Once diagnosed, the best course of management is a matter of debate. Many support periodic endoscopy with biopsy, for dysplasia surveillance. However, randomized trials have failed to demonstrate that surveillance improves patient survival. Furthermore, uncertainties regarding the potential of dysplasia, particularly low grade, to regress spontaneously and limited information on the risk of progression complicate clinical decisions.

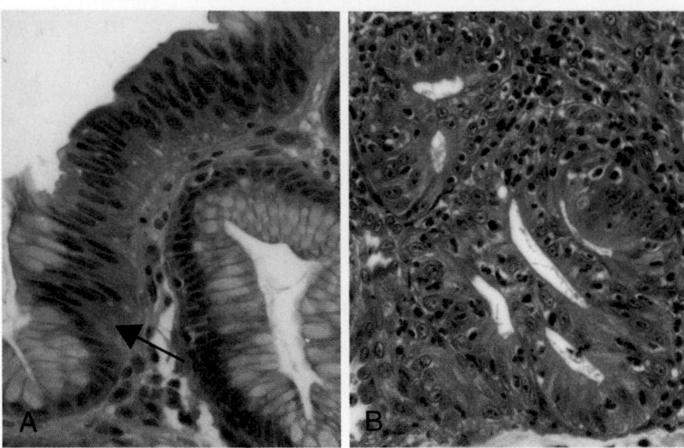

Figure 17-8 Dysplasia in Barrett esophagus. **A,** Abrupt transition from Barrett metaplasia to low-grade dysplasia *(arrow)*. Note the nuclear stratification and hyperchromasia. **B,** Architectural irregularities, including gland-within-gland, or cribriform, profiles in high-grade dysplasia.

Intramucosal or invasive carcinoma requires therapeutic intervention. Treatment options include surgical resection, or esophagectomy, as well as newer modalities such as photodynamic therapy, laser ablation, and endoscopic mucosectomy. Multifocal high-grade dysplasia, which carries a significant risk of progression to intramucosal or invasive carcinoma, is treated as intramucosal carcinoma. Many physicians follow low-grade dysplasia or a single focus of high-grade dysplasia with endoscopy and biopsy at frequent intervals. However, management of esophageal dysplasia is evolving, and it is hoped that improved molecular understanding of neoplastic progression may allow development of chemopreventive approaches that reduce the incidence of esophageal adenocarcinoma.

Esophageal Tumors

The vast majority of esophageal cancers fall into one of two types, adenocarcinoma and squamous cell carcinoma. Squamous cell carcinoma is more common worldwide, but adenocarcinoma is on the rise in the United States and other Western countries. Other malignancies of the esophagus are far less common and include unusual forms of adenocarcinoma, undifferentiated carcinoma, carcinoid tumor, melanoma, lymphoma, and sarcoma; these are not discussed here. Benign tumors of the esophagus are generally mesenchymal, and arise within the esophageal wall, with leiomyomas being most common. Fibromas, lipomas, hemangiomas, neurofibromas, and lymphangiomas also occur.

Adenocarcinoma

Most esophageal adenocarcinomas arise from Barrett esophagus. Thus, increased rates of esophageal adenocarcinoma may be partly due to the increased incidence of obesity-related gastroesophageal reflux and Barrett esophagus. Additional risk factors include tobacco use and exposure to radiation. Conversely, risk is reduced by diets rich in fresh fruits and vegetables. Some serotypes of *Helicobacter pylori* are associated with decreased risk of esophageal adenocarcinoma, because they cause gastric atrophy, which in turn leads to reduced acid secretion and reflux, and reduced incidence of Barrett esophagus. Thus, reduced rates of *Helicobacter pylori* infection may also be a factor in the increasing incidence of esophageal adenocarcinoma.

Esophageal adenocarcinoma occurs most frequently in Caucasians and shows a strong gender bias, being sevenfold more common in men. However, the incidence varies widely worldwide, with rates being highest in countries that include the United States, the United Kingdom, Canada, Australia, the Netherlands, and Brazil, and lowest in Korea, Thailand, Japan, and Ecuador. In countries where esophageal adenocarcinoma is more common, the incidence has increased markedly since 1970, more rapidly than almost any other cancer. For unknown reasons, these increases have been restricted to white and Hispanic men and white women in the United States. As a result, esophageal adenocarcinoma, which represented less than 5% of esophageal cancers before 1970, now accounts for more than half of all esophageal cancers in the United States.

Pathogenesis. **Molecular studies suggest that the progression of Barrett esophagus to adenocarcinoma occurs over an extended period through the stepwise acquisition of genetic and epigenetic changes.** This model is supported by the observation that epithelial clones identified in nondysplastic Barrett metaplasia persist and accumulate mutations during progression to dysplasia and invasive carcinoma. Chromosomal abnormalities, mutation of *TP53*, and downregulation of the cyclin-dependent kinase inhibitor *CDKN2A*, also known as *p16/INK4a*, are detected at early stages. In the case of *CDKN2A*, both allelic loss and hypermethylation-induced epigenetic silencing have been described. Later during progression there is amplification of *EGFR, ERBB2, MET, cyclin D1*, and *cyclin E* genes.

MORPHOLOGY

Esophageal adenocarcinoma usually occurs in the distal third of the esophagus and may invade the adjacent gastric cardia (Fig. 17-9*A*). Initially appearing as flat or raised patches in otherwise intact mucosa, large masses of 5 cm or more in diameter may develop. Alternatively, tumors may infiltrate diffusely or ulcerate and invade deeply. Microscopically, Barrett esophagus is frequently present adjacent to the tumor. Tumors most commonly produce mucin and form glands (Fig. 17-10*A*), often with intestinal-type morphology; less frequently tumors are composed of diffusely infiltrative signet-ring cells (similar to those seen in diffuse gastric cancers) or, in rare cases, small poorly differentiated cells (similar to small-cell carcinoma of the lung).

Clinical Features. Although esophageal adenocarcinomas are occasionally discovered in evaluation of GERD or surveillance of Barrett esophagus, they more commonly present with pain or difficulty in swallowing, progressive weight loss, hematemesis, chest pain, or vomiting. By the time symptoms appear, the tumor has usually spread to submucosal lymphatic vessels. As a result of the advanced stage at diagnosis, overall 5-year survival is less than 25%. In contrast, 5-year survival approximates 80% in the few patients with adenocarcinoma limited to the mucosa or submucosa.

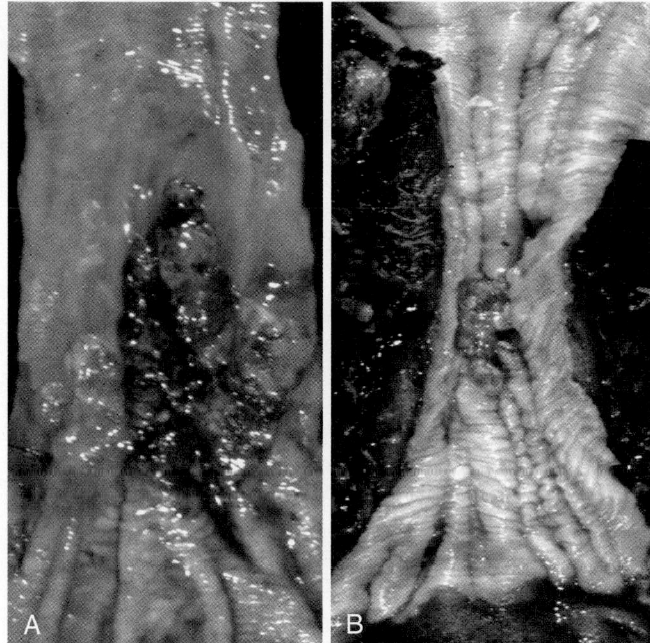

Figure 17-9 Esophageal cancer. **A,** Adenocarcinoma usually occurs distally and, as in this case, often involves the gastric cardia. **B,** Squamous cell carcinoma is most frequently found in the mid-esophagus, where it commonly causes strictures.

Squamous Cell Carcinoma

In the United States, esophageal squamous cell carcinoma occurs in adults older than age 45 and affects males four times more frequently than females. Risk factors include alcohol and tobacco use, poverty, caustic esophageal injury, achalasia, tylosis, Plummer-Vinson syndrome, diets that are deficient in fruits or vegetables, and frequent consumption of very hot beverages. Previous radiation to the mediastinum also predisposes individuals to esophageal carcinoma, with most cases occurring 5 to 10 or more years after exposure. Esophageal squamous cell carcinoma is nearly eight-fold more common in African Americans than Caucasians, a striking risk disparity that reflects differences in rates of alcohol and tobacco use as well as other poorly understood factors.

Esophageal squamous cell carcinoma incidence varies up to 180-fold between and within countries, being more common in rural and underdeveloped areas. The regions with highest incidence are Iran, central China, Hong Kong, Brazil, and South Africa. A pocket of extremely high esophageal squamous cell carcinoma incidence in western Kenya includes patients younger than 30 years of age and has been linked to consumption of a traditional fermented milk, termed mursik, which contains the carcinogen acetaldehyde (Chapter 9).

Pathogenesis. The majority of esophageal squamous cell carcinomas in Europe and the United States are linked to the use of alcohol and tobacco, which synergize to increase the risk. However, esophageal squamous cell carcinoma is also common in some regions where alcohol and tobacco use is uncommon. Thus, nutritional deficiencies, as well as polycyclic hydrocarbons, nitrosamines, and other mutagenic compounds, such as those found in fungus-contaminated foods, must also be considered. Human papillomavirus (HPV) infection has also been implicated in esophageal squamous cell carcinoma in high-risk areas but not in low-risk regions. The molecular pathogenesis of esophageal squamous cell carcinoma remains incompletely defined, but recurrent abnormalities include amplification of the transcription factor gene *SOX2* (believed to be involved in cancer stem cell self-renewal and survival); overexpression of the cell cycle regulator cyclin D1; and loss-of-function mutations in the tumor suppressors *TP53, E-cadherin,* and *NOTCH1.*

MORPHOLOGY

In contrast to adenocarcinoma, half of squamous cell carcinomas occur in the middle third of the esophagus (Fig. 17-9B). Squamous cell carcinoma begins as an in situ lesion termed **squamous dysplasia** (this lesion is referred to as intraepithelial neoplasia or carcinoma in situ at other sites). Early lesions appear as small, gray-white, plaque-like thickenings. Over months to years they grow into tumor masses that may be

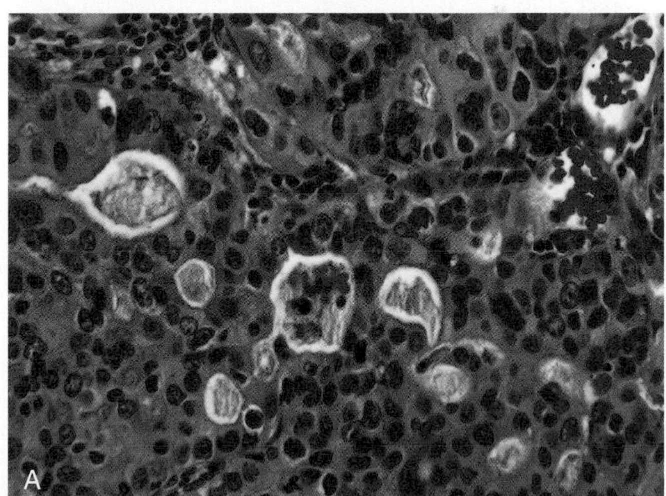

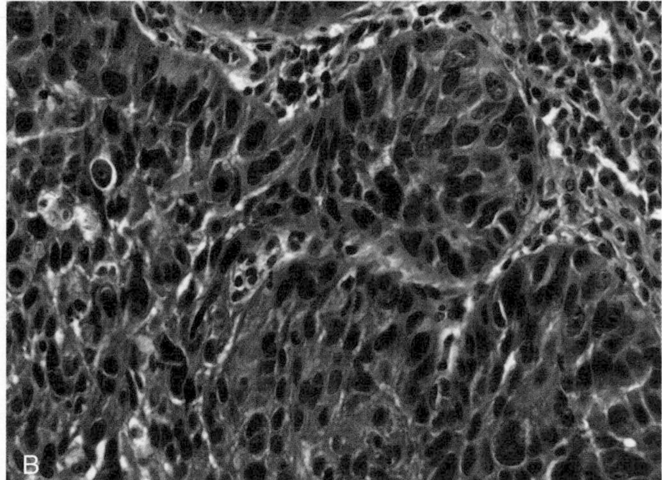

Figure 17-10 Esophageal cancer. **A,** Esophageal adenocarcinoma organized into back-to-back glands. **B,** Squamous cell carcinoma composed of nests of malignant cells that partially recapitulate the organization of squamous epithelium.

polypoid, or exophytic, and protrude into and obstruct the lumen. Other tumors are either ulcerated or diffusely infiltrative lesions that spread within the esophageal wall and cause thickening, rigidity, and luminal narrowing. They may invade surrounding structures including the respiratory tree, causing pneumonia; the aorta, causing catastrophic exsanguination; or the mediastinum and pericardium.

Most squamous cell carcinomas are moderately to well-differentiated (Fig. 17-10*B*). Less common histologic variants include verrucous squamous cell carcinoma, spindle cell carcinoma, and basaloid squamous cell carcinoma. Regardless of histology, symptomatic tumors are generally very large at diagnosis and have already invaded the esophageal wall. The rich lymphatic network promotes circumferential and longitudinal spread, and intramural tumor nodules may be present several centimeters away from the principal mass. The sites of lymph node metastases vary with tumor location: cancers in the upper third of the esophagus favor cervical lymph nodes; those in the middle third favor mediastinal, paratracheal, and tracheobronchial nodes; and those in the lower third spread to gastric and celiac nodes.

Clinical Features. The onset of esophageal squamous cell carcinoma is insidious and it most commonly presents with dysphagia, odynophagia (pain on swallowing), or obstruction. Patients subconsciously adjust to the progressively increasing obstruction by altering their diet from solid to liquid foods. Prominent weight loss and debilitation result from both impaired nutrition and effects of the tumor itself. Hemorrhage and sepsis may accompany tumor ulceration, and symptoms of iron deficiency are often present. Occasionally, the first symptoms are caused by aspiration of food via a tracheoesophageal fistula.

Increased prevalence of endoscopic screening has led to earlier detection of esophageal squamous cell carcinoma. This is critical, because 5-year survival rates are 75% in individuals with superficial esophageal squamous cell carcinoma but much lower in patients with more advanced tumors. Lymph node metastases, which are common, are associated with poor prognosis. The overall 5-year survival rate in the United States remains less than 20%, and varies by tumor stage and patient age, race, and gender.

KEY CONCEPTS

Esophageal Diseases

- Abnormalities of esophageal motility include **nutcracker esophagus** and **diffuse esophageal spasm**.
- **Achalasia**, characterized by incomplete lower esophageal sphincter (LES) relaxation, increased LES tone, and esophageal aperistalsis, is a common form of functional esophageal obstruction. It can be primary or secondary, with the latter form most commonly due to *Trypanosoma cruzi* infection.
- **Mallory-Weiss tears** of mucosa at the gastroesophageal junction develop as a result of severe retching or vomiting.
- **Esophagitis** can result from chemical or infectious mucosal injury. Infection is most common in immunocompromised individuals.
- The most prevalent cause of esophagitis is **gastroesophageal reflux disease** (GERD).
- **Eosinophilic esophagitis** is strongly associated with food allergy, allergic rhinitis, asthma, or modest peripheral eosinophilia. It is a common cause of GERD-like symptoms in children living in developed countries.
- **Gastroesophageal varices** are a consequence of portal hypertension and are present in nearly half of cirrhosis patients.
- **Barrett esophagus** develops in patients with chronic GERD and represents columnar metaplasia of the esophageal squamous mucosa.
- Barrett esophagus is a risk factor for development of **esophageal adenocarcinoma**.
- **Esophageal squamous cell carcinoma** is associated with alcohol and tobacco use, poverty, caustic esophageal injury, achalasia, tylosis, and Plummer-Vinson syndrome.

STOMACH

Disorders of the stomach are a frequent cause of clinical disease, with inflammatory and neoplastic lesions being particularly common. In the United States, diseases related to the stomach account for nearly one third of all health care spending on GI disease. In addition, despite decreasing incidence in certain locales such as the United States, gastric cancer remains a leading cause of death worldwide.

The stomach is divided into four major anatomic regions: the cardia, fundus, body, and antrum. The cardia and antrum are lined mainly with mucin-secreting foveolar cells that form small glands. The antral glands are similar but also contain endocrine cells, such as G cells, that release gastrin to stimulate luminal acid secretion by parietal cells within the gastric fundus and body. The well-developed glands of the body and fundus also contain chief cells that produce and secrete digestive enzymes such as pepsin.

Gastropathy and Acute Gastritis

Gastritis is a mucosal inflammatory process. When neutrophils are present, the lesion is referred to as acute gastritis. When inflammatory cells are rare or absent, the term *gastropathy* is applied; it includes a diverse set of disorders marked by gastric injury or dysfunction. Agents that cause gastropathy include NSAIDs, alcohol, bile, and stress induced injury. Acute mucosal erosion or hemorrhage, such as Curling ulcers or lesions following disruption of gastric blood flow, for example, in portal hypertension, can also cause gastropathy that typically progress to gastritis. The term *hypertrophic gastropathy* is applied to a specific group of diseases exemplified by Ménétrier disease and Zollinger-Ellison Syndrome (discussed later).

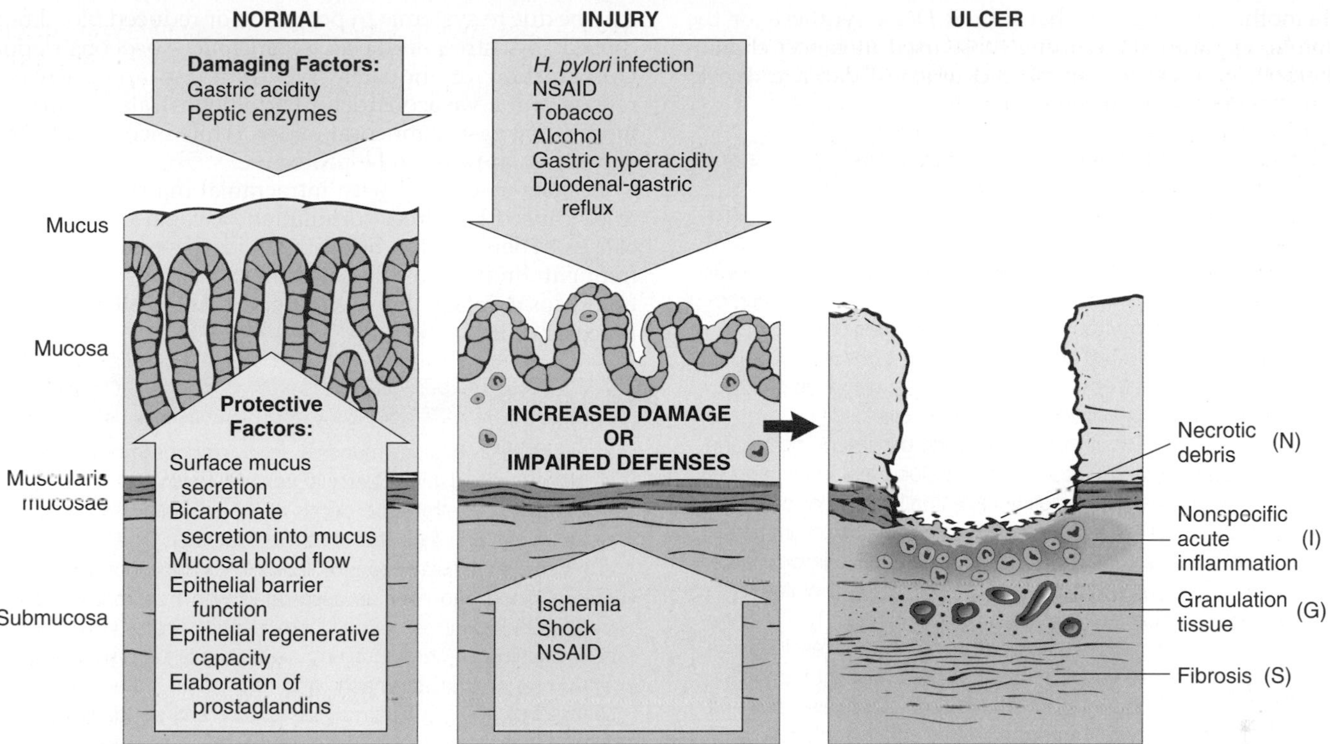

Figure 17-11 Mechanisms of gastric injury and protection. This diagram illustrates the progression from more mild forms of injury to ulceration that may occur with acute or chronic gastritis. Ulcers include layers of necrosis (N), inflammation (I), and granulation tissue (G), but a fibrotic scar (S), which takes time to develop, is only present in chronic lesions.

Both gastropathy and acute gastritis may be asymptomatic or cause variable degrees of epigastric pain, nausea, and vomiting. In more severe cases there may be mucosal erosion, ulceration, hemorrhage, hematemesis, melena, or, rarely, massive blood loss.

Pathogenesis. The gastric lumen has a pH of close to 1, more than a million times more acidic than the blood. This harsh environment contributes to digestion but also has the potential to damage the gastric mucosa. Multiple mechanisms have evolved to protect the gastric mucosa (Fig. 17-11). Mucin secreted by surface foveolar cells forms a thin layer of mucus and phospholipids that prevents large food particles from directly touching the epithelium. The mucus covering also promotes formation of an "unstirred" layer of fluid over the epithelium that protects the mucosa and has a neutral pH as a result of bicarbonate ion secretion by surface epithelial cells. Beneath the mucus, a continuous layer of gastric epithelial cells forms a physical barrier that limits back diffusion of acid and leakage of other luminal materials, including pepsin, into the lamina propria. Complete replacement of the surface foveolar cells every 3 to 7 days is essential for both the maintenance of the epithelial layer and the secretion of mucus and bicarbonate from these cells. In acid-secreting parts of the stomach, a capillary "alkaline tide" is generated as parietal cells secrete hydrochloric acid into the gastric lumen and bicarbonate into the vessels. In addition to delivering bicarbonate, the rich mucosal vasculature delivers oxygen and nutrients while washing away acid that has back-diffused into the lamina propria.

Gastropathy, acute gastritis, and chronic gastritis can occur following disruption of any of these protective mechanisms.

- Nonsteroidal antiinflammatory drugs (NSAIDs) inhibit cyclooxygenase- (COX) dependent synthesis of prostaglandins E_2 and I_2, which stimulate nearly all of the above defense mechanisms including mucus, bicarbonate, and phospholipid secretion, mucosal blood flow, and epithelial restitution while reducing acid secretion. Although COX-1 plays a larger role than COX-2, both isoenzymes contribute to mucosal protection. Thus, while the risk of NSAID-induced gastric injury is greatest with non-selective inhibitors, for example, aspirin, ibuprofen, and naproxen, selective COX-2 inhibition, for example, by celecoxib, can also result in gastropathy or gastritis.
- The gastric injury that occurs in uremic patients and those infected with urease-secreting *H. pylori* may be due to inhibition of gastric bicarbonate transporters by ammonium ions.
- Reduced mucin and bicarbonate secretion have been suggested as factors that explain the increased susceptibility of older adults to gastritis.
- Decreased oxygen delivery may account for an increased incidence of acute gastritis at high altitudes.

Ingestion of harsh chemicals, particularly acids or bases, either accidentally or as a suicide attempt, also results in severe gastric injury, predominantly as a result of direct injury to mucosal epithelial and stromal cells. Direct cellular damage also contributes to gastritis induced by excessive alcohol consumption, NSAIDs, radiation therapy, and chemotherapy. Agents that inhibit DNA synthesis or the mitotic apparatus, including those used in cancer chemotherapy, may cause generalized mucosal damage due to insufficient epithelial renewal.

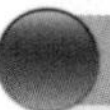

MORPHOLOGY

Histologically, gastropathy and mild acute gastritis may be difficult to recognize, since the lamina propria shows only moderate edema and slight vascular congestion. The surface epithelium is intact, but foveolar cell hyperplasia, with characteristic corkscrew profiles and epithelial proliferation are typically present. Neutrophils are not abundant, but a few may be found among the epithelial cells or within mucosal glands in gastritis. There are few lymphocytes and plasma cells.

The presence of neutrophils above the basement membrane in direct contact with epithelial cells is abnormal in all parts of the GI tract and signifies active inflammation, or, in this case, gastritis (rather than gastropathy). The term active inflammation is preferred over acute inflammation, since active inflammation may be present in both acute and chronic disease states. With more severe mucosal damage, erosions and hemorrhage develop. Erosion denotes loss of the epithelium, resulting in a superficial mucosal defect. It is accompanied by a pronounced mucosal neutrophilic infiltrate and a fibrin-containing purulent exudate in the lumen. Hemorrhage may occur and cause dark punctae in hyperemic mucosa. Concurrent erosion and hemorrhage is termed **acute erosive hemorrhagic gastritis.** Large areas of the gastric surface may be denuded, although the involvement is typically superficial. When erosions extend deeply, they may progress to ulcers, as described later.

Clinical Features. The presentation of gastropathy and acute gastritis varies according to etiology, and the two cannot be distinguished on clinical grounds. Patients with NSAID-induced gastropathy may be asymptomatic or have persistent epigastric pain that responds to antacids or proton pump inhibitors. In contrast, pain associated with bile reflux is typically refractory to such therapies and may be accompanied by occasional bilious vomiting.

Stress-Related Mucosal Disease

Stress-related mucosal disease occurs in patients with severe trauma, extensive burns, intracranial disease, major surgery, serious medical disease, and other forms of severe physiologic stress. More than 75% of critically ill patients develop endoscopically visible gastric lesions during the first 3 days of their illness. In some cases, the associated ulcers are given specific names based on location and clinical associations. For example:

- *Stress ulcers* are most common in individuals with shock, sepsis, or severe trauma.
- Ulcers occurring in the proximal duodenum and associated with severe burns or trauma are called *Curling ulcers.*
- Gastric, duodenal, and esophageal ulcers arising in persons with intracranial disease are termed *Cushing ulcers* and carry a high incidence of perforation.

Pathogenesis. The pathogenesis of stress-related gastric mucosal injury is most often related to local ischemia. This may be due to systemic hypotension or reduced blood flow caused by stress-induced splanchnic vasoconstriction. Upregulation of inducible NO synthase and increased release of the vasoconstrictor endothelin-1 also contribute to ischemic gastric mucosal injury, while increased COX-2 expression appears to be protective.

Lesions associated with intracranial injury are thought to be caused by direct stimulation of vagal nuclei, which causes hypersecretion of gastric acid. Systemic acidosis, a frequent finding in these settings, may also contribute to mucosal injury by lowering the intracellular pH of mucosal cells.

MORPHOLOGY

Stress-related gastric mucosal injury ranges from shallow erosions caused by superficial epithelial damage to deeper lesions that penetrate the depth of the mucosa. Acute ulcers are rounded and less than 1 cm in diameter. The ulcer base is frequently stained brown to black by acid digestion of extravasated blood and may be associated with transmural inflammation and local serositis. Unlike peptic ulcers, which arise in the setting of chronic injury, acute stress ulcers are found anywhere in the stomach and are most often multiple. Microscopically, acute stress ulcers are sharply demarcated, with essentially normal adjacent mucosa. There may be a suffusion of blood into the mucosa and submucosa and an associated inflammatory reaction. Conspicuously absent are the scarring and blood vessel thickenings that characterize chronic peptic ulcers. Healing with complete re-epithelialization occurs within days to several weeks after removal of the injurious factors.

Clinical Features. **Most critically ill patients admitted to hospital intensive care units have histologic evidence of gastric mucosal damage.** Bleeding from superficial gastric erosions or ulcers that may require transfusion develops in 1% to 4% of these patients. Other complications, including perforation, can also occur. Prophylactic proton pump inhibitors may blunt the impact of stress ulceration, but the most important determinant of clinical outcome is the ability to correct the underlying condition. The gastric mucosa can recover completely if the patient does not succumb to the primary disease.

Other, non-stress-related causes of gastric bleeding include the *Dieulafoy lesion* and *gastric antral vascular ectasia* (GAVE).

- Dieulafoy lesion is caused by a submucosal artery that does not branch properly within the wall of the stomach. This results in a mucosal artery with a diameter of up to 3 mm, or 10 times the size of mucosal capillaries. Dieulafoy lesions are most commonly found along the lesser curvature, near the gastroesophageal junction. Erosion of the overlying epithelium can cause gastric bleeding that, while usually self-limited, can be copious. Bleeding is often associated with NSAID use and may be recurrent.
- GAVE is responsible for 4% of non-variceal upper gastrointestinal bleeding. It can be recognized endoscopically as longitudinal stripes of edematous erythematous mucosa that alternate with less severely injured, paler mucosa, and is sometimes referred to as watermelon

stomach. The erythematous stripes are created by ectatic mucosal vessels. Histologically, the antral mucosa shows reactive gastropathy with dilated capillaries containing fibrin thrombi. While most often idiopathic, GAVE can also be associated with cirrhosis and systemic sclerosis. Patients may present with occult fecal blood or iron deficiency anemia.

Chronic Gastritis

The most common cause of chronic gastritis is infection with the bacillus *H. pylori*. Autoimmune gastritis, the most common cause of diffuse atrophic gastritis, represents less than 10% of cases of chronic gastritis, but is the most common form of chronic gastritis in patients without *H. pylori* infection. However, it is important to recognize that longstanding *H. pylori* infection can also result in atrophic gastritis, typically in a multifocal rather than diffuse pattern. Less common causes of chronic gastritis include radiation injury, chronic bile reflux, mechanical injury (e.g. an indwelling nasogastric tube), and involvement by systemic diseases, such as Crohn disease, amyloidosis, or graft-versus-host disease.

In contrast to acute gastritis, the symptoms associated with chronic gastritis are typically less severe but more persistent. Nausea and upper abdominal pain are typical, sometimes with vomiting, but hematemesis is uncommon.

Helicobacter pylori Gastritis

H. pylori are spiral-shaped or curved bacilli present in gastric biopsy specimens of almost all patients with duodenal ulcers as well as most individuals with gastric ulcers or chronic gastritis. Acute *H. pylori* infection does not produce sufficient symptoms to come to medical attention in most cases; it is the chronic gastritis that ultimately causes the individual to seek treatment. *H. pylori* organisms are present in 90% of individuals with chronic gastritis affecting the antrum.

Epidemiology. In the United States, *H. pylori* infection is associated with poverty, household crowding, limited education, African American or Mexican American ethnicity, residence in rural areas, and birth outside of the United States. Humans are the primary carriers, suggesting that transmission is primarily by the fecal-oral route. Infection is typically acquired in childhood and persists for life without treatment. Improved sanitation in the United States likely explains the marked reduction in *H. pylori* infection rates among younger people that has resulted in a cohort effect. For example, the prevalence of *H. pylori* infection in those younger than 12 years old is less than 15% relative to the 50% to 60% prevalence in those older than 60 years of age. Accordingly, colonization rates vary from less than 10% to more than 80% worldwide, as a function of age and geography.

***Pathogenesis.* *H. pylori* infection most often presents as a predominantly antral gastritis with normal or increased acid production.** Local gastrin production may be increased, but hypergastrinemia (increased serum gastrin) is uncommon. When inflammation remains limited to the antrum, increased acid production results in greater risk of duodenal peptic ulcer (see later). In other patients gastritis may progress to involve the gastric body and fundus. This *multifocal atrophic gastritis* is associated with patchy mucosal atrophy, reduced parietal cell mass and acid secretion, intestinal metaplasia, and increased risk of gastric adenocarcinoma. Thus, there is an inverse relationship between duodenal ulcer and gastric adenocarcinoma that correlates with the pattern of gastritis. The bacterial and host factors that determine which pattern develops in an individual patient are discussed later.

H. pylori organisms have adapted to the ecologic niche provided by gastric mucus. Its virulence is linked to the following factors:

- *Flagella*, which allow the bacteria to be motile in viscous mucus
- *Urease*, which generates ammonia from endogenous urea and thereby elevates local gastric pH and enhances bacterial survival
- *Adhesins* that enhance bacterial adherence to surface foveolar cells
- *Toxins*, such as cytotoxin-associated gene A *(CagA)*, that may be involved in disease progression

Variation in these and other bacterial factors are strongly linked to outcome. For example, *CagA* gene and the associated 20 gene pathogenicity islands are present in 50% of *H. pylori* isolates overall but in 90% of *H. pylori* isolates found in populations with elevated gastric cancer risk. This may, in part, be because CagA expressing strains can effectively colonize the gastric body and cause multifocal atrophic gastritis.

Host factors also play an important role in the outcome of *H. pylori* infection. Genetic polymorphisms that lead to increased expression of the proinflammatory cytokines tumor necrosis factor (TNF) and interleukin-1β (IL-1β) or decreased expression of the antiinflammatory cytokine interleukin-10 (IL-10) are associated with development of pangastritis, atrophy, and gastric cancer. Iron deficiency may also be a risk factor for *H. pylori*–associated gastric cancer. The course of *H. pylori* gastritis is, therefore, the result of interplay between gastroduodenal mucosal defenses, inflammatory responses, and bacterial virulence factors.

MORPHOLOGY

Gastric biopsy specimens generally demonstrate *H. pylori* in infected individuals. The organism is concentrated within the superficial mucus overlying epithelial cells in the surface and neck regions. The distribution can be irregular, with areas of heavy colonization adjacent to those with few organisms. In extreme cases, the organisms carpet the luminal surfaces of foveolar and mucous neck cells, and can even extend into the gastric pits. Organisms are most easily demonstrated with special stains (Fig. 17-12A). *H. pylori* display tropism for gastric epithelia and are generally not found in association with intestinal metaplasia or duodenal epithelium.

Within the stomach, *H. pylori* are most often found in the antrum (Table 17-2). Although there is often concordance between colonization of the antrum and cardia, infection of the

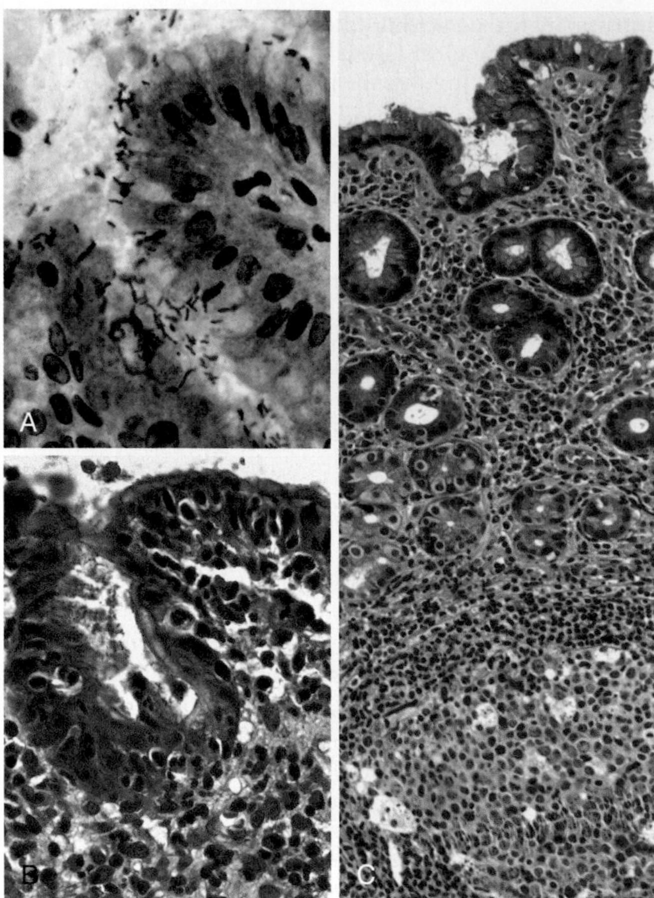

Figure 17-12 *Helicobacter pylori* gastritis. **A,** Spiral-shaped *H. pylori* are highlighted in this Warthin-Starry silver stain. Organisms are abundant within surface mucus. **B,** Intraepithelial and lamina propria neutrophils are prominent. **C,** Lymphoid aggregates with germinal centers and abundant subepithelial plasma cells within the superficial lamina propria are characteristic of *H. pylori* gastritis.

cardia occurs at somewhat lower rates. *H. pylori* are less common in oxyntic (acid-producing) mucosa of the fundus and body. Thus, an antral biopsy is preferred for evaluation of *H. pylori* gastritis. When viewed endoscopically, *H. pylori*-infected antral mucosa is usually erythematous and has a coarse or even nodular appearance. The inflammatory infiltrate generally includes variable numbers of neutrophils within the lamina propria, including some that cross the basement membrane to assume an intraepithelial location (Fig. 17-12*B*) and accumulate in the lumen of gastric pits to create pit abscesses. In addition, the superficial lamina propria contains large numbers of plasma cells, often in clusters or sheets, and increased numbers of lymphocytes and macrophages. Intraepithelial neutrophils and subepithelial plasma cells are characteristic of *H. pylori* gastritis. When intense, inflammatory infiltrates may create thickened rugal folds, mimicking the appearance of early cancers. Lymphoid aggregates, some with germinal centers, are frequently present (Fig. 17-12*C*) and represent an induced form of mucosa-associated lymphoid tissue, or MALT, that has the potential to transform into lymphoma.

Long-standing *H. pylori* gastritis may extend to involve the body and fundus, and the mucosa can become atrophic, with loss of parietal and chief cells. As a result, the oxyntic mucosa can take on the appearance of antral mucosa. In contrast to autoimmune gastritis, this is typically a patchy process, and biopsies of the gastric body can show intact oxyntic glands adjacent to antral-type glands. The development of atrophy is typically associated with the presence of intestinal metaplasia and increased risk of gastric adenocarcinoma.

Clinical Features. In addition to histologic identification of the organism, several diagnostic tests have been developed including a noninvasive serologic test for antibodies to *H. pylori*, fecal bacterial detection, and the urea breath test based on the generation of ammonia by the bacterial urease. Gastric biopsy specimens can also be analyzed by the rapid urease test, bacterial culture, or bacterial DNA detection by PCR.

Effective treatments for *H. pylori* infection include combinations of antibiotics and proton pump inhibitors. Individuals with *H. pylori* gastritis usually improve after treatment, although relapses can occur after incomplete eradication or reinfection, which is common in regions with high endemic colonization rates. Prophylactic and therapeutic vaccines are still at an early stage of development.

Autoimmune Gastritis

Autoimmune gastritis accounts for less than 10% of cases of chronic gastritis. In contrast to *H. pylori*–associated gastritis, autoimmune gastritis typically spares the antrum and is associated with hypergastrinemia (Table 17-2). Autoimmune gastritis is characterized by:

- Antibodies to parietal cells and intrinsic factor that can be detected in serum and gastric secretions
- Reduced serum pepsinogen I concentration
- Endocrine cell hyperplasia
- Vitamin B_{12} deficiency
- Defective gastric acid secretion (achlorhydria)

Table 17-2 Characteristics of *Helicobacter pylori*–Associated and Autoimmune Gastritis

	H. pylori–Associated	Autoimmune
Location	Antrum	Body
Inflammatory infiltrate	Neutrophils, subepithelial plasma cells	Lymphocytes, macrophages
Acid production	Increased to slightly decreased	Decreased
Gastrin	Normal to decreased	Increased
Other lesions	Hyperplastic/inflammatory polyps	Neuroendocrine hyperplasia
Serology	Antibodies to *H. pylori*	Antibodies to parietal cells (H^+,K^+-ATPase, intrinsic factor)
Sequelae	Peptic ulcer, adenocarcinoma, MALToma	Atrophy, pernicious anemia, adenocarcinoma, carcinoid tumor
Associations	Low socioeconomic status, poverty, residence in rural areas	Autoimmune disease; thyroiditis, diabetes mellitus, Graves disease

Pathogenesis. **Autoimmune gastritis is associated with loss of parietal cells, which are responsible for secretion of gastric acid and intrinsic factor.** The absence of acid production stimulates gastrin release, resulting in hypergastrinemia and hyperplasia of antral gastrin-producing G cells. Lack of intrinsic factor disables ileal vitamin B_{12} absorption, which ultimately leads to vitamin B_{12} deficiency and a slow-onset megaloblastic anemia *(pernicious anemia)*. Reduced serum pepsinogen I concentration results from chief cell destruction. Although *H. pylori* infection can cause gastric atrophy and hypochlorhydria, it is not associated with achlorhydria or pernicious anemia. This is because, in contrast to the diffuse atrophy of autoimmune gastritis, the damage in *H. pylori* gastritis is multifocal and leaves patches of residual parietal and chief cells.

CD4+ T cells directed against parietal cell components, including the H+,K+-ATPase, are considered to be the principal agents of injury in autoimmune gastritis. This is supported by the observation that transfer of H+,K+-ATPase-reactive CD4+ T cells into naïve mice results in gastritis and production of H+,K+-ATPase autoantibodies. There is no evidence of an autoimmune reaction to chief cells, suggesting that these may be lost through gastric gland destruction during autoimmune attack on parietal cells. If autoimmune destruction is controlled by immunosuppression, the glands can repopulate, demonstrating that gastric stem cells survive and are able to differentiate into parietal and chief cells.

Autoantibodies to parietal cell components, most prominently the H+,K+-ATPase, or proton pump, and intrinsic factor are present in up to 80% of patients with autoimmune gastritis. However, these antibodies are not thought to be pathogenic because neither secreted intrinsic factor nor the luminally oriented proton pump are accessible to circulating antibodies, and passive transfer of these antibodies does not produce gastritis in experimental animals. Nevertheless, the presence of these autoantibodies is a useful diagnostic tool.

MORPHOLOGY

Autoimmune gastritis is characterized by diffuse mucosal damage of the oxyntic (acid-producing) mucosa within the body and fundus. Damage to the antrum and cardia is typically absent or mild. With diffuse atrophy, the oxyntic mucosa of the body and fundus appears markedly thinned, and rugal folds are lost. If vitamin B_{12} deficiency is severe, nuclear enlargement (megaloblastic change) occurs within epithelial cells. Neutrophils may be present, but the inflammatory infiltrate is typically composed of lymphocytes, macrophages, and plasma cells, often in association with lymphoid aggregates and follicles. The superficial lamina propria plasma cells typical of *H. pylori* gastritis are absent, and the inflammatory reaction is deeper and centered on the gastric glands (Fig. 17-13*A*). Loss of parietal and chief cells can be extensive. When atrophy is incomplete, residual islands of oxyntic mucosa may give the appearance of multiple small polyps or nodules. In other areas, small surface elevations may represent sites of intestinal metaplasia, characterized by the presence of goblet cells and columnar absorptive cells (Fig. 17-13B). Although present in most patients, endocrine cell hyperplasia can be difficult to appreciate on hematoxylin and eosin-stained sections. This hyperplasia, which can be clearly demonstrated with immunostains for proteins such as chromogrannin A, parallels the degree of mucosal atrophy and is a physiologic response to decreased acid production. Over time, hypergastrinemia can stimulate endocrine cell hyperplasia in the fundus and body. Rarely, this may progress to form small, multicentric, low-grade neuroendocrine (carcinoid) tumors.

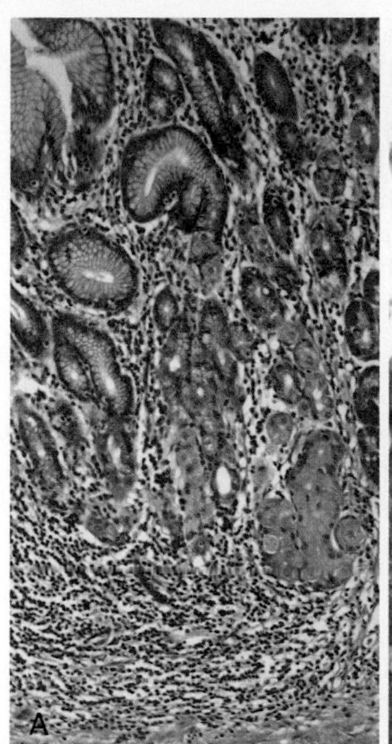

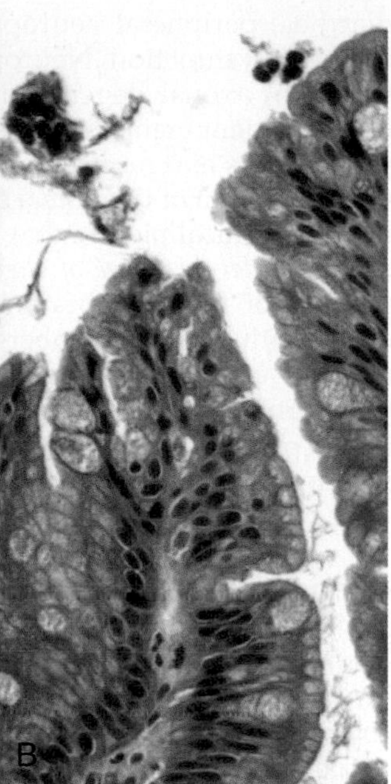

Figure 17-13 Autoimmune gastritis. **A,** Low-magnification image of gastric body demonstrating deep inflammatory infiltrates, primarily composed of lymphocytes, and glandular atrophy. **B,** Intestinal metaplasia, recognizable as the presence of goblet cells admixed with gastric foveolar epithelium.

Clinical Features. Antibodies to parietal cells and to intrinsic factor are present early in the disease course. Progression to gastric atrophy probably occurs over 2 to 3 decades, and anemia is seen in only a few patients. Because of the slow onset and variable progression, patients are generally diagnosed only after being affected for many years; the median age at diagnosis is 60. Slightly more women than men are affected. Pernicious anemia and autoimmune gastritis are often associated with other autoimmune diseases including Hashimoto thyroiditis, insulin-dependent (type I) diabetes mellitus, Addison disease, primary ovarian failure, primary hypoparathyroidism, Graves disease, vitiligo, myasthenia gravis, and Lambert-Eaton syndrome. These associations, along with concordance in some monozygotic twins and clustering of disease in families, support a genetic predisposition. In general, about 20% of relatives of individuals with pernicious anemia also have autoimmune gastritis, although they may be asymptomatic. Despite this strong genetic influence, autoimmune gastritis stands apart from many other autoimmune diseases in that there is little evidence of linkage to specific HLA alleles.

Clinical presentation may be linked to symptoms of anemia (Chapter 14). Vitamin B_{12} deficiency may also cause atrophic glossitis, in which the tongue becomes smooth and beefy red, epithelial megaloblastosis, malabsorptive diarrhea, peripheral neuropathy, spinal cord lesions, and cerebral dysfunction. Neuropathic changes include demyelination, axonal degeneration, and neuronal death. The most frequent manifestations of peripheral neuropathy are paresthesias and numbness. The spinal lesions result from demyelination of the dorsal and lateral spinal tracts, giving rise to a clinical picture that is often referred to as *subacute combined degeneration of the cord.* It is associated with a mixture of loss of vibration and position sense, sensory ataxia with positive Romberg sign, limb weakness, spasticity, and extensor plantar responses. Cerebral manifestations range from mild personality changes and memory loss to psychosis. In contrast to anemia, neurologic changes are not reversed by vitamin B_{12} replacement therapy.

Uncommon Forms of Gastritis

Eosinophilic Gastritis. This form of gastritis is characterized by tissue damage associated with dense infiltrates of eosinophils in the mucosa and muscularis, usually in the antral or pyloric region. The lesion may also be present at other sites within the GI tract and is associated with peripheral eosinophilia and increased serum IgE levels. Allergic reactions are one cause of eosinophilic gastritis, with cow's milk and soy protein being the most common allergens in children. Eosinophilic gastritis can also occur in association with immune disorders such as systemic sclerosis and polymyositis, parasitic infections, and even *H. pylori* infection.

Lymphocytic Gastritis. This disease preferentially affects women and produces nonspecific abdominal symptoms. It is idiopathic, but approximately 40% of cases are associated with celiac disease, suggesting an immune-mediated pathogenesis. Lymphocytic gastritis typically affects the entire stomach and is often referred to as *varioliform gastritis* based on the distinctive endoscopic appearance (thickened folds covered by small nodules with central aphthous ulceration). Histologically there is a marked increase in the number of intraepithelial T lymphocytes.

Granulomatous Gastritis. This descriptive term is applied to any gastritis that contains well-formed granulomas or aggregates of epithelioid macrophages. It encompasses a diverse group of diseases with widely varying clinical and pathologic features. Many cases are idiopathic. In Western populations, gastric involvement by Crohn disease is the most common specific cause of granulomatous gastritis, followed by sarcoidosis and infections (including mycobacteria, fungi, CMV, and *H. pylori*). In addition to the presence of histologically evident granulomas, narrowing and rigidity of the gastric antrum may occur secondary to transmural granulomatous inflammation.

Complications of Chronic Gastritis

Peptic Ulcer Disease

Peptic ulcer disease (PUD) refers to chronic mucosal ulceration affecting the duodenum or stomach. Nearly all peptic ulcers are associated with *H. pylori* infection, NSAIDs, or cigarette smoking. The most common form of peptic ulcer disease (PUD) occurs within the gastric antrum or duodenum as a result of chronic, *H. pylori*-induced antral gastritis, which is associated with increased gastric acid secretion, and decreased duodenal bicarbonate secretion. In contrast, PUD within the gastric fundus or body is usually accompanied by lesser acid secretion as a result of mucosal atrophy (associated with some cases of *H. pylori*-induced or autoimmune chronic gastritis, as discussed earlier). While these patients still secrete more acid than normal individuals, they are incapable of secreting the much larger amounts needed to overcome the defense mechanisms that "protect" the antral and duodenal mucosa. Thus, individuals with gastric mucosal atrophy are generally protected from antral and duodenal ulcers. PUD may also be caused by acid secreted by ectopic gastric mucosa within the duodenum or an ileal Meckel diverticulum. PUD may also occur in the esophagus as a result of GERD or acid secretion by esophageal ectopic gastric mucosa (an inlet patch).

Table 17-3 Risk factors for Peptic Ulcer Disease

- *H. pylori* infection
- Cigarette use (synergizes with *H. pylori* for gastric PUD)
- Chronic obstructive pulmonary disease
- Illicit drugs, e.g. cocaine, that reduce mucosal blood flow
- NSAIDs (potentiated by corticosteroids)
- Alcoholic cirrhosis (primarily duodenal PUD)
- Psychological stress (can increase gastric acid secretion)
- Endocrine cell hyperplasia (can stimulate parietal cell growth and gastric acid secretion)
- Zollinger-Ellison Syndrome (PUD of stomach, duodenum, and jejunum)
- Viral infection (CMV, herpes simplex virus)

Epidemiology. The incidence of PUD is falling in developed countries along with reduced prevalence of *H. pylori*, infection. However, a new group of duodenal PUD patients older than 60 years of age has emerged as a result of increased NSAID use. This is particularly true when low-dose aspirin (for cardiovascular benefits) is combined with other NSAIDs. This is facilitated if concurrent *H. pylori* infection is also present. PUD has been associated with cigarette use and cardiovascular disease, likely due to reduced mucosal blood flow, oxygenation, and healing. Other risk factors for PUD are listed in Table 17-3.

Pathogenesis. **PUD results from imbalances between mucosal defense mechanisms and damaging factors that cause chronic gastritis** (discussed earlier). Thus, PUD generally develops on a background of chronic gastritis. The reasons why some people develop only chronic gastritis while others develop PUD are poorly understood. However, as with *H. pylori* gastritis, it is likely that host factors as well as variation between bacterial strains are involved.

MORPHOLOGY

Peptic ulcers occur in the context of chronic gastritis, but are most common in the proximal duodenum, where they occur within a few centimeters of the pyloric valve and involve the anterior duodenal wall. Gastric peptic ulcers are predominantly located along the lesser curvature near the interface of the body and antrum.

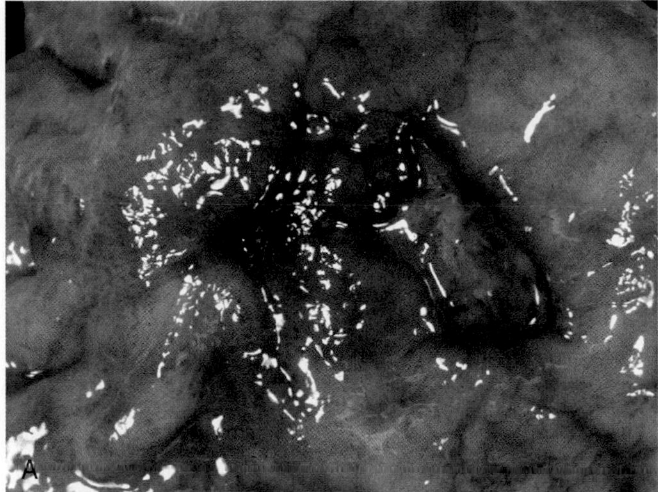

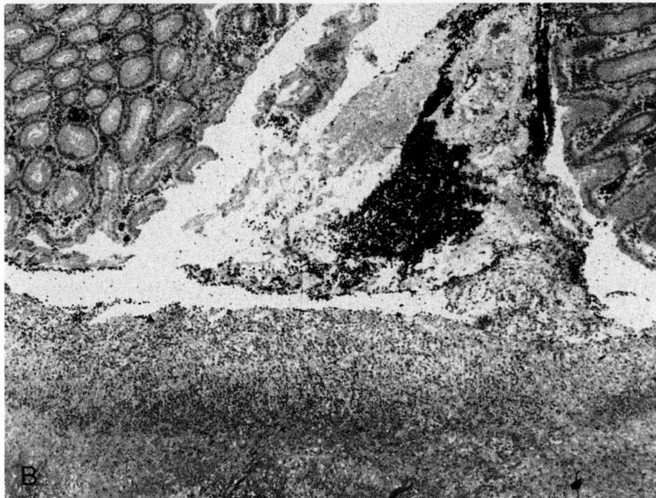

Figure 17-14 Acute gastric perforation in a patient presenting with free air under the diaphragm. **A,** Mucosal defect with clean edges. **B,** The necrotic ulcer base is composed of granulation tissue.

Peptic ulcers are solitary in more than 80% of patients. Lesions less than 0.3 cm in diameter tend to be shallow while those greater than 0.6 cm are likely to be deeper. The classic peptic ulcer is a round to oval, **sharply punched-out defect** (Fig. 17-14*A*). The mucosal margin may overhang the base slightly, particularly on the upstream side, but is usually level with the surrounding mucosa. In contrast, **heaped-up margins are more characteristic of cancers**. The depth of ulcers may be limited by the thick gastric muscularis propria or by adherent pancreas, omental fat, or the liver. Hemorrhage and fibrin deposition are often present on the gastric serosa. **Perforation** into the peritoneal cavity is a surgical emergency that may be identified by detection of free air under the diaphragm on upright radiographs of the abdomen.

The base of peptic ulcers is smooth and clean as a result of peptic digestion of exudate. Active ulcers may be lined by a thin layer of fibrinoid debris underlaid by a predominantly neutrophilic inflammatory infiltrate. Beneath this, granulation tissue infiltrated with mononuclear leukocytes and a fibrous or collagenous scar forms the ulcer base (Fig. 17-14*B*). Vessel walls within the scarred area are typically thickened and are occasionally thrombosed. Bleeding from damaged vessels within the ulcer base may cause life-threatening **hemorrhage.** Scarring may involve the entire thickness of the wall and pucker the surrounding mucosa into folds that radiate outward.

Size and location do not differentiate between benign and malignant ulcers. However, the gross appearance of chronic peptic ulcers is virtually diagnostic. **Malignant transformation of peptic ulcers occurs rarely**, if ever, and reports of transformation probably represent cases in which a lesion thought to be a chronic peptic ulcer was actually an ulcerated carcinoma from the start.

Clinical Features. Peptic ulcers can be chronic, recurring lesions with significant morbidity. The majority of peptic ulcers come to clinical attention because of *epigastric burning or aching pain,* although a significant fraction present with complications such as *iron deficiency anemia, hemorrhage,* or *perforation* (Table 17-4). The pain tends to occur 1 to 3 hours after meals during the day, is worse at night (usually between 11 PM and 2 AM), and is relieved by alkali or food. Nausea, vomiting, bloating, belching, and significant weight loss are additional manifestations. With penetrating ulcers the pain is occasionally referred to the back, the left upper quadrant, or the chest, where it may be misinterpreted as cardiac in origin.

Current therapies for PUD are aimed at *H. pylori* eradication and neutralization of gastric acid, primarily with proton pump inhibitors. It is also important to withdraw other offending agents, such as NSAIDs, including selective COX-2 inhibitors, that may interfere with mucosal healing. While peptic ulcers were previously notorious for their recurrence, the recurrence rate is now less than 20% following successful clearance of *H. pylori.*

A variety of surgical approaches were formerly used to treat PUD, including antrectomy to remove gastrin-producing cells and vagotomy to prevent the acid-stimulatory effects mediated by the vagus nerve. However, the success of proton pump inhibitors and *H. pylori* eradication has relegated surgical intervention to treatment of bleeding or perforated peptic ulcers.

Table 17-4 Complications of Peptic Ulcer Disease

Bleeding
Occurs in 15% to 20% of patients Most frequent complication May be life-threatening Accounts for 25% of ulcer deaths May be the first indication of an ulcer
Perforation
Occurs in up to 5% of patients Accounts for two thirds of ulcer deaths Is rarely first indication of an ulcer
Obstruction
Mostly in chronic ulcers Secondary to edema or scarring Occurs in about 2% of patients Most often associated with pyloric channel ulcers May occur with duodenal ulcers Causes incapacitating, crampy abdominal pain Can rarely cause total obstruction and intractable vomiting

KEY CONCEPTS

Gastritis

- **Gastritis** is a mucosal inflammatory process. When inflammatory cells are absent or rare, the term **gastropathy** can be applied.
- The spectrum of **acute gastritis** ranges from asymptomatic disease to mild epigastric pain, nausea, and vomiting. Causative factors include any agent or disease that interferes with gastric mucosal protective mechanisms.
- Severe acute gastritis can result in **acute gastric ulceration**.
- The most common cause of chronic gastritis is ***H. pylori* infection**. Other agents include NSAIDs and alcohol.
- ***H. pylori* gastritis** typically affects the antrum and is associated with increased gastric acid production. In later disease, the body can be involved and the resulting glandular atrophy can lead to mildly reduced acid production. Host immune responses and bacterial characteristics determine whether the infection remains antral or progresses to **pangastritis**.
- ***H. pylori* gastritis induces mucosa-associated lymphoid tissue (MALT)** that can give rise to B cell lymphomas (MALTomas).
- **Autoimmune gastritis** is the most frequent etiology of noninfectious chronic gastritis. It results in atrophy of the gastric body oxyntic glands, which leads to decreased gastric acid production, antral G cell hyperplasia, achlorhydria, and vitamin B_{12} deficiency. Anti-parietal cell and anti-intrinsic factor antibodies are typically present.
- **Intestinal metaplasia** develops in both forms of chronic gastritis and is a risk factor for gastric adenocarcinoma.
- **Peptic ulcer disease** is usually secondary to *H. pylori* chronic gastritis and the resulting hyperchlorhydria. Ulcers can develop in the stomach or duodenum, and usually heal after suppression of gastric acid production and eradication of *H. pylori*.

Mucosal Atrophy and Intestinal Metaplasia

Long-standing chronic gastritis that involves the body and fundus may ultimately lead to significant loss of parietal cell mass. This oxyntic atrophy may be associated with intestinal metaplasia, recognized by the presence of goblet cells, and is strongly associated with increased risk of gastric adenocarcinoma. The risk of adenocarcinoma is greatest in autoimmune gastritis. This may be because achlorhydria of gastric mucosal atrophy permits overgrowth of bacteria that produce carcinogenic nitrosamines. Intestinal metaplasia also occurs in chronic *H. pylori* gastritis and may regress after clearance of the organism.

Dysplasia

Chronic gastritis exposes the epithelium to inflammation-related free radical damage and proliferative stimuli. Over time this combination of stressors can lead to the accumulation of genetic alterations that result in carcinoma. Preinvasive in situ lesions can be recognized histologically as dysplasia. The morphologic hallmarks of dysplasia are variations in epithelial size, shape, and orientation along with coarse chromatin texture, hyperchromasia, and nuclear enlargement. The distinction between dysplasia and regenerative epithelial changes induced by active inflammation can be a challenge for the pathologist, since increased epithelial proliferation and mitotic figures may be prominent in both. However, reactive epithelial cells mature as they reach the mucosal surface, while dysplastic lesions remain cytologically immature.

Gastritis Cystica

Gastritis cystica is an exuberant reactive epithelial proliferation associated with entrapment of epithelial-lined cysts. These may be found within the submucosa (gastritis cystica polyposa) or deeper layers of the gastric wall (gastritis cystica profunda). Because of the association with chronic gastritis and partial gastrectomy, it is presumed that gastritis cystica is trauma-induced, but the reasons for the development of epithelial cysts within deeper portions of the gastric wall are not clear. Regenerative epithelial changes can be prominent in the entrapped epithelium, and gastritis cystica can therefore mimic invasive adenocarcinoma.

Hypertrophic Gastropathies

Hypertrophic gastropathies are uncommon diseases characterized by giant "cerebriform" enlargement of the rugal folds due to epithelial hyperplasia without inflammation. As might be expected, the hypertrophic gastropathies are linked to excessive growth factor release. Two well-defined examples are Ménétrier disease and Zollinger-Ellison syndrome, the morphologic features of which are compared with other gastric proliferations in Table 17-5.

Ménétrier Disease

Ménétrier disease is a rare disorder associated with excessive secretion of transforming growth factor α (TGF-α). It is characterized by diffuse hyperplasia of the foveolar epithelium of the body and fundus and hypoproteinemia due to protein-losing enteropathy. Secondary symptoms, such as weight loss, diarrhea, and peripheral edema, are commonly present. Symptoms and pathologic features of Ménétrier disease in children are similar to those in adults, but pediatric disease is usually self-limited and often follows a respiratory infection. Risk of gastric adenocarcinoma is increased in adults with Ménétrier disease.

MORPHOLOGY

Ménétrier disease is characterized by irregular enlargement of the gastric rugae. Some areas may appear polypoid. Enlarged rugae are present in the body and fundus (Fig. 17-15*A*), but the antrum is generally spared. Histologically, the most characteristic feature is hyperplasia of foveolar mucous cells. The glands are elongated with a corkscrew-like appearance and cystic dilation is common (Fig. 17-15*B*). Inflammation is usually modest, although some cases show marked intraepithelial lymphocytosis. Diffuse or patchy glandular atrophy, evident as hypoplasia of parietal and chief cells, is typical.

Table 17-5 Hypertrophic Gastropathies and Gastric Polyps

Parameter	Ménétrier Disease (adult)	Zollinger-Ellison Syndrome	Inflammatory and Hyperplastic Polyps	Gastritis Cystica	Fundic Gland Polyps	Gastric Adenomas
Mean patient age (yr)	30-60	50	50-60	Variable	50	50-60
Location	Body and fundus	Fundus	Antrum > body	Body	Body and fundus	Antrum > body
Predominant cell type	Mucous	Parietal > mucous, endocrine	Mucous	Mucous, cyst-lining	Parietal and chief	Dysplastic, intestinal
Inflammatory infiltrate	Limited, lymphocytes	Neutrophils	Neutrophils and lymphocytes	Neutrophils and lymphocytes	None	Variable
Symptoms	Hypoproteinemia, weight loss, diarrhea	Peptic ulcers	Similar to chronic gastritis	Similar to chronic gastritis	None, nausea	Similar to chronic gastritis
Risk factors	None	Multiple endocrine neoplasia	Chronic gastritis, *H. pylori*	Trauma, prior surgery	PPIs, FAP	Chronic gastritis, atrophy, intestinal metaplasia
Association with adenocarcinoma	Yes	No	Occasional	No	Syndromic (FAP) only	Frequent

FAP, Familial adenomatous polyposis; PPIs, proton pump inhibitors.

Treatment of Ménétrier disease is supportive, with intravenous albumin and parenteral nutritional supplementation. In severe cases gastrectomy may be needed. More recently, agents that block TGF-α-mediated activation of the epidermal growth factor receptor have shown promise.

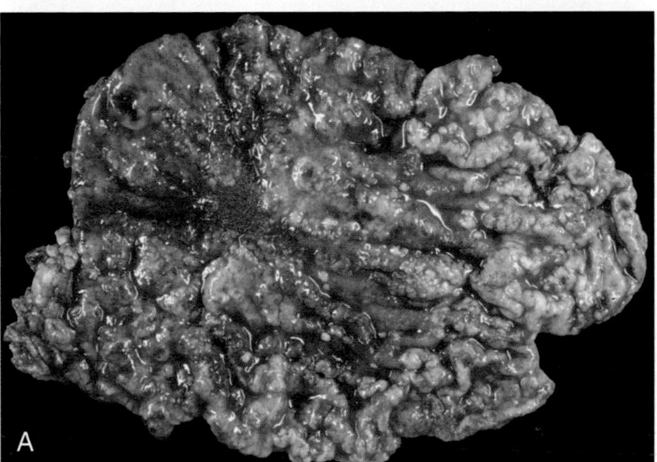

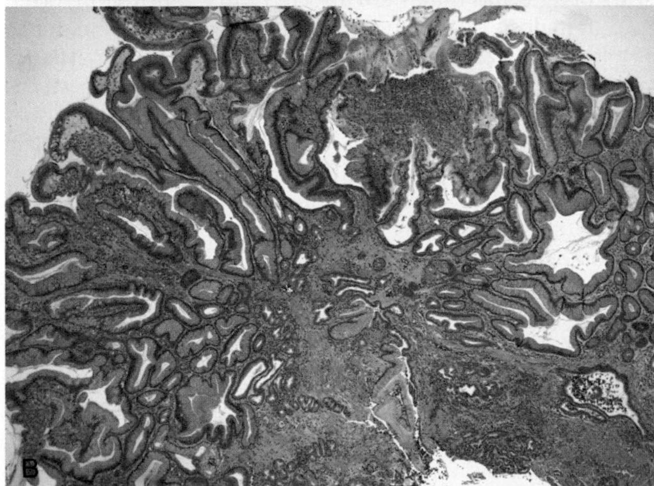

Figure 17-15 Ménétrier disease. **A,** Marked hypertrophy of rugal folds. **B,** Foveolar hyperplasia with elongated and focally dilated glands. (Courtesy Dr. M. Kay Washington, Vanderbilt University, Nashville, Tenn.)

Zollinger-Ellison Syndrome

Zollinger-Ellison syndrome is caused by gastrin-secreting tumors. These gastrinomas are most commonly found in the small intestine or pancreas. Patients often present with duodenal ulcers or chronic diarrhea. Within the stomach, the most remarkable feature is a doubling of oxyntic mucosal thickness due to a five-fold increase in the number of parietal cells. Gastrin also induces hyperplasia of mucous neck cells, mucin hyperproduction, and proliferation of endocrine cells within oxyntic mucosa. In some cases these endocrine cells can form small dysplastic nodules or, rarely, true carcinoid tumors.

Treatment of individuals with Zollinger-Ellison syndrome includes blockade of acid hypersecretion. This can be accomplished in almost all patients with proton pump inhibitors. Acid suppression allows peptic ulcers to heal and prevents gastric perforation, allowing treatment to focus on the gastrinoma, which becomes the main determinant of long-term survival.

Although they grow slowly, 60% to 90% of gastrinomas are malignant. Tumors are sporadic in 75% of patients. These tend to be solitary and can be surgically resected. The remaining 25% of patients with gastrinomas have multiple endocrine neoplasia type I (MEN I). These individuals often have multiple tumors or metastatic disease and may benefit from treatment with somatostatin analogues. Detection of tumors may be enhanced by using somatostatin receptor scintigraphy or endoscopic ultrasonography.

Gastric Polyps and Tumors

Polyps, nodules or masses that project above the level of the surrounding mucosa, are identified in up to 5% of upper GI endoscopies. Polyps may develop as a result of epithelial or stromal cell hyperplasia, inflammation, ectopia, or neoplasia. Only the most common types of polyps will be discussed here (Peutz-Jeghers and juvenile polyps are discussed with intestinal polyps). This is followed by a presentation of gastric tumors, including adenocarcinomas, lymphomas, carcinoid tumors, and stromal tumors.

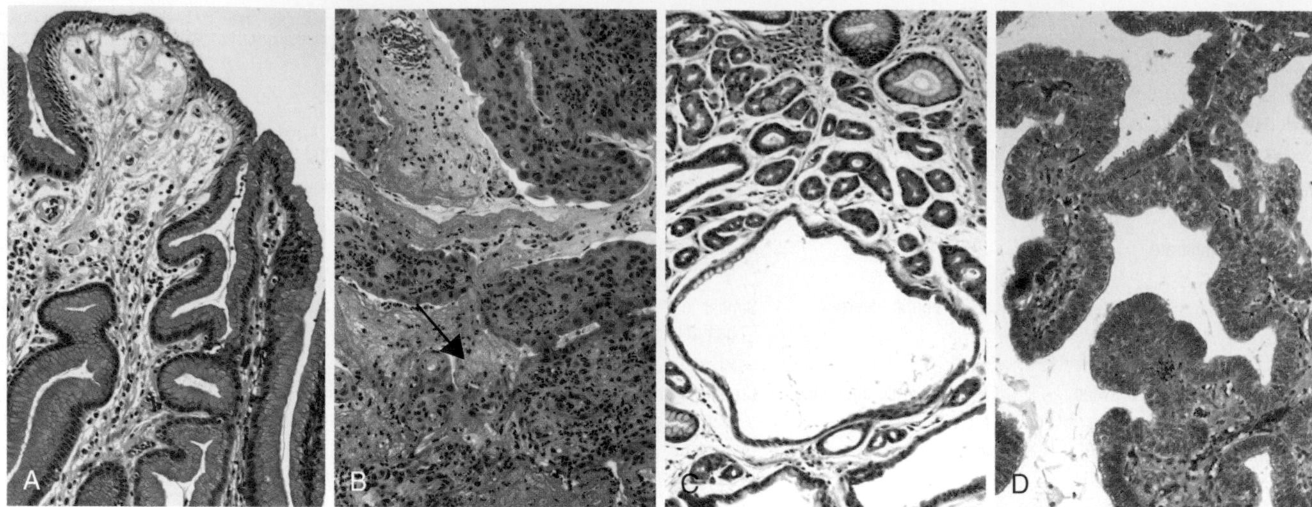

Figure 17-16 Gastric polyps. **A,** Hyperplastic polyp containing corkscrew-shaped foveolar glands. **B,** Hyperplastic polyp with ulceration *(arrow)*. **C,** Fundic gland polyp composed of cystically dilated glands lined by parietal, chief, and foveolar cells. **D,** Gastric adenoma recognized by the presence of epithelial dysplasia.

Inflammatory and Hyperplastic Polyps

Up to 75% of all gastric polyps are inflammatory or hyperplastic polyps. Since chronic inflammation drives the development of such polyps, the incidence depends partly on the regional prevalence of *H. pylori* infection. These polyps are most common in individuals between 50 and 60 years of age, and usually develop in association with chronic gastritis, which initiates the injury that leads to reactive hyperplasia and polyp growth. Among individuals with *H. pylori* gastritis, polyps may regress after bacterial eradication. Because the risk of dysplasia correlates with size, polyps larger than 1.5 cm should be resected and examined histologically.

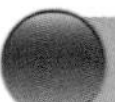

MORPHOLOGY

The majority of inflammatory or hyperplastic polyps are smaller than 1 cm in diameter and are frequently multiple, particularly in individuals with atrophic gastritis. These polyps are ovoid in shape and have a smooth surface, though superficial erosions are common. Microscopically, polyps have irregular, cystically dilated, and elongated foveolar glands (Fig. 17-16*A*). The lamina propria is typically edematous with variable degrees of acute and chronic inflammation, and surface ulceration may be present (Fig. 17-16*B*).

Fundic Gland Polyps

Fundic gland polyps occur sporadically and in individuals with familial adenomatous polyposis (FAP). The prevalence of fundic gland polyps has increased markedly in recent years as a result of increasing use of proton pump inhibitor therapy. These drugs inhibit acid production, which leads to increased gastrin secretion and, in turn, oxyntic gland growth. Fundic gland polyps may be asymptomatic or associated with nausea, vomiting, or epigastric pain.

MORPHOLOGY

Fundic gland polyps occur in the gastric body and fundus and are well-circumscribed lesions with a smooth surface. They may be single or multiple and are composed of cystically dilated, irregular glands lined by flattened parietal and chief cells. Inflammation is typically absent or minimal (Fig. 17-16*C*). Dysplasia and even cancer may occur in FAP-associated fundic gland polyps, but sporadic fundic gland polyps carry no cancer risk.

Gastric Adenoma

Gastric adenomas represent up to 10% of all gastric polyps (Table 17-5). Their frequency increases progressively with age, and there is a marked variation in prevalence among different populations that parallels the incidence of gastric adenocarcinoma. Patients are usually between 50 and 60 years of age, and males are affected three times more often than females. Like fundic gland polyps, the incidence of adenomas is increased in individuals with FAP. *Similar to other forms of gastric dysplasia, adenomas almost always occur on a background of chronic gastritis with atrophy and intestinal metaplasia.* The risk of adenocarcinoma in gastric adenomas is related to the size of the lesion and is particularly increased in lesions greater than 2 cm in diameter. Overall, carcinoma may be present in up to 30% of gastric adenomas.

MORPHOLOGY

Gastric adenomas are usually solitary lesions less than 2 cm in diameter, most commonly located in the antrum. The majority of adenomas are composed of intestinal-type columnar epithelium that exhibits varying degrees of dysplasia (Fig. 17-16*D*). Dysplasia can be classified as low or high grade, and both grades may include enlargement, elongation, pseudostratification, and hyperchromasia of epithelial cell nuclei, and epithelial crowding. High-grade dysplasia is characterized by more severe cytologic atypia and irregular architecture, including glandular budding and gland-within-gland, or cribriform, structures. Like intestinal adenomas, gastric adenomas are premalignant neoplastic lesions. However, the risk of transformation to invasive cancer is much higher in gastric adenomas.

Gastric Adenocarcinoma

Adenocarcinoma is the most common malignancy of the stomach, comprising more than 90% of all gastric cancers. As discussed in more detail later, gastric adenocarcinoma is often separated morphologically into intestinal type, which tends to form bulky masses, and a diffuse type, which infiltrates the wall diffusely, thickens it, and is typically composed of signet ring cells. Early symptoms of both types of gastric adenocarcinoma resemble those of chronic gastritis and peptic ulcer disease, including dyspepsia, dysphagia, and nausea. As a result, these tumors are often discovered at advanced stages, when symptoms such as weight loss, anorexia, early satiety (primarily in diffuse cancers), anemia, and hemorrhage trigger further diagnostic evaluation.

Epidemiology. Gastric cancer incidence varies markedly with geography. In Japan, Chile, Costa Rica, and Eastern Europe, the incidence is up to 20-fold higher than in North America, northern Europe, Africa, and Southeast Asia. Mass endoscopic screening programs have been successful in regions where the incidence is high, such as Japan, where 35% of newly detected cases are early gastric cancers, limited to the mucosa and submucosa. Unfortunately, mass screening programs are not cost-effective in regions where the incidence is low, and fewer than 20% of cases are detected at an early stage in North America and northern Europe. Metastases are often detected at time of diagnosis. Sites most commonly involved include the supraclavicular sentinel lymph node (Virchow node), periumbilical lymph nodes (Sister Mary Joseph nodule), the left axillary lymph node (Irish node), the ovary (Krukenberg tumor), or the pouch of Douglas (Blumer shelf).

Gastric cancer is more common in lower socioeconomic groups and in individuals with multifocal mucosal atrophy and intestinal metaplasia. *Gastric dysplasia and adenomas are recognizable precursor lesions associated with gastric adenocarcinoma.* PUD does not impart an increased risk of gastric cancer, but patients who have had partial gastrectomies for PUD have a slightly higher risk of developing cancer in the residual gastric stump, possibly due to hypochlorhydria, bile reflux, and chronic gastritis.

In the United States, gastric cancer rates dropped by more than 85% during the twentieth century. Adenocarcinoma of the stomach was the most common cause of cancer death in the United States in 1930 and remains a leading cause of cancer death worldwide, but now accounts for fewer than 2.5% of cancer deaths in the United States. Similar declines have been reported in many other Western countries, suggesting that environmental and dietary factors contribute to the development of gastric cancers. Consistent with this conclusion, studies of migrants from high-risk to low-risk regions have shown that gastric cancer rates in second-generation immigrants are similar to those in their new country of residence.

The cause of the overall reduction in gastric cancer is most closely linked to decreases in H. pylori prevalence. Another possible contributor is the decreased consumption of dietary carcinogens, such as N-nitroso compounds and benzo[*a*]pyrene, because of the reduced use of salt and smoking for food preservation and the widespread availability of food refrigeration.

Although overall incidence of gastric adenocarcinoma is falling, cancer of the gastric cardia is on the rise. This is probably related to Barrett esophagus and may reflect the increasing incidence of chronic GERD and obesity. Consistent with this presumed common pathogenesis, distal esophageal adenocarcinomas and gastric cardia adenocarcinomas are similar in morphology, clinical behavior, and therapeutic response.

Pathogenesis. While the majority of gastric cancers are not hereditary, the mutations identified in familial gastric cancer have provided important insights into mechanisms of carcinogenesis in sporadic cases. Familial gastric cancer is strongly associated with germline loss-of-function mutations in the tumor suppressor gene *CDH1*, which encodes the cell adhesion protein E-cadherin (discussed in Chapter 7). Loss-of-function mutations in *CDH1* are also present in about 50% of sporadic diffuse gastric tumors, while E-cadherin expression is drastically decreased in the rest, often by hyper methylation and silencing of the *CDH1* promoter. *Thus, the loss of E-cadherin is a key step in the development of diffuse gastric cancer. CDH1* mutations are also common in sporadic and familial lobular carcinoma of the breast, which, like diffuse gastric cancer (see later), tends to infiltrate as single cells, and individuals with *BRCA2* mutations are at increased risk of developing diffuse gastric cancer. Mutation of *TP53* is also found in the majority of sporadic gastric cancers of both diffuse and intestinal types.

In contrast to diffuse gastric cancers, sporadic intestinal-type gastric cancers are strongly associated with mutations that result in increased signaling via the Wnt pathway. These include loss-of-function mutations in the adenomatous polyposis coli (APC) tumor suppressor gene and gain-of-function mutations in the gene encoding β-catenin. Loss-of-function mutations or silencing of a number of other tumor suppressor genes have also been identified, including those involved in TGFβ signaling (TGFβRII), regulation of apoptosis (BAX), and cell cycle control (CDKN2A), all of which are discussed in more detail in Chapter 7. As expected, FAP patients, who carry germline *APC* mutations, have an increased risk of intestinal-type gastric cancer. This is particularly true in Japan and other high-risk areas, as compared to individuals with FAP residing in areas of low gastric cancer incidence. Thus, both host genetic background and environmental factors affect risk. As discussed in the context of *H. pylori* gastritis, genetic variants of proinflammatory and immune response genes, including those that encode IL-1β, TNF, IL-10, IL-8, and Toll-like receptor 4 (TLR4), are associated with elevated risk of gastric cancer when accompanied by *H. pylori* infection. Thus, it is clear that chronic inflammation promotes gastric neoplasia. Other associations between chronic inflammation and cancer are discussed in Chapter 7.

MORPHOLOGY

Gastric adenocarcinomas are classified according to their location and gross and histologic morphology. Most gastric adenocarcinomas involve the gastric antrum; the lesser curvature is involved more often than the greater curvature. **Gastric tumors with an intestinal morphology,** which tend to form bulky tumors (Fig. 17-17*A*), are composed of glandular structures (Fig. 17-18*A*), while cancers with a **diffuse infiltrative growth pattern** (Fig. 17-17*B*) are more often composed of signet-ring cells (Fig. 17-18*B*). Although intestinal-type adenocarcinomas may penetrate the gastric wall, they more frequently grow along broad cohesive fronts to form either an exophytic mass or an ulcerated tumor. The neoplastic cells often contain apical mucin vacuoles, and abundant mucin may be present in gland lumina. In contrast, diffuse gastric cancer is generally composed of discohesive cells, likely as a result of E-cadherin loss. These cells do not form glands but instead have large mucin vacuoles that expand the cytoplasm and push the nucleus to the periphery, creating a signet-ring cell morphology. They permeate the mucosa and stomach wall individually or in small clusters, and may be mistaken for inflammatory cells, such as macrophages, at low magnification. Release of extracellular mucin in either type of gastric cancer can result in formation of large mucin lakes that dissect tissue planes.

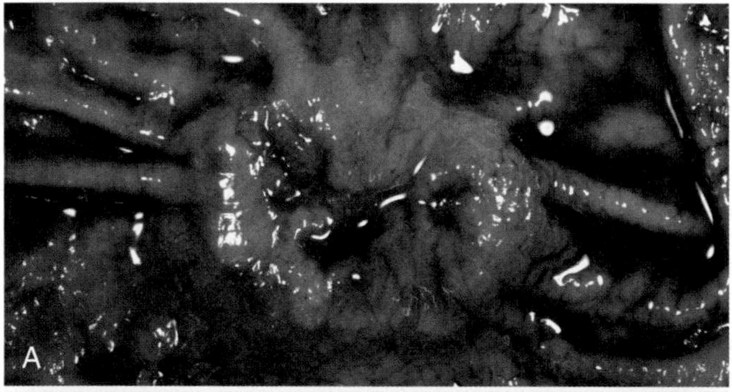

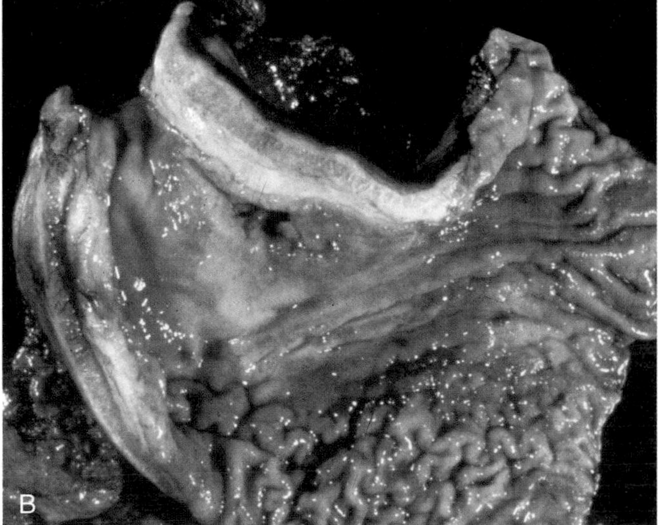

Figure 17-17 Gastric adenocarcinoma. **A,** Intestinal-type adenocarcinoma consisting of an elevated mass with heaped-up borders and central ulceration. Compare to the peptic ulcer in Figure 17-14*A*. **B,** Linitis plastica. The gastric wall is markedly thickened and rugal folds are partially lost.

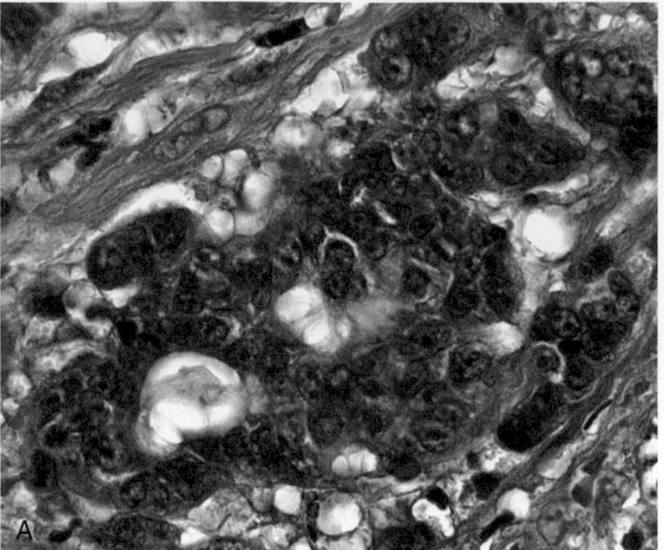

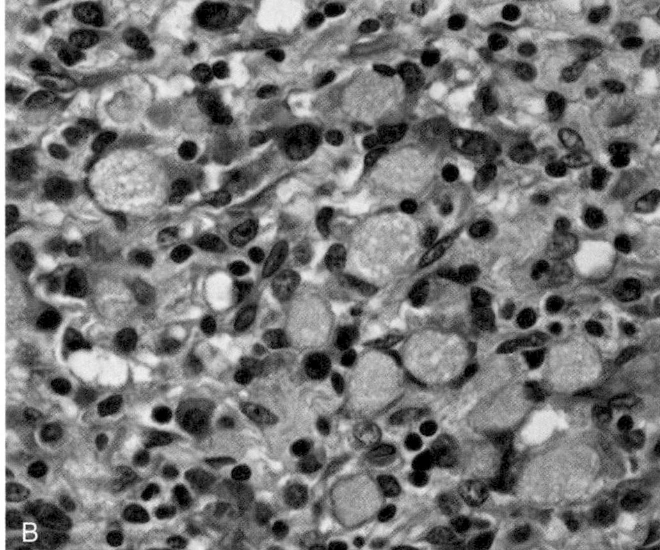

Figure 17-18 Gastric adenocarcinoma. **A,** Intestinal-type adenocarcinoma composed of columnar, gland-forming cells infiltrating through desmoplastic stroma. **B,** Signet-ring cells can be recognized by their large cytoplasmic mucin vacuoles and peripherally displaced, crescent-shaped nuclei.

A mass may be difficult to appreciate in diffuse gastric cancer, but these infiltrative tumors often evoke a **desmoplastic** reaction that stiffens the gastric wall and may provide a valuable diagnostic clue. When there are large areas of infiltration, diffuse rugal flattening and a rigid, thickened wall may impart a **leather bottle** appearance termed **linitis plastica** (Fig. 17-17*B*).

Clinical Features. **Intestinal-type gastric cancer predominates in high-risk areas and develops from precursor lesions, including flat dysplasia and adenomas.** The mean age of presentation is 55 years, and the male-to-female ratio is 2:1. In contrast, the incidence of diffuse gastric cancer is relatively uniform across countries, there are no identified precursor lesions, and the disease occurs at similar frequencies in males and females. Notably, the remarkable decrease in gastric cancer incidence applies only to the intestinal type, which is most closely associated with atrophic gastritis and intestinal metaplasia. As a result, the incidence of diffuse type gastric cancer, which was previously low, is now similar to intestinal type gastric cancer.

The depth of invasion and the extent of nodal and distant metastases at the time of diagnosis remain the most powerful prognostic indicators in gastric cancer. Local invasion into the duodenum, pancreas, and retroperitoneum is common. In such cases efforts are usually focused on chemotherapy or radiation therapy and palliative care. However, when possible, surgical resection remains the preferred treatment for gastric adenocarcinoma. With surgical resection, the 5-year survival rate of early gastric cancer can exceed 90%, even if lymph node metastases are present. In contrast, the 5-year survival rate for advanced gastric cancer remains less than 20%. Because of the advanced stage at which most gastric cancers are discovered in the United States, the overall 5-year survival is less than 30%.

Lymphoma

Although extranodal lymphomas can arise in virtually any tissue, they do so most commonly in the GI tract, particularly the stomach. In allogeneic hematopoietic stem cell and organ transplant recipients, the bowel is also the most frequent site for Epstein-Barr virus-positive B-cell lymphoproliferations. This preferential location is most likely because the deficits in T-cell function caused by oral immunosuppressive agents (e.g., cyclosporine) are greatest at intestinal sites of drug absorption. Nearly 5% of all gastric malignancies are primary lymphomas, the most common of which are indolent extranodal marginal zone B-cell lymphomas. *In the gut these tumors are often referred to as lymphomas of mucosa-associated lymphoid tissue (MALT), or MALTomas.* This and other lymphomas of the gut are discussed in Chapter 13.

Pathogenesis. Extranodal marginal zone B-cell lymphomas usually arise at sites of chronic inflammation. They can originate in the GI tract at sites of preexisting MALT, such as the Peyer patches of the small intestine, but more commonly arise within tissues that are normally devoid of organized lymphoid tissue. *In the stomach, MALT is induced, typically as a result of chronic gastritis. H. pylori* infection is the most common inducer in the stomach and, therefore, is found in association with most cases of gastric MALToma. Remarkably, *H. pylori* eradication results in durable remissions with low rates of recurrence in most MALToma patients.

Three translocations are associated with gastric MALToma, the t(11;18)(q21;q21) and the less common t(1;14)(p22;q32) and t(14;18)(q32;q21). The t(11;18)(q21;q21) translocation brings together the apoptosis inhibitor 2 *(API2)* gene on chromosome 11 with the "mutated in MALT lymphoma," or *MLT*, gene on chromosome 18. This creates a chimeric *API2-MLT* fusion gene that encodes an API2-MLT fusion protein. The t(14;18)(q32;q21) and t(1;14)(p22;q32) translocations cause increased expression of intact MALT1 and BCL-10 proteins, respectively.

Each of the three translocations has the same net effect, the constitutive activation of NF-κB, a transcription factor that promotes B-cell growth and survival. Antigen-dependent activation of NF-κB in normal B and T cells requires both BCL-10 and MLT, which work together in a pathway downstream of the B- and T-cell antigen receptors. Thus, *H. pylori*–induced inflammation may trigger NF-κB activation through the MLT/BCL-10 pathway in MALTomas that lack these translocations. Removal of this stimulus may explain why these tumors tend to respond to *H. pylori* eradication. In contrast, NF-κB is constitutively active in tumors bearing translocations involving *MLT* or *BCL10*, and *H. pylori* treatment is ineffective. Other tumor characteristics, including invasion to the muscularis propria or beyond and lymph node involvement, also correlate with failure of *H. pylori* eradication to induce remission.

As with other low-grade lymphomas, MALTomas can transform into more aggressive tumors that are histologically identical to diffuse large B-cell lymphomas. This is often associated with additional genetic changes, such as inactivation of the tumor suppressor genes that encode p53 and p16. As one might guess, MALTomas that have undergone such transformation are not responsive to *H. pylori* eradication.

MORPHOLOGY

Histologically, gastric MALToma takes the form of a dense lymphocytic infiltrate in the lamina propria (Fig. 17-19*A*). Characteristically, the neoplastic lymphocytes infiltrate the gastric glands focally to create **diagnostic lymphoepithelial lesions** (Fig. 17-19*A*, inset). Reactive-appearing B-cell follicles may be present, and, in about 40% of tumors, plasmacytic differentiation is observed. At other sites GI lymphomas may disseminate as discrete small nodules (Fig. 17-19*B*) or infiltrate the wall diffusely (Fig. 17-19*C*).

Like other tumors of mature B cells, MALTomas express the B-cell markers CD19 and CD20. They do not express CD5 or CD10, but are positive for CD43 in about 25% of cases, an unusual feature that can be diagnostically helpful. In cases lacking lymphoepithelial lesions, monoclonality may be demonstrated by restricted expression of either κ or λ immunoglobulin light chains or by molecular detection of clonal IgH rearrangements. Molecular analysis is being used increasingly to identify tumors with translocations that predict resistance to therapy.

Clinical Features. The most common presenting symptoms are dyspepsia and epigastric pain. Hematemesis, melena, and constitutional symptoms such as weight loss can also be present. Because gastric MALTomas and *H. pylori* gastritis often coexist and have overlapping clinical symptoms and endoscopic appearances, diagnostic difficulties may arise, particularly in small biopsy specimens.

Carcinoid Tumor

Carcinoid tumors arise from the diffuse components of the endocrine system and are now properly referred to as *well-differentiated neuroendocrine tumors.* The term carcinoid, or "carcinoma-like," was applied because these tumors tend to have a more indolent clinical course than GI carcinomas. Most are found in the GI tract, and more than 40% occur in the small intestine (Table 17-6). The tracheobronchial tree and lungs are the next most

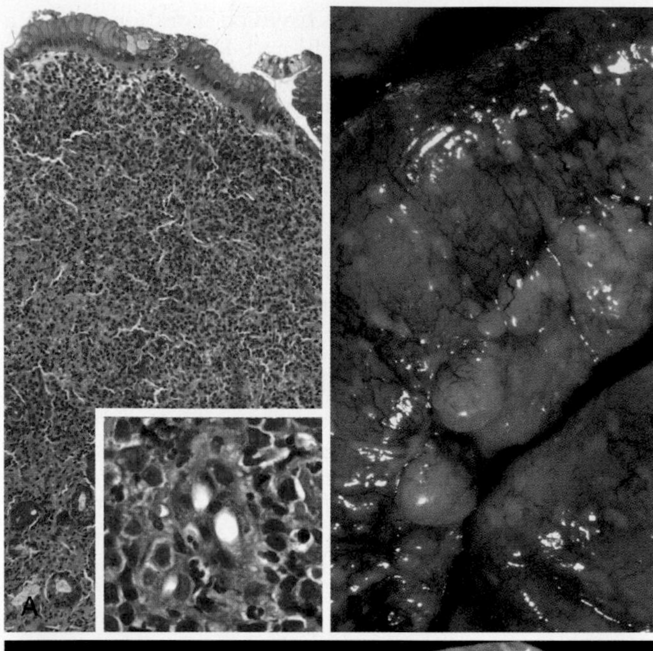

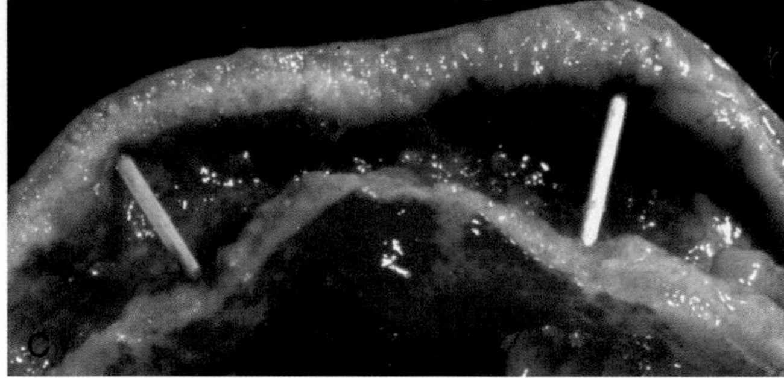

Figure 17-19 Lymphoma. **A,** Gastric MALT lymphoma replacing much of the gastric epithelium. Inset shows lymphoepithelial lesions with neoplastic lymphocytes surrounding and infiltrating gastric glands. **B,** Disseminated lymphoma within the small intestine with numerous small serosal nodules. **C,** Large B-cell lymphoma infiltrating the small intestinal wall and producing diffuse thickening.

commonly involved sites. Gastric carcinoid tumors may be associated with endocrine cell hyperplasia, autoimmune chronic atrophic gastritis, MEN-I, and Zollinger-Ellison syndrome. In addition to autoimmune chronic atrophic gastritis, as already discussed, gastric endocrine cell hyperplasia has been linked to proton pump inhibitor therapy, but the risk of progression to a neuroendocrine neoplasm in this circumstance is extremely low.

MORPHOLOGY

Grossly, carcinoids are intramural or submucosal masses that create small polypoid lesions (Fig. 17-20*A*). In the stomach they typically arise within oxyntic mucosa. At all GI sites, the overlying mucosa may be intact or ulcerated, and in the intestines the tumors may invade deeply to involve the mesentery. Carcinoids tend to be yellow or tan in color and are very firm as a consequence of an intense desmoplastic reaction, which may cause kinking and obstruction of the bowel. Histologically, carcinoids are composed of islands, trabeculae, strands, glands, or sheets of uniform cells with scant, pink granular cytoplasm and a round to oval stippled nucleus (Fig. 17-20). In most tumors there is minimal pleomorphism, but anaplasia, mitotic activity, and necrosis may be present in rare cases. Immunohistochemical stains are typically positive for endocrine granule markers, such as synaptophysin and chromogranin A.

Clinical Features. The peak incidence of carcinoid tumors is in the sixth decade, but they may appear at any age. Symptoms are determined by the hormones produced. For example, *tumors that produce gastrin may cause Zollinger-Ellison syndrome, while ileal tumors may cause carcinoid syndrome,* which is characterized by cutaneous flushing, sweating, bronchospasm, colicky abdominal pain, diarrhea, and right-sided cardiac valvular fibrosis. Carcinoid syndrome occurs in fewer than 10% of patients and is caused by vasoactive substances secreted by the tumor into the systemic circulation. When tumors are confined to the

Table 17-6 Features of Gastrointestinal Carcinoid Tumors

Feature	Esophagus	Stomach	Proximal Duodenum	Jejunum and Ileum	Appendix	Colorectum
Fraction of GI carcinoids	<1%	<10%	<10%	>40%	<25%	<25%
Mean patient age (yr)	Rare	55	50	65	All ages	60
Location	Distal	Body and fundus	Proximal third, peri-ampullary	Throughout	Tip	Rectum > cecum
Size	Limited data	1-2 cm, multiple; >2 cm, solitary	0.5-2 cm	<3.5 cm	0.2-1 cm	>5 cm (cecum); <1 cm (rectum)
Secretory product(s)	Limited data	Histamine, somatostatin, serotonin	Gastrin, somatostatin, cholecystokinin	Serotonin, substance P, polypeptide YY	Serotonin, polypeptide YY	Serotonin, polypeptide YY
Symptoms	Dysphagia, weight loss, reflux	Gastritis, ulcer, incidental	Peptic ulcer, biliary obstruction, abdominal pain	Asymptomatic, obstruction, metastatic disease	Asymptomatic, incidental	Abdominal pain, weight loss, incidental
Behavior	Limited data	Variable	Variable	Aggressive	Benign	Variable
Disease associations	None	Atrophic gastritis, MEN-I	Zollinger-Ellison syndrome, NF-1, sporadic	None	None	None

MEN-I, Multiple endocrine neoplasia type I; NF-1, neurofibromatosis type I.

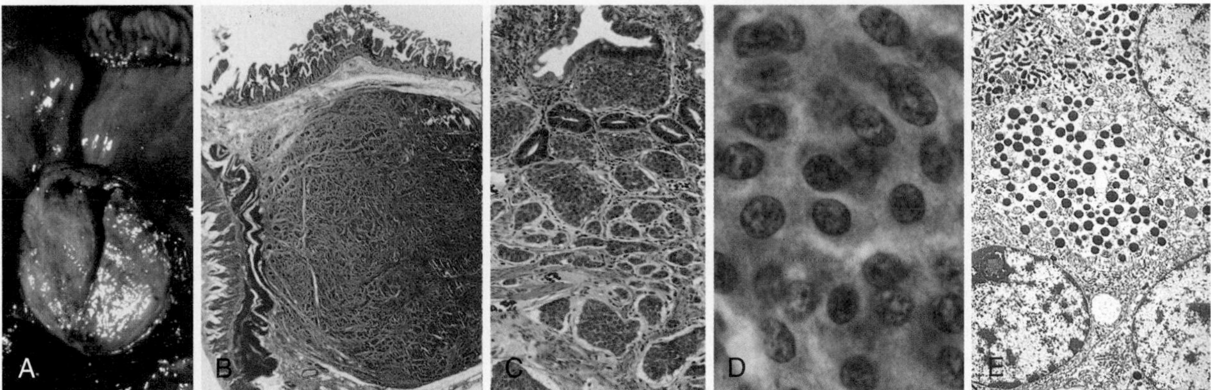

Figure 17-20 GI carcinoid tumor (neuroendocrine carcinoma). **A,** Gross cross-section of a submucosal tumor nodule. **B,** Microscopically the nodule is composed of tumor cells embedded in dense fibrous tissue. **C,** In other areas, the tumor has spread extensively within mucosal lymphatic channels. **D,** High magnification shows the bland cytology of carcinoid tumors. The chromatin texture, with fine and coarse clumps, is frequently described as a "salt and pepper" pattern. Despite their innocuous appearance, carcinoids can be clinically aggressive. **E,** Electron microscopy reveals cytoplasmic dense core neurosecretory granules.

intestine, the vasoactive substances released are metabolized to inactive forms by the liver, a "first-pass" effect similar to that exerted on oral drugs. This can be overcome by a large tumor burden or, more commonly, when tumors secrete hormones into a nonportal venous circulation. The carcinoid syndrome is therefore strongly associated with metastatic disease in the liver since the bioactive products can be released directly into systemic circulation.

The most important prognostic factor for GI carcinoid tumors is location.

- *Foregut carcinoid tumors*, those found within the stomach, duodenum proximal to the ligament of Treitz, and esophagus, rarely metastasize and are generally cured by resection. This is particularly true for gastric carcinoid tumors that arise in association with atrophic gastritis, while gastric carcinoid tumors without predisposing factors are often more aggressive.
- *Midgut carcinoid tumors* that arise in the jejunum and ileum are often multiple and tend to be aggressive. In these tumors, greater depth of local invasion, increased size, and the presence of necrosis and mitoses are associated with a worse outcome.
- *Hindgut carcinoids* arising in the appendix and colorectum are typically discovered incidentally. Those in the appendix occur at any age and are generally located at the tip. These tumors are rarely more than 2 cm in diameter and are almost always benign. Rectal carcinoid tumors tend to produce polypeptide hormones and, when symptomatic, present with abdominal pain and weight loss. Because they are usually discovered when small, metastasis of rectal carcinoid tumors is uncommon.

Gastrointestinal Stromal Tumor

A wide variety of mesenchymal neoplasms may arise in the stomach. Many are named according to the cell type they most resemble; for example, smooth muscle tumors are called *leiomyomas* or *leiomyosarcomas,* nerve sheath tumors are termed *schwannomas,* and those resembling glomus bodies in the nail beds and at other sites are termed *glomus tumors.* These are all rare and are discussed in greater detail in Chapter 26. ***GI stromal tumor (GIST)* is the most common mesenchymal tumor of the abdomen,** with annual incidences between 11 and 20 per million people. More than half of these tumors occur in the stomach. The term stromal reflects historical confusion about the origin of this tumor, which is now recognized to arise from the interstitial cells of Cajal, or pacemaker cells, of the gastrointestinal muscularis propria.

Epidemiology. Clinically silent, microscopic proliferations that may represent precursors to GIST are present in 10% to 30% of resected stomachs. These have a low mitotic index and lack pleomorphism and other features suggesting malignancy. The risk of of these benign proliferations becoming a GIST is estimated to be 1 in 2000.

The peak age at which clinically evident GISTs are recognized is approximately 60 years, with fewer than 10% occurring in individuals younger than 40 years of age. Of the uncommon GISTs in children, some are related to the *Carney triad*, a nonhereditary syndrome of unknown etiology seen primarily in young females that includes gastric GIST, paraganglioma, and pulmonary chondroma. There is also an increased incidence of GIST in individuals with neurofibromatosis type 1.

Pathogenesis. **Approximately 75% to 80% of all GISTs have oncogenic, gain-of-function mutations in the receptor tyrosine kinase KIT.** Approximately 8% of GISTs have mutations that activate a closely related receptor tyrosine kinase, platelet-derived growth factor receptor α (PDGFRA). For unknown reasons, GISTs bearing PDGFRA mutations are overrepresented in the stomach. *KIT* and *PDGFRA* gene mutations are mutually exclusive, reflecting their activities within the same signal transduction pathway. Germline mutations in these same genes are present in rare familial GISTs, in which patients develop multiple GISTs and may also have diffuse hyperplasia of Cajal cells. Both sporadic and germline mutations result in constitutively active KIT or PDGFRA receptor tyrosine kinases and produce intracellular signals that promote tumor cell proliferation and survival (Chapter 7). Some GISTs without mutated *KIT* or *PDGFRA* have mutations in other genes that function in these pathways (*NF1, BRAF, HRAS,* or *NRAS*). However, more common are mutations in genes encoding components of the mitochondrial succinate dehydrogenase complex (*SDHA, SDHB, SDHC, SDHD*). These mutations, which cause loss of SDH function, are often inherited in the germline and confer an increased risk for GIST and paraganglioma (*Carney-Stratakis syndrome*, not to be confused with Carney triad); with the second copy of the affected gene being either mutated or lost in the tumor. The mechanisms by which SDH mutations lead to GIST are unclear; one hypothesis is that the accumulation of succinate leads to dysregulation of hypoxia inducible factor-1α (HIF-1α), which results in increased transcription of the vascular endothelial growth factor (*VEGF*) and insulin-like growth factor-1 (*IGF1R*) genes.

Mutation of KIT or PDGFRA is an early event in sporadic GISTs and is detectable in lesions as small as 3 mm. Therefore, *KIT* or *PDGFRA* mutations alone are insufficient for tumorigenesis. Changes associated with progression to overt GIST are not well-defined, but loss or partial deletion of chromosomes 14 and 22 is common and losses and gains at other chromosomes also occur. In particular, deletion of 9p results in loss of the cell cycle regulator *CDKN2A*, a tumor suppressor that is involved in many cancers. In addition to potentially being related to progression, increased numbers of chromosomal alterations correlate with poor prognosis.

MORPHOLOGY

Primary gastric GISTs can be quite large, as much as 30 cm in diameter. They usually form a solitary, well-circumscribed, fleshy mass (Fig. 17-21*A*) covered by ulcerated or intact mucosa (Fig. 17-21*B*), but can also project outward toward the serosa. The cut surface shows a whorled appearance. Metastases may take the form of multiple serosal nodules throughout the peritoneal cavity or as one or more nodules in the liver; spread outside of the abdomen is uncommon, but can occur. GISTs composed of thin elongated cells are classified as **spindle cell type** (Fig. 17-21*C*), whereas tumors dominated by epithelial-appearing cells are termed **epithelioid type**; mixtures of the two patterns also occur. The most useful diagnostic marker is KIT, which is detectable in Cajal cells and 95% of gastric GISTs by immunohistochemical stains.

Clinical Features. Symptoms of GISTs at presentation may be related to mass effects. Mucosal ulceration can cause blood loss, and approximately half of individuals with GIST present with anemia or related symptoms. GISTs may also be discovered as an incidental finding during radiologic imaging, endoscopy, or abdominal surgery performed for other reasons. Complete surgical resection is the primary treatment for localized gastric GIST. The prognosis correlates with tumor size, mitotic index, and location, with gastric GISTs being less aggressive than those arising in the small intestine. Recurrence or metastasis is rare for gastric GISTs smaller than 5 cm but common for mitotically active tumors larger than 10 cm. Many tumors fall into an intermediate category where the malignant potential of the lesion cannot be predicted with certainty on the basis of histology alone.

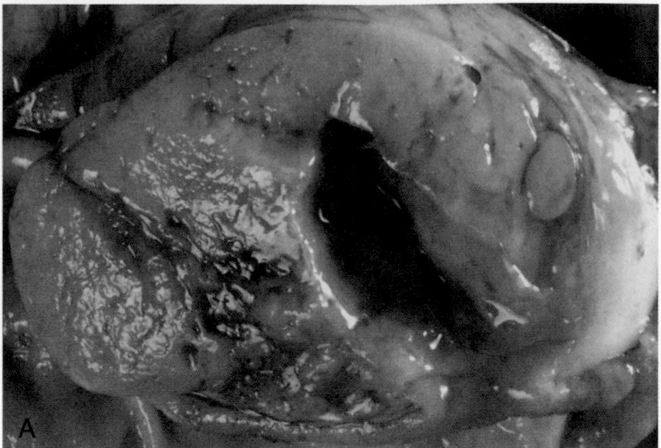

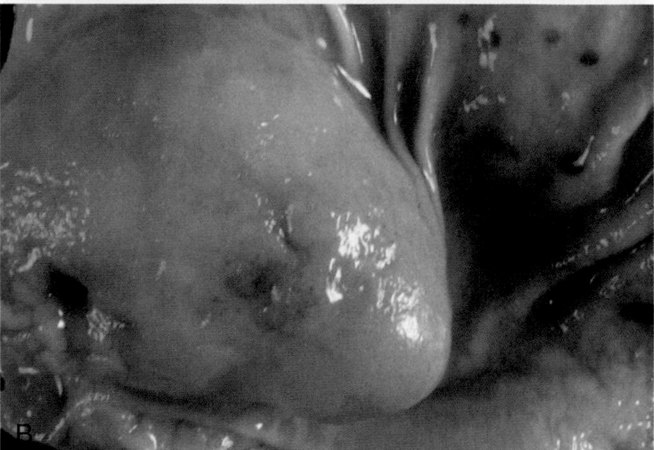

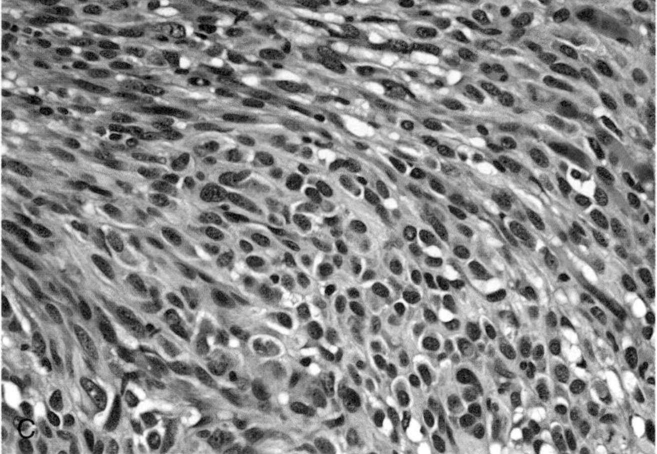

Figure 17-21 GI stromal tumor. **A,** On cross-section a whorled texture is evident within the white, fleshy tumor. **B,** The mass is covered by intact mucosa. **C,** Histologically the tumor is primarily composed of bundles, or fascicles, of spindle-shaped tumor cells. (Courtesy Dr. Christopher Weber, The University of Chicago, Chicago, Ill.)

The molecular phenotype is an important consideration in the treatment of patients with unresectable, recurrent, or metastatic GISTs. Those with mutations in *KIT* or *PDGFRA* often respond to the tyrosine kinase inhibitor imatinib. In contrast, tumors without these mutations are generally resistant. Further, specific *KIT* or *PDGFRA* mutations are associated with different drug sensitivities. In treated patients, development of imatinib-resistance is common.

This is due to secondary *KIT* or *PDGFRA* mutations. Tumors with secondary mutations may respond to other tyrosine kinase inhibitors as well as experimental therapies that target other pathways.

KEY CONCEPTS

Neoplastic and Non neoplastic proliferations of the stomach

- **Ménétrier disease** is a rare disorder caused by excessive secretion of transforming growth factor α (TGF-α) and characterized by diffuse foveolar hyperplasia and protein-losing enteropathy.
- **Zollinger-Ellison syndrome** is caused by gastrin-secreting tumors that cause parietal cell hyperplasia and acid hyper secretion; 60% to 90% of gastrinomas are malignant.
- The majority of gastric polyps are **inflammatory or hyperplastic polyps,** reactive lesions that are associated with chronic gastritis.
- **Fundic gland polyps** occur sporadically, most often as a consequence of proton pump inhibitor therapy, and in familial adenomatous polyposis (FAP) patients.
- **Gastric adenomas** develop in a background of chronic gastritis and are particularly associated with intestinal metaplasia and mucosal (glandular) atrophy. Adenocarcinoma is frequent in gastric adenomas, which therefore require more aggressive therapy than adenomas of the colon.
- **Gastric adenocarcinoma** incidence varies markedly with geography. Individual tumors are classified according to location, gross, and histologic morphology. Gastric tumors with an **intestinal histology tend to form bulky tumors** and may be ulcerated, while those composed of **signet-ring cells typically display a diffuse infiltrative growth pattern** that may thicken the gastric wall without forming a discrete mass. Gastric adenocarcinomas are linked to *H. pylori* induced chronic gastritis.
- **Primary gastric lymphomas** are most often derived from mucosa-associated lymphoid tissue (MALT), whose development is induced by chronic gastritis that is most often induced by *H. pylori*.
- **Carcinoid tumors** (well-differentiated neuroendocrine tumors) arise from diffuse components of the endocrine system and are most common in the GI tract, particularly the small intestine. Prognosis is based on location; tumors of the small intestine tend to be most aggressive, while those of the appendix are typically benign.
- **Gastrointestinal stromal tumor (GIST)** is the most common mesenchymal tumor of the abdomen, occurs most often in the stomach, and is related to benign pacemaker cells, or interstitial cells of Cajal. Tumors generally have activating mutations in either KIT or PDGFRA tyrosine kinases and respond to specific kinase inhibitors.

SMALL INTESTINE AND COLON

The small intestine and colon make up the majority of the GI tract and are the sites of a broad array of diseases. Some of these relate to nutrient and water transport. Perturbation of these processes can cause malabsorption and diarrhea. The intestines are also the principal site where the immune system interfaces with a diverse array of antigens present in food and gut microbes. Indeed, intestinal bacteria outnumber eukaryotic cells in our bodies by tenfold. Thus, it is not surprising that the small intestine and colon are frequently affected by infectious and inflammatory disorders. Finally, the colon is the most common site of GI neoplasia in Western populations.

Intestinal Obstruction

Obstruction of the GI tract may occur at any level, but the small intestine is most often involved because of its relatively narrow lumen. Collectively, *hernias, intestinal adhesions, intussusception, and volvulus* account for 80% of mechanical obstructions (Fig. 17-22), while tumors, infarction, and other causes of strictures, for example, Crohn disease, account for an additional 10% to 15%. **The clinical manifestations of intestinal obstruction include abdominal pain and distention, vomiting, and constipation.** Surgical intervention is usually required in cases where the obstruction has a mechanical basis or is associated with bowel infarction.

Hernias

Any weakness or defect in the abdominal wall may permit protrusion of a serosa-lined pouch of peritoneum called a hernia sac. Acquired hernias typically occur anteriorly, via the inguinal and femoral canals, umbilicus, or at sites of surgical scars, and are common, occurring in up to 5% of the population. *Hernias are the most frequent cause of intestinal obstruction worldwide* and the third most common cause of obstruction in the U.S. Obstruction usually occurs because of visceral protrusion (external herniation) and is most frequently-associated with inguinal hernias, which tend to have narrow orifices and large sacs. Small bowel loops are typically involved, but omentum or large bowel may also protrude, and any of these may become entrapped. Pressure at the neck of the pouch may impair venous drainage of the entrapped viscus. The resultant stasis and edema increase the bulk of the herniated loop, leading to permanent entrapment (incarceration) and, over time, arterial and venous compromise (strangulation), and infarction (Fig. 17-23*A*).

Adhesions

Surgical procedures, infection, or other causes of peritoneal inflammation, such as endometriosis, may result in development of adhesions between bowel segments, the abdominal wall, or operative sites. These fibrous bridges can

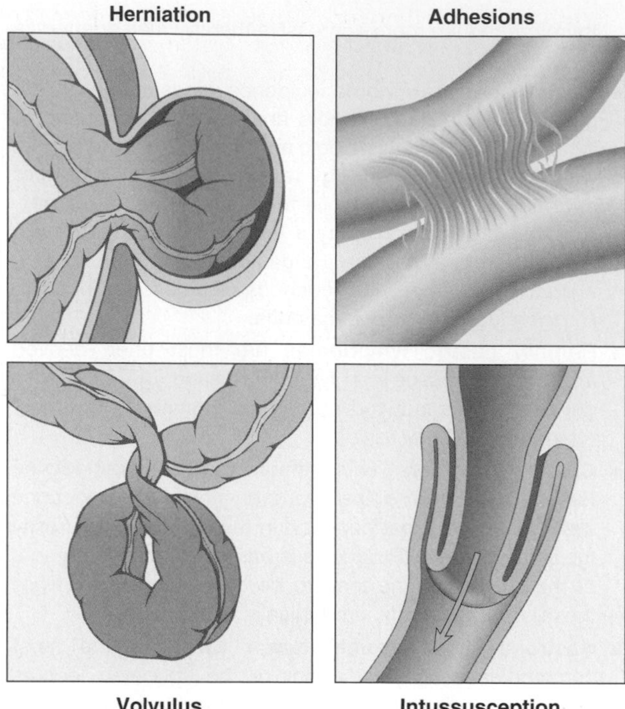

Figure 17-22 Intestinal obstruction. The four major causes of intestinal obstruction are (1) herniation of a segment in the umbilical or inguinal regions, (2) adhesion between loops of intestine, (3) volvulus, and (4) intussusception.

create closed loops through which other viscera may slide and become entrapped, resulting in internal herniation. Sequelae, including obstruction and strangulation, are much the same as with external hernias; *adhesions are the most common cause of intestinal obstruction in the United States.* Fibrous adhesions are most often acquired, but can be congenital in rare cases. Therefore, internal herniation must be considered even in the absence of a history of peritonitis or surgery.

Volvulus

Twisting of a loop of bowel about its mesenteric point of attachment is termed volvulus; it results in both luminal and vascular compromise. Thus, volvulus presents with features of both obstruction and infarction. It occurs most often in large redundant loops of sigmoid colon, followed in frequency by the cecum, small bowel, stomach, or, rarely, transverse colon. Because it is rare, volvulus can be overlooked clinically.

Intussusception

Intussusception occurs when a segment of the intestine, constricted by a wave of peristalsis, telescopes into the immediately distal segment. Once trapped, the invaginated segment is propelled by peristalsis and pulls the mesentery along. Untreated intussusception may progress to intestinal obstruction, compression of mesenteric vessels, and infarction.

Intussusception is the most common cause of intestinal obstruction in children younger than 2 years of age. In these idiopathic cases there is usually no underlying anatomic defect and the patient is otherwise healthy. Other cases have been associated with viral infection and rotavirus vaccines, perhaps due to reactive hyperplasia of Peyer patches and other mucosa-associated lymphoid tissue which can act as the leading edge of the intussusception. Intussusception is rare in older children and adults, and is generally caused by an intraluminal mass or tumor that serves as the initiating point of traction (Fig. 17-23*B*). Contrast enemas can be used both diagnostically and therapeutically for idiopathic intussusception in infants and young children, in whom air enemas may also effectively reduce the intussusception. However, surgical intervention is necessary when a mass is present, as is generally the case in older children and adults.

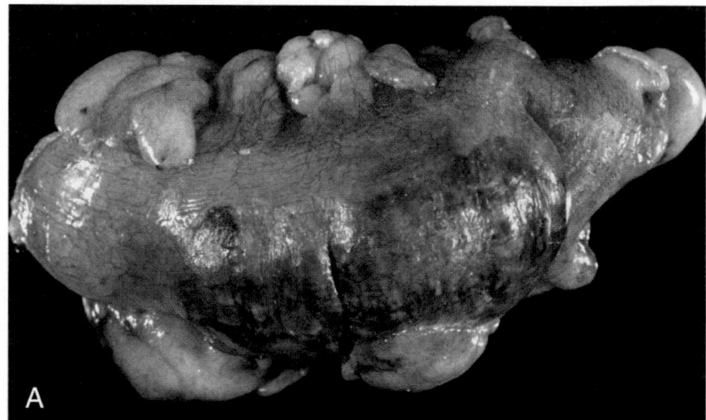

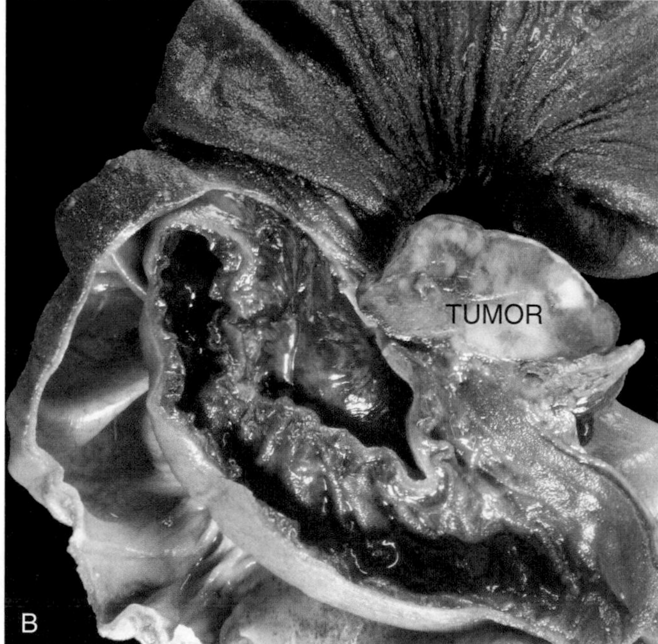

Figure 17-23 Intestinal obstruction. **A,** Portion of bowel incarcerated within an inguinal hernia. Note dusky serosa and hemorrhage that indicate ischemic damage. **B,** Intussusception caused by a tumor. The outermost layer of intestine with external serosa has been removed, leaving the mucosa of the second layer exposed. The serosa of the second layer is apposed to the serosa of the intussuscepted intestine. A tumor mass (right, labeled tumor) is present at the leading edge of the intussusception. Compare to Figure 17-22. (**B,** Courtesy Dr. Christopher Weber, The University of Chicago, Chicago, Ill.)

Ischemic Bowel Disease

The majority of the GI tract is supplied by the celiac, superior mesenteric, and inferior mesenteric arteries. As they approach the intestinal wall the superior and inferior mesenteric arteries ramify into the mesenteric arcades. Interconnections between arcades, as well as collateral supplies from the proximal celiac and distal pudendal and iliac circulations, make it possible for the small intestine and colon to tolerate slowly progressive loss of blood supply from one artery.

In contrast to chronic, progressive hypoperfusion, acute compromise of any major vessel can lead to infarction of several meters of intestine. Damage can range from mucosal infarction, extending no deeper than the muscularis mucosae, to mural infarction of mucosa and submucosa; to transmural infarction involving all three wall layers. While mucosal or mural infarctions can follow acute or chronic hypoperfusion, transmural infarction is typically caused by acute vascular obstruction. Important causes of acute arterial obstruction include severe atherosclerosis (which is often prominent at the origin of mesenteric vessels), aortic aneurysm, hypercoagulable states, oral contraceptive use, and embolization of cardiac vegetations or aortic atheromas. Intestinal hypoperfusion can be associated with cardiac failure, shock, dehydration, or use of vasoconstrictive drugs. Systemic vasculitides, such as polyarteritis nodosa, Henoch-Schönlein purpura, or granulomatosis with polyangiitis (Wegener granulomatosis), may also damage intestinal arteries. Mesenteric venous thrombosis, which can also lead to ischemic disease, is uncommon but can result from inherited or acquired hypercoagulable states, invasive neoplasms, cirrhosis, trauma, or abdominal masses that compress the portal drainage.

Pathogenesis. Intestinal responses to ischemia occur in two phases. The initial *hypoxic injury* occurs at the onset of vascular compromise. While some damage occurs during this phase, the epithelial cells lining the intestine are relatively resistant to transient hypoxia. The second phase, *reperfusion injury,* is initiated by restoration of the blood supply and it is at this time that the greatest damage occurs. In severe cases this may trigger multiorgan failure. While the underlying mechanisms of reperfusion injury are incompletely understood, they include leakage of gut lumen bacterial products, e.g. lipopolysaccharide, into the systemic circulation, free radical production, neutrophil infiltration, and release of additional inflammatory mediators (Chapter 2).

The severity of vascular compromise, the time frame during which it develops, and the vessels affected are the major variables in ischemic bowel disease. Two aspects of intestinal vascular anatomy also contribute to the distribution of ischemic damage and are worthy of note:

- Intestinal segments at the end of their respective arterial supplies are particularly susceptible to ischemia. These *watershed zones* include the splenic flexure, where the superior and inferior mesenteric arterial circulations terminate, and, to a lesser extent, the sigmoid colon and rectum where inferior mesenteric, pudendal, and iliac arterial circulations end. Generalized hypotension or hypoxemia can therefore cause localized injury, and ischemic disease should be considered in the differential diagnosis of focal colitis of the splenic flexure or rectosigmoid colon.
- Intestinal capillaries run alongside the glands, from crypt to surface, before making a hairpin turn to empty into the post-capillary venules. This arrangement makes the surface epithelium particularly vulnerable to ischemic injury, relative to the crypts. Organization of the blood supply in this patterns has advantages, as it protects the epithelial stem cells, which are located within the crypts and are necessary for recovery from epithelial injury. This pattern of surface epithelial atrophy, or even necrosis and sloughing, with normal or hyperproliferative crypts is a morphologic signature of ischemic intestinal disease.

MORPHOLOGY

Although the colon is the most common site of gastrointestinal ischemia, mucosal and mural infarction may involve any level of the gut from stomach to anus. The lesions can be continuous but are most often segmental and patchy (Fig. 17-24*A*). The mucosa is hemorrhagic and may be ulcerated (Fig. 17-24*B*). The bowel wall is also thickened by edema that may involve the mucosa or extend into the submucosa and muscularis propria.

Substantial portions of the bowel are generally involved in **transmural infarction** due to acute arterial obstruction. The demarcation between normal and ischemic bowel is sharply defined and the infarcted bowel is initially intensely congested and dusky to purple-red. Later, blood-tinged mucus or frank blood accumulates in the lumen and the wall becomes edematous, thickened, and rubbery. There is coagulative necrosis of the muscularis propria within 1 to 4 days, and perforation may occur. Serositis, with purulent exudates and fibrin deposition, may be prominent.

In mesenteric venous thrombosis, arterial blood continues to flow for a time, resulting in a less abrupt transition from affected to normal bowel. However, propagation of the thrombus may lead to secondary involvement of the splanchnic bed. The ultimate result is similar to that produced by acute arterial obstruction because impaired venous drainage eventually prevents oxygenated arterial blood from entering the capillaries.

Microscopic examination of ischemic intestine demonstrates the characteristic atrophy or sloughing of surface epithelium (Fig. 17-24*C*). In contrast, crypts may be hyperproliferative. Inflammatory infiltrates are initially absent in acute ischemia, but neutrophils are recruited within hours of reperfusion. Chronic ischemia is accompanied by fibrous scarring of the lamina propria (Fig. 17-24*D*) and, uncommonly, stricture formation. In both acute and chronic ischemia, bacterial superinfection and enterotoxin release may induce **pseudomembrane formation** that resembles *Clostridium difficile*–associated pseudomembranous colitis (discussed later).

Clinical Features. Ischemic disease of the colon is most common in patients older than 70 years of age, and occurs slightly more often in women. While frequently associated with coexisting cardiac or vascular disease ischemia can also be precipitated by therapeutic vasoconstrictors, some illicit drugs, for example, cocaine, endothelial damage and small vessel occlusion after cytomegalovirus or *Escherichia*

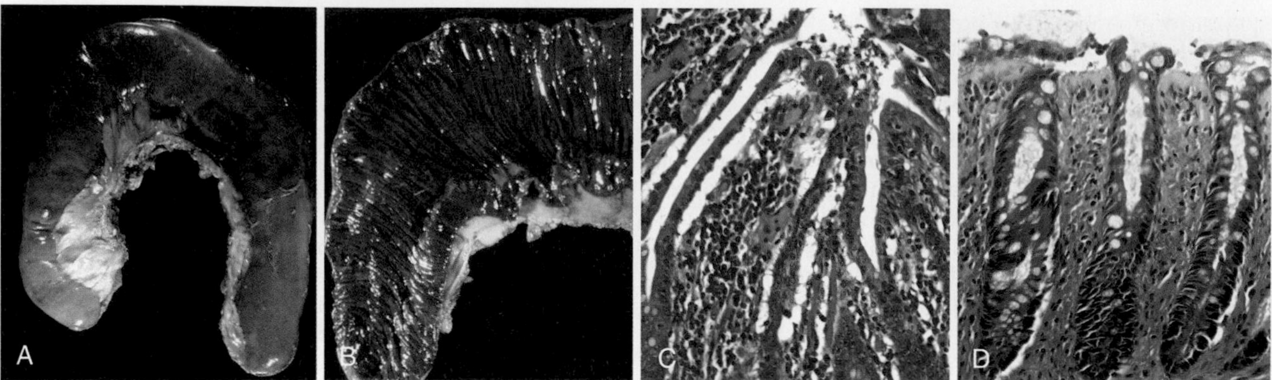

Figure 17-24 Ischemic bowel disease. **A,** Jejunal resection with dusky serosa of acute ischemia (mesenteric thrombosis). **B,** Mucosa is stained with blood after hemorrhage. **C,** Characteristic attenuated villous epithelium in this case of acute mesenteric thrombosis. **D,** Chronic colonic ischemia with atrophic surface epithelium and fibrotic lamina propria.

coli O157:H7 infection, strangulated hernia, or vascular compromise due to prior surgery.

Acute colonic ischemia typically presents with sudden onset of cramping, left lower abdominal pain, a desire to defecate, and passage of blood or bloody diarrhea. The blood loss is usually insufficient to require transfusion, but patients may progress to shock and vascular collapse within hours in severe cases. Surgical intervention, which is necessary in approximately 10% of cases, should be considered if peristaltic sounds diminish or disappear, that is, paralytic ileus, or other features of infarction, such as guarding and rebound tenderness develop. Because these physical signs overlap with those of other abdominal emergencies, including acute appendicitis, perforated ulcer, and acute cholecystitis, the diagnosis of intestinal necrosis may be delayed or missed, with disastrous consequences.

With appropriate management, mortality in the first 30 days is approximately 10%. Mortality is doubled in patients with right sided colonic disease, who have a more severe course in general. This may be because the right side of the colon is supplied by the superior mesenteric artery, which also supplies much of the small intestine. Thus, right sided colonic ischemia may be the initial presentation of more severe disease, including that caused by acute occlusion of the superior mesenteric artery (Fig. 17-24). Other poor prognostic indicators include co-existing chronic obstructive pulmonary disease (COPD) and persistence of symptoms for more than 2 weeks. Happily, most patients recover fully and colonic ischemia does not recur in the majority of cases. Listed below are some additional forms of bowel ischemia, their antecedents and outcomes.

- *Mucosal and mural infarctions* by themselves may not be fatal. However, these often progress to more extensive infarction if the vascular supply is not restored by correction of the insult or, in chronic disease, by development of in adequate collateral supplies. The diagnosis of nonocclusive ischemic enteritis and colitis can be particularly difficult because there may be a confusing array of nonspecific abdominal symptoms, including intermittent bloody diarrhea and intestinal obstruction.
- *Chronic ischemia* may masquerade as inflammatory bowel disease, with episodes of bloody diarrhea interspersed with periods of healing.
- *CMV infection* causes ischemic GI disease due to viral tropism for endothelial cells. CMV infection, which can be a complication of immunosuppressive therapy, is discussed further in Chapter 8.
- *Radiation enterocolitis* occurs when the GI tract is irradiated. In addition to epithelial damage, radiation-induced vascular injury may be significant and produce changes that are similar to ischemic disease. Beyond clinical history, the presence of highly atypical "radiation fibroblasts" within the stroma may provide an important clue to the etiology. Acute radiation enteritis manifests as anorexia, abdominal cramps, and malabsorptive diarrhea, while chronic radiation enteritis or colitis is often more indolent and may present as an inflammatory entero colitis.
- *Necrotizing enterocolitis* (NEC) is an acute disorder of the small and large intestines that can result in transmural necrosis. It is the most common acquired GI emergency of neonates, particularly those who are premature or of low birth weight, and frequently presents when oral feeding is initiated. NEC is discussed in more detail in Chapter 10, but is noted here because ischemic injury is thought to contribute to the pathogenesis.

Angiodysplasia

Angiodysplasia, a lesion characterized by malformed submucosal and mucosal blood vessels, occurs most often in the cecum or right colon and usually presents after the sixth decade of life. Although the prevalence of angiodysplasia is less than 1% in the adult population, it accounts for 20% of major episodes of lower intestinal bleeding; intestinal hemorrhage may be chronic and intermittent or acute and massive.

The pathogenesis of angiodysplasia remains undefined but has been attributed to mechanical and congenital factors. Normal distention and contraction may intermittently occlude the submucosal veins that penetrate through the muscularis propria and can lead to focal dilation and tortuosity of overlying submucosal and mucosal vessels. Because the cecum has the largest diameter of any colonic segment, it develops the greatest wall tension. This may explain the preferential distribution of angiodysplastic lesions in the cecum and right colon. Finally, some data link angiodysplasia with Meckel diverticulum, suggesting the possibility of a developmental component.

Morphologically, angiodysplastic lesions are characterized by ectatic nests of tortuous veins, venules, and capillaries. The vascular channels may be separated from the intestinal lumen by only the vascular wall and a layer of attenuated epithelial cells; limited injury may therefore result in significant bleeding.

Malabsorption and Diarrhea

Malabsorption, which presents most commonly as chronic diarrhea, is characterized by defective absorption of fats, fat- and water-soluble vitamins, proteins, carbohydrates, electrolytes and minerals, and water. Chronic malabsorption can be accompanied by weight loss, anorexia, abdominal distention, borborygmi, and muscle wasting. A hallmark of malabsorption is *steatorrhea*, characterized by excessive fecal fat and bulky, frothy, greasy, yellow or clay-colored stools. The chronic malabsorptive disorders most commonly encountered in the United States are pancreatic insufficiency, celiac disease, and Crohn disease (Table 17-7). Intestinal graft-versus-host disease is an important cause of malabsorption and diarrhea after allogeneic hematopoietic stem cell transplantation.

Malabsorption results from disturbance in at least one of the four phases of nutrient absorption:

- *Intraluminal digestion,* in which proteins, carbohydrates, and fats are broken down into forms suitable for absorption;
- *Terminal digestion,* which involves the hydrolysis of carbohydrates and peptides by disaccharidases and peptidases in the brush border of the small intestinal mucosa;
- *Transepithelial transport,* in which nutrients, fluid, and electrolytes are transported across and processed within the small intestinal epithelium; and
- *Lymphatic transport of absorbed lipids.*

In many malabsorptive disorders a defect in one of these processes predominates, but more than one usually contributes. As a result, malabsorption syndromes resemble each other more than they differ. General symptoms include diarrhea (from nutrient malabsorption and excessive intestinal secretion), flatus, abdominal pain, and weight loss. Inadequate absorption of vitamins and minerals can result in anemia and mucositis due to pyridoxine, folate, or vitamin B_{12} deficiency; bleeding, due to vitamin K deficiency; osteopenia and tetany due to calcium, magnesium, or vitamin D deficiencies; or peripheral neuropathy due to vitamin A or B_{12} deficiencies. A variety of endocrine and skin disturbances may also occur.

Diarrhea is defined as an increase in stool mass, frequency, or fluidity, typically greater than 200 gm per day. In severe cases stool volume can exceed 14 L per day and, without fluid resuscitation, result in death. Painful, bloody, small-volume diarrhea is known as *dysentery*. Diarrhea can be classified into four major categories:

- *Secretory diarrhea* is characterized by isotonic stool and persists during fasting.
- *Osmotic diarrhea*, such as that which occurs with lactase deficiency, is due to the excessive osmotic forces exerted by unabsorbed luminal solutes. The diarrhea fluid is more than 50 mOsm more concentrated than plasma and abates with fasting.
- *Malabsorptive diarrhea* follows generalized failure of nutrient absorption, is associated with steatorrhea, and is relieved by fasting.
- *Exudative diarrhea* due to inflammatory disease is characterized by purulent, bloody stools that continue during fasting.

Table 17-7 Defects in Malabsorptive and Diarrheal Disease

Disease	Intraluminal Digestion	Terminal Digestion	Transepithelial Transport	Lymphatic Transport
Celiac disease		+	+	
Environmental enteropathy		+	+	
Chronic pancreatitis	+			
Cystic fibrosis	+			
Primary bile acid malabsorption	+		+	
Carcinoid syndrome			+	
Autoimmune enteropathy		+	+	
Disaccharidase deficiency		+		
Whipple disease				+
Abetalipoproteinemia			+	
Viral gastroenteritis		+	+	
Bacterial gastroenteritis		+	+	
Parasitic gastroenteritis		+	+	
Inflammatory bowel disease	+	+	+	

+ indicates that the process is abnormal in the disease indicated. Other processes are not affected.

Cystic Fibrosis

Cystic fibrosis affects many organ systems, primarily the lungs, and is discussed in greater detail elsewhere (Chapter 10). Only the malabsorption associated with cystic fibrosis is considered here. Due to the absence of the epithelial cystic fibrosis transmembrane conductance regulator (CFTR), individuals with cystic fibrosis have defects in chloride and, in certain tissues, bicarbonate ion secretion. This interferes with bicarbonate, sodium, and water secretion, ultimately resulting in defective luminal hydration. Reduced hydration can occasionally lead to intestinal obstruction, but commonly results in formation of pancreatic intraductal concretions. The latter can begin in utero, and result in duct obstruction, low-grade chronic autodigestion of the pancreas, and eventual exocrine pancreatic insufficiency in more than 80% of patients. The result is failure of the intraluminal phase of nutrient absorption, which can be effectively treated in most patients with oral enzyme supplementation.

Celiac Disease

Celiac disease is also known as celiac sprue or gluten-sensitive enteropathy. It is an immune-mediated enteropathy triggered by the ingestion of gluten-containing foods, such as wheat, rye, or barley, in genetically predisposed individuals. Celiac disease has an overall worldwide incidence of 0.6% to 1%, but its prevalence varies widely between countries and regions. Some of these differences correlate with variation in wheat consumption, but the reasons for other disparities are not defined. While previously uncommon, the incidence of celiac disease in developing countries is growing, possibly as a result of adoption of Western diets.

Pathogenesis. Celiac disease is triggered by ingestion of gluten, which is the major storage protein of wheat and similar grains. The alcohol-soluble fraction of gluten, *gliadin,* contains most of the disease-producing components. Gluten is digested by luminal and brush-border enzymes into amino acids and peptides, including a 33-amino acid α-gliadin peptide that is resistant to degradation by gastric, pancreatic, and small intestinal proteases (Fig. 17-25). Some gliadin peptides may induce epithelial cells to express IL-15, which in turn triggers activation and proliferation of CD8+ intraepithelial lymphocytes. These lymphocytes express NKG2D, a natural killer cell marker and receptor for MIC-A. Enterocytes that have been induced to express surface MIC-A, in response to stress, are then attacked by NKG2D-expressing intraepithelial lymphocytes. The resulting epithelial damage may enhance passage of other gliadin peptides into the lamina propria where they are deamidated by tissue transglutaminase. These gliadin peptides interact with HLA-DQ2 or HLA-DQ8 on antigen-presenting cells and, in turn, can stimulate CD4+ T cells to produce cytokines that contribute to tissue damage.

While nearly all people eat grain and are exposed to gluten and gliadin, most do not develop celiac disease. Thus, host factors determine whether disease develops. Among these, HLA proteins seem to be critical, since almost all people with celiac disease carry the class II HLA-DQ2 or HLA-DQ8 allele. However, the HLA locus accounts for less than half of the genetic component of celiac disease. Remaining genetic factors may include polymorphisms of genes involved in immune regulation and epithelial function. These genetic variables may also contribute to associations between celiac disease and other immune diseases, including type 1 diabetes, thyroiditis, and Sjögren syndrome, IgA nephropathy, as well as neu-

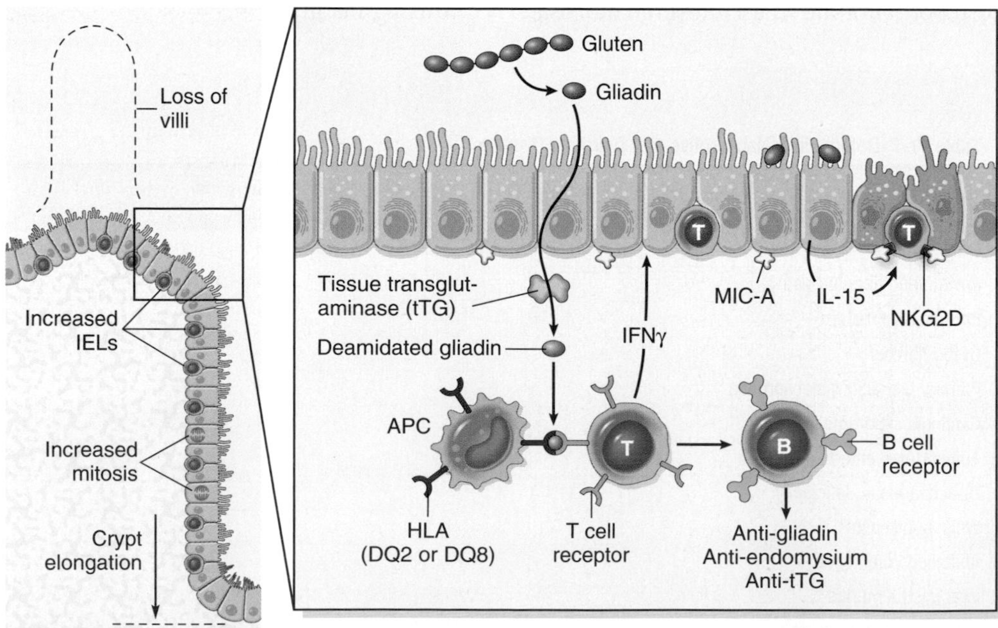

Figure 17-25 The left panel illustrates the morphologic alterations that may be present celiac disease, including villous atrophy, increased numbers of intraepithelial lymphocytes (IELs), and epithelial proliferation with crypt elongation (compare to Fig. 17-26). The right panel depicts a model for the pathogenesis of celiac disease. Note that both innate (CD8+ intraepithelial T cells, activated by IL 15) and adaptive (CD4+ T cells, and B cells sensitization to gliadin) immune mechanisms are involved in the tissue responses to gliadin.

rologic disorders, such as ataxia, autism, depression, epilepsy, Down syndrome, and Turner syndrome.

MORPHOLOGY

Biopsy specimens from the second portion of the duodenum or proximal jejunum, which are exposed to the highest concentrations of dietary gluten, are generally diagnostic in celiac disease. The histopathology is characterized by increased numbers of intraepithelial CD8+ T lymphocytes (intraepithelial lymphocytosis), crypt hyperplasia, and villous atrophy (Fig. 17-26). This loss of mucosal and brush-border surface area probably accounts for the malabsorption. In addition, increased rates of epithelial turnover, reflected in increased crypt mitotic activity, may limit the ability of absorptive enterocytes to fully differentiate and express proteins necessary for terminal digestion and transepithelial transport. Other features of fully developed celiac disease include increased numbers of plasma cells, mast cells, and eosinophils, especially within the upper part of the lamina propria. With increased frequency of serologic screening and early detection of disease-associated antibodies, it is now appreciated that an increase in the number of intraepithelial lymphocytes, particularly within the villus, is a sensitive marker of celiac disease, even in the absence of epithelial damage and villous atrophy. However, intraepithelial lymphocytosis and villous atrophy are not specific for celiac disease and can be present in other diseases, including viral enteritis. The combination of histology and serology, therefore, is most specific for diagnosis of celiac disease.

Adherence to a gluten-free diet typically results in resolution of symptoms, decreasing titers of anti-tissue transglutaminase or other celiac disease-associated antibodies, and restoration of normal or near normal mucosal histology within 6 to 24 months.

Clinical Features. In adults, celiac disease presents most commonly between the ages of 30 and 60. Many cases of celiac disease escape clinical attention for extended periods because of atypical presentations. Other patients may have silent celiac disease, defined as positive serology and villous atrophy without symptoms, or latent celiac disease, in which positive serology is not accompanied by villous atrophy. Celiac disease may be associated with chronic diarrhea, bloating, or chronic fatigue, but is often asymptomatic. These cases may present with anemia due to chronic iron and vitamin malabsorption. In adults, celiac disease is detected twice as frequently in women, perhaps because monthly menstrual bleeding accentuates the effects of impaired absorption.

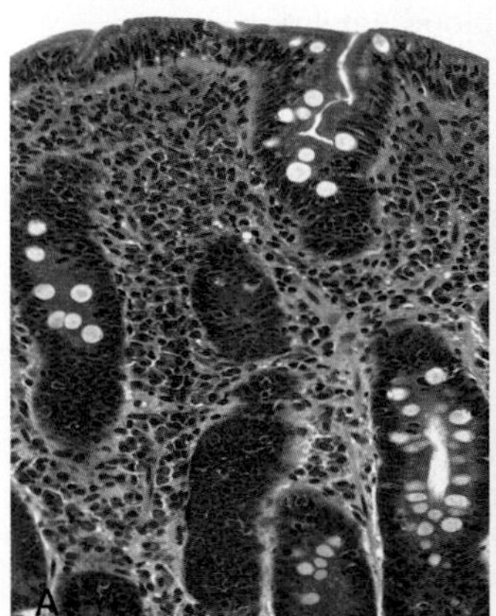

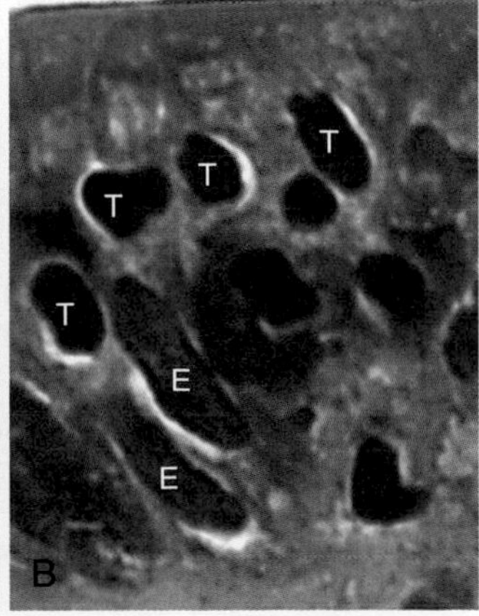

Figure 17-26 Celiac disease. **A,** Advanced cases of celiac disease show complete loss of villi, or total villous atrophy. Note the dense plasma cell infiltrates in the lamina propria. **B,** Infiltration of the surface epithelium by T lymphocytes, which can be recognized by their densely stained nuclei (labelled **T**). Compare to elongated, pale-staining epithelial nuclei (labeled **E**).

Pediatric celiac disease, which affects males and females equally, may present with malabsorption or atypical symptoms affecting almost any organ. In those with classic symptoms, disease typically begins after introduction of gluten to the diet, between ages of 6 and 24 months, and manifests as irritability, abdominal distention, anorexia, chronic diarrhea, failure to thrive, weight loss, or muscle wasting. Children with nonclassic symptoms tend to present at older ages with complaints of abdominal pain, nausea, vomiting, bloating, or constipation. Common extraintestinal complaints include arthritis or joint pain, aphthous stomatitis, iron deficiency anemia, delayed puberty, and short stature.

A characteristic itchy, blistering skin lesion, dermatitis herpetiformis (Chapter 25), can be present in as many as 10% of patients. Unfortunately, the only treatment currently available for celiac disease is a gluten-free diet. While adhering to this diet can be challenging, it does result in symptomatic improvement for most patients. A gluten-free diet may also reduce the risk of long-term complications including anemia, female infertility, osteoporosis, and cancer (discussed bellow).

Noninvasive serologic tests are generally performed prior to biopsy. The most sensitive tests are the measurement of IgA antibodies against tissue transglutaminase. IgA anti-endomysial antibodies can also be present. IgG anti-tissue transglutaminase antibodies may be detected in patients with IgA deficiency. The absence of HLA-DQ2 and HLA-DQ8 is useful for its high negative predictive value, but the presence of these alleles is not helpful in confirming the diagnosis.

Individuals with celiac disease have a higher than normal rate of malignancy. The most common celiac disease-associated cancer is enteropathy-associated T-cell lymphoma, an aggressive lymphoma of intraepithelial T lymphocytes. Small intestinal adenocarcinoma is also more frequent in individuals with celiac disease. Thus, when symptoms such as abdominal pain, diarrhea, and weight loss develop despite a strict gluten-free diet, cancer or refractory sprue, in which the response to a gluten-free diet is lost, must be considered.

Environmental Enteropathy

Environmental enteropathy, which has also been referred to as *tropical enteropathy* or *tropical sprue*, is a disorder prevalent in areas and populations with poor sanitation and hygiene, such as those in developing countries, including many parts of sub-Saharan Africa, such as Gambia; aboriginal populations within northern Australia; and some groups within South America and Asia, such as residents of impoverished communities within Brazil, Guatemala, India, and Pakistan. Affected individuals often suffer from malabsorption and malnutrition, stunted growth, and defective intestinal mucosal immune function. The relatively high oral vaccine failure rates in regions where environmental enteropathy is endemic has been proposed to be due to defective mucosal immune function.

There are presently no accepted clinical, laboratory, or histopathologic criteria that allow diagnosis of environmental enteropathy. Intestinal biopsy specimens have been examined in a small number of cases, and reported histologic features are more similar to severe celiac disease than infectious enteritis.

The underlying causes of environmental enteropathy are unknown, but defective intestinal barrier function, chronic exposure to fecal pathogens and other microbial contaminants, and repeated bouts of diarrhea within the first 2 or 3 years of life are likely involved. Many pathogens are endemic in these communities, but no single infectious agent has been linked to environmental enteropathy. Neither oral antibiotics nor nutritional supplementation, with calorie-dense foods, vitamins, or minerals, are able to correct these deficits. Moreover, recent data suggest that irreversible losses in physical development may be accompanied by uncorrectable cognitive deficits. Thus, the global impact of environmental enteropathy, which is estimated to affect more than 150 million children worldwide and may contribute to a very large number of childhood deaths, is difficult to overstate.

Autoimmune Enteropathy

Autoimmune enteropathy is an X-linked disorder characterized by severe persistent diarrhea and autoimmune disease that occurs most often in young children. A particularly severe familial form, termed *IPEX*, an acronym denoting immune dysregulation, polyendocrinopathy, enteropathy, and X-linkage, is due to a germline mutation in the *FOXP3* gene, which is located on the X chromosome. FOXP3 is a transcription factor expressed in CD4+ regulatory T cells, and individuals with IPEX and *FOXP3* mutations have defective function of these cells. Other defects in regulatory T cell function have also been linked to less severe forms of autoimmune enteropathy. Autoantibodies to enterocytes and goblet cells are common, and some patients may have antibodies to parietal or islet cells. Within the small intestine, intraepithelial lymphocytes may be increased, but not to the extent seen in celiac disease, and neutrophils are often present. Therapy includes immunosuppressive drugs such as cyclosporine and, in rare cases, hematopoietic stem cell transplantation.

Lactase (Disaccharidase) Deficiency

The disaccharidases, including lactase, are located in the apical brush-border membrane of the villus absorptive epithelial cells. Because the defect is biochemical, biopsy histology is generally unremarkable. Lactase deficiency is of two types:

- *Congenital lactase deficiency*, caused by a mutation in the gene encoding lactase, is an autosomal recessive disorder. The disease is rare and presents as explosive diarrhea with watery, frothy stools and abdominal distention upon milk ingestion. Symptoms abate when exposure to milk and milk products is terminated, thus removing the osmotically active but unabsorbable lactose from the lumen. As a result, congenital lactase deficiency was often fatal prior to the availability of soy-based infant formula.
- *Acquired lactase deficiency* is caused by down-regulation of lactase gene expression and is particularly common among Native American, African American, and Chinese populations. Acquired lactase deficiency can develop following enteric viral or bacterial infections and may resolve over time. Symptoms of acquired lactase deficiency, including abdominal fullness, diarrhea, and flatulence, due to fermentation of the unabsorbed sugars by colonic bacteria, are triggered by ingestion of lactose-containing dairy products.

Abetalipoproteinemia

Abetalipoproteinemia is a rare autosomal recessive disease characterized by an inability to secrete triglyceride-rich lipoproteins. It is caused by a mutation in the microsomal triglyceride transfer protein (MTP) that catalyzes transfer of lipids to specialized domains of the nascent apolipoprotein B polypeptide within the rough endoplasmic reticulum. MTP also promotes production of triglyceride droplets within the smooth endoplasmic reticulum. Without MTP, enterocytes cannot assemble or export lipoproteins. This results in intracellular lipid accumulation. The malabsorption of abetalipoproteinemia is therefore a failure of intraepithelial processing and transport. Because of the triglyceride accumulation, vacuolization of small intestinal epithelial cells is evident and can be highlighted by special stains, such as oil red-O, particularly after a fatty meal.

Abetalipoproteinemia presents in infancy and the clinical picture is dominated by failure to thrive, diarrhea, and steatorrhea. Patients also have a complete absence of all plasma lipoproteins containing apolipoprotein B, although the gene that encodes apolipoprotein B itself is not affected. Failure to absorb essential fatty acids leads to deficiencies of fat-soluble vitamins as well as lipid membrane defects that can be recognized by the presence of *acanthocytic red cells (burr cells)* in peripheral blood smears.

KEY CONCEPTS

Congenital and acquired (non infectious) disorders of the intestines

- **Abdominal hernias** may occur through any weakness or defect in the wall of the peritoneal cavity, including inguinal and femoral canals, the umbilicus, and sites of surgical scars.
- **Intussusception** occurs when a segment of intestine telescopes into the immediately distal segment. It is the most common cause of intestinal obstruction in children younger than 2 years of age.
- **Ischemic bowel disease** of the colon is most common at the splenic flexure, sigmoid colon, and rectum; these

are watershed zones where two arterial circulations terminate.

- **Angiodysplasia** is a malformation of submucosal and mucosal blood vessels and a common cause of lower intestinal bleeding in those older than 60 years of age.
- **Diarrhea** can be characterized as secretory, osmotic, malabsorptive, or exudative.
- The malabsorption associated with **cystic fibrosis** is the result of pancreatic insufficiency, leading to inadequate pancreatic digestive enzymes, and deficient luminal breakdown of nutrients.
- **Celiac disease** is an immune-mediated enteropathy triggered by the ingestion of gluten-containing grains. The malabsorptive diarrhea in celiac disease is due to loss of brush border surface area, including villous atrophy, and, possibly, deficient enterocyte maturation as a result of immune-mediated epithelial damage.
- **Environmental enteropathy** is prevalent in areas with poor sanitation. It is estimated to affect more than 150 million children worldwide and may contribute to a very large number of childhood deaths.
- **Lactase deficiency** causes an osmotic diarrhea due to the inability to break down or absorb lactose. The autosomal recessive form is rare and severe; the acquired form usually presents in adulthood and is common.
- **Autoimmune enteropathy** is an X-linked disorder characterized by severe persistent diarrhea and autoimmune disease that is caused by mutation in *FOXP3* gene, resulting in defective function of regulatory T cells.
- **Abetalipoproteinemia** is a rare autosomal recessive disease due to a mutation in microsomal triglyceride transfer protein that is required for enterocytes to process and secrete triglyceride-rich lipoproteins.

Infectious Enterocolitis

Enterocolitis can present with a broad range of symptoms including diarrhea, abdominal pain, urgency, perianal discomfort, incontinence, and hemorrhage (Table 17-8). This global problem is responsible for more than 2000 deaths each day among children in developing countries and greater than 10% of all deaths before age 5 worldwide. Bacterial infections, such as enterotoxigenic *Escherichia coli*, are frequently responsible, but the etiology varies with age, nutrition, and host immune status as well as environmental influences (Table 17-8). For example, epidemics of cholera are common in areas with poor sanitation, as a result of inadequate public health measures, natural disasters, such as floods and earthquakes, or war. Pediatric infectious diarrhea, which may result in severe dehydration and metabolic acidosis, is commonly caused by enteric viruses.

Cholera

***Vibrio cholerae* are comma-shaped, gram-negative bacteria that cause cholera, a disease that has been endemic in the Ganges Valley of India and Bangladesh** for almost all of recorded history. Since 1817, seven great pandemics have spread along trade routes to large parts of Europe, Australia, and the Americas, but, for unknown reasons these pandemics resolved and cholera retreated back to the Ganges Valley. Cholera also persists within the Gulf of Mexico but causes only rare cases of seafood-associated disease; this occurs because shellfish and plankton can be reservoirs of *Vibrio* bacteria.

There is a marked seasonal variation in the incidence of cholera in most climates due to rapid growth of *Vibrio* bacteria at warm temperatures. While the bacteria can be present in food, the infection is primarily transmitted by contaminated drinking water. Thus, cholera can become rampant in areas devastated by natural or man-made disasters, such as earthquakes or war, that threaten sewage systems and drinking water supplies. For example, the January 2010 Haitian earthquake led to a cholera epidemic that began in October 2010. At the end of the first year, more than 5% of the population was affected. More than half of the cases required hospitalization and approximately 1% were fatal. In all, the cholera epidemic in Haiti accounted for more than half of worldwide cholera cases and deaths reported to the World Health Organization in 2010 and 2011.

Pathogenesis. *Despite the severe diarrhea, Vibrio organisms are noninvasive and remain within the intestinal lumen.* While cholera toxin, encoded by a virulence phage and released by the *Vibrio* organism, causes disease, the flagellar proteins, which are involved in motility and attachment, are necessary for efficient bacterial colonization. Hemagglutinin, a metalloproteinase, is important for bacterial detachment and shedding in the stool. The mechanism by which cholera toxin induces diarrhea is well understood (Fig. 17-27). Cholera toxin is composed of five B subunits and a single A subunit. The B subunit binds GM1 ganglioside on the surface of intestinal epithelial cells, and is carried by endocytosis to the endoplasmic reticulum, a process called retrograde transport. Here, the A subunit is reduced by protein disulfide isomerase, and a fragment of the A subunit is unfolded and released. This peptide fragment is then transported into the cytosol using host cell machinery that moves misfolded proteins from the endoplasmic reticulum to the cytosol. Such unfolded proteins are normally disposed of via the proteasome, but the A subunit refolds to avoid degradation. The refolded A subunit peptide then interacts with cytosolic ADP ribosylation factors (ARFs) to ribosylate and activate the stimulatory G protein $G_s\alpha$. This stimulates adenylate cyclase and the resulting increase in intracellular cAMP opens the cystic fibrosis transmembrane conductance regulator, CFTR, which releases chloride ions into the lumen. Chloride and sodium absorption are also inhibited by cAMP. The resulting accumulation of chloride, bicarbonate, and sodium within the intestinal lumen creates an osmotic driving force that draws water into the lumen and causes massive diarrhea. Remarkably, mucosal biopsies show only minimal histologic alterations.

Clinical Features. Most individuals exposed to *V. cholerae* are asymptomatic or develop only mild diarrhea. In those with severe disease there is an abrupt onset of watery diarrhea and vomiting following an incubation period of 1 to 5 days. The voluminous stools resemble rice water and are sometimes described as having a fishy odor. The rate of diarrhea may reach 1 liter per hour, leading to

Table 17-8 Features of Bacterial Enterocolitides

Infection Type	Geography	Reservoir	Transmission	Epidemiology	Affected GI Sites	Symptoms	Complications
Cholera	India, Africa	Shellfish	Fecal-oral, water	Sporadic, endemic, epidemic	Small intestine	Severe watery diarrhea	Dehydration, electrolyte imbalances
Campylobacter spp.	Developed countries	Chickens, sheep, pigs, cattle	Poultry, milk, other foods	Sporadic; children, travelers	Colon	Watery or bloody diarrhea	Arthritis, Guillain-Barré syndrome
Shigellosis	Worldwide, endemic in developing countries	Humans	Fecal-oral, food, water	Children, migrant workers, travelers,nursing homes	Left colon, ileum	Bloody diarrhea	Reactive arthritis, urethritis, conjunctivitis, hemolytic-uremic syndrome
Salmonellosis	Worldwide	Poultry, farm animals, reptiles	Meat, poultry, eggs, milk	Children, older adults	Colon and small intestine	Watery or bloody diarrhea	Sepsis, abscess
Enteric (typhoid) fever	India, Mexico, Philippines	Humans	Fecal-oral, water	Children. adolescents, travelers	Small intestine	Bloody diarrhea, fever	Chronic infection, carrier state, encephalopathy, myocarditis, intestinal perforation
Yersinia spp.	Northern and central Europe	Pigs, cows, puppies, cats	Pork, milk, water	Clustered cases	Ileum, appendix, right colon	Abdominal pain, fever, diarrhea	Reactive arthritis, erythema nodosum
Escherichia coli							
Enterotoxigenic (ETEC)	Developing countries	Unknown	Food or fecal-oral	Infants, adolescents, travelers	Small intestine	Severe watery diarrhea	Dehydration, electrolyte imbalances
Enteropathogenic (EPEC)	Worldwide	Humans	Fecal-oral	Infants	Small intestine	Watery diarrhea	Dehydration, electrolyte imbalances
Enterohemorrhagic (EHEC)	Worldwide	Widespread, includes cattle	Beef, milk, produce	Sporadic and epidemic	Colon	Bloody diarrhea	Hemolytic-uremic syndrome
Enteroinvasive (EIEC)	Developing countries	Unknown	Cheese, other foods, water	Young children	Colon	Bloody diarrhea	Unknown
Enteroaggregative (EAEC)	Worldwide	Unknown	Unknown	Children, adults, travelers	Colon	Nonbloody diarrhea, afebrile	Poorly defined
Pseudomembranous colitis (*C. difficile*)	Worldwide	Humans, hospitals	Antibiotics allow emergence	Immunosuppressed, antibiotic-treated	Colon	Watery diarrhea, fever	Relapse, toxic megacolon
Whipple disease	Rural > urban	Unknown	Unknown	Rare	Small intestine	Malabsorption	Arthritis, CNS disease
Mycobacterial infection	Worldwide	Unknown	Unknown	Immunosuppressed, endemic	Small intestine	Malabsorption	Pneumonia, infection at other sites

CNS, Central nervous system; GI, gastrointestinal.

dehydration, hypotension, muscular cramping, anuria, shock, loss of consciousness, and death. Most deaths occur within the first 24 hours after presentation. Although the mortality for severe cholera is about 50% without treatment, timely fluid replacement can save more than 99% of patients. Oral rehydration is often sufficient. Because of an improved understanding of the host and *Vibrio* proteins involved, new therapies are being developed, including CFTR inhibitors that block chloride secretion and prevent diarrhea. Prophylactic vaccination is a long-term goal, and data from trials of new cholera vaccines have prompted the WHO to recommend vaccination with other prevention and control strategies in endemic regions and during outbreaks. However, it should be noted that variant strains that cause more severe clinical disease may be displacing earlier strains as the major cause of disease. Thus, vaccines may need to be modified to keep pace with changes in pathogenic cholera strains.

Campylobacter Enterocolitis

***Campylobacter jejuni* is the most common bacterial enteric pathogen in developed countries and is an important cause of traveler's diarrhea.** Most infections are associated with ingestion of improperly cooked chicken, but outbreaks can also be caused by unpasteurized milk or contaminated water. It is an important bacterial cause of food poisoning.

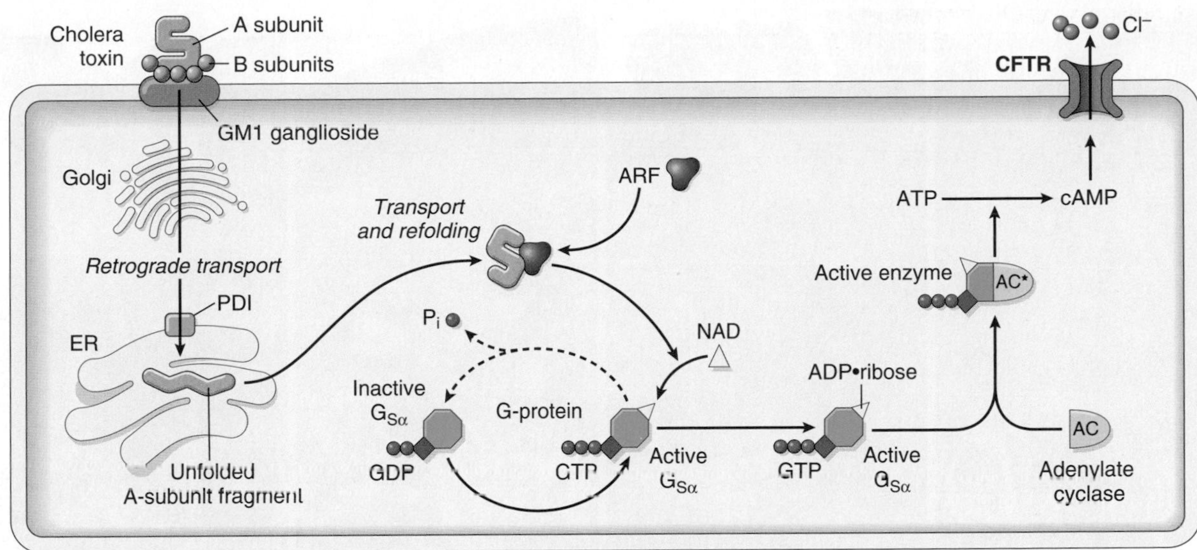

Figure 17-27 Cholera toxin transport and signaling. After retrograde toxin transport to the endoplasmic reticulum (ER), the A subunit is released by the action of protein disulfide isomerase (PDI) and is then able to access the epithelial cell cytoplasm. In concert with an ADP-ribosylation factor (ARF), the A subunit then ADP-ribosylates $G_s\alpha$, which locks it in the active, GTP-bound state. This leads to adenylate cyclase (AC) activation, and the cAMP produced opens CFTR to drive chloride secretion and diarrhea.

Pathogenesis. The pathogenesis of *Campylobacter* infection remains poorly defined, but the four major properties that contribute to virulence are: motility, adherence, toxin production, and invasion. Flagella allow *Campylobacter* to be motile. This facilitates adherence and colonization, which are necessary for mucosal invasion. Cytotoxins that cause epithelial damage and a cholera toxin-like enterotoxin are also released by some *C. jejuni* isolates. Dysentery, i.e. bloody diarrhea, is generally associated with invasion and only occurs with a small minority of *Campylobacter* strains. Enteric fever occurs when bacteria proliferate within the lamina propria and mesenteric lymph nodes.

Campylobacter infection can result in reactive arthritis, primarily in patients with HLA-B27. Other extraintestinal complications, including erythema nodosum and Guillain-Barré syndrome, a flaccid paralysis caused by immunologically mediated inflammation of peripheral nerves, are not HLA-linked (Chapter 27). Molecular mimicry has been implicated in the pathogenesis of Guillain-Barré syndrome, as serum antibodies to *C. jejuni* lipopolysaccharide cross-react with peripheral and central nervous system gangliosides. Up to 40% of Guillain-Barré syndrome cases are associated with *Campylobacter* infection in the preceding 1 to 2 weeks and up to 50% have positive stool cultures or circulating antibodies to *Campylobacter*. Guillain-Barré syndrome develops in 0.1% or less of those infected with *Campylobacter*.

MORPHOLOGY

Campylobacter are comma-shaped, flagellated, gram-negative organisms. Diagnosis is primarily by stool culture, since biopsy findings are nonspecific, and reveal acute self-limited colitis with features common to many forms of infectious colitis. Mucosal and intraepithelial neutrophil infiltrates are prominent, particularly within the superficial mucosa (Fig. 17-28*A*); cryptitis (neutrophil infiltration of the crypts) and crypt abscesses (crypts with accumulations of luminal neutrophils) may also be present. Importantly, crypt architecture is preserved (Fig. 17-28*D*), although this can be difficult to assess in cases with severe mucosal damage.

Clinical Features. Ingestion of as few as 500 *C. jejuni* organisms can cause disease after an incubation period of up to 8 days. Watery diarrhea, either acute or following an influenza-like prodrome, is the primary symptom, but dysentery develops in 15% of adults and more than 50% of children. Patients may shed bacteria for 1 month or more after clinical resolution. Antibiotic therapy is generally not required.

Shigellosis

Shigella are gram-negative unencapsulated, nonmotile, facultative anaerobes that belong to the Enterobacteriaceae family and are closely related to enteroinvasive E. coli. Although humans are the only known reservoir, *Shigella* spp. remain one of the most common causes of bloody diarrhea. It is estimated that 165 million cases occur worldwide each year. Given the infective dose of fewer than several hundred organisms and the presence of as many as 10^9 organisms in each gram of stool during acute disease, *Shigella* are highly transmissible by the fecal-oral route or via contaminated water and food.

In the United States and Europe, children in daycare centers, migrant workers, travelers to developing countries, and those in nursing homes are most commonly affected. Most *Shigella* infections and deaths occur in children younger than 5 years of age. In countries where *Shigella* is endemic it is responsible for approximately 10% of pediatric diarrheal disease and as many as 75% of diarrheal deaths.

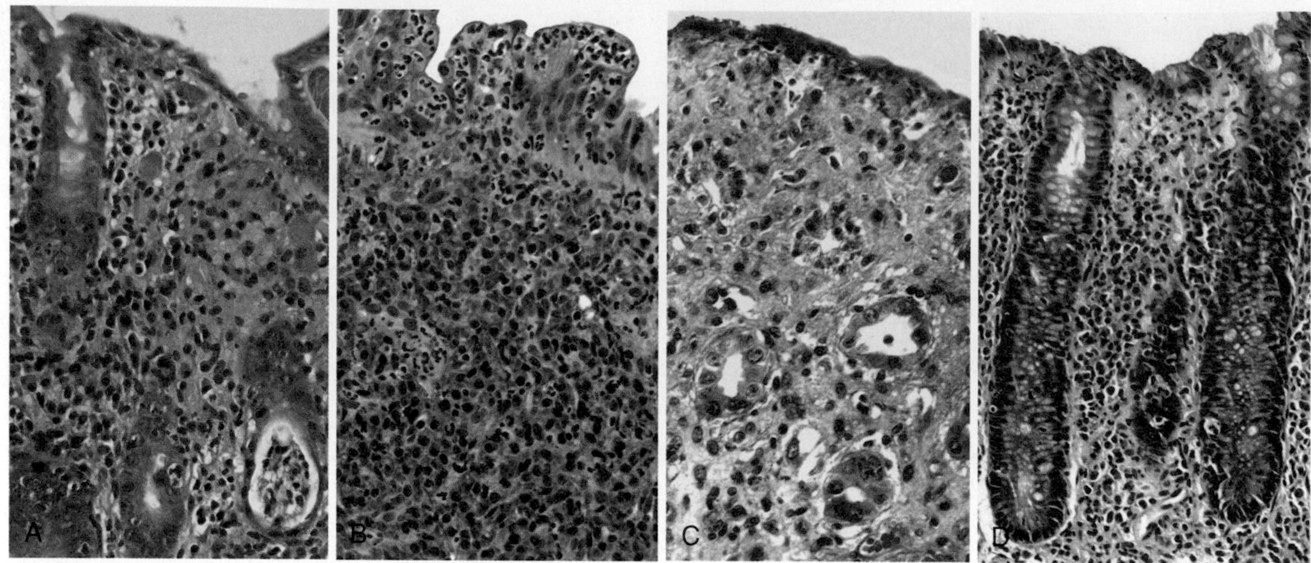

Figure 17-28 Bacterial enterocolitis. **A,** *Campylobacter jejuni* infection produces acute, self-limited colitis. Neutrophils can be seen within the surface and crypt epithelia and a crypt abscess is present at the lower right. **B,** In *Yersinia* infection the surface epithelium can be eroded by neutrophils and the lamina propria is densely infiltrated by sheets of plasma cells admixed with lymphocytes and neutrophils. **C,** Enterohemorrhagic *E. coli* O157:H7 results in an ischemia-like morphology with surface atrophy and erosion. **D,** Enteroinvasive *E. coli* infection is similar to other acute, self-limited colitides such as those caused by *Campylobacter jejuni*. Note the maintenance of normal crypt architecture and spacing, despite abundant intraepithelial neutrophils.

Pathogenesis. *Shigella are resistant to the harsh acidic environment of the stomach, thereby explaining the extremely low infective dose.* Once in the intestine, organisms are taken up by M, or microfold cells. These are epithelial cells, which are specialized for sampling and presentation of luminal antigens. *Shigella* proliferate intracellularly, escape into the lamina propria, and are phagocytosed by macrophages, in which they induce apoptosis. The ensuing inflammatory response damages surface epithelia and allows *Shigella* within the intestinal lumen to gain access to the basolateral membranes of colonic epithelial cells, which is the preferred domain for invasion. All *Shigella* spp. carry virulence plasmids, some of which encode a type III secretion system capable of directly injecting bacterial proteins into the host cytoplasm. *S. dysenteriae* serotype 1 also release the Shiga toxin Stx, which inhibits eukaryotic protein synthesis, resulting in host cell damage and death.

MORPHOLOGY

Shigella infections are most prominent in the left colon, but the ileum may also be involved, perhaps reflecting the abundance of M cells in the dome epithelium over the Peyer patches. The mucosa is hemorrhagic and ulcerated, and pseudomembranes may be present. The histology of early cases is similar to other acute self-limited colitides, such as *Campylobacter* colitis, but because of the tropism for M cells, aphthous-appearing ulcers similar to those seen in Crohn disease may occur. The potential for confusion with chronic inflammatory bowel disease is significant, particularly if there is distortion of crypt architecture.

Clinical Features. After an incubation period of up to 1 week, *Shigella* causes self-limited disease characterized by about 1 week of diarrhea, fever, and abdominal pain. The initially watery diarrhea progresses to a dysenteric phase in approximately 50% of patients, and constitutional symptoms can persist for as long as 1 month. The subacute presentation that develops in a minority of adults is characterized by several weeks of waxing and waning diarrhea that can mimic new-onset ulcerative colitis. While duration is typically shorter in children, severity is often much greater. Confirmation of *Shigella* infection requires stool culture.

Complications of *Shigella* infection are uncommon and include a triad of sterile reactive arthritis, urethritis, and conjunctivitis that preferentially affects HLA-B27-positive men between 20 and 40 years of age. Hemolytic-uremic syndrome, which is typically associated with *enterohemorrhagic E. coli* (EHEC), may also occur after infection with *S. dysenteriae* serotype 1 that secrete Shiga toxin (Chapter 20). Toxic megacolon and intestinal obstruction are uncommon complications. Antibiotic treatment shortens the clinical course and reduces the duration of organism shedding in stools, but antidiarrheal medications are contraindicated because they can prolong symptoms and delay *Shigella* clearance.

Salmonella

Salmonella, which are classified within the Enterobacteriaceae family of gram-negative bacilli, are divided into *Salmonella typhi*, the causative agent of typhoid fever (discussed in the next section) and nontyphoid *Salmonella*. The latter are the causative agent of salmonellosis, which is usually due to *S. enteritidis;* more than 1 million cases occur each year in the United States, and the prevalence is even greater in developing countries. Infection is most common in young children and older adults, with peak incidence in the summer and fall. Salmonella may also cause food poisoning by ingestion of contaminated food, particularly raw or undercooked meat, poultry, eggs, and milk. Centralized food processing can lead to large outbreaks. Vaccines are available for both humans and farm animals, e.g. egg-laying hens.

Pathogenesis. Very few viable *Salmonella* are necessary to cause infection, and the absence of gastric acid, in individuals with atrophic gastritis or those on acid-suppressive therapy, further reduces the required inoculum. *Salmonella* possess virulence genes that encode a type III secretion system capable of transferring bacterial proteins into M cells and enterocytes. The transferred proteins activate host Rho GTPases, thereby triggering actin rearrangement and bacterial endocytosis which, in turn, allows bacterial growth within endosomes. In addition, flagellin, the core protein of bacterial flagellae, activates TLR5 on host cells and increases the local inflammatory response. Similarly, bacterial lipopolysaccharide activates TLR4, although some *Salmonella* strains express a virulence factor that prevents TLR4 activation. *Salmonella* also secrete a molecule that induces epithelial cell release of the eicosanoid hepoxilin A3, thereby drawing neutrophils into the intestinal lumen and potentiating mucosal damage. Both T_H1 and T_H17 immune responses limit infection and explain why those with genetic defects in T_H17 immunity are at risk for disseminated salmonellosis.

The gross and microscopic features of *Salmonella* enteritis are nonspecific and are similar to the acute self-limited colitis of *Campylobacter* and *Shigella*. Stool cultures are essential for diagnosis.

Clinical Features. Salmonella infections are clinically indistinguishable from those caused by other enteric pathogens, and symptoms range from loose stools to cholera-like profuse diarrhea to dysentery. Fever often resolves within 2 days, but diarrhea can persist for a week and organisms can be shed in the stool for several weeks after resolution. Antibiotic therapy is not recommended in uncomplicated cases because it can prolong the carrier state or even cause relapse and does not typically shorten the duration of diarrhea. Most *Salmonella* infections are self-limited, but deaths do occur. The risk of severe illness and complications is increased in patients with malignancies, immunosuppression, alcoholism, cardiovascular dysfunction, sickle cell disease, and hemolytic anemia.

Typhoid Fever

Typhoid fever, also referred to as enteric fever, affects up to 30 million individuals worldwide each year. The disease is caused by *Salmonella enterica,* and its two subtypes, *typhi* and *paratyphi. The majority of cases in endemic countries are due to S. typhi, while infection by S. paratyphi is more common among travelers, perhaps because travelers tend to be vaccinated against S. typhi.* In endemic areas, children and adolescents are affected most often, but there is no age preference in developed countries. Infection is strongly associated with travel to India, Mexico, the Philippines, Pakistan, El Salvador, and Haiti. Humans are the sole reservoir for *S. typhi* and *S. paratyphi* and transmission occurs from person to person or via food or contaminated water. Gallbladder colonization with *S. typhi* or *S. paratyphi* may be associated with gallstones and the chronic carrier state.

Pathogenesis. *S. typhi* are able to survive in gastric acid and, once in the small intestine, they are taken up by and invade M cells. Bacteria are then engulfed by mononuclear cells in the underlying lymphoid tissue. Unlike *S. enteritidis, S. typhi* can then disseminate via lymphatic and blood vessels. This causes reactive hyperplasia of phagocytes and lymphoid tissues throughout the body.

MORPHOLOGY

Infection causes **Peyer patches in the terminal ileum** to enlarge into sharply delineated, plateau-like elevations up to 8 cm in diameter. Draining mesenteric lymph nodes are also enlarged. Neutrophils accumulate within the superficial lamina propria, and macrophages containing bacteria, red cells, and nuclear debris mix with lymphocytes and plasma cells in the lamina propria. Mucosal damage creates oval ulcers, oriented along the axis of the ileum, that may perforate. The draining lymph nodes also harbor organisms and are enlarged due to phagocyte accumulation.

The spleen is enlarged and soft, with uniformly pale red pulp, obliterated follicular markings, and prominent phagocyte hyperplasia. The liver shows small, randomly scattered foci of parenchymal necrosis in which hepatocytes are replaced by macrophage aggregates, called **typhoid nodules**; such nodules may also develop in the bone marrow and lymph nodes.

Clinical Features. Patients experience anorexia, abdominal pain, bloating, nausea, vomiting, and bloody diarrhea followed by a short asymptomatic phase that gives way to bacteremia and fever with flulike symptoms. *Blood cultures are positive in more than 90% of affected individuals during the febrile phase. Antibiotic treatment can prevent further disease progression.* In patients who do not receive antibiotics, the initial febrile phase continues for up to 2 weeks; patients have sustained high fevers and abdominal tenderness that may mimic appendicitis. *Rose spots*, small erythematous maculopapular lesions, are seen on the chest and abdomen. Symptoms abate after several weeks in those who survive, although relapse can occur. Systemic dissemination may cause *extraintestinal complications* including encephalopathy, meningitis, seizures, endocarditis, myocarditis, pneumonia, and cholecystitis. Patients with sickle cell disease are particularly susceptible to *Salmonella* osteomyelitis.

Yersinia

Three *Yersinia* species are human pathogens. *Y. enterocolitica* and *Y. pseudotuberculosis* cause GI disease and are discussed here; *Y. pestis*, the agent of pulmonic and bubonic plague, is discussed in Chapter 8. *Yersinia* infections of the GI system are more common in Europe than North America and are most frequently linked to ingestion of pork, raw milk, and contaminated water. *Y. enterocolitica* is far more common than *Y. pseudotuberculosis*, and infections tend to cluster in the winter, possibly related to inadequately cooked foods.

Pathogenesis. *Yersinia* invade M cells and use specialized bacterial proteins, called adhesins, to bind to host cell β_1

integrins. A pathogenicity island encodes an iron uptake system that mediates iron capture and transport; similar iron transport systems are also present in *E. coli*, *Klebsiella*, *Salmonella*, and enterobacteria. In *Yersinia*, iron enhances virulence and stimulates systemic dissemination, explaining why individuals with increased non-heme iron, such as those with certain chronic forms of anemia or hemochromatosis, are more likely to develop sepsis and are at greater risk for death.

MORPHOLOGY

Yersinia infections preferentially involve the ileum, appendix, and right colon (Fig. 17-28*B*). The organisms multiply extracellularly in lymphoid tissue, resulting in regional lymph node and Peyer patch hyperplasia as well as bowel wall thickening. The mucosa overlying lymphoid tissue may become hemorrhagic, and aphthous-like erosions and ulcers may develop, along with neutrophil infiltrates (Fig. 17-28*B*) and granulomas. This can result in diagnostic confusion with Crohn disease.

Clinical Features. People infected with *Yersinia* generally present with abdominal pain, but fever and diarrhea may also occur. Nausea, vomiting, and abdominal tenderness are common, and Peyer patch invasion with subsequent involvement of regional lymphatics can mimic acute appendicitis in teenagers and young adults. Enteritis and colitis predominate in younger children. *Extraintestinal symptoms of pharyngitis, arthralgia, and erythema nodosum occur frequently. Yersinia* can be detected by stool culture on *Yersinia*-selective agar. In cases with extraintestinal disease, cultures of lymph nodes or blood may also be positive. Postinfectious complications include reactive arthritis with urethritis and conjunctivitis, myocarditis, erythema nodosum, and kidney disease.

Escherichia coli

E. coli are gram-negative bacilli that colonize the healthy GI tract; most are nonpathogenic, but a subset cause human disease. The latter are classified according to morphology, mechanism of pathogenesis, and in vitro behavior. Subgroups with major clinical relevance include enterotoxigenic *E. coli* (ETEC), enteropathogenic *E. coli* (EPEC), enterohemorrhagic *E. coli* (EHEC), enteroinvasive *E. coli* (EIEC), and enteroaggregative *E. coli* (EAEC).

***Enterotoxigenic* E. coli. ETEC organisms are the principal cause of traveler's diarrhea and spread via contaminated food or water.** In developing countries, children younger than 2 years of age are particularly susceptible. ETEC produce heat-labile toxin (LT) and heat-stable toxin (ST), both induce chloride and water secretion while inhibiting intestinal fluid absorption. The LT toxin is similar to cholera toxin and activates adenylate cyclase, resulting in increased intracellular cAMP. This stimulates chloride secretion and, simultaneously, inhibits absorption. ST toxins, which have homology to the mammalian regulatory protein guanylin, bind to guanylate cyclase and increase intracellular cGMP with resulting effects on transport that are similar to those produced by LT. Like cholera, the histopathology induced by ETEC infection is limited. The patients have secretory, noninflammatory diarrhea, dehydration, and, in severe cases, shock.

***Enteropathogenic* E. coli.** EPEC are prevalent in developed and developing countries, where they are an important cause of endemic diarrhea as well as diarrheal outbreaks particularly in children less than 2 years of age. EPEC are characterized by their ability to produce attaching and effacing (A/E) lesions in which bacteria attach tightly to the enterocyte apical membranes and cause local loss, i.e. effacement, of the microvilli. The proteins necessary for creating A/E lesions are all encoded by large genomic pathogenicity island, the locus of enterocyte effacement (LEE), which is also present in many EHEC strains. These proteins include Tir, which is inserted into the intestinal epithelial cell plasma membrane. Tir acts as a receptor for the bacterial outer membrane protein intimin, which is encoded by the *espE* gene and is used for molecular detection and diagnosis of EPEC infection. The locus of enterocyte effacement also encodes a type III secretion system, similar to that in *Shigella*, that injects bacterial effector proteins into the epithelial cell cytoplasm. All EPEC strains lack genes to produce Shiga toxin.

***Enterohemorrhagic* E. coli. EHEC are categorized as *E. coli* O157:H7 and non-O157:H7 serotypes.** Because cows are a natural reservoir, it is not surprising that large outbreaks of *E. coli* O157:H7 infection in developed countries are often associated with the consumption of inadequately cooked ground beef. However, contaminated milk and vegetables are also vehicles for infection. Both O157:H7 and non-O157:H7 serotypes produce Shiga-like toxins, and therefore lesions (Fig. 17-28*C*) and clinical symptoms are similar to those resulting from *S. dysenteriae* infection. O157:H7 strains of EHEC are more likely than non-O157:H7 serotypes to cause large outbreaks, bloody diarrhea, *hemolytic-uremic syndrome,* and ischemic colitis. Importantly, antibiotics are not recommended for treatment because killing the bacteria can lead to increased release of Shiga-like toxins that enhance the risk of hemolytic uremic syndrome, especially in children.

***Enteroinvasive* E. coli. EIEC organisms are bacteriologically similar to *Shigella* and are transmitted via food, water, or by person-to-person contact.** While EIEC do not produce toxins, they invade epithelial cells and cause nonspecific features of acute self-limited colitis (Fig. 17-28*D*). EIEC infections are most common among young children in developing countries and are occasionally associated with outbreaks in developed countries.

***Enteroaggregative* E. coli. EAEC organisms were identified on the basis of their unique pattern of adherence to epithelial cells.** These organisms are now recognized as a cause of diarrhea in children and adults in developed as well as developing countries. EAEC can also cause traveler's diarrhea. The organisms attach to enterocytes via adherence fimbriae and are aided by dispersin, a bacterial surface protein that neutralizes the negative surface charge of lipopolysaccharide. While the bacteria do produce enterotoxins related to *Shigella* enterotoxin and ETEC ST toxin, histologic damage is minimal and the characteristic adherence lesions are only visible by electron microscopy.

EAEC organisms cause nonbloody diarrhea that may be prolonged in individuals with the acquired immunodeficiency syndrome.

Pseudomembranous Colitis

Pseudomembranous colitis, generally caused by *C. difficile*, can also be referred to as antibiotic-associated colitis or antibiotic-associated diarrhea. While antibiotic-associated diarrhea may also be caused by other organisms such as *Salmonella*, *C. perfringens* type A, or *Staphylococcus aureus* only *C. difficile* causes pseudomembranous colitis.

Pathogenesis. It is likely that disruption of the normal colonic microbiota by antibiotics allows *C. difficile* overgrowth. Almost any antibiotic may be responsible; the most important determinants of the disease are frequency of use and the affect on colonic microbiota. Immunosuppression is also a predisposing factor for *C. difficile* colitis. Toxins released by *C. difficile* cause the ribosylation of small GTPases, such as Rho, and lead to disruption of the epithelial cytoskeleton, tight junction barrier loss, cytokine release, and apoptosis. The mechanisms by which these processes lead to pseudomembranous colitis are incompletely understood.

MORPHOLOGY

Fully developed *C. difficile*–associated colitis is accompanied by formation of **pseudomembranes** (Fig. 17-29*A, B*), made up of an adherent layer of inflammatory cells and debris at sites of colonic mucosal injury. While pseudomembranes are not specific and may occur with ischemia or necrotizing infections, the histopathology of *C. difficile*-associated colitis is pathognomonic. The surface epithelium is denuded, and the superficial lamina propria contains a dense infiltrate of neutrophils and occasional fibrin thrombi within capillaries. Superficially damaged crypts are distended by a mucopurulent exudate that forms an eruption reminiscent of a volcano (Fig. 17-29*C*). These exudates coalesce to form pseudomembranes.

Clinical Features. *Risk factors for C. difficile–associated colitis include advanced age, hospitalization, and antibiotic treatment.* The organism is particularly prevalent in hospitals; as many as 30% of hospitalized adults are colonized with *C. difficile* (a rate tenfold greater than the general population), but most colonized patients are free of disease. Individuals with *C. difficile*–associated colitis present with fever, leukocytosis, abdominal pain, cramps, watery diarrhea, and dehydration. Protein loss can give rise to hypoalbuminemia. Fecal leukocytes and occult blood may be present, but grossly bloody diarrhea is uncommon. Diagnosis of *C. difficile*–associated colitis is usually accomplished by detection of *C. difficile* toxin, rather than culture, and is supported by the characteristic histopathology. Metronidazole or vancomycin are generally effective therapies, but antibiotic-resistant and hypervirulent *C. difficile* strains are increasingly common. Another major challenge in *C. difficile*–associated colitis is recurrent infection, which occurs in up to 40% of patients. New antibiotics, monoclonal antibodies against toxins A and B, and fecal microbial transplants can be effective therapies for recurrent *C. difficile* infection, but are not yet in widespread use.

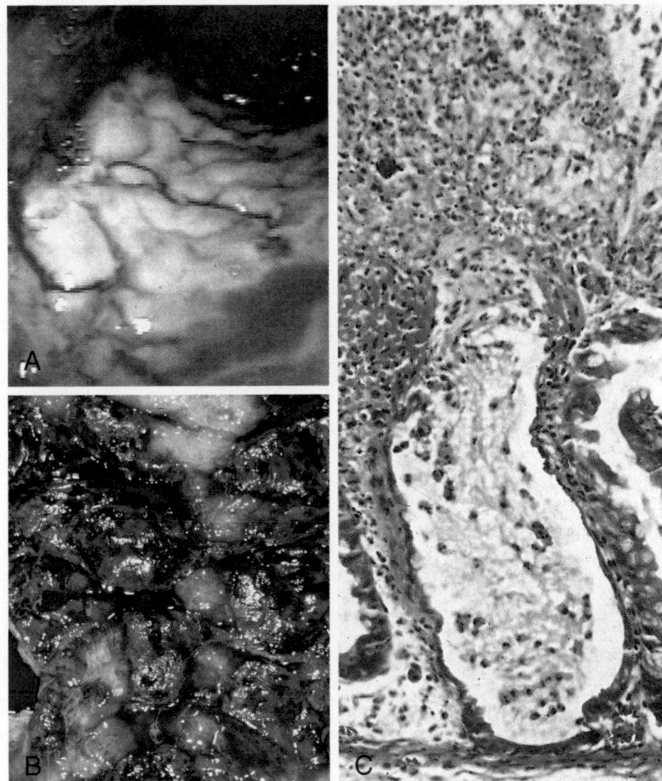

Figure 17-29 *Clostridium difficile* colitis. **A,** The colon is coated by tan pseudomembranes composed of neutrophils, dead epithelial cells, and inflammatory debris (endoscopic view). **B,** Pseudomembranes are easily appreciated on gross examination. **C,** Typical pattern of neutrophils emanating from a crypt is reminiscent of a volcanic eruption.

Whipple Disease

Whipple disease is a rare, multivisceral chronic disease first described as intestinal lipodystrophy in 1907 by George Hoyt Whipple. A mere 27 years later the pathologist went on to win the Nobel Prize for his work on pernicious anemia. He was a contemporary, but not a relative, of Allen Oldfather Whipple, the surgeon who pioneered the pancreatoduodenectomy.

Pathogenesis. Whipple's original case report described an individual with malabsorption, lymphadenopathy, and arthritis of undefined origin. Postmortem examination demonstrated the presence of foamy macrophages and large numbers of argyrophilic rods in the lymph nodes, suggesting that the disease was caused by a microbe. The gram-positive actinomycete, named *Tropheryma whippelii*, which is responsible for Whipple disease, was identified by PCR in 1992 and finally cultured in 2000. Clinical symptoms occur because organism-laden macrophages accumulate within the small intestinal lamina propria and mesenteric lymph nodes, causing lymphatic obstruction. Thus, *the malabsorptive diarrhea of Whipple disease is due to impaired lymphatic transport.*

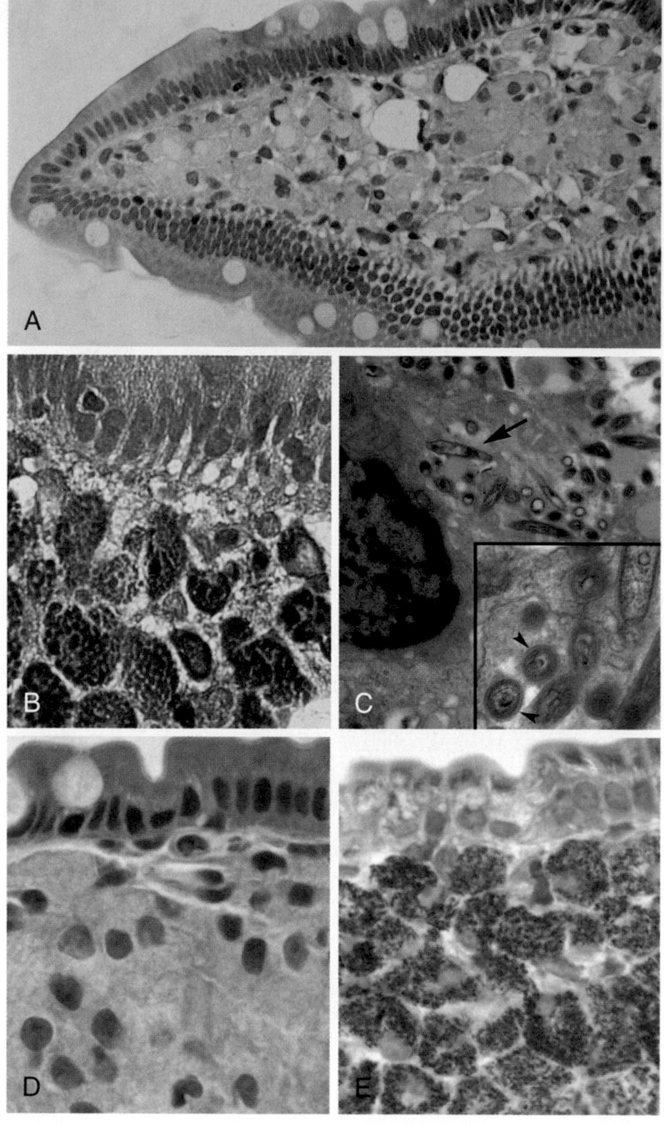

Figure 17-30 Whipple disease and mycobacterial infection. **A,** hematoxylin and eosin staining shows effacement of normal lamina propria by a sheet of swollen macrophages. **B,** PAS stain highlights macrophage lysosomes full of bacilli. Note the positive staining of mucous vacuoles in the overlying goblet cells. **C,** An electron micrograph of part of a macrophage shows bacilli within the cell (top arrow); also seen at higher magnification (inset). **D,** The morphology of mycobacterial infection can be similar to Whipple disease, particularly in the immunocompromised host. Compare with **A.** **E,** Mycobacteria are positive with stains for for acid-fast bacteria. (**C,** Courtesy George Kasnic and Dr. William Clapp, University of Florida, Gainesville, Fla.)

MORPHOLOGY

The morphologic hallmark of Whipple disease is a **dense accumulation of distended, foamy macrophages in the small intestinal lamina propria** (Fig. 17-30*A*). The macrophages contain periodic acid–Schiff (PAS)-positive, diastase-resistant granules that represent lysosomes stuffed with partially digested bacteria (Fig. 17-30*B*). Intact rod-shaped bacilli can also be identified by electron microscopy (Fig. 17-30*C*). A similar infiltrate of foamy macrophages is present in intestinal tuberculosis (Fig. 17-30*D*), and the organisms are PAS-positive in both diseases. The acid-fast stain can be helpful, since mycobacteria stain positively (Fig. 17-30E) while *T. whippelii* do not.

The **villous expansion** caused by the dense macrophage infiltrate imparts a shaggy gross appearance to the mucosal surface. Lymphatic dilatation and mucosal lipid deposition account for the common endoscopic detection of white to yellow mucosal plaques. In Whipple disease, bacteria-laden macrophages can accumulate within **mesenteric lymph nodes, synovial membranes of affected joints, cardiac valves, the brain,** and other sites.

Whipple disease is most common in Caucasian men, particularly farmers and others with occupational exposure to soil or animals. While there is no consistent familial clustering, the rarity of infection despite a large number of healthy carriers suggests that genetic risk factors may exist.

The clinical presentation of Whipple disease is usually a triad of diarrhea, weight loss, and arthralgia. Extraintestinal symptoms, which can exist for months or years before malabsorption, include arthritis, arthralgia, fever, lymphadenopathy, and neurologic, cardiac, or pulmonary disease.

Mycobacterial infections are considered in detail in Chapter 8.

Viral Gastroenteritis

Symptomatic human infection is caused by several distinct groups of viruses. The most common are discussed here.

Norovirus. This was previously known as Norwalk-like virus and is a common cause of nonbacterial gastroenteritis. These are small icosahedral viruses with a single-stranded RNA genome that forms a genus within the Caliciviridae family. **Norovirus causes approximately half of all gastroenteritis outbreaks worldwide and is a common cause of sporadic gastroenteritis in developed countries.** In the United States, noroviruses are the most common cause of acute gastroenteritis requiring medical attention and are second only to rotavirus as a cause of severe diarrhea in infants and young children. In developing countries, noroviruses cause more than 200,000 childhood deaths annually. Norovirus is expected to become the most common cause of diarrhea worldwide in all age groups as rotavirus vaccination becomes widespread.

Local norovirus outbreaks are usually related to contaminated food or water, but person-to-person transmission underlies most sporadic cases. Infections spread easily within schools, hospitals, nursing homes, and other large groups in close quarters, such as those on cruise ships. In these environments, vehicles of infection include airborne droplets, environmental surfaces and fomites.

Following a short incubation period, affected individuals develop nausea, vomiting, watery diarrhea, and abdominal pain. Biopsy morphology is nonspecific. When present, abnormalities are most evident in the small intestine and include mild villous shortening, epithelial vacuolization, loss of the microvillus brush border, crypt hypertrophy, and lamina propria infiltration by lymphocytes (Fig. 17-31*A*). The disease is self-limited in immunocompetent hosts.

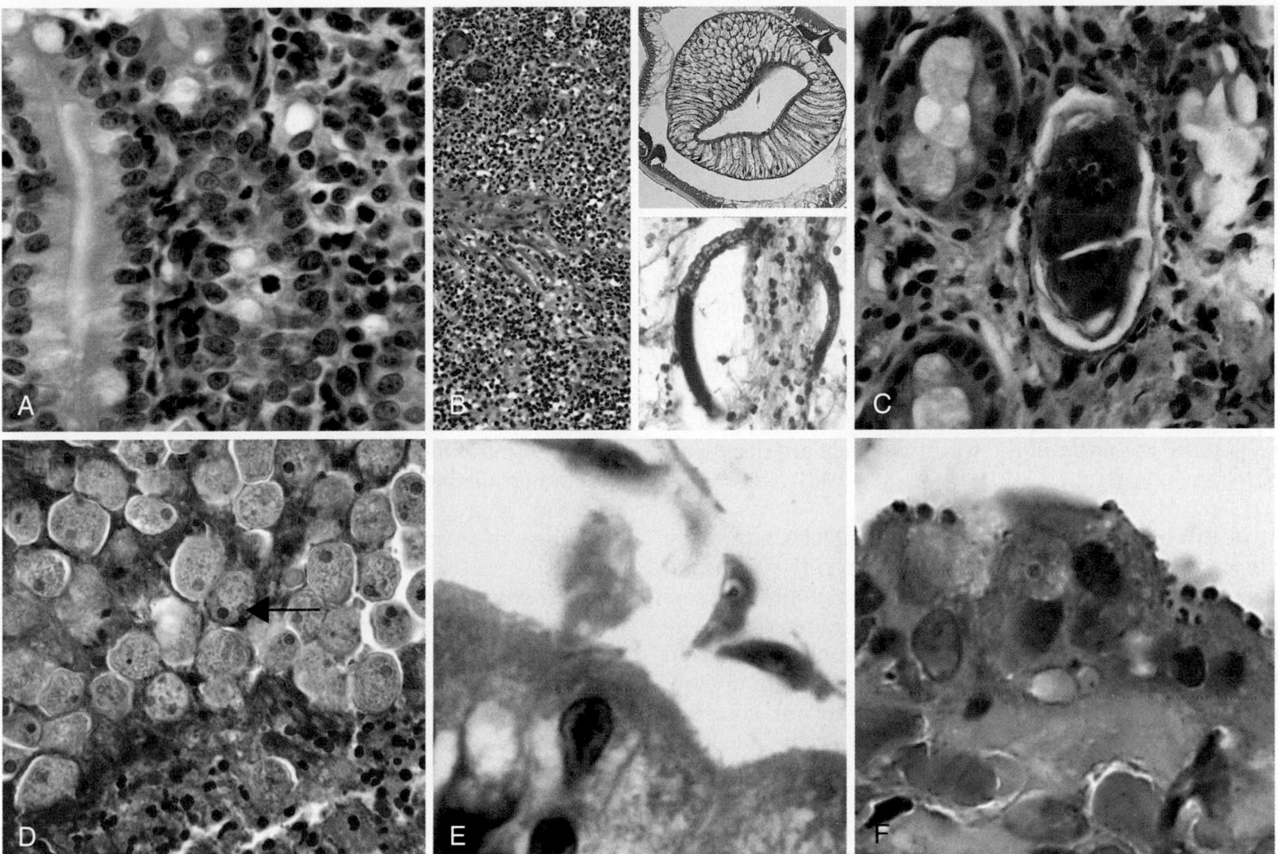

Figure 17-31 Infectious enteritis. **A,** Histologic features of viral enteritis include increased numbers of intraepithelial and lamina propria lymphocytes and crypt hypertrophy. **B,** Diffuse eosinophilic infiltrates in parasitic infection. This case was caused by *Ascaris* (upper inset), but a similar tissue reaction could be caused by *Strongyloides* (lower inset). **C,** Schistosomiasis can induce an inflammatory reaction to eggs trapped within the lamina propria. **D,** *Entamoeba histolytica* in a colon biopsy specimen. Note some organisms ingesting red blood cells *(arrow)*. **E,** *Giardia lamblia*, which are present in the luminal space over nearly normal-appearing villi, are easily overlooked. **F,** *Cryptosporidia* organisms are seen as small blue spheres that appear to lie on top of the brush border but are actually enveloped by a thin layer of host cell cytoplasm.

Norovirus infection in immunocompromised patients is a significant problem. Some data suggest that nearly 20% of patients on immunosuppression after renal transplantation or as treatment for graft-versus-host disease after hematopoietic stem cell transplantation are infected with norovirus and have intermittent diarrhea. Many of these patients fail to clear the infection, and diarrhea persists for an average of 9 months. The resulting malnutrition and dehydration can increase morbidity of the underlying disease.

Rotavirus. **This encapsulated virus with a segmented, double-stranded RNA genome infects 140 million people and causes 1 million deaths each year, making rotavirus a common cause of severe childhood diarrhea and diarrheal mortality worldwide.** Children between 6 and 24 months of age are most vulnerable. Protection in the first 6 months of life is probably due to the presence of antibodies in breast milk, while protection beyond 2 years is due to immunity that develops following the first or second infection. However, protection conferred by maternal antibodies seems to be less effective in India, Asia and Africa. Thus, in these locales infections are common in those younger than 6 months of age, hence early vaccination has been suggested. Because live, attenuated virus is used, vaccination is contraindicated in patients with immunodeficiency. Vaccination has also been associated with intussusception, as discussed earlier.

Rotavirus outbreaks in hospitals and daycare centers are common, and infection spreads easily; the estimated minimal infective inoculum is only 10 viral particles. Rotavirus selectively infects and destroys mature enterocytes in the small intestine, and the villus surface is repopulated by immature secretory cells. Enterocyte damage may be mediated by a viral factor called nonstructural protein 4 (NSP4), which can induce epithelial apoptosis. The loss of absorptive function and net secretion of water and electrolytes is compounded by an osmotic diarrhea caused by the incomplete absorption of nutrients. Like norovirus, rotavirus has a short incubation period followed by several days of vomiting and watery diarrhea.

Adenovirus. A common cause of pediatric diarrhea, adenovirus also affects immunocompromised patients. Small intestinal biopsy specimens can show epithelial degeneration but more often exhibit nonspecific villous atrophy and compensatory crypt hyperplasia. Viral nuclear inclusions are uncommon. Disease typically presents after an incubation period of 1 week with nonspecific symptoms that include diarrhea, vomiting, and abdominal pain. Fever and weight loss may also be present. Symptoms generally resolve within 10 days.

Parasitic Enterocolitis

Although viruses and bacteria are the predominant enteric pathogens in the United States, parasitic disease and protozoal infections affect more than one half of the world's population on a chronic or recurrent basis. The small intestine can harbor as many as 20 species of parasites, including nematodes, such as the roundworms *Ascaris* and *Strongyloides*; hookworms and pinworms; cestodes, including flatworms and tapeworms; trematodes, or flukes; and protozoa. Parasitic infections are covered in Chapter 8; those that are common in the intestinal tract are discussed briefly here.

Ascaris lumbricoides. This nematode infects more than a billion individuals worldwide as a result of human fecal-oral contamination. Ingested eggs hatch in the intestine and larvae penetrate the intestinal mucosa. Larvae then migrate from splanchnic to systemic circulation and, finally, enter the lungs to grow within the alveoli. Approximately 3 weeks later, the larvae are coughed up and swallowed. Upon return to the small intestine, the larvae mature into adult worms, which induce an eosinophil-rich inflammatory reaction (Fig. 17-31*B*) that can cause physical obstruction of the intestine or biliary tree. Larvae can also form hepatic abscesses and cause *Ascaris* pneumonitis. Diagnosis is usually made by detection of eggs in stool samples.

Strongyloides. The larvae of *Strongyloides* live in fecally contaminated ground soil and can penetrate unbroken skin. They migrate through the lungs, where they induce inflammatory infiltrates, and then reside in the intestine while maturing into adult worms. Unlike other intestinal worms, which require an ova or larval stage outside the human, the eggs of *Strongyloides* can hatch within the intestine and release larvae that penetrate the mucosa, causing autoinfection (Fig. 17-31*B*). Hence, *Strongyloides* infection can persist for life, and immunosuppressed individuals can develop overwhelming autoinfection. *Strongyloides* incite a strong tissue reaction and induce peripheral eosinophilia.

Necator duodenale *and* Ancylostoma duodenale. These hookworms infect 1 billion people worldwide and cause significant morbidity. Infection is initiated by larval penetration through the skin and, after further development in the lungs the larvae migrate up the trachea and are swallowed. Once in the duodenum the worms attach to the mucosa, suck blood, and reproduce. This causes multiple superficial erosions, focal hemorrhage, and inflammatory infiltrates and, in chronic infection, iron deficiency anemia. Diagnosis can be made by detection of the eggs in fecal smears.

Enterobius vermicularis. Also known as pinworms, these parasites infect people in industrialized and developing countries; in the United States as many as 40 million people have pinworms. Because they do not invade host tissue and live their entire life within the intestinal lumen, they rarely cause serious illness. Infection by *E. vermicularis*, or enterobiasis, is primarily by the fecal-oral route. Adult worms living in the intestine migrate to the anal orifice at night, where the female deposits eggs on the perirectal mucosa. The eggs cause intense irritation. Rectal and perineal pruritus ensues. The intense itching leads to contamination of the fingers, which promotes human-to-human transmission. Both eggs and adult pinworms remain viable outside the body, and repeat infection is common. Diagnosis can be made by applying cellophane tape to the perianal skin and examining the tape for eggs under a microscope.

Trichuris trichiura. Whipworms primarily infect young children. Similar to *E. vermicularis*, *Trichuris trichiura* does not penetrate the intestinal mucosa and rarely cause serious disease. Heavy infections, however, may cause bloody diarrhea and rectal prolapse.

Schistosomiasis. This disease involving the intestines most commonly takes the form of adult worms residing within the mesenteric veins. Symptoms of intestinal schistosomiasis are caused by trapping of eggs within the mucosa and submucosa (Fig. 17-31*C*). The resulting immune reaction is often granulomatous and can cause bleeding and even obstruction. More details are presented in Chapter 8.

Intestinal Cestodes. The three primary species of cestodes that affect humans are *Diphyllobothrium latum*, fish tapeworms; *Taenia solium*, pork tapeworms; and *Hymenolepis nana*, dwarf tapeworms. They reside exclusively within the intestinal lumen and are transmitted by ingestion of raw or undercooked fish, meat, or pork that contains encysted larvae. Release of the larvae allows attachment to the intestinal mucosa through its head, or scolex. The worm derives its nutrients from the food stream and enlarges by formation of egg-filled segments termed proglottids. Humans are usually infected by a single worm, and since the worm does not penetrate the intestinal mucosa, peripheral eosinophilia does not generally occur. Nevertheless, the parasite burden can be staggering, since adult worms can grow to many meters in length. Large numbers of proglottids and eggs are shed in the feces. Clinical symptoms include abdominal pain, diarrhea, and nausea, but the majority of cases are asymptomatic. Occasionally, *D. latum* causes B_{12} deficiency and megaloblastic anemia because it competes with the host for dietary B_{12}. Identification of proglottids and eggs in stools is the most efficient method of diagnosis.

Entamoeba histolytica. This protozoan causes amebiasis and is spread by fecal-oral transmission. *E. histolytica* infects approximately 500 million people in countries such as India, Mexico, and Colombia, and causes 40 million cases of dysentery and liver abscess annually. *E. histolytica* cysts, which have a chitin wall and four nuclei, are resistant to gastric acid, a characteristic that allows them to pass through the stomach without harm. Cysts then colonize the epithelial surface of the colon and release trophozoites, ameboid forms that reproduce under anaerobic conditions.

While amebiasis affects the cecum and ascending colon, most often, the sigmoid colon, rectum, and appendix can also be involved. Dysentery develops when the amebae attach to the colonic epithelium, induce apoptosis, invade crypts, and burrow laterally into the lamina propria. This recruits neutrophils, causes tissue damage, and creates a flask-shaped ulcer with a narrow neck and broad base. Histologic diagnosis can be difficult, since amebae are similar to macrophages in size and general appearance (Fig. 17-31*D*). Parasites may penetrate splanchnic vessels and embolize to the liver to produce abscesses in about 40% of patients with amebic dysentery. Amebic liver abscesses, which can exceed 10 cm in diameter, have a scant inflammatory reaction at their margins and a shaggy fibrin lining. The abscesses persist after the acute intestinal illness has passed and may, rarely, reach the lung and the heart by direct extension. Amebae may also spread to the kidneys and brain via the bloodstream.

Individuals with amebiasis may present with abdominal pain, bloody diarrhea, or weight loss. Occasionally, acute necrotizing colitis and megacolon occur, and both are associated with significant mortality. The parasites lack mitochondria or Krebs cycle enzymes and are thus obligate fermenters of glucose. Metronidazole, which inhibits pyruvate oxidoreductase, an enzyme required for fermentation, is the most effective treatment for systemic disease.

Giardia lamblia. These organisms, also referred to as *G. duodenalis* or *G. intestinalis,* were initially described by van Leeuwenhoek, the inventor of the microscope, who discovered the pathogen in his own stool. *Giardia lamblia* are the most common parasitic pathogen in humans and are spread by fecally contaminated water or food. Infection may occur after ingestion of as few as 10 cysts. Because cysts are resistant to chlorine, *Giardia* are endemic in unfiltered public water supplies. They are commonly present in rural streams, explaining infection in campers who use these as a water source. Infection may also occur by the fecal-oral route and, because the cysts are stable, they may be accidentally swallowed while swimming in contaminated water.

Giardia are flagellated protozoans that cause decreased expression of brush-border enzymes, including lactase. In addition they cause microvillous damage and apoptosis of small intestinal epithelial cells. Secretory IgA and mucosal IL-6 responses are important for clearance of *Giardia* infections. Immunosuppressed, agammaglobulinemic, or malnourished individuals are often severely affected. *Giardia* can evade immune clearance through continuous modification of the major surface antigen, variant surface protein, and can persist for months or years while causing intermittent symptoms.

Giardia trophozoites can be identified in duodenal biopsies based on their characteristic pear shape and the presence of two equally sized nuclei. Despite large numbers of trophozoites, which are tightly bound to the brush border of villous enterocytes, there is no invasion and small intestinal morphology may be normal (Fig. 17-31*E*). However, villous blunting with increased numbers of intraepithelial lymphocytes and mixed lamina propria inflammatory infiltrates can develop in patients with heavy infections.

Giardiasis may be subclinical or accompanied by acute or chronic diarrhea, malabsorption, and weight loss. Infection is usually documented by immunofluorescent detection of cysts in stool samples. Although oral antimicrobial therapy is effective, recurrence is common.

Cryptosporidium. Like *Giardia,* cryptosporidia are an important cause of diarrhea worldwide. Cryptosporidiosis was first discovered in the 1980s as an agent of *chronic diarrhea in AIDS patients* and is now recognized as a cause of acute, self-limited disease in immunologically normal hosts. Cryptosporidiosis also causes persistent diarrhea in residents of developing countries. The organisms are present worldwide, with the exception of Antarctica, perhaps because the oocysts are killed by freezing. The oocysts are resistant to chlorine and may, therefore, persist in treated, but unfiltered, water. Contaminated drinking water continues to be the most common means of transmission. The largest documented outbreak, a result of inadequate water purification, occurred in 1993 in Milwaukee, Wisconsin, and affected more than 400,000 people. Like giardiasis, cryptosporidiosis can be spread to water sport participants via contaminated water. Food-borne infection occurs less frequently.

Humans are infected by several different *Cryptosporidium* species, including *C. hominis* and *C. parvum*. All are able to go through an entire life cycle, with asexual and sexual reproductive phases, in a single host. The ingested encysted oocyte, of which 10 are sufficient to cause symptomatic infection, releases sporozoites following activation of proteases by gastric acid. The sporozoites are motile and have a specialized organelle that attaches to the brush border and causes changes in the enterocyte cytoskeleton. These changes induce the enterocyte to engulf the parasite, which takes up residence in an endocytic vacuole within the microvilli. The presence of the parasite leads to sodium malabsorption, chloride secretion, and increased tight junction permeability, which are responsible for the nonbloody, watery diarrhea that ensues.

Mucosal histology is often only minimally altered, but persistent cryptosporidiosis in children and heavy infection in immunosuppressed patients can result in villous atrophy, crypt hyperplasia, and inflammatory infiltrates. Although the sporozoite is intracellular, it appears, by light microscopy, to sit on top of the epithelial apical membrane (Fig. 17-31*F*). Organisms are typically most concentrated in the terminal ileum and proximal colon, but can be present throughout the gut, biliary tract, and even the respiratory tract of immunodeficient hosts. Diagnosis is based on finding oocysts in the stool.

KEY CONCEPTS

Infectious Enterocolitis

- ***Vibrio cholerae*** secrete a preformed toxin that causes massive chloride secretion. Water follows the resulting osmotic gradient, leading to *secretory diarrhea*.
- ***Campylobacter jejuni*** is the most common bacterial enteric pathogen in developed countries and also causes traveler's diarrhea. Most isolates are noninvasive.
- ***Salmonella* and *Shigella* spp.** are invasive and associated with and exudative bloody diarrhea (dysentery).
- ***Salmonella* infection** is a common cause of food poisoning.

- ***S. typhi*** can cause systemic disease (typhoid fever).
- **Pseudomembranous colitis** is often triggered by antibiotic therapy that allows colonization by ***Clostridium difficile***. The organism releases toxins that disrupt epithelial function. The associated inflammatory response includes characteristic volcano-like eruptions of neutrophils from colonic crypts that spread to form mucopurulent pseudomembranes.
- **Norovirus** is a very common cause of self limited diarrhea both in adults and children. It spreads from person to person in sporadic cases and by water in epidemic cases.
- **Rotavirus** is the most common cause of severe childhood diarrhea and diarrheal mortality worldwide. The diarrhea is caused by loss of mature enterocytes, resulting in malabsorption as well as secretion.
- **Parasitic and protozoal infections** affect more than one half of the world's population on a chronic or recurrent basis. Each parasite has a distinctive life cycle and tissue reaction. Most are associated with tissue and systemic eosinophilia.

Irritable Bowel Syndrome

Irritable bowel syndrome (IBS) is characterized by chronic, relapsing abdominal pain, bloating, and changes in bowel habits. Despite very real symptoms, the gross and microscopic evaluation is normal in most IBS patients. Thus, the diagnosis depends on clinical symptoms and functional testing. It should be recognized that IBS is a syndrome, and that multiple illnesses are represented under this global descriptor. IBS is currently divided into several subtypes, as defined by successive revisions of the Rome criteria.

Pathogenesis. The pathogenesis of IBS remains poorly defined, although there is clearly interplay between psychologic stressors, diet, perturbation of the gut microbiome, increased enteric sensory responses to gastrointestinal stimuli, and abnormal GI motility. For example, patients with *constipation-predominant* or *diarrhea-predominant* IBS tend to have decreased or increased colonic contractions and transit rates, respectively. Excess bile acid synthesis or bile acid malabsorption has been identified as one cause of diarrhea-predominant IBS, likely due to the effects of bile acids on intestinal motility.

Other data link disturbances in enteric nervous system function to IBS, suggesting a role for defective brain-gut axis signaling. Consistent with this, deep sequencing and genome wide association studies have linked several candidate genes to IBS, including serotonin reuptake transporters, cannabinoid receptors, and TNF-related inflammatory mediators. Further, 5-HT3 receptor anatagonists are effective in many cases of diarrhea-predominant IBS. Opioids and psychoactive drugs with anti-cholinergic effects are also commonly used to treat diarrhea-predominant IBS.

A separate group of IBS patients, relate onset to a bout of infectious gastroenteritis, suggesting that immune activation or, alternatively, a shift in the gut microbiome may trigger some cases. While unproven, this could explain the efficacy of fecal transplantation in some IBS cases.

There may be some overlap in mechanisms underlying constipation-predominant and diarrhea-predominant IBS. For example, single nucleotide polymorphisms in immune mediators have been detected in both.

Clinical Features. The peak prevalence of IBS is between 20 and 40 years of age, and there is a significant female predominance. Variability in diagnostic criteria makes it difficult to establish the incidence, but most authors report prevalence in developed countries of between 5% and 10%. IBS is presently diagnosed using clinical criteria that require the occurrence of abdominal pain or discomfort at least 3 days per month over 3 months with improvement following defecation and a change in stool frequency or form. Other causes, such as enteric infection or inflammatory bowel disease, must be excluded.

IBS is not associated with serious long-term sequelae, but affected patients may undergo unnecessary abdominal surgery due to chronic pain and their ability to function socially may be compromised. The prognosis of IBS is most closely related to symptom duration, with longer duration correlating with reduced likelihood of improvement.

Inflammatory Bowel Disease

Inflammatory bowel disease (IBD) is a chronic condition resulting from inappropriate mucosal immune activation. The two disorders that comprise IBD are *ulcerative colitis* and *Crohn disease.* Descriptions of ulcerative colitis and Crohn disease date back to antiquity and at least the sixteenth century, respectively, but it took modern microbiologic techniques to exclude conventional infectious etiologies for these diseases. As will be discussed later, however, the luminal microbiota likely play a role in the pathogenesis of IBD.

The distinction between ulcerative colitis and Crohn disease is based, in large part, on the distribution of affected sites (Fig. 17-32) and the morphologic expression of disease (Table 17-9) at those sites. **Ulcerative colitis is limited to the colon and rectum and extends only into the mucosa and submucosa. In contrast, Crohn disease, which has also been referred to as regional enteritis (because of frequent ileal involvement) may involve any area of the GI tract and is typically transmural.**

Epidemiology. Ulcerative colitis and Crohn disease frequently present in the teens and early 20s, with the former being slightly more common in females. IBD is most common among Caucasians and, in the United States, occurs 3 to 5 times more often among eastern European (Ashkenazi) Jews than the general population. This is at least partly due to genetic factors, as discussed later. The geographic distribution of IBD is highly variable, but it is most common in North America, northern Europe, and Australia. However, IBD incidence worldwide is on the rise, and it is becoming more common in regions such as Africa, South America, and Asia where its prevalence was historically low. The hygiene hypothesis suggests that this increasing incidence is related to improved food storage conditions, decreased food contamination, and changes in

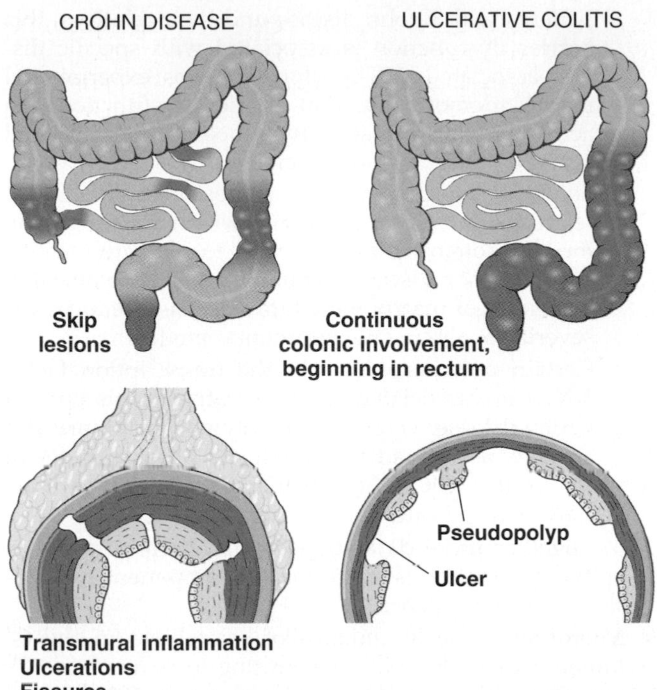

Figure 17-32 Distribution of lesions in inflammatory bowel disease. The distinction between Crohn disease and ulcerative colitis is primarily based on morphology.

gut microbiome composition. Apparently this results in inadequate development of regulatory processes that limit mucosal immune responses. This in turn allows some mucosa-associated microbial organisms to trigger persistent and chronic inflammation in susceptible hosts. Although many details to support this hypothesis are lacking, the observation that helminth infections, which are endemic in regions where IBD incidence is low, can prevent IBD development in animal models and even reduce disease in some patients, lends support to this idea.

Pathogenesis. Although precise causes are not yet defined **most investigators believe that IBD results from the combined effects of alterations in host interactions with intestinal microbiota, intestinal epithelial dysfunction, aberrant mucosal immune responses, and altered composition of the gut microbiome.** This view is supported by epidemiologic, genetic, and clinical studies as well as data from laboratory models of IBD (Fig. 17-33).

- **Genetics.** There is compelling evidence that genetic factors contribute to IBD. Risk of disease is increased when there is an affected family member and, in Crohn disease, the concordance rate for monozygotic twins approaches 50%. Genetic factors may also contribute to phenotypic expression of the disease, because twins affected by Crohn disease tend to present within a few years of each other and develop disease in similar regions of the GI tract. The concordance of monozygotic twins for ulcerative colitis is only about 15%, suggesting that genetic factors are less dominant than in Crohn disease. Concordance for dizygotic twins is less than 10% for both forms of IBD.

Population based genome wide association studies have identified over 160 IBD-associated genes. Most of these are shared between Crohn disease and ulcerative colitis, as well as other complex immune-mediated diseases. Interestingly, several IBD associated genes overlap with genes involved in responses to mycobacteria, including *Mycobacterium tuberculosis* and *Mycobacterium leprae*. This supports the idea that host-microbial interactions are critical to the pathogenesis of IBD and may explain some overlap in the histopathology of Crohn disease and mycobacterial infection. One of genes most strongly associated with Crohn disease is *NOD2* (nucleotide oligomerization binding domain 2), which encodes an intracellular protein that binds to bacterial peptidoglycans and activates signaling events, including the NF-κB pathway. Despite the increase in risk attributable to *NOD2* polymorphisms, it should be remembered that fewer than 10% of individuals carrying risk associated *NOD2* variants develop disease. Thus, as is the case with all IBD-associated genes, any one gene confers only a small increase in the risk of developing these diseases.

In addition to *NOD2,* two Crohn disease–related genes of particular interest are *ATG16L1* (autophagy-related 16-like), and *IRGM* (immunity-related GTPase M). Both are part of the autophagy pathways that are critical for cellular responses to intracellular bacteria; *ATG16L1* may also regulate epithelial homeostasis.

NOD2, ATG16L1, and *IRGM* are expressed in multiple cell types, and their precise roles in the pathogenesis of Crohn disease have yet to be defined. However, all

Table 17-9 Features That Differ between Crohn Disease and Ulcerative Colitis

Feature	Crohn Disease	Ulcerative Colitis
Macroscopic		
Bowel region	Ileum ± colon	Colon only
Distribution	Skip lesions	Diffuse
Stricture	Yes	Rare
Wall appearance	Thick	Thin
Microscopic		
Inflammation	Transmural	Limited to mucosa
Pseudopolyps	Moderate	Marked
Ulcers	Deep, knife-like	Superficial, broad-based
Lymphoid reaction	Marked	Moderate
Fibrosis	Marked	Mild to none
Serositis	Marked	Mild to none
Granulomas	Yes (~35%)	No
Fistulae/sinuses	Yes	No
Clinical		
Perianal fistula	Yes (in colonic disease)	No
Fat/vitamin malabsorption	Yes	No
Malignant potential	With colonic involvement	Yes
Recurrence after surgery	Common	No
Toxic megacolon	No	Yes

All features may not be present in a single case.

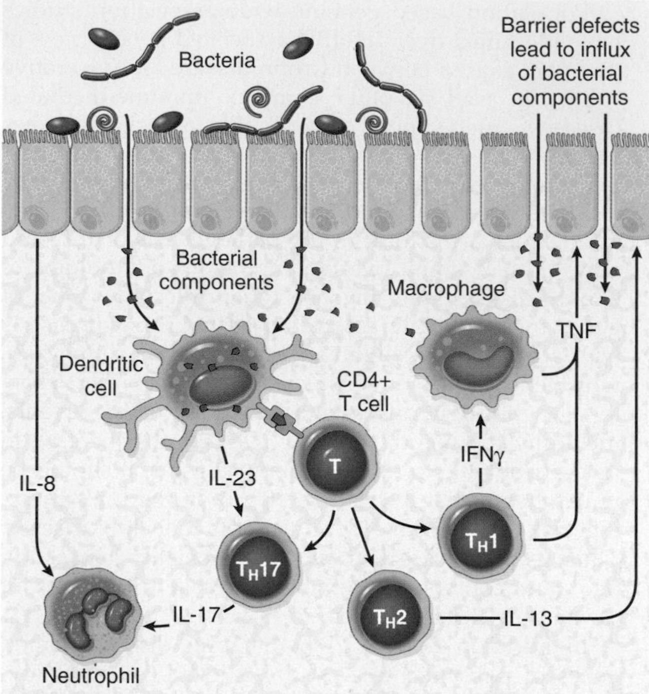

Figure 17-33 One model of IBD pathogenesis. Aspects of both Crohn disease and ulcerative colitis are shown. See text for details.

three are involved in recognition and response to intracellular pathogens, supporting the hypothesis that inappropriate immune reactions to luminal bacteria are an important component of IBD pathogenesis.

- **Mucosal immune responses.** Several observations support a role for mucosal immune responses in the pathogenesis of IBD. Some of these are:
  - T helper cells are activated in Crohn disease and the response is polarized to the T_H1 type (see Chapter 6)
  - T_H17 T cells most likely contribute to disease pathogenesis. Consistent with this, certain polymorphisms of the IL-23 receptor, which is involved in the development and maintenance of T_H17 cells, confer marked reductions in the risk of both Crohn disease and ulcerative colitis.
  - Many other pro-inflammatory cytokines, including TNF, interferon-γ and IL-13, as well as immunoregulatory molecules such as IL-10 and TGF-β, appear to be play a role the pathogenesis of IBD. The role of IL-10 is supported by the observations that autosomal recessive mutations of the IL-10 and IL-10 receptor genes are linked to severe, early onset IBD.

  Overall, while details remain to be defined, it is clear that deranged mucosal immune activation and defective immunoregulation contribute to the development of ulcerative colitis and Crohn disease. Immunosuppresive agents remain the mainstay of treatment for these conditions.
- **Epithelial defects.** A variety of epithelial defects have been described in both Crohn disease and ulcerative colitis. Some examples follow:
  - Defects in intestinal epithelial tight junction barrier function are present in Crohn disease patients and a subset of their healthy first-degree relatives. In patients with Crohn disease and their relatives, this barrier dysfunction is associated with specific disease-associated *NOD2* polymorphisms; experimental models demonstrate that barrier dysfunction can activate innate and adaptive mucosal immunity and sensitize subjects to disease.
  - Some polymorphisms, such as those involving *ECM1* (extracellular matrix protein 1), which inhibits matrix metalloproteinase 9, are linked to ulcerative colitis but not Crohn disease. In this context it is notable that inhibition of matrix metalloproteinase 9 reduces the severity of colitis in experimental models.
  - Certain polymorphisms in the transcription factor *HNFA* are associated with ulcerative colitis but not Crohn disease. These *HNFA* polymorphisms are also strongly associated with maturity onset diabetes of the young (MODY), which like IBD, is associated with reduced intestinal barrier function.

  Together these data suggest that, derangements in epithelial function is an important component are critical to IBD pathogenesis.
- **Microbiota.** The abundance of microbiota in the GI lumen is overwhelming, amounting to as much as 10^{12} organisms per milliliter in the colon and 50% of fecal mass. In total, these organisms greatly outnumber human cells in our bodies, a sober reminder that at a cellular level, we may be only about 10% human. A sampling of data that supports the notion that microbiota play a role in the evolution of IBD follows:
  - As mentioned earlier, linkage to NOD2, points to the involvement of microbes in the causation of Crohn disease.
  - The presence of antibodies against the bacterial protein flagellin are most common in Crohn disease patients who have disease associated *NOD2* variants, stricture formation, perforation, and small-bowel involvement. In contrast, anti-flagellin antibodies are uncommon in ulcerative colitis patients.
  - Microbial transfer studies are able to induce or reduce disease in animal models of IBD, and clinical trials suggest that probiotic (or beneficial) bacteria or even fecal microbial transplants from healthy individuals may benefit IBD patients.

One model that unifies the roles of intestinal microbiota, epithelial function, and mucosal immunity suggests a cycle by which transepithelial flux of luminal bacterial components activates innate and adaptive immune responses. In a genetically susceptible host, the subsequent release of TNF and other immune-mediated signals direct epithelia to increase tight junction permeability, which causes further increases in the in flux of luminal material. These events may establish a self-amplifying cycle that gives rise to maladaptative and injurious immune responses.

Crohn Disease

Crohn disease, an eponym based on the 1932 description by Crohn, Ginzburg, and Oppenheimer, has existed for centuries. Louis XIII of France (1601-1643) suffered relapsing bloody diarrhea, fever, rectal abscess, small intestinal and colonic ulcers, and fistulae beginning at age 20 years, most likely due to Crohn disease.

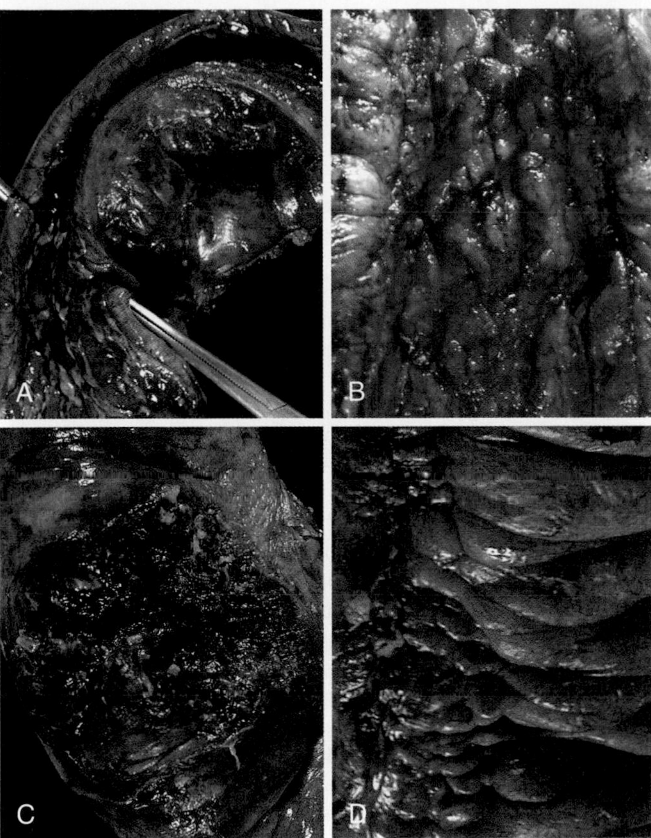

Figure 17-34 Gross pathology of Crohn disease. **A,** Small-intestinal stricture. **B,** Linear mucosal ulcers, which impart a cobblestone appearance to the mucosa, and thickened intestinal wall. **C,** Perforation and associated serositis. **D,** Creeping fat.

MORPHOLOGY

Crohn disease may occur in any area of the GI tract, but the most common sites involved at presentation are the terminal ileum, ileocecal valve, and cecum. Disease is limited to the small intestine alone in about 40% of cases; the small intestine and colon are both involved in 30% of patients; the remainder have only colonic involvement. The presence of multiple, separate, sharply delineated areas of disease, resulting in **skip lesions**, is characteristic of Crohn disease and may help in the differentiation from ulcerative colitis. Strictures are common in Crohn disease, but do not generally develop in ulcerative colitis (Fig. 17-34*A*).

The earliest lesion, the **aphthous ulcer**, may progress, and multiple lesions often coalesce into elongated, serpentine ulcers oriented along the axis of the bowel (Fig. 17-34*B*). Edema and loss of the normal mucosal texture are common. Sparing of interspersed mucosa, a result of the patchy distribution of Crohn disease, results in a coarsely textured, **cobblestone** appearance in which diseased tissue is depressed below the level of normal mucosa (Fig. 17-34*B*). **Fissures** frequently develop between mucosal folds and may extend deeply to become fistula tracts or sites of perforation (Fig. 17-34*C*). The intestinal wall is thickened and rubbery as a consequence of transmural edema, inflammation, submucosal fibrosis, and hypertrophy of the muscularis propria, all of which contribute to stricture formation (Fig. 17-34*A*). In cases with extensive transmural disease, mesenteric fat frequently extends around the serosal surface **(creeping fat)** (Fig. 17-34*D*).

The microscopic features of active Crohn disease include abundant neutrophils that infiltrate and damage crypt epithelium. Clusters of neutrophils within a crypt are referred to as **crypt abscesses** and are often associated with crypt destruction. Ulceration is common in Crohn disease, and there may be an abrupt transition between ulcerated and adjacent normal mucosa. Even in areas where gross examination suggests diffuse disease, microscopic pathology can appear patchy. Repeated cycles of crypt destruction and regeneration lead to **distortion of mucosal architecture**; the normally straight and parallel crypts take on bizarre branching shapes and unusual orientations to one another (Fig. 17-35*A*). Epithelial metaplasia, another consequence of chronic relapsing injury, often takes the form of gastric antral-appearing glands, and is called pseudopyloric metaplasia. **Paneth cell metaplasia** may also occur in the left colon, where Paneth cells are normally absent. These architectural and metaplastic changes may persist even when active inflammation has resolved. Mucosal atrophy, with loss of crypts, may occur after years of disease. **Noncaseating granulomas** (Fig. 17-35*B*), a hallmark of Crohn disease, are found in approximately 35% of cases and may occur in areas of active disease or uninvolved regions in any layer of the intestinal wall (Fig. 17-35*C*). Granulomas may also be present in mesenteric lymph nodes. Cutaneous granulomas form nodules that are referred to as **metastatic Crohn disease** (a misnomer since there is no cancer). The absence of granulomas does not preclude a diagnosis of Crohn disease.

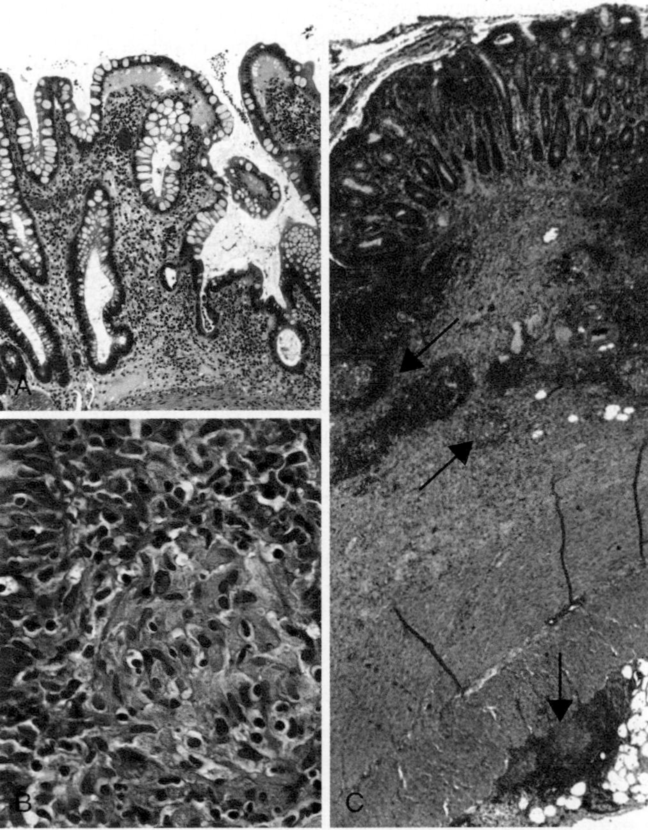

Figure 17-35 Microscopic pathology of Crohn disease. **A,** Haphazard crypt organization results from repeated injury and regeneration. **B,** Noncaseating granuloma. **C,** Transmural Crohn disease with submucosal and serosal granulomas (arrows).

Clinical Features. The clinical manifestations of Crohn disease are extremely variable. In most patients disease begins with intermittent attacks of relatively mild diarrhea, fever, and abdominal pain. Approximately 20% of patients present acutely with right lower quadrant pain, fever, and bloody diarrhea that may mimic acute appendicitis or bowel perforation. Periods of active disease are typically interrupted by asymptomatic periods that last for weeks to many months. Disease re-activation can be associated with a variety of external triggers, including physical or emotional stress, specific dietary items, and cigarette smoking. The latter is a strong exogenous risk factor for development of Crohn disease and, in some cases, disease onset is associated with initiation of smoking. Unfortunately, smoking cessation does not result in disease remission.

Iron-deficiency anemia may develop in individuals with colonic disease, while extensive small bowel disease may result in serum protein loss and hypoalbuminemia, generalized nutrient malabsorption, or malabsorption of vitamin B_{12} and bile salts. *Fibrosing strictures,* particularly of the terminal ileum, are common and require surgical resection. Disease often recurs at the site of anastomosis, and as many as 40% of patients require additional resections within 10 years. *Fistulae* develop between loops of bowel and may also involve the urinary bladder, vagina, and abdominal or perianal skin. *Perforations* and peritoneal abscesses are common. Anti-TNF antibodies have revolutionized treatment of Crohn disease, and other biologic therapies are becoming available.

Extraintestinal manifestations of Crohn disease include uveitis, migratory polyarthritis, sacroiliitis, ankylosing spondylitis, erythema nodosum, and clubbing of the fingertips, any of which may develop before intestinal disease is recognized. Pericholangitis and primary sclerosing cholangitis occur in Crohn disease with a higher frequency than in those without Crohn disease, but are even more common in those who have ulcerative colitis (see below and Chapter 18). As discussed later, risk of colonic adenocarcinoma is increased in patients with long-standing IBD affecting the colon.

Ulcerative Colitis

Ulcerative colitis is closely related to Crohn disease. However, the disease in ulcerative colitis is limited to the colon and rectum. Common extraintestinal manifestations of ulcerative colitis overlap with those of Crohn disease and include migratory polyarthritis, sacroiliitis, ankylosing spondylitis, uveitis, and skin lesions. Approximately 2.5% to 7.5% of individuals with ulcerative colitis also have primary sclerosis cholangitis (Chapter 18). The long-term outlook for ulcerative colitis patients depends on the severity of active disease and disease duration.

MORPHOLOGY

Grossly, ulcerative colitis always involves the rectum and extends proximally in a continuous fashion to involve part or all of the colon. Disease of the entire colon is termed pancolitis (Fig. 17-36*A*), while left-sided disease extends no farther than the transverse colon. Limited distal disease may be referred to descriptively as ulcerative proctitis or ulcerative proctosigmoiditis. The small intestine is normal, although mild mucosal inflammation of the distal ileum, termed backwash ileitis, may be present in severe cases of pancolitis. Skip lesions are not seen (although focal appendiceal or cecal inflammation may occasionally be present in left-sided ulcerative colitis).

Grossly, involved colonic mucosa may be slightly red and granular or have extensive, **broad-based ulcers**. There can be an abrupt transition between diseased and uninvolved colon (Fig. 17-36*B*). Ulcers are aligned along the long axis of the colon but do not typically replicate the serpentine ulcers of Crohn disease. Isolated islands of regenerating mucosa often bulge into the lumen to create **pseudopolyps** (Fig. 17-36*C*), and the tips of these polyps may fuse to create **mucosal bridges** (Fig. 17-36*D*). Chronic disease may lead to **mucosal atrophy** with a flat and smooth mucosal surface that lacks normal folds. Unlike Crohn disease, **mural thickening is not present, the serosal surface is normal, and strictures do not occur**. However, inflammation and inflammatory mediators can damage the muscularis propria and disturb neuromuscular function leading to colonic dilation and **toxic megacolon**, which carries a significant risk of perforation.

Histologic features of mucosal disease in ulcerative colitis are similar to colonic Crohn disease and include inflammatory infiltrates, crypt abscesses (Fig. 17-37*A*), crypt distortion, and pseudopyloric epithelial metaplasia (Fig. 17-37*B*). However, **the inflammatory process is diffuse and generally limited to the mucosa and superficial submucosa** (Fig. 17-37*C*). In severe cases, extensive mucosal destruction may be accompanied by ulcers that extend more deeply into the submucosa, but the muscularis propria is rarely involved. Submucosal fibrosis, mucosal atrophy, and distorted mucosal architecture remain as residua of healed disease but histology may also revert to near normal after prolonged remission. **Granulomas are not present** in ulcerative colitis.

Clinical Features. Ulcerative colitis is a relapsing disorder characterized by attacks of bloody diarrhea with stringy, mucoid material, lower abdominal pain, and cramps that are temporarily relieved by defecation. These symptoms may persist for days, weeks, or months before they subside. The initial attack may, in some cases, be severe enough to constitute a medical or surgical emergency. More than half of patients have clinically mild disease, although almost all experience at least one relapse during a 10-year period, and up to 30% require colectomy within the first 3 years after presentation because of uncontrollable symptoms. Colectomy effectively cures intestinal disease in ulcerative colitis, but extraintestinal manifestations may persist.

The factors that trigger ulcerative colitis are not known, but infectious enteritis precedes disease onset in some cases. In other cases the first attack is preceded by psychologic stress, which may also be linked to relapse during remission. The initial onset of symptoms has also been reported to occur shortly after smoking cessation in some patients, and smoking may partially relieve symptoms. Unfortunately, studies of nicotine as a therapeutic agent have been disappointing.

Indeterminate Colitis

Because of the extensive pathologic and clinical overlap between ulcerative colitis and Crohn disease (Table 17-9),

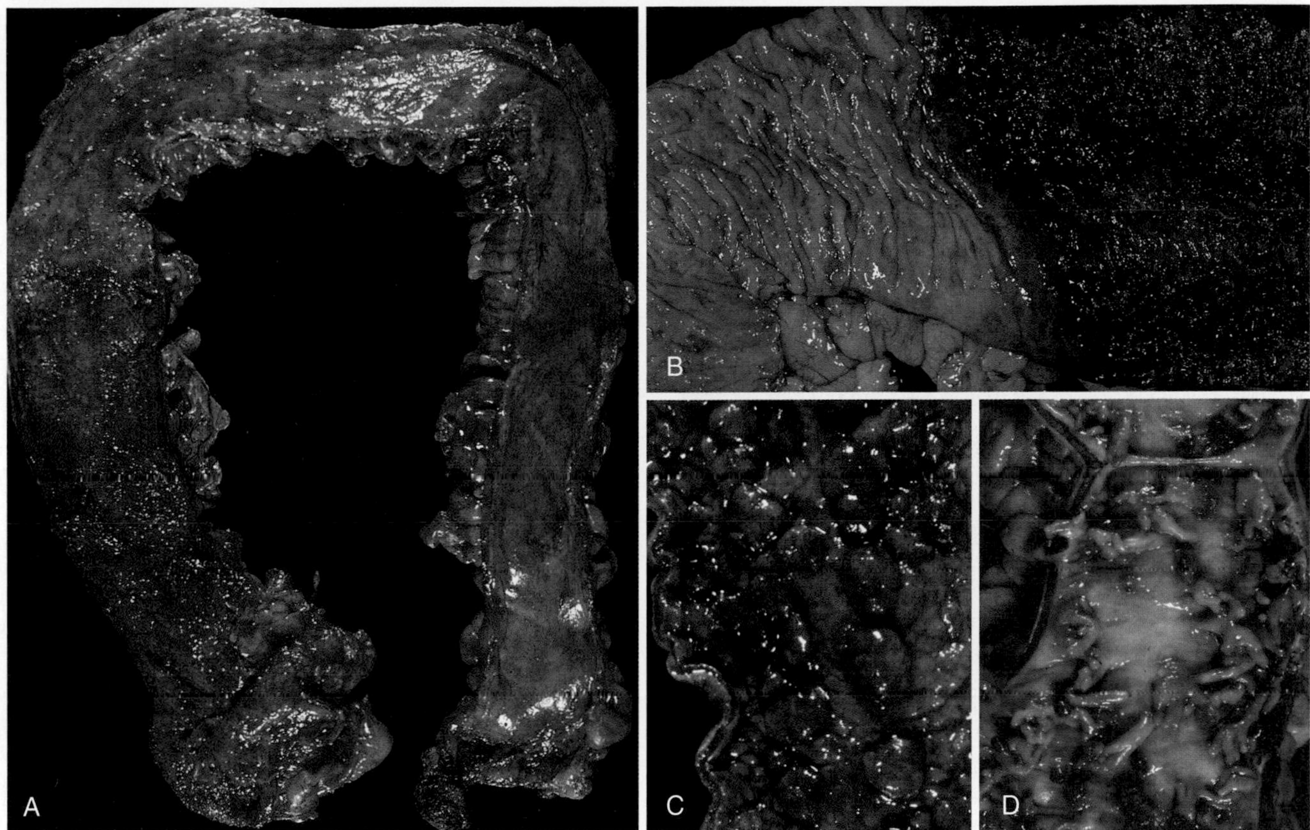

Figure 17-36 Gross pathology of ulcerative colitis. **A,** Total colectomy with pancolitis showing active disease, with red, granular mucosa in the cecum (left) and smooth, atrophic mucosa distally (right). **B,** Sharp demarcation between active ulcerative colitis (right) and normal mucosa (left). **C,** Inflammatory polyps. **D,** Mucosal bridges.

definitive diagnosis is not possible in approximately 10% of IBD patients. These cases, termed indeterminate colitis, do not involve the small bowel and have colonic disease in a continuous pattern that would typically indicate ulcerative colitis. However, patchy histologic disease, fissures, a family history of Crohn disease, perianal lesions, onset after initiating use of cigarettes, or other features that are not typical of ulcerative colitis may prompt more detailed endoscopic, radiographic, and histologic examination. Serologic studies can be useful in these cases because perinuclear anti-neutrophil cytoplasmic antibodies are found in 75% of individuals with ulcerative colitis but only 11% with Crohn disease. In contrast, ulcerative colitis patients tend to lack antibodies to *Saccharomyces cerevisiae,* which are often present in those with Crohn disease. However, even the serologic results can be ambiguous in cases that are indeterminate on clinical grounds. Despite diagnostic uncertainty, extensive overlap in medical management of ulcerative colitis and Crohn disease allows patients carrying a diagnosis of indeterminate colitis to be treated effectively.

Colitis-Associated Neoplasia

One of the most feared long-term complications of ulcerative colitis and colonic Crohn disease is the development of neoplasia. The risk of dysplasia is related to several factors:

- *Duration of the disease.* Risk increases sharply 8 to 10 years after disease onset.
- *Extent of the disease.* Patients with pancolitis are at greater risk than those with only left-sided disease.
- *Nature of the inflammatory response.* Greater frequency and severity of active inflammation (characterized by the presence of neutrophils) confers increased risk.

To facilitate early detection of neoplasia, patients are typically enrolled in surveillance programs approximately 8 years after diagnosis of IBD. The major exception to this is patients with IBD and primary sclerosing cholangitis, who have an even greater risk of developing cancer and are generally enrolled for surveillance at the time of diagnosis. Surveillance requires regular and extensive mucosal biopsies, making it a costly practice. Research efforts are therefore focused on discovery of molecular markers of dysplasia.

The goal of surveillance biopsies is to identify dysplastic epithelium, which is a precursor to colitis-associated carcinoma. Dysplasia can develop in flat areas of mucosa that are not grossly recognized as abnormal. Thus, advanced endoscopic imaging techniques including chromoendoscopy and confocal endoscopy are beginning to be used to increase the sensitivity of detection. IBD-associated dysplasia is classified histologically as low grade or high grade (Fig. 17-38*A, B*) and may be multifocal. High-grade dysplasia may be associated with invasive carcinoma at the same site (Fig. 17-38*C*) or elsewhere in the colon and, therefore, often prompts colectomy. Low-grade dysplasia may be treated with colectomy or followed closely, depending on a variety of factors including patient age and the number of dysplastic foci present. Colonic

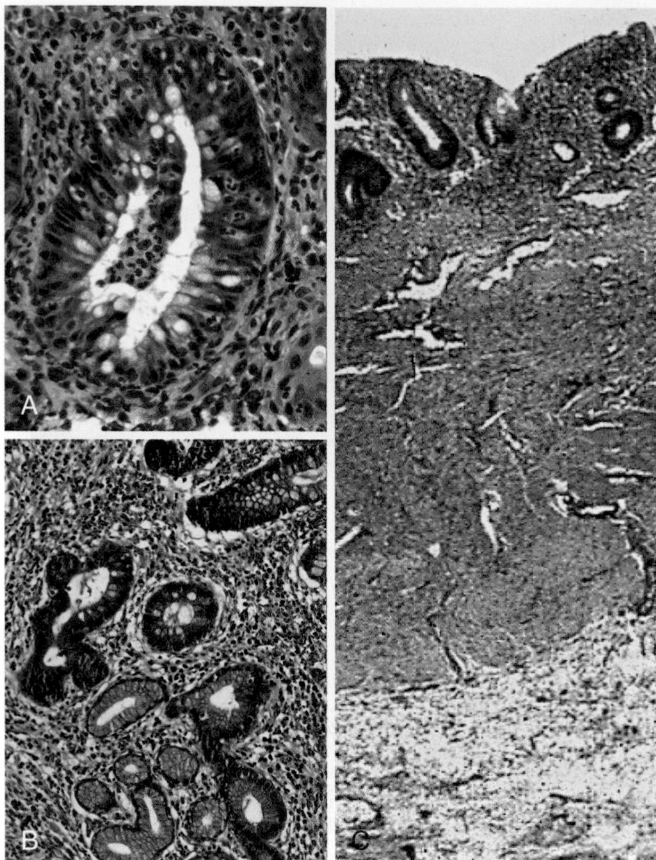

Figure 17-37 Microscopic pathology of ulcerative colitis. **A,** Crypt abscess. **B,** Pseudopyloric metaplasia (bottom). **C,** Disease is limited to the mucosa. Compare to Figure 17-35*C*.

adenomas (discussed later) also occur in IBD patients, and in some cases these may be difficult to differentiate from a polypoid focus of IBD-associated dysplasia.

Other Causes of Chronic Colitis

Diversion Colitis

Surgical treatment of ulcerative colitis, Hirschsprung disease and other intestinal disorders sometimes require creation of a temporary or permanent ostomy and a blind distal segment of colon, from which the normal fecal flow is diverted. Colitis can develop within the diverted segment, particularly in ulcerative colitis patients. Besides mucosal erythema and friability, the most striking feature of diversion colitis is the development of numerous mucosal lymphoid follicles (Fig. 17-39*A*). Increased numbers of lamina propria lymphocytes, monocytes, macrophages, and plasma cells may also be present. In severe cases the histopathology may resemble IBD and include crypt abscesses, mucosal architectural distortion, or, rarely, granulomas. The mechanisms responsible for diversion colitis are not well understood, but changes in the luminal microbiota and diversion of the fecal stream that provides nutrients to colonic epithelial cells have been proposed. Consistent with this, enemas containing short-chain fatty acids, a product of bacterial digestion in the colon and an important energy source for colonic epithelial cells, can promote mucosal recovery in some cases. The ultimate cure is reanastomosis of the diverted segment.

Microscopic Colitis

Microscopic colitis encompasses two entities, *collagenous colitis* and *lymphocytic colitis*. These idiopathic diseases both present with chronic, nonbloody, watery diarrhea without weight loss. Radiologic and endoscopic studies are typically normal. Collagenous colitis, which occurs primarily in middle-aged and older women, is characterized by the presence of a dense subepithelial collagen layer, increased numbers of intraepithelial lymphocytes, and a mixed inflammatory infiltrate within the lamina propria (Fig. 17-39*B*). Lymphocytic colitis is histologically similar, but the subepithelial collagen layer is of normal thickness and the increase in intraepithelial lymphocytes is greater, frequently exceeding one T lymphocyte per five colonocytes (Fig. 17-39*C*). Lymphocytic colitis shows a strong association with celiac disease and autoimmune diseases, including Graves disease, rheumatoid arthritis, and autoimmune or lymphocytic gastritis.

Graft-Versus-Host Disease

Graft-versus-host disease occurs following hematopoietic stem cell transplantation. The small bowel and colon are involved in most cases. Although graft-versus-host disease is secondary to donor T cells targeting antigens on the recipient's GI epithelial cells, the lamina propria lymphocytic infiltrate is typically sparse. Epithelial apoptosis,

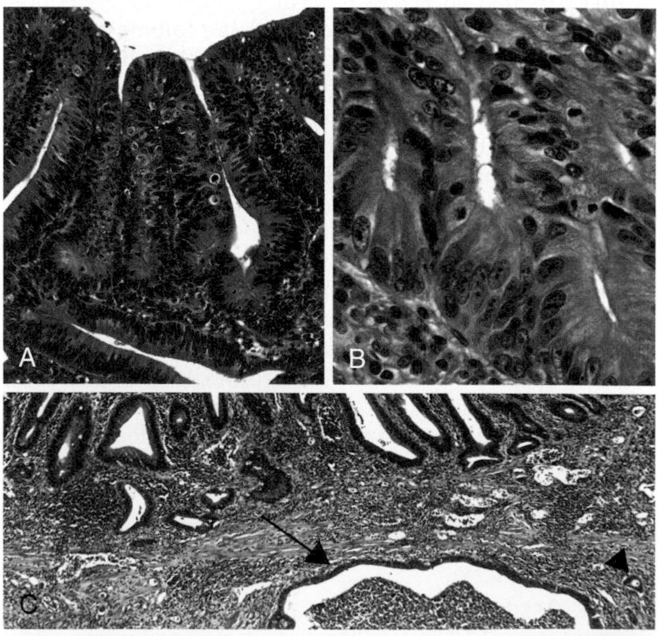

Figure 17-38 Colitis-associated dysplasia. **A,** Dysplasia with extensive nuclear stratification and marked nuclear hyperchromasia. **B,** Cribriform glandular arrangement in high-grade dysplasia. **C,** Colectomy specimen with high-grade dysplasia on the surface and underlying invasive adenocarcinoma. A large cystic, neutrophil-filled space lined by invasive adenocarcinoma is apparent *(arrow)* beneath the muscularis mucosae. Also seen are small invasive glands *(arrowhead).*

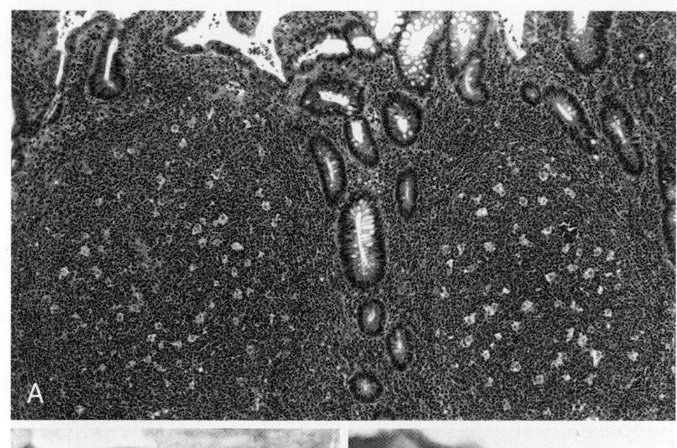

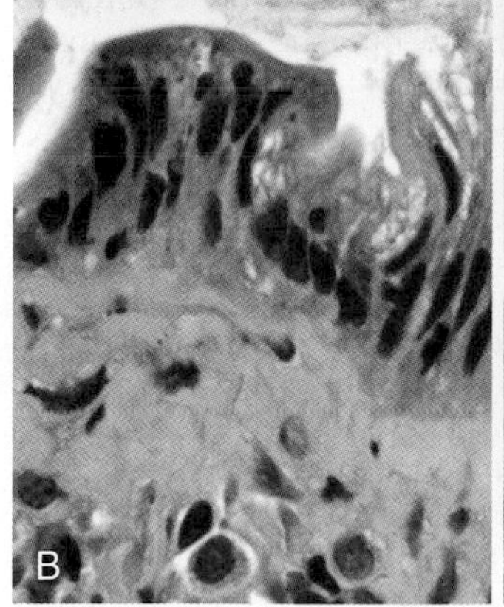

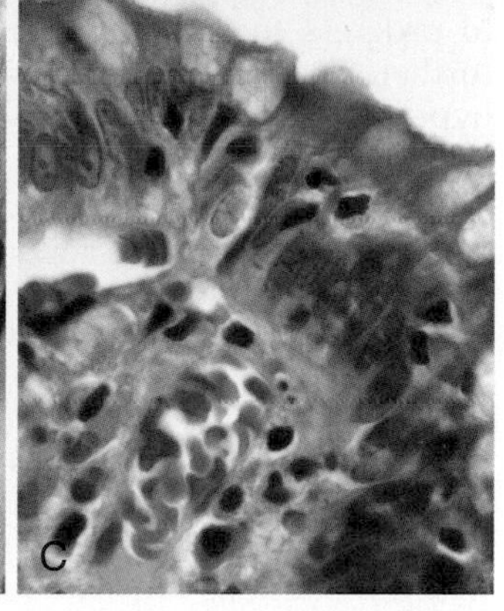

Figure 17-39 Uncommon causes of colitis. **A,** Diversion colitis. Note the large lymphoid aggregates with germinal centers. **B,** Collagenous colitis with intraepithelial lymphocytes and a dense subepithelial collagen band. **C,** Lymphocytic colitis.

particularly of crypt cells, is the most common histologic finding. Rarely, total gland destruction occurs, although endocrine cells may persist. Intestinal graft-versus-host disease often presents as a watery diarrhea but may become bloody in severe cases.

Sigmoid Diverticular Disease

Diverticular disease generally refers to acquired pseudo-diverticular outpouchings of the colonic mucosa and submucosa. Unlike true diverticula, such as Meckel diverticulum, they are not invested by all three layers of the colonic wall. Colonic diverticula are rare in persons younger than age 30, but the prevalence approaches 50% in Western adult populations older than age 60. Diverticula are generally multiple and the condition is referred to as diverticulosis. This disease is much less common in Japan as well as developing countries, probably because of dietary differences. Moreover, most diverticula in Asia and Africa occur in the right colon, while right-sided diverticula are uncommon in Western countries. The reasons for this difference in distribution are not well-defined.

Pathogenesis. Colonic diverticula result from the unique structure of the colonic muscularis propria and elevated intraluminal pressure in the sigmoid colon. Where nerves, arterial vasa recta, and their connective tissue sheaths penetrate the inner circular muscle coat, focal discontinuities in the muscle wall are created. In other parts of the intestine these gaps are reinforced by the external longitudinal layer of the muscularis propria, but, in the colon, this muscle layer is gathered into the three bands termed taeniae coli. Increased intraluminal pressure is probably due to exaggerated peristaltic contractions, with spasmodic sequestration of bowel segments, and may be enhanced by diets low in fiber, which reduce stool bulk, particularly in the sigmoid colon.

MORPHOLOGY

Anatomically, colonic diverticula are small, flask-like outpouchings, usually 0.5 to 1 cm in diameter, that occur in a regular distribution alongside the taeniae coli (Fig. 17-40*A*). These are most common in the sigmoid colon, but more extensive areas may be affected in severe cases. Because diverticula are compressible, easily emptied of fecal contents, and often surrounded by the fat-containing epiploic appendices on the surface of the colon, they may be missed on casual inspection. Colonic diverticula have a thin wall composed of a flattened or atrophic mucosa, compressed submucosa, and attenuated or, most often, totally absent muscularis propria (Fig. 17-40*B, C*). Hypertrophy of the circular layer of the muscularis propria in the affected bowel segment is common. Obstruction of diverticula leads to inflammatory changes, producing diverticulitis and peri-diverticulitis. Because the wall of the diverticulum is supported only by the muscularis mucosae and a thin layer of subserosal adipose tissue, inflammation and increased pressure within an obstructed diverticulum can lead to perforation. With or without perforation, diverticulitis may cause segmental diverticular disease-associated colitis, fibrotic thickening in and around the colonic wall, or stricture formation. Perforation is uncommon but it can result in pericolonic abscesses, sinus tracts, and, occasionally, peritonitis.

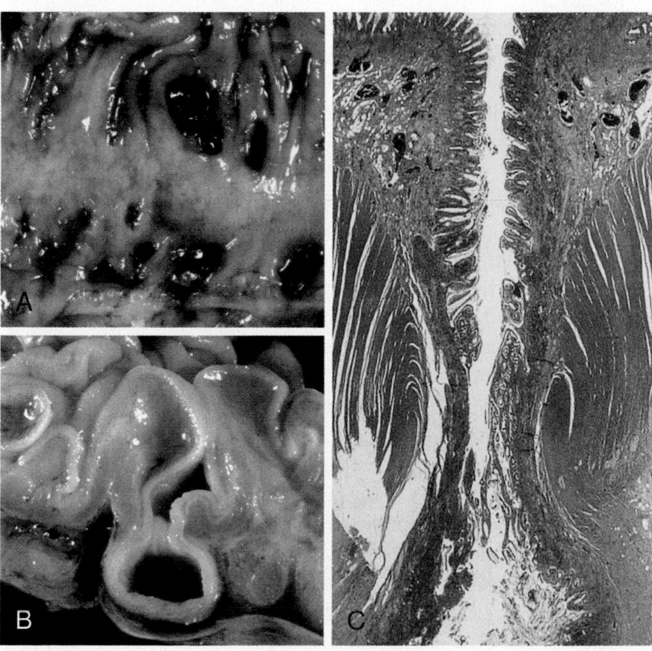

Figure 17-40 Sigmoid diverticular disease. **A,** Stool-filled diverticula are regularly arranged. **B,** Cross-section showing the outpouching of mucosa beneath the muscularis propria. **C,** Low-power photomicrograph of a sigmoid diverticulum showing protrusion of the mucosa and submucosa through the muscularis propria.

Clinical Features. Most individuals with diverticular disease remain asymptomatic throughout their lives. However, about 20% of individuals with diverticuli develop manifestations of diverticular disease, such as intermittent cramping, continuous lower abdominal discomfort, constipation, distention, or a sensation of never being able to completely empty the rectum. Patients sometimes experience alternating constipation and diarrhea that can mimic IBS. Occasionally there may be minimal chronic or intermittent blood loss, and, rarely, massive hemorrhage. When present, bleeding is macroscopically visible in the stools. Whether a high-fiber diet prevents such progression or protects against diverticulitis is unclear, but diets supplemented with fiber may provide symptomatic improvement. Even when diverticulitis occurs, it most often resolves spontaneously and relatively few patients require surgical intervention.

KEY CONCEPTS

- **Irritable bowel syndrome (IBS)** is characterized by chronic, relapsing abdominal pain, bloating, and changes in bowel habits without obvious gross or histologic pathology. The pathogenesis of IBS is not defined, but includes contributions by psychologic stressors, diet, the gut microbiome, abnormal GI motility, and increased enteric sensory responses to gastrointestinal stimuli.
- **Inflammatory bowel disease (IBD)** is an umbrella term for **ulcerative colitis** and **Crohn disease**. **Indeterminate colitis** is used for cases of IBD without definitive features of either ulcerative colitis or Crohn disease.
- **Ulcerative colitis is limited to the colon**, is **continuous from the rectum**, and ranges from only rectal disease to pancolitis; neither skip lesions nor granulomas are present.
- **Crohn disease** most commonly affects the **terminal ileum and cecum**, but any site within the gastrointestinal tract can be involved; **skip lesions** are common and **noncaseating granulomas** also occur.
- Both forms of IBD typically present in the **teens and early 20s** and are associated with **extraintestinal manifestations**.
- IBD is thought to arise from a combination of alterations in host interactions with intestinal microbiota, intestinal epithelial dysfunction, and aberrant mucosal immune responses. Molecular analyses have identified more than 160 IBD-associated genes, of which the function of only a few is understood.
- The risk of colonic **epithelial dysplasia and adenocarcinoma** is increased in IBD patients who have had colonic disease for more than 8 to 10 years.
- The two forms of microscopic colitis, **collagenous colitis** and **lymphocytic colitis**, both cause chronic watery diarrhea. The intestines are grossly normal, and the diseases are identified by their characteristic histologic features.
- **Diverticular disease** of the sigmoid colon is common in western populations older than age 60. The causes include low fiber diets, colonic spasm, and the unique anatomy of the colon. Inflammation of diverticula, **diverticulitis**, affects a minority of those with **diverticulosis**, but can cause perforation in its most severe form.

Polyps

Polyps are most common in the colo-rectal region but may occur in the esophagus, stomach, or small intestine. Most, if not all, polyps begin as small elevations of the mucosa. These are referred to as sessile, a term borrowed from botanists who use it to describe flowers and leaves that grow directly from the stem without a stalk. As sessile polyps enlarge, proliferation of cells adjacent to the mass and the effects of traction on the luminal protrusion, may combine to create a stalk. Polyps with stalks are termed pedunculated. In general, intestinal polyps can be classified as nonneoplastic or neoplastic in nature. The most common neoplastic polyp is the adenoma, which has the potential to progress to cancer. The nonneoplastic polyps can be further classified as inflammatory, hamartomatous, or hyperplastic.

Hyperplastic Polyps

Colonic hyperplastic polyps are benign epithelial proliferations that are typically discovered in the sixth and seventh decades of life. The pathogenesis of hyperplastic polyps is incompletely understood, but they are thought to result from decreased epithelial cell turnover and delayed shedding of surface epithelial cells, leading to a "piling up" of goblet cells and absorptive cells. It is now appreciated that these lesions are without malignant potential. **Their chief significance is that they must be distinguished from sessile serrated adenomas, that are histologically similar but have malignant potential, as described later**. It is also important to remember that epithelial hyperplasia can occur as a nonspecific reaction adjacent to or overlying any mass or inflammatory lesion and, therefore, can be a clue to the presence of an adjacent, clinically important lesion.

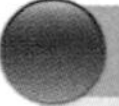

MORPHOLOGY

Hyperplastic polyps are most commonly found in the left colon and are typically less than 5 mm in diameter. They are smooth, nodular protrusions of the mucosa, often on the crests of mucosal folds. They may occur singly but are more frequently multiple, particularly in the sigmoid colon and rectum. Histologically, hyperplastic polyps are composed of mature goblet and absorptive cells. The delayed shedding of these cells leads to crowding that creates the serrated surface architecture that is the morphologic hallmark of these lesions (Fig. 17-41). Serration is typically restricted to the upper third, or less, of the crypt.

Inflammatory Polyps

Polyps that form as part of the solitary rectal ulcer syndrome are examples of purely inflammatory lesions. Patients present with a clinical triad of rectal bleeding, mucus discharge, and an inflammatory lesion of the anterior rectal wall. The underlying cause is impaired relaxation of the anorectal sphincter that creates a sharp angle at the anterior rectal shelf and leads to recurrent abrasion and ulceration of the overlying rectal mucosa. An inflammatory polyp may ultimately form as a result of chronic cycles of injury and healing. Entrapment of this polyp in

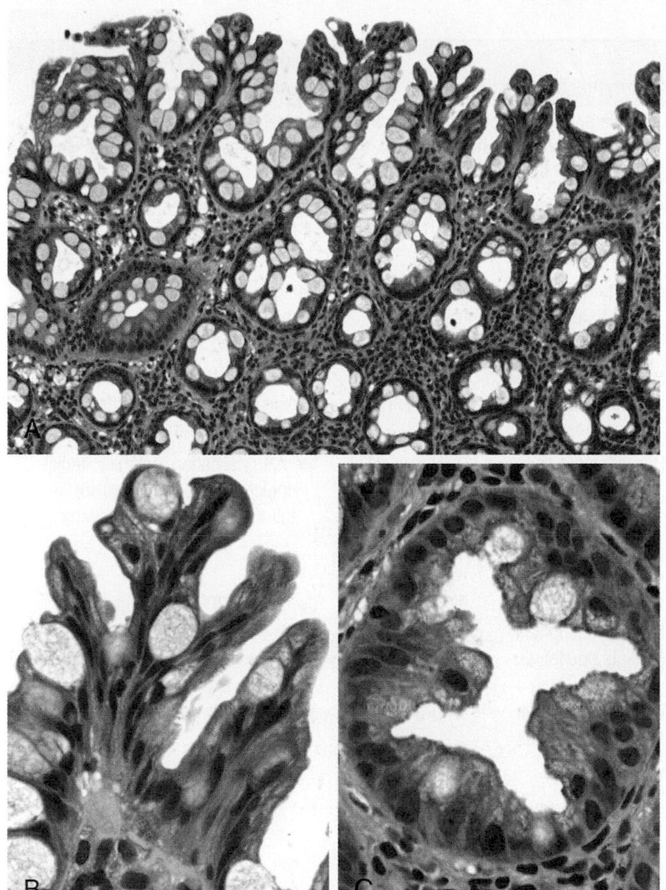

Figure 17-41 Hyperplastic polyp. **A,** Polyp surface with irregular tufting of epithelial cells. **B,** Tufting results from epithelial overcrowding. **C,** Epithelial crowding produces a serrated architecture when crypts are cut in cross-section.

the fecal stream leads to mucosal prolapse. The distinctive histologic features of a typical inflammatory polyp include mixed inflammatory infiltrates, erosion, and epithelial hyperplasia together with lamina propria fibromuscular hyperplasia (Fig. 17-42).

Hamartomatous Polyps

Hamartomatous polyps occur sporadically or as components of various genetically determined or acquired syndromes (Table 17-10).

Although they were originally thought to be caused by developmental abnormalities, it is now appreciated that many hamartomatous polyp syndromes are caused by germline mutations in tumor suppressor genes or proto-oncogenes. Some of these syndromes are associated with increased cancer risk, either within the polyps or at other intestinal or extra-intestinal sites. Thus, in some hamartomatous polyp syndromes, the polyps can be considered to be pre-malignant, neoplastic lesions, much like adenomas. In addition, it is important to recognize these polyps because of associated extraintestinal manifestations and the possibility that other family members are affected. Several of these syndromes are discussed below, while other syndromes are summarized in Table 17-10.

Juvenile Polyps

Juvenile polyps are focal malformations of the epithelium and lamina propria. These may be sporadic or syndromic, but the morphology of the two forms is often indistinguishable. The vast majority of juvenile polyps occur in children younger than 5 years of age but they can present at older ages as well. Most juvenile polyps are located in the rectum and typically present with rectal bleeding. In some cases intussusception, intestinal obstruction, or polyp prolapse (through the anal sphincter) may occur.

Sporadic juvenile polyps are usually solitary lesions and may also be referred to as retention polyps. In contrast, individuals with the autosomal dominant syndrome of juvenile polyposis have from 3 to as many as 100 hamartomatous polyps and may require colectomy to limit the chronic and sometimes severe hemorrhage associated with polyp ulceration. A minority of patients also have polyps in the stomach and small bowel that can undergo malignant transformation. Pulmonary arteriovenous malformations and other congenital malformations are recognized extraintestinal manifestation of juvenile polyposis.

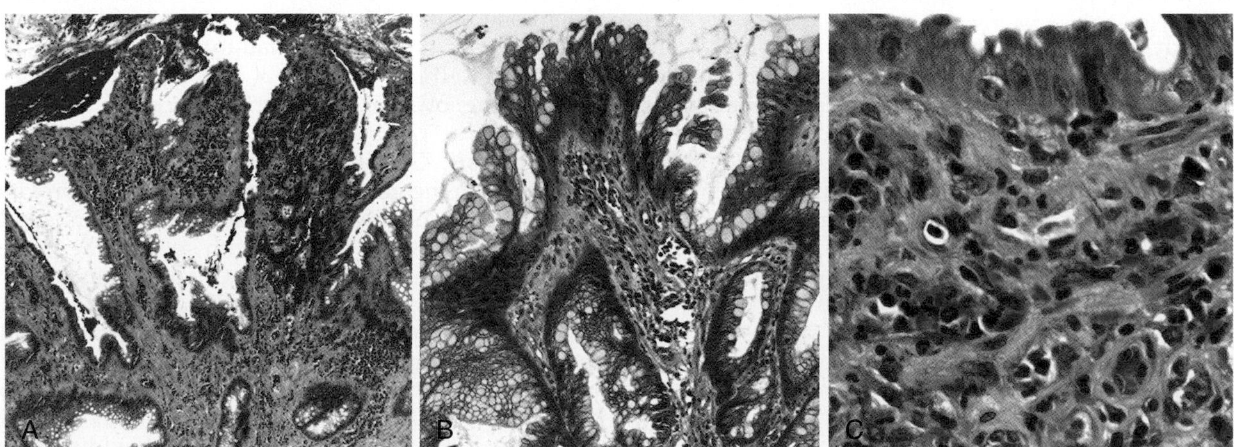

Figure 17-42 Solitary rectal ulcer syndrome. **A,** The dilated glands, proliferative epithelium, superficial erosions, and inflammatory infiltrate are typical of an inflammatory polyp. However, the smooth muscle hyperplasia within the lamina propria suggests that mucosal prolapse has also occurred. **B,** Epithelial hyperplasia. **C,** Granulation tissue-like capillary proliferation within the lamina propria caused by repeated erosion.

Table 17-10 Gastrointestinal Polyposis Syndromes

Syndrome	Mean Age at Presentation (yr)	Mutated Gene(s); Pathway	Gastrointestinal Lesions	Selected Extra-Gastrointestinal Manifestations
Juvenile polyposis	<5	*SMAD4,BMPR1A*; TGF-β signaling pathway	Juvenile polyps; risk of gastric, small intestinal, colonic, and pancreatic adenocarcinoma	Congenital malformations, digital clubbing
Peutz-Jeghers syndrome	10-15	*STK11*; AMP kinase-related pathways	Arborizing polyps; Small intestine > colon > stomach; colonic adenocarcinoma	Pigmented macules; risk of colon, breast, lung, pancreatic, and thyroid cancer
Cowden syndrome, Bannayan-Ruvalcaba-Riley syndrome*	<15	*PTEN*: PI3K/AKT pathway	Hamartomatous/ inflammatory intestinal polyps, lipomas, ganglioneuromas	Benign skin tumors, benign and malignant thyroid and breast lesions; no increase in GI cancers
Cronkhite-Canada syndrome	>50	Nonhereditary, unknown cause	Hamartomatous polyps of stomach, small intestine colon; abnormalities in nonpolypoid mucosa	Nail atrophy, hair loss, abnormal skin pigmentation, cachexia, and anemia. Fatal in up to 50%.
Tuberous sclerosis		*TSC1* (hamartin), *TSC2* (tuberin); mTOR pathway	Hamartomatous polyps	Mental retardation, epilepsy. facial angiofibroma, cortical (CNS) tubers, renal angiomyolipoma
Familial adenomatous polyposis (FAP)				
Classic FAP	10-15	*APC*	Multiple adenomas	Congenital RPE hypertrophy
Attenuated FAP	40-50	*APC*	Multiple adenomas	
Gardner syndrome	10-15	*APC*	Multiple adenomas	Osteomas, thyroid and desmoid tumors, skin cysts
Turcot syndrome	10-15	*APC*	Multiple adenomas	Medulloblastoma, glioblastoma
MYH-associated polyposis	30-50	*MYH*	Multiple adenomas	

CNS, Central nervous system; mTOR, mammalian target of rapamycin; RPE, retinal pigmented epithelium.
*Also called PTEN Hamartoma-Tumor Syndromes.

MORPHOLOGY

Most juvenile polyps are less than 3 cm in diameter. They are typically pedunculated, smooth-surfaced, reddish lesions with characteristic cystic spaces apparent after sectioning. Microscopic examination shows these cysts to be dilated glands filled with mucin and inflammatory debris (Fig. 17-43). The remainder of the polyp is composed of lamina propria expanded by mixed inflammatory infiltrates. The muscularis mucosae may be normal or attenuated.

Although the morphogenesis of juvenile polyps is incompletely understood, it has been proposed that mucosal hyperplasia is the initiating event. This hypothesis is consistent with the discovery that mutations in pathways that regulate cellular growth cause autosomal dominant juvenile polyposis. The most common mutation identified is of *SMAD4*, which encodes a cytoplasmic intermediate in the TGF-β signaling pathway. *BMPR1A*, a kinase that is a member of the TGF-β superfamily, may be mutated in other cases (Table 17-10). However, these mutations account for fewer than half of patients, suggesting that other genes responsible for autosomal dominant juvenile polyposis remain to be discovered.

Dysplasia is extremely rare in sporadic juvenile polyps. In contrast juvenile polyposis syndrome is associated with dysplasia, both within the juvenile polyps and in separate adenomas. As a result, 30% to 50% of patients with juvenile polyposis develop colonic adenocarcinoma by age 45.

Peutz-Jeghers Syndrome

This rare autosomal dominant syndrome presents at a median age of 11 years with multiple GI hamartomatous polyps and mucocutaneous hyperpigmentation. The latter takes the form of dark blue to brown macules on the lips, nostrils, buccal mucosa, palmar surfaces of the hands, genitalia, and perianal region. These lesions are similar to freckles but are distinguished by their presence in the buccal mucosa. Peutz-Jeghers polyps can initiate intussusception, which is occasionally fatal. Of greater importance, *Peutz-Jeghers syndrome is associated with a markedly increased risk of several malignancies.* Lifetime risk is approximately 40% for these, and regular surveillance is recommended beginning at birth, for sex cord tumors of the testes; late childhood for gastric and small intestinal cancers; and the second and third decades of life for colon, pancreatic, breast, lung, ovarian, and uterine cancers.

Pathogenesis. Germline heterozygous loss-of-function mutations in the gene *STK11* are present in approximately half of individuals with familial Peutz-Jeghers syndrome as well as a subset of patients with sporadic Peutz-Jeghers syndrome. You will recall from Chapter 7 that *STK11* is a tumor suppressor gene that encodes a kinase that regulates cell polarization and acts as a brake on growth and anabolic metabolism. As is common with other tumor suppressor genes, the function of the second "normal" copy of *STK11* is often lost through somatic mutation in cancers occurring in Peutz-Jeghers syndrome, providing an explanation for the high risk of neoplasia in affected patients. Importantly, colon cancers can also develop at sites without Peutz-Jeghers polyps.

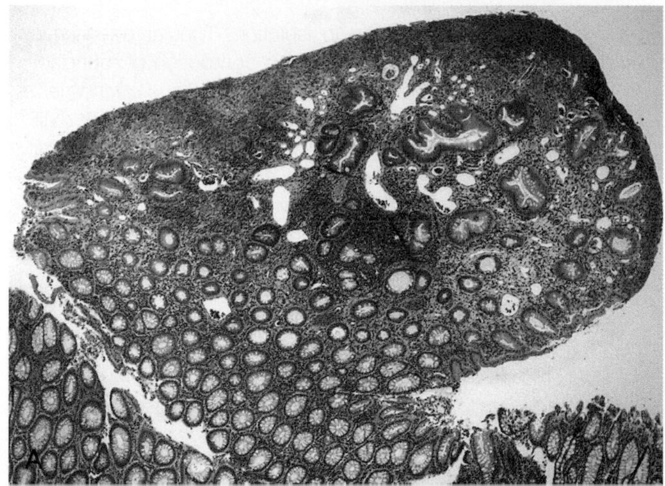

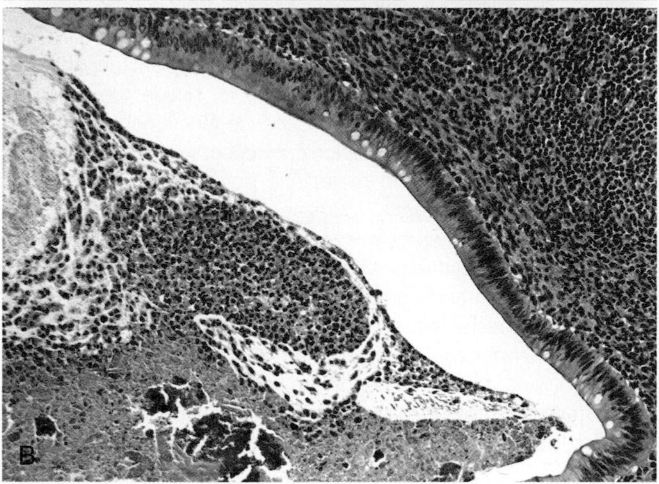

Figure 17-43 Juvenile polyposis. **A,** Juvenile polyp. Note the surface erosion and cystically dilated crypts. **B,** Inspissated mucous, neutrophils, and inflammatory debris can accumulate within dilated crypts.

MORPHOLOGY

The polyps of Peutz-Jeghers syndrome are most common in the small intestine, although they may occur in the stomach and colon, and, with much lower frequency, in the bladder and lungs. Grossly, the polyps are large and pedunculated with a lobulated contour. Histologic examination demonstrates a characteristic arborizing network of connective tissue, smooth muscle, lamina propria, and glands lined by normal-appearing intestinal epithelium (Fig. 17-44). The arborization and presence of smooth muscle intermixed with lamina propria are helpful in distinguishing polyps of Peutz-Jeghers syndrome from juvenile polyps.

Clinical Features. Because the morphology of Peutz-Jeghers polyps can overlap with that of sporadic hamartomatous polyps, the presence of multiple polyps in the small intestine, mucocutaneous hyperpigmentation, and a positive family history are critical to the diagnosis. Detection of *STK11* mutations can be helpful diagnostically in patients with polyps who lack mucocutaneous hyperpigmentation. However, the absence of *STK11* mutations does not exclude the diagnosis, since mutations in other presently unknown genes can also cause the syndrome.

Neoplastic Polyps

Any neoplastic mass lesion in the GI tract may produce a mucosal protrusion, or polyp. This includes adenocarcinomas, neuroendocrine (carcinoid) tumors, stromal tumors, lymphomas, and even metastatic cancers from distant sites. *The most common neoplastic polyps are colonic adenomas, which are precursors to the majority of colorectal adenocarcinomas.*

Adenomas are intraepithelial neoplasms that range from small, often pedunculated, polyps to large sessile lesions. There is a small male predominance, and they are present in approximately 30% of adults living in the Western world by age 60. Because these polyps are precursors to colorectal adenocarcinoma, it is recommended that all adults in the United States undergo surveillance by age 50. Patients at increased risk, including those with a family history of colorectal adenocarcinoma, are typically screened colonoscopically at least 10 years before the youngest age at which a relative was diagnosed. The preferred approach to surveillance varies, but colonoscopy is most common.

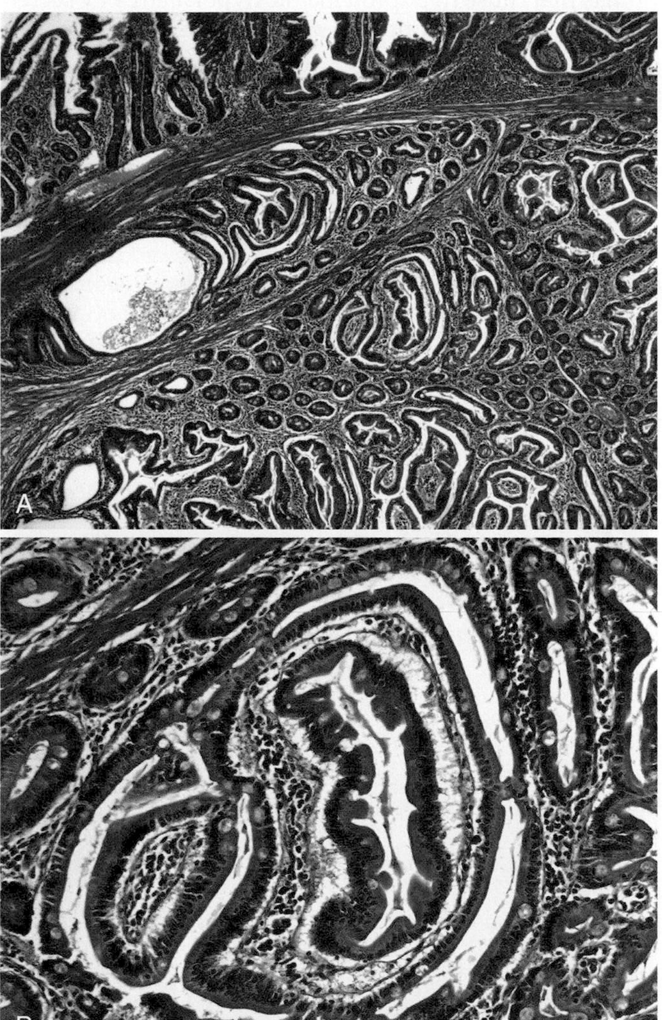

Figure 17-44 Peutz-Jeghers polyp. **A,** Polyp surface (top) overlies stroma composed of smooth muscle bundles cutting through the lamina propria. **B,** Complex glandular architecture and the presence of smooth muscle are features that distinguish Peutz-Jeghers polyps from juvenile polyps. Compare to Figure 17-42.

While adenomas are less common in Asia, their frequency has risen (in parallel with an increasing incidence of colorectal adenocarcinoma) in these populations as Western diets and lifestyles become more common.

Colorectal adenomas are characterized by the presence of epithelial dysplasia. Consistent with their being precursor lesions, the prevalence of colorectal adenomas correlates with that of colorectal adenocarcinoma and the distributions of adenomas and adenocarcinoma within the colon are similar. Large studies have demonstrated that regular surveillance colonoscopy and polyp removal reduces the incidence of colorectal adenocarcinoma. Despite this strong relationship, it must be emphasized that majority of adenomas do not progress to become adenocarcinomas. There are no tools presently available to distinguish between adenomas that will or will not undergo malignant transformation, and indeed it may be that transformation is stochastic, being dependent on acquisition of oncogenic mutations merely by chance. Most adenomas are clinically silent, with the exception of large polyps that produce occult bleeding and anemia and rare villous adenomas that cause hypoproteinemic hypokalemia by secreting large amounts of protein and potassium.

MORPHOLOGY

Typical adenomas range from 0.3 to 10 cm in diameter and can be pedunculated (Fig. 17-45*A*) or sessile, with the surface of both types having a texture resembling velvet or a raspberry (Fig. 17-45*B*). Histologically, the hallmark of epithelial dysplasia is nuclear hyperchromasia, elongation, and stratification (see Fig. 17-46*C*). These changes are most easily appreciated at the surface of the adenoma and are often accompanied by prominent nucleoli, eosinophilic cytoplasm, and a reduction in the number of goblet cells. Notably, epithelial cells fail to mature as they migrate from crypt to surface. Pedunculated adenomas have slender fibromuscular stalks (Fig. 17-45*C*) containing prominent blood vessels derived from the submucosa. The stalk is usually covered by nonneoplastic epithelium, but dysplastic epithelium is sometimes present.

Adenomas can be classified as **tubular, tubulovillous,** or **villous** based on their architecture. These categories, however, have little clinical significance in isolation. Tubular adenomas tend to be small, pedunculated polyps composed of rounded, or tubular, glands (Fig. 17-46*A*). In contrast, villous adenomas, which are often larger and sessile, are covered by slender villi (Fig. 17-46*B*). Tubulovillous adenomas have a mixture of tubular and villous elements. Although villous adenomas contain foci of invasion more frequently than tubular adenomas, villous architecture alone does not increase cancer risk when polyp size is considered.

Sessile serrated adenomas overlap histologically with hyperplastic polyps, but are more commonly found in the right colon. Despite their malignant potential, sessile serrated adenomas lack typical cytologic features of dysplasia that are present in other adenomas, prompting some to refer to these lesions as sessile serrated polyps. Histologic criteria for these lesions include serrated architecture throughout the full length of the glands, including the crypt base, crypt dilation, and lateral growth (Fig. 17-46*D*).

Intramucosal carcinoma occurs when dysplastic epithelial cells breach the basement membrane to invade the lamina propria or muscularis mucosae. Because functional lymphatic channels are absent in the colonic mucosa, intramucosal carcinomas have little or no metastatic potential and complete polypectomy is generally curative (Fig. 17-47*A*). Invasion beyond the muscularis mucosae, including into the submucosal stalk of a pedunculated polyp (Fig. 17-47*B*), constitutes invasive adenocarcinoma and carries a risk of spread to other sites. In such cases several factors, including the histologic grade of the invasive component, the presence of vascular or lymphatic invasion, and the distance of the invasive component from the margin of resection, must be considered in planning further therapy.

Although most colorectal adenomas are benign lesions, a small proportion may harbor invasive cancer at the time of detection. *Size is the most important characteristic that correlates with risk of malignancy.* For example, while cancer is extremely rare in adenomas less than 1 cm in diameter, some studies suggest that nearly 40% of lesions larger than 4 cm in diameter contain foci of cancer. High-grade dysplasia is also a risk factor for cancer in an individual polyp,

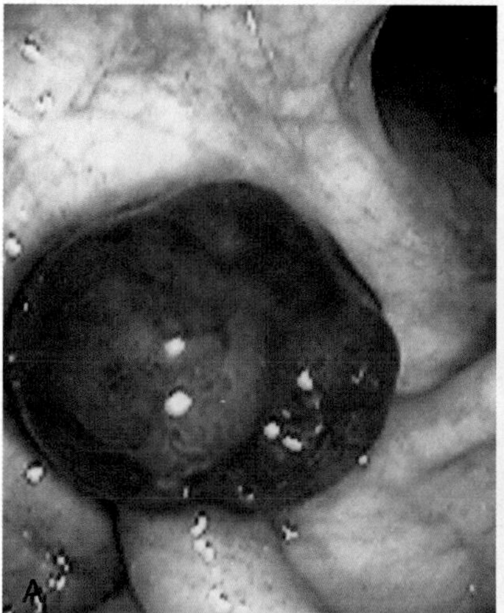

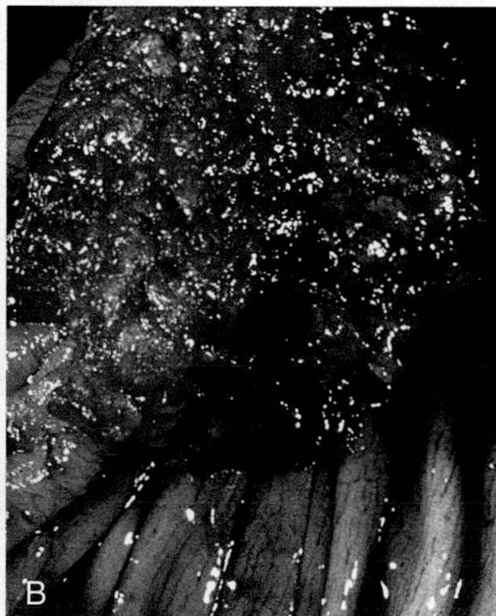

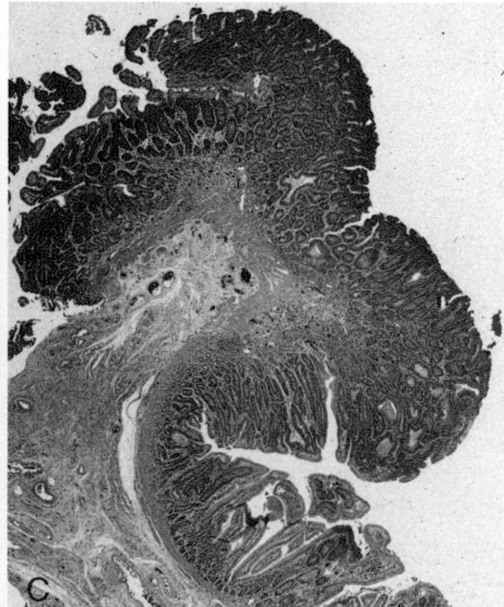

Figure 17-45 Colonic adenomas. **A,** Pedunculated adenoma (endoscopic view). **B,** Adenoma with a velvety surface. **C,** Low-magnification photomicrograph of a pedunculated tubular adenoma.

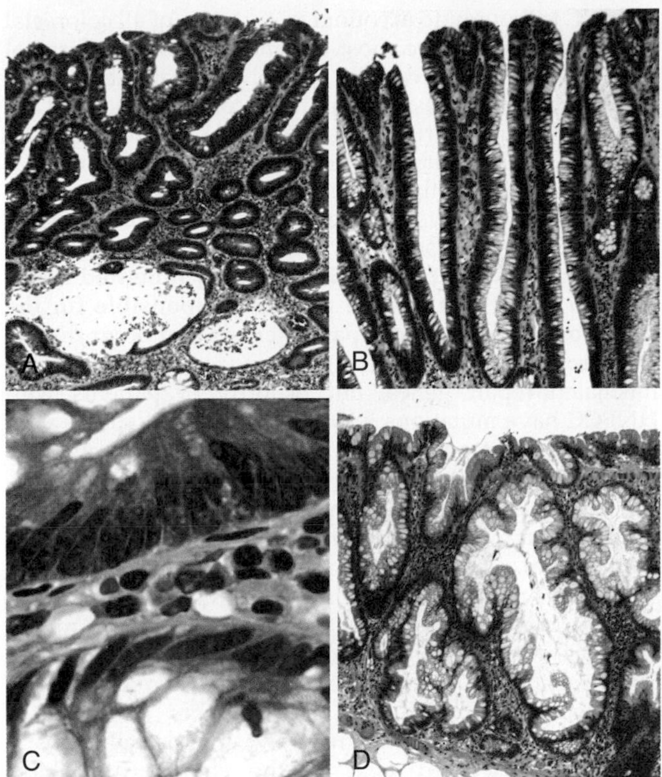

Figure 17-46 Histologic appearance of colonic adenomas. **A,** Tubular adenoma with a smooth surface and rounded glands. Active inflammation is occasionally present in adenomas, in this case, crypt dilation and rupture can be seen at the bottom of the field. **B,** Villous adenoma with long, slender projections that are reminiscent of small intestinal villi. **C,** Dysplastic epithelial cells (top) with an increased nuclear-to-cytoplasmic ratio, hyperchromatic and elongated nuclei, and nuclear pseudostratification. Compare to the non-dysplastic epithelium below. **D,** Sessile serrated adenoma lined by goblet cells without cytologic features of dysplasia. This lesion is distinguished from a hyperplastic polyp by extension of the neoplastic process to the crypts, resulting in lateral growth. Compare to the hyperplastic polyp in Figure 17-44A.

but does not confer an increased risk of cancer in other polyps within the same patient.

Adenomatous Polyposis

Familial adenomatous polyposis (FAP) is an autosomal dominant disorder in which patients develop numerous colorectal adenomas as teenagers. It is caused by mutations of the adenomatous polyposis coli, or *APC*, gene, which you will recall is a key negative regulator of the Wnt signaling pathway (Chapter 7). Approximately 75% of cases are inherited, while the remaining appear to be caused by de novo mutations.

At least 100 polyps are necessary for a diagnosis of classic FAP, but as many as several thousand may be present (Fig. 17-48). Except for their remarkable numbers, these growths are morphologically indistinguishable from sporadic adenomas. In addition, however, flat or depressed adenomas are also prevalent in FAP, and microscopic adenomas, consisting of only one or two dysplastic crypts, are frequently observed in otherwise normal-appearing mucosa.

Colorectal adenocarcinoma develops in 100% of untreated FAP patients, often before age 30 and nearly always by age 50. As a result, prophylactic colectomy is the standard therapy for individuals carrying *APC* mutations. Colectomy prevents colorectal cancer, but patients remain at risk for neoplasia at other sites. Adenomas may develop elsewhere in the GI tract, particularly adjacent to the ampulla of Vater and in the stomach.

FAP is associated with a variety of extraintestinal manifestations including congenital hypertrophy of the retinal pigment epithelium, which can generally be detected at birth, and therefore may be an adjunct to early screening. Specific *APC* mutations have been associated with the development of other manifestations of FAP and partly explain variants such as Gardner syndrome and Turcot syndrome (Table 17-11).

Some polyposis patients without *APC* loss have bi-allelic mutations of the base-excision repair gene *MYH* (also referred to as *MUTYH*). This autosomal recessive disorder is termed *MYH*-associated polyposis. The colonic phenotype is similar to attenuated FAP, with polyp development at later ages, the presence of fewer than 100 adenomas, and the delayed appearance of colon cancer, often at ages of 50 or older. In addition, serrated polyps, often with *KRAS*

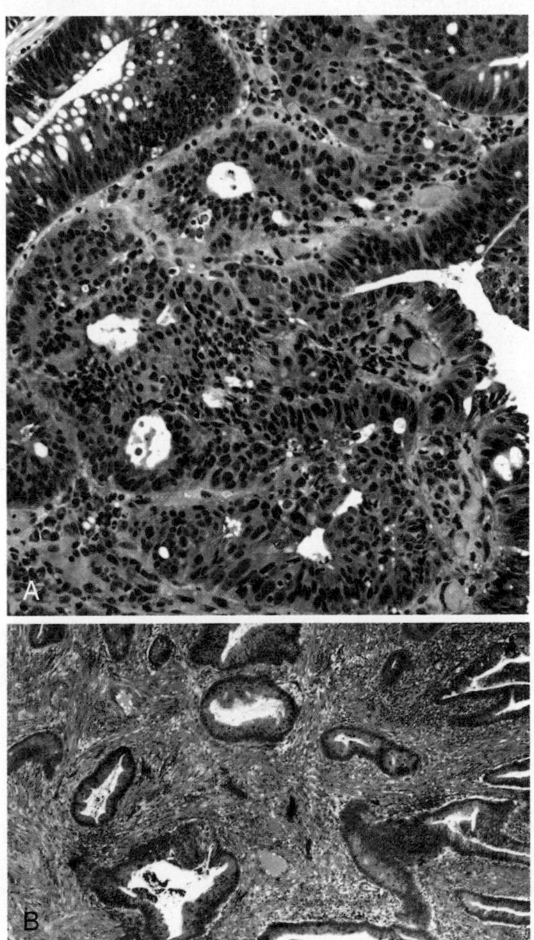

Figure 17-47 Adenoma with intramucosal carcinoma. **A,** Cribriform glands interface directly with the lamina propria without an intervening basement membrane. **B,** Invasive adenocarcinoma (left) beneath a villous adenoma (right). Note the desmoplastic response to the invasive components.

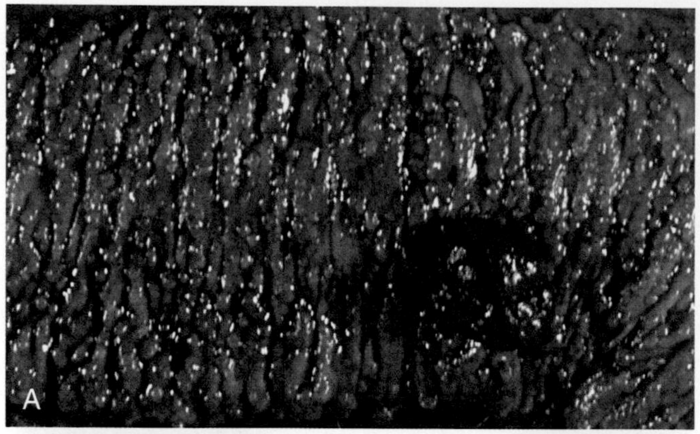

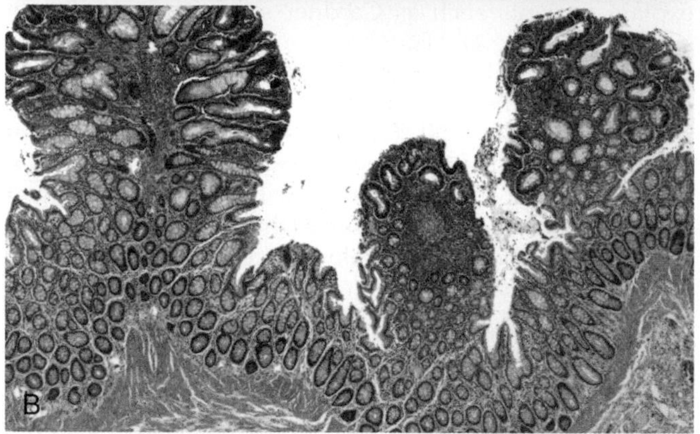

Figure 17-48 Familial adenomatous polyposis. **A,** Hundreds of small polyps are present throughout this colon with a dominant polyp (right). **B,** Three tubular adenomas are present in this single microscopic field.

mutations, are frequently present in MUTYH-associated polyposis.

Hereditary Non-Polyposis Colorectal Cancer

Hereditary non-polyposis colorectal cancer (HNPCC), also known as Lynch syndrome, was originally described based on familial clustering of cancers at several sites including the colorectum, endometrium, stomach, ovary, ureters, brain, small bowel, hepatobiliary tract, pancreas, and skin. HNPCC is thought to account for 2% to 4% of all colorectal cancers, making it the most common syndromic form of colon cancer. Colon cancers in HNPCC patients tend to occur at younger ages than sporadic colon cancers and are often located in the right colon (Table 17-11). Just as identification of *APC* mutations in FAP has provided molecular insights into the pathogenesis of the majority of sporadic colon cancers, unraveling the defects in HNPCC has shed light on the mechanisms responsible for most of the remaining sporadic cases. **HNPCC is caused by inherited mutations in genes that encode proteins responsible for the detection, excision, and repair of errors that occur during DNA replication** (Chapter 7). There are at least five such mismatch repair genes, but majority of patients with HNPCC have mutations in *MSH2* or *MLH1*. Patients with HNPCC inherit one mutant gene and one normal allele. When the second copy is lost through mutation or epigenetic silencing, defects in mismatch repair lead to the accumulation of mutations at rates up to 1000 times higher than normal, mostly in regions containing short repeatings sequences referred to as microsatellites. The human genome contains approximately 50,000 to 100,000 microsatellites, which are prone to undergo expansion during DNA replication and represent the most frequent sites of mutations in HNPCC. The consequences of mismatch repair deficiency and the resulting microsatellite instability are discussed next in the context of colonic adenocarcinoma.

Adenocarcinoma

Adenocarcinoma of the colon is the most common malignancy of the GI tract and is a major cause of morbidity and mortality worldwide. In contrast, the small intestine, which accounts for 75% of the overall length of the GI tract, is an uncommon site for benign and malignant tumors. Among malignant small intestinal tumors, adenocarcinomas and well-differentiated neuroendocrine (carcinoid) tumors have roughly equal incidence, followed by lymphomas and sarcomas.

Epidemiology. Approximately 1.2 million new cases of colorectal adenocarcinoma, and 600,000 associated deaths, occur each year worldwide. Thus, colorectal adenocarcinoma is responsible for nearly 10% of all cancer deaths. The

Table 17-11 Common Patterns of Sporadic and Familial Colorectal Neoplasia

Etiology	Molecular Defect	Target Gene(s)	Transmission	Predominant Site(s)	Histology
Familial adenomatous polyposis	APC/WNT pathway	*APC*	Autosomal dominant	None	Tubular, villous; typical adenocarcinoma
MYH-associated polyposis	DNA mismatch repair	*MYH*	Autosomal recessive	None	Sessile serrated adenoma; mucinous adenocarcinoma
Hereditary nonpolyposis colorectal cancer	DNA mismatch repair	*MSH2, MLH1*	Autosomal dominant	Right side	Sessile serrated adenoma; mucinous adenocarcinoma
Sporadic colon cancer (70%-80%)	APC/WNT pathway	*APC*	None	Left side	Tubular, villous; typical adenocarcinoma
Sporadic colon cancer (10%-15%)	DNA mismatch repair	*MSH2, MLH1*	None	Right side	Sessile serrated adenoma; mucinous adenocarcinoma
Sporadic colon cancer (5%-10%)	Hypermethylation	*MLH1, BRAF*	None	Right side	Sessile serrated adenoma; mucinous adenocarcinoma

incidence of these tumors is highest in North America, with the United States accounting for approximately 10% of worldwide cases and cancer deaths. This represents nearly 15% of all cancer-related deaths in the United States, second only to lung cancer. Australia, New Zealand, Europe, and, with changes in lifestyle and diet, Japan, also have high incidences of colorectal adenocarcinoma. In contrast, rates are lower in South America, India, Africa, and South Central Asia. Colorectal cancer incidence peaks at 60 to 70 years of age, with fewer than 20% of cases occuring before age 50.

The *dietary factors* most closely associated with increased rates of colorectal cancer are low intake of unabsorbable vegetable fiber and high intake of refined carbohydrates and fat. Although these associations are clear, the mechanistic relationship between diet and risk remains poorly understood. It is theorized that reduced fiber content leads to decreased stool bulk and altered composition of the intestinal microbiota. This change may increase synthesis of potentially toxic oxidative by-products of bacterial metabolism, which would be expected to remain in contact with the colonic mucosa for longer periods of time as a result of reduced stool bulk. High fat intake also enhances hepatic synthesis of cholesterol and bile acids, which can be converted into carcinogens by intestinal bacteria.

In addition to dietary modification, *pharmacologic chemoprevention* has become an area of great interest. Several epidemiologic studies suggest that aspirin or other NSAIDs have a protective effect. This is consistent with studies showing that some NSAIDs cause polyp regression in FAP patients in whom the rectum was left in place after colectomy. It is suspected that this effect is mediated by inhibition of the enzyme cyclooxygenase-2 (COX-2), which is highly expressed in 90% of colorectal carcinomas and 40% to 90% of adenomas. COX-2 is necessary for production of prostaglandin E_2, which promotes epithelial proliferation, particularly after injury. Of further interest, COX-2 expression is regulated by TLR4, which recognizes lipopolysaccharide and is also overexpressed in adenomas and carcinomas.

Pathogenesis. Studies of colorectal carcinogenesis have provided fundamental insights into the general mechanisms of cancer evolution. These were discussed in Chapter 7; concepts that pertain specifically to colorectal carcinogenesis will be reviewed here.

The combination of molecular events that lead to colonic adenocarcinoma is heterogeneous and includes genetic and epigenetic abnormalities. At least two genetic pathways have been described. In simplest terms, these are the *APC/β-catenin pathway,* which is activated in the classic adenoma-carcinoma sequence; and the *microsatellite instability pathway,* which is associated with defects in DNA mismatch repair and accumulation of mutations in microsatellite repeat regions of the genome (Table 17-11). Both pathways involve the stepwise accumulation of multiple mutations, but differ in the genes involved and the mechanisms by which mutations accumulate. Epigenetic events, the most common of which is methylation-induced gene silencing, may enhance progression along either pathway.

- **The classic adenoma-carcinoma sequence, accounts for up to 80% of sporadic colon tumors and typically includes mutation of *APC* early in the neoplastic process** (Fig. 17-49). Both copies of the *APC* gene must be functionally inactivated, either by mutation or epigenetic events, for adenomas to develop. *APC is a key negative regulator of β-catenin, a component of the Wnt signaling pathway* (Chapter 7). The APC protein normally binds to and promotes degradation of β-catenin. With loss of APC function, β-catenin accumulates and

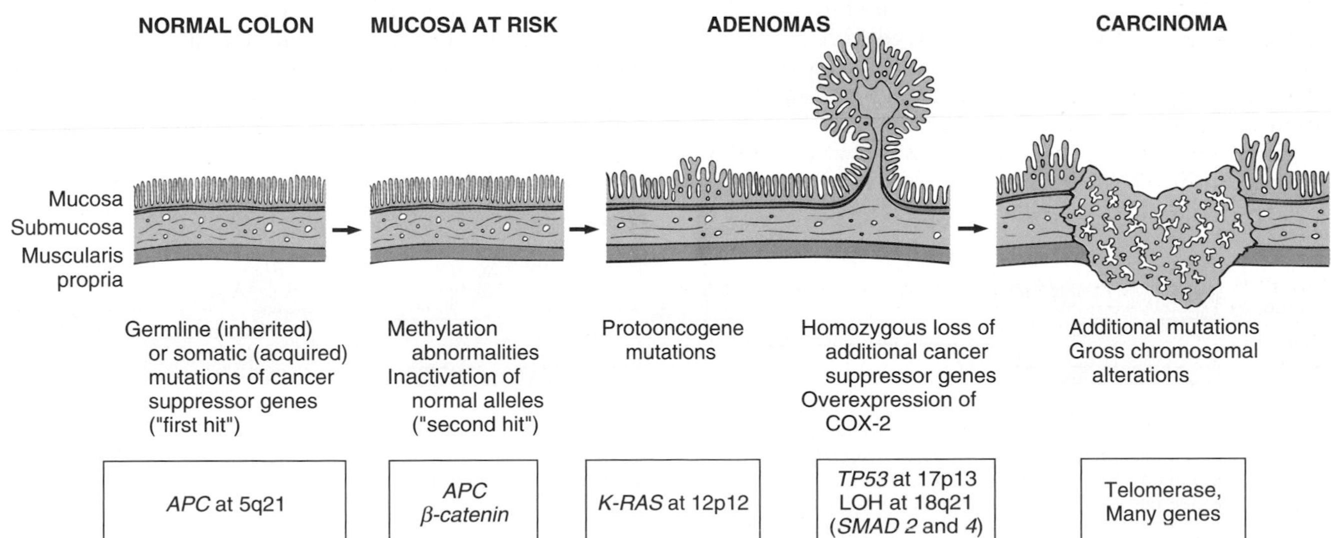

Figure 17-49 Morphologic and molecular changes in the adenoma-carcinoma sequence. Loss of one normal copy of the tumor suppressor gene *APC* occurs early. Individuals born with one mutant allele are therefore at increased risk of developing colon cancer. Alternatively, inactivation of *APC* in colonic epithelium may occur later in life. This is the "first hit" according to the Knudson hypothesis (Chapter 7). The loss of the intact second copy of *APC* follows ("second hit"). Other changes, including mutation of *KRAS*, losses at 18q21 involving *SMAD2* and *SMAD4*, and inactivation of the tumor suppressor gene *TP53*, lead to the emergence of carcinoma, in which further mutations occur. Although there seems to be a temporal sequence of changes, the accumulation of mutations, rather than their occurrence in a specific order, is most critical.

translocates to the nucleus, where it forms a complex with the DNA-binding factor TCF and activates the transcription of genes, including MYC and cyclin D1, that promote proliferation. The critical role of β-catenin in this pathway is demonstrated by the fact that many colon cancers without *APC* mutations harbor β-catenin mutations that allow them to avoid APC-dependent degradation, thereby having the same impact as loss of APC function. Additional mutations accumulate, including activating mutations in *KRAS* that promote growth and prevent apoptosis. The idea that mutation of *KRAS* is a late event in carcinoma development is supported by the observation that such mutations are present in fewer than 10% of adenomas less than 1 cm in diameter but are found in 50% of adenomas greater than 1 cm in diameter and in 50% of invasive adenocarcinomas. Neoplastic progression is also associated with mutations in other tumor suppressor genes such as those encoding SMAD2 and SMAD4, which are effectors of TGF-β signaling. Because TGF-β signaling normally inhibits the cell cycle, loss of these genes may allow unrestrained cell growth. The tumor suppressor gene *TP53* is mutated in 70% to 80% of colon cancers, but is uncommonly affected in adenomas, suggesting that *TP53* mutations also occur at later stages of tumor progression. Loss of function of *TP53* and other tumor suppressor genes is often caused by chromosomal deletions, supporting the idea that chromosomal instability is a hallmark of the APC/β-catenin pathway. Alternatively, tumor suppressor genes may be silenced by methylation of a CpG-rich zone, or CpG island, a 5′ region of some genes that frequently includes the promoter and transcriptional start site. Expression of telomerase also increases as lesions become more advanced.

- **In patients with DNA mismatch repair deficiency, mutations accumulate in microsatellite repeats, a condition referred to as microsatellite instability (MSI).** These are referred to as MSI high, or MSI-H, tumors. Some microsatellite sequences are located in the coding or promoter regions of genes involved in regulation of cell growth, such as those encoding the type II TGF-β receptor and the pro-apoptotic protein BAX (Fig. 17-50). Because TGF-β inhibits colonic epithelial cell proliferation, mutation of type II TGF-β receptor can contribute to uncontrolled cell growth, while loss of *BAX* may enhance the survival of genetically abnormal clones.
- **A subset of microsatellite unstable colon cancers without mutations in DNA mismatch repair enzymes demonstrate the CpG island hypermethylation phenotype (CIMP).** In these tumors, the *MLH1* promoter region is typically hypermethylated, thereby reducing MLH1 expression and repair function. Activating mutations in the oncogene *BRAF* are common in these cancers. In contrast, *KRAS* and *TP53* are not typically mutated. Thus, the combination of microsatellite instability, *BRAF* mutation, and methylation of specific targets, such as *MLH1*, is the signature of this pathway of carcinogenesis.
- **A small group of colon cancers display increased CpG island methylation in the absence of microsatellite instability.** Many of these tumors harbor *KRAS* mutations, but *TP53* and *BRAF* mutations are uncommon. In contrast, *TP53* mutations are common in colon cancers that do not display a CpG island methylator phenotype.

While morphology cannot reliably define the underlying molecular events that lead to carcinogenesis, certain correlations have been associated with mismatch repair deficiency and microsatellite instability. These molecular alterations are common in sessile serrated adenomas and cancers that arise from them. In addition, invasive carcinomas with microsatellite instability often have prominent mucinous differentiation and peritumoral lymphocytic infiltrates. These tumors, as well as those with a CpG island hypermethylation phenotype, are frequently located in the right colon. Tumors with microsatellite instability can be recognized by the absence of immunohistochemical staining for mismatch repair proteins or by molecular genetic analysis of microsatellite sequences. It is important to identify patients with HNPCC because of the implications for genetic counseling, the elevated risk of a second malignancy of the colon or other organs, and, in some settings, differences in prognosis and therapy.

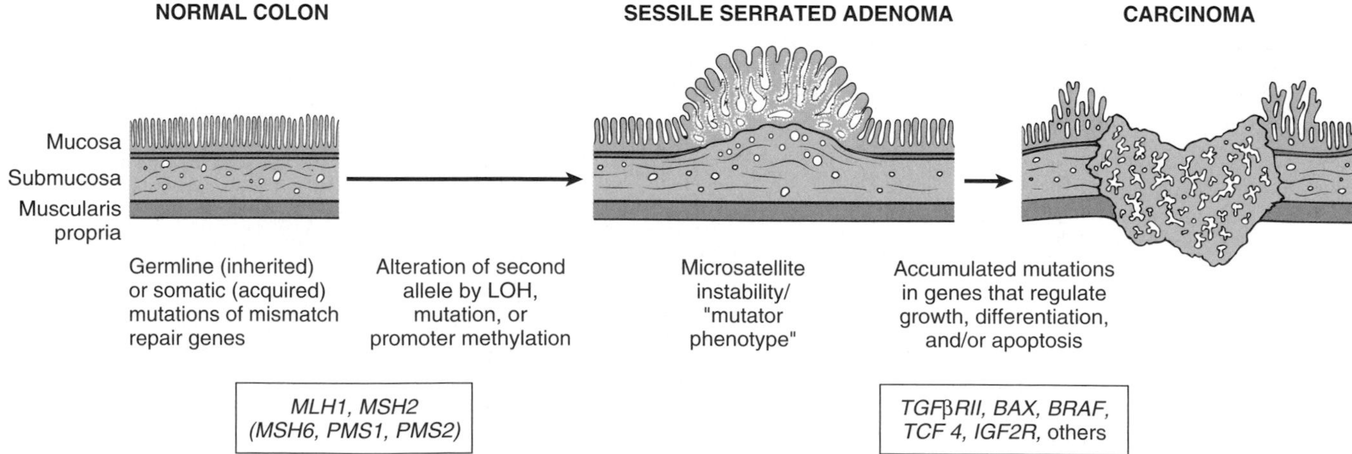

Figure 17-50 Morphologic and molecular changes in the mismatch repair pathway of colon carcinogenesis. Defects in mismatch repair genes result in microsatellite instability and permit accumulation of mutations in numerous genes. If these mutations affect genes involved in cell survival and proliferation, cancer may develop.

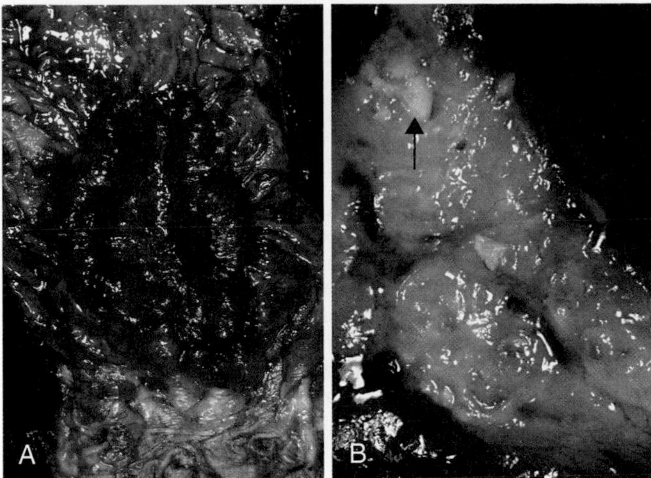

Figure 17-51 Colorectal carcinoma. **A,** Circumferential, ulcerated rectal cancer. Note the anal mucosa at the bottom of the image. **B,** Cancer of the sigmoid colon that has invaded through the muscularis propria and is present within subserosal adipose tissue (left). Areas of chalky necrosis are present within the colon wall *(arrow)*.

MORPHOLOGY

Overall, adenocarcinomas are distributed approximately equally over the entire length of the colon. Tumors in the **proximal colon often grow as polypoid, exophytic masses** that extend along one wall of the large-caliber cecum and ascending colon; these tumors rarely cause obstruction. In contrast, **carcinomas in the distal colon tend to be annular lesions** that produce "napkin-ring" constrictions and luminal narrowing (Fig. 17-51), sometimes to the point of obstruction. Both forms grow into the bowel wall over time. The general microscopic characteristics of right- and left-sided colonic adenocarcinomas are similar. Most tumors are composed of tall columnar cells that resemble dysplastic epithelium found in adenomas (Fig. 17-52*A*). The invasive component of these tumors elicits a strong stromal desmoplastic response, which is responsible for their characteristic firm consistency. Some poorly differentiated tumors form few glands (Fig. 17-52*B*). Others may produce abundant mucin that accumulates within the intestinal wall, and these are associated with poor prognosis. Tumors may also be composed of signet-ring cells that are similar to those in gastric cancer (Fig. 17-52*C*) or may display features of neuroendocrine differentiation.

Clinical Features. The availability of endoscopic screening combined with the knowledge that most carcinomas arise within adenomas presents a unique opportunity for cancer prevention. Unfortunately, colorectal cancers develop insidiously and may go undetected for long periods. Cecal and other *right-sided colon cancers* are most often called to clinical attention by the appearance of *fatigue and weakness due to iron deficiency anemia*. Thus, it is a clinical maxim that the underlying cause of iron deficiency anemia in an older man or postmenopausal woman is GI cancer until proven otherwise. *Left-sided colorectal adenocarcinomas* may produce *occult bleeding*, *changes in bowel habits*, or *cramping* and *left lower quadrant discomfort*.

Although poorly differentiated and mucinous histologies are associated with poor prognosis, *the two most important prognostic factors are depth of invasion and the presence of lymph node metastases*. Invasion into the muscularis propria confers significantly reduced survival that is decreased further by the presence of lymph node metastases (Fig. 17-53*A*). Metastases may involve regional lymph nodes, lungs (Fig. 17-53*B*) and bones, but as a result of portal drainage of the colon, the liver is the most common site of metastatic lesions (Fig. 17-53*C*). The rectum does not drain via the portal circulation, hence carcinomas of the anal region that metastasize often circumvent the liver.

The prognostic factors were originally recognized by Dukes and Kirklin and form the core of the TNM (tumor-nodes-metastasis) classification (Table 17-12). The American Joint Committee on Cancer (AJCC) staging system is compared to the Astler-Coller modification of the Dukes system in Table 17-13. Regardless of stage, it must be remembered that some patients with small numbers of metastases do well for years following resection of distant tumor nodules.

Five-year survival rates vary widely worldwide. The overall 5-year survival rate in the United States is 65%, and ranges from 90% to 40% depending on stage. Survival rates in Europe, Japan and Australia are similar, ranging

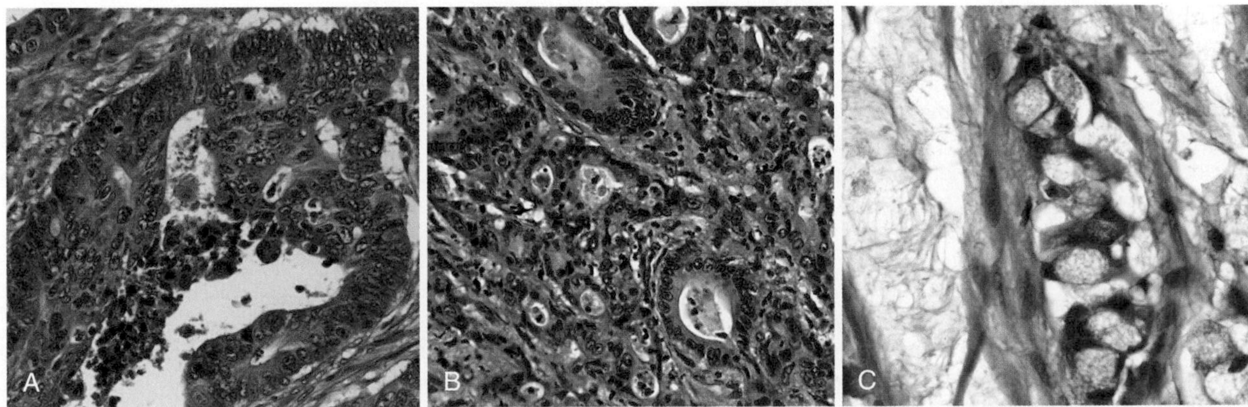

Figure 17-52 Histologic appearance of colorectal carcinoma. **A,** Well-differentiated adenocarcinoma. Note the elongated, hyperchromatic nuclei. Necrotic debris, present in the gland lumen, is typical. **B,** Poorly differentiated adenocarcinoma forms a few glands but is largely composed of infiltrating nests of tumor cells. **C,** Mucinous adenocarcinoma with signet-ring cells and extracellular mucin pools.

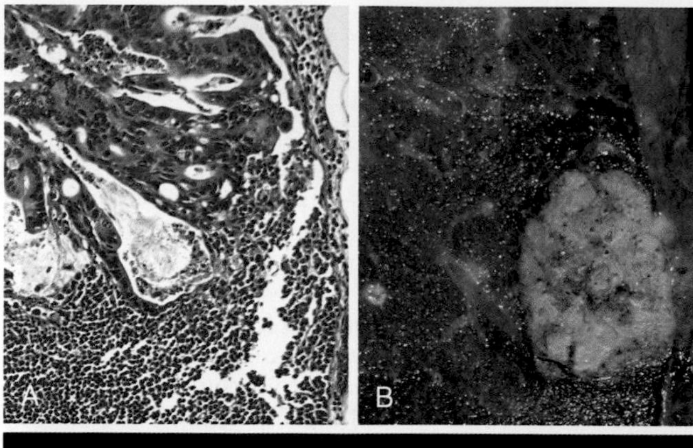

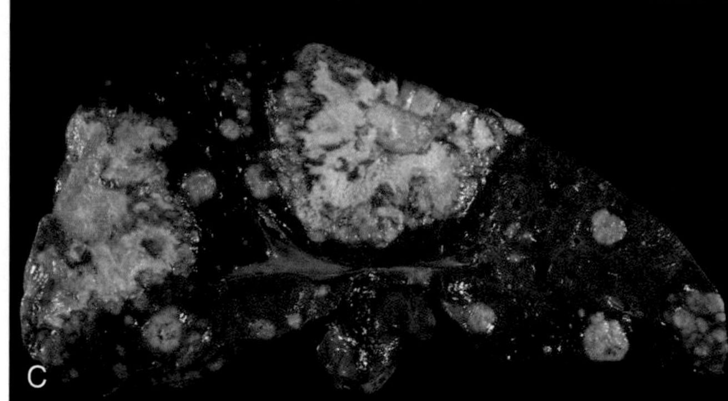

Figure 17-53 Metastatic colorectal carcinoma. **A,** Lymph node metastasis. Note the glandular structures within the subcapsular sinus. **B,** Solitary subpleural nodule of colorectal carcinoma metastatic to the lung. **C,** Liver containing two large and many smaller metastases. Note the central necrosis within metastases.

from 60% (Switzerland, Japan) to (40%) Poland. Overall survival rates are somewhat lower in other countries, such as China, India, the Philippines, and Thailand (30% to 42%). Sadly, the 5-year survival rate in Gambia is only 4%.

Table 17-12 American Joint Committee on Cancer (AJCC) TNM Classification of Colorectal Carcinoma

TNM	
Tumor	
Tis	In situ dysplasia or intramucosal carcinoma
T1	Tumor invades submucosa
T2	Tumor invades into, but not through, muscularis propria
T3	Tumor invades through muscularis propria
T3a	Invasion < 0.1 cm beyond muscularis propria
T3b	Invasion 0.1 to 0.5 cm beyond muscularis propria
T3c	Invasion > 0.5 to 1.5 cm beyond muscularis propria
T3d	Invasion > 1.5 cm beyond muscularis propria
T4	Tumor penetrates visceral peritoneum or invades adjacent organs
T4a	Penetration into visceral peritoneum
T4b	Invasion into other organs or structures
Regional Lymph Nodes	
NX	Lymph nodes cannot be assessed
N0	No regional lymph node metastasis
N1	Metastasis in one to three regional lymph nodes
N1a	Metastasis in one regional lymph nodes
N1b	Metastasis in two or three regional lymph nodes
N1c	Tumor deposit(s) in the subserosa, mesentery, or nonperitonealized pericolic or perirectal tissues without regional nodal metastasis
N2	Metastasis in four or more regional lymph nodes
N2a	Metastasis in four to six regional lymph nodes
N2b	Metastasis in seven or more regional lymph nodes
Distant Metastasis	
MX	Distant metastasis cannot be assessed
M0	No distant metastasis
M1	Distant metastasis
M1a	Metastasis confined to one organ or site
M1b	Metastases in more than one organ/site or the peritoneum

Table 17-13 Colorectal Cancer Staging Systems

	American Joint Committee on Cancer (AJCC) Stage			Astler-Coller Modification of Dukes Classification
	T	N	M	
I	T1	N0	M0	A
	T2	N0	M0	B1
IIA	T3	N0	M0	B2
IIB	T4a	N0	M0	B2
IIC	T4b	N0	M0	B3
IIIA	T1-T2	N1/N1c	M0	C1
	T1	N2a	M0	C1
IIIB	T3, T4a	N1 (any)	M0	C2
	T2, T3	N2a	M0	C1/C2
	T1, T2	N2b	M0	C1
IIIC	T4a	N2a	M0	C2
	T3, T4a	N2b	M0	C2
	T4b	N1, N2	M0	C3
IVA	Any T	Any N	M1a	D*
IVB	Any T	Any N	M1b	D*

*Stages not included in original Dukes classification; added later for comparison with AJCC staging.

KEY CONCEPTS

Benign and malignant proliferative lesions of the colon

- **Intestinal polyps** can be classified as nonneoplastic or neoplastic. The nonneoplastic polyps can be further defined as hyperplastic, inflammatory, or hamartomatous.
- **Hyperplastic polyps** are benign epithelial proliferations most commonly found in the left colon and rectum. They have no malignant potential, and must be distinguished from sessile serrated adenomas.
- **Inflammatory polyps** form as a result of chronic cycles of injury and healing.
- **Hamartomatous polyps** occur sporadically or as a part of genetic diseases. The latter include **juvenile polyposis** and **Peutz-Jeghers Syndrome**, which are associated with **increased risk of malignancy**.
- Benign epithelial neoplastic polyps of the intestines are termed **adenomas**. The hallmark of these lesions, which are the precursors of colonic adenocarcinomas, is cytologic dysplasia.
- In contrast to traditional adenomas, **sessile serrated adenomas** lack cytologic dysplasia and share morphologic features with hyperplastic polyps.

- **Familial adenomatous polyposis** (FAP) and **hereditary non-polyposis colorectal cancer** (HNPCC) are the most common forms of familial colon cancer.
- **FAP** is caused by *APC* mutations. Patients typically have more than 100 adenomas and develop colon cancer before 30 years of age.
- **HNPCC** is caused by mutations in DNA mismatch repair enzymes. HNPCC patients have far fewer polyps and develop cancer at older ages than FAP patients but younger ages than those with sporadic colon cancer.
- FAP and HNPCC typify **distinct pathways of neoplastic transformation and progression** that also contribute to the majority of **sporadic colon cancers**.
- Nearly all colonic cancers are **adenocarcinomas.** The two most important prognostic factors are **depth of invasion** and the presence or absence of **lymph node metastases**.

Tumors of the Anal Canal

The anal canal can be divided into thirds. The upper zone is lined by columnar rectal epithelium; the middle third by transitional epithelium; and the lower third by stratified squamous epithelium. Carcinomas of the anal canal may have typical glandular or squamous patterns of differentiation, recapitulating the normal epithelium of the upper and lower thirds, respectively (Fig. 17-54*A*). An additional differentiation pattern, termed basaloid, is present in tumors populated by immature cells derived from the basal layer of transitional epithelium (Fig. 17-54*B*). When the entire tumor displays a basaloid pattern, the archaic term cloacogenic carcinoma is still often applied. Alternatively, basaloid differentiation may be mixed with squamous or mucinous differentiation. All are considered variants of anal canal carcinoma. Pure squamous cell carcinoma of the anal canal is frequently associated with HPV infection, which also causes precursor lesions such as condyloma acuminatum (Fig. 17-54*C*).

Hemorrhoids

Hemorrhoids affect about 5% of the general population and develop secondary to persistently elevated venous pressure within the hemorrhoidal plexus. The most frequent predisposing influences are straining at defecation, because of constipation, and the venous stasis of pregnancy. Hemorrhoids may also develop in association with portal hypertension. The pathogenesis of hemorrhoids (anal varices) in portal hypertension is similar to that of esophageal varices, although anal varices are both more common and much less serious. Variceal dilations of the anal and perianal venous plexuses form collaterals that connect the portal and caval venous systems, thereby relieving the venous hypertension.

MORPHOLOGY

Collateral vessels within the inferior hemorrhoidal plexus are located below the anorectal line and are termed **external hemorrhoids**, while those that result from dilation of the superior hemorrhoidal plexus within the distal rectum are referred to as **internal hemorrhoids.** Histologically, hemorrhoids consist of thin-walled, dilated, submucosal vessels that protrude beneath the anal or rectal mucosa. In their exposed position, they are subject to trauma and tend to become inflamed, thrombosed, and, in the course of time, recanalized. Superficial ulceration may occur.

Hemorrhoids often present with pain and rectal bleeding, particularly bright red blood seen on toilet tissue. Except for pregnant women, hemorrhoids are rarely encountered in persons younger than age 30. Hemorrhoidal bleeding is not generally a medical emergency and can be treated by sclerotherapy, rubber band ligation, or infrared coagulation. Extensive or severe internal or external hemorrhoids may be removed surgically by hemorrhoidectomy.

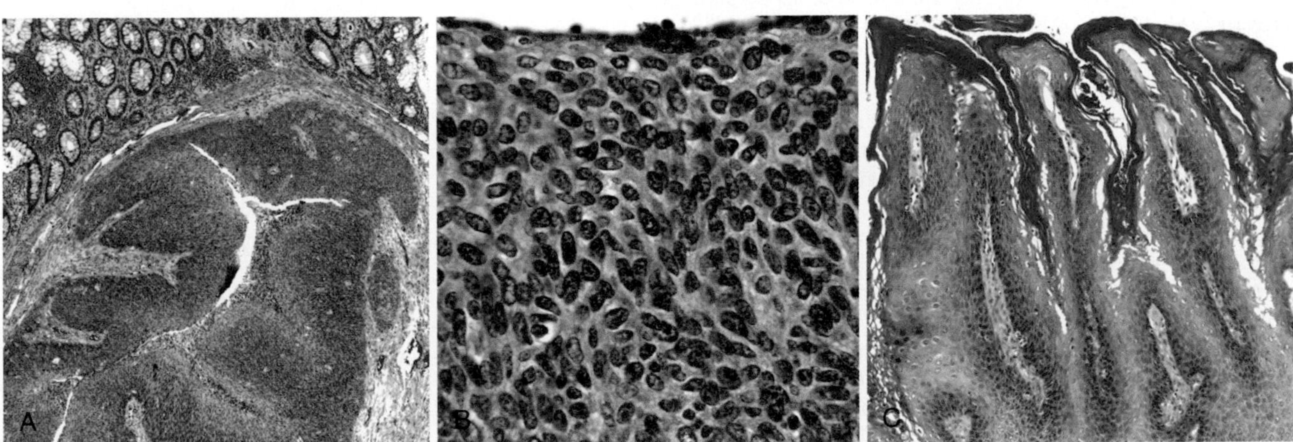

Figure 17-54 Anal tumors. **A,** This anal transition zone carcinoma demonstrates a multilayered organization reminiscent of benign squamous mucosa. The adjacent rectal mucosa is intact. **B,** This basaloid anal transition zone tumor is composed of hyperchromatic cells that resemble the basal layer of normal squamous mucosa. **C,** Condyloma acuminatum with verrucous architecture.

Acute Appendicitis

The appendix is a normal true diverticulum of the cecum that is prone to acute and chronic inflammation. Acute appendicitis is most common in adolescents and young adults, with a lifetime risk of 7%; males are affected slightly more often than females. Despite the prevalence of acute appendicitis, the diagnosis can be difficult to confirm preoperatively and may be confused with mesenteric lymphadenitis (often secondary to unrecognized *Yersinia* infection or viral enterocolitis), acute salpingitis, ectopic pregnancy, mittelschmerz (pain caused by minor pelvic bleeding at the time of ovulation), and Meckel diverticulitis.

Pathogenesis. Acute appendicitis is thought to be initiated by progressive increases in intraluminal pressure that compromise venous outflow. In 50% to 80% of cases, acute appendicitis is associated with overt luminal obstruction, usually caused by a small stone-like mass of stool, or fecalith, or, less commonly, a gallstone, tumor, or mass of worms (oxyuriasis vermicularis). Stasis of luminal contents, which favors bacterial proliferation, triggers ischemia and inflammatory responses, resulting in tissue edema and neutrophilic infiltration of the lumen, muscular wall, and periappendiceal soft tissues.

MORPHOLOGY

In early acute appendicitis subserosal vessels are congested and there is a modest perivascular neutrophilic infiltrate within all layers of the wall. The inflammatory reaction transforms the normal glistening serosa into a dull, granular, erythematous surface. Although mucosal neutrophils and focal superficial ulceration are often present, these are not specific markers of acute appendicitis. Diagnosis of acute appendicitis requires **neutrophilic infiltration of the muscularis propria.** In more severe cases a prominent neutrophilic exudate generates a serosal fibrinopurulent reaction. As the process continues, focal abscesses may form within the wall (acute suppurative appendicitis). Further compromise of appendiceal vessels leads to large areas of hemorrhagic ulceration and gangrenous necrosis that extends to the serosa creating acute gangrenous appendicitis, which can be followed by rupture and suppurative peritonitis.

Clinical Features. Typically, early acute appendicitis produces periumbilical pain that ultimately localizes to the right lower quadrant, followed by nausea, vomiting, low-grade fever, and a mildly elevated peripheral white cell count. A classic physical finding is the *McBurney sign,* deep tenderness located two thirds of the distance from the umbilicus to the right anterior superior iliac spine (McBurney point).

Regrettably, classic signs and symptoms of acute appendicitis are often absent. In some cases, a retrocecal appendix may generate right flank or pelvic pain, while a malrotated colon may give rise to appendicitis in the left upper quadrant. As with other causes of acute inflammation there is neutrophilic leukocytosis. In some cases the peripheral leukocytosis may be minimal or, alternatively, so great that other causes are considered. The diagnosis of acute appendicitis in young children and the very old is particularly problematic, since other causes of abdominal emergencies are prevalent in these populations, and the very young and old are also more likely to have atypical clinical presentations.

Given these diagnostic challenges, it should be no surprise that even highly skilled surgeons remove normal appendices. This is preferred to delayed resection of a diseased appendix, given the significant morbidity and mortality associated with appendiceal perforation. Other complications of appendicitis include pyelophlebitis, portal venous thrombosis, liver abscess, and bacteremia.

Tumors of the Appendix

The most common tumor of the appendix is the well-differentiated neuroendocrine (carcinoid) tumor. It is usually discovered incidentally at the time of surgery or examination of a resected appendix. This neoplasm, which is almost always benign, most frequently forms a solid bulbous swelling at the distal tip of the appendix, where it can reach 2 to 3 cm in diameter. Although intramural and transmural extension may be evident, nodal metastases are very infrequent, and distant spread is exceptionally rare. Conventional adenomas or non–mucin-producing adenocarcinomas also occur in the appendix and may cause obstruction and enlargement that mimics acute appendicitis. Mucocele, a dilated appendix filled with mucin, may simply represent an obstructed appendix containing inspissated mucin or be a consequence of mucinous cystadenoma or mucinous cystadenocarcinoma. In the latter instance, invasion through the appendiceal wall can lead to intraperitoneal seeding and spread. In women the resulting peritoneal implants may be mistaken for mucinous ovarian tumors. In the most advanced cases the abdomen fills with tenacious, semisolid mucin, a condition called *pseudomyxoma peritonei* (Chapter 22). This disseminated intraperitoneal disease may be held in check for years by repeated debulking but, in most instances, follows an inexorably fatal course.

KEY CONCEPTS

- **Hemorrhoids** are collateral vessels that develop secondary to persistently elevated venous pressure within the hemorrhoidal plexus. They also occur in portal hypertension.
- **Acute appendicitis** is most common in children and adolescents. It is thought to be initiated by increased intraluminal pressure and compromised venous outflow
- The most common tumor of the appendix is the **benign carcinoid.**
- Peritoneal dissemination of mucinous tumors can cause **pseudomyxoma peritonei**.

PERITONEAL CAVITY

The peritoneal cavity houses the abdominal viscera and is lined by a single layer of mesothelial cells; these cover the visceral and parietal surfaces and are supported by a thin layer of connective tissue to form the peritoneum. Here we discuss inflammatory, infectious, and neoplastic disorders of the peritoneal cavity and retroperitoneal space. Although they are less common than inflammatory and infectious processes, tumors can carry a grave prognosis and, thus, also deserve discussion.

Inflammatory Disease

Peritonitis may result from bacterial invasion or chemical irritation and is most often due to:

- Leakage of bile or pancreatic enzymes, which produces *sterile peritonitis*
- *Perforation or rupture of the biliary system* that evokes a highly irritating peritonitis, usually complicated by bacterial superinfection
- *Acute hemorrhagic pancreatitis* (Chapter 19), which is associated with leakage of pancreatic enzymes and fat necrosis. Damage to the bowel wall may allow bacteria to spread to the peritoneal cavity.
- *Foreign material*, including that introduced surgically (e.g., talc and sutures), that induces foreign body-type granulomas and fibrous scarring
- *Endometriosis*, which causes hemorrhage into the peritoneal cavity, where it acts as an irritant
- *Ruptured dermoid cysts* that release keratins and induce an intense granulomatous reaction
- *Perforation* of abdominal viscera.

Peritoneal Infection

Bacterial peritonitis occurs when bacteria from the gastrointestinal lumen are released into the abdominal cavity, most commonly following perforation. *E. coli*, streptococci, *S. aureus*, enterococci, and *C. perfringens* are implicated most often.

Spontaneous bacterial peritonitis develops in the absence of an obvious source of contamination. It is seen most often in patients with cirrhosis and ascites and less frequently in children with nephrotic syndrome.

MORPHOLOGY

The cellular inflammatory response is composed primarily of dense collections of neutrophils and fibrinopurulent debris that coat the viscera and abdominal wall. Serous or slightly turbid fluid begins to accumulate and becomes suppurative as infection progresses. Subhepatic and subdiaphragmatic abscesses may be formed. With the exception of tuberculous peritonitis, the reaction usually remains superficial.

Sclerosing Retroperitonitis

Sclerosing retroperitonitis, also known as idiopathic retroperitoneal fibrosis or Ormond disease, is characterized by dense fibrosis that may extend to involve the mesentery. Although the cause of sclerosing retroperitonitis is unknown, many cases are now thought to fall within the spectrum of IgG4-related sclerosing disease, an immunoinflammatory disorder that can lead to fibrosis in a wide variety of tissues. Because the process frequently compresses the ureters, this entity is described in more detail in Chapters 6 and 21.

Tumors

Primary malignant tumors arising from peritoneal lining are mesotheliomas that are similar to tumors of the pleura and pericardium. Peritoneal mesotheliomas are almost always associated with significant asbestos exposure. Rarely, primary benign and malignant soft-tissue tumors may also develop within the peritoneum and retroperitoneum. The most common of these is desmoplastic small round cell tumor. This is an aggressive tumor that occurs in children and young adults and bears resemblance to Ewing sarcoma and other small round cell tumors. It is characterized by a reciprocal translocation, t(11;22)(p13;q12) that results in the formation of a fusion gene involving *EWS* and *WT1* genes.

Secondary tumors may involve the peritoneum by direct spread or metastatic seeding, resulting in peritoneal carcinomatosis. Mucinous carcinomas, particularly those of the appendix may cause pseudomyxoma peritonei.

SUGGESTED READINGS

Congenital Abnormalities

Amin SC, Pappas C, Iyengar H, et al: Short bowel syndrome in the NICU. *Clin Perinatol* 40:53, 2013. *[A comprehensive discussion of the epidemiology and management of short bowel syndrome in neonates.]*

Kapur RP: Practical pathology and genetics of Hirschsprung's disease. *Semin Pediatr Surg* 18:212, 2009. *[A review of Hirschsprung disease etiology and diagnosis.]*

Peeters B, Benninga MA, Hennekam RC: Infantile hypertrophic pyloric stenosis–genetics and syndromes. *Nat Rev Gastroenterol Hepatol* 9:646, 2012. *[A review that focuses on disease mechanisms and clinical associations.]*

Esophagus

Esophageal Obstruction

Clarke JO, Pandolfino JE: Esophageal motor disorders: how to bridge the gap between advanced diagnostic tools and paucity of therapeutic modalities? *J Clin Gastroenterol* 46:442, 2012. *[A diagnosis-based discussion of esophageal motor disorders.]*

Richter JE, Boeckxstaens GE: Management of achalasia: surgery or pneumatic dilation. *Gut* 60:869, 2011. *[A therapy-focused discussion of the etiology, pathophysiology, and management of achalasia.]*

Esophagitis

Abonia JP, Rothenberg ME: Eosinophilic esophagitis: rapidly advancing insights. *Annu Rev Med* 63:421, 2012. *[Comprehensive review of pathobiology and treatment of eosinophilic esophagitis.]*

Coss-Adame E, Erdogan A, Rao SS: Treatment of Esophageal (Noncardiac) Chest Pain: Review. *Clin Gastroenterol Hepatol* 2013. *[A careful consideration of the approach to a patient with esophageal symptoms.]*

Kandulski A, Malfertheiner P: Gastroesophageal reflux disease–from reflux episodes to mucosal inflammation. *Nat Rev Gastroenterol Hepatol* 9:15, 2012. *[A mechanism-based update on gastroesophageal reflux.]*

Barrett Esophagus

Jankowski JA, Satsangi J: Barrett's esophagus: evolutionary insights from genomics. *Gastroenterol* 144:667, 2013. *[A detailed discussion of Barrett esophagus pathogenesis.]*

Kahrilas PJ: The problems with surveillance of Barrett's esophagus. *N Engl J Med* 365:1437, 2011. *[Analysis of the utility of current surveillance protocols for esophageal glandular dysplasia.]*

Shaheen NJ, Sharma P, Overholt BF, et al.: Radiofrequency ablation in Barrett's esophagus with dysplasia. *N Engl J Med* 360:2277, 2009. *[Clinical trial report for radiofrequency ablation of Barrett esophagus.]*

Sharma P: Clinical practice. Barrett's esophagus, *N Engl J Med* 361:2548, 2009. *[A comprehensive discussion of Barrett esophagus.]*

Spechler SJ, Fitzgerald RC, Prasad GA, et al: History, molecular mechanisms, and endoscopic treatment of Barrett's esophagus. *Gastroenterol* 138:854, 2010. *[Overarching review of Barrett esophagus.]*

Spechler SJ, Sharma P, Souza RF, et al: American Gastroenterological Association technical review on the management of Barrett's esophagus. *Gastroenterol* 140:e18, 2011. *[Practice-based focus on management of Barrett esophagus.]*

Esophageal Tumors

Cook MB, Shaheen NJ, Anderson LA, et al: Cigarette smoking increases risk of Barrett's esophagus: an analysis of the Barrett's and Esophageal Adenocarcinoma Consortium. *Gastroenterol* 142:744, 2012. *[Analysis of risk factors associated with Barrett esophagus.]*

Fleischer DE: Comparing apples with apples and oranges: the role of radiofrequency ablation alone versus radiofrequency ablation plus EMR for endoscopic management of Barrett's esophagus with advanced neoplasia. *Gastrointest Endosc* 76:740, 2012. *[Comparison of therapeutic options in Barrett esophagus with neoplasia.]*

Hvid-Jensen F, Pedersen L, Drewes AM, et al: Incidence of adenocarcinoma among patients with Barrett's esophagus. *N Engl J Med* 365:1375, 2011. *[Analysis of adenocarcinoma risk for Barrett esophagus patients.]*

Stomach

Gastropathy and Acute Gastritis

Ali T, Harty RF: Stress-induced ulcer bleeding in critically ill patients. *Gastroenterol Clin North Am* 38:245, 2009. *[Historically and clinically focused discussion of stress-related erosive syndrome.]*

Camilleri M, Bharucha AE, Farrugia G: Epidemiology, mechanisms, and management of diabetic gastroparesis. *Clin Gastroenterol Hepatol* 9:5, 2011. *[Comprehensive discussion of diabetic gastroparesis.]*

Fourmy D, Gigoux V, Reubi JC: Gastrin in gastrointestinal diseases. *Gastroenterol* 141:814, 2011. *[Discussion of gastrin contributions to gastric physiology and disease.]*

Sostres C, Lanas A: Gastrointestinal effects of aspirin. *Nat Rev Gastroenterol Hepatol* 8:385, 2011. *[Mechanisms and management of NSAID toxicities are explored.]*

Tang SJ, Daram SR, Wu R, et al: Pathogenesis, Diagnosis, and Management of Gastric Ischemia. *Clin Gastroenterol Hepatol* 2013. *[All-encompassing review of gastric ischemic disease.]*

Chronic Gastritis

Arnold IC, Lee JY, Amieva MR, et al.: Tolerance rather than immunity protects from Helicobacter pylori-induced gastric preneoplasia. *Gastroenterol* 140:199, 2011. *[Consideration of host factors that contribute to outcomes of H. pylori infection.]*

Neumann WL, Coss E, Rugge M, et al: Autoimmune atrophic gastritis-pathogenesis, pathology and management. *Nat Rev Gastroenterol Hepatol* 10:529, 2013. *[All-encompassing review of atrophic gastritis.]*

Sonnenberg A, Lash RH, Genta RM: A national study of Helicobactor pylori infection in gastric biopsy specimens. *Gastroenterol* 139:1894, 2010. *[Pathology-based review of nearly 80,000 gastric biopsies.]*

Complications of Chronic Gastritis

Malfertheiner P, Chan FK, McColl KE: Peptic ulcer disease. *Lancet* 374:1449, 2009. *[Summary of current understanding of peptic ulcer disease.]*

Park JY, Cornish TC, Lam-Himlin D, et al: Gastric lesions in patients with autoimmune metaplastic atrophic gastritis (AMAG) in a tertiary care setting. *Am J Surg Pathol* 34:1591, 2010. *[Review of over 40,000 gastric biopsies and analysis of the incidence of autoimmune metaplastic atrophic gastritis and associated lesions.]*

Hypertrophic Gastropathies

Fiske WH, Tanksley J, Nam KT, et al: Efficacy of cetuximab in the treatment of Menetrier's disease. *Sci Transl Med* 1:8ra18, 2009. *[Analysis of series of patients treated for Menetrier's disease.]*

Nalle SC, Turner JR: Menetrier's disease therapy: rebooting mucosal signaling. *Sci Transl Med* 1:8ps10, 2009. *[Review of mechanisms of Menetrier's disease.]*

Rich A, Toro TZ, Tanksley J, et al: Distinguishing Menetrier's disease from its mimics. *Gut* 59:1617, 2010. *[Discussion of the differential diagnostic features of Menetrier's disease.]*

Simmons LH, Guimaraes AR, Zukerberg LR: Case records of the Massachusetts General Hospital. Case 6-2013. A 54-year-old man with recurrent diarrhea. *N Engl J Med* 368:757, 2013. *[Case report and discussion of Zollinger-Ellison syndrome.]*

Gastric Polyps and Tumors

Carmack SW, Genta RM, Graham DY, et al: Management of gastric polyps: a pathology-based guide for gastroenterologists. *Nat Rev Gastroenterol Hepatol* 6:331, 2009. *[Discussion of endoscopic characteristics, histopathology, pathogenesis, and clinical management gastric polyps.]*

Corless CL, Barnett CM, Heinrich MC: Gastrointestinal stromal tumours: origin and molecular oncology. *Nat Rev Cancer* 11:865, 2011. *[Comprehensive review of gastrointestinal stromal tumor biology.]*

Lei Z, Tan IB, Das K, et al: Identification of Molecular Subtypes of Gastric Cancer With Different Responses to PI3-Kinase Inhibitors and 5-Fluorouracil. *Gastroenterol* 145:554, 2013. *[Expression profiling-based detection of gastric cancer subtypes and permanent characterization of chemotherapeutic responses.]*

Polk DB, Peek RM Jr: Helicobacter pylori: gastric cancer and beyond. *Nat Rev Cancer* 10:403, 2010. *[A good review of H. pylori and mechanisms by which it is linked to gastric cancer.]*

Sagaert X, Van Cutsem E, De Hertogh G, et al: Gastric MALT lymphoma: a model of chronic inflammation-induced tumor development. *Nat Rev Gastroenterol Hepatol* 7:336, 2010. *[A discussion of gastric MALT lymphoma pathogenesis.]*

Turner ES, Turner JR: Expanding the Lauren Classification: A New Gastric Cancer Subtype? *Gastroenterol* 2013. *[Commentary exploring the interactions between molecular and morphologic analysis in gastric cancer characterization.]*

Small Intestine and Colon

Intestinal Obstruction

Hellebrekers BW, Kooistra T: Pathogenesis of postoperative adhesion formation. *Br J Surg* 98:1503, 2011. *[Review of adhesion pathogenesis and consideration of therapies to prevent adhesion formation.]*

Justice FA, Nguyen LT, Tran SN, et al: Recurrent intussusception in infants. *J Paediatr Child Health* 47:802, 2011. *[Review of over 600 cases of pediatric intussusception.]*

Osiro SB, Cunningham D, Shoja MM, et al: The twisted colon: a review of sigmoid volvulus. *Am Surg* 78:271, 2012. *[Review of colonic volvulus.]*

Patel MM, Lopez-Collada VR, Bulhoes MM, et al: Intussusception risk and health benefits of rotavirus vaccination in Mexico and Brazil. *N Engl J Med* 364:2283, 2011. *[Epidemiologic analysis of intussusception risk following rotavirus vaccination.]*

Ischemic Bowel Disease and Angiodysplasia

Barnert J, Messmann H: Diagnosis and management of lower gastrointestinal bleeding. *Nat Rev Gastroenterol Hepatol* 6:637, 2009. *[Discussion of clinical approaches to lower GI bleeding.]*

Brandt LJ, Feuerstadt P, Blaszka MC: Anatomic patterns, patient characteristics, and clinical outcomes in ischemic colitis: a study of 313 cases supported by histology. *Am J Gastroenterol* 105:2245, 2010. *[Study of disease associations and clinical outcomes in colonic ischemia.]*

Longstreth GF, Yao JF: Diseases and drugs that increase risk of acute large bowel ischemia. *Clin Gastroenterol Hepatol* 8:49, 2010. *[Detailed clinical analysis of nearly 400 cases of colonic ischemia in older adults.]*

Swanson E, Mahgoub A, Macdonald R, et al: Medical and Endoscopic Therapies for Angiodysplasia and Gastric Antral Vascular Ectasia: a Systematic Review. *Clin Gastroenterol Hepatol* 2013. *[Comprehensive review of angiodysplasia and gastric antral vascular ectasia (GAVE).]*

Malabsorption and Diarrhea

Gelfond D, Borowitz D: Gastrointestinal complications of cystic fibrosis. *Clin Gastroenterol Hepatol* 11:333, 2013. *[Clinical review of cystic fibrosis associated lesions of the gastrointestinal tract.]*

Guerrant RL, DeBoer MD, Moore SR, et al: The impoverished gut–a triple burden of diarrhoea, stunting and chronic disease. *Nat Rev Gastroenterol Hepatol* 10:220, 2013. *[Review of mechanisms underlying growth failure (stunting).]*

Hammer HF, Hammer J: Diarrhea caused by carbohydrate malabsorption. *Gastroenterol Clin North Am* 41:611, 2012. *[Pathophysiology focused review of carbohydrate malabsorption-induced diarrhea.]*

Ludvigsson JF, Leffler DA, Bai JC, et al: The Oslo definitions for coeliac disease and related terms. *Gut* 62:43, 2013. *[Presentation of accepted terminology in diagnosis of celiac disease.]*

Meresse B, Malamut G, Cerf-Bensussan N: Celiac disease: an immunological jigsaw. *Immunity* 36:907, 2012. *[Immunology-focused review of disease mechanisms associated with celiac disease.]*

Moore SR, Lima NL, Soares AM, et al: Prolonged episodes of acute diarrhea reduce growth and increase risk of persistent diarrhea in children. *Gastroenterology* 139:1156, 2010. *[A detailed study of environmental enteropathy.]*

Infectious Enterocolitis

Barton Behravesh C, Mody RK, Jungk J, et al: 2008 outbreak of Salmonella Saintpaul infections associated with raw produce. *N Engl J Med* 364:918, 2011. *[Analysis of a Salmonella epidemic.]*

Barzilay EJ, Schaad N, Magloire R, et al: Cholera surveillance during the Haiti epidemic–the first 2 years. *N Engl J Med* 368:599, 2013. *[Study of cholera outbreak following following the 2010 Haitian earthquake.]*

de Jong HK, Parry CM, van der Poll T, et al: Host-pathogen interaction in invasive Salmonellosis. *PLoS Pathog* 8:e1002933, 2012. *[Mechanism-based review of salmonella pathobiology.]*

Kuehne SA, Cartman ST, Heap JT, et al: The role of toxin A and toxin B in Clostridium difficile infection. *Nature* 467:711, 2010. *[A detailed analysis of toxin function in C. difficile pathogenesis.]*

Madhi SA, Cunliffe NA, Steele D, et al: Effect of human rotavirus vaccine on severe diarrhea in African infants. *N Engl J Med* 362:289, 2010. *[Clinical trial demonstrating reduced efficacy of rotavirus vaccine in some patient groups.]*

Irritable Bowel Syndrome

Ford AC, Bercik P, Morgan DG, et al: Validation of the Rome III Criteria for the Diagnosis of Irritable Bowel Syndrome in Secondary Care. *Gastroenterol* 2013. *[Analysis of the sensitivity and specificity of current diagnostic criteria for IBS.]*

Sperber AD, Drossman DA, Quigley EM: The global perspective on irritable bowel syndrome: a Rome Foundation-World Gastroenterology Organisation symposium. *Am J Gastroenterol* 107:1602, 2012. *[An analysis of IBS from a global perspective.]*

Vazquez-Roque MI, Camilleri M, Smyrk T, et al: A controlled trial of gluten-free diet in patients with irritable bowel syndrome-diarrhea: effects on bowel frequency and intestinal function. *Gastroenterol* 144:903, 2013. *[An analysis of gluten sensitivity in diarrhea predominant IBS patients.]*

Inflammatory Bowel Disease

Abraham C, Medzhitov R: Interactions between the host innate immune system and microbes in inflammatory bowel disease. *Gastroenterol* 140:1729, 2011. *[Immunology-focused review considering host microbe interactions in IBD.]*

Glocker EO, Kotlarz D, Boztug K, et al: Inflammatory bowel disease and mutations affecting the interleukin-10 receptor. *N Engl J Med* 361:2033, 2009. *[Identification of IL-10 receptor mutations in a subset of ulcerative colitis patients.]*

Jostins L, Ripke S, Weersma RK, et al: Host-microbe interactions have shaped the genetic architecture of inflammatory bowel disease. *Nature* 491:119, 2012. *[A comprehensive analysis of 163 IBD-associated genes with new insight into the relationship to pathogen responses.]*

Marchiando AM, Graham WV, Turner JR: Epithelial barriers in homeostasis and disease. *Annu Rev Pathol* 5:119, 2010. *[Review of intestinal epithelial barrier function and its implications in IBD and other disorders.]*

Other Causes of Colitis

Pardi DS, Kelly CP: Microscopic colitis. *Gastroenterology* 140:1155, 2011. *[Review of collagenous and lymphocytic colitis pathobiology and diagnosis.]*

Turner JR: Intestinal mucosal barrier function in health and disease. *Nat Rev Immunol* 9:799, 2009. *[Analysis of epithelial-immune interactions in gastrointestinal disease.]*

Sigmoid Diverticulitis

Strate LL, Modi R, Cohen E, et al: Diverticular disease as a chronic illness: evolving epidemiologic and clinical insights. *Am J Gastroenterol* 107:1486, 2012. *[Review of emerging epidemiology and pathophysiology of chronic diverticular disease.]*

Polyps

Beggs AD, Latchford AR, Vasen HF, et al: Peutz Jeghers syndrome: a systematic review and recommendations for management. *Gut* 59:975, 2010. *[Review of Peutz-Jeghers disease etiology and management.]*

Rex DK, Ahnen DJ, Baron JA, et al: Serrated lesions of the colorectum: review and recommendations from an expert panel. *Am J Gastroenterol* 107:1315, 2012. *[Clinical perspective on management of sessile serrated adenomas.]*

Adenocarcinoma

Boland CR, Goel A: Microsatellite instability in colorectal cancer. *Gastroenterology* 138:2073, 2010. *[Discussion of the microsatellite instability pathway of colon cancer.]*

Corley DA, Jensen CD, Marks AR, et al: Adenoma detection rate and risk of colorectal cancer and death. *N Engl J Med* 370:1298, 2014. *[Large study of the relationship between adenoma detection rates and colon cancer incidence.]*

Jasperson KW, Tuohy TM, Neklason DW, et al: Hereditary and familial colon cancer. *Gastroenterology* 138:2044, 2010. *[Comprehensive review of colon cancer syndromes.]*

Pino MS, Chung DC: The chromosomal instability pathway in colon cancer. *Gastroenterology* 138:2059, 2010. *[Review of colon cancer genetics.]*

Hemorrhoids

Sneider EB, Maykel JA: Diagnosis and management of symptomatic hemorrhoids. *Surg Clin North Am* 90:17, 2010. *[Clinically oriented review of hemorrhoids.]*

Acute Appendicitis and Tumors of the Appendix

Cartwright SL, Knudson MP: Evaluation of acute abdominal pain in adults. *Am Fam Physician* 77:971, 2008. *[Clinically oriented approach to the acute abdomen.]*

Deschamps L, Couvelard A: Endocrine tumors of the appendix: a pathologic review. *Arch Pathol Lab Med* 134:871, 2010. *[Pathology-focused review of appendiceal carcinoid tumors.]*

Peritoneal Cavity

Baratti D, Kusamura S, Deraco M: Diffuse malignant peritoneal mesothelioma: systematic review of clinical management and biological research. *J Surg Oncol* 103:822, 2011. *[Overarching review of diffuse malignant peritoneal mesothelioma.]*

Li PK, Chow KM: Infectious complications in dialysis–epidemiology and outcomes. *Nat Rev Nephrol* 8:77, 2012. *[A review of that includes discussion of peritoneal infections occurring in association with peritoneal dialysis.]*

See TARGETED THERAPY available online at www.studentconsult.com

CHAPTER 18

Liver and Gallbladder

Neil D. Theise

CHAPTER CONTENTS

THE LIVER AND BILE DUCTS

The normal adult liver weighs 1400 to 1600 gm. It has a dual blood supply, with the portal vein providing 60% to 70% of hepatic blood flow and the hepatic artery supplying the remaining 30% to 40%. The portal vein and the hepatic artery enter the inferior aspect of the liver through the hilum, or *porta hepatis*. Within the liver, the branches of the portal veins, hepatic arteries, and bile ducts travel in parallel within *portal tracts*, ramifying variably through 17 to 20 orders of branches.

The most common terminology of the hepatic microarchitecture is based on the lobular model (Fig. 18-1). Accordingly the liver is divided into 1- to 2-mm in diameter *lobules* that are oriented around the terminal tributaries of the hepatic vein *(terminal hepatic veins)*, with portal tracts at the lobule's periphery. These are often drawn as hexagonal structures, although in humans the shapes are far more variable; nonetheless, it is a useful oversimplification. The hepatocytes in the vicinity of the terminal hepatic vein are

*The contributions of Dr James Crawford to this chapter in the last several editions of this book are gratefully acknowledged.

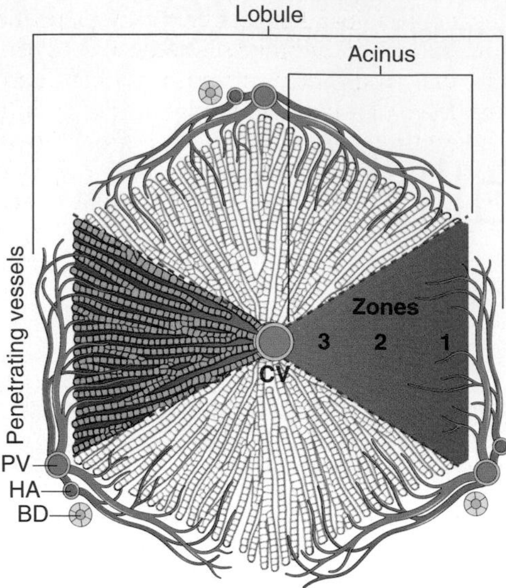

Figure 18-1 Models of liver anatomy. In the lobular model, the terminal hepatic vein (CV) is at the center of a "lobule," while the portal tracts (PV) are at the periphery. Pathologists often refer to the regions of the parenchyma as "periportal" and "centrilobular." In the acinar model, on the basis of blood flow, three zones can be defined, zone 1 being the closest to the blood supply and zone 3 being the farthest. BD, Bile duct; HA, hepatic artery.

called "centrilobular"; those near the portal tract are "periportal." *Division of the parenchyma into zones is a useful concept since certain types of hepatic injury tend to preferentially affect particular zones.* This results in part from the zonal gradient of oxygenation and metabolic activities.

Within the lobule, hepatocytes are organized into anastomosing sheets or "plates" extending from portal tracts to the terminal hepatic veins. Between the trabecular plates of hepatocytes are vascular *sinusoids.* Blood traverses the sinusoids and exits into the terminal hepatic veins through numerous orifices in the vein wall. Hepatocytes are thus bathed on two sides by well-mixed, portal venous and hepatic arterial blood. The sinusoids are lined by fenestrated endothelial cells. Beneath the endothelial cells lies the *space of Disse,* into which protrude abundant hepatocyte microvilli. Scattered *Kupffer cells* of the mononuclear phagocyte system are attached to the luminal face of endothelial cells, and fat-containing myofibroblastic *hepatic stellate cells* are found in the space of Disse. Between abutting hepatocytes are *bile canaliculi,* which are channels 1 to 2 μm in diameter, formed by grooves in the plasma membranes of facing hepatocytes and separated from the vascular space by tight junctions. These channels drain into the *canals of Hering* that, in turn, connect to *bile ductules* in the periportal region. The ductules empty into the *terminal bile ducts* within the portal tracts. Large numbers of lymphocytes are also present in normal liver, comprising as much as 22% of cells other than hepatocytes.

General Features of Liver Disease

The liver is vulnerable to a wide variety of metabolic, toxic, microbial, circulatory, and neoplastic insults. The major primary diseases of the liver are viral hepatitis, nonalcoholic fatty liver disease (NAFLD), alcoholic liver disease, and hepatocellular carcinoma (HCC). Hepatic damage also occurs secondary to some of the most common diseases in humans, such as heart failure, disseminated cancer, and extrahepatic infections. The enormous functional reserve of the liver masks the clinical impact of mild liver damage, but with progression of diffuse disease or disruption of bile flow, the consequences of deranged liver function may become life-threatening.

With the exception of acute liver failure failure, liver disease is an insidious process in which clinical detection and symptoms of hepatic decompensation may occur weeks, months, or many years after the onset of injury. The ebb and flow of hepatic injury may be imperceptible to the patient and detectable only by abnormal laboratory tests (Table 18-1); liver injury and healing may also occur without clinical detection. Hence, individuals with hepatic abnormalities who are referred to hepatologists most frequently have chronic liver disease.

Mechanisms of Injury and Repair

Hepatocyte and Parenchymal Responses

Hepatocytes can undergo a number of degenerative, but potentially reversible changes, such as accumulation of fat (steatosis) and bilirubin (cholestasis). When injury is not reversible, hepatocytes die principally by two mechanisms: necrosis or apoptosis.

In *hepatocyte necrosis,* the cell swells due to defective osmotic regulation at the cell membrane: fluid flows into the cell, which swells and ruptures. Even before rupture, membrane blebs form, carrying off cytoplasmic contents (without organelles) into the extracellular compartment. Macrophages cluster at such sites of injury and mark the sites of hepatocyte necrosis since the dying cells essentially burst and disappear (Fig. 18-2). This form of injury is the

Table 18-1 Laboratory Evaluation of Liver Disease

Test Category	Serum Measurement
Hepatocyte integrity	Cytosolic hepatocellular enzymes†
	Serum aspartate aminotransferase (AST)
	Serum alanine aminotransferase (ALT)
	Serum lactate dehydrogenase (LDH)
Biliary excretory function	Substances normally secreted in bile†
	Serum bilirubin
	Total: unconjugated plus conjugated
	Direct: conjugated only
	Urine bilirubin
	Serum bile acids
	Plasma membrane enzymes (from damage to bile canaliculus)†
	Serum alkaline phosphatase
	Serum γ-glutamyl transpeptidase (GGT)
Hepatocyte synthetic function	Proteins secreted into the blood
	Serum albumin‡
	Coagulation factors:
	Prothrombin (PT) and partial thromboplastin (PTT) times (fibrinogen, prothrombin,factors V, VII, IX,and X)
	Hepatocyte metabolism
	Serum ammonia†
	Aminopyrine breath test (hepatic demethylation)‡

†Increased in liver disease.
‡Decreased in liver disease.

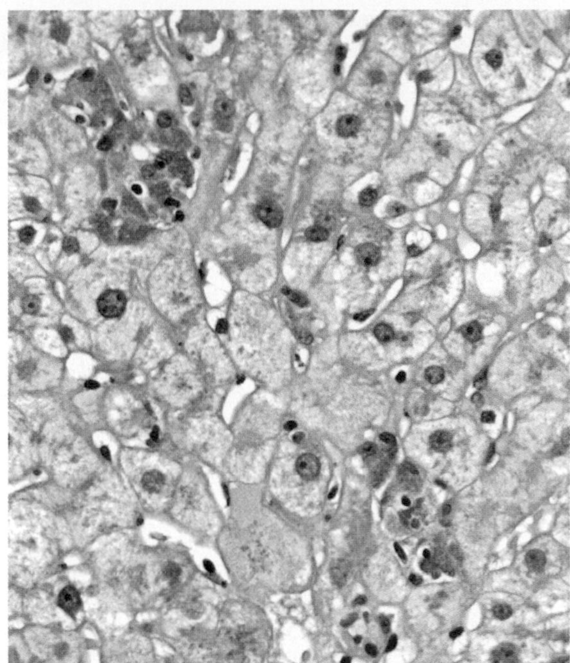

Figure 18-2 Acute hepatitis B. In this PAS-D stained slide, clusters of macrophages with eosinophilic cytoplasm indicate foci where hepatocytes have undergone necrosis. PAS-D, Periodic acid–Schiff after diastase digestion.

predominant mode of death in ischemic/hypoxic injury and a significant part of the response to oxidative stress.

Hepatocyte apoptosis is an active form of "programmed" cell death resulting in hepatocyte shrinkage, nuclear chromatin condensation (*pyknosis*), fragmentation (*karyorrhexis*), and cellular fragmentation into acidophilic *apoptotic bodies*. These changes are a result of caspase cascades described in detail in Chapter 2. Apoptotic hepatocytes were first clearly described in yellow fever by William Thomas Councilman and therefore have often been referred to as *Councilman bodies;* while apoptosis occurs in many forms of liver disease, by convention this eponym is restricted to that disease. In the more frequent settings in which apoptotic hepatocytes are seen, (e.g., acute and chronic hepatitis), the term *acidophil bodies* is used, due to their deeply eosinophilic staining characteristics (Fig. 18-3).

When there is widespread parenchymal loss there is often evidence of *confluent necrosis*, a severe, zonal loss of hepatocytes. This may be seen in acute toxic or ischemic injuries or in severe viral or autoimmune hepatitis. Confluent necrosis may begin as a zone of hepatocyte dropout around the central vein. The resulting space is filled by cellular debris, macrophages, and remnants of the reticulin meshwork. In *bridging necrosis* this zone may link central veins to portal tracts or bridge adjacent portal tracts (often with an inapparent central vein within the zone of injury). Even in diseases such as viral hepatitis in which hepatocytes are the principal targets of attack, vascular insults—via inflammation or thrombosis—lead to parenchymal extinction due to large areas of contiguous hepatocyte death (Fig. 18-4). The process depicted in Fig. 18-4 occurs in many types of liver diseases in which there is extensive hepatocyte loss and collapse of the supporting framework. The resultant cirrhosis is a common form of liver disease. In some cases there is scar regression as depicted in the figure and described in the next section.

Regeneration of lost hepatocytes occurs primarily by mitotic replication of hepatocytes adjacent to those that have died, even when there is significant confluent necrosis. *Hepatocytes are almost stem cell-like in their ability to continue to replicate even in the setting of years of chronic injury and thus stem cell replenishment is usually not a significant part of parenchymal repair.* In the most severe forms of acute liver failure, there is activation of the primary intrahepatic stem cell niche, namely the canal of Hering, but the contribution of stem cells to the replenishment of hepatocytes in such a setting setting remains unclear. Eventually, however, in many individuals with chronic disease the hepatocytes do reach replicative senescence and then there is clear evidence of stem cell activation seen in the form of *ductular reactions*. These duct like structures, sometimes without any lumens develop from stem cells and contribute significantly to parenchymal restoration. Interestingly, in biliary diseases, the "ductular" progeny of stem cells can give rise to cholangiocytes.

Scar Formation and Regression

The principal cell type involved in scar deposition is the hepatic stellate cell. In its quiescent form, it is a lipid (vitamin A) storing cell. However, in several forms of acute and chronic injury, the stellate cells can become activated and are converted into highly fibrogenic myofibroblasts. Proliferation of hepatic stellate cells and their activation into myofibroblasts is initiated by a series of changes that include an increase in the expression of platelet-derived growth factor receptor β (PDGFR-β) in the stellate cells. At the same time, Kupffer cells and lymphocytes release cytokines and chemokines that modulate the expression of genes in stellate cells that are involved in fibrogenesis. These, include transforming growth factor β (TGF-β) and its receptors, metalloproteinase 2 (MMP-2),

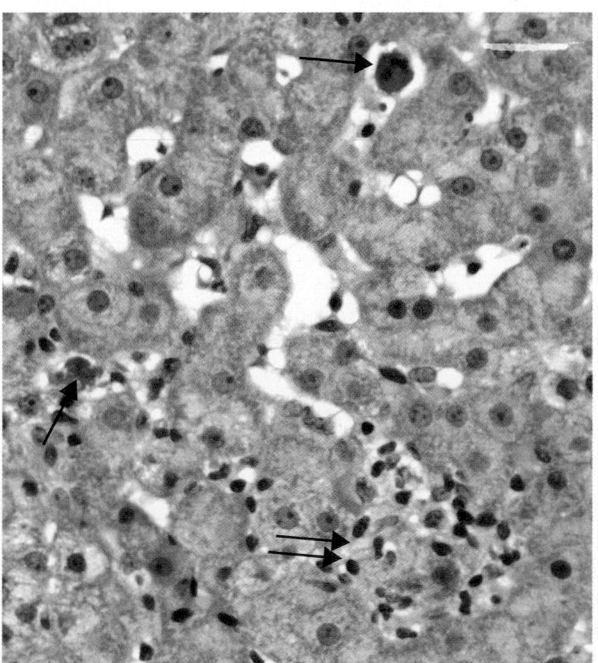

Figure 18-3 Foci of lobular hepatitis in chronic hepatitis C show apoptotic hepatocytes ("acidophil bodies"; *arrows*) and a focus of mononuclear infiltration surrounding a more darkly stained, injured hepatocyte (double arrows).

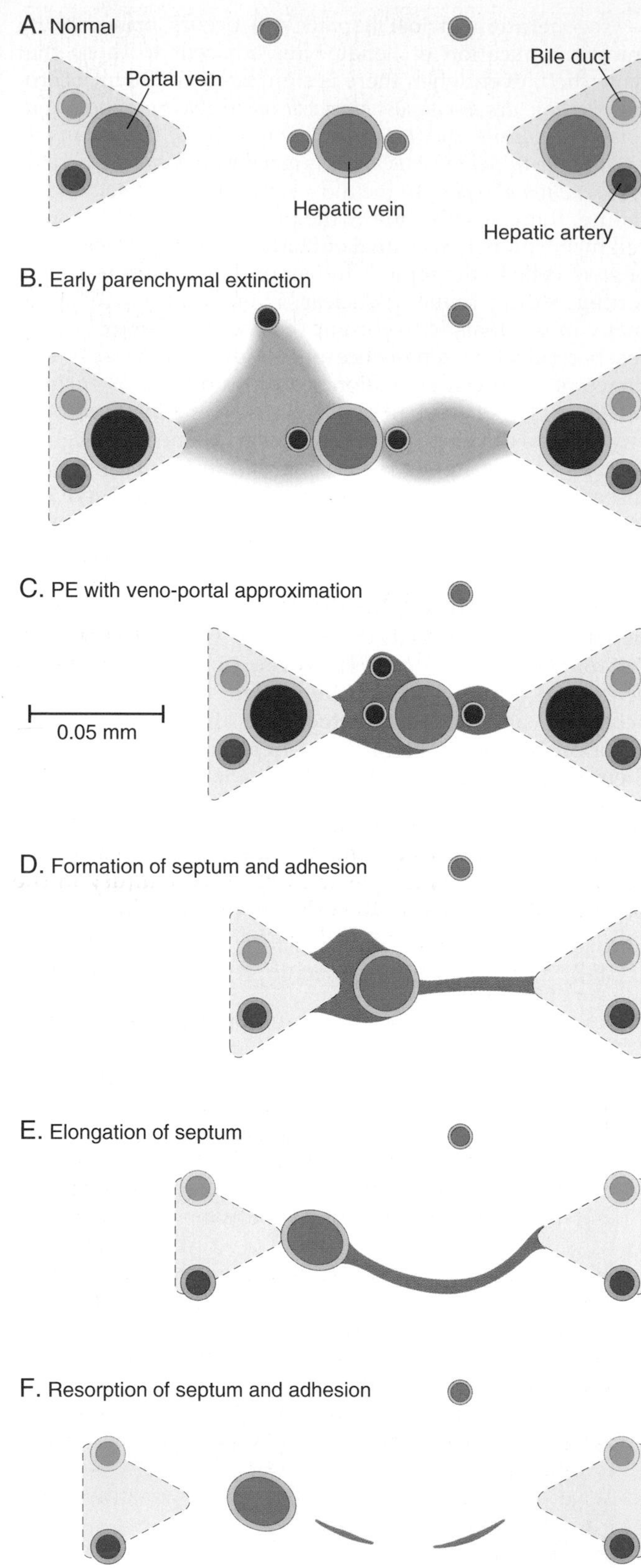

Figure 18-4 Diagrammatic representation of the natural history of small regions of hepatocelleular extinction and the related scarring. **A,** Normal liver with patent portal and hepatic veins (blue). **B,** Extinction occurs when contiguous hepatocytes die, usually after inflammatory injury to their blood supply (ischemic hepatocytes are shown in orange; obstructed veins are black). **C,** Empty parenchyma collapses and begins to scar (brown) and adjacent portal tracts and hepatic veins become approximated. **D,** Scars in regions of extinction contract and condense, becoming fibrous septa. The larger region of extinction (on the left) has formed a short adhesion between the adjacent portal tract and hepatic vein. Obliterated small veins have disappeared. **E,** Septa elongate by the traction caused by hyperplasia of adjacent hepatocytes. Portal tract collagen (light gray) is less than normal as resorption begins. **F,** Septa are resorbed. The resulting tissue has either venoportal fibrous adhesions or hepatic veins that are closely approximated to portal tracts. Portal tracts are remnants, often with no portal vein. (From Wanless IR, et al: Regression of Human Cirrhosis: Morphologic Features and the Genesis of Incomplete Septal Cirrhosis, Arch Pathol Lab Med Vol. 124, page 1606, 2000.)

and tissue inhibitors of metalloproteinases 1 and 2 (TIMP-1 and -2). As they are converted into myofibroblasts, the cells release chemotactic and vasoactive factors, cytokines, and growth factors. Myofibroblasts are contractile cells; their contraction is stimulated by endothelin-1 (ET-1). The stimuli for stellate cell activation may originate from several sources (Fig. 18-5): (1) chronic inflammation, with production of inflammatory cytokines such as tumor necrosis factor (TNF), lymphotoxin, and interleukin-1β (IL-1β), and lipid peroxidation products; (2) cytokine and chemokine production by Kupffer cells, endothelial cells, hepatocytes, and bile duct epithelial cells; (3) in response to disruption of the extracellular matrix (ECM); and (4) direct stimulation of stellate cells by toxins. If injury persists, scar deposition begins, often in the space of Disse. This is particularly important in alcoholic and nonalcoholic fatty liver diseases, but is also a generalized mechanism of scar formation in other forms of chronic liver injury.

Zones of parenchymal loss transform into dense *fibrous septa* through a combination of the collapse of the underlying reticulin where large swaths of hepatocytes have irrevocably disappeared and hepatic stellate cells have been activated. Eventually, these fibrous septa encircle surviving, regenerating hepatocytes in the late stages of chronic liver diseases that give rise to diffuse scarring described as cirrhosis.

Other cells probably contribute significantly to scar deposition in different settings, including portal fibroblasts. Ductular reactions also play a role, both through activation and recruitment of all these fibrogenic cells, but also, perhaps, through *epithelial-mesenchymal transition*. The relative roles played by these other cells and processes are less well understood.

If the chronic injury leading to scar formation is interrupted (e.g. clearance of hepatitis virus infection, cessation of alcohol use), then stellate cell activation ceases, scars condense, becoming more dense and thin, and then, due to metalloproteinases produced by hepatocytes, begin to break apart. In this way, scar formation can be reversed. It should be kept in mind that in any chronic liver disease there are probably areas of both fibrotic progression and regression, but the balance in active disease favors the former and with remission of disease the latter is favored.

Inflammation and Immunity

Innate and adaptive immune systems are, not surprisingly, involved in all manner of liver injury and repair. Antigens in the liver are taken up by antigen presenting cells,

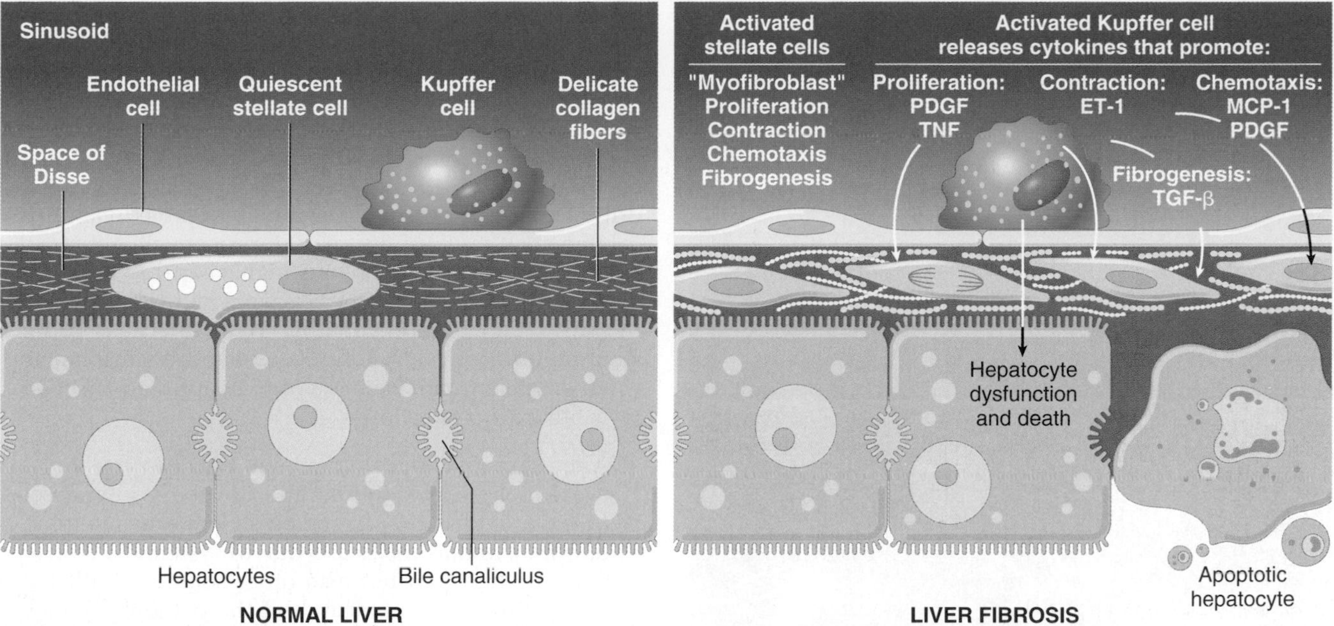

Figure 18-5 Stellate cell activation and liver fibrosis. Kupffer cell activation leads to secretion of multiple cytokines. Platelet-derived growth factor (PDGF) and tumor necrosis factor (TNF) activate stellate cells, and contraction of the activated stellate cells is stimulated by endothelin-1 (ET-1). Fibrosis is stimulated by transforming growth factor β (TGF-β). Chemotaxis of activated stellate cells to areas of injury is promoted by PDGF and monocyte chemotactic protein-1 (MCP-1). See text for details.

including, Kupffer cells and blood-derived dendritic cells, and presented to lymphocytes. Toll-like receptors detect host molecules, and also those derived from foreign invaders such as bacteria and viruses. These processes lead to elaboration of proinflammatory cytokines, which have diverse effects on the liver, including recruitment of inflammatory cells, hepatocyte injury, vascular disturbances, promotion of scarring, and perhaps even malignant transformation. Adaptive immunity plays an even more critical role in viral hepatitis. Antigen-specific and CD8+ T cells are involved in eradication of hepatitis B and C, the primary causes of chronic viral hepatitis, largely through elimination of infected hepatocytes. Lymphocytes, however, not only play a destructive role, but also help induce local hepatocyte replication through secretion of cytokines.

Liver Failure

The most severe clinical consequence of liver disease is liver failure. It may be the result of sudden and massive hepatic destruction, *acute liver failure*, which occurs in about 2000 people per year in the United States, or, more often, *chronic liver failure*, which follows upon years or decades of insidious, progressive liver injury. In some cases, individuals with chronic liver disease develop *acute-on-chronic liver failure*, in which an unrelated acute injury supervenes on a well-compensated late-stage chronic disease or the chronic disease itself has a flare of activity that leads directly to liver failure. Whatever the sequence, 80% to 90% of hepatic functional capacity must be lost before hepatic failure ensues. When the liver can no longer maintain homeostasis, transplantation offers the best hope for survival; the mortality rate in persons with hepatic failure without liver transplantation is about 80%.

Acute Liver Failure

Acute liver failure is defined as an acute liver illness associated with encephalopathy and coagulopathy that occurs within 26 weeks of the initial liver injury in the absence of pre-existing liver disease. Within this 26 week window, it is useful to know the interval between the onset of symptoms and liver failure, since this may provide helpful clues to the etiology as we shall describe below. Here we should clarify some terminology. Acute liver failure has been referred to as "fulminant liver failure" until recently. The term "acute liver failure" is preferred but since the older term remains entrenched in the literature, these terms are often used interchangeably. Acute liver failure is caused by *massive hepatic necrosis*, most often induced by drugs or toxins. Accidental or deliberate ingestion of acetaminophen (Chapter 9) accounts for almost 50% of cases in the United States, while autoimmune hepatitis, other drugs/toxins, and acute hepatitis A and B infections account for rest of cases. In Asia, acute hepatitis B and E predominate. With acetoaminophen toxicity, the liver failure occurs within a week of the onset of symptoms, whereas failure due to hepatitis viruses takes longer to develop. The mechanism of hepatocellular necrosis may be direct toxic damage (as with acetaminophen), but more often is a variable combination of toxicity and immune-mediated hepatocyte destruction (e.g., hepatitis virus infection).

MORPHOLOGY

Acute liver failure usually displays **massive hepatic necrosis**, with broad regions of parenchymal loss surrounding islands of regenerating hepatocytes (Fig. 18-6). These livers are small and shrunken. The prominence of scar and of ductular reactions in

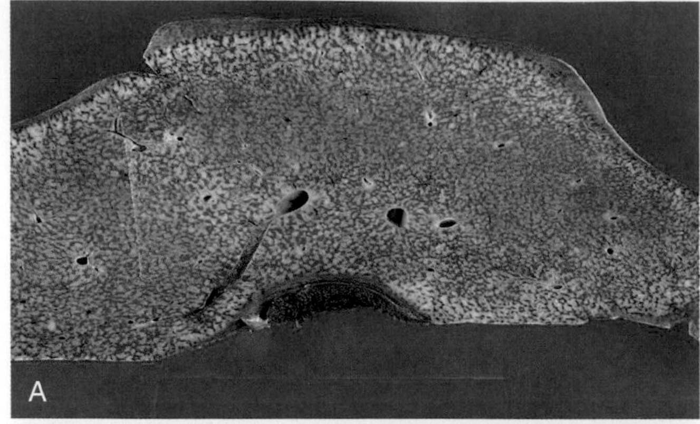

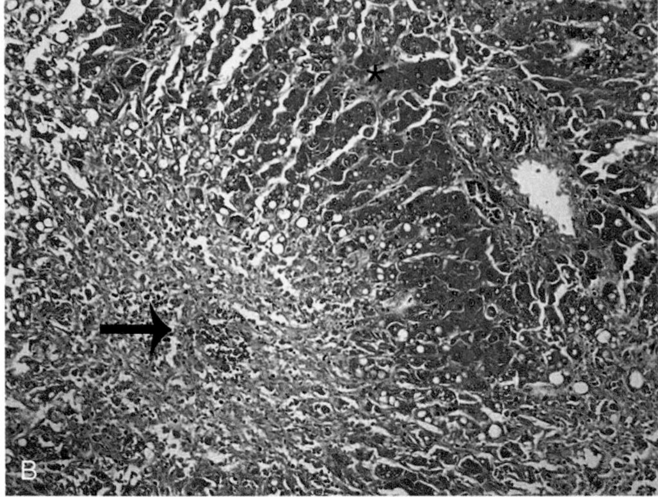

Figure 18-6 **A,** Massive necrosis, cut section of liver. The liver is small (700 g), bile-stained, soft, and congested. **B,** Hepatocellular necrosis caused by acetaminophen overdose. Confluent necrosis is seen in the perivenular region (zone 3) *(large arrow)*. Residual normal tissue is indicated by the asterisk. (Courtesy Dr. Matthew Yeh, University of Washington, Seattle, Wash.)

these livers depends on the nature and duration of the insult. Toxic injuries, such as acetaminophen overdoses, usually take place within hours to days, too brief a period to allow time for scar formation or regeneration. Acute viral infections may cause failure over weeks to a few months, so that while hepatocyte injury continues to outpace repair, regeneration is often demonstrable. Also, this time scale allows for early scarring in areas of parenchymal loss.

Rarely, there may be diffuse poisoning of liver cells without obvious cell death and parenchymal collapse, such as in **diffuse microvesicular steatosis** related to fatty liver of pregnancy or idiosyncratic reactions to toxins (e.g., valproate, tetracycline). In these settings, usually related to primary mitochondrial dysfunction, hepatocytes are unable to perform their usual metabolic functions. In states of immunodeficiency, such as untreated infection with human immunodeficiency virus (HIV) or posttransplant immunosuppression, non-hepatotropic viruses, particularly cytomegalovirus, herpes simplex viruses, and adenovirus, can cause fulminant liver failure with histologic features specific to each of those viruses. With better treatments for HIV infection, these are declining as a cause of acute liver failure.

Clinical Course. **Acute liver failure manifests first with nausea, vomiting, and jaundice, followed by life-threatening encephalopathy, and coagulation defects.** Typically, serum liver transaminases are markedly elevated. The liver is initially enlarged due to hepatocyte swelling, inflammatory infiltrates, and edema; as parenchyma is destroyed, however, the liver shrinks dramatically. Decline of serum transaminases as the liver shrinks is often not, therefore, a sign of improvement, but is rather an indication that there are few viable hepatocytes left; this suspicion is confirmed if there is worsening jaundice, coagulopathy, and encephalopathy. With unabated progression, multiorgan system failure occurs and, if transplantation is not possible, death ensues. Other manifestations of acute liver failure are as follows:

- Alterations of bile formation and flow become clinically evident as yellow discoloration of the skin and sclera (*jaundice* and *icterus*, respectively) due to retention of bilirubin, and as *cholestasis* due to systemic retention of not only bilirubin but also other solutes eliminated in bile. Bilirubin metabolism and the pathophysiology of jaundice are discussed in detail later under cholestatic diseases. In the setting of acute liver failure, there is classic yellowing of skin, sclerae, and mucous membranes; cholestasis increases the risk of life-threatening bacterial infection.
- *Hepatic encephalopathy* is a spectrum of disturbances in consciousness, ranging from subtle behavioral abnormalities, to marked confusion and stupor, to deep coma and death. Encephalopathy may progress over days, weeks, or months following acute injury. Associated fluctuating, neurologic signs include rigidity and hyperreflexia. *Asterixis,* a particularly characteristic sign, is manifested as nonrhythmic, rapid extension-flexion movements of the head and extremities, best seen when the arms are held in extension with dorsiflexed wrists. Hepatic encephalopathy is regarded as a disorder of neurotransmission in the central nervous system and neuromuscular system. Elevated ammonia levels in blood and the central nervous system correlate with impaired neuronal function and cerebral edema.
- The liver is responsible for production of vitamin K-dependent and -independent clotting factors (Chapter 4). Thus, with massively impaired hepatic synthetic function, *coagulopathy* develops. Easy bruisability is an early sign of this process, which can lead to life-threatening or fatal intracranial bleeding. The liver is also responsible for helping to remove activated coagulation factors from the circulation, and loss of this function in some instances can lead to disseminated intravascular coagulation (Chapter 14), further exacerbating the bleeding tendency.
- *Portal hypertension* arises when there is diminished flow through the portal venous system, which may occur because of obstruction at the prehepatic, intrahepatic, or posthepatic level. While it can occur in acute live failure, portal hypertension is more commonly seen with chronic liver failure and is described later. In acute liver failure, if portal hypertension develops within days to weeks, obstruction is predominantly intrahepatic and the major clinical consequences are *ascites* and *hepatic encephalopathy*. In chronic liver disease, portal

hypertension develops over months to years, and its effects are more complex and widespread (see later).

- *Hepatorenal syndrome* is a form of renal failure occurring in individuals with liver failure in whom there are no intrinsic morphologic or functional causes for kidney dysfunction. Sodium retention, impaired free-water excretion, and decreased renal perfusion and glomerular filtration rate are the main renal functional abnormalities. There is decreased renal perfusion pressure due to systemic vasodilation, activation of the renal sympathetic nervous system with vasoconstriction of the afferent renal arterioles, and increased activation of the renin/angiotensin axis, causing vasoconstrition that further decreases glomerular filtration. The syndrome's onset begins with a drop in urine output and rising blood urea nitrogen and creatinine levels.

Chronic Liver Failure and Cirrhosis

The leading causes of chronic liver failure worldwide include chronic hepatitis B, chronic hepatitis C, non-alcoholic fatty liver disease, and alcoholic liver disease. In the United States, chronic liver disease is the twelfth most common cause of mortality, accounting for most liver-related deaths. **Liver failure in chronic liver disease is most often associated with cirrhosis, a condition marked by the diffuse transformation of the entire liver into regenerative parenchymal nodules surrounded by fibrous bands and variable degrees of vascular (often portosystemic) shunting.**

However, not all cirrhosis leads inexorably to chronic liver failure and not all end-stage chronic liver disease is cirrhotic. For example, chronic diseases such as primary biliary cirrhosis, primary sclerosing cholangitis, nodular regenerative hyperplasia, chronic schistosomiasis, and fibropolycystic liver disease are often not accompanied by fully established cirrhosis, even at end stage. On the other hand, patients with well-treated autoimmune hepatitis or those with suppressed hepatitis B or cured hepatitis C often do not progress to end stage, even though they are cirrhotic. *The Child-Pugh classification of cirrhosis* distinguishes between class A (well compensated), B (partially decompensated), and C (decompensated), which correlate with different morphologic features histologically. The utility of such a system is that it helps monitor the decline of patients on the path to chronic liver failure.

Even in diseases that are likely to give rise to cirrhosis, such as untreated viral hepatitis, alcoholic liver disease, non-alcoholic fatty liver disease, metabolic diseases—the morphology and pathophysiology of cirrhosis may be different. Thus, while the term cirrhosis implies the presence of severe chronic disease, it is not a specific diagnosis and it lacks clear prognostic implications. The term *cryptogenic cirrhosis* is sometimes used to describe cirrhosis when there is no clear cause.

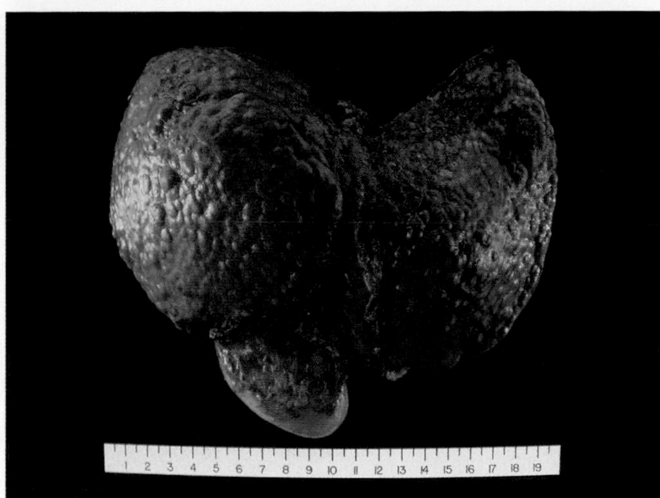

Figure 18-7 Cirrhosis resulting from chronic viral hepatitis. Note the depressed areas of dense scar separating bulging regenerative nodules over the liver surface.

MORPHOLOGY

As described, **cirrhosis occurs diffusely throughout the liver, which is comprised of regenerating parenchymal nodules surrounded by dense bands of scar and variable degrees of vascular shunting** (Fig. 18-7). The size of the nodules, the pattern of scarring (linking portal tracts to each other vs. linking portal tracts to central veins), the degree of parenchymal collapse in which no viable liver tissue is present, the range of macroscopic vascular thrombosis (particularly of the portal vein) all vary between diseases and even, in some cases, between individuals with the same disease. Again, to re-emphasize, there is no single cirrhosis, but many cirrhoses. The important details distinguishing cirrhosis of different causes as they pertain to each disease are described in subsequent disease specific sections.

It is becoming increasingly clear that changes identifiable on biopsy in different cirrhotic patients correlate with the prognostically useful Child-Pugh classification mentioned earlier and with portal venous wedge pressures—a new, important, albeit not yet universal method for assessing the presence and degree of portal hypertension. Biopsy specimens demonstrating narrow, densely compacted fibrous septa separated by large islands of intact hepatic parenchyma are likely to have less portal hypertension. Those with broad bands of dense scar, often with dilated lymphatic spaces, with less intervening parenchyma are likely to be progressing toward portal hypertension and, therefore, to end-stage disease.

Clinical implications of these histologic findings and the clinical implications of increased hepatic venous wedge pressures are in the process of being defined. They are expected to play an increasingly important roles in coming years, particularly in patients with chronic hepatitis B and C infections, for whom distinguishing the ebb and flow of cirrhotic features may be essential for determining prognosis as anti-viral treatments improve.

As mentioned earlier stem cell activation is seen in the form of ductular reactions. **In chronic liver disease ductular reactions increase with advancing stage of disease and are usually most prominent in cirrhosis.** There are two correlates of ductular reactions:

- The role of liver stem cells in parenchymal regeneration increases as the preexisting hepatocytes undergo replicative senescence after years to decades of high turnover.
- Ductular reactions may incite some of the scarring in chronic liver disease and thus may have a negative effect on progressive liver disease.

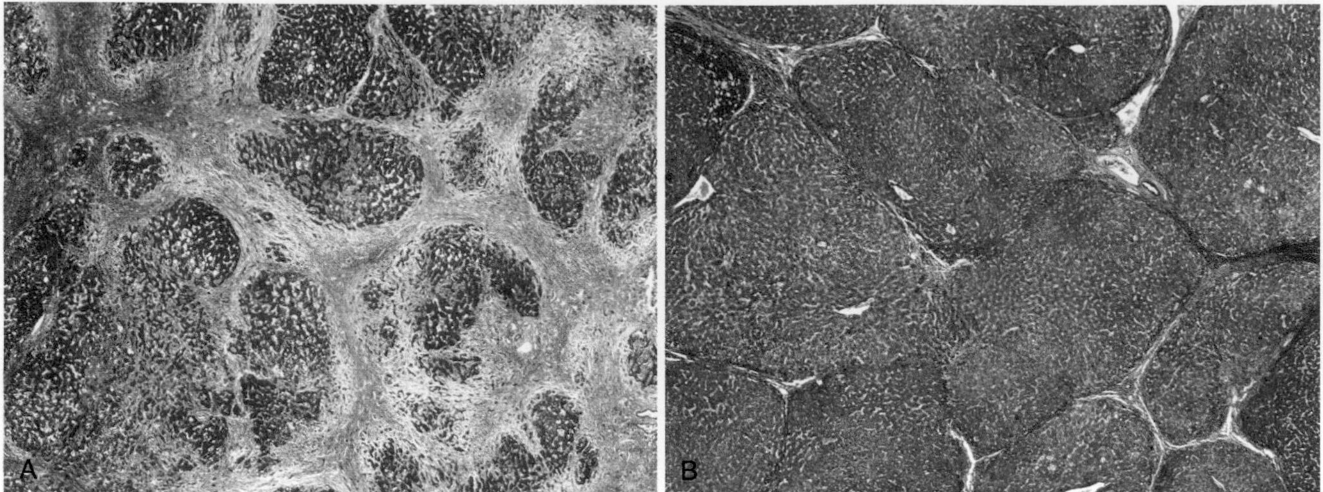

Figure 18-8 Alcoholic cirrhosis in an active drinker (A) and following long-term abstinence (B). **A,** Thick bands of collagen separate rounded cirrhotic nodules. **B,** After a year of abstinence, most scars are gone. (Masson trichrome stain) (Courtesy Drs. Hongfa Zhu and Isabel Fiel, Mount Sinai School of Medicine, New York.)

Although uncommon, regression of fibrosis, albeit rarely, in fully established cirrhosis, does occur; this is another reason why cirrhosis should not be automatically equated with end stage disease. In the past when there were no reliable ways to cure any chronic liver disease, there were no opportunities to see whether cirrhosis could regress. With increasing numbers of effective treatments for cirrhosis-causing conditions, however, we now understand that regression of scars can take place (Figs. 18-4 and 18-8). Scars can become thinner, more densely compacted, and eventually fragment. As fibrous septa break apart, adjacent nodules of regenerating parenchyma coalesce into larger islands. All cirrhotic livers show elements of both progression and regression, the balance determined by the severity and persistence of the underlying disease.

Clinical Features. **About 40% of individuals with cirrhosis are asymptomatic until the most advanced stages of the disease.** When symptomatic, they present with nonspecific manifestations: anorexia, weight loss, weakness, and, in advanced disease, symptoms and signs of liver failure discussed earlier. *The ultimate causes of death in chronic liver failure, whether cirrhotic or not, include those seen in acute liver failure, and additional grim outcomes, such as development of hepatocellular carcinoma in the context of cirrhosis.* Hepatic encephalopathy, bleeding from esophageal varices and bacterial infections (resulting from damage to mucosal barrier in the gut and Kupffer cell dysfunction) are often the the terminal events.

The course and severity of clinical manifestations of cirrhosis vary from patient to patient. In a small number of cases, as noted earlier, cessation of liver injury may give the necessary time for resorption of the fibrous tissue and "regression" of the cirrhosis. Even in such instances, the portal hypertension (from irreversible vascular shunts) and risk of hepatocellular carcinoma usually remain.

Jaundice, encephalopathy, and coagulopathy are very much the same as in acute liver failure. However, there are some significant additional features. Jaundice, when chronic, can lead to *pruritus*, that is, itching, the intensity of which can be profound. Some patients may even scratch their skin raw and risk repeated bouts of potentially life-threatening infection. Pruritus can be so severe that it can be relieved only by liver transplantation.

Impaired estrogen metabolism and consequent *hyperestrogenemia* in male patients with chronic liver failure can give rise to *palmar erythema* (a reflection of local vasodilatation) and *spider angiomas* of the skin. Each angioma is a central, pulsating, dilated arteriole from which small vessels radiate. In men, hyperestrogenemia also leads to *hypogonadism* and *gynecomastia*. Hypogonadism can also occur in women from disruption of hypothalamic-pituitary axis function, either through nutritional deficiencies associated with the chronic liver disease or primary hormonal alterations.

We next turn to a discussion of portal hypertension which as alluded to earlier can develop in acute liver failure but is much more common in chronic liver failure with cirrhosis.

Portal Hypertension

Increased resistance to portal blood flow may develop in a variety of circumstances, which can be divided into *prehepatic, intrahepatic, and posthepatic* (Table 18-2). The major *prehepatic conditions* are obstructive thrombosis, narrowing of the portal vein before it ramifies within the liver or massive splenomegaly with increased splenic vein blood flow. The main post-hepatic causes are severe right-sided heart failure, constrictive pericarditis, and hepatic vein outflow obstruction. **The dominant intrahepatic cause is cirrhosis, accounting for most cases of portal hypertension.** Far less frequent intrahepatic causes are schistosomiasis, massive fatty change, diffuse fibrosing granulomatous disease such as sarcoidosis, and diseases affecting the portal microcirculation such as nodular regenerative hyperplasia (discussed later). The pathophysiology of portal hypertension is complex and involves resistance to portal flow at the level of sinusoids and an increase in portal flow caused by hyperdynamic circulation.

The increased resistance to portal flow at the level of the sinusoids is caused by contraction of vascular smooth

Table 18-2 Location and Causes of Portal Hypertension

Prehepatic causes
Obstructive thrombosis of portal vein
Structural abnormalities such as narrowing of the portal vein before it ramifies in the liver
Intrahepatic causes
Cirrhosis from any cause
Nodular regenerative hyperplasia
Primary biliary cirrhosis (even in the absence of cirrhosis)
Schistosomiasis
Massive fatty change
Diffuse, fibrosing granulomatous disease (e.g., sarcoid)
Infiltrative malignancy, primary or metastatic
Focal malignancy with invasion into portal vein (particularly hepatocellular carcinoma)
Amyloidosis
Posthepatic causes
Severe right-sided heart failure
Constrictive pericarditis
Hepatic vein outflow obstruction

muscle cells and myofibroblasts, and disruption of blood flow by scarring and the formation of parenchymal nodules. Alterations in sinusoidal endothelial cells that contribute to the intrahepatic vasoconstriction associated with portal hypertension include a decrease in nitric oxide production, and increased release of endothelin-1 (ET-1), angiotensinogen, and eicosanoids. Sinusoidal remodeling and anastomosis between the arterial and portal system in the fibrous septa contribute to portal hypertension by imposing arterial pressures on the low pressure portal venous system. Sinusoidal remodeling and intrahepatic shunts also interfere with the metabolic exchange between sinusoidal blood and hepatocytes.

Another major factor in the development of portal hypertension is an *increase in portal venous blood flow resulting from a hyperdynamic circulation*. This is caused by arterial vasodilation, primarily in the splanchnic circulation. The increased splanchnic arterial blood flow in turn leads to increased venous efflux into the portal venous system. While various mediators such as prostacyclin and TNF have been implicated in the causation of the splanchnic arterial vasodilation, NO has emerged as the most significant one.

The four major clinical consequences of portal hypertension are (1) ascites, (2) the formation of portosystemic venous shunts, (3) congestive splenomegaly, and (4) hepatic encephalopathy (discussed earlier). These are illustrated in Figure 18-9.

Ascites. The accumulation of excess *fluid in the peritoneal cavity is called ascites.* In 85% of cases, ascites is caused by cirrhosis. Ascites usually becomes clinically detectable when at least 500 mL have accumulated. The fluid is generally serous, having less than 3 gm/dL of protein (largely albumin), and a serum to ascites albumin gradient of ≥1.1 gm/dL. The fluid may contain a scant number of mesothelial cells and mononuclear leukocytes. Influx of neutrophils suggests infection, whereas the presence of blood cells points to possible disseminated intra-abdominal cancer. With long-standing ascites, seepage of peritoneal fluid through trans-diaphragmatic lymphatics may produce hydro-thorax, more often on the right side. The pathogenesis of ascites is complex, involving the following mechanisms:

Sinusoidal hypertension, altering Starling's forces and driving fluid into the space of Disse, from where it is removed by hepatic lymphatics; this movement of fluid is also promoted by *hypoalbuminemia.*

Percolation of hepatic lymph into the peritoneal cavity: Normal thoracic duct lymph flow approximates 800 to 1000 mL/day. With cirrhosis, hepatic lymphatic flow may approach 20 L/day, exceeding thoracic duct capacity. Hepatic lymph is rich in proteins and low in triglycerides, which explains the presence of protein in the ascitic fluid.

Splanchnic vasodilation and hyperdynamic circulation. These conditions were described earlier, in relationship to the pathogenesis of portal hypertension. Arterial vasodilation in the splanchnic circulation tends to reduce arterial blood pressure. With worsening of the vasodilation, the heart rate and cardiac output are unable to maintain the blood pressure. This triggers the activation of

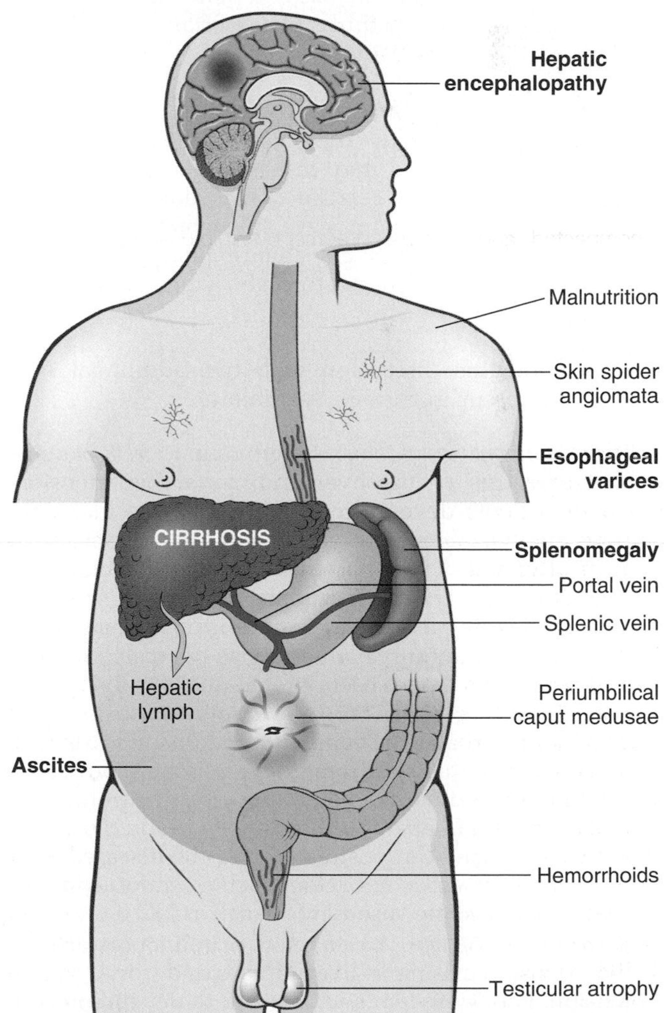

Figure 18-9 Major clinical consequences of portal hypertension in the setting of cirrhosis, shown for the male. In women, oligomenorrhea, amenorrhea, and sterility as a result of hypogonadism are frequent. Clinically significant findings are bold faced.

vasoconstrictors, including the renin-angiotensin system, and also increases the secretion of antidiuretic hormone. The combination of portal hypertension, vasodilation, and sodium and water retention increases the perfusion pressure of interstitial capillaries, causing extravasation of fluid into the abdominal cavity.

Portosystemic Shunts. With the rise in portal system pressure, the flow is reversed from portal to systemic circulation by dilation of collateral vessels and development of new vessels. Venous bypasses develop wherever the systemic and portal circulation share common capillary beds (Fig. 18-9). Principal sites are veins around and within the rectum (manifest as hemorrhoids), the esophagogastric junction (producing varices), the retroperitoneum, and the falciform ligament of the liver (involving periumbilical and abdominal wall collaterals). Although hemorrhoidal bleeding may occur, it is rarely massive or life-threatening. Much more important are the esophagogastric varices that appear in about 40% *of individuals with advanced cirrhosis of the liver and cause massive hematemesis and death in about half of them. Each episode of bleeding is associated with a 30% mortality. Abdominal wall collaterals appear as dilated subcutaneous veins extending from the umbilicus toward the rib margins (caput medusae)* and constitute an important clinical hallmark of portal hypertension.

Splenomegaly. Long-standing congestion may cause congestive splenomegaly. The degree of splenic enlargement varies widely and may reach as much as 1000 gm, but it is not necessarily correlated with other features of portal hypertension. The massive splenomegaly may secondarily induce hematologic abnormalities attributable to hypersplenism, such as thrombocytopenia or even pancytopenia.

We conclude this discussion with two additional syndromes that occur in chronic liver failure:

- *Hepatopulmonary syndrome* is seen in up to 30% patients with cirrhosis of the liver and portal hypertension. These patients develop intrapulmonary vascular dilations involving capillary and pre-capillary vessels up to 100 μM in size. The blood flows rapidly through such dilated vessels, giving inadequate time for oxygen diffusion and leading to ventilation-perfusion mismatch and right-to-left shunting, manifesting as hypoxia. Hypoxia and resultant dyspnea occur preferentially in an upright position rather than in the recumbent position, as gravity exacerbates the ventilation-perfusion mismatch. Patients with this syndrome have a poorer prognosis than patients without hepatopulmonary syndrome. The pathogenesis of hepatopulmonary syndrome is unclear, although it has been postulated that the diseased liver may not clear vasoconstrictors such as endothelin-1 or may produce some vasodilators such as NO.
- *Portopulmonary hypertension* refers to pulmonary arterial hypertension arising in liver disease and portal hypertension. Poorly understood, it seems to depend on concomitant portal hypertension and excessive pulmonary vasoconstriction and vascular remodeling. The most common clinical manifestations are dyspnea on exertion and clubbing of the fingers.

Acute-on-Chronic Liver Failure

Some individuals with stable but well-compensated, advanced chronic liver disease, suddenly develop signs of acute liver failure. In such patients there is often established cirrhosis with extensive vascular shunting. Thus, large volumes of functioning liver parenchyma have a borderline vascular supply, leaving them vulnerable to superimposed, potentially lethal insults. The short-term mortality of patients with this form of liver failure is around 50%.

Patients with chronic hepatitis B infection who become superinfected with hepatitis D may undergo sudden decompensation, as can patients with medically suppressed hepatitis B infection in whom viral mutants arise that are resistant to therapy. In either case there is an acute flare of disease. Ascending cholagitis in a patient with primary sclerosing cholangitis or fibropolycystic liver disease (described later) could have the same effect, rapidly propelling a well-compensated yet chronically sick individual into someone facing death or transplant.

Other causes may be systemic rather than primarily intrahepatic. For example, sepsis and its attendant hypotension may further undermine insufficiently vascularized parenchyma leading to superimposed, sometimes severe, acute injury. Likewise, acute cardiac failure or a superimposed drug or toxic injury might tip a well compensated cirrhotic patient to failure. Finally, there is the possibility of malignancy, either an unrelated extrahepatic malignancy metastatic to the chronically diseased liver or secondary to the liver disease itself, particularly hepatocellular carcinoma or cholangiocarcinoma.

KEY CONCEPTS

Liver Failure

- Liver failure may follow acute injury or chronic injury, but may also occur as an acute insult superimposed on an otherwise well-compensated chronic liver disease.
- Mnemonic for causes of acute liver failure:
  - A: Acetaminophen, hepatitis A, autoimmune hepatitis
  - B: Hepatitis B
  - C: Hepatitis C, cryptogenic
  - D: Drugs/toxins, hepatitis D
  - E: Hepatitis E, esoteric causes (Wilson disease, Budd-Chiari)
  - F: Fatty change of the microvesicular type (fatty liver of pregnancy, valproate, tetracycline, Reye syndrome)
- Serious and sometimes fatal sequelae of liver failure include coagulopathy, encephalopathy, portal hypertension, bleeding esophageal varices, hepatorenal syndrome, and portopulmonary hypertension.

Infectious Disorders

Viral Hepatitis

The terminology for acute and chronic viral hepatitis can be confusing, because the same word, *hepatitis*, can be used for several things; careful attention to context can clarify its meaning in any situation. First, "hepatitis" is the name of each of the *hepatotropic viruses* (hepatitis A, B, C, D, and E) that have a specific affinity for the liver. Second, "hepatitis" stands for the histologic patterns of hepatitic injury, both acute and chronic (depending on the specific virus), that are seen in the livers infected by hepatotropic viruses (and in autoimmune and drug or toxin induced hepatitis, as well). Third, to a more minor degree, it is any form of hepatocellular injury due to infection by other, usually systemic viruses, such as (1) mild Epstein-Barr virus hepatitis sometimes seen in infectious mononucleosis; (2) cytomegalovirus, herpes virus, and adenovirus infections, particularly in the newborn or immunosuppressed patient; and (3) yellow fever (yellow fever virus), a major and serious cause of hepatitis in tropical countries. We first present the main features of each hepatotropic virus, followed by a discussion of the clinicopathologic characteristics of acute and chronic viral hepatitis.

Hepatitis A Virus

Hepatitis A virus (HAV) is a usually benign, self-limited disease with an incubation period of 2 to 6 weeks. HAV does not cause chronic hepatitis or a carrier state and only uncommonly causes acute hepatic failure, so the fatality rate associated with HAV is only about 0.1-0.3%. HAV occurs throughout the world and is endemic in countries with poor hygiene and sanitation. Many individuals in these countries have detectable anti-HAV antibodies by the time they are 10 years old. Clinical disease tends to be mild or asymptomatic and is rare after childhood.

In developed countries, the prevalence of seropositivity (indicative of previous exposure) increases gradually with age, reaching 50% by age 50 years in the United States. In this population, acute HAV tends to be a sporadic febrile illness. Affected individuals have nonspecific symptoms such as fatigue and loss of appetite, and often develop jaundice. Overall, HAV accounts for about 25% of clinically evident acute hepatitis worldwide and an estimated 2000 new cases per year in the United States.

Discovered in 1973, HAV is a small, nonenveloped, positive-strand RNA picornavirus that occupies its own genus, *Hepatovirus*. Ultrastructurally, HAV is an icosahedral capsid 27 nm in diameter. The receptor for HAV is HAVcr-1, a 451–amino acid class I integral-membrane mucin-like glycoprotein. HAV is spread by ingestion of contaminated water and foods and is shed in the stool for 2 to 3 weeks before and 1 week after the onset of jaundice. Thus, close personal contact with an infected individual or fecal-oral contamination during this period accounts for most cases and explains the outbreaks in institutional settings such as schools and nurseries, and the water-borne epidemics in places where people live in overcrowded, unsanitary conditions. HAV vaccine, available since 1992, is effective in preventing infection. Immunization of toddlers in Israel has eliminated outbreaks in day care centers.

HAV can also be detected in serum and saliva. *Because HAV viremia is transient, blood-borne transmission of HAV occurs only rarely; therefore, donated blood is not specifically screened for this virus.* In developed countries, sporadic infections may be contracted by the consumption of raw or steamed shellfish (oysters, mussels, clams), which concentrate the virus from seawater contaminated with human sewage. Infected workers in the food industry may also be the source of outbreaks. HAV itself does not seem to be cytopathic. Cellular immunity, particularly CD8+ T cells, plays a key role in hepatocellular injury during HAV infection.

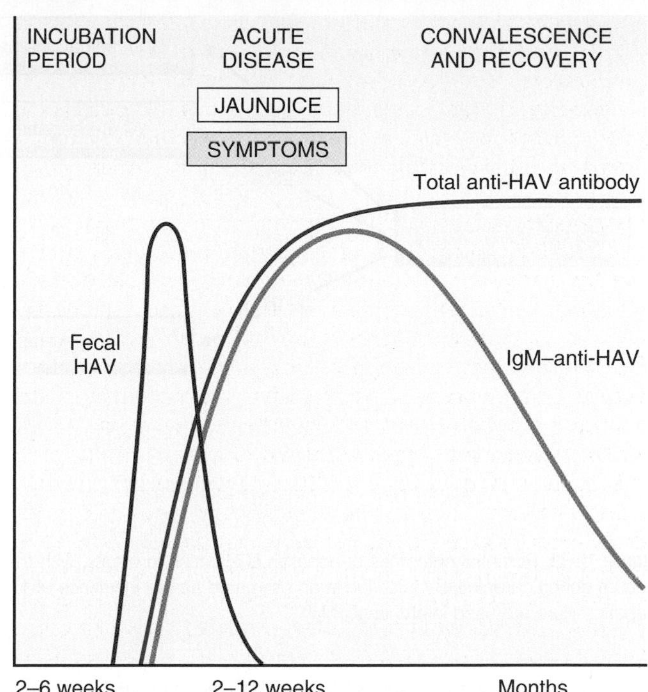

Figure 18-10 Temporal changes in serologic markers in acute hepatitis A infection. HAV, Hepatitis A virus.

Specific IgM antibody against HAV appears with the onset of symptoms, constituting a reliable marker of acute infection (Fig. 18-10). Fecal shedding of the virus ends as the IgM titer rises. The IgM response usually begins to decline in a few months and is followed by the appearance of IgG anti-HAV. The latter persists for years, perhaps conferring lifelong immunity against reinfection by all strains of HAV. Since there are no routinely available tests for IgG anti-HAV, the presence of IgG anti-HAV is inferred from the difference between total and IgM anti-HAV.

Hepatitis B Virus

Hepatitis B virus (HBV) can produce (1) acute hepatitis followed by recovery and clearance of the virus, (2) nonprogressive chronic hepatitis, (3) progressive chronic disease ending in cirrhosis, (4) acute hepatic failure with massive liver necrosis, and (5) an asymptomatic, "healthy" carrier state. HBV-induced chronic liver disease is also an important precursor for the development of hepatocellular carcinoma even in the absence of cirrhosis. The approximate frequencies of clinical outcomes of HBV infection are depicted in Figure 18-11.

Liver disease due to HBV is an enormous global health problem. One third of the world population (2 billion people) have been infected with HBV and 400 million people have chronic infection. Seventy-five percent of all chronic carriers live in Asia and the Western Pacific rim. The global prevalence of chronic hepatitis B infection varies widely, from high (>8%) in Africa, Asia, and the Western Pacific to intermediate (2% to 7%) in southern and eastern Europe, to low (<2%) in Western Europe, North America,

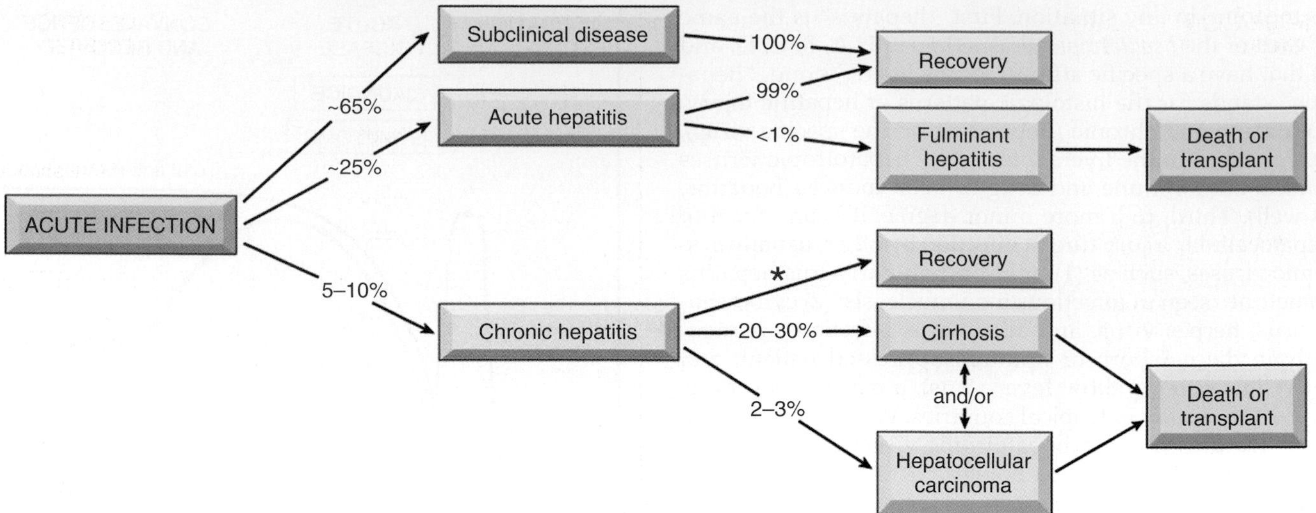

Figure 18-11 Potential outcomes of hepatitis B infection in adults, with their approximate frequencies in the United States. *Spontaneous HBsAg clearance occurs during chronic HBV infection at an estimated annual incidence of 1 to 2% in Western countries. As mentioned in the text, fulminant hepatitis and acute hepatic failure are used interchangeably

and Australia. As discussed later, the carrier rate is largely dictated by the age at infection, being the highest when infection occurs in children perinatally and the lowest when adults are infected.

The mode of transmission of HBV also varies with geographic areas. In high prevalence regions of the world, transmission during childbirth accounts for 90% of cases. In areas with intermediate prevalence, horizontal transmission, especially in early childhood, is the dominant mode of transmission. Such spread occurs through minor breaks in the skin or mucous membranes among children with close bodily contact. In low prevalence areas, unprotected sex and intravenous drug abuse (sharing of needles and syringes) are the chief modes of spread. The incidence of transfusion-related spread has dwindled greatly in recent decades due to screening of donated blood for HBsAg and exclusion of paid blood donors. Vaccination induces a protective anti-HBs antibody response in 95% of infants, children, and adolescents. Universal vaccination has had notable success in Taiwan and Gambia, but unfortunately, has not been adopted worldwide. Broad childhood population vaccination programs in endemic countries (e.g., Taiwan) are expected to curtail the disease in coming years.

HBV has a prolonged incubation period (2 to 26 weeks). Unlike HAV, HBV remains in the blood until and during active episodes of acute and chronic hepatitis. Approximately 65% of adults newly acquiring HBV have mild or no symptoms and do not develop jaundice. The remaining 25% have nonspecific constitutional symptoms such as anorexia, fever, jaundice, and upper right quadrant pain. In almost all cases the infection is self-limited and resolves without treatment. Chronic disease occurs in 5%-10% of infected individuals. Fulminant hepatitis (acute hepatic failure) is rare, occurring in approximately 0.1% to 0.5% of acutely infected individuals.

HBV was first linked to hepatitis in the 1960s when Australia antigen (later known as HBV surface antigen) was identified. The virus is a member of the *Hepadnaviridae*, a family of DNA viruses that cause hepatitis in multiple animal species. There are eight HBV genotypes that are distributed around the globe. The mature HBV virion is a 42-nm, spherical double-layered "Dane particle" that has an outer surface envelope of protein, lipid, and carbohydrate enclosing an electron-dense, 28-nm, slightly hexagonal core. The genome of HBV is a partially double-stranded circular DNA molecule having 3200 nucleotides with four open reading frames coding for:

- A nucleocapsid "core" protein (HBcAg, hepatitis B core antigen) and a longer polypeptide transcript with a precore and core region, designated HBeAg (hepatitis B e antigen). The precore region directs the secretion of the HBeAg polypeptide, whereas HBcAg remains in hepatocytes, where it participates in the assembly of complete virions.
- Envelope glycoproteins (HBsAg, hepatitis B surface antigen), which consist of three related proteins: large, middle, and small HBsAg. Infected hepatocytes are capable of synthesizing and secreting massive quantities of noninfective surface protein (mainly small HBsAg).
- A polymerase (Pol) that exhibits both DNA polymerase activity and reverse transcriptase activity. Replication of the viral genome occurs via an intermediate RNA template, through a unique replication cycle: DNA $\rightarrow$ RNA $\rightarrow$ DNA
- HBx protein, which is necessary for virus replication and may act as a transcriptional transactivator of both viral genes and a subset of host genes. It has been implicated in the pathogenesis of hepatocellular carcinoma in HBV infection.

The natural course of the disease can be followed by serum markers (Fig. 18-12)

- HBsAg appears before the onset of symptoms, peaks during overt disease, and then often declines to undetectable levels in 12 weeks, although it may persist in some individuals for as long as 24 weeks.
- Anti-HBs antibody does not rise until the acute disease is over, concomitant with the disappearance of HBsAg

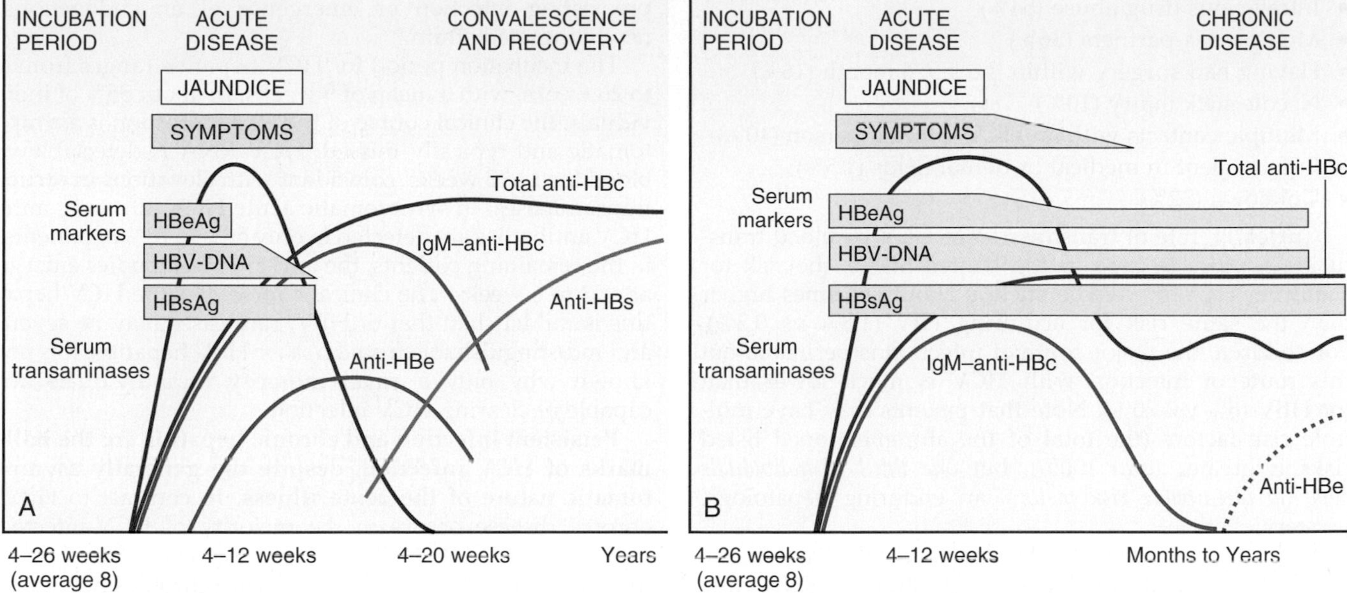

Figure 18-12 Temporal changes in serologic markers in hepatitis B viral infection. **A,** Acute infection with resolution. **B,** progression to chronic infection. Note in some cases of chronic HBV, serum transaminases may become normal.

(Fig. 18-12*A*). In some cases, however, Anti-HBs antibody is not detectable for a few weeks to several months after the disappearance of HBsAg. During this window period, serologic diagnosis can be made by detection of IgM anti-HBc antibody (see below and Fig. 18-12). Anti-HBs may persist for life, conferring protection; this is the basis for current vaccination strategies using noninfectious HBsAg.

- HBeAg, HBV-DNA, and DNA polymerase appear in serum soon after HBsAg, and all signify active viral replication. Persistence of HBeAg is an important indicator of continued viral replication, infectivity, and probable progression to chronic hepatitis. The appearance of anti-HBe antibodies implies that an acute infection has peaked and is on the wane.
- IgM anti-HBc antibody becomes detectable in serum shortly before the onset of symptoms, concurrent with the onset of elevated serum aminotransferase levels (indicative of hepatocyte destruction). Over a period of months the IgM anti-HBc antibody is replaced by IgG anti-HBc. As in the case of anti-HAV, there is no direct assay for IgG anti-HBc; its presence is inferred from decline of IgM anti-HBc in the face of rising total anti-HBc.

Occasionally, mutated strains of HBV emerge that do not produce HBeAg but are replication competent and express HBcAg. In such patients, the HBeAg may be low or undetectable despite the presence of serum HBV DNA. A second, ominous development is the appearance of vaccine-induced escape mutants, which replicate in the presence of vaccine-induced immunity.

The host immune response to the virus is the main determinant of the outcome of the infection. Innate immune mechanisms protect the host during the initial phases of the infection, and a strong response by virus-specific CD4+ and CD8+ interferon (IFN)-γ-producing cells is associated with the resolution of acute infection. HBV generally does not cause direct hepatocyte injury. Instead, injury is caused by CD8+ cytotoxic T cells attacking infected cells.

Age at the time of infection is the best predictor of chronicity. The younger the age at the time of HBV infection, the higher the probability of chronicity. Despite progress in the treatment of chronic HBV infection, complete cure is extremely difficult to achieve even when treated with highly effective antiviral agents. The difficulty in achieving cure has been attributed to the ability of the virus to insert itself in the host DNA, thus limiting the development of an effective immune response (HBsAb development). This allows the virus to persist in the face of drugs that impair its replication. Hence, the goal of the treatment of chronic hepatitis B is to slow disease progression, reduce liver damage, and prevent liver cirrhosis or liver cancer.

Hepatitis B can be prevented by vaccination and by the screening of donor blood, organs, and tissues. Vaccination induces a protective anti-HBs antibody response in 95% of infants, children, and adolescents.

Hepatitis C Virus

Hepatitis C Virus (HCV) is a major cause of liver disease worldwide, with approximately 170 million people affected. Approximately 3.6 million Americans, or 1.3% of the population, have antibodies to HCV, indicative of past or current infection. Of these, 2.7 million have chronic HCV based on presence of HCV RNA. Notably, there has been a decrease in the annual incidence of infection from its mid-1980s peak of more than 230,000 new infections per year to a current 17,000 new infections per year, due primarily to a marked reduction in transfusion-associated cases as a result of donor blood screening. Nevertheless, the number of patients with chronic infection will continue to increase, as a result of potential lifelong persistence of HCV infection.

According to data from the USA Centers for Disease Control, the most common risk factors for HCV infection are:

- Intravenous drug abuse (54%)
- Multiple sex partners (36%)
- Having had surgery within the last 6 month (16%)
- Needle stick injury (10%)
- Multiple contacts with an HCV-infected person (10%)
- Employment in medical or dental fields (1.5%)
- Unknown (32%)

Currently, rate of transmission of HCV by blood transfusion is close to zero in the United States; the risk for acquiring HCV by needle stick is about six times higher than the same risk for acquiring HIV (1.8% vs 0.3%). For children, the major route of infection is perinatal, but this route of infection with HCV is much lower than for HBV (6% vs. 20%). Note that patients may have multiple risk factors (the total of the aforementioned listed risks is greater than 100%), but *one third of individuals have no identifiable risk factors*, an enduring hepatologic mystery.

HCV, discovered in 1989, is a member of the Flaviviridae family. It is a small, enveloped, single-stranded RNA virus with a 9.6-kilobase (kb) genome that codes for a single polyprotein with one open reading frame, which is subsequently processed into functional proteins. Because of the low fidelity of the HCV RNA polymerase, the virus is inherently unstable, giving rise to multiple genotypes and subtypes. Indeed, *within any given individual, HCV exists as closely related genetic variants known as quasispecies.*

Over time, dozens of quasispecies can be detected within one individual all derived from the original HCV strain that infected the patient. The E2 protein of the envelope is the target of many anti-HCV antibodies but is also the most variable region of the entire viral genome, enabling emergent virus strains to escape from neutralizing antibodies. This genomic instability and antigenic variability have seriously hampered efforts to develop an HCV vaccine. In particular, *elevated titers of anti-HCV IgG occurring after an active infection do not confer effective immunity.* A characteristic feature of HCV infection, therefore, is repeated bouts of hepatic damage, the result of reactivation of a preexisting infection or emergence of an endogenous, newly mutated strain.

The incubation period for HCV hepatitis ranges from 4 to 26 weeks, with a mean of 9 weeks. In about 85% of individuals, the clinical course of the acute infection is asymptomatic and typically missed. HCV RNA is detectable in blood for 1 to 3 weeks, coincident with elevations in serum transaminases. In symptomatic acute HCV infection, anti-HCV antibodies are detected in only 50% to 70% of patients; in the remaining patients, the anti-HCV antibodies emerge after 3 to 6 weeks. The clinical course of acute HCV hepatitis is milder than that of HBV; rare cases may be severe and indistinguishable from HAV or HBV hepatitis. It is not known why only a small minority of individuals are capable of clearing HCV infection.

Persistent infection and chronic hepatitis are the hallmarks of HCV infection, despite the generally asymptomatic nature of the acute illness. In contrast to HBV, chronic disease occurs in the majority of HCV-infected individuals (80% to 90%) and cirrhosis eventually occurs in as many as a 20% of individuals with chronic HCV infection. The mechanisms that lead to the chronicity of HCV infection are not well understood, but it is clear that the virus has developed multiple strategies to evade host antiviral immunity. HCV is able to actively inhibit the IFN-mediated cellular antiviral response at multiple steps, including toll-like receptor signaling in response to viral RNA recognition and signaling downstream of IFN receptors that would otherwise have antiviral effects.

In more than 90% of individuals with chronic HCV infection, circulating HCV RNA persists despite the presence of antibodies (Fig. 18-13). Hence, in persons with chronic hepatitis, HCV RNA testing must be performed to assess viral replication and to confirm the diagnosis of HCV infection. A clinical feature that is quite characteristic of chronic HCV infection is persistent elevations in serum aminotransferases. Their levels wax and wane but almost never become normal. Even rare patients with normal transaminases are at risk for developing permanent liver damage. Therefore, any individual with detectable HCV

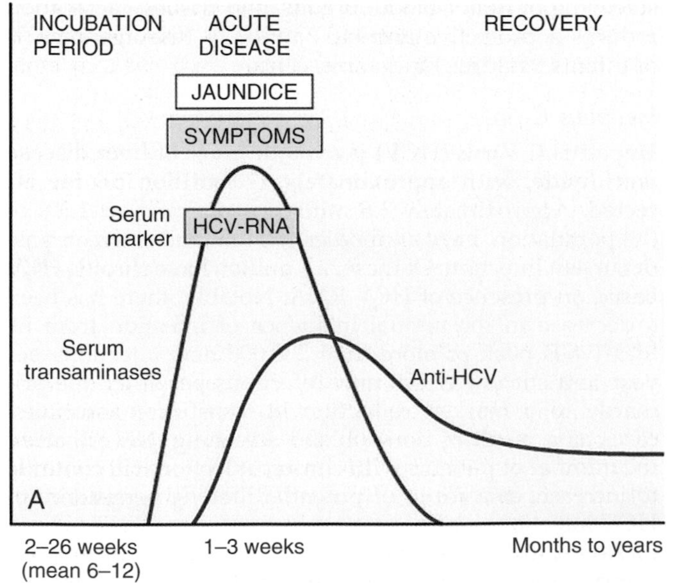

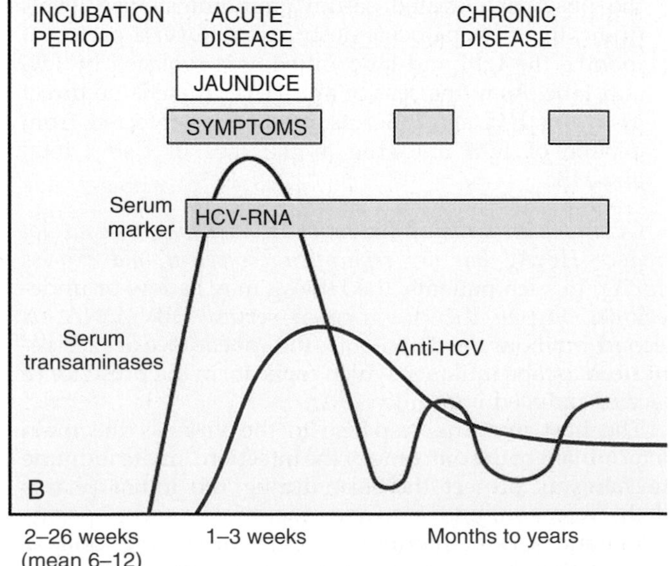

Figure 18-13 Temporal changes in serologic markers in hepatitis C viral infection. **A,** Acute infection with resolution. **B,** progression to chronic infection.

RNA in the serum needs close clinical follow-up. *A feature unique to hepatitis C infection is the association with the metabolic syndrome,* in particular with HCV genotype 3. Apparently, HCV can give rise to insulin resistance and non alcoholic fatty liver disease.

HCV infection is potentially curable. Until recently, treatment has been based on combination of pegylated IFN-α and ribavirin and cure rates depended on the viral genotype; patients with genotype 2 or 3 infection generally have had the best responses. Interestingly, host genotype also influences the response. Certain polymorphism in the IL-28B gene are associated with better response to interferon-alpha and ribavarin. IL-28B encodes interferon lambda, which is involved in resistance to HCV. New drugs targeting viral protease and polymerase have now been approved or are in development. With currently available drugs sustained virologic response (defined as undetectable HCV RNA in the patient's blood 24 weeks after the end of treatment) can be achieved in 50% to 80% of patients. Thus there is every reason to believe that newer regimens, based on principles similar to those used in highly active antiretroviral therapy (HAART) for HIV infection, will change the course of chronic hepatitis C in the coming decade.

Hepatitis D Virus

Also called "the delta agent," hepatitis D virus (HDV) is a unique RNA virus that is dependent for its life cycle on HBV. Infection with HDV arises in the following settings.

- *Co-infection* occurs following exposure to serum containing both HDV and HBV. The HBV must become established first to provide the HBsAg necessary for development of complete HDV virions. Co-infection of HBV and HDV results in acute hepatitis that is indistinguishable from acute hepatitis B. It is self -limited and is usually followed by clearance of both viruses. However, there is a higher rate of acute hepatic failure, in intravenous drug users.
- *Superinfection* occurs when a chronic carrier of HBV is exposed to a new inoculum of HDV. This results in disease 30 to 50 days later presenting either as severe acute hepatitis in a previously unrecognized HBV carrier or as an exacerbation of preexisting chronic hepatitis B infection. Chronic HDV infection occurs in almost all of such patients. The superinfection may have two phases: an acute phase with active HDV replication and suppression of HBV with high transaminase levels, and a chronic phase in which HDV replication decreases, HBV replication increases, transferase levels fluctuate, and the disease progresses to cirrhosis and sometimes hepatocellular carcinoma.

Worldwide, 15 million people are estimated to be infected with HDV (about 5% of 300 million of HBV infected persons). Prevalence varies, being high in the Amazon basin, and in central Africa, the Middle East, and the Mediterranean basin, where 20% to 40% of HbsAg carriers may have anti-HDV antibody; the rate has been declining in recent years. Surprisingly, HDV infection is uncommon in the large population of HBsAg carriers in Southeast Asia and China. In western countries it is largely restricted to intravenous drug abusers and those who have had multiple blood transfusions.

HDV, discovered in 1977, is a 35-nm, double-shelled particle. The external coat antigen of HBsAg surrounds an internal polypeptide assembly, designated delta antigen (HDAg), the only protein produced by the virus. Associated with HDAg is a small circular molecule of single-stranded RNA, whose length is smaller than the genome of any known animal virus. Replication of the virus is through RNA-directed RNA synthesis by host RNA polymerase.

HDV RNA is detectable in the blood and liver just before and in the early days of acute symptomatic disease. IgM anti-HDV antibody is the most reliable indicator of recent HDV exposure, although its appearance is late and frequently short-lived. Nevertheless, acute co-infection by HDV and HBV is best indicated by detection of IgM against both HDAg and HBcAg (denoting new infection with hepatitis B). With chronic delta hepatitis arising from HDV superinfection, HBsAg is present in serum, and anti-HDV antibodies (IgG and IgM) persist for months or longer. Vaccination for HBV also prevents HDV infection.

Hepatitis E Virus

Hepatitis E virus (HEV) is an enterically transmitted, water-borne infection that occurs primarily in young to middle-aged adults. HEV is a zoonotic disease with animal reservoirs, such as monkeys, cats, pigs, and dogs. Epidemics have been reported in Asia and the Indian subcontinent, sub-Saharan Africa, Middle East, China and Mexico, although sporadic cases are seen in industrialized nations, particularly in regions where pig farming is common. Sporadic infection may also occur in travelers to these regions, but, most importantly, HEV infection accounts for more than 30% to 60% of cases of sporadic acute hepatitis in India, exceeding the frequency of HAV. *A characteristic feature of HEV infection is the high mortality rate among pregnant women, approaching 20%.* In most cases the disease is self-limiting; HEV is not associated with chronic liver disease or persistent viremia in immunocompetent patients. Chronic HEV infection does occur in patients with AIDS and immunosuppressed transplant patients. The average incubation period following exposure is 4 to 5 weeks.

Discovered in 1983, HEV is an unenveloped, positive-stranded RNA virus in the *Hepevirus* genus. Viral particles are 32 to 34 nm in diameter, and the RNA genome is approximately 7.3 kb in size. Virions are shed in stool during the acute illness.

Before the onset of clinical illness, HEV RNA and HEV virions can be detected by PCR in stool and serum. The onset of rising serum aminotransferases, clinical illness, and elevated IgM anti-HEV titers are virtually simultaneous. Symptoms resolve in 2 to 4 weeks, during which time the IgM is replaced with a persistent IgG anti-HEV antibodies.

Clinicopathologic Syndromes of Viral Hepatitis

Several clinical syndromes may develop following exposure to hepatitis viruses: (1) acute asymptomatic infection with recovery (serologic evidence only), (2) acute symptomatic hepatitis with recovery, anicteric or icteric, (3) chronic hepatitis, with or without progression to cirrhosis, and (4) acute liver failure with massive to submassive hepatic necrosis. Table 18-3 provides a summary of the salient features of infection by various hepatitis viruses. All of the hepatotropic viruses can cause acute

Table 18-3 The Hepatitis Viruses

Virus	Hepatitis A	Hepatitis B	Hepatitis C	Hepatitis D	Hepatitis E
Type of virus	ssRNA	partially dsDNA	ssRNA	Circular defective ssRNA	ssRNA
Viral family	Hepatovirus; related to picornavirus	Hepadnavirus	Flaviviridae	Subviral particle in Deltaviridae family	Hepevirus
Route of transmission	Fecal-oral (contaminated food or water)	Parenteral, sexual contact, perinatal	Parenteral; intranasal cocaine use is a risk factor	Parenteral	Fecal-oral
Mean incubation period	2 to 6 weeks	2 to 26 weeks (mean 8 weeks)	4 to 26 weeks (mean 9 weeks)	Same as HBV	4 to 5 weeks
Frequency of chronic liver disease	Never	5%-10%	>80%	10% (co-infection); 90%-100% for superinfection	In immunocompromised hosts only
Diagnosis	Detection of serum IgM antibodies	Detection of HBsAg or antibody to HBcAg; PCR for HBV DNA	3rd-generation ELISA for antibody detection; PCR for HCV RNA	Detection of IgM and IgG antibodies; HDV RNA serum; HDAg in liver	Detection of serum IgM and IgG antibodies; PCR for HEV RNA

dsDNA, Double-stranded DNA; ELISA, enzyme-linked immunosorbent assay; HBcAg, hepatitis B core antigen; HBsAg, hepatitis B surface antigen; HBV, hepatitis B virus; HCV, hepatitis C virus; HDAg, hepatitis D antigen; HDV, hepatitis D virus; HEV, hepatitis E virus; IV, intravenous; PCR, polymerase chain reaction; ssRNA, single stranded RNA.
From Washington K: Inflammatory and infectious diseases of the liver. In Iacobuzio-Donahue CA, Montgomery EA (eds): Gastrointestinal and Liver Pathology. Philadelphia, Churchill Livingstone; 2005.

asymptomatic or symptomatic infection. HAV and HEV (in immunocompetent hosts) do not cause chronic hepatitis and only a small number of HBV-infected adult patients develop chronic hepatitis. In contrast, HCV is notorious for chronic infection. Fulminant hepatitis (acute liver failure) is unusual and is seen primarily with HAV, HBV, or HDV infection depending on region. HEV can cause fulminant hepatitis in pregnant women. Although HBV and HCV are responsible for most cases of chronic hepatitis, there are many other causes of similar clinicopathologic presentation, especially autoimmunity and drug/toxin-induced hepatitis, described later. Therefore, *serologic and molecular studies are essential for the diagnosis of viral hepatitis and for distinguishing between the various types.*

Acute Asymptomatic Infection with Recovery. Patients in this group are identified only incidentally on the basis of minimally elevated serum transaminases or, after the fact, by the presence of antiviral antibodies. Worldwide, HAV and HBV infection are frequently subclinical events in childhood, verified only in adulthood by the presence of anti-HAV or anti-HBV antibodies.

Acute Symptomatic Infection with Recovery. Regardless of the virus, the disease is more or less the same and can be divided into four phases: (1) an incubation period, (2) a symptomatic preicteric phase, (3) a symptomatic icteric phase, and (4) convalescence. The incubation period for the different viruses is given in Table 18-3. Peak infectivity occurs during the last asymptomatic days of the incubation period and the early days of acute symptoms.

Acute Liver Failure. Viral hepatitis is responsible for about 10% of cases of acute hepatic failure. The causative virus differs depending on the geographic location. Globally, hepatitis A and E are the most common causes; HBV is more common in Asian and Mediterranean countries. Morphologic details of massive necrosis under these circumstance were previously described in the section on Acute Liver Failure. There are no specific histologic findings which are indicative of hepatotropic virus causation.

Survival for more than a week may permit the replication of residual hepatocytes. Activation of the stem/progenitor cells in the canals of Hering gives rise to very prominent ductular reactions, although these are usually insufficient to accomplish full restitution; recovery depends on surviving hepatocytes undergoing cell division to restore missing parenchyma. The treatment for acute hepatic failure that follows acute viral hepatitis is to provide supportive care. Liver transplantation is the only option for patients whose disease does not resolve before secondary infection and other organ failure develop.

Chronic Hepatitis. **Chronic hepatitis is defined as symptomatic, biochemical, or serologic evidence of continuing or relapsing hepatic disease for more than 6 months.** Etiology rather than the histologic pattern is the most important determinant of the probability of developing progressive chronic hepatitis. The clinical features of chronic hepatitis are extremely variable and are not predictive of outcome. In some patients the only signs of chronic disease are persistent elevations of serum transaminases. Laboratory studies may also reveal prolongation of the prothrombin time and, in some instances, hyperglobulinemia, hyperbilirubinemia, and mild elevations in alkaline phosphatase levels. In symptomatic individuals, the most common finding is fatigue; less common symptoms are malaise, loss of appetite, and occasional bouts of mild jaundice. In precirrhotic chronic hepatitis, physical findings are few, the most common being mild hepatomegaly, hepatic tenderness, and mild splenomegaly. Occasionally, in cases of HBV and HCV infection, immune complex disease may develop secondary to the presence of circulating antibody-antigen complexes, in the form of vasculitis (Chapter 11) and glomerulonephritis (Chapter 20). Cryoglobulinemia is found in about 35% of individuals with chronic hepatitis C infection.

The Carrier State. A "carrier" is an individual who harbors and can transmit an organism, but has no manifest symptoms. In the case of hepatotropic virus this definition is somewhat confusing, as it can be interpreted to mean: (1) individuals who carry one of the viruses but have no liver disease; (2) those who harbor one of the viruses and have non-progressive liver damage, but are essentially free of symptoms or disability. In both cases, particularly the latter, these individuals constitute reservoirs for infection. In the case of HBV infection an older, but still often used term is the so called "healthy carrier". It is defined as an individual with HBsAg, without HBeAg, but with presence of anti-HBe; these patients have normal aminotransferases, low or undetectable serum HBV DNA, and a liver biopsy showing a lack of significant inflammation and necrosis (Fig. 18-11). In non-endemic areas such as the United States, between 5 and 10% of adults who acquire HBV infections become chronically infected, a very small number of whom become such "healthy carriers"; the rest have active disease, with consistent or intermittent signs and symptoms of active hepatitis, 20% of whom will go on to develop cirrhosis. In contrast, HBV infection acquired early in life in endemic areas (such as Southeast Asia, China, and Sub-Saharan Africa) gives rise to carrier states of the two types described above, in more than 90% of cases. It should be kept in mind that "healthy carrier" is probably not a stable state and that re-activation of hepatitis can occur in response to co-infection or alterations of immune function related to age or co-morbid diseases. Because of the confusion generated by the term "healthy carriers" many authorities prefer to use the term "inactive carrier".

HCV infection in the United States is quite different. Equivalent states to the HBV "healthy carrier" are not recognized. Acute HCV infection progresses to chronic hepatitis in 80% or more of infected individuals, one third of whom may progress to cirrhosis.

HIV and Chronic Viral Hepatitis. Because of the similar transmission mode and the similar high-risk patient population, co-infection of HIV and hepatitis viruses has become a common clinical problem. For example, in the United States, 10% of HIV-infected individuals are co-infected with HBV and 25% with HCV. In fact, chronic HBV and HCV infection are now leading causes of morbidity and mortality for HIV-infected individuals, even those who are on successful anti-HIV therapy. In individuals who are untreated or resistant to treatment and who therefore progress to acquired immunodeficiency syndrome (AIDS), liver disease is the second most common cause of death. It is clear that untreated HIV infection significantly exacerbates the severity of liver disease caused by HBV or HCV. In immunocompetent individuals with HIV infection, the differences in severity and progression of either HBV or HCV may not differ greatly from those who are HIV negative.

MORPHOLOGY

The general morphologic features of viral hepatitis are depicted schematically in Fig. 18-14. **The morphologic changes in acute and chronic viral hepatitis are shared among the hepatotropic viruses and can be mimicked by drug reactions or autoimmune hepatitis.**

Acute viral hepatitis. On gross inspection, livers involved by mild acute hepatitis appear normal or slightly mottled. At the other end of the spectrum, in massive hepatic necrosis the liver may shrink greatly as described earlier under acute liver failure (Fig. 18-6).

Microscopically, both acute and chronic hepatitis evoke a lymphoplasmacytic (mononuclear) infiltrate. Portal inflammation in acute hepatitis is minimal or absent. Most parenchymal injury is scattered throughout the hepatic lobule as "spotty necrosis" or **lobular hepatitis**. As described earlier, the hepatocyte injury may result in necrosis or apoptosis. In the former, the cytoplasm appears empty with only scattered wisps of cytoplasmic remnants. Eventually there is rupture of cell membranes leading to "dropout" of hepatocytes, leaving collapsed sinusoidal collagen reticulin framework behind; scavenger macrophages mark sites of dropout (Fig. 18-2). With apoptosis, hepatocytes shrink, becoming intensely eosinophilic, and their nuclei become pyknotic and fragmented; effector T cells may be present in the immediate vicinity (Figs. 18-3 and 18-14).

In severe acute hepatitis, confluent necrosis of hepatocytes is seen around central veins (Fig. 18-6*B*). In these areas there may be cellular debris, collapsed reticulin fibers, congestion/hemorrhage, and variable inflammation. With increasing severity, there is central-portal bridging necrosis, followed by, even worse, parenchymal collapse (Fig. 18-4*B*). In some cases massive hepatic necrosis and acute liver failure ensue, as described previously. In occasional cases, the injury is not severe enough to cause death (or necessitate transplantation), and the liver survives, although with abundant scarring, usually with replacement of areas of confluent necrosis. In such cases, some patients rapidly develop posthepatitic cirrhosis.

There is considerable morphologic overlap in acute hepatitis caused by various hepatotropic viruses. However, subtle differences may be seen, for example the mononuclear infiltrate in hepatitis A may be especially rich in plasma cells.

Chronic viral hepatitis. The defining histologic feature of chronic viral hepatitis is mononuclear portal infiltration. It may be mild to severe and variable from one portal tract to the next (Fig. 18-14). There is often **interface hepatitis** as well, in addition to lobular hepatitis, distinguished by its location at the interface between hepatocellular parenchyma and portal tract stroma. The hallmark of progressive chronic liver damage is scarring. At first, only portal tracts exhibit fibrosis, but in some patients, with time, fibrous septa—bands of dense scar—extend between portal tracts. In parallel with increasing scarring there is also increasing ductular reaction, reflecting stem cell activation. In the most severe cases, continued scarring and nodule formation leads to the development of cirrhosis as described earlier (Fig. 18-8).

Clinical assessment of chronic hepatitis often requires liver biopsy in addition to clinical and serologic data. Liver biopsy is helpful in confirming the clinical diagnosis, excluding common concomitant conditions (e.g., fatty liver disease, hemochromatosis), assessing histologic features associated with an increased risk of malignancy (e.g., small and large cell change, described later), grading the extent of hepatocyte injury and inflammation, and staging the progression of scarring. Histologic grading and staging of chronic hepatitis in liver biopsy specimens are often central to determinations of whether to treat the underlying disease.

A somewhat greater range of histologic features distinguish one viral infection from another in chronic hepatitis. In chronic hepatitis B, **"ground-glass" hepatocytes**—cells with endoplasmic reticulum swollen by HBsAg—is a diagnostic hallmark. Immunostaining can confirm the presence of viral antigen (Fig. 18-15). Chronic hepatitis C quite commonly shows lymphoid aggregates or fully formed lymphoid follicles (Fig. 18-16). Often, hepatitis C, particularly genotype 3, shows fatty change of scattered hepatocytes, although the infection may also cause systemic alterations leading to metabolic syndrome and, therefore,

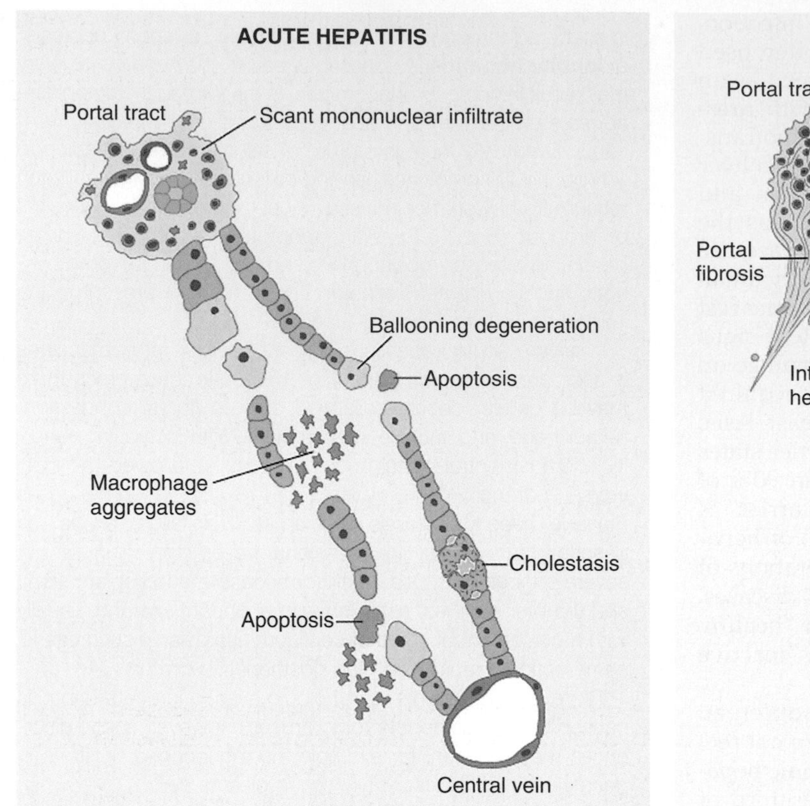

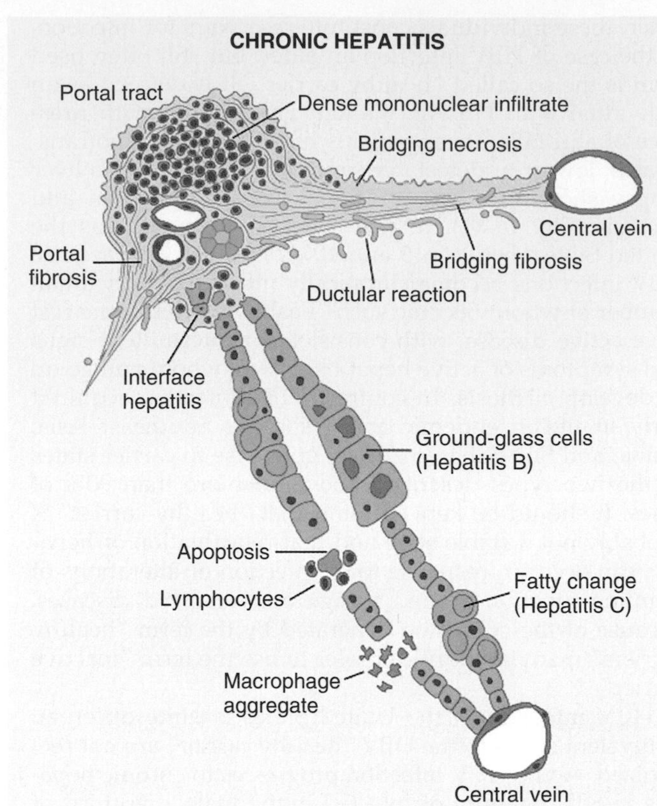

Figure 18-14 Diagrammatic representation of the morphologic features of acute and chronic hepatitis. Notice that there is very little portal mononuclear infiltration in acute hepatitis (or sometimes none at all), while in chronic hepatitis the portal infiltrates are dense and prominent—the defining change of chronic hepatitis. Bridging necrosis and fibrosis is shown only for chronic hepatitis, but bridging necrosis may also occur in more severe acute hepatitis. Ductular reactions in chronic hepatitis are minimal in early stages of scarring, but become extensive in late stage disease.

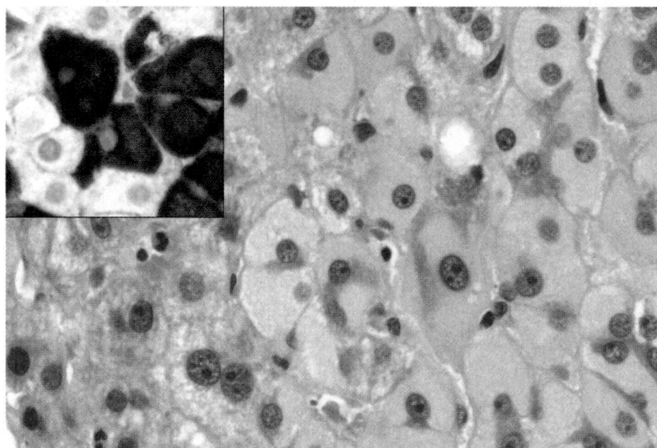

Figure 18-15 Ground-glass hepatocytes in chronic hepatitis B infection caused by accumulation of hepatitis B surface antigen. Note the large pale, finely granular pink cytoplasmic inclusions on hematoxylin and eosin staining; immunostaining (inset) confirms the presence of surface antigen (brown).

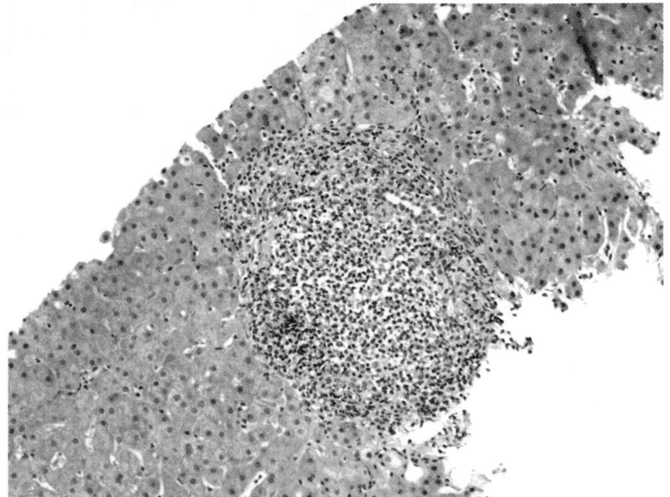

Figure 18-16 Chronic viral hepatitis due to HCV showing characteristic portal tract expansion by a lymphoid follicle.

a superimposed non-alcoholic fatty liver disease in the liver (see later). Bile duct injury is also prominent in some individuals with hepatitis C infection, potentially mimicking primary biliary cirrhosis (see later); clinical parameters distinguish these two diseases easily, however.

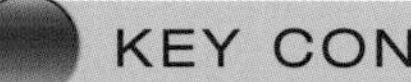

KEY CONCEPTS

Viral Hepatitis

- In the alphabet of hepatotropic viruses, some easy mnemonic devices may be useful:

- The vowels (hepatitis A and E) never cause chronic hepatitis, only *AcutE* hepatitis, except HEV in immunocompromised hosts and pregnant females.
- Only the consonants (hepatitis B, C, D) have the potential to cause chronic disease (C for consonant and for chronic).
- Hepatitis B can be transmitted by blood, birthing, and "bonking" (as they say in the United Kingdom).
- Hepatitis C is the single virus that is more often chronic than not (almost never detected acutely; 80% or more of patients develop chronic hepatitis, 20% of whom will develop cirrhosis).
- Hepatitis D, the delta agent, is a defective virus, requiring hepatitis B co-infection for its own capacity to infect and replicate.
- Hepatitis E is endemic in equatorial regions and frequently epidemic.

- The inflammatory cells in both acute and chronic viral hepatitis are mainly T cells; it is the pattern of injury that is different between the two time courses, not the nature of the infiltrate.
- Biopsy assessment in chronic viral hepatitis is most important for grading and staging of disease, which are used to decide whether a patient undergoes often arduous antiviral treatments.
- Patients with long-standing HBV or HCV related cirrhosis are at increased risk for the development of hepatocellular carinoma.

Bacterial, Parasitic, and Helminthic Infections

A multitude of organisms can infect the liver and biliary tree, including bacteria, fungi, helminths and other parasites, and protozoa. Several bacteria can infect the liver directly, including *Staphylococcus aureus* in toxic shock syndrome, *Salmonella typhi* in typhoid fever, and *Treponema pallidum* in secondary or tertiary syphilis. Bacteria may also proliferate in the biliary tree especially when outflow is compromised by partial or complete obstruction. The intrabiliary bacterial composition reflects the gut flora, and the acute inflammatory response within the intrahepatic biliary tree is called *ascending cholangitis*.

Bacteria may give rise to abscesses by spreading from extrahepatic sites, through the vascular supply, or from adjacent infected tissues. Liver abscesses are associated with fever and, in many instances, right upper quadrant pain and tender hepatomegaly. Jaundice may result from extrahepatic biliary obstruction. Although antibiotic therapy may control smaller lesions, surgical drainage is often necessary for the larger lesions. In the past almost 90% of the patients succumbed to the disease, but with early recognition and management, as many as 90% of patients can survive. Extrahepatic bacterial infections, particularly sepsis, can induce mild hepatic inflammation and varying degrees of hepatocellular cholestasis (see later).

Fungi (e.g., histoplasmosis) and mycobacteria can also infect the liver in disseminated disease, with histology showing classical granulomas. Organisms are usually not visible histologically, even with special stains, although serologic studies and tissue or blood cultures can often identify the causative agent.

Parasitic and helminthic infections are major causes of morbidity worldwide, and the liver is frequently involved (Chapter 8). These diseases include malaria, schistosomiasis, strongyloidiasis, cryptosporidiosis, leishmaniasis, echinococcosis, amebiasis, and infections by the liver flukes *Fasciola hepatica, Opisthorchis* species, and *Clonorchis sinensis*. *Schistosomiasis*, most commonly found in Asia, Africa, and South America, especially in those areas where the water contains numerous freshwater snails as a vector, is particularly associated with insidious sequelae of chronic liver disease. The liver flukes, most common in Southeast Asia, are notorious for causing a very high rate of cholangiocarcinoma. *Hydatid cysts* are usually caused by echinococcal infections (Chapter 8). They often have calcifications in the cyst walls which may aid radiologic diagnosis. In developed countries, hydatid cysts are uncommon. Cystic liver degeneration or abscesses can be caused by amebas and other protozoal and helminthic organisms. The incidence of amebic infections is low in developed countries and is usually found in immigrants from endemic regions.

Autoimmune Hepatitis

Autoimmune hepatitis is a chronic, progressive hepatitis with all the features of autoimmune diseases in general: genetic predisposition, association with other autoimmune diseases, presence of autoantibodies, and therapeutic response to immunosuppression. Strong HLA-associations for autoimmune hepatitis support a genetic predisposition. In Caucasians, there is a frequent association with DRB1* alleles. As with most other autoimmune diseases , the mechanistic basis of the HLA association are not clear. Triggers for the immune reaction may include viral infections or drug or toxin exposures.

Clinicopathologic Features. The annual incidence is highest among white northern Europeans at 1.9 per 100,000, but all ethnic groups are susceptible. There is a *female predominance* (78%). The diagnostic features are summarized in Table 18-4. As can be seen, a point system is used for the diagnosis of definite and probable autoimmune hepatitis. *Autoimmune hepatitis is classified into types 1 and 2, based on the patterns of circulating antibodies.* Type 1, more common in middle-aged to older individuals, is characterized by the presence of antinuclear (ANA), anti–smooth muscle actin (SMA), anti–soluble liver antigen/liver-pancreas antigen (anti-SLA/LP) antibodies, and less commonly, anti-mitochondrial (AMA) antibodies. In type 2, usually seen in children and teenagers, the main serologic markers are anti–liver kidney microsome-1 (anti-LKM-1) antibodies, which are mostly directed against CYP2D6, and anti–liver cytosol-1 (ACL-1) antibodies.

MORPHOLOGY

Although autoimmune hepatitis shares patterns of injury with acute or chronic viral hepatitis, the time course of histologic progression differs. In viral hepatitis, fibrosis typically follows many years of slowly accumulating parenchymal injury, whereas in autoimmune hepatitis, there is an early phase of severe

Table 18-4 Simplified Diagnostic Criteria (2008) of the International Autoimmune Hepatitis Group

		Points*
Autoantibodies	ANA or ASMA or LKM > 1:80	2
	ANA or ASMA or LKM > 1:40	1
	SLA/LP Positive (>20 units)	0
IgG (or gamma-globulins)	>1.10 times normal limit	2
	Upper normal limit	1
Liver histology†	Typical for autoimmune hepatitis	2
	Compatible with autoimmune hepatitis	1
	Atypical for autoimmune	0
Absence of viral hepatitis	Yes	2
	No	0

*Definite autoimmune hepatitis (AIH): P7; probable AIH: P6.

†Typical: (1) Interface hepatitis, lymphocytic/lymphoplasmacytic infiltrates in portal tracts and extending in the lobule; (2) emperipolesis (active penetration by one cell into and through larger cell); (3) hepatic rosette formation.

Compatible: Chronic hepatitis with lymphocytic infiltration without features considered typical.

Atypical: Showing signs of another diagnosis like NAFLD.

ANA, antinuclear antibody; ASMA, anti–smooth muscle actin; LP, liver pancreas; LKM, anti-liver kidney microsomal antibodies; SLA, soluble liver antigen; IgG, immunoglobulin G; AIH, autoimmune hepatitis.

Adapted from Hennes EM, et al. Simplified criteria for the diagnosis of autoimmune hepatitis. Hepatology 48:169-176; 2008.

parenchymal destruction followed rapidly by scarring. Features considered typical of autoimmune hepatitis include:

- Severe necroinflammatory activity indicated by extensive interface hepatitis or foci of confluent (perivenular or bridging necrosis) or parenchymal collapse
- Plasma cell predominance in the mononuclear inflammatory infiltrates (Fig. 18-17)
- Hepatocyte "rosettes" in areas of marked activity

The disease may be rapidly progressive or indolent, both giving rise eventually to liver failure. Clinical evolution correlates with a limited number of histologic patterns, any of which may be seen at the time of initial diagnosis:

- Very severe hepatocyte injury with widespread confluent necrosis, but little scarring; this pattern is often seen as symptomatic acute hepatitis and represents the first sign of disease.
- A mix of marked inflammation and some degree of scarring, seen in early or later stage disease
- Burned-out cirrhosis, with little necroinflammatory activity, that has been preceded, presumably, by years of subclinical disease

An acute appearance of clinical illness is common (40%) and a fulminant presentation with hepatic encephalopathy within 8 weeks of disease onset may also occur. The mortality of patients with severe untreated autoimmune hepatitis is approximately 40% within 6 months of diagnosis and cirrhosis develops in at least 40% of survivors. In general, prognosis is better in adults than in children, possibly due to delay in diagnosis in the pediatric population. Hence, diagnosis and intervention are imperative. Immunosuppressive therapy is usually successful, leading to remissions in 80% of patients that permits long term survival. In end stage disease, liver transplantation is indicated. Ten-year survival rate after liver transplant is 75%, but recurrence in the transplanted organ may affect 20% of transplanted patients.

In a small subset of patients, there may be overlap with other autoimmune liver diseases, in particular primary biliary cirrhosis or, less commonly, primary sclerosing cholangitis. *Diagnosis of "overlap" syndromes requires full display of both clinical and histologic features of autoimmune hepatitis and the other, concomitant disease.*

KEY CONCEPTS

Autoimmune Hepatitis

- There are two primary types of autoimmune hepatitis:
  - Type 1 autoimmune hepatitis is most often seen in middle-aged women and is most characteristically associated with antinuclear and anti–smooth muscle antibodies (ANA and ASMA)
  - Type 2 autoimmune hepatitis is most often seen in children or teenagers and is associated with anti-liver kidney microsomal autoantibodies (anti-LKM1)
- Autoimmune hepatitis may either develop with a rapidly progressive acute disease or follow a more indolent path; if untreated, both are likely to lead to liver failure.
- Plasma cells are a prominent and characteristic component of the inflammatory infiltrate in biopsy specimens showing autoimmune hepatitis.

Drug- and Toxin-Induced Liver Injury

As the major drug metabolizing and detoxifying organ in the body, the liver is subject to injury from an enormous array of therapeutic and environmental agents. Injury may result from direct toxicity, occur through hepatic conversion of a xenobiotic to an active toxin, or be produced by immune mechanisms, such as by the drug or a metabolite acting as a hapten to convert a cellular protein into an immunogen. A diagnosis of drug- or toxin-induced liver injury may be made on the basis of a temporal

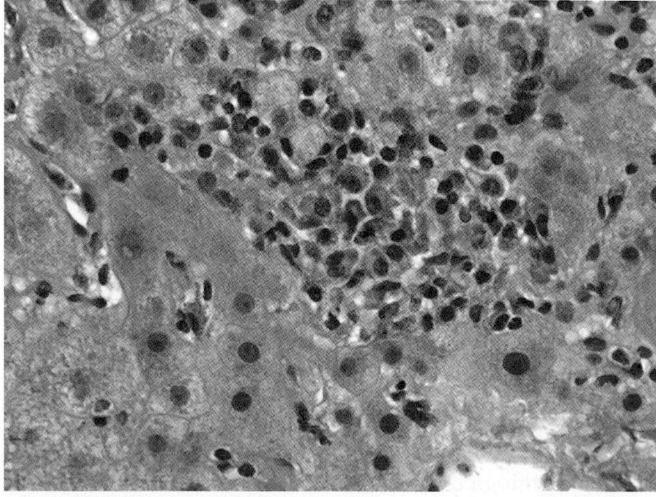

Figure 18-17 Autoimmune hepatitis. A focus of lobular hepatitis with prominent plasma cells typical for this disease.

Table 18-5 Patterns of Drug- and Toxin-Induced Hepatic Injury

Pattern of Injury	Morphologic Findings	Examples of Associated Agents
Cholestatic	Bland hepatocellular cholestasis, without inflammation	Contraceptive and anabolic steroids, antibiotics, HAART
Cholestatic hepatitis	Cholestasis with lobular necroinflammatory activity; may show bile duct destruction	Antibiotics, phenothiazines, statins
Hepatocellular necrosis	Spotty hepatocyte necrosis	Methyldopa, phenytoin
	Massive necrosis	Acetaminophen, halothane
	Chronic hepatitis	Isoniazid
Fatty liver disease	Large and small droplet fat	Ethanol, corticosteroids, methotrexate, total parenteral nutrition
	"Microvesicular steatosis" (diffuse small droplet fat)	Valproate, tetracycline, aspirin (Reye syndrome), HAART
	Steatohepatitis with Mallory-Denk bodies	Ethanol, amiodarone
Fibrosis and cirrhosis	Periportal and pericellular fibrosis	Alcohol, methotrexate, enalapril, vitamin A and other retinoids
Granulomas	Noncaseating epithelioid granulomas	Sulfonamides, amiodarone, isoniazid
	Fibrin ring granulomas	Allopurinol
Vascular lesions	Sinusoidal obstruction syndrome (veno-occlusive disease): obliteration of central veins	High-dose chemotherapy, bush teas
	Budd-Chiari syndrome	Oral contraceptives
	Peliosis hepatis: blood-filled cavities, not lined by endothelial cells	Anabolic steroids, tamoxifen
Neoplasms	Hepatocellular adenoma	Oral contraceptives, anabolic steroids
	Hepatocellular carcinoma	Alcohol, thorotrast
	Cholangiocarcinoma	Thorotrast
	Angiosarcoma	Thorotrast, vinyl chloride

HAART, highly active anti-retroviral therapy. Adapted from Washington K: Metabolic and toxic conditions of the liver. In Iacobuzio-Donahue CA, Montgomery EA (eds): Gastrointestinal and Liver Pathology. Philadelphia, Churchill Livingstone; 2005.

association of liver damage with drug or toxin exposure, recovery (usually) upon removal of the inciting agent, and exclusion of other potential causes. *Exposure to a toxin or therapeutic agent should always be included in the differential diagnosis of any form of liver disease.*

Drug-induced liver injury has a global incidence of 1 to 14 per 100,000. Reactions may be mild to very serious, including acute liver failure or chronic liver disease. A large number of drugs and chemicals can produce liver injury (Table 18-5). Alcohol produces more toxic liver injury than any other agent; it is discussed separately later in this chapter. It is also important to keep in mind that not only compounds normally thought of as drugs or medicines may be implicated, but that careful, detailed history taking may identify other potential toxins such as herbal remedies, dietary supplements, topical applications (e.g., ointments, perfumes, shampoo), and environmental exposures (e.g., cleaning solvents, pesticides, fertilizers).

Principles of drug and toxic injury are discussed in Chapter 9. Drug toxic reactions may be classified as *predictable* (intrinsic) or *unpredictable* (idiosyncratic). Predictable reactions affect all people in a dose-dependent fashion. Unpredictable reactions depend on idiosyncrasies of the host, particularly the propensity to mount an immune response to the antigenic stimulus or the rate at which the agent can be metabolized. Both classes of injury may be immediate or take weeks to months to develop.

A classic, predictable hepatotoxin is acetaminophen, now the most common cause of acute liver failure necessitating transplantation in the United States. The toxic agent is not acetaminophen itself but rather a toxic metabolite produced by the cytochrome P-450 system in acinus zone 3 hepatocytes (Fig. 18-1). As these hepatocytes die, the zone 2 hepatocytes take over this metabolic function, in turn becoming injured. In severe overdoses, the zone of injury extends to the periportal hepatocytes, resulting in acute hepatic failure (Fig. 18-6). While suicide attempts with acetaminophen are common, so are accidental overdoses. This is because the cytotoxicity is dependent on the cytochrome P-450 system, which may be upregulated by other agents taken in combination with acetaminophen, such as alcohol (beware acetaminophen as a hangover prophylactic) or codeine in acetaminophen compound tablets.

Examples of drugs that can cause idiosyncratic reactions include *chlorpromazine,* an agent that causes cholestasis in patients who are slow to metabolize it to an innocuous byproduct, and *halothane,* which can cause a fatal immune-mediated hepatitis in some patients exposed to this anesthetic on multiple occasions. Often, idiosyncratic drug reactions involve a variable combination of direct cytotoxicity and immune-mediated hepatocyte or bile duct destruction. Table 18-5 lists the more common drugs and toxins that cause liver injury according to the type of morphologic changes produced. As will be evident from the table, a single agent can produce more than one pattern of injury.

KEY CONCEPTS

Drug- or Toxin-Induced Liver Injury

- Most drugs or toxins affecting the liver may be classified as:
  - Predictable hepatotoxins, acting in a dose-dependent manner and occurring in most individuals.
  - Unpredictable or idiosyncratic hepatotoxins, which happen in rare individuals and which are often independent of dose
- Hepatotoxins may cause harm from direct cell toxicity, through hepatic conversion of a xenobiotic to an active toxin, or by immune mechanisms, such as by the drug or a metabolite acting as a hapten to convert a cellular protein into an immunogen.
- The most common hepatotoxin causing acute liver failure is acetaminophen.
- The most common hepatotoxin causing chronic liver disease is alcohol.

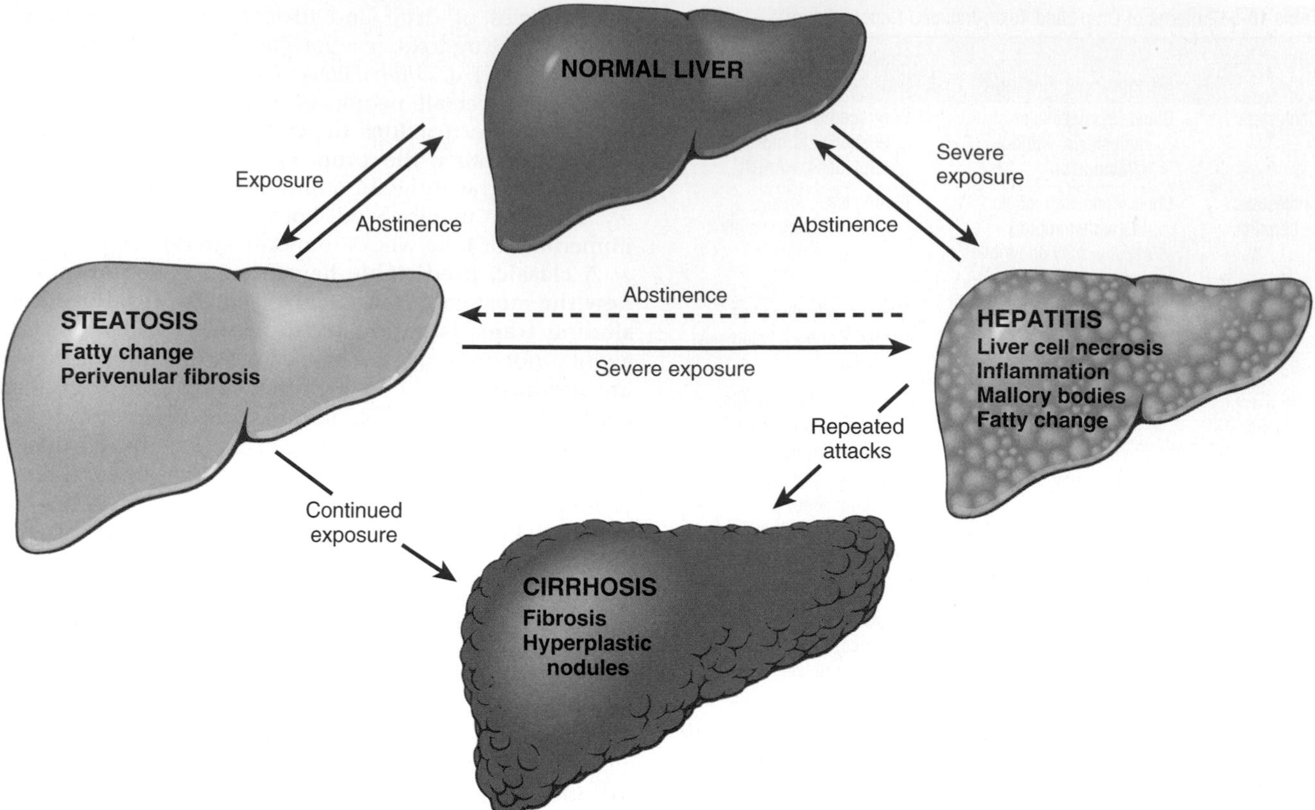

Figure 18-18 Alcoholic liver disease. The interrelationships among hepatic steatosis, alcoholic hepatitis, and alcoholic cirrhosis are shown, along with depictions of key morphologic features. It should be noted that steatosis, alcoholic hepatitis, and steatofibrosis may also develop independently. In particular some patients present initially with cirrhosis without any of the other forms of alcoholic liver disease.

Alcoholic Liver Disease

Excessive alcohol (ethanol) consumption is the leading cause of liver disease in most Western countries. Alcohol accounts for 3.8% of deaths globally, making it the eighth highest risk factor for death (fifth in middle-income countries and ninth in high-income countries). There are three distinctive, albeit overlapping forms of alcoholic liver injury: (1) hepatocellular steatosis or fatty change, (2) alcoholic (or steato-) hepatitis, and (3) steatofibrosis (patterns of scarring typical for all fatty liver diseases including alcohol) up to and including cirrhosis in the late stages of disease (Fig. 18-18). For some unknown reason, cirrhosis develops in only a small fraction of chronic alcoholics. The morphology of the three interrelated forms of alcoholic liver disease is presented first, to facilitate the later discussion of their pathogenesis.

MORPHOLOGY

All changes in alcoholic liver disease begin in acinus zone 3 and extend outward toward the portal tracts with increasing severity of injury.

Hepatic Steatosis (Fatty Liver). After even moderate intake of alcohol, lipid droplets accumulate in hepatocytes increasing with amount and chronicity of alcohol intake. The lipid begins as small droplets that coalesce into large droplets which distend the hepatocyte and push the nucleus aside (Fig. 18-19). Macroscopically, the fatty liver in individuals with chronic alcoholism is a large (as heavy as 4 to 6 kg), soft organ that is yellow and greasy. **Fatty change is completely reversible if there is abstention from further intake of alcohol.**

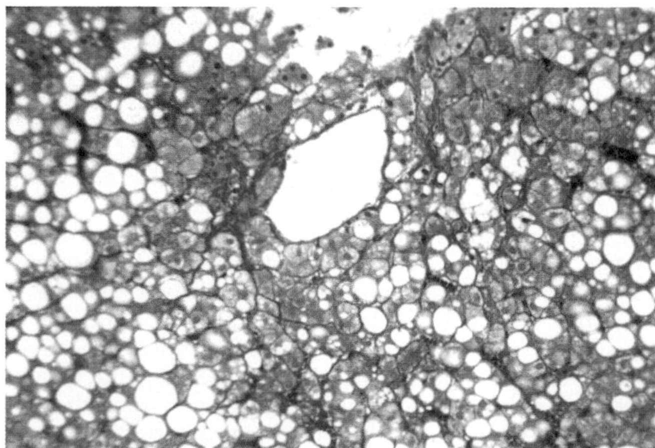

Figure 18-19 Alcoholic steatosis and steatofibrosis. A mix of small and large fat droplets (seen as clear vacuoles) is most prominent around the central vein and extends outward to the portal tracts. Some fibrosis (stained blue) is present in a characteristic perisinusoidal chicken wire fence pattern. (Masson trichrome stain). (Courtesy Dr. Elizabeth Brunt, Washington University, St. Louis, Mo.)

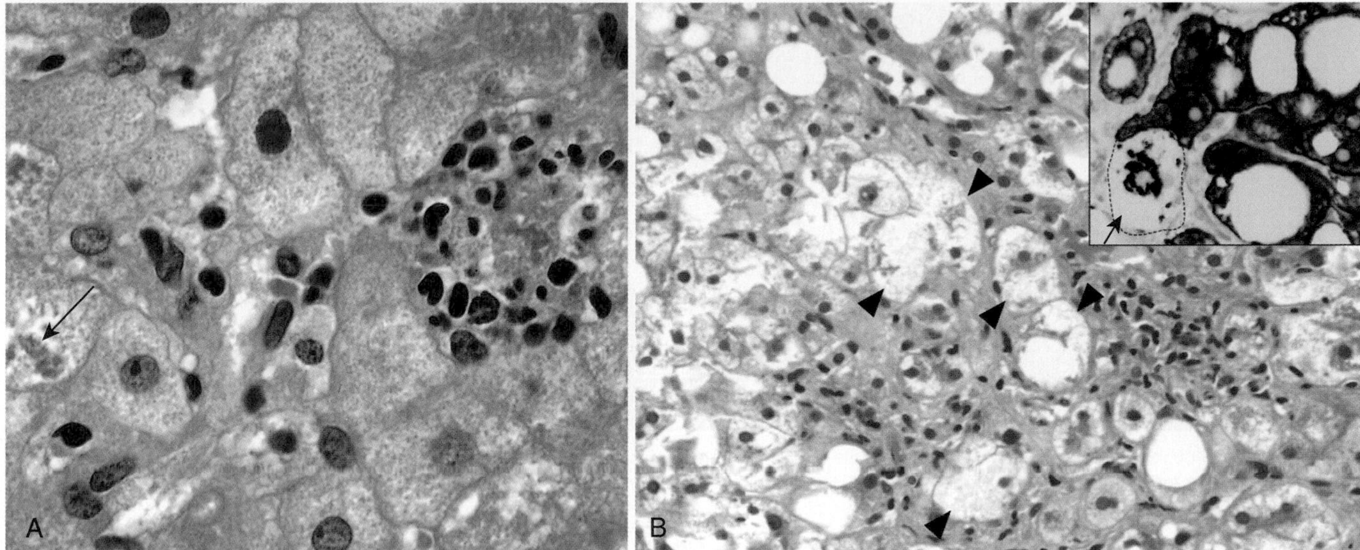

Figure 18-20 **A,** Alcoholic hepatitis with clustered inflammatory cells marking the site of a necrotic hepatocyte. A Mallory Denk body is present in another hepatocyte (arrow). **B,** Alcoholic steatohepatitis with many ballooned hepatocytes (arrowheads). Clusters of inflammatory cells are also present; inset shows immunostaining for keratins 8 and 18 (brown), with most hepatocytes, including those with fat vacuoles, showing normal cytoplasmic staining, but in the ballooned cell (arrow) the ubiquinated keratins are collapsed into the Mallory-Denk body, leaving the cytoplasm "empty." (Courtesy Dr. Elizabeth Brunt, Washington University, St. Louis, Mo.)

Alcoholic (Steato-) Hepatitis. Alcoholic hepatitis is characterized by:

1. Hepatocyte swelling and necrosis: Single or scattered foci of cells undergo swelling (ballooning) and necrosis (Fig. 18-20). The swelling results from the accumulation of fat and water, as well as proteins that are normally exported.

2. Mallory-Denk bodies: These are usually present as clumped, amorphous, eosinophilic material in ballooned hepatocytes. They are made up of tangled skeins of intermediate filaments such as keratins 8 and 18 in complex with other proteins such as ubiquitin (Fig. 18-20*B*). These inclusions are a characteristic but not specific feature of alcoholic liver disease, since they are also present in non-alcoholic fatty liver disease and in periportal distributions in Wilson disease and in chronic biliary tract diseases.

3. Neutrophilic reaction: Neutrophils permeate the hepatic lobule and accumulate around degenerating hepatocytes, particularly those having Mallory-Denk bodies. They may be more or less admixed with mononuclear cells (Fig. 18-20*B*).

Alcoholic steatofibrosis. Alcoholic hepatitis is often accompanied by prominent activation of sinusoidal stellate cells and portal fibroblasts, giving rise to fibrosis. Fibrosis begins with sclerosis of central veins. Perisinusoidal scar then accumulates in the space of Disse of the centrilobular region, spreading outward, encircling individual or small clusters of hepatocytes in a **chicken wire fence pattern** (Fig. 18-19). These webs of scar eventually link to portal tracts and then begin to condense into central-portal fibrous septa. With developing nodularity, cirrhosis becomes established. When alcohol use continues without interruption over the long term, the continual subdivision of established nodules by new webs of, perisinusoidal scarring leads to a classic micronodular or **Laennec cirrhosis** first described for end-stage alcoholic liver disease (Fig. 18-21). Early stages of scarring can regress with cessation of alcohol use, but the farther along toward cirrhosis the liver gets, the more vascular derangements prevent a full restoration of normal. Complete regression of alcoholic cirrhosis, while reported, is rare (Fig. 18-8).

Pathogenesis. Short-term ingestion of as much as 80 gm of alcohol (six beers or 8 ounces of 80-proof liquor) over one to several days generally produces mild, reversible hepatic steatosis. Daily intake of 80 gm or more of ethanol generates significant risk for severe hepatic injury, and daily ingestion of 160 gm or more for 10 to 20 years is associated more consistently with severe injury. *Only 10% to 15% of alcoholics, however, develop cirrhosis.* Thus, other factors must also influence the development and severity of alcoholic liver disease. These include:

- *Gender.* Women seem to be more susceptible to hepatic injury than men, although the majority of patients are men. This difference may be related to alcohol pharmacokinetics and metabolism, and the estrogen-dependent response to gut-derived endotoxin (LPS) in the liver. Although exact mechanisms are not known, it appears that estrogen increases gut permeability to endotoxins, which, in turn, increase the expression of the LPS receptor CD14 in Kupffer cells. This predisposes to increased production of proinflammatory cytokines and chemokines.
- *Ethnic and genetic differences.* In the United States, cirrhosis rates are higher for African American drinkers than for white Americans drinker. The difference cannot be explained by the amount of alcohol consumption, since there is no significant difference in consumption among the ethnic groups. Studies with twins suggest that there is a genetic component in alcohol-induced liver disease, although it remains difficult to separate genetic from environmental influences. Genetic polymorphisms in detoxifying enzymes and some cytokine promoters may play significant roles and contribute to ethnic differences. ALDH*2, a variant of aldehyde-dehydrogenase (ALDH), found in 50% of Asians, has a very low activity. Individuals homozygous for ALDH*2 are unable to oxidize acetaldehyde and do not tolerate alcohol, leading to alcohol intolerance characterized by upper body flushing and, variably, nausea or lethargy.

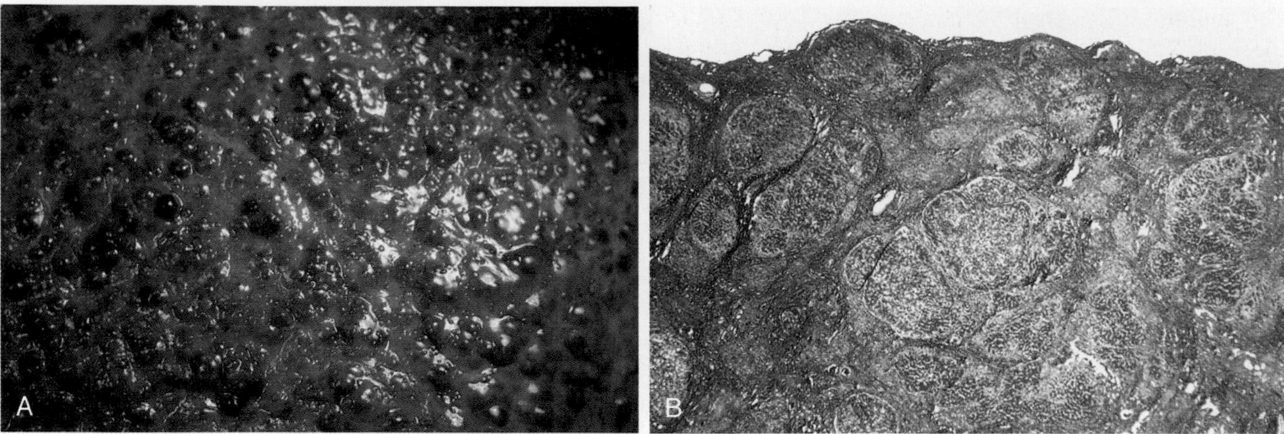

Figure 18-21 Alcoholic cirrhosis. **A,** The characteristic diffuse nodularity of the surface is induced by the underlying fibrous scarring. The average nodule size is 3 mm in this close-up view, typical of the "micronodular" cirrhosis of alcoholic liver disease. The greenish tint is caused by cholestasis. **B,** Microscopically, this cirrhosis is marked by small nodules entrapped in blue-staining fibrous tissue; fatty accumulation is no longer seen in this "burned out" stage. (Masson trichrome stain.)

- *Comorbid conditions.* Iron overload and infections with HCV and HBV synergize with alcohol, leading to increased severity of liver disease.

The pharmacokinetics and metabolism of alcohol are described in Chapter 9. Pertinent to this discussion are the detrimental effects of alcohol and its byproducts on hepatocellular function. *Exposure to alcohol causes steatosis, dysfunction of mitochondrial and cellular membranes, hypoxia, and oxidative stress.* At millimolar concentrations, alcohol directly affects microtubular and mitochondrial function and membrane fluidity.

Hepatocellular steatosis results from (1) shunting of normal substrates away from catabolism and toward lipid biosynthesis, as a result of increased generation of reduced nicotinamide adenine dinucleotide (NADH) by the two major enzymes of alcohol metabolism, alcohol dehydrogenase and acetaldehyde dehydrogenase; (2) impaired assembly and secretion of lipoproteins; and (3) increased peripheral catabolism of fat, thus releasing free fatty acids into the circulation.

The causes of alcoholic hepatitis are uncertain, but some of the factors that likely play important roles are discussed next. *Acetaldehyde* (the major intermediate metabolite of alcohol) induces lipid peroxidation and acetaldehyde-protein adduct formation, further disrupting cytoskeletal and membrane function. Cytochrome P-450 metabolism produces *reactive oxygen species* (ROS) that react with cellular proteins, damage membranes, and alter hepatocellular function. In addition, alcohol impairs hepatic metabolism of methionine, which *decreases glutathione levels,* thereby sensitizing the liver to oxidative injury. The induction of cytochrome P-450 enzymes in the liver by alcohol increases alcohol catabolism in the endoplasmic reticulum and enhances the conversion of other drugs (e.g., acetaminophen) to toxic metabolites. Alcohol causes the *release of bacterial endotoxin* from the gut into the portal circulation, inducing inflammatory responses in the liver, due to the activation of NF-κB, and release of TNF, IL-6, and TGF-α. In addition, alcohol stimulates the release of endothelins from sinusoidal endothelial cells, causing vasoconstriction and *contraction of activated, myofibroblastic stellate cells,* leading to a decrease in hepatic sinusoidal perfusion (already discussed under "Portal Hypertension").

Alcoholic liver disease, thus, is a chronic disorder featuring steatosis, hepatitis, progressive fibrosis, and marked derangement of vascular perfusion. In essence, alcoholic liver disease can be a regarded as a maladaptive state in which cells in the liver respond in an increasingly pathologic manner to a stimulus (alcohol) that originally was only marginally harmful.

Clinical Features. Hepatic steatosis may cause hepatomegaly, with mild elevation of serum bilirubin and alkaline phosphatase levels. Severe hepatic dysfunction is unusual. Alcohol withdrawal and the provision of an adequate diet are sufficient treatment. In contrast, alcoholic hepatitis tends to appear acutely, usually following a bout of heavy drinking. Symptoms and laboratory manifestations may range from minimal to those that mimic acute liver failure. Between these two extremes are the nonspecific symptoms of malaise, anorexia, weight loss, upper abdominal discomfort, and tender hepatomegaly, and the laboratory findings of hyperbilirubinemia, elevated serum aminotransferases and alkaline phosphatase, and often a neutrophilic leukocytosis. In contrast to other chronic liver diseases where serum ALT tends to be higher than serum AST, serum AST levels tend to be higher than serum ALT levels in a 2:1 ratio or higher in alcoholic liver disease. This can be helpful in differential diagnosis of chronic liver injury when adequate history is not available. An acute cholestatic syndrome may appear, resembling large bile duct obstruction.

The outlook is unpredictable; each bout of hepatitis incurs about a 10% to 20% risk of death. With repeated bouts, cirrhosis develops in about one third of patients within a few years. Alcoholic hepatitis also may be superimposed on established cirrhosis. With proper nutrition and total cessation of alcohol consumption, the alcoholic hepatitis may clear slowly. However, in some patients, the hepatitis persists, despite abstinence, and progresses to cirrhosis.

The manifestations of alcoholic cirrhosis are similar to those of other forms of cirrhosis. Laboratory findings reflect hepatic dysfunction, with elevated serum aminotransferases, hyperbilirubinemia, variable elevation of serum alkaline phosphatase, hypoproteinemia (globulins, albumin, and clotting factors), and anemia. In some instances, liver biopsy may be indicated, since in about 10% to 20% of cases of presumed alcoholic cirrhosis, another disease process is found. Finally, cirrhosis may be clinically silent, discovered only at autopsy or when stress such as infection or trauma tips the balance toward hepatic insufficiency.

The long-term outlook for alcoholics with liver disease is variable. Five-year survival approaches 90% in abstainers who are free of jaundice, ascites, or hematemesis; it drops to 50% to 60% in those who continue to imbibe. In the end-stage alcoholic the proximate causes of death are (1) hepatic coma, (2) massive gastrointestinal hemorrhage, (3) intercurrent infection (to which these patients are predisposed), (4) hepatorenal syndrome following a bout of alcoholic hepatitis, and (5) hepatocellular carcinoma (the risk of developing this tumor in alcoholic cirrhosis is 1% to 6% of cases annually).

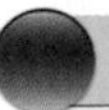

KEY CONCEPTS

Alcoholic Liver Disease

- Alcoholic liver disease is a chronic disorder that can give rise to steatosis, alcoholic hepatitis, progressive steatofibrosis and marked derangement of vascular perfusion leading eventually to cirrhosis.
- Consumption of 80 gm/day of alcohol is considered to be the threshold for the development of alcoholic liver disease.
- It may take 10 to 15 years of drinking for the development of cirrhosis, which occurs only in a small proportion of chronic alcoholics.
- The multiple pathologic effects of alcohol include changes in lipid metabolism, decreased export of lipoproteins, and cell injury caused by reactive oxygen species and cytokines.

Metabolic Liver Disease

A distinct group of liver diseases is attributable to disorders of metabolism, either acquired or inherited. The most common acquired metabolic disorder is non-alcoholic fatty liver disease. Among inherited metabolic diseases, hemochromatosis, Wilson disease, and α_1-antitrypsin deficiency are most prominent. Also included among liver metabolic diseases is neonatal hepatitis, a broad disease category encompassing rare inherited diseases and neonatal infections.

Nonalcoholic Fatty Liver Disease (NAFLD)

NAFLD represents a spectrum of disorders that have in common the presence of hepatic steatosis (fatty liver) in individuals who do not consume alcohol or do so in very small quantities (less than 20 g of ethanol/week). NAFLD has become the most common cause of chronic liver disease in the United States and in its various forms probably affects 3 to 5% of the population. However, these estimates are approximate, because fatty liver without other complications may not be detected clinically. The term "nonalcoholic steatohepatitis" (or its common acronym *NASH*) is often used to denote overt clinical features of liver injury, such as elevated serum transaminases, but the designation NAFLD is preferred, with *steatohepatitis* reserved for histologic features of hepatocyte injury already described in the section on alcoholic liver disease.

Table 18-6 World Health Organization Criteria for the Metabolic Syndrome

One of	Diabetes mellitus *or* impaired glucose tolerance *or* impaired fasting glucose *or* insulin resistance
and two of:	Blood pressure: ≥ 140/90 mm Hg Dyslipidemia: triglycerides (TG): ≥ 1.695 mmol/L and high-density lipoprotein cholesterol (HDL-C) ≤ 0.9 mmol/L (male), ≤ 1 mmol/L (female) Central obesity: waist-hip ratio > 0.90 (male); > 0.85 (female), or body mass index > 30 kg/m^2 Microalbuminuria: urinary albumin excretion rate of ≥ 20 μg/min or albumin-to-creatinine ratio ≥ 30 mg/gm

The histologic hallmarks of NAFLD are most consistently associated with the *metabolic syndrome* (Table 18-6). The epidemic of obesity in the United States and, and its overall, dramatic global increase, has resulted in increasing rates of NAFLD. Prevalence in children has also registered a steady rise. NAFLD contributes to the progression of other liver diseases such as HCV and HBV infection. Increasingly, NAFLD is found to increase the risk for hepatocellular carcinoma, although, unlike in chronic viral hepatitis and alcoholic liver disease, it may often do so in the absence of significant scarring.

The prevalence of NAFLD varies among ethnic groups and probably relates, at least in part, to genetic differences. For example, in the United States, Hispanics have the highest prevalence of NAFLD/NASH, followed by African Americans and Caucasians.

Pathogenesis. Currently available data suggests a two hit model for NAFLD.

- Insulin resistance gives rise to hepatic steatosis.
- Hepatocellular oxidative injury resulting in liver cell necrosis and the inflammatory reactions to it.

The interplay of these two factors is discussed below.

Hepatic steatosis, like obesity in general, arises from an overabundance of calorie rich food, diminished exercise, and genetic/epigenetic mechanisms. Data indicate that individuals with NAFLD eat more fast food and exercise less. High fructose corn syrup, a nearly ubiquitous, inexpensive sweetener in manufactured foods, also appears to promote insulin resistance.

In individuals with established insulin resistance and metabolic syndrome, the visceral adipose tissue not only increases, but also becomes dysfunctional, with reduced production of the lipid hormone,adiponectin, and increased production of inflammatory cytokines such as TNF-α and IL-6. These changes in turn promote hepatocyte apoptosis. Fat laden cells are highly sensitive to lipid peroxidation products generated by oxidative stress which can damage mitochondrial and plasma membranes, causing apoptosis.

Diminished autophagy also contributes to mitochondrial injury and formation of Mallory-Denk bodies. Kupffer cell production of TNF-α and TGF-β activate stellate cells directly leading to deposition of scar tissue (Fig. 18-5). Stellate cell activation also occurs through the hedgehog signaling pathway in part through natural killer T-cell activation. In fact, the level of hedgehog pathway activity correlates with stage of fibrosis in NAFLD.

MORPHOLOGY

Pathologic steatosis is defined as involving more than 5% of hepatocytes. Small, medium, and large droplets of fat, predominantly triglycerides, accumulate within hepatocytes just as they do in alcoholic steatosis. At the most clinically benign end of the spectrum, there is no appreciable hepatic inflammation, hepatocyte death, or scarring, despite persistent elevation of serum liver enzymes. **NASH almost completely overlaps in its histologic features with alcoholic hepatitis** (Fig. 18-22). In NASH, compared with alcoholic hepatitis, mononuclear cells may be more prominent than neutrophis and Mallory-Denk bodies are often less prominent. Steatofibrosis in NAFLD shows precisely the same features and progression as it does in alcoholic liver disease, although portal fibrosis may be more prominent. Cirrhosis may develop, is often subclinical for years, and, when established, the steatosis or steatohepatitis may be reduced or absent. **Greater than 90% of previously described "cryptogenic cirrhosis" (i.e., cirrhosis of unknown cause) is now thought to represent such "burned out" NAFLD.**

Pediatric NAFLD differs significantly from that seen in adults. Typically children show more diffuse steatosis, portal rather than central fibrosis, and portal and parenchymal mononuclear infiltration, rather than parenchymal neutrophils.

Clinical Features. Clinical course of individuals with NAFLD/NASH are summarized in Figure 18-23. Individuals with simple steatosis are generally asymptomatic. Clinical presentation is often related to other signs and symptoms of the metabolic syndrome, in particular insulin resistance or diabetes mellitus. Imaging studies may reveal fat accumulation in the liver. However, liver biopsy is the most reliable diagnostic tool for NAFLD and NASH, and for assessment of scarring. Viral, autoimmune and other metabolic diseases of the liver must be excluded before the diagnosis can be made. Serum AST and ALT are elevated in about 90% of patients with NASH. Despite the enzyme elevations, patients may be asymptomatic. Others have general symptoms such as fatigue or right-sided abdominal discomfort caused by hepatomegaly. Because of the association between NASH and the metabolic syndrome, cardiovascular disease is a frequent cause of death in patients with NASH. The goal of treating individuals with NASH is to reverse the steatosis and prevent cirrhosis by correcting the underlying risk factors, such as obesity and hyperlipidemia, and to treat insulin resistance. NASH also increases the risk of hepatocellular carcinoma as do other metabolic diseases (discussed later).

KEY CONCEPTS

Nonalcoholic Fatty Liver Disease

- The most common metabolic disorder is nonalcoholic fatty liver disease, which is associated with the metabolic syndrome, obesity, type 2 diabetes mellitus or other impairments of insulin responsiveness, dyslipidemia, and hypertension.
- Nonalcoholic fatty liver disease may show all the changes associated with alcoholic liver disease: steatosis, steatohepatitis, and steatofibrosis, even though the features of steatohepatitis (e.g., hepatocyte ballooning, Mallory-Denk bodies, and neutrophilic infiltration) are often less prominent than they are in alcohol-related injury.

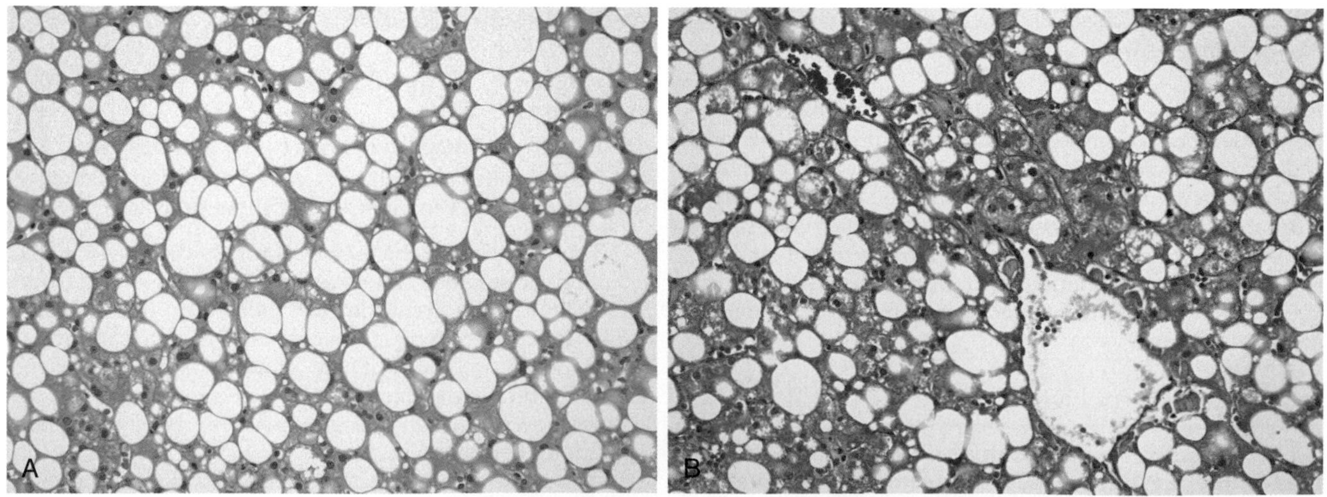

Figure 18-22 Nonalcoholic fatty liver disease. **A,** Liver with mixed small and large fat droplets. **B,** Steatosis and steatofibrosis extending along sinusoids in a chicken wire fence pattern in which individual and clustered hepatocytes are surrounded by thin scars (blue fibers). Note the resemblance to alcoholic steatohepatitis depicted in Fig. 18-19. (Masson trichrome stain.)

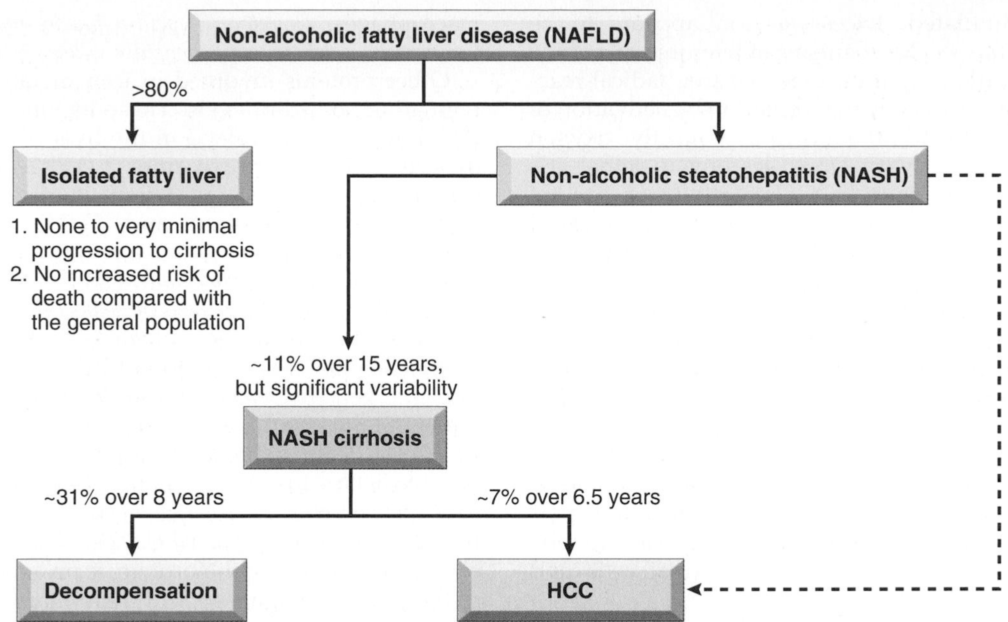

Figure 18-23 Natural history of NAFLD phenotypes. Isolated fatty liver, shows minimal risk for progression to cirrhosis or increased mortality, while non-alcoholic steatohepatitis shows increased overall mortality as well as increased risk for cirrhosis and hepatocellular carcinoma (HCC). DM, Diabetes mellitus.

- Pediatric NAFLD is being increasingly recognized as the obesity epidemic spreads to pediatric age groups, although its histologic features differ somewhat from that seen in adults.

Hemochromatosis

Hemochromatosis is caused by excessive iron absorption, most of which is deposited in parenchymal organs such as the liver and pancreas, followed by heart, joints, and endocrine organs. When hemochromatosis results from an inherited disorder, it is referred to as *hereditary hemochromatosis,* of which there are many forms, some more likely than others to lead to overwhelming iron overload. When accumulation occurs as a consequence of parenteral administration of iron, usually in the form of transfusions, or other causes (Table 18-7), it is called as *secondary hemochromatosis.*

As discussed in Chapter 14, the total body iron pool ranges from 2 to 6 gm in normal adults; about 0.5 gm is stored in the liver, 98% of which is in hepatocytes. In the most severe forms of hemochromatosis, total iron accumulation may exceed 50 gm, more than one third of which accumulates in the liver. The following features characterize severe iron overload in the body:

- Fully developed cases exhibit (1) micronodular cirrhosis in all patients; (2) diabetes mellitus in 75% to 80% of patients; and (3) abnormal skin pigmentation in 75% to 80% of patients.
- Iron accumulation in hereditary forms is lifelong but the injury caused by excessive iron is slow and progressive; hence *symptoms usually first appear in the fourth to fifth decades of life in men and later in women since menstrual bleeding counterbalances the accumulation until menopause.*
- Because many women do not accumulate clinically relevant amounts of iron within their lifetime, hereditary hemochromatosis affects more males than females (ratio of 5 to 7:1).

Pathogenesis. Because there is no regulated iron excretion from the body, the total body content of iron is tightly regulated by intestinal absorption. *In hereditary hemochromatosis, regulation of intestinal absorption of dietary iron is abnormal, leading to net iron accumulation of 0.5 to 1 gm/year.* The disease manifests itself typically after 20 gm of stored

Table 18-7 Classification of Iron Overload

I. Hereditary hemochromatosis
Mutations of genes encoding HFE, transferrin receptor 2 (TfR2), or hepcidin
Mutations of genes encoding HJV (hemojuvelin: juvenile hemochromatosis)
(Neonatal hemochromatosis)*
II. Hemosiderosis (secondary hemochromatosis)
A. Parenteral iron overload
Transfusions
Long-term hemodialysis
Aplastic anemia
Sickle cell disease
Myelodysplastic syndromes
Leukemias
Iron-dextran injections
B. Ineffective erythropoiesis with increased erythroid activity
β-Thalassemia
Sideroblastic anemia
Pyruvate kinase deficiency
C. Increased oral intake of iron
African iron overload (Bantu siderosis)
D. Congenital atransferrinemia
E. Chronic liver disease
Alcoholic liver disease
Porphyria cutanea tarda
F. Neonatal hemochromatosis

*Neonatal hemochromatosis develops in utero and does not appear to be a hereditary condition.

iron have accumulated. Excessive iron appears to be directly toxic to tissues. Mechanisms of liver injury include (1) lipid peroxidation via iron-catalyzed free radical reactions, (2) stimulation of collagen formation by activation of hepatic stellate cells, and (3) interaction of reactive oxygen species and iron itself with DNA, leading to lethal cell injury and predisposition to HCC. The actions of iron are reversible in cells that are not fatally injured, and removal of excess iron with therapy promotes recovery of tissue function.

The main regulator of iron absorption is the protein hepcidin, encoded by the *HAMP* gene and secreted by the liver (Fig. 18-24). Hepcidin is named for its originally elucidated properties as a *hep*atocellular protein with bacbactericidal activities. Transcription of hepcidin is increased by inflammatory cytokines and iron, and decreased by iron deficiency, hypoxia, and ineffective erythropoiesis. Hepcidin binds to the cellular iron efflux channel ferroportin, causing its internalization and proteolysis, thereby inhibiting the release of iron from intestinal cells and macrophages. *Therefore, hepcidin lowers plasma iron levels. Conversely, a deficiency in hepcidin causes iron overload.*

Other proteins involved in iron metabolism, do so by regulating hepcidin levels. These include (1) hemojuvelin (HJV), which is expressed in the liver, heart, and skeletal muscle, (2) transferrin receptor 2 (TFR2), which is highly expressed in hepatocytes, where it mediates the uptake of transferrin-bound iron, and (3) HFE, the product of the hemochromatosis gene. *Decreased hepcidin synthesis caused by mutations in hepcidin, HJV, TFR2, and HFE has a central role in the pathogenesis of hemochromatosis.*

The adult form of hemochromatosis is almost always caused by mutations of HFE; mutation of *TFR2* is far less common. The *HFE* gene is located on the short arm of chromosome 6 at 6p21.3, close to the *HLA* gene locus; it encodes an HLA class I-like molecule that governs intestinal absorption of dietary iron by regulating hepcidin synthesis. *The most common HFE mutation is a cysteine-to-tyrosine substitution at amino acid 282 (called C282Y).* This mutation, which causes inactivation of the protein, is present in 70% to 100% of the patients diagnosed with hereditary hemochromatosis. *The other common mutation is H63D (histidine at position 63 to aspartate).* The H63D homozygous state and C282Y/H63D compound heterozygous mutations often cause only mild iron accumulation.

The C282Y mutation of the HFE gene is largely confined to white populations of European origin, while the H63D has a worldwide distribution. The frequency of C282Y homozygosity is 0.45% (1 of every 220 persons), and the heterozygous frequency is 11%, making hereditary hemochromatosis one of the most common genetic disorders in humans. However, the penetrance of this disorder is low in patients with the homozygous C282Y mutation, so the genetic change does not lead to clinical disease in all individuals.

Adult hemochromatosis is generally a milder disease than the juvenile form. Mutations of HAMP and HJV cause severe juvenile hemochromatosis.

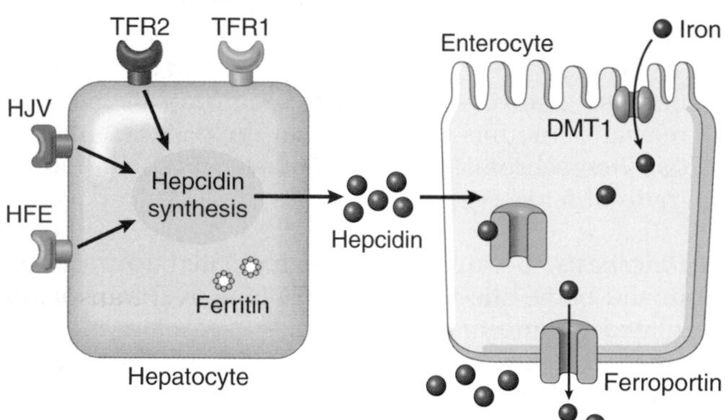

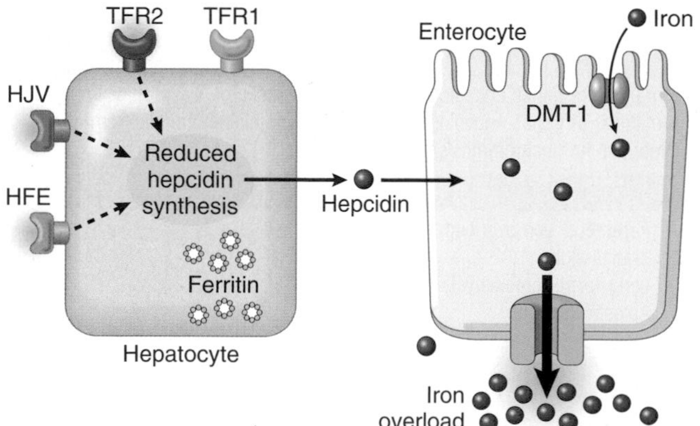

Figure 18-24 A: In normal state HFE, HJV, and TFR2 regulate hepcidin synthesis by hepatocytes maintaining normal circulating hepcidin levels. Hepcidin binds to ferroportin on enterocytes leading to internalization of the complex and ferroportin degradation.This in turn reduces efflux of iron from enterocytes Through these regulatory interactions normal iron absorption is maintained. **B:** In hereditary hemochromatosis HFE or HJV or TFR2 gene mutations reduce hepcidin synthesis thus diminishing circulating hepcidin. The resulting decreased hepcidin-ferroportin interaction allows for increased ferroportin activity, increased iron efflux from enterocytes, giving rise to systemic iron overload in hereditary hemochromatosis. HFE, HFE protein; HJV, hemojuvelin, TFR1, transferrin receptor 1; TFR2: transferrin receptor 2; DMT1: divalent metal transporter 1.

MORPHOLOGY

Severe hemochromatosis (hereditary or secondary) is characterized principally by (1) **deposition of hemosiderin** in the following organs (in decreasing order of severity) the liver, pancreas, myocardium, pituitary gland, adrenal gland, thyroid and parathyroid glands, joints, and skin; (2) cirrhosis; and (3) pancreatic fibrosis. In the **liver,** iron becomes evident first as golden-yellow hemosiderin granules in the cytoplasm of periportal hepatocytes that stain with Prussian blue (Fig. 18-25). With increasing iron load, there is progressive involvement of the rest of the lobule, along with bile duct epithelium and Kupffer cell pigmentation. Iron is a direct hepatotoxin and inflammation is characteristically absent. In early stages of accumulation, the liver is typically slightly larger than normal, dense, and chocolate brown. Fibrous septa develop slowly, leading ultimately to a small, shrunken liver with a micronodular pattern of cirrhosis. The liver parenchyma in later stages is often dark brown to nearly black due to overwhelming iron accumulation.

Biochemical determination of hepatic tissue iron concentration has been the gold standard for quantitating hepatic iron

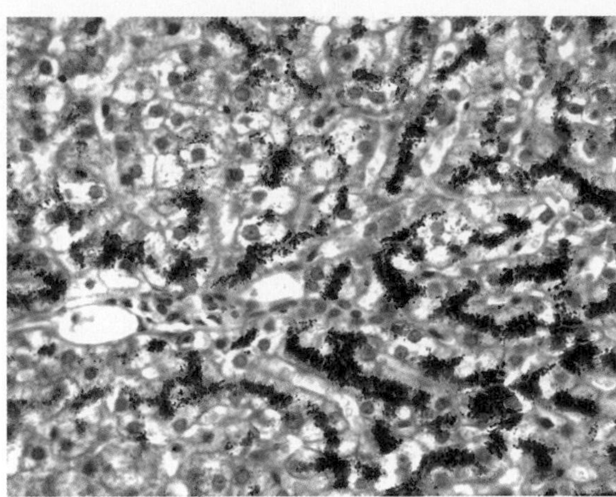

Figure 18-25 Hereditary hemochromatosis. In this Prussian blue–stained section, hepatocellular iron appears blue. The parenchymal architecture is normal.

content. In normal individuals, the iron content of liver tissue is less than 1000 μg per gram dry weight of liver. Adult patients with hereditary hemochromatosis exhibit more than 10,000 μg iron per gram dry weight; hepatic iron concentrations in excess of 22,000 μg per gram dry weight are associated with the development of fibrosis and cirrhosis. However, **with newly available genetic testing for these diseases, quantitative assessment of tissue iron content is no longer necessary for confirmation of a suspected diagnosis.**

The **pancreas** becomes intensely pigmented, has diffuse interstitial fibrosis, and may exhibit some parenchymal atrophy. Hemosiderin is found in both the acinar and the islet cells, and sometimes in the interstitial fibrous stroma. The **heart** is often enlarged and has hemosiderin granules within the myocardial fibers, producing a striking brown coloration to the myocardium. A delicate interstitial fibrosis may appear.

Although skin pigmentation is partially attributable to hemosiderin deposition in dermal macrophages and fibroblasts, most of the pigmentation results from increased epidermal melanin production, the mechanism of which in unknown. The combination of these pigments imparts a characteristic slate-gray color to the skin. With hemosiderin deposition in the synovial joint linings, an **acute synovitis** may develop. Excessive deposition of calcium pyrophosphate damages the articular cartilage, producing a disabling polyarthritis referred to as **pseudogout**. The **testes may be small and atrophic**, secondary to a derangement in the hypothalamic-pituitary axis resulting in reduced gonadotropin and testosterone levels.

Clinical Features. **The principal manifestations of classic hemochromatosis include hepatomegaly, abdominal pain, abnormal skin pigmentation (particularly in sun-exposed areas), deranged glucose homeostasis or diabetes mellitus due to destruction of pancreatic islets, cardiac dysfunction (arrhythmias, cardiomyopathy), and atypical arthritis.** In some patients, the presenting complaint is hypogonadism (e.g., amenorrhea in the female, impotence and loss of libido in the male). It is more often a disease of males, for reasons described earlier, and rarely becomes evident before age 40. The classic tetrad of cirrhosis with hepatomegaly, abnormal skin pigmentation, diabetes mellitus, and cardiac dysfunction might not develop until late in the course of the disease. Death may result from cirrhosis or cardiac disease. *A significant cause of death is hepatocellular carcinoma; the risk is 200-fold greater than in the general population.* Treatment for iron overload does not fully remove the cancer risk presumably because of DNA alterations that occur prior to the time of diagnosis and treatment initiation.

Fortunately, hemochromatosis can be diagnosed long before irreversible tissue damage has occurred. Screening involves demonstration of very high levels of serum iron and ferritin, exclusion of secondary causes of iron overload, and liver biopsy if indicated. *Screening of family members of probands is important.* Heterozygotes also accumulate excessive iron, but not to a level that causes significant tissue damage. Currently most patients with hemochromatosis are diagnosed in the subclinical, precirrhotic stage due to routine serum iron measurements (as part of other diagnostic workup). Treatment by regular phlebotomy steadily depletes tissue iron stores. With treatment, life expectancy is normal.

Neonatal hemochromatosis (also called congenital hemochromatosis) is a disease of unknown origin manifested by severe liver disease and extrahepatic hemosiderin deposition. Neonatal hemochromatosis is not an inherited disease; liver injury, leading to hemosiderin accumulation, occurs in utero, and might be related to maternal alloimmune injury to the fetal liver. Extrahepatic hemosiderin deposition, detected by buccal biopsy, needs to be documented for the correct diagnosis. There is no specific treatment, except for supportive care and liver transplantation in severe cases.

The most common causes of secondary (or acquired) hemochromatosis are disorders associated with ineffective erythropoiesis, such as severe forms of thalassemia (Chapter 14) and myelodysplastic syndromes (Chapter 13). In these disorders, the excess iron results not only from transfusions, but also from increased absorption. Transfusions alone, when given repeatedly over a period of years (e.g., in patients with chronic hemolytic anemias), can also lead to systemic hemosiderosis and parenchymal organ injury.

Cirrhosis caused by chronic liver diseases in which hepatitis is the predominant form of injury (e.g., chronic viral hepatitis, autoimmune hepatitis) can lead to diminished hepcidin production from loss of hepatocyte mass and, therefore, to cirrhosis-associated increased iron uptake from the gut. However, the increase in stainable iron in alcoholic cirrhosis, cannot be readily explained by decrease in hepcidin production alone. It is suspected that other, yet to be discovered, mechanisms are involved.

Wilson Disease

Wilson disease is an autosomal recessive disorder caused by mutation of the *ATP7B* gene, resulting in impaired copper excretion into bile and a failure to incorporate copper into ceruloplasmin. This disorder is marked by the accumulation of toxic levels of copper in many tissues and organs, principally the liver, brain, and eye. Normally, 40% to 60% of ingested copper (2 to 5 mg/day) is absorbed in the duodenum and proximal small intestine, and is transported to the portal circulation complexed with albumin and histidine. Free copper dissociates and is taken up by hepatocytes. In the liver copper binds to an α_2-globulin (apoceruloplasmin) to form *ceruloplasmin*, which is secreted into the blood. Excess copper is transported into the bile. Ceruloplasmin accounts for 90% to 95% of plasma copper. Circulating ceruloplasmin is eventually desialylated, endocytosed by the liver, and degraded within lysosomes, after which the released copper is excreted into bile. This degradation/excretion pathway is the primary route for copper elimination. The estimated total body copper is only 50 to 150 mg.

Pathogenesis. Wilson disease results from mutations in the *ATP7B* gene. Located on chromosome 13, the *ATP7B* gene, encodes a transmembrane copper-transporting ATPase, expressed on the hepatocyte canalicular membrane. More than 300 mutations in the *ATP7B* gene have been identified, but not all cause the disease. *The overwhelming majority of patients are compound heterozygotes containing different mutations on each ATP7B allele.* The overall frequency of mutated alleles is 1:100, and the prevalence of the disease is approximately 1:30,000 to 1:50,000 (approximately 9000 patients in the United States). Deficiency in the ATP7B protein causes a decrease in copper transport into bile, impairs its incorporation into ceruloplasmin, and inhibits ceruloplasmin secretion into the blood. These changes cause copper accumulation in the liver and a decrease in circulating ceruloplasmin. The accumulated copper causes toxic liver injury by three mechanisms: 1) Promoting the formation of free radicals by the Fenton reaction (Chapter 2); 2) binding to sulfhydryl groups of cellular proteins; and 3) displacing other metals from hepatic metalloenzymes. Although there is a latent period of variable duration, there may be sudden onset of a severe systemic illness. This is triggered by spillage of non–ceruloplasmin-bound copper from the liver into the circulation, causing hemolysis and pathologic changes at other sites such as the brain, corneas, kidneys, bones, joints, and parathyroids. Concomitantly, urinary excretion of copper markedly increases from its normal miniscule levels.

MORPHOLOGY

The liver often bears the brunt of injury, but the disease may also present as a neurologic disorder. The hepatic changes are variable, ranging from relatively minor to massive damage, and mimic many other disease processes. **Fatty change (steatosis)** may be mild to moderate with focal hepatocyte necrosis. An acute, fulminant hepatitis can mimic acute viral hepatitis. Chronic hepatitis in Wilson disease exhibits moderate to severe inflammation and hepatocyte necrosis, admixed with fatty change and features of steatohepatitis (hepatocyte ballooning with prominent Mallory-Denk bodies). Eventually cirrhosis supervenes.

Excess copper deposition can often be demonstrated by special stains (rhodamine stain for copper, orcein stain for copper-associated protein). Because copper also accumulates in chronic obstructive cholestasis and because histology cannot reliably distinguish Wilson disease from viral- and drug-induced hepatitis, demonstration of hepatic copper content in excess of 250 μg per gram dry weight is most helpful for making a diagnosis. Unlike in hereditary hemochromatosis, where genetic testing has lessened the need for quantitative metal assessment, the vast range of genetic alterations in Wilson disease means that genetic testing is not yet a primary diagnostic modality; with the advent of next generation sequencing, however, this is likely to change in the near future.

Toxic injury to the brain primarily affects the basal ganglia, particularly the putamen, which shows atrophy and even cavitation. Nearly all patients with neurologic involvement develop eye lesions called **Kayser-Fleischer rings**, green to brown deposits of copper in Descemet membrane in the limbus of the cornea.

Clinical Features. The age at onset and the clinical presentation of Wilson disease are extremely variable (average age is 11.4 years), but the disorder usually manifests in affected individuals between 6 and 40 years of age. Initial presentation may either be with acute or chronic liver disease. Neurologic involvement presents as movement disorders (tremor, poor coordination, chorea or choreoathetosis) or rigid dystonia (spastic dystonia, mask like facies, rigidity and gait disturbances); these symptoms may be confused with Parkinsonism. Patients may also have psychiatric symptoms such as depression, phobias, compulsive behavior, and labile mood. Hemolytic anemia may occur due to toxicity of copper to red cell membranes. *The biochemical diagnosis of Wilson disease is based on a decrease in serum ceruloplasmin, an increase in hepatic copper content (the most sensitive and accurate test), and increased urinary excretion of copper (the most specific screening test).* Serum copper levels are of no diagnostic value, since they may be low, normal, or elevated, depending on the stage of evolution of the disease. Demonstration of Kayser-Fleischer rings further favors the diagnosis. Early recognition and long-term copper chelation therapy (with D-penicillamine or Trientine) or zinc-based therapy (which blocks uptake of copper in the gut) has dramatically altered the usual progressive downhill course. Individuals with hepatitis or unmanageable cirrhosis require liver transplantation, which can be curative.

α_1-Antitrypsin Deficiency

α_1-Antitrypsin deficiency is an autosomal recessive disorder of protein folding marked by very low levels of circulating α_1-Antitrypsin (α_1AT). The major function of this protein is the inhibition of proteases, particularly neutrophil elastase, cathepsin G, and proteinase 3, which are normally released from neutrophils at sites of inflammation. α_1AT deficiency leads to the development of pulmonary emphysema, because the activity of destructive proteases is not inhibited (Chapter 15). It also causes liver disease as a consequence of hepatocellular accumulation of the misfolded protein. Cutaneous necrotizing panniculits also occurs in a minor subset of patients.

α_1AT is a small 394–amino acid plasma glycoprotein synthesized predominantly by hepatocytes. It is a member of the serine protease inhibitor (serpin) family. The gene, located on chromosome 14, is very polymorphic, and at

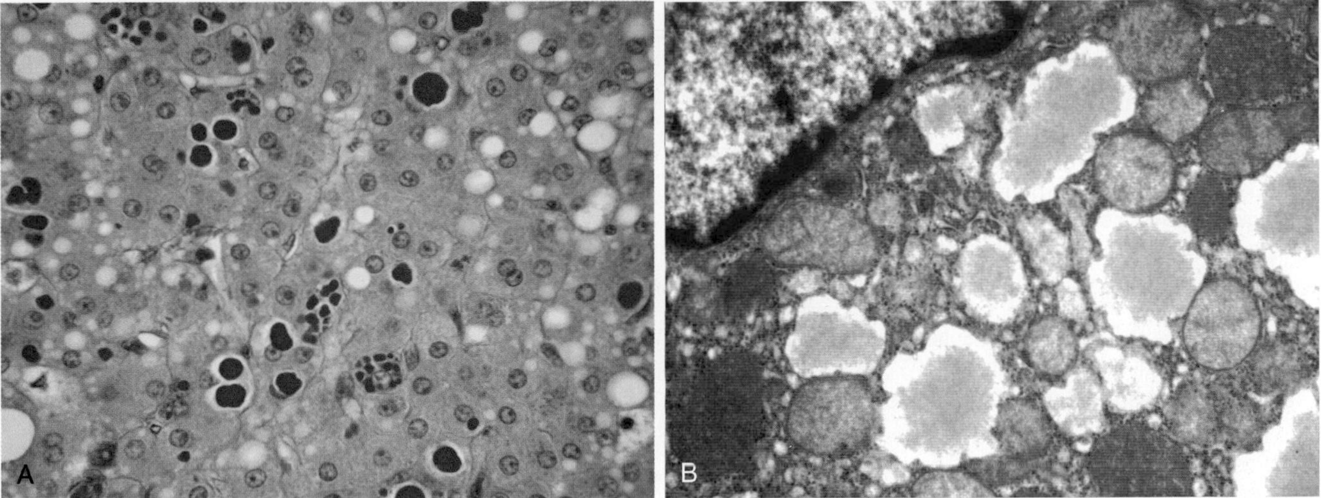

Figure 18-26 α_1-Antitrypsin deficiency. **A,** Periodic acid–Schiff (PAS) stain after diastase digestion of the liver, highlighting the characteristic magenta cytoplasmic granules. **B,** Electron micrograph showing endoplasmic reticulum dilated by aggregates of misfolded protein.

least 75 α_1AT forms have been identified, denoted alphabetically by their relative migration on an isoelectric gel. The general notation is "Pi" for "protease inhibitor" and an alphabetic letter for the position on the gel; two letters denote the genotype of an individual's two alleles. The most common genotype is PiMM, occurring in 90% of individuals (the "wild-type"). Most allelic variants show substitutions in the polypeptide chain but produce normal levels of functional α_1AT. Some deficiency variants, including the PiS variant, result in a moderate reduction in serum concentrations of α_1AT without clinical manifestations. Rare variants termed *Pi-null* have no detectable serum α_1AT.

The most common clinically significant mutation is PiZ; homozygotes for the PiZZ protein have circulating α_1AT levels that are only 10% of normal. These individuals are at high risk for developing clinical disease. Expression of alleles is autosomal codominant, and consequently, PiMZ heterozygotes have intermediate plasma levels of α_1AT. Among people of northern European descent, the PiS frequency is 6% and the PiZ frequency is 4%; the PiZZ state affects 1 in 1800 live births. Because of its early presentation with liver disease, α_1AT deficiency is the most commonly diagnosed inherited hepatic disorder in infants and children.

Pathogenesis. With most allelic variants, the protein is synthesized and secreted normally. Deficiency variants show a selective defect in migration of protein from endoplasmic reticulum to Golgi apparatus; this is particularly characteristic of the PiZ polypeptide, resulting from a single amino acid substitution of Glu342 to Lys342. *The mutant polypeptide (α_1AT-Z) is abnormally folded and polymerized, creating endoplasmic reticulum stress and triggering the unfolded protein response, a signaling cascade that may lead to apoptosis* (Chapter 2). *All individuals with the PiZZ genotype accumulate α_1AT-Z in the endoplasmic reticulum of hepatocytes, but only 10% to 15% of PiZZ individuals develop overt clinical liver disease.* Other genetic factors or environmental factors are thus posited to play a role in the development of liver disease.

MORPHOLOGY

α_1AT deficiency is characterized by the presence of round-to-oval **cytoplasmic globular inclusions in hepatocytes,** which on routine hematoxylin and eosin stains are acidophilic, but are strongly periodic acid–Schiff (PAS)-positive and diastase-resistant (Fig. 18-26). The globules are also present, but in diminished size and number in the PiMZ and PiSZ genotypes. Periportal hepatocytes contain the mutant proteins in early and mild forms of the disease with accumulation involving progressively more central hepatocytes with duration and more severe forms like the PiZZ variant. However, the number of globule-containing hepatocytes in a patient's liver is not correlated with the severity of pathologic findings.

The hepatic pathology associated with PiZZ homozygosity is extremely varied, ranging from neonatal hepatitis without or with cholestasis and fibrosis (discussed later), to childhood cirrhosis, to a smoldering chronic hepatitis or cirrhosis that becomes apparent only late in life. The diagnostic α_1AT globules may be absent in the young infant, although steatosis may be present as a tip-off to the possibility of α_1AT deficiency.

Clinical Features. Neonatal hepatitis with cholestatic jaundice appears in 10% to 20% of newborns with the deficiency. In adolescence, presenting symptoms may be related to hepatitis, cirrhosis or pulmonary disease. Attacks of hepatitis may subside with apparent complete recovery, or they may become chronic and lead progressively to cirrhosis. Alternatively, the disease may remain silent until cirrhosis appears in middle to later life. Hepatocellular carcinoma develops in 2% to 3% of PiZZ adults, usually, but not always, in the setting of cirrhosis. The treatment, indeed the cure, for severe hepatic disease is orthotopic liver transplantation. In patients with pulmonary disease the single most important preventive measure is avoidance of cigarette smoking, because smoking markedly accelerates emphysema and the destructive lung disease associated with α_1AT deficiency.

KEY CONCEPTS

Inherited Metabolic Liver Disease

- The inherited metabolic diseases include hemochromatosis, Wilson disease, and α_1-antitrypsin deficiency.
- **Hereditary hemochromatosis** is caused by a mutation in the *HFE* gene, whose product is involved in intestinal iron uptake by its effect on hepcidin levels. It is characterized by accumulation of iron in liver and pancreas.
- **Wilson disease** is caused by a mutation in the metal ion transporter *ATP7B*, which results in accumulation of copper in the liver, brain (particularly basal ganglia), and eyes ("Kayser-Fleisher rings").
  - Wilson disease effects on the liver are protean, presenting as acute massive hepatic necrosis, fatty liver disease, or chronic hepatitis and cirrhosis.
- **α_1-Antitrypsin deficiency** is a disease of protein misfolding that results in impaired secretion of α_1 Antitrypsin into the serum.
  - The Z variant of α_1-Antitrypsin is the most likely to impair secretion by hepatocytes and cause disease, particularly when homozygous, that is, the *PiZZ* genotype; the main consequences are pulmonary emphysema caused by increased elastase activity and liver injury caused by the accumulation of abnormal α_1-Antitrypsin.

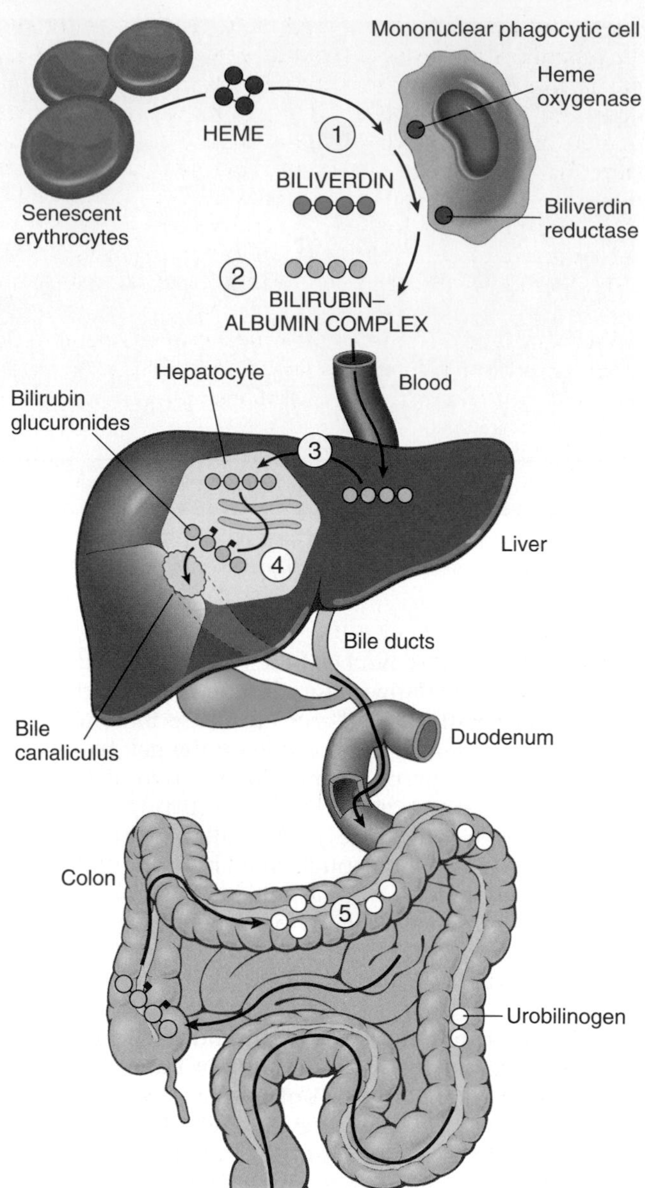

Figure 18-27 Bilirubin metabolism and elimination. (1) Normal bilirubin production from heme (0.2 to 0.3 gm/day) is derived primarily from the breakdown of senescent circulating erythrocytes. (2) Extrahepatic bilirubin is bound to serum albumin and delivered to the liver. (3) Hepatocellular uptake and (4) glucuronidation in the endoplasmic reticulum generates bilirubin monoglucuronides and diglucuronides, which are water soluble and readily excreted into bile. (5) Gut bacteria deconjugate the bilirubin and degrade it to colorless urobilinogens. The urobilinogens and the residue of intact pigments are excreted in the feces, with some reabsorption and excretion into urine.

Cholestatic Diseases

Hepatic bile serves two major functions: (1) the emulsification of dietary fat in the lumen of the gut through the detergent action of bile salts, and (2) the elimination of bilirubin, excess cholesterol, xenobiotics, and other waste products that are insufficiently water-soluble to be excreted into urine. Tissue deposition of bile becomes clinically evident as yellow discoloration of the skin and sclera (*jaundice* and *icterus*, respectively) due to retention of bilirubin, and as *cholestasis*, when there is systemic retention of not only bilirubin but also other solutes eliminated in bile.

Jaundice occurs when there is bilirubin overproduction, hepatitis, or obstruction of the flow of bile, any of which can disturb the equilibrium between bilirubin production and clearance. To understand the pathophysiology of jaundice it is important first to become familiar with the major aspects of bile formation and metabolism. The metabolism of bilirubin by the liver consists of four separate but interrelated events: uptake from the circulation; intracellular storage; conjugation with glucuronic acid; and biliary excretion. These are described next.

Bilirubin and Bile Formation

Bilirubin is the end product of heme degradation (Fig. 18-27). The majority of daily production (0.2 to 0.3 gm, 85%) is derived from breakdown of senescent red cells by the mononuclear phagocytic system, especially in the spleen, liver, and bone marrow. Most of the remainder (15%) of bilirubin is derived from the turnover of hepatic heme or hemoproteins (e.g., the P-450 cytochromes) and from premature destruction of red cell precursors in the bone marrow (Chapter 13). Whatever the source, intracellular heme oxygenase converts heme to biliverdin (step 1 in Fig. 18-27), which is immediately reduced to bilirubin by biliverdin reductase. Bilirubin thus formed outside the liver is released and bound to serum albumin (step 2). Albumin binding is necessary to transport bilirubin because bilirubin is virtually insoluble in aqueous solutions at physiologic pH. Hepatic processing of bilirubin involves carrier-mediated uptake at the sinusoidal membrane (step 3), conjugation with one or two molecules of glucuronic acid by bilirubin uridine diphosphate (UDP) glucuronyl transferase (UGT1A1, step 4) in the endoplasmic reticulum, and excretion of the water-soluble, nontoxic bilirubin glucuronides into bile. Most bilirubin glucuronides are deconjugated in the gut lumen by bacterial β-glucuronidases and degraded to colorless urobilinogens (step 5). The urobilinogens and the residue of intact pigment are largely excreted in feces. Approximately 20% of the urobilinogens formed are reabsorbed in the ileum and colon, returned to the liver, and reexcreted into bile. A small amount of reabsorbed urobilinogen is excreted in the urine.

Two thirds of the organic materials in bile are bile salts, which are formed by the conjugation of bile acids with taurine or glycine. Bile acids, the major catabolic products of cholesterol, are a family of water-soluble sterols with carboxylated side chains. The primary human bile acids are cholic acid and chenodeoxycholic acid. Bile acids in bile salts are highly effective detergents. Their primary physiologic role is to solubilize water-insoluble lipids secreted by hepatocytes into bile, and also to solubilize dietary lipids in the gut lumen. Ninety-five percent of secreted bile acids, conjugated or unconjugated, are reabsorbed from the gut lumen and recirculate to the liver *(enterohepatic circulation)*, thus helping to maintain a large endogenous pool of bile acids for digestive and excretory purposes.

Pathophysiology of Jaundice

Both unconjugated bilirubin and conjugated bilirubin (bilirubin glucuronides) may accumulate systemically. There are two important pathophysiologic differences between the two forms of bilirubin. Unconjugated bilirubin is virtually insoluble in water at physiologic pH and exists in tight complexes with serum albumin. This form cannot be excreted in the urine even when blood levels are high. Normally, a very small amount of unconjugated bilirubin is present as an albumin-free anion in plasma. This fraction of unbound bilirubin may diffuse into tissues, particularly the brain in infants, and produce toxic injury. The unbound plasma fraction may increase in severe hemolytic disease or when drugs displace bilirubin from albumin. Hence, hemolytic disease of the newborn (erythroblastosis fetalis) may lead to accumulation of unconjugated bilirubin in the brain, which can cause severe neurologic damage, referred to as *kernicterus* (Chapter 10). In contrast, conjugated bilirubin is water-soluble, nontoxic, and only loosely bound to albumin. Because of its solubility and weak association with albumin, excess conjugated bilirubin in plasma can be excreted in urine.

Serum bilirubin levels in the normal adult vary between 0.3 and 1.2 mg/dL, and the rate of systemic bilirubin production is equal to the rates of hepatic uptake, conjugation, and biliary excretion. Jaundice becomes evident when the serum bilirubin levels rise above 2 to 2.5 mg/dL; levels as high as 30 to 40 mg/dL can occur with severe disease. Mechanisms underlying jaundice are summarized in Table 18-8. Although more than one mechanism may be operative, generally one predominates, so knowledge of the major form of plasma bilirubin is of value in evaluating possible causes of hyperbilirubinemia.

The following two conditions result from specific defects in hepatocellular bilirubin metabolism.

Table 18-8 Causes of Jaundice

Predominantly Unconjugated Hyperbilirubinemia
Excess production of bilirubin
Hemolytic anemias
Resorption of blood from internal hemorrhage (e.g., alimentary tract bleeding, hematomas)
Ineffective erythropoiesis (e.g., pernicious anemia, thalassemia)
Reduced hepatic uptake
Drug interference with membrane carrier systems
Some cases of Gilbert syndrome
Impaired bilirubin conjugation
Physiologic jaundice of the newborn (decreased UGT1A1 activity, decreased excretion)
Breast milk jaundice (β-glucuronidases in milk)
Genetic deficiency of UGT1A1 activity (Crigler-Najjar syndrome types I and II)
Gilbert syndrome
Diffuse hepatocellular disease (e.g., viral or drug-induced hepatitis, cirrhosis)
Predominantly Conjugated Hyperbilirubinemia
Deficiency of canalicular membrane transporters (Dubin-Johnson syndrome, Rotor syndrome)
Impaired bile flow from duct obstruction or autoimmune cholangiopathies

UGT1A1, Uridine diphosphate-glucuronyltransferase family, peptide A1

Neonatal Jaundice. Because the hepatic machinery for conjugating and excreting bilirubin does not fully mature until about 2 weeks of age, almost every newborn develops transient and mild unconjugated hyperbilirubinemia, termed neonatal jaundice or *physiologic jaundice of the newborn*. This may be exacerbated by breastfeeding, as a result of the presence of bilirubin-deconjugating enzymes in breast milk. Nevertheless, sustained jaundice in the newborn is abnormal (discussed later).

Hereditary Hyperbilirubinemias. Multiple genetic mutations can cause hereditary hyperbilirubinemia (Table 18-9). For example, the hepatic conjugating enzyme UGT1A1 is a product of the *UGT1A1* gene located on chromosome 2q37. It is a member of a family of enzymes that catalyze the glucuronidation of an array of substrates such as steroid hormones, carcinogens, and drugs. In humans, UGT1A1, generated from the *UGT1A1* gene, is the only isoform responsible for bilirubin glucuronidation. Mutations of *UGT1A1* cause hereditary unconjugated hyperbilirubinemias: *Crigler-Najjar syndrome types I and II* and *Gilbert syndrome*. Crigler-Najjar syndrome type 1 is caused by severe UGT1A1 deficiency and is fatal around the time of birth, while in Crigler-Najjar type II and Gilbert syndrome there is some UGT1A1 activity and the phenotypes are much milder. In contrast, *Dubin-Johnson syndrome* and *Rotor syndrome* result from other defects that lead to conjugated hyperbilirubinemia. Both are autosomal recessive disorders and innocuous.

Cholestasis

Cholestasis is caused by impaired bile formation and bile flow that gives rise to accumulation of bile pigment in the hepatic parenchyma. It can be caused by extrahepatic or intrahepatic obstruction of bile channels, or by defects in hepatocyte bile secretion. Patients may have jaundice, pruritus, skin xanthomas (focal accumulation of

Table 18-9 Hereditary Hyperbilirubinemias

Disorder	Inheritance	Defects in Bilirubin Metabolism	Liver Pathology	Clinical Course
Unconjugated Hyperbilirubinemia				
Crigler-Najjar syndrome type I	Autosomal recessive	Absent UGT1A1 activity	None	Fatal in neonatal period
Crigler-Najjar syndrome type II	Autosomal dominant with variable penetrance	Decreased UGT1A1 activity	None	Generally mild, occasional kernicterus
Gilbert syndrome	Autosomal recessive	Decreased UGT1A1 activity	None	Innocuous
Conjugated Hyperbilirubinemia				
Dubin-Johnson syndrome	Autosomal recessive	Impaired biliary excretion of bilirubin glucuronides due to mutation in canalicular multidrug resistance protein 2 (MRP2)	Pigmented cytoplasmic globules	Innocuous
Rotor syndrome	Autosomal recessive	Decreased hepatic uptake and storage? Decreased biliary excretion?	None	Innocuous

UGT1A1, Uridine diphosphate-glucuronyltransferase family, peptide A1

cholesterol), or symptoms related to intestinal malabsorption, including nutritional deficiencies of the fat-soluble vitamins A, D, or K. A characteristic laboratory finding is elevated serum alkaline phosphatase and γ-glutamyl transpeptidase (GGT), enzymes present on the apical (canalicular) membranes of hepatocytes and bile duct epithelial cells.

MORPHOLOGY

The morphologic features of cholestasis depend on its severity, duration, and underlying cause. Common to both obstructive and nonobstructive cholestasis is the accumulation of bile pigment within the hepatic parenchyma (Fig. 18-28*A, B*). Elongated green-brown plugs of bile are visible in dilated bile canaliculi (Fig. 18-28*C*). Rupture of canaliculi leads to extravasation of bile, which is quickly phagocytosed by Kupffer cells. Droplets of bile pigment also accumulate within hepatocytes, which can take on a fine, foamy appearance, so called "feathery degeneration."

Large Bile Duct Obstruction

The most common cause of bile duct obstruction in adults is extrahepatic cholelithiasis (gallstones) followed by malignancies of the biliary tree or head of the pancreas, and strictures resulting from previous surgical procedures. Obstructive conditions in children include biliary atresia, cystic fibrosis, choledochal cysts and syndromes in which there are insufficient intrahepatic bile ducts. The initial morphologic features of cholestasis (described below) are entirely reversible with correction of the obstruction. Prolonged obstruction can lead to biliary cirrhosis, described later.

Subtotal or intermittent obstruction may promote *ascending cholangitis*, a secondary bacterial infection of the biliary tree that aggravates the inflammatory injury. Enteric organisms such as coliforms and enterococci are common culprits. Cholangitis usually presents with fever, chills, abdominal pain, and jaundice. *The most severe form of cholangitis is suppurative cholangitis, in which purulent bile fills and distends bile ducts.* Since sepsis rather than cholestasis tends to dominate this potentially grave process, prompt diagnostic evaluation and intervention are imperative.

MORPHOLOGY

Acute biliary obstruction, either intrahepatic or extrahepatic, causes distention of upstream bile ducts, which often become dilated. In addition, bile ductules proliferate at the portal-parenchymal interface, accompanied by stromal edema and infiltrating neutrophils (Fig. 18-28*B* and 18-29). These labyrinthine ductules reabsorb secreted bile salts, serving to protect the downstream obstructed bile ducts from their toxic detergent action. Indeed, **the histologic hallmark of ascending cholangitis is the influx of these periductular neutrophils directly into the bile duct epithelium and lumen** (Fig. 18-30).

Left uncorrected, secondary inflammation resulting from **chronic biliary obstruction** and ductular reactions initiate periportal fibrosis, eventually leading to hepatic scarring and nodule formation, generating **secondary or obstructive biliary cirrhosis** (Fig. 18-31). Cholestatic features in the parenchyma may be severe, with extensive **feathery degeneration of periportal hepatocytes**, cytoplasmic swelling often with **Mallory-Denk bodies** (differing from those in alcohol-induced liver disease and non-alcoholic fatty liver disease by their periportal predominance), and formation of **bile infarcts** from detergent effects of extravasated bile. However, once regenerative nodules have formed, bile stasis may become less conspicuous. **Ascending cholangitis may be superimposed on this chronic process as well, sometimes triggering acute-on-chronic liver failure.**

Since extrahepatic biliary obstruction is frequently amenable to surgical alleviation, correct and prompt diagnosis is imperative. In contrast, cholestasis due to diseases of the intrahepatic biliary tree or hepatocellular secretory failure (collectively termed intrahepatic cholestasis) is not benefited by surgery (short of transplantation), and the patient's condition may be worsened by an operative procedure. *There is thus some urgency in making a correct diagnosis of the cause of jaundice and cholestasis.*

Cholestasis of Sepsis

Sepsis may affect the liver by several mechanisms (1) through direct effects of intrahepatic bacterial infection (e.g., abscess formation or bacterial cholangitis), (2)

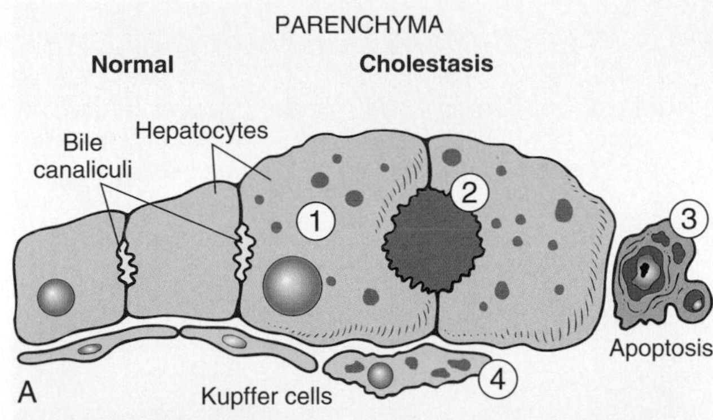

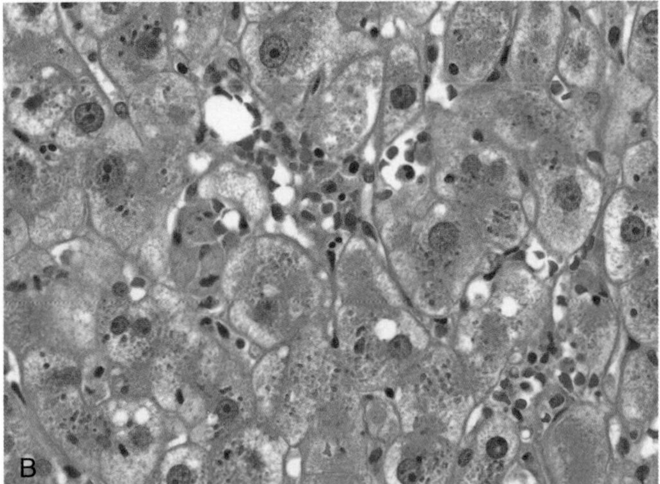

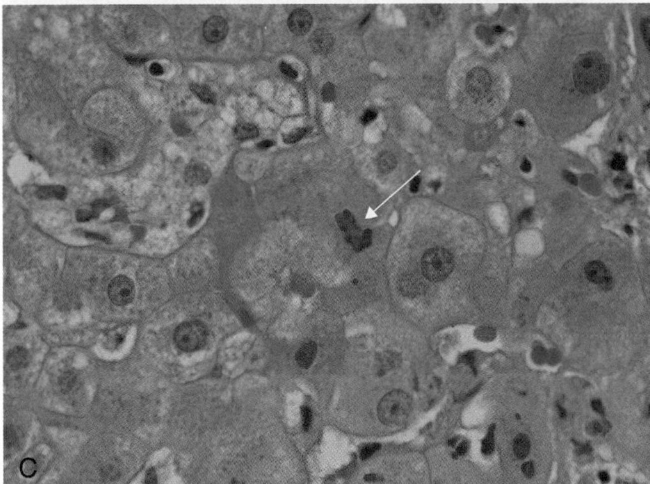

Figure 18-28 Cholestasis. **A,** Morphologic features of cholestasis (right) and comparison with normal liver (left). Cholestatic hepatocytes (1) are enlarged with dilated canalicular spaces (2). Apoptotic cells (3) may be seen, and Kupffer cells (4) frequently contain regurgitated bile pigments. **B,** Intracellular cholestasis showing the bile pigments in the cytoplasm. **C,** Bile plug (arrow) showing the expansion of bile canaliculus by bile.

ischemia relating to hypotension caused by sepsis (particularly when the liver is cirrhotic), or (3) in response to circulating microbial products. The last mentioned is most likely to lead to the cholestasis of sepsis, particularly when the systemic infection is due to gram-negative organisms. The most common form is *canalicular cholestasis,* with bile plugs within predominantly centrilobular canaliculi. This entity may be associated with activated Kupffer cells and mild portal inflammation, but hepatocyte necrosis is scant or absent. *Ductular cholestasis* is a more ominous finding, wherein dilated canals of Hering and bile ductules at the interface of portal tracts and parenchyma become dilated and contain obvious bile plugs (Fig. 18-32). This change, which is not a typical feature of biliary obstruction, despite the appearance of bile in large, dilated ductules, often accompanies or even precedes the development of septic shock.

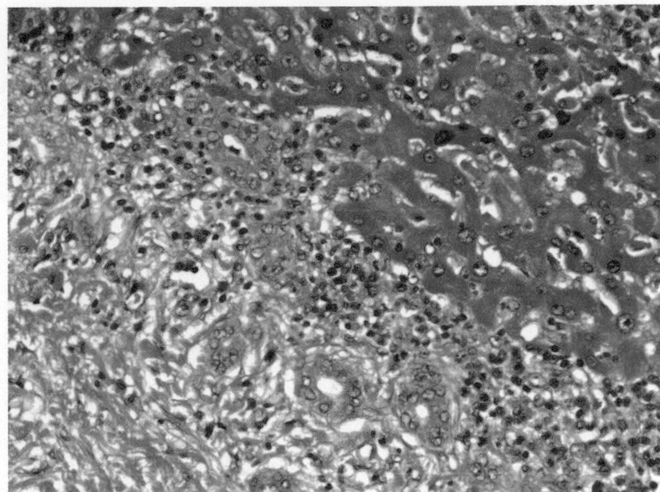

Figure 18-29 Acute large duct obstruction. There is marked edema of the portal tract stroma (white spaces) and a ductular reaction with admixed neutrophils at the interface between portal tract and hepatocellular parenchyma.

Primary Hepatolithiasis

Hepatolithiasis is a disorder of intrahepatic gallstone formation that leads to repeated bouts of ascending cholangitis, progressive inflammatory destruction of hepatic parenchyma, and predisposes to biliary neoplasia. The disease has a high prevalence in East Asia, but elsewhere is rare. Previously this disease has been called *recurrent*

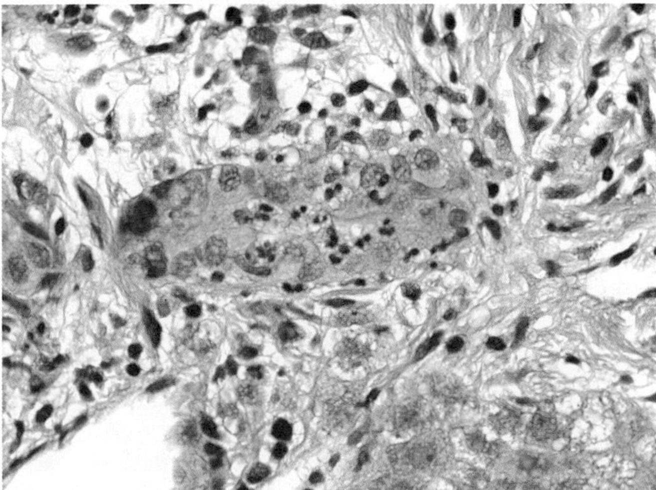

Figure 18-30 Ascending cholangitis. Individuals with large bile duct obstruction risk bacterial infections of the static bile within the biliary tree. Neutrophils are then seen within the bile duct epithelial lining and within the lumen.

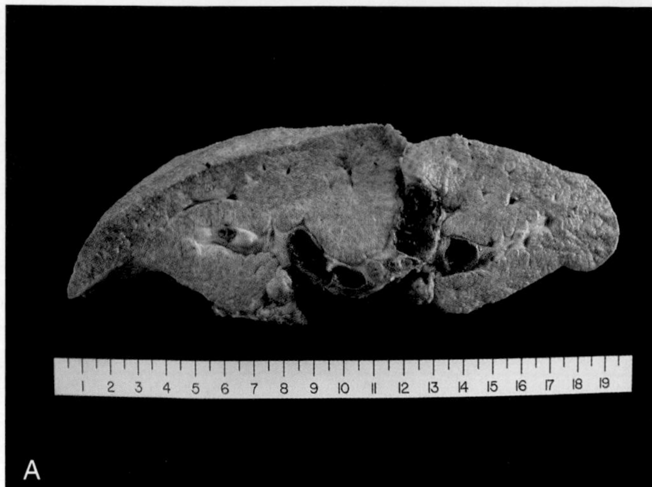

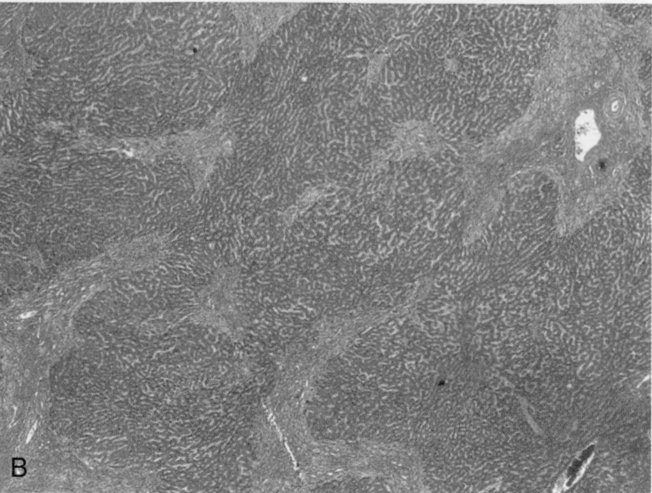

Figure 18-31 Biliary cirrhosis. **A,** Sagittal section through the liver demonstrates the nodularity (most prominent at the right) and bile staining of end-stage biliary cirrhosis. **B,** Unlike other forms of cirrhosis, nodules of liver cells in biliary cirrhosis are often not round but irregular, like jigsaw puzzle shapes.

pyogenic cholangitis focusing on its most common clinical findings and *oriental cholangitis* based on its ethnic predilection, but the underlying disease is one of stone formation, thus the currently accepted name, *hepatolithiasis.* There are regional differences regarding the composition of stones, but the consequences are largely the same.

MORPHOLOGY

Hepatolithiasis has **pigmented calcium bilirubinate stones** in distended intrahepatic bile ducts (Fig. 18-33). The ducts show chronic inflammation, mural fibrosis, and peribiliary gland hyperplasia, all in the absence of extrahepatic duct obstruction. Biliary dysplasia may be seen and may evolve to invasive cholangiocarcinoma.

Clinical Features. Individuals may present with repeated episodes of cholangitis due to secondary infections of the involved ducts, marked by fever and abdominal pain. Due to repeated rounds of inflammation, parenchymal collapse and scarring, the disease sometimes presents with a mass-like lesion mistaken for malignancy and is thus sometimes diagnosed at resection. This disease seems to increase the risk of cholangiocarcinoma by unknown mechanisms.

Neonatal Cholestasis

Prolonged conjugated hyperbilirubinemia in the neonate, termed neonatal cholestasis affects approximately 1 in 2500 live births. Since physiologic jaundice of the new born abates by two weeks, infants who have jaundice beyond 14-21 days after birth should be evaluated for neonatal cholestasis. The major causes are (1) cholangiopathies, primarily *biliary atresia* (discussed later), and (2) a variety of disorders causing conjugated hyperbilirubinemia in the neonate, collectively referred to as *neonatal hepatitis.*

Neonatal hepatitis is not a specific entity, nor are the disorders necessarily inflammatory. Instead, the finding of

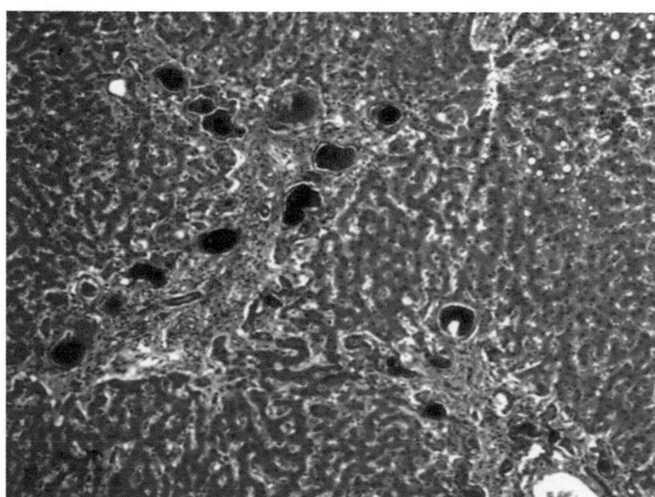

Figure 18-32 Ductular cholestasis of sepsis. Large, dark, bile concretions within markedly dilated canals of Hering and ductules at the portal-parenchymal interface. (Courtesy Dr. Jay Lefkowitch, Columbia University College of Physicians and Surgeons, New York.)

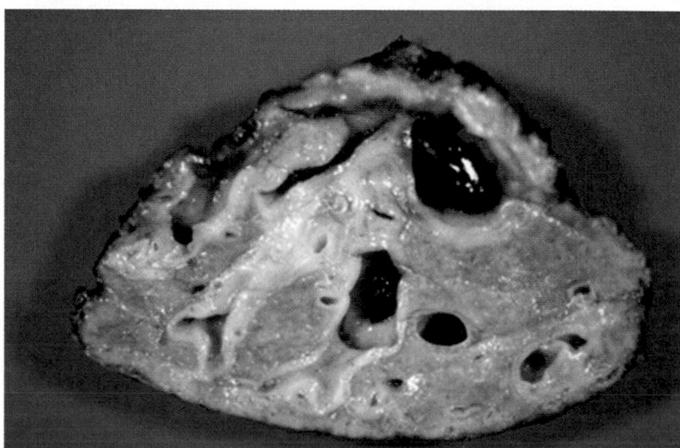

Figure 18-33 Hepatolithiasis. A resected, atrophic right hepatic lobe with characteristic findings including markedly dilated and distorted bile ducts containing large pigment stones and broad areas of collapsed liver parenchyma. (Courtesy Dr. Wilson M.S. Tsui, Caritas Medical Centre, Hong Kong.)

Table 18-10 Major Causes of Neonatal Cholestasis

Bile duct obstruction
Extrahepatic biliary atresia
Neonatal infection
Cytomegalovirus
Bacterial sepsis
Urinary tract infection
Syphilis
Toxic
Drugs
Parenteral nutrition
Genetic disorders
Tyrosinemia
Niemann-Pick disease
Galactosemia
Defective bile acid synthetic pathways
α_1-Antitrypsin deficiency
Cystic fibrosis
Alagille syndrome (paucity of bile ducts)
Miscellaneous
Shock/hypoperfusion
Indian childhood cirrhosis
Idiopathic neonatal hepatitis

neonatal cholestasis should evoke a diligent search for recognizable toxic, metabolic, and infectious liver diseases (Table 18-10). With greater awareness of etiology and better diagnostic tools, *idiopathic neonatal hepatitis* constitutes only 10% to 15% of cases of neonatal hepatitis.

Differentiation of biliary atresia from nonobstructive neonatal cholestasis is very important, since definitive treatment of biliary atresia requires surgical intervention (Kasai procedure), whereas surgery may adversely affect the clinical course of a child with other disorders. Fortunately, discrimination can be made with clinical data in about 90% of cases, without liver biopsy. In 10% of cases, liver biopsy may be critical for distinguishing neonatal hepatitis from an identifiable cholangiopathy. Affected infants have jaundice, dark urine, light or acholic stools, and hepatomegaly. Variable degrees of hepatic synthetic dysfunction, such as hypoprothrombinemia, may be present.

MORPHOLOGY

The morphologic features of neonatal hepatitis (Fig. 18-34) include lobular disarray with focal liver cell apoptosis and necrosis. There is panlobular **giant-cell transformation** of hepatocytes; prominent hepatocellular and canalicular cholestasis; mild mononuclear infiltration of the portal areas; reactive changes in Kupffer cells; and extramedullary hematopoiesis. This predominantly parenchymal pattern of injury may blend imperceptibly into a ductal pattern of injury, with ductular reaction and fibrosis of portal tracts. In these cases distinction from an obstructive biliary atresia may therefore be difficult.

Biliary Atresia

Biliary atresia is defined as a complete or partial obstruction of the lumen of the extrahepatic biliary tree within the first 3 months of life. A major contributor to neonatal cholestasis, worthy of separate mention, it represents one third of infants with neonatal cholestasis. Although the definition for the disease is based on extrahepatic biliary obstruction, progressive inflammation and fibrosis are not necessarily confined to these locales; in some patients there is also progressive loss of intrahepatic ducts. Biliary atresia is the single most frequent cause of death from liver disease in early childhood and accounts for 50% to 60% of children referred for liver transplantation.

Pathogenesis. Two major forms of biliary atresia are recognized based on the presumed timing of luminal obliteration. The *fetal form* accounts for as many as 20% of cases and is commonly associated with other anomalies resulting from ineffective establishment of laterality of thoracic and abdominal organs during development. These include situs inversus malrotation of abdominal viscera, interrupted inferior vena cava, polysplenia, and congenital heart disease. The presumed cause is aberrant intrauterine development of the extrahepatic biliary tree.

Much more common is the *perinatal form* of biliary atresia, in which a presumed normally developed biliary tree is destroyed following birth. The etiology of perinatal biliary atresia remains unknown; viral infection and autoimmune reactions are leading suspects. Reovirus, rotavirus, and cytomegalovirus have been implicated in some cases. Biliary atresia with organ malformations has genetic basis.

MORPHOLOGY

The salient features of biliary atresia include **inflammation and fibrosing stricture of the hepatic or common bile ducts**; in some individuals, periductular inflammation also progresses into the intrahepatic bile ducts leading, additionally, to progressive destruction of the intrahepatic biliary tree. On liver biopsy, florid features of extrahepatic biliary obstruction as described earlier are evident in about two thirds of cases. In the remainder, inflammatory destruction of intrahepatic ducts leads to duct paucity, often without the accompanying ductular reactions, edema and neutrophils characteristic of obstruction. When biliary atresia is unrecognized or uncorrected, cirrhosis develops within 3 to 6 months of birth.

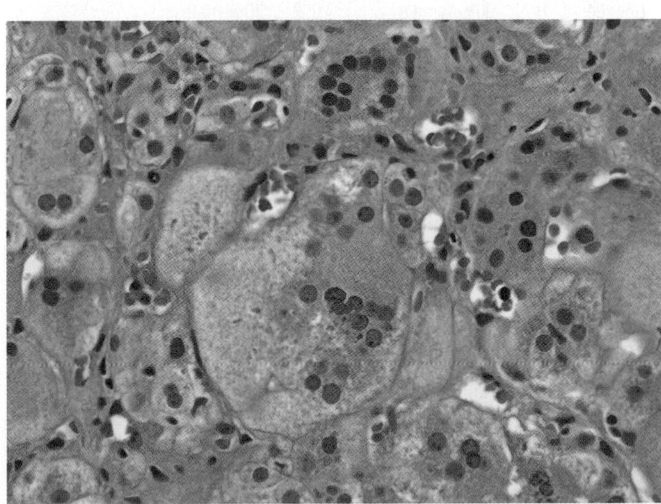

Figure 18-34 Neonatal hepatitis. Note the multinucleated giant hepatocytes.

There is considerable variability in the anatomy of biliary atresia. When the disease is limited to the common duct (type I) or right and/or left hepatic bile ducts (type II), the disease is surgically correctable (Kasai procedure). Unfortunately, 90% of patients have type III biliary atresia, in which there is also obstruction of bile ducts at or above the porta hepatis. These cases are not correctable, since there are no patent bile ducts amenable to surgical anastomosis. Moreover, in most patients, bile ducts within the liver are initially patent, but then are progressively destroyed.

Clinical Features. Infants with biliary atresia present with neonatal cholestasis, but exhibit normal birth weight and postnatal weight gain. There is a slight female preponderance. Initially normal stools change to acholic stools as the disease evolves. At the time of presentation, serum bilirubin values are usually in the range of 6 to 12 mg/dL, with only moderately elevated aminotransferase and alkaline phosphatase levels. The success of surgical resection and bypass of the biliary tree is limited by ascending cholangitis and/or intrahepatic progression of the disease. Liver transplantation remains the primary hope for salvage of these young patients. Without surgical intervention, death usually occurs within 2 years of birth.

Autoimmune Cholangiopathies

This section discusses the two main autoimmune disorders of intrahepatic bile ducts: primary biliary cirrhosis (PBC) and primary sclerosing cholangitis (PSC). The features of these two conditions are contrasted in Table 18-11. It should be noted that intrahepatic bile ducts are frequently damaged as part of other liver diseases, including viral hepatitis, drug- or toxin-induced liver injury, liver transplantation, and graft-versus-host disease that follows hematopoietic stem cell transplantation.

Table 18-11 Main Features of Primary Biliary Cirrhosis and Primary Sclerosing Cholangitis

Parameter	Primary Biliary Cirrhosis	Primary Sclerosing Cholangitis
Age	Median age 50 years (30 to 70)	Median age 30 years
Gender	90% female	70% male
Clinical course	Progressive	Unpredictable but progressive
Associated conditions	Sjögren syndrome (70%) Scleroderma (5%) Thyroid disease (20%)	Inflammatory bowel disease (70%) Pancreatitis (≤25%) Idiopathic fibrosing diseases (retroperitoneal fibrosis)
Serology	95% AMA-positive 50% ANA-positive 40% ANCA-positive	0-5% AMA-positive (low titer) 6% ANA-positive 65% ANCA-positive
Radiology	Normal	Strictures and beading of large bile ducts; pruning of smaller ducts
Duct lesion	Florid duct lesions and loss of small ducts only	Inflammatory destruction of extrahepatic and large intrahepatic ducts; fibrotic obliteration of medium and small intrahepatic ducts

AMA, Antimitochondrial antibody; ANA, antinuclear antibody; ANCA, antineutrophil cytoplasmic antibody.

Primary Biliary Cirrhosis (PBC)

PBC is an autoimmune disease characterized by nonsuppurative, inflammatory destruction of small and medium-sized intrahepatic bile ducts. Large intrahepatic ducts and the extrahepatic biliary tree are not involved. Most patients are diagnosed in the early stages of disease when cirrhosis is a distant possibility. Moreover, not all end-stage PBC is fully cirrhotic. Thus, the name is a misnomer for many patients. At best this name leads to confusion, at worst patients think they have an imminently fatal disease requiring transplantation, a fate that is not, in fact, the norm.

PBC is primarily a disease of middle-aged women, with a female predominance of 9:1. Occurring between the ages of 30 and 70 years, its peak incidence is between 40 and 50 years of age. The disease is most prevalent in Northern European countries (England and Scotland) and the Northern United States (Minnesota) where the prevalence is as high as 400 cases per million. Recent increases in incidence and prevalence along with geographic clustering suggest that genetic and environmental factors are important in its pathogenesis. Family members of PBC patients have an increased risk for development of the disease.

Pathogenesis. PBC is thought to be an autoimmune disorder, but as with other autoimmune diseases, the triggers that initiate PBC are unknown. *Antimitochondrial antibodies are the most characteristic laboratory finding in PBC.* They recognize the E2 component of the pyruvate dehydrogenase complex (PDC-E2). PDC-E2–specific T cells are also present in these patients, further supporting the notion of an immune-mediated process. Other findings suggestive of altered immunity include aberrant expression of MHC class II molecules on bile duct epithelial cells, accumulation of autoreactive T cells around bile ducts, and antibodies against other cellular components (nuclear pore proteins, and centromeric proteins, among others).

MORPHOLOGY

Interlobular bile ducts are actively destroyed by lymphoplasmacytic inflammation with or without granulomas (the *florid duct lesion*) (Fig. 18-35). Some biopsy specimens, however, show only absence of bile ducts in portal tracts. The disease is quite patchy in distribution; it is common to see a single bile duct under immune attack in one level of a biopsy specimen, while deeper levels, less than a millimeter away, remain unaffected. Ductular reactions follow duct injury, and these in turn participate in the development of portal-portal septal fibrosis (Fig. 18-36).

In patients who follow a classic path to end stage, there is increasingly widespread duct loss, slowly leading to cirrhosis and, in the end stages, to profound cholestasis (Fig. 18-37). The bile accumulation in such cholestasis is not centrilobular, unlike in drug-induced or sepsis-associated cholestatsis, but is periportal/periseptal. It is associated with feathery degeneration and ballooned, bile-stained hepatocytes, often with prominent

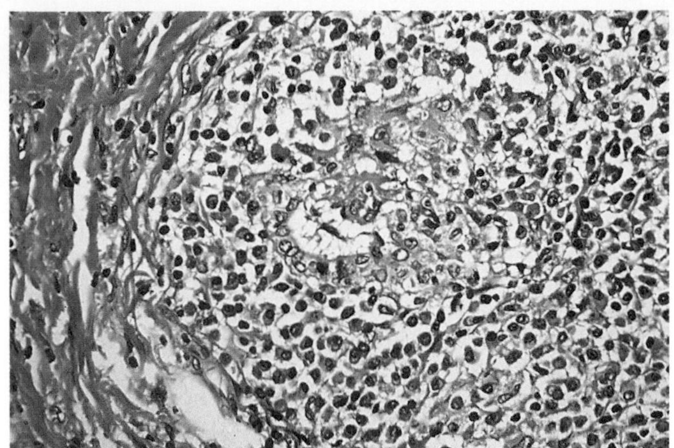

Figure 18-35 Primary biliary cirrhosis. A portal tract is markedly expanded by an infiltrate of lymphocytes and plasma cells surrounding a destructive granulomatous reaction centered on a bile duct (the "florid duct lesion").

Mallory-Denk bodies, as seen in chronic duct obstruction. Such end-stage livers show established cirrhosis and intense green pigmentation, matching the patient's icteric state.

Alternatively, some patients develop prominent portal hypertension rather than severe cholestasis. In these individuals there is widespread nodularity without the surrounding scar tissue seen in cirrhosis—a feature called nodular regenerative hyperplasia. Why this takes place in a disease that appears to be primarily biliary in nature is not understood.

In both cases, with little hepatocyte loss and often regenerative hyperplasia, there is **marked hepatomegaly**, a point of distinction from the shrunken, end-stage cirrhotic livers of chronic hepatitis, alcoholism, and non-alcoholic fatty liver disease.

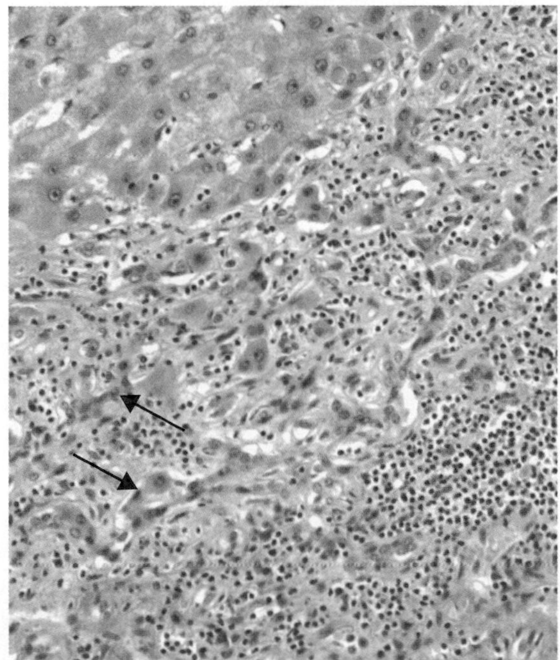

Figure 18-36 Ductular reaction (arrows) in primary biliary cirrhosis. In the earlier stages of disease, these structures may help maintain bile flow past destroyed segments of biliary tree, but later they may contribute to subsequent scarring.

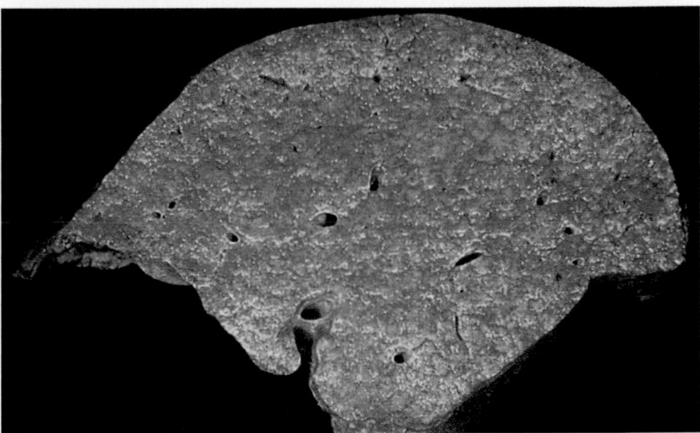

Figure 18-37 Primary biliary cirrhosis. This sagittal section demonstrates liver enlargement, nodularity indicative of cirrhosis, and green discoloration due to cholestasis.

Clinical Features. Most cases are diagnosed when asymptomatic, with elevated serum alkaline phosphatase and γ-glutamyltransferase. Both of these are markers of cholestasis and indicate the need for a liver disease work-up. Hypercholesterolemia is common. Antimitochondrial antibodies are present in 90% to 95% of patients. They are highly characteristic of PBC, although other autoantibodies may be seen in a small number of cases. *The disease is confirmed by liver biopsy, which is considered diagnostic if a florid duct lesion is present.* When symptomatic, the onset is insidious, presenting with fatigue and pruritus, which increase slowly over time.

Over a period of two or more decades, untreated patients follow one of two pathways to end-stage disease, one in which hyperbilirubinemia predominates and another with prominent portal hypertension. However, treatment of early stage disease with oral ursodeoxycholic acid greatly slows progression. Its mechanism of action is uncertain, but is presumably related to the ability of ursodeoxycholate to enter the bile acid pool and alter the biochemical composition of bile.

With progression, secondary features may emerge: skin hyperpigmentation, xanthelasmas, steatorrhea, and vitamin D malabsorption–related osteomalacia and/or osteoporosis. Individuals with PBC may also have extrahepatic manifestations of autoimmunity, including the sicca complex of dry eyes and mouth (Sjögren syndrome), systemic sclerosis, thyroiditis, rheumatoid arthritis, Raynaud phenomenon, and celiac disease. Ursodeoxycholate is not effective in advanced disease, and for these patients liver transplantation is the best form of treatment.

Primary Sclerosing Cholangitis (PSC)

PSC is characterized by inflammation and obliterative fibrosis of intrahepatic and extrahepatic bile ducts with dilation of preserved segments. Characteristic "beading" on radiographs of the intrahepatic and extrahepatic biliary tree is attributable to these irregular, biliary strictures and dilations (Fig. 18-38). *Inflammatory bowel disease* (Chapter 17), *particularly ulcerative colitis, coexists in approximately 70% of individuals with PSC.* Conversely, the prevalence of PSC in persons with ulcerative colitis is about 4%. Like inflammatory bowel disease, PSC tends to occur in the third through fifth decades of life and males predominate 2:1 (Table 18-11).

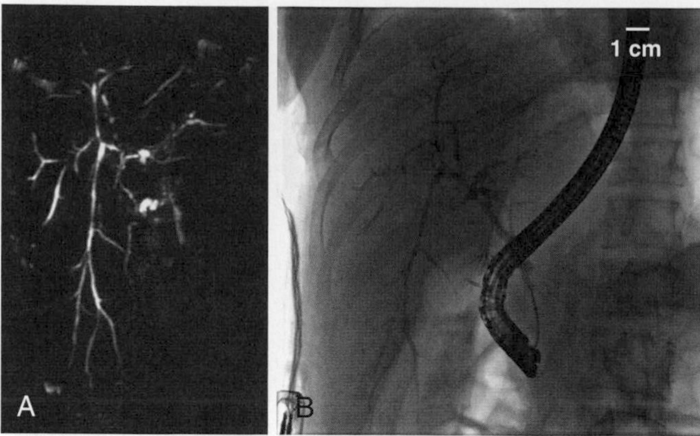

Figure 18-38 Imaging studies of a patient with primary sclerosing cholangitis. **A,** Magnetic resonance cholangiography shows focal dilatation in some bile ducts (bright, broad areas) and stricturing of others (thinning or absence). **B,** Endoscopic retrograde cholangiography of the same patient shows nearly identical features as in **A.** The endoscope is visible, giving a sense of scale. (Courtesy Dr. M. Edwyn Harrison, MD, Mayo Clinic, Scottsdale, Ariz.)

Pathogenesis. Several features of PSC suggest immunologically mediated injury to bile ducts, even though environmental triggers presumably also play a role. First degree relatives of patients with PSC have an increased risk of developing the disease suggesting a genetic component. T cells in the periductal stroma, the presence of circulating autoantibodies, association with HLA-B8 and other MHC antigens, and linkage to ulcerative colitis all support an inherent immunologic process.

It has been proposed that T cells activated in the damaged mucosa of patients with ulcerative colitis migrate to the liver where they recognize a cross-reacting bile duct antigen. Autoantibody profiles in PSC are not as characteristic as they are in PBC, although atypical perinuclear antineutrophil cytoplasmic antibodies (pANCA) targeting a nuclear envelope protein are found in approximately 65% of patients; however, the pathogenic relationship of pANCA to PSC is unknown.

MORPHOLOGY

Morphologic changes differ between the large ducts (intrahepatic and extrahepatic) and the smaller intrahepatic ducts. **Large duct inflammation** is similar to that seen in ulcerative colitis: acute, neutrophilic infiltration of the epithelium superimposed on a chronic inflammatory background. Inflamed areas develop strictures because edema and inflammation narrows the lumen or because of subsequent scarring. The **smaller ducts,** however, often have little inflammation and show a striking **circumferential "onion skin" fibrosis** around an increasingly atrophic duct lumen (Fig. 18-39), eventually leading to obliteration by a "tombstone" scar. Because the likelihood of sampling smaller duct lesions on a random needle biopsy is miniscule, diagnosis depends on radiologic imaging of the extrahepatic and larger intrahepatic ducts. As the disease progresses the liver becomes markedly cholestatic, culminating in biliary cirrhosis much like that seen with chronic obstruction and primary biliary cirrhosis. Biliary intraepithelial neoplasia may develop and cholangiocarcinoma appears usually with a fatal outcomes.

Clinical Features. **Asymptomatic patients may come to attention only because of persistent elevation of serum alkaline phosphatase, particularly in patients with ulcerative colitis who are being routinely screened.** Alternatively, progressive fatigue, pruritus, and jaundice may develop. Acute bouts of ascending cholangitis may also signal the development of PSC. The disease follows a protracted course of 5 to 17 years, and the severely afflicted patients have the usual symptoms of chronic cholestatic liver disease including steatorrhea. Approximately 25 % of the patients develop cholelithiasis in the dilated ducts. The annual risk of developing cholangiocarcinoma is 0.6 to 1.5 % with a lifetime risk of 20%.

Chronic pancreatitis and chronic cholecystitis from involvement of pancreatic ducts and gallbladder are also seen. A distinctive type of sclerosing cholangitis, with elevated IgG4 levels in association with autoimmune pancreatitis, has been recognized recently. There is no specific medical therapy for PSC. Cholestyramine has been used for pruritus and endoscopic dilation with sphincterotomy or stenting is used for relieving symptoms. Ursodeoxycholic acid has not yet been shown to be effective. Liver transplantation is the definitive treatment for persons with end-stage liver disease.

KEY CONCEPTS

Cholestatic Diseases

- **Cholestasis** occurs with impaired bile flow, leading to accumulation of bile pigment in the hepatic parenchyma. Causes include mechanical or inflammatory obstruction or destruction of the bile ducts or by metabolic defects in hepatocyte bile secretion.
- **Large bile duct obstruction** is most commonly associated with gallstones and malignancies involving the head of the pancreas. Chronic obstruction can lead to cirrhosis. Ascending cholangitis may develop.
- **Cholestasis in sepsis** may arise through direct effects of intrahepatic bacterial infection, ischemia relating to hypotension caused by sepsis, or in response to circulating microbial products.
- **Primary hepatolithiasis** is a disorder of *intrahepatic* gallstone formation, most common in East Asia, that

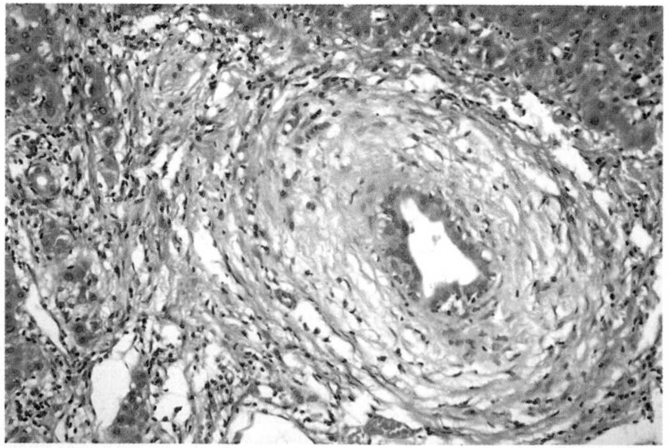

Figure 18-39 Primary sclerosing cholangitis. A degenerating bile duct is entrapped in a dense, "onion-skin" concentric scar.

leads to repeated bouts of ascending cholangitis and inflammatory parenchymal destruction. It predisposes to cholangiocarcinoma.

- **Neonatal cholestasis** is not a specific entity; it is variously associated with cholangiopathies such as primarily *biliary atresia* and a variety of inherited or acquired disorders causing conjugated hyperbilirubinemia in the neonate, collectively referred to as *neonatal hepatitis*.
- **Primary biliary cirrhosis** is an autoimmune disease with progressive, inflammatory, often granulomatous, destruction of small to medium sized intrahepatic bile ducts.
  - Primary biliary cirrhosis occurs most often in middle aged women, is associated with autoantibodies (particularly AMA), and with other autoimmune diseases such as Sjögren syndrome and Hashimoto thyroiditis.
- **Primary sclerosing cholangitis** is an autoimmune disease with progressive inflammatory and sclerosing destruction of bile ducts of all sizes, intrahepatic and extrahepatic; diagnosis is made not by biopsy, but by radiologic imaging of the biliary tree. It occurs most often in younger men and has strong associations with inflammatory bowel disease, particularly ulcerative colitis.

Structural Anomalies of the Biliary Tree

Choledochal Cysts

Choledochal cysts are congenital dilations of the common bile duct. They present most often in children before age 10 as jaundice and/or recurrent abdominal pain, symptoms that are typical of biliary colic. Approximately 20% of cases become symptomatic only in adulthood. In some cases choledochal cysts occur in conjunction with cystic dilation of the intrahepatic biliary tree (Caroli disease, discussed later). The female-to-male ratio is 3:1 to 4:1. These uncommon cysts may take the form of segmental or cylindric dilation of the common bile duct, diverticula of the extrahepatic ducts, or choledochoceles, which are cystic lesions that protrude into the duodenal lumen. Choledochal cysts predispose to stone formation, stenosis and stricture, pancreatitis, and obstructive biliary complications within the liver. In older patients the risk of bile duct carcinoma is elevated.

Fibropolycystic Disease

Fibropolycystic disease of the liver is a heterogeneous group of lesions in which the primary abnormalities are congenital malformations of the biliary tree. Lesions may be found incidentally during radiographic studies, surgery, or at autopsy. The most severe forms of fibropolycystic disease may become manifest as hepatosplenomegaly or portal hypertension in the absence of hepatic dysfunction, starting in late childhood or adolescence. Three sets of pathologic findings may be seen, sometimes overlapping with each other:

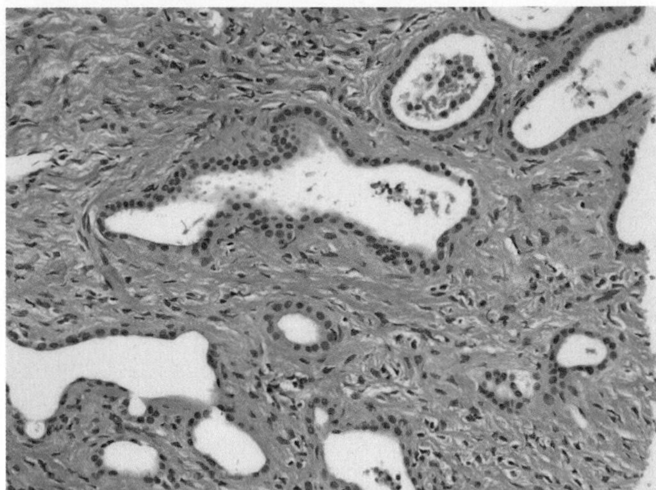

Figure 18-40 Von Meyenburg complex. This bile duct hamartoma is always associated with portal tracts. Note the dilated and irregularly shaped bile ducts.

- *Von Meyenburg complexes* are small bile duct hamartomas (Fig. 18-40). Occasional von Meyenburg complexes are common in otherwise normal individuals. When they are diffuse they signal the underlying, more clinically important fibropolycystic disease.
- *Single or multiple, intrahepatic or extrahepatic biliary cysts.* When present in isolation these may be symptomatic due to ascending cholangitis and are referred to as *Caroli disease*. When biliary cysts occur along with congenital hepatic fibrosis, the term *Caroli syndrome* is used (Fig. 18-41). Ducts may be cystically dilated, but true cysts are also present. These may be intrahepatic cysts or choledochal cysts, as already described.
- In *congenital hepatic fibrosis*, portal tracts are enlarged by irregular, broad bands of collagenous tissue, forming septa that divide the liver into irregular islands. Variable numbers of abnormally shaped bile ducts are embedded in the fibrous tissue, although they remain in continuity with the biliary tree (Fig. 18-42). Individuals

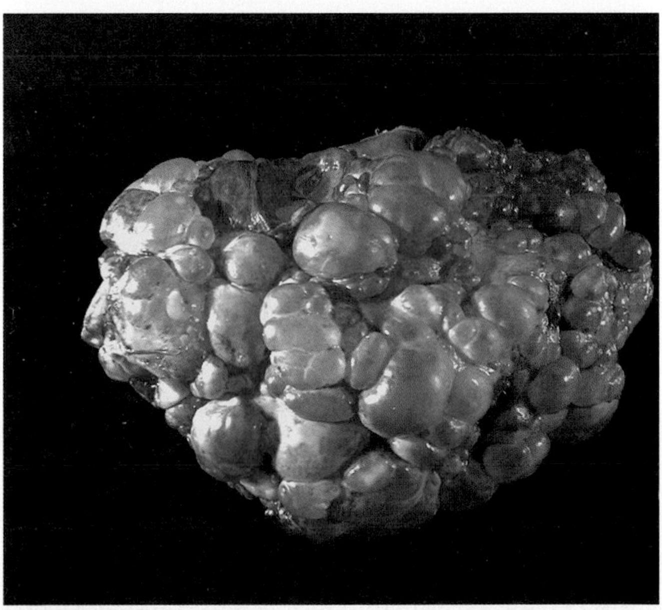

Figure 18-41 Congenital hepatic fibrosis with multiple biliary cysts.

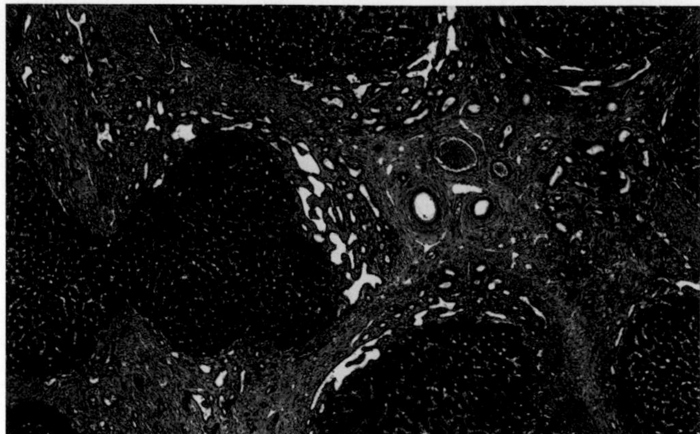

Figure 18-42 Congenital hepatic fibrosis. Broad bands of stroma are seen coursing through this liver, which is involved by a variant of fibropolycystic disease. Note the dilated remnants of ductal plates along the margins of the stroma. The intervening parenchyma is comprised of relatively normal parenchyma (Masson Trichrome stain).

with congenital hepatic fibrosis are not truly cirrhotic, despite the serpiginous scarring separating the hepatic parenchyma, but they may still face complications of portal hypertension, particularly bleeding varices.

All of these lesions are related to abnormal development of the biliary tree representing *ductal plate malformations* associated with persistence of the periportal ductal plates from fetal development. The caliber of involved portal tracts determines the different size, morphology, and distributions of lesions. Fibropolycystic liver disease often occurs with autosomal recessive polycystic renal disease. The involved gene encodes a protein called polycystin which is expressed in fetal kidney as well as liver (Chapter 20). Persons with fibropolycystic liver disease have an increased risk for cholangiocarcinoma.

Circulatory Disorders

Given the enormous flow of blood through the liver, it is not surprising that circulatory disturbances have considerable impact on the liver. In most instances, however, clinically significant liver function abnormalities do not develop, but hepatic morphology may be strikingly affected. These disorders can be grouped according to whether blood flow into, through, or from the liver is impaired (Fig. 18-43).

Impaired Blood Flow into the Liver

Hepatic Artery Compromise

Liver infarcts are rare, thanks to the double blood supply to the liver. Nonetheless, thrombosis or compression of an intrahepatic branch of the hepatic artery by embolism (Fig. 18-44), neoplasia, polyarteritis nodosa (Chapter 11), or sepsis may result in a localized infarct that is either pale and anemic or hemorrhagic if there is suffusion with portal blood. Interruption of the main hepatic artery does not always produce ischemic necrosis of the organ, particularly if the liver is otherwise normal. Retrograde arterial flow through accessory vessels, when coupled with the portal venous supply, is usually sufficient to sustain the liver parenchyma. The one exception is hepatic artery thrombosis in a transplanted liver, which generally leads to infarction of the major ducts of the biliary tree, since their blood supply is entirely arterial.

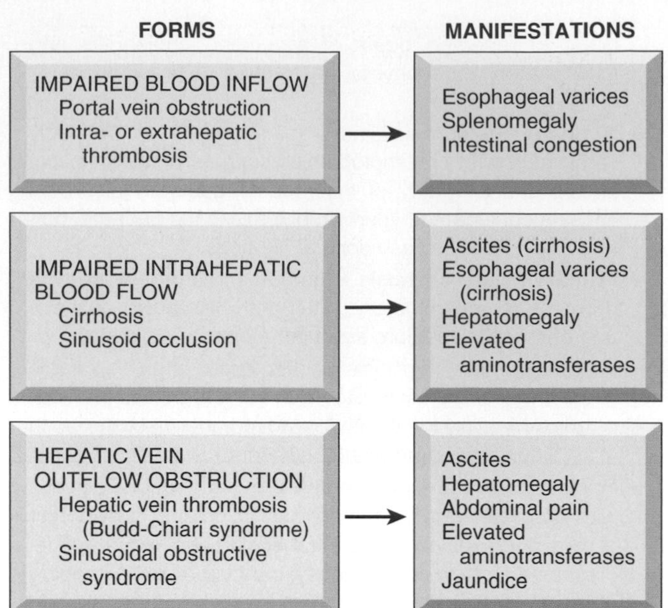

FORMS	MANIFESTATIONS
IMPAIRED BLOOD INFLOW Portal vein obstruction Intra- or extrahepatic thrombosis	Esophageal varices Splenomegaly Intestinal congestion
IMPAIRED INTRAHEPATIC BLOOD FLOW Cirrhosis Sinusoid occlusion	Ascites (cirrhosis) Esophageal varices (cirrhosis) Hepatomegaly Elevated aminotransferases
HEPATIC VEIN OUTFLOW OBSTRUCTION Hepatic vein thrombosis (Budd-Chiari syndrome) Sinusoidal obstructive syndrome	Ascites Hepatomegaly Abdominal pain Elevated aminotransferases Jaundice

Figure 18-43 Forms and clinical manifestations of hepatic circulatory disorders.

Portal Vein Obstruction and Thrombosis

Blockage of the extrahepatic portal vein may be insidious and well tolerated or may be a catastrophic and potentially lethal event; most cases fall somewhere in between. Occlusive disease of the portal vein or its major radicles typically produces abdominal pain and, in most instances, other manifestations of portal hypertension, principally esophageal varices that are prone to rupture. Ascites is not common (because the block is presinusoidal), but when present is often massive and intractable.

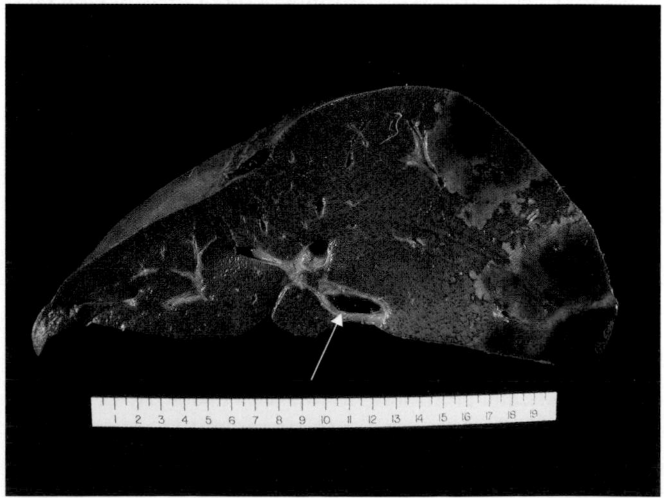

Figure 18-44 Liver infarct. A thrombus is lodged in a peripheral branch of the hepatic artery (arrow) and compresses the adjacent portal vein; the distal hepatic tissue is pale, with a hemorrhagic margin.

Extrahepatic portal vein obstruction may be may idiopathic (approximately one-third of cases) or may arise from the following conditions:

- Subclinical occlusion of the portal vein, from neonatal umbilical sepsis or umbilical vein catheterization, presenting as variceal bleeding and ascites years later.
- Intraabdominal sepsis, caused by acute diverticulitis or appendicitis, leading to pyelophlebitis in the splanchnic circulation
- Inherited or acquired hypercoagulable disorders, including those arising in myeloproliferative disorders such as polycythemia vera (Chapter 13)
- Trauma, surgical or otherwise
- Pancreatitis and pancreatic cancer that initiate splenic vein thrombosis, which propagates into the portal vein
- Invasion of the portal vein by hepatocellular carcinoma
- Cirrhosis, which is associated with portal vein thrombosis in about 25% of patients. Many such patients have an underlying thrombophilic genotype

Intrahepatic portal vein radicles may be obstructed by acute thrombosis. The thrombosis does not cause ischemic infarction but instead results in a sharply demarcated area of red-blue discoloration called *infarct of Zahn*. There is no necrosis, only severe hepatocellular atrophy and marked stasis in distended sinusoids.

Small portal vein branch diseases include a variety of pathogenetically distinct conditions that are characterized by noncirrhotic portal hypertension with portal fibrosis and obliteration of small portal vein branches. *The most common cause of small portal vein branch obstruction is schistosomiasis;* the eggs of the parasites lodge in and obstruct the smallest portal vein branches. The other diseases in this group are now collectively referred to as *obliterative portal venopathy*, although regional and clinical differences suggest several related but independent diseases. In India, non cirrhotic portal fibrosis has been reported to account for approximately 23 % of cases of portal hypertension but the incidence seems to be declining. The patients often present with upper gastrointestinal bleeding. In East Asia, particularly Japan, there is a female predominance and patients present with splenomegaly, often in association with rheumatologic diseases. The disease is seen in untreated HIV disease and in those being treated with anti-retroviral therapy, in whom it may represent a complication of treatment. Liver transplantation may be necessary to avoid fatal sequelae of the portal hypertension in all these forms.

Impaired Blood Flow Through the Liver

The most common intrahepatic cause of blood flow obstruction is cirrhosis, as described earlier. In addition, physical sinusoidal occlusion occurs in a small group of diseases: *sickle cell disease* (Fig. 18-45), *disseminated intravascular coagulation*, *eclampsia* (discussed later), and diffuse intrasinusoidal *metastatic tumor*. In all of these, obstruction of blood flow may lead to massive necrosis of hepatocytes and acute hepatic failure.

Peliosis hepatis is a peculiar form of sinusoidal dilation that occurs in any condition in which efflux of hepatic blood is impeded. The liver contains blood-filled cystic spaces, either unlined or lined with sinusoidal endothelial cells. The pathogenesis of peliosis hepatis is unknown.

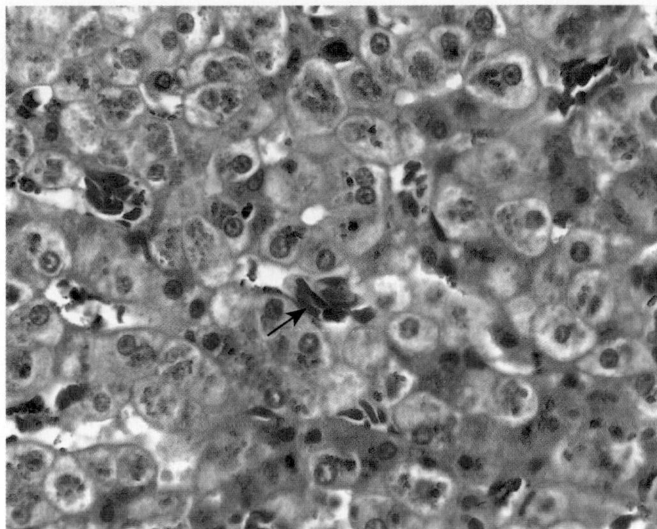

Figure 18-45 Sickle cell crisis in liver. The photomicrograph shows several sinusoids containing "sickled" red cells *(arrow)*.

Bartonella species have been seen in the sinusoidal endothelial cells in AIDS-associated peliosis, but peliosis is also seen in cancer, tuberculosis, and posttransplantation immunodeficiency. Sex hormone administration (e.g., anabolic steroids, oral contraceptives, danazol) sometimes causes peliosis as well. While clinical signs are generally absent, potentially fatal intraabdominal hemorrhage or hepatic failure may occur. Lesions usually disappear after correction of the underlying causes.

Hepatic Venous Outflow Obstruction

Hepatic Vein Thrombosis

The obstruction of two or more major hepatic veins produces liver enlargement, pain, and ascites, a condition known as Budd-Chiari syndrome. Obstruction of a single main hepatic vein by thrombosis is clinically silent. Hepatic damage is the consequence of increased intrahepatic blood pressure. Hepatic vein thrombosis is associated with myeloproliferative disorders such as polycythemia vera (Chapter 13), inherited disorders of coagulation (Chapter 4), antiphospholipid antibody syndrome, paroxysmal nocturnal hemoglobinuria (Chapter 14), and intraabdominal cancers, particularly hepatocellular carcinoma. In pregnancy or with oral contraceptive use, it occurs through interaction with an underlying thrombogenic disorder.

MORPHOLOGY

In the Budd-Chiari syndrome, the liver is swollen and red-purple and has a tense capsule (Fig. 18-46). There may be differential areas of hemorrhagic collapse alternating with areas of preserved or regenerating parenchyma, the patterns are dependent on which small and large hepatic veins are obstructed. Microscopically the affected hepatic parenchyma reveals severe centrilobular congestion and necrosis. Centrilobular fibrosis develops in instances in which the thrombosis is more slowly developing. The major veins may contain totally occlusive fresh thrombi, subtotal occlusion, or, in chronic cases, organized adherent thrombi.

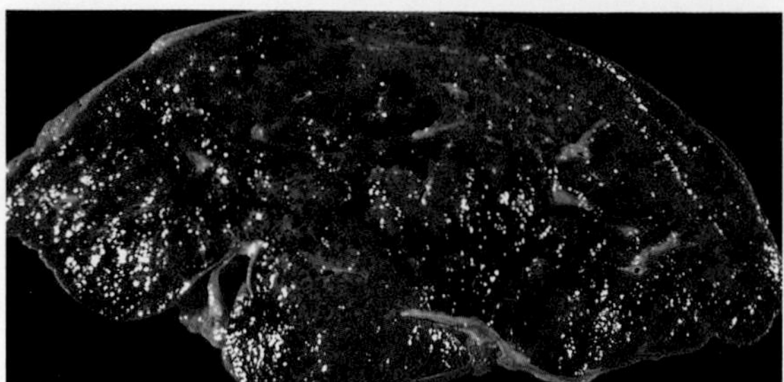

Figure 18-46 Budd-Chiari syndrome. Thrombosis of the major hepatic veins has caused hemorrhagic liver necrosis.

The mortality of untreated acute hepatic vein thrombosis is high. Prompt surgical creation of a portosystemic venous shunt permits reverse flow through the portal vein and improves the prognosis. The chronic form is far less lethal, and more than two thirds of patients are alive after 5 years.

Sinusoidal Obstruction Syndrome

Originally described in Jamaican drinkers of pyrrolizidine alkaloid–containing bush tea and named *veno-occlusive disease*, the disease is now called *sinusoidal obstruction syndrome*. It now occurs primarily in two settings: (1) following allogeneic hematopoietic stem cell transplantation, usually within the first 3 weeks; (2) in cancer patients receiving chemotherapy. The mortality rates can be higher than 30%.

Pathogenesis. **Sinusoidal obstruction syndrome arises from toxic injury to the sinusoidal endothelium.** Injured, sloughed endothelium obstructs sinusoidal blood flow. Erythrocytes enter into the space of Disse followed by necrosis of perivenular hepatocytes and downstream accumulation of cellular debris in the terminal hepatic vein.

MORPHOLOGY

Sinusoidal obstruction syndrome is characterized by obliteration of the terminal hepatic venules by subendothelial swelling and collagen deposition. In acute disease, there is centrilobular congestion, hepatocellular necrosis, and accumulation of hemosiderin-laden macrophages. As the disease progresses, obliteration of the lumen of the venule is easily identified with special stains for connective tissue (Fig. 18-47). In chronic or healed sinusoidal obstruction syndrome, fibrous obliteration of the venule may follow.

Although histology is the gold standard for diagnosis, in typical settings, diagnosis is frequently made on clinical grounds (tender hepatomegaly, ascites, weight gain, and jaundice), because of the high risk associated with liver biopsy. Early results suggest that treatment with anticoagulants and ursodeoxycholate may lower the incidence and severity of sinusoidal obstruction syndrome in patients undergoing hematopoieitic stem cell transplantation.

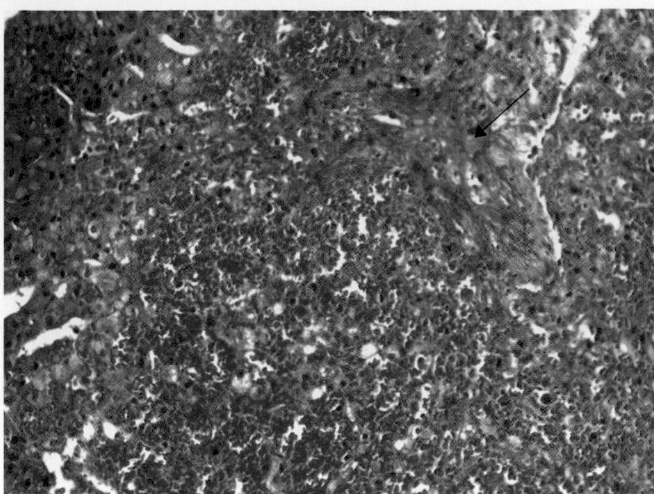

Figure 18-47 Sinusoidal obstruction syndrome. Collagen stain reveals marked sinusoidal congestion, hepatocyte atrophy and loss, and organizing thrombus within the vein lumen (arrow). (Masson trichrome stain.)

Passive Congestion and Centrilobular Necrosis

These hepatic manifestations of systemic circulatory compromise—passive congestion and centrilobular necrosis—are considered together because they represent a morphologic continuum. Both changes are commonly seen at autopsy because there is an element of preterminal circulatory failure with virtually every nontraumatic death. Components of both left and right sided heart failure can contribute to the injury variably in different clinical settings and with different forms of possibly underlying cardiac disease.

MORPHOLOGY

Right-sided cardiac decompensation leads to passive congestion of the liver. The liver is slightly enlarged, tense, and cyanotic, with rounded edges. Microscopically there is **congestion of centrilobular sinusoids.** With time, centrilobular hepatocytes become atrophic, resulting in markedly attenuated liver cell plates. Left-sided cardiac failure or shock may lead to hepatic hypoperfusion and hypoxia, causing ischemic coagulative necrosis of hepatocytes in the central region of the lobule (centrilobular necrosis). In most instances the only clinical evidence of centrilobular necrosis or its variants is transient elevation of serum aminotransferases, but the parenchymal damage may be sufficient to induce mild to moderate jaundice.

The combination of hypoperfusion and retrograde congestion acts synergistically to cause centrilobular hemorrhagic necrosis. The liver takes on a variegated mottled appearance, reflecting hemorrhage and necrosis in the centrilobular regions (Fig. 18-48*A*). This finding is known as **nutmeg liver** due to its resemblance to the cut surface of a nutmeg.

By microscopy there is a sharp demarcation of viable periportal and necrotic or atrophic pericentral hepatocytes, with suffusion of blood through the centrilobular region (Fig. 18-48*B*). Uncommonly, with sustained chronic severe congestive heart failure, **cardiac sclerosis** develops with centrilobular fibrosis, sometimes with central-central linking fibrous septa.

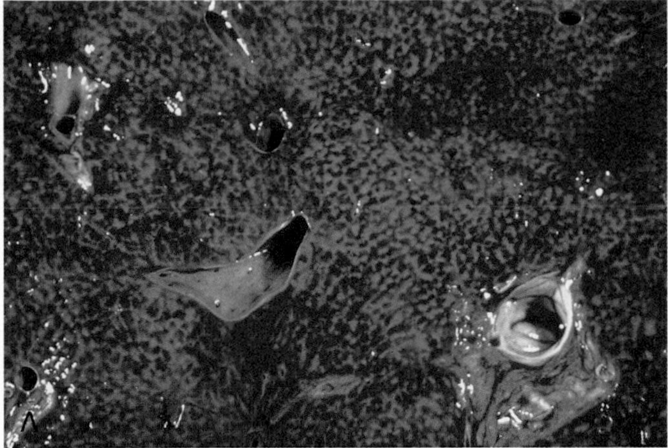

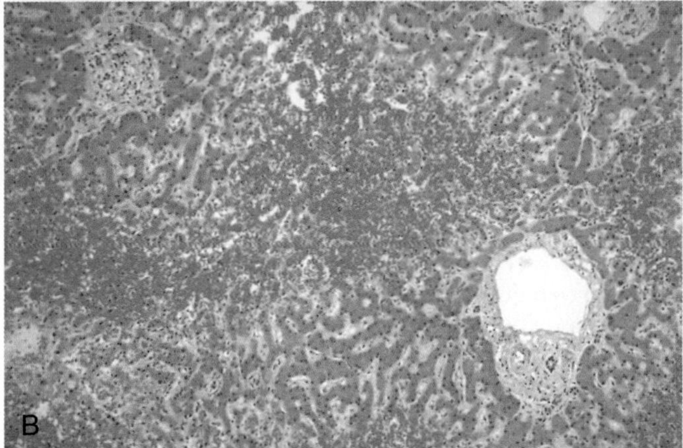

Figure 18-48 Acute passive congestion ("nutmeg liver"). **A,** The cut surface of the liver has a variegated mottled red appearance, representing congestion and hemorrhage in the centrilobular regions of the parenchyma. **B,** On microscopic examination, the centrilobular region is suffused with red blood cells and atrophied hepatocytes are not easily seen. Portal tracts and the periportal parenchyma are intact.

KEY CONCEPTS

Circulatory Disorders

- Circulatory disorders of the liver can be caused by impaired blood inflow, defects in intrahepatic blood flow, and obstruction of blood outflow.
- Portal vein obstruction by intrahepatic or extrahepatic thrombosis may cause portal hypertension, esophageal varices, and ascites.
- The most common cause of impaired intrahepatic blood flow is cirrhosis.
- Obstructions of blood outflow include hepatic vein thrombosis (Budd-Chiari syndrome) and sinusoidal obstruction syndrome, previously known as veno-occlusive disease.

Hepatic Complications of Organ or Hematopoietic Stem Cell Transplantation

The use of transplantation for bone marrow, renal, hepatic and other organ disorders has generated a challenging group of hepatic complications. Although the clinical settings are obviously different for each patient population, defined by underlying disease and the organ transplanted, the common themes of toxic or immunologically mediated liver damage, opportunistic infection of immunosuppressed hosts, recurrent disease, and posttransplant lymphoproliferative disorder are shared by all.

Graft-Versus-Host Disease and Liver Graft Rejection

The liver has the unenviable position of being attacked by graft-versus-host and host-versus-graft mechanisms, in the setting of bone marrow transplantation and liver transplantation, respectively. These processes are discussed in detail in Chapter 6. More than other solid organs, liver transplants are reasonably well tolerated by recipients. That being said, the hepatic morphologic features that are peculiar to immunological attack after transplantation deserve comment.

MORPHOLOGY

Liver damage after hematopoietic stem cell transplantation is the consequence of acute or chronic **graft-versus-host disease.** In acute graft-versus-host disease, which occurs 10 to 50 days after hematopoietic stem cell transplantation, donor lymphocytes attack the epithelial cells of the liver. This results in hepatitis with necrosis of hepatocytes and bile duct epithelial cells, and inflammation of the parenchyma and portal tracts. In chronic hepatic graft-versus-host disease (usually more than 100 days after transplantation), there is portal tract inflammation, selective bile duct destruction, and eventual fibrosis. Portal vein and hepatic vein radicles may show endothelitis with subendothelial lymphocytes lifting the endothelium from its basement membrane. Cholestasis may be observed in both acute and chronic graft-versus-host disease.

In **transplanted livers, acute (cellular) rejection** is characterized by infiltration of a mixed portal inflammatory infiltrated associated with bile duct injury and endothelitis (Fig. 18-49). With **chronic rejection** an obliterative arteriopathy of small and large arteries leads to ischemic changes in the liver parenchyma. This includes destruction of bile ducts both by immunologic attack and interruption of blood flow; the resulting **vanishing bile duct syndrome** often requires retransplantation.

Hepatic Disease Associated with Pregnancy

Hepatic diseases may occur in women with chronic liver disease who become pregnant, or develop during pregnancy in women who were not affected by liver disease. Abnormal liver tests occur in 3% to 5% of pregnancies. Viral hepatitis (HAV, HBV, HCV, or HBV + HDV) is the most common cause of jaundice in pregnancy. While these women require careful clinical management, pregnancy does not specifically alter the course of the liver disease. The one exception is HEV infection, which, for unknown reasons, runs a more severe course in pregnant patients, with fatality approaching 20%.

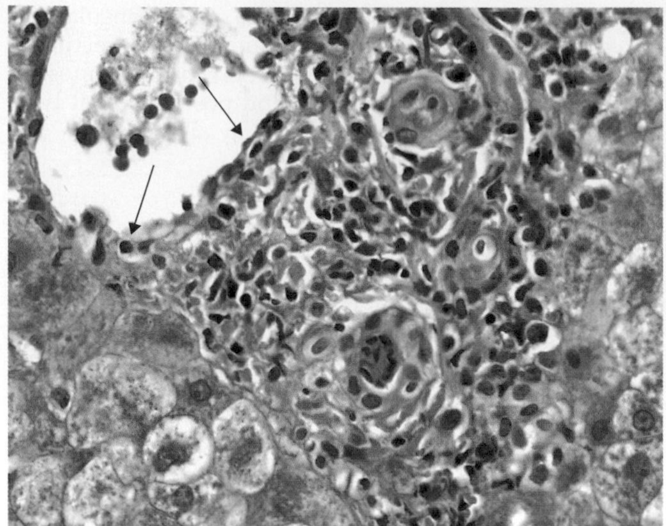

Figure 18-49 Transplanted liver with acute cellular rejection. Note the mixed inflammatory cell infiltration including eosinophils in portal tracts, bile duct damage, and endotheliitis. Arrows show subendothelial lymphocytes.

In a very small subgroup of pregnant women (0.1%), hepatic complications develop that are directly attributable to pregnancy. These disorders include preeclampsia and eclampsia, acute fatty liver of pregnancy, and intrahepatic cholestasis of pregnancy. In extreme cases, eclampsia and acute fatty liver of pregnancy may be fatal.

Preeclampsia and Eclampsia

Preeclampsia affects 3% to 5% of pregnancies and is characterized by maternal hypertension, proteinuria, peripheral edema, and coagulation abnormalities (Chapter 22). When hyperreflexia and convulsions occur, the condition is called *eclampsia* and may be life-threatening. Alternatively, subclinical hepatic disease may be the primary manifestation of preeclampsia, as part of a syndrome of *h*emolysis, *e*levated *l*iver enzymes, and *l*ow *p*latelets, dubbed the *HELLP syndrome*.

MORPHOLOGY

In preeclampsia, the periportal sinusoids contain fibrin deposits associated with hemorrhage into the space of Disse, leading to periportal hepatocellular coagulative necrosis. Blood under pressure may coalesce and expand to form a hepatic hematoma; dissection of blood under Glisson capsule may lead to catastrophic hepatic rupture in eclampsia (Fig. 18-50). Patients with hepatic involvement in preeclampsia may show modest to severe elevation of serum aminotransferases and mild elevation of serum bilirubin. Hepatic dysfunction sufficient to cause a coagulopathy signifies far advanced and potentially lethal disease. Mild cases may be managed conservatively. Termination of pregnancy is required in severe cases. Women who survive mild or severe preeclampsia recover without sequelae.

Acute Fatty Liver of Pregnancy

Acute fatty liver of pregnancy presents with a spectrum of disorders ranging from subclinical or modest hepatic dysfunction (evidenced by elevated serum aminotransferase levels) to hepatic failure, coma, and death. It is a rare disease affecting 1 in 13,000 deliveries. Affected women present in the latter half of pregnancy, usually in the third trimester. Symptoms are directly attributable to incipient hepatic failure, including bleeding, nausea and vomiting, jaundice, and coma. In 20% to 40% of cases, the presenting symptoms may be those of coexistent preeclampsia.

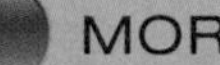

MORPHOLOGY

The diagnosis of acute fatty liver of pregnancy rests on biopsy identification of the characteristic diffuse microvesicular steatosis of hepatocytes. In severe cases there may be lobular disarray with hepatocyte dropout, reticulin collapse, and portal tract inflammation, making distinction from viral hepatitis difficult.

While this condition most commonly runs a mild course, women with acute fatty liver of pregnancy can progress within days to hepatic failure and death. The primary treatment is termination of the pregnancy. The pathogenesis of this disease is unknown, but mitochondrial dysfunction has been implicated. In a subset of patients, both mother and father carry a heterozygous deficiency in mitochondrial long-chain 3-hydroxyacyl coenzyme A (CoA) dehydrogenase. The homozygous-deficient fetuses fare well during pregnancy but cause hepatic dysfunction in the mother, because long-chain 3-hydroxylacyl metabolites produced by the fetus or placenta enter the maternal circulation and cause hepatic toxicity. This is a rare instance of the fetus causing metabolic disease in the mother.

Intrahepatic Cholestasis of Pregnancy

The onset of pruritus in the third trimester, followed in some cases (10-25%) by darkening of the urine and occasionally light stools and jaundice, heralds the development of this enigmatic syndrome. Serum bilirubin (mostly conjugated) rarely exceeds 5 mg/dL; alkaline phosphatase may be slightly elevated. The level of bile salts is increased greatly. The altered hormonal state of pregnancy seems to combine with biliary defects in the secretion of bile salts or sulfated progesterone metabolites to engender cholestasis.

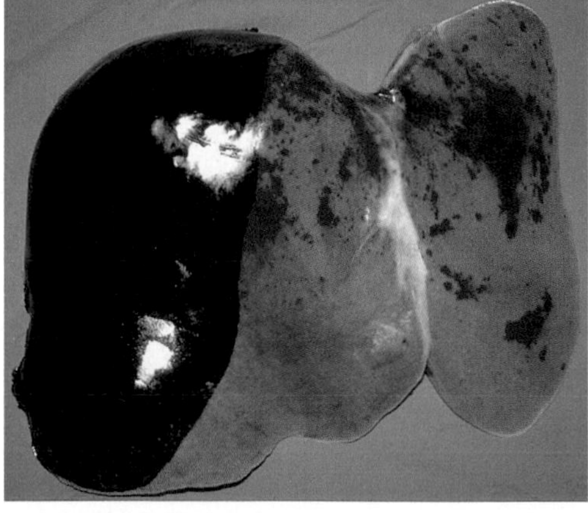

Figure 18-50 Eclampsia. Subcapsular hematoma dissecting under Glisson capsule in a fatal case. (Courtesy Dr. Brian Blackbourne, Office of the Medical Examiner, San Diego, Calif.)

Although this is generally a benign condition, the incidence of fetal distress, stillbirths, and prematurity is modestly increased. Perhaps most importantly, the pruritus resulting from retention of bile salts can be extremely distressing for the pregnant mother.

Nodules and Tumors

Hepatic masses may come to attention for a variety of reasons. They may generate epigastric fullness and discomfort or be detected by routine physical examination or radiographic studies for other indications. Hepatic masses include nodular hyperplasias and true neoplasms.

Nodular Hyperplasias

Solitary or multiple hyperplastic hepatocellular nodules may develop in the noncirrhotic liver. Two such conditions are *focal nodular hyperplasia* and *nodular regenerative hyperplasia.* The common factor in both types of nodules seems to be either focal or diffuse alterations in hepatic blood supply, arising from obliteration of portal vein radicles and compensatory augmentation of arterial blood supply.

MORPHOLOGY

Focal nodular hyperplasia appears as a well-demarcated but poorly encapsulated nodule, ranging up to many centimeters in diameter (Fig. 18-51*A*). It presents as a spontaneous mass lesion in an otherwise normal liver, most frequently in young to middle-aged adults. The lesion is generally lighter than the surrounding liver and is sometimes yellow indicating steatosis. Typically, there is a central gray-white, depressed stellate scar from which fibrous septa radiate to the periphery.

The central scar contains large vessels, usually arterial, that typically show fibromuscular hyperplasia with eccentric or concentric narrowing of the lumen. The radiating septa show variable ductular reactions along septal margins. The parenchyma between septa is comprised of normal hepatocytes separated by thickened sinusoidal plates (Fig. 18-51*B*). The vascular lesion, congenital or acquired, is probably the initiating insult. Resulting areas of hypoperfused parenchyma collapse to become the septa, while hyperperfused regions undergo hyperplasia.

Nodular regenerative hyperplasia denotes a liver entirely transformed into nodules—grossly similar to micronodular cirrhosis—but without fibrosis. Microscopically, plump hepatocytes are surrounded by rims of atrophic hepatocytes. **Nodular regenerative hyperplasia can lead to the development of portal hypertension** and occurs in association with conditions affecting intrahepatic blood flow, including solid-organ (particularly renal) transplantation, hematopoetic stem cell transplantation, and vasculitis. It also occurs in HIV-infected persons and in association with rheumatologic diseases such as SLE. Most such patients are asymptomatic and the condition is found at autopsy.

Benign Neoplasms

Cavernous hemangiomas, blood vessel tumors identical to those occurring elsewhere, are the most common benign liver tumors (Chapter 11). They appear as discrete red-blue, soft nodules, usually less than 2 cm in diameter, generally located directly beneath the capsule. Histologically, the tumor consists of vascular channels in a bed of fibrous connective tissue (Fig. 18-52). Their chief clinical significance is that they might be mistaken radiographically or intraoperatively for metastatic tumors.

Hepatocellular Adenomas

Benign neoplasms developing from hepatocytes are called hepatocellular adenomas (Fig. 18-53). They may be detected incidentally with abdominal imaging or when they cause abdominal pain from their rapid growth, causing pressure on the liver capsule, or following hemorrhagic necrosis as the lesion outstrips its blood supply. Rupture of hepatocellular adenomas may lead to intraabdominal bleeding that is a surgical emergency. Three large subtypes have been defined on the basis of molecular analysis and associated clinical and pathologic findings, each

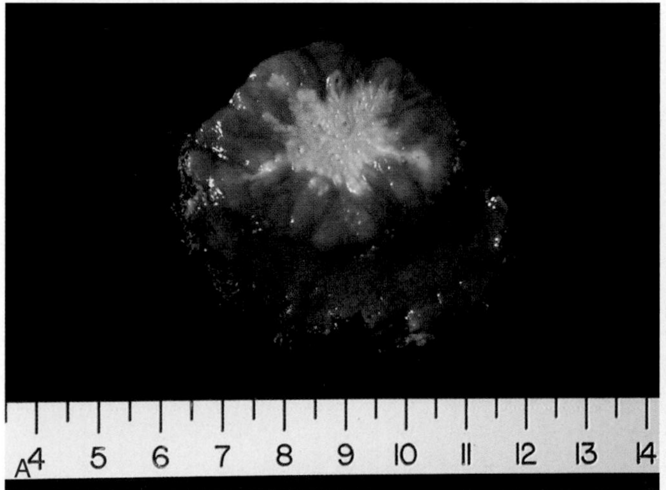

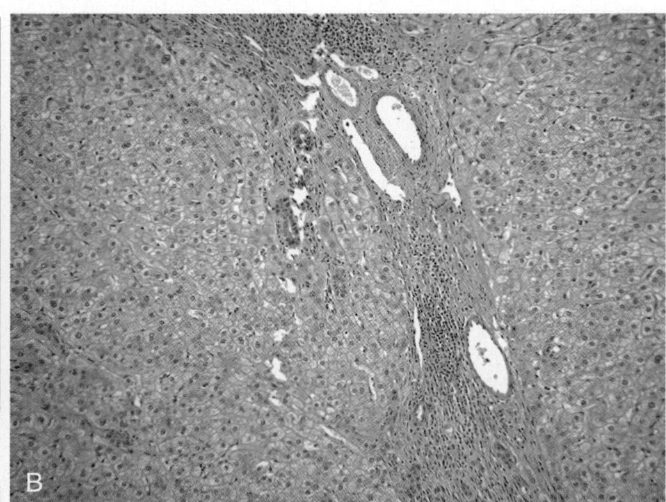

Figure 18-51 Focal nodular hyperplasia. **A,** Resected specimen showing lobulated contours and a central stellate scar. **B,** Low-power micrograph showing a broad fibrous scar with hepatic arterial and bile duct elements and chronic inflammation present within parenchyma that lacks normal architecture due to hepatocyte regeneration.

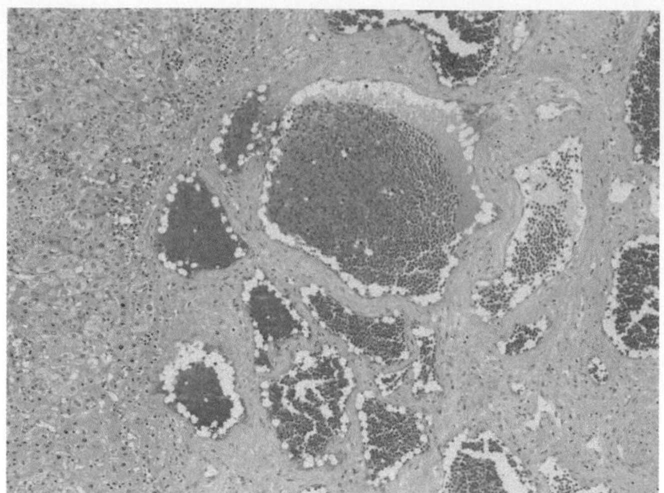

Figure 18-52 Hemangioma. Blood-filled vascular channels separated by a dense fibrous stroma.

with a different relative risk of malignant transformation. Both oral contraceptives and anabolic steroids are associated with the development of these adenomas. In fact before the advent of oral contraceptives, hepatocellular adenomas were virtually unknown. The risk of developing these tumors is increased 30-40 fold in users of oral contraceptives. The highest risk is from prolonged use of estrogen rich oral contraceptives. If surgery is not possible or is ill-advised, cessation of exposure to sex hormones often can lead to full regression.

Pathogenesis. Three large subtypes have been defined on the basis of molecular analysis and associated clinical and pathologic findings, each with a different relative risk of malignant transformation.

HNF1-α Inactivated hepatocellular adenomas. Ninety percent of these tumors have inactivating mutations of HNF1-α that are somatic, while 10% have germline mutations. HNF1-α encodes a transcription factor. Heterozygous germline mutations are responsible for autosomal dominant MODY-3 (maturity onset diabetes of the young, type 3). Patients with MODY-3 who develop hepatocellular adenomas have acquired a second somatic mutation. These lesions are most commonly found in women. Oral contraceptive pills are implicated in some.

β-Catenin Activated Hepatocellular Adenomas. Activating mutations of β-catenin are associated with neoplasia and malignancy in many organs. In the liver they may give rise to hepatocellular adenomas that are considered at very high risk for malignant transformation and should be resected even when asymptomatic. They are associated with oral contraceptive and anabolic steroid use. They are found in men and women.

Inflammatory hepatocellular adenomas. These lesions are found in both men and women and are associated with non-alcoholic fatty liver disease; thus, their incidence seems to be increasing. They have a small but definite risk of malignant transformation and should probably be resected even when asymptomatic. They are characterized by activating mutations in gp130, a co-receptor for IL-6, that lead to constitutive JAK-STAT signaling and overexpression of acute phase reactants, which you will recall are normally upregulated in systemic inflammatory states. As will be discussed later, IL-6 mediated JAK-STAT signaling has also been linked to the pathogenesis of hepatocellular carcinoma, and undoubtedly explains the inflammatory background that characterizes this subtype of hepatocellular adenoma. Ten percent of inflammatory hepatocellular adenomas also have concomitant β-catenin activating mutations and these tumors have a higher risk of malignant transformation.

MORPHOLOGY

The tumors resulting from **HNF1-α mutations** are often fatty and devoid of cellular or architectural atypia. They have almost no risk of malignant transformation. Liver fatty acid binding protein (LFABP), a downstream regulated protein of HNF1-α, is constitutively expressed in all normal hepatocytes, but is

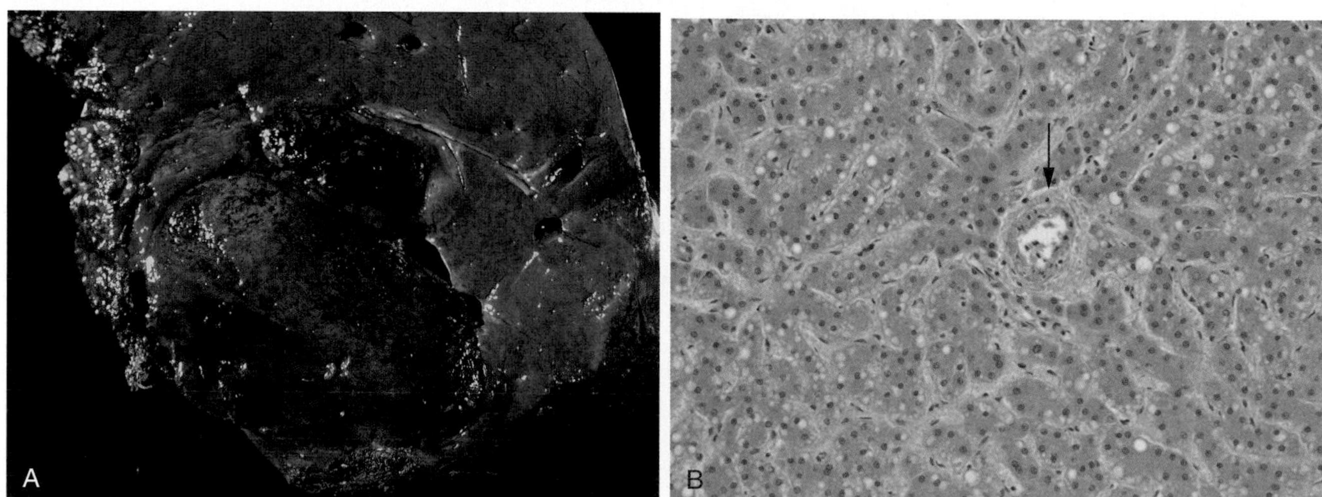

Figure 18-53 Liver cell adenoma. **A,** Resected specimen presenting as a pendulous mass arising from the liver. **B,** Microscopic view showing cords of hepatocytes, with an arterial vascular supply *(arrow)* and no portal tracts.

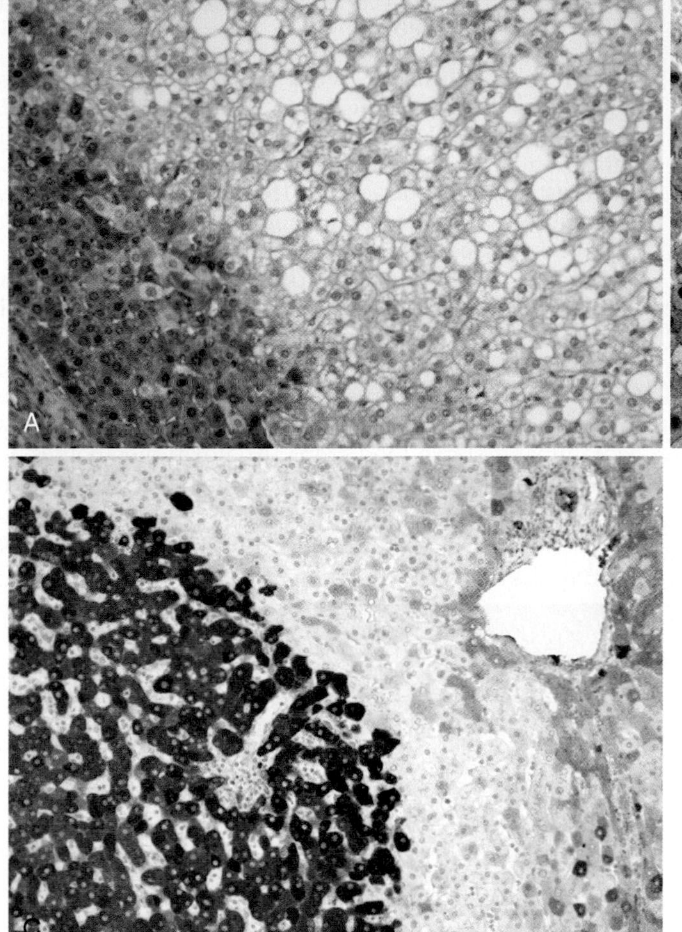

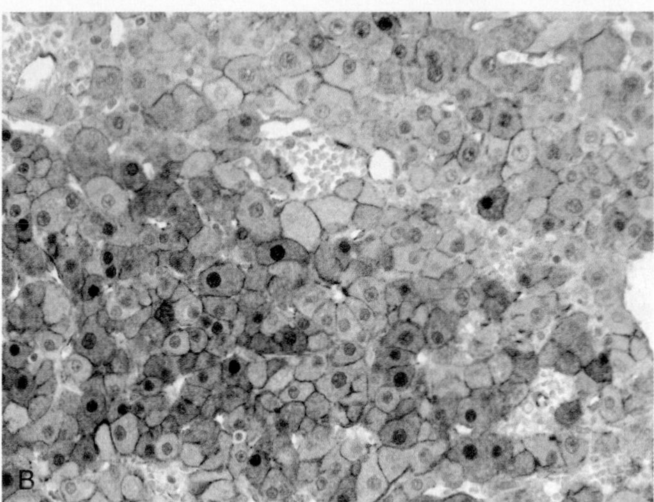

Figure 18-54 Molecular subtypes of hepatocellular adenoma. **A,** HNF1α-inactivated hepatocellular adenoma. Liver fatty acid binding protein (LFABP, expression of which depends on HNF1α) is absent in the tumor by immunostain and present in nearby normal hepatocytes (lower left). **B,** An hepatocellular adenoma with β-catenin mutation. Note nuclear immunostaining for the mutant protein in some tumor hepatocytes (compared to other tumor hepatocytes that maintain normal membranous staining). **C,** Inflammatory hepatocellular adenoma. There is marked up-regulation of C-reactive protein in neoplastic hepatocytes, compared to the highly variable and usually low-level expression in adjacent hepatic parenchyma. (Immunostain with DAB [brown] and hematoxylin counterstain.) (**A,** Courtesy Dr. Valerie Paradis, Beaujon Hospital, Paris, France.)

absent in these tumors due to the inactivating mutation of HNF1-α. Thus, immunostaining for LFABP demonstrating its absence in the tumor is diagnostic of the mutation (Fig. 18-54*A*).

β-Catenin mutated hepatocellular adenomas often have a high degree of cytologic or architectural dysplasia or even overt areas of hepatocellular carcinoma. Immunostain for β-catenin usually shows nuclear translocation indicative of its activated state (Fig. 18-54*B*). This change is diagnostic. Glutamine synthetase, a target of beta-catenin, (normally only positive in perivenular hepatocytes) is also diffusely positive in these tumors, a change that may be seen even when the activating β-catenin mutation doesn't result in nuclear staining. In such tumors, molecular analysis is necessary for definitive confirmation.

Inflammatory hepatocellular adenomas. Unlike the other hepatocellular adenomas, which are comprised of only hepatocytes and vessels with minor amounts of stroma, these lesions characteristically have in addition areas of fibrotic stroma, mononuclear inflammation, ductular reactions, dilated sinusoids, and telangiectatic vessels. Most of these tumors overexpress acute phase reactants such as C-reactive protein and serum amyloid A (Fig. 18-54*C*). These molecules may also be elevated in the serum. 10% of these HCAs that also have β-catenin activating mutations and, as would be anticipated, also show increased nuclear levels of b-catenin by immunohistochemistry.

Malignant Tumors

Malignant tumors occurring in the liver can be primary or metastatic. Most of the discussion in this section deals with primary hepatic tumors. Most primary liver cancers arise from hepatocytes and are termed *hepatocellular carcinoma* (HCC). Much less common are carcinomas of bile duct origin, *cholangiocarcinomas*.

Before embarking on a discussion of the major forms of malignancy affecting the liver, a rare form of primary liver cancer, hepatoblastoma deserves a brief discussion.

Hepatoblastoma

Hepatoblastoma is the most common liver tumor of early childhood. It is rarely occurs over the age of 3 years. Its incidence, which is increasing, is approximately 1 to 2 in 1 million births. Two primary anatomic variants are recognized:

- The *epithelial type*, composed of small polygonal fetal cells or smaller embryonal cells forming acini, tubules, or papillary structures vaguely recapitulating liver development (Fig. 18-55)
- The *mixed epithelial and mesenchymal type*, which contains foci of mesenchymal differentiation that may consist of primitive mesenchyme, osteoid, cartilage, or striated muscle

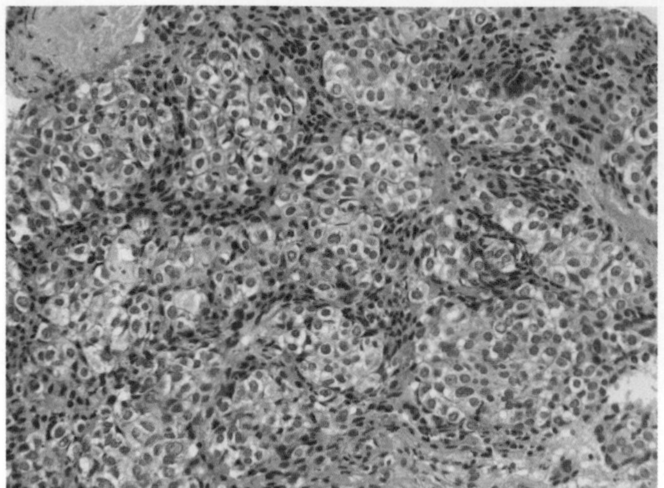

Figure 18-55 Hepatoblastoma. The photograph shows proliferating hepatoblasts consisting mostly of round "epithelial" type cells.

A characteristic feature of hepatoblastomas is the frequent activation of the WNT signaling pathway. This occurs by a variety of mechanisms involving mutations in molecules downstream of WNT signaling, including mutations in APC gene. Patients with Familial adenomatous polyposis frequently develop hepatoblastomas. Sporadic cases have activation of the beta-catenin signaling through other mechanisms. Chromosomal abnormalities are common in hepatoblastomas, and FOXG1, a regulator of the TGF-β pathway, is highly expressed in some tumors. Hepatoblastoma may be associated Beckwith-Wiedemann syndrome as well. The treatment is sugical resection and chemotherapy. Untreated, the tumor is usually fatal within a few years, but therapy has raised the 5-year survival to 80%.

Hepatocellular Carcinoma (HCC)

Worldwide, HCC (also known erroneously as *hepatoma*) accounts for approximately 5.4% of all cancers, but its incidence varies widely in different parts of the world. *More than 85% of cases occur in countries with high rates of chronic HBV infection.* The highest incidences of HCC are found in Asian countries (southeast China, Korea, Taiwan) and sub-Saharan African countries. In these locales, HBV is transmitted vertically and, as already discussed, the carrier state starts in infancy. The peak incidence of HCC in these areas is between 20 and 40 years of age, and in almost 50% of cases, the tumor appears in the absence of cirrhosis. As discussed later, many of these populations are exposed to aflatoxin, which is also a carcinogen (Chapter 7). The risk of HCC is decreasing in China, Singapore and Hong Kong, most likely due to institution of hepatitis B vaccination.

In Western counties, the incidence of HCC is rapidly increasing, largely owing to the hepatitis C epidemic. It tripled in the United States in recent decades, but it is still eightfold to 30-fold lower than the incidence in some Asian countries. In Western populations, HCC rarely manifests before the age of 60, and, in almost 90% of cases, the malignancy emerges after cirrhosis becomes established. There is a pronounced male preponderance throughout the world, about 3:1 in low-incidence areas and as high as 8:1 in high incidence areas. The reason for the gender imbalance is not known. Worldwide, liver cell cancer is the fifth leading cause of death in males.

Pathogenesis. **Chronic liver diseases are the most common setting for emergence of HCC.** While usually identified in a background of cirrhosis, cirrhosis per se is not a premalignant lesion. Indeed, cirrhosis is not required for hepatocarcinogenesis (Fig. 18-56). Rather, progression to cirrhosis and hepatocarcinogenesis take place *in parallel* over years to decades.

The most important underlying factors in hepatocarcinogenesis are viral infections (HBV, HCV) and toxic injuries (aflatoxin, alcohol). Thus where HBV and HCV are endemic, there is a very high incidence of HCC. Co-infection further increases risk. In Africa and Asia, aflatoxin, produced by *Aspergillus* species, is a mycotoxin that contaminates staple food crops. Aflatoxin metabolites are present in the urine of affected individuals as are aflatoxin-albumin adducts in serum. This helps to identify the populations at risk and confirm the important influence of

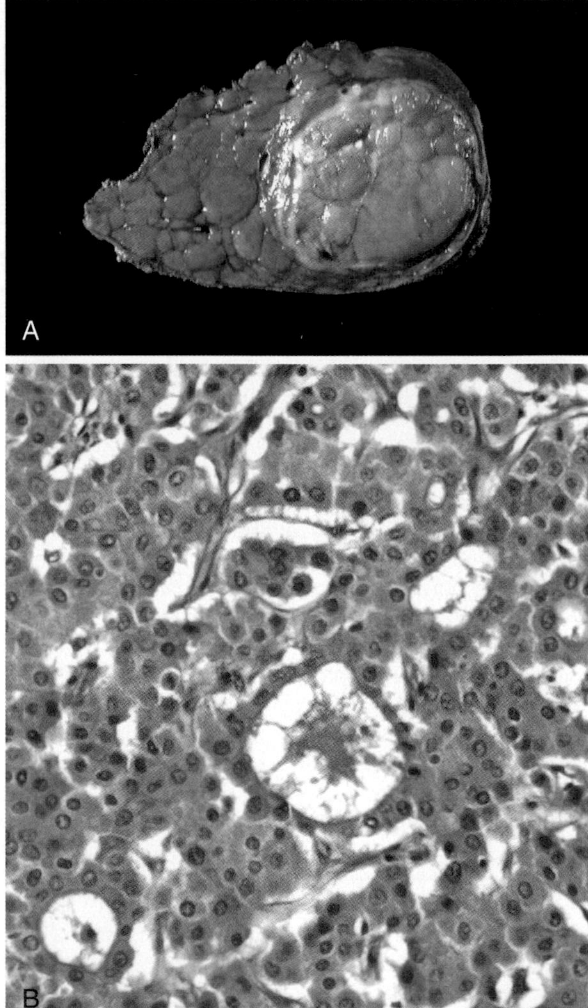

Figure 18-56 Hepatocellular carcinoma. **A,** Liver removed at autopsy showing a unifocal neoplasm replacing most of the right hepatic lobe. **B,** Malignant hepatocytes growing in distorted versions of normal architecture, including large pseudoacinar spaces (malformed, dilated bile canaliculi) and thickened hepatocyte trabeculae.

aflatoxin for hepatocarcinogenesis. Aflatoxin also synergizes with HBV (perhaps also with HCV) to increase risk further. Alcohol is another toxin which probably, by itself, is a risk factor for HCC, but it also synergizes with HBV and HCV, and even, possibly, cigarette smoking.

Metabolic diseases such as hereditary hemochromatosis and α_1AT deficiency markedly increase the risk of HCC. Wilson disease probably does so with much less frequency. Of probably greater import is the metabolic syndrome associated with obesity, diabetes mellitus, and nonalcoholic fatty liver disease, all of which increase the risk of HCC.

No single, universal sequence of molecular or genetic alterations leads to emergence of HCC. *Activation of β-catenin and inactivation of p53 are the two most common early mutational events.* Activating β-catenin mutations are identified in up to 40% of persons with HCC. These tumors are more likely to be unrelated to HBV and to demonstrate genetic instability. Inactivation of p53 is present in up to 60% of HCC cases. These tumors are strongly associated with aflatoxin. Neither of these alterations, however, is found in premalignant lesions.

Recent evidence has provided some novel insights into the role of HBV, HCV, alcoholic liver disease and other states of chronic inflammation in the pathogenesis of HCC. Traditional thinking has been that cycles of cell death and regeneration in chronic inflammatory states increases the risk of mutations in regenerating hepatocytes. But the precise molecular mechanisms of such changes have remained obscure. More recent studies implicate a role for signaling through the IL-6/JAK/STAT pathway in the causation of HCC. IL-6 is an inflammatory cytokine that is overproduced in many chronic hepatitides. Based on some preliminary experiments, it has been proposed that IL-6 can suppress hepatocyte differentiation and promote their proliferation by regulating the function of the transcription factor HNF4-α. In keeping with this, hepatic carcinogenesis can be suppressed by uncoupling HNF4-α from the control of IL-6, in experimental animals. More studies are needed to determine the significance of IL-6/HNF4-α signaling axis in human HCC.

Precursor Lesions of HCC

Several cellular and nodular precursor lesions to HCC have been identified (Table 18-12). Hepatocellular adenoma has already been discussed, in particular those with β-catenin activating mutations. In chronic liver disease there are cellular dysplasias, called *large cell change* and *small cell change* (Fig. 18-57). These may be found at any stage of chronic liver disease, before or after development of cirrhosis, and serve as markers in biopsy specimens to indicate which patients need more aggressive cancer surveillance. *Small cell change is thought to be directly premalignant. Large cell change is at least a marker of increased risk of HCC in the liver as a whole, but in hepatitis B they may also be directly premalignant.*

Dysplastic nodules are usually detected in cirrhosis, either radiologically or in resected specimens (including explants). These are nodules that have a different appearance from the surrounding cirrhotic nodules (Fig. 18-58). The differences are in size or vascular supply (increasingly arterial with increasingly high grade, a defining feature in contrast radiologic studies) or other aspects of appearance (color, texture). *Low-grade dysplastic nodules,* may or may not

Table 18-12 Precursor Lesions of Hepatocellular Carcinoma and Cholangiocarcinoma

	Hepatocellular Carcinoma					Cholangiocarcinoma		
	Hepatocellular Adenoma	Small Cell Change	Large Cell Change	Low Grade Dysplastic Nodule	High Grade Dysplastic Nodule	BilIN-3	Mucinous Cystic Neoplasm	Intraductal Papillary Biliary Neoplasia
Focality in liver	Single or multiple (adenomatosis)	Diffuse	Diffuse	Single or multiple	Single or multiple	Diffuse or multifocal	Single	Focal or diffuse
Premalignant	Yes	Yes	In some HBV*	Uncertain*	Yes	Yes	Yes	Yes
Association with cirrhosis	Rare	Common	Common	Usual	Usual	Sometimes	No	No
Commonly associated diseases	NAFLD, Sex hormone exposures Glycogen storage diseases	HBV, HCV, Alcohol, NAFLD, A1AT, HH, PBC	HBV, HCV, Alcohol, NAFLD, A1AT, HH PBC	HBV, HCV, Alcohol, NAFLD, A1AT, HH PBC	HBV, HCV, Alcohol, NAFLD, A1AT, HH PBC	PSC, Hepatolithiasis, Liver flukes	None	None
Occurrence without identified predisposing condition	Occasional	No	No	No	No	Yes	Yes	Yes
Need for surveillance cancer screening	± depending on presence of predisposing condition	Yes	Yes	Yes	Yes	Yes	No	Yes

*While these are not certain to be directly premalignant, they are always at least an indication of increased risk for malignancy in the liver as a whole.

BilIN-3, Biliary intraepithelial neoplasia, high grade; NAFLD, nonalcoholic fatty liver disease; HBV, hepatitis B virus; HCV, hepatitis C virus; A1AT, α_1-antitrypsin deficiency; HH, hereditary hemochromatosis; PBC, primary biliary cirrhosis; PSC, primary sclerosing cholangitis.

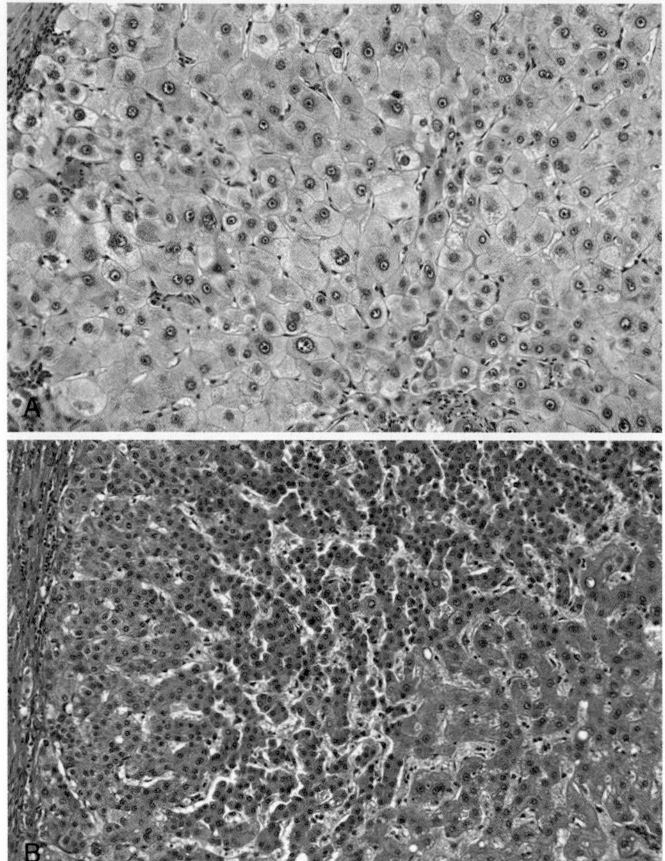

Figure 18-57 A, Large cell change. Large hepatocytes with large, often atypical nuclei are scattered among normal-size hepatocytes with round, typical nuclei. **B,** Small cell change. The abnormal cells have a high nuclear-to-cytoplasmic ratio and are separated by thickened plates. Normal-appearing hepatocytes are in the lower right corner. (Courtesy Dr. Young Nyun Park, Yonsei Medical College, Seoul, South Korea.)

undergo transformation to higher grade lesions, but they at least indicate a higher risk for HCC in the liver as a whole. *High-grade dysplastic nodules* are probably the most important primary pathway for emergence of HCC in viral hepatitis and alcoholic liver disease. Subnodules of HCC are often found in high-grade dysplastic nodules in biopsy or resection specimens.

MORPHOLOGY

Large cell change shows scattered hepatocytes, usually near portal tracts or septa, that are larger than normal hepatocytes and with large, often multiple, often moderately pleomorphic nuclei; however, the nuclear-cytoplasmic ratio is normal since both nuclei and the cell as a whole become larger (Fig. 18-57*A*). In **small cell change** the hepatocytes have high nuclear-cytoplasmic ratio and mild nuclear hyperchromasia and/or pleomorphism (Fig. 18-57*B*). Hepatocytes exhibiting small cell change often form tiny expansile nodules within a single parenchymal lobule.

Low-grade dysplastic nodules are devoid of cytologic or architectural atypia, but have been shown to be clonal and are probably neoplastic, rather than simply large cirrhotic nodules. Portal tracts are still present within these nodules, often in near normal distribution. Thus, the blood supply remains a mix of portal venous and hepatic arterial blood. **High grade dysplastic nodules** have cytologic (e.g., small cell change) or architectural features (occasional pseudoglands, trabecular thickening) suggestive of, but still insufficient for diagnosis of overt HCC. Such atypia often presents as a subnodule within the larger nodule. Portal tracts are fewer in these higher grade nodules and arteries feeding the growing lesion gradually come to predominate over the portal veinous flow. Overt HCC may then arise within the dysplastic nodules (Fig. 18-58*B*), eventually overgrowing it.

Overall, **HCC may appear grossly as (1) a unifocal (usually large) mass, (2) multifocal, widely distributed nodules of variable size, or (3) a diffusely infiltrative**

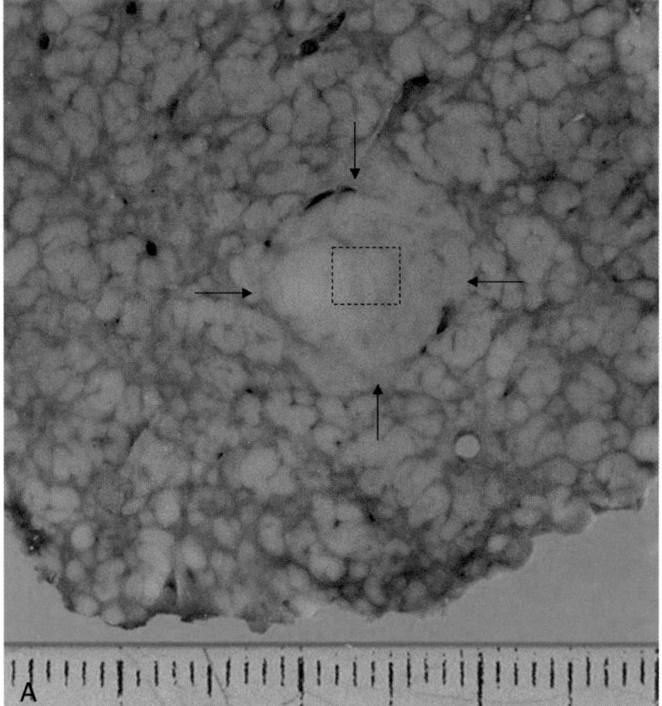

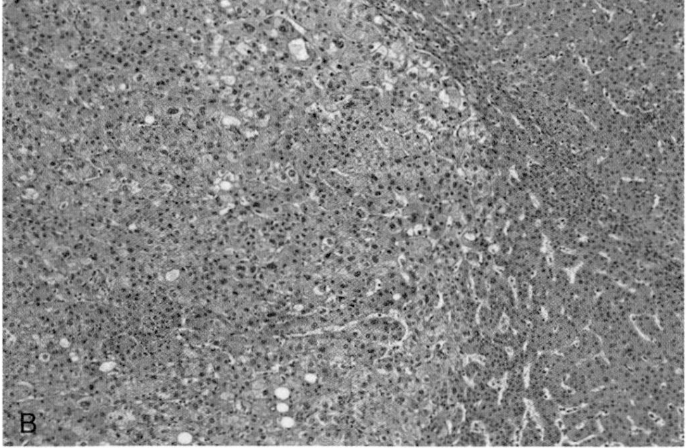

Figure 18-58 A, Hepatitis C–related cirrhosis with a distinctively large nodule *(arrows)*. Nodule-in-nodule growth suggests an evolving cancer. **B,** Histologically the region with in the box in **A** shows a well-differentiated hepatocellular carcinoma (HCC) (right side) and a subnodule of moderately differentiated HCC within it (center, left). (Courtesy Dr. Masamichi Kojiro, Kurume University, Kurume, Japan.)

cancer, permeating widely and sometimes involving the entire liver. All three patterns may cause liver enlargement. The diffusely infiltrative tumor may blend so imperceptibly into a background of cirrhosis that it might not be apparent by imaging, even though most of the liver is replaced. HCCs may be pale compared to surrounding liver or they may have a variegated appearance reflecting different differentiation states (white when there is abundant stroma, yellow when fatty change predominates, green when well-differentiated malignant hepatocytes make abundant bile).

Intrahepatic metastases, by either vascular invasion or direct extension, become more likely once tumors reach 3 cm in size. These metastases are usually small, satellite tumor nodules around the larger, primary mass. The vascular route is also the most likely route for extrahepatic metastasis, especially by the hepatic venous system. Hematogenous metastases, especially to the lung, tend to occur late in the disease. Occasionally, long, snakelike masses of tumor invade the portal vein (causing portal hypertension) or inferior vena cava. The latter can even extend into the right side of the heart. Lymph node metastases are less common routes of extrahepatic spread. If venous invasion is identified in HCC-bearing explanted livers at the time of transplantation, tumor recurrence is likely to occur in the transplanted liver due to seeding of circulating tumor cells in the transplant recipient. Such lesions may appear months after the operation.

HCCs range from well-differentiated to highly anaplastic lesions. The better differentiated HCCs are comprised of cells that look much like normal hepatocytes and grow in structures that are distortions of normal: thickened trabecular structures (recapitulating liver cell plates) or pseudoglandular structures that are poorly formed, ectatic bile canaliculi (Fig. 18-56).

A distinctive variant of HCC is **fibrolamellar carcinoma**, constituting less than 5% of HCCs. 85% occur under the age of 35 years and without gender predilection or identifiable predisposing conditions. It usually presents as single large, hard "scirrhous" tumor with fibrous bands coursing through it. Microscopically, they are composed of well-differentiated cells rich in mitochondria (oncocytes) growing in nests or cords separated by parallel lamellae of dense collagen bundles (hence the name) (Fig. 18-59).

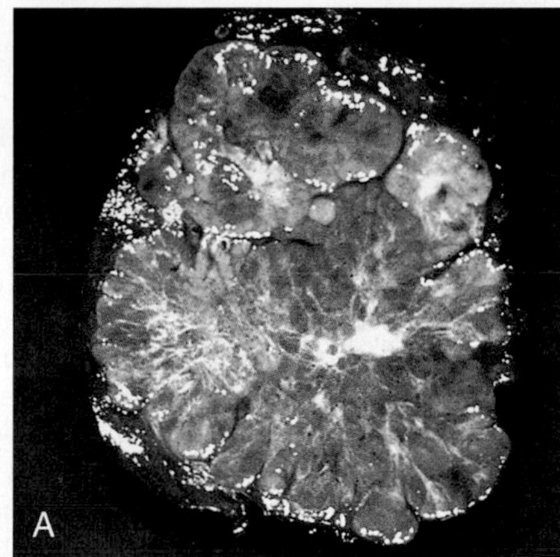

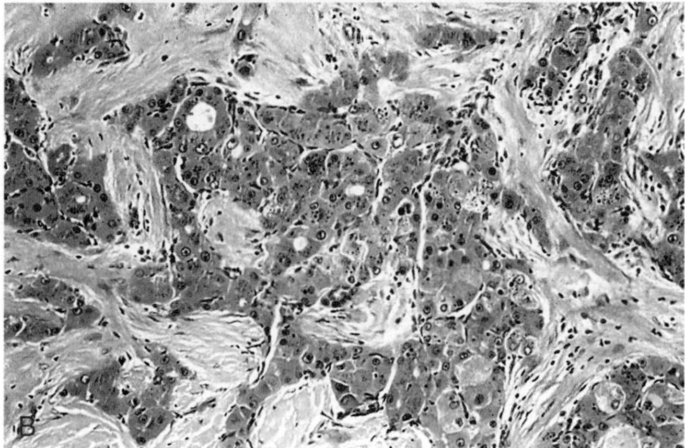

Figure 18-59 Fibrolamellar carcinoma. **A,** Resected specimen showing a well demarcated nodule. **B,** Microscopic view showing nests and cords of malignant-appearing, oncocytic hepatocytes separated by dense bundles of collagen.

Clinical Features. The clinical manifestations of HCC are seldom characteristic and, in the Western population, often are masked by those related to the underlying cirrhosis or chronic hepatitis. In areas of high incidence such as tropical Africa, in particular where aflatoxin exposure is common, patients usually have no clinical history of liver disease, although cirrhosis may be detected at autopsy. In both populations most patients have ill-defined upper abdominal pain, malaise, fatigue, weight loss, and sometimes awareness of hepatomegaly or an abdominal mass or abdominal fullness. Jaundice, fever, and gastrointestinal or esophageal variceal bleeding are inconstant findings.

Laboratory studies may be helpful but are rarely conclusive. Rising or elevated levels of *serum α-fetoprotein* are found in 50% of persons with advanced HCC. However, it is insensitive as a screening test for premalignant or early lesions as these usually do not produce particularly high levels of the protein.

Most valuable for detection of small tumors are imaging studies: ultrasonography to identify distinctive nodules of all kinds, and computed tomography and magnetic resonance imaging with vascular/contrast studies. The increasing arterialization in the process of conversion from high grade dysplastic nodule to early HCC and then to fully developed HCC, form the basis of diagnostic imaging. HCC, even when small, has such characteristic vascular changes that imaging can be diagnostic.

The natural course of HCC involves the progressive enlargement of the primary mass until it disturbs hepatic function or metastasizes to the lungs or to other sites. Death usually occurs from (1) cachexia, (2) gastrointestinal or esophageal variceal bleeding, (3) liver failure with hepatic coma, or, rarely, (4) rupture of the tumor with fatal hemorrhage. The 5-year survival of large tumors is dismal, the majority of patients dying within the first 2 years.

With implementation of screening procedures and advances in imaging, the detection of HCCs less than 2 cm in diameter has increased in countries where such facilities are available. These small tumors can be removed surgically or ablated (e.g., through embolization or with microwave radiation or freezing) with good outcomes. Radiofrequency ablation is used for local control of large tumors, and chemoembolization can also be used.

Cholangiocarcinoma (CCA)

Cholangiocarcinoma (CCA), the second most common primary malignant tumor of the liver after HCC, is a malignancy of the biliary tree, arising from bile ducts within and outside of the liver. It accounts for 7.6% of cancer deaths worldwide and 3% of cancer deaths in the United States. However, in some regions of Southeast Asia such as northeastern Thailand, Laos, and Cambodia where infestation with liver flukes is endemic, cholangiocarcinoma is more common than hepatocellular carcinoma.

All risk factors for cholangiocarcinomas cause chronic inflammation and cholestasis, which presumably promote occurrence of somatic mutations or epigenetic alterations in cholangiocytes. The risk factors include infestation by liver flukes (particularly Opisthorchis and Clonorchis species), chronic inflammatory disease of the large bile ducts, such as primary sclerosing cholangitis, hepatolithiasis, and fibropolycystic liver disease. It should be noted that patients with hepatitis B and C, and non alcoholic fatty liver disease, not only have a higher risk of developing HCC, but also of cholangiocarcinoma. Globally, cholangiocarcinomas are most often sporadic and not associated with any preexisting condition.

Cholangiocarcinoma may be either intrahepatic or extrahepatic. The extrahepatic forms include perihilar tumors known as *Klatskin tumors*, which are located at the junction of the right and left hepatic ducts. Fifty percent to 60% of all cholangiocarcinomas are perihilar (Klatskin) tumors, 20% to 30% are distal tumors, arising in the common bile duct where it lies posterior to the duodenum. The remaining 10% are intrahepatic. Regardless of site, the prognosis is dismal, with survival rates of about 15% at 2 years after diagnosis for extrahepatic tumors. The median time from diagnosis to death for intrahepatic CCAs is 6 months, even after surgery because intrahepatic CCAs are not usually detected until late in their course. They come to the attention because of obstruction of bile flow or as a symptomatic liver mass. In contrast, hilar and distal tumors present with symptoms of biliary obstruction, cholangitis, and right upper quadrant pain.

Premalignant lesions for cholangiocarcinoma are also known, the most important of which are biliary intraepithelial neoplasias (low to high grade, BilIN-1, -2, or -3). BilIN-3, the highest grade lesion, incurs the highest risk of malignant transformation. More rare are *mucinous cystic neoplasms* and intraductal *papillary biliary neoplasia* (Table 18-12).

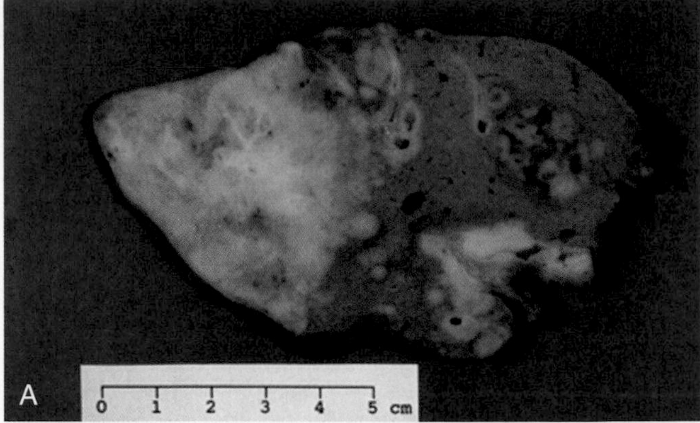

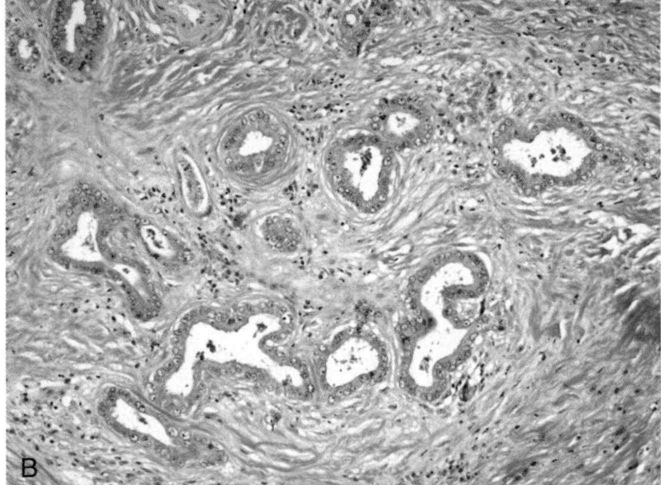

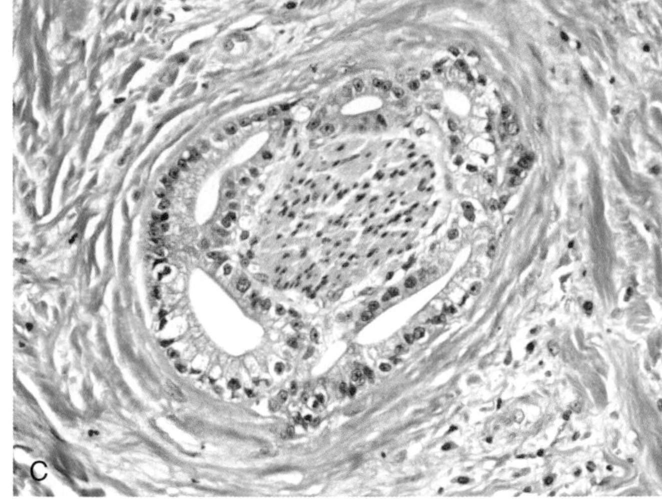

Figure 18-60 Cholangiocarcinoma. **A,** Multifocal cholangiocarcinoma in a liver from a patient with infestation by the liver fluke *Clonorchis sinensis*. **B,** Invasive malignant glands in a reactive, sclerotic stroma. **C,** Perineural invasion by malignant glands, forming a wreathlike pattern around the central, trapped nerve. (**A,** Courtesy Dr. Wilson M.S. Tsui, Caritas Medical Centre, Hong Kong.)

MORPHOLOGY

Extrahepatic cholangiocarcinomas are generally small lesions at the time of diagnosis as they rapidly cause obstructive features. Most tumors appear as firm, gray nodules within the bile duct wall; some may be diffusely infiltrative lesions; others are papillary, polypoid lesions. Intrahepatic cholangiocarcinomas occur in the noncirrhotic liver (Fig. 18-60) and may track along the intrahepatic portal tract system creating a branching tumor within a portion of the liver. Alternatively, a massive tumor nodule may develop.

Regardless of site, cholangiocarcinomas are typical adenocarcinomas. They often produce mucin. Most are well- to moderately differentiated with clearly defined glandular/tubular structures lined by malignant epithelial cells (Fig. 18-60*B*). They typically incite marked desmoplasia. Lymphovascular invasion and perineural invasion (Fig. 18-60*C*) are both common, each a path to extensive intrahepatic and extrahepatic metastases.

Other Primary Hepatic Malignant Tumors

Other primary liver malignancies are rare, but noteworthy. Some tumors show *combined hepatocellular and cholangiocarcinoma,* suggesting an origin from a multipotent stem cell. *Mucinous cystic neoplasms* and *intraductal papillary biliary neoplasia* may occur as in situ lesions or as invasive cholangiocarcinoma.

Angiosarcoma of the liver resembles those occurring elsewhere and has historical associations with vinyl chloride, arsenic, or Thorotrast (Chapters 9 and 11), although with reduced exposures to these compounds in recent decades, this malignancy is becoming very rare. *Epithelioid hemangioendothelioma,* another form of endothelial malignancy, has a much more variable prognosis than the almost uniformly fatal angiosarcoma. Hepatic lymphomas are primarily diseases of middle aged men and are seen, albeit rarely, in association with hepatitis B and C, HIV, and PBC. Most are *diffuse large B-cell lymphomas,* followed by *MALT lymphomas. Hepatosplenic delta-gamma T cell lymphoma,* most common in young adult males, has a predilection for hepatic and splenic sinusoids as well as the marrow.

Metastasis

Involvement of the liver by metastatic malignancy is far more common than primary hepatic neoplasia. Although the most common primary sources are the colon, breast, lung, and pancreas, any cancer in any site of the body may spread to the liver. Typically, multiple nodular metastases are found that often cause striking hepatomegaly and replace much of the normal liver parenchyma. The liver weight can exceed several kilograms. Metastasis may also appear as a single nodule, in which case it may be resected surgically. Always surprising is the amount of metastatic involvement that may be present in the absence of clinical or laboratory evidence of hepatic functional insufficiency. Often the only telltale clinical sign is hepatomegaly. However, with massive destruction of liver substance or direct obstruction of major bile ducts, jaundice and elevations of liver enzymes may appear.

KEY CONCEPTS

Liver Tumors

- The liver is the most common site of **metastatic cancers** from primary tumors of the colon, lung, and breast.
- **Hepatocellular adenomas** are benign tumors of neoplastic hepatocytes. Most can be subclassified on the basis of molecular changes:
  - **HNF1-α inactivated adenomas,** with virtually no risk of malignant transformation, often associated with oral contraceptive pill use or in individuals with MODY-3
  - **β-Catenin activated adenoma,** with mutations in the β-catenin gene leading to marked atypia and associated with a very high risk for malignant transformation
  - **Inflammatory adenomas,** the hallmark of which is up-regulation of C-reactive protein and serum amyloid A (often derived from gp130 mutations); 10% of these have concomitant β-catenin activating mutations. Risk for malignant transformation is intermediate.
- The main **primary malignancies are HCCs and cholangiocarcinomas;** HCCs are by far the most common.
  - HCC is a common tumor in regions of Asia and Africa, and its incidence is increasing in the United States.
  - The main etiologic agents for HCC are chronic hepatitis B and C, alcoholic cirrhosis, non-alcoholic fatty liver disease, and hemochromatosis. In the Western population, about 90% of HCCs develop in cirrhotic livers; in Asia, almost 50% of cases develop in noncirrhotic livers.
  - The chronic inflammation and cellular regeneration associated with viral hepatitis or the activation of IL-6/JAK STAT pathway may be predisposing factors for the development of carcinomas.
  - HCCs may be unifocal or multifocal, tend to invade blood vessels, and recapitulate normal liver architecture to varying degrees.
- **Cholangiocarcinoma** is endemic in areas where liver flukes such as *Opisthorchis* and *Clonorchis* species are endemic. Chronic inflammatory diseases of bile ducts are also risk factors. The tumors may arise from extra hepatic or intrahepatic bile ducts. They have uniformly poor prognosis.

GALLBLADDER

As much as 1 L of bile is secreted by the liver per day. Between meals, bile is stored in the gallbladder, where it is concentrated. The adult gallbladder has a capacity of about 50 mL. The organ is not essential for biliary function, since humans do not suffer from indigestion or malabsorption of fat after cholecystectomy. **More than 95% of biliary tract disease is attributable to cholelithiasis (gallstones).** In the United States, gallstones affect 20 million people, and more than 700,000 cholecystectomies are performed annually at a cost of approximately $6 billion.

Congenital Anomalies

The gallbladder may be congenitally absent, or there may be gallbladder duplication with conjoined or independent cystic ducts. A longitudinal or transverse septum may create a bilobed gallbladder. Aberrant locations of the gallbladder occur in 5% to 10% of the population, most commonly partial or complete embedding in the liver substance. A folded fundus is the most common anomaly, creating a *phrygian cap* (Fig. 18-61). *Agenesis* of all or any portion of the hepatic or common bile ducts and hypoplastic narrowing of biliary channels (true "biliary atresia") may also occur. *Choledochal cysts,* described earlier, may be isolated findings in the gallbladder or associated with other cysts in the extrahepatic biliary tree or with fibropolycystic disease.

Cholelithiasis (Gallstones)

Gallstones afflict 10% to 20% of adult populations in developed countries. It is estimated that more than 20 million

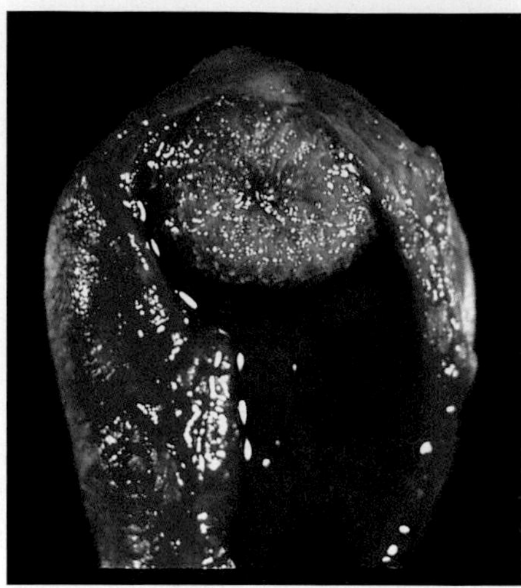

Figure 18-61 Phrygian cap of the gallbladder; the fundus is folded inward.

persons in the United States have gallstones, totaling some 25 to 50 tons in weight. The vast majority of gallstones (>80%) are "silent," and most individuals remain free of biliary pain or other complications for decades. There are two general classes of gallstones: *cholesterol stones*, containing more than 50% of crystalline cholesterol monohydrate, and *pigment stones* composed predominantly of bilirubin calcium salts.

Prevalence and Risk Factors. Certain populations are far more prone than others to develop gallstones. Cholesterol gallstones are more prevalent in the United States and Western Europe (90%) and uncommon in developing countries. The prevalence rates of cholesterol gallstones approach 75% in Native Americans of the Pima, Hopi,and Navajo groups; pigment stones are rare in these populations. Pigment gallstones, the predominant type of gallstone in non-Western populations, arise primarily in the setting of bacterial infections of the biliary tree and parasitic infestations.

The major risk factors associated with the development of gallstones are listed in Table 18-13 and are briefly described here:

- *Age and sex.* The prevalence of cholesterol gallstones increases throughout life but they predominantly affect individuals of middle to older age. Prevalence is higher in females in any region or ethnicity; in Caucasian women it is about twice as high as in men. Hypersecretion of biliary cholesterol seems to play the major role in both age and gender differences. Significant associations are also seen with the metabolic syndrome and obesity.
- *Environmental factors.* Estrogen exposure, including through oral contraceptive use and during pregnancy, increases the expression of hepatic lipoprotein receptors and stimulates hepatic HMG-CoA reductase activity, enhancing both cholesterol uptake and biosynthesis, respectively. The net result is excess biliary secretion of cholesterol. Obesity and rapid weight loss also are strongly associated with increased biliary cholesterol secretion.
- *Acquired disorders.* Gallbladder stasis, either neurogenic or hormonal, fosters a local environment that is favorable for both cholesterol and pigment gallstone formation.
- *Hereditary factors.* Genes encoding hepatocyte proteins that transport biliary lipids, known as ATP-binding cassette (ABC) transporters have associations with gallstone formation. In particular, a common variant of the sterol transporter encoded by the *ABCG8* gene is associated with an increased risk for the development of cholesterol gallstones.

Pathogenesis of Cholesterol Stones. Cholesterol is rendered soluble in bile by aggregation with water-soluble bile salts and water-insoluble lecithins, both of which act as detergents. *When cholesterol concentrations exceed the solubilizing capacity of bile (supersaturation), cholesterol can no longer remain dispersed and nucleates into solid cholesterol monohydrate crystals.* Four conditions appear to contribute to formation of cholesterol gallstones (1) supersaturation of bile with cholesterol; (2) hypomotility of the gallbladder; (3) accelerated cholesterol crystal nucleation; (4) and hypersecretion of mucus in the gallbladder, which traps the nucleated crystals, leading to accretion of more cholesterol and the appearance of macroscopic stones.

Pathogenesis of Pigment Stones. Pigment gallstones are complex mixtures of insoluble calcium salts of unconjugated bilirubin along with inorganic calcium salts. Disorders that are associated with elevated levels of unconjugated bilirubin in bile, such as chronic hemolytic anemias, severe ileal dysfunction or bypass, and bacterial contamination of the biliary tree, increase the risk of developing pigment stones. Unconjugated bilirubin is normally a minor component of bile, but it increases when infection of the biliary tract leads to release of microbial β-glucuronidases, which hydrolyze bilirubin glucuronides. Thus, infection of the biliary tract with *Escherichia coli*, *Ascaris lumbricoides*, or the liver fluke *C. sinensis*, increases the likelihood of pigment stone formation. In hemolytic anemias the secretion of conjugated bilirubin into the bile increases. About 1% of bilirubin glucuronides are deconjugated in the biliary tree, and in the setting of chronically increased secretion of conjugated bilirubin, there is

Table 18-13 Risk Factors for Gallstones

Cholesterol Stones
Demography: northern Europeans, North and South Americans, Native Americans, Mexican Americans
Advancing age
Female sex hormones
Female gender
Oral contraceptives
Pregnancy
Obesity and metabolic syndrome
Rapid weight reduction
Gallbladder stasis
Inborn disorders of bile acid metabolism
Hyperlipidemia syndromes
Pigment Stones
Demography: Asians more than Westerners, rural more than urban
Chronic hemolytic syndromes
Biliary infection
Gastrointestinal disorders: ileal disease (e.g., Crohn disease), ileal resection or bypass, cystic fibrosis with pancreatic insufficiency

sufficiently large amount of deconjugated bilirubin left to allow pigment stones to form.

MORPHOLOGY

Cholesterol stones arise exclusively in the gallbladder and range from 100% pure (which is rare) down to around 50% cholesterol. Pure cholesterol stones are pale yellow, round to ovoid, and have a finely granular, hard external surface (Fig. 18-62), which on transection reveals a glistening radiating crystalline palisade. With increasing proportions of calcium carbonate, phosphates, and bilirubin, the stones take on a gray-white to black color and may be lamellated. Multiple stones are usually present that range up to several centimeters in diameter. Rarely, a very large stone may virtually fill the fundus. Surfaces of multiple stones may be rounded or faceted, because of tight apposition. Stones composed largely of cholesterol are radiolucent; sufficient calcium carbonate is found in 10% to 20% of cholesterol stones to render them radiopaque.

Pigment gallstones are brown to black. In general, black pigment stones are found in sterile gallbladder bile and brown stones are found in infected large bile ducts. Black stones contain oxidized polymers of the calcium salts of unconjugated bilirubin, small amounts of calcium carbonate, calcium phosphate, and mucin glycoprotein, and some cholesterol monohydrate crystals. Brown stones contain similar compounds along with some cholesterol and calcium salts of palmitate and stearate. The black stones are rarely greater than 1.5 cm in diameter, are almost invariably present in great number (with an inverse relationship between size and number; Fig. 18-63), and are quite friable. Their contours are usually spiculated and molded. Brown stones tend to be laminated and soft and may have a soaplike or greasy consistency. Approximately 50% to 75% of black stones are radiopaque due to calcium salts while brown stones, containing calcium soaps, are radiolucent. Mucin glycoproteins constitute the scaffolding and interparticle cement of all types of stones.

Clinical Features. Gallstones may be present for decades before symptoms develop, and 70% to 80% of patients remain asymptomatic throughout their lives. Asymptomatic individuals probably convert to being symptomatic at a rate of up to 4% per year, although the risk diminishes with time. Prominent among symptoms is *biliary colic* that may be excruciating. Despite its characterization as "colic" it is usually constant and not colicky. It usually follows a fatty meal which forces a stone against the gall bladder outlet leading to increased pressure in the gall bladder causing pain. Pain is localized to right upper quadrant or epigastrium that may radiate to the right shoulder or the back. Inflammation of the gallbladder (cholecystitis, discussed later), in association with stones, also generates pain. More severe complications include *empyema, perforation, fistulas, inflammation of the biliary tree (cholangitis), obstructive cholestasis* and *pancreatitis.* The larger the calculi, the less likely they are to enter the cystic or common ducts to produce obstruction; it is the very small stones, or "gravel," that are more dangerous. Occasionally a large stone may erode directly into an adjacent loop of small bowel, generating intestinal obstruction (*"gallstone ileus"* or *Bouveret syndrome*). Lastly (but not least), gallstones are associated with an increased risk of gallbladder carcinoma, discussed later.

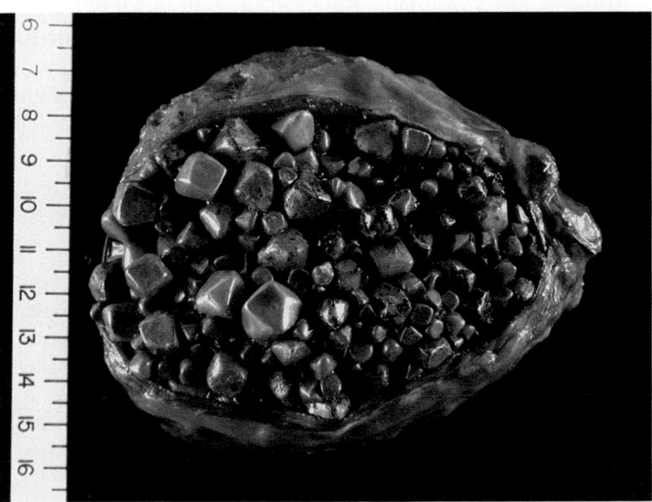

Figure 18-62 Cholesterol gallstones. The wall of the gallbladder is thickened and fibrotic due to chronic cholecystitis.

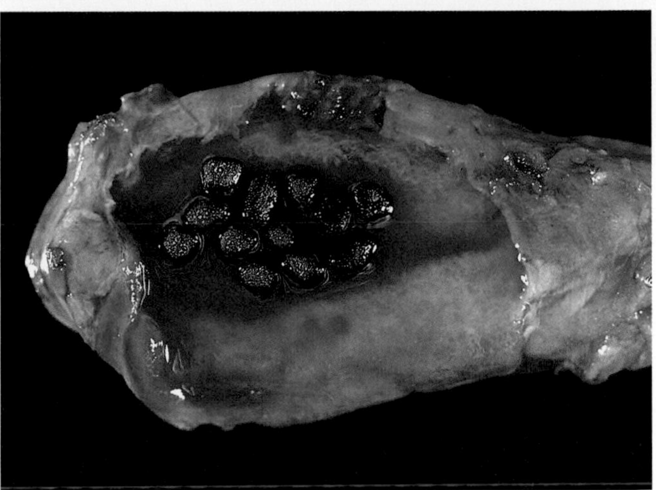

Figure 18-63 Pigment gallstones. Several faceted black gallstones are present in this otherwise unremarkable gallbladder from a patient with a mechanical mitral valve prosthesis, leading to chronic intravascular hemolysis.

Cholecystitis

Inflammation of the gallbladder may be acute, chronic, or acute superimposed on chronic. It almost always occurs in association with gallstones. In the United States cholecystitis is one of the most common indications for abdominal surgery. Its epidemiologic distribution closely parallels that of gallstones.

Acute Cholecystitis

Acute calculous cholecystitis is precipitated in 90% of cases by obstruction of the neck or the cystic duct by a stone. It is the primary complication of gallstones and the most common reason for emergency cholecystectomy. *Cholecystitis without gallstones (acalculous cholecystitis) may occur in severely ill patients and accounts for about 10% of patients with cholecystitis.*

Pathogenesis. *Acute calculous cholecystitis results from chemical irritation and inflammation of a gallbladder obstructed by stones.* The action of mucosal phospholipases hydrolyzes luminal lecithins to toxic lysolecithins. The normally protective glycoprotein mucus layer is disrupted, exposing the mucosal epithelium to the direct detergent action of bile salts. Prostaglandins released within the wall of the distended gallbladder contribute to mucosal and mural inflammation; distention and increased intraluminal pressure compromise blood flow to the mucosa. *These events occur in the absence of bacterial infection; only later in the course may bacterial contamination develop.* Acute calculous cholecystitis frequently develops in diabetic patients who have symptomatic gallstones.

Acute acalculous cholecystitis, without stone involvement, is thought to result from ischemia. The cystic artery is an end artery with no collateral circulation. Contributing factors may include inflammation and edema of the wall compromising blood flow, gallbladder stasis, and accumulation of microcrystals of cholesterol (biliary sludge), viscous bile, and gallbladder mucus, causing cystic duct obstruction in the absence of stones. It occurs in patients who are hospitalized for unrelated conditions. Risk factors for acute acalculous cholecystitis include: (1) sepsis with hypotension and multisystem organ failure; (2) immunosuppression; (3) major trauma and burns; (4) diabetes mellitus; (5) infections.

MORPHOLOGY

In **acute cholecystitis** the gallbladder is usually enlarged and tense, and it may assume a bright red or blotchy, violaceous to green-black discoloration, imparted by subserosal hemorrhages. The serosal covering is frequently covered by a fibrinous exudate that may be fibrinopurulent in severe cases. There are no specific morphologic differences between acute acalculous and calculous cholecystitis, save the absence of stones in the acalculous form. In **calculous cholecystitis**, an obstructing stone is usually present in the neck of the gallbladder or the cystic duct. The gallbladder lumen may contain one or more stones and is filled with a cloudy or turbid bile that may contain large amounts of fibrin, pus, and hemorrhage. When the exudate is virtually pure pus, the condition is referred to as **gallbladder empyema**. In mild cases the gallbladder wall is thickened, edematous, and hyperemic. In more severe cases it is transformed into a green-black necrotic organ, termed **gangrenous cholecystitis**, with small-to-large perforations. Inflammation is predominantly neutrophilic. The invasion of gas-forming organisms, notably clostridia and coliforms, may cause an **acute "emphysematous" cholecystitis**.

Clinical Features. Individuals with acute calculous cholecystitis usually, but not always, have experienced previous episodes of pain. An attack of acute cholecystitis begins with progressive right upper quadrant or epigastric pain that lasts for more than six hours. It is frequently associated with mild fever, anorexia, tachycardia, sweating, nausea, and vomiting. Most patients are free of jaundice; the presence of hyperbilirubinemia suggests obstruction of the common bile duct. Mild to moderate leukocytosis may be accompanied by mild elevations in serum alkaline phosphatase values. *Acute calculous cholecystitis may appear with remarkable suddenness and constitute an acute surgical emergency or may present with mild symptoms that resolve without medical intervention.* In the absence of medical attention, the attack usually subsides in 7 to 10 days and frequently within 24 hours. However, as many as 25% of patients progressively develop more severe symptoms and require immediate surgical intervention. Recurrence is common in patients who recover without surgery.

Clinical symptoms of acute acalculous cholecystitis tend to be more insidious, since they are obscured by the underlying conditions precipitating the attacks. A higher proportion of patients have no symptoms referable to the gallbladder; diagnosis therefore rests on a high index of suspicion. In the severely ill patient, early recognition of the condition is crucial, since failure to do so almost ensures a fatal outcome. As a result of either delay in diagnosis or the disease itself, the incidence of gangrene and perforation is much higher in acalculous than in calculous cholecystitis. In rare instances, primary bacterial infection can give rise to acute acalculous cholecystitis, by agents such as *Salmonella typhi* and staphylococci. A more indolent form of acute acalculous cholecystitis may occur in the setting of systemic vasculitis, severe atherosclerotic ischemic disease in the elderly, in patients with AIDS, and with biliary tract infection.

Chronic Cholecystitis

Chronic cholecystitis may be a sequel to repeated bouts of mild to severe acute cholecystitis, but in many instances it develops in the apparent absence of antecedent attacks. Since it is associated with *cholelithiasis in more than 90% of cases*, the at-risk patient population is the same as that for gallstones. The evolution of chronic cholecystitis is obscure; it is not clear that gallstones play a direct role in the initiation of inflammation or the development of pain, particularly since chronic acalculous cholecystitis shows symptoms and histology similar to those of the calculous form. Rather, supersaturation of bile predisposes to both chronic inflammation and, in most instances, stone formation. Microorganisms, usually *E. coli* and enterococci, can be cultured from the bile in about one third of cases. Unlike acute calculous cholecystitis, obstruction of gallbladder outflow is not a requisite. Since most gallbladders that are removed at elective surgery for gallstones show features of chronic cholecystitis, one must conclude that biliary symptoms often emerge following long-term coexistence of gallstones and low-grade inflammation.

MORPHOLOGY

The morphologic changes in chronic cholecystitis are extremely variable and sometimes minimal. The serosa is usually smooth and glistening but may be dulled by **subserosal fibrosis**. Dense fibrous adhesions may remain as sequelae of preexistent acute inflammation. On sectioning, the wall is variably thickened, and has an opaque gray-white appearance. In the uncomplicated case the lumen contains green-yellow, mucoid bile and usually stones. The mucosa itself is generally preserved.

On histologic examination the degree of inflammation is variable. In the mildest cases, only scattered lymphocytes, plasma

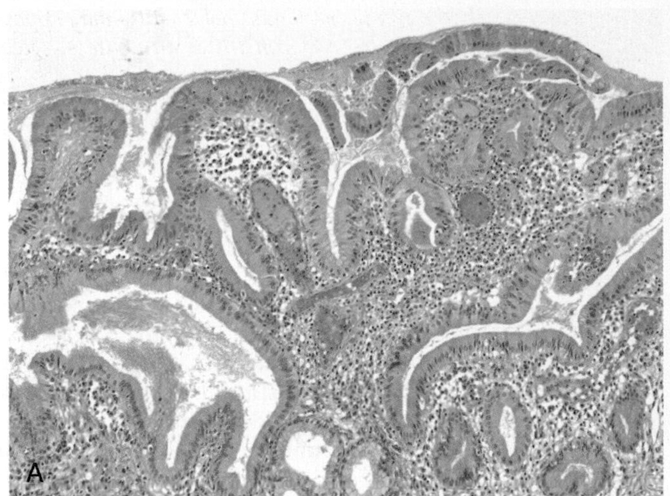

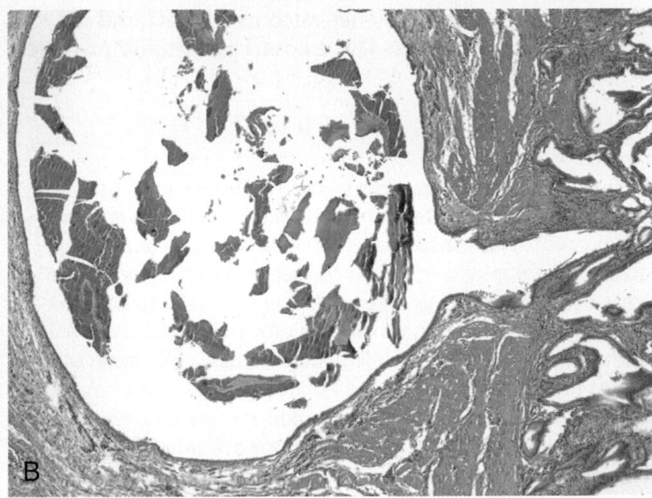

Figure 18-64 Chronic cholecystitis. **A,** The gallbladder mucosa is infiltrated by inflammatory cells. **B,** Outpouching of the mucosa through the wall forms Rokitansky-Aschoff sinus (contains bile).

cells, and macrophages are found in the mucosa and in the subserosal fibrous tissue (Fig. 18-64*A*). In more advanced cases there is marked subepithelial and subserosal fibrosis, accompanied by mononuclear cell infiltration. Reactive proliferation of the mucosa and fusion of the mucosal folds may give rise to buried crypts of epithelium within the gallbladder wall. Outpouchings of the mucosal epithelium through the wall (**Rokitansky-Aschoff sinuses**) may be quite prominent (Fig. 18-64*B*). Presence of acute inflammatory changes implies acute exacerbation of an already chronically injured gallbladder.

In rare instances extensive dystrophic calcification within the gallbladder wall may yield a **porcelain gallbladder**, notable for a markedly increased incidence of associated cancer. In **xanthogranulomatous cholecystitis**, the gallbladder has a massively thickened wall and is shrunken, nodular, and chronically inflamed with foci of necrosis and hemorrhage. It is triggered by rupture of Rokitansky-Aschoff sinuses into the wall of the gall bladder followed by an accumulation of macrophages that have ingested biliary phospholipids. Such lipid containing cells with foamy cytoplasm are called xanthoma cells and hence the name of this condition. Finally, an atrophic, chronically obstructed, often dilated gallbladder, may contain only clear secretions, a condition known as **hydrops of the gallbladder**.

Clinical Features. Chronic cholecystitis does not have the striking manifestations of the acute forms and is usually characterized by recurrent attacks of either steady epigastric or right upper quadrant pain. Nausea, vomiting, and intolerance for fatty foods are frequent accompaniments.

Diagnosis of both acute and chronic cholecystitis is important because of the following complications:

- Bacterial superinfection with cholangitis or sepsis
- Gallbladder perforation and local abscess formation
- Gallbladder rupture with diffuse peritonitis
- Biliary enteric (cholecystenteric) fistula, with drainage of bile into adjacent organs, entry of air and bacteria into the biliary tree, and potentially, gallstone-induced intestinal obstruction (ileus)
- Aggravation of preexisting medical illness, with cardiac, pulmonary, renal, or liver decompensation
- Porcelain gallbladder, with increased risk of cancer, although surveys of this risk have yielded widely discrepant frequencies

Carcinoma

Carcinoma of the gallbladder is the most common malignancy of the extrahepatic biliary tract. Approximately 6,000 new cases of gallbladder cancer are diagnosed each year in the United States. There are wide variations in the incidence of gallbladder cancer worldwide, with some regions such as Chile, Bolivia and Northern India, harboring the highest numbers of cases. Even within the United States, areas with large numbers of Native American or Hispanic populations, such as the southwest, have a higher incidence of gallbladder cancer than the rest of the country. *Gallbladder cancer is at least twice as common in women than in men;* this gender disparity can be several fold greater in regions of highest incidence. The overwhelming majority of patients are diagnosed at an advanced, surgically unresectable, stage, and the mean 5-year survival for these patients remains at less than 10%.

Pathogenesis. *The most important risk factor for gallbladder cancer (besides gender and ethnicity) is gallstones* which are present in 95% of cases. However, it should be noted that only 1-2% of patients with gallstones develop gallbladder cancer. In Asia, chronic bacterial or parasitic infections have been implicated as risk factors, and the coexistence of gallstones with gallbladder cancer is much lower. Nonetheless, the common thread that ties gallstones or chronic infections together with gallbladder cancer is chronic inflammation. Gallbladder cancers harbor recurrent molecular alterations that might be "actionable" targets of therapy. One example is the oncoprotein ERBB2 (Her-2/neu) that is overexpressed in a third to two-thirds of cases, and therefore might be targeted with small molecule inhibitors or monoclonal antibodies. Recent deep sequencing of gallbladder cancers has revealed mutations of chromatin remodeling genes such as *PBRM1* and *MLL3* in up to a quarter of cases. These could potentially provide targets for therapy.

MORPHOLOGY

Carcinomas of the gallbladder show two patterns of growth: **infiltrating** and **exophytic**. The infiltrating pattern is more common and usually appears as a poorly defined area of diffuse mural thickening and induration. Deep ulceration can cause direct penetration into the liver or fistula formation to adjacent viscera into which the neoplasm has grown. These tumors are scirrhous and have a very firm consistency. The exophytic pattern grows into the lumen as an irregular, cauliflower mass, but at the same time invades the underlying wall (Fig. 18-65*A*).

Most carcinomas of the gallbladder are adenocarcinomas. Some of the carcinomas are papillary in architecture and are well to moderately differentiated; others are infiltrative and poorly differentiated to undifferentiated (Fig. 18-65*B*). About 5% are squamous cell carcinomas or have adenosquamous differentiation. A minority may show carcinoid or a variety of mesenchymal features (carcinosarcoma). Papillary tumors generally have a better prognosis than other tumors. By the time these neoplasms are discovered, most have invaded the liver centrifugally, and many have extended to the cystic duct and adjacent bile ducts and portal-hepatic lymph nodes. The peritoneum, gastrointestinal tract, and lungs are common sites of seeding.

It is not uncommon to find preneoplastic (dysplastic) lesions in the epithelium adjacent to invasive cancer, or in gallbladders with long-standing cholelithiasis. These are nearly always flat dysplasias, with varying grades of cellular atypia, including carcinoma-in-situ. Although polypoid adenomas of the gallbladder have been reported, these are uncommon precursors to invasive adenocarcinomas, and harbor distinct genetic alterations.

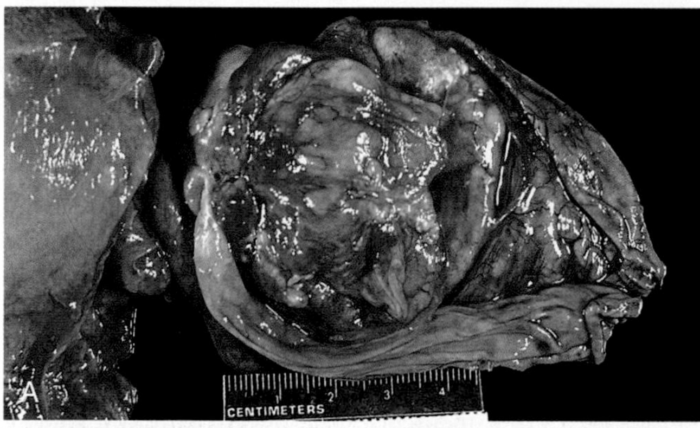

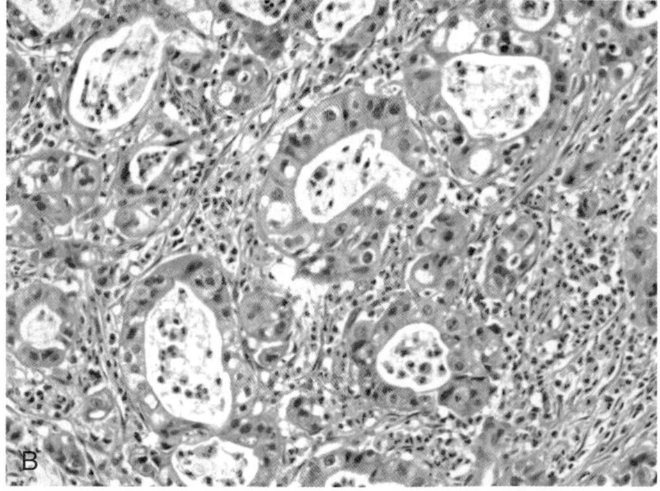

Figure 18-65 Gallbladder adenocarcinoma. **A,** The opened gallbladder contains a large, exophytic tumor that virtually fills the lumen. **B,** Malignant glands are seen infiltrating a densely fibrotic gallbladder wall.

Clinical Features. Preoperative diagnosis of carcinoma of the gallbladder is the exception rather than the rule, occurring in fewer than 20% of patients. Presenting symptoms are insidious and typically indistinguishable from those associated with cholelithiasis: abdominal pain, jaundice, anorexia, and nausea and vomiting. Early detection of the tumor may be possible in patients who develop a palpable gallbladder and acute cholecystitis before extension of the tumor into adjacent structures, or when the carcinoma is an incidental finding during a cholecystectomy for symptomatic gallstones. Surgical resection, often including adjacent liver, is the only effective treatment, when possible, but chemotherapy regimens are also used.

KEY CONCEPTS

Diseases of the Gallbladder

- Gallbladder diseases include cholelithiasis and acute and chronic cholecystitis and gall bladder cancer.
- Gallstones are common in Western countries. The great majority are cholesterol stones. Pigmented stones containing bilirubin and calcium are most common in Asian countries.
- Risk factors for the development of cholesterol stones are advancing age, female gender, estrogen use, obesity, and heredity.
- Cholecystitis almost always occurs in association with cholelithiasis, although in about 10% of cases it occurs in the absence of gallstones. Gall stones are also a risk factor for gall bladder cancer.
- Acute calculous cholecystitis is the most common reason for emergency cholecystectomy.
- Gall bladder cancers are associated with gall stones in the vast majority of cases. Typically they are detected late because of non specific symptoms and hence carry a poor prognosis.

SUGGESTED READINGS

Mechanisms of Liver Injury and Repair

Gouw ASW, Clouston AD, Theise ND: Ductular reactions in human livers: diversity at the interface. *Hepatology* 54:1853, 2011. *[A review of ductular reactions, the stem cell response of human livers in all liver diseases, that are related to mechanisms of regeneration, fibrogenesis and neoplasia.]*

Kocabayoglu P, Friedman SL: Cellular basis of hepatic fibrosis and its role in inflammation and cancer. *Front Biosci (Schol Ed)* 5:217, 2013. *[Interweaving what is known about hepatic stellate cells and other myofibroblastic cells of the liver with inflammatory, fibrosing, and neoplastic disease processes.]*

Iwaisako K, Brenner DA, Kisseleva T: What's new in liver fibrosis? The origin of myofibroblasts in liver fibrosis. *J Gastroenterol Hepatol* 27(Suppl 2):65, 2012.

Wanless IR, Nakashima E, Sherman M: Regression of human cirrhosis. Morphologic features and the genesis of incomplete septal cirrhosis. *Arch Pathol Lab Med* 124:1599, 2000. *[The revolutionary paper which began the reassessment of whether fibrosis/cirrhosis could regress; take a look also, in the same volume of the journal, at the critiques by the original reviewers of the paper (published despite their objections) and the authors' response to these. Pathology history happening before your eyes.]*

Acute, Chronic, Acute-On-Chronic Liver Failure

Berzigotti A, Seijo S, Reverter E, et al: Assessing portal hypertension in liver diseases. *Expert Rev Gastroenterol Hepatol* 7:141, 2013. *[Evolving definitions and methodologies for evaluating portal hypertension are at the leading edge of advances in Hepatology.]*

Chun LJ, Tong MJ, Busuttil RW, et al: Acetaminophen hepatotoxicity and acute liver failure. *J Clin Gastroenterol* 43:342, 2009. *[About the most common cause of acute liver failure leading to transplantation.]*

Hytiroglou P, Snover DC, Alves V: Beyond "cirrhosis": a proposal from the International Liver Pathology Study Group. *Am J Clin Pathol* 137:5, 2012. *[New understandings of diverse cirrhoses and a new look at the old concept of cirrhosis and advanced stage liver disease.]*

Khungar V, Poordad F: Hepatic encephalopathy. *Clin Liver Dis* 16:301, 2012. *[A good overview of the one of the most ominous sequelae of all forms of liver failure.]*

Laleman W, Verbeke L, Meersseman P: Acute-on-chronic liver failure: current concepts on definition, pathogenesis, clinical manifestations and potential therapeutic interventions. *Expert Rev Gastroenterol Hepatol* 5:523, 2011.

Bernal W, Wendon J: Acute Liver Failure. *New Engl J Med* 369:2525, 2013. *[An excellent clinical review.]*

Viral Hepatitis

Chung RT, Baumert TF: Curing chronic hepatitis C—The arc of medical triumph. *New Engl J Med* 370:1576, 2014. *[An excellent perspective on why and how hepatitis C can be cured.]*

Joyce MA, Tyrrell DL: The cell biology of hepatitis C virus. *Microbes Infect* 12:263, 2010. *[What we understand and don't understand about hepatitis C virus and the cells it infects.]*

Lai M, Liaw YF: Chronic hepatitis B: past, present, and future. *Clin Liver Dis* 14:531, 2010. *[A thorough look at the continually evolving nature of hepatitis B and of our attempts to prevent and treat it.]*

Ward JW, Lok AS, Thomas DL: Report on a single-topic conference on "Chronic viral hepatitis–strategies to improve effectiveness of screening and treatment". *Hepatology* 55:307, 2012. *[Overview of all aspects of chronic viral hepatitis and the relationship of pathology to disease course and management.]*

Autoimmune Liver Diseases

Czaja AJ, Manns MP: Advances in the diagnosis, pathogenesis, and management of autoimmune hepatitis. *Gastroenterology* 139:58, 2010.

Eisenmann de Torres B and members of the International Autoimmune Hepatitis Group: Simplified criteria for the diagnosis of autoimmune hepatitis. *Hepatology* 48:169, 2008.

Imam MH, Talwalkar JA, Lindor KD: An update on primary sclerosing cholangitis:from pathogenesis to treatment. *Minerva Gastroenterol Dietol* 59:49, 2013. *[A comprehensive review of all aspects of this disease.]*

Uibo R, Kisand K, Yang CY: Primary biliary cirrhosis: a multi-faced interactive disease involving genetics, environment and the immune response. *APMIS* 120:857, 2012. *[A classic liver disease whose origins remain obscure - the latest in what is understood or hypothesized.]*

Drug- and Toxin-Induced Liver Injury

Beier JI, Arteel GE, McClain CJ: Advances in alcoholic liver disease. *Curr Gastroenterol Rep* 13:56, 2011.

Crawford JM: Histologic findings in alcoholic liver disease. *Clin Liver Dis* 16:699, 2012. *[A thorough look at the morphologic changes in alcoholic liver disease and the underlying mechanisms that produce them.]*

Gunawan B, Kaplowitz N: Clinical perspectives on xenobiotic-induced hepatotoxicity. *Drug Metab Rev* 36:301, 2004. *[A comprehensive and current review.]*

Kleiner DE: The pathology of drug-induced liver injury. *Semin Liver Dis* 29:364, 2009.

Metabolic Liver Diseases

Kleiner DE, Brunt EM: Nonalcoholic fatty liver disease: pathologic patterns and biopsy evaluation in clinical research. *Semin Liver Dis* 32:3, 2012. *[As authoritative as one can be on the topic.]*

Perlmutter DH, Silverman GA: Hepatic fibrosis and carcinogenesis in α1-antitrypsin deficiency: a prototype for chronic tissue damage in gain-of-function disorders. *Cold Spring Harb Perspect Biol* 1:3, 2011. *[A broader perspective on some chronic hereditary diseases using alpha-1-antitrypsin as the paradigmatic example.]*

Pietrangelo A: Hereditary hemochromatosis: pathogenesis, diagnosis, and treatment. *Gastroenterology* 139:393, 2010.

Rosencrantz R, Schilsky M: Wilson disease: pathogenesis and clinical considerations in diagnosis and treatment. *Semin Liver Dis* 31:245, 2011.

Santos PC, Krieger JE, Pereira AC: Molecular diagnostic and pathogenesis of hereditary hemochromatosis. *Int J Mol Sci* 13:1497, 2012.

Cholestatic Syndromes

Desmet VJ: Congenital diseases of intrahepatic bile ducts: variations on the theme "ductal plate malformation". *Hepatology* 16:1069, 1992. *[A classic paper in liver pathology.]*

Hirschfield GM, Heathcote EJ, Gershwin ME: Pathogenesis of cholestatic liver disease and therapeutic approaches. *Gastroenterology* 139:1481, 2010. *[Thorough overview of the most common features of liver disease.]*

Paumgartner G: Biliary physiology and disease: reflections of a physician-scientist. *Hepatology* 51:1095, 2010. *[How bench top work comes to exert an impact on clinical medicine, sometimes, slowly, over decades.]*

Tsui WM, Lam PW, Lee WK: Primary hepatolithiasis, recurrent pyogenic cholangitis, and oriental cholangiohepatitis: a tale of 3 countries. *Adv Anat Pathol* 18:318, 2011. *[A review that reveals much about the diseases discussed as well as the variable histories of medical understanding in different regions of the globe.]*

Benign and Malignant Liver Tumors

Bioulac-Sage P, Cubel G, Balabaud C: Revisiting the pathology of resected benign hepatocellular nodules using new immunohistochemical markers. *Semin Liver Dis* 31:91, 2011. *[From the team largely responsible for the new molecular subclassifications of hepatocellular adenomas.]*

Bosman F, Carneiro F, Hruban R, et al, editors: *WHO Classification of Tumours of the Digestive System*, ed 4, Geneva, Switzerland, 2010, WHO Press. *[Current bible for tumors of the liver and biliary tree – and the rest of the digestive tract as well.]*

El-Serag HB: Epidemiology of Viral Hepatitis and Hepatocellular Carcinoma. *Gastroenterology* 142:1264, 2012. *[Trends in the incidence of hepatocellular carcinoma with a good discussion about the causes of the increased incidence.]*

Forner A, Llovet JM, Bruix J: Hepatocellular carcinoma. *Lancet* 379:1245, 2012. *[Clinical, radiological, pathological, and oncologic perspectives all woven together.]*

Gatto M, Alvaro D: New insights on cholangiocarcinoma. *World J Gastrointest Oncol* 2:136, 2010.

International Consensus Group for Hepatocellular Neoplasia: Pathologic diagnosis of early hepatocellular carcinoma. *Hepatology* 49:658, 2009. *[A good example of how change comes to medicine, individual efforts combining, over years, to achieve a new consensus.]*

Razumilava N, Gores GJ: Classification, diagnosis, and management of cholangiocarcinoma. *Clin Gastroenterol Hepatol* 11:13, 2013.

See TARGETED THERAPY available online at www.studentconsult.com

CHAPTER 19

The Pancreas

Ralph H. Hruban • Christine A. Iacobuzio-Donahue

CHAPTER CONTENTS

The adult pancreas is a transversely oriented retroperitoneal organ extending from the C-loop of the duodenum to the hilum of the spleen (Fig. 19-1*A*). Although the organ gets its name from the Greek *pankreas* ("all flesh"), it is in fact a complex lobulated organ with distinct exocrine and endocrine components.

The *exocrine pancreas* constitutes 80% to 85% of the organ and is composed of acinar cells that secrete enzymes needed for digestion. Acinar cells are pyramidally shaped epithelial cells containing membrane-bound granules rich in proenzymes (zymogens), including trypsinogen, chymotrypsinogen, procarboxypeptidase, proelastase, kallikreinogen, and prophospholipase A and B. Upon secretion, these proenzymes and enzymes are carried by a series of ductules and ducts to the duodenum, where they are activated by proteolytic cleavage in the gastrointestinal tract (described later).

The *endocrine pancreas* is composed of about 1 million clusters of cells, the islets of Langerhans, scattered throughout the gland. The islet cells secrete insulin, glucagon, and somatostatin and constitute only 1% to 2% of the organ. Diseases of the endocrine pancreas are described in detail in Chapter 24.

Congenital Anomalies

The complex process by which the dorsal and ventral pancreatic primordia fuse during pancreatic development is prone to "imperfections" that frequently gives rise to congenital variations in pancreatic anatomy. The pancreas normally arises from the fusion of dorsal and ventral outpouchings of the foregut. The body, the tail, and the superior/anterior aspect of the head of the pancreas, as well as the accessory duct of Santorini, are derived from the dorsal primordium. Normally, the ventral primordium gives rise to the posterior/inferior part of the head of the pancreas and drains through the main pancreatic duct into the papilla of Vater.

Pancreas Divisum. **Pancreas divisum is the most common congenital anomaly of the pancreas,** with an incidence of 3% to 10%. In most individuals, the main pancreatic duct (the duct of Wirsung) joins the common bile duct just proximal to the papilla of Vater, and the accessory pancreatic duct (the duct of Santorini) drains into the duodenum through a separate minor papilla (Fig. 19-1*A*). Pancreas divisum is caused by a failure of fusion of the fetal duct systems of the dorsal and ventral pancreatic primordia. As a result, the bulk of the pancreas (formed by the dorsal pancreatic primordium) drains into the duodenum through the small-caliber minor papilla (Fig. 19-1*B*). The duct of Wirsung in persons with divisum drains only a small portion of the head of the gland through the papilla of Vater. Although controversial, it has been suggested that inadequate drainage of the pancreatic secretions through the minor papilla, especially when combined with genetic defects that also increases susceptibility to pancreatitis (described later), predisposes individuals with pancreatic divisum to chronic pancreatitis.

Annular Pancreas. Annular pancreas is a band-like ring of normal pancreatic tissue that completely encircles the second portion of the duodenum. Annular pancreas can produce duodenal obstruction.

Ectopic Pancreas. Pancreatic tissue that is aberrantly situated, or ectopic, is found in about 2% of careful routine postmortem examinations. The favored sites for ectopia are the stomach and duodenum, followed by the jejunum,

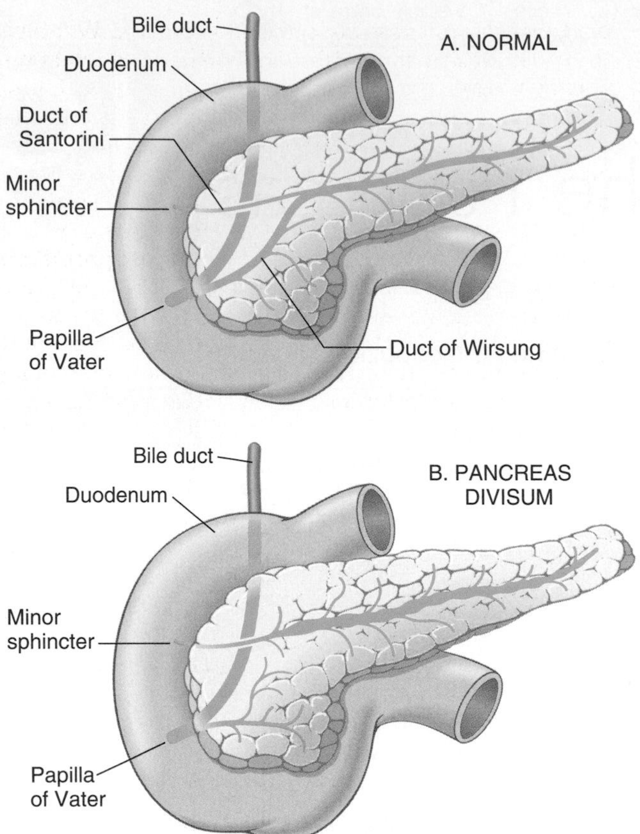

Figure 19-1 Pancreatic ductal anatomy. **A,** The normal ductal anatomy. **B,** The ductal anatomy in pancreatic divisum. (Adapted from Gregg JA, et al: Pancreas divisum: results of surgical intervention. Am J Surg 1983; 145:488-492.)

Meckel diverticula, and ileum. Although usually incidental findings, these embryologic rests, composed of normal-appearing pancreatic acini, glands, and sometimes islets of Langerhans, may cause pain from localized inflammation, or, rarely, may incite mucosal bleeding.

Agenesis. Very rarely the pancreas fails to develop (agenesis). Some cases of agenesis are caused by homozygous germline mutations involving *PDX1*, a gene encoding a homeobox transcription factor that is critical for pancreatic development.

Pancreatitis

Pancreatitis is divided into two forms, acute and chronic, each with its own characteristic pathologic and clinical features. As we will discuss, both are initiated by injuries that lead to autodigestion of the pancreas by its own enzymes. Under normal circumstances, the following mechanisms protect the pancreas from self-digestion by its secreted enzymes:

- Most digestive enzymes are synthesized as inactive proenzymes (zymogens), which are packaged within secretory granules.
- Most proenzymes are activated by trypsin, which itself is activated by duodenal enteropeptidase (enterokinase) in the small bowel; thus, intrapancreatic activation of proenzymes is normally minimal.
- Acinar and ductal cells secrete trypsin inhibitors, including serine protease inhibitor Kazal type 1 (SPINK1), which further limit intrapancreatic trypsin activity.

Table 19-1 Etiologic Factors in Acute Pancreatitis

Metabolic
Alcoholism
Hyperlipoproteinemia
Hypercalcemia
Drugs (e.g., azathioprine)
Genetic
Mutations in genes encoding trypsin, trypsin regulators, or proteins that regulate calcium metabolism
Mechanical
Gallstones
Trauma
Iatrogenic injury
Operative injury
Endoscopic procedures with dye injection
Vascular
Shock
Atheroembolism
Vasculitis
Infectious
Mumps

Pancreatitis occurs when these protective mechanisms are deranged or overwhelmed. As discussed later, the clinical manifestations of pancreatitis vary widely. Acute attacks may be mild and self-limited or present as a life-threatening acute inflammatory process; with recurrent or persistent pancreatitis, there may be permanent loss of pancreatic function.

Acute Pancreatitis

Acute pancreatitis is characterized by *reversible* pancreatic parenchymal injury associated with inflammation and has diverse etiologies, including toxic exposures (e.g., alcohol), pancreatic duct obstruction (e.g., biliary calculi), inherited genetic defects, vascular injury, and infections. Acute pancreatitis is relatively common; the annual incidence in Western countries is 10 to 20 cases per 100,000 people. Biliary tract disease and alcoholism account for approximately 80% of cases of acute pancreatitis in Western countries (Table 19-1). Gallstones are present in 35% to 60% of cases, and pancreatitis develops in about 5% of patients with gallstones. The proportion of cases of acute pancreatitis caused by excessive alcohol intake varies from 65% in the United States to 20% in Sweden to 5% or less in southern France and the United Kingdom. The male-to-female ratio is 1:3 in the group with biliary tract disease and 6:1 in those with alcoholism.

Pathogenesis. **Acute pancreatitis results from inappropriate release and activation of pancreatic enzymes, which destroy pancreatic tissue and elicit an acute**

inflammatory reaction. As we discussed, pancreatic enzymes, including trypsin, are synthesized in an inactive proenzyme form. Inappropriate intrapancreatic activation of trypsin can in turn cause the activation of other proenzymes such as prophospholipase and proelastase, which then degrade fat cells and damage the elastic fibers of blood vessels, respectively. Trypsin also converts prekallikrein to its activated form, thus bringing into play the kinin system and, by activation of coagulation factor XII, the clotting and complement systems as well (Chapters 3 and 4). The resulting inflammation and small-vessel thromboses (which may lead to congestion and rupture of already weakened vessels) damage acinar cells, further amplifying intrapancreatic activation of digestive enzymes.

How inappropriate activation of pancreatic enzymes occurs in sporadic forms of acute pancreatitis is not entirely clear, but there is evidence for at least three major initiating events (Fig. 19-2):

- **Pancreatic duct obstruction.** Obstruction is most commonly caused by *gallstones* and biliary sludge, but can also stem from *periampullary neoplasms* (e.g., pancreatic cancer), *choledochoceles* (congenital cystic dilatation of the common bile duct), *parasites* (particularly the *Ascaris lumbricoides* and *Clonorchis sinensis* organisms), and possibly pancreas divisum. Whatever the cause, obstruction raises intrapancreatic ductal pressure and leads to the accumulation of enzyme-rich fluid in the interstitium. Although most pancreatic enzymes are secreted as inactive zymogens, lipase is produced in an active form and has the potential to cause local fat necrosis. The death of adipocytes is hypothesized to produce "danger" signals locally that stimulate periacinar myofibroblasts and leukocytes to release proinflammatory cytokines and other inflammatory mediators that initiate local inflammation and promote the development of interstitial edema through a leaky microvasculature. Edema may further compromise local blood flow, causing vascular insufficiency and ischemic injury to acinar cells.
- **Primary acinar cell injury,** leading to release of digestive enzymes, inflammation, and autodigestion of pancreatic tissues. As described later, acinar cells can be damaged by a variety of endogenous, exogenous, and iatrogenic insults. Oxidative stress may generate free radicals in acinar cells, leading to membrane lipid oxidation and the activation of transcription factors, including AP1 and NF-κB, which in turn induce the expression of chemokines that attract mononuclear

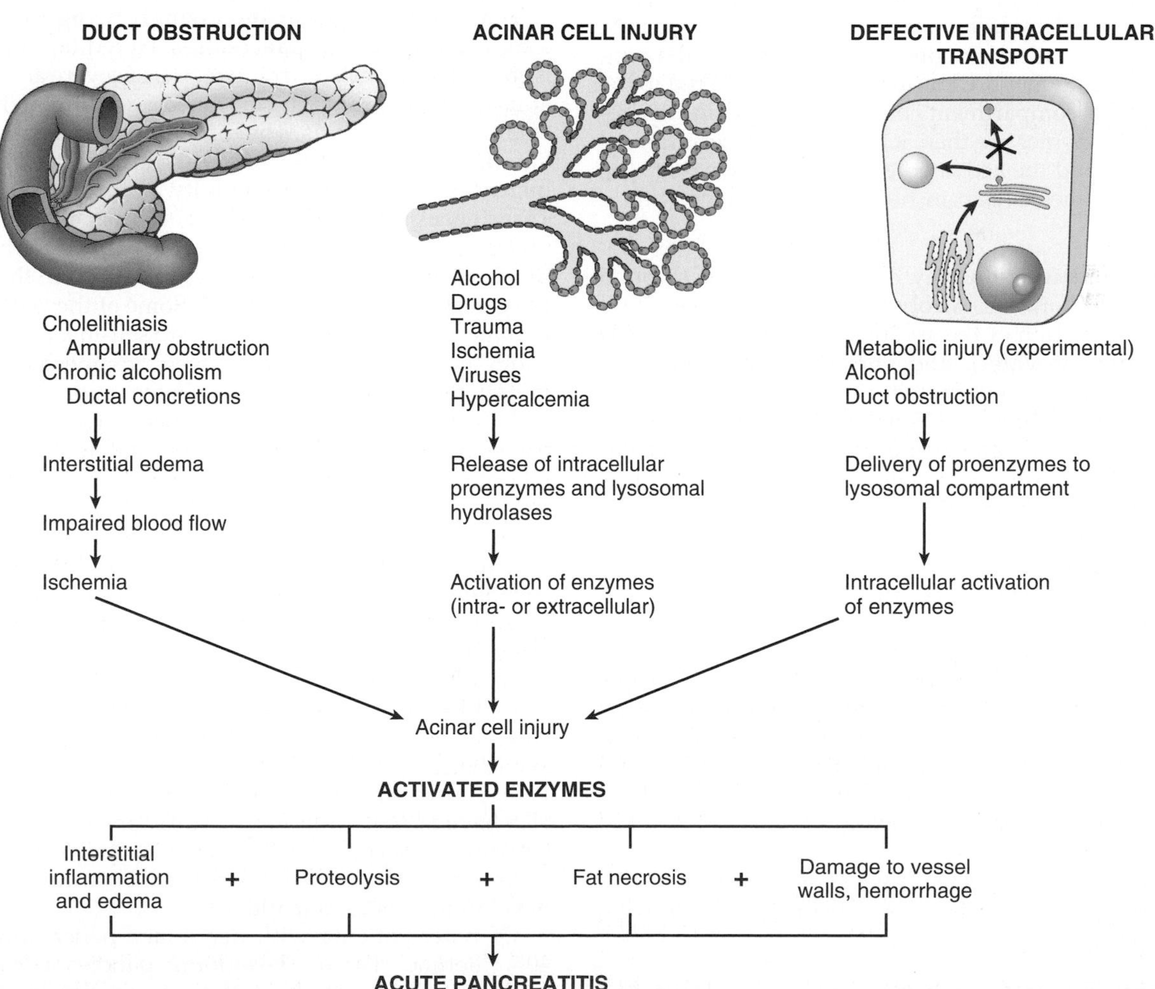

Figure 19-2 Three proposed pathways in the pathogenesis of acute pancreatitis.

Table 19-2 Inherited Predisposition to Pancreatitis

Gene (Chromosome Location)	Protein Product	Function
CFTR (7q31)	Cystic fibrosis transmembrane conductance regulator	Epithelial anion channel. Loss-of-function mutations alter fluid pressure and limit bicarbonate secretion, leading to inspissation of secreted fluids and duct obstruction
PRSS1 (7q34)	Serine protease 1 (trypsinogen 1)	Cationic trypsin. Gain-of-function mutations prevent self-inactivation of trypsin
SPINK1 (5q32)	Serine peptidase inhibitor, Kazal type 1	Inhibitor of trypsin. Mutations cause loss-of-function, increasing trypsin activity
CASR (3q13)	Calcium-sensing receptor	Membrane-bound receptor that senses extracellular calcium levels and controls luminal calcium levels. Mutations may alter calcium concentrations and activate trypsin.
CTRC (1p36)	Chymotrypsin C (caldecrin)	Degrades trypsin, protects the pancreas from trypsin-related injury
CPA1 (7q32)	Carboxypeptidase A1	Exopeptidase involved in regulating zymogen activation

cells. Increased calcium flux appears to be another important trigger for inappropriate activation of digestive enzymes. Calcium has a key role in regulating trypsin activation. When calcium levels are low, trypsin tends to cleave and inactivate itself, but when calcium levels are high autoinhibition is abrogated and activation of trypsinogen by trypsin is favored. It is suspected that any factor that causes calcium levels to rise in acinar cells may trigger excessive activation of trypsin, including certain inherited abnormalities that affect calcium levels (Table 19-2).

- **Defective intracellular transport of proenzymes within acinar cells.** In normal acinar cells, digestive enzymes and lysosomal hydrolases are transported in separate pathways. In animal models of acinar injury, the pancreatic proenzymes are inappropriately delivered to the intracellular compartment containing lysosomal hydrolases. Proenzymes are then activated, the lysosomes are disrupted, and the activated enzymes are released. The role of this mechanism in human acute pancreatitis is not clear.

Alcohol consumption may cause pancreatitis through all of these mechanisms. Alcohol consumption transiently increases contraction of the sphincter of Oddi (the muscle at the Papilla of Vater), and chronic alcohol ingestion results in the secretion of protein-rich pancreatic fluid that leads to the deposition of inspissated protein plugs and obstruction of small pancreatic ducts. Alcohol also has direct toxic effects on acinar cells. Alcohol-induced oxidative stress may generate free radicals in acinar cells, leading to membrane lipid oxidation and free radical production, which as already mentioned has been linked to activation of the pro-inflammatory transcription factors AP1 and NF-κB. Oxidative stress also may promote the fusion of lysosomes and zymogen granules and alter intracellular calcium levels, possibly through mitochondrial damage, promoting the intraacinar activation of trypsin and other digestive enzymes. Nevertheless, it should be noted that most drinkers never develop pancreatitis and those who do usually do so after many years of alcohol abuse. Thus, key aspects of the pathophysiology of alcohol-induced pancreatitis remain obscure.

Other proven or suspected triggers of acute pancreatitis in the remaining sporadic cases include the following (Table 19-1):

- **Metabolic disorders,** such as hypertriglyceridemia, and hypercalcemic states, such as hyperparathyroidism
- **Genetic lesions,** described below
- **Medications**. More than 85 drugs have been implicated, including furosemide, azathioprine, 2′,3′-dideoxyinosine, estrogens, and many others. In most cases the mechanism of drug-induced pancreatitis is unknown.
- **Traumatic injury of acinar cells,** either by blunt abdominal trauma or by iatrogenic injury during surgery or endoscopic retrograde cholangiopancreatography
- **Ischemic injury of acinar cells,** caused by shock, vascular thrombosis, embolism, and vasculitis
- **Infections,** including mumps, can lead to acute pancreatitis through direct acinar cell injury

Hereditary factors are increasingly being recognized as a significant cause of pancreatitis. Hereditary pancreatitis is characterized by recurrent attacks of severe acute pancreatitis often beginning in childhood and ultimately leading to chronic pancreatitis. The disorder is genetically diverse, but **the shared feature of most forms is a defect that increases or sustains the activity of trypsin** (Table 19-2). Three genes implicated in hereditary pancreatitis deserve special note: *PRSS1, SPINK1,* and *CFTR*. Most hereditary cases are due to gain-of-function mutations in the *trypsinogen* gene (also known as *PRSS1*). Some of these *PRSS1* gene mutations make trypsin resistant to self-inactivation, abrogating an important negative feedback mechanism; other mutations appear to make trypsinogen more prone to proteolytic activation. Hereditary pancreatitis associated with trypsinogen mutation has an autosomal dominant mode of inheritance, as is typically true of disorders associated with gain-of-function mutations.

Hereditary pancreatitis can also be caused by loss-of-function mutations in *SPINK1*, already described as a gene encoding a trypsin inhibitor. As expected, this form of hereditary pancreatitis has an autosomal recessive mode of inheritance.

As discussed in detail in Chapter 5, cystic fibrosis is caused by mutations in the cystic fibrosis transmembrane conductance regulator (*CFTR*) gene, and homozygous and even heterozygous *CFTR* gene mutations are associated with pancreatitis, the latter particularly in patients who also have *SPINK1* mutations. Mutations in *CFTR* decrease bicarbonate secretion by pancreatic ductal cells, thereby promoting protein plugging, duct obstruction, and the development of pancreatitis.

Of note, patients with hereditary pancreatitis have a 40% lifetime risk of developing pancreatic cancer, yet another example of the nefarious association of chronic tissue injury and inflammation with neoplasia.

MORPHOLOGY

The morphology of acute pancreatitis ranges from trivial inflammation and edema to severe extensive necrosis and hemorrhage. The basic alterations are **(1) microvascular leak and edema, (2) fat necrosis, (3) acute inflammation, (4) destruction of pancreatic parenchyma, and (5) destruction of blood vessels and interstitial hemorrhage.** The extent of each of these alterations depends on the duration and severity of the process.

In the milder form, **acute interstitial pancreatitis,** histologic alterations are limited to mild inflammation, interstitial edema, and focal areas of fat necrosis in the pancreas and the peripancreatic fat (Fig. 19-3). Fat necrosis, as we have seen, results from enzymatic activity of lipase. The released fatty acids combine with calcium to form insoluble salts that impart a granular blue microscopic appearance to the fat cells (Chapter 2).

In the more severe form, **acute necrotizing pancreatitis,** there is necrosis of acinar and ductal tissues as well as islets of Langerhans. Vascular injury can lead to hemorrhage into the pancreatic parenchyma. Macroscopically, the pancreatic substance is red-black from hemorrhage and contains interspersed foci of yellow-white, chalky fat necrosis (Fig. 19-4). Focal fat necrosis may also occur adjacent to the pancreas in the omentum and the mesentery of the bowel, and even outside the abdominal cavity, such as in the subcutaneous fat. In most cases the peritoneal cavity contains a serous, slightly turbid, brown-tinged fluid containing globules of fat (derived from the action of enzymes on adipose tissue). In its most severe form, **hemorrhagic pancreatitis,** extensive parenchymal necrosis is accompanied by dramatic hemorrhage within the substance of the gland.

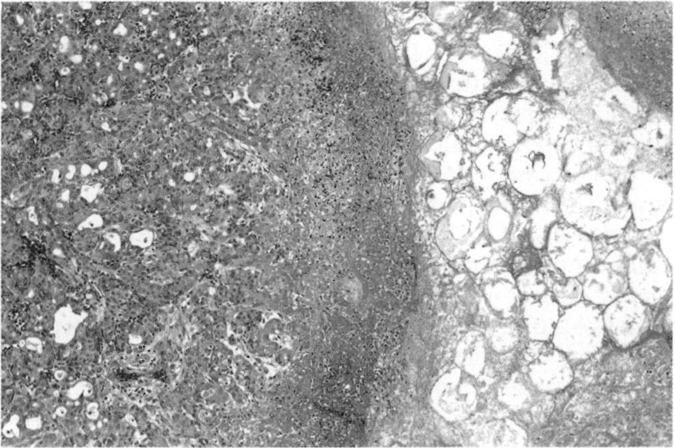

Figure 19-3 The microscopic field shows a region of fat necrosis on the right and focal pancreatic parenchymal necrosis *(center)*.

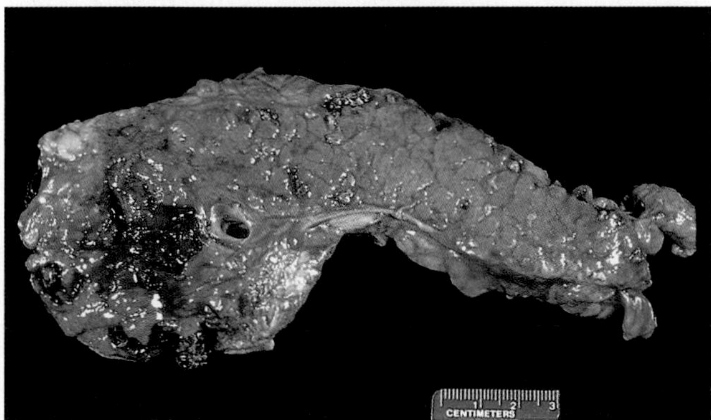

Figure 19-4 The pancreas has been sectioned longitudinally to reveal dark areas of hemorrhage in the head of the pancreas and a focal area of pale fat necrosis in the peripancreatic fat *(upper left)*.

Clinical Features. *Abdominal pain* is the cardinal manifestation of acute pancreatitis. Characteristically, the pain is constant and intense and is referred to the upper back and occasionally to the left shoulder. Its severity varies from mild and uncomfortable to severe and incapacitating. Anorexia, nausea, and vomiting frequently accompany the pain. Elevated plasma levels of amylase and lipase support the diagnosis of acute pancreatitis, as does the exclusion of other causes of abdominal pain.

Full-blown acute pancreatitis is a medical emergency. Patients usually have the sudden calamitous onset of an "acute abdomen." Many of the systemic features of severe acute pancreatitis can be attributed to release of toxic enzymes, cytokines, and other mediators into the circulation and explosive activation of a systemic inflammatory response, resulting in *leukocytosis, disseminated intravascular coagulation, edema, and acute respiratory distress syndrome.* Shock, due to the systemic inflammatory response syndrome (Chapters 4), and acute renal tubular necrosis may occur.

Laboratory findings include *marked elevation of serum amylase* levels during the first 24 hours, followed by a rising serum lipase level by 72 to 96 hours after the beginning of the attack. *Glycosuria* occurs in 10% of cases. *Hypocalcemia* may result from precipitation of calcium soaps in necrotic fat. Direct visualization of the enlarged inflamed pancreas by CT scanning is useful in the diagnosis of pancreatitis.

The key to the management of acute pancreatitis is "resting" the pancreas by total restriction of oral intake and by supportive therapy with intravenous fluids and analgesia. Although most individuals with acute pancreatitis recover fully, about 5% with severe acute pancreatitis die in the first week of illness. Acute respiratory distress syndrome and acute renal failure are ominous complications. Sequelae can include a sterile *pancreatic abscess* and a *pancreatic pseudocyst* (discussed later). In 40% to 60% of patients with acute necrotizing pancreatitis the necrotic debris becomes infected, usually by gram-negative organisms from the alimentary tract, further complicating the clinical course. Systemic organ failure and necrosis in the pancreas are both poor prognostic findings.

KEY CONCEPTS

- Acute pancreatitis is a form of *reversible* pancreatic parenchymal injury associated with inflammation.
- Acute pancreatitis may be caused by
  - Excessive alcohol intake
  - Pancreatic duct obstruction (e.g., gallstones)
  - Genetic factors (e.g., *PRSS1*, *SPINK1*)
  - Traumatic injuries
  - Medications
  - Infections (e.g., mumps)
  - Metabolic disorders leading to hypercalcemia
  - Ischemia

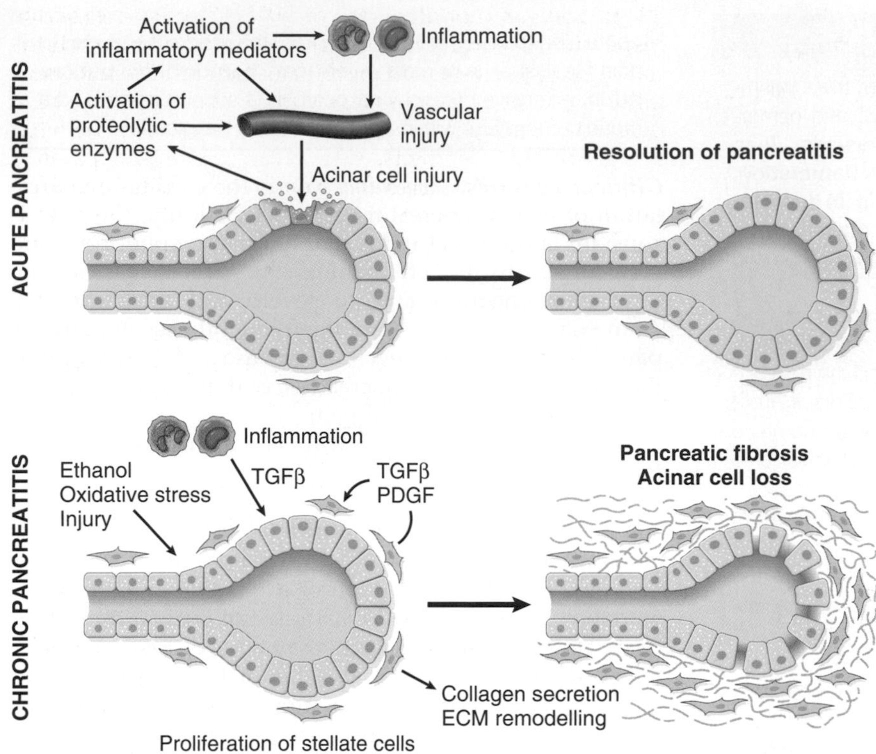

Figure 19-5 Comparison of the mediators in acute and chronic pancreatitis. In acute pancreatitis acinar injury results in release of proteolytic enzymes, leading to a cascade of events including activation of the clotting cascade, acute and chronic inflammation, vascular injury, and edema. In most patients, complete resolution of the acute injury occurs with restoration of acinar cell mass. In chronic pancreatitis, repeated episodes of acinar cell injury lead to the production of profibrogenic cytokines such as transforming growth factor β (TGF-β) and platelet-derived growth factor (PDGF), resulting in the proliferation of myofibroblasts, the secretion of collagen, and remodeling of the extracellular matrix (ECM). Repeated injury produces irreversible loss of acinar cell mass, fibrosis, and pancreatic insufficiency.

- The key feature of all of these causes is that they promote the inappropriate activation of digestive enzymes within the substance of the pancreas
- Clinical features include acute abdominal pain, systemic inflammatory response syndrome, and elevated serum lipase and amylase levels

Chronic Pancreatitis

Chronic pancreatitis is defined as prolonged inflammation of the pancreas associated with *irreversible* destruction of exocrine parenchyma, fibrosis, and, in the late stages, the destruction of endocrine parenchyma. The prevalence of chronic pancreatitis ranges between 0.04% and 5%; most affected patients are middle-aged males. **The most common cause of chronic pancreatitis by far is long-term alcohol abuse.** In addition to alcohol, chronic pancreatitis has been associated with the following conditions:

- Long-standing *obstruction* of the pancreatic duct by calculi or neoplasms
- *Autoimmune injury* to the gland
- *Hereditary pancreatitis,* as discussed under acute pancreatitis; up to 25% of chronic pancreatitis has a genetic basis

Pathogenesis. Chronic pancreatitis most often follows repeated episodes of acute pancreatitis. It has been proposed that acute pancreatitis initiates a sequence of perilobular fibrosis, duct distortion, and altered pancreatic secretions. Over time and with multiple episodes, this can lead to loss of pancreatic parenchyma and fibrosis.

Chronic pancreatic injury, whatever its cause, leads to local production of inflammatory mediators that promote fibrosis and acinar cell loss. While the cytokines produced during chronic and acute pancreatitis are similar, fibrogenic factors tend to predominate in chronic pancreatitis. These fibrogenic cytokines include transforming growth factor β (TGF-β) and platelet-derived growth factor, which induce the activation and proliferation of periacinar myofibroblasts (pancreatic stellate cells), resulting in the deposition of collagen and fibrosis (Fig. 19-5).

Autoimmune pancreatitis is a pathogenically distinct form of chronic pancreatitis that is associated with the presence of IgG4-secreting plasma cells in the pancreas. Autoimmune pancreatitis is one manifestation of IgG-related disease (Chapter 6), which may involve multiple tissues. Autoimmune pancreatitis may mimic the signs and symptoms of pancreatic carcinoma. It is important to recognize because it responds to steroid therapy.

MORPHOLOGY

Chronic pancreatitis is characterized by fibrosis, atrophy and dropout of acini, and variable dilation of pancreatic ducts (Fig. 19-6*A*). Grossly, the gland is hard, sometimes with visibly dilated ducts containing calcified concretions. These changes are typically accompanied by a chronic inflammatory infiltrate around lobules and ducts. The ductal epithelium may be atrophied or hyperplastic or may show squamous metaplasia. Acinar loss is a constant feature. There is usually relative sparing of the islets of Langerhans, which become embedded in the sclerotic tissue and may fuse and appear enlarged, but in advanced disease the islets also are lost. Chronic pancreatitis caused by alcohol abuse is characterized by ductal dilatation and intraluminal protein plugs and calcifications (Fig. 19-6*B*). **Autoimmune pancreatitis** is characterized by a duct-centric mixed inflammatory cell infiltrate, venulitis, and increased numbers of IgG4-secreting plasma cells.

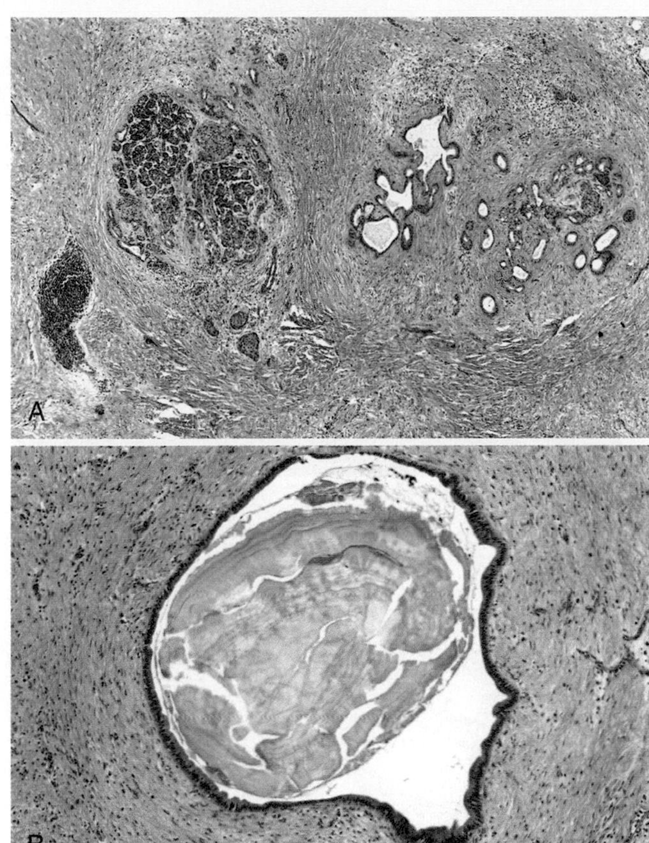

Figure 19-6 Chronic pancreatitis. **A,** Extensive fibrosis and atrophy has left only residual islets *(left)* and ducts *(right)*, with a sprinkling of chronic inflammatory cells and a few islands of acinar tissue. **B,** A higher power view demonstrating dilated ducts with inspissated eosinophilic ductal concretions in a person with alcoholic chronic pancreatitis.

Clinical Features. Chronic pancreatitis may present in many different ways. It may follow repeated bouts of acute pancreatitis. There may be repeated attacks of mild to moderately severe abdominal pain, or persistent abdominal and back pain. Attacks may be precipitated by alcohol abuse, overeating (which increases demand on the pancreas), or the use of opiates and other drugs that increase the tone of the sphincter of Oddi. In other patients the disease may be entirely silent until pancreatic insufficiency and diabetes mellitus develop due to destruction of the exocrine and endocrine pancreas.

The diagnosis of chronic pancreatitis requires a high degree of suspicion. During an attack of abdominal pain there may be mild fever and mild-to-moderate elevations of serum amylase. When the disease has been present for a long time, however, the dropout of acinar cells may be so great as to eliminate these diagnostic clues. Gallstone-induced obstruction may be evident as jaundice or elevations in serum levels of alkaline phosphatase. A very helpful finding is visualization of calcifications within the pancreas by computed tomography and ultrasonography. Weight loss and edema due to low albumin from malabsorption caused by pancreatic exocrine insufficiency also support the diagnosis.

Although chronic pancreatitis is usually not an immediately life-threatening condition, the long-term outlook for individuals with chronic pancreatitis is poor, with a 20- to 25-year mortality rate of 50%. Pancreatic exocrine insufficiency, chronic malabsorption, and diabetes mellitus can all lead to significant morbidity and contribute to mortality. In other patients **severe chronic pain** is a dominant problem. **Pancreatic pseudocysts** (described later) develop in about 10% of patients. As already mentioned, patients with hereditary pancreatitis have a 40% lifetime risk of developing pancreatic cancer; whether this increased cancer risk extends to other forms of chronic pancreatitis is unclear.

KEY CONCEPTS

- Chronic pancreatitis is characterized by *irreversible injury* of the pancreas leading to fibrosis, loss of pancreatic parenchyma, loss of exocrine and endocrine function, and high risk of developing pseudocysts
- Chronic pancreatitis is most often caused by
  - Repeated bouts of acute pancreatitis
  - Chronic alcohol abuse
  - Germline mutations in genes such as *CFTR* (the gene encoding the transporter that is defective in cystic fibrosis), particularly when combined with environmental stressors
  - Clinical features include intermittent or persistent abdominal pain, intestinal malabsorption, and diabetes

Nonneoplastic Cysts

A variety of cysts can arise in the pancreas. Most are nonneoplastic pseudocysts (discussed later), but congenital cysts and neoplastic cysts also occur.

Congenital Cysts

Congenital cysts are unilocular, thin-walled cysts that are believed to result from anomalous development of the pancreatic ducts. They range in size from microscopic lesions to 5 cm in diameter, and are lined by a glistening, uniform cuboidal epithelium or, if the intracystic pressure is high, by a flattened and attenuated cell layer. Congenital cysts are enclosed in a thin, fibrous capsule and are filled with a clear serous fluid. Congenital cysts may be sporadic, or part of inherited conditions such as *autosomal-dominant polycystic kidney disease* (Chapter 20) and *von Hippel-Lindau disease* (Chapter 28). Cysts in the kidney, liver, and pancreas frequently coexist in polycystic kidney disease. In von Hippel-Lindau disease vascular neoplasms are found in the retina and cerebellum or brain stem in association with congenital cysts (and also neoplasms) in the pancreas, liver, and kidney.

Pseudocysts

Pseudocysts are localized collections of necrotic and hemorrhagic material that are rich in pancreatic enzymes and lack an epithelial lining (hence the prefix "pseudo"). Pseudocysts account for approximately 75% of cysts in the pancreas. They usually arise following a bout of acute pancreatitis, particularly one superimposed on chronic alcoholic pancreatitis. Traumatic injury to the pancreas can also give rise to pseudocysts.

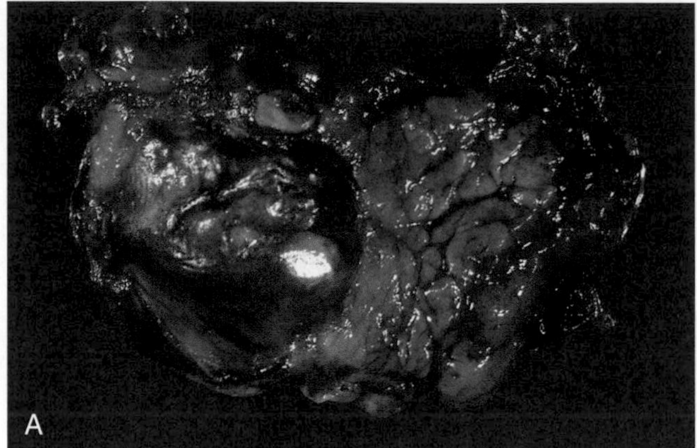

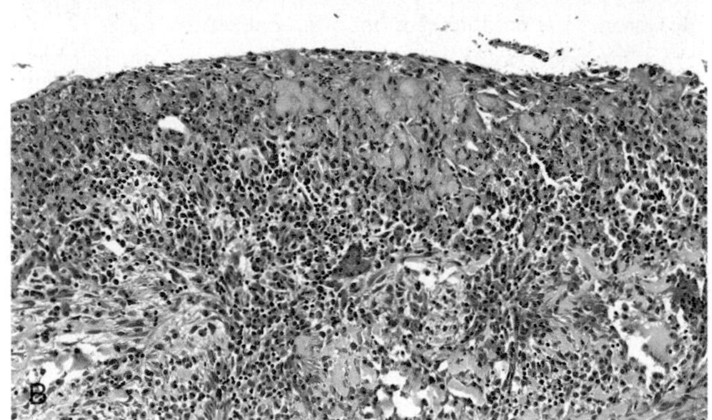

Figure 19-7 Pancreatic pseudocyst. **A,** Cross-section revealing a poorly defined cyst with a necrotic brown-black wall. **B,** The cyst lacks a true epithelial lining and instead is lined by fibrin and granulation tissue.

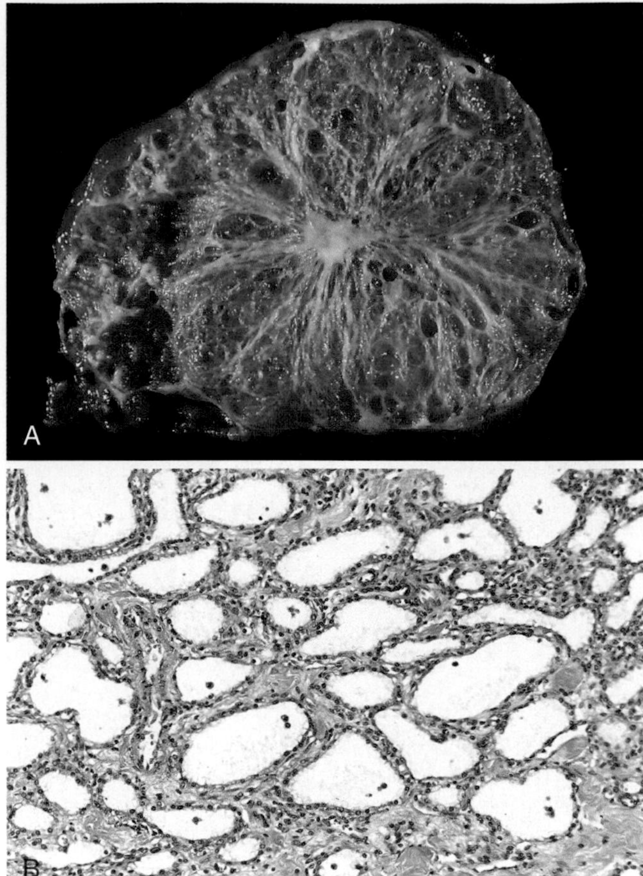

Figure 19-8 Serous cystic neoplasm (serous cystadenoma). **A,** Cross-section through a serous cystic neoplasm. Only a thin rim of normal pancreatic parenchyma remains. The cysts are relatively small and contain clear, straw-colored fluid. **B,** The cysts are lined by cuboidal epithelium without atypia.

MORPHOLOGY

Pseudocysts are usually solitary and may be situated within the pancreas, or, more commonly, in the lesser omental sac or in the retroperitoneum between the stomach and transverse colon or between the stomach and liver. They can even be subdiaphragmatic (Fig. 19-7*A*). Pseudocysts are formed when areas of intrapancreatic or peripancreatic hemorrhagic fat necrosis are walled off by fibrous tissue and granulation tissue (Fig. 19-7*B*). They range in size from 2 to 30 cm in diameter.

While many pseudocysts spontaneously resolve, they may become secondarily infected, and larger pseudocysts may compress or even perforate into adjacent structures.

Neoplasms

A broad spectrum of exocrine neoplasms arises in the pancreas. Such neoplasms may be cystic or solid; some are benign, while others are among the most lethal of all malignancies. Neuroendocrine tumors also occur in the pancreas and are discussed in Chapter 24.

Cystic Neoplasms

Cystic neoplasms are diverse tumors that range from harmless benign cysts to lesions that may be precursors to invasive, potentially lethal, cancers. Only 5% to 15% of all pancreatic cysts are neoplastic (most are pseudocysts; see the previous section), and cystic neoplasms make up fewer than 5% of all pancreatic neoplasms. Serous cystic neoplasms are entirely benign, whereas others, such as intraductal papillary mucinous neoplasms and mucinous cystic neoplasms, are precancerous. Recent whole-exome sequencing has identified genetic alterations specific for each type of cystic neoplasm.

Serous cystic neoplasms are multicystic neoplasms that usually occur in the tail of the pancreas. The cysts are small (1 to 3 mm), lined by glycogen-rich cuboidal cells, and contain clear, thin, straw-colored fluid (Fig. 19-8). They account for about 25% of all cystic neoplasms of the pancreas. These neoplasms arise twice as often in women as in men and typically present in the sixth to seventh decade of life with nonspecific symptoms such as abdominal pain. Many are now being detected incidentally during imaging for another indication. Serous cystic neoplasms, called serous cystadenomas, are almost always benign and, if small, can be safely observed. Surgical resection is curative in the vast majority of patients. Inactivation of the *VHL* tumor suppressor gene is the most common genetic abnormality in serous cystic neoplasms.

Close to 95% of *mucinous cystic neoplasms* arise in women, and, in contrast to serous cystic neoplasms, they

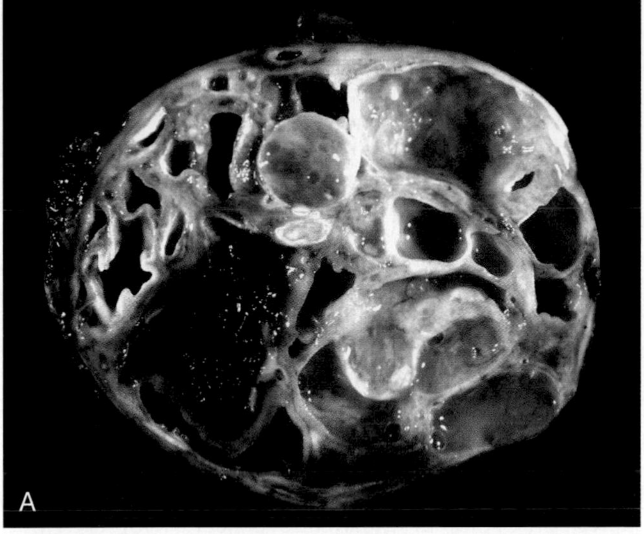

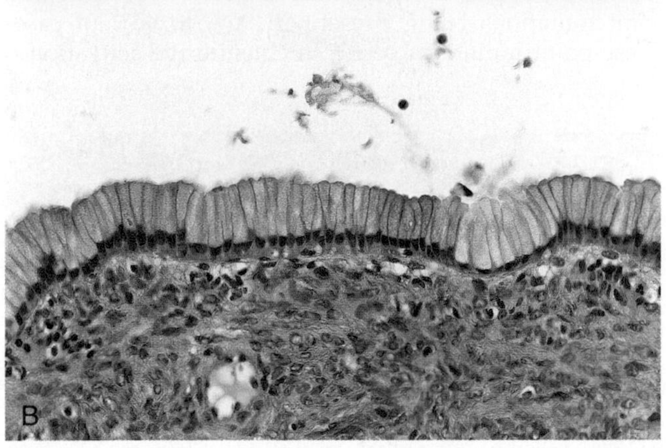

Figure 19-9 Pancreatic mucinous cystic neoplasm with low-grade dysplasia. **A,** Cross-section through a mucinous multiloculated cyst in the tail of the pancreas. The cysts are large and filled with tenacious mucin. **B,** The cysts are lined by columnar mucinous epithelium, and a dense "ovarian" stroma is noted.

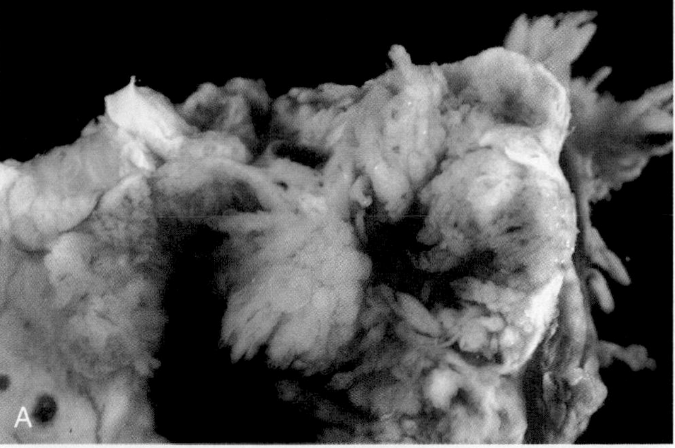

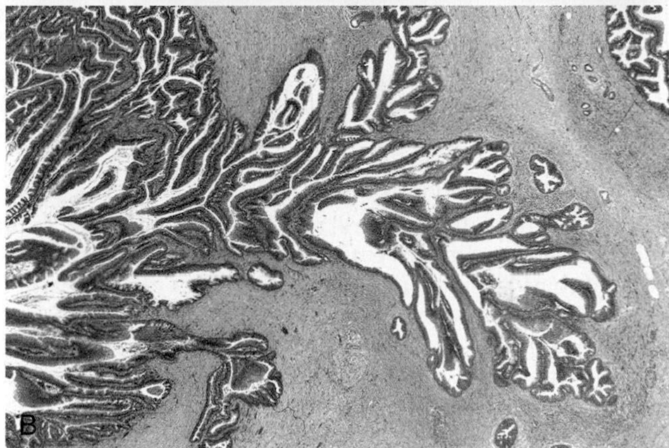

Figure 19-10 Intraductal papillary mucinous neoplasm. **A,** Cross-section through the head of the pancreas showing a prominent papillary neoplasm distending the main pancreatic duct. **B,** The neoplasm involves the main pancreatic duct *(left)* and extends down into the smaller ducts and ductules *(right)*.

can be precursors to invasive carcinomas. These neoplasms usually arise in the tail of the pancreas and present as painless, slow-growing masses. The cystic cavities are larger than those in serous cystic neoplasms. They are filled with thick, tenacious mucin and lined by a columnar mucin-producing epithelium associated with a dense stroma similar to ovarian stroma (Fig. 19-9). Up to one third of surgically resected mucinous cystic neoplasms harbor an associated invasive adenocarcinoma. While surgical resection is curative for noninvasive mucinous cystic neoplasms, half of patients with an invasive carcinoma arising in a mucinous cystic neoplasm will die of their disease. Early detection and treatment before an invasive cancer develops is therefore critical. The *KRAS* oncogene and the *TP53* and *RNF43* tumor suppressor genes are frequently mutated in these neoplasms.

Intraductal papillary mucinous neoplasms (IPMNs) are mucin-producing neoplasms that involve the larger ducts of the pancreas. In contrast to mucinous cystic neoplasms, IPMNs arise more frequently in men than in women, and they involve the head of the pancreas more often than the tail. Ten to twenty percent are multifocal. Two features are useful in distinguishing IPMNs from mucinous cystic neoplasms: (1) absence of the dense "ovarian" stroma seen in mucinous cystic neoplasms and (2) involvement of a pancreatic duct (Fig. 19-10). Just as with mucinous cystic neoplasms, IPMNs can progress to an invasive cancer. Early detection and treatment of IPMNs before they progress to an invasive cancer is therefore critical. Frequent mutations in the *GNAS* and *KRAS* oncogenes and the *TP53*, *SMAD4*, and *RNF43* tumor suppressor genes have been reported in these neoplasms.

The unusual *solid-pseudopapillary neoplasm* is seen mainly in young women. These large, well-circumscribed malignant neoplasms have solid and cystic components filled with hemorrhagic debris. The neoplastic cells grow in solid sheets or, as the name suggests, as pseudopapillary projections, and often appear to be poorly cohesive. These neoplasms often cause abdominal discomfort because of their large size. Of note, this neoplasm is virtually always associated with hyperactivation of the Wnt signaling pathway due to acquired activating mutations of the *CTNNB1* (β-catenin) oncogene. Surgical resection is the treatment of choice. Although some solid-pseudopapillary neoplasms are locally aggressive, most patients are cured following complete surgical resection of the neoplasm.

KEY CONCEPTS

- Virtually all serous cystic neoplasms are benign.
- Intraductal papillary mucinous neoplasms and mucinous cystic neoplasms are curable noninvasive cystic neoplasms that can progress to incurable invasive carcinoma.
- Each of the major cystic neoplasms has a relatively specific mutational profile.

Pancreatic Carcinoma

Infiltrating ductal adenocarcinoma of the pancreas, more commonly known as pancreatic cancer, is the fourth leading cause of cancer deaths in the United States, trailing only lung, colon, and breast cancers, and has one of the highest mortality rates of any cancer. It was estimated that in 2013 pancreatic cancer would strike approximately 44,000 Americans, virtually all of whom would die of their disease. The 5-year survival rate is dismal, less than 5%.

Precursors to Pancreatic Cancer

Invasive pancreatic cancers are believed to arise from well-defined noninvasive precursor lesions in small ducts referred to as *pancreatic intraepithelial neoplasia* (PanIN, Fig. 19-11). Just as there is a progression in the colorectum from nonneoplastic epithelium to adenoma to invasive carcinoma (Chapters 7 and 17), there is a progression in the pancreas from nonneoplastic epithelium to PanIN to invasive carcinoma. The PanIN-invasive carcinoma sequence is supported by the following observations:

- The genetic and epigenetic alterations identified in PanIN are similar to those found in invasive cancers (described later).
- PanIN is often found in pancreatic parenchyma adjacent to infiltrating carcinoma.
- PanIN precedes the development of invasive cancer in genetically engineered mouse models of pancreatic cancer.
- Isolated case reports have documented individuals with PanIN who later developed an invasive pancreatic cancer.

The epithelial cells in PanIN show dramatic telomere shortening. A critical shortening of telomere length in PanIN may predispose these lesions to accumulate progressive chromosomal abnormalities and to develop invasive carcinoma (Chapter 7).

Based on these observations, a model for progression of PanINs has been proposed (Fig. 19-12).

Pathogenesis

Multiple genes are somatically mutated or epigenetically silenced in each pancreatic carcinoma, consistent with their stepwise evolution from precursor lesions, and the patterns of genetic alterations in pancreatic carcinoma as a group differs from those seen in other malignancies. Molecular alterations in pancreatic carcinogenesis are summarized in Table 19-3 and include the following:

KRAS. *KRAS* (chromosome 12p) is the most frequently altered oncogene in pancreatic cancer, with activating point mutations being present in 90% to 95% of cases. These point mutations result in constitutive activation of

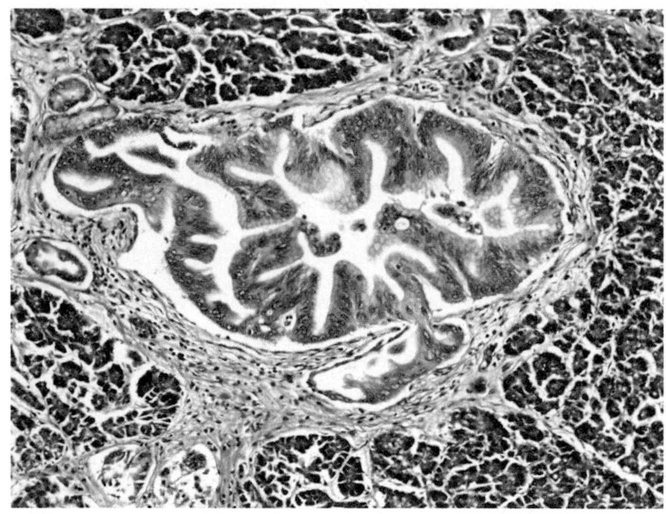

Figure 19-11 Pancreatic intraepithelial neoplasia grade 3 (PanIN-3) involving a small pancreatic duct.

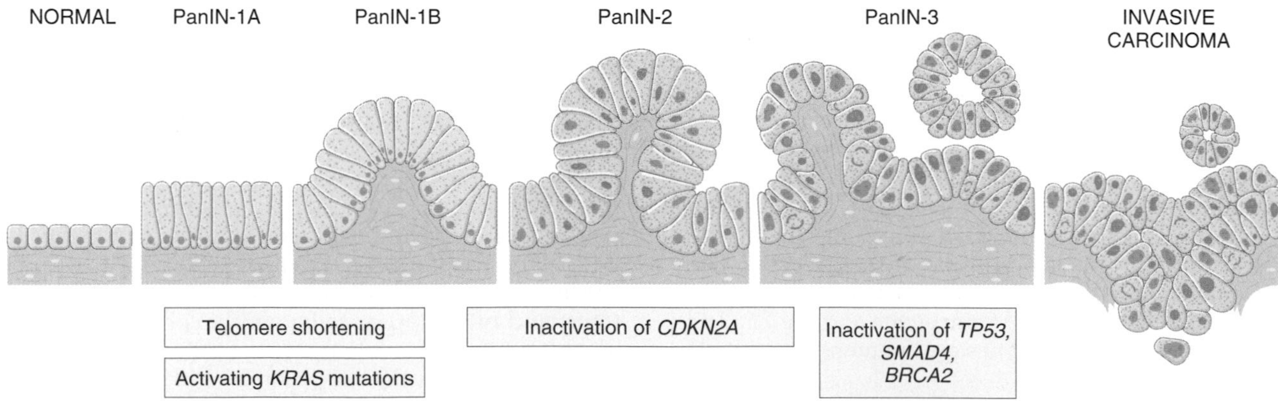

Figure 19-12 Model for the progression from normal ducts *(far left)* through PanINs *(center)* to invasive carcinoma *(far right)*. It is postulated that telomere shortening and mutations of the oncogene *KRAS* occur early, that inactivation of the *CDKN2A* tumor suppressor gene that encodes the cell cycle regulator p16 sta occurs in intermediate grade lesions, and that the inactivation of the *TP53*, *SMAD4*, and *BRCA2* tumor suppressor genes occur in higher grade (PanIN-3) lesions. It is important to note that while there is a general temporal sequence of changes, the accumulation of multiple mutations is more important than their occurrence in a specific order. (Adapted from Wilentz RE, et al: Loss of expression of DPC4 in pancreatic intraepithelial neoplasia: evidence that *DPC4* inactivation occurs late in neoplastic progression. Cancer Res 2000;60:2002.)

Table 19-3 Somatic Molecular Alterations in Invasive Pancreatic Adenocarcinoma

Gene	Chromosomal Region	Percentage of Carcinoma with Genetic Alteration	Gene Function
Oncogenes			
KRAS	12p	90	Growth factor signal transducer
AKT2	19q	10-20	Growth factor signal transducer
MYB	6q	10	Transcription factor
NCOA3/AIB1	20q	10	Chromatin regulator
MAP2K4/MKK4	17p	5	Growth factor signal transducer
Tumor Suppressor and DNA Repair Genes			
p16/CDKN2A	9p	95	Negative cell-cycle regulator
TP53	17p	50-70	Response to DNA damage
SMAD4	18q	55	TGFβ pathway
GATA-6	18q	10	Transcription factor
RB	13q	5	Negative cell-cycle regulator
STK11	19p	5	Regulation of cellular metabolism
ATM	11q	5	DNA damage response
ARID1A	1p	4	Chromatin regulator
TGFBR1	9q	2	TGFβ pathway
TGFBR2	3p	2	TGFβ pathway

KRAS, which is a small, GTP-binding protein that normally participates in signaling events downstream of growth factor receptors with intrinsic tyrosine kinase activity (Chapters 1 and 7). KRAS signaling activates a number of downstream pathways that augment cell growth and survival, most notably the MAPK and PI3K/AKT pathways (Chapter 7).

CDKN2A. The *CDKN2A* gene (chromosome 9p) is inactivated in 95% of pancreatic cancers, making it the most frequently inactivated tumor suppressor gene in these tumors. This complex locus encodes two tumor suppressor proteins (Chapter 7): p16/INK4a, a cyclin-dependent kinase inhibitor that antagonizes cell cycle progression, and ARF, a protein that augments the function of the p53 tumor suppressor protein.

SMAD4. The *SMAD4* tumor suppressor gene (chromosome 18q) is inactivated in 55% of pancreatic cancers. *SMAD4* encodes a protein that plays an important role in signal transduction from the TGF-β family of cell surface receptors. *SMAD4* is only rarely inactivated in other cancer types.

TP53. Inactivation of the *TP53* tumor suppressor gene (chromosome 17p) occurs in 70% to 75% of pancreatic cancers. This gene encodes p53, a nuclear DNA-binding protein that can respond to DNA damage by arresting cell growth, inducing cell death (apoptosis) or causing cellular senescence (Chapter 7).

Other Genes. A growing number of less common, but nonetheless important, genetic loci have been reported to be damaged in pancreatic cancer (Table 19-3).

DNA Methylation Abnormalities. Several DNA methylation abnormalities also occur in pancreatic cancer. Hypermethylation of the promoter of several tumor suppressor genes, including *CDKN2A*, is associated with transcriptional silencing of these genes and loss of their function.

Gene Expression. In addition to DNA alterations, global analyses of gene expression have identified several pathways that seem to be abnormally active in pancreatic cancers. These pathways and their downstream consequences are potential targets for novel therapies and may form the basis of future screening tests. For example, the Hedgehog signaling pathway has been shown to be activated in pancreatic cancer and represents a potential therapeutic target.

Epidemiology and Inheritance. Pancreatic cancer is primarily a disease of older adults, with 80% of cases occurring in people aged 60 to 80 years. It is more common in blacks than in whites, and it is slightly more common in individuals of Ashkenazi Jewish descent.

The strongest environmental influence is *cigarette smoking*, which is believed to double the risk of pancreatic cancer. Even though the magnitude of this increased risk is not great, the impact of smoking on pancreatic cancer is significant because of the large number of people who smoke. Consumption of a diet rich in fats has also been implicated, but less consistently. Chronic pancreatitis and diabetes mellitus are both risk factors for, and complications of, pancreatic cancer. In an individual patient it can be difficult to sort out whether chronic pancreatitis is the cause of pancreatic cancer or an effect of the disease, since small pancreatic cancers may block the pancreatic duct and produce chronic pancreatitis. A similar argument applies to the association of diabetes mellitus with pancreatic cancer, in that diabetes may develop as a consequence of pancreatic cancer and new-onset diabetes mellitus in an older patient may be the first sign that the patient has pancreatic cancer.

Familial clustering of pancreatic cancer has been reported, and a growing number of inherited genetic defects are recognized to increase pancreatic cancer risk (Table 19-4). Germline *BRCA2* mutations account for approximately 10% of pancreatic cancer cases in Ashkenazi Jews. Patients with these mutations may not have a family history of breast or ovarian cancers. Germline mutations in *CDKN2A* are associated with pancreatic cancer and are almost always observed in individuals from families with an increased incidence of melanoma, which also frequently harbors *CDKN2A* loss-of-function mutations.

MORPHOLOGY

Approximately 60% of cancers of the pancreas arise in the head of the gland, 15% in the body, and 5% in the tail; in 20% the neoplasm diffusely involves the entire gland. Carcinomas of the

Table 19-4 Inherited Predisposition to Pancreatic Cancer

Disorder	Gene	Increased Risk of Pancreatic Cancer (Fold)	Risk of Pancreatic Cancer by Age 70 (%)
Peutz-Jeghers syndrome	*STK11*	130	30-60
Hereditary pancreatitis	*PRSS1*, *SPINK1*	50-80	25-40
Familial atypical multiple-mole melanoma syndrome	*CDKN2A*	20-35	10-17
Strong family history (3 or more relatives with pancreatic cancer)	Unknown	14-32	8-16
Hereditary breast and ovarian cancer	Multiple, including *BRCA1*, *BRCA2*, *PALP2*, *BRCA2*	4-10	5
Hereditary non-polyposis colorectal cancer (HNPCC)	Multiple, including *MLH1*, *MSH2* (2p21)	8-10	4

pancreas are usually hard, stellate, gray-white, poorly defined masses (Fig. 19-13*A*).

The vast majority of carcinomas are ductal adenocarcinomas that recapitulate to some degree normal ductal epithelium by forming glands and secreting mucin. Two features are characteristic of pancreatic cancer; it is highly invasive (even "early" invasive pancreatic cancers extensively invade peripancreatic tissues), and it elicits an intense host reaction in the form of dense fibrosis ("desmoplastic response"), described later.

Most carcinomas of the head of the pancreas obstruct the distal common bile duct as it courses through the head of the pancreas. As a consequence there is marked distention of the biliary tree in about 50% of patients with carcinoma of the head of the pancreas, and most develop jaundice. In marked contrast, **carcinomas of the body and tail of the pancreas do not impinge on the biliary tract and hence remain silent for some time. They may be quite large and most are widely disseminated by the time they are discovered.** Pancreatic cancers often grow along nerves and invade into blood vessels and the retroperitoneum. They can directly invade the spleen, adrenals, transverse colon, and stomach. Peripancreatic, gastric, mesenteric, omental, and portohepatic lymph nodes are frequently involved. Distant metastases occur, principally to the liver and lungs.

Microscopically, there is no difference between carcinomas of the head of the pancreas and those of the body and tail of the pancreas. The appearance is usually that of a **moderately to poorly differentiated adenocarcinoma forming abortive tubular structures or cell clusters and showing an aggressive, deeply infiltrative growth pattern** (Fig. 19-13*B*). The malignant glands are poorly formed and are usually lined by pleomorphic cuboidal-to-columnar epithelial cells. Well-differentiated carcinomas are the exception. As noted earlier, a characteristic feature of these cancers is that they elicit an intense desmoplastic reaction with dense stromal fibrosis. The marked degree of desmoplasia can hinder the interpretation of diagnostic biopsies, as much of the tissue present is nonneoplastic. Perineural invasion within and beyond the organ is common, as are lymphatic and large vessel invasion.

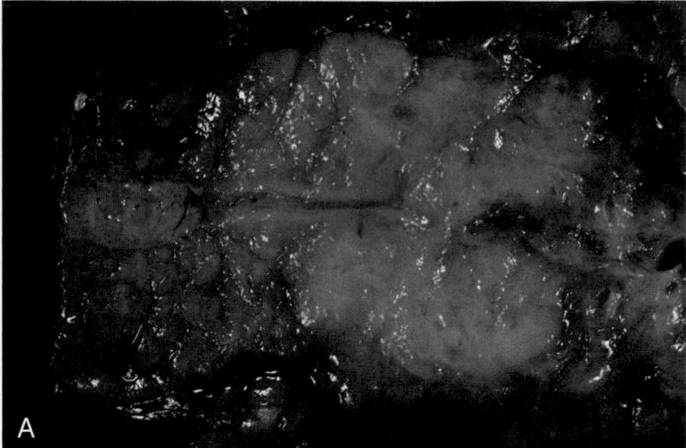

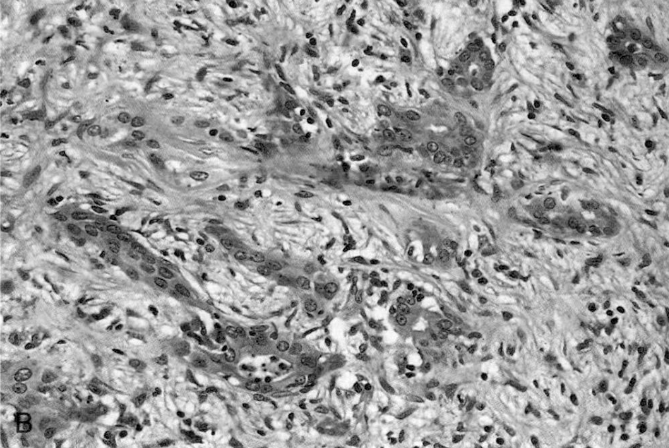

Figure 19-13 Carcinoma of the pancreas. **A,** A cross-section through the tail of the pancreas showing normal pancreatic parenchyma and a normal pancreatic duct *(left)*, an ill-defined mass in the pancreatic substance *(center)* with narrowing of the pancreatic duct, and dilatation of the pancreatic duct upstream *(right)* from the mass. **B,** Poorly formed glands are present in densely fibrotic stroma within the pancreatic substance; some inflammatory cells are also present.

Less common morphologic variants of pancreatic cancer include adenosquamous carcinomas, colloid carcinoma, hepatoid carcinoma, medullary carcinoma, signet-ring cell carcinoma, undifferentiated carcinoma, and undifferentiated carcinoma with osteoclast-like giant cells.

Clinical Features. From the preceding discussion it should be evident that **carcinomas of the pancreas remain silent until they invade into adjacent structures**. *Pain* is usually the first symptom, but by the time pain appears these cancers are usually beyond cure. *Obstructive jaundice* is associated with most cases of carcinoma of the head of the pancreas, but it rarely draws attention to the invasive cancer soon enough. Weight loss, anorexia, and generalized malaise and weakness tend to be signs of advanced disease. *Migratory thrombophlebitis*, known as the *Trousseau sign*, occurs in about 10% of patients and is attributable to the elaboration of platelet-activating factors and procoagulants from the carcinoma or its necrotic products (Chapter 4). On a sad note, Armand Trousseau (1801-1867, physician at Hotel Dieu, Paris), for whom this sign is named, correctly suspected that he had carcinoma when he developed spontaneously appearing and disappearing (migratory) thromboses.

The course of pancreatic carcinoma is typically brief and progressive. Despite the tendency of lesions of the head of the pancreas to obstruct the biliary system, fewer than 20% of pancreatic cancers overall are resectable at the time of diagnosis. Most have invaded vessels and other structures that cannot be removed surgically, or have metastasized to distant organs. There has long been a search for tests that could be useful in the early detection of pancreatic cancer. Serum levels of several antigens (e.g., carcinoembryonic antigen and CA19-9 antigen) are often elevated in individuals with pancreatic cancer. These markers, while useful in following an individual patient's response to treatment, are relatively nonspecific and also lack the sensitivity needed to be used as tests to screen the wider population. Several imaging techniques, such as endoscopic ultrasonography and computed tomography, have proved of great value in establishing the diagnosis once it is suspected, but are also not useful as screening tests.

KEY CONCEPTS

- Cigarette smoking is the leading preventable cause of pancreatic cancer.
- Pancreatic cancer is one of the most aggressive of the solid malignancies.
- Many invasive pancreatic cancer arises from histologically well-defined precursor lesions called *pancreatic intraepithelial neoplasia* (PanIN).
- Ductal adenocarcinomas elicit an intense desmoplastic response.
- The genes most frequently mutated or otherwise altered in pancreatic cancer include *KRAS*, *p16/CDKN2A*, *TP53*, and *SMAD4*
- Clinically, most patients present with abdominal pain and weight loss, sometimes accompanied by jaundice and deep vein thrombosis, and succumb to the disease within 1 to 2 years.

Acinar Cell Carcinoma

Like normal acinar cells, acinar cell carcinomas form zymogen granules and produce exocrine enzymes such as trypsin and lipase. Fifteen percent of individuals with acinar cell carcinoma develop the syndrome of metastatic fat necrosis caused by the release of lipase into the circulation.

Pancreatoblastoma

Pancreatoblastomas are rare neoplasms that occur primarily in children aged 1 to 15 years. They have a distinct microscopic appearance consisting of squamous islands admixed with acinar cells. They are malignant neoplasms, but survival is better with these tumors than it is for pancreatic ductal adenocarcinomas.

SUGGESTED READINGS

Congenital Anomalies

Cano DA, Hebrok M, Zenker M: Pancreatic development and disease. *Gastroenterology* 132:745-62, 2007. *[A review of the normal development of the pancreas and how development explains anomalies.]*

Acute Pancreatitis

Cappell MS: Acute pancreatitis: etiology, clinical presentation, diagnosis, and therapy. *Med Clin North Am* 92:889-923, ix–x, 2008. *[A review of acute pancreatitis.]*

Frossard JL, Steer ML, Pastor CM: Acute pancreatitis. *Lancet* 371:143-52, 2008. *[An overview of acute pancreatitis.]*

Giakoustidis A, Mudan SS, Giakoustidis D: Dissecting the stress activating signaling pathways in acute pancreatitis. *Hepatogastroenterology* 57:653-6, 2010. *[Reviews the role of nuclear factors NF-kappaB and AP-1, TNFalpha, and TLR-4 in acute pancreatitis.]*

Papachristou GI, Clermont G, Sharma A, et al: Risk and markers of severe acute pancreatitis. *Gastroenterol Clin North Am* 36:277-96, 2007. *[A review of the pathogenesis, immunology, and genetics of severe acute pancreatitis by a leading expert in the field.]*

Vonlaufen A, Wilson JS, Apte MV: Molecular mechanisms of pancreatitis: current opinion. *J Gastroenterol Hepatol* 23:1339-48, 2008. *[An overview of the pathogenesis of pancreatitis.]*

Yadav D, Whitcomb DC: The role of alcohol and smoking in pancreatitis. *Nat Rev Gastroenterol Hepatol* 7:131-45, 2010. *[Highlights the importance of alcohol abuse in pancreatitis.]*

Chronic Pancreatitis

Apte M, Pirola R, Wilson J: The fibrosis of chronic pancreatitis: new insights into the role of pancreatic stellate cells. *Antioxid Redox Signal* 15:2711-22, 2011. *[A discussion of the role of stellate cells in pancreatitis.]*

Braganza JM, Lee SH, McCloy RF, et al: Chronic pancreatitis. *Lancet* 377:1184-97, 2011. *[An overview of chronic pancreatitis.]*

Klöppel G: Chronic pancreatitis, pseudotumors and other tumor-like lesions. *Mod Pathol* 20(Suppl 1):S113-31, 2007. *[A review of the pathology of chronic pancreatitis.]*

LaRusch J, Whitcomb DC: Genetics of pancreatitis. *Curr Opin Gastroenterol* 27:467-74, 2011. *[Highlights the growing recognition of genetics in the etiology of pancreatitis.]*

Lowenfels AB, Maisonneuve P, Whitcomb DC: Risk factors for cancer in hereditary pancreatitis. International Hereditary Pancreatitis Study Group. *Med Clin North Am* 84:565-73, 2000. *[Demonstrates that patients with familial pancreatitis have an increased risk of developing pancreatic cancer.]*

Sah RP, Chari ST: Autoimmune pancreatitis: an update on classification, diagnosis, natural history and management. *Curr Gastroenterol Rep* 14:95-105, 2012. *[Autoimmune pancreatitis is an important treatable form of the disease.]*

Witt H, Apte MV, Keim V, et al: Chronic pancreatitis: challenges and advances in pathogenesis, genetics, diagnosis, and therapy. *Gastroenterology* 132:1557-73, 2007. *[Review of chronic pancreatitis.]*

Pseudocysts

Klöppel G: Pseudocysts and other non-neoplastic cysts of the pancreas. *Semin Diagn Pathol* 17:7-15, 2000. *[Discussion of pseudocysts by a leading expert in pancreatic pathology.]*

Cystic Neoplasms

Hruban RH, Takaori K, Klimstra DS, et al: An illustrated consensus on the classification of pancreatic intraepithelial neoplasia and intraductal papillary mucinous neoplasms. *Am J Surg Pathol* 28:977-87, 2004. *[Guidelines defining the difference between two common precursor lesions.]*

Tanaka M, Fernandez-Del Castillo C, Adsay V, et al: International consensus guidelines 2012 for the management of IPMN and MCN of the pancreas. *Pancreatology* 12:183-97, 2012. *[Guidelines on the clinical management of cysts.]*

Wu J, Jiao Y, Dal Molin M, et al: Whole-exome sequencing of neoplastic cysts of the pancreas reveals recurrent mutations in components of ubiquitin-dependent pathways. *Proc Natl Acad Sci U S A* 108:21188-93, 2011. *[Sequencing the exomes of the most common cystic neoplasms of the pancreas reveals a mutation profile specific for each type of cyst.]*

Wu J, Matthaei H, Maitra A, et al: Recurrent GNAS mutations define an unexpected pathway for pancreatic cyst development. *Sci Transl Med* 3:92ra66, 2011. *[Discovery of a gene specific for intraductal papillary mucinous neoplasms.]*

Pancreatic Carcinoma

Chari ST, Leibson CL, Rabe KG, et al: Pancreatic cancer-associated diabetes mellitus: prevalence and temporal association with diagnosis of cancer. *Gastroenterology* 134:95-101, 2008. *[Study showing that new onset diabetes can be the first sign of pancreatic cancer.]*

Feldmann G, Beaty R, Hruban RH, et al: Molecular genetics of pancreatic intraepithelial neoplasia. *J Hepatobiliary Pancreat Surg* 14:224-32, 2007. *[Review of the most common precancerous lesion in the pancreas.]*

Habbe N, Koorstra JB, Mendell JT, et al: MicroRNA miR-155 is a biomarker of early pancreatic neoplasia. *Cancer Biol Ther* 8:340-6, 2009. *[Highlights the role of microRNAs in pancreatic cancer.]*

Hahn SA, Schutte M, Hoque AT, et al: DPC4, a candidate tumor suppressor gene at human chromosome 18q21.1. *Science* 271:350-3, 1996. *[Classic paper on the discovery of a major pancreatic cancer gene.]*

Hruban RH, Canto MI, Goggins M, et al: Update on familial pancreatic cancer. *Adv Surg* 44:293-311, 2010. *[Review of familial pancreatic cancer.]*

Iacobuzio-Donahue CA, Velculescu VE, Wolfgang CL, et al: Genetic basis of pancreas cancer development and progression: Insights from whole-exome and whole-genome sequencing. *Clin Can Res* 18:4257-65, 2012. *[Overview of the genetic alterations in neoplasms of the pancreas.]*

Jones S, Zhang X, Parsons DW, et al: Core signaling pathways in human pancreatic cancers revealed by global genomic analyses. *Science* 321:1801-6, 2008. *[Sequencing the exomes of ductal adenocarcinoma of the pancreas defines targeted pathways.]*

Lowenfels AB, Maisonneuve P: Epidemiology and risk factors for pancreatic cancer. *Best Pract Res Clin Gastroenterol* 20:197-209, 2006. *[Review of the risk factors for pancreatic cancer by an expert in the field.]*

Sato N, Fukushima N, Maitra A, et al: Discovery of novel targets for aberrant methylation in pancreatic carcinoma using high-throughput microarrays. *Cancer Res* 63:3735-42, 2003. *[Highlights the role of abbarent methylation in pancreatic cancer.]*

See TARGETED THERAPY available online at www.studentconsult.com

CHAPTER 20

The Kidney

Charles E. Alpers • Anthony Chang

CHAPTER CONTENTS

What is a human but an ingenious machine designed to turn, with "infinite artfulness, the red wine of Shiraz into urine?" So said the storyteller in Isak Dinesen's *Seven Gothic Tales*. More accurately but less poetically, human kidneys serve to convert more than 1700 L of blood per day into about 1 L of a highly concentrated fluid called *urine*. In so doing, the kidney excretes the waste products of metabolism, precisely regulates the body's concentration of water, salt, calcium, phosphorus, and other anions and cations, and maintains the appropriate acid balance of plasma. The kidney also serves as an endocrine organ, secreting such hormones as erythropoietin, renin, and prostaglandins, and regulating vitamin D metabolism. The physiologic mechanisms that the kidney has developed to carry out these functions require a high degree of structural complexity.

Renal diseases are responsible for a great deal of morbidity and mortality. When last surveyed in 2009, more than 570,000 Americans had end-stage renal disease (ESRD), of whom two thirds are maintained on dialysis, at a cost of approximately $42.5 billion. The 1-year mortality rate of ESRD, when the enhanced risk for cardiovascular disease conferred by ESRD is considered, exceeds that of most newly diagnosed cancers. Acute kidney injury occurs in more than 2 million people worldwide, and is a major risk factor for the development of chronic kidney disease (CKD) and ESRD. In addition, millions of people are affected annually by nonfatal kidney diseases, most notably infections of the kidney or lower urinary tract, kidney stones, and urinary obstruction. The availability of dialysis and the success of renal transplantation have improved the outlook for patients.

The study of kidney diseases is facilitated by dividing them into those that affect the four basic morphologic components: glomeruli, tubules, interstitium, and blood vessels. This approach is useful, since the early manifestations of disease affecting each of these components tend to be distinct. Further, some components seem to be more vulnerable to specific forms of renal injury; for example, **most glomerular diseases are immunologically mediated, whereas tubular and interstitial disorders are frequently caused by toxic or infectious agents**. However, some disorders affect more than one structure, and the anatomic and functional interdependence of the components of the kidney means that damage to one almost always secondarily affects the others. Primary disorders of the blood vessels, for example, inevitably affect all the structures supplied by these vessels. Severe glomerular damage impairs the flow through the peritubular vascular system; conversely, tubular destruction, by increasing intraglomerular pressure, may induce glomerular injury. Thus, whatever the origin, all forms of chronic kidney disease ultimately damage all four components of the kidney, culminating in what has been called *end-stage kidneys*. The functional reserve of the kidney is large, and much damage may occur before there is evident functional impairment. For these reasons the early signs and symptoms are of particular clinical importance.

Clinical Manifestations of Renal Diseases

The clinical manifestations of renal disease can be grouped into reasonably well-defined syndromes. Some are unique to glomerular diseases, and others are present in diseases that affect any one of the components.

- *Azotemia* is a biochemical abnormality that refers to an elevation of blood urea nitrogen (BUN) and creatinine levels, and is related largely to a decreased glomerular filtration rate (GFR). Azotemia is a consequence of many renal disorders, but it also arises from extrarenal disorders. It is a typical feature of both acute and chronic kidney injury. *Prerenal azotemia* is encountered when there is hypoperfusion of the kidneys (e.g., hypotension or excessive fluid losses from any cause, or if the effective intravascular volume is decreased due to shock, volume depletion, congestive heart failure or cirrhosis of the liver) that impairs renal function in the absence of parenchymal damage. *Postrenal azotemia* is seen whenever urine flow is obstructed distal to the kidney. Relief of the obstruction is followed by correction of the azotemia.

  When azotemia becomes associated with a constellation of clinical signs and symptoms and biochemical abnormalities, it is termed *uremia*. Uremia is characterized not only by failure of renal excretory function but also by a host of metabolic and endocrine alterations resulting from renal damage. Uremic patients frequently manifest secondary involvement of the gastrointestinal system (e.g., uremic gastroenteritis), peripheral nerves (e.g., peripheral neuropathy), and heart (e.g., uremic fibrinous pericarditis).
- *Nephritic syndrome* is a clinical entity caused by glomerular disease and is dominated by the acute onset of either grossly visible hematuria (red blood cells in urine) or microscopic hematuria with dysmorphic red cells and red cell casts on urinalysis, diminished GFR, mild to moderate proteinuria, and hypertension. It is the classic presentation of acute poststreptococcal glomerulonephritis. *Rapidly progressive glomerulonephritis* is characterized as a nephritic syndrome with rapid decline in GFR (within hours to days).
- The *nephrotic syndrome*, also due to glomerular disease, is characterized by heavy proteinuria (more than 3.5 gm/day), hypoalbuminemia, severe edema, hyperlipidemia, and lipiduria (lipid in the urine).
- *Asymptomatic hematuria or proteinuria*, or a combination of these two, is usually a manifestation of subtle or mild glomerular abnormalities.
- *Acute kidney injury* is characterized by rapid decline in GFR (within hours to days), with concurrent dysregulation of fluid and electrolyte balance, and retention of metabolic waste products normally excreted by the kidney including urea and creatinine. In its most severe forms, it is manifested by *oliguria* or *anuria* (reduced or no urine flow). It can result from glomerular, interstitial, vascular or acute tubular injury.
- *Chronic kidney disease* (previously called chronic renal failure) is defined as the presence of a diminished GFR that is persistently less than 60 mL/minute/1.73 m^2 for at least 3 months, from any cause, and/or persistent albuminuria. It may present with clinically silent decline in renal excretory function in milder forms, and in more severe cases, by prolonged symptoms and signs of uremia. It is the end result of all chronic renal parenchymal diseases.
- *In end-stage renal disease (ESRD)* the GFR is less than 5% of normal; this is the terminal stage of uremia.
- *Renal tubular defects* are dominated by polyuria (excessive urine formation), nocturia, and electrolyte disorders (e.g., metabolic acidosis). They are the result of diseases that either directly affect tubular structures (e.g., the nephronophthisis-medullary cystic disease complex) or cause defects in specific tubular functions. The latter can be inherited (e.g., familial nephrogenic

diabetes, cystinuria, renal tubular acidosis) or acquired (e.g., lead nephropathy).

- *Urinary tract obstruction* and *renal tumors* have varied clinical manifestations based on the specific anatomic location and nature of the lesion. *Urinary tract infection* is characterized by bacteriuria and pyuria (bacteria and leukocytes in the urine). The infection may be symptomatic or asymptomatic, and it may affect the kidney *(pyelonephritis)* or the bladder *(cystitis).*
- *Nephrolithiasis (renal stones)* is manifested by spasms of severe pain (renal colic) and hematuria, often with recurrent stone formation.

Chronic kidney disease is estimated to affect 11% of all adults in the United States, with a particular predominance amongst older adults. It is the end result of a variety of renal diseases, but most commonly diabetes and hypertension, and the major cause of death from renal disease. The evolution from normal renal function to symptomatic chronic kidney injury progresses through a series of stages that are defined by measures of serum creatinine from which estimates of reduction in GFR are derived. Chronic kidney disease causes significant systemic abnormalities, which are listed in Table 20-1.

Table 20-1 Principal Systemic Manifestations of Chronic Kidney Disease and Uremia

Fluid and Electrolytes
Dehydration
Edema
Hyperkalemia
Metabolic acidosis
Calcium Phosphate and Bone
Hyperphosphatemia
Hypocalcemia
Secondary hyperparathyroidism
Renal osteodystrophy
Hematologic
Anemia
Bleeding diathesis
Cardiopulmonary
Hypertension
Congestive heart failure
Cardiomyopathy
Pulmonary edema
Uremic pericarditis
Gastrointestinal
Nausea and vomiting
Bleeding
Esophagitis, gastritis, colitis
Neuromuscular
Myopathy
Peripheral neuropathy
Encephalopathy
Dermatologic
Sallow color
Pruritus
Dermatitis

KEY CONCEPTS

Clinical Manifestations of Renal Diseases

- Azotemia is the biochemical manifestation of acute or chronic kidney injury and is characterized by elevated blood urea nitrogen (BUN) or alternately by an elevated serum creatinine. It reflects a reduction in the glomerular filtration rate.
- Kidney injury that results in azotemia can be either acute or chronic. Acute kidney injury can be reversible or progress to chronic kidney disease; chronic kidney disease is generally irreversible.
- One major manifestation of kidney injury is the nephrotic syndrome, in which injury to the glomerulus results in abnormal filtration, leading to heavy proteinuria, edema and metabolic disturbances.
- Nephritic syndromes are those in which hematuria, azotemia, hypertension, and sub-nephrotic proteinuria are the major manifestations.
- Diseases involving the tubules and interstitium may have clinical manifestations of the nephritic syndrome, or of specific defects in tubular function, or of acute or chronic kidney disease without more specific defining features.

Glomerular Diseases

Glomerular diseases constitute some of the major problems in nephrology; indeed, chronic glomerulonephritis is one of the most common causes of chronic kidney disease in humans. Glomeruli may be injured by a variety of factors and in the course of several systemic diseases. Systemic immunologic diseases such as systemic lupus erythematosus (SLE), vascular disorders such as hypertension, metabolic diseases such as diabetes mellitus, and some hereditary conditions such as Fabry disease often affect the glomerulus. These are termed *secondary glomerular diseases*. Disorders in which the kidney is the only or predominant organ involved constitute the various types of *primary glomerulonephritis* or, because some do not have a cellular inflammatory component, *glomerulopathy.* However, both the clinical manifestations and glomerular histologic changes in primary and secondary forms can be similar.

In the following sections we discuss the various types of primary glomerulopathies and briefly review the secondary forms covered in other parts of this book. Table 20-2 lists the most common forms of glomerulonephritis that have reasonably well defined morphologic and clinical characteristics. The clinical manifestations of glomerular disease are clustered into the five major glomerular syndromes summarized in Table 20-3. Both the primary glomerulopathies and the systemic diseases affecting the glomerulus can result in these syndromes. Because glomerular diseases are often associated with systemic disorders, mainly *diabetes mellitus, SLE, vasculitis,* and *amyloidosis,* in any patient with manifestations of glomerular disease it is essential to consider these systemic conditions.

Table 20-2 Glomerular Diseases

Primary Glomerulopathies
Acute proliferative glomerulonephritis
Postinfectious
Other
Rapidly progressive (crescentic) glomerulonephritis
Membranous nephropathy
Minimal-change disease
Focal segmental glomerulosclerosis
Membranoproliferative glomerulonephritis
Dense deposit disease
IgA nephropathy
Chronic glomerulonephritis
Systemic Diseases with Glomerular Involvement
Systemic lupus erythematosus
Diabetes mellitus
Amyloidosis
Goodpasture syndrome
Microscopic polyarteritis/polyangiitis
Wegener granulomatosis
Henoch-Schönlein purpura
Bacterial endocarditis
Hereditary Disorders
Alport syndrome
Thin basement membrane disease
Fabry disease

Structure of the Glomerulus

Many clinical manifestations of glomerular diseases result from perturbations of specific components of the glomerular tuft, so we before discussing these diseases we describe the key anatomic structures of glomeruli. The glomerulus consists of an anastomosing network of capillaries lined by fenestrated endothelium invested by two layers of epithelial cells (Fig. 20-1). The visceral epithelial cells (commonly referred to as *podocytes*) are incorporated into and become an intrinsic part of the capillary wall, separated from endothelial cells by a basement membrane. The parietal epithelium, situated on the Bowman capsule, lines the urinary space, the cavity in which plasma filtrate first collects.

The glomerular capillary wall is the filtering membrane and consists of the following structures (Fig. 20-2):

- There is a thin layer of fenestrated *endothelial cells*, with each fenestra being about 70 to 100 nm in diameter.
- A *glomerular basement membrane* (GBM) with a thick electron-dense central layer, the *lamina densa*, and thinner electron-lucent peripheral layers, the *lamina rara interna* and *lamina rara externa*. The GBM consists of collagen (mostly type IV), laminin, polyanionic proteoglycans (mostly heparan sulfate), fibronectin, entactin, and several other glycoproteins. Type IV collagen forms a network suprastructure to which other glycoproteins attach. The building block (monomer) of this network is a triple-helical molecule composed of one or more of six types of α chains (α_1 to α_6 or COL4A1 to COL4A6). Each molecule consists of a 7S domain at the N terminus, a triple-helical domain in the middle, and a globular noncollagenous domain (NC1) at the C terminus. The NC1 domain is important for helix formation and for assembly of collagen monomers into the basement membrane suprastructure. Glycoproteins (laminin, entactin) and proteoglycans (heparan sulfate, perlecan) attach to the collagenous suprastructure. The biochemical properties of these structural components are critical to understanding glomerular diseases. For example, antigens in the NC1 domain are the targets of antibodies in anti-GBM nephritis; genetic defects in the α-chains underlie some forms of hereditary nephritis; and the proteoglycan content of the GBM may contribute to its permeability characteristics.
- The *visceral epithelial cells* (podocytes) possess interdigitating processes embedded in and adherent to the lamina rara externa of the basement membrane (Fig. 20-1). Adjacent *foot processes* are separated by 20- to 30-nm–wide *filtration slits*, which are bridged by a thin diaphragm (Fig. 20-2).
- The entire glomerular tuft is supported by *mesangial cells* lying between the capillaries. Basement membrane–like *mesangial matrix* forms a meshwork in which the mesangial cells are embedded (Fig. 20-1). These cells, of mesenchymal origin, are contractile, phagocytic, and capable of proliferation, of laying down both matrix and collagen, and of secreting several biologically active mediators. Biologically, they are most akin to vascular smooth muscle cells and pericytes. They are important in many forms of glomerulonephritis.

The normal glomerulus is highly permeable to water and small solutes, because of the fenestrated nature of the endothelium, and impermeable to proteins of the size of albumin (~3.6-nm radius; 70 kilodaltons [kD] molecular weight) or larger. The permeability characteristics of the *glomerular filtration barrier* allow discrimination among various protein molecules, depending on their size (the larger, the less permeable) and charge (the more cationic, the more permeable). This size- and charge-dependent barrier function is accounted for by the structure of the capillary wall. The charge-dependent restriction is important in the virtually complete exclusion of albumin from the filtrate, because albumin is an anionic molecule.

The visceral epithelial cell is important for the maintenance of glomerular barrier function; its slit diaphragm presents a size-selective distal diffusion barrier to the filtration of proteins, and it is the cell type that is largely responsible for synthesis of GBM components. Proteins located in the slit diaphragm or present in assemblies of molecules within visceral epithelial cells that are attached

Table 20-3 Glomerular Syndromes

Syndrome	Manifestations
Nephritic syndrome	Hematuria, azotemia, variable proteinuria, oliguria, edema, and hypertension
Rapidly progressive glomerulonephritis	Acute nephritis, proteinuria, and acute renal failure
Nephrotic syndrome	>3.5 gm/day proteinuria, hypoalbuminemia, hyperlipidemia, lipiduria
Chronic renal failure	Azotemia → uremia progressing for months to years
Isolated urinary abnormalities	Glomerular hematuria and/or subnephrotic proteinuria

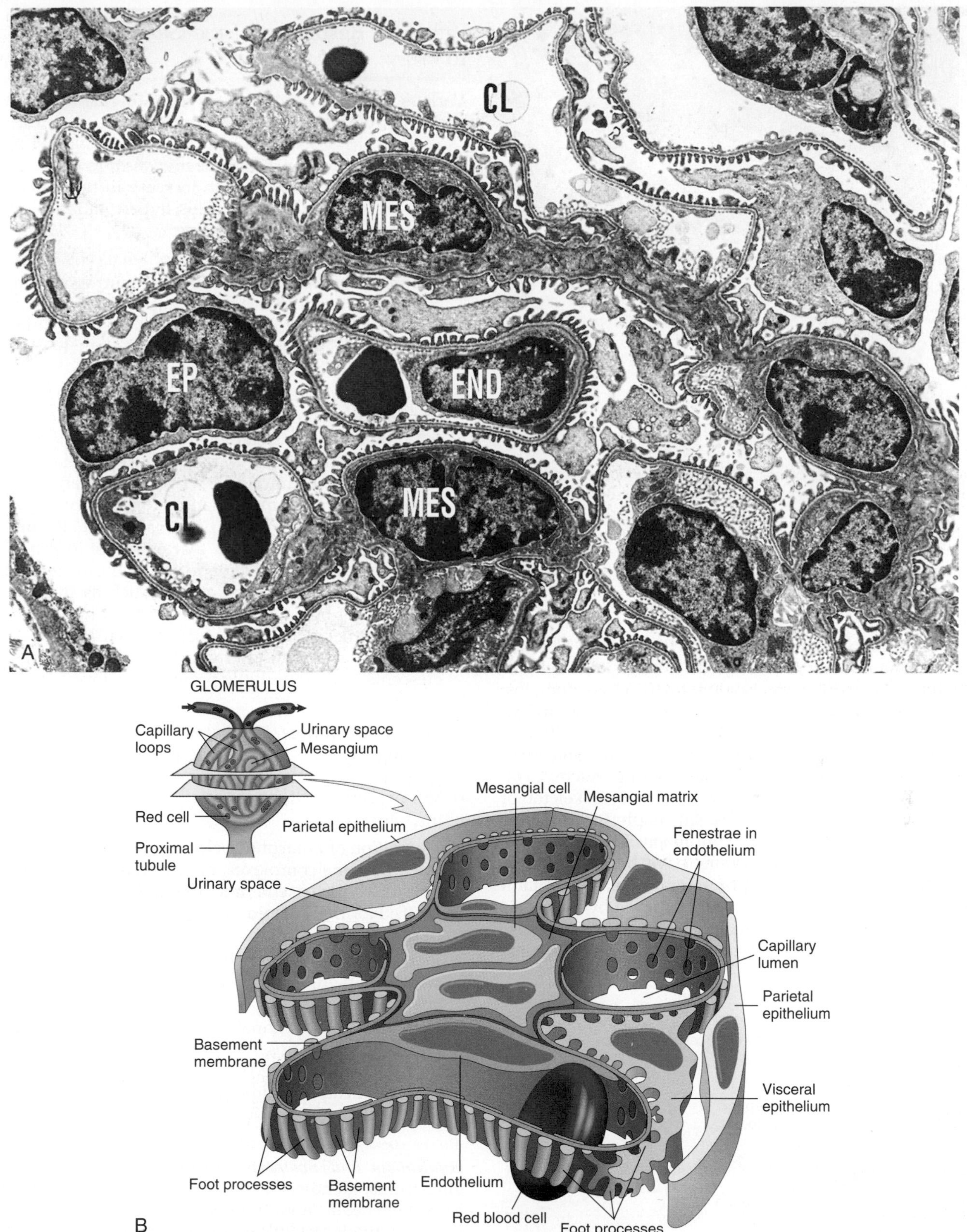

Figure 20-1 **A,** Low-power electron micrograph of renal glomerulus. CL, Capillary lumen; EP, visceral epithelial cells with foot processes; END, endothelium; MES, mesangium. **B,** Schematic representation of a glomerular lobe. (**A,** Courtesy Dr. Vicki Kelley, Brigham and Women's Hospital, Boston, Mass.)

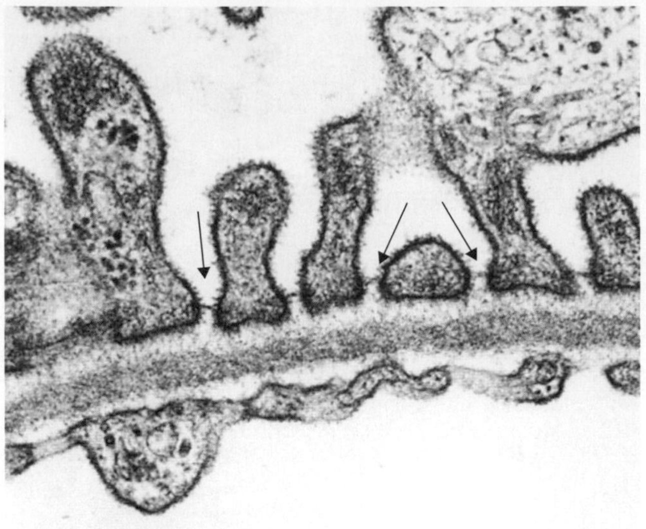

Figure 20-2 Glomerular filter consisting, from bottom to top, of fenestrated endothelium, basement membrane, and foot processes of epithelial cells. Note the filtration slits *(arrows)* and diaphragm situated between the foot processes. Note also that the basement membrane consists of a central lamina densa, sandwiched between two looser layers, the lamina rara interna and lamina rara externa. (Courtesy Dr. Helmut Rennke, Brigham and Women's Hospital, Boston, Mass.)

to the slit diaphragm are illustrated in Figure 20-3. Nephrin is a transmembrane protein with a large extracellular portion made up of immunoglobulin (Ig)-like domains. Nephrin molecules extend toward each other from neighboring foot processes and dimerize across the slit diaphragm. Within the cytoplasm of the foot processes, nephrin forms molecular connections with podocin, CD2-associated protein, and ultimately the actin cytoskeleton of the visceral epithelial cells. More slit diaphragm proteins continue to be identified, and comprehensive descriptions of their structure and interactions have been published. The importance of the slit diaphragm proteins in maintaining glomerular permeability is demonstrated by the observation that mutations in the genes encoding them give rise to defects in permeability and the nephrotic syndrome (discussed later).

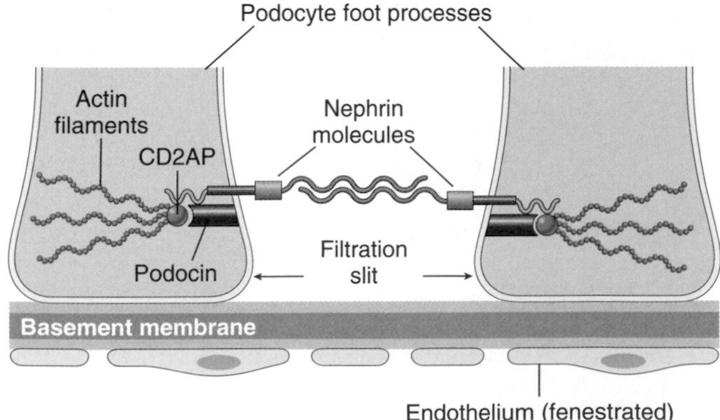

Figure 20-3 A simplified schematic diagram of some of the best-studied proteins of the glomerular slit diaphragm. CD2AP, CD2-associated protein.

Pathologic Responses of the Glomerulus to Injury

Various types of glomerulopathies are characterized by one or more of four basic tissue reactions.

Hypercellularity. Some *inflammatory diseases* of the glomerulus are characterized by an increase in the number of cells in the glomerular tufts. This hypercellularity results from one or more of the following:

- *Proliferation* of mesangial or endothelial cells.
- *Infiltration of leukocytes,* including neutrophils, monocytes, and, in some diseases, lymphocytes. The combination of infiltration of leukocytes and swelling and proliferation of mesangial and/or endothelial cells is often referred to as *endocapillary proliferation.*
- *Formation of crescents.* These are accumulations of cells composed of proliferating glomerular epithelial cells (predominately parietal but including some visceral cells) and infiltrating leukocytes. The epithelial cell proliferation that characterizes crescent formation occurs following an immune/inflammatory injury involving the capillary walls. Plasma proteins leak into the urinary space, where it is believed that exposure to procoagulants such as tissue factor leads to fibrin deposition. Activation of coagulation factors such as thrombin is suspected of being a trigger for crescent formation, but the actual mechanisms are still unknown. Molecules that have been implicated in recruitment of leukocytes into crescents include multiple proinflammatory cytokines.

Basement Membrane Thickening. By light microscopy, this change appears as thickening of the capillary walls, best seen in sections stained with periodic acid-Schiff (PAS). By electron microscopy such thickening takes one of three forms:

- Deposition of amorphous electron-dense material, most often immune complexes, on the endothelial or epithelial side of the basement membrane or within the GBM itself. Fibrin, amyloid, cryoglobulins, and abnormal fibrillary proteins may also deposit in the GBM.
- Increased synthesis of the protein components of the basement membrane, as occurs in diabetic glomerulosclerosis.
- Formation of additional layers of basement membrane matrices, which most often occupy subendothelial locations and may range from poorly organized matrix to fully duplicated lamina densa, as occurs in membranoproliferative glomerulonephritis.

Hyalinosis and Sclerosis. *Hyalinosis,* as applied to the glomerulus, denotes the accumulation of material that is homogeneous and eosinophilic by light microscopy. *Hyalin* is an extracellular, amorphous material composed of plasma proteins that have insudated from the circulation into glomerular structures. When extensive, these deposits may obliterate the capillary lumens of the glomerular tuft. Hyalinosis is usually a consequence of endothelial or capillary wall injury and typically the end result of various forms of glomerular damage.

Sclerosis is characterized by deposition of extracellular collagenous matrix. It may be confined to mesangial areas, as is often the case in diabetic glomerulosclerosis, involve the capillary loops, or both. The sclerosing process may also result in obliteration of some or all of the capillary lumens in affected glomeruli.

Many primary glomerulopathies are classified by their histology, as seen in Table 20-2. The histologic changes can be further subdivided by their distribution into the following categories: *diffuse*, involving all of the glomeruli in the kidney; *global*, involving the entirety of individual glomeruli; *focal*, involving only a fraction of the glomeruli in the kidney; *segmental*, affecting a part of each glomerulus; and *capillary loop* or *mesangial*, affecting predominantly capillary or mesangial regions.

KEY CONCEPTS

Injury of Glomerular Structures

- The glomerular basement membrane is composted of type IV collagen molecules and other matrix proteins. These proteins can be the target of antibodies in some types of glomerulonephritis; genetic abnormalities in their composition are the basis for some forms of hereditary nephritis.
- Visceral epithelial cells (podocytes) are a critical component of the glomerular filtration barrier, and injury to these cells leads to leakage of proteins into the urinary space, clinically manifest as proteinuria.
- The acute glomerular response to injury includes hypercellularity with proliferation of mesangial and/or endothelial cells, influx of leukocytes, and, in severe injuries, formation of crescents.
- Chronic glomerular responses to injury include basement membrane thickening, hyalinosis, and sclerosis.

Pathogenesis of Glomerular Injury

Although much remains unknown about etiologic agents and triggering events, it is clear that **immune mechanisms underlie most forms of primary glomerulopathy and many of the secondary glomerular disorders** (Table 20-4). Glomerulonephritis can be readily induced experimentally by antigen-antibody reactions. Furthermore, glomerular deposits of immunoglobulins, often with components of complement, are found in the majority of individuals with glomerulonephritis. Cell-mediated immune reactions also may play a role, usually in concert with antibody-mediated events. We begin this discussion with a review of antibody-instigated injury.

Two forms of antibody-associated injury have been established: (1) injury by *antibodies reacting in situ within the glomerulus,* either binding to insoluble fixed (intrinsic) glomerular antigens or extrinsic molecules planted within the glomerulus, and (2) injury resulting from *deposition of circulating antigen-antibody complexes in the glomerulus.* It is clear that the major cause of glomerulonephritis resulting from formation of antigen-antibody complexes is the consequence of in situ immune complex formation, and not deposition of circulating complexes as was once thought.

Table 20-4 Immune Mechanisms of Glomerular Injury

Antibody-Mediated Injury
In Situ Immune Complex Deposition
Fixed intrinsic tissue antigens
NC1 domain of type IV collagen antigen (anti-GBM nephritis)
PLA_2R antigen (membranous glomerulopathy)
Mesangial antigens
Others
Planted antigens
Exogenous (infectious agents, drugs)
Endogenous (DNA, nuclear proteins, immunoglobulins, immune complexes, IgA)
Circulating Immune Complex Deposition
Endogenous antigens (e.g., DNA, tumor antigens)
Exogenous antigens (e.g., infectious products)
Cell-Mediated Immune Injury
Activation of Alternative Complement Pathway

GBM, glomerular basement membrane.

Diseases Caused by In Situ Formation of Immune Complexes

In this form of injury, immune complexes are formed locally by antibodies that react with intrinsic tissue antigen or with extrinsic antigens "planted" in the glomerulus from the circulation. Membranous nephropathy is the classic example of glomerular injury resulting from local formation of immune complexes. It has a well-studied experimental counterpart in the Heymann nephritis rat model, from which much of the underlying pathophysiology of glomerular immune complex–mediated diseases has been deduced.

The Heymann model of glomerulonephritis is induced by immunizing rats with an antigen, now known to be *megalin*, that is present in epithelial cell foot processes (Fig. 20-4C). The rats develop antibodies to this antigen, and disease develops from the reaction of antibody with the megalin-containing protein complex located on the basal surface of visceral epithelial cells, leading to localized immune complex formation. A major advance in our understanding of glomerulonephritis came from the identification of the M-type phospholipase A_2 receptor (PLA_2R) as the antigen that underlies most cases of primary human membranous nephropathy. Antibody binding to PLA_2R present in the glomerular epithelial cell membrane is followed by complement activation and then shedding of the immune aggregates from the cell surface to form characteristic deposits of immune complexes along the *subepithelial aspect* of the basement membrane (Fig. 20-4C). On electron microscopy the glomerulopathy is characterized by the presence of numerous discrete subepithelial electron-dense deposits (made up largely of immune reactants). **The pattern of immune deposition by immunofluorescence microscopy is granular rather than linear, reflective of the very localized antigen-antibody interaction.** These subepithelial complexes, with resultant host responses, can result in a thickened basement membrane appearance by light microscopy; hence the term *membranous nephropathy* has been applied to both the experimental model and human disease.

In humans, primary membranous nephropathy is an autoimmune disease, caused by antibodies to endogenous

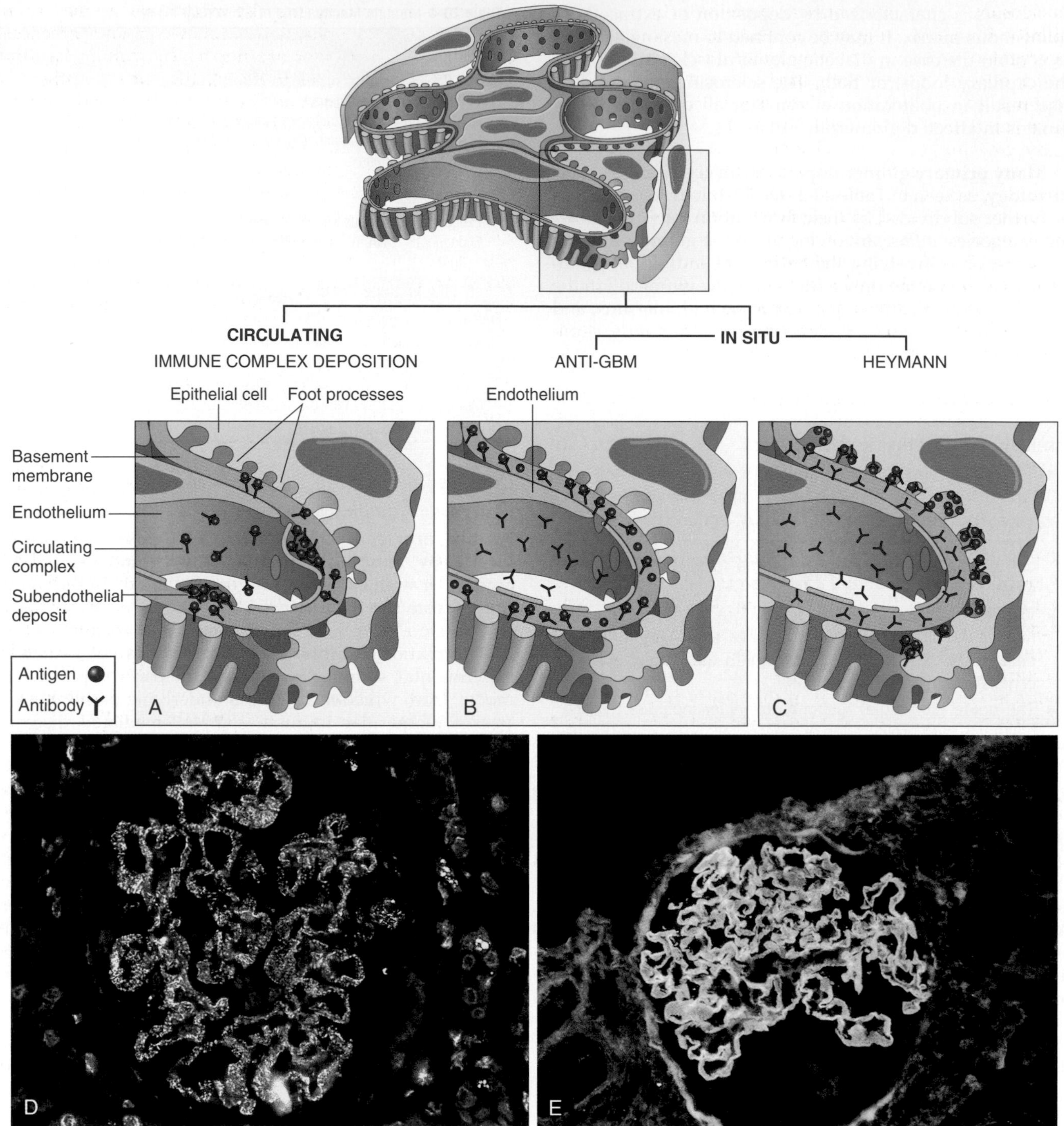

Figure 20-4 Antibody-mediated glomerular injury can result either from the deposition of circulating immune complexes **(A)** or, more commonly, from in situ formation of complexes exemplified by anti-GBM disease **(B)** or Heymann nephritis **(C)**. **D** and **E,** Two patterns of deposition of immune complexes as seen by immunofluorescence microscopy: granular, characteristic of circulating and in situ immune complex nephritis **(D),** and linear, characteristic of classic anti-GBM disease **(E).**

tissue components. What triggers these autoantibodies is unclear. Secondary forms of membranous nephropathy can be experimentally induced by drugs (e.g., mercuric chloride), and graft-versus-host disease (Chapter 6). In some of these situations there may be uncontrolled B-cell activation, leading to the production of autoantibodies that react with renal antigens.

Antibodies Against Planted Antigens

Antibodies can react in situ with antigens that are not normally present in the glomerulus but are "planted" there. Such antigens may localize in the kidney by interacting with various intrinsic components of the glomerulus. Planted antigens include cationic molecules that bind to anionic components of the glomerulus; DNA, nucleosomes, and other nuclear proteins, which have an affinity for GBM components; bacterial products; large aggregated proteins (e.g., aggregated immunoglobulins), which deposit in the mesangium because of their size; and immune complexes themselves, since they continue to have reactive sites for further interactions with free antibody, free antigen, or complement.

There is no dearth of other possible planted antigens, including viral, bacterial, and parasitic products and drugs. As an example, membranous nephropathy develops in a small number of infants fed cow's milk. These children have been found to have antibodies to bovine albumin and their lesions contain bovine milk antigens, which presumably become lodged in the glomerular basement membrane following intestinal absorption, where they serve as the substrate for immune complex formation in situ. Antibodies that bind to these planted antigens induce a discrete pattern of Ig deposition detected as granular staining by immunofluorescence microscopy that is indistinguishable from the pattern of staining observed with immune complexes formed from intrinsic antigens.

Disease Caused by Antibodies Directed Against Normal Components of the Glomerular Basement Membrane

In anti-GBM antibody induced glomerulonephritis, antibodies bind to intrinsic antigens homogeneously distributed along the entire length of the GBM, resulting in a diffuse linear pattern of staining for the antibodies by immunofluorescence techniques (Fig. 20-4*B* and *E*). This contrasts with the granular pattern of immunofluorescence staining corresponding to the discrete immune complexes seen in membranous nephropathy, or other glomerular diseases in which large complexes of antigens and antibodies form in situ. These intrinsic, fixed antigens cannot be mobilized to form large, discrete complexes.

Often the anti-GBM antibodies cross-react with other basement membranes, especially those in the lung alveoli, resulting in simultaneous lung and kidney lesions *(Goodpasture syndrome)*. The GBM antigen that is responsible for classic anti-GBM antibody-induced glomerulonephritis and Goodpasture syndrome is a component of the noncollagenous domain (NC1) of the α_3 chain of type IV collagen that is critical for maintenance of GBM suprastructure. Although anti-GBM antibody-induced glomerulonephritis accounts for fewer than 5% of cases of human glomerulonephritis, it causes severe necrotizing and crescentic glomerular damage and the clinical syndrome of rapidly progressive glomerulonephritis.

Glomerulonephritis Resulting from Deposition of Circulating Immune Complexes

In this type of nephritis, glomerular injury is caused by the trapping of circulating antigen-antibody complexes within glomeruli. The antibodies have no immunologic specificity for glomerular constituents, and the complexes localize within the glomeruli because of their physicochemical properties and the hemodynamic factors peculiar to the glomerulus (Fig. 20-4*A*).

The antigens that trigger the formation of circulating immune complexes may be of endogenous origin, as in the glomerulonephritis associated with SLE or in IgA nephropathy, **or they may be exogenous**, as may occur in the glomerulonephritis that follows certain infections. Microbial antigens that are implicated include bacterial products (streptococcal proteins), the surface antigen of hepatitis B virus, hepatitis C virus antigens, and antigens of *Treponema pallidum*, *Plasmodium falciparum*, and several viruses. Some tumor antigens are also thought to cause immune complex-mediated nephritis. In many cases the inciting antigen is unknown. In most instances of immune complex–mediated glomerulonephritis associated with these systemic disorders, evidence is strongest that the inciting event underlying the glomerulonephritis is deposition of the antigens with subsequent formation of immune complexes in situ rather than deposition of preformed immune complexes from the circulation.

Mechanisms of Glomerular Injury Following Immune Complex Formation

The pathogenesis of immune complex diseases is discussed in Chapter 6. Here we briefly review the salient features that relate to glomerular injury. **Whatever the antigen may be, antigen-antibody complexes formed or deposited in the glomeruli may elicit a local inflammatory reaction that produces injury.** It has long been thought that the inflammation and injury are mediated and amplified by the binding of complement, but recent studies in knockout mice also point to the importance of engagement of Fc receptors on leukocytes and perhaps glomerular mesangial or other cells as mediators of the injury process. The glomerular lesions may exhibit leukocytic infiltration and proliferation of mesangial and endothelial cells.

Electron microscopy reveals electron-dense deposits, presumably containing immune complexes, that may lie in the mesangium, between the endothelial cells and the GBM (subendothelial deposits), or between the outer surface of the GBM and the podocytes (subepithelial deposits). Deposits may be located at more than one site in a given case. By immunofluorescence microscopy the immune complexes are seen as granular deposits along the basement membrane (Fig. 20-4*D*), in the mesangium, or in both locations. Once deposited in the kidney, immune complexes may eventually be degraded, mostly by infiltrating neutrophils and monocytes/macrophages, mesangial cells, and endogenous proteases, and the inflammatory reaction may then subside. Such a course occurs when the exposure to the inciting antigen is short-lived and limited, as in most cases of poststreptococcal glomerulonephritis. However, if immune complexes are deposited for prolonged periods, as may be seen in SLE or viral hepatitis, repeated cycles of injury may occur, leading to a more chronic membranous or membranoproliferative type of glomerulonephritis.

Several factors affect glomerular localization of antigen, antibody or immune complexes. The molecular charge and size of these reactants are clearly important. Highly cationic antigens tend to cross the GBM, and the resultant complexes eventually reside in a subepithelial location. Highly anionic macromolecules are excluded from the GBM and are trapped subendothelially or are not nephritogenic at all. Molecules of neutral charge and immune complexes containing these molecules tend to accumulate in the mesangium. Large circulating complexes are not

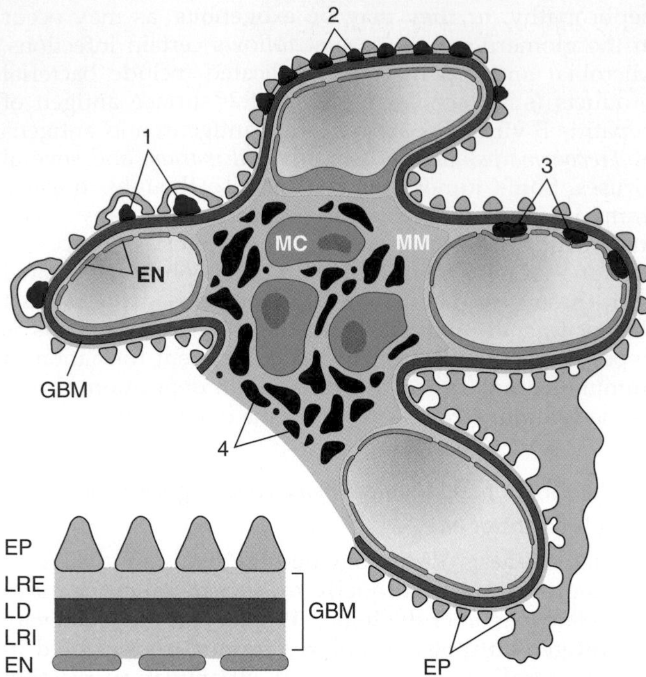

Figure 20-5 Localization of immune complexes in the glomerulus: (1) subepithelial humps, as in acute glomerulonephritis; (2) epimembranous deposits, as in membranous nephropathy and Heymann nephritis; (3) subendothelial deposits, as in lupus nephritis and membranoproliferative glomerulonephritis; (4) mesangial deposits, as in IgA nephropathy. *EN,* Endothelium; *EP,* epithelium; *GBM,* glomerular basement membrane; *LD,* lamina densa; *LRE,* lamina rara externa; *LRI,* lamina rara interna; *MC,* mesangial cell; *MM,* mesangial matrix. (Modified from Couser WG: Mediation of immune glomerular injury. J Am Soc Nephrol 1:13, 1990.)

usually nephritogenic, because they are cleared by the mononuclear phagocyte system and do not enter the GBM in significant quantities. The pattern of localization is also affected by changes in glomerular hemodynamics, mesangial function, and integrity of the charge-selective barrier in the glomerulus. These influences may underlie the variable pattern of immune reactant deposition in various forms of glomerulonephritis (Fig. 20-5). In turn, the distinct patterns of localization of immune complexes is a key determinant of the injury response and the histologic features that subsequently develop. Immune complexes located in subendothelial portions of capillaries and in mesangial regions are accessible to the circulation and more likely to be involved in inflammatory processes that require interaction and activation of circulating leukocytes. Diseases in which immune complexes are confined to the subepithelial locations and for which the capillary basement membranes may be a barrier to interaction with circulating leukocytes, as in the case of membranous nephropathy, typically have a noninflammatory pathology.

In summary, **most cases of immune complex mediated glomerulonephritis are a consequence of deposition of discrete immune complexes, which give rise to granular immunofluorescence staining along the basement membranes or in the mesangium.** However, it may be difficult to determine whether the deposition has occurred in situ, by circulating complexes, or by both mechanisms because, as we discussed earlier, trapping of circulating immune complexes can initiate further in situ complex formation. Single etiologic agents, such as hepatitis B and C viruses, can cause either a membranous pattern of glomerulonephritis, with subepithelial in situ deposition of antigens, or a membranoproliferative pattern, more indicative of subendothelial deposition of antigens or deposition of circulating complexes. It is best then to consider that **antigen-antibody deposition in the glomerulus is a major pathway of glomerular injury and that in situ immune reactions, trapping of circulating complexes, interactions between these two events, and local hemodynamic and structural determinants in the glomerulus all contribute to the diverse morphologic and functional alterations in glomerulonephritis.**

Cell-Mediated Immunity in Glomerulonephritis

Although antibody-mediated mechanisms may initiate many forms of glomerulonephritis, there is evidence that sensitized T cells cause glomerular injury and are involved in the progression of some glomerulonephritides. Clues to the role of cellular immunity include the presence of activated macrophages and T cells and their products in the glomerulus in some forms of human and experimental glomerulonephritis; in vitro and in vivo evidence of lymphocyte activation on exposure to antigen in human and experimental glomerulonephritis; abrogation of glomerular injury by lymphocyte depletion; and experiments in which glomerular injury may be induced by transfer of T cells from nephritic animals to normal recipients. The evidence is most compelling for certain types of experimental crescentic glomerulonephritis in which antibodies to GBM initiate glomerular injury and activated T lymphocytes then propagate the inflammation. Despite this body of suggestive evidence, proof of glomerulonephritis in humans resulting primarily from T-cell activation remains lacking.

KEY CONCEPTS

Pathogenesis of Immune-mediated Glomerular Injury

- Antibody-mediated immune injury is an important mechanism of glomerular damage, mainly via complement- and leukocyte-mediated pathways. Antibodies may also be directly cytotoxic to cells in the glomerulus.
- The most common forms of antibody-mediated glomerulonephritis are caused by the formation of immune complexes, which may involve either endogenous antigens (e.g., PLA_2R in membranous nephropathy) or exogenous (e.g., microbial) antigens. Immune complexes show a granular pattern of deposition by immunofluorescence.
- Autoantibodies against components of the GBM are the cause of anti–GBM antibody–mediated disease, often associated with severe injury. The pattern of antibody deposition is linear by immunofluorescence.

Activation of Alternative Complement Pathway

Alternative complement pathway activation occurs in the clinicopathologic entity called *dense-deposit disease,* until recently referred to as *membranoproliferative glomerulone-*

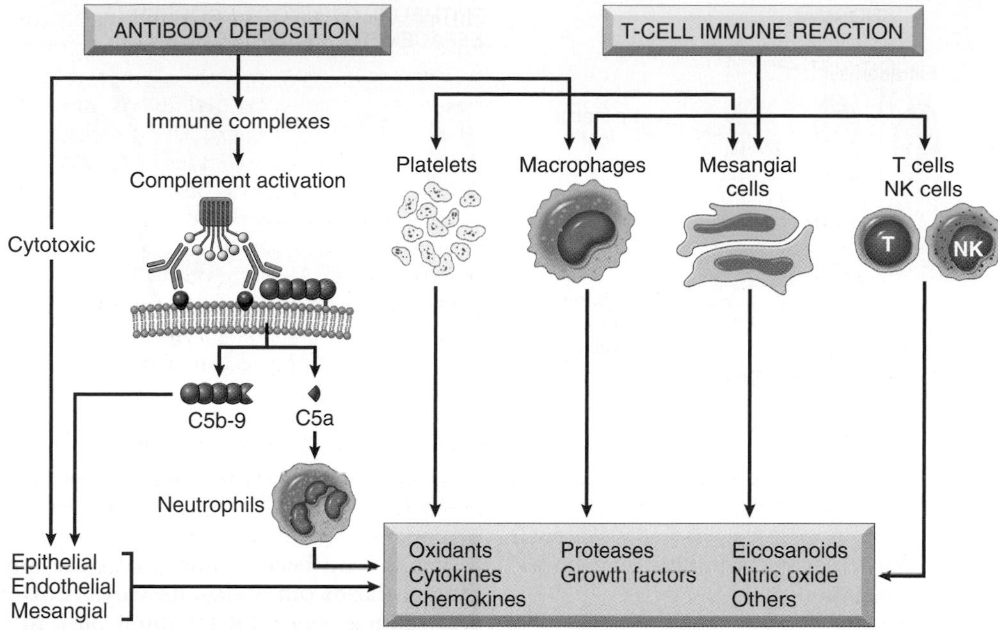

Figure 20-6 Mediators of immune glomerular injury.

phritis (MPGN type II), and in an emerging diagnostic category of diseases broadly termed *C3 glomerulopathies.* This is discussed later in the sections describing these diseases.

Mediators of Glomerular Injury

Once immune reactants or sensitized T cells have localized in the glomerulus, how does the glomerular damage ensue? The mediators—both cells and molecules—are the usual suspects involved in acute and chronic inflammation, described in Chapter 3, and only a few are highlighted here (Fig. 20-6).

Cells

- *Neutrophils* and *monocytes* infiltrate the glomerulus in certain types of glomerulonephritis, largely as a result of activation of complement, resulting in generation of chemotactic agents (mainly C5a), but also by Fc-mediated adherence and activation. Neutrophils release proteases, which cause GBM degradation; oxygen-derived free radicals, which cause cell damage; and arachidonic acid metabolites, which contribute to the reductions in GFR.
- *Macrophages and T lymphocytes,* which infiltrate the glomerulus in antibody- and cell-mediated reactions, when activated, release a vast number of biologically active molecules.
- *Platelets* may aggregate in the glomerulus during immune-mediated injury. Their release of eicosanoids, growth factors and other mediators may contribute to vascular injury and proliferation of glomerular cells. Antiplatelet agents have beneficial effects in both human and experimental glomerulonephritis.
- *Resident glomerular cells,* particularly mesangial cells, can be stimulated to produce several inflammatory mediators, including reactive oxygen species (ROS), cytokines, chemokines, growth factors, eicosanoids, nitric oxide, and endothelin. They may initiate inflammatory responses in the glomerulus even in the absence of leukocytic infiltration.

Soluble Mediators

Virtually all the known inflammatory chemical mediators (Chapter 3) have been implicated in glomerular injury.

- *Complement activation* leads to the generation of chemotactic products that induce leukocyte influx (complement-neutrophil–dependent injury) and the formation of C5b-C9, the membrane attack complex. C5b-C9 causes cell lysis but, in addition, stimulates mesangial cells to produce oxidants, proteases, and other mediators. Thus, even in the absence of neutrophils, C5b-C9 can cause proteinuria, as has been demonstrated in experimental membranous glomerulopathy.
- *Eicosanoids, nitric oxide, angiotensin,* and *endothelin* are involved in the hemodynamic changes.
- *Cytokines,* particularly IL-1 and TNF, which may be produced by infiltrating leukocytes and resident glomerular cells, induce leukocyte adhesion and a variety of other effects.
- *Chemokines* such as monocyte chemoattractant protein 1 promote monocyte and lymphocyte influx. *Growth factors* such as platelet-derived growth factor (PDGF) are involved in mesangial cell proliferation. TGF-β, connective tissue growth factor, and fibroblast growth factor seem to be critical in the ECM deposition and hyalinization leading to glomerulosclerosis in chronic injury. Vascular endothelial growth factor (VEGF) seems to maintain endothelial integrity and may help regulate capillary permeability.
- The *coagulation system* is also a mediator of glomerular damage. Fibrin is frequently present in the glomeruli and Bowman space in glomerulonephritis, indicative of coagulation cascade activation, and activated

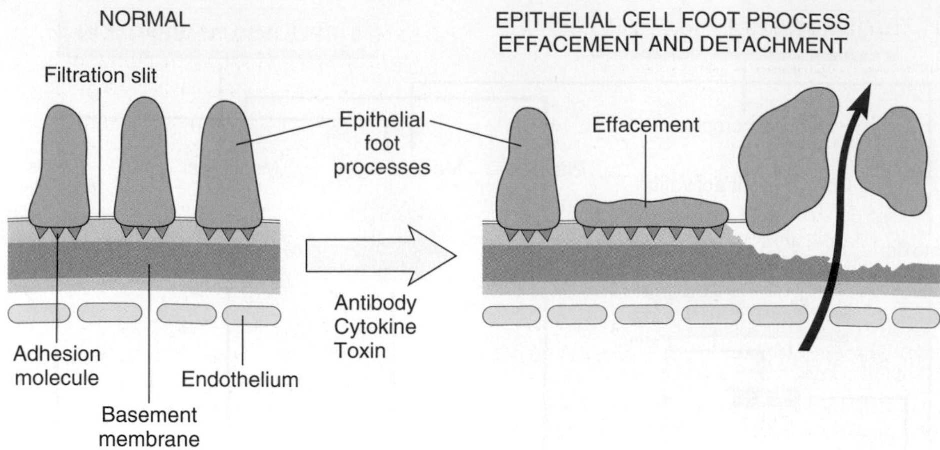

Figure 20-7 Epithelial cell injury. The postulated sequence is a consequence of antibodies specific to epithelial cell antigens, toxins, cytokines, or other factors causing injury; this results in foot process effacement and sometimes detachment of epithelial cells and protein leakage through defective GBM and filtration slits.

coagulation factors, particularly thrombin, may be a stimulus for crescent formation.

Epithelial Cell Injury

Podocyte injury is common to many forms of both primary and secondary glomerular diseases, of both immune and non-immune etiologies. The term *podocytopathy* has been applied to diseases with disparate etiologies whose principal manifestation is injury to podocytes. This can be induced by antibodies to podocyte antigens; by toxins, as in an experimental model of proteinuria induced by puromycin aminonucleoside; conceivably by certain cytokines; by certain viral infections such as human immunodeficiency virus (HIV) or by still inadequately characterized circulating factors, as in some cases of focal segmental glomerulosclerosis. Such injury is reflected by stereotypic morphologic changes in the podocytes, which include effacement of foot processes, vacuolization, and retraction and detachment of cells from the GBM, and functionally by proteinuria (Fig. 20-7).

Loss of podocytes, which have only a very limited capacity for replication and repair, may be a feature of multiple types of glomerular injury including focal and segmental glomerulosclerosis and diabetic nephropathy. Such loss typically cannot be recognized in pathologic specimens unless specialized morphologic techniques are applied. In most forms of glomerular injury, loss of normal slit diaphragms is a key event in the development of proteinuria (Fig. 20-6). Functional abnormalities of the slit diaphragm may also result from mutations in its components, such as nephrin and podocin, without actual inflammatory damage to the glomerulus. Such mutations are the cause of rare hereditary forms of the nephrotic syndrome.

Mechanisms of Progression in Glomerular Diseases

Thus far, the immunologic mechanisms and mediators that *initiate* glomerular injury have been discussed. The outcome of such injury depends on several factors, including the severity of renal damage, the nature and persistence of the antigens, and the immune status, age, and genetic predisposition of the host.

It has long been known that **once any renal disease, glomerular or otherwise, destroys functioning nephrons and reduces the GFR to about 30% to 50% of normal, progression to end-stage renal failure proceeds at a steady rate, independent of the original stimulus or activity of the underlying disease.** The secondary factors that lead to progression are of great clinical interest, since they can be targets of therapy that delays or even prevents the inexorable journey to dialysis or transplantation.

The two major histologic characteristics of such progressive renal damage are *focal segmental glomerulosclerosis* (FSGS) and *tubulointerstitial fibrosis*.

Focal Segmental Glomerulosclerosis (FSGS). **Progressive fibrosis involving portions of some glomeruli develops after many types of renal injury and leads to proteinuria and increasing functional impairment.** FSGS may be seen even in cases in which the primary disease was nonglomerular. The glomerulosclerosis seems to be initiated by the *adaptive change* that occurs in the relatively unaffected glomeruli of diseased kidneys. Such a mechanism is suggested by experiments in rats subjected to subtotal nephrectomy. *Compensatory hypertrophy* of the remaining glomeruli initially maintains renal function in these animals, but proteinuria and segmental glomerulosclerosis soon develop, leading eventually to total glomerular sclerosis and uremia. The glomerular hypertrophy is associated with *hemodynamic changes*, including increases in glomerular blood flow, filtration, and transcapillary pressure (glomerular hypertension), and often with systemic hypertension.

The sequence of events (Fig. 20-8) that is thought to lead to sclerosis in this setting entails endothelial and visceral epithelial cell injury, visceral epithelial cell loss leading to segments of GBM denuded of overlying foot processes and consequently increased glomerular permeability to proteins, and accumulation of proteins in the mesangial matrix. This is followed by proliferation of mesangial cells, infiltration by macrophages, increased accumulation of extracellular matrix (ECM), and segmental and eventually global sclerosis of glomeruli. With increasing reductions in nephron mass and ongoing compensatory changes, a vicious cycle of continuing glomerulosclerosis sets in. Most of the mediators of chronic inflammation and fibrosis, particularly TGF-β, play a role in the induction of

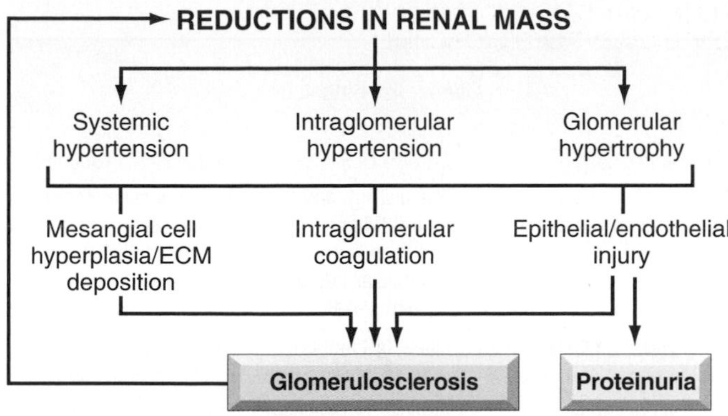

Figure 20-8 Focal segmental glomerulosclerosis associated with loss of renal mass. The adaptive changes in glomeruli (hypertrophy and glomerular capillary hypertension), as well as systemic hypertension, cause epithelial and endothelial injury and resultant proteinuria. The mesangial response, involving mesangial cell proliferation and ECM production, together with intraglomerular coagulation, causes the glomerulosclerosis. This results in further loss of functioning nephrons and a vicious circle of progressive glomerulosclerosis.

sclerosis. Currently, the most successful interventions to interrupt these mechanisms of progressive glomerulosclerosis involve treatment with inhibitors of the renin-angiotensin system, which not only reduce intraglomerular hypertension, but also have direct effects on each of the mechanisms identified above. Importantly, these agents have been shown to ameliorate progression of sclerosis in both animal and human studies.

Tubulointerstitial Fibrosis. **Tubulointerstitial injury, manifested by tubular damage and interstitial inflammation, is a component of many acute and chronic glomerulonephritides.** Tubulointerstitial fibrosis contributes to progression in both immune and nonimmune glomerular diseases, for example, diabetic nephropathy. Indeed, **there is often a much better correlation of decline in renal function with the extent of tubulointerstitial damage than with the severity of glomerular injury.** Many factors may lead to such tubulointerstitial injury, including ischemia of tubule segments downstream from sclerotic glomeruli, acute and chronic inflammation in the adjacent interstitium, and damage or loss of the peritubular capillary blood supply. Current work also points to the effects of *proteinuria* on tubular cell structure and function. It appears that proteinuria can cause *direct injury to and activation of tubular cells*. Activated tubular cells in turn express adhesion molecules and elaborate pro-inflammatory cytokines, chemokines, and growth factors that contribute to interstitial fibrosis. Filtered proteins that may produce these tubular effects include cytokines, complement products, the iron in hemoglobin, immunoglobulins, lipid moieties, and oxidatively modified plasma proteins.

KEY CONCEPTS

Progression of Glomerular Disease

- Progressive glomerular injury can be the result of either primary or secondary glomerular injuries, of diseases that are either renal limited or systemic, and of diseases that initially involve renal structures other than glomeruli.
- The principal glomerular manifestation of progressive injury is focal segmental glomerulosclerosis, eventually leading to global glomerular involvement and glomerular obsolescence.
- Progressive injury ensues from a cycle of glomerular and nephron loss, compensatory changes that lead to further glomerular injury and glomerulosclerosis, and eventually end-stage renal disease.
- Progressive glomerular injury is accompanied by chronic injuries to other renal structures, typically manifest as tubulointerstitial fibrosis.

Having discussed the factors involved in the initiation and progression of glomerular injury, we now turn to a discussion of individual glomerular diseases. Table 20-5 summarizes the main clinical and pathologic features of the major forms of primary glomerulopathies.

Nephritic Syndrome

Glomerular diseases presenting with a nephritic syndrome are often characterized by inflammation in the glomeruli. The nephritic patient usually presents with hematuria, red cell casts in the urine, azotemia, oliguria, and mild to moderate hypertension. Proteinuria and edema are common, but these are not as severe as those encountered in the nephrotic syndrome, discussed later. The acute nephritic syndrome may occur in such multisystem diseases as SLE and microscopic polyangiitis. Typically, however, it is characteristic of acute proliferative and exudative glomerulonephritis and is an important component of crescentic glomerulonephritis, which is described later.

Acute Proliferative (Poststreptococcal, Postinfectious) Glomerulonephritis

As the name implies, **this cluster of diseases is characterized histologically by diffuse proliferation of glomerular cells associated with influx (exudation) of leukocytes. These lesions are typically caused by immune complexes.** The inciting antigen may be exogenous or endogenous. The prototypic exogenous antigen-induced disease pattern is postinfectious glomerulonephritis, whereas an example of an endogenous antigen-induced disease is the nephritis of SLE, described in Chapter 6. The most common underlying infections are streptococcal, but the disorder may also be associated with other infections.

Poststreptococcal Glomerulonephritis

This is a prototypical glomerular disease of immune complex etiology, which is decreasing in frequency in the United States but continues to be a fairly common disorder worldwide. It usually appears 1 to 4 weeks after a streptococcal infection of the pharynx or skin (impetigo). Skin infections are commonly associated with overcrowding and poor hygiene. Poststreptococcal glomerulonephritis occurs most frequently in children 6 to 10 years of age, but children and adults of any age can also be affected.

Table 20-5 Summary of Major Primary Glomerulonephritides

Disease	Most Frequent Clinical Presentation	Pathogenesis	Glomerular Pathology		
			Light Microscopy	Fluorescence Microscopy	Electron Microscopy
Postinfectious glomerulonephritis	Nephritic syndrome	Immune complex mediated; circulating or planted antigen	Diffuse endocapillary proliferation; leukocytic infiltration	Granular IgG and C3 in GBM and mesangium; Granular IgA in some cases	Primarily subepithelial humps; subendothelial deposits in early disease stages.
Goodpasture syndrome	Rapidly progressive glomerulonephritis	Anti-GBM COL4-A3 antigen	Extracapillary proliferation with crescents; necrosis	Linear IgG and C3; fibrin in crescents	No deposits; GBM disruptions; fibrin
Chronic glomerulonephritis	Chronic renal failure	Variable	Hyalinized glomeruli	Granular or negative	
Membranous nephropathy	Nephrotic syndrome	In situ immune complex formation; PLA_2Rantigen in most cases of primary disease mostly unknown	Diffuse capillary wall thickening	Granular IgG and C3; diffuse	Subepithelial deposits
Minimal change disease	Nephrotic syndrome	Unknown; loss of glomerular polyanion; podocyte injury	Normal; lipid in tubules	Negative	Loss of foot processes; no deposits
Focal segmental glomerulosclerosis	Nephrotic syndrome; nonnephrotic proteinuria	Unknown Ablation nephropathy Plasma factor (?); podocyte injury	Focal and segmental sclerosis and hyalinosis	Focal; IgM + C3 in many cases	Loss of foot processes; epithelial denudation
Membranoproliferative glomerulonephritis (MPGN) type I	Nephrotic/nephrotic syndrome	Immune complex	Mesangial proliferative or membranoproliferative patterns of proliferation; GBM thickening; splitting	IgG ++ C3; C1q ++ C4	Subendothelial deposits
Dense-deposit disease (MPGN type II)	Hematuria Chronic renal failure	Autoantibody; alternative complement pathway	Mesangial proliferative or membranoproliferative patterns of proliferation; GBM thickening; splitting	C3; no C1q or C4	Dense deposits
IgA nephropathy	Recurrent hematuria or proteinuria	Unknown	Focal mesangial proliferative glomerulonephritis; mesangial widening	IgA ± IgG, IgM, and C3 in mesangium	Mesangial and paramesangial dense deposits

GBM, Glomerular basement membrane.

Etiology and Pathogenesis. **Poststreptococcal GN is caused by immune complexes containing streptococcal antigens and specific antibodies, which are formed in situ.** Only certain strains of group A β-hemolytic streptococci are nephritogenic, more than 90% of cases being traced to types 12, 4, and 1, which can be identified by typing of the M protein of the bacterial cell walls.

Many lines of evidence support an immunologic basis for poststreptococcal glomerulonephritis. The latent period between infection and onset of nephritis is compatible with the time required for the production of antibodies and the formation of immune complexes. Elevated titers of antibodies against one or more streptococcal antigens are present in a great majority of patients. Serum complement levels are low, compatible with activation of the complement system and consumption of complement components. There are granular immune deposits in the glomeruli, indicative of an immune complex–mediated mechanism.

The streptococcal antigenic component responsible for the immune reaction had long eluded identification, but the preponderance of evidence identifies streptococcal pyogenic exotoxin B (SpeB) as the principal antigenic determinant in most but not all cases of poststreptococcal glomerulonephritis. This protein can directly activate complement, is commonly secreted by nephritogenic strains of streptococci, and has been localized to the "hump-like" deposits characteristic of this disease (described later). At the outset, the inciting antigens are exogenously planted from the circulation in subendothelial locations in glomerular capillary walls, leading to in situ formation of immune complexes, where they elicit an inflammatory response. Subsequently, through mechanisms that are not well understood, the antigen-antibody complexes dissociate, migrate across the GBM, and re-form on the subepithelial side of the GBM.

MORPHOLOGY

The classic histologic picture is one of **enlarged, hypercellular glomeruli** (Fig. 20-9). The hypercellularity is caused by (1) infiltration by leukocytes, both neutrophils and monocytes; (2) proliferation of endothelial and mesangial cells; and (3) in severe cases by crescent formation. The proliferation and leukocyte infiltration are typically global and diffuse, that is, involving all lobules of all glomeruli. There is also swelling of endothelial cells, and the combination of proliferation, swelling, and leukocyte infiltration obliterates the capillary lumens. There may be

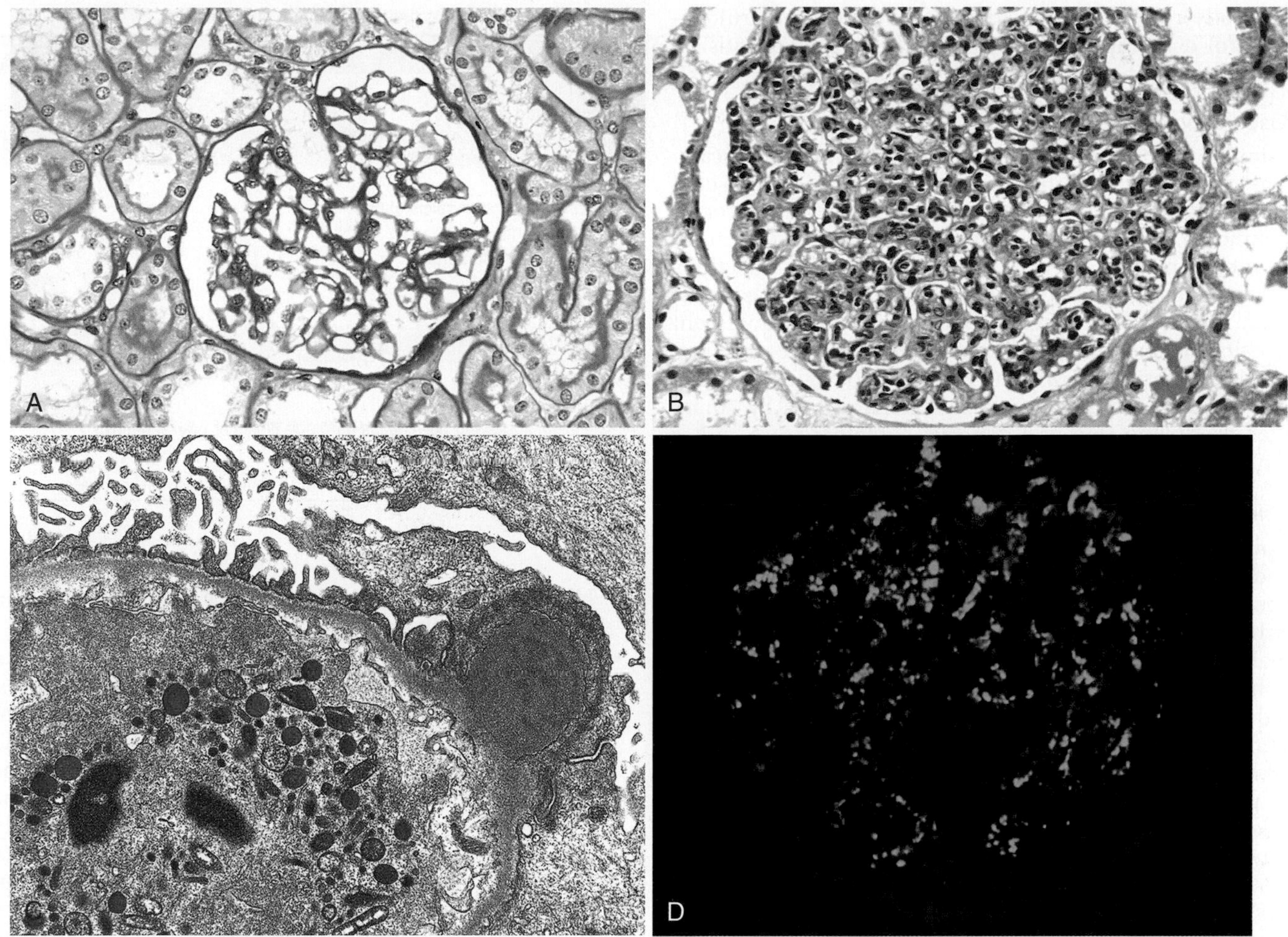

Figure 20-9 Acute proliferative glomerulonephritis. **A,** Normal glomerulus. **B,** Glomerular hypercellularity is due to intracapillary leukocytes and proliferation of intrinsic glomerular cells. **C,** Typical electron-dense subepithelial "hump" and a neutrophil in the lumen. **D,** Immunofluorescent stain demonstrates discrete, coarsely granular deposits of complement protein C3 (stain for IgG was similar), corresponding to "humps" illustrated in part **C.** (**A-C,** Courtesy Dr. H. Rennke, Brigham and Women's Hospital, Boston, Mass. **D,** Courtesy D. J. Kowaleska, Cedars-Sinai Medical Center, Los Angeles, Calif.)

interstitial edema and inflammation, and the tubules often contain red cell casts.

By **immunofluorescence microscopy,** there are granular deposits of IgG, and C3, and sometimes IgM in the mesangium and along the GBM (Fig. 20-9*D*). Although immune complex deposits are almost universally present, they are often focal and sparse. The characteristic **electron microscopic findings** are discrete, amorphous, electron-dense deposits on the epithelial side of the membrane, often having the appearance of "humps" (Fig. 20-9*C*), presumably representing the antigen-antibody complexes at the subepithelial cell surface. Subendothelial deposits are also commonly seen, typically early in the disease course, and mesangial and intramembranous deposits may be present.

Clinical Course. In the typical case, a young child abruptly develops malaise, fever, nausea, oliguria, and hematuria (smoky or cola-colored urine) 1 to 2 weeks after recovery from a sore throat. The patients have dysmorphic red cells or red cell casts in the urine, mild proteinuria (usually less than 1 gm/day), periorbital edema, and mild to moderate hypertension. In adults the onset is more likely to be atypical, such as the sudden appearance of hypertension or edema, frequently with elevation of BUN. The glomerulonephritis is subclinical in some infected individuals, and is discovered only on screening for microscopic hematuria carried out during epidemic outbreaks. Important laboratory findings include elevations of antistreptococcal antibody titers and a decline in the serum concentration of C3 and other components of the complement cascade.

More than 95% of affected children eventually recover renal function with conservative therapy aimed at maintaining sodium and water balance. A small minority of children (perhaps fewer than 1%) do not improve, become severely oliguric, and develop a rapidly progressive form of glomerulonephritis (described later). Some of the remaining patients may undergo slow progression to chronic glomerulonephritis with or without recurrence of an active nephritic picture. Prolonged and persistent heavy proteinuria and abnormal GFR mark patients with an unfavorable prognosis.

In adults the disease is less benign. Although the overall prognosis in epidemics is good, in only about 60% of sporadic cases do the patients recover promptly. In the remainder the glomerular lesions fail to resolve quickly, as manifested by persistent proteinuria, hematuria, and hypertension. In some of these patients, the lesions eventually clear, but others develop chronic glomerulonephritis or even rapidly progressive glomerulonephritis.

Nonstreptococcal Acute Glomerulonephritis (Postinfectious Glomerulonephritis)

A similar form of glomerulonephritis occurs sporadically in association with other infections, including those of bacterial (e.g., staphylococcal endocarditis, pneumococcal pneumonia, and meningococcemia), viral (e.g., hepatitis B, hepatitis C, mumps, HIV infection, varicella, and infectious mononucleosis), and parasitic (malaria, toxoplasmosis) origin. In these settings, granular immunofluorescent deposits and subepithelial humps characteristic of immune complex nephritis are present. Postinfectious glomerulonephritis due to staphylococcal infections differs by sometimes producing immune deposits containing IgA rather than IgG.

Table 20-6 Rapidly Progressive Glomerulonephritides

Type I (Anti-GBM Antibody)
Renal limited Goodpasture syndrome
Type II (Immune Complex)
Idiopathic Postinfectious glomerulonephritis Lupus nephritis Henoch-Schönlein purpura IgA nephropathy Others
Type III (Pauci-Immune)
ANCA-associated Idiopathic Granulomatosis with polyangiitis (formerly Wegener granulomatosis) Microscopic polyangiitis

ANCA, Antineutrophil cytoplasmic antibodies; GBM, glomerular basement membrane.

Rapidly Progressive (Crescentic) Glomerulonephritis

Rapidly progressive glomerulonephritis (RPGN) is a syndrome associated with severe glomerular injury, but does not denote a specific etiologic form of glomerulonephritis. It is characterized by rapid and progressive loss of renal function associated with severe oliguria and signs of nephritic syndrome; if untreated, death from renal failure occurs within weeks to months. *The most common histologic picture is the presence of crescents in most of the glomeruli (crescentic glomerulonephritis).* As discussed earlier, these are produced predominantly by the proliferation of the parietal epithelial cells lining Bowman capsule and by the infiltration of monocytes and macrophages.

Classification and Pathogenesis. RPGN may be caused by a number of different diseases, some restricted to the kidney and others systemic. Although no single mechanism can explain all cases, there is little doubt that **in most cases the glomerular injury is immunologically mediated**. A practical classification divides RPGN into three groups on the basis of immunologic findings (Table 20-6). In each group the disease may be associated with a known disorder, or it may be idiopathic. The common denominator in all types of RPGN is severe glomerular injury. Several distinct pathogenic mechanisms have been described, as follows:

- *Anti-GBM antibody-mediated disease, characterized by linear deposits of IgG and, in many cases, C3 in the GBM.* In some of these patients, the anti-GBM antibodies cross-react with pulmonary alveolar basement membranes to produce the clinical picture of pulmonary hemorrhage associated with renal failure *(Goodpasture syndrome)*. Plasmapheresis to remove the pathogenic circulating antibodies is usually part of the treatment, which also includes therapy to suppress the underlying immune response.

  The antigen common to the alveoli and GBM is a peptide within the noncollagenous portion of the α_3 chain of collagen type IV. What triggers the formation of these antibodies is unclear in most patients. Exposure to viruses or hydrocarbon solvents (found in paints and dyes) has been implicated in some patients, as have various drugs and cancers. There is a high prevalence of certain HLA subtypes and haplotypes (e.g., HLA-DRB1) in affected patients, a finding consistent with the genetic predisposition to autoimmunity.
- *Diseases caused by immune complex deposition. RPGN can be a complication of any of the immune complex nephritides, including postinfectious glomerulonephritis, lupus nephritis, IgA nephropathy, and Henoch-Schönlein purpura.* In all these cases, immunofluorescence studies reveal the granular pattern of staining characteristic of immune complex deposition. This type of RPGN frequently demonstrates cellular proliferation and influx of leukocytes within the glomerular tuft, in addition to crescent formation. These patients usually cannot be helped by plasmapheresis, and they require treatment for the underlying disease.
- *Pauci-immune RPGN, defined by the lack of detectable anti-GBM antibodies or immune complexes by immunofluorescence and electron microscopy.* Most patients with this type of RPGN have circulating *antineutrophil cytoplasmic antibodies* (ANCAs) that produce cytoplasmic (c) or perinuclear (p) staining pattern and are known to play a role in some vasculitides (Chapter 11). This type of RPGN may be a component of a systemic vasculitis such as granulomatosis with polyangiitis (formerly called *Wegener granulomatosis*) or microscopic polyangiitis. In many cases, however, pauci-immune crescentic glomerulonephritis is limited to the kidneys and hence *idiopathic*. More than 90% of such idiopathic cases have c-ANCAs or p-ANCAs in the sera. The presence of circulating ANCAs in both idiopathic crescentic glomerulonephritis and cases of crescentic glomerulonephritis that occur as a component of systemic vasculitis, and the similar pathologic features in either setting, have led to the idea that these disorders are pathogenetically related. According to this concept, all cases of crescentic glomerulonephritis of the pauci-immune type are manifestations of small-vessel vasculitis or polyangiitis, which is limited to glomerular and perhaps peritubular capillaries in cases of idiopathic crescentic glomerulonephritis. Since these entities are viewed as part of a spectrum of vasculitic disease, the clinical distinction between systemic vasculitis with pauci-immune renal involvement and idiopathic crescentic

glomerulonephritis has been de-emphasized. ANCAs have proved to be invaluable as a highly sensitive diagnostic marker for pauci-immune crescentic glomerulonephritis, but proof of their role as a direct cause of this glomerulonephritis has been elusive. Recent evidence of their pathogenic potential has been obtained by studies in mice showing that transferring antibodies against myeloperoxidase (the target antigen of most p-ANCAs) induces a form of RPGN.

To summarize, about one fifth of patients with RPGN have anti-GBM antibody-mediated glomerulonephritis without lung involvement; another one fourth have immune complex-mediated crescentic glomerulonephritis; and the remainder are of the pauci-immune type.

MORPHOLOGY

The kidneys are enlarged and pale, often with petechial hemorrhages on the cortical surfaces. Depending on the underlying cause, the glomeruli often show focal and segmental necrosis, and variably show diffuse or focal endothelial proliferation, and mesangial proliferation. Segmental glomerular necrosis adjacent to glomerular segments uninvolved by inflammatory or proliferative changes is the feature most typical of pauci-immune RPGN. The histologic picture, however, is dominated by distinctive **crescents** (Fig. 20-10). Crescents are formed by proliferation of parietal cells and by migration of monocytes and macrophages into the urinary space. Neutrophils and lymphocytes may be present. The crescents may obliterate the urinary space and compress the glomerular tuft. **Fibrin strands are frequently prominent between the cellular layers in the crescents;** indeed, as discussed earlier, the escape of procoagulant factors, fibrin and cytokines into Bowman space may contribute to crescent formation. By immunofluorescence microscopy, immune complex-mediated cases show granular immune deposits; Goodpasture syndrome cases show linear GBM fluorescence for Ig and complement, and pauci-immune cases have little or no deposition of immune reactants. Electron microscopy discloses deposits in those cases due to immune complex deposition (type II). Regardless of type, electron microscopy may show **ruptures in the GBM,** a severe injury that allows leukocytes, plasma proteins such as coagulation factors and complement, and inflammatory mediators to reach the urinary space, where they trigger crescent formation (Fig. 20-11). In time, most crescents undergo organization and foci of segmental necrosis resolve as segmental scars (a type of segmental sclerosis), but restoration of normal glomerular architecture may be achieved with early aggressive therapy.

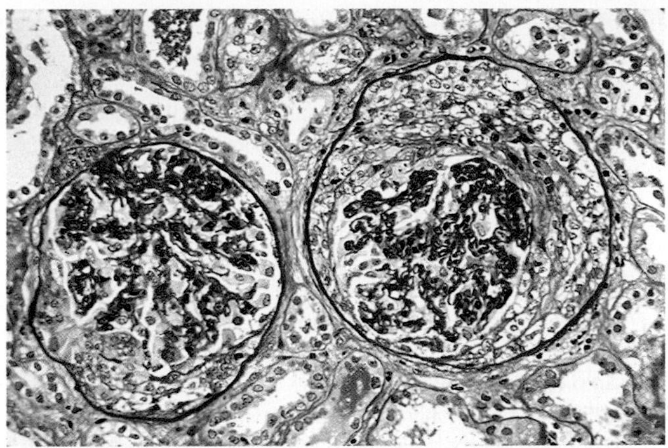

Figure 20-10 Crescentic glomerulonephritis (PAS stain). Note the collapsed glomerular tufts and the crescent-shaped mass of proliferating parietal epithelial cells and leukocytes internal to Bowman capsule. (Courtesy Dr. M.A. Venkatachalam, University of Texas Health Sciences Center, San Antonio, Tex.)

Clinical Course. The renal manifestations of all forms of crescentic glomerulonephritis include hematuria with red blood cell casts in the urine, moderate proteinuria occasionally reaching the nephrotic range, and variable hypertension and edema. In Goodpasture syndrome the course may be dominated by recurrent hemoptysis or even life-threatening pulmonary hemorrhage. Serum analyses for anti-GBM antibodies, antinuclear antibodies, and ANCAs are helpful in the diagnosis of specific subtypes. Although milder forms of glomerular injury may subside, the renal involvement is usually progressive over a matter of weeks and culminates in severe oliguria. Recovery of renal function may follow early intensive plasmapheresis (plasma exchange) combined with steroids and cytotoxic agents in Goodpasture syndrome. This therapy can reverse both pulmonary hemorrhage and renal failure. Other forms of RPGN also respond well to steroids and cytotoxic agents. However, despite therapy, many patients eventually require chronic dialysis or transplantation, particularly if the disease is discovered at a late stage.

KEY CONCEPTS

The Nephritic Syndrome

- The nephritic syndrome is characterized by hematuria, oliguria with azotemia, proteinuria, and hypertension.

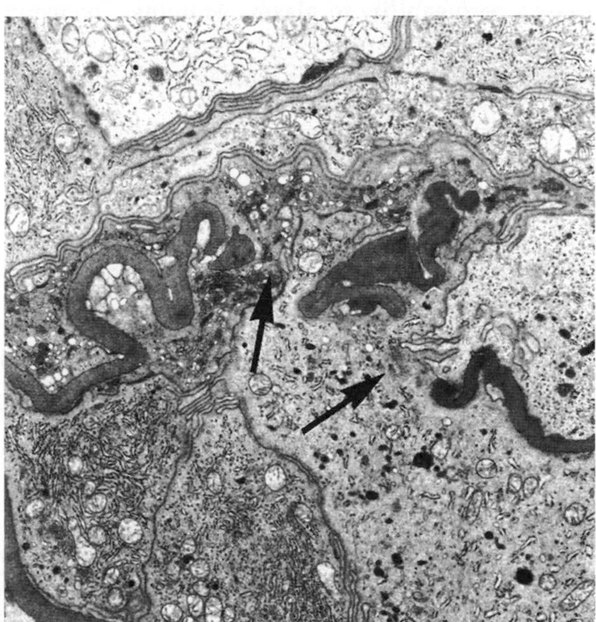

Figure 20-11 Crescentic glomerulonephritis. Electron micrograph showing characteristic wrinkling of glomerular basement membrane with focal disruptions *(arrows)*.

- The most common causes are immunologically mediated glomerular injury; lesions are characterized by proliferative changes and leukocyte infiltration.
- **Acute postinfectious glomerulonephritis** typically occurs after streptococcal infection in children and young adults but may occur following infection with many other organisms; it is caused by deposition of immune complexes, mainly in the subepithelial spaces, with abundant neutrophils and proliferation of glomerular cells. Most affected children recover; the prognosis is worse in adults.
- **Rapidly progressive glomerulonephritis** (RPGN) is a clinical entity with features of the nephritic syndrome and rapid loss of renal function.
- RPGN is commonly associated with severe glomerular injury with necrosis and GBM breaks and subsequent proliferation of parietal epithelial cells (forming crescents).
- RPGN may be antibody mediated, caused by autoantibodies to the GBM or as a result of immune complex deposition. It can also occur in the absence of significant antibody deposition, although most affected patients with this type of RPGN have circulating antineutrophil cytoplasmic antibodies (ANCAs).

Nephrotic Syndrome

Certain glomerular diseases virtually always produce the nephrotic syndrome. In addition, many other forms of primary and secondary glomerulopathies discussed in this chapter may underlie the syndrome. Before the major diseases associated with nephrotic syndrome are presented, the causes and pathophysiology of this clinical complex are briefly discussed.

Pathophysiology. **Nephrotic syndrome is caused by a derangement in glomerular capillary walls resulting in increased permeability to plasma proteins.** The manifestations of the syndrome include:

- *Massive proteinuria*, with the daily loss of 3.5 gm or more of protein (less in children)
- *Hypoalbuminemia*, with plasma albumin levels less than 3 gm/dL
- *Generalized edema*
- *Hyperlipidemia and lipiduria*

The various components of nephrotic syndrome bear a logical relationship to one another. The glomerular capillary wall, with its endothelium, GBM, and visceral epithelial cells, acts as a size and charge barrier through which the plasma filtrate passes. Increased permeability resulting from either structural or physicochemical alterations in this barrier allows proteins to escape from the plasma into the urinary space, resulting in proteinuria.

Heavy proteinuria depletes serum albumin levels at a rate beyond the compensatory synthetic capacity of the liver, resulting in hypoalbuminemia. Increased renal catabolism of filtered albumin also contributes to the hypoalbuminemia. The generalized edema is a direct consequence of *decreased intravascular colloid osmotic pressure.* There is also *sodium and water retention*, which aggravates the edema (Chapter 4). This seems to be due to several factors, including compensatory secretion of aldosterone, mediated by the hypovolemia-enhanced renin secretion; stimulation of the sympathetic system; and a reduction in the secretion of natriuretic factors such as atrial peptides. Edema is characteristically soft and pitting, and is most marked in the periorbital regions and dependent portions of the body. If severe, it may also lead to pleural effusions and ascites.

The largest proportion of protein lost in the urine is albumin, but globulins are also excreted in some diseases. The ratio of low- to high-molecular-weight proteins in the urine in various cases of nephrotic syndrome is a manifestation of the *selectivity* of proteinuria. A *highly selective proteinuria* consists mostly of low-molecular-weight proteins (albumin, 70 kD; transferrin, 76 kD molecular weight), whereas a *poorly selective proteinuria* consists of higher molecular-weight globulins in addition to albumin.

The genesis of the hyperlipidemia is complex. Most patients with nephrotic syndrome have increased blood levels of cholesterol, triglyceride, very-low-density lipoprotein, low-density lipoprotein, Lp(a) lipoprotein, and apoprotein, and there is a decrease in high-density lipoprotein concentration in some patients. These defects seem to be due to a combination of increased synthesis of lipoproteins in the liver, abnormal transport of circulating lipid particles, and decreased lipid catabolism. Lipiduria follows the hyperlipidemia, because lipoproteins also leak across the glomerular capillary wall. The lipid appears in the urine either as free fat or as *oval fat bodies*, representing lipoprotein resorbed by tubular epithelial cells and then shed along with injured tubular cells that have detached from the basement membrane.

Nephrotic patients are particularly vulnerable to *infection*, especially staphylococcal and pneumococcal infections, probably due to loss of immunoglobulins in the urine. *Thrombotic and thromboembolic complications* are also common in nephrotic syndrome, due in part to loss of endogenous anticoagulants (e.g., antithrombin III) in the urine. *Renal vein thrombosis*, once thought to be a cause of nephrotic syndrome, is most often a *consequence* of this hypercoagulable state, particularly in patients with membranous nephropathy (see later).

Causes. The incidences of the several causes of the nephrotic syndrome vary according to age and geography. In children younger than 17 years in North America, for example, nephrotic syndrome is almost always caused by a lesion primary to the kidney; among adults, in contrast, it is often associated with a systemic disease. Table 20-7 represents a composite derived from several studies of the causes of the nephrotic syndrome and is therefore only approximate. The most frequent *systemic causes* of the nephrotic syndrome are diabetes, amyloidosis, and SLE. The most important of the *primary glomerular lesions* are *minimal-change disease, membranous glomerulopathy*, and *focal segmental glomerulosclerosis*. The first is most common in children in North America, the second is most common in older adults, and focal segmental glomerulosclerosis occurs at all ages. These three lesions are discussed individually in the following sections. Other less common causes of nephrotic syndrome include the various proliferative glomerulonephritides such as MPGN and IgA nephropathy.

Table 20-7 Cause of Nephrotic Syndrome

Causes	Approximate Prevalence (%)*	
	Children	Adults
Primary Glomerular Disease		
Membranous nephropathy	3	30
Minimal-change disease	75	8
Focal segmental glomerulosclerosis	10	35
Membranoproliferative glomerulonephritis and dense deposit disease†	10	10
Other proliferative glomerulonephritides (focal, "pure mesangial," IgA nephropathy)†	2	17
Systemic Diseases		
Diabetes mellitus		
Amyloidosis		
Systemic lupus erythematosus		
Drugs (nonsteroidal anti-inflammatory, penicillamine, heroin)		
Infections (malaria, syphilis, hepatitis B and C, HIV)		
Malignant disease (carcinoma, lymphoma)		
Miscellaneous (bee-sting allergy, hereditary nephritis)		

*Approximate prevalence of primary disease = 95% of nephrotic syndrome in children, 60% in adults. Approximate prevalence of systemic disease = 5% in children, 40% in adults.
†Membranoproliferative and other proliferative glomerulonephritides may result in mixed nephrotic/nephritic syndromes.

Membranous Nephropathy

Membranous nephropathy is characterized by diffuse thickening of the glomerular capillary wall due to the accumulation of deposits containing Ig along the subepithelial side of the basement membrane. Approximately 75% of cases of membranous nephropathy are primary. The remaining cases occur in association with other systemic diseases and have identifiable etiologic agents, and hence are referred to as secondary membranous nephropathy. The most notable of these associations are as follows:

- *Drugs* (penicillamine, captopril, gold, nonsteroidal anti-inflammatory drugs (NSAIDs). From 1% to 7% of patients with rheumatoid arthritis treated with penicillamine or gold (drugs now used infrequently for this purpose) develop membranous nephropathy.
- *Underlying malignant tumors*, particularly carcinomas of the lung and colon, and melanoma. According to some studies, these are present in as many as 5% to 10% of adults with membranous nephropathy.
- *SLE.* About 10% to 15% of glomerulonephritis in SLE is of the membranous type.
- *Infections* (chronic hepatitis B, hepatitis C, syphilis, schistosomiasis, malaria)
- *Other autoimmune disorders* such as thyroiditis can be associated with secondary membranous nephropathy.

Pathogenesis. Membranous nephropathy is a form of chronic immune complex-mediated disease. In secondary membranous nephropathy, the inciting antigens can sometimes be identified in the immune complexes. The antigens may be endogenous or exogenous. The endogenous antigens may be renal or non renal. For example, membranous nephropathy in SLE is associated with deposition of complexes of self nuclear proteins and autoantibodies. Another example of an endogenous antigen is neutral endopeptidase, a membrane protein recognized by placentally transferred maternal antibodies in cases of neonatal membranous nephropathy. Exogenous antigens include those derived from hepatitis B virus and *Treponema pallidum* in patients infected with these microbes.

Primary (also called idiopathic) membranous nephropathy, long thought to be of unknown cause, is now considered to be an *autoimmune disease linked to certain HLA alleles such as HLA-DQA1 and caused in most cases by antibodies to a renal autoantigen.* In many adult cases the autoantigen is the phospholipase A_2 receptor. The lesions bear a striking resemblance to those of experimental Heymann nephritis, which, as you might recall, is induced by antibodies to the megalin antigenic complex present in the rat podocyte, which is the antigenic counterpart of the human phospholipase A_2 receptor.

How does the glomerular capillary wall become leaky in membranous nephropathy? There is a paucity of neutrophils, monocytes, or platelets in glomeruli. The virtually uniform presence of complement and corroborating experimental work suggest that the complement C5b-C9 membrane attack complex has an important role. It is postulated that C5b-C9 activates glomerular epithelial and mesangial cells, inducing them to liberate proteases and oxidants, which cause capillary wall injury and increased protein leakage. A subclass of IgG, IgG4, which differs from other IgG subclasses in being a poor activator of the classical complement pathway, is the principal immunoglobulin deposited in cases of primary membranous nephropathy. How IgG4 may activate the complement system is not clear. Perhaps other modes of complement activation may be harnessed.

MORPHOLOGY

By light microscopy the glomeruli either appear normal in the early stages of the disease or exhibit **uniform, diffuse thickening of the glomerular capillary wall** (Fig. 20-12*A*). By electron microscopy the thickening is seen to be caused by irregular electron dense also deposits containing immune complexes between the basement membrane and the overlying epithelial cells, with effacement of podocyte foot processes (Fig. 20-12*B* and *D*). Basement membrane material is laid down between these deposits, appearing as irregular spikes protruding from the GBM. These spikes are best seen by silver stains, which color the basement membrane, but not the deposits, black. In time, these spikes thicken to produce domelike protrusions and eventually close over the immune deposits, burying them within a markedly thickened, irregular membrane. Immunofluorescence microscopy demonstrates that the granular deposits contain both immunoglobulins and complement (Fig. 20-12*C*). As the disease advances segmental sclerosis may occur; in the course of time glomeruli may become totally sclerosed. The epithelial cells of the proximal tubules contain protein reabsorption droplets, and there may be considerable interstitial mononuclear cell inflammation.

Clinical Features. This disorder usually presents with the insidious onset of the nephrotic syndrome or, in 15% of patients, with nonnephrotic proteinuria. Hematuria and mild hypertension are present in 15% to 35% of cases. It is necessary in any patient to first rule out the secondary causes described earlier, since treatment of the underlying

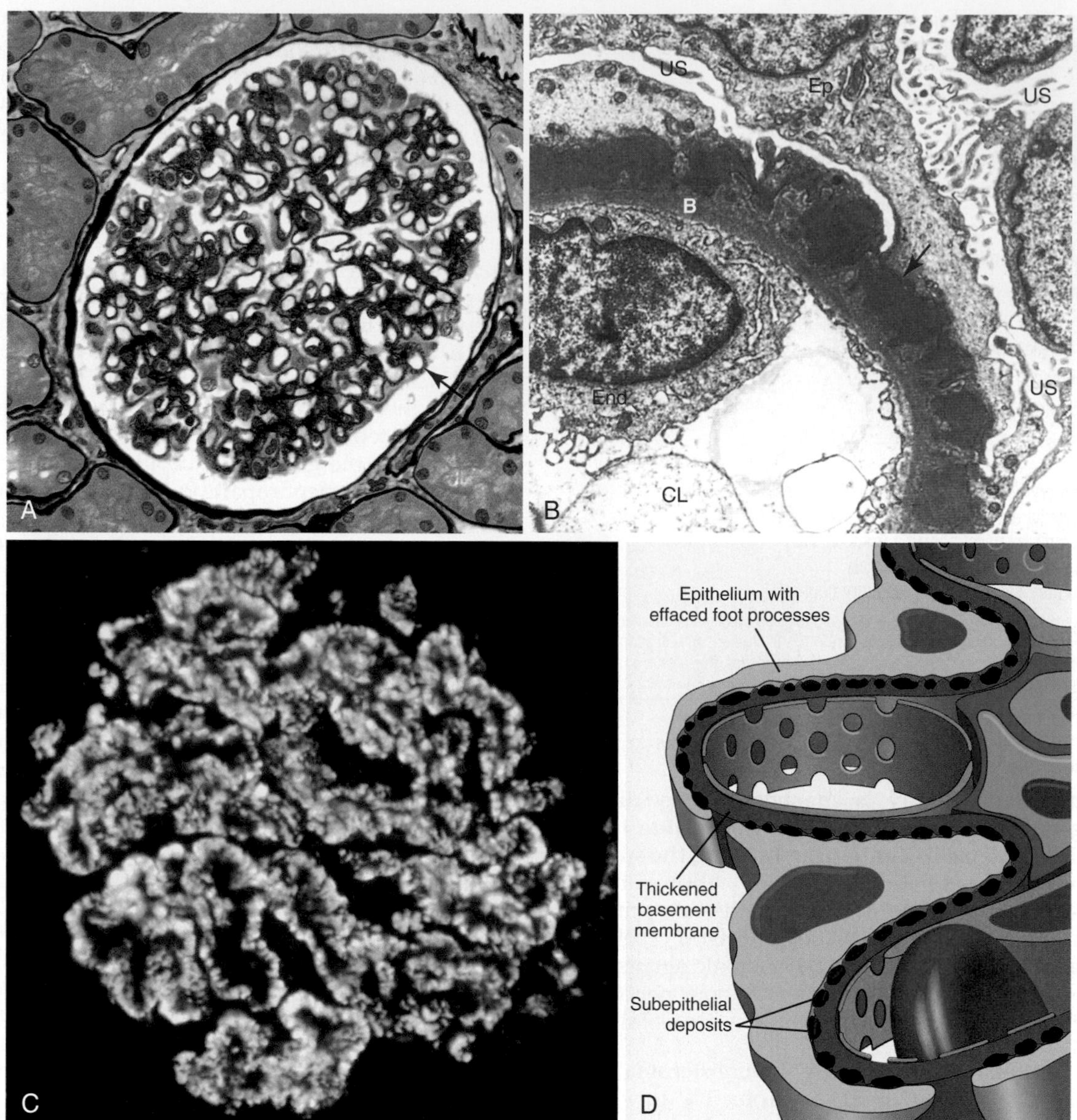

Figure 20-12 Membranous nephropathy. **A,** Silver methenamine stain. Note the marked diffuse thickening of the capillary walls without an increase in the number of cells. There are prominent "spikes" of silver-staining matrix *(arrow)* projecting from the basement membrane lamina densa toward the urinary space, which separate and surround deposited immune complexes that lack affinity for the silver stain. **B,** Electron micrograph showing electron-dense deposits *(arrow)* along the epithelial side of the basement membrane (B). Note the effacement of foot processes overlying deposits. CL, Capillary lumen; End, endothelium; Ep, epithelium; US, urinary space. **C,** Characteristic granular immunofluorescent deposits of IgG along glomerular basement membrane. **D,** Diagrammatic representation of membranous nephropathy. (**A,** Courtesy Dr. Charles Lassman, UCLA School of Medicine, Los Angeles, Calif.)

condition (malignant neoplasm, infection, or SLE) or discontinuance of the offending drug can reverse or ameliorate the injury.

The course of the disease is variable but generally indolent. In contrast to minimal-change disease, described later, the proteinuria is nonselective and usually does not respond well to corticosteroid therapy. Complete or partial remissions may occur in up to 40% of patients, even in some patients without therapy. Progression is associated with increasing sclerosis of glomeruli, rising serum creatinine reflecting renal insufficiency, and development of hypertension. Although proteinuria persists in more than 60% of patients, only about 10% die or progress to renal failure within 10 years, and no more than 40% eventually develop severe chronic kidney disease or end-stage renal disease. The disease recurs in up to 40% of patients who undergo transplantation for end-stage renal disease. Spontaneous remissions and a relatively benign outcome occur more commonly in women and in those with proteinuria in the nonnephrotic range.

Because of the variable course of the disease, it has been difficult to evaluate the overall effectiveness of corticosteroids or other immunosuppressive therapy in controlling the proteinuria or progression. It is thought that circulating antibodies to PLA_2 receptor may be a useful biomarker of disease activity and thereby aid in the diagnosis and management of primary membranous nephropathy in the future.

Minimal-Change Disease

This relatively benign disorder is characterized by diffuse effacement of foot processes of visceral epithelial cells (podocytes), detectable only by electron microscopy, in glomeruli that appear virtually normal by light microscopy. It is the most frequent cause of nephrotic syndrome in children, but it is less common in adults (Table 20-7). The peak incidence is between 2 and 6 years of age. The disease sometimes follows a respiratory infection or routine prophylactic immunization.

Etiology and Pathogenesis. Although the absence of immune deposits in the glomerulus excludes classic immune complex mechanisms, several features of the disease point to an immunologic basis, including (1) the clinical association with respiratory infections and prophylactic immunization; (2) the response to corticosteroids and/or other immunosuppressive therapy; (3) the association with other atopic disorders (e.g., eczema, rhinitis); (4) the increased prevalence of certain HLA haplotypes in patients with minimal-change disease associated with atopy (suggesting a genetic predisposition); and (5) the increased incidence of minimal-change disease in patients with Hodgkin lymphoma, in whom defects in T cell-mediated immunity are well recognized.

The current leading hypothesis is that minimal-change disease involves some immune dysfunction that results in the elaboration of factors that damage visceral epithelial cells and cause proteinuria. Candidate pathogenic factors such as angiopoietin-like-4 have been identified in animal models but none have been proven to cause the human disease. The ultrastructural changes point to a primary *visceral epithelial cell injury* (podocytopathy), and studies in animal models suggest the loss of glomerular polyanions. Thus, defects in the charge barrier may contribute to the proteinuria. The actual route by which protein traverses the epithelial cell portion of the capillary wall remains an enigma. Possibilities include transcellular passage through the epithelial cells, passage through residual spaces between remaining but damaged foot processes or through abnormal spaces developing underneath the portion of the foot process that directly abuts the basement membrane, or leakage through foci in which the epithelial cells have become detached from the basement.

MORPHOLOGY

The glomeruli are normal by light microscopy (Fig. 20-13). By electron microscopy the GBM appears normal, and no electron-dense material is deposited. **The principal lesion is in the visceral epithelial cells, which show a uniform and diffuse effacement of foot processes,** these being reduced to a rim of cytoplasm with loss of recognizable intervening slit diaphragms (Fig. 20-13). This change, often incorrectly termed "fusion" of foot processes, actually represents simplification of the epithelial cell architecture with flattening, retraction, and swelling of foot processes. Foot process effacement is also present in other proteinuric states (e.g., membranous glomerulopathy, diabetic nephropathy); it is only when effacement is associated with normal glomeruli by light microscopy that the diagnosis of minimal-change disease can be made. The visceral epithelial changes are completely reversible after corticosteroid therapy, concomitant with remission of the proteinuria. The cells of the proximal tubules are often laden with lipid and protein, reflecting tubular reabsorption of lipoproteins passing through diseased glomeruli (thus, the historical name **lipoid nephrosis** for this disease). Immunofluorescence studies show no Ig or complement deposits.

Clinical Features. Despite massive proteinuria, renal function remains good, and there is commonly no hypertension or hematuria. The proteinuria usually is highly selective, most of the protein being albumin. **A characteristic feature is its usually dramatic response to corticosteroid therapy.** Most children (>90%) with minimal-change disease respond rapidly to this treatment. However, proteinuria may recur, and some patients may become

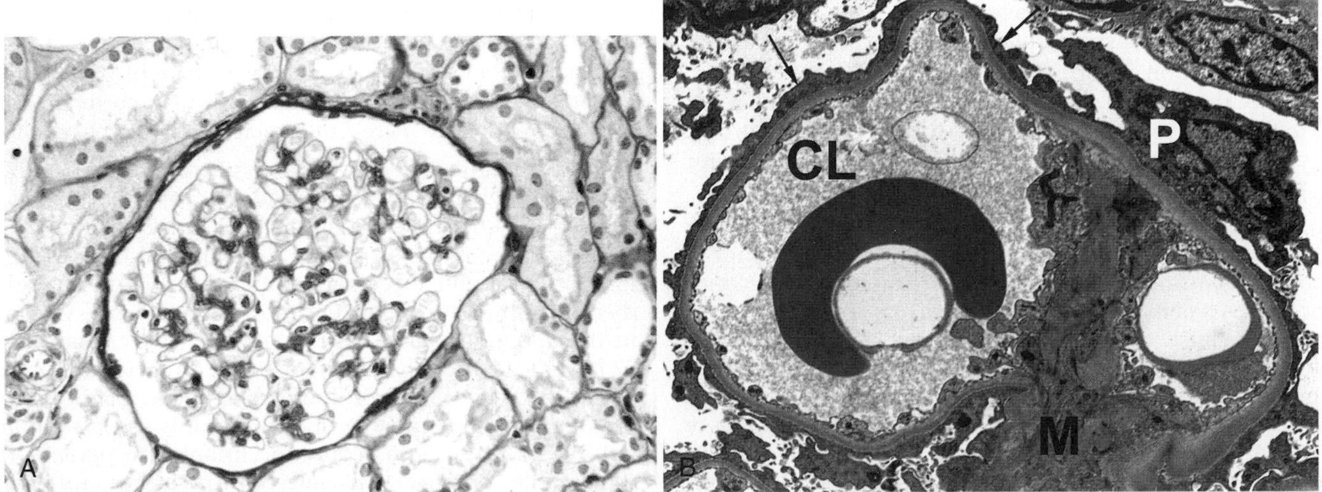

Figure 20-13 Minimal-change disease. **A,** Glomerulus stained with PAS. Note normal basement membranes and absence of proliferation. **B,** Ultrastructural characteristics of minimal-change disease include effacement of foot processes *(arrows)* and absence of deposits. *CL,* Capillary lumen; *M,* mesangium; *P,* podocyte cell body.

steroid-dependent or resistant. Nevertheless, the long-term prognosis for patients is excellent, and even steroid-dependent disease usually resolves when children reach puberty. Although adults are slower to respond, their long-term prognosis is also excellent.

As has been noted, minimal-change disease in adults can be associated with Hodgkin lymphoma and, less frequently, other lymphomas and leukemias. In addition, secondary minimal-change disease may follow NSAID therapy, usually in association with acute interstitial nephritis, to be described later in this chapter.

Focal Segmental Glomerulosclerosis (FSGS)

Primary focal segmental glomerulosclerosis is the most common cause of nephrotic syndrome in adults in the United States. It is sometimes considered to be a primary disorder of podocytes, like minimal change disease. As the name implies, this lesion is characterized by sclerosis of some, but not all, glomeruli (thus, it is focal); and in the affected glomeruli, only a portion of the capillary tuft is involved (thus, it is segmental). Focal segmental glomerulosclerosis is frequently manifest clinically by the acute or subacute onset of nephrotic syndrome or nonnephrotic proteinuria. Hypertension, microscopic hematuria, and some degree of azotemia are commonly present when the disease is first clinically recognized.

Classification and Types. Focal segmental glomerulosclerosis occurs in the following settings:

- As a primary disease (idiopathic focal segmental glomerulosclerosis)
- In association with other known conditions, such as HIV infection (HIV-associated nephropathy), heroin addiction (heroin nephropathy), sickle-cell disease, and massive obesity
- As a secondary event, reflecting scarring of previously active necrotizing lesions, in cases of focal glomerulonephritis (e.g., IgA nephropathy)
- As a component of the adaptive response to loss of renal tissue (renal ablation, described earlier), whether from congenital anomalies (e.g., unilateral renal agenesis or renal dysplasia) or acquired causes (e.g., reflux nephropathy), or in advanced stages of other renal disorders, such as hypertensive nephropathy.
- In uncommon inherited forms of nephrotic syndrome where the disease may be caused by mutations in genes that encode proteins localized to the slit diaphragm, e.g., podocin, α-actinin 4, and TRPC6 (transient receptor potential calcium channel-6)

Idiopathic focal segmental glomerulosclerosis accounts for 10% and 35% of cases of nephrotic syndrome in children and adults, respectively. FSGS (both primary and secondary forms) has increased in incidence and is now the most common cause of nephrotic syndrome in adults in the United States, particularly in Hispanic and African-American patients. The clinical signs differ from those of minimal-change disease in the following respects: (1) there is a higher incidence of hematuria, reduced GFR, and hypertension; (2) proteinuria is more often nonselective; (3) there is poor response to corticosteroid therapy; and (4) there is progression to chronic kidney disease, with at least 50% developing ESRD within 10 years.

Pathogenesis. The characteristic degeneration and focal disruption of visceral epithelial cells with effacement of foot processes resemble the diffuse epithelial cell change typical of minimal-change disease and other podocytopathies. *It is this epithelial damage that is the hallmark of FSGS.* Multiple different mechanisms can cause such epithelial damage, including circulating factors and genetically determined defects affecting components of the slit diaphragm complex. The hyalinosis and sclerosis stem from entrapment of plasma proteins in extremely hyperpermeable foci and increased ECM deposition. The recurrence of proteinuria after transplantation, sometimes within 24 hours, with subsequent progression to overt lesions of FSGS, suggests that an unknown circulating factor is the cause of the epithelial damage in some patients.

The discovery of a genetic basis for some cases of FSGS and other causes of the nephrotic syndrome has improved the understanding of the pathogenesis of proteinuria in the nephrotic syndrome and has provided new methods for diagnosis and prognosis of affected patients. Leading examples of this include:

- The first relevant gene to be identified, *NPHS1*, maps to chromosome 19q13 and encodes the protein *nephrin*. Nephrin is a key component of the slit diaphragm (Fig. 20-3), the structure that controls glomerular permeability. Several mutations of the *NPHS* gene have been identified that give rise to *congenital nephrotic syndrome* of the Finnish type, producing a minimal-change disease like glomerulopathy with extensive foot process effacement.
- A distinctive pattern of autosomal recessive FSGS results from mutations in the *NPHS2* gene, which maps to chromosome 1q25-q31 and encodes the protein product *podocin*. Podocin has also been localized to the slit diaphragm. Mutations in *NPHS2* result in a syndrome of steroid-resistant nephrotic syndrome of childhood onset.
- A third set of mutations in the gene encoding the podocyte actin-binding protein α-actinin 4 underlies some cases of autosomal dominant FSGS, which can be insidious in onset but has a high rate of progression to renal insufficiency.
- A fourth type of mutation was found in some kindreds with adult-onset FSGS, in the gene encoding TRPC6. This protein is widely expressed, including in podocytes, and the pathogenic mutations may perturb podocyte function by increasing calcium flux in these cells.

What these proteins have in common is their localization to the slit diaphragm and to adjacent podocyte cytoskeletal structures. Their specific functions and interactions are incompletely understood, but it is clear that the integrity of each is necessary to maintain the normal glomerular filtration barrier. Recently two sequence variants in the apolipoprotein L1 gene (APOL1) on chromosome 22 have been strongly associated with an increased risk of FSGS and renal failure in individuals of African descent, although the mechanisms underlying this association are not yet known. These sequence variants are particularly remarkable because the selective pressures for their conservation in people of African descent is a result of resistance to trypanosome infection conferred by these polymorphisms.

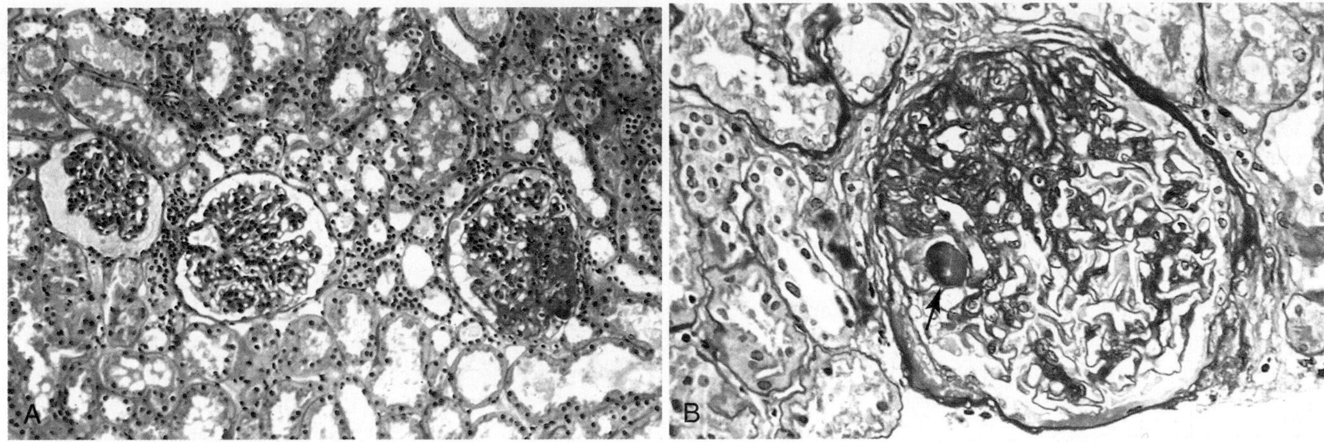

Figure 20-14 Focal segmental glomerulosclerosis, PAS stain. **A,** Low-power view showing segmental sclerosis in one of three glomeruli (at 3 o'clock). **B,** High-power view showing hyaline insudation *(arrow)* and lipid (small vacuoles) in sclerotic area.

Renal ablation FSGS, a secondary form of FSGS, occurs as a complication of glomerular and nonglomerular diseases causing reduction in functioning renal tissue. Particularly striking examples where this occurs are reflux nephropathy and unilateral agenesis. These may lead to progressive glomerulosclerosis and renal failure. The pathogenesis of FSGS in this setting is described earlier in this chapter.

MORPHOLOGY

By light microscopy the **focal and segmental lesions may involve only a minority of the glomeruli** and may be missed if the biopsy specimen contains an insufficient number of glomeruli (Fig. 20-14*A*). In the sclerotic segments there is collapse of capillary loops, increase in matrix and segmental deposition of plasma proteins along the capillary wall (hyalinosis), which may become so pronounced as to occlude capillary lumens. Lipid droplets and foam cells are often present (Fig. 20-14*B*). Glomeruli that do not show segmental lesions usually appear normal on light microscopy but may show increased mesangial matrix. On electron microscopy both sclerotic and nonsclerotic areas show **diffuse effacement of foot processes**, and there may also be focal detachment of the epithelial cells and denudation of the underlying GBM. By immunofluorescence microscopy IgM and C3 may be present in the sclerotic areas and/or in the mesangium. In addition to the focal sclerosis, there may be pronounced hyalinosis and thickening of afferent arterioles. With the progression of the disease, increased numbers of glomeruli become involved and sclerosis spreads within each glomerulus. In time, this leads to total (i.e., global) sclerosis of glomeruli, with pronounced tubular atrophy and interstitial fibrosis.

A morphologic variant of FSGS, called **collapsing glomerulopathy,** is characterized by retraction and/or collapse of the entire glomerular tuft, with or without additional FSGS lesions of the type described above (Fig. 20-15). A characteristic feature is proliferation and hypertrophy of glomerular visceral epithelial cells. This lesion may be idiopathic, but it also has been associated with some drug toxicities (e.g., pamidronate), and it is the most characteristic lesion of HIV-associated nephropathy. Collapsing glomerulopathy is typically associated with prominent tubular injury with formation of microcysts. It has a particularly poor prognosis.

Clinical Course. There is little tendency for spontaneous remission in idiopathic FSGS, and responses to corticosteroid therapy are variable. In general, children have a better prognosis than adults do. Progression to renal failure occurs at variable rates. About 20% of patients follow an unusually rapid course, with intractable massive proteinuria ending in renal failure within 2 years. Factors associated with rapid progression include the degree of proteinuria, the degree of renal insufficiency at diagnosis, and histologic subtype (the collapsing variant has an unfavorable course; the tip variant has a relatively good prognosis). Recurrences are seen in 25% to 50% of patients receiving allografts.

HIV-Associated Nephropathy

HIV infection can directly or indirectly cause several renal complications, including acute renal failure or acute

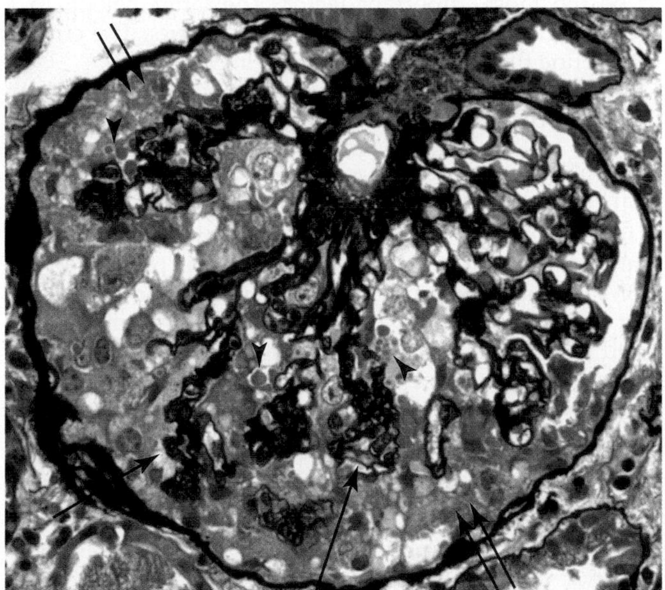

Figure 20-15 Collapsing glomerulopathy. Visible are retraction of the glomerular tuft *(arrows),* narrowing of capillary lumens, proliferation and swelling of visceral epithelial cells *(double arrows),* and prominent accumulation of intracellular protein absorption droplets in the visceral epithelial cells *(arrowheads).* Silver methenamine stain. (Courtesy Dr. Jolanta Kowalewska, Cedars-Sinai Medical Center, Los Angeles, Calif.)

interstitial nephritis induced by drugs or the infection, thrombotic microangiopathies, postinfectious glomerulonephritis, and, most commonly, a severe form of the collapsing variant of FSGS, termed *HIV-associated nephropathy*. The latter has been reported in 5% to 10% of HIV-infected individuals in some older series, more frequently in blacks than in whites. With the advent of highly active antiretroviral therapy for HIV infection, the incidence of this lesion has been much reduced. The morphologic features of HIV-associated nephropathy are:

- A high frequency of the collapsing variant of FSGS (Fig. 20-15)
- A striking focal cystic dilation of tubule segments, which are filled with proteinaceous material, and inflammation and fibrosis
- The presence of large numbers of tubuloreticular inclusions within endothelial cells, detected by electron microscopy. Such inclusions, also present in SLE, have been shown to be modifications of endoplasmic reticulum induced by circulating interferon-α. They are not usually present in idiopathic FSGS and therefore may have diagnostic value in a biopsy specimen.

The pathogenesis of HIV-associated FSGS is unclear. There is some data to suggest that HIV can infect tubular epithelial cells and podocytes, but much remains to be known.

Membranoproliferative Glomerulonephritis (MPGN)

MPGN is best considered a pattern of immune-mediated injury rather than a specific disease. An emerging consensus on classification separates one group of disorders MPGN into two groups, one (type I) characterized by deposition of immune complexes containing IgG and complement, and a second (type II, often called *dense deposit disease*) in which activation of complement appears to be the most important factor. The latter belong to a group of disorders called *C3 glomerulopathies*. The criteria that define this group are still evolving.

MPGN is characterized histologically by alterations in the glomerular basement membrane, proliferation of glomerular cells, leukocyte infiltration, and the presence of deposits in mesangial regions and glomerular capillary walls. As will be described later, these deposits are made up of immune complexes in Type 1 MPGN and some unknown material in type II MPGN. In type II, C3 is present on the GBM but not in the dense deposits. This difference is important and suggests that while morphologically similar, type I and II MPGN are pathogenically distinct. In both types, because the proliferation is predominantly in the mesangium but also may involve the capillary loops, a frequently used synonym is *mesangiocapillary glomerulonephritis*.

MPGN accounts for up to 10% of cases of nephrotic syndrome in children and young adults. Some patients present only with hematuria or proteinuria in the nonnephrotic range, but many others have a combined nephrotic-nephritic picture. MPGN is increasingly recognized to be associated with other systemic disorders and known etiologic agents (secondary MPGN), but there is still a residue of cases of unknown etiology (primary MPGN).

Pathogenesis. **In most cases of type I MPGN there is evidence of immune complexes in the glomerulus and activation of both classical and alternative complement pathways.** The antigens involved in idiopathic MPGN are unknown. In many cases they are believed to be proteins derived from infectious agents such as hepatitis C and B viruses, which presumably behave either as "planted" antigens after first binding to or becoming trapped within glomerular structures or are contained in preformed immune complexes deposited from the circulation.

MORPHOLOGY

The **glomeruli are large and hypercellular**. The hypercellularity is produced both by proliferation of cells in the mesangium and so-called endocapillary proliferation involving capillary endothelium and infiltrating leukocytes. The glomeruli have an accentuated "lobular" appearance due to the **proliferating mesangial cells and increased mesangial matrix** (Fig. 20-16). The GBM is thickened, and often shows a **"double-contour" or "tram-track" appearance**, especially evident in silver or PAS stains. This is caused by **"duplication" of the basement membrane** (also commonly referred to as splitting), usually as the result of new basement membrane synthesis in response to subendothelial deposits of immune complexes. Between the duplicated basement membranes there is inclusion or interposition of cellular elements, which can be of mesangial, endothelial, or leukocytic origin. Such interposition also gives rise to the appearance of "split" basement membranes (Fig. 20-17*A*). Crescents are present in many cases.

Type I MPGN is characterized by the presence of discrete **subendothelial electron-dense deposits.** Mesangial and occasional subepithelial deposits may also be present (Fig. 20-17*A*). By immunofluorescence, IgG and C3 are deposited in a granular pattern, and early complement components (C1q and C4) are often also present, indicative of an immune complex pathogenesis.

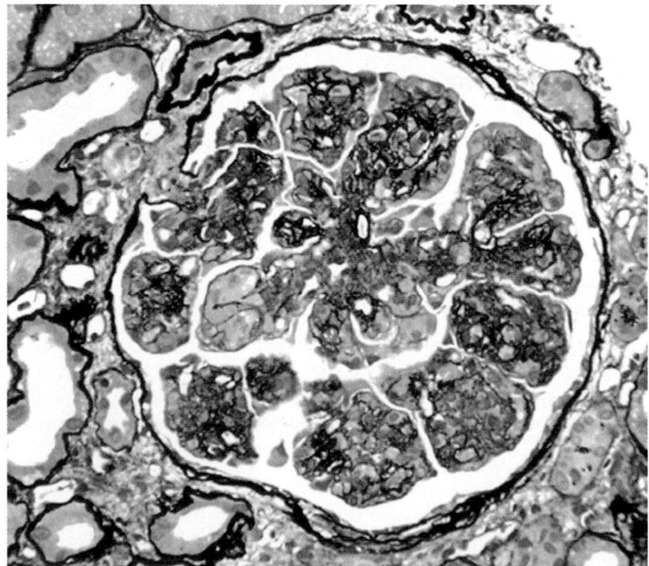

Figure 20-16 Membranoproliferative glomerulonephritis, showing mesangial cell proliferation, increased mesangial matrix (staining black with silver stain), basement membrane thickening with segmental splitting, accentuation of lobular architecture, swelling of cells lining peripheral capillaries, and influx of leukocytes (endocapillary proliferation).

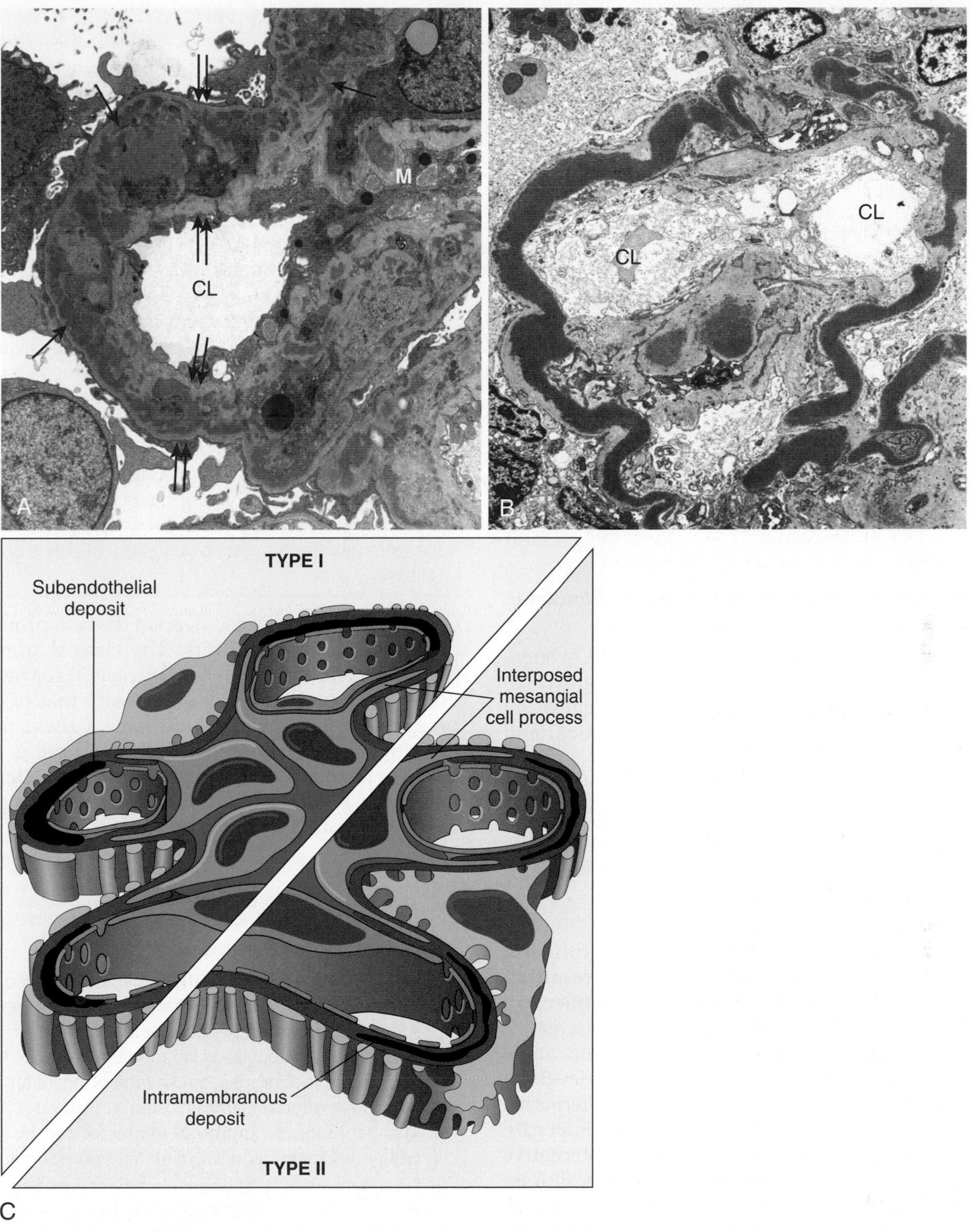

Figure 20-17 A, Membranoproliferative glomerulonephritis, type I. Note discrete electron-dense deposits *(arrows)* incorporated into the glomerular capillary wall between duplicated (split) basement membranes *(double arrows)*, and in mesangial regions (M); CL, Capillary lumen. **B,** Dense-deposit disease (type II membranoproliferative glomerulonephritis). There are dense homogeneous deposits within the basement membrane. CL, Capillary lumen. In both, mesangial interposition gives the appearance of split basement membranes when viewed in the light microscope. **C,** Schematic representation of patterns in the two types of membranoproliferative glomerulonephritis. In type I there are subendothelial deposits; type II is characterized by intramembranous dense deposits (dense-deposit disease). In both, the basement membranes appear split when viewed in the light microscope. (**A,** Courtesy Dr. Jolanta Kowalewska, Cedars-Sinai Medical Center, Los Angeles, Calif.)

Clinical Features. Most patients with primary MPGN present in adolescence or as young adults with nephrotic syndrome and a nephritic component manifested by hematuria or, more insidiously, as mild proteinuria. Few remissions occur spontaneously in either type, and the disease follows a slowly progressive but unremitting course. Some patients develop numerous crescents and a clinical picture of RPGN. About 50% develop chronic renal failure within 10 years. Treatments with steroids, immunosuppressive agents, and antiplatelet drugs have not proven to be of any benefit.

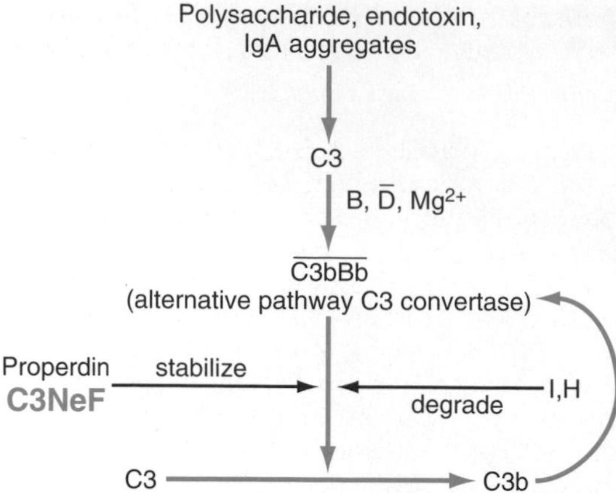

Figure 20-18 The alternative complement pathway in dense deposit disease (Type II MPGN). Note that C3NeF, an antibody present in the serum of individuals with membranoproliferative glomerulonephritis, acts at the same step as properdin, serving to stabilize the alternative pathway C3 convertase, thus enhancing C3 activation and consumption, causing hypocomplementemia.

Secondary MPGN

Secondary MPGN (invariably type I) is more common in adults and arises in the following settings:

- Chronic immune complex disorders, such as SLE; hepatitis B infection; hepatitis C infection, usually with cryoglobulinemia; endocarditis; infected ventriculoatrial shunts; chronic visceral abscesses; HIV infection; and schistosomiasis
- α_1-Antitrypsin deficiency
- Malignant diseases, particularly lymphoid tumors such as chronic lymphocytic leukemia, which are commonly complicated by development of autoantibodies

Dense Deposit Disease

Most patients with dense-deposit disease (formerly called type II MPGN) have abnormalities resulting in excessive activation of the alternative complement pathway. These patients have a consistently decreased serum C3 but normal C1 and C4, the early components of complement. They also have diminished serum levels of Factor B and properdin, components of the alternative complement pathway. In the glomeruli, C3 and properdin are deposited, but IgG is not. Recall that in the alternative complement pathway, C3 is directly cleaved to C3b (Fig. 20-18; see also Chapter 3, Fig. 3-12). The reaction depends on the initial activation of C3 by such substances as bacterial polysaccharides, endotoxin, and aggregates of IgA via a pathway involving Factors B and D. This leads to the generation of C3bBb, the alternative pathway C3 convertase. Normally, this C3 convertase is labile, but more than 70% of patients with dense-deposit disease have a circulating autoantibody termed *C3 nephritic factor (C3NeF)* that binds the alternative pathway C3 convertase and protects it from inactivation (Fig. 20-18). This favors persistent C3 activation and hypocomplementemia. There is also decreased C3 synthesis by the liver, further contributing to the profound hypocomplementemia. The precise nature of the dense deposits is unknown. Mutations in components of the alternate pathway such as Factor H have also been associated with dense deposit disease.

MORPHOLOGY

While some cases of dense deposit disease share histologic features with MPGN, there is a wider spectrum of histologic alterations in dense deposit disease. Many cases have a predominately mesangial proliferative pattern of injury, while others have an inflammatory and focally crescentic appearance. In some cases, dense deposits of a cellular material can be seen permeating the glomerular basement membranes in histologic sections. The defining feature is revealed by election microscopy, which demonstrates permeation of the lamina densa of the GBM by a ribbon-like, homogeneous, extremely electron-dense material of unknown composition (Fig. 20-17*B*). By immunofluorescence C3 is present in irregular granular or linear foci in the basement membranes on either side but not within the dense deposits. C3 is also present in the mesangium in characteristic circular aggregates (mesangial rings). IgG is usually absent, as are components of the classical pathway of complement activation (such as C1q and C4). C3 glomerlopathies other than dense deposit disease can have a similar distribution, with mesangial and capillary wall involvement, but lack the extremely electron dense deposits that define dense deposit disease.

Clinical Features. Dense deposit disease primarily affects children and young adults. The clinical presentation of nephritic syndrome with hematuria and/or nephrotic syndrome with proteinuria overlaps with that of MPGN. The prognosis is poor, with about half of these patients progressing to end-stage renal disease. There is a high incidence of recurrence in transplant recipients; dense deposits may recur in 90% of such patients, although renal failure in the allograft is much less common.

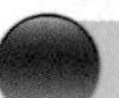

KEY CONCEPTS

The Nephrotic Syndrome

- **Membranous nephropathy** is caused by an autoimmune response, most often directed against the phospholipase A2 receptor on podocytes; it is characterized by granular subepithelial deposits of antibodies with GBM thickening and loss of foot processes but little or no inflammation; the disease is often resistant to steroid therapy.
- The nephrotic syndrome is characterized by proteinuria, which results in hypoalbuminemia and edema.
- Podocyte injury is an underlying mechanism of proteinuria, and may be the result of nonimmune causes (as in minimal-change disease and FSGS) or immune mechanisms (as in membranous nephropathy).
- **Minimal change disease** is the most frequent cause of nephrotic syndrome in children; it is manifested by proteinuria and effacement of glomerular foot processes without antibody deposits; the pathogenesis is unknown; the disease responds well to steroid therapy.
- **Focal and segmental glomerulosclerosis** (FSGS) may be primary (podocyte injury by unknown mechanisms) or secondary (e.g., as a consequence of prior glomerulonephritis, hypertension or infection such as HIV); glomeruli show focal and segmental obliteration of capillary lumens, and loss of foot processes; the disease is often resistant to therapy and may progress to end-stage renal disease.

- **Membranoproliferative glomerulonephritis** (MPGN) in most cases is the result of immune complex deposition in both mesangial regions and capillary walls. It may be associated with systemic infections.
- **Dense deposit disease (type II MPGN),** defined by a unique permeation of glomerular basement membranes by electron dense material, primarily affects children and young adults. It is associated with acquired or genetic dysregulation of the alternate pathway of complement.

Isolated Glomerular Abnormalities

IgA Nephropathy (Berger Disease)

IgA nephropathy, characterized by the presence of prominent IgA deposits in the mesangial regions and recurrent hematuria, is the most common type of glomerulonephritis worldwide. The disease can be suspected by light microscopic examination, but the diagnosis is made only by the detection of glomerular IgA deposition (Fig. 20-19). Mild proteinuria is usually present, and the nephrotic syndrome may occasionally develop. Rarely, patients may present with crescentic RPGN.

Whereas IgA nephropathy is typically an isolated renal disease, similar IgA deposits are present in a systemic disorder of children, *Henoch-Schönlein purpura,* to be discussed later, which has many overlapping features with IgA nephropathy. In addition, *secondary IgA nephropathy* occurs in patients with liver and intestinal diseases, as discussed later.

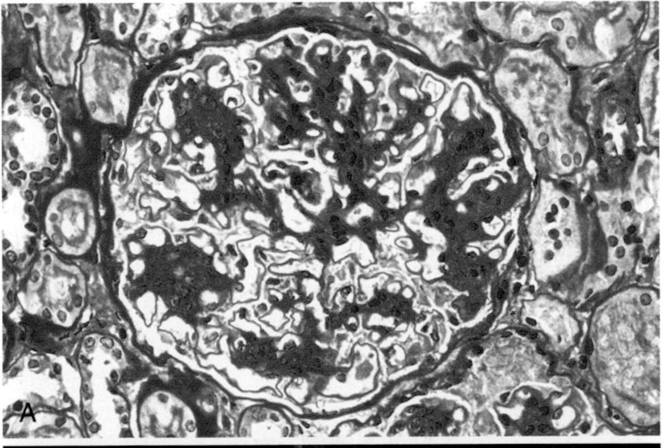

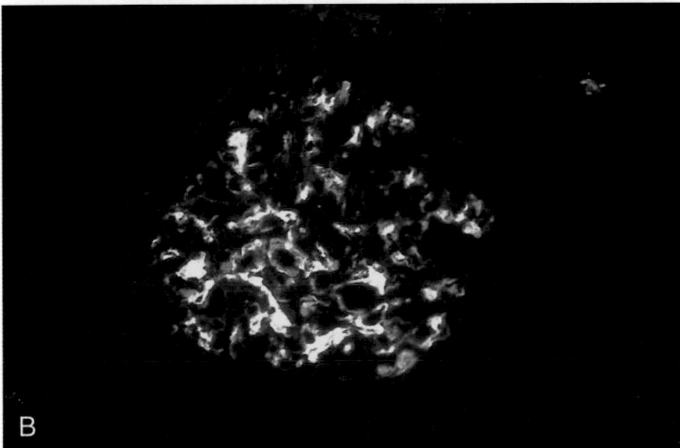

Figure 20-19 IgA nephropathy. **A,** Light microscopy showing mesangial proliferation and matrix increase. **B,** Characteristic deposition of IgA, principally in mesangial regions, detected by immunofluorescence.

Pathogenesis. Current evidence favors a "multi-hit" etiology for this disorder involving several steps. IgA, the main Ig in mucosal secretions, is present in plasma at low concentrations, mostly in monomeric form, the polymeric forms being catabolized in the liver. In patients with IgA nephropathy, levels of plasma polymeric IgA are increased, but increased production is not sufficient to cause this disease. A clue comes from the observation that in IgA nephropathy, the glomerular deposits consist predominantly of polymeric IgA molecules with aberrant glycosylation. It is believed that a key facet of IgA nephropathy is a hereditary or acquired defect in the normal formation or attachment of galactose-containing sugar chains called O-linked glycans to the hinge region of the IgA molecule (particularly to those of the IgA1 subclass) prior to their secretion by B cells. This aberrantly glycosylated IgA1 is either deposited by itself in glomeruli or it elicits an autoimmune response and forms immune complexes in the circulation with IgG autoantibodies directed against the abnormal IgA molecules. The immune complexes are deposited in the mesangium; alternatively, the abnormal IgA1 is deposited in the mesangium with subsequent formation of immune complexes in situ. The mesangial immune deposits then activate mesangial cells to proliferate, produce increased amounts of extracellular matrix, and secrete numerous cytokines and growth factors. These secreted mediators may not only participate in further mesangial cell activation but may also recruit inflammatory cells into the glomeruli. The recruited leukocytes contribute to glomerular injury and also to a reparative response, which can include opsonization and removal of the immune complexes. The deposited IgA and IgA-containing immune complexes activate the complement system via the alternate pathway, and hence the presence of C3 and the absence of C1q and C4 in glomeruli are typical of this disorder. A genetic influence is suggested by the occurrence of this condition in families and in HLA-identical siblings, the increased frequency of certain HLA and complement genotypes in some populations, and the findings of genome wide association studies linking specific MHC Class II loci to disease susceptibility.

Epidemiologic features of this disorder indicate that the increased synthesis of abnormal IgA may occur in response to respiratory or gastrointestinal exposure to environmental agents (e.g., viruses, bacteria, food proteins). The specific initiating antigens are unknown, and several infectious agents and food products have been implicated. IgA nephropathy occurs with increased frequency in individuals with *gluten enteropathy* (celiac disease), in whom intestinal mucosal defects are well defined, and in *liver disease,* in which there is defective hepatobiliary clearance of IgA complexes *(secondary IgA nephropathy).*

MORPHOLOGY

On histologic examination the lesions vary considerably. The glomeruli may be normal or may show mesangial widening and endocapillary proliferation (mesangioproliferative glomerulonephritis), segmental proliferation confined to some glomeruli (focal proliferative glomerulonephritis), or rarely, overt crescentic glomerulonephritis. The presence of leukocytes within glomerular capillaries is a variable feature. The mesangial widening may be the result of cell proliferation, accumulation of matrix, immune deposits, or some combination of these abnormalities. Healing of the focal proliferative lesion may lead to secondary focal segmental sclerosis. The characteristic immunofluorescent picture is of **mesangial deposition of IgA** (Fig. 20-19*B*), often with C3 and properdin and lesser amounts of IgG or IgM. Early complement components are usually absent. Electron microscopy confirms the presence of electron-dense deposits predominantly in the mesangium; capillary wall deposits, if present, are usually sparse.

Clinical Features. The disease affects people of any age, most commonly older children and young adults. Many patients present with gross hematuria after an infection of the respiratory or, less commonly, gastrointestinal or urinary tract; 30% to 40% have only microscopic hematuria, with or without proteinuria; and 5% to 10% develop acute nephritic syndrome, including some with rapidly progressive glomerulonephritis. The hematuria typically lasts for several days and then subsides, only to return every few months. The subsequent course is highly variable. Many patients maintain normal renal function for decades. Slow progression to chronic renal failure occurs in 15% to 40% of cases over a period of 20 years. Onset in old age, heavy proteinuria, hypertension, and the extent of glomerulosclerosis on biopsy are clues to an increased risk of progression. Recurrence of IgA deposits in transplanted kidneys is frequent, and in approximately 15% of those with recurrent IgA deposits, the disease runs the same slowly progressive course as that of primary IgA nephropathy.

Hereditary Nephritis

Hereditary nephritis refers to a group of heterogeneous familial renal diseases associated with mutations in collagen genes that manifest primarily with glomerular injury. Two deserve discussion: *Alport syndrome*, because the lesions and genetic defects have been well studied, and *thin basement membrane lesion*, the most common cause of *benign familial hematuria*.

Alport Syndrome

Alport syndrome, when fully developed, is manifest by hematuria with progression to chronic renal failure, accompanied by nerve deafness and various eye disorders, including lens dislocation, posterior cataracts, and corneal dystrophy. The disease is inherited as an X-linked trait in approximately 85% of cases. In the X-linked form, males express the full syndrome, while female heterozygotes typically present with hematuria. Approximately 90% of affected males progress to ESRD before 40 years of age. Autosomal recessive and autosomal dominant pedigrees also exist, in which males and females are equally susceptible to the full syndrome.

Pathogenesis. The disease manifestations are due to mutations in one of several genes coding for subunits of the collagen IV molecule. More than 500 mutations resulting in disease have been identified, resulting in defective assembly of type IV collagen, which is crucial for function of the GBM, the lens of the eye, and the cochlea. Because the GBM consists of networks of trimeric collagen IV molecules composed of α_3, α_4, and α_5 chains, mutations affecting any one chain result in defective assembly of the collagen network. Since type IV collagen chains are encoded on autosomes (chromosomes 2 and 13) and the X-chromosome, the inheritance pattern can be autosomal or X-linked. Mutations of missense, splice site, insertions, and deletion types have all been identified. Genetic analysis has shown that in patients with X-linked disease, large deletions in the collagen IV α5 chain (COL4A5) are associated with end stage renal disease at an earlier age.

MORPHOLOGY

Fully developed Alport syndrome has characteristic electron microscopic findings. The GBM shows irregular foci of thickening alternating with attenuation (thinning), and pronounced splitting and lamination of the lamina densa, often producing a distinctive basket-weave appearance (Fig. 20-20). Similar alterations can be found in the tubular basement membranes.

Immunohistochemistry can be helpful in cases with absent or borderline basement membrane lesions, because antibodies to α_3, α_4, and α_5 collagen fail to stain both glomerular and tubular basement membranes in the classic X-linked form. There is also absence of α_5 staining in skin biopsy specimens from these patients. As the disease progresses there is development of focal segmental and global glomerulosclerosis and other changes of progressive renal injury, including vascular sclerosis, tubular atrophy, and interstitial fibrosis.

Clinical Features. The most common presenting sign is gross or microscopic hematuria, frequently accompanied by red cell casts. Proteinuria may develop later, and rarely, the nephrotic syndrome develops. Symptoms appear at ages 5 to 20 years, and the onset of overt renal failure is between ages 20 and 50 years in men. The auditory defects may be subtle, requiring sensitive testing.

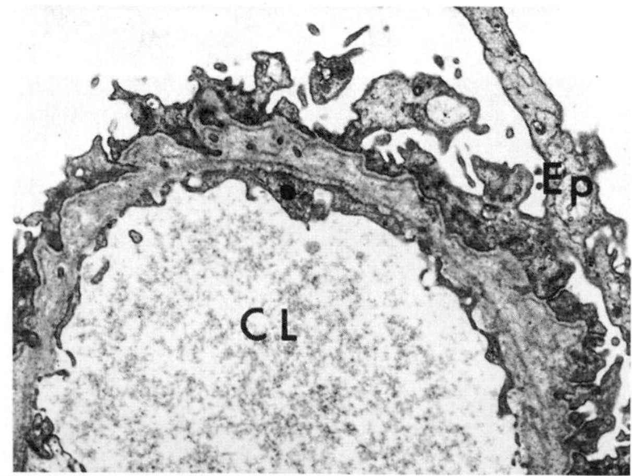

Figure 20-20 Hereditary nephritis (Alport syndrome). Electron micrograph of glomerulus with irregular thickening of the basement membrane, lamination of the lamina densa, and foci of rarefaction. Such changes may be present in other diseases but are most pronounced and widespread in hereditary nephritis. *CL*, Capillary lumen; *Ep*, epithelium.

Thin Basement Membrane Lesion (Benign Familial Hematuria)

This is a fairly common hereditary entity manifested *clinically by familial asymptomatic hematuria* – usually uncovered on routine urinalysis—*and morphologically by diffuse thinning of the GBM* to widths between 150 and 225 nm (compared with 300 to 400 nm in healthy adults). Although mild or moderate proteinuria may also be present, renal function is normal and prognosis is excellent. The abnormality is estimated to affect 1% of the general population.

The disorder should be distinguished from IgA nephropathy, another common cause of hematuria, and X-linked Alport syndrome. In contrast to Alport syndrome, hearing loss, ocular abnormalities, and a family history of renal failure are absent.

The anomaly in thin basement membrane lesion has also been traced to mutations in genes encoding α_3 or α_4 chains of type IV collagen. The disease most often has an autosomal inheritance and most patients are heterozygous for the defective gene. The disorder in homozygotes resembles autosomal recessive Alport syndrome. Homozygotes or compound heterozygotes may progress to renal failure. Thus, these diseases illustrate a continuum of changes resulting from mutations in collagen type IV genes.

KEY CONCEPTS

Isolated Glomerular Abnormalities

- **IgA nephropathy,** characterized by mesangial deposits of IgA-containing immune complexes, is the most common cause of glomerulonephritis worldwide. It is a common cause of both a nephritic syndrome and of isolated and frequently recurrent hematuria; it commonly affects children and young adults and has a variable course.
- **Alport syndrome**, a form of **hereditary nephritis,** is caused by mutations in genes encoding GBM type IV collagen. It manifests as hematuria and slowly progressing proteinuria and declining renal function; glomeruli appear normal by light microscopy until late in the disease course.
- **Thin basement membrane lesion** has a benign clinical course and is also the result of mutations in genes coding for GBM type IV collagen and hence may be considered as part of a spectrum of diseases that includes hereditary nephritis.

Chronic Glomerulonephritis

Chronic glomerulonephritis refers to end-stage glomerular disease that may result from specific types of glomerulonephritis or may develop without antecedent history of any of the well-recognized forms of acute glomerulonephritis. Poststreptococcal glomerulonephritis is a rare antecedent of chronic glomerulonephritis, except in adults. Patients with crescentic glomerulonephritis, if they survive the acute episode, usually progress to chronic glomerulonephritis. Membranous nephropathy, MPGN, IgA nephropathy, and FSGS all may progress to chronic renal failure. Nevertheless, **in any series of individuals with chronic glomerulonephritis, a variable percentage of cases arise mysteriously with no antecedent history of acute glomerulonephritis.** These cases may represent the end result of relatively asymptomatic forms of glomerulonephritis, either known or still unrecognized, that progress to uremia. Predictably, the proportion of such unexplained cases depends on the availability of renal biopsy material from patients early in their disease.

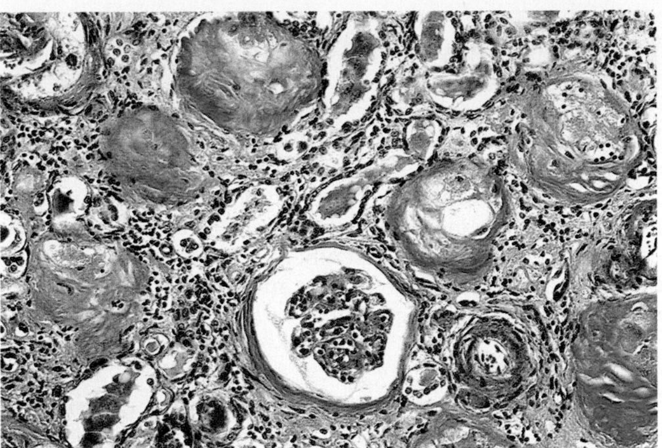

Figure 20-21 Chronic glomerulonephritis. A Masson trichrome preparation shows complete replacement of virtually all glomeruli by blue-staining collagen. (Courtesy Dr. M.A. Venkatachalam, Department of Pathology, University of Texas Health Sciences Center, San Antonio, Tex.)

MORPHOLOGY

The kidneys are symmetrically contracted and have diffusely granular cortical surfaces. On section, **the cortex is thinned,** and there is an increase in peripelvic fat. The glomerular histology depends on the stage of the disease. In early cases, the glomeruli may still show evidence of the primary disease (e.g., membranous nephropathy or MPGN). However, there eventually ensues **obliteration of glomeruli,** transforming them into acellular eosinophilic masses, representing a combination of trapped plasma proteins, increased mesangial matrix, basement membrane-like material, and collagen (Fig. 20-21). Because hypertension is an accompaniment of chronic glomerulonephritis, **arterial and arteriolar sclerosis may be conspicuous.** Marked atrophy of associated tubules, irregular interstitial fibrosis, and mononuclear leukocytic infiltration of the interstitium also occur.

Clinical Course. In most individuals, chronic glomerulonephritis develops insidiously and slowly progresses to renal insufficiency or death from uremia during a span of years or possibly decades (see the discussion of chronic renal failure). Not infrequently, patients present with such nonspecific complaints as loss of appetite, anemia, vomiting, or weakness. In some, the renal disease is suspected with the discovery of proteinuria, hypertension, or azotemia on routine medical examination. In others, the underlying renal disorder is discovered in the course of investigation of edema. Most patients are hypertensive, and sometimes the dominant clinical manifestations relate to cerebral or cardiovascular disease. In all, the disease is relentlessly progressive, though at widely varying rates. In nephrotic patients, as glomeruli become obliterated and therefore the GFR decreases, the protein loss in the urine diminishes. If patients with chronic glomerulonephritis do not receive dialysis or if they do not receive a renal transplant, they invariably succumb to their disease.

Glomerular Lesions Associated with Systemic Diseases

Many immunologically mediated, metabolic, or hereditary systemic disorders are associated with glomerular injury; in some (e.g., SLE and diabetes mellitus), the glomerular involvement is a major clinical manifestation. Most of these diseases are discussed elsewhere in this book. Here we briefly recall some of the lesions and discuss only those not considered in other sections.

Lupus Nephritis

The various types of lupus nephritis were described in Chapter 6. As discussed, SLE gives rise to a wide variety of renal lesions and clinical presentations. The clinical manifestations can include recurrent microscopic or gross hematuria, the nephritic syndrome, rapidly progressive glomerulonephritis, the nephrotic syndrome, acute and chronic renal failure, and hypertension.

Henoch-Schönlein Purpura

This childhood syndrome consists of purpuric skin lesions, abdominal pain and intestinal bleeding, and arthralgias along with renal abnormalities. Skin lesions characteristically involve the extensor surfaces of arms and legs as well as buttocks; abdominal manifestations include pain, vomiting, and intestinal bleeding. The renal manifestations occur in one third of patients and include gross or microscopic hematuria, nephritic syndrome, nephrotic syndrome, or some combination of these. A small number of patients, mostly adults, develop a rapidly progressive form of glomerulonephritis with many crescents. Not all components of the syndrome need to be present for the diagnosis, and individual patients may have purpura, abdominal pain, or urinary abnormalities as the dominant feature. The disease is most common in children 3 to 8 years old, but it also occurs in adults, in whom the renal manifestations are usually more severe. There is a strong background of atopy in about one third of patients, and onset often follows an upper respiratory infection. IgA is deposited in the glomerular mesangium in a distribution similar to that of IgA nephropathy. This has led to the concept that *IgA nephropathy and Henoch-Schönlein purpura are manifestations of the same disease.* The finding of Ig and C3 deposits in glomeruli suggests that immune complexes are involved in the disease.

MORPHOLOGY

On histologic examination, the renal lesions vary from mild focal mesangial proliferation to diffuse mesangial proliferation and/or endocapillary proliferation to crescentic glomerulonephritis. Whatever the histologic lesions, the pathognomonic feature by fluorescence microscopy is the **deposition of IgA, sometimes with IgG and C3, in the mesangial region**, sometimes with deposits extending to the capillary loops. The skin lesions consist of subepidermal hemorrhages and a necrotizing vasculitis involving the small vessels of the dermis. Deposits of IgA, along with IgG and C3, are also present in such vessels. Vasculitis also occurs in other organs, such as the gastrointestinal tract, but is rare in the kidney.

The course of the disease is variable, but recurrences of hematuria may persist for many years after onset. Most children have an excellent prognosis. Patients with the more diffuse lesions, crescents, or the nephrotic syndrome have a somewhat poorer prognosis.

Glomerulonephritis Associated with Bacterial Endocarditis and Other Systemic Infections

Glomerular lesions occurring in the course of bacterial endocarditis or other systemic infections, such as infected atrioventricular shunts, represent a type of immune complex nephritis initiated by complexes of bacterial antigen and antibody. Hematuria and proteinuria of various degrees characterize this entity clinically, but an acute nephritic presentation is not uncommon, and even RPGN may occur in rare instances. The histologic lesions, when present, generally reflect these clinical manifestations. The histologic features may vary from a focal and segmental necrotizing glomerulonephritis to a diffuse and more global exudative and proliferative glomerulonephritis, which may have a MPGN pattern. More severe forms show a diffuse proliferative glomerulonephritis. The lesions may be acute (influx of neutrophils) or chronic (fully developed MPGN pattern with basement membrane changes); the rapidly progressive forms show large numbers of crescents. Immunofluorescence and electron microscopy show the presence of glomerular immune deposits.

Diabetic Nephropathy

Diabetes mellitus is a major cause of renal morbidity and mortality, and diabetic nephropathy is the leading cause of chronic kidney failure in the United States. Advanced or end-stage kidney disease occurs in as many as 40% of both insulin-dependent 1 diabetics and type 2 diabetics. The pathology and pathogenesis of this disorder is discussed in Chapter 24.

Fibrillary Glomerulonephritis

Fibrillary glomerulonephritis is a morphologic variant of glomerulonephritis associated with characteristic fibrillar deposits in the mesangium and glomerular capillary walls that resemble amyloid fibrils superficially but differ ultrastructurally and do not stain with Congo red. The glomerular lesions usually show membranoproliferative or mesangioproliferative patterns by light microscopy. By immunofluorescence microscopy, there is selective deposition of polyclonal IgG, often of the IgG4 subclass, complement C3, and Igκ and Igλ light chains. Clinically, patients develop nephrotic syndrome, hematuria, and progressive renal insufficiency. The disease recurs in kidney transplants. The pathogenesis of this entity is unknown.

Other Systemic Disorders

Goodpasture syndrome (Chapter 15), *microscopic polyangiitis*, and *granulomatosis with polyangiitis (formally called Wegener granulomatosis)* (Chapter 11) are commonly associated with glomerular lesions, as described in the discussion of these diseases. Suffice it to say here that the glomerular lesions in these three conditions can be histologically similar and are principally characterized by foci of glomerular necrosis and crescent formation. In the early or mild forms of renal involvement, there is focal and segmental, sometimes necrotizing, glomerulonephritis, and most of these patients will have hematuria with mild decline in GFR. In the more severe cases, which may be associated with RPGN, there is more extensive necrosis, fibrin deposition, and extensive formation of epithelial (cellular) crescents, which can become organized to form fibrocellular and fibrous crescents if the glomerular injury evolves into segmental or global scarring (sclerosis).

Essential mixed cryoglobulinemia is another systemic condition in which deposits of cryoglobulins composed principally of IgG-IgM complexes induce cutaneous vasculitis, synovitis, and a proliferative glomerulonephritis, typically MPGN. Most cases of essential mixed cryoglobulinemia have been associated with infection with hepatitis C virus, and this condition in particular is associated with glomerulonephritis, usually MPGN type I.

Immunoglobulins secreted by plasma cell neoplasms may also induce glomerular lesions, including amyloidosis.

Tubular and Interstitial Diseases

Most forms of tubular injury involve the interstitium as well; therefore, diseases affecting these two components are discussed together. Under this heading we consider two major processes: (1) ischemic or toxic tubular injury, and (2) inflammatory reactions of the tubules and interstitium *(tubulointerstitial nephritis)*.

Acute Tubular Injury/Necrosis

Acute tubular injury (ATI) is a clinicopathologic entity characterized clinically by acute renal failure and often, but not invariably, morphologic evidence of tubular injury, in the form of necrosis of tubular epithelial cells. Since necrosis is not invariable, the term ATI is now preferred over the older term acute tubular necrosis (ATN). It is the most common cause of acute kidney injury (acute renal failure). ATI can be caused by a variety of conditions, including

- *Ischemia, due to decreased or interrupted blood flow*, examples of which include diffuse involvement of the intrarenal blood vessels such as in microscopic polyangiitis, malignant hypertension, microangiopathies and systemic conditions associated with thrombosis (e.g., hemolytic uremic syndrome [HUS], thrombotic thrombocytopenic purpura [TTP], and disseminated intravascular coagulation [DIC]), or decreased effective circulating blood volume, as occurs in hypovolemic shock (Chapter 4)
- *Direct toxic injury to the tubules by endogenous* (e.g., myoglobin, hemoglobin, monoclonal light chains, bile/bilirubin) *or exogenous agents* (e.g., drugs, radiocontrast dyes, heavy metals, organic solvents)

ATI accounts for some 50% of cases of acute kidney injury in hospitalized patients. Other causes of acute renal failure are discussed elsewhere in this chapter.

ATI is a reversible process that arises in a variety of clinical settings. Most of these, ranging from severe trauma to acute pancreatitis, have in common a period of inadequate blood flow to the peripheral organs, usually accompanied by marked hypotension and shock. This pattern is called *ischemic ATI*. The second pattern, called *nephrotoxic ATI*, is caused by a multitude of drugs, such as gentamicin; radiographic contrast agents; poisons, including heavy metals (e.g., mercury); and organic solvents (e.g., carbon tetrachloride). Combinations of ischemic and nephrotoxic ATI also can occur, exemplified by mismatched blood transfusions and other hemolytic crises causing *hemoglobinuria* and skeletal muscle injuries causing *myoglobinuria*. Such injuries result in characteristic intratubular hemoglobin or myoglobin casts, respectively; the toxic iron content of these globin molecules contributes to the ATI. In addition to its frequency, the potential reversibility of ATI adds to its clinical importance. Proper management can make the difference between recovery and death.

Pathogenesis. **The critical events in both ischemic and nephrotoxic ATI are believed to be (1) tubular injury and (2) persistent and severe disturbances in blood flow** (Fig. 20-22).

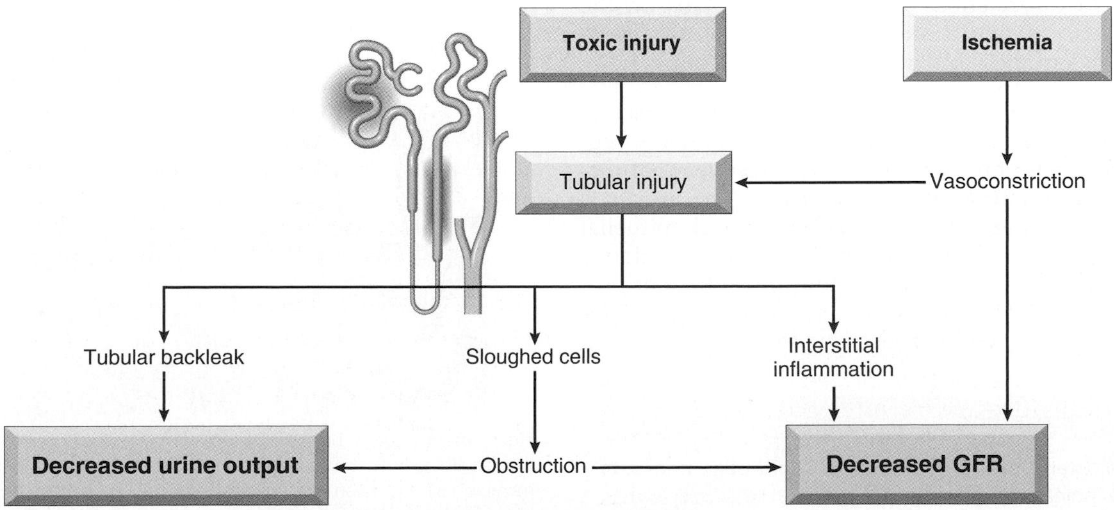

Figure 20-22 Postulated sequence in ischemic or toxic acute tubular injury.

- *Tubule cell injury:* Tubular epithelial cells are particularly sensitive to ischemia and are also vulnerable to toxins. Several factors predispose the tubules to toxic injury, including an increased surface area for tubular reabsorption, active transport systems for ions and organic acids, a high rate of metabolism and oxygen consumption that is required to perform these transport and reabsorption functions, and the capability for resorption and concentration of toxins.

  Ischemia causes numerous structural and functional alterations in epithelial cells, as discussed in Chapter 2. One early reversible result of ischemia is *loss of cell polarity* due to redistribution of membrane proteins (e.g., the enzyme Na,K^+-ATPase) from the basolateral to the luminal surface of the tubular cells, resulting in abnormal ion transport across the cells and *increased sodium delivery to distal tubules*. The latter incites vasoconstriction via *tubuloglomerular feedback*. In addition, ischemic tubular cells express cytokines and adhesion molecules, thus recruiting leukocytes that appear to participate in the subsequent injury. In time, injured cells detach from the basement membranes and cause *luminal obstruction*, increased intratubular pressure, and decreased GFR. In addition, glomerular filtrate in the lumen of the damaged tubules can leak back into the interstitium, resulting in interstitial edema, increased interstitial pressure, and further damage to the tubule. All these effects, as shown in Figure 20-22, contribute to the decreased GFR.
- *Disturbances in blood flow:* Ischemic renal injury is also characterized by *hemodynamic alterations* that cause reduced GFR. The major one is *intrarenal vasoconstriction*, which results in both reduced glomerular blood flow and reduced oxygen delivery to the functionally important tubules in the outer medulla (thick ascending limb and straight segment of the proximal tubule). Several vasoconstrictor pathways have been implicated, including the renin-angiotensin system, stimulated by increased distal sodium delivery (via *tubuloglomerular feedback*), and *sublethal endothelial injury*, leading to increased release of the vasoconstrictor *endothelin* and decreased production of the vasodilators *nitric oxide* and *prostacyclin (prostaglandin I_2)*. There is also some evidence of a direct effect of ischemia or toxins on the glomerulus, causing a reduced glomerular ultrafiltration coefficient, possibly due to mesangial contraction.

The patchiness of tubular necrosis and maintenance of the integrity of the basement membrane along many segments allow repair of the injured foci and recovery of function if the precipitating cause is removed. This repair is dependent on the capacity of reversibly injured epithelial cells to proliferate and differentiate. Re-epithelialization is mediated by a variety of growth factors and cytokines produced locally by the tubular cells themselves or by inflammatory cells in the vicinity of necrotic foci.

MORPHOLOGY

ATI is characterized by **focal tubular epithelial necrosis** at multiple points along the nephron, with large skip areas in between, often accompanied by rupture of basement membranes (tubulorrhexis) and **occlusion of tubular lumens by casts** (Figs. 20-23 and 20-24). The distinct patterns of tubular injury in ischemic and toxic ATI are shown in Figure 20-23. The straight portion of the proximal tubule and the ascending thick limb in the renal medulla are especially vulnerable, but focal lesions may also occur in the distal tubule, often in conjunction with casts. It should be noted that the severity

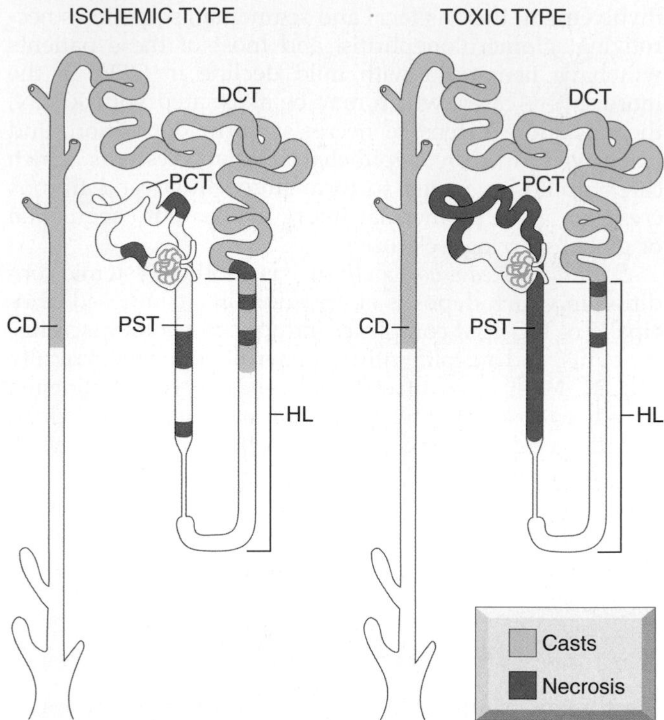

Figure 20-23 Patterns of tubular damage in ischemic and toxic acute tubular injury. In the ischemic type, tubular necrosis is patchy, relatively short lengths of tubules are affected, and straight segments of proximal tubules (PST) and ascending limbs of Henle's loop (HL) are most vulnerable. In toxic acute tubular injury, extensive necrosis is present along the proximal convoluted tubule segments (PCT) with many toxins (e.g., mercury), but necrosis of the distal tubule, particularly ascending HL, also occurs. In both types, lumens of the distal convoluted tubules (DCT) and collecting ducts (CD) contain casts.

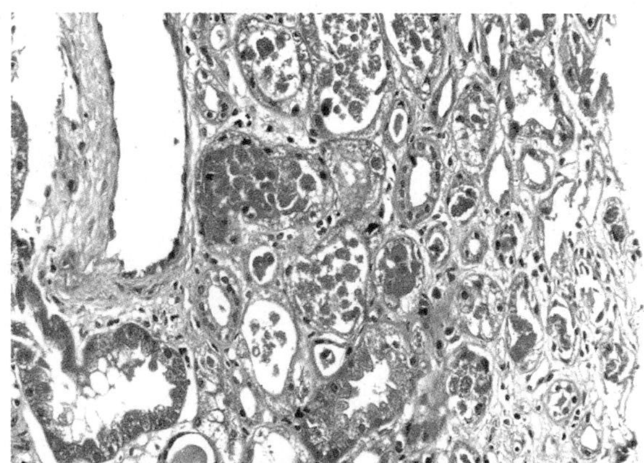

Figure 20-24 Acute tubular injury. Some of the tubular epithelial cells in the tubules are necrotic, and many have become detached (from their basement membranes) and been sloughed into the tubular lumens, whereas others are swollen, vacuolated, and regenerating. (Courtesy Dr. Agnes Fogo, Vanderbilt University, Nashville, Tenn.)

of the morphologic findings often do not correlate well with the severity of the clinical manifestations.

Eosinophilic hyaline casts, as well as pigmented granular casts, are common, particularly in distal tubules and collecting ducts. These casts consist principally of Tamm-Horsfall protein (a urinary glycoprotein normally secreted by the cells of ascending thick limb and distal tubules) in conjunction with other plasma proteins. Other findings in ischemic ATI are interstitial edema and accumulations of leukocytes within dilated vasa recta. There is also evidence of epithelial regeneration in the form of flattened epithelial cells with hyperchromatic nuclei and mitotic figures. In the course of time this regeneration repopulates the tubules so that no residual evidence of damage is seen.

Toxic ATI is manifested by acute tubular injury, most obvious in the proximal convoluted tubules. On histologic examination the tubular necrosis may be nonspecific, but it is somewhat distinctive in poisoning with certain agents. With mercuric chloride, for example, severely injured cells may contain large acidophilic inclusions. Later, these cells become necrotic, are desquamated into the lumen, and may undergo calcification. Carbon tetrachloride poisoning, in contrast, is characterized by the accumulation of neutral lipids in injured cells; again, such fatty change is followed by necrosis. Ethylene glycol produces marked ballooning and hydropic or vacuolar degeneration of proximal convoluted tubules. Calcium oxalate crystals are often also found in the tubular lumens in ethylene glycol poisoning.

Clinical Course. The clinical course of ATI is highly variable, but the classic case may be divided into *three* stages.

- *Initiation phase*, lasting about 36 hours, is dominated by the inciting medical, surgical, or obstetric event. The only indication of renal involvement is a slight decline in urine output with a rise in BUN. At this point, oliguria could be explained by a transient decrease in blood flow and declining GFR.
- *Maintenance phase* is characterized by sustained decreases in urine output to between 40 and 400 mL/day (oliguria), salt and water overload, rising BUN concentrations, hyperkalemia, metabolic acidosis, and other manifestations of uremia. With appropriate management, the patient can overcome this oliguric crisis.
- *Recovery phase* is ushered in by a steady increase in urine volume that may reach up to 3 L/day. The tubules are still damaged, so large amounts of water, sodium, and potassium are lost in the flood of urine. *Hypokalemia, rather than hyperkalemia, becomes a clinical problem.* There is a peculiar increased vulnerability to infection at this stage. Eventually, renal tubular function is restored and concentrating ability improves. At the same time, BUN and creatinine levels begin to return to normal. Subtle tubular functional impairment may persist for months, but most patients who reach this phase eventually recover completely.

The prognosis of ATI depends on the magnitude and duration of injury. Recovery is expected with nephrotoxic ATI when the toxin has not caused serious damage to other organs, such as the liver or heart. With current supportive care, 95% of those who do not succumb to the precipitating cause recover. Conversely, in shock related to sepsis, extensive burns, or other causes of multi-organ failure, the mortality rate can be more than 50%.

KEY CONCEPTS

Acute Tubular Injury

- Acute tubular injury is the most common cause of acute kidney injury and attributed to ischemia and/or toxicity from an endogenous or exogenous substance.
- Tubular epithelial cell injury and altered intrarenal hemodynamics are the primary contributors to acute tubular injury.
- The clinical outcome is determined by the magnitude and duration of acute tubular injury.

Tubulointerstitial Nephritis

This group of renal diseases involves inflammatory injuries of the tubules and interstitium that are often insidious in onset and are principally manifest by azotemia. We have previously seen that chronic tubulointerstitial damage is an important consequence of progression in diseases that primarily affect the glomerulus (Fig. 20-21). *Secondary tubulointerstitial nephritis* is also present in a variety of vascular, cystic (polycystic kidney disease), and metabolic (diabetes) renal disorders, in which it may also contribute to progressive damage. Here we discuss primary causes of tubulointerstitial injury (Table 20-8). Glomerular

Table 20-8 Causes of Tubulointerstitial Nephritis

Infections
Acute bacterial pyelonephritis
Chronic pyelonephritis (including reflux nephropathy)
Other infections (e.g., viruses, parasites)
Toxins
Drugs
Acute-hypersensitivity interstitial nephritis
Analgesics
Heavy metals
Lead, cadmium
Metabolic Diseases
Urate nephropathy
Nephrocalcinosis (hypercalcemic nephropathy)
Acute phosphate nephropathy
Hypokalemic nephropathy
Oxalate nephropathy
Physical Factors
Chronic urinary tract obstruction
Neoplasms
Multiple myeloma (light-chain cast nephropathy)
Immunologic Reactions
Transplant rejection
Sjögren syndrome
Sarcoidosis
Vascular Diseases
Miscellaneous
Balkan nephropathy
Nephronophthisis-medullary cystic disease complex
"Idiopathic" interstitial nephritis

and vascular abnormalities may also be present in advanced stages of these diseases.

Tubulointerstitial nephritis can be acute or chronic. *Acute tubulointerstitial nephritis* has a rapid clinical onset and is characterized histologically by interstitial edema, often accompanied by leukocytic infiltration of the interstitium and tubules, and tubular injury. In *chronic interstitial nephritis* there is infiltration with predominantly mononuclear leukocytes, prominent interstitial fibrosis, and widespread tubular atrophy. Morphologic features that are helpful in separating acute from chronic tubulointerstitial nephritis include edema and, when present, eosinophils and neutrophils in the acute form, while fibrosis and tubular atrophy characterize the chronic form.

These conditions are distinguished clinically from the glomerular diseases by the following hallmarks:

- Absence of nephritic or nephrotic syndrome
- The presence of defects in tubular function. The latter may be subtle and include impaired ability to concentrate urine, evidenced clinically by polyuria or nocturia; salt wasting; diminished ability to excrete acids (metabolic acidosis); and isolated defects in tubular reabsorption or secretion. Advanced forms, however, may be difficult to distinguish clinically from other causes of renal insufficiency.

Specific conditions are listed in Table 20-8 and are discussed elsewhere in this book. This section deals principally with pyelonephritis and interstitial diseases induced by drugs.

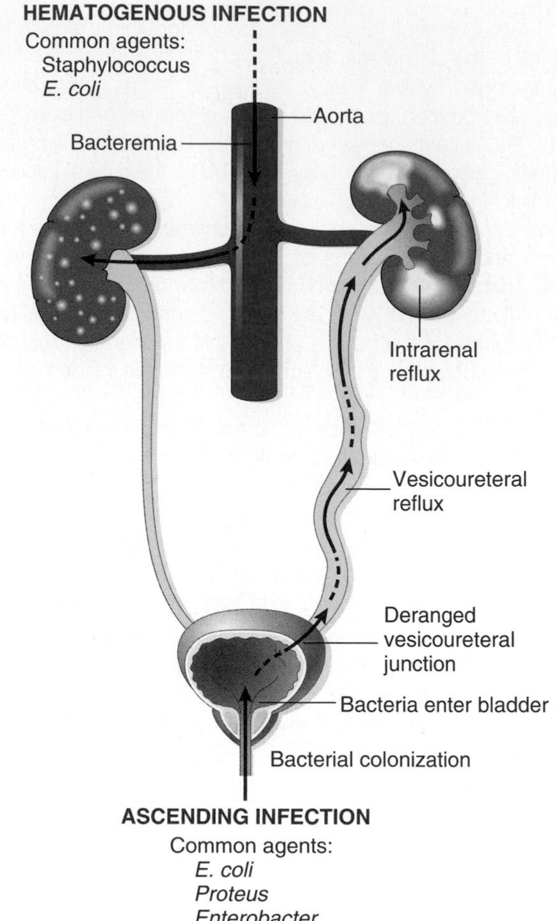

Figure 20-25 Schematic representation of pathways of renal infection. Hematogenous infection results from bacteremic spread. More common is ascending infection, which results from a combination of urinary bladder infection, vesicoureteral reflux, and intrarenal reflux.

Pyelonephritis and Urinary Tract Infection

Pyelonephritis is one of the most common diseases of the kidney and is defined as inflammation affecting the tubules, interstitium, and renal pelvis. It occurs in two forms. *Acute pyelonephritis* is generally caused by bacterial infection and is associated with urinary tract infection. *Chronic pyelonephritis* is a more complex disorder; bacterial infection plays a dominant role, but other factors (vesicoureteral reflux, obstruction) predispose to repeat episodes of acute pyelonephritis.

Pyelonephritis is a serious complication of *urinary tract infections* that affect the bladder (cystitis), the kidneys and their collecting systems (pyelonephritis), or both. Bacterial infections of the lower urinary tract may be asymptomatic (asymptomatic bacteriuria) and often remain localized to the bladder without the development of renal infection. However, lower urinary tract infection can potentially spread to the kidney.

Etiology and Pathogenesis. **More than 85% of cases of urinary tract infection are caused by the gram-negative bacilli that are normal inhabitants of the intestinal tract.** For most urinary tract infections, the infecting organisms are derived from the patient's own fecal flora. By far the most common is *Escherichia coli*, followed by *Proteus*, *Klebsiella*, and *Enterobacter*. *Streptococcus faecalis*, also of enteric origin, staphylococci, and virtually every other bacterial and fungal agent can also cause lower urinary tract and renal infection. Mycobacterial and fungal organisms induce caseating and non-caseating granulomatous inflammation, respectively. In immunocompromised persons, particularly those with transplanted organs, viruses such as *polyomavirus*, cytomegalovirus, and adenovirus can also be a cause of renal infection.

There are two routes by which bacteria can reach the kidneys: (1) through the bloodstream (hematogenous infection) and (2) from the lower urinary tract (ascending infection) (Fig. 20-25). The hematogenous route is less common and results from seeding of the kidneys by bacteria from distant foci in the course of septicemia or localized infections such as infective endocarditis. Hematogenous infection is more likely to occur in the presence of ureteral obstruction, and in debilitated patients. Typically, in patients receiving immunosuppressive therapy, nonenteric organisms, such as staphylococci and certain fungi and viruses, are involved.

Ascending infection is the most common cause of clinical pyelonephritis. Normal human bladder and bladder urine are sterile; therefore, a number of steps must occur for renal infection to occur:

- The first step in ascending infection is the *colonization of the distal urethra and introitus* (in the female) by coliform bacteria. This colonization is influenced by the degree of bacterial adherence to urethral mucosal epithelial, as discussed in Chapter 8, which involves adhesive molecules (adhesins) on the P-fimbriae (pili) of bacteria that interact with receptors on the surface of urothelial cells. Specific adhesins (e.g., those encoded by the pyelonephritis-associated pili [*pap*] gene) are associated with infection. In addition, certain types of fimbriae promote renal tropism, persistence of infection, or an enhanced inflammatory response.

- *From the urethra to the bladder*, organisms gain entrance during urethral catheterization or other instrumentation. Long-term catheterization, in particular, carries a risk of infection. In the absence of instrumentation, *urinary infections are much more common in females*, and this has been ascribed to the shorter urethra in females, as well as the absence of antibacterial properties found in prostatic fluid, hormonal changes affecting adherence of bacteria to the mucosa, and urethral trauma during sexual intercourse, or a combination of these factors.

The mechanisms by which microbes move *from the bladder to the kidneys* are described below.

- *Urinary tract obstruction and stasis of urine.* Ordinarily, organisms introduced into the bladder are cleared by continual voiding and by antibacterial mechanisms. However, outflow obstruction or bladder dysfunction results in incomplete emptying and residual urine. In the presence of stasis, bacteria introduced into the bladder can multiply unhindered. Accordingly, urinary tract infection is frequent among patients with lower urinary tract obstruction, such as may occur with benign prostatic hypertrophy, tumors, or calculi, or with neurogenic bladder dysfunction caused by diabetes or spinal cord injury.
- *Vesicoureteral reflux.* Although obstruction is an important predisposing factor in ascending infection, it is *incompetence of the vesicoureteral valve* that allows bacteria to ascend the ureter into the renal pelvis. The normal ureteral insertion into the bladder is a one-way valve that prevents retrograde flow of urine when the intravesical pressure rises, as in micturition. An incompetent vesicoureteral orifice allows the reflux of bladder urine into the ureters *(vesicoureteral reflux)* (Fig. 20-26). Reflux is most often due to a congenital absence or shortening of the intravesical portion of the ureter, such that the ureter is not compressed during micturition. In addition, it may be acquired by bladder infection itself. It is postulated that bacteria themselves or the associated inflammation can promote reflux by affecting ureteral contractility, particularly in children. Vesicoureteral reflux is estimated to affect 1% to 2% of otherwise normal children. *Acquired vesicoureteral reflux* in adults can result from persistent bladder atony caused by spinal cord injury. The effect of vesicoureteral reflux is similar to that of an obstruction in that there is residual urine in the urinary tract after voiding, which favors bacterial growth.
- *Intrarenal reflux.* Vesicoureteral reflux also affords a ready mechanism by which the infected bladder urine can be propelled up to the renal pelvis and deep into the renal parenchyma through open ducts at the tips of the papillae (intrarenal reflux). Intrarenal reflux is most common in the upper and lower poles of the kidney, where papillae tend to have flattened or concave tips rather than the convex pointed type present in the midzones of the kidney (and depicted in most textbooks). Reflux can be demonstrated radiographically by a voiding cystourethrogram, in which the bladder is filled with a radiopaque dye and films are taken during micturition. Vesicoureteral reflux can be demonstrated by this method in about 30% of infants and children with urinary tract infection (Fig. 20-26).

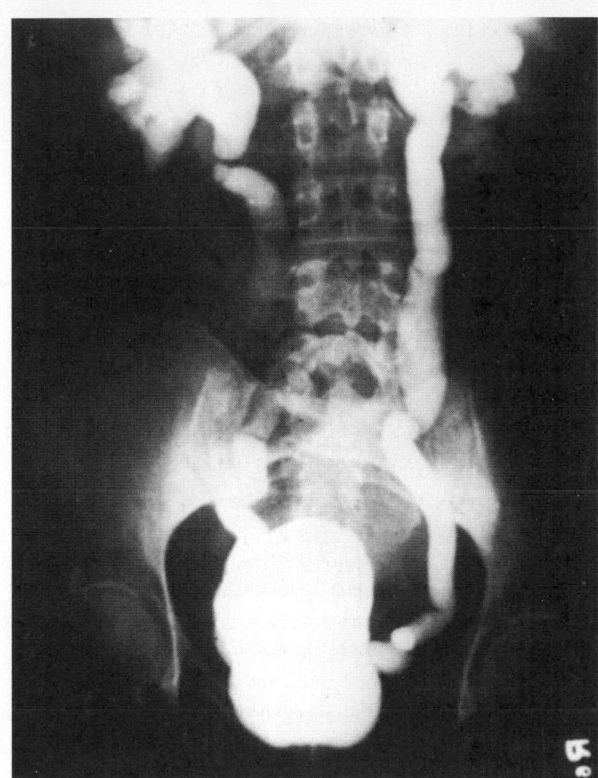

Figure 20-26 Vesicoureteral reflux demonstrated by a voiding cystourethrogram. Dye injected into the bladder refluxes into both dilated ureters, filling the pelvis and calyces.

In the absence of vesicoureteral reflux, infection usually remains localized in the bladder. Thus, the majority of individuals with repeated or persistent bacterial colonization of the urinary tract suffer from cystitis and urethritis *(lower urinary tract infection)* rather than pyelonephritis.

Acute Pyelonephritis

Acute pyelonephritis is a suppurative inflammation of the kidney caused by bacterial and sometimes viral (e.g., polyomavirus) infection, which can reach the kidney by hematogenous spread or, more commonly, through the ureters in association with vesicoureteral reflux.

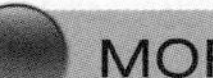

MORPHOLOGY

The hallmarks of acute pyelonephritis are **patchy interstitial suppurative inflammation, intratubular aggregates of neutrophils, neutrophilic tubulitis and tubular necrosis**. The suppuration may occur as discrete focal abscesses or large wedge-like areas and can involve one or both kidneys (Fig. 20-27).

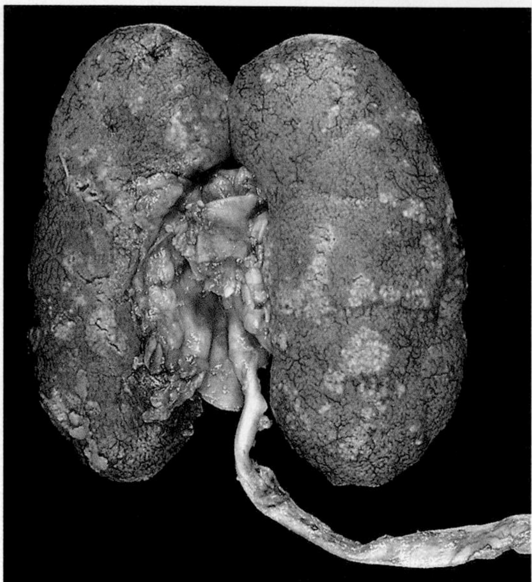

Figure 20-27 Acute pyelonephritis. Cortical surface shows grayish white areas of inflammation and abscess formation.

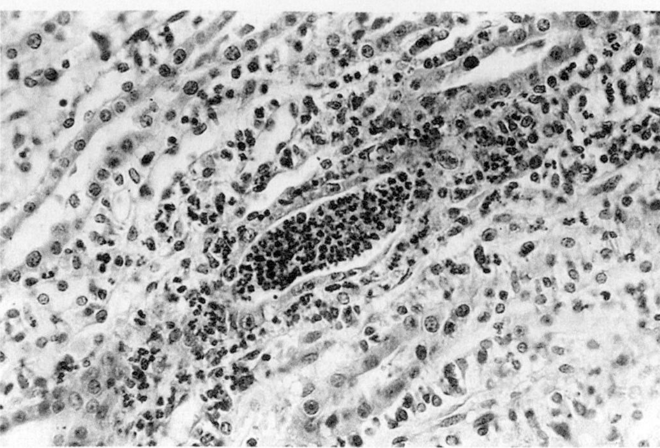

Figure 20-28 Acute pyelonephritis marked by an acute neutrophilic exudate within tubules and interstitial inflammation.

In the early stages, the neutrophilic infiltration is limited to the tubules. The tubular lumens are a conduit for the extension of the infection, and soon, the infection extends to the interstitium and produces abscesses that destroy the involved tubules (Fig. 20-28). Characteristically, glomeruli are relatively resistant to the infection. Extensive disease, however, eventually also destroys the glomeruli, and fungal pyelonephritis (e.g., *Candida*) often affects glomeruli and results in granulomatous interstitial inflammation.

Three complications of acute pyelonephritis can be encountered.

- **Papillary necrosis** is seen mainly in diabetics, sickle cell disease, and in those with urinary tract obstruction. Papillary necrosis is usually bilateral but may be unilateral. One or all of the pyramids of the affected kidney may be involved. On cut section, the tips or distal two thirds of the pyramids have areas of gray-white to yellow necrosis (Fig. 20-29). On microscopic examination the necrotic tissue shows characteristic ischemic coagulative necrosis, with preservation of outlines of tubules. The leukocytic response is limited to the junctions between preserved and destroyed tissue.
- **Pyonephrosis** is seen when there is total or almost complete obstruction, particularly when it is high in the urinary tract. The suppurative exudate is unable to drain and thus fills the renal pelvis, calyces, and ureter with pus.
- **Perinephric abscess** is an extension of suppurative inflammation through the renal capsule into the perinephric tissue.

After the acute phase of pyelonephritis, healing occurs. The neutrophilic infiltrate is replaced by one that is predominantly composed of macrophages, plasma cells, and lymphocytes. The inflammatory foci are eventually replaced by irregular scars that can be seen on the cortical surface as fibrous depressions. Such scars are characterized microscopically by tubular atrophy, interstitial fibrosis, and a lymphocytic infiltrate in a characteristic patchy, jigsaw pattern with intervening preserved parenchyma. **The pyelonephritic scar is almost always associated with inflammation, fibrosis, and deformation of the underlying calyx and pelvis,** reflecting the role of ascending infection and vesicoureteral reflux in the pathogenesis of the disease.

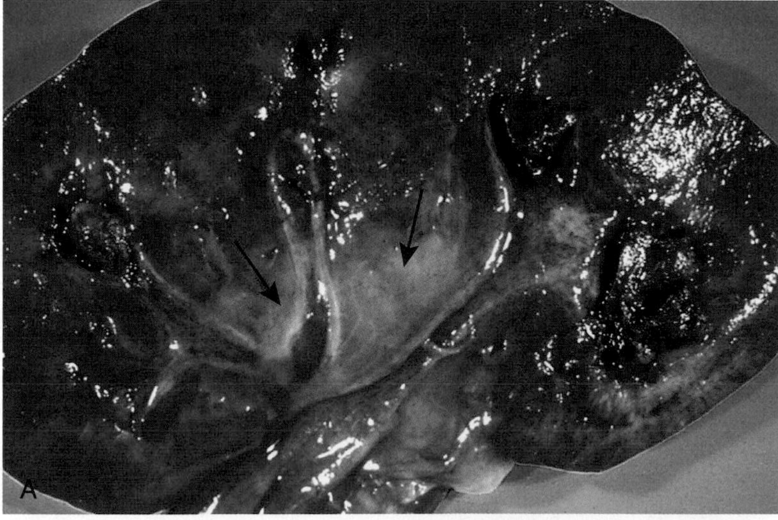

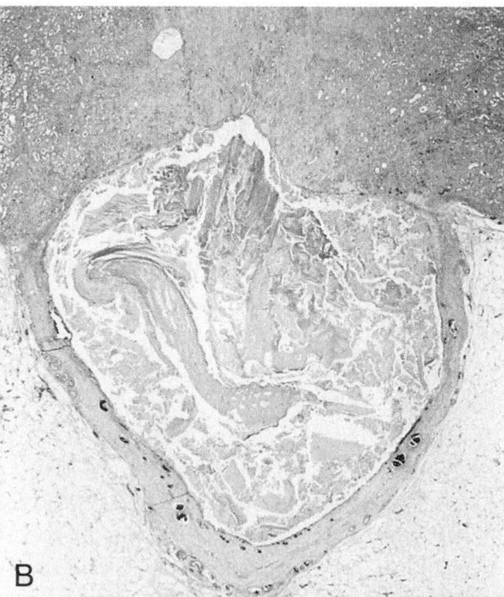

Figure 20-29 Papillary necrosis. Areas of pale-gray necrosis involve the papillae *(arrows)*.

Clinical Features. Acute pyelonephritis is often associated with the following:

- *Urinary tract obstruction,* either congenital or acquired
- *Instrumentation* of the urinary tract, most commonly catheterization
- *Vesicoureteral reflux*
- *Pregnancy.* Between 4% and 6% of pregnant women develop bacteriuria sometime during pregnancy, and 20% to 40% of these eventually develop symptomatic urinary infection if not treated.
- *Gender and age.* After the first year of life (when congenital anomalies in males commonly become evident) and up to around age 40 years, infections are much more frequent in females. With increasing age the incidence in males rises as a result of prostatic hypertrophy and instrumentation.
- *Preexisting renal lesions,* causing intrarenal scarring and obstruction
- *Diabetes mellitus,* in which increased susceptibility to infection, neurogenic bladder dysfunction, and more frequent instrumentation are predisposing factors
- *Immunosuppression and immunodeficiency*

Acute pyelonephritis usually presents with a sudden onset of pain at the costovertebral angle and systemic evidence of infection, such as fever and malaise. There are often indications of bladder and urethral irritation, such as dysuria, frequency, and urgency. The urine contains many leukocytes (pyuria) derived from the inflammatory infiltrate, but pyuria does not differentiate upper from lower urinary tract infection. The finding of leukocyte *casts,* typically rich in neutrophils (pus casts), indicates renal involvement, because casts are formed only in tubules. The diagnosis of infection is established by quantitative urine culture.

Uncomplicated acute pyelonephritis follows a benign course, and symptoms disappear within a few days after the institution of appropriate antibiotic therapy. Bacteria, however, may persist in the urine, or there may be recurrence of infection with new serologic types of *E. coli* or other organisms. Such bacteriuria then either disappears or may persist, sometimes for years. In the presence of unrelieved urinary obstruction, diabetes mellitus, or immunodeficiency, acute pyelonephritis may be more serious, leading to repeated septicemic episodes. The superimposition of *papillary necrosis* may lead to acute renal failure.

An emerging viral pathogen causing pyelonephritis in kidney allografts is *polyomavirus.* Latent infection with polyomavirus is widespread in the general population, and immunosuppression of the allograft recipient can lead to reactivation of latent infection and the development of nephropathy resulting in allograft failure in up to 5% of kidney transplant recipients. This form of pyelonephritis, now referred to as polyomavirus nephropathy, is characterized by infection of tubular epithelial cell nuclei, leading to nuclear enlargement and intranuclear inclusions visible by light microscopy (viral cytopathic effect). The inclusions are composed of virions arrayed in distinctive crystalline-like lattices when visualized by electron microscopy (Fig. 20-30). An interstitial inflammatory response is invariably present. Treatment consists of a reduction in immunosuppression.

Chronic Pyelonephritis and Reflux Nephropathy

Chronic pyelonephritis is a disorder in which chronic tubulointerstitial inflammation and scarring involve the calyces and pelvis (Fig. 20-31). Although several diseases produce chronic tubulointerstitial alterations (Table 20-8), only chronic pyelonephritis and analgesic nephropathy affect the calyces, making pelvocalyceal damage an important diagnostic clue. Chronic pyelonephritis at one time accounted for 10% to 20% of patients in renal transplant or dialysis units, until predisposing conditions such as reflux became better recognized. This condition remains an important cause of kidney destruction in children with severe lower urinary tract abnormalities.

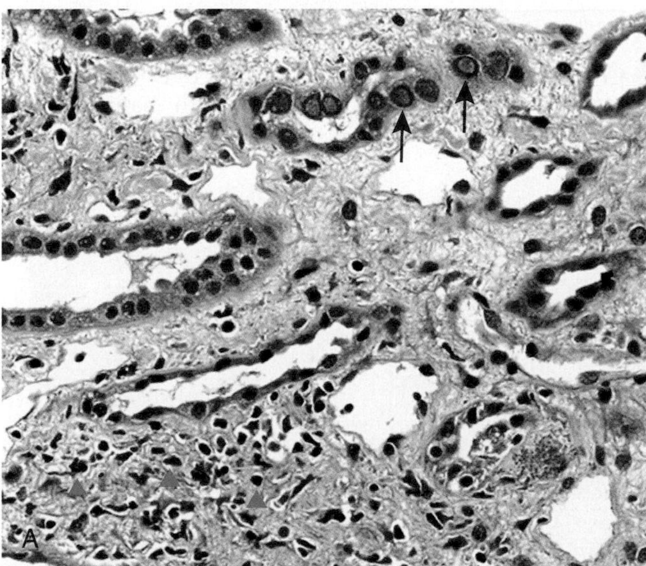

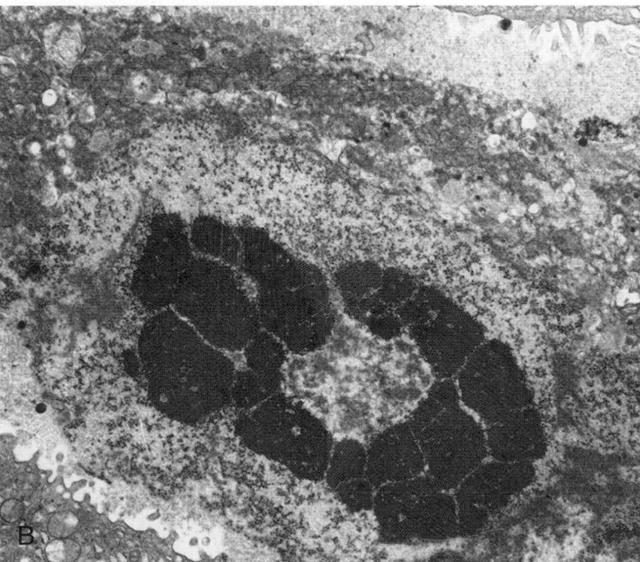

Figure 20-30 Polyomavirus nephropathy. **A,** The kidney shows enlarged tubular epithelial cells with nuclear inclusions *(arrows)* and interstitial inflammation *(arrowheads).* **B,** Intranuclear viral inclusions visualized by electron microscopy. (Courtesy Dr. Jean Olson, Department of Pathology, University of California San Francisco, San Francisco, Calif.)

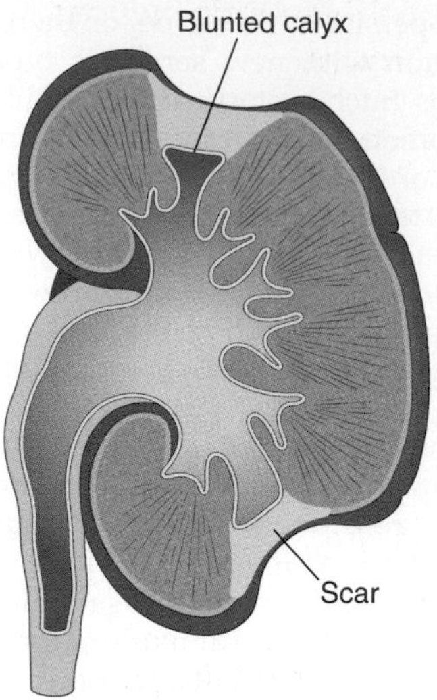

Figure 20-31 Typical coarse scars of chronic pyelonephritis associated with vesicoureteral reflux. The scars are usually polar and are associated with underlying blunted calyces.

Chronic pyelonephritis can be divided into two forms:

- *Reflux nephropathy.* This is by far the more common form of chronic pyelonephritic scarring. Reflux nephropathy occurs early in childhood as a result of superimposition of a urinary infection on congenital vesicoureteral reflux and intrarenal reflux. Reflux may be unilateral or bilateral; thus, the continuous renal damage may cause scarring and atrophy of one kidney or involve both, leading to renal insufficiency. Vesicoureteral reflux occasionally causes renal damage in the absence of infection (sterile reflux), but only when obstruction is severe.
- *Chronic obstructive pyelonephritis.* We have seen that obstruction predisposes the kidney to infection. Recurrent infections superimposed on diffuse or localized obstructive lesions lead to repeated bouts of renal inflammation and scarring, resulting in chronic pyelonephritis. In this condition, the effects of obstruction contribute to the parenchymal atrophy; indeed, it is sometimes difficult to differentiate the effects of bacterial infection from those of obstruction alone. The disease can be bilateral, as with posterior urethral valves, resulting in renal insufficiency unless the anomaly is corrected, or unilateral, as occurs with calculi and unilateral obstructive anomalies of the ureter.

MORPHOLOGY

The characteristic changes of chronic pyelonephritis are seen on gross examination (Figs. 20-31 and 20-32*A*). The kidneys usually are irregularly scarred; if bilateral, the involvement is asymmetric. In contrast, both kidneys in chronic glomerulonephritis are diffusely and symmetrically scarred. The hallmarks of chronic pyelonephritis are **coarse, discrete, corticomedullary scars overlying dilated, blunted, or deformed calyces, and flattening of the papillae** (Fig. 20-33*B*). The scars vary from one to several and most are in the upper and lower poles, consistent with the frequency of reflux in these sites.

The microscopic changes involve predominantly tubules and interstitium. The tubules show atrophy in some areas and hypertrophy or dilation in others. Dilated tubules with flattened epithelium may be filled with casts resembling thyroid colloid (thyroidization). There are varying degrees of chronic interstitial inflammation and fibrosis in the cortex and medulla. Arcuate and interlobular vessels demonstrate obliterative intimal sclerosis in the scarred areas; and in the presence of hypertension, hyaline arteriolosclerosis is seen in the entire kidney. There is often fibrosis around the calyceal epithelium as well as a marked chronic inflammatory infiltrate. Glomeruli may appear normal except for a variety of ischemic changes, including periglomerular fibrosis, fibrous obliteration and secondary changes related to hypertension. Individuals with chronic pyelonephritis and reflux nephropathy who develop proteinuria in advanced stages show secondary focal segmental glomerulosclerosis, as described later.

Xanthogranulomatous pyelonephritis is a relatively rare form of chronic pyelonephritis characterized by accumulation of foamy macrophages intermingled with plasma cells, lymphocytes, polymorphonuclear leukocytes, and occasional giant cells. Often associated with *Proteus* infections and obstruction, the lesions sometimes produce large, yellowish orange nodules that may be grossly confused with renal cell carcinoma.

Clinical Features. Chronic obstructive pyelonephritis may have a silent onset or present with manifestations of

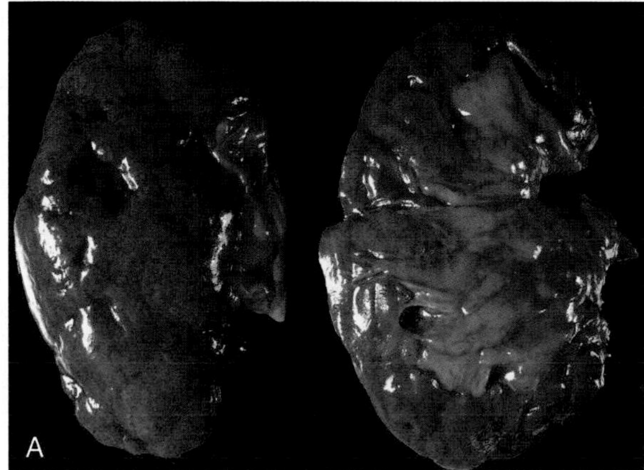

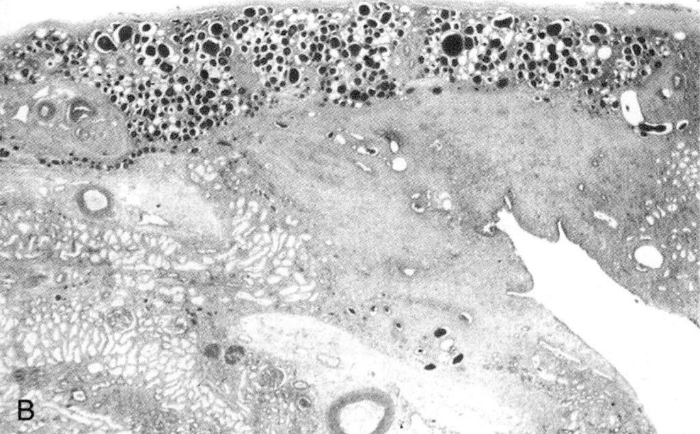

Figure 20-32 A, Chronic pyelonephritis. The surface *(left)* is irregularly scarred. The cut section *(right)* reveals blunting and loss of several papillae. **B,** Low-power view showing a corticomedullary renal scar with an underlying dilated deformed calyx. Note the thyroidization of tubules in the cortex.

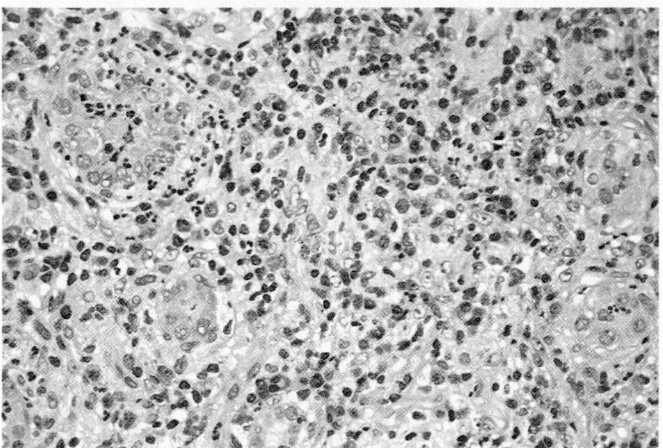

Figure 20-33 Drug-induced interstitial nephritis, with prominent eosinophilic and mononuclear cell infiltrate. (Courtesy Dr. H. Rennke, Brigham and Women's Hospital, Boston, Mass.)

acute recurrent pyelonephritis, such as back pain, fever, pyuria, and bacteriuria. These patients receive medical attention relatively late in their disease course because of the gradual onset of renal insufficiency and hypertension. Reflux nephropathy is often discovered in children when the cause of hypertension is investigated. Loss of tubular function—in particular of concentrating ability—gives rise to polyuria and nocturia. Radiographic studies show asymmetrically contracted kidneys with characteristic coarse scars and blunting and deformity of the calyceal system. Significant bacteriuria may be present, but it is often absent in the late stages.

Although proteinuria is usually mild, some individuals with pyelonephritic scars develop secondary *focal segmental glomerulosclerosis* with significant proteinuria, even in the nephrotic range, usually several years after the scarring has occurred and often in the absence of continued infection or persistent vesicoureteral reflux. The onset of proteinuria and focal segmental glomerulosclerosis is a poor prognostic sign, which may progress to ESRD. The glomerulosclerosis, as discussed, is attributable to the adaptive glomerular alterations secondary to loss of renal mass caused by pyelonephritic scarring (renal ablation nephropathy).

KEY CONCEPTS

Pyelonephritis

- Both acute and chronic pyelonephritis may be caused by infection via the ascending (more common) or hematogenous route. Obstructive lesions of the urinary tract are important predisposing factors.
- Bacteria are the most common infectious agent in acute pyelonephritis and induce a prominent neutrophilic inflammatory response; granulomatous interstitial inflammation is characteristic of fungal or mycobacterial infections.
- Chronic pyelonephritis ensues when anatomic anomalies result in urine reflux or urine outflow obstruction; multiple episodes of this injury leads to irregular scarring of the kidney that is typically more prominent at the upper or lower poles where reflux is more common.

Tubulointerstitial Nephritis Induced by Drugs and Toxins

Drug and toxin-induced tubulointerstitial nephritis is the second most common cause of acute kidney injury (after pyelonephritis). Toxins and drugs can injure kidneys in at least three ways: (1) trigger an interstitial immunologic reaction, exemplified by the acute hypersensitivity nephritis induced by drugs such as methicillin; (2) cause acute tubular injury, as described earlier; and (3) cause subclinical but cumulative injury to tubules that takes years to result in chronic renal insufficiency. The last type of damage is especially worrisome, because it may be unrecognized until irreversible renal damage has occurred.

Acute Drug-Induced Interstitial Nephritis

First reported after the use of sulfonamides, acute tubulointerstitial nephritis most frequently occurs with synthetic penicillins (methicillin, ampicillin), other synthetic antibiotics (rifampin), diuretics (thiazides), NSAIDs, and miscellaneous drugs (allopurinol, cimetidine). The chronic tubulointerstitial nephritis caused by phenacetin-containing analgesics, termed *analgesic nephropathy*, is mostly of historical importance as its incidence has substantially diminished due to the withdrawal or restriction of phenacetin in most countries.

Drug-induced acute interstitial nephritis begins about 15 days (range: 2-40) after drug exposure and is characterized by *fever*, *eosinophilia* (which may be transient), *a rash* in about 25% of patients, and *renal abnormalities*. The latter takes the form of hematuria, mild proteinuria, and leukocyturia (often including eosinophils). A rising serum creatinine or acute kidney injury with oliguria develops in about 50% of cases, particularly in older patients.

Pathogenesis. Many features of the disease suggest an idiosyncratic immune mechanism that is not dose-related. Clinical evidence of hypersensitivity includes the latent period, the eosinophilia and rash, the fact that the onset of nephropathy is not dose-related, and the recurrence of clinical and pathologic manifestations after re-exposure to the same or a chemically related drug. In some patients, serum IgE levels are increased, and IgE-containing plasma cells and basophils are present in the lesions, suggesting that the *late-phase reaction of an IgE-mediated (type I) hypersensitivity* may be involved in the pathogenesis (Chapter 6). In other cases, a mononuclear or granulomatous reaction, together with positive results of skin tests to drug haptens, suggest a T cell-mediated (type IV) delayed-hypersensitivity reaction.

The most likely sequence of events is that the drugs function as haptens and covalently bind to some plasma membrane or extracellular component of tubular cells. These modified self antigens then become immunogenic. The resultant injury is due to IgE or cell-mediated immune reactions to tubular cells or their basement membranes.

MORPHOLOGY

On histologic examination the interstitium shows variable but frequently pronounced **edema and infiltration by mononuclear cells,** principally lymphocytes and macrophages.

Eosinophils and neutrophils may be present (Fig. 20-33), often in clusters and large numbers, and smaller numbers of plasma cells and mast cells are sometimes also present. Inflammation may be more prominent in the medulla where the inciting agent is often concentrated. With some drugs (e.g., methicillin, thiazides), interstitial nonnecrotizing granulomas may be seen. Tubulitis, the infiltration of tubules by lymphocytes, is common. Variable degrees of tubular necrosis and regeneration are present. The glomeruli are normal except in some cases caused by NSAIDs, when minimal-change disease and the nephrotic syndrome develop concurrently (see below). In analgesic nephropathy, papillae can show various stages of necrosis, calcification, fragmentation, and sloughing.

Clinical Features. It is important to recognize drug-induced acute interstitial nephritis because withdrawal of the offending drug is followed by recovery, although it may take several months, and irreversible damage can occur. It is also important to remember that while drugs are the leading identifiable cause of acute interstitial nephritis, in many affected patients (approximately 30% to 40%) an offending drug or mechanism cannot be identified.

On occasion, necrotic papillae are excreted, and may cause gross hematuria or renal colic due to ureteric obstruction. Papillary necrosis is not specific for analgesic nephropathy, and is also seen in diabetes mellitus, as well as in urinary tract obstruction, sickle cell disease or trait (described later), and focally in renal tuberculosis. In all cases it is caused by ischemia resulting from compression or obstruction of small blood vessels in the medulla. Such compression may be caused by interstitial edema (as in inflammatory reactions and urinary tract obstruction) or microvascular disease (as in diabetes). Table 20-9 lists the main features of papillary necrosis in these conditions. A small percentage of patients with analgesic nephropathy develop *urothelial carcinoma of the renal pelvis.*

Nephropathy Associated with NSAIDs

NSAIDs, one of the most commonly used classes of drugs, produce several forms of renal injury. Although these complications are uncommon, they should be kept in mind since NSAIDs are frequently administered to patients with other potential causes of renal disease. Many NSAIDs are nonselective cyclooxygenase inhibitors, and their adverse renal effects are related to their ability to inhibit cyclooxygenase-dependent prostaglandin synthesis. The selective COX-2 inhibitors, while sparing the gastrointestinal tract, do affect the kidneys because COX-2 is expressed in human kidneys. NSAID-associated renal syndromes include

- *Acute kidney injury,* due to the decreased synthesis of vasodilatory prostaglandins and resultant ischemia. This is particularly likely to occur in the setting of other renal diseases or conditions causing volume depletion.
- *Acute hypersensitivity interstitial nephritis,* resulting in renal failure, as described earlier.
- *Acute interstitial nephritis and minimal-change disease.* This curious association of two diverse renal conditions, one leading to renal failure and the other to nephrotic syndrome, suggests a hypersensitivity reaction affecting the interstitium and possibly the glomeruli, but also is consistent with injury to podocytes mediated by cytokines released as part of the inflammatory process.
- *Membranous nephropathy,* with the nephrotic syndrome, is a recently appreciated association, also of unclear pathogenesis.

KEY CONCEPTS

Tubulointerstitial Nephritis Induced by Drugs and Toxins

- Drug-induced tubulointerstitial nephritis is the second most common cause of acute kidney injury.
- Prominent interstitial inflammation with associated tubular injury, which may or may not be accompanied by eosinophils or granulomatous inflammation, can be induced by almost any pharmacologic agent.
- NSAIDs can cause tubulointerstitial nephritis and/or glomerular injury, such as minimal change disease or membranous nephropathy.

Other Tubulointerstitial Diseases

Urate Nephropathy

Three types of nephropathy can occur in persons with hyperuricemic disorders:

- *Acute uric acid nephropathy* is caused by the precipitation of uric acid crystals in the renal tubules, principally in collecting ducts, leading to obstruction of nephrons and the development of acute renal failure. This is particularly likely to occur in individuals with leukemias or lymphomas who are undergoing chemotherapy (tumor lysis syndrome); the drugs kill tumor cells, and uric acid is produced as released nucleic acids are broken down. Precipitation of uric acid is favored by the acidic pH in collecting tubules.
- *Chronic urate nephropathy,* or gouty nephropathy, occurs in a subset of patients with protracted forms of

Table 20-9 Causes of Papillary Necrosis

	Diabetes Mellitus	Analgesic Nephropathy	Sickle-Cell Disease	Obstruction
Male-to-female ratio	1:3	1:5	1:1	9:1
Time course	10 years	7 years of abuse	Variable	Variable
Infection	80%	25%	±	90%
Calcification	Rare	Frequent	Rare	Frequent
Number of papillae affected	Several; all of same stage	Almost all; different stages of necrosis	Few	Variable

Data from Seshan S, et al. (eds): Classification and Atlas of Tubulointerstitial and Vascular Diseases. Baltimore, Williams & Wilkins, 1999.

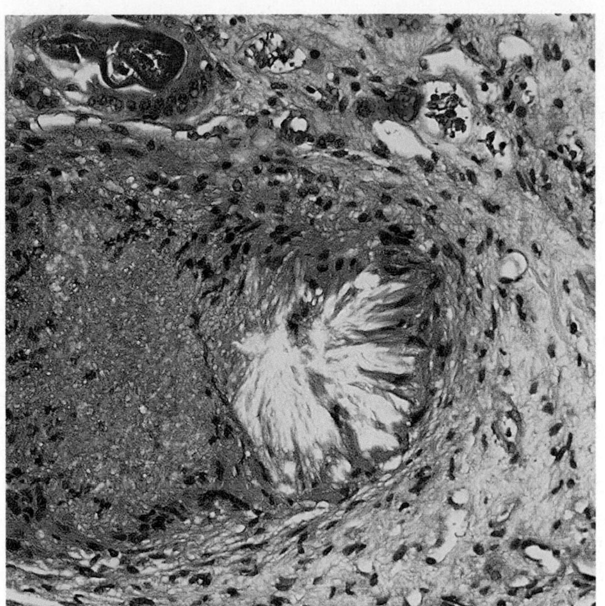

Figure 20-34 Granulomatous inflammation and fibrosis outline the slender urate crystals in the renal medulla.

hyperuricemia. The monosodium urate crystals deposit in the acidic milieu of the distal tubules and collecting ducts as well as in the interstitium, and form distinct birefringent needle-like crystals either in the tubular lumens or in the interstitium (Fig. 20-34). The urate deposits evoke a mononuclear response that contains foreign-body giant cells. This lesion is called a *tophus* (Chapter 26). Tubular obstruction by the urates causes cortical atrophy and scarring. Clinically, urate nephropathy is a subtle disease associated with tubular defects that may progress slowly. Some individuals with gout who develop a chronic nephropathy have evidence of increased exposure to lead.

- *Nephrolithiasis:* uric acid stones are present in 22% of individuals with gout and 42% of those with secondary hyperuricemia (see later discussion of renal stones).

Hypercalcemia and Nephrocalcinosis

Disorders associated with hypercalcemia, such as hyperparathyroidism, multiple myeloma, vitamin D intoxication, metastatic cancer, or excess calcium intake (milk-alkali syndrome), may induce the formation of calcium stones and deposition of calcium in the kidney (nephrocalcinosis). Extensive degrees of calcinosis, under certain conditions, may lead to chronic tubulointerstitial disease and renal insufficiency.

The earliest functional defect is an inability to concentrate the urine. Other tubular defects, such as tubular acidosis and salt-losing nephritis, may also occur. With further damage, a slowly progressive renal insufficiency develops. This is usually due to nephrocalcinosis, but many of these patients also have calcium stones and secondary pyelonephritis.

Acute Phosphate Nephropathy

Extensive accumulations of calcium phosphate crystals in tubules can occur in patients consuming high doses of select oral phosphate solutions in preparation for colonoscopy. These patients are not hypercalcemic, but the excess phosphate load, perhaps complicated by dehydration, causes marked precipitation of calcium phosphate, typically presenting as renal insufficiency several weeks after the exposure. Patients with acute and reversible injury typically recover partial renal function.

Light-Chain Cast Nephropathy ("Myeloma Kidney")

Nonrenal malignant tumors, particularly those of hematopoietic origin, affect the kidneys in several ways (Table 20-10). The most common involvements are tubulointerstitial, caused by complications of the tumor (hypercalcemia, ureteral obstruction) or therapy (irradiation, hyperuricemia, chemotherapy, hematopoietic cell transplantation, infections in immunosuppressed patients). We limit the discussion here to the tubulointerstitial lesions in *multiple myeloma* patients.

Overt renal insufficiency occurs in half of those with multiple myeloma and related lymphoplasmacytic disorders. Several factors contribute to renal damage:

- *Bence-Jones proteinuria and cast nephropathy.* The main cause of renal dysfunction is related to Bence-Jones (light-chain) proteinuria, and correlates with the degree of proteinuria. Two mechanisms seem to account for the renal toxicity of Bence-Jones proteins. First, some Ig light chains are directly toxic to epithelial cells, apparently because of their intrinsic physicochemical properties. Second, Bence-Jones proteins combine with the urinary glycoprotein (Tamm-Horsfall protein) under acidic conditions to form large, histologically distinct tubular casts that obstruct the tubular lumens and induce a characteristic inflammatory reaction (light-chain cast nephropathy).
- *Amyloidosis* of AL type, formed from free light chains (usually of λ type), which occurs in 6% to 24% of individuals with myeloma.
- *Light-chain deposition disease.* In some patients, light chains (usually of κ type) deposit in GBMs and mesangium in nonfibrillar forms, causing a glomerulopathy (described earlier), and in tubular basement membranes, which may cause tubulointerstitial nephritis.
- *Hypercalcemia* and *hyperuricemia* are often present in these patients.

Table 20-10 Renal Disease Related to Nonrenal Neoplasms

Direct or Metastatic Tumor Invasion of Renal Parenchyma
Ureters (obstruction) Artery (renovascular hypertension)
Hypercalcemia
Hyperuricemia
Amyloidosis (Al, Light-Chain Type)
Excretion of Abnormal Proteins (Multiple Myeloma)
Glomerulopathies
Membranous nephropathy, secondary (carcinomas) Minimal-change disease (Hodgkin disease) Membranoproliferative glomerulonephritis (leukemias and lymphomas) Monoclonal immunoglobin/light-chain deposition disease (multiple myeloma)
Effects of Radiation Therapy, Chemotherapy, Hematopoietic Cell Transplantation, Secondary Infection

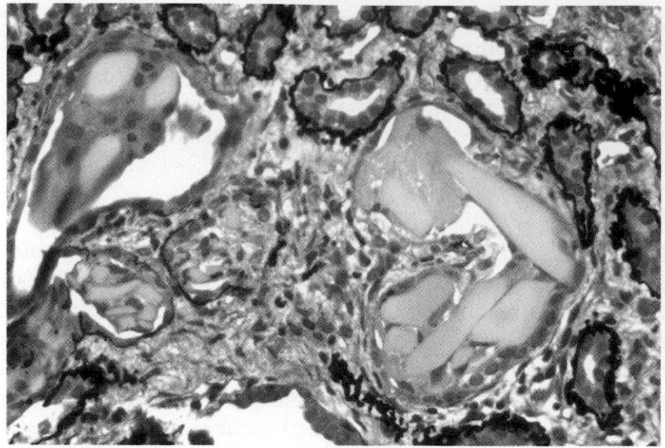

Figure 20-35 Light-chain cast nephropathy. Note the angulated and tubular casts, surrounded by macrophages, including multinucleate cells.

MORPHOLOGY

The tubulointerstitial changes in light-chain cast nephropathy are characteristic. The Bence-Jones tubular casts appear as pink to blue amorphous masses, sometimes concentrically laminated and often fractured, which fill and distend the tubular lumens. Some casts are surrounded by multinucleate giant cells that are derived from activated macrophages (Fig. 20-35). The adjacent interstitial tissue usually shows an inflammatory response and fibrosis. On occasion, the casts rupture the tubules, evoking a granulomatous inflammatory reaction. Amyloidosis, light-chain deposition disease, nephrocalcinosis, and infection may also be present.

Clinical Features. Clinically, the renal manifestations are of several types. In the most common form, *chronic kidney disease* develops insidiously and progresses slowly during a period of several months to years. Another form occurs suddenly and is manifested by *acute kidney injury* with oliguria. Precipitating factors include dehydration, hypercalcemia, acute infection, and treatment with nephrotoxic antibiotics. *Bence-Jones proteinuria* occurs in 70% of individuals with multiple myeloma; the presence of significant non-light-chain proteinuria (e.g., albuminuria) suggests AL amyloidosis or light-chain deposition disease.

Bile Cast Nephropathy

Hepatorenal syndrome refers to impairment of renal function in patients with acute or chronic liver disease with advanced liver failure. In this setting, serum bilirubin levels can be markedly elevated, particularly in jaundiced patients, with bile cast formation (also known as cholemic nephrosis) in distal nephron segments. The casts can extend to proximal tubules, resulting in both direct toxic effects on tubular epithelial cells and obstruction of the involved nephron. This mechanism of injury is analogous to that with myeloma protein and myoglobin casts. The tubular bile casts can range from yellowish-green to pink and contain variable degrees of sloughed cells or cellular debris. The reversibility of the renal injury depends upon the severity and duration of the liver dysfunction.

Vascular Diseases

Nearly all diseases of the kidney involve the renal blood vessels secondarily. Systemic vascular diseases, such as various forms of vasculitis, also affect renal vessels, and their effects on the kidney are often clinically important. Hypertension, as we discussed in Chapter 11, is intimately linked with the kidney, because kidney disease can be both a cause and consequence of increased blood pressure. In this chapter we discuss nephrosclerosis and renal artery stenosis, lesions associated with hypertension, and sundry lesions involving mostly smaller vessels of the kidney.

Nephrosclerosis

***Nephrosclerosis* is the term used for the renal pathology associated with sclerosis of renal arterioles and small arteries and is strongly associated with hypertension, which can be both a cause and a consequence of nephrosclerosis.** The affected vessels have thickened walls and consequently narrowed lumens, changes that result in focal parenchymal ischemia. Ischemia leads to glomerulosclerosis and chronic tubulointerstitial injury, and produces a reduction in functional renal mass. Nephrosclerosis at autopsy is associated with advanced age, is more frequent in blacks than whites, and may be seen in the absence of hypertension. Hypertension and diabetes mellitus, however, increase the incidence and severity of the lesions.

Pathogenesis. Two processes participate in the arterial lesions:

- Medial and intimal thickening, as a response to hemodynamic changes, aging, genetic defects, or some combination of these
- Hyalinization of arteriolar walls, caused by extravasation of plasma proteins through injured endothelium and by increased deposition of basement membrane matrix

MORPHOLOGY

The kidneys are either normal or moderately reduced in size, with average weights between 110 and 130 gm. The cortical surfaces have a fine, even granularity that resembles grain leather (Fig. 20-36). The loss of mass is due mainly to **cortical scarring and shrinking.**

On histologic examination there is narrowing of the lumens of arterioles and small arteries, caused by thickening and hyalinization of the walls **(hyaline arteriolosclerosis)** (Fig. 20-37). Corresponding to the finely granular surface are microscopic subcapsular scars with sclerotic glomeruli and tubular dropout, alternating with better preserved parenchyma. In addition, the interlobular and arcuate arteries show medial hypertrophy, replication of the internal elastic lamina, and increased myofibroblastic tissue in the intima, all of which narrow the lumen. This change, called fibroelastic hyperplasia, often accompanies hyaline arteriolosclerosis and increases in severity with age and in the presence of hypertension.

Consequent to the vascular narrowing, there is patchy ischemic atrophy, which consists of (1) foci of **tubular atrophy and interstitial fibrosis** and (2) a variety of **glomerular**

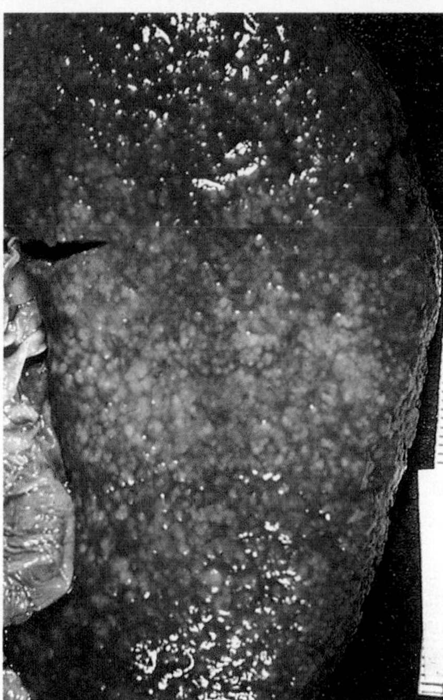

Figure 20-36 Close-up of the gross appearance of the cortical surface in benign nephrosclerosis illustrating the fine, leathery granularity of the surface.

alterations. The latter include collapse of the GBM, deposition of collagen within Bowman space, periglomerular fibrosis, and total sclerosis of glomeruli. When the ischemic changes are pronounced and affect large areas of parenchyma, they can produce wedge shaped infarcts or regional scars with histologic alterations that may resemble those in renal ablation injury, mentioned earlier.

Clinical Features. It is unusual for uncomplicated nephrosclerosis to cause renal insufficiency or uremia. However, three groups of hypertensive patients with nephrosclerosis are at increased risk of developing renal failure: people of African descent, people with severe blood pressure elevations, and persons with a second underlying disease, especially diabetes. In these groups renal insufficiency may supervene after prolonged hypertension, but rapid renal failure results from the development of the malignant or accelerated phase of hypertension, discussed next.

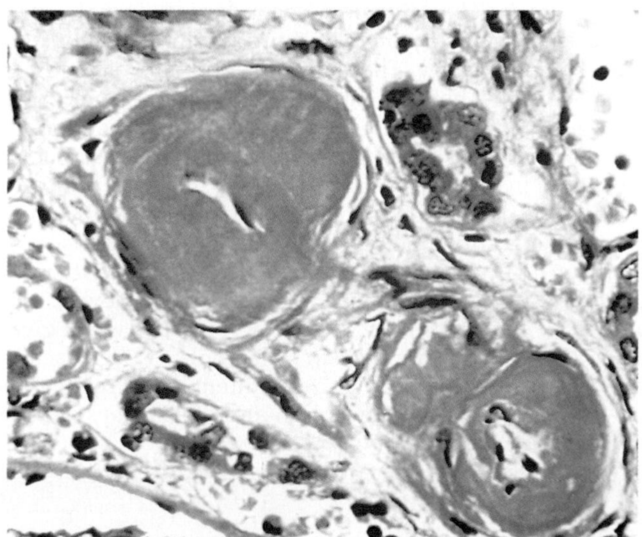

Figure 20-37 Hyaline arteriolosclerosis. High-power view of two arterioles with hyaline deposition, marked thickening of the walls, and a narrowed lumen. (Courtesy Dr. M.A. Venkatachalam, Department of Pathology, University of Texas Health Sciences Center, San Antonio, Tex.)

Malignant Nephrosclerosis

Malignant nephrosclerosis is a renal vascular disorder associated with malignant or accelerated hypertension. It occasionally develops suddenly in previously normotensive individuals but more often is superimposed on preexisting essential hypertension, secondary forms of hypertension, or an underlying chronic renal disease, particularly glomerulonephritis or reflux nephropathy. It is also a frequent cause of renal failure in individuals with systemic sclerosis. Malignant hypertension is relatively uncommon, occurring in 1% to 5% of all people with elevated blood pressure. In its pure form it usually affects younger individuals, and occurs more often in men and in blacks.

Pathogenesis. **The fundamental lesion in malignant nephrosclerosis is vascular injury.** The initial insult seems to be some form of vascular damage to the kidneys that might result from a variety of disorders, including longstanding hypertension, arteritis, or a coagulopathy, alone or in combination. The initiating event injures endothelium and results in increased permeability of the small vessels to fibrinogen and other plasma proteins, focal death of cells of the vascular wall, and platelet deposition. This can lead to *fibrinoid necrosis* of arterioles and small arteries, with activation of platelets and coagulation factors causing intravascular thrombosis. Mitogenic factors from platelets (e.g., PDGF), plasma, and other cells cause hyperplasia of intimal smooth muscle of vessels, resulting in the hyperplastic arteriolosclerosis that is typical of malignant hypertension and responsible for further narrowing of the lumens. The kidneys become markedly ischemic. With severe involvement of the renal afferent arterioles, the renin-angiotensin system receives a powerful stimulus; indeed, **patients with malignant hypertension have markedly elevated levels of plasma renin**. This sets up a self-perpetuating cycle in which angiotensin II causes intrarenal vasoconstriction, and the attendant renal ischemia perpetuates renin secretion.

MORPHOLOGY

The kidney size varies depending on the duration and severity of the hypertensive disease. Small, pinpoint **petechial hemorrhages** may appear on the cortical surface from rupture of arterioles or glomerular capillaries, giving the kidney a peculiar "flea-bitten" appearance.

Two histologic alterations characterize blood vessels in malignant hypertension (Fig. 20-38):

- **Fibrinoid necrosis of arterioles.** In this form of necrosis, cytologic detail is lost and the vessel wall takes on a smudgy eosinophilic appearance due to fibrin deposition. Inflammation is usually not seen or is minimal. Sometimes the glomeruli become necrotic and infiltrated with neutrophils, and the glomerular capillaries may thrombose.

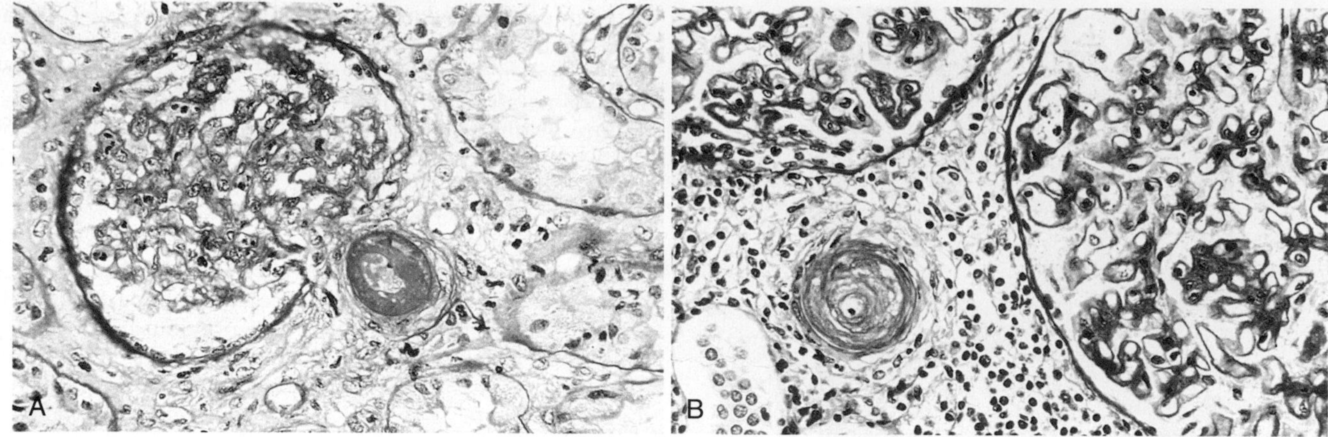

Figure 20-38 Accelerated hypertension. **A,** Fibrinoid necrosis of afferent arteriole (PAS stain). **B,** Hyperplastic arteriolitis (onion-skin lesion). (Courtesy Dr. H. Rennke, Brigham and Women's Hospital, Boston, Mass.)

- In the interlobular arteries and arterioles, there is intimal thickening caused by a proliferation of elongated, concentrically arranged smooth muscle cells, together with fine concentric layering of collagen and accumulation of pale-staining material that probably represents deposition of proteoglycans and plasma proteins. This alteration has been referred to as **onion-skinning** because of its concentric appearance. The lesion, also called **hyperplastic arteriolitis**, correlates with renal failure. There may be superimposed intraluminal thrombosis. The arteriolar and arterial lesions result in considerable narrowing of all vascular lumens, ischemic atrophy and, at times, infarction distal to the abnormal vessels.

Clinical Features. The full-blown syndrome of malignant hypertension is characterized by systolic pressures greater than 200 mm Hg and diastolic pressures greater than 120 mm Hg, papilledema, retinal hemorrhages, encephalopathy, cardiovascular abnormalities, and renal failure. Most often, the early symptoms are related to increased intracranial pressure and include headaches, nausea, vomiting, and visual impairments, particularly scotomas or spots before the eyes. "Hypertensive crises" are sometimes encountered, characterized by loss of consciousness or even convulsions. At the onset, there may only be marked proteinuria and microscopic or macroscopic hematuria, but renal failure soon ensues. The syndrome is a medical emergency requiring aggressive and prompt antihypertensive therapy to prevent irreversible renal injury. Before the development of current antihypertensive drugs, malignant hypertension was associated with a 50% mortality rate within 3 months of onset, progressing to 90% within a year. At present, however, about 75% of patients survive 5 years, and 50% survive with restoration of pre-crisis renal function.

KEY CONCEPTS

Nephrosclerosis

- Nephrosclerosis, which is commonly associated with hypertension, is defined by the presence of varying degrees of glomerulosclerosis, interstitial fibrosis and tubular atrophy, arteriosclerosis, and arteriolosclerosis.
- Luminal reduction of the renal vasculature (arteries and arterioles) contributes to glomerulosclerosis (both global and segmental), which can subsequently cause interstitial fibrosis and tubular atrophy.
- Malignant nephrosclerosis is associated with malignant hypertension. The renal lesions manifest as fibrinoid necrosis of arterioles and hyperplastic arteriolosclerosis. The latter lesion affects interlobular arteries and arterioles and is characterized by proliferation of smooth muscle cells of the arterial wall that are arranged concentrically.

Renal Artery Stenosis

Unilateral renal artery stenosis is responsible for 2% to 5% of hypertension cases, and is important to recognize because it is potentially curable by surgery. Furthermore, important insights into renal mechanisms of hypertension came from studies of experimental and human renal artery stenosis.

Pathogenesis. **Hypertension secondary to renal artery stenosis is caused by increased production of renin from the ischemic kidney.** The classic experiments of Goldblatt and colleagues showed that constriction of one renal artery in dogs results in hypertension and that the magnitude of the effect is proportional to the amount of narrowing. Elevation in blood pressure, at least initially, is due to stimulation of renin secretion by the juxtaglomerular apparatus and the subsequent production of the vasoconstrictor angiotensin II. A large proportion of individuals with renovascular hypertension have elevated renin levels, and almost all show a reduction of blood pressure when given drugs that block angiotensin II activity. Other factors, however, may contribute to the maintenance of renovascular hypertension after the renin-angiotensin system has initiated it, including *sodium retention.*

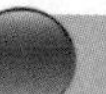

MORPHOLOGY

The most common cause of renal artery stenosis (70% of cases) is narrowing at the origin of the renal artery by an atheromatous plaque. This occurs more frequently in men, and the incidence increases with advancing age and diabetes mellitus.

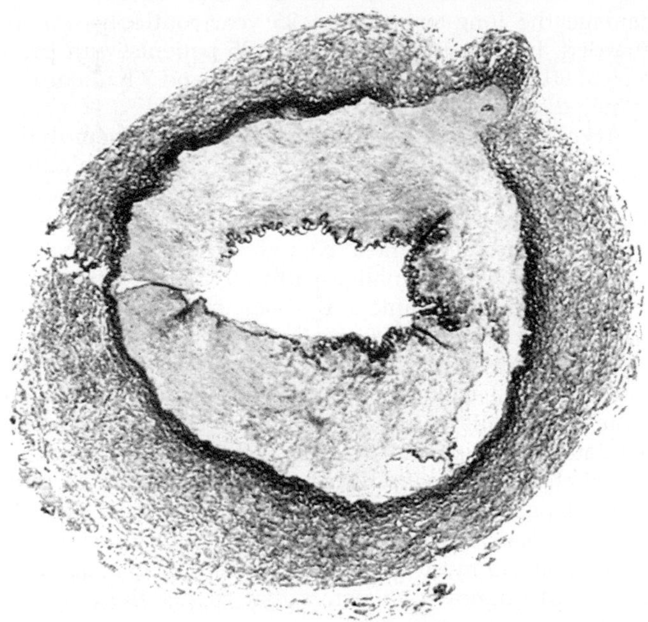

Figure 20-39 Fibromuscular dysplasia of the renal artery, medial type (elastic tissue stain). The media shows marked fibrous thickening, and the lumen is stenotic. (Courtesy Dr. Seymour Rosen, Beth Israel Hospital, Boston, Mass.)

The plaque is usually concentrically placed, and superimposed thrombosis often occurs.

The second most frequent cause of stenosis is **fibromuscular dysplasia** of the renal artery. This heterogeneous entity is characterized by fibrous or fibromuscular thickening that may involve the intima, the media, or the adventitia of the artery (Fig. 20-39). The stenoses, as a whole, are more common in women and tend to occur in younger age groups (i.e., in the third and fourth decades).

The ischemic kidney is reduced in size and shows signs of **diffuse ischemic atrophy**, with crowded glomeruli, atrophic tubules, interstitial fibrosis, and focal inflammatory infiltrates. The arterioles in the ischemic kidney are usually protected from the effects of high pressure, thus showing only mild arteriolosclerosis. In contrast, the contralateral nonischemic kidney may show more severe arteriolosclerosis, depending on the severity of the hypertension.

Clinical Course. Few distinctive features suggest the presence of renal artery stenosis, and in general, these patients resemble those with essential hypertension. On occasion, a bruit can be heard on auscultation of the affected kidneys. Elevated plasma or renal vein renin, response to angiotensin-converting enzyme inhibitor, renal scans, and intravenous pyelography may aid with diagnosis, but arteriography is required to localize the stenotic lesion. The cure rate after surgery is 70% to 80% in well-selected cases.

Thrombotic Microangiopathies

The term *thrombotic microangiopathy* encompasses a spectrum of clinical syndromes that includes thrombotic thrombocytopenic purpura (TTP) and hemolytic-uremic syndrome (HUS). As already discussed in Chapter 14, **HUS and TTP are caused by diverse insults that lead to the excessive activation of platelets, which deposit as thrombi in capillaries and arterioles in various tissue beds, including those of the kidney** (Fig. 20-40). Widespread "consumption" of platelets leads to thrombocytopenia, and the resulting thrombi create flow abnormalities that shear red cells, producing a microangiopathic hemolytic anemia. Of even greater importance, the thrombi produce microvascular occlusions that cause tissue ischemia and organ dysfunction.

This group of disorders is now classified according to the current understanding of their causes or associations, as follows:

- *Typical HUS (synonyms: epidemic, classic, diarrhea-positive)*, most frequently associated with consumption of food contaminated by bacteria producing Shiga-like toxins
- *Atypical HUS (synonyms: non-epidemic, diarrhea-negative)*, associated with:
  - Inherited mutations of complement-regulatory proteins
  - Diverse acquired causes of endothelial injury, including: antiphospholipid antibodies; complications of pregnancy and oral contraceptives; vascular renal diseases such as scleroderma and hypertension; chemotherapeutic and immunosuppressive drugs; and radiation
- *TTP*, which is often associated with inherited or acquired deficiencies of ADAMTS13, a plasma metalloprotease that regulates the function of von Willebrand factor (vWF)

Pathogenesis. Within the thrombotic microangiopathies, two pathogenetic triggers dominate: (1) *endothelial injury*, and (2) *excessive platelet activation and aggregation*. As will be discussed, endothelial injury appears to be the primary cause of HUS, whereas platelet activation may be the inciting event in TTP.

Endothelial injury. In typical (epidemic, classic, diarrhea-positive) HUS, the trigger for endothelial injury and activation is usually a Shiga-like toxin, while for inherited forms of atypical HUS the cause of the endothelial injury appears to be excessive, inappropriate activation of complement. Many other exposures and conditions can occasionally precipitate a HUS-like picture, presumably also by injuring the endothelium. The endothelial injury in

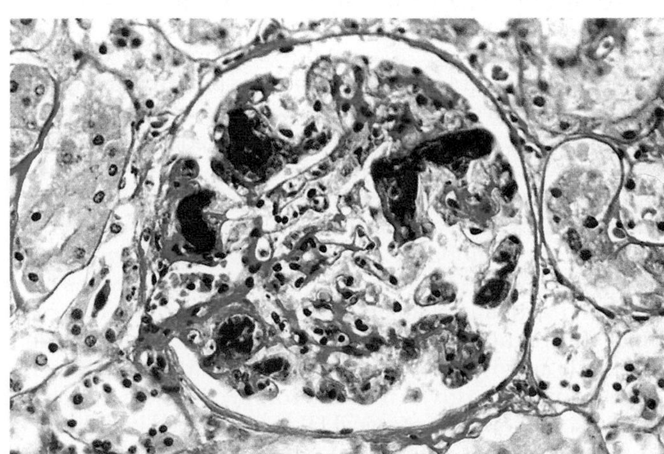

Figure 20-40 Fibrin stain showing platelet-fibrin thrombi (*red*) in the glomerular capillaries, characteristic of thrombotic microangiopathic disorders.

HUS appears to cause platelet activation and thrombosis within microvascular beds. There is evidence that reduced endothelial production of prostaglandin I_2 and NO (both inhibitors of platelet aggregation) contributes to thrombosis. The reduction in these two factors and increased production of endothelium-derived endothelin may also promote vasoconstriction, exacerbating the hypoperfusion of tissues.

Platelet aggregation. In contrast to HUS, in TTP the initiating event appears to be platelet aggregation induced by very large multimers of vWF, which accumulate due to a deficiency of ADAMTS13, a plasma protease that cleaves vWF multimers into smaller sizes. The deficiency of ADAMTS13 is most often caused by autoantibodies that inhibit ADAMTS13 function. Less commonly, a chronic relapsing and remitting form of TTP is associated with inherited deficiencies of ADAMTS13. Very large vWF multimers can bind platelet surface glycoproteins and activate platelets spontaneously, providing a pathophysiologic explanation for the microthrombi that are observed in vascular beds.

With this as an introduction, we will now briefly delve into the various subtypes of HUS/TTP and then return to the morphologic features that are common to all.

Typical (epidemic, classic, diarrhea-positive) hemolytic uremic syndrome. This is the best-characterized form of HUS. Most cases occur following intestinal infection with strains of *E. coli* (the most common being O157:H7) that produce Shiga-like toxins, so-called because they resemble those made by *Shigella dysenteriae* (Chapter 17). Epidemics have been traced to various sources, most commonly the ingestion of contaminated ground meat (as in hamburgers), but also drinking water, raw milk, and person-to-person transmission. However, most cases of typical HUS caused by *E. coli* are sporadic. Less commonly, infections by other agents, including *Shigella dysenteriae*, can give rise to a similar clinical picture.

Typical HUS can occur at any age, but children and older adults are at highest risk. Following a prodrome of influenza-like or diarrheal symptoms, there is a sudden onset of bleeding manifestations (especially hematemesis and melena), severe oliguria, and hematuria, associated with microangiopathic hemolytic anemia, thrombocytopenia, and (in some patients) prominent neurologic changes. Hypertension is present in about half the patients.

Precisely how Shiga-like toxin exposure causes HUS is not well understood. According to one model the toxin "activates" endothelial cells, which respond by increasing their expression of leukocyte adhesion molecules and endothelin and decreasing nitric oxide production. In the presence of cytokines such as TNF, Shiga-like toxin may cause endothelial apoptosis. These alterations lead to platelet activation and induce vasoconstriction, resulting in the characteristic microangiopathy. But other possibilities remain. For example, there is some evidence that Shiga-like toxins may bind and activate platelets directly; or alternatively, may bind the regulatory complement protein Factor H and inhibit its activity, causing hyperactivation of complement, an intriguing idea given the clear role of complement activation in some forms of atypical HUS (described below).

In typical HUS, if the renal failure is managed properly with dialysis, most patients recover normal renal function in a matter of weeks. However, due to underlying renal damage the long-term (15 to 25 year) outlook is more guarded. In one study, only 10 of 25 patients with prior typical HUS had normal renal function, and 7 had chronic kidney disease.

Atypical (non-epidemic, diarrhea-negative) hemolytic-uremic syndrome. Atypical HUS occurs mainly in adults in a number of different settings. More than half of those affected have an inherited deficiency of complement-regulatory proteins, most commonly Factor H, which breaks down the alternative pathway C3 convertase and protects cells from damage by uncontrolled complement activation (Chapter 3). A small number of patients have mutations in two other proteins that regulate complement, complement Factor I and CD46 (membrane cofactor protein). Patients with genetic mutations in complement-regulatory proteins may develop HUS at any age. Roughly half of affected individuals have a course marked by multiple relapses and progression to end-stage renal disease. As the deficiencies in complement-regulatory factors are life-long, it is a mystery why the onset of HUS is delayed; additional unknown co-factors that trigger the development of HUS are suspected.

The remaining cases of atypical HUS arise in association with a variety of miscellaneous conditions or exposures. These include:

- The *antiphospholipid syndrome*, either primary or secondary to SLE (lupus anticoagulant). The syndrome is described in detail in Chapter 4. In this setting the microangiopathy tends to follow a chronic course.
- Complications of pregnancy or the postpartum period. So-called *postpartum renal failure* is a form of HUS that usually occurs after an uneventful pregnancy, 1 day to several months after delivery. The condition has a grave prognosis, although recovery can occur in milder cases.
- *Vascular diseases affecting the kidney*, such as systemic sclerosis and malignant hypertension.
- Chemotherapeutic and immunosuppressive drugs, such as mitomycin, cyclosporine, cisplatin, gemcitabine, and antagonists of VEGF.
- Irradiation of the kidney.

Patients with atypical HUS do not fare as well as those with typical HUS, in large part because the underlying conditions may be chronic and difficult to treat. As in typical HUS, some patients have neurologic symptoms; the disease in these patients can be distinguished from TTP by the presence of normal ADAMTS13 levels in the plasma (see later).

Thrombotic Thrombocytopenic Purpura. TTP is classically manifested by the pentad of fever, neurologic symptoms, microangiopathic hemolytic anemia, thrombocytopenia, and renal failure. The most common cause of deficient ADAMTS13 activity is inhibitory autoantibodies, and the majority with such antibodies are women. Regardless of cause, most patients present as adults at ages younger than 40. Less commonly, patients inherit an inactivating mutation in *ADAMTS13*. In those with hereditary ADAMTS13 deficiency, the onset is often delayed until adolescence and the symptoms are episodic. Thus, factors other than ADAMTS13 (e.g., some superimposed vascular injury or prothrombotic state) must be involved in triggering full-blown TTP.

For unknown reasons, in TTP, central nervous system involvement is the dominant feature, whereas renal involvement is seen in about 50% of patients. The clinical findings are dictated by the distribution of the microthrombi, which are found in arterioles throughout the body. With plasma exchange, which removes autoantibodies and provides functional ADAMTS13, TTP (which once was uniformly fatal) can be treated successfully in more than 80% of patients.

MORPHOLOGY

The morphologic findings in the various forms of HUS/TTP show considerable overlap, and vary mainly according to chronicity rather than cause. In acute, active disease the kidney may show patchy or diffuse cortical necrosis (described later) and subcapsular petechiae. On microscopic examination, the glomerular capillaries are occluded by thrombi composed of aggregated platelets and to a lesser extent fibrin. The capillary walls are thickened due to endothelial cell swelling and subendothelial deposits of cell debris and fibrin. Disruption of the mesangial matrix and damage to the mesangial cells often results in mesangiolysis. Interlobular arteries and arterioles often show fibrinoid necrosis of the wall and occlusive thrombi. Chronic disease is confined to patients with atypical HUS or TTP, and has features that stem from continued injury and attempts at healing. The renal cortex reveals various degrees of scarring. By light microscopy the glomeruli are mildly hypercellular and have marked thickening of the capillary walls associated with splitting or reduplication of the basement membrane (so called double contours or tram tracks). The walls of arteries and arterioles often exhibit increased layers of cells and connective tissue ("onion-skinning") that narrow the vessel lumens. These changes lead to persistent hypoperfusion and ischemic atrophy of the parenchyma, which manifests clinically as renal failure and hypertension.

KEY CONCEPTS

Thrombotic Microangiopathy

- Thrombotic microangiopathy encompasses a diverse set of conditions that all lead to platelet activation and deposition of thrombi in the microvasculature, accompanied by red cell hemolysis, tissue ischemia and organ dysfunction, and a consumptive thrombocytopenia.
- In typical HUS, Shiga-like toxin produced by bacteria, most commonly *E. coli* strain O157:H7, is responsible for producing platelet activation and thrombosis.
- In most cases of atypical HUS, aberration activation of complement due to inherited mutations or acquired autoantibodies is the key pathogenic abnormality.
- In TTP, deficiencies of ADAMTS13, a negative regulator of vWF, permits the formation of abnormally large multimers of vWF that are capable of activating platelets.

Other Vascular Disorders

Atherosclerotic Ischemic Renal Disease

We have seen that atherosclerotic unilateral renal artery stenosis can lead to hypertension. *Bilateral renal artery disease*, usually diagnosed definitively by arteriography, is a fairly common cause of chronic ischemia with renal insufficiency in older individuals, sometimes in the absence of hypertension. The importance of recognizing this condition is that surgical revascularization can prevent further decline in renal function.

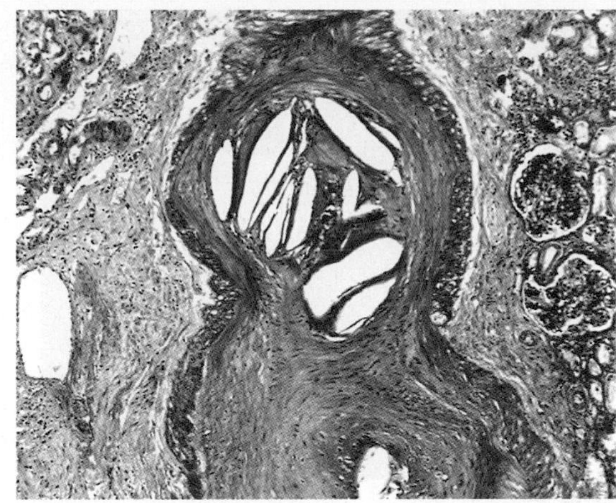

Figure 20-41 Atheroemboli with typical cholesterol clefts in an interlobar artery.

Atheroembolic Renal Disease

Embolization of fragments of atheromatous plaques from the aorta or renal artery into intrarenal vessels occurs in older adults with severe atherosclerosis, especially after surgery on the abdominal aorta, aortography, or intra-aortic cannulization. These emboli can be recognized in the lumens of arcuate and interlobular arteries by their content of cholesterol crystals, which appear as rhomboid clefts (Fig. 20-41). The clinical consequences of atheroemboli vary according to the number of emboli and the preexisting state of renal function. Frequently they are of no significance. However, acute renal injury or failure may develop in older adults in whom renal function is already compromised.

Sickle-Cell Nephropathy

Sickle-cell disease (homozygous) or trait (heterozygous) may lead to a variety of alterations in renal morphology and function, some of which produce clinically significant abnormalities. The various manifestations are grouped under *sickle-cell nephropathy*.

The most common abnormalities are *hematuria* and a *diminished concentrating ability* (hyposthenuria). These are thought to be due to accelerated sickling in the hypertonic hypoxic milieu of the renal medulla; the hyperosmolarity dehydrates red cells and increases intracellular HbS concentrations, which likely explains why even those with sickle trait are affected. Patchy *papillary necrosis* may occur in both homozygotes and heterozygotes; this is sometimes associated with cortical scarring. *Proteinuria* is also common in sickle-cell disease, occurring in about 30% of patients. It is usually mild to moderate, but on occasion the overt nephrotic syndrome arises, associated with sclerosing glomerular lesions.

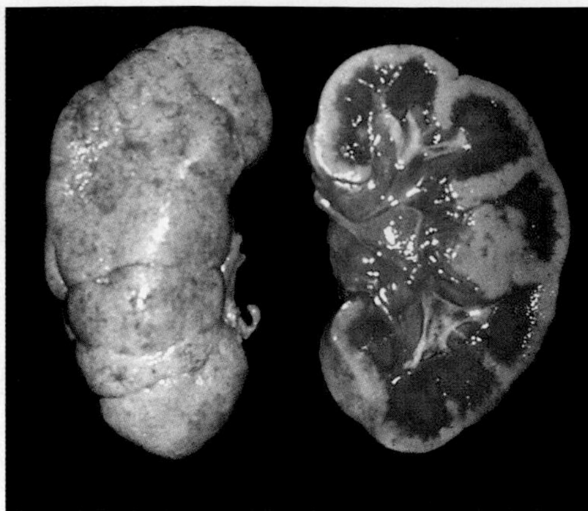

Figure 20-42 Diffuse cortical necrosis. The pale ischemic necrotic areas are confined to the cortex and columns of Bertin.

Diffuse Cortical Necrosis

This uncommon condition occurs most frequently after an obstetric emergency, such as abruptio placentae (premature separation of the placenta), septic shock, or extensive surgery. The cortical destruction has the features of ischemic necrosis. Glomerular and arteriolar microthrombi are often found and contribute to the necrosis and renal damage. The morphologic features considerably overlap with thrombotic microangiopathy and disseminated intravascular coagulation, but the pathogenic sequence of events remains obscure.

MORPHOLOGY

The gross alterations of massive ischemic necrosis are sharply limited to the cortex (Fig. 20-42). The histologic appearance is that of acute ischemic infarction. The lesions may be patchy, with areas of coagulative necrosis and apparently better preserved cortex. Intravascular and intraglomerular thromboses may be prominent but are usually focal, and acute necroses of small arterioles and capillaries may occasionally be present. Hemorrhages occur into the glomeruli, together with the formation of fibrin plugs in the glomerular capillaries.

Massive acute cortical necrosis is of grave significance, since it gives rise to sudden anuria, terminating rapidly in uremic death. Instances of unilateral or patchy involvement are compatible with survival.

Renal Infarcts

The kidneys are common sites for the development of infarcts. Contributing to this predisposition is the extensive blood flow to the kidneys (one fourth of the cardiac output), but probably more important is the limited collateral circulation from extrarenal sites (small blood vessels penetrating from the renal capsule supply only the very outer rim of the cortex). Although thrombosis in advanced atherosclerosis and the acute vasculitis of polyarteritis nodosa may occlude arteries, most infarcts are due to embolism. A major source of such emboli is mural thrombosis in the left atrium and ventricle as a result of myocardial infarction. Vegetative endocarditis, aortic aneurysms, and aortic atherosclerosis are less frequent sources of emboli.

MORPHOLOGY

Because of the lack of a collateral blood supply, most renal infarcts are of the "white" anemic variety. Within 24 hours infarcts become sharply demarcated, pale, yellow-white areas that may contain small irregular foci of hemorrhagic discoloration. They are usually ringed by a zone of intense hyperemia.

The infarcts are wedge-shaped, with the base against the cortical surface and the apex pointing toward the medulla. In time these acute areas of ischemic necrosis undergo progressive fibrous scarring, giving rise to depressed, pale, gray-white scars that assume a V-shape on section. The histologic changes in renal infarcts are those of ischemic coagulative necrosis, described in Chapter 2.

Many renal infarcts are clinically silent. Sometimes, pain with tenderness localized to the costovertebral angle occurs, associated with showers of red cells in the urine. Large infarcts of one kidney are probably associated with narrowing of the renal artery or one of its major branches, which in turn may cause hypertension.

Congenital and Developmental Anomalies

About 10% of people are born with significant malformations of the urinary system. Renal dysplasias and hypoplasias account for 20% of chronic kidney disease in children.

Congenital renal disease can be hereditary but most often results from an acquired developmental defect during gestation. As discussed in Chapter 10, defects in genes involved in normal renal development, including the Wilms tumor-associated genes, understandably cause urogenital anomalies. As a rule, the resulting developmental abnormalities involve structural components of both the kidney and urinary tract. Other genetic defects primarily produce functional abnormalities in tubular transport, such as cystinuria and renal tubular acidosis. Here, we restrict the discussion to structural anomalies involving primarily the kidney. All except horseshoe kidney are uncommon. Anomalies of the lower urinary tract are discussed in Chapter 21.

Agenesis of the Kidney. Bilateral agenesis is incompatible with life, and usually encountered in stillborn infants. It is often associated with other congenital disorders (e.g., limb defects, hypoplastic lungs). Unilateral agenesis is uncommon and compatible with normal life if no other abnormalities exist. The solitary kidney enlarges as a result of compensatory hypertrophy. Some patients eventually develop progressive glomerular sclerosis in the remaining kidney as a result of the adaptive changes in hypertrophied nephrons, discussed earlier in the chapter, and in time, chronic kidney disease ensues.

Hypoplasia. Hypoplasia refers to failure of the kidneys to develop to a normal size. This anomaly may occur bilaterally, resulting in renal failure in early childhood, but it is more commonly encountered as a unilateral defect. True renal hypoplasia is observed in low birth weight infants and may contribute to their increased lifetime risk for chronic kidney disease. Differentiation between congenital and acquired atrophic kidneys may be impossible, but a truly hypoplastic kidney shows no scars and has a reduced number of renal lobes and pyramids, usually six or fewer.

Ectopic Kidneys. The development of the metanephros into the kidneys may occur in ectopic foci. These kidneys lie either just above the pelvic brim or sometimes within the pelvis. They are usually normal or slightly small in size but otherwise are not remarkable. Because of their abnormal position, kinking or tortuosity of the ureters may cause obstruction to urinary flow, which predisposes to bacterial infections.

Horseshoe Kidneys. Fusion of the upper (10%) or lower poles (90%) of the kidneys produces a horseshoe-shaped structure that is continuous across the midline anterior to the great vessels. This anomaly is found in 1 in 500 to 1000 autopsies.

Cystic Diseases of the Kidney

Cystic diseases of the kidney are heterogeneous, comprising hereditary, developmental, and acquired disorders. They are important for several reasons: (1) They are reasonably common and often represent diagnostic problems for clinicians, radiologists, and pathologists; (2) some forms, such as adult polycystic kidney disease, are major causes of chronic kidney disease; and (3) they can occasionally be confused with malignant tumors. A useful classification of renal cysts is as follows:

- Polycystic kidney disease
  - Autosomal dominant (adult) polycystic disease
  - Autosomal recessive (childhood) polycystic disease
- Medullary cystic disease
  - Medullary sponge kidney
  - Nephronophthisis
- Multicystic renal dysplasia
- Acquired (dialysis-associated) cystic disease
- Localized (simple) renal cysts
- Renal cysts in hereditary malformation syndromes (e.g., tuberous sclerosis)
- Glomerulocystic disease
- Extraparenchymal renal cysts (pyelocalyceal cysts, hilar lymphangitic cysts)

Only the more important of the cystic diseases are discussed later. Table 20-11 summarizes the characteristic features of the principal renal cystic diseases.

Autosomal Dominant (Adult) Polycystic Kidney Disease

Autosomal dominant (adult) polycystic kidney disease is a hereditary disorder characterized by multiple expanding cysts of both kidneys that ultimately destroy the renal parenchyma and cause renal failure. It is a common condition affecting roughly 1 of every 400 to 1000 live births and accounting for about 5% to 10% of cases of end-stage renal disease requiring transplantation or dialysis. The inheritance pattern is autosomal dominant with high

Table 20-11 Summary of Renal Cystic Diseases

Disease	Inheritance	Pathologic Features	Clinical Features or Complications	Typical Outcome	Diagrammatic Representation
Adult polycystic kidney disease	Autosomal dominant	Large multicystic kidneys, liver cysts, berry aneurysms	Hematuria, flank pain, urinary tract infection, renal stones, hypertension	Chronic renal failure beginning at age 40-60 years	
Childhood polycystic kidney disease	Autosomal recessive	Enlarged, cystic kidneys at birth	Hepatic fibrosis	Variable, death in infancy or childhood	
Medullary sponge kidney	None	Medullary cysts on excretory urography	Hematuria, urinary tract infection, recurrent renal stones	Benign	
Familial juvenile nephronophthisis	Autosomal recessive	Corticomedullary cysts, shrunken kidneys	Salt wasting, polyuria, growth retardation, anemia	Progressive renal failure beginning in childhood	
Adult-onset medullary cystic disease	Autosomal dominant	Corticomedullary cysts, shrunken kidneys	Salt wasting, polyuria	Chronic renal failure beginning in adulthood	
Multicystic renal dysplasia	None	Irregular kidneys with cysts of variable size	Association with other renal anomalies	Renal failure if bilateral, surgically curable if unilateral	
Acquired renal cystic disease	None	Cystic degeneration in end-stage kidney disease	Hemorrhage, erythrocytosis, neoplasia	Dependence on dialysis	
Simple cysts	None	Single or multiple cysts in normal-sized kidneys	Microscopic hematuria	Benign	

penetrance. Although the susceptibility to develop this disease is inherited as an autosomal dominant trait, as with tumor suppressor genes, both alleles of the involved genes have to be nonfunctional for development of the disease. Thus, individuals prone to autosomal dominant polycystic kidney disease inherit one copy of a mutated APKD gene, and mutation of the other allele is acquired in the somatic cells of the kidney. The disease is bilateral; reported unilateral cases probably represent multicystic dysplasia. The cysts initially involve a minority of the nephrons, so renal function is retained until about the fourth or fifth decade of life.

Genetics and Pathogenesis. A wide range of different mutations in *PKD1* and *PKD2* has been described, and this allelic heterogeneity has complicated genetic diagnosis of this disorder.

- The *PKD1* gene is located on chromosome 16p13.3. It encodes a large (460-kD) integral membrane protein named *polycystin-1,* which has a large extracellular region, multiple transmembrane domains, and a short cytoplasmic tail. Polycystin-1 is expressed in tubular epithelial cells, particularly those of the distal nephron. At present its precise function is not known, but it contains domains that are usually involved in cell-cell and cell-matrix interactions. Mutations in *PKD1* account for about 85% of cases. In individuals with these mutations, the likelihood of developing renal failure is less than 5% by 40 years of age, rising to more than 35% by 50 years, more than 70% at 60 years of age, and more than 95% by 70 years of age.
- The *PKD2* gene, located on chromosome 4q21, accounts for most of the remaining cases of polycystic disease. Its product, *polycystin-2,* is an integral membrane protein that is expressed in all segments of the renal tubules and in many extrarenal tissues. Polycystin-2 functions as a Ca2+-permeable cation channel. Overall, the disease is less severe than that associated with *PKD1* mutations. Renal failure occurs in less than 5% of patients with *PKD2* mutations at 50 years of age, but this rises to 15% at 60 years of age, and 45% at 70 years of age.

The pathogenesis of polycystic disease is not established, but the currently favored hypothesis places the cilia-centrosome complex of tubular epithelial cells at the center of the disorder (Fig. 20-43). The tubular epithelial cells of the kidney contain a single nonmotile primary cilium, a 2- to 3-μm long hairlike organelle that projects into the tubular lumen from the apical surface of the cells. The cilium is made up of microtubules, and arises from and is attached to a basal body derived from the centriole. The cilia are part of a system of organelles and cellular structures that sense mechanical signals. The apical cilia function in the kidney tubule as a mechanosensor to monitor changes in fluid flow and shear stress, while intercellular junctional complexes monitor forces between cells, and focal adhesions sense attachment to extracellular matrices. In response to external signals, these sensors regulate ion flux (cilia can induce Ca2+ flux in cultured kidney epithelial cells) and cellular behavior, including cell polarity and proliferation. The idea that defects in mechanosensing, Ca2+ flux, and signal transduction underlie cyst formation is supported by several observations.

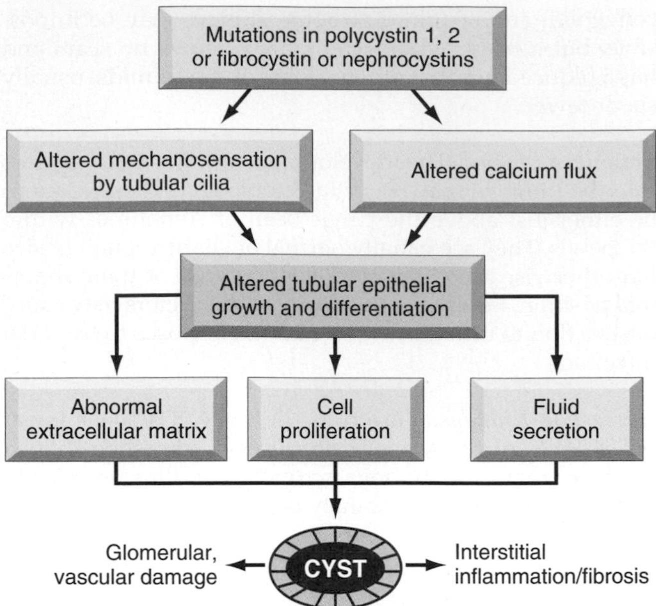

Figure 20-43 Possible mechanisms of cyst formation in cystic kidney diseases (see text).

- Both polycystin-1 and polycystin-2 are localized to the primary cilium.
- Other genes that are mutated in cystic diseases (e.g., the nephrocystin genes, described later) encode proteins that are also localized to cilia and/or basal bodies.
- Knockout of the *PKD1* gene in one model organism (the worm *Caenorhabditis elegans*) results in ciliary abnormalities and cyst formation.
- Tubular cells obtained from mice with a deletion of the *PKD1* gene (which causes embryonic lethality in this species) retain normal architecture of cilia but lack the flow-induced Ca2+ flux that occurs in normal tubular cells.

Polycystin-1 and polycystin-2 appear to form a protein complex that regulates intracellular Ca2+ in response to fluid flow, perhaps because fluid moving through the kidney tubules causes ciliary bending that opens Ca2+ channels. Mutation of either of the *PKD* genes leads to loss of the polycystin complex or formation of an aberrant complex. The consequent disruption of normal polycystin activity results in alterations of intracellular Ca2+, which (you will recall) regulates many downstream signaling events, including pathways that directly or indirectly impact cellular proliferation, apoptosis, and secretory functions. The increase in calcium is thought to stimulate proliferation and secretion from epithelial cells lining the cysts, which together result in progressive cyst formation and enlargement. In addition, cyst fluids have been shown to harbor mediators, derived from epithelial cells that enhance fluid secretion and induce inflammation. Finally, the calcium-induced signals also alter the interaction of epithelial cells with extracellular matrix, and this too is thought to contribute to the cyst formation and interstitial fibrosis that are characteristic of progressive polycystic kidney disease.

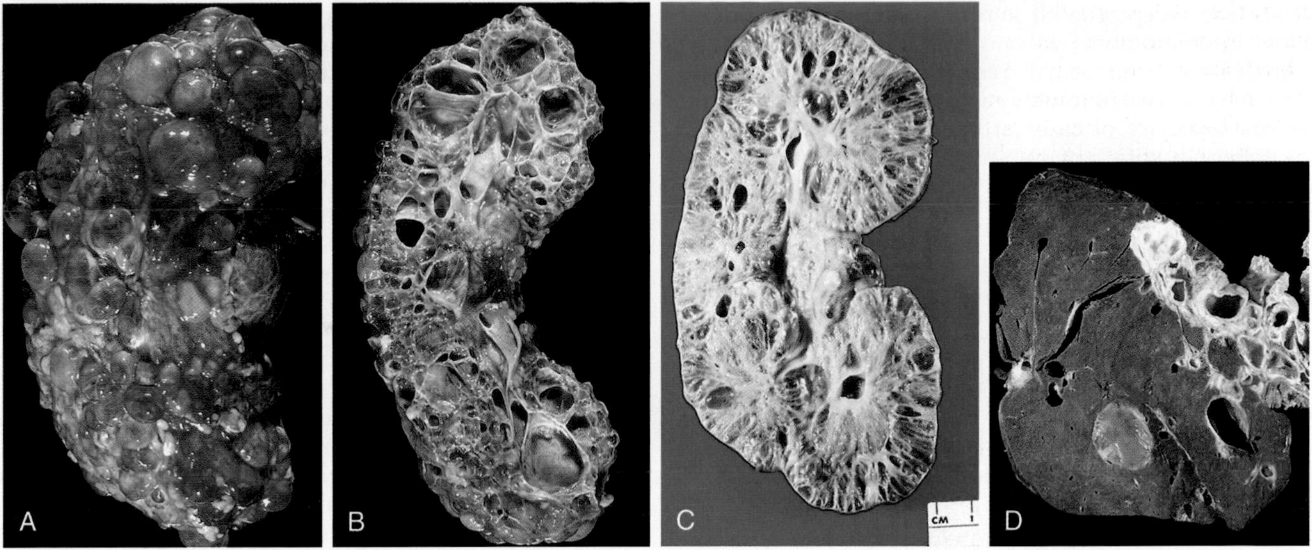

Figure 20-44 **A** and **B,** Autosomal dominant adult polycystic kidney disease (ADPKD) viewed from the external surface and bisected. The kidney is markedly enlarged and contains numerous dilated cysts. **C,** Autosomal recessive childhood PKD, showing smaller cysts and dilated channels at right angles to the cortical surface. **D,** Liver cysts in adult PKD.

MORPHOLOGY

In gross appearance, the kidneys are bilaterally enlarged and may achieve enormous sizes; weights as much as 4 kg for each kidney have been reported. The external surface appears to be composed solely of a mass of cysts, up to 3 to 4 cm in diameter, with no intervening parenchyma (Fig. 20-44*A* and *B*). However, microscopic examination reveals functioning nephrons dispersed between the cysts. The cysts may be filled with a clear, serous fluid or with turbid, red to brown, sometimes hemorrhagic fluid. As these cysts enlarge, they may encroach on the calyces and pelvis to produce pressure defects. The cysts arise from the tubules throughout the nephron and therefore have variable lining epithelia. On occasion, papillary epithelial formations and polyps project into the lumen. Bowman capsules are occasionally involved in cyst formation, and glomerular tufts may be seen within the cystic space.

Clinical Features. Many patients remain asymptomatic until renal insufficiency announces the presence of the disease. In others, hemorrhage or progressive dilation of cysts may produce pain. Excretion of blood clots causes renal colic. The enlarged kidneys, usually apparent on abdominal palpation, may induce a dragging sensation. The disease occasionally begins with the insidious onset of hematuria, followed by other features of progressive chronic kidney disease, such as proteinuria (rarely more than 2 gm/day), polyuria, and hypertension. Patients with *PKD2* mutations tend to have an older age at onset and later development of renal failure. Both genetic and environmental factors influence disease severity. Progression is accelerated in blacks (particularly in those with sickle-cell trait), in males, and in the presence of hypertension.

Individuals with polycystic kidney disease also tend to have extrarenal congenital anomalies. About 40% have one to several cysts in the liver (polycystic liver disease) that are usually asymptomatic. The cysts are derived from biliary epithelium. Cysts occur much less frequently in the spleen, pancreas, and lungs. Intracranial berry aneurysms, presumably from altered expression of polycystin in vascular smooth muscle, arise in the circle of Willis, and subarachnoid hemorrhages from these account for death in 4% to 10% of individuals. *Mitral valve prolapse* and other cardiac valvular anomalies occur in 20% to 25% of patients, but most are asymptomatic. The diagnosis is made by radiologic imaging techniques.

This form of chronic kidney disease is remarkable in that patients may survive for many years with azotemia slowly progressing to uremia. Ultimately, about 40% of adult patients die of coronary or hypertensive heart disease, 25% of infection, 15% of a ruptured berry aneurysm or hypertensive intracerebral hemorrhage, and the rest of other causes.

Autosomal Recessive (Childhood) Polycystic Kidney Disease

Autosomal recessive (childhood) polycystic kidney disease is genetically distinct from adult polycystic kidney disease. *Perinatal*, *neonatal*, *infantile*, and *juvenile* subcategories have been defined, depending on the time of presentation and presence of associated hepatic lesions. The first two are the most common; serious manifestations are usually present at birth, and the young infant might succumb rapidly to renal failure.

Genetics and Pathogenesis. In most cases, the disease is caused by mutations of the *PKHD1* gene, which maps to chromosome region 6p21-p23. The gene is highly expressed in adult and fetal kidney and also in liver and pancreas. The *PKHD1* gene encodes *fibrocystin*, a 447-kD integral membrane protein with a large extracellular region, a single transmembrane component, and a short cytoplasmic tail. The extracellular region contains multiple copies of a domain forming an Ig-like fold. Like polycystins 1 and 2, fibrocystin also has been localized to the primary cilium of tubular cells. The function of fibrocystin is unknown, but its putative conformational structure indicates it may be a cell surface receptor with a role in collecting duct and biliary differentiation.

Analysis of autosomal recessive polycystic disease patients has revealed a wide range of different mutations. The vast majority of cases are compound heterozygotes (i.e., inherit a different mutant allele from each of the two parents). This complicates molecular diagnosis of the disorder.

MORPHOLOGY

The kidneys are enlarged and have a smooth external appearance. On cut section, numerous small cysts in the cortex and medulla give the kidney a spongelike appearance. Dilated elongated channels are present at right angles to the cortical surface, completely replacing the medulla and cortex (Fig. 20-44*C*). On microscopic examination, there is cylindrical or, less commonly, saccular dilation of all collecting tubules. The cysts have a uniform lining of cuboidal cells, reflecting their origin from the collecting ducts. In almost all cases the liver has cysts associated with portal fibrosis (Fig. 20-44*D*) and proliferation of portal bile ducts.

Patients who survive infancy (infantile and juvenile forms) may develop a peculiar hepatic injury characterized by bland periportal fibrosis and proliferation of well-differentiated biliary ductules, now termed *congenital hepatic fibrosis*. In older children, hepatic disease is the predominant clinical concern. Such patients may develop portal hypertension with splenomegaly. Curiously, congenital hepatic fibrosis sometimes occurs in the absence of polycystic kidneys or has been reported in the presence of adult polycystic kidney disease.

Cystic Diseases of Renal Medulla

The three major types of medullary cystic disease are *medullary sponge kidney*, a relatively common and usually innocuous structural change, *nephronophthisis* and *adult-onset medullary cystic disease*, which are almost always associated with renal dysfunction.

Medullary Sponge Kidney

The term *medullary sponge kidney* is restricted to multiple cystic dilations of the collecting ducts in the medulla. The condition occurs in adults and is usually discovered radiographically. Renal function is usually normal. On gross inspection the papillary ducts in the medulla are dilated, and small cysts may be present. The cysts are lined by cuboidal epithelium or occasionally by transitional epithelium. Unless there is superimposed pyelonephritis, cortical scarring is absent. The pathogenesis is unknown.

Nephronophthisis and Adult-Onset Medullary Cystic Disease

This group of progressive renal disorders is characterized by variable number of cysts in the medulla, usually concentrated at the corticomedullary junction. Initial injury probably involves the distal tubules with tubular basement membrane disruption, followed by chronic and progressive tubular atrophy involving both medulla and cortex and interstitial fibrosis. Although the medullary cysts are important, the **cortical tubulointerstitial damage is the cause of the eventual renal insufficiency.**

Three variants of the nephronophthisis disease complex are recognized: (1) sporadic, nonfamilial; (2) familial juvenile nephronophthisis (most common); and (3) renal-retinal dysplasia (15%) in which the kidney disease is accompanied by ocular lesions. The familial forms are inherited as autosomal recessive traits and usually become manifest in childhood or adolescence. As a group, the nephronophthisis complex is now the most common genetic cause of end-stage renal disease in children and young adults.

Children affected with nephronophthisis present first with polyuria and polydipsia, which reflect a marked defect in the concentrating ability of renal tubules. Sodium wasting and tubular acidosis are also prominent. Some syndromic variants of nephronophthisis (e.g., Senior-Loken syndrome, Joubert syndrome, Bardet Biedl syndrome, Jeune syndrome, Meckel Gruber syndrome, Mainzer-Saldino syndrome, Sensenbrenner syndrome) can have extrarenal associations, including ocular motor abnormalities, retinal dystrophy, liver fibrosis, and cerebellar abnormalities. The expected course is progression to ESRD in 5 to 10 years.

Genetics and Pathogenesis. Sixteen responsible gene loci, *NPHP1* to *NPHP11* (that encode proteins called nephrocystins, *JBTS2, JBTS3, JBTS9,* and *JBTS11,* are mutated in the juvenile forms of nephronophthisis and the list continually expands as additional loci that contribute to this ciliopathy are identified. These proteins are present in the primary cilia, basal bodies attached to these cilia, or the centrosome organelle from which the basal bodies originate.

The NPHP2 gene product has been identified as *inversin,* which mediates left-right patterning during embryogenesis. Adult-onset medullary cystic disease has an autosomal dominant pattern of transmission. At one time it was considered to be part of the nephronophthisis spectrum, but based on its distinctive genetics it is now considered a separate entity. Mutations in two genes (*MCKD1* and *MCKD2*) have been identified as causing medullary cystic disease, which is characterized by progression to end-stage kidney disease in adult life.

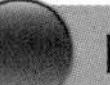

MORPHOLOGY

In nephronopthisis, the kidneys are small, have contracted granular surfaces, and show cysts in the medulla, most prominently at the corticomedullary junction (Fig. 20-45). Small cysts are also seen in the cortex. The cysts are lined by flattened or cuboidal epithelium and are usually surrounded by either inflammatory cells or fibrous tissue. In the cortex there is widespread atrophy and thickening of the tubular basement membranes, together with interstitial fibrosis. In general, glomerular structure is preserved.

There are few specific clues to diagnosis, because the medullary cysts might be too small to be visualized radiographically. The disease should be strongly considered in children or adolescents with otherwise unexplained chronic

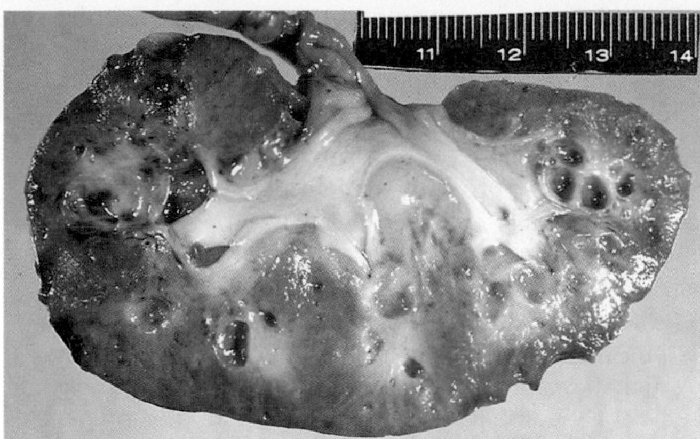

Figure 20-45 Medullary cystic disease. Cut section of kidney showing cysts at the corticomedullary junction and in the medulla.

renal failure, a positive family history, and chronic tubulointerstitial nephritis on biopsy.

Multicystic Renal Dysplasia

Dysplasia is a sporadic disorder that can be unilateral or bilateral and is almost always cystic. The kidney is usually enlarged, extremely irregular, and multicystic (Fig. 20-46*A*).

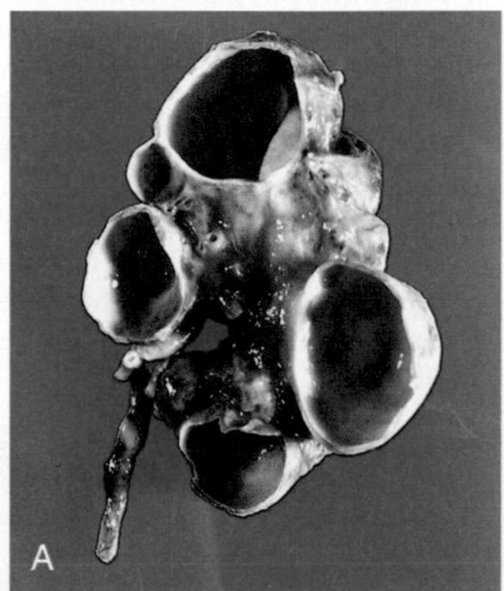

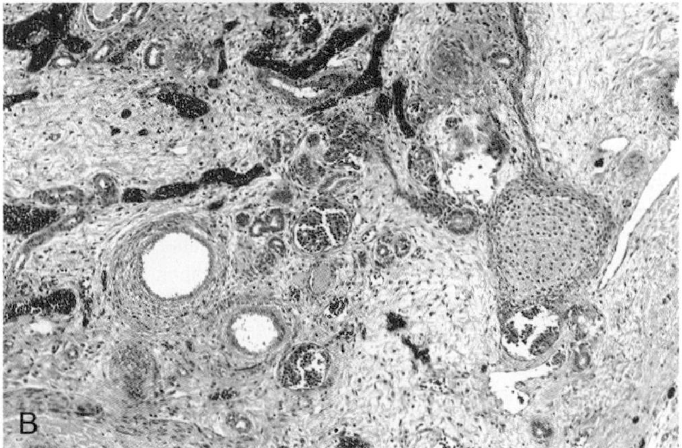

Figure 20-46 Multicystic renal dysplasia. **A,** Gross appearance. **B,** Histologic section showing disorganized architecture, dilated tubules with cuffs of primitive stroma, and an island of cartilage (Hematoxylin and eosin stain). (**A,** Courtesy Dr. D. Schofield, Children's Hospital, Los Angeles, Calif.; **B,** courtesy Dr. Laura Finn, Children's Hospital, Seattle, Wash.)

The cysts vary in size from several millimeters to centimeters in diameter. On histologic examination, they are lined by flattened epithelium. Although normal nephrons are present, many have immature collecting ducts. The characteristic histologic feature is the presence of islands of undifferentiated mesenchyme, often with cartilage, and immature collecting ducts (Fig. 20-46*B*). Most cases are associated with ureteropelvic obstruction, ureteral agenesis or atresia, and other anomalies of the lower urinary tract.

When unilateral, the dysplasia may mimic a neoplasm and lead to surgical exploration and nephrectomy. The opposite kidney functions normally, and such patients have an excellent prognosis after surgical removal of the affected kidney. In bilateral multicystic renal dysplasia, renal failure may ultimately result.

Acquired (Dialysis-Associated) Cystic Disease

Patients with end-stage renal disease who have undergone prolonged dialysis sometimes show numerous cortical and medullary renal cysts. The cysts measure 0.1 to 4 cm in diameter, contain clear fluid, are lined by either hyperplastic or flattened tubular epithelium, and often contain calcium oxalate crystals. They probably form as a result of obstruction of tubules by interstitial fibrosis or by oxalate crystals. Most are asymptomatic, but sometimes the cysts bleed, causing hematuria. There is a 12- to 18-fold increased risk of renal cell carcinoma, which develops in 7% of dialyzed patients observed for 10 years.

Simple Cysts

Simple cysts may be single or multiple and usually involve the cortex. They are commonly 1 to 5 cm but may reach 10 cm or more in size. They are translucent, lined by a gray, glistening, smooth membrane, and filled with clear fluid. On microscopic examination these membranes are composed of a single layer of cuboidal or flattened cuboidal epithelium, which in many instances may be completely atrophic.

Simple cysts are common postmortem findings without clinical significance. On occasion, hemorrhage into them may cause sudden distention and pain, and calcification of the hemorrhage may give rise to bizarre radiographic shadows. The main importance of cysts lies in their differentiation from kidney tumors. Radiologic studies show that in contrast to renal tumors, renal cysts have smooth contours, are almost always avascular, and give fluid rather than solid signals on ultrasonography.

KEY CONCEPTS

Cystic Diseases

- Autosomal dominant polycystic kidney disease accounts for a small yet significant subset of end stage renal disease.
- Ciliopathies or abnormalities of the cilium-centrosome complex underlie the major cystic kidney diseases, including polycystic kidney disease (both autosomal dominant and autosomal recessive forms), medullary cystic kidney disease, and nephronophthisis.

- Dysfunction of the primary cilium of tubular epithelial cells results in alterations in ion flux and changes in cell proliferation and function, culminating in renal cyst formation.

Urinary Tract Obstruction (Obstructive Uropathy)

Obstructive lesions of the urinary tract increase susceptibility to infection and to stone formation, and unrelieved obstruction almost always leads to permanent renal atrophy, termed *hydronephrosis* or *obstructive uropathy*. Fortunately, many causes of obstruction are surgically correctable or medically treatable.

Obstruction may be sudden or insidious, partial or complete, unilateral or bilateral; it may occur at any level of the urinary tract from the urethra to the renal pelvis. It can be caused by *intrinsic* lesions of the urinary tract or *extrinsic* lesions that compress the ureter. The common causes are as follows (Fig. 20-47):

- *Congenital anomalies:* posterior urethral valves and urethral strictures, meatal stenosis, bladder neck obstruction; ureteropelvic junction narrowing or obstruction; severe vesicoureteral reflux
- *Urinary calculi*
- *Benign prostatic hypertrophy*
- *Tumors:* carcinoma of the prostate, bladder tumors, contiguous malignant disease (retroperitoneal lymphoma), carcinoma of the cervix or uterus
- *Inflammation:* prostatitis, ureteritis, urethritis, retroperitoneal fibrosis
- *Sloughed papillae or blood clots*
- *Pregnancy*
- *Uterine prolapse and cystocele*
- *Functional disorders:* neurogenic (spinal cord damage or diabetic nephropathy) and other functional abnormalities of the ureter or bladder (often termed *dysfunctional obstruction*)

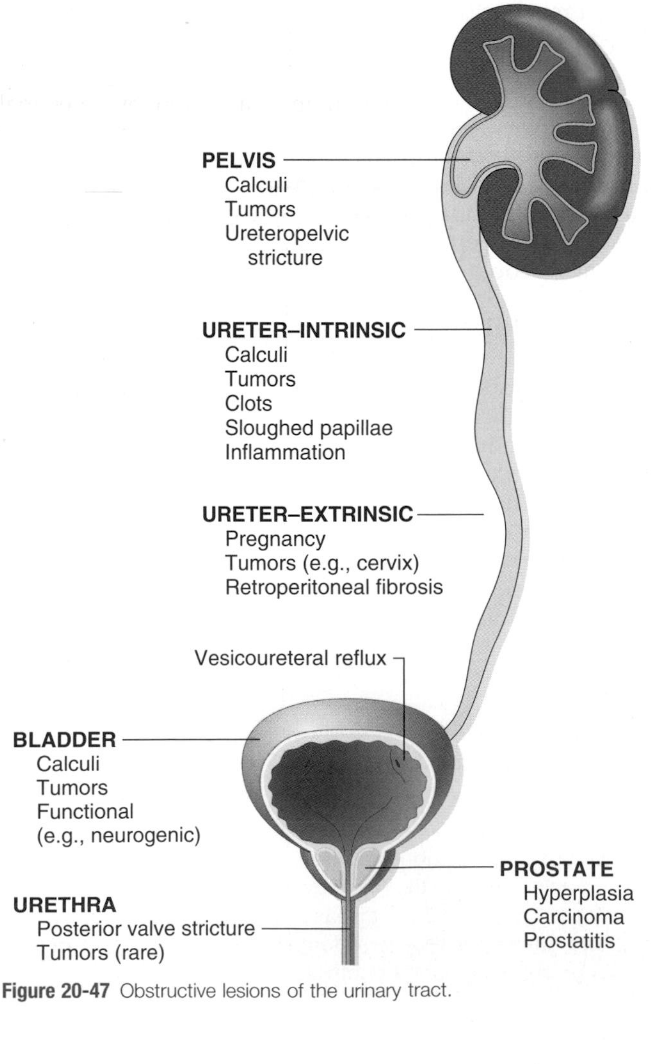

Figure 20-47 Obstructive lesions of the urinary tract.

***Hydronephrosis* is the term used to describe dilation of the renal pelvis and calyces associated with progressive atrophy of the kidney due to obstruction to the outflow of urine.** Even with complete obstruction, glomerular filtration persists for some time because the filtrate subsequently diffuses back into the renal interstitium and perirenal spaces, from where it ultimately returns to the lymphatic and venous systems. Because of this continued filtration, the affected calyces and pelvis become dilated, often markedly so. The high pressure in the pelvis is transmitted back through the collecting ducts into the cortex, causing renal atrophy, but it also compresses the renal vasculature of the medulla, causing a diminution in inner medullary blood flow. The medullary vascular defects are initially reversible, but lead to medullary functional disturbances. Accordingly, the initial functional alterations caused by obstruction are largely tubular, manifested primarily by impaired concentrating ability. Only later does the GFR begin to fall. Obstruction also triggers an interstitial inflammatory reaction, leading eventually to interstitial fibrosis, by mechanisms similar to those discussed earlier (Fig. 20-9).

MORPHOLOGY

When the obstruction is sudden and complete, it leads to mild dilation of the pelvis and calyces and sometimes to atrophy of the renal parenchyma. When the obstruction is subtotal or intermittent, progressive dilation ensues, giving rise to hydronephrosis (Fig. 20-48). Depending on the level of urinary block, the dilation may affect the bladder first, or the ureter and then the kidney.

The kidney may be slightly to massively enlarged, depending on the degree and the duration of the obstruction. The earlier features are those of simple dilation of the pelvis and calyces, but in addition there is often significant interstitial inflammation, even in the absence of infection. In chronic cases the picture is one of cortical tubular atrophy with marked diffuse interstitial fibrosis. Progressive blunting of the apices of the pyramids occurs, and these eventually become cupped. In far-advanced cases the kidney may become transformed into a thin-walled cystic structure having a diameter of up to 15 to 20 cm (Fig. 20-48) with striking parenchymal atrophy, total obliteration of the pyramids, and thinning of the cortex.

Clinical Features. *Acute obstruction* may provoke pain attributed to distention of the collecting system or renal

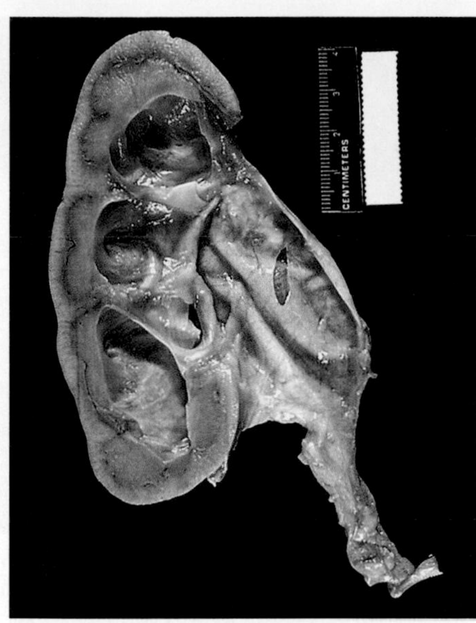

Figure 20-48 Hydronephrosis of the kidney, with marked dilation of the pelvis and calyces and thinning of the renal parenchyma.

capsule. Most of the early symptoms are produced by the underlying cause of the hydronephrosis. Thus, calculi lodged in the ureters may give rise to renal colic, and prostatic enlargements may give rise to bladder symptoms.

Unilateral complete or partial hydronephrosis may remain silent for long periods, since the unaffected kidney can maintain adequate renal function. Sometimes its existence first becomes apparent in the course of imaging studies. In its early stages, perhaps the first few weeks, relief of obstruction leads to reversion to normal function. *Ultrasonography* is a useful noninvasive technique in the diagnosis of obstructive uropathy.

In *bilateral partial obstruction* the earliest manifestation is inability to concentrate urine, reflected by polyuria and nocturia. Some patients develop distal tubular acidosis, renal salt wasting, secondary renal calculi, and chronic tubulointerstitial nephritis with scarring and atrophy of the papilla and medulla. Hypertension is common.

Complete bilateral obstruction of rapid onset results in oliguria or anuria and is incompatible with survival unless the obstruction is relieved. Curiously, after relief of complete urinary tract obstruction, postobstructive *diuresis* occurs. This can often be massive, with the kidney excreting large amounts of urine that is rich in sodium chloride.

Urolithiasis (Renal Calculi, Stones)

Urolithiasis affects 5% to 10% of Americans in their lifetime and the stones may form anywhere in the urinary tract, but most arise in the kidney. Men are affected more often than women, and the peak age at onset is between 20 and 30 years. Familial and hereditary predisposition to stone formation has long been known. Many inborn errors of metabolism, such as cystinuria and primary hyperoxaluria, provide examples of hereditary disease characterized by excessive production and excretion of stone-forming substances.

Etiology and Pathogenesis. There are four main types of calculi (Table 20-12): (1) *calcium stones* (about 70%), composed largely of calcium oxalate or calcium oxalate mixed with calcium phosphate; (2) another 15% are so-called *triple stones* or *struvite stones*, composed of magnesium ammonium phosphate; (3) 5% to 10% are *uric acid stones*; and (4) 1% to 2% are made up of cystine. An organic mucoprotein matrix, making up 1% to 5% of the stone by weight, is present in all calculi. **Although there are many causes for the initiation and propagation of stones, the most important determinant is an increased urinary concentration of the stones' constituents, such that it exceeds their solubility (supersaturation).** A low urine volume in some metabolically normal patients may also favor supersaturation.

- *Calcium oxalate stones* (Table 20-12) are associated in about 5% of patients with hypercalcemia and hypercalciuria, such as occurs with hyperparathyroidism, diffuse bone disease, sarcoidosis, and other hypercalcemic states. About 55% have hypercalciuria without hypercalcemia. This is caused by several factors, including hyperabsorption of calcium from the intestine (absorptive hypercalciuria), an intrinsic impairment in renal tubular reabsorption of calcium (renal hypercalciuria), or idiopathic fasting hypercalciuria with normal parathyroid function. As many as 20% of calcium oxalate stones are associated with increased uric acid secretion *(hyperuricosuric calcium nephrolithiasis)*, with or without hypercalciuria. The mechanism of stone formation in this setting involves "nucleation" of calcium oxalate by uric acid crystals in the collecting ducts. Five percent are associated with *hyperoxaluria*, either hereditary (primary oxaluria) or, more commonly, acquired by intestinal overabsorption in patients with enteric diseases. *Hypocitraturia,* which can be idiopathic or associated with acidosis and chronic diarrhea of unknown cause, may produce calcium stones. In a variable proportion of

Table 20-12 Prevalence of Various Types of Renal Stones

Stone Type	Percentage of All Stones
Calcium Oxalate and Phosphate	70
Idiopathic hypercalciuria (50%)	
Hypercalciuria and hypercalcemia (10%)	
Hyperoxaluria (5%)	
Enteric (4.5%)	
Primary (0.5%)	
Hyperuricosuria (20%)	
Hypocitraturia	
No known metabolic abnormality (15% to 20%)	
Magnesium Ammonium Phosphate (Struvite)	5-10
Uric Acid	5-10
Associated with hyperuricemia	
Associated with hyperuricosuria	
Idiopathic (50% of uric stones)	
Cystine	1-2
Others or Unknown	±5

individuals with calcium stones, no cause can be found (idiopathic calcium stone disease).

- *Magnesium ammonium phosphate stones* are formed largely after infections by urea-splitting bacteria (e.g., *Proteus* and some staphylococci) that convert urea to ammonia. The resultant alkaline urine causes the precipitation of magnesium ammonium phosphate salts. These form some of the largest stones, as the amount of urea excreted normally is very large. Indeed, so-called *staghorn calculi* occupying large portions of the renal pelvis are frequently a consequence of infection.
- *Uric acid stones* are common in individuals with hyperuricemia, such as patients with gout, and diseases involving rapid cell turnover, such as the leukemias. However, **more than half of all patients with uric acid calculi have neither hyperuricemia nor increased urinary excretion of uric acid.** In this group, it is thought that a tendency to excrete urine of pH below 5.5 may predispose to uric acid stones, because uric acid is insoluble in acidic urine. In contrast to the radiopaque calcium stones, uric acid stones are radiolucent.
- *Cystine stones* are caused by genetic defects in the renal reabsorption of amino acids, including cystine, leading to cystinuria. These stones also form at low urinary pH.

It can therefore be appreciated that **increased concentration of stone constituents, changes in urinary pH, decreased urine volume, and the presence of bacteria influence the formation of calculi.** However, many calculi occur in the absence of these factors; conversely, individuals with hypercalciuria, hyperoxaluria, and hyperuricosuria often do not form stones. It has been postulated that stone formation is enhanced by a deficiency in inhibitors of crystal formation in urine. The list of such inhibitors is long, including pyrophosphate, diphosphonate, citrate, glycosaminoglycans, osteopontin, and a glycoprotein called nephrocalcin.

MORPHOLOGY

Stones are unilateral in about 80% of patients. The favored sites for their formation are within the renal calyces and pelves (Fig. 20-49) and in the bladder. If formed in the renal pelvis they tend to remain small, having an average diameter of 2 to 3 mm. These may have smooth contours or may take the form of an irregular, jagged mass of spicules. Often many stones are found within one kidney. On occasion, progressive accretion of salts leads to the development of branching structures known as staghorn calculi, which create a cast of the pelvic and calyceal system.

Clinical Features. Urolithiasis may be asymptomatic, produce severe renal colic and abdominal pain, or may cause significant renal damage. Larger stones often manifest themselves by hematuria. Stones also predispose to superimposed infection, both by their obstructive nature and by the trauma they produce.

Neoplasms of the Kidney

Both benign and malignant neoplasms occur in the kidney. Malignant neoplasms are of great importance clinically. By far the most common malignant tumor is renal cell carcinoma, followed by Wilms tumor, which is found in children and is described in Chapter 10, and finally urothelial carcinomas of the calyces and pelves.

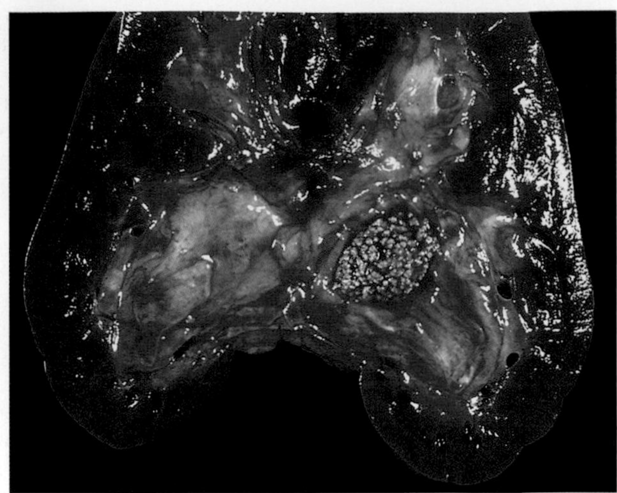

Figure 20-49 Nephrolithiasis. A large stone impacted in the renal pelvis. (Courtesy Dr. E. Mosher, Brigham and Women's Hospital, Boston, Mass.)

Benign Neoplasms

Renal Papillary Adenoma

Small, discrete adenomas arising from the renal tubular epithelium are found commonly (7% to 22%) at autopsy. They are most frequently papillary and are therefore called *papillary adenomas*.

MORPHOLOGY

These are small tumors, usually less than 0.5 cm in diameter. They are present invariably within the cortex and appear grossly as pale yellow-gray, discrete, well-circumscribed nodules. On microscopic examination, they are composed of complex, branching, papillomatous structures with numerous complex fronds. Cells may also grow as tubules, glands, cords, and sheets of cells. The cells are cuboidal to polygonal in shape and have regular, small central nuclei, scanty cytoplasm, and no atypia.

By histologic criteria, these tumors do not differ from low-grade papillary renal cell carcinoma and indeed share some immunohistochemical and cytogenetic features (trisomies 7 and 17) with papillary cancers, to be discussed later. The size of the tumor is used as a prognostic feature, with a cutoff of 3 cm separating those that metastasize from those that rarely do. However, because of occasional reports of small tumors that have metastasized, the current view is to regard all adenomas, regardless of size, as potentially malignant.

Angiomyolipoma

This is a benign neoplasm consisting of vessels, smooth muscle, and fat originating from perivascular epithelioid cells. **Angiomyolipomas are present in 25% to 50% of patients with tuberous sclerosis,** a disease caused by loss-of-function mutations in the *TSC1* or *TSC2* tumor suppressor genes. Tuberous sclerosis is characterized by lesions of the cerebral cortex that produce epilepsy and mental retardation, a variety of skin abnormalities, and unusual benign tumors at other sites, such as the heart (Chapters 12 and 28). The clinical importance of angiomyolipoma is due largely to their susceptibility to spontaneous hemorrhage.

Oncocytoma

This is an epithelial neoplasm composed of large eosinophilic cells having small, round, benign-appearing nuclei that have large nucleoli. It is thought to arise from the intercalated cells of collecting ducts, and accounts for approximately 5% to 15% of renal neoplasms. Ultrastructurally the eosinophilic cells have numerous mitochondria. In gross appearance, the tumors are tan or mahogany brown, relatively homogeneous, and usually well encapsulated with a central scar in one-third of cases. However, they may achieve a large size (up to 12 cm in diameter). There are some familial cases in which these tumors are multicentric rather than solitary.

Malignant Neoplasms

Renal Cell Carcinoma

Renal cell carcinomas represent about 3% of all newly diagnosed cancers in the United States and account for 85% of renal cancers in adults. There are approximately 65,000 new cases per year and 13,000 deaths from the disease. The tumors occur most often in older individuals, usually in the sixth and seventh decades of life, and show a 2:1 male preponderance.

Epidemiology. Tobacco is the most significant risk factor. Cigarette smokers have double the incidence of renal cell carcinoma, and pipe and cigar smokers are also more susceptible. An international study has identified additional risk factors, including obesity (particularly in women); hypertension; unopposed estrogen therapy; and exposure to asbestos, petroleum products, and heavy metals. There is also an increased risk in patients with end-stage renal disease, chronic kidney disease, acquired cystic disease (see earlier) and tuberous sclerosis.

Most renal cancer is sporadic, but unusual forms of autosomal dominant familial cancers occur, usually in younger individuals. Although they account for only 4% of renal cancers, familial variants have been instructive in understanding renal carcinogenesis.

- *Von Hippel-Lindau (VHL) syndrome:* Half to two thirds of individuals with VHL (nearly all, if they live long enough) (Chapter 28) develop renal cysts and bilateral, often multiple, renal cell carcinomas. *Current studies implicate the VHL gene in the development of both familial and sporadic clear cell carcinomas.*
- *Hereditary leiomyomatosis and renal cell cancer syndrome:* This autosomal dominant disease is caused by mutations of the *FH* gene, which expresses fumarate hydratase, and is characterized by cutaneous and uterine leiomyomata and an aggressive type of papillary carcinoma with increased propensity for metastatic spread.
- *Hereditary papillary carcinoma.* This autosomal dominant form is manifested by multiple bilateral tumors with papillary histology. These tumors show a series of cytogenetic abnormalities and, as will be described, mutations in the *MET* proto-oncogene.
- *Birt-Hogg-Dubé syndrome:* The autosomal dominant inheritance pattern of this disease is due to mutations involving the *BHD* gene, which expresses folliculin. The syndrome features a constellation of skin (fibrofolliculomas, trichodiscomas, and acrochordons), pulmonary (cysts or blebs), and renal tumors with a wide range of histologic subtypes.

Classification of renal cell carcinoma: histology, cytogenetics, and genetics. The classification of renal cell carcinoma is based on correlative cytogenetic, genetic, and histologic studies of both familial and sporadic tumors. The major types of tumor are as follows (Fig. 20-50):

- *Clear cell carcinoma.* This is the most common type, accounting for 70% to 80% of renal cell cancers. The tumors are made up of cells with clear or granular cytoplasm and are *nonpapillary*. They can be familial, but in most cases (95%) are sporadic. In 98% of these tumors, whether familial, sporadic, or associated with VHL syndrome, there is loss of sequences on the short arm of chromosome 3. The deleted region harbors the *VHL* gene (3p25.3). A second nondeleted allele of the *VHL* gene shows somatic mutations or hypermethylation-induced inactivation in up to 80% of clear cell cancers, indicating that the *VHL* gene acts as a tumor suppressor gene in both sporadic and familial cancers (Chapter 7). The *VHL* gene encodes a protein that is part of a ubiquitin ligase complex involved in targeting other proteins for degradation. Important among the targets of the VHL protein is the transcription factor hypoxia-inducible factor-1 (HIF-1). When *VHL* is inactive, HIF-1 levels remain high, even under normoxic conditions, causing inappropriate expression of a number of genes that are turned on by HIF. These include genes that promote angiogenesis, such as VEGF, and genes that stimulate cell growth, such as insulin-like growth factor-1 (IGF-1). In addition, HIF collaborates in complex ways with the oncogenic factor MYC to "reprogram" cellular metabolism in a way that favors growth. Deep sequencing of renal carcinoma genomes has revealed frequent mutations in a number of genes that regulate histone modifications, indicating that dysregulation of the epigenome also has an important role in clear cell carcinoma.
- *Papillary carcinoma* accounts for 10% to 15% of renal cancers. It is characterized by a papillary growth pattern and also occurs in both familial and sporadic forms. These tumors are not associated with 3p deletions. The most common cytogenetic abnormalities are trisomies 7 and 17 and loss of Y in male patients in the sporadic form, and trisomy 7 in the familial form. The gene on chromosome 7 for the familial form has been mapped to *MET*, a proto-oncogene that encodes the tyrosine kinase receptor for *hepatocyte growth factor. MET* is also mutated in a small proportion of sporadic papillary carcinomas. Described in Chapter 3, hepatocyte growth factor (also called *scatter factor*) mediates growth, cell

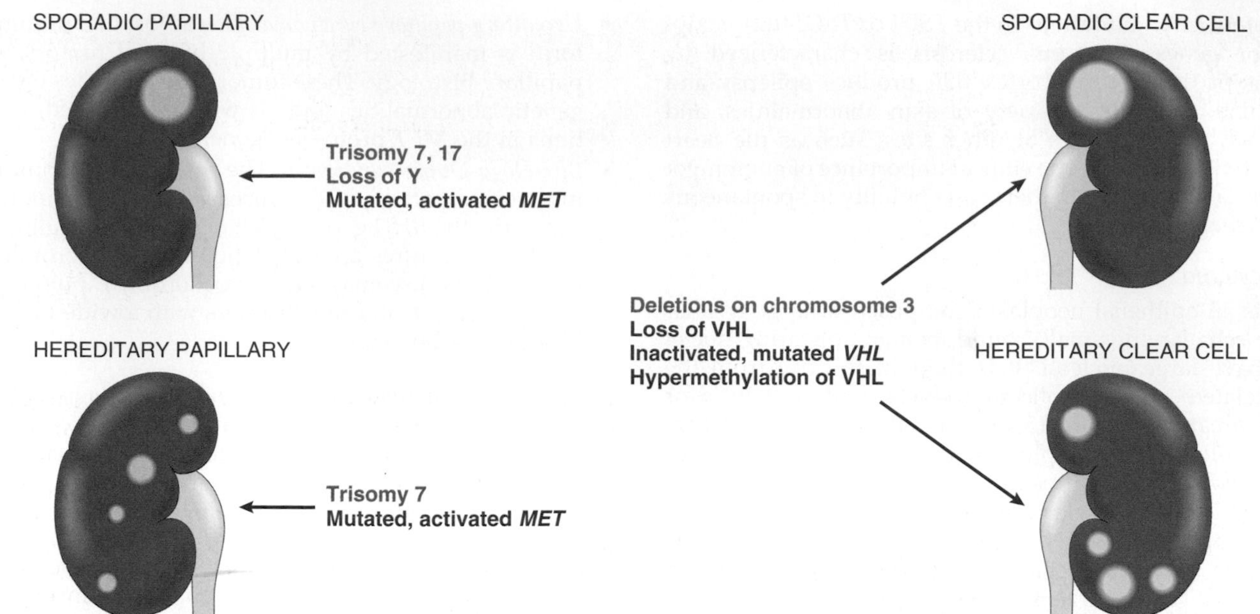

Figure 20-50 Cytogenetics (blue) and genetics (red) of clear cell versus papillary renal cell carcinoma. (Courtesy Dr. Keith Ligon, Brigham and Women's Hospital, Boston, Mass.)

mobility, invasion, and morphogenetic differentiation. Unlike clear cell carcinomas, papillary carcinomas are frequently multifocal in origin.

- *Chromophobe carcinoma* represents 5% of renal cell cancers and is composed of cells with prominent cell membranes and pale eosinophilic cytoplasm, usually with a halo around the nucleus. On cytogenetic examination these tumors show multiple chromosome losses and extreme hypodiploidy. Like the benign oncocytoma, they are thought to grow from intercalated cells of collecting ducts and have an excellent prognosis compared with that of the clear cell and papillary cancers. Histologic distinction from oncocytoma can be difficult.
- *Xp11 translocation carcinoma* is a genetically distinct subtype of renal cell carcinoma. It often occurs in young patients and is defined by translocations of the *TFE3* gene located at Xp11.2 with a number of partner genes, all of which result in overexpression of the TFE3 transcription factor. The neoplastic cells consist of clear cytoplasm with a papillary architecture.
- *Collecting duct (Bellini duct) carcinoma* represents approximately 1% or less of renal epithelial neoplasms. They arise from collecting duct cells in the medulla. Several chromosomal losses and deletions have been described, but a distinct pattern has not been identified. Histologically these tumors are characterized by malignant cells forming glands enmeshed within a prominent fibrotic stroma, typically in a medullary location. *Medullary carcinoma* is a morphologically similar neoplasm that is seen in patients with sickle cell trait.

MORPHOLOGY

Renal cell carcinomas may arise in any portion of the kidney, but more commonly affects the poles. **Clear cell carcinomas** most likely arise from proximal tubular epithelium, and usually occur as solitary unilateral lesions. They are bright yellow-gray-white spherical masses of variable size that distort the renal outline. The yellow color is a consequence of the prominent lipid accumulations in tumor cells. There are commonly large areas of gray-white necrosis and foci of hemorrhagic discoloration. The margins are usually sharply defined and confined within the renal capsule (Fig. 20-51). In clear cell carcinoma the growth pattern varies from solid to trabecular (cordlike) or tubular (resembling tubules). The tumor cells have a rounded or polygonal shape and abundant clear or granular cytoplasm, which contains glycogen and lipids (Fig. 20-52*A*). The tumors have

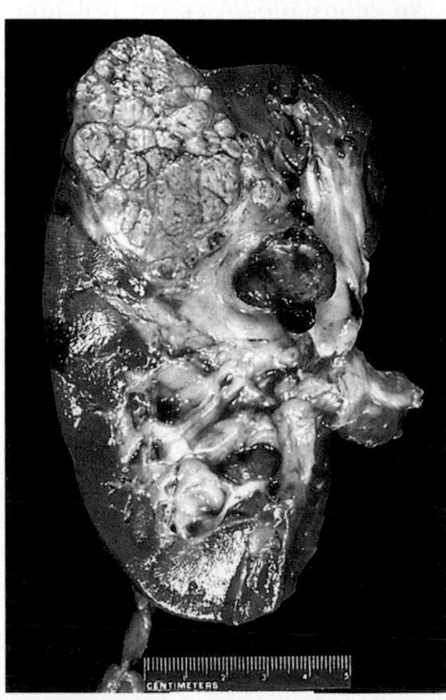

Figure 20-51 Renal cell carcinoma. Typical cross-section of yellowish, spherical neoplasm in one pole of the kidney. Note the tumor in the dilated thrombosed renal vein.

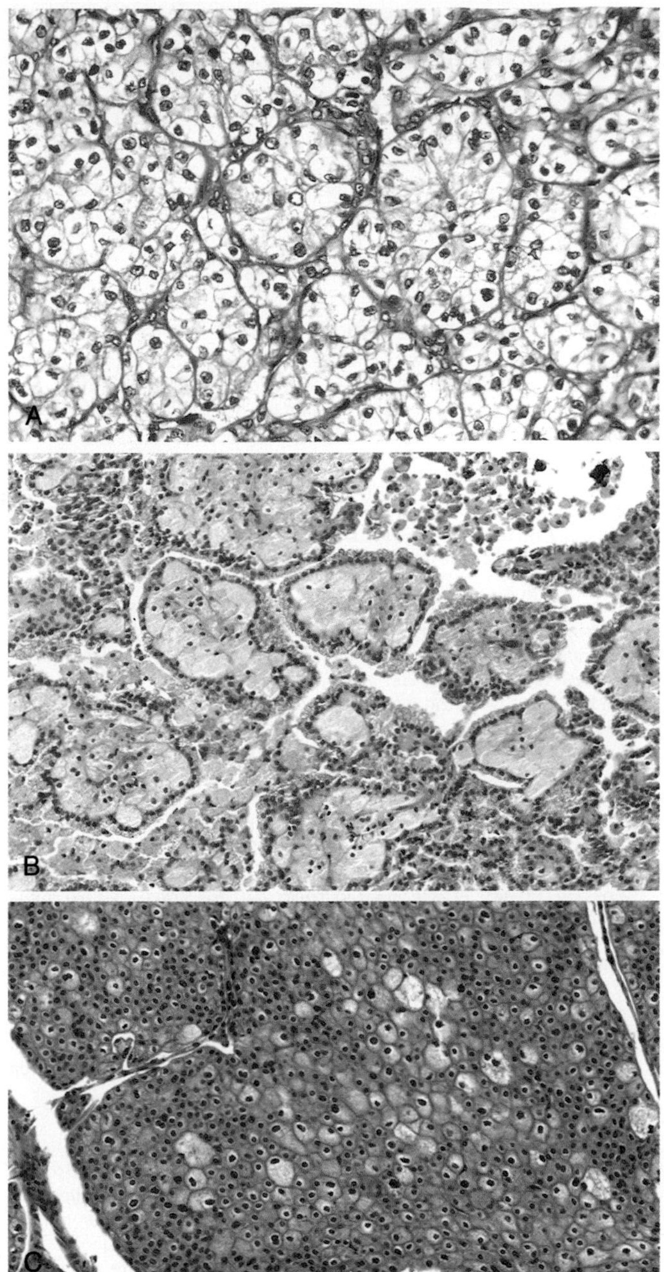

Figure 20-52 Renal cell carcinoma. **A,** Clear cell type. **B,** Papillary type. Note the papillae and foamy macrophages in the stalk. **C,** Chromophobe type. (Courtesy Dr. A. Renshaw, Baptist Hospital, Miami, Fla.)

delicate branching vasculature and may show cystic as well as solid areas. Most tumors are well differentiated, but some show nuclear atypia with bizarre nuclei and giant cells.

As tumors enlarge they may bulge into the calyces and pelvis and eventually fungate through the walls of the collecting system to extend into the ureter. **One of the striking characteristics of renal cell carcinoma is its tendency to invade the renal vein** (Fig. 20-51), in which it may grow as a solid column of cells that extends up the inferior vena cava, sometimes as far as the right side of the heart.

Papillary carcinomas, thought to arise from distal convoluted tubules, can be multifocal and bilateral. They are typically hemorrhagic and cystic, especially when large. The tumor is composed of cuboidal or low columnar cells arranged in papillary formations. Interstitial foam cells are common in the papillary cores (Fig. 20-52*B*). Psammoma bodies may be present. The stroma is usually scanty but highly vascularized. **Chromophobe renal carcinoma** is made up of pale eosinophilic cells, often with a perinuclear halo, arranged in solid sheets with a concentration of the largest cells around blood vessels (Fig. 20-52*C*). **Collecting duct carcinoma** is a rare variant showing irregular channels lined by highly atypical epithelium with a hobnail pattern. Sarcomatoid changes arise infrequently in all types of renal cell carcinoma and are a decidedly ominous feature.

Clinical Features. The classic clinical features of renal cell carcinoma are *costovertebral pain, palpable mass,* and *hematuria,* but all three are seen in only 10% of cases. The most reliable clue is hematuria, but it is usually intermittent and may be microscopic; thus, the tumor may remain silent until it attains a large size, often greater than 10 cm. At this time it is often associated with generalized constitutional symptoms, such as fever, malaise, weakness, and weight loss. This pattern of asymptomatic growth occurs in many patients, so the tumor may have reached a diameter of more than 10 cm when it is discovered. Currently, an increasing number of tumors are being discovered in the asymptomatic state by incidental radiologic studies (e.g., computed tomographic scan or magnetic resonance imaging) performed for other indications.

Renal cell carcinoma is considered one of the great mimics in medicine, because it tends to produce a diversity of systemic symptoms not related to the kidney. In addition to fever and constitutional symptoms mentioned earlier, renal cell carcinomas produce a number of syndromes ascribed to abnormal hormone production, including *polycythemia, hypercalcemia, hypertension, hepatic dysfunction, feminization or masculinization, Cushing syndrome, eosinophilia, leukemoid reactions, and amyloidosis.*

A particularly troublesome feature of renal cell carcinoma is its tendency to metastasize widely before giving rise to any local symptoms or signs. In 25% of new patients with renal cell carcinoma, there is radiologic evidence of metastases at the time of presentation. The most common locations of metastasis are the lungs (more than 50%) and bones (33%), followed in frequency by the regional lymph nodes, liver, adrenal, and brain.

The average 5-year survival rate of persons with renal cell carcinoma is about 70% and as high as 95% in the absence of distant metastases. With renal vein invasion or extension into the perinephric fat, the figure is reduced to approximately 60%. Radical nephrectomy has been the treatment of choice, but partial nephrectomy to preserve renal function is recommended for T1a tumors (<4 cm) as well as larger tumors when technically feasible. Drugs that inhibit VEGF and various tyrosine kinases are used as an adjunct to therapy in patients with metastatic disease.

Urothelial Carcinoma of the Renal Pelvis

Approximately 5% to 10% of primary renal tumors originate from the urothelium of the renal pelvis (Fig. 20-53). These tumors range from apparently benign papillomas to invasive urothelial (transitional cell) carcinomas.

Renal pelvic tumors usually become clinically apparent within a relatively short time, because they lie within the

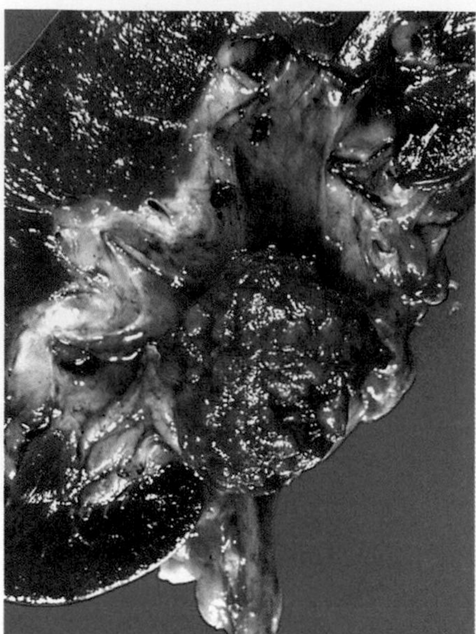

Figure 20-53 Urothelial carcinoma of the renal pelvis. The pelvis has been opened to expose the nodular irregular neoplasm, just proximal to the ureter.

pelvis and, by fragmentation, produce noticeable hematuria. They are almost invariably small when discovered. These tumors may block the urinary outflow and lead to palpable hydronephrosis and flank pain. On histologic examination, pelvic tumors are the exact counterpart of those found in the urinary bladder; further details are in Chapter 21.

Urothelial tumors may occasionally be multiple, involving the pelvis, ureters, and bladder. In 50% of renal pelvic tumors there is a preexisting or concomitant bladder urothelial tumor. On histologic examination, there are also foci of atypia or carcinoma in situ in grossly normal urothelium remote from the pelvic tumor. There is an increased incidence of urothelial carcinomas of the renal pelvis in individuals with Lynch syndrome and analgesic nephropathy.

Infiltration of the wall of the pelvis and calyces is common. For this reason, despite their apparently small, deceptively benign appearance, the prognosis for these tumors is not good. Reported 5-year survival rates vary from 50% to 100% for low-grade noninvasive lesions to 10% with high-grade infiltrating tumors.

KEY CONCEPTS

Kidney Neoplasms

- Clear cell renal cell carcinoma is the most common subtype of malignant renal neoplasms, which often involves *VHL*, a tumor suppressor gene.
- Papillary renal cell carcinoma is the second most common subtype of malignant renal neoplasms, which may involve the *MET* proto-oncogene.
- Hereditary forms of renal cell carcinoma have led to the discovery of important genes (e.g., *VHL, BHD*) in renal carcinogenesis.
- Urothelial tumors resembling similar tumors in the urinary bladder can also originate in the renal pelvis. These tumors have a poor prognosis.

SUGGESTED READINGS

Pathogenesis of Immune-Mediated Glomerular Injury

Couser WG: Basic and translational concepts of immune-mediated glomerular diseases. *J Am Soc Nephrol* 23:381–99, 2012. *[An outstanding and comprehensive review of the immunopathogensis of glomerular diseases.]*

Pickering M, Cook HT: Complement and glomerular disease: new insights. *Curr Opin Nephrol Hypertens* 20:271–7, 2011. *[An insightful review into newly emerging concepts of the contribution of complement to renal disease, with an emphasis on dysregulation of the alternate pathway of complement activation.]*

Mechanisms of Progression in Glomerular Diseases

Schlondorff DO: Overview of factors contributing to the pathophysiology of progressive renal disease. *Kidney Int* 74:860–6, 2008. *[An excellent summary of complex and interacting pathways that lead to progressive chronic kidney injury.]*

Nephrotic Syndrome

D'Agati VD, Kaskel FJ, Falk RJ: Focal segmental glomerulosclerosis. *N Engl J Med* 365:2398–411, 2011. *[An excellent and well-illustrated review of pathologic and clinical characteristics of this group of diseases.]*

Jefferson JA, Nelson PJ, Najafian B, et al: Podocyte disorders: Core Curriculum 2011. *Am J Kidney Dis* 58:666–77, 2011. *[An excellent clinically oriented synopsis of alternations in podocytes that underly multiple types of glomerular disease.]*

Ronco P, Debiec H: Pathogenesis of membranous nephropathy: recent advances and future challenges. *Nat Rev Nephrol* 8:203–13, 2012. *[Comprehensive review of the immunopathology of membranous nephropathy by two of the foremost investigators in the identification of the target antigens in this disease.]*

Sethi S, Fervenza FC: Membranoproliferative glomerulonephritis–a new look at an old entity. *N Engl J Med* 366:1119–31, 2012. *[An excellent reassessment of traditional classifications of this entity with a review of new classification schema that are based on underlying pathogenesis.]*

Nephritic Syndrome

Nast CC: Infection-related glomerulonephritis: changing demographics and outcomes. *Adv Chronic Kidney Dis* 19:68–75, 2012. *[A thoughtful review that integrates long established concepts in infection related glomerulonephritis with changing patterns of disease expression in both first and third world societies.]*

Rapidly Progressive (Crescentic) Glomerulonephritis

Jennette JC, Falk RJ, Gasim AH: Pathogenesis of antineutrophil cytoplasmic autoantibody vasculitis. *Curr Opin Nephrol Hypertens* 20:263–70, 2011. *[A short but thorough review of this major form of vasculitis with an emphasis on underlying pathophysiology.]*

Kambham N: Crescentic Glomerulonephritis: an update on Pauci-immune and Anti-GBM diseases. *Adv Anat Pathol* 19(2):111–24, 2012. *[A current review of the clinico-pathologic manifestations of these diseases.]*

Tarzi RM, Cook HT, Pusey CD: Crescentic glomerulonephritis: new aspects of pathogenesis. *Semin Nephrol* 31:361–8, 2011. *[An excellent consideration of pathogenesis of crescentic glomerulonephritis that complements the review of vasculitis by Jennette, et al.]*

Isolated Urinary Abnormalities

Gubler MC: Inherited diseases of the glomerular basement membrane. *Nat Clin Pract Nephrol* 4:24–37, 2008. *[A detailed review of the pathophysiology of hereditary nephritides and a clear guide to their identification and differential diagnosis.]*

Suzuki H, Kiryluk K, Novak J, et al: J The pathophysiology of IgA nephropathy. *Am Soc Nephrol* 22:1795–803, 2011. *[An excellent review that details emerging concepts of the pathophysiology of this disorder.]*

Acute Tubular Injury/Necrosis

Bellomo R, Kellum JA, Ronco C: Acute kidney injury. *Lancet* 380:756–66, 2012. *[An excellent review of acute kidney injury with an emphasis on the clinical aspects and management issues.]*

Bonventre JV, Yang LJ: Cellular pathophysiology of ischemic acute kidney injury. *Clin Invest* 121:4210–21, 2011. *[A comprehensive review of the cellular components and various mechanisms that contribute to ischemic kidney injury.]*

Tubulointerstitial Nephritis

Montini G, Tullus K, Hewitt I: Febrile urinary tract infectiouns in children. *N Engl J Med* 365:239–50, 2011. *[A review of the clinical and pathologic aspects of pediatric pyelonephritis.]*

Perazella MA, Markowitz GS: Drug-induced acute interstitial nephritis. *Nat Rev Nephrol* 6:461–70, 2010. *[A review of the various drugs that can induce acute interstitial nephritis along with the relevant clinical and pathologic issues.]*

Vascular Diseases

Hill GS. Hypertensive nephrosclerosis. *Curr Opin Nephrol Hypertens* 17:266–70, 2008. *[A review of the pathophysiologic underpinning of hypertensive nephrosclerosis.]*

Keir L, Coward RJM: Advances in our understanding of the pathogenesis of glomerular thrombotic microangiopathy. *Pediatr Nephrol* 26:523–33, 2011. *[An update of the dysregulation of the alternative pathway of complement cascade and other mechanisms that contribute to thrombotic microangiopathy.]*

Cystic Diseases of the Kidney

Benoit G, Machuca E, Heidet L, et al: Hereditary kidney diseases: highlighting the importance of classical Mendelian phenotypes. *Ann NY Acad Sci* 1214:83–98, 2010. *[A review of the genetic mutations that affect a variety of kidney structures ranging from the podocyte to glomerular basement membranes to mitochrondria.]*

Hildebrandt F, Benzing T, Katsanis N. Ciliopathies. *N Engl J Med* 364:1533–43, 2011. *[An excellent review of the spectrum of single gene mutations involving cilia and their clinical manifestations and underlying disease mechanisms.]*

Neoplasms of the Kidney

Algaba F, Akaza H, Lopez-Beltran A, et al: Current pathology keys of renal cell carcinoma. *Eur Urol* 60:634–43, 2011. *[A comprehensive review of the pathologic classification of renal cell carcinoma.]*

Jonasch E, Futreal A, Davis I, et al: State of the science: an update on renal cell carcinoma. *Mol Cancer Res* 10:859–80, 2012. *[An excellent review of the molecular basis of renal cell carcinoma and their subtypes with an emphasis on potential therapeutic implications.]*

See TARGETED THERAPY available online at www.studentconsult.com

CHAPTER 21

The Lower Urinary Tract and Male Genital System

Jonathan I. Epstein • Tamara L. Lotan

CHAPTER CONTENTS

THE LOWER URINARY TRACT

The renal pelves, ureters, bladder, and urethra (except the terminal portion) are lined by a special form of transitional epithelium called *urothelium*. Urothelium is composed of five to six layers of cells with oval nuclei, often with linear nuclear grooves, and a surface layer consisting of large, flattened "umbrella cells" with abundant cytoplasm. This epithelium rests on a well-developed basement membrane, beneath which is a lamina propria. The lamina propria in the urinary bladder contains wisps of smooth muscle that form discontinuous muscularis mucosae. It is important to differentiate the muscularis mucosae from the deeper well-defined larger muscle bundles of the detrusor muscle (muscularis propria), since bladder cancers are staged on the basis of invasion of the latter. If urine flow is obstructed and intravesical pressures rise, the bladder musculature undergoes hypertrophy.

The ureters lie throughout their course in a retroperitoneal position. Retroperitoneal tumors or fibrosis may entrap the ureters, sometimes obstructing them. As ureters enter the pelvis, they pass anterior to either the common iliac or the external iliac artery. In the female pelvis they lie close to the uterine arteries and are therefore vulnerable to injury in operations on the female genital tract. There are three points of slight narrowing—at the ureteropelvic junction, where they enter the bladder, and where they cross the iliac vessels—all locales where renal calculi may become impacted when they pass from the kidney to the bladder. As the ureters enter the bladder they pursue an oblique course, terminating in a slitlike orifice. The obliquity of this intramural segment of the ureteral orifice permits the enclosing bladder musculature to act like a sphincteric valve, blocking the upward reflux of urine even in the presence of marked distention of the urinary bladder. As discussed in Chapter 20, a defect in the intravesical portion of the ureter leads to vesicoureteral reflux.

The close relationship of the female genital tract to the bladder makes possible the spread of disease from one tract to the other. In middle-aged and older women, relaxation of pelvic support leads to prolapse (descent) of the uterus, pulling with it the floor of the bladder. In this fashion the bladder is protruded into the vagina, creating a pouch *(cystocele)* that fails to empty readily with micturition. In males, the seminal vesicles and prostate have similar close relationships, being situated just posterior and inferior to the neck of the bladder. Thus, enlargement of the prostate, so common in middle to later life, constitutes an important cause of urinary tract obstruction. Subsequent sections discuss the major pathologic lesions of the ureters, urinary bladder, and urethra.

Ureters

Congenital Anomalies

Congenital anomalies of the ureters are found in about 2% or 3% of all autopsies. Although most have little clinical significance, certain anomalies may contribute to obstruction of the flow of urine and thus cause clinical disease. Anomalies of the ureterovesical junction that potentiate reflux are discussed with pyelonephritis in Chapter 20.

- **Double and bifid ureters**. Double ureters are almost invariably associated with totally distinct double renal pelves or with the anomalous development of a large kidney having a partially bifid pelvis terminating in separate ureters. Double ureters may pursue separate courses to the bladder but commonly are joined within the bladder wall and drain through a single ureteral orifice. Most are unilateral and of no clinical significance.
- **Ureteropelvic junction (UPJ) obstruction** is a congenital disorder that is the most common cause of hydronephrosis in infants and children. Cases that present early in life are bilateral in 20% of cases, are often associated with other congenital anomalies, and preferentially occur in males. There is agenesis of the contralateral kidney in a minority of cases. In adults, UPJ obstruction is more common in women and is most often unilateral. The condition has been ascribed to abnormal organization of smooth muscle bundles at the UPJ, to excess stromal deposition of collagen between smooth muscle bundles, or rarely to congenitally extrinsic compression of the UPJ by renal vessels.
- **Diverticula**, saccular outpouchings of the ureteral wall, are uncommon lesions that may be congenital or acquired. Most are asymptomatic, but urinary stasis within diverticula sometimes leads to recurrent infections. Dilation *(hydroureter)*, elongation, and tortuosity of the ureters may occur as congenital anomalies or as acquired defects.

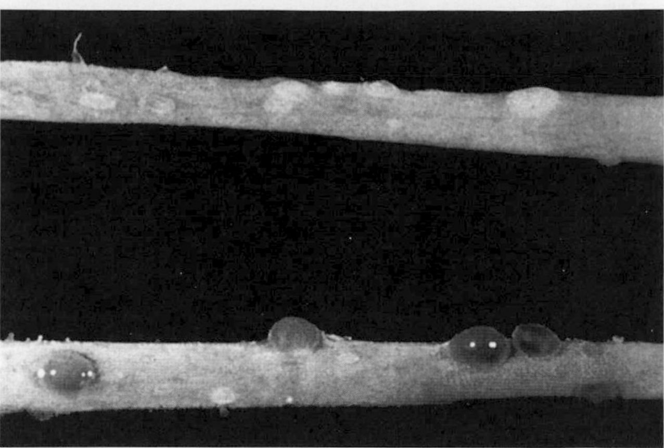

Figure 21-1 Opened ureters showing ureteritis cystica. Note smooth cysts projecting from the mucosa.

Inflammation

Ureteritis, though associated with inflammation, is typically not associated with infection and is of little clinical consequence.

MORPHOLOGY

The accumulation or aggregation of lymphocytes forming germinal centers in the subepithelial region may cause slight elevations of the mucosa and produce a fine granular mucosal surface **(ureteritis follicularis).** At other times the mucosa may become sprinkled with fine cysts varying in diameter from 1 to 5 mm lined by flattened urothelium **(ureteritis cystica)** (Fig. 21-1).

Tumors and Tumor-like Lesions

Primary tumors of the ureter are rare. Small benign tumors of the ureter are generally of mesenchymal origin. *Fibroepithelial polyp* is a tumor-like lesion that presents as a small mass projecting into the lumen, often in children. This lesion occurs more commonly in the ureters but may also involve the bladder, renal pelves, and urethra. The polyp is composed of loose, vascularized connective tissue overlaid by urothelium.

Primary malignant tumors of the ureter resemble those arising in the renal pelvis, calyces, and bladder. The majority are *urothelial carcinomas* (Fig. 21-2). They occur most frequently during the sixth and seventh decades of life and cause obstruction of the ureteral lumen. They are sometimes multifocal and commonly occur concurrently with similar neoplasms in the bladder or renal pelvis.

Obstructive Lesions

A great variety of lesions may obstruct the ureters and give rise to *hydroureter, hydronephrosis,* and sometimes *pyelonephritis* (Chapter 20). It is not the ureteral dilation that is of significance in these cases, but the consequent involvement of the kidneys. The more important causes, divided into those of intrinsic or extrinsic origin, are listed in Table 21-1.

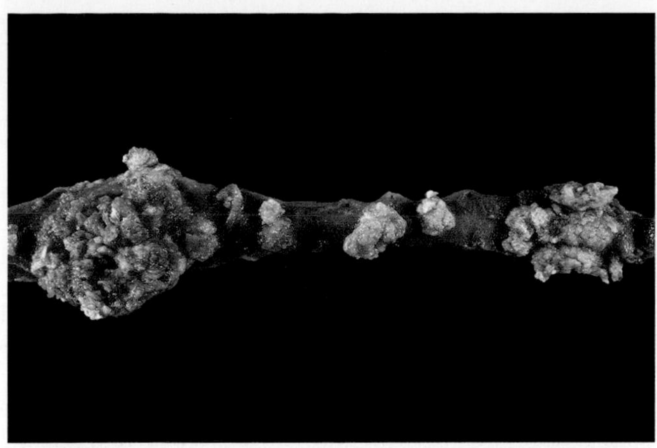

Figure 21-2 Papillary transitional cell carcinoma extensively involving the ureter. (Courtesy Dr. Cristina Magi-Galluzzi, The Johns Hopkins Hospital, Baltimore, Md.)

Unilateral obstruction typically results from proximal causes, whereas bilateral obstruction arises from distal causes, such as nodular hyperplasia of the prostate. Only sclerosing retroperitoneal fibrosis is discussed further.

Sclerosing Retroperitoneal Fibrosis. This uncommon cause of ureteral narrowing or obstruction is characterized by a fibrotic proliferative inflammatory process encasing the retroperitoneal structures and causing hydronephrosis. The disorder occurs in middle to late age and is more common in males than females. At least a subset of these cases is related to *IgG4-related disease*, a recently described entity associated with elevated levels serum IgG4 and fibroinflammatory lesions rich in IgG4-secreting plasma cells (Chapter 6). In addition to the retroperitoneum, this disorder often involves other tissues as well, particularly exocrine organs such as the pancreas and salivary glands. Other cases of retroperitoneal fibrosis are associated with drug exposures (ergot derivatives, β-adrenergic blockers), adjacent inflammatory conditions (vasculitis, diverticulitis, Crohn disease), or malignant disease (lymphomas, urinary tract carcinomas). Most, however, have no obvious cause and are considered primary or idiopathic (Ormond disease).

Microscopic examination typically reveals fibrous tissue containing a prominent infiltrate of lymphocytes, often with germinal centers, plasma cells (frequently IgG4-positive), and eosinophils. Treatment initially involves corticosteroids, although many patients eventually become resistant and require ureteral stents or surgical extrication of the ureters from the surrounding fibrous tissue (ureterolysis).

Table 21-1 Major Causes of Ureteral Obstruction

Type of Obstruction	Cause
Intrinsic	
Calculi	Of renal origin, rarely more than 5 mm in diameter Larger renal stones cannot enter ureters Impact at loci of ureteral narrowing—ureteropelvic junction, where ureters cross iliac vessels, and where they enter bladder—and cause excruciating "renal colic"
Strictures	Congenital or acquired (inflammations)
Tumors	Transitional cell carcinomas arising in ureters Rarely, benign tumors or fibroepithelial polyps
Blood clots	Massive hematuria from renal calculi, tumors, or papillary necrosis
Neurogenic	Interruption of the neural pathways to the bladder
Extrinsic	
Pregnancy	Physiologic relaxation of smooth muscle or pressure on ureters at pelvic brim from enlarging fundus
Periureteral inflammation	Salpingitis, diverticulitis, peritonitis, sclerosing retroperitoneal fibrosis
Endometriosis	With pelvic lesions, followed by scarring
Tumors	Cancers of the rectum, bladder, prostate, ovaries, uterus, cervix; lymphomas, sarcomas

KEY CONCEPTS

Disorders of the Ureters

- Ureteral obstruction is clinically significant because it can subsequently involve the kidney (hydronephrosis or even pyelonephritis), compromising renal function.
- In children, congenital ureteropelvic junction (UPJ) obstruction is the most common obstructive lesion in the ureter.
- In adults, ureteral obstruction may be acute (e.g., due to obstructing calculi), or chronic (e.g., due to intrinsic or extrinsic tumors or rarely idiopathic conditions such as sclerosing retroperitoneal fibrosis).

Urinary Bladder

Diseases of the bladde are often disabling but rarely lethal. Cystitis is particularly common in young women of reproductive age. Tumors of the bladder are an important source of both morbidity and mortality.

Congenital Anomalies

- **Vesicoureteral reflux** is the most common and serious congenital anomaly. As a major contributor to renal infection and scarring, it was discussed earlier, in Chapter 20, in the consideration of pyelonephritis. Abnormal connections between the bladder and the vagina, rectum, or uterus may create *congenital vesicouterine fistulae.*
- **Diverticula** are pouchlike evaginations of the bladder wall that vary from less than 1 cm to 5 to 10 cm in diameter and may be congenital or acquired. *Congenital diverticula* may be due to a focal failure of development of the normal musculature or to some urinary tract obstruction during fetal development. *Acquired diverticula* are most often seen with prostatic enlargement (hyperplasia or neoplasia), producing obstruction to urine outflow and marked muscle thickening of the bladder wall. The increased intravesical pressure causes outpouching of the bladder wall and the formation of diverticula. They are frequently multiple and have narrow necks located

between the interweaving hypertrophied muscle bundles.

Although most diverticula are small and asymptomatic, they may be clinically significant, since they constitute sites of urinary stasis and predispose to infection and the formation of bladder calculi. They may also predispose to vesicoureteral reflux as a result of impingement on the ureter. Rarely, a carcinoma may arise in a bladder diverticulum; such tumors tend to be more advanced in stage as a result of the thin or absent muscle wall of diverticula.

- **Exstrophy of the bladder** is a developmental failure in the anterior wall of the abdomen and the bladder, so that the bladder either communicates directly through a large defect with the surface of the body or lies as an opened sac (Fig. 21-3). The exposed bladder mucosa may undergo colonic glandular metaplasia and is subject to infections that often spread to upper levels of the urinary system. Patients have an increased risk of adenocarcinoma arising in the bladder remnant. These lesions are amenable to surgical correction, and long-term survival is possible.
- **Urachal anomalies.** The urachus (the canal that connects the fetal bladder with the allantois) is normally obliterated after birth, but it sometimes remains patent in part or in whole. When totally patent, a *fistulous urinary tract* connects the bladder with the umbilicus. In other instances, only the central region of the urachus persists, giving rise to *urachal cysts*, lined by either urothelium or metaplastic glandular epithelium. **Carcinomas**, mostly glandular tumors, may arise from such cysts (see "Neoplasms"). These account for only a minority of all bladder cancers (0.1% to 0.3%) but 20% to 40% of bladder adenocarcinomas.

Inflammation

Acute and Chronic Cystitis

Bacterial pyelonephritis is frequently preceded by infection of the urinary bladder, with retrograde spread of microorganisms into the kidneys and their collecting systems (discussed in Chapter 20). The common etiologic agents of cystitis are the coliforms: *Escherichia coli*, followed by *Proteus, Klebsiella*, and *Enterobacter*. Women are more likely to develop cystitis as a result of their shorter urethras. *Tuberculous cystitis* is almost always a sequel to renal tuberculosis. *Candida albicans* and, much less often, cryptococcal agents cause cystitis, particularly in immunosuppressed patients or those receiving long-term antibiotics. Schistosomiasis *(Schistosoma haematobium)* is rare in the United States but is common in certain Middle Eastern countries, notably Egypt. Viruses (e.g., adenovirus), *Chlamydia*, and *Mycoplasma* may also cause cystitis. Predisposing factors include bladder calculi, urinary obstruction, diabetes mellitus, instrumentation, and immune deficiency. Finally, irradiation of the bladder region gives rise to *radiation cystitis*.

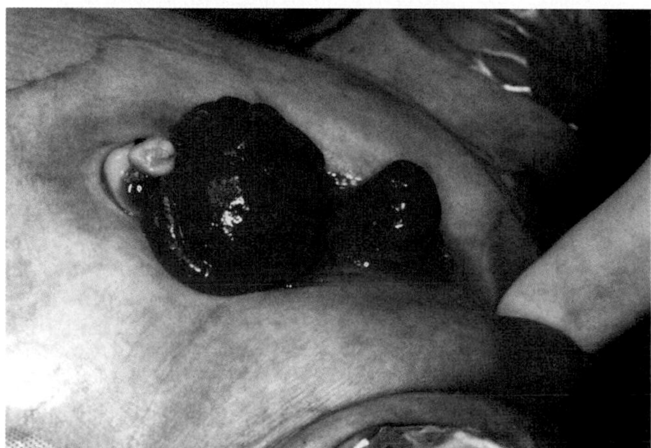

Figure 21-3 Exstrophy of the bladder in a newborn boy. The tied umbilical cord is seen above the hyperemic mucosa of the everted bladder. Below is an incompletely formed penis with marked epispadias. (Courtesy of Dr. John Gearhart, The Johns Hopkins Hospital, Baltimore, MD.)

MORPHOLOGY

Most cases of cystitis produce nonspecific acute or chronic inflammation of the bladder. In acute cystitis there is hyperemia of the mucosa and neutrophilic infiltrate, sometimes associated with exudate. Patients receiving **cytotoxic antitumor drugs**, such as cyclophosphamide, may develop **hemorrhagic cystitis.** Adenovirus infection also causes a hemorrhagic cystitis. Persistence of the bacterial infection leads to **chronic cystitis** associated with mononuclear inflammatory infiltrates.

Other patterns of chronic cystitis worthy of brief mention are not always related to infection. **Follicular cystitis** is characterized by the presence of lymphoid follicles within the bladder mucosa and underlying wall. **Eosinophilic cystitis**, manifested by infiltration with submucosal eosinophils, typically is a nonspecific subacute inflammation but may also be a manifestation of a systemic allergic disorder.

All forms of cystitis are characterized by a triad of symptoms: (1) frequency, which in acute cases may necessitate urination every 15 to 20 minutes; (2) lower abdominal pain localized over the bladder region or in the suprapubic region; and (3) dysuria—pain or burning on urination.

The local symptoms of cystitis may be merely disturbing, but these infections may also be antecedents to pyelonephritis, a more serious disorder (Chapter 20). Cystitis is sometimes a secondary complication of an underlying disorder associated with urinary stasis, such as prostatic enlargement, cystocele of the bladder, calculi, or tumors. These primary diseases must be corrected before the cystitis can be relieved.

Special Forms of Cystitis

Several variants of cystitis have distinctive causes or morphologic appearances.

Interstitial Cystitis (Chronic Pelvic Pain Syndrome). This form of chronic cystitis occurs most frequently in women and is characterized by intermittent, often severe, suprapubic pain, urinary frequency, urgency, hematuria and dysuria, and cystoscopic findings of fissures and punctate hemorrhages (glomerulations) in the bladder mucosa after luminal distention. The etiology of this troubling condition is unknown, its evaluation and diagnosis remain controversial, and its treatment is largely empiric. Some cases are associated with chronic mucosal ulcers *(Hunner ulcers)*; this is termed the *late (classic, ulcerative) phase*. Increased numbers of mucosal mast cells are characteristic of this disease, but their pathogenic significance and diagnostic utility are uncertain. Late in the course, transmural fibrosis may appear, leading to a contracted bladder. The pathologic findings are nonspecific, and the main role of biopsy is to rule out carcinoma in situ, which may mimic interstitial cystitis clinically.

Malakoplakia. A distinctive chronic inflammatory reaction that appears to stem from acquired defects in phagocyte function, malakoplakia arises in the setting of chronic bacterial infection, mostly by *E. coli* or occasionally *Proteus* species. It occurs with increased frequency in immunosuppressed transplant recipients.

MORPHOLOGY

In the bladder, malakoplakia takes the form of soft, yellow, slightly raised mucosal plaques, 3 to 4 cm in diameter (Fig. 21-4), that are filled with large, foamy macrophages mixed with occasional multinucleate giant cells and lymphocytes. The **macrophages have an abundant granular cytoplasm** due to phagosomes stuffed with particulate and membranous debris of bacterial origin. In addition, laminated mineralized concretions resulting from deposition of calcium in enlarged lysosomes, known as **Michaelis-Gutmann bodies,** are typically present within the macrophages (Fig. 21-5). The unusual-appearing macrophages and giant phagosomes point to defects in the phagocytic function of macrophages, which become overloaded with undigested bacterial products. Similar lesions have been described in the colon, lungs, bones, kidneys, prostate, and epididymis.

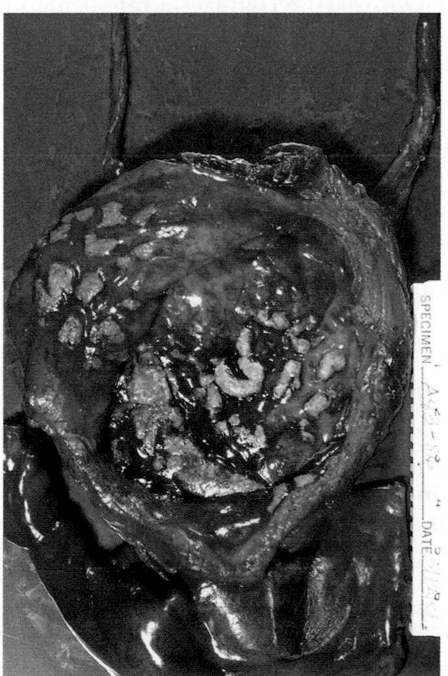

Figure 21-4 Cystitis with malakoplakia showing inflammatory exudate and broad, flat plaques.

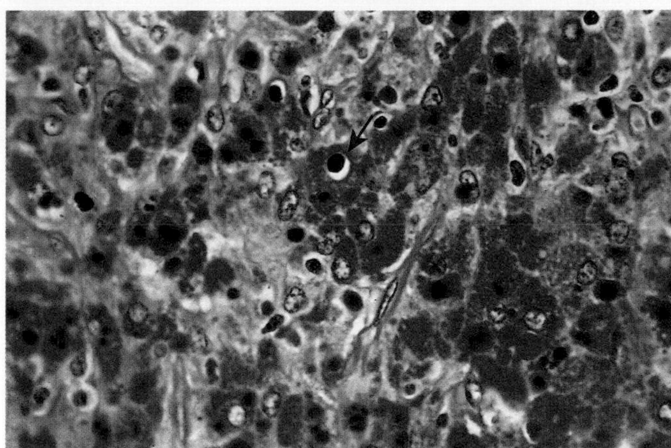

Figure 21-5 Malacoplakia, periodic acid–Schiff (PAS) stain. Note the large macrophages with granular PAS-positive cytoplasm and several dense, round Michaelis-Gutmann bodies surrounded by artifactual cleared holes in the upper middle field *(arrow)*.

Polypoid Cystitis. Polypoid cystitis is an inflammatory lesion resulting from irritation of the bladder mucosa. Although indwelling catheters are the most commonly cited culprits, any injurious agent may give rise to this lesion. The urothelium is thrown into broad bulbous polypoid projections as a result of marked submucosal edema. Polypoid cystitis may be confused with papillary urothelial carcinoma both clinically and histologically.

Metaplastic Lesions

- **Cystitis glandularis and cystitis cystica.** These are common lesions of the urinary bladder in which nests of urothelium (Brunn nests) grow downward into the lamina propria. Here, epithelial cells in the center of the nest undergo metaplasia and take on a cuboidal or columnar appearance *(cystitis glandularis)*, or retract to produce cystic spaces lined by flattened urothelium *(cystitis cystica)*. Because the two processes often coexist, the condition is typically referred to as *cystitis cystica et glandularis*. In a variant of cystitis glandularis goblet cells are present, and the epithelium resembles intestinal mucosa *(intestinal* or *colonic metaplasia)*. Both variants are common incidental findings in normal bladders, but they can also arise in the setting of inflammation and metaplasia.
- **Squamous metaplasia.** As a response to injury, the urothelium is often replaced by nonkeratinizing squamous epithelium, which is a more durable lining. This should be distinguished from glycogenated squamous epithelium that is normally found in women at the trigone.
- **Nephrogenic adenoma.** Nephrogenic adenoma is an unusual lesion that results from implantation of shed renal tubular cells at sites of injured urothelium. The overlying urothelium may be focally replaced by cuboidal epithelium, which can assume a papillary growth pattern. Although the lesions are typically less than a centimeter in size, larger lesions have been reported that can produce signs and symptoms that raise a suspicion of cancer. In addition, the tubular proliferation can

infiltrate the underlying lamina propria and superficial detrusor muscle, mimicking a malignant process.

KEY CONCEPTS

Inflammatory disorders and metaplasias of the bladder

- The bladder can be involved by a number of inflammatory lesions, many of which manifest with frequency and dysuria.
- Acute or chronic bacterial cystitis is extremely common, particularly in women, and results from retrograde spread of colonic bacteria in most cases.
- Other forms of cystitis have iatrogenic causes, such as radiation cystitis and hemorrhagic cystitis due to antitumor chemotherapeutics.
- Some inflammatory or metaplastic bladder lesions are significant in that they may clinically mimic bladder cancer, including malakoplakia, polypoid cystitis, cystitis cystica et glandularis and nephrogenic adenoma.

Neoplasms

Bladder cancer accounts for approximately 7% of cancers and 3% of cancer mortality in the United States. About 95% of bladder tumors are of epithelial origin, the remainder being mesenchymal tumors (Table 21-2). Most epithelial tumors are urothelial (transitional cell) type and are thus interchangeably called *urothelial or transitional tumors,* but squamous and glandular carcinomas also occur. Here we focus on urothelial tumors and touch briefly on the others.

Urothelial Tumors

Urothelial tumors represent about 90% of all bladder tumors and run the gamut from small benign lesions that do not recur to aggressive cancers that are often fatal. Many of these tumors are multifocal at presentation. Though most common in the bladder, all of the urothelial lesions described here may be seen at any site where there is urothelium, from the renal pelvis to the distal urethra.

There are two distinct precursor lesions to invasive urothelial carcinoma: noninvasive papillary tumors and flat noninvasive urothelial carcinoma. The most common precursor lesions are the noninvasive papillary tumors, which originate from papillary urothelial hyperplasia. These tumors have a range of atypical changes, and are graded according to their biologic behavior. The other precursor lesion to invasive carcinoma, flat noninvasive urothelial carcinoma is referred to as carcinoma in situ, or CIS.

Table 21-2 Tumors of the Urinary Bladder

Urothelial (transitional) tumors
Exophytic papilloma
Inverted papilloma
Papillary urothelial neoplasms of low malignant potential
Low-grade and high-grade papillary urothelial cancers
Carcinoma in situ (CIS, or flat noninvasive urothelial carcinoma)
Mixed carcinoma
Adenocarcinoma
Small-cell carcinoma
Sarcomas

Table 21-3 Grading of Urothelial (Transitional Cell) Tumors

WHO/ISUP Grades
Urothelial papilloma
Urothelial neoplasm of low malignant potential
Papillary urothelial carcinoma, low grade
Papillary urothelial carcinoma, high grade
WHO Grades
Urothelial papilloma
Urothelial neoplasm of low malignant potential
Papillary urothelial carcinoma, grade 1
Papillary urothelial carcinoma, grade 2
Papillary urothelial carcinoma, grade 3

ISUP, International Society of Urological Pathology; WHO, World Health Organization.

As discussed in Chapter 7, CIS is a term used to describe epithelial lesions that have the cytologic features of malignancy but are confined to the epithelium, showing no evidence of basement membrane invasion. Such lesions are considered to be high grade. In about one half of individuals with invasive bladder cancer, the tumor has already invaded the bladder wall at the time of presentation, and precursor lesions are not detected. It is presumed in such cases that the precursor lesion was destroyed by the high-grade invasive component, which typically appears as a large, frequently ulcerated mass. Although invasion into the lamina propria worsens the prognosis, the major decrease in survival is associated with invasion of the muscularis propria (detrusor muscle). Once muscularis propria invasion occurs, there is a 30% 5-year mortality rate.

Table 21-3 lists two of the most common grading systems of these tumors. The World Health Organization (WHO) 1973 classification grades tumors into a rare totally benign papilloma and three grades of transitional cell carcinoma (grades I, II, and III). A more recent classification, based on a consensus reached at a conference by the International Society of Urological Pathology (ISUP) in 1998 and adopted by the WHO in 2004, recognizes a rare benign papilloma, a group of papillary urothelial neoplasms of low malignant potential, and two grades of carcinoma (low and high grade).

Epidemiology and Pathogenesis. The incidence of carcinoma of the bladder is higher in men than in women, in developed than in developing nations, and in urban than in rural dwellers. The male-to-female ratio for urothelial tumors is approximately 3:1. About 80% of patients are between 50 and 80 years of age. Bladder cancer, with rare exceptions, is not familial.

Several factors have been implicated in the causation of urothelial carcinoma. Some of the more important contributors include the following:

- **Cigarette smoking is clearly the most important influence, increasing the risk threefold to sevenfold, depending on the duration and type of tobacco use.** Between 50% and 80% of all bladder cancers among men are associated with the use of cigarettes. Cigars, pipes, and smokeless tobacco are associated with a smaller risk.
- **Industrial exposure to aryl amines**, particularly 2-naphthylamine and related compounds, as pointed out in our earlier discussion of chemical carcinogenesis

(Chapter 7). The cancers appear 15 to 40 years after the first exposure.

- ***Schistosoma haematobium*** infections in endemic areas (Egypt, Sudan) are an established risk. The ova are deposited in the bladder wall and incite a brisk chronic inflammatory response that induces progressive mucosal squamous metaplasia and dysplasia and, in some instances, neoplasia. Seventy percent of the cancers are squamous, the remainder being urothelial or, least commonly, glandular.
- **Long-term use of analgesics** is implicated, as it is in analgesic nephropathy (Chapter 20).
- **Heavy long-term exposure to cyclophosphamide**, an immunosuppressive agent, induces, as noted, hemorrhagic cystitis, and increases the risk of bladder cancer.
- **Irradiation**, often administered for other pelvic malignancies, increases the risk of urothelial carcinoma. In this setting, bladder cancer occurs many years after the irradiation.

Several acquired genetic alterations have been observed in urothelial carcinoma, many of which lead to constitutive activation of growth factor receptor signaling cascades (Chapter 7). Some of these alterations are strongly associated with tumor histopathology. These include gain-of-function mutations in *FGFR3*, which are found predominantly in noninvasive low-grade papillary carcinomas and result in constitutive activation of the FGFR3 receptor tyrosine kinase. In contrast, loss-of-function mutations in the *TP53* and *RB* tumor suppressor genes are almost always seen in high-grade and, frequently, muscle invasive tumors. Other genetic alterations are not as tightly associated with tumor histologic features. Activating mutations in the *HRAS* oncogene are freqeuntly found, particularly in low-grade, noninvasive tumors. Recalling that RAS signal transducers act downstream of receptor tyrosine kinases such as FGFR3, it is not surprising that *HRAS* and *FGFR3* mutations are generally mutually exclusive in bladder cancer.

Particularly common (occurring in 30% to 60% of tumors) are losses of genetic material on chromosome 9 (including monosomy or deletions of 9p and 9q). These abnormalities are often the only chromosomal changes present in superficial noninvasive papillary tumors and occasionally in noninvasive flat tumors, suggesting that these are early events in the evolution of bladder carcinomas. The 9p deletions (9p20) span a region that includes the tumor suppressor gene *CDKN2A*, which encodes the cyclin-dependent kinase inhibitor p16/INK4a and ARF, a protein that augments p53 function (Chapter 7). Several different tumor suppressor genes have been proposed to be the target of deletions on chromosome 9q, including *PTCH*, which encodes a negative regulator of the Hedgehog signaling pathway, and *TSC1*, which encodes a negative regulator of mTOR signaling. On the basis of these findings, a model for bladder carcinogenesis has been proposed. In this two-pathway model, low-grade superficial papillary tumors are characterized by *FGFR3* and *RAS* mutations and chromosome 9 deletions. Of these, a minority may then lose *TP53* and/or *RB* function and progress to invasion. In the second more aggressive pathway, noninvasive high-grade flat or papillary lesions are initiated by *TP53* mutations and, with loss of chromosome 9 and acquisition of other, still to be characterized mutations, progression to invasion ensues (Chapter 7).

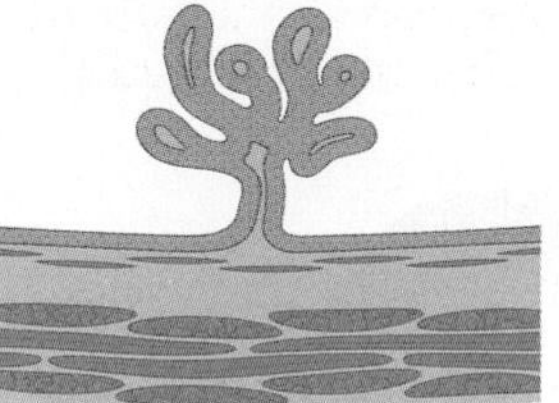

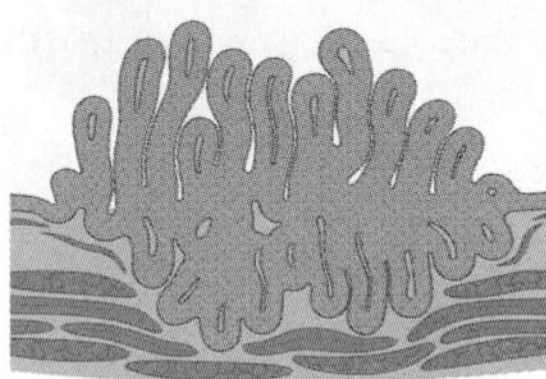

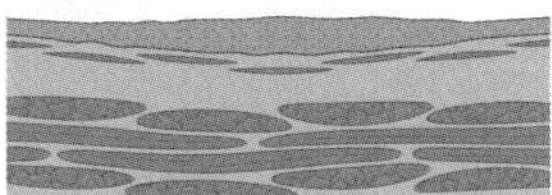

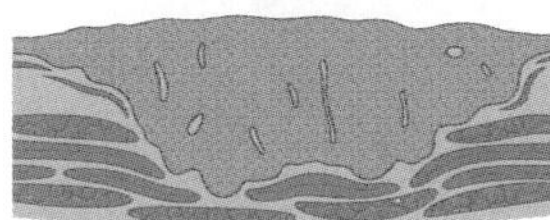

Figure 21-6 Four morphologic patterns of bladder tumors. CIS, Carcinoma in situ.

MORPHOLOGY

The appearance of urothelial tumors varies from purely papillary to nodular or flat (Fig. 21-6). Most arise from the lateral or posterior walls at the bladder base. Papillary lesions are red, elevated excrescences ranging in size from less than 1 cm in diameter to large masses up to 5 cm in diameter (Fig. 21-7). Multiple discrete tumors are often present. As noted, the histologic features encompass a spectrum from benign papilloma to highly aggressive anaplastic cancers. Overall, the majority of papillary tumors are low grade.

- **Papillomas** represent 1% or less of bladder tumors, and are usually seen in younger patients. These tumors typically arise singly as small (0.5 to 2 cm), delicate, structures, superficially

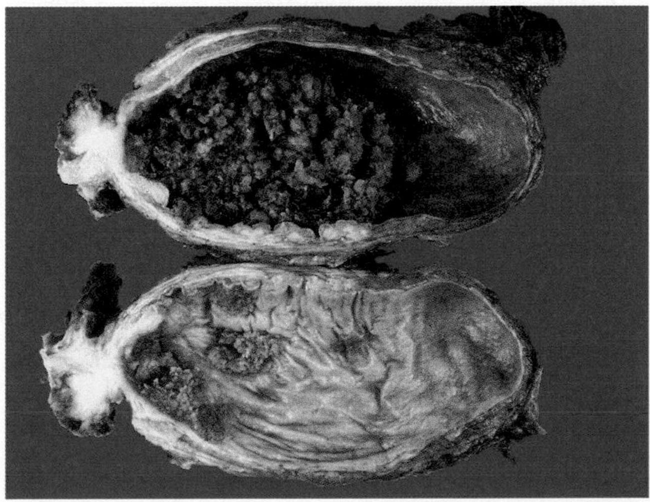

Figure 21-7 Cross-section of bladder with upper section showing a large papillary tumor. The lower section demonstrates multifocal smaller papillary neoplasms. (Courtesy Dr. Fred Gilkey, Sinai Hospital, Baltimore, Md.)

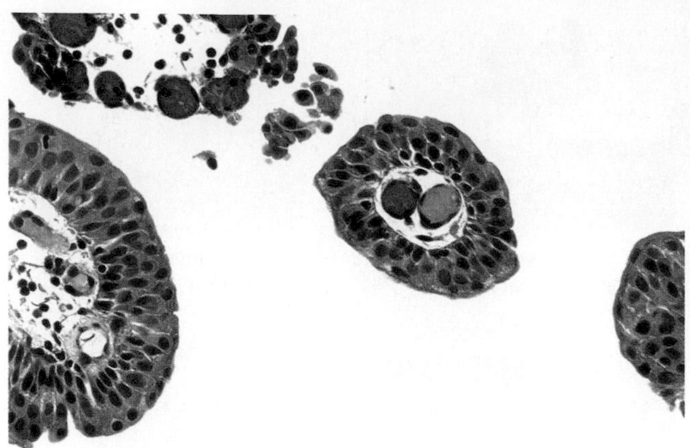

Figure 21-8 Papilloma consisting of small papillary fronds lined by normal-appearing urothelium.

attached to the mucosa by a stalk and are referred to as **exophytic papillomas**. The individual finger-like papillae have a central core of loose fibrovascular tissue covered by epithelium that is **histologically identical to normal urothelium** (Fig. 21-8). Recurrences and progression are rare but may occur. In contrast to exophytic papillomas, **inverted papillomas** are completely benign lesions consisting of inter-anastomosing cords of cytologically bland urothelium that extend down into the lamina propria.

- **Papillary urothelial neoplasms of low malignant potential** share many histologic features with papilloma, differing only in having thicker urothelium. At cystoscopy, these tumors tend to be larger than papillomas and may be indistinguishable from low- and high-grade papillary cancers. Recurrent tumors usually show the same morphology; progression to tumors of higher grade may occur but is rare.
- **Low-grade papillary urothelial carcinomas** have an orderly architectural and cytologic appearance. The cells are evenly spaced (i.e., maintain polarity) and cohesive. There is a mild degree of nuclear atypia consisting of scattered hyperchromatic nuclei, infrequent mitotic figures predominantly toward the base, and slight variation in nuclear size and shape (Fig. 21-9). These low-grade cancers may recur and, although infrequent, may also invade. Only rarely do these tumors pose a threat to the patient's life.

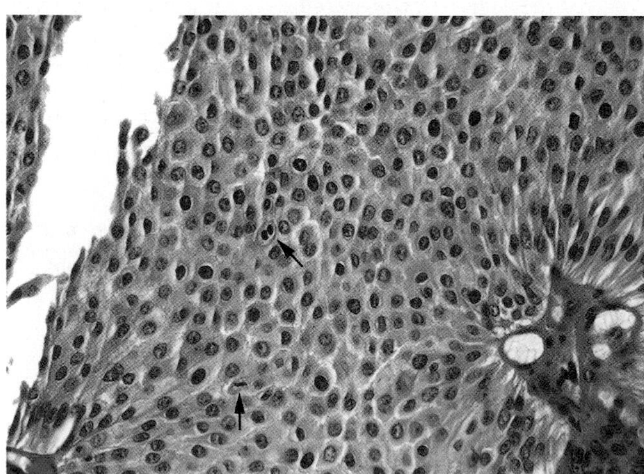

Figure 21-9 Low-grade papillary urothelial carcinoma with an overall orderly appearance, with a thicker lining than papilloma and scattered hyperchromatic nuclei and mitotic figures *(arrows)*.

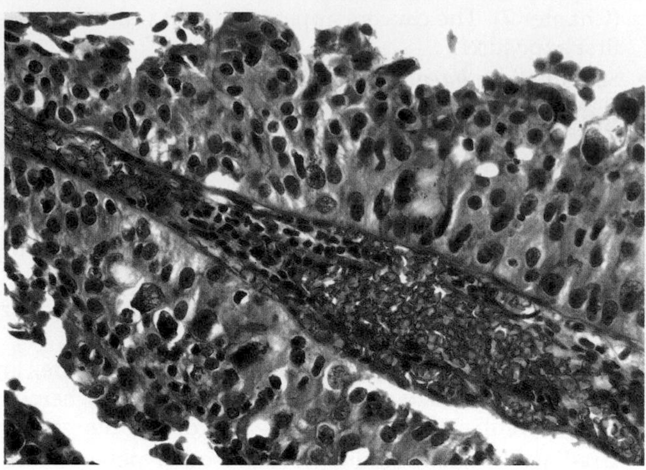

Figure 21-10 High-grade papillary urothelial carcinoma with marked cytologic atypia.

- **High-grade papillary urothelial cancers** contain dyscohesive cells with large hyperchromatic nuclei. Some of the tumor cells are highly anaplastic (Fig. 21-10). Mitotic figures, including atypical ones, are frequent. Architecturally, there is disarray and loss of polarity. As compared to low-grade lesions, these tumors have a much higher incidence of invasion into the muscular layer, a higher risk of progression, and, when associated with invasion, a significant metastatic potential.

In most series, less than 10% of low-grade cancers invade, but as many as 80% of high-grade urothelial carcinomas are invasive. Aggressive tumors may extend into the bladder wall, and, in more advanced stages, invade the adjacent prostate, seminal vesicles, ureters, and retroperitoneum. Some tumors produce fistulous communications to the vagina or rectum. About 40% of these deeply invasive tumors metastasize to regional lymph nodes. Hematogenous dissemination, principally to the liver, lungs, and bone marrow, may result.

Carcinoma in situ (CIS, or flat urothelial carcinoma) is defined by the presence of cytologically malignant cells within a flat urothelium. CIS may range from full-thickness cytologic atypia to scattered malignant cells in an otherwise normal urothelium, the latter termed **pagetoid spread** (Fig. 21-11). A common feature shared with high-grade papillary urothelial carcinoma is a lack of cohesiveness, which leads to the shedding of malignant cells into the urine. When shedding is extensive, only a few CIS cells may be left clinging to a largely denuded basement membrane. CIS usually appears as an area of mucosal reddening, granularity, or thickening without an evident intraluminal mass. It is commonly multifocal and may involve most of the bladder surface and extend into the ureters and urethra. If untreated, 50% to 75% of CIS cases progress to invasive cancer.

Invasive urothelial cancer (Fig. 21-12) may be associated with papillary urothelial cancer, usually high grade, or adjacent CIS. The extent of the invasion into the muscularis mucosae is of prognostic significance, and understaging on biopsy is a significant problem. The extent of spread **(staging)** at the time

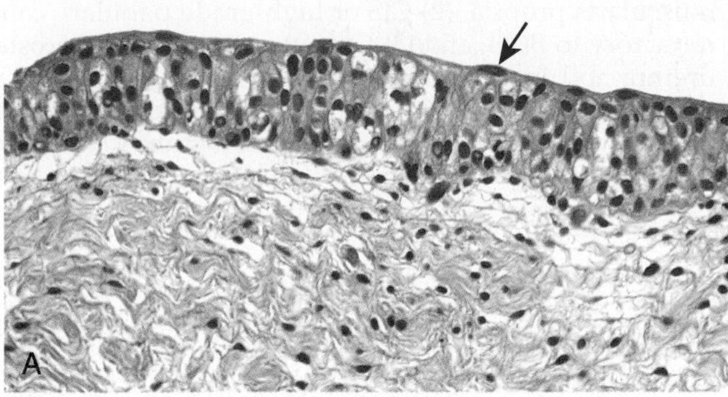

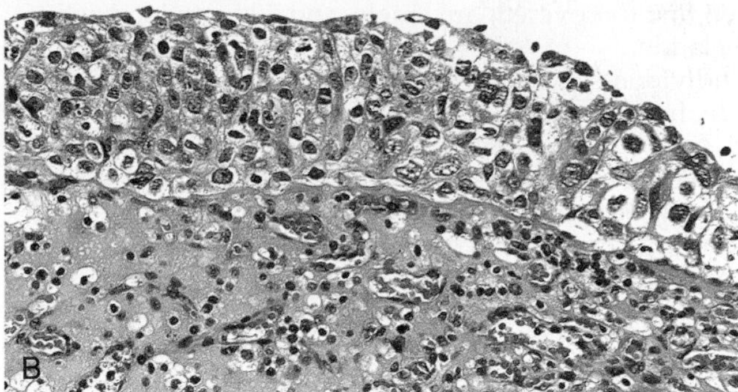

Figure 21-11 **A,** Normal urothelium with uniform nuclei and well-developed umbrella cell layer *(arrow)*. **B,** Flat carcinoma in situ with numerous cells having enlarged and pleomorphic nuclei.

of initial diagnosis is the most important factor in determining the outlook for a patient (Table 21-4). Almost all infiltrating urothelial carcinomas are high grade, and as a result grading of the infiltrating component is not critical, as opposed to the importance of grading noninvasive papillary urothelial carcinoma.

Figure 21-12 Opened bladder showing a high-grade invasive transitional cell carcinoma at an advanced stage. The aggressive multinodular neoplasm has fungated into the bladder lumen and spread over a wide area. The yellow areas represent areas of ulceration and necrosis.

Variants of Urothelial Carcinoma. Unusual variants of urothelial cancer include a nested variant with deceptively bland cytology, lymphoepithelioma-like carcinoma, and micropapillary carcinoma.

Other Epithelial Bladder Tumors. *Squamous cell carcinomas* resembling squamous cancers occurring at other sites make up 3% to 7% of bladder cancers in the United States, but are much more frequent in countries where urinary schistosomiasis is endemic. Pure squamous cell carcinomas are nearly always associated with chronic bladder irritation and infection. *Mixed urothelial carcinomas with areas of squamous carcinoma* are more frequent than pure squamous cell carcinomas. Most are invasive, fungating tumors or are infiltrative and ulcerative. The level of cellular differentiation varies widely, from well differentiated lesions producing abundant keratin to anaplastic tumors with only focal evidence of squamous differentiation.

Adenocarcinomas of the bladder are rare and histologically identical to adenocarcinomas seen in the gastrointestinal tract. Some arise from urachal remnants or in association with extensive intestinal metaplasia (discussed earlier).

Small-cell carcinomas, indistinguishable from small-cell carcinomas of the lung, arise in the bladder often in association with urothelial, squamous, or adenocarcinoma.

Clinical Course of Bladder Cancer. Bladder tumors classically produce *painless hematuria.* This is their dominant and sometimes only clinical manifestation. Frequency, urgency, and dysuria occasionally accompany the hematuria. When the ureteral orifice is involved, pyelonephritis or hydronephrosis may follow. About 60% of neoplasms,

Table 21-4 Pathologic T (Primary Tumor) Staging of Bladder Carcinoma

Depth of Invasion	AJCC/UICC
Ta	Noninvasive, papillary
Tis	Carcinoma in situ (noninvasive, flat)
T1	Lamina propria invasion
T2	Muscularis propria invasion
T3a	Microscopic extravesicle invasion
T3b	Grossly apparent extravesicle invasion
T4	Invades adjacent structures

AJCC/UICC, American Joint Commission on Cancer/Union Internationale Contre le Cancer.

when first discovered, are single, and 70% are localized to the bladder.

Individuals with urothelial tumors, whatever their grade, have a tendency to develop new tumors after excision, and *recurrences* may show a higher grade. The risk of recurrence and progression is related to several variables, including tumor size, stage, grade, multifocality, prior recurrence rate, and associated dysplasia and/or CIS in the surrounding mucosa. Although the term recurrence is used, most of the subsequent tumors arise at different sites from the original lesion. In some instances the recurrences may be entirely independent new tumors, but in other cases they share the same clonal abnormalities as the initial tumor and represent a true recurrence caused (presumably) by shedding and implantation of the original tumor cells at a new anatomic site.

Prognosis depends on the histologic grade and the stage at diagnosis. Papillomas, papillary urothelial neoplasms of low malignant potential, and low-grade papillary urothelial cancer yield a 98% 10-year survival rate regardless of the number of recurrences; only a few patients (<10%) have progression of their disease to higher grade lesions. High-grade papillary urothelial carcinomas invade and lead to death in about 25% of cases. Patients with primary (de novo) CIS, as opposed to CIS associated with infiltrating urothelial carcinoma, are less likely to progress to muscle-invasive cancer (28% versus 59%) or die of disease (7% versus 45%). Invasive urothelial carcinoma is associated with a 30% mortality rate once tumor invades into the lamina propria. Overall, squamous cell carcinoma and adenocarcinoma are associated with a worse prognosis than urothelial carcinoma, yet stage for stage they are all similar.

The clinical challenge with these neoplasms is early detection and adequate follow-up. A significant issue is that 50% of invasive bladder cancers present with muscle-invasive disease and have a relatively poor prognosis despite therapy. For tumors detected at an earlier stage, cystoscopy and biopsy are the mainstays of diagnosis. Subsequently, patients are typically followed with additional surveillance cystoscopies to look for tumor recurrence. Additionally, cytologic examination of cells obtained from urine samples and tests performed on urine to detect chromosomal abnormalities (aneuploidy of chromosome 3, 7, and 17 and 9p deletions) by fluorescent in situ hybridization (FISH) are also helpful screening measures, particularly for CIS that might be missed by cytoscopy. The major limitation of both FISH and cytologic screening is that they often fail to identify low-grade neoplasms.

The selection of treatment for bladder cancer depends on the grade, stage, and whether the lesion is flat or papillary. For small, localized low-grade papillary tumors, the diagnostic transurethral resection is the only surgical procedure done. Patients are followed with cystoscopy and urine cytology for the rest of their lives to detect recurrence. Patients at high risk of recurrence and/or progression (CIS; papillary tumors that are high grade, multifocal, have a history of recurrence, or are associated with lamina propria invasion) receive intravesical instillation of an attenuated strain of *Mycobacterium bovis* called bacillus Calmette-Guérin (BCG). The bacteria elicit a local inflammatory reaction that destroys the tumor. Radical cystectomy is typically reserved for (1) tumor invading the muscularis propria, (2) CIS or high-grade papillary cancer refractory to BCG, and (3) CIS extending into the prostatic urethra and into the prostatic ducts, where BCG will not come into contact with the neoplastic cells. Metastatic bladder cancer responds to chemotherapy, but is not curable with current agents.

Mesenchymal Tumors

Benign Tumors. A great variety of benign mesenchymal tumors may arise in the bladder, having the histologic features of their counterparts elsewhere. Collectively, they are rare. The most common is *leiomyoma.* They all tend to grow as isolated, intramural, encapsulated, oval-to-spherical masses, varying in diameter up to several centimeters.

Sarcomas. True sarcomas are distinctly uncommon in the bladder. Inflammatory myofibroblastic tumors and various carcinomas may assume sarcomatoid growth patterns and be mistaken histologically for sarcomas. As a group, sarcomas tend to produce large masses (varying up to 10 to 15 cm in diameter) that protrude into the vesicle lumen. Their soft, fleshy, gray-white gross appearance suggests their sarcomatous nature. The most common sarcoma in infancy or childhood is *embryonal rhabdomyosarcoma.* In some of these cases they manifest as a polypoid grapelike mass *(sarcoma botryoides).* The most common sarcoma in the bladder in adults is leiomyosarcoma (Chapter 26).

Secondary Tumors

Secondary malignant involvement of the bladder is most often by direct extension from primary lesions in nearby organs, cervix, uterus, prostate, and rectum. Lymphomas may involve the bladder as a component of systemic disease, but also, rarely, as primary bladder lymphoma.

KEY CONCEPTS

Bladder Tumors

- Bladder cancer is more common in males than in females and cigarette smoking constitutes one of the most important risk factors.
- Painless hematuria is a common presenting symptom of bladder cancer and requires clinical investigation by cystoscopy and/or urine cytology specimens to rule out urothelial neoplasia.
- There are two different noninvasive precursor lesions to invasive urothelial carcinoma: papillary urothelial carcinoma (which may be low- or high-grade) and flat urothelial carcinoma in situ (uniformly high grade).
- Noninvasive high-grade urothelial carcinoma (either papillary or flat) is associated with loss of the *TP53* and *RB* tumor suppressor genes and frequently progresses to muscle-invasive disease with the potential for systemic spread.
- Noninvasive low-grade papillary urothelial carcinoma is associated with gain of function *FGFR3* and *HRAS* mutations. While these tumors are infrequently life-threatening, they may locally recur and a subset may progress to high grade disease.

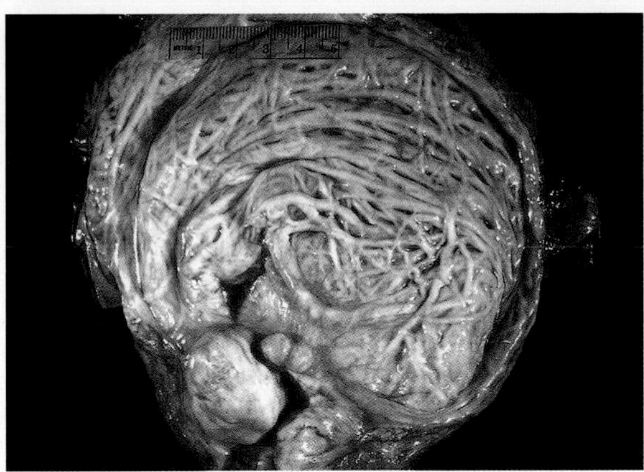

Figure 21-13 Hypertrophy and trabeculation of bladder wall secondary to polypoid hyperplasia of the prostate.

- Other epithelial bladder tumor variants may occur, either alone or mixed with urothelial carcinoma, including squamous cell carcinoma, adenocarcinoma and small cell carcinoma.

Obstruction

Obstruction of the bladder outlet is of major clinical importance because of its eventual effect on the kidney. In males, the most common cause is enlargement of the prostate gland due to nodular hyperplasia (Fig. 21-13). Bladder obstruction is less common in females and is most often caused by cystocele of the bladder. Infrequent causes are (1) congenital urethral strictures, (2) inflammatory urethral strictures, (3) inflammatory fibrosis and contraction of the bladder, (4) bladder tumors, either benign or malignant, (5) invasion of the bladder neck by tumors arising in contiguous organs, (6) mechanical obstructions caused by foreign bodies and calculi, and (7) injury of nerves controlling bladder contraction (neurogenic bladder).

MORPHOLOGY

In the early stages there is only thickening of the bladder wall due to smooth muscle hypertrophy. With progressive hypertrophy the individual muscle bundles greatly enlarge and produce trabeculation of the bladder wall. In the course of time, crypts form and may be converted into diverticula.

In some cases of acute obstruction or in terminal disease when the patient's normal reflex mechanisms are depressed, the bladder may become extremely dilated. The enlarged bladder may reach the brim of the pelvis or even the level of the umbilicus. In these cases the bladder wall is markedly thinned and lacks trabeculations.

Urethra

Inflammation

Urethritis is classically divided into gonococcal and nongonococcal causes. *Gonococcal urethritis* is one of the earliest manifestations of this venereal infection. *Nongonococcal urethritis* is common and can be caused by several different organisms. Various strains of *Chlamydia* (e.g., *C. trachomatis*) are the cause of 25% to 60% of nongonococcal urethritis in men and about 20% in women. *Mycoplasma (Ureaplasma urealyticum)* also accounts for the symptoms of urethritis in many cases. Urethritis is often accompanied by cystitis in women and by prostatitis in men. In many instances of suspected bacterial urethritis, no organism can be isolated. Some urethritis is truly noninfectious in origin. An example of such an inflammatory urethritis is a disorder known as *reactive arthritis*, which is associated with the clinical triad of arthritis, conjunctivitis, and urethritis (Chapter 26).

The morphologic changes are entirely typical of inflammation in other sites within the urinary tract. The urethral involvement is not itself a serious clinical problem but may cause considerable local pain, itching, and frequency, and may warn of more serious disease at higher levels of the urogenital tract.

Tumors and Tumor-like Lesions

Urethral caruncle is an inflammatory lesion that presents as a small, red, painful mass about the external urethral meatus, typically in older females. It consists of inflamed granulation tissue covered by an intact but extremely friable mucosa, which may ulcerate and bleed with the slightest trauma. Surgical excision affords prompt relief and cure.

Benign epithelial tumors of the urethra include squamous and urothelial papillomas, inverted urothelial papillomas, and condylomas.

Primary carcinoma of the urethra is an uncommon lesion (Fig. 21-14). Tumors arising within the proximal urethra tend to show urothelial differentiation and are analogous to those occurring within the bladder, whereas lesions found within the distal urethra are more often squamous cell carcinomas. Adeno carcinomas are infrequent in the urethra and generally occur in women. Some neoplastic lesions of the urethra are similar to those described in the bladder, arising through metaplasia or, less commonly, from periurethral glands. Cancers arising within the prostatic urethra are dealt with in the section on the prostate.

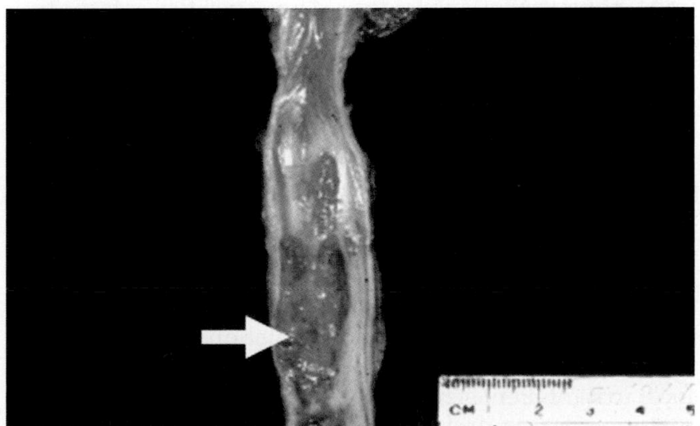

Figure 21-14 Carcinoma of urethra with typical fungating growth.

THE MALE GENITAL TRACT

Penis

The penis can be affected by congenital anomalies, inflammations, and tumors, inflammations and tumors being the most important.

Congenital Anomalies

The penis is involved by many congenital anomalies; only those that are clinically significant are discussed here.

Hypospadias and Epispadias

Malformation of the urethral groove and urethral canal may create an abnormal urethral opening either on the ventral surface of the penis (*hypospadias*) or on the dorsal surface (*epispadias*). Either of these two anomalies may be associated with failure of normal descent of the testes and with malformations of the urinary tract. Hypospadias, the more common of the two, occurs in approximately 1 in 300 live male births. Even when isolated, these urethral defects may have clinical significance, because the abnormal opening is often constricted, resulting in urinary tract obstruction and an increased risk of ascending urinary tract infections. When the orifices are situated near the base of the penis, normal ejaculation and insemination are hampered and may be a cause of sterility.

Phimosis

When the orifice of the prepuce is too small to permit its normal retraction, the condition is designated *phimosis*. An abnormally small orifice may result from anomalous development but is more frequently the result of repeated attacks of infection that cause scarring of the preputial ring. Phimosis is important because it interferes with cleanliness and permits the accumulation of secretions and detritus under the prepuce, favoring the development of secondary infections and possibly carcinoma.

Inflammation

Inflammations of the penis almost invariably involve the glans and prepuce and include a wide variety of specific and nonspecific infections. The specific infections—syphilis, gonorrhea, chancroid, granuloma inguinale, lymphopathia venerea, genital herpes—are sexually transmitted and are discussed in Chapter 8. Only the nonspecific infections causing so-called balanoposthitis are described here.

Balanoposthitis refers to infection of the glans and prepuce caused by a wide variety of organisms. Among the more common agents are *Candida albicans*, anaerobic bacteria, *Gardnerella*, and pyogenic bacteria. Most cases occur as a consequence of poor local hygiene in uncircumcised males, in whom the accumulation of desquamated epithelial cells, sweat, and debris, termed *smegma*, acts as local irritant. Persistence of such infections leads to inflammatory scarring and, as mentioned earlier, is a common cause of phimosis.

Tumors

Tumors of the penis are, on the whole, uncommon. The most frequent neoplasms are carcinomas and a benign epithelial tumor, condyloma acuminatum. Benign proliferations of fibroblasts (Peyronie disease) are also worthy of brief mention.

Benign Tumors

Condyloma Acuminatum

Condyloma acuminatum is a benign sexually transmitted wart caused by human papillomavirus (HPV). It is related to the common wart and may occur on any moist mucocutaneous surface of the external genitals in either sex. HPV type 6, and less frequently type 11, are the most frequent agents that cause condylomata acuminata.

MORPHOLOGY

Condylomata acuminata may occur on the external genitalia or perineal areas. On the penis these lesions occur most often about the coronal sulcus and inner surface of the prepuce. They consist of **single or multiple sessile or pedunculated, red papillary excrescences** that may be up to several millimeters in diameter (Fig. 21-15). Histologically, a branching, villous, papillary connective tissue stroma is covered by epithelium that may have considerable superficial hyperkeratosis and thickening of the underlying epidermis (**acanthosis**) (Fig. 21-16). The normal orderly maturation of the epithelial cells is preserved; dysplasia is not evident. Cytoplasmic vacuolization of the squamous cells (**koilocytosis**), characteristic of HPV infection, is noted in these lesions (Fig. 21-17). Condylomata acuminata tend to recur but only rarely progress into in situ or invasive cancers.

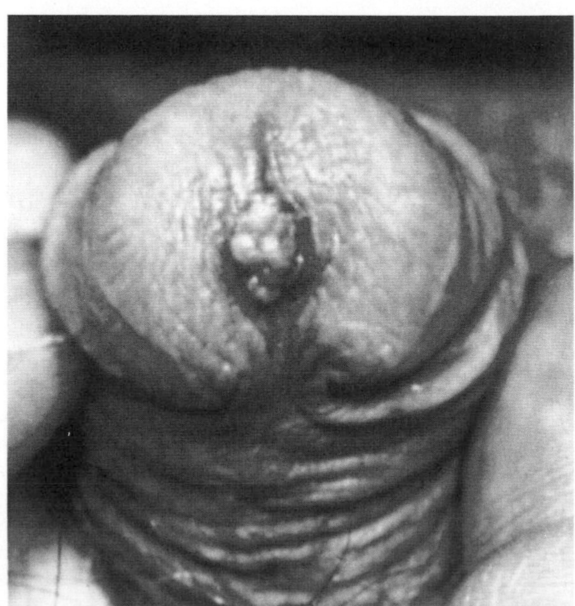

Figure 21-15 Condyloma acuminatum of the penis.

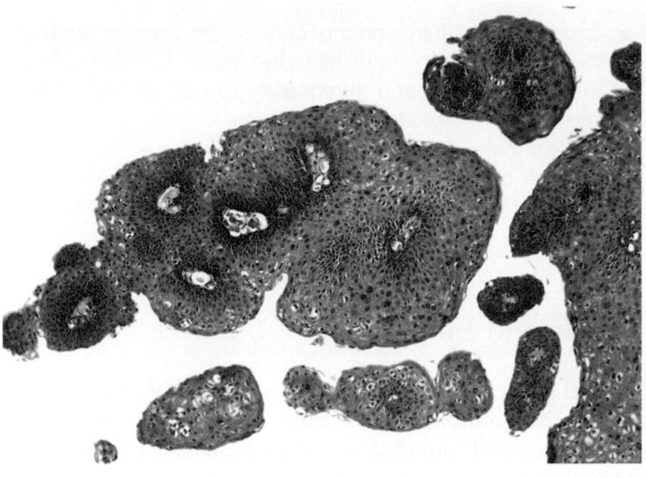

Figure 21-16 Condyloma acuminatum of the penis. Low magnification reveals the papillary (villous) architecture and thickening of the epidermis.

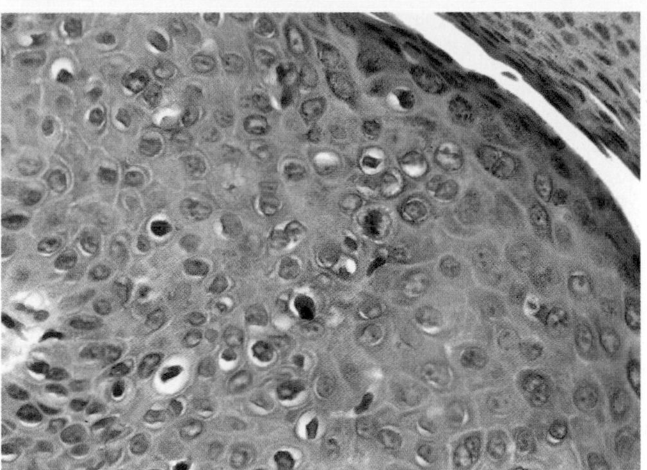

Figure 21-18 Bowen disease (carcinoma in situ) of the penis. Note the hyperchromatic, dysplastic dyskeratotic epithelial cells with scattered mitoses above the basal layer. The intact basement membrane is not readily seen in this picture.

Peyronie Disease

This disorder results in fibrous bands involving the corpus cavernosum of the penis. Although some classify it as a variant of fibromatosis, its etiology remains an enigma. Clinically, the lesion results in penile curvature and pain during intercourse.

Malignant Tumors

Carcinoma in Situ (CIS)

In the external male genitalia, two distinct lesions display histologic features of CIS: Bowen disease and bowenoid papulosis. These lesions have a strong association with infection by high-risk HPV, most commonly type 16.

- *Bowen disease* occurs in the genital region of both men and women, usually in those older than age 35 years. In men it tends to involve the skin of the shaft of the penis and the scrotum. Grossly it appears as a solitary, thickened, gray-white, opaque plaque. It can also manifest on the glans and prepuce as single or multiple shiny red, sometimes velvety plaques. Histologically the epidermis is hyperproliferative, containing numerous mitoses, some atypical. The cells are markedly dysplastic with large hyperchromatic nuclei and lack of orderly maturation (Fig. 21-18). Nevertheless, the dermal-epidermal border is sharply delineated by an intact basement membrane. Bowen disease transforms into infiltrating squamous cell carcinoma in approximately 10% of patients, usually over a span of many years.
- *Bowenoid papulosis* occurs in sexually active adults. It is distinguished from Bowen disease by the younger age of affected patients and its presentation as multiple (rather than solitary) reddish brown papular lesions. Although bowenoid papulosis is histologically indistinguishable from Bowen disease and is also related to HPV type 16, it virtually never develops into an invasive carcinoma and in many cases regresses spontaneously.

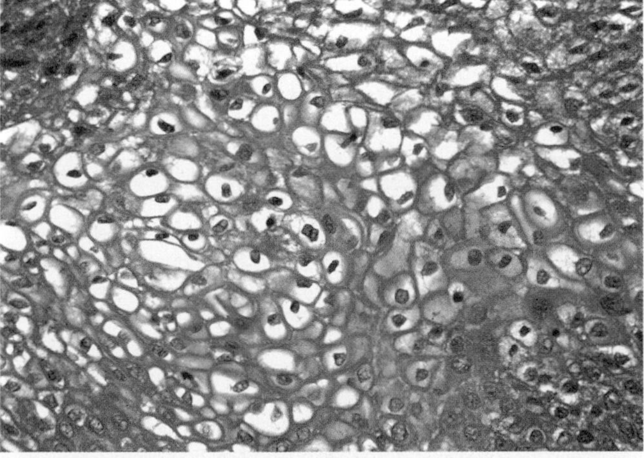

Figure 21-17 Condyloma acuminatum of the penis. The epithelium shows vacuolization (koilocytosis) characteristic of human papillomavirus infection.

Invasive Carcinoma

Squamous cell carcinoma of the penis is associated with poor genital hygiene and with high-risk HPV infection. Carcinomas are usually found in patients between the ages of 40 and 70 years. It accounts for less than 1% of cancers in males in the United States. In contrast, in some parts of Asia, Africa, and South America, squamous cell carcinoma of the penis makes up from 10% to 20% of male malignancies. Circumcision confers protection, and hence this cancer is extremely rare among Jews and Muslims and is correspondingly more common in populations in which circumcision is not practiced routinely. It is postulated that circumcision reduces exposure to carcinogens that may be concentrated in smegma and decreases the likelihood of infection with potentially oncogenic types of HPV. HPV DNA can be detected in penile squamous cancer in approximately 50% of patients. HPV type 16 is the most frequent culprit, but HPV 18 is also implicated. The recent availability of a vaccine to both the low-risk (6, 11) and high-risk (16, 18) subtypes of HPV may help reduce the incidence of this tumor, as well as condyloma acuminatum. Cigarette smoking also elevates the risk of developing penile cancer.

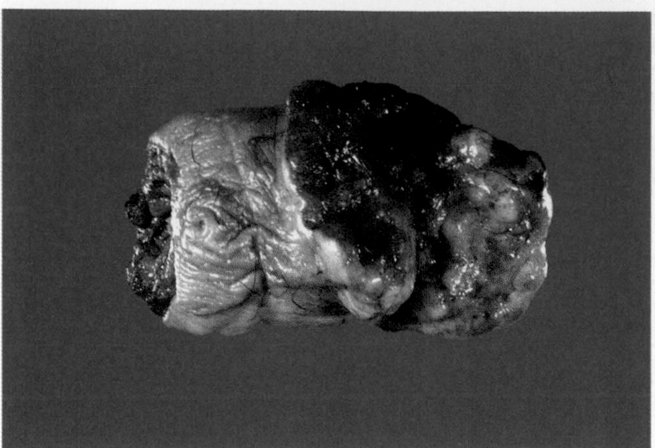

Figure 21-19 Carcinoma of the penis. The glans penis is deformed by a firm, ulcerated, infiltrative mass.

MORPHOLOGY

Squamous cell carcinoma of the penis usually begins on the glans or inner surface of the prepuce near the coronal sulcus. Two macroscopic patterns are seen—papillary and flat. The papillary lesions simulate condylomata acuminata and may produce a cauliflower-like fungating mass. Flat lesions appear as areas of epithelial thickening accompanied by graying and fissuring of the mucosal surface. With progression, an ulcerated papule develops (Fig. 21-19). Histologically, both the papillary and the flat lesions are squamous cell carcinomas with varying degrees of differentiation. **Verrucous carcinoma** is an exophytic well-differentiated variant of squamous cell carcinoma that are locally invasive, but rarely metastasize. Other, less common, subtypes of penile squamous carcinoma include basaloid, warty, and papillary variants.

Clinical Features. Invasive squamous cell carcinoma of the penis is a slowly growing, locally invasive lesion that often has been present for a year or more before it is brought to medical attention. The lesions are nonpainful until they undergo secondary ulceration and infection. Metastases to inguinal lymph nodes may occur early in its course, but widespread dissemination is extremely uncommon until the lesion is far advanced. Clinical assessment of regional lymph node involvement is notoriously inaccurate; only 50% of enlarged inguinal nodes detected in men with penile squamous cell carcinoma contain cancer, with the remainder showing only reactive lymphoid hyperplasia when examined histologically. The prognosis is related to the stage of the tumor. Without spread to lymph nodes, the 5-year survival rate is 66%, whereas metastasis to the lymph nodes carries a grim 27% 5-year survival.

KEY CONCEPTS

Lesions of the Penis

- Squamous cell carcinoma and its precursor lesions are the most important penile lesions. Many are associated with HPV infection.
- Squamous cell carcinoma occurs on the glans or shaft of the penis as an ulcerated infiltrative lesion that may spread to inguinal nodes and infrequently to distant sites. Most cases occur in uncircumcised males.
- Other important penile disorders include congenital abnormalities involving the position of the urethra (epispadias, hypospadias) and inflammatory disorders (balanitis, phimosis).

Testis and Epididymis

Distinct pathologic conditions affect the testis and epididymis. In the epididymis, the most important and frequent conditions are inflammatory diseases, whereas in the testis the major lesions are tumors.

Congenital Anomalies

With the exception of undescended testes (cryptorchidism), congenital anomalies are extremely rare and include absence of one or both testes and fusion of the testes (so-called *synorchism*).

Cryptorchidism

Cryptorchidism is a complete or partial failure of the intra-abdominal testes to descend into the scrotal sac and is associated with testicular dysfunction and an increased risk of testicular cancer. It is found in approximately 1% of 1-year-old boys. It usually occurs as an isolated anomaly but may be accompanied by other malformations of the genitourinary tract, such as hypospadias.

Testicular descent occurs in two morphologically and hormonally distinct phases. During the first transabdominal, phase, the testis comes to lie within the lower abdomen or brim of the pelvis. This phase is believed to be controlled by a hormone called *müllerian-inhibiting substance.* In the second inguinoscrotal, phase, the testes descend through the inguinal canal into the scrotal sac. This phase is androgen-dependent and is possibly mediated by androgen-induced release of calcitonin gene-related peptide from the genitofemoral nerve. Although testes may arrest anywhere along their pathway of descent, the most common site is in the inguinal canal; arrest within the abdomen is uncommon, accounting for approximately 5% to 10% of cases. Even though testicular descent is controlled by hormonal factors, cryptorchidism is only rarely associated with a well-defined hormonal disorder.

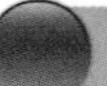

MORPHOLOGY

Cryptorchidism is unilateral in most cases, being bilateral in 25% of patients. Histologic changes in the malpositioned testis begin as early as 2 years of age. They are characterized by **arrested germ cell development** associated with **marked hyalinization and thickening of the basement membrane** of the spermatic tubules (Fig. 21-20). Eventually the tubules appear as dense cords of hyaline connective tissue outlined by prominent basement membranes. There is concomitant increase in interstitial stroma. Because Leydig cells are spared, they appear to be prominent. As might be expected with

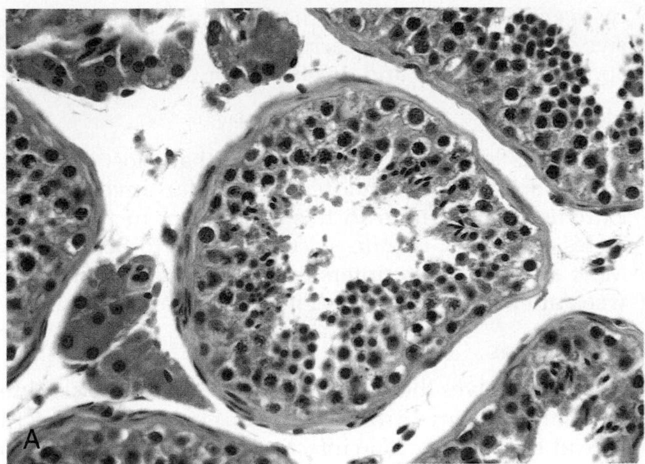
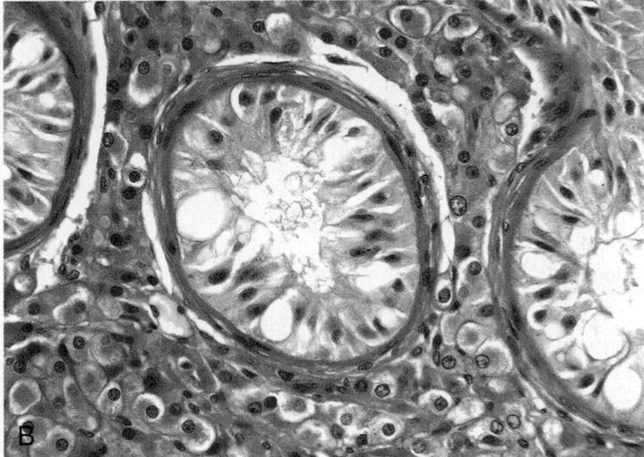

Figure 21-20 A, Normal testis shows tubules with active spermatogenesis. **B,** Testicular atrophy in cryptorchidism. The tubules show Sertoli cells but no spermatogenesis. There is thickening of basement membranes and an apparent increase in interstitial Leydig cells.

progressive tubular atrophy, the cryptorchid testis is small in size and is firm in consistency as a result of fibrotic changes. Similar histologic changes may also be seen in the contralateral (descended) testis in males with unilateral cryptorchidism, suggesting that cryptorchidism is a marker of some intrinsic defect in testicular development or function.

Cryptorchidism is completely asymptomatic, and comes to attention when the scrotal sac is discovered to be empty by the patient or an examining physician. In addition to sterility, cryptorchidism may be associated with other morbidity. When the testis lies in the inguinal canal, it is particularly prone to trauma and crushing injuries. A concomitant inguinal hernia accompanies the undescended testis in about 10% to 20% of cases. In addition, the undescended testis is at a greater risk of developing testicular cancer than is the descended testis.

During the first year of life the majority of inguinal cryptorchid testes descend spontaneously into the scrotum. Those that remain undescended require surgical correction, preferably before histologic deterioration sets in at around 2 years of age. Orchiopexy (placement in the scrotal sac) does not guarantee fertility; deficient spermatogenesis has been reported in 10% to 60% of patients in whom surgical repositioning was performed. To what extent the risk of cancer is reduced after orchiopexy is also unclear, and the risk is changing over time as orchiopexy has been offered at an increasingly younger age over the past few decades (current recommendations are for correction at 6 to 12 months of age). Cancer may also develop in the contralateral, normally descended testis, further supporting the idea that cryptorchidism signals the presence of a defect in testicular development and cellular differentiation that is unrelated to anatomic position.

KEY CONCEPTS

Cryptorchidism

- Cryptorchidism refers to incomplete descent of the testis from the abdomen to the scrotum and is present in about 1% of 1-year-old male infants.
- Bilateral or, in some cases, even unilateral cryptorchidism is associated with tubular atrophy and sterility.
- The cryptorchid testis carries a 3- to 5-fold higher risk for testicular cancer, which arises from foci of intratubular germ cell neoplasia within the atrophic tubules. Orchiopexy reduces the risk of sterility and cancer.

Regressive Changes

Atrophy and Decreased Fertility

Testicular atrophy may be caused by one of several conditions, including (1) progressive atherosclerotic narrowing of the blood supply in old age, (2) the end stage of an inflammatory orchitis, (3) cryptorchidism, (4) hypopituitarism, (5) generalized malnutrition or cachexia, (6) irradiation, (7) prolonged administration of antiandrogens (treatment for advanced carcinoma of the prostate), and (8) exhaustion atrophy, which may follow persistent stimulation by high levels of follicle-stimulating pituitary hormone. The gross and microscopic alterations follow the pattern already described for cryptorchidism. Atrophy occasionally occurs as a primary failure of genetic origin, such as in Klinefelter syndrome (Chapter 5).

Inflammation

Inflammations are distinctly more common in the epididymis than in the testis. Of the three major specific inflammatory states that affect the testis and epididymis, gonorrhea and tuberculosis almost invariably arise in the epididymis, whereas syphilis affects the testis first.

Nonspecific Epididymitis and Orchitis

Epididymitis and possible subsequent orchitis are commonly related to infections in the urinary tract (cystitis, urethritis, prostatitis), which reach the epididymis and the testis through either the vas deferens or the lymphatics of the spermatic cord. The cause of epididymitis varies with the age of the patient. Though uncommon in children, epididymitis in childhood is usually associated with a congenital genitourinary abnormality and infection with

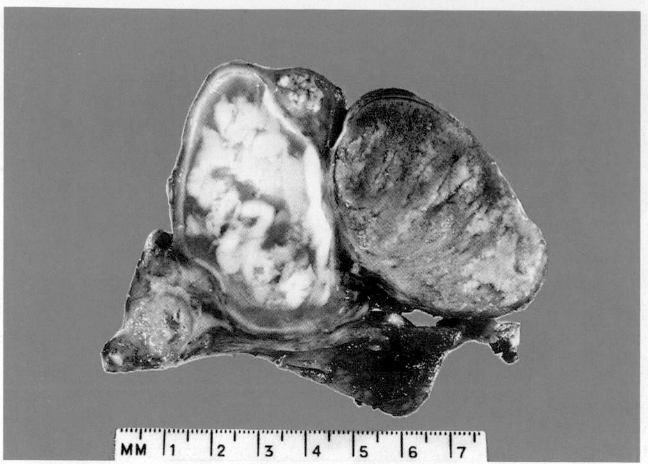

Figure 21-21 Acute epididymitis caused by gonococcal infection. The epididymis is replaced by an abscess. Normal testis is seen on the *right*.

gram-negative rods. In sexually active men younger than age 35 years, the sexually transmitted pathogens *C. trachomatis* and *Neisseria gonorrhoeae* are the most frequent culprits. In men older than age 35 the common urinary tract pathogens, such as *E. coli* and *Pseudomonas*, are responsible for most infections.

MORPHOLOGY

The bacterial invasion induces nonspecific acute inflammation characterized by congestion, edema, and infiltration by neutrophils, macrophages, and lymphocytes. Although the infection, in the early stage, is more or less limited to the interstitial connective tissue, it rapidly extends to involve the tubules and may progress to abscess formation or complete suppurative necrosis of the entire epididymis (Fig. 21-21). Usually, having involved the epididymis, the infection extends into the testis to evoke a similar inflammatory reaction. Such inflammatory involvement of the epididymis and testis is often followed by fibrous scarring, which in many cases leads to sterility. Usually the Leydig cells are not totally destroyed, and as a result androgen production by the testis may be relatively unaffected.

Granulomatous (Autoimmune) Orchitis

Idiopathic granulomatous orchitis presents in middle age as a moderately tender testicular mass of sudden onset sometimes associated with fever. It may appear insidiously, however, as a painless testicular mass mimicking a testicular tumor, hence its importance. Histologically the orchitis is distinguished by granulomas restricted to spermatic tubules. The lesions closely resemble tubercles but differ in that the granulomatous reaction is present diffusely throughout the testis and is confined to the seminiferous tubules. Although an autoimmune basis is suspected, the cause of these lesions remains unknown.

Specific Inflammations

Gonorrhea

Extension of infection from the posterior urethra to the prostate, seminal vesicles, and then to the epididymis is the usual course of a neglected gonococcal infection. In severe cases epididymal abscesses may develop, leading to extensive destruction and scarring. The infection may also spread to the testis and produce suppurative orchitis.

Mumps

Mumps is a systemic viral disease that most commonly affects school-aged children. Testicular involvement is extremely uncommon in this age group. In postpubertal males, however, orchitis occurs in 20% to 30% of cases. Most often, an acute interstitial orchitis develops about 1 week after the onset of swelling of the parotid glands.

Tuberculosis

When it involves the male genital tract, tuberculosis almost invariably begins in the epididymis, from where it may spread to the testis. The infection invokes the classic morphologic reactions of caseating granulomatous inflammation characteristic of tuberculosis elsewhere.

Syphilis

The testis and epididymis may be affected in both acquired and congenital syphilis, but almost invariably the testis is involved first, and in many cases the epididymis is spared altogether. The morphologic pattern of the reaction takes two forms: (1) the production of gummas or (2) a diffuse interstitial inflammation that produces the histologic hallmark of syphilitic infections, obliterative endarteritis associated with perivascular cuffs of lymphocytes and plasma cells.

Vascular Disorders

Torsion

Twisting of the spermatic cord typically cuts off the venous drainage of the testis. If untreated, it frequently leads to testicular infarction and thus represents one of the few true urologic emergencies. The thick-walled arteries remain patent, producing intense vascular engorgement followed by hemorrhagic infarction.

There are two settings in which testicular torsion occurs. Neonatal torsion occurs either in utero or shortly after birth. It lacks any associated anatomic defect to account for its occurrence. "Adult" torsion is typically seen in adolescence and presents with the sudden onset of testicular pain. It often occurs without any inciting injury and may even occur during sleep. If the testis is manually untwisted within approximately 6 hours of the onset of torsion, there is a good chance that the testis will remain viable. In contrast to neonatal torsion, adult torsion results from a bilateral anatomic defect that leads to increased mobility of the testes (*bell-clapper abnormality*). To prevent the catastrophic recurrence of torsion in the contralateral testis, the testis unaffected by torsion is surgically fixed to the scrotum (*orchiopexy*).

MORPHOLOGY

Depending on the duration of the process, the morphologic changes range from intense congestion to widespread hemorrhage to testicular infarction (Fig. 21-22). In advanced stages the testis is markedly enlarged and consists entirely of soft, necrotic, hemorrhagic tissue.

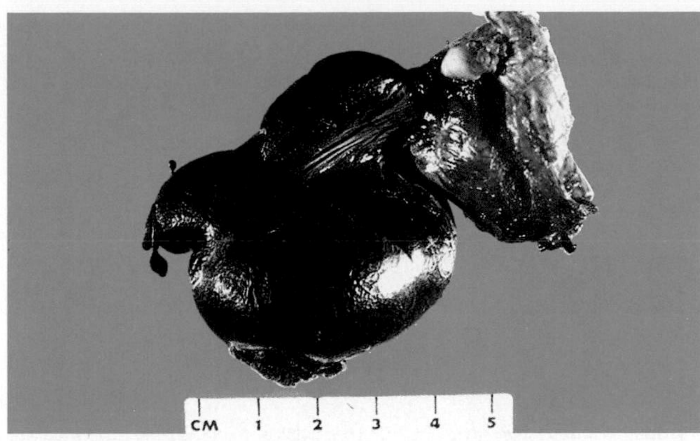

Figure 21-22 Torsion of testis.

Spermatic Cord and Paratesticular Tumors

Lipomas are common lesions involving the proximal spermatic cord, identified at the time of inguinal hernia repair. Although diagnosed as "lipomas," many of these lesions probably represent retroperitoneal adipose tissue that has been pulled into the inguinal canal along with the hernia sac, rather than a true neoplasm.

The most common benign paratesticular tumor is *adenomatoid tumor*. Although these lesions are mesothelial in nature, they are not referred to as mesotheliomas to distinguish them from other mesothelial lesions that may occur at this site. Adenomatoid tumors are usually small nodules, typically occurring near the upper pole of the epididymis. Although grossly well circumscribed, microscopically they may be minimally invasive into the adjacent testis. The importance of this lesion is that it is one of the few benign tumors that occur near the testis. If the pathologist can identify the nature of this lesion in intraoperative frozen sections, local excision of the adenomatoid tumor can spare the patient from an orchiectomy.

The most common malignant paratesticular tumors are rhabdomyosarcomas in children and liposarcomas in adults.

Testicular Tumors

Testicular neoplasms span an amazing gamut of anatomic types and can be divided into two major categories: germ cell tumors (95%) and sex cord-stromal tumors (Table 21-5). Germ cell tumors are subdivided into seminomas and nonseminomas. Most germ cell tumors are aggressive cancers capable of rapid, wide dissemination, although with current therapy most can be cured. Sex cord-stromal tumors, in contrast, are generally benign.

Table 21-5 Pathologic Classification of Common Testicular Tumors

Germ Cell Tumors

- Seminomatous tumors
  - Seminoma
  - Spermatocytic seminoma
- Nonseminomatous tumors
  - Embryonal carcinoma
  - Yolk sac (endodermal sinus) tumor
  - Choriocarcinoma
- Teratoma
- Sex Cord-Stromal Tumors
  - Leydig cell tumor
  - Sertoli cell tumor

Germ Cell Tumors

In the 15- to 34-year age group, testicular germ cell tumors constitute the most common tumor of men and cause approximately 10% of all cancer deaths. The incidence of testicular tumors in the United States is approximately 6 per 100,000, resulting in approximately 300 deaths per year. For unexplained reasons there has been worldwide increase in the incidence of these tumors in recent years. In the United States these tumors are much more common in whites than in blacks (ratio 5:1).

Environmental Factors. Environmental factors play a role in testicular germ cell tumors, as demonstrated by population migration studies. For example, the incidence of testicular germ cell tumors in Finland is about two times lower than in Sweden, but second generation Finnish immigrants to Sweden have a tumor incidence that approaches that of the Swedish population. Testicular germ cell tumors are associated with a spectrum of disorders collectively known as *testicular dysgenesis syndrome (TDS)*. Components of this syndrome include cryptorchidism, hypospadias, and poor sperm quality. It has been proposed that these conditions are increased by in utero exposures to pesticides and nonsteroidal estrogens. The most important association is with cryptorchidism, which is seen with approximately 10% of testicular germ cell tumors. Curiously, Klinefelter syndrome is associated with a greatly increased risk (50 times normal) for development of mediastinal germ cell tumors, but these patients do not develop testicular tumors.

Genetic Factors. There is a strong familial predisposition associated with the development of testicular germ cell tumors. The relative risk of these tumors is four times higher than normal in fathers and sons of affected patients and is 8 to 10 times higher in brothers. Several genetic loci have been linked to familial germ cell tumor risk, including the genes encoding the ligand for the receptor tyrosine kinase KIT and BAK, which you will recall is an important inducer of apoptotic cell death (Chapter 1). Interestingly, these genes are also thought to play a role in gonadal development.

Classification. A simple classification of the most common types of testicular tumors is presented in Table 21-5. Two broad groups are recognized. *Seminomatous tumors* are composed of cells that resemble primordial germ cells or early gonocytes. The *nonseminomatous tumors* may be composed of undifferentiated cells that resemble embryonic stem cells, as in the case of embryonal carcinoma, but the malignant cells may also differentiate along other lineages, generating yolk sac tumors, choriocarcinomas and teratomas. Germ cell tumors may have a single tissue component, but in approximately 60% of cases the tumors contain mixtures of seminomatous and nonseminomatous components and multiple tissues.

Pathogenesis. **Most testicular germ cell tumors originate from a precursor lesion called intratubular germ cell neoplasia (ITGCN).** The exceptions to this rule are pediatric yolk sac tumors and teratomas, and adult spermatocytic seminomas, all of which are of uncertain origin. ITGCN is believed to arise in utero and stay dormant until puberty, after which it may progress to seminoma or nonseminomatous tumors. The lesion consists of atypical primordial germ cells with large nuclei and clear cytoplasm, which are about twice the size of normal germ cells. These cells retain the expression of the transcription factors OCT3/4 and NANOG, which are important in maintenance of pluripotent stem cells. ITGCN shares some of the genetic alterations that are found in germ cell tumors. One that is particularly important is the reduplication of the short arm of chromosome 12 (12p) in the form of an isochromosome i(12p), a cytogenetic alteration that is invariably found in invasive germ cell tumors regardless of histological type. Activating mutations in the gene encoding the KIT receptor tyrosine kinase, which may be present in seminomas, are also freqeuntly present in ITGCN. About 50% of individuals with ITGCN develop invasive germ cell tumors within five years after diagnosis, and it may be that practically all patients with ITGCN will eventually develop invasive tumors.

Seminoma

Seminomas are the most common type of germ cell tumor, making up about 50% of these tumors. The peak incidence is the third decade and they almost never occur in infants. An identical tumor arises in the ovary, where it is called *dysgerminoma* (Chapter 22). Seminomas contain isochromosome 12p and express OCT3/4 and NANOG. Approximately 25% of these tumors have *KIT* activating mutations. *KIT* amplification and *KIT* overexpression through other unknown mechanisms have also been reported.

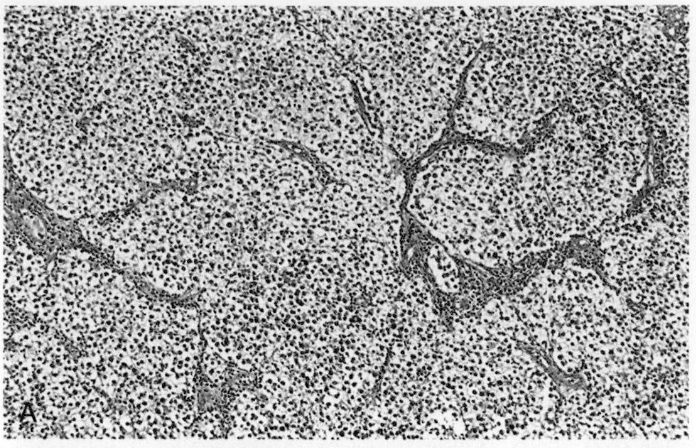

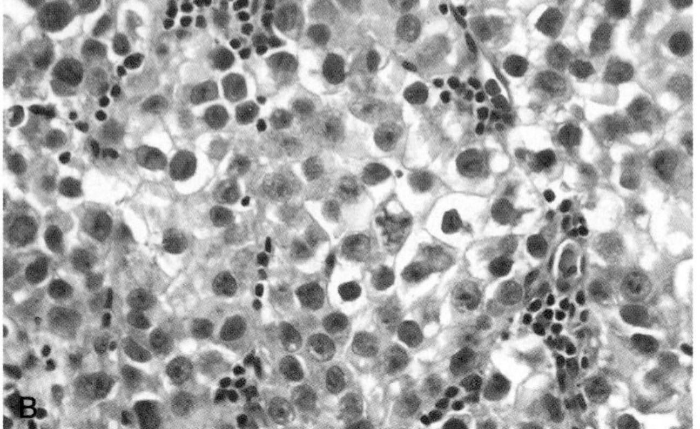

Figure 21-24 Seminoma. **A,** Low magnification shows clear seminoma cells divided into poorly demarcated lobules by delicate septa. **B,** Microscopic examination reveals large cells with distinct cell borders, pale nuclei, prominent nucleoli, and a sparse lymphocytic infiltrate.

MORPHOLOGY

If not otherwise specified, "seminoma" refers to "classic" or "typical" seminoma. Spermatocytic seminoma, despite its similar name, is a distinct tumor discussed later. Seminomas produce bulky masses, sometimes ten times the size of the normal testis. The typical seminoma has a homogeneous, gray-white, lobulated cut surface, usually devoid of hemorrhage or necrosis (Fig. 21-23). Generally the tunica albuginea is not penetrated, but occasionally extension to the epididymis, spermatic cord, or scrotal sac occurs.

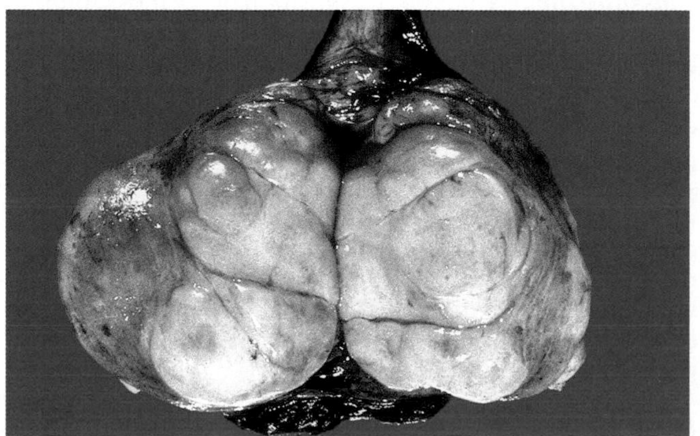

Figure 21-23 Seminoma of the testis appears as a fairly well-circumscribed, pale, fleshy, homogeneous mass.

Microscopically the typical seminoma is composed of sheets of uniform cells divided into poorly demarcated lobules by delicate fibrous septa containing a lymphocytic infiltrate (Fig. 21-24*A*). **The classic seminoma cell is large and round to polyhedral and has a distinct cell membrane; clear or watery-appearing cytoplasm; and a large, central nucleus with one or two prominent nucleoli** (Fig. 21-24*B*). Mitoses vary in frequency. The cytoplasm contains varying amounts of glycogen. Some tumors have anaplastic features (anaplastic seminoma), including frequent tumor giant cells and greater mitotic activity, but this does not appear to portend a worse prognosis when matched for stage with classic seminoma. By immunohistochemistry, seminoma cells stain positively for KIT, (regardless of KIT mutational status), OCT4, and placental alkaline phosphatase (PLAP). A few scattered keratin-positive cells may also be present.

Approximately 15% of seminomas contain syncytiotrophoblasts. In this subset of patients, serum human chorionic gonadotropin (HCG) levels are elevated, though not to the extent seen in patients with choriocarcinoma. Seminomas may also be accompanied by an ill-defined granulomatous reaction, in contrast to the well-formed discrete granulomas seen with tuberculosis.

Spermatocytic Seminoma

In contrast to the classic seminoma described earlier, spermatocytic seminoma is a rare, slow-growing germ cell tumor predominantly affecting older men. Though related by name to seminoma, spermatocytic seminoma is a distinctive tumor both clinically and histologically. Spermatocytic seminoma is uncommon, representing 1% to 2% of all testicular germ cell neoplasms. The age of involvement is much later than for most testicular tumors: Affected individuals are generally older than age 65 years. Becuase it is a slow-growing tumor that does not produce metastases, the prognosis is excellent.

MORPHOLOGY

Spermatocytic seminoma tends to have a soft, pale gray, cut surface that sometimes reveal mucoid cysts. Spermatocytic seminomas contain three cell populations, all intermixed: (1) medium-sized cells, the most numerous, containing a round nucleus and eosinophilic cytoplasm; (2) smaller cells with a narrow rim of eosinophilic cytoplasm resembling secondary spermatocytes; and (3) scattered giant cells, either uninucleate or multinucleate. The chromatin in some intermediate-sized cells is similar to that seen in the meiotic phase of nonneoplastic spermatocytes (spireme chromatin). In contrast to typical seminomas, spermatocytic seminomas lack lymphocytes, granulomas, syncytiotrophoblasts, extra-testicular sites of origin, admixture with other germ cell tumors, and association with ITGCN.

Embryonal Carcinoma

Embryonal carcinomas occur mostly in the 20- to 30-year age group. These tumors are more aggressive than seminomas.

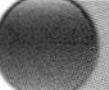

MORPHOLOGY

Most primary tumors are smaller than seminoma and do not replace the entire testis. However, extension through the tunica albuginea into the epididymis or cord frequently occurs. On cut surfaces the tumor is often variegated, poorly demarcated at the margins, and punctuated by foci of hemorrhage or necrosis (Fig. 21-25). **Histologically the cells grow in alveolar or tubular patterns, sometimes with papillary convolutions** (Fig. 21-26). **More undifferentiated lesions may display sheets of cells.** Well formed glands are absent. The neoplastic cells have an epithelial appearance, are large and anaplastic, and have hyperchromatic nuclei with prominent nucleoli. The cell borders are usually indistinct, and there is considerable variation in cell and nuclear size and shape. Mitotic figures and tumor giant cells are frequently seen. Embryonal carcinomas share some markers with seminomas such as OCT 3/4 and PLAP, but differ by being positive for cytokeratin and CD30, and negative for KIT.

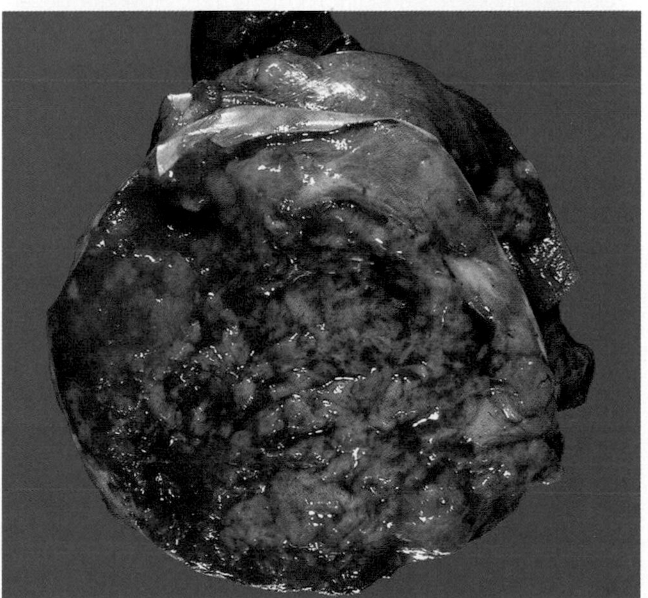

Figure 21-25 Embryonal carcinoma. In contrast to the seminoma illustrated in Figure 21-23, embryonal carcinoma is a hemorrhagic mass.

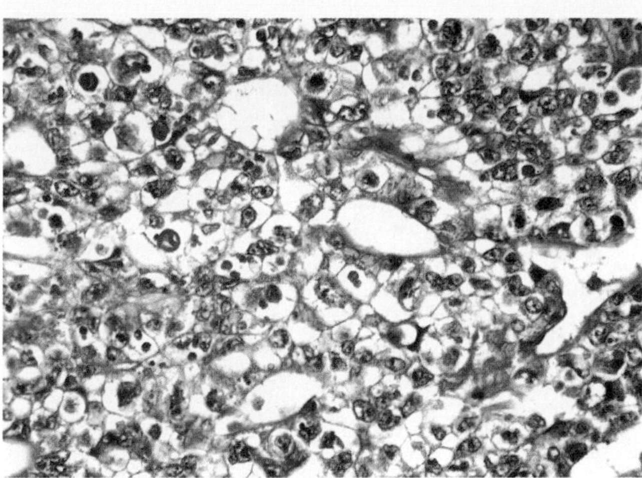

Figure 21-26 Embryonal carcinoma shows sheets of undifferentiated cells as well as primitive glandular differentiation. The nuclei are large and hyperchromatic.

Yolk Sac Tumor

Also known as *endodermal sinus tumor*, yolk sac tumor is of interest because it is the most common testicular tumor in infants and children up to 3 years of age. In this age group it has a very good prognosis. In adults the pure form of this tumor is rare; instead, yolk sac elements frequently occur in combination with embryonal carcinoma.

MORPHOLOGY

These tumors are nonencapsulated and have a homogeneous, yellow-white, mucinous appearance. They are composed of a lacelike (reticular) network of medium-sized cuboidal or flattened cells. In addition, papillary structures, solid cords of cells, and a multitude of other less common patterns may be found. In approximately 50% of tumors, structures resembling endodermal sinuses (**Schiller-Duval** bodies) may be seen; these consist of a mesodermal core with a central capillary and a visceral and parietal layer of cells resembling primitive glomeruli. Present within and outside the cytoplasm are eosinophilic, hyaline-like globules in which α-fetoprotein (AFP) and α_1-antitrypsin can be demonstrated by immunocytochemical staining. The presence of AFP in the tumor cells is highly characteristic, and underscores resemblance to yolk sac cells.

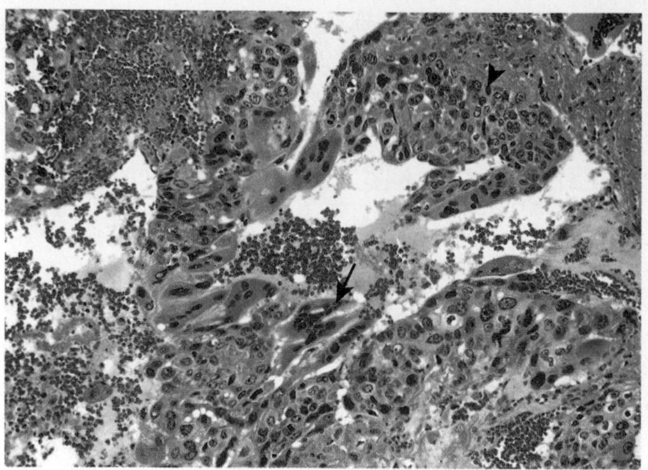

Figure 21-27 Choriocarcinoma shows cytotrophoblastic cells *(arrowhead)* with central nuclei and syncytiotrophoblastic cells *(arrow)* with multiple dark nuclei embedded in eosinophilic cytoplasm. Hemorrhage and necrosis are seen in the *upper right field*.

Choriocarcinoma

Choriocarcinoma is a highly malignant form of testicular tumor. In its "pure" form, choriocarcinoma is rare, constituting less than 1% of all germ cell tumors.

MORPHOLOGY

Choriocarcinomas often cause no testicular enlargement and are detected only as a small palpable nodule. Typically, these tumors are small, rarely larger than 5 cm in diameter. Hemorrhage and necrosis are extremely common. Histologically the tumors contain two cell types, **syncytiotrophoblasts** and **cytotrophoblasts** (Fig. 21-27). Syncytiotrophoblasts are large multinucleated cells with abundant eosinophilic vacuolated cytoplasm containing HCG, which is readily detected by immunohistochemistry. Cytotrophoblasts are more regular and tend to be polygonal, with distinct borders and clear cytoplasm; they grow in cords or masses and have a single, fairly uniform nucleus. This neoplasm can also arise in the female genital tract (Chapter 21).

Teratoma

The designation *teratoma* refers to testicular tumors having various cellular or organoid components reminiscent of the normal derivatives of more than one germ layer. They may occur at any age from infancy to adult life. Pure forms of teratoma are fairly common in infants and children, second in frequency only to yolk sac tumors. In adults, pure teratomas are rare, constituting 2% to 3% of germ cell tumors. However, the frequency of teratomas mixed with other germ cell tumors is approximately 45%.

MORPHOLOGY

Grossly, teratomas are usually large, ranging from 5 to 10 cm in diameter. Because they are composed of various tissues, the gross appearance is heterogeneous with solid, sometimes cartilaginous, and cystic areas (Fig. 21-28). Hemorrhage and necrosis usually indicate admixture with embryonal carcinoma, choriocarcinoma, or both.

Teratomas are composed of a heterogeneous, helter-skelter collection of differentiated cells or organoid structures, such as **neural tissue, muscle bundles, islands of cartilage, clusters of squamous epithelium, structures reminiscent of thyroid gland, bronchial or bronchiolar epithelium, and bits of intestinal wall or brain substance,** all embedded in a fibrous or myxoid stroma (Fig. 21-29). Elements may be mature (resembling various adult tissues) or immature (sharing histologic features with fetal or embryonal tissue).

Rarely, malignant non–germ cell tumors arise in teratomas, a phenomenon that is referred to as "teratoma with malignant transformation". Transformation may take the form of a squamous cell carcinoma, mucin-secreting adenocarcinoma, sarcoma, or other cancers. The importance of recognizing a non–germ cell malignancy arising in a teratoma is that these secondary tumors are chemoresistant; thus, the only hope for cure resides in the resectability of the tumor. These non–germ cell malignancies retain isochromosome 12p, proving a clonal relationship to the preceding teratoma.

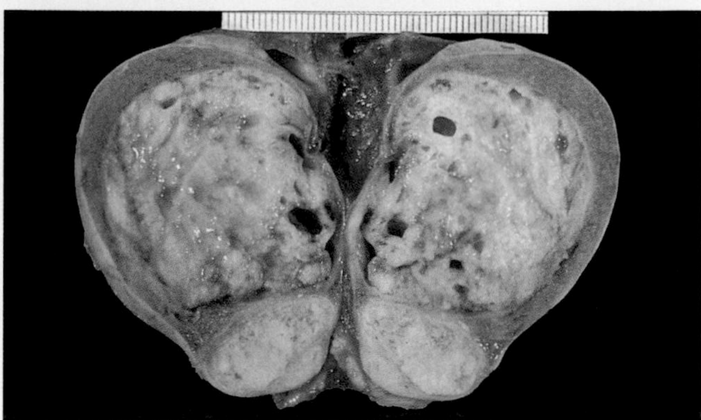

Figure 21-28 Teratoma of testis. The variegated cut surface with cysts reflects the multiplicity of tissue types found histologically.

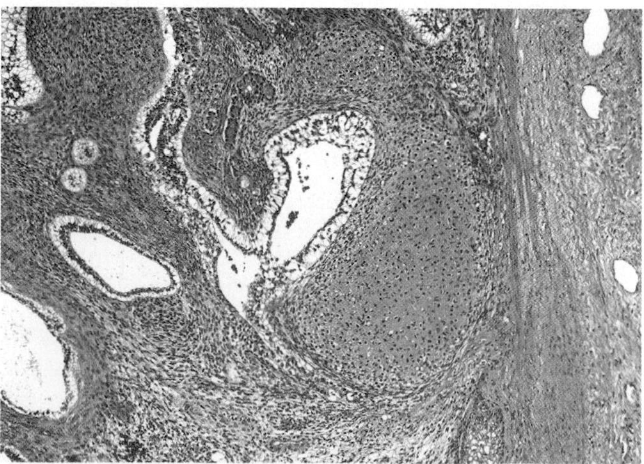

Figure 21-29 Teratoma of the testis consisting of a disorganized collection of glands, cartilage, smooth muscle, and immature stroma.

In the child, differentiated mature teratomas usually follow a benign course. **In the postpubertal male all teratomas are regarded as malignant**, capable of metastatic behavior whether the elements are mature or immature. Consequently, it is not critical to detect immaturity in a testicular teratoma of a postpubertal male.

Mixed Tumors

About 60% of testicular tumors are composed of more than one of the "pure" patterns. Common mixtures include: teratoma, embryonal carcinoma, and yolk sac tumor; seminoma with embryonal carcinoma; and embryonal carcinoma with teratoma *(teratocarcinoma)*. In most instances the prognosis is worsened by the presence of the more aggressive element.

Clinical Features of Testicular Germ Cell Tumors. Although painless enlargement of the testis is a characteristic feature of germ cell neoplasms, any solid testicular mass should be considered neoplastic until proven otherwise. Biopsy of a testicular neoplasm is associated with a risk of tumor spillage, which would necessitate excision of the scrotal skin in addition to orchiectomy. Consequently, the standard management of a solid testicular mass is radical orchiectomy based on the presumption of malignancy.

Testicular tumors have a characteristic mode of spread. *Lymphatic spread* is common to all forms of testicular tumors. In general, retroperitoneal para-aortic nodes are the first to be involved. Subsequent spread may occur to mediastinal and supraclavicular nodes. *Hematogenous spread* is primarily to the lungs, but liver, brain, and bones may also be involved. The histology of metastases may differ from that of the testicular lesion. For example, an embryonal carcinoma may present a teratomatous picture in the secondary deposits. As discussed earlier, because all these tumors are derived from pluripotent germ cells, the apparent "forward" and "backward" differentiation seen in different locations is not entirely surprising. Another explanation for the differing morphologic patterns in the primary and metastatic site is that minor components in the primary tumor that were unresponsive to chemotherapy survive and subsequently become the dominant metastatic pattern.

Because of differing behaviors, tumors of the testis are segregated clinically into two broad categories: seminoma and nonseminomatous germ cell tumors (NSGCTs).

- Seminomas tend to remain localized to the testis for a long time, and hence approximately 70% present in clinical stage I (see later). In contrast, approximately 60% of males with NSGCTs present with advanced clinical disease (stages II and III).
- Metastases from seminomas typically involve lymph nodes. Hematogenous spread occurs later in the course of dissemination. NSGCTs not only metastasize earlier but also use the hematogenous route more frequently.
- The rare pure choriocarcinoma is the most aggressive NSGCT. It may not cause any testicular enlargement but instead spreads predominantly and rapidly by the bloodstream. Therefore, lungs and liver are involved early in virtually every case.

To summarize, as compared with seminomas, NSGCTs are biologically more aggressive and in general have a poorer prognosis.

In the United States, three clinical stages of testicular tumors are defined:

- Stage I: tumor confined to the testis, epididymis, or spermatic cord
- Stage II: distant spread confined to retroperitoneal nodes below the diaphragm
- Stage III: metastases outside the retroperitoneal nodes or above the diaphragm

Biomarkers. Germ cell tumors of the testis often secrete polypeptide hormones and certain enzymes that can be detected in blood by sensitive assays. Such biologic markers include HCG, AFP, and lactate dehydrogenase, which are valuable in the diagnosis and management of testicular cancer. The elevation of lactate dehydrogenase correlates with the mass of tumor cells, and provides a tool to assess tumor burden. Marked elevation of serum AFP or HCG levels are produced by yolk sac tumor and choriocarcinoma elements, respectively. Both of these markers are elevated in more than 80% of individuals with NSGCT at the time of diagnosis. As stated earlier, approximately 15% of seminomas have syncytiotrophoblastic giant cells and minimal elevation of HCG levels, which does not affect prognosis. In the context of testicular tumors, the value of serum markers is fourfold:

- In the evaluation of testicular masses
- In the staging of testicular germ cell tumors. For example, after orchiectomy, persistent elevation of HCG or AFP concentrations indicates stage II disease even if the lymph nodes appear of normal size by imaging studies.
- In assessing tumor burden
- In monitoring the response to therapy. After eradication of tumors there is a rapid fall in serum AFP and HCG. With serial measurements it is often possible to predict recurrence before the patients become symptomatic or develop any other clinical signs of relapse.

The therapy and prognosis of testicular tumors depend largely on clinical stage and on the histologic type. Seminoma, which is radiosensitive and tends to remain localized for long periods, has the best prognosis. More than 95% of patients with stage I and II disease can be cured. Among NSGCTs, the histologic subtype does not influence the prognosis significantly, and hence these are treated as a group. Approximately 90% of patients with NSGCTs can achieve complete remission with aggressive chemotherapy, and most can be cured. Pure choriocarcinoma has a poor prognosis. However, when it is a minor component of a mixed germ cell tumor, the prognosis is less adversely affected. With all testicular tumors, distant metastases, if present, usually occur within the first 2 years after treatment.

Tumors of Sex Cord-Gonadal Stroma

As indicated in Table 21-5, sex cord-gonadal stroma tumors are subclassified based on their presumed histogenesis and differentiation. The two most important members of this group—Leydig cell tumors and Sertoli cell tumors—are described here.

Leydig Cell Tumors

Tumors of Leydig cells are particularly interesting, because they may elaborate androgens and in some cases both androgens and estrogens, and even corticosteroids. They may arise at any age, although most cases occur between 20 and 60 years of age. As with other testicular tumors, the most common presenting feature is testicular swelling, but in some patients gynecomastia may be the first symptom. In children, hormonal effects, manifested primarily as sexual precocity, are the dominant features.

MORPHOLOGY

These neoplasms form circumscribed nodules, usually less than 5 cm in diameter. They have a distinctive golden brown, homogeneous cut surface. Histologically, neoplastic Leydig cells have an appearance that is similar to their normal counterparts. They are large in size and have round or polygonal cell outlines, abundant granular eosinophilic cytoplasm, and a round central nucleus. The cytoplasm frequently contains lipid droplets, vacuoles, or lipofuscin pigment, and, most characteristically, rod-shaped **crystalloids of Reinke**, which are seen in about 25% of the tumors. Approximately 10% of the tumors in adults are invasive and produce metastases; most are benign.

Sertoli Cell Tumors

Most Sertoli cell tumors are hormonally silent and present as a testicular mass. These neoplasms appear as firm, small nodules with a homogeneous gray-white to yellow cut surface. Histologically the tumor cells are arranged in distinctive trabeculae that tend to form cordlike structures and tubules. Most Sertoli cell tumors are benign, but approximately 10% pursue a malignant course.

Gonadoblastoma

Gonadoblastomas are rare neoplasms comprised of a mixture of germ cells and gonadal stromal elements that almost always arise in gonads with some form of testicular dysgenesis (discussed earlier). In some cases the germ cell component becomes malignant, giving rise to seminoma.

Testicular Lymphoma

Aggressive non–Hodgkin lymphomas account for 5% of testicular neoplasms, and are the most common form of testicular neoplasms in men older than age 60 years. Although an uncommon tumor of the testis, testicular lymphoma is included here because affected patients may present with only a testicular mass, mimicking other, more common, testicular tumors. In most cases, the disease is already disseminated at the time of detection. The most common testicular lymphomas, in decreasing order of frequency, are diffuse large B-cell lymphoma, Burkitt lymphoma, and EBV-positive extranodal NK/T cell lymphoma (Chapter 13). Testicular lymphomas have a higher propensity for central nervous system involvement than do similar tumors arising at other sites.

KEY CONCEPTS

Testicular Tumors

- Testicular tumors are the most common cause of painless testicular enlargement. They occur with increased frequency in association with undescended testis and with testicular dysgenesis.
- Germ cells are the source of 95% of testicular tumors; most the remainder arise from Sertoli or Leydig cells. Germ cell tumors may be composed of a single histologic pattern (60% of cases) or mixed patterns (40%).
- The most common "pure" histologic patterns of germ cell tumors are seminoma, embryonal carcinoma, yolk sac tumors, choriocarcinoma, and teratoma. Mixed tumors contain more than one element, most commonly embryonal carcinoma, teratoma, and yolk sac tumor.
- Clinically, testicular germ cell tumors can be divided into two groups: seminomas and nonseminomatous tumors. Seminomas remain confined to the testis for a long time and spread mainly to paraaortic nodes—distant spread is rare. Nonseminomatous tumors tend to spread earlier, by both lymphatics and blood vessels.
- HCG is produced by syncytiotrophoblasts and is always elevated in patients with choriocarcinomas or seminomas containing syncytiotrophoblasts. AFP is elevated when there is a yolk sac tumor component.
- Non–germ cell tumors include sex cord-gonadal stroma tumors and non–Hodgkin lymphomas.
- Non–Hodgkin lymphoma is the most common testicular tumor in men older than 60 years.

Miscellaneous Lesions of Tunica Vaginalis

Brief mention should be made of the tunica vaginalis, which is a mesothelial-lined surface exterior to the testis that may accumulate serous fluid *(hydrocele)* causing considerable enlargement of the scrotal sac. By transillumination it is usually possible to define the clear, translucent character of the contained fluid. Hydrocele sacs are frequently lined by mesothelial cells. Rarely, malignant mesotheliomas also can also arise from the tunica vaginalis.

Hematocele indicates the presence of blood in the tunica vaginalis. It is an uncommon condition usually encountered following testicular trauma or torsion, or in individuals with systemic bleeding disorders. *Chylocele* refers to the accumulation of lymph in the tunica and is almost always found in patients with elephantiasis who have widespread, severe lymphatic obstruction caused, for example, by filariasis (Chapter 8). *Spermatocele* refers to a small cystic accumulation of semen in dilated efferent ducts or ducts of the rete testis. *Varicocele* is a dilated vein in the spermatic cord. Varicoceles may be asymptomatic but have also been implicated in some men as a contributing factor to infertility. They can be corrected by surgical repair.

Prostate

In the normal adult the prostate weighs approximately 20 gm. The prostate is a retroperitoneal organ encircling the

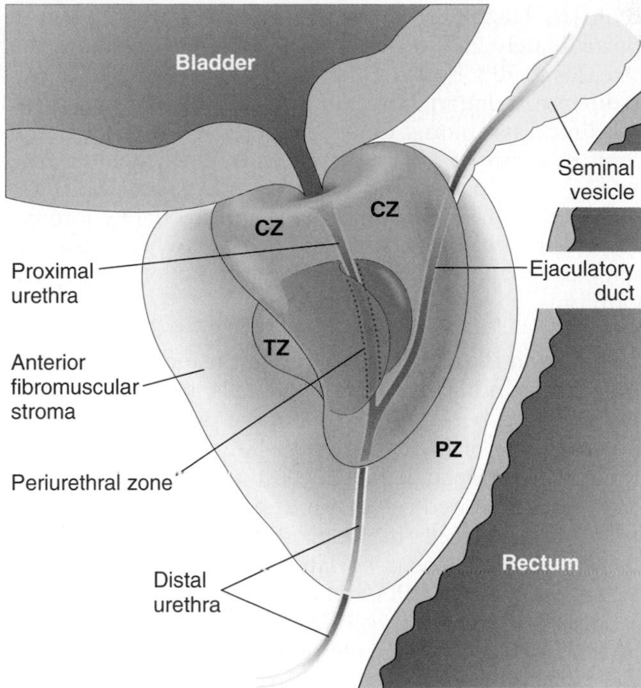

Figure 21-30 Adult prostate. The normal prostate contains several distinct regions, including a central zone (CZ), a peripheral zone (PZ), a transitional zone (TZ), and a periurethral zone. Most carcinomas arise from the peripheral zone and may be palpable during digital examination of the rectum. Nodular hyperplasia, in contrast, arises from the more centrally situated transitional zone and often produces urinary obstruction.

neck of the bladder and urethra, and is devoid of a distinct capsule. In the adult, prostatic parenchyma can be divided into four biologically and anatomically distinct zones or regions: the peripheral, central, transitional, and periurethral zones (Fig. 21-30). The types of proliferative lesions are different in each region. For example, most hyperplasias arise in the transitional zone, whereas most carcinomas originate in the peripheral zone.

Histologically the prostate is composed of glands lined by two layers of cells: a basal layer of low cuboidal epithelium covered by a layer of columnar secretory cells (Fig. 21-31). In many areas there are small papillary infoldings of the epithelium. These glands are separated by abundant fibromuscular stroma. Testicular androgens control the growth and survival of prostatic cells. Castration leads to atrophy of the prostate caused by widespread apoptosis.

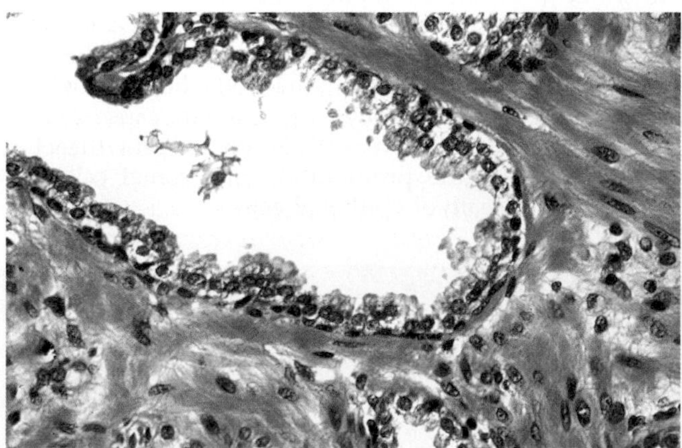

Figure 21-31 Benign prostate gland with basal cell and secretory cell layer.

Only three pathologic processes affect the prostate gland with sufficient frequency to merit discussion: inflammation, benign nodular enlargement, and tumors. Of these three, the benign nodular enlargements are by far the most common and occur so often in advanced age that they can almost be construed as a "normal" aging process. Prostatic carcinoma is also an extremely common lesion in men and therefore merits careful consideration. We begin our discussion with consideration of the inflammatory processes.

Inflammation

Prostatitis may be divided into several categories: acute and chronic bacterial prostatitis, chronic abacterial prostatitis, and granulomatous prostatitis.

- **Acute bacterial prostatitis** typically results from bacteria similar to those that cause urinary tract infections. Thus, most cases are caused by various strains of *E. coli*, other gram-negative rods, enterococci, and staphylococci. The organisms become implanted in the prostate usually by intraprostatic reflux of urine from the posterior urethra or from the urinary bladder, but occasionally they seed the prostate by lymphohematogenous routes from distant foci of infection. Prostatitis sometimes follows surgical manipulation of the urethra or prostate gland itself, such as catheterization, cystoscopy, urethral dilation, or resection procedures on the prostate. Clinically, acute bacterial prostatitis is associated with fever, chills, and dysuria. On rectal examination the prostate is exquisitely tender and boggy. The diagnosis can be established by urine culture and clinical features.
- **Chronic bacterial prostatitis** is difficult to diagnose and treat. It may present with low back pain, dysuria, and perineal and suprapubic discomfort. Alternatively, it may be virtually asymptomatic. Patients often have a history of recurrent urinary tract infections (cystitis, urethritis) caused by the same organism. Because most antibiotics penetrate the prostate poorly, bacteria find safe haven in the parenchyma and constantly seed the urinary tract. Diagnosis of chronic bacterial prostatitis depends on the demonstration of leukocytosis in the expressed prostatic secretions, along with positive bacterial cultures. In most cases, there is no antecedent acute attack, and the disease appears insidiously and without obvious provocation. The implicated organisms are the same as those cited as causes of acute prostatitis.
- **Chronic abacterial prostatitis** is the most common form of prostatitis seen today. It is indistinguishable from chronic bacterial prostatitis in terms of signs and symptoms, but there is no history of recurrent urinary tract infection. Expressed prostatic secretions contain more than 10 leukocytes per high-power field, but bacterial cultures are uniformly negative.
- **Granulomatous prostatitis** may be specific, where an etiologic infectious agent may be identified, or nonspecific. In the United States the most common cause is instillation of BCG within the bladder for treatment of

superficial bladder cancer, discussed earlier in this chapter. BCG is an attenuated mycobacterial strain that gives rise to a histologic picture indistinguishable from that seen with systemic tuberculosis. However, in the setting of BCG treatment the finding of granulomas in the prostate is of no clinical significance and requires no treatment. Fungal granulomatous prostatitis is typically seen only in immunocompromised hosts. Nonspecific granulomatous prostatitis is relatively common and represents a reaction to secretions from ruptured prostatic ducts and acini. Although some of these men have a recent history of urinary tract infection, bacteria are not seen within the tissue in nonspecific granulomatous prostatitis.

MORPHOLOGY

Acute prostatitis may appear as minute, disseminated abscesses; as large, coalescent focal areas of necrosis; or as diffuse edema, congestion, and boggy suppuration of the entire gland.

In men with symptoms of acute or chronic prostatitis, biopsy or surgical specimens are usually not obtained, because the diagnosis is made on clinical and laboratory findings. In fact biopsy in suspected acute prostatitis is contraindicated, as it may lead to sepsis. It is common in prostate specimens removed surgically to find histologic evidence of acute or chronic inflammation in men with no clinical symptoms of acute or chronic prostatitis. In these instances etiologic infectious agents have yet to be identified. So as not to be confused with the clinical syndromes of acute and chronic prostatitis, these prostate specimens are instead diagnosed using descriptive terms such as "acute inflammation" or "chronic inflammation" and not as "prostatitis."

KEY CONCEPTS

Prostatitis

- Bacterial prostatitis may be acute or chronic; the responsible organism usually is *E. coli* or another gram-negative rod.
- Chronic abacterial prostatitis, despite sharing symptomatology with chronic bacterial prostatitis, is of unknown etiology and does not respond to antibiotics.
- Granulomatous prostatitis has a multifactorial etiology, including infectious and noninfectious causes.

Benign Enlargement

Benign Prostatic Hyperplasia or Nodular Hyperplasia

BPH is the most common benign prostatic disease in men older than age 50 years. It results from nodular hyperplasia of prostatic stromal and epithelial cells and often leads to urinary obstruction. It is characterized by the formation of large, fairly discrete nodules in the periurethral region of the prostate, which, when sufficiently large, compress and narrow the urethral canal to cause partial, or sometimes virtually complete, obstruction of the urethra. Nodular hyperplasia is not considered to be a premalignant lesion.

Incidence. Histologic evidence of BPH can be seen in approximately 20% of men 40 years of age, a figure that increases to 70% by age 60 and to 90% by age 80. There is no direct correlation, however, between histologic changes and clinical symptoms. Only 50% of those who have microscopic evidence of BPH have clinically detectable enlargement of the prostate, and of these individuals, only 50% develop clinical symptoms. BPH is a problem of enormous magnitude, with approximately 30% of white American men older than 50 years of age having moderate to severe symptoms.

Etiology and Pathogenesis. Despite the fact that there are an increased number of epithelial cells and stromal components in the periurethral area of the prostate, there is no clear evidence of increased epithelial cell proliferation in human BPH. Instead, it is believed that hyperplasia mainly stems from impaired cell death, resulting in the accumulation of senescent cells in the prostate. In keeping with this idea, androgens (discussed later), which are required for the development of BPH, not only increase cellular proliferation, but also inhibit cell death.

The main androgen in the prostate, constituting 90% of total prostatic androgens, is dihydrotestosterone (DHT). DHT is formed in the prostate from testosterone through the action of an enzyme called type 2 5α-reductase. This enzyme is located almost entirely in stromal cells; with the exception of a few basal cells, prostatic epithelial cells do not express type 2 5α-reductase. Thus, stromal cells are responsible for androgen-dependent prostatic growth. Type 1 5α-reductase is not detected in the prostate, or is present at very low levels. However this enzyme may produce DHT from testosterone in liver and skin, and circulating DHT may act in the prostate by an endocrine mechanism.

DHT binds to the nuclear androgen receptor (AR) present in both stromal and epithelial prostate cells. DHT is more potent than testosterone because it has a higher affinity for AR and forms a more stable complex with the receptor. Binding of DHT to AR stimulates the transcription of androgen-dependent genes, which includes several growth factors and their receptors. Most important among these are members of the fibroblast growth factor (FGF) family and transforming growth factor (TGF)-β (Chapter 3). FGFs, produced by stromal cells, are paracrine regulators of androgen-stimulated epithelial growth during embryonic prostatic development, and some of these pathways may be "reawakened" in adulthood to produce prostatic growth in BPH. TGF-β serves as a mitogen for fibroblasts and other mesenchymal cells, but inhibits epithelial proliferation. Although the ultimate cause of BPH is unknown, it is believed that DHT-induced growth factors act by increasing the proliferation of stromal cells and decreasing the death of epithelial cells.

MORPHOLOGY

In the usual case of benign prostatic enlargement, the prostate weighs between 60 and 100 gm. Nodular hyperplasia of the prostate originates almost exclusively in the inner aspect of the prostate gland (transition zone). The early nodules are composed almost entirely of stromal cells, and later predominantly

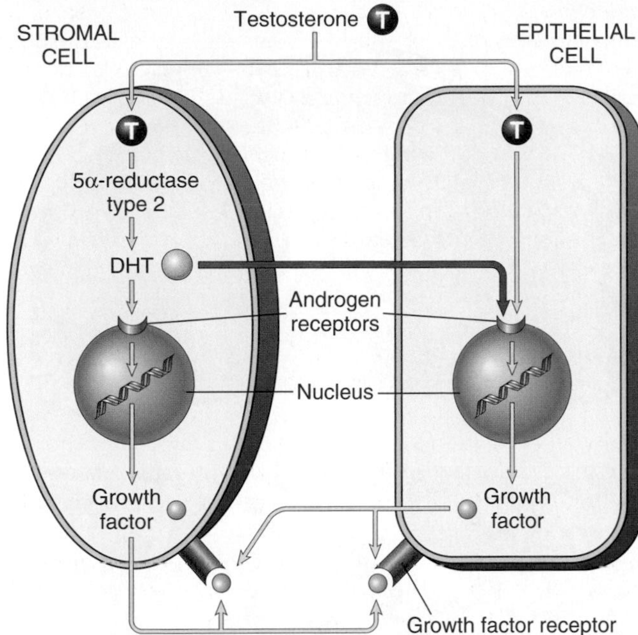

Figure 21-32 Simplified scheme of the pathogenesis of prostatic hyperplasia. The central role of the stromal cells in generating dihydrotestosterone (DHT) should be noted. DHT may also be produced in skin and liver by both type 1 and 2 5α-reductase.

epithelial nodules arise. From their origin in this strategic location the nodular enlargements may encroach on the lateral walls of the urethra to compress it to a slitlike orifice (Fig. 21-33). In some cases, nodular enlargement may project up into the floor of the urethra as a hemispheric mass directly beneath the mucosa of the urethra, which is termed **median lobe hypertrophy**.

On cross-section, the nodules vary in color and consistency depending on their cellular content (Fig. 21-33*B*). Nodules that contain mostly glands are yellow-pink and soft, and exude a milky white prostatic fluid. Nodules composed primarily of fibromuscular stroma are pale gray and tough; these nodules do not exude fluid and are less clearly demarcated from the surrounding prostatic tissue. Although the nodules do not have true capsules, the compression of surrounding prostatic tissue creates a plane of cleavage about them.

Microscopically, glandular proliferation takes the form of aggregations of small to large to cystically dilated glands lined by two layers of cells, an inner columnar layer and an outer layer of cuboidal or flattened epithelium (Fig. 21-33*C*). Occasionally foci of reactive squamous metaplasia mimicking urothelial carcinoma are seen adjacent to prostatic infarcts in prostates with prominent BPH. The diagnosis of BPH cannot usually be made on needle biopsy because such biopsies are too small to appreciate the nodularity of the process and do not usually sample the transition zone where BPH occurs.

Clinical Features. **The major clinical problem in those with BPH is urinary obstruction, which stems from the increased size of the prostate and the smooth muscle-mediated prostatic contraction.** The increased resistance to urinary outflow leads to bladder hypertrophy and distention, accompanied by urine retention. The inability to empty the bladder completely creates a reservoir of residual urine that is a common source of infection. Patients experience increased urinary frequency, nocturia, difficulty in starting and stopping the stream of urine, overflow dribbling, dysuria (painful micturition), and have an increased risk of developing bacterial infections of the bladder and kidney. In many cases, sudden, acute urinary retention occurs that requires emergency catheterization for relief.

Mild cases of BPH may be treated without medical or surgical therapy, such as by decreasing fluid intake, especially before bedtime; moderating the intake of alcohol and caffeine-containing products; and following timed voiding schedules. The most commonly used and effective medical therapy for symptoms relating to BPH are α-blockers, which decrease prostate smooth muscle tone via inhibition of α_1-adrenergic receptors. Another common pharmacologic therapy aims to decrease symptoms by physically shrinking the prostate with an agent that inhibits the synthesis of DHT. Inhibitors of 5-α-reductase fall into this category. For moderate to severe cases recalcitrant to medical therapy, a wide range of more invasive procedures exist. Transurethral resection of the prostate (TURP) has been the gold standard in terms of reducing symptoms, improving flow rates, and decreasing post-voiding residual urine. It is indicated as a first line of therapy in certain circumstances, such as recurrent urinary retention. As a result of its morbidity and cost, alternative procedures have been developed. These include high-intensity focused ultrasound, laser therapy, hyperthermia, transurethral electrovaporization, and transurethral needle ablation using radiofrequency.

KEY CONCEPTS

Benign Prostatic Hyperplasia

- BPH is characterized by proliferation of benign stromal and glandular elements. DHT, an androgen derived from testosterone, is the major hormonal stimulus for proliferation.
- BPH most commonly affects the inner periurethral zone of the prostate, producing nodules that compress the prostatic urethra. On microscopic examination, the nodules exhibit variable proportions of stroma and glands. Hyperplastic glands are lined by two cell layers, an inner columnar layer and an outer layer composed of flattened basal cells.
- Clinical symptoms and signs are reported by 10% of affected patients and include hesitancy, urgency, nocturia, and poor urinary stream. Chronic obstruction predisposes to recurrent urinary tract infections. Acute urinary obstruction may occur.

Tumors

Adenocarcinoma

Adenocarcinoma of the prostate is the most common form of cancer in men, accounting for 29% of cancer in the United States in 2012. Prostate cancer is tied with colorectal cancer in terms of cancer mortality, causing 9% of cancer deaths in the United States in 2012. There is a one in six lifetime probability of being diagnosed with prostate cancer. It demonstrates a remarkably wide range of clinical

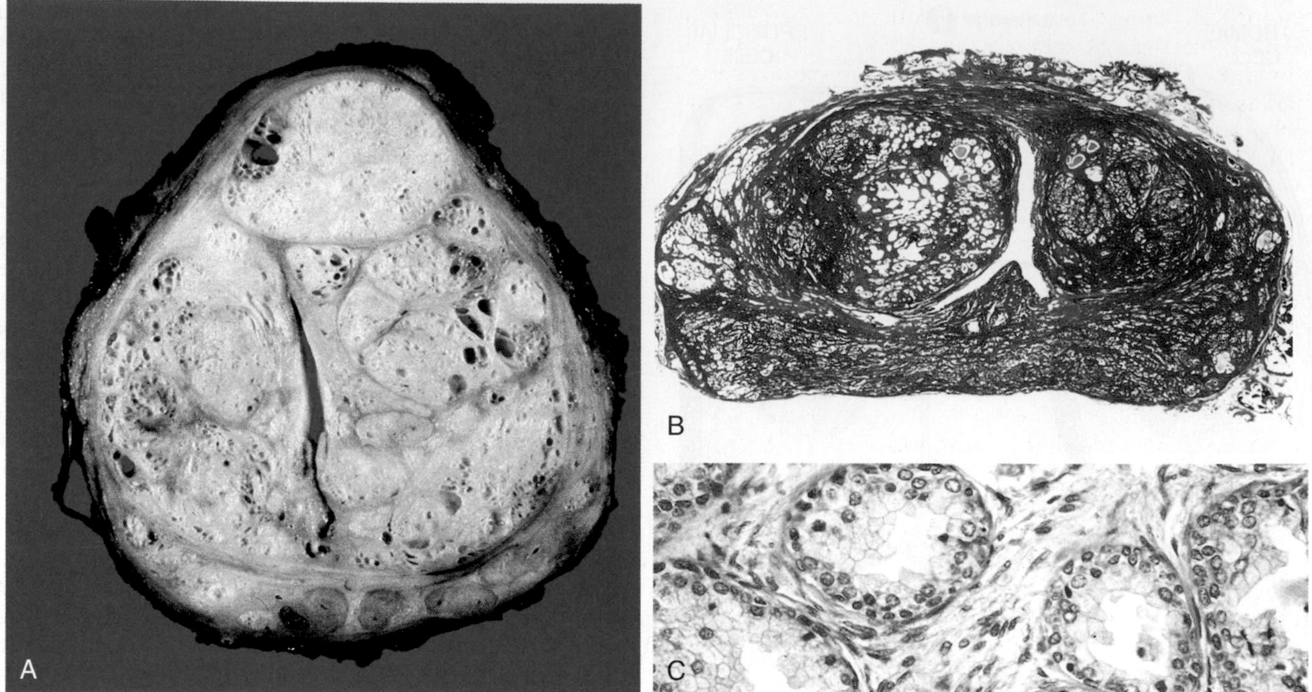

Figure 21-33 Nodular prostatic hyperplasia. **A,** Well-defined nodules of benign prostatic hypertrophy compress the urethra into a slitlike lumen. **B,** A microscopic view of a whole mount of the prostate shows nodules of hyperplastic glands on both sides of the urethra. **C,** Under high power the characteristic dual cell population: the inner columnar and outer flattened basal cell can be seen.

behaviors, from very aggressive lethal cancers to incidentally discovered clinically insignificant cancers.

Incidence. Cancer of the prostate is typically a disease of men older than age 50 years, in whom it is quite common. Based on autopsy studies, its incidence increases from 20% in men in their 50s to approximately 70% in men between the ages of 70 and 80 years. There are some remarkable and puzzling national and racial differences in the incidence of the disease. Prostatic cancer is uncommon in Asians and occurs most frequently among blacks. In addition to hereditary factors, environment plays a role, as evidenced by the rise in the incidence of the disease in Japanese immigrants to the United States, though not nearly to the level of that of native-born Americans. Also, as the diet in Asia becomes more westernized, the incidence of clinically significant prostate cancer in this region of the world seems to be increasing. Whether this is due to dietary factors or other lifestyle changes is not clear.

Etiology and Pathogenesis. Our knowledge of the causes of prostate cancer is far from complete. Several factors, including age, race, family history, hormone levels, and environmental influences are suspected to play a role. The increased incidence of this disease upon migration from a low-incidence region to one with a high incidence is consistent with a role for environmental influences. There are many candidate environmental factors, but none has been proven to be causative. For example, increased consumption of fats or carcinogens present in charred red meats has been implicated. Other dietary products suspected of preventing or delaying prostate cancer development include lycopenes (found in tomatoes), soy products, and vitamin D.

Androgens play an important role in prostate cancer. Like their normal counterparts, the growth and survival of prostate cancer cells depends on androgens, which bind to the androgen receptor (AR) and induce the expression of pro-growth and pro-survival genes. Of interest with respect to differences in prostate cancer risk among races, the X-linked AR gene contains a polymorphic sequence composed of repeats of the codon CAG (which codes for glutamine). Very large expansions of this stretch of CAGs cause a rare neurodegenerative disorder, Kennedy disease, characterized by muscle cramping and weakness. However, even in normal individuals, there is sufficient variation in the length of the CAG repeats to affect AR function. ARs with the shortest stretches of polyglutamine have the highest sensitivity to androgens. The shortest polyglutamine repeats on average are found in African Americans, while Caucasians have an intermediate length and Asians have the longest, paralleling the incidence and mortality of prostate cancer in these groups. More directly, the length of the repeats is inversely related to rate at which prostate cancer develops in mouse models.

The importance of androgens in maintaining the growth and survival of prostate cancer cells can be seen in the therapeutic effect of castration or treatment with antiandrogens, which usually induce disease regression. Unfortunately, most tumors eventually become resistant to androgen blockade. Tumors escape through a variety of mechanisms, including acquisition of hypersensitivity to low levels of androgen (e.g., through AR gene amplification); ligand-independent AR activation (e.g., via splice variants that lack the ligand binding domain); mutations in AR that allow it to be activated by non-androgen ligands; and other mutations or epigenetic changes that activate alternative signaling pathways, which may bypass the need for AR altogether. Among the latter are changes that lead to increased activation of the PI3K/AKT signaling pathway (such loss of the *PTEN* tumor suppressor gene), which is observed most often in tumors that have become resistant to antiandrogen therapy.

There is much interest in the role of other inherited polymorphisms in the development of prostate cancer. Compared with men with no family history, men with one first-degree relative with prostate cancer have twice the risk and those with two first-degree relatives have five times the risk of developing prostate cancer. Men with a strong family history of prostate cancer also tend to develop the disease at an earlier age. Men with germline mutations of the tumor suppressor *BRCA2* have a 20-fold increased risk of prostate cancer, and a germline mutation in *HOXB13*, a homeobox gene encoding a transcription factor that regulates prostatic development, also confers substantially increased risk in the small percentage of families that carry it. However, the vast majority of familial prostate cancers are due to variation in other loci that confer a small increase in cancer risk. Family and genome-wide association studies have identified more than 40 risk-associated loci, which explain approximately 25% of the familial risk. Of possible interest, a number of the candidate genes in these regions are involved in innate immunity, leading to speculation that inflammation, an emerging hallmark of cancer (Chapter 7) may set the stage for the development of prostate carcinoma.

Other work is focused on the role of tumor-specific acquired mutations and epigenetic changes. **One very common structural genetic change in prostate cancer is chromosomal rearrangements that juxtapose the coding sequence of an ETS family transcription factor gene (most commonly *ERG* or *ETV1*) next to the androgen-regulated *TMPRSS2* promoter.** These rearrangements, which occur in approximately half of prostate cancer cases in Caucasian cohorts, place the involved ETS gene under the control of the *TMPRSS2* promoter and lead to its overexpression in an androgen-dependent fashion. Overexpression of ETS transcription factors does not directly transform prostate epithelial cells, but it does make normal prostate epithelial cells more invasive, possibly through the upregulation of matrix metalloproteases. The clinical significance of these gene rearrangements remains unclear, as most studies show that in surgically treated cohorts, the presence of ETS gene rearrangement alone does not portend a worse prognosis.

In contrast to breast and colon cancer, recent whole genome sequencing efforts have demonstrated that genomic deletions and amplifications are more common in prostate cancer than point mutations involving oncogenes. Common genetic alterations in prostate cancer include amplification of the 8q24 locus containing the *MYC* oncogene, and deletions involving the *PTEN* tumor suppressor. In late stage disease, loss of *TP53* (by deletion or mutation), and deletions involving *RB* are common, as are amplifications of the androgen receptor gene locus.

The most common epigenetic alteration in prostate cancer is hypermethylation of the glutathione *S*-transferase (*GSTP1*) gene, which down-regulates *GSTP1* expression. The *GSTP1* gene is located on chromosome 11q13 and is an important part of the pathway that prevents damage from a wide range of carcinogens. Other genes silenced by epigenetic modifications in a subset of prostate cancers include a number of tumor suppressor genes, including genes involved in cell cycle regulation (*RB*, *CDKN2A*, maintenance of genomic stability (*MLH1*, *MSH2*), and suppression of Wnt pathway signaling (*APC*).

As can be surmised from the multiplicity of abnormalities, prostate carcinoma (like other cancers) is the product of some critical combination of acquired genomic structural changes, somatic mutations and epigenetic changes. A putative precursor lesion, prostatic intraepithelial neoplasia (PIN), has been described. There are several lines of evidence relating PIN to invasive cancer. First, both PIN and cancer typically predominate in the peripheral zone and are relatively uncommon in other zones. Prostates containing cancer have a higher frequency and a greater extent of PIN, which is also often seen in proximity to cancer. Studies have revealed that many of the molecular changes seen in invasive cancers are present in PIN (for example, rearrangements involving *ETS* genes are found in a subset), strongly supporting the argument that PIN is a precursor of invasive cancer. Despite all this evidence, we do not know the natural history of PIN, and in particular how often it progresses to cancer. Thus, unlike in cancer of the cervix, the term "carcinoma in situ" is not used for PIN.

MORPHOLOGY

When the terms **"prostate cancer"** or **"prostate adenocarcinoma"** are used without qualifications it refers to the common or acinar variant of prostate cancer. In approximately 70% of cases, carcinoma of the prostate arises in the peripheral zone of the gland, classically in a posterior location, where it may be palpable on rectal examination (Fig. 21-34). Characteristically, on cross-section of the prostate **the neoplastic tissue is gritty and firm, but when embedded within the prostatic substance it may be extremely difficult to visualize and be more readily apparent on palpation**. Local extension most commonly involves periprostatic tissue, seminal vesicles, and the base of the urinary bladder, which in advanced disease may produce ureteral obstruction. Metastases spread via lymphatics to the obturator nodes and eventually to the para-aortic

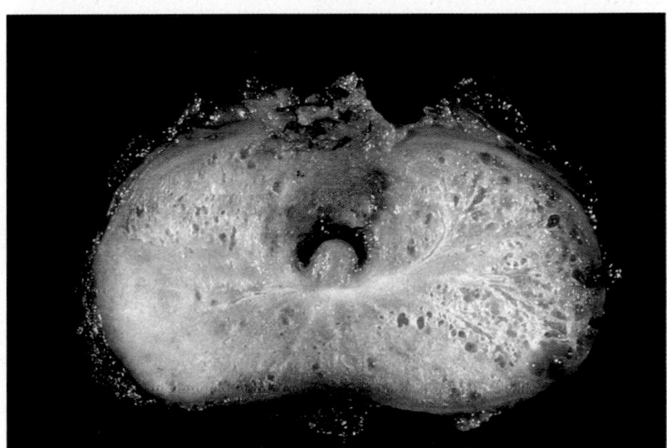

Figure 21-34 Adenocarcinoma of the prostate. Carcinomatous tissue is seen on the posterior aspect *(lower left)*. Note solid whiter tissue of cancer in contrast to spongy appearance of benign peripheral zone in the contralateral side.

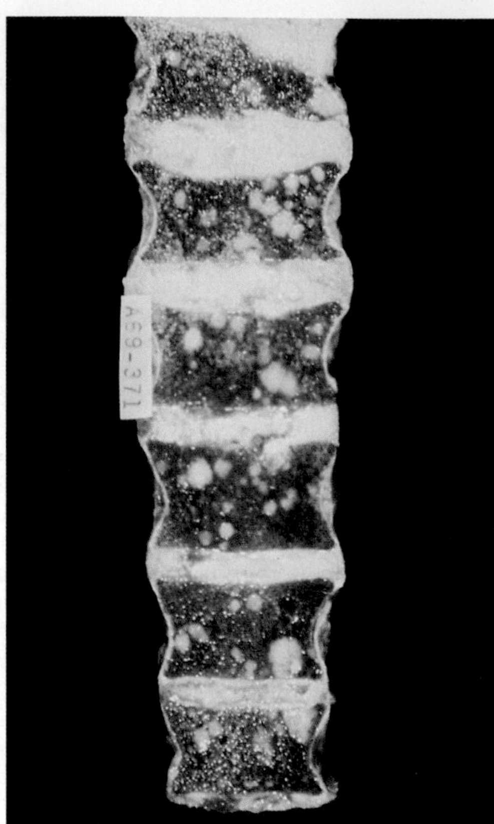

Figure 21-35 Metastatic osteoblastic prostatic carcinoma within vertebral bodies.

nodes. Hematogenous spread occurs chiefly to the bones, particularly the axial skeleton, but some lesions spread widely to viscera. Massive visceral dissemination is an exception rather than the rule. The bony metastases are typically osteoblastic, a feature that in men points strongly to a prostatic origin (Fig. 21-35). The bones commonly involved, in descending order of frequency, are lumbar spine, proximal femur, pelvis, thoracic spine, and ribs.

Histologically, most lesions are adenocarcinomas that produce well-defined, readily demonstrable gland patterns. The glands are typically smaller than benign glands and are lined by a single uniform layer of cuboidal or low columnar epithelium. In contrast to benign glands, prostate cancer glands are more crowded, and characteristically lack branching and papillary infolding. **The outer basal cell layer typical of benign glands is absent.** The cytoplasm of the tumor cells ranges from pale-clear to a distinctive amphophilic appearance. Nuclei are large and often contain one or more large nucleoli. There is some variation in nuclear size and shape, but in general pleomorphism is not marked. Mitotic figures are uncommon.

The diagnosis of prostate cancer on biopsy specimens can be challenging due to several factors. There is often only a scant amount of tissue available for histologic examination in needle biopsies, and malignant glands may be admixed with numerous benign glands (Fig. 21-36). Moreover, the histologic findings pointing to malignancy may be subtle (leading to underdiagnosis), and there are also benign mimickers of cancer that can lead to a misdiagnosis of cancer. A few histologic findings on biopsy are specific for prostate cancer, such as perineural invasion, but in general the diagnosis is made based on a constellation of architectural, cytologic, and ancillary findings (Fig. 21-37). As discussed earlier, one distinguishing feature between benign and malignant prostate glands is that benign glands contain basal cells, which are absent in cancer (compare benign and malignant glands in Fig. 21-36*A*, and benign glands in Fig. 21-33*C* with cancerous glands in Fig. 21-36*B*). This distinction can be brought out by using various immunohistologic markers to label basal cells. Another useful immunohistochemical marker is α-methylacyl-coenzyme A-racemase (AMACR), which is up-regulated in prostate cancer. The majority of prostate cancers are positive for AMACR, the sensitivity varying among studies from 82% to 100%. Such markers, while improving diagnostic accuracy, are still prone to false-positive and false-negative results and must be used in conjunction with the routine hematoxylin and eosin–stained sections.

In approximately 80% of cases, prostatic tissue removed for carcinoma also harbors presumptive precursor lesions, referred to as **high-grade prostatic intraepithelial neoplasia (PIN)**. PIN consists of architecturally benign large, branching prostatic acini lined by cytologically atypical cells with prominent nucleoli. Cytologically PIN and carcinoma may be identical. Unlike malignant glands, PIN glands are surrounded by a patchy layer of basal cells and an intact basement membrane.

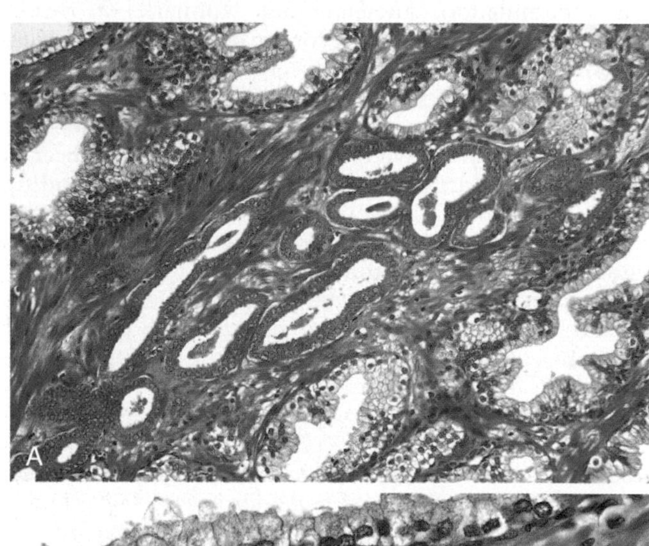

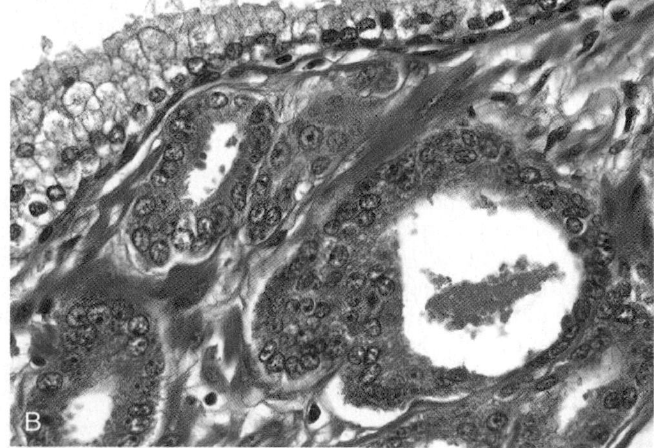

Figure 21-36 A, Photomicrograph of small focus of adenocarcinoma of the prostate demonstrating small glands crowded in between larger benign glands. **B,** Higher magnification shows several small malignant glands with enlarged nuclei, prominent nucleoli, and dark cytoplasm, compared with larger benign gland *(top)*.

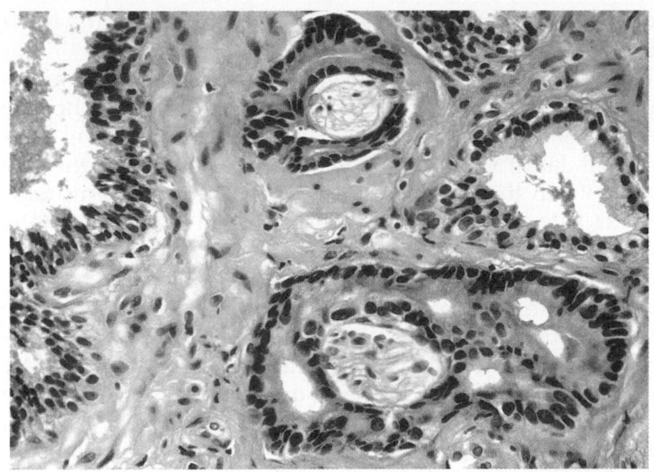

Figure 21-37 Carcinoma of prostate showing perineural invasion by malignant glands. Compare to benign gland *(left)*.

Grading and Staging. **Grading is of particular importance in prostatic cancer, because grade and stage (discussed below) are the best prognostic predictors.** Prostate cancer is graded using the Gleason system, which stratifies prostate cancer into five grades on the basis of glandular patterns of differentiation. Grade 1 represents the most well differentiated tumors, in which the neoplastic glands are uniform and round in appearance and are packed into well-circumscribed nodules (Fig. 21-38*A*). In contrast, grade 5 tumors show no glandular differentiation, with tumor cells infiltrating the stroma in the form of cords, sheets, and nests (Fig. 21-38*C*). The other grades fall in between these extremes. Most tumors contain more than one pattern; in such instances, a primary grade is assigned to the dominant pattern and a secondary grade to the second most frequent pattern. The two numeric grades are then added to obtain a combined Gleason grade or score. Thus, for example, a tumor with a dominant grade 3 and a secondary grade 4 has a Gleason score of 7. Tumors with only one pattern are treated as if their primary and secondary grades are the same, and hence, the number is doubled. An exception to the rule is if three patterns are present on biopsy, the most common and highest grades are added together to arrive at the Gleason score. Thus, under this schema the most well-differentiated tumors have a Gleason score of 2 (1 + 1), and the least-differentiated tumors merit a score of 10 (5 + 5). Gleason scores are often combined into groups with similar biologic behavior, with grades 2 through 6 representing well-differentiated tumors with an excellent prognosis, 3 + 4 = 7 moderately differentiated tumors, 4 + 3 = 7 moderately to poorly differentiated tumors, and 8 through 10 poorly to undifferentiated tumors with aggressive biologies. In surgical specimens, Gleason scores of 2 through 4 are typically small tumors found incidentally in TURP performed for symptoms of BPH. The majority of potentially treatable cancers detected on needle biopsy as a result of screening have Gleason scores of 6 through 7. Tumors with Gleason scores 8 through 10 tend to be advanced cancers that are less likely to be cured. Although there is some evidence that prostate cancers can become more aggressive with time, most

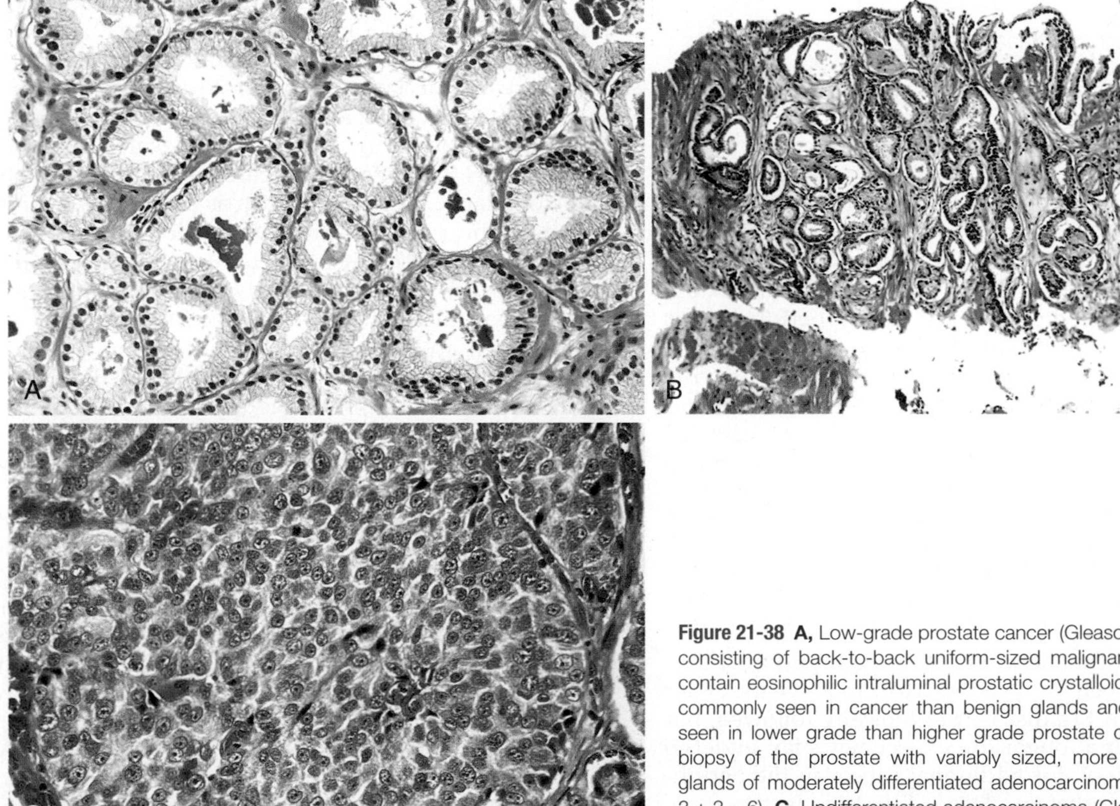

Figure 21-38 A, Low-grade prostate cancer (Gleason score 1 + 1 = 2) consisting of back-to-back uniform-sized malignant glands. Glands contain eosinophilic intraluminal prostatic crystalloids, a feature more commonly seen in cancer than benign glands and more frequently seen in lower grade than higher grade prostate cancer. **B,** Needle biopsy of the prostate with variably sized, more widely dispersed glands of moderately differentiated adenocarcinoma (Gleason score 3 + 3 = 6). **C,** Undifferentiated adenocarcinoma (Gleason score 5 + 5 = 10) composed of sheets of malignant cells.

Table 21-6 Staging of Prostatic Adenocarcinoma Using the TNM System

TNM Designation	Anatomic Findings
Extent of Primary Tumor (T)	
T1	Clinically inapparent lesion (by palpation/imaging studies)
T1a	Involvement of ≤ 5% of resected tissue
T1b	Involvement of > 5% of resected tissue
T1c	Carcinoma present on needle biopsy (following elevated PSA)
T2	Palpable or visible cancer confined to prostate
T2a	Involvement of ≤ 5% of one lobe
T2b	Involvement of > 5% of one lobe, but unilateral
T2c	Involvement of both lobes
T3	Local extraprostatic extension
T3a	Extracapsular extension
T3b	Seminal vesical invasion
T4	Invasion of contiguous organs and/or supporting structures including bladder neck, rectum, external sphincter, levator muscles, or pelvic floor
Status of Regional Lymph Nodes (N)	
N0	No regional nodal metastases
N1	Metastasis in regional lymph nodes
Distant Metastases (M)	
M0	No distant metastases
M1	Distant metastases present
M1a	Metastases to distant lymph nodes
M1b	Bone metastases
M1c	Other distant sites

PSA, Prostate-specific antigen.

commonly, the Gleason score remains stable over a period of several years.

Staging of prostatic cancer is also important in the selection of the appropriate form of therapy (Table 21-6). Stage T1 refers to incidentally found cancer, either on TURP done for BPH symptoms (T1a and T1b depending on the extent and grade) or on needle biopsy typically performed for elevated serum prostate-specific antigen (PSA) levels (stage T1c). Stage T2 is organ-confined cancer. Stage T3a and T3b tumors show extra-prostatic extension, with and without seminal vesicle invasion, respectively. Stage T4 reflects direct invasion of contiguous organs. Any spread of tumor to the lymph nodes regardless of extent is eventually associated with a fatal outcome, such that the staging system merely records the presence or absence of this finding (N0/N1).

Clinical Course. It is generally accepted that most incidentally discovered focal (stage T1a) cancers found on TURP do not progress when followed for 10 or more years. Older patients with stage T1a disease are typically followed, but younger men with a longer life expectancy may undergo needle biopsy to look for additional cancer in the peripheral zone of the prostate. Stage T1b lesions are more ominous and are treated the same as tumors that are found on needle biopsy, since they have a mortality of 20% if left untreated.

Localized prostate cancer is asymptomatic, and is usually discovered by the detection of a suspicious nodule on rectal examination or elevated serum PSA level (discussed later). Most prostatic cancers arise peripherally away from the urethra, and therefore urinary symptoms occur late. Patients with clinically advanced prostatic cancer may present with urinary symptoms, such as difficulty in starting or stopping the stream, dysuria, frequency, or hematuria. Today it is uncommon for patients to come to attention because of back pain caused by vertebral metastases. As already mentioned, **the finding of osteoblastic metastases by skeletal surveys or the much more sensitive radionuclide bone scanning is virtually diagnostic of this form of cancer in men**. These cancers pursue a universally fatal course.

Digital rectal examination may detect some early prostatic carcinomas because of their posterior location, but the test suffers from both low sensitivity and specificity. Likewise, while transrectal ultrasonography and other imaging modalities show characteristic findings in those with cancerous prostates, the poor sensitivity and specificity of these tests also limit their diagnostic utility. Typically a transrectal needle biopsy is required to confirm the diagnosis.

Measurement of serum PSA levels is widely used to assist with the diagnosis and management of prostate cancer. PSA is a product of prostatic epithelium and is normally secreted in the semen. It is an androgen-regulated serine protease whose function is to cleave and liquefy the seminal coagulum formed after ejaculation. In normal men, only minute amounts of PSA circulate in the serum. Elevated blood levels of PSA occur in association with localized as well as advanced cancer. However, as a screening test for prostate cancer, the use of PSA remains controversial in that it lacks both sensitivity and specificity. Importantly, PSA is organ specific, but not cancer specific. Although serum levels of PSA are elevated to a lesser extent in BPH than in prostatic carcinomas, there is considerable overlap. Other factors such as prostatitis, infarction of nodular hyperplasias, instrumentation of the prostate, and ejaculation also increase serum PSA levels. If the cut-off between normal and abnormal PSA levels is too low, this may falsely indicate the need for a prostate biopsy in some men and result in the detection and potentially unnecessary treatment of indolent and non–life-threatening tumors. In most laboratories, a serum level of 4 ng/mL is reported as the cut-off between normal and abnormal; however, this cut-off may be too high because 20% to 40% of patients with organ-confined prostate cancer have a PSA value of 4 ng/mL or less, which is not detected by this simple screening test. Thus, some guidelines consider PSA values above 2.5 ng/mL abnormal.

Several refinements in the estimation and interpretation of PSA values are currently used. These include the ratio between the serum PSA value and volume of prostate gland (*PSA density*), the rate of change in PSA value with time (*PSA velocity*), the use of age-specific reference ranges, and the ratio of free and bound PSA in the serum. Men with enlarged hyperplastic prostate glands have higher total serum PSA levels than men with small glands. The measurement of serum PSA density factors out the contribution of benign prostatic tissue to serum PSA levels. It is calculated by dividing the total serum PSA level by the estimated gland volume (usually determined by transrectal ultrasound measurements) to estimate the PSA produced per gram of prostate tissue. As men age, their prostates tend to enlarge with BPH. One would then anticipate that, overall, older men would have higher serum PSA levels than younger men. The upper *age-specific PSA* reference ranges are 2.5 ng/mL for men 40 to 49 years of age, 3.5 ng/mL for men 50 to 59 years, 4.5 ng/mL for men 60 to 69 years, and 6.5 ng/mL for men 70 to 79 years. Consequently, a serum PSA value of 3.5, while it will appear as a normal value on a laboratory test, is a worrisome finding in a man in his 40s, warranting additional evaluation. Another means of interpreting serum PSA tests is to assess PSA velocity or the rate of change of PSA. Men with prostate cancer demonstrate a more rapid increase in PSA levels over time than do men who do not have prostate cancer. The rate of change in PSA that best distinguishes between men with and without prostate cancer is 0.75 ng/mL per year. For this measurement to be valid, at least three PSA measurements must be performed over a period of 1.5 to 2 years, as there is substantial short-term variability (up to 20%) between repeat PSA measurements. A man who has a significant increase in serum PSA levels, even if the latest serum PSA test is below the normal cut-off (<4 ng/mL), should undergo additional work-up. Studies have revealed that immunoreactive PSA (the form detected by the widely used antibody test) exists in two forms: a major fraction bound to α_1-antichymotrypsin and a minor free fraction. The percentage of free PSA (free PSA/total PSA × 100) is lower in men with prostate cancer than in men with benign prostatic diseases.

Because many small cancers localized to the prostate may never progress to clinically significant invasive cancers, there is considerable uncertainty regarding the management of small lesions that are detected because of an elevated PSA level. This has created controversy about the role of widespread screening for prostate cancer. Much effort is therefore focused in devising criteria by which those localized lesions most likely to advance can be distinguished from those that remain innocuous.

In contrast to its role in screening, there is no controversy about the value of serial measurements of PSA in assessing the response to therapy. For example, a rising PSA level after radical prostatectomy or radiotherapy for localized disease is indicative of recurrent or disseminated disease. Immunohistochemical localization of PSA on tissue sections can also help the pathologist to determine whether a metastatic tumor originated in the prostate.

In addition to prostate specific antigen, other genes that may serve as biomarkers in prostate cancer have emerged. *PCA3* is a noncoding RNA which is overexpressed in 95% of prostate cancers. A diagnostic test that quantifies urine PCA3 is currently used as an additional biomarker in patients suspected to have prostate cancer because of elevated PSA, but who have had a negative prostate biopsy. Elevated urine PCA3 scores have been shown to be associated with an increased risk of a positive repeat biopsy in this setting. The combination of urinary PCA3 with screening of urine for *TMPRSS2-ERG* fusion DNA (see earlier) may have increased sensitivity and specificity compared to PSA screening alone.

Cancer of the prostate is treated by surgery, radiation therapy, and hormonal manipulations. More than 90% of patients who receive such therapy can expect to live for 15 years. Currently, the most common treatment for clinically localized prostate cancer is radical prostatectomy. The prognosis following radical prostatectomy is based on the pathologic stage, margin status, and Gleason grade. Alternative treatments for localized prostate cancer are either external-beam radiation therapy or interstitial radiation therapy, the latter consisting of placing radioactive seeds throughout the prostate (brachytherapy). External-beam radiation therapy is also used to treat prostate cancer that is too locally advanced to be cured by surgery. Since some prostate cancers have a relatively indolent course, wherein it may take 10 years to see benefit from surgery or radiation therapy, active surveillance is appropriate for many older men or those with significant co-morbidity or even some younger men with low serum PSA values and limited lower grade cancer on biopsy. Advanced, metastatic carcinoma is treated by androgen deprivation therapy. Androgen deprivation may be achieved by orchiectomy, or by administration of synthetic analogs of luteinizing hormone-releasing hormone (LHRH) which suppress normal LHRH, achieving, in effect, a pharmacologic orchiectomy. Other agents decrease levels of local and circulating androgens by inhibiting systemic steroid hormone synthesis. Finally, pharmacologic blockade of the androgen receptor constitutes an additional means of treatment. Although androgen deprivation therapy induces remissions, eventually tumors become resistant to testosterone withdrawal, an event that is a harbinger of disease progression and death.

KEY CONCEPTS

Carcinoma of the Prostate

- Carcinoma of the prostate is a common cancer of older men between 65 and 75 years of age. Aggressive, clinically significant disease is more common in American blacks than in whites, while clinically insignificant occult lesions appear to occur at equal frequencies in these two races.
- Prostate carcinomas range from indolent lesions that will never cause harm to aggressive fatal tumors.
- The most common acquired genetic lesions in prostatic carcinomas are *TPRSS2-ETS* fusion genes and mutations or deletions that activate the PI3K/AKT signaling pathway.
- Carcinomas of the prostate arise most commonly in the outer, peripheral gland and may be palpable by rectal examination.
- Microscopically, they are adenocarcinomas with variable differentiation. Neoplastic glands are lined by a single layer of cells.
- Grading of prostate cancer by the Gleason system correlates with pathologic stage and prognosis.
- Most localized cancers are clinically silent and are detected by routine monitoring of PSA concentrations in older men. Bone metastases, often osteoblastic, typify advanced prostate cancer.

- Serum PSA measurement is a useful but imperfect cancer-screening test, with significant rates of false-negative and false-positive results. Evaluation of PSA concentrations after treatment has great value in monitoring progressive or recurrent disease.

Miscellaneous Tumors and Tumor-like Conditions

Prostate adenocarcinomas may also arise from prostatic ducts. Ductal adenocarcinomas arising in peripheral ducts may present in a fashion similar to ordinary prostate cancer, whereas those arising in the larger periurethral ducts may show signs and symptoms similar to urothelial cancer, causing hematuria and urinary obstructive symptoms. Ductal adenocarcinomas are associated with a relatively poor prognosis. Prostate cancers may show squamous differentiation, either following hormone therapy or de novo, resulting in either adenosquamous or pure squamous cancer. Prostate cancer that reveal abundant mucinous secretions are termed *colloid carcinoma of the prostate*. The most aggressive variant of prostate cancer is small-cell cancer (also known as neuroendocrine carcinoma). Almost all cases of small-cell carcinoma are rapidly fatal.

The most common tumor to secondarily involve the prostate is urothelial cancer. Two distinct patterns of involvement exist. Large invasive urothelial cancers can directly invade from the bladder into the prostate. Alternatively, carcinoma in situ of the bladder can extend into the prostatic urethra and down into the prostatic ducts and acini.

The same mesenchymal tumors described earlier that involve the bladder may also manifest in the prostate. In addition, there exist unique mesenchymal tumors of the prostate derived from the prostatic stroma. Although lymphomas may appear to first arise in the prostate, most patients shortly thereafter demonstrate systemic disease.

SUGGESTED READINGS

Penile Disorders

Bleeker MC, Heideman DA, Snijders PJ, et al: Penile cancer: epidemiology, pathogenesis, and prevention. *World J Urol* 27:141, 2009. *[A systematic review of the literature evaluating penile carcinogenesis, risk factors, and molecular mechanisms involved.]*

Lee PK, Wilkins KB: Condyloma and other infections including human immunodeficiency virus. *Surg Clin North Am* 90:99, 2010.

Testicular Disorders

Bahrami A, Ro JY, Ayala AG: An overview of testicular germ cell tumors. *Arch Pathol Lab Med* 131:1267, 2007.

Greene MH, Kratz CP, Mai PL, et al: Familial testicular germ cell tumors in adults: 2010 summary of genetic risk factors and clinical phenotype. *Endocr Relat Cancer* 17:R109, 2010. *[An update on inherited risk factors in germ cell tumors.]*

Winter C, Albers P: Testicular germ cell tumors: pathogenesis, diagnosis and treatment. *Nat Rev Endocrinol* 7:43, 2011.

Bladder Disorders

Cheng L, Zhang S, MacLennan GT, et al: Bladder cancer: translating molecular genetic insights into clinical practice. *Hum Pathol* 42:455, 2011.

Goebell PJ, Knowles MA: Bladder cancer or bladder cancers? Genetically distinct malignant conditions of the urothelium. *Urol Oncol* 28:409, 2010.

Morgan TM, Keegan KA, Clark PE: Bladder cancer. *Curr Opin Oncol* 23:275, 2011. *[Reviews the diagnosis and management of both more superficial and advanced bladder cancer.]*

Prostatic Disorders

Barbieri CE, Demichelis F, Rubin MA: Molecular genetics of prostate cancer: emerging appreciation of genetic complexity. *Histopathology* 60:187, 2012.

Barbieri CE, Baca SC, Lawrence MS, et al: Exome sequencing identifies recurrent SPOP, FOXA1, and MED12 mutations in prostate cancer, *Nat Genet* 44:685, 2012. *[A primary paper describing heterogeneity in the genetic underpinnings of prostate cancer.]*

Bushman W: Etiology, epidemiology, and natural history of benign prostatic hyperplasia. *Urol Clin N Am* 36:403, 2009.

Epstein JI: An update of the Gleason grading system. *J Urol* 183:433, 2010.

Gjertson CK, Albertsen PC: Use and assessment of PSA in prostate cancer. *Med Clin North Am* 95:191, 2011. *[An excellent summary of clinical use of PSA and current controversies.]*

Ewing CM, Ray AM, Lange EM, et al: Germline mutations in HOXB13 and prostate cancer risk. *NEJM* 12:141, 2012.

Haffner MC, Aryee MJ, Toubaji A, et al: Androgen-induced TOP2B-mediated double-strand breaks and prostate cancer gene rearrangements. *Nat Genet* 42:668, 2010. *[A paper pointing to possible mechanisms of chromosomal rearrangements that drive prostate carcinogenesis.]*

Hsing AW, Chokkalingam AP: Prostate cancer epidemiology. *Front Biosci* 11:1388, 2006.

Le BV, Schaeffer AJ: Genitourinary pain syndromes, prostatitis and lower urinary tract symptoms. *Urol Clin North Am* 36:527, 2009. *[A recent review of the etiology, diagnosis, symptoms, and treatment of prostatitis and interstitial cystitis along with pelvic pain syndromes.]*

Nelson WG, De Marzo AM, Yegnasubramanian S: Epigenetic alterations in human prostate cancers. *Endocrinology* 150:3991, 2009.

Patel AK, Chapple CR: Medical management of lower urinary tract symptoms in men: current treatment and future approaches. *Nat Clin Pract Urol* 5:211, 2008. *[This article also clarifies the terminology used to evaluate men with lower urinary tract symptoms.]*

Pettersson A, Graff RE, Bauer SR, et al: The TMPRSS2:ERG rearrangement, ERG expression and prostate cancer outcomes: a cohort study and meta-analysis. *Cancer Epidemiol Biomarkers Prev* 21:1497, 2012.

Prensner JR, Rubin MA, Wei JT, et al: Beyond PSA: the next generation of prostate cancer biomarkers. *Sci Transl Med* 4:127rv3, 2012. *[A review covering PSA and possible new prostate cancer biomarkers that are under evaluation.]*

See TARGETED THERAPY available online at www.studentconsult.com

CHAPTER 22

The Female Genital Tract

Lora Hedrick Ellenson • Edyta C. Pirog

CHAPTER CONTENTS

A brief review of the development and anatomy of the female genital tract is fundamental to understanding the diseases that affect this complex organ system. Normal development of the female genital tract proceeds through a series of tightly choreographed events involving the primordial germ cells, the müllerian (paramesonephric) ducts, the wolffian (mesonephric) ducts, and the urogenital sinus (Fig. 22-1).

- *Germ cells* arise in the wall of the yolk sac by the fourth week of gestation. By the fifth or sixth week they migrate into the urogenital ridge and induce proliferation of the mesodermal epithelium, which gives rise to the epithelium and stroma of the ovary.
- The lateral *müllerian ducts* form at about the sixth week of development through invagination and fusion of the coelomic lining epithelium. The ducts progressively grow caudally into the pelvis, where they swing medially to fuse with the urogenital sinus at the müllerian tubercle (Fig. 22-1*A*). Further caudal growth brings these fused ducts into contact with the urogenital sinus. The unfused upper portions of the müllerian ducts mature into the fallopian tubes, while the fused lower portion develops into the uterus, cervix and upper vagina.
- The *urogenital sinus* develops when the cloaca is subdivided by the urorectal septum; it eventually forms the lower part of the vagina and the vestibule of the external genitalia (Fig. 22-1*B*).
- The *mesonephric ducts* normally regress in the female, but remnants may persist into adult life as epithelial inclusions adjacent to the ovaries, tubes, and uterus. In the cervix and vagina these rests may be cystic and are termed *Gartner duct cysts*.

The epithelial lining of the female genital tract as well as the ovarian surface share a common origin from coelomic epithelium (mesothelium), which may explain why morphologically similar benign and malignant lesions arise in various sites within the female genital tract and the adjacent peritoneal surfaces.

Diseases of the female genital tract are extremely common and include complications of pregnancy, infections, tumors, and hormonally induced abnormalities. The following discussion presents the pathology of the major diseases that result in clinical problems. Additional details can be found in current textbooks of gynecologic pathology and clinical obstetrics and gynecology. We will discuss the pathologic conditions peculiar to each segment of the female genital tract separately, but before doing so will briefly review infections and pelvic inflammatory disease because they can affect many of the various anatomic structures concomitantly.

Infections

A large variety of organisms can infect the female genital tract. Some infections with microorganisms such as *Candida, Trichomonas,* and *Gardnerella* are very common and may cause significant discomfort, but are without serious sequelae. Others, such as *Neisseria gonorrhoeae* and *Chlamydia* infections, are major causes of female infertility, and others still, such as *Ureaplasma urealyticum* and *Mycoplasma hominis* infections, are implicated in preterm deliveries. Viruses, especially herpes simplex viruses (HSVs) and human papillomaviruses (HPVs), also account for considerable morbidity; HSVs cause painful genital ulcerations, whereas HPVs are involved in the pathogenesis of cervical, vaginal, and vulvar cancers.

Many of these infections are sexually transmitted, including trichomoniasis, gonorrhea, chancroid, granuloma inguinale, lymphogranuloma venereum, syphilis, *Mycoplasma, Chlamydia,* HSV, and HPV. Most of these conditions are considered in Chapter 8; HPV is also discussed

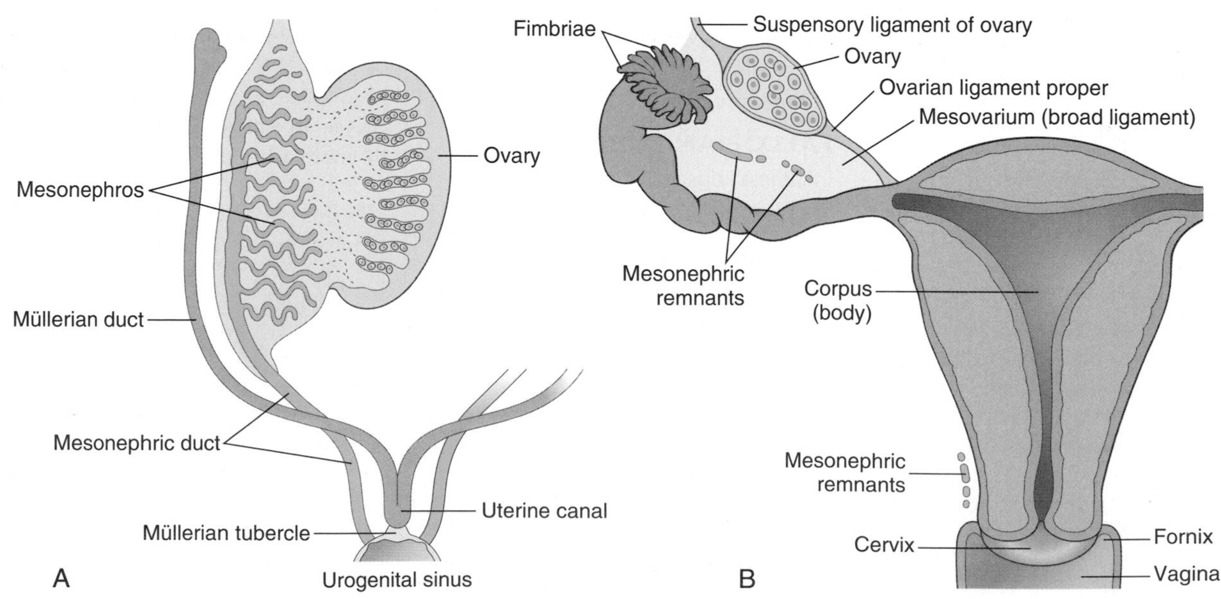

Figure 22-1 Embryology and anatomy of the female genital tract. **A,** Early in development, the mesonephric *(blue)* and müllerian *(red)* ducts merge at the urogenital sinus to form the müllerian tubercle. **B,** By birth, the müllerian ducts have fused to form the fallopian tubes, uterus, and endocervix *(red)*, merging with the vaginal squamous mucosa. The mesonephric ducts regress, but may be found as a remnant in the ovary, adnexa, and cervix (Gartner duct). (Adapted from Langman J: Medical Embryology. Baltimore, Williams and Wilkins, 1981.)

in Chapter 7 due to its important role as a transforming virus. Here we touch only on aspects relevant to the female genital tract, including pathogens confined to the lower genital tract (vulva, vagina, and cervix) and those that involve the entire genital tract and are implicated in pelvic inflammatory disease.

Infections of the Lower Genital Tract

Herpes Simplex Virus. Genital herpes simplex virus (HSV) infection is common and involves, in order of frequency, the cervix, vagina, and vulva. HSVs are DNA viruses that include two serotypes, HSV-1 and HSV-2. HSV-1 typically results in oropharyngeal infection, whereas HSV-2 usually involves genital mucosa and skin; however, depending on the sexual practices HSV-1 may be detected in the genital region and HSV-2 may cause oral infections as well (Chapter 8). By age 40 years, approximately 30% of women are seropositive for antibodies against HSV-2.

About one third of newly infected individuals are symptomatic. Lesions typically develop 3 to 7 days after transmission and are often associated with systemic symptoms such as fever, malaise, and tender inguinal lymph nodes. The earliest lesions usually consist of red papules that progress to vesicles and then to painful coalescent ulcers. The lesions are easily visible on vulvar skin and mucosa, while cervical or vaginal lesions present with severe purulent discharge and pelvic pain. Lesions around the urethra may cause painful urination and urinary retention. The vesicles and ulcers contain numerous viral particles, accounting for the high transmission rate during active infection. The mucosal and skin lesions heal spontaneously in 1 to 3 weeks, but during the acute infection the virus migrates to the regional lumbosacral nerve ganglia and establishes a latent infection. Because of viral latency, HSV infections persist indefinitely and any decrease in immune function, as well as stress, trauma, ultraviolet radiation, and hormonal changes, can trigger reactivation of the virus and recurrence of the skin and mucosal lesions. As expected, recurrences are much more common in immunosuppressed individuals.

MORPHOLOGY

By the time an HSV lesion is biopsied it is typically in the phase of an ulcer. The epithelium is desquamated and marked acute inflammation is present at the ulcer bed. Smears of the inflammatory exudate from the active lesions show characteristic HSV cytopathic changes consisting of multinucleated squamous cells containing eosinophilic to basophilic viral inclusions with a "ground-glass" appearance (Fig. 22-2).

Transmission of HSV takes place mainly during the active phase, but occasionally may also occur during the latent phase due to subclinical virus shedding. Condoms and antiviral therapies can reduce the risk of transmission, but do not prevent it. As with other sexually transmitted diseases, women are more susceptible to transmission than men. Previous infection with HSV-1 seems to reduce susceptibility to HSV-2 infection. The gravest consequence of HSV infection is transmission to the neonate during birth. This risk is highest if the infection is active during delivery and particularly if it is a primary (initial) infection in the mother. Cesarean section is warranted in such cases. In addition, HSV-2 infection enhances HIV-1 acquisition and transmission.

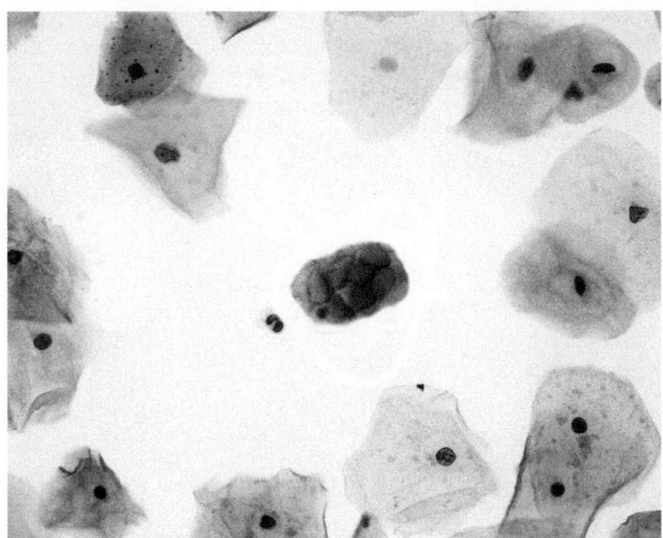

Figure 22-2 Herpes simplex virus infection (cervical smear). The cell in the center shows HSV cytopathic effect. Infected cells become multinucleated and contain intranuclear viral inclusions with a characteristic "ground-glass" appearance.

The diagnosis is based on typical clinical findings and HSV detection. The purulent exudate is aspirated from the lesions and inoculated into a tissue culture. After 48 to 72 hours the viral cytopathic effect can be seen and the virus may then be serotyped. In addition, some laboratories offer more sensitive polymerase chain reaction, enzyme-linked immunosorbent assays, and direct immunofluorescent antibody tests for detection of HSV in the lesional secretions. Individuals with primary, acute-phase HSV infection do not have serum anti-HSV antibodies. Detection of anti-HSV antibodies in the serum is indicative of recurrent/latent infection.

There is no effective treatment for latent HSV; however, antiviral agents like acyclovir or famciclovir may shorten the length of the initial and recurrent symptomatic phase. The ultimate solution is an effective vaccine, a tantalizing goal that is yet to be realized.

Other Lower Female Genital Tract Infections. As mentioned, a variety of other viruses, fungi, and bacteria can also cause symptomatic infections of the lower genital tract. Those that are most common include the following:

- *Molluscum contagiosum* is a skin or mucosal lesion caused by poxvirus (Fig. 22-3*A*). There are four types of molluscum contagiosum viruses (MCVs), MCV-1 to -4, with MCV-1 being the most prevalent and MCV-2 being most often sexually transmitted. The infections are common in young children between 2 and 12 years of age and are transmitted through direct contact or shared articles (e.g., towels). Molluscum may affect any area of the skin but is most common on the trunk, arms, and legs. In adults, molluscum infections are typically sexually transmitted and affect the genitals, lower abdomen, buttocks, and inner thighs. The average incubation period is 6 weeks. Diagnosis is based on the characteristic clinical appearance of pearly, dome-shaped papules with a

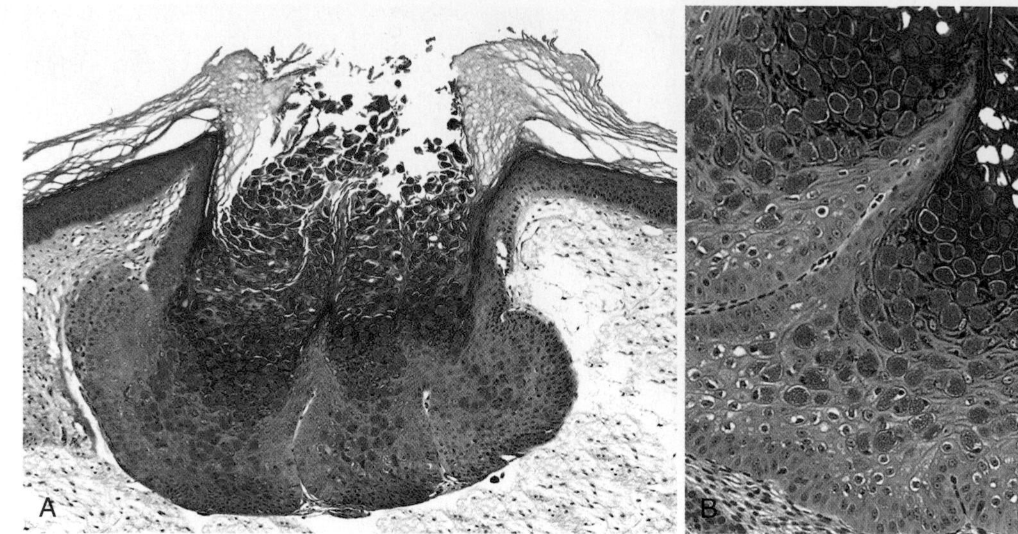

Figure 22-3 Molluscum contagiosum infection. **A,** Low power appearance of a dome-shaped papule with dimpled center. **B,** High power magnification reveals intracytoplasmic viral inclusions.

dimpled center. The papules measure 1 to 5 mm in diameter, and their central waxy core contains cells with *cytoplasmic viral inclusions* (Fig. 22-3*B*).

- *Fungal infections*, especially those caused by yeast (*Candida*), are extremely common; in fact, **yeast are part of many women's normal vaginal microflora and the development of symptomatic candidiasis is typically a result of a disturbance in the patient's vaginal microbial ecosystem.** Diabetes mellitus, antibiotics, pregnancy, and conditions resulting in compromised neutrophil or T_H17 T-cell function are permissive to symptomatic fungal infection, which manifests itself by marked vulvovaginal pruritus, erythema, swelling, and curdlike vaginal discharge. Severe infection may result in mucosal ulcerations. The diagnosis is made by finding the pseudospores or filamentous fungal hyphae in wet KOH mounts of the discharge or on Papanicolaou (Pap) smear. Even though sexual transmission of yeast infection has been documented, candidiasis is not considered a sexually transmitted disease.
- *Trichomonas vaginalis* is a large, flagellated ovoid protozoan that is usually transmitted by sexual contact and develops within 4 days to 4 weeks. The patients may be asymptomatic or may complain of yellow, frothy vaginal discharge, vulvovaginal discomfort, dysuria (painful urination), and dyspareunia (painful intercourse). The vaginal and cervical mucosa typically has a fiery-red appearance, with marked dilatation of cervical mucosal vessels resulting in characteristic colposcopic appearance of "*strawberry cervix.*"
- *Gardnerella vaginalis* is a gram-negative bacillus that is implicated as the main cause of *bacterial vaginosis* (vaginitis). Patients typically present with thin, green-gray, malodorous (fishy) vaginal discharge. Pap smears reveal superficial and intermediate squamous cells covered with a shaggy coating coccobacilli. Bacterial cultures in such cases reveal *G. vaginalis* and other bacteria, including anaerobic peptostreptococci and aerobic α-hemolytic streptococci. In pregnant patients, bacterial vaginosis has been implicated in premature labor.
- *Ureaplasma urealyticum* and *Mycoplasma hominis* species account for some cases of vaginitis and cervicitis, and have been implicated in chorioamnionitis and premature delivery in pregnant patients.
- *Chlamydia trachomatis* infections mainly take the form of cervicitis. However, in some patients the infection may ascend to the uterus and fallopian tubes, resulting in endometritis and salpingitis; thus Chlamydia is one of the causes of pelvic inflammatory disease, as discussed later.

Infections Involving the Lower and Upper Genital Tract

Pelvic Inflammatory Disease

Pelvic inflammatory disease (PID) is an infection that begins in the vulva or vagina and spreads upward to involve most of the structures in the female genital system, resulting in pelvic pain, adnexal tenderness, fever, and vaginal discharge. *Neisseria gonorrhoeae* continues to be a common cause of PID, the most serious complication of gonorrhea in women. *Chlamydia* infection is another well-recognized cause of PID. Infections after spontaneous or induced abortions and normal or abnormal deliveries (called *puerperal infections*) are also important causes of PID. In these situations the infections are typically polymicrobial and may be caused by staphylococci, streptococci, coliforms, and *Clostridium perfringens*.

With gonococcus, inflammatory changes start to appear approximately 2 to 7 days after inoculation. The initial infection most commonly involves the endocervical mucosa, but it may also begin in the Bartholin gland and other vestibular, or periurethral, glands. From these sites the organisms may spread upward to involve the fallopian tubes and tubo-ovarian region. The non-gonococcal bacterial infections that follow induced abortion, dilation and curettage of the uterus, and other surgical procedures are thought to spread upwards from the uterus through the lymphatics or venous channels rather than on the mucosal

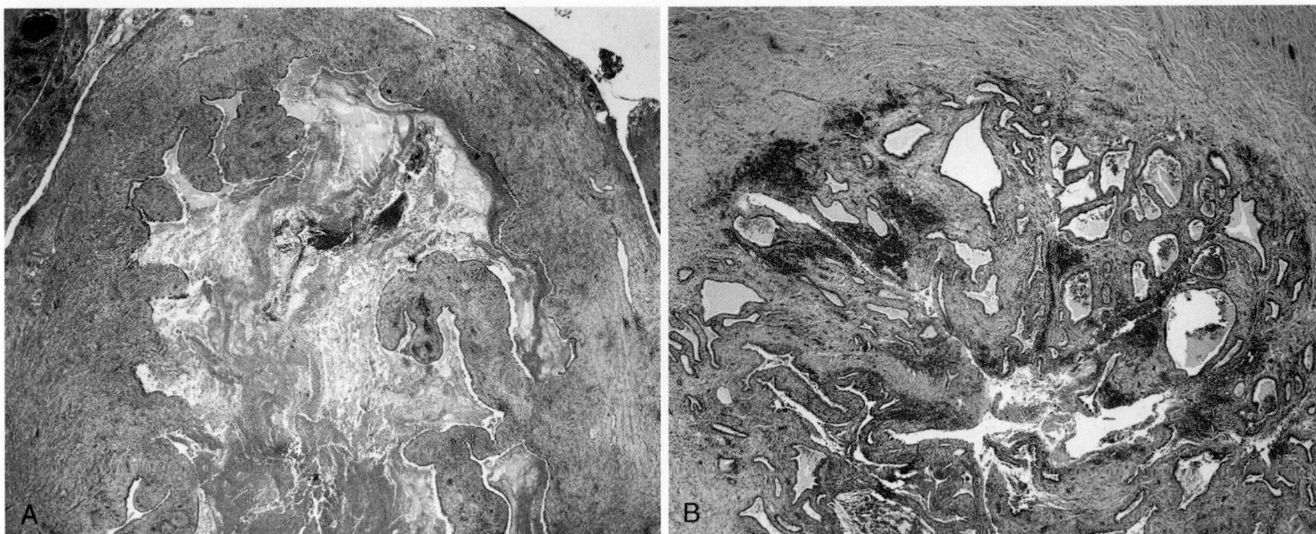

Figure 22-4 Acute salpingitis. **A,** Note the dilated tube lumen and edematous tubal plicae expanded by inflammatory cell infiltrates. Pus fills the center of the fallopian tube. **B,** Chronic salpingitis showing scarring and fusion of the plicae. Such scarring may cause infertility or ectopic tubal pregnancy.

surfaces. Therefore, these infections tend to produce more inflammation within the deeper layers of the organs than gonococcal infections.

MORPHOLOGY

Gonococcal infection is characterized by marked acute inflammation of involved mucosal surfaces. Smears of the inflammatory exudate disclose phagocytosed gram-negative diplococci within neutrophils; however, definitive diagnosis requires culture or detection of gonococcal RNA or DNA. If infection spreads, the endometrium is usually spared (for unclear reasons), but within the fallopian tubes, an **acute suppurative salpingitis** ensues (Fig. 22-4*A*). The tubal mucosa becomes congested and diffusely infiltrated by neutrophils, plasma cells, and lymphocytes, resulting in epithelial injury and sloughing of the plicae. The tubal lumen fills with purulent exudate that may leak out of the fimbriated end. The infection may then spread to the ovary to create a **salpingo-oophoritis**. Collections of pus may accumulate within the ovary and tube **(tubo-ovarian abscesses)** or tubal lumen **(pyosalpinx) (Fig. 22-4*A*)**. With time the infecting organisms may disappear, but the tubal plicae, denuded of epithelium, adhere to one another and slowly fuse in a reparative, scarring process that forms glandlike spaces and blind pouches, referred to as **chronic salpingitis (Fig. 22-4*B*)**. The scarring of the tubal lumen and fimbriae may prevent the uptake and passage of oocytes, leading to infertility or ectopic pregnancy. **Hydrosalpinx** may also develop as a consequence of the fusion of the fimbriae and the subsequent accumulation of the tubal secretions and tubal distention.

As compared to gonococcal infections, PID caused by staphylococci, streptococci, and the other puerperal invaders tends to show less involvement of the mucosa and the tube lumen, and more inflammation within the deeper tissue layers. These infections often spread throughout the wall to involve the serosa and the broad ligaments, pelvic structures, and peritoneum. Bacteremia is a more frequent complication of streptococcal or staphylococcal PID than of gonococcal infections.

The acute complications of PID include peritonitis and bacteremia, which in turn may result in endocarditis, meningitis, and suppurative arthritis. The chronic sequelae of PID include infertility and tubal obstruction, ectopic pregnancy, pelvic pain, and intestinal obstruction due to adhesions between the bowel and pelvic organs.

In the early stages, gonococcal infections are readily controlled with antibiotics, although penicillin-resistant strains have regrettably emerged. Infections that become walled off in tubo-ovarian abscesses are difficult to eradicate with antibiotics, and it sometimes becomes necessary to remove the organs surgically. Postabortion and postpartum PIDs may also be amenable to treatment with antibiotics, but are far more difficult to control because of the broad spectrum of pathogens that may be involved.

VULVA

Diseases of the vulva in the aggregate constitute only a small fraction of gynecologic practice. Many inflammatory diseases that affect skin elsewhere on the body also occur on the vulva, such as psoriasis, eczema, and allergic dermatitis. Because it is constantly exposed to secretions and moisture, the vulva is more prone to superficial infections than skin elsewhere on the body. Nonspecific vulvitis is particularly likely to occur in the setting of immunosuppression. Most skin cysts (epidermal inclusion cysts) and skin tumors such as squamous cell carcinoma, basal cell carcinoma and melanoma can also occur in the vulva. Here we discuss relatively specific and common vulvar disorders, including Bartholin cyst, nonneoplastic epithelial disorders, benign exophytic lesions, and tumors of the vulva.

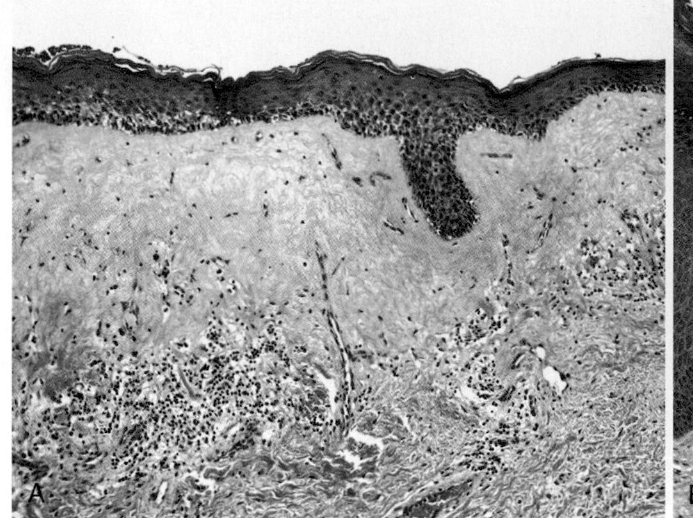

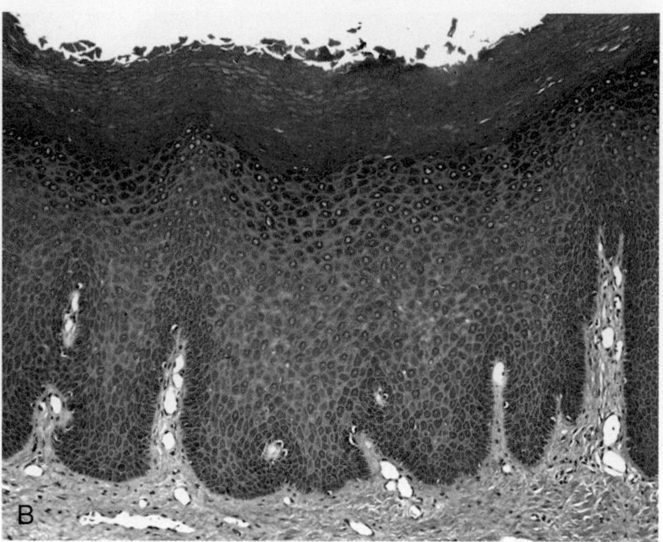

Figure 22-5 Nonneoplastic epithelial vulvar disorders. **A,** Lichen sclerosus. There is marked thinning of the epidermis, sclerosis of the superficial dermis and chronic inflammatory cells in deeper dermis. **B,** Squamous cell hyperplasia, displaying thickened epidermis and hyperkeratosis.

Bartholin Cyst

Infection of the Bartholin gland produces an acute inflammation (adenitis) and may result in an abscess. Bartholin duct cysts are relatively common, occur at all ages, and result from obstruction of the duct by an inflammatory process. These cysts are usually lined by transitional or squamous epithelium. They may become large, up to 3 to 5 cm in diameter, and produce pain and local discomfort. Bartholin duct cysts are either excised or opened permanently (marsupialization).

Nonneoplastic Epithelial Disorders

Leukoplakia is a descriptive clinical term for opaque, white, plaquelike epithelial thickening that may produce pruritus and scaling. Leukoplakia (literally, *white plaques*) may be caused by a variety of benign, premalignant, or malignant disorders, including:

- Inflammatory dermatoses (e.g., psoriasis, chronic dermatitis)
- Lichen sclerosus and squamous cell hyperplasia
- Neoplasias, such as vulvar intraepithelial neoplasia (VIN), Paget disease, and invasive carcinoma

Inflammatory dermatoses associated with leukoplakia are described in Chapter 25, while neoplastic disorders are discussed later in this chapter. Here the major nonneoplastic causes of leukoplakia—lichen sclerosis and squamous cell hyperplasia—are briefly discussed.

Lichen Sclerosus

Lichen sclerosis presents as smooth, white plaques or macules that in time may enlarge and coalesce, producing a surface that resembles porcelain or parchment. When the entire vulva is affected, the labia become atrophic and agglutinated, and the vaginal orifice constricts. Histologically the lesion is characterized by marked thinning of the epidermis (Fig. 22-5*A*); degeneration of the basal cells; excessive keratinization (hyperkeratosis); sclerotic changes of the superficial dermis; and a bandlike lymphocytic infiltrate in the underlying dermis. The disease occurs in all age groups but is most common in postmenopausal women. It may also be encountered elsewhere on the skin. Its pathogenesis is uncertain, but the presence of activated T cells in the subepithelial inflammatory infiltrate and the increased frequency of autoimmune disorders in affected women suggest that an autoimmune reaction is involved. Although lichen sclerosus is not itself a premalignant lesion, women with symptomatic lichen sclerosus have a slightly increased chance of developing squamous cell carcinoma of the vulva.

Squamous Cell Hyperplasia

Previously called hyperplastic dystrophy or *lichen simplex chronicus*, squamous cell hyperplasia is a nonspecific condition resulting from rubbing or scratching of the skin to relieve pruritus. Clinically it presents as leukoplakia and histologic examination reveals thickening of the epidermis (acanthosis), and hyperkeratosis (Fig. 22-5*B*). Lymphocytic infiltration of the dermis is sometimes present. The hyperplastic epithelium may show mitotic activity but lacks cellular atypia. While squamous cell hyperplasia is not considered premalignant, it is sometimes present at the margins of vulvar cancers.

Benign Exophytic Lesions

Benign raised (exophytic) or wartlike lesions of the vulva may be caused by infection or may be reactive conditions of unknown etiology. *Condyloma acuminatum*, a papillomavirus-induced lesion, also called a *genital wart*, and syphilitic *condyloma latum* (described in Chapter 21) are consequences of sexually transmitted infections. Vulvar

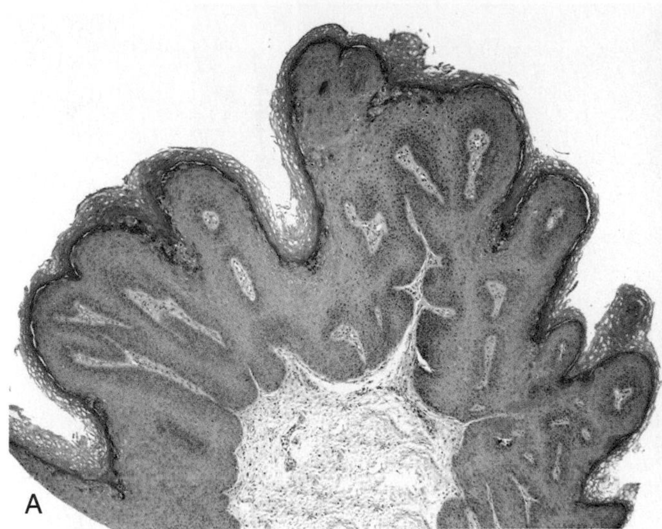

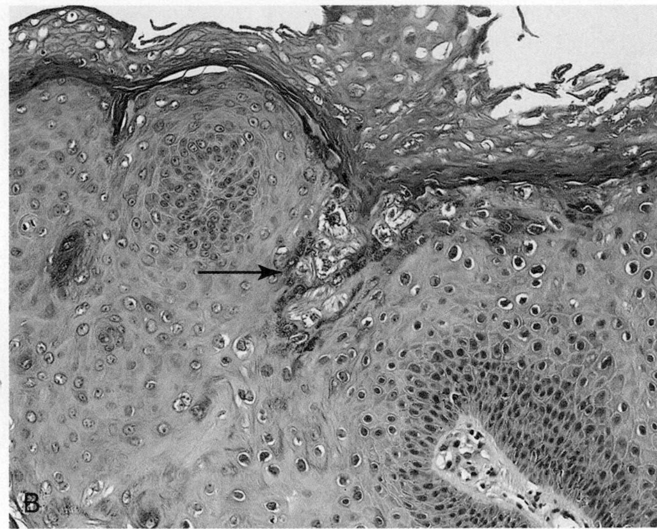

Figure 22-6 Condyloma acuminatum. **A,** Low-power view showing exophytic, papillary architecture. **B,** High-power view reveals HPV cytopathic effect (koilocytic atypia) characterized by atypical, enlarged, hyperchromatic nuclei with perinuclear halos *(arrow).*

fibroepithelial polyps, or skin tags, are similar to skin tags occurring elsewhere on the skin. Vulvar *squamous papillomas* are benign exophytic proliferations covered by nonkeratinized squamous epithelium, which develop on vulvar surfaces and may be single or numerous (vulvar papillomatosis). The etiology of fibroepithelial polyps and squamous papillomas is unknown.

Condyloma Acuminatum

Condylomata acuminata are benign genital warts caused by low oncogenic risk HPVs, mainly types 6 and 11. They may be solitary, but are more frequently multifocal, and may involve vulvar, perineal, and perianal regions as well as the vagina and, less commonly, the cervix. The lesions are identical to those found on the penis and around the anus in males (Chapter 21). On histologic examination, they consist of papillary, exophytic, treelike cores of stroma covered by thickened squamous epithelium (Fig. 22-6*A*). The surface epithelium shows characteristic viral cytopathic changes referred to as *koilocytic atypia* (Fig. 22-6*B*), which manifest as nuclear enlargement, hyperchromasia and a cytoplasmic perinuclear halo (see also "Cervix"). Condylomata acuminata are not precancerous lesions.

Squamous Neoplastic Lesions

Vulvar Intraepithelial Neoplasia and Vulvar Carcinoma

Carcinoma of the vulva is an uncommon malignant neoplasm (approximately one eighth as frequent as cervical cancer) representing about 3% of all genital cancers in the female; approximately two thirds occur in women older than 60 years. Squamous cell carcinoma is the most common histologic type of vulvar cancer. In terms of etiology, pathogenesis, and histologic features, vulvar squamous cell carcinomas are divided into two groups:

- Basaloid and warty carcinomas related to infection with high risk HPVs (30% of cases), most commonly HPV-16. These are less common and occur at younger ages.
- Keratinizing squamous cell carcinomas unrelated to HPV infection (70% of cases). These are more common and occur in older women.

Basaloid and warty carcinomas develop from an in situ precursor lesion called *classic vulvar intraepithelial neoplasia* (VIN). This form of VIN occurs mainly in reproductive age women and includes lesions designated formerly as carcinoma in situ or Bowen disease. The risk factors for VIN are the same as those associated with cervical squamous intraepithelial lesions (e.g., young age at first intercourse, multiple sexual partners, male partner with multiple sexual partners), as both are related to HPV infection. VIN is frequently multicentric, and 10% to 30% of patients with VIN also have vaginal or cervical HPV-related lesions. Spontaneous regression of classic VIN has been reported, usually in younger women. The risk of progression to invasive carcinoma is higher in women older than 45 years of age or in women who are immunosuppressed. The peak age for basaloid and warty vulvar cancer is in the sixth decade.

Keratinizing squamous cell carcinoma occurs most often in individuals with long-standing lichen sclerosus or squamous cell hyperplasia and is not related to HPV. The peak occurrence is in the eighth decade. It arises from a precursor lesion referred to as *differentiated vulvar intraepithelial neoplasia* (differentiated VIN) or *VIN simplex*. It is postulated that chronic epithelial irritation in lichen sclerosus or squamous cell hyperplasia may contribute to a gradual evolution to the malignant phenotype, presumably through acquisition of driver mutations in oncogenes and tumor suppressors. In line with this idea, some investigators have reported a high frequency of *TP53* mutations in differentiated VIN.

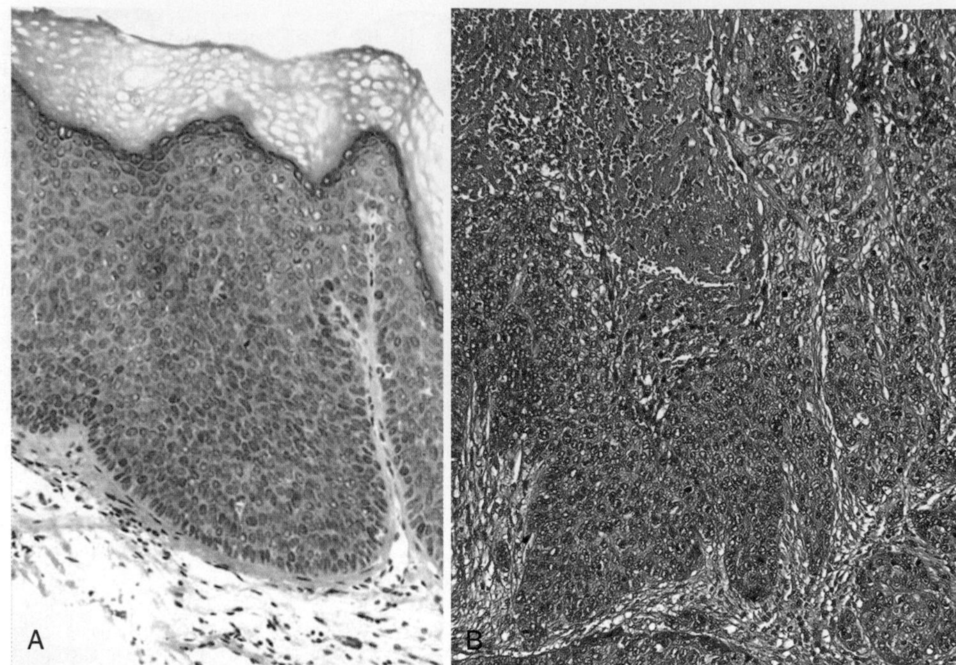

Figure 22-7 Variants of vulvar intraepithelial neoplasia. **A,** Classic vulvar intraepithelial neoplasia (HPV positive), showing nuclear enlargement, hyperchromasia, and small immature basaloid cells extending up to the epithelial surface. **B,** Basaloid vulvar carcinoma (HPV positive), composed of small, immature (basaloid) cells. This invasive tumor has an area of central necrosis.

MORPHOLOGY

Classic VIN presents either as a discrete white (hyperkeratotic) or a slightly raised, pigmented lesion. Microscopically, it is characterized by epidermal thickening, nuclear atypia, increased mitoses, and lack of cellular maturation (Fig. 22-7*A*), features analogous to those seen in cervical squamous intraepithelial lesions (SILs, see under "Cervix"). Invasive carcinomas that arise from classic VIN may be exophytic or indurated with central ulceration. On histologic examination, basaloid carcinoma (Fig. 22-7*B*) consists of nests and cords of small, tightly packed cells that lack maturation and resemble the basal layer of the normal epithelium. The tumor may have foci of central necrosis. By contrast, warty carcinoma is characterized by exophytic, papillary architecture and prominent koilocytic atypia.

Differentiated VIN is characterized by marked atypia of the basal layer of the squamous epithelium and normal-appearing differentiation of the more superficial layers (Fig. 22-8*A*). Invasive keratinzing squamous cell carcinomas that arise in differentiated VIN contain nests and tongues of malignant squamous epithelium with prominent central keratin pearls (Fig. 22-8*B*).

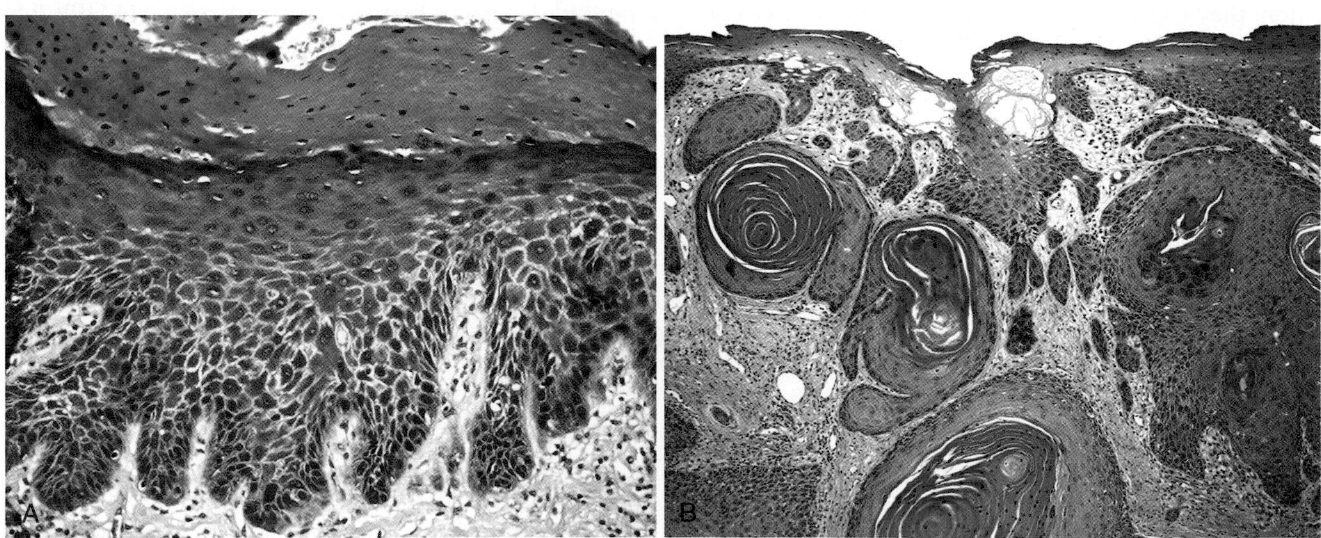

Figure 22-8 A, Differentiated vulvar intraepithelial neoplasia (HPV negative), showing maturation of the superficial layers, hyperkeratosis, and basal cell atypia. This is in-situ lesion; no invasion is present. **B,** Well-differentiated, keratinizing squamous cell carcinoma of the vulva (HPV negative).

The risk of cancer development in VIN depends on duration and extent of disease, and the immune status of the patient. Invasive carcinomas associated with lichen sclerosus, squamous cell hyperplasia, and differentiated VIN may develop in an insidious fashion and may be misinterpreted as dermatitis or leukoplakia for long periods. Once invasive cancer develops, the risk of metastatic spread is linked to the size of tumor, depth of invasion, and involvement of lymphatic vessels. The initial spread is to inguinal, pelvic, iliac, and periaortic lymph nodes. Ultimately, lymphohematogenous dissemination to the lungs, liver, and other internal organs may occur. Patients with lesions less than 2 cm in diameter have a 90% 5-year survival after treatment with vulvectomy and lymphadenectomy; however, larger lesions with lymph node involvement have poor prognosis.

Glandular Neoplastic Lesions

Like the breast, the vulva contains modified apocrine sweat glands. Presumably because of these "breastlike" features, the vulva may be involved by two tumors with counterparts in the breast, namely papillary hidradenoma and extramammary Paget disease.

Papillary Hidradenoma

Papillary hidradenoma presents as a sharply circumscribed nodule, most commonly on the labia majora or interlabial folds, and may be confused clinically with carcinoma because of its tendency to ulcerate. *Its histologic appearance is identical to that of intraductal papilloma of the breast* and consists of papillary projections covered with two layers of cells: an upper layer of columnar secretory cells covering a deeper layer of flattened myoepithelial cells. These myoepithelial elements are characteristic of sweat glands and sweat gland tumors (Fig. 22-9).

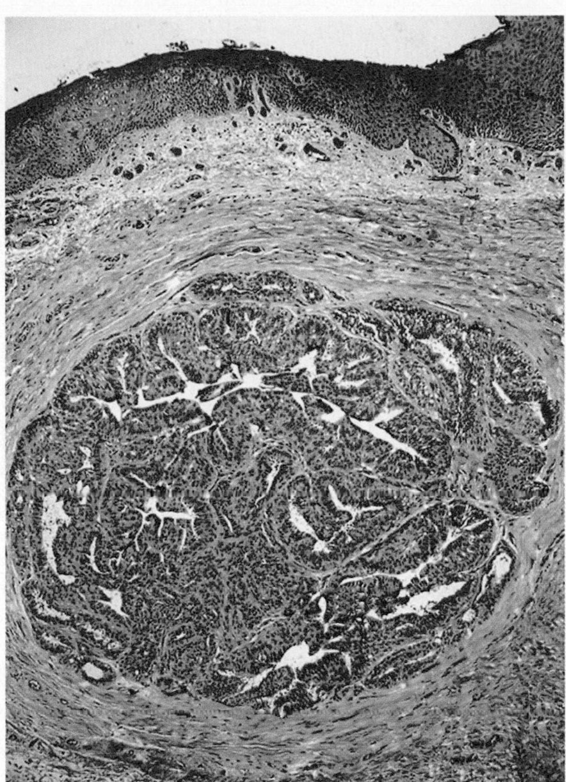

Figure 22-9 Papillary hidradenoma of the vulva, a well-circumscribed tumor composed of benign papillary projections covered with columnar secretory epithelium and underlying myoepithelial cells.

Extramammary Paget Disease

This curious and rare lesion of the vulva is *similar in its manifestations to Paget disease of the breast* (Chapter 23). In the vulva, it presents as a pruritic, red, crusted, maplike area, usually on the labia majora.

MORPHOLOGY

Paget disease is a distinctive intraepithelial proliferation of malignant cells. Paget cells are larger than surrounding keratinocytes and are seen singly or in small clusters within the epidermis (Fig. 22-10*A*). The cells have pale cytoplasm containing mucopolysaccharide that stains with periodic acid–Schiff (PAS), Alcian blue, or mucicarmine stains. In addition, the cells express cytokeratin 7 (Fig. 22-10*B*). Ultrastructurally, Paget cells display apocrine, eccrine, and keratinocyte differentiation and presumably arise from multipotent cells found within the mammary-like gland ducts of the vulvar skin.

In contrast to Paget disease of the nipple, in which 100% of patients have an underlying ductal breast carcinoma, vulvar Paget is typically not associated with underlying cancer and is confined to the epidermis of vulvar skin. The treatment consists of wide local excision. Paget cells spread laterally within the epidermis and may be present beyond the confines of the grossly visible lesion. As a result, the tumor cells may not be completely excised and the disease can recur. Intraepidermal Paget disease may persist for many years or even decades without invasion or metastases. In the rare instances when invasion develops, the prognosis is poor.

KEY CONCEPTS

- Approximately 30% of vulvar cancers are caused by infection with high risk HPVs, principally HPV-16. These cancers develop from an in situ lesion termed *classic vulvar intraepithelial neoplasia* (classic VIN).
- Most vulvar cancers (70%) are not related to HPV and develop in a background of lichen sclerosus or squamous cell hyperplasia from the premalignant lesion called *differentiated vulvar intraepithelial neoplasia* (differentiated VIN).

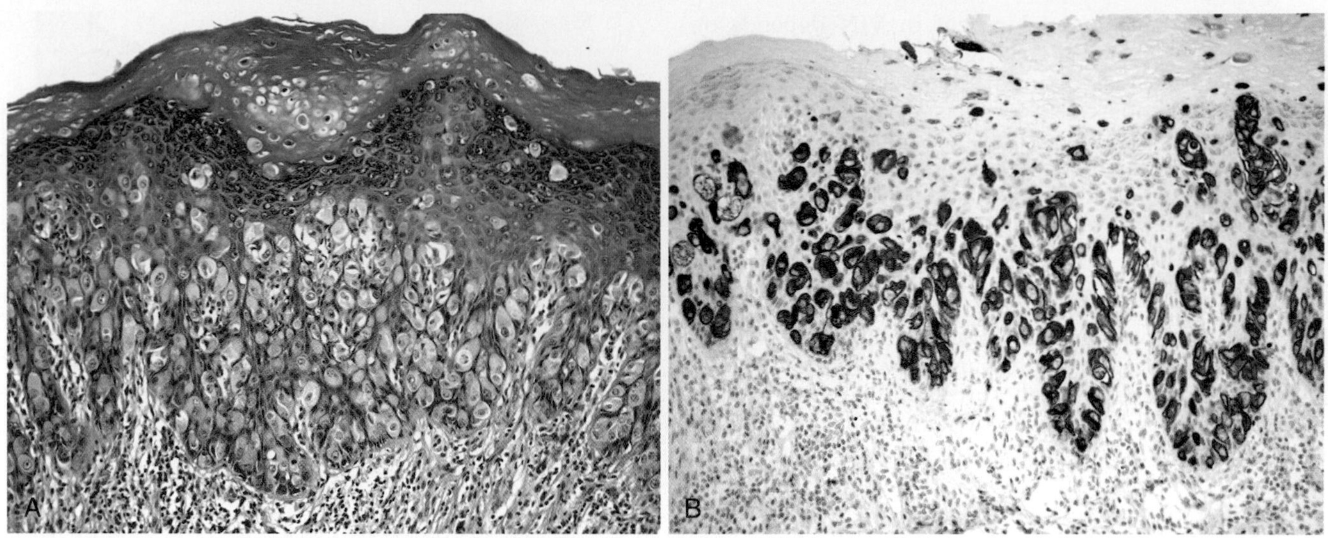

Figure 22-10 Paget disease of the vulva. **A,** The epidermis is infiltrated by large cells with pale-pink cytoplasm that are spreading along the basal portion of the squamous epithelium. There is inflammation in the underlying dermis. **B,** Immunostaining for cytokeratin 7 highlights the intraepidermal Paget cells.

VAGINA

The vagina is a portion of the female genital tract that is remarkably free from primary disease. In the adult, inflammation often affects the vulva and perivulvar structures and spreads to the cervix without significant involvement of the vagina. Primary lesions of the vagina are rare, the most serious being vaginal squamous cell carcinoma; they are discussed only briefly here.

Developmental Anomalies

Septate, or double, vagina is an uncommon anomaly that arises from a failure of müllerian duct fusion and is accompanied by a double uterus (uterus didelphys). These and other anomalies of the external genitalia may be the manifestations of genetic syndromes, in utero exposure to diethylstilbestrol (DES, used to prevent threatened abortions in the 1940s through 1960s), or other unknown factors that perturb reciprocal epithelial-stromal signaling during fetal development.

During embryonal development , the vagina is initially covered by columnar, endocervical-type epithelium. This is normally replaced by squamous epithelium advancing upwards from the urogenital sinus. Small patches of residual glandular epithelium may persist into adult life and is recognized as *vaginal adenosis*. It presents clinically as red, granular areas that stand out from the surrounding normal pale-pink vaginal mucosa. On microscopic examination, adenosis consists of columnar mucinous epithelium indistinguishable from endocervical epithelium. Adenosis is found in only a small percentage of adult women, but has been reported in 35% to 90% of women exposed to DES in utero. Rare cases of clear cell carcinoma arising in DES-related adenosis were recorded in teenagers and young adult women in the 1970s and 1980s, resulting in discontinuation of DES treatment.

Gartner duct cysts are relatively common lesions found along the lateral walls of the vagina and are derived from wolffian (mesonephric) duct rests. They are 1- to 2-cm fluid-filled cysts that occur in the submucosal location. Other cysts, including mucus cysts, which occur in the proximal vagina, are derived from müllerian epithelium. Another müllerian-derived lesion, endometriosis (described later), may occur in the vagina and clinically simulate a neoplasm.

Premalignant and Malignant Neoplasms of the Vagina

Most of the benign tumors of the vagina occur in reproductive-age women and include stromal tumors (stromal polyps), leiomyomas, and hemangiomas. The most common malignant tumor to involve the vagina is carcinoma spreading from the cervix, followed by primary squamous cell carcinoma of the vagina. Infants may develop a unique, rare malignancy—embryonal rhabdomyosarcoma (sarcoma botryoides).

Vaginal Intraepithelial Neoplasia and Squamous Cell Carcinoma

Virtually all primary carcinomas of the vagina are squamous cell carcinomas associated with high risk HPVs. It is an extremely uncommon cancer (about 0.6 per 100,000 women yearly) that accounts for about 1% of malignant neoplasms in the female genital tract. The greatest risk factor is a previous carcinoma of the cervix or vulva; 1% to 2% of women with an invasive cervical carcinoma eventually develop a vaginal squamous cell carcinoma. Squamous cell carcinoma of the vagina arises from a premalignant lesion, *vaginal intraepithelial neoplasia*, analogous to cervical squamous intraepithelial lesions (SILs, see under "Cervix"). Most often the invasive tumor affects the upper vagina, particularly the posterior wall at the junction with the ectocervix. The lesions in the lower two thirds of the vagina metastasize to the inguinal nodes, whereas lesions in the upper vagina tend to spread to regional iliac nodes.

Embryonal Rhabdomyosarcoma

Also called *sarcoma botryoides,* this uncommon vaginal tumor composed of malignant embryonal rhabdomyoblasts is most frequently found in infants and in children younger than 5 years of age. These tumors tend to grow as polypoid, rounded, bulky masses that have the appearance and consistency of grapelike clusters (hence the designation *botryoides,* or grapelike) (Fig. 22-11). The tumor cells are small and have oval nuclei, with small protrusions of cytoplasm from one end, resembling a tennis racket. Rarely, striations (indicative of muscle differentiation) can be seen within the cytoplasm. Beneath the vaginal epithelium, the tumor cells are crowded in a so-called cambium layer, but in the deep regions they lie within a loose fibromyxomatous stroma that is edematous and may contain many inflammatory cells. Such lesions can be mistaken for benign inflammatory polyps. The tumors tend to invade locally and cause death by penetration into the peritoneal cavity or by obstruction of the urinary tract. Conservative surgery coupled with chemotherapy offer the best hope, particularly in cases diagnosed sufficiently early.

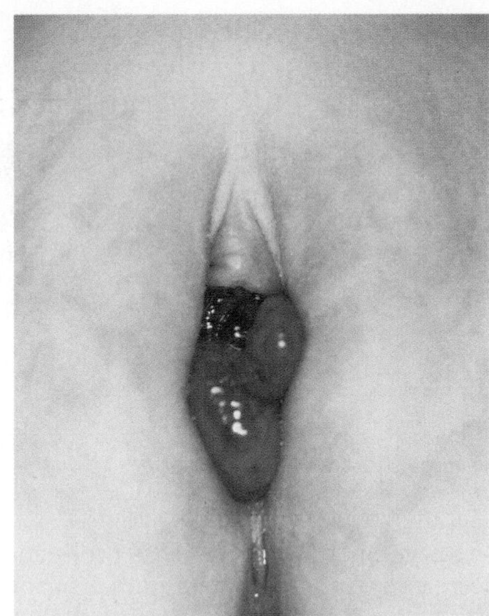

Figure 22-11 Sarcoma botryoides (embryonal rhabdomyosarcoma) of the vagina appearing as a polypoid mass protruding from the vagina. (Courtesy Dr. Michael Donovan, Children's Hospital, Boston, Mass.)

CERVIX

Anatomically the cervix consists of the external vaginal portio (ectocervix) and the endocervical canal. The ectocervix is visible on vaginal examination and is covered by a mature squamous epithelium that is continuous with the vaginal wall. The squamous epithelium converges centrally at a small opening termed the *external os* that leads to the endocervical canal. The endocervix is lined by columnar, mucus-secreting epithelium. The point where the squamous and columnar epithelium meet is referred to as the *squamocolumnar junction* (Fig. 22-12). The position of the junction is variable and changes with age and hormonal influence, but in general the junction moves upwards into the endocervical canal with time. The replacement of the glandular epithelium by advancing squamous epithelium is a process called squamous metaplasia. The area of the cervix where the columnar epithelium abuts the squamous epithelium is termed the "*transformation zone*." The unique epithelial environment of the cervix renders it highly susceptible to infections with HPV, the main cause of cervical cancer. Immature squamous metaplastic epithelial cells in the transformation zone are most susceptible to HPV infection, and as a result this is where cervical precursor lesions and cancers develop.

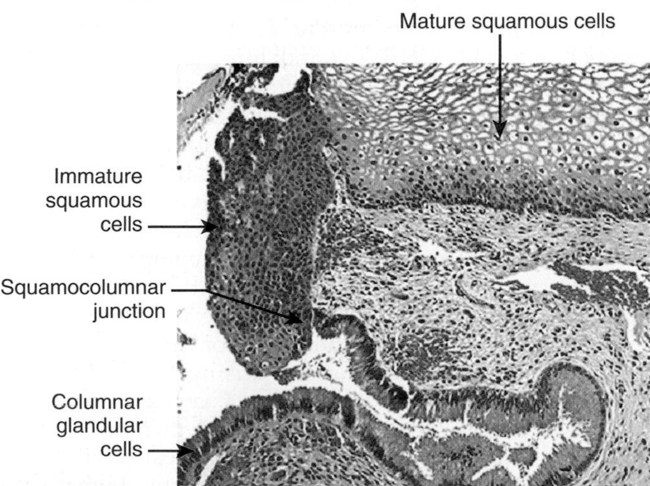

Figure 22-12 Cervical squamocolumnar junction showing mature, glycogenized squamous epithelium, immature squamous metaplastic cells, and columnar endocervical glandular epithelium.

Inflammations

Acute and Chronic Cervicitis

At the onset of menarche, the production of estrogens by the ovary stimulates maturation of the cervical and vaginal squamous mucosa and formation of intracellular glycogen vacuoles in the squamous cells. As these cells are shed, the glycogen provides a substrate for various endogenous vaginal aerobes and anaerobes, but particularly lactobacilli, which are the dominant microbial species in the normal vagina. Lactobacilli produce lactic acid, which maintains the vaginal pH below 4.5, suppressing the growth of other saprophytic and pathogenic organisms. In addition, at low pH, lactobacilli produce bacteriotoxic hydrogen peroxide (H_2O_2). If the pH becomes alkaline due to bleeding, sexual

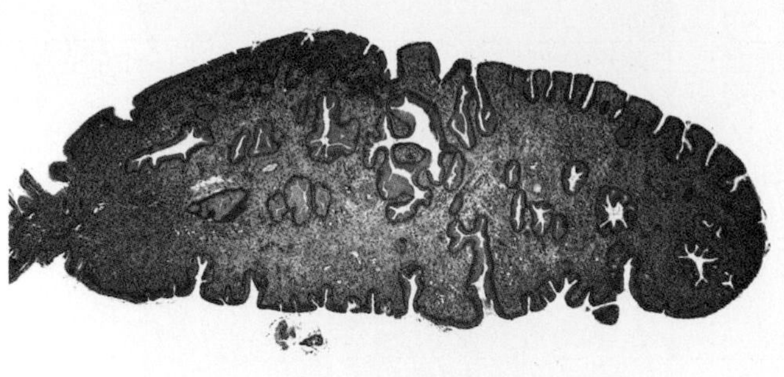

Figure 22-13 Endocervical polyp composed of a dense fibrous stroma covered with endocervical columnar epithelium.

intercourse, or vaginal douching, H_2O_2 production by lactobacilli decreases. Antibiotic therapy that suppress lactobacilli can also cause the pH to rise. In each of these settings the altered vaginal environment promotes the overgrowth of other microorganisms, which may result in cervicitis or vaginitis. Some degree of cervical inflammation may be found in virtually all women, and it is usually of little clinical consequence. However, *infections by gonococci, chlamydiae, mycoplasmas, and HSV may produce significant acute or chronic cervicitis* and are important to identify due to their association with upper genital tract disease, complications during pregnancy, and sexual transmission. Marked cervical inflammation produces reparative and reactive changes of the epithelium and shedding of atypical-appearing squamous cells, and therefore may cause an abnormal Pap test result.

Endocervical Polyps

Endocervical polyps are common benign exophytic growths that arise within the endocervical canal. They vary from small, sessile "bumps" to large polypoid masses that may protrude through the cervical os. Histologically, they are composed of a loose fibromyxomatous stroma covered by mucus-secreting endocervical glands, often accompanied by inflammation (Fig. 22-13). Their main significance is that they may be the source of irregular vaginal "spotting" or bleeding that arouses suspicion of some more ominous lesion. Simple curettage or surgical excision is curative.

Premalignant and Malignant Neoplasms of the Cervix

Worldwide, cervical carcinoma is the third most common cancer in women, with an estimated 530,000 new cases in 2008, of which more than half are fatal. In the United States, 12,410 women were diagnosed with cervical cancer and 4000 women died of the disease in 2008. Fifty years ago, carcinoma of the cervix was the leading cause of cancer deaths in women in the United States, but the death rate has declined by two thirds to its present rank as the thirteenth cause of cancer mortality. No form of cancer better documents the remarkable benefits of effective screening, early diagnosis, and curative therapy than does cancer of the cervix. Much credit for these dramatic gains belongs to the effectiveness of the Pap test in detecting cervical precursor lesions, some of which would have progressed to cancer if not treated; in addition, the Pap test can also detect low-stage, highly curable cancers. The accessibility of the cervix to Pap testing and visual exam (colposcopy) as well as the slow progression from precursor lesions to invasive carcinoma (typically over the course of years) provides ample time for screening, detection, and preventive treatment.

Pathogenesis. **High-risk HPVs are by far the most important factor in the development of cervical cancer.** HPVs are DNA viruses that are typed based on their DNA sequence and grouped into those of high and low oncogenic risk. There are 15 high risk HPVs that are currently identified, but HPV-16 alone accounts for almost 60% of cervical cancer cases, and HPV-18 accounts for another 10% of cases; other HPV types contribute to less than 5% of cases, individually. *High risk HPVs are also implicated in squamous cell carcinomas arising at many other sites, including the vagina, vulva, penis, anus, tonsil, and other oropharyngeal locations* (Chapter 16). As noted earlier, low oncogenic risk HPVs are the cause of the sexually transmitted vulvar, perineal, and perianal warts (condyloma acuminatum).

Genital HPV infections are extremely common; most of them are asymptomatic, do not cause any tissue changes, and therefore are not detected on Pap test. The prevalence of HPV in cervical smears in women with normal Pap test results peaks between the ages of 20 and 24 years, a relationship that is related to the onset of sexual activity, while the subsequent decrease in prevalence reflects acquisition of immunity and entry into monogamous relationships with age. Most HPV infections are transient and are eliminated by the immune response in the course of months. *On average, 50% of HPV infections are cleared within 8 months, and 90% of infections are cleared within 2 years.* The duration of the infection is related to HPV type; on average, infections with high-risk HPVs last longer than infections with low oncogenic risk HPVs (13 months versus 8 months, respectively). Persistent infection increases the risk of the development of cervical precursor lesions and subsequent carcinoma.

HPVs infect immature basal cells of the squamous epithelium in areas of epithelial breaks, or immature metaplastic squamous cells present at the squamocolumnar junction (Fig. 22-11). HPVs cannot infect the mature superficial squamous cells that cover the ectocervix, vagina, or vulva. Establishment of HPV infection in these sites requires damage to the surface epithelium, which allows the virus access to the immature cells in the basal layer of the epithelium. The cervix, with its relatively large areas of immature squamous metaplastic epithelium, is particularly vulnerable to HPV infection as compared to, for example, vulvar skin and mucosa that are covered by mature squamous cells. This difference in epithelial susceptibility to HPV infection accounts for the wide range in incidence of HPV-related cancers arising in various sites, and explains the high frequency of cervical cancer in women and anal cancer in homosexual men and a relatively low frequency of vulvar and penile cancer.

The ability of HPV to act as a carcinogen depends on the viral proteins E6 and E7, which interfere with the activity of tumor suppressor proteins that regulate cell growth and survival. Although HPV infects immature squamous cells, viral replication occurs in maturing squamous cells. Normally, these more mature cells are arrested in the G_1 phase of the cell cycle, but they continue to actively progress through the cell cycle when infected with HPV, which uses the host cell DNA synthesis machinery to replicate its own genome. As you will recall from Chapter 7, viral E7 protein binds the hypophosphorylated (active) form of RB and promotes its degradation via the proteasome pathway, and also binds and inhibits p21 and p27, two important cyclin-dependent kinase inhibitors. Removal of these controls not only enhances cell cycle progression, but also impairs the ability of cells to repair DNA damage. This defect in DNA repair is exacerbated by the viral E6 proteins of high-risk HPV subtypes, which bind to the tumor suppressor protein p53 and promote its degradation by the proteasome. In addition, E6 up-regulates the expression of telomerase, which leads to cellular immortalization. The net effect is increased proliferation of cells that are prone to acquire additional mutations that may lead to cancer development. By contrast to high-risk HPVs, the E7 proteins of low risk HPVs bind RB with lower affinity, while the E6 proteins of low-risk HPVs fail to bind p53 altogether and instead appear to dysregulate growth and survival by interfering with the Notch signaling pathway.

Another factor that contributes to malignant transformation by HPV is the physical state of the virus. The viral DNA is integrated into the host cell genome in most cancers. This configuration increases the expression of E6 and E7 genes, and may also dysregulate oncogenes near the sites of viral insertion, such as *MYC*. By contrast, viral DNA is extrachromosomal (episomal) in precursor lesions associated with high risk HPVs and in condylomata associated with low risk HPVs.

Even though HPV has been firmly established as a common cause of cervical cancer, it is not sufficient to cause cancer. This conclusion is supported by the fact that a high percentage of young women are infected with one or more HPV types during their reproductive years, but only a few develop cancer. Thus, other factors, such as exposure to co-carcinogens and host immune status, influence whether an HPV infection regresses or persists and eventually progresses to cancer.

Cervical Intraepithelial Neoplasia (Squamous Intraepithelial Lesions)

The classification of cervical precursor lesions has evolved over time and the terms from the different classification systems are currently used interchangeably. Hence a brief review of the terminology is warranted. The oldest classification system grouped lesions as having mild dysplasia on one end and severe dysplasia/carcinoma in situ on the other. This was followed by the *cervical intraepithelial neoplasia* (CIN) classification, with mild dysplasia termed *CIN I*, moderate dysplasia *CIN II*, and severe dysplasia termed *CIN III*. Because the decision with regard to patient management is two-tiered (observation versus surgical treatment), the three-tier classification system has been recently simplified to a two-tiered system, with CIN I renamed low-grade squamous intraepithelial lesion (LSIL) and CIN II and CIN III combined into one category referred to as high-grade squamous intraepithelial lesion (HSIL) (Table 22-1).

Table 22-1 Classification Systems for Squamous Cervical Precursor Lesions

Dysplasia/Carcinoma in Situ	Cervical Intraepithelial Neoplasia (CIN)	Squamous Intraepithelial Lesion (SIL), Current Classification
Mild dysplasia	CIN I	Low-grade SIL (LSIL)
Moderate dysplasia	CIN II	High-grade SIL (HSIL)
Severe dysplasia	CIN III	High-grade SIL (HSIL)
Carcinoma in situ	CIN III	High-grade SIL (HSIL)

CIN, Cervical intraepithelial neoplasia; SIL, squamous intraepithelial lesion.

LSIL is associated with a productive HPV infection. In LSIL, there is a high level of viral replication and only mild alterations in the growth of host cells. *LSIL does not progress directly to invasive carcinoma and in fact most cases regress spontaneously; only a small percentage progress to HSIL*. For these reasons, LSIL is not treated like a premalignant lesion. In HSIL, on the other hand, there is a progressive deregulation of the cell cycle by HPV, which results in increased cellular proliferation, decreased or arrested epithelial maturation, and a lower rate of viral replication, as compared with LSIL. Derangement of the cell cycle in HSIL may become irreversible and lead to a fully transformed malignant phenotype, and thus *all HSILS are considered to be at high risk for progression to carcinoma*. LSILs are ten times more common than HSILs.

MORPHOLOGY

The diagnosis of SIL is based on identification of nuclear atypia characterized by nuclear enlargement, hyperchromasia (dark staining), coarse chromatin granules, and variation in nuclear size and shape (Fig. 22-14). The nuclear changes are often accompanied by cytoplasmic "halos." At an ultrastructural level, these "halos" consist of perinuclear vacuoles, a cytopathic change created in part by an HPV-encoded protein called E5 that localizes to the membranes of the endoplasmic reticulum. Nuclear alterations with an associated perinuclear halo are termed **koilocytic atypia**. The grading of SIL into low or high grade is based on expansion of the immature cell layer from its normal, basal location. If the immature squamous cells are confined to the lower one third of the epithelium, the lesion is graded as LSIL; if they expand to the upper two thirds of the epithelial thickness, it is graded as HSIL.

The histologic features of LSIL correlate with HPV replication and changes in host cell growth and gene expression (Fig. 22-15).

- The highest viral loads (assessed by HPV DNA in situ hybridization, Fig. 22-15*B*) are found in maturing keratinocytes in the upper half of the epithelium.
- HPV E6 and E7 proteins prevent cell cycle arrest. As a result, cells in the upper portion of the epithelium express markers of actively dividing cells, such as Ki-67 (Fig. 22-15*C*), that are normally are confined to the basal layer of the epithelium. Disturbed growth regulation also leads to overexpression of p16, a cyclin-dependent kinase inhibitor (Fig. 22-15*D*).
- Both Ki-67 and p16 staining are highly correlated with HPV infection and are useful for confirmation of the diagnosis in equivocal cases of SIL.

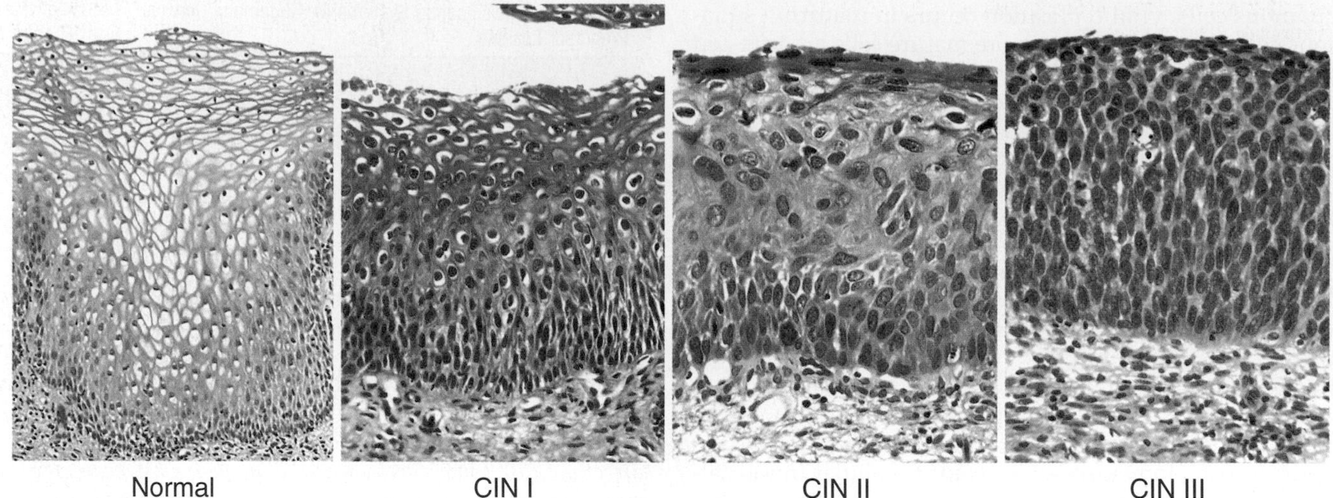

Figure 22-14 Spectrum of cervical intraepithelial neoplasia: normal squamous epithelium for comparison; LSIL (CIN I) with koilocytic atypia; HSIL (CIN II) with progressive atypia and expansion of the immature basal cells above the lower third of the epithelial thickness; HSIL (CIN III) with diffuse atypia, loss of maturation, and expansion of the immature basal cells to the epithelial surface.

More than 80% of LSILs and 100% of HSILs are associated with high-risk HPVs, with HPV-16 being the most common HPV type in both categories of lesions. Table 22-2 shows rates of regression and progression of SILs within 2-year follow-up. Although the majority of HSILs develop from LSILs, approximately 20% of cases of HSIL develop de novo, independent of any preexisting LSIL. The rates of progression are by no means uniform, and although HPV type—especially HPV 16—is associated with increased risk, it is difficult to predict the outcome in an individual patient. These findings underscore that the risk of developing precursor lesions and cancer is conferred only in part by HPV type. Progression to invasive carcinoma, when it occurs, takes place over a period of a few years to more than a decade.

Cervical Carcinoma

The average age of patients with invasive cervical carcinoma is 45 years. Squamous cell carcinoma is the most common histologic subtype, accounting for approximately 80% of cases. The second most common tumor type is adenocarcinoma, which constitutes about 15% of cervical cancer cases and develops from a precursor lesion called *adenocarcinoma in situ.* Adenosquamous and neuroendocrine carcinomas are rare cervical tumors that account for the remaining 5% of cases. All of the aforementioned tumor types are caused by high-risk HPVs. The progression time from in situ to invasive adenosquamous and neuroendocrine carcinomas is shorter than in squamous cell carcinoma, and patients with these tumors often

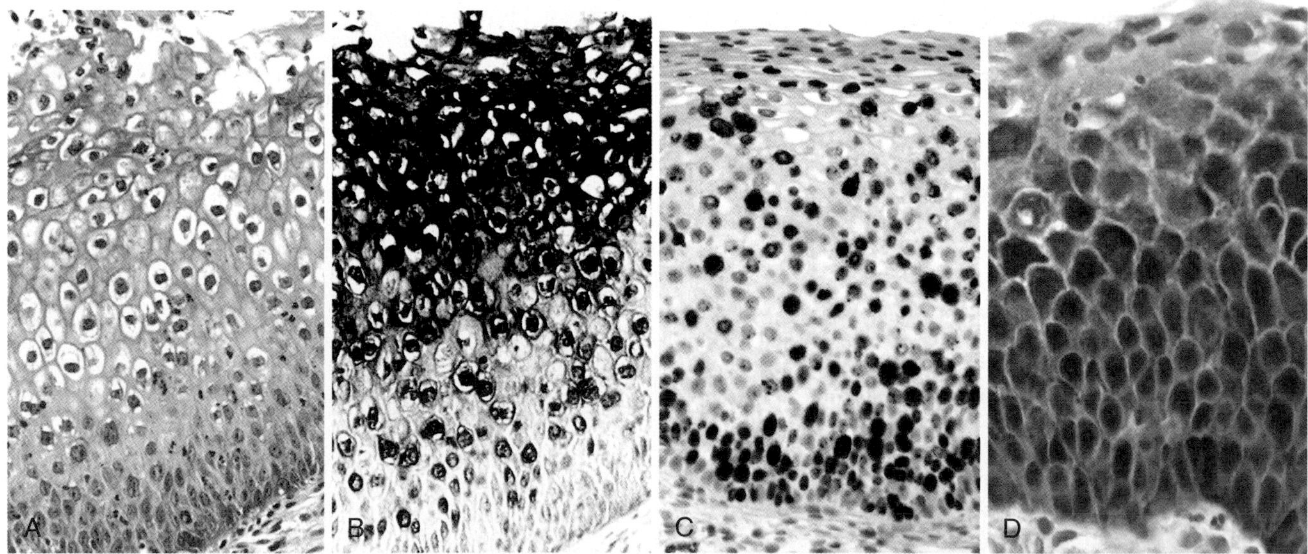

Figure 22-15 **A,** Low-grade squamous intraepithelial lesion (LSIL)—Routine hematoxylin and eosin staining shows marked koilocytic change, seen as perinuclear "halos" in suprabasilar cells. **B,** In situ hybridization test for HPV DNA. The dark granular staining denotes HPV DNA, which is typically most abundant in the koilocytes. **C,** Diffuse positivity for the proliferation marker Ki-67 (seen as brown nuclear staining), illustrates abnormal expansion of the proliferating cells from the normal basal location to the superficial layers of the epithelium. **D,** Upregulation of the cyclin-dependent kinase inhibitor p16 (seen here as brown staining) characterizes high-risk HPV infections.

Table 22-2 Natural History of Squamous Intraepithelial Lesions with Approximate 2-Year Follow-up

Lesion	Regress	Persist	Progress
LSIL	60%	30%	10% to HSIL
HSIL	30%	60%	10% to carcinoma*

HSIL, High-grade squamous intraepithelial lesion; LSIL, low-grade squamous intraepithelial lesion.
*Progression within 2 to 10 years.

present with advanced disease and have a less favorable prognosis.

MORPHOLOGY

Invasive cervical carcinoma may manifest as either fungating (exophytic) or infiltrative masses. **Squamous cell carcinoma** is composed of nests and tongues of malignant squamous epithelium, either keratinizing or nonkeratinizing, which invade the underlying cervical stroma (Fig. 22-16*A,B*). **Adenocarcinoma** is characterized by proliferation of glandular epithelium composed of malignant endocervical cells with large, hyperchromatic nuclei and relatively mucin-depleted cytoplasm, resulting in a dark appearance of the glands, as compared to the normal endocervical epithelium (Fig. 22-17*A,B*). Adenosquamous carcinoma is composed of intermixed malignant glandular and squamous epithelium. Neuroendocrine cervical carcinoma has an appearance similar to small cell carcinoma of the lung (Chapter 15), but differs in being positive for high risk HPVs.

Advanced cervical carcinoma spreads by direct extension to contiguous tissues, including paracervical soft tissue, urinary bladder, ureters (resulting in hydronephrosis), rectum, and vagina. Lymphvascular invasion results in local and distant lymph nodes metastases. Distant metastases may also be found in the liver, lungs, bone marrow, and other organs.

Cervical cancer is staged as follows:

Stage 0—Carcinoma in situ (CIN III, HSIL)

Stage I—Carcinoma confined to the cervix

Ia—Preclinical carcinoma, that is, diagnosed only by microscopy

Ia1—Stromal invasion no deeper than 3 mm and no wider than 7 mm (so-called microinvasive carcinoma)

Ia2—Maximum depth of invasion of stroma deeper than 3 mm and no deeper than 5 mm taken from base of epithelium; horizontal invasion not more than 7 mm

Ib—Histologically invasive carcinoma confined to the cervix and greater than stage Ia2

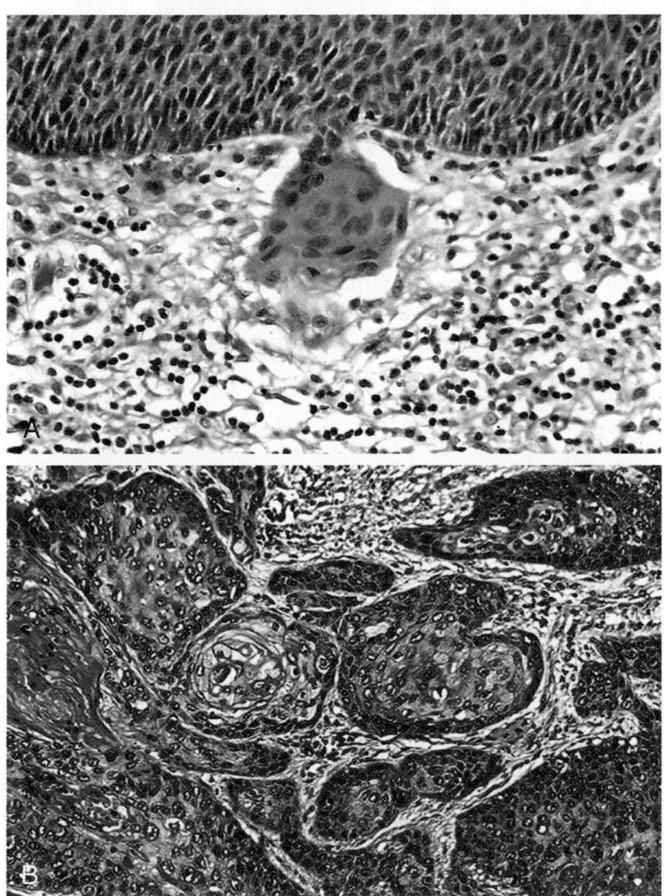

Figure 22-16 Squamous cell carcinoma of the cervix. **A,** Microinvasive squamous cell carcinoma with invasive nest breaking through the basement membrane of high-grade squamous intraepithelial lesion. **B,** Invasive squamous cell carcinoma.

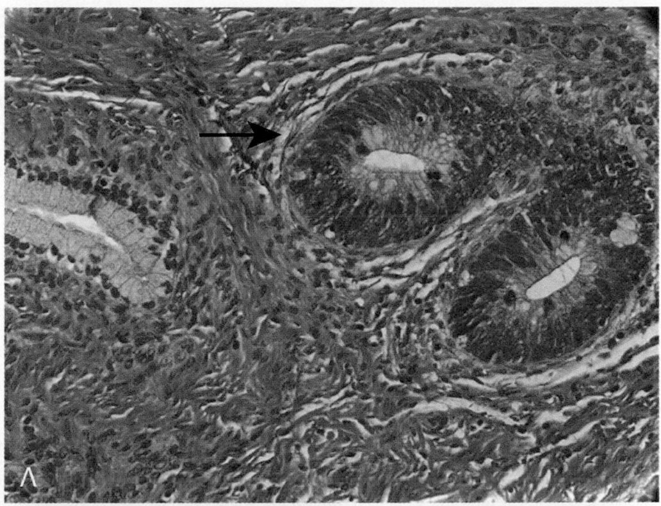

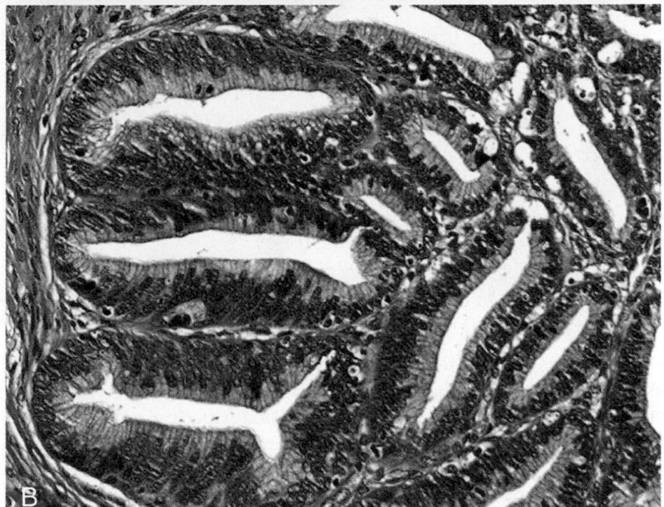

Figure 22-17 Adenocarcinoma of the cervix. **A,** Adenocarcinoma in situ *(arrow)* showing dark glands adjacent to normal pale endocervical glands. **B,** Invasive adenocarcinoma.

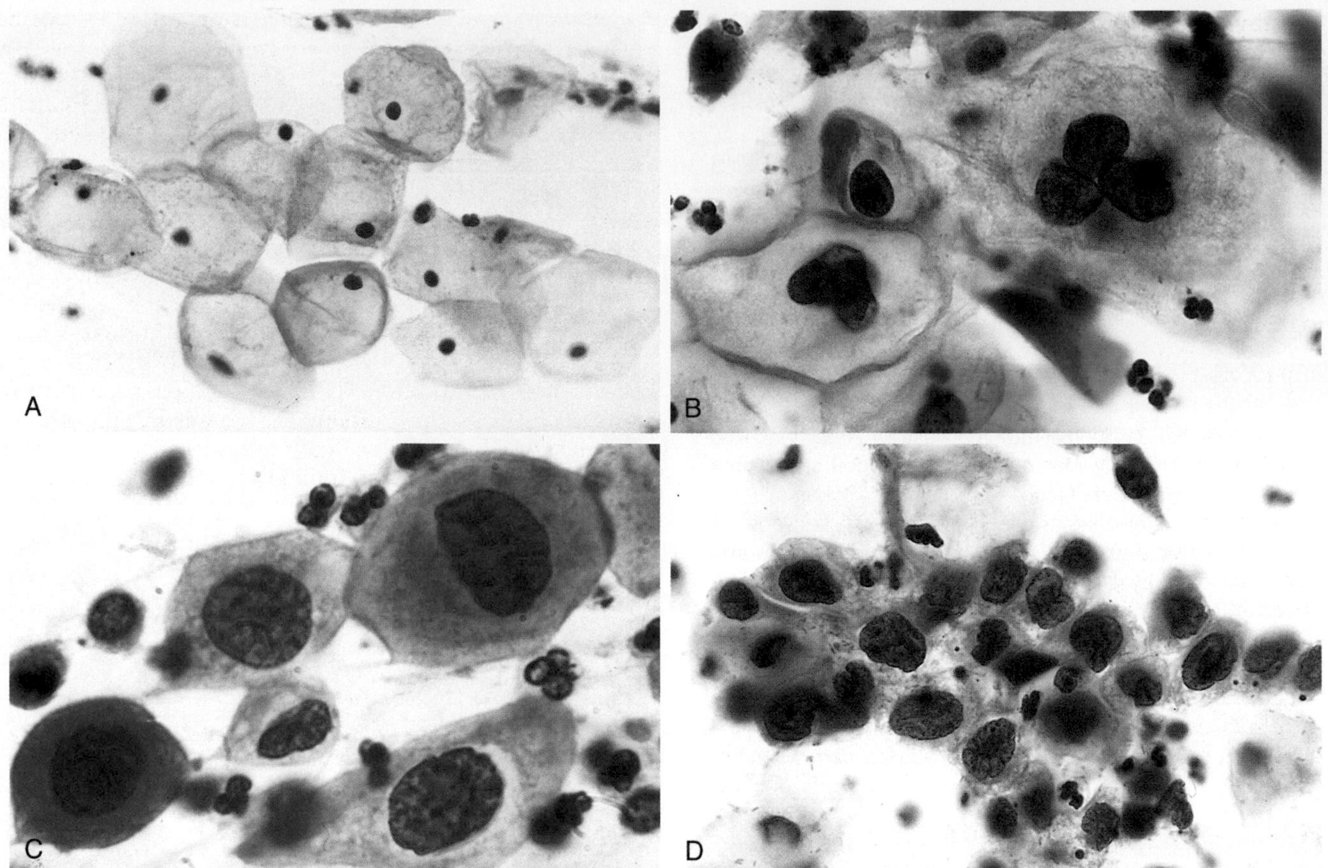

Figure 22-18 The cytology of cervical intraepithelial neoplasia as seen on the Papanicolaou smear. Normal cytoplasmic staining in superficial cells (**A** and **B**) may be either red or blue. **A,** Normal exfoliated superficial squamous cells. **B,** Low-grade squamous intraepithelial lesion (LSIL)—koilocytes. **C,** High-grade squamous intraepithelial lesion (HSIL; CIN II). **D,** HSIL (CIN III). Note the reduction in cytoplasm and the increase in the nucleus-to-cytoplasm ratio, which occurs as the grade of the lesion increases. This reflects the progressive loss of cellular differentiation on the surface of the lesions from which these cells are exfoliated. (Courtesy Dr. Edmund S. Cibas, Brigham and Women's Hospital, Boston, Mass.)

Stage II—Carcinoma extends beyond the cervix but not to the pelvic wall. Carcinoma involves the vagina but not the lower third.

Stage III—Carcinoma has extended to the pelvic wall. On rectal examination there is no cancer-free space between the tumor and the pelvic wall. The tumor involves the lower third of the vagina.

Stage IV—Carcinoma has extended beyond the true pelvis or has involved the mucosa of the bladder or rectum. This stage also includes cancers with metastatic dissemination.

Clinical Features. More than half of invasive cervical cancers are detected in women who did not participate in regular screening. While early invasive cancers of the cervix (microinvasive carcinomas) may be treated by cervical cone excision alone, most invasive cancers are managed by hysterectomy with lymph node dissection and, for advanced lesions, radiation and chemotherapy. The prognosis and survival for invasive carcinomas depend on the stage of the cancer at diagnosis and to some degree on histologic subtype, with small-cell neuroendocrine tumors having a very poor prognosis. With current treatments the 5-year survival rate is 100% for microinvasive carcinomas and less than 50% for tumors extending beyond pelvis. Most patients with advanced cervical cancer die of the consequences of local tumor invasion (e.g., ureteral obstruction, pyelonephritis, and uremia) rather than distant metastases.

Cervical Cancer Screening and Prevention

As is well known, cytologic cancer screening has significantly reduced mortality from cervical cancer. In countries where such screening is not widely practiced, cervical cancer continue to exact a high toll. The reason that cytologic screening is so effective in preventing cervical cancer is that most cancers arise from precursor lesions over the course of years. These lesions shed abnormal cells that can be detected on cytologic examination. Using a spatula or brush, the transformation zone of the cervix is circumferentially scraped and the cells are smeared or spun down onto a slide. Following fixation and staining with the Papanicolaou method, the smears are screened microscopically by eye or (increasingly) with automated image analysis systems. The cellular changes seen on the Pap test, illustrating the spectrum from LSIL to HSIL, are shown in Figure 22-18.

Testing for the presence of HPV DNA in the cervical scrape is a molecular method of cervical cancer screening. HPV testing has a higher sensitivity but lower specificity, as compared to Pap test. HPV DNA testing may be added to cervical cytology for screening in women aged 30 years or older. HPV testing of women younger than 30 is not recommended because of the high incidence of infection, and thus the particularly low specificity of HPV test results in this age group.

- Cervical cancer screening and preventive measures are carried out in a step wise fashion. Recommendations for the frequency of Pap screening vary, but in general the first smear should be at age 21 years or within 3 years of onset of sexual activity, and thereafter every 3 years. After age 30, women who have had normal cytology results and are negative for HPV may be screened every 5 years. Women with a normal cytology result, but test positive for high-risk HPV DNA, should have cervical cytology repeated every 6 to 12 months.
- When the result of a Pap test is abnormal, a colposcopic examination of the cervix and vagina is performed to identify the lesion. The mucosa is examined with a magnifying glass following application of acetic acid, which highlights abnormal epithelium as white spots (*acetowhite areas*). Abnormal appearing areas are biopsied. Women with biopsy confirmed LSIL can be followed in a conservative fashion. Some gynecologists will perform local ablation (e.g., cryotherapy) of LSIL, particularly if there is concern about the reliability of patient follow-up. HSILs are treated with cervical conization (superficial excision).
- **A new aspect of cervical cancer prevention is vaccination against high-risk oncogenic HPVs, which is now recommended for all girls and boys by age 11 to 12 years, as well as young men and women up to age 26 years.** Two HPV vaccines are now FDA-licensed. Both provide nearly complete protection against high-risk oncogenic HPV types 16 and 18 (together accounting for approximately 70% of cervical cancers), and one also provides protection against HPV types 6 and 11, which are responsible for genital warts. Vaccination is now recommended for boys as well as girls due to the role of that males play in the spread of HPV to women and the toll that HPV-related anal and oropharyngeal cancers take in men. The vaccines offer protection for up to 10 years; longer follow-up studies are still pending. Since the HPV vaccine does not protect against all high-risk HPV types, current guidelines recommend that cervical cancer screening be continued as in the past.

KEY CONCEPTS

- Cervical low-grade squamous intraepithelial lesions (LSILs) are productive HPV infections that usually regress spontaneously, but occasionally progress to high-grade squamous intraepithelial lesions (HSILs).
- HSILs are characterized by progressive deregulation of the cell cycle and increasing cellular atypia. HSILs may progress to invasive carcinoma.
- Almost all cervical precursor lesions and cervical carcinomas are caused by high-risk HPV types, most commonly HPV-16.

BODY OF UTERUS AND ENDOMETRIUM

The uterus has two major components: the myometrium and the endometrium. The myometrium is composed of tightly interwoven bundles of smooth muscle that form the wall of the uterus. The internal cavity of the uterus is lined by the endometrium, which is composed of glands embedded in a cellular stroma. The uterus is affected by a variety of disorders, the most common of which results from endocrine imbalances, complications of pregnancy, and neoplastic proliferation.

Endometrial Histology in the Menstrual Cycle

The endometrium undergoes dynamic physiologic and morphologic changes during the menstrual cycle in response to sex steroid hormones coordinately produced in the ovary. The ovary is influenced by hormones produced by the pituitary due to signals from the hypothalamus. Together the hypothalamic, pituitary, and ovarian factors and their interactions regulate maturation of ovarian follicles, ovulation, and menstruation.

"Dating" the endometrium by its histologic appearance may be used to assess hormonal status, document ovulation, and determine causes of endometrial bleeding and infertility (Fig. 22-19). Progression through a normal menstrual cycle is correlated with the following histologic features:

- The cycle commences with *menses*, during which the superficial portion of the endometrium, referred to as the functionalis, is shed.
- The *proliferative phase* is marked by rapid growth of glands and stroma arising from the deeper portion of the endometrium (basalis). During the proliferative phase the glands are straight, tubular structures lined by regular, tall, pseudostratified columnar cells. Mitotic figures are numerous, and there is no evidence of mucus secretion or vacuolation. The endometrial stroma is composed of spindle cells with scant cytoplasm that are also actively proliferating (Fig. 22-19*A*).
- At *ovulation*, endometrial proliferation ceases and differentiation commences in response to the effects of progesterone made by the corpus luteum in the ovary.
- *Postovulation* is initially marked by the appearance of *secretory vacuoles* beneath the nuclei in the glandular epithelium (Fig. 22-19*B*). Secretory activity is most prominent during the third week of the menstrual cycle, when the basal vacuoles progressively move to the apical surface. When secretion is maximal, between 18 and 24 days, the glands are dilated. By the fourth week

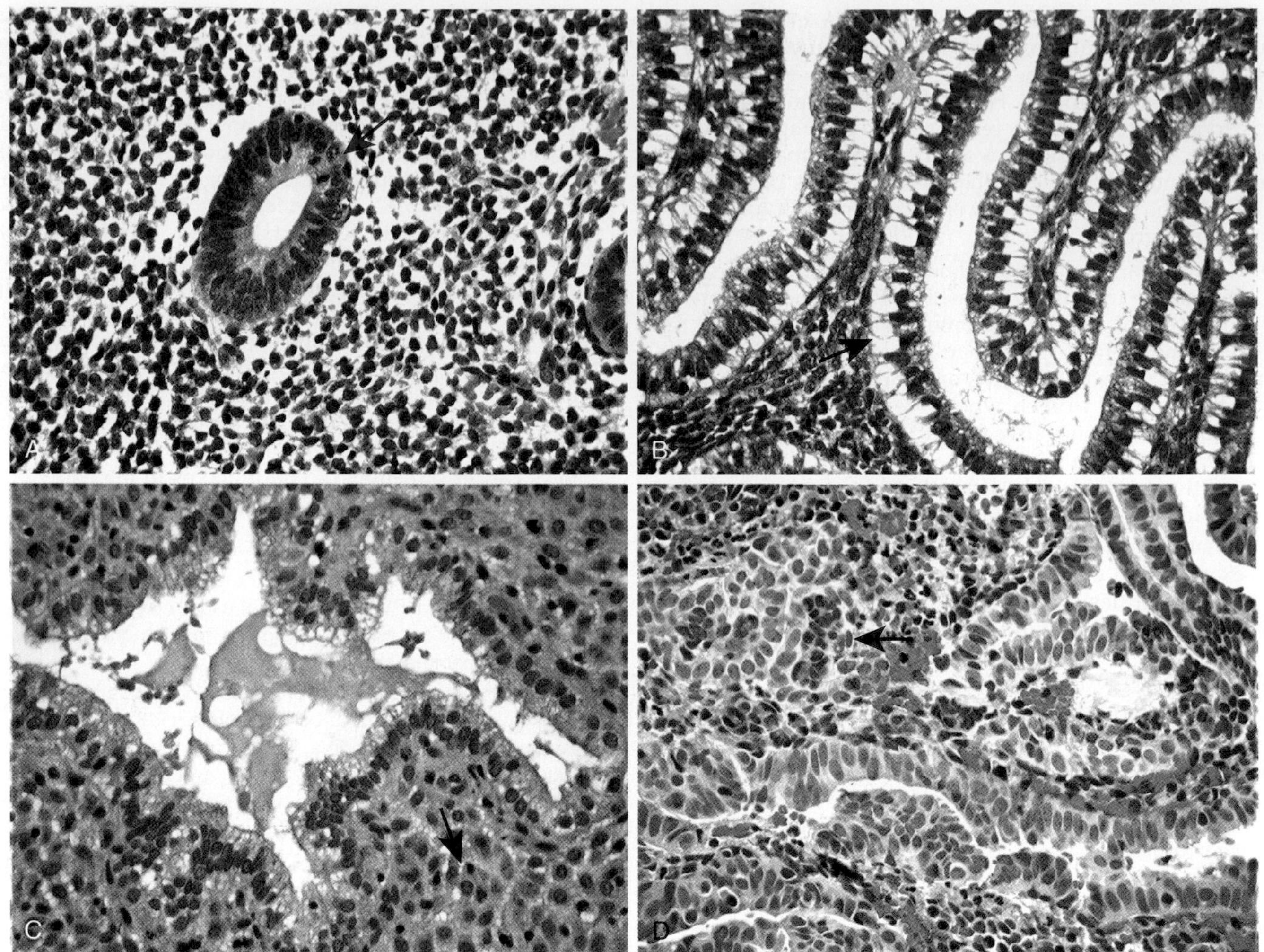

Figure 22-19 Histology of the menstrual cycle. **A,** Proliferative phase with mitoses *(arrow)*. **B,** Early secretory phase with subnuclear vacuoles *(arrow)*. **C,** Late secretory exhaustion and predecidual changes *(arrow)*. **D,** Menstrual endometrium with stromal breakdown *(arrow)* (see text).

the glands are tortuous, producing a serrated appearance. This serrated or "saw-toothed" appearance is accentuated by secretory exhaustion and shrinkage of the glands.

- *Stromal changes in the late secretory phase*, due predominantly to progesterone, are important for dating the endometrium. Prominent spiral arterioles appear by days 21 to 22 accompanied by an increase in ground substance and edema between the stromal cells. By days 23 to 24, stromal cell hypertrophy, increased cytoplasmic eosinophilia (*predecidual change*) and a resurgence of stromal mitoses appear (Fig. 22-19*C*). Predecidual changes spread throughout the functionalis during days 24 to 28 and are accompanied by a sparse infiltrate of neutrophils and lymphocytes, which in this context are considered normal.
- With the dissolution of the corpus luteum and the subsequent drop in progesterone levels, the functionalis degenerates and bleeding into the stroma occurs, followed by stromal breakdown and onset of the next menstrual cycle (Fig. 22-19*D*).

Much of the action of the ovarian hormones on the endometrium occurs through their cognate nuclear receptors and perhaps even by receptor-independent mechanisms. During the proliferative phase, estrogen drives the proliferation of both glands and stroma, sometimes by promoting "cross-talk" between these two cell types. For example, much of the effect of estrogen on glandular proliferation occurs via stromal cells, which in response to estrogen produce growth factors (e.g., insulin-like growth factor 1 and epidermal growth factor) that bind receptors expressed on the epithelial cells. During the secretory phase, progesterone down-regulates the expression of estrogen receptor in both the glands and the stroma, and as a result endometrial proliferation is suppressed. Progesterone also promotes the differentiation of the glands and causes functional changes in the stromal cells. Endometrial stem cells have been identified and there is recent data to suggest that they play a central role in the regeneration of the endometrium after menses. They may also contribute to the development of ectopic endometrial tissue and endometrial cancer.

Functional Endometrial Disorders (Dysfunctional Uterine Bleeding)

Although abnormal uterine bleeding can be caused by well-defined pathologic conditions, such as chronic endometritis, endometrial polyps (Fig. 22-20*C*), submucosal

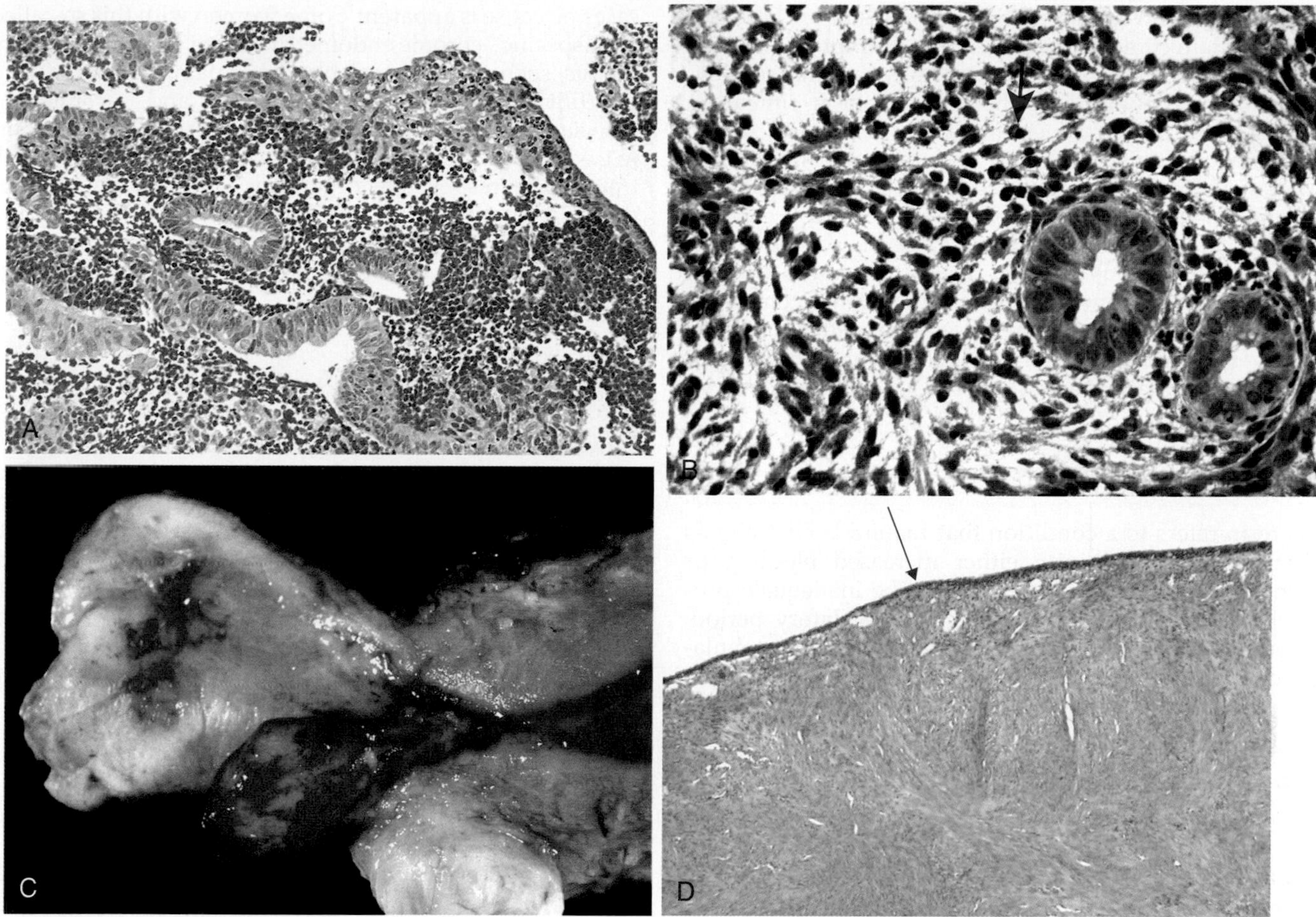

Figure 22-20 Common causes of abnormal uterine bleeding. **A,** The most common is dysfunctional uterine bleeding, seen here as anovulatory endometrium with stromal breakdown. Note breakdown associated with proliferative glands. **B,** Chronic endometritis with numerous plasma cells *(arrow)*. **C,** Endometrial polyp. **D,** Submucosal leiomyoma with attenuation of the endometrial lining *(arrow)*.

leiomyomas (Fig. 22-20*D*), or endometrial neoplasms, it most commonly stems from hormonal disturbances that produce *dysfunctional uterine bleeding* (Table 22-3). This is a clinical term for uterine bleeding that lacks an underlying organic (structural) abnormality. As discussed earlier, the normal cyclical proliferation, differentiation, and shedding of the endometrium requires that all the involved pituitary and ovarian hormones be released at the proper time in the right amounts. Any disturbance of this finely tuned system may result in dysfunctional uterine bleeding, the most common causes of which are discussed in the following sections.

Table 22-3 Causes of Abnormal Uterine Bleeding by Age Group

Age Group	Causes
Prepuberty	Precocious puberty (hypothalamic, pituitary, or ovarian origin)
Adolescence	Anovulatory cycle, coagulation disorders
Reproductive age	Complications of pregnancy (abortion, trophoblastic disease, ectopic pregnancy) Anatomic lesions (leiomyoma, adenomyosis, polyps, endometrial hyperplasia, carcinoma) Dysfunctional uterine bleeding Anovulatory cycle Ovulatory dysfunctional bleeding (e.g., inadequate luteal phase)
Perimenopausal	Dysfunctional uterine bleeding Anovulatory cycle Anatomic lesions (carcinoma, hyperplasia, polyps)
Postmenopausal	Endometrial atrophy Anatomic lesions (carcinoma, hyperplasia, polyps)

Anovulatory Cycle

The most frequent cause of dysfunctional bleeding is anovulation (failure to ovulate). Anovulatory cycles result from subtle hormonal imbalances and are most common at menarche and in the perimenopausal period. Less commonly, anovulation is the result of:

- *Endocrine disorders,* such as thyroid disease, adrenal disease, or pituitary tumors
- *Ovarian lesions,* such as a functioning ovarian tumor (granulosa cell tumors) or polycystic ovaries (see "Ovaries")
- *Generalized metabolic disturbances,* such as obesity, malnutrition, or other chronic systemic diseases

Failure of ovulation results in excessive endometrial stimulation by estrogens that is unopposed by progesterone. Under these circumstances the endometrial glands undergo mild architectural changes, including cystic dilation, that usually resolve due to a subsequent ovulatory cycle.

However, repeated anovulation may result in bleeding that, in certain clinical situations, may prompt an endometrial biopsy. In this setting biopsies reveal stromal condensation and eosinophilic epithelial metaplasia similar to those seen in menstrual endometrium. However, unlike menstrual endometrium, the endometrium of women with anovulatory cycles lacks progesterone-dependent morphologic features (e.g., glandular secretory changes and stromal pre-decidualization), since the source of progesterone, the corpus luteum, does not develop without ovulation. Most commonly the endometrium is comprised of pseudostratified glands and contains scattered mitotic figures (Fig. 22-20*A*). More severe consequences of repeated anovulation are discussed under "Endometrial Hyperplasia."

Inadequate Luteal Phase

This term refers to a condition that manifests clinically as infertility associated with either increased bleeding or amenorrhea. The cause is believed to be inadequate progesterone production during the post-ovulatory period. Endometrial biopsy performed at an estimated postovulatory date shows secretory endometrium with features that lag behind those expected for the estimated date.

Inflammatory Disorders

The endometrium and myometrium are relatively resistant to infections, primarily because the endocervix forms a barrier to ascending infection. Thus, although chronic inflammation in the cervix is an expected and frequently insignificant finding, it is of concern in the endometrium, excluding the menstrual phase.

Acute Endometritis

Acute endometritis is uncommon and limited to bacterial infections that arise after delivery or miscarriage. Retained products of conception are the usual predisposing influence; the causative agents include group A hemolytic streptococci, staphylococci, and other bacteria. The inflammatory response is chiefly limited to the stroma and is entirely nonspecific. Removal of the retained gestational fragments by curettage, accompanied by antibiotic therapy, promptly clears the infection.

Chronic Endometritis

Chronic endometritis occurs in association with the following disorders:

- Chronic pelvic inflammatory disease (PID)
- Retained gestational tissue, postpartum or postabortion
- Intrauterine contraceptive devices
- Tuberculosis, either from miliary spread or, more often, from drainage of tuberculous salpingitis. Both are rare in Western countries.

The diagnosis of chronic endometritis rests on the identification of plasma cells in the stroma, which are not seen in normal endometrium (Fig. 22-20*B*). In about 15% of cases no cause is apparent. Some women with this so-called "nonspecific" chronic endometritis have gynecologic complaints such as abnormal bleeding, pain, discharge, and infertility. *Chlamydia* may be involved and is commonly associated with both acute (e.g., neutrophils) and chronic (e.g., lymphocytes, plasma cells) inflammatory cell infiltrates. The responsible organisms may or may not be detected by culture. If infection is suspected on clinical grounds, antibiotic therapy is indicated even in the face of negative cultures, as it may prevent other sequelae (e.g., salpingitis).

Endometriosis and Adenomyosis

Endometriosis is defined by the presence of "ectopic" endometrial tissue at a site outside of the uterus. The abnormal tissue most commonly includes both endometrial glands and stroma, but may consist only of stroma in some cases. It occurs in the following sites, in descending order of frequency: (1) ovaries, (2) uterine ligaments, (3) rectovaginal septum, (4) cul de sac, (5) pelvic peritoneum, (6) large and small bowel and appendix, (7) mucosa of the cervix, vagina, and fallopian tubes, and (8) laparotomy scars.

Endometriosis takes a significant toll on the afflicted; it often causes *infertility, dysmenorrhea* (painful menstruation), *pelvic pain*, and other problems. The disorder is principally a disease of women in active reproductive life, most often in the third and fourth decades, and affects approximately 6% to 10% of women. Uncommonly endometriosis may "invade" and "spread," behaviors that often contribute to significant complications. For example, involvement of the muscular wall of the bowel by endometriosis can result in intestinal symptoms (Fig. 22-21).

Pathogenesis. The pathogenesis of endometriosis remains elusive. Proposed origins of endometriotic lesions fall into two main categories: (1) those that propose an origin from the uterine endometrium and (2) those that propose an origin from cells outside the uterus that have the capacity to give rise to endometrial tissue. The leading theories are as follows:

- *The regurgitation theory* proposes that endometrial tissue implants at ectopic sites via retrograde flow of menstrual endometrium. Retrograde menstruation through the fallopian tubes occurs regularly even in normal women and can explain the distribution of endometriosis within the peritoneal cavity.
- *The benign metastases theory* holds that endometrial tissue from the uterus can "spread" to distant sites (e.g., bone, lung, and brain) via blood vessels and lymphatic channels.
- *The metaplastic theory* suggests that endometrium arises directly from coelomic epithelium (mesothelium of pelvis or abdomen), from which the müllerian ducts and ultimately the endometrium itself originate during embryonic development. In addition, mesonephric remnants may undergo endometrial differentiation and give rise to ectopic endometrial tissue.
- *The extrauterine stem/progenitor cell theory* is a recent idea that proposes that stem/progenitor cells from the bone marrow differentiate into endometrial tissue.

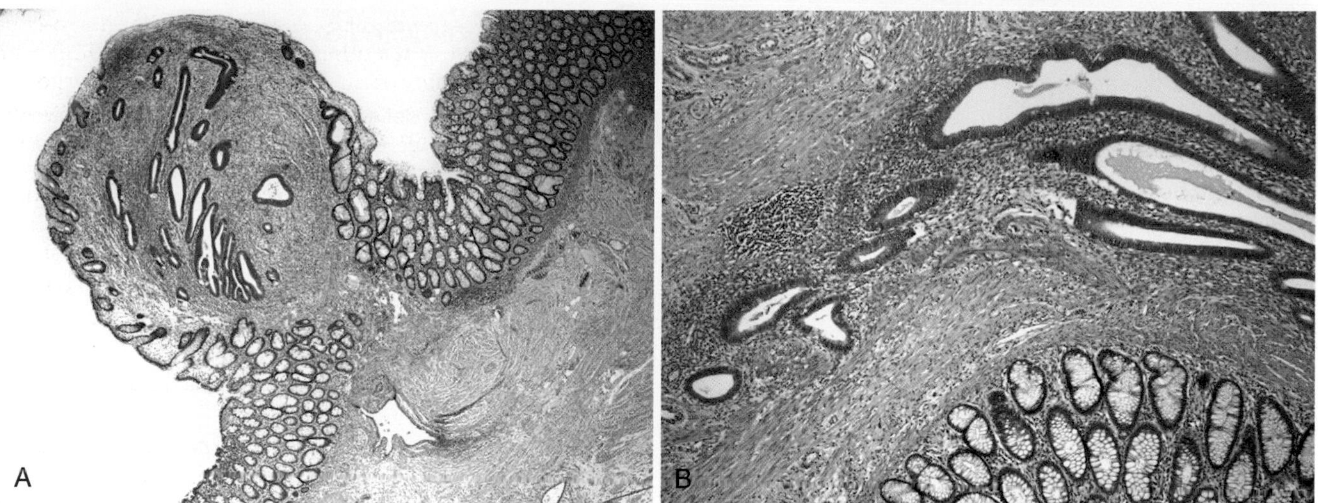

Figure 22-21 Endometriosis. **A,** Endometriosis involving the mucosa of the colon. **B,** Higher magnification reveals endometrial glands and stroma adjacent to normal colonic mucosa.

The regurgitation theory provides a plausible explanation for the anatomic location of ectopic endometrial tissue in the vast majority of cases. However, it cannot explain all cases, such as endometriosis in women who are amenorrheic because of a variety of underlying etiologies (e.g., gonadal dysgenesis); endometriosis in the urogenital tract of men treated with high-dose estrogens for prostate cancer; and endometriosis in distant sites like the brain, lung and bone. In addition, the relatively low incidence of endometriosis, despite the common occurrence of retrograde menstruation (up to 90% of women), suggests that additional factors must be involved in the pathogenesis of the disorder.

Molecular analyses have provided additional insights into the pathogenesis of endometriosis. The endometriotic implants show certain differences when compared to the endometria of women without endometriosis (Fig. 22-22). These include the following:

- *Release of proinflammatory and other factors,* including PGE2, IL-1β, TNFα, IL-6 and -8, NGF, VEGF, MCP-1, MMPs, and TIMPs.
- *Increased estrogen production by endometriotic stromal cells,* due in large part to high levels of the key steroidogenic enzyme aromatase, which is absent in normal endometrial stroma. Estrogen enhances the survival and persistence of endometriotic tissue, and inhibitors of aromatase are beneficial in the treatment of endometriosis. A link between inflammation and estrogen production is made plausible by the ability of prostaglandin E_2 to stimulate local synthesis of estrogen.

The expression of these factors contributes to the survival of ectopic endometrial tissue by promoting invasion and the establishment of neurovascular networks and by decreasing immune clearance. In addition, epigenetic alterations have been described that lead to increase responsiveness to estrogen and decreased responsiveness to progesterone, alterations that promote endometrial proliferation and survival. These abnormalities are present not only in ectopic endometriotic tissue, but also, albeit to a lesser degree, in the uterine endometrium of patients with endometriosis, suggesting that there is a fundamental defect in the endometrium.

- An association between endometriosis and ovarian cancer of the endometrioid and clear cell types (discussed later) has been noted in a number of epidemiologic studies with an approximate threefold increase in women with endometriosis. More recent molecular studies have demonstrated shared mutations in specific genes (*PTEN* and *ARID1A*) in endometriotic cysts, atypical endometriosis (see later) and associated carcinomas. These studies suggest a common origin of abnormal

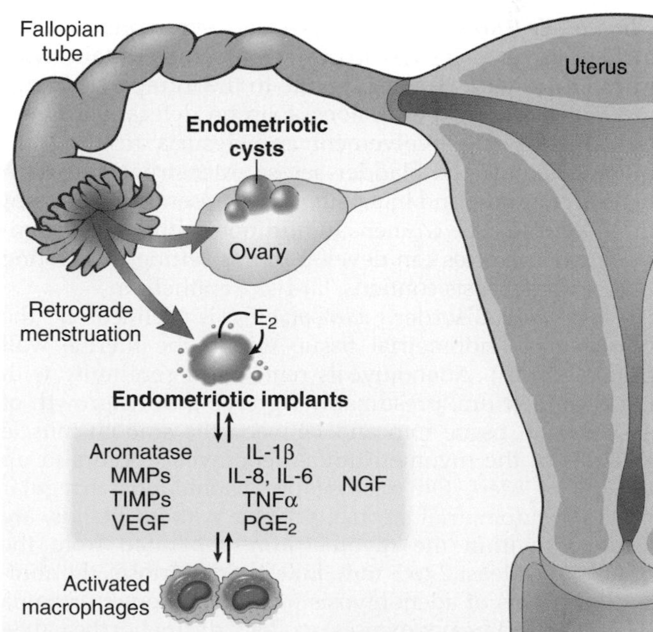

Figure 22-22 Pathogenesis of endometriosis. The factors expressed in endometriotic implants, eutopic endometrium and activated macrophages that play a role in the establishment and maintenance of endometriotic implants.

endometriotic tissue and ovarian cancers in some cases, as described below.

MORPHOLOGY

Endometriotic lesions bleed periodically in response to both extrinsic cyclic (ovarian) and intrinsic hormonal stimulation. This bleeding produces nodules with a red-blue to yellow-brown appearance on or just beneath the mucosal and/or serosal surfaces at sites of involvement. When lesions are extensive, organizing hemorrhage causes extensive fibrous adhesions between tubes, ovaries, and other structures and obliterates the pouch of Douglas. The ovaries may become markedly distorted by large cystic masses (3 to 5 cm in diameter) filled with brown fluid resulting from previous hemorrhage; these are often referred to clinically as **chocolate cysts** or **endometriomas**. Aggressive forms of endometriosis can invade tissues and cause fibrosis and subsequent adhesions.

The histologic diagnosis of endometriosis is usually straightforward but may be difficult in long-standing cases in which the endometrial tissue is obscured by secondary fibrosis. The diagnosis is readily made when both endometrial glands and stroma are present (Fig. 22-21*B*), with or without the presence of hemosiderin. In rare cases only stroma is identified. If only glands are present, other diagnoses with different clinical ramifications, such as endosalpingiosis, must be considered.

Atypical endometriosis, the likely precursor to endometriosis-related ovarian carcinoma, has two morphologic appearances. One consists of cytologic atypia of the epithelium lining the endometriotic cyst without major architectural changes. The second is marked by glandular crowding due to excessive epithelial proliferation, often associated with cytologic atypia, producing an appearance that resembles complex atypical endometrial hyperplasia (discussed later).

Clinical Features. Clinical signs and symptoms usually include severe dysmenorrhea, dyspareunia (pain with intercourse), and pelvic pain due to the intrapelvic bleeding and periuterine adhesions. Pain on defecation occurs with rectal wall involvement and dysuria results from involvement of the bladder serosa. Menstrual irregularities are common, and infertility is the presenting complaint in 30% to 40% of women. In addition, although uncommon, malignancies can develop in this setting, suggesting that endometriosis contains "at-risk" epithelium.

A related disorder, *adenomyosis*, is defined as the presence of endometrial tissue within the uterine wall (myometrium). Adenomyosis remains in continuity with the endometrium, presumably signifying downgrowth of endometrial tissue into and between the smooth muscle fascicles of the myometrium. Adenomyosis occurs in up to 20% of uteri. On microscopic examination, irregular nests of endometrial stroma, with or without glands, are arranged within the myometrium, separated from the basalis by at least 2 to 3 mm. Like endometriosis, the clinical symptoms of adenomyosis include menometrorrhagia (irregular and heavy menses), colicky dysmenorrhea, dyspareunia, and pelvic pain, particularly during the premenstrual period. It can coexist with endometriosis.

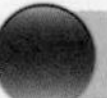

KEY CONCEPTS

Endometriosis

- Endometriosis is defined as endometrial glands and stroma outside of the uterus. The "ectopic" endometrial tissue may undergo cyclic bleeding.
- Most common sites of endometriosis are within the abdominal cavity, but occasionally it is found at distant sites.
- Several theories (regurgitation, metaplasia, metastasis, and stem cell origin) are proposed to explain the distribution of endometriosis.
- It commonly results in dysmenorrhea, pelvic pain, and infertility.
- Endometriosis may be a precursor to carcinoma (endometrioid and clear cell carcinoma).

Endometrial Polyps

Endometrial polyps are exophytic masses of variable size that project into the endometrial cavity. They may be single or multiple and are usually sessile, measuring from 0.5 to 3 cm in diameter, but are occasionally large and pedunculated. Polyps may be asymptomatic or may cause abnormal bleeding (intramenstrual, menometrorrhagia, or postmenopausal) if they ulcerate or undergo necrosis.

Cytogenetic studies indicate that the stromal cells in endometrial polyps contain certain chromosomal rearrangements that are similar to those found in other benign mesenchymal tumors. These findings suggest that the polyp stroma is neoplastic, and that the associated glands are reactive, merely "coming along for the ride." The glands in polyps may be hyperplastic or atrophic, and may occasionally demonstrate secretory changes (functional polyps). Polyps may by become hyperplastic in association with generalized endometrial hyperplasia and are responsive to estrogen but show little or no response to progesterone (Fig. 22-20C). Endometrial polyps have been observed in association with the administration of tamoxifen, which is often used in the therapy of breast cancer due to its anti-estrogenic activity on the breast. However, tamoxifen has weak pro-estrogenic effects in the endometrium. Atrophic polyps, which mainly occur in postmenopausal women, likely represent the atrophic remnants of previously hyperplastic polyps. Rarely, adenocarcinomas arise within endometrial polyps.

Endometrial Hyperplasia

Endometrial hyperplasia is an important cause of abnormal bleeding and a frequent precursor to the most common type of endometrial carcinoma. It is defined as an increased proliferation of the endometrial glands relative to the stroma, resulting in an increased gland-to-stroma ratio when compared with normal proliferative endometrium. Clinicopathologic and epidemiologic studies have supported the malignant potential of endometrial hyperplasia and the concept of a continuum of proliferative glandular lesions culminating, in some cases, in carcinoma. Molecular studies have confirmed this relationship, since endometrial hyperplasia and carcinoma share specific acquired genetic alterations in genes linked to oncogenesis (described later).

Endometrial hyperplasia is associated with *prolonged estrogenic stimulation of the endometrium*, which can be due to anovulation, increased estrogen production from endogenous sources, or exogenous estrogen. Associated conditions include:

- Obesity (peripheral conversion of androgens to estrogens)
- Menopause
- Polycystic ovarian syndrome
- Functioning granulosa cell tumors of the ovary
- Excessive ovarian cortical function (cortical stromal hyperplasia)
- Prolonged administration of estrogenic substances (estrogen replacement therapy)

These are the same influences postulated to be of pathogenic significance in some endometrial carcinomas, discussed later.

Inactivation of the *PTEN* tumor suppressor gene is a common genetic alteration in both endometrial hyperplasias and endometrial carcinomas. As discussed in Chapter 7, *PTEN* encodes a lipid phosphatase that is an important negative regulator of phosphatidylinositol 3-kinase (PI3K)/AKT growth-regulatory pathway. When PTEN function is lost, the PI3K/AKT pathway becomes overactive. Mutations in *PTEN* are found in more than 20% of hyperplasias, both with and without atypia, and in 30% to 80% of endometrial carcinomas, suggesting that alterations in *PTEN* occur at an early stage in endometrial tumorigenesis (although they are not predictive of progression of hyperplasia to carcinoma). Of note, patients with Cowden syndrome, which is caused by germline mutations in *PTEN*, have a high incidence of endometrial carcinoma and certain other tumors, particular breast cancer. As with many other tumor suppressors, it is not entirely clear why the loss of *PTEN* (which is expressed in many tissues) is so highly associated with particular tumors. It is interesting to note, however, that PI3K/AKT signaling enhances the ability of the estrogen receptor to turn on the expression of its target genes. Thus, loss of PTEN function may stimulate estrogen-dependent gene expression, leading to overgrowth of cell types that depend on estrogen for trophic signals, such as endometrial and mammary epithelial cells.

The classification of endometrial hyperplasia has undergone a number of changes over the years to keep pace with new insights into the disorder. In the recent past, the most widely used system divided endometrial hyperplasia into four categories: simple hyperplasia without atypia; complex hyperplasia without atypia; simple atypical hyperplasia; and complex atypical hyperplasia. However, the most current World Health Organization (WHO) classification recommends collapsing the four categories into two major categories: Non-atypical hyperplasia and atypical hyperplasia (also referred to as *endometrial intraepithelial neoplasia*), which differ in appearance and in their propensity to progress to carcinoma.

MORPHOLOGY

Non-atypical hyperplasia has a wide-range of appearances, but the cardinal feature is an increase in the gland-to-stroma ratio. The glands show variation in size and shape and may be dilated (Fig. 22-23*A*). Although there may be back-to-back glands focally, some intervening stroma is usually retained (Fig. 22-23*B*). These lesions reflect an endometrial response to persistent estrogen stimulation and rarely progress to adenocarcinoma (approximately 1% to 3%). Non-atypical hyperplasia may evolve into cystic atrophy when estrogen is withdrawn.

Atypical hyperplasia (endometrial intraepithelial neoplasia) is composed of complex patterns of proliferating glands displaying nuclear atypia. The glands are commonly back-to-back and often have complex outlines due to branching structures. Individual cells are rounded and lose the normal perpendicular orientation to the basement membrane. In addition, the nuclei have open (vesicular) chromatin and conspicuous nucleoli. The features of atypical hyperplasia have considerable overlap with those of well-differentiated endometrioid adenocarcinoma (discussed later), and accurate distinction from cancer may not be possible without hysterectomy (Fig. 22-23*C* and *D*). Indeed, approximately 23% to 48% of women with a diagnosis of atypical hyperplasia are found to have carcinoma when a hysterectomy is performed.

A proportion of endometrial hyperplasias are less easily classified, including complex lesions without cellular atypia (uncommon) and those with altered cellular differentiation, such as squamous, ciliated cell, eosinophilic, and mucinous metaplasias. Metaplastic epithelium is benign and the diagnosis of hyperplasia is based on the appearance of the nonmetaplastic areas.

Currently, atypical hyperplasia is managed by hysterectomy or, in young women who desire fertility, a trial of progestin therapy and close follow-up. Most often, hopefully after a successful pregnancy, lack of regression prompts removal of the uterus.

KEY CONCEPTS

Endometrial Hyperplasia

- Endometrial hyperplasia is defined as an increase in the number of glands relative to the stroma, appreciated as crowded glands, often with abnormal shapes.
- It is most commonly caused by unopposed estrogen stimulation and is an important cause of abnormal vaginal bleeding.
- It is divided into non-atypical and atypical hyperplasia based on nuclear atypia. Atypical hyperplasia is associated with an increased risk of endometrial carcinoma.
- The *PTEN* tumor suppressor gene is mutated in approximately 20% of endometrial hyperplasias.

Malignant Tumors of the Endometrium

Carcinoma of the Endometrium

Endometrial carcinoma is the most common invasive cancer of the female genital tract. It accounts for 7% of

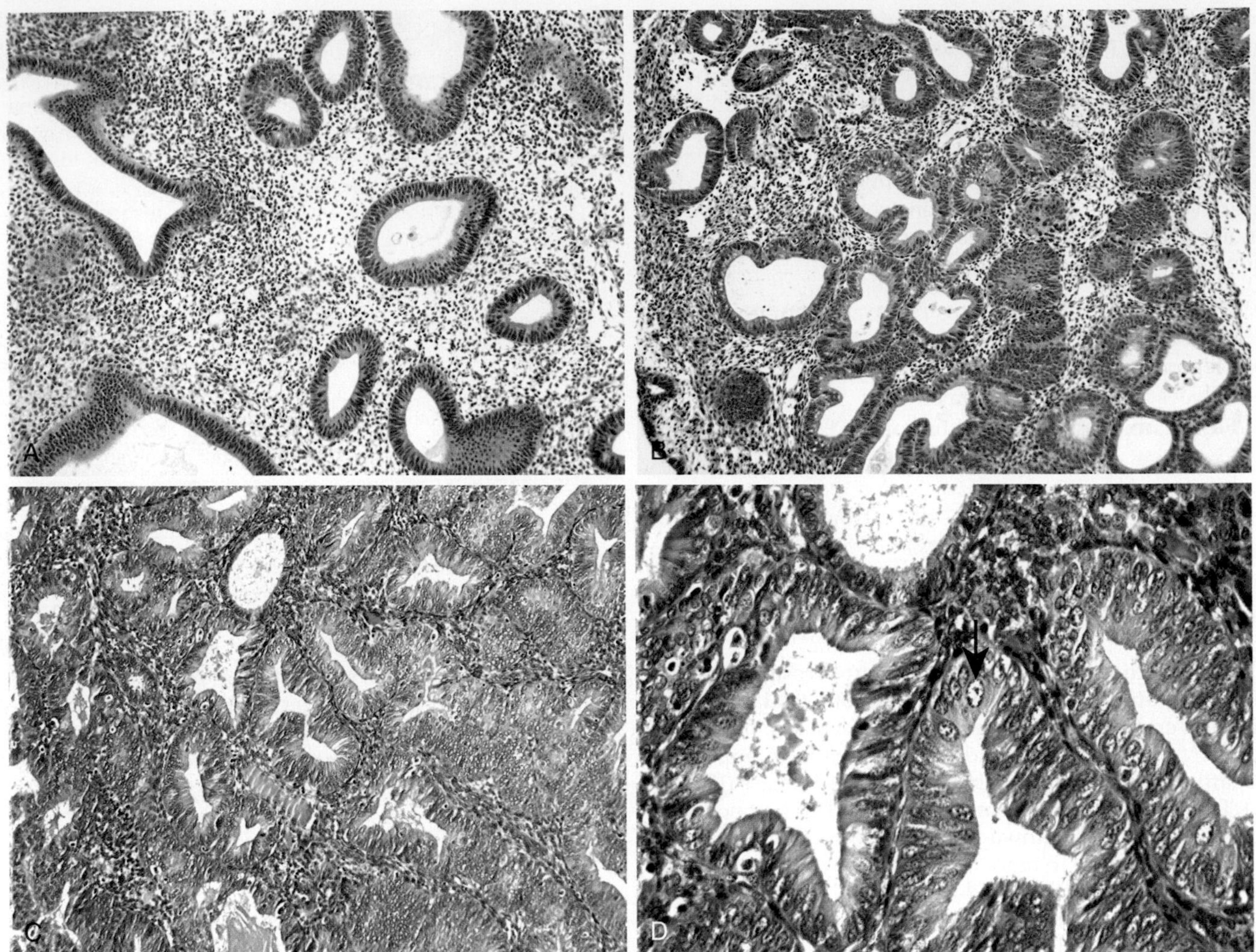

Figure 22-23 Endometrial hyperplasia. **A,** Hyperplasia without atypia. Note architectural abnormalities including mild glandular crowding and cystic glandular dilatation. **B,** Hyperplasia without atypia demonstrating increased glandular crowding with areas of back-to-back glands and cytologic features similar to proliferative endometrium. **C,** Atypical hyperplasia with further increase in glandular crowding and abnormal cytologic features. **D,** High magnification of atypical hyperplasia showing rounded, vesicular nuclei with prominent nucleoli *(arrow).*

all invasive cancer in women, excluding skin cancer. At one time endometrial carcinoma was far less common than cancer of the cervix, but earlier detection and eradication of the precursor lesions of cervical carcinoma, coupled with an increase in endometrial carcinomas in younger women, have reversed this ratio. In 2012 in the United States, 47,130 new endometrial cancers and 8010 deaths were predicted. Worldwide there are approximately 280,000 new cases of endometrial cancer per year.

Pathogenesis. Clinicopathologic studies and molecular analyses support the classification of endometrial carcinoma into two broad categories referred to as type I and type II (summarized in Table 22-4). Because of their distinct pathogenesis, they are discussed separately.

Type I (Endometrial) Carcinoma. These are the most common type, accounting for approximately 80% of cases. Most are well differentiated and mimic proliferative endometrial glands and, as such, are referred to as *endometrioid carcinoma*. As discussed earlier, they typically arise in the setting of endometrial hyperplasia and like endometrial hyperplasia they are associated with (1) obesity, (2) diabetes (abnormal glucose tolerance is found in more than 60%), (3) hypertension, (4) infertility, and (5) unopposed estrogen stimulation.

As with other cancers, development of endometrial carcinoma involves the stepwise acquisition of several genetic alterations in tumor suppressor genes and oncogenes. In hysterectomy specimens containing both atypical hyperplasia and carcinoma, identical *PTEN* mutations have been identified in each component, supporting the view that atypical hyperplasia is a precursor to carcinoma and that *PTEN* mutations occur before the development of overt carcinoma (Fig. 22-24*A*).

Sequencing of the genomes of type I endometrioid carcinomas has shown that the most common mutations act to increase signaling through the PI3K/AKT pathway, which is a hallmark of this particular tumor type. As mentioned earlier, PI3K/AKT signaling somehow augments expression of estrogen receptor-dependent target genes in endometrial cells. Type I endometrial carcinomas

Table 22-4 Characteristics of Type I and Type II Endometrial Carcinoma

Characteristics	Type I	Type II
Age	55-65 yr	65-75 yr
Clinical setting	Unopposed estrogen Obesity Hypertension Diabetes	Atrophy Thin physique
Morphology	Endometrioid	Serous Clear cell Mixed müllerian tumor
Precursor	Hyperplasia	Serous endometrial intraepithelial carcinoma
Mutated genes/ genetic abnormalities	*PTEN* *ARID1A* (regulator of chromatin) *PIK3CA* (PI3K) *KRAS* *FGF2* (growth factor) MSI* *CTNNB1* (Wnt signaling) *TP53*	*TP53* Aneuploidy *PIK3CA* (PI3K) *FBXW7* (regulator of MYC, cyclin E) *CHD4* (regulator of chromatin) *PPP2R1A* (PP2A)
Behavior	Indolent Spreads via lymphatics	Aggressive Intraperitoneal and lymphatic spread

*MSI, Microsatellite instability; CTNNB1, beta-catenin gene

are somewhat unique in that individual tumors may harbor multiple mutations that increase PI3K/AKT signaling, suggesting that tumor development and progression is fostered by successive increases in signal strength. Among the mutations that impact the PI3K/AKT pathway in endometrial carcinomas are the following:

- Mutations in the *PTEN* tumor suppressor gene have been identified in 30% to 80% of endometrioid carcinomas.
- *PIK3CA*, an oncogene that encodes the catalytic subunit of PI3K, harbors activating mutations in approximately 40% of endometrioid carcinomas. *PIK3CA* mutations rarely occur in atypical hyperplasias, suggesting that mutations in *PIK3CA* play a role in invasion.
- Mutations that activate *KRAS*, which also stimulates PI3K/AKT signaling, are found in approximately 25% of cases.
- Loss-of-function mutations in *ARID1A*, a regulator of chromatin structure, occur in approximately one-third of tumors. Of interest, *ARID1A* is also frequently mutated in ovarian endometrioid and clear cell carcinomas, tumors that arise within endometriosis. Although the mechanisms are not yet clear, loss of ARID1A function also enhances PI3K/AKT signaling.

Defects involving *DNA mismatch repair genes* are found in about 20% of sporadic tumors and are particularly prevalent in endometrial carcinomas arising in women from

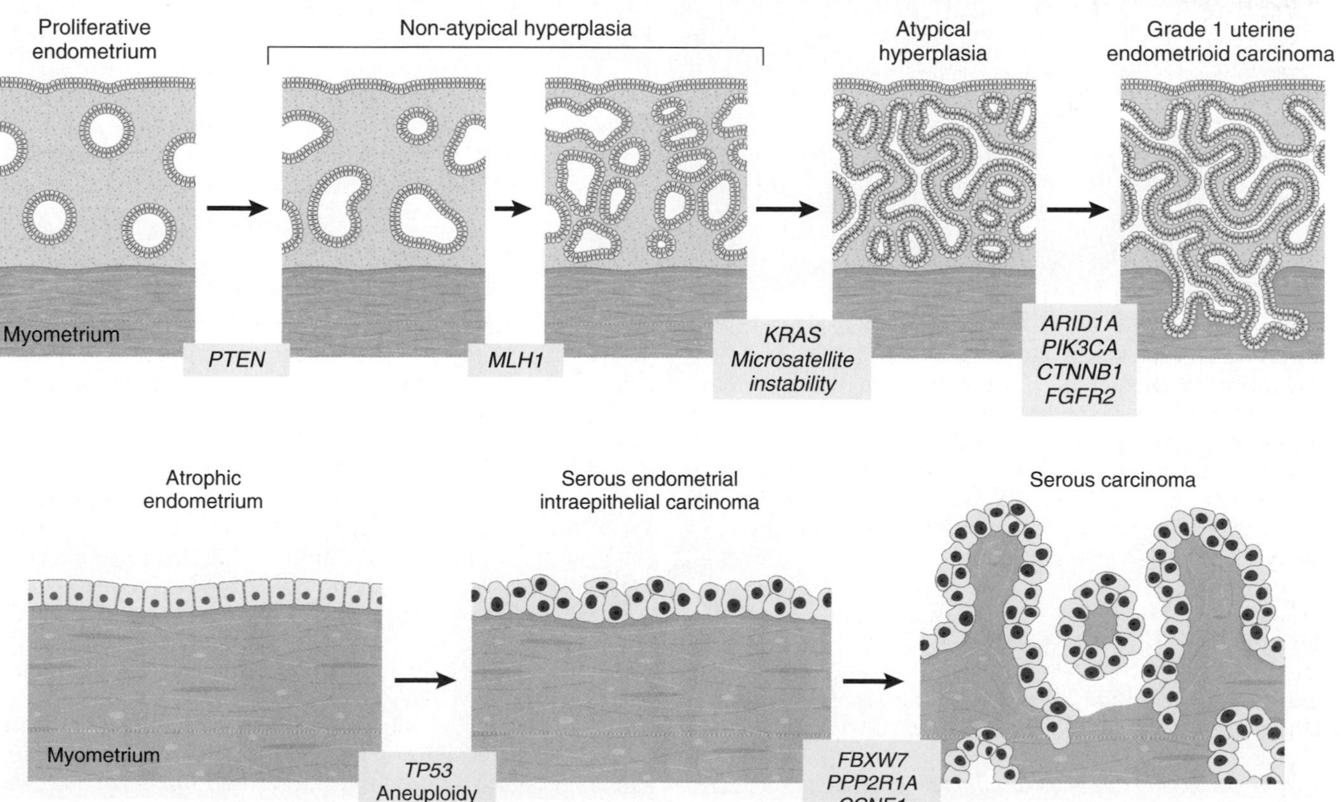

Figure 22-24 A, Schematic depicting the development of type I endometrial carcinoma arising in the setting of hyperplasia. **B,** Schematic diagram of the development of type II endometrial carcinoma. The most common molecular genetic alterations are shown at the time they are most likely to occur during the progression of the disease. *MI, Microsatellite instability. *CTNNB1*, beta-catenin gene; *PPP2R1A*, PP2A gene; *CCNE1*, cyclin E gene.

families with hereditary nonpolyposis colorectal carcinoma (HNPCC, discussed in Chapter 17). This defect creates a mutator phenotype, leading to more rapid accumulation of mutations that may by chance alter the function of cancer genes and thereby drive tumor development. In sporadic endometrioid carcinomas, loss of expression of DNA mismatch repair genes is commonly caused by epigenetic silencing (via promoter hypermethylation). Finally, loss-of-function mutations in *TP53* are present in approximately 50% of poorly differentiated carcinomas. Since *TP53* mutations are lacking in well-differentiated endometrioid carcinomas, these mutations are thought to be late events involved in tumor progression.

MORPHOLOGY

Endometrioid carcinoma can take the form of a localized polypoid tumor or a tumor that diffusely infiltrates the endometrial lining (Fig. 22-25*A*). Spread generally occurs by myometrial invasion followed by direct extension to adjacent structures/organs. Invasion of the broad ligaments may create a palpable mass. Dissemination to the regional lymph nodes eventually occurs, and in the late stages, the tumor may metastasize to the lungs, liver, bones, and other organs.

Endometrioid adenocarcinomas demonstrate glandular growth patterns resembling normal endometrial epithelium. There are three histologic grades: **well differentiated** (grade 1) (Fig. 22-25*B*), composed almost entirely of well-formed glands; **moderately differentiated** (grade 2) (Fig. 22-25*C*), showing well-formed glands mixed with areas composed of solid sheets of cells, which by definition make up 50% or less of the tumor; and **poorly differentiated** (grade 3) (Fig. 22-25*D*), characterized by greater than 50% solid growth pattern. Well differentiated tumors may be distinguished from hyperplasias by lack of intervening stroma.

Up to 20% of endometrioid carcinomas contain foci of squamous differentiation. Squamous elements may be histologically benign-appearing when they are associated with well-differentiated adenocarcinomas. Less commonly, moderately or poorly differentiated endometrioid carcinomas contain squamous elements that appear frankly malignant. Current classification systems grade the carcinomas based on glandular differentiation alone and ignore areas of solid squamous differentiation.

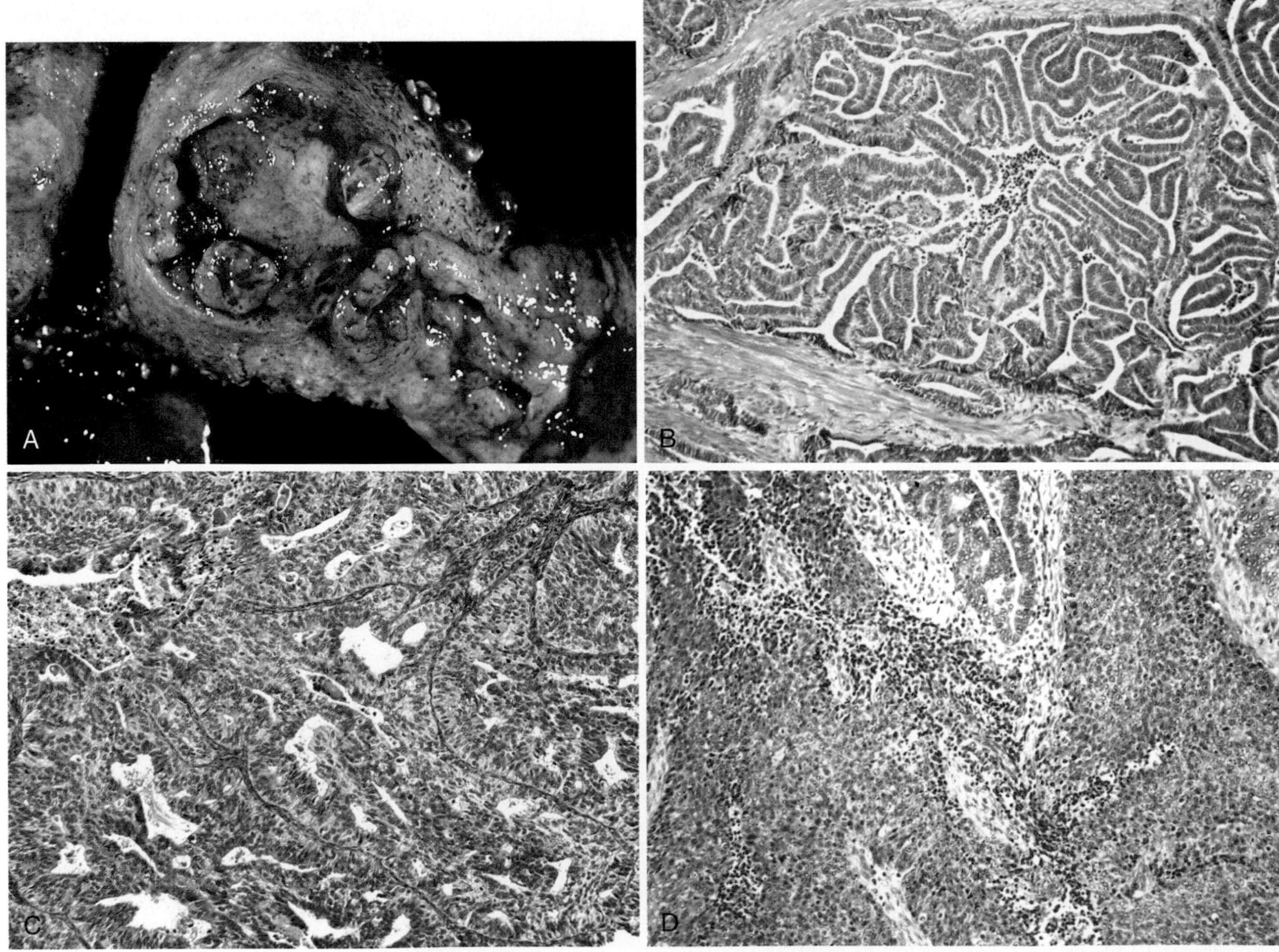

Figure 22-25 Type I endometrial carcinoma. **A,** Endometrial adenocarcinoma presenting as a fungating mass in the fundus of the uterus. **B,** Well-differentiated (grade 1) endometrioid adenocarcinoma with preserved glandular architecture but lack of intervening stroma. **C,** Moderately differentiated (grade 2) endometrioid adenocarcinoma with glandular architecture admixed with solid areas. **D,** Poorly differentiated (grade 3) endometrioid adenocarcinoma with a predominantly solid growth pattern.

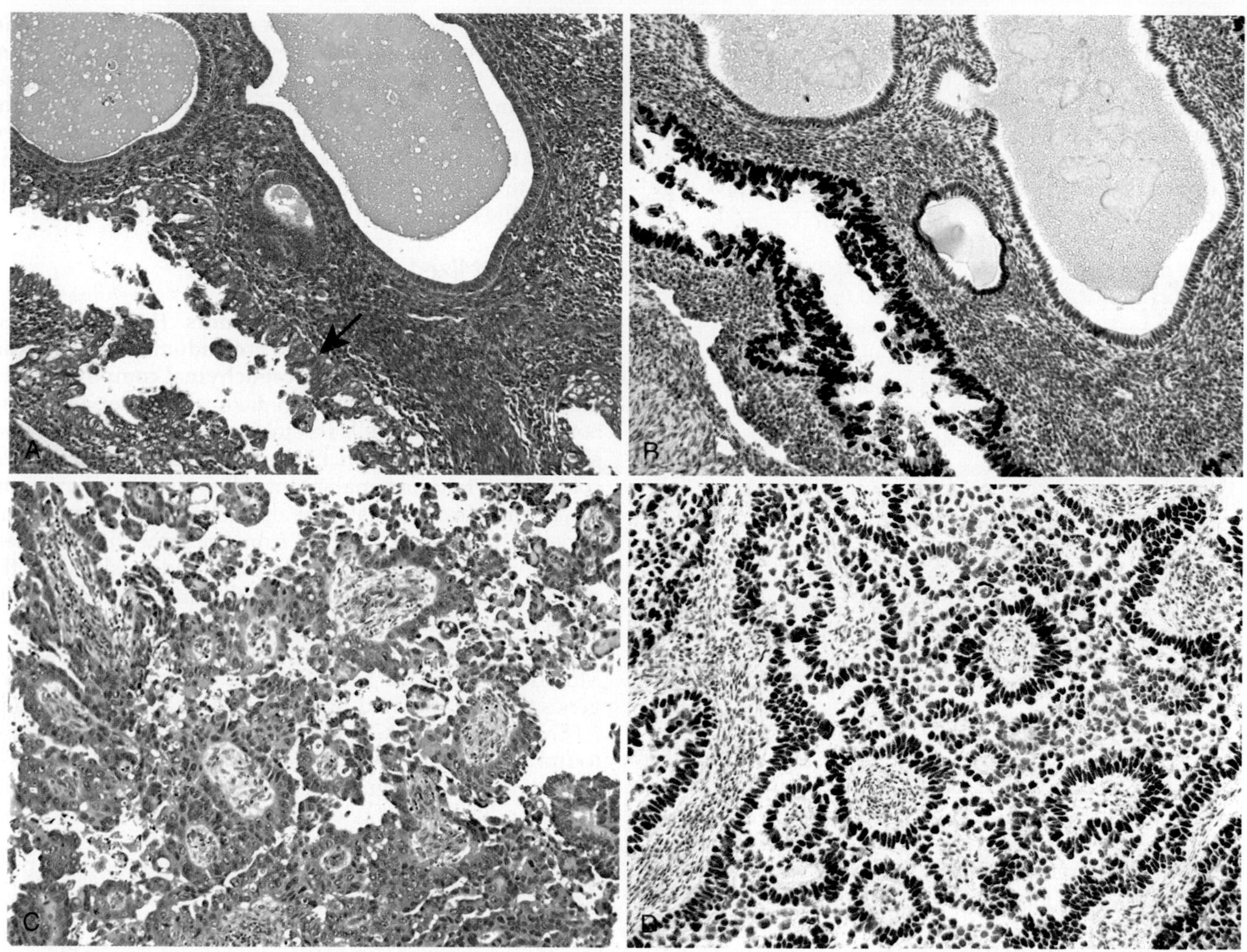

Figure 22-26 Type II endometrial carcinoma. **A,** Endometrial intraepithelial carcinoma, the precursor to serous carcinoma showing malignant cells *(arrow)* with morphologic features identical to serous carcinoma lining the surfaces of the endometrial glands without obvious stromal invasion. **B,** Strong, diffuse expression of p53 as detected by immunohistochemistry in endometrial intraepithelial carcinoma. **C,** Serous carcinoma of the endometrium with papillary growth pattern consisting of malignant cells with marked cytologic atypia including high nuclear-to-cytoplasmic ratio, atypical mitotic figures, and hyperchromasia. **D,** As with the previous lesion, there is an accumulation of p53 protein in the nucleus.

Pathologic staging of both type I and II endometrial adenocarcinoma and malignant mixed müllerian tumors (described later) is as follows:

Stage I—Carcinoma is confined to the corpus uteri itself.

Stage II—Carcinoma involves the corpus and the cervix.

Stage III—Carcinoma extends outside the uterus but not outside the true pelvis.

Stage IV—Carcinoma extends outside the true pelvis or involves the mucosa of the bladder or the rectum.

Type II (Serous) Carcinoma. These generally occur in women who are about 10 years older than those with type I carcinomas, and in contrast to type I carcinoma they usually arise in the setting of *endometrial atrophy* (Fig. 22-24*B*). Type II tumors are by definition poorly differentiated (grade 3) tumors and account for approximately 15% of cases of endometrial carcinoma. The most common subtype is *serous carcinoma*, referred to as such because of morphologic and biologic overlap with ovarian serous carcinoma. Several less common histologic subtypes (clear cell carcinoma and malignant mixed müllerian tumor) are also included within this category.

Mutations in the tumor suppressor *TP53* are present in at least 90% of serous endometrial carcinoma. The majority are missense mutations that result in an accumulation of the altered protein (Fig. 22-26*B* and *D*). The precursor of serous carcinoma, serous endometrial intraepithelial carcinoma, consists of cells identical to those of serous carcinoma but lacks identifiable stromal invasion. Mutations in *TP53* are also found in approximately 75% of endometrial intraepithelial carcinoma, suggesting that mutation of *TP53* is an early event in the evolution of serous endometrial carcinoma. Thus, serous carcinoma presumably begins as a surface epithelial neoplasm that extends into adjacent gland structures and later invades endometrial stroma. Their generally poorer prognosis is thought to be a consequence of a propensity to exfoliate, travel through the fallopian tubes, and implant on peritoneal surfaces like their ovarian counterparts. They have often spread outside of the uterus at the time of diagnosis. Recent whole-exome sequencing studies have detected mutations in a number of additional genes, including those encoding PI3K and PP2A (a tumor suppressive phosphatase that is the target of the certain viral oncoproteins), in a significant number of serous carcinomas. Mutations in the genes encoding these two proteins are also found in serous endometrial intraepithelial carcinoma, suggesting that (like *TP53* mutations) they occur early in the development of this aggressive type of endometrial carcinoma.

MORPHOLOGY

Generally, serous carcinomas arise in small atrophic uteri and are often large bulky tumors or deeply invasive into the myometrium. The precursor lesion, **serous endometrial intraepithelial carcinoma,** consists of malignant cells identical to those of serous carcinoma that are confined to the epithelial surfaces (Fig. 22-26*A* and *B*). The invasive lesions may have a papillary growth pattern composed of cells with marked cytologic atypia including high nuclear-to-cytoplasmic ratio, atypical mitotic figures, hyperchromasia, and prominent nucleoli (Fig. 22-26*C* and *D*). However, they can also have a predominantly glandular growth pattern; in such cases they are distinguished from endometrioid carcinoma by the marked cytologic atypia. All of the tumors in this category are classified as grade 3 irrespective of histologic pattern. Serous carcinoma, despite relatively superficial endometrial involvement, may be associated with extensive peritoneal disease, suggesting spread by routes (i.e., tubal or lymphatic transmission) other than direct invasion.

Clinical Features. Carcinoma of the endometrium is uncommon in women younger than 40 years of age; the peak incidence is in postmenopausal women 55 to 65 years of age. There is no currently available screening test for carcinoma of the endometrium. Although it may be asymptomatic for a period of time, it usually produces irregular or postmenopausal vaginal bleeding with excessive leukorrhea. Fortunately, postmenopausal bleeding often leads to early detection, and cures are possible in most patients. Uterine enlargement may be absent in the early stages. The diagnosis of endometrial cancer must be established by histologic examination of tissue obtained by biopsy or curettage.

As would be anticipated, the prognosis depends heavily on the clinical stage at diagnosis, as well as histologic grade and subtype. In the United States, most tumors (about 80%) are stage I well-differentiated or moderately differentiated endometrioid carcinomas. Surgery, alone or in combination with irradiation, gives about 90% 5-year survival in stage I (grade 1 or 2) disease. This rate drops to approximately 75% for grade 3/stage I tumors and to 50% or less for stage II and III endometrial carcinomas.

As mentioned, serous carcinoma has a propensity for extrauterine (lymphatic or transtubal) spread, even when apparently confined to the endometrium or its surface epithelium. For unknown reasons, serous carcinoma occurs more frequently in women of African American descent, a difference that accounts for a two fold higher mortality rate in African American women compared with Caucasian women. Overall, the 5-year survival for women with serous carcinoma is 18% to 27% and even when it is confined to the uterus the recurrence rate is as high as 80%. Adjuvant radiation is often used to reduce local recurrence and chemotherapy is given to women with endometrioid carcinoma when it has spread beyond the uterus. However, because of the aggressive nature of serous carcinoma, women may be treated with chemotherapy even in the absence of detectable extrauterine spread. Inhibitors of the PI3K/AKT pathway are being tested in clinical trials and the continued identification of biologic targets is likely to expand the roster of rational therapies in the future.

Malignant Mixed Müllerian Tumors

Malignant mixed müllerian tumors (MMMTs) (also referred to as *carcinosarcomas*) are endometrial adenocarcinomas with a malignant mesenchymal component. The mesenchymal component can take a number of forms. Some contain tumor cells resembling uterine mesenchymal elements (stromal sarcoma, leiomyosarcoma), while others contain heterologous malignant cell types (rhabdomyosarcoma, chondrosarcoma). The epithelial and stromal components appear to be derived from the same founding cell, a concept supported by molecular studies showing the presence of shared mutations. Both clinicopathologic and molecular studies suggest that the vast majority of these tumors are carcinomas with sarcomatous differentiation. Mutations found in MMMTs tend to involve the same genes that are mutated in endometrial carcinoma, such as *PTEN*, *TP53*, and *PIK3CA*, while alterations typical of those found in sarcomas are absent. At present, the mechanisms underlying the sarcomatous transformation are unknown, but some abnormality of epigenetic regulation seems likely.

MORPHOLOGY

MMMTs are often bulky and polypoid, and may protrude through the cervical os. On histology, the tumors usually consist of adenocarcinoma (endometrioid, serous, or clear cell) mixed with the malignant mesenchymal (sarcomatous) elements (Fig. 22-27A); alternatively, the tumor may contain two distinct and separate epithelial and mesenchymal components. Sarcomatous components may also mimic extrauterine tissues (e.g., striated muscle, cartilage, adipose tissue, and bone). Metastases usually contain only epithelial components (Fig. 22-27*B*).

MMMTs occur in postmenopausal women and present with bleeding. Outcome is determined primarily by depth of invasion and stage. The only other known prognostic factor is the differentiation of the mesenchymal component; patients with tumors that have heterologous mesenchymal components do worse than those whose tumors do not. Overall 5-year survival rates are 25% to 30% for patients with high-stage disease.

KEY CONCEPTS

Endometrial Carcinoma

- Endometrial carcinoma is the most common malignancy of the female genital tract.
- There are two major types of endometrial carcinoma: type I and type II. Type I tumors are low-grade and usually indolent; type II tumors are high-grade aggressive tumors and have a poor prognosis.

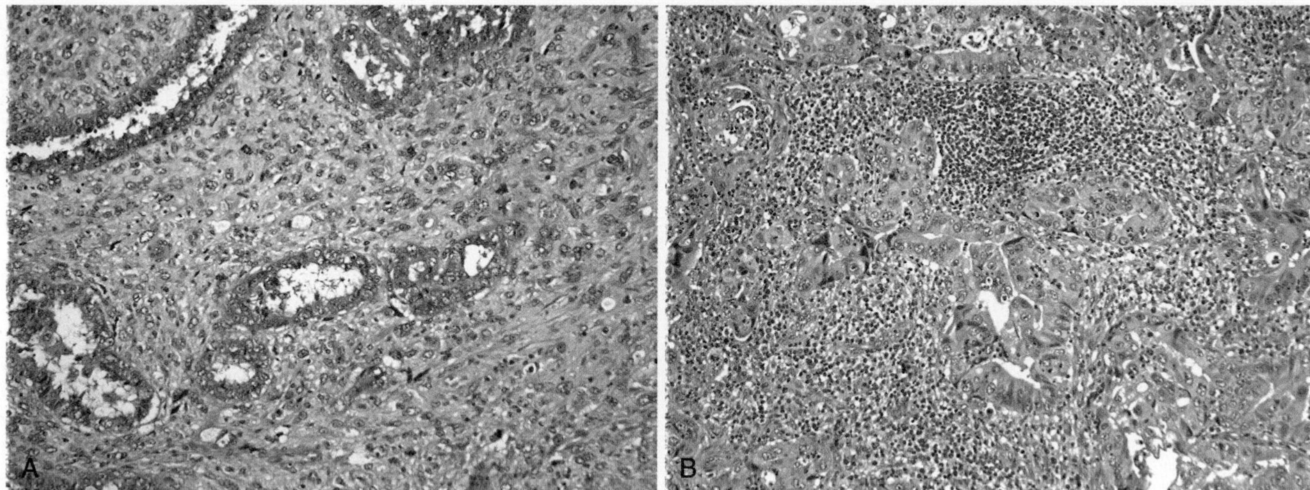

Figure 22-27 Malignant mixed müllerian tumor (MMMT). **A,** Micrograph showing both malignant epithelial and stromal components. **B,** Lymph node metastasis from a MMMT showing only the epithelial component, as is typically the case.

- Endometrioid (type I) carcinoma is often preceded by atypical hyperplasia and commonly has mutations in the *PTEN*, *PIK3CA*, *KRAS*, and *ARID1A* genes.
- Serous (type II) carcinoma is associated with serous endometrial intraepithelial carcinoma and the most common mutations are in *TP53*. *TP53* mutations are also found in precursor lesions.
- Stage remains the most important factor in outcome; serous tumors are much more likely to present at advanced stage and have a decidedly worse prognosis.
- Malignant mixed müllerian tumors (MMMTs) are carcinosarcomas that resemble endometrial carcinoma genetically and have poor outcomes with current therapies.

Tumors of Endometrial Stroma

These relatively uncommon tumors comprise less than 5% of endometrial cancers and include stromal neoplasms admixed with benign glands (adenosarcomas) and pure stromal neoplasms.

Adenosarcomas

Adenosarcomas present most commonly as large broad-based endometrial polypoid growths that may prolapse through the cervical os. The diagnosis is based on the presence of malignant-appearing stroma, which coexists with benign but abnormally shaped endometrial glands. These tumors predominate in women between the fourth and fifth decades and are generally considered to be a low-grade malignancy; recurrences develop in one fourth of cases and are nearly always confined to the pelvis. The principal diagnostic dilemma is distinguishing these tumors from large benign polyps. The distinction is important, because adenosarcoma is estrogen-sensitive and responds to oophorectomy.

Stromal Tumors

The endometrium occasionally gives rise to neoplasms that resemble normal stromal cells. Endometrial stromal neoplasms are divided into two categories: (1) benign stromal nodules and (2) endometrial stromal sarcomas. The stromal sarcomas may be further divided into low-grade and high-grade types depending on their differentiation.

Clues to the pathogenesis of stromal sarcomas have come from the identification of several recurrent chromosomal aberrations that are quite specific for these malignancies. As with many sarcomas, stromal sarcomas are associated with chromosomal translocations that create fusion genes. Low-grade endometrial stromal sarcomas usually have translocations in which portions of the *JAZF1* gene, which encode a transcriptional repressor, is fused to a second gene belonging to the polycomb gene family, such as *SUZ12*. Polycomb proteins participate in complexes that introduce repressive histone marks into chromatin, thereby silencing genes, and it is hypothesized that the JAZF1 fusion proteins act by disrupting the function of the polycomb complex, leading to misexpression of oncogenic genes. Recently, high-grade endometrial stromal sarcomas have been observed to contain different chromosomal translocations that also result in the formation of fusion genes, which are presumed to be pathogenically significant but are currently of unknown function.

About half of stromal sarcomas recur; relapse rates range from 36% to more than 80% for stage I and stage III/IV tumors, respectively. Unfortunately, relapse is not reliably predicted by either mitotic index or the degree of cytologic atypia. Distant metastases may announce their presence decades after the initial diagnosis, and death from metastatic tumor occurs in about 15% of cases. Five-year survival rates average 50% for low-grade tumors and are even lower for high-grade tumors.

Tumors of the Myometrium

Leiomyomas

Uterine leiomyoma (commonly called *fibroids*) is perhaps the most common tumor in women. They are benign smooth muscle neoplasms that may occur singly, but more often are multiple. Most leiomyomas have normal karyotypes, but approximately 40% have a simple chromosomal abnormality. Several cytogenetic subgroups are recognized, including tumors with rearrangements of chromosomes 12q14 and 6p involving the *HMGIC* and *HMGIY* genes, respectively, which are also implicated in a variety of other benign neoplasms. Both genes encode closely related DNA-binding factors that regulate chromatin structure. Recently, mutations in the *MED12* gene have been identified in up to 70% of uterine leiomyomas. The *MED12* gene encodes a component of Mediator, a multiprotein complex that stimulates gene expression by serving as a bridge between long-range DNA regulatory elements (so-called enhancers) and gene promoters. The effect of *MED12* mutations on gene expression in leiomyomas is an area of active investigation.

MORPHOLOGY

Leiomyomas are sharply circumscribed, discrete, round, firm, gray-white tumors varying in size from small, barely visible nodules to massive tumors that fill the pelvis. Except in rare instances, they are found within the myometrium of the corpus. Only infrequently do they involve the uterine ligaments, lower uterine segment, or cervix. They can occur within the myometrium (intramural), just beneath the endometrium (submucosal) or beneath the serosa (subserosal) (Fig. 22-28*A*).

Whatever their size, the characteristic whorled pattern of smooth muscle bundles on cut section usually makes these lesions readily identifiable. Large tumors may develop areas of yellow-brown to red softening.

Leiomyomas are typically composed of bundles of smooth muscle cells that resemble the uninvolved myometrium (Fig. 22-28*B*). Usually, the individual muscle cells are uniform in size and shape and have the characteristic oval nucleus and long, slender bipolar cytoplasmic processes. Mitotic figures are scarce. Benign variants of leiomyoma include atypical or bizarre (symplastic) tumors with nuclear atypia and giant cells, and cellular leiomyomas. Both have a low mitotic index, helping to distinguish these benign tumors from leiomyosarcomas. An extremely rare variant, **benign metastasizing leiomyoma**, is a uterine leiomyoma that extends into vessels and spreads hematogenously to other sites, most commonly the lung. Another variant, **disseminated peritoneal leiomyomatosis**, presents as multiple small peritoneal nodules. Both are considered benign despite their unusual behavior.

Leiomyomas of the uterus, even when large or numerous, may be asymptomatic. Common signs and symptoms include abnormal bleeding, urinary frequency due to compression of the bladder, sudden pain from infarction of a large or pedunculated tumor, and impaired fertility. Myomas in pregnant women increase the frequency of spontaneous abortion, fetal malpresentation, uterine inertia (failure to contract with sufficient force), and postpartum hemorrhage. Malignant transformation to leiomyosarcoma, if it occurs at all, is extremely rare.

Leiomyosarcomas

These uncommon malignant neoplasms are thought to arise from the myometrium or endometrial stromal precursor cells, rather than leiomyomas. In contrast to leiomyomas, leiomyosarcomas have complex, highly variable karyotypes that frequently include deletions. Like leiomyomas, a subset contains *MED12* mutations, a genetic aberration that appears to be virtually unique to uterine smooth muscle tumors.

MORPHOLOGY

Leiomyosarcomas grow within the uterus in two somewhat distinctive patterns: (1) bulky, fleshy masses that invade the uterine wall or (2) polypoid masses that project into the uterine lumen (Fig. 22-29*A*). They exhibit a wide range of cytologic atypia, from extremely well differentiated to highly anaplastic (Fig. 22-29*B*). The distinction from leiomyoma is based on nuclear atypia, mitotic index, and zonal necrosis. With few

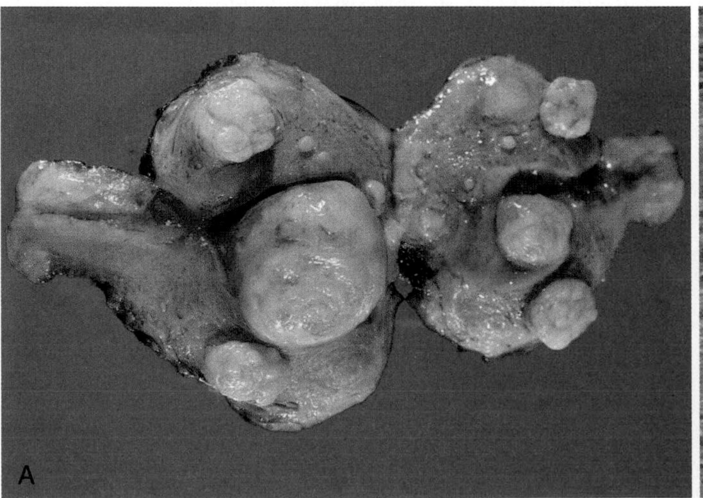

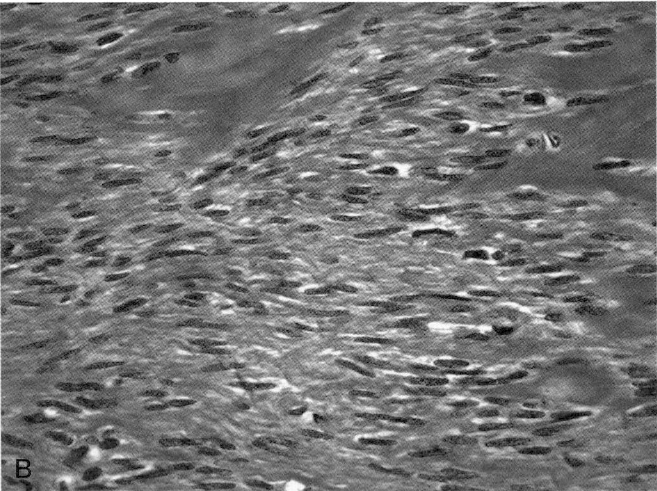

Figure 22-28 Leiomyomas of the uterine myometrium **A,** The uterus is opened to reveal multiple tumors in submucosal (bulging into the endometrial cavity), intramural, and subserosal locations that display a firm white appearance on sectioning. **B,** Leiomyoma showing well-differentiated, regular, spindle-shaped smooth muscle cells associated with hyalinization.

exceptions, the presence of 10 or more mitoses per 10 high-power (400×) fields indicates malignancy, particularly if accompanied by cytologic atypia and/or necrosis. If the tumor contains nuclear atypia or large (epithelioid) cells, five mitoses per 10 high-power (400×) fields are sufficient to justify a diagnosis of malignancy. Rare exceptions include mitotically active leiomyomas in young or pregnant women, and caution should be exercised in interpreting such neoplasms as malignant. A proportion of smooth muscle neoplasms may be impossible to classify and are called smooth muscle tumors of "uncertain malignant potential."

Leiomyosarcomas occur both before and after menopause, with a peak incidence at 40 to 60 years of age. These tumors often recur following surgery, and more than half eventually metastasize hematogenously to distant organs, such as lungs, bone, and brain. Dissemination throughout the abdominal cavity is also encountered. The overall 5-year survival rate is about 40%, but the anaplastic lesions have a 5-year survival rate of only 10% to 15%.

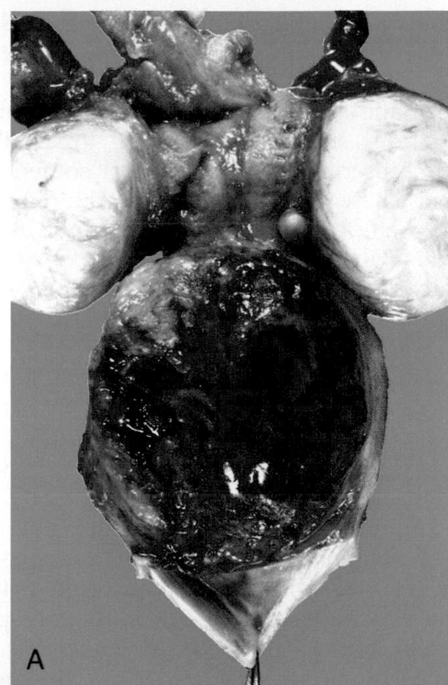

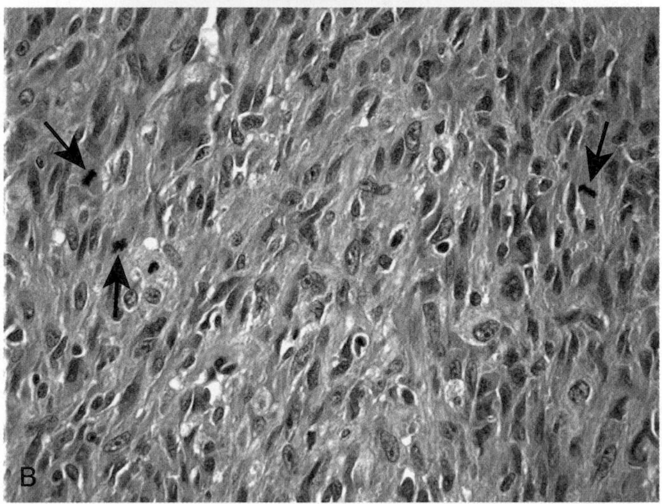

Figure 22-29 Leiomyosarcoma. **A,** A large hemorrhagic tumor mass distends the lower corpus and is flanked by two leiomyomas. **B,** The tumor cells are irregular in size and have hyperchromatic nuclei. Numerous mitotic figures are present *(arrows)*.

KEY CONCEPTS

- Endometrial stromal tumors include stromal nodules, low-grade stromal sarcomas, and high-grade stromal sarcomas.
  - Stromal nodules are benign, well-circumscribed tumors.
  - Low-grade stromal sarcomas resemble stromal nodules, but infiltrate into the surrounding myometrium. They are associated with fusion of the *JAZF1* gene and various polycomb factor genes, usually *SUZ12*.
  - High-grade stromal sarcomas show marked atypia and are associated with other gene fusions.
  - Both low- and high-grade stromal sarcomas are prone to late recurrences.
- Leiomyomas are common benign smooth muscle tumors that cause significant morbidity and are often associated with *MED12* mutations.
- Leiomyosarcomas (malignant smooth muscle tumors) are uncommon, highly malignant myometrial tumors that usually arise de novo

FALLOPIAN TUBES

The most common disorders affecting the fallopian tube are infections and associated inflammatory conditions, followed in frequency by ectopic (tubal) pregnancy and endometriosis.

Inflammations

Suppurative salpingitis may be caused by any pyogenic organism, and in some cases more than one organism is involved. *Gonococcus* is the causative organism in more than 60% of cases of this disorder, with *Chlamydiae* being responsible for many of the remaining cases. These tubal infections are a part of pelvic inflammatory disease, described earlier in this chapter.

Tuberculous salpingitis is rare in the United States, accounting for not more than 1% to 2% of all forms of salpingitis. It is more common, however, in parts of the world where tuberculosis is prevalent and is an important cause of infertility in these areas.

Tumors and Cysts

The most common primary lesions of the fallopian tube (excluding endometriosis) are minute, 0.1- to 2-cm translucent cysts filled with clear serous fluid, called *paratubal cysts*. Larger varieties are found near the fimbriated end of the tube or in the broad ligaments and are referred to as *hydatids of Morgagni*. These cysts, lined by benign serous (tubal type) epithelium, are presumed to arise in remnants of the müllerian duct and are of little significance.

Tumors of the fallopian tube are uncommon. Benign tumors include *adenomatoid tumors* (mesotheliomas), which occur subserosally on the tube or sometimes in the mesosalpinx. These small nodules are the exact counterparts of the adenomatoid tumors that occur in the testes or epididymis (Chapter 21). Primary *adenocarcinoma* of the fallopian tubes is rare. It usually presents as a dominant tubal mass that may be detected by pelvic examination. Other fallopian adenocarcinomas come to attention due to abnormal discharge, bleeding, or (occasionally) abnormal cells in a Pap smear. Approximately one half of tumors are stage I at diagnosis, but nearly 40% of affected patients are dead within 5 years, with higher stage tumors pursuing an even more aggressive course. Patients are typically treated with ovarian cancer chemotherapy protocols. Recently, data have accumulated to suggest that at least a subset of "serous ovarian cancers" actual arise from the epithelium of the fallopian tube (discussed later).

OVARIES

The most common lesions encountered in the ovary are functional or benign cysts and tumors. Neoplastic disorders can be grouped according to their origin from each of the three main ovarian cell types: (1) müllerian epithelium, (2) germ cells, and (3) sex cord-stromal cells. Primary inflammations of the ovary (oophoritis) are uncommon, and on rare occasions may have an autoimmune basis (autoimmune oophoritis); the autoimmune reactions affect the ovarian follicles and may lead to infertility.

Nonneoplastic and Functional Cysts

Follicle and Luteal Cysts

Cystic follicles are very common in the ovary. They originate from unruptured graafian follicles or in follicles that have ruptured and immediately sealed.

MORPHOLOGY

These cysts are usually multiple. They range in size up to 2 cm in diameter, are filled with a clear serous fluid, and are lined by a gray, glistening membrane. On occasion, larger cysts exceeding 2 cm (follicle cysts) may be diagnosed by palpation or ultrasonography; these may cause pelvic pain. Granulosa lining cells are present if the intraluminal pressure has not been so great as to cause their atrophy. The outer theca cells may be conspicuous due to increased amounts of pale cytoplasm (a change referred to as luteinization). As discussed subsequently, when luteinization is pronounced (hyperthecosis), it may be associated with increased estrogen production and endometrial abnormalities.

Luteal cysts (corpora lutea) are present in the normal ovaries of women of reproductive age. These cysts are lined by a rim of bright yellow tissue containing luteinized granulosa cells. They occasionally rupture and cause a peritoneal reaction. Sometimes the combination of old hemorrhage and fibrosis may make their distinction from endometriotic cysts difficult.

Polycystic Ovaries and Stromal Hyperthecosis

Polycystic ovarian syndrome **(PCOS) is a complex endocrine disorder characterized by hyperandrogenism, menstrual abnormalities, polycystic ovaries, chronic anovulation, and decreased fertility.** Formerly called Stein Leventhal syndrome, it affects 6-10% of reproductive age women worldwide. It is also associated with obesity, type 2 diabetes, and premature atherosclerosis, all of which may be indicative of an underlying metabolic disorder. The etiology of PCOS remains incompletely understood. It is marked by a dysregulation of enzymes involved in androgen biosynthesis and excessive androgen production, which is considered to be a central feature of this disorder. In addition, women with PCOS show insulin resistance and altered adipose tissue metabolism, which contribute to the development of both diabetes and obesity.

The central morphologic abnormality of PCOS is numerous cystic follicles or follicle cysts that enlarge the ovaries. However, polycystic ovaries are detected in 20% to 30% of all women, so this finding is not specific. In addition, due to an increase in free serum estrone levels, women with PCOS are at risk for endometrial hyperplasia and carcinoma.

Stromal hyperthecosis, also called cortical stromal hyperplasia, is a disorder of ovarian stroma most often seen in postmenopausal women, but it may overlap with PCOS in younger women. The disorder is characterized by uniform enlargement of the ovary (up to 7 cm), which has a white to tan appearance on sectioning. The involvement is usually bilateral and microscopically shows hypercellular stroma and luteinization of the stromal cells, which are visible as discrete nests of cells with vacuolated cytoplasm. The clinical presentation and effects on the endometrium are similar to those of PCOS, although virilization may be even more striking.

A physiologic condition mimicking the aforementioned syndromes is *theca lutein hyperplasia of pregnancy*. In response to pregnancy hormones (gonadotropins), theca cells proliferate and the perifollicular zone expands. As the follicles regress, the concentric theca-lutein hyperplasia may appear nodular. This change is not to be confused with true luteomas of pregnancy (see later).

Ovarian Tumors

There are numerous types of ovarian tumors. About 80% are benign, and these occur mostly in young women between the ages of 20 and 45 years. Borderline tumors occur at slightly older ages. Malignant tumors are more common in older women, between the ages of 45 and 65 years. Ovarian cancer accounts for 3% of all cancers in females and is the fifth most common cause of death due to cancer in women in the United States. **Because most ovarian cancers have spread beyond the ovary by the time of diagnosis, they account for a disproportionate number of deaths from cancer of the female genital tract.**

Classification. The classification of ovarian tumors given in Table 22-5 is a simplified version of the World Health Organization Histological Classification, which separates ovarian neoplasms according to the most probable tissue of origin. It is now believed that most tumors of the ovary arise ultimately from one of three ovarian components:

- surface/fallopian tube epithelium and endometriosis
- germ cells, which migrate to the ovary from the yolk sac and are pluripotent
- stromal cells, including the sex cords, which are forerunners of the endocrine apparatus of the postnatal ovary

There is also a group of tumors that defy classification, and finally there are secondary or metastatic tumors to the ovary.

Although some of the specific tumors have distinctive features and are hormonally active, most are nonfunctional and tend to produce relatively mild symptoms until they reach a large size. Some of these tumors, principally epithelial tumors, tend to be bilateral. Table 22-6 lists the tumors and their subtypes. Abdominal pain and distention, urinary and gastrointestinal tract symptoms due to compression by the tumor or cancer invasion, and vaginal bleeding are the most common symptoms. The benign forms may be entirely asymptomatic and occasionally are found unexpectedly on abdominal or pelvic examination or during surgery.

Table 22-5 WHO Classification of Ovarian Neoplasms

Surface Epithelial-Stromal Tumors
Serous tumors
Benign (cystadenoma, cystadenofibroma)
Borderline (serous borderline tumor)
Malignant (low- and high-grade serous adenocarcinoma)
Mucinous tumors, endocervical-like and intestinal type
Benign (cystadenoma, cystadenofibroma)
Borderline (mucinous borderline tumor)
Malignant (mucinous adenocarcinoma)
Endometrioid tumors
Benign (cystadenoma, cystadenofibroma)
Borderline (endometrioid borderline tumor)
Malignant (endometrioid adenocarcinoma)
Clear cell tumors
Benign
Borderline
Malignant (clear cell adenocarcinoma)
Transitional cell tumors
Benign Brenner tumor
Brenner tumor of borderline malignancy
Malignant Brenner tumor
Epithelial-stromal
Adenosarcoma
Malignant mixed müllerian tumor
Sex Cord-Stromal Tumors
Granulosa tumors
Fibromas
Fibrothecomas
Thecomas
Sertoli-Leydig cell tumors
Steroid (lipid) cell tumors
Germ Cell Tumors
Teratoma
Immature
Mature
Solid
Cystic (dermoid cyst)
Monodermal (e.g., struma ovarii, carcinoid)
Dysgerminoma
Yolk sac tumor
Mixed germ cell tumors
Metastatic Cancer From Non-ovarian Primary
Colonic, appendiceal
Gastric
Pancreaticobiliary
Breast

Table 22-6 Frequency of Major Ovarian Tumors

Type	Percentage of Malignant Ovarian Tumors	Percentage That Are Bilateral
Serous		
Benign (60%)		25
Borderline (15%)	47	30
Malignant (25%)		65
Mucinous		
Benign (80%)		5
Borderline (10%)	3	10
Malignant (10%)		<5
Endometrioid carcinoma	20	40
Undifferentiated carcinoma	10	—
Clear cell carcinoma	6	40
Granulosa cell tumor	5	5
Teratoma		15
Benign (96%)	1	Rare
Malignant (4%)		
Metastatic	5	>50
Others	3	—

Epithelial Tumors

Most primary ovarian neoplasms arise from müllerian epithelium. The classification of these tumors is based on both differentiation and extent of proliferation of the epithelium. There are three major histologic types based on the differentiation of the neoplastic epithelium: *serous, mucinous,* and *endometrioid tumors*. These epithelial proliferations are classified as benign, borderline, and malignant. The benign tumors are often further subclassified based on the components of the tumors, which may include cystic areas (cystadenomas), cystic and fibrous areas (cystadenofibromas), and predominantly fibrous areas (adenofibromas). The borderline tumors and the malignant tumors can also have a cystic component, and when malignant they are sometimes referred to as *cystadenocarcinomas*.

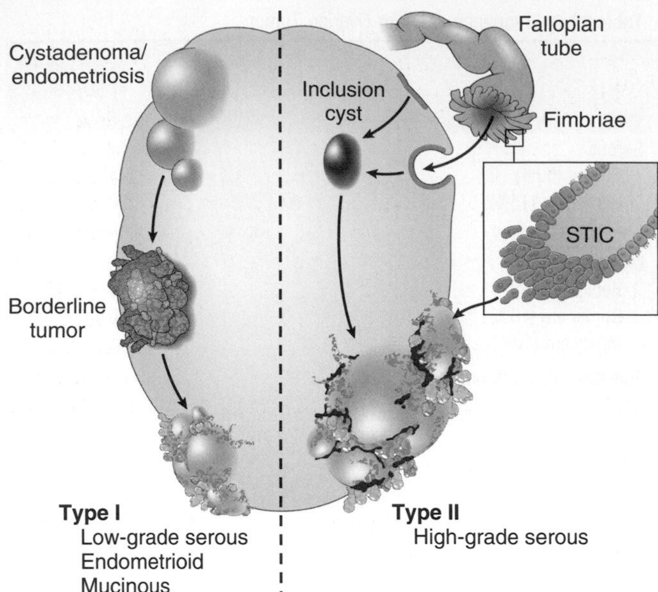

Figure 22-30 Schematic diagram of the pathogenesis of ovarian epithelial tumors. Type I tumors progress from benign tumors through borderline tumors that may give rise to a low-grade carcinoma. These include low-grade serous, endometrioid and mucinous carcinomas. Type II tumors arise from inclusions cysts/fallopian tube epithelium via intraepithelial precursors that are often not identified. They demonstrate high-grade features and are most commonly of serous histology. STIC, serous tubal intraepithelial carcinoma.

The tumors can be relatively small, or they can grow to fill the entire pelvis before they are detected.

Clinicopathologic and molecular studies have suggested that ovarian carcinomas may be broadly categorized into two different types, referred to as type I and type II (Fig. 22-30). Type I carcinomas are low-grade tumors that often arise in association with borderline tumors or endometriosis. These tumors demonstrate several different histologic subtypes including low-grade serous, endometrioid, and mucinous tumors, as discussed later. Type II tumors are most often high-grade serous carcinomas that arise from serous intraepithelial carcinoma (see later).

Serous Tumors

These cystic neoplasms include the most common malignant ovarian tumors and account for approximately 40% of all cancers of the ovary. Although the term *serous* appropriately describes the cyst fluid, it has become synonymous with the tubal-like epithelium in these tumors. Together the benign, borderline, and malignant types account for about 30% of all ovarian tumors and just over 50% of ovarian epithelial tumors. About 70% are benign or borderline, and 30% are malignant. Benign and borderline tumors are most common between the ages of 20 and 45 years. Serous carcinomas occur later in life on average, but often occur at earlier ages in familial cases.

Pathogenesis. Little is known about the risk factors for benign and borderline tumors. Risk factors for malignant serous tumors (serous carcinomas) are also incompletely understood, *but nulliparity, family history, and heritable mutations play a role in tumor development.* There is a higher frequency of carcinoma in women with low parity. Women 40 to 59 years of age who have taken oral contraceptives or undergone tubal ligation have a reduced risk of developing ovarian cancer. The most intriguing risk factors are genetic. As discussed in Chapters 7 and 23, inherited germline mutations in both *BRCA1* and *BRCA2* increase susceptibility to ovarian cancer. *BRCA1* mutations are present in about 5% of patients younger than 70 years of age with ovarian cancer. The estimated risk of ovarian cancer in women bearing *BRCA1* or *BRCA2* mutations is 20% to 60% by the age of 70 years.

Serous ovarian carcinoma is divided into two major groups: (1) low-grade (well-differentiated) carcinoma and (2) high-grade (moderately to poorly differentiated) carcinoma. This distinction is made based on the degree of nuclear atypia and correlates with patient survival. Low-grade carcinomas may arise in association with serous borderline tumors, while high-grade carcinomas arise from in situ lesions in the fallopian tube fimbriae or from serous inclusion cysts within the ovary.

The concept of a fallopian tube origin for high-grade serous carcinomas arose initially from studies on women with *BRCA1/2* germline mutations who were discovered at the time of prophylactic salpingo-oophorectomy to have areas of marked epithelial atypia in their fallopian tubes. The lesions, called serous tubal intraepithelial carcinoma (STIC), have since been described in association with sporadic high-grade serous ovarian cancers, leading to the idea that at least some high-grade serous carcinomas arise from the fallopian tube. What then is the origin of high-grade serous carcinomas that involve the ovary, without concomitant involvement of the fallopian tube? Historically it was thought that the vast majority of serous ovarian carcinomas arose from cortical inclusion cysts (Fig. 22-31). These cysts were thought to arise through invagination of the surface epithelium, followed by serous metaplasia. A recent alternative hypothesis is that the cysts arise from implantation of detached fallopian tube epithelium at sites where ovulation has disrupted the surface of the ovary (Fig. 22-30).

The percentage of sporadic high-grade serous carcinomas that arise in the fallopian tube or from ovarian inclusion cysts is currently unknown, as is the origin of the cortical inclusion cysts. Studies attempting to address these unsettled issues are being pursued. However, this paradigm shift has already altered the management of

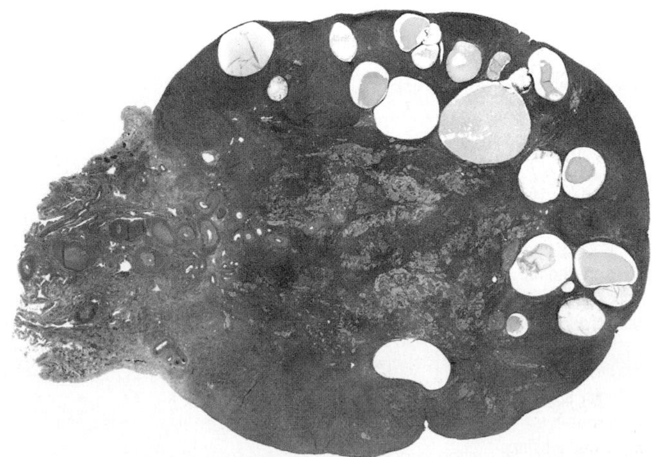

Figure 22-31 Cortical inclusion cysts of the ovary.

women at high-risk for ovarian carcinoma (*BRCA* mutation carriers and women with a strong family history of breast/ovarian cancer), as these women now undergo salpingo-oophorectomy, instead of simple oophorectomy.

Regardless of their origin, studies have shown that low- and high-grade serous carcinomas have distinct mutational profiles, as follows:

- Low-grade tumors arising in serous borderline tumors have mutations in the *KRAS, BRAF,* or *ERBB2* oncogenes, and usually have wild type *TP53* genes.
- High-grade tumors have a high frequency of *TP53* mutations and lack mutations in either *KRAS* or *BRAF*. Genomic imbalances are very common and include amplifications of a number of oncogenes (e.g., *PIK3CA*, the gene encoding the catalytic subunit of PI3K) and deletions of tumor suppressor genes (e.g., *RB*). Almost all ovarian carcinomas arising in women with *BRCA1* or *BRCA2* mutations are high-grade serous carcinomas with *TP53* mutations. Interestingly, *BRCA1/2* mutations are rare in sporadic high-grade serous carcinoma.

MORPHOLOGY

Serous tumors may present as either a multicystic lesion in which papillary epithelium is contained within a few fibrous walled cysts (intracystic) (Fig. 22-32*A*) or as a mass projecting from the ovarian surface. Benign tumors typically have a smooth glistening cyst wall with no epithelial thickening or with small papillary projections. Borderline tumors contain an increased number of papillary projections (Fig. 22-32*A* and *C*). Larger areas of solid or papillary tumor mass, tumor irregularity, and fixation or nodularity of the capsule are features associated with malignancy (Fig. 22-32*B*). Bilaterality is common, occurring in 20% of benign serous cystadenomas, 30% of serous borderline tumors, and approximately 66% of serous carcinomas. A significant proportion of both serous borderline tumors and malignant serous tumors involve the surface of the ovary (Fig. 22-32*C*).

Microscopically, the cysts are lined by columnar epithelium, which has abundant cilia in benign tumors (Fig. 22-33*A*). Microscopic papillae may be found. **Serous borderline tumors** exhibit increased complexity of the stromal papillae, stratification of the epithelium and mild nuclear atypia, but invasion of the stroma is not seen (Fig. 22-33*B*). This epithelial proliferation often grows in a delicate, papillary pattern referred to as "micropapillary carcinoma," which is thought to be the precursor to **low-grade serous carcinoma** (Fig. 22-33*C*). **High-grade serous carcinomas** are distinguished from low-grade tumors by having more complex growth patterns and widespread infiltration or frank effacement of the underlying stroma (Fig. 22-33*D*). The individual tumor cells display marked nuclear atypia, including pleomorphism, atypical mitotic figures, and multinucleation. The serous tubal intraepithelial carcinomas consist of cells morphologically identical to high-grade serous carcinomas but are distinguished by the lack of invasion. The cells of invasive high-grade serous carcinoma can even become so undifferentiated that serous features are no longer recognizable. Concentric calcifications (psammoma bodies) characterize serous tumors, but are not specific for neoplasia. Ovarian serous tumors, both low- and high-grade, have a propensity to spread to the peritoneal surfaces and omentum and are commonly associated with the presence of ascites. As with other tumors, the extent of the spread outside the ovary determines the stage of the disease.

The biologic behavior of serous tumors depends on the degree of differentiation and the distribution and characteristics of the disease in the peritoneum, if present. Importantly, serous tumors may occur on the surface of the ovaries and, rarely, as primary tumors of the peritoneal surface, which are referred to as primary peritoneal serous carcinoma. As discussed, at least some of these carcinomas may originate from the fallopian tube. Predictably, unencapsulated serous tumors of the ovarian surface are more likely to spread to the peritoneal surfaces, and prognosis is closely related to the histologic appearance of the tumor and its growth pattern on the peritoneum. Borderline serous tumors may arise from or extend to the peritoneal surfaces as noninvasive implants, remaining localized and causing no symptoms, or slowly spread, producing intestinal obstruction or other complications after many years. As discussed earlier, low-grade serous carcinomas can arise in borderline serous tumors and may be associated with spread to the peritoneal surfaces. However, low-grade carcinomas, even after spread outside the ovary, often progress slowly, and patients may survive for relatively long periods before dying of disease. In contrast, high-grade tumors are often widely metastatic throughout the abdomen at the time of presentation, a picture

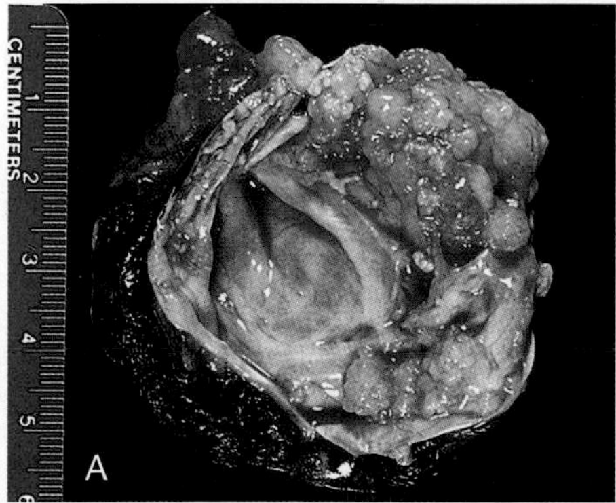

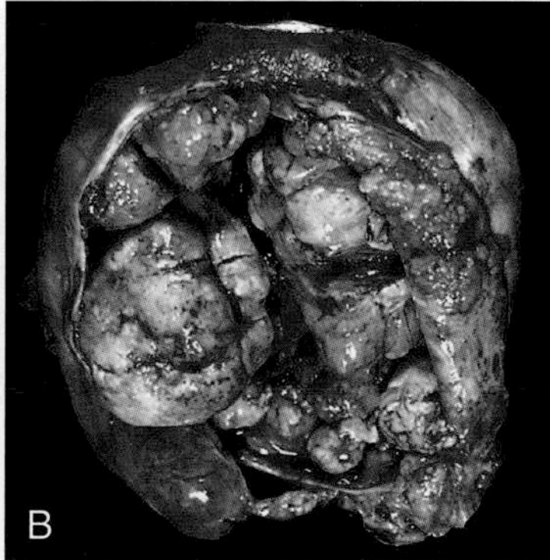

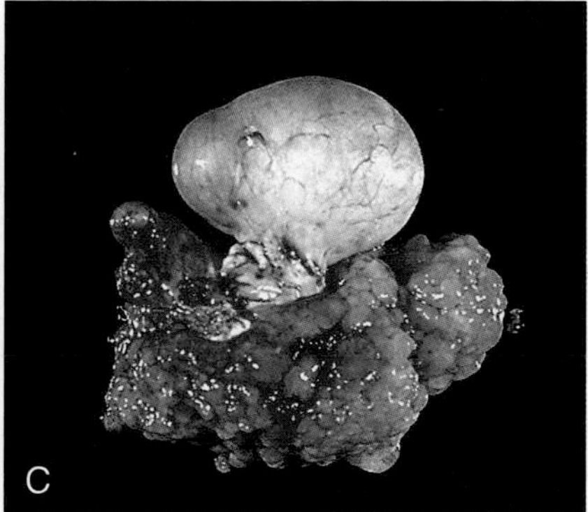

Figure 22-32 Gross appearances of serous tumors of the ovary. **A,** Serous borderline tumor opened to display a cyst cavity lined by delicate papillary tumor growths. **B,** Carcinoma. The cyst is opened to reveal a large, bulky tumor mass. **C,** Another borderline tumor growing on the ovarian surface *(lower)*.

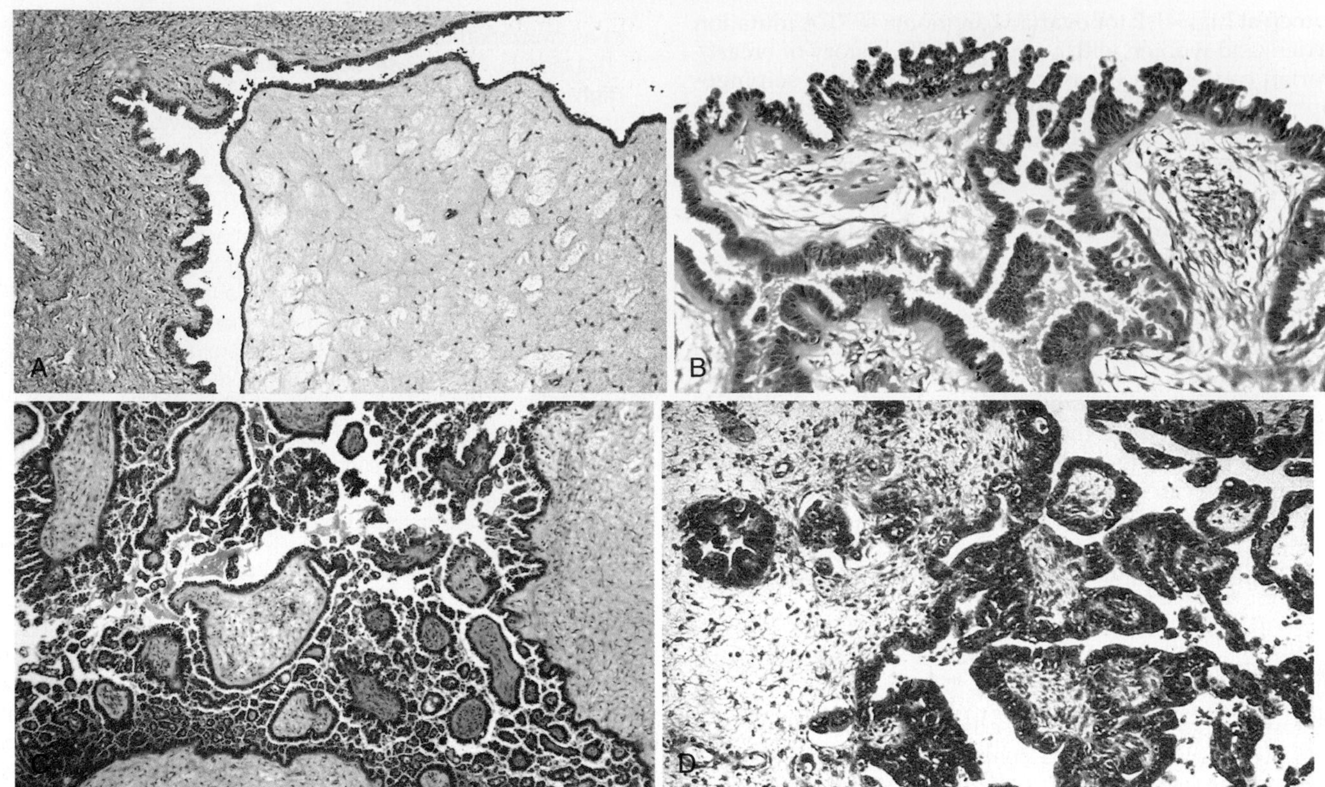

Figure 22-33 Microscopic appearances of serous tumors of the ovary. **A,** Serous cystadenoma revealing stromal papillae with a columnar epithelium. **B,** Borderline serous tumor showing increased architectural complexity and epithelial cell stratification. **C,** Complex micropapillary growth defines a low-grade "micropapillary" serous carcinoma. **D,** High-grade serous carcinoma of the ovary with invasion of underlying stroma.

associated with rapid clinical deterioration. Consequently, pathologic classification of the tumor, even if it has extended to the peritoneum, is relevant to both prognosis and selection of therapy. The 5-year survival rate for borderline and malignant tumors confined to the ovary is, respectively, 100% and 70%, whereas the 5-year survival rate for the same tumors involving the peritoneum is about 90% and 25%, respectively. Because of their protracted course, borderline tumors may recur after many years, and 5-year survival is not synonymous with cure.

Mucinous Tumors

Mucinous tumors account for about 20% to 25% of all ovarian neoplasms. They occur principally in middle adult life and are rare before puberty and after menopause. The vast majority are benign or borderline tumors. Primary ovarian mucinous carcinomas are uncommon and account for approximately 3% of all ovarian cancers.

Pathogenesis. **Mutation of the *KRAS* proto-oncogene is a consistent genetic alteration in mucinous tumors of the ovary**, including the majorities of benign mucinous cystadenomas (58%), mucinous borderline tumors (75% to 86%), and ovarian mucinous carcinomas (85%). Interestingly, one study showed that several tumors with distinct areas of epithelium showing benign, borderline, and carcinoma had identical *KRAS* mutations in each area. Thus, *KRAS* mutations may initiate the development of these neoplasms. The mutations that collaborate with *KRAS* mutations to generate mucinous tumors are largely unknown.

MORPHOLOGY

Mucinous tumors differ from the serous variety in several ways. The surface of the ovary is rarely involved and only 5% of primary mucinous cystadenomas and mucinous carcinomas are bilateral. Mucinous tumors also tend to produce larger cystic masses; some have been recorded with weights of more than 25 kg. They are multiloculated tumors filled with sticky, gelatinous fluid rich in glycoproteins (Fig. 22-34*A*).

Microscopically, benign mucinous tumors are characterized by a lining of tall, columnar epithelial cells with apical mucin that lack cilia. The vast majority demonstrates gastric or intestinal type differentiation, with uncommon tumors showing endocervical type mucinous differentiation instead (Fig. 22-34*B*). Mucinous borderline tumors are distinguished from cystadenomas by epithelial stratification, tufting, and/or papillary intraglandular growth, often producing an appearance strikingly similar to tubular adenomas or villous adenomas of the intestine. **Mucinous carcinomas** characteristically demonstrate confluent glandular growth that is now recognized as a form of "expansile" invasion. Some authors use the term intraepithelial carcinomas for tumors with marked epithelial atypia that lack invasive features. Approximate 10-year survival rates for stage I, noninvasive "intraepithelial carcinomas" and for frankly invasive malignant tumors are greater than 95% and 90%, respectively. Mucinous carcinomas that have spread beyond the ovary are usually fatal, but as previously stated, these tumors are uncommon and must be distinguished from metastatic mucinous adenocarcinomas.

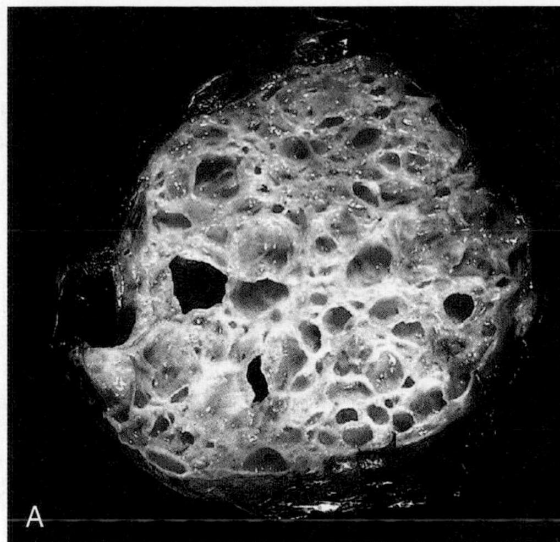

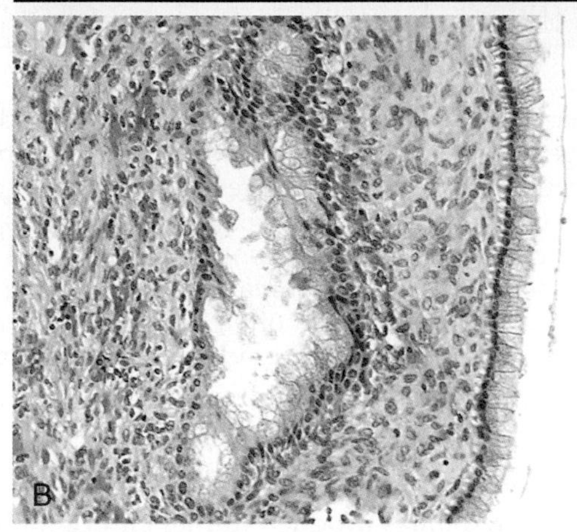

Figure 22-34 Mucinous cystadenoma **A,** Note the multicystic appearance, delicate septa, and the presence of glistening mucin within the cysts. **B,** Columnar cells lining the cysts.

A clinical condition referred to as *pseudomyxoma peritonei* is marked by extensive mucinous ascites, cystic epithelial implants on the peritoneal surfaces, adhesions, and frequent involvement of the ovaries (Fig. 22-35). Pseudomyxoma peritonei, if extensive, may result in intestinal obstruction and death. Historically, it was thought that many cases in women were due to the spread of primary ovarian mucinous neoplasms. However, recent evidence points to the source being, in almost all cases, extraovarian (usually appendiceal) (Chapter 18). Because the majority of primary mucinous ovarian tumors are unilateral, bilateral presentation of mucinous tumors always requires exclusion of a nonovarian origin.

Endometrioid Ovarian Tumors

Endometrioid carcinoma accounts for approximately 10% to 15% of all ovarian cancers. Benign endometrioid tumors, called *endometrioid adenofibromas,* and borderline endometrioid tumors also occur, but are uncommon. Endometrioid tumors are distinguished from serous and mucinous tumors by the presence of tubular glands resembling benign or malignant endometrium. Endometrioid carcinomas may arise in the setting of endometriosis and are occasionally associated with areas of borderline tumor. Although these tumors are less common than either serous or mucinous tumors, more is known about the molecular genetic alterations associated with their development. This is due to the recent development of mouse models that closely mimic the human disease and molecular genetic overlap with endometrioid carcinomas of the endometrium. In fact, 15% to 30% of ovarian endometrioid carcinomas are accompanied by carcinoma of the endometrium, and the relatively good prognosis in such cases suggests that the two arise independently rather than by metastatic spread.

Pathogenesis. **About 15% to 20% of cases with endometrioid carcinoma coexist with endometriosis**. The peak incidence of tumors associated with endometriosis occurs a decade earlier than that of endometrioid carcinomas that are not associated with endometriosis. Molecular studies have found striking similarities to endometrial endometrioid carcinoma; shared features include relatively frequent alterations that increase PI3K/AKT pathway signaling (mutations in *PTEN, PIK3CA, ARID1A,* and *KRAS*) and mutations in mismatch DNA repair genes and *CTNNB1* (β-catenin). As mentioned earlier, mutations in *PTEN* have also been found in atypical endometriosis suggesting that it occurs early in the pathogenesis of ovarian endometrioid carcinoma, as it does in endometrioid carcinoma of the endometrium. Also similar to endometrioid carcinomas of the endometrium, *TP53* mutations are common in poorly differentiated tumors.

MORPHOLOGY

Endometrioid carcinomas typically present with solid and cystic areas of growth. Forty percent involve both ovaries, and such bilaterality usually implies extension of the neoplasm beyond the genital tract. These are low-grade tumors that reveal glandular patterns bearing a strong resemblance to those of endometrial origin. The 5-year survival rate for patients with stage I tumors is approximately 75%.

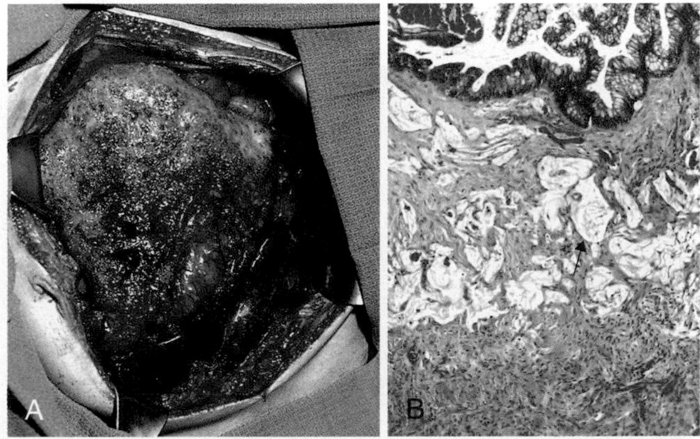

Figure 22-35 Pseudomyxoma peritonei. **A,** View at laparotomy revealing massive overgrowth of a gelatinous metastatic tumor. **B,** Histology of peritoneal implants from an appendiceal tumor, showing mucin-producing epithelium and free mucin *(arrow)*. (**A,** Courtesy Dr. Paul H. Sugarbaker, Washington Hospital Cancer Center, Washington, D.C.)

Clear Cell Carcinoma

Benign and borderline clear cell tumors are exceedingly rare, and clear cell carcinomas are uncommon. They are composed of large epithelial cells with abundant clear cytoplasm, an appearance that resembles hypersecretory gestational endometrium. Because these tumors sometimes occur in association with endometriosis or endometrioid carcinoma of the ovary and resemble clear cell carcinoma of the endometrium, they are now thought to be variants of endometrioid adenocarcinoma. In line with this idea, the most common genetic aberrations (*PIK3CA, ARID1A, KRAS, PTEN,* and *TP53*) are shared with endometrioid carcinoma, albeit at somewhat different frequencies. Clear cell tumors of the ovary can be predominantly solid or cystic. In the solid neoplasms, the clear cells are arranged in sheets or tubules, while in the cystic variety, the neoplastic cells line the spaces. Clear cell carcinoma confined to the ovaries has a 90% 5-year survival, but in advanced stage disease it appears that clear cell morphology portends a poor outcome. Clear cell carcinoma is treated like other types of ovarian carcinoma.

Cystadenofibroma

Cystadenofibromas are uncommon variants in which there is more pronounced proliferation of the fibrous stroma that underlies the columnar lining epithelium. These benign tumors are usually small and multilocular and have simple papillary processes that do not become as complicated and branching as those found in the ordinary cystadenoma. They may contain mucinous, serous, endometrioid, and transitional (Brenner tumors) epithelium. Borderline lesions with cellular atypia and, rarely, tumors with focal areas of carcinoma occur, but metastatic spread of either is extremely uncommon.

Transitional Cell Tumors

Transitional cell tumors contain neoplastic epithelial cells resembling urothelium and are usually benign. They comprise roughly 10% of ovarian epithelial tumors and are also referred to as Brenner tumors. Uncommon transitional cell carcinomas also occur in the ovary.

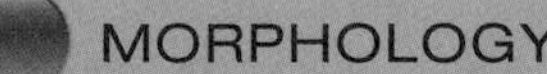

MORPHOLOGY

These neoplasms may be solid or cystic, are usually unilateral (approximately 90%), and vary in size from small lesions less than 1 cm in diameter to massive tumors up to 20 to 30 cm in diameter (Fig. 22-36*A*). The fibrous stroma, resembling that of the normal ovary, is marked by sharply demarcated nests of epithelial cells resembling the epithelium of the urinary tract, often with mucinous glands in their center (Fig. 22-36*B*). Infrequently, the stroma is composed of somewhat plump fibroblasts resembling theca cells; such neoplasms may have hormonal activity. Most Brenner tumors are benign, but borderline (atypical proliferative Brenner tumor) and malignant counterparts have been reported. Tumors with benign Brenner nests admixed with malignant tumor cells are referred to as malignant Brenner tumors, while tumors with greater than 50% malignant transitional type epithelium are considered transitional cell carcinomas of the ovary.

Brenner tumors are often detected incidentally and even when large behave in a benign fashion. Malignant Brenner tumors generally present in stage 1 and for prognostic purposes are considered to be equivalent to low-grade (type 1) carcinomas. The uncommon transitional cell carcinomas are considered to be equivalent to high-grade (type II) ovarian carcinomas; these often present at advanced stage and are treated like high-grade serous carcinomas.

Clinical Course, Detection, and Prevention of Ovarian Epithelial Tumors

All ovarian carcinomas produce similar clinical manifestations, most commonly lower abdominal pain and abdominal enlargement. Gastrointestinal complaints, urinary frequency, dysuria, pelvic pressure, and many other symptoms may appear. Benign lesions are easily resected and cured. The malignant forms tend to cause progressive weakness, weight loss, and cachexia. If the carcinomas extend through the capsule of the tumor to seed the peritoneal cavity, massive ascites is common. Characteristically, the ascitic fluid is filled with exfoliated

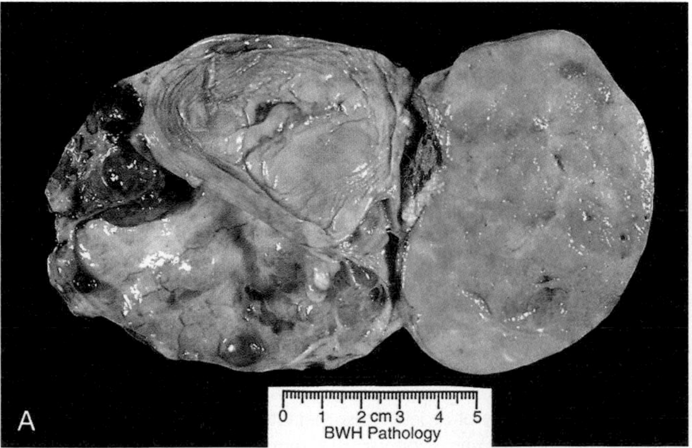

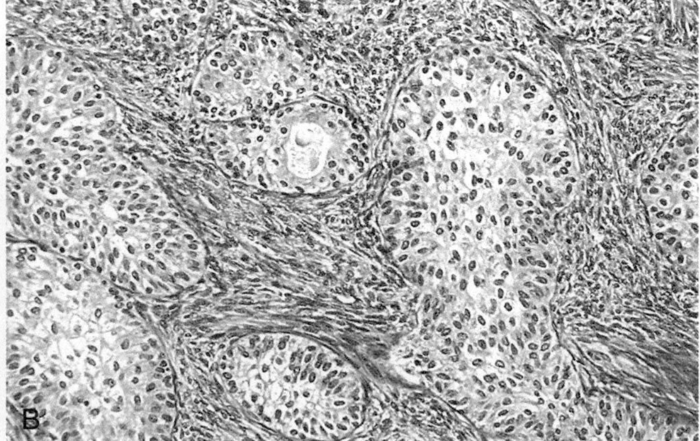

Figure 22-36 Brenner tumor **A,** Brenner tumor *(right)* associated with a benign cystic teratoma *(left)*. **B,** Histologic detail of characteristic epithelial nests within the ovarian stroma. (Courtesy Dr. M. Nucci, Brigham and Women's Hospital, Boston, Mass.)

tumor cells. The peritoneal pattern of spread is distinctive: all serosal surfaces are diffusely seeded with 0.1- to 0.5-cm nodules of tumor that only rarely invade deeply into the underlying parenchyma. The regional nodes are often involved, and metastases may be found in the liver, lungs, gastrointestinal tract, and elsewhere. Metastasis across the midline to the opposite ovary is discovered in about half the cases at surgery and heralds a progressive downhill course and death within a few months or years.

Most women with ovarian carcinoma present with high stage disease. This is the primary reason for the relatively poor 5- and 10-year survival rates of patients with these tumors, compared with rates for patients with cervical or endometrial carcinoma. For these reasons, development of new assays that permit early diagnosis is a top priority. Biochemical tests for tumor antigens or tumor products in the plasma of these patients are being sought vigorously, but none proposed to date has sufficient sensitivity and specificity to be useful. The serum marker CA-125 is used in patients with known disease to monitor disease recurrence/progression.

Prevention of ovarian cancer also remains an elusive goal. Screening to identify women at risk (positive for *BRCA* mutations or with strong family histories) and treatment with prophylactic salpingo-oophorectomy are currently standard, but the long-term impact of these approaches remains to be determined.

KEY CONCEPTS

- Epithelial ovarian tumors are classified into benign, borderline or malignant.
- About 80% of all ovarian epithelial tumors are benign and occur in young women. The malignant tumors occur most commonly in older women and account for approximately 3% of all cancers in women in the United States.
- The majority of the malignant epithelial tumors are high-grade serous carcinomas, which have a poor prognosis in large part due to the fact that they are detected after they have spread beyond the ovary.
- There are three major histologic types of epithelial ovarian tumors: serous, mucinous and endometrioid, all of which have a benign, borderline and malignant category.
- Benign tumors are composed of well-differentiated epithelial cells with minimal proliferation. Borderline tumors show increased cell proliferation, but lack stromal invasion. Malignant tumors show increased epithelial atypia and are defined by the presence of stromal invasion.
- Ovarian carcinomas are currently divided into Type I (low grade) and Type II (high-grade) tumors.
- The origin of ovarian tumors is still under investigation, but it is clear that *BRCA1*- and *BRCA2*-related tumors as well as a subset of sporadic, ovarian serous tumors are likely to arise from fallopian tube epithelium instead of ovarian epithelium.

Germ Cell Tumors

Germ cell tumors constitute 15% to 20% of all ovarian tumors. *Most are benign cystic teratomas*, but others, found principally in children and young adults, may show

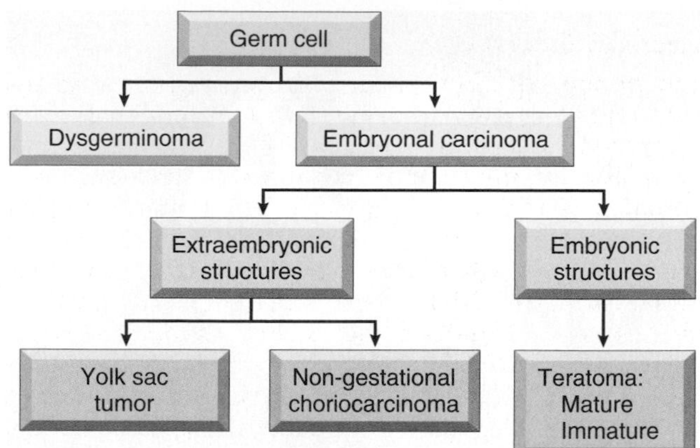

Figure 22-37 Histogenesis and interrelationships of tumors of germ cell origin.

malignant behavior and pose problems in histologic diagnosis and in therapy. They bear a remarkable similarity to germ cell tumors in the male testis (Chapter 21) and arise in a similar manner (Fig. 22-37).

Teratomas

Teratomas are divided into three categories: (1) mature (benign), (2) immature (malignant), and (3) monodermal or highly specialized.

Mature (Benign) Teratomas. Most benign teratomas are cystic and are often referred to as *dermoid cysts*, because they are almost always lined by skin-like structures. Cystic teratomas are usually found in young women during the active reproductive years. They may be discovered incidentally, but are occasionally associated with clinically important paraneoplastic syndromes, such as inflammatory limbic encephalitis, which may remit upon removal of the tumor.

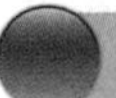

MORPHOLOGY

Benign teratomas are bilateral in 10% to 15% of cases. Characteristically they are unilocular cysts containing hair and sebaceous material (Fig. 22-38). Sectioning reveals a thin wall lined by an opaque, gray-white, wrinkled epidermis, frequently with protruding hair shafts. Within the wall, it is common to find grossly evident tooth structures and areas of calcification.

Microscopically, the cyst wall is composed of stratified squamous epithelium with underlying sebaceous glands, hair shafts, and other skin adnexal structures (Fig. 22-39). In most cases tissues from other germ layers can be identified, such as cartilage, bone, thyroid, and neural tissue. Dermoid cysts are sometimes incorporated within the wall of a mucinous cystadenoma. **About 1% of the dermoids undergo malignant transformation, most commonly to squamous cell carcinoma, but also to other cancers as well (e.g., thyroid carcinoma, melanoma).**

In rare instances a benign teratoma is solid and composed entirely of benign-looking heterogeneous collections of tissues and organized structures derived from all three germ layers. These tumors presumably have the same histogenetic origin as dermoid cysts but lack preponderant differentiation into ectodermal derivatives. These neoplasms may be difficult to distinguish, on gross inspection, from malignant immature teratomas.

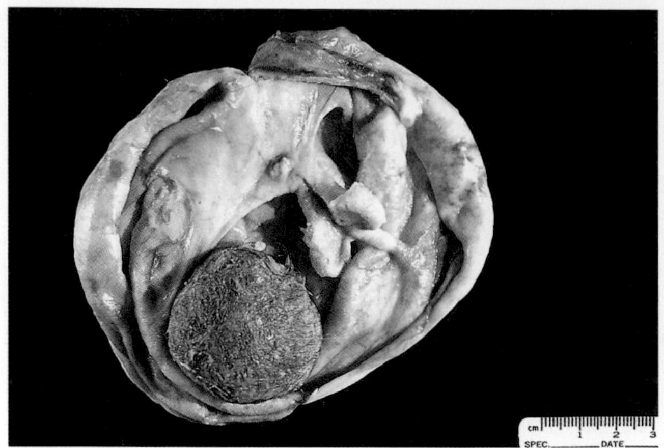

Figure 22-38 Opened mature cystic teratoma (dermoid cyst) of the ovary. Hair *(bottom)* and a mixture of tissues are evident.

The origin of teratomas has been a matter of fascination for centuries. Some common beliefs blamed witches, nightmares, or adultery with the devil. The karyotype of almost all benign ovarian teratomas is 46,XX. Genetic analyses indicate that the majority of teratomas arise from an ovum after the first meiotic division, while a minority arises before the first division.

Monodermal or Specialized Teratomas. The specialized teratomas are a remarkable, rare group of tumors, the most common of which are *struma ovarii* and *carcinoid*. They are always unilateral, although a contralateral teratoma may be present. Struma ovarii is composed entirely of mature thyroid tissue, which may be functional and cause hyperthyroidism. The ovarian carcinoid, which presumably arises from intestinal tissue found in teratomas, may also be functional; particularly if large (>7 cm), they can produce sufficient 5-hydroxytryptamine to cause the carcinoid syndrome even in the absence of hepatic metastases, since ovarian veins are directly connected to systemic circulation. Primary ovarian carcinoid must be distinguished from metastatic intestinal carcinoid, which is virtually always bilateral. Even rarer is the strumal carcinoid, a combination of struma ovarii and carcinoid in the same ovary. Only about 2% of carcinoids in teratomas metastasize.

Immature Malignant Teratomas. These are rare tumors that differ from benign teratomas in that the component tissues resemble embryonal and immature fetal tissue. The tumor is found chiefly in prepubertal adolescents and young women, the mean age being 18 years.

MORPHOLOGY

The tumors are bulky and have a smooth external surface and tend to be solid on sectioning. Hair, sebaceous material, cartilage, bone, and calcification may be present, along with areas of necrosis and hemorrhage. On microscopic examination there are varying amounts of immature neuroepithelium, cartilage, bone, muscle, and other elements. An important risk for subsequent extraovarian spread is the histologic grade of tumor (I through III), which is based on the proportion of tissue containing immature neuroepithelium (Fig. 22-40).

Immature teratomas grow rapidly, frequently penetrate the capsule, and spread either locally or distantly. Stage I tumors, however, particularly those with low-grade (grade 1) histology, have an excellent prognosis. Higher-grade tumors confined to the ovary are generally treated with prophylactic chemotherapy. Most recurrences develop in the first 2 years, and absence of disease beyond this period carries an excellent chance of cure.

Dysgerminoma

Dysgerminoma is the ovarian counterpart of testicular seminoma. Dysgerminomas account for about 2% of ovarian cancers and roughly 50% of malignant ovarian germ cell tumors. They may occur in childhood, but 75% occur in the second and third decades. Some occur in patients with gonadal dysgenesis, including pseudohermaphroditism. Most of these tumors have no endocrine function. A few produce elevated levels of chorionic gonadotropin, a finding that correlates with the presence of syncytiotrophoblastic giant cells. Like seminomas, dysgerminomas express OCT-3, OCT4, and NANOG. These transcription factors are implicated in maintenance of pluripotency. They also express the receptor tyrosine kinase KIT and approximately one third have activating mutations in the *KIT* gene. These proteins are useful diagnostic

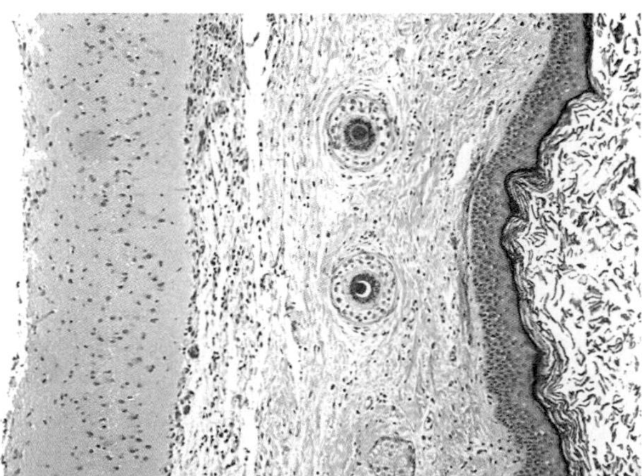

Figure 22-39 Benign cystic teratoma. Low-power view of skin *(right edge)*, beneath which there is brain tissue *(left edge)*.

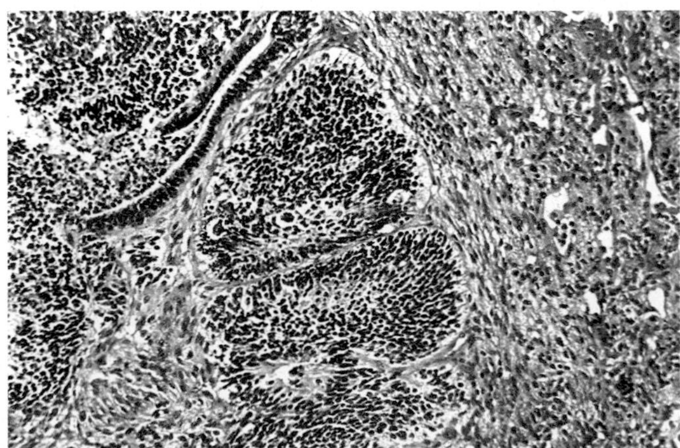

Figure 22-40 Immature teratoma of the ovary illustrating primitive neuroepithelium.

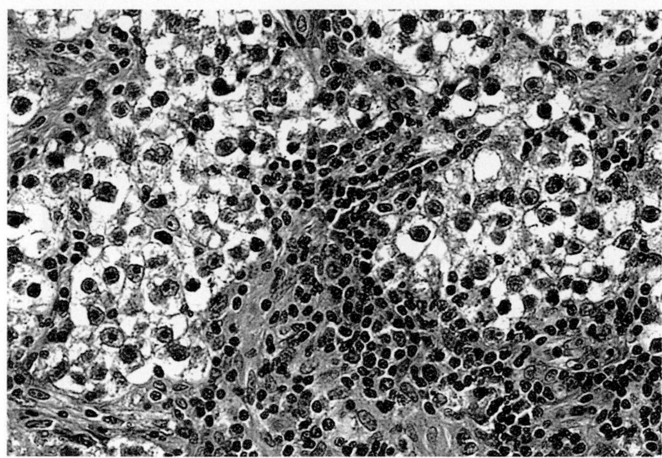

Figure 22-41 Dysgerminoma showing polyhedral tumor cells with round nuclei and adjacent inflammation.

markers and, in the case of KIT, may also serve as a therapeutic target.

MORPHOLOGY

Most dysgerminomas (80% to 90%) are unilateral tumors ranging in size from barely visible nodules to masses that virtually fill the entire abdomen. On cut surface they have a solid yellow-white to gray-pink appearance and are often soft and fleshy. Like seminoma, it is composed of large vesicular cells having a clear cytoplasm, well-defined cell boundaries, and centrally placed regular nuclei. The tumor cells grow in sheets or cords separated by scant fibrous stroma (Fig. 22-41), which is infiltrated by mature lymphocytes and may contain occasional granulomas. On occasion, small nodules of dysgerminoma are encountered in the wall of an otherwise benign cystic teratoma; conversely, a predominantly dysgerminomatous tumor may contain a small cystic teratoma.

All dysgerminomas are malignant, but the degree of histologic atypia is variable, and only about one third are aggressive. A unilateral tumor that has not broken through the capsule or spread outside the ovary has an excellent prognosis (up to 96% cure rate) after simple salpingo-oophorectomy. These neoplasms are responsive to chemotherapy, and even those that have extended beyond the ovary can often be cured. Overall survival exceeds 80%.

Yolk Sac Tumor

Though rare, yolk sac tumor (also known as *endodermal sinus tumor*) still ranks as the second most common malignant tumor of germ cell origin. It is thought that to be derived from malignant germ cells that are differentiating along the extraembryonic yolk sac lineage (Fig. 22-37). Similar to the normal yolk sac, the tumor cells elaborate *α-fetoprotein*. Its characteristic histologic feature is a glomerulus-like structure composed of a central blood vessel enveloped by tumor cells within a space that is also lined by tumor cells (*Schiller-Duval body*) (Fig. 22-42). Conspicuous intracellular and extracellular hyaline droplets are present in all tumors, and some of these stain for α-fetoprotein by immunoperoxidase techniques.

Most patients are children or young women presenting with abdominal pain and a rapidly growing pelvic mass that usually appears to involve a single ovary. With combination chemotherapy, there is greater than 80% survival independent of disease stage.

Choriocarcinoma

More commonly of placental origin, choriocarcinoma, like the yolk sac tumor, is an example of extraembryonic differentiation of malignant germ cells. It is generally held that a germ cell origin can be confirmed only in prepubertal females, because after this age an origin from an ovarian ectopic pregnancy cannot be excluded.

Most ovarian choriocarcinomas exist in combination with other germ cell tumors, and pure choriocarcinoma is extremely rare. They are histologically identical to the more common placental lesions (described later). The ovarian tumors are aggressive and have usually metastasized hematogenously to the lungs, liver, bone, and other sites by the time of diagnosis. Like all choriocarcinomas they elaborate high levels of *chorionic gonadotropins*, which may be helpful in establishing the diagnosis or detecting recurrences. In contrast to choriocarcinomas arising in placental tissue, those arising in the ovary are generally unresponsive to chemotherapy and are often fatal.

Other Germ Cell Tumors

These include (1) embryonal carcinoma, a highly malignant tumor of primitive embryonal elements that is histologically similar to embryonal carcinoma arising in the testes (Chapter 21); (2) polyembryoma, a malignant tumor containing so-called embryoid bodies; and (3) mixed germ cell tumors containing various combinations of dysgerminoma, teratoma, yolk sac tumor, and choriocarcinoma.

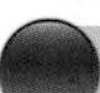

KEY CONCEPTS

Germ Cell Tumors

- Germ cell tumors constitute 15% to 20% of ovarian tumors.
- The majority are mature cystic teratomas (dermoid cysts) in women of reproductive age.

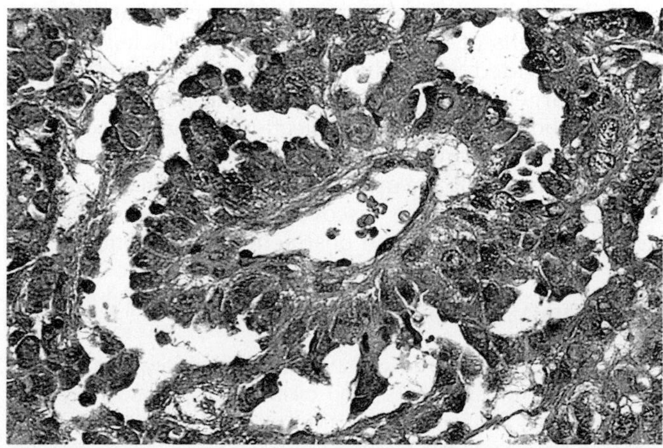

Figure 22-42 A Schiller-Duval body in yolk sac carcinoma.

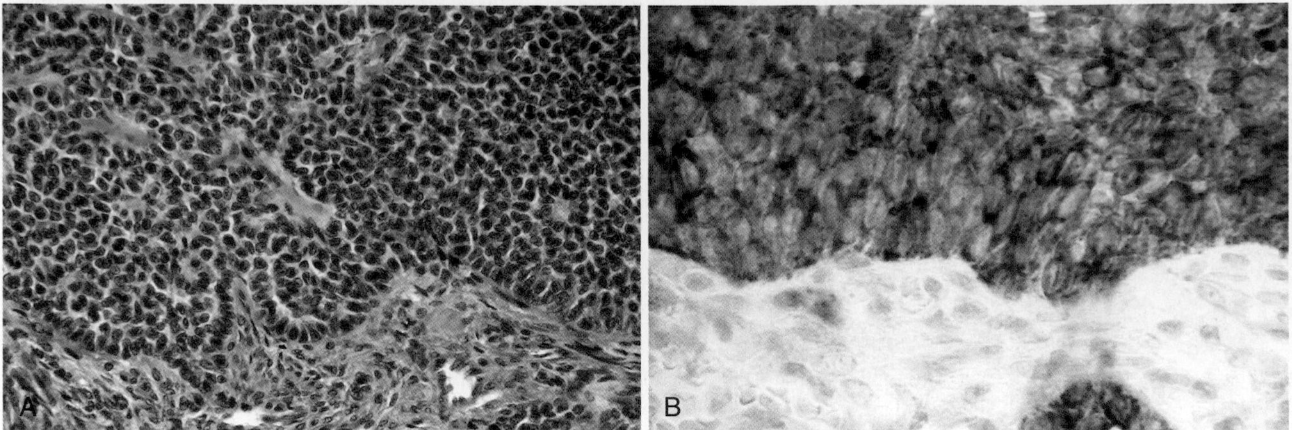

Figure 22-43 Granulosa cell tumor. **A,** The tumor cells are arranged in sheets punctuated by small follicle-like structures (Call-Exner bodies). **B,** Strong immunohistochemical positivity with an antibody to inhibin characterizes these tumors.

- The remainder occur in young women and children; in these age groups, malignant tumor dominate.
- Immature teratomas are distinguished from mature teratomas by the presence of immature elements, most often consisting of primitive neuroepithelium.
- Germ cell tumors show various lines of differentiation toward oogonia (dysgerminoma), extraembryonic yolk sac (yolk sac tumors), placenta (choriocarcinoma), or multiple germ layers (teratoma).

Sex Cord-Stromal Tumors

These ovarian neoplasms are derived from the ovarian stroma, which in turn is derived from the sex cords of the embryonic gonad. The undifferentiated gonadal mesenchyme eventually produces specific types of cells in both male (Sertoli and Leydig) and female (granulosa and theca) gonads, and tumors resembling all of these cell types can be identified in the ovary. Moreover, because some of these cells normally secrete estrogens (granulosa and theca cells) or androgens (Leydig cells), their corresponding tumors may be either feminizing (granulosa/theca cell tumors) or masculinizing (Leydig cell tumors).

Granulosa Cell Tumors

Granulosa cell tumors are composed of cells that resemble granulosa cells of a developing ovarian follicle. They are broadly divided into adult and juvenile granulosa cell tumors largely based on the age of the patient, but also on morphologic findings. Collectively, these neoplasms account for about 5% of all ovarian tumors and adult granulosa cell tumors make up 95% of all granulosa cell tumors. Although they may be discovered at any age, approximately two thirds occur in postmenopausal women.

MORPHOLOGY

Granulosa cell tumors are usually unilateral and vary from microscopic foci to large, solid, and cystic encapsulated masses. Tumors that are hormonally active have a yellow coloration to their cut surfaces, due to intracellular lipids.

The granulosa cell component of these tumors has many histologic patterns. The small, cuboidal to polygonal cells may grow in anastomosing cords, sheets, or strands (Fig. 22-43*A*). In occasional cases, small, distinctive, glandlike structures filled with an acidophilic material recall immature follicles (**Call-Exner bodies**). When these structures are evident, the diagnosis is straightforward. Occasionally, there is a predominant thecoma component that consists of clusters or sheets of cuboidal to polygonal cells (see later). In some tumors, the granulosa or theca cells may appear plumper and have ample cytoplasm characteristic of luteinization (i.e., luteinized granulosa-theca cell tumors).

Granulosa cell tumors are of clinical importance for two reasons: (1) they may elaborate large amounts of estrogen, and (2) they may behave like low-grade malignancies. Functionally active tumors in prepubertal girls (juvenile granulosa cell tumors) may produce precocious sexual development. In adult women they may be associated with proliferative breast disease, endometrial hyperplasia, and endometrial carcinoma, which eventually develops in about 10% to 15% of women with steroid-producing tumors. Occasionally, granulosa cell tumors produce androgens, masculinizing the patient.

All granulosa cell tumors are potentially malignant. It is difficult to predict their biologic behavior from histology. The likelihood of malignant behavior (recurrence, extension) ranges from 5% to 25%. In general, malignant tumors pursue an indolent course in which local recurrences may be amenable to surgical therapy. Recurrences within the pelvis and abdomen may appear 10 to 20 years after removal of the original tumor. The 10-year survival rate is approximately 85%. Tumors composed predominantly of theca cells are almost never malignant.

Elevated tissue and serum levels of *inhibin*, a product of granulosa cells, are associated with granulosa cell tumors. This biomarker may be useful for identifying granulosa and other sex cord-stromal tumors, and for monitoring patients being treated for these neoplasms (Fig. 22-43*B*). Recent studies reported mutations of the *FOXL2* gene in 97% of adult granulosa cell tumors. Although details remain to be worked out, *FOXL2* encodes a transcription

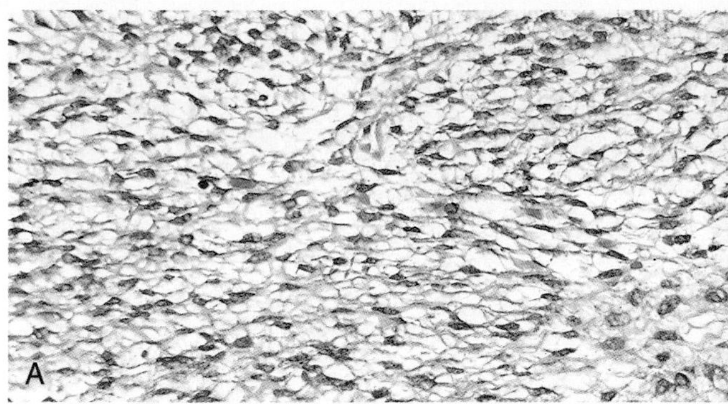

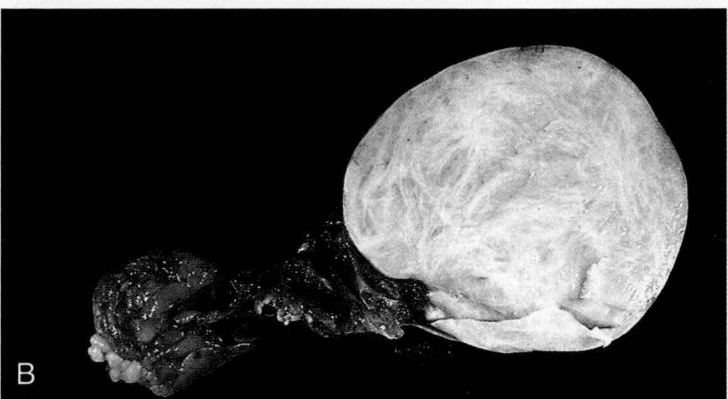

Figure 22-44 Ovarian fibromas **A,** Thecoma-fibroma composed of plump, differentiated stromal cells with thecal appearance. **B,** Large bisected fibroma of the ovary apparent as a white, firm mass *(right)*. The fallopian tube is attached.

factor that is important in granulosa cell development, which presumably explains its strong association with this tumor type. Interestingly, mutations in *FOXL2*, in one small study, were uncommon in juvenile granulosa tumor, suggesting that it is genetically distinct from the adult type.

Fibromas, Thecomas, and Fibrothecomas

Tumors arising in the ovarian stroma that are composed of either fibroblasts (fibromas) or plump spindle cells with lipid droplets (thecomas) are relatively common and account for about 4% of all ovarian tumors (Fig. 22-44*A*). Many tumors contain a mixture of these cells and are termed *fibrothecomas*. Pure thecomas are rare, but tumors in which these cells predominate may be hormonally active. By contrast, fibromas as a rule are hormonally inactive.

Fibromas of the ovary are unilateral in about 90% of cases and are usually solid, spherical or slightly lobulated, encapsulated, hard, gray-white masses covered by glistening, intact ovarian serosa (Fig. 22-44*B*). On histologic examination, they are composed of well-differentiated fibroblasts and a scant interspersed collagenous stroma. Focal areas of thecal differentiation may be identified.

Most of these tumors come to attention as a pelvic mass, sometimes accompanied by pain and two decidedly curious associations. The first is ascites, found in about 40% of cases in which the tumors measure more than 6 cm in diameter. Uncommonly there is also a hydrothorax, usually only on the right side. This combination of findings (ovarian tumor, hydrothorax, and ascites) is designated *Meigs syndrome*. Its genesis is unknown. The second association is with the basal cell nevus syndrome, described in Chapter 25. The vast majority of fibromas, fibrothecomas, and thecomas are benign. Rarely, cellular fibromas with mitotic activity and increased nuclear-to-cytoplasmic ratio are identified; because they may pursue a malignant course, they are termed *fibrosarcomas*.

Sertoli-Leydig Cell Tumors

These tumors are often functional and commonly produce masculinization or defeminization, but a few have estrogenic effects. The tumor cells recapitulate, to a certain extent, testicular sertoli or Leydig cells at various stages of development. They occur in women of all ages, although the peak incidence is in the second and third decades. In over half of cases, the tumor cells have mutations in *DICER1*, a gene that you will recall encodes an endonuclease that is essential for proper processing of micro-RNAs (Chapter 1). The presence of *DICER1* mutations suggests the genesis of male-directed stromal cells may involve abnormalities of gene expression related to dysregulation of micro-RNAs.

MORPHOLOGY

These tumors are unilateral and may resemble granulosa cell tumors grossly. The cut surface is usually solid and varies from gray to golden brown in appearance (Fig. 22-45A). Microscopically, a range of differentiation is seen. Well-differentiated tumors show tubules composed of Sertoli cells or Leydig cells interspersed with stroma (Fig. 22-45*B*). The intermediate forms show only outlines of immature tubules and large eosinophilic Leydig cells. The poorly differentiated tumors have a sarcomatous pattern with a disorderly disposition of epithelial cell cords. Leydig cells may be absent. Heterologous elements, such as mucinous glands, bone, and cartilage, may be present in some tumors.

The incidence of recurrence or metastasis by Sertoli-Leydig cell tumors is less than 5%. These neoplasms may block normal female sexual development in children and may cause defeminization of women, manifested by atrophy of the breasts, amenorrhea, sterility, and loss of hair. The syndrome may progress to striking virilization (hirsutism) associated with male distribution of hair, hypertrophy of the clitoris, and voice changes.

Other Sex Cord-Stromal Tumors

There are several other uncommon but distinctive ovarian tumors of sex cord or stromal origin that often produce steroid hormones.

- *Hilus cell tumors (pure Leydig cell tumors)* are usually derived from clusters of polygonal cells arranged around hilar vessels. These rare, unilateral tumors are comprised of large lipid-laden Leydig cells with distinct borders and characteristic cytoplasmic structures called Reinke crystalloids. Women with hilus cell tumors usually present with evidence of masculinization in the form of

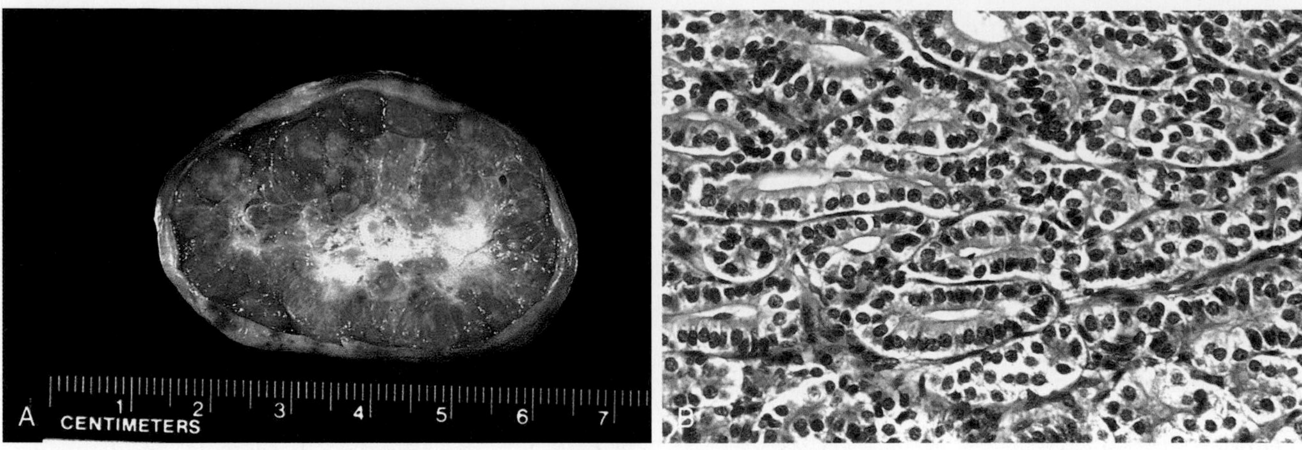

Figure 22-45 Sertoli cell tumor. **A,** Gross photograph illustrating characteristic golden-yellow appearance of the tumor. **B,** Photomicrograph showing well-differentiated Sertoli cell tubules. (Courtesy Dr. William Welch, Brigham and Women's Hospital, Boston, Mass.)

hirsutism, voice changes, and clitoral enlargement, but these changes are milder than those seen in association with Sertoli-Leydig cell tumors. The tumors produce predominantly testosterone. Treatment is surgical excision. True hilus cell tumors are almost always benign.

- *Pregnancy luteoma* refers to a rare tumor that closely resembles the corpus luteum of pregnancy. These tumors may produce virilization in pregnant patients and their female infants.
- *Gonadoblastoma* is an uncommon tumor composed of germ cells and sex cord-stroma derivatives resembling immature Sertoli and granulosa cells. It occurs in individuals with abnormal sexual development and in gonads of indeterminate nature. Eighty percent of patients are phenotypic females, and 20% are phenotypic males with undescended testicles and female internal secondary organs. A coexistent dysgerminoma occurs in 50% of the cases. The prognosis is excellent if the tumor is completely excised.

KEY CONCEPTS

Sex Cord-Stromal Tumors

- Granulosa cells tumors are the most common malignant tumor in this category. They are indolent tumors, but can recur 10 to 20 years after resection of the primary tumor. They are often hormonally active and are associated with endometrial hyperplasia/cancer.
- Fibromas are relatively common benign tumors composed of fibroblasts. They are predominantly unilateral and are generally hormonally inactive.
- Pure thecomas are rare but may be hormonally active.
- Sertoli-Leydig cell tumors commonly present with masculinization and less than 5% recur or metastasize.

Metastatic Tumors

The most common metastatic tumors of the ovary are derived from tumors of müllerian origin: the uterus, fallopian tube, contralateral ovary, or pelvic peritoneum. The most common extra-müllerian tumors metastatic to the ovary are carcinomas of the breast and gastrointestinal tract, including colon, stomach, biliary tract, and pancreas. Also included in this group are the rare cases of pseudomyxoma peritonei, derived from appendiceal tumors. A classic metastatic gastrointestinal carcinoma involving the ovaries is termed *Krukenberg tumor*, characterized by bilateral metastases composed of mucin-producing, signet-ring cancer cells, most often of gastric origin.

GESTATIONAL AND PLACENTAL DISORDERS

Diseases of pregnancy and pathologic conditions of the placenta are important causes of fetal intrauterine or perinatal death, congenital malformations, intrauterine growth retardation, maternal death, and morbidity for both mother and child. Only those disorders for which recognition of morphologic features contribute to an understanding of the clinical problem are discussed here. These include selected disorders of early pregnancy, late pregnancy, and trophoblastic neoplasia.

Understanding placental disorders requires a working knowledge of normal placental anatomy. The placenta is composed of chorionic villi (Fig. 22-46*A, B*) that sprout from the chorion to provide a large contact area between the fetal and maternal circulations. In the mature placenta, the maternal blood enters the intervillous space through endometrial arteries (spiral arteries) and circulates around the villi to allow gas and nutrient exchange (Fig. 22-47). The deoxygenated blood flows back from the intervillous space to the decidua and enters the endometrial veins. Deoxygenated fetal blood enters the placenta through two umbilical arteries that branch radially to form chorionic arteries. Chorionic arteries branch further as they enter the

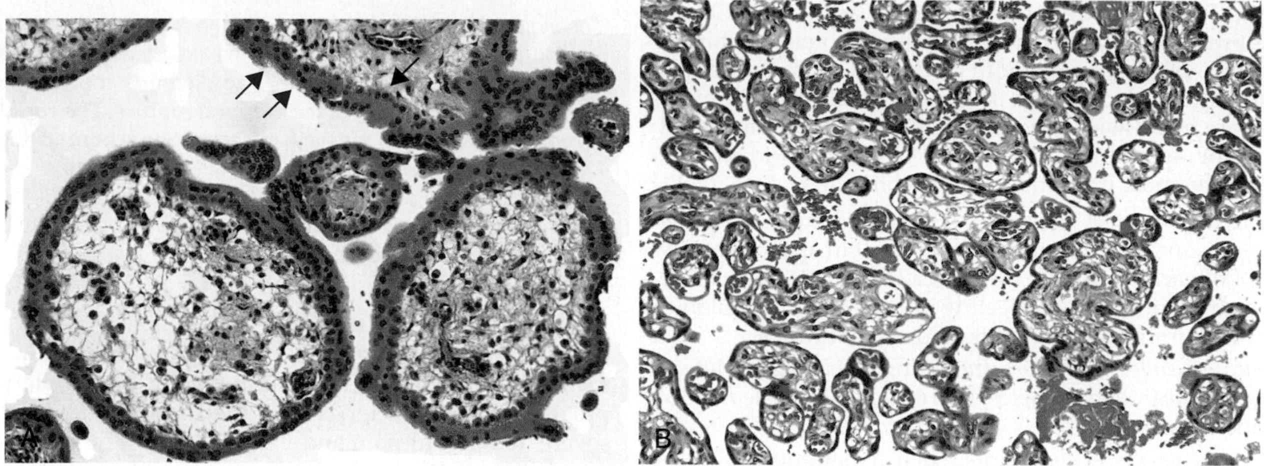

Figure 22-46 Normal placenta. **A,** First-trimester chorionic villi composed of delicate mesh of central stroma surrounded by two discrete layers of epithelium—the outer layer consisting of syncytiotrophoblast *(two arrows)* and the inner layer consisting of cytotrophoblast *(arrow)*. **B,** Third-trimester chorionic villi composed of stroma with dense network of dilated capillaries surrounded by markedly thinned-out syncytiotrophoblast and cytotrophoblast (same magnification as **A.**)

villi. In the chorionic villi they form an extensive capillary system, bringing fetal blood in close proximity to maternal blood. The gas and nutrient diffusion occurs through the villous capillary endothelial cells and thinned-out syncytiotrophoblast and cytotrophoblast. Under normal circumstances there little or no mixing between the fetal and maternal blood, though sufficient free fetal DNA reaches the maternal circulation to permit prenatal genetic testing (Chapter 5). Blood oxygenated in the placenta returns to the fetus through the single umbilical vein.

Disorders of Early Pregnancy

Spontaneous Abortion

Spontaneous abortion, or "miscarriage," is defined as pregnancy loss before 20 weeks of gestation. Most of these occur before 12 weeks. Ten to fifteen percent of clinically recognized pregnancies terminate in spontaneous abortion. However, using sensitive chorionic gonadotropin

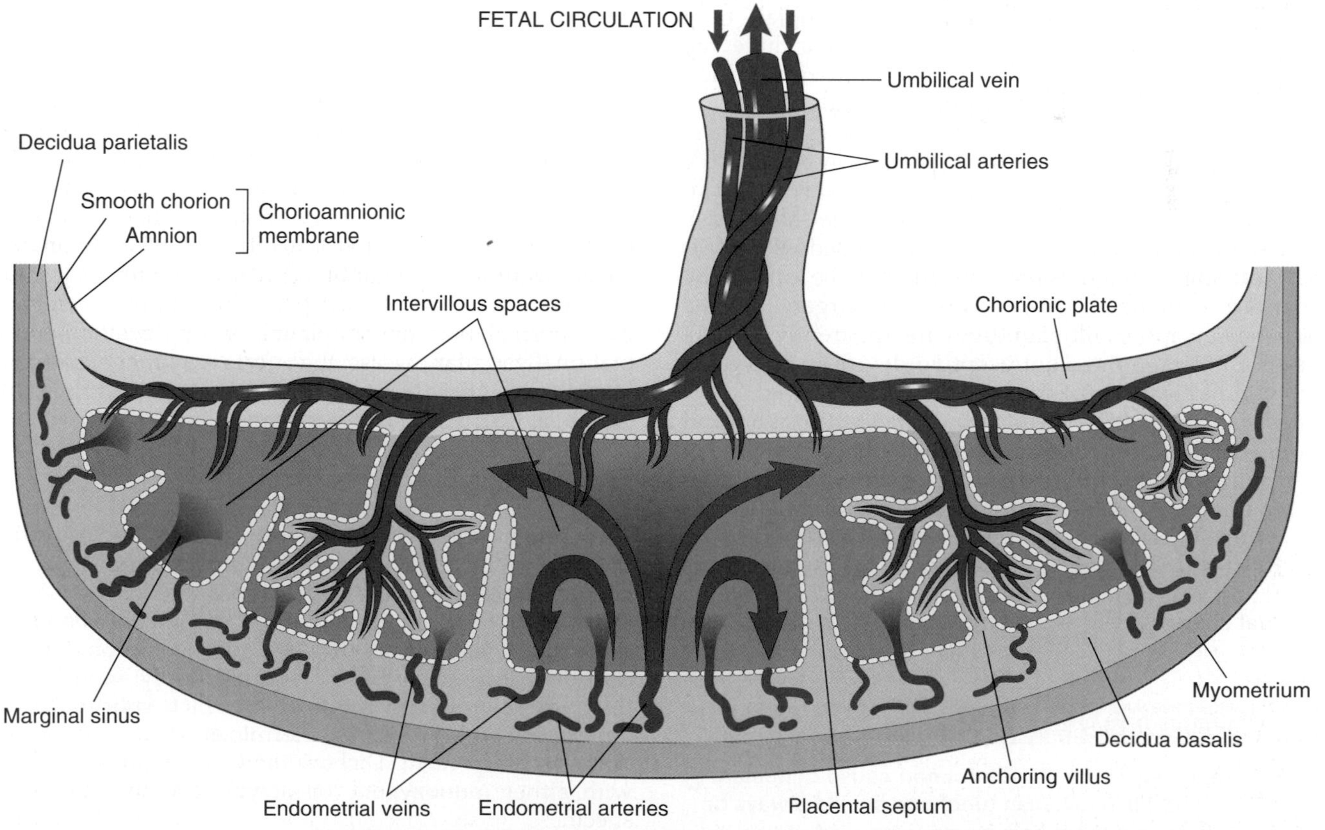

Figure 22-47 Diagram of placental anatomy. Within the outer boundary of myometrium is a layer of decidua, from which the maternal vessels originate and deliver blood to and from the intervillous spaces. Umbilical vessels branch and terminate in placental villi, where nutrient exchange takes place.

assays, it has been determined that an additional 20% of early pregnancies in otherwise healthy women terminate spontaneously, many without notice. In most individual instances, the mechanisms leading to early loss of pregnancy are unknown. However, multiple fetal and maternal causes of spontaneous abortion have been identified. Among the most important are the following:

- *Fetal chromosomal anomalies*, such as aneuploidy, polyploidy, and translocations, are present in approximately 50% of early abortuses. More subtle genetic defects, for which routine genetic testing is not readily available, account for an additional fraction of abortions.
- *Maternal endocrine factors*, including luteal-phase defect, poorly controlled diabetes, and other uncorrected endocrine disorders
- *Physical defects of the uterus*, such as submucosal leiomyomas, uterine polyps, or uterine malformations, may prevent or disrupt implantation
- *Systemic disorders affecting the maternal vasculature*, such as antiphospholipid antibody syndrome, coagulopathies, and hypertension
- *Infections* with protozoa (Toxoplasma), bacteria (Mycoplasma, Listeria), or a number of viruses. Ascending infection is particularly common in second-trimester losses.

Ectopic Pregnancy

Ectopic pregnancy refers to implantation of the fetus in a site other than the normal intrauterine location; the most common site is the extrauterine fallopian tube (approximately 90% of cases). Other sites include the ovary, the abdominal cavity, and the intrauterine portion of the fallopian tube (cornual pregnancy). Ectopic pregnancies account for 2% of confirmed pregnancies. The most important predisposing condition, present in 35% to 50% of patients, is prior *pelvic inflammatory disease* resulting in intralumenal fallopian tube scarring (chronic salpingitis). The risk of ectopic pregnancy is also increased with peritubal scarring and adhesions, which may be caused by appendicitis, endometriosis, and previous surgery. In some cases, however, the fallopian tubes are apparently normal. Use of an intrauterine contraceptive device is associated with twofold increase of ectopic pregnancy.

Ovarian pregnancy results from the fertilization and trapping of the ovum within the follicle just at the time of its rupture. Abdominal pregnancies occur when the fertilized ovum fails to enter or drops out of the fimbriated end of the tube. In each abnormal location, the fertilized ovum develops as usual, forming placental tissue, amniotic sac, and fetus. The host implantation site may also develop decidual changes.

MORPHOLOGY

Tubal pregnancy is the most common cause of hematosalpinx (blood-filled fallopian tube) and should always be suspected when a tubal hematoma is present. Initially the embryonal sac, surrounded by immature chorionic villi, implants within the lumen of the fallopian tube. Trophoblastic cells and chorionic villi then invade the wall of the fallopian tube as they would do in the uterus during normal pregnancy. **With time the growth of the gestational sac distends the fallopian tube, causing thinning of the wall and rupture. The rupture frequently results in massive intraperitoneal hemorrhage, which sometimes is fatal.** Less commonly the tubal pregnancy may undergo spontaneous regression and resorption, or be extruded through the fimbriated end of the tube into the abdominal cavity (tubal abortion).

Clinical Features. **Rupture of a tubal pregnancy is a medical emergency**. The clinical course of ectopic tubal pregnancy is characterized by the onset of moderate to severe abdominal pain and vaginal bleeding 6 to 8 weeks after last menstrual period, correlating with distention and then rupture of the fallopian tube. In such cases the patient may rapidly develop *hemorrhagic shock* with signs of an acute abdomen, and therefore early diagnosis is critical. Diagnosis is based on determination of chorionic gonadotropin titers, pelvic sonography, endometrial biopsy (which shows decidua without chorionic villi or implantation site) and/or laparoscopy. Despite advances in early diagnosis, ectopic pregnancy still accounts for 4% to 10% of pregnancy-related deaths.

Disorders of Late Pregnancy

Disorders that occur in the third trimester of pregnancy are related to the complex anatomy of the maturing placenta. Complete interruption of blood flow through the umbilical cord from any cause (e.g., constricting knots or compression) can be lethal to the fetus. Ascending infections involving the chorioamnionic membranes may lead to premature rupture of amniotic membranes and delivery. Retroplacental hemorrhage at the interface of placenta and myometrium (*abruptio placentae*) threatens both mother and fetus. Disruption of the fetal vessels in terminal villi may produce a significant loss of fetal blood with resultant fetal injury or death. Uteroplacental malperfusion can be precipitated by abnormal placental implantation or development, or maternal vascular disease; the effects may range from mild intrauterine growth retardation to severe uteroplacental ischemia, and maternal preeclampsia.

Twin Placentas

Twin pregnancies arise from fertilization of two ova (dizygotic) or from division of one fertilized ovum (monozygotic). There are three basic types of twin placentas (Fig. 22-48): diamnionic dichorionic (which may be fused), diamnionic monochorionic, and monoamnionic monochorionic. Monochorionic placentas imply monozygotic (identical) twins, and the time at which splitting of the developing embryo occurs determines whether one or two amnions are present. Dichorionic placentation may occur with either monozygotic or dizygotic twins and is not specific.

One complication of monochorionic twin pregnancy is *twin-twin transfusion syndrome*. Monochorionic twin placentas have vascular anastomoses that connect the

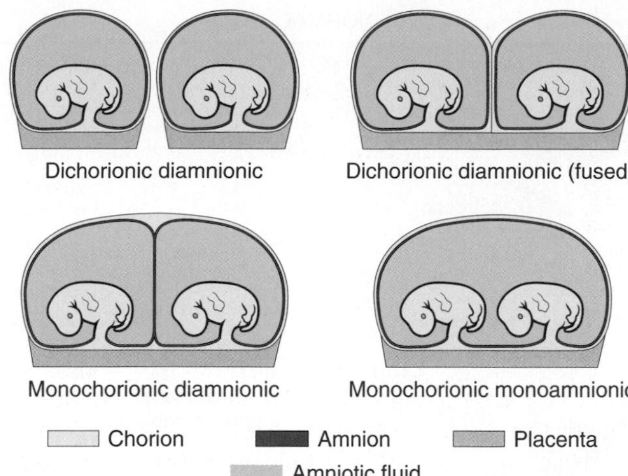

Figure 22-48 Diagrammatic representation of the various types of twin placentation and their membrane relationships. (Adapted from Gersell D, et al: Diseases of the placenta. In Kurman R (ed): Blaustein's Pathology of the Female Genital Tract. New York, Springer-Verlag, 1994.)

circulations of the twins, and in some cases these connections include one or more arteriovenous shunts. If these shunts preferentially increase blood flow to one twin at the expense of the second, one twin will be underperfused, while the second will be fluid overloaded. It is this phenomenon that constitutes the twin-twin transfusion syndrome, which if severe may result in the death of one or both fetuses.

Abnormalities of Placental Implantation

Several types of abnormal placental implantations are associated with significant complications. *Placenta previa* is a condition in which the placenta implants in the lower uterine segment or cervix, often leading to serious third-trimester bleeding. A complete placenta previa covers the internal cervical os and thus requires delivery via cesarean section to avert placental rupture and fatal maternal hemorrhage during vaginal delivery. *Placenta accreta* is caused by partial or complete absence of the decidua, such that the placental villous tissue adheres directly to the myometrium, which leads to a failure of placental separation at birth. It is an important cause of severe, potentially life-threatening postpartum bleeding. Common predisposing factors are placenta previa (in up to 60% of cases) and history of previous cesarean section.

Placental Infections

Infections in the placenta develop by two pathways: (1) ascending infection through the birth canal and (2) hematogenous (transplacental) infection. Ascending infections are by far the most common and are virtually always bacterial; in many such instances, localized infection of the membranes produces premature rupture of membranes and preterm delivery. The amniotic fluid may be cloudy with purulent exudate, and histologically the chorion-amnion contains an infiltrate of neutrophils accompanied by edema and congestion of the vessels (Fig. 22-49*A*, *B*). The infection frequently elicits a fetal response consisting of a "vasculitis" of the umbilical and fetal chorionic plate vessels. Uncommonly, bacterial infections may result from hematogenous spread to the placenta, leading to acute villitis (Fig. 22-49*C*).

Several hematogenous infections, classically components of the TORCH group (*t*oxoplasmosis and *o*thers [syphilis, tuberculosis, listeriosis], *r*ubella, *c*ytomegalovirus, *h*erpes simplex), can affect the placenta. They give rise to chronic inflammatory cell infiltrates in the chorionic villi (chronic villitis) and are described in Chapter 10.

Preeclampsia and Eclampsia

Preeclampsia is a systemic syndrome characterized by widespread maternal endothelial dysfunction that presents during pregnancy with hypertension, edema, and

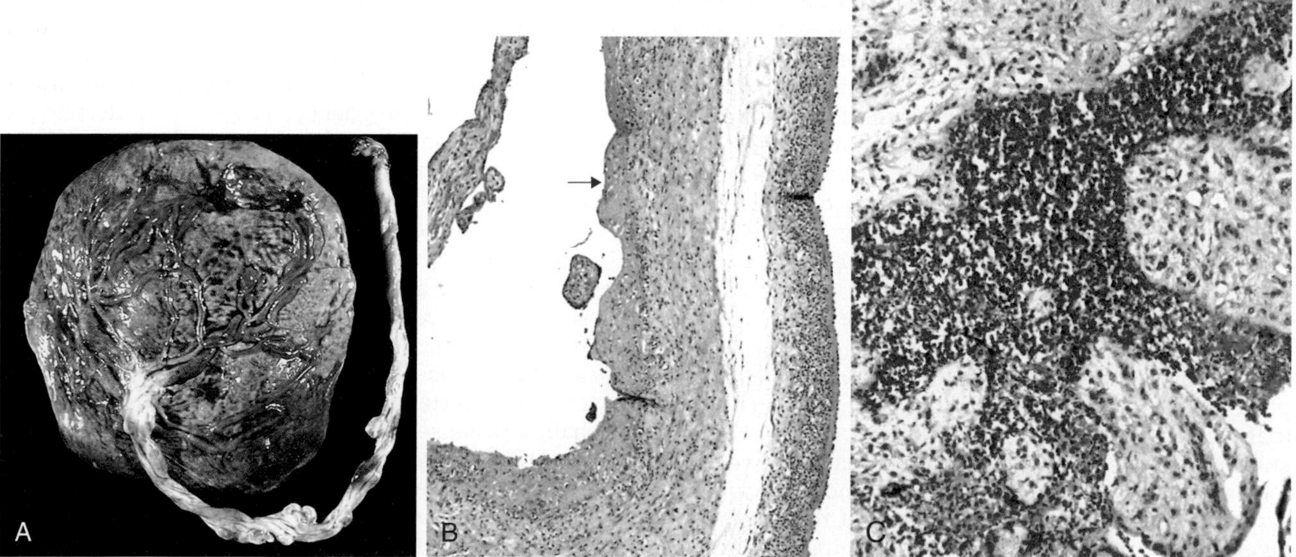

Figure 22-49 Placental infections derived from ascending and blood-borne routes. Acute chorioamnionitis. **A,** On gross examination the placenta contains greenish opaque membranes. **B,** A photomicrograph illustrates a dense bandlike inflammatory exudate on the amniotic surface *(arrow)*. **C,** Acute necrotizing intervillositis, from a fetal-maternal infection by *Listeria*.

proteinuria. It occurs in about 3% to 5% of pregnant women, usually in the last trimester and more commonly in primiparas (women pregnant for the first time). Some of these women become more seriously ill, developing convulsions; this more severe form of the disorder is termed *eclampsia*. Other complications stemming from systemic endothelial dysfunction include hypercoagulability, acute renal failure, and pulmonary edema. Approximately 10% of women with severe preeclampsia develop microangiopathic hemolytic anemia, elevated liver enzymes, and low platelets, referred to as the HELLP syndrome (Chapter 17). Preeclampsia should be distinguished from gestational hypertension that can develop in pregnancy without proteinuria.

Pathogenesis. **While the exact mechanisms leading to development of preeclampsia are still being investigated, it is clear that the placenta plays a central role in the pathogenesis of the syndrome, since the symptoms disappear rapidly after delivery of the placenta.** The critical abnormalities in preeclampsia are diffuse endothelial dysfunction, vasoconstriction (leading to hypertension), and increased vascular permeability (resulting in proteinuria and edema). Recent work has demonstrated that these effects are most likely mediated by placenta-derived factor(s) released into the maternal circulation. Although the release of these factors and the clinical syndrome develop late in gestation, the pathogenesis of the disease appears to be closely tied to the earliest events of pregnancy and placentation. The principal pathophysiologic aberrations appear to be the following:

- *Abnormal placental vasculature.* The precipitating events in the pathogenesis of preeclampsia are abnormal trophoblastic implantation and a failure of physiologic remodeling of the maternal vessels, which is required for adequate perfusion of the placental bed. In normal pregnancy, fetal extravillous trophoblastic cells (trophoblastic cells not associated with chorionic villi) at the implantation site invade the maternal decidua and decidual vessels, destroy the vascular smooth muscle, and replace the maternal endothelial cells with fetal trophoblastic cells (forming hybrid fetomaternal blood vessels). This process converts the decidual spiral arteries from small-caliber resistance vessels to large capacity uteroplacental vessels lacking a smooth muscle coat (Fig. 22-50). In preeclampsia, this remodeling fails to occur, leaving the placenta ill equipped to meet the increased circulatory demands of late gestation and setting the stage for the development of placental ischemia.
- *Endothelial dysfunction and imbalance of angiogenic and antiangiogenic factors.* Although not formally proven, it is postulated that in response to hypoxia, the ischemic placenta releases factors into the maternal circulation that cause an imbalance in circulating angiogenic and anti-angiogenic factors; this in turn leads to systemic maternal endothelial dysfunction and the clinical symptoms of the disease. In support of this, the blood levels of two placenta-derived antiangiogenic factors, soluble FMS-like tyrosine kinase (sFltl) and endoglin, which antagonize the effects of VEGF and TGFβ, respectively, are several orders of magnitude higher in women

NORMAL

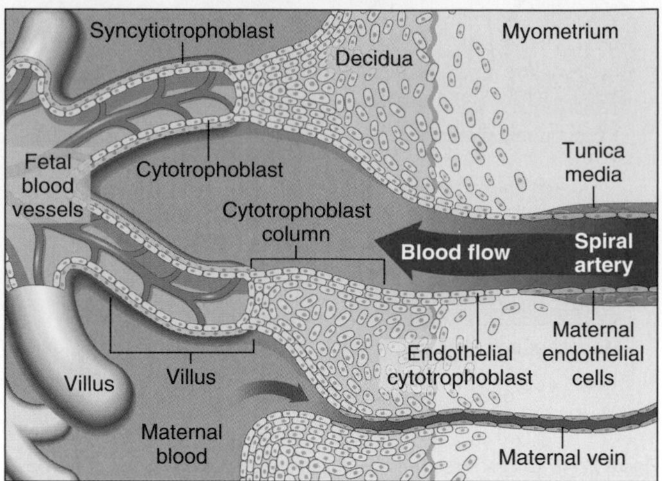

PREECLAMPSIA

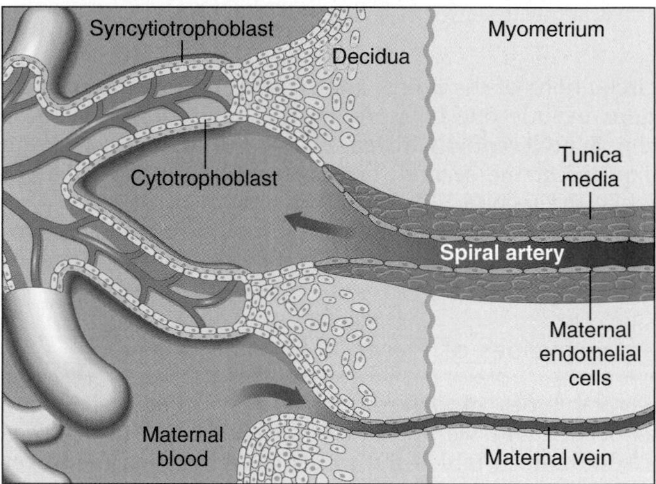

Figure 22-50 The physiologic alterations in the uterine spiral arteries and the failure of their remodeling in preeclampsia. (Modified from Maynard S, et al: Preeclampsia and angiogenic imbalance. Ann Rev Med 59:61, 2008.)

with preeclampsia than in healthy controls. In preeclampsia, high levels of sFlt1 and soluble endoglin bring about a decrease in angiogenesis much earlier than in normal pregnancy. The result is defective vascular development in the placenta. Furthermore, TGFβ induces endothelial production of NO, a potent vasodilator; thus, inhibition of TGFβ by endoglin may directly contribute to systemic vasoconstriction, hypertension, and tissue hypoperfusion.

Studies in animal models also implicate sFltl and soluble endoglin in the pathogenesis of endothelial dysfunction. When sFlt and endoglin are overexpressed together, rats develop nephrotic-range proteinuria, severe hypertension, and fetal growth restriction, the hallmarks of severe preeclampsia, as well as features of the HELLP syndrome, including elevated liver enzymes, decreased platelet counts, and hemolysis. Thus, it seems that sFlt1 and soluble endoglin are key mediators that link the placenta to the characteristic maternal endothelial dysfunction of preeclampsia.

- *Coagulation abnormalities.* Preeclampsia is associated with a hypercoagulable state that may lead to the formation of thrombi in arterioles and capillaries throughout the body, but particularly in the liver, kidneys, brain, and pituitary. Hypercoagulability is likely related to the reduced endothelial production of PGI_2, a potent antithrombotic factor, and increased release of procoagulant factors. Production of PGI_2 is stimulated by VEGF, and women with preeclampsia have decreased endothelial production of PGI_2, presumably due to antagonism of VEGF by sFlt1.

MORPHOLOGY

The **placenta** reveals various microscopic changes, most of which reflect malperfusion, ischemia, and vascular injury. These include (1) **infarcts**, which are larger and more numerous that those that may be seen in normal full-term placentas, (2) **exaggerated ischemic changes** in the chorionic villi and trophoblast, consisting of increased syncytial knots, (3) frequent **retroplacental hematomas** due to bleeding and instability of uteroplacental vessels, and (4) **abnormal decidual vessels**, which may show thrombi, lack of normal physiologic conversion (described earlier), fibrinoid necrosis, or intraintimal lipid deposition (acute atherosis) (Fig. 22-51).

The **liver** lesions, when present, take the form of irregular, focal, subcapsular, and intraparenchymal hemorrhages. On histologic examination there are fibrin thrombi in the portal capillaries and foci of hemorrhagic necrosis.

The **kidney** lesions are variable. The glomeruli show marked swelling of endothelial cells, amorphous dense deposits on the endothelial side of the basement membrane, and mesangial cell hyperplasia. Immunofluorescent studies show an abundance of fibrin in glomeruli. In advanced cases, fibrin thrombi are present in the glomeruli and capillaries of the cortex. If widespread and severe, these thrombi may produce complete destruction of the cortex in the pattern referred to as bilateral renal cortical necrosis (Chapter 20). The **brain** may have gross or microscopic foci of hemorrhage along with small-vessel thromboses. Similar changes are often found in the **heart** and the **anterior pituitary**.

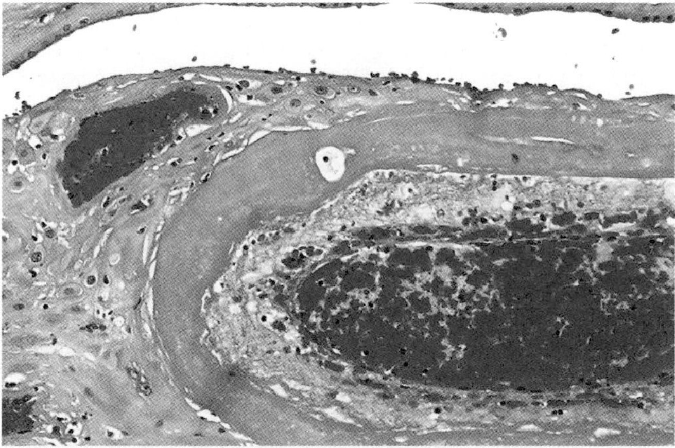

Figure 22-51 Acute atherosis of uterine vessels in eclampsia. Note fibrinoid necrosis of the vessel walls, subendothelial macrophages, and perivascular lymphocytic infiltrate. (Courtesy Dr. Drucilla J. Roberts, Massachusetts General Hospital, Boston, Mass.)

Clinical Features. *Preeclampsia* most commonly starts after 34 weeks of gestation but begins earlier in women with hydatidiform mole (discussed later) or preexisting kidney disease, hypertension, or coagulopathies. The onset is typically insidious, characterized by hypertension and edema, with proteinuria following within several days. Headaches and visual disturbances are serious events and are indicative of severe preeclampsia, often requiring delivery. *Eclampsia* is heralded by central nervous system involvement, including convulsions and eventual coma.

Management of preeclampsia differs depending on the gestational age and severity of disease. For term pregnancies, delivery is the treatment of choice regardless of disease severity. In preterm pregnancies, where delivery may not be in the best interest of the fetus, patients with mild disease can be managed expectantly by closely monitoring the mother and fetus. However, eclampsia, severe preeclampsia with maternal end-organ dysfunction, fetal compromise, or the HELLP syndrome are indications for delivery regardless of gestational age. Antihypertensive therapy does not affect the disease course or improve outcomes. Proteinuria and hypertension usually disappear within 1 to 2 weeks after delivery except when they predate the pregnancy. Although in most instances preeclampsia has no lasting sequelae, recent studies indicate that about 20% of affected women develop hypertension and microalbuminuria within 7 years of a pregnancy complicated by preeclampsia. There is also a twofold increase in the long-term risk of vascular diseases of the heart and the brain.

Gestational Trophoblastic Disease

Gestational trophoblastic disease encompasses a spectrum of tumors and tumor-like conditions characterized by proliferation of placental tissue, either villous or trophoblastic. The major disorders of this type are hydatidiform mole (complete and partial), invasive mole, choriocarcinoma, and placental site trophoblastic tumor (PSTT).

Hydatidiform Mole

Hydatidiform moles are important to recognize because they are associated with an increased risk of persistent trophoblastic disease (invasive mole) or choriocarcinoma. Moles are characterized histologically by cystic swelling of the chorionic villi, accompanied by variable trophoblastic proliferation. They are usually diagnosed during early pregnancy (average 9 weeks) by pelvic sonogram. Molar pregnancy can develop at any age, but the risk is higher at the two ends of reproductive life, in teenagers and between the ages of 40 and 50 years. For poorly explained reasons, the incidence varies considerably in different parts of the world. Hydatidiform mole occurs about once in every 1000 to 2000 pregnancies in the United States, but it is twice as common in Southeast Asia. Two types of benign, noninvasive moles—complete and partial—can be identified by cytogenetic and histologic studies.

Complete Mole

Complete mole results from fertilization of an egg that has lost its female chromosomes, and as a result the genetic material is completely paternally derived (Fig. 22-52*A, B*).

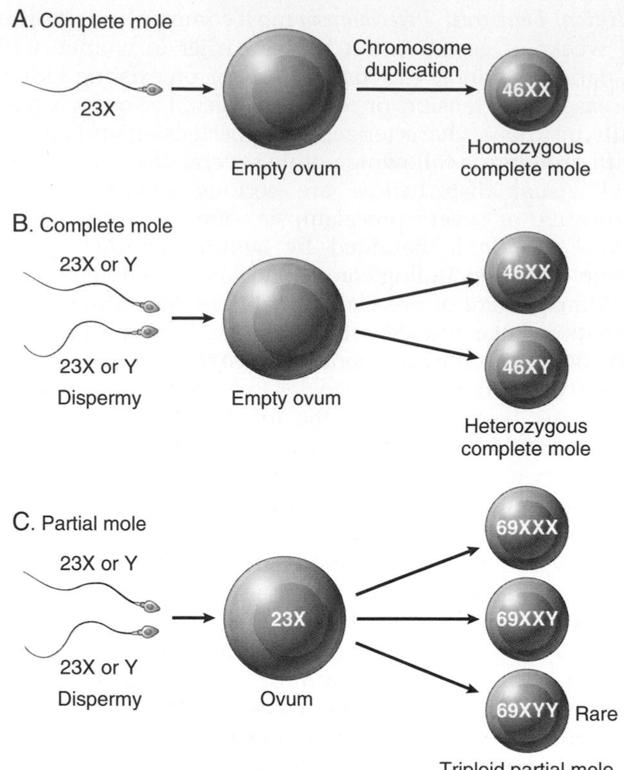

Figure 22-52 Origin of complete and partial hydatidiform moles. **A,** Complete moles most commonly arise from fertilization of an empty ovum by a single sperm that undergoes duplication of its chromosomes. **B,** Less commonly, complete moles arise from dispermy in which two sperm fertilize an empty ovum. **C,** Partial moles arise from two sperm fertilizing a single ovum.

Ninety percent have a 46,XX karyotype stemming from the duplication of the genetic material of one sperm (a phenomenon called androgenesis). The remaining 10% result from the fertilization of an empty egg by two sperm; these may have 46,XX or 46,XY karyotype. In complete moles the embryo dies very early in development and therefore is usually not identified. Patients have 2.5% risk of subsequent choriocarcinoma and 15% risk of persistent or invasive mole.

Partial Mole

Partial moles result from fertilization of an egg with two sperm (Fig. 22-52C). In these moles the karyotype is triploid (e.g., 69,XXY) or occasionally tetraploid (92,XXXY). Fetal tissues are typically present. Partial moles have an increased risk of persistent molar disease, but are not associated with choriocarcinoma.

MORPHOLOGY

The classic appearance of hydatidiform moles is that of a delicate, friable mass of thin-walled, translucent, cystic, grapelike structures consisting of swollen edematous (hydropic) villi (Figs. 22-53 and 22-54). In complete mole, the microscopic abnormalities involve all or most of the villous tissue. The chorionic villi are enlarged, scalloped in shape with central cavitation (cisterns), and are covered by extensive trophoblast proliferation that involves the entire circumference of the villi. In contrast, in partial moles, only a fraction of the villi are enlarged and edematous. The trophoblastic hyperplasia is focal and less marked than in complete moles.

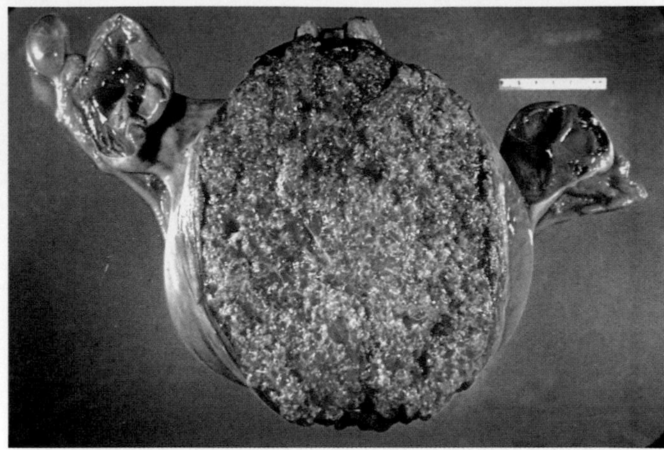

Figure 22-53 Complete hydatidiform mole. Note marked distention of the uterus by vesicular chorionic villi. Adnexa (ovaries and fallopian tubes) are visible on the *left* and *right side* of the uterus.

Clinical Features. Most women with partial and early complete moles present with spontaneous miscarriage or undergo curettage because of ultrasound findings of abnormal villous enlargement. In complete moles, human chorionic gonadotropin (HCG) levels greatly exceed those of a normal pregnancy of similar gestational age. In addition, the rate at which HCG levels rise over time in molar pregnancies exceeds those seen with normal single or even multiple pregnancies. Most moles are successfully removed by curettage. The patients are subsequently monitored for 6 months to a year to ensure that HCG levels decrease to non-pregnant levels. Continuous elevation of HCG may be indicative of *persistent or invasive mole*, which develops in up to 15% of molar pregnancies and is seen more frequently with complete moles. In addition, 2.5% of complete moles give rise to gestational choriocarcinoma.

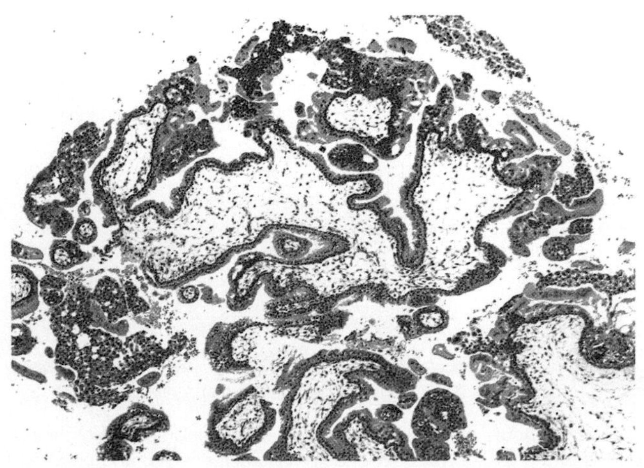

Figure 22-54 Complete hydatidiform mole demonstrating marked villous enlargement, edema, and circumferential trophoblast proliferation.

Invasive Mole

Invasive mole is defined as a mole that penetrates or even perforates the uterine wall. There is invasion of the myometrium by hydropic chorionic villi, accompanied by proliferation of both cytotrophoblasts and syncytiotrophoblasts. The tumor is locally destructive and may invade parametrial tissue and blood vessels. Hydropic villi may embolize to distant sites, such as lungs and brain, but do not grow in these organs as true metastases, and even without chemotherapy they eventually regress. The tumor is manifested clinically by vaginal bleeding and irregular uterine enlargement. It is always associated with a persistently elevated serum HCG. The tumor responds well to chemotherapy but may result in uterine rupture and necessitate hysterectomy.

Choriocarcinoma

Gestational choriocarcinoma is a malignant neoplasm of trophoblastic cells derived from a previously normal or abnormal pregnancy, such as an extrauterine ectopic pregnancy. Choriocarcinoma is rapidly invasive and metastasizes widely, but once identified responds well to chemotherapy.

Incidence. Gestational choriocarcinoma is an uncommon condition that arises in 1 in 20,000 to 30,000 pregnancies in the United States. It may be preceded by several conditions; 50% arise in complete hydatidiform moles, 25% in previous abortions, approximately 22% follow normal pregnancies, with the remainder occurring in ectopic pregnancies. Very rarely, a nongestational choriocarcinoma may develop from germ cells in the ovaries or the mediastinum.

MORPHOLOGY

Choriocarcinoma is a soft, fleshy, yellow-white tumor that usually has large pale areas of necrosis and extensive hemorrhage (Fig. 22-55*A*). Histologically, it does not produce chorionic villi and consists entirely of proliferating syncytiotrophoblasts and cytotrophoblasts (Fig. 22-55*B*). Mitoses are abundant and sometimes abnormal. The tumor invades the underlying myometrium, frequently penetrates blood vessels, and in some cases extends out onto the uterine serosa and into adjacent structures.

Clinical Features. Uterine choriocarcinoma usually manifests as irregular vaginal spotting of a bloody, brown fluid. This discharge may appear in the course of an apparently normal pregnancy, after a miscarriage, or after curettage. Sometimes the tumor does not appear until months after these events. This tumor has high propensity for hematogenous spread, and by the time it is discovered, radiographs of the chest and bones may disclose the presence of metastatic lesions. The HCG levels are typically elevated to levels above those encountered in hydatidiform moles, but occasional tumors produce little hormone, and some tumors are so necrotic that HCG levels are low. Widespread metastases are characteristic; the most common sites are the lungs (50%) and vagina (30% to 40%), followed by, in descending order of frequency, the brain, liver, bone and kidney.

The treatment of gestational choriocarcinoma depends on the stage of the tumor and usually consists of evacuation of the contents of the uterus and chemotherapy. The results of chemotherapy are spectacular and result in nearly 100% remission and a high rate of cures. Many of the cured patients have had normal subsequent pregnancies and deliveries. By contrast, nongestational choriocarcinomas that arise outside of the uterus are much more resistant to therapy.

Placental Site Trophoblastic Tumor (PSTT)

PSTTs comprise less than 2% of gestational trophoblastic neoplasms. They are neoplastic proliferations of extravillous trophoblasts, also called *intermediate trophoblasts.* In normal pregnancy, extravillous (intermediate) trophoblasts are found in nonvillous sites such as the implantation site, in islands of cells within the placental parenchyma, and in the placental membranes. Normal extravillous

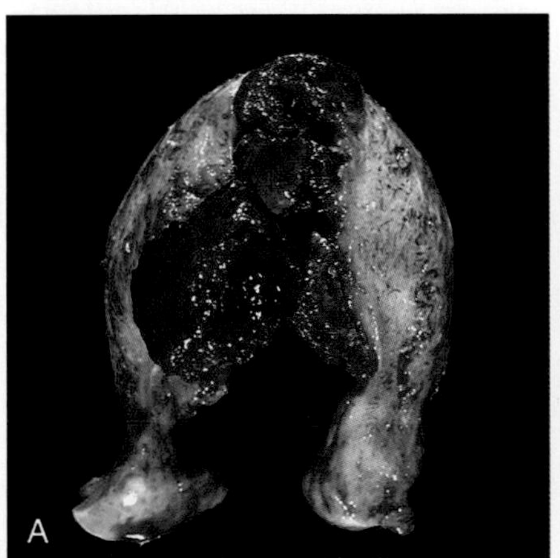

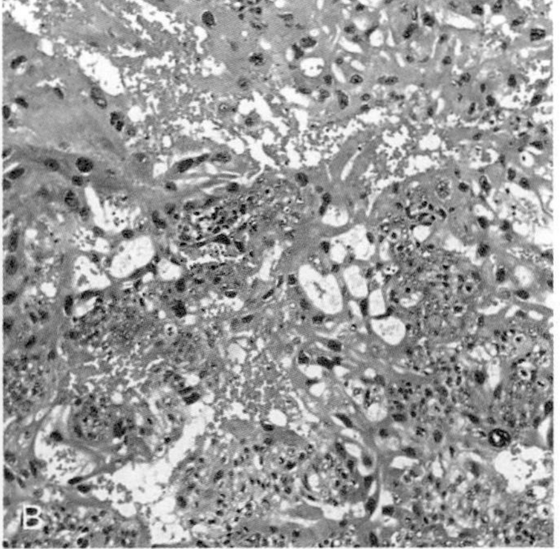

Figure 22-55 Choriocarcinoma. **A,** Choriocarcinoma presenting as a bulky hemorrhagic mass invading the uterine wall. **B,** Photomicrograph illustrating neoplastic cytotrophoblasts and syncytiotrophoblasts. (Courtesy Dr. David R. Genest, Brigham and Women's Hospital, Boston, Mass.)

trophoblasts are polygonal mononuclear cells that have abundant cytoplasm and produce human placental lactogen. PSTT presents as a uterine mass, accompanied by either abnormal uterine bleeding or amenorrhea and moderately elevated HCG. Histologically, PSTT is composed of malignant trophoblastic cells diffusely infiltrating the endomyometrium. It may follow a normal pregnancy (half of the cases), spontaneous abortion, or hydatidiform mole. Patients with localized disease have an excellent prognosis, however about 10% to 15% of women die of disseminated disease.

SUGGESTED READINGS

Infectious Diseases of Lower Genital Tract

Lee AJ, Ashkar AA: Herpes simplex virus-2 in the genital mucosa: insights into the mucosal host response and vaccine development. *Curr Opin Infect Dis* 25:92, 2012. *[Overview of HSV immunopathology.]*

Vulva

de Koning MN, Quint WGV, Pirog EC, et al: Prevalence of mucosal and cutaneous human papillomaviruses in different histologic subtypes of vulvar carcinoma. *Mod Pathol* 21:334, 2008. *[Comprehensive study of HPV in vulvar cancer.]*

Vagina

Schrager S, Potter BE: Diethylstilbestrol exposure. *Am Fam Physician* 69:2395, 2004. *[Review of clinical outcomes in patient with intrauterine DES exposure.]*

Cervix

Cutts FT, Francheschi S, Goldie S, et al: Human papillomavirus and HPV vaccines: a review. *Bull World Health Organ* 85:719, 2007. *[Review of HPV vaccines development.]*

Munoz N, Bosch FX, de Sanjose S, et al: Epidemiologic classification of human papillomavirus types associated with cervical cancer. *N Engl J Med* 348:518, 2003. *[Seminal study of HPV detection in cervical carcinoma.]*

Ostor AG: Natural history of cervical intraepithelial neoplasia: a critical review. *Int J Gynecol Pathol* 12:186, 1993. *[Comprehensive literature review of natural history of cervical intraepithelial neoplasia.]*

Saslow D, Runowicz CD, Solomon D, et al: American Cancer Society guideline for the early detection of cervical neoplasia and cancer. *J Low Genit Tract Dis* 7:67, 2003. *[Current recommendations for Pap screening.]*

Schiffman M, Castle PE, Jeronimo J, et al: Human papillomavirus and cervical cancer. *Lancet* 370:890, 2007. *[Review of HPV-related cervical carcinogenesis.]*

Wright TC Jr, Schiffman M, Solomon D, et al: Interim guidance for the use of human papillomavirus DNA testing as an adjunct to cervical cytology for screening. *Obstet Gynecol* 103:304, 2004. *[Current recommendations for HPV testing.]*

Uterus and Endometrium

Bulun SE: Endometriosis, *N Engl J Med* 360(3):268–79, 2009. *[Seminal review of endomtriosis pathogenesis.]*

Gargett CE, Nguyen HP, Ye L: Endometrial regeneration and endometrial stem/progenitor cells. *Rev Endocr Metab Disord* 13:235–51, 2012. *[Review of endometrial regeneration.]*

Giudice LC: Endometriosis. *N Engl J Med* 362(25):2389–98, 2010. *[Review of pathophysiology of endometriosis.]*

Kuhn E, Wu RC, Guan B, et al: Identification of Molecular Pathway Aberrations in Uterine Serous Carcinoma by Genome-wide Analyses. *J Natl Cancer Inst* 104(19):1503–13, 2012. *[First manuscript to describe novel mutations in serous carcinoma.]*

Le Gallo M, O'Hara AJ, Rudd ML, et al: Exome sequencing of serous endometrial tumors identifies recurrent somatic mutations in chromatin-remodeling and ubiquitin ligase complex genes. *Nat Genet* 44:1310–5, 2012. *[Comprehensive sequence analysis of serous endometrial carcinoma.]*

Makinen N, Mehine M, Tolvanen J, et al: MED12, the mediator complex subunit 12 gene is mutated at high frequency in uterine leiomyomas. *Science* 334:252–5, 2011. *[Landmark finding of a common intragenic mutation in leiomyomas.]*

Yeramian A, Moreno-Bueno G, Dolcet X, et al: Endometrial carcinoma: molecular alterations involved in tumor development and progression. *Oncogene* 32:403–13, 2013. *[Recent overview of the molecular biology of endometrial carcinoma.]*

Ovary

Cheng L, Roth M, Zhang S, et al: KIT gene mutation and amplification in dysgerminoma of the ovary. *Cancer* 117:2096–103, 2011. *[Clinicopathologica study of KIT alterations in dysgerminomas.]*

Cho KR, Shih IeM: Ovarian cancer. *Annu Rev Pathol* 4:287-313, 2009. *[Comprehensive review of the molecular genetics of ovarian carcinoma.]*

Diaz-Padilla I, Malpica AL, Minig L, et al: Ovarian low-grade serous carcinoma: a comprehensive update. *Gynecol Oncol* 126:279–85, 2012. *[Review of pathogenesis of low grade serous carcinoma of the ovary.]*

Goodarzi MO, Dumesic DA, Chazenbalk G, et al: Polycystic ovary syndrome: etiology, pathogenesis and diagnosis. *Nat Rev Endocrinol* 7:219–31, 2011. *[Overview of polycystic ovarian syndrome.]*

Heravi-Moussavi A, Anglesio MS, Cheng SW, et al: Recurrent somatic dicer mutations in nonepithelial ovarian cancers. *N Engl J Med* 366:234–42, 2012. *[Landmark study of mutations in non-epithelial ovarian tumors.]*

Weigand KC, Shah SP, Al-Agha OM, et al: ARID1A Mutations in Endometriosis-Associated Ovarian Carcinomas. *N Engl J Med* 363:1532–43, 2010. *[Discovery of ARID1A mutation in ovarian cancer].*

Placenta

Baumwell S, Karumanchi SA: Pre-eclampsia: clinical manifestations and molecular mechanisms. *Nephron Clin Pract* 106:72, 2007. *[Review of clinical and molecular correlates in pre-eclampsia pathophysiology.]*

Lurain JR: Gestational trophoblastic disease I: epidemiology, pathology, clinical presentation and diagnosis of gestational trophoblastic disease, and management of hydatidiform mole. *Am J Obstet Gynecol* 203:531, 2010. *[Review of clinicopathologic characteristics of molar pregnancies.]*

Maynard S, Epstein FH, Karumanchi SA: Preeclampsia and angiogenic imbalance. *Ann Rev Med* 59:61, 2008. *[Review of angiogenic alterations pre-eclampsia.]*

Wilcox AJ, Weinberg CR, O'Connor JF, et al: Incidence of early loss of pregnancy. *N Engl J Med* 319:189, 1988. *[Older but still useful paper on early pregnancy loss.]*

See TARGETED THERAPY available online at www.studentconsult.com

CHAPTER 23

The Breast

Susan C. Lester

CHAPTER CONTENTS

Three important features distinguish the breast from other organs. First, the major function is the nutritional support of another individual, the infant. Second, the structure of the organ undergoes marked periodic changes during adulthood, particularly during pregancy, before involuting with age. Finally, breasts are visible and, as a result, have a social, cultural, and personal significance not shared by other organs. All of these features play a role when considering the origins, presentations, and treatment of breast disease.

Understanding diseases of the breast requires a working knowledge of its normal anatomy and cellular constituents, which include two major structures (ducts and lobules), two types of epithelial cells (luminal and myoepithelial), and two types of stroma (interlobular and intralobular). Each element is the source of both benign and malignant lesions (Fig. 23-1). Six to 10 major duct orifices open onto the skin surface at the nipple. The superficial portions are lined by keratinizing squamous cells that abruptly change to the double-layered epithelium (luminal and myoepithelial cells) of the remainder of the duct/lobular system. Successive branching of the large ducts eventually leads to the terminal duct lobular unit. In adult women, the terminal duct branches into a grapelike cluster of small acini to form a lobule (Figs. 23-1 and 23-2*B*). In some women, ducts extend into the subcutaneous tissue of the chest wall and into the axilla.

In the prepubertal female breast and in males, the large duct system ends in terminal ducts. Changes in the breast are most dynamic and profound during the reproductive years of females (Fig. 23-2). Just as the endometrium grows and ebbs with each menstrual cycle, so does the breast. In the first half of the menstrual cycle the lobules are relatively quiescent. After ovulation, under the influence of estrogen and rising progesterone levels, cell proliferation increases, as does the number of acini per lobule. The intralobular stroma becomes markedly edematous. Upon menstruation, the fall in hormone levels induces the regression of the lobules and the disappearance of edema.

Only with the onset of pregnancy does the breast become completely mature and functional. Lobules increase progressively in number and size. By the end of the pregnancy the breast is composed almost entirely of lobules separated by relatively scant stroma (Fig. 23-2*C*). Immediately after parturition, the lobules produce

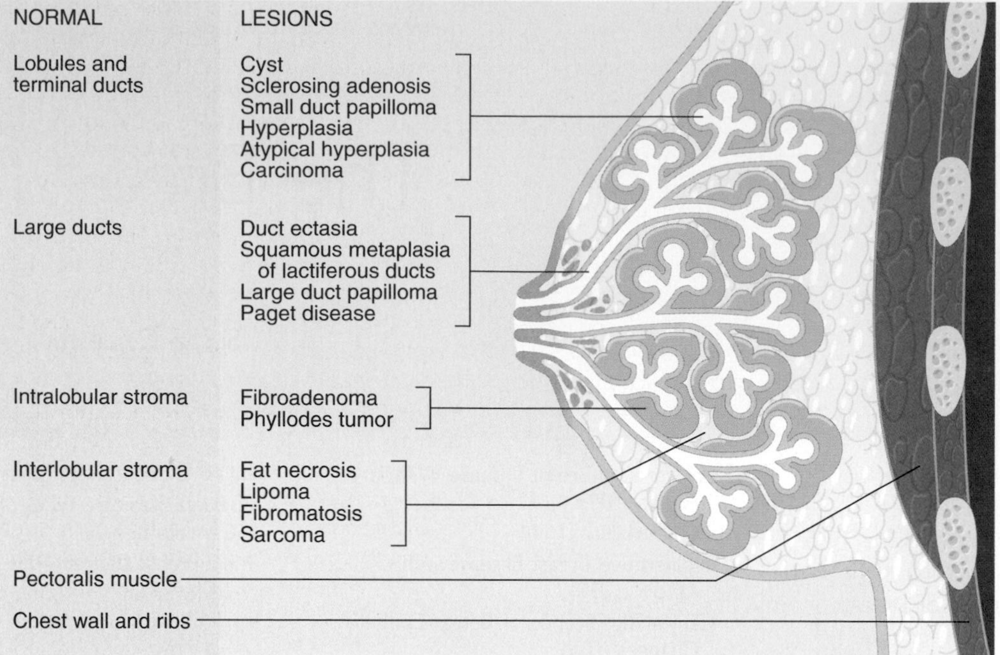

Figure 23-1 Anatomic origins of common breast lesions.

colostrum (high in protein), changing to milk (higher in fat and calories) over the next 10 days as progesterone levels drop. The permanent changes produced by pregnancy may explain the reduction in breast cancer risk that is observed in women who give birth to children at young ages. Upon the cessation of lactation, epithelial cells undergo apoptosis and lobules regress. However, full regression does not occur, and as a result pregnancy causes a permanent increase in the size and number of lobules.

After the third decade, long before menopause, lobules and their specialized stroma start to involute (Fig. 23-2*D*) and the interlobular stroma converts from radiodense fibrous stroma (Fig. 23-2*A*) to radiolucent adipose tissue (Fig. 23-2*E*). To some extent, these changes are obscured by either endogenous sources of hormones (e.g., estrogen from fat stores in obese women) or exogenous sources (e.g., menopausal hormone replacement therapy).

Disorders of Development

Milk Line Remnants

Supernumerary nipples or breasts result from the persistence of epidermal thickenings along the milk line, which extends from the axilla to the perineum. The disorders that affect the normally situated breast rarely arise in these heterotopic, hormone-responsive foci, which most commonly come to attention as a result of painful premenstrual enlargements.

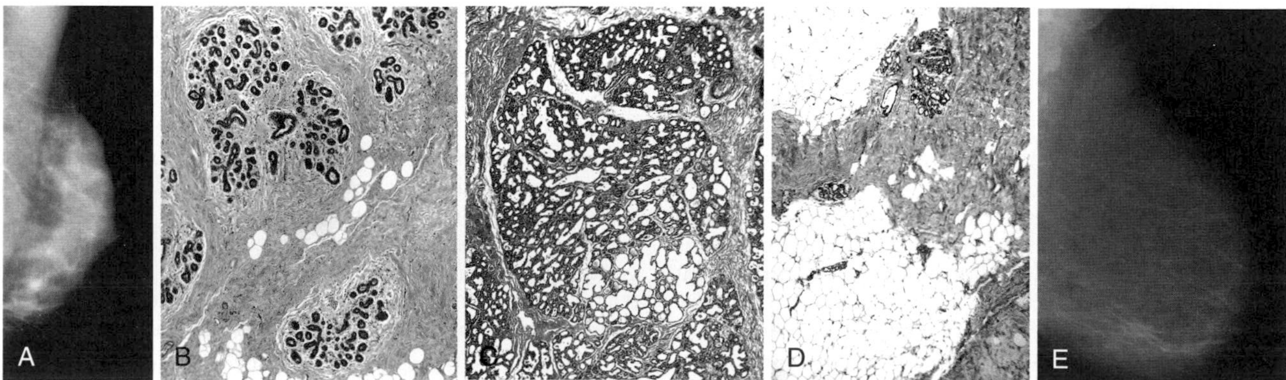

Figure 23-2 Life cycle changes. **A,** Mammograms in young women are typically radiodense or white in appearance, making mass-forming lesions or calcifications (which are also radiodense) difficult to detect. **B,** The density of a young woman's breast stems from the predominance of fibrous interlobular stroma and the paucity of adipose tissue. Before pregnancy the lobules are small and are invested by loose cellular intralobular stroma. **C,** During pregnancy, branching of terminal ducts produces more numerous, larger lobules. Luminal cells within lobules undergo lactational change, a precursor to milk formation. **D,** With increasing age the lobules decrease in size and number, and the interlobular stroma is replaced by adipose tissue. **E,** Mammograms become more radiolucent with age as a result of the increase in adipose tissue, which facilitates the detection of radiodense mass-forming lesions and calcifications. (**A, E,** Courtesy of Dr. Darrell Smith, Brigham and Women's Hospital, Boston, MA.)

Accessory Axillary Breast Tissue

In some women the normal ductal system extends into the subcutaneous tissue of the chest wall or the axillary fossa (the "axillary tail of Spence"), outside of the area clinically identified as breast tissue. Because breast tissue may not be removed in these areas, prophylactic mastectomies markedly reduce, but do not completely eliminate, the risk of breast cancer.

Congenital Nipple Inversion

The failure of the nipple to evert during development is common and may be unilateral. Congenitally inverted nipples are usually of little significance since they correct spontaneously during pregnancy, or can sometimes be everted by simple traction. Acquired nipple retraction is of more concern, since it may indicate the presence of an invasive cancer or an inflammatory nipple disease.

Clinical Presentations of Breast Disease

The most common symptoms reported by women with disorders of the breast are pain, a palpable mass, "lumpiness" (without a discrete mass), or nipple discharge (Fig. 23-3*A*). All are nonspecific but must be evaluated because of the possibility of malignancy.

- *Pain* (mastalgia or mastodynia) is a common symptom that may be cyclic with menses or noncyclic. Diffuse cyclic pain may be due to premenstrual edema. Noncyclic pain is usually localized to one area of the breast and may be caused by ruptured cysts, physical injury, and infections, but often no specific lesion is identified. Although almost all painful masses are benign, about 10% of breast cancers present with pain.
- *Palpable masses* are also common and must be distinguished from the normal nodularity (or "lumpiness") of the breast. **The most common palpable lesions are cysts, fibroadenomas, and invasive carcinomas.** Benign palpable masses are most common in premenopausal women and the likelihood of a malignancy increases with age. Only 10% of breast masses in women younger than age 40 are malignant as compared with 60% of masses in women older than age 50. Approximately 50% of carcinomas are located in the upper outer quadrant, 10% in each of the remaining quadrants, and about 20% in the central or subareolar region. Although about one third of cancers are first detected as a palpable mass, screening by breast examination has little effect on reducing breast cancer mortality. Unfortunately, the majority of cancers that have the capacity to metastasize will have done so by the time they reach a size that can be palpated—generally around 2 to 3 cm.
- *Nipple discharge* is a less common finding that is most worrisome for carcinoma when it is spontaneous and unilateral. A small discharge is often produced by the manipulation of normal breasts. Milky discharges (galactorrhea) are associated with elevated prolactin levels (e.g., by a pituitary adenoma), hypothyroidism, or endocrine anovulatory syndromes, and also occur in patients taking oral contraceptives, tricyclic antidepressants, methyldopa, or phenothiazines. Repeated nipple stimulation can also induce lactation. Galactorrhea is not associated with malignancy. Bloody or serous discharges are most commonly due to large duct papillomas and cysts. During pregnancy, a bloody discharge can result from the rapid growth and remodeling of the breast. The risk of malignancy in a woman with nipple discharge increases with age; it is associated with carcinoma in 7% of women younger than age 60 but in 30% of older women.

Mammographic screening was introduced in the 1980s as a means to detect small, nonpalpable, asymptomatic breast carcinomas and is currently the most common means to detect breast cancer (Fig 23-3*B*). The sensitivity and specificity of mammography increase with age, as a result of replacement of the fibrous, radiodense tissue of youth with the fatty, radiolucent tissue of older women (Fig. 23-2). At age 40, the probability that a mammographic

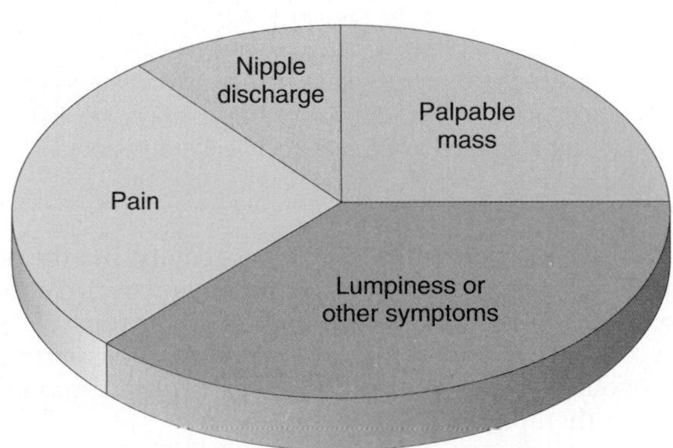

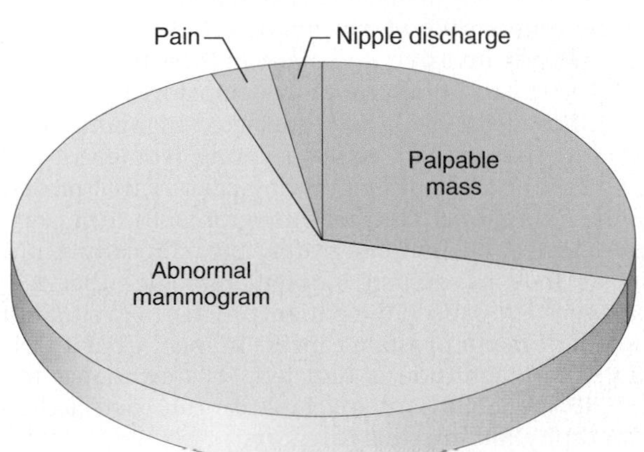

Figure 23-3 Symptoms of breast disease and presentations of breast cancer. **A,** Common symptoms of breast disease. Although pain, "lumpiness," and nipple discharge often cause concern, these symptoms are associated with cancer in less than 10% of affected women. **B,** Presentations of breast cancer. In the United States, more than half of cancers are asymptomatic and are detected by mammographic screening and about another one third present as palpable masses—almost all discovered by the patient.

lesion is cancer is only 10%, but this rises to greater than 25% in women older than 50. **The principal mammographic signs of breast carcinoma are densities and calcifications:**

- *Densities.* Breast lesions that replace adipose tissue with radiodense tissue form mammographic densities. Rounded densities are most commonly benign lesions such as fibroadenomas or cysts (see Fig. 23-27), whereas invasive carcinomas generally form irregular masses (see Fig. 23-22). Mammography can identify small, nonpalpable cancers that are, on average, about half the size of invasive carcinomas detected by palpation (i.e., 1 cm rather than 2 to 3 cm).
- *Calcifications.* Calcifications form on secretions, necrotic debris, or hyalinized stroma. Calcifications are often associated with benign lesions such as clusters of apocrine cysts, hyalinized fibroadenomas, and sclerosing adenosis (see Fig. 23-6). Calcifications associated with malignancy are usually small, irregular, numerous, and clustered. Screening has increased the diagnosis of ductal carcinoma in situ (DCIS), since it is most commonly detected as mammographic calcifications (see Figs. 23-14 and 23-17).

Approximately 10% of invasive carcinomas are not detected by mammography. The principal causes are the presence of surrounding radiodense tissue obscuring the tumor (especially in younger women), small size, a diffuse infiltrative pattern with little or no desmoplastic response, or a location close to the chest wall or in the periphery of the breast. The inability to image a palpable mass does not indicate that it is benign, and all palpable masses require further investigation. Other imaging modalities can be useful adjuncts. For example, ultrasonography distinguishes between solid and cystic lesions and defines more precisely the borders of solid lesions, while magnetic resonance imaging (MRI) detects cancers by the rapid uptake of contrast agents due to increased tumor vascularity and blood flow.

Although the recent downward trend in deaths from breast cancer is partially attributed to earlier diagnosis due to mammography, the beneficial effect of screening has been smaller than originally anticipated for several reasons. Seventy percent to 80% of cancers detected by mammography are already invasive, and many of these have already metastasized. In addition, the cancers most likely to cause death are those least likely to be detected by mammography. These lethal cancers arise in young women of prescreening age, or are rapidly growing cancers that present during the interval between mammograms. In turn, some cancers detected by mammography are clinically unimportant, as they have such indolent biologies that they would never have caused the patient any harm (a situation reminiscent of many prostate cancers in men, Chapter 21). Although the magnitude is debated, it is estimated that between 10% and 30% of invasive cancers detected by mammography fall into this category.

Inflammatory Disorders

Inflammatory diseases of the breast are rare (accounting for less than 1% of breast symptoms) and are caused by infections, autoimmune disease, or by foreign body type reactions to extravasated keratin or secretions. "Inflammatory breast cancer" mimics inflammation by obstructing dermal vasculature with tumor emboli, and should always be considered in women with an erythematous swollen breast.

Acute Mastitis

Acute bacterial mastitis typically occurs during the first month of breastfeeding and is caused by a local bacterial infection when the breast is most vulnerable due to cracks and fissures in the nipples. From this portal of entry, *Staphylococcus aureus* or, less commonly, streptococci invade the breast tissue. The breast is erythematous and painful, and fever is often present. At the outset only one duct system or sector of the breast is involved. If not treated the infection may spread to the entire breast. Staphylococcal abscesses may be single or multiple whereas Streptococci cause spreading infection in the form of cellulitis.

Most cases of lactational mastitis are easily treated with appropriate antibiotics and continued expression of milk from the breast. Rarely, surgical drainage is required.

Squamous Metaplasia of Lactiferous Ducts

Squamous metaplasia of lactiferous ducts is known by a variety of names, including recurrent subareolar abscess, periductal mastitis, and Zuska disease. Women, and sometimes men, present with a painful erythematous subareolar mass that clinically appears to be a bacterial abscess. In recurrent cases, a characteristic fistula tract often tunnels under the smooth muscle of the nipple and opens onto the skin at the edge of the areola. Many women have an inverted nipple, most likely as a secondary effect of the underlying inflammation. More than 90% of the afflicted are smokers. It has been suggested that a relative deficiency of vitamin A associated with smoking or toxic substances in tobacco smoke alter the differentiation of the ductal epithelium.

MORPHOLOGY

The key feature is **keratinizing squamous metaplasia** of the nipple ducts (Fig. 23-4). Keratin shed from these cells plugs the ductal system, causing dilation and eventually rupture of the duct. An intense chronic granulomatous inflammatory response develops once keratin spills into the surrounding periductal tissue. With recurrences, a secondary anaerobic bacterial infection may supervene and cause acute inflammation.

Simple incision drains the abscess cavity, but the offending keratinizing epithelium remains and recurrences are common. In most cases, en bloc surgical removal of the involved duct and contiguous fistula tract is curative. If secondary bacterial infection is present, antibiotics also have a therapeutic role.

Duct Ectasia

Duct ectasia presents as a palpable periareolar mass that is often associated with thick, white nipple secretions and occasionally with skin retraction. Pain and erythema are

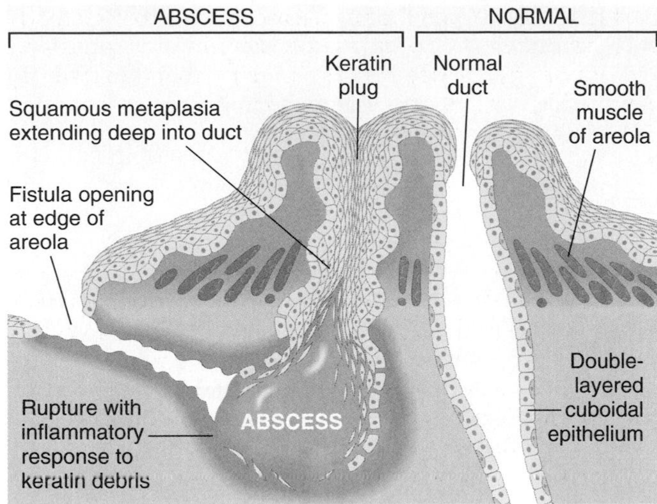

Figure 23-4 Squamous metaplasia of lactiferous ducts. When squamous metaplasia extends deep into a nipple duct, keratin becomes trapped and accumulates. If the duct ruptures, the ensuing intense inflammatory response to keratin results in an erythematous painful mass. A fistula tract may burrow beneath the smooth muscle of the nipple to open at the edge of the areola.

uncommon. This disorder tends to occur in the fifth or sixth decade of life, usually in multiparous women. Unlike squamous metaplasia of lactiferous ducts, it is not associated with cigarette smoking.

MORPHOLOGY

Ectatic dilated ducts are filled with inspissated secretions and numerous lipid-laden macrophages. When ruptured, a marked periductal and interstitial chronic inflammatory reaction ensues, consisting of lymphocytes, macrophages, and variable numbers of plasma cells (Fig. 23-5). Granulomas may form around cholesterol deposits and secretions. Subsequent fibrosis produces an irregular mass with skin and nipple retraction.

The principal significance of this disorder is that the irregular palpable mass mimics the clinical and radiographic appearance of invasive carcinoma.

Fat Necrosis

The presentations of fat necrosis are protean and can closely mimic cancer—as a painless palpable mass, skin thickening or retraction, or mammographic densities or calcifications. About half of affected women have a history of breast trauma or prior surgery.

MORPHOLOGY

Acute lesions may be hemorrhagic and contain central areas of liquefactive fat necrosis with neutrophils and macrophages. Over the next few days proliferating fibroblasts and chronic inflammatory cells surround the injured area. Subsequently, giant cells, calcifications, and hemosiderin make their appearance, and eventually the focus is replaced by scar tissue or is encircled and walled off by fibrous tissue. Ill-defined, firm, gray-white nodules containing small chalky-white foci are seen grossly.

Lymphocytic Mastopathy (Sclerosing Lymphocytic Lobulitis)

This condition presents with single or multiple hard palpable masses or mammographic densities. It can be difficult to obtain tissue with a needle biopsy due to the dense collagenized stroma. Atrophic ducts and lobules have thickened basement membranes and are surrounded by a prominent lymphocytic infiltrate. This condition is most common in women with type 1 (insulin-dependent) diabetes or autoimmune thyroid disease and is hypothesized to have an autoimmune basis. Its only clinical significance is that it must be distinguished from breast cancer.

Granulomatous Mastitis

Granulomatous inflammation of the breast can be a manifestation of systemic granulomatous diseases (e.g., granulomatosis with polyangiitis, sarcoidosis, tuberculosis) or of disorders that are localized to the breast (granulomatous lobular mastitis, rare infections). *Granulomatous lobular mastitis* is an uncommon disease that only occurs in parous women. The granulomas are closely associated with lobules, suggesting that the disease may be caused by a hypersensitivity reaction to antigens expressed during lactation. Treatment with steroids is sometimes effective. A similar histologic pattern is seen in *cystic neutrophilic granulomatous mastitis* caused by *Corynebacteria*. Localized infections by mycobacteria or fungi are very rare and are most common in immunocompromised patients or adjacent to foreign objects such as breast prostheses or nipple piercings.

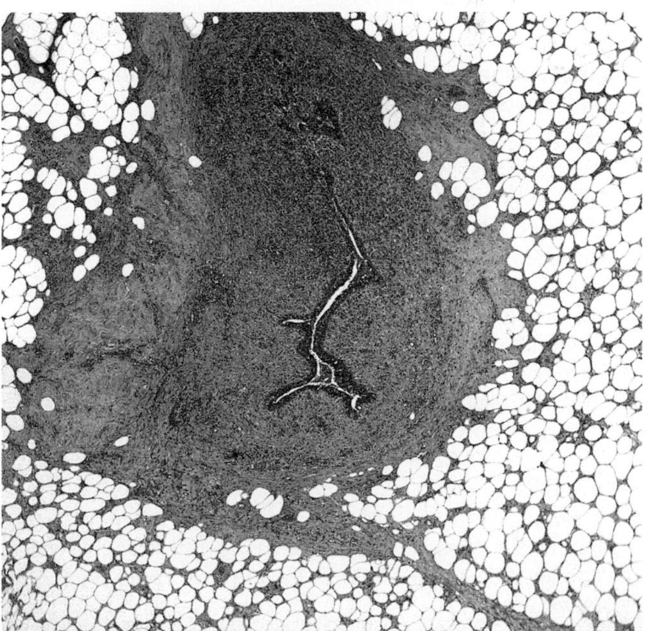

Figure 23-5 Duct ectasia. Chronic inflammation and fibrosis surround an ectatic duct filled with inspissated debris. The fibrotic response can produce a firm irregular mass that mimics invasive carcinoma on palpation or mammogram.

KEY CONCEPTS

Inflammatory Disorders

- Inflammatory diseases of the breast are rare outside of the lactational period.
- The specific cause must be determined as appropriate treatment may be antibiotics, steroids, or surgery.
- The possibility of inflammatory carcinoma mimicking a non-neoplastic inflammatiory disorder should always be considered.

Benign Epithelial Lesions

Benign epithelial lesions are classified into three groups, according to the subsequent risk of developing breast cancer: (1) *nonproliferative breast changes,* (2) *proliferative breast disease,* and (3) *atypical hyperplasia.* Most come to clinical attention when detected by mammography or as incidental findings in surgical specimens.

Nonproliferative Breast Changes (Fibrocystic Changes)

This group includes common morphologic alterations that are often grouped under the term *fibrocystic changes.* To the clinician the term might mean "lumpy bumpy" breasts on palpation; to the radiologist, a dense breast with cysts; and to the pathologist, benign histologic findings. These lesions are termed *nonproliferative* to indicate that they are not associated with an increased risk of breast cancer.

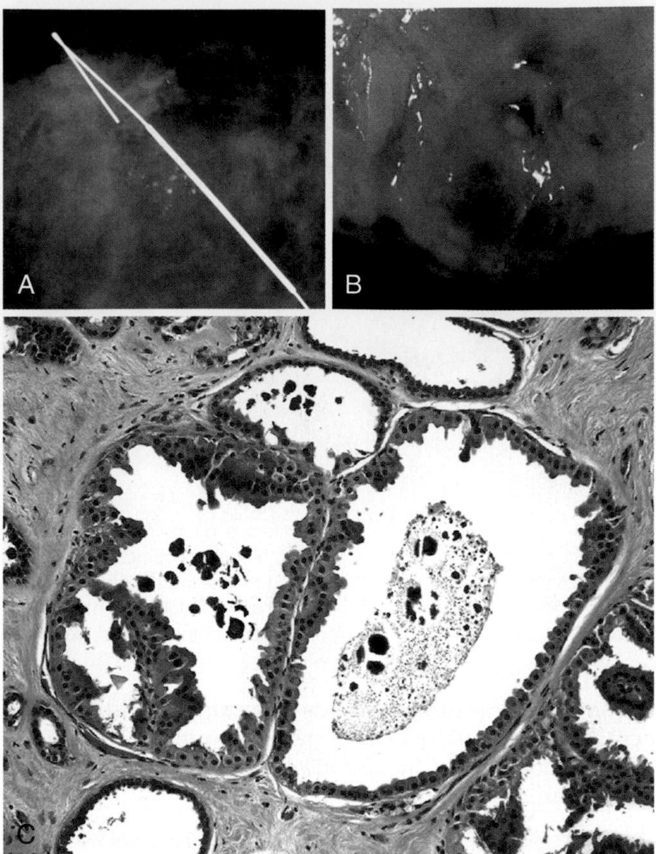

Figure 23-6 Apocrine cysts. **A,** Clustered, rounded calcifications are seen in a specimen radiograph. **B,** Gross appearance of typical cysts filled with dark, turbid fluid contents. **C,** Cysts are lined by apocrine cells with round nuclei and abundant granular cytoplasm. Note the luminal calcifications, which form on secretory debris.

MORPHOLOGY

There are three principal morphologic changes: (1) cystic change, often with apocrine metaplasia, (2) fibrosis, and (3) adenosis.

- ***Cysts.*** Small cysts form by the dilation of lobules and in turn may coalesce to form larger cysts. Unopened cysts contain turbid, semi-translucent fluid of a brown or blue color (blue-dome cysts) (Fig. 23-6*B*). Cysts are lined either by a flattened atrophic epithelium or by metaplastic apocrine cells. The latter cells have abundant granular, eosinophilic cytoplasm and round nuclei and closely resemble the normal apocrine epithelium of sweat glands (Fig. 23-6*C*). Calcifications are common and may be detected by mammography (Fig. 23-6*A*). Cysts may cause concern when they are solitary and firm to palpation. The diagnosis is confirmed by the disappearance of the mass after fine-needle aspiration of its contents.
- ***Fibrosis.*** Cysts frequently rupture, releasing secretory material into the adjacent stroma. The resulting chronic inflammation and fibrosis contribute to the palpable nodularity of the breast.
- ***Adenosis.*** Adenosis is defined as an increase in the number of acini per lobule. It is a normal feature of pregnancy. In nonpregnant women, adenosis can occur as a focal change. Calcifications are occasionally present within the lumens. The acini are lined by columnar cells, which may appear benign or show nuclear atypia (**"flat epithelial atypia"**). Flat epithelial atypia is a clonal proliferation associated with deletions of chromosome 16q. This lesion is thought to be the earliest recognizable precursor of low-grade breast cancers, but does not convey an increased cancer risk, presumably because other steps in cancer development are rate limiting.

Lactational adenomas present as palpable masses in pregnant or lactating women. They consist of normal-appearing breast tissue with lactational changes. These lesions are not proven to be neoplastic and may simply represent an exaggerated local response to gestational hormones.

Proliferative Breast Disease Without Atypia

Lesions characterized by proliferation of epithelial cells, without atypia, are associated with a small increase in the risk of subsequent carcinoma in either breast. They are commonly detected as mammographic densities, calcifications, or as incidental findings in biopsies performed for other reasons. These lesions are not clonal and are not commonly found to have genetic changes. Thus they are predictors of risk but unlikely to be true precursors of carcinoma.

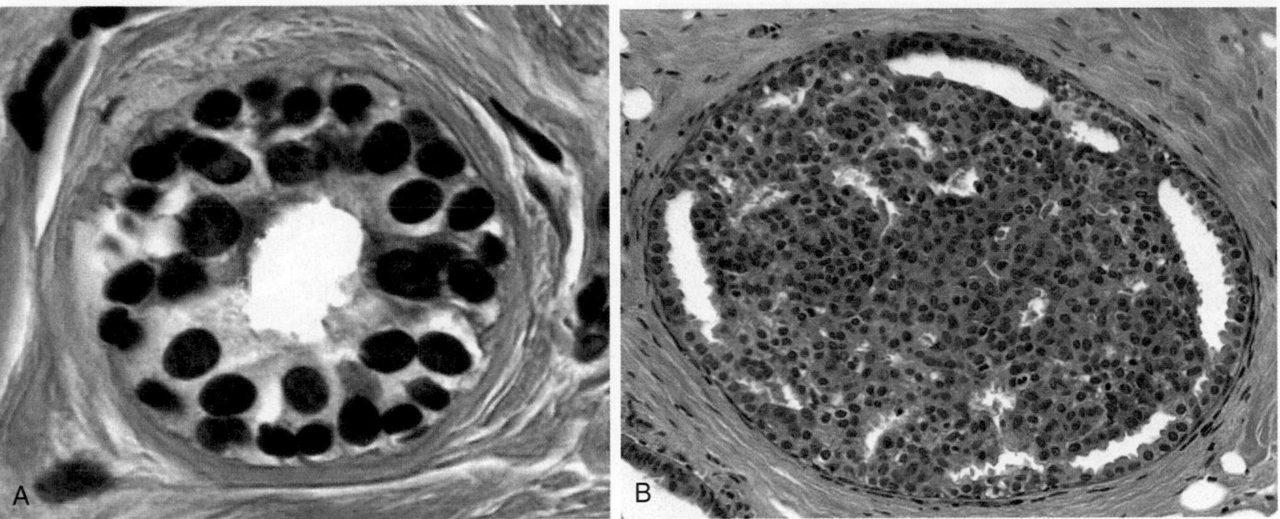

Figure 23-7 A, A normal duct or acinus with a single basally located myoepithelial cell layer (cells with dark, compact nuclei and scant cytoplasm) and a single luminal cell layer (cells with larger open nuclei, small nucleoli, and more abundant cytoplasm). **B,** Epithelial hyperplasia. The lumen is filled by a heterogeneous, mixed population of luminal and myoepithelial cell types. Irregular slitlike fenestrations are prominent at the periphery.

MORPHOLOGY

Epithelial Hyperplasia. Normal breast ducts and lobules are lined by a double-layer of myoepithelial cells and luminal cells (Fig. 23-7*A*). In epithelial hyperplasia, increased numbers of both luminal and myoepithelial cell types fill and distend ducts and lobules. Irregular lumens can often be discerned at the periphery of the cellular masses (Fig. 23-7*B*). Epithelial hyperplasia is usually an incidental finding.

Sclerosing Adenosis. There are an increased number of acini that are compressed and distorted in the central portion of the lesion. On occasion, stromal fibrosis may completely compress the lumens to create the appearance of solid cords or double strands of cells lying within dense stroma, a histologic pattern that at times closely mimics invasive carcinoma (Fig. 23-8). Sclerosing adenosis can come to attention as a palpable mass, a radiologic density, or calcifications.

Complex Sclerosing Lesion. These lesions have components of sclerosing adenosis, papillomas, and epithelial hyperplasia. One member of this group, the radial sclerosing lesion ("radial scar"), has an irregular shape and can closely mimic invasive carcinoma mammographically, grossly, and histologically (Fig. 23-9). A central nidus of entrapped glands in a hyalinized stroma is surrounded by long radiating projections into stroma. The term *radial scar* is a misnomer, as these lesions are not associated with prior trauma or surgery.

Papilloma. Papillomas grow within a dilated duct and are composed of multiple branching fibrovascular cores (Fig. 23-10). Epithelial hyperplasia and apocrine metaplasia are frequently present. Large duct papillomas are situated in the lactiferous sinuses of the nipple and are usually solitary. Small duct papillomas are commonly multiple and located deeper within the ductal system.

More than 80% of large duct papillomas produce a nipple discharge. Some discharges are bloody if the stalk undergoes torsion causing infarction. Serous discharge results from intermittent blockage and release of normal breast secretions or irritation of the duct by the papilloma. Most small duct papillomas come to clinical attention as small palpable masses, or as densities or calcifications seen on mammograms.

Gynecomastia

Gynecomastia (enlargement of the male breast) is the only benign lesion seen with any frequency in the male breast. It presents as a button-like subareolar enlargement and may be unilateral or bilateral. Microscopically, there is an increase in dense collagenous connective tissue associated with epithelial hyperplasia of the duct lining with characteristic tapering micropapillae (Fig. 23-11). Lobule formation is almost never observed.

Gynecomastia occurs as a result of an imbalance between estrogens, which stimulate breast tissue, and androgens, which counteract these effects. It may appear during

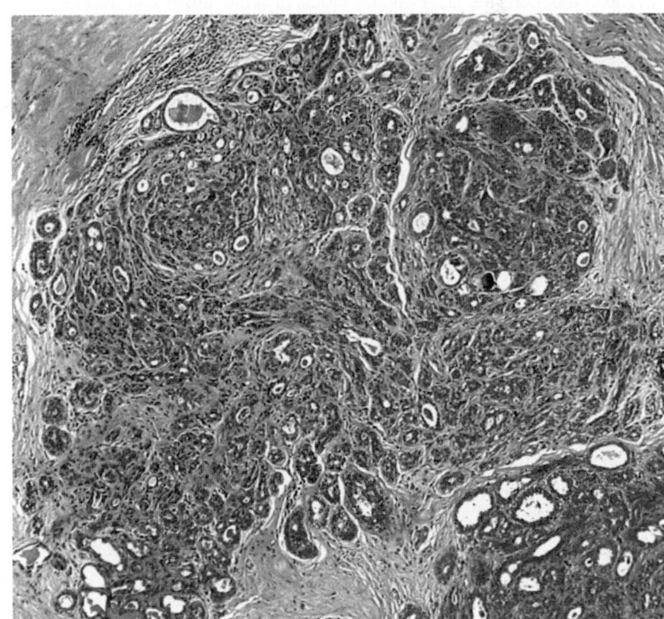

Figure 23-8 Sclerosing adenosis. The involved terminal duct lobular unit is enlarged, and the acini are compressed and distorted by dense stroma. Calcifications are present within some of the lumens. Unlike carcinomas, the acini are arranged in a swirling pattern, and the outer border is well circumscribed.

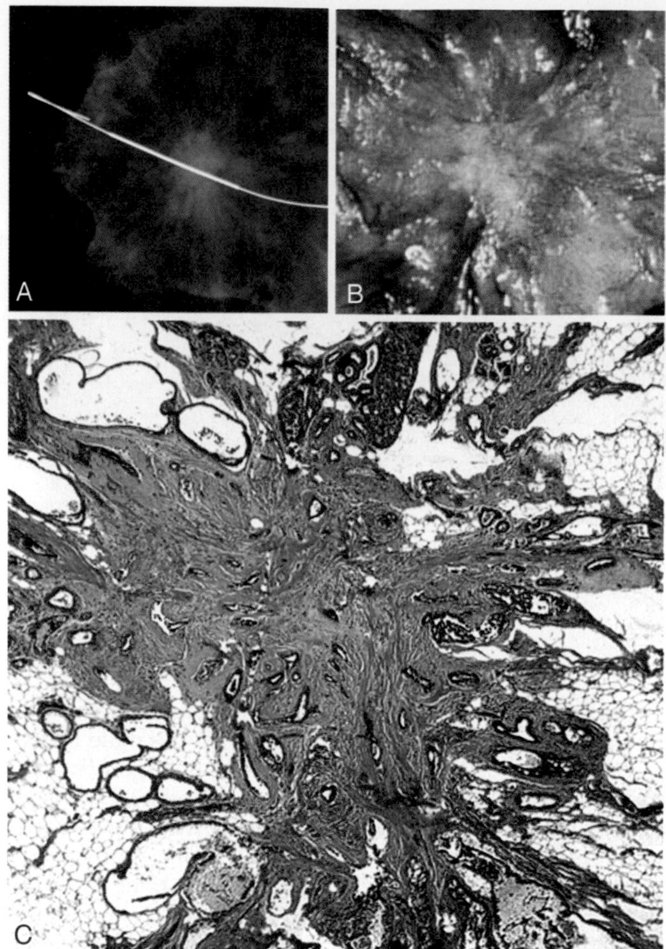

Figure 23-9 Radial sclerosing lesion. **A,** The radiograph shows an irregular central mass with long radiodense projections. **B,** Grossly the mass appears solid and has irregular borders, but it is not as firm as an invasive carcinoma. **C,** The mass consists of a central nidus of small tubules entrapped in a densely fibrotic stroma and numerous projections containing epithelium with varying degrees of cyst formation and hyperplasia.

puberty, in the very aged, or at any time during adult life when there is cause for hyperestrinism. The most important of these is cirrhosis of the liver, since this organ is responsible for metabolizing estrogen. In older males, gynecomastia may stem from a relative increase in estrogens as testicular androgen production falls. Drugs such as alcohol, marijuana, heroin, antiretroviral therapy, and anabolic steroids have been associated with gynecomastia. Rarely, gynecomastia occurs as part of Klinefelter syndrome (XXY karyotype) or in association with functioning testicular neoplasms, such as Leydig cell or Sertoli cell tumors. Similar to proliferative disease in women, gynecomastia may be associated with a small increased risk of breast cancer.

Proliferative Breast Disease with Atypia

Atypical hyperplasia is a clonal proliferation having some, but not all, of the histologic features that are required for the diagnosis of carcinoma in situ. It is associated with a moderately increased risk of carcinoma and includes two forms, atypical ductal hyperplasia and atypical lobular hyperplasia. Atypical ductal hyperplasia is

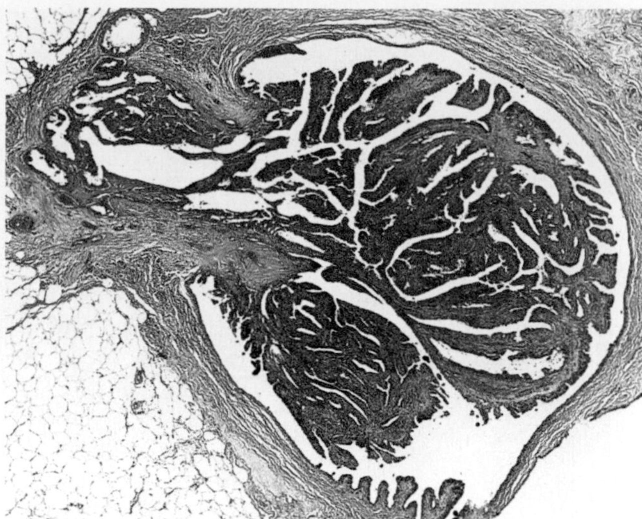

Figure 23-10 Intraductal papilloma. A central fibrovascular core extends from the wall of a duct. The papillae arborize within the lumen and are lined by myoepithelial and luminal cells.

present in 5% to 17% of specimens from biopsies performed for calcifications. Atypical lobular hyperplasia is an incidental finding and is found in fewer than 5% of biopsies.

MORPHOLOGY

Atypical ductal hyperplasia is recognized by its histologic resemblance to ductal carcinoma in situ (DCIS). It consists of a relatively monomorphic proliferation of regularly spaced cells, sometimes with cribriform spaces. It is distinguished from DCIS in that it only partially fills involved ducts (Fig. 23-12*A*).

Atypical lobular hyperplasia consists of cells identical to those of lobular carcinoma in situ (described later), but the cells do not fill or distend more than 50% of the acini within a lobule (Fig. 23-12*B*). In atypical lobular hyperplasia, atypical lobular cells may lie between the ductal basement membrane and overlying normal luminal cells.

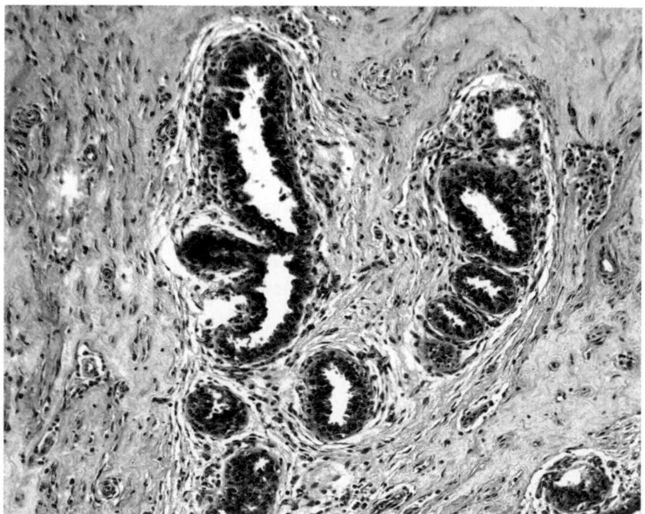

Figure 23-11 Gynecomastia. Breast enlargement in males is due to an increase in the number of ducts accompanied by loose cellular stroma. Lobule formation is absent.

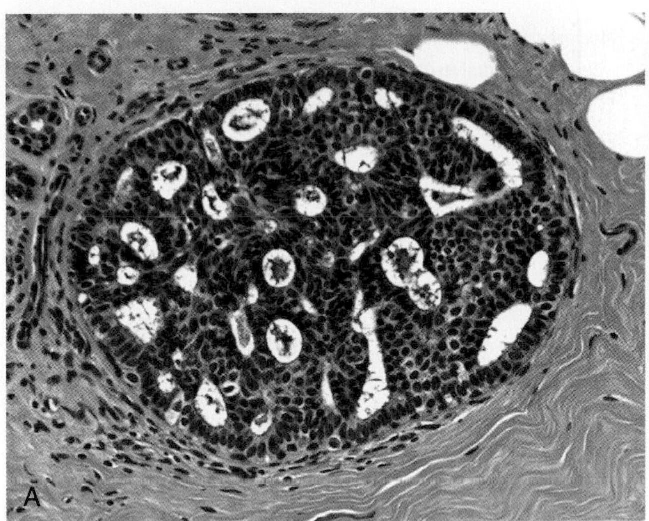

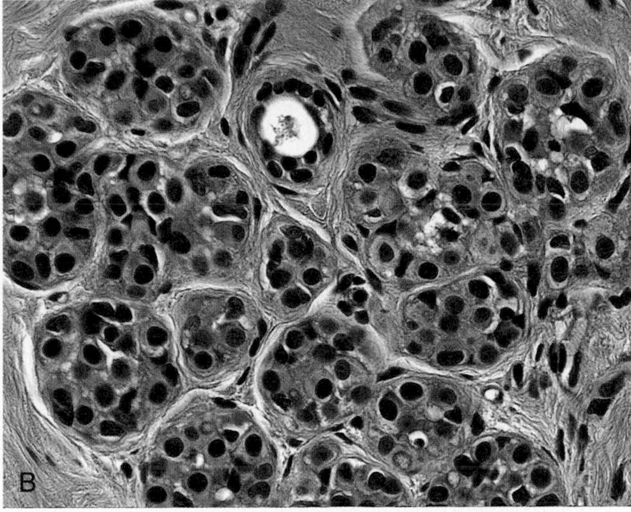

Figure 23-12 A, Atypical ductal hyperplasia. A duct is filled with a mixed population of cells consisting of oriented columnar cells at the periphery and more rounded cells within the central portion. Although some of the spaces are round and regular, the peripheral spaces are irregular and slitlike. These features are highly atypical, but fall short of a diagnosis of ductal carcinoma in situ. **B,** Atypical lobular hyperplasia. A population of monomorphic small, round, loosely cohesive cells partially fills a lobule. Although the cells are morphologically identical to the cells of lobular carcinoma in situ, the extent of involvement is not sufficient for this diagnosis.

Atypical ductal and atypical lobular hyperplasias may have acquired chromosomal aberrations such as loss of 16q or gain of 17p, changes also found in carcinoma in situ. Atypical lobular hyperplasia also shows loss of E-cadherin expression, a feature it shares with lobular carcinoma in situ (discussed later). This form of intraepithelial spread is called "pagetoid" because of its resemblance to Paget disease, described later.

Clinical Significance of Benign Epithelial Changes

Epidemiologic studies have established the association of benign histologic changes with the later development of invasive cancer (Table 23-1). Nonproliferative changes do not increase the risk of cancer. Proliferative disease is associated with a 1.5- to two-fold increased risk, while proliferative disease with atypia confers a four- to five-fold increased risk. Both breasts are at increased risk, although the risk to the ipsilateral breast may be slightly higher. Risk reduction can be achieved by bilateral prophylactic mastectomy or treatment with estrogen antagonists, such as tamoxifen. However, fewer than 20% of women with atypical hyperplasia develop breast cancer, and therefore many choose careful clinical and radiologic surveillance over intervention.

KEY CONCEPTS

Benign Epithelial Lesions

- Benign epithelial lesions usually do not cause symptoms but are frequently detected as mammographic calcifications or densities.
- These lesions are classified according to the subsequent risk of cancer in either breast.
- The majority are not precursors of cancer.
- Although risk reduction can be achieved by surgery or chemoprevention, the majority of women will not develop cancer and many women choose surveillance instead of intervention.

Carcinoma of the Breast

Carcinoma of the breast is the most common non-skin malignancy in women and is second only to lung cancer as a cause of cancer deaths. A woman who lives to age 90 has a one in eight chance of developing breast cancer. In 2012, approximately 226,000 women in the United States were diagnosed with invasive breast cancer, 63,000 with carcinoma in situ, and almost 40,000 women died of the

Table 23-1 Epithelial Breast Lesions and the Risk of Developing Invasive Carcinoma

Pathologic Lesion	Relative Risk (Absolute Lifetime Risk)*
Nonproliferative Breast Changes (Fibrocystic changes)	1 (3%)
Duct ectasia Cysts Apocrine change Mild hyperplasia Adenosis Fibroadenoma without complex features	
Proliferative Disease Without Atypia	1.5 to 2 (5%-7%)
Moderate or florid hyperplasia Sclerosing adenosis Papilloma Complex sclerosing lesion (radial scar) Fibroadenoma with complex features	
Proliferative Disease with Atypia	4 to 5 (13%-17%)
Atypical ductal hyperplasia (ADH) Atypical lobular hyperplasia (ALH)	
Carcinoma in Situ	8 to 10 (25%-30%)
Lobular carcinoma in situ (LCIS) Ductal carcinoma in situ (DCIS)	

*Relative risk is the risk compared to women without any risk factors. Absolute lifetime risk is the percentage of patients expected to develop invasive carcinoma if untreated.

disease (Surveillance Epidemiology and End Results [SEER] data at http://seer.cancer.gov/). It is both ironic and tragic that a neoplasm arising in an exposed organ, readily accessible to self-examination and clinical surveillance, continues to exact such a heavy toll.

Almost all breast malignancies are adenocarcinomas and based on the expression of estrogen receptor and HER2 can be divided into three major biologic subgroups: *estrogen receptor (ER)-positive, HER2-negative* (50% to 65% of tumors); *HER2-positive* (10% to 20% of tumors, which may either be ER-positive or ER-negative); and *ER-negative, HER2-negative* (10% to 20% of tumors). These groups (described in detail later) show striking differences with regard to patient characteristics, pathologic features, treatment response, and outcome.

Incidence and Epidemiology

Breast cancer is rare in women younger than age 25, but the incidence increases rapidly after age 30 (Fig. 23-13). ER-positive cancers continue to increase with age whereas the incidence of ER-negative cancers and HER2-positive cancers remains relatively constant. The number of ER-positive cancers detected in older women has risen as a result of mammographic screening (which preferentially detects ER-positive cancers) and menopausal hormone therapy (which is associated with an increase in these cancers). As a result, ER-negative and HER2-positive cancers comprise almost half of cancers in young women but fewer than 20% of cancers in older women.

Ductal carcinoma in situ (DCIS) is rarely palpable and is almost always detected by mammography. The increased diagnosis of invasive carcinoma and DCIS after 1980 is related to the introduction of mammographic screening and is confined to older women (Fig. 23-14). Rates of screening levelled off recently at 65% to 75% of eligible women, and the number of new breast cancer diagnoses has also plateaued. In the age of screening, the number of stage I cancers (small node-negative carcinomas) has increased in frequency, while the number of large node-positive or advanced-stage breast carcinomas (stages II to IV) has fallen.

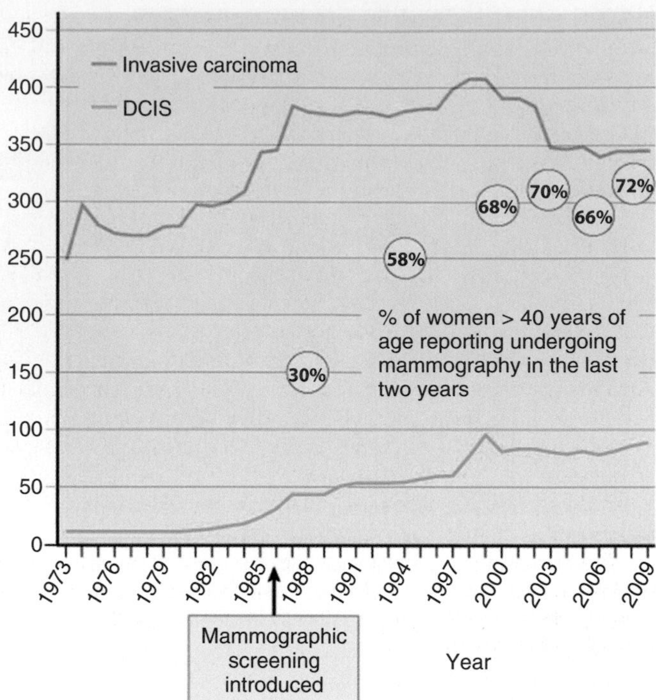

Figure 23-14 Changing incidences of ductal carcinoma in situ (DCIS) and invasive carcinoma during the years 1973 to 2009 in women older than 50 years of age. Rates are per 100,000 women and are age-adjusted to the 2000 US standard million population. (Data from SEER Cancer Statistics Review; http://seer.cancer.gov.) Following introduction of mammographic screening in the 1980s, the number of cases of DCIS and invasive carcinoma increased in older women. The number of women screened has recently plateaued, as has the incidence of breast cancer.

Invasive cancer is less common overall in non-white women, especially in older women (Fig. 23-15). The average age at diagnosis is 61 years for white women, 56 for

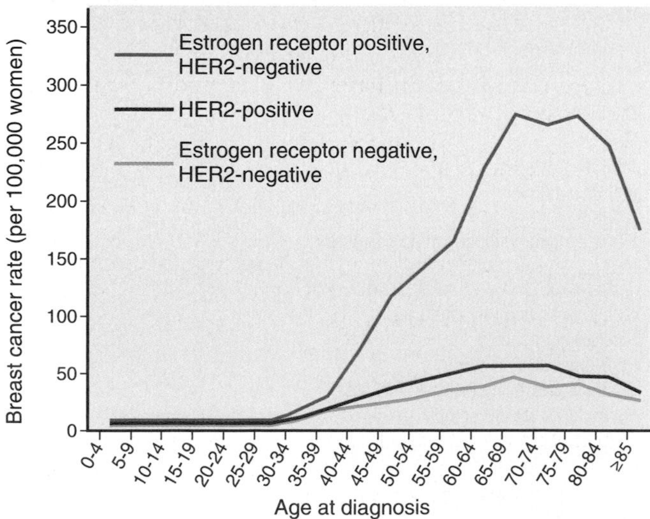

Figure 23-13 Incidence of ER-positive, ER-negative, and HER2-positive breast cancers according to age. Rates are per 100,000 women. ER-negative and HER2-positive cancers have a relatively constant incidence after age 40 years. In contrast, ER-positive cancers show a marked increase in incidence starting at around age 40 that peaks between the ages of 70 and 80.

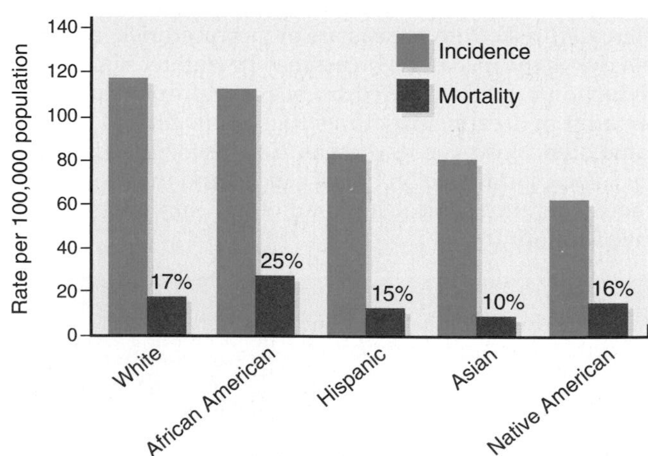

Figure 23-15 Breast cancer incidence and mortality in different ethnic groups (Data from North American Association of Central Cancer Registries). White women have the highest incidence of breast cancer, while African American women have the highest mortality rate. Likely contributors to these differences include socioeconomic factors (better access to care in white women) and biologic factors, particularly the higher incidence of aggressive, high grade, ER-negative tumors in younger African American women.

Hispanic women, and 46 for African American women. Only 20% of non-Hispanic white women are diagnosed at ages younger than 50 years, compared with 35% of African American women and 31% of Hispanic women. The incidence of ER-negative and HER2-positive cancers is relatively constant in all ethnic groups, but the number of ER-positive cancers is lower in non-white women.

The risk of death from breast cancer in those diagnosed with the disease remained constant for many years, but since 1994 has gradually declined from 30% to about 20%. This decrease is attributed to mammographic screening as well as more effective treatment modalities. However, the decline in the death rate has been less impressive for African American women, who have the highest mortality rate (Fig. 23-15). Although this difference is explained partly by unequal access to care, breast cancers in African American women are also on average more biologically aggressive, as they are more likely to be ER-negative and to have a high nuclear grade.

The incidence of breast cancer is four to seven times higher in the United States and Europe than in other countries, but rates are rising worldwide and by 2020 it is estimated that 70% of cases will be in developing countries. This change in incidence likely stems from adoption of Western social lifestyles, including delayed pregnancy, fewer pregnancies, and decreased breastfeeding.

Risk Factors. Beyond female sex (99% of those affected are female), the major risk factors are related to hereditary factors, lifetime exposure to estrogen and, to a lesser extent, environmental or lifestyle factors. Among the large number of identified risk factors are the following:

- ***Germline mutations.*** Approximately 5% to 10% of breast cancers occur in persons with germline mutations in tumor suppressor genes (discussed later). For these individuals, the lifetime risk of breast cancer can be more than 90%.
- ***First-degree relatives with breast cancer.*** About 15% to 20% of women with breast cancer have an affected first-degree relative (mother, sister, or daughter), but do not carry an identified breast cancer gene mutation. This increased risk is probably due to the interaction of low-risk susceptibility genes and shared environmental factors. Genome-wide association studies are being used to identify candidate genetic variants. It is important to note that risk is not increased if the only affected relative is a postmenopausal mother with cancer.
- ***Race/ethnicity.*** Ethnic background is correlated with breast cancer risk. Non-Hispanic white women have the highest incidence in the United States (Fig. 23-15). Variation in the frequency of breast cancer genes across ethnic groups is partly responsible for these differences. For example, germline *BRCA1* and *BRCA2* mutations are particularly prevalent in Ashkenazi Jewish populations.
- ***Age.*** Breast cancer risk rises throughout a woman's lifetime, peaking at 70 to 80 years and then declining slightly thereafter (Fig. 23-13).
- ***Age at menarche.*** Menarche at ages younger than 11 years increases risk by 20% compared to menarche at ages greater than 14. Late menopause also increases risk.
- ***Age at first live birth.*** A full-term pregnancy before the age of 20 halves the risk compared to nulliparous women or women who are older than the age of 35 at the time of their first birth.
- ***Benign breast disease.*** A prior breast biopsy revealing atypical hyperplasia or proliferative changes increases the risk of invasive carcinoma (Table 23-1).
- ***Estrogen exposure.*** Menopausal hormone therapy increases the risk of breast cancer, particularly when estrogen and a progestin are given together for a period of years. Most excess cancers are small ER-positive carcinomas. In contrast, oral contraceptives do not appear to increase the risk of breast cancer. Reducing endogenous estrogens by oophorectomy decreases the risk of developing breast cancer by up to 75%. Drugs that block estrogenic effects (e.g., tamoxifen) or block the formation of estrogen (e.g., aromatase inhibitors) also decrease the risk of ER-positive breast cancer.
- ***Breast density.*** Women with very dense breasts on mammography have a four- to six-fold higher risk of both ER-positive and ER-negative breast cancer compared to women with the lowest density. High breast density clusters in families and is correlated with other risk factors such as older age at first birth, fewer children, and menopausal hormone therapy. Persistently high breast density in older women may stem from a failure of normal breast involution.
- ***Radiation exposure.*** Radiation to the chest, whether for cancer therapy, due to atomic bomb exposure, or nuclear accidents, results in a higher rate of breast cancer. The risk is greatest with exposure at young ages and with high radiation doses. For example, women in their teens and early 20s who received radiation to the chest for Hodgkin lymphoma have a 20% to 30% risk of developing breast cancer over 10 to 30 years. Older women undergoing radiation do not incur this risk.
- ***Carcinoma of the contralateral breast or endometrium.*** Approximately 1% of women with breast cancer develop a second contralateral breast carcinoma per year. Breast and endometrial carcinomas have several risk factors in common, the most important of which is exposure to prolonged estrogenic stimulation.
- ***Diet.*** Large studies have failed to find strong correlations between breast cancer risk and dietary intake of any specific type of food. Moderate or heavy alcohol consumption increases risk.
- ***Obesity.*** Obese women under the age of 40 have a decreased risk as a result of anovulatory cycles and lower progesterone levels. In contrast, postmenopausal obese women are a increased risk, which is attributed to the synthesis of estrogens in fat depots.
- ***Exercise.*** There is a probable small protective effect for women who are physically active.
- ***Breastfeeding.*** The longer women breastfeed, the greater the reduction in risk. Lactation suppresses ovulation and may trigger terminal differentiation of luminal cells. The lower incidence of breast cancer in developing countries can largely be explained by the more frequent and longer nursing of infants.
- ***Environmental toxins.*** There is concern that environmental contaminants, such as organochlorine pesticides, have estrogenic effects on humans. Possible links to

breast cancer risk are being investigated intensively, but definitive associations have yet to be made.

Etiology and Pathogenesis

Like other cancers, breast cancers are clonal proliferations that arise from cells with multiple genetic aberrations, acquisition of which is influenced by hormonal exposures and inherited susceptibility genes. Breast cancers may be hereditary, arising in women with germline mutations in tumor suppressor genes, or sporadic. However, environmental factors clearly influence the penetrance of hereditary forms of breast cancer, and both genetic and environmental factors contribute to sporadic forms of breast cancer. The identification of breast cancer susceptibility genes has provided important insights into the pathogenesis of both familial and sporadic forms of breast cancer. We begin our discussion with hereditary breast cancer and the major susceptibility genes.

Familial Breast Cancer

Approximately 12% of breast cancers occur due to inheritance of an identifiable susceptibility gene or genes. The probability of a hereditary etiology increases when there are multiple affected first-degree relatives, early onset cancers, multiple cancers, or family members with other specific cancers. As with other familial forms of cancer (Chapter 7), in some instances cancer risk is an autosomal dominant trait that is conferred by inheritance of a defective copy of a tumor suppressor gene. In such instances, a single sporadic mutation in the remaining normal allele is all that is required to completely lose tumor suppressor function, which is likely to be the initiating driver mutation in these forms of breast cancer. The major known susceptibility genes for familial breast cancer—*BRCA1, BRCA2, TP53,* and *CHEK2*—are all tumor suppressor genes that have normal roles in DNA repair and maintenance of genomic integrity (Chapter 7 and Table 23-2). It is likely that complete loss-of-function of these proteins creates a "mutator" phenotype, an increased propensity to accumulate genetic damage that speeds cancer development.

Mutations in *BRCA1* and *BRCA2* are responsible for 80% to 90% of "single gene" familial breast cancers and about 3% of all breast cancers. Penetrance (the percentage of carriers who develop breast cancer) varies from 30% to 90% depending on the specific mutation present. Mutations in *BRCA1* also markedly increase the risk of developing ovarian carcinoma, which occurs in as many as 20% to 40% of carriers. *BRCA2* confers a smaller risk for ovarian carcinoma (10% to 20%) but is associated more frequently with male breast cancer. *BRCA1* and *BRCA2* carriers are also at higher risk for other epithelial cancers, such as prostatic and pancreatic carcinomas.

BRCA1 (on chromosome 17q21) and *BRCA2* (on chromosome 13q12.3) are both large genes, and hundreds of different mutations distributed throughout their coding regions have been associated with familial breast cancers. The frequency of mutations that increase breast cancer risk is only about 1 in 400 persons in the general population,

Table 23-2 Most Common "Single Gene" Mutations Associated with Hereditary Susceptibility to Breast Cancer

Gene (Location) Syndrome (Incidence)*	% of "Single Gene" Hereditary Cancers†	Breast Cancer Risk by Age 70‡	Changes in Sporadic Breast Cancer	Other Associated Cancers	Functions	Comments
BRCA1 (17q21) Familial breast and ovarian cancer (1 in 860)	52% (~2% of all breast cancers)	40%- 90%	Mutations rare; inactivated in 50% of some subtypes (e.g., medullary and metaplastic) by methylation	Ovarian, male breast cancer (but lower than *BRCA2*), prostate, pancreas, fallopian tube	Tumor suppressor, transcriptional regulation, repair of double-stranded DNA breaks	Breast carcinomas are commonly poorly differentiated and triple negative (basal-like), and have *TP53* mutations
BRCA2 (13q12-13) Familial breast and ovarian cancer (1 in 740)	32% (~1% of all breast cancers)	30%-90%	Mutations and loss of expression rare	Ovarian, male breast cancer, prostate, pancreas, stomach, melanoma, gallbladder, bile duct, pharynx	Tumor suppressor, transcriptional regulation, repair of double-stranded DNA breaks	Biallelic germline mutations cause a rare form of Fanconi anemia
TP53 (17p13.1) Li-Fraumeni (1 in 20,000)	3% (~1% of all breast cancers)	>90%	Mutations in 20%, LOH in 30%-42%; most frequent in triple negative cancers	Sarcoma, leukemia, brain tumors, adrenocortical carcinoma, others	Tumor suppressor with critical roles in cell cycle control, DNA replication, DNA repair, and apoptosis	*TP53* is the most commonly mutated gene in sporadic breast cancers 53% ER- and HER2-positive
CHEK2 (22q12.1) (1 in 100)	5% (~1% of all breast cancers)	10%-20%	Mutations in 5%	Prostate, thyroid, kidney, colon	Cell cycle checkpoint kinase, recognition and repair of DNA damage, activates BRCA1 and p53 by phosphorylation	May increase risk for breast cancer after radiation exposure 70%-80% ER-positive

*Frequency of heterozygotes in the U.S. population; the incidence of gene mutations is higher in some ethnic populations (e.g., *BRCA1* and *BRCA2* mutations occur at high frequencies in Ashkenazi Jews).
†Defined as familial breast cancers showing a pattern of inheritance consistent with a major effect of a single gene.
‡Risk varies with specific mutations and is likely modified by other genes. *LOH,* loss of heterozygosity.

and inconsequential polymorphisms are common. As a result, genetic testing is difficult and generally restricted to individuals with a strong family history or those belonging to certain ethnic groups. For example, in Ashkenazi Jewish populations, about 1 in 40 individuals carry one of three specific mutations, two in *BRCA1* and one in *BRCA2*. Identification of carriers is important, since increased surveillance, prophylactic mastectomy, and salpingo-oophorectomy can reduce cancer-related morbidity and mortality.

BRCA1-associated breast cancers are commonly poorly differentiated, have "medullary features" (a syncytial growth pattern with pushing margins and a lymphocytic response, described later), and are biologically very similar to ER-negative/HER2-negative breast cancers identified as "basal-like" by gene expression profiling (described later), as well as to serous ovarian carcinomas (Chapter 22). *BRCA2*-associated breast carcinomas also tend to be relatively poorly differentiated, but are more often ER-positive than *BRCA1* cancers.

The remaining known susceptibility genes accounts for fewer than 10% of hereditary breast carcinomas (Table 23-2). Germline mutations in *TP53* (Li-Fraumeni syndrome) and mutations in *CHEK2* together account for about 8% of breast cancers caused by single genes. Three other tumor suppressor genes—*PTEN* (Cowden syndrome), *STK11* (Peutz-Jeghers syndrome), and *ATM* (ataxia telangiectasia)—are mutated in less than 1% of all familial breast cancers.

Most of these genes play complex and interrelated roles in maintaining genomic integrity. After a cell sustains DNA damage, it must undergo cell cycle arrest and either repair its DNA or die by apoptosis. ATM senses DNA damage and with p53 and CHEK2 induces cell cycle arrest. BRCA1, BRCA2, and CHEK2 all have important functions in repair of double stranded DNA breaks. If any of these functions are impaired, the likelihood that cells with permanent DNA damage will survive is increased and the mutation will be propagated.

Yet it must be admitted that it is unknown why malfunction of these genes, particularly *BRCA1* and *BRCA2*, is more highly associated with breast cancer than other cancers. BRCA1 and BRCA2 are part of a large complex of proteins that are required to repair double stranded DNA breaks through a process called homologous recombination, in which a normal sister chromatid is used as a template for repairing the broken stretch of DNA. BRCA1 and BRCA2 are expressed ubiquitously, so the link to breast cancer is not obviously explained by tissue-specific patterns of gene expression. An alternative possibility is that breast (and ovarian) epithelial cells may be particularly prone to suffer the type of DNA damage that BRCA1 and BRCA2 are required to repair. BRCA1 also interacts with protein complexes that regulate chromatin structure, and it remains possible that its tumor suppressive role involves functions that are independent of DNA repair.

Sporadic Breast Cancer

The major risk factors for sporadic breast cancer are related to hormone exposure: gender, age at menarche and menopause, reproductive history, breastfeeding, and exogenous estrogens. Other environmental risk factors, proven or suspected, include radiation exposure (discussed under risk factors) and exposure to chemicals with estrogen-like effects (Chapter 9).

Estrogen clearly functions as a promoter of breast cancers (Chapter 7), probably through several different effects on the breast. Hormonal exposure stimulates breast growth during puberty, menstrual cycles, and pregnancy, thereby increasing the number of cells that can potentially give rise to a cancer. The proliferation of breast epithelium during the menstrual cycle is also conducive to the accumulation of DNA damage, and the temporary lull in cell division that occurs during the latter part of the menstrual cycle may allow time for defective DNA repair to occur and for mutations to become "fixed" in the genome. Repeated rounds of this process during each cycle may underlie the association between the cumulative number of menstrual cycles a woman experiences and her risk of developing breast cancer. Once premalignant or malignant cells are present, hormones can stimulate their growth as well as the growth of normal stromal cells that may aid and abet tumor development.

Molecular Mechanisms of Carcinogenesis and Tumor Progression

The diverse histologic appearances of breast carcinomas and putative precursor lesions are the outward manifestations of the complex genetic and epigenetic changes that drive carcinogenesis. As with other cancers, resident breast tissue stem cells have been hypothesized to be the cell of origin for all breast cancers. Once the process is initiated in such cells by a driver mutation, there appear to be three major genetic pathways of carcinogenesis (Fig. 23-16).

- **ER-positive, HER2-negative cancers arise via the dominant pathway of breast cancer development, constituting 50% to 65% of cases.** This is the most common subtype of breast cancer in individuals who inherit germline mutations in *BRCA2*. They are often associated with gains of chromosome 1q, losses of chromosome 16q, and activating mutations in *PIK3CA*, a gene that encodes phosphoinositide-3 kinase (PI3K), which is an important component of signaling pathways downstream of growth factor receptors (Chapter 7). These same genetic lesions are often found in flat epithelial atypia and atypical ductal hyperplasia, which are hypothesized to be precursor lesions for this subtype of breast cancer. ER-positive cancers are termed "luminal," as these cancers most closely resemble normal breast luminal cells in terms of their mRNA expression pattern, which is dominated by genes that are regulated by estrogen. As discussed later, tumors arising through this pathway include at least two major molecular subtypes that differ in their proliferation rate and response to therapy.
- **HER2-positive cancers arise through a pathway that is strongly associated with amplifications of the HER2 gene on chromosome 17q.** They constitute approximately 20% of all breast cancers and may be either ER-positive or ER-negative. This is the most common subtype of breast cancer in patients with germline mutations in *TP53* (Li-Fraumeni syndrome). A putative precursor lesion termed atypical apocrine adenosis has

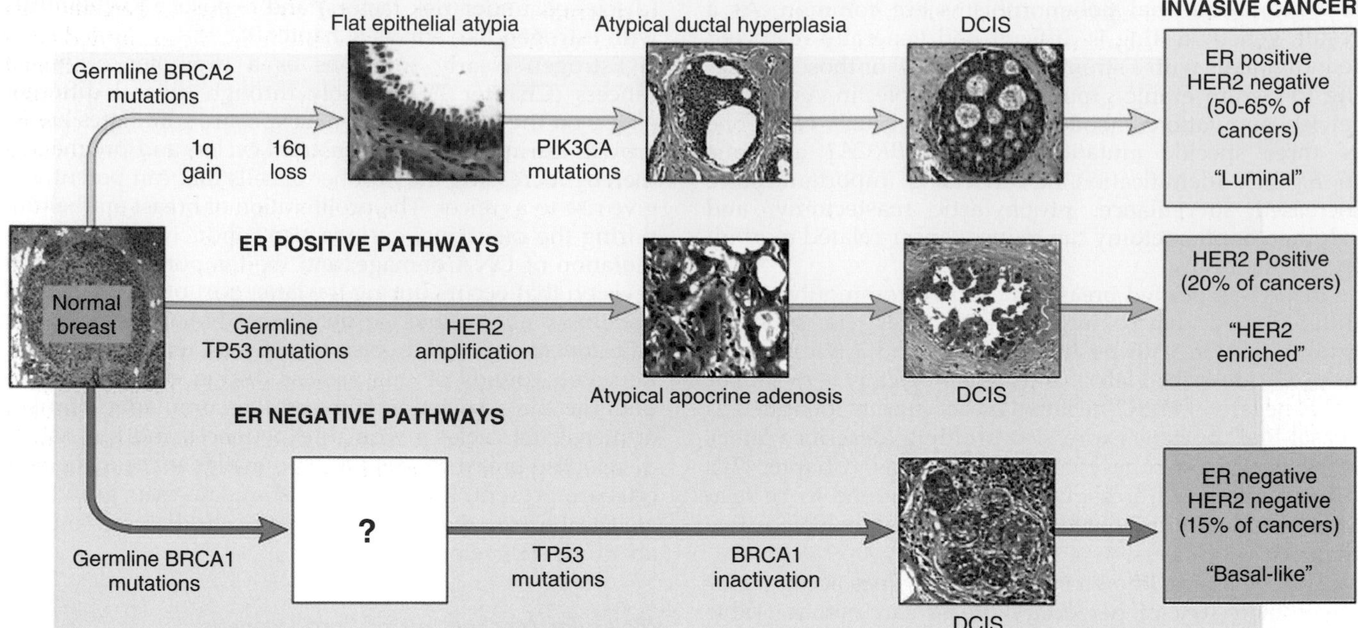

Figure 23-16 Major pathways of breast cancer development. Three main pathways have been identified. The most common pathway *(yellow arrow)* leads to ER-positive carcinomas. Recognizable precursor lesions include flat epithelial atypia and atypical hyperplasia. A less common pathway *(blue arrow)* leads to carcinomas that are negative for ER and HER2. The box with the question mark indicates that no precursor lesions have been identified—perhaps because lesions progress quickly to carcinoma. The third pathway *(green arrow)* consists of HER2-positive cancers, which may be ER-positive or ER-negative. Amplification of the *HER2* gene is also present in a subset of atypical apocrine lesions, which may represent a precursor lesion. Each molecular subtype has a characteristic gene expression profile termed luminal, HER2 enriched, and basal-like, respectively. See text for other details.

been described. These cancers have a distinct gene expression pattern that is dominated by genes related to proliferation that are regulated by signaling pathways lying downstream of the HER2 receptor tyrosine kinase.

- **ER-negative, HER2-negative cancers arise through a distinct pathway that is independent of ER-mediated changes in gene expression and HER2 gene amplifications.** Precursor lesions have yet to be described and as a result this is the least understood of the pathways. These tumors comprise about 15% of breast cancers overall, but are the most common tumor type observed in patients with germline *BRCA1* mutations; they also occur with increased frequency in African American women. Sporadic tumors of this type often have loss-of-function mutations in *TP53*; mutations in *BRCA1* are uncommon, but *BRCA1* may be silenced in sporadic tumors through epigenetic mechanisms. These tumors have a "basal-like" pattern of mRNA expression that includes many genes that are expressed in normal myoepithelial cells.

Deep sequencing of breast cancer genomes has been used to reconstruct the genetic events that occur during tumor development and progression. The most common driver mutations involve the proto-oncogenes *PIK3CA*, *HER2*, *MYC*, and *CCND1* (which encodes cyclin D1), and the tumor suppressor genes *TP53* and (in familial cancers) *BRCA1* and *BRCA2*. Once a founding tumor clone is established, subclonal heterogeneity arising by chance due to genomic instability undoubtedly contributes to both tumor progression and resistance to therapy. As with many solid tumors, the profound genetic heterogeneity of breast cancer is a major challenge to the success of therapy, as it increases the likelihood of emergence of more aggressive, therapy-resistant subclones.

Neoplastic epithelial cells do not develop in isolation, but are dependent on interactions with stromal cells in the local microenvironment. Cancers occur in the areas of greatest mammographic density, suggesting that increased amounts of fibrous stroma is both a marker of risk and biologically important for tumorigenesis. The role of stroma is not yet completely understood. The stroma is a complex mixture of fibroblasts, blood vessels, lymphatics, inflammatory cells, and extracellular matrix. Focal alterations in the stroma may play a direct role by creating a microenvironment conducive to tumor development and growth. Angiogenesis and tumor-associated inflammation are commonly associated with carcinoma, starting at the in situ stage. With better understanding of the role played by stroma, it may be possible to develop therapies that target stromal components.

The final step of carcinogenesis, the transition of carcinoma in situ to invasive carcinoma, is both the most important and the least understood. The majority of genetic changes observed in invasive carcinomas are already present in the associated carcinoma in situ (Fig. 23-16). It is possible that the same molecular events that allow for the normal formation of new ductal branch points and lobules during pregnancy—abrogation of the basement membrane, increased proliferation, escape from growth inhibition, angiogenesis, and invasion of stroma—may be replicated during invasion. Remodeling of the breast during post-pregnancy involution, which involves inflammatory and "wound healing-like" tissue reactions and is known to increase the risk of tumor invasion, may also facilitate the transition of carcinoma in situ to invasive carcinoma.

As can be surmised from this discussion, breast cancer is not one disease, but many, each with its own clinical characteristics and optimal prevention and treatment strategies. This recognition has led to the introduction of new molecular classification systems, which are discussed later.

KEY CONCEPTS

Breast Cancer Incidence, Epidemiology, and Etiology

- Breast cancer is the most common non-skin malignancy in women and the second most common cause of cancer deaths.
- The most important risk factors are estrogenic stimulation and age.
- All cancers arise by the accumulation of DNA alterations and epigenetic changes.
- Tumorigenesis also requires changes in the normal supporting cells—alteration of the normal crosstalk and function of stromal cells may be an important determinant of stromal invasion.
- The hormonal milieu of the breast plays an important role in expanding populations of potential precursor cells, altering stroma during pregnancy, and driving the proliferation of cancers.

Types of Breast Carcinoma

Almost all (>95%) of breast malignancies are adenocarcinomas that first arise in the duct/lobular system as carcinoma in situ; at the time of clinical detection the majority (at least 70%) will have breached the basement membrane and invaded the stroma. Carcinoma in situ refers to a neoplastic proliferation of epithelial cells that is confined to ducts and lobules by the basement membrane. Invasive carcinoma (synonymous with "infiltrating" carcinoma) has penetrated through the basement membrane and grows within stroma. Here, the cells have the potential to invade into the vasculature and thereby reach regional lymph nodes and distant sites.

The terms *ductal* and *lobular* are still used to describe subsets of both in situ and invasive carcinomas, but most evidence suggests all breast carcinomas actually arise from cells in the terminal duct lobular unit. Carcinoma in situ was originally classified as DCIS or lobular carcinoma in situ (LCIS) based on the resemblance of the involved spaces to normal ducts or lobules. It is now recognized that these growth patterns are not related to the cell of origin, but rather reflect differences in tumor cell genetics and biology. By current convention, "lobular" refers to invasive carcinomas that are biologically related to LCIS, and "ductal" is used more generally for adenocarcinomas that cannot be classified as a special histologic type.

Carcinoma in Situ

Ductal Carcinoma in Situ (DCIS)

DCIS is a malignant clonal proliferation of epithelial cells limited to ducts and lobules by the basement membrane. The term "ductal" was used to describe this lesion because when it involves lobules, the expanded acini take on an appearance resembling small ducts. Myoepithelial cells are preserved in involved ducts/lobules, although they may be diminished in number. DCIS can spread throughout the ductal system and produce extensive lesions involving an entire sector of a breast.

DCIS is almost always detected by mammography. Without screening, fewer than 5% of all carcinomas are detected when in situ, but DCIS comprises 15% to 30% of carcinomas in screened populations (Fig. 23-14). Most are identified as a result of calcifications associated with secretory material or necrosis; less commonly, periductal fibrosis surrounding DCIS forms a mammographic density or a vaguely palpable mass. Rarely, DCIS (often of micropapillary or papillary types) produces a nipple discharge or is detected as an incidental finding upon biopsy for another lesion.

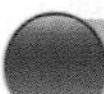

MORPHOLOGY

DCIS can be divided into two major architectural subtypes, comedo and noncomedo (Fig. 23-17). Some cases of DCIS have a single growth pattern, but most are comprised of a mixture of patterns. Nuclear grade and necrosis are better predictors of local recurrence and progression to invasion than architectural type.

Comedo DCIS may occasionally produce vague nodularity, but more often it is detected on mammography as clustered or linear and branching areas of calcification (Fig. 23-17*A*). It is defined by two features: (1) tumor cells with pleomorphic, high-grade nuclei and (2) areas of central necrosis (Fig. 23-17*B*).

Noncomedo DCIS lacks either high-grade nuclei or central necrosis. Several patterns may be seen. Cribriform DCIS may have rounded (cookie cutter–like) spaces (Fig. 23-17*C*) within the ducts, or a solid DCIS pattern. Micropapillary DCIS produces bulbous protrusions without a fibrovascular core, often arranged in complex intraductal patterns (Fig. 23-17*D*). In other cases, DCIS produces true papillae with fibrovascular cores that lack a myoepithelial cell layer. Calcifications may also be seen in noncomedo forms of DCIS in association with focal necrosis or intraluminal secretions.

Paget disease of the nipple is a rare manifestation of breast cancer (1% to 4% of cases) that presents as a unilateral erythematous eruption with a scale crust. Pruritus is common, and the lesion may be mistaken for eczema. Malignant cells (Paget cells) extend from DCIS within the ductal system via the lactiferous sinuses into nipple skin without crossing the basement membrane (Fig. 23-18). The tumor cells disrupt the normal epithelial barrier, allowing extracellular fluid to seep out onto the nipple surface. The Paget cells are readily detected by nipple biopsy or cytologic preparations of the exudate.

A palpable mass is present in 50% to 60% of women with Paget disease, and almost all of these women have an underlying invasive carcinoma. The carcinomas are usually poorly differentiated, ER-negative, and overexpress HER2. In contrast, the majority of women without a palpable mass have only DCIS. Prognosis of Paget disease depends on the features of the underlying carcinoma and is not affected by the presence or absence of DCIS involving the skin when matched for other prognostic factors.

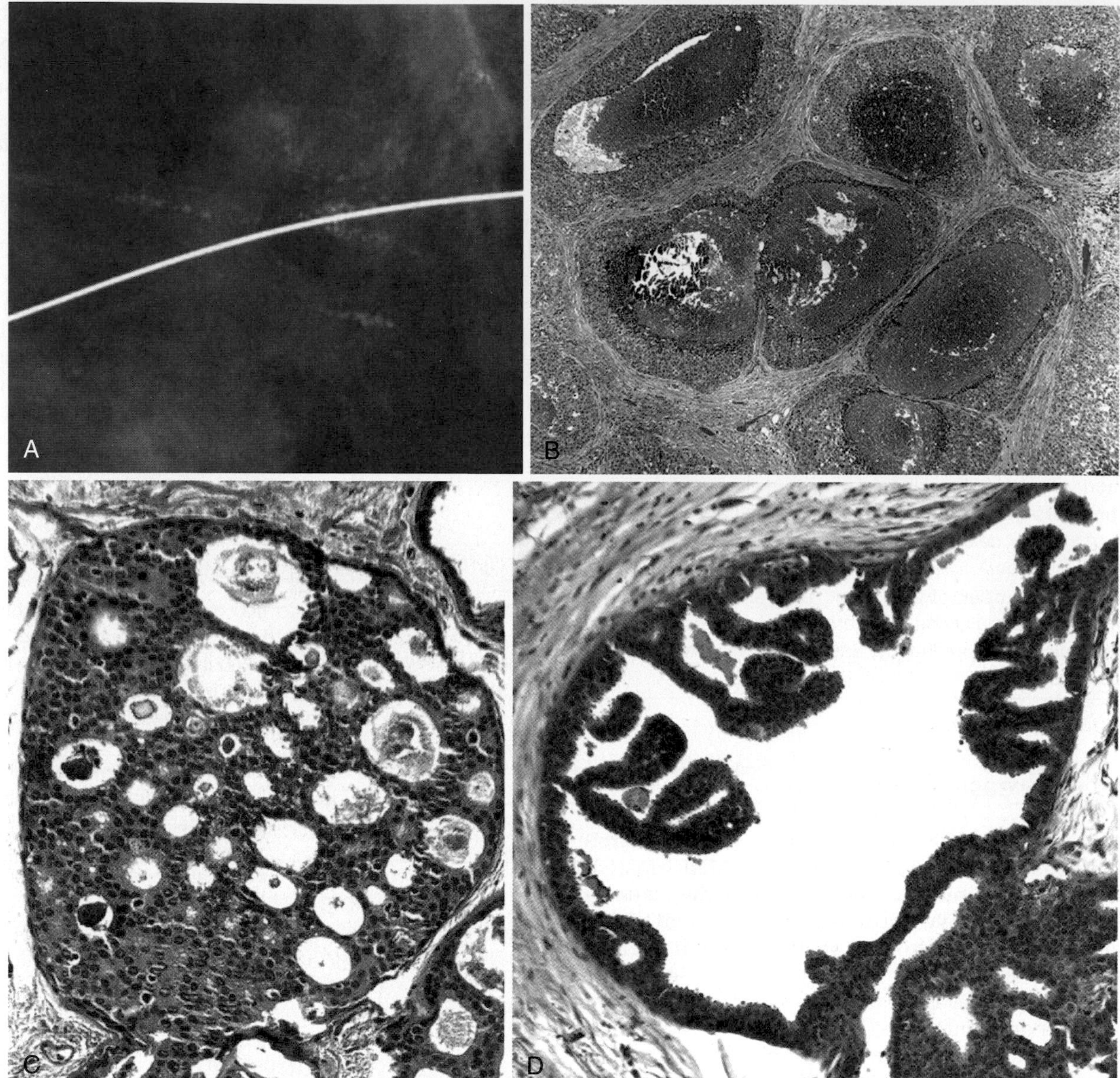

Figure 23-17 Ductal carcinoma in situ (DCIS). **A** and **B,** Comedo type. **A,** The specimen radiogram reveals linear and branching calcifications within the ductal system. **B,** A high-grade proliferation associated with large central zones of necrosis and calcifications fills several ducts. **C** and **D,** Noncomedo types. **C,** Cribriform DCIS. Note the round, regular ("cookie cutter") spaces containing calcifying secretory material. **D,** Micropapillary DCIS. The papilllary projections lack fibrovascular cores.

The natural history of DCIS has been difficult to determine because, until recently, all women were treated with mastectomy, and the current practice of surgical excision, usually followed by radiation, is largely curative. If untreated, women with small, low-grade DCIS develop invasive cancer at a rate of about 1% per year. The majority of these invasive cancers occurs in the same quadrant and have a similar grade and expression pattern of ER and HER2 as the associated DCIS. Tumors with high-grade or extensive DCIS are believed to have a higher risk for progression to invasive carcinoma.

Remarkably, the overall death rate for women with DCIS is lower than that for women in the population as a whole, possibly because mammographic screening is a "marker" for better access to medical care or other socioeconomic factors that are associated with longevity. Death from metastatic breast cancer after a diagnosis of DCIS occurs in 1% to 3% of women. The origin of metastatic disease may be a second invasive carcinoma in the ipsilateral or contralateral breast or occult foci of invasion that were not detected at the time of DCIS diagnosis.

Mastectomy is curative in greater than 95% of women. Breast conservation is appropriate for most women but has a slightly higher risk of recurrence—about half of which are DCIS and half invasive carcinoma. The major risk factors for recurrence are (1) high nuclear grade and necrosis, (2) extent of disease, and (3) positive surgical margins. Ensuring complete excision of DCIS is not straightforward, since its distribution in the breast is not reliably predicted by imaging and it is usually not grossly evident at surgery. Postoperative radiation therapy and tamoxifen also reduce the risk of recurrence.

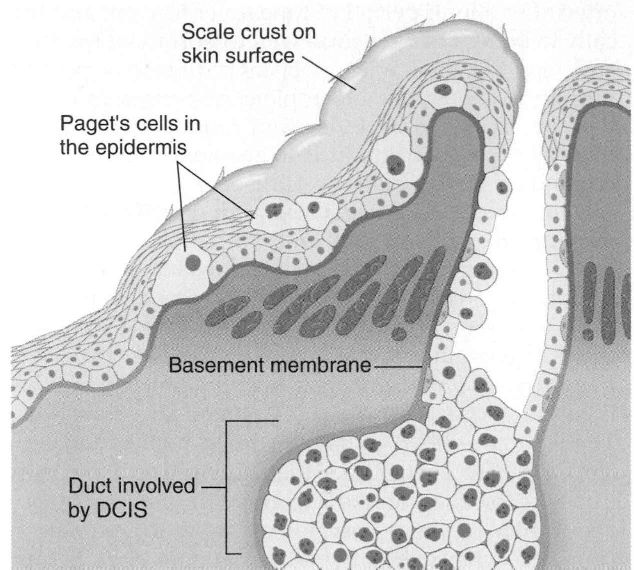

Figure 23-18 Paget disease of the nipple. Ductal carcinoma in situ arising within the ductal system of the breast can extend up the lactiferous ducts and into the skin of the nipple without crossing the basement membrane. The malignant cells disrupt the normally tight squamous epithelial cell barrier, allowing extracellular fluid to seep out and form an oozing scaly crust.

Lobular Carcinoma in Situ

LCIS is a clonal proliferation of cells within ducts and lobules that grow in a discohesive fashion, usually due to an acquired loss of the tumor suppressive adhesion protein E-cadherin. The term "lobular" was used to describe this lesion because the cells expand but do not distort involved spaces and, thus, the underlying lobular architecture is preserved. LCIS is always an incidental biopsy finding, since it is not associated with calcifications or stromal reactions that produce mammographic densities. As a result, its incidence (1% to 6% of all carcinomas) did not increase after the introduction of mammographic screening. When both breasts are biopsied, LCIS is bilateral in 20% to 40% of cases, compared with 10% to 20% of cases of DCIS.

The cells of atypical lobular hyperplasia, LCIS, and invasive lobular carcinoma are morphologically identical. In most cases, loss of cellular adhesion is due to dysfunction of E-cadherin, a transmembrane protein that contributes to the cohesion of normal epithelial cells in the breast and other glandular tissues. E-cadherin functions as a tumor suppressor protein in such tissues, and may be lost in neoplastic proliferations through a variety of mechanisms, including mutation of the E-cadherin gene (*CDH1*). In rare cases, there is dysregulation of other proteins, such as catenins, that are also needed for E-cadherin–mediated cellular cohesion.

MORPHOLOGY

LCIS consists of a uniform population of cells with oval or round nuclei and small nucleoli involving ducts and lobules (Fig. 23-19*A*). Mucin-positive signet-ring cells are commonly present. The lack of E-cadherin results in a rounded shape without attachment to adjacent cells (Fig. 23-19*B*). The cells cannot form cribriform spaces or papillae, such as are seen in DCIS. Pagetoid spread, the presence of neoplastic cells between the basement membrane and overlying luminal cells, is commonly seen in the breast, but LCIS does not involve nipple skin (Fig. 23-19*B*). Necrosis and secretory activity are not seen with classic LCIS and, thus, substrates for calcification are not present. LCIS almost always expresses ER and PR. Overexpression of HER2 is not observed.

LCIS is a risk factor for invasive carcinoma. Invasive carcinoma develops in 25% to 35% of women over 20 to 30 years time, or at a rate of about 1% per year, similar to that observed for untreated DCIS. However, unlike DCIS, the risk is almost as high in the contralateral breast as in the ipsilateral breast. Invasive carcinomas developing in women after LCIS are three-fold more likely to be lobular carcinoma; however, most are of other morphologies. Treatment choices include bilateral prophylactic mastectomy, tamoxifen, or, more typically, close clinical follow-up and mammographic screening.

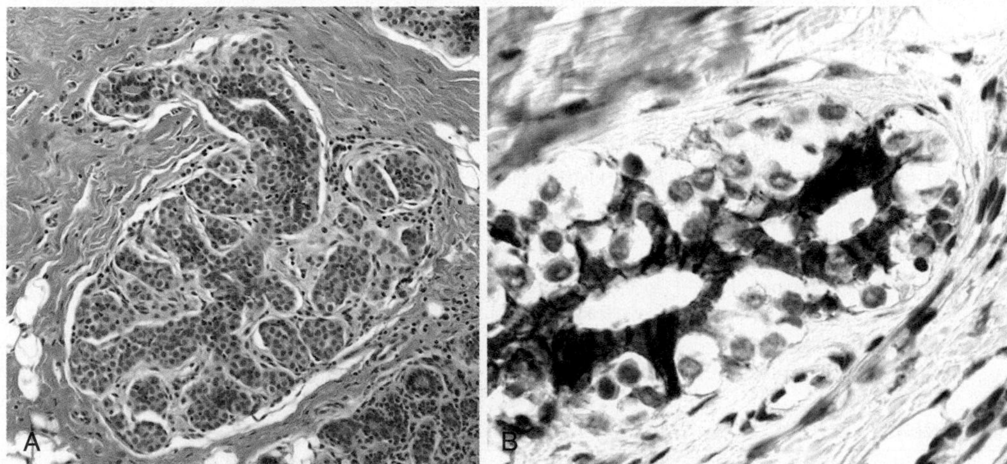

Figure 23-19 Lobular carcinoma in situ. **A,** A monomorphic population of small, rounded, loosely cohesive cells fills and expands the acini of a lobule. The underlying lobular architecture can still be recognized. The cells extend into the adjacent lobule by pagetoid spread. **B,** An immunoperoxidase study shows E-cadherin–positive normal luminal cells that have been undermined by E-cadherin-negative LCIS cells spreading along the basement membrane.

Rare variants of LCIS have high-grade nuclei and/or central necrosis. The cells may be ER negative and some overexpress HER2. The natural history of this type of LCIS is not well known and may well be different from typical LCIS.

Invasive (Infiltrating) Carcinoma

Invasive carcinomas can be divided based on molecular and morphologic characteristics into several clinically important subgroups. Breast carcinomas have a wide variety of morphologic appearances. One third can be classified morphologically into special histologic types, some of which are strongly associated with clinically relevant biologic characteristics (discussed later). The remainder are grouped together and called "ductal" or no special type (NST). Recent detailed description of genomic alterations and gene and protein expression in large cohorts of breast cancers has provided a framework for a molecular classification for this group of breast cancers (Fig. 23-20 and Table 23-3). These breast cancers fall into three major molecular subtypes, each with important associations with clinical features, response to treatment, and outcome (Table 23-3).

ER-positive, HER- negative (also termed "luminal," 50% to 65% of cancers) is the most common form of invasive breast cancer. Based on proliferation rates, it is further divided into two subgroups.

- **ER-positive, HER2-negative, low proliferation (40% to 55% of cancers): This group of breast cancers makes up the majority of cancers in older women and in men.** It is also the most common type detected by mammographic screening and in women treated with menopausal hormone therapy. The gene expression signature of this group of cancers is dominated by genes that are directly regulated by estrogen receptor. Many of these cancers are detected at an early stage. They have the lowest incidence of local recurrence and are often cured by surgery. When these carcinomas do metastasize, it is often after a long period of time (over 6 years) and typically to bone. They respond well to hormonal treatment and long survival with metastatic disease is possible, despite the fact that incomplete responses to chemotherapy are the rule. Indeed, in most patients chemotherapy appears to add little to hormone therapy, which is standard in this subtype of disease.
- **ER-positive, HER2-negative, high proliferation (approximately 10% of cancers):** Although these tumors are ER-positive, ER levels may be low and progesterone receptor expression may be low or absent. This is the most common type of carcinoma associated with *BRCA2* germline mutations. The mRNA expression pattern is similar to other ER-positive cancers, but there is higher expression of genes related to proliferation. These tumors tend to have a much higher burden of chromosomal aberrations than low-grade ER-positive tumors. However, unlike low-grade ER-positive cancers, about 10% of these carcinomas show a complete response to chemotherapy; such patients have a much better prognosis than patients with cancers that do not respond.

HER2-positive (approximately 20% of cancers) is the second most common molecular subtype of invasive breast cancer. About half of these cancers are ER-positive. When present, ER expression is usually low; progesterone receptor expression is often absent. These cancers are relatively more common in young women and in non-white women. More than half (53%) of familial breast cancers in patients with germline *TP53* mutations (Li-Fraumeni syndrome) develop carcinomas that are positive for both ER and HER2. The mRNA profile shows increased expression of *HER2* and flanking genes on the same amplicon, as well as genes related to proliferation. These cancers characteristically have complex interchromosomal translocations, high-level amplifications of *HER2*, and a high mutational load. Identification of cancers belonging to this subtype is achieved through assays of HER2 protein overexpression or *HER2* gene amplification (Fig. 23-21). Cancers in this

Table 23-3 Molecular Subtypes of Invasive Breast Cancer

Defining Features	ER-positive, HER2-negative		HER2-Positive (ER-Positive or Negative*)	ER-Negative† HER2-Negative
Frequency	~40-55% (Low proliferation)	~10% (High proliferation)	~20%	~15%
Included special histologic types	Well or moderately differentiated lobular, tubular, mucinous	Poorly differentiated lobular	Some apocrine	Medullary,‡ adenoid cystic,‡ secretory,‡ metaplastic
Typical patient groups	Older women, men, cancers detected by mammographic screening	*BRCA2* mutation carriers	Young women, non-white women, *TP53* mutation carriers (ER positive)	Young women, *BRCA1* mutation carriers, African American and Hispanic women
Metastatic pattern	Bone (70%), more common than visceral (25%) or brain (<10%)	Bone (80%) more common than visceral (30%) or brain (10%)	Bone (70%), visceral (45%),and brain (30%) are all common	Bone (40%), visceral (35%), brain (25%) are all common
Relapse pattern	Late, >10 years, long survival possible with metastases	Intermediate	Usually short, <10 years, survival with metastases rare	Usually short, <5 years, survival with metastases rare
Complete response to chemotherapy	<10%	~10%	ER positive—15% ER negative—>30%	~30%

*About half of HER2-positive cancers are ER positive and half ER negative. ER and PR levels tend to be low in this group.
†This group is also referred to as "triple negative" carcinoma.
‡Some special histologic types have a more favorable prognosis than this group as a whole.

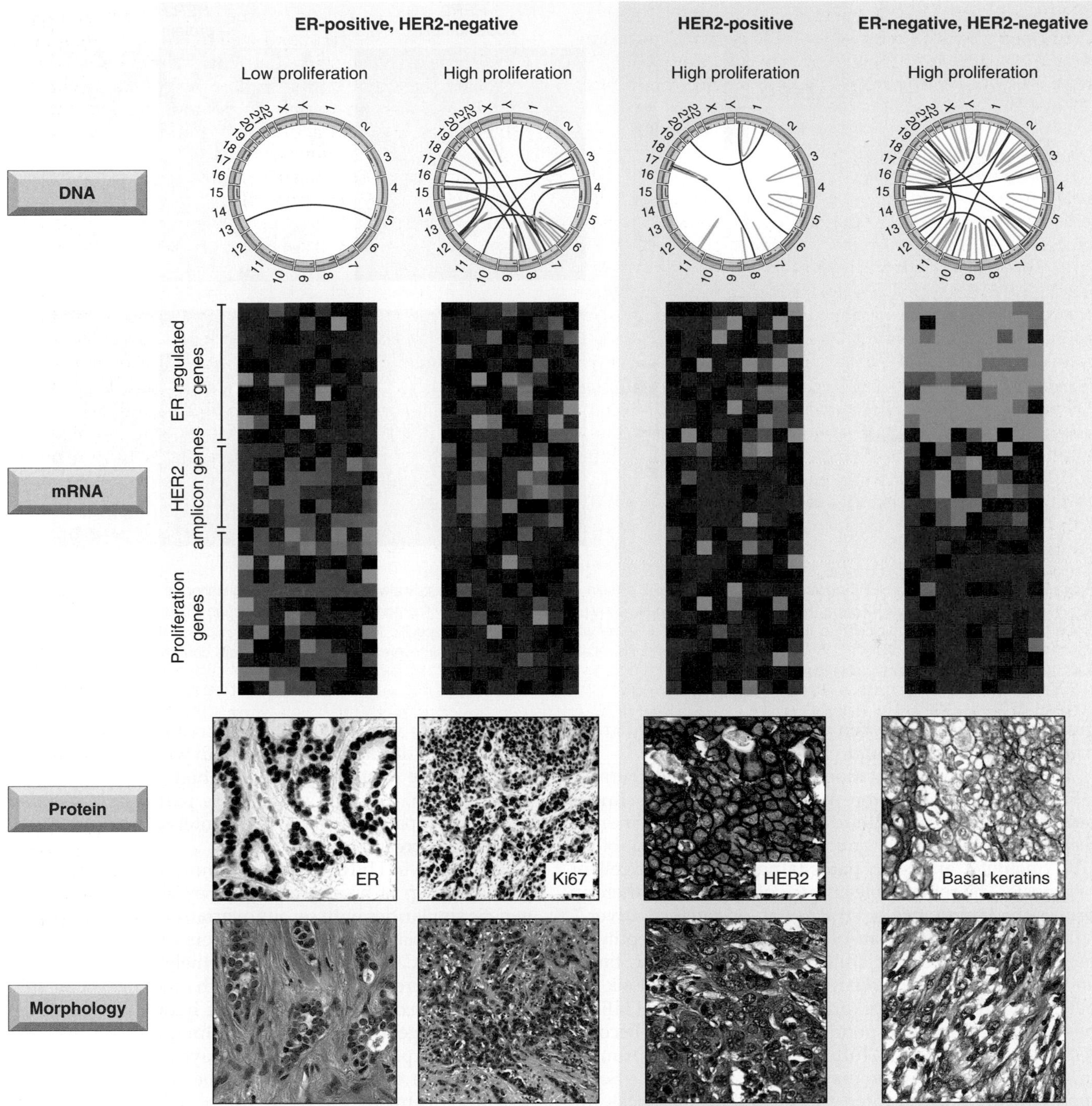

Figure 23-20 Major molecular subtypes of invasive breast cancer. Three major subtypes of breast cancer are distinguished by characteristic changes in genomic DNA, mRNA, protein, and morphology. Genomic abnormalities are shown in circos plots (Chapter 7), which present a snapshot of all of the genomic abnormalities within a particular tumor; these abnormalities are mapped onto the chromosomes, which are displayed at the periphery of a circle. Green loops show intrachromosomal rearrangements, while red loops show interchromosomal rearrangements. Gene expression profiling measures relative levels of mRNA expression. Red indicates a relative increase, green a relative decrease, and black no change in levels. Genes are arrayed from top to bottom and tumors from left to right. Immunohistochemical studies detect proteins using specific antibodies visualized by a brown chromogen. *ER-positive HER2-negative tumors* are diverse, ranging from well-differentiated cancers with low proliferative rates and few chromosomal changes to poorly differentiated cancers with high proliferative rates and large numbers of chromosomal rearrangements. All of these cancers express ER (an estrogen-dependent transcription factor). Proliferation is estimated by counting mitoses or by staining for cell cycle-specific proteins such as Ki-67. *HER2-positive cancers* may be ER-positive or ER-negative, but when ER is present, levels are typically low. HER2 positivity can be detected as an increase in HER2 gene copy number, an increase in HER2 mRNA, or an increase in HER2 protein, as shown here. *ER-negative, HER2-negative ("triple negative" or "basal-like") carcinomas* are characterized by genomic instability (denoted by numerous chromosomal changes), a high proliferative rate, and expression of many proteins typical of myoepithelial cells (e.g., basal keratins).

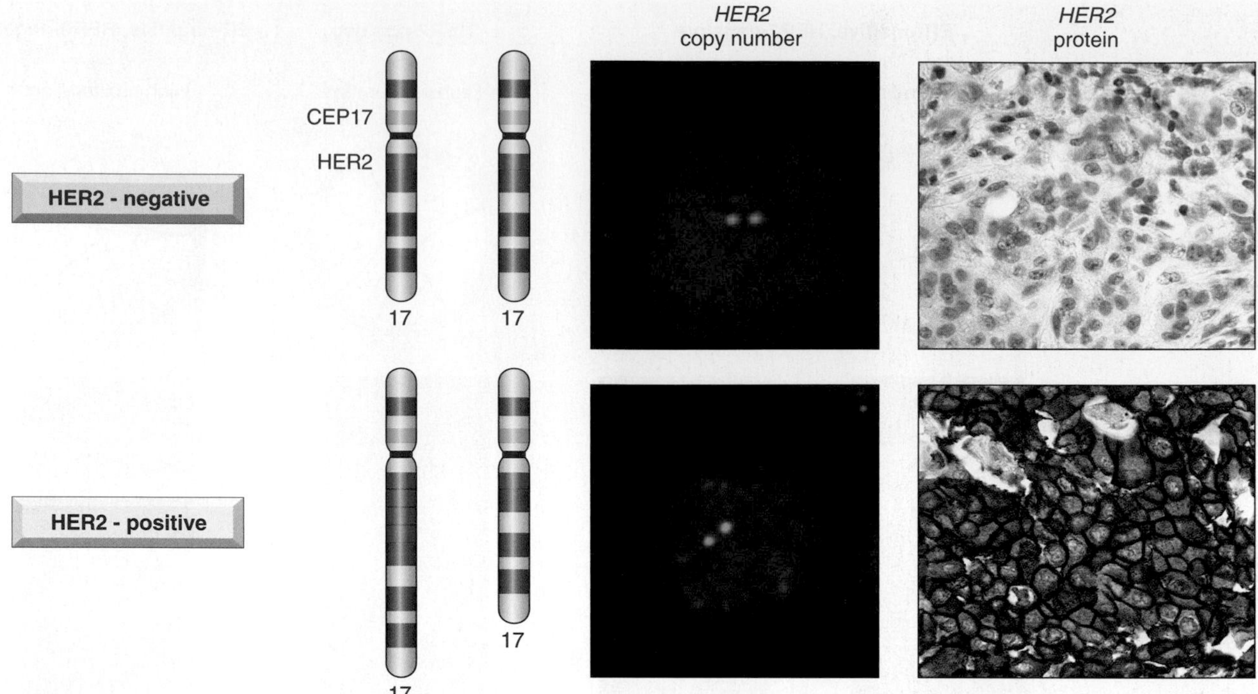

Figure 23-21 Identification of HER2-positive breast cancer. HER2 protein overexpression is virtually always caused by amplification of the region of chromosome 17q that contains the *HER2* gene. The increase in *HER2* gene copy number is detected by fluorescence in situ hybridization (FISH) using a *HER2*-specific probe (red signal), which is typically co-hybridized to tumor cell nuclei with a second probe specific for the centromeric region of chromosome 17 (green signal), allowing the chromosome 17 copy number to be determined. Alternatively, HER2 protein overexpression in tumor cells can be detected by immunohistochemical staining with antibodies specific for HER2.

group can metastasize when small in size and early in the course, often to viscera and brain.

Before the implementation of HER2-targeted therapy, HER2-positive cancers were associated with a poor clinical outcome. However, one third or more of these carcinomas respond completely to antibodies that bind and block HER2 activity, and such patients now have an excellent prognosis. The remarkable efficacy of this form of therapy proves the importance of HER2 as an oncogenic "driver."

While the introduction of trastuzumab (Herceptin), a humanized monoclonal antibody that specifically binds and inhibits HER2, markedly improved the outlook for patients with HER2 overexpressing cancers, not all HER2-positive carcinomas respond and some that do become resistant to treatment. Multiple mechanisms of primary or acquired resistance have been described. Some tumors express a truncated form of HER2 that lacks the trastuzumab-binding site but retains kinase activity, while others upregulate downstream pathways, such as the PI-3 kinase pathway. Numerous therapeutic agents are under investigation to improve response and overcome resistance to trastuzumab, including new antibodies that bind different HER2 epitopes; dual tyrosine kinase inhibitors that target both EGFR and HER2; antibody-toxin conjugates (one of which is now approved for use); and inhibitors of downstream signaling components, such as PI-3 kinase and AKT.

ER-negative, HER2-negative tumors ("basal-like" triple negative carcinoma; approximately 15% of cancers) are the third major molecular subtype. These cancers are more common in young premenopausal women as well as African American (20% to 25% of carcinomas in this group) and Hispanic women (17% of carcinomas in this group). The majority of carcinomas arising in women with *BRCA1* mutations are of this type. Due to high proliferation and rapid growth, this type of cancer is particularly likely to present as a palpable mass in the interval between mammographic screenings.

ER-negative, HER2-negative tumors are the most distinctive group of breast cancers. They share a number of genetic similarities with serous ovarian carcinomas, including the association of familial cancers of both types with germline *BRCA1* mutations. Nevertheless, in some cases features are present that overlap with other molecular subgroups. For example, about 10% of basal-like cancers (as defined by gene expression profiling) express ER and about 15% express HER2. Thus, assays for protein expression or gene amplification must be done to determine whether treatment targeting ER or HER2 is indicated. These cancers can metastasize when small in size, frequently to viscera and to the brain. However, approximately 30% completely respond to chemotherapy and cure may be possible in this chemosensitive subgroup. Recurrences are generally diagnosed within 5 years of treatment. Local recurrence is common, even after mastectomy. Prolonged survival after distant metastasis is rare.

MORPHOLOGY

Invasive carcinomas presenting on mammography as calcifications without an associated density are generally less than 1 cm in size. In the absence of mammographic screening, invasive carcinoma usually presents as a mass of at

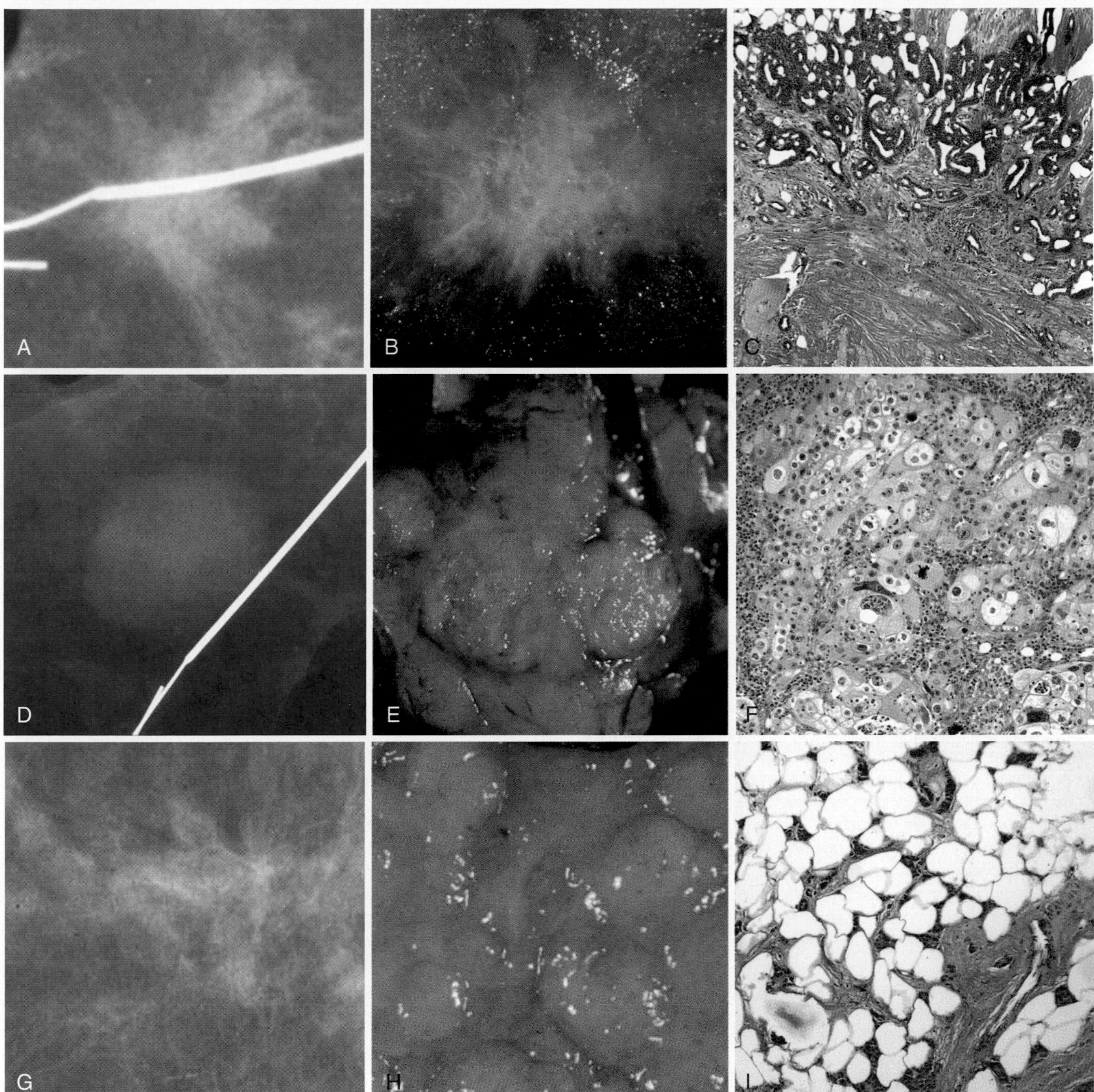

Figure 23-22 Invasive carcinoma of no special type. The majority of invasive carcinomas have a haphazard pattern of stromal invasion that produce masses with irregular margins on imaging (**A**) and gross examination (**B**). Microscopically, such tumors are marked by an exuberant desmoplastic stromal response (**C**). A subset of carcinomas grows as masses that appear to be well circumscribed or lobulated by imaging (**D**) and by gross inspection (**E**). Microscopically, such cancers typically take on the appearance of expansile masses of cells with pushing borders; stromal response is often limited to a narrow zone of fibrosis at the tumor margin (**F**). Rarely, invasive cancers produce little or no stromal response. Such cancers may only show subtle architectural distortion on mammography (**G**) and may not produce palpable masses or be identifiable grossly (**H**). Microscopically, tumor cells are found scattered within normal appearing fibroadipose tissue (**I**). (**B,** Courtesy of Dr. David Hicks, University of Rochester Medical Center, Rochester, NY.)

least 2 to 3 cm in size. The mammographic and gross appearance of invasive carcinoma varies widely depending on the stromal reaction to the tumor (Fig. 23-22). They most commonly present as a hard, irregular radiodense mass (Fig. 23-22*A, B*) associated with a desmoplastic stromal reaction (Fig. 23-22*C*). When cut or scraped, such tumors typically produce a characteristic grating sound (similar to cutting a water chestnut) due to small, central pinpoint foci or streaks of chalky-white desmoplastic stroma and occasional foci of calcification. Less commonly, tumors present as deceptively well-circumscribed (Fig. 23-22*D, E*) masses composed of sheets of tumor cells with scant stromal reaction (Fig. 23-22*F*), or may be almost

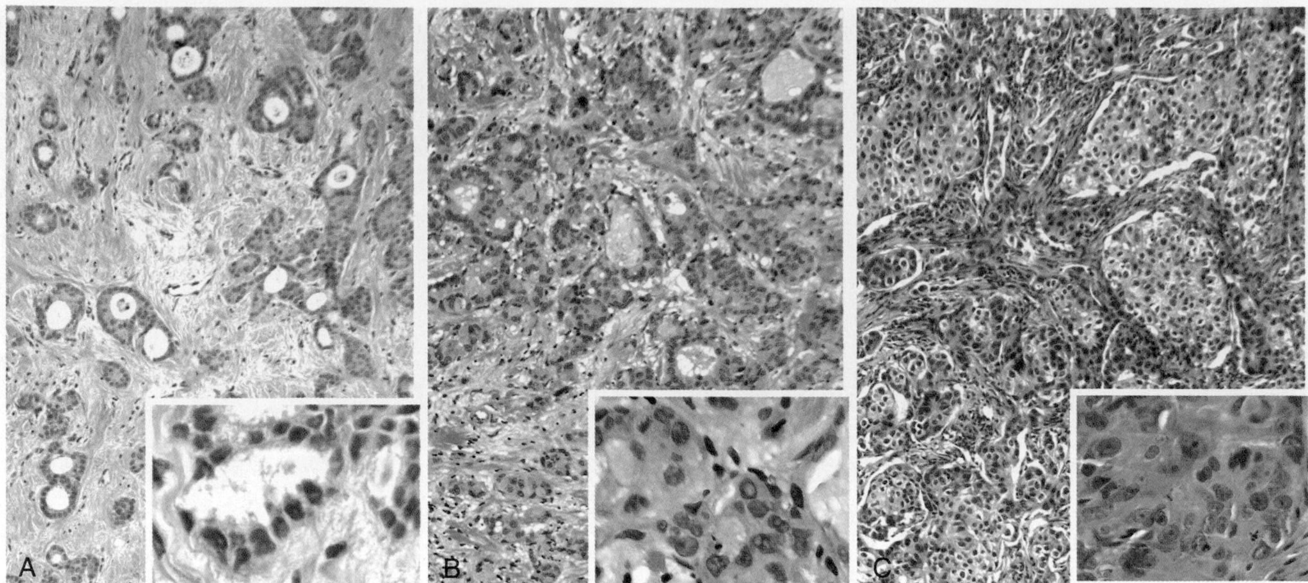

Figure 23-23 Grading of invasive carcinoma. **A,** A well-differentiated carcinoma of no special type consists of tubules or a cribriform pattern of cells with small monomorphic nuclei. **B,** A moderately differentiated carcinoma of no special type shows less tubule formation and more solid nests of cells and pleomorphic nuclei. **C,** A poorly differentiated carcinoma of no special type infiltrates as ragged sheets of pleomorphic cells and contains numerous mitotic figures and central areas of tumor necrosis.

imperceptible (Fig. 23-22*G, H*), being comprised of scattered neoplastic glands or single tumor cells infiltrating otherwise unremarkable fibrofatty tissue (Fig. 23-22*I*).

Larger carcinomas may invade the pectoralis muscle and be fixed to the chest wall or invade into the dermis and cause dimpling of the skin. When the tumor involves the central portion of the breast, retraction of the nipple may develop. Rarely, breast cancer presents as metastasis to an axillary node or distant metastasis before cancer is detected in the breast. In such cases, the primary carcinoma may be small, or be obscured by dense breast tissue, or fail to produce a desmoplastic response, making it difficult to detect by palpation or mammography. In most cases, these "occult" primary tumors can now be detected by imaging studies using ultrasound or MRI.

All types of invasive carcinoma are graded using the Nottingham Histologic Score. Carcinomas are scored for tubule formation, nuclear pleomorphism, and mitotic rate and the points added to divide carcinomas into grade I (well differentiated), grade II (moderately differentiated), and grade III (poorly differentiated) types. **Grade I** carcinomas grow in a tubular pattern with small round nuclei and have a low proliferative rate (Fig. 23-23*A*). **Grade II** carcinomas may also show some tubule formation, but solid clusters or single infiltrating cells are also present. There is a greater degree of nuclear pleomorphism and mitotic figures are present (Fig. 23-23*B*). **Grade III** carcinomas invade as ragged nests or solid sheets of cells with enlarged irregular nuclei. A high proliferative rate and areas of tumor necrosis are common (Fig. 23-23*C*).

ER-positive, HER2-negative carcinoma. Many morphologic patterns are possible, with grades ranging from well to poorly differentiated. Essentially all well differentiated carcinomas are in this group. Mucinous, papillary, cribriform, and lobular patterns may be present and may be so prominent as to prompt classification as a special histologic type (described later).

HER2-positive carcinoma. The majority of these carcinomas are poorly differentiated with only a few classified as moderately differentiated. There is no specific morphologic pattern associated with this cell type. About 50% of apocrine carcinomas and 40% of micropapillary carcinomas (described later) are in this group. The associated DCIS is often more extensive than that associated with other types of invasive carcinoma.

ER-negative, HER2-negative carcinomas. Almost all of these tumors are poorly differentiated and several typical histologic patterns are recognized. Many have circumscribed pushing borders with a central fibrotic or necrotic center. Others have a similar appearance but with a prominent lymphocytic infiltrate and fall into the group of "carcinomas with medullary features" (described later). Spindle cell, squamous, and matrix producing patterns can also be seen. DCIS is generally very limited or not present.

Special Histologic Types of Invasive Carcinoma

Multiple subtypes of invasive carcinoma are recognized with distinctive morphologies and relatively unique biologic characteristics. Like breast cancers of "no special type," these special tumors can be organized into groups based on expression of ER and HER2, which carry their usual therapeutic implications. However, special histologic types of breast cancer often harbor unique genetic aberrations, sometimes have distinct gene signatures, and frequently show associations with clinical behavior and prognosis that break the "rules" that have been established for breast cancers of no special type. Although relatively uncommon, study of these tumors has also provided important insights into breast cancer pathogenesis, some of which merit brief discussion.

Lobular carcinoma is the subtype with the clearest association of phenotype and genotype. Most cases show biallelic loss of expression of *CDH1*, the gene that encodes E-cadherin. Due to loss of E-cadherin, lobular carcinomas are discohesive and often fail to incite a desmoplastic response. They also have characteristic patterns of metastatic spread, often involving the peritoneum and retroperitoneum, the leptomeninges (carcinomatous meningitis), the gastrointestinal tract, and the ovaries and uterus. Males and females with heterozygous germline mutations in *CDH1* also have a greatly increased risk of gastric signet ring cell carcinoma.

Medullary carcinoma is of great interest due to the finding that many tumors of this type have features that are characteristic of *BRCA1*-associated carcinomas. Among cancers arising in *BRCA1* carriers, 13% are of medullary type, and up to 60% have a subset of medullary features (Table 23-3). Although the majority of medullary carcinomas are not associated with germline *BRCA1* mutations, hypermethylation of the *BRCA1* promoter leading to downregulation of *BRCA1* expression is observed in 67% of these tumors. The basis for the relatively good prognosis of this subtype compared to other poorly differentiated carcinomas is not known, but it has been noted that the presence of lymphocytic infiltrates within the tumors is associated with higher survival rates and a greater response to chemotherapy, suggesting that improved outcomes may be related to a host immune response to tumor antigens.

Micropapillary carcinoma shows a characteristic pattern of anchorage-independent growth. Although the cells are adherent to each other and express E-cadherin, they lack adhesion to the stroma.

Many of the other special histologic types of breast cancer (too numerous to list) also have unique biologic, genetic and clinical features. There is much that remains to be learned about the biology and pathogenesis of these tumors, some of which are described below.

MORPHOLOGY

Some special histologic types of cancer are almost always ER-positive and have gene expression profiles that resemble luminal cancers. These include lobular carcinoma, mucinous carcinoma, tubular carcinoma, and papillary carcinoma.

Lobular carcinoma most commonly forms hard irregular masses similar to other breast cancers, but (as already mentioned) may also have a diffuse infiltrative pattern with minimal desmoplasia. Such cancers can be difficult to palpate or detect by imaging. This is the most common type of breast carcinoma to present as an occult primary. The histologic hallmark is the presence of discohesive infiltrating tumor cells, often including signet-ring cells containing intracytoplasmic mucin droplets (Fig. 23-24*A*). Tubule formation is absent. Alveolar and solid variants consist of circumscribed clusters of tumor cells.

Mucinous (colloid) carcinoma is soft or rubbery and has the consistency and appearance of pale gray-blue gelatin. The borders are pushing or circumscribed. The tumor cells are arranged in clusters and small islands of cells within large lakes of mucin (Fig. 23-24*B*).

Tubular carcinoma consists exclusively of well-formed tubules and is sometimes mistaken for a benign sclerosing lesion (Fig. 23-24*C*). A cribriform pattern may also be present. Apocrine snouts are typical, and calcifications may be present within the lumens. Tubular carcinomas are frequently associated with flat epithelial atypia, atypical lobular hyperplasia, LCIS, or low-grade DCIS.

Papillary carcinoma, as the name implies, produces true papillae, fronds of fibrovascular tissue lined by tumor cells (Fig. 23-24*D*).

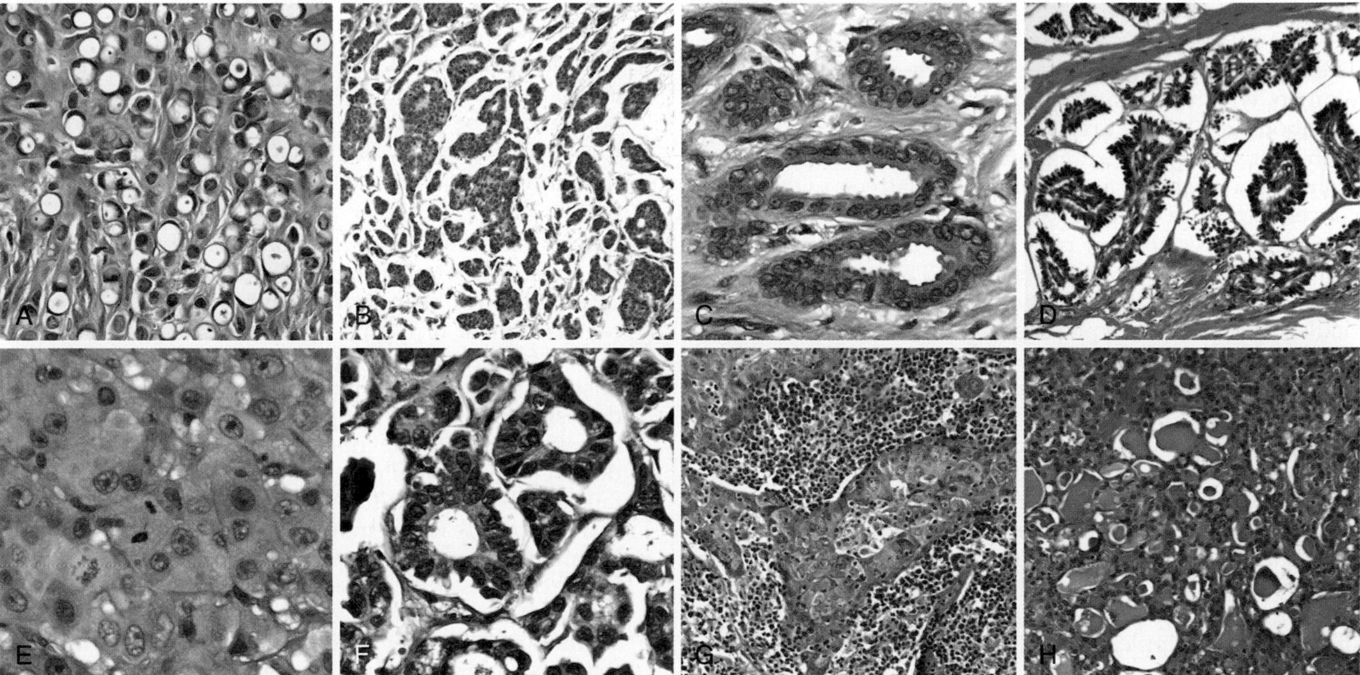

Figure 23-24 Special histologic types of invasive carcinoma. **A,** Lobular carcinoma. **B,** Mucinous carcinoma. **C,** Tubular carcinoma. **D,** Papillary carcinoma. **E,** Apocrine carcinoma. **F,** Micropapillary carcinoma. **G,** Medullary carcinoma. **H,** Secretory carcinoma. See text for morphologic descriptions.

Two special histologic types frequently overexpress HER2. The tumor cells of **apocrine carcinoma** resemble the cells that line sweat glands. These cells have enlarged round nuclei with prominent nucleoli and abundant eosinophilic, occasionally granular, cytoplasm (Fig. 23-24*E*). **Micropapillary carcinoma** (a misnomer) forms hollow balls of cells that float within intercellular fluid, creating structures that mimic the appearance of true papillae (Fig. 23-24*F*).

ER-negative, HER2-negative tumors often correspond to one of several special histologic types. Chief among these is **medullary carcinoma**. Medullary carcinoma is softer than other carcinomas (*medulla* is Latin for "marrow") due to minimal desmoplasia, and often presents as a well-circumscribed mass. It is characterized by (1) solid, syncytium-like sheets of large cells with pleomorphic nuclei, and prominent nucleoli, which compose more than 75% of the tumor mass; (2) frequent mitotic figures; (3) a moderate to marked lymphoplasmacytic infiltrate surrounding and within the tumor; and (4) a pushing (noninfiltrative) border (Fig. 23-24*G*). DCIS is minimal or absent. Due to difficulties in defining this subtype, the current World Health Organization classification system recommends grouping medullary carcinomas with similar carcinomas into one group termed "carcinomas with medullary features."

Other ER-negative, HER2-negative special histologic types include secretory carcinoma, spindle cell carcinoma, low-grade adenosquamous carcinoma, and adenoid cystic carcinoma. **Secretory carcinoma** mimics lactating breast by forming dilated spaces filled with eosinophilic material (Fig. 23-24*H*).

Another clinical and morphologic subtype that merits brief mention is **inflammatory carcinoma**. As discussed earlier, these tumors show extensive invasion and proliferation within lymphatic channels, causing swelling that mimics non-neoplastic inflammatory lesions. These tumors are usually of high grade, but do not belong to any particular molecular subtype.

Male Breast Cancer

The incidence in breast cancer in men is only 1% of that in women, which translates to a lifetime risk of 0.11%. There are about 2000 cases and 400 deaths in the United States each year. Risk factors are similar to those in women and include increasing age, first-degree relatives with breast cancer, exposure to exogenous estrogens or ionizing radiation, infertility, obesity, prior benign breast disease, and residency in Western countries. From 3% to 8% of cases are associated with Klinefelter syndrome and decreased testicular function. The typical age at diagnosis is between 60 and 70 years. From 4% to 14% of cases in males are attributed to germline *BRCA2* mutations. There is a 60% to 76% chance of a *BRCA2* mutation in families with at least one affected male. Male breast cancer is also observed in *BRCA1* families, although not as frequently (Table 23-2).

The pathology of male breast cancer is remarkably similar to that of cancers seen in women. However, ER positivity is more common (81% of tumors). Prognostic factors are similar in men and women.

Because breast epithelium in men is limited to large ducts near the nipple, carcinomas usually present as a palpable subareolar mass, 2 to 3 cm in size and/or as nipple discharge. The carcinoma is situated close to the overlying skin and underlying thoracic wall, and even small carcinomas can invade these structures and cause ulceration. Dissemination follows the same pattern as in women, and axillary lymph node involvement is present in about half of cases at the time of diagnosis. Distant metastases to the lungs, brain, bone, and liver are common. Although men present at higher stages, prognosis is similar in men and women when they are matched stage for stage. Most cancers are treated locally with mastectomy and axillary node dissection. The same systemic treatment guidelines are used for men and women, and response rates are similar.

Prognostic and Predictive Factors

The outcome for women with breast cancer depends on the biologic features of the carcinoma (molecular or histologic type) and the extent to which the cancer has spread (stage) at the time of diagnosis. Many women with breast cancer have a normal life expectancy, whereas others have only a 10% chance of being alive in 5 years. Tumors that present with distant metastasis (<10% of breast cancer cases) or with inflammatory carcinoma (<5%) have a particularly poor prognosis. For all other women, prognosis is determined by pathologic examination of the primary carcinoma and the axillary lymph nodes.

Prognostic information is important in counseling patients about the likely outcome of their disease, choosing appropriate treatment, and the design of clinical trials. Prognostic factors fall into two groups—those related to the extent of carcinoma (tumor burden or stage) and those related to the underlying biology of the cancer. Prognostic factors related to extent of carcinoma are as follows:

- ***Invasive carcinoma versus carcinoma in situ.*** Women with in situ carcinoma understandably have an excellent prognosis. Only rarely do such patients die due to the subsequent development of invasive carcinoma or areas of invasion that were not detected at the time of diagnosis.
- ***Distant metastases.*** Once distant metastases are present, cure is unlikely, although long-term remissions and palliation can be achieved, especially in women with ER-positive tumors. As discussed earlier, the tumor type influences the timing and location of metastases (Table 23-3).
- ***Lymph node metastases.*** **Axillary lymph node status is the most important prognostic factor for invasive carcinoma in the absence of distant metastases.** The clinical assessment of lymph node status is unreliable due to both false positives (e.g., palpable reactive nodes) and false negatives (e.g., lymph nodes with small metastatic deposits). Therefore, biopsy is necessary for accurate assessment. With no nodal involvement, the 10-year disease-free survival rate is close to 70% to 80%; the rate falls to 35% to 40% with one to three positive nodes, and to 10% to 15% when more than 10 nodes are positive. Lymphatic vessels in most breast carcinomas drain first to one or two *sentinel nodes*, which can be identified with radiotracer or colored dyes. If a biopsy restricted to the sentinel nodes is negative for metastasis, it is unlikely that other more distant nodes will be involved and the patient can be spared the morbidity of a complete axillary dissection. Approximately 10% to 20% of women

without axillary lymph node metastases recur with distant metastasis. In these patients, metastasis may occur via the internal mammary lymph nodes or hematogenously. Up until recently, nodal status has been a major determinant of treatment choice. As this decision shifts to being based on the molecular type of carcinoma (discussed below), the information gained from nodal status is becoming less important. It is likely that in the future many women will not undergo node sampling.

- ***Tumor size.*** The risk of axillary lymph node metastases increases with the size of the primary tumor, but both are independent prognostic factors. Women with node-negative carcinomas less than 1 cm in size have a 10-year survival rate of more than 90%, whereas survival drops to 77% for cancers greater than 2 cm. Size is less important for HER2-positive and ER-negative carcinomas, as these carcinomas can metastasize even when quite small.
- ***Locally advanced disease.*** Carcinomas invading into skin or skeletal muscle are usually large and may be difficult to treat surgically. With increased awareness of breast cancer detection, such cases have fortunately decreased in frequency and are now rare at presentation.
- ***Inflammatory carcinoma.*** Breast cancers presenting with breast erythema and skin thickening have a very poor prognosis, as most patients prove to have distant metastases. The edematous skin is tethered to the breast by Cooper ligaments and mimics the surface of an orange peel, an appearance referred to as *peau d'orange*. These clinical signs are caused by dermal lymphatics filled with metastatic carcinoma that blocks lymphatic drainage. The 3-year survival rate is only 3% to 10%. Fewer than 3% of cancers are in this group, but the incidence is higher in African American women and younger women. The underlying carcinoma is usually diffusely infiltrative and typically does not form a discrete palpable mass. The presentation of a swollen breast without a mass can be confused with a breast infection, leading to delayed diagnosis. These carcinomas are not of a uniform specific histologic or molecular type, and thus are classified as "inflammatory" based on the clinical presentation. More than half (60%) are ER-negative and 40% to 50% overexpress HER2.
- ***Lymphovascular invasion.*** Tumor cells are present within vascular spaces (either lymphatics or small capillaries) in about half of all invasive carcinomas. This finding is strongly associated with the presence of lymph node metastases. It is a poor prognostic factor for overall survival in women without lymph node metastases and a risk factor for local recurrence. As already mentioned, extensive plugging of the lymphovascular spaces of the dermis with carcinoma cells (inflammatory carcinoma) bodes a very poor prognosis.

Other prognostic factors are related to tumor biology, as follows:

- ***Molecular subtype.*** The molecular subtype, determined by expression of ER and HER2 and proliferation, is an important prognostic factor
- ***Special histologic types.*** The survival rate of women with some special types of invasive carcinomas (tubular, mucinous, lobular, papillary, adenoid cystic) is greater than that of women with cancers of no special type. Alternatively, women with metaplastic carcinoma or micropapillary carcinoma have a poorer prognosis. In other special subtypes, particularly adenoid cystic carcinoma, low-grade adenosquamous carcinoma, and secretory carcinoma in young women, the histologic

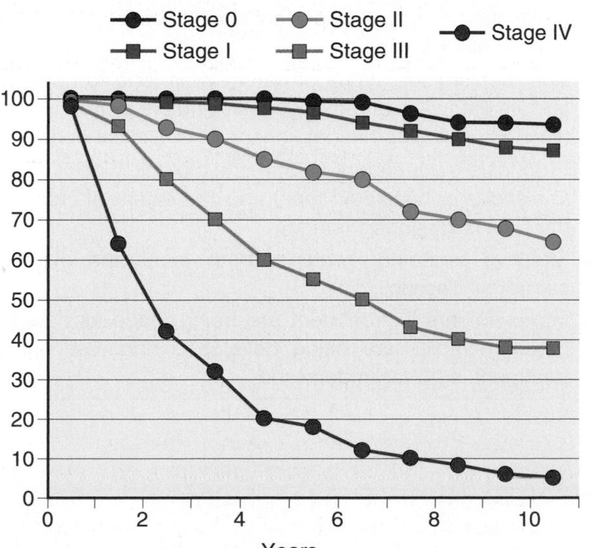

Figure 23-25 Ten-year survival according to AJCC/UICC stage (Table 23-4). Survival is strongly correlated with the extent of disease at the time of diagnosis.

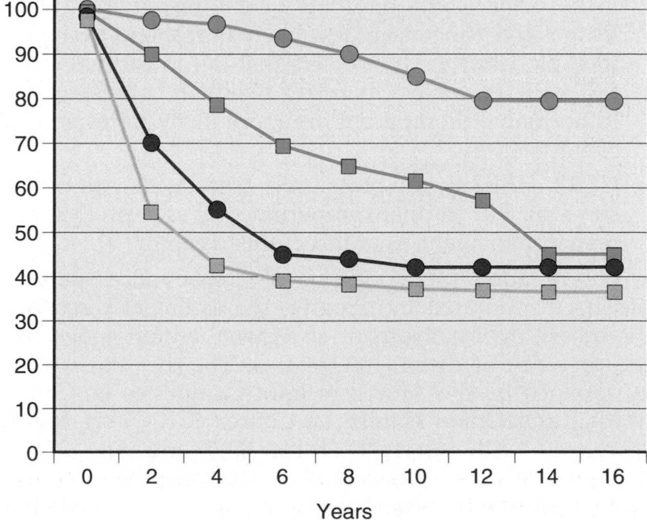

Figure 23-26 Biologic (intrinsic) breast cancer type predicts clinical outcome. Overall survival and disease-free survival are shown for the most favorable biologic type (well-differentiated, ER-positive, HER2-negative, low proliferation) and least favorable biologic type (poorly differentiated, ER-negative and/or HER2-positive). See text for other details.

Table 23-4 American Joint Committee on Cancer and Union Contre Le Cancer Staging*

Stage	T: Primary Cancer	N: Lymph Nodes	M: Distant Metastasis	10-Year Survival (%)
0	DCIS or LCIS	No metastases	Absent	92
I	Invasive carcinoma ≤2 cm	No metastases or only micrometastases	Absent	87
II	Invasive carcinoma >2 cm Invasive carcinoma >5 cm but ≤5 cm	1 to 3 positive LNs 0 to 3 positive LNs	Absent Absent	65
III	Invasive carcinoma >5 cm Any size invasive carcinoma Invasive carcinoma with skin or chest wall involvement or inflammatory carcinoma	Negative or positive LNs ≥4 positive LNs Negative or positive LNs	Absent Absent Absent	40
IV	Any size invasive carcinoma	Negative or positive lymph nodes	Present	5

DCIS, Ductal carcinoma in situ; LCIS, lobular carcinoma in situ.

*The groups listed in the table are based on the characteristics of the primary carcinoma and the axillary lymph nodes. For rare women with involved internal mammary lymph nodes or supraclavicular lymph nodes, there are additional staging criteria.

type is more strongly correlated with prognosis than the molecular type.

- ***Histologic grade.*** All invasive carcinomas are graded using the Nottingham Histologic Score (already described). Nuclear grade, tubule formation, and mitotic rate classify invasive carcinomas into three groups that are highly correlated with disease free and overall survival.
- ***Proliferative rate.*** Proliferation can be measured by mitotic counts (e.g., as part of histologic grading), by immunohistochemical detection of proteins that are specifically expressed by actively dividing cells (e.g., cyclins, Ki-67). Proliferation is primarily important for ER-positive, HER2-negative carcinomas, as the majority of ER-negative and/or HER2 positive carcinomas have high proliferative rates. Carcinomas with high proliferation rates have a poorer prognosis but may respond better to chemotherapy.
- ***Estrogen and progesterone receptors.*** Eighty percent of carcinomas that are both ER- and PR-positive respond to hormonal manipulation, whereas only about 40% of those positive for only ER or PR respond. Strongly ER-positive cancers are less likely to respond to chemotherapy. Conversely, cancers that fail to express either ER or PR have a less than 10% likelihood of responding to hormonal therapy but are more likely to respond to chemotherapy.
- ***HER2.*** HER2 overexpression is associated with poorer survival, but its main importance is as a predictor of response to agents that target this receptor.

For decades, the prognosis of breast cancer patients has been estimated by gauging the extent of disease in the breast, the involvement of regional lymph nodes, and the presence of distant metastases. The five stages (0 to IV) defined by the American Joint Committee on Cancer (AJCC) and Union Contre Le Cancer (UICC) are highly correlated with survival (Table 23-4 and Fig. 23-25). More recently, insights gained by studying the molecular biology of breast cancers has improved outcome prediction (Fig. 23-26).

In the absence of adequate surgery, the majority of patients with breast cancer die with extensive local disease causing ulceration of the skin. *Carcinoma en cuirasse* (literally "carcinoma of the breastplate") is a dreaded complication that must be prevented in order to maintain the best possible quality of life, even in women with distant metastatic disease. Unfortunately, it remains a common presentation for women living in areas with limited resources. With earlier detection, local control of the disease can be achieved in the majority of women with breast conserving surgery and radiation. Carcinoma in situ and small node negative invasive carcinomas are often cured by this treatment alone. For those who require mastectomy, skin- and nipple-sparing procedures provide cosmetically superior results.

KEY CONCEPTS

Types of Carcinoma, Prognostic Factors

- DCIS is treated locally, as subsequent invasive carcinomas usually occur at the same site, whereas LCIS confers bilateral risk.
- Invasive carcinomas can be classified into molecular types based on expression of hormone receptors and HER2 along with proliferative rate.
- Molecular types have important clinical, biologic, and therapeutic associations.
- Special histologic types of carcinomas tend to have distinctive pathways of tumorigenesis and are providing additional clues linking biologic changes to clinical behavior.
- Prognosis is dependent on both the biologic type of cancer (molecular or histologic type) and the extent of cancer at the time of diagnosis (stage).
- Effective treatment requires both local and systemic control of disease.
- Improvements in treatment are being made as new targeted therapies are being developed and response to treatment is better understood.

Stromal Tumors

The two types of stroma in the breast, intralobular and interlobular give rise to distinct types of neoplasms. The breast-specific biphasic tumors fibroadenoma and phyllodes tumor arise from intralobular stroma. This specialized stroma may elaborate growth factors for epithelial cells, resulting in the proliferation of the non-neoplastic epithelial component of these tumors. Interlobular stroma is the source of the same types of tumors found in connective tissue in other sites of the body (e.g., lipomas and angiosarcomas) as well as tumors arising more commonly in the breast (e.g., pseudoangiomatous stromal hyperplasia, myofibroblastomas, and fibrous tumors).

Fibroadenoma

Fibroadenomas are the most common benign tumor of the female breast. Most occur in women in their 20s and 30s, and they are frequently multiple and bilateral. Young women usually present with a palpable mass and older women with a mammographic density (Fig. 23-27*A*) or clustered calcifications. The epithelial component is hormonally responsive and there is typically an increase in size due to lactational changes during pregnancy. Such increases in size may be complicated by infarction and inflammation, and may raise a false suspicion of carcinoma.

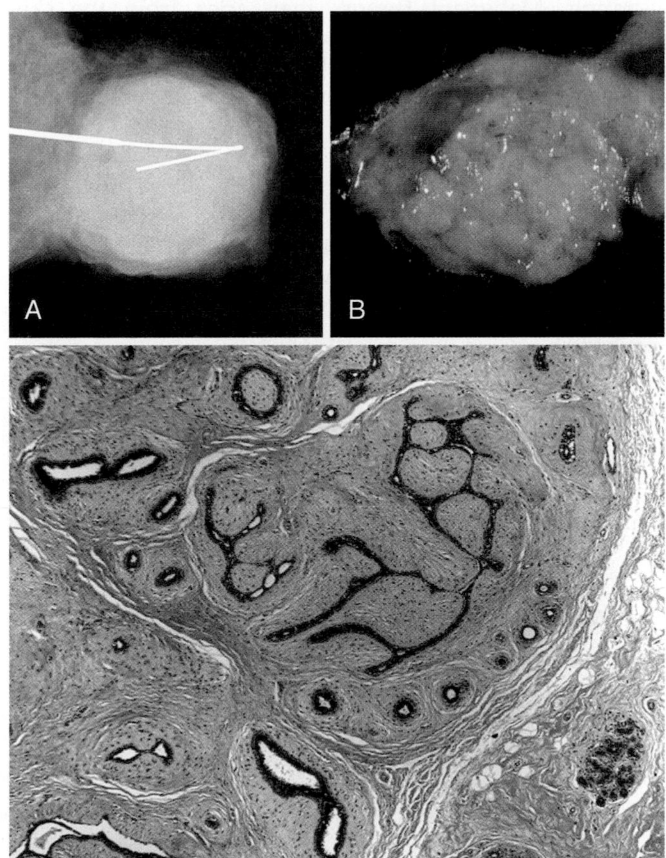

Figure 23-27 Fibroadenoma. **A,** The radiograph shows a characteristically well-circumscribed mass. **B,** Grossly, a rubbery, white, well-circumscribed mass is clearly demarcated from the surrounding yellow adipose tissue. The absence of adipose tissue accounts for the radiodensity of the lesion. **C,** The proliferation of intralobular stroma surrounds, pushes, and distorts the associated epithelium. The border is sharply delimited from the surrounding tissue.

MORPHOLOGY

Fibroadenomas vary in size from less than 1 cm to large tumors that replace most of the breast. The tumors are well-circumscribed, rubbery, grayish white nodules that bulge above the surrounding tissue and often contain slitlike spaces (Fig. 23-27*B*).

The delicate and often myxoid stroma resembles normal intralobular stroma. The epithelium may be surrounded by stroma (pericanicular pattern) or compressed and distorted by it (intracanicular pattern) (Fig. 23-27*C*). In older women, the stroma typically becomes densely hyalinized and the epithelium atrophic.

Many fibroadenomas are polyclonal hyperplasias of lobular stroma. For example, almost half of women receiving cyclosporin A after renal transplantation develop multiple and bilateral fibroadenomas that regress after cessation of treatment. Other fibroadenomas are benign neoplasms associated with clonal cytogenetic aberrations that are confined to the stromal component. No consistent cytogenetic changes have been found.

Fibroadenomas are grouped with "proliferative changes without atypia" in conferring a mildly increased risk of subsequent cancer. However, in one study the increased risk was limited to fibroadenomas associated with cysts larger than 0.3 cm, sclerosing adenosis, epithelial calcifications, or papillary apocrine change ("complex fibroadenomas") (Table 23-1).

Phyllodes Tumor

Phyllodes tumors, like fibroadenomas, arise from intralobular stroma, but are much less common. Although they can occur at any age, most present in the sixth decade, 10 to 20 years later than the peak age for fibroadenomas. The majority are detected as palpable masses, but a few are found by mammography. *Cystosarcoma phyllodes* is a term sometimes used for these lesions. However, *phyllodes tumor* is preferred, since most behave in a relatively benign fashion and are not cystic.

Phyllodes tumors are associated with clonal acquired chromosomal changes, with gains in chromosome 1q being the most frequent. Increased numbers of chromosomal aberrations and overexpression of the homeobox transcription factor HOXB13 are associated with higher tumor grade and more aggressive clinical behavior.

MORPHOLOGY

The tumors vary in size from a few centimeters to massive lesions involving the entire breast. The larger lesions often have bulbous protrusions (*phyllodes* is Greek for "leaflike") due to the presence of nodules of proliferating stroma covered by epithelium (Fig. 23-28). In some tumors these protrusions extend into a cystic space. This growth pattern can also occasionally be seen in larger fibroadenomas and is not an indication of malignancy. Phyllodes tumors are distinguished from fibroadenomas on the basis of higher cellularity, higher mitotic rate, nuclear pleomorphism, stromal overgrowth, and infiltrative borders. Low-grade lesions resemble fibroadenomas but are more

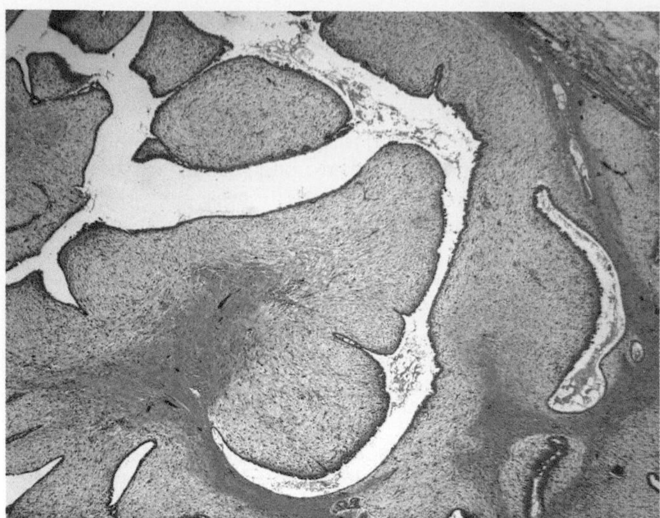

Figure 23-28 Phyllodes tumor. Compared to a fibroadenoma, there is increased stromal cellularity and overgrowth, giving rise to the typical leaflike architecture.

cellular and are mitotically active. High-grade lesions may be difficult to distinguish from malignant sarcomas and may have foci of mesenchymal differentiation (e.g., resembling rhabdomyosarcoma or liposarcoma).

Most phyllodes tumors are low-grade; these occasionally recur locally but do not metastasize. In contrast, intermediate and high-grade phyllodes tumors often recur locally unless they are treated with wide excision or mastectomy. Regardless of grade, lymphatic spread is rare and axillary lymph node dissection is contraindicated. The uncommon high-grade lesions give rise to distant hematogenous metastases in about one third of cases. Only the stromal component metastasizes.

Lesions of Interlobular Stroma

Tumors of the interlobular stroma of the breast are composed of stromal cells without an accompanying epithelial component. These include benign tumors as well as malignant tumors, all uncommon and hence considered briefly. *Myofibroblastoma* consists of myofibroblasts and is unusual in that it is the only breast tumor that is equally common in males. *Lipomas* are often palpable but can also be detected mammographically as fat-containing lesions. The only importance of these lesions is to distinguish them from malignancies.

Fibromatosis is a clonal proliferation of fibroblasts and myofibroblasts. It presents as an irregular, infiltrating mass that can involve both skin and muscle. Though locally aggressive, this lesion does not metastasize. Some cases are associated with prior trauma or surgery. Other cases occur as part of familial adenomatous polyposis, hereditary desmoid syndrome, and Gardner syndrome.

Malignant Tumors of Interlobular Stroma

Malignant stromal tumors include angiosarcoma, rhabdomyosarcoma, liposarcoma, leiomyosarcoma, chondrosarcoma, and osteosarcoma. The only sarcoma that occurs with any frequency in the breast is angiosarcoma—however, it accounts for less than 0.05% of breast malignancies. *Angiosarcomas of the breast* can be sporadic or arise as a complication of therapy. Most sporadic angiosarcomas occur in the breast parenchyma of young women (mean age 35), are of high grade, and have a poor prognosis. Treatment related tumors arise secondary to radiation or edema. After radiation therapy, approximately 0.3% of women develop angiosarcomas in breast skin, with most cases being diagnosed 5 to 10 years after treatment.

Other Malignant Tumors of the Breast

Malignancies of the breast arising from lymphocytes or skin, or metastatic from another site, comprise less than 5% of breast cancers. *Non-Hodgkin lymphoma* may arise primarily in the breast, or the breasts may be secondarily involved by systemic disease. Most primary breast lymphomas are of B-cell type, while rare T cell lymphomas may arise in the scar capsule that is associated with breast implants, possibly due to chronic inflammation, which is known to stimulate lymphoma development in other contexts. Young women with Burkitt lymphoma may present with massive bilateral breast involvement and are often pregnant or lactating. Malignant tumors may arise from the skin and dermis of the breast; these tumors are identical to their counterparts found in skin elsewhere (Chapter 25). Metastases to the breast are rare and most commonly arise from melanomas and ovarian cancers.

KEY CONCEPTS

Stromal Lesions and Other Malignant Tumors

- Intralobular stroma is the origin of the biphasic tumors, fibroadenoma and phyllodes tumor.
- Fibroadenomas are the most common benign tumor of the breast.
- Tumors of interlobular stroma consist only of stromal cells and include both benign and malignant lesions.
- Angiosarcoma is the most common stromal malignancy and can either be sporadic or associated with radiation exposure or lymphedema.

SUGGESTED READINGS

Benign Breast Disease

Ellis IO: Intraductal proliferative lesions of the breast: morphology, associated risk and molecular biology. *Mod Pathol* 23(Suppl 2):S1-7, 2010. *[Benign lesions of the breast have been classified according to the subsequent risk of cancer based on large epidemiologic studies. This is a comprehensive review on the diagnosis, clinical management, and underlying biology of these common findings in breast biopsies.]*

Howard BA: In the beginning: the establishment of the mammary lineage during embryogenesis. *Semin Cell Dev Biol* 23:574, 2012. *[Early mammary mesenchyme and epithelium work together to form the mammary primordium – this fundamental interaction has a key role in the pathogenesis of stromal tumors and carcinomas.]*

Raouf A, Sun Y, Chatterjee S, et al: The biology of human breast epithelial progenitors. *Semin Cell Dev Biol* 23:606, 2012. *[Stem or progenitor cells that give rise to mature breast cells persist into adulthood and are active during expansion of the epithelium during pregnancy. This review discusses the current state of knowledge about this difficult-to-study cell population.]*

Yalom M: *History of the breast*, 1998, Ballantine Books. *[A scholarly work on the cultural, political, psychologic, artistic, physical, and religious significance of the breast.]*

Risk Factors for Developing Carcinoma

Benson JR, Jatoi I: The global breast cancer burden. *Future Oncol* 8:697, 2012. *[The incidence of breast cancer is increasing rapidly in developing countries. This review discusses possible etiologic factors and the challenge of diagnosing and treating cancer in areas with limited resources.]*

Fanale D, Amodeo V, Corsini LR, et al: Breast cancer genome-wide association studies: there is strength in numbers. *Oncogene* 31:2121, 2012. *[In addition to known high-risk genes, additional genes confer a smaller but appreciable risk for breast cancer. This review describes some of the "suspects".]*

Gage N, Wattendorf D, Henry LR: Translational advances regarding hereditary breast cancer syndromes. *J Surg Oncol* 105:444, 2012. *[The major germline mutations conferring a high risk for developing breast cancer are discussed along with guidelines for testing and interpretation.]*

Hopper JL, Jenkins MA, Dowty JG, et al: Using tumour pathology to identify people at high genetic risk of breast and colorectal cancers. *Pathology* 44:89, 2012. *[Describes how the use of histologic characteristics of cancers can be used to help identify kindreds with germline mutations associated with high breast cancer risk.]*

Kurian AW, Fish K, Shema SJ, et al: Lifetime risks of specific breast cancer subtypes among women in four racial/ethnic groups. *Breast Cancer Research* 12:R99, 2010. *[Breast cancer must now be investigated as a group of related, but distinct, diseases. In this study, the risk of different subtypes of cancers is shown to vary for different racial groups.]*

Peres J: Understanding breast density and breast cancer risk. *J Natl Cancer Inst* 104:1345, 2012. *[Density as defined by mammography has been identified as predictor of increased risk and underscores the importance of the tumor environment in the biology of cancer.]*

Biology of Breast Carcinoma

Bombonati A and Sgroi DC: The molecular pathology of breast cancer progression. *J Pathol* 223:307, 2011. *[New techniques allow the breast cancer precursor lesions to be identified and studied; this review describes the early events in breast cancer development.]*

Boudreau A, van't Veer LJ, Bissell MJ: An "elite hacker": breast tumors exploit the normal microenvironment program to instruct their progression and biological diversity. *Cell Adh Migr* 6:236, 2012. *[Stroma is an important partner in cancer progression, but has been difficult to study. This paper reviews the stromal changes during breast development that might be co-opted by cancer cells and the contribution of the microenvironment to clinical outcomes.]*

Gray J, Druker B: Genomics: the breast cancer landscape. *Nature* 486:328, 2012. *[This paper summarizes the results of five important papers on genomic analysis of breast cancer; findings include the identification of new breast cancer subtypes, mutations in triple negative cancers, additional driver mutations, and genomic changes associated with resistance to aromatase inhibitors.]*

Hernandez L, Wilkerson PM, Lambros MB, et al: Genomic and mutational profiling of ductal carcinomas in situ and matched adjacent invasive breast cancers reveals intra-tumour genetic heterogeneity and clonal selection. *J Pathol* 227:42, 2012. *[A detailed study showing that the genetic heterogeneity in breast cancers is present at the in situ stage.]*

Nik-Zainal S, Alexandrov LB, Wedge DC, et al: Mutational processes molding the genomes of 21 breast cancers. *Cell* 149:979, 2012. *[This study from the Cancer Genome Project analyzes specific patterns of mutation and describes the phenomenon of "kataegis" or localized hypermutation.]*

Nik-Zainal S, Van Loo P, Wedge DC, et al: The life history of 21 breast cancers. *Cell* 149:994, 2012. *[Another study from the Cancer Genome Project uses DNA sequencing of multiple subclones within a cancer to reconstruct the order in which mutations accumulated over time.]*

Stephens PJ, Tarpey PS, Davies H, et al: The landscape of cancer genes and mutational processes in breast cancer. *Nature* 486:400, 2012. *[The Welcome Trust Sanger Institute in the United Kingdom has created the Cancer Genome Project, which is analogous to the Cancer Genome Atlas Network in the U.S. This study of 100 breast cancers uses exome sequencing in order to identify the most important driver mutations.]*

The Cancer Genome Atlas Network: Comprehensive molecular portraits of human breast tumours. *Nature* 490:61, 2012. *[In this report, data on over 400 invasive breast cancers including genomic DNA copy number arrays, DNA methylation, exome sequencing, messenger RNA arrays, microRNA sequencing, and reverse-phase protein arrays are described.]*

Breast Cancer Classification

Caddo KA, McArdle O, O'Shea AM, et al: Management of unusual histologic types of breast cancer. *Oncologist* 17:1135, 1012. *[This study presents a compilation of information on rare subtypes of breast cancer.]*

International Agency for Research on Cancer: *World Health Organization Classification of Tumours of the Breast*, July, 2012. *[Over 100 experts from around the world collaborate with W.H.O. to issue guidelines on the classification of breast cancers.]*

Masuda S: Breast cancer pathology: the impact of molecular taxonomy on morphological taxonomy. *Pathol Internat* 62:295, 2012. *[The most useful classification systems combine information from morphology as well as gene expression.]*

Clinical Aspects of Breast Carcinoma

American Joint Committee on Cancer: *AJCC Cancer Staging Manual*, ed 7, New York, 2009, Springer. *[The AJCC, in cooperation with the Union Internationale Contre le Cancer, issues international guidelines on cancer staging.]*

Kaufmann M, et al: Recommendations from an international consensus conference on the current status and future of neoadjuvant systemic therapy in primary cancer. *Ann Surg Oncol* 19:1508, 2012. *[Neoadjuvant therapy is a powerful tool for both patient care and research, as it is currently the only method to directly measure the degree to which carcinomas respond to different types of therapy.]*

Lester SC, Bose S, Chen YY, et al: Protocol for the examination of specimens from patients with invasive carcinoma of the breast. *Arch Pathol Lab Med* 133:1515, 2009. *[The College of American Pathologists has developed national standards for the reporting of breast carcinoma and is currently working on developing a worldwide consensus.]*

Mukherjee S: The Emperor of All Maladies: A biography of cancer. *Scribner* 2011. *[This look back at the evolution of our understanding of cancer includes the story of the discovery of HER2 and the remarkable impact of HER2 targeted therapy.]*

Murphy CG, Morris PG: Recent advances in novel targeted therapies for HER2-positive breast cancer. *Anticancer Drugs* 23:765, 2012. *[New treatments for HER2 overexpressing carcinomas include antibodies to different epitopes, antibody-drug conjugates, targeting of downstream pathway components, and combination therapies.]*

Olson JS: *Bathsheba's breast: women, cancer, and history*, 2002, The Johns Hopkins University Press. *[This book is a 2,000-year chronicle of breast cancer as told by the women who suffered from the disease as well as an informative history of the important milestones in cancer treatment.]*

Reis-Filho JS, Pusztai L: Gene expression profiling in breast cancer: classification, prognostication, and prediction. *Lancet* 378:1812, 2011. *[Gene-expression profiling has been a method to classify the biologic types of cancers and have primarily been of use to help identify patients with hormone receptor positive cancers who do not benefit from chemotherapy.]*

Shah-Khan M, Boughey JC: Evolution of axillary nodal staging in breast cancer: clinical implications of the ACOSOG Z0011 trial. *Cancer Control* 19:267, 2012. *[This paper discusses the diminishing need to sample nodes in women with breast cancer who receive systemic therapy.]*

Sharma K, et al: A systematic review of barriers to breast cancer care in developing countries resulting in delayed patient presentation. *J Oncol* 1012, Epub Aug 22 2012. *[This study describes the challenges to basic health interventions such as local control and systemic treatment with hormonal agents in developing countries.]*

Other Tumors

Karim RZ, O'Toole SA, Scolyer RA: Recent insights into the molecular pathogenesis of mammary phyllodes tumours, *J Clin Pathol* 2013 Feb 12 [Epub ahead of print]. *[Molecular studies of phyllodes tumors, as described in this article, may enable pathologists to predict recurrences or rare metastases with greater accuracy.]*

Lucas DR: Angiosarcoma, radiation-associated angiosarcoma, and atypical vascular lesion, *Arch Pathol Lab Med* 133:1804, 2009. *[This review describes the most important malignancy of the breast after carcinoma and the association of some cases with prior treatment.]*

See TARGETED THERAPY available online at
www.studentconsult.com

CHAPTER 24

The Endocrine System

Anirban Maitra

CHAPTER CONTENTS

The endocrine system consists of a highly integrated and widely distributed group of organs that orchestrate a state of metabolic equilibrium among the various organs of the body. Signaling by secreted molecules can be classified into three types—autocrine, paracrine, or endocrine—on the basis of the distance over which the signal acts. **In endocrine signaling, the secreted molecules, also known as hormones, act on target cells that are distant from their sites of synthesis.** An endocrine hormone is frequently carried by the blood from its site of release to its target. In response, the target tissue often secretes factors that down-regulate the activity of the gland that produces the stimulating hormone, a process known as *feedback inhibition*.

Several processes can disturb the normal activity of the endocrine system, including impaired synthesis or release of hormones, abnormal interactions between hormones and their target tissues, and abnormal responses of target organs. Endocrine diseases can be generally classified as (1) diseases of *underproduction or overproduction* of hormones and their resulting biochemical and clinical consequences, and (2) diseases associated with the development of *mass lesions*. Such lesions might be nonfunctional, or they might be associated with overproduction or underproduction of hormones. The study of endocrine diseases requires integration of morphologic findings with biochemical measurements of the levels of hormones, their regulators, and other metabolites.

PITUITARY GLAND

The pituitary gland is composed of two morphologically and functionally distinct components: the anterior lobe (adenohypophysis) and the posterior lobe (neurohypophysis). The *anterior pituitary* constitutes about 80% of the gland. The production of most pituitary hormones is controlled in large part by positively and negatively acting factors from the hypothalamus (Fig. 24-1), which are carried to the anterior pituitary by a portal vascular system.

In routine histologic sections of the anterior pituitary, a colorful array of cells is present that contain eosinophilic cytoplasm (*acidophil*), basophilic cytoplasm (*basophil*), or poorly staining cytoplasm (*chromophobe*) cells (Fig. 24-2). There are six terminally differentiated cell types in the anterior pituitary, including:

- Somatotrophs, producing growth hormone (GH)
- Mammosomatotrophs, producing GH and prolactin (PRL)
- Lactotrophs, producing PRL
- Corticotrophs, producing adrenocorticotropic hormone (ACTH) and pro-opiomelanocortin (POMC), melanocyte-stimulating hormone (MSH)
- Thyrotrophs, producing thyroid-stimulating hormone (TSH), and
- Gonadotrophs, producing follicle-stimulating hormone (FSH) and luteinizing hormone (LH). FSH stimulates the formation of graafian follicles in the ovary, and LH induces ovulation and the formation of corpora lutea in the ovary. The same two hormones also regulate spermatogenesis and testosterone production in males

Specific *transcription factors* have been identified that regulate the differentiation of pluripotent stem cells within the Rathke's pouch into these terminally differentiated cell types. For example, somatotrophs, mammosomatotrophs, and lactotrophs are derived from stem cells that express the pituitary transcription factor, PIT-1. By contrast steroidogenic factor -1 (SF-1) and GATA-2 are factors that are required for gonadotroph differentiation.

The *posterior pituitary* consists of modified glial cells (termed *pituicytes*) and axonal processes extending from the hypothalamus through the pituitary stalk to the posterior lobe (*axon terminals*). Two peptide hormones are secreted from the posterior pituitary, *oxytocin* and *antidiuretic hormone* (ADH, also called *vasopressin*). These are actually synthesized in the hypothalamus and stored within the axon terminals residing in the posterior pituitary. In response to appropriate stimuli, the preformed hormones are released directly into the systemic circulation through the venous channels of the pituitary. For example, dilation of the cervix in pregnancy results in massive oxytocin release, leading to contraction of the

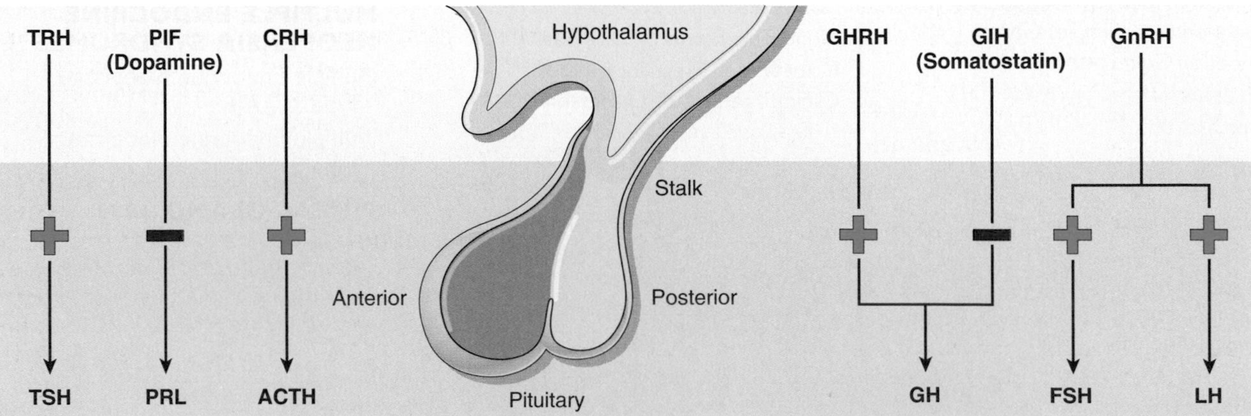

Figure 24-1 Hormones released by the anterior pituitary. The adenohypophysis (anterior pituitary) releases five hormones that are in turn under the control of various stimulatory and inhibitory hypothalamic releasing factors. TSH, Thyroid-stimulating hormone (thyrotropin); PRL, prolactin; ACTH, adrenocorticotropic hormone (corticotropin); GH, growth hormone (somatotropin); FSH, follicle-stimulating hormone; LH, luteinizing hormone. The stimulatory releasing factors are TRH (thyrotropin-releasing hormone), CRH (corticotropin-releasing hormone), GHRH (growth hormone-releasing hormone), GnRH (gonadotropin-releasing hormone). The inhibitory hypothalamic influences comprise PIF (prolactin inhibitory factor or dopamine) and growth hormone inhibitory factor (GIH or somatostatin).

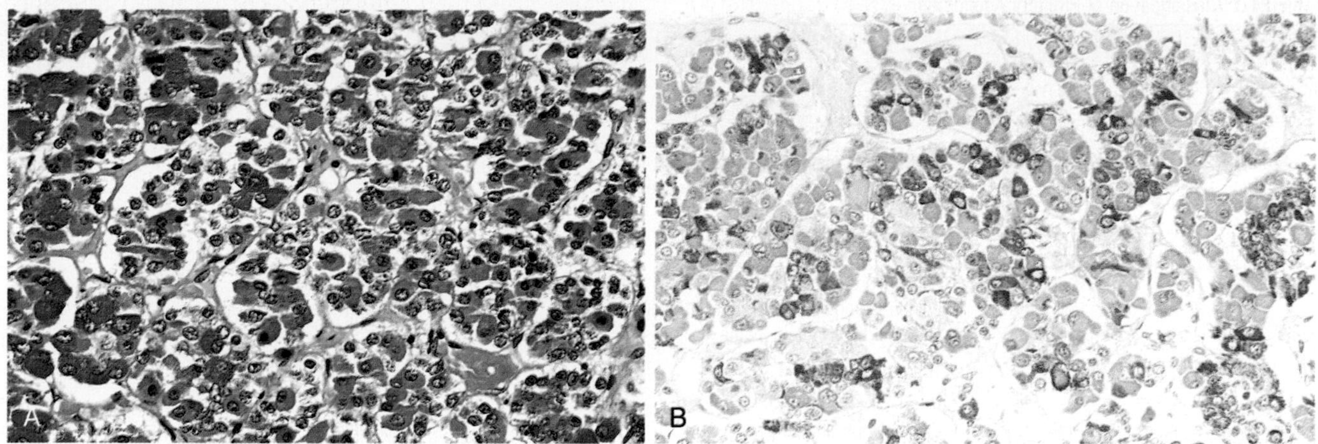

Figure 24-2 A, Photomicrograph of normal pituitary. The gland is populated by several distinct cell populations containing a variety of stimulating (tropic) hormones. Each of the hormones has different staining characteristics, resulting in a mixture of cell types in routine histologic preparations. **B,** Immunostain for human growth hormone.

uterine smooth muscle, facilitating parturition (uterine labor). Similarly, oxytocin released upon nipple stimulation in the postnatal period acts on the smooth muscles surrounding the lactiferous ducts of the mammary glands and facilitates lactation. Synthetic oxytocin can be given to pregnant women to induce labor. The most important function of ADH is to conserve water by restricting diuresis during periods of dehydration and hypovolemia. Decreased blood pressure, sensed by *baroreceptors* (pressure-sensing receptors) in the cardiac atria and carotids, stimulates ADH release. An increase in plasma osmotic pressure detected by *osmoreceptors* also triggers ADH secretion. In contrast, states of hypervolemia and increased atrial distention result in inhibition of ADH secretion.

Clinical Manifestations of Pituitary Disease

The manifestations of pituitary disorders are related to either excess or deficiency of pituitary hormones, or to mass effects.

Hyperpituitarism: Arising from excess secretion of trophic hormones. The causes of hyperpituitarism include pituitary adenoma, hyperplasia and carcinomas of the anterior pituitary, secretion of hormones by nonpituitary tumors, and certain hypothalamic disorders. The symptoms of hyperpituitarism are discussed later in the context of individual tumors.

Hypopituitarism: Arising from deficiency of trophic hormones. This may be caused by destructive processes, including ischemic injury, surgery or radiation, inflammatory reactions, and nonfunctional pituitary adenomas.

Local mass effects: Among the earliest changes referable to mass effect are radiographic abnormalities of the sella turcica, including sellar expansion, bony erosion, and disruption of the diaphragma sella. Because of the close proximity of the optic nerves and chiasm to the sella, expanding pituitary lesions often compress decussating fibers in the optic chiasm. This gives rise to *visual field abnormalities*, classically in the form of defects in both lateral (temporal) visual fields, so-called *bitemporal hemianopsia*. In addition, a variety of other visual field abnormalities may be caused by asymmetric growth of many tumors. Like any expanding intracranial mass, pituitary adenomas can produce signs and symptoms of *elevated intracranial pressure*, including headache, nausea, and vomiting. On occasion, acute hemorrhage into an adenoma is associated with clinical evidence of rapid enlargement of the lesion, a situation appropriately termed *pituitary apoplexy*. Acute pituitary apoplexy is a neurosurgical emergency, in that it can cause sudden death (see later).

Diseases of the posterior pituitary often come to clinical attention because of increased or decreased secretion of ADH.

Pituitary Adenomas and Hyperpituitarism

The most common cause of hyperpituitarism is an adenoma arising in the anterior lobe. These benign tumors are classified on the basis of the hormones that are produced by the neoplastic cells, which are detected by immunohistochemical stains (Table 24-1). Some pituitary adenomas can secrete two hormones (GH and prolactin being the most common combination), and rarely, pituitary adenomas are plurihormonal. Pituitary adenomas can be *functional* (i.e., associated with hormone excess and clinical manifestations thereof) or *nonfunctioning* (i.e., without clinical symptoms of hormone excess). Less common causes of hyperpituitarism include pituitary carcinomas and some hypothalamic disorders. Large pituitary adenomas, and particularly nonfunctioning ones, may cause hypopituitarism by encroaching on and destroying the adjacent anterior pituitary parenchyma.

Pituitary adenomas are usually found in adults; the peak incidence is from 35 to 60 years of age. They are designated, somewhat arbitrarily, *microadenomas* if they are less than 1 cm in diameter and *macroadenomas* if they

Table 24-1 Classification of Pituitary Adenomas

Pituitary Cell Type	Hormone	Adenoma Subtypes	Associated Syndrome*
Lactotroph	Prolactin	Lactotroph adenoma Silent lactotroph adenoma	Galactorrhea and amenorrhea (in females) Sexual dysfunction, infertility
Somatotroph	GH	Densely granulated somatotroph adenoma Sparsely granulated somatotroph adenoma Silent somatotroph adenoma	Gigantism (children) Acromegaly (adults)
Mammosomatotroph	Prolactin, GH	Mammosomatotroph adenomas	Combined features of GH and prolactin excess
Corticotroph	ACTH and other POMC-derived peptides	Densely granulated corticotroph adenoma Sparsely granulated corticotroph adenoma Silent corticotroph adenoma	Cushing syndrome Nelson syndrome
Thyrotroph	TSH	Thyrotroph adenomas Silent thyrotroph adenomas	Hyperthyroidism
Gonadotroph	FSH, LH	Gonadotroph adenomas Silent gonadotroph adenomas ("null cell," oncocytic adenomas)	Hypogonadism, mass effects, and hypopituitarism

ACTH, Adrenocorticotrophic hormone; FSH, follicle-stimulating hormone; GH, growth hormone; LH, luteinizing hormone; POMC, pro-opiomelanocortin; TSH, thyroid-stimulating hormone.
*Note that nonfunctional (silent) adenomas in each category express the corresponding hormone(s) within the neoplastic cells, as determined by special immunohistochemical staining on tissues. However, these adenomas do not produce the associated clinical syndrome, and typically present with *mass effects* accompanied by *hypopituitarism* due to destruction of normal pituitary parenchyma. These features are particularly common with gonadotroph adenomas.
Partially adapted from Asa SL, Essat S: The pathogenesis of pituitary tumors. Annu Rev Pathol Medch Dis 4:97; 2009.

exceed 1 cm in diameter. Non-functional adenomas are likely to come to clinical attention at a later stage than those associated with endocrine abnormalities and are therefore more likely to be macroadenomas. Based on autopsy studies, the prevalence of pituitary adenomas in the population is estimated to be about 14%, but the vast majority of these lesions are clinically silent microadenomas ("pituitary incidentaloma").

With recent advances in molecular techniques, substantial insight has been gained into *the genetic abnormalities associated with pituitary adenomas* (Table 24-2):

- **G-protein mutations are one of the most common alterations in pituitary adenomas**. G proteins are described in Chapter 1; here their function in the context of endocrine neoplasms is reviewed. G proteins play a

Table 24-2 Genetic Alterations in Pituitary Tumors

Gene	Protein Function	Mechanism of Alteration	Most Commonly Associated Pituitary Tumor
Gain of Function			
GNAS	GNAS encodes for alpha subunit of stimulatory G-protein, Gsα. Oncogenic mutation of GNAS constitutively activates Gsα, leading to upregulation of intracellular cyclic AMP (cAMP) activity	Activating mutation	GH adenomas
Protein kinase A, regulatory subunit 1 (PRKAR1A)*	*PRKAR1A* encodes for a negative regulator of protein kinase A (PKA), a downstream mediator of cAMP signaling. Loss of PKA regulation leads to inappropriate cAMP activity	Germline inactivating mutations of *PRKARIA* are present in autosomal dominant Carney complex	GH and prolactin adenomas
Cyclin D1	Cell cycle regulatory protein; promotes G1-S transition	Overexpression	Aggressive adenomas
HRAS	Ras regulates multiple oncogenic pathways including proliferation, cell survival and metabolism	Activating mutation	Pituitary carcinomas
Loss of Function			
MEN1*	MEN1 encodes for menin, a protein with protean roles in tumor suppression, including repression of oncogenic transcription factor JunD, and in histone modification.	Germline inactivating mutations of *MEN1* (multiple endocrine neoplasia, type 1)	GH, prolactin, and ACTH adenomas
CDKN1B (p27/KIP1)*	The p27 protein is a negative regulator of the cell cycle	Germline inactivating mutations of CDKN1B ("MEN-1-like" syndrome)	ACTH adenomas
Aryl hydrocarbon receptor interacting protein (AIP)*	Receptor for aryl hydrocarbons and a ligand-activated transcription factor	Germline mutations of *AIP* cause pituitary adenoma predisposition [PAP] syndrome	GH adenomas (especially in patients younger than 35 years of age)
Retinoblastoma (RB)	Retinoblastoma protein is a negative regulator of the cell cycle (Chapter 7)	Methylation of *RB* gene promoter	Aggressive adenomas

ACTH, Adrenocorticotrophic hormone; GH, growth hormone.
*Genetic alterations associated with *familial* predisposition to pituitary adenomas.
Partially adapted from Boikos SA, Stratakis CA: Molecular genetics of the cAMP-dependent protein kinase pathway and of sporadic pituitary tumorigenesis. Hum Mol Genet 16:R80-R87, 2007.

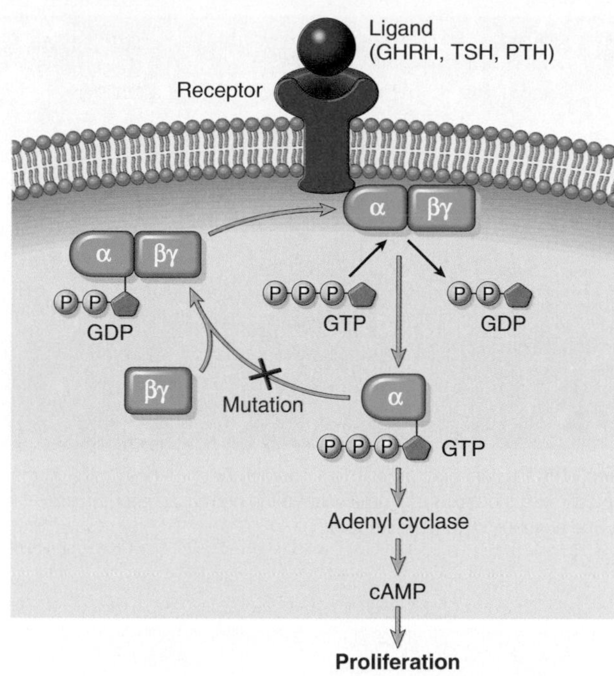

Figure 24-3 G-protein signaling in endocrine neoplasia. Mutations that lead to G-protein hyperactivity are seen in a variety of endocrine neoplasms, including pituitary, thyroid, and parathyroid adenomas. G proteins (composed of α and βγ subunits) play a critical role in signal transduction, transmitting signals from cell surface receptors (GHRH, TSH, or PTH receptor) to intracellular effectors (e.g., adenyl cyclase), which then generate second messengers (cAMP, cyclic adenosine monophosphate) that stimulate cellular responses. GDP, guanosine diphosphate; GTP, guanosine triphosphate; P_i, inorganic phosphate. See Figure 24-1 for other abbreviations.

critical role in signal transduction, transmitting signals from particular *cell surface receptors* (e.g., GHRH receptor) to *intracellular effectors* (e.g., adenyl cyclase), which then generate *second messengers* (e.g., cyclic adenosine monophosphate, cAMP). These are heterotrimeric proteins, composed of a specific α-subunit that binds guanine nucleotide and interacts with both cell surface receptors and intracellular effectors (Fig. 24-3); the β- and γ-subunits are noncovalently bound to the specific α-subunit. G_s is a stimulatory G protein that has a pivotal role in signal transduction in several endocrine organs, including the pituitary. The α-subunit of G_s ($G_s\alpha$) is encoded by the *GNAS* gene, located on chromosome 20q13.

In the basal state, G_s exists in an inactive state, with guanosine diphosphate (GDP) bound to the guanine nucleotide-binding site of $G_s\alpha$. On interaction with the ligand-bound cell surface receptor, GDP dissociates, and guanosine triphosphate (GTP) binds to $G_s\alpha$, activating the G protein. The activation of $G_s\alpha$ results in the generation of cAMP, which is a potent mitogen for a variety of endocrine cell types (e.g., pituitary somatotrophs and corticotrophs, thyroid follicular cells, parathyroid cells), promoting cellular proliferation and hormone synthesis and secretion. Normally, $G_s\alpha$ activation is *transient* because of an intrinsic GTPase activity in the α-subunit, which hydrolyzes GTP into GDP.

Approximately 40% of somatotroph cell adenomas bear GNAS mutations that abrogate the GTPase activity of Gsα, leading to constitutive activation of Gsα, persistent generation of cAMP, and unchecked cellular proliferation (Table 24-2). *GNAS* mutations have also been described in a minority of corticotroph adenomas; in contrast, *GNAS* mutations are absent in thyrotroph, lactotroph, and gonadotroph adenomas, because their respective hypothalamic release hormones do not act via cAMP-dependent pathways.

- The overwhelming majority of pituitary adenomas are sporadic in nature, but approximately 5% of cases arise as a result of an inherited genetic defect. Four causative genes have been identified thus far: *MEN1*, *CDKN1B*, *PRKAR1A*, and *AIP* (see Table 24-2 for a summary of these aberrrations and most commonly associated pituitary tumor subtypes). Of note, somatic mutations of these four genes are rarely encountered in sporadic pituitary adenomas.
- Molecular abnormalities associated with aggressive behavior include aberrations in cell cycle checkpoint proteins, such as overexpression of cyclin D1, mutations of *TP53*, and epigenetic silencing of the retinoblastoma gene (*RB*). In addition, activating mutations of the *HRAS* oncogene are observed in rare *pituitary carcinomas* (Table 24-2).

MORPHOLOGY

The **typical pituitary adenoma** is soft and well-circumscribed. Small adenomas may be confined to the sella turcica, but with expansion they frequently erode the sella turcica and anterior clinoid processes. Larger lesions usually extend superiorly through the diaphragm sella into the suprasellar region, where they often compress the optic chiasm and adjacent structures, such as some of the cranial nerves (Fig. 24-4). In as many as 30% of cases, the adenomas are not grossly encapsulated and infiltrate neighboring tissues such as the cavernous and sphenoid sinuses, dura, and on occasion, the brain itself. Such lesions are termed **invasive adenomas**. Not unexpectedly, macroadenomas are invasive more frequently than smaller tumors. Foci of hemorrhage and necrosis are also more common in these larger adenomas.

Histologically, typical pituitary adenomas are composed of uniform, polygonal cells arrayed in sheets or cords. Supporting connective tissue, or reticulin, is sparse, accounting for the soft, gelatinous consistency of many of these tumors. Mitotic activity is usually sparse. The cytoplasm of the tumor cells may be acidophilic, basophilic, or chromophobic, depending on the type and amount of secretory product within the cells, but it is generally uniform throughout the tumor. **This cellular monomorphism and the absence of a significant reticulin network distinguish pituitary adenomas from nonneoplastic anterior pituitary parenchyma** (Fig. 24-5). The biologic behavior of the adenoma cannot always be reliably predicted from its histologic appearance. A subset of pituitary adenomas demonstrates elevated mitotic activity and nuclear p53 expression, a feature that correlates with the presence of *TP53* mutations. These tumors have a higher propensity for aggressive behavior, including invasion and recurrence, and are termed **atypical adenomas**.

Clinical Course. The signs and symptoms of pituitary adenomas are related to endocrine abnormalities and mass effects. The effects of excessive secretion of anterior

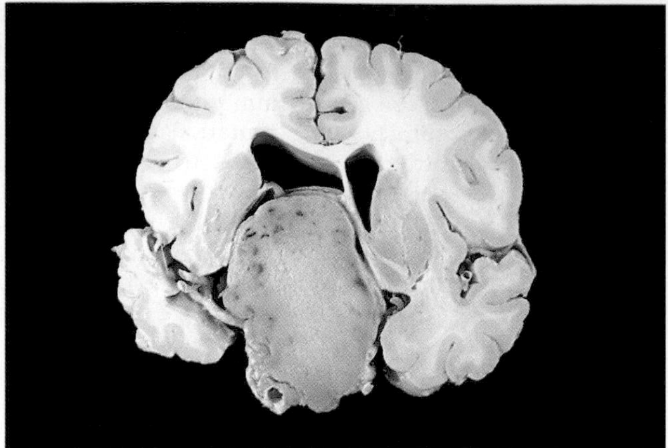

Figure 24-4 Pituitary adenoma. This massive, nonfunctional adenoma has grown far beyond the confines of the sella turcica and has distorted the overlying brain. Nonfunctional adenomas tend to be larger at the time of diagnosis than those that secrete a hormone.

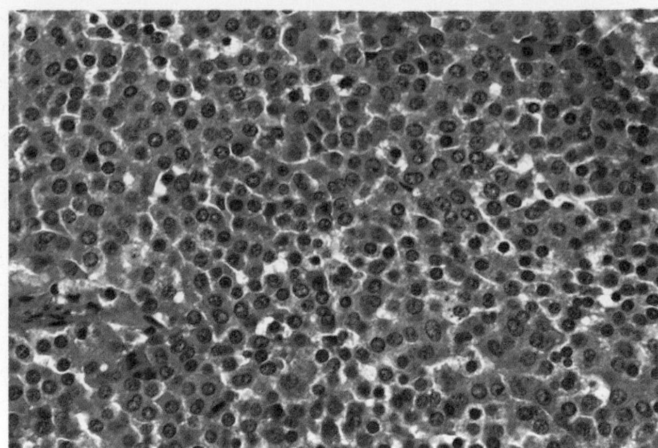

Figure 24-5 Pituitary adenoma. The monomorphism of these cells contrasts markedly with the mixture of cells seen in the normal anterior pituitary. Note also the absence of reticulin network.

pituitary hormones are mentioned later, when the specific types of pituitary adenoma are described. Local mass effects may be produced by any type of pituitary tumor. As already mentioned, these effects include *radiographic abnormalities of the sella turcica, visual field abnormalities,* signs and symptoms of *elevated intracranial pressure,* and occasionally *hypopituitarism.* Acute hemorrhage into an adenoma is sometimes associated with *pituitary apoplexy,* as noted earlier.

The following is a discussion of the individual types of tumors.

Lactotroph Adenoma

Prolactin-secreting lactotroph adenomas are the most frequent type of hyperfunctioning pituitary adenoma, accounting for about 30% of all clinically recognized cases. These lesions range from small microadenomas to large, expansile tumors associated with substantial mass effect.

MORPHOLOGY

The overwhelming majority of lactotroph adenomas are comprised of chromophobic cells with juxtanuclear localization of the transcription factor PIT-1; these are known as **sparsely granulated lactotroph adenomas** (Fig. 24-6*A*). Much rarer are the acidophilic **densely granulated lactotroph adenomas**, characterized by diffuse cytoplasmic PIT-1 expression localization (Fig. 24-6*B*). Prolactin can be demonstrated within the secretory granules in the cytoplasm of the cells using immunohistochemical stains. Lactotroph adenomas have a propensity to undergo dystrophic calcification, ranging from isolated psammoma bodies to extensive calcification of virtually the entire tumor mass ("pituitary stone"). Prolactin secretion by functioning adenomas is usually efficient (even microadenomas secrete sufficient prolactin to cause hyperprolactinemia) and proportional, in that serum prolactin concentrations tend to correlate with the size of the adenoma.

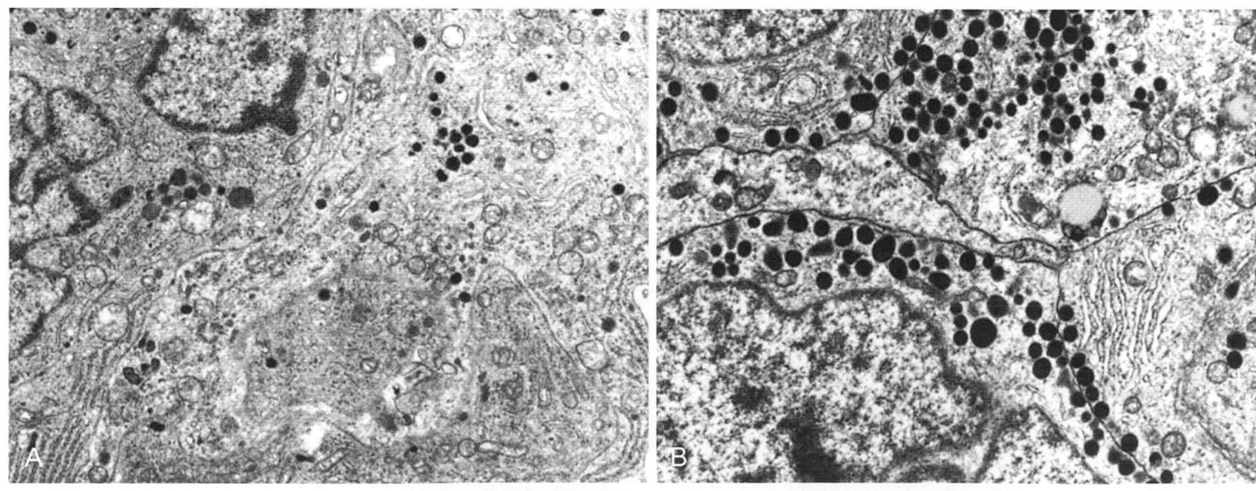

Figure 24-6 Ultrastructural features of prolactinomas. **A,** Electron micrograph of a sparsely granulated prolactinoma. The tumor cells contain abundant granular endoplasmic reticulum (indicative of active protein synthesis) and small numbers of electron-dense secretory granules. **B,** Electron micrograph of densely granulated growth hormone-secreting adenoma. The tumor cells are filled with numerous large, electron-dense secretory granules. (Courtesy Dr. Eva Horvath, St. Michael's Hospital, Toronto, Ont. Canada.)

Clinical Course. Increased serum levels of prolactin, or *prolactinemia,* cause amenorrhea, galactorrhea, loss of libido, and infertility. The diagnosis of an adenoma is made more readily in women than in men, especially between the ages of 20 and 40 years, presumably because of the sensitivity of menses to disruption by hyperprolactinemia. Lactotroph adenoma underlies almost a quarter of cases of amenorrhea. In contrast, in men and older women, the hormonal manifestations may be subtle, allowing the tumors to reach considerable size (macroadenomas) before being detected clinically.

Hyperprolactinemia may result from causes other than prolactin-secreting pituitary adenomas. Physiologic hyperprolactinemia occurs in pregnancy. Prolactin levels are also elevated by nipple stimulation, as occurs during suckling in lactating women, and as a response to many types of stress. Pathologic hyperprolactinemia can also result from *lactotroph hyperplasia* caused by loss of dopamine-mediated inhibition of prolactin secretion. This may occur with damage of the dopaminergic neurons of the hypothalamus, damage of the pituitary stalk (e.g., due to head trauma), or exposure to drugs that block dopamine receptors on lactotroph cells. Any mass in the suprasellar compartment (e.g., a pituitary adenoma) may disturb the normal inhibitory influence of the hypothalamus on prolactin secretion, resulting in hyperprolactinemia. Therefore, a mild elevation in serum prolactin in a person with a pituitary adenoma does not necessarily indicate a prolactin-secreting tumor. Other causes of hyperprolactinemia include renal failure and hypothyroidism. Lactotroph adenomas are treated by surgery or, more commonly, with bromocriptine, a dopamine receptor agonist that causes the lesions to diminish in size.

Somatotroph Adenomas

Growth hormone (GH)-secreting somatotroph adenomas are the second most common type of functioning pituitary adenoma, and cause gigantism in children and acromegaly in adults. Somatotroph adenomas may be quite large by the time they come to clinical attention because the manifestations of excessive GH may be subtle.

MORPHOLOGY

Histologically, pure somatotroph adenomas are also classified into **densely granulated** and **sparsely granulated subtypes**. Densely granulated adenomas are composed of monomorphic, acidophilic cells that have strong cytoplasmic GH reactivity on immunohistochemistry. In contrast, the sparsely granulated variants are composed of chromophobe cells with considerable nuclear and cytologic pleomorphism and focal, weak staining for GH. Bihormonal **mammosomatotroph** adenomas that synthesize both GH and prolactin are being increasingly recognized; morphologically, most bihormonal adenomas resemble the densely granulated pure somatotroph adenomas, but are distinguished by having immunohistochemical reactivity for prolactin as well as GH.

Clinical Course. Persistently elevated levels of GH stimulate the hepatic secretion of insulin-like growth factor 1 (IGF-1), which causes many of the clinical manifestations.

- If a somatotroph adenoma appears in children before the epiphyses have closed, the elevated levels of GH (and IGF-1) result in *gigantism*. This is characterized by a generalized increase in body size with disproportionately long arms and legs.
- If the increased levels of GH are present after closure of the epiphyses, *acromegaly* develops. In this condition, growth is most conspicuous in skin and soft tissues, viscera (thyroid, heart, liver, and adrenals), and the bones of the face, hands, and feet. Bone density may increase (hyperostosis) in both the spine and the hips. Enlargement of the jaw results in its protrusion (prognathism), and broadening of the lower face. The feet and hands are enlarged, and the fingers become thickened and sausage-like. In most instances gigantism is also accompanied by evidence of acromegaly. These changes may develop slowly over decades before being recognized, hence the opportunity for the adenomas to reach substantial size.
- GH excess can also be associated with a variety of other disturbances, including gonadal dysfunction, diabetes mellitus, generalized muscle weakness, hypertension, arthritis, congestive heart failure, and an increased risk of gastrointestinal cancers.

The diagnosis of pituitary GH excess relies on documentation of elevated serum GH and IGF-1 levels. In addition, failure to suppress GH production in response to an oral load of glucose is one of the most sensitive tests for acromegaly. The underlying pituitary adenoma can be either removed surgically or treated via pharmacologic means. The latter includes somatostatin analogs (recall that somatostatin inhibits pituitary GH secretion) or the use of GH receptor antagonists, which prevent hormone binding to target organs such as the liver. When effective control of high GH levels is achieved, the characteristic tissue overgrowth and related symptoms gradually recede, and the metabolic abnormalities improve.

Corticotroph Adenomas

Excess production of ACTH by functioning corticotroph adenomas leads to adrenal hypersecretion of cortisol and the development of *hypercortisolism* (also known as *Cushing syndrome*).

MORPHOLOGY

Corticotroph adenomas are usually microadenomas at the time of diagnosis. These tumors are most often basophilic **(densely granulated)** and occasionally chromophobic **(sparsely granulated)**. Both variants stain positively with periodic acid-Schiff (PAS) because of the presence of carbohydrate in proopiomelanocortin (POMC), the ACTH precursor molecule; in addition, they demonstrate variable immunoreactivity for POMC and its derivatives, including ACTH and β-endorphin.

Clinical Course. The clinical manifestations of Cushing syndrome are discussed in more detail later with the diseases of the adrenal gland. The syndrome can be caused by a wide variety of conditions in addition to ACTH-producing pituitary tumors. When the hypercortisolism is due to excessive production of ACTH by the pituitary, it is designated *Cushing disease*. Large destructive pituitary adenomas can develop in patients after surgical removal of the adrenal glands for treatment of Cushing syndrome. This condition, known as *Nelson syndrome*, occurs most often because of a loss of the inhibitory effect of adrenal corticosteroids on a preexisting corticotroph microadenoma. Because the adrenals are absent in persons with this disorder, hypercortisolism does not develop, and patients present with mass effects due to the pituitary tumor, and there can be hyperpigmentation because of the stimulatory effect of other products of the ACTH precursor molecule on melanocytes.

Other Anterior Pituitary Adenomas

Pituitary adenomas may elaborate more than one hormone (e.g., mammosomatotroph adenomas). Other unusual "plurihormonal" adenomas secrete multiple hormones; these tumors are usually aggressive. A few comments are made about several of the less frequent functioning tumors.

- *Gonadotroph (LH-producing and FSH-producing) adenomas* can be difficult to recognize because they secrete hormones inefficiently and variably, and the secretory products usually do not cause a recognizable clinical syndrome (*nonfunctioning adenomas*, see later). Gonadotroph adenomas are most frequently found in middle-aged men and women when they become large enough to cause neurologic symptoms, such as impaired vision, headaches, diplopia, or pituitary apoplexy. Pituitary hormone deficiencies can also be found, most commonly impaired secretion of LH. This causes decreased energy and libido in men (due to reduced testosterone) and amenorrhea in premenopausal women. The neoplastic cells usually demonstrate immunoreactivity for the common gonadotropin α-subunit and the specific β-FSH and β-LH subunits; FSH is usually the predominant secreted hormone. Gonadotroph adenomas usually express steroidogenic factor-1 (SF-1) and GATA-2, transcription factors associated with normal gonadotroph differentiation.
- *Thyrotroph (TSH-producing)* adenomas are uncommon, accounting for approximately 1% of all pituitary adenomas. Thyrotroph adenomas are a rare cause of *hyperthyroidism*.
- *Nonfunctioning pituitary adenomas* are a heterogeneous group that constitutes approximately 25% to 30% of all pituitary tumors. Their lineage can be established by immunohistochemical staining for hormones or by biochemical demonstration of cell type-specific transcription factors. In the past, many such tumors have been called *silent variants* or *null-cell adenomas*. Not surprisingly, nonfunctioning adenomas typically present with symptoms stemming from mass effects. These lesions may also compromise the residual anterior pituitary sufficiently to cause hypopituitarism, which may appear slowly due to gradual enlargement of the adenoma or abruptly because of acute intratumoral hemorrhage (pituitary apoplexy).

Pituitary carcinoma is rare, accounting for less than 1% of pituitary tumors. The presence of craniospinal or systemic metastases is a sine qua non of a pituitary carcinoma. Most pituitary carcinomas are functional, with prolactin and ACTH being the most common secreted products. Metastases usually appear late in the course, following multiple local recurrences.

KEY CONCEPTS

Hyperpituitarism

- The most common cause of hyperpituitarism is an anterior lobe pituitary adenoma.
- Pituitary adenomas can be *macroadenomas* (greater than 1 cm in diameter) or *microadenomas*.
- Functioning adenomas are associated with distinct endocrine signs and symptoms, while nonfunctioning (silent) adenomas typically present with mass effects, including visual disturbances.
- Lactotroph adenomas secrete prolactin and can present with amenorrhea, galactorrhea, loss of libido, and infertility
- Somatotroph adenomas secrete GH and present with gigantism in children and acromegaly in adults, impaired glucose tolerance, and diabetes mellitus.
- Corticotroph adenomas secrete ACTH and present with Cushing syndrome and hyperpigmentation.
- The two distinctive morphologic features of most adenomas are their cellular monomorphism and absence of a reticulin network.

Hypopituitarism

***Hypopituitarism* refers to decreased secretion of pituitary hormones, which can result from diseases of the hypothalamus or of the pituitary.** Hypofunction of the anterior pituitary occurs when approximately 75% of the parenchyma is lost or absent. This may be congenital or the result of a variety of acquired abnormalities that are intrinsic to the pituitary. Hypopituitarism accompanied by evidence of posterior pituitary dysfunction in the form of diabetes insipidus (see later) is almost always of hypothalamic origin.

Most cases of hypopituitarism arise from destructive processes directly involving the anterior pituitary. The causes include the following:

- *Tumors and other mass lesions:* Pituitary adenomas, other benign tumors arising within the sella, primary and metastatic malignancies, and cysts can cause hypopituitarism. Any mass lesion in the sella can cause damage by exerting pressure on adjacent pituitary cells.
- *Traumatic brain injury and subarachnoid hemorrhage* are among the most common causes of pituitary hypofunction.
- *Pituitary surgery or radiation:* Surgical excision of a pituitary adenoma may inadvertently extend to the nonadenomatous pituitary. Radiation of the pituitary, used to prevent regrowth of residual tumor after surgery, can damage the nonadenomatous pituitary.
- *Pituitary apoplexy:* As mentioned earlier, this is caused by a sudden hemorrhage into the pituitary gland, often occurring into a pituitary adenoma. In its most dramatic presentation, apoplexy causes the sudden onset of

excruciating headache, diplopia due to pressure on the oculomotor nerves, and hypopituitarism. In severe cases, it can cause cardiovascular collapse, loss of consciousness, and even sudden death. The combination of mass effects from the hemorrhage and the acute hypopituitarism makes pituitary apoplexy a true neurosurgical emergency.

- *Ischemic necrosis of the pituitary and Sheehan syndrome:* Sheehan syndrome, also known as postpartum necrosis of the anterior pituitary, is the most common form of clinically significant ischemic necrosis of the anterior pituitary. During pregnancy the anterior pituitary enlarges to almost twice its normal size. This physiologic expansion of the gland is not accompanied by an increase in blood supply from the low-pressure venous system; hence, there is relative hypoxia. Any further reduction in blood supply caused by obstetric hemorrhage or shock may precipitate infarction of the anterior lobe. Because the posterior pituitary receives its blood directly from arterial branches, it is much less susceptible to ischemic injury and is therefore usually not affected. Pituitary necrosis may also be encountered in other conditions, such as disseminated intravascular coagulation and (more rarely) sickle cell anemia, elevated intracranial pressure, traumatic injury, and shock of any origin. Whatever the pathogenesis, the ischemic area is resorbed and replaced by a nubbin of fibrous tissue attached to the wall of an empty sella.
- *Rathke cleft cyst:* These cysts, lined by ciliated cuboidal epithelium with occasional goblet cells and anterior pituitary cells, can accumulate proteinaceous fluid and expand, compromising the normal gland.
- *Empty sella syndrome:* Any condition or treatment that destroys part or all of the pituitary gland, such as ablation of the pituitary by surgery or radiation, can result in an *empty sella* and the *empty sella syndrome*. There are two types: (1) In a *primary* empty sella, a defect in the diaphragma sella allows the arachnoid mater and cerebrospinal fluid to herniate into the sella, expanding the sella and compressing the pituitary. Classically, this occurs in obese women with a history of multiple pregnancies. Affected individuals often present with visual field defects and occasionally with endocrine anomalies, such as *hyperprolactinemia*, due to interruption of inhibitory hypothalamic inputs. Sometimes the loss of functioning parenchyma is sufficient to produce hypopituitarism. (2) In *secondary* empty sella, a mass, such as a pituitary adenoma, enlarges the sella and is then either surgically removed or undergoes infarction, leading to loss of pituitary function.
- *Hypothalamic lesions*: As mentioned earlier, hypothalamic lesions can also affect the pituitary by interfering with the delivery of pituitary hormone-releasing factors. In contrast to diseases that involve the pituitary directly, hypothalamic abnormalities can also diminish the secretion of ADH, resulting in diabetes insipidus (discussed later). Hypothalamic lesions that cause hypopituitarism include *tumors*, which may be benign (e.g., craniopharyngioma) or malignant; most of the latter are metastases from tumors such as breast and lung carcinoma. Hypothalamic insufficiency can also appear following irradiation of brain or nasopharyngeal tumors.
- *Inflammatory disorders and infections*, such as sarcoidosis or tuberculous meningitis, can involve the hypothalamus and cause deficiencies of anterior pituitary hormones and diabetes insipidus.
- *Genetic defects:* Congenital deficiency of transcription factors required for normal pituitary function is a rare cause of hypopituitarism. For example, mutation of the pituitary-specific gene *PIT-1* results in combined pituitary hormone deficiency, characterized by deficiencies of GH, prolactin, and TSH.

The clinical manifestations of anterior pituitary hypofunction vary depending on the specific hormones that are lacking.

- Children can develop growth failure *(pituitary dwarfism)* due to growth hormone deficiency.
- Gonadotropin (LH and FSH) deficiency leads to amenorrhea and infertility in women and decreased libido, impotence, and loss of pubic and axillary hair in men.
- TSH and ACTH deficiencies result in symptoms of hypothyroidism and hypoadrenalism, respectively, and are discussed later in the chapter.
- Prolactin deficiency results in failure of postpartum lactation.
- The anterior pituitary is also a rich source of MSH, synthesized from the same precursor molecule that produces ACTH; therefore, one of the manifestations of hypopituitarism includes pallor due to a loss of stimulatory effects of MSH on melanocytes.

Posterior Pituitary Syndromes

The clinically relevant posterior pituitary syndromes involve ADH and include *diabetes insipidus* and *secretion of inappropriately high levels of ADH.*

- ***Diabetes insipidus.* ADH deficiency causes *diabetes insipidus*, a condition characterized by excessive urination (polyuria) due to an inability of the kidney to resorb water properly from the urine.** Diabetes insipidus can occur in a variety of conditions, including head trauma, tumors, inflammatory disorders of the hypothalamus and pituitary, and surgical complications. The condition can also arise spontaneously, in the absence of an identifiable underlying disorder. Diabetes insipidus from ADH deficiency is designated as *central* to differentiate it from *nephrogenic* diabetes insipidus, which is a result of renal tubular unresponsiveness to circulating ADH. The clinical manifestations of these two disorders are similar and include the excretion of large volumes of dilute urine with a lower than normal specific gravity. Serum sodium and osmolality are increased by the excessive renal loss of free water, resulting in thirst and polydipsia. Patients who can drink water generally compensate for the urinary losses, but patients who are obtunded, bedridden, or otherwise limited in their ability to obtain water may develop life-threatening dehydration.
- ***Syndrome of inappropriate ADH (SIADH) secretion.* ADH excess causes resorption of excessive amounts of free water, resulting in *hyponatremia*.** The most

frequent causes of SIADH are the secretion of ectopic ADH by malignant neoplasms (particularly small-cell carcinoma of the lung), drugs that increase ADH secretion, and a variety of central nervous system disorders, including infections and trauma. The clinical manifestations of SIADH are dominated by hyponatremia, cerebral edema, and resultant neurologic dysfunction. Although total body water is increased, blood volume remains normal, and peripheral edema does not develop.

Hypothalamic Suprasellar Tumors

Neoplasms in this location may induce hypofunction or hyperfunction of the anterior pituitary, diabetes insipidus, or combinations of these manifestations. The most commonly implicated tumors are *gliomas* (sometimes arising in the chiasm; Chapter 28) and *craniopharyngiomas.* The craniopharyngioma is thought to arise from vestigial remnants of Rathke pouch. These slow-growing tumors account for 1% to 5% of intracranial tumors. A small minority of these lesions occurs within the sella, but most are suprasellar, with or without intrasellar extension. A bimodal age distribution is observed, with one peak in childhood (5 to 15 years) and a second peak in adults 65 years or older. Patients usually come to attention because of headaches and visual disturbances, while children sometimes present with growth retardation due to pituitary hypofunction and GH deficiency. Abnormalities of the *WNT signaling pathway,* including activating mutations of the gene encoding β-catenin, have been reported in craniopharyngiomas.

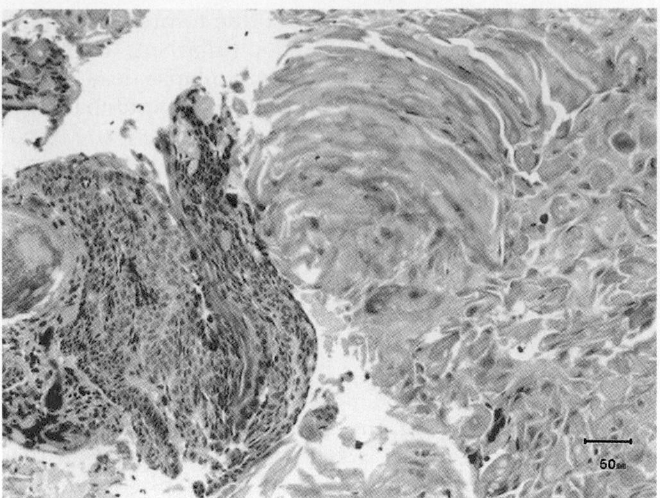

Figure 24-7 Adamantinomatous craniopharyngioma, demonstrating characteristic compact, lamellar "wet" keratin (right half of photomicrograph) and cords of squamous epithelium with peripheral palisading on the left. (Courtesy Dr. Charles Eberhart, Department of Pathology, Johns Hopkins University, Baltimore, Md.)

MORPHOLOGY

Craniopharyngiomas average 3 to 4 cm in diameter; they may be encapsulated and solid, but more commonly they are cystic and sometimes multiloculated. They often encroach on the optic chiasm or cranial nerves, and not infrequently they bulge into the floor of the third ventricle and base of the brain. Two distinct histologic variants are recognized: **adamantinomatous craniopharyngioma** (most often observed in children) and **papillary craniopharyngioma** (most often observed in adults). The adamantinomatous type frequently contains radiologically demonstrable calcifications; the papillary variant calcifies only rarely.

Adamantinomatous craniopharyngioma consists of nests or cords of stratified squamous epithelium embedded in a spongy "reticulum" that becomes more prominent in the internal layers. "Palisading" of the squamous epithelium is frequently observed at the periphery. Compact, lamellar keratin formation ("wet keratin") is a diagnostic feature of this tumor (Fig. 24-7). As mentioned earlier, **dystrophic calcification** is a frequent finding. Additional features include cyst formation, fibrosis, and chronic inflammation. The cysts of adamantinomatous craniopharyngiomas often contain a cholesterol-rich, thick brownish-yellow fluid that has been compared to "machine oil." These tumors extend fingerlets of epithelium into adjacent brain, where they elicit a brisk glial reaction.

Papillary craniopharyngiomas contain both solid sheets and papillae lined by well-differentiated squamous epithelium. These tumors usually lack keratin, calcification, and cysts. The squamous cells of the solid sections of the tumor lack the peripheral palisading and do not typically generate a spongy reticulum in the internal layers.

Patients with craniopharyngiomas, especially those less than 5 cm in diameter, have an excellent recurrence-free and overall survival. Larger lesions are more invasive but this does not impact on the prognosis. Malignant transformation of craniopharyngiomas into squamous carcinomas is exceptionally rare and usually occurs after irradiation.

THYROID GLAND

The thyroid gland, usually located below and anterior to the larynx, consists of two bulky lateral lobes connected by a relatively thin isthmus. The thyroid is divided by thin fibrous septae into lobules composed of about 20 to 40 evenly dispersed follicles, lined by a cuboidal to low columnar epithelium, and filled with PAS-positive thyroglobulin. In response to hypothalamic factors, TSH *(thyrotropin)* is released by thyrotrophs in the anterior pituitary into the circulation. The binding of TSH to its receptor on the thyroid follicular epithelium results in activation of the receptor, allowing it to associate with a G_s protein (Fig. 24-8). Activation of the G protein stimulates downstream

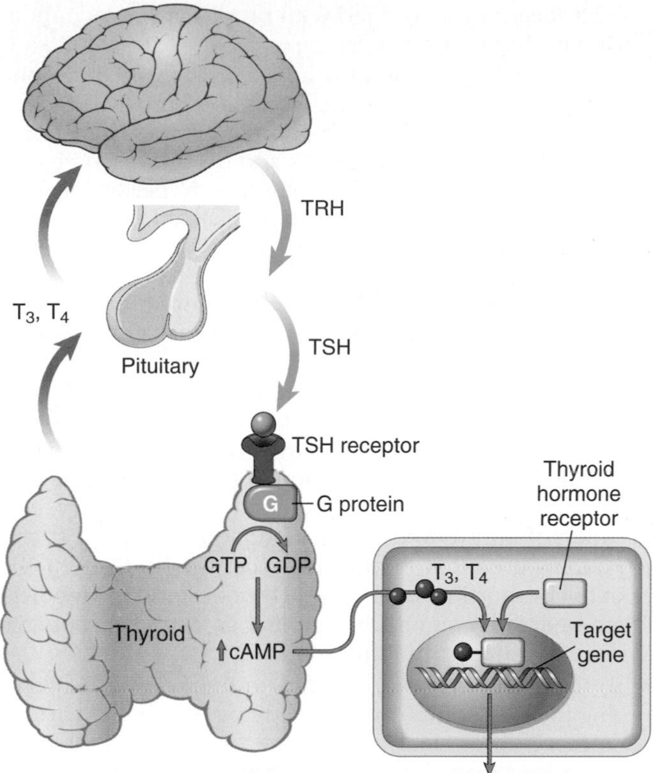

Figure 24-8 Homeostasis in the hypothalamus-pituitary-thyroid axis and mechanism of action of thyroid hormones. Secretion of thyroid hormones (T_3 and T_4) is controlled by trophic factors secreted by both the hypothalamus and the anterior pituitary. Decreased levels of T_3 and T_4 stimulate the release of thyrotropin-releasing hormone (TRH) from the hypothalamus and thyroid-stimulating hormone (TSH) from the anterior pituitary, causing T_3 and T_4 levels to rise. Elevated T_3 and T_4 levels, in turn, feed back to suppress the secretion of both TRH and TSH. TSH binds to the TSH receptor on the thyroid follicular epithelium, which causes activation of G proteins, and cAMP-mediated synthesis and release of thyroid hormones (T_3 and T_4). In the periphery, T_3 and T_4 interact with the thyroid hormone receptor (TR) to form a hormone-receptor complex that translocates to the nucleus and binds to so-called thyroid response elements (TREs) on target genes to initiate transcription.

events that result in an increase in intracellular cAMP levels, which stimulates thyroid growth and thyroid hormone synthesis and release via cAMP-dependent protein kinases.

Thyroid follicular epithelial cells convert thyroglobulin into *thyroxine (T_4)* and lesser amounts of *triiodothyronine (T_3)*. T_4 and T_3 are released into the systemic circulation, where most of these peptides are reversibly bound to circulating plasma proteins, such as thyroxine-binding globulin and transthyretin. The binding proteins act as a buffer that maintains the serum unbound ("free") T_3 and T_4 concentrations within narrow limits, while ensuring that the hormones are readily available to the tissues. In the periphery, the majority of free T_4 is deiodinated to T_3; the latter binds to thyroid hormone nuclear receptors in target cells with tenfold greater affinity than does T_4 and has proportionately greater activity. Binding of thyroid hormone to its nuclear thyroid hormone receptor (TR) results in the assembly of a multiprotein hormone-receptor complex on thyroid hormone response elements (TREs) in target genes, up regulating their transcription (Fig. 24-8). Thyroid hormone has diverse cellular effects, including the stimulation of carbohydrate and lipid catabolism and protein synthesis in a wide range of cells. The net result is an increase in the basal metabolic rate. In addition, thyroid hormone has a critical role in brain development in the fetus and neonate (see later).

The function of the thyroid gland can be inhibited by a variety of chemical agents, collectively referred to as *goitrogens*. Because they suppress T_3 and T_4 synthesis, the level of TSH increases, and subsequent hyperplastic enlargement of the gland (*goiter*) follows. The antithyroid agent *propylthiouracil* inhibits the oxidation of iodide and thus blocks the production of thyroid hormones; parenthetically, propylthiouracil also inhibits the peripheral deiodination of circulating T_4 into T_3, thus ameliorating symptoms of thyroid hormone excess (see later). Iodide, when given in large doses to individuals with thyroid hyperfunction, also blocks the release of thyroid hormones by inhibiting the proteolysis of thyroglobulin. Thus, thyroid hormone is synthesized and incorporated into colloid, but it is not released into the blood.

The thyroid gland follicles also contain a population of *parafollicular cells*, or C cells, which synthesize and secrete the hormone *calcitonin*. This hormone promotes the absorption of calcium by the skeletal system and inhibits the resorption of bone by osteoclasts.

Diseases of the thyroid include conditions associated with excessive release of thyroid hormones (hyperthyroidism), thyroid hormone deficiency (hypothyroidism), and mass lesions of the thyroid. We will first consider the clinical consequences of disturbed thyroid function, and then turn to the disorders that generate these problems.

Hyperthyroidism

***Thyrotoxicosis* is a hypermetabolic state caused by elevated circulating levels of free T_3 and T_4.** Because it is caused most commonly by hyperfunction of the thyroid gland, it is often referred to as *hyperthyroidism*. However, in certain conditions the oversupply is related to either excessive release of preformed thyroid hormone (e.g., in thyroiditis) or to an extrathyroidal source, rather than hyperfunction of the gland (Table 24-3). Thus, strictly speaking, hyperthyroidism is only one (albeit the most common) cause of thyrotoxicosis. The terms *primary* and *secondary hyperthyroidism* are sometimes used to designate hyperthyroidism arising from an intrinsic thyroid abnormality and that arising from processes outside of the thyroid, such as a TSH-secreting pituitary tumor, respectively. With this caveat, we follow the common practice of using the terms *thyrotoxicosis* and *hyperthyroidism* interchangeably. **The three most common causes of thyrotoxicosis are associated with hyperfunction of the gland and include the following:**

- *Diffuse hyperplasia* of the thyroid associated with Graves disease (approximately 85% of cases)
- Hyperfunctional *multinodular goiter*
- Hyperfunctional thyroid *adenoma*

Clinical Course. The clinical manifestations of hyperthyroidism are protean and include changes referable to the

Table 24-3 Disorders Associated with Thyrotoxicosis

Associated with Hyperthyroidism
Primary
Diffuse hyperplasia (Graves disease) Hyperfunctioning ("toxic") multinodular goiter Hyperfunctioning ("toxic") adenoma Iodine-induced hyperthyroidism Neonatal thyrotoxicosis associated with maternal Graves disease
Secondary
TSH-secreting pituitary adenoma (rare)*
Not Associated with Hyperthyroidism
Granulomatous (de Quervain) thyroiditis (*painful*) Subacute lymphocytic thyroiditis (*painless*) Struma ovarii (ovarian teratoma with ectopic thyroid) Factitious thyrotoxicosis (exogenous thyroxine intake)

*Associated with increased thyroid-stimulating hormone (TSH); all other causes of thyrotoxicosis associated with decreased TSH.

hypermetabolic state induced by excess thyroid hormone and to overactivity of the *sympathetic nervous system* (i.e., an increase in the β-adrenergic "tone").

- Excessive levels of thyroid hormone result in *an increase in the basal metabolic rate*. The *skin* of thyrotoxic patients tends to be soft, warm, and flushed because of increased blood flow and peripheral vasodilation, adaptations that serve to increase heat loss. *Heat intolerance* is common. Sweating is increased because of higher levels of calorigenesis. Heightened catabolic metabolism results in *weight loss despite increased appetite*.
- *Cardiac manifestations are among the earliest and most consistent features*. Individuals with hyperthyroidism can have elevated cardiac contractility and cardiac output, in response to increased peripheral oxygen requirements. Tachycardia, palpitations, and cardiomegaly are common. Arrhythmias, particularly atrial fibrillation, occur frequently and are more common in older patients. Congestive heart failure may develop, especially in older patients with preexisting cardiac disease. Myocardial changes, such as focal lymphocytic and eosinophilic infiltrates, mild fibrosis, myofibril fatty change, and an increase in size and number of mitochondria, have been described. Some individuals with thyrotoxicosis develop reversible *left ventricular dysfunction* and "low-output" heart failure, so-called *thyrotoxic or hyperthyroid cardiomyopathy*.
- *Overactivity of the sympathetic nervous system* produces tremor, hyperactivity, emotional lability, anxiety, inability to concentrate, and insomnia. Proximal muscle weakness and decreased muscle mass are common *(thyroid myopathy)*. In the *gastrointestinal system*, sympathetic hyperstimulation of the gut results in hypermotility, diarrhea, and malabsorption.
- *Ocular changes* often call attention to hyperthyroidism. A wide, staring gaze and lid lag are present because of sympathetic overstimulation of the superior tarsal muscle (also known as *Müller's muscle*), which functions alongside the levator palpebrae superioris muscle to raise the upper eyelid (Fig. 24-9). However, true *thyroid ophthalmopathy* associated with proptosis occurs only in Graves disease (see later).
- The *skeletal system* is also affected. Thyroid hormone stimulates bone resorption, increasing porosity of cortical bone and reducing the volume of trabecular bone. The net effect is osteoporosis and an increased risk of fractures in patients with chronic hyperthyroidism. Other findings include atrophy of skeletal muscle, with fatty infiltration and focal interstitial lymphocytic infiltrates; minimal liver enlargement due to fatty changes in the hepatocytes; and generalized lymphoid hyperplasia and lymphadenopathy in patients with Graves disease.
- *Thyroid storm* refers to the abrupt onset of severe hyperthyroidism. This condition occurs most commonly in patients with underlying Graves disease and probably results from an acute elevation in catecholamine levels, as might be encountered during infection, surgery, cessation of antithyroid medication, or any form of stress. Patients are often febrile and present with tachycardia out of proportion to the fever. Thyroid storm is a medical emergency. A significant number of untreated patients die of cardiac arrhythmias.
- *Apathetic hyperthyroidism* refers to thyrotoxicosis occurring in older adults, in whom advanced age and various co-morbidities may blunt the features of thyroid hormone excess that typically bring younger patients to attention. The diagnosis of thyrotoxicosis in these individuals is often made during laboratory work-up for unexplained weight loss or worsening cardiovascular disease.

A diagnosis of hyperthyroidism is made using both clinical and laboratory findings. The measurement of serum TSH concentration is the most useful single screening test for hyperthyroidism, because its levels are decreased even at the earliest stages, when the disease may still be subclinical. A low TSH value is usually confirmed with measurement of free T_4, which is predictably increased. In occasional patients, hyperthyroidism results

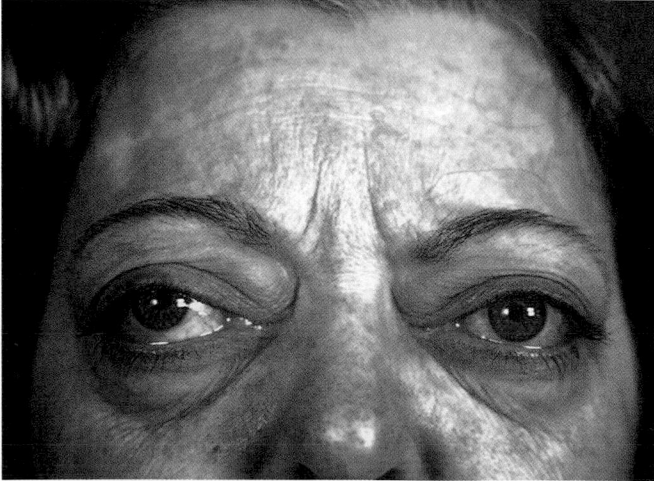

Figure 24-9 A person with hyperthyroidism. A wide-eyed, staring gaze, caused by overactivity of the sympathetic nervous system, is one of the features of this disorder. In Graves disease, one of the most important causes of hyperthyroidism, accumulation of loose connective tissue behind the eyeballs, also adds to the protuberant appearance of the eyes.

predominantly from increased circulating levels of T_3 ("T_3 toxicosis"). In these cases, free T_4 levels may be decreased, and direct measurement of serum T_3 may be useful. In rare cases of pituitary-associated (secondary) hyperthyroidism, TSH levels are either normal or raised. Determining TSH levels after the injection of thyrotropin-releasing hormone (TRH stimulation test) is used in the evaluation of cases of suspected hyperthyroidism with equivocal changes in the baseline serum TSH level. A normal rise in TSH after administration of TRH excludes secondary hyperthyroidism. Once the diagnosis of thyrotoxicosis has been confirmed by a combination of TSH assays and free thyroid hormone levels, measurement of radioactive iodine uptake by the thyroid gland can help to determine the etiology. For example, there may be diffusely increased uptake in the whole gland (Graves disease), increased uptake in a solitary nodule (toxic adenoma), or decreased uptake (thyroiditis).

The therapeutic options for hyperthyroidism include several medications, each with a different mechanism of action. Typically, these include a β-blocker to control symptoms induced by increased adrenergic tone, a thionamide to block new hormone synthesis, an iodine solution to block the release of thyroid hormone, and agents that inhibit peripheral conversion of T_4 to T_3. Radioiodine, which is incorporated into thyroid tissues, resulting in ablation of thyroid function over a period of 6 to 18 weeks, may also be used.

Table 24-4 Causes of Hypothyroidism

Primary
Genetic defects in thyroid development (*PAX8, FOXE1*, TSH receptor mutations) (rare)
Thyroid hormone resistance syndrome (*THRB* mutations) (rare)
Postablative
Surgery, radioiodine therapy, or external irradiation
Autoimmune hypothyroidism
Hashimoto thyroiditis*
Iodine deficiency*
Drugs (lithium, iodides, *p*-aminosalicylic acid)*
Congenital biosynthetic defect (dyshormonogenetic goiter) (rare) *
Secondary (Central)
Pituitary failure (rare)
Hypothalamic failure (rare)

*Associated with enlargement of thyroid ("goitrous hypothyroidism"). Hashimoto thyroiditis and postablative hypothyroidism account for the majority of cases of hypothyroidism in developed countries. *FOXE1*, forkhead box E1; *PAX8*, paired box 8; *THRB*, thyroid hormone receptor β.

Hypothyroidism

***Hypothyroidism* is a condition caused by a structural or functional derangement that interferes with the production of thyroid hormone.** Hypothyroidism is a fairly common disorder. By some estimates the population prevalence of overt hypothyroidism is 0.3%, while subclinical hypothyroidism can be found in greater than 4%. The prevalence increases with age, and it is nearly tenfold more common in women than in men. It can result from a defect anywhere in the hypothalamic-pituitary-thyroid axis. As in the case of hyperthyroidism, this disorder is divided into *primary* and *secondary* forms, depending on whether the hypothyroidism arises from an intrinsic abnormality in the thyroid itself, or occurs as a result of pituitary and hypothalamic disease (Table 24-4). Primary hypothyroidism accounts for the vast majority of cases, and may be accompanied by an enlargement in the size of the thyroid gland (goiter).

Primary hypothyroidism can be congenital, autoimmune, or iatrogenic.

***Congenital hypothyroidism.* Worldwide, congenital hypothyroidism is most often the result of *endemic iodine deficiency* in the diet** (see later). Other rare forms of congenital hypothyroidism include *inborn errors of thyroid metabolism (dyshormonogenetic goiter),* wherein any one of the multiple steps leading to thyroid hormone synthesis may be defective, such as (1) iodide transport into thyrocytes, (2) "organification" of iodine (binding of iodine to tyrosine residues of the storage protein, thyroglobulin), and (3) iodotyrosine coupling to form hormonally active T_3 and T_4. In rare instances there may be complete absence of thyroid parenchyma *(thyroid agenesis),* or the gland may be greatly reduced in size *(thyroid hypoplasia)* due to germline mutations in genes responsible for thyroid development (Table 24-4).

***Autoimmune hypothyroidism.* Autoimmune hypothyroidism is the most common cause of hypothyroidism in iodine-sufficient areas of the world.** The vast majority of cases of autoimmune hypothyroidism are due to Hashimoto thyroiditis. Circulating autoantibodies, including *antimicrosomal, antithyroid peroxidase,* and *antithyroglobulin* antibodies, are found in this disorder, and the thyroid is typically enlarged (goitrous). Autoimmune hypothyroidism can occur in isolation or in conjunction with autoimmune polyendocrine syndrome (APS), types 1 and 2 (see discussion in "Adrenal Glands").

Iatrogenic hypothyroidism. This can be caused by either *surgical or radiation-induced ablation*. A large resection of the gland (total thyroidectomy) for the treatment of hyperthyroidism or a primary neoplasm can lead to hypothyroidism. The gland may also be ablated by radiation, whether in the form of radioiodine administered for the treatment of hyperthyroidism, or exogenous irradiation, such as external radiation therapy to the neck. *Drugs* given intentionally to decrease thyroid secretion (e.g., methimazole and propylthiouracil) can also cause acquired hypothyroidism, as can agents used to treat nonthyroid conditions (e.g., lithium, *p*-aminosalicylic acid).

Secondary (or central) hypothyroidism is caused by deficiencies of TSH or, far more uncommonly, TRH. Any of the causes of hypopituitarism (for example, pituitary tumor, postpartum pituitary necrosis, trauma, and nonpituitary tumors), or of hypothalamic damage from tumors, trauma, radiation therapy, or infiltrative diseases can cause central hypothyroidism.

Cretinism

***Cretinism* refers to hypothyroidism that develops in infancy or early childhood.** The term *cretin* was derived from the French *chrétien,* meaning "Christian" or

"Christlike," and was applied to these unfortunates because they were considered to be so mentally retarded as to be incapable of sinning. In the past this disorder occurred fairly commonly in regions of the world where dietary iodine deficiency is endemic, such as the Himalayas, inland China, Africa, and other mountainous areas. It is now much less prevalent as a result of the widespread supplementation of foods with iodine. On rare occasions, cretinism may also result from genetic defects that interfere with the biosynthesis of thyroid hormone (dyshormonogenetic goiter, see earlier).

Clinical features of cretinism include impaired development of the skeletal system and central nervous system, manifested by severe mental retardation, short stature, coarse facial features, a protruding tongue, and umbilical hernia. The severity of the mental impairment seems to be related to the time at which thyroid deficiency occurs in utero. Normally, maternal T_3 and T_4 cross the placenta and are critical for fetal brain development. If there is maternal thyroid deficiency before the development of the fetal thyroid gland, mental retardation is severe. In contrast, maternal thyroid hormone deficiency later in pregnancy, after the fetal thyroid has become functional, does not affect normal brain development.

Myxedema

The term *myxedema* is applied to hypothyroidism developing in the older child or adult. Myxedema was first linked with thyroid dysfunction in 1873 by Sir William Gull in an article addressing the development of a "cretinoid state" in adults. The clinical manifestations vary with the age of onset of the deficiency. Older children show signs and symptoms intermediate between those of the cretin and those of the adult with hypothyroidism. In the adult the condition appears insidiously and may take years before arousing clinical suspicion.

Myxedema is marked by a slowing of physical and mental activity. The initial symptoms include generalized fatigue, apathy, and mental sluggishness, which may mimic depression. Speech and intellectual functions are slowed. Patients with myxedema are listless, cold intolerant, and frequently overweight. Decreased sympathetic activity results in constipation and decreased sweating. The skin is cool and pale because of decreased blood flow. Reduced cardiac output probably contributes to shortness of breath and decreased exercise capacity, two frequent complaints. Thyroid hormones regulate the transcription of several sarcolemmal genes, such as calcium ATPases and the β adrenergic receptor, and lowered expression of these genes results in a decrease in cardiac output. In addition, hypothyroidism promotes an atherogenic profile—an increase in total cholesterol and low-density lipoprotein (LDL) levels—that probably contributes to the increased cardiovascular mortality in this disease. Histologically, there is an accumulation of matrix substances, such as glycosaminoglycans and hyaluronic acid, in skin, subcutaneous tissue, and a number of visceral sites. This results in nonpitting edema, a broadening and coarsening of facial features, enlargement of the tongue, and deepening of the voice.

Laboratory evaluation plays a vital role in the diagnosis of suspected hypothyroidism because of the nonspecific nature of symptoms. Patients with unexplained increases in body weight or hypercholesterolemia should be assessed for potential hypothyroidism. **Measurement of the serum TSH level is the most sensitive screening test for this disorder.** The TSH level is increased in primary hypothyroidism as a result of a loss of feedback inhibition of TRH and TSH production by the hypothalamus and pituitary, respectively. The TSH level is not increased in persons with hypothyroidism due to primary hypothalamic or pituitary disease. T_4 levels are decreased in individuals with hypothyroidism of any origin.

Thyroiditis

Thyroiditis, or inflammation of the thyroid gland, encompasses a diverse group of disorders characterized by some form of thyroid inflammation.

Although multiple entities exist under the diagnostic umbrella of "thyroiditis," this discussion focuses on the three most common and clinically significant subtypes: (1) Hashimoto thyroiditis, (2) granulomatous (de Quervain) thyroiditis, and (3) subacute lymphocytic thyroiditis.

Hashimoto Thyroiditis

Hashimoto thyroiditis is an autoimmune disease that results in destruction of the thyroid gland and gradual and progressive thyroid failure. It is the most common cause of hypothyroidism in areas of the world where iodine levels are sufficient. The name is derived from the 1912 report by Hashimoto describing patients with goiter and intense lymphocytic infiltration of the thyroid *(struma lymphomatosa)*. It is most prevalent between 45 and 65 years of age and is more common in women than in men, with a female predominance of 10:1 to 20:1. It can also occur in children and is a major cause of nonendemic goiter in the pediatric population.

Pathogenesis. **Hashimoto thyroiditis is caused by a breakdown in self-tolerance to thyroid autoantigens.** This is exemplified by the presence of circulating autoantibodies against thyroglobulin and thyroid peroxidase in the vast majority of Hashimoto patients. The inciting events have not been elucidated, but possibilities include abnormalities of regulatory T cells (Tregs), or exposure of normally sequestered thyroid antigens (Chapter 6). Similar to other autoimmune diseases, Hashimoto thyroiditis has a strong genetic component. Increased susceptibility to Hashimoto thyroiditis is associated with polymorphisms in immune regulation-associated genes, including *cytotoxic T lymphocyte-associated antigen-4 (CTLA4)* and *protein tyrosine phosphatase-22 (PTPN22)*, both of which code for regulators of T-cell responses. Susceptibility to other autoimmune diseases, such as type 1 diabetes (see later), is also associated with polymorphisms in both *CTLA4* and *PTPN22*.

Induction of thyroid autoimmunity is accompanied by a progressive depletion of thyroid epithelial cells by apoptosis and replacement of the thyroid parenchyma by mononuclear cell infiltration and fibrosis. Multiple immunologic mechanisms may contribute to thyroid cell death, including (Fig. 24-10):

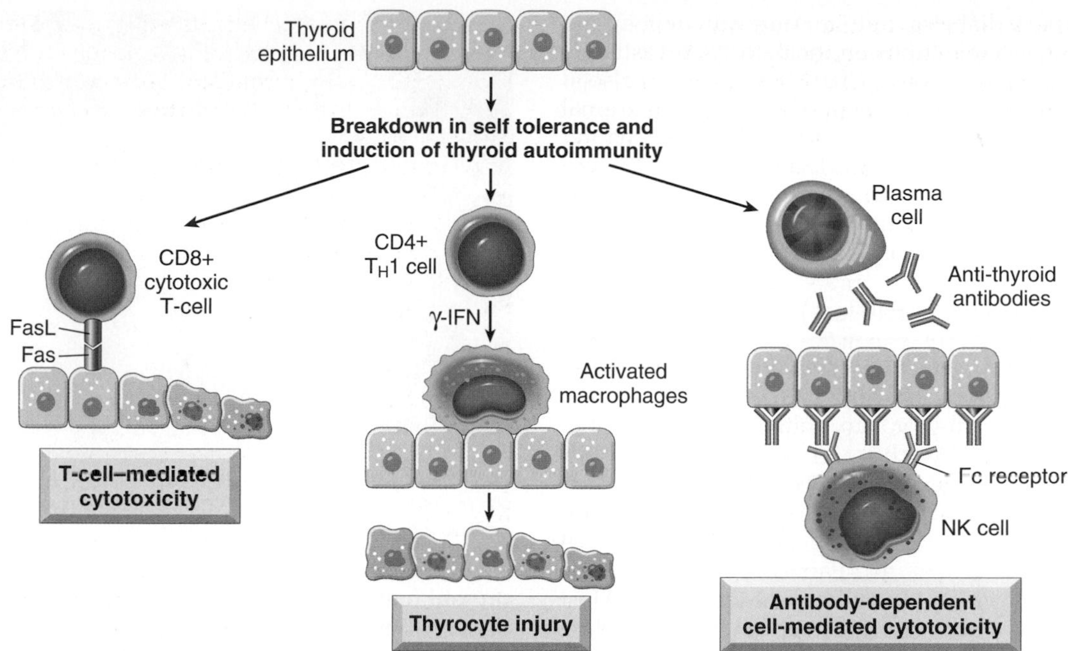

Figure 24-10 Pathogenesis of Hashimoto thyroiditis. Breakdown of peripheral tolerance to thyroid autoantigens, results in progressive autoimmune destruction of thyroid cells by infiltrating cytotoxic T cells, locally released cytokines, or by antibody-dependent cytotoxicity.

- *CD8+ cytotoxic T cell-mediated cell death:* CD8+ cytotoxic T cells may destroy thyroid follicular cells.
- *Cytokine-mediated cell death:* Activation of CD4+ T cells leads to the production of inflammatory cytokines such as interferon-γ in the thyroid gland, with resultant recruitment and activation of macrophages and damage to follicles.
- A less likely mechanism involves binding of antithyroid antibodies (antithyroglobulin, and antithyroid peroxidase antibodies) followed by antibody-dependent cell-mediated cytotoxicity (Chapter 6).

MORPHOLOGY

The thyroid is often diffusely enlarged, although more localized enlargement may be seen in some cases. The capsule is intact, and the gland is well demarcated from adjacent structures. The cut surface is pale, yellow-tan, firm, and somewhat nodular. There is extensive infiltration of the parenchyma by a **mononuclear inflammatory infiltrate** containing small lymphocytes, plasma cells, and well-developed **germinal centers** (Fig. 24-11). The thyroid follicles are atrophic and are lined in many areas by epithelial cells distinguished by the presence of abundant eosinophilic, granular cytoplasm, termed **Hürthle cells**. This is a metaplastic response of the normally low cuboidal follicular epithelium to ongoing injury. In fine-needle aspiration biopsy samples, the presence of Hürthle cells in conjunction with a heterogeneous population of lymphocytes is characteristic of Hashimoto thyroiditis. In "classic" Hashimoto thyroiditis, interstitial connective tissue is increased and may be abundant. Unlike Reidel thyroiditis (see later), the fibrosis does not extend beyond the capsule of the gland.

Clinical Course. Hashimoto thyroiditis most often comes to clinical attention as painless enlargement of the thyroid, usually associated with some degree of hypothyroidism, in a middle-aged woman. The enlargement of the gland is usually symmetric and diffuse, but in some cases it may be sufficiently localized to raise the suspicion of a neoplasm. In the usual case, hypothyroidism develops gradually. In some patients, however, it may be preceded by transient thyrotoxicosis caused by disruption of thyroid follicles, leading to release of thyroid hormones ("*hashitoxicosis*"). During this phase, free T_4 and T_3 levels are elevated, TSH is diminished, and radioactive iodine uptake is decreased. As hypothyroidism supervenes, T_4 and T_3 levels fall, accompanied by a compensatory increase in TSH.

Individuals with Hashimoto thyroiditis are at increased risk for developing other autoimmune diseases, both

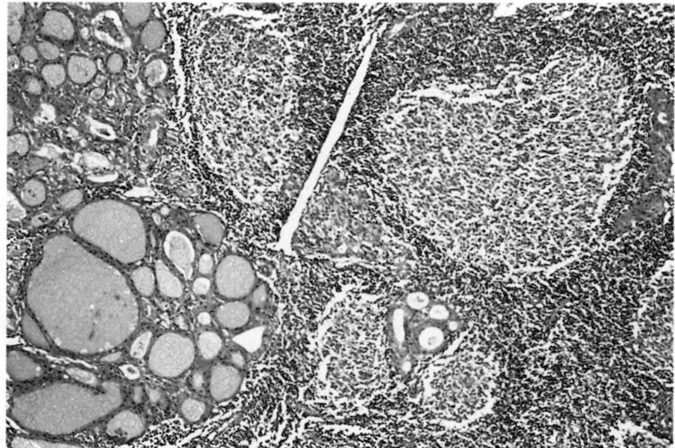

Figure 24-11 Hashimoto thyroiditis. The thyroid parenchyma contains a dense lymphocytic infiltrate with germinal centers. Residual thyroid follicles lined by deeply eosinophilic Hürthle cells are also seen.

endocrine (type 1 diabetes, autoimmune adrenalitis) and nonendocrine (systemic lupus erythematosus, myasthenia gravis, and Sjögren syndrome; Chapter 6). They are also at increased risk for the development of extranodal marginal zone B-cell lymphomas within the thyroid gland (Chapter 13). The relationship between Hashimoto disease and thyroid epithelial cancers remains controversial, with some morphologic and molecular studies suggesting a predisposition to papillary carcinomas.

Subacute Lymphocytic (Painless) Thyroiditis

Subacute lymphocytic thyroiditis, which is also referred to as *painless thyroiditis,* usually comes to clinical attention because of mild hyperthyroidism, goitrous enlargement of the gland, or both. Although it can occur at any age, it is most often seen in middle-aged adults and is more common in women. A disease process resembling painless thyroiditis can occur during the postpartum period in up to 5% of women *(postpartum thyroiditis).* Painless and postpartum thyroiditides are variants of autoimmune thyroiditis. Most of the patients have circulating antithyroid peroxidase antibodies or a family history of other autoimmune disorders. As many as a third of cases can evolve into overt hypothyroidism over time, and the thyroid histology may resemble Hashimoto thyroiditis.

MORPHOLOGY

Except for possible mild symmetric enlargement, the thyroid appears grossly normal. Microscopic examination reveals lymphocytic infiltration with large germinal centers within the thyroid parenchyma and patchy disruption and collapse of thyroid follicles. Unlike Hashimoto thyroiditis, however, fibrosis and Hürthle cell metaplasia are not prominent.

Clinical Course. Affected individuals may present with a painless goiter, transient overt hyperthyroidism, or both. Some patients transition from hyperthyroidism to hypothyroidism before recovery. As stated, as many as a third of affected individuals eventually progress to overt hypothyroidism over a 10-year period.

Granulomatous Thyroiditis

Granulomatous thyroiditis (also called *De Quervain thyroiditis*) occurs much less frequently than does Hashimoto disease. The disorder is most common between the ages of 40 and 50 and, like other forms of thyroiditis, affects women considerably more often than men (4:1).

Pathogenesis. Granulomatous thyroiditis is believed to be triggered by a viral infection. The majority of patients have a history of an upper respiratory infection just before the onset of thyroiditis. The disease has a seasonal incidence, with occurrences peaking in the summer, and clusters of cases have been reported in association with coxsackievirus, mumps, measles, adenovirus, and other viral infections. Although the pathogenesis of the disease is unclear, one model suggests that it results from a viral infection that leads to exposure to a viral or thyroid antigen secondary to virus-induced host tissue damage. This antigen stimulates cytotoxic T lymphocytes, which then damage thyroid follicular cells. In contrast to autoimmune thyroid disease, the immune response is virus-initiated and not self-perpetuating, so the process is limited.

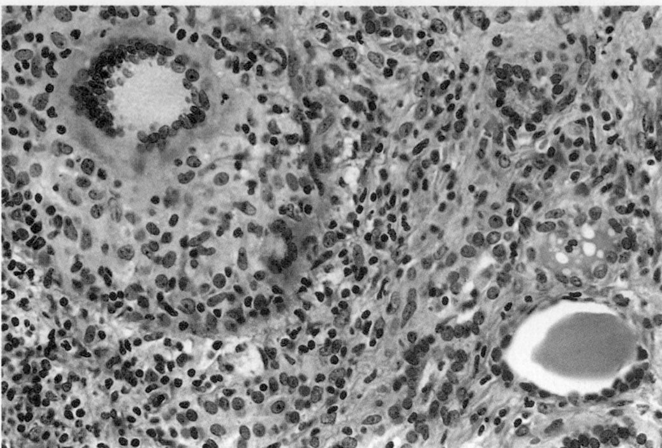

Figure 24-12 Granulomatous thyroiditis. The thyroid parenchyma contains a chronic inflammatory infiltrate with a multinucleate giant cell *(above left)* and a colloid follicle *(bottom right).*

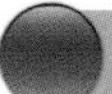

MORPHOLOGY

The gland may be unilaterally or bilaterally enlarged and firm, with an intact capsule that may adhere to surrounding structures. On cut section, the involved areas are firm and yellow-white and stand out from the more rubbery, normal brown thyroid substance. Histologic changes are patchy and depend on the stage of the disease. Early in the active inflammatory phase, scattered follicles may be disrupted and replaced by neutrophils forming microabscesses. Later, more characteristic features appear in the form of aggregates of lymphocytes, activated macrophages, and plasma cells associated with collapsed and damaged thyroid follicles. **Multinucleate giant cells** enclose naked pools or fragments of colloid (Fig. 24-12), hence the designation **granulomatous thyroiditis**. In later stages of the disease a chronic inflammatory infiltrate and fibrosis may replace the foci of injury. Different histologic stages are sometimes found in the same gland, suggesting waves of destruction over a period of time.

Clinical Course. Granulomatous thyroiditis is the most common cause of *thyroid pain.* There is a variable enlargement of the thyroid. Inflammation of the thyroid and hyperthyroidism are transient, usually diminishing in 2 to 6 weeks, even if the patient is not treated. Nearly all patients have high serum T_4 and T_3 levels and low serum TSH levels during this phase. However, unlike in hyperthyroid states such as Graves disease, radioactive iodine uptake is diminished. After recovery, generally in 6 to 8 weeks, normal thyroid function returns.

Other, less common forms of thyroiditis include *Riedel thyroiditis,* a rare disorder characterized by extensive fibrosis involving the thyroid and contiguous neck structures. The presence of a hard and fixed thyroid mass clinically simulates a thyroid carcinoma. It may be associated with fibrosis in other sites in the body, such as the retroperitoneum, and appears to be another manifestation of a systemic autoimmune IgG4-related disease, which is associated with fibrosis and tissue infiltration by plasma cells producing IgG4 (Chapter 6).

KEY CONCEPTS

Thyroiditis

- Hashimoto thyroiditis is the most common cause of hypothyroidism in regions where dietary iodine levels are sufficient.
- Hashimoto thyroiditis is an *autoimmune* thyroiditis characterized by progressive destruction of thyroid parenchyma, Hürthle cell change, and mononuclear (lymphoplasmacytic) infiltrates, with germinal centers and with or without extensive fibrosis.
- Subacute lymphocytic thyroiditis often occurs after a pregnancy (*postpartum thyroiditis*), typically is painless, and is characterized by lymphocytic inflammation in the thyroid. It is also a type of autoimmune thyroiditis.
- Granulomatous (de Quervain) thyroiditis is a self-limited disease, probably secondary to a viral infection, and is characterized by pain and the presence of a granulomatous inflammation in the thyroid.

Graves Disease

Graves disease is the most common cause of endogenous hyperthyroidism. Graves reported in 1835 his observations of a disease characterized by "violent and long continued palpitations in females" associated with enlargement of the thyroid gland. The disease is characterized by a *triad* of clinical findings:

- *Hyperthyroidism* associated with diffuse enlargement of the gland
- Infiltrative *ophthalmopathy* with resultant exophthalmos
- Localized, infiltrative *dermopathy*, sometimes called *pretibial myxedema*, which is present in a minority of patients

Graves disease has a peak incidence between 20 and 40 years of age. Women are affected as much as 10 times more frequently than men. This disorder is said to affect 1.5% to 2% of women in the United States.

Pathogenesis. **Graves disease is an autoimmune disorder characterized by the production of autoantibodies against multiple thyroid proteins, most importantly the TSH receptor.** A variety of antibodies that can either stimulate or block the TSH receptor are detected in the circulation. The most common antibody subtype, known as *thyroid-stimulating immunoglobulin* (TSI), is observed in approximately 90% of patients with Graves disease. In contrast to antibodies reactive with thyroglobulin and thyroid peroxidase, TSI is almost never observed in other autoimmune diseases of the thyroid. TSI binds to the TSH receptor and mimics its actions, stimulating adenyl cyclase and increasing the release of thyroid hormones. As stated, some patients also have TSH receptor *blocking antibodies* in the circulation, and in a minority of patients these may lead to hypothyroidism.

Graves disease (hyperthyroidism) and Hashimoto thyroiditis (hypothyroidism) represent two extremes of autoimmune thyroid disorders, and not surprisingly share many underlying features. For example, as with Hashimoto thyroiditis, genetic factors are important in the etiology of Graves disease. The concordance rate in monozygotic twins is 30% to 40%, compared with less than 5% among dizygotic twins, and like Hashimoto thyroiditis, genetic susceptibility is linked to polymorphisms in immune-function genes like *CTLA4* and *PTPN22* and the HLA-DR3 allele.

Autoimmunity also plays a role in the development of the *infiltrative ophthalmopathy* that is characteristic of Graves disease. In Graves ophthalmopathy, the protrusion of the eyeball (exopthalmos) is associated with increased volume of the retroorbital connective tissues and extraocular muscles, for several reasons. These include (1) marked infiltration of the retroorbital space by mononuclear cells, predominantly T cells; (2) inflammation with edema and swelling of extraocular muscles; (3) accumulation of extracellular matrix components, specifically hydrophilic glycosaminoglycans such as hyaluronic acid and chondroitin sulfate; and (4) increased numbers of adipocytes (fatty infiltration). These changes displace the eyeball forward and can interfere with the function of the extraocular muscles. Studies performed in animal models suggest that orbital preadipocyte fibroblasts, which express the TSH receptor, appear to stimulate the autoimmune reaction. Activated CD4+ helper T cells secrete cytokines that stimulate fibroblast proliferation and synthesis of extracellular matrix proteins (glycosaminoglycans), leading to progressive infiltration of the retroorbital space and ophthalmopathy.

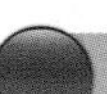

MORPHOLOGY

The thyroid gland is usually symmetrically enlarged due to **diffuse hypertrophy and hyperplasia** of thyroid follicular epithelial cells (Fig. 24-13*A*). Increases in weight to over 80 gm are not uncommon. On cut section, the parenchyma has a soft, meaty appearance resembling muscle. Histologically, the follicular epithelial cells in untreated cases are tall and more crowded than usual. This crowding often results in the formation of small papillae, which project into the follicular lumen and encroach on the colloid, sometimes filling the follicles (Fig. 24-13*B*). Such papillae lack fibrovascular cores, in contrast to those of papillary carcinoma (see later). The colloid within the follicular lumen is pale, with scalloped margins. Lymphoid infiltrates, consisting predominantly of T cells, along with scattered B cells and mature plasma cells, are present throughout the interstitium. Germinal centers are common.

Preoperative therapy alters the morphology of the thyroid in Graves disease. Administration of iodine causes involution of the epithelium and the accumulation of colloid by blocking thyroglobulin secretion. Treatment with the antithyroid drug propylthiouracil exaggerates the epithelial hypertrophy and hyperplasia by stimulating TSH secretion.

Changes in extrathyroidal tissue include lymphoid hyperplasia, especially enlargement of the thymus in younger patients. The heart may be hypertrophied, and ischemic changes may be present, particularly in patients with preexisting coronary artery disease. In patients with ophthalmopathy, the tissues of the orbit are edematous because of the presence of hydrophilic

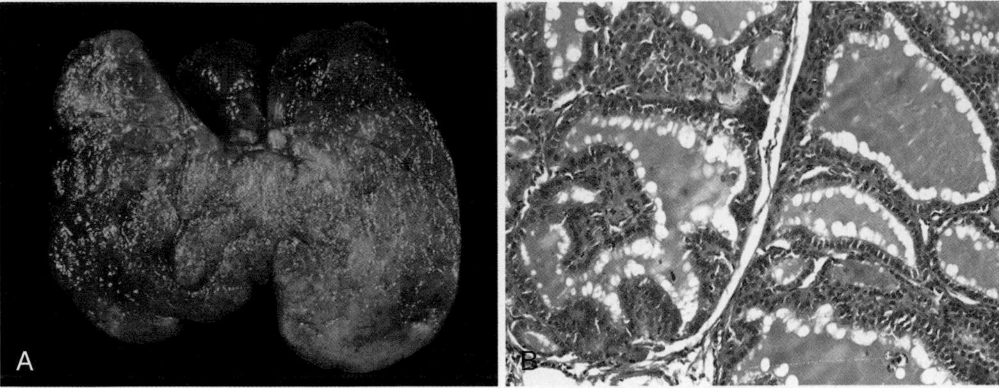

Figure 24-13 Graves disease. **A,** There is diffuse symmetric enlargement of the gland and a beefy deep red parenchyma. Compare with gross photograph of multinodular goiter in Figure 24-15. **B,** Diffusely hyperplastic thyroid in a case of Graves disease. The follicles are lined by tall, columnar epithelium. The crowded, enlarged epithelial cells project into the lumens of the follicles. These cells actively resorb the colloid in the centers of the follicles, resulting in the scalloped appearance of the edges of the colloid. (**A,** Reproduced with permission from Lloyd RV, et al (eds): Atlas of Nontumor Pathology: Endocrine Diseases. Washington, DC, American Registry of Pathology, 2002.)

mucopolysaccharides. In addition, there is infiltration by lymphocytes and fibrosis. Orbital muscles are edematous initially but may undergo fibrosis late in the course of the disease. The dermopathy, if present, is characterized by thickening of the dermis due to deposition of glycosaminoglycans and lymphocyte infiltration.

Clinical Course. The clinical findings in Graves disease include some changes associated with *thyrotoxicosis* and others associated uniquely with Graves disease, such as *diffuse hyperplasia of the thyroid, ophthalmopathy,* and *dermopathy*. The degree of thyrotoxicosis varies from case to case and is sometimes less conspicuous than other manifestations of the disease. Diffuse enlargement of the thyroid is present in all cases. The *thyroid enlargement* may be accompanied by increased flow of blood through the hyperactive gland, often producing an audible "bruit." *Sympathetic overactivity* produces a characteristic wide, staring gaze and lid lag. The ophthalmopathy of Graves disease results in abnormal protrusion of the eyeball (*exophthalmos*). The extraocular muscles are often weak. The exophthalmos may persist or progress despite successful treatment of the thyrotoxicosis, sometimes resulting in corneal injury. The infiltrative dermopathy, or *pretibial myxedema*, is most common in the skin overlying the shins, where it presents as scaly thickening and induration. The basis of such localization is not clear, and it is present only in a minority of patients. Sometimes individuals spontaneously develop thyroid hypofunction. Patients are at increased risk for other autoimmune diseases, such as systemic lupus erythematosus, pernicious anemia, type 1 diabetes, and Addison disease.

Laboratory findings in Graves disease include *elevated free T_4 and T_3* levels and *depressed TSH* levels. Because of ongoing stimulation of the thyroid follicles by thyroid-stimulating immunoglobulins, radioiodine scans show a diffusely increased uptake of iodine.

Graves disease is treated with β-blockers, which address symptoms related to the increased β-adrenergic tone (e.g., tachycardia, palpitations, tremulousness, and anxiety), and by measures aimed at decreasing thyroid hormone synthesis, such as the administration of thionamides (e.g., propylthiouracil), radioiodine ablation, and thyroidectomy. Surgery is used mostly in patients who have large goiters that are compressing surrounding structures.

KEY CONCEPTS

Graves Disease

- Graves disease, the most common cause of endogenous hyperthyroidism, is characterized by the triad of thyrotoxicosis, ophthalmopathy, and dermopathy.
- Graves disease is an autoimmune disorder caused by activation of thyroid epithelial cells by autoantibodies to the TSH receptor that mimic TSH action (*thyroid-stimulating immunoglobulins*).
- The thyroid in Graves disease is characterized by diffuse hypertrophy and hyperplasia of follicles and lymphoid infiltrates; glycosaminoglycan deposition and lymphoid infiltrates are responsible for the ophthalmopathy and dermopathy.
- Laboratory features include elevations in serum free T_3 and T_4 and decreased serum TSH.

Diffuse and Multinodular Goiters

Enlargement of the thyroid, or *goiter* is caused by impaired synthesis of thyroid hormone, which is most often the result of dietary iodine deficiency. Impairment of thyroid hormone synthesis leads to a compensatory rise in the serum TSH level, which, in turn, causes hypertrophy and hyperplasia of thyroid follicular cells and, ultimately, gross enlargement of the thyroid gland. The compensatory increase in functional mass of the gland overcomes the hormone deficiency, ensuring a *euthyroid* metabolic state in most individuals. If the underlying disorder is sufficiently severe (e.g., a congenital biosynthetic defect or endemic iodine deficiency, discussed later), the compensatory responses may be inadequate, resulting in *goitrous hypothyroidism*. The degree of thyroid enlargement is proportional to the level and duration of thyroid hormone deficiency. Goiters can broadly be divided into two types: *diffuse nontoxic* and *multinodular*.

Diffuse Nontoxic (Simple) Goiter

Diffuse nontoxic (simple) goiter causes enlargement of the entire gland without producing nodularity. Because the enlarged follicles are filled with colloid, the term *colloid goiter* has been applied to this condition. This disorder occurs in both an endemic and a sporadic distribution.

- *Endemic goiter* occurs in geographic areas where the soil, water, and food supply contain low levels of iodine. The term endemic is used when goiters are present in more than 10% of the population in a given region. Such conditions are particularly common in mountainous areas of the world, including the Andes and Himalayas, where iodine deficiency is widespread. The lack of iodine leads to decreased synthesis of thyroid hormone and a compensatory increase in TSH, leading to follicular cell hypertrophy and hyperplasia and goitrous enlargement. With increasing dietary iodine supplementation, the frequency and severity of endemic goiter have declined significantly, although as many as 200 million people worldwide continue to be at risk for severe iodine deficiency.

  Variations in the prevalence of endemic goiter in regions with similar levels of iodine deficiency point to the existence of other causative influences, particularly dietary substances, referred to as *goitrogens*. The ingestion of substances that interfere with thyroid hormone synthesis at some level, such as vegetables belonging to the Brassicaceae (Cruciferae) family (e.g., cabbage, cauliflower, Brussels sprouts, turnips, and cassava), has been documented to be goitrogenic. Native populations subsisting on cassava root are particularly at risk. Cassava contains a thiocyanate that inhibits iodide transport within the thyroid, worsening any possible concurrent iodine deficiency.
- *Sporadic goiter* occurs less frequently than does endemic goiter. There is a striking female preponderance and a peak incidence at puberty or in young adult life. Sporadic goiter can be caused by several conditions, including the ingestion of substances that interfere with thyroid hormone synthesis. In other instances, goiter may result from hereditary enzymatic defects that interfere with thyroid hormone synthesis, all transmitted as autosomal-recessive conditions (dyshormonogenetic goiter; see earlier). In most cases, however, the cause of sporadic goiter is not apparent.

MORPHOLOGY

Two phases can be identified in the evolution of diffuse nontoxic goiter: the **hyperplastic phase** and the phase of **colloid involution.** In the hyperplastic phase, the thyroid gland is diffusely and symmetrically enlarged, although the increase is usually modest, and the gland rarely exceeds 100 to 150 gm. The follicles are lined by crowded columnar cells, which may pile up and form projections similar to those seen in Graves disease. The accumulation is not uniform throughout the gland, and some follicles are hugely distended, whereas others remain small. If dietary iodine subsequently increases or if the demand for thyroid hormone decreases, the stimulated follicular epithelium involutes to form an enlarged, colloid-rich gland **(colloid goiter).** In these cases the cut surface of the thyroid is usually brown, somewhat glassy, and translucent. Histologically the follicular epithelium is flattened and cuboidal, and colloid is abundant during periods of involution.

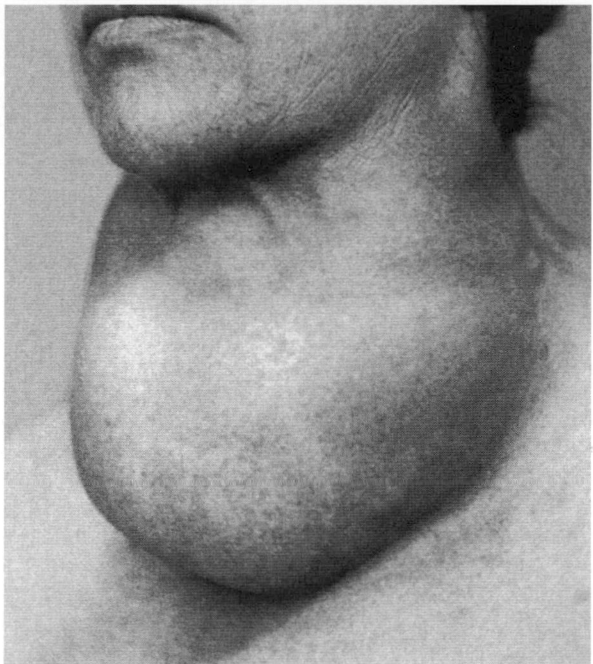

Figure 24-14 A 52-year-old woman with a huge colloid goiter who developed compressive symptoms. (Reproduced with permission from Lloyd RV, et al (eds): Atlas of Nontumor Pathology: Endocrine Diseases. Washington, DC, American Registry of Pathology, 2002.)

Clinical Course. As stated earlier, the vast majority of persons with simple goiters are clinically euthyroid. Therefore, the clinical manifestations are primarily related to *mass effects* from the enlarged thyroid gland (Fig. 24-14). Although serum T_3 and T_4 levels are normal, the serum TSH is usually elevated or at the upper range of normal, as is expected in marginally euthyroid individuals. In children, dyshormonogenetic goiter, caused by a congenital biosynthetic defect, may induce cretinism.

Multinodular Goiter

With time, recurrent episodes of hyperplasia and involution combine to produce a more irregular enlargement of the thyroid, termed *multinodular goiter*. Virtually all long-standing simple goiters convert into multinodular goiters. **Multinodular goiters produce the most extreme thyroid enlargements and are more frequently mistaken for neoplasms than any other form of thyroid disease**. Because they derive from simple goiter, they occur in both sporadic and endemic forms, having the same female-to-male distribution and presumably the same origins but affecting older individuals because they are late complications.

It is believed that multinodular goiters arise because of variations among follicular cells in their response to external stimuli, such as trophic hormones. If some cells in a follicle have a growth advantage, perhaps because of intrinsic genetic abnormalities similar to those that give

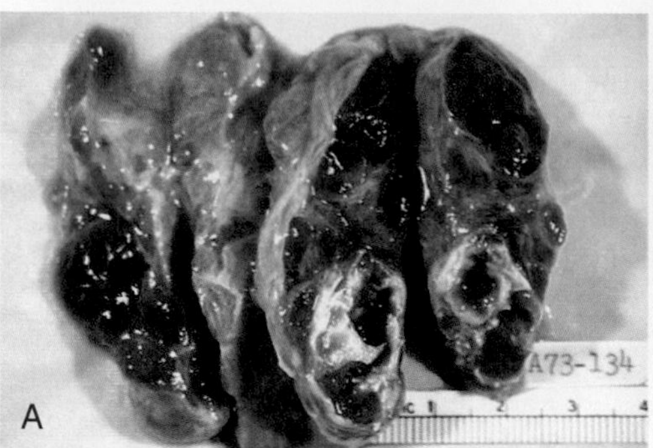

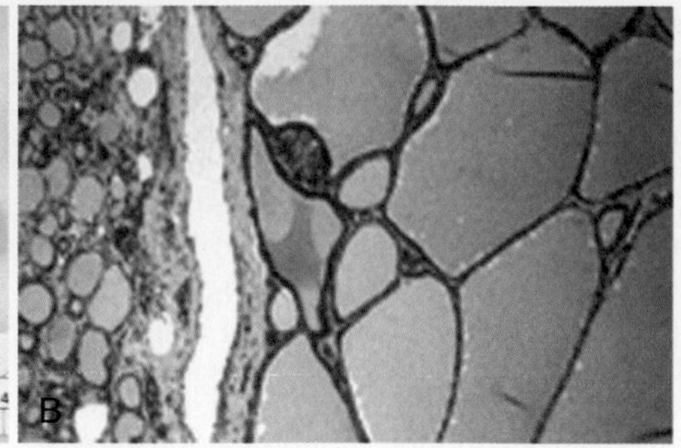

Figure 24-15 Multinodular goiter. **A,** Gross morphology demonstrating a coarsely nodular gland, containing areas of fibrosis and cystic change. **B,** Photomicrograph of a hyperplastic nodule, with compressed residual thyroid parenchyma on the periphery. Note absence of a prominent capsule, a distinguishing feature from follicular neoplasms. (**B,** Courtesy Dr. William Westra, Department of Pathology, Johns Hopkins University, Baltimore, Md.)

rise to adenomas, such cells can give rise to clones of proliferating cells. This may result in the formation of a nodule whose continued growth is autonomous, without the external stimulus. Consistent with this model, both polyclonal and monoclonal nodules coexist within the same multinodular goiter, the latter presumably having arisen because of the acquisition of a genetic abnormality favoring growth. Not surprisingly, activating mutations affecting proteins of the TSH-signaling pathway have been identified in a subset of autonomous thyroid nodules (TSH-signaling pathway mutations and their implications are discussed under "Adenomas"). The uneven follicular hyperplasia, generation of new follicles, and accumulation of colloid produce physical stress that may lead to rupture of follicles and vessels followed by hemorrhages, scarring, and sometimes calcifications. With scarring, nodularity appears, which may be accentuated by the preexisting stromal framework of the gland.

MORPHOLOGY

Multinodular goiters are multilobulated, asymmetrically enlarged glands that can reach weights of more than 2000 gm. The pattern of enlargement is quite unpredictable and may involve one lobe far more than the other, producing lateral pressure on midline structures, such as the trachea and esophagus. In other instances the goiter grows behind the sternum and clavicles to produce the so-called **intrathoracic** or **plunging goiter.** Occasionally, most of it is hidden behind the trachea and esophagus; in other instances one nodule may stand out, imparting the clinical appearance of a solitary nodule. On cut section, irregular nodules containing variable amounts of brown, gelatinous colloid are present (Fig. 24-15A). Older lesions have areas of hemorrhage, fibrosis, calcification, and cystic change. The microscopic appearance includes colloid-rich follicles lined by flattened, inactive epithelium and areas of **follicular hyperplasia**, accompanied by degenerative changes related to physical stress. In contrast to follicular neoplasms, a prominent capsule between the hyperplastic nodules and residual compressed thyroid parenchyma is not present (Fig. 24-15*B*).

Clinical Course. The dominant clinical features of multinodular goiter are those caused by *mass effects*. In addition to the obvious cosmetic effects, goiters may cause airway obstruction, dysphagia, and compression of large vessels in the neck and upper thorax *(superior vena cava syndrome)*. Most patients are euthyroid or have subclinical hyperthyroidism (identified only by reduced TSH levels), but in a substantial minority of patients an autonomous nodule may develop within a long-standing goiter and produce hyperthyroidism *(toxic multinodular goiter)*. This condition, known as *Plummer syndrome,* is not accompanied by the infiltrative ophthalmopathy and dermopathy of Graves disease. It is estimated that clinically apparent autonomous nodules develop in approximately 10% of multinodular goiters over a 10-year follow-up. The incidence of malignancy in long-standing multinodular goiters is low (<5%) but not zero, and concern for malignancy arises in goiters that demonstrate sudden changes in size or symptoms (e.g., hoarseness). Dominant nodules in a multinodular goiter can present as a "solitary thyroid nodule", mimicking a thyroid neoplasm. A radioiodine scan demonstrates uneven iodine uptake (including the occasional "hot" autonomous nodule) consistent with the diffuse parenchymal involvement, and an admixture of hyperplastic and involuting nodules. A fine-needle aspiration biopsy is helpful and can often, albeit not always, facilitate the distinction of follicular hyperplasia from a thyroid neoplasm (see later).

Neoplasms of the Thyroid

The solitary thyroid nodule is a palpably discrete swelling within an otherwise apparently normal thyroid gland. The estimated incidence of solitary palpable nodules in the adult population of the United States varies between 1% and 10%, but is significantly higher in endemic goitrous regions. Single nodules are about four times more common in women than in men. The incidence of thyroid nodules increases throughout life.

From a clinical standpoint, the major concern in persons who present with thyroid nodules is the possibility of a malignant neoplasm. Fortunately, the overwhelming majority of solitary nodules of the thyroid prove to be localized, nonneoplastic lesions (e.g., a dominant nodule in multinodular goiter, simple cysts, or foci of thyroiditis) or benign neoplasms such as follicular adenoma. In fact, *benign neoplasms outnumber thyroid carcinomas by a ratio of nearly 10:1*. While less than 1% of solitary thyroid nodules are malignant, this still represents about 15,000 new cases of thyroid carcinoma per year in the United States. Fortunately, most of these cancers are indolent; more than 90% of affected patients are alive 20 years after being diagnosed.

Several clinical criteria provide clues to the nature of a thyroid nodule:

- *Solitary nodules,* in general, are more likely to be neoplastic than are multiple nodules.
- *Nodules in younger patients* are more likely to be neoplastic than are those in older patients.
- *Nodules in males* are more likely to be neoplastic than are those in females.
- A history of *radiation* treatment to the head and neck region is associated with an increased incidence of thyroid malignancy.
- Functional nodules that take up radioactive iodine in imaging studies *(hot nodules)* are much more likely to be benign than malignant.

These associations and statistics, however, are of little comfort to a patient, in whom the timely recognition of a malignancy can be lifesaving. Ultimately, morphologic evaluation of a given thyroid nodule, by fine-needle aspiration and surgical resection, provides the most definitive information about its nature. The following sections consider the major thyroid tumors, including adenoma and carcinoma in its various forms.

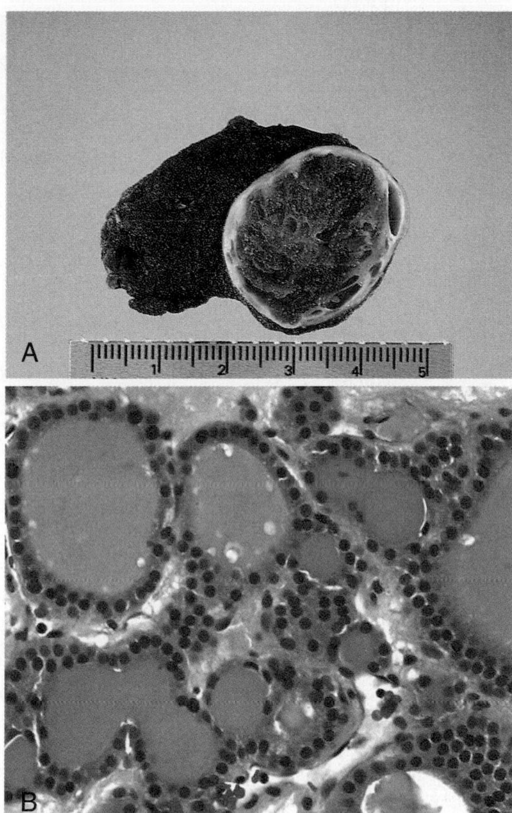

Figure 24-16 Follicular adenoma of the thyroid. **A,** A solitary, well-circumscribed nodule is seen. **B,** The photomicrograph shows well-differentiated follicles resembling normal thyroid parenchyma.

Adenomas

Adenomas of the thyroid are typically discrete, solitary masses, derived from follicular epithelium, and hence they are also known as *follicular adenomas.* Clinically, follicular adenomas can be difficult to distinguish from dominant nodules of follicular hyperplasia or from the less common follicular carcinomas. In general, follicular adenomas are *not* forerunners to carcinomas; nevertheless, shared genetic alterations support the possibility that at least of subset of follicular carcinomas arises in preexisting adenomas (see later). Although the vast majority of adenomas are nonfunctional, a small subset produces thyroid hormones and causes clinically apparent thyrotoxicosis. Hormone production in functional adenomas ("toxic adenomas") is independent of TSH stimulation.

Pathogenesis. **Somatic mutations of the *TSH receptor signaling pathway* are found in toxic adenomas, as well as in toxic multinodular goiter.** Gain-of-function mutations in one of two components of this signaling system—most often the gene encoding the TSH receptor (TSHR) or the α-subunit of G_s (*GNAS*)—cause follicular cells to secrete thyroid hormone independent of TSH stimulation ("thyroid autonomy"). This leads to symptoms of hyperthyroidism and produces a functional "hot" nodule on imaging. Overall, mutations in the TSH receptor signaling pathway are present in slightly over half of toxic thyroid nodules. Notably, *TSHR* and *GNAS* mutations are rare in follicular carcinomas; thus, toxic adenomas and toxic multinodular goiter do not seem to be forerunners of malignancy.

A minority (<20%) of *nonfunctioning* follicular adenomas have mutations of *RAS or PIK3CA,* which encodes a subunit of the PI-3 kinase, or bear a *PAX8-PPARG* fusion gene, genetic alterations that are shared with follicular carcinomas. These are discussed in further detail under "Carcinomas" (see later).

MORPHOLOGY

The typical thyroid adenoma is a solitary, spherical, encapsulated lesion that is demarcated from the surrounding thyroid parenchyma by a well-defined, intact capsule (Fig. 24-16A). **These features are important in making the distinction from multinodular goiters,** which contain multiple nodules even in patients presenting clinically with a solitary dominant nodule. Follicular adenomas average about 3 cm in diameter, but some are much larger (≥10 cm in diameter). In freshly resected specimens the adenoma bulges from the cut surface and compresses the adjacent thyroid. The color ranges from gray-white to red-brown, depending on the cellularity of the adenoma and its colloid content. Areas of hemorrhage, fibrosis, calcification, and cystic change, similar to those encountered in multinodular goiters, are common in follicular adenomas, particularly within larger lesions.

Microscopically, the constituent cells often form uniform-appearing follicles that contain colloid (Fig. 24-16*B*). The follicular growth pattern is usually quite distinct from the adjacent nonneoplastic thyroid. The neoplastic cells show little variation in cell size, cell shape, or nuclear morphology, and mitotic figures are rare. Occasionally the neoplastic cells acquire brightly eosinophilic granular cytoplasm (*oxyphil* or *Hürthle cell change*) (Fig. 24-17). The hallmark of all follicular adenomas is

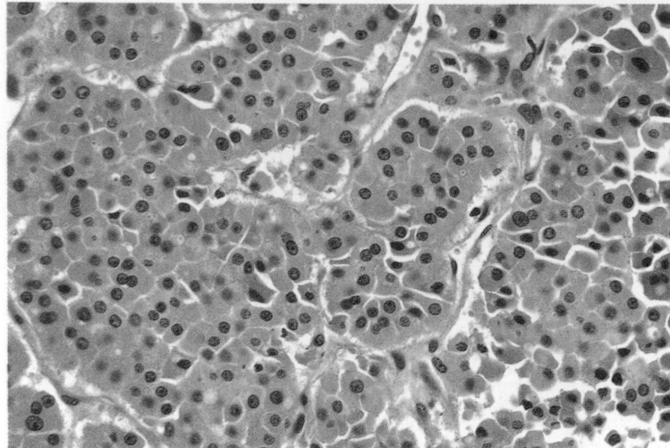

Figure 24-17 Hürthle cell (oxyphil) adenoma. A high-power view showing that the tumor is composed of cells with abundant eosinophilic cytoplasm and small regular nuclei. (Courtesy Dr. Mary Sunday, Duke University, Durham, N.C.)

the presence of an intact, well-formed capsule encircling the tumor. **Careful evaluation of the integrity of the capsule is therefore critical in distinguishing follicular adenomas from follicular carcinomas,** which demonstrate capsular and/or vascular invasion (see later). Extensive mitotic activity, necrosis, or high cellularity also warrants close inspection to exclude follicular carcinoma and the follicular variant of papillary carcinoma (see later).

Clinical Features. Many follicular adenomas present as unilateral painless masses that are discovered during a routine physical examination. Larger masses may produce local symptoms, such as difficulty in swallowing. Nonfunctioning adenomas take up less radioactive iodine than does normal thyroid parenchyma. On radionuclide scanning, therefore, nonfunctioning adenomas appear as *cold* nodules relative to the adjacent thyroid tissue. However, as many as 10% of cold nodules are malignant. Other techniques used to evaluate suspected adenomas are ultrasonography and fine-needle aspiration biopsy. **Because of the need for evaluating capsular integrity, the definitive diagnosis of adenomas can be made only after careful histologic examination of the resected specimen.** Suspected adenomas of the thyroid are therefore removed surgically to exclude malignancy. Follicular adenomas do not recur or metastasize and have an excellent prognosis.

Carcinomas

Carcinomas of the thyroid are relatively uncommon in the United States, accounting for about 1.5% of all cancers. A female predominance has been noted among patients who develop thyroid carcinoma in the early and middle adult years. In contrast, cases presenting in childhood and late adult life are distributed equally among males and females.

The major subtypes of thyroid carcinoma and their relative frequencies are as follows:

- Papillary carcinoma (>85% of cases)
- Follicular carcinoma (5% to 15% of cases)
- Anaplastic (undifferentiated) carcinoma (<5% of cases)
- Medullary carcinoma (5% of cases)

Most thyroid carcinomas (except medullary carcinomas) are derived from the thyroid follicular epithelium, and of these, the vast majority are well-differentiated lesions. Because of the unique clinical, molecular and biologic features associated with each variant of thyroid carcinoma, these subtypes are described separately. We begin with a discussion of the molecular pathogenesis of all thyroid cancers.

Pathogenesis

Genetic Factors. Distinct genetic events are involved in the pathogenesis of the four major histologic variants of thyroid cancer. As stated, medullary carcinomas do not arise from the follicular epithelium. **Genetic alterations in the three follicular cell–derived malignancies are in growth factor receptor signaling pathways** (Fig. 24-18). You will recall that in normal cells, these pathways are transiently activated by binding of soluble growth factor ligands to the extracellular domain of receptor tyrosine kinases, which results in autophosphorylation of the cytoplasmic domain of the receptor. This in turn sets in motion events that lead to activation of RAS and two downstream signaling arms involving MAP kinase (MAPK) and PI-3 kinase (PI3K). In thyroid carcinomas, as with many cancers (Chapter 7), gain-of-function mutations in components of these pathways lead to their constitutive activation, driving excessive cellular proliferation and increased cell survival.

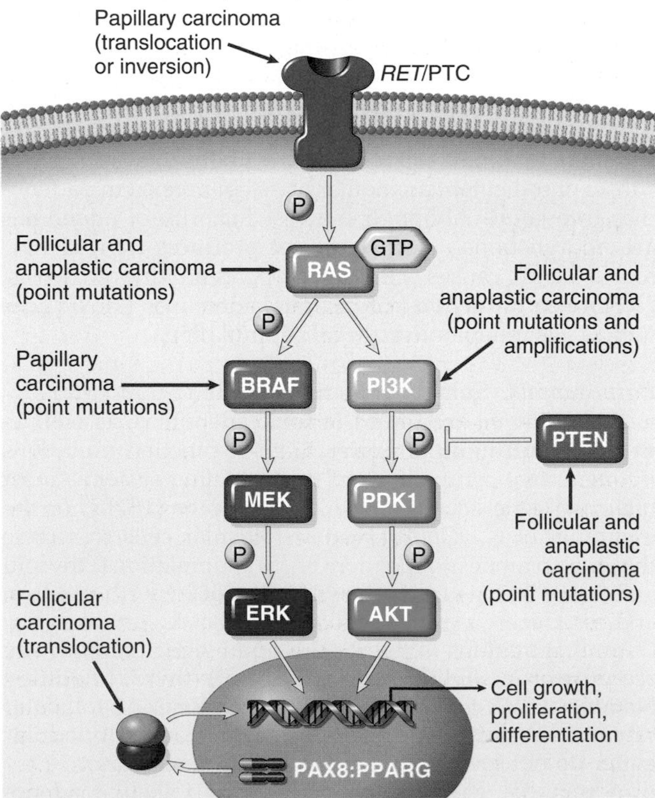

Figure 24-18 Genetic alterations in follicular cell-derived malignancies of the thyroid gland.

Papillary Carcinomas. Most papillary carcinomas have gain-of-function mutations involving the genes encoding the RET or NTRK1 receptor tyrosine kinases, or in the serine/threonine kinase BRAF, which you will recall lies in the MAPK pathway (Fig. 24-18).

- The *RET* gene is located on chromosome 10q11, and the receptor tyrosine kinase it encodes is normally not expressed in thyroid follicular cells. In papillary cancers, either a paracentric inversion of chromosome 10 or a reciprocal translocation between chromosomes 10 and 17 places the tyrosine kinase domain of RET under the transcriptional control of genes that are constitutively expressed in the thyroid epithelium. The novel fusion genes that are so formed are known as *RET/PTC* (RET/papillary thyroid carcinoma) and are present in approximately 20% to 40% of papillary thyroid cancers. There are more than 15 fusion partners of *RET*, and two—designated as *PTC1* and *PTC2*—are most commonly observed in sporadic papillary cancers. The frequency of *RET/PTC* rearrangements is significantly higher in papillary cancers arising in the backdrop of radiation exposure. The *RET/PTC* rearrangements produce genes that encode fusion proteins with constitutive tyrosine kinase activity. Similarly, paracentric inversions or translocations of *NTRK1* on chromosome 1q21 are present in 5% to 10% of papillary thyroid cancers. These genetic events also produce constitutively active NTRK1 fusion proteins.
- *BRAF* encodes an intermediate signaling component in the MAP kinase pathway. One third to one half of papillary thyroid carcinomas harbor a gain-of-function mutation in the *BRAF* gene, which is most commonly a valine-to-glutamate change in codon 600 ($BRAF^{V600E}$). The presence of *BRAF* mutations in papillary carcinomas correlates with adverse prognostic factors like metastatic disease and extrathyroidal extension. As discussed in other chapters, a similar BRAF mutation is found in some other cancers as well, including melanomas, hairy cell leukemia and a subset of colon cancers, suggesting that diverse tumors may share a similar pathway to malignancy.

Because chromosomal rearrangements of the *RET* or *NTRK1* genes and mutations of *BRAF* have redundant effects on MAP kinase signaling, it is not surprising that they are usually (but not always) mutually exclusive events. The histologic variants of papillary carcinoma demonstrate some unique characteristics vis-à-vis the frequency or nature of *BRAF* mutation (see later). Of further interest, *RET/PTC* rearrangements and *BRAF* point mutations are not observed in follicular adenomas or carcinomas.

Follicular Carcinomas. **In contrast to papillary carcinomas, follicular carcinomas are associated with acquired mutations that activate RAS or the PI-3K/AKT arm of the receptor tyrosine kinase signaling pathway.** It is evident from Figure 24-18 that activated mutations in RAS would be expected to stimulate both the MAPK and PI3K signaling pathways. Why RAS mutations produce follicular neoplasms, rather than papillary neoplasms, is not understood, a point that highlights our lack of insight into the nuances of intracellular signaling. Approximately one third to one half of follicular thyroid carcinomas harbor gain-of-function point mutations of *RAS* or *PIK3CA* (the gene that encodes PI-3 kinase), *PIK3CA* amplifications, or loss-of-function mutations of *PTEN*, a tumor suppressor gene and negative regulator of this pathway (Fig. 24-18). These genetic alterations are almost always mutually exclusive in follicular carcinomas, in line with their functional equivalence. The progressive increase in the prevalence of *RAS* and *PIK3CA* mutations from benign follicular adenomas to follicular carcinomas to anaplastic carcinomas (see later) suggests a shared histogenesis and molecular evolution among these follicular tumors.

A unique (2;3)(q13;p25) translocation has been described in one third to one half of follicular carcinomas. This translocation creates a fusion gene composed of portions of *PAX8*, a paired homeobox gene that is important in thyroid development, and the peroxisome proliferator-activated receptor gene (*PPARG*), whose gene product is a nuclear hormone receptor implicated in terminal differentiation of cells. Fewer than 10% of follicular adenomas harbor *PAX8-PPARG* fusion genes, and these have not been documented thus far in other thyroid neoplasms.

Anaplastic (Undifferentiated) Carcinomas. These highly aggressive and lethal tumors can arise de novo, or more commonly, by "dedifferentiation" of a well-differentiated papillary or follicular carcinoma. Molecular alterations present in anaplastic carcinomas include those also seen in well-differentiated carcinomas (e.g., *RAS* or *PIK3CA* mutations). Other genetic "hits," such as inactivation of *TP53* or activating mutations of β-catenin, are essentially restricted to anaplastic carcinomas and may contribute to their aggressive behavior.

Medullary Thyroid Carcinomas. Familial medullary thyroid carcinomas occur in multiple endocrine neoplasia type 2 (MEN-2, see later) and are associated with germline *RET* mutations that lead to constitutive activation of the receptor. *RET* mutations are also seen in approximately one half of nonfamilial (sporadic) medullary thyroid cancers. Chromosomal rearrangements involving *RET*, such as the *RET/PTC* translocations reported in papillary cancers, are not seen in medullary carcinomas.

Environmental Factors. The major risk factor predisposing to thyroid cancer is exposure to *ionizing radiation*, particularly during the first 2 decades of life. In keeping with this, there was a marked increase in the incidence of papillary carcinomas among children exposed to ionizing radiation after the Chernobyl nuclear disaster in 1986. *Deficiency of dietary iodine* (and by extension, an association with goiter) is linked with a higher frequency of follicular carcinomas.

Papillary Carcinoma

Papillary carcinomas are the most common form of thyroid cancer, accounting for nearly 85% of primary thyroid malignancies in the United States. They occur throughout life but most often between the ages of 25 and 50, and account for the majority of thyroid carcinomas associated with previous exposure to ionizing radiation. The diagnosis of papillary carcinoma has increased markedly in the last 30 years, partly because of the recognition of follicular variants (see later) that were misclassified in the past.

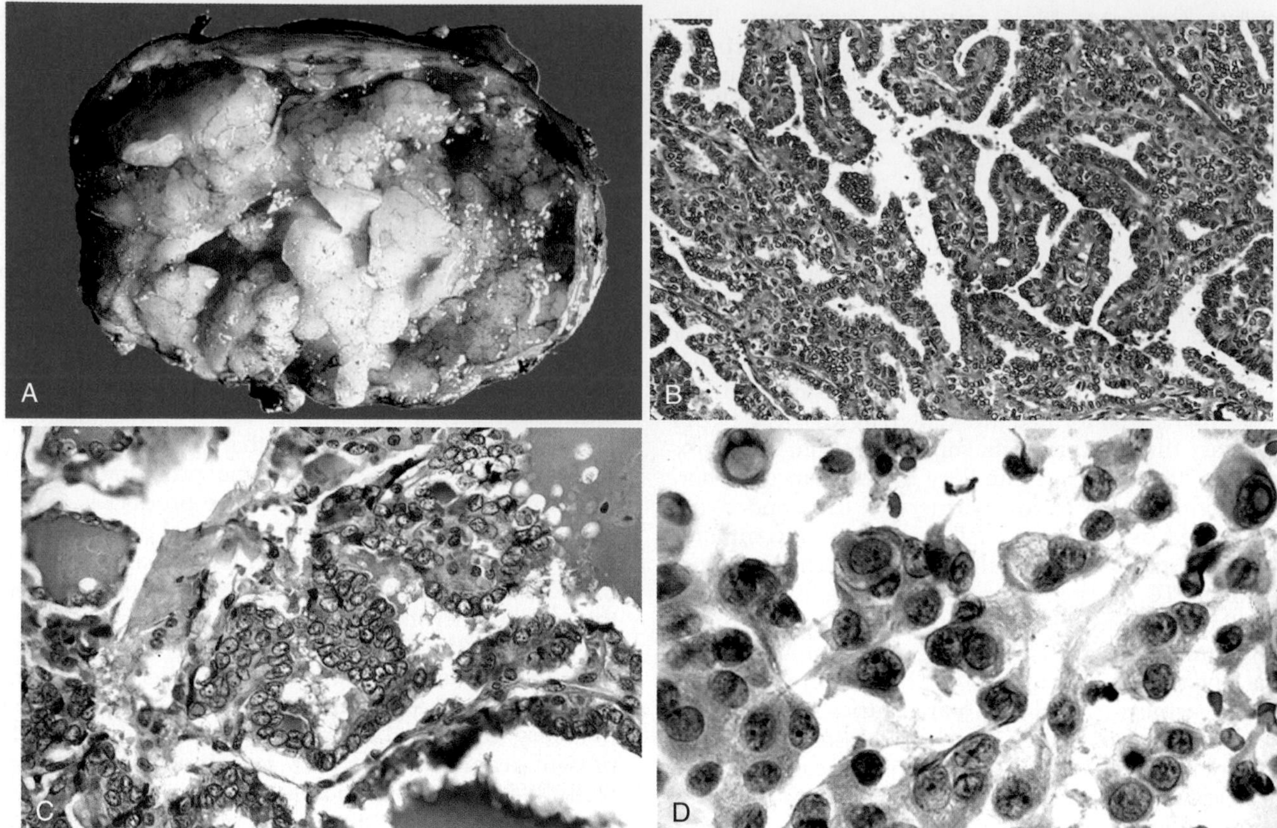

Figure 24-19 Papillary carcinoma of the thyroid. **A,** The macroscopic appearance of a papillary carcinoma with grossly discernible papillary structures. **B,** This particular example contains well-formed papillae. **C,** High power shows cells with characteristic empty-appearing nuclei, sometimes called "Orphan Annie eye" nucle. **D,** Cells obtained by fine-needle aspiration of a papillary carcinoma. Characteristic intranuclear inclusions are visible in some of the aspirated cells.

MORPHOLOGY

Papillary carcinomas may be solitary or multifocal. Some tumors are well circumscribed and even encapsulated; others infiltrate the adjacent parenchyma and have ill-defined margins. The tumors may contain areas of fibrosis and calcification and are often cystic. The cut surface sometimes reveals papillary foci that point to the diagnosis. The microscopic hallmarks of papillary neoplasms include the following (Fig. 24-19):

- Papillary carcinomas may contain branching **papillae** having a fibrovascular stalk covered by a single to multiple layers of cuboidal epithelial cells. In most neoplasms, the epithelium covering the papillae consists of well-differentiated, uniform, orderly cuboidal cells, but at the other extreme are those with fairly anaplastic epithelium showing considerable variation in cell and nuclear morphology. When present, the papillae of papillary carcinoma differ from those seen in areas of hyperplasia in being more complex and having dense fibrovascular cores.
- The nuclei of papillary carcinoma cells contain finely dispersed chromatin, which imparts an **optically clear** or **empty** appearance, giving rise to the designation **ground-glass** or **Orphan Annie eye nuclei**. In addition, invaginations of the cytoplasm may give the appearance of intranuclear inclusions ("pseudo-inclusions") or intranuclear grooves. **The diagnosis of papillary carcinoma can be made based on these nuclear features,** even in the absence of papillary architecture.
- Concentrically calcified structures termed **psammoma bodies** are often present, usually within the cores of papillae. These structures are almost never found in follicular and medullary carcinomas, and so, when present in fine-needle aspiration material, they are a strong indication that the lesion is a papillary carcinoma.
- Foci of lymphatic invasion by tumor are often present, but involvement of blood vessels is relatively uncommon, particularly in smaller lesions. Metastases to adjacent cervical lymph nodes occur in up to half of cases.

There are over a dozen histologic variants of papillary carcinoma that can mimic other thyroid lesions or harbor distinct prognostic implications; most are beyond the scope of this book. The most common variant, and the one most liable to misdiagnosis, is the **follicular variant,** which has the characteristic nuclear features of papillary carcinoma and an almost totally follicular architecture. Follicular variant papillary carcinomas can be either encapsulated or poorly circumscribed and infiltrative. The encapsulated follicular variant of papillary carcinoma has a generally favorable prognosis, while the poorly circumscribed and infiltrative lesions need to be treated more aggressively. The genetic alterations in the follicular variant, especially the encapsulated tumors, demonstrate several distinctions from conventional papillary carcinomas, including a lower frequency of *RET/PTC* rearrangements, a lower frequency and different spectrum of *BRAF* mutations, and a significantly higher frequency of *RAS* mutations. When considered in conjunction with their higher propensity for angioinvasion and lower incidence of lymph node metastases, it has become evident that at least a subset of the encapsulated follicular variant display biological features that are more comparable to minimally invasive follicular carcinomas (see later) than conventional papillary carcinomas.

The **tall-cell variant** has tall columnar cells with intensely eosinophilic cytoplasm lining the papillary structures. These tumors tend to occur in older individuals and have higher frequencies of vascular invasion, extrathyroidal extension, and cervical and distant metastases than conventional papillary thyroid carcinoma. Tall-cell variant papillary carcinomas harbor *BRAF* mutations in most (55% to 100%) cases, and often have *RET/PTC* translocations as well. The occurrence of these two aberrations together may synergistically enhance MAPK signaling, contributing to the aggressive behavior of this variant.

An unusual **diffuse sclerosing variant** of papillary carcinoma occurs in younger individuals, including children. The tumor has a prominent papillary growth pattern intermixed with solid areas containing nests of squamous metaplasia. As the name suggests, there is extensive, diffuse fibrosis throughout the thyroid gland, often associated with a prominent lymphocytic infiltrate, simulating Hashimoto thyroiditis. Lymph node metastases are present in almost all cases. The diffuse sclerosing variant carcinomas lack *BRAF* mutations, but *RET/PTC* translocations are found in approximately half the cases.

Finally, the **papillary microcarcinoma** is defined as an otherwise conventional papillary carcinoma less than 1 cm in size. These lesions most commonly come to attention as an incidental finding in patients undergoing surgery, and may be precursors of typical papillary carcinomas.

Clinical Course. Most conventional papillary carcinomas present as asymptomatic thyroid nodules, but the first manifestation may be a mass in a cervical lymph node. Interestingly, the presence of isolated cervical nodal metastases does not have a significant influence on prognosis, which is generally good. Most carcinomas are single nodules that move freely with the thyroid gland during swallowing and are not distinguishable on examination from benign nodules. Hoarseness, dysphagia, cough, or dyspnea suggests advanced disease. In a minority of patients, hematogenous metastases are present at the time of diagnosis, most commonly in the lung.

A variety of diagnostic tests have been used to help separate benign from malignant thyroid nodules, including radionuclide scanning and fine-needle aspiration. Papillary carcinomas are *cold* masses on scintiscans. Improvements in cytologic analysis have made fine-needle aspiration cytology a reliable test for distinguishing between benign and malignant nodules. The nuclear features are often demonstrated nicely in aspirated specimens.

Papillary thyroid cancers have an excellent prognosis, with a 10-year survival rate in excess of 95%. Between 5% and 20% of patients have local or regional recurrences, and 10% to 15% have distant metastases. The prognosis of someone with papillary thyroid cancers is dependent on several factors including age (in general, being less favorable among patients older than 40 years), the presence of extrathyroidal extension, and presence of distant metastases (stage).

Follicular Carcinoma

Follicular carcinomas account for 5% to 15% of primary thyroid cancers, but are more frequent in areas with dietary iodine deficiency, where they constitute 25% to 40% of thyroid cancers. They are more common in women (3:1) and present more often in older patients than do papillary carcinomas; the peak incidence is between 40 and 60 years of age.

MORPHOLOGY

Follicular carcinomas are single nodules that may be well circumscribed or widely infiltrative (Fig. 24-20*A*). Sharply demarcated lesions may be exceedingly difficult to distinguish from follicular adenomas by gross examination. Larger lesions may penetrate the capsule and infiltrate well beyond the thyroid capsule into the adjacent neck. They are gray to tan to pink on cut section and may be somewhat translucent due to the presence of large, colloid-filled follicles. Degenerative changes, such as central fibrosis and foci of calcification, are sometimes present.

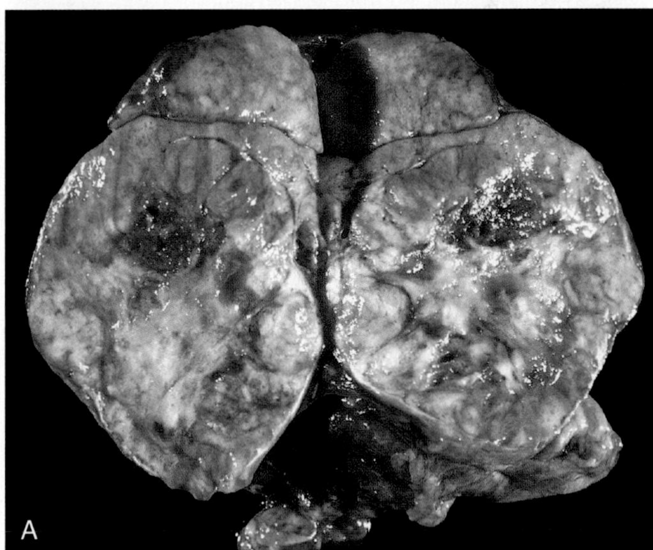

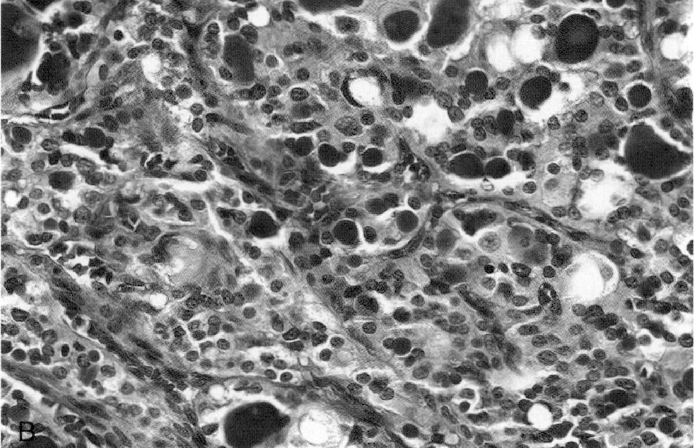

Figure 24-20 Follicular carcinoma. **A,** Cut surface of a follicular carcinoma with substantial replacement of the lobe of the thyroid. The tumor has a light-tan appearance and contains small foci of hemorrhage. **B,** A few of the glandular lumens contain recognizable colloid.

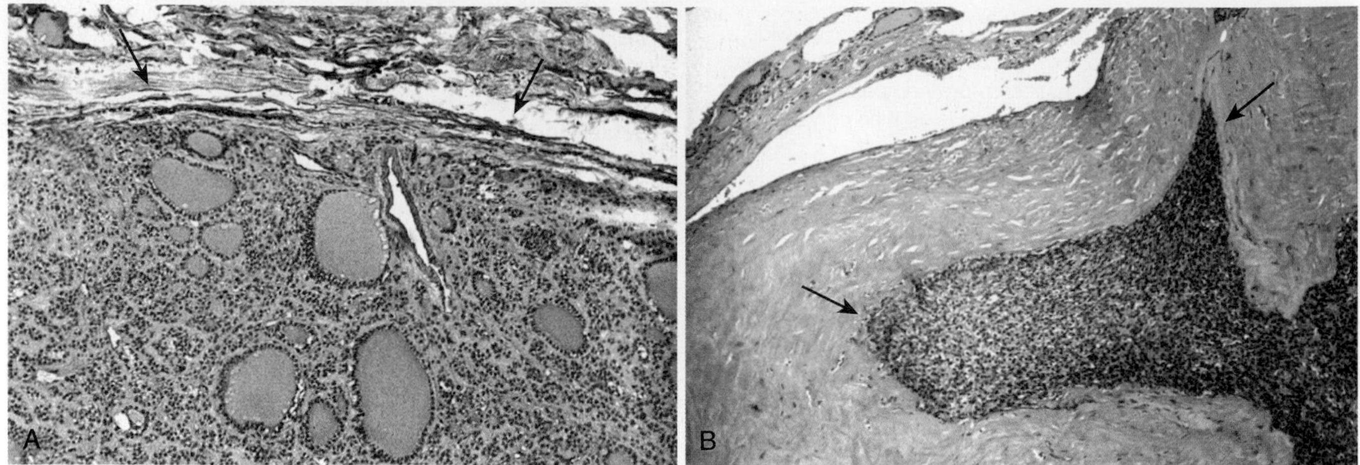

Figure 24-21 Capsular integrity in follicular neoplasms. In adenomas (**A**), a fibrous capsule, usually thin but occasionally more prominent, circumferentially surrounds the neoplastic follicles and no capsular invasion is seen *(arrows)*; compressed normal thyroid parenchyma is usually present external to the capsule *(top of the panel)*. In contrast, follicular carcinomas demonstrate capsular invasion (**B,** *arrows*) that may be minimal, as in this case, or widespread. The presence of vascular invasion is another feature of follicular carcinomas.

Microscopically, most follicular carcinomas are composed of fairly uniform cells forming small follicles containing colloid, quite reminiscent of normal thyroid (Fig. 24-20*B*). In other cases follicular differentiation may be less apparent, and there may be nests or sheets of cells without colloid. Occasional tumors are dominated by cells with abundant granular, eosinophilic cytoplasm **(Hürthle cell or oncocytic variant of follicular carcinoma)**. Whatever the pattern, the nuclei lack the features typical of papillary carcinoma, and psammoma bodies are not present. While nuclear features (optically clear nuclei, nuclear grooves) are helpful in distinguishing papillary from follicular neoplasms, **there is no reliable cytologic difference between follicular adenomas and minimally invasive follicular carcinomas**. Making this distinction requires extensive histologic sampling of the tumor-capsule-thyroid interface to exclude capsular and/or vascular invasion (Fig. 24-21). The criterion for vascular invasion is applicable only to capsular vessels and vascular spaces beyond the capsule; the presence of tumor plugs within intra-tumoral blood vessels has little prognostic significance. Unlike in papillary cancers, lymphatic spread is uncommon in follicular cancers.

In contrast to minimally invasive follicular cancers, the diagnosis of carcinoma is obvious in **widely invasive follicular carcinomas,** which infiltrate the thyroid parenchyma and extrathyroidal soft tissues. Histologically, these cancers tend to have a greater proportion of solid or trabecular growth pattern, less evidence of follicular differentiation, and increased mitotic activity.

Clinical Course. Follicular carcinomas present as slowly enlarging painless nodules. Most frequently they are *cold nodules* on scintigrams, although rare, better-differentiated lesions may be hyperfunctional, take up radioactive iodine and appear *warm* on scintiscan. Because follicular carcinomas have little propensity for invading lymphatics, regional lymph nodes are rarely involved, but vascular (hematogenous) dissemination is common, with metastases to bone, lungs, liver, and elsewhere.

The prognosis depends largely on the extent of invasion and stage at presentation. Widely invasive follicular carcinoma often presents with systemic metastases, and as many as half of affected patients succumb to their disease within 10 years. This is in sharp contrast to minimally invasive follicular carcinomas, which have a 10-year survival rate of greater than 90%. Most follicular carcinomas are treated with total thyroidectomy followed by the administration of radioactive iodine, which can be used to identify metastases and to ablate such lesions. In addition, because any residual follicular carcinoma may respond to TSH stimulation, patients are usually treated with thyroid hormone after surgery to suppress endogenous TSH levels. Serum thyroglobulin levels are used for monitoring tumor recurrence, because this thyroid protein should be barely detectable in a patient who is free of disease.

Anaplastic (Undifferentiated) Carcinoma

Anaplastic carcinomas are undifferentiated tumors of the thyroid follicular epithelium, accounting for less than 5% of thyroid tumors. They are aggressive, with a mortality rate approaching 100%. Patients with anaplastic carcinoma are older than those with other types of thyroid cancer, with a mean age of 65 years. Approximately a quarter of patients with anaplastic thyroid carcinomas have a past history of a well-differentiated thyroid carcinoma, and another quarter harbors a concurrent well-differentiated tumor in the resected specimen.

MORPHOLOGY

Microscopically, these neoplasms are composed of highly anaplastic cells, with variable morphology, including (1) large, pleomorphic **giant** cells, including occasional osteoclast-like multinucleate giant cells; (2) **spindle** cells with a sarcomatous appearance; and (3) **mixed** spindle and giant cells. Foci of papillary or follicular differentiation may be present in some tumors, suggesting an origin from a better-differentiated carcinoma. The neoplastic cells express epithelial markers like cytokeratin, but are usually negative for markers of thyroid differentiation, like thyroglobulin.

Clinical Course. Anaplastic carcinomas usually present as a rapidly enlarging bulky neck mass. In most cases, the disease has already spread beyond the thyroid capsule into adjacent neck structures or has metastasized to the lungs at the time of presentation. Symptoms related to compression and invasion, such as dyspnea, dysphagia, hoarseness, and cough, are common. There are no effective therapies, and the disease is almost uniformly fatal. Although metastases to distant sites are common, in most cases death occurs in less than 1 year as a result of aggressive growth and compromise of vital structures in the neck.

Medullary Carcinoma

Medullary carcinomas of the thyroid are neuroendocrine neoplasms derived from the parafollicular cells, or C cells, of the thyroid, and account for approximately 5% of thyroid neoplasms. Medullary carcinomas, similar to normal C cells, secrete *calcitonin*, the measurement of which plays an important role in the diagnosis and postoperative follow-up of patients. In some instances the tumor cells elaborate other polypeptide hormones, such as serotonin, ACTH, and vasoactive intestinal peptide (VIP). About 70% of tumors arise sporadically. The remainder occurs in the setting of MEN syndrome 2A or 2B or as familial tumors without an associated MEN syndrome (familial medullary thyroid carcinoma, or FMTC; see "Multiple Endocrine Neoplasia Syndromes"). Recall that *activating point mutations in the RET proto-oncogene* play an important role in the development of both familial and sporadic medullary carcinomas. Cases associated with MEN types 2A or 2B occur in younger patients, and may even arise during the first decade of life. In contrast, sporadic as well as familial medullary carcinomas are lesions of adulthood, with a peak incidence in the 40s and 50s.

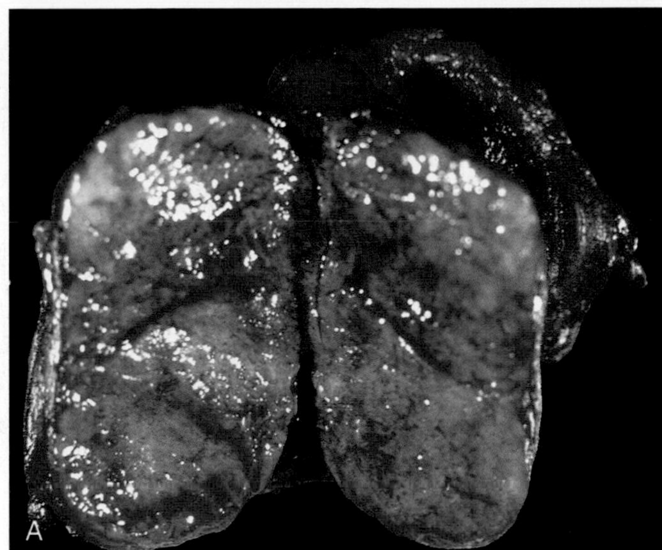

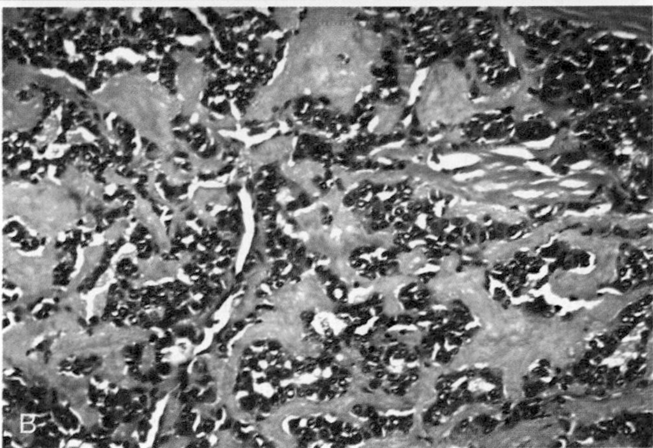

Figure 24-22 Medullary carcinoma of thyroid. **A,** These tumors typically show a solid pattern of growth and do not have connective tissue capsules. **B,** Histology demonstrates abundant deposition of amyloid, visible here as homogeneous extracellular material, derived from calcitonin molecules secreted by the neoplastic cells. (**A,** Courtesy Dr. Joseph Corson, Brigham and Women's Hospital, Boston, Mass.)

MORPHOLOGY

Sporadic medullary thyroid carcinomas present as a solitary nodule (Fig. 24-22*A*). In contrast, **bilaterality and multicentricity are common in familial cases**. Larger lesions often contain areas of necrosis and hemorrhage and may extend through the capsule of the thyroid. The tumor tissue is firm, pale gray to tan, and infiltrative. There may be foci of hemorrhage and necrosis in the larger lesions.

Microscopically, medullary carcinomas are composed of polygonal to spindle-shaped cells, which may form nests, trabeculae, and even follicles. Small, more anaplastic cells are present in some tumors and may be the predominant cell type. Acellular **amyloid deposits** derived from calcitonin polypeptides are present in the stroma in many cases (Fig. 24-22*B*). Calcitonin is readily demonstrable within the cytoplasm of the tumor cells as well as in the stromal amyloid by immunohistochemical methods. As with all neuroendocrine tumors, electron microscopy reveals variable numbers of membrane-bound electron-dense granules within the cytoplasm of the neoplastic cells (Fig. 24-23). One of the features of familial medullary cancers is the presence of multicentric **C-cell hyperplasia** in the surrounding thyroid parenchyma, a feature that is usually absent in sporadic lesions, and that is believed to be a precursor lesion in familial cases. Thus, the presence of multiple prominent clusters of C cells scattered throughout the parenchyma should raise the specter of an inherited predisposition, even if a family history is not present.

Clinical Course. *Sporadic* cases of medullary carcinoma come to medical attention most often as a mass in the neck, sometimes associated with dysphagia or hoarseness. In some instances, the initial manifestations are those of a paraneoplastic syndrome caused by the secretion of a peptide hormone (e.g., diarrhea due to the secretion of VIP, or Cushing syndrome due to ACTH). Notably, hypocalcemia is not a prominent feature, despite the presence of raised calcitonin levels. In addition to circulating calcitonin, secretion of carcinoembryonic antigen by the neoplastic cells is a useful biomarker, especially for presurgical assessment of tumor load and in calcitonin-negative tumors.

Patients with *familial syndromes* may come to attention because of symptoms localized to the thyroid or as a result of endocrine neoplasms in other organs (e.g., adrenal or

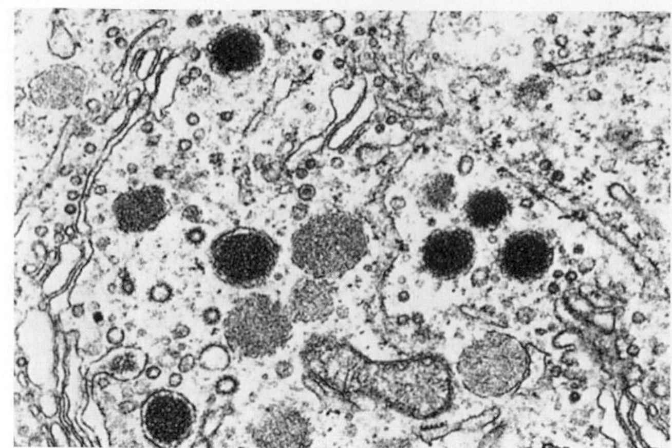

Figure 24-23 Electron micrograph of medullary thyroid carcinoma. These cells contain membrane-bound secretory granules that are the sites of storage of calcitonin and other peptides.

parathyroid glands). Medullary carcinomas arising in the context of MEN-2B are generally more aggressive and metastasize more frequently than those occurring in patients with sporadic tumors, MEN-2A, or FMTC. As will be discussed later, asymptomatic MEN-2 patients carrying germline *RET* mutations are offered prophylactic thyroidectomy as early as possible to prevent the otherwise inevitable development of medullary carcinomas, the major risk factor for poor outcome in these individuals. Sometimes the only histologic finding in the resected thyroid of asymptomatic carriers is the presence of C-cell hyperplasia or small (<1 cm) "micromedullary" carcinomas. Several small-molecule inhibitors of RET tyrosine kinase have recently been developed, and are being tested in individuals with medullary carcinomas.

KEY CONCEPTS

Thyroid Neoplasms

- Most thyroid neoplasms manifest as *solitary thyroid nodules*; only 1% of all thyroid nodules are neoplastic.
- *Follicular adenomas* are the most common benign neoplasms, while papillary carcinoma is the most common malignancy.
- Multiple genetic pathways are involved in *thyroid carcinogenesis.* Some of the genetic abnormalities that are fairly unique to thyroid cancers include *PAX8/PPARG* fusion genes or mutations that activate RAS or PI-3K (in follicular carcinomas), chromosomal rearrangements involving the *RET* oncogene or mutations in *BRAF* (in papillary carcinomas), and mutations of *RET* (in medullary carcinomas).
- *Follicular adenomas and carcinomas* both are composed of well-differentiated follicular epithelial cells; the latter are distinguished by evidence of capsular and/or vascular invasion.
- *Papillary carcinomas* are recognized based on nuclear features (ground-glass nuclei, pseudoinclusions) even in the absence of papillae. Psammoma bodies are a characteristic feature of papillary cancers; these neoplasms often metastasize by way of lymphatics, but the prognosis is excellent.
- *Anaplastic carcinomas* are thought to arise by dedifferentiation of more differentiated neoplasms. They are highly aggressive, uniformly lethal cancers.
- *Medullary cancers* are neoplasms arising from the parafollicular C cells and can occur in either sporadic (70%) or familial (30%) settings. Multicentricity and C cell hyperplasia are features of familial cases. Amyloid deposits are a characteristic histologic finding.

Congenital Anomalies

Thyroglossal duct cyst is the most common clinically significant congenital anomaly of the thyroid. A sinus tract may persist as a vestige of the tubular development of the thyroid gland. Parts of this tube may be obliterated, leaving small segments to form cysts. These occur at any age and might not become evident until adult life. Mucinous, clear secretions may collect within the cysts to form either spherical masses or fusiform swellings, rarely over 2 to 3 cm in diameter, that present in the midline of the neck anterior to the trachea. Segments of the duct and cysts that occur high in the neck are lined by stratified squamous epithelium resembling the covering of the posterior portion of the tongue in the region of the foramen cecum. Anomalies that occur in the lower neck more proximal to the thyroid gland are lined by epithelium resembling the thyroidal acinar epithelium. Characteristically, subjacent to the lining epithelium, there is an intense lymphocytic infiltrate. Superimposed infection may convert these lesions into abscess cavities, and rarely, they give rise to cancers.

PARATHYROID GLANDS

The four parathyroid glands are composed of two cell types: chief cells and oxyphil cells. Chief cells predominate; they are are polygonal, 12 to 20 μm in diameter, and have central, round, uniform nuclei and light to dark pink cytoplasm. Sometimes these cells take on a *water-clear* appearance due to the presence of large amounts of cytoplasmic glycogen. In addition, they have secretory granules containing *parathyroid hormone (PTH). Oxyphil cells* and transitional oxyphils are found throughout the normal parathyroid, either singly or in small clusters. They are slightly larger than the chief cells, have acidophilic cytoplasm, and are tightly packed with mitochondria. Glycogen granules are also present in these cells, but secretory granules are sparse or absent. In early infancy and childhood, the parathyroid glands are composed almost entirely of solid sheets of chief cells. The amount of stromal fat increases up to age 25, reaching a maximum of approximately 30% of the gland, and then plateaus.

The function of the parathyroid glands is to regulate calcium homeostasis. The activity of the parathyroid glands is controlled by the level of free (ionized) calcium in the bloodstream. Normally, decreased levels of free calcium stimulate the synthesis and secretion of PTH. The metabolic functions of PTH that regulate serum calcium levels are several. Specifically, PTH:

- Increases the renal tubular reabsorption of calcium, thereby conserving free calcium
- Increases the conversion of vitamin D to its active dihydroxy form in the kidneys
- Increases urinary phosphate excretion, thereby lowering serum phosphate levels
- Augments gastrointestinal calcium absorption

The net result of these activities is to elevate the level of free calcium, which, in turn, inhibits further PTH secretion in a classic feedback loop. Similar to the other endocrine organs, abnormalities of the parathyroid glands include both hyperfunction and hypofunction. Tumors of the parathyroid glands, in contrast to thyroid tumors, usually come to attention because of excessive secretion of PTH rather than mass effects.

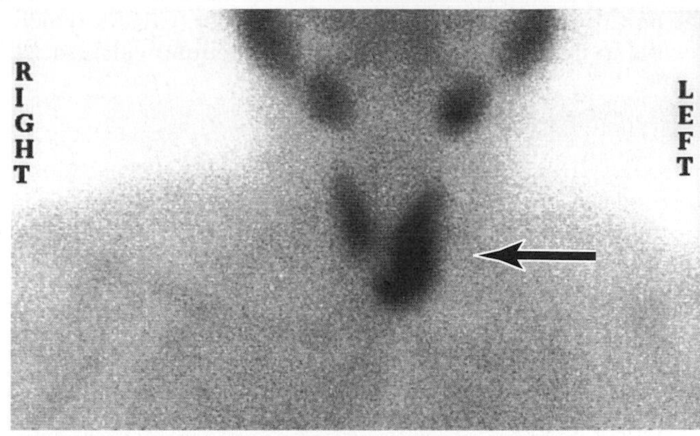

Figure 24-24 Parathyroid adenoma imaging. Technetium-^{99}m-sestamibi radionuclide scan demonstrates an area of increased uptake corresponding to the left inferior parathyroid gland *(arrow)*, which contained a parathyroid adenoma. Preoperative scintigraphy is useful in localizing and distinguishing adenomas from parathyroid hyperplasia, where more than one gland would demonstrate increased uptake.

Hyperparathyroidism

Hyperparathyroidism is caused by elevated parathyroid hormone and is classified into primary, secondary, and least commonly, tertiary types.

- *Primary hyperparathyroidism*: an autonomous overproduction of parathyroid hormone (PTH), usually resulting from an adenoma or hyperplasia of parathyroid tissue
- *Secondary hyperparathyroidism*: compensatory hypersecretion of PTH in response to prolonged hypocalcemia, most commonly from chronic renal failure
- *Tertiary hyperparathyroidism*: persistent hypersecretion of PTH even after the cause of prolonged hypocalcemia is corrected, for example after renal transplant

Primary Hyperparathyroidism

Primary hyperparathyroidism is one of the most common endocrine disorders, and it is an important cause of hypercalcemia. The frequency of the various parathyroid lesions underlying the hyperfunction is as follows:

- Adenoma: 85% to 95%
- Primary hyperplasia (diffuse or nodular): 5% to 10%
- Parathyroid carcinoma: ~1%

Primary hyperparathyroidism is usually a disease of adults and is more common in women than in men by a ratio of nearly 4:1. The annual incidence is now estimated to be about 25 cases per 100,000 in the United States and Europe; as many as 80% of patients with this condition are identified in the outpatient setting, when hypercalcemia is discovered incidentally on a serum electrolyte panel. Most cases occur in the 50s or later in life.

The most common cause of primary hyperparathyroidism is a solitary parathyroid adenoma arising sporadically (Fig. 24-24). Most, if not all, sporadic parathyroid adenomas are monoclonal, consistent with their being neoplasms. As with nodules in goitrous thyroids, sporadic parathyroid "hyperplasia" is also monoclonal in many instances, particularly when associated with a persistent stimulus for parathyroid growth (refractory secondary or tertiary parathyroidism; see later), suggesting that these lesions lie in the gray zone between reactive hyperplasias and neoplasia. There are two molecular defects that have an established role in the development of sporadic adenomas:

- *Cyclin D1 gene inversions leading to overexpression of cyclin D1,* a major regulator of the cell cycle. A pericentromeric inversion on chromosome 11 results in relocation of the *cyclin D1* gene (normally on 11q), so that it is positioned adjacent to the 5′-flanking region of the *PTH* gene (on 11p). As a consequence of these changes, a regulatory element from the *PTH* gene 5′-flanking sequence directs overexpression of cyclin D1 protein, causing the cells to proliferate. Between 10% and 20% of adenomas have this clonal rearrangement. In addition, cyclin D1 is overexpressed in approximately 40% of parathyroid adenomas, suggesting that mechanisms other than *cyclin D1* gene inversion can lead to its overexpression.
- *MEN1 mutations:* Approximately 20% to 30% of sporadic parathyroid tumors have mutations in both copies of the *MEN1* gene, a tumor suppressor gene on chromosome 11q13. Germline mutations of *MEN1* are also found in patients with familial parathyroid adenomas (see later). The spectrum of *MEN1* mutations in sporadic tumors is virtually identical to that in familial parathyroid adenomas.

Familial syndromes are a distant second to sporadic adenomas as causes of primary hyperparathyroidism. The genetic syndromes associated with *familial parathyroid adenomas* include Multiple Endocrine Neoplasia, types 1 and 2, caused by germline mutations of *MEN1* and *RET*, respectively (both are discussed in further detail later), and familial hypocalciuric hypercalcemia, a rare autosomal-dominant disorder caused by loss-of-function mutations in the parathyroid *calcium-sensing receptor gene* (*CASR*), which results in decreased sensitivity to extracellular calcium.

MORPHOLOGY

The morphologic changes seen in primary hyperparathyroidism include those in the parathyroid glands as well as those in other organs affected by elevated levels of PTH and calcium. Parathyroid **adenomas** are almost always solitary and, similar to the normal parathyroid glands, may lie in close proximity to the thyroid gland or in an ectopic site (e.g., the mediastinum). The typical parathyroid adenoma averages 0.5 to 5 gm and consists of a well-circumscribed, soft, tan to reddish-brown nodule invested by a delicate capsule. In contrast to primary hyperplasia, the glands outside the adenoma are usually normal in size or somewhat shrunken because of feedback inhibition by elevated levels of serum calcium. Microscopically, parathyroid adenomas are mostly composed of uniform, polygonal chief cells with small, centrally placed nuclei (Fig. 24-25). At least a few nests of larger oxyphil cells are present as well; uncommonly, adenomas are composed entirely of this cell type **(oxyphil adenomas)**. These may resemble Hürthle cell tumors in the thyroid. A rim of compressed, nonneoplastic parathyroid tissue, generally separated by a fibrous capsule, is often visible at the edge of the adenoma. Mitotic figures are rare, but it is not uncommon to find bizarre and pleomorphic nuclei even within adenomas (so-called **endocrine atypia**); this is not a criterion for malignancy. In contrast to the normal parathyroid parenchyma, adipose tissue is inconspicuous.

Primary hyperplasia may occur sporadically or as a component of MEN syndrome. Although classically all four glands are involved, there is frequently asymmetry with apparent sparing of one or two glands, making the distinction between hyperplasia and adenoma difficult. The combined weight of all glands rarely exceeds 1 gm and is often less. Microscopically, the most common pattern seen is that of chief cell hyperplasia, which may involve the glands in a diffuse or multinodular pattern. Less commonly, the constituent cells contain abundant water-clear cells ("water-clear cell hyperplasia"). In many instances there are islands of oxyphils, and poorly developed, delicate fibrous strands may envelop the nodules. As in the case of adenomas, stromal fat is inconspicuous within hyperplastic glands.

Parathyroid carcinomas may be circumscribed lesions that are difficult to distinguish from adenomas, or they may be clearly invasive neoplasms. These tumors enlarge cne parathyroid gland and consist of gray-white, irregular masses that sometimes exceed 10 gm in weight. The cells are usually uniform and resemble normal parathyroid cells, and are arrayed in nodular or trabecular patterns. The mass is usually enclosed by a dense, fibrous capsule. **Diagnosis of carcinoma based on cytologic detail is unreliable, and invasion of surrounding tissues and metastasis are the only reliable criteria.** Local recurrence occurs in one third of cases, and more distant dissemination occurs in another third.

Morphologic changes of hyperparathyroidism in the skeletal system (Chapter 26) and the urinary tract deserve special mention. Symptomatic, untreated primary hyperparathyroidism manifests with three interrelated skeletal abnormalities: osteoporosis, brown tumors and osteitis fibrosa cystica. The osteoporosis results in decreased bone mass, with preferential involvement of the phalanges, vertebrae and proximal femur. For unknown reasons, the increased osteoclast activity in hyperparathyroidism affects cortical bone (subperiosteal and endosteal surfaces) more severely than medullary bone. In medullary bone, osteoclasts tunnel into and dissect centrally along the length of the trabeculae, creating the appearance of railroad tracks and producing what is known as dissecting osteitis (Fig. 24-26). The marrow spaces around the affected surfaces are replaced by fibrovascular tissue. The correlative radiographic finding is a decrease in bone density or osteoporosis.

The bone loss predisposes to microfractures and secondary hemorrhages that elicit an influx of macrophages and an ingrowth of reparative fibrous tissue, creating a mass of reactive tissue, known as a **brown tumor** (Fig. 26-16, Chapter 26). The brown color is the result of the vascularity, hemorrhage, and hemosiderin deposition, and it is not uncommon for the lesions to undergo cystic degeneration. The combination of increased osteoclast activity, peritrabecular fibrosis, and cystic brown tumors is the hallmark of severe hyperparathyroidism and is known as **generalized osteitis fibrosa cystica (von Recklinghausen disease of bone**). Osteitis fibrosa cystica is now rarely encountered because hyperparathyroidism is usually diagnosed on routine blood tests and treated at an early, asymptomatic stage (see later).

PTH-induced hypercalcemia favors formation of **urinary tract stones** (nephrolithiasis) as well as calcification of the renal interstitium and tubules (nephrocalcinosis). Metastatic

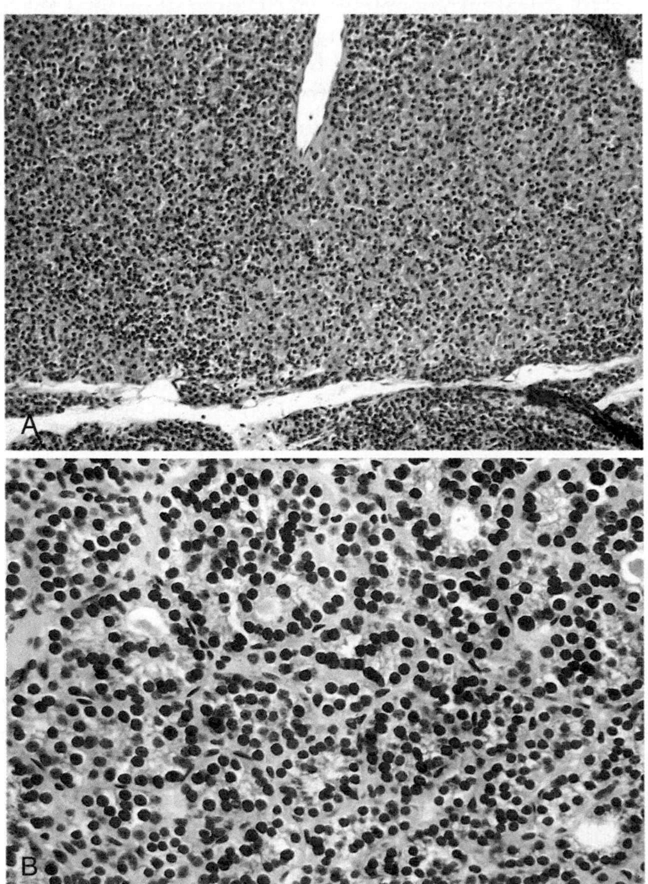

Figure 24-25 Parathyroid adenoma. **A,** Solitary chief cell parathyroid adenoma (low-power photomicrograph) revealing clear delineation from the residual gland below. **B,** High-power detail of a chief cell parathyroid adenoma. There is some slight variation in nuclear size but no anaplasia and some slight tendency to follicular formation.

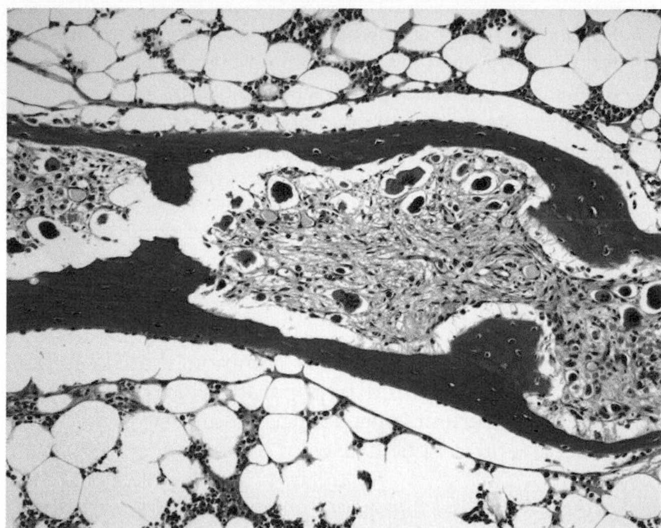

Figure 24-26 Hyperparathyroidism with osteoclasts boring into the center of the trabeculum (dissecting osteitis). (Photomicrograph reproduced from Horvai A: Bone and Soft Tissue Pathology: A Volume in the High Yield Pathology Series, Elsevier, Philadelphia, 2012.)

calcification secondary to hypercalcemia may also be seen in other sites, including the stomach, lungs, myocardium, and blood vessels.

Clinical Course. Primary hyperparathyroidism may be (1) asymptomatic and identified on routine blood chemistry profile, or (2) associated with the classic clinical manifestations of primary hyperparathyroidism.

Asymptomatic Hyperparathyroidism. Because serum calcium levels are routinely assessed, most patients with primary hyperparathyroidism are diagnosed incidentally, on the basis of clinically silent hypercalcemia. In fact, primary hyperparathyroidism is the most common cause of *asymptomatic* hypercalcemia. Hence, many of the classic manifestations, particularly those referable to bone and renal disease, are now seen infrequently in clinical practice. Among other causes of hypercalcemia (Table 24-5), *malignancy* stands out as the most frequent cause of *symptomatic* hypercalcemia in adults, and must be excluded by appropriate clinical and laboratory investigations. As discussed in Chapter 7, hypercalcemia can occur both with solid tumors, such as lung, breast, head and neck, and renal cancers, and with hematologic malignancies, notably multiple myeloma. The most common mechanism (in ~80% of cases) through which osteolytic tumors induce hypercalcemia is by secretion of PTH-related peptide (PTHrP), whose functions are similar to PTH in inducing osteoclastic bone resorption and hypercalcemia; the remaining 20% induce hypercalcemia through metastases to the bone and subsequent cytokine-induced bone resorption. In individuals with primary hyperparathyroidism, serum PTH levels are inappropriately elevated for the level of serum calcium, whereas PTH levels are low to undetectable in hypercalcemia caused by of nonparathyroid diseases (Table 24-5). Radioimmunoassays specific for PTH and PTHrP are available and can be useful in distinguishing primary hyperparathyroidism and malignancy-associated hypercalcemia. Other laboratory alterations referable to PTH excess include hypophosphatemia and increased urinary excretion of both calcium and phosphate. Secondary renal disease may lead to phosphate retention with normalization of serum phosphate levels.

Table 24-5 Causes of Hypercalcemia

Raised [PTH]	Decreased [PTH]
Hyperparathyroidism	Hypercalcemia of malignancy*
Primary (adenoma > hyperplasia)*	Vitamin D toxicity
Secondary†	Immobilization
Tertiary†	Thiazide diuretics
Familial hypocalciuric hypercalcemia	Granulomatous disease (sarcoidosis)

[PTH], Parathyroid hormone concentration.
*Primary hyperparathyroidism is the most common cause of hypercalcemia overall. Malignancy is the most common cause of *symptomatic* hypercalcemia. Primary hyperparathyroidism and malignancy account for nearly 90% of cases of hypercalcemia.
†Secondary and tertiary hyperparathyroidism are most commonly associated with progressive renal failure.

Symptomatic Primary Hyperparathyroidism. The signs and symptoms of hyperparathyroidism reflect the combined effects of increased PTH secretion and hypercalcemia. Primary hyperparathyroidism is associated with "painful bones, renal stones, abdominal groans, and psychic moans." The constellation of symptoms includes:

- *Bone disease* and bone pain secondary to fractures of bones weakened by osteoporosis or osteitis fibrosa cystica.
- *Nephrolithiasis* (renal stones) in 20% of newly diagnosed patients, with attendant pain and obstructive uropathy. Chronic renal insufficiency and abnormalities in renal function lead to polyuria and secondary polydipsia.
- Gastrointestinal disturbances, including constipation, nausea, peptic ulcers, pancreatitis, and gallstones.
- Central nervous system alterations, including depression, lethargy, and eventually seizures.
- Neuromuscular abnormalities, including weakness and fatigue.
- Cardiac manifestations, including aortic or mitral valve calcifications (or both).

The abnormalities most directly related to hyperparathyroidism are nephrolithiasis and bone disease, whereas those attributable to hypercalcemia include fatigue, weakness, pancreatitis, metastatic calcifications, and constipation.

Secondary Hyperparathyroidism

Secondary hyperparathyroidism is caused by any condition that gives rise to chronic hypocalcemia, which in turn leads to compensatory overactivity of the parathyroid glands. Renal failure is by far the most common cause of secondary hyperparathyroidism, although several other diseases, including inadequate dietary intake of calcium, steatorrhea, and vitamin D deficiency, may also cause this disorder. The mechanisms by which chronic renal failure induces secondary hyperparathyroidism are complex and not fully understood. Chronic renal insufficiency is associated with decreased phosphate excretion, which in turn results in hyperphosphatemia. The elevated serum phosphate levels directly depress serum calcium levels and thereby stimulate parathyroid gland activity. In addition, loss of renal substance reduces the availability of α-1-hydroxylase necessary for the synthesis of the active form of vitamin D, which in turn reduces intestinal absorption of calcium (Chapter 9). Because vitamin D has suppressive effects on parathyroid growth and PTH secretion, its relative deficiency compounds the hyperparathyroidism in renal failure.

MORPHOLOGY

The **parathyroid glands in secondary hyperparathyroidism are hyperplastic.** As in primary hyperparathyroidism, the degree of glandular enlargement is not necessarily symmetric. Microscopically, the hyperplastic glands contain an increased number of chief cells, or cells with more abundant, clear cytoplasm (so-called water-clear cells) in a diffuse or multinodular distribution. Fat cells are decreased in number. **Metastatic calcification** may be seen in many tissues, including lungs, heart, stomach, and blood vessels.

Clinical Course. The clinical features of secondary hyperparathyroidism are usually dominated by the inciting chronic renal failure. Secondary hyperparathyroidism *per se* is usually not as severe or as prolonged as primary hyperparathyroidism, hence the skeletal abnormalities (referred to as *renal osteodystrophy)* tend to be milder. Control of the hyperparathyroidism allows the bony changes to regress significantly or disappear completely. The vascular calcification associated with secondary hyperparathyroidism may occasionally result in significant ischemic damage to skin and other organs, a process sometimes referred to as *calciphylaxis.* Patients with secondary hyperparathyroidism often respond to dietary vitamin D supplementation, as well as phosphate binders, which decrease the prevailing hyperphosphatemia.

In a minority of patients, parathyroid activity may become autonomous and excessive, with resultant hypercalcemia, a process that is sometimes termed *tertiary hyperparathyroidism.* Parathyroidectomy may be necessary to control the hyperparathyroidism in such patients.

KEY CONCEPTS

Hyperparathyroidism

- Primary hyperparathyroidism is the most common cause of asymptomatic hypercalcemia.
- In a majority of cases, primary hyperparathyroidism is caused by a sporadic parathyroid adenoma and, less commonly, by parathyroid hyperplasia.
- Parathyroid adenomas are solitary, while hyperplasia typically is a multiglandular process.
- Skeletal manifestations of hyperparathyroidism include bone resorption, *osteitis fibrosa cystica,* and *brown tumors.* Renal changes include nephrolithiasis (stones) and nephrocalcinosis.
- The clinical manifestations of hyperparathyroidism can be summarized as "painful bones, renal stones, abdominal groans, and psychic moans."
- Secondary hyperparathyroidism most often is caused by renal failure, which lowers serum calcium levels, resulting in reactive hyperplasia of parathyroid glands.
- Malignancies are the most important cause of symptomatic hypercalcemia, which results from osteolytic metastases or release of PTH-related protein from nonparathyroid tumors.

Hypoparathyroidism

Hypoparathyroidism is far less common than is hyperparathyroidism. Acquired hypoparathyroidism is almost always an inadvertent consequence of surgery; in addition, there are several genetic causes of hypoparathyroidism.

- *Surgically induced hypoparathyroidism* occurs with inadvertent removal of all the parathyroid glands during thyroidectomy, excision of the parathyroid glands in the mistaken belief that they are lymph nodes during radical neck dissection for some form of malignant disease, or removal of too large a proportion of parathyroid tissue in the treatment of primary hyperparathyroidism.
- *Autoimmune hypoparathyroidism* is often associated with chronic mucocutaneous candidiasis and primary adrenal insufficiency; this syndrome is known as autoimmune polyendocrine syndrome type 1 (APS1) and is caused by mutations in the *autoimmune regulator (AIRE)* gene. The syndrome typically presents in childhood with the onset of candidiasis, followed several years later by hypoparathyroidism and then adrenal insufficiency during adolescence. APS1 is discussed further under "Adrenal Glands."
- *Autosomal-dominant hypoparathyroidism* is caused by gain-of-function mutations in the *calcium-sensing receptor* (*CASR*) gene. Inappropriate CASR activity due to heightened calcium sensing suppresses PTH, resulting in *hypocalcemia* and *hypercalciuria.* Recall that loss-of-function CASR mutations are a rare cause of familial parathyroid adenomas.
- *Familial isolated hypoparathyroidism* (FIH) is a rare condition with either autosomal dominant or autosomal recessive patterns of inheritance. Autosomal-dominant FIH is caused by a mutation in the gene encoding PTH precursor peptide, which impairs its processing to the mature hormone. Autosomal-recessive FIH is caused by loss-of-function mutations in the transcription factor gene *glial cells missing-2* (*GCM2*), which is essential for development of the parathyroid.
- *Congenital absence* of parathyroid glands can occur in conjunction with other malformations, such as thymic aplasia and cardiovascular defects, or as a component of the 22q11 deletion syndrome. As discussed in Chapter 6, when thymic defects are present, the condition is called *DiGeorge syndrome.*

Clinical Features. The major clinical manifestations of hypoparathyroidism are related to the severity and chronicity of the hypocalcemia.

- The hallmark of hypocalcemia is *tetany,* which is characterized by *neuromuscular irritability,* resulting from decreased serum calcium levels. The symptoms range from circumoral numbness or paresthesias (tingling) of the distal extremities and carpopedal spasm, to life-threatening laryngospasm and generalized seizures. The classic findings on physical examination are *Chvostek sign* and *Trousseau sign*. Chvostek sign is elicited in subclinical disease by tapping along the course of the facial nerve, which induces contractions of the muscles of the eye, mouth, or nose. Trousseau sign refers to carpal spasms produced by occlusion of the circulation to the forearm and hand with a blood pressure cuff for several minutes.

- *Mental status changes* include emotional instability, anxiety and depression, confusional states, hallucinations, and frank psychosis.
- *Intracranial manifestations* include calcifications of the basal ganglia, parkinsonian-like movement disorders, and increased intracranial pressure with resultant papilledema. The paradoxical association of hypocalcemia with calcifications may be because of an increase in phosphate levels, resulting in tissue deposits with calcium that exists in local extracellular milieu.
- *Ocular disease* takes the form of calcification of the lens and cataract formation.
- *Cardiovascular manifestations* include a conduction defect that produces a characteristic prolongation of the QT interval in the electrocardiogram.
- *Dental abnormalities* occur when hypocalcemia is present during early development. These findings are highly characteristic of hypoparathyroidism and include dental hypoplasia, failure of eruption, defective enamel and root formation, and abraded carious teeth.

Pseudohypoparathyroidism

In this condition, hypoparathyroidism occurs because of end-organ resistance to the actions of PTH. Indeed, serum PTH levels are normal or elevated. In one form of pseudohypoparathyroidism, there is end-organ resistance to TSH and FSH/LH as well as PTH. All of these hormones signal via G-protein–coupled receptors, and the disorder results from genetic defects in components of this pathway that are shared across endocrine tissues. PTH resistance is the most obvious clinical manifestation. It presents as hypocalcemia, hyperphosphatemia, and elevated circulating PTH. TSH resistance is generally mild, while LH/FSH resistance manifests as hypergonadotropic hypogonadism in females.

THE ENDOCRINE PANCREAS

The endocrine pancreas consists of about 1 million clusters of cells, the *islets of Langerhans*, which contain four major and two minor cell types. The four main types are β, α, δ, and PP (pancreatic polypeptide) cells. They can be differentiated by the ultrastructural characteristics of their granules, and by their hormone content (Fig. 24-27). *The β cells produce insulin*, which regulates glucose utilization in tissues and reduces blood glucose levels, as will be detailed in the discussion of diabetes. *α cells secrete glucagon*, which stimulates glycogenolysis in the liver and thus increases blood sugar. *δ cells secrete somatostatin*, which suppresses both insulin and glucagon release. *PP cells secrete pancreatic polypeptide*, which exerts several gastrointestinal effects, such as stimulation of secretion of gastric and intestinal enzymes and inhibition of intestinal motility. These cells not only are present in islets but also are scattered in the exocrine pancreas. The two rare cell types are *D1 cells* and *enterochromaffin cells*. D1 cells elaborate vasoactive intestinal polypeptide (*VIP*), a hormone that induces glycogenolysis and hyperglycemia; it also stimulates gastrointestinal fluid secretion and causes secretory diarrhea. *Enterochromaffin cells synthesize serotonin* and are the source of pancreatic tumors that cause the carcinoid syndrome (Chapter 19).

The following discussion focuses on the two main disorders of islet cells: diabetes mellitus and pancreatic endocrine tumors.

Diabetes Mellitus

Diabetes mellitus is a group of metabolic disorders sharing the common feature of hyperglycemia. Hyperglycemia in diabetes results from defects in insulin secretion, insulin action, or, most commonly, both. The chronic hyperglycemia and attendant metabolic dysregulation may be associated with secondary damage in multiple organ systems, especially the kidneys, eyes, nerves, and blood vessels. **In the United States, diabetes is the leading cause of end-stage renal disease, adult-onset blindness and non-traumatic lower extremity amputations resulting from atherosclerosis of the arteries**.

Diabetes and related disorders of glucose metabolism are extremely common. According to the American Diabetes Association, diabetes affects more than 25 million children and adults, or more than 8% of the population, in the United States, nearly a third of whom are currently unaware that they have hyperglycemia. Approximately 1.9 million new cases of adult diabetes are diagnosed each year in the United States. Furthermore, a staggering 79 million adults in this country have impaired glucose tolerance or "prediabetes," which is defined as elevated blood sugar that does not reach the criterion accepted for an outright diagnosis of diabetes (see later), and individuals with prediabetes are at high risk for developing frank diabetes. Compared to non-Hispanic whites, Native Americans, African Americans, and Hispanics are 1.5 to 2 times more likely to develop diabetes in their lifetimes. The World Health Organization estimates that as many as 346 million people suffer from diabetes worldwide, with India and China being the largest contributors to the world's diabetic load. Increasingly sedentary life styles and poor eating habits have contributed to the simultaneous escalation of diabetes and obesity, which some have called the *diabesity epidemic*. Sadly, obesity and diabetes have now extended even to

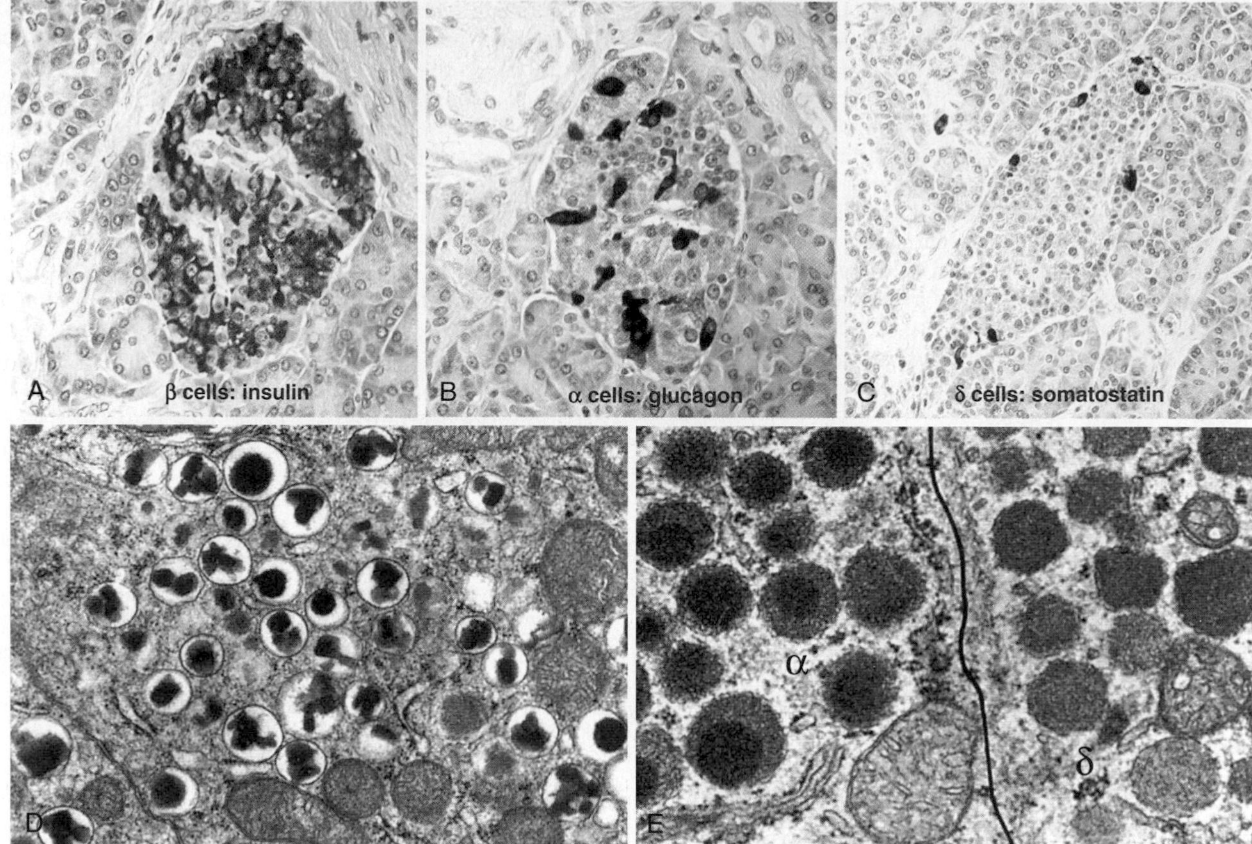

Figure 24-27 Hormone production in pancreatic islet cells**.** Immunoperoxidase staining shows a dark reaction product for insulin in β cells (**A**), glucagon in α cells (**B**), and somatostatin in δ cells (**C**). **D,** Electron micrograph of a β cell shows the characteristic membrane-bound granules, each containing a dense, often rectangular core and distinct halo. **E,** Portions of an α cell *(left)* and a δ cell *(right)* also show granules, but with closely apportioned membranes. The α-cell granule shows a dense, round center. (Electron micrographs courtesy Dr. Arthur Like, University of Massachusetts Medical School, Worcester, Mass.)

children who subsist on "junk" food and lack adequate exercise.

The mortality rate from diabetes varies across countries, with middle- and low-income nations accounting for almost 80% of diabetes-related deaths and nearly double the mortality rates observed in developed nations. Nonetheless, diabetes continues to be one of the top 10 "killers" in the United States. The total yearly costs related to diabetes in the United States are estimated to be an astounding 174 billion dollars, including $116 billion in direct medical costs and the additional $58 billion in indirect costs such as disability, work loss, and premature mortality.

Diagnosis

Blood glucose is normally maintained in a very narrow range of 70 to 120 mg/dL. According to the ADA and WHO, **diagnostic criteria for diabetes include**:

1. A fasting plasma glucose ≥ 126 mg/dL,
2. A random plasma glucose ≥ 200 mg/dL (in a patient with classic hyperglycemic signs, as discussed later),
3. 2-hour plasma glucose ≥ 200 mg/dL during an oral glucose tolerance test (OGTT) with a loading dose of 75 gm, and
4. A glycated hemoglobin (Hb_{A1C}) level ≥ 6.5% (glycated hemoglobin is further discussed under chronic complications of diabetes)

All tests, except the random blood glucose test in a patient with classic hyperglycemic signs, need to be repeated and confirmed on a separate day. If there is discordance between two assays (e.g., fasting glucose and Hb_{A1C} level), then the result with greater degree of abnormality is considered the "readout." Of note, many acute stresses, such as severe infections, burns or trauma, can lead to transient hyperglycemia due to secretion of hormones like catecholamines and cortisol that oppose the action of insulin. The diagnosis of diabetes requires persistence of hyperglycemia following resolution of the acute illness.

Impaired glucose tolerance (prediabetes) is defined as:

1. A fasting plasma glucose between 100 and 125 mg/dL ("impaired fasting glucose"),
2. 2-hour plasma glucose between 140 and 199 mg/dL following a 75-gm glucose OGTT, and/or
3. A glycated hemoglobin (Hb_{A1C}) level between 5.7% and 6.4%

As many as one-fourth of individuals with impaired glucose tolerance will develop overt diabetes over 5 years, with additional factors such as obesity and family history compounding the risk. In addition, individuals with prediabetes also harbor a significant risk for cardiovascular complications.

Classification

Although all forms of diabetes mellitus share hyperglycemia as a common feature, the underlying abnormalities involved in the development of hyperglycemia vary widely. The previous classification schemes of diabetes mellitus were based on the age at onset of the disease or on the mode of therapy; in contrast, the current etiologic classification reflects our greater understanding of the pathogenesis of each variant (Table 24-6). The vast majority of cases of diabetes fall into one of two broad classes:

- ***Type 1 diabetes* is an autoimmune disease characterized by pancreatic β cell destruction and an absolute deficiency of insulin**. It accounts for approximately 5% to 10% of all cases, and is the most common subtype diagnosed in patients younger than 20 years of age.
- ***Type 2 diabetes* is caused by a combination of peripheral resistance to insulin action and an inadequate secretory response by the pancreatic β cells ("relative insulin deficiency").** Approximately 90% to 95% of diabetic patients have type 2 diabetes, and the vast majority of such individuals are overweight. Although classically considered "adult-onset," the prevalence of type 2 diabetes in children and adolescents has been increasing at an alarming pace due to the increasing rates of obesity in these age groups. One piece of encouraging news is that the incidence of obesity in the U.S. in children ages 2-5 years fell by over 40% during the period of 2004 to 2012, a tipping of the scales that may signal a reversal of a troubling trend.

The important similarities and differences between types 1 and 2 diabetes are summarized in Table 24-7.

A variety of monogenic and secondary causes are responsible for the remaining cases (discussed later). It should be stressed that while the major types of diabetes have different pathogenic mechanisms, the long-term complications affecting the kidneys, eyes, nerves, and blood vessels are the same, as are the principal causes of morbidity and death. The pathogenesis of the two major types is discussed separately. We will first briefly review normal insulin secretion and the mechanism of insulin action since these are critical to understanding the pathogenesis of diabetes.

Glucose Homeostasis

Normal glucose homeostasis is tightly regulated by three interrelated processes: glucose production in the liver; glucose uptake and utilization by peripheral tissues, chiefly skeletal muscle; and actions of insulin and counterregulatory hormones, including glucagon, on glucose uptake and metabolism.

Insulin and glucagon have opposing regulatory effects on glucose homeostasis. During fasting states, low insulin and high glucagon levels facilitate hepatic gluconeogenesis and glycogenolysis (glycogen breakdown) while decreasing glycogen synthesis, thereby preventing hypoglycemia.

Table 24-6 Classification of Diabetes Mellitus

Type 1 diabetes (β-cell destruction, usually leading to absolute insulin deficiency)
Immune-mediated
Idiopathic
Type 2 diabetes (combination of insulin resistance and β-cell dysfunction)
Genetic defects of β-cell function
Maturity-onset diabetes of the young (MODY), caused by mutations in:
Hepatocyte nuclear factor 4α (*HNF4A*), MODY1
Glucokinase (*GCK*), MODY2
Hepatocyte nuclear factor 1α (*HNF1A*), MODY3
Pancreatic and duodenal homeobox 1 (*PDX1*), MODY4
Hepatocyte nuclear factor 1β (*HNF1B*), MODY5
Neurogenic differentiation factor 1 (*NEUROD1*), MODY6
Neonatal diabetes (activating mutations in *KCNJ11* and *ABCC8*, encoding Kir6.2 and SUR1, respectively)
Maternally inherited diabetes and deafness (MIDD) due to mitochondrial DNA mutations (m.3243A→G)
Defects in proinsulin conversion
Insulin gene mutations
Genetic defects in insulin action
Type A insulin resistance
Lipoatrophic diabetes
Exocrine pancreatic defects
Chronic pancreatitis
Pancreatectomy/trauma
Neoplasia
Cystic fibrosis
Hemochromatosis
Fibrocalculous pancreatopathy
Endocrinopathies
Acromegaly
Cushing syndrome
Hyperthyroidism
Pheochromocytoma
Glucagonoma
Infections
Cytomegalovirus
Coxsackie B virus
Congenital rubella
Drugs
Glucocorticoids
Thyroid hormone
Interferon-α
Protease inhibitors
β-adrenergic agonists
Thiazides
Nicotinic acid
Phenytoin (Dilantin)
Vacor
Genetic syndromes associated with diabetes
Down syndrome
Klinefelter syndrome
Turner syndrome
Prader-Willi syndrome
Gestational diabetes mellitus

American Diabetes Association: Position statement from the American Diabetes Association on the diagnosis and classification of diabetes mellitus. Diabetes Care 31 (Suppl. 1): S55-S60, 2008.

Table 24-7 Type 1 Versus Type 2 Diabetes Mellitus

Type 1 Diabetes Mellitus	Type 2 Diabetes Mellitus
Clinical	
Onset: usually childhood and adolescence	Onset: usually adult; increasing incidence in childhood and adolescence
Normal weight or weight loss preceding diagnosis	Vast majority are obese (80%)
Progressive decrease in insulin levels	Increased blood insulin (early); normal or moderate decrease in insulin (late)
Circulating islet autoantibodies (anti-insulin, anti-GAD, anti-ICA512)	No islet autoantibodies
Diabetic ketoacidosis in absence of insulin therapy	Nonketotic hyperosmolar coma more common
Genetics	
Major linkage to MHC class II genes; also linked to polymorphisms in *CTLA4* and *PTPN22*, and insulin gene VNTRs	No HLA linkage; linkage to candidate diabetogenic and obesity-related genes (*TCF7L2*, *PPARG*, *FTO*, etc.)
Pathogenesis	
Dysfunction in T cell selection and regulation leading to breakdown in self-tolerance to islet autoantigens	Insulin resistance in peripheral tissues, failure of compensation by β-cells
	Multiple obesity-associated factors (circulating nonesterified fatty acids, inflammatory mediators, adipocytokines) linked to pathogenesis of insulin resistance
Pathology	
Insulitis (inflammatory infiltrate of T cells and macrophages) β-cell depletion, islet atrophy	No insulitis; amyloid deposition in islets Mild β-cell depletion

HLA, Human leukocyte antigen; MHC, major histocompatibility complex; VNTRs, variable number of tandem repeats.

Thus, fasting plasma glucose levels are determined primarily by hepatic glucose output. Following a meal, insulin levels rise and glucagon levels fall in response to the large glucose load. Insulin promotes glucose uptake and utilization in tissues (discussed later). The skeletal muscle is the major insulin-responsive site for postprandial glucose utilization, and is critical for preventing hyperglycemia and maintaining glucose homeostasis.

Regulation of Insulin Release

Insulin is produced in the β cells of the pancreatic islets (Fig. 24-27) as a precursor protein and is proteolytically cleaved in the Golgi complex to generate the mature hormone and a peptide byproduct, *C-peptide*. Both insulin and C-peptide are then stored in secretory granules and secreted in equimolar quantities after physiologic stimulation; thus, C-peptide levels serve as a surrogate for β-cell function, decreasing with loss of β-cell mass in type 1 diabetes, or increasing with insulin resistance-associated hyperinsulinemia.

The most important stimulus for insulin synthesis and release is glucose itself. An increase in blood glucose levels results in glucose uptake into pancreatic β cells, facilitated by an insulin-independent glucose-transporter, GLUT-2 (Fig. 24-28). β cells express an ATP-sensitive K^+ channel on the membrane, which comprises two subunits: an ATP-sensitive K^+ channel and the sulfonylurea receptor, the latter being the binding site for oral hypoglycemic agents (sulfonylureas), one of the several classes of drugs used in the treatment of diabetes (see later). Metabolism of glucose generates ATP, which inhibits the activity of the ATP-sensitive K^+ channel, leading to membrane depolarization and the influx of Ca^{2+}. The resultant increase in intracellular Ca^{2+} stimulates secretion of insulin, presumably from stored hormone within the β-cell granules. This is the phase of *immediate release of insulin*. If the secretory stimulus persists, a delayed and protracted response follows that involves *active synthesis of insulin*.

Oral intake of food leads to secretion of multiple hormones that play a role in glucose homeostasis and satiety. Of these, the most important class of hormones responsible for promoting insulin secretion from pancreatic β cells following feeding is the incretins. Two incretins have been identified: *glucose-dependent insulinotropic polypeptide (GIP)*, secreted by enteroendocrine "K cells" in the proximal small bowel, and *glucagon-like peptide-1 (GLP-1)*, secreted by "L cells" in the distal ileum and colon. The elevation in GIP and GLP-1 levels following oral food intake is known as the "incretin effect." In addition to increased insulin secretion from β cells, these hormones also reduce glucagon secretion and delay gastric emptying, which promotes satiety. Once released, circulating GIP and GLP-1 are degraded in circulation by a class of enzymes known as dipeptidyl peptidase (DPPs), especially DPP-4. The "incretin effect" is significantly blunted in patients with type 2 diabetes, and efforts to restore incretin function can lead to improved glycemic control and loss of weight (through restoration of satiety). These observations have resulted in the development of two new classes of drugs for patients with type 2 diabetes: *GLP-1 receptor agonists*, which are synthetic GLP-1 mimetics that bind to, and activate the GLP-1 receptor on islet and extrapancreatic sites, and DPP-4 inhibitors, which enhance levels of endogenous incretins by delaying their degradation.

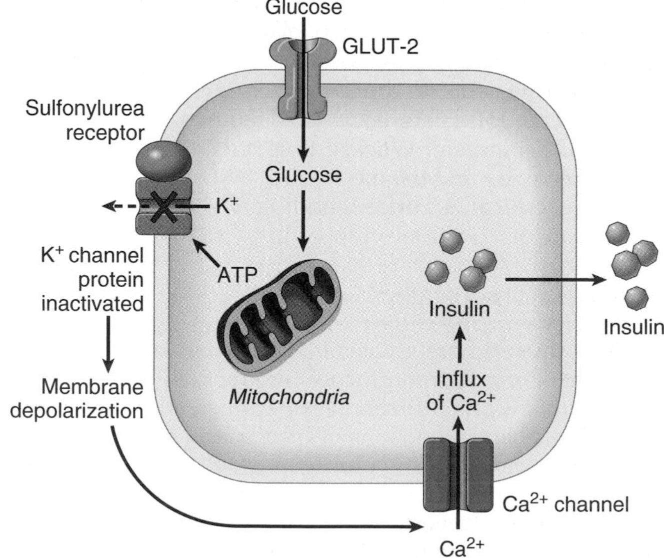

Figure 24-28 Insulin synthesis and secretion. The influx of glucose into β cells through the GLUT-2 receptors initiates a cascade of signaling events that culminates in Ca^{2+}-induced release of stored insulin (see text for details).

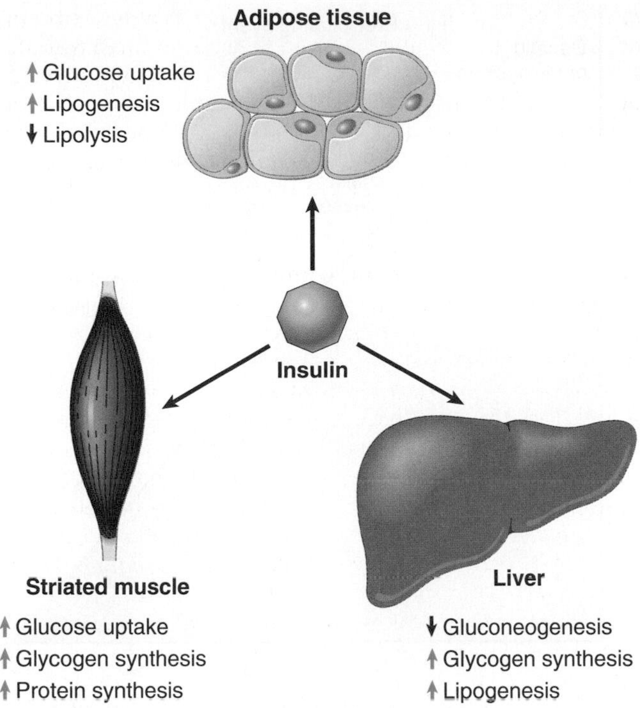

Figure 24-29 Metabolic actions of insulin in striated muscle, adipose tissue, and liver.

Insulin Action and Insulin Signaling Pathways

Insulin is the most potent anabolic hormone known, with multiple synthetic and growth-promoting effects (Fig. 24-29). The principal metabolic function of insulin is to increase the rate of glucose transport into certain cells in the body, thus increasing a major source of energy as well as metabolic intermediates that are used in the biosynthesis of cellular building blocks such as lipids, nucleotides, and amino acids. These cells are the *striated muscle cells* (including myocardial cells) and, to a lesser extent, *adipocytes,* which together represent about two thirds of the entire body weight. Glucose uptake in other peripheral tissues, most notably the brain, is insulin independent. In muscle cells, glucose is then either stored as glycogen or oxidized to generate ATP. In adipose tissue, glucose is primarily stored as lipid. Besides promoting lipid synthesis, insulin also inhibits lipid degradation in adipocytes. Similarly, insulin promotes amino acid uptake and protein synthesis, while inhibiting protein degradation. Thus, the anabolic effects of insulin are attributable to increased synthesis and reduced degradation of glycogen, lipids, and proteins. In addition, insulin has several *mitogenic* functions, including initiation of DNA synthesis in certain cells and stimulation of their growth and differentiation.

The molecular basis of insulin signaling is complex; the more pertinent mediators are summarized in Fig. 24-30. The *insulin receptor* is a tetrameric protein composed of two α- and two β-subunits. The β-subunit cytosolic domain possesses tyrosine kinase activity. Insulin binding to the α-subunit extracellular domain activates the β-subunit tyrosine kinase, resulting in autophosphorylation of the receptor and the phosphorylation (activation) of several intracellular substrate proteins, such as the family of insulin receptor substrates (IRS), which includes IRS1-IRS4 and GAB1. The substrate proteins, in turn, activate multiple downstream signaling cascades, including the PI3K and the MAP kinase pathways, which mediate the metabolic and mitogenic activities of insulin on the cell. Insulin signaling also facilitates the trafficking and docking of vesicles containing the insulin-sensitive glucose transporter protein GLUT-4 to the plasma membrane, which promotes glucose uptake. This process is mediated by AKT, the principal effector of the PI3K pathway, but also independently by the cytoplasmic protein CBL, which is a direct phosphorylation target of the insulin receptor.

Pathogenesis of Type I Diabetes Mellitus

Type 1 diabetes is an autoimmune disease in which islet destruction is caused primarily by immune effector cells reacting against endogenous β-cell antigens. Type 1 diabetes most commonly develops in childhood, becomes manifest at puberty, and progresses with age. Because the disease can develop at any age, including late adulthood, the previously used appellation "juvenile diabetes" is now considered inaccurate. Similarly, the older moniker "insulin-dependent diabetes mellitus" has been excluded from the current classification of diabetes because all forms of diabetes may be treated with insulin. Nevertheless, most patients with type 1 diabetes require insulin for survival; without insulin they develop serious metabolic complications such as ketoacidosis and coma.

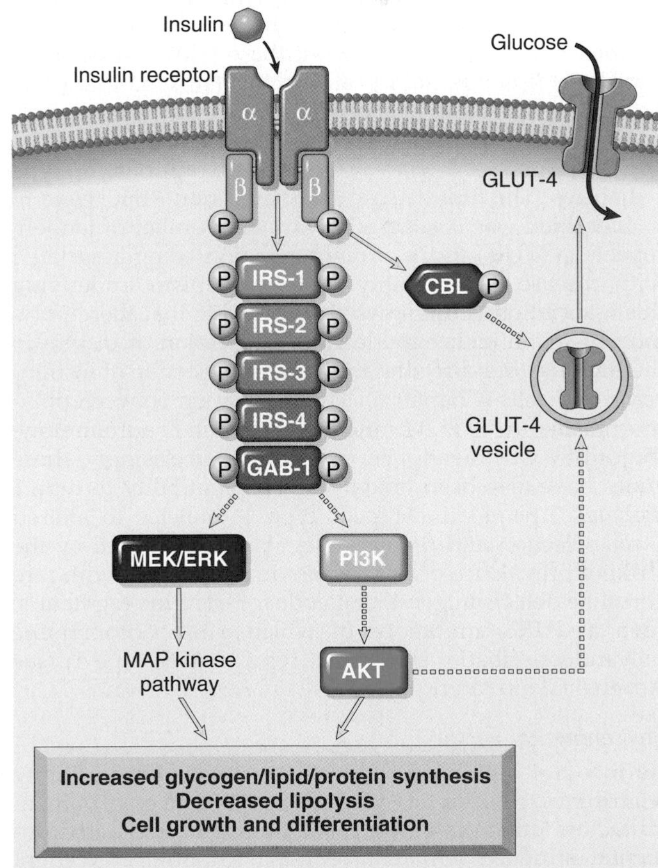

Figure 24-30 Insulin action on a target cell. The metabolic actions of insulin include promoting glycogen synthesis by activating glycogen synthase, and enhancing protein synthesis and lipogenesis while inhibiting lipolysis (see text). Dashed arrows represent intermediate proteins and binding partners that are not shown in this overview diagram.

As with most autoimmune diseases, the pathogenesis of type 1 diabetes involves an interplay of genetic and environmental factors.

Genetic Susceptibility

Epidemiologic studies, such as those demonstrating higher concordance rates for disease in monozygotic vs dizygotic twins, have convincingly established a genetic basis for type 1 diabetes. More recently, genome-wide association studies have identified multiple genetic susceptibility loci for type 1 diabetes, as well as for type 2 diabetes (see later). More than 30 susceptibility loci for type 1 diabetes are now known. **Of these, the most important locus is the *HLA* gene cluster on chromosome 6p21, which according to some estimates contributes as much as 50% of the genetic susceptibility to type 1 diabetes**. Ninety percent to 95% of Caucasians with this disease have either an HLA-DR3 or HLA-DR4 haplotype, in contrast to about 40% of normal subjects; moreover, 40% to 50% of patients with type 1 diabetes are combined DR3/DR4 heterozygotes, in contrast to 5% of normal subjects. Individuals who have either DR3 or DR4 concurrently with a DQ8 haplotype (which corresponds to *DQA1*0301-DQB1*0302* alleles) demonstrate one of the highest inherited risks for type 1 diabetes in sibling studies. Predictably, the polymorphisms in the HLA molecules are located in or adjacent to the peptide-binding pockets, consistent with the notion that disease-associated alleles code for molecules that have the capacity to display particular antigens. However, as discussed in Chapter 6, it is still not known if these HLA-disease associations reflect the ability of specific HLA molecules to present self islet antigens or if they are related to the role of HLA molecules in T-cell selection and tolerance.

Several *non-HLA genes* also confer susceptibility to type 1 diabetes. The first disease-associated non-MHC gene to be identified was *insulin*, with variable number of tandem repeats (VNTRs) in the promoter region being associated with disease susceptibility. The mechanism underlying this association is unknown. It is possible that these polymorphisms influence the level of expression of insulin in the thymus, thus affecting the negative selection of insulin-reactive T cells (Chapter 6). The association between polymorphisms in *CTLA4* and *PTPN22* and autoimmune thyroiditis was mentioned earlier; not surprisingly, these genes have also been linked with susceptibility to type 1 diabetes. The relationship of type 1 diabetes to altered T-cell selection and regulation is also underscored by the striking prevalence of this disease in individuals with rare germline defects in genes that code for immune regulators, such as *AIRE*, mutations of which cause autoimmune polyendocrinopathy syndrome, type 1 (APS, type 1) (see Adrenal Gland later).

Environmental Factors

As in other autoimmune diseases, genetic susceptibility contributes to only a part of diabetes risk, and environmental factors must play a role. The nature of these environmental influences remains an enigma. Although antecedent *viral infections* have been suggested as triggers for development of the disease, neither the type of virus nor how it promotes islet-specific autoimmunity is established. Some studies suggest that viruses might share epitopes with islet antigens, and the immune response to the virus results in cross-reactivity and destruction of islet tissues, a phenomenon known as *molecular mimicry*. On the other hand, infections are also known to be protective against type 1 diabetes.

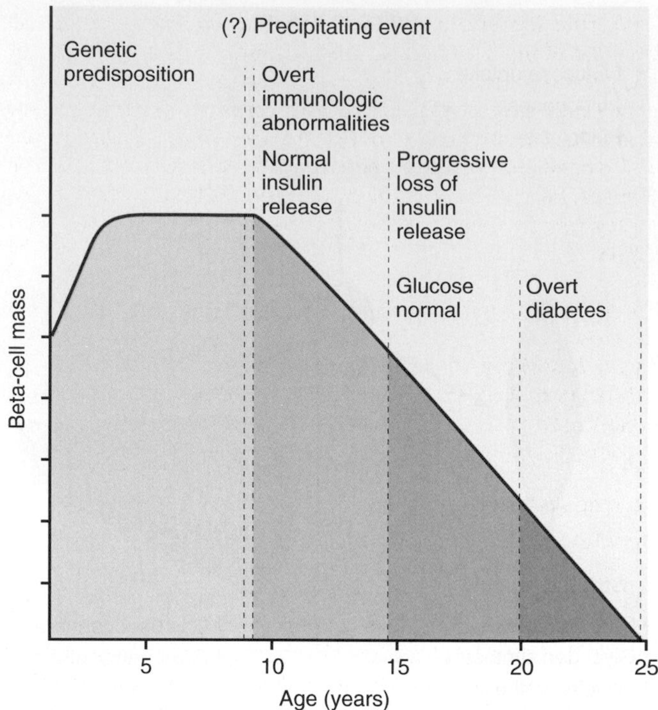

Figure 24-31 Stages in the development of type 1 diabetes mellitus. The stages are listed from left to right, and hypothetical β-cell mass is plotted against age. (From Eisenbarth GE: Type 1 diabetes: a chronic autoimmune disease. N Engl J Med 314:1360, 1986. Copyright © 1986, Massachusetts Medical Society. All rights reserved.)

Mechanisms of β Cell Destruction

Although the clinical onset of type 1 diabetes is often abrupt, there is a lengthy lag period between initiation of the autoimmune process and the appearance of disease, during which there is progressive loss of insulin reserves (Fig. 24-31). The classic manifestations of the disease (hyperglycemia and ketosis) occur late in its course, after more than 90% of the β cells have been destroyed.

The fundamental immune abnormality in type 1 diabetes is a failure of self-tolerance in T cells specific for islet antigens. This failure of tolerance may be a result of some combination of defective clonal deletion of self-reactive T cells in the thymus, as well as defects in the functions of regulatory T cells or resistance of effector T cells to suppression by regulatory cells. Thus, autoreactive T cells not only survive but are poised to respond to self-antigens. The initial activation of these cells is thought to occur in the peripancreatic lymph nodes, perhaps in response to antigens that are released from damaged islets. The activated T cells then traffic to the pancreas, where they cause β-cell injury. Multiple T-cell populations have been implicated in this damage, including T_H1 cells (which may secrete cytokines, including IFN-γ and TNF, that injure β cells), and CD8+ CTLs (which kill β cells directly). The islet autoantigens that are the targets of immune attack may include insulin, the β cell enzyme glutamic acid decarboxylase (GAD), and islet cell autoantigen 512 (ICA512).

A role for antibodies in type 1 diabetes is suspected because of the observation that autoantibodies against islet antigens are found in the vast majority of patients with type 1 diabetes, as well as in asymptomatic family members at risk for progression to overt disease; in fact, the presence of islet cell antibodies is used as a predictive marker for the disease. However, it is not clear if the autoantibodies cause injury or are merely produced as a consequence of islet injury.

Pathogenesis of Type 2 Diabetes Mellitus

Type 2 diabetes is a complex disease that involves an interplay of genetic and environmental factors and a pro-inflammatory state. Unlike type 1 diabetes, there is no evidence of an autoimmune basis.

Genetic Factors

Genetic susceptibility contributes to the pathogenesis, as evidenced by the disease concordance rate of greater than 90% in monozygotic twins. Furthermore, first-degree relatives have 5- to 10-fold higher risk of developing type 2 diabetes than those without a family history, when matched for age and weight. Genome-wide association studies (GWAS) performed over the last decade have identified at least 30 loci that individually confer a minimal to modest increase in the lifetime risk for type 2 diabetes. The detailed description of these susceptibility loci is beyond the scope of this chapter, although many of the polymorphisms identified are in genes associated with *insulin secretion*. Elucidating the biochemical mechanisms through which these and other linked genes contribute to diabetes pathogenesis is a work in progress.

Environmental Factors

The most important environmental risk factor for type 2 diabetes is obesity, particularly central or visceral obesity. Greater than 80% of individuals with type 2 diabetes are obese, and the incidence of diabetes worldwide has risen in proportion to obesity. Obesity contributes to the cardinal metabolic abnormalities of diabetes (see later) and to insulin resistance early in disease. In fact, even modest weight loss through dietary modifications can reduce insulin resistance and improve glucose tolerance. A sedentary lifestyle (typified by lack of exercise) is another risk factor for diabetes, independent of obesity. Weight loss and exercise usually have additive effects on improving insulin sensitivity and are often the first non-pharmacological measures attempted in patients with milder type 2 diabetes.

Metabolic Defects in Diabetes

The two cardinal metabolic defects that characterize type 2 diabetes are:

- Decreased response of peripheral tissues, especially skeletal muscle, adipose tissue, and liver, to insulin (**insulin resistance**)
- Inadequate insulin secretion in the face of insulin resistance and hyperglycemia (**β-cell dysfunction**)

Insulin resistance predates the development of hyperglycemia and is usually accompanied by compensatory β-cell hyperfunction and hyperinsulinemia in the early stages of the evolution of diabetes (Fig. 24-32). Over time, the inability of β cells to adapt to increasing secretory needs for maintaining a euglycemic state results in chronic hyperglycemia and the resulting long-standing complications of diabetes.

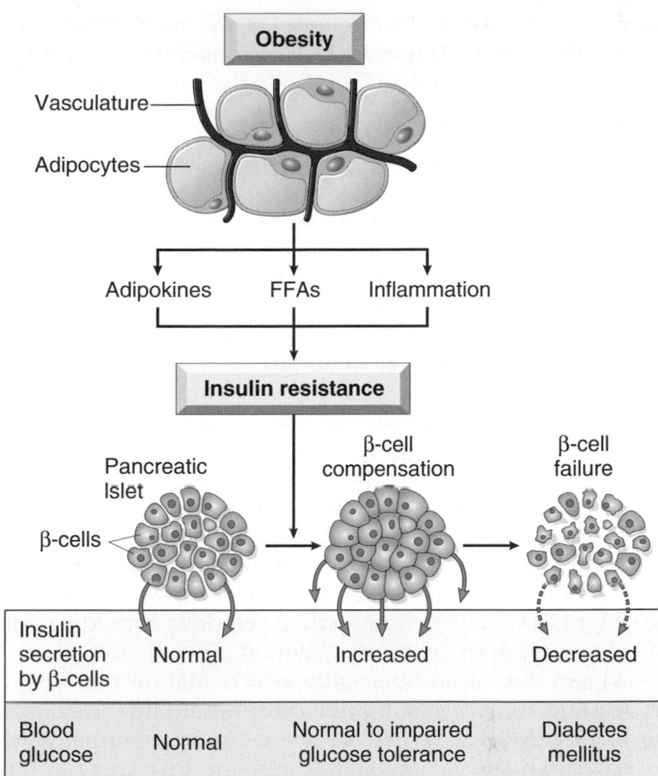

Figure 24-32 Development of type 2 diabetes. Insulin resistance associated with obesity is induced by adipokines, free fatty acids, and chronic inflammation in adipose tissue. Pancreatic β cells compensate for insulin resistance by hypersecretion of insulin. However, at some point, β-cell compensation is followed by β-cell failure, and diabetes ensues. (Reproduced with permission from Kasuga M: Insulin resistance and pancreatic β-cell failure. J Clin Invest 116:1756, 2006.)

Insulin Resistance

Insulin resistance is the failure of target tissues to respond normally to insulin. The liver, skeletal muscle and adipose tissue are the major tissues where insulin resistance manifests in abnormal glucose tolerance. Insulin resistance results in:

- Failure to inhibit endogenous glucose production (gluconeogenesis) in the liver, which contributes to high fasting blood glucose levels
- Failure of glucose uptake and glycogen synthesis to occur in skeletal muscle following a meal, which contributes to high post-prandial blood glucose level
- Failure to inhibit lipoprotein lipase in adipose tissue, leading to excess circulating free fatty acids (FFAs), which in turn, amplify the state of insulin resistance

A variety of functional defects have been reported in the insulin signaling pathway in states of insulin resistance. For example, reduced tyrosine phosphorylation of the insulin receptor and IRS proteins is observed in peripheral tissues, which compromises insulin signaling and reduces the level of the glucose transporter GLUT-4 on the cell surface (Fig. 24-30). In fact, one of the mechanisms by which exercise can improve insulin sensitivity is through increased translocation of GLUT-4 to the surface of skeletal muscle cells.

Obesity and Insulin Resistance. Multiple factors contribute to insulin resistance, of which obesity is probably the most important. The risk for diabetes increases as the body mass index (a measure of body fat content) increases. It is not only the absolute amount but also the distribution of body fat that has an effect on insulin sensitivity: central obesity (abdominal fat) is more likely to be linked with insulin resistance than are peripheral (gluteal/subcutaneous) fat depots.

Obesity can adversely impact insulin sensitivity in numerous ways (Fig. 24-32):

- *Free fatty acids (FFAs).* Cross-sectional studies have demonstrated an inverse correlation between fasting plasma FFAs and insulin sensitivity. Central adipose tissue is more "lipolytic" than peripheral sites, which might explain the particularly deleterious consequences of this pattern of fat distribution. Excess FFAs overwhelm the intracellular fatty acid oxidation pathways, leading to accumulation of cytoplasmic intermediates like diacylglycerol (DAG). These "toxic" intermediates can attenuate signaling through the insulin receptor pathway. In liver cells, insulin normally inhibits gluconeogenesis by blocking the activity of phosphoenolpyruvate carboxykinase, the first enzymatic step in this process. Attenuated insulin signaling allows phosphoenolpyruvate carboxykinase to "ramp up" gluconeogenesis. Excess FFAs also compete with glucose for substrate oxidation, leading to feedback inhibition of glycolytic enzymes, thereby further exacerbating the existing glucose imbalance.
- *Adipokines.* You will recall that adipose tissue is not merely a passive storage depot for fat but is a functional endocrine organ that releases hormones in response to changes in metabolic status (Chapter 9). A variety of proteins secreted into the systemic circulation by adipose tissue have been identified, and these are collectively termed *adipokines* (or adipose cytokines). Some of these promote hyperglycemia, and other adipokines (such as leptin and adiponectin) decrease blood glucose, in part by increasing insulin sensitivity in peripheral tissues. Adiponectin levels are reduced in obesity, thus contributing to insulin resistance.
- *Inflammation:* Over the past several years, inflammation has emerged as an important factor in the pathogenesis of type 2 diabetes. It is now known that an inflammatory milieu—mediated not by an autoimmune process such as type 1 diabetes but rather by proinflammatory cytokines that are secreted in response to excess nutrients such as free fatty acid (FFAs) and glucose—results in both insulin resistance and β-cell dysfunction. Excess FFAs within macrophages and β cells can activate the inflammasome, a multiprotein cytoplasmic complex that leads to secretion of the cytokine interleukin IL-1β (Chapter 3). IL-1β, in turn, mediates the secretion of additional pro-inflammatory cytokines from macrophages, islet cells, and other cells. IL-1 and other cytokines are released into the circulation and act on the major sites of insulin action to promote insulin resistance. Thus, excess FFAs can impede insulin signaling directly within peripheral tissues, as well as indirectly through the release of pro-inflammatory cytokines.

β-Cell Dysfunction

While insulin resistance by itself can lead to impaired glucose tolerance, **β-cell dysfunction is virtually a requirement for the development of overt diabetes.** In contrast to the severe genetic defects in β-cell function that occur in monogenic forms of diabetes (see later), β-cell function actually increases early in the disease process in most patients with "sporadic" type 2 diabetes, mainly as a compensatory measure to counter insulin resistance and maintain euglycemia. Eventually, however, β cells seemingly exhaust their capacity to adapt to the long-term demands of peripheral insulin resistance, and the hyperinsulinemic state gives way to a state of relative insulin deficiency.

Several mechanisms have been implicated in promoting β-cell dysfunction in type 2 diabetes, including:

- Excess free fatty acids that compromise β cell function and attenuate insulin release ("*lipotoxicity*")
- The impact of chronic hyperglycemia ("*glucotoxicity*")
- An abnormal "*incretin effect,*" leading to reduced secretion of GIP and GLP-1, hormones that promote insulin release (see earlier)
- Amyloid deposition within islets. This is a characteristic finding in individuals with long-standing type 2 diabetes, being present in more than 90% of diabetic islets examined, but it is unclear whether it is a cause or an effect of β-cell "burnout."
- Finally, the impact of genetics cannot be discounted, as many of the polymorphisms associated with an increased lifetime risk for type 2 diabetes occur in genes that control insulin secretion (see earlier).

Monogenic Forms of Diabetes

Although genetically defined causes of diabetes are uncommon, they have been intensively studied in the hope of gaining insights into the disease. As Table 24-6 illustrates, monogenic forms of diabetes are classified separately from types 1 and 2. These forms of diabetes result from either a primary defect in β-cell function or a defect in insulin receptor signaling (described later).

Genetic Defects in β-Cell Function. Approximately 1% to 2% of patients with diabetes harbor a primary defect in β-cell function that occurs without β-cell loss, affecting either β-cell mass and/or insulin production. This form of monogenic diabetes is caused by a heterogeneous group of genetic defects. The largest subgroup of patients in this category was traditionally designated as having "maturity-onset diabetes of the young" (MODY) because of its superficial resemblance to type 2 diabetes and its occurrence in younger patients. MODY can result from germline loss-of-function mutations in one of six genes (Table 24-6), of which mutations of *glucokinase* (*GCK*) are the most common. Glucokinase is a rate limiting step in oxidative glucose metabolism, which in turn, is coupled to insulin secretion within islet β cells (Fig. 24-28). Other rare genetic causes for primary defects in β cell function include mutations of genes that code for the two subunits of the ATP-sensitive K^+-channel, defects in mitochondrial DNA (which can impede ATP synthesis), and mutations of the insulin gene itself.

Genetic Defects that Impair Tissue Response to Insulin. Rare *insulin receptor mutations* that affect receptor synthesis, insulin binding, or receptor tyrosine kinase activity can cause severe insulin resistance, accompanied by hyperinsulinemia and diabetes (type A insulin resistance). Such patients often show a velvety hyperpigmentation of the skin, known as *acanthosis nigricans*. Females with type A insulin resistance frequently have polycystic ovaries and elevated androgen levels. *Lipoatrophic diabetes,* as the name suggests, is hyperglycemia accompanied by loss of adipose tissue, the latter occurring selectively in the subcutaneous fat. This rare group of genetic disorders has in common insulin resistance, diabetes, hypertriglyceridemia, acanthosis nigricans, and abnormal fat deposition in the liver (hepatic steatosis). Multiple subtypes of lipoatrophic diabetes, each ascribed to a different causal mutation, have been reported.

Diabetes and Pregnancy

Pregnancy can be complicated by diabetes in one of two settings: when women with preexisting diabetes become pregnant ("pregestational" or overt diabetes), or women who were previously euglycemic develop impaired glucose tolerance and diabetes for the first time during pregnancy ("gestational" diabetes). Approximately 5% of pregnancies occurring in the United States are complicated by hyperglycemia, and the incidence of both pregestational and gestational diabetes is rising in parallel with the rising incidence of obesity and diabetes in the general population. Pregnancy is a "diabetogenic" state in which the prevailing hormonal milieu favors a state of insulin resistance. In a previously euglycemic woman who is otherwise susceptible due to concurrent genetic and environmental factors, the consequence may be gestational diabetes. Women with pregestational diabetes (where hyperglycemia is already present in the periconception period) have an increased risk of *stillbirth* and *congenital malformations* in the fetus. Poorly controlled diabetes that arises later in pregnancy, regardless of prior history, can lead to excessive birth weight in the newborn (*macrosomia*), as well as long-term sequelae for the child exposed to a diabetic environment in utero, including obesity and diabetes later in life. Gestational diabetes typically resolves following delivery; however, the majority of women with this condition will develop overt diabetes over the next 10 to 20 years.

Clinical Features of Diabetes

It is difficult to sketch with brevity the diverse clinical presentations of diabetes mellitus. We will discuss the most common initial presentation or mode of diagnosis for each of the two major subtypes, followed by a discussion of acute, and then chronic (long-term) complications of diabetes.

Type 1 diabetes was formerly thought to occur primarily in persons younger than age 18 but is now known to occur at any age. In the initial 1 or 2 years following the onset of overt type 1 diabetes, the exogenous insulin requirements may be minimal because of ongoing endogenous insulin secretion (referred to as the *honeymoon period*). Thereafter, any residual β-cell reserve is exhausted and insulin requirements increase dramatically. Although β-cell destruction is a prolonged process, the transition from impaired glucose tolerance to overt diabetes may be abrupt and is often brought on by an event, such as infection, that is also associated with increased insulin requirements.

In contrast to type 1 diabetes, patients with **type 2 diabetes** are typically older than 40 years and frequently obese. However, with the increase in obesity and sedentary lifestyle in this society, type 2 diabetes is being seen in children and adolescents with increasing frequency. In some cases, medical attention is sought because of unexplained fatigue, dizziness, or blurred vision. **Most frequently, however, the diagnosis of type 2 diabetes is made after routine blood testing in asymptomatic persons.** In fact, in light of the large number of asymptomatic individuals with undiagnosed hyperglycemia in the United States, routine glucose testing is recommended for everyone older than 45 years of age.

The Classic Triad of Diabetes

The onset of type 1 diabetes is usually marked by the triad of polyuria, polydipsia, polyphagia, and, when severe, diabetic ketoacidosis, all resulting from metabolic derangements. Because insulin is a major anabolic hormone, its deficiency results in a *catabolic* state that affects not only glucose metabolism but also fat and protein metabolism. Unopposed secretion of counterregulatory hormones (glucagon, growth hormone, epinephrine) also plays a role in these metabolic derangements. The assimilation of glucose into muscle and adipose tissue is sharply diminished or abolished. Not only does storage of glycogen in liver and muscle cease, but also reserves are depleted by glycogenolysis. The resultant hyperglycemia exceeds the renal threshold for reabsorption, and glycosuria ensues. The glycosuria induces an osmotic diuresis and thus *polyuria,* causing a profound loss of water and electrolytes (Fig. 24-33). The obligatory renal water loss combined with the hyperosmolarity resulting from the increased levels of glucose in the blood tends to deplete intracellular water, triggering the osmoreceptors of the thirst centers of the brain. In this manner, intense thirst (*polydipsia*) appears. With a deficiency of insulin the scales swing from insulin-promoted anabolism to catabolism of proteins and fats. Proteolysis follows, releasing gluconeogenic amino acids that are removed by the liver and used as building blocks for glucose. The catabolism of proteins and fats tends to induce a negative energy balance, which in turn leads to increasing appetite (*polyphagia*), thus completing the classic triad of diabetes: polyuria, polydipsia, and polyphagia. Despite the increased appetite, catabolic effects prevail, resulting in weight loss and muscle weakness. The combination of polyphagia and weight loss is paradoxical and should always raise the suspicion of diabetes.

Acute Metabolic Complications of Diabetes

Diabetic ketoacidosis is a severe acute metabolic complication of type 1 diabetes, but may also occur in type 2 diabetes, though not as commonly and not to as marked an

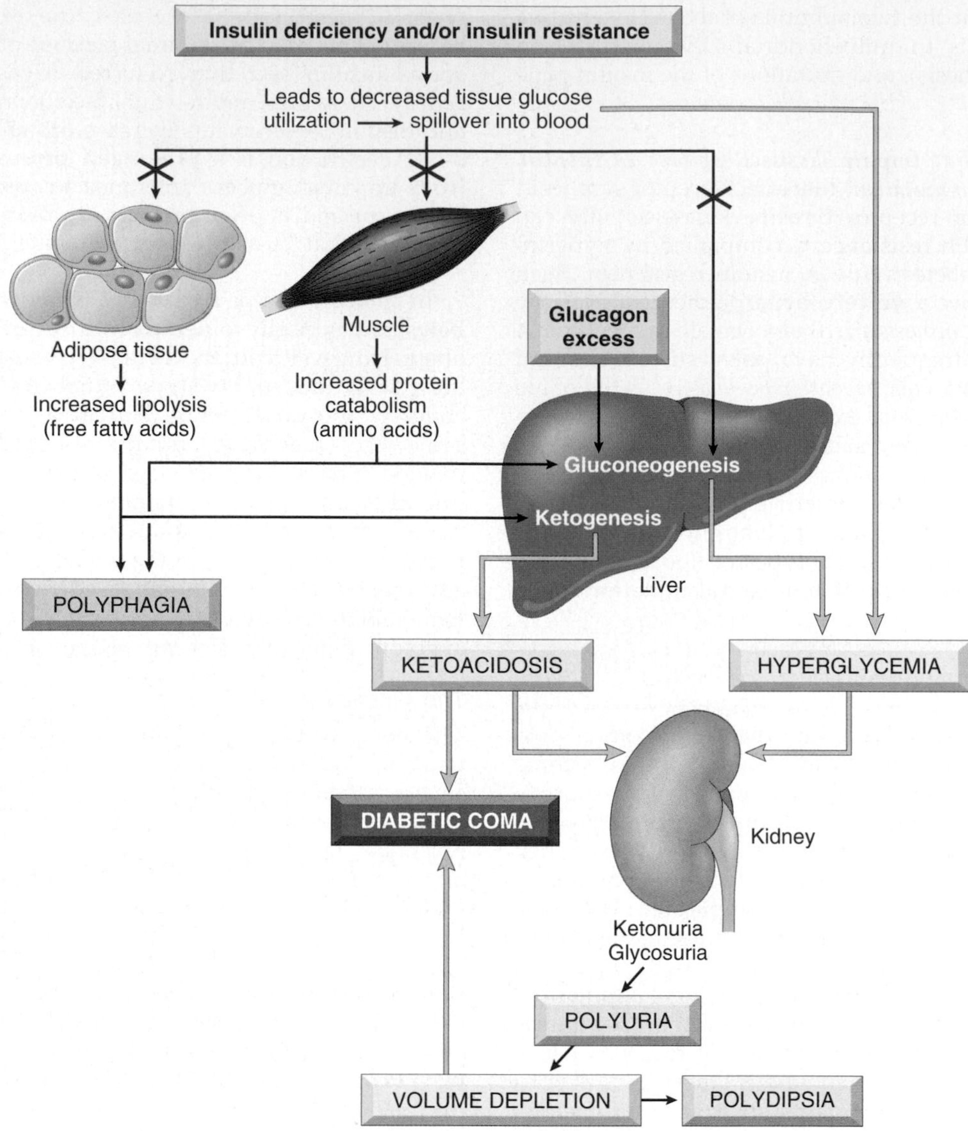

Figure 24-33 Sequence of metabolic derangements underlying the clinical manifestations of diabetes. An absolute insulin deficiency leads to a catabolic state, culminating in ketoacidosis and severe volume depletion. These cause sufficient central nervous system compromise to lead to coma and eventual death if left untreated.

extent. The most common precipitating factor is a failure to take insulin, although other stressors such as intercurrent infections, illness, trauma and certain drugs might also lead to this complication. Many of these factors are associated with the release of the catecholamine *epinephrine*, which blocks any residual insulin action and stimulates the secretion of glucagon. The insulin deficiency coupled with glucagon excess decreases peripheral utilization of glucose while increasing gluconeogenesis, severely exacerbating hyperglycemia (the plasma glucose levels are usually in the range of 250 to 600 mg/dL). The hyperglycemia causes an osmotic diuresis and dehydration characteristic of the ketoacidotic state.

The second major effect of insulin deficiency is activation of the ketogenic machinery. Insulin deficiency stimulates lipoprotein lipase, with resultant breakdown of adipose stores and an increase in levels of free fatty acids. When these free fatty acids reach the liver, they are esterified to fatty acyl coenzyme A. Oxidation of fatty acyl coenzyme A molecules within the hepatic mitochondria produces *ketone bodies* (acetoacetic acid and β-hydroxybutyric acid). The rate at which ketone bodies are formed may exceed the rate at which acetoacetic acid and β-hydroxybutyric acid can be utilized by peripheral tissues, leading to *ketonemia* and *ketonuria*. If the urinary excretion of ketones is compromised by dehydration, the result is a systemic *metabolic ketoacidosis*. Release of ketogenic amino acids by protein catabolism aggravates the ketotic state.

The clinical manifestations of diabetic ketoacidosis include fatigue, nausea and vomiting, severe abdominal pain, a characteristic fruity odor, and deep, labored breathing (also known as *Kussmaul breathing*). Persistence of the ketotic state eventually leads to depression in cerebral consciousness and coma. Reversal of ketoacidosis requires administration of insulin, correction of metabolic acidosis, and treatment of the underlying precipitating factors such as infection.

In contrast to type 1 diabetes, the frequency of ketoacidosis is significantly lower in type 2 diabetes, presumably because of higher portal vein insulin levels in these patients, which prevents unrestricted hepatic fatty acid oxidation and keeps the formation of ketone bodies in check. Instead, **type 2 diabetics may develop a condition known as hyperosmolar hyperosmotic syndrome** (HHS) due to severe dehydration resulting from sustained osmotic diuresis (particularly in patients who do not drink enough water to compensate for urinary losses from chronic hyperglycemia). Typically, the patient is an older diabetic who is disabled by a stroke or an infection and is unable to maintain adequate water intake. Furthermore, the absence of ketoacidosis and its symptoms (nausea, vomiting, Kussmaul breathing) delays the seeking of medical attention until severe dehydration and impairment of mental status occur. The hyperglycemia is usually more severe than in diabetic ketoacidosis, in the range of 600 to 1200 mg/dL.

Ironically, the most common acute metabolic complication in either type of diabetes is *hypoglycemia*, usually as a result of having missed a meal, excessive physical exertion, an excess insulin administration, or during the phase of dose finding for antidiabetic agents. The signs and symptoms of hypoglycemia include dizziness, confusion, sweating, palpitations, and tachycardia; if hypoglycemia persists, loss of consciousness may occur. Reversal of hypoglycemia through oral or intravenous glucose intake prevents the onset of permanent neurological damage.

Chronic Complications of Diabetes

The morbidity associated with longstanding diabetes of either type is due to damage induced in large- and medium-sized muscular arteries (*diabetic macrovascular disease*) and in small vessels (*diabetic macrovascular disease*) by chronic hyperglycemia. Macrovascular disease causes accelerated atherosclerosis among diabetics, resulting in increased risk of myocardial infarction, stroke, and lower extremity ischemia. The effects of microvascular disease are most profound in the retina, kidneys, and peripheral nerves, resulting in *diabetic retinopathy, nephropathy, and neuropathy,* respectively (see later).

Pathogenesis of Chronic Complications. **Persistent hyperglycemia ("glucotoxicity") seems to be responsible for the long term complications of diabetes**. Much of the evidence supporting a role for glycemic control in ameliorating the long-term complications of diabetes has come from large randomized trials. The assessment of glycemic control in these trials has been based on the percentage of *glycated hemoglobin*, also known as Hb_{A1C}, which is formed by nonenzymatic covalent addition of glucose moieties to hemoglobin in red cells. Unlike blood glucose levels, Hb_{A1C} provides a measure of glycemic control over the lifespan of a red cell (120 days) and is affected little by day-to-day variations. *It is recommended that Hb_{A1C} be maintained below 7% in diabetic patients.* It is important to stress that hyperglycemia is not the only factor responsible for the long-term complications of diabetes, and that other underlying abnormalities, such as insulin resistance, and co-morbidities like obesity, also play an important role.

At least four distinct mechanisms have been implicated in the deleterious effects of persistent hyperglycemia on peripheral tissues, although the primacy of any one over the others is unclear. **In each of the proposed mechanisms, increased glucose flux through various intracellular metabolic pathways is thought to generate harmful precursors that contribute to end organ damage**.

Formation of Advanced Glycation End Products. *Advanced glycation end products* (AGEs) are formed as a result of nonenzymatic reactions between intracellular glucose-derived dicarbonyl precursors (glyoxal, methylglyoxal, and 3-deoxyglucosone) with the amino groups of both intracellular and extracellular proteins. The natural rate of AGE formation is greatly accelerated in the presence of hyperglycemia. AGEs bind to a specific receptor (RAGE) that is expressed on inflammatory cells (macrophages and T cells), endothelium, and vascular smooth muscle. The detrimental effects of the AGE-RAGE signaling axis within the vascular compartment include:

- Release of *cytokines and growth factors*, including *transforming growth factor β* (TGFβ), which leads to deposition of excess basement membrane material, and *vascular endothelial growth factor* (VEGF), implicated in diabetic retinopathy (see later)
- Generation of *reactive oxygen species* (ROS) in endothelial cells
- Increased *procoagulant activity* on endothelial cells and macrophages
- Enhanced *proliferation of vascular smooth muscle cells* and *synthesis of extracellular matrix*

Not surprisingly, endothelium specific overexpression of RAGE in diabetic mice accelerates large vessel injury and microangiopathy, while RAGE-null mice show attenuation of these features. Antagonists of RAGE have emerged as a therapeutic strategy in diabetes and are being tested in clinical trials.

In addition to receptor-mediated effects, AGEs can directly cross-link extracellular matrix proteins. Cross-linking of collagen type I molecules in large vessels decreases their elasticity, which may predispose these vessels to shear stress and endothelial injury (Chapter 11). Similarly, AGE-induced cross-linking of type IV collagen in basement membrane decreases endothelial cell adhesion and increases extravasation of fluid. Proteins cross-linked by AGEs are resistant to proteolytic digestion. Thus, cross-linking decreases protein removal while enhancing protein deposition. AGE-modified matrix components also trap nonglycated plasma or interstitial proteins. In large vessels, trapping of LDL, for example, retards its efflux from the vessel wall and enhances the deposition of cholesterol in the intima, thus accelerating atherogenesis (Chapter 11). In capillaries, including those of renal glomeruli, plasma proteins such as albumin bind to the glycated basement membrane, accounting in part for the basement membrane thickening that is characteristic of diabetic microangiopathy.

Activation of Protein Kinase C. Calcium-dependent activation of intracellular protein kinase C (PKC) and the second messenger diacyl glycerol (DAG) is an important signal transduction pathway. Intracellular hyperglycemia stimulates the *de novo* synthesis of DAG from glycolytic intermediates, and hence causes excessive PKC activation. The downstream effects of PKC activation are numerous, including production of VEGF, TGF-β, and the procoagulant protein plasminogen activator inhibitor-1 (PAI-1) (Chapter 4) by the vascular endothelium.

It should be evident that some effects of AGEs and activated PKC are overlapping, and both likely contribute to diabetic microangiopathy.

Oxidative Stress and Disturbances in Polyol Pathways. Even in some tissues that do not require insulin for glucose transport (e.g., nerves, lenses, kidneys, blood vessels), persistent hyperglycemia in the extracellular milieu leads to an increase in intracellular glucose. This excess glucose is metabolized by the enzyme *aldose reductase* to sorbitol, a polyol, and eventually to fructose, in a reaction that uses NADPH (the reduced form of nicotinamide dinucleotide phosphate) as a cofactor. NADPH is also required by the enzyme glutathione reductase in a reaction that regenerates reduced glutathione (GSH). GSH is one of the important antioxidant mechanisms in the cell (Chapter 2), and any reduction in GSH increases cellular susceptibility to ROS ("oxidative stress"). In the face of sustained hyperglycemia, progressive depletion of intracellular NADPH by aldol reductase compromises GSH regeneration, increasing cellular susceptibility to oxidative stress. Sorbitol accumulation in the lens contributes to cataract formation.

Hexosamine Pathways and Generation of Fructose-6-Phosphate. Finally, it is postulated that hyperglycemia-induced flux through the hexosamine pathway increases intracellular levels of *fructose-6-phosphate*, which is a substrate for glycosylation of proteins, leading to generation of excess proteoglycans. These glycosylation changes are accompanied by abnormal expression of TGFβ or PAI-1, which further exacerbate the end-organ damage.

Morphology and Clinical Features of Chronic Complications of Diabetes

The important morphologic changes are related to the many late systemic complications of diabetes. As previously discussed, these changes are seen in both type 1 and type 2 diabetes (Fig. 24-34). We will first discuss the morphologic changes and then describe the clinical manifestations resulting from the altered morphology.

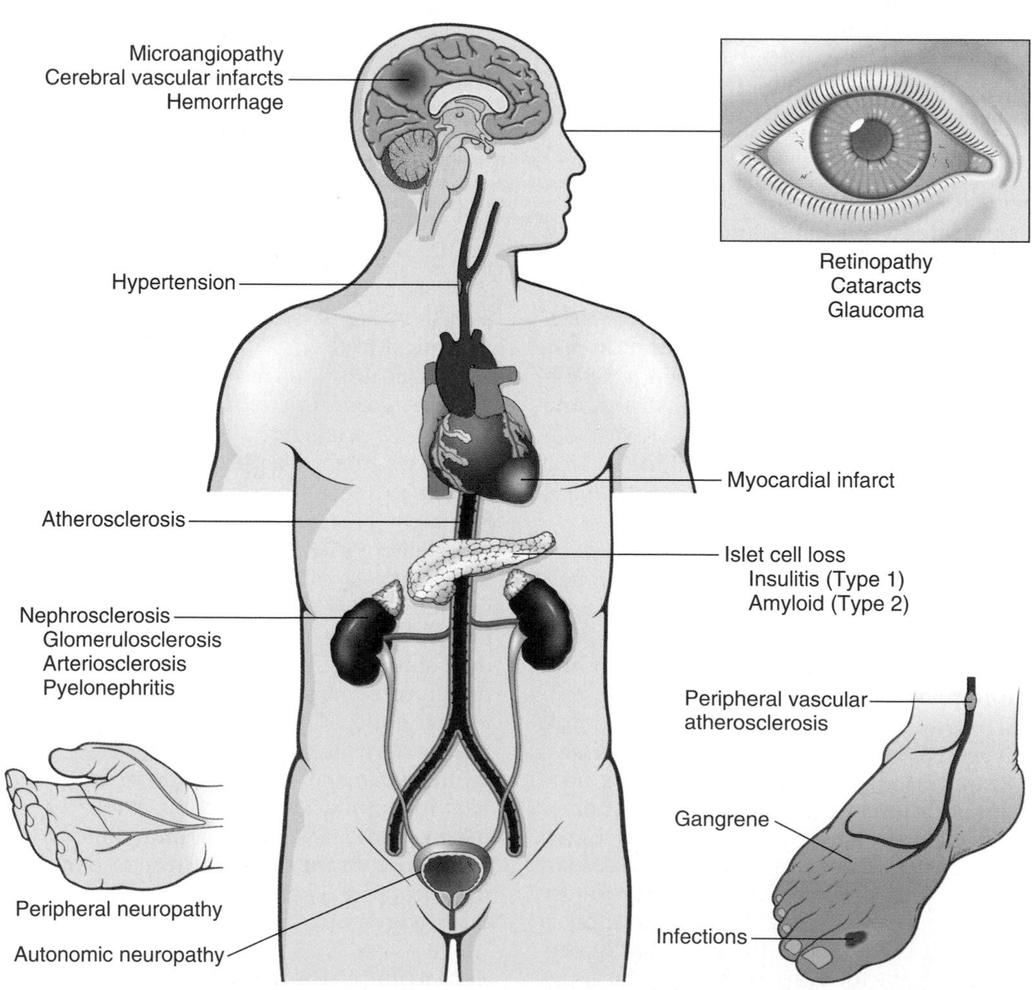

Figure 24-34 Long-term complications of diabetes.

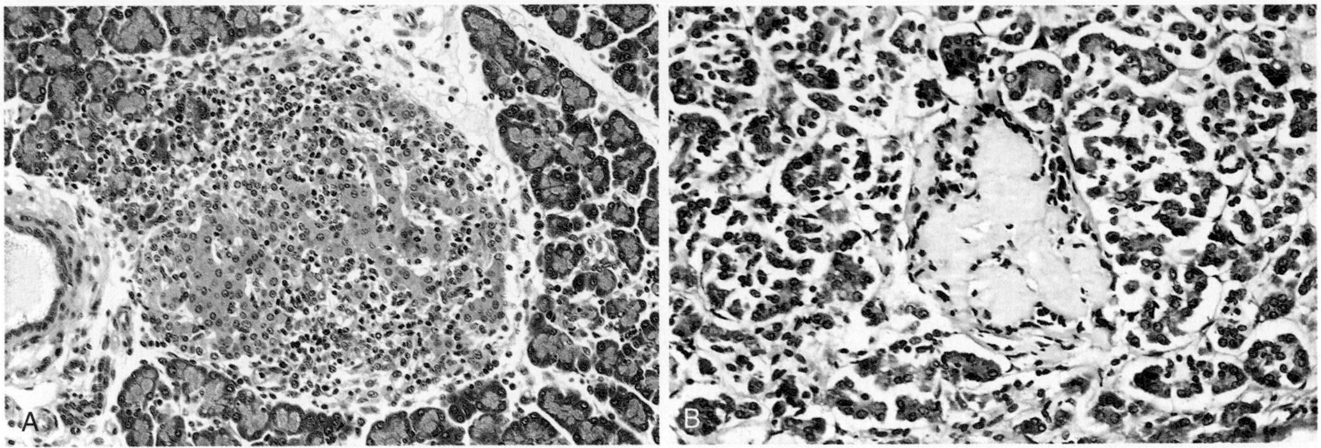

Figure 24-35 A, Insulitis, shown here from a rat (BB) model of autoimmune diabetes, also seen in type 1 human diabetes. **B,** Amyloidosis of a pancreatic islet in type 2 diabetes. (**A,** Courtesy Dr. Arthur Like, University of Massachusetts, Worchester, Mass.)

MORPHOLOGY

Pancreas

Lesions in the pancreas are inconstant and rarely of diagnostic value. Distinctive changes are more commonly associated with type 1 than with type 2 diabetes. One or more of the following alterations may be present:

- **Reduction in the number and size of islets.** This is most often seen in type 1 diabetes, particularly with rapidly advancing disease. Most of the islets are small and inconspicuous.
- **Leukocytic infiltrates in the islets** (insulitis) are principally composed of T lymphocytes, and are also seen in animal models of autoimmune diabetes (Fig. 24-35*A*). Lymphocytic infiltrates may be present in type 1 diabetics at the time of clinical presentation. The distribution of insulitis may be strikingly uneven in infants who fail to survive the immediate postnatal period.
- **In type 2 diabetes there may be a subtle reduction in islet cell mass,** demonstrated only by special morphometric studies.
- **Amyloid deposition within islets in type 2 diabetes** begins in and around capillaries and between cells. At advanced stages, the islets may be virtually obliterated (Fig. 24-35*B*); fibrosis may also be observed. Similar lesions may be found in older nondiabetics, apparently as part of normal aging.
- **An increase in the number and size of islets** is especially characteristic of nondiabetic newborns of diabetic mothers. Presumably, fetal islets undergo hyperplasia in response to the maternal hyperglycemia.

Diabetic Macrovascular Disease

Diabetes exacts a heavy toll on the vascular system. **Endothelial dysfunction** (Chapter 11), which predisposes to atherosclerosis and other cardiovascular morbidities, is widespread in diabetes, as a consequence of the deleterious effects of persistent hyperglycemia and insulin resistance on the vascular compartment. The hallmark of diabetic macrovascular disease is **accelerated atherosclerosis** involving the aorta and large- and medium-sized arteries. Except for its greater severity and earlier age at onset, atherosclerosis in diabetics is indistinguishable from that in nondiabetics (Chapter 11). **Myocardial infarction, caused by atherosclerosis of the coronary arteries, is the most common cause of death in diabetics. Gangrene of the lower extremities,** as a result of advanced vascular disease, is about 100 times more common in diabetics than in the general population. The larger renal arteries are also subject to severe atherosclerosis, but the most damaging effect of diabetes on the kidneys is exerted at the level of the glomeruli and the microcirculation. This is discussed later.

Hyaline arteriolosclerosis, the vascular lesion associated with hypertension (Chapters 11 and 20), is both more prevalent and more severe in diabetics than in nondiabetics, but it is not specific for diabetes and may be seen in older nondiabetics without hypertension. It takes the form of an amorphous, hyaline thickening of the wall of the arterioles, which causes narrowing of the lumen (Fig. 24-36). Not surprisingly, in diabetics it is related not only to the duration of the disease but also to the level of blood pressure.

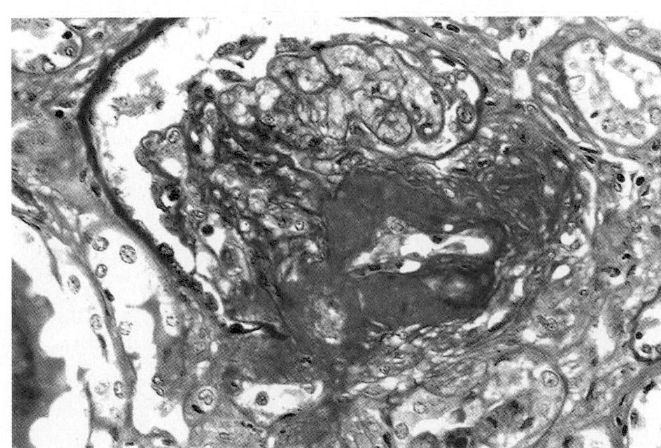

Figure 24-36 Severe renal hyaline arteriolosclerosis. Note a markedly thickened, tortuous afferent arteriole. The amorphous nature of the thickened vascular wall is evident. (PAS stain). (Courtesy M.A. Venkatachalam, MD, Department of Pathology, University of Texas Health Science Center at San Antonio, Texas.)

Diabetic Microangiopathy

One of the most consistent morphologic features of diabetes is **diffuse thickening of basement membranes**. The thickening is most evident in the capillaries of the skin, skeletal muscle, retina, renal glomeruli, and renal medulla. However, it may also be seen in such nonvascular structures as renal tubules, the Bowman capsule, peripheral nerves, and placenta. It should be noted that despite the increase in the thickness of basement membranes, **diabetic capillaries are more leaky than normal to plasma proteins. The microangiopathy underlies the development of diabetic nephropathy, retinopathy, and some forms of neuropathy.** An indistinguishable microangiopathy can be found in aged nondiabetic patients but rarely to the extent seen in patients with long-standing diabetes.

Diabetic Nephropathy

The kidneys are prime targets of diabetes. Renal failure is second only to myocardial infarction as a cause of death from this disease. **Three lesions are encountered: (1) glomerular lesions; (2) renal vascular lesions, principally arteriolosclerosis; and (3) pyelonephritis, including necrotizing papillitis.**

The most important glomerular lesions are capillary basement membrane thickening, diffuse mesangial sclerosis, and nodular glomerulosclerosis.

Capillary Basement Membrane Thickening. Widespread thickening of the glomerular capillary basement membrane (GBM) occurs in virtually all cases of diabetic nephropathy and is part and parcel of the diabetic microangiopathy. Pure capillary basement membrane thickening can be detected only by electron microscopy (Fig. 24-37). Careful morphometric studies demonstrate that this thickening begins as early as 2 years after the onset of type 1 diabetes and by 5 years amounts to about a 30% increase. The thickening continues progressively and usually concurrently with mesangial widening. Simultaneously, there is thickening of the tubular basement membranes (Fig. 24-38).

Diffuse Mesangial Sclerosis. This lesion consists of **diffuse increase in mesangial matrix**. There can be mild proliferation of mesangial cells early in the disease process, but cell proliferation is not a prominent part of this injury. The mesangial increase is typically associated with the overall thickening of the GBM. The matrix depositions are PAS-positive (Fig. 24-39). As the disease progresses, the expansion of mesangial areas can extend to nodular configurations. The progressive expansion of the mesangium has been shown to correlate well with measures of deteriorating renal function such as increasing proteinuria.

Nodular Glomerulosclerosis. This is also known as **intercapillary glomerulosclerosis or Kimmelstiel-Wilson disease**. The glomerular lesions take the form of ovoid or spherical, often laminated, nodules of matrix situated in the periphery of the glomerulus. The nodules are PAS-positive. They lie within the mesangial core of the glomerular lobules and can be surrounded by patent peripheral capillary loops (Fig. 24-39) or loops that are markedly dilated. The nodules often show features of mesangiolysis with fraying of the mesangial/capillary lumen interface and disruption of sites at which the capillaries are anchored into the mesangial stalks. The latter may produce capillary microaneurysms as the untethered capillaries distend outward due to force imparted by intracapillary blood pressure and flow. Usually, not all the lobules in individual glomeruli are

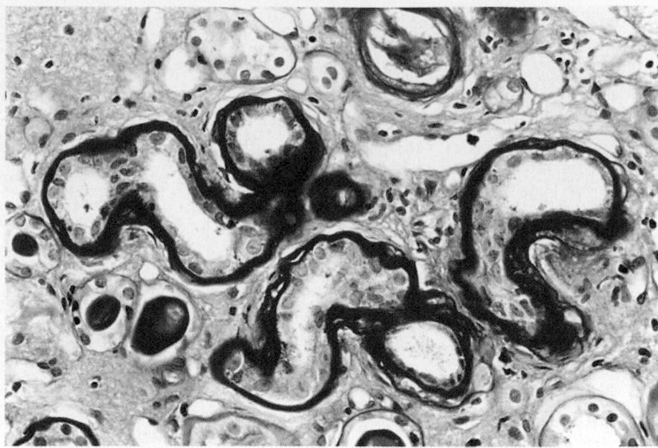

Figure 24-38 Renal cortex showing thickening of tubular basement membranes in a diabetic patient (PAS stain).

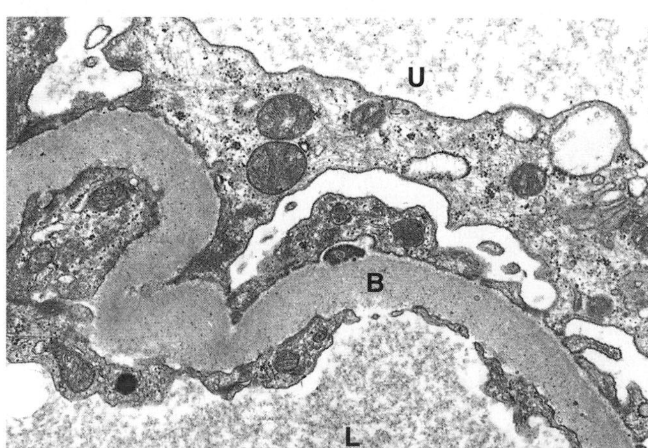

Figure 24-37 Electron micrograph of a renal glomerulus showing markedly thickened glomerular basement membrane (B) in a diabetic. L, glomerular capillary lumen; U, urinary space. (Courtesy Dr. Michael Kashgarian, Department of Pathology, Yale University School of Medicine, New Haven, Conn.)

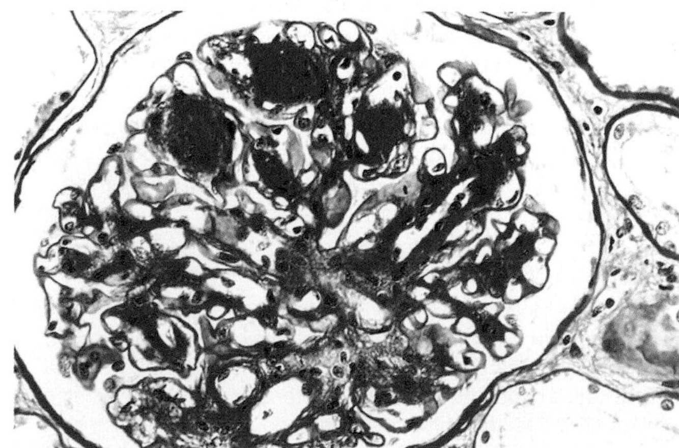

Figure 24-39 Diffuse and nodular diabetic glomerulosclerosis (PAS stain). Note the diffuse increase in mesangial matrix and characteristic acellular PAS-positive nodules.

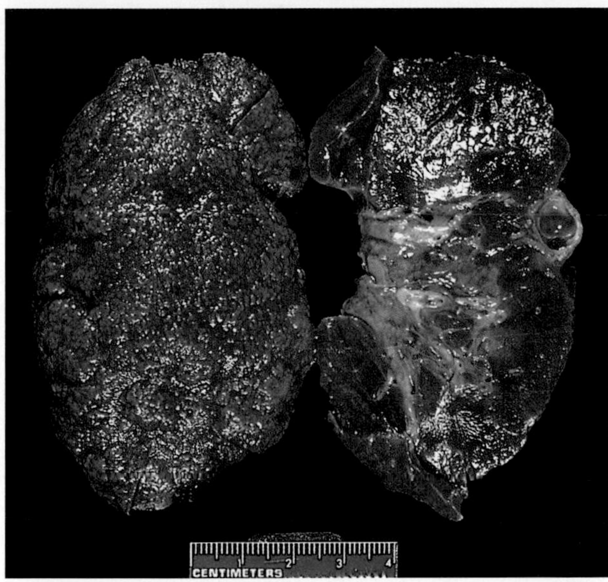

Figure 24-40 Nephrosclerosis in a patient with long-standing diabetes. The kidney has been bisected to demonstrate both diffuse granular transformation of the surface *(left)* and marked thinning of the cortical tissue *(right)*. Additional features include some irregular depressions, the result of pyelonephritis, and an incidental cortical cyst *(far right)*.

involved by nodular lesions, but even uninvolved lobules and glomeruli show striking diffuse mesangial sclerosis. As the disease advances, the individual nodules enlarge and may eventually compress and engulf capillaries, obliterating the glomerular tuft. These nodular lesions are frequently accompanied by prominent accumulations of hyaline material in capillary loops ("**fibrin caps**") or adherent to Bowman capsules ("**capsular drops**"). Both afferent and efferent glomerular hilar arterioles show hyalinosis. As a consequence of the glomerular and arteriolar lesions, the kidney suffers from ischemia, develops tubular atrophy and interstitial fibrosis, and usually undergoes overall contraction in size (Fig. 24-40). Approximately 15% to 30% of individuals with long-term diabetes develop nodular glomerulosclerosis, and in most instances it is associated with renal failure.

Renal atherosclerosis and arteriolosclerosis constitute part of the macrovascular disease in diabetics. The kidney is one of the most frequently and severely affected organs; however, the changes in the arteries and arterioles are similar to those found in other tissues. Hyaline arteriolosclerosis affects not only the afferent but also the efferent arteriole. Such efferent arteriolosclerosis is rarely, if ever, encountered in individuals who do not have diabetes.

Pyelonephritis is an acute or chronic inflammation of the kidneys that usually begins in the interstitial tissue and then spreads to affect the tubules. Both the acute and chronic forms of this disease are more common in diabetics than in the general population, and, once affected, diabetics tend to have more severe involvement. One special pattern of acute pyelonephritis, **necrotizing papillitis** (or papillary necrosis), is much more prevalent in diabetics than in nondiabetics.

Diabetic Ocular Complications

The eye is profoundly affected by diabetes mellitus. The architecture and microanatomy of the eye are discussed in Chapter 29.

Diabetes-induced hyperglycemia leads to acquired opacification of the lens, a condition known as *cataract*. Long-standing diabetes is also associated with increased intraocular pressure (**glaucoma**) (see later), and resulting damage to the optic nerve.

The most profound histopathologic changes of diabetes are seen in the retina. The retinal vasculopathy of diabetes mellitus can be classified into *background (preproliferative) diabetic retinopathy* and *proliferative diabetic retinopathy* (Chapter 29).

Diabetic Neuropathy

The prevalence of peripheral neuropathy in individuals with diabetes depends on the duration of the disease; up to 50% of diabetics overall have peripheral neuropathy clinically, and up to 80% of those who have had the disease for more than 15 years. This is discussed further in Chapter 27.

Clinical Manifestations of Chronic Diabetes

Table 24-7 summarizes some of the pertinent clinical, genetic, and histopathologic features that distinguish type 1 and type 2 diabetes. **In both types it is the long-term effects of diabetes, more than the acute metabolic complications, that are responsible for the overwhelming majority of the morbidity and mortality**. In most instances these complications appear approximately 15 to 20 years after the onset of hyperglycemia. The severity of chronic complications is related to both the degree and the duration of hyperglycemia, as evidenced by the attenuation of end-organ damage by effective glycemic control in prospective studies.

- **Macrovascular complications such as myocardial infarction, renal vascular insufficiency, and cerebrovascular accidents are the most common causes of mortality in long-standing diabetes**. Diabetics have a two to four times greater incidence of coronary artery disease, and a fourfold higher risk of dying from cardiovascular complications than nondiabetics. An elevated risk for cardiovascular disease is even observed in prediabetics. Significantly, myocardial infarction is almost as common in diabetic women as in diabetic men. In contrast, myocardial infarction is uncommon in nondiabetic women of reproductive age. Diabetes is often accompanied by underlying conditions that favor the development of adverse cardiovascular events. For example, *hypertension* is found in approximately 75% of individuals with type 2 diabetes and potentiates the effects of hyperglycemia and insulin resistance on endothelial dysfunction and atherosclerosis. Another cardiovascular risk frequently seen in diabetics is *dyslipidemia,* which includes both increased triglycerides and LDL levels and decreased levels of the "protective" lipoprotein, high-density lipoprotein (Chapter 11). Insulin resistance is believed to contribute to "diabetic dyslipidemia" by favoring the hepatic production of atherogenic lipoproteins and by suppressing the uptake of circulating lipids in peripheral tissues. Finally, diabetics have elevated levels of PAI-1, which is an inhibitor of fibrinolysis and therefore acts as a procoagulant in the formation of atherosclerotic plaques.

- ***Diabetic nephropathy* is a leading cause of end-stage renal disease in the United States.** Approximately 30% to 40% of all diabetics develop clinical evidence of nephropathy, but a considerably smaller fraction of patients with type 2 diabetes progress to end-stage renal disease. However, because of the much greater prevalence of type 2 diabetes, these patients constitute slightly over half the diabetic patients starting dialysis each year.

  The frequency of diabetic nephropathy is greatly influenced by the genetic makeup of the population in question; for example, Native Americans, Hispanics, and African Americans have a greater risk of developing end-stage renal disease than do non-Hispanic whites with type 2 diabetes. The earliest manifestation of diabetic nephropathy is the appearance of low amounts of albumin in the urine (>30 mg/day, but <300 mg/day), that is, *microalbuminuria*. Notably, microalbuminuria is also a marker for greatly increased cardiovascular morbidity and mortality for persons with either type 1 or type 2 diabetes. Therefore, all patients with microalbuminuria should be screened for macrovascular disease, and aggressive intervention should be undertaken to reduce cardiovascular risk factors. Without specific interventions, approximately 80% of type 1 diabetics and 20% to 40% of type 2 diabetics will develop *overt nephropathy with macroalbuminuria* (>300 mg of urinary albumin per day) over 10 to 15 years, usually accompanied by the appearance of hypertension. The progression from overt nephropathy to end-stage renal disease is highly variable, but by 20 years, more than 75% of type 1 diabetics and approximately 20% of type 2 diabetics with overt nephropathy will develop end-stage renal disease, requiring dialysis or renal transplantation.
- ***Visual impairment*, sometimes even total blindness, is one of the more feared consequences of long-standing diabetes.** Approximately 60% to 80% of patients develop some form of *diabetic retinopathy* approximately 15 to 20 years after diagnosis. The fundamental lesion of retinopathy—neovascularization—is attributable to hypoxia-induced overexpression of VEGF in the retina. Current treatment for this condition includes administration of antiangiogenic agents. As stated earlier, diabetics also have an increased propensity for *glaucoma* and *cataract formation*, both of which contribute to visual impairment in diabetes.
- *Diabetic neuropathy* can elicit a variety of clinical syndromes, afflicting the central nervous system, peripheral sensorimotor nerves, and the autonomic nervous system. **The most frequent pattern of involvement is a *distal symmetric polyneuropathy* of the lower extremities that affects both motor and sensory function.** Over time the upper extremities may be involved as well, thus approximating a "glove and stocking" pattern of polyneuropathy. Other forms include *autonomic neuropathy*, which produces disturbances in bowel and bladder function and sometimes erectile dysfunction, and *diabetic mononeuropathy*, which may manifest as sudden footdrop, wristdrop, or isolated cranial nerve palsies.
- **Diabetics are plagued by enhanced susceptibility to infections of the skin and to tuberculosis, pneumonia, and pyelonephritis.** Such infections cause the deaths of about 5% of diabetics. In an individual with diabetic neuropathy, a trivial infection in a toe may be the first event in a long succession of complications (gangrene, bacteremia, pneumonia) that may ultimately lead to death. The basis of enhanced susceptibility is multifactorial, and includes decreased neutrophil functions (chemotaxis, adherence to the endothelium, phagocytosis, and microbicidal activity), and impaired cytokine production by macrophages. The vascular compromise also reduces delivery of circulating cells and molecules that are required for host defense.

The staggering numbers and the societal and economic impact of diabetes have already been discussed. For the most part, diabetes remains a lifelong diagnosis, although pancreatic islet cell transplantation has the potential to ameliorate type 1 diabetes for many patients. For some individuals with type 2 diabetes, dietary modifications, exercise and weight loss regimens can reduce insulin resistance and hyperglycemia at least early in the disease. However, all patients will ultimately require some form of therapeutic intervention to maintain glycemic control.

KEY CONCEPTS

Diabetes Mellitus: Pathogenesis and Long-Term Complications

- Type 1 diabetes is an *autoimmune disease* characterized by progressive destruction of islet β cells, leading to absolute insulin deficiency. The fundamental immune abnormality in type 1 diabetes is a failure of self-tolerance in T cells, and circulating autoantibodies to islet cell antigens (including insulin) often are detected in affected patients.
- Type 2 diabetes has no autoimmune basis; instead, features central to its pathogenesis are *insulin resistance* and *β-cell dysfunction*, resulting in relative insulin deficiency.
- *Obesity* has an important relationship with insulin resistance (and hence type 2 diabetes), mediated through multiple factors including excess free fatty acids, cytokines released from adipose tissues (adipocytokines), and inflammation.
- Monogenic forms of diabetes are uncommon and are caused by single-gene defects that result in primary β-cell dysfunction (e.g., *glucokinase* mutation) or lead to abnormalities of insulin-insulin receptor signaling (e.g., insulin receptor gene mutations).
- The long-term complications of diabetes are similar in both types and involve four potential mechanisms resulting from sustained hyperglycemia: formation of advanced glycation end products (AGEs), activation of protein kinase C (PKC), disturbances in the polyol pathways leading to oxidative stress, and overload of the hexosamine pathway.
- Long term complications of diabetes include both large vessel disease (*macroangiopathy*), such as atherosclerosis, ischemic heart disease and lower extremity ischemia, as well as small vessel disease (*microangiopathy*), the latter manifesting mainly as retinopathy, nephropathy and neuropathy.

Pancreatic Neuroendocrine Tumors

The preferred term for tumors of the pancreatic islet cells ("islet cell tumors") is *pancreatic neuroendocrine tumors or PanNETs*. They are rare in comparison with tumors of the exocrine pancreas, accounting for only 2% of all pancreatic neoplasms. PanNETs can occur anywhere along the length of the pancreas, embedded in the substance of the pancreas or arising in the immediate peripancreatic tissues. They resemble their counterparts, carcinoid tumors, found elsewhere in the alimentary tract (Chapter 17). These tumors may be single or multiple and benign or malignant. Pancreatic endocrine neoplasms often elaborate pancreatic hormones, or may be nonfunctional.

Like other endocrine neoplasms, it is difficult to predict the behavior of a pancreatic endocrine neoplasm based on their light microscopic appearance. Unequivocal criteria for malignancy include metastases, vascular invasion, and local infiltration. The functional status of the tumor has some impact on prognosis, in that approximately 90% of insulin producing tumors are benign, while 60% to 90% of other functioning and nonfunctioning pancreatic endocrine neoplasms are malignant. Fortunately, insulinomas are the most common subtype of pancreatic endocrine neoplasms.

The genome of sporadic PanNETs recently has been sequenced, with identification of recurrent somatic alterations in three major genes or pathways:

- *MEN1*, which causes familial MEN syndrome, type 1, also is mutated in a number of sporadic neuroendocrine tumors
- Loss-of-function mutations in tumor suppressor genes such *PTEN* and *TSC2* (Chapter 7), which result in activation of the oncogenic mammalian TOR (mTOR) signaling pathway.
- Inactivating mutations in two genes, *alpha-thalassemia/mental retardation syndrome, X-linked* (*ATRX*) and death-domain associated protein (*DAXX*), which have multiple cellular functions, including telomere maintenance. Of note, nearly half of PanNETs have a somatic mutation in either *ATRX* or *DAXX*, but not both, suggesting that the encoded proteins function in a critical common pathway.

The three most common and distinctive clinical syndromes associated with functional pancreatic endocrine neoplasms are (1) *hyperinsulinism*, (2) *hypergastrinemia and the Zollinger-Ellison syndrome*, and (3) *multiple endocrine neoplasia (MEN)* (described in detail later).

Hyperinsulinism (Insulinoma)

β-cell tumors (insulinomas) are the most common of pancreatic endocrine neoplasms, and may produce sufficient insulin to induce clinically significant hypoglycemia. The characteristic clinical picture is dominated by hypoglycemic episodes, which occur if the blood glucose level falls below 50 mg/dL of serum. The clinical manifestations include confusion, stupor, and loss of consciousness. These episodes are precipitated by fasting or exercise and are promptly relieved by feeding or parenteral administration of glucose.

MORPHOLOGY

Insulinomas are most often found within the pancreas and are generally benign. Most are solitary, although multiple tumors may be encountered. *Bona fide* carcinomas, making up only about 10% of cases, are diagnosed on the basis of local invasion and distant metastases. On rare occasions an insulinoma may arise in ectopic pancreatic tissue. In such cases, electron microscopy reveals the distinctive granules of β-cells (Fig. 24-27).

Solitary tumors are usually small (often < 2 cm in diameter), encapsulated, pale to red-brown nodules located anywhere in the pancreas. Histologically, these benign tumors look remarkably like giant islets, with preservation of the regular cords of monotonous cells and their orientation to the vasculature. Not even the malignant lesions present much evidence of anaplasia, and they may be deceptively encapsulated. **Deposition of amyloid** is a characteristic feature of many insulinomas (Fig. 24-41).

Hyperinsulinism may also be caused by **focal or diffuse hyperplasia of the islets**. This change is found occasionally in adults but is far more commonly encountered as congenital hyperinsulinism with hypoglycemia in neonates and infants. Several clinical scenarios may result in islet hyperplasia (previously known as *nesidioblastosis*), including maternal diabetes, Beckwith-Wiedemann syndrome (Chapter 10), and rare mutations in the β-cell K^+-channel protein or sulfonylurea receptor. In maternal diabetes, the fetal islets respond to hyperglycemia by increasing their size and number. In the postnatal period, these hyperactive islets may be responsible for serious episodes of hypoglycemia. This phenomenon is usually transient.

Clinical Features. While up to 80% of islet cell tumors demonstrate excessive insulin secretion, the hypoglycemia is mild in all but about 20%, and many cases never become clinically symptomatic. The critical laboratory findings in insulinomas are high circulating levels of insulin and a high insulin-to-glucose ratio. Surgical removal of the tumor is usually followed by prompt reversal of the hypoglycemia.

It is important to note that there are many other causes of hypoglycemia besides insulinomas. The differential diagnosis of this metabolic abnormality includes such conditions as abnormal insulin sensitivity, diffuse liver disease, inherited glycogenoses, and ectopic production of insulin by certain retroperitoneal fibromas and fibrosarcomas. Depending on the clinical circumstances, hypoglycemia induced by self-injection of insulin should also be considered.

Zollinger-Ellison Syndrome (Gastrinomas)

Marked hypersecretion of gastrin usually has its origin in gastrin-producing tumors *(gastrinomas)*, which are just as likely to arise in the duodenum and peripancreatic soft tissues as in the pancreas (so-called gastrinoma triangle). There has been lack of agreement regarding the cell of origin of these tumors, although it seems likely that endocrine cells of either the gut or the pancreas could be the source. Zollinger and Ellison first called attention to the **association of pancreatic islet cell lesions, hypersecretion of gastric acid and severe peptic ulceration**, which are present in 90% to 95% of patients.

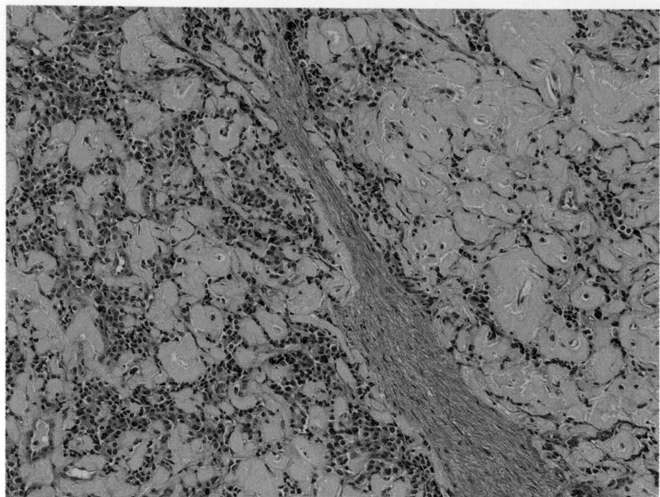

Figure 24-41 Pancreatic endocrine neoplasm ("islet cell tumor"). The neoplastic cells are monotonous and demonstrate minimal pleomorphism or mitotic activity. There is abundant amyloid deposition, characteristic of an insulinoma. Clinically, the patient had episodic hypoglycemia.

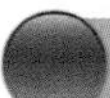

MORPHOLOGY

More than half of gastrin-producing tumors are locally invasive or have already metastasized at the time of diagnosis. In approximately 25% of patients, gastrinomas arise in conjunction with other endocrine tumors, as part of the MEN-1 syndrome (see later); MEN-1-associated gastrinomas are frequently multifocal, while sporadic gastrinomas are usually single. As with insulin-secreting tumors of the pancreas, gastrin-producing tumors are histologically bland and rarely show marked anaplasia.

In the Zollinger-Ellison syndrome, hypergastrinemia gives rise to extreme gastric acid secretion, which in turn causes **peptic ulceration** (Chapter 17). The duodenal and gastric ulcers are often multiple; although they are identical to those found in the general population, they are often unresponsive to therapy. In addition, ulcers may occur in unusual locations such as the jejunum; **when intractable jejunal ulcers are found, Zollinger-Ellison syndrome should be considered**.

Clinical Features. More than 50% of the patients have diarrhea; in 30%, it is the presenting symptom. Treatment of Zollinger-Ellison syndrome involves control of gastric acid secretion by use of H^+K^+-ATPase inhibitors and excision of the neoplasm. Total resection of the neoplasm, when possible, eliminates the syndrome. Patients with hepatic metastases have a shortened life expectancy, with progressive tumor growth leading to liver failure usually within 10 years.

Other Rare Pancreatic Endocrine Neoplasms

α-cell tumors (glucagonomas) are associated with increased serum levels of glucagon and a syndrome consisting of mild diabetes mellitus, a characteristic skin rash (necrolytic migratory erythema), and anemia. They occur most frequently in perimenopausal and postmenopausal women and are characterized by extremely high plasma glucagon levels.

δ-cell tumors (somatostatinomas) are associated with diabetes mellitus, cholelithiasis, steatorrhea, and hypochlorhydria. They are exceedingly difficult to localize preoperatively. High plasma somatostatin levels are required for diagnosis.

VIPoma (watery diarrhea, hypokalemia, achlorhydria, or WDHA syndrome) induces a characteristic syndrome that is caused by release of vasoactive intestinal peptide (VIP) from the tumor. Some of these tumors are locally invasive and metastatic. A VIP assay should be performed on all patients with severe secretory diarrhea. Neural crest tumors, such as neuroblastomas, ganglioneuroblastoma, and ganglioneuromas (Chapter 10) and pheochromocytomas (see later) can also be associated with the VIPoma syndrome.

Pancreatic carcinoid tumors producing serotonin and an atypical carcinoid syndrome are exceedingly rare. *Pancreatic polypeptide-secreting endocrine tumors* present as mass lesions as even high plasma levels of this hormone fail to cause symptoms.

Some pancreatic and extra-pancreatic endocrine tumors produce two or more hormones. In addition to insulin, glucagon, and gastrin, pancreatic endocrine tumors may produce ACTH, MSH, ADH, serotonin, and norepinephrine. These *multihormonal tumors* are to be distinguished from the MEN syndromes (discussed later), in which a multiplicity of hormones is produced by tumors in several different glands.

ADRENAL GLANDS

Adrenal Cortex

The *adrenal glands* are paired endocrine organs consisting of a cortex and a medulla, which differ in their development, structure, and function. In essence the cortex and medulla are two glands packaged as one structure. The adrenal cortex has three zones. Beneath the capsule is the narrow layer of zona glomerulosa. An equally narrow zona reticularis abuts the medulla. Intervening is the broad zona fasciculata, which makes up about 75% of the total cortex. The *adrenal cortex* synthesizes three different types of steroids: (1) *glucocorticoids* (principally cortisol), which are synthesized primarily in the zona fasciculata and to a lesser degree in the zona reticularis; (2) *mineralocorticoids*, the most important being aldosterone, which is generated in the zona glomerulosa; and (3) *sex steroids* (estrogens and androgens), which are produced largely in the zona reticularis. The *adrenal medulla* is composed of chromaffin cells, which synthesize and secrete *catecholamines*, mainly epinephrine. Catecholamines have many effects that allow rapid adaptations to changes in the environment.

Diseases of the adrenal cortex can be conveniently divided into those associated with hyperfunction and those associated with hypofunction.

Adrenocortical Hyperfunction (Hyperadrenalism)

The syndromes of adrenal hyperfunction are caused by overproduction of the three major hormones of the adrenal cortex (1) *Cushing syndrome,* characterized by an excess of cortisol; (2) *hyperaldosteronism* as a result of excessive aldosterone; and (3) *adrenogenital or virilizing syndromes* caused by an excess of androgens. The clinical features of these syndromes overlap somewhat because of the overlapping functions of some of the adrenal steroids.

Hypercortisolism (Cushing Syndrome)

Pathogenesis. **This disorder is caused by conditions that produce elevated glucocorticoid levels.** Cushing syndrome can be broadly divided into *exogenous* and *endogenous* causes. The vast majority of cases of Cushing syndrome are the result of the administration of exogenous glucocorticoids ("iatrogenic" Cushing syndrome). The endogenous causes can, in turn, be divided into those that are *ACTH dependent* and those that are *ACTH independent* (Table 24-8).

ACTH-secreting pituitary adenomas account for approximately 70% of cases of endogenous hypercortisolism. In recognition of Harvey Cushing, the neurosurgeon who first published the full description of this syndrome, the pituitary form is referred to as *Cushing disease*. The disorder affects women about four times more frequently than men and occurs most frequently in young adults. In the vast majority of cases it is caused by an *ACTH-producing pituitary microadenoma*. In some cases there is an underlying macroadenoma and rarely there is *corticotroph cell hyperplasia* without a discrete adenoma. Corticotroph cell hyperplasia may be primary or arise secondarily from excessive stimulation of ACTH release by a hypothalamic corticotrophin-releasing hormone (CRH)-producing tumor. The adrenal glands in individuals with Cushing disease are characterized by variable degrees of nodular cortical hyperplasia (discussed later), caused by the elevated levels of ACTH. The cortical hyperplasia, in turn, is responsible for hypercortisolism.

Secretion of ectopic ACTH by nonpituitary tumors accounts for about 10% of ACTH-dependent Cushing syndrome. In many instances the responsible tumor is a *small-cell carcinoma of the lung*, although other neoplasms, including carcinoids, medullary carcinomas of the thyroid, and islet cell tumors, have been associated with the syndrome. In addition to tumors that elaborate ectopic ACTH, occasionally a neuroendocrine neoplasm may produce ectopic corticotrophin releasing hormone (CRH), which, in turn, causes ACTH secretion and hypercortisolism. As in the pituitary variant, the adrenal glands undergo bilateral cortical hyperplasia, but the rapid downhill course of patients with these cancers often limits the extent of the adrenal enlargement. This variant of Cushing syndrome is more common in men and usually occurs in the 40s and 50s.

Primary adrenal neoplasms, such as adrenal adenoma (~10%) and carcinoma (~5%) are the most common underlying causes for ACTH-independent Cushing syndrome. The biochemical *sine qua non* of ACTH-independent Cushing syndrome is elevated serum levels of cortisol with low levels of ACTH. Cortical carcinomas tend to produce more marked hypercortisolism than adenomas or hyperplasias. In instances of a unilateral neoplasm, the uninvolved adrenal cortex and the cortex in the opposite gland undergo atrophy because of suppression of ACTH secretion.

The overwhelming majority of hyperplastic adrenals are ACTH dependent, and *primary cortical hyperplasia* (i.e., ACTH-independent hyperplasia) is uncommon. In *macronodular hyperplasia* the nodules are usually greater than 3 mm in diameter. Macronodular hyperplasia is typically a sporadic (nonsyndromic) condition observed in adults. It is now known that, although the condition is ACTH independent, it is not entirely "autonomous." Specifically, cortisol production is regulated by non-ACTH circulating hormones, because of ectopic overexpression of their corresponding receptors in the adrenocortical cells. Such non-ACTH hormones include gastric inhibitory peptide, LH and ADH; their receptors are overexpressed on hyperplastic adrenal cortical cells. The mechanism by which these receptors for non-ACTH hormones are overexpressed in adrenocortical tissues is not known. A subset of macronodular hyperplasia arises in the setting of McCune-Albright syndrome (Chapter 26), characterized by somatic mutations that activate *GNAS*, which encodes a stimulatory $G_s\alpha$. This $G_s\alpha$ mutation causes hyperplasia by increasing intracellular levels of cAMP, which you will recall is an important second messenger in many endocrine cell types. Given this, it is not surprising that mutations in several other proteins that are involved in cAMP signaling, such as the regulatory subunit of cAMP-dependent protein kinase (encoded by the *PRKAR1A* gene) and a phosphodiesterase (an enzyme that breaks down cAMP, encoded by the *PDE11A* gene), are also associated with primary cortical hyperplasia.

Table 24-8 Endogenous Causes of Cushing Syndrome

Cause	Relative Frequency (%)	Ratio of Females to Males
ACTH-Dependent		
Cushing disease (pituitary adenoma; rarely CRH	70	3.5:1
Ectopic corticotropin syndrome (ACTH)	10	1:1
ACTH-Independent		
Adrenal adenoma	10	4:1
Adrenal carcinoma	5	1:1
Macronodular hyperplasia (ectopic expression of hormone receptors, including GIPR, LHR, vasopressin and serotonin receptors)	<2	1:1
Primary pigmented nodular adrenal disease (*PRKARIA* and *PDE11* mutations)	<2	1:1
McCune-Albright syndrome (*GNAS* mutations)	<2	1:1

ACTH, Adrenocorticotropic hormone; GIPR, gastric inhibitory polypeptide receptor; LHR, luteinizing hormone receptor; *PRKAR1A*, protein kinase A regulatory subunit 1α; *PDE11*, phosphodiesterase 11A.
Note: These etiologies are responsible for endogenous Cushing syndrome. The most common overall cause of Cushing syndrome is exogenous glucocorticoid administration (iatrogenic Cushing syndrome).
Adapted with permission from Newell-Price J, et al: Cushing syndrome. Lancet 367:1605-1616, 2006.

MORPHOLOGY

The main lesions of Cushing syndrome are found in the pituitary and adrenal glands. The **pituitary** shows changes regardless of the cause. The most common alteration, resulting from high levels of endogenous or exogenous glucocorticoids, is termed **Crooke hyaline change.** In this condition the normal granular, basophilic cytoplasm of the ACTH-producing cells in the anterior pituitary becomes homogeneous and paler. This alteration is the result of the accumulation of intermediate keratin filaments in the cytoplasm.

Depending on the cause of the hypercortisolism the **adrenals** show one of the following abnormalities: (1) cortical atrophy, (2) diffuse hyperplasia, (3) macronodular or micronodular hyperplasia, and (4) an adenoma or carcinoma. In patients in whom the syndrome results from exogenous glucocorticoids, suppression of endogenous ACTH results in bilateral **cortical atrophy,** due to a lack of stimulation of the zonae fasciculata and reticularis by ACTH. The zona glomerulosa is of normal thickness in such cases, because this portion of the cortex functions independently of ACTH. In contrast, in cases of endogenous hypercortisolism, the adrenals either are hyperplastic or contain a cortical neoplasm. **Diffuse hyperplasia** is found in individuals with ACTH-dependent Cushing syndrome (Fig. 24-42). Both glands are enlarged, either subtly or markedly, weighing up to 30 gm. The adrenal cortex is diffusely thickened and variably nodular, although the latter is not as pronounced as seen in cases of ACTH-independent nodular hyperplasia. Microscopically, the hyperplastic cortex demonstrates an expanded "lipid-poor" zona reticularis, comprising compact, eosinophilic cells, surrounded by an outer zone of vacuolated "lipid-rich" cells, resembling those seen in the zona fasciculata. Any nodules present are usually composed of vacuolated "lipid-rich" cells, which account for the yellow color of diffusely hyperplastic glands. In contrast, in **macronodular hyperplasia** the adrenals are almost entirely replaced by prominent nodules of varying sizes (≤3 cm), which contain an admixture of lipid-poor and lipid-rich cells. Unlike diffuse hyperplasia, the areas between the macroscopic nodules also demonstrate evidence of microscopic nodularity. **Micronodular hyperplasia** is composed of 1- to 3-mm darkly pigmented (brown to black) micronodules, with atrophic intervening areas (Fig. 24-43). The pigment is believed to be lipofuscin, a wear-and-tear pigment (Chapter 2).

Primary adrenocortical neoplasms causing Cushing syndrome may be malignant or benign. Functional adenomas or carcinomas of the adrenal cortex as the source of cortisol are not morphologically distinct from nonfunctioning adrenal neoplasms (described later). Both the benign and the malignant lesions are more common in women in their 30s to 50s. Adrenocortical **adenomas** are yellow tumors surrounded by thin or well-developed capsules, and most weigh less than 30 gm. Microscopically, they are composed of cells that are similar to those encountered in the normal zona fasciculata. The **carcinomas** associated with Cushing syndrome, by contrast, tend to be larger than the adenomas. These tumors (detailed later) are unencapsulated masses frequently exceeding 200 to 300 gm in weight that have all of the anaplastic characteristics of cancer. With functioning tumors, both benign and malignant, the adjacent adrenal cortex and that of the contralateral adrenal gland are atrophic, as a result of suppression of endogenous ACTH by high cortisol levels.

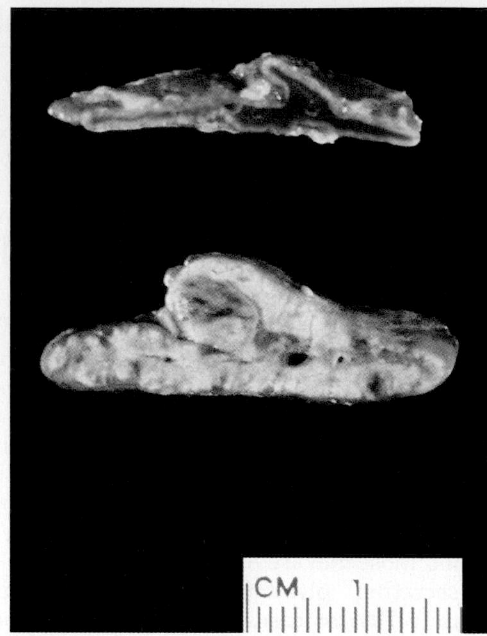

Figure 24-42 Diffuse hyperplasia of the adrenal contrasted with normal adrenal gland. In cross-section the adrenal cortex is yellow and thickened, and a subtle nodularity is seen (contrast with Fig. 24-46). Both adrenal glands were diffusely hyperplastic in this patient with ACTH-dependent Cushing syndrome.

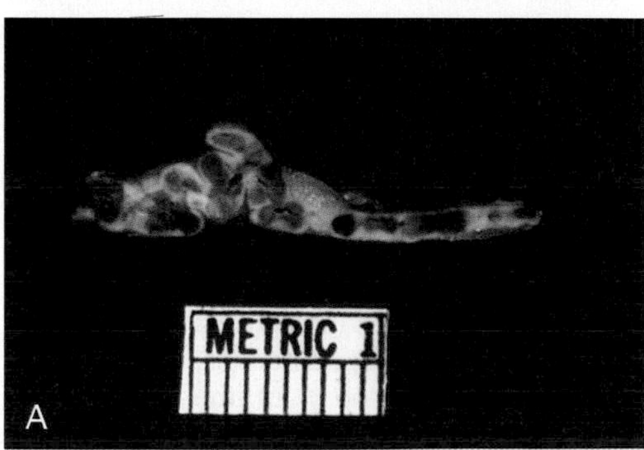

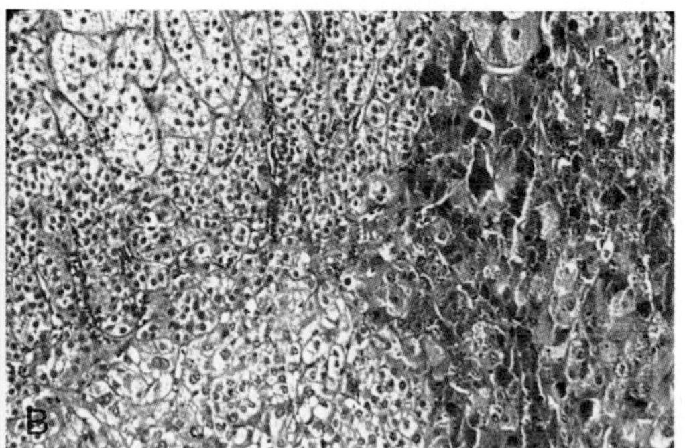

Figure 24-43 **A,** Micronodular adrenocortical hyperplasia with prominent pigmented nodules in the adrenal gland. **B,** On histologic examination the nodules are composed of cells containing lipofuscin pigment, seen in the right part of the field. (Photographs courtesy Dr. Aidan Carney, Department of Medicine, Mayo Clinic, Rochester, Minn.)

Table 24-9 Clinical Features of Cushing Syndrome

Feature	Percent
Obesity or weight gain	95%*
Facial plethora	90%
Rounded face	90%
Decreased libido	90%
Thin skin	85%
Decrease in linear growth in children	70-80%
Menstrual irregularity	80%
Hypertension	75%
Hirsutism	75%
Depression/emotional liability	70%
Easy bruising	65%
Glucose intolerance	60%
Weakness	60%
Osteopenia or fracture	50%
Nephrolithiasis	50%

*100% in children.
Adapted from Newell-Price J, et al: Cushing syndrome. Lancet 367:1605-1616, 2006.

Clinical Course. Cushing syndrome develops slowly and can be quite subtle in its early manifestations. Early stages of the disorder may present with hypertension and weight gain (Table 24-9). With time the more characteristic central pattern of adipose tissue deposition becomes apparent in the form of truncal obesity, moon facies, and accumulation of fat in the posterior neck and back *(buffalo hump).* Hypercortisolism causes selective atrophy of fast-twitch (type 2) myofibers, resulting in decreased muscle mass and proximal limb weakness. Glucocorticoids induce gluconeogenesis and inhibit the uptake of glucose by cells, with resultant *hyperglycemia, glucosuria* and *polydipsia (secondary diabetes).* The catabolic effects cause loss of collagen and resorption of bones. Consequently the *skin is thin, fragile, and easily bruised;* wound healing is poor; and cutaneous striae are particularly common in the abdominal area (Fig. 24-44). Bone resorption results in the development of *osteoporosis,* with consequent backache and increased susceptibility to fractures. Persons with Cushing syndrome are at increased risk for a variety of infections, because glucocorticoids suppress the immune response. Additional manifestations include several *mental disturbances,* including mood swings, depression, and frank psychosis, as well as *hirsutism* and *menstrual abnormalities.*

The laboratory diagnosis of Cushing syndrome is based on the following: (1) the 24-hour urine free-cortisol concentration, which is increased, and (2) loss of normal diurnal pattern of cortisol secretion. Determining the cause of Cushing syndrome depends on the serum ACTH and measurement of urinary steroid excretion after administration of dexamethasone (dexamethasone suppression test). The results of these tests fall into three general patterns:

- In pituitary Cushing syndrome, the most common form, ACTH levels are elevated and cannot be suppressed by the administration of a low dose of dexamethasone. Hence, there is no reduction in urinary excretion of 17-hydroxycorticosteroids. After higher doses of injected dexamethasone, however, the pituitary responds by reducing ACTH secretion, which is reflected by suppression of urinary steroid secretion.
- Ectopic ACTH secretion results in an elevated level of ACTH, but its secretion is completely insensitive to low or high doses of exogenous dexamethasone.
- When Cushing syndrome is caused by an adrenal tumor, the ACTH level is quite low because of feedback inhibition of the pituitary. As with ectopic ACTH secretion, both low-dose and high-dose dexamethasone fail to suppress cortisol excretion.

KEY CONCEPTS

Hypercortisolism (Cushing Syndrome)

- The most common cause of hypercortisolism is exogenous administration of steroids.
- Endogenous hypercortisolism most often is secondary to an ACTH-producing pituitary microadenoma (*Cushing disease*), followed by primary adrenal neoplasms (*ACTH-independent* hypercortisolism) and paraneoplastic ACTH production by tumors (e.g., small cell lung cancer).
- The morphologic features in the adrenal vary from bilateral cortical atrophy (in exogenous steroid-induced disease), to bilateral diffuse or nodular hyperplasia (most common finding in endogenous Cushing syndrome), to an adrenocortical neoplasm.

Primary Hyperaldosteronism

Hyperaldosteronism is the generic term for a group of closely related conditions characterized by chronic excess aldosterone secretion. Hyperaldosteronism may be primary, or it

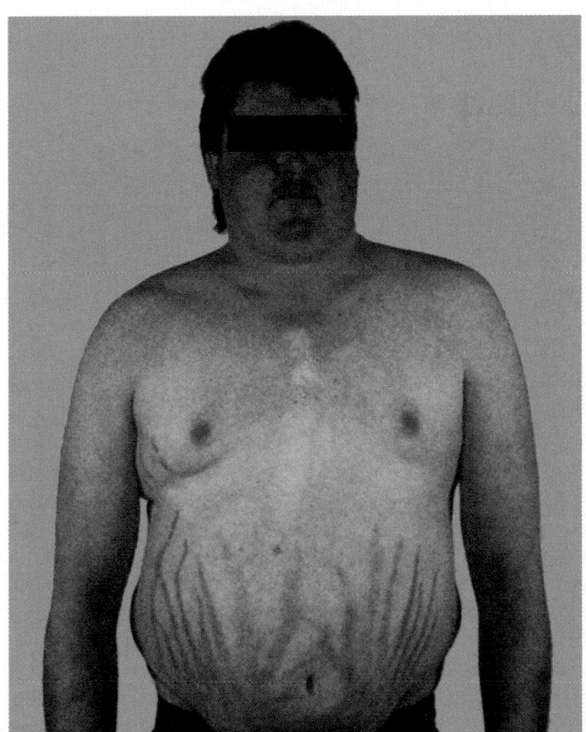

Figure 24-44 A patient with Cushing syndrome demonstrating central obesity, "moon facies," and abdominal striae. (Reproduced with permission from Lloyd RV, et al (eds): Atlas of Nontumor Pathology: Endocrine Diseases. Washington, DC, American Registry of Pathology, 2002.)

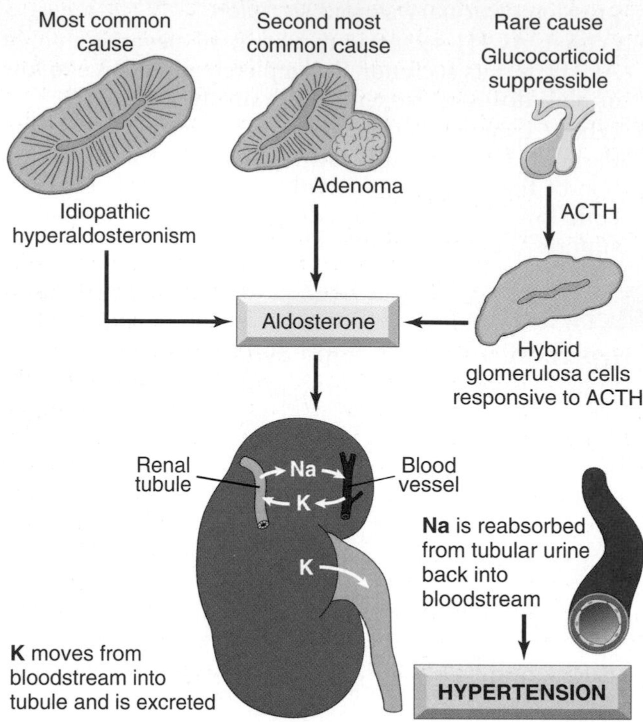

Figure 24-45 The major causes of primary hyperaldosteronism and its principal effects on the kidney.

may be secondary to an extra-adrenal cause. *Primary hyperaldosteronism* stems from an autonomous overproduction of aldosterone, with resultant suppression of the renin-angiotensin system and *decreased plasma renin activity*. **Blood pressure elevation is the most common manifestation of primary hyperaldosteronism**, which is caused by one of three mechanisms (Fig. 24-45):

- *Bilateral idiopathic hyperaldosteronism* (IHA), characterized by bilateral nodular hyperplasia of the adrenal glands, is the most common underlying cause of primary hyperaldosteronism, accounting for about 60% of cases. Individuals with idiopathic hyperaldosteronism tend to be older and to have less severe hypertension than those presenting with adrenal neoplasms. The pathogenesis of idiopathic hyperaldosteronism remains unclear, although recent studies suggest that a subset of patients with familial idiopathic hyperaldosteronism harbor germline mutations of *KCNJ5*, encoding a potassium channel.
- *Adrenocortical neoplasm*, either an aldosterone-producing adenoma (the most common cause) or, rarely, an adrenocortical carcinoma. In approximately 35% of cases, primary hyperaldosteronism is caused by a solitary aldosterone-secreting adenoma, a condition referred to as *Conn syndrome*. This syndrome occurs most frequently in adult middle life and is more common in women than in men (2:1). Multiple adenomas may be present in an occasional patient. Somatic mutations of *KCNJ5* are also present in a subset of aldosterone-secreting adenomas.
- *Glucocorticoid-remediable hyperaldosteronism* is an uncommon cause of primary familial hyperaldosteronism. In some families, it stems from a rearrangement involving chromosome 8 that places *CYP11B2* (the gene that encodes *aldosterone synthase*) under the control of the ACTH responsive *CYP11B1* gene promoter. ACTH thus stimulates the production of aldosterone synthase, the enzyme that is responsible for the last step in aldosterone synthesis. Because in this unusual circumstance aldosterone production is under the control of ACTH, it is suppressible by dexamethasone.

In *secondary hyperaldosteronism*, in contrast, aldosterone release occurs in response to activation of the renin-angiotensin system (Chapter 11). It is characterized by *increased levels of plasma renin* and is encountered in conditions such as the following:

- Decreased renal perfusion (arteriolar nephrosclerosis, renal artery stenosis)
- Arterial hypovolemia and edema (congestive heart failure, cirrhosis, nephrotic syndrome)
- Pregnancy (due to estrogen-induced increases in plasma renin substrate)

MORPHOLOGY

Aldosterone-producing adenomas are almost always solitary, small (<2 cm in diameter), well-circumscribed lesions, more often found on the left than on the right. They tend to occur in the 30s and 40s, and in women more often than in men. They are often buried within the gland and do not produce visible enlargement, a point to be remembered in interpreting sonographic or scanning images. They are bright yellow on cut section and, surprisingly, are composed of lipid-laden cortical cells that more closely resemble fasciculata cells than glomerulosa cells (the normal source of aldosterone). In general, the cells tend to be uniform in size and shape; occasionally, there is modest nuclear and cellular pleomorphism (see Fig. 24-51). A characteristic feature of aldosterone-producing adenomas is the presence of eosinophilic, laminated cytoplasmic inclusions, known as **spironolactone bodies**, found after treatment with the antihypertensive drug spironolactone. In contrast to cortical adenomas associated with Cushing syndrome, those associated with hyperaldosteronism do not usually suppress ACTH secretion. Therefore, the adjacent adrenal cortex and that of the contralateral gland are not atrophic.

Bilateral idiopathic hyperplasia is marked by diffuse and focal hyperplasia of cells resembling those of the normal zona glomerulosa. The hyperplasia is often wedge-shaped, extending from the periphery toward the center of the gland. The enlargement may be subtle, and as a rule an adrenocortical adenoma must be carefully excluded as the cause for hyperaldosteronism.

Clinical Course. **The most important clinical consequence of hyperaldosteronism is hypertension**. With an estimated prevalence rate of 5% to 10% among nonselected hypertensive patients, primary hyperaldosteronism may be the most common cause of secondary hypertension (i.e., hypertension secondary to an identifiable cause). The prevalence of hyperaldosteronism increases with the severity of hypertension, reaching nearly 20% in patients who are classified as having treatment-resistant hypertension.

Through its effects on the renal mineralocorticoid receptor, aldosterone promotes sodium reabsorption, which secondarily increases the reabsorption of water, expanding the extracellular fluid volume and elevating cardiac output.

The long-term effects of hyperaldosteronism-induced hypertension are cardiovascular compromise (e.g., left ventricular hypertrophy and reduced diastolic volumes) and an increase in the prevalence of adverse events such as stroke and myocardial infarction. *Hypokalemia* was considered a mandatory feature of primary hyperaldosteronism, but increasing numbers of normokalemic patients are now diagnosed. Hypokalemia results from renal potassium wasting and, when present, can cause a variety of neuromuscular manifestations, including weakness, paresthesias, visual disturbances, and occasionally frank tetany.

The diagnosis of primary hyperaldosteronism is confirmed by elevated ratios of plasma aldosterone concentration to plasma renin activity; if this screening test is positive, a confirmatory *aldosterone suppression test* must be performed, because many unrelated causes can alter the plasma aldosterone and renin ratios.

In primary hyperaldosteronism, the therapy varies according to cause. Adenomas are amenable to surgical excision. In contrast, surgical intervention is not very beneficial in patients with primary hyperaldosteronism due to bilateral hyperplasia, which often occurs in children and young adults. These patients are best managed medically with an aldosterone antagonist such as spironolactone. The treatment of secondary hyperaldosteronism rests on correcting the underlying cause stimulating the renin-angiotensin system.

Adrenogenital Syndromes

Disorders of sexual differentiation, such as *virilization* or *feminization*, can be caused by primary gonadal disorders (Chapter 22) and several primary adrenal disorders. The adrenal cortex secretes two compounds—dehydroepiandrosterone and androstenedione—that can be converted to testosterone in peripheral tissues. Unlike gonadal androgens, ACTH regulates adrenal androgen formation (Fig. 24-46); thus, excess secretion can occur either as a "pure" syndrome or as a component of Cushing disease. The adrenal causes of androgen excess include *adrenocortical neoplasms* and a group of disorders that have been designated *congenital adrenal hyperplasia (CAH)*.

Adrenocortical neoplasms associated with virilization are more likely to be *androgen-secreting adrenal carcinomas* than adenomas. Such tumors are often also associated with hypercortisolism ("mixed syndrome"). They are

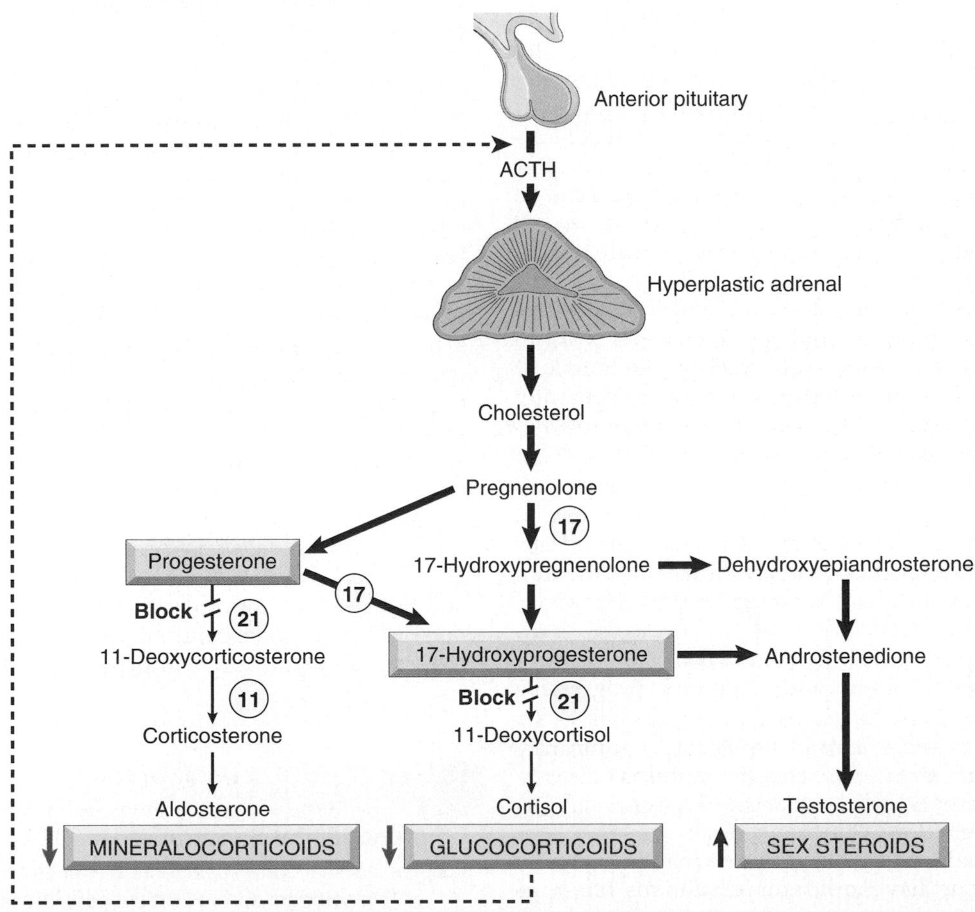

Figure 24-46 Consequences of C-21 hydroxylase deficiency. 21-Hydroxylase deficiency impairs the synthesis of both cortisol and aldosterone at different steps (shown as "Block" in the biosynthesis pathway). The resultant decrease in feedback inhibition *(dashed line)* causes increased secretion of ACTH, resulting ultimately in adrenal hyperplasia and increased synthesis of testosterone. The sites of action of 11-, 17-, and 21-hydroxylase are shown by the numbers in circles.

morphologically identical to other cortical neoplasms and will be discussed later.

***Congenital adrenal hyperplasia* stems from several autosomal-recessive, inherited metabolic errors, each characterized by a deficiency or total lack of a particular enzyme involved in the biosynthesis of cortical steroids, particularly cortisol** (Fig. 24-46)**.** Steroid precursors that build behind the defective step in the pathway are channeled into other pathways, resulting in increased production of androgens, which accounts for virilization. Simultaneously, the deficiency of cortisol leads to increased secretion of ACTH, culminating in adrenal hyperplasia. Certain enzyme defects may also impair aldosterone secretion, adding *salt wasting* to the virilizing syndrome. Other enzyme deficiencies may be incompatible with life or, in rare instances, may involve only the aldosterone pathway without involving cortisol synthesis.

21-hydroxylase deficiency (caused by mutations of *CYP21A2*) is by far the most common, accounting for over 90% of cases. Figure 24-46 illustrates normal adrenal steroidogenesis and the consequences of 21-hydroxylase deficiency, which may range from a total lack to a mild loss, depending on the nature of the *CYP21A2* mutation. Three distinctive syndromes have been described: (1) salt-wasting ("classic") adrenogenitalism, (2) simple virilizing adrenogenitalism, and (3) "nonclassic" adrenogenitalism.

- The *salt-wasting syndrome* results from an inability to convert progesterone into deoxycorticosterone because of a total lack of the hydroxylase. Thus, there is virtually no synthesis of mineralocorticoids, and concomitantly, there is a block in the conversion of hydroxyprogesterone into deoxycortisol resulting in deficient cortisol synthesis. This pattern usually comes to light soon after birth, because in utero the electrolytes and fluids can be maintained by the maternal kidneys. There is *salt wasting, hyponatremia,* and *hyperkalemia,* which induce acidosis, *hypotension*, cardiovascular collapse, and possibly death. The concomitant block in cortisol synthesis and excess production of androgens, however, lead to virilization, which is easily recognized in the female at birth or in utero. Males with this disorder are generally unrecognized at birth but come to clinical attention 5 to 15 days later because of some salt-losing crisis.
- *Simple virilizing adrenogenital syndrome without salt wasting* (presenting as genital ambiguity) occurs in approximately a third of patients with 21-hydroxylase deficiency. These patients generate sufficient mineralocorticoid to prevent a salt-wasting "crisis." However, the lowered glucocorticoid level fails to cause feedback inhibition of ACTH secretion. Thus, the level of testosterone is increased, with resultant progressive virilization.
- *Nonclassic or late-onset adrenal virilism* is significantly more common than the classic patterns already described. There is only a partial deficiency in 21-hydroxylase function, which accounts for the later onset. Individuals with this syndrome may be virtually asymptomatic or have mild manifestations, such as hirsutism, acne, and menstrual irregularities. Nonclassic CAH cannot be diagnosed on routine newborn screening, and the diagnosis is usually rendered by demonstration of biosynthetic defects in steroidogenesis.

MORPHOLOGY

In all cases of CAH the adrenals are bilaterally hyperplastic, sometimes increasing to 10 to 15 times their normal weights because of the sustained elevation in ACTH. The adrenal cortex is thickened and nodular, and on cut section the widened cortex appears brown, because of total depletion of all lipid. The proliferating cells are mostly compact, eosinophilic, lipid-depleted cells, intermixed with lipid-laden clear cells. Hyperplasia of corticotroph (ACTH-producing) cells is present in the anterior pituitary in most persons with CAH.

Clinical Course. The clinical features of these disorders are determined by the specific enzyme deficiency and include abnormalities related to *androgen excess*, with or without *aldosterone* and *glucocorticoid deficiency*. CAH affects not only adrenal cortical enzymes but also products synthesized in the medulla. High levels of intra-adrenal glucocorticoids are required to facilitate medullary catecholamine (epinephrine and norepinephrine) synthesis. In patients with severe salt-wasting 21-hydroxylase deficiency, a combination of low cortisol levels and developmental defects of the medulla *(adrenomedullary dysplasia)* profoundly affects catecholamine secretion, further predisposing these individuals to hypotension and circulatory collapse.

Depending on the nature and severity of the enzymatic defect, the onset of clinical symptoms may occur in the perinatal period, later childhood, or, less commonly, adulthood. For example, in 21-hydroxylase deficiency excessive androgenic activity causes signs of masculinization in females, ranging from clitoral hypertrophy and pseudohermaphroditism in infants, to oligomenorrhea, hirsutism, and acne in postpubertal females. In males, androgen excess is associated with enlargement of the external genitalia and other evidence of precocious puberty in prepubertal patients and oligospermia in older males.

CAH should be suspected in any neonate with ambiguous genitalia. Severe enzyme deficiency in infancy can be a life-threatening condition with vomiting, dehydration, and salt wasting. Individuals with CAH are treated with exogenous glucocorticoids, which, in addition to providing adequate levels of glucocorticoids, also suppress ACTH levels and thus decrease the excessive synthesis of the steroid hormones responsible for many of the clinical abnormalities. Mineralocorticoid supplementation is required in the salt-wasting variants of CAH. With the availability of routine neonatal metabolic screens for CAH and the feasibility of molecular testing for antenatal detection of 21-hydroxylase mutations, the outcome for even the most severe variants has improved significantly.

KEY CONCEPTS

Adrenogenital Syndromes

- The adrenal cortex can secrete excess androgens in either of two settings: adrenocortical neoplasms (usually *virilizing* carcinomas) or congenital adrenal hyperplasia (CAH).
- CAH consists of a group of autosomal recessive disorders characterized by defects in steroid biosynthesis, usually

cortisol; the most common subtype is caused by deficiency of the enzyme 21-hydroxylase.

- Reduction in cortisol production causes a compensatory increase in ACTH secretion, which in turn stimulates androgen production. Androgens have virilizing effects, including masculinization in females (ambiguous genitalia, oligomenorrhea, hirsutism), precocious puberty in males, and in some instances, salt (sodium) wasting and hypotension.
- Bilateral hyperplasia of the adrenal cortex is characteristic, and a subset of 21-hydroxylase-deficient patients also demonstrates *adrenomedullary dysplasia.*

Adrenocortical Insufficiency

Adrenocortical insufficiency, or hypofunction, may be caused by either primary adrenal disease (primary hypoadrenalism) or decreased stimulation of the adrenals due to a deficiency of ACTH (secondary hypoadrenalism) (Table 24-10). The patterns of adrenocortical insufficiency can be considered under the following headings: (1) primary *acute* adrenocortical insufficiency (adrenal crisis), (2) primary *chronic* adrenocortical insufficiency *(Addison disease)*, and (3) secondary adrenocortical insufficiency.

Primary Acute Adrenocortical Insufficiency

Acute adrenal cortical insufficiency occurs in a variety of clinical settings.

Table 24-10 Adrenocortical Insufficiency

Primary Insufficiency
Loss of Cortical Cells
Congenital adrenal *hypo*plasia
X-linked adrenal hypoplasia (*DAX1* gene on Xp21)
"Miniature"-type adrenal hypoplasia (unknown cause)
Adrenoleukodystrophy (*ALD* gene on Xq28)
Autoimmune adrenal insufficiency
Autoimmune polyendocrinopathy syndrome type 1 (*AIRE1* gene on 21q22)
Autoimmune polyendocrinopathy syndrome type 2 (polygenic)
Isolated autoimmune adrenalitis (polygenic)
Infection
Acquired immune deficiency syndrome
Tuberculosis
Fungi
Acute hemorrhagic necrosis (*Waterhouse-Friderichsen syndrome*)
Amyloidosis, sarcoidosis, hemochromatosis
Metastatic carcinoma
Metabolic Failure in Hormone Production
Congenital adrenal *hyper*plasia (cortisol and aldosterone deficiency with virilization)
Drug- and steroid-induced inhibition of ACTH or cortical cell function
Secondary Insufficiency
Hypothalamic Pituitary Disease
Neoplasm, inflammation (sarcoidosis, tuberculosis, pyogens, fungi)
Hypothalamic Pituitary Suppression
Long-term steroid administration
Steroid-producing neoplasms

ACTH, Adrenocorticotropic hormone.

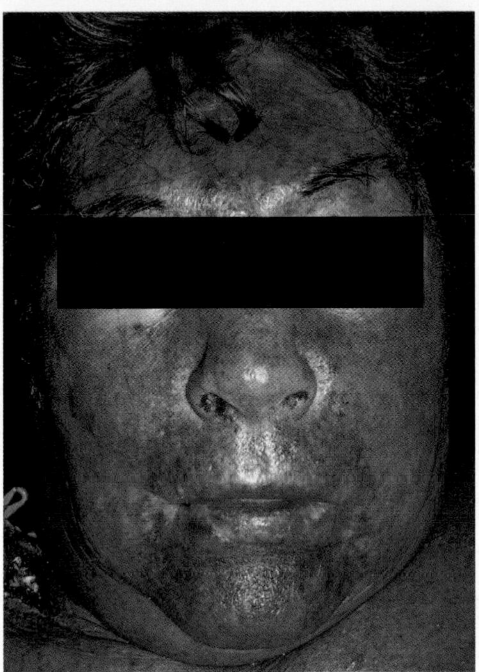

Figure 24-47 Diffuse purpuric rash in a patient with Waterhouse-Friderichsen syndrome. (Reproduced with permission from C. Vincentelli et al, Am J Emerg Med, 27:751, 2009).

- As a *crisis* in individuals with chronic adrenocortical insufficiency precipitated by any form of stress that requires an immediate increase in steroid output from glands incapable of responding
- In patients maintained on exogenous corticosteroids, in whom *rapid withdrawal of steroids* or failure to increase steroid doses in response to an acute stress may precipitate an adrenal crisis, because of the inability of the atrophic adrenals to produce glucocorticoid hormones
- As a result of *massive adrenal hemorrhage*, which damages the adrenal cortex sufficiently to cause acute adrenocortical insufficiency—as occurs in newborns following prolonged and difficult delivery with considerable trauma and hypoxia. It also occurs in some patients maintained on anticoagulant therapy, in postsurgical patients who develop disseminated intravascular coagulation and consequent hemorrhagic infarction of the adrenals, and as a complication of disseminated bacterial infection; in this last setting, it is called *Waterhouse-Friderichsen syndrome.*

Waterhouse-Friderichsen Syndrome

This uncommon but catastrophic syndrome is characterized by the following:

- Overwhelming bacterial infection, classically *Neisseria meningitidis* septicemia but occasionally caused by other highly virulent organisms, such as *Pseudomonas* species, pneumococci, *Haemophilus influenzae,* or even staphylococci
- Rapidly progressive hypotension leading to shock
- Disseminated intravascular coagulation associated with widespread purpura, particularly of the skin (Fig. 24-47)

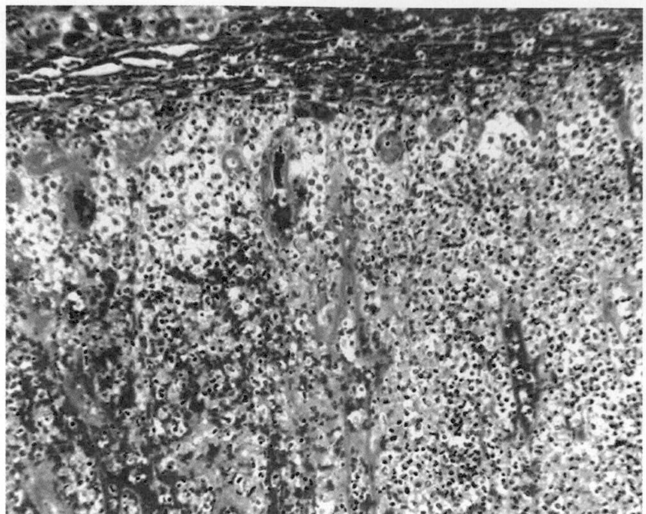

Figure 24-48 Waterhouse-Friderichsen syndrome. At autopsy, the adrenals were grossly hemorrhagic and shrunken; microscopically, little residual cortical architecture is discernible.

- Rapidly developing adrenocortical insufficiency associated with massive bilateral adrenal hemorrhage

Waterhouse-Friderichsen syndrome can occur at any age but is more common in children. The basis for the adrenal hemorrhage is uncertain but could be due to direct bacterial seeding of small vessels in the adrenal, the development of disseminated intravascular coagulation, or endothelial dysfunction caused by microbial products and inflammatory mediators. Whatever the basis, the adrenals are converted to sacs of clotted blood, which obscures virtually all of the underlying detail. Histologic examination reveals that the hemorrhage starts within the medulla near thin-walled venous sinusoids, then suffuses peripherally into the cortex, often leaving islands of recognizable cortical cells (Fig. 24-48). Prompt recognition and appropriate therapy must be instituted immediately, or death follows within hours to a few days.

Primary Chronic Adrenocortical Insufficiency (Addison Disease)

In an article published in 1855, Thomas Addison described a group of patients suffering from a constellation of symptoms, including "general languor and debility, remarkable feebleness of the heart's action, and a peculiar change in the color of the skin" associated with disease of the "supra-renal capsules" or, in more modern parlance, the adrenal glands. Addison disease, or chronic adrenocortical insufficiency, is an uncommon disorder resulting from progressive destruction of the adrenal cortex. In general, clinical manifestations of adrenocortical insufficiency do not appear until at least 90% of the adrenal cortex has been compromised. The causes of chronic adrenocortical insufficiency are listed in Table 24-10. Although all races and both sexes may be affected, certain causes of Addison disease (e.g., autoimmune adrenalitis) are much more common in whites and in women.

Pathogenesis. A large number of diseases may affect the adrenal cortex, including lymphomas, amyloidosis, sarcoidosis, hemochromatosis, fungal infections, and adrenal hemorrhage, but more than 90% of all cases are attributable to one of four disorders: autoimmune adrenalitis, tuberculosis, AIDS, or metastatic cancers.

- *Autoimmune adrenalitis* accounts for 60% to 70% of cases; it is by far the most common cause of primary adrenal insufficiency in developed countries. As the name implies, there is autoimmune destruction of steroidogenic cells. Autoantibodies to several key steroidogenic enzymes (21-hydroxylase, 17-hydroxylase) have been detected in these patients. Autoimmune adrenalitis can occur in one of two clinical settings:
  - *Autoimmune polyendocrine syndrome type 1* (APS1), also known as autoimmune polyendocrinopathy, candidiasis, and ectodermal dystrophy (APECED), is characterized by chronic mucocutaneous candidiasis and abnormalities of skin, dental enamel, and nails (ectodermal dystrophy) in association with a combination of organ-specific autoimmune disorders (autoimmune adrenalitis, autoimmune hypoparathyroidism, idiopathic hypogonadism, pernicious anemia) that result in immune destruction of target organs. APS1 is caused by mutations in the autoimmune regulator *(AIRE)* gene on chromosome 21q22. AIRE is expressed primarily in the thymus, where it functions as a transcription factor that promotes the expression of many peripheral tissue antigens. Self-reactive T cells that recognize these antigens are eliminated (Chapter 6). In the absence of AIRE function, central T-cell tolerance to peripheral tissue antigens is compromised, promoting autoimmunity. Individuals with APS1 develop autoantibodies against IL-17 and IL-22, which are the principal effector cytokines secreted by T_H17 T-cells (Chapter 6). Because these two T_H17-derived cytokines are crucial for defense against fungal infections, it is not surprising that patients develop chronic mucocutaneous candidiasis.
  - *Autoimmune polyendocrine syndrome type 2* (APS2) usually starts in early adulthood and presents as a combination of adrenal insufficiency and autoimmune thyroiditis or type 1 diabetes. Unlike in APS1, mucocutaneous candidiasis, ectodermal dysplasia, and autoimmune hypoparathyroidism do not develop.
- *Infections*, particularly tuberculosis and those produced by fungi, may also cause primary chronic adrenocortical insufficiency. *Tuberculous adrenalitis,* which once accounted for as much as 90% of cases of Addison disease, has become less common with the development of antituberculous agents. With the resurgence of tuberculosis in most urban centers and the persistence of the disease in developing countries, however, this cause of adrenal insufficiency must be kept in mind. When present, tuberculous adrenalitis is usually associated with active infection in other sites, particularly in the lungs and genitourinary tract. Among fungi, disseminated infections caused by *Histoplasma capsulatum* and *Coccidioides immitis* may result in chronic adrenocortical insufficiency. AIDS sufferers are at risk for developing adrenal insufficiency from several infectious (cytomegalovirus, *Mycobacterium*

avium-intracellulare) and noninfectious (Kaposi sarcoma) complications.
- *Metastatic neoplasms* involving the adrenals are another cause of adrenal insufficiency. The adrenals are a fairly common site for metastases in patients with disseminated carcinomas. Although adrenal function is preserved in most such patients, the metastatic tumors occasionally destroy enough adrenal cortex to produce a degree of adrenal insufficiency. Carcinomas of the lung and breast are the source of a majority of metastases, although many other neoplasms, including gastrointestinal carcinomas, malignant melanoma, and hematopoietic neoplasms, may also metastasize to the adrenals.
- *Genetic causes of adrenal insufficiency* include congenital adrenal hypoplasia (*adrenal hypoplasia congenita*) and *adrenoleukodystrophy*. Adrenoleukodystrophy is described in Chapter 28. Congenital adrenal hypoplasia is a rare X-linked disease caused by mutations in a gene that encodes a transcription factor implicated in adrenal development.

MORPHOLOGY

The anatomic changes in the adrenal glands depend on the underlying disease. **Primary autoimmune adrenalitis** is characterized by irregularly shrunken glands, which may be difficult to identify within the suprarenal adipose tissue. Histologically the cortex contains only scattered residual cortical cells in a collapsed network of connective tissue. A variable lymphoid infiltrate is present in the cortex and may extend into the adjacent medulla, although the medulla is otherwise preserved (Fig. 24-49). In cases of **tuberculous and fungal disease** the adrenal architecture is effaced by a granulomatous inflammatory reaction identical to that encountered in other sites of infection. When hypoadrenalism is caused by **metastatic carcinoma**, the adrenals are enlarged and the normal architecture is obscured by the infiltrating neoplasm.

Clinical Course. Addison disease begins insidiously and does not come to attention until the levels of circulating glucocorticoids and mineralocorticoids are significantly decreased. The initial manifestations include *progressive weakness and easy fatigability*, which may be dismissed as nonspecific complaints. *Gastrointestinal* disturbances are common and include anorexia, nausea, vomiting, weight loss, and diarrhea. In individuals with primary adrenal disease, *hyperpigmentation* of the skin, particularly of sun-exposed areas and at pressure points, such as the neck, elbows, knees, and knuckles, is quite characteristic. This is caused by elevated levels of pro-opiomelanocortin (POMC), which is derived from the anterior pituitary and is a precursor of both ACTH and melanocyte stimulating hormone (MSH). By contrast, hyperpigmentation is not seen in persons with adrenocortical insufficiency caused by primary pituitary or hypothalamic disease. Decreased mineralocorticoid activity in persons with primary adrenal insufficiency results in potassium retention and sodium loss, with consequent *hyperkalemia, hyponatremia, volume depletion, and hypotension*. Hypoglycemia may occasionally occur as a result of glucocorticoid deficiency and impaired gluconeogenesis. Stresses such as infections, trauma, or surgical procedures in such patients can precipitate an acute adrenal crisis, manifested by intractable vomiting, abdominal pain, hypotension, coma, and vascular collapse. Death occurs rapidly unless corticosteroid therapy begins immediately.

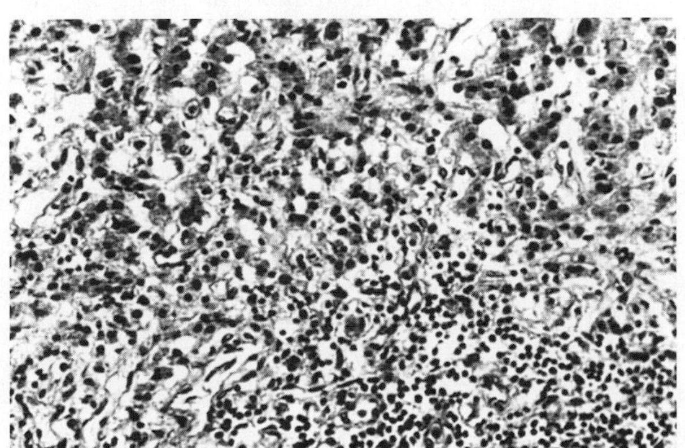

Figure 24-49 Autoimmune adrenalitis. In addition to loss of all but a subcapsular rim of cortical cells, there is an extensive mononuclear cell infiltrate.

KEY CONCEPTS

Adrenocortical Insufficiency (Hypoadrenalism)

- Primary adrenocortical insufficiency can be acute (Waterhouse-Friderichsen syndrome) or chronic (Addison disease)
- Chronic adrenal insufficiency in the developed world most often is secondary to *autoimmune adrenalitis*, which occurs in the context of one of two autoimmune polyendocrine syndromes: APS1 (caused by mutations in the *AIRE* gene) or APS2. APS1 is characterized by autoimmune attack against multiple endocrine organs and autoantibodies against IL-17.
- Tuberculosis and infections due to opportunistic pathogens associated with the human immunodeficiency virus and tumors metastatic to the adrenals are the other important causes of chronic hypoadrenalism.
- Patients typically present with fatigue, weakness, and gastrointestinal disturbances. Primary adrenocortical insufficiency also is characterized by high ACTH levels with associated skin pigmentation.

Secondary Adrenocortical Insufficiency

Any disorder of the hypothalamus and pituitary, such as metastatic cancer, infection, infarction, or irradiation, that reduces the output of ACTH leads to a syndrome of hypoadrenalism that has many similarities to Addison disease. Analogously, prolonged administration of exogenous glucocorticoids suppresses the output of ACTH and adrenal function. With secondary disease the hyperpigmentation of primary Addison disease is lacking, because levels of melanocyte-stimulating hormone are not elevated. The manifestations also differ in that secondary hypoadrenalism is characterized by deficient cortisol and androgen output but normal or near-normal aldosterone synthesis. Thus, in adrenal insufficiency secondary to pituitary malfunction, marked hyponatremia and hyperkalemia are not seen.

ACTH deficiency can occur alone, but in some instances, it is only one component of panhypopituitarism, associated with multiple trophic hormone deficiencies. Secondary disease can be differentiated from Addison disease by demonstration of low levels of plasma ACTH in the former. In patients with primary disease the destruction of the adrenal cortex reduces the response to exogenously administered ACTH, whereas in those with secondary hypofunction there is a prompt rise in plasma cortisol levels.

MORPHOLOGY

In cases of hypoadrenalism secondary to hypothalamic or pituitary disease **(secondary hypoadrenalism)**, depending on the severity of ACTH deficiency, the adrenals may be moderately to markedly decreased in size. The small, flattened glands usually retain their yellow color as a result of a small amount of residual lipid. The cortex may be reduced to a thin ribbon composed largely of zona glomerulosa. The medulla is unaffected.

Adrenocortical Neoplasms

It should be evident from the preceding sections that functional adrenal neoplasms may be responsible for any of the various forms of hyperadrenalism. Adenomas and carcinomas are about equally common in adults; in children, carcinomas predominate. While most cortical neoplasms are sporadic, two familial cancer syndromes are associated with a predisposition for developing adrenocortical carcinomas: Li-Fraumeni syndrome, in patients who harbor germline *TP53* mutations (Chapter 7), and Beckwith-Wiedemann syndrome, a disorder of epigenetic imprinting (Chapter 10).

Functional adenomas are most commonly associated with hyperaldosteronism and Cushing syndrome, whereas a virilizing neoplasm is more likely to be a carcinoma. However, not all adrenocortical neoplasms elaborate steroid hormones. *Functional and nonfunctional adrenocortical neoplasms cannot be distinguished on the basis of morphologic features.* Determination of functionality is based on clinical evaluation, and measurement of hormones or hormone metabolites in the blood.

MORPHOLOGY

Most **adrenocortical adenomas** are clinically silent and are usually incidental findings at autopsy or during abdominal imaging for an unrelated cause (see the discussion of adrenal "incidentalomas" later). The typical cortical adenoma is a well-circumscribed, nodular lesion up to 2.5 cm in diameter that expands the adrenal (Fig. 24-50). In contrast to functional adenomas, which are associated with atrophy of the adjacent cortex, the cortex adjacent to nonfunctional adenomas is normal. On cut surface, adenomas are usually yellow to yellow-brown because of the presence of lipid.

Microscopically, adenomas are composed of cells similar to those populating the normal adrenal cortex. The nuclei tend to be small, although some degree of pleomorphism may be encountered even in benign lesions ("endocrine atypia"). The cytoplasm of the neoplastic cells ranges from eosinophilic to vacuolated, depending on their lipid content (Fig. 24-51). Mitotic activity is generally inconspicuous.

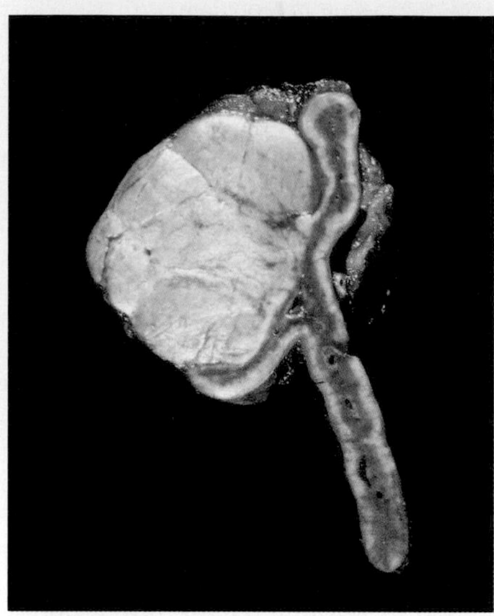

Figure 24-50 Adrenal cortical adenoma. The adenoma is distinguished from nodular hyperplasia by its solitary, circumscribed nature. The functional status of an adrenal cortical adenoma cannot be predicted from its gross or microscopic appearance.

Adrenocortical carcinomas are rare neoplasms that can occur at any age, including childhood. They are more likely to be functional than adenomas and are often associated with virilism or other clinical manifestations of hyperadrenalism. In most cases adrenocortical carcinomas are large, invasive lesions, many exceeding 20 cm in diameter, which efface the native adrenal gland (Fig. 24-52). The less common, smaller, and better-circumscribed lesions may be difficult to distinguish from an adenoma. On cut surface, adrenocortical carcinomas are typically variegated, poorly demarcated lesions containing areas of necrosis, hemorrhage, and cystic change. Adrenal cancers have a strong tendency to invade the adrenal vein, vena cava, and lymphatics. Metastases to regional and periaortic nodes are common, as is distant hematogenous spread to

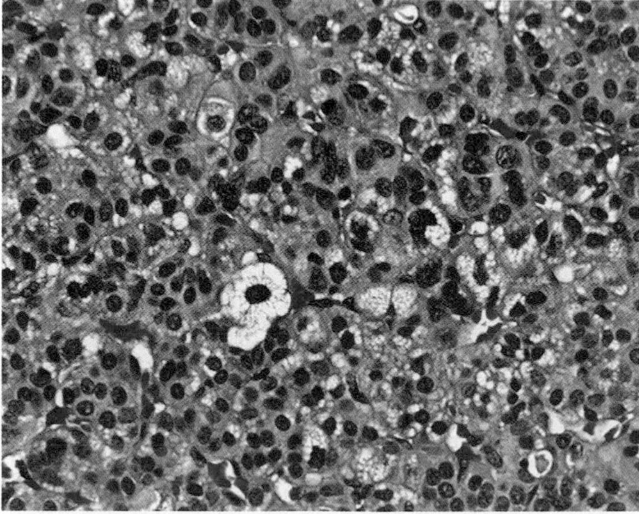

Figure 24-51 Histologic features of an adrenal cortical adenoma. The neoplastic cells are vacuolated because of the presence of intracytoplasmic lipid. There is mild nuclear pleomorphism. Mitotic activity and necrosis are not seen.

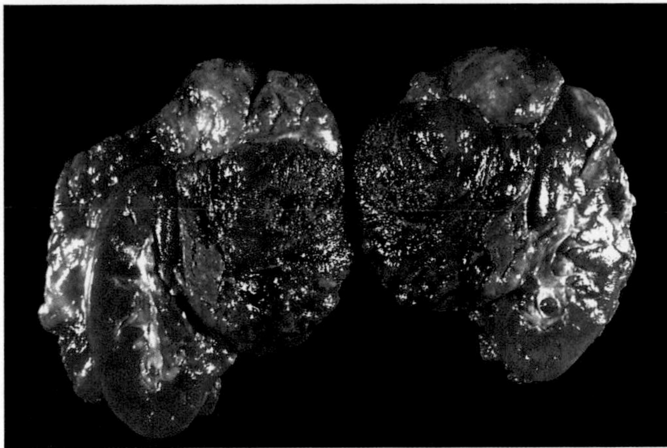

Figure 24-52 Adrenal carcinoma. The hemorrhagic and necrotic tumor dwarfs the kidney and compresses the upper pole.

the lungs and other viscera. The median patient survival is about 2 years.

Microscopically, adrenocortical carcinomas may be composed of well-differentiated cells, resembling those seen in cortical adenomas, or bizarre, monstrous giant cells (Fig. 24-53), which may be difficult to distinguish from those of an undifferentiated carcinoma metastatic to the adrenal. Between these extremes are found cancers with moderate degrees of anaplasia, some composed predominantly of spindle cells. Carcinomas, particularly those of bronchogenic origin, may metastasize to the adrenals, and may be difficult to differentiate from primary cortical carcinomas. Of note, metastases to the adrenal cortex are significantly more common than primary adrenocortical carcinomas.

Other Adrenal Lesions

Adrenal cysts are relatively uncommon; however, with the use of sophisticated abdominal imaging techniques, the frequency of detection of these lesions is increasing. Larger cysts may produce an abdominal mass and flank pain. Both cortical and medullary neoplasms may undergo necrosis and cystic degeneration and may present as "nonfunctional cysts."

Adrenal myelolipomas are unusual benign lesions composed of mature fat and hematopoietic cells. Although most of these lesions represent incidental findings, occasional myelolipomas may reach massive proportions. Histologically, mature adipocytes are admixed with aggregates of hematopoietic cells belonging to all three lineages. Foci of myelolipomatous change may be seen in cortical tumors and in adrenals with cortical hyperplasia.

The term *adrenal incidentaloma* is a half-facetious moniker that has crept into the medical lexicon as advancements in medical imaging have led to the incidental discovery of adrenal masses in asymptomatic individuals or in individuals in whom the presenting complaint is not directly related to the adrenal gland. The estimated population prevalence of "incidentalomas" discovered by imaging is approximately 4%, with an age-dependent increase in prevalence. Fortunately, the vast majority of adrenal incidentalomas are small nonsecreting cortical adenomas of no clinical importance.

Adrenal Medulla

The adrenal medulla is developmentally, functionally, and structurally distinct from the adrenal cortex. It is composed of specialized neural crest (neuroendocrine) cells, termed *chromaffin* cells, and their supporting (sustentacular) cells. The adrenal medulla is the major source of catecholamines (epinephrine, norepinephrine) in the body. Neuroendocrine cells similar to chromaffin cells are widely dispersed in an extra-adrenal system of clusters and nodules that, together with the adrenal medulla, make up the *paraganglion system*. These extra-adrenal paraganglia are closely associated with the autonomic nervous system and can be divided into three groups based on their anatomic distribution: (1) branchiomeric, (2) intravagal, and (3) aorticosympathetic. The branchiomeric and intravagal paraganglia associated with the parasympathetic system are located close to the major arteries and cranial nerves of the head and neck and include the carotid bodies (Chapter 16). The intravagal

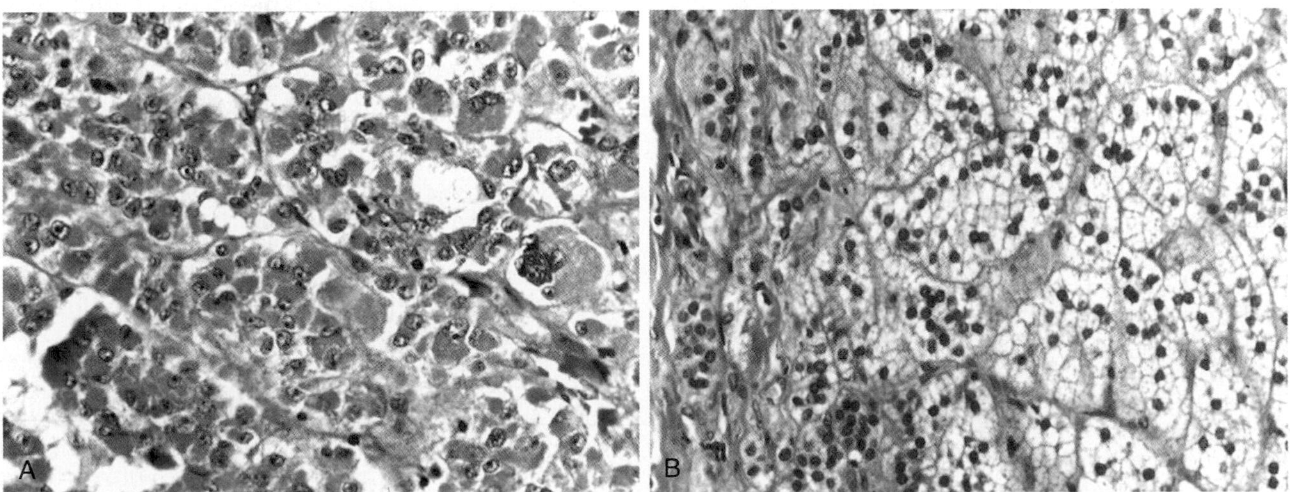

Figure 24-53 Adrenal carcinoma (**A**) revealing marked anaplasia, contrasted with normal adrenal cortical cells (**B**).

Table 24-11 Familial Syndromes Associated with Pheochromocytoma and Extra-adrenal Paragangliomas

Syndrome	Gene	Associated Lesion	Other Features
Multiple endocrine neoplasia, type 2A (MEN-2A)	*RET*	Pheochromocytoma	Medullary thyroid carcinoma Parathyroid hyperplasia
Multiple endocrine neoplasia, type 2B (MEN-2B)	*RET*	Pheochromocytoma	Medullary thyroid carcinoma Marfanoid habitus Mucocutaneous GNs
Neurofibromatosis, type 1 (NF1)	*NF1*	Pheochromocytoma	Neurofibromatosis Café-au-lait spots Optic nerve glioma
Von Hippel-Lindau (VHL)	*VHL*	Pheochromocytoma, paraganglioma *(uncommon)*	Renal cell carcinoma Hemangioblastoma Pancreatic endocrine neoplasm
Familial paraganglioma 1	*SDHD*	Pheochromocytoma, paraganglioma	
Familial paraganglioma 3	*SDHC*	Paraganglioma	
Familial paraganglioma 4	*SDHB*	Pheochromocytoma, paraganglioma	

GN, Ganglioneuroma; *NF1*, neurofibromin; *SDHB*, succinate dehydrogenase complex, subunit B; *SDHC*, succinate dehydrogenase complex, subunit C; *SDHD*, succinate dehydrogenase complex, subunit D.
Adapted with permission from Elder EE, et al: Pheochromocytoma and functional paraganglioma syndrome: no longer the 10% tumor. J Surg Oncol 89:193-201, 2005.

paraganglia, as the term implies, are distributed along the vagus nerve. The aorticosympathetic chain is found in association with segmental ganglia of the sympathetic system and therefore is distributed mainly alongside of the abdominal aorta. The organs of Zuckerkandl, close to the aortic bifurcation, belong to this group.

The most important diseases of the adrenal medulla are neoplasms, which include neoplasms of chromaffin cells *(pheochromocytomas)* and neuronal neoplasms *(neuroblastic tumors)*. Neuroblastomas and other neuroblastic tumors are discussed in Chapter 10.

Pheochromocytoma

Pheochromocytomas are neoplasms composed of chromaffin cells, which synthesize and release catecholamines and in some instances peptide hormones. It is important to recognize these tumors because they are a rare cause of surgically correctable hypertension. Traditionally, the features of pheochromocytomas have been summarized by the "rule of 10s".

- *Ten percent of pheochromocytomas are extra-adrenal*, occurring in sites such as the organs of Zuckerkandl and the carotid body. Pheochromocytomas that develop in extra-adrenal paraganglia are designated *paragangliomas* and are discussed in Chapter 16.
- *Ten percent of sporadic adrenal pheochromocytomas are bilateral*; this figure may rise to as high as 50% in cases that are associated with familial tumor syndromes (see later).
- *Ten percent of adrenal pheochromocytomas are biologically malignant*, defined by the presence of metastatic disease. Malignancy is more common (20% to 40%) in extra-adrenal paragangliomas, and in tumors arising in the setting of certain germline mutations (see later).
- *Ten percent of adrenal pheochromocytomas are not associated with hypertension*. Of the 90% that present with hypertension, approximately two thirds have "paroxysmal" episodes associated with sudden rise in blood pressure and palpitations, which can, on occasion, be fatal.

One "traditional" 10% rule that has now been modified pertains to familial cases. It is now recognized that *as many as 25% of individuals with pheochromocytomas and paragangliomas harbor a germline mutation* in one one of at least six known genes (Table 24-11). Patients with germline mutations are typically younger at presentation than those with sporadic tumors and more often harbor bilateral disease. The affected genes fall into two broad classes, those that enhance growth factor receptor pathway signaling (e.g., *RET, NF1*), and those that increase the activity of the transcription factor HIF-1α. You will recall that the VHL gene encodes a tumor suppressor protein that is needed for the oxygen-dependent degradation of HIF-1α and is mutated in patients with von Hippel-Lindau (VHL) syndrome, which is associated with a number of tumors, including pheochromocytoma. Other familial cases of pheochromocytoma are associated with germline mutations in genes encoding components of the succinate dehydrogenase complex (*SDHB, SDHC,* and *SDHD*). This complex is involved in mitochondrial electron transport and oxygen sensing, and it is believed that these mutations also lead to upregulation of HIF-1α, which appears to be a key oncogenic driver in this type of tumor.

MORPHOLOGY

Pheochromocytomas range from small, circumscribed lesions confined to the adrenal (Fig. 24-54) to large hemorrhagic masses weighing kilograms. The average weight of a pheochromocytoma is 100 gm, but weights from just over 1 gm to almost 4000 gm have been reported. The larger tumors are well demarcated by either connective tissue or compressed cortical or medullary tissue. Richly vascularized fibrous trabeculae within the tumor produce a lobular pattern. In many tumors, remnants of the adrenal gland can be seen, stretched over the surface or attached at one pole. On section, the cut surfaces of smaller pheochromocytomas are yellow-tan. Larger lesions tend to be hemorrhagic, necrotic, and cystic and typically efface the adrenal gland. Incubation of fresh tissue with a potassium dichromate solution turns the tumor a dark brown color

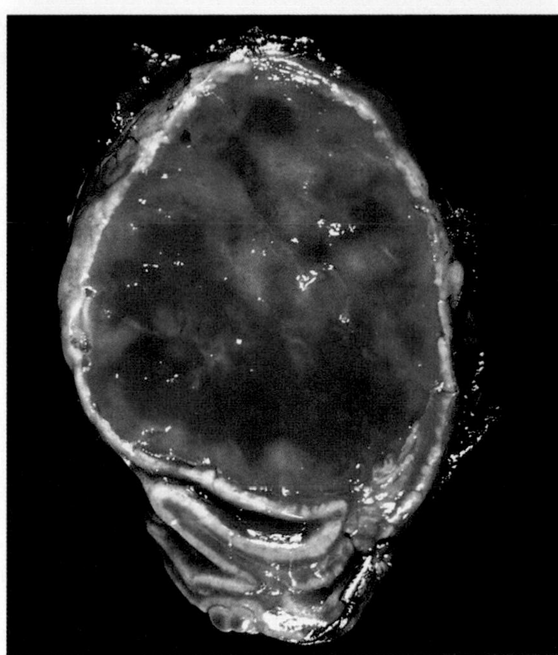

Figure 24-54 Pheochromocytoma. The tumor is enclosed within an attenuated cortex and demonstrates areas of hemorrhage. The comma-shaped residual adrenal is seen below. (Courtesy Dr. Jerrold R. Turner, Department of Pathology, University of Chicago Hospitals, Chicago, Ill.)

due to oxidation of stored catecholamines, thus the term **chromaffin**.

The histologic pattern in pheochromocytoma is quite variable. The tumors are composed of clusters of polygonal to spindle-shaped chromaffin cells or chief cells that are surrounded by supporting sustentacular cells, creating small nests or alveoli **(zellballen)** that are supplied by a rich vascular network (Fig. 24-55). Uncommonly, the dominant cell type is a spindle or small cell; various patterns can be found in any one tumor. The cytoplasm has a finely granular appearance, best demonstrated with silver stains, due to the presence of granules containing catecholamines. The nuclei are usually round to ovoid, with a stippled "salt and pepper" chromatin that is characteristic of neuroendocrine tumors. Electron microscopy reveals variable numbers of membrane-bound, electron-dense secretory granules (Fig. 24-56). Immunoreactivity for neuroendocrine markers (chromogranin and synaptophysin) is seen in the chief cells, while the peripheral sustentacular cells stain with antibodies against S-100, a calcium-binding protein expressed by a variety of mesenchymal cell types.

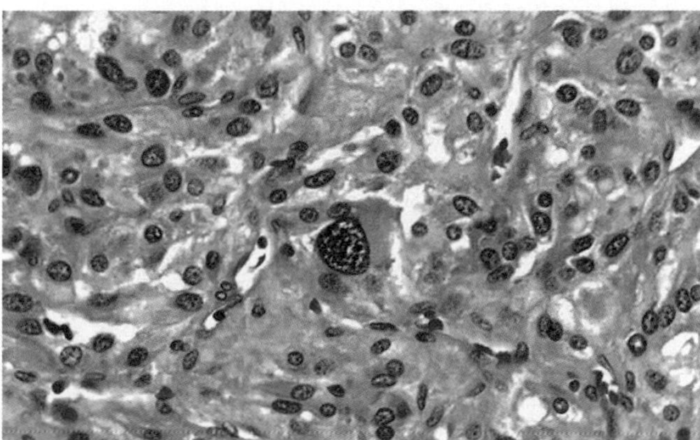

Figure 24-55 Pheochromocytoma demonstrating characteristic nests of cells ("zellballen") with abundant cytoplasm. Granules containing catecholamine are not visible in this preparation. It is not uncommon to find bizarre cells even in pheochromocytomas that are biologically benign. (Courtesy Dr. Jerrold R. Turner, Department of Pathology, University of Chicago Hospitals, Chicago, Ill.)

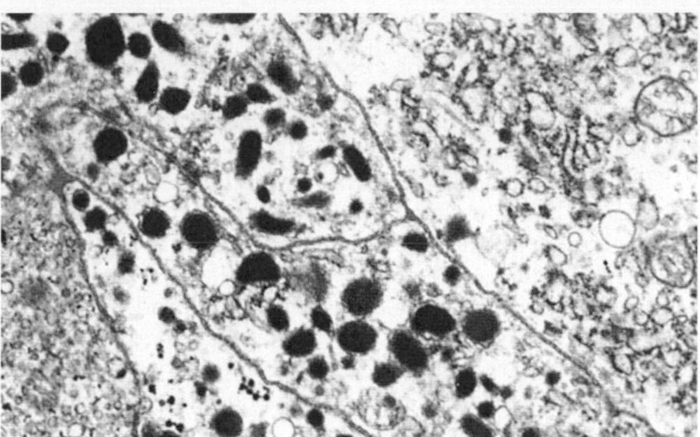

Figure 24-56 Electron micrograph of pheochromocytoma. This tumor contains membrane-bound secretory granules in which catecholamines are stored (30,000×).

Determining malignancy in pheochromocytomas can be vexing. **There is no histologic feature that reliably predicts clinical behavior.** Several histologic features, such as numbers of mitoses, confluent tumor necrosis, and spindle cell morphology, have been associated with an aggressive behavior and increased risk of metastasis, but are not entirely reliable. Tumors with "benign" histologic features may metastasize, while bizarrely pleomorphic tumors may remain confined to the adrenal gland. In fact, cellular and nuclear pleomorphism, including the presence of giant cells, and mitotic figures are often seen in benign pheochromocytomas, while cellular monotony is paradoxically associated with an aggressive behavior. Even capsular and vascular invasion may be encountered in benign lesions. **Therefore, the definitive diagnosis of malignancy in pheochromocytomas is based exclusively on the presence of metastases.** These may involve regional lymph nodes as well as more distant sites, including liver, lung, and bone.

Clinical Course. The dominant clinical manifestation of pheochromocytoma is *hypertension*, observed in 90% of patients. Approximately two thirds of patients with hypertension demonstrate *paroxysmal episodes*, which are described as an abrupt, precipitous elevation in blood pressure, associated with tachycardia, palpitations, headache, sweating, tremor, and a sense of apprehension. These episodes may also be associated with pain in the abdomen or chest, nausea, and vomiting. *Isolated* paroxysmal episodes of hypertension occur in fewer than half of patients; more commonly, patients demonstrate chronic, sustained elevation in blood pressure punctuated by the aforementioned paroxysms. The paroxysms may be precipitated by emotional stress, exercise, changes in posture, and palpation in the region of the tumor; patients with urinary bladder paragangliomas occasionally precipitate a paroxysm during micturition. The elevations of blood pressure are induced by the sudden release of catecholamines that may acutely precipitate congestive heart failure, pulmonary edema, myocardial infarction, ventricular fibrillation, and cerebrovascular accidents.

The cardiac complications have been attributed to what has been called *catecholamine cardiomyopathy*, or catecholamine-induced myocardial instability and ventricular arrhythmias. Nonspecific myocardial changes, such as focal necrosis, mononuclear infiltrates, and interstitial fibrosis, have been attributed either to ischemic damage secondary to catecholamine-induced constriction of myocardial blood vessels or to direct catecholamine toxicity. In some cases pheochromocytomas secrete other hormones, such as ACTH and somatostatin, and may therefore be associated with clinical features related to the secretion of these or other peptide hormones. The laboratory diagnosis of pheochromocytoma is based on the demonstration of increased urinary excretion of free catecholamines and their metabolites, such as vanillylmandelic acid and metanephrines.

Isolated benign tumors are treated with surgical excision, after preoperative and intraoperative medication of patients with adrenergic-blocking agents to prevent a hypertensive crisis. Multifocal lesions require long-term medical treatment for hypertension.

MULTIPLE ENDOCRINE NEOPLASIA SYNDROMES

The MEN syndromes are a group of inherited diseases resulting in proliferative lesions (hyperplasia, adenomas, and carcinomas) of multiple endocrine organs. Like other inherited cancer disorders (Chapter 7), endocrine tumors arising in the context of MEN syndromes have certain distinct features that contrast with their sporadic counterparts.

- Tumors occur at a *younger age* than sporadic tumors.
- They arise in *multiple endocrine organs*, either *synchronously* (at the same time) or *metachronously* (at different times).
- Even in one organ, the tumors are often *multifocal*.
- The tumors are usually preceded by an *asymptomatic stage of hyperplasia* involving the cell of origin. For example, individuals with MEN-2 almost universally demonstrate C-cell hyperplasia in the thyroid parenchyma adjacent to medullary thyroid carcinomas.
- These tumors are usually *more aggressive* and *recur* in a higher proportion of cases than do similar sporadic endocrine tumors.

Multiple Endocrine Neoplasia, Type 1

MEN-1, or *Wermer syndrome*, is a rare heritable disorder with a prevalence of about 2 per 100,000. MEN-1 is characterized by abnormalities involving the *parathyroid, pancreas,* and *pituitary glands*; thus the mnemonic device, the *3Ps*:

- *Parathyroid: Primary hyperparathyroidism* is the most common manifestation of MEN-1 (80% to 95% of patients) and is the initial manifestation of the disorder in most patients, appearing in almost all patients by age 40 to 50. Parathyroid abnormalities include both hyperplasia and adenomas.
- *Pancreas: Endocrine tumors of the pancreas* are a leading cause of morbidity and mortality in persons with MEN-1. These tumors are usually aggressive and often present with metastatic disease. It is not uncommon to find multiple "microadenomas" scattered throughout the pancreas in conjunction with one or two dominant lesions. MEN-1-associated pancreatic endocrine tumors are often functional; however, because pancreatic polypeptide is the most commonly secreted product, many tumors fail to produce an endocrine hypersecretion syndrome. Among those that do, Zollinger-Ellison syndrome (associated with gastrinomas) and hypoglycemia and neurologic manifestations (associated with insulinomas) are most common.
- *Pituitary:* The most frequent anterior pituitary tumor encountered in MEN-1 is a *prolactinoma*; some patients develop acromegaly from somatotrophin-secreting tumors.
- It is now recognized that the spectrum of this disease extends beyond the *3Ps*. The *duodenum is the most common site of gastrinomas in individuals with MEN-1* (far in excess of the frequency of pancreatic gastrinomas), and synchronous duodenal and pancreatic tumors may be present in the same individual. In addition, carcinoid tumors, thyroid and adrenocortical adenomas, and lipomas are more frequent than in the general population.

MEN-1 syndrome is caused by germline mutations in the *MEN1* tumor suppressor gene, which encodes a protein called menin. Menin is a component of several different transcription factor complexes, which (depending on the specific binding partner) may either promote or inhibit tumorigenesis. This dichotomy in menin function is best exemplified in the interactions of menin with two oncogenic transcription factors—JunD and the mixed-lineage leukemia (MLL) protein. When menin partners with JunD, it blocks transcriptional activation by JunD; in fact, loss of this tumor suppressor interaction is believed to contribute to the multiple endocrine neoplasia observed in the setting of MEN1 inactivating mutations. On the contrary, the association of wild-type menin with MLL leads to the formation of a tumor promoting transcriptional complex in a subset of leukemias (Chapter 13).

The dominant clinical manifestations of MEN-1 usually result from the peptide hormones that are overproduced and include such abnormalities as recurrent hypoglycemia due to insulinomas, intractable peptic ulcers in persons with Zollinger-Ellison syndrome, nephrolithiasis caused by PTH-induced hypercalcemia, or symptoms of prolactin excess from a pituitary tumor. As expected, malignant behavior by one or more of the endocrine tumors arising in these patients is often the proximate cause of death.

Multiple Endocrine Neoplasia, Type 2

MEN-2 is subclassified into three distinct syndromes: MEN-2A, MEN-2B, and familial medullary thyroid cancer.

- *MEN-2A*, or *Sipple syndrome*, is characterized by *pheochromocytoma, medullary carcinoma of the thyroid*, and *parathyroid hyperplasia* (Table 24-11). Medullary carcinomas of the thyroid occur in almost 100% of patients. They are usually multifocal and are virtually always associated with foci of C-cell hyperplasia in the adjacent thyroid. The medullary carcinomas may elaborate calcitonin and other active products and are usually clinically aggressive. Among individuals with MEN-2A, 40% to 50% have pheochromocytomas, which are often bilateral and may arise in extra-adrenal sites. Parathyroid hyperplasia and evidence of hypercalcemia or renal stones occur in 10% to 20% of patients. **MEN-2A is clinically and genetically distinct from MEN-1 and is caused by germline gain-of-function mutations in the *RET* proto-oncogene on chromosome 10q11.2**. As was noted earlier, the *RET* proto-oncogene encodes a receptor tyrosine kinase that binds *glial-derived neurotrophic factor* (GDNF) and other ligands in the GDNF family and transmits growth and differentiation signals (Chapter 7). *Loss-of-function* mutations in *RET* result in intestinal aganglionosis and Hirschsprung disease (Chapter 17). In contrast, in MEN-2A (as well as in MEN-2B), germline mutations constitutively activate the RET receptor.
- *MEN-2B* has significant clinical overlap with MEN-2A. Patients develop medullary thyroid carcinomas, which are usually multifocal and more aggressive than in MEN-2A, and pheochromocytomas. However, unlike in MEN-2A, primary hyperparathyroidism is not present. In addition, MEN-2B is accompanied by *neuromas* or ganglioneuromas involving the skin, oral mucosa, eyes, respiratory tract, and gastrointestinal tract, and a *marfanoid habitus*, with long axial skeletal features and hyperextensible joints (Table 24-11). A germline mutation leading to a single amino acid change in RET, distinct from the mutations that are seen in MEN-2A, seems to be responsible for virtually all cases of MEN-2B. This point substitution affects a critical region of the tyrosine kinase domain of the protein and leads to constitutive activation of RET in the absence of ligand. Of note, approximately a third of sporadic medullary thyroid carcinomas harbor the identical mutation, and these cases are associated with aggressive disease and an adverse prognosis.
- *Familial medullary thyroid cancer* is a variant of MEN-2A, in which there is a strong predisposition to medullary thyroid cancer but not the other clinical manifestations of MEN-2A or MEN-2B. A substantial majority of cases of medullary thyroid cancer are sporadic, but as many as 20% may be familial. Familial medullary thyroid cancers develop at an older age than those occurring in the full-blown MEN-2 syndrome and follow a more indolent course.

In contrast to MEN-1, in which the long-term benefit of early diagnosis by genetic screening is not well established, diagnosis via screening of at-risk family members in MEN-2A kindred is important because medullary thyroid carcinoma is a life-threatening disease that can be prevented by early thyroidectomy. Now, routine genetic testing identifies *RET* mutation carriers earlier and more reliably in MEN-2 kindreds; all individuals carrying germline RET mutations are advised to undergo prophylactic thyroidectomy to prevent the inevitable development of medullary carcinomas.

PINEAL GLAND

The rarity of clinically significant lesions (virtually only tumors) justifies brevity in the consideration of the pineal gland. It is a minute, pinecone-shaped organ (hence its name), weighing 100 to 180 mg and lying between the superior colliculi at the base of the brain. It is composed of a loose, neuroglial stroma enclosing nests of epithelial-appearing *pineocytes*, cells with photosensory and neuroendocrine functions (hence the designation of the pineal gland as the "third eye"). Silver impregnation stains reveal that these cells have long, slender processes reminiscent of primitive neuronal precursors intermixed with the processes of astrocytic cells. The principal secretory product of the pineal gland is melatonin, which is involved in the control of circadian rhythms, including the sleep-wake cycle; hence the popular use of melatonin for the treatment of jet lag.

All tumors involving the pineal are rare; most (50% to 70%) arise from sequestered embryonic germ cells (Chapter 28). They most commonly take the form of so-called *germinomas*, resembling testicular seminoma (Chapter 21) or ovarian dysgerminoma (Chapter 22). Other lines of germ cell differentiation include embryonal carcinomas; choriocarcinomas; mixtures of germinoma, embryonal carcinoma, and choriocarcinoma; and, uncommonly, typical teratomas (usually benign). Whether to characterize these germ cell neoplasms as pinealomas is debated, but most "pinealophiles" favor restricting the term *pinealoma* to neoplasms arising from the pineocytes.

Pinealomas

These neoplasms are divided into two categories, pineoblastomas and pineocytomas, based on their level of differentiation, which, in turn, correlates with their aggressiveness. These tumors are rare, and are described in specialized texts.

SUGGESTED READINGS

Pituitary

Asa SL, Ezzat S: The pathogenesis of pituitary tumors. *Annu Rev Pathol* 4:97–126, 2009. [*A somewhat dated but excellent review on the molecular genetics of pituitary tumors by two foremost experts in this area*]

Cushing HW: The basophil adenomas of the pituitary body and their clinical manifestations (pituitary basophilism). *Bull Johns Hopkins Hosp* 50:137–95, 1932. [*Harvey Cushing's original description of the eponymous eyndrome*]

Thyroid

Bahn RS: Graves' ophthalmopathy. *N Engl J Med* 362:726–38, 2010. [*An outstanding review on Graves opthalmopathy that encompasses pathogenesis, clinical features and treatment*]

Franklyn JA, Boelaert K: Thyrotoxicosis. *Lancet* 379:1155–66, 2012. [*A clinically oriented review on causes and main therapeutic avenues in hyperthyroidism*]

Graves RJ: A newly observed affection of the thyroid gland in females. *London Med Surg J* 7:516–17, 1835. [*A classic publication describing the index case of the disease named after the author*]

Gull WW: On a cretinoid state supervening in adult life in women. *Trans Clin Soc Lond* 7:180–5, 1873. [*The original description of myxedema, hence also known as "Gull's disease"*]

Hashimoto H: Zur Kenntnis der lymphomatösen Veränderung der Schilddrüse (Struma lymphomatosa). *Arch Klin*, 97, 1912. [*Dr. Hashimoto, a Japanese physician, also trained in Pathology in Germany, which might explain why his paper describing the eponymously named condition in four patients was originally published in German*]

Iyer S, Bahn R: Immunopathogenesis of Graves' ophthalmopathy: the role of the TSH receptor. *Best Pract Res Clin Endocrinol Metab* 26:281–9, 2012. [*A comprehensive review of the autoimmune deregulation targeted against the TSH receptor in Graves opthalmopathy*]

LiVolsi VA: Papillary thyroid carcinoma: an update. *Mod Pathol* 24(Suppl 2):S1–9, 2011. [*A primer on papillary thyroid carcinoma from one of the foremost thyroid pathologists in the world*]

Nikiforov YE, Nikiforova MN: Molecular genetics and diagnosis of thyroid cancer. *Nat Rev Endocrinol* 7:569–80, 2011. [*An excellent review on the molecular abnormalities in thyroid cancer and how to translate these to clinical diagnostics*]

Parathyroid

Al-Azem H, Khan AA: Hypoparathyroidism. *Best Pract Res Clin Endocrinol Metab* 26:517–22, 2012. [*A clinically oriented review on parathyroid hypofunction*]

Sharretts JM, Simonds WF: Clinical and molecular genetics of parathyroid neoplasms. *Best Pract Res Clin Endocrinol Metab* 24:491–502, 2010. [*A review on underlying genetic abnormalities contributing to parathyroid neoplasia, and clinical manifestations thereof*]

Pancreas—Diabetes

Antonetti DA, Klein R, Gardner TW: Diabetic retinopathy. *N Engl J Med* 366:1227–39, 2012. [*A comprehensive review on the most common underlying cause of blindness in the United States, with discussions on pathophysiology, symptoms, diagnosis, and treatment*]

Danaei G, Finucane MM, Lu Y, et al: National, regional, and global trends in fasting plasma glucose and diabetes prevalence since 1980: systematic analysis of health examination surveys and epidemiological studies with 370 country-years and 2.7 million participants. *Lancet* 378:31–40, 2011. [*An epidemiological treatise on global trends in impaired glucose tolerance and diabetes*]

Ferrannini E, Cushman WC: Diabetes and hypertension: the bad companions. *Lancet* 380:601–10, 2012. [*A well balanced review that begins with a discussion of the pathogenetic mechanisms underlying the significant associations between these two conditions, and the impact of hypertension as co-morbidity on the natural history of type 2 diabetes*]

Inzucchi SE: Clinical practice. Diagnosis of diabetes. *N Engl J Med* 367:542–50, 2012. [*An informative paper that tabulates the diagnostic criteria for diabetes in the clinic*]

Jellinger PS: Focus on incretin-based therapies: targeting the core defects of type 2 diabetes. *Postgrad Med* 123:53–65, 2011. [*A insightful review on this new class of therapeutics that is increasingly being utilized as a mainstay in type 2 diabetes*]

McCarthy MI: Genomics, type 2 diabetes, and obesity. *N Engl J Med* 363:2339–50, 2010. [*Informative review on genome-wide susceptibility loci that contribute to the risk of type 2 diabetes, as well as those linked to body mass index and obesity*]

Neale GA, Hooiveld GJ, Hijmans A, et al: Inflammasome is a central player in the induction of obesity and insulin resistance. *Proc Natl Acad Sci U S A* 108:15324–9, 2011. [*An excellent review on the role of the inflammosome in the pathogenesis of insulin resistance and type 2 diabetes, underscoring the rising importance of inflammation in this disease*]

Rodbard HW, Jellinger PS, Davidson JA, et al: Statement by an American Association of Clinical Endocrinologists/American College of Endocrinology consensus panel on type 2 diabetes mellitus: an algorithm for glycemic control. *Endocr Pract* 15:540–59, 2009. [*An algorithm based consensus statement from two of the major academic groups on how to treat hyperglycemia in diabetes, using the available armamentarium of therapies*]

Samuel VT, Shulman GI: Mechanisms for insulin resistance: common threads and missing links. *Cell* 148:852–71, 2012. [*A mechanism heavy, yet lucid review on the pathogenesis of insulin resistance, with outsanding self-explanatory color illustrations*]

Tabak AG, Herder C, Rathmann W, et al: Prediabetes: a high-risk state for diabetes development. *Lancet* 379:2279–90, 2012. [*A timely review on impaired glucose tolerance, a.k.a. prediabetes, and its natural history in progression to eventual diabetes*]

Tahrani AA, Bailey CJ, Del Prato S, et al: Management of type 2 diabetes: new and future developments in treatment. *Lancet* 378:182–97, 2011. [*A clinical review on current and emerging treatment modalities available for control of type 2 diabetes*]

Vaxillaire M, Bonnefond A, Froguel P: The lessons of early-onset monogenic diabetes for the understanding of diabetes pathogenesis. *Best Pract Res Clin Endocrinol Metab* 26:171–87, 2012. [*A review on monogenic forms of diabetes, and how these rare variants might inform the pathogenesis and management of the significantly more common multigenic type 2 diabetes*]

Pancreas—Neuroendocrine Tumors

de Wilde RF, Edil BH, Hruban RH, et al: Well-differentiated pancreatic neuroendocrine tumors: from genetics to therapy. *Nat Rev Gastroenterol Hepatol* 9:199–208, 2012. [*An up-to-date review on newly identified genomic aberrations in pancreatic neuroendocrine tumors and how these can form the basis for personalized therapy*]

Adrenal Cortex

Addison T: *On the constitutional and local effects of disease of the suprarenal capsules*. London, 1855, Samuel Highley. [*The original description of Addison disease*]

Almeida MQ, Stratakis CA: Carney complex and other conditions associated with micronodular adrenal hyperplasias. *Best Pract Res Clin Endocrinol Metab* 24:907–14, 2010. [*An excellent review on the genetic bases of Carnex complex from one of the most prolific research groups in this entity*]

Arnaldi G, Boscaro M: Adrenal incidentaloma. *Best Pract Res Clin Endocrinol Metab* 26:405–19, 2012. [*A clinically oriented review on incidental lesions of the adrenal glands*]

Bornstein SR: Predisposing factors for adrenal insufficiency. *N Engl J Med* 360:2328–39, 2009. [*An outstanding review on etiological bases for adrenal insufficiency, with a discussion of etiopathogenesis, clinical features and treatment*]

Carroll TB, Findling JW: The diagnosis of Cushing's syndrome. *Rev Endocr Metab Disord* 11:147–53, 2010. [*A clinically oriented review on Cushing syndrome, including relevant laboratory tests that establish diagnosis*]

Choi M, Scholl UI, Yue P, et al: K+ channel mutations in adrenal aldosterone-producing adenomas and hereditary hypertension. *Science* 331:768–72, 2011. [*Original research study on the genetic basis for a subset of aldosterone-producing adenomas which cause severe hypertension to run in some families*]

Kisand K, Boe Wolff AS, Podkrajsek KT, et al: Chronic mucocutaneous candidiasis in APECED or thymoma patients correlates with autoimmunity to Th17-associated cytokines. *J Exp Med* 207:299–308, 2010. [*Original research study describing the role of neutralizing autoantibodies against Th17-associated cytokines like IL-17 and IL-22 in the pathogenesis of chronic mucocutaneous candidiasis*]

Adrenal Medulla

Friderichsen C: Nebennierenapoplexie bei kleinen Kindern. *Jahrbuch für Kinderhilkunde* 87:109–25, 1918. [*One of the two original descriptions of the eponymously named Waterhouse-Friderichsen syndromFre; Carl Friderichsen was a Danish pediatrician*]

Lowery AJ, Walsh S, McDermott EW, et al: Molecular and therapeutic advances in the diagnosis and management of malignant pheochromocytomas and paragangliomas. *Oncologist* 18:391–407, 2013. [*A recent review on genetic susceptibility to pheochromocytomas and paragangliomas, including rarer variants not discussed in the text, as well as therapeutic opportunities in this calss of neoplasms*]

Waterhouse R: A case of suprarenal apoplexy. *Lancet* 1:577–8, 1911. [*The second of two papers, this one authored by Rupert Waterhouse, an English physician, which led to recognition of the eponymous syndrome*]

Multiple Endocrine Neoplasia

Huang J, Gurung B, Wan B, et al: The same pocket in menin binds both MLL and JUND but has opposite effects on transcription. *Nature* 482:542–6, 2012. [*Seminal paper elucidating how menin demonstrates a context specific function in tumorigenesis based on the nature of its binding partner*]

Thakker RV: Multiple endocrine neoplasia type 1 (MEN1). *Best Pract Res Clin Endocrinol Metab* 24:355–70, 2010. [*A detailed treatise on MEN1, which incorporates both genetics and clinical descriptions for this syndrome*]

See TARGETED THERAPY available online at www.studentconsult.com 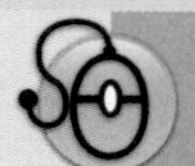

CHAPTER 25

The Skin

Alexander J.F. Lazar • George F. Murphy

CHAPTER CONTENTS

The Skin: More Than a Mechanical Barrier

More than a century and a half ago, the noted pathologist Rudolph Virchow described the skin as a mere protective covering for more delicate and functionally sophisticated internal viscera. Then, and for most of the time that followed, the skin was viewed as a necessary but rather uninteresting barrier to fluid loss and mechanical injury. Over the last several decades, however, the skin has come to be appreciated as a surprisingly complicated organ—the largest in the body—in which precisely regulated cellular and molecular interactions govern many essential processes.

Although the human integument may appear drab compared with the skin and pelage of other members of the animal kingdom, it is extraordinarily vibrant with regard to the diversity of functions that it carries out. Chief among these is its role as one of the first lines of defense against potentially harmful infectious and physical agents. However, the skin is also a highly sophisticated sensory organ, and even has important endocrine roles, particularly the synthesis of vitamin D (Chapter 9), which is "powered" by sun exposure. It is composed of several cell types and structures that function interdependently and cooperatively (Fig. 25-1).

- *Squamous epithelial cells (keratinocytes)* are normally "glued" tightly together by cell junctions known as desmosomes and produce abundant amounts of keratin protein, both of which serve to create a tough, durable physical barrier. In addition, keratinocytes secrete soluble molecules such as cytokines and defensins that augment and regulate cutaneous immune responses (described later).
- *Melanocytes* within the epidermis are responsible for the production of melanin, a brown pigment that absorbs and protects against potentially injurious ultraviolet (UV) radiation in sunlight.

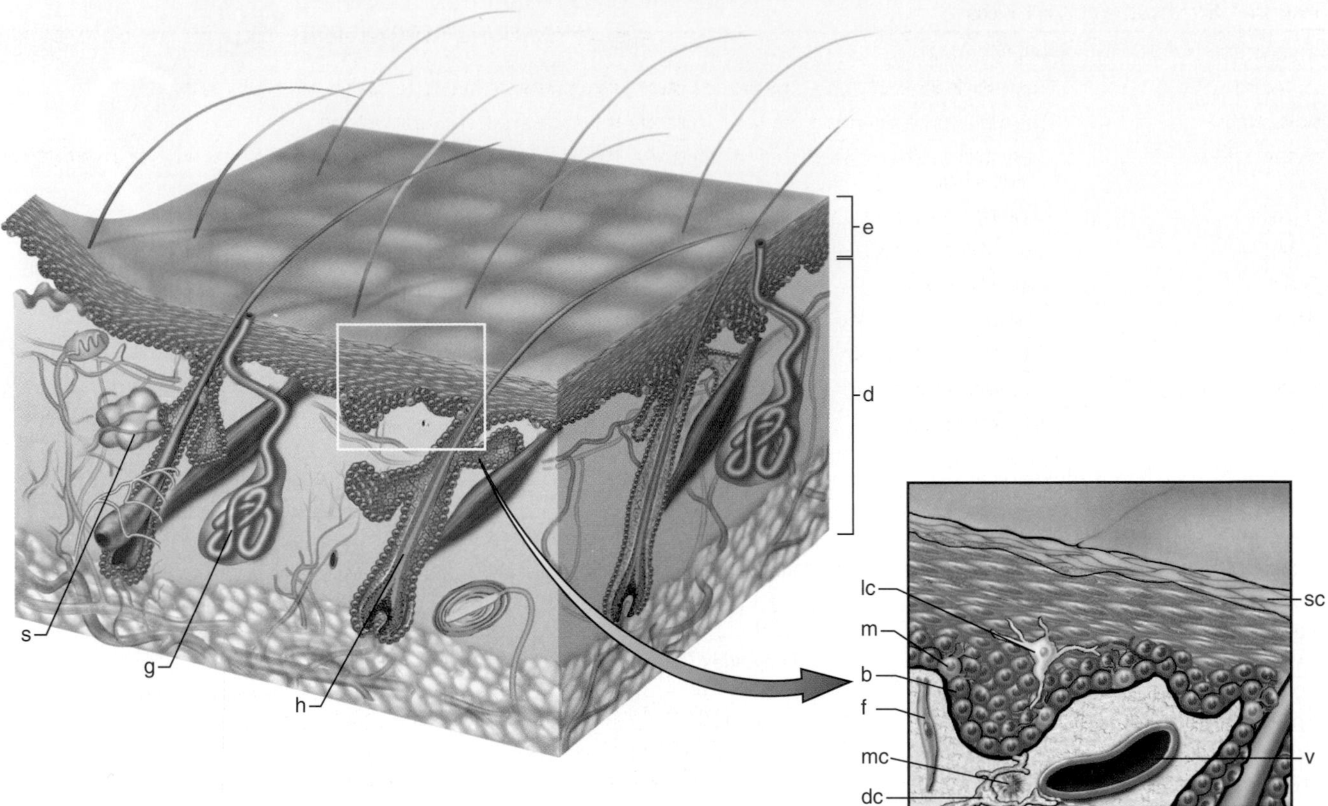

Figure 25-1 *Left,* The skin is composed of an epidermal layer (e) from which specialized adnexa (hair follicles, h; sweat glands, g; and sebaceous glands, s) descend into the underlying dermis (d). *Inset,* This projection of the epidermal layer (e) and underlying superficial dermis demonstrates the progressive upward maturation of basal cells (b) into cornified squamous epithelial cells of the stratum corneum (sc). Melanin-containing dendritic melanocytes (m) (and rare Merkel cells containing neurosecretory granules) and mid-epidermal dendritic Langerhans cells (lc) are also present. The underlying dermis contains small vessels (v), fibroblasts (f), perivascular mast cells (mc), and dendrocytes (dc), which participate in dermal immune responses and repair.

- *Dendritic cells.* Skin serves as one of the first lines of defense against microorganisms and is constantly exposed to microbial and nonmicrobial antigens, which are processed by intraepidermal dendritic cells known as *Langerhans cells.* Langerhans cells secrete factors that augment innate immune responses, and migrate from the skin to regional lymph nodes where they present their antigenic cargoes to T lymphocytes, thereby stimulating the adaptive immune system. Specialized *dendrocytes,* another type of dendritic cell found within the dermis, perform similar functions.
- *Lymphocytes.* Following their stimulation by dendritic cells in regional lymph nodes, T cells expressing an adhesion molecule called cutaneous lymphocyte-associated antigen (CLA) and chemokine receptors such as CCR4 and CCR10 leave the lymph node and home back to the dermis, a process that is directed in part by chemokines secreted by activated keratinocytes. The infiltrating T cells usually include helper (CD4+), cytotoxic (CD8+), and regulatory (Treg) T cells (Chapter 6). Cytokines produced by these T cells mediate the microscopic patterns and clinical expressions of cutaneous inflammatory and infectious diseases. In addition, small numbers of B cells are found in the dermis that can participate in humoral responses to antigens encountered in the skin.
- Like the gut (Chapter 17), there is increasing appreciation that the skin is a large and complex ecosystem that provides niches for a broad spectrum of organisms, including bacteria, fungi, viruses, and mites. These organisms have evolved symbiotic relationships with their human hosts and appear to contribute to health in a number of ways. By occupying skin niches, the normal "zoo" of skin organisms prevents colonization of the skin by other potentially harmful organisms. In addition, the skin fauna primes and "educates" the cutaneous immune system in a manner that is believe to enhance immune responses to potential pathogens. This story is just in its infancy, and it is likely that the role of the skin microbiome in health and disease will continue to expand in the coming years.
- *Afferent nerve fibers* and a diverse set of associated specialized structures referred to as *neural end organs* are responsible for physical sensations that run that gamut from pleasurable to painful, including touch, vibration, itchiness, cold, and heat. In addition, *autonomic efferent nerve fibers* regulate adnexal components such as sweat glands and effector pili muscles (see later) and can also influence the function of innate and adaptive immune cells in the dermis. Another cell type found in skin that remains cloaked in mystery is the *Merkel cell;* these cells are located in epithelial basal cell layer and may have neuroendocrine or mechanoreceptor functions.
- *Adnexal components. Sweat glands* guard against deleterious variations in body temperature, and *hair follicles,* in addition to manufacturing hair shafts, have protected

Table 25-1 Nomenclature of Skin Lesions

Macroscopic Lesions	Definition
Excoriation	Traumatic lesion breaking the epidermis and causing a raw linear area (i.e., deep scratch); often self-induced
Lichenification	Thickened, rough skin (similar to a lichen on a rock); usually the result of repeated rubbing
Macule, Patch	Circumscribed, flat lesion distinguished from surrounding skin by color. Macules are 5 mm in diameter or less, patches are greater than 5 mm.
Onycholysis	Separation of nail plate from nail bed
Papule, Nodule	Elevated dome-shaped or flat-topped lesion. Papules are 5 mm or less across, while nodules are greater than 5 mm in size.
Plaque	Elevated flat-topped lesion, usually greater than 5 mm across (may be caused by coalescent papules)
Pustule	Discrete, pus-filled, raised lesion
Scale	Dry, horny, platelike excrescence; usually the result of imperfect cornification
Vesicle, Bulla, Blister	Fluid-filled raised lesion 5 mm or less across (vesicle) or greater than 5 mm across (bulla). Blister is the common term for either.
Wheal	Itchy, transient, elevated lesion with variable blanching and erythema formed as the result of dermal edema
Microscopic Lesions	**Definition**
Acanthosis	Diffuse epidermal hyperplasia
Dyskeratosis	Abnormal, premature keratinization within cells below the stratum granulosum
Erosion	Discontinuity of the skin showing incomplete loss of the epidermis
Exocytosis	Infiltration of the epidermis by inflammatory cells
Hydropic swelling (ballooning)	Intracellular edema of keratinocytes, often seen in viral infections
Hypergranulosis	Hyperplasia of the stratum granulosum, often due to intense rubbing
Hyperkeratosis	Thickening of the stratum corneum, often associated with a qualitative abnormality of the keratin
Lentiginous	A linear pattern of melanocyte proliferation within the epidermal basal cell layer
Papillomatosis	Surface elevation caused by hyperplasia and enlargement of contiguous dermal papillae
Parakeratosis	Keratinization with retained nuclei in the stratum corneum. On mucous membranes, parakeratosis is normal.
Spongiosis	Intercellular edema of the epidermis
Ulceration	Discontinuity of the skin showing complete loss of the epidermis revealing dermis or subcutis
Vacuolization	Formation of vacuoles within or adjacent to cells; often refers to basal cell-basement membrane zone area

niches harboring epithelial stem cells capable of regenerating superficial epithelial skin structures, which may be disrupted by trauma, burns, and other types of injuries.

Imbalances in factors affecting the delicate homeostasis that exists among skin cells may result in conditions as diverse as wrinkles and hair loss, blisters and rashes, and life-threatening cancers and disorders of immune regulation. For example, long-term exposure to sunlight fosters premature cutaneous aging, blunts immunologic responses to environmental antigens, and favors the development of a variety of premalignant and malignant cutaneous neoplasms. Ingested agents, such as therapeutic drugs, can cause an enormous number of rashes or exanthems. Systemic disorders, such as diabetes mellitus, amyloidosis, and lupus erythematosus, may also have important manifestations in the skin.

Skin conditions are very common, affecting about one third of the United States population each year. Since skin is uniquely accessible to visual examination, for the experienced observer it can yield numerous insights into the functional state of the body (if not the very soul of a patient). Close attention to the appearance and distribution of skin lesions is critical, as these characteristics are essential in formulating diagnoses and in understanding pathogenesis. To underscore this point, special emphasis is placed on the gross appearance of skin lesions under each specific entity.

Thousands of diseases affect the skin. Only those that are common or that illustrate important pathologic mechanisms are described here. Dermatologists and dermatopathologists have developed a set of terms to describe the gross and microscopic appearance of skin lesions that every student must be familiar with in order to be fluent in dermatopathology; the most important of these terms and definitions are given in Table 25-1.

Disorders of Pigmentation and Melanocytes

Focal or widespread loss of normal protective pigmentation can make individuals extraordinarily vulnerable to the harmful effects of sunlight (as in albinism). Changes in preexisting skin pigmentation may signify important primary skin disorders (e.g., malignant transformation of a mole) or point to the existence of an underlying systemic disorder (e.g., Addison disease, Chapter 24).

Freckle (Ephelis)

Freckles are the most common pigmented lesions of childhood in lightly pigmented individuals. It is unclear whether freckles result from a focal abnormality in pigment production in a discrete field of melanocytes, enhanced melanin transfer to adjacent basal keratinocytes, or some

Table 25-2 Representative Variant Forms of Melanocytic Nevi

Nevus Variant	Diagnostic Architectural Features	Cytologic Features	Clinical Significance
Congenital nevus	Deep dermal and sometimes subcutaneous growth around adnexa, neurovascular bundles, and blood vessel walls	Identical to ordinary acquired nevi	Present at birth; large variants have increased melanoma risk
Blue nevus	Non-nested dermal infiltration, often with associated fibrosis	Highly dendritic, heavily pigmented nevus cells	Black-blue nodule; often confused with melanoma clinically
Spindle and epithelioid cell nevus (Spitz nevus)	Fascicular growth	Large, plump cells with pink-blue cytoplasm; fusiform cells	Common in children; red-pink nodule; often confused with hemangioma clinically
Halo nevus	Lymphocytic infiltration surrounding nevus cells	Identical to ordinary acquired nevi	Host immune response against nevus cells and surrounding normal melanocytes
Dysplastic nevus	Coalescent intraepidermal nests	Cytologic atypia	Potential marker or precursor of melanoma

combination thereof. The *café au lait* spots seen in neurofibromatosis (Chapter 27) are similar to freckles histologically, but differ in that they are larger, arise independently of sun exposure, and contain aggregated melanosomes (macromelanosomes), which can be seen within the cytoplasm of melanocytes in electron micrographs.

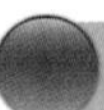

MORPHOLOGY

Freckles are generally small (1 to several mm in diameter), tan-red or light brown macules that appear after sun exposure. Once present, freckles fade and darken in a cyclic fashion during winter and summer, respectively. This is not because of changes in the number of melanocytes, but in the degree of pigmentation. Hyperpigmentation of freckles results from increased amounts of melanin pigment within basal keratinocytes. Associated melanocytes may be slightly enlarged but are normal in density.

Lentigo

The term lentigo (plural, lentigines) refers to a common benign localized hyperplasia of melanocytes occurring at all ages, but often initiated in infancy and childhood. There is no sex or racial predilection, and the cause and pathogenesis are unknown.

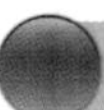

MORPHOLOGY

Lentigines may involve mucous membranes as well as the skin and consist of small (5 to 10 mm across), oval, tan-brown macules or patches. Unlike freckles, lentigines do not darken when exposed to sunlight. The essential histologic feature is **linear (nonnested) melanocytic hyperplasia** restricted to the cell layer immediately above the basement membrane that produces a hyperpigmented basal cell layer. So characteristic is this pattern that the term *lentiginous* is used to describe similar cellular proliferations within the basal cell layer in melanocytic tumors, such as in lentiginous nevi and in certain melanomas (termed *acral lentiginous melanomas*). Elongation and thinning of the rete ridges are also commonly seen in a lentigo.

Melanocytic Nevus (Pigmented Nevus, Mole)

Melanocytic nevi (known colloquially as moles) are common benign neoplasms caused in most cases by acquired activating mutations in components of the Ras signaling pathway. Most of us have at least a few "moles" and probably regard them as mundane and uninteresting. However, in truth moles (or melanocytic nevi) are diverse, dynamic, and biologically fascinating neoplasms. There are numerous subtypes of melanocytic nevi that are distinguished based on their clinical and histologic features; Table 25-2 provides a summary of salient features of some commonly encountered forms. Acquired melanocytic nevi are the most common type and are found in virtually all individuals.

Pathogenesis. Proof that nevi are neoplasms comes from studies showing that many have acquired mutations that lead to constitutive activation of NRAS or the serine/threonine kinase BRAF, which lies immediately downstream of RAS (described in Chapter 7 and later under Melanoma). Given that RAS signals have potent transforming activity and are thought to have key roles in many full-blown cancers, it is reasonable to ask why nevi only rarely give rise to melanomas. One answer appears to lie in the phenomenon referred to as oncogene-induced senescence. Expression of either activated RAS or BRAF in normal human melanocytes causes only a limited period of proliferation that is followed by a permanent growth arrest mediated by the accumulation of p16/INK4a, a potent inhibitor of several cyclin-dependent kinases, including CDK4 and CDK6 (Chapter 7). This protective response is disrupted in melanoma and some precursor lesions that give rise to melanoma.

MORPHOLOGY

Common acquired melanocytic nevi are tan to brown, uniformly pigmented, small (usually less than 6 mm across), relatively flat macules or elevated papules with well-defined, rounded borders (Figs. 25-2*A* and 25-3*A*). They may become more prominent during pregnancy, indicating a degree of hormone sensitivity. Melanocytic nevi are thought to progress through a series of morphologic changes over time. The earliest lesions are believed to be **junctional nevi**, which consist of aggregates or nests of round cells that grow along the dermoepidermal junction (Fig. 25-2*B*). Nuclei of nevus cells are uniform and rounded in contour, contain inconspicuous nucleoli, and show little or no mitotic activity. Eventually, most junctional nevi grow into the underlying dermis as nests or cords of cells to form **compound nevi** (Fig. 25-3*B*). In older lesions the epidermal nests may be lost entirely to form pure **intradermal nevi.**

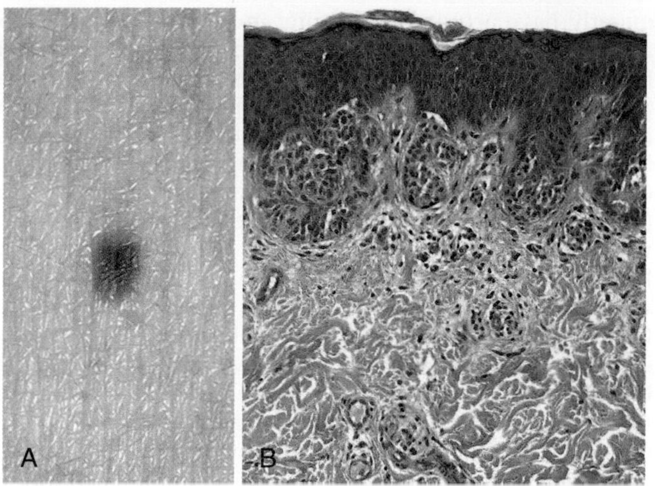

Figure 25-2 Melanocytic nevus, junctional type. **A,** Grossly, lesions are small, relatively flat, symmetric, and uniform. **B,** On histologic examination, junctional nevi are characterized by rounded nests of nevus cells originating at the tips of rete ridges along the dermoepidermal junction.

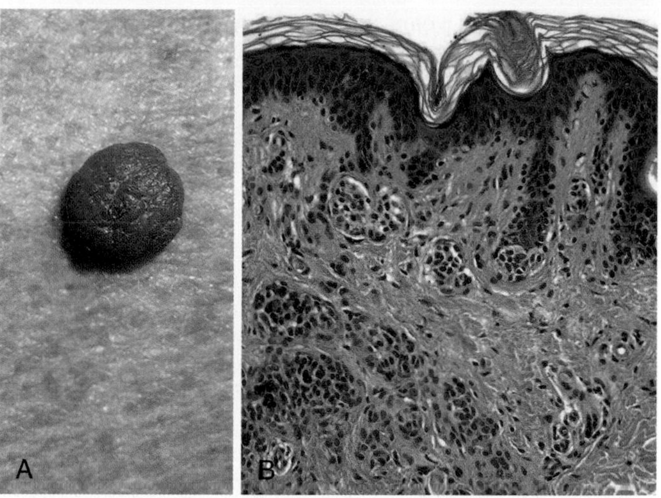

Figure 25-3 Melanocytic nevus, compound type. In contrast to the junctional nevus, the compound nevus **(A)** is raised and dome-shaped. The symmetry and uniform pigment distribution suggest a benign process. Histologically **(B),** compound nevi combine the features of junctional nevi (intraepidermal nevus cell nests) with nests and cords of dermal nevus cells.

Clinically, compound and dermal nevi are often more elevated than junctional nevi.

Progressive growth of nevus cells from the dermoepidermal junction into the underlying dermis is accompanied by morphologic changes that are taken to be a reflection of oncogene-induced senescence (Fig. 25-4). Whereas superficial nevus cells are larger, tend to produce melanin, and grow in nests, deeper nevus cells are smaller, produce little or no pigment, and appear as cords and single cells. At the deepest extent of the lesions, these cells often acquire fusiform contours and grow in fascicles resembling neural tissue (neurotization; Fig. 25-4*E*). This striking metamorphosis correlates with enzymatic changes (progressive loss of tyrosinase activity and acquisition of cholinesterase activity) in deeper, nonpigmented "nervelike" nevus cells. **These changes are helpful in distinguishing benign nevi from melanomas, which lack such features.**

Although melanocytic nevi are common, their clinical and histologic diversity necessitates thorough knowledge of their appearance and natural evolution, lest they be confused with other skin conditions, most notably melanoma. The biologic importance of some nevi, however, resides in their possible transformation to melanoma or as markers of increased risk for melanoma (as described below).

Dysplastic Nevi

Dysplastic nevi are important because they may be direct precursors of melanoma and when multiple in number are a marker of an increased risk for melanoma. The association of melanocytic nevi with melanoma was

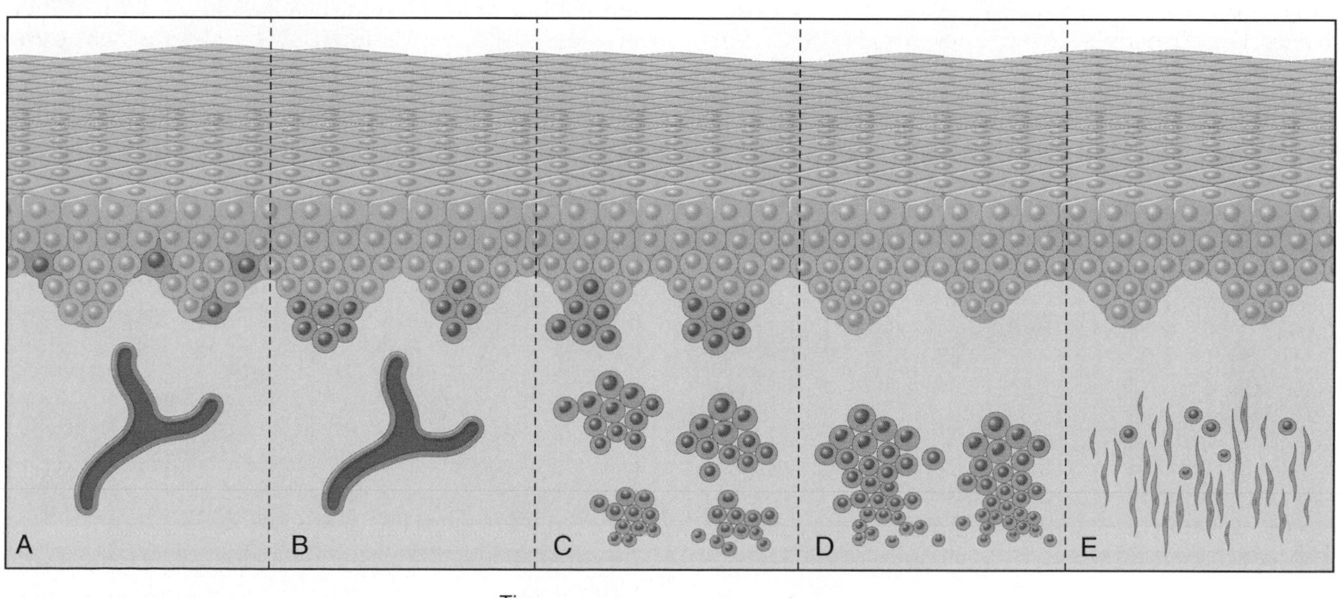

Figure 25-4 Maturation sequence of nondysplastic melanocytic nevi. **A,** Normal skin shows only scattered dendritic melanocytes within the epidermal basal cell layer. **B,** Junctional nevus. **C,** Compound nevus. **D,** Dermal nevus. **E,** Dermal nevus with neurotization, a change that is also referred to as maturation. Nevi may exist at any stage in this sequence for variable periods of time, although many are believed to progress through this sequence.

made almost 200 years ago, but a potential precursor of melanoma was not identified until 1978 when Clark and colleagues described the lesions that are now referred to as *dysplastic nevi.* Several lines of evidence support the concept that some dysplastic nevi are precursors of melanoma. One of the most compelling pieces of evidence involves studies of families affected by *dysplastic nevus syndrome*, an autosomal dominant disorder in which a tendency to develop multiple dysplastic nevi and melanoma are co-inherited. The probability that a person with dysplastic nevus syndrome will develop melanoma is over 50% by age 60, and at-risk individuals sometimes develop several melanomas at multiple sites. Even more directly, apparent transformation of dysplastic nevi to melanoma has been documented histologically.

Although dysplastic nevi can give rise to melanoma, the vast majority of such lesions are clinically stable and never progress. Conversely, not all melanomas in individuals with dysplastic nevus syndrome arise from dysplastic nevi, suggesting that these lesions may be best viewed as indicators of increased melanoma risk. Indeed, melanoma may arise in individuals completely lacking in dysplastic nevi. Dysplastic nevi may also occur as isolated lesions in otherwise normal individuals, in which case the risk of malignant transformation is very low.

Pathogenesis. Clark and associates have proposed stages in the development of dysplastic nevi and their eventual progression to melanoma (Fig. 25-5), presumably through stepwise acquisition of mutations or epigenetic changes. Indeed, like conventional nevi, dysplastic nevi also frequently have acquired activating mutations in the *NRAS* and *BRAF* genes. What then distinguishes dysplastic nevi from typical melanocytic nevi? An important clue comes from individuals with dysplastic nevus syndrome. Such individuals often have inherited loss of function mutations in *CDKN2A*. As discussed further under melanoma, *CDKN2A* encodes several proteins including p16/INK4a (described in more detail under melanoma), which you will recall is a negative regulator of cyclin-dependent kinase 4 (CDK4) and cyclin-dependent kinase 6. Other affected families have mutations in *CDK4* that make the CDK4 protein resistant to inhibition by p16/INK4a. Thus, it appears that RAS or BRAF activation and increased CDK4 activity contributes to the development of dysplastic nevi. However, not all patients with germline mutations in *CDKN2A* or *CDK4* have dysplastic nevi, and not all familial dysplastic nevi are associated with mutations in these genes. As a result it is suspected that additional genes influence whether dysplastic nevi occur in a particular individual; the identities of these modifier genes, as well as the other genes that are responsible for the syndrome, are being sought. One possible suspect is germline mutations that increase the expression of *TERT*, the gene that encodes the catalytic subunit of telomerase (described later under Melanoma).

MORPHOLOGY

Dysplastic nevi are **larger than most acquired nevi (often greater than 5 mm across) and may number in the**

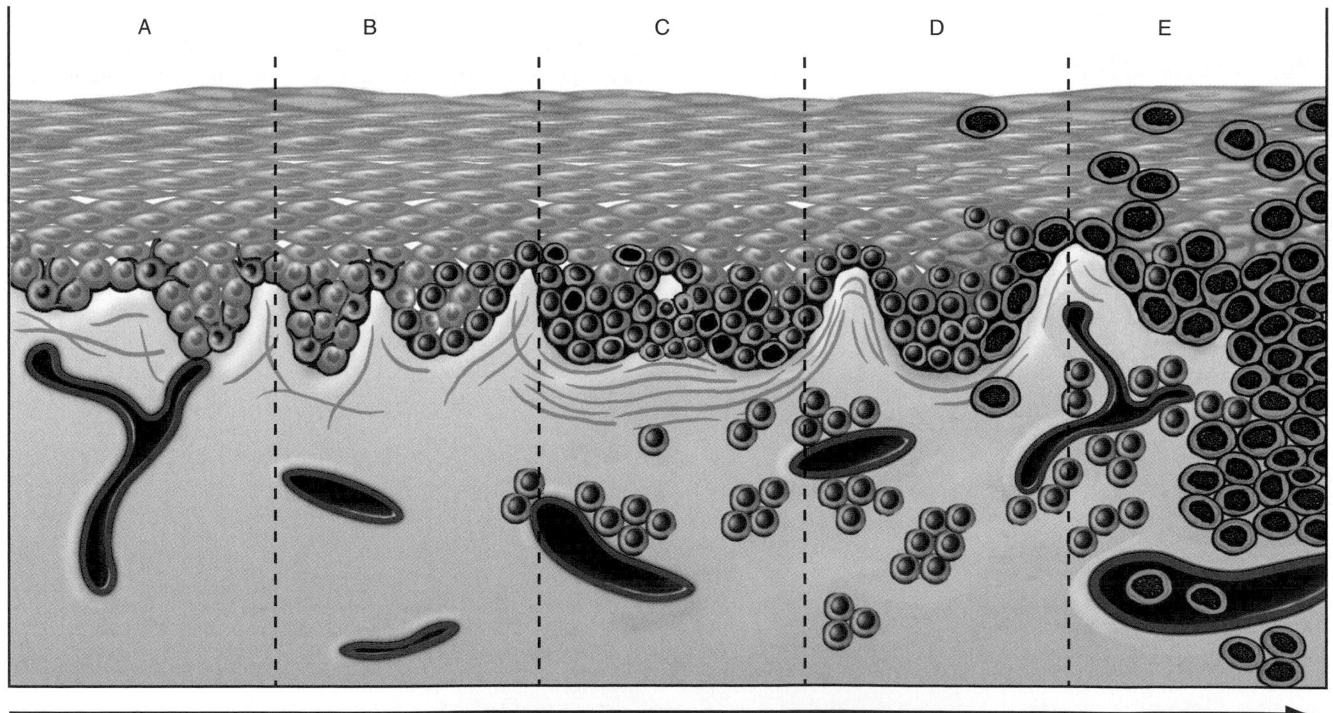

Figure 25-5 Potential steps of tumor progression in dysplastic nevi. **A,** Lentiginous melanocytic hyperplasia. **B,** Lentiginous junctional nevus. **C,** Lentiginous compound nevus with abnormal architectural and cytologic features (dysplastic nevus). **D,** Early melanoma, or melanoma in radial growth phase (large dark cells in epidermis). **E,** Advanced melanoma (vertical growth phase) with malignant spread into the dermis and vessels. The risk of malignant transformation of any single dysplastic nevus is small, but appears to be higher than that of typical nevi.

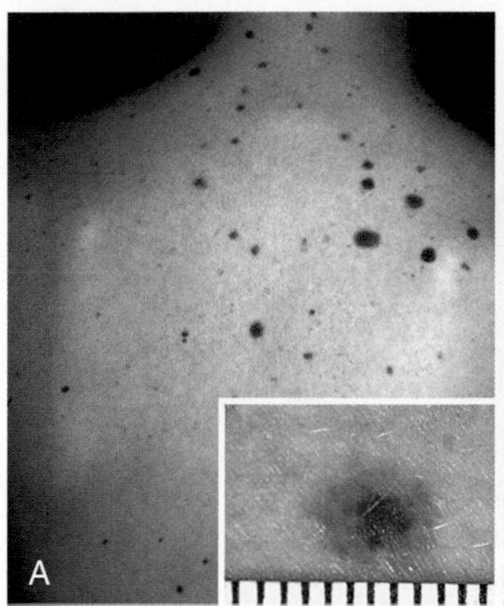

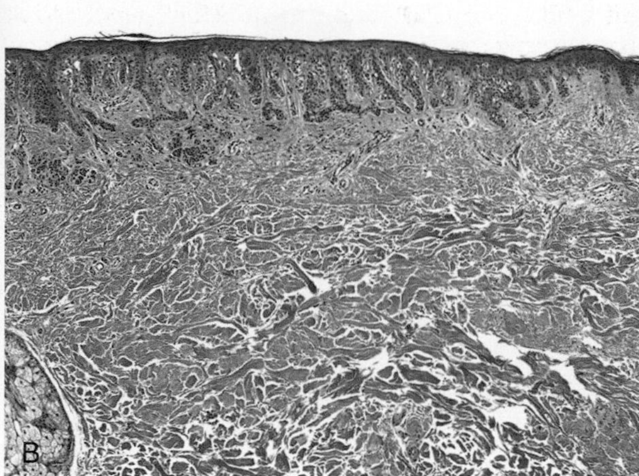

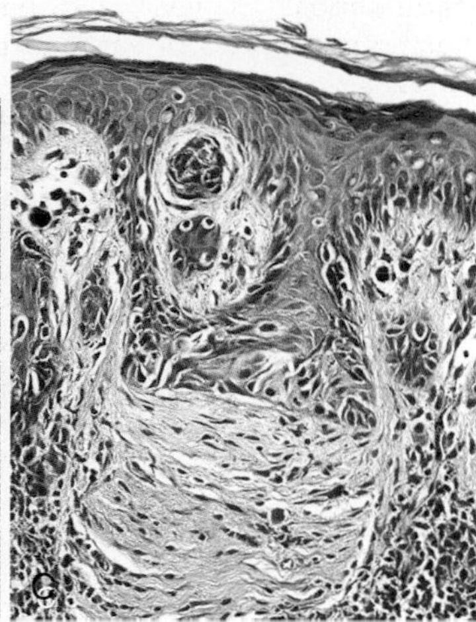

Figure 25-6 Dysplastic nevus. **A,** Numerous atypical nevi on the back. **B,** One such lesion (*inset A*) has a compound nevus component (*left*) and an asymmetric junctional nevus component (*right*). The former corresponds to the more pigmented and raised central zone and the latter to the less pigmented, flat peripheral rim of the lesion shown in **A. C,** An important feature is the presence of cytologic atypia (irregularly shaped, dark-staining nuclei). The dermis underlying the atypical cells characteristically shows linear, or lamellar, fibrosis.

hundreds in those with the dysplastic nevus syndrome (Fig. 25-6*A*). They are flat macules, slightly raised plaques with a "pebbly" surface, or target-like lesions with a darker raised center and irregular flat periphery. They can be recognized by their size, variability in pigmentation (variegation), and irregular borders. Most seem to be acquired rather than congenital. Unlike ordinary moles, dysplastic nevi occur on both sun-exposed and protected body surfaces.

Microscopically, dysplastic nevi usually involve both the epidermis and the dermis and exhibit architectural and cytologic atypia (Fig. 25-6*A, B*). **Nevus cell nests within the epidermis may be enlarged and often fuse or coalescence with adjacent nests.** As part of this process, single nevus cells begin to replace the normal basal cell layer along the dermo-epidermal junction, producing **lentiginous hyperplasia.** Cytologic atypia takes the form of nuclear enlargement, irregular, often angulated, nuclear contours, and hyperchromasia (Fig. 25-6*C*). Associated alterations in the superficial dermis include lymphocytic infiltrates (usually sparse); release of melanin from dead nevus cells into the dermis (**melanin incontinence**), where it is phagocytosed by dermal macrophages; and a peculiar **linear fibrosis** surrounding the epidermal rete ridges that are involved by the nevus. The diagnosis is based on this constellation of features, rather than any single finding.

Melanoma

Melanoma is the most deadly of all skin cancers and is strongly linked to acquired mutations caused by exposure to UV radiation in sunlight. Melanoma is a relatively common neoplasm that can be cured if it is detected and treated when it is in its earliest stages. The great preponderance of melanoma arises in the skin; other sites of origin include the oral and anogenital mucosal surfaces (i.e., oropharynx, gastrointestinal and genitourinary tracts), esophagus, meninges, and the uvea of the eye (Chapter 29). The following comments apply to cutaneous melanomas.

Today, as a result of increased public awareness of the signs of cutaneous melanoma, most are cured surgically. Nevertheless, the reported incidence of melanoma is increasing; more than 76,000 cases and more than 9,700 deaths are expected in the United States in 2014.

Pathogenesis. About 10% to 15% of melanomas are inherited as an autosomal dominant trait with variable penetrance; as mentioned when discussing dysplastic nevi, some of these familial cases are associated with germline mutations affecting the genes that regulate cell-cycle progression or telomerase (described later). The overwhelming majority of melanoma is sporadic and is related to a single predisposing environmental factor: ultraviolet radiation (UVR) damage from sun exposure. UVR is associated strongly with DNA damage. Consistent with a pathogenic role in this disease, sequencing of melanoma genomes has demonstrated a very high rate of point mutations that bear the signature of the damaging effects of UV radiation on DNA. In line with this molecular evidence, melanomas most commonly arise on sun-exposed surfaces, particularly the upper back in men and the back and legs in women, and lightly pigmented individuals are at higher risk than are darkly pigmented individuals. Other inherited genetic variants linked to a modestly increased risk of melanoma in fair-skinned populations act by diminishing melanin production in skin, thus presumably increasing the amount of damage that sun-exposure wreaks on melanocytes.

Nevertheless, the relationship between sun exposure and melanoma is not as straightforward as with other skin cancers (discussed later). Some studies suggest that periodic severe sunburns early in life are the most important risk factor. Furthermore, since melanomas sometimes occur in dark-skinned individuals and at body sites that are not sun-exposed, sunlight is not always an essential predisposing factor, and other environmental factors may also contribute to risk.

The most frequent "driver" mutations in melanoma affect cell cycle control, pro-growth pathways, and telomerase. Some of the more common mutations are as follows:

- *Mutations that disrupt cell cycle control genes.* The *CDKN2A* gene is mutated in approximately 40% of pedigrees with

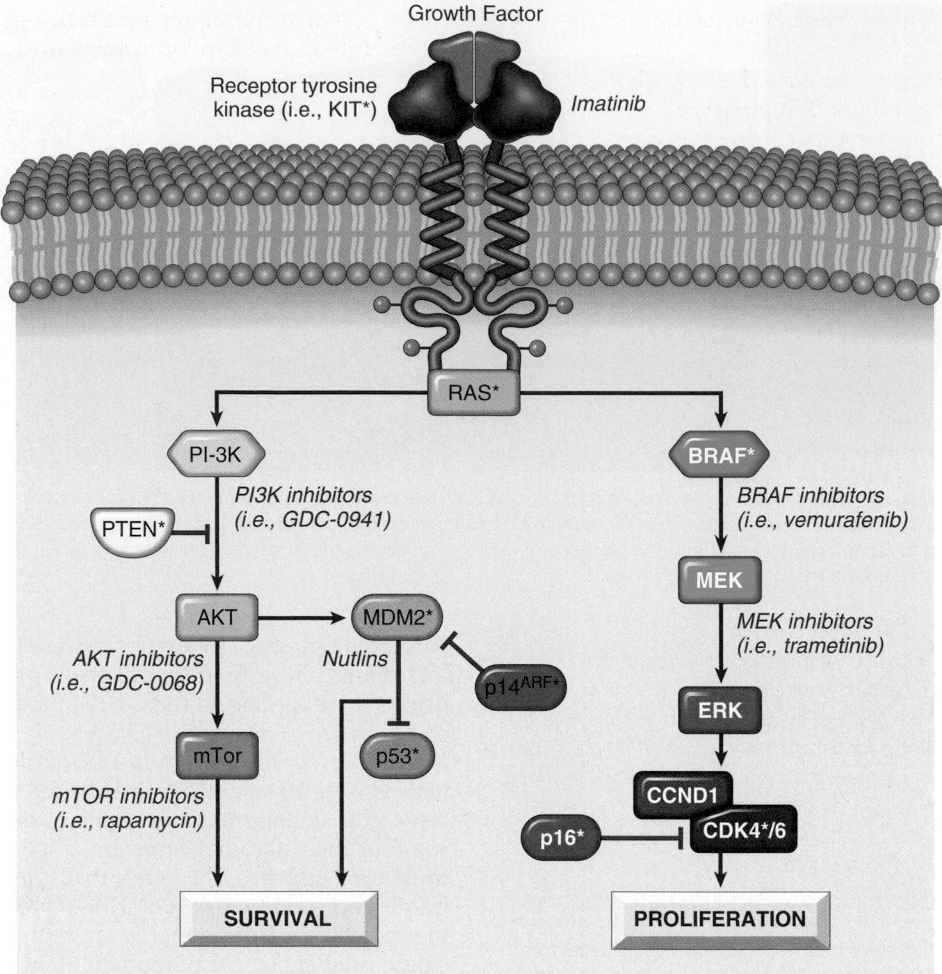

Figure 25-7 Pathways important in melanoma. Growth factors activate signaling circuits involving receptor tyrosine kinases (e.g., KIT), RAS, and two key downstream pathways that include the serine/threonine kinase BRAF and the phospholipid kinase PI3K. Proteins indicated by asterisks are mutated in melanoma. Components of these pathways that are being targeted by drugs are indicated.

autosomal dominant familial melanoma. *CDKN2A* is a complex locus that encodes three different tumor suppressors, p15/INK4b, p16/INK4a, and p14/ARF. Of these, loss of p16/INK4a is clearly implicated in human melanoma, and experimental evidence also supports a role for loss of p14/ARF. As already mentioned, p16/INK4a inhibits cyclin-dependent kinase 4 (CDK4) and cyclin-dependent kinase 6 (CDK6), thus reinforcing the ability of the RB tumor suppressor to block cells in the G_1 phase of the cell cycle. By contrast, p14/ARF enhances the activity of the p53 tumor suppressor by inhibiting MDM2, an oncoprotein that stimulates p53 degradation. *CDKN2A* is mutated in approximately 10% of sporadic melanomas, and these mutations uniformly abolish the production of p16/INK4a and more variably affect p14/ARF. However, it is suspected that these mutations are the tip of the "oncogenic iceberg" with respect to molecular lesions affecting the G_1 checkpoint. For example, 30% to 70% of melanomas show loss of p16/INK4a expression though varied mechanisms, and other familial and sporadic melanomas have mutations in CDK4 that prevent its inhibition by p16/INK4a. The net effect of all of these alterations is the same; increased melanocytic proliferation due to loss of cell-cycle control and escape from oncogene-induced cellular senescence.

- *Mutations that activate pro-growth signaling pathways.* A second common group of molecular lesions in sporadic melanoma leads to aberrant increases in RAS and PI3K/AKT signaling (Fig. 25-7), which you will recall promote cell growth and survival (Chapter 7). Activating mutations in BRAF, a serine/threonine kinase that is downstream of RAS, are seen in 40% to 50% of melanomas, while activating mutations in NRAS occur in an additional 15% to 20% of tumors. Melanomas with BRAF mutations also often show loss of the PTEN tumor suppressor, leading to heightened activation of the PI3K/AKT pathway. For reasons that are unclear, melanomas arising in non-sun exposed cutaneous sites rarely have mutations in BRAF or NRAS and are more likely to have activating mutations in the receptor tyrosine kinase KIT, which sits upstream of both RAS and PI3K/AKT. PTEN is also silenced in 20% of melanomas arising at in non-sun exposed sites. Other melanomas have loss-of-function mutations in the tumor suppressor neurofibromin 1 (NF1), a negative regulator of RAS, which represents yet another mechanism of unleashing RAS signaling.

- *Mutations that activate telomerase.* Reactivation of telomerase, the enzyme activity that preserves telomeres and protects cells from senescence, has long been known to be important in cancer (Chapter 7), but how this occurs has been mysterious. Recently, sequencing of sporadic melanomas identified mutations in the promoter of *TERT*, the gene that encodes the catalytic subunit of telomerase, in roughly 70% of tumors, making *TERT* the most commonly mutated gene yet identified in this cancer. As might be anticipated, the mutations increase *TERT* expression, suggesting that they act as an antidote to senescence. The *TERT* promoter mutations create new binding sites for Ets family transcription factors, which are known to be up-regulated by BRAF signaling, providing a mechanistic link between these two oncogenic events. These findings strongly suggest that mutations that turn on telomerase have a key role in the development of most melanomas.

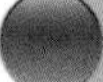

MORPHOLOGY

Unlike benign nevi, melanomas show striking **variations in color**, appearing in shades of black, brown, red, dark blue, and gray (Fig. 25-8*A*). On occasion, zones of white or flesh-colored hypopigmentation also appear, sometimes due to focal regression of the tumor. **The borders of melanomas are irregular and often notched**, unlike the smooth, round, and uniform borders of melanocytic nevi.

Central to understanding the progression of melanoma is the concept of radial and vertical growth phases. **Radial growth** describes the horizontal spread of melanoma within the epidermis and superficial dermis (Fig. 25-8*B*). During this initial stage

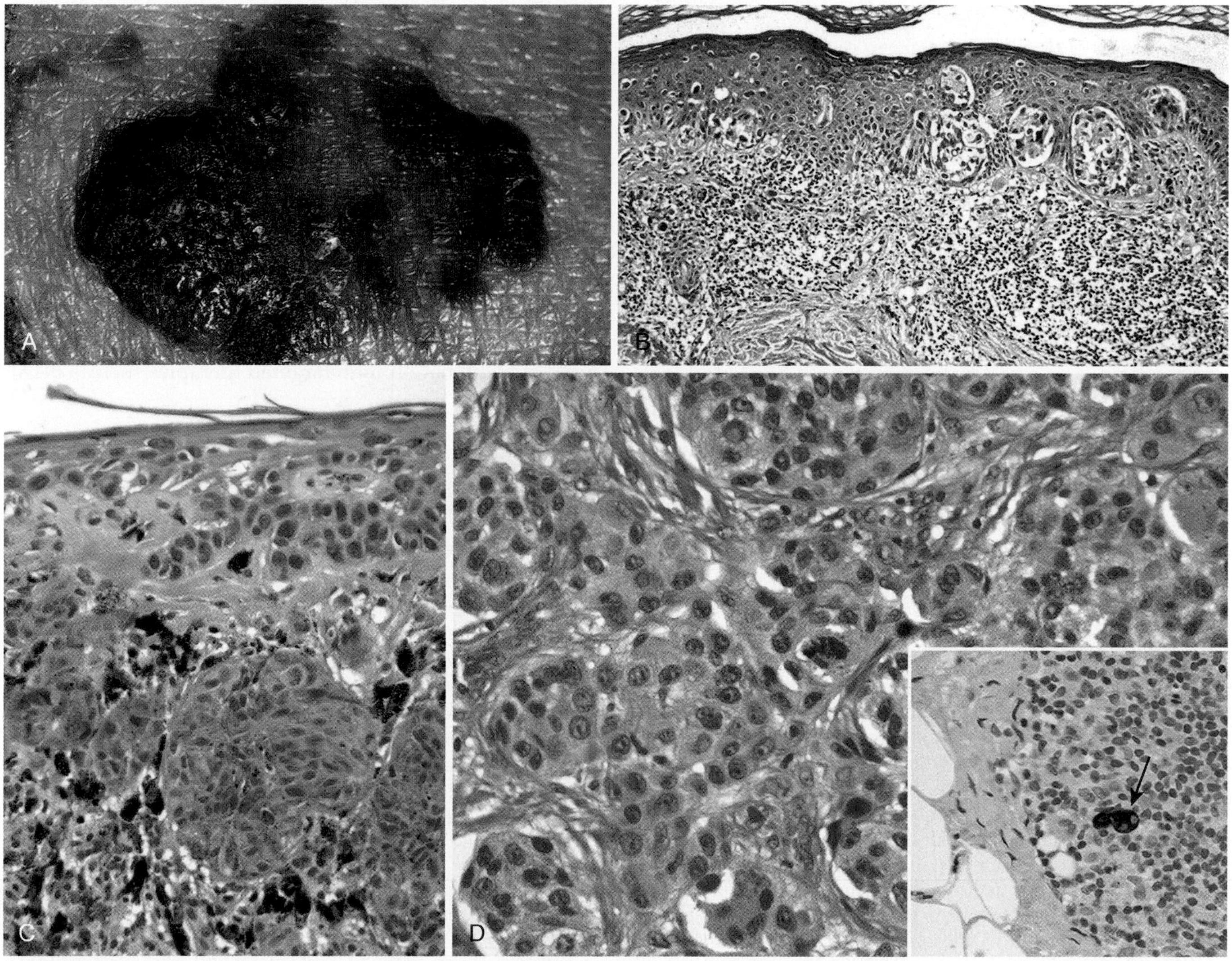

Figure 25-8 Melanoma. **A,** Typical lesions are irregular in contour and pigmentation. Macular areas correlate with the radial growth phase, while raised areas correspond to nodular aggregates of malignant cells in vertical growth phase. **B,** Radial growth phase, showing irregular nested and single-cell growth of melanoma cells within the epidermis and an underlying inflammatory response within the dermis. **C,** Vertical growth phase, demonstrating nodular aggregates of infiltrating cells. **D,** High-power view of melanoma cells. The *inset* shows a sentinel lymph node with a tiny cluster of melanoma cells *(arrow)* staining for the melanocytic marker HMB-45. Even small numbers of malignant cells in a draining lymph node may confer a worse prognosis.

the tumor cells seem to lack the capacity to metastasize. Tumors in radial growth phase fall into several clinicopathologic classes, including: **lentigo maligna**, usually presenting as an indolent lesion on the face of older men that may remain in the radial growth phase for several decades; **superficial spreading**, the most common type of melanoma, usually involving sun-exposed skin; and **acral/mucosal lentiginous** melanoma that is unrelated to sun exposure.

After a variable (and unpredictable) period of time, melanoma shifts from the radial phase to a **vertical growth phase**, during which the tumor cells invade downward into the deeper dermal layers as an expansile mass (Fig. 25-8*C*). **The vertical growth phase is often heralded by the appearance of a nodule and correlates with the emergence of a tumor subclone with metastatic potential.** Unlike melanocytic nevi, "neurotization" is absent from the deep invasive portion of melanoma. The probability of metastasis in such lesions correlates with the depth of invasion, which by convention is the distance from the superficial epidermal granular cell layer to the deepest intradermal tumor cells; this measurement is known as the **Breslow thickness**. Other histologic features that correlate with outcome include the number of mitoses and the presence of ulceration; these and other prognostic factors are discussed later.

Individual melanoma cells are usually considerably larger than normal melanocytes or cells found in melanocytic nevi. They have large nuclei with irregular contours, chromatin that is characteristically clumped at the periphery of the nuclear membrane, and prominent red (eosinophilic) nucleoli (Fig. 25-8*D*). The appearance of the tumor cells is similar in the radial and vertical phases of growth. While most nevi and melanomas are easily distinguished based on their appearance, a tiny fraction of "atypical" lesions fall in a histologic gray zone and have been termed melanocytic tumors of uncertain malignant potential; such lesions require complete excision and close clinical follow-up.

Clinical Features. **The most important warning signs, sometimes called the ABCDEs of melanoma, are (1)** ***a*****symmetry; (2) irregular** ***b*****orders; and (3) variegated** ***c*****olor, (4) increasing** ***d*****iameter, and (5)** ***e*****volution or change over time, especially if rapid.** Because locally advanced melanomas often metastasize, early recognition and complete excision are critical. Melanoma of the skin is usually asymptomatic, although itching or pain may be early manifestations. The majority of lesions are greater than 10 mm in diameter at diagnosis. The most consistent clinical signs are changes in the color, size, or shape of a pigmented lesion. Other features of pigmented lesions that should raise concern are a diameter greater than 6 mm, any change in appearance, and new onset of itching or pain.

Molecular insights into the pathogenesis of melanoma have spawned attempts to treat this cancer with drugs that target the RAS and PI3K/AKT pathways (Fig. 25-8). Such approaches are urgently needed, as metastatic melanoma is resistant to both conventional chemotherapy and radiation treatment. Ultimately, it is likely that these types of targeted therapies will be used in combinations tailored to fit the oncogenic molecular lesions found in individual tumors. This idea is based on the observation that a high fraction of tumors with BRAF mutations respond to BRAF inhibitors, whereas tumors belonging to other molecular subtypes do not.

More recently, recognition that melanoma is inherently immunogenic has spawned interest in therapies such as anti-CTLA4 blocking antibodies or, even more promising, anti-PD1 blocking antibodies that enhance host recognition of melanoma-specific antigens. Such treatments have produced encouraging results in early clinical trials. This clinical paradigm of taking the brakes off the immune system is one that may be applicable to other cancers as well (Chapter 7). Ultimately, it may be that such agents will be used in combination with targeted therapies such as BRAF antagonists.

Prognostic Factors. Once a melanoma is excised, a number of clinical and pathologic features are used to gauge the probability of metastatic spread and prognosis. One model used to predict outcome is based on the following variables: (1) tumor depth (the Breslow thickness); (2) number of mitoses; (3) evidence of tumor regression (presumably due to the host immune response); (4) ulceration of overlying skin; (5) the presence and number of tumor infiltrating lymphocytes; (6) gender; and (7) location (central body or extremity). Determinants of a more favorable prognosis in this model include thinner tumor depth, no or very few mitoses (< 1 per mm^2), a brisk tumor infiltrating lymphocyte response, absence of regression, and lack of ulceration. Since most melanomas initially metastasize to regional lymph nodes, additional prognostic information may be obtained by performing a sentinel lymph node biopsy; as in breast cancer (Chapter 23), this involves the identification, removal, and careful examination of the lymph node (or nodes) that is the initial site of drainage of intratumoral lymphatic vessels. Microscopic involvement of a sentinel node by even a small number of melanoma cells (micrometastases) confers a worse prognosis (Fig. 25-7*D*, *inset*). The degree of involvement and the total number of lymph nodes involved correlate well with overall survival.

KEY CONCEPTS

Melanocytic Lesions, Benign and Malignant

- Most *melanocytic nevi* have activating mutations in *BRAF* or less often *NRAS*, but the vast majority never undergo malignant transformation
- Most sporadic *dysplastic nevi* are best regarded as markers of melanoma risk rather than premalignant lesions. They are characterized by architectural and cytologic atypia and are associated with germline mutations in genes encoding cell cycle regulators (p16/INK4a, CDK4) and telomerase.
- *Melanoma* is a highly aggressive malignancy linked to sun exposure; risk of spread is predicted by a number of tumor characteristics, particularly the vertical thickness of excised tumors
- Melanoma is associated with mutations in cell cycle regulators (p16/INK4a, CDK4), pro-growth signaling factors (growth factor receptors [e.g., KIT], RAS, BRAF), and telomerase
- Melanoma often incites a host immune response and sometimes shows dramatic responses to antibody therapies that enhance T-cell immunity

Benign Epithelial Tumors

Benign cutaneous epithelial neoplasms are common tumors that are derived from the keratinizing stratified squamous epithelium of the epidermis and hair follicles and the ductular epithelium of cutaneous glands. They often recapitulate the structures from which they arise. Their appearance sometime raises a concern of malignancy, particularly when they are pigmented or inflamed, and biopsy is frequently required to establish a definitive diagnosis. In very rare instances they are a telltale sign of syndromes associated with potentially life-threatening visceral malignancies, such as multiple trichilemmomas in Cowden syndrome or multiple sebaceous neoplasms in Muir-Torre syndrome. Diagnosis of epithelial tumors in these instances may facilitate recognition of the underlying syndrome and implementation of appropriate clinical interventions.

Seborrheic Keratoses

These common epidermal tumors occur most frequently in middle-aged or older individuals. They arise spontaneously and are particularly numerous on the trunk, although the extremities, head, and neck may also be involved. In people of color, multiple small lesions on the face are termed *dermatosis papulosa nigra.*

Pathogenesis. Activating mutations in the fibroblast growth factor receptor-3 (FGFR3), a receptor tyrosine kinase, are found in many sporadic seborrheic keratoses and are thought to drive the growth of the tumor. Seborrheic keratoses may suddenly appear in large numbers as part of a paraneoplastic syndrome *(Leser-Trélat sign)*, possibly due to stimulation of keratinocytes by transforming growth factor-α produced by tumor cells, most commonly carcinomas of the gastrointestinal tract.

MORPHOLOGY

Seborrheic keratoses characteristically appear as round, flat, coinlike, waxy plaques that vary in diameter from millimeters to several centimeters (Fig. 25-9, *inset*). They are uniformly tan to dark brown and usually have a velvety to granular surface. Inspection with a hand lens usually reveals small, round, porelike ostia impacted with keratin, a feature helpful in differentiating these pigmented lesions from melanomas.

On histologic examination, these neoplasms are exophytic and sharply demarcated from the adjacent epidermis. They are composed of sheets of small cells that most resemble basal cells of the normal epidermis (Fig. 25-9). Variable melanin pigmentation is present within these basaloid cells, accounting for the brown coloration. Exuberant keratin production (hyperkeratosis) occurs at the surface, and small keratin-filled cysts (horn cysts) and invaginations of keratin into the main mass (invagination cysts) are characteristic features. If irritated and inflamed, seborrheic keratoses develop whirling foci of squamous differentiation resembling eddy currents in a stream.

Acanthosis Nigricans

Acanthosis nigricans may be an important cutaneous sign of several underlying benign and malignant conditions. It is a condition marked by thickened, hyperpigmented skin with a "velvet-like" texture that most commonly appears in the flexural areas (axillae, skin folds of the neck, groin, and anogenital regions). It is divided into two types based on the underlying condition.

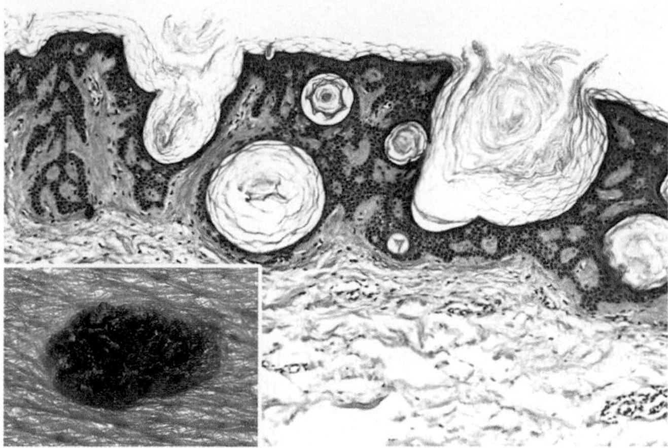

Figure 25-9 Seborrheic keratosis. A well-demarcated coinlike pigmented lesion containing dark keratin-filled surface plugs *(inset)* is composed of benign basaloid cells associated with prominent keratin-filled "horn" cysts, some of which communicate with the surface (pseudohorn cysts).

- In 80% of cases, acanthosis nigricans is associated with benign conditions and develops gradually, usually during childhood or puberty. It may occur (1) as an autosomal dominant trait with variable penetrance, (2) in association with obesity or endocrine abnormalities (particularly with pituitary or pineal tumors and diabetes), and (3) as part of several rare congenital syndromes. The most common associations are with obesity and diabetes.
- In the remaining cases, acanthosis nigricans arises in association with cancers, most commonly *gastrointestinal adenocarcinomas*, usually in middle-aged and older individuals. In this setting, acanthosis nigricans is best viewed as a paraneoplastic phenomenon that is likely caused by growth factors released from tumors.

Pathogenesis. **The unifying feature in all types of acanthosis nigricans is a disturbance that leads to increased growth factor receptor signaling in the skin.** The familial form is associated with germline activating mutations in the receptor tyrosine kinase FGFR3, the same receptor that is frequently mutated in seborrheic keratoses. Depending on the mutation, acanthosis may be an isolated finding or be seen together with skeletal deformities, including achondroplasia and thanatophoric dysplasia. Why in some cases FGFR3 mutation gives rise to seborrhic keratosis and in others acanthosis nigricans is not clear. In those with type 2 diabetes, hyperinsulinemia is believed to provoke increased stimulation of insulin-like growth factor receptor-1 (IGFR1), another receptor tyrosine kinase that activates the same signaling pathways as FGFR3. Factors responsible for paraneoplastic acanthosis nigricans are uncertain; some cases have been linked to high levels of transforming growth factor-alpha (TGF-α), which may result in excessive activation of epidermal growth factor receptor (EGFR), yet another receptor tyrosine kinase, in the skin.

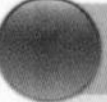

MORPHOLOGY

All forms of acanthosis nigricans have similar histologic features. The epidermis and underlying enlarged dermal papillae undulate sharply to form numerous repeating peaks and valleys. Variable hyperplasia may be seen, along with hyperkeratosis and slight basal cell layer hyperpigmentation (but no melanocytic hyperplasia).

Fibroepithelial Polyp

The fibroepithelial polyp has many names (acrochordon, squamous papilloma, skin tag) and is one of the most common cutaneous lesions. It usually comes to attention in middle-aged and older individuals on the neck, trunk, face, and intertriginous areas. Rarely, fibroepithelial polyps and tumors of perifollicular mesenchyme (specialized fibroblasts associated with the hair bulb) are seen together in *Birt-Hogg-Dubé syndrome,* but the vast majority of polyps are sporadic.

MORPHOLOGY

Fibroepithelial polyps are soft, flesh-colored, bag-like tumors that are often attached to the surrounding skin by a slender stalk. On histologic examination these tumors consist of fibrovascular cores covered by benign squamous epithelium. It is not uncommon for the polyps to undergo ischemic necrosis due to torsion, which may cause pain and precipitate their removal.

Fibroepithelial polyps are usually inconsequential, but can occasionally be associated with diabetes, obesity, and intestinal polyposis. Of interest, like melanocytic nevi and hemangiomas, they often become more numerous or prominent during pregnancy, presumably related to hormonal stimulation.

Epithelial or Follicular Inclusion Cyst (Wen)

Epithelial cysts are common lesions formed by the invagination and cystic expansion of the epidermis or, perhaps more commonly, a hair follicle. The lay term, *wen,* derives from the Anglo-Saxon *wenn,* meaning a lump or tumor. When large they may be subject to traumatic rupture, which can spill keratin into the dermis and lead to an extensive and often painful granulomatous inflammatory response.

Adnexal (Appendage) Tumors

There are literally hundreds of neoplasms arising from or showing differentiation toward cutaneous appendages. Their significance varies according to type and clinical context.

- Some are entirely benign, but may be confused with cutaneous cancers such as basal cell carcinoma.
- Other appendage tumors are associated with mendelian patterns of inheritance and occur as multiple disfiguring lesions.
- In some instances, these lesions warn of a predisposition for internal malignancy; such is the relationship between multiple *trichilemmomas* and *Cowden syndrome,* a disorder caused by germline loss of function mutations in the tumor suppressor gene *PTEN* that is associated with an increased risk of endometrial cancer, breast cancer, and many other tumors.

Appendage tumors are often nondescript, flesh-colored solitary or multiple papules and nodules. Some have a predisposition to occur on specific body surfaces. Selected examples are provided here to illustrate neoplasms of hair follicles and sebaceous, eccrine, and apocrine glands.

- *Eccrine poroma* occurs predominantly on the palms and soles where sweat glands are numerous.
- *Cylindroma,* an appendage tumor with ductal (apocrine or eccrine) differentiation, usually occurs on the forehead and scalp (Fig. 25-10*A*), where coalescence of nodules with time may produce a hatlike growth, hence the name *turban tumor.* These lesions may be dominantly inherited; in such cases they appear early in life and are associated with inactivating mutations in the tumor suppressor gene *CYLD*, which encodes a deubiquitinating enzyme that negatively regulates the oncogenic transcription factor NF-κB and other factors that contribute to cell cycle progression. In addition to familial cylindromatosis, germline mutations in *CYLD* are associated with two other genetic syndromes marked by the occurrence of multiple adnexal tumors, multiple *familial trichoepithelioma* (a follicular tumor) and *Brooke-Spiegler syndrome* (associated with both trichoepithelioma and cylindroma).
- *Syringomas,* lesions with eccrine differentiation, usually occur as multiple, small, tan papules in the vicinity of the lower eyelids.
- *Sebaceous adenomas* can be associated with internal malignancy in the *Muir-Torre syndrome,* a subset of the hereditary nonpolyposis colorectal carcinoma syndrome (Chapter 17) associated with germline deficits in DNA mismatch repair proteins.
- *Pilomatricomas,* showing follicular differentiation, are associated with activating mutations in *CTNNB1*, the gene encoding β-catenin. Mutations in this gene are seen in numerous neoplasms but are of interest here since Wnt signaling through β-catenin is critical for early hair development and regulates hair growth and maintenance.
- Adnexal tumors can also show primarily apocrine differentiation; these usually arise in body areas where apocrine glands are most prevalent, such as the axilla and scalp. Some skin adnexal tumors may arise from multipotent cutaneous stem cells, which are believed to reside in a specialized niche associated with hair follicles.

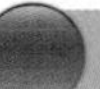

MORPHOLOGY

The **cylindroma** is composed of islands of cells resembling those of the normal epidermal or adnexal basal cell layer (basaloid cells). These islands fit together like pieces of a jigsaw puzzle within a fibrous dermal matrix (Fig. 25-10*B*).

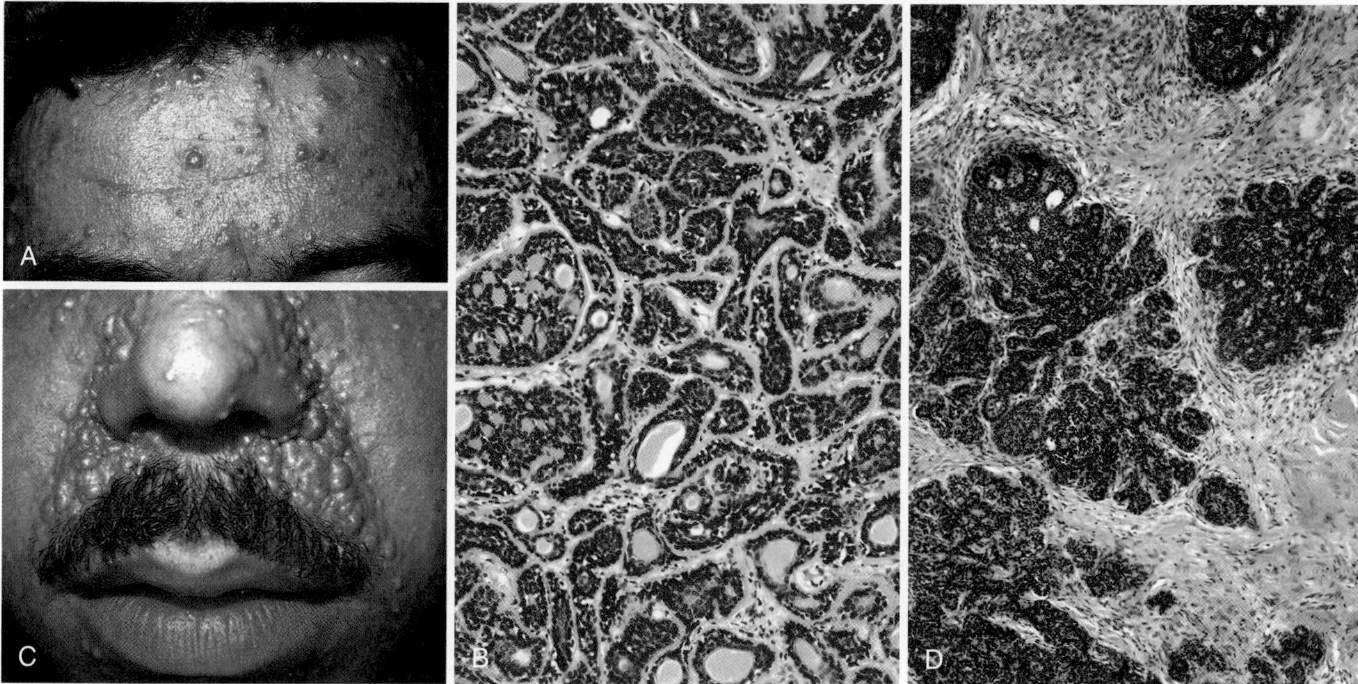

Figure 25-10 Cylindroma and trichoepithelioma. **A,** Multiple cylindromas (papules) on the forehead are composed (**B**) of islands of basaloid cells containing occasional ducts that fit together like pieces of a jigsaw puzzle. **C,** Perinasal papules and small nodules of trichoepithelioma are composed (**D**) of buds of basaloid cells that resemble primitive hair follicles.

Trichoepithelioma is a proliferation of basaloid cells that forms primitive structures resembling hair follicles (Fig. 25-10*C, D*). **Sebaceous adenoma** shows a lobular proliferation of sebocytes with increased peripheral basaloid cells and more mature sebocytes in the central portion, characterized by frothy or bubbly cytoplasm due to lipid vesicle content (Fig. 25-11*A*). **Pilomatrixomas** are composed of basaloid cells that show trichilemmal or hairlike differentiation similar to that seen in the germinal portion of the normal hair bulb in the anagen growth phase (Fig. 25-11*B*). **Apocrine carcinoma** shows ductal differentiation with prominent decapitation secretion similar to that seen in the normal apocrine gland (Fig. 25-11*C*). The infiltrative growth pattern is a hint of malignancy in this otherwise well-differentiated tumor.

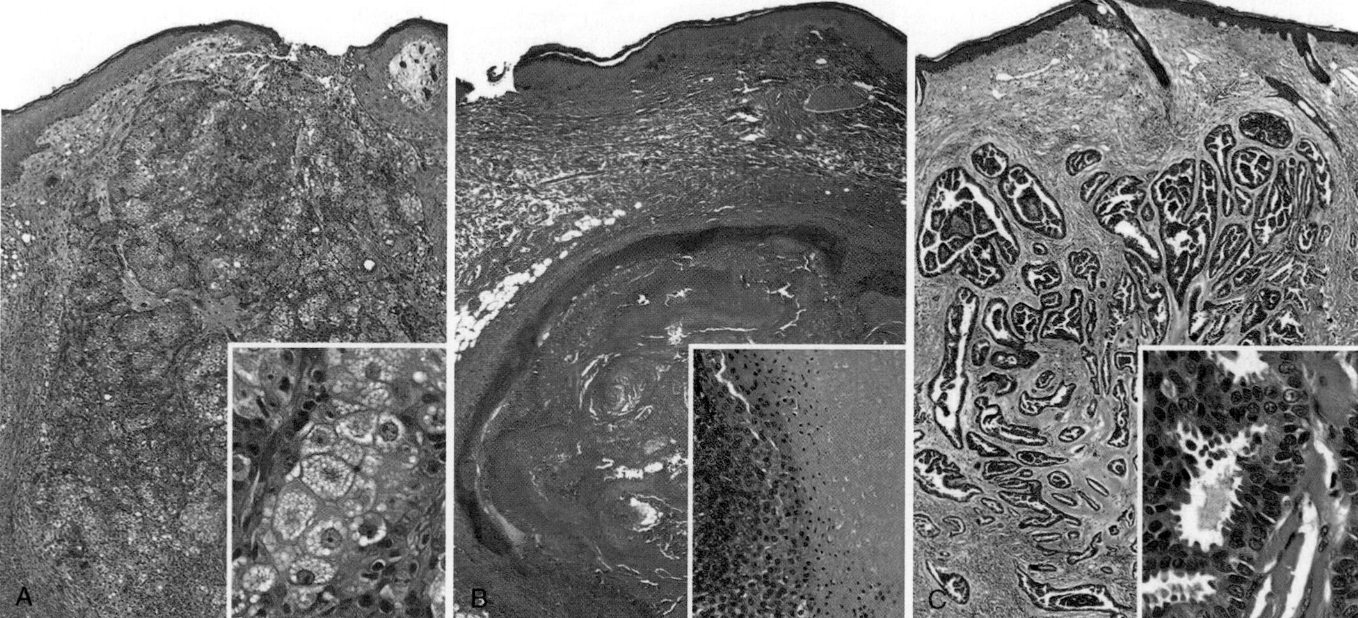

Figure 25-11 Diverse adnexal tumors. **A,** Sebaceous adenoma; *inset* demonstrates sebaceous differentiation. **B,** Pilomatrixoma; *inset* shows hair matrix differentiation to anucleate "ghost cells." **C,** Apocrine carcinoma (well-differentiated); *inset* shows apocrine differentiation and luminal secretions produced by "decapitation" of the lining cells.

Although most appendage tumors are benign, malignant variants do exist. Apocrine tumors are unusual in that malignant forms seem to be more common than benign forms. *Sebaceous carcinoma* arises from the meibomian glands of the eyelid and may follow an aggressive course replete with systemic metastases. *Eccrine* and *apocrine carcinomas* can be confused with metastatic adenocarcinoma because of their tendency to form gland-like structures.

Premalignant and Malignant Epidermal Tumors

Actinic Keratosis

Actinic keratoses; as the name implies, usually occur in sun-damaged skin and exhibit hyperkeratosis. As expected, they occur with particularly high incidence in lightly pigmented individuals. Exposure to ionizing radiation, industrial hydrocarbons, and arsenicals may induce similar lesions. These lesions may show progressively worsening dysplastic changes that culminate in cutaneous squamous cell carcinoma, and are analogous in this regard to the precursor lesions that give rise to squamous carcinomas of the uterine cervix (Chapter 22).

MORPHOLOGY

Actinic keratoses are usually less than 1 cm in diameter. They are typically tan-brown, red, or skin-colored and have a rough, sandpaper-like consistency. Some lesions produce so much keratin that a "cutaneous horn" develops (Fig. 25-12*A*), which in extreme cases may become so prominent that they resemble the actual horns of animals! Sun-exposed sites (face, arms, dorsum of hands) are most frequently affected. The lips may also develop similar lesions (termed **actinic cheilitis**).

Cytologic atypia is seen in the lowermost layers of the epidermis and may be associated with hyperplasia of basal cells (Fig. 25-12*B*) or, alternatively, with atrophy that results in thinning of the epidermis. The atypical basal cells usually have pink or reddish cytoplasm due to dyskeratosis. Intercellular bridges are present, in contrast to basal cell carcinoma, in which they are not visible. The superficial dermis contains thickened, blue-gray elastic fibers (**elastosis**), a probable result of abnormal elastic fiber synthesis by sun-damaged fibroblasts. The stratum corneum is thickened, and unlike normal skin, the cells in this layer often retain their nuclei (**parakeratosis**).

Whether all actinic keratoses progress to skin cancer (usually squamous cell carcinoma) if given enough time is conjectural. Lesions may regress or remain stable during a normal life span, but enough do become malignant that local eradication is warranted. This can usually be accomplished by gentle curettage, freezing, or topical application of chemotherapeutic agents. Of interest, topical administration of imiquimod, a drug that activates Toll-like receptors (TLRs), eradicates up to 50% of lesions, a rate considerably higher than the spontaneous regression rate of approximately 5%. By stimulating TLR signaling, imiquimod activates cutaneous innate immune cells, which may recognize and eradicate precancerous lesions. Direct pro-apoptotic effects of the imiquimod on lesional keratinocytes have also been proposed, but these are poorly understood at present.

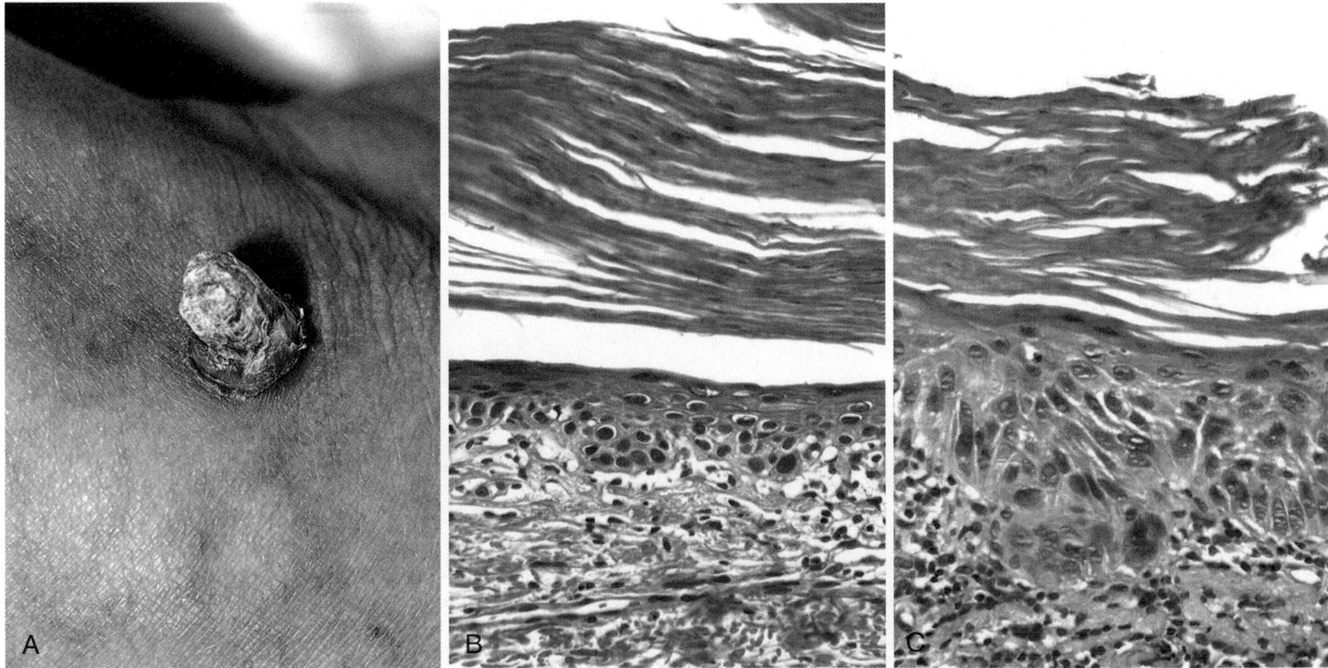

Figure 25-12 Actinic keratosis. **A,** Excessive keratotic scale in this lesion has produced a "cutaneous horn." **B,** Basal cell layer atypia (dysplasia) is associated with marked hyperkeratosis and parakeratosis. **C,** Progression to full-thickness nuclear atypia, with or without the presence of superficial epidermal maturation, heralds the development of squamous cell carcinoma in situ.

Squamous Cell Carcinoma

Squamous cell carcinoma is the second most common tumor arising on sun-exposed sites in older people, exceeded only by basal cell carcinoma. Except for lesions on the lower legs, these tumors have a higher incidence in men than in women. Invasive squamous cell carcinomas are usually discovered while they are small and resectable. Less than 5% of these tumors metastasize to regional nodes; these lesions are generally deeply invasive and involve the subcutis.

Pathogenesis. **The most important cause of cutaneous squamous cell carcinoma is DNA damage induced by exposure to UV light.** Tumor incidence is proportional to the degree of lifetime sun exposure. A second common association is with immunosuppression, most notably chronic immunosuppression as a result of chemotherapy or organ transplantation. Immunosuppression may contribute to carcinogenesis by reducing host surveillance and increasing the susceptibility of keratinocytes to infection and transformation by oncogenic viruses, particularly human papilloma virus (HPV) subtypes 5 and 8. These same HPVs have been implicated in tumors arising in patients with a rare autosomal recessive condition, *epidermodysplasia verruciformis*, which is marked by a high susceptibility to cutaneous squamous cell carcinomas. In addition to its damaging effect on DNA, sunlight, through uncertain mechanisms, seems to cause a transient defect in cutaneous innate immunity that may diminish immune-mediated elimination of sun-damaged cells. Other risk factors for squamous cell carcinoma include industrial carcinogens (tars and oils), chronic ulcers and draining osteomyelitis, old burn scars, ingestion of arsenicals, ionizing radiation, and (in the oral cavity) tobacco and betel nut chewing.

Most studies on the genetics of squamous cell carcinoma have focused on acquired defects in sporadic tumors and their precursors (actinic keratoses), and the relationships between these defects and sun-exposure. The incidence of *TP53* mutations in actinic keratoses found in Caucasians is high, suggesting that p53 dysfunction is an early event in the development of tumors induced by sunlight. Normally, DNA damaged by UV light is sensed by checkpoint kinases such as ATM and ATR, which send out signals that up-regulate the expression and stability of p53. p53 in turn arrests cells in the G_1 phase of the cell cycle and promotes either "high-fidelity" DNA repair or the elimination by apoptosis of cells that are damaged beyond repair (Chapter 7). When these protective functions of p53 are lost, DNA damage induced by UV light is more likely to be "repaired" by error-prone mechanisms, creating mutations that are passed down to daughter cells. Of note, the mutations that are seen in *TP53* often occur at pyrimidine dimers, indicating that they, too, stem from damage caused by UV light. A similar story underlies the remarkable susceptibility of patients with *xeroderma pigmentosum* to squamous cell carcinoma. This disorder is caused by inherited mutations in genes in the nucleotide excision repair pathway, which is required for accurate repair of pyrimidine dimers; when this pathway is defective, error-prone repair pathways take over, leading to the rapid accumulation of mutations and eventual carcinogenesis.

As with all other forms of cancer, cutaneous squamous cell carcinoma stems from multiple driver mutations. In addition to defects in p53, mutations that increase RAS signaling and decrease Notch signaling are common and are also likely to contribute to the transformation process.

MORPHOLOGY

Squamous cell carcinomas that have not invaded through the basement membrane of the dermoepidermal junction (termed in situ carcinoma) appear as sharply defined, red, scaling plaques. More advanced, invasive lesions are nodular, show variable keratin production (appreciated grossly as hyperkeratotic scale), and may ulcerate (Fig. 25-13*A*).

Unlike actinic keratoses, in squamous cell carcinoma in situ, cells with atypical (enlarged and hyperchromatic) nuclei involve all levels of the epidermis (Fig. 25-12*C*). Invasive squamous cell carcinoma (Fig. 25-13*B, C*) shows variable degrees of differentiation, ranging from tumors composed of polygonal cells arranged in orderly lobules and having numerous large areas of keratinization, to neoplasms consisting of highly anaplastic cells that exhibit only abortive, single-cell keratinization (dyskeratosis). The latter tumors may be so poorly differentiated that immunohistochemical stains for keratins are needed to confirm the diagnosis.

Basal Cell Carcinoma

Basal cell carcinoma is a distinctive locally aggressive cutaneous tumor that is associated with mutations that activate the Hedgehog pathway signaling. Basal cell carcinoma is the most common invasive cancer in humans, numbering nearly 1 million cases per year in the United States. These are slow-growing tumors that rarely metastasize. The vast majority is recognized at an early stage and is cured by local excision. However, a small number of tumors (<0.5%) are locally aggressive and potentially disfiguring, or exceedingly rarely may metastasize to distant sites. They occur at sun-exposed sites in lightly pigmented elderly adults. As with squamous cell carcinoma, the incidence of basal cell carcinoma is increased in the setting of immunosuppression and in disorders of DNA repair, such as xeroderma pigmentosum (Chapter 7).

Pathogenesis. **Most basal cell carcinomas have mutations that lead to unbridled Hedgehog signaling.** As is often the case in biology and medicine, study of a rare genetic syndrome associated with a high risk of a common disease (basal cell carcinoma) has led to the elucidation of pathogenic mechanisms of general importance. The syndrome in question, *nevoid basal cell carcinoma syndrome* (NBCCS; also known as *basal cell nevus* or *Gorlin syndrome*), is an autosomal dominant disorder characterized by the development of multiple basal cell carcinomas, often before age 20, accompanied by various other tumors (especially medulloblastomas and ovarian fibromas), odontogenic keratocysts, pits of the palms and soles, and certain developmental abnormalities. NBCCS is one of a number of cancer syndromes associated with skin manifestations (Table 25-3). The gene associated with NBCCS is *PTCH*, a tumor suppressor that is the human homologue of the *Drosophila* developmental gene *patched*. Individuals with

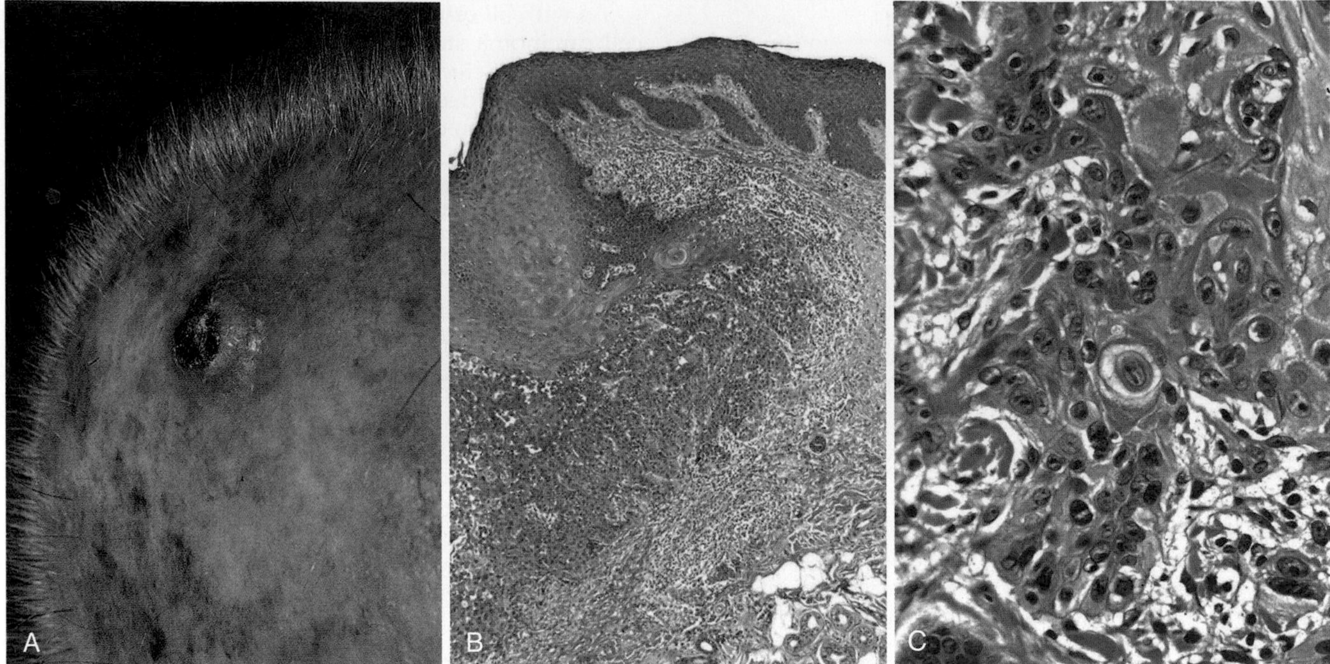

Figure 25-13 Invasive squamous cell carcinoma. **A,** Lesions are often nodular and ulcerated, as seen in this scalp tumor. **B,** Tongues of atypical squamous epithelium have transgressed the basement membrane and invaded deeply into the dermis. **C,** Invasive tumor cells show enlarged nuclei with angulated contours and prominent nucleoli.

NBCCS are born with a germline loss of function mutation in one *PTCH* allele; the second normal allele is inactivated in tumors by a mutation acquired by chance or due to exposure to mutagens (particularly UV light).

PTCH protein is a receptor for *sonic hedgehog (SHH),* a component of the Hedgehog signaling pathway, which determines polarity during embryonic development and also regulates hair follicle formation and hair growth. In the "off" state, PTCH exists in a complex with another transmembrane protein called SMO (for "smoothened"). Binding of SHH to PTCH releases SMO, which in turn activates the transcription factor GLI1 (Fig. 25-14), thus turning on the expression of genes that support tumor cell growth and survival. Mice engineered to have excessive GLI1 activation are prone to development of skin tumors resembling basal cell carcinomas. Similarly, in NBCCS the loss of PTCH function causes constitutive activation of SMO and GLI1, leading to the development of basal cell carcinoma.

Mutations that activate Hedgehog signaling are also prevalent in sporadic basal cell carcinomas. Loss of function *PTCH* mutations are common, and about one third

Table 25-3 Survey of Familial Cancer Syndromes with Cutaneous Manifestations

Disease	Inheritance	Chromosomal Location	Gene/Protein	Normal Function/Manifestation of Loss
Ataxia-telangiectasia	AR	11q22.3	*ATM*/ATM	DNA repair after radiation injury/neurologic and vascular lesions
Nevoid basal cell carcinoma syndrome	AD	9q22	*PTCH*/PTCH	Developmental patterning gene/multiple basal cell carcinomas; medulloblastoma, jaw cysts
Cowden syndrome	AD	10q23	*PTEN*/PTEN	Lipid phosphatase/benign follicular appendage tumors (trichilemmomas); internal adenocarcinoma (often breast or endometrial)
Familial melanoma syndrome	AD	9p21	*CDKN2*/p16/INK4 *CDKN2*/p14/ARF	Inhibits CDK4/6 phosphorylation of RB, promoting cell cycle arrest/melanoma; pancreatic carcinoma Binds MDM2, promoting p53 function/melanoma; pancreatic carcinoma
Muir-Torre syndrome	AD	2p22 3p21	*MSH2*/MSH2 *MLH1*/MLH1	Involved in DNA mismatch repair/sebaceous neoplasia; internal malignancy (colon and others)
Neurofibromatosis I	AD	17q11	*NF1*/neurofibromin	Negatively regulates RAS signaling/neurofibromas
Neurofibromatosis II	AD	22q12	*NF2*/merlin	Integrates cytoskeletal signaling/neurofibromas and acoustic neuromas
Tuberous sclerosis	AD	9q34 16p13	*TSC1*/hamartin *TSC2*/tuberin	Work together in a complex that negatively regulates mTOR/angiofibromas/mental retardation
Xeroderma pigmentosum	AR	9q22 and others	*XPA*/XPA and others	Nucleotide excision repair/melanoma and nonmelanoma skin cancers

AD, Autosomal dominant; AR, autosomal recessive.
From Tsai KY, Tsao H: The genetics of skin cancer. Am J Med Genet C Semin Med Genet 131C:82, 2004.

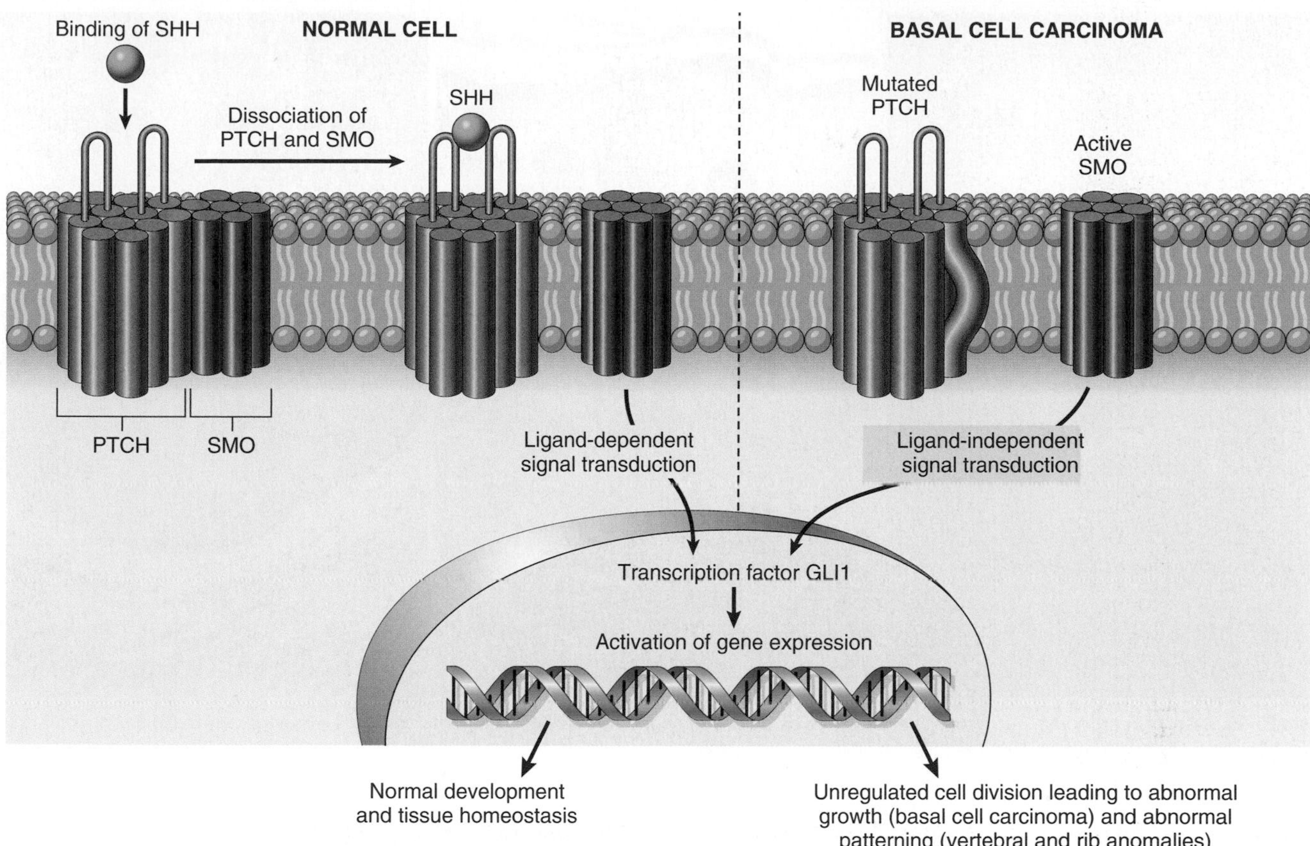

Figure 25-14 Normal and oncogenic hedgehog signaling. *Left,* Normally, PTCH and SMO form a receptor complex that can bind sonic hedgehog (SHH). In the absence of SHH, PTCH blocks SMO activity. When SHH binds PTCH, SMO is released to trigger a signal transduction cascade that leads to activation of GLI1 and other transcription factors. *Right,* Mutations in *PTCH*, and less often in *SMO*, allow SMO to signal without SHH binding and produce constitutive activation of GLI1. GLI signaling is a characteristic feature of sporadic basal cell carcinomas and tumors associated with the nevoid basal cell carcinoma (Gorlin) syndrome.

of these mutations consist of C→T transitions that are considered hallmarks of UV damage. Other tumors have activating mutations in *SMO*. This insight has paved the way for the development of small molecule inhibitors of the Hedgehog pathway, which produce excellent clinical responses in patients with locally aggressive or metastatic basal cell carcinoma.

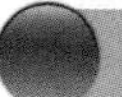

MORPHOLOGY

Basal cell carcinomas usually present as **pearly papules** containing prominent dilated subepidermal blood vessels (**telangiectasias**) (Fig. 25-15*A*). Some tumors contain melanin and superficially resemble melanocytic nevi or melanomas. Advanced lesions may ulcerate, and extensive local invasion of bone or facial sinuses may occur after many years of neglect or in unusually aggressive tumors, explaining the archaic designation **rodent ulcers**. One common and important variant, the superficial basal cell carcinoma, presents as an erythematous, occasionally pigmented plaque that may resemble early forms of melanoma.

Histologically, the tumor cells resemble those in the normal basal cell layer of the epidermis. They arise from the epidermis or follicular epithelium and do not occur on mucosal surfaces. Two patterns are seen: **multifocal growths** originating from the epidermis and sometimes extending over several square centimeters or more of skin surface (multifocal superficial type) and **nodular lesions** growing downward deeply into the dermis as cords and islands of variably basophilic cells with hyperchromatic nuclei, embedded in a mucinous matrix, and often surrounded by many fibroblasts and lymphocytes (Fig. 25-15*B*). The cells at the periphery of the tumor cell islands tend to be arranged radially with their long axes in parallel alignment **(palisading)**. In sections, the stroma retracts away from the carcinoma (Fig. 25-15*C*), creating clefts or separation artifacts that assist in differentiating basal cell carcinomas from certain appendage tumors that are also characterized by proliferation of basaloid cells, such as trichoepithelioma.

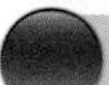

KEY CONCEPTS

Malignant Epidermal Tumors

- The incidence of both basal cell and squamous cell carcinoma is strongly correlated with increasing lifetime sun exposure.
- Cutaneous squamous cell carcinoma can progress from actinic keratoses but also arises from chemical exposure, at thermal burn sites, or in association with HPV infection in the setting of immunosuppression.
- Cutaneous squamous cell carcinoma has potential for metastasis but is much less aggressive than squamous cell carcinoma at mucosal sites.

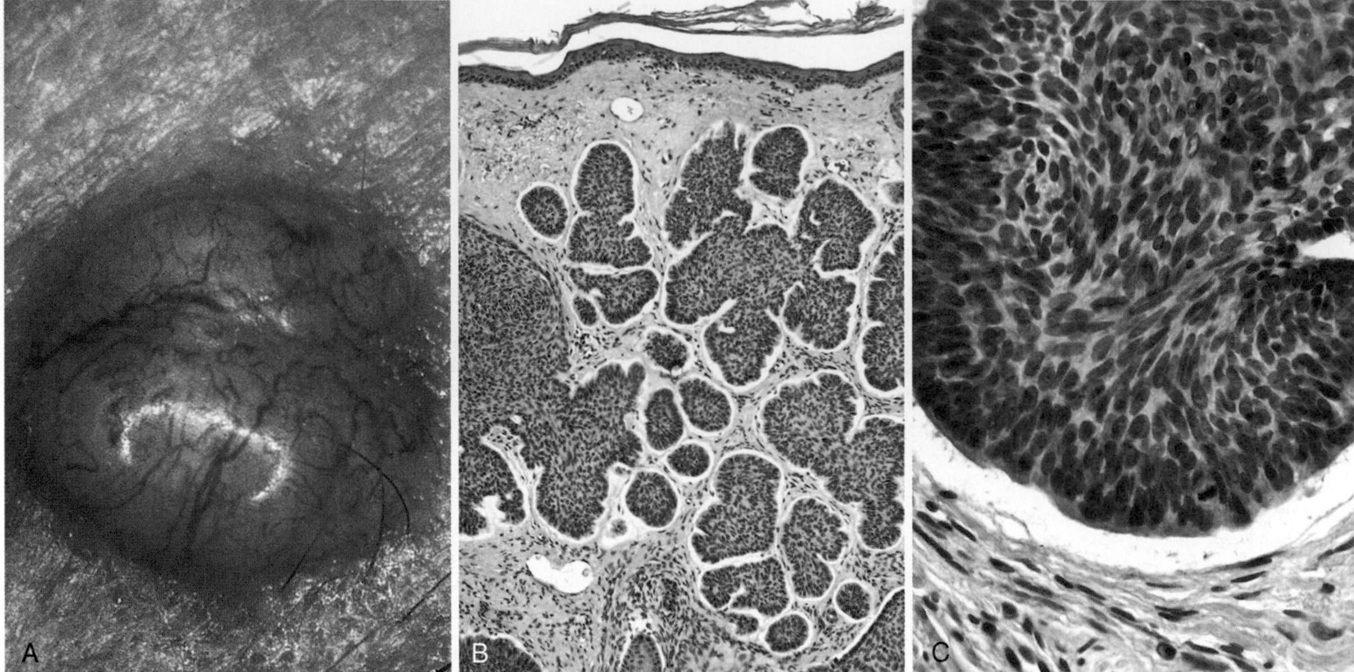

Figure 25-15 Basal cell carcinoma. Pearly, telangiectatic nodules **(A)** are composed of nests of uniform basaloid cells within the dermis **(B)** that are often separated from the adjacent stroma by thin clefts **(C),** an artifact of sectioning.

- Basal cell carcinoma, the most common malignancy worldwide, is a locally aggressive tumor associated with mutations that activate Hedgehog signaling. Metastasis is very rare.

Tumors of the Dermis

The dermis contains a variety of elements such as smooth muscle, pericytes, fibroblasts, neural tissue, and endothelium. Neoplasms comprised of cells resembling all of these elements occur in the skin, but most also involve other soft tissues and viscera and are discussed elsewhere, or are too rare to merit mention. This section discusses two dermal neoplasms—one benign, one malignant—that arise primarily in the skin.

Benign Fibrous Histiocytoma (Dermatofibroma)

Benign fibrous histiocytoma refers to a heterogeneous family of morphologically and histogenetically related benign dermal neoplasms of uncertain lineage. These tumors are usually seen in adults and often occur on the legs of young and middle-aged women. Lesions are asymptomatic or tender and may increase and decrease slightly in size over time. Their biologic behavior is indolent.

The cause of fibrous histiocytomas remains a mystery. Many cases have a history of antecedent trauma, suggesting an abnormal response to injury and inflammation, perhaps analogous to the deposition of increased amounts of altered collagen in a hypertrophic scar or keloid. These common yet curious tumors appear to be composed at least partially of factor XIIIa-positive dermal dendritic cells.

MORPHOLOGY

These neoplasms appear as firm, tan to brown papules (Fig. 25-16*A*). Most are less than 1 cm in diameter, but actively growing lesions may reach several centimeters in diameter; with time they often become flattened.

The most common form of fibrous histiocytoma is referred to as a **dermatofibroma.** These tumors consist of benign, spindle-shaped cells that are usually arranged in a well-defined, nonencapsulated mass within the mid-dermis (Fig. 25-16*B, C*). Extension of these cells into the subcutaneous fat is sometimes observed. Many cases demonstrate a peculiar form of overlying epidermal hyperplasia, characterized by downward elongation of hyperpigmented rete ridges (**pseudoepitheliomatous hyperplasia**). Numerous histologic variants are noted, such as more cellular forms or tumors with pools of extravascular blood and hemosiderin (aneurysmal).

Dermatofibrosarcoma Protuberans

Dermatofibrosarcoma protuberans is best regarded as a well-differentiated, primary fibrosarcoma of the skin. These tumors are slow growing, and although they are locally aggressive and can recur, they rarely metastasize.

Pathogenesis. **The molecular hallmark of dermatofibrosarcoma protuberans is a translocation involving the genes encoding collagen 1A1 *(COL1A1)* and platelet-derived growth factor-β *(PDGFB).*** The resulting rearrangement juxtaposes the *COL1A1* promoter sequences and the coding region of *PDGFB* and leads to overexpression and increased secretion of PDGFβ, which drives tumor cell growth through an autocrine loop. While the primary mode of treatment is wide local excision, rare cases that are

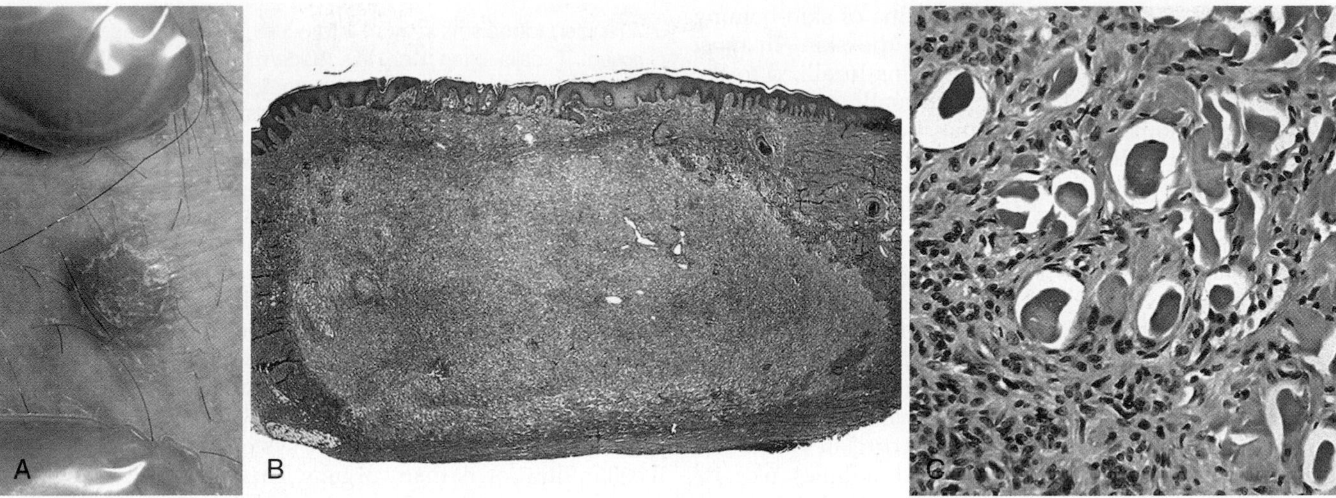

Figure 25-16 Benign fibrous histiocytoma (dermatofibroma). This firm, tan papule on the leg **(A)** contains a circumscribed dermal proliferation of benign-appearing spindle cells **(B).** Note the characteristic overlying epidermal hyperplasia **(B)** and the tendency of fibroblasts to surround individual collagen bundles **(C)**.

unresectable due to their location or because of metastatic spread can be treated with inhibitors of the PDGFβ receptor tyrosine kinase. Included in this class of drugs is imatinib mesylate, which first came to fame for its efficacy in treatment of chronic myeloid leukemia (CML). As in CML patients, withdrawal of the drug is followed by regrowth of the tumor, so use of this agent is lifelong.

MORPHOLOGY

Dermatofibrosarcoma protuberans usually appears as a "protuberant" nodule, most often on the trunk, within a firm (indurated) plaque that may sometimes ulcerate (Fig. 27-17*A*). These neoplasms are composed of closely packed fibroblasts arranged radially, reminiscent of blades of a pinwheel, a pattern referred to as **storiform.** Mitoses are rare. In contrast to dermatofibroma, the overlying epidermis is generally thinned. Deep extension from the dermis into subcutaneous fat, producing a characteristic "honeycomb" pattern, is frequently seen (Fig. 25-17*B, C*). These tumors may extend down into the subcutis and thus require wide excision to prevent local recurrence.

Tumors of Cellular Migrants to the Skin

Aside from tumors that arise directly from epidermal and dermal cells, several proliferative disorders of the skin involve cells whose progenitors arise elsewhere and then specifically home to the cutaneous microenvironment.

Mycosis Fungoides (Cutaneous T-Cell Lymphoma)

Cutaneous T-cell lymphoma (CTCL) spans a spectrum of lymphoproliferative disorders affecting the skin (Chapter 13), many with distinctive presentations. This section

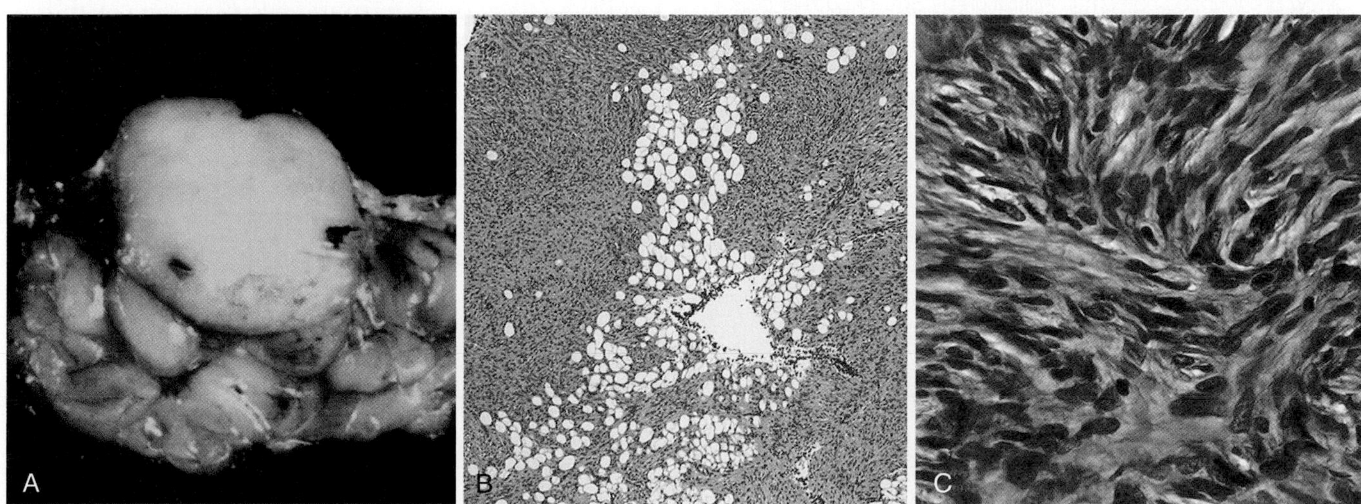

Figure 25-17 Dermatofibrosarcoma protuberans. **A,** The tumor consists of a flesh-colored fibrotic nodule on sectioning. **B,** The lesion often infiltrates the subcutis in a manner reminiscent of "Swiss cheese" to aficionados. **C,** A characteristic storiform (swirling) alignment of the spindled cells is apparent.

focuses on *mycosis fungoides*, a lymphoma of skin-homing CD4+ T helper cells that presents in the skin. In most affected individuals, the disease remains localized to the skin for many years, but it may eventually evolve into a systemic lymphoma. This tumor may occur at any age, but most commonly afflicts persons older than age 40.

Lesions of mycosis fungoides usually involve truncal areas and include scaly, red-brown *patches*; raised, scaling *plaques* that may even be confused with psoriasis; and fungating *nodules*. Prognosis is related to the percentage of body surface involved and progression from patch to plaque to nodular forms. Eczema-like lesions typify early stages of disease when obvious visceral or nodal spread has not occurred. Raised, indurated, irregularly outlined, erythematous plaques may then supervene. Development of multiple, large red-brown nodules correlates with systemic spread. Sometimes plaques and nodules ulcerate (Fig. 25-18*A*). Ultimately, lesions may affect numerous body surfaces, including the trunk, extremities, face, and scalp. In some individuals, seeding of the blood by malignant T cells is accompanied by diffuse erythema and scaling of the entire body surface (erythroderma), a condition known as *Sézary syndrome* (Chapter 13).

The proliferating cells in CTCL are clonal populations of CD4-positive T helper cells that home to the skin due expression of cutaneous lymphocyte antigen. The neoplastic cells have clonal T-cell receptor gene rearrangements and sometimes express aberrant combinations of T-cell surface antigens. Topical therapy with steroids or UV light is often used for early skin lesions, whereas more aggressive systemic chemotherapy is indicated for advanced disease.

MORPHOLOGY

The histologic hallmark of CTCL of the mycosis fungoides type is the presence of the **Sézary-Lutzner cells**, which characteristically form bandlike aggregates within the superficial dermis (Fig. 25-18*B*) and invade the epidermis as single cells and small clusters **(Pautrier microabscesses).** These cells have markedly infolded nuclear membranes, imparting a hyperconvoluted or cerebriform contour. Although patches and plaques show pronounced epidermal infiltration by Sézary-Lutzner cells (epidermotropism), in more advanced nodular lesions the malignant T cells often lose this epidermotropic tendency, grow deeply into the dermis, and eventually spread systemically.

Mastocytosis

The term *mastocytosis* encompasses a spectrum of rare disorders characterized by increased numbers of mast cells in the skin and, in some instances, in other organs as well. A cutaneous form of the disease that affects predominantly children and accounts for more than 50% of all cases is termed *urticaria pigmentosa.* The cutaneous lesions are usually multiple, although solitary mastocytomas may also occur in very young children. About 10% of individuals with mast cell disease have systemic disease, with mast cell infiltration of many organs. These individuals are often adults, and unlike localized cutaneous disease, the prognosis may be poor.

Many of the signs and symptoms of mastocytosis are due to the effects of histamine, heparin, and other substances released when mast cells degranulate. *Darier sign* refers to a localized area of dermal edema and erythema (wheal) that occurs when lesional skin is rubbed. *Dermatographism* refers to an area of dermal edema resembling a hive that occurs as a result of localized stroking of apparently normal skin with a pointed instrument. In systemic disease, all of the following may be seen: pruritus and flushing, variously triggered by certain foods, temperature changes, alcohol, and certain drugs (morphine, codeine, aspirin); watery nasal discharge (rhinorrhea); rarely, gastrointestinal or nasal bleeding, possibly due to the anticoagulant effects of heparin; and bone pain, which may be caused by mast cell infiltration or by pathologic fractures stemming from osteoporosis. Osteoporosis is caused by excessive histamine release in the marrow microenvironment and can be a clue to the diagnosis, particularly in premenopausal women and in men.

Pathogenesis. Many cases of mastocytosis have acquired activating point mutations in the KIT receptor tyrosine kinase. The resulting increase in KIT signaling drives mast cell growth and survival. This insight has led to trials of KIT kinase inhibitors in patients with disseminated disease.

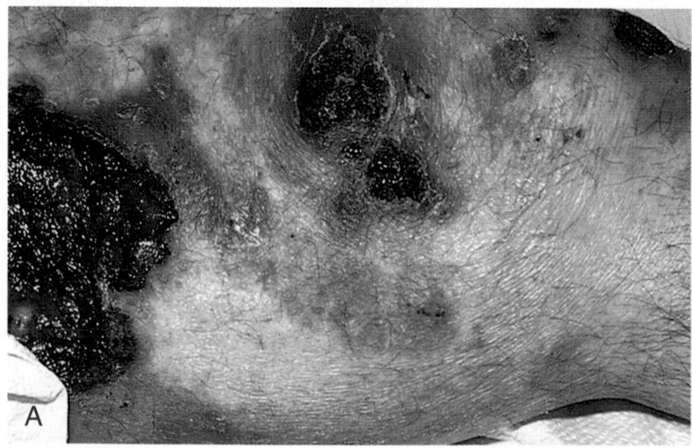

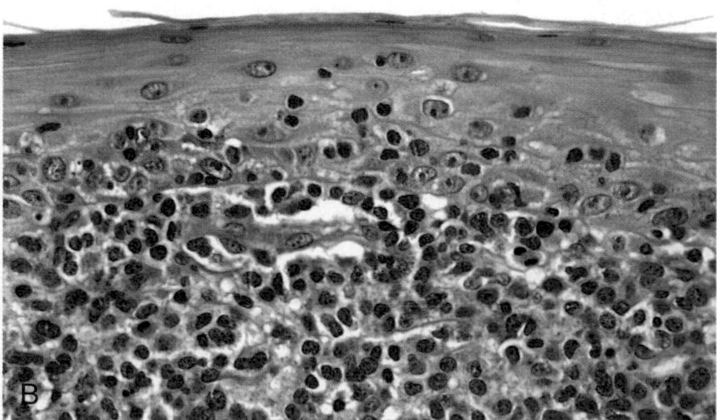

Figure 25-18 Cutaneous T-cell lymphoma. **A,** Several erythematous plaques with scaling and ulceration are evident. **B,** Microscopically, there is an infiltrate of atypical lymphocytes that accumulates beneath and invades the epidermis.

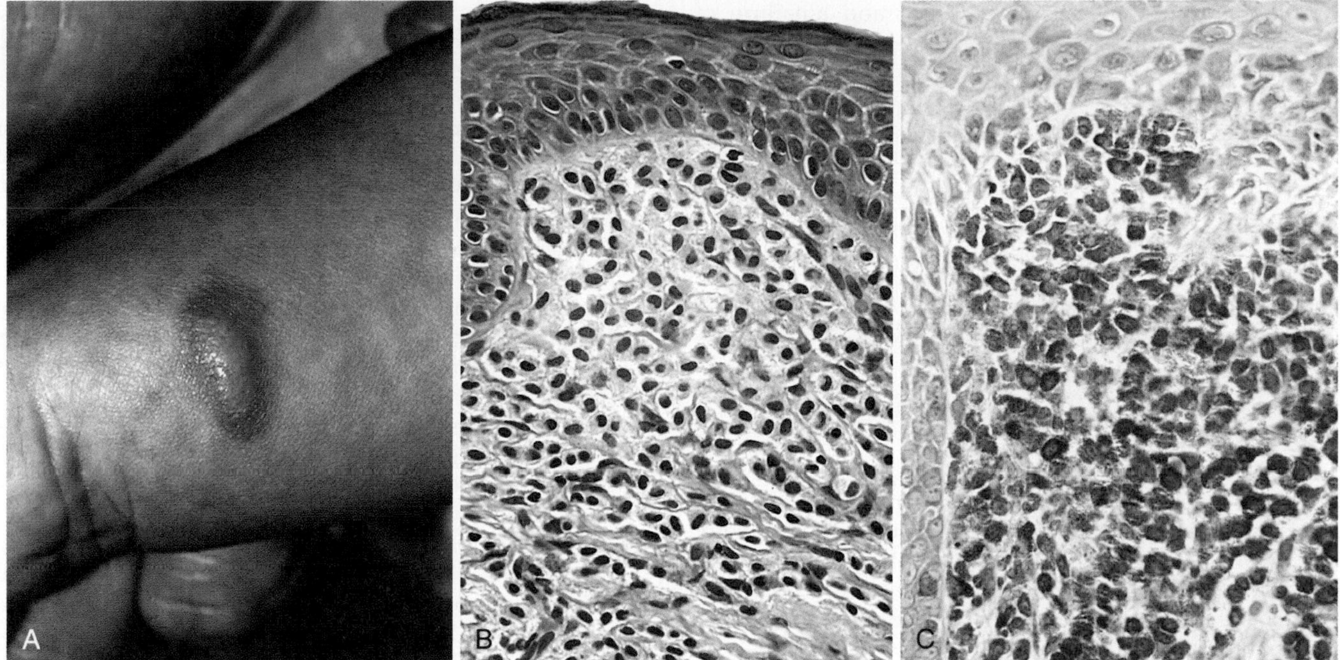

Figure 25-19 Mastocytosis. **A,** Solitary mastocytoma in a 1-year-old child. **B,** By histology, numerous ovoid cells with uniform, centrally located nuclei are observed in the dermis. **C,** Giemsa staining reveals purple "metachromatic" granules within the cytoplasm of the mast cells.

MORPHOLOGY

The pathologic findings are highly variable. In **urticaria pigmentosa**, lesions are multiple and widely distributed, consisting of round to oval, red-brown, nonscaling papules and small plaques. Solitary **mastocytoma** presents as a pink to tan-brown nodule that may be pruritic or show blister formation (Fig. 25-19*A*). The histologic picture in urticaria pigmentosa or solitary mastocytoma varies from a subtle increase in the numbers of spindle-shaped and stellate mast cells around superficial dermal blood vessels, to large numbers of tightly packed, round to oval mast cells in the upper to mid-dermis (Fig. 25-19*B*). Fibrosis, edema, and small numbers of eosinophils may also be present. Mast cells may be difficult to differentiate from lymphocytes in routine, hematoxylin and eosin–stained sections, and special metachromatic stains (toluidine blue or Giemsa) must be used to visualize their granules (Fig. 25-19*C*). Even with these stains, extensive degranulation may result in failure to recognize these cells by light microscopy, but their identity can be readily confirmed with immunohistochemical stains for mast cell markers, such as mast cell tryptase and KIT.

Disorders of Epidermal Maturation

Ichthyosis

Of the numerous disorders that impair epidermal maturation, ichthyosis is perhaps one of the most striking. The term is derived from the Greek root *ichthy,* meaning "fishy," and accordingly, this group of inherited disorders is associated with chronic, excessive keratin buildup (hyperkeratosis) that results clinically in fishlike scales (Fig. 25-20*A*). The clinical types of ichthyosis vary according to the mode of inheritance, histology, and clinical features; the primary categories include *ichthyosis vulgaris* (autosomal dominant or acquired), *congenital ichthyosiform erythroderma* (autosomal recessive), *lamellar ichthyosis* (autosomal recessive), and *X-linked ichthyosis.* Most ichthyoses become apparent either at or around the time of birth. Acquired (noninherited) variants also exist; one such variant, *ichthyosis vulgaris,* may be associated with lymphoid and visceral malignancies.

Pathogenesis. The primary abnormality in some forms of ichthyosis is defective desquamation, leading to retention of abnormally formed scale. For example, X-linked ichthyosis is caused by a deficiency of steroid sulfatase, an enzyme helps to remove proadhesive cholesterol sulfate from intercellular spaces. In its absence cholesterol sulfate accumulates, resulting in persistent cell-to-cell

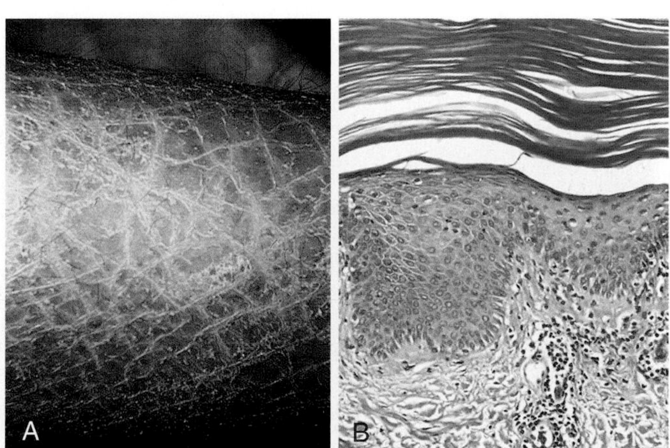

Figure 25-20 Ichthyosis. Note prominent fishlike scales (**A**) and compacted, thickened stratum corneum (**B**).

adhesion within the stratum corneum and a failure of desquamation.

MORPHOLOGY

All forms of ichthyosis exhibit a buildup of compacted stratum corneum that is associated with loss of the normal basket-weave pattern (Fig. 25-20*B*). There is generally little or no inflammation. Variations in the thickness of the epidermis and the stratum granulosum and the gross appearance and distribution of lesions are used to subclassify these disorders.

Acute Inflammatory Dermatoses

Literally thousands of inflammatory dermatoses have been described. In general, acute lesions last from days to weeks and are characterized by inflammatory infiltrates (usually composed of lymphocytes and macrophages rather than neutrophils), edema, and variable degrees of epidermal, vascular, or subcutaneous injury. Chronic lesions, on the other hand, persist for months to years and are often associated with changes in epidermal growth (atrophy or hyperplasia) or dermal fibrosis. The lesions discussed here are examples of the more commonly encountered acute dermatoses.

Urticaria

Urticaria (hives) is a common disorder of the skin characterized by localized mast cell degranulation and resultant dermal microvascular hyperpermeability. This combination of effects produces pruritic edematous plaques called *wheals.* Angioedema is closely related to urticaria and is characterized by edema of the deeper dermis and the subcutaneous fat.

Urticaria most often occurs between ages 20 and 40, but all age groups are susceptible. Individual lesions develop and fade within hours (usually less than 24 hours), and episodes may last for days or persist for months. Sites of predilection for urticarial eruptions include any area exposed to pressure, such as the trunk, distal extremities, and ears. Persistent episodes of urticaria may herald an underlying disease (e.g., collagen vascular disorders, Hodgkin lymphoma), but in the majority of cases no underlying cause is identified.

Pathogenesis. **Urticaria is most commonly the result of antigen-induced release of vasoactive mediators from mast cells but there are other less common causes as well.**

- *Mast cell-dependent, IgE-dependent.* Urticaria of this type follows exposure to many different antigens (pollens, foods, drugs, insect venom), and is an example of a localized immediate hypersensitivity (type I) reaction triggered by the binding of antigen to IgE antibodies that are attached to mast cells through Fc receptors (Chapter 6).
- *Mast cell-dependent, IgE-independent.* This subset results from substances that directly incite the degranulation of mast cells, such as opiates, certain antibiotics, curare, and radiographic contrast media.
- *Mast cell-independent, IgE-independent.* These forms of urticaria are triggered by local factors that increase vascular permeability. One form is initiated by exposure to chemicals or drugs, such as aspirin, that inhibit cyclooxygenase and arachidonic acid production. The precise mechanism of aspirin-induced urticaria is unknown. A second form is *hereditary angioneurotic edema* (Chapter 6), caused by an inherited deficiency of C1 inhibitor that results in excessive activation of the early components of the complement system and production of vasoactive mediators.

MORPHOLOGY

Lesions vary from small, pruritic papules to large edematous plaques (Fig. 25-21*A*). Individual lesions may coalesce to form annular, linear, or arciform configurations. The histologic features of urticaria may be very subtle. There is usually a sparse superficial perivenular infiltrate consisting of mononuclear cells and rare neutrophils. Eosinophils may also be present. Collagen bundles are more widely spaced than in normal skin, a result of superficial dermal edema (Fig. 25-21*B*). Superficial lymphatic channels are dilated due to increased absorption of edema fluid. There are no changes in the epidermis.

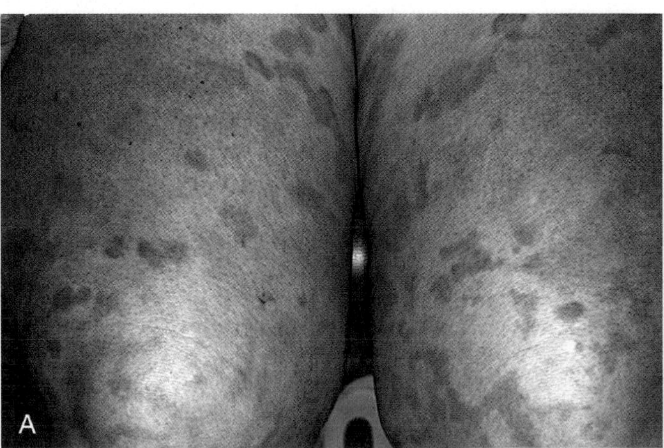

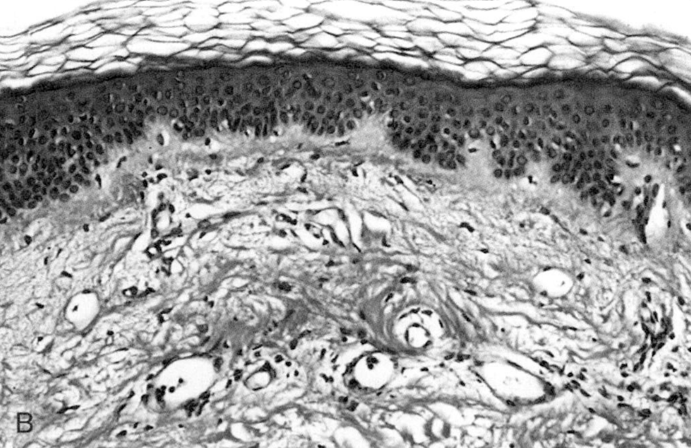

Figure 25-21 Urticaria. **A,** Erythematous, edematous, often circular plaques are characteristic. **B,** Histologically, there is superficial dermal edema, manifested by spaces between collagen bundles, and dilated lymphatic and blood-filled vascular spaces; the epithelium is normal.

Acute Eczematous Dermatitis

The Greek word *eczema*, meaning "to boil over," vividly describes the appearance of acute eczematous dermatitis one of the most common skin disorders. Based on initiating factors, eczematous dermatitis can be subdivided into the following categories: (1) allergic contact dermatitis, (2) atopic dermatitis, (3) drug-related eczematous dermatitis, (4) photoeczematous dermatitis, and (5) primary irritant dermatitis.

The causes of eczema are sometimes broadly separated into "inside" and "outside" types: disease resulting from external application of an antigen (e.g., poison ivy) or a reaction to an internal circulating antigen (which may be derived from ingested food or a drug). Treatment involves a search for offending substances that can be removed from the environment. Topical steroids nonspecifically block the inflammatory response. While such treatments are only palliative and do not cure, they are nevertheless helpful in interrupting acute exacerbations of eczema that can become self-perpetuating if unchecked.

***Pathogenesis.* Eczematous dermatitis typically results from T cell-mediated inflammatory reactions (type IV hypersensitivity).** This has been well studied in dermatitis triggered by contact antigens (e.g., uroshiol from poison ivy). It is believed that reactive chemicals introduced at the epidermal surface modify self proteins, acting as "haptens", and these proteins become neoantigens. The antigens are taken up by Langerhans cells, which then migrate by way of dermal lymphatics to draining lymph nodes. Here the antigens are presented to naive CD4+ T cells, which are activated and develop into effector and memory cells (Chapter 6). On antigen reexposure, memory T cells expressing homing molecules such as common lymphocyte antigen and particular chemokine receptors migrate to skin sites of antigen localization. Here they release the cytokines and chemokines that recruit the numerous inflammatory cells characteristic of eczema. This process occurs within 24 hours and accounts for the initial erythema and pruritus that characterize cutaneous delayed hypersensitivity in the acute, spongiotic phase.

Langerhans cells within the epidermis play a central role in contact dermatitis, and understandably factors that affect Langerhans cell function impact the inflammatory reaction. Chronic exposure to UV light is injurious to epidermal Langerhans cells and can prevent sensitization to contact antigens, although UV light can also alter antigens and generate forms that are more likely to induce sensitivity reactions.

MORPHOLOGY

All types of eczematous dermatitis are characterized by red, papulovesicular, oozing, and crusted lesions that, if persistent, develop reactive **acanthosis** and **hyperkeratosis** that produce raised scaling plaques (Fig. 25-22). A striking example of

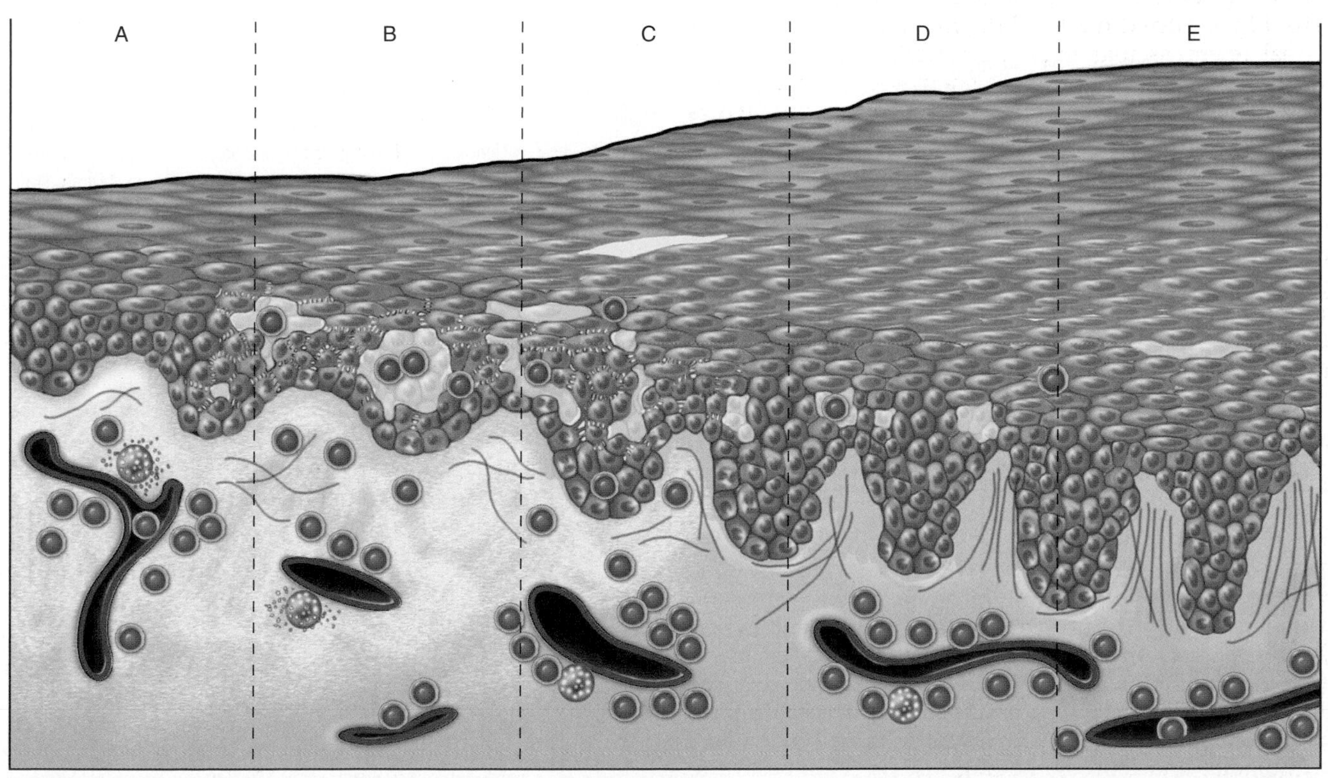

Figure 25-22 Stages of eczema development. **A,** Initial dermal edema and perivascular infiltration by inflammatory cells is followed within 24 to 48 hours by **(B)** epidermal spongiosis and microvesicle formation. **C,** Abnormal scale, including parakeratosis, along with progressive acanthosis **(D)** and hyperkeratosis **(E)** appear as the lesion becomes chronic.

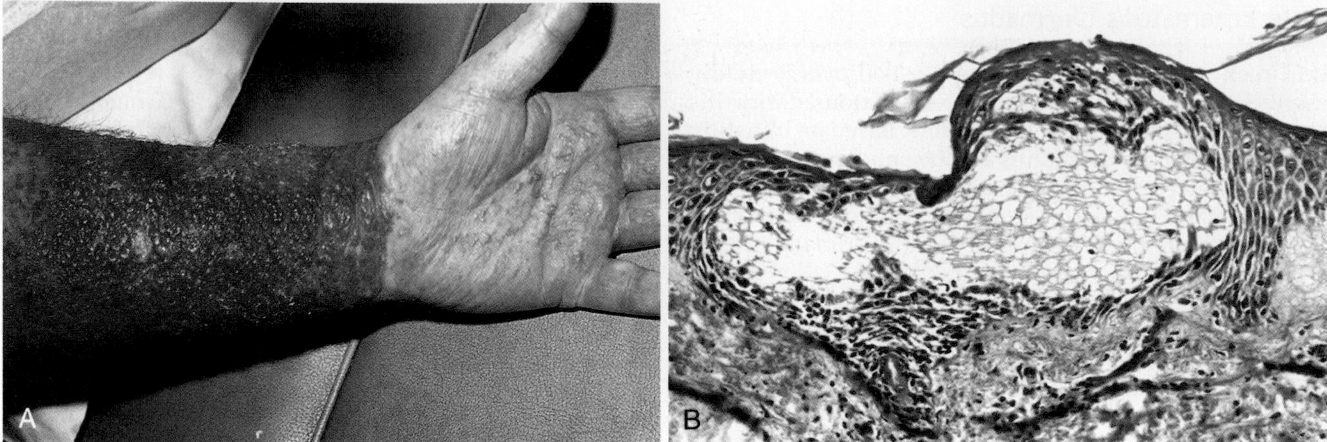

Figure 25-23 Eczematous dermatitis. **A,** Acute allergic contact dermatitis due to antigen exposure (in this case, laundry detergent in clothing) marked by numerous vesicular lesions on erythematous skin. **B,** Edema within the epidermis creates small fluid-filled intraepidermal vesicles.

eczema is an acute contact reaction to topical antigens such as urushiol in poison ivy/oak *(Rhus toxicodendron)*, characterized by pruritic, edematous, oozing plaques, often containing small and large blisters (vesicles and bullae) (Fig. 25-23*A*). Such lesions are prone to bacterial superinfection, which produces a yellow crust (impetiginization). With time, persistent lesions become less "wet" (fail to ooze or form vesicles) and become progressively (hyperkeratotic and acanthotic). **Spongiosis** characterizes acute eczematous dermatitis, hence the histologic synonym spongiotic dermatitis. Unlike urticaria, in which edema is restricted to the superficial dermis, edema seeps into the intercellular spaces of the epidermis, splaying apart keratinocytes, particularly in the stratum spinosum. Mechanical shearing of intercellular attachment sites (desmosomes) and cell membranes by progressive accumulation of intercellular fluid may result in the formation of intraepidermal vesicles (Fig. 25-23*B*).

During the earliest stages of eczematous dermatitis, there is a superficial, perivascular, lymphocytic infiltrate associated with papillary dermal edema and mast cell degranulation. The pattern and composition of this infiltrate may provide clues to the underlying cause. For example, eczema resulting from certain ingested drugs is marked by a lymphocytic infiltrate, often containing eosinophils**,** around deep as well as superficial dermal vessels. By contrast, eczematous dermatitis resulting from contact antigens tends to produce a mononuclear inflammatory reaction that preferentially affects the superficial dermal layer.

Erythema Multiforme

Erythema multiforme is an uncommon self-limited hypersensitivity reaction to certain infections and drugs. It affects individuals of any age and is associated with the following conditions: (1) infections such as herpes simplex, mycoplasmal infections, histoplasmosis, coccidioidomycosis, typhoid, and leprosy, among others; (2) exposure to certain drugs (sulfonamides, penicillin, barbiturates, salicylates, hydantoins, and antimalarials); (3) cancer (carcinomas and lymphomas); and (4) collagen vascular diseases (lupus erythematosus, dermatomyositis, and polyarteritis nodosa).

Pathogenesis. **Erythema multiforme is characterized by keratinocyte injury mediated by skin-homing CD8+ cytotoxic T lymphocytes.** This mechanism of injury is shared with a number of other conditions, including acute graft-versus-host disease, skin allograft rejection, and fixed drug eruptions. In erythema multiforme, CD8+ cytotoxic T cells are more prominent in the central portion of the lesions, while CD4+ helper T cell and Langerhans cells are more prevalent in the peripheral portions. The epidermal antigens that are recognized by the infiltrating T cells in erythema multiforme remain unknown.

MORPHOLOGY

Affected individuals present with a diverse array of lesions (hence the term multiforme), including macules, papules, vesicles, bullae, and characteristic targetoid (target-like) lesions (Fig. 25-24*A*). The lesions may occur in a variety of distributions. Cases that are limited in extent often show symmetric involvement of the extremities. A febrile form associated with extensive involvement of the skin is called **Stevens-Johnson syndrome**, which is often (but not exclusively) seen in children. In Stevens-Johnson syndrome, lesions involve not only the skin but also the lips and oral mucosa, conjunctiva, urethra, and genital and perianal areas. Secondary infection of involved areas due to loss of skin integrity may result in life-threatening sepsis. Another variant termed **toxic epidermal necrolysis** is characterized by diffuse necrosis and sloughing of cutaneous and mucosal epithelial surfaces. The widespread epidermal damage produces a clinical picture similar to that seen in patients with extensive burns.

On histologic examination, the "targetoid" lesions show a superficial perivascular, lymphocytic infiltrate associated with dermal edema and accumulation of lymphocytes along the dermoepidermal junction, where they are intimately associated with degenerating and necrotic keratinocytes, a pattern termed *interface dermatitis* (Fig. 25-24*B*). With time there is upward migration of lymphocytes into the epidermis. Discrete and confluent zones of epidermal necrosis occur with concomitant blister formation. Epidermal sloughing leads to shallow erosions.

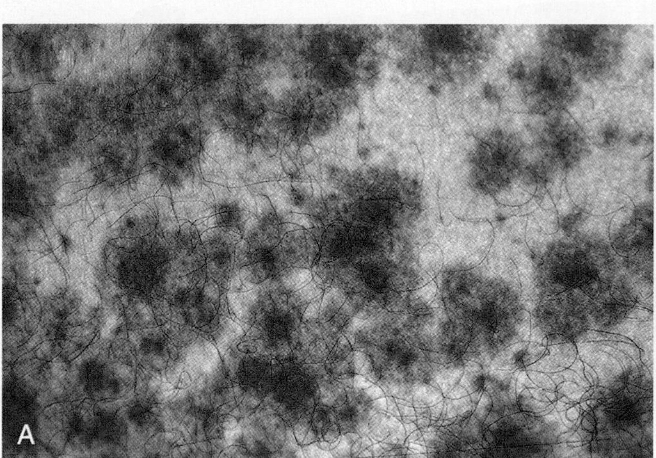
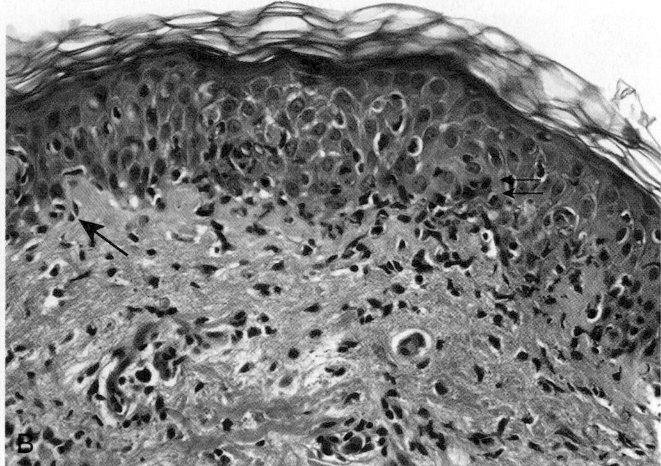

Figure 25-24 Erythema multiforme. **A,** The target-like lesions consist of a central blister or zone of epidermal necrosis surrounded by macular erythema. **B,** An early lesion shows lymphocytes accumulating along the dermoepidermal junction where basal keratinocytes have begun to become vacuolated (arrow). With time, necrotic/apoptotic keratinocytes appear in the overlying epithelium (double arrow).

Chronic Inflammatory Dermatoses

This category includes inflammatory skin disorders that persist for many months to years. The skin surface in some chronic inflammatory dermatoses is roughened as a result of excessive or abnormal scale formation and shedding. However, not all scaling lesions are inflammatory; witness the hereditary ichthyoses, described earlier, with extensive scale due to defects in desquamation.

Psoriasis

Psoriasis is a chronic inflammatory dermatosis that appears to have an autoimmune basis. It is a common disorder, affecting as many as 1% to 2% of people in the United States. Persons of all ages may develop the disease. Approximately 15% of the patients with psoriasis have associated arthritis. Psoriatic arthritis may be mild or may produce severe deformities resembling the joint changes seen in rheumatoid arthritis. It can affect any joint in the body and may be symmetrical or affect one side only. In addition, psoriasis may also be associated with myopathy, enteropathy, and AIDS.

Pathogenesis. Psoriasis results from interactions of genetic and environmental factors. As in the case of many autoimmune diseases it is linked to genes within the HLA locus. There is a strong association with HLA-C, particularly with the *HLA-Cw*0602* allele. About two thirds of affected individuals carry this allele, and homozygotes for *HLA-Cw*0602* have a 2.5-fold higher risk for developing psoriasis than do heterozygotes. Conversely, only about 10% of *HLA-Cw*0602* heterozygotes develop psoriasis, indicating that other factors interact with this MHC molecule to cause disease susceptibility. The culprit antigens remain elusive, but it appears that sensitized populations of CD4+ T_H1 and T_H17 cells and activated CD8+ cytotoxic effector T cells enter the skin and accumulate in the epidermis. These T cells may create an abnormal microenvironment by stimulating the secretion of cytokines and growth factors that induce keratinocyte proliferation, resulting in the characteristic lesions. The interactions between CD4+ T cells, CD8+ T cells, dendritic cells, and keratinocytes give rise to a cytokine "soup" dominated by T_H1-type and T_H17-type cytokines such as IL-12, interferon-γ, tumor necrosis factor (TNF), and IL-17. The importance of these factors is highlighted by the generally excellent clinical responses that are observed in patients treated with therapies that block TNF function. Lymphocytes also produce growth factors for keratinocytes that may contribute to epidermal thickening. Psoriatic lesions can be induced in susceptible individuals by local trauma, a process known as the *Koebner phenomenon*, presumably because trauma sets in motion a local inflammatory response that becomes self-perpetuating.

MORPHOLOGY

Psoriasis most frequently affects the skin of the elbows, knees, scalp, lumbosacral areas, intergluteal cleft, and glans penis. The typical lesion is a well-demarcated, **pink to salmon-colored plaque covered by loosely adherent silver-white scale** (Fig. 25-25*A*). Variations exist, with some lesions occurring in annular, linear, gyrate, or serpiginous configurations. Psoriasis is one cause of total body erythema and scaling known as erythroderma. **Nail changes** occur in 30% of cases of psoriasis and consist of yellow-brown discoloration (often likened to an oil slick), with pitting, dimpling, separation of the nail plate from the underlying bed (onycholysis), thickening, and crumbling.

Established lesions of psoriasis have a characteristic histologic picture. Increased epidermal cell proliferation results in marked epidermal thickening (acanthosis), with regular downward elongation of the rete ridges sometimes described as appearing like test tubes in a rack (Fig. 25-25*B*). Mitotic figures are easily identified well above the basal cell layer, where mitotic activity is confined in normal skin. **The stratum granulosum is thinned or absent, and extensive overlying parakeratotic scale is seen.** Typical of psoriatic plaques is thinning of the portion of the epidermal cell layer that overlies the tips of dermal papillae (suprapapillary plates) and dilated, tortuous blood vessels within these papillae. This constellation of changes results in abnormal proximity of vessels within the dermal papillae to the overlying parakeratotic scale, and accounts for

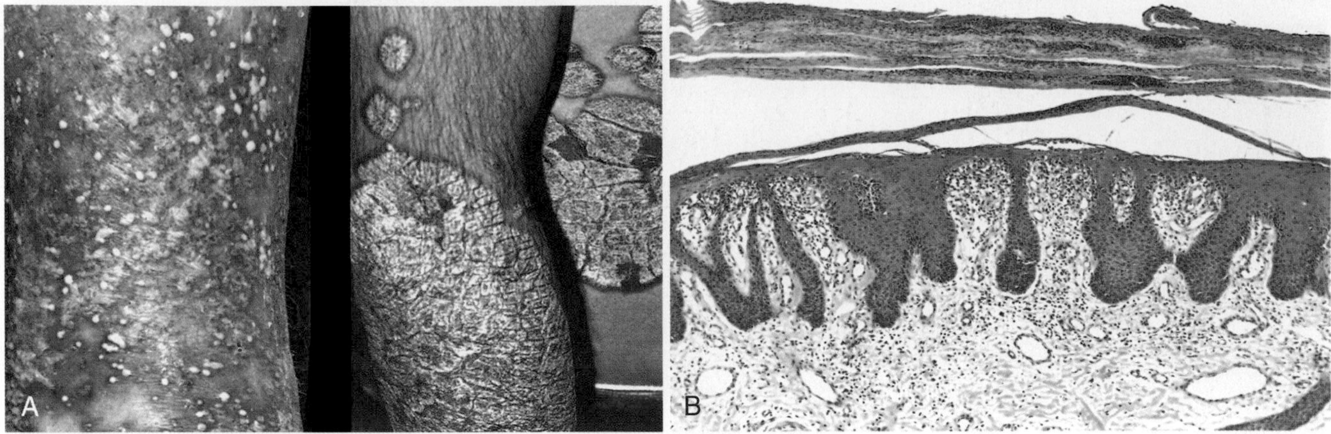

Figure 25-25 Psoriasis. **A,** Early lesions may be dominated by inflammation, marked by the presence of small pustules and erythema *(left).* Established chronic lesions are erythematous and covered by a characteristic silver-white scale *(right).* **B,** Microscopically there is epidermal hyperplasia, parakeratotic scale, and accumulation of neutrophils within the superficial epidermis.

the characteristic clinical phenomenon of multiple, minute, bleeding points when the scale is lifted from the plaque **(Auspitz sign).** Neutrophils form small aggregates within slightly spongiotic foci of the superficial epidermis **(spongiform pustules)** and within the parakeratotic stratum corneum **(Munro microabscesses).** In pustular psoriasis, larger abscess-like accumulations of neutrophils are present directly beneath the stratum corneum.

Seborrheic Dermatitis

Seborrheic dermatitis is a chronic inflammatory dermatosis that is even more common than psoriasis, affecting up to 5 % of the general population. It classically involves regions with a high density of sebaceous glands, such as the scalp, forehead (especially the glabella), external auditory canal, retroauricular area, nasolabial folds, and the presternal area. Despite this association and its name, however, seborrheic dermatitis is associated with inflammation of the epidermis and is not a disease of the sebaceous glands per se.

Pathogenesis. The precise etiology of seborrheic dermatitis is unknown. Increased sebum production, often in response to androgens, is one possible contributory factor. Involvement of sebum is supported by clinical observations of patients with Parkinson disease, who typically show increased sebum production secondary to dopamine deficiency and have a markedly increased incidence of seborrheic dermatitis. Once treated with levodopa, the oiliness of the skin decreases and the seborrheic dermatitis improves. However, other conditions associated with increased sebum production such as acne (discussed later) are not associated with seborrheic dermatitis, and sebum production is probably best viewed as being necessary but not sufficient to cause the disorder. Other work has suggested a relationship with colonization of the skin by certain fungal species of the genus *Malassezia*, but there is no definitive evidence of a cause and effect relationship. A severe form of seborrheic dermatitis that is difficult to treat is seen in many HIV-infected individuals with low CD4 counts; as with other forms of the disorder, its etiology is also unknown.

MORPHOLOGY

The individual lesions are macules and papules on an erythematous-yellow, often greasy base, typically in association with extensive scaling and crusting. Fissures may also be present, particularly behind the ears. Dandruff is the common clinical expression of seborrheic dermatitis of the scalp. Microscopically, seborrheic dermatitis shares features with both spongiotic dermatitis and psoriasis, with earlier lesions being more spongiotic and later ones more acanthotic. Typically, mounds of parakeratosis containing neutrophils and serum are present at the ostia of hair follicles (so-called **follicular lipping**). A superficial perivascular inflammatory infiltrate generally consists of an admixture of lymphocytes and neutrophils. With human immunodeficiency virus infection, apoptotic keratinocytes and plasma cells may also be present.

Lichen Planus

"Pruritic, purple, polygonal, planar, papules, and plaques" are the tongue-twisting "six Ps" of lichen planus, a disorder of skin and mucosa. Lichen planus is usually self-limited, most commonly resolving spontaneously 1 to 2 years after onset. Resolution often leaves a residuum of postinflammatory hyperpigmentation. Oral lesions, however, may persist for years. Squamous cell carcinoma has been noted to occur in chronic mucosal and paramucosal lesions of lichen planus, and could be an example of carcinogenesis in the setting of a chronic inflammatory process. As in psoriasis, the Koebner phenomenon may be seen in lichen planus.

Pathogenesis. The pathogenesis of lichen planus is not known. It is plausible that expression of altered antigens in basal epidermal cells or the dermoepidermal junction elicit a cell-mediated cytotoxic (CD8+) T cell response. In support of this notion, T-lymphocyte infiltrates and hyperplasia of Langerhans cells are characteristic features of this disorder.

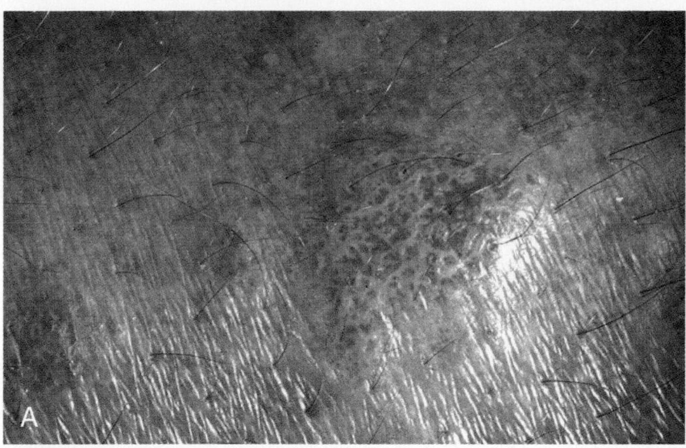

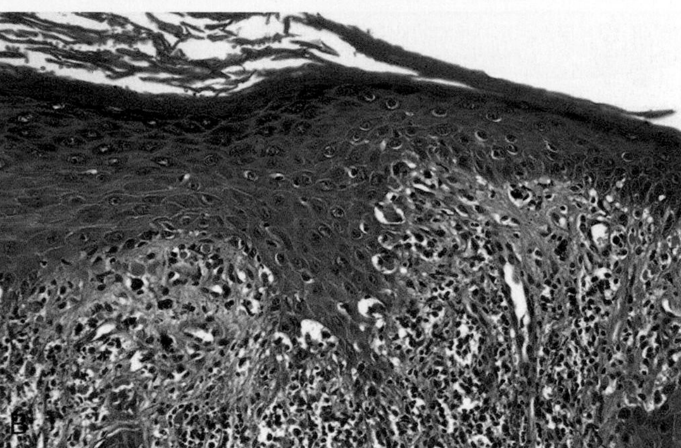

Figure 25-26 Lichen planus. **A,** This flat-topped pink-purple, polygonal papule has a white lacelike pattern of lines that are referred to as Wickham stria. **B,** There is a bandlike infiltrate of lymphocytes at the dermoepidermal junction, hyperkeratosis, and pointed rete ridges (sawtoothing), the latter as a result of chronic basal cell layer injury.

MORPHOLOGY

Cutaneous lesions consist of itchy, violaceous, flat-topped papules that may coalesce focally to form plaques (Fig. 25-26*A*). These papules are often highlighted by white dots or lines called **Wickham striae**, which are created by areas of hypergranulosis. In darkly pigmented individuals, lesions may acquire a dark-brown color due to release of melanin into the dermis as the basal cell layer is destroyed. Lesions are usually multiple and symmetrically distributed, particularly on the extremities and often about the wrists and elbows. The glans penis is another common site of involvement. In 70% of cases, oral lesions are present as white, reticulated, or netlike areas involving the mucosa.

Lichen planus is characterized histologically by a dense, continuous infiltrate of lymphocytes along the dermoepidermal junction, a prototypic example of **interface dermatitis** (Fig. 25-26*B*). The lymphocytes are intimately associated with basal keratinocytes, which show degeneration, necrosis, and a resemblance in size and contour to more mature cells of the stratum spinosum (squamatization). As a consequence of this destructive lymphocytic infiltrate, the dermoepidermal interface takes on an angulated zigzag contour (sawtoothing). Anucleate, necrotic basal cells may become incorporated into the inflamed papillary dermis, where they are referred to as **colloid** or **Civatte bodies.** Though characteristic of lichen planus, these bodies may be detected in any chronic dermatitis in which basal keratinocytes are destroyed. Although the lesions bear some similarities to those in erythema multiforme, lichen planus shows changes of chronicity, namely, epidermal hyperplasia (or rarely atrophy) and thickening of the granular cell layer and stratum corneum (hypergranulosis and hyperkeratosis, respectively).

KEY CONCEPTS

Inflammatory Dermatoses

- Many specific inflammatory dermatoses exist, which can be mediated by IgE antibodies (urticaria) or antigen-specific T cells (eczema, erythema multiforme, and psoriasis)
- These disorders are diagnosed based on the distribution and gross appearance of skin lesions and the microscopic patterns of inflammation (e.g., interface dermatitis in lichen planus and erythema multiforme)

Blistering (Bullous) Diseases

Although vesicles and bullae (blisters) occur in several unrelated conditions such as herpesvirus infection, spongiotic dermatitis, erythema multiforme, and thermal burns, there exists a group of disorders in which blisters are the primary and most distinctive features. These *bullous diseases*, as they are called, produce dramatic lesions and in some instances are fatal if untreated. Blisters in the various disorders occur at different levels within the skin (Fig. 25-27); histologic assessment is essential for accurate diagnosis and provides insight into the pathogenic mechanisms. Knowledge of the structure of desmosomes and hemidesmosomes (described in Chapter 1), which you will recall provide the skin with mechanical stability, is helpful in understanding these diseases, as they are often caused by acquired or inherited defects in proteins that make up or bind to these structures (Fig. 25-28).

Inflammatory Blistering Disorders

Pemphigus

Pemphigus is a blistering disorder caused by autoantibodies that result in the dissolution of intercellular attachments within the epidermis and mucosal epithelium. The pathobiology of blistering disorders provides important insights into the molecular underpinnings of keratinocyte adhesion. The majority of individuals who develop pemphigus are in the fourth to sixth decades of life, and men and women are affected equally. There are multiple variants: (1) pemphigus vulgaris, (2) pemphigus vegetans, (3) pemphigus foliaceus, (4) pemphigus erythematosus, and (5) paraneoplastic pemphigus. These disorders are usually benign, but in extreme cases can be fatal without treatment.

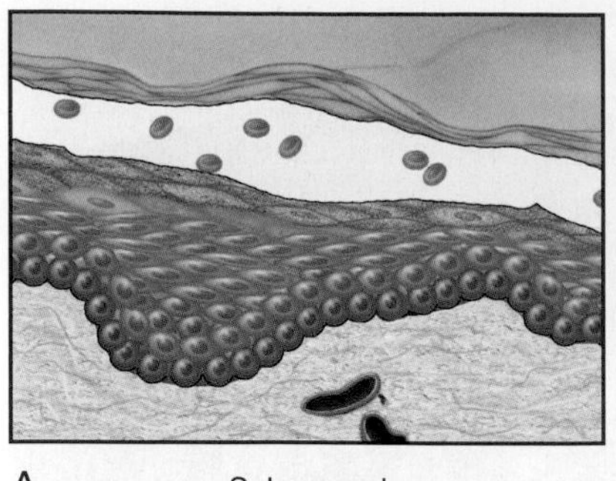

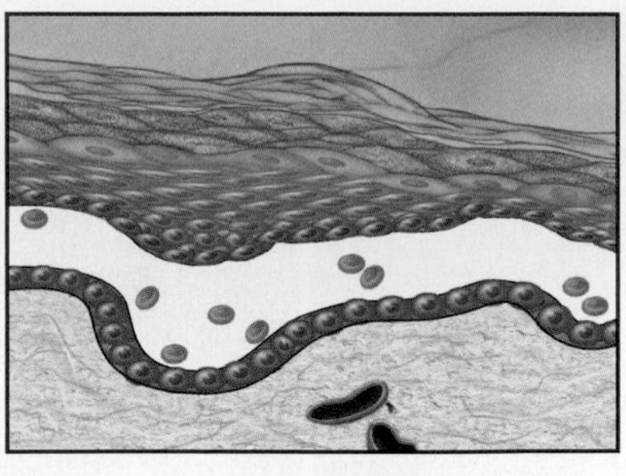

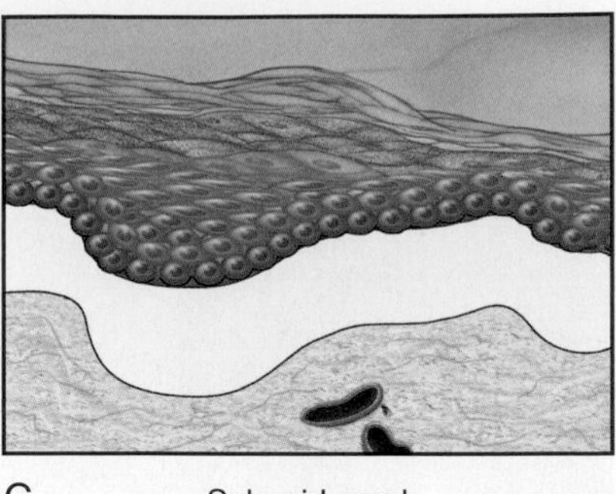

Figure 25-27 Schematic representation of different types of blisters. **A,** In subcorneal blisters, the stratum corneum forms the roof of the bulla (as in pemphigus foliaceus). **B,** In a suprabasilar blister, a portion of the epidermis, including the stratum corneum, forms the roof (as in pemphigus vulgaris). **C,** In a subepidermal blister, the entire epidermis separates from the dermis (as in bullous pemphigoid).

- *Pemphigus vulgaris,* by far the most common type (accounting for more than 80% of cases worldwide), involves the mucosa and skin, especially on the scalp, face, axilla, groin, trunk, and points of pressure. It may present as oral ulcers that may persist for months before skin involvement appears. Primary lesions are superficial vesicles and bullae that rupture easily, leaving shallow erosions covered with dried serum and crust (Fig. 25-29*A*).
- *Pemphigus vegetans* is a rare form that usually presents not with blisters but with large, moist, verrucous (wartlike), vegetating plaques studded with pustules on the groin, axillae, and flexural surfaces.
- *Pemphigus foliaceus* is a more benign form that is endemic in Brazil (where it is called *fogo selvagem*) and occurs sporadically in other geographic regions. Sites of predilection are the scalp, face, chest, and back, and the mucous membranes are only rarely affected. Bullae are so superficial that they mainly present as areas of erythema and crusting; these represent superficial erosions at sites of previous blister rupture (Fig. 25-30*A*).
- *Pemphigus erythematosus* is considered to be a localized, less severe form of pemphigus foliaceus that may selectively involve the malar area of the face in a lupus erythematosus-like fashion.

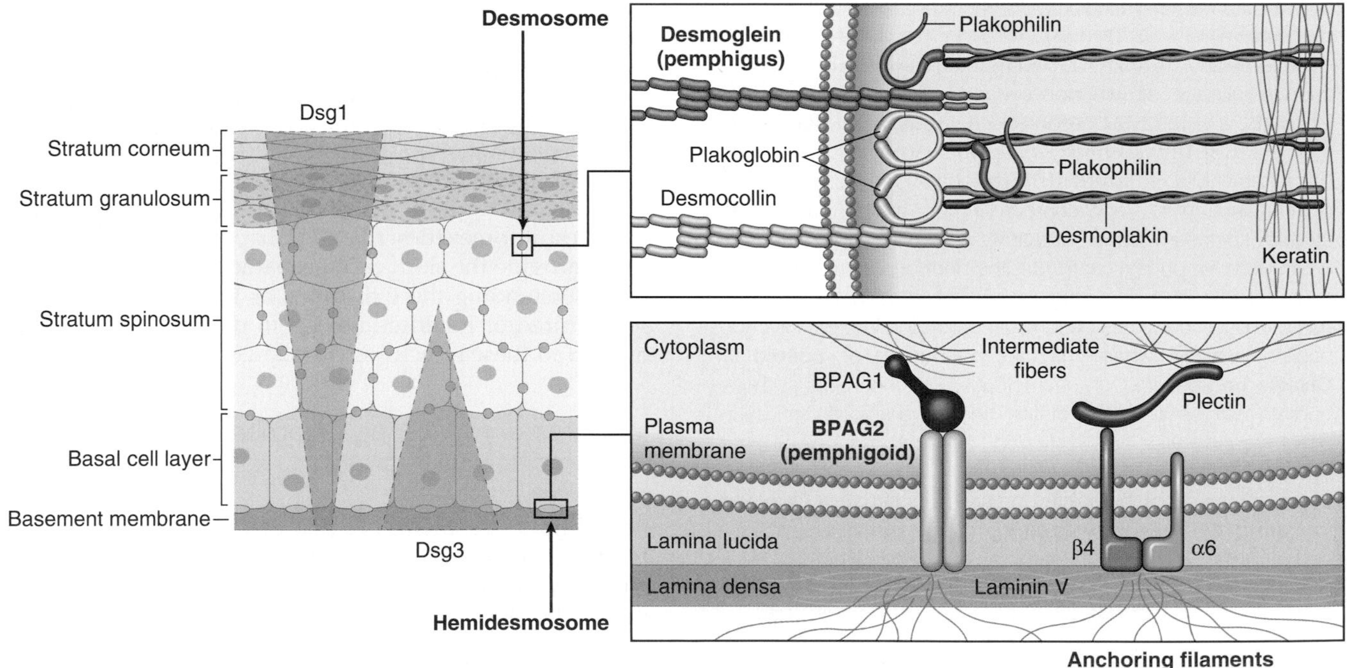

Figure 25-28 Keratinocyte adhesion molecules and blistering inflammatory disorders. Knowledge of the proteins composing desmosomes and hemidesmosomes is key to understanding blistering disorders. Desmogleins 1 and 3 (Dsg1, Dsg3) are functionally interchangeable components of desmosomes, but have different distributions within the epidermis *(left panel)*. The major structural proteins of desmosomes and hemidesmosomes are shown at *right*. In pemphigus vulgaris autoantibodies against Dsg1 and Dsg3 cause blisters in the deep suprabasal epidermis, whereas in pemphigus foliaceus the autoantibodies are against Dsg1 alone, leading to superficial, subcorneal blisters. In bullous pemphigoid autoantibodies bind BPAG2, a component of the hemidesmosomes, leading to blister formation at the level of the lamina lucida of the basement membrane. Dermatitis herpetiformis is caused by IgA autoantibodies to the fibrils that anchor hemidesmosomes to the dermis.

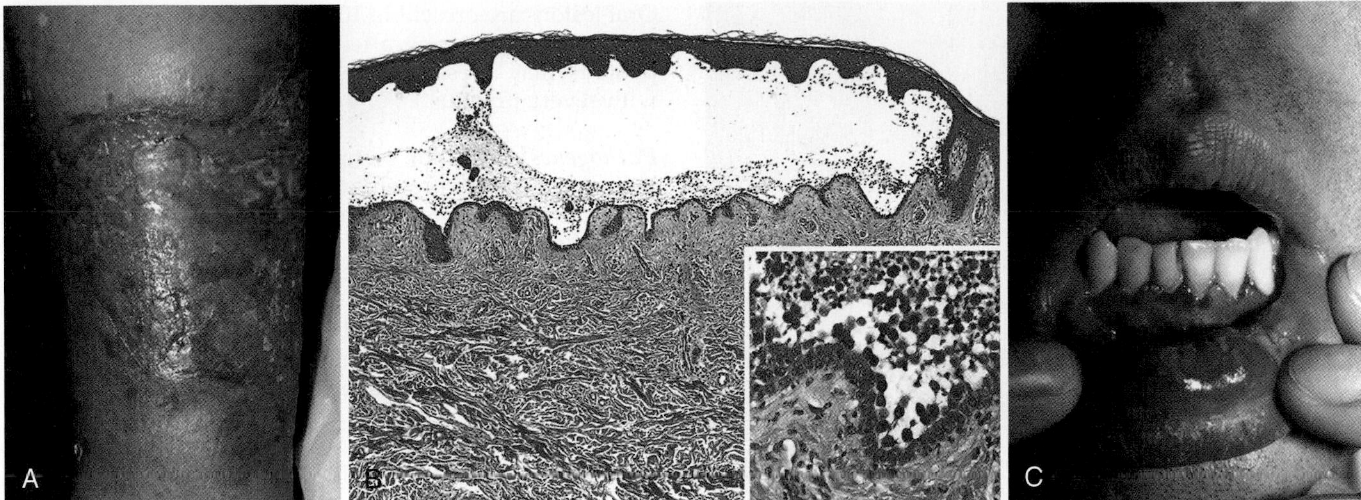

Figure 25-29 Pemphigus vulgaris. **A,** Eroded plaques are formed following the rupture of confluent, thin-roofed bullae, here affecting axillary skin. **B,** Suprabasal acantholysis results in an intraepidermal blister in which dyscohesive (acantholytic) epidermal cells are present *(inset)*. **C,** Ulcerated blisters in the oral mucosa are also common, as seen here on the lip.

- *Paraneoplastic pemphigus* occurs in association with various malignancies, most commonly non-Hodgkin lymphoma.

Pathogenesis. All forms of pemphigus are autoimmune diseases caused by IgG autoantibodies against desmogleins that disrupt intercellular adhesions and result in the formation of blisters. By direct immunofluorescence, lesions show a characteristic net-like pattern of intercellular IgG deposits. IgG is usually seen at all levels of the epithelium in pemphigus vulgaris, but tends to be more superficial in pemphigus foliaceus (Fig. 25-31). The distribution of desmoglein 1 and 3 in the epidermis and the presence of autoantibodies to one or both proteins appear to explain the position and severity of the blisters (Fig. 25-28). The antibodies cause these lesions primarily by disrupting the intercellular adhesive function of the desmosomes; they may also act indirectly by activating intercellular proteases. Paraneoplastic pemphigus arises most often in the setting of lymphoid neoplasms, and is also caused by autoantibodies that recognize desmogleins or other proteins involved in intercellular adhesion.

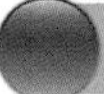

MORPHOLOGY

The common histologic denominator in all forms of pemphigus is **acantholysis**, the dissolution or lysis of the intercellular bridges that connect squamous epithelial cells. Acantholytic cells dissociate from one another, lose their polyhedral shape and become rounded. In pemphigus vulgaris and pemphigus vegetans, acantholysis selectively involves the cells immediately above the basal cell layer. In the vegetans variant, there is also overlying epidermal hyperplasia. An immediately **suprabasal acantholytic blister** is characteristic of pemphigus vulgaris (Fig. 25-29*B*). The single layer of intact basal cells that forms the blister base has been likened to a row of tombstones. In pemphigus foliaceus, blisters form by similar mechanisms but,

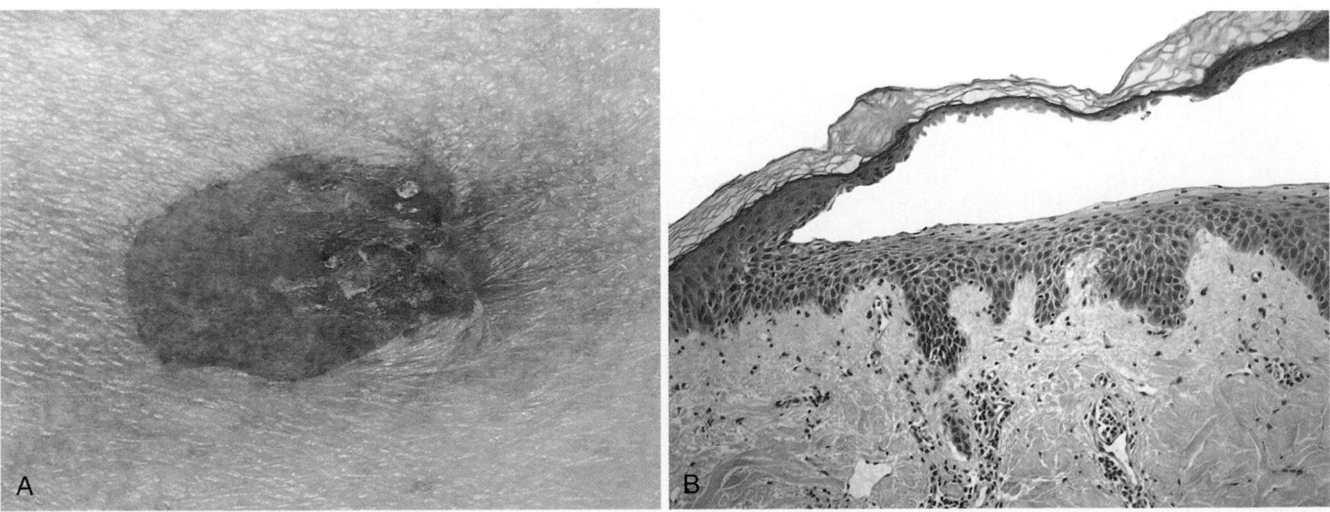

Figure 25-30 Pemphigus foliaceus. **A,** The delicate superficial (subcorneal) blisters are much less erosive than those seen in pemphigus vulgaris. **B,** Subcorneal separation of the epithelium is seen.

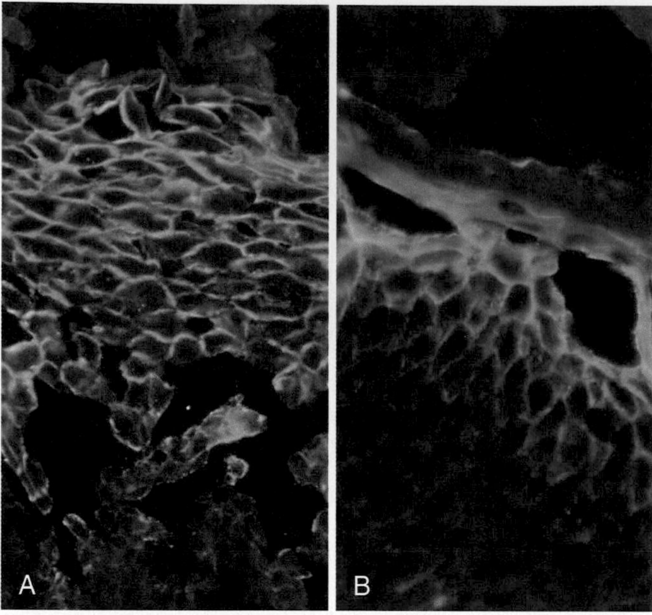

Figure 25-31 Direct immunofluorescence staining for immunoglobulin of epidermis involved by pemphigus. **A,** In pemphigus vulgaris there is deposition of immunoglobulin along the plasma membranes of keratinocytes in a reticular or fishnet-like pattern accompanied by suprabasalar loss of cell-to-cell adhesion (acantholysis). **B,** In pemphigus foliaceus the immunoglobulin deposits and acantholysis are more superficial.

unlike pemphigus vulgaris, are found in the superficial epidermis at the level of the stratum granulosum (Fig. 25-30*B*). Variable superficial dermal infiltration by lymphocytes, macrophages, and eosinophils accompanies each type of pemphigus.

The mainstay of treatment in all forms of pemphigus is immunosuppressive agents, which decrease the titers of the pathogenic antibodies.

Bullous Pemphigoid

Generally affecting elderly individuals, bullous pemphigoid shows a wide range of clinical presentations. Sites of involvement include the inner aspects of the thighs, flexor surfaces of the forearms, axillae, groin, and lower abdomen. Oral lesions are present in 10% to 15% of affected individuals, usually appearing after the cutaneous lesions. Some patients may present with urticarial plaques associated with severe pruritus.

Pathogenesis. Bullous pemphigoid is caused by autoantibodies that bind to proteins that are required for adherence of basal keratinocytes to the basement membrane. Most antibody deposition occurs in a continuous linear pattern at the dermoepidermal junction (Fig. 25-33*A*), which contains specialized structures called hemidesmosomes that link basal keratinocytes to the underlying basement membrane (Fig. 25-33*B*). The so-called bullous pemphigoid antigens (BPAGs) are components of hemidesmosomes (Fig. 25-29). Antibodies against one such component called BPAG2 are proven to cause blistering. Pathogenic autoantibodies also activate complement, leading to the recruitment of neutrophils and eosinophils, inflammation, and disruption of epidermal attachments.

MORPHOLOGY

The lesions are tense bullae filled with clear fluid involving erythematous or normal-appearing skin (Fig. 25-32*A*). The bullae are usually less than 2 cm in diameter but occasionally may reach 4 to 8 cm in diameter. They do not rupture easily, unlike the blisters seen in pemphigus, and heal without scarring unless they become infected secondarily. The separation of bullous pemphigoid from pemphigus is based on the identification of **subepidermal, nonacantholytic** blisters. Early lesions show a superficial and sometimes deep perivascular infiltrate of lymphocytes and variable numbers of eosinophils, occasional neutrophils, superficial dermal edema, and associated basal cell layer vacuolization (Fig. 25-32*B*). Eosinophils showing degranulation are typically detected directly beneath the epidermal basal cell layer. The vacuolated basal cell layer eventually lifts away, allowing space for a fluid-filled blister to form.

Dermatitis Herpetiformis

Dermatitis herpetiformis is a rare disorder characterized by urticaria and grouped vesicles. The disease affects predominantly males, most often in the third and fourth

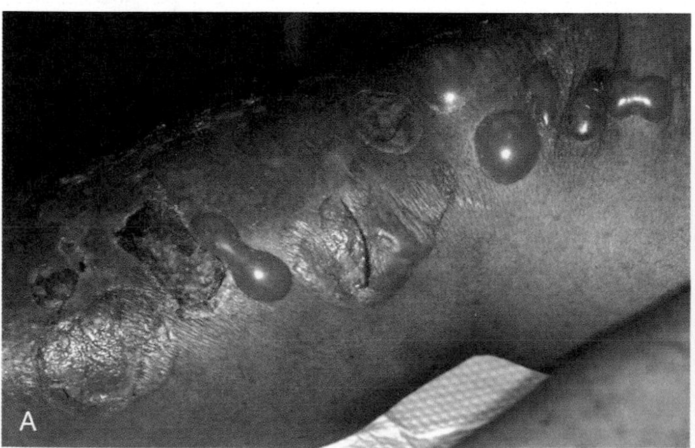

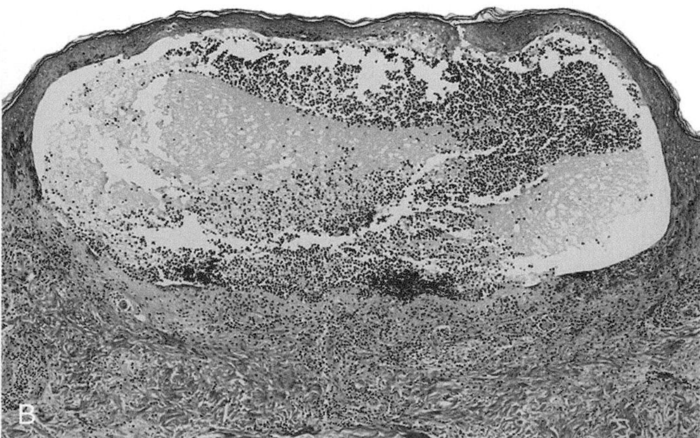

Figure 25-32 Bullous pemphigoid. **A,** Bullae consist of tense subepidermal blisters that usually fail to rupture, as their roof consists of the full epidermal thickness. Ulcers form when the blisters are rupture. **B,** An intact sub-basilar blister associated with eosinophils, lymphocytes and occasional neutrophils.

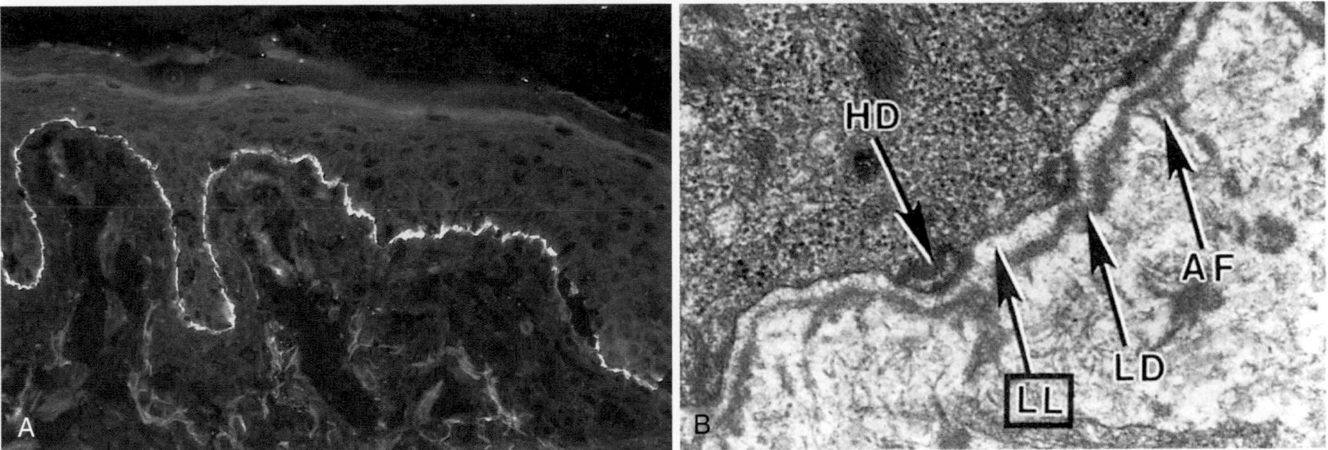

Figure 25-33 A, Linear deposition of complement along the dermoepidermal junction in bullous pemphigoid. **B,** Electron micrograph showing the ultrastructural features of the dermoepidermal junction. The bullous pemphigoid antigen (BPAG) is located in the basal portion of basal keratinocytes in association with hemidesmosomes (HD), which attach the epidermis to the lamina lucida (LL) of the basement membrane. AF, Anchoring fibrils; LD, lamina densa. (See also Fig. 25-31.)

decades of life. In some cases it occurs in association with intestinal celiac disease and responds to a gluten-free diet (Chapter 17). The plaques and vesicles are extremely pruritic.

Pathogenesis. The association of dermatitis herpetiformis with celiac disease provides a clue to its pathogenesis. Genetically predisposed individuals develop IgA antibodies to dietary gluten (derived from the wheat protein *gliadin*). The antibodies cross-react with reticulin, a component of the anchoring fibrils that tether the epidermal basement membrane to the superficial dermis. The resultant injury and inflammation produce a subepidermal blister. In some people with dermatitis herpetiformis and gluten-sensitive enteropathy, both disorders respond to a gluten-free diet.

MORPHOLOGY

The lesions are bilateral, symmetric and grouped, involving preferentially the extensor surfaces, elbows, knees, upper back, and buttocks (Fig. 25-34*C*). Fibrin and neutrophils accumulate selectively at the **tips of dermal papillae**, forming small microabscesses (Fig. 25-34*A*). The basal cells overlying these microabscesses show vacuolization and focal dermoepidermal separation that ultimately coalesce to form a true **subepidermal blister**. By direct immunofluorescence, dermatitis herpetiformis shows discontinuous, **granular deposits of IgA** that selectively localize in the tips of dermal papillae (Fig. 25-34*B*).

Noninflammatory Blistering Disorders

Epidermolysis Bullosa and Porphyria

Some disorders characterized by vesicles and bullae are mediated by inherited or in some cases acquired defects involving structural proteins that maintain the normal organization of the skin. Two such disorders are epidermolysis bullosa and porphyria.

Epidermolysis Bullosa. Epidermolysis bullosa is a blanket term for a group of disorders caused by inherited defects in structural proteins that lend mechanical stability to the skin. The common feature is a proclivity to form blisters at sites of pressure, rubbing, or trauma, at or soon after birth. The histologic changes in all forms are so subtle that electron microscopy may be required to differentiate among the various types.

- In the *simplex type,* defects of the basal cell layer of the epidermis almost always result from mutations in the genes encoding keratin 14 or keratin 5. These two proteins normally pair with one another to make a functional keratin fiber, thus explaining the similar phenotype resulting from mutations in either gene. The mutated proteins have a dominant negative activity, and as a result the disorder shows an autosomal dominant mode of inheritance. This is the most common type of epidermolysis bullosa, encompassing 75% to 85% of cases.
- In the *junctional type,* blisters occur in otherwise histologically normal skin at precisely the level of the lamina lucida (Figs. 25-35 and 25-28). Most cases are caused by autosomal recessive defects in one of the subunits of laminin, a multicomponent protein located in the lamina lucida that binds to both hemidesmosomes and anchoring filaments. Some of the remaining cases are caused by mutations in BPAG2, the same protein that is targeted by autoantibodies in bullous pemphigoid.
- In the scarring *dystrophic types,* blisters develop beneath the lamina densa in association with rudimentary or defective anchoring fibrils. Dystrophic epidermolysis bullosa usually results from mutations in the *COL7A1* gene, which encodes type VII collagen (Chapter 3), a major component of the basement membrane anchoring fibrils. Depending on the mutation, the disorder may follow an autosomal dominant or autosomal recessive mode of inheritance.
- *Mixed types,* marked by defects at several levels, are also recognized.

Porphyria. *Porphyria* refers to a group of uncommon inborn or acquired disturbances of porphyrin metabolism.

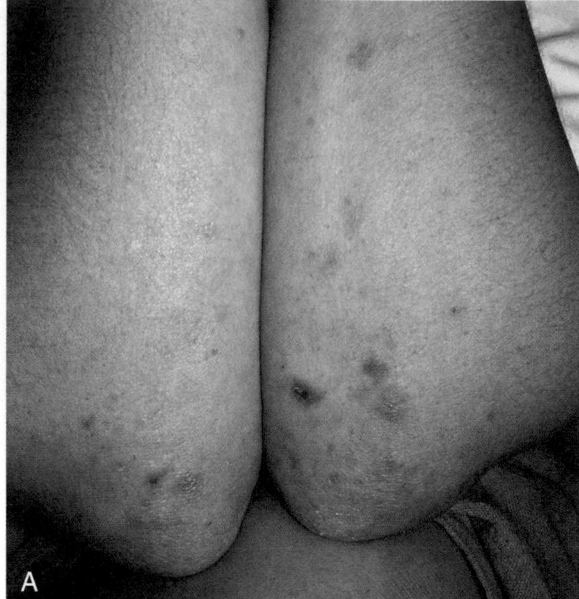

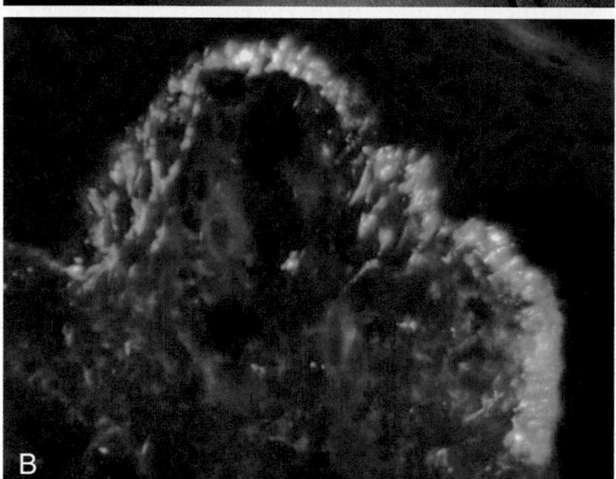

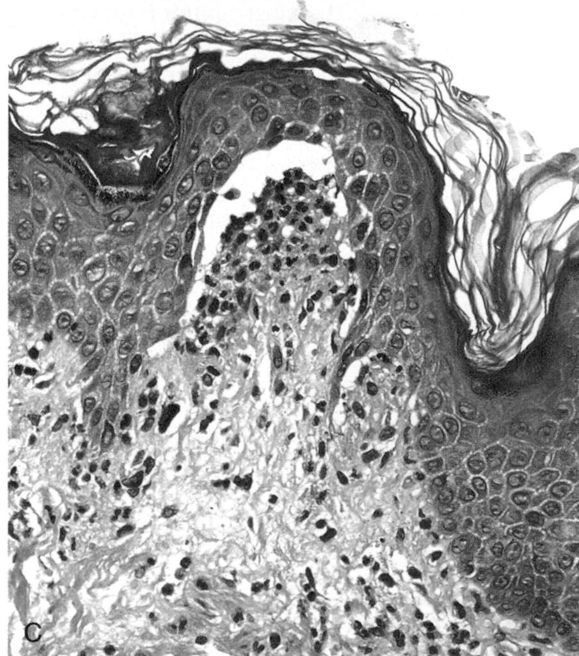

Figure 25-34 Dermatitis herpetiformis. **A,** Lesions consist of intact and eroded (usually scratched) erythematous blisters, often grouped (seen here on elbows and arms). **B,** Selective deposition of IgA autoantibody at the tips of dermal papillae is characteristic. **C,** The blisters are associated with the accumulation of neutrophils (microabscesses) at the tips of dermal papillae. (**B,** Courtesy Dr. Victor G. Prieto, Houston, Texas.)

Porphyrins are pigments that are normally present in hemoglobin, myoglobin, and cytochromes. The classification of porphyrias is based on both clinical and biochemical features. The five major types are (1) congenital erythropoietic porphyria, (2) erythrohepatic protoporphyria, (3) acute intermittent porphyria, (4) porphyria cutanea tarda, and (5) mixed porphyria. Cutaneous manifestations consist of urticaria and vesicles associated with scarring that are exacerbated by exposure to sunlight. The vesicles are subepidermal in location and the adjacent dermis contains vessels with walls that are thickened by glassy deposits of serum proteins, including immunoglobulins (Fig. 25-36). The pathogenesis of these alterations is not understood.

KEY CONCEPTS

Blistering Disorders

- Blistering disorders are classified based on the level of epidermal separation.
- These disorders are often caused by autoantibodies specific for epithelial or basement membrane proteins that lead to unmooring of keratinocytes (acantholysis).
- Pemphigus is associated with IgG autoantibodies to various intercellular desmogleins, resulting in bullae that are either subcorneal (pemphigus foliaceus) or suprabasilar (pemphigus vulgaris).
- Bullous pemphigoid is associated with IgG autoantibodies to basement membrane proteins and produces a subepidermal blister.
- Dermatitis herpetiformis is associated with IgA autoantibodies to fibrils that bind the epidermal basement membrane to the dermis, and also produces subepidermal blisters.
- None inflammatory blistering disorders include inherited defects in proteins that stabilize the epidermis (e.g., epidermolysis bullosa) and inherited defects in porphyrin synthesis (the porphrias) that lead to sun-induced skin damage through uncertain mechanisms.

Disorders of Epidermal Appendages

Acne Vulgaris

Virtually universal in the middle to late teenage years, acne vulgaris affects both males and females, although males tend to have more severe disease. Acne is seen in all races but is usually milder in people of Asian descent. It may be induced or exacerbated by drugs (corticosteroids, adrenocorticotropic hormone, testosterone, gonadotropins, contraceptives, trimethadione, iodides, and bromides), occupational exposures (cutting oils, chlorinated hydrocarbons, and coal tars), and conditions that favor occlusion of

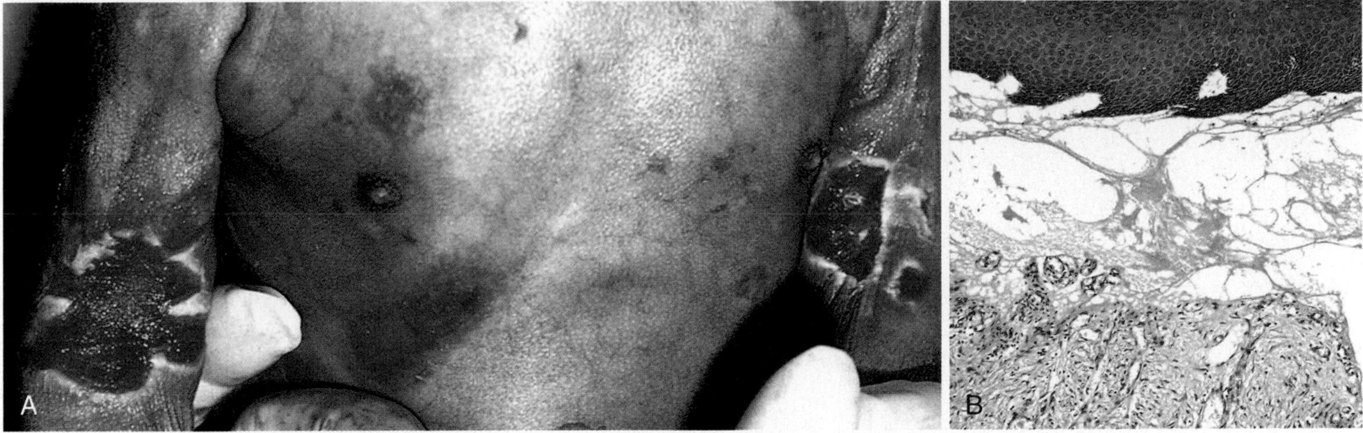

Figure 25-35 Epidermolysis bullosa. **A,** Junctional epidermolysis bullosa showing typical erosions in flexural creases. **B,** A subepidermal blister at the level of the lamina lucida. There is no associated inflammation.

sebaceous glands, such as heavy clothing, cosmetics, and tropical climates. Some families seem to be particularly prone to acne, suggesting a hereditary component.

Acne is divided into noninflammatory and inflammatory types, although both types may coexist. Noninflammatory acne may take the form of open and closed comedones.

- *Open comedones* are small follicular papules containing a central black keratin plug. This color is the result of oxidation of melanin pigment (not dirt).
- *Closed comedones* are follicular papules without a visible central plug. Because the keratin plug is trapped beneath the epidermal surface, these lesions are potential sources of follicular rupture and inflammation.

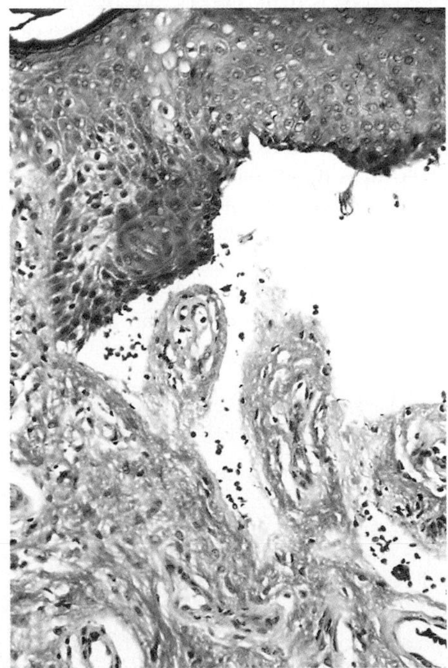

Figure 25-36 Porphyria. A noninflammatory blister at the dermoepidermal junction; note the seemingly rigid dermal papillae at the base that contain abnormal superficial vessels.

Pathogenesis. The pathogenesis of acne is incompletely understood and is likely multifactorial. At least four factors contribute to its development: (1) keratinization of the lower portion of the follicular infundibulum and development of a keratin plug that blocks outflow of sebum to the skin surface, (2) hypertrophy of sebaceous glands during puberty under the influence of androgens, (3) lipase-synthesizing bacteria *(Propionibacterium acnes)* colonizing the upper and midportion of the hair follicle, converting lipids within sebum to proinflammatory fatty acids, and (4) secondary inflammation of the involved follicle. Androgens, which increase sebum production, were first implicated in times past when it was noted that young castrated males generally did not develop the condition (a questionable tradeoff). Elimination of *P. acnes* is the rationale for administration of antibiotics to individuals with inflammatory acne. The synthetic vitamin A derivative 13-*cis*-retinoic acid (isotretinoin) brings about remarkable improvement in some cases of severe acne through its strong antisebaceous action.

MORPHOLOGY

Inflammatory acne is marked by erythematous papules, nodules, and pustules (Fig. 25-37*A*). Severe variants (e.g., **acne conglobata**) result in sinus tract formation and dermal scarring. Depending on the stage of the disease, open or closed comedones, papules, pustules, or deep inflammatory nodules may develop. **Open comedones** have large, patulous orifices, whereas those of **closed comedones** are identifiable only microscopically (Fig. 25-37*B*, *C*). Variable infiltrates of lymphocytes and macrophages are present in and around affected follicles, and extensive acute inflammation accompanies follicular rupture. Dermal abscesses may form in association with rupture (Fig. 25-37*B*) and lead to scarring.

Rosacea

Rosacea is a common disease of middle age and beyond, affecting up to 3% of the US population, with a predilection for females. Four stages are recognized: (1) flushing episodes (pre-rosacea), (2) persistent erythema and

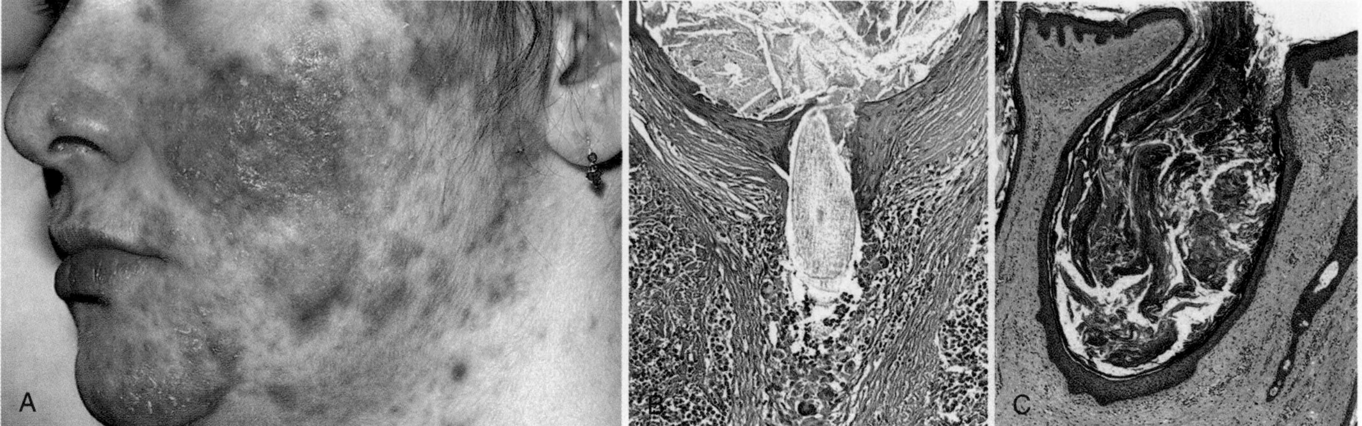

Figure 25-37 Acne. **A,** Inflammatory acne associated with erythematous papules and pustules. **B,** A hair shaft pierces the follicular epithelium, eliciting inflammation and fibrosis. **C,** An open comedone.

telangiectasia, (3) pustules and papules, and (4) rhinophyma—permanent thickening of the nasal skin by confluent erythematous papules and prominent follicles.

Pathogenesis. Individuals with rosacea have high cutaneous levels of the antimicrobial peptide cathelicidin, an important mediator of the cutaneous innate immune response. *The cathelicidin peptides present are qualitatively distinct from those seen in individuals without rosacea as a result of alternative processing by proteases such as kallikrein 5* (also known as stratum corneum tryptic enzyme). Injection of cathelicidin peptides from patients into mice induces some of the cutaneous changes seen in rosacea, including inflammation and vascular dilation. In addition, it has been noted that activation of Toll-like receptor 2 (TLR2) up-regulates kallikrein 5 expression in keratinocytes, suggesting that factors that stimulate TLR2 are involved. Several microbial triggers have been proposed, but none are proven.

MORPHOLOGY

Rosacea is characterized by a nonspecific perifollicular infiltrate composed of lymphocytes surrounded by dermal edema and telangiectasia. In the pustular phase neutrophils may colonize the follicles, and follicular rupture may cause a granulomatous dermal response. The development of rhinophyma is associated with hypertrophy of sebaceous glands and follicular plugging by keratotic debris.

Panniculitis

Erythema Nodosum and Erythema Induratum

Panniculitis is an inflammatory reaction in the subcutaneous adipose tissue that may preferentially affect (1) the lobules of fat, or (2) the connective tissue that separates fat into lobules. Panniculitis often involves the lower legs. *Erythema nodosum* is the most common form and usually has a subacute presentation. A second somewhat distinctive form, erythema induratum, also merits brief discussion.

- *Erythema nodosum* presents as poorly defined, exquisitely tender, erythematous plaques and nodules that may be more readily palpated than seen. Its occurrence is often associated with infections (β-hemolytic streptococcal infection, tuberculosis and, less commonly, coccidioidomycosis, histoplasmosis, and leprosy), drug administration (sulfonamides, oral contraceptives), sarcoidosis, inflammatory bowel disease, and certain malignant neoplasms, but many times a cause cannot be identified. Fever and malaise may accompany the cutaneous signs. It is considered to be caused by a delayed hypersensitivity reaction to microbial or drug related antigens. In some cases immune complexes have been implicated but in many cases the pathogenesis remains mysterious. Over the course of weeks, lesions usually flatten and become bruiselike, leaving no residual clinical scars, while new lesions develop. Biopsy of a deep wedge of tissue to generously sample the subcutis is usually required for histologic diagnosis.
- *Erythema induratum* is an uncommon type of panniculitis that affects primarily adolescents and menopausal women. Although the cause is not known, most observers regard this as a primary vasculitis of deep vessels supplying the fat lobules of the subcutis; the associated vascular compromise leads to fat necrosis and inflammation. Erythema induratum presents as an erythematous, slightly tender nodule that usually goes on to ulcerate. Originally considered a hypersensitivity response to tuberculosis, erythema induratum today most commonly occurs without an associated underlying disease.

MORPHOLOGY

The histopathology of **erythema nodosum** is distinctive. In early lesions, the connective tissue septae are widened by edema, fibrin exudation, and neutrophilic infiltration. Later, infiltration by lymphocytes, histiocytes, multinucleated giant cells, and occasional eosinophils is associated with septal fibrosis. Vasculitis is not present. In **erythema induratum**, on the other hand, granulomatous inflammation and zones of caseous necrosis involve the fat lobule. Early lesions show necrotizing vasculitis affecting small- to medium-sized arteries and veins in the deep dermis and subcutis.

Many other types of panniculitis have also been described, a few of which merit brief mention.

- *Weber-Christian disease (relapsing febrile nodular panniculitis)* is a rare form of lobular, nonvasculitic panniculitis seen in children and adults. It is marked by crops of erythematous plaques or nodules, predominantly on the lower extremities, created by deep-seated foci of inflammation containing aggregates of foamy macrophages admixed with lymphocytes, neutrophils, and giant cells.
- *Factitial panniculitis* is a form of secondary panniculitis caused by self-inflicted trauma or injection of foreign or toxic substances.
- Rare types of *T-cell lymphoma* home to fat lobules, producing fat necrosis and superimposed inflammation that mimics panniculitis.
- *Lupus erythematosus* may occasionally cause inflammation of the subcutis and an associated panniculitis.

Infection

The skin frequently succumbs to the attack of microorganisms, parasites, and insects. We have already discussed the possible role of bacteria in the pathogenesis of common acne, and the dermatoses resulting from viruses are too numerous to list. In the setting of the immunocompromised individual, ordinarily trivial cutaneous infections may become life threatening. Many disorders, such as herpes simplex and herpes zoster, the viral exanthems, deep fungal infections, and immune reactions in skin provoked by infectious agents, are discussed in Chapter 8. Here we cover a representative sampling of common infections whose primary clinical manifestations are in the skin.

Verrucae (Warts)

Verrucae are squamoproliferative disorders caused by human papillomaviruses. They are common lesions of children and adolescents, although they may be encountered at any age. Transmission of disease usually involves direct contact between individuals or autoinoculation. Verrucae are generally self-limited, regressing spontaneously within 6 months to 2 years.

Pathogenesis. More than 150 types of papillomavirus have been identified, many of them capable of producing warts in humans. The clinical variants of warts are often associated with distinct HPV subtypes. For example, anogenital warts are caused predominantly by HPV types 6 and 11. HPV type 16 has been associated with in situ squamous cell carcinoma of the genitalia and with *bowenoid papulosis* (genital lesions of young adults with the histologic appearance of carcinoma in situ, but which usually regress spontaneously; see also Chapter 21). The relationship of HPV subtypes 5 and 8 to squamous cell carcinomas, particularly in individuals affected by the rare condition epidermodysplasia verruciformis, was mentioned earlier. These patients develop multiple flat warts that contain HPV genomes, some of which progress to carcinoma. Viral typing can be accomplished by either in situ hybridization (Fig. 25-38*D*) or polymerase chain reaction.

You will recall that HPVs that are associated with a high risk of cancer produce E6 proteins that abolish p53 function (Chapter 7). By contrast, HPV subtypes 5 and 8 produce variant E6 proteins that do not affect p53, probably explaining why these forms of HPV have low oncogenic potential. Some recent studies suggest that the E6 proteins of low-risk HPVs interfere with Notch signaling, which is known to be required for the normal maturation of keratinocytes, and this effect may contribute to the epidermal hyperplasia that characterizes warts.

MORPHOLOGY

The classification of verrucae is based largely on appearance and location. **Verruca vulgaris** is the most common type of wart. The lesions of verruca vulgaris occur anywhere but most frequently on the hands, particularly on the dorsal surfaces and periungual areas, where they appear as gray-white to tan, flat to convex, 0.1- to 1-cm papules with a rough, pebble-like surface (Fig. 25-38*A*). **Verruca plana**, or **flat wart**, is common on the face or the dorsal surfaces of the hands. The warts are slightly elevated, flat, smooth, tan papules that are generally smaller than verruca vulgaris. **Verruca plantaris** and **verruca palmaris** occur on the soles and palms, respectively. Rough, scaly lesions may reach 1 to 2 cm in diameter, coalesce, and be confused with ordinary calluses. **Condyloma acuminatum (venereal wart)** occurs on the penis, female genitalia, urethra, perianal areas, and rectum. Venereal warts appear as soft, tan, cauliflower-like masses that occasionally reach many centimeters in diameter.

Histologic features common to verrucae include epidermal hyperplasia that is often undulant in character, termed **verrucous or papillomatous epidermal hyperplasia** (Fig. 25-38*B*); and cytoplasmic vacuolization (koilocytosis) involving the more superficial epidermal layers, producing haloes of pallor surrounding infected nuclei. Electron microscopy of these zones reveals numerous HPV virions within nuclei. Infected cells may also demonstrate prominent and apparently condensed keratohyaline granules and jagged eosinophilic intracytoplasmic keratin aggregates as a result of viral cytopathic effects (Fig. 25-38*C*). These cellular alterations are not as prominent in condylomas; hence, their diagnosis is based primarily on hyperplastic papillary architecture containing wedge-shaped zones of koilocytosis.

Molluscum Contagiosum

Molluscum contagiosum is a common, self-limited viral disease of the skin caused by a poxvirus. The virus is characteristically brick shaped, has a dumbbell-shaped DNA core, and measures 300 nm in maximal dimension, and thus represents the largest pathogenic poxvirus in humans and one of the largest viruses in nature. Infection is usually spread by direct contact, particularly among children and young adults.

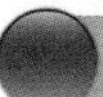

MORPHOLOGY

Multiple lesions may occur on the skin and mucous membranes, with a predilection for the trunk and anogenital areas. Individual lesions are firm, often pruritic, pink to skin-colored

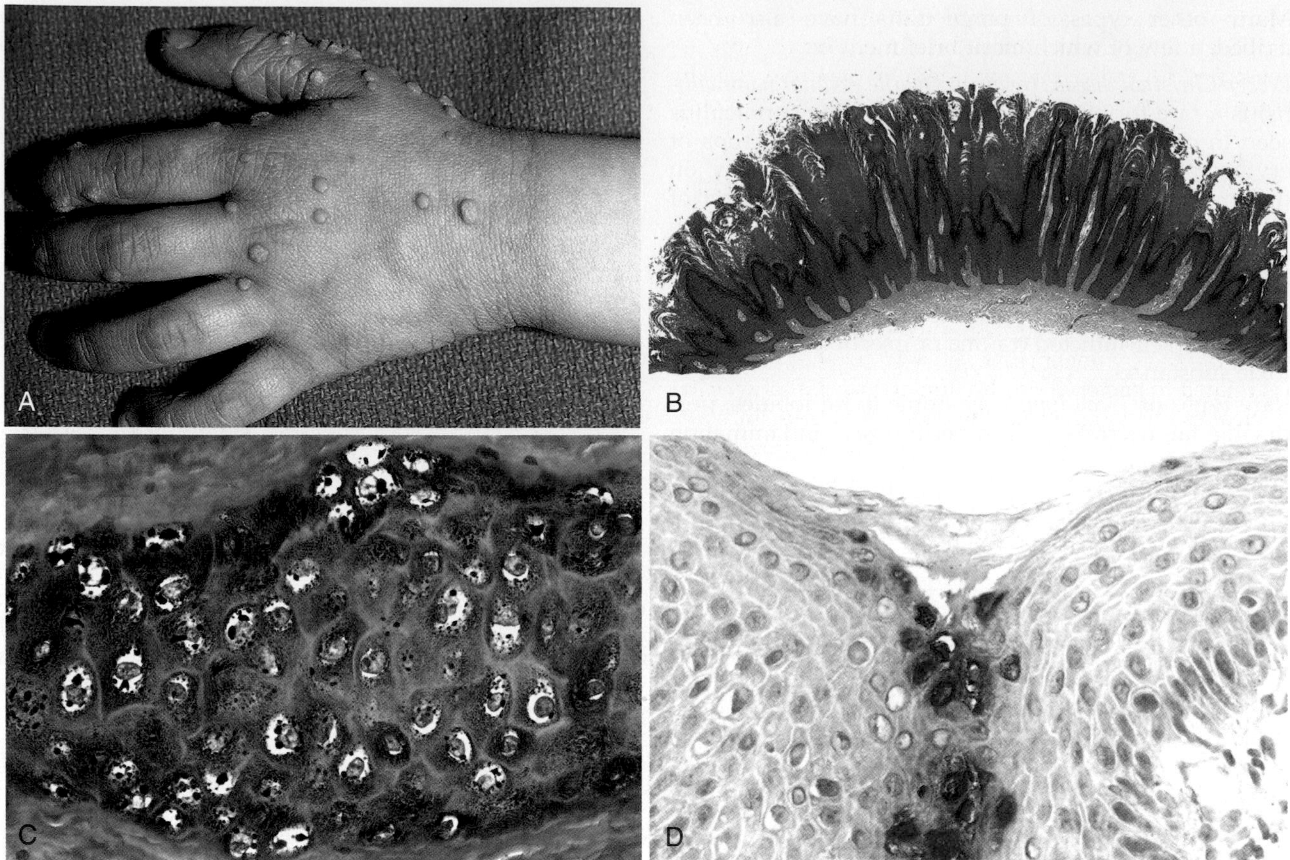

Figure 25-38 Verruca vulgaris. **A,** Multiple papules with rough pebble-like surfaces. Low power **(B)** and high power **(C)** lesions showing papillomatous epidermal hyperplasia and cytopathic alterations, including nuclear pallor and prominent keratohyaline granules. **D,** In situ hybridization demonstrating HPV DNA within epidermal cells.

umbilicated papules, generally ranging in diameter from 0.2 cm to 0.4 cm. Rarely, "giant" forms occur measuring up to 2 cm in diameter. A curd-like material can be expressed from the central umbilication. Smearing this material onto a glass slide and staining with Giemsa often shows diagnostic molluscum bodies.

On microscopic examination, lesions show cuplike verrucous epidermal hyperplasia. The diagnostically specific structure is the **molluscum body**, which occurs as a large (up to 35 μm), ellipsoid, homogeneous, cytoplasmic inclusion in cells of the stratum granulosum and the stratum corneum (Fig. 25-39). In the hematoxylin and eosin stain, these inclusions are eosinophilic in the blue-purple stratum granulosum and acquire a pale blue hue in the red stratum corneum. Numerous virions are present within molluscum bodies.

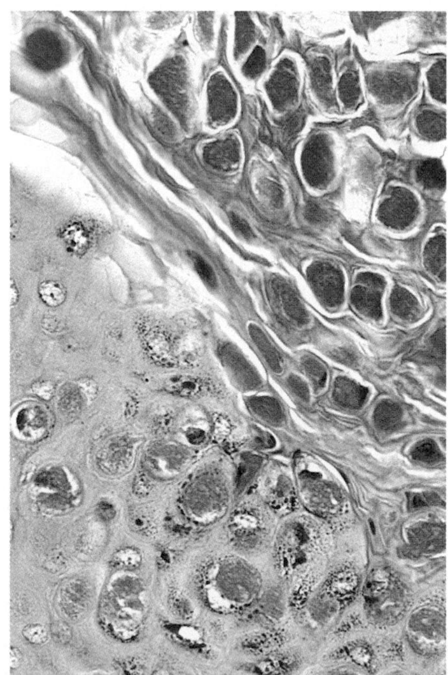

Figure 25-39 Molluscum contagiosum. A focus of verrucous epidermal hyperplasia contains numerous cells with ellipsoid cytoplasmic inclusions (molluscum bodies) within the stratum granulosum and stratum corneum.

Impetigo

Impetigo is a common superficial bacterial infection of skin. It is highly contagious and is frequently seen in otherwise healthy children as well as occasionally in adults in poor health. The infection usually involves exposed skin, particularly that of the face and hands. Two forms exist, classically referred to as *impetigo contagiosa* and *impetigo bullosa;* they differ from each other simply by the size of the pustules. Over the past decade a remarkable shift in etiology has been observed. Whereas in the past impetigo contagiosa was almost exclusively caused by group A β-hemolytic streptococci and impetigo bullosa by *Staphylococcus aureus,* both are now usually caused by *Staphylococcus aureus.*

Pathogenesis. Bacterial species in the epidermis evoke an innate immune response that causes epidermal injury, leading to local serous exudate and formation of a scale crust (scab). The pathogenesis of blister formation in impetigo is related to bacterial production of a toxin that specifically cleaves desmoglein 1, the protein responsible for cell-to-cell adhesion within the uppermost epidermal layers. Recall that in pemphigus foliaceus, which has a similar plane of blister formation, desmoglein 1 is compromised not by a toxin but by an autoantibody (Fig. 25-28). Because there is virtually no involvement of the dermis, once the bacteria are eliminated the lesions heal without scarring.

MORPHOLOGY

Impetigo presents as an erythematous macule, but multiple small pustules rapidly supervene. As pustules break, shallow erosions form, covered with drying serum, giving the characteristic appearance of **honey-colored crust**. If the crust is not removed, new lesions form about the periphery and extensive epidermal damage may ensue. A bullous form of impetigo mainly occurs in children.

The characteristic microscopic feature of impetigo is **accumulation of neutrophils beneath the stratum corneum,** often producing a subcorneal pustule containing serum proteins and inflammatory cells. Special stains reveal the presence of bacteria in these foci. Nonspecific, reactive epidermal alterations and superficial dermal inflammation accompany these findings. Rupture of pustules releases serum, neutrophils, and cellular debris, which layer out and dry to form the characteristic crust.

Superficial Fungal Infections

As opposed to deep fungal infections of the skin, where the dermis or subcutis is primarily involved, superficial fungal infections of the skin are confined to the stratum corneum, and are caused primarily by dermatophytes. These organisms grow in the soil and on animals and produce a number of diverse lesions with characteristic distributions, as follows:

- *Tinea capitis* usually occurs in children and is only rarely seen in infants and adults. It is a dermatophytosis of the scalp characterized by asymptomatic, often hairless patches of skin associated with mild erythema, crust formation, and scaling.
- *Tinea barbae* is a dermatophyte infection of the beard area that affects adult men; it is a relatively uncommon disorder.
- *Tinea corporis,* on the other hand, is a common superficial fungal infection of the body surface that affects persons of all ages, but particularly children. Predisposing factors include excessive heat and humidity, exposure to infected animals, and chronic dermatophytosis of the feet or nails. The most common type of tinea corporis is an expanding, round, slightly erythematous plaque with an elevated scaling border (Fig. 25-40*A*).
- *Tinea cruris* occurs most frequently in the inguinal areas of obese men during warm weather. Heat, friction, and maceration all predispose to its development. The infection usually first appears on the upper inner thighs as moist, red patches with raised scaly borders.
- *Tinea pedis (athlete's foot)* affects 30% to 40% of the population at some time in their lives. There is diffuse erythema and scaling, often initially localized to the web spaces. Most of the inflammatory reaction, however, appears to be the result of bacterial superinfection and is not directly related to the primary dermatophytosis. Spread to (or primary infection of the nails) is referred to as *onychomycosis.* This produces discoloration, thickening, and deformity of the nail plate.
- *Tinea versicolor* usually occurs on the upper trunk and is highly distinctive in appearance. Caused by *Malassezia furfur* (a yeast, not a dermatophyte), the lesions consist

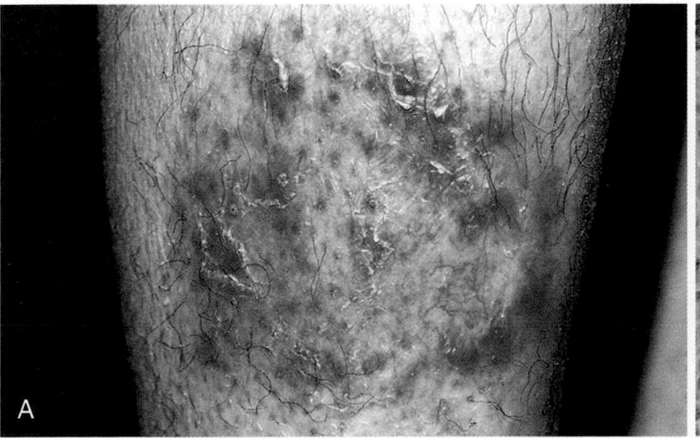

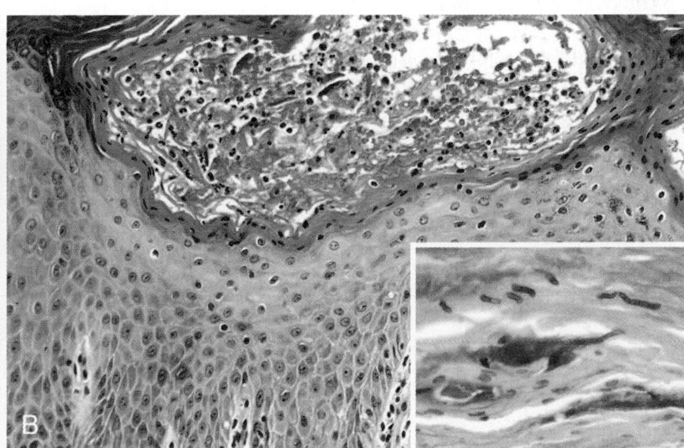

Figure 25-40 Tinea. **A,** Characteristic plaque of tinea corporis. **B,** Routine histology shows a mild eczematous (spongiotic) dermatitis and focal neutrophilic abscesses. A periodic acid–Schiff stain *(inset)* reveals deep red hyphae within the stratum corneum.

of groups of macules of varied size and color with a fine peripheral scale.

MORPHOLOGY

The histologic features of dermatophytoses are variable, depending on the properties of the organism, the host response, and the degree of bacterial superinfection. There may be mild eczematous dermatitis associated with intraepidermal neutrophils (Fig. 25-40*B*). Due to cell walls rich in mucopolysaccharides, fungi stain bright pink to red with periodic acid–Schiff stain. They are found in the anucleate cornified layer of lesional skin, hair, or nails (Fig. 25-40*B*, *inset*). Culture of material scraped from these areas usually permits the identification of the offending species.

SUGGESTED READINGS

Melanoma and Dysplastic Nevi

Breslow A: Prognosis in cutaneous melanoma: tumor thickness as a guide to treatment. *Pathol Annu* 15:1, 1980. *[Paper describing the importance of vertical growth of melanoma, which remains the best predictor of outcome in this disease.]*

Clark WH Jr, Remmer RR, Greene M, et al: Origin of familial malignant melanomas from heritable melanocytic lesions. "The B-K mole syndrome." *Arch Dermatol* 114:732, 1978. *[Classic paper describing familial dysplastic nevi and their possible relationship to melanoma.]*

Elder DE: Dysplastic nevi: an update. *Histopathology* 56:112, 2010. *[Updated discussion of the histology and pathogenesis of dysplastic nevi and their relationship to melanoma.]*

Horn S, Figl A, Rachakonda PS, et al: TERT promoter mutations in familial and sporadic melanoma. *Science* published on-line on 1/24/2013.

Huang FW, Hodis E, Xu MJ, et al: Highly recurrent TERT promoter mutations in human melanoma. *Science* published on-line on 1/24/2013. *[Two landmark papers documenting frequent mutations in the promoter of the gene encoding the catalytic subunit of telomerase in melanoma.]*

Ibrahim N, Haluska FG: Molecular pathogenesis of cutaneous melanocytic neoplasms. *Annu Rev Pathol* 4:551, 2009. *[The genetic pathways relevant to melanoma suggest future therapeutic interventions.]*

Mellman I, Coukos G, Dranoff G: Cancer immunotherapy comes of age. *Nature* 480:480, 2012. *[Update on exciting progress in treating melanoma with immunotherapeutic agents.]*

Ribas A, Flaherty KT: BRAF targeted therapy changes the treatment paradigm in melanoma. *Nat Rev Clin Oncol* 8:426, 2011. *[Impact of inhibitors of mutated BRAF kinase on treatment of melanoma.]*

Epidermal Skin Tumors

Epstein EH: Basal cell carcinomas: attack of the hedgehog. *Nat Rev Cancer* 8:743, 2008. *[Epidemiology, clinical presentation, molecular pathogenesis, and novel treatment options are succinctly reviewed.]*

Hafner C, Hartmann H, Vogt T, et al: High frequency of FGFR3 mutations in adenoid seborrheic keratoses. *J Invest Dermatol* 126:2404, 2006. *[Description of activating mutations in FGFR3 in seborrheic keratoses.]*

Ratushny V, Gober MD, Hick R, et al: From keratinocyte to cancer: the pathogenesis and modeling of cutaneous squamous cell carcinoma. *J Clin Invest* 112:464, 2012. *[Discussion of clinical and molecular features of cutaneous neoplasia and experimental approaches used to study this disease.]*

Mastocytosis and Cutaneous T Cell Lymphoma

George TI, Horny HP: Systemic mastocytosis. *Hematol Oncol Clin North Am* 25:1067, 2011. *[Discussion of clinical features, diagnosis, pathogenesis, and treatment of systemic mast cell disease.]*

Wong HK, Mishra A, Hake T, et al: Evolving insights into the pathogenesis and therapy of cutaneous T-cell lymphoma (mycosis fungoides and Sezary syndrome). *Br J Haematol* 155:150, 2011. *[A summary of the epidemiology, staging, natural history, and immunopathogenesis of cutaneous T-cell lymphoma.]*

Autoimmune and Inflammatory Skin Disorders

Coenraads PJ: Hand eczema. *N Eng J Med* 367:1829, 2012. *[A thorough discussion of the causes and management of a common form of eczema.]*

Nestle FO, Kaplan DH, Barker J: Psoriasis. *N Engl J Med* 361:496, 2009. *[Pathogenesis, clinical features, and targeted treatment options are discussed.]*

Schaefer P: Urticaria: evaluation and treatment. *Am Fam Physician* 83:1078, 2011. [A practical discussion of the clinical evaluation and treatment of urticaria.]

Sharma A, Bialynicki-Birula R, Schwatz RA, et al: Lichen planus: an update and review. *Cutis* 90:17, 2012. *[Review of pathology and clinical features, natural history, and treatment.]*

Blistering Disorders

Bonciani D, Verdelli A, Bonciolini V, et al: Dermatitis herpetiformis: from genetics to the development of skin lesions. *Clin Dev Immunol* 2012, in press. *[Description of factors and disease mechanisms underlying this rare disorder.]*

Ujiie H, Shibaki A, Nishie W, et al: What's new in bullous pemphigoid. *J Dermatol* 37:194, 2010. *[Review of bullous pemphigoid pathogenesis.]*

Yokoyama T, Amagai M: Immune dysregulation of pemphigus in humans and mice. *J Dermatol* 37:205, 2010. *[Review of immune disturbances that may underlie pemphigus.]*

Disorders of Skin Appendages and Subcutis

Knutsen-Larson S, Dawson AL, Dunnick CA, et al: Acne vulgaris: pathogenesis, treatment, and needs assessment. *Dermatol Clin* 30:99, 2012. *[Review of the epidemiology, pathogenesis, and treatment of acne in the United States.]*

Nakatsuji T, Gallo RL: Antimicrobial peptides: old molecules with new ideas. *J Invest Dermatol* 132:887, 2012. *[Discussion of the possible role of antimicrobial peptides such as campthelicidin in rosacea, psoriasis, and atopic dermatitis.]*

See TARGETED THERAPY available online at www.studentconsult.com

CHAPTER 26

Bones, Joints, and Soft Tissue Tumors

Andrew Horvai

CHAPTER CONTENTS

*The contributions of Dr. Andrew Rosenberg to this chapter over the past many editions are gratefully acknowledged.

BONE

Basic Structure and Function of Bone

The adult human skeleton is composed of 206 bones and accounts for approximately 12% of body weight. The functions of bone include mechanical support, transmission of forces generated by muscles, protection of viscera, mineral homeostasis, and providing a niche for production of blood cells. The constituents of bone include an extracellular matrix and specialized cells responsible for production and maintenance of the matrix.

Matrix

Bone matrix is the extracellular component of bone. It is composed of an organic component known as osteoid (35%) and a mineral component (65%). Osteoid is made up of predominantly type I collagen with smaller amounts of glycosaminoglycans and other proteins, which are grouped according to function in Table 26-1. Of these, only osteopontin (also called osteocalcin) is unique to bone. It is produced by osteoblasts and plays a role in bone formation and mineralization and in calcium homeostasis. It is measurable in the serum and serves as a sensitive and specific marker for osteoblast activity. Several cytokines and growth factors also control bone cell proliferation, maturation, and metabolism, thereby playing a crucial role in translating mechanical and metabolic signals into local bone cell activity and eventual skeletal adaptation.

The unique feature of bone matrix, its hardness, is imparted by the inorganic moiety hydroxyapatite [$Ca_{10}(PO_4)_6(OH)_2$], which also serves as a repository for 99% of the body's calcium and 85% of its phosphorus. The bone matrix is synthesized in one of two histologic forms, woven or lamellar (Fig. 26-1). Woven bone is produced rapidly, such as during fetal development or fracture repair, but the haphazard arrangement of collagen fibers imparts less structural integrity than the parallel collagen fibers in slowly produced lamellar bone. In an adult, the presence of woven bone is always abnormal, but it is not specific for any particular bone disease since it can be found in a variety of pathologic settings (discussed later). A cross-section of a typical long bone shows a dense outer cortex and a central medulla composed of bony trabeculae separated by marrow.

Table 26-1 Proteins of Bone Matrix

Osteoblast-Derived Proteins
Type I collagen
Calcium-binding proteins
Osteonectin, bone sialoprotein
Cell adhesion proteins
Osteopontin, fibronectin, thrombospondin
Cytokines
IL-1, IL-6, RANKL
Enzymes
Collagenase, alkaline phosphatase
Growth factors
IGF-1, TGF-β, PDGF
Proteins involved in mineralization
Osteocalcin
Proteins Concentrated from Serum
Albumin
β_2-microglobulin

IGF, linsulin-like growth factor; *TGF*, transforming growth factor; *PDGF*, platelet-derived growth factor; *IL*, interleukin; *RANKL*, receptor activator of nuclear factor-κB ligand.

Cells

The cellular component of mature bone consists of bone synthesizing osteoblasts, osteocytes, and bone-resorbing osteoclasts.

- **Osteoblasts,** located on the surface of the matrix, synthesize, transport and assemble the matrix and regulate its mineralization (Fig. 26-2*A*). The synthesis of matrix is tightly regulated by hormonal and local mediators as described in detail later. Over time, osteoblasts may become inactive, indicated by a decrease in cytoplasm. Some inactive cells remain on the surface of

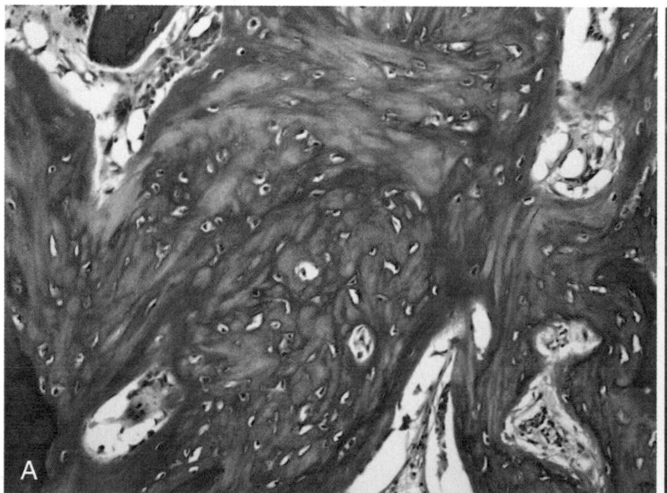

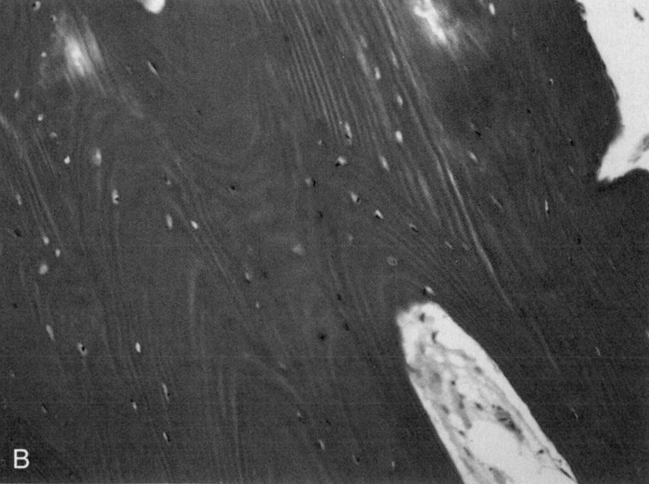

Figure 26-1 Woven bone **(A)** is more cellular and disorganized than lamellar bone **(B)**.

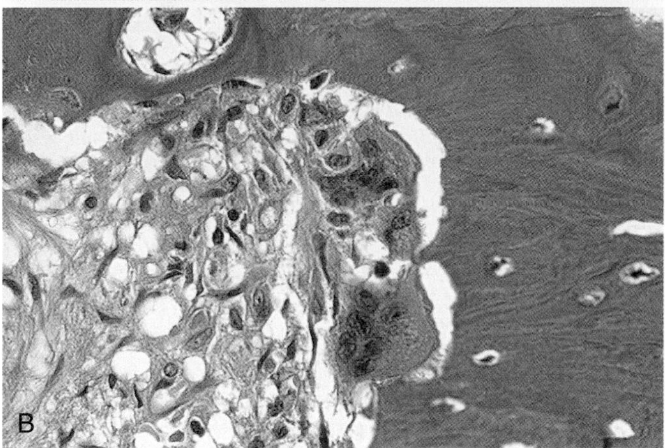

Figure 26-2 **A,** Active osteoblasts synthesizing bone matrix. The surrounding spindle cells represent osteoprogenitor cells. **B,** Two osteoclasts resorbing bone.

trabecula. Alternatively, they may become embedded within the matrix (osteocytes).

- **Osteocytes** are interconnected by an intricate network of dendritic cytoplasmic processes through tunnels known as canaliculi. Osteocytes help to control calcium and phosphate levels in the microenvironment, and detect mechanical forces and translate them into biologic activity—a process called mechanotransduction.
- **Osteoclasts** are specialized multinucleated macrophages derived from circulating monocytes that are responsible for bone resorption (Fig. 26-2*B*). By means of cell surface integrins, osteoclasts attach to bone matrix and create a sealed extracellular trench (resorption pit). Secretion of acid and neutral proteases (predominantly matrix metalloproteases, [MMPs]) into the pit results in dissolution of the inorganic and organic components of bone.

Development

During embryogenesis, most bones develop from a cartilage mold by the process of endochondral ossification. The cartilage mold *(anlagen)* is synthesized by mesenchymal precursor cells. At approximately 8 weeks' gestation, a putative mononuclear cell known as the chondroclast removes the central portion of the mold creating the medullary canal. Simultaneously, at midshaft *(diaphysis)*, osteoblasts begin to deposit the cortex beneath the nascent periosteum. The resulting *primary center of ossification* produces radial growth of bone. At each longitudinal end *(epiphysis)*, endochondral ossification proceeds in a centrifugal fashion *(secondary center of ossification)*. Eventually, a plate of the cartilage anlage becomes entrapped between the two expanding centers of ossification forming the *physis* or *growth plate* (Fig. 26-3). The chondrocytes within the growth plate undergo sequential proliferation, hypertrophy and apoptosis. In the region of apoptosis the matrix mineralizes and is invaded by capillaries, providing the nutrients for osteoblasts to be activated and synthesize osteoid. Although the calcified cartilage matrix is resorbed, remnant struts persist and act as scaffolding for the deposition of bone on their surfaces. These structures are known as *primary spongiosa* and are the first bony trabeculae (Fig. 26-3). The above process progressively deposits new bone at the bottom of the growth plate resulting in longitudinal bone growth.

Intramembranous ossification, by contrast, is responsible for the development of flat bones. Bones of the cranium, for example, are formed by osteoblasts directly from a fibrous layer of tissue that is derived from mesenchyme, without a cartilage anlagen. Because bone is made only by osteoblasts, the enlargement of bones is achieved by the deposition of new bone on a preexisting surface. This mechanism of appositional growth is instrumental in bone development and modeling.

The development of bone is controlled by a number of local and systemic factors:

- Growth hormone (GH) is secreted by the anterior pituitary. It acts on resting chondrocytes to induce and maintain proliferation.

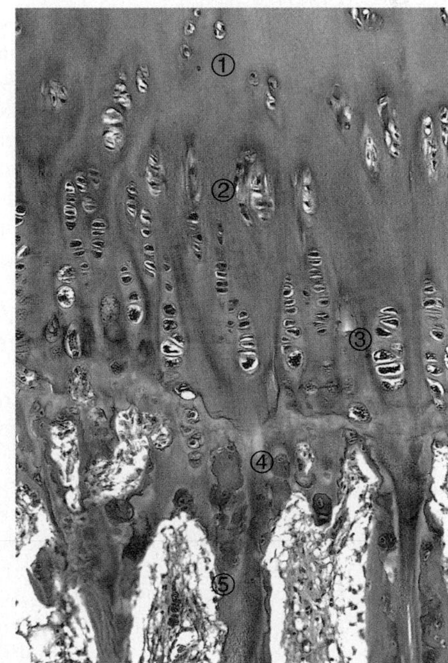

Figure 26-3 Active growth plate with ongoing enchondral ossification. 1, Reserve zone. 2, Zone of proliferation. 3, Zone of hypertrophy. 4, Zone of mineralization. 5, Primary spongiosa.

- Thyroid hormone (T3) is secreted by the thyroid gland, and acts on proliferating chondrocytes to induce hypertrophy.
- Indian hedgehog (Ihh) is a locally secreted regulator, made by prehypertrophic chondrocytes, that coordinates chondrocyte proliferation and differentiation and osteoblasts proliferation.
- Parathyroid hormone related protein (PTHrP) is a local factor, expressed by perichondrial stromal cells and early proliferating chondrocytes, that activates the PTH receptor and maintains proliferation of chondrocytes.
- Wnt is a family of secreted factors that are expressed at highest levels in the proliferating zone and bind to the receptors Frizzled and LRP5/6 to activate β-catenin signaling. They can promote both proliferation and maturation of chondrocytes.
- SOX9 is a transcription factor expressed by proliferating but not hypertrophic chondrocytes that is essential for differentiation of precursor cells into chondrocytes.
- RUNX2 is a transcription factor involved in chondrocyte and osteoblast differentiation. It is expressed in early hypertrophic chondrocytes and immature mesenchymal cells and controls terminal chondrocyte and osteoblast differentiation, respectively.
- Fibroblast growth factors (FGFs) are secreted by a variety of mesenchymal cells. FGF (most notably FGF3) acts on hypertrophic chondrocytes to inhibit proliferation and promote differentiation.
- Bone morphogenic proteins (BMPs) are members of the TGF-β family. They are expressed at various stages of chondrocyte development in the growth plate and have diverse effects on chondrocyte proliferation and hypertophy.

Homeostasis and Remodeling

The adult skeleton appears static but is actually constantly turning over in a tightly regulated process known as remodeling. Approximately 10% of the skeleton is replaced annually. This process can repair microdamage or change the shape of bones in response to structural and mechanical demands. Remodeling takes place at a microscopic locus known as the bone (or basic) multicellular unit (BMU), which consists of a unit of coupled osteoblast and osteoclast activity on the bone surface. An orderly sequence of osteoclast attachment, resorption, osteoblast attachment and proliferation and, finally, matrix synthesis proceeds at the BMU.

The events at the bone multicellular unit are regulated by cell-cell interactions and cytokines. The control mechanisms are not known completely, but several signaling pathways of particular importance have emerged (Fig. 26-4). One such pathway involves three factors: (1) the transmembrane receptor RANK (receptor activator for NF-κB), which is expressed on osteoclast precursors; (2) RANK ligand, (RANKL) which is expressed on osteoblasts and marrow stromal cells; and (3) osteoprotegerin (OPG), a secreted "decoy" receptor made by osteoblasts and several other types of cells that can bind RANKL and thus prevent its interaction with RANK. When stimulated by RANKL, RANK signaling activates the transcription factor

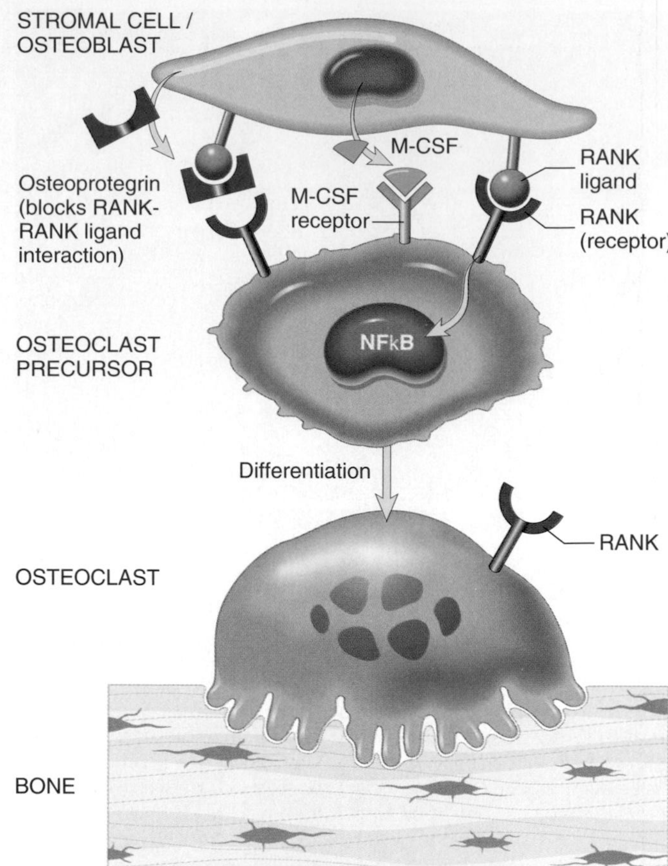

Figure 26-4 Paracrine molecular mechanisms that regulate osteoclast formation and function. Osteoclasts are derived from the same mononuclear cells that differentiate into macrophages. Osteoblast/stromal cell membrane-associated RANKL binds to its receptor RANK located on the cell surface of osteoclast precursors. This interaction in the background of macrophage colony-stimulating factor (M-CSF) causes the precursor cells to produce functional osteoclasts. Stromal cells also secrete osteoprotegerin (OPG), which acts as a "decoy" receptor for RANKL, preventing it from binding the RANK receptor on osteoclast precursors. Consequently, OPG prevents bone resorption by inhibiting osteoclast differentiation.

NF-κB, which is essential for the generation and survival of osteoclasts. A second important pathway involves monocyte colony stimulating factor (M-CSF) produced by osteoblasts. Activation of the M-CSF receptor on osteoclast precursors stimulates a tyrosine kinase cascade that is also crucial for the generation of osteoclasts. Also notable is the WNT/β-catenin pathway. WNT proteins produced by osteoprogenitor cells bind to the LRP5 and LRP6 receptors on osteoblasts and thereby trigger the activation of β-catenin and the production of OPG (Fig. 26-5). Conversely, sclerostin, which is produced by osteocytes, inhibits the WNT/β-catenin pathway. The importance of these pathways is proven by rare but informative germline mutations in the *OPG, RANK, RANKL,* and *LRP5* genes, which cause severe disturbances of bone metabolism (described later).

The balance between net bone formation and resorption is modulated by the signals that connect to the RANK and WNT signaling pathways. For example, because OPG and RANKL oppose one another, either bone resorption or bone formation can be favored by tipping the RANK-to-OPG ratio. Systemic factors that affect this balance include hormones (parathyroid hormone, estrogen, testosterone,

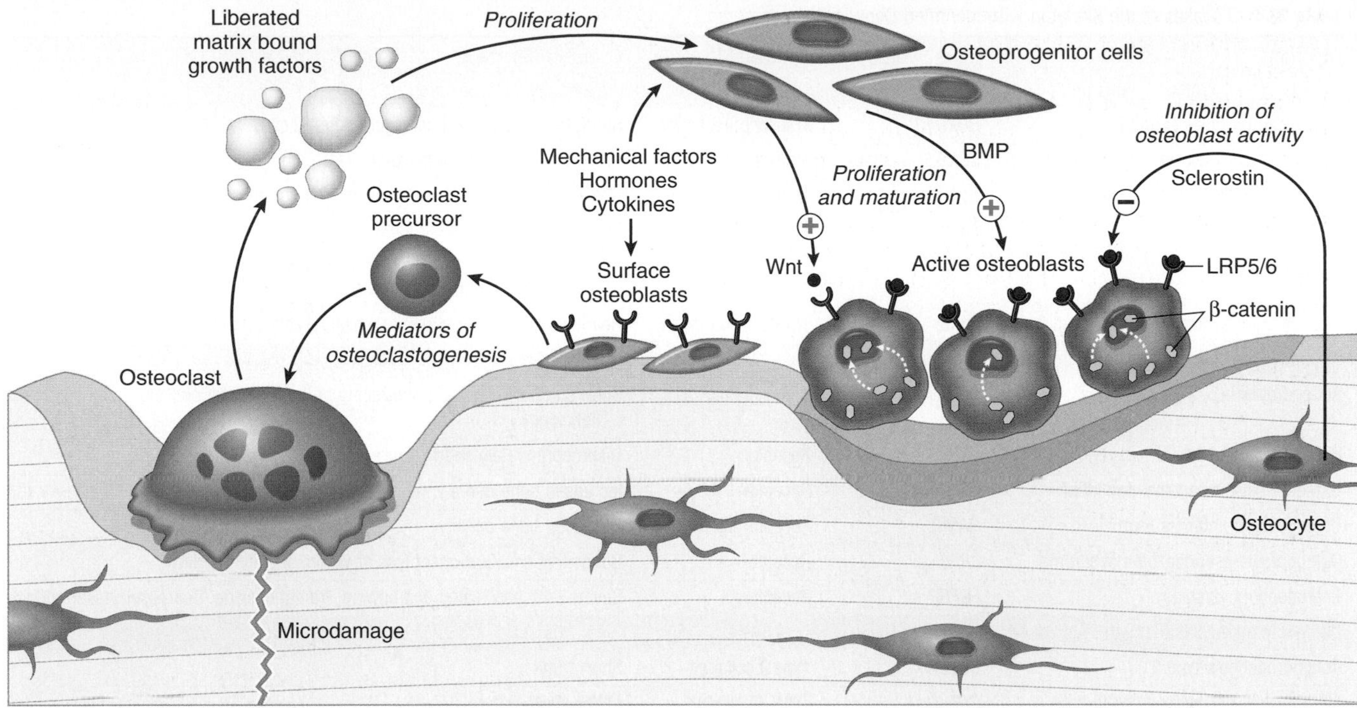

Figure 26-5 Bone cells and their interrelated activities. Hormones, cytokines, growth factors, and signal-transducing molecules are instrumental in their formation and maturation, and allow communication between osteoblasts and osteoclasts. Bone resorption and formation in remodeling are coupled processes that are controlled by systemic factors and local cytokines, some of which are deposited in the bone matrix. BMP, bone morphogenic protein; LRP5/6, LDL receptor related proteins 5 and 6.

and glucocorticoids), vitamin D, inflammatory cytokines (e.g., IL-1), and growth factors (e.g., bone morphogenetic factors). Each of the above presumably acts by altering the levels of RANK/NF-κB and WNT/β-catenin signaling in osteoblasts. The mechanisms are complex, but parathyroid hormone, IL-1 and glucocorticoids promote osteoclast differentiation and bone turnover. In contrast, bone morphogenic proteins and sex hormones generally block osteoclast differentiation or activity by favoring OPG expression.

Another level of control involves paracrine crosstalk between osteoblasts and osteoclasts. Breakdown of matrix by osteoclasts liberates and activates matrix proteins, growth factors, cytokines, and enzymes (e.g., collagenase), including some that stimulate osteoblasts. Thus, as bone is broken down to its elemental units, substances are released into the microenvironment that initiate its renewal (Fig. 26-5).

Peak bone mass is achieved in early adulthood after the cessation of skeletal growth. This set point is determined by a variety of factors, including polymorphisms in the receptors for vitamin D and LRP5/6, nutrition, physical activity, age, and hormonal status. Beginning in the fourth decade, however resorption exceeds formation, so there is a steady decline in skeletal mass.

Developmental Disorders of Bone and Cartilage

Developmental abnormalities of the skeleton are frequently the result of inherited mutations and first become manifest during the earliest stages of bone formation. In contrast, acquired diseases are usually detected in adulthood. The complexity of the skeleton's growth, development, maintenance, and relationships with other organ systems makes it unusually vulnerable to adverse influences. The spectrum of disorders of bone development is broad and the classification system is not standardized. Here we will categorize the major diseases according to their perceived pathogenesis.

Developmental anomalies can result from localized problems in the migration and condensation of mesenchyme (dysostosis) or global disorganization of bone and/or cartilage (dysplasia). Dysostoses are usually limited to defined embryologic structures and may occur in isolation or as part of more complex syndromes. They result from defects in the formation of the mesenchymal condensations and their differentiation into the cartilage anlage. The most common forms include complete absence of a bone or entire digit *(aplasia)*, extra bones or digits *(supernumerary digit)*, and abnormal fusion of bones (e.g., *syndactyly, craniosynostosis*). Genetic alterations that affect transcription factors, especially those encoded by the homeobox genes, cytokines and cytokine receptors, are especially common among the dysostoses. In contrast, dysplasias arise from mutations in genes that control development or remodeling of the entire skeleton. It is important to note that the term dysplasia in this context simply implies abnormal growth rather than a premalignant lesion as used in the context of neoplasia (Chapter 7).

More than 350 skeletal dysostoses and dysplasias, most extremely rare, have been recognized. The classification has evolved from purely clinical and radiographic

Table 26-2 Diseases of the Skeleton with Identified Genetic Defects

Disorder	Gene Symbol	Affected Molecule	Clinical Phenotype
Defects in transcription factors producing abnormalities in mesenchymal condensation and related cell differentiation			
Brachydactyly types D and E	*HOXD13*	Transcription factor	Short, broad terminal phalanges of first digits
Camptomelic dysplasia	*SOX9*	Transcription factor	Sex reversal, abnormal skeletal development
Cleidocranial dysplasia	*RUNX2*	Transcription factor	Abnormal clavicles, Wormian bones, supernumerary teeth
Holt-Oram syndrome	*TBX5*	Transcription factor	Congenital abnormalities, forelimb anomalies
Nail-patella syndrome	*LMX1B*	Transcription factor	Hypoplastic nails, hypoplastic or aplastic patellas, dislocated radial head, progressive nephropathy
Waardenburg syndrome types 1 and 3	*PAX3*	Transcription factor	Hearing loss, abnormal pigmentation, craniofacial abnormalities
Defects in hormones and signal transduction proteins producing abnormal proliferation or maturation of osteoblasts, osteoclasts or chondrocytes			
Achondroplasia	*FGFR3*	Receptor	Short stature, rhizomelic shortening of limbs, frontal bossing, midface deficiency
Hypochondroplasia	*FGFR3*	Receptor	Disproportionately short stature, micromelia, relative macrocephaly
Osteopetrosis, autosomal dominant	*LRP5*	Receptor	Increased bone density, hearing loss, skeletal fragility
Osteopetrosis, infantile form	*RANKL*	Receptor ligand	Increased bone density
Osteoporosis-pseudoglioma syndrome	*LRP5*	Receptor	Congenital or infant-onset loss of vision, skeletal fragility
Thanatophoric dysplasia	*FGFR3*	Receptor	Severe limb shortening and bowing, frontal bossing, depressed nasal bridge
Defects in extracellular structural proteins			
Achondrogenesis type 2	*COL2A1*	Type II collagen	Short trunk
Metaphyseal dysplasia, Schmid type	*COL10A1*	Type X collagen	Mildly short stature
Osteogenesis imperfecta types 1-4	*COL1A1, COL1A2*	Type I collagen	Bone fragility
Defects in metabolic enzymes and transporters			
Osteopetrosis with renal tubular acidosis	*CA2*	Carbonic anhydrase	Increased bone density, fragility, renal tubular acidosis
Osteopetrosis, late onset type 2	*CLCN7*	Chloride channel	Increased bone density, fragility

Modified from Mundlos S, Olsen BR: Heritable diseases of the skeleton. Part I: Molecular insights into skeletal development—transcription factors and signaling pathways. FASEB J 11:125-132, 1997; Mundlos S, Olsen BR: Heritable diseases of the skeleton. Part II: Molecular insights into skeletal development—matrix components and their homeostasis. FASEB J 11:227-233, 1997; Superti-Furga A, et al.: Molecular-pathogenetic classification of genetic disorders of the skeleton. Am J Med Genet 106:262-293, 2001; Krakow D, Rimoin DL: The skeletal dysplasias. Genet Med 2010:12(6):327-341.

descriptions to one that also includes recently identified genetic defects. Table 26-2 lists some of the better characterized developmental abnormalities based on the nature of the genetic defect. The relationships between genes and phenotypes illustrate that various point mutations in a single gene (e.g., *COL2A1*) can result in different phenotypes while mutations in diverse genes (e.g., *LRP5, RANKL*) can give rise to similar clinical phenotypes.

Defects in Nuclear Proteins and Transcription Factors

Defects in nuclear proteins and transcription factors, especially homeobox proteins, cause disorganized mesenchymal condensation and abnormal differentiation of osteoblasts and chondrocytes. These defects manifest as abnormally developed bones.

- *Brachydactyly types D and E,* caused by mutation in the homeobox *HOXD13* gene, produces shortening of the terminal phalanges of the thumb and big toe.
- Loss-of-function mutations in the *RUNX2* gene result in *cleidocranial dysplasia*, an autosomal dominant disorder characterized by patent fontanelles, delayed closure of cranial sutures, Wormian bones (extra bones that occur within a cranial suture), delayed eruption of secondary teeth, primitive clavicles, and short height.

Defects in Hormones and Signal Transduction Proteins

Achondroplasia is the most common skeletal dysplasia and a major cause of dwarfism. It is an autosomal dominant disorder resulting in retarded cartilage growth. Affected individuals have shortened proximal extremities, a trunk of relatively normal length, and an enlarged head with bulging forehead and conspicuous depression of the root of the nose. The skeletal abnormalities are usually not associated with changes in longevity, intelligence, or reproductive status. It is caused by gain-of-function mutations in the FGF receptor 3 (FGFR3). Normally, FGF-mediated activation of FGFR3 inhibits endochondral growth. Constitutive activation of FGFR3 exaggerates this effect, suppressing growth. Approximately 90% of cases stem from new mutations, almost all of which occur in the paternal allele.

Thanatophoric dysplasia is the most common lethal form of dwarfism, affecting about 1 in every 20,000 live births. Affected individuals have micromelic shortening of the limbs, frontal bossing, relative macrocephaly, a small chest cavity, and a bell-shaped abdomen. The underdeveloped thoracic cavity leads to respiratory insufficiency, and these individuals frequently die at birth or soon after. The histologic changes in the growth plate show diminished proliferation of chondrocytes and disorganization

Table 26-3 Subtypes of Osteogenesis Imperfecta

Subtype	Collagen Defect	Inheritance	Major Clinical Features	Prognosis
I	Decreased synthesis of pro-α1(1) chain Abnormal pro-α1(1) or pro-α2(1) chains	Autosomal dominant	Postnatal fractures, blue sclera Normal stature Skeletal fragility Dentinogenesis imperfecta Hearing impairment Joint laxity Blue sclerae	Compatible with survival
II	Abnormally short pro-α1(1) chain Unstable triple helix Abnormal or insufficient pro-α2(1)	Most autosomal recessive Some autosomal dominant New mutations	Death in utero or within days of birth Skeletal deformity with excessive fragility and multiple fractures Blue sclera	Perinatal lethal
III	Altered structure of pro-peptides of pro-α2(1) Impaired formation of triple helix	Autosomal dominant (75%) Autosomal recessive (25%)	Compatible with survival Growth retardation Multiple fractures Progressive kyphoscoliosis Blue sclera at birth that become white Hearing impairment Dentinogenesis imperfecta	Progressive, deforming
IV	Short pro-α2(1) chain Unstable triple helix	Autosomal dominant	Postnatal fractures, normal sclerae Moderate skeletal fragility Short stature Sometimes dentinogenesis imperfecta	Compatible with survival

OI, Osteogenesis imperfecta.

in the zone of proliferation. It is also caused by gain-of-function mutations in FGFR3 that differ from those in achondroplasia.

Abnormal bone density can result from mutations in genes that regulate osteoclast differentiation or osteoclast function. Such mutations can cause either osteoporosis (too little bone) or osteopetrosis (too much), which are described in more detail in separate sections. Interestingly, specific mutations in the gene for the receptor *LPR5* can manifest as either osteoporosis or osteopetrosis in adults, depending on the gene defect. One infantile form of osteopetrosis is associated with mutation of *RANKL*, resulting in decreased or absent osteoclasts. In animals, osteopetrosis can also be caused by mutations in *M-CSF* and *OPG*, which (as already discussed) regulate osteoclast formation and function.

Defects in Extracellular Structural Proteins

The interaction of the organic components of bone matrix is complex and a focus of intense scientific investigation. The importance of the structural bone proteins is exemplified by the diseases associated with deranged metabolism of the major bone and cartilage collagens (types I, II, IX, X, and XI). Their clinical manifestations are highly variable, ranging from lethal disease to premature osteoarthritis.

Type I Collagen Diseases (Osteogenesis Imperfecta)

Osteogenesis imperfecta (OI), or brittle bone disease, is a phenotypically diverse disorder caused by deficiencies in the synthesis of type I collagen. It is the most common inherited disorder of connective tissue. OI principally affects bone, but also impacts other tissues rich in type I collagen (joints, eyes, ears, skin, and teeth). It usually results from autosomal dominant mutations (more than 800 have been identified) in the genes that encode the α1 and α2 chains of type I collagen. Many of these mutations lead to replacement of a glycine residue with another amino acid in the triple-helical domain, resulting in defective assembly of higher order collagen polypeptides. Collagen synthesis and extracellular transport require triple helix formation, and these defects not only cause the misfolding of the mutated collagen polypeptides, but also interfere with the proper assembly of wild type collagen chains (a dominant negative loss of function activity).

The fundamental abnormality in OI is too little bone, resulting in extreme skeletal fragility. Other findings include blue sclerae caused by decreased collagen content, making the sclera translucent and allowing partial visualization of the underlying choroid; hearing loss related to both a sensorineural deficit and impeded conduction due to abnormalities in the bones of the middle and inner ear; and dental imperfections (small, misshapen, and blue-yellow teeth) secondary to a deficiency in dentin.

Osteogenesis imperfecta can be separated into four major clinical subtypes that vary widely in severity (Table 26-3). The severity of the disease is based on the location of the mutation within the protein. Mutations resulting in decreased synthesis of qualitatively normal collagen are associated with mild skeletal abnormalities. More severe or lethal phenotypes have abnormal polypeptide chains that cannot be arranged in a triple helix. The type 2 variant is at one end of the spectrum and is uniformly fatal in utero or during the perinatal period. It is characterized by extraordinary bone fragility with multiple intrauterine fractures (Fig. 26-6). In contrast, individuals with the type 1 form have a normal life span but experience childhood fractures that decrease in frequency following puberty.

Diseases Associated with Mutations of Types II, IX, X, and XI Collagen

Types II, IX, X, and XI collagens are important structural components of hyaline cartilage. Although uncommon, mutations in the genes encoding these proteins produce an

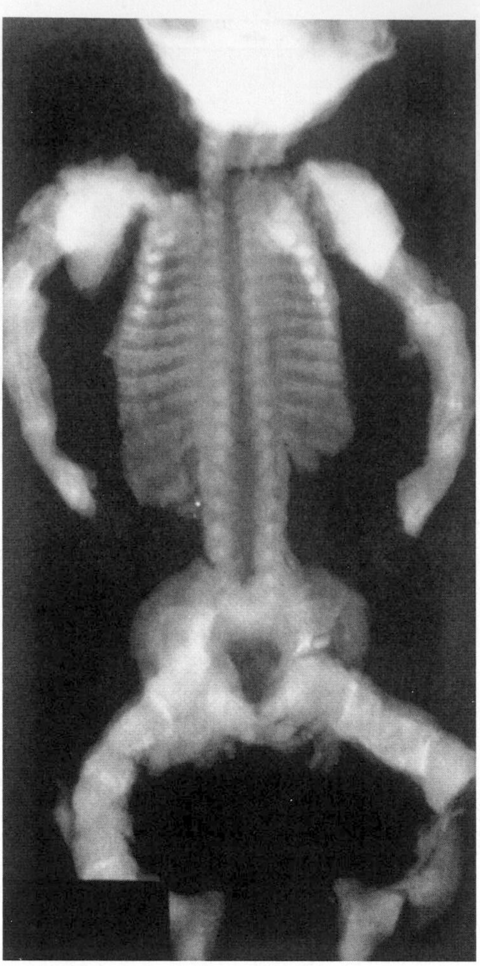

Figure 26-6 Skeletal radiograph of a fetus with lethal type 2 osteogenesis imperfecta. Note the numerous fractures of virtually all bones, resulting in accordion-like shortening of the limbs.

array of disorders of varying severity (Table 26-2). In the severe disorders, the type II collagen molecules are not secreted by the chondrocytes, and insufficient bone formation occurs. In the milder disorders there is reduced synthesis of normal type II collagen.

Defects in Metabolic Pathways (Enzymes, Ion Channels, and Transporters)

Osteopetrosis

Osteopetrosis, also known as *marble bone disease* and *Albers-Schönberg disease*, refers to a group of rare genetic diseases that are characterized by reduced bone resorption and diffuse symmetric skeletal sclerosis due to impaired formation or function of osteoclasts. The term *osteopetrosis* reflects the stone-like quality of the bones. However, the bones are abnormally brittle and fracture easily, like a piece of chalk. Osteopetrosis is classified into variants based on both the mode of inheritance and the severity of clinical findings.

Pathogenesis. Most of the mutations underlying osteopetrosis interfere with the process of acidification of the osteoclast resorption pit, which is required for the dissolution of the calcium hydroxyapatite within the matrix. Examples include autosomal recessive defects in the gene for the enzyme carbonic anhydrase 2 (*CA2*). CA2 is required by osteoclasts and renal tubular cells to generate protons from carbon dioxide and water. The absence of CA2 prevents osteoclasts from acidifying the resorption pit and solubilizing hydroxyapatite, and also blocks the acidification of urine by the renal tubular cells. Other forms of the disease are caused by mutations in *CLCN7*, which encodes a proton pump located on the surface of osteoclasts.

MORPHOLOGY

Due to deficient osteoclast activity, bones involved by osteopetrosis lack a medullary canal, and the ends of long bones are bulbous (Erlenmeyer flask deformity) and misshapen (Fig. 26-7). The neural foramina are small and compress exiting nerves. The primary spongiosa, which is normally removed during growth, persists and fills the medullary cavity, leaving no room for the hematopoietic marrow and preventing the formation of mature trabeculae (Fig. 26-8). Deposited bone is not remodeled and tends to be woven in architecture. Depending on the underlying genetic defect, the number of osteoclasts may be normal, increased, or decreased.

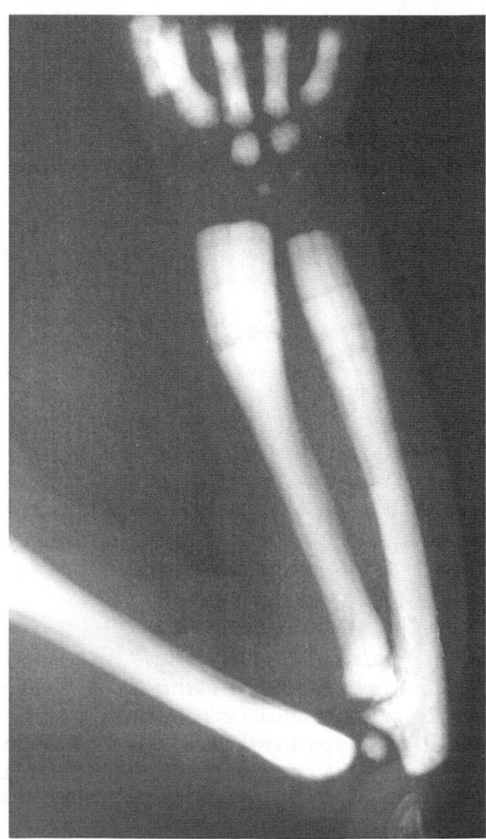

Figure 26-7 Radiograph of the upper extremity in an individual with osteopetrosis. The bones are diffusely sclerotic, and the distal metaphyses of the ulna and radius are poorly formed.

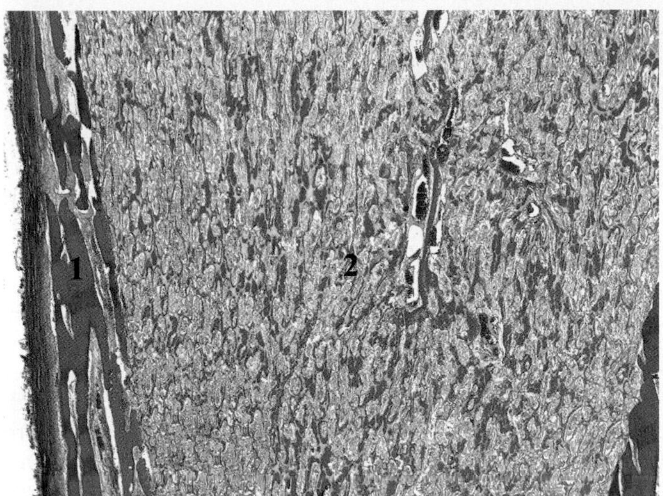

Figure 26-8 Section of proximal tibial diaphysis from a fetus with osteopetrosis. The cortex (1) is present, but the medullary cavity (2) is filled with primary spongiosa, which replaces the hematopoietic elements.

Clinical Features. Severe infantile osteopetrosis is autosomal recessive and usually becomes evident in utero or soon after birth. Fracture, anemia, and hydrocephaly are often seen, resulting in postpartum mortality. Affected individuals who survive into their infancy have cranial nerve defects (optic atrophy, deafness, and facial paralysis) and repeated—often fatal—infections because of leukopenia, despite extensive extramedullary hematopoiesis that can lead to prominent hepatosplenomegaly. The mild autosomal dominant form may not be detected until adolescence or adulthood, when it is discovered on x-ray studies performed because of repeated fractures. These individuals may also have mild cranial nerve deficits and anemia.

Osteopetrosis was the first genetic disease treated with hematopoietic stem cell transplantation, which is effective because osteoclasts are derived from hematopoietic precursors. The normal osteoclasts produced from donor stem cells reverse many of the skeletal abnormalities.

Diseases Associated with Defects in Degradation of Macromolecules

Mucopolysaccharidoses

The mucopolysaccharidoses, discussed in Chapter 5, are a group of lysosomal storage diseases that are caused by deficiencies in the enzymes that degrade dermatan sulfate, heparan sulfate, and keratan sulfate. The affected enzymes are mainly acid hydrolases. Mesenchymal cells, especially chondrocytes, normally degrade extracellular matrix mucopolysaccharides. In these diseases, mucopolysaccharides accumulate inside the chondrocytes, causing apoptotic death of the cells, and also in the extracellular space, resulting in structural defects in articular cartilage. Consequently, many of the skeletal manifestations of the mucopolysaccharidoses result from abnormalities in hyaline cartilage, including the cartilage anlage, growth plates, costal cartilages, and articular surfaces. Affected individuals are frequently of short stature and have chest wall abnormalities, and malformed bones.

KEY CONCEPTS

Developmental Disorders of Bone and Cartilage

Abnormalities in a single bone or a localized group of bones are called **dysostoses** and arise from defects in the migration and condensation of mesenchyme. They manifest as absent, supernumerary or abnormally fused bones. Global disorganization of bone and/or cartilage is called a **dysplasia**. Developmental abnormalities can be categorized by the associated genetic defect.

- Transcription factors: Homeobox genes, such as *HOXD13*, are frequently mutated in some cases of brachydactyly syndromes.
- Hormones and signal transduction molecules: *FGFR3* mutations are responsible for achondroplasia and thanatophoric dysplasia, both of which manifest as dwarfism.
- Structural proteins: Mutations in the genes for type I collagen underlie most types of osteogenesis imperfecta (brittle bone disease), characterized by defective bone formation and skeletal fragility.
- Metabolic enzymes and transporters: Mutations in *CA2* result in osteopetrosis (marble bone disease, in which bones are hard but brittle) and renal tubular acidosis.

Acquired Disorders of Bone and Cartilage

Osteopenia and Osteoporosis

The term osteopenia refers to decreased bone mass, and osteoporosis is defined as osteopenia that is severe enough to significantly increase the risk of fracture. Radiographically, osteoporosis is considered bone mass at least 2.5 standard deviations below mean peak bone mass in young adults and osteopenia as 1 to 2.5 standard deviations below the mean. Alternatively, the presence of an atraumatic or vertebral compression fracture signifies osteoporosis. The disorder may be localized to a certain bone or region, as in disuse osteoporosis of a limb, or may involve the entire skeleton, as a manifestation of a metabolic bone disease. Generalized osteoporosis, in turn, may be primary or secondary to a large variety of conditions (Table 26-4).

The most common forms of osteoporosis are the senile and postmenopausal types. An estimated one million Americans experience a fracture related to osteoporosis each year, at a cost of more than 14 billion dollars. Effective treatment and prevention are imperative. The following discussion relates largely to these dominant forms of osteoporosis.

Pathogenesis. Peak bone mass is achieved during young adulthood. Its magnitude is determined largely by hereditary factors, especially polymorphisms in the genes that influence bone metabolism (discussed later). Physical activity, muscle strength, diet, and hormonal state also make important contributions. Once maximal skeletal mass is attained, a small deficit in bone formation accrues with every resorption and formation cycle of each bone

Table 26-4 Categories of Generalized Osteoporosis

Primary
Idiopathic
Postmenopausal
Senile
Secondary
Endocrine Disorders
Addison disease
Diabetes, type 1
Hyperparathyroidism
Hyperthyroidism
Hypothyroidism
Pituitary tumors
Neoplasia
Carcinomatosis
Multiple myeloma
Gastrointestinal
Hepatic insufficiency
Malabsorption
Malnutrition
Vitamin C, D deficiencies
Drugs
Alcohol
Anticoagulants
Anticonvulsants
Chemotherapy
Corticosteroids
Miscellaneous
Anemia
Homocystinuria
Immobilization
Osteogenesis imperfecta
Pulmonary disease

metabolic unit. Accordingly, age-related bone loss, which may average 0.7% per year, is a normal and predictable biologic phenomenon. Both sexes are affected equally and whites more so than blacks. Gender and racial differences in peak bone mass may partially explain why certain populations are prone to develop this disorder. Although much remains unknown, discoveries in the molecular biology of bone formation and resorption have provided new insights into the pathogenesis of osteoporosis (Fig. 26-9):

- **Age-related changes** in bone cells and matrix have a strong impact on bone metabolism. Osteoblasts from older individuals have reduced proliferative and biosynthetic potential when compared with osteoblasts from younger individuals. Also, the cellular response to growth factors bound to the extracellular matrix becomes attenuated in older individuals. The net result is a diminished capacity to make bone. This form of osteoporosis, known as *senile osteoporosis*, is categorized as a *low-turnover variant.*
- **Reduced physical activity** increases the rate of bone loss in experimental animals and humans, because mechanical forces stimulate normal bone remodeling. Bone loss in an immobilized or paralyzed extremity, the reduction of skeletal mass in astronauts in a zero gravity environment for prolonged periods, and the higher bone density in athletes exemplify the role of physical activity in preventing bone loss. The type of exercise is important, as load magnitude influences bone density more than the number of load cycles. Because muscle contraction is the dominant source of skeletal loading, resistance exercises such as weight training are more effective stimuli for increasing bone mass than repetitive endurance activities such as bicycling. The decreased physical activity that is associated with normal aging contributes to senile osteoporosis.
- **Genetic factors.** Single gene defects (e.g., *LRP5*, discussed above) account for only a small fraction of cases. Polymorphisms in other genes may account for the variation in peak bone density within a population. In genome-wide association studies, the top associated genes include *RANKL*, *OPG*, and *RANK*, all of which encode key regulators of osteoclasts. Also associated are the HLA locus (perhaps reflecting the effects of inflammation on calcium metabolism) and the estrogen receptor gene (discussed later). Some studies have also implicated genetic variants of the vitamin D receptor and genes involved in Wnt signaling as risk factors.
- **Calcium nutritional state** contributes to peak bone mass. Adolescent girls (more than boys) tend to have insufficient calcium intake in the diet. This calcium deficiency occurs during a period of rapid bone growth, restricting the peak bone mass ultimately achieved. Thus, these individuals are at greater risk of developing osteoporosis. Calcium deficiency, increased PTH concentrations, and reduced levels of vitamin D may also have a role in the development of senile osteoporosis.
- **Hormonal influences.** Postmenopausal osteoporosis is characterized by an acceleration of bone loss. In the decade after menopause, yearly reductions in bone mass may reach up to 2% of cortical bone and 9% of cancellous bone. Women may lose as much as 35% of their cortical bone and 50% of their cancellous bone by 30 to 40 years after menopause. It is thus no surprise that post-menopausal women suffer osteoporotic fractures more commonly than men of the same age. *Estrogen deficiency* plays the major role in this phenomenon and close to 40% of postmenopausal women are affected by

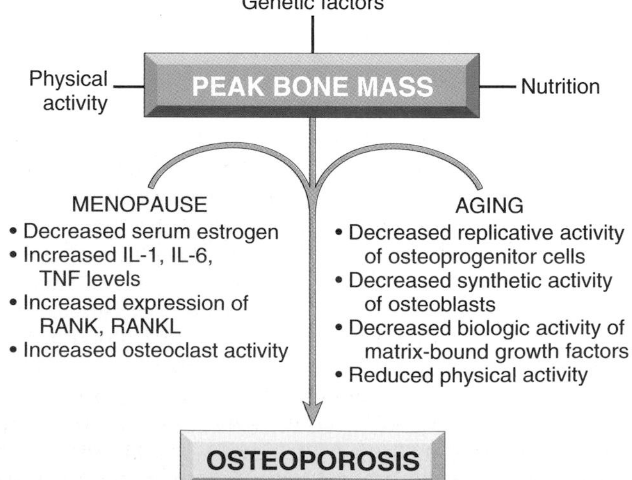

Figure 26-9 Pathophysiology of postmenopausal and senile osteoporosis (see text).

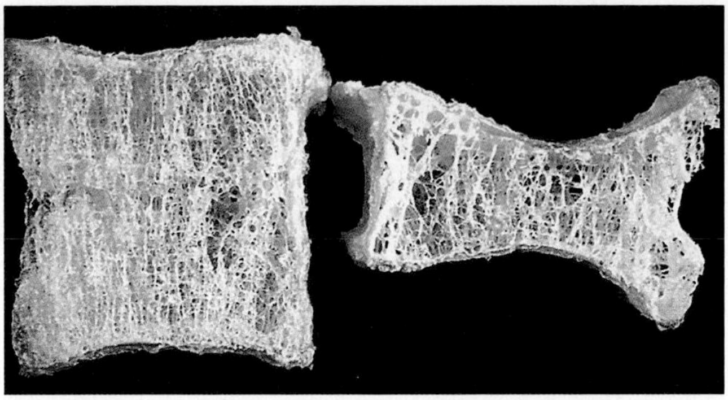

Figure 26-10 Osteoporotic vertebral body *(right)* shortened by compression fractures compared with a normal vertebral body *(left)*. Note that the osteoporotic vertebra has a characteristic loss of horizontal trabeculae and thickened vertical trabeculae.

osteoporosis. Decreased estrogen levels after menopause actually increase *both* bone resorption and formation but the latter does not keep up with the former, leading to **high-turnover** osteoporosis. The decreased estrogen appears to increase secretion of inflammatory cytokines by blood monocytes and bone marrow cells. These cytokines stimulate osteoclast recruitment and activity by increasing the levels of RANKL, diminishing the expression of OPG, decreasing osteoclast proliferation and preventing osteoclast apoptosis. Cytokines such as IL-6, TNF-α, and IL-1 have also been implicated in postmenopausal osteoporosis, either independently or as downstream mediators of estrogen signaling.

MORPHOLOGY

The hallmark of osteoporosis is histologically normal bone that is decreased in quantity. The entire skeleton is affected in postmenopausal and senile osteoporosis (Fig. 26-10), but certain bones tend to be more severely impacted. In postmenopausal osteoporosis the increase in osteoclast activity affects mainly bones or portions of bones that have increased surface area, such as the cancellous compartment of vertebral bodies. The trabecular plates become perforated, thinned, and lose their interconnections (Fig. 26-11), leading to progressive microfractures and eventual vertebral collapse. In senile osteoporosis the cortex is thinned by subperiosteal and endosteal resorption and the Haversian systems are widened. In severe cases the Haversian systems are so enlarged that the cortex mimics cancellous bone.

Clinical Course. The clinical manifestations of osteoporosis depend on which bones are involved. Vertebral fractures that frequently occur in the thoracic and lumbar regions are painful, and, when multiple, can cause significant loss of height and various deformities, including lumbar lordosis and kyphoscoliosis. Complications of fractures of the femoral neck, pelvis, or spine, such as pulmonary embolism and pneumonia, are frequent and result in 40,000 to 50,000 deaths per year.

Osteoporosis cannot be reliably detected in plain radiographs until 30% to 40% of the bone mass is lost, and measurement of blood levels of calcium, phosphorus, and alkaline phosphatase are not diagnostic. Osteoporosis is thus a difficult condition to screen for in asymptomatic people. The best estimates of bone loss, aside from biopsy (which is rarely performed), are specialized radiographic imaging techniques, such as dual-energy x-ray absorptiometry and quantitative computed tomography, both of which measure bone density.

The prevention and treatment of senile and postmenopausal osteoporosis includes exercise, appropriate calcium and vitamin D intake, and pharmacologic agents, most commonly bisphosphonates, which reduce osteoclast activity and induce apoptosis. Although menopausal hormone therapy has been used to prevent fracture, complications, particularly deep venous thrombosis and stroke, have prompted search for more selective estrogen receptor modulators. Denosumab, an anti-RANKL antibody, has shown promise in treating some forms of postmenopausal osteoporosis. Other novel investigational therapeutic approaches include anti-sclerostin antibodies and cathepsin K inhibitors.

Paget Disease (Osteitis Deformans)

Paget disease is a disorder of increased, but disordered and structurally unsound, bone mass. This unique skeletal disease can be divided into three sequential phases: (1) an initial osteolytic stage, (2) a mixed osteoclastic-osteoblastic stage, which ends with a predominance of osteoblastic activity and evolves ultimately into (3) a final burned-out quiescent osteosclerotic stage (Fig. 26-12).

Paget disease usually begins in late adulthood (average age at diagnosis, 70 years) and becomes progressively more common thereafter. An intriguing aspect is the striking geographic variation in its prevalence. Paget disease is relatively common in whites in England, France, Austria, regions of Germany, Australia, New Zealand, and the United States. In contrast, the disease is rare in the native populations of Scandinavia, China, Japan, and Africa. The exact incidence is hard to determine because many affected individuals are asymptomatic; it is estimated that 1% of the US population older than age 40 is affected and the prevalence in England is 2.5% for men and 1.6% for women 55 years or older. Recent surveys show that there has been a decrease in new cases in some countries over the past 25 to 30 years.

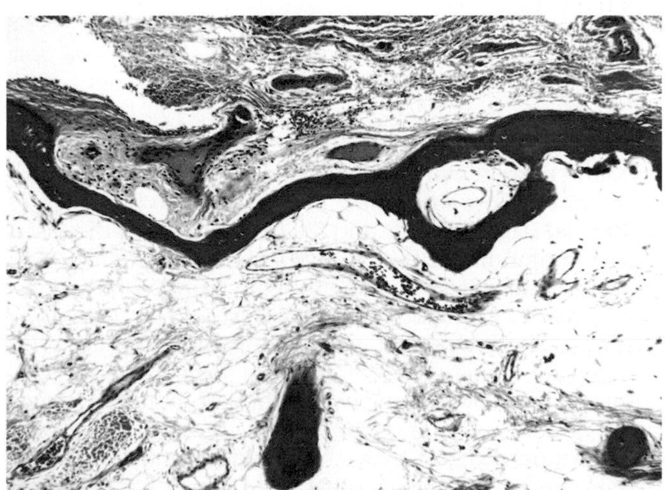

Figure 26-11 In advanced osteoporosis, both the trabecular bone of the medulla (*bottom*) and the cortical bone (*top*) are markedly thinned.

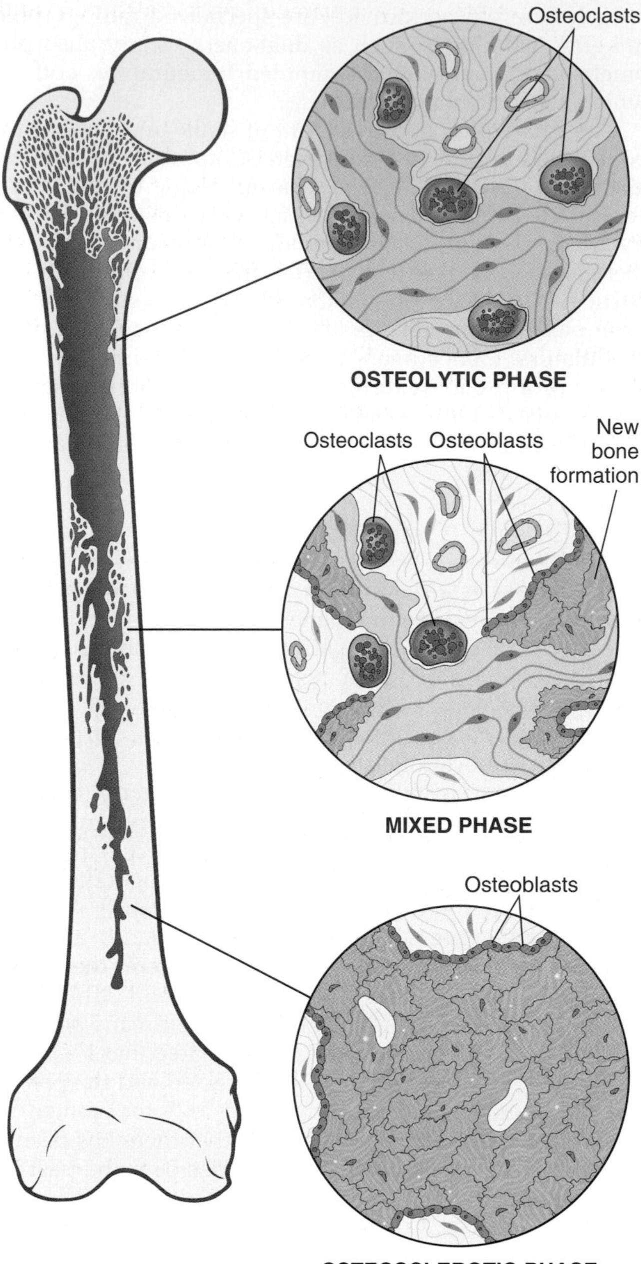

Figure 26-12 Diagrammatic representation of Paget disease of bone demonstrating the three phases in the evolution of the disease.

Pathogenesis. The cause of Paget disease remains uncertain, and current evidence suggests both genetic and environmental factors contribute. Forty percent to 50% of cases of familial Paget disease, and 5% to 10% of sporadic cases, harbor mutations in the *SQSTM1* gene. The net effect of these mutations is to increase the activity of NF-κB, which as already discussed increases osteoclast activity. Activating mutations in *RANK* and inactivating mutations in *OPG* account for some cases of juvenile Paget disease. Cell culture studies have show modulation of vitamin D sensitivity and IL-6 secretion by virally infected osteoclasts. These results suggest that chronic infection of osteoclast precursors by measles or other RNA viruses may play a role in the disease. The geographic distribution is also consistent with some environmental influence.

MORPHOLOGY

Paget disease shows remarkable histologic variation over time and from site to site. **The hallmark is a mosaic pattern of lamellar bone, seen in the sclerotic phase**. This jigsaw puzzle-like appearance is produced by unusually **prominent cement lines**, which join haphazardly oriented units of lamellar bone (Fig. 26-13). The findings during the other phases are less specific. In the initial lytic phase there are waves of osteoclastic activity and numerous resorption pits. The osteoclasts are abnormally large and have many more than the normal 10 to 12 nuclei; sometimes 100 nuclei are present. Osteoclasts persist in the mixed phase, but now many of the bone surfaces are lined by prominent osteoblasts. The marrow adjacent to the bone-forming surface is replaced by loose connective tissue that contains osteoprogenitor cells and numerous blood vessels. The newly formed bone may be woven or lamellar, but eventually all of it is remodeled into lamellar bone. As the mosaic pattern unfolds and the cell activity decreases, the periosseous fibrovascular tissue recedes and is replaced by normal marrow. In the end, the bone is composed of coarsely thickened trabeculae and cortices that are soft and porous and lack structural stability. These aspects make the bone vulnerable to deformation under stress; consequently, it fractures easily.

Clinical Course. Clinical findings are extremely variable and depend on the extent and site of the disease. Most cases are asymptomatic and are discovered as an incidental radiographic finding. Paget disease is *monostotic* in about 15% of cases and *polyostotic* in the remainder. The axial skeleton or proximal femur is involved in up to 80% of cases. Pain localized to the affected bone is common. It is caused by microfractures or by bone overgrowth that compresses spinal and cranial nerve roots. Enlargement of the craniofacial skeleton may produce *leontiasis ossea* (lion face) and a cranium so heavy that is difficult for the person to hold the head erect. The weakened Pagetic bone may lead to invagination of the skull base *(platybasia)* and compression of the posterior fossa. Weight bearing causes anterior bowing of the femurs and tibiae and distorts the femoral

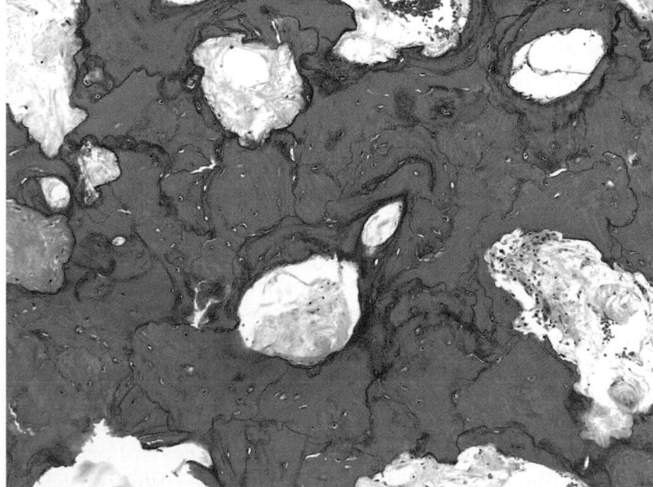

Figure 26-13 Mosaic pattern of lamellar bone pathognomonic of Paget disease.

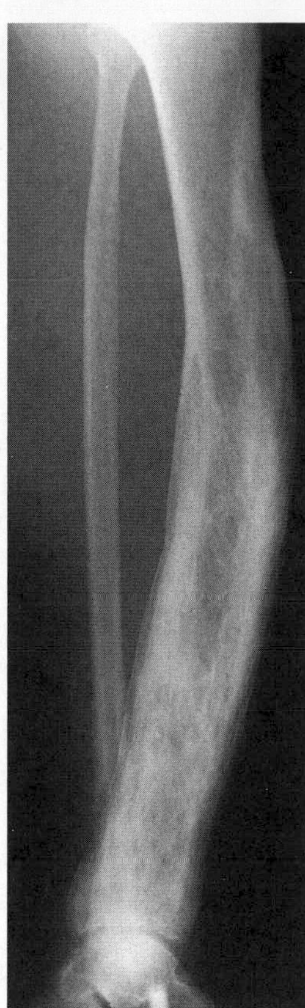

Figure 26-14 Severe Paget disease. The tibia is bowed and the affected portion is enlarged, sclerotic, and exhibits irregular thickening of both the cortical and cancellous bone.

heads, resulting in the development of severe *secondary osteoarthritis*. *Chalk stick-type fractures* are another frequent complication and usually occur in the long bones of the lower extremities. Compression fractures of the spine result in spinal cord injury and the development of kyphosis. The hypervascularity of Pagetic bone warms the overlying skin, and in severe polyostotic disease the increased blood flow acts like an arteriovenous shunt, leading to high-output heart failure or exacerbation of underlying cardiac disease.

A variety of tumor and tumor-like conditions develop in Pagetic bone. The benign lesions include giant cell tumor, giant cell reparative granuloma, and extra-osseous masses of hematopoietic tissue. The most dreaded complication is sarcoma, which occurs in less than 1% of all individuals with Paget disease, and in 5% to 10% of those with severe polyostotic disease. The sarcomas are usually osteosarcoma or fibrosarcoma, and they arise in Paget lesions in the long bones, pelvis, skull, and spine.

The diagnosis can frequently be made from the radiographic findings. Pagetic bone is typically enlarged with thick, coarsened cortices and cancellous bone (Fig. 26-14). Active disease has a wedge-shaped lytic leading edge that may progress along the length of the bone at a rate of 1 cm per year. Many affected individuals have elevated serum alkaline phosphatase levels but normal serum calcium and phosphorus.

In the absence of malignant transformation, Paget disease is usually not a serious or life-threatening disease. Most affected individuals have mild symptoms that are readily suppressed by treatment with calcitonin and bisphosphonates.

Rickets and Osteomalacia

Both rickets and osteomalacia are manifestations of vitamin D deficiency or its abnormal metabolism (and are detailed in Chapter 9). The fundamental defect is an impairment of mineralization and a resultant accumulation of unmineralized matrix. This contrasts with osteoporosis, in which the mineral content of the bone is normal and the total bone mass is decreased. *Rickets* refers to the disorder in children, in whom it interferes with the deposition of bone in the growth plates. *Osteomalacia* is the adult counterpart, in which bone formed during remodeling is undermineralized, resulting in predisposition to fractures.

Hyperparathyroidism

As discussed in Chapter 24, parathyroid hormone (PTH) plays a central role in calcium homeostasis through the following effects:

- Osteoclast activation, increasing bone resorption and calcium mobilization. PTH mediates the effect indirectly by increased RANKL expression on osteoblasts.
- Increased resorption of calcium by the renal tubules
- Increased urinary excretion of phosphates
- Increased synthesis of active vitamin D, 1,25$(OH)_2$-D, by the kidneys, which in turn enhances calcium absorption from the gut and mobilizes bone calcium by inducing RANKL on osteoblasts

The net result of the actions of PTH is an elevation in serum calcium, which, under normal circumstances, inhibits further PTH production. However, excessive or inappropriate levels of PTH can result from autonomous parathyroid secretion *(primary hyperparathyroidism)* or can occur in the setting of underlying renal disease *(secondary hyperparathyroidism)* (see also Chapter 24).

In either setting, **hyperparathyroidism leads to significant skeletal changes related to unabated osteoclast activity**. The entire skeleton is affected, although some sites can be more severely affected than others. PTH is directly responsible for the bone changes seen in primary hyperparathyroidism, but additional alterations contribute to the development of bone disease in secondary hyperparathyroidism. In chronic renal insufficiency there is inadequate 1,25-$(OH)_2$-D synthesis, which ultimately affects gastrointestinal calcium absorption. The hyperphosphatemia of renal failure also suppresses renal α1-hydroxylase, further impairing vitamin D synthesis; additional influences include metabolic acidosis and aluminum deposition in bone. As bone mass decreases, affected patients are increasingly susceptible to fractures, bone deformation, and joint problems. Fortunately, a reduction in PTH levels to normal can completely reverse the bone changes.

MORPHOLOGY

Symptomatic, untreated primary hyperparathyroidism manifests with three interrelated skeletal abnormalities: **osteoporosis, brown tumors** and **osteitis fibrosa cystica.** Osteoporosis is

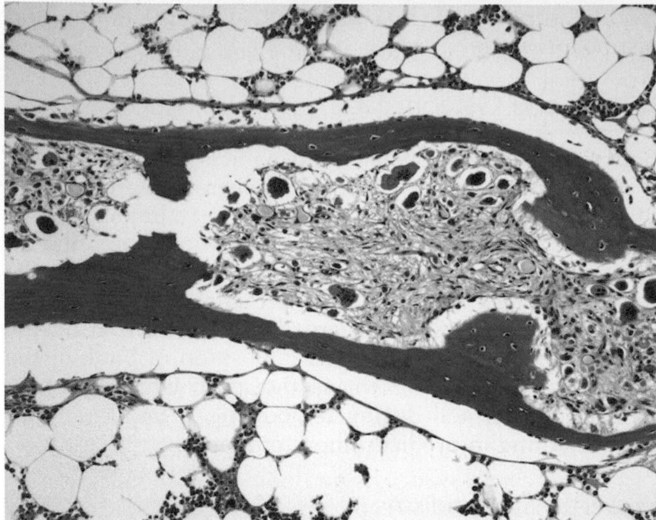

Figure 26-15 Hyperparathyroidism with osteoclasts boring into the center of the trabeculum (dissecting osteitis).

generalized, but is most severe in the phalanges, vertebrae and proximal femur. The increased osteoclast activity in hyperparathyroidism is most prominent in cortical bone (subperiosteal and endosteal surfaces) but medullary bone is not spared. Indeed, osteoclasts may tunnel into and dissect centrally along the length of the trabeculae, creating the appearance of railroad tracks and producing what is known as **dissecting osteitis** (Fig. 26-15). The marrow spaces around the affected surfaces are replaced by fibrovascular tissue. The correlative radiographic finding is a decrease in bone density or osteoporosis.

The bone loss predisposes to microfractures and secondary hemorrhages that elicit an influx of macrophages and an ingrowth of reparative fibrous tissue, creating a mass of reactive tissue, known as a **brown tumor** (Fig. 26-16). The brown color is the result of the vascularity, hemorrhage, and hemosiderin deposition, and it is not uncommon for the lesions to undergo cystic degeneration. The combination of increased bone cell activity, peritrabecular fibrosis, and cystic brown tumors is the hallmark of severe hyperparathyroidism and is known as **generalized osteitis fibrosa cystica (von Recklinghausen disease of bone)**.

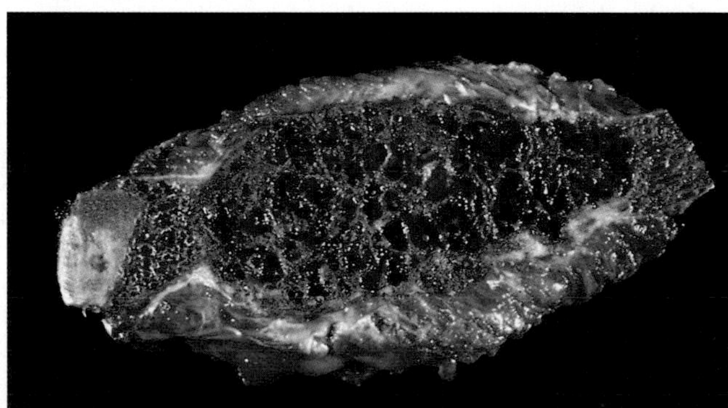

Figure 26-16 Resected rib, harboring an expansile brown tumor adjacent to the costal cartilage.

Osteitis fibrosa cystica is now rarely encountered because hyperparathyroidism is usually diagnosed on routine blood tests and treated at an early stage. Secondary hyperparathyroidism is usually not as severe or as prolonged as primary hyperparathyroidism, hence the skeletal abnormalities tend to be milder. Control of hyperparathyroidism allows the bony changes to regress or disappear completely.

Renal Osteodystrophy

The term *renal osteodystrophy* describes collectively the skeletal changes that occur in chronic renal disease, including those associated with dialysis. The manifestations are not unique, but include many of the entities described above including (1) osteopenia/osteoporosis (2) osteomalacia, (3) secondary hyperparathyroidism, and (4) growth retardation. As advances in medical technology have prolonged the lives of individuals with renal disease, its impact on skeletal homeostasis has assumed greater clinical importance. The various histologic bone changes in individuals with end-stage renal failure can be divided into three major types of disorders:

- *High-turnover osteodystrophy* is characterized by increased bone resorption and bone formation, with the former predominating.
- *Low-turnover or aplastic disease* is manifested by adynamic bone (little osteoclastic and osteoblastic activity) and, less commonly, osteomalacia.
- *Mixed pattern of disease* with areas of high turnover and low turnover.

Pathogenesis. Kidney disease causes skeletal abnormalities through three mechanisms (Fig. 26-17).

- **Tubular dysfunction.** The major tubular disease that affects the skeleton is renal tubular acidosis. The associated low pH dissolves hydroxyappatite, resulting in demineralization of the matrix and osteomalacia.
- **Generalized renal failure**, affecting glomerular and tubular function, leads to reduced phosphate excretion, chronic hyperphosphatemia, hypocalcemia and, ultimately *secondary hyperparathyroidism*. The resulting metabolic state is not completely analogous to primary

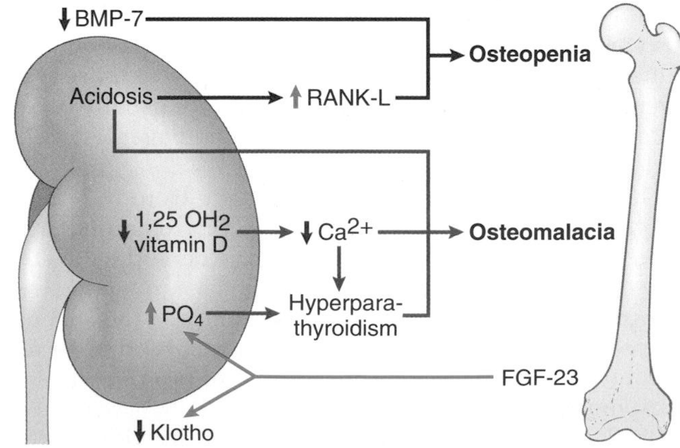

Figure 26-17 Mechanisms of renal osteodystrophy involves electrolyte levels and endocrine signaling between bone and kidney.

hyperparathyroidism in that bone volume, turnover, and mineralization can vary independently.

- **Decreased production of secreted factors.** The kidney converts vitamin D to its active form (1,25-OH_2-vitamin D_3) and secretes the proteins BMP-7 and Klotho. Decreased vitamin D_3 results in hypocalcemia and contributes to secondary hyperparathyroidism. A hormonal feedback loop between kidney and bone that regulates calcium and phosphate homeostasis involves secreted BMP-7 and FGF-23 and the membrane protein Klotho. BMP-7, produced by renal renal tubular cells, induces osteoblast differentiation and proliferation, whereas FGF-23, made by osteocytes, acts on the kidney to regulate phosphate homeostasis and vitamin D production, which are dependent on production of membrane-bound Klotho in the kidney. The mechanism of action of Klotho is not understood. The levels of these signals change in chronic renal failure, interrupting the steady state and resulting in osteopenia and osteomalacia.

Other factors, such as aluminum from dialysis, oral phosphate binders, iron deposition, and diabetes mellitus may indirectly contribute to bone disease in the setting of renal failure.

KEY CONCEPTS

Acquired Disorders of Bone and Cartilage

- **Osteopenia** and **osteoporosis** represent histologically normal bone that is decreased in quantity, but osteoporosis is sufficiently severe to significantly increase risk of fracture. The disease is very common with marked morbidity and mortality from fractures. Multiple factors including peak bone mass, age, activity, genetics, nutrition and hormonal influences contribute to its pathogenesis.
- **Paget disease** is a disorder of locally increased but disordered bone. Typically asymptomatic, it is usually discovered incidentally. A mosaic pattern of mineralization is the histologic hallmark at the late stage of the disease. Genetic and possibly viral infectious etiologies have been proposed.
- **Osteomalacia** is characterized by bone that is insufficiently mineralized. In the developing skeleton, the manifestations are characterized by a condition known as rickets.
- **Hyperparathyroidism** arises from either autonomous or compensatory hypersecretion of PTH and can lead to **osteoporosis**, **brown tumors,** and **osteitis fibrosa cystica**. However, in developed countries, where early diagnosis is the norm, these manifestations are rarely seen.
- **Renal osteodystrophy** represents the constellation of bone abnormalities (osteopenia, osteomalacia, hyperparathyroidism, and growth retardation) from chronic renal failure. The mechanisms are complex but stem from decreased tubular, glomerular, and hormonal functions of the kidney.

Fractures

A fracture is defined as loss of bone integrity due to mechanical injury and/or diminished bone strength. Fractures are some of the most common pathologic conditions affecting bone. The following qualifiers describe fracture types and affect treatment:

- **Simple:** the overlying skin is intact.
- **Compound:** the bone communicates with the skin surface.
- **Comminuted:** the bone is fragmented.
- **Displaced:** the ends of the bone at the fracture site are not aligned.
- **Stress:** a slowly developing fracture that follows a period of increased physical activity in which the bone is subjected to repetitive loads
- **"Greenstick"**: extending only partially through the bone, common in infants when bones are soft
- **Pathologic**: involving bone weakened by an underlying disease process, such as a tumor

Healing of Fractures

Bone has a remarkable capacity for repair. This process involves regulated expression of a multitude of genes and can be separated into overlapping stages with particular molecular, biochemical, histologic, and biomechanical features.

Immediately after fracture, rupture of blood vessels results in a hematoma, which fills the fracture gap and surrounds the area of bone injury. The clotted blood provides a fibrin mesh, sealing off the fracture site and at the same time creates a framework for the influx of inflammatory cells and ingrowth of fibroblasts and new capillaries. Simultaneously, degranulated platelets and migrating inflammatory cells release PDGF, TGF-β, FGF, and other factors, which activate osteoprogenitor cells in the periosteum, medullary cavity, and surrounding soft tissues and stimulate osteoclastic and osteoblastic activity. Thus, by the end of the first week, the major changes are organization of the hematoma, matrix production in adjacent tissues, and remodeling of the fractured ends of the bone. This fusiform and predominantly uncalcified tissue—called *soft tissue callus* or *procallus*—provides some anchorage between the ends of the fractured bones but not structural rigidity for weight bearing.

After approximately 2 weeks, the soft tissue callus is transformed into a *bony callus*. The activated osteoprogenitor cells deposit subperiosteal trabeculae of **woven bone** that are oriented perpendicular to the cortical axis and within the medullary cavity. In some cases, the activated mesenchymal cells in the soft tissues and bone surrounding the fracture line also differentiate into chondrocytes that make fibrocartilage and hyaline cartilage. The bony callus reaches its maximal girth at the end of the second or third week and helps to stabilize the fracture site. The newly formed cartilage along the fracture line undergoes enchondral ossification, forming a contiguous network of bone with newly deposited bone trabeculae in the medulla and beneath the periosteum. In this fashion, the fractured ends are bridged, and as it mineralizes, the stiffness and strength of the callus increases to the point that controlled weight bearing is tolerated (Fig. 26-18).

In the early stages of callus formation, an excess of fibrous tissue, cartilage, and woven bone is produced. As the callus matures and is subjected to weight-bearing

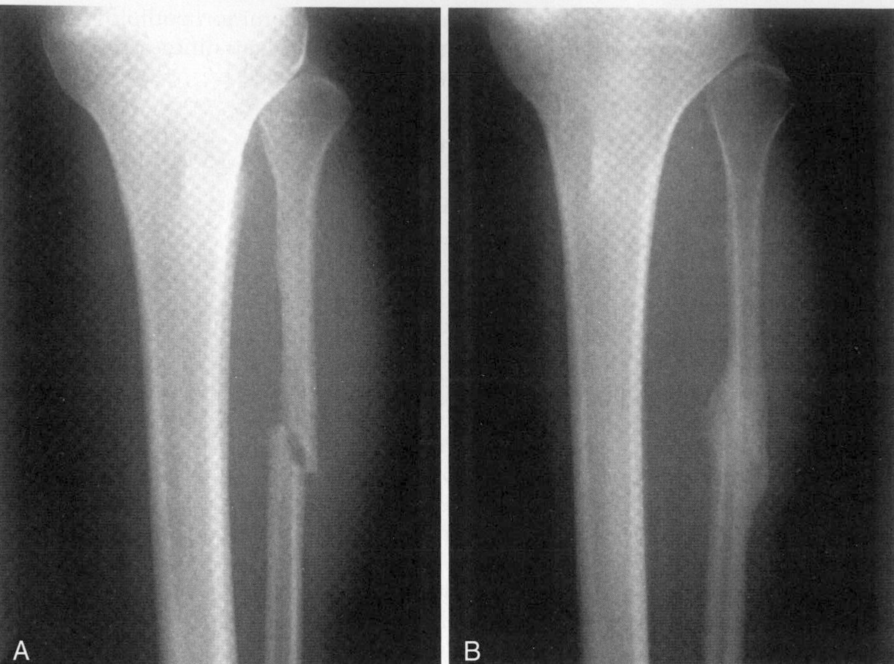

Figure 26-18 A, Recent fracture of the fibula. **B,** Marked callus formation 6 weeks later. (Courtesy Dr. Barbara Weissman, Brigham and Women's Hospital, Boston, Mass.)

forces, the portions that are not physically stressed are resorbed. In this manner the callus is reduced in size and the shape and outline of the fractured bone are reestablished as *lamellar bone*. The healing process is complete with restoration of the medullary cavity.

The sequence of events in the healing of a fracture can be easily impeded or even blocked. For example, displaced and comminuted fractures frequently result in some deformity. Inadequate immobilization permits movement of the callus and prevents its normal formation, resulting in *delayed union* or *nonunion*. If a nonunion persists, the malformed callus undergoes cystic degeneration, and the luminal surface can actually become lined by synovial-like cells, creating a false joint or *pseudoarthrosis*. A serious obstacle to healing is infection of the fracture site, which is especially common in open fractures. Malnutrition and skeletal dysplasia also hinder fracture healing. In children and young adults, near perfect union is the norm. In older adults, fractures often occur in the background of other bone disorders (e.g., osteoporosis and osteomalacia). In such settings, surgical immobilization is often needed for adequate repair.

Osteonecrosis (Avascular Necrosis)

Infarction of bone and marrow is a relatively common event that can occur in the medullary cavity or involve both the medulla and cortex. Most cases of bone necrosis stem from fractures or corticosteroid administration. A diverse set of other conditions also predispose to osteonecrosis (Table 26-5). All are believed to lead to vascular insufficiency through mechanical injury to blood vessels, thromboembolism, external pressure on vessels, or venous occlusion.

MORPHOLOGY

Regardless of etiology, medullary infarcts are geographic and involve the trabecular bone and marrow. The cortex is usually not affected because of its collateral blood flow. In subchondral infarcts, a triangular or wedge-shaped segment of tissue that has the subchondral bone plate as its base undergoes necrosis. The overlying articular cartilage remains viable, as it can access nutrients that are present in synovial fluid. Microscopically, dead bone is recognized by empty lacunae surrounded by necrotic adipocytes that frequently rupture. The released fatty acids bind calcium and form insoluble calcium soaps that may persist for life. In the healing response, osteoclasts resorb the necrotic trabeculae. Trabeculae that remain act as scaffolding for the deposition of new bone in a process known as creeping substitution. In subchondral infarcts the pace of this substitution is too slow to be effective, so there is collapse of the necrotic bone and distortion, fracture, and even sloughing of the articular cartilage (Fig. 26-19).

Table 26-5 Conditions Associated with Osteonecrosis

Alcohol abuse
Bisphosphonate therapy (especially jawbones)
Connective tissue disorders
Corticosteroid administration
Chronic pancreatitis
Dysbarism (the "bends")
Gaucher disease
Infection
Pregnancy
Radiation therapy
Sickle cell crisis (Chapter 14)
Trauma
Tumors

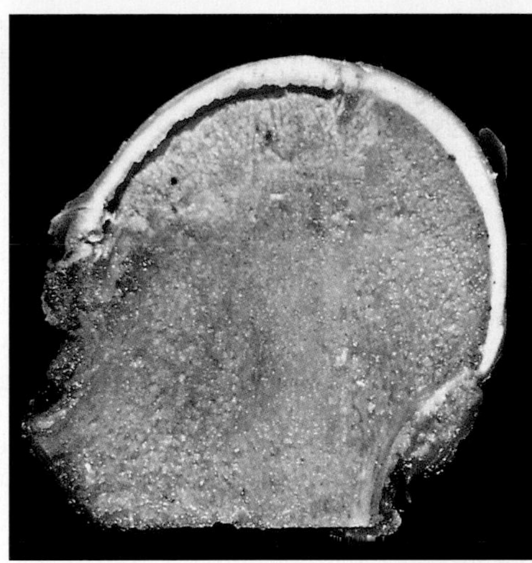

Figure 26-19 Femoral head with a subchondral, wedge-shaped pale yellow area of osteonecrosis. The space between the overlying articular cartilage and bone is caused by trabecular compression fractures without repair.

Clinical Course. **The symptoms depend on the location and extent of infarction.** Typically, subchondral infarcts cause pain that is initially associated only with activity but then becomes constant as secondary changes supervene. Subchondral infarcts often collapse and may lead to severe, secondary osteoarthritis. In contrast, medullary infarcts are usually small and clinically silent except when they occur in the setting of Gaucher disease, dysbarism (e.g., the "bends", Chapter 4), and sickle cell anemia. More than 10% of the 500,000 joint replacements performed annually in the United States are for treatment of complications of osteonecrosis.

Osteomyelitis

Osteomyelitis denotes inflammation of bone and marrow, virtually always secondary to infection. Osteomyelitis may be a complication of any systemic infection but frequently manifests as a primary solitary focus of disease. All types of organisms, including viruses, parasites, fungi, and bacteria, can produce osteomyelitis, but infections caused by certain pyogenic bacteria and mycobacteria are the most common. Currently in the United States, exotic infections in immigrants from developing countries and opportunistic infections in immunosuppressed individuals have made the diagnosis and treatment of osteomyelitis challenging.

Pyogenic Osteomyelitis

Pyogenic osteomyelitis is almost always caused by bacterial infections. Organisms may reach the bone by (1) hematogenous spread, (2) extension from a contiguous site, and (3) direct implantation. In otherwise healthy children, most osteomyelitis is hematogenous in origin and develops in the long bones. The initiating bacteremia may stem from seemingly trivial mucosal injuries, such as may occur during defecation or vigorous chewing of hard foods, or from minor infections of the skin. In adults, however, osteomyelitis more often occurs as a complication of open fractures, surgical procedures, and diabetic infections of the feet.

Staphylococcus aureus is responsible for 80% to 90% of the cases of culture-positive pyogenic osteomyelitis. These organisms express cell wall proteins that bind to bone matrix components such as collagen, which facilitates adherence of the bacteria to bone. *Escherichia coli*, *Pseudomonas*, and *Klebsiella* are more frequently isolated from individuals with genitourinary tract infections or who are intravenous drug abusers. Mixed bacterial infections are seen in the setting of direct spread or inoculation of organisms during surgery or into open fractures. In the neonatal period, *Haemophilus influenzae* and group B streptococci are frequent pathogens, and individuals with sickle cell disease are predisposed to *Salmonella* infection. In almost 50% of suspected cases, no organisms can be isolated.

The location of the bone infections is influenced by the osseous vascular circulation, which varies with age. In the neonate the metaphyseal vessels penetrate the growth plate, resulting in frequent infection of the metaphysis, epiphysis, or both. In children, localization of microorganisms in the metaphysis is typical. After growth plate closure, the metaphyseal vessels reunite with their epiphyseal counterparts and provide a route for the bacteria to seed the epiphyses and subchondral regions, which are common sites of infection in the adult.

MORPHOLOGY

Changes associated with osteomyelitis depend on the stage (acute, subacute, or chronic) and location of the infection. In the acute phase, bacteria proliferate and induce a neutrophilic inflammatory reaction. Necrosis of bone cells and marrow ensues within the first 48 hours. The bacteria and inflammation spread longitudinally and may percolate throughout the Haversian systems to reach the periosteum. In children the periosteum is loosely attached to the cortex. Thus, a sizable subperiosteal abscesses may form that can dissect for long distances along the bone surface. Lifting of the periosteum further impairs the blood supply to the affected region, contributing to the necrosis. The dead bone is known as a **sequestrum**. Rupture of the periosteum leads to a soft tissue abscess which can channel to the skin as a draining sinus. Sometimes the sequestrum crumbles, releasing fragments that pass through the sinus tract.

In infants, but uncommonly in adults, epiphyseal infection spreads through the articular surface or along capsular and tendoligamentous insertions into a joint, producing septic or suppurative arthritis, which can cause destruction of the articular cartilage and permanent disability. An analogous process involves the vertebrae, in which the infection destroys the hyaline cartilage end plate and intervertebral disc and spreads into adjacent vertebrae.

After the first week, chronic inflammatory cells release cytokines that stimulates osteoclastic bone resorption, ingrowth of fibrous tissue, and the deposition of reactive bone at the periphery. The newly deposited bone can form a shell of living tissue, known as an **involucrum,** around the segment of devitalized infected bone (Fig. 26-20). Several morphologic variants of osteomyelitis have eponyms. **Brodie abscess** is a small intraosseous abscess that frequently involves the cortex and is walled off by reactive bone. **Sclerosing osteomyelitis of Garré** typically develops in the jaw and is associated with extensive new bone formation that obscures much of the underlying osseous structure.

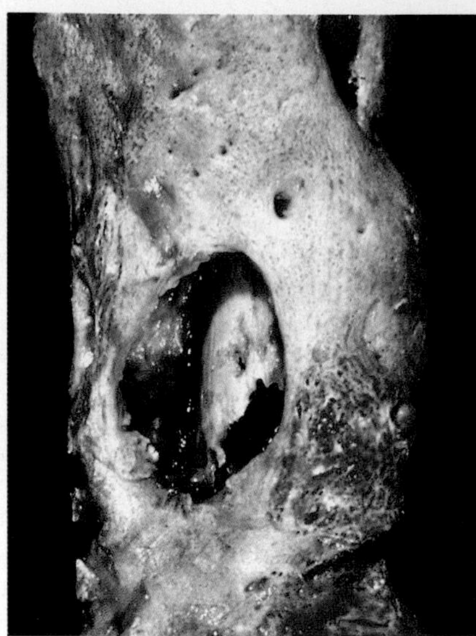

Figure 26-20 Resected femur in a person with draining osteomyelitis. The drainage tract in the subperiosteal shell of viable new bone (involucrum) reveals the inner native necrotic cortex (sequestrum).

Clinical Course. Hematogenous osteomyelitis sometimes manifests as an acute systemic illness with malaise, fever, chills, leukocytosis, and marked-to-intense throbbing pain over the affected region. In other instances, the presentation is subtle, with only unexplained fever (most often in infants) or localized pain (most often in adults). The diagnosis is strongly suggested by the characteristic radiographic findings of a lytic focus of bone destruction surrounded by a zone of sclerosis. In some untreated cases blood cultures are positive, but biopsy and bone cultures are required to identify the pathogen in most instances. The combination of antibiotics and surgical drainage is usually curative.

In 5% to 25% of cases, acute osteomyelitis fails to resolve and persists as chronic infection. Chronic infections may develop when there is delay in diagnosis, extensive bone necrosis, inadequate antibiotic therapy or surgical debridement, or weakened host defenses. The course of chronic infections may be punctuated by acute flare-ups; these are usually spontaneous and may occur after years of dormancy. Other complications of chronic osteomyelitis include pathologic fracture, secondary amyloidosis, endocarditis, sepsis, and development of squamous cell carcinoma in the draining sinus tracts and sarcoma in the infected bone.

Mycobacterial Osteomyelitis

Mycobacterial osteomyelitis, historically a problem in developing countries, has increased in incidence in the developed world due to immigration patterns and immunocompromised patients. Overall, approximately 1% to 3% of individuals with pulmonary or extrapulmonary tuberculosis have osseous infection.

The organisms are usually blood borne and originate from a focus of active visceral disease during the initial stages of primary infection. Direct extension (e.g., from a pulmonary focus into a rib or from tracheobronchial nodes into adjacent vertebrae) or spread via the circulation may also occur. The bone infection may persist for years before being recognized. Typically, affected individuals present with localized pain, low-grade fevers, chills, and weight loss. Infection is usually solitary except in immunocompromised individuals. The histologic findings, namely caseous necrosis and granulomas, are typical of tuberculosis elsewhere (Chapter 8). Mycobacterial osteomyelitis tends to be more destructive and resistant to control than pyogenic osteomyelitis.

Tuberculous spondylitis (Pott disease) is particularly destructive. The spine is involved in 40% of cases of mycobacterial osteomyelitis. The infection breaks through intervertebral discs to affect multiple vertebrae and extends into the soft tissues. Destruction of discs and vertebrae frequently results in permanent compression fractures that produce scoliosis or kyphosis and neurologic deficits secondary to spinal cord and nerve compression. Other complications of tuberculous osteomyelitis include tuberculous arthritis, sinus tract formation, psoas abscess, and amyloidosis.

Skeletal Syphilis

Syphilis (*Treponema pallidum*) and yaws (*Treponema pertenue*) can involve bone. Currently, syphilis is experiencing resurgence; however, bone involvement remains infrequent because the disease is usually diagnosed and treated before this complication develops.

In congenital syphilis, the bone lesions appear about the fifth month of gestation and are fully developed at birth. The spirochetes tend to localize in areas of active enchondral ossification (osteochondritis) and in the periosteum (periostitis). The syphilitic *saber shin* is produced by massive reactive periosteal bone deposition on the medial and anterior surfaces of the tibia. In acquired syphilis, bone disease may begin early in the tertiary stage, usually 2 to 5 years after the initial infection. The bones most frequently involved are those of the nose, palate, skull, and extremities, especially the long tubular bones such as the tibia.

MORPHOLOGY

Syphilitic bone infection is characterized by edematous granulation tissue containing numerous plasma cells and necrotic bone. The spirochetes can be demonstrated in the inflammatory tissue with silver histochemical stains or immunohistochemistry. Typical gummas may also form in both congenital and acquired syphilis (Chapter 8).

Bone Tumors and Tumor-Like Lesions

The rarity of primary bone tumors and the often disfiguring surgery required to treat a malignancy make this group of disorders especially challenging. Although metastases and hematopoietic tumors far outnumber primary bone neoplasms, about 2400 new cases of bone sarcoma are diagnosed annually, accounting for less than 1% of all bone disease in the United States. While not very common, bone sarcomas are lethal in 50% of cases. Therapy aims to optimize survival while maintaining the function of affected

Table 26-6 Classification of Major Primary Tumors Involving Bones

Category and fraction (%)	Behavior	Tumor type	Common locations	Age (yr)	Morphology
Hematopoietic (20)	Malignant	Myeloma Lymphoma	Vertebrae, pelvis	50-60	Malignant plasma cells or lymphocytes replacing marrow space
Cartilage forming (30)	Benign	Osteochondroma	Metaphysis of long bones	10-30	Bony excrescence with cartilage cap
		Chondroma	Small bones of hands and feet	30-50	Circumscribed hyaline cartilage nodule in medulla
		Chondroblastoma	Epiphysis of long bones	10-20	Circumscribed, pericellular calcification
		Chondromyxoid fibroma	Tibia, pelvis	20-30	Collagenous to myxoid matrix, stellate cells
	Malignant	Chondrosarcoma (conventional)	Pelvis, shoulder	40-60	Extends from medulla through cortex into soft tissue, chondrocytes with increased cellularity and atypia
Bone forming (26)	Benign	Osteoid osteoma	Metaphysis of long bones	10-20	Cortical, interlacing microtrabeculae of woven bone
		Osteoblastoma	Vertebral column	10-20	Posterior elements of vertebra, histology similar to osteoid osteoma
	Malignant	Osteosarcoma	Metaphysis of distal femur, proximal tibia	10-20	Extends from medulla to lift periosteum, malignant cells producing woven bone
Unknown origin (15)	Benign	Giant cell tumor	Epiphysis of long bones	20-40	Destroys medulla and cortex, sheets of osteoclasts
		Aneurysmal bone cyst	Proximal tibia, distal femur, vertebra	10-20	Vertebral body, hemorrhagic spaces separated by cellular, fibrous septae
	Malignant	Ewing sarcoma	Diaphysis of long bones	10-20	Sheets of primitive small round cells
		Adamantinoma	Tibia	30-40	Cortical, fibrous , bone matrix with epithelial islands
Notochordal (4)	Malignant	Chordoma	Clivus, sacrum	30-60	Destroys medulla and cortex, foamy cells in myxoid matrix

Adapted from Unni KK, Inwards CY: Dahlin's Bone Tumors, 6th ed. Philadelphia, Lippincott-Williams & Wilkins, 2010, p 5; by permission of Mayo Foundation.

body parts. Most bone neoplasms develop during the first several decades of life and have a propensity for the long bones of the extremities. The occurrence in certain age groups and predilection for particular anatomic sites provides important diagnostic clues about specific types of tumors. For example, osteosarcoma peaks during adolescence and most frequently involves the knee whereas chondrosarcoma affects older adults and involves the pelvis and proximal extremities.

Bone tumors may present in a number of ways. The more common benign lesions are often asymptomatic incidental findings. Many tumors, however, produce pain or a slow-growing mass. In some circumstances the first hint of a tumor's presence is a pathologic fracture. Radiographic imaging studies have an important role in diagnosing these lesions. In addition to providing the exact location and extent of the tumor, imaging studies can detect features that narrow the diagnostic possibilities. Ultimately, in almost all instances biopsy is necessary for definitive diagnosis.

When possible, bone tumors are classified according to the normal cell or matrix they produce. Lesions that do not have normal tissue counterparts are grouped according to their clinicopathologic features (Table 26-6). **Benign tumors greatly outnumber their malignant counterparts** and occur with greatest frequency within the first three decades of life, whereas in older adults, a bone tumor is likely to be malignant. Excluding neoplasms originating from hematopoietic cells (myeloma, lymphoma, and leukemia), osteosarcoma is the most common primary cancer of bone, followed by chondrosarcoma and Ewing sarcoma.

Insults that induce chronic injury and inflammation, such as bone infarcts, chronic osteomyelitis, Paget disease, radiation, and metal prostheses, increase the risk of bone neoplasia, possibly because proliferation associated with chronic inflammation and repair set the stage for acquisition of oncogenic mutations. As we will describe, some of the causative mutations involve classic oncogenes and tumor suppressors that are implicated in many other tumors, whereas others involve genes that are specifically involved in bone development and are mutated only in bone tumors.

Bone-Forming Tumors

Tumors in this category all produce unmineralized osteoid or mineralized woven bone.

Osteoid Osteoma and Osteoblastoma

Osteoid osteoma and osteoblastoma are benign bone-producing tumors that have identical histologic features but differ in size, sites of origin, and symptoms. Osteoid osteomas are, by definition less than 2 cm in diameter, and usually occur in young men in their teens and 20s. These tumors can arise in any bone but have a predilection for the appendicular skeleton. About 50% of cases involve the femur or tibia, wherein they typically arise in the cortex and less frequently within the medullary cavity. Usually, there is a thick rind of reactive cortical bone that may be the only clue radiographically. Despite the small size, they present with severe nocturnal pain that is relieved by aspirin and other non-steroidal anti-inflammatory agents. The pain is probably caused by prostaglandin E_2 (PGE_2) produced by the proliferating osteoblasts. Osteoblastoma is larger than 2 cm and involves the posterior spine (laminae and pedicles) more frequently; the pain is unresponsive to aspirin, and the tumor usually does not induce a marked bony reaction. Osteoid osteoma is frequently treated by radiofrequency ablation, whereas osteoblastoma is usually curetted or excised en bloc. Malignant transformation is rare.

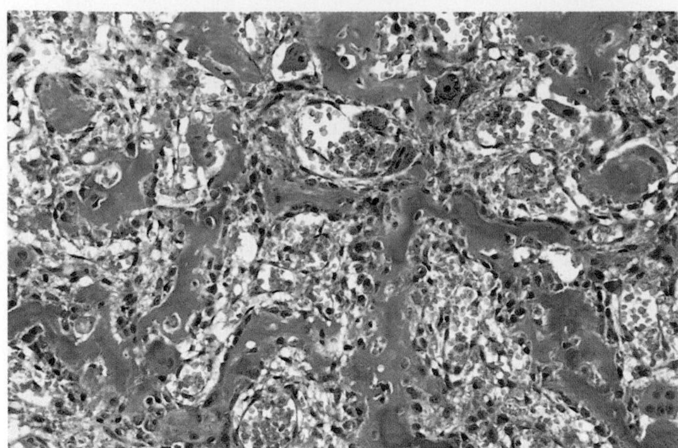

Figure 26-21 Osteoid osteoma composed of haphazardly interconnecting trabeculae of woven bone that are rimmed by prominent osteoblasts. The intertrabecular spaces are filled by vascularized loose connective tissue.

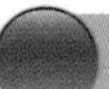

MORPHOLOGY

Osteoid osteoma and osteoblastoma are round-to-oval masses of hemorrhagic gritty tan tissue. They are well circumscribed and composed of randomly interconnecting trabeculae of woven bone that are prominently rimmed by a single layer of osteoblasts (Fig. 26-21). The stroma surrounding the neoplastic bone consists of loose connective tissue that contains many dilated and congested capillaries. The relatively small size, well-defined margins, and benign cytologic features of the neoplastic osteoblasts help distinguish these tumors from osteosarcoma. Osteoid osteomas elicit the formation of a tremendous amount of reactive bone, which encircles the lesion. The actual neoplasm (known as the nidus) manifests radiographically as a small round lucency that may be centrally mineralized (Fig. 26-22).

Osteosarcoma

Osteosarcoma is a malignant tumor in which the cancerous cells produce osteoid matrix or mineralized bone. It is the most common primary malignant tumor of bone, exclusive of myeloma and lymphoma, and accounts for approximately 20% of primary bone cancers. Osteosarcoma occurs in all age groups but has a bimodal age distribution; 75% occur in persons younger than 20 years of age. The smaller second peak occurs in older adults, who frequently suffer from conditions known to predispose to osteosarcoma—Paget disease, bone infarcts, and prior radiation. Overall, men are more commonly affected than women (1.6 : 1). Any bone can be involved. The tumors usually arise in the metaphyseal region of the long bones of the extremities, and almost 50% occur about the knee (i.e., distal femur or proximal tibia).

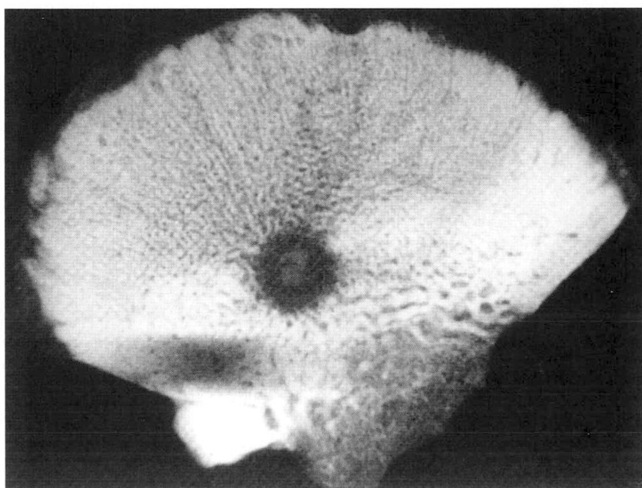

Figure 26-22 Specimen radiograph of intracortical osteoid osteoma. The round radiolucency with central mineralization represents the lesion and is surrounded by abundant reactive bone that has massively thickened the cortex.

Osteosarcomas typically present as painful, progressively enlarging masses. Sometimes a sudden fracture of the bone is the first symptom. Radiographs usually show a large destructive, mixed lytic and blastic mass with infiltrative margins (Fig. 26-23). The tumor frequently breaks through the cortex and lifts the periosteum, resulting in reactive periosteal bone formation. The triangular shadow between the cortex and raised ends of periosteum, known radiographically as *Codman triangle,* is indicative of an aggressive tumor. It is characteristic but not diagnostic of osteosarcoma.

Pathogenesis. Approximately 70% of osteosarcomas have acquired genetic abnormalities such as complex structural and numerical chromosomal aberrations. Molecular studies have shown that these tumors usually have mutations in

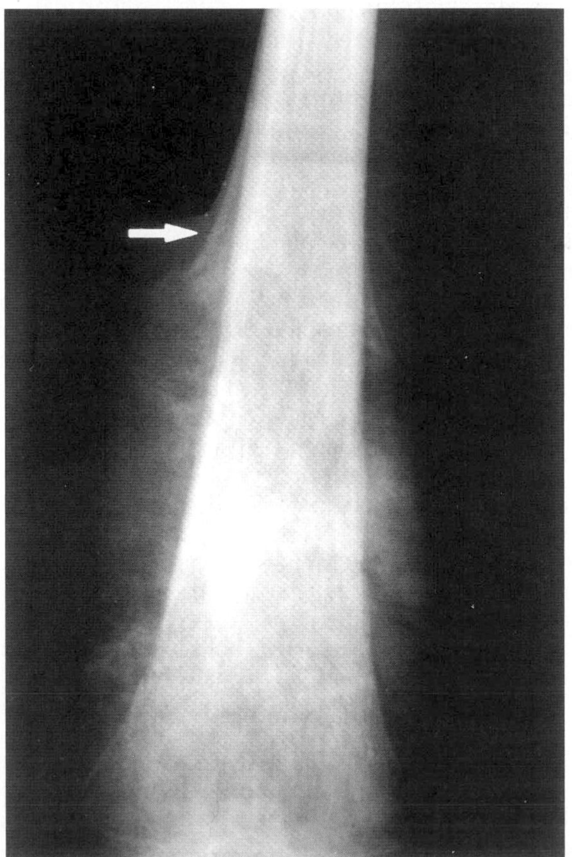

Figure 26-23 Distal femoral osteosarcoma with prominent bone formation extending into the soft tissues. The periosteum, which has been lifted, has laid down a proximal triangular shell of reactive bone known as a Codman triangle *(arrow)*.

well-known tumor suppressors and oncogenes, including the following:

- *RB*, which you will recall is a critical negative regulator of the cell cycle. Patients with germline mutations in *RB* have a 1000-fold increased risk of osteosarcoma and *RB* mutations are present in up to 70% of sporadic osteosarcomas.
- *TP53*, a gene whose product functions as the guardian of genomic integrity by promoting DNA repair and apoptosis of irreversibly damaged cells (Chapter 7): Patients with Li-Fraumeni syndrome, who have germline *TP53* gene mutations, have greatly elevated incidence of this tumor, and abnormalities that interfere with p53 function are common in sporadic tumors.
- *INK4a* is inactivated in many osteosarcomas. You will recall that this gene encodes two tumor suppressors, p16 (a negative regulator of cyclin-dependent kinases) and p14 (which augments p53 function).
- *MDM2* and *CDK4*, which are cell cycle regulators that inhibit into p53 and RB function, respectively, are overexpressed in many low-grade osteosarcomas, often through chromosomal amplification of region 12q13-q15.

It is also noteworthy that osteosarcomas peak in incidence around the time of the adolescent growth spurt and occur most frequently in the region of the growth plate in bones with the fastest growth. The increased proliferation at these sites may predispose to mutations that drive osteosarcoma development.

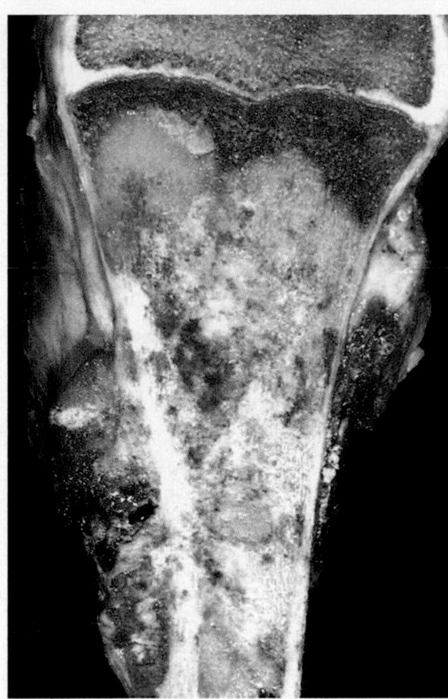

Figure 26-24 Osteosarcoma of the proximal tibia. The tan-white tumor fills most of the medullary cavity of the metaphysis and proximal diaphysis. It has infiltrated through the cortex, lifted the periosteum, and formed soft tissue masses on both sides of the bone.

MORPHOLOGY

Several subtypes of osteosarcoma are recognized and are grouped according to:

- Site of origin (intramedullary, intracortical, or surface)
- Histologic grade (low, high)
- Primary (underlying bone is unremarkable) or secondary to preexisting disorders (benign tumors, Paget disease, bone infarcts, previous radiation)
- Histologic features (osteoblastic, chondroblastic, fibroblastic, telangiectatic, small cell, and giant cell)

The most common subtype arises in the metaphysis of long bones and is primary, intramedullary, osteoblastic, and high grade.

Osteosarcomas are bulky tumors that are gritty, gray-white, and often contain areas of hemorrhage and cystic degeneration (Fig. 26-24). The tumors frequently destroy the surrounding cortices and produce soft tissue masses. They spread extensively in the medullary canal, infiltrating and replacing hematopoietic marrow. Infrequently, they penetrate the epiphyseal plate or enter the joint. When joint invasion occurs, the tumor grows into it along tendoligamentous structures or through the attachment site of the joint capsule.

The tumor cells vary in size and shape and frequently have large hyperchromatic nuclei. Bizarre tumor giant cells are common, as are mitoses, some of them abnormal (e.g. tripolar). Vascular invasion is usually conspicuous, and some tumors also exhibit extensive necrosis. **The formation of bone by the tumor cells is diagnostic** (Fig. 26-25). The neoplastic bone usually has a fine, lace-like architecture but also may be deposited in broad sheets or as primitive trabeculae. In addition to bone, tumor cells may produce cartilage or fibrous tissue, but these are not required for diagnosis. When malignant cartilage is abundant, the tumor is called **chondroblastic osteosarcoma**.

Clinical Course. Osteosarcoma is treated with a multimodality approach that includes neoadjuvant chemotherapy, which is given under the assumption that all patients have occult metastases at the time of diagnosis, followed by surgery. The prognosis of osteosarcoma has improved substantially since the advent of chemotherapy, with 5-year survival rates reaching 60% to 70% in patients without overt metastases at initial diagnosis. These aggressive neoplasms spread hematogenously to the lungs. At the time of diagnosis, approximately 10% to 20% of affected individuals have demonstrable pulmonary metastases; of

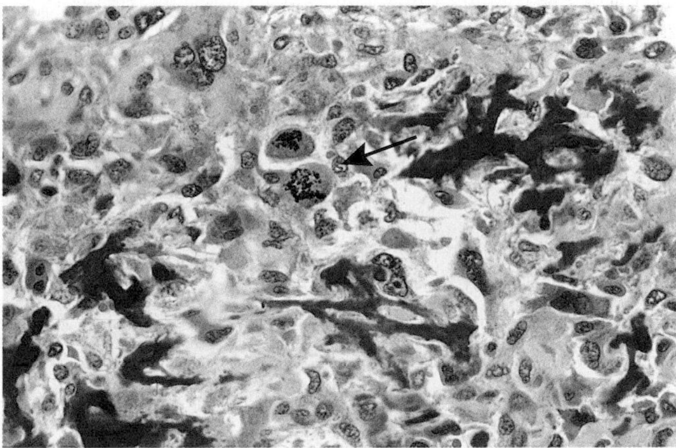

Figure 26-25 Fine, lacelike pattern of neoplastic bone produced by anaplastic malignant tumor cells in an osteosarcoma. Note the abnormal mitotic figures (arrow).

those who die of the neoplasm, 90% have metastases to the lungs, bones, brain, and elsewhere. Unfortunately, the outcome for patients with metastases, recurrent disease or secondary osteosarcoma is still poor (<20% 5-year survival rate).

Cartilage-Forming Tumors

Although osteosarcoma is the most common primary malignant tumor of the bones, cartilage tumors account for the majority of primary bone tumors (both benign and malignant). They are characterized by the formation of hyaline or myxoid cartilage; fibrocartilage and elastic cartilage are rare components. As in most types of bone tumors, benign cartilage tumors are much more common than malignant ones.

Osteochondroma

Osteochondroma, also known as an *exostosis*, is a benign cartilage-capped tumor that is attached to the underlying skeleton by a bony stalk. It is the most common benign bone tumor; about 85% are solitary. The remainder is seen as part of the *multiple hereditary exostosis syndrome*, which is an autosomal dominant hereditary disease. Solitary osteochondromas are usually first diagnosed in late adolescence and early adulthood, but multiple osteochondromas become apparent during childhood. Men are affected three times more often than women. Osteochondromas develop only in bones of endochondral origin and arise from the metaphysis near the growth plate of long tubular bones, especially near the knee. Occasionally, they develop from bones of the pelvis, scapula, and ribs, and in these sites they are frequently sessile and have short stalks. Osteochondromas present as slow-growing masses, which can be painful if they impinge on a nerve or if the stalk is fractured. In many cases they are detected incidentally. In multiple hereditary exostosis the underlying bones may be bowed and shortened, reflecting an associated disturbance in epiphyseal growth.

Pathogenesis. Hereditary exostoses are associated with germline loss-of-function mutations in either the *EXT1* or the *EXT2* gene and subsequent loss of the remaining wild type allele in chondrocytes of the growth plate. Reduced expression of EXT1 or EXT2 has also been observed in sporadic osteochondromas. These genes encode enzymes that synthesize heparan sulfate glycosaminoglycans. The reduced or abnormal glycosaminoglycans may prevent normal diffusion of the factor Indian hedgehog (Ihh), a local regulator of cartilage growth, thereby disrupting chondrocyte differentiation and local skeletal development.

MORPHOLOGY

Osteochondromas are sessile or pedunculated, and range in size from 1 to 20 cm. The cap is composed of benign hyaline cartilage varying in thickness (Fig. 26-26) and is covered peripherally by perichondrium. The cartilage has the appearance of disorganized growth plate and undergoes enchondral ossification, with the newly made bone forming the inner portion of the head and stalk. The cortex of the stalk merges with the cortex of the host bone, so that the medullary cavity of the osteochondroma and bone from which it arises are in continuity.

Clinical Course. Osteochondromas usually stop growing at the time of growth plate closure (Fig. 26-27). Symptomatic tumors are cured by simple excision. Rarely in sporadic cases, but more commonly in those with multiple hereditary exostosis (5% to 20%), osteochondromas progress to chondrosarcoma.

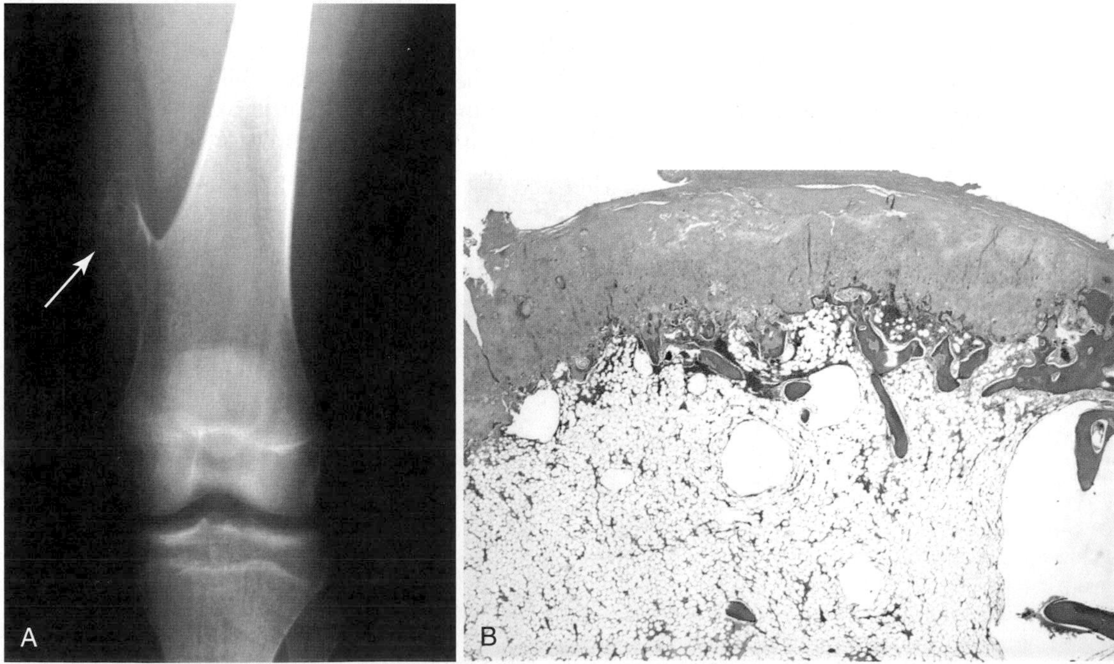

Figure 26-26 Osteochondroma. **A,** Radiograph of an osteochondroma arising from the distal femur (arrow). **B,** The cartilage cap has the histologic appearance of disorganized growth plate-like cartilage.

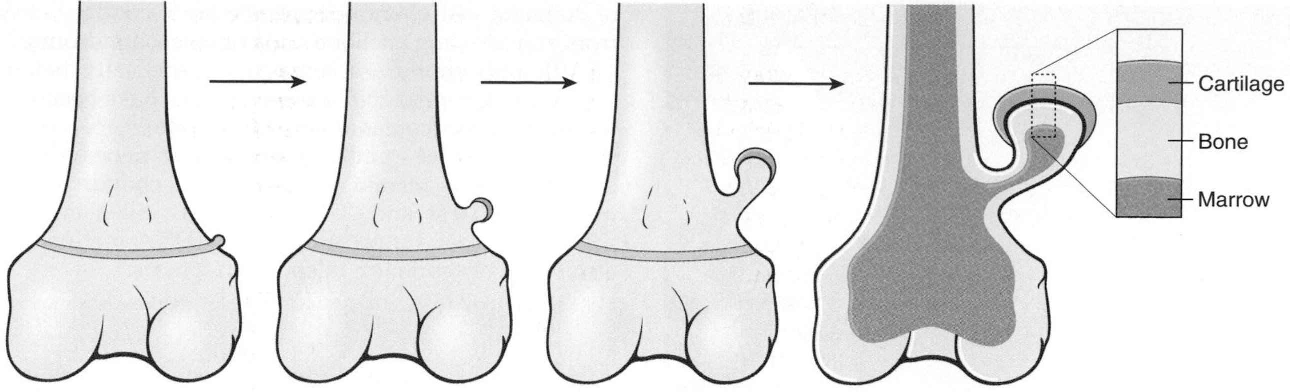

Figure 26-27 The development of an osteochondroma, beginning with an outgrowth from the epiphyseal cartilage.

Chondromas

Chondromas are benign tumors of hyaline cartilage that usually occur in bones of enchondral origin. They can arise within the medullary cavity, where they are known as *enchondromas*, or on the surface of bone, where they are called *juxtacortical chondromas*. Enchondromas are the most common of the intraosseous cartilage tumors and are usually diagnosed in individuals 20 to 50 years of age. Typically, they appear as solitary metaphyseal lesions of tubular bones of the hands and feet. The radiographic features consist of circumscribed lucencies with central irregular calcifications, a sclerotic rim and an intact cortex (Fig. 26-28). *Ollier disease* and *Maffucci syndrome* are nonhereditary disorders characterized by multiple enchondromas. *Maffucci syndrome* is, in addition, distinguished by presence of spindle cell hemangiomas.

Most enchondromas of large bones are asymptomatic and are detected incidentally. Occasionally, they are painful and cause pathologic fracture. The tumors in enchondromatosis may be numerous and large, producing severe deformities.

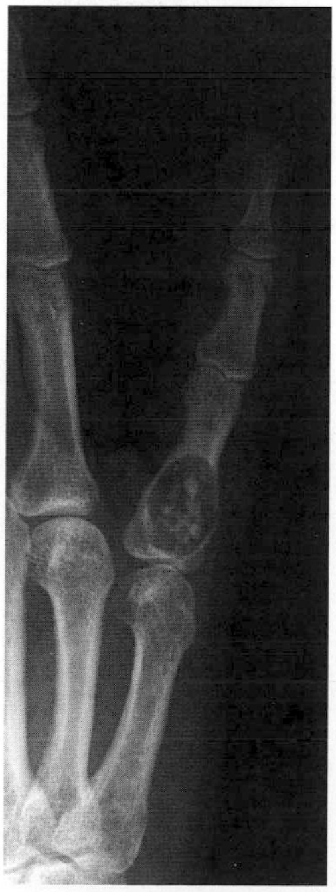

Figure 26-28 Enchondroma of the proximal phalanx. The radiolucent nodule of cartilage with central calcification thins but does not penetrate the cortex.

Pathogenesis. Heterozygous mutations in the *IDH1* and *IDH2* genes have been identified in the chondrocytes of syndromic and solitary enchondromas. Patients with enchondroma syndromes are mosaics, harboring IDH mutations in only a subset of otherwise normal cells throughout their bodies. Similarly, IDH mutations are found in only a subset of tumor cells in both syndromic and sporadic enchondromas. This unusual situation may be explained by the functional consequences of the IDH1 and IDH2 mutations. Both cause the encoded proteins, two isoforms of the enzyme isocitrate dehydrogenase, to acquire a new enzymatic activity that leads to the synthesis of 2-hydroxyglutarate. You will recall from Chapter 7 that this so-called "oncometabolite" interferes with regulation of DNA methylation. It is hypothesized that the 2-hydroxyglutarate produced by the subset of IDH-mutated cells in enchondromas diffuses into neighboring cells with normal IDH genes, thereby causing oncogenic epigenetic changes in genetically normal neighbors (transformation by association).

MORPHOLOGY

Enchondromas are usually smaller than 3 cm and are gray-blue and translucent. They are composed of well-circumscribed nodules of hyaline cartilage containing cytomorphologically benign chondrocytes (Fig. 26-29). The peripheral portion of the nodules may undergo enchondral ossification, and the center can calcify and infarct. The enchondromas in Ollier disease and Maffucci syndrome are sometimes more cellular than sporadic enchondromas and exhibit cytologic atypia, making them more difficult to distinguish from chondrosarcomas.

Clinical Course. The growth potential of chondromas is limited. Treatment depends on the clinical situation and is usually observation or curettage. Solitary chondromas rarely undergo sarcomatous transformation, but those associated with enchondromatosis do so more frequently. Individuals with Maffucci syndrome are also at risk of developing other types of malignancies, including ovarian carcinomas and brain gliomas.

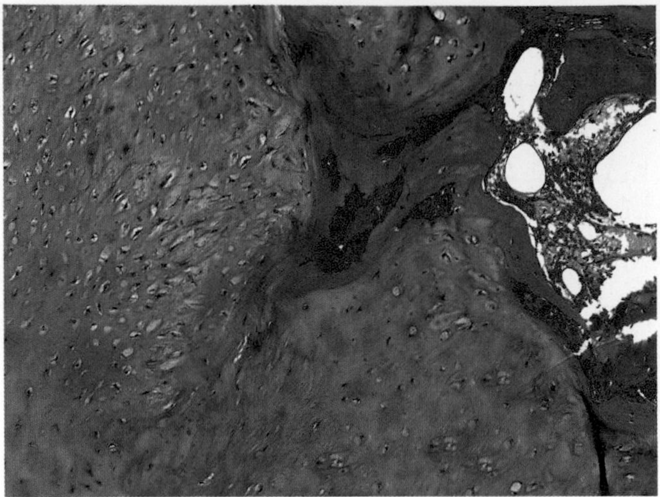

Figure 26-29 Enchondroma composed of a nodule of hyaline cartilage encased by a thin layer of reactive bone.

Chondrosarcoma

Chondrosarcomas are malignant tumors that produce cartilage. They are subclassified histologically as *conventional* (hyaline cartilage producing), *clear cell*, *dedifferentiated*, and *mesenchymal* variants. Conventional tumors are further subdivided by site as *central* (intramedullary) and *peripheral* (juxtacortical). Conventional central tumors constitute about 90% of chondrosarcomas. Chondrosarcoma is about half as common as osteosarcoma and is the second most common malignant matrix-producing tumor of bone. Individuals with chondrosarcoma are usually in their 40s or older. The clear cell and especially the mesenchymal variants occur in younger patients, in their teens or 20s. These tumors affect men twice as frequently as women. Chondrosarcomas commonly arise in the axial skeleton, especially the pelvis, shoulder, and ribs. Unlike benign enchondroma, the distal extremities are rarely involved. On imaging, the calcified matrix appears as foci of flocculent densities. A slow-growing, low-grade tumor causes reactive thickening of the cortex, whereas a more aggressive high-grade neoplasm destroys the cortex and forms a soft tissue mass. The clear cell variant is unique in that it originates in the epiphyses of long tubular bones. About 15% of conventional chondrosarcomas are secondary, arising from a preexisting enchondroma or osteochondroma.

Although chondrosarcomas are genetically heterogeneous, a few reproducible abnormalities have been identified. Chondrosarcomas arising in multiple osteochondroma syndrome exhibit mutations in the *EXT* genes, and both chondromatosis-related and sporadic chondrosarcomas may have *IDH1* and *IDH2* mutations. Silencing of the *CDKN2A* tumor suppressor gene by DNA methylation is also relatively common in sporadic tumors.

MORPHOLOGY

Conventional chondrosarcomas are large bulky tumors made up of nodules of glistening gray-white, translucent cartilage but matrix is often gelatinous or myxoid (Fig. 26-30*A*). The myxoid matrix can ooze from the cut surface. Spotty calcifications are typically present, and central necrosis may create cystic spaces. The tumor spreads through the cortex into surrounding muscle or fat. Histologically, the cartilage infiltrates the marrow space and surrounds pre-existing bony trabeculae. The tumors vary in cellularity, cytologic atypia, and mitotic activity and are assigned a grade from 1 to 3. Grade 1 tumors have relatively low cellularity, and the chondrocytes have plump vesicular nuclei with small nucleoli. By contrast, grade 3 chondrosarcomas are characterized by high cellularity, extreme pleomorphism with bizarre tumor giant cells, and mitoses (Fig. 26-30*B*).

Dedifferentiated chondrosarcoma is defined as a low-grade chondrosarcoma with a second, high-grade component that does not produce cartilage. **Clear cell chondrosarcoma** contains sheets of large, malignant chondrocytes that have abundant clear cytoplasm, numerous osteoclast-type giant cells, and intralesional reactive bone formation, which often causes confusion with osteosarcoma. **Mesenchymal chondrosarcoma** is composed of islands of well-differentiated hyaline cartilage surrounded by sheets of small round cells, which can mimic Ewing sarcoma.

Clinical Course. Chondrosarcomas usually present as painful, progressively enlarging masses. There is a direct correlation between the grade and the biologic behavior of the tumor. Fortunately, most conventional chondrosarcomas are grade 1 tumors with 5-year survival rates of 80% to 90% (versus 43% for grade 3 tumors). Grade 1

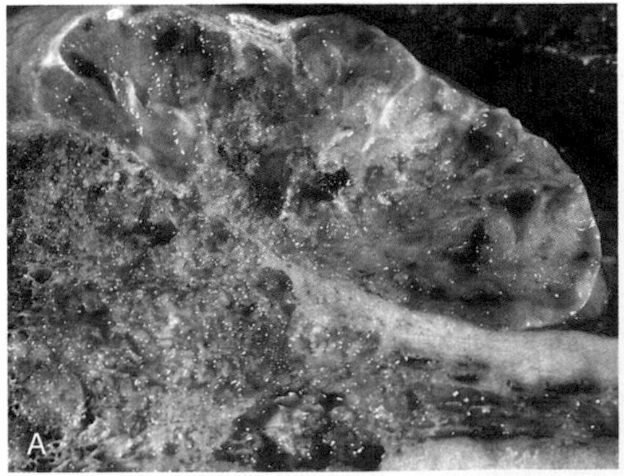

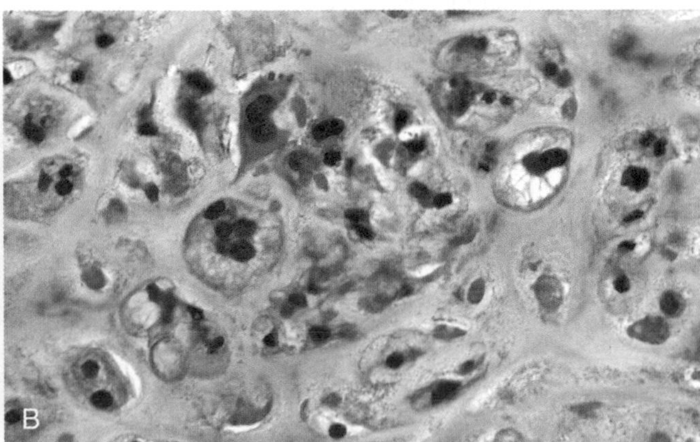

Figure 26-30 Chondrosarcoma. **A,** Nodules of hyaline and myxoid cartilage permeating throughout the medullary cavity, growing through the cortex, and forming a relatively well-circumscribed soft tissue mass. **B,** Anaplastic chondrocytes amid hyaline cartilage matrix in a grade 3 chondrosarcoma.

chondrosarcomas rarely metastasize, whereas 70% of grade 3 tumors spread hematogenously, especially to the lungs. The treatment of conventional chondrosarcoma is wide surgical excision. The mesenchymal and dedifferentiated tumors are also excised and additionally treated with chemotherapy because of their more aggressive clinical course.

Tumors of Unknown Origin

Ewing Sarcoma Family Tumors

Ewing sarcoma is a malignant bone tumor characterized by primitive round cells without obvious differentiation. Recently, Ewing sarcoma and **primitive neuroectodermal tumor** (PNET) have been unified into a single category: the **Ewing sarcoma family tumors** (ESFT) based on shared clinical, morphologic, biochemical and molecular features (discussed later). Although PNET demonstrates more neuroectodermal differentiation than Ewing sarcoma, the distinction is not clinically significant.

Ewing sarcoma family tumors account for approximately 6% to 10% of primary malignant bone tumors and follow osteosarcoma as the second most common group of bone sarcomas in children. Of all bone sarcomas, ESFT have the youngest average age at presentation, since approximately 80% are younger than 20 years. Boys are affected slightly more frequently than girls, and there is a striking predilection for whites; blacks and Asians are rarely afflicted. ESFT usually arise in the diaphysis of long tubular bones, especially the femur and the flat bones of the pelvis. They present as painful enlarging masses, and the affected site is frequently tender, warm, and swollen. Some affected individuals have systemic findings that mimic infection, including fever, elevated sedimentation rate, anemia, and leukocytosis. Plain radiographs show a destructive lytic tumor with permeative margins that extends into the surrounding soft tissues. The characteristic periosteal reaction produces layers of reactive bone deposited in an *onion-skin* fashion.

Pathogenesis. Most ESFT contain a (11;22) (q24;q12) translocation generating in-frame fusion of the *EWS* gene on chromosome 22 to the *FLI1* gene. Variant translocations fuse *EWS* to other members of the ETS transcription factor family. The exact fusion sites vary between tumors, leading to different downstream effects. How EWS fusion proteins contribute to transformation remains unsettled; effects on transcription, RNA splicing, and the cell cycle machinery have all been proposed. Similarly, the cell of origin still remains to be identified; the leading candidates are mesenchymal stem cells and primitive neurectodermal cells.

MORPHOLOGY

Arising in the medullary cavity, Ewing sarcoma usually invades the cortex, periosteum, and soft tissue. The tumor is soft, tan-white, and frequently contains areas of hemorrhage and necrosis. It is composed of sheets of uniform small, round cells that are slightly larger and more cohesive than lymphocytes (Fig. 26-31). They have scant cytoplasm, which may appear clear because it is rich in glycogen. The presence of Homer-Wright rosettes (round groupings of cells with a central fibrillary core) indicate a greater degree of neuroectodermal differentiation.

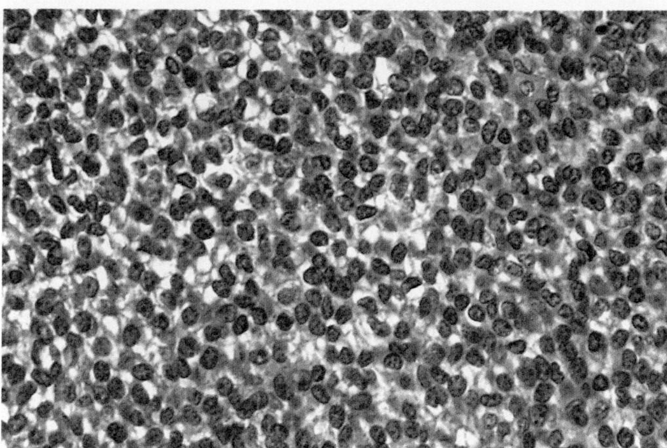

Figure 26-31 Ewing sarcoma composed of sheets of small round cells with small amounts of clear cytoplasm.

Although the tumor contains fibrous septae, there is generally little stroma. Geographic necrosis may be prominent, and there are relatively few mitotic figures in relation to the dense cellularity of the tumor.

Clinical Course. ESFT are aggressive malignancies treated with neoadjuvant chemotherapy followed by surgical excision with or without irradiation. The advent of effective chemotherapy has achieved 5-year survival of 75% and long-term cure in 50%. The amount of chemotherapy-induced necrosis is an important prognostic finding.

Giant Cell Tumor

Giant cell tumor is so named because the histology is dominated by multinucleated osteoclast-type giant cells, giving rise to the synonym **osteoclastoma**. It is a relatively uncommon benign, but locally aggressive, neoplasm. It usually arises in individuals in their 20s to 40s.

Pathogenesis. Current evidence suggests that the neoplastic cells of giant cell tumor are primitive osteoblast precursors but they represent only a minority of the tumor cells. The bulk of the tumor consists of non-neoplastic osteoclasts and their precursors. The neoplastic cells express high levels of RANKL, which promotes the proliferation of osteoclast precursors and their differentiation into mature osteoclasts via RANK expressed by these cells. However, the feedback between osteoblasts and osteoclasts that normally regulates this process during bone remodeling is absent. What results is a localized but highly destructive resorption of bone matrix by reactive osteoclasts.

Giant cell tumors arise in the epiphysis but may extend into the metaphysis. The majority arise around the knee (distal femur and proximal tibia), but virtually any bone can be involved. The typical location of these tumors near joints frequently causes arthritis-like symptoms. Occasionally, they present with pathologic fractures. Most are solitary; however, multicentric tumors do occur, especially in the distal extremities.

MORPHOLOGY

Giant cell tumors often destroy the overlying cortex, producing a bulging soft tissue mass delineated by a thin shell of reactive

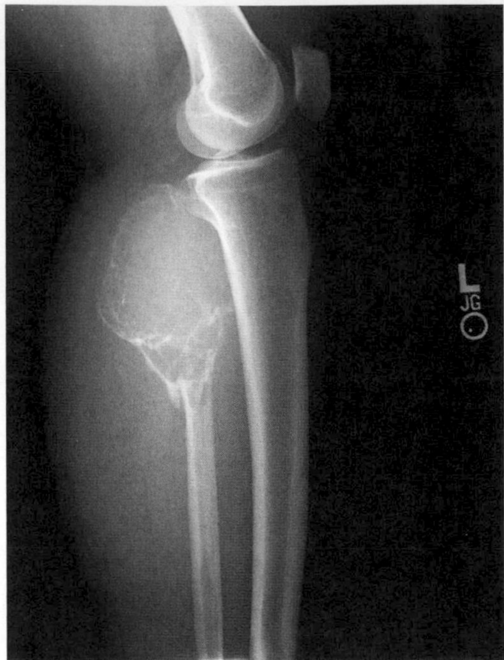

Figure 26-32 Giant cell tumor of the proximal fibula is predominantly lytic, expansile with destruction of the cortex. A pathologic fracture is also present.

bone (Fig. 26-32). These are large, red-brown masses that frequently undergo cystic degeneration. Histologically, the tumor consists of sheets of uniform oval mononuclear cells and numerous osteoclast-type giant cells with 100 or more nuclei (Fig. 26-33). The nuclei of the mononuclear cells and the osteoclasts are similar, ovoid with prominent nucleoli. Thus, the neoplastic population of osteoblast precursors is difficult to identify on routine histology. Necrosis and mitotic activity may be prominent. Although reactive bone, especially at the periphery of a lesion, may be present, the tumor cells do not synthesize bone or cartilage.

Clinical Course. Giant cell tumors are typically treated with curettage, but 40% to 60% recur locally. Up to 4% of tumors metastasize to the lungs, but these sometimes spontaneously regress and they are seldom fatal. Recently, the RANKL inhibitor, denosumab has shown promise as an adjuvant therapy in giant cell tumor.

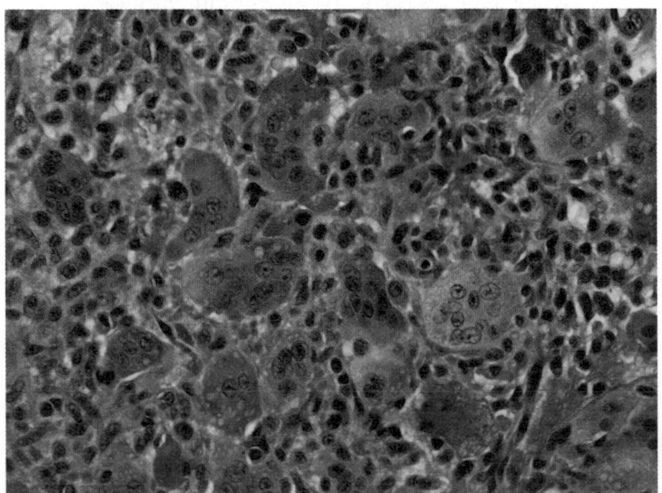

Figure 26-33 Benign giant cell tumor illustrating an abundance of multinucleated giant cells with background mononuclear stromal cells.

Aneurysmal Bone Cyst

Aneurysmal bone cyst (ABC) is a tumor characterized by multiloculated blood-filled cystic spaces. Interestingly, radiographic and histologic findings typical of ABC can also be seen as a secondary reaction to other primary bone tumors. Primary ABC affects all age groups but generally occurs during the first 2 decades of life and has no sex predilection. It most frequently develops in the metaphysis of long bones and the posterior elements of vertebral bodies. The most common signs and symptoms are pain and swelling. When an ABC involves the vertebrae, it can compress nerves and cause neurologic symptoms. Rarely, pathologic fractures occur. Secondary ABC can be present in the setting of a number of primary neoplasms, especially giant cell tumor and chondroblastoma.

Radiographically, ABC is usually an eccentric, expansile lesion with well-defined margins (Fig. 26-34*A*). Most lesions are completely lytic and often contain a thin shell of reactive bone at the periphery. Computed tomography and magnetic resonance imaging may demonstrate internal septa and characteristic fluid-fluid levels (Fig. 26-34*B*).

Pathogenesis. The spindle cells of ABC frequently demonstrate rearrangements of chromosome 17p13 resulting in fusion of the coding region of *USP6* to the promoters of genes that are highly expressed in osteoblasts, leading to USP6 overexpression. *USP6* encodes an ubiquitin specific protease that regulates the activity of the transcription factor NFκB. Increased NFκB activity appears to upregulate genes such as matrix metalloproteases that lead to cystic resorption of bone. Secondary ABCs do not have *USP6* rearrangements and appear to be triggered by epigenetic mechanisms.

MORPHOLOGY

Aneurysmal bone cyst consists of multiple blood-filled cystic spaces separated by thin, tan-white septa (Fig. 26-35). The septa are composed of plump uniform fibroblasts, multinucleated osteoclast-like giant cells, and reactive woven bone. The bone is lined by osteoblasts, and its deposition typically follows the contours of the fibrous septa. Approximately one third of cases contain an unusual densely calcified matrix called "blue bone." Necrosis is uncommon unless a pathologic fracture is present.

Clinical Course. The treatment of aneurysmal bone cyst is surgical, usually curettage or, in certain situations, en bloc resection. The recurrence rate is low, and spontaneous regression may occur following incomplete removal.

Lesions Simulating Primary Neoplasms

Fibrous Cortical Defect and Nonossifying Fibroma

Fibrous cortical defects (also known as **metaphyseal fibrous defects**) are extremely common, present in 30% to 50% of children older than 2 years. The vast majority arise eccentrically in the metaphysis of the distal femur and proximal tibia, and almost half are bilateral or multiple. Often they are small, about 0.5 cm in diameter. Those that

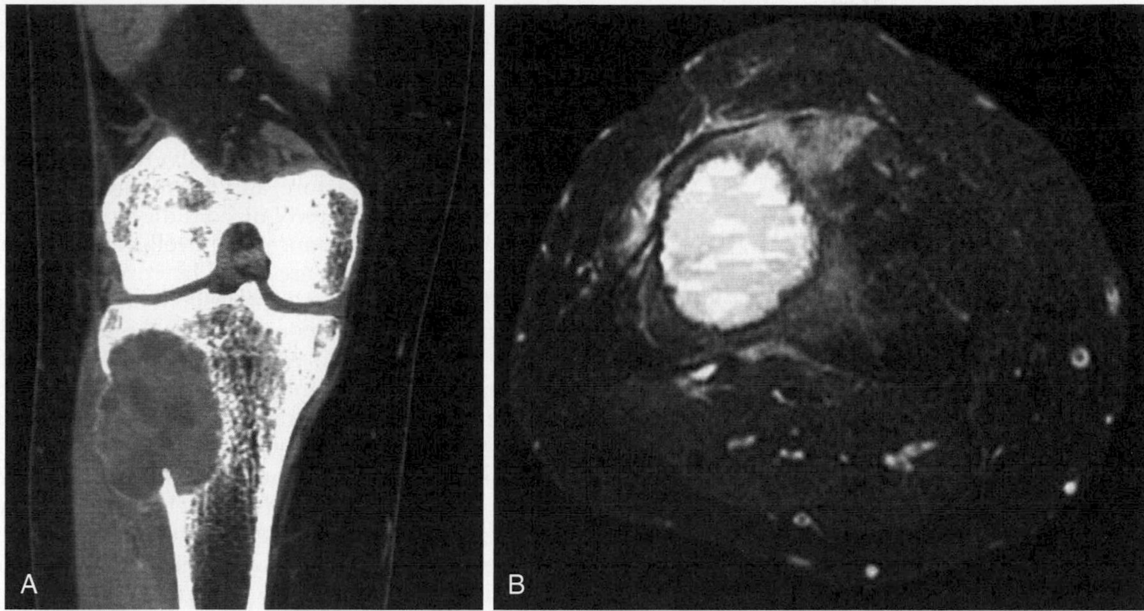

Figure 26-34 **A,** Coronal computed axial tomography scan showing eccentric aneurysmal bone cyst of tibia. The soft tissue component is delineated by a thin rim of reactive subperiosteal bone. **B,** Axial magnetic resonance image demonstrating characteristic fluid-fluid levels.

grow to 5 or 6 cm in size are classified as **nonossifying fibromas**; these are usually not detected until adolescence or adulthood.

MORPHOLOGY

Both fibrous cortical defect and nonossifying fibroma produce sharply demarcated radiolucencies with a long axis of a bone parallel to the cortex, surrounded by a thin rim of sclerosis (Fig. 26-36). They consist of gray to yellow-brown cellular lesions containing fibroblasts and macrophages. The cytologically bland fibroblasts are frequently arranged in a storiform (pinwheel) pattern, and the macrophages may take the form of clustered cells with foamy cytoplasm or multinucleated giant cells (Fig. 26-37). Hemosiderin is commonly present.

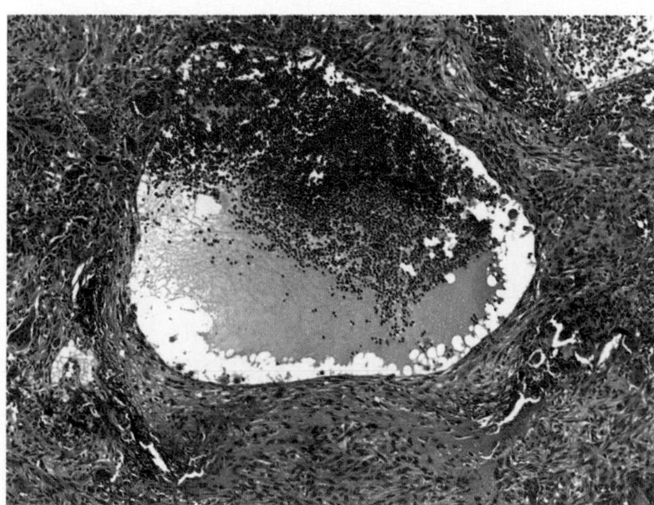

Figure 26-35 Aneurysmal bone cyst with blood-filled cystic space surrounded by a fibrous wall containing proliferating fibroblasts, reactive woven bone, and osteoclast-type giant cells.

Fibrous cortical defects are asymptomatic and are detected incidentally on radiographic studies. The findings are sufficiently specific on plain radiography that biopsy is rarely necessary. Most fibrous cortical defects have limited growth potential and undergo spontaneous resolution within several years, being replaced by normal cortical bone. The few that progressively enlarge into nonossifying fibromas may present with pathologic fracture or require biopsy and curettage to exclude other types of tumors.

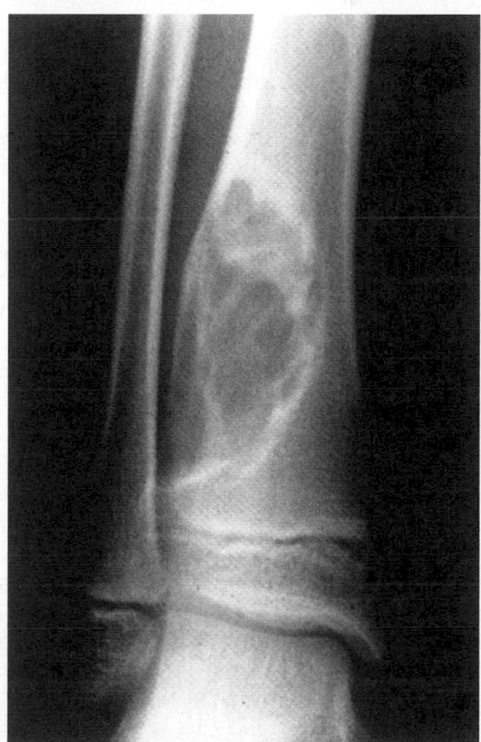

Figure 26-36 Nonossifying fibroma of the distal tibial metaphysis producing an eccentric lobulated radiolucency surrounded by a sclerotic margin.

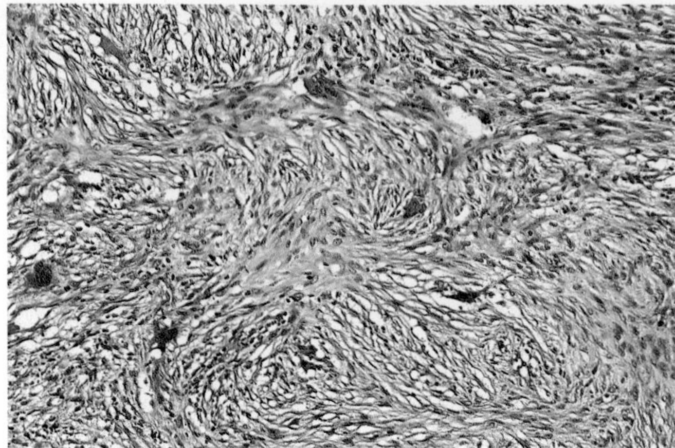

Figure 26-37 Storiform pattern created by benign spindle cells with scattered osteoclast-type giant cells characteristic of a fibrous cortical defect and nonossifying fibroma.

Fibrous Dysplasia

Fibrous dysplasia is a benign tumor that has been likened to a localized developmental arrest; all of the components of normal bone are present, but they do not differentiate into mature structures. The lesions arise during skeletal development, and appear in several distinctive but sometimes overlapping clinical patterns:

- Monostotic: involvement of a single bone
- Polyostotic: involvement of multiple bones
- *Mazabraud syndrome*: fibrous dysplasia (usually polyostotic) and soft tissue myxomas
- *McCune-Albright syndrome*: polyostotic disease, associated with café-au-lait skin pigmentations and endocrine abnormalities, especially precocious puberty.

Pathogenesis. All of the above manifestations result from a somatic gain-of-function mutation during development in *GNAS1*, the gene that is also mutated in pituitary adenomas (Chapter 24). The mutations produce a constitutively active G_s-protein that promotes cellular proliferation. The extent of phenotype depends on (1) the stage of embryogenesis when the mutation is acquired and (2) the fate of the cell harboring the mutation. At one extreme, a mutation during embryogenesis produces the McCune-Albright syndrome while a mutation in an osteoblast precursor, during or after formation of the skeleton, results in monostotic fibrous dysplasia. The skeletal manifestations arise from G_s-cAMP mediated interruption of normal osteoblast differentiation from precursors.

MORPHOLOGY

The lesions of fibrous dysplasia are well circumscribed, intramedullary, and vary greatly in size. Larger lesions expand and distort the bone. The lesional tissue is tan-white and gritty and is composed of curvilinear trabeculae of woven bone surrounded by a moderately cellular fibroblastic proliferation. The curvilinear shapes of the trabeculae mimic Chinese characters, and the bone lacks prominent osteoblastic rimming (Fig. 26-38). Nodules of hyaline cartilage with the appearance of disorganized growth plate are also present in approximately 20% of cases. Cystic degeneration, hemorrhage, and foamy macrophages are other common findings.

Clinical Course. Monostotic fibrous dysplasia occurs equally in boys and girls, usually in early adolescence, and often stops enlarging at the time of growth plate closure. The femur, tibia, ribs, jawbones, calvarium, and humerus are most commonly affected. The lesion is frequently asymptomatic and usually discovered incidentally but it may cause pain, fracture, and discrepancies in limb length. The lesion is readily recognized radiologically by its typical ground-glass appearance and well-defined margination. Symptomatic lesions are cured by curettage.

Polyostotic fibrous dysplasia manifests at a slightly earlier age than the monostotic type and may continue to cause problems into adulthood. The bones affected, in descending order of frequency, are the femur, skull, tibia, humerus, ribs, fibula, radius, ulna, mandible, and vertebrae. Craniofacial involvement is present in 50% of those who have a moderate number of bones affected and in 100% of those with extensive skeletal disease. Polyostotic disease has a propensity to involve the shoulder and pelvic girdles, resulting in severe, progressive disease including crippling deformities and fractures. Patients may require multiple corrective orthopedic surgical procedures. Bisphosphonates can be used to reduce the severity of the bone pain. A rare complication, usually in the setting of polyostotic involvement, is malignant transformation of a lesion into a sarcoma.

Mazabraud syndrome presents with skeletal features of polyostotic fibrous dysplasia with multiple skeletal deformities identified in childhood. The intramuscular myxomas present in adulthood often in the same anatomic region as existing fibrous dysplasia. Although benign, these tumors can cause local compression symptoms or further deformity to a limb but are cured by surgical excision.

The most common clinical presentation of *McCune-Albright syndrome* is precocious sexual development, which occurs most often in girls. The syndrome can include other endocrinopathies such as hyperthyroidism, pituitary adenomas that secrete growth hormone, and primary adrenal hyperplasia. The bone lesions are often unilateral, and the skin pigmentation is usually limited to the same side of the body. The cutaneous macules are classically large; dark to

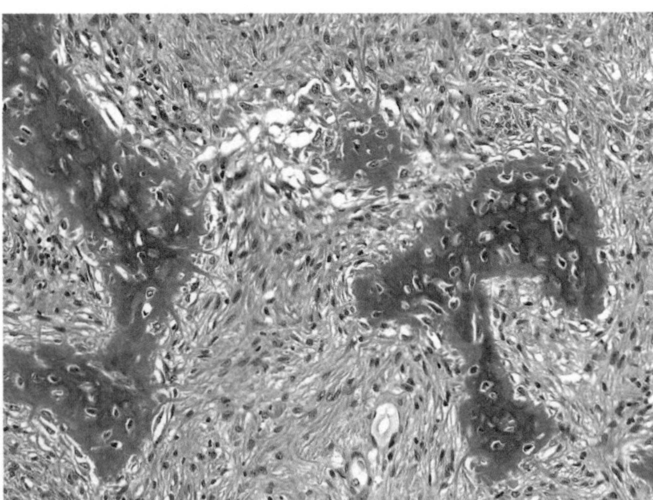

Figure 26-38 Fibrous dysplasia composed of curvilinear trabeculae of woven bone that lack conspicuous osteoblastic rimming and arise in a background of fibrous tissue.

café-au-lait in color; have irregular serpiginous borders; and are found primarily on the neck, chest, back, shoulder, and pelvic region. The skeletal manifestations are managed as for other polyostotic fibrous dysplasia while the endocrinopathies are treated medically, for example with aromatase inhibitors for precocious puberty.

Metastatic Tumors

Metastatic tumors are the most common form of skeletal malignancy, greatly outnumbering primary bone cancers. The pathways of spread include (1) direct extension, (2) lymphatic or hematogenous dissemination, and (3) intraspinal seeding (via the Batson plexus of veins). Any cancer can spread to bone, but in adults more than 75% of skeletal metastases originate from cancers of the prostate, breast, kidney, and lung. In children, metastases to bone originate from neuroblastoma, Wilms tumor, osteosarcoma, Ewing sarcoma, and rhabdomyosarcoma.

Skeletal metastases are typically multifocal. However, carcinomas of the kidney and thyroid may present with solitary lesions. Most metastases involve the axial skeleton (vertebral column, pelvis, ribs, skull, and sternum). The red marrow in these areas, with its rich capillary network and slow blood flow, facilitates implantation and growth of the tumor cells. Metastases to the small bones of the hands and feet are uncommon and usually originate from cancers of the lung, kidney, or colon.

The radiographic appearance of metastases may be purely *lytic* (bone destroying), purely *blastic* (bone forming), or *mixed* lytic and blastic. Furthermore, some cancers are associated with predominantly one pattern or the other. For example, prostatic adenocarcinoma is predominantly blastic whereas carcinomas of the kidney, lung, and gastrointestinal tract and malignant melanoma produce lytic lesions. Bidirectional interactions between metastatic cancer cells and native bone cells account for the changes that manifest in the bone matrix. Tumor cells do not directly resorb bone in lytic lesions. Rather, they secrete substances such as prostaglandins, cytokines, and PTHrP that upregulate RANKL on osteoblasts and stromal cells thereby stimulating osteoclast activity. At the same time, tumor cell growth is supported by the release of matrix-bound growth factors (e.g., TGF-β, IGF-1, and FGF) as bone is resorbed. Sclerotic metastases may be produced by tumor cells secreting WNT proteins that stimulate osteoblastic bone formation.

The presence of bone metastases unfortunately carries a dim prognosis since it indicates wide dissemination of the cancer. Treatment strategies aim at managing symptoms and limiting further spread. Therapeutic options include systemic chemotherapy, localized radiation and bisphosphonates. Surgery may be necessary to stabilize pathologic fractures.

KEY CONCEPTS

Bone Tumors and Tumor-Like Lesions

Primary bone tumors are classified according to the normal cell or matrix they produce. The remainder is grouped according to clinicopathologic features. Most primary bone tumors are benign. Metastases, especially adenocarcinomas, are more common than primary bone neoplasms.

Major categories of primary bone tumors include:

- **Bone forming:** Osteoblastoma and osteoid osteoma consist of benign osteoblasts that synthesize osteoid. Osteosarcoma is a tumor of malignant osteoblasts, predominantly involving adolescents with an aggressive clinical course.
- **Cartilage forming:** Osteochondroma is a polypoid exostosis with a cartilage cap. Sporadic and syndromic forms arise from mutations in the *EXT* genes. Chondromas are benign intramedullary tumors producing hyaline cartilage, usually arising in the digits. Chondrosarcomas are malignant tumors of cartilage, involving the axial skeleton in adults.
- **Ewing sarcoma family of tumors** consists of are aggressive malignant small round cell tumors most often associated with t(11;22).
- **Fibrous cortical defect** and **fibrous dysplasia** are unusual examples of disorders caused by gain-of-function mutations that occur during development

JOINTS

Joints allow movement while providing mechanical stability. They are classified as *solid (nonsynovial)* and *cavitated (synovial)*. The solid joints, also known as *synarthroses*, provide structural integrity and allow only minimal movement. They lack a joint space and are grouped according to the type of connective tissue (fibrous tissue or cartilage) that bridges the ends of the bones. Fibrous synarthroses include the cranial sutures and the bonds between roots of teeth and the jawbones. Cartilaginous synarthroses (synchondroses) are represented by the symphyses (manubriosternalis and pubic). Synovial joints, in contrast, have a joint space that allows for a wide range of motion. Situated between the ends of bones formed via enchondral ossification, they are strengthened by a dense fibrous capsule reinforced by ligaments and muscles. The boundary of the joint space consists of the synovial membrane, which is firmly anchored to the underlying capsule and does not cover the articular surface. Its contour is smooth except near the osseous insertion, where it is thrown into numerous villous folds. Synovial membranes are lined by two types of cells that are arranged one to four layers deep. Type A synoviocytes are specialized macrophages with phagocytic activity. Type B synoviocytes are similar to fibroblasts and synthesize hyaluronic acid and various proteins. The synovial lining lacks a basement membrane, which allows for efficient exchange of nutrients, wastes, and gases between blood and synovial fluid. Synovial fluid is a plasma filtrate containing hyaluronic acid that acts as a viscous lubricant and provides nutrition for the articular hyaline cartilage.

Hyaline cartilage is a unique connective tissue ideally suited to serve as an elastic shock absorber and wear-resistant surface. It lacks a blood supply and does not have lymphatic drainage or innervation. Hyaline cartilage is composed of water (70%), type II collagen (10%), proteoglycans (8%), and chondrocytes. The collagen fibers enable the cartilage to resist tensile stresses and transmit vertical loads. The water and proteoglycans give hyaline cartilage its resistance to compression and have an important role in limiting friction. The chondrocytes synthesize the matrix as well as enzymatically digest it, with the half-life of the different components ranging from weeks (proteoglycans) to years (type II collagen). Chondrocytes secrete degradative enzymes in inactive forms and enrich the matrix with enzyme inhibitors. Diseases that destroy articular cartilage do so by activating the catabolic enzymes and decreasing the production of inhibitors, thereby accelerating the rate of matrix breakdown. Cytokines such as IL-1 and TNF trigger the degradative process; their sources include chondrocytes, synoviocytes, fibroblasts, and inflammatory cells. Destruction of articular cartilage by indigenous cells is an important mechanism in many joint diseases.

Osteoarthritis

Osteoarthritis, also called degenerative joint disease, is characterized by degeneration of cartilage that results in structural and functional failure of synovial joints. It is the most common type of joint disease. Annual costs from lost productivity and treatment of osteoarthritis in the United States are estimated to be more than 65 billion dollars. Although the term osteoarthritis implies an inflammatory disease, it is considered to be an intrinsic disease of cartilage in which chondrocytes respond to biochemical and mechanical stresses resulting in breakdown of the matrix.

In most instances osteoarthritis appears insidiously, without apparent initiating cause, as an aging phenomenon *(idiopathic* or *primary osteoarthritis)*. In these cases the disease is usually oligoarticular (affects few joints) but may be generalized. In about 5% of cases, osteoarthritis appears in younger individuals with some predisposing condition, such as joint deformity, a previous joint injury, or an underlying systemic disease such as diabetes, ochronosis, hemochromatosis, or marked obesity that places joints at risk. In these settings the disease is called *secondary osteoarthritis*. Gender has some influence on distribution. The knees and hands are more commonly affected in women and the hips in men.

Pathogenesis. **The lesions of osteoarthritis (OA) stem from degeneration of the articular cartilage and its disordered repair.** The articular cartilage contributes to the virtually frictionless movement of the joint while providing resistance to tension and compression, from type II collagen and proteoglycans, respectively, both synthesized by chondrocytes. Although historically OA was considered an inevitable process of wear and tear, this is an oversimplification, as the disease actually involves complex pathologic changes in chondrocytes and matrix.

The changes to chondrocytes can be divided into three phases: (1) chondrocyte injury, related to genetic and biochemical factors; (2) early OA, in which chondrocytes proliferate and secrete inflammatory mediators, collagens, proteoglycans, and proteases, which act together to remodel the cartilaginous matrix and initiate secondary inflammatory changes in the synovium and subchondral bone; and (3) late OA, in which repetitive injury and chronic inflammation lead to chondrocyte drop out, marked loss of cartilage, and extensive subchondral bone changes.

Virtually every extracellular component of articular cartilage is affected in OA. Collagen type II is degraded by matrix metalloproteinases. Although chondrocytes continuously synthesize and secrete proteoglycans during disease progression, degradation ultimately exceeds synthesis, and the composition of proteoglycans changes. Inflammatory cells are sparse, but cytokines and diffusible factors associated with other inflammatory conditions, particularly TGF-β (which induces matrix metalloproteinases), TNF, prostaglandins and nitric oxide, have been implicated in osteoarthritis.

Environmental and genetic influences contribute to the pathogenesis of OA. The major environmental factors relate to aging and biomechanical stress. The association with aging is strong; the prevalence of OA increases exponentially beyond the age of 50, and about 40% of people older than 70 are affected. Studies of families and twins have suggested that the risk of OA is the sum of multiple genes, each with a small effect. Candidate gene studies and genome-wide association studies show that OA is genetically heterogeneous.

MORPHOLOGY

In the early stages of osteoarthritis, the chondrocytes proliferate, forming clusters (so-called cloning). Concurrently, the water content of the matrix increases and the concentration of proteoglycans decreases. The normally horizontally arranged collagen type II fibers in the superficial zone are cleaved, yielding fissures and clefts at the articular surface (Fig. 26-39*A*). This manifests as a granular soft articular surface. Eventually, chondrocytes die and full-thickness portions of the cartilage are sloughed. The dislodged pieces of cartilage and subchondral bone tumble into the joint, forming loose bodies (joint mice). The exposed subchondral bone plate becomes the new articular surface, and friction with the opposing surface smooths and burnishes the exposed bone, giving it the appearance of polished ivory (bone eburnation) (Fig. 26-39*B*). There is rebuttressing and sclerosis of the underlying cancellous bone. Small fractures through the articulating bone are common, and the fracture gaps allow synovial fluid to be forced into the subchondral regions in a one-way, ball valve-like mechanism. The loculated fluid collection increases in size, forming fibrous-walled cysts. Mushroom-shaped osteophytes (bony outgrowths) develop at the margins of the articular surface and are capped by fibrocartilage and hyaline cartilage that gradually ossify. The synovium is usually only mildly congested and fibrotic, and may have scattered chronic inflammatory cells.

Clinical Course. Osteoarthritis is an insidious disease. Patients with primary disease are usually asymptomatic until they are in their 50s. If a young person has significant manifestations of osteoarthritis, a search for some underlying cause should be made. Characteristic symptoms include deep, achy pain that worsens with use, morning stiffness, crepitus, and limitation of range of movement. Impingement on spinal foramina by osteophytes results in cervical and lumbar nerve root compression and radicular pain, muscle

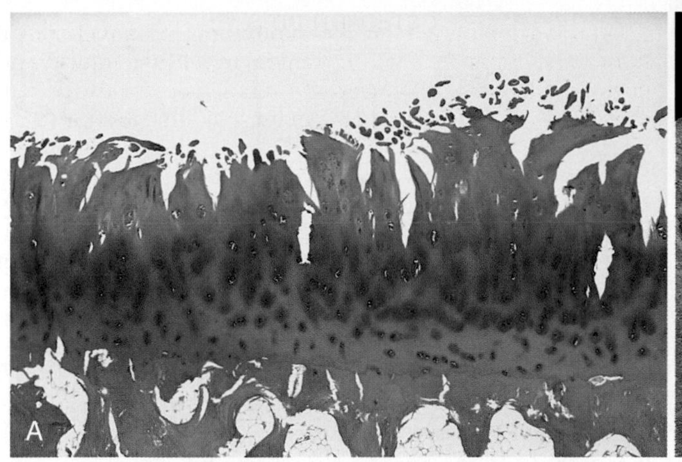

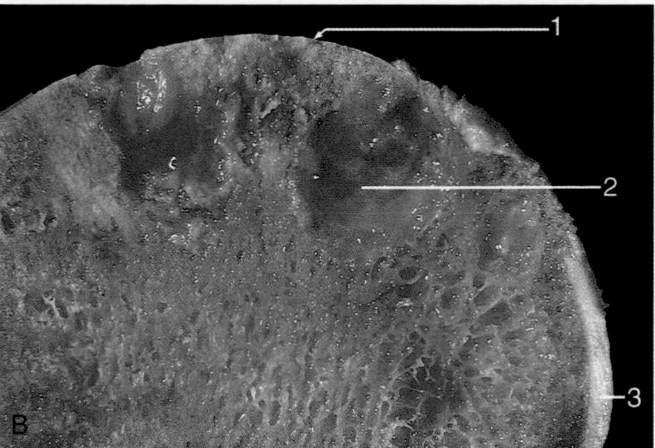

Figure 26-39 Osteoarthritis. **A,** Histologic demonstration of the characteristic fibrillation of the articular cartilage. **B,** Eburnated articular surface exposing subchondral bone (1), subchondral cyst (2) and residual articular cartilage (3).

spasms, muscle atrophy, and neurologic deficits. Typically, only one or a few joints are involved except in the uncommon generalized variant. The joints commonly involved include the hips (Fig. 26-40), knees, lower lumbar and cervical vertebrae, proximal and distal interphalangeal joints of the fingers, first carpometacarpal joints, and first tarsometatarsal joints. *Heberden nodes*, prominent osteophytes at the distal interphalangeal joints, are common in women (but not men). The wrists, elbows, and shoulders are usually spared. With time, joint deformity can occur, but unlike rheumatoid arthritis (discussed next), fusion does not take place (Fig. 26-41). The level of disease severity detected radiographically, however, does not correlate well with pain and disability. There are still no satisfactory means of preventing primary osteoarthritis, and there are no effective methods of halting its progression. Therapy includes management of pain, activity modification and, for severe cases, arthroplasty.

Figure 26-40 Severe osteoarthritis of the hip. The joint space is narrowed, and there is subchondral sclerosis with scattered oval radiolucent cysts and peripheral osteophyte lipping *(arrows)*.

Rheumatoid Arthritis

Rheumatoid arthritis (RA) is a chronic inflammatory disorder of autoimmune origin that may affect many tissues and organs but principally attacks the joints, producing a nonsuppurative proliferative and inflammatory synovitis. RA often progresses to destruction of the articular cartilage and ankylosis of the joints. Extraarticular lesions may involve skin, heart, blood vessels and lungs and, therefore, the clinical manifestations can resemble other systemic autoimmune disorders such as systemic lupus erythematosus or scleroderma. The prevalence in the United States is approximately 1%. The disease peaks in the second to fourth decades and is three times more common in women than men.

Pathogenesis. As in other autoimmune diseases, genetic predisposition and environmental factors contribute to the development, progression, and chronicity of the disease. The pathologic changes are mediated by antibodies against self-antigens and cytokine-mediated inflammation, predominantly secreted by CD4+ T-cells (Fig. 26-42).

CD4+ T helper (T_H) cells may initiate the autoimmune response in RA by reacting with an arthritogenic agent, perhaps microbial or a self-antigen. The T cells produce cytokines that stimulate other inflammatory cells to effect tissue injury. Although a large number of cytokines can be isolated from inflamed joints, the most important ones include:

- IFN-γ from T_H1 cells activates macrophages and resident synovial cells.
- IL-17 from T_H17 cells recruits neutrophils and monocytes.
- TNF and IL-1 from macrophages stimulates resident synovial cells to secrete proteases that destroy hyaline cartilage.
- RANKL expressed on activated T cells stimulates bone resorption.

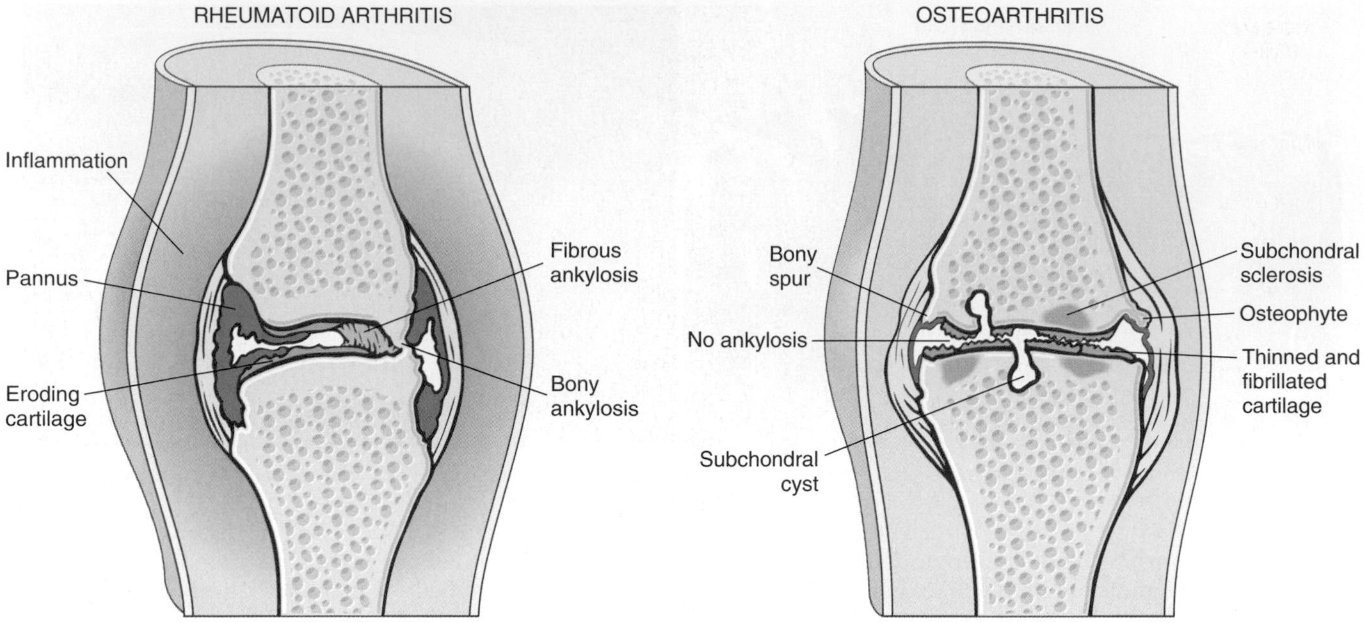

Figure 26-41 Comparison of the morphologic features of rheumatoid arthritis and osteoarthritis.

Of these, TNF has been most firmly implicated in the pathogenesis of RA and TNF antagonists have proved to be remarkable effective therapies for the disease (see later).

The synovium of RA contains germinal centers with secondary follicles and abundant plasma cells which produce antibodies, some of which are against self-antigens. Many of the autoantibodies produced in lymphoid organs and in the synovium are specific for *citrullinated peptides* (CCPs) in which arginine residues are post-translationally converted to citrulline. In RA, antigen-antibody complexes containing citrullinated fibrinogen, type II collagen, α-enolase and vimentin deposit in the joints. Antibodies against these peptides are diagnostic markers for the disease and may mediate joint injury. Evidence suggests that the raised levels of anti-CCP antibodies in combination with a T-cell response to the citrullinated proteins contribute to the disease becoming chronic. Additionally, about 80% of patients have serum IgM or IgA autoantibodies that bind to the F_c portions of their own IgG. These autoantibodies are called *rheumatoid factor* and may also deposit in joints as immune complexes although they are not uniformly present in all patients with RA and can be found in patients without the disease, so the link to pathogenesis is questionable.

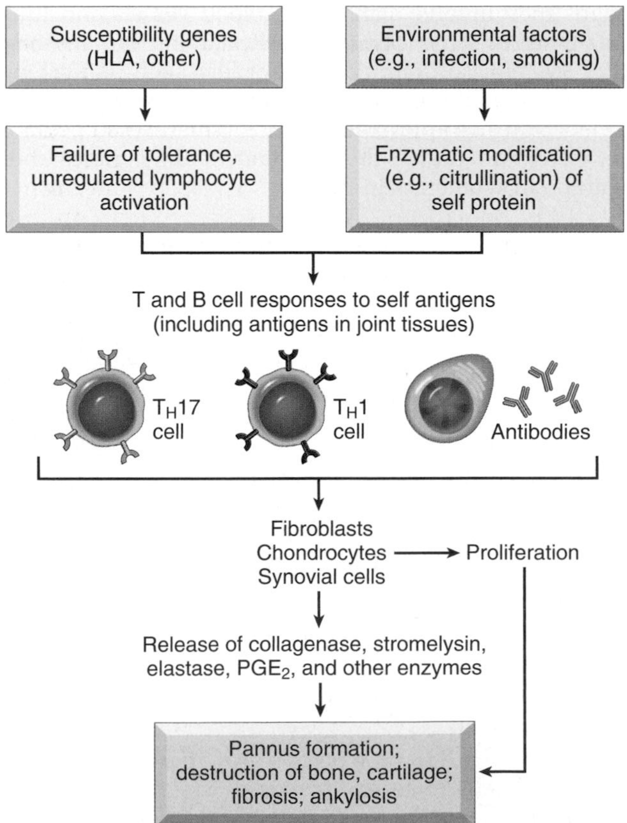

Figure 26-42 Major processes involved in the pathogenesis of rheumatoid arthritis.

It is estimated that 50% of the risk of developing RA is related to inherited genetic susceptibility. Specific *HLA-DRB1* alleles are linked to rheumatoid arthritis, and these alleles share a common sequence of amino acids in a polymorphic region of the β chain, which is designated the *shared epitope*. The shared epitope is located in the antigen-binding cleft of the DR molecule. This location is presumably the specific binding site of the arthritogen(s) that initiates the inflammatory synovitis. Linkage and genome wide association studies have also implicated the *PTPN22* gene. *PTPN22* encodes a protein tyrosine phosphatase that is postulated to inhibit T-cell activation.

The environmental arthritogen whose antigens initiate RA by activating T or B cells remains uncertain. CCPs are produced during inflammation, so insults such as infection and smoking may promote citrullination of self-proteins, creating new epitopes that trigger autoimmune reactions. The robust immune reaction to these autoantigens suggests that they may be important arthritogenic agents.

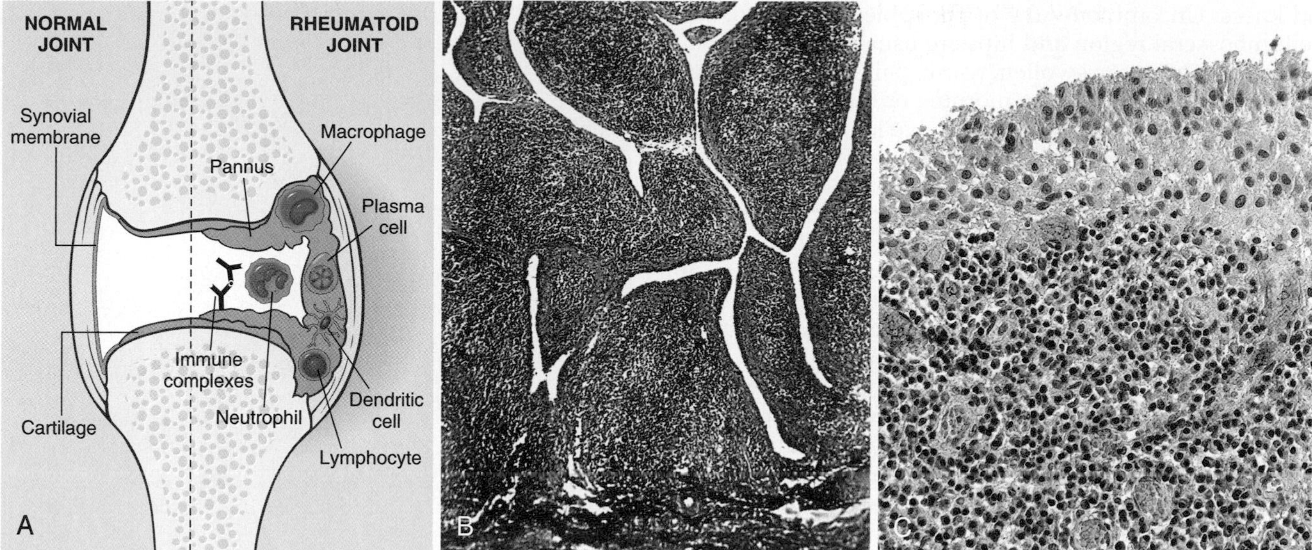

Figure 26-43 Rheumatoid arthritis. **A,** Schematic view of the joint lesion. **B,** Low magnification reveals marked synovial hypertrophy with formation of villi. **C,** At higher magnification, subsynovial tissue containing a dense lymphoid aggregate. (**A,** Modified from Feldmann M: Development of anti-TNF therapy for rheumatoid arthritis. Nat Rev Immunol 2:364, 2002.)

MORPHOLOGY

Joints. RA typically manifests as a symmetric arthritis principally affecting the small joints of the hand and feet. The synovium becomes grossly edematous, thickened, and hyperplastic, transforming its smooth contour to one covered by delicate and bulbous villi (Fig. 26-43*A, B)*. The characteristic histologic features include (1) **synovial cell hyperplasia** and proliferation; (2) **dense inflammatory infiltrates** (frequently forming lymphoid follicles) of CD4+ helper T cells, B cells, plasma cells, dendritic cells, and macrophages (Fig. 26-43*C*); (3) increased vascularity due to angiogenesis; (4) fibrinopurulent exudate on the synovial and joint surfaces; (5) osteoclastic activity in underlying bone, allowing the synovium to penetrate into the bone and cause periarticular erosions and subchondral cysts. Together, the above changes produce a **pannus:** a mass of edematous synovium, inflammatory cells, granulation tissue, and fibroblasts that grows over the articular cartilage and causes its erosion. In time, after the cartilage has been destroyed, the pannus bridges the apposing bones to form a **fibrous ankylosis**, which eventually ossifies and results in fusion of the bones, called **bony ankylosis** (Fig. 26-41).

Skin. **Rheumatoid subcutaneous nodules** are the most common cutaneous lesions. They occur in approximately 25% of affected individuals, usually those with severe disease, and arise in regions of the skin that are subjected to pressure, including the ulnar aspect of the forearm, elbows, occiput, and lumbosacral area. Less commonly they form in the lungs, spleen, pericardium, myocardium, heart valves, aorta, and other viscera. Rheumatoid nodules are firm, nontender, and round to oval, and in the skin arise in the subcutaneous tissue. Microscopically they resemble necrotizing granulomas with a central zone of fibrinoid necrosis surrounded by a prominent rim activated macrophages and numerous lymphocytes and plasma cells (Fig. 26-44).

Blood Vessels. Affected individuals with severe erosive disease, rheumatoid nodules, and high titers of rheumatoid factor are at risk of developing **vasculitis** (Chapter 11). The acute necrotizing vasculitis involves small and large arteries. It may involve the pleura, pericardium or lung evolving into chronic fibrosing processes. Frequently, segments of small arteries such as vasa nervorum and the digital arteries are obstructed by an obliterating endarteritis resulting in peripheral neuropathy, ulcers, and gangrene. Leukocytoclastic vasculitis produces purpura, cutaneous ulcers, and nail bed infarction. Ocular changes such as uveitis and keratoconjunctivitis (similar to Sjögren syndrome, Chapter 6) may be prominent.

Clinical Course. In about half of patients, RA may begin slowly and insidiously with malaise, fatigue, and generalized musculoskeletal pain, likely mediated by IL-1 and TNF. After several weeks to months the joints become involved. The pattern of joint involvement varies, but it is generally symmetrical and the small joints are affected before the larger ones. Symptoms usually develop in the hands (metacarpophalangeal and proximal interphalangeal joints) and feet, followed by the wrists, ankles, elbows,

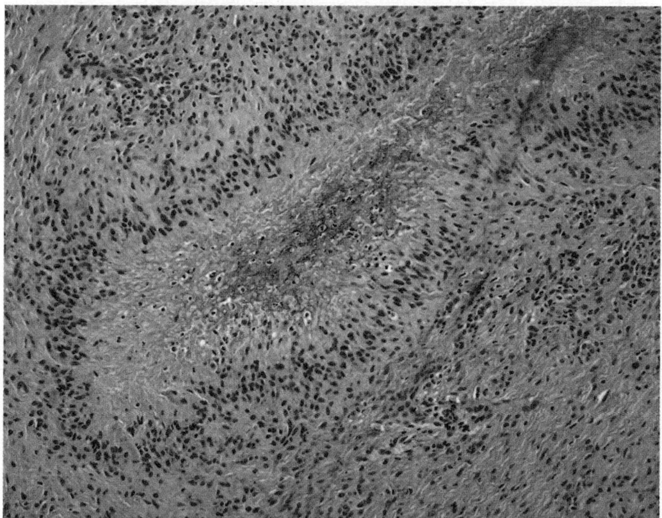

Figure 26-44 Rheumatoid nodule composed of central necrosis rimmed by palisaded histiocytes.

and knees. Uncommonly the upper spine is involved, but the lumbosacral region and hips are usually spared.

Involved joints are swollen, warm, painful, and particularly stiff when rising in the morning or following inactivity. The typical patient has progressive joint enlargement, decreased range of motion evolving to complete ankylosis, with the greatest damage occurring in the first 4 or 5 years. Approximately 20% of affected individuals enjoy periods of partial or complete remission, but the symptoms inevitably return and involve previously unaffected joints. A minority of individuals (10%) have an acute onset over several days with severe symptoms and polyarticular involvement.

Inflammation in the tendons, ligaments, and occasionally the adjacent skeletal muscle frequently accompanies the arthritis and produces the characteristic radial deviation of the wrist, ulnar deviation of the fingers and flexion-hyperextension of the fingers (swan-neck deformity, boutonnière deformity). The end result is a joint that has no stability and minimal or no range of motion. Large synovial cysts, like the *Baker cyst* in the posterior knee, may develop as the increased intra-articular pressure causes herniation of the synovium. Radiographic hallmarks are joint effusions and juxta-articular osteopenia with erosions and narrowing of the joint space and loss of articular cartilage (Fig. 26-45).

The presence of multisystem involvement must be distinguished from other forms of chronic arthritis (lupus, scleroderma, Lyme disease). The diagnosis of RA is supported by (1) characteristic radiographic findings, (2) sterile, turbid synovial fluid with decreased viscosity, poor mucin clot formation, and inclusion-bearing neutrophils, and (3) the combination of rheumatoid factor and anti-CCP antibody (80% of patients).

The treatment of rheumatoid arthritis is aimed at relieving the pain and inflammation, and slowing or arresting the relentless joint destruction. Therapies include corticosteroids, synthetic and biologic disease-modifying drugs such as methotrexate, and, most notably, antagonists of TNF. Such drugs prevent or slow joint destruction, which is the greatest source of disability, and have altered the natural history of the disease for the better. However, anti-TNF agents are not curative, and patients must be maintained on TNF antagonists to avoid disease flares. Other biologic agents that interfere with T and B lymphocyte responses are also approved therapies.

Long-term complications include *systemic amyloidosis* (Chapter 6) in 5% to 10% of patients and infection with opportunistic organisms in patients who receive long-term anti-TNF or other immunosuppressive agents.

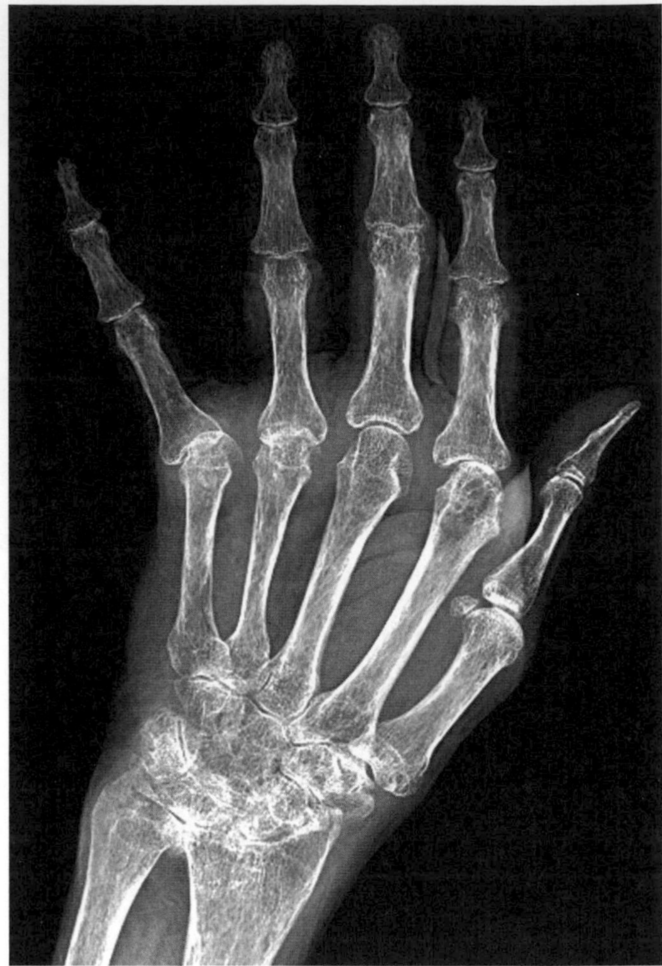

Figure 26-45 Rheumatoid arthritis of the hand. Characteristic features include diffuse osteopenia, marked loss of the joint spaces of the carpal, metacarpal, phalangeal, and interphalangeal joints, periarticular bony erosions, and ulnar drift of the fingers.

Juvenile Idiopathic Arthritis

Juvenile idiopathic arthritis (JIA) is a heterogeneous group of disorders of unknown cause that present with arthritis before age 16 and persist for at least 6 weeks. The prevalence is 30,000 to 50,000 in the United States. Compared to RA, in JIA (1) oligoarthritis is more common, (2) systemic disease is more frequent, (3) large joints are affected more often than small joints, (4) rheumatoid nodules and rheumatoid factor are usually absent, and (5) antinuclear antibody (ANA) seropositivity is common. The pathogenesis is unknown but similar to adult RA; risk factors include *HLA* and *PTPN22* variants. Also like adult RA, damage in JIA appears to be caused by T_H1 and T_H17 cells and the mediators IL-1, IL-17, TNF, and IFN-γ.

Attempts at subclassification of JIA are based on clinical (e.g., oligoarticular, systemic) and laboratory (ANA, rheumatoid factor titers) variables. Some of these subgroups (e.g., systemic, polyarticular rheumatoid factor positive; enthesitis-related, which refers to involvement of sites of ligament and cartilage insertion into bone; oligoarticular) seem to represent defined entities while others (e.g., polyarticular rheumatoid factor negative; psoriatic) remain heterogeneous. Treatment consists of similar regimens as adult RA with some success using an IL-6 receptor antibody in the systemic form. Long-term prognosis of JIA is very variable. Although many affected individuals may have chronic disease, only about 10% develop serious functional disability.

Seronegative Spondyloarthropathies

The spondyloarthropathies are also a heterogeneous group of disorders that are unified by the following features:

- Pathologic changes in the ligamentous attachments rather than synovium

- Involvement of sacroiliac joints, with or without other joints
- Absence of rheumatoid factor
- Association with HLA-B27

The manifestations are immune mediated and are triggered by a T-cell response presumably directed against an undefined antigen, likely infectious, that may cross-react with native molecules of the musculoskeletal system.

Ankylosing Spondylitis

Ankylosing spondylitis causes destruction of articular cartilage and bony ankylosis, especially of the sacroiliac and apophyseal joints (between tuberosities and processes). It is also known as *rheumatoid spondylitis* and *Marie-Strümpell disease*. Disease involving the sacroiliac joints and vertebrae becomes symptomatic in the second and third decades of life as lower back pain and spinal immobility. Involvement of peripheral joints, such as the hips, knees, and shoulders, occurs in at least one third of affected individuals. Approximately 90% of patients are HLA-B27 positive; associations have also been found with the IL-23 receptor gene.

Reactive Arthritis

Reactive arthritis is defined by a triad of arthritis, nongonococcal urethritis or cervicitis, and conjunctivitis. Most affected individuals are men in their 20s or 30s, and more than 80% are HLA-B27 positive. This form of arthritis also affects individuals infected with the human immunodeficiency virus (HIV). The disease is probably caused by an autoimmune reaction initiated by prior infection of the genitourinary system (*Chlamydia*) or the gastrointestinal tract (*Shigella, Salmonella, Yersinia, Campylobacter*).

Arthritic symptoms develop within several weeks of the inciting bout of urethritis or diarrhea. Joint stiffness and low back pain are common early symptoms. The ankles, knees, and feet are affected most often, frequently in an asymmetric pattern. Synovitis of a digital tendon sheath produces the sausage finger or toe, and ossification of tendoligamentous insertion sites leads to calcaneal spurs and bony outgrowths. Patients with severe chronic disease have involvement of the spine that is indistinguishable from ankylosing spondylitis. Extraarticular involvement manifests as inflammatory balanitis, conjunctivitis, cardiac conduction abnormalities, and aortic regurgitation. The episodes of arthritis usually wax and wane over several weeks to 6 months. Almost 50% of affected individuals have recurrent arthritis, tendonitis and lumbosacral pain.

Enteritis Associated Arthritis

Enteritis-associated arthritis is caused by gastrointestinal infection by Yersinia, Salmonella, Shigella, and Campylobacter, among others. The outer cell membranes of these organisms have lipopolysaccharides as a major component, and they stimulate a range of immunological responses. The arthritis appears abruptly and tends to involve the knees and ankles but sometimes also the wrists, fingers, and toes. Unlike reactive arthritis, it lasts for about a year, then generally clears and only rarely is accompanied by ankylosing spondylitis.

Psoriatic Arthritis

Psoriatic arthritis is a chronic inflammatory arthropathy associated with psoriasis that affects peripheral and axial joints and entheses (ligaments and tendons). Susceptibility to the disease is genetically determined and related to HLA-B27 and HLA-Cw6 alleles. Symptoms manifest between the ages of 30 and 50. It develops in more than 10% of the psoriatic population, usually concurrently or following the onset of skin disease. Although the sacroiliac joints are involved in 20% of patients, this is predominantly a peripheral arthritis of the hands and feet. The distal interphalangeal joints of the hands and feet are first affected in an asymmetric distribution in more than 50% of patients, producing the characteristic "pencil in cup" deformity (unlike RA, which you will recall typically involves the proximal interphalangeal joints). Histologically, psoriatic arthritis is similar to rheumatoid arthritis. Psoriatic arthritis, however, is usually not as severe, remissions are more frequent, and joint destruction is less frequent.

Infectious Arthritis

Microorganisms of all types can seed joints during hematogenous dissemination. Articular structures can also become infected by direct inoculation or from contiguous spread from a soft tissue abscess or focus of osteomyelitis. Infectious arthritis is potentially serious, because it can cause rapid joint destruction leading to permanent deformities.

Suppurative Arthritis

Bacterial infections that cause acute suppurative arthritis usually enter the joints from distant sites by hematogenous spread. In neonates there is an increased incidence of contiguous spread from underlying epiphyseal osteomyelitis. *H. influenza* arthritis predominates in children younger than 2 years of age, *S. aureus* is the main causative agent in older children and adults, and gonococcus is prevalent during late adolescence and young adulthood. Individuals with sickle cell disease are prone to infection with *Salmonella* at any age. These joint infections affect the sexes equally except for gonococcal arthritis, which is seen mainly in sexually active women. Individuals with deficiencies of components of the complement membrane attack complex (C5, C6, and C7) are susceptible to disseminated gonococcal infections and hence arthritis. Other predisposing conditions include immune deficiencies (congenital and acquired), debilitating illness, joint trauma, chronic arthritis of any cause, and intravenous drug abuse.

The classic presentation is the sudden development of an acutely painful and swollen joint that has a restricted range of motion. Systemic findings of fever, leukocytosis, and elevated sedimentation rate are common. In disseminated gonococcal infection the symptoms are more subacute. In 90% of nongonococcal cases, the infection involves only a single joint, most commonly the knee followed in frequency by the hip, shoulder, elbow, wrist, and sternoclavicular joints. The axial joints are more often involved in drug users. Joint aspiration is diagnostic if it yields purulent fluid in which the causal agent can be identified. Prompt recognition and effective antimicrobial therapy can prevent joint destruction.

Mycobacterial Arthritis

Mycobacterial arthritis is a chronic progressive monoarticular infection caused by *M. tuberculosis,* which occurs in all age groups, especially adults. It usually develops as a complication of adjoining osteomyelitis or after hematogenous dissemination from a visceral (usually pulmonary) site of infection. Onset is insidious and causes gradual progressive pain. Systemic symptoms may or may not be present. Mycobacterial seeding of the joint induces the formation of confluent granulomas with central caseous necrosis. The affected synovium may grow as a pannus over the articular cartilage and erode the bone along the joint margins. Chronic disease results in fibrous ankylosis and obliteration of the joint space. The weight-bearing joints are usually affected, especially the hips, knees, and ankles in descending order of frequency.

Lyme Arthritis

Lyme arthritis is caused by infection with the spirochete *Borrelia burgdorferi*, which is transmitted by deer ticks of the *Ixodes ricinus* complex. It is the leading arthropod borne disease in the United States. In its classic form, Lyme disease progressively involves multiple organ systems, as outlined in Chapter 8. The initial infection of the skin is followed within several days or weeks by dissemination of the organism to other sites, especially the joints.

Approximately 60% to 80% of untreated individuals with the disease develop arthritis during the late stage. The arthritis primarily involves large joints, especially the knees, shoulders, elbows, and ankles in descending order of frequency. Usually one or two joints are affected at a time, and the attacks last for a few weeks to months, migrating to new sites. Spirochetes can only be identified in about 25% of joints with arthritis but the diagnosis can be confirmed by serologic testing for anti-*Borrelia* antibodies. The majority of individuals respond to antibiotic therapy.

A chronic arthritis that is antibiotic refractory develops in approximately 10% of affected individuals. In many of these patients, *Borrelia* cannot be detected in the joint fluid even by PCR. It has been proposed that cellular (especially T_H1) and humoral responses to *Borrelia* outer surface protein A may initiate an autoimmune arthritis, but this is not proven.

Infected synovium exhibits a chronic synovitis marked by synoviocyte hyperplasia, fibrin deposition, mononuclear cell infiltrates (especially CD4+ T cells), and onion-skin thickening of arterial walls. The morphology in severe cases can closely resemble that of rheumatoid arthritis.

Viral Arthritis

Arthritis can occur in the setting of a variety of viral infections, including alphavirus, parvovirus B19, rubella, Epstein-Barr virus, and hepatitis B and C viruses. The manifestations of the arthritis range from acute to subacute symptoms. The joint symptoms may be caused by direct infection of the joint by the virus, as seen in rubella and some alphavirus infections, or by an autoimmune reaction generated by the infection, as is seen in other forms of reactive or post-infectious arthritides. A variety of rheumatic conditions, including reactive arthritis, psoriatic arthritis, and septic arthritis, may develop in individuals infected with HIV. The pathogenesis of some of these forms of HIV-associated chronic arthritis is probably autoimmune. Antiretroviral therapies for HIV have reduced the severity of HIV-associated arthritis.

Crystal-Induced Arthritis

Articular crystal deposits are associated with a variety of acute and chronic joint disorders. Endogenous crystals shown to be pathogenic include monosodium urate *(gout)*, calcium pyrophosphate dehydrate *(pseudogout)*, and basic calcium phosphate. Exogenous crystals, such as corticosteroid ester crystals and talcum, and the biomaterials polyethylene and methyl methacrylate, may also induce joint disease. Silicone, polyethylene, and methyl methacrylate are used in prosthetic joints, and their debris that accumulates with long use and wear may result in local arthritis and failure of the prosthesis. Endogenous and exogenous crystals produce disease by triggering a cytokine-mediated cascade that destroys cartilage.

Gout

Gout is marked by transient attacks of acute arthritis initiated by crystallization of monosodium urate within and around joints. Gout can be divided into primary and secondary forms (Table 26-7), both sharing the common feature of hyperuricemia. In the primary form (90% of cases), gout is the major manifestation of the disease and the cause is usually unknown. In secondary gout (10% of cases), uric acid is increased because of a known underlying disease that usually dominates the clinical picture.

Table 26-7 Classification of Gout

Clinical Category	Uric Acid Production	Uric Acid Excretion
Primary Gout (90%)		
Unknown enzyme defects (85%-90%)	↑ (majority) ↑↑ (minority) Normal	Normal ↑ ↓
Known enzyme defects (e.g., partial HGPRT deficiency)	↑	Normal
Secondary Gout (10%)		
Increased nucleic acid turnover (e.g., leukemia)	↑↑	↑
Chronic renal disease	Normal	↓
Congenital (e.g., Lesch-Nyhan syndrome HGPRT deficiency)	↑↑	↑

HGPRT, Hypoxanthine guanine phosphoribosyl transferase.

Pathogenesis. **Hyperuricemia (plasma urate level above 6.8 mg/dL) is necessary, but not sufficient, for the development of gout.** Elevated uric acid can result from overproduction or reduced excretion or both (Table 26-7). Uric acid metabolism can be summarized as follows:

- Synthesis: Uric acid is the end product of purine catabolism. Increased urate synthesis typically reflects some abnormality in purine production. The synthesis of purine nucleotides, in turn, involves two interlinked pathways. In the de novo pathway, purine nucleotides are synthesized from nonpurine precursors, and in salvage pathways they are synthesized from free purine bases from dietary intake and catabolism of purine nucleotides.
- Excretion: Uric acid is filtered from the circulation by the glomerulus and virtually completely resorbed by the proximal tubule of the kidney. A small fraction of the resorbed uric acid is secreted by the distal nephron and excreted in the urine.

Hyperuricemia can result from either overproduction or reduced excretion. The vast majority of *primary gout* is caused by increased uric acid biosynthesis for unknown reasons. A small minority of patients have overproduction because of identifiable enzymatic defects. For example, partial deficiency of hypoxanthine guanine phosphoribosyl transferase (HGPRT) interrupts the salvage pathway, so purine metabolites cannot be savaged and are, instead, degraded into uric acid. Complete absence of HGPRT also results in hyperuricemia, but the significant neurologic manifestations of this condition (*Lesch-Nyhan syndrome*) dominate the clinical picture so it is classified as *secondary gout.* Secondary gout can also be caused by increased production (e.g., rapid cell lysis during chemotherapy for leukemia) or decreased excretion (chronic renal disease).

The inflammation in gout is triggered by precipitation of monosodium urate (MSU) crystals into the joints, which result in the production of cytokines that recruit leukocytes (Fig. 26-46). Macrophages phagocytose the MSU and the intracellular sensor, the inflammasome (Chapter 3), recognizes the crystals. The inflammasome activates caspase-1, which is involved in the production of some biologically active cytokines, most notably IL-1. IL-1 is proinflammatory, and promotes accumulation of neutrophils and macrophages in the joint. These cells, in turn, release other cytokines, free radicals, proteases and arachidonic acid metabolites, all of which recruit more leukocytes and damage the joint. Urate crystals may also activate the complement system, leading to the generation of chemotactic complement byproducts. These cascades trigger an acute arthritis, which typically remits spontaneously in days to weeks.

The solubility of MSU in a joint is modulated by temperature and the chemical composition of the fluid. Synovial fluid is inherently a poorer solvent for monosodium urate than plasma. The lower temperature of the peripheral joints also favors precipitation. Crystallization is dependent on the presence of nucleating agents such as insoluble collagen fibers, chondroitin sulfate, proteoglycans and cartilage fragments.

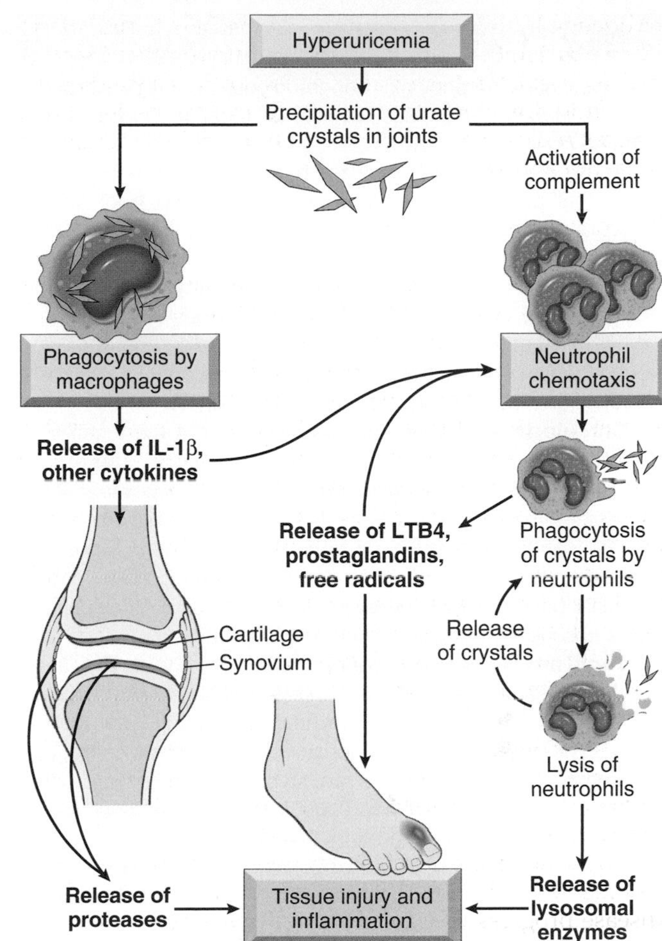

Figure 26-46 Pathogenesis of acute gouty arthritis. LTB4, Leukotriene B4; IL-1β, interleukin 1β.

Hyperuricemia does not necessarily lead to gouty arthritis. Many factors contribute to the conversion of asymptomatic hyperuricemia into primary gout, including the following:

- Age of the individual and duration of the hyperuricemia. Gout usually appears after 20 to 30 years of hyperuricemia.
- Genetic predisposition. In addition to the well-defined X-linked abnormalities of HGPRT, primary gout follows multifactorial inheritance and runs in families. Polymorphisms in genes involved in urate transport and homeostasis (URAT1 and GLUT9) are also associated with gout.
- Heavy alcohol consumption
- Obesity
- Drugs (e.g., thiazides) that reduce excretion of urate
- Lead toxicity (so-called saturnine gout)

Repeated attacks of acute arthritis lead eventually to chronic tophaceous arthritis and the formation of tophi in the inflamed synovial membranes and periarticular tissue. Severe damage to the cartilage develops and the function of the joints is compromised.

MORPHOLOGY

The distinctive morphologic changes in gout are (1) acute arthritis, (2) chronic tophaceous arthritis, (3) tophi in various sites, and (4) gouty nephropathy.

Acute arthritis is characterized by a dense neutrophilic infiltrate that permeates the synovium and synovial fluid. MSU crystals are frequently found in the cytoplasm of the neutrophils and are arranged in small clusters in the synovium. They are long, slender, and needle-shaped, and are negatively birefringent. The synovium is edematous and congested, and also contains scattered lymphocytes, plasma cells, and macrophages. When the episode of crystallization abates and the crystals are resolubilized, the acute attack remits.

Chronic tophaceous arthritis evolves from the repetitive precipitation of urate crystals during acute attacks. The MSU encrusts the articular surface and forms visible deposits in the synovium (Fig. 26-47*A*). The synovium becomes hyperplastic, fibrotic, and thickened by inflammatory cells and forms a pannus that destroys the underlying cartilage and lead to juxta-articular bone erosions. In severe cases, fibrous or bony ankylosis ensues, resulting in loss of joint function.

Tophi are the pathognomonic hallmark of gout. They are formed by large aggregations of urate crystals surrounded by an intense inflammatory reaction of foreign body giant cells. (Fig. 26-47*B,C*). Tophi may appear in the articular cartilage, ligaments, tendons, and bursae. Less frequently they may occur in soft tissues (earlobes, fingertips) or kidneys. Superficial tophi can ulcerate through the overlying skin.

Gouty nephropathy (Chapter 20) refers to the renal complications caused by MSU crystals or tophi in the renal medullary interstitium or tubules. Complications include uric acid nephrolithiasis and pyelonephritis, particularly when the urates induce urinary obstruction.

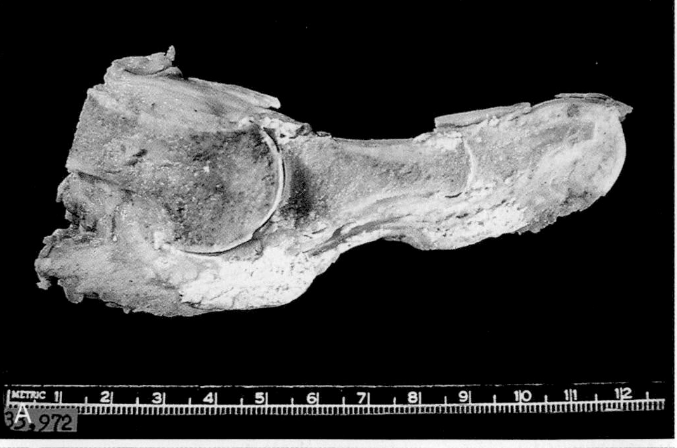

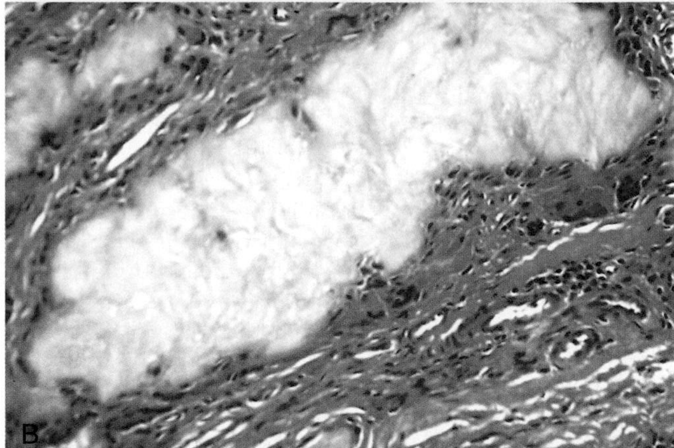

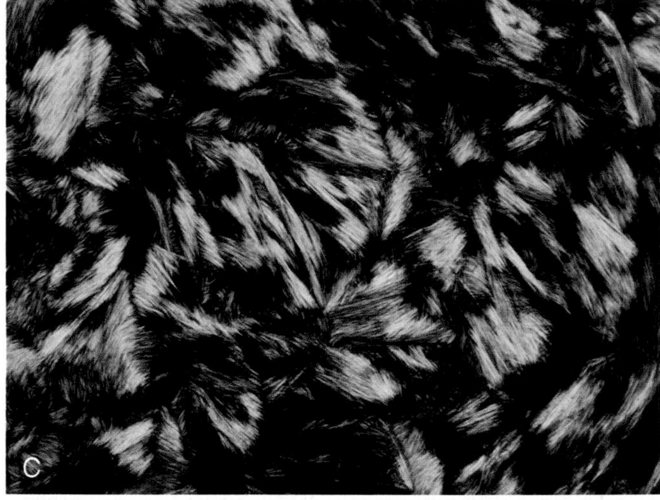

Figure 26-47 Gout. **A,** Amputated great toe with white tophi involving the joint and soft tissues. **B,** Gouty tophus—an aggregate of dissolved urate crystals is surrounded by reactive fibroblasts, mononuclear inflammatory cells, and giant cells. **C,** Urate crystals are needle shaped and negatively birefringent under polarized light.

Clinical Course. Gout is more common in men and after the age of 30. Patients with obesity, metabolic syndrome, excess alcohol intake and renal failure are at increased risk.

Four clinical stages are recognized:

- *Asymptomatic hyperuricemia* appears around puberty in males and after menopause in females.
- *Acute arthritis* presents after several years as sudden onset of excruciating joint pain associated with localized hyperemia, warmth. Constitutional symptoms are uncommon except for occasional mild fever. Most first attacks are monoarticular; 50% occur in the first metatarsophalangeal joint. Eventually, about 90% of affected individuals experience acute attacks in the following locations (in descending order of frequency): insteps, ankles, heels, knees, wrists, fingers, and elbows. Untreated, acute gouty arthritis may last for hours to weeks, but gradually there is complete resolution.
- *Asymptomatic intercritical period*: Resolution of the acute arthritis leads to a symptom free interval. Although some patients never have another attack, most experience a second acute episode within months to a few years. In the absence of appropriate therapy, the attacks recur at shorter intervals and frequently become polyarticular.
- *Chronic tophaceous gout* develops on average about 12 years after the initial acute attack and the appearance of chronic tophaceous arthritis. At this stage, radiographs show characteristic juxta-articular bone erosion caused by osteoclastic bone resorption and loss of the joint space. Progression leads to severe crippling disease.

Renal manifestations sometimes appear in the form of renal colic associated with the passage of gravel and stones and may proceed to chronic gouty nephropathy. About 20% of those with chronic gout die of renal failure.

Numerous drugs are available to abort or prevent acute attacks of arthritis and mobilize tophaceous deposits. Their use is important, because many aspects of the disease are related to the duration and severity of the hyperuricemia. Generally, gout does not materially shorten the life span, but it may impair the quality of life.

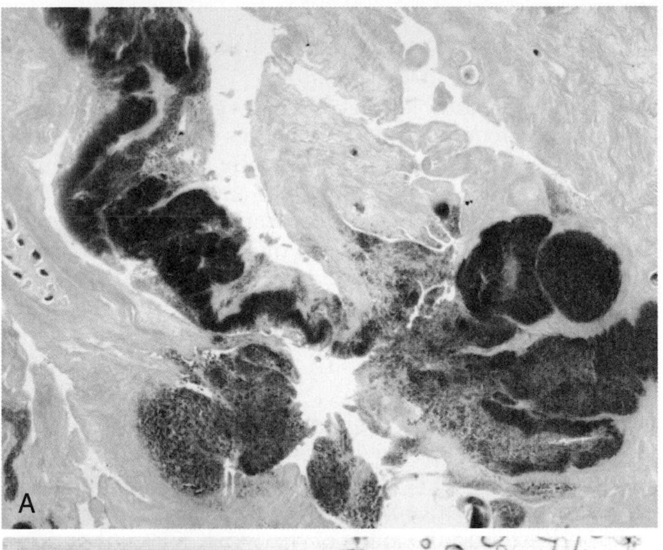

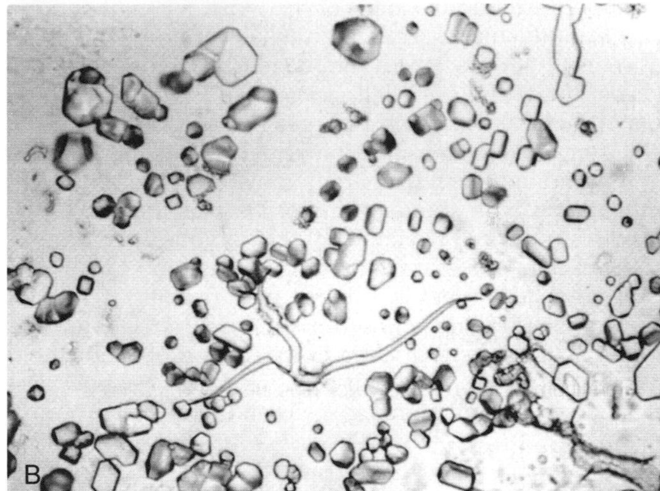

Figure 26-48 Pseudogout. **A,** Deposits are present in cartilage and consist of amorphous basophilic material. **B,** Smear preparation of calcium pyrophosphate crystals.

Calcium Pyrophosphate Crystal Deposition Disease (Pseudo-Gout)

Calcium pyrophosphate crystal deposition disease (CPPD), also known as *pseudo-gout* and *chondrocalcinosis*, usually occurs in individuals older than 50 years of age and becomes more common with increasing age, rising to a prevalence of 30% to 60% in those 85 years or older. The sexes and races are equally affected. CPPD is divided into sporadic (idiopathic), hereditary, and secondary types. In an autosomal dominant variant the crystals develop relatively early in life and are associated with severe osteoarthritis. The disease is caused by germline mutations in the pyrophosphate transport channel. The secondary form is associated with various disorders, including previous joint damage, hyperparathyroidism, hemochromatosis, hypomagnesemia, hypothyroidism, ochronosis, and diabetes.

Pathophysiology. The basis for crystal formation is not known but studies suggest that articular cartilage proteoglycans, which normally inhibit mineralization, are degraded allowing crystallization around chondrocytes. As in gout, inflammation is caused by activation of the inflammasome in macrophages (Fig. 26-46).

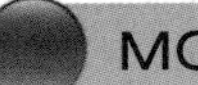

MORPHOLOGY

The crystals first develop in the articular cartilage, menisci, and intervertebral discs, and as the deposits enlarge they may rupture and seed the joint. The crystals form chalky, white friable deposits, which are seen histologically in stained preparations as oval blue-purple aggregates (Fig. 26-48*A*). Individual crystals are rhomboid, 0.5 to 5 μm in greatest dimension (Fig. 26-48*B*) and are positively birefringent. Inflammation, if present, is usually milder than in gout.

CPPD is frequently asymptomatic. However, it may produce acute, subacute, or chronic arthritis that can be confused with osteoarthritis or rheumatoid arthritis. The joint involvement may last from several days to weeks and may be monoarticular or polyarticular; the knees, followed by the wrists, elbows, shoulders, and ankles, are most commonly affected. Ultimately, approximately 50% of affected individuals experience significant joint damage. Therapy is supportive. There is no known treatment that prevents or slows crystal formation.

KEY CONCEPTS

Arthritis

- **Osteoarthritis (degenerative joint disease)**, the most common disease of joints, is a degenerative process of articular cartilage in which matrix breakdown exceeds synthesis. Inflammation is minimal and typically secondary. Local production of inflammatory cytokines may contribute to the progression of joint degeneration.
- **Rheumatoid arthritis (RA)** is a chronic autoimmune inflammatory disease that affects mainly small joints, but can be systemic. RA is caused by a cellular and humoral immune response against self-antigens, particularly citrullinated proteins. TNF plays a central role and antagonists against TNF are of clinical benefit.
- **Seronegative spondyloarthropathies** are a heterogeneous group of likely autoimmune arthritides that preferentially involve the sacroiliac and vertebral joints and are associated with HLA-B27.
- **Suppurative arthritis** describes direct infection of a joint space by bacterial organisms.
- **Lyme disease** is a systemic infection by *Borrelia burgdorferi* which manifests, in part, as an infectious arthritis, possibly with an autoimmune component in chronic stages.
- **Gout and pseudogout** result from inflammatory responses triggered by precipitation of urate or calcium pyrophosphate, respectively.

Joint Tumors and Tumor-Like Conditions

Reactive tumor-like lesions, such as ganglions, synovial cysts, and osteochondral loose bodies commonly involve joints and tendon sheaths. They usually result from trauma or degenerative processes and are much more common than neoplasms. Primary neoplasms are rare, usually benign and tend to recapitulate the cells and tissue types (synovial membrane, fat, blood vessels, fibrous tissue, and cartilage) native to joints and related structures. Malignant tumors are rare; these are discussed later with soft tissue tumors.

Ganglion and Synovial Cysts

A *ganglion* is a small (1 to 1.5 cm) cyst that is almost always located near a joint capsule or tendon sheath. A common location is around the joints of the wrist, where it appears as a firm, fluctuant, pea-sized translucent nodule. It arises as a result of cystic or myxoid degeneration of connective tissue; hence the cyst wall lacks a cell lining. The lesion may be multilocular and enlarges through coalescence of adjacent areas of myxoid change. The fluid that fills the cyst is similar to synovial fluid; however, there is no communication with the joint space. Despite the name, the lesion is unrelated to ganglia of the nervous system.

Herniation of synovium through a joint capsule or massive enlargement of a bursa may produce a *synovial cyst*. A well-recognized example is the synovial cyst that forms in the popliteal space in the setting of rheumatoid arthritis (*Baker cyst*). The synovial lining may be hyperplastic and contain inflammatory cells and fibrin.

Tenosynovial Giant Cell Tumor

Tenosynovial giant cell tumor is the term for several closely related benign neoplasms that develop in the synovial lining of joints, tendon sheaths, and bursae. Clinical variants of tenosynovial giant cell tumor include the *diffuse type* (previously known as *pigmented villonodular synovitis*), and the *localized type* (also known as *giant cell tumor of tendon sheath*). Whereas the diffuse form tends to involve large joints, the localized type usually occurs as a discrete nodule attached to a tendon sheath, commonly in the hand. Both variants usually are diagnosed in the 20s to 40s and affect the sexes equally.

Pathogenesis. These tumors harbor a reciprocal somatic chromosomal translocation, t(1;2)(p13;q37), resulting in fusion of the type VI collagen α-3 promoter upstream of the coding sequence of the monocyte colony-stimulating factor (M-CSF) gene. As a result, the tumor cells overexpress M-CSF, which, through autocrine and paracrine effects, stimulates proliferation of macrophages, in a manner similar to giant cell tumor of bone (described previously).

MORPHOLOGY

Tenosynovial giant cell tumors are red-brown to orange-yellow. In diffuse tumors the normally smooth joint synovium is converted into a tangled mat by red-brown folds, finger-like projections, and nodules (Fig. 26-49*A*). In contrast, localized tumors are well circumscribed. The neoplastic cells, which account for only 2% to 16% of the cells in the mass, are polygonal, moderately sized, and resemble synoviocytes (Fig. 26-49*B*). In the diffuse variant they spread along the surface and infiltrate the subsynovial issue. In nodular tumors, the cells grow in a solid aggregate that may be attached to the synovium by a pedicle. Both variants are heavily infiltrated by macrophages, and may contain hemosiderin or foamy lipid. Scattered multinucleated giant cells and patchy fibrosis are commonly present.

Clinical Features. Diffuse tenosynovial giant cell tumor presents in the knee in 80% of cases, followed in frequency by the hip, ankle, and calcaneocuboid joints. Affected individuals typically complain of pain, locking, and recurrent swelling similar to monoarticular arthritis. Tumor progression limits the range of movement of the joint and causes it to become stiff and firm. Sometimes a palpable mass is appreciated. Aggressive tumors erode into adjacent bones and soft tissues, causing confusion with other types of

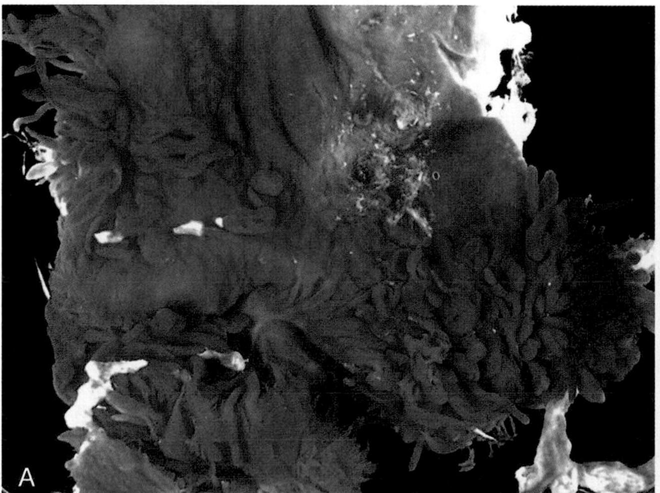

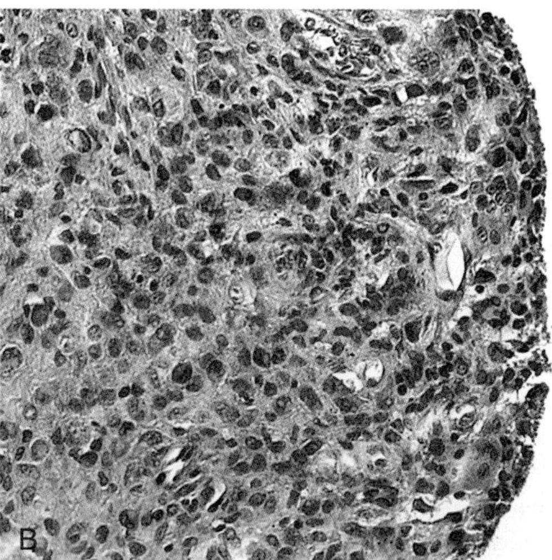

Figure 26-49 Tenosynovial giant cell tumor, diffuse type. **A,** Excised synovium with fronds and nodules typical of pigmented villonodular synovitis *(arrow)*. **B,** Sheets of proliferating cells in tenosynovial giant cell tumor bulging the synovial lining.

neoplasms. In contrast, the localized variant manifests as a solitary, slow-growing, painless mass that frequently involves the tendon sheaths along the wrists and fingers; it is the most common mesenchymal neoplasm of the hand. Cortical erosion of adjacent bone occurs in approximately 15% of cases. Both types are amenable to surgical excision, but recurrence is common. Clinical trials using antagonists of M-CSF signaling have produced encouraging responses.

SOFT TISSUE

In terms of clinical and pathologic entities, soft tissue refers to non-epithelial tissue excluding the skeleton, joints, central nervous system, hematopoietic and lymphoid tissues. Although nonneoplastic conditions can involve soft tissue, they are seldom confined to this compartment so the area of soft tissue pathology is restricted to neoplasms. With the exception of skeletal muscle neoplasms, benign soft tissue tumors outnumber their malignant counterparts, the sarcomas, by 100 fold. In the United States, the incidence of soft tissue sarcomas is approximately 12,000 per year, which is less than 1% of all cancers. Sarcomas, however, cause 2% of all cancer mortality, reflecting their aggressive behavior. Most soft tissue tumors arise in the extremities, especially the thigh. Approximately 15% arise in children but the incidence increases with age.

Pathogenesis. The majority of sarcomas are sporadic and have no known predisposing cause. A small minority of soft tissue neoplasms are associated with germline mutations in tumor suppressor genes (neurofibromatosis 1, Gardner syndrome, Li-Fraumeni syndrome, Osler-Weber Rendu syndrome). A few tumors can be linked to known environmental exposures such as radiation, burns or toxins.

Unlike tumors such as colonic carcinoma that usually arises from easily recognized precursor lesions, the origin of sarcomas is unknown. The best guess is that the tumors arise from pluripotent mesenchymal stem cells, which acquire somatic "driver" mutations in oncogenes and tumor suppressor genes. Despite heterogeneous mechanisms of tumorigenesis among sarcomas, some generalizations can be made based on their karyotypic complexity:

- Simple karyotype (15% to 20%): Like many leukemias and lymphomas, sarcomas are often euploid tumors with a single, or limited number, of chromosomal changes (Table 26-8) that occur early in tumorigenesis and are specific enough to serve as diagnostic markers. Tumors with these features most commonly arise in younger patients and tend to have a monomorphic appearance microscopically. Examples include the Ewing sarcoma, described earlier, and synovial sarcoma. In some cases, the oncogenic effect of these rearrangements is reasonably well understood, but in other cases it remains unknown (Table 26-8).
- Complex karyotype (80% to 85%): These tumors are usually aneuploid or polyploid and demonstrate multiple, severe chromosomal gains and losses, none of which are recurrent, a feature that probably speaks to an underlying abnormality producing genomic instability. Examples include leiomyosarcomas and undifferentiated sarcomas. Such tumors are more common in adults and tend to be morphologically pleomorphic.

Classification of soft tissue tumors continues to evolve as new molecular genetic abnormalities are identified. Clinically, soft tissue tumors range from benign, self-limited lesions that require minimal treatment to intermediate grade, locally aggressive tumors with minimal metastatic risk to highly aggressive malignancies with significant metastatic risk and mortality. The term *sarcoma* is applied somewhat inconsistently such that some, but not all, locally aggressive tumors fall into this category. Tumors with significant metastatic potential are, of course, considered sarcomas. Pathologic classification integrates morphology (e.g., muscle differentiation), immunohistochemistry and molecular diagnostics (Table 26-9). In addition to accurate diagnosis, grade (degree of differentiation)

Table 26-8 Chromosomal Abnormalities in Soft tissue Tumors

Tumor	Cytogenetic Abnormality	Gene fusion	Proposed function
Ewing sarcoma family tumors	t(11;22)(q24;q12) t(21;22)(q22;q12)	*EWS-FLI1* *EWS-ERG*	Disordered protein with multiple functions, including aberrant transcription, cell cycle regulation, RNA splicing and telomerase
Extraskeletal myxoid chondrosarcoma	t(9;22)(q22;q12)	*EWS-CHN*	
Desmoplastic small round-cell tumor	t(11;22)(p13;q12)	*EWS-WT1*	
Clear-cell sarcoma	t(12;22)(q13;q12)	*EWS-ATF1*	
Liposarcoma—myxoid and round-cell type	t(12;16)(q13;p11)	*FUS-DDIT3*	Arrests adipocytic differentiation
Synovial sarcoma	t(x;18)(p11;q11)	*SS18-SSX1* *SS18-SSX2* *SS18-SSX4*	Chimeric transcription factors, interrupts cell cycle control
Rhabdomyosarcoma—alveolar type	t(2;13)(q35;q14) t(1;13)(p36;q14)	*PAX3-FOXO1* *PAX7-FOXO1*	Chimeric transcription factors, disrupt skeletal muscle differentiation
Dermatofibrosarcoma protuberans	t(17;22)(q22;q15)	*COLA1-PDGFB*	Promoter driven overexpression of PDGF-β, autocrine stimulation
Alveolar soft-part sarcoma	t(X;17)(p11.2;q25)	*TFE3-ASPL*	unknown
Infantile fibrosarcoma	t(12;15)(p13;q23)	*ETV6-NTRK3*	Chimeric tyrosine kinase leads to constitutively active Ras/MAPK pathway
Nodular fasciitis	t(22;17)	*MYH9-USP6*	Unknown

Table 26-9 Soft Tissue Tumors

Category	Behavior	Tumor Type	Common Locations	Age (yr)	Morphology
Adipose	Benign	Lipoma	Superficial extremity, trunk	40-60	Mature adipose tissue
	Malignant	Well-differentiated Liposarcoma	Deep extremity, retroperitoneum	50-60	Adipose tissue with scattered atypical spindle cells
		Myxoid liposarcoma	Thigh, leg	30s	Myxoid matrix, "chicken wire" vessels, round cells, lipoblasts
Fibrous	Benign	Nodular fasciitis	Arm, forearm	20-30	Tissue culture growth, extravasated erythrocytes,
		Deep fibromatosis	Abdominal wall	30-40	Dense collagen, long, unidirectional fascicles
Skeletal muscle	Benign	Rhabdomyoma	Head and neck	0-60	Polygonal rhabdomyoblasts, "spider" cells
	Malignant	Alveolar rhabdomyosarcoma	Extremities, sinuses	5-15	Uniform round discohesive cells between septae
		Embryonal rhabdomyosarcoma	Genitourinary tract	1-5	Primitive spindle cells, "strap" cells
Smooth muscle	Benign	Leiomyoma	Extremity	20s	Uniform, plump eosinophilic cells in fascicles
	Malignant	Leiomyosarcoma	Thigh, retroperitoneum	40-60	Pleomorphic eosinophilic cells
Vascular	Benign	Hemangioma	Head and neck	0-10	Circumscribed mass of capillary or venous channels
	Malignant	Angiosarcoma	Skin, deep lower extremity	50-80	Infiltrating capillary channels
Nerve sheath	Benign	Schwannoma	Head and neck	20-50	Encapsulated, fibrillar stroma, nuclear palisading
		Neurofibroma	Wide, cutaneous, subcutis	10-20+	Myxoid, ropy collagen, loose fascicles, mast cells
	Malignant	Malignant peripheral nerve sheath tumor	Extremities, shoulder girdle	20-50	Tight fascicles, atypia, mitotic activity, necrosis
Uncertain histotype	Benign	Solitary fibrous tumor	Pelvis, pleura	20-70	Branching ectatic vessels,
	Malignant	Synovial sarcoma	Thigh, leg	15-40	Tight fascicles of uniform basophilic spindle cells, Pseudoglandular structures
		Undifferentiated pleomorphic sarcoma	Thigh	40-70	High grade anaplastic polygonal, round or spindle cells Bizarre nuclei, atypical mitoses, necrosis
		Alveolar soft part sarcoma	Trunk, extremities	15-35	Multiple nodules of eosinophilic round cells, septae
		Clear cell sarcoma	Tendons, extremities	20-40	Sheets of pale or clear spindle cells, wreath-like giant cells

and stage (size and depth) are important prognostic indicators.

With this as a primer, we will next consider representative or especially illustrative soft tissue tumors.

Tumors of Adipose Tissue

Lipoma

Lipoma, a benign tumor of fat, is the most common soft tissue tumor of adulthood. These tumors are subclassified according to morphologic and/or characteristic molecular features as conventional lipoma, fibrolipoma, angiolipoma, spindle cell lipoma and myelolipoma.

MORPHOLOGY

The conventional lipoma, the most common subtype, is a well-encapsulated mass of mature adipocytes. It usually arises in the subcutis of the proximal extremities and trunk, most frequently during middle adulthood. Infrequently, lipomas are large, intramuscular, and poorly circumscribed.

Lipomas are soft, mobile, and painless (except angiolipoma) and are usually cured by simple excision.

Liposarcoma

Liposarcoma is one of the most common sarcomas of adulthood. It occurs mainly in people in their 50s to 60s in the deep soft tissues of the proximal extremities and in the retroperitoneum. Amplification of 12q13-q15 and t(12;16) are characteristic of well-differentiated and myxoid liposarcomas, respectively. One of the key genes in the amplified region of chromosome 12q is *MDM2*, which you will recall encodes a potent inhibitor of p53. Pleomorphic liposarcomas contain complex karyotypes without reproducible genetic abnormalities.

MORPHOLOGY

Liposarcomas are histologically divided into three morphologic subtypes:

- Well-differentiated liposarcoma contains adipocytes with scattered atypical spindle cells (Fig. 26-50*A*).
- Myxoid liposarcoma contains abundant basophilic extracellular matrix, arborizing capillaries and primitive cells at various stages of adipocyte differentiation reminiscent of fetal fat (Fig. 26-50*B*).
- Pleomorphic liposarcoma consists of sheets of anaplastic cells, bizarre nuclei and variable amounts of immature adipocytes (lipoblasts).

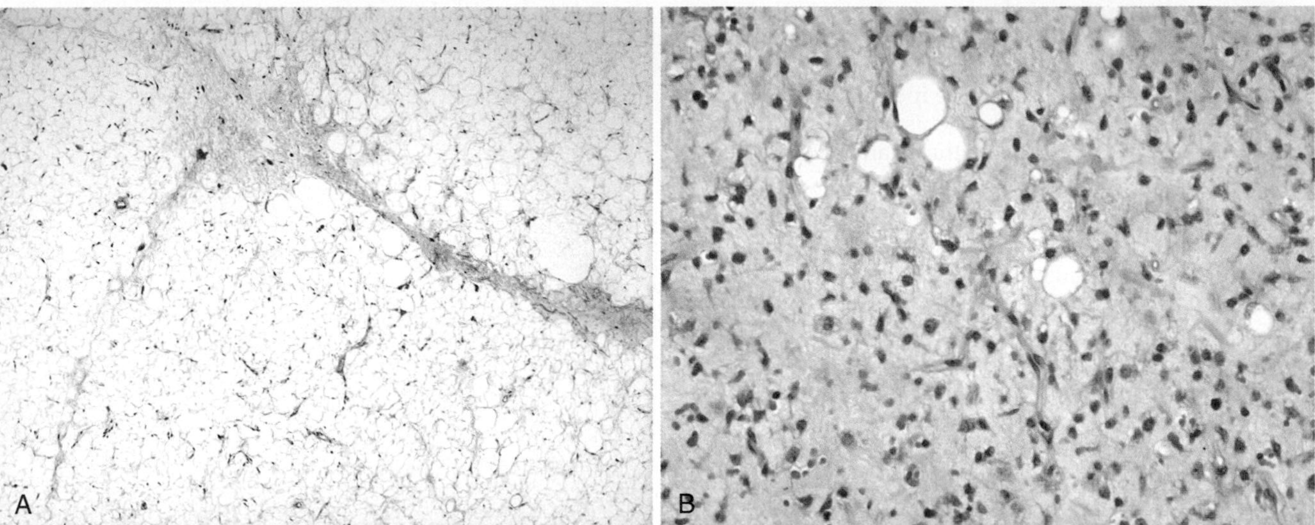

Figure 26-50 Liposarcoma. **A,** the well- differentiated subtype consists of mature adipocytes and scattered spindle cells with hyperchromatic nuclei. **B,** Myxoid liposarcoma with abundant ground substance and a rich capillary network in which are scattered immature adipocytes and more primitive round to stellate cells.

All types of liposarcoma recur locally and often repeatedly unless adequately excised. The well-differentiated variant is relatively indolent, the myxoid/round cell type is intermediate in its malignant behavior, while the pleomorphic variant usually is aggressive and frequently metastasizes.

Fibrous Tumors

Nodular Fasciitis

Nodular fasciitis is a self-limited fibroblastic and myofibroblastic proliferation that typically occurs in young adults in the upper extremity. A history of trauma is present in approximately 25% of cases and the tumors grow rapidly over a period of several weeks or months, typically no larger than 5 cm. Whereas nodular fasciitis was historically considered a reactive inflammatory lesion, identification of t(17;22) that produces a *MYH9-USP6* fusion gene indicates that it is a clonal, but self-limited, proliferation. It appears that the proliferating cells lack some key hallmark of cancer, perhaps the ability to avoid senescence. Intriguingly, ABC (discussed earlier), another tumor that sits in a gray zone between reactive and neoplastic proliferations, also contains *USP6* fusion genes. Nodular fasciitis typically spontaneously regresses and if excised, it rarely recurs.

MORPHOLOGY

Nodular fasciitis arises in the deep dermis, subcutis, or muscle. Grossly the lesion is less than 5 cm, circumscribed, or slightly infiltrative. The lesion is richly cellular and contains plump, immature-appearing fibroblasts and myofibroblasts arranged randomly or in short fascicles reminiscent of tissue culture fibroblasts (Fig. 26-51). A gradient of maturation (zonation) from cellular, loose, and myxoid to organized and fibrous is typical. The cells vary in size and shape (spindle to stellate) and have conspicuous nucleoli; mitotic figures are abundant. Lymphocytes and extravasated red blood cells are common but neutrophils are unusual.

Fibromatoses

Superficial Fibromatosis

Superficial fibromatosis is an infiltrative fibroblastic proliferation that can cause local deformity but has an innocuous clinical course. All forms of superficial fibromatosis affect males more frequently than females. They are characterized by nodular or poorly defined broad fascicles of fibroblasts in long, sweeping fascicles, surrounded by abundant dense collagen. Several clinical subtypes have been identified:

- Palmar *(Dupuytren contracture):* Irregular or nodular thickening of the palmar fascia either unilaterally or bilaterally (50%). Over a span of years, attachment to the overlying skin causes puckering and dimpling. At the same time a slowly progressive flexion contracture develops that mainly affects the fourth and fifth fingers of the hand.

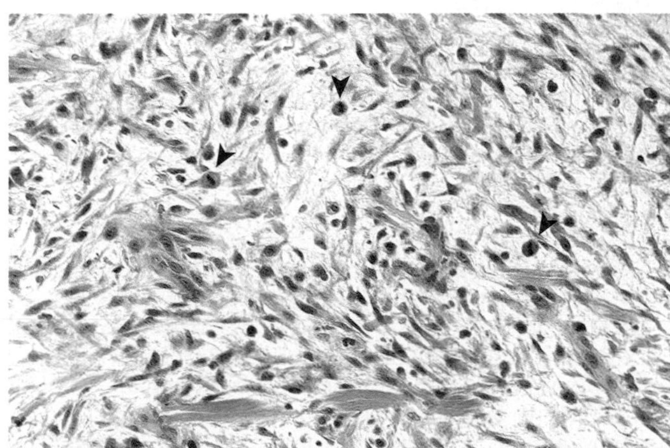

Figure 26-51 Nodular fasciitis with plump, randomly oriented spindle cells surrounded by myxoid stroma. Note the mitotic activity (*arrowheads*) and extravasated red blood cells.

- Plantar: Common in young patients, unilateral and without contractures.
- Penile *(Peyronie disease):* Palpable induration or mass on the dorsolateral aspect of the penis. Eventually, it may cause abnormal curvature of the shaft, constriction of the urethra, or both.

In about 20% to 25% of cases, the palmar and plantar fibromatoses stabilize and do not progress, in some instances resolving spontaneously. Some recur after excision, particularly the plantar variant.

Deep Fibromatosis (Desmoid Tumors)

Deep fibromatoses are large, infiltrative masses that frequently recur but do not metastasize. They are most frequent in the teens to 30s, predominantly in women. Abdominal fibromatosis generally arises in the musculoaponeurotic structures of the anterior abdominal wall but tumors can arise in the limb girdles or the mesentery. Deep fibromatoses contain mutations in the *APC* or β-catenin genes, both of which lead to increased Wnt signaling. The majority of tumors are sporadic, but individuals with familial adenomatous polyposis (Gardner syndrome, Chapter 17) who have germline *APC* mutations are predisposed to deep fibromatosis.

MORPHOLOGY

Fibromatoses are gray-white, firm, poorly demarcated masses varying from 1 to 15 cm in greatest diameter. They are rubbery and tough, and have marked infiltration of surrounding muscle, nerve and fat. Cytologically bland fibroblasts arranged in broad sweeping fascicles amid dense collagen are the characteristic histologic pattern (Fig. 26-52). The histology resembles scar.

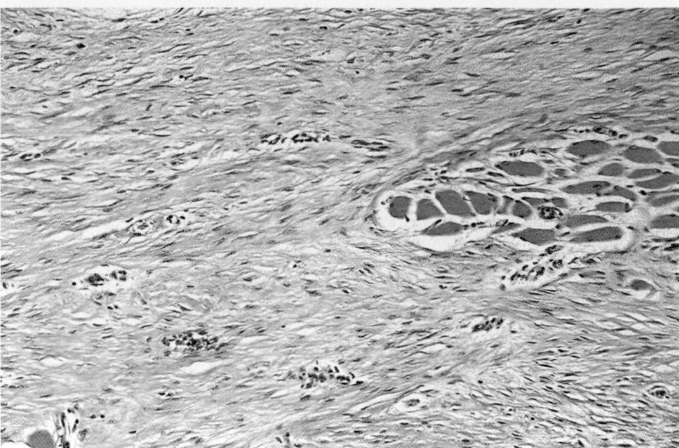

Figure 26-52 Fibromatosis infiltrating between skeletal muscle cells.

In addition to possibly being disfiguring or disabling, deep-seated fibromatosis is occasionally painful. Because of the extensively infiltrative nature, complete excision is often difficult. Recent efforts have concentrated on medical therapy with cyclooxygenase 2 inhibitors, tyrosine kinase inhibitors, or hormonal blockade (tamoxifen).

Skeletal Muscle Tumors

Skeletal muscle neoplasms, in contrast to other mesenchymal histotypes, are almost all malignant. The benign variant, rhabdomyoma, is frequent in individuals with tuberous sclerosis and is discussed in Chapter 28.

Rhabdomyosarcoma

Rhabdomyosarcoma is a malignant mesenchymal tumor with skeletal muscle differentiation. Three subtypes are recognized: *alveolar* (20%), *embryonal* (60%) and *pleomorphic* (20%). Rhabdomyosarcoma (alveolar and embryonal) is the most common soft tissue sarcoma of childhood and adolescence, usually appearing before age 20. Pleomorphic rhabdomyosarcoma is seen predominantly in adults. The pediatric forms often arise in the sinuses, head and neck and genitourinary tract, locations that do not normally contain much skeletal muscle, underscoring the notion that arcomas do not arise from mature, terminally differentiated muscle cells. The embryonal and pleomorphic subtypes are genetically heterogeneous. Alveolar rhabdomyosarcoma frequently contains fusions of the *FOXO1* gene to either the *PAX3* or the *PAX7* gene, rearrangements marked by the presence of (2;13) or(1;13) translocations, respectively. PAX3 is a transcription factor that initiates skeletal muscle differentiation, and it appears that the chimeric PAX3-FOXO1 fusion protein interferes with the gene expression program that drives differentiation, a mechanism similar to many of the transcription factor fusion proteins that are found in various forms of acute leukemia.

MORPHOLOGY

Embryonal rhabdomyosarcoma presents as soft gray infiltrative mass. The tumor cells mimic skeletal muscle at various stages of embryogenesis and consist of sheets of both primitive round and spindled cells in a myxoid stroma (Fig. 26-53*A*). Rhabdomyoblasts with visible cross-striations may be present. **Sarcoma botryoides**, described in Chapter 22, is a variant of embryonal rhabdomyosarcoma that develops in the walls of hollow, mucosal-lined structures, such as the nasopharynx, common bile duct, bladder, and vagina. Where the tumors abut the mucosa of an organ, they form a submucosal zone of hypercellularity called the **cambium layer.**

Alveolar rhabdomyosarcoma is traversed by a network of fibrous septae that divide the cells into clusters or aggregates, creating a crude resemblance to pulmonary alveoli. Those in the center of the aggregates are discohesive, while those at the periphery adhere to the septae. The tumor cells are uniform round, with little cytoplasm—cross striations are not a common feature (Fig. 26-53*B*).

Pleomorphic rhabdomyosarcoma is characterized by numerous large, sometimes multinucleated, bizarre eosinophilic tumor cells and can resemble other pleomorphic sarcomas histologically. Immunohistochemistry (e.g., myogenin) is usually necessary to confirm rhabdomyoblastic differentiation.

Rhabdomyosarcomas are aggressive neoplasms that are usually treated with surgery and chemotherapy, with or without radiation therapy. The histologic type and location of the tumor influence survival. The botryoid variant of embryonal rhabdomyosarcoma has the best prognosis, while the pleomorphic subtype is often fatal.

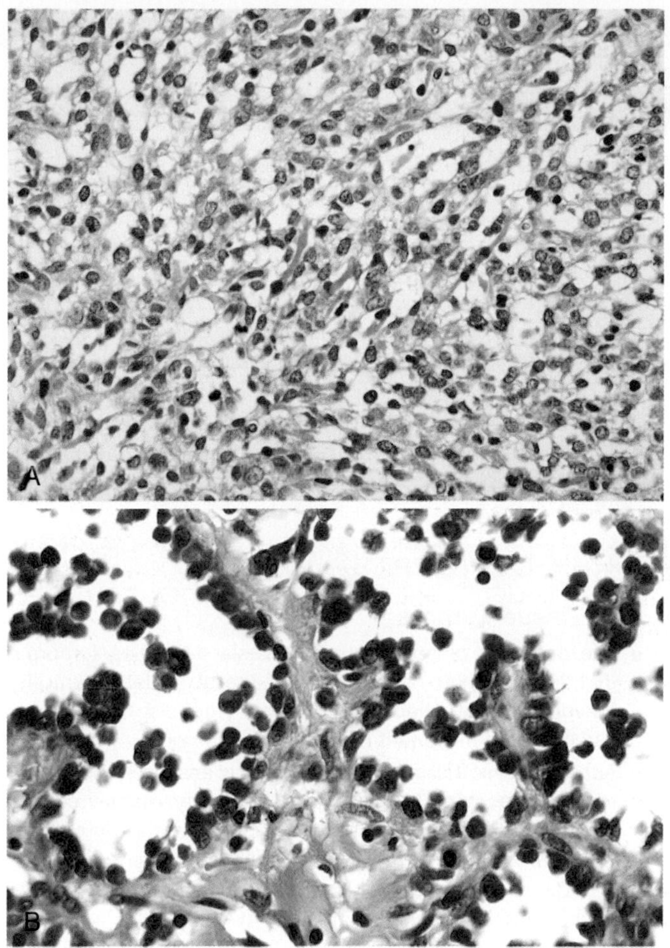

Figure 26-53 Rhabdomyosarcoma. **A,** Embryonal subtype composed of malignant cells ranging from primitive and round to densely eosinophilic with skeletal muscle differentiation. **B,** Alveolar rhabdomyosarcoma with numerous spaces lined by discohesive, uniform round tumor cells.

Smooth Muscle Tumors

Leiomyoma

Leiomyoma, a benign tumor of smooth muscle, often arises in the uterus; in fact, uterine leiomyomas are the most common neoplasm in women (Chapter 22). They develop in 77% of women and, depending on their number, size, and location, may cause a variety of symptoms including infertility. Leiomyomas may also arise from the erector pili muscles *(pilar leiomyomas)* found in the skin, nipples, scrotum, and labia and rarely in the deep soft tissues and the muscularis of the gut. Pilar leiomyomas may be multiple and painful. The phenotype of multiple cutaneous leiomyomas may be transmitted as an autosomal dominant trait that is also associated with uterine leiomyomas and renal cell carcinoma—*hereditary leiomyomatosis and renal cell cancer syndrome*. This disorder is associated with a germline loss-of-function mutation in the fumarate hydratase gene located on chromosome 1q42.3. Fumarate hydratase is an enzyme that participates in the Krebs cycle, and this association thus constitutes another intriguing example of the link between metabolic abnormalities and certain forms of neoplasia.

Soft tissue leiomyomas are usually 1 to 2 cm and are composed of fascicles of densely eosinophilic spindle cells that tend to intersect each other at right angles. The tumor cells have blunt-ended, elongated nuclei and show minimal atypia and few mitotic figures. Solitary lesions are easily cured. However, multiple tumors may be so numerous that complete surgical removal is impractical.

Leiomyosarcoma

Leiomyosarcoma accounts for 10% to 20% of soft tissue sarcomas. They occur in adults and afflict women more frequently than men. Most develop in the deep soft tissues of the extremities and retroperitoneum. A particularly deadly form arises from the great vessels, especially the inferior vena cava. Leiomyosarcomas have complex genotypes that stem from underlying defects that lead to profound genomic instability.

MORPHOLOGY

Leiomyosarcomas present as painless firm masses. Retroperitoneal tumors may be large and bulky and cause abdominal symptoms. They consist of eosinophilic spindle cells with blunt-ended, hyperchromatic nuclei arranged in interweaving fascicles. Ultrastructurally, the tumor cells contain bundles of thin filaments with dense bodies and pinocytic vesicles, and individual cells are surrounded by basal lamina. Immunohistochemically, they stain with antibodies to smooth muscle actin and desmin.

Treatment depends on tumor size, location, and grade. Superficial or cutaneous leiomyosarcomas are usually small and have a good prognosis, whereas those of the retroperitoneum are large, cannot be entirely excised, and cause death by both local extension and metastatic spread, especially to the lungs.

Tumors of Uncertain Origin

Although many soft tissue tumors can be assigned to recognizable histological types, a large proportion of tumors do not recapitulate any known mesenchymal lineage. This group includes examples with simple and complex karyotypes; one of each type is described later.

Synovial Sarcoma

Synovial sarcoma was so-named because the first described cases arose in the soft tissues near the knee joint and a morphologic relationship to synovium was postulated. However, this name is a misnomer, as these tumors can present in locations (chest wall, head and neck) that lack synovium and their morphologic features are inconsistent with an origin from synoviocytes. Synovial sarcomas account for approximately 10% of all soft tissue sarcomas and rank as the fourth most common sarcoma. Most occur in people in their 20s to 40s. Patients usually present with a deep-seated mass that has been present for several years. Most synovial sarcomas show a characteristic chromosomal translocation t(x;18)(p11;q11) producing *SS18-SSX1*,

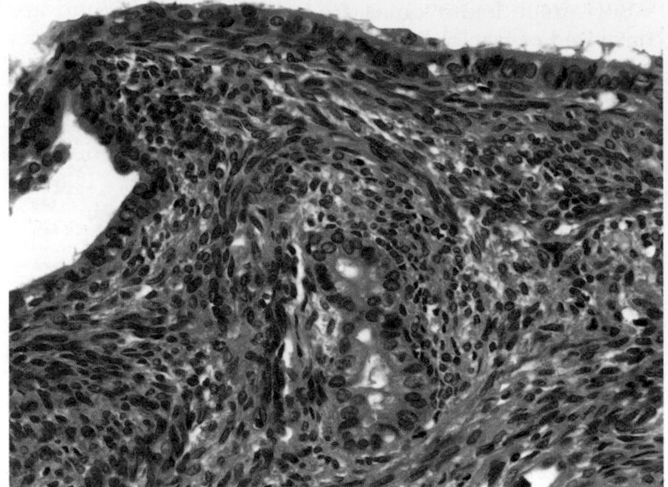

Figure 26-54 Synovial sarcoma revealing the classic biphasic spindle cell and glandlike histologic appearance.

-*SSX2*, or -*SSX4* fusion genes that encode chimeric transcription factors.

MORPHOLOGY

Synovial sarcomas are morphologically monophasic or biphasic. Monophasic synovial sarcoma consists of uniform spindle cells with scant cytoplasm and dense chromatin growing in short, tightly packed fascicles. Many tumors historically classified as fibrosarcoma likely would be classified as synovial sarcoma today. The tumors may calcify. The biphasic type contains, in addition to the spindle cell component above, gland-like structures composed of cuboidal to columnar epithelioid cells (Fig. 26-54). Immunohistochemistry is helpful in identifying these tumors, since the tumor cells, especially in the biphasic type, are positive for epithelial markers (e.g., keratins), differentiating them from most other sarcomas.

Synovial sarcomas are treated aggressively with limb-sparing surgery and frequently chemotherapy. The 5-year survival varies from 25% to 62%, related to stage and patient age. Common sites of metastases are the lung and occasionally the regional lymph nodes.

Undifferentiated Pleomorphic Sarcoma

Undifferentiated pleomorphic sarcoma (UPS) includes malignant mesenchymal tumors with high-grade, pleomorphic cells that cannot be classified into another category by a combination of histomorphology, immunophenotype, ultrastructure or molecular genetics. Despite advances in molecular characterization of sarcomas, UPS represents the largest category of adult sarcomas. Most arise in the deep soft tissues of the extremity, especially the thigh of middle aged or older adults. The diagnosis of *malignant fibrous histiocytoma* (MFH), sometimes used interchangeably with UPS, has fallen out of usage because (1) the category included both undifferentiated tumors and others that were reclassified with immunohistochemistry or molecular methods, and (2) no consensus exists for the morphologic definition of fibrohistiocytic. Not surprisingly, reproducible genetic changes are not typical of UPS. Most tumors are aneuploid with multiple structural and numerical chromosomal changes.

MORPHOLOGY

UPS are usually large, grey-white fleshy masses and can grow quite large (10 to 20 cm) depending on the anatomic compartment. Necrosis and hemorrhage are common. They consist of sheets of large, anaplastic spindled to polygonal cells with hyperchromatic irregular, sometimes bizarre nuclei (Fig. 26-55). Mitotic figures, including atypical non-symmetric forms, are abundant as is coagulative necrosis. By definition, tumor cells lack differentiation along recognized lineages.

UPS are aggressive malignancies that are treated with surgery and adjuvant chemotherapy and/or radiation. The prognosis is generally poor, with metastases arising in 30% to 50% of cases.

KEY CONCEPTS

Soft Tissue Tumors

- The category of soft tissue neoplasia describes tumors that do not fall into categories of epithelial, skeletal, central nervous system, hematopoietic or lymphoid tissues. A sarcoma is a malignant mesenchymal tumor.
- Although all soft tissue tumors probably arise from pluripotent mesenchymal stem cells, rather than mature cells, tumors can be classified into:
  - Tumors that recapitulate a mature mesenchymal tissue (e.g., skeletal muscle) can be further subdivided into benign and malignant forms.
  - Tumors composed of cells for which there is no normal counterpart (e.g., synovial sarcoma, undifferentiated pleomorphic sarcoma)
- Sarcomas with simple karyotypes demonstrate reproducible, chromosomal and molecular abnormalities which contribute to pathogenesis and are sufficiently specific to have diagnostic utility.
- Most adult sarcomas have complex karyotypes, tend to be pleomorphic and genetically heterogeneous with a poor prognosis.

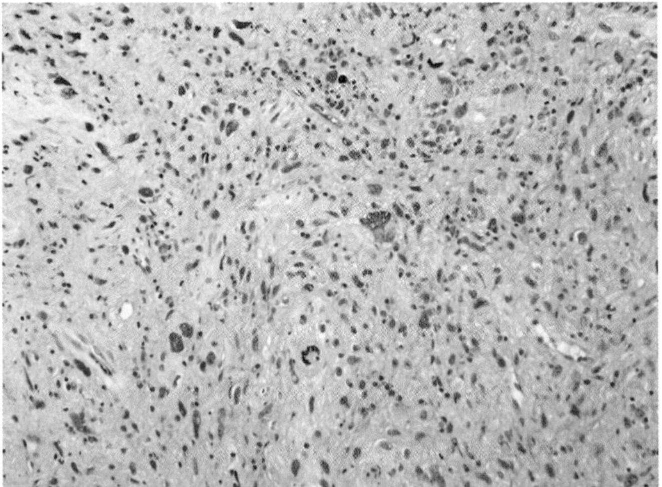

Figure 26-55 Undifferentiated pleomorphic sarcoma revealing anaplastic spindled to polygonal cells.

Acknowledgement

We would like to thank Dr. Andrew Rosenberg for his outstanding contribution to previous editions of this chapter.

SUGGESTED READINGS

Basic Structure and Biology of Bone

Cohen MM Jr: The new bone biology: pathologic, molecular, and clinical correlates. *Am J Med Genet A* 140:2646–706, 2006.

Kogianni G, Noble BS: The biology of osteocytes. *Curr Osteoporos Rep* 5:81–6, 2007.

Olsen BR, Reginato AM, Wang W: Bone development. *Annu Rev Cell Dev Biol* 16:191–220, 2000.

Raisz LG: Physiology and pathophysiology of bone remodeling. *Clin Chem* 45:1353–8, 1999.

Zaidi M: Skeletal remodeling in health and disease. *Nat Med* 13:791–801, 2007.

Skeletal Dysplasias

Askmyr MK, Fasth A, Richter J: Towards a better understanding and new therapeutics of osteopetrosis. *Br J Haematol* 140:597–609, 2008.

Kornak U, Kasper D, BÃpsl MR, et al: Loss of the ClC-7 Chloride Channel Leads to Osteopetrosis in Mice and Man. *Cell* 104:205–15, 2001.

Krakow D, Rimoin DL: The skeletal dysplasias. *Genet Med* 12:327–41, 2010.

Martin E, Shapiro JR: Osteogenesis imperfecta:epidemiology and pathophysiology. *Curr Osteoporos Rep* 5:91–7, 2007.

Van Dijk FS, Pals G, Van Rijn RR, et al: Classification of Osteogenesis Imperfecta revisited. *Eur J Med Genet* 53:1–5, 2010.

Osteoporosis

Anderson GL, Limacher M, Assaf AR, et al: Effects of conjugated equine estrogen in postmenopausal women with hysterectomy: the Women's Health Initiative randomized controlled trial. *JAMA* 291:1701–12, 2004.

Mosekilde L: Mechanisms of age-related bone loss. *Novartis Found Symp* 235:150–66; discussion 66–71, 2001.

Russell RG, Watts NB, Ebetino FH, et al: Mechanisms of action of bisphosphonates: similarities and differences and their potential influence on clinical efficacy. *Osteoporos Int* 19:733–59, 2008.

Styrkarsdottir U, Halldorsson BV, Gretarsdottir S, et al: Multiple genetic loci for bone mineral density and fractures. *N Engl J Med* 358:2355–65, 2008.

Paget Disease

Roodman GD, Windle JJ: Paget disease of bone. *J Clin Invest* 115:200–8, 2005.

Singer FR: The Etiology of Paget's Disease of Bone: Viral and Genetic Interactions. *Cell Metabolism* 13:5–6, 2011.

Whyte MP: Clinical practice. Paget's disease of bone. *N Engl J Med* 355:593–600, 2006.

Metabolic Bone Diseases

Mazzaferro S, Pasquali M, Pirrò G, et al: The bone and the kidney. *Archives of Biochemistry and Biophysics* 503:95–102, 2010.

Schwarz C, Sulzbacher I, Oberbauer R: Diagnosis of renal osteodystrophy. *Eur J Clin Invest* 36(Suppl 2):13–22, 2006.

Osteogenic Tumors

Klein MJ, Siegal GP: Osteosarcoma: anatomic and histologic variants.*Am J Clin Pathol* 125:555–81, 2006.

Lee EH, Shafi M, Hui JH: Osteoid osteoma: a current review. *J Pediatr Orthop* 26:695–700, 2006.

Wagner ER, Luther G, Zhu G, et al: Defective osteogenic differentiation in the development of osteosarcoma. *Sarcoma* 2011:325238, 2011.

Chondrogenic Tumors

Bovee JV, Hogendoorn PC, Wunder JS, et al: Cartilage tumours and bone development: molecular pathology and possible therapeutic targets. *Nat Rev Cancer* 10:481–8, 2010.

Pansuriya TC, van Eijk R, d'Adamo P, et al: Somatic mosaic IDH1 and IDH2 mutations are associated with enchondroma and spindle cell hemangioma in Ollier disease and Maffucci syndrome. *Nat Genet* 43:1256–61, 2011.

Wuyts W, Van Hul W: Molecular basis of multiple exostoses: mutations in the EXT1 and EXT2 genes. *Human Mutation* 15:220–7, 2000.

Ewing Sarcoma

Erkizan HV, Uversky VN, Toretsky JA: Oncogenic partnerships: EWS-FLI1 protein interactions initiate key pathways of Ewing's sarcoma. *Clin Cancer Res* 16:4077–83, 2010.

Liang H, Mao X, Olejniczak ET, et al: Solution structure of the ets domain of Fli-1 when bound to DNA. *Nat Struct Biol* 1:871–5, 1994.

Pinto A, Dickman P, Parham D: Pathobiologic markers of the ewing sarcoma family of tumors: state of the art and prediction of behaviour. *Sarcoma* 2011:856190, 2011.

Giant Cell Tumor of Bone

Robinson D, Einhorn TA: Giant cell tumor of bone: a unique paradigm of stromal-hematopoietic cellular interactions. *J Cell Biochem* 55:300–3, 1994.

Salerno M, Avnet S, Alberghini M, et al: Histogenetic characterization of giant cell tumor of bone. *Clin Orthop Relat Res* 466:2081–91, 2008.

Aneurysmal Bone Cyst

Oliveira AM, Chou MM: The TRE17/USP6 oncogene: a riddle wrapped in a mystery inside an enigma. *Front Biosci (Schol Ed)* 4:321–34, 2012.

Fibrous Dysplasia

Riminucci M, Robey PG, Saggio I, et al: Skeletal progenitors and the GNAS gene: fibrous dysplasia of bone read through stem cells. *J Mol Endocrinol* 45:355–64, 2010.

Osteoarthritis

Goldring MB, Goldring SR: Articular cartilage and subchondral bone in the pathogenesis of osteoarthritis. *Ann N Y Acad Sci* 1192:230–7, 2010.

Valdes AM, Spector TD: Genetic epidemiology of hip and knee osteoarthritis. *Nat Rev Rheumatol* 7:23–32, 2011.

Yelin E, Callahan LF: The economic cost and social and psychological impact of musculoskeletal conditions. National Arthritis Data Work Groups. *Arthritis Rheum* 38:1351–62, 1995.

Rheumatoid Arthritis and Related Conditions

Fox DA, Gizinski A, Morgan R, et al: Cell-cell interactions in rheumatoid arthritis synovium. *Rheum Dis Clin North Am* 36:311–23, 2010.

Imboden JB: The immunopathogenesis of rheumatoid arthritis. *Annu Rev Pathol* 4:417–34, 2009.

Petty RE, Southwood TR, Manners P, et al: International League of Associations for Rheumatology classification of juvenile idiopathic arthritis: second revision, Edmonton, 2001. *J Rheumatol* 31:390–2, 2004.

Scott DL, Wolfe F, Huizinga TW: Rheumatoid arthritis. *Lancet* 376:1094–108, 2011.

Thomas GP, Brown MA: Genetics and genomics of ankylosing spondylitis. *Immunol Rev* 233:162–80, 2010.

Infectious Arthritis

Iliopoulou BP, Huber BT: Infectious arthritis and immune dysregulation: lessons from Lyme disease. *Curr Opin Rheumatol* 22:451–5, 2010.

Rosenberg AE, Nielsen GP, Reith J: Surgical pathology of joint prostheses. *Semin Diagn Pathol* 28:65–72, 2011.

Steere AC, Drouin EE, Glickstein LJ: Relationship between immunity to Borrelia burgdorferi outer-surface protein A (OspA) and Lyme arthritis. *Clin Infect Dis* 52(Suppl 3):S259–65, 2011.

Gout and Pseudogout

Rosenthal AK: Update in calcium deposition diseases. *Curr Opin Rheumatol* 19:158–62, 2007.

VanItallie TB: Gout: epitome of painful arthritis. *Metabolism* 59(Suppl 1):S32–6, 2010.

Tenosynovial Giant Cell Tumor

Moller E, Mandahl N, Mertens F, et al: Molecular identification of COL6A3-CSF1 fusion transcripts in tenosynovial giant cell tumors. *Genes Chromosomes Cancer* 47:21–5, 2008.

Soft Tissue Sarcomas

Bovee JV, Hogendoorn PC: Molecular pathology of sarcomas: concepts and clinical implications. *Virchows Arch* 456:193–9, 2010.

Fletcher CD, Gustafson P, Rydholm A, et al: Clinicopathologic re-evaluation of 100 malignant fibrous histiocytomas: prognostic relevance of subclassification. *J Clin Oncol* 19:3045–50, 2001.

Jain S, Xu R, Prieto VG, et al: Molecular classification of soft tissue sarcomas and its clinical applications. *Int J Clin Exp Pathol* 3:416–28, 2010.

Saito T, Nagai M, Ladanyi M: SYT-SSX1 and SYT-SSX2 interfere with repression of E-cadherin by snail and slug: a potential mechanism for aberrant mesenchymal to epithelial transition in human synovial sarcoma. *Cancer Res* 66:6919–27, 2006.

West RB: Expression profiling in soft tissue sarcomas with emphasis on synovial sarcoma, gastrointestinal stromal tumor, and leiomyosarcoma. *Adv Anat Pathol* 17:366–73, 2010.

See TARGETED THERAPY available online at www.studentconsult.com

CHAPTER 27

Peripheral Nerves and Skeletal Muscles

Peter Pytel • Douglas C. Anthony

CHAPTER CONTENTS

Neuromuscular diseases are a complex group of disorders with numerous inherited and acquired causes that typically present with weakness, muscle pain, or sensory deficits. They can be grouped according to anatomy, the tempo of the disease course, and pathogenesis. Physicians keep all these characteristics in mind when evaluating a patient. This chapter uses an anatomical approach, grouping neuromuscular disorders into those that preferentially affect the peripheral nerves, the neuromuscular junction, or the skeletal muscles. A discussion of neoplasms that arise from peripheral nerves ends the chapter. Conditions that can produce similar clinical presentations but are caused by disorders of the central nervous system are discussed in Chapter 28.

Diseases of Peripheral Nerves

The two main components of peripheral nerves are axons and myelin sheaths made by Schwann cells. Injuries to either of these components may result in a peripheral neuropathy. Before discussing the pathology of these disorders, a brief review of peripheral nerve structure and function is in order. *Somatic motor function* is carried out by the motor unit, which consists of (1) a lower motor neuron located in the anterior horn of the spinal cord or in the brainstem; (2) an axon that travels to a target muscle as part of a nerve; (3) the neuromuscular junctions; and (4) multiple innervated myofibers (muscle fibers). *Somatic sensory function* depends on (1) the distal nerve endings, which may contain specialized structures that serve to register specific sensory modalities; (2) an axon that travels as part of a peripheral nerve to the dorsal root ganglia; and (3) a proximal axon segment that synapses on neurons in the spinal cord or the brainstem. *Autonomic nerve fibers* outnumber somatic fibers in the peripheral nervous system, but signs and symptoms related to their involvement are generally not prominent features of peripheral neuropathies, with a few important exceptions (e.g., in some cases of diabetic neuropathy, discussed later).

Specific sensations (pain, temperature, touch) and motor signals are each conveyed by axons that can be distinguished based on their diameter. Axonal diameters are in turn correlated with the thickness of their myelin sheaths

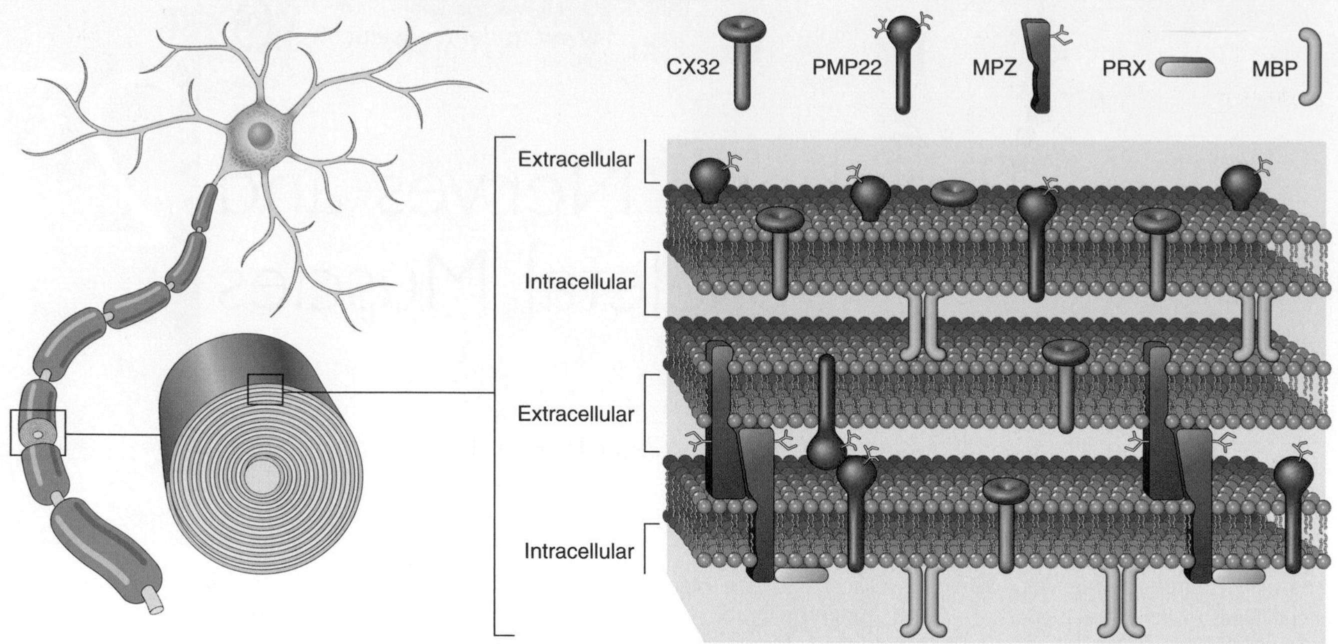

Figure 27-1 Relationship between lipid bilayers and associated proteins in myelin within internodes. Myelin basic protein (MBP) is an intracellular protein that has a role in myelin compaction. Mutant forms of myelin protein zero (MPZ), peripheral myelin protein 22 (PMP22), and periaxin (PRX) cause some forms of Charcot-Marie-Tooth disease, a hereditary demyelinating neuropathy.

and with their conduction speeds. Thin unmyelinated fibers mediate autonomic functions as well as pain and temperature sensation and have the slowest conduction speeds. Large diameter axons with thick myelin sheaths transmit light touch and motor signals and have fast conduction speeds. In the case of myelinated axons, individual Schwann cells make exactly one myelin sheath that wraps around a single axon to create a myelinated segment called an *internode*. Internodes are separated by unmyelinated gaps referred to as *nodes of Ranvier*, which are uniformly spaced along the length of the axon. A number of specialized proteins are essential for normal assembly and function of myelin within internodes (Fig. 27-1). Unmyelinated axons are also intimately associated with Schwann cells but in a different arrangement in which one cell surrounds segments of multiple axons.

Most peripheral nerves carry out both motor and sensory functions and thus contain axons of varying diameter and myelin thickness. The axons are bundled together by three major connective tissue components: the *epineurium*, which encloses the entire nerve; the *perineurium*, a multilayered concentric connective tissue sheath that groups subsets of axons into fascicles; and the *endoneurium*, which surrounds individual nerve fibers.

General Types of Peripheral Nerve Injury

Axonal Neuropathies

Axons are the primary target of the damage in this large group of peripheral neuropathies (Fig. 27-2). The morphologic hallmarks of axonal neuropathies can be produced experimentally by cutting a peripheral nerve, which results in a prototypical pattern of injury described as *Wallerian degeneration*. Portions of axons that are distal to the point of transsection are disconnected from the central neuron and degenerate. Within a day of injury, the distal axons begin to fragment and the associated myelin sheaths unravel (Fig. 27-3) and disintegrate into spherical structures (*myelin ovoids*). Macrophages are recruited and they participate in the removal of axonal and myelin debris. Regeneration starts at the site of transsection with the formation of a growth cone and the outgrowth of new branches from the stump of the proximal axon. Schwann cells and their associated basement membranes guide the sprouting axons, which grow at about 1 mm per day, toward their distal target. Continuous pruning of the sprouting axons removes misguided branches. The Schwann cells create new myelin sheaths around the regenerating axons, but these myelin internodes tend to be thinner and shorter than in the original ones. The repair process is successful only if the two transected ends remain closely approximated. A failure of the outgrowing axons to find their distal target can produce a "pseudotumor" termed *traumatic neuroma*– a nonneoplastic haphazard whorled proliferation of axonal processes and associated Schwann cells that results in a painful nodule (Fig. 27-4).

The changes observed following experimental nerve transsections only partially resemble those seen in various axonal neuropathies. One key difference is that in these disease states (unlike nerve transection) damage occurs over an extended period of time. As a result, degenerating and regenerating axons co-exist in a single biopsy. With time, damage tends to outpace repair, resulting in progressive loss of axons. Consequently, the electrophysiologic hallmark of axonal neuropathies is a reduction in signal strength owing to the dropout of axons from affected peripheral nerves.

Demyelinating Neuropathies

In these disorders, Schwann cells with their myelin sheaths are the primary targets of damage (Fig. 27-2),

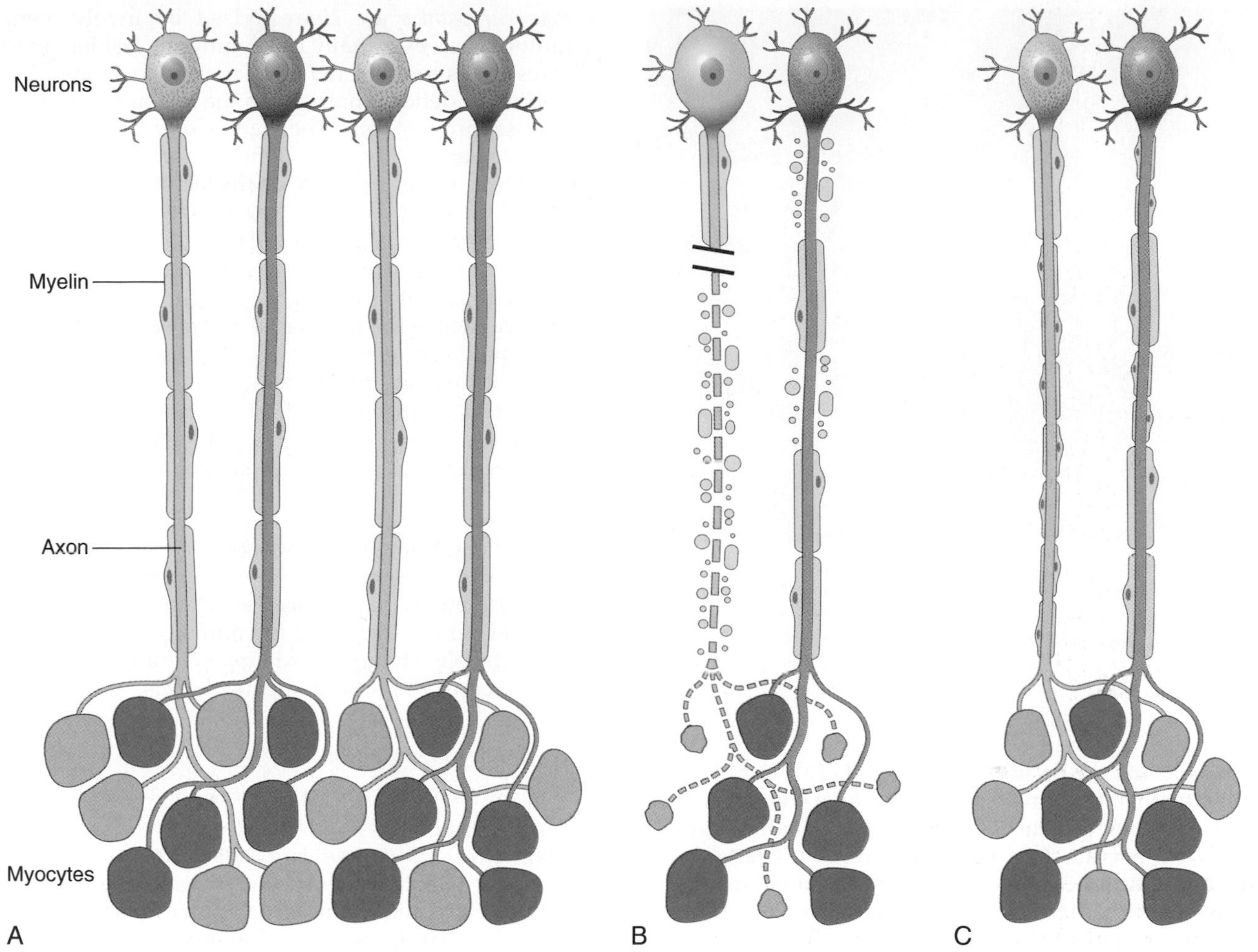

Neurons

Myelin

Axon

Myocytes

A B C

Figure 27-2 Patterns of peripheral nerve damage. **A,** In normal motor units, type I and type II myofibers are arranged in a "checkerboard" distribution, and the internodes along the motor axons are uniform in thickness and length. **B,** Acute axonal injury (*left axon*) results in degeneration of the distal axon and its associated myelin sheath, with atrophy of denervated myofibers. In contrast, acute demyelinating disease (*right axon*) produces random segmental degeneration of individual myelin internodes, while sparing the axons. **C,** Regeneration of axons after injury (*left axon*) allows reinnervation of myofibers. The regenerated axon is myelinated by proliferating Schwann cells, but the new internodes are shorter and the myelin sheaths are thinner than the original ones. Remission of demyelinating disease (*right axon*) allows remyelination to take place, but the new internodes also are shorter and have thinner myelin sheaths than flanking normal undamaged internodes. See Table 27-1 and Fig. 27-7 for comparison.

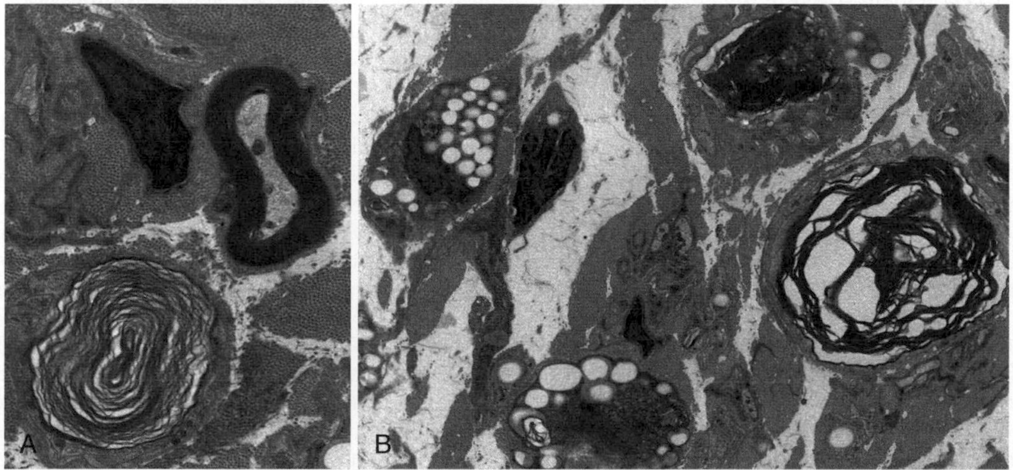

Figure 27-3 Electron micrographs illustrating features of axonal degeneration. **A,** Degenerating myelin with loosened myelin layers is seen in the degenerating axon in the lower left corner, to be contrasted with a normal myelin sheath with tightly packed myelin and intact axon in the upper right corner. **B,** In addition to an unraveling myelin sheath, several cells contain lipid droplets (seen as vacuoles) derived from degenerating myelin.

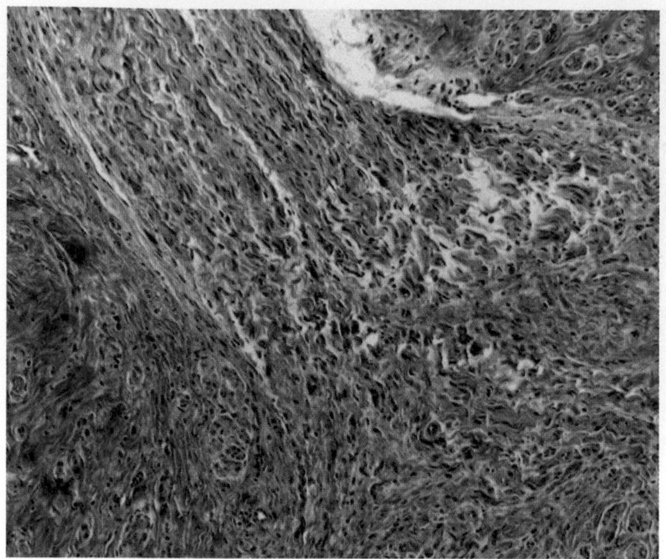

Figure 27-4 Trichrome-stained section of a traumatic neuroma showing the transition from normal nerve containing a parallel arrangement of axons (*upper left corner*) to a haphazard swirl of red stained axons associated with admixture of Schwann cells and blue-staining connective tissue.

whereas axons are relatively preserved. This definition is similar to that of demyelinating diseases that affect the central nervous system (Chapter 28). Individual myelin sheaths degenerate in a seemingly random pattern, resulting in discontinuous damage of myelin segments. In response to this damage, Schwann cells or Schwann cell precursors proliferate and initiate repair through the formation of new myelin sheaths, but these again tend to be shorter and thinner than the original ones. The electrophysiologic hallmark of these disorders is slowed nerve conduction velocity, reflective of the loss of myelin.

Neuronopathies

Neuronopathies result from destruction of neurons, leading to secondary degeneration of axonal processes. Infections like herpes zoster and toxins like platinum compounds are examples of insults that may lead to neuronopathies. Because the damage is at the level of the neuronal cell body, peripheral nerve dysfunction caused by neuronopathies is equally likely to affect proximal and distal parts of the body (unlike peripheral axonopathies which preferentially affect the distal extremities).

Anatomic Patterns of Peripheral Neuropathies

Peripheral neuropathies can be separated into several groups according to the anatomic distribution of involvement and the associated neurological deficits. This approach can be helpful clinically, since each pattern has a different set of potential underlying causes. These anatomic patterns of injury are as follows:

- *Mononeuropathies* affect a single nerve and result in deficits in a restricted distribution dictated by normal anatomy. Trauma, entrapment, and infections are common causes of mononeuropathy.
- *Polyneuropathies* are characterized by involvement of multiple nerves, usually in a symmetric fashion. In most cases axons are affected in a length dependent fashion leading to deficits that start in the feet and ascend with disease progression. The hands often start to show involvement by the time deficits extend to the level of the knee, resulting in a characteristic "stocking and glove" distribution of sensory deficits.
- *Mononeuritis multiplex* describes a disease process that damages several nerves in a haphazard fashion. An affected patient might have a right wrist drop from involvement of the right radial nerve and a left foot drop from peroneal nerve damage. Vasculitis is a common cause of this pattern of injury.
- *Polyradiculoneuropathies* affect nerve roots as well as peripheral nerves, leading to diffuse symmetric symptoms in proximal and distal parts of the body.

Specific Peripheral Neuropathies

Many different types of disease processes can damage peripheral nerves, including inflammatory diseases, infections, metabolic changes, toxic injury, trauma, (para)neoplastic disease, and inherited gene defects.

Inflammatory Neuropathies

Guillain-Barré Syndrome (Acute Inflammatory Demyelinating Polyneuropathy)

Guillain-Barré syndrome is a demyelinating peripheral neuropathy that may lead to life-threatening respiratory paralysis. The overall annual incidence is approximately one case per 100,000 persons. The disease is characterized clinically by weakness beginning in the distal limbs that rapidly advances to affect proximal muscle function ("ascending paralysis"). Histologic features are inflammation and demyelination of spinal nerve roots and peripheral nerves (radiculoneuropathy).

Pathogenesis. **In most cases, Guillain-Barré syndrome is thought to be an acute-onset *immune-mediated demyelinating neuropathy.*** Approximately two thirds of cases are preceded by an acute, influenza-like illness from which the affected individual has recovered by the time the neuropathy becomes symptomatic. Infections with *Campylobacter jejuni*, cytomegalovirus, Epstein-Barr virus, and *Mycoplasma pneumoniae*, or prior vaccination, have significant epidemiologic associations with Guillain-Barré syndrome. No infectious agent has been demonstrated in affected nerves, and an immunologic reaction is favored as the underlying cause. A similar inflammatory disease of peripheral nerves can be reproduced in experimental animals by immunization with a peripheral nerve myelin protein. A T-cell–mediated immune response ensues, accompanied by segmental demyelination induced by activated macrophages. Transfer of these T cells to a naive animal results in comparable lesions. Moreover, lymphocytes from individuals with Guillain-Barré syndrome have been shown to produce demyelination in tissue cultures of myelinated nerve fibers. Circulating antibodies that cross-react with components of peripheral nerves may also play a role.

MORPHOLOGY

The dominant histopathologic finding is **inflammation of peripheral nerves**, manifested as perivenular and endoneurial infiltration by lymphocytes, macrophages, and a few plasma cells. Segmental demyelination affecting peripheral nerves is the most prominent lesion, but damage to axons is also seen, particularly when the disease is severe. Electron microscopy has identified an early effect on myelin sheaths. The cytoplasmic processes of macrophages penetrate the basement membrane of Schwann cells, particularly in the vicinity of the nodes of Ranvier, and extend between the myelin lamellae, stripping the myelin sheath from the axon. Ultimately, the remnants of the myelin sheath are engulfed by the macrophages. Inflammation and demyelination can be widespread in the peripheral nervous system but are typically most prominent proximally, close to the nerve roots.

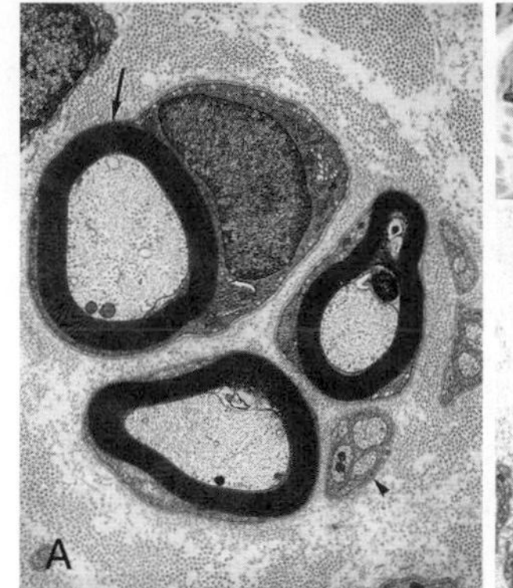

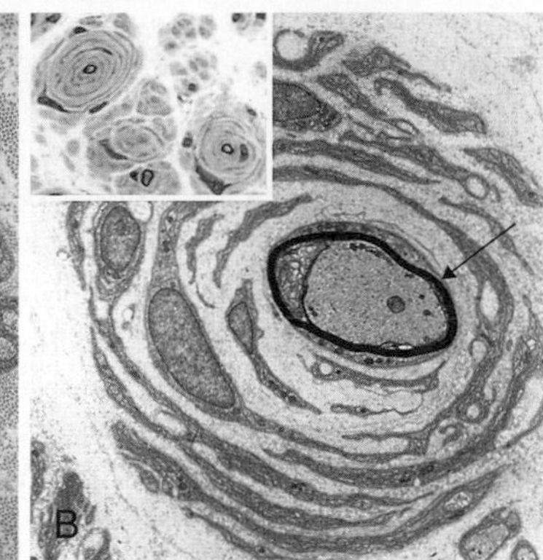

Figure 27-5 Onion bulb neuropathy. Compared with the normal ultrastructure of axons in a nerve **(A),** an "onion bulb" **(B)** is composed of a thinly myelinated axon (*arrow*) surrounded by multiple concentrically arranged Schwann cells. *Inset*, Light-microscopic appearance of an onion bulb neuropathy, characterized by "onion bulbs" surrounding axons. (**B,** Courtesy G. Richard Dickersin, MD, from Diagnostic Electron Microscopy: A Text Atlas. New York, Igaku-Shoin Medical Publishers, 2000, p 984.)

Clinical Features. The clinical picture is dominated by ascending paralysis and areflexia. Deep tendon reflexes disappear early in the process. Sensory involvement, including loss of pain sensation, is often present but is usually not a prominent feature. Nerve conduction velocities are slowed because of multifocal destruction of myelin segments in many axons within a nerve. Cerebrospinal fluid (CSF) protein levels are elevated due to inflammation and altered permeability of the microcirculation within the spinal roots as they traverse the subarachnoid space. Inflammatory cells, on the other hand, remain confined to the roots, therefore, there is little or no CSF pleocytosis. Many patients spend weeks in hospital intensive-care units before recovering normal function. With improved supportive respiratory care, cardiovascular monitoring, and prophylaxis against deep venous thrombosis, the mortality rate has fallen. Plasmapheresis and intravenous immunoglobulin appear to be beneficial, apparently because these remove pathogenic antibodies and suppress immune function, respectively. However, 2% to 5% of affected patients still die of respiratory paralysis, autonomic instability, cardiac arrest, or related complications, and up to 20% of hospitalized survivors suffer long-term disability.

Chronic Inflammatory Demyelinating Poly(radiculo)neuropathy

This is the most common chronic acquired inflammatory peripheral neuropathy, characterized by symmetrical mixed sensorimotor polyneuropathy that persists for 2 months or more. By definition, signs and symptoms must be present for at least 2 months but often the disease evolves over years, usually with relapses and remissions. While typically there is a symmetric, mixed sensorimotor polyneuropathy, some patients may present with predominantly sensory or motor impairment. Clinical remissions can often be achieved with immunosuppressive therapies, such as glucocorticoids, intravenous immunoglobulin, plasmapheresis, and biologic agents directed against T cells or B cells. The time course and the response to steroids distinguish chronic inflammatory demyelinating polyradiculoneuropathy from Guillain-Barré syndrome.

Pathogenesis. T cells as well as humoral factors are implicated in the inflammatory process. Molecules expressed at the Schwann cell-axon junction and in noncompact areas of myelin appear to be the target of the immune response. Complement-fixing IgG and IgM can be found on the myelin sheath, and the deposition of these opsonins leads to recruitment of macrophages that strip myelin from axons. Sural nerve biopsies show evidence of recurrent demyelination and remyelination associated with proliferation of Schwann cells. When excessive, this proliferation leads to the formation of so-called *onion-bulbs* – structures in which multiple layers of Schwann cells wrap around an axon like the layers of an onion (Fig. 27-5).

Neuropathy Associated with Systemic Autoimmune Diseases

Systemic autoimmune diseases like rheumatoid arthritis, Sjögren syndrome, or systemic lupus erythematosus (SLE) can be associated with peripheral neuropathies that often take the form of distal sensory or sensorimotor polyneuropathies. These neuropathies are distinct from vasculitic peripheral neuropathies, which can arise as secondary manifestations of these same diseases.

Neuropathy Associated with Vasculitis

Vasculitis is a noninfectious inflammation of blood vessels that can involve and damage peripheral nerves. About one third of patients with vasculitis have peripheral nerve involvement, and neuropathy may be the presenting feature. Vasculitis often presents as mononeuritis multiplex, but mononeuritis and polyneuropathy are also encountered.

Peripheral nerves involved by vasculitis typically show patchy axonal degeneration and loss, with some fascicles being more severely affected than others. Perivascular inflammatory infiltrates are often present. Identification of blood vessels with characteristic forms of acute or chronic damage (Chapter 11) helps establish the diagnosis.

Infectious Neuropathies

Many infectious processes affect peripheral nerves. Among these, leprosy, diphtheria, and varicella-zoster cause relatively specific pathologic changes in nerves that are the point of focus here. Each of these disorders is also discussed in more detail in Chapter 8.

Leprosy (Hansen Disease)

Peripheral nerves are involved in both lepromatous and tuberculoid leprosy (discussed in Chapter 8).

- In *lepromatous leprosy,* Schwann cells are invaded by *Mycobacterium leprae,* which proliferate and eventually infect other cells. There is evidence of segmental demyelination and remyelination and loss of both myelinated and unmyelinated axons. As the infection advances, endoneurial fibrosis and multilayered thickening of the perineurial sheaths occur. Affected individuals develop a symmetric polyneuropathy that is most severe in the relatively cool distal extremities and in the face because lower temperatures favor mycobacterial growth. The infection prominently involves pain fibers, and the resulting loss of sensation contributes to injury, since the patient is rendered unaware of injurious stimuli and damaged tissues. Thus, large traumatic ulcers may develop.
- *Tuberculoid leprosy* is characterized by an active cell-mediated immune response to *M. leprae* that is usually manifest as dermal nodules containing granulomatous inflammation. The inflammation injures cutaneous nerves in the vicinity; axons, Schwann cells, and myelin are lost, and there is fibrosis of the perineurium and endoneurium. In tuberculoid leprosy, affected individuals have much more localized nerve involvement.

Lyme Disease

Lyme disease causes various neurologic manifestations in the second and third stage of the disease. These include polyradiculoneuropathy and unilateral or bilateral facial nerve palsies.

HIV/AIDS

Patients infected with human immunodeficiency virus (HIV) develop several patterns of peripheral neuropathy that are poorly understood, but all appear to be related in some way to immune dysregulation. Early stage HIV infection can be associated with mononeuritis multiplex and demyelinating disorders that may resemble Guillain-Barré syndrome or chronic inflammatory demyelinating polyradiculoneuropathy. More commonly, later stages of HIV infection are associated with a distal sensory neuropathy that is often painful.

Diphtheria

Diphtheria is most commonly found in the developing world and is a continuing medical problem because of incomplete immunization or waning immunity in adults. *Peripheral nerve dysfunction results from the effects of the diphtheria exotoxin.* It produces an acute peripheral neuropathy associated with prominent bulbar and respiratory muscle dysfunction, which can lead to death or long-term disability. The mechanism of action of diphtheria toxin is described in Chapter 8.

Varicella-Zoster Virus

Varicella-zoster is one of the most common viral infections of the peripheral nervous system. Following chickenpox, a latent infection persists within neurons of sensory ganglia. If the virus is reactivated, sometimes many years later, it may be transported along the sensory nerves to the skin. Here it infects keratinocytes, leading to a *painful, vesicular skin eruption (shingles) in a distribution that follows sensory dermatomes.* Most common is the involvement of thoracic or trigeminal nerve dermatomes. The factors underlying reactivation of the virus are not fully understood, but decreased cell-mediated immunity is suspected to play a role. In a small proportion of patients, weakness is also apparent in the same distributions. Affected ganglia show neuronal death, usually accompanied by abundant mononuclear inflammatory cell infiltrates; focal necrosis and hemorrhage may also be found. Peripheral nerves show degeneration of the axons that belong to the dead sensory neurons. Focal destruction of the large motor neurons of the anterior horns or cranial nerve motor nuclei may be seen at the corresponding levels. Intranuclear inclusions generally are not found in the peripheral nervous system.

Metabolic, Hormonal, and Nutritional Neuropathies

Diabetes

Diabetes is the most common cause of peripheral neuropathy. The prevalence of this complication depends on the duration of the disease; up to 50% of patients with diabetes overall and up to 80% of those who have had the disease for more than 15 years have clinical evidence of peripheral neuropathy. Patients with type 1 and type 2 diabetes are affected (Chapter 24). Several distinct clinicopathologic patterns of diabetes-related peripheral neuropathy are recognized (described later), but the most common by far is an ascending distal symmetric sensorimotor polyneuropathy.

Pathogenesis. The mechanism of diabetic neuropathy is complex and not completely resolved; both metabolic and secondary vascular changes are believed to contribute to the damage of neurons and Schwann cells. Hyperglycemia causes the nonenzymatic glycosylation of proteins, lipids, and nucleic acids. The resulting advanced glycosylation end products (AGEs) may interfere with normal protein function and activate inflammatory signaling through the receptor for AGE. Excess glucose within cells is reduced to sorbitol, a process that depletes NADPH and increases intracellular osmolality. These and other metabolic disturbances may predispose peripheral nerves to injury by reactive oxygen species. In addition, the vascular injuries that occur in chronic diabetes due to hyperlipidemia and other metabolic alterations may cause ischemic damage of the nerves.

MORPHOLOGY

In individuals with a **distal symmetric sensorimotor neuropathy,** the predominant pathologic finding is an axonal neuropathy. Nerve biopsies show reduced numbers of axons. Variable degrees of ongoing axonal damage, marked by degenerating myelin sheaths and regenerative axonal clusters, may be present. Endoneurial arterioles show thickening, hyalinization, and intense periodic acid–Schiff positivity of their walls and extensive reduplication of basement membranes (Fig. 27-6).

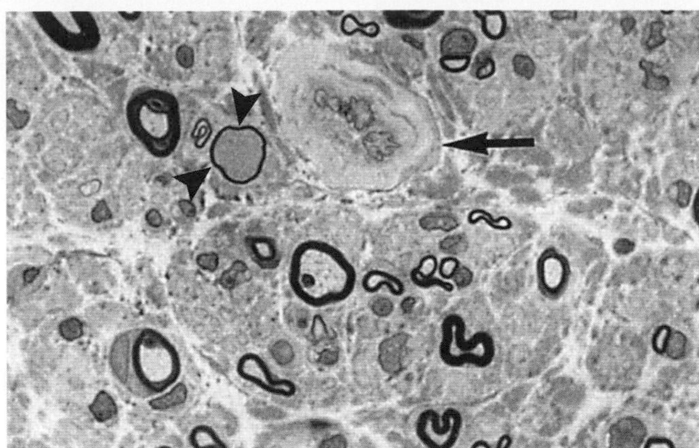

Figure 27-6 Diabetic neuropathy with marked loss of myelinated fibers, a thinly myelinated fiber (*arrowheads*), and thickening of endoneurial vessel wall (*arrow*).

Clinical Features. *Distal symmetric diabetic polyneuropathy* typically presents with sensory symptoms, like numbness, loss of pain sensation, difficulty with balance, and paresthesias or dysesthesias. Paresthesias or dysesthesias are so called "positive" symptoms—painful sensations that result from abnormal discharges of damaged nerves. Neuropathy leads to considerable morbidity, in particular an increased susceptibility to foot and ankle fractures and chronic skin ulcers, which may eventually lead to amputations.

Another manifestation is *dysfunction of the autonomic nervous system*; this affects 20% to 40% of individuals with diabetes mellitus, nearly always in association with a distal sensorimotor neuropathy. Diabetic autonomic neuropathy has protean manifestations, including postural hypotension, incomplete emptying of the bladder (resulting in recurrent infections), and sexual dysfunction. Some affected individuals, especially older adults with a long history of diabetes, develop a peripheral neuropathy that manifests with asymmetric presentations, including *mononeuropathy, cranial neuropathy* and *radiculoplexus neuropathy*. The latter is a devastatingly painful acute disorder that presents in the distribution of the brachial or lumbosacral nerve plexus. It is often monophasic and can improve over several months. These asymmetric manifestations may be caused by microvascular disease.

Other Metabolic, Hormonal, and Nutritional Neuropathies

A diverse group of metabolic, hormonal, and nutritional disorders are associated with peripheral neuropathy, including the following:

- *Uremic neuropathy*. Most individuals with renal failure have a peripheral neuropathy. Typically this is a distal, symmetric neuropathy that may be asymptomatic or may be associated with muscle cramps, distal dysesthesias, and diminished deep tendon reflexes. In these patients axonal degeneration is the primary event; occasionally there is secondary demyelination. Regeneration and recovery are common after dialysis.
- *Thyroid dysfunction*. Hypothyroidism can lead to compression mononeuropathies such as carpal tunnel syndrome or cause a distal symmetric predominantly sensory polyneuropathy. In rare cases, hyperthyroidism is associated with a neuropathy resembling Guillain-Barré syndrome.
- *Vitamin B_{12} (cyanocobalamin) deficiency* classically results in subacute combined degeneration with damage to long tracts in the spinal cord (Chapter 28), and also peripheral nerves.
- *Deficiencies of vitamin B_1 (thiamine), vitamin B_6 (pyridoxine), folate, vitamin E, copper, and zinc* have all been associated with peripheral neuropathy.

Toxic Neuropathies

Peripheral neuropathies may appear after *exposure to industrial or environmental chemicals, biologic toxins, or therapeutic drugs*. Important causes of toxic peripheral nerve damage include alcohol (independent of associated nutritional deficiencies), heavy metals (lead, mercury, arsenic, and thallium), and organic solvents. Various medications can cause toxic nerve damage, but the most notorious are chemotherapeutic agents. These include vinca alkaloids and taxanes, microtubule inhibitors that interfere with axonal transport, and cisplatin, which may cause a neuronopathy.

Neuropathies Associated with Malignancy

Neuropathies associated with cancers may stem from local effects, complications of therapy, paraneoplastic effects, or (in the case of B-cell tumors) tumor-derived immunoglobulins.

- *Direct infiltration or compression of peripheral nerves* by tumor is a common cause of mononeuropathy and may be a presenting symptom of cancer. These neuropathies include *brachial plexopathy* from neoplasms of the apex of the lung, *obturator palsy* from pelvic malignant neoplasms, and *cranial nerve palsies* from intracranial tumors or tumors of the base of the skull. A *polyradiculopathy* involving the lower extremity may develop when the cauda equina is involved by meningeal carcinomatosis.
- In addition to complications of chemotherapy (discussed earlier), damage to nerves in cancer patients may be caused by *radiation, poor nutrition* and *infection*.
- *Paraneoplastic neuropathies*. These can occur at any time during the patient's course, but often precede the diagnosis of the underlying tumor. *Sensorimotor neuronopathy is the most common paraneoplastic form,* but a chronic inflammatory demyelinating polyradiculoneuropathy-like picture, plexopathy, and autonomic neuropathy may also be seen. Paraneoplastic sensorimotor neuronopathy is most commonly associated with small cell lung cancer. Antibodies that recognize proteins expressed by cancer cells and normal neurons (for example anti-Hu antibodies) are often present, but the damage appears to be mediated by a CD8+ cytotoxic T-cell attack on dorsal root ganglion cells. Sensory symptoms usually start distally in an asymmetric and multifocal pattern. Other patients with so-called anti-CV2 autoantibodies (which recognize CRMP5, an intracellular signaling protein) tend to present with a mixed axonal and demyelinating sensorimotor neuropathy.

- *Neuropathies associated with monoclonal gammopathies.* Neoplastic B cells may secrete monoclonal immunoglobulins or immunoglobulin fragments (so-called paraproteins) that damage nerves. For example, tumors that secrete IgM immunoglobulin may be associated with a demyelinating peripheral neuropathy. In most cases, the pathogenic IgM paraprotein is thought to bind directly to myelin-associated antigens such as myelin associated glycoprotein (MAG). Deposition of IgM can be seen ultrastructurally between the membrane layers of the myelin sheath. IgG or IgA paraproteins may also be associated with peripheral neuropathy. One distinctive presentation is *POEMS syndrome* (polyneuropathy, organomegaly, endocrinopathy, monoclonal gammopathy, and skin changes), in which patients often develop a demyelinating neuropathy associated with deposition of paraprotein between noncompacted myelin lamellae. Finally, excess immunoglobulin light chain may deposit as amyloid (Chapter 6), which can lead to peripheral neuropathy due to vascular insufficiency or a direct toxic effects.

Neuropathies Caused by Physical Forces

Peripheral nerves are commonly injured by trauma or entrapment. *Lacerations* result from cutting injuries and from sharp fragments of fractured bone, both of which may sever a nerve. *Avulsion* of a nerve may occur when tension is applied, often to one of the limbs. *Compression neuropathy (entrapment neuropathy)* occurs when a peripheral nerve is chronically subjected to increased pressure, often within an anatomic compartment. *Carpal tunnel syndrome*, the most common entrapment neuropathy, results from compression of the median nerve at the level of the wrist within the compartment delimited by the transverse carpal ligament. Women are more commonly affected than men, and the problem is frequently bilateral. The disorder may be observed in association with many conditions including tissue edema, pregnancy, inflammatory arthritis, hypothyroidism, amyloidosis (especially that related to β_2-microglobulin deposition in individuals on renal dialysis), acromegaly, diabetes mellitus, and excessive repetitive motions of the wrist. Symptoms are limited to dysfunction of the median nerve and typically include numbness and paresthesias of the tips of the thumb and first two digits. Other nerves prone to compression neuropathies include the ulnar nerve at the level of the elbow, the peroneal nerve at the level of the knee, and the radial nerve in the upper arm; the latter occurs from sleeping with the arm in an awkward position ("Saturday night palsy"). Another form of compression neuropathy is found in the foot, affecting the interdigital nerve at intermetatarsal sites. This problem, which occurs more often in women than in men, leads to foot pain (metatarsalgia) and is associated with a histologic lesion called a *Morton neuroma*, which is marked by perineural fibrosis.

Inherited Peripheral Neuropathies

Inherited peripheral neuropathies are a group of genetically diverse disorders with overlapping clinical phenotypes that often present in adults. Even with delayed onset, the possibility of an inherited neuropathy has to be considered in the differential diagnosis for any patient that presents with a peripheral neuropathy. The major types of inherited peripheral neuropathies include (1) hereditary motor and sensory neuropathies, also known as *Charcot-Marie-Tooth* (CMT) disease, (2) hereditary motor neuropathies, (3) hereditary sensory neuropathies, with or without autonomic neuropathy, and (4) other inherited conditions causing neuropathy, including familial amyloidosis and inherited metabolic diseases.

Historically, these diseases were classified based on their inheritance pattern and clinical features. Now there is a continuously growing list of genetic defects that are linked to these. The complexity of the genetics of inherited neuropathies is no doubt a reflection of the complicated homeostatic mechanisms that sustain normal peripheral nerve function. There is no simple unifying concept tying all the implicated genes together, but subsets of involved genes can be clustered into the following functionally related groups:

- Genes encoding myelin-associated proteins (Fig. 27-1)
- Genes encoding growth factors and growth factor receptors
- Genes encoding proteins that regulate mitochondrial function
- Genes encoding proteins that are involved in vesicle and axonal transport
- Genes encoding heat shock proteins, which may prevent protein aggregation
- Genes encoding proteins that are involved in cell membrane structure or function

Many areas of the classification are muddy, and genotype/phenotype relationships are not always clear-cut. For example, mutations in the *HSPB1* gene, which encodes the heat shock protein HSP27, may be associated with a clinical picture resembling CMT disease or a hereditary motor neuron disorder. Below, some of the more common and distinctive types of inherited peripheral neuropathies are described in brief.

Hereditary motor and sensory neuropathies/ Charcot-Marie-Tooth (CMT) disease

These are by far the most common inherited peripheral neuropathies, affecting up to 1 in 2500 people. The initial description of these disorders, based on clinical features, was deceptively simple—an inherited disease associated with distal muscle atrophy, sensory loss, and foot deformities. It is now appreciated that this clinical phenotype encompasses mutations in more than 50 different genes, some with relatively distinctive clinical features. Current systems classify hereditary motor and sensory neuropathies based on the mode of inheritance and the pattern of injury (e.g., axonal, demyelinating, or mixed). Demyelinating forms of CMT are associated with morphologic features of demyelination and remyelination including Schwann cell hyperplasia and onion bulb formation, which may be so severe that the involved nerve is palpably enlarged. Listed are a few more common variants:

- CMT1 encompasses a group of autosomal dominant disorders that collectively are the most common subtype of hereditary motor and sensory neuropathy. CMT1A accounts for some 55% of genetically defined CMT cases and 37% of all CMT disease. It is caused by a duplication of a region on chromosome 17 that includes the peripheral myelin protein 22 (*PMP22*) gene. The disease usually presents in the second decade of life as a slowly progressive distal demyelinating motor and sensory neuropathy. CMT1B is caused by mutations in the myelin protein zero gene and accounts for about 9% of genetically defined cases of CMT.

- CMTX encompasses X-linked forms of CMT disease. CMT1X is the most common of these, accounting for 15% of genetically defined cases of CMT. It is linked to mutations in the *GJB1* gene, which encodes connexin32, a gap junction component that is expressed in Schwann cells.
- CMT2 includes autosomal dominant neuropathies associated with axonal rather than demyelinating injury. CMT2A is the most common subtype, accounting for 4% of all CMT disease. It is caused by mutations in the *MFN2* gene, which is required for normal mitochondrial fusion. The phenotype is typically severe, with disease onset in early childhood.

Hereditary sensory neuropathies with or without autonomic neuropathy

This is a diverse group of diseases marked by loss of sensation and variable autonomic disturbances. Loss of pain and temperature sensation is the most common symptom. The inability to sense pain leads to traumatic injury to affected portions of the body. These are typically axonal neuropathies.

Hereditary neuropathy with pressure palsy

This disorder is caused by deletion of the gene encoding *PMP22* (the same gene that is duplicated in CMT1A). It is marked by transient motor and sensory mononeuropathies that are triggered by compression of individual nerves at sites that are prone to entrapment (e.g., the carpal tunnel or the fibular head). Symptoms related to the neuropathy usually resolve within days or weeks, but in some patients the disease eventually progresses to a chronic neuropathy. Swollen, bulbous myelin sheaths at the end of internodes (referred to as *tomaculi*, Latin for a type of sausage) are a characteristic morphologic feature that can be appreciated on special teased fiber preparations of affected nerves.

Familial amyloid polyneuropathies

These are hereditary disorders characterized by amyloid deposition within peripheral nerves. Most are caused by germ line mutations of the transthyretin gene. The mutated transthyretin protein, which is normally involved in serum binding and transport of thyroid hormone, is prone to deposit as amyloid fibrils in a number of tissues, including peripheral nerve (Chapter 6). The clinical presentation is similar to that of hereditary sensory and autonomic neuropathies.

Peripheral neuropathy accompanying inherited metabolic disorders

Several hereditary metabolic disorders are accompanied by peripheral neuropathy during the course of the disease. These include leukodystrophies such as adrenoleukodystrophy (Chapter 28), porphyria (Chapter 25), and Refsum disease, a disorder caused by deficiency of a peroxisomal enzyme.

KEY CONCEPTS

Peripheral Neuropathies

- Anatomic patterns include mononeuropathy, mononeuritis multiplex, polyneuropathy, and polyradiculoneuropathy.
- Damage may occur primarily in Schwann cells (demyelinating neuropathy), axons (axonal neuropathy), or central neurons (neuronopathy); mixed patterns of injury occur.
- Inflammatory disease, infections, metabolic changes, toxic injury, trauma, paraneoplastic disorders, and inherited gene defects can all cause peripheral neuropathy.
- Diabetes mellitus is the most common cause of peripheral neuropathy, which most often presents as a distal symmetric neuropathy.
- Guillain-Barré syndrome and chronic inflammatory demyelinating polyradiculoneuropathy are the major acute and chronic acquired demyelinating peripheral neuropathies.
- Inherited peripheral neuropathies are genetically and phenotypically diverse disorders that often present in adulthood and may be marked by sensory, motor, or autonomic dysfunction, alone or in combination.

Diseases of the Neuromuscular Junction

The neuromuscular junction is a complex specialized structure located at the interface of motor nerve axons and skeletal muscle that serves to control muscle contraction. Neuromuscular junctions are found midway along the length of myofibers. Here, the distal ends of peripheral motor nerves branch into small processes that terminate in bulbous synaptic boutons. Upon depolarization, these presynaptic nerve terminals release acetylcholine (ACh) into the synaptic cleft, the space separating the nerve endings from the myofiber membrane (referred to as the *sarcolemma*). The postsynaptic sarcolemma is characterized by complex infoldings and exhibits distinct specializations with localized clustering of acetylcholine receptors (AChR). These receptors are responsible for the initiation of signals leading to muscle contraction.

Regardless of cause, disorders that impair the function of neuromuscular junctions tend to present with painless weakness. Autoantibodies that inhibit key neuromuscular junction proteins are the most common cause of disrupted neuromuscular transmission, as found in myasthenia gravis (literally, *grave weakness*). Understandably, inherited defects in specialized neuromuscular junction proteins are also associated with myasthenic syndromes. Disorders caused by toxins that alter neuromuscular transmission are rarely encountered, but had an important role historically in elucidating how the neuromuscular junction functions.

Antibody-Mediated Diseases of the Neuromuscular Junction

Myasthenia Gravis

Myasthenia gravis is an autoimmune disease that is usually associated with autoantibodies directed against acetylcholine receptors. It has a prevalence of 150 to 200 per million and shows a bimodal age distribution. The female-to-male ratio is 2:1 in the young adults, but in older adults there is a male predominance.

Pathogenesis. About 85% of patients have autoantibodies against postsynaptic acetylcholine receptors, while most of the remaining patients have antibodies against the sarcolemmal protein *muscle-specific receptor tyrosine kinase.* These autoantibodies appear to be pathogenic, as the disease can be passively transferred to animals with serum from affected individuals, and therapeutic maneuvers that decrease autoantibody levels are associated with a reduction in symptoms.

The mechanism of action of the various autoantibodies appears to differ. Anti-acetylcholine receptor antibodies are thought to lead to the aggregation and degradation of the receptors, and also to damage of the postsynaptic membrane through complement fixation. As a result, postsynaptic membranes show alterations in morphology and are depleted of acetylcholine receptors. This limits the ability of myofibers to respond to acetylcholine. Autoantibodies directed against muscle-specific receptor tyrosine kinase do not fix complement. Instead, these antibodies seem to interfere with the trafficking and clustering of acetylcholine receptor within the sarcolemmal membrane, the net effect again being decreased acetylcholine receptor function.

There is a strong association between pathogenic anti-acetylcholine receptor autoantibodies and thymic abnormalities. Approximately 10% of patients with myasthenia gravis have a *thymoma*, a tumor of thymic epithelial cells (Chapter 13). An additional 30% of patients (and particularly those who are young) have a different thymic abnormality called *thymic hyperplasia*. This peculiar condition is marked by the appearance of B-cell follicles in the thymus. The thymus normally contains small numbers of myoid cells, stromal cells that express skeletal muscle antigens. It is hypothesized that both thymoma and thymic hyperplasia disrupt normal thymic function in a manner that promotes autoimmunity against acetylcholine receptors expressed on thymic myoid cells. In contrast, thymic abnormalities are usually absent in cases of myasthenia gravis that occur in older patients or that are not associated with anti-acetylcholine receptor autoantibodies; the basis for the development of autoantibodies in such cases is unknown.

Clinical Features. Patients with anti-acetylcholine receptor antibodies typically present with fluctuating weakness that worsens with exertion and often over the course of the day. *Diplopia* and *ptosis* due to involvement of extraocular muscles are common and distinguish myasthenia gravis from myopathies, in which involvement of extraocular muscles is unusual. In some patients, symptoms are confined to ocular muscles, while others develop generalized weakness that can be so severe as to require mechanical ventilation. Cases with antibodies against muscle-specific receptor tyrosine kinase differ from typical cases by exhibiting more focal muscle involvement (neck, shoulder, facial, respiratory, and bulbar muscles).

Diagnosis is based on clinical history, physical findings, the identification of autoantibodies, and electrophysiologic studies. The latter reveal a decrement in muscle response with repeated stimulation, a characteristic of this disorder. Overall mortality has dropped from over 30% in the 1950s to less than 5% with current therapies. Acetylcholinesterase inhibitors that increase the half-life of acetylcholine are the first line of treatment. Other treatments, such as plasmapheresis and immunosuppressive drugs (e.g., glucocorticoids, cyclosporine, rituximab), can bring symptoms under control by decreasing autoantibody titers. Thymectomy is often effective in patients with thymoma, but is of uncertain benefit in those with thymic hyperplasia or lacking thymic abnormalities.

Lambert-Eaton Myasthenic Syndrome

Lambert-Eaton myasthenic syndrome is an autoimmune disorder caused by antibodies that block acetylcholine release by inhibiting a presynaptic calcium channel. In contrast to myasthenia gravis, rapid repetitive stimulation increases muscle response. Muscle strength is augmented after a few seconds of muscle activity. Patients typically present with weakness of their extremities. In about half of cases there is an underlying malignancy, most often neuroendocrine carcinoma of the lung. Symptoms may precede the diagnosis of cancer, sometimes by years. It is thought that the stimulus for autoantibody formation in paraneoplastic cases may be the expression of the same calcium channel in the neoplastic cells. Patients without cancer often have other autoimmune diseases, such as vitiligo or thyroid disease. Treatment consists of drugs that increase acetylcholine release by depolarizing synaptic membranes and immunosuppressive agents, such as those used to treat myasthenia gravis.

Congenital Myasthenic Syndromes

Rare disorders falling into this group most commonly have an autosomal recessive mode of inheritance and are marked by varying degrees of muscle weakness. Causative mutations have been identified in genes encoding several different presynaptic, synaptic, or postsynaptic proteins. The most common of these are loss-of-function mutations in the gene encoding the ε-subunit of the acetylcholine receptor. Another group of mutations affect proteins that are important in normal clustering of acetylcholine receptors on postsynaptic membranes. Many patients with congenital myasthenic syndromes present in the perinatal period with poor muscle tone, external eye muscle weakness, and breathing difficulties, but others have milder forms of the disease and may not come to clinical attention until adolescence or adulthood. The clinical presentation, response to drugs such as acetylcholinesterase inhibitors, and prognosis depend largely on the underlying mutation.

Disorders Caused by Toxins

Botulism is caused by exposure to a neurotoxin (popularly known as *Botox*) that is produced by the anaerobic Gram-positive organism *Clostridium botulinum*. Botox acts by blocking the release of acetylcholine from presynaptic neurons (Chapter 8). *Curare* is a common name for related muscle relaxants that block acetylcholine receptors, resulting in flaccid paralysis. It was initially discovered and used as poison on arrow tips by indigenous people in the Amazon rain forest. At one time it was used as a muscle relaxant during certain forms of surgery, but has now been supplanted by other related drugs with a similar mechanism of action.

KEY CONCEPTS

Diseases of the Neuromuscular Junction

- Disorders of neuromuscular junctions present with painless weakness.
- Myasthenia gravis and Lambert-Eaton myasthenic syndrome, the most common forms, are both immune mediated, being caused by antibodies to postsynaptic acetylcholine receptors and presynaptic calcium channels, respectively.
- **Myasthenia gravis** is often associated with thymic hyperplasia or thymoma, frequently involves ocular muscles, and is marked by fluctuating weakness that worsens with exertion.
- **Lambert-Eaton** myasthenic presents with weakness in the extremities that improves with repetitive stimulation and is often a paraneoplastic disorder associated with lung cancer.
- Genetic defects in neuromuscular junction proteins give rise to **congenital myasthenic syndromes.**
- **Bacterial toxins** such as Botox can block neuromuscular transmission by blocking the release of acetylcholine from presynaptic neurons.

Diseases of Skeletal Muscle

Skeletal muscle has unique structural, cellular, and molecular characteristics and accordingly unique patterns of injury and repair. During embryogenesis, skeletal muscle develops through the fusion of mononucleated precursor cells (myoblasts) into multinucleated myotubes. These subsequently mature into myofibers (muscle fibers) of varying length that contain thousands of nuclei. In adult tissues, these myofibers are arranged in fascicles, each associated with a small pool of tissue stem cells referred to as satellite cells, which can contribute to muscle regeneration following injury (outlined later). Myofibers are of two main types, type I and type II (Table 27-1), which are admixed in a checkerboard pattern in normal skeletal muscle. Fiber type is determined by signals received from innervating motor neurons and, as a result, all fibers that are part of a motor unit are of the same type.

Skeletal Muscle Atrophy

Skeletal muscle atrophy is a common feature of many disorders. Loss of innervation, disuse, cachexia, old age, and primary myopathies can all produce muscle atrophy and, if the atrophy is severe, loss of muscle mass. Certain patterns of atrophy are suggestive of specific underlying etiologies:

- Clusters or groups of atrophic fibers are seen in neurogenic disease (Fig. 27-7).
- Perifascicular atrophy is seen in dermatomyositis (see later).
- Type II fiber atrophy with sparing of type I fibers is seen with prolonged corticosteroid therapy or disuse.

Table 27-1 Muscle fiber types

	Type I	Type II
Action	Sustained force	Fast movement
Activity type	Aerobic exercise	Anaerobic exercise
Power produced	Low	High
Resistance to fatigue	High	Low
Lipid content	High	Low
Glycogen content	Low	High
Energy metabolism	Low glycolytic capacity, high oxidative capacity	High glycolytic capacity, low oxidative capacity
Mitochondrial density	High	Low
Enzyme activity	NADH-TR, dark staining ATPase at pH 4.3, dark staining ATPase at pH 9.4, light staining	NADH-TR, light staining ATPase at pH 4.3, light staining ATPase at pH 9.4, dark staining
Myosin heavy chain gene expressed	*MYH7*	*MYH2, MYH4, MYH1*
Color	Red (high myoglobin content)	Pale red / tan (low myoglobin content)
Prototype	Soleus (pigeon)	Pectoral (pigeon)

ATPase, Adenosine triphosphatase; NADH-TR, nicotinamide adenine dinucleotide, reduced form, tetrazolium reductase.

Neurogenic and Myopathic Changes in Skeletal Muscle

Disorders impacting skeletal muscle may do so by damaging myofibers directly (myopathic injury) or by disrupting muscle innervation (neurogenic injury). Neurogenic injuries lead to *fiber type grouping* and *grouped atrophy* (Fig. 27-7), both of which stem from the disruption of muscle innervation. The key to understanding these abnormalities is to recognize that muscle fiber type is determined by the innervating motor neuron and can switch if the innervating motor neuron changes from one type to the other. Following denervation, myofibers undergo atrophy, often assuming a flattened, angulated shape. Reinnervation restores fiber size and shape, but may make a denervated myofiber part of a different motor unit and that may lead to a switch in fiber type. In the face of ongoing axonal or neuronal damage and drop out, residual motor axons may innervate increasingly larger numbers of myofibers, leading to enlargement of motor units, each comprised of a single type of muscle fiber (fiber type grouping). These large motor units are also susceptible to grouped atrophy if the innervating axon is damaged.

In contrast, most primary myopathic processes are associated with a distinct set of morphologic changes that include the following:

- *Segmental myofiber degeneration and regeneration* is seen when only part of a myofiber undergoes necrosis. Degeneration is associated with release of cytoplasmic enzymes into the blood such as creatine kinase, making these useful markers of muscle damage. The sarcomeres and other components of the damaged myofiber segment are removed by macrophages in a process termed *myophagocytosis*. This sets the stage for

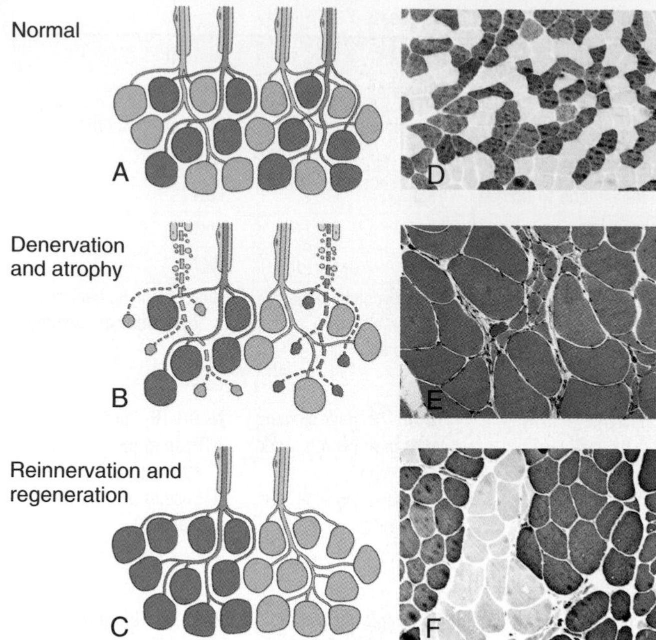

Figure 27-7 A, This diagrammatic representation of four normal motor units shows a normal checkerboard type admixture of light and dark stained fibers of opposite type. **B,** Damage to innervating axons leads to loss of trophic input and atrophy of myofibers. **C,** Reinnervation of myofibers can lead to a switch in fiber type and segregation of fibers of like type. As illustrated here, reinnervation is also often associated with an increase in motor unit size, with more myofibers innervated by an individual axon. **D,** Normal muscle has a checkerboard type distribution of type I (light) and type II (dark) fibers on this ATPase reaction (pH9.4) corresponding to findings in **A. E,** Clustered flattened "angulated" atrophic fibers (*group atrophy*) are a typical finding associated with disrupted innervation. **F,** With ongoing denervation and reinnervation, large clusters of fibers appear that all share the same fiber type (*type grouping*).

regeneration. Fusion of activated satellite cells to damaged myofibers is an important step for regeneration. Eventually, new sarcomeres are generated and the continuity of the original myofiber is restored. *Regenerating myofibers* are rich in RNA and therefore blue (basophilic) in hematoxylin and eosin stained sections. They have enlarged nuclei with prominent nucleoli that are often randomly distributed in the cytoplasm, instead of being in their normal subsarcolemmal location. Depending on the nature of the primary insult, atrophic myofibers may also be seen. Regeneration can restore muscle to normal following an acute, transient injury, but in chronic disease states regeneration often fails to keep pace with damage. In this setting, muscles often show endomysial fibrosis (collagen deposition), dropout of myofibers, and fatty replacement.

- *Myofiber hypertrophy* can be seen as a physiologic adaptation to exercise or in association with certain chronic myopathic conditions.
- *Cytoplasmic inclusions* in the form of vacuoles, aggregates of proteins, or clustered organelles are characteristic of several primary forms of myopathy.

Inflammatory Myopathies

Historically, polymyositis, dermatomyositis, and inclusion body myositis have been considered the three main primary inflammatory myopathies; however, inclusion body myositis is an enigmatic condition (discussed later) in which the role of inflammation is uncertain. In contrast, polymyositis and dermatomyositis show typical features of autoimmune inflammatory diseases, including associations with certain autoantibodies, particular HLA-DR genotypes, and other autoimmune disorders. In addition to prototypical presentations, there are overlapping forms and cases that defy precise classification. Other immune-mediated disorders, such as systemic lupus erythematosus, systemic sclerosis, and sarcoidosis (Chapter 6), as well as certain infectious agents (Chapter 8), can also cause myositis and are discussed elsewhere.

Dermatomyositis

Dermatomyositis is a systemic autoimmune disease that typically presents with proximal muscle weakness and skin changes.

Pathogenesis. **Dermatomyositis is an immunologic disease in which damage to small blood vessels contributes to muscle injury.** The vasculopathic changes can be seen as *telangiectasias* (dilated capillary loops) in the nail folds, eyelids, and gums, and as dropout of capillary vessels in skeletal muscle. Biopsies of muscle and skin may show deposition of the complement membrane attack complex (C5b-9) within capillary beds in both tissues. An inflammatory signature enriched for genes that are upregulated by type I interferons is seen in muscle and in leukocytes. The prominence of this signature appears to correlate with disease activity. Various autoantibodies are often detected by serologic studies, and B lymphocytes as well as plasma cells are part of the inflammatory infiltrate that is seen in muscles. Certain autoantibodies tend to be associated with specific clinical features:

- *Anti-Mi2 antibodies* (directed against a helicase implicated in nucleosome remodeling) show a strong association with prominent Gottron papules and heliotrope rash (described later).
- *Anti-Jo1 antibodies* (directed against the enzyme histidyl t-RNA synthetase) are associated with interstitial lung disease, nonerosive arthritis, and a skin rash described as "mechanic's hands."
- *Anti-P155/P140 antibodies* (directed against several transcriptional regulators) are associated with paraneoplastic and juvenile cases of dermatomyositis.

A direct link between these autoantibodies and disease pathogenesis has not yet been established.

MORPHOLOGY

Muscle biopsies of affected patients show infiltrates of mononuclear inflammatory cells that tend to be most pronounced in the perimysial connective tissue and around blood vessels. Sometimes there is a distinctive pattern in which myofiber atrophy is accentuated at the edges of the fascicles—**perifascicular atrophy** (Fig. 27-8*B*). Segmental fiber necrosis and regeneration may also be seen. Immunohistochemical

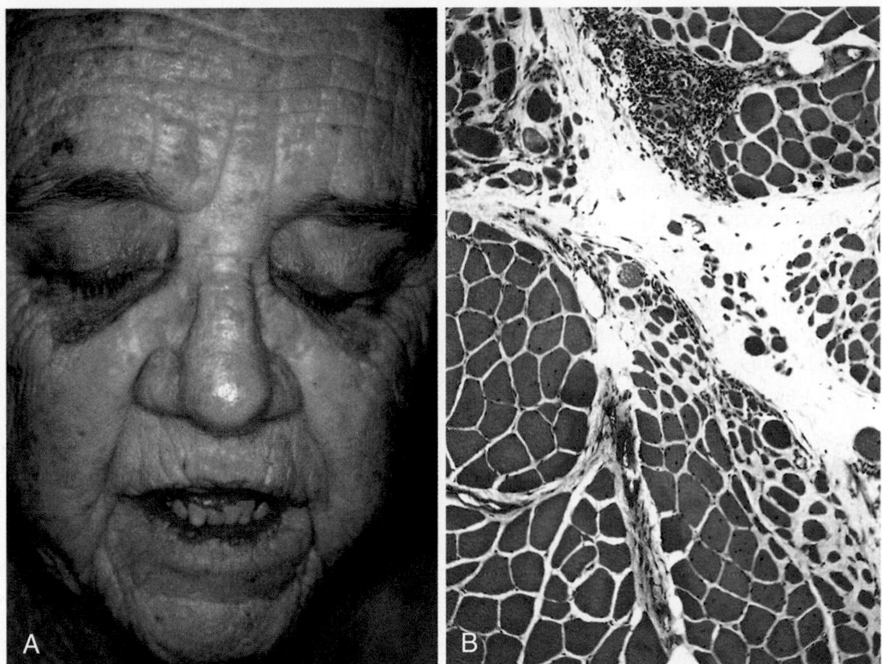

Figure 27-8 A, Dermatomyositis. Note the heliotrope rash affecting the eyelids. **B,** Dermatomyositis. The histologic appearance of muscle shows perifascicular atrophy of muscle fibers and inflammation. (Courtesy Dr. Dennis Burns, Department of Pathology, University of Texas Southwestern Medical School, Dallas, Texas.)

studies may identify an infiltrate rich in CD4+ T-helper cells and the deposition of C5b-9 in capillary vessels. Electron microscopic studies may show tubuloreticular endothelial cell inclusions, a feature of a number of inflammatory disorders that are linked to a type I interferon response.

Clinical Features. Muscle weakness is slow in onset, symmetric, and often accompanied by myalgias. It typically affects the proximal muscles first. As a result, tasks such as getting up from a chair and climbing steps become increasingly difficult. Fine movements controlled by distal muscles are affected only late in the disease. Associated myopathic changes on electrophysiologic studies and elevation in serum creatine kinase levels are reflective of muscle damage. Various rashes are described in dermatomyositis, but the most characteristic ones are a lilac colored discoloration of the upper eyelids *(heliotrope rash)* associated with periorbital edema (Fig. 27-8*A*) and a scaling erythematous eruption or dusky red patches over the knuckles, elbows, and knees (*Gottron papules*). *Dysphagia* resulting from involvement of oropharyngeal and esophageal muscles occurs in one third of the affected individuals, and another 10% of patients have *interstitial lung disease*, which can sometimes be rapidly progressive and lead to death. Cardiac involvement is common, but rarely leads to cardiac failure.

Juvenile and adult forms are recognized. The average age of onset of juvenile dermatomyositis is 7 years, whereas adult cases tend to present from the fourth to sixth decade of life. Dermatomyositis is the most common inflammatory myopathy in children. Compared to adult disease, childhood disease is more likely to be associated with calcinosis and lipodystrophy and less likely to be associated myositis-specific antibodies, cardiac involvement, interstitial lung disease, or an underlying malignancy. As might be expected based on these differences, the overall prognosis is better in children than in adults. From 15% to 24% of adult patients have an associated malignancy, and in such patients dermatomyositis may be viewed as a paraneoplastic disorder.

Polymyositis

Polymyositis is an adult-onset inflammatory myopathy that shares myalgia and weakness with dermatomyositis but lacks its distinctive cutaneous features and is therefore to some degree a diagnosis of exclusion. As in dermatomyositis, patients typically develop symmetric proximal muscle involvement, and there may be inflammatory involvement of the heart and the lungs, as well as similar autoantibodies.

Pathogenesis. The pathogenesis of polymyositis is uncertain, but it is believed to have an immunologic basis. CD8-positive cytotoxic T cells are a prominent part of the inflammatory infiltrate in affected muscle, and it is hypothesized that these cells are the mediators of tissue damage. Unlike dermatomyositis, vascular injury is not believed to have a major role in polymyositis.

MORPHOLOGY

Mononuclear inflammatory cell infiltrates are present, but in contrast to dermatomyositis, these are usually endomysial in location. Sometimes myofibers with otherwise normal morphology appear to be invaded by mononuclear inflammatory cells. Degenerating necrotic, regenerating, and atrophic myofibers are typically found in a random or patchy distribution. The perifascicular pattern of atrophy that is characteristic of dermatomyositis is absent.

Inclusion Body Myositis

Inclusion body myositis is a disease of late adulthood that typically affects patients older than 50 years and is the most common inflammatory myopathy in patients older than age 65 years. Most affected individuals present with slowly progressive muscle weakness that tends to be most severe in the quadriceps and the distal upper extremity muscles. Dysphagia from esophageal and pharyngeal muscle involvement is not uncommon. Laboratory studies usually show modestly elevated creatine kinase levels; most myositis-associated autoantibodies are absent, although an antibody to cN1A has recently been described.

MORPHOLOGY

Inclusion body myositis has a number of features that are similar to those found in polymyositis, including:

- Patchy often endomysial mononuclear inflammatory cell infiltrates rich in CD8+ T-cells
- Increased sarcolemmal expression of MHC class I antigens
- Focal invasion of normal appearing myofibers by inflammatory cells
- Admixed degenerating and regenerating myofibers

Other associated changes, however, are more typical or even specific for inclusion body myositis, as follows:

- Abnormal cytoplasmic inclusions described as "rimmed vacuoles" (Fig. 27-9)
- Tubolofilamentous inclusions in myofibers, seen by electron microscopiy
- Cytoplasmic inclusions containing proteins typically associated with neurodegenerative diseases, like beta-amyloid, TDP-43, and ubiquitin
- Endomysial fibrosis and fatty replacement, reflective of a chronic disease course

Whether inclusion body myositis is indeed an inflammatory condition or a degenerative process with secondary inflammatory changes remains an unresolved question. It has certain features in common with polymyositis, as discussed earlier. On the other hand, it shares some features with neurodegenerative diseases, such as the presence of abnormal protein aggregates. Furthermore, there are several familial inclusion body myopathies that are also associated with chronic myopathic changes and rimmed vacuoles. These typically lack any associated inflammation—hence the designation *inclusion body "myopathy"* rather than *"myositis."*

Treatment of Inflammatory Myopathies

The prognosis for patients with dermatomyositis and polymyositis was poor before the use of corticosteroids, with mortality rates as high as 50% or more. Corticosteroids remain the first-line of treatment for polymyositis and dermatomyositis. Immunosuppressive drugs are used in steroid-resistant disease or as steroid-sparing agents and include azathioprine and methotrexate. Intravenous immunoglobulin (IVIG), cyclophosphamide, cyclosporine, and rituximab (an antibody that targets B cells) are third-line therapies. Inclusion body myositis usually responds poorly to steroids or immunosuppressive therapies, another feature that argues against an inflammatory or immune origin for this disorder.

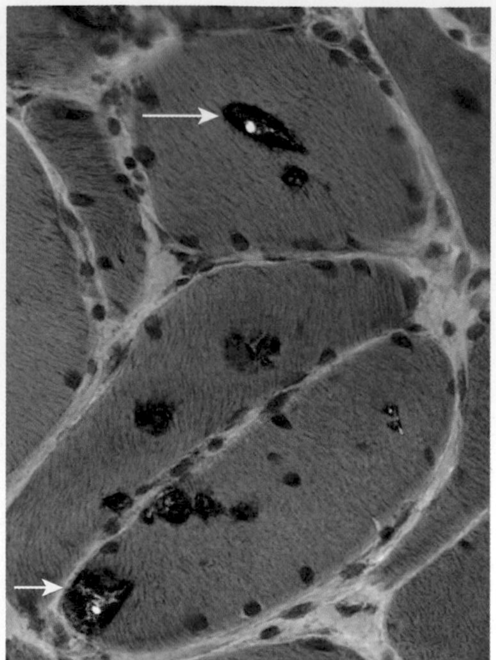

Figure 27-9 Inclusion body myositis, showing myofibers containing rimmed vacuoles—inclusions with reddish granular rimming (*arrows*). Modified Gomori trichrome stain.

Toxic Myopathies

Toxic myopathies can be caused by prescription or recreational drugs, or by certain hormonal imbalances. Among prescription drugs, *statins* are among the leading culprits. Statins are cholesterol-lowering drugs that are widely used to reduce the risks of acute ischemic cardiac events and stroke. *Myopathy is the most common complication of statins* (e.g., atorvastatin, simvastatin, pravastatin). It occurs in approximately 1.5% of users, and is unrelated to dose, cumulative dose, or statin subtype. Genetic variants that influence statin metabolism, on the other hand, may help identify those who are at risk.

Chloroquine and *hydroxychloroquine* were originally used as antimalarial agents and are currently given as long-term therapy to some patients with systemic autoimmune diseases. These drugs interfere with normal lysosomal function and can cause a drug-induced lysosomal storage myopathy that presents with slowly progressive muscle weakness. The muscle tissue shows myopathic changes including vacuolation that predominantly affects type I fibers. Ultrastructural studies identify aggregates of whorled, lamellar membranous structures, including curvilinear bodies that mimic those seen in ceroid lipofuscinoses (Chapter 28).

ICU myopathy or *myosin deficient myopathy* is a neuromuscular disorder seen in patients during the course of treatment for critical illness (usually in an intensive care unit) especially with corticosteroid therapy. There may be relatively selective degradation of sarcomeric myosin thick filaments, producing profound weakness that can complicate the clinical course (e.g., by interfering with the weaning of a patient from a mechanical respirator).

Thyroid dysfunction can lead to several types of myopathy. *Thyrotoxic myopathy* presents most commonly as an acute or chronic proximal muscle weakness that may precede other signs of hyperthyroidism. Such patients may also present with *exophthalmic ophthalmoplegia*, characterized by swelling of the eyelids, edema of the conjunctiva, and diplopia. *Hypothyroidism* can cause cramping or aching of muscles, and decreased movement. Reflexes may be slowed. Findings in skeletal muscle include fiber atrophy, an increased number of abnormally localized nuclei, glycogen aggregates, and (occasionally) deposition of mucopolysaccharides in connective tissue.

Alcohol can also be myopathic. Most notably, binge drinking may produce an acute toxic syndrome of rhabdomyolysis, myoglobinuria, and renal failure. The affected individual may complain of acute myalgias that are generalized or confined to a single muscle group.

Inherited Diseases of Skeletal Muscle

Inherited mutations are responsible for a diverse collection of disorders marked by defects in skeletal muscle. In some of these disorders, skeletal muscle is the main site of disease, but in others multiple organs are involved. Of the other organs involved, the heart is of particular importance, since cardiac involvement is common and often life-limiting.

Historically, inherited myopathies have been subdivided into several broad categories based on inheritance pattern, anatomic pattern of muscle involvement, onset age, clinical course, and underlying pathogenesis.

Congenital myopathies (Table 27-2) typically present in infancy with muscle defects that tend to be static or to even improve over time. They are often associated with distinct structural abnormalities of the muscle.

Muscular dystrophies are characterized by progressive muscle damage that typically comes to attention after infancy. Exceptions to this rule are the *congenital muscular dystrophies*; these tend to present in infancy and are often associated with developmental abnormalities of the CNS as well as progressive muscle damage. These include two important groups:

- *Conditions with defects in extracellular matrix surrounding myofibers.* These are exemplified by Ullrich congenital musclar dystrophy (UCMD) and merosin deficiency. In the former the causative mutations involve one of three collagen VI alpha genes; in the case of merosin deficiency, the gene encoding merosin is disrupted. UCMD is characterized by hypotonia, proximal contractures and distal hyperextensibility. A morphologic hallmark is mismatched expression of normally co-localized matrix proteins perlecan and collagen VI.

Table 27-2 Congenital myopathies

Disease and Inheritance	Gene and Locus	Clinical Findings	Pathologic Findings
Central-core disease; autosomal dominant	Ryanodine receptor-1 (*RYR1*) gene; 19q13.1	Early-onset hypotonia and weakness; "floppy infant"; associated skeletal abnormalities like scoliosis, hip dislocation, or foot deformities; some RYR1 mutations cause central core disease, some malignant hyperthermia, and some both	Cytoplasmic cores represent demarcated central zones in which the normal arrangement of sarcomeres is disrupted and mitochondria are decreased in number
Nemaline myopathy (NEM)	AD NEM1—α-tropomyosin 3 (*TPM3*) gene; 1q22–q23 AR NEM2—nebulin (*NEB*) gene; 2q22 AR NEM3—α-actin-1 (*ACTA*) gene; 1q42 AR NEM4—tropomyosin-2 (*TPM2*) gene; 19p13.2–p13.1 AR NEM5—troponin T1 (*TNNT1*) gene; 19q13.4 AR NEM7—coffilin-2 (*CFL2*) gene; 14q12	Childhood weakness; some with more severe weakness, hypotonia at birth ("floppy infant")	Aggregates of spindle-shaped particles *(nemaline rods)*; occur predominantly in type 1 fibers; derived from Z-band material (α-actinin) and best seen on modified Gomori stain or by electron microscopy
Centronuclear myopathy	XL—myotubularin (*MTM1*) gene; Xq28 AD—dynamin-2 (and others) *DNM2* gene; 19p13.2 AR—amphiphysin-2(*BIN1*) gene; 2q14)	Severe congenital hypotonia, "floppy infant" and poor prognosis in X-linked form ("myotubular myopathy") Childhood onset or young adult onset with other variants with weakness and hypotonia	Many fibers contain nuclei in the geometric center of the myofiber; central nuclei are more common in type 1 fibers, which are small in diameter, but can occur in both fiber types
Congenital fiber type disproportion	Selenoprotein 1 *(SEPN1)* gene; 1p36.11 Alpha-actin-1 *(ACTA1)* gene; 1q42.13 Tropomyosin 3 *(TPM3)* gene; 1q21.3	Hypotonia, weakness, failure to thrive, facial and resp. weakness, contractures Wide phenotypic spectrum Mutations in SEPN1 are also associated with protein aggregate myopathy and rigid spine muscular dystrophy; mutations in ACTA1 are also associated with nemaline myopathy and protein aggregate myopathy; mutations in TPM3 are also associated with nemaline myopathy	Predominance and atrophy of type I fibers (not specific)

AD, Autosomal dominant; AR, autosomal recessive; XL, X-linked.

- *Conditions with abnormalities in receptors for extracellular matrix.* In this group are diseases that disrupt the post-translational modification of alpha-dystroglycan (Fig. 27-10) by O-linked glycosylation. Mutations of alpha-dystroglycan itself result in fetal demise but defects in its post-translational modification result in milder forms of dystroglycan deficiency. Alpha-dystroglycan expression is important for CNS and eye development. Severe cases exhibit features of congenital muscular dystrophy as well as developmental defects of the CNS and eyes that cause seizures, mental retardation and blindness. Milder forms may only cause skeletal muscle disease. Some of these mutations are also linked to a presentation described as limb girdle muscular dystrophy (see below).

The following section focuses on the most common and best understood forms of inherited myopathies.

Muscular Dystrophies

Muscular dystrophies include several inherited disorders of skeletal muscle that have in common progressive muscle damage that typically manifests itself between childhood and adulthood. As mentioned earlier, with the exception of congenital muscular dystrophies, these diseases do not present in infancy.While our focus is on X-linked muscular dystrophies, other forms in which the disease pathogenesis is reasonably well understood are also briefly discussed.

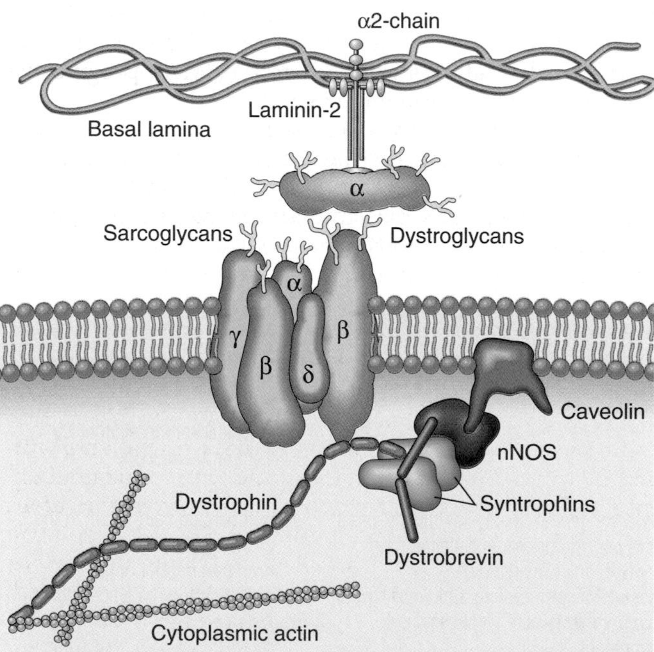

Figure 27-10 Relationship between the cell membrane (sarcolemma) and the sarcolemmal associated proteins. Dystrophin, an intracellular protein, forms an interface between the cytoskeletal proteins and a group of transmembrane proteins, the dystroglycans and the sarcoglycans. These transmembrane proteins have interactions with the extracellular matrix, including the laminin proteins. Dystrophin also interacts with dystrobrevin and the syntrophins, which form a link with neuronal type nitric oxide synthetase (nNOS) and caveolin. Mutations in dystrophin are associated with the X-linked muscular dystrophies; mutations in caveolin and the sarcoglycan proteins with the limb-girdle muscular dystrophies, which can be autosomal dominant or recessive disorders; and mutations in the α_2-laminin (merosin) with autosomal recessive congenital muscular dystrophy.

X-Linked Muscular Dystrophy with Dystrophin Mutation/ Duchenne and Becker Muscular Dystrophy

The most common muscular dystrophies are X-linked and stem from mutations that disrupt the function of a large structural protein called *dystrophin*. As a result, these diseases are sometimes referred to as *dystrophinopathies*. The most common early onset form is referred to as *Duchenne muscular dystrophy*. It has an incidence of 1 per 3500 live male births and has a severe progressive phenotype. Becker muscular dystrophy is a second relatively common dystrophinopathy that is characterized by later disease onset and a milder phenotype. Other rare dystrophinopathies may present with isolated cardiomyopathy, asymptomatic elevations of creatine kinase levels, or exercise intolerance because of myalgias and cramps. As with many X-linked diseases, female carriers of dystrophin mutations may be mildly symptomatic due to unfavorable X-chromosome inactivation.

Pathogenesis. **Duchenne and Becker muscular dystrophy are caused by loss-of-function mutations in the dystrophin gene on the X chromosome.** Dystrophin is one of the largest human genes, spanning 2.3 million base pairs and composed of 79 exons. The encoded protein, dystrophin, is a key component of the dystrophin glycoprotein complex (DGC) (Fig. 27-10). This complex spans the plasma membrane and serves as a link between the cytoskeleton inside the myofiber and the basement membrane outside of the cell. The amino terminus of dystrophin binds actin filaments in the cytoplasm of myofibers, while the carboxy terminus binds β-dystroglycan, one of the transmembrane proteins of the DGC. By doing so, dystrophin is thought to provide mechanical stability to the myofiber and its cell membrane during muscle contraction. Defects in the complex may lead to small membrane tears that permit influx of calcium, triggering events that result in myofiber degeneration. In addition to its mechanical function, dystrophin may have a role in signaling pathways; for example, its carboxy terminus interacts with nitric oxide synthase, which generates NO.

Identification and characterization of specific dystrophin mutations has provided an explanation for some of the phenotypic variation in patients with dystrophinopathies. Duchenne muscular dystrophy is typically associated with deletions or frame shift mutations that result in total absence of dystrophin. In contrast, the mutations in Becker muscular dystrophy typically permit the synthesis of a truncated version of dystrophin, which presumably retains some function.

MORPHOLOGY

The changes in Duchenne and Becker muscular dystrophy are similar, but differ in degree. Both are marked by chronic muscle damage that outpaces the capacity for repair (Fig. 27-11). Muscle biopsies in young boys show ongoing damage in the form of **segmental myofiber degeneration and regeneration** associated with an admixture of **atrophic myofibers**. The fascicular architecture is preserved at this stage of the disease,

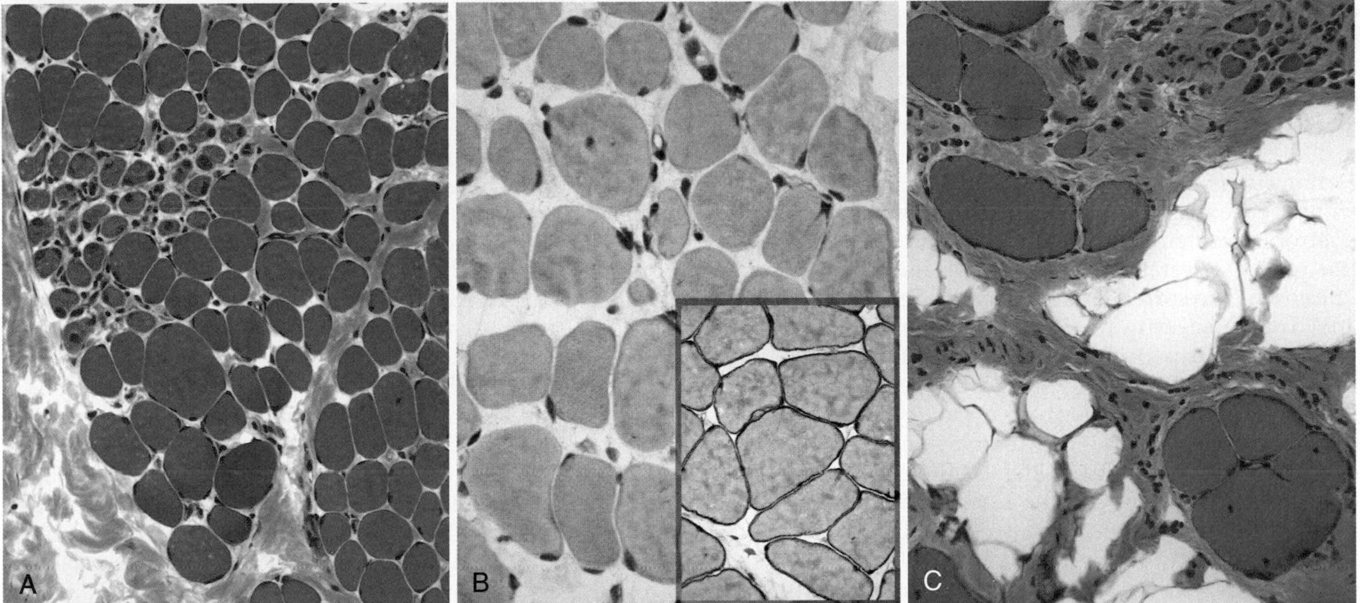

Figure 27-11 Duchenne muscular dystrophy. Histologic images of muscle biopsy specimens from two brothers. **A** and **B,** Specimens from a 3-year-old boy. **C,** Specimen from his 9-year old brother. As seen in **A,** at a younger age fascicular muscle architecture is maintained, but myofibers show variation in size. Additionally, there is a cluster of basophilic regenerating myofibers (*left side*) and slight endomysial fibrosis, seen as focal pink-staining connective tissue between myofibers. In **B,** immunohistochemical staining shows complete absence of membrane-associated dystrophin, seen as a brown stain in normal muscle (*inset*). In **C,** the biopsy from the older brother illustrates disease progression, which is marked by extensive variation in myofiber size, fatty replacement, and endomysial fibrosis.

and there is usually no inflammation except for the presence of myophagocytosis. As the disease progresses, muscle tissue is replaced by collagen and fat cells (**"fatty replacement"** or "fatty infiltration"). The remaining myofibers at this point in the course show prominent variation in size, from small atrophic fibers to large hypertrophied fibers. This remodeling distorts the fascicular architecture of the muscle, which becomes markedly abnormal over time. **Immunohistochemical studies for dystrophin show absence of the normal sarcolemmal staining pattern in Duchenne muscular dystrophin and reduced staining in Becker muscular dystrophy.**

Clinical Features. Boys with Duchenne muscular dystrophy are normal at birth. Very early motor milestones are met, but walking is often delayed. The first indications of muscle weakness are clumsiness and inability to keep up with peers. Weakness begins in the pelvic girdle muscles and then extends to the shoulder girdle. Enlargement of the muscles of the lower leg associated with weakness, termed *pseudohypertrophy,* is often present. The mean age of wheel chair dependence is around 9.5 years. Patients develop joint contractures, scoliosis, worsening respiratory reserve, and sleep hypoventilation.

Dystrophin is also expressed in the heart and the central nervous system, hence both are affected. Dystrophin deficiency in cardiac muscle often leads to the development of cardiomyopathy and arrhythmias, particulary in older patients. Cognitive impairment, presumably due to a functional role for dystrophin in the brain, is also common and sometimes produces frank mental retardation. Despite supportive care, the mean age of death for patients with Duchenne muscular dystrophy is 25 to 30 years of age, with most patients succumbing to respiratory insufficiency, pulmonary infection, or heart failure. In contrast, Becker muscular dystrophy presents in later childhood, adolescence or adult life. Its course is more slowly progressive often with a near normal life expectancy.

The diagnosis is based on the history, physical exam, and laboratory studies. Serum creatine kinase is markedly elevated during the first decade of life due to ongoing muscle damage, and then falls as the disease progresses and muscle mass is lost. The presence of a dystrophin mutation can be confirmed by genetic studies.

Treatment of patients with dystrophinopathies is challenging. Current treatment consists primarily of supportive care. Definitive therapy requires restoration of dystrophin levels in skeletal and cardiac muscle fibers. Work in this area is emboldened by the recognition that expression of some dystrophin protein (as in patients with Becker muscular dystrophy) is sufficient to substantially ameliorate the disease phenotype. One approach involves the expression of antisense RNAs that alter RNA splicing so as to cause "skipping" of exons containing deleterious mutations, thus permitting the expression of a truncated, but partially functional, dystrophin protein. A second strategy is exploring the use of drugs that promote ribosomal "read-through" of stop codons, another ploy that may enable the expression of some dystrophin protein. Both of these approaches are mutation-specific and thus need to be tailored to individual patients. Gene therapy (introduction of a normal dystrophin gene) is being investigated, but gene delivery to skeletal muscle cells remains a daunting hurdle.

Myotonic Dystrophy

Myotonic dystrophy is an autosomal dominant multisystem disorder associated with skeletal muscle weakness,

cataracts, endocrinopathy, and cardiomyopathy. It affects about 1 in 10,000 individuals. Myotonia, a sustained involuntary contraction of muscles, is a key feature of the disease. Some patients present with "*congenital myotonia,*" marked by severe manifestations in infancy.

Pathogenesis. The disease is caused by expansions of CTG triplet repeats in the 3′-noncoding region of the myotonic dystrophy protein kinase (*DMPK*) gene, but precisely how this genetic aberration produces the disease phenotype is unknown. The correlation between the length of expansion and disease severity is variable compared to some other triplet repeat expansion disorders like Huntington disease (Chapter 28). Experimental studies suggest that the skeletal muscle phenotype stems from a "toxic" gain-of-function caused by the triplet repeat expansion. Specifically, the expanded CUG-repeats in the *DMPK* mRNA transcript appear to bind and sequester a protein called *muscleblind-like-1,* which has an important role in RNA splicing. This inhibits muscleblind-like-1 function, leading to missplicing of other RNA transcripts, including the transcript for a chloride channel called *CLC1*. It is believed that the resulting deficiency of CLC1 is responsible for the characteristic myotonia. In support of this scenario, one rare form of congenital myotonia is caused by germ line loss-of-function mutations in *CLC1,* indicating that CLC1 is required for normal muscle relaxation.

Emery-Dreifuss Muscular Dystrophy

Emery-Dreifuss muscular dystrophy (EMD) is caused by mutations in genes that encode nuclear lamina proteins. Clinically, it is marked by a triad consisting of slowly progressive humeroperoneal weakness, cardiomyopathy associated with conduction defects, and early contractures of the Achilles tendon, spine, and elbows. The X-linked form (EMD1) and the autosomal form (EMD2) are caused by mutations in the genes encoding emerin and lamin A/C, respectively, both of which localize to the inner face of the nuclear membrane. It is hypothesized that these proteins help maintain the shape and mechanical stability of the nucleus during muscle contraction. They may also influence gene expression by affecting chromatin organization in the nucleus. How defects in these proteins produce the observed phenotypes is unknown.

Fascioscapulohumeral Dystrophy

Fascioscapulohumeral dystrophy is associated with a characteristic pattern of muscle involvement that includes prominent weakness of facial muscles and muscles of the shoulder girdle. It is an autosomal dominant disease affecting about 1 in 20,000 individuals.

Pathogenesis. The pathogenesis of fascioscapulohumeral dystrophy is complex and only partly understood. It is established that the disease involves overexpression of a gene called *DUX4* that is located in a region of subtelomeric repeats on the long arm of chromosome 4. What remains unclear is the mechanism and consequences of *DUX4* overexpression. Some individuals with fascioscapulohumeral dystrophy inherit an abnormally small number of subtelomeric repeats. Each repeat carries a copy of the *DUX4* gene, and it appears that deletion of flanking repeats causes changes in chromatin that "derepress" the remaining copies of *DUX4* thus leading to its overexpression. However, the reduction in repeats by itself is not sufficient to produce the disease; instead, the disease is confined to those who also inherit certain single nucleotide polymorphisms (SNPs) at positions immediately 3′ of the *DUX4* coding sequence. Only when the SNPs and the repeat contractions are both present is *DUX4* expressed at high enough levels to be pathogenic. Other individuals have a normal number of repeats and possibly have other mechanisms of *DUX4* overexpression. *DUX4* encodes a transcription factor, suggesting that the disease ultimately results from the overexpression of DUX4 target genes.

Limb-Girdle Muscular Dystrophy

Limb-girdle muscular dystrophies are a heterogeneous group of at least six autosomal dominant and 15 autosomal recessive entities. Their overall incidence is 1 in 25,000 to 50,000 individuals. **As indicated by the name, all forms are characterized by muscle weakness that preferentially involves proximal muscle groups.** Both the age of onset and the disease severity are highly variable. The causative mutations involve genes that participate in diverse cellular functions, making it difficult to discern a unifying mechanism of disease pathogenesis. Based on current knowledge, the implicated genes can be grouped according to function as follows:

- Genes encoding structural components (sarcoglycans) of the dystrophin glycoprotein complex
- Genes encoding enzymes that are responsible for glycosylation of α-dystroglycan, a component of the dystrophin glycoprotein complex
- Genes encoding proteins that associate with the Z-disks of sarcomeres
- Genes encoding proteins involved in vesicle trafficking and cell signaling
- Genes that seemingly stand alone, such as those encoding the protease calpain 3 and lamin A/C (which is also mutated in some patients with Emery-Dreifuss muscular dystrophy)

Diseases of Lipid or Glycogen Metabolism

Many inborn errors of lipid or glycogen metabolism affect skeletal muscle. These disorders tend to produce one of two general patterns of muscle dysfunction. In some, patients become symptomatic only with exercise or fasting, which may produce severe muscle cramping and pain, or even extensive muscle necrosis (*rhabdomyolysis*). Other disorders of this type result in slowly progressive muscle damage, without episodic manifestations. Listed below are some examples in this group of muscle diseases:

- *Carnitine palmitoyltransferase II deficiency* is the most common disorder of lipid metabolism to cause episodic muscle damage with exercise or fasting. The defect in this disorder impairs the transport of free fatty acids into mitochondria.
- *Myophosphorylase deficiency (McArdle disease)* is one of the more common glycogen storage diseases affecting skeletal muscle; it also results in episodic muscle damage with exercise.
- *Acid maltase deficiency* results in impaired lysosomal conversion of glycogen to glucose, causing glycogen to

accumulate within lysosomes. Severe deficiency results in the generalized glycogenosis of infancy, *Pompe disease* (Chapter 5). Milder deficiency can cause a progressive adult onset myopathy that preferentially involves the respiratory and truncal muscles. Enzyme replacement therapy is now being used to treat affected patients.

Mitochondrial Myopathies

Mitochondrial diseases are complex systemic conditions that can involve many organ systems, including skeletal muscle. The genetics of these disorders are varied and unusually complex (discussed later), but many of the causative mutations appear to impair the ability of mitochondria to generate ATP. As a result, these diseases tend to affect skeletal muscles and other tissues rich in cell types with high ATP requirements, particularly cardiac muscle cells and neurons.

Skeletal muscle involvement can manifest as weakness, elevations in serum creatine kinase levels, or rhabdomyolysis. Although the anatomic pattern of muscle weakness is variable, involvement of extraocular eye muscles is common and can be a clue to the diagnosis. Indeed, *chronic progressive external ophthalmoplegia* is a common feature of mitochondrial disorders, and may occur as an isolated phenomenon or a part of a multisystem syndrome. The reason that extraocular eye muscles are particularly sensitive to mitochondrial disease is uncertain, but it may be that these muscles have exceptionally high requirements for ATP. In line with this idea, extraocular eye muscles have the most mitochondria per mass of any of the body's muscles.

Mitochondrial proteins and tRNAs may be encoded by either the nuclear genome or the mitochondrial genome (mtDNA). While mutations in nuclear mitochondrial genes follow Mendelian inheritance patterns, mutations in mtDNA are maternally inherited, since all of the mitochondria in the embryo are contributed by the oocyte (Chapter 5). In addition, unlike nuclear DNA, which is present in only two copies and is evenly distributed from a mother cell to daughter cells during cell division, each cell contains thousands of mtDNA copies, which are distributed in a random fashion to daughter cells at the time of cell division. It is believed that disease results only when a certain threshold of mutated mtDNA copies is exceeded within a substantial fraction of "at-risk" cells (e.g., skeletal muscle cells) in a tissue.

MORPHOLOGY

The most consistent pathologic change in skeletal muscle is abnormal aggregates of mitochondria that are seen preferentially in the subsarcolemmal area of affected myofibers, producing an appearance that is referred to as "ragged red fibers" (Fig. 27-12). By electron microscopy, morphologically abnormal mitochondria are seen. Loss of particular mitochondrial enzyme activities characterizes some mitochondrial diseases and may be appreciated by histochemical staining for cytochrome oxidase. Some mitochondrial diseases lack morphologic changes and can only be diagnosed through enzymatic assays or genetic analyses.

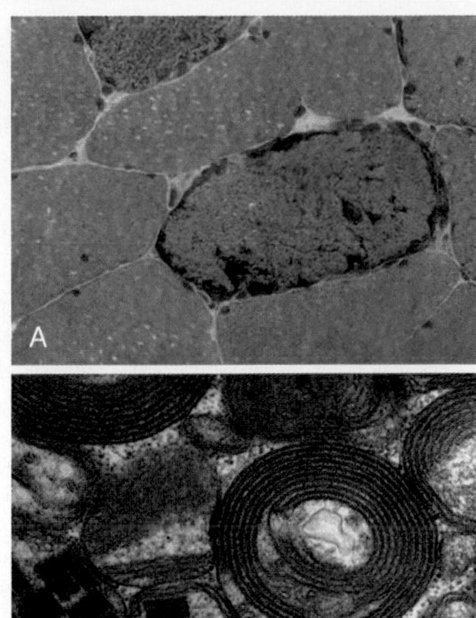

Figure 27-12 A, Ragged red fiber with increased reddish granular subsarcolemmal staining reflective of abnormal aggregation of mitochondria. **B,** Electron micrograph showing morphologically abnormal mitochondria with concentric membranous rings (so-called "phonograph records") and rhomboid paracrystalline inclusions (*lower left side*).

Clinical Features. Due to the complexity of mitochondrial genetics, genotype/phenotype relationships in mitochondrial disorders are not straightforward. For example, a single point mutation in the mitochondrial leucine tRNA gene may produce isolated chronic progressive external ophthalmoplegia in one patient and a much more severe phenotype, *mitochondrial encephalomyopathy with lactic acidosis and strokelike episodes*, in a second. Similarly, deletions in mtDNA may lead to either isolated ophthalmoplegia or to *Kearns-Sayre syndrome*, characterized by ophthalmoplegia, pigmentary degeneration of the retina, and complete heart block. *Myoclonic epilepsy with ragged red fibers* and *Leber hereditary optic neuropathy* are other examples of mitochondrial disease caused by point mutations in mtDNA. Many mitochondrial disorders, such as subacute necrotizing encephalopathy (*Leigh syndrome*), are remarkably heterogeneous genetically and may be caused by mutations in either mtDNA or the nuclear genome. In the case of Leigh syndrome, at last count causative mutations have been identified in more than 30 different genes, the common feature being that all of the affected genes encode proteins with essential roles in mitochondrial metabolism.

Spinal Muscular Atrophy and the Differential Diagnosis of a Hypotonic Infant

Spinal muscular atrophy is a neuropathic disorder in which loss of motor neurons leads to muscle weakness and atrophy. Infants with neurologic or neuromuscular disease may present with generalized hypotonia ("floppy infant"). The differential diagnosis of infantile hypotonia includes primary diseases of skeletal muscle (e.g., congenital myasthenic syndrome, congenital myotonia, congenital myopathies, and congenital muscular dystrophies),

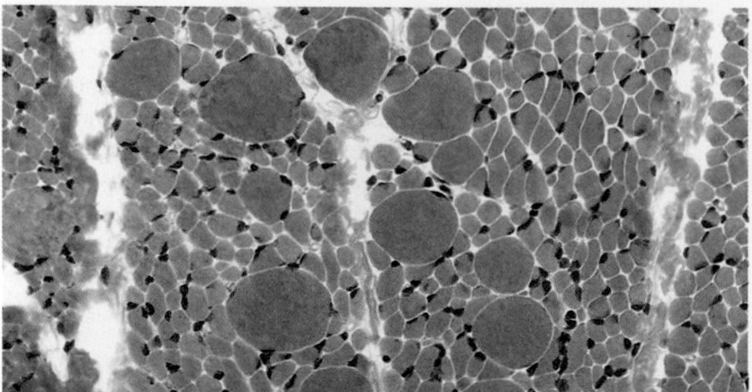

Figure 27-13 Spinal muscular atrophy with only rare hypertrophied myofibers admixed with numerous atrophic rounded myofibers. The larger fibers are those that are innervated and have undergone compensatory hypertrophy.

abnormalities of the brain (e.g. encephalopathy), and neuronopathies, of which spinal muscular atrophy is a prototypic example.

Spinal muscular atrophy is an autosomal recessive disorder with an incidence of 1 in 6,000 births, and is caused by loss-of-function mutations in the *SMN1* (survival of motor neuron-1) gene. The function of the gene is uncertain—the encoded protein may have a role in RNA splicing—but SMN1 deficiency has a dramatic effect on motor neuron survival, sometimes leading to loss of motor neurons in utero. The resulting denervation of skeletal muscle may lead to characteristic morphologic changes consisting of large zones of severely atrophic myofibers mixed with scattered normal sized or hypertrophied myofibers, found individually or in small groups (Fig. 27-13). These normal or hypertrophied fibers are those that retain innervation from remaining motor neurons.

Ion Channel Myopathies (Channelopathies)

Channelopathies are a group of inherited diseases caused by mutations affecting the function of ion channel proteins. Most channelopathies are autosomal dominant disorders with variable penetrance. Depending on the channel that is affected, clinical manifestations may include epilepsy, migraine, movement disorders with cerebellar dysfunction, peripheral nerve disease, and muscle disease.

Different ion channel myopathies may cause decreased or increased excitability resulting in hypotonia or hypertonia. Disorders associated with hypotonia can be further sub-classified based on whether symptomatic patients have elevated, depressed, or normal serum potassium levels and are called *hyperkalemic, hypokalemic,* and *normokalemic periodic paralysis*, respectively. Examples of mutated gene products that are associated with muscle dysfunction are the following:

- KCNJ2—Mutations affecting this potassium channel cause *Andersen-Twail syndrome,* an autosomal disorder associated with periodic paralysis, heart arrhythmias, and skeletal abnormalities.
- SCN4A—Mutations affecting this sodium channel cause several autosomal disorders with presentations ranging from myotonia to periodic paralysis.
- CACNA1S—Missense mutations in this protein, a subunit of a muscle calcium channel, are the most common cause of *hypokalemic paralysis.*
- CLC1—Mutations affecting this chloride channel cause myotonia congenita. As already discussed, CLC1 expression is decreased in myotonic dystrophy.
- RYR1—Mutations in the *RYR1* gene disrupt the function of the ryanodine receptor, which regulates calcium release from the sarcoplasmic reticulum. *RYR1* mutations are linked to a congenital myopathy (central core disease) and to *malignant hyperthermia*. The latter is characterized by a hypermetabolic state (tachycardia, tachypnea, muscle spasms, and later hyperpyrexia) that can be triggered by anesthetics, most commonly halogenated inhalational agents and succinylcholine. Upon exposure to anesthetic, the mutated receptor allows increased efflux of calcium from the sarcoplasmic reticulum, leading to tetany and excessive heat production.

KEY CONCEPTS

Disorders of Skeletal Muscle

- Altered muscle function may stem from neurogenic or primary myopathic processes.
- Myopathic processes are often marked by degeneration and regeneration of myofibers.
- The three main inflammatory myopathies are polymyositis, dermatomyositis, and inclusion body myositis.
  - **Inclusion body myositis** is a chronic progressive disease of older patients associated with rimmed vacuoles.
  - **Dermatomyositis** occurs in children and adults, the latter frequently as a paraneoplastic disorder. Immune damage to small blood vessels and perifascicular atrophy are common features.
  - **Polymyositis** is an adult onset myopathy caused by CD8+ T cells.
- **Muscular dystrophies** and **congenital myopathies** result from mutations that disrupt the function of proteins that are important for various aspects of muscle development, function, and regeneration. Some of these diseases present in infancy, others in adulthood. They may be relentlessly progressive or cause relatively static deficits.
- Myopathy can result from toxic injury or be the result of metabolic diseases including those of lipid metabolism, glycogen metabolism, and mitochondria.

Peripheral Nerve Sheath Tumors

A number of benign and malignant neoplasms are grouped together as peripheral nerve sheath tumors. *The vast majority of these are composed of cells that show evidence of Schwann cell differentiation.* These include the three common types, schwannoma, neurofibroma, and malignant peripheral nerve sheath tumor (MPNST). Other rare tumors arising from nerves may show evidence of perineurial cell differentiation. There is an abrupt transition between myelination by oligodendrocytes (central myelin) and myelination by Schwann cells (peripheral myelin) that occurs as nerves extend out from the substance of the brain. Thus, peripheral nerve tumors sometimes arise within the dura as well as along the distal course of peripheral nerves.

Peripheral nerve sheath tumors have several unique features. One is their association with relatively common familial tumor syndromes, including neurofibromatosis type 1 (NF1), neurofibromatosis type 2 (NF2), and schwannomatosis. Furthermore MPNSTs seen in the context of NF1 are thought to arise through malignant transformation of preexisting benign plexiform neurofibromas. Although malignant transformation of a preexisting benign lesion is a common origin for certain carcinomas (e.g., colon cancer), it is unusual in soft tissue tumors. Tumors with skeletal muscle differentiation are discussed in Chapter 26.

Schwannomas

These are benign tumors that exhibit Schwann cell differentiation and often arise directly from peripheral nerves. Schwannomas are a component of NF2, and even sporadic schwannomas are commonly associated with inactivating mutations in the *NF2* gene on chromosome 22. Loss of expression of the *NF2* gene product, *merlin*, is a consistent finding in all schwannomas. Merlin normally restricts the cell-surface expression of growth factor receptors, such as EGFR, through interactions involving the actin cytoskeleton; in its absence, cells hyperproliferate in response to growth factors.

MORPHOLOGY

Schwannomas are well-circumscribed, encapsulated masses that abut the associated nerve without invading it, a feature that simplifies surgical excision. Grossly, these tumors form firm, gray masses. Microscopically, they are comprised of an admixture of dense and loose areas referred to as **Antoni A** and **Antoni B** areas, respectively (Fig. 27-14*A*). The dense eosinophilic Antoni A areas often contain spindle cells arranged into cellular intersecting fascicles. Palisading of nuclei is common and "nuclear-free zones" that lie between the regions of nuclear palisading are termed **Verocay bodies** (Fig. 27-14*B*). In the loose, hypocellular **Antoni B** areas the spindle cells are spread apart by a prominent myxoid extracellular matrix that may be associated with microcyst formation. Schwann cells are characterized by the presence of a spindled elongated nucleus with a wavy or buckled shape. Electron microscopy shows basement membrane deposits encasing single cells and collagen fibers. Because the lesion displaces the nerve of origin as it grows, silver stains or immunostains for neurofilament proteins demonstrate that axons are largely excluded from the tumor, although they may become entrapped in the capsule. The Schwann cell origin of these tumors is borne out by their uniform immunoreactivity for S-100. A variety of degenerative changes may be found in schwannomas, including nuclear pleomorphism, xanthomatous change, vascular hyalinization, cystic change, necrosis and mitotic activity. Some large mitotically active Schwannomas lacking Antoni B areas may mimic a sarcoma. Schwannomas may recur locally if incompletely resected, but malignant transformation is extremely rare (in contrast to plexiform neurofibromas, discussed later).

Clinical Features. Most Schwannomas cause symptoms by local compression of the involved nerve or adjacent structures (e.g., brainstem or spinal cord). Within the cranial vault, most schwannomas occur at the cerebellopontine angle, where they are attached to the vestibular branch of the eighth nerve. Affected individuals often present with tinnitus and hearing loss; the tumor is commonly referred to as an *acoustic neuroma*—a double misnomer, since the tumor neither arises from the acoustic portion of the nerve nor is it a neuroma. Elsewhere within the dura, sensory nerves are preferentially involved, including branches of the trigeminal nerve and dorsal roots. When extradural, schwannomas can arise in association with large nerve trunks or as soft tissue lesions without an identifiable associated nerve. Surgical removal is curative.

Neurofibromas

Neurofibromas are benign nerve sheath tumors that are more heterogeneous in composition than schwannomas. *The neoplastic Schwann cells are admixed with perineurial-like cells, fibroblasts, mast cells, and CD34+ spindle cells.* Neurofibromas may be either sporadic or NF1-associated. Different types of neurofibroma can be distinguished depending on their growth pattern.

- *Superficial cutaneous neurofibromas* often present as pedunculated nodules that can be seen isolated (if sporadic) or multiple (if NF1-associated).
- *Diffuse neurofibromas* often present as a large plaquelike elevation of skin and are typically NF1-associated.
- *Plexiform neurofibromas* can be found in deep or superficial locations in association with nerve roots or large nerves and are uniformly NF1-associated.

Pathogenesis. Only the Schwann cells in neurofibromas show complete loss of the *NF1* gene product, neurofibromin, indicating that these are the neoplastic cells. You will recall from Chapter 7 that neurofibromin is a tumor suppressor that inhibits RAS activity by stimulating the activity of a GTPase (RAS is active only when bound to GTP). Haploinsufficiency for the NF1 gene in other associated cells may also contribute to the growth of NF1-associated tumors. For example, there is evidence that NF1-haploinsufficient mast cells are hypersensitive to KIT ligand produced by Schwann cells and in response secrete factors that stimulate Schwann cell growth. This form of tumor/stromal cell cross-talk may be targetable with inhibitors of the KIT receptor tyrosine kinase. Other studies suggest that plexiform neurofibromas and dermal neurofibromas arise from different neural crest derived precursor cells. With rare exceptions, transformation to MPNST is only seen in plexiform neurofibromas. The overall incidence of MPNST in NF1 patients is about 5% to 10%, but patients with large numbers of plexiform neurofibromas and large deletions in the NF1 gene are at higher risk.

MORPHOLOGY

Localized cutaneous neurofibroma. These are small, well-delineated but unencapsulated nodular lesions that arise in the dermis and subcutaneous fat. They have relatively low cellularity and contain bland Schwann cells admixed with stromal cells such as mast cells, perineurial cells, CD34+ spindle cells, and fibroblasts. Adnexal structures are sometimes entrapped at the edges of the lesion. The stroma of these tumors contains loose collagen.

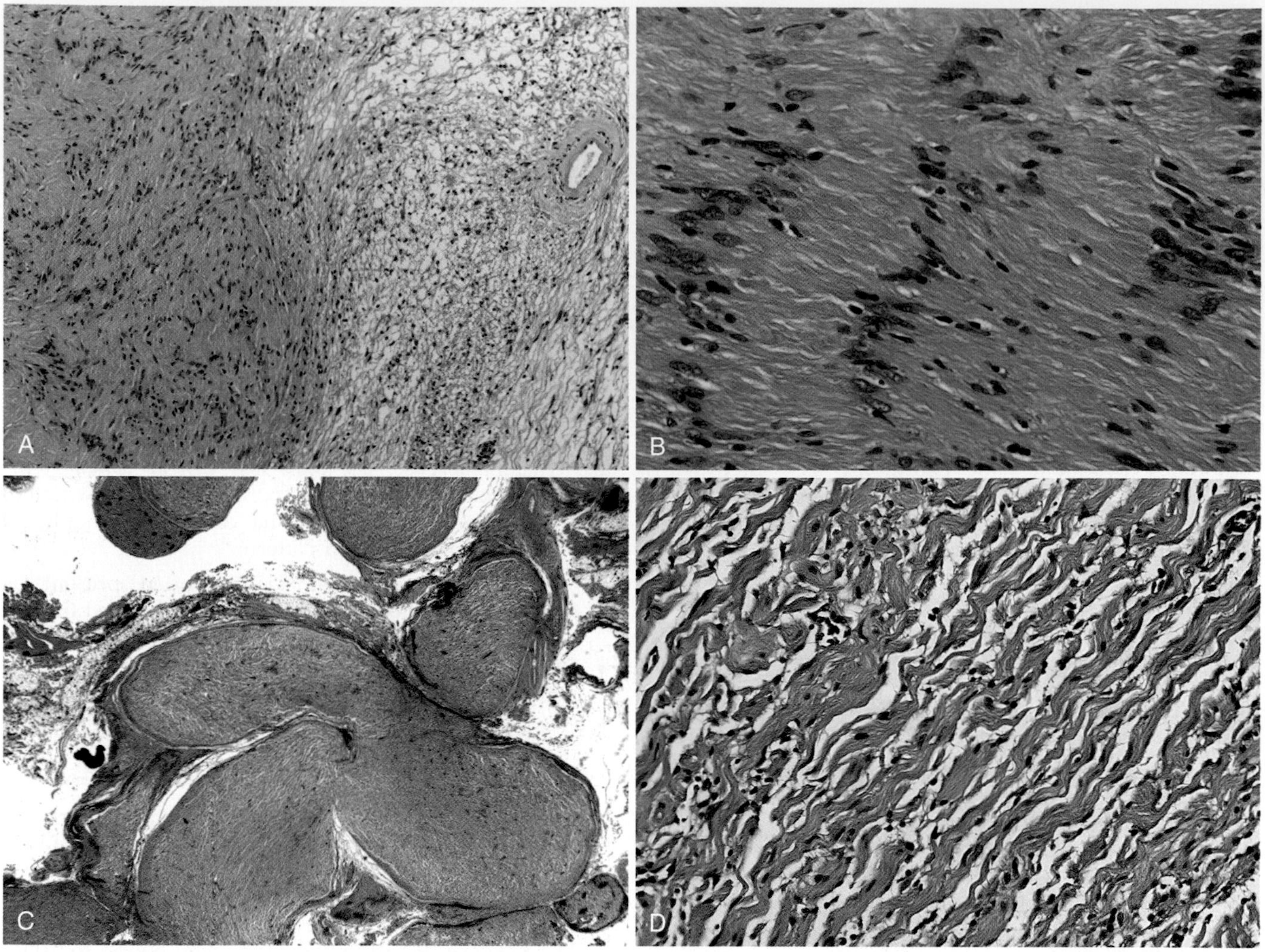

Figure 27-14 Schwannoma and plexiform neurofibroma. **A** and **B,** Schwannoma. As seen in **A,** schwannomas often contain dense eosinophilic Antoni A areas (*left*) and loose, pale Antoni B areas (*right*), as well as hyalinized blood vessels (*right*). **B,** Antoni A area with the tumor cell nuclei aligned in palisading rows leaving anuclear zones and resulting in the formation of structures termed *Verocay bodies*. **C** and **D,** Plexiform neurofibroma. **C,** Multiple nerve fascicles are expanded by infiltrating tumor cells. **D,** At high power bland spindle cells are admixed with wavy collagen bundles resembling carrot shavings.

Diffuse neurofibroma. This tumor has morphologic features similar to those seen in localized cutaneous neurofibromas, but exhibits a distinctly different growth pattern. The tumor diffusely infiltrates the dermis and subcutaneous connective tissue, entrapping fat and appendage structures and producing a plaque-like appearance. Some of these neurofibromas can grow to large sizes. Focal collections of cells mimicking the appearance of Meissner corpuscles (so-called **pseudo-Meissner corpuscles** or **tactile-like bodies**) are an associated feature.

Plexiform neurofibroma. These tumors grow within and expand nerve fascicles (Fig. 27-14*C*), entrapping associated axons. The external perineurial layer of the nerve is preserved, giving individual nodules an encapsulated appearance. The expanded, ropy thickening of multiple nerve fascicles results in what is sometimes referred to as a "bag of worms" appearance. The tumor has cellular composition similar to that of other neurofibromas. The extracellular matrix varies from loose and myxoid to more collagenous and fibrous. Often the collagen is seen in bundles likened to "shredded carrot" (Fig. 27-14*D*).

Malignant Peripheral Nerve Sheath Tumors (MPNST)

Most MPNSTs (approximately 85%) are high-grade tumors, but low-grade variants are recognized. About half arise in NF1 patients and are assumed to result from malignant transformation of a plexiform neurofibroma. Sporadic cases may arise de novo. Most are associated with larger peripheral nerves in the chest, abdomen, pelvis, neck or limb-girdle. MPNSTs exhibit complex chromosomal aberrations, including chromosome gains, losses, and rearrangements. The molecular alterations driving malignant transformation of a neurofibroma to MPNST are still poorly understood.

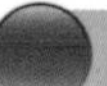

MORPHOLOGY

The lesions are poorly defined tumor masses that frequently infiltrate along the axis of the parent nerve and invade adjacent soft tissues. A wide range of histologic appearance can be encountered. Typical cases show a fasciculated arrangement of spindle cells. At low power the tumor often appears "marble-ized" due to variations in cellularity. Mitoses, necrosis, and nuclear anaplasia are common. An interesting phenomenon observed in MPNST is described as "divergent differentiation." This term refers to the presence of focal areas that exhibit other lines of differentiation, including glandular, cartilaginous, osseous, or rhabdomyoblastic morphology. A tumor exhibiting the latter is referred to as **Triton tumor**. Due to the poorly differentiated nature of MPNST, the distinction from an undifferentiated sarcoma may not be straightforward. Helpful clues include a diagnosis of NF1 in the affected patient and a clearly demonstrated anatomic relationship to a nerve or to a preexisting neurofibroma.

Neurofibromatosis Type I and Type 2

Neurofibromatosis Type I

This is a common autosomal dominant disorder with a frequency of 1 in 3000. It is a systemic disease associated with nonneoplastic manifestations and with a variety of tumors, including neurofibromas of all types, malignant peripheral nerve sheath tumors, gliomas of the optic nerve, other glial tumors and hamartomatous lesions, and pheochromocytomas. Other features include mental retardation or seizures, skeletal defects pigmented nodules of the iris (*Lisch nodules*), and cutaneous hyperpigmented macules *(café au lait spots)*. The disease is caused by loss-of-function mutations in the *NF1* gene, located at 17q11.2, which encodes the tumor suppressor neurofibromin. The neoplastic cells in NF1-related tumors lack neurofibromin due to biallelic defects in the *NF1* gene. As has been mentioned earlier, NF-1 protein has GTPase activity that restrains RAS function. In the absence of NF-1, RAS remains trapped in its active state.

The disease has a high penetrance but variable expressivity. Some patients exhibit only subtle features, while others show disease that is restricted to certain parts of the body, a distribution that is attributable to mosaicism. An unfortunate subset has severe disease. Large chromosomal deletions that span *NF1* and extend to involve adjacent genes tend to be associated with more severe phenotypes.

Neurofibromatosis Type 2

This is an autosomal dominant disorder resulting in a range of tumors, most commonly bilateral eighth-nerve schwannomas and multiple meningiomas. Gliomas, typically ependymomas of the spinal cord, also occur in these patients. Many individuals with NF2 also have nonneoplastic lesions, which include nodular ingrowth of Schwann cells into the spinal cord (schwannosis), meningioangiomatosis (a proliferation of meningeal cells and blood vessels that grows into the brain), and glial hamartia (microscopic nodular collections of glial cells at abnormal locations, often in the superficial and deep layers of cerebral cortex). This disorder is much less common than NF1, having a frequency of 1 in 40,000 to 50,000. Certain other rare familial syndromes are also associated with multiple schwannomas, such as schwannomatosis and Carney complex.

The *NF2* gene is located on chromosome 22q12, and is also commonly mutated in sporadic meningiomas and schwannomas. The *NF2* gene product, merlin, is a cytoskeletal protein that appears to regulate membrane receptor signaling. Its tumor suppressive function may be related to a role in contact inhibition of cell growth. There is some correlation between the type of mutation and clinical symptoms, with nonsense and frameshift mutations causing more severe phenotypes than missense mutations.

KEY CONCEPTS

Peripheral Nerve Sheath Tumors

- The three common peripheral nerve sheath tumors—Schwannoma, neurofibroma, and malignant peripheral nerve sheath tumor—all likely arise from cells of Schwann cell lineage.
- Schwannomas are encapsulated benign tumors that can be associated with NF2.
- Neurofibromas are benign peripheral nerve sheath tumors sometimes associated with NF1 that can be subtyped as localized cutaneous, diffuse, or plexiform.
- Malignant peripheral nerve sheath tumors can be de novo sporadic neoplasms or NF1-associated tumors arising through malignant transformation of a (plexiform) neurofibroma.

SUGGESTED READINGS

Neuropathies and Other Non-Neoplastic Disorders of Peripheral Nerves

Dalakas MC: Advances in the diagnosis, pathogenesis and treatment of chronic inflammatory demyelinating polyneuropathy. *Nat Rev Neurol* 7:507, 2011. *[Review of CIDP with discussion of immune-pathogenesis.]*

Espinos C, Calpena E, Martinez-Rubio D, et al: Autosomal recessive Charcot-Marie-Tooth neuropathy. *Adv Exp Med Biol* 724:61, 2012. *[review of Charco-Marie-Tooth disease discussing the classification and genetic diversity.]*

Grantz M, Huan MC: Unusual peripheral neuropathies. Part I: extrinsic causes. *Semin Neurol* 30:387, 2010. *[Review of acquired extrnisic neuropathies including toxic, infectious and metabolic forms from a pragmatic clinical persepctive.]*

Koike H, Tanaka F, Sobue G: Paraneoplastic neuropathy: wide-ranging clinicopathological manifestations. *Curr Opin Neurol* 24:504, 2011. *[Review of paraneoplastic neuropathies with focus on clinical presentation and management.]*

Manji H: Toxic neuropathy. *Curr Opin Neurol* 24:484, 2011. *[Review of mechanisms of toxic neuropathies and their clinical manifestations with focus on chemotherapy induced forms.]*

Robinson-Papp J, Simpson DM: Neuromuscular diseases associated with HIV-1 infection. *Muscle Nerve* 40:1043, 2009. *[Discussion of peripheral neuropathy and myopathy as they develop at different stages of HIV.]*

Vallat JM, Funalot B, Magy L: Nerve biopsy: requirements for diagnosis and clinical value. *Acta Neuropathol* 121:313, 2011. *[Review of the pathologist's approach to peripheral nerve biopsies.]*

Muscular Dystrophies and Other Disorders of Muscle

Broglio L, Tentorio M, Cotelli MS, et al: Limb-girdle muscular dystrophy-associated protein diseases. *Neurologist* 16:340, 2010. *[Review of the classification of limb girdle mucular dystrophies.]*

Dimachkie MM: Idiopathic inflammatory myopathies. *J Neuroimmunol* 231:32, 2011. *[Review of inflammatory myopathies including clinical features and pathobiology.]*

DiMauro S: Pathogenesis and treatment of mitochondrial myopathies: recent advances. *Acta Myol* 29:333, 2010. *[Review of myopathy as manifestation of mitochondrial disease.]*

Hoffman EP, Bronson A, Levin AA, et al: Restoring dystrophin expression in duchenne muscular dystrophy muscle progress in exon skipping and stop codon read through. *Am J Pathol* 179:12, 2011. *[Discussion of new treatment strategies for patients with Duchenn muscular dystrophy.]*

Kullmann DM: Neurological channelopathies. *Annu Rev Neurosci* 33:151, 2010. *[General review of channelopathies as cause of neurologic disease including myasthenic syndromes and myopathies.]*

Lemmers RJ, van der Vliet PJ, Klooster R, et al: A unifying genetic model for facioscapulohumeral muscular dystrophy. *Science* 329:1650, 2010. *[Key study suggesting a complex two-hit genetic mechanism of FSHD.]*

Mendell JR, Boue DR, Martin PT: The congenital muscular dystrophies: recent advances and molecular insights. *Pediatr Dev Pathol* 9:427, 2006. *[Review of congenital muscular dystrophies and their classification.]*

Nagaraju K, Lundberg IE: Polymyositis and dermatomyositis: pathophysiology. *Rheum Dis Clin North Am* 37:159, 2011. *[Discussion of immune mechanisms in the pathobiology of polymyositis and dermatomyositis.]*

Richards M, Coppee F, Thomas N, et al: Facioscapulohumeral muscular dystrophy (FSHD): an enigma unravelled? *Hum Genet* 131:325, 2012. *[Review of new insights into the complex genetics underlying FSHD.]*

Robinson AB, Reed AM: Clinical features, pathogenesis and treatment of juvenile and adult dermatomyositis. *Nat Rev Rheumatol* 7:664, 2011. *[Review of outlining differences and similarities between adult and juvenile cases of deramatomyositis.]*

Sicot G, Gourdon G, Gomes-Pereira M: Myotonic dystrophy, when simple repeats reveal complex pathogenic entities: new findings and future challenges. *Hum Mol Genet* 20:R116, 2011. *[Review of myotoinc dystrophy focused on the current model of its pathogenesis.]*

Tumors of Peripheral Nerves

Carroll SL: Molecular mechanisms promoting the pathogenesis of Schwann cell neoplasms. *Acta Neuropathol* 132:321, 2012. *[Review of the molecular changes driving the growth of nerve sheath tumors including those arising associated with familial syndromes.]*

Rodriguez FJ, Folpe AL, Giannini C, et al: Pathology of peripheral nerve sheath tumors: diagnostic overview and update on selected diagnostic problems. *Acta Neuropathol* 123:295, 2012. *[Review of the pathologic classification and features of peripheral nerve sheath tumors.]*

See TARGETED THERAPY available online at www.studentconsult.com

CHAPTER 28

The Central Nervous System

Matthew P. Frosch • Douglas C. Anthony • Umberto De Girolami

CHAPTER CONTENTS

The principal functional unit of the central nervous system (CNS) is the neuron. Of all the cells in the body, neurons have the unique ability to receive and transmit information. Neurons of different types and in different locations have distinct properties, including functional roles, distribution of their connections, neurotransmitters used, metabolic requirements, and levels of electrical activity at a given moment. A set of neurons, not necessarily clustered together in a region of the brain, may thus show *selective vulnerability* to various insults because it shares one or more of these properties. Since different regions of the brain participate in different functions, the pattern of clinical signs and symptoms that follow injury depend as much on the region of brain involved as on the pathologic process. Mature neurons are incapable of cell division, so destruction of even a small number of neurons essential for a specific function may leave the individual with a neurologic deficit. Neural progenitor populations are present in certain regions of the brain and have been shown to respond to injury by generating new neurons. For this reason, there is continuing interest in whether expansion of endogenous progenitors or delivery of exogenously derived progenitor cells might be a useful therapeutic approach for repair after injury or in the setting of degenerative diseases.

In addition to neurons the CNS contains other cells, such as *astrocytes* and *oligodendrocytes*, which make up the *glia*. The components of the CNS are affected by a number of unique neurologic disorders and also respond to common insults (e.g., ischemia, infection) in a manner that is distinct from other tissues. We start our discussion of diseases of the CNS with an overview of the patterns of injury of different cells and the reactions of these cells to various insults.

Cellular Pathology of the Central Nervous System

Neurons and glia of the CNS undergo a range of functional and morphologic changes in the setting of injury. Understanding these patterns can be informative about the mechanism of cellular injury and type of disease.

Reactions of Neurons to Injury

Neuronal injury may be an acute process, often a consequence of depletion of oxygen or glucose or trauma, or a slower process, often associated with accumulation of abnormal protein aggregates, as occurs in degenerative disorders of the brain. Neurons require a continuous supply of oxygen and glucose to meet metabolic needs. This satisfies essential physiologic and anatomic requirements of the cells, including maintaining membrane gradients that are essential for action potentials, and supporting the extensive cytoplasmic dendritic arborization of neurons and of axons, which may extend over great distances from the cell body (up to a meter in adults). As most mature neurons are maintained for the life span of an individual, protein turnover and quality have to be carefully regulated to ensure cellular integrity. Not surprisingly, many neurologic diseases result from the injurious effects of accumulated misfolded proteins (*proteinopathies*) (see discussion of protein misfolding and the unfolded protein response in Chapter 2).

MORPHOLOGY

Acute neuronal injury ("red neurons") refers to a spectrum of changes that accompany acute CNS hypoxia/ischemia or other acute insults and reflect the earliest morphologic markers of neuronal cell death (see Fig. 28-13*B*). "Red neurons" are evident by about 12 to 24 hours after an irreversible hypoxic/ischemic insult. The morphologic features consist of shrinkage of the cell body, pyknosis of the nucleus, disappearance of the nucleolus, and loss of Nissl substance, with intense eosinophilia of the cytoplasm.

Subacute and chronic neuronal injury ("degeneration") refers to neuronal death occurring as a result of a progressive disease of some duration, as is seen in certain slowly evolving neurodegenerative diseases such as amyotrophic lateral sclerosis and Alzheimer disease. The characteristic histologic feature is cell loss, often selectively involving functionally related groups of neurons, and reactive gliosis. At an early stage, the cell loss is difficult to detect; the associated reactive glial changes are often the best indicator of neuronal injury. For many of these diseases, there is evidence that cell loss occurs via apoptotic death.

Axonal reaction is a change observed in the cell body during regeneration of the axon; it is best seen in anterior horn cells of the spinal cord when motor axons are cut or seriously damaged. There is increased protein synthesis associated with axonal sprouting. This is reflected in enlargement and rounding up of the cell body, peripheral displacement of the nucleus, enlargement of the nucleolus, and dispersion of Nissl substance from the center to the periphery of the cell (central chromatolysis).

Neuronal damage may be associated with a wide range of subcellular alterations in the neuronal organelles and cytoskeleton. **Neuronal inclusions** may occur as a manifestation of aging, when there are intracytoplasmic accumulations of complex lipids (lipofuscin), proteins, or carbohydrates. Abnormal cytoplasmic deposition of complex lipids and other substances also occurs in genetically determined disorders of metabolism in which substrates or intermediates accumulate (Chapter 5). Viral infection can lead to abnormal intranuclear inclusions, as seen in herpetic infection (Cowdry body), cytoplasmic inclusions, as seen in rabies (Negri body), or both nucleus and cytoplasm as in cytomegalovirus infection.

Some degenerative diseases of the CNS are associated with neuronal intracytoplasmic inclusions, such as neurofibrillary tangles of Alzheimer disease and Lewy bodies of Parkinson disease; others cause abnormal vacuolization of the perikaryon and neuronal cell processes in the neuropil (Creutzfeldt-Jakob disease).

Reactions of Astrocytes to Injury

Gliosis is the most important histopathologic indicator of CNS injury, regardless of etiology, and is characterized by both hypertrophy and hyperplasia of astrocytes. The astrocyte derives its name from its star-shaped appearance. These cells have multipolar, branching cytoplasmic processes that emanate from the cell body and contain glial fibrillary acidic protein (GFAP), a cell type-specific intermediate filament (Fig. 28-1). Astrocytes act as metabolic buffers and detoxifiers within the brain. Additionally, through the foot processes, which surround capillaries or extend to the subpial and subependymal zones, they contribute to barrier functions controlling the flow of macromolecules between the blood, the cerebrospinal fluid (CSF), and the brain. In gliosis, the nuclei of astrocytes, which are typically round to oval (10 μm wide) with evenly dispersed, pale chromatin, enlarge, become vesicular, and develop prominent nucleoli. The previously scant cytoplasm expands to a bright pink, somewhat irregular swath around an eccentric nucleus, from which emerge numerous stout, ramifying processes; these cells are called *gemistocytic astrocytes*.

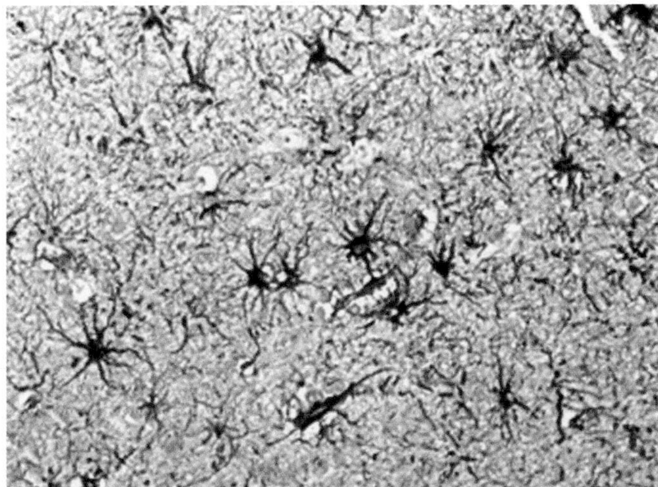

Figure 28-1 Astrocytes and their processes. Immunohistochemical staining for glial fibrillary acidic protein reveals astrocytic perinuclear cytoplasm and well-developed processes *(brown)*.

Acute cell injury, as occurs in hypoxia, hypoglycemia, and toxic injuries, is manifested by cellular swelling, as in other cells (Chapter 2). The *Alzheimer type II astrocyte* (unrelated to Alzheimer disease but first described by the same individual) is a gray matter cell with a large (two to three times normal) nucleus, pale-staining central chromatin, an intranuclear glycogen droplet, and a prominent nuclear membrane and nucleolus. This type of change is mainly seen in individuals with long-standing hyperammonemia due to chronic liver disease, Wilson disease, or hereditary metabolic disorders of the urea cycle.

Other types of cell injury lead to the formation of cytoplasmic inclusion bodies. *Rosenthal fibers* are thick, elongated, brightly eosinophilic, irregular structures that occur within astrocytic processes, and contain two heat-shock proteins (αB-crystallin and hsp27) as well as ubiquitin. Rosenthal fibers are typically found in regions of long-standing gliosis; they are also characteristic of one type of glial tumor, pilocytic astrocytoma. In *Alexander disease*, a leukodystrophy associated with mutations in the gene encoding GFAP, abundant Rosenthal fibers are found in periventricular, perivascular, and subpial locations. More commonly seen are *corpora amylacea*, or polyglucosan bodies. These are round, faintly basophilic, periodic acid-Schiff (PAS)-positive, concentrically lamellated structures of 5 to 50 μm in diameter that are located wherever there are astrocytic end processes, especially in the subpial and perivascular zones. They consist primarily of glycosaminoglycan polymers, as well as heat-shock proteins and ubiquitin. They occur in increasing numbers with advancing age and are thought to represent a degenerative change in the astrocyte. The *Lafora bodies* that are seen in the cytoplasm of neurons (as well as hepatocytes, myocytes, and other cells) in myoclonic epilepsy (Lafora body myoclonus with epilepsy) have a similar structure and biochemical composition.

Reactions of Microglia to Injury

Microglia are mesoderm-derived phagocytic cells that serve as the resident macrophages of the CNS. They share many surface markers with peripheral monocytes/macrophages (e.g., CR3 and CD68). They respond to injury by (1) proliferating; (2) developing elongated nuclei *(rod cells)*, as in neurosyphilis; (3) forming aggregates around small foci of tissue necrosis *(microglial nodules)*; or (4) congregating around cell bodies of dying neurons *(neuronophagia)*. In addition to resident microglia, blood-derived macrophages may also be present in inflammatory foci.

Reactions of Other Glial Cells to Injury

Oligodendrocytes are cells that wrap their cytoplasmic processes around axons and form myelin. Each oligodendrocyte myelinates numerous internodes on multiple axons, in contrast to the myelinating Schwann cell in peripheral nerve, which has a one-to-one correspondence between cells and internodes. Injury or apoptosis of oligodendroglial cells is a feature of acquired demyelinating disorders and leukodystrophies. Oligodendroglial nuclei may harbor viral inclusions in progressive multifocal leukoencephalopathy. *Glial cytoplasmic inclusions*, primarily composed of α-synuclein, are found in oligodendrocytes in multiple system atrophy (MSA).

Ependymal cells, the ciliated columnar epithelial cells lining the ventricles, do not have specific patterns of reaction. When there is inflammation or marked dilation of the ventricular system, disruption of the ependymal lining is paired with proliferation of subependymal astrocytes to produce small irregularities on the ventricular surfaces *(ependymal granulations)*. Certain infectious agents, particularly CMV, may produce extensive ependymal injury, with viral inclusions in ependymal cells. However, neither oligodendrocytes nor ependymal cells mediate significant responses to most forms of injury in the CNS.

KEY CONCEPTS

Cellular Pathology of the Central Nervous System

- Each cellular component of the nervous system has a distinct set of patterns of response to injury.
- Neuronal injury commonly results in cell death, either by apoptosis or necrosis. Loss of neurons that is difficult to detect without formal quantification may still contribute to dysfunction.
- Astrocytes show morphologic changes including hypertrophy of the cytoplasm, accumulation of intermediate filament protein (GFAP), and hyperplasia.
- Microglia, the resident monocyte-lineage population of the CNS, proliferate and accumulate in response to injury.

Cerebral Edema, Hydrocephalus, and Raised Intracranial Pressure and Herniation

The brain and the spinal cord are encased and protected by the rigid skull and the bony spinal canal. The pressure within the cranial cavity may rise in one of three commonly observed clinical settings: generalized brain edema, increased CSF volume (hydrocephalus), and focally expanding mass lesions. Depending on the degree and rapidity of the pressure increase and the nature of the underlying lesion, the consequences range from subtle neurologic deficits to death.

Cerebral Edema

Cerebral edema (more precisely, brain parenchymal edema) is the result of increased fluid leakage from blood vessels or injury to various cells of the CNS. There are two main pathways of edema formation in the brain.

- *Vasogenic edema* is an increase in extracellular fluid caused by blood-brain barrier disruption and increased vascular permeability, allowing fluid to shift from the intravascular compartment to the intercellular spaces of the brain. The paucity of lymphatics greatly impairs the resorption of excess extracellular fluid. Vasogenic edema may be either localized (e.g., adjacent to inflammation or neoplasms) or generalized, as can follow ischemic injury.
- *Cytotoxic edema* is an increase in intracellular fluid secondary to neuronal, glial, or endothelial cell membrane injury, as might be encountered in someone with a generalized hypoxic/ischemic insult or with a metabolic derangement that prevents maintenance of the normal membrane ionic gradient.

In practice, conditions associated with generalized edema often have elements of both vasogenic and cytotoxic edema. In generalized edema, the gyri are flattened, the intervening sulci are narrowed, and the ventricular cavities are compressed. As the brain expands, herniation may occur.

Interstitial edema (hydrocephalic edema) occurs especially around the lateral ventricles when an increase in intravascular pressure causes an abnormal flow of fluid from the intraventricular CSF across the ependymal lining to the periventricular white matter.

Hydrocephalus

Hydrocephalus is the accumulation of excessive CSF within the ventricular system (Fig. 28-2). The choroid plexus within the ventricular system produces CSF, which normally circulates through the ventricular system and enters the cisterna magna at the base of the brain stem through the foramina of Luschka and Magendie. Subarachnoid CSF bathes the superior cerebral convexities and is absorbed by the arachnoid granulations. Most cases of hydrocephalus are a consequence of impaired flow and resorption of CSF; overproduction is a rare cause that can accompany tumors of the choroid plexus. An increased volume of CSF within the ventricles expands them and can elevate the intracranial pressure.

When hydrocephalus develops in infancy before closure of the cranial sutures, there is enlargement of the head,

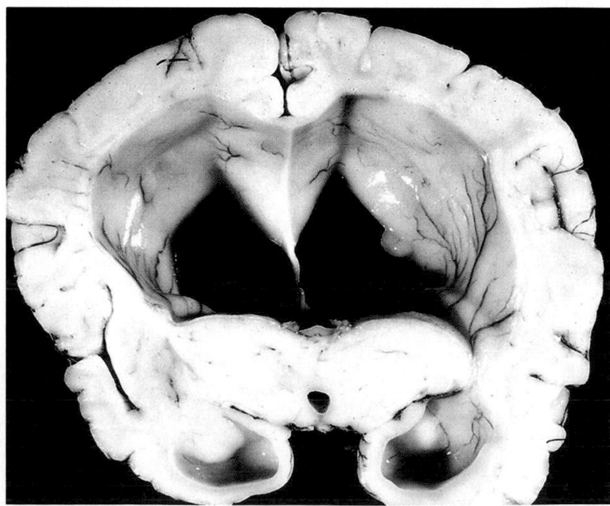

Figure 28-2 Hydrocephalus. Dilated lateral ventricles seen in a coronal section through the midthalamus.

manifested by an increase in head circumference. Hydrocephalus developing after this period, in contrast, is associated with expansion of the ventricles and increased intracranial pressure, without a change in head circumference. If the ventricular system is obstructed and does not communicate with the subarachnoid space, as may occur because of a mass in the third ventricle, it is called *noncommunicating, or obstructive, hydrocephalus.* In *communicating hydrocephalus,* the ventricular system is in communication with the subarachnoid space, and there is enlargement of the entire ventricular system. The term *hydrocephalus ex vacuo* refers to a compensatory increase in ventricular volume secondary to a loss of brain parenchyma.

Raised Intracranial Pressure and Herniation

Herniation is the displacement of brain tissue past rigid dural folds (the falx and tentorium) or through openings in the skull because of increased intracranial pressure. As the volume of the brain increases, CSF is displaced and the vasculature is compressed, leading to increasing pressure within the cranial cavity. When the increase is beyond the limit permitted by compression of veins and displacement of CSF, tissue herniates between compartments across the pressure gradient. Herniation is mostly associated with mass effect, either diffuse (generalized brain edema) or focal (tumors, abscesses, or hemorrhages). Elevated intracranial pressure may also reduce perfusion of the brain, further exacerbating cerebral edema. If the expansion is sufficiently severe, herniation may occur in multiple anatomic locations (Fig. 28-3).

- *Subfalcine (cingulate) herniation* occurs when unilateral or asymmetric expansion of a cerebral hemisphere displaces the cingulate gyrus under the falx. This may lead to compression of the anterior cerebral artery and its branches.
- *Transtentorial (uncinate, mesial temporal) herniation* occurs when the medial aspect of the temporal lobe is compressed against the free margin of the tentorium. With increasing displacement of the temporal lobe, the third cranial nerve is compromised, resulting in pupillary dilation and impairment of ocular movements on the side of the lesion. The posterior cerebral artery may also be compressed, resulting in ischemic injury to the territory supplied by that vessel, including the primary visual cortex. When the extent of herniation is large enough the contralateral cerebral peduncle may be compressed, resulting in hemiparesis ipsilateral to the side of the herniation; the compression in the peduncle in this setting is known as the *Kernohan notch*. Progression of transtentorial herniation is often accompanied by secondary hemorrhagic lesions in the midbrain and pons, termed *Duret hemorrhages* (Fig. 28-4). These linear or flame-shaped lesions usually occur in the midline and paramedian regions and are believed to be due to distortion or tearing of penetrating veins and arteries supplying the upper brainstem.
- *Tonsillar herniation* refers to displacement of the cerebellar tonsils through the foramen magnum. This pattern of herniation is life-threatening because it causes brainstem compression and compromises vital respiratory and cardiac centers in the medulla.

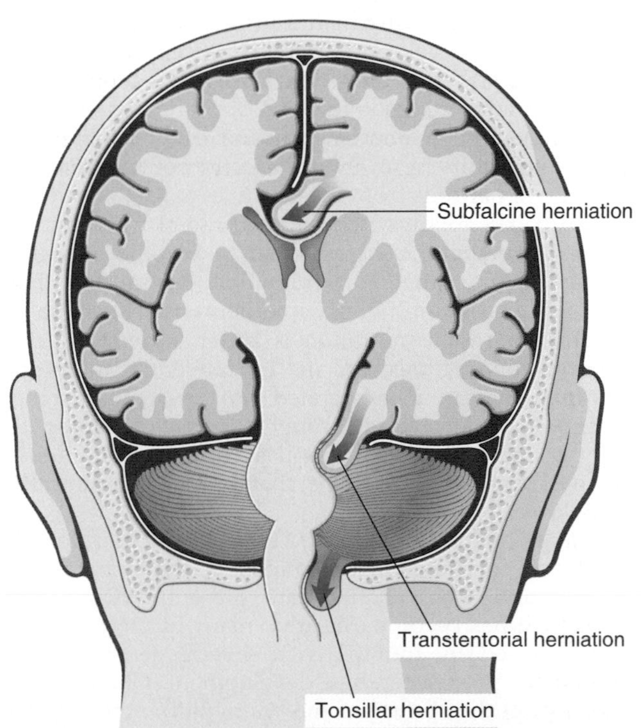

Figure 28-3 Major herniation syndromes of the brain: subfalcine, transtentorial, and tonsillar.

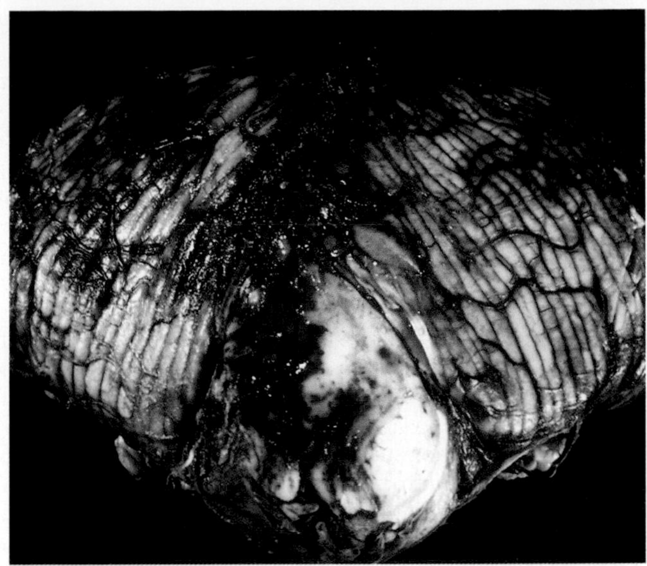

Figure 28-4 Duret hemorrhage involving the brainstem at the junction of the pons and midbrain.

KEY CONCEPTS

Cerebral Edema, Hydrocephalus, and Raised Intracranial Pressure and Herniation

- Cerebral edema is the accumulation of excess fluid within the brain parenchyma. Hydrocephalus is an increase in CSF volume within all or part of the ventricular system.

- Increases in the volume of intracranial contents (as a result of increased CSF volume, edema, hemorrhage, or tumor) raise the pressure inside the fixed capacity of the skull.
- Increases in pressure may result in decreased perfusion (leading to ischemia). The increased pressure may also result in displacement of tissue past the edges of dural partitions inside the skull or through openings in the skull (herniations).

Malformations and Developmental Disorders

Although the pathogenesis and etiology of many CNS malformations remain unknown, both genetic and environmental influences appear to be involved. Newer genetic methods, including whole exome and whole genome sequencing, have begun to uncover a range of alterations that may cause many of these malformations. The causal relationship between the genetic alterations and the pathogenesis of the malformations is the subject of active research. Besides genetic factors, many toxic compounds and infectious agents also have teratogenic effects and may cause brain malformations.

Neural Tube Defects

Failure of a portion of the neural tube to close, or reopening of a region of the tube after successful closure, may lead to malformations involving some combination of neural tissue, meninges, and overlying bone or soft tissues. Collectively, neural tube defects account for most CNS malformations, with the most common neural tube defects involving the spinal cord.

- *Spinal dysraphism* or *spina bifida* may be an asymptomatic bony defect (spina bifida occulta) or a severe malformation with a flattened, disorganized segment of spinal cord, associated with an overlying meningeal outpouching.
- *Myelomeningocele* (or meningomyelocele) refers to extension of CNS tissue through a defect in the vertebral column; the term *meningocele* applies when there is only a meningeal extrusion. Myelomeningoceles occur most commonly in the lumbosacral region. Affected individuals have motor and sensory deficits in the lower extremities as well as disturbances of bowel and bladder control. These are often complicated by superimposed infection that extends into the cord from the thin, overlying skin.
- *Encephalocele* refers to a diverticulum of malformed brain tissue extending through a defect in the cranium. It most often occurs in the posterior fossa, although comparable extensions of brain occur through the cribriform plate in the anterior fossa (sometimes misleadingly referred to as a "nasal glioma").

The frequency of neural tube defects varies widely among different ethnic groups. Evidence for a genetic basis includes the high concordance rate among monozygotic twins. The overall recurrence rate for a neural tube defect in subsequent pregnancies has been estimated at 4% to 5%. Folate deficiency during the first several weeks of gestation is a well established risk factor; differences in rates of neural tube defects between populations can be attributed in part to polymorphisms in enzymes involved in folic acid metabolism. Folate supplementation can lower the risk of neural tube defects, but because neural tube closure is normally complete by day 28 of embryonic development (before most pregnancies are recognized), it must be given to women throughout their reproductive years to be fully effective. Precisely how folate deficiency increases the risk is uncertain; defects in the timing of DNA synthesis and effects on DNA methylation (an important epigenetic mode of gene regulation) are suspected.

Anencephaly is a malformation of the anterior end of the neural tube, with absence of most of the brain and calvarium. Forebrain development is disrupted at approximately 28 days of gestation, and all that remains in its place is the *area cerebrovasculosa*, a flattened remnant of disorganized brain tissue with admixed ependyma, choroid plexus, and meningothelial cells. The posterior fossa structures may be spared, depending on the extent of the skull deficit; descending tracts associated with disrupted structures are, as expected, absent.

Forebrain Anomalies

Abnormalities in the generation and migration of neurons result in malformations of the forebrain that may be focal or involve entire structures. The pool of proliferating precursor cells in the developing brain lies adjacent to the ventricular system. Overall neuronal number is determined by the fraction of proliferating cells that undergo transition into migrating cells with each cell cycle. Early on, most cell divisions yield two more progenitor cells, while as development progresses there are more asymmetric divisions yielding both a progenitor cell and a cell directed to the developing cortex. If excess cells exit the proliferating pool too early, then the overall generation of neurons is reduced; if too few exit during early rounds of division, then the geometric expansion of the proliferating population results in an overproduction of neurons. The migration of neurons from the germinal matrix zone to the cerebral cortex follows two paths: a radial migration for neuronal progenitor cells destined to become excitatory neurons and a tangential migration course for those which will become inhibitory interneurons. The signaling that governs radial migration is better understood than the corresponding mechanisms for tangential migration. For radial migration, a secreted protein (reelin) signals to migrating neuroblasts through a surface receptor; the ability of these cells to respond appropriately is dependent on cytoskeletal proteins that propel the migrating neuroblasts.

A range of malformation patterns have been defined, initially by focusing on the region of the brain that is involved and what changes are present. With genetic advances, it has become clear that many of these patterns can be caused by mutations in several genes that are required for proper cerebral development. Changes may be seen from the surface of the brain, with either too few or too many gyri, in the organization of the brain into normal lobes, in the structure of the cerebral cortex or in the distribution of neurons within the brain.

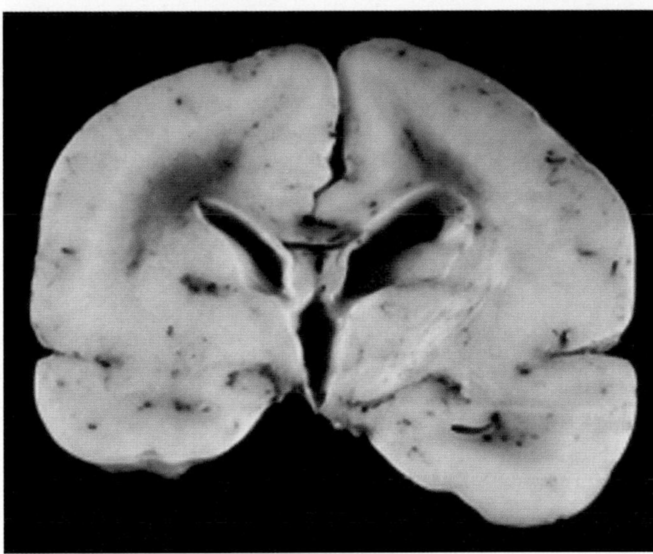

Figure 28-5 Lissencephaly. The absence of cortical gyri defines this abnormality, seen here in the brain from a full-term infant.

- The volume of brain may be abnormally large *(megalencephaly)* or abnormally small *(microencephaly)*. Microencephaly, by far the more common of the two, is typically accompanied by a small head circumference. It can be associated with a number of conditions, including chromosome abnormalities, fetal alcohol syndrome, and human immunodeficiency virus 1 (HIV-1) infection acquired in utero. It is postulated that the underlying anomaly is a reduction in the number of neurons that reach the neocortex and this leads to a simplification of the gyral folding, a model supported by experimental results in mouse models.
- *Lissencephaly* is a malformation characterized by reduction in the number of gyri, which in the extreme case may show no gyral pattern *(agyria)* (Fig. 28-5). Two general patterns are observed, a smooth surfaced form (type 1), and a rough or cobblestoned surfaced form (type 2). In general, type 1 forms are associated with mutations that disrupt the signaling for migration and the cytoskeletal "motor" proteins that drive migration of neuroblasts. In contrast, type 2 lissencephaly is most commonly associated with genetic alterations that disrupt the "stop signal" for migration. This signal depends on a set of specifically glycosylated proteins, and mutations in the enzymes that place the sugars onto the proteins are the most common causes of this form of lissencephaly.
- *Polymicrogyria* is characterized by small, unusually numerous, irregularly formed cerebral convolutions. The gray matter is composed of four layers (or fewer), with entrapment of apparent meningeal tissue at points of fusion that would otherwise be the cortical surface. Polymicrogyria can be induced by localized tissue injury toward the end of neuronal migration, although genetically determined forms, which are typically bilateral and symmetric, are also recognized.
- *Neuronal heterotopias* are a group of migrational disorders that are commonly associated with epilepsy. They are defined by the presence of collections of neurons in inappropriate locations along the pathway of migration. As might be expected, one location in which heterotopias can be found is along the ventricular surface—as though the cells never managed to leave their place of birth. Periventricular heterotopias can be caused by mutations in the gene encoding filamin A, an actin-binding protein responsible for assembly of complex meshworks of filaments. This gene is on the X chromosome, and the mutant allele causes male lethality; in females the process of X inactivation separates neurons into those with a normal allele (in the correct location) and those with the mutant allele (in the heterotopia). Another microtubule-associated protein, doublecortin (DCX), is also encoded by a gene on the X chromosome; mutations in this gene result in lissencephaly in males and in subcortical band heterotopias in females. These heterotopias may consist of discrete nodules of neurons sitting in the subcortical white matter or complete ribbons that parody the overlying cortex.
- *Holoprosencephaly* is a spectrum of malformations characterized by incomplete separation of the cerebral hemispheres across the midline. Severe forms manifest midline facial abnormalities, including cyclopia; less severe variants (*arrhinencephaly*) show absence of the olfactory cranial nerves and related structures. Intrauterine diagnosis of severe forms by ultrasound examination is now possible. Holoprosencephaly is associated with trisomy 13 as well as other genetic syndromes. Mutations in genes that encode components of the sonic hedgehog signaling pathway may result in holoprosencephaly.
- *Agenesis of the corpus callosum*, a relatively common malformation, refers to the absence of the white matter bundles that carry cortical projections from one hemisphere to the other (Fig. 28-6). Radiologic imaging studies show misshapen lateral ventricles ("bat-wing" deformity); on coronal whole-mount sections of the brain, bundles of anteroposteriorly oriented white

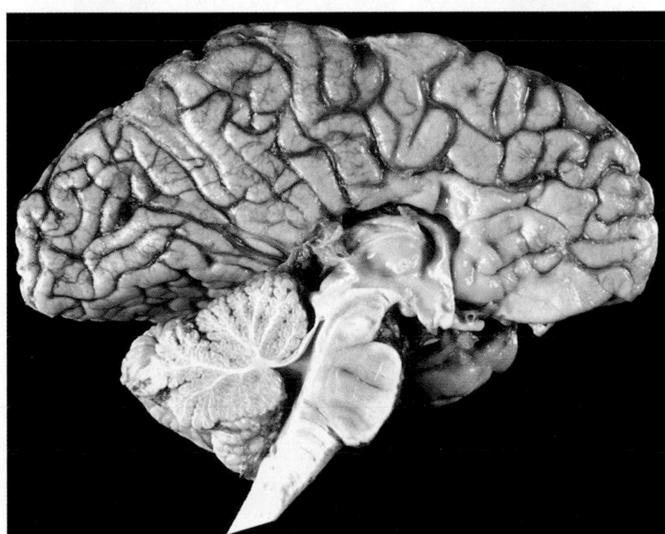

Figure 28-6 Agenesis of the corpus callosum. The midsagittal view of the left hemisphere shows the lack of a corpus callosum and cingulate gyrus above the third ventricle.

matter can be demonstrated. Agenesis of the corpus callosum is commonly associated with mental retardation but may occur in clinically normal individuals. It can be present in isolation or associated with a wide range of other malformations.

Posterior Fossa Anomalies

A distinct set of malformations primarily affect the brainstem and the cerebellum, which often show dramatic changes in size and shape. These may be accompanied by morphologic changes in other regions of the brain.

- *Arnold-Chiari malformation* (Chiari type II malformation) consists of a small posterior fossa, a misshapen midline cerebellum with downward extension of vermis through the foramen magnum (Fig. 28-7), and, almost invariably, hydrocephalus and a lumbar myelomeningocele. Other associated changes may include caudal displacement of the medulla, malformation of the tectum, aqueductal stenosis, cerebral heterotopias, and hydromyelia (see later).
- *Chiari type I malformation* is a less severe disorder in which low-lying cerebellar tonsils extend down into the vertebral canal. This may be a silent abnormality or may become symptomatic because of impaired CSF flow and medullary compression; if present, these symptoms can usually be corrected by neurosurgical intervention.
- *Dandy-Walker malformation* is characterized by an enlarged posterior fossa. The cerebellar vermis is absent or present only in rudimentary form in its anterior portion. In its place is a large midline cyst that is lined by ependyma and is contiguous with leptomeninges on its outer surface. This cyst represents the expanded, roofless fourth ventricle in the absence of a normally formed vermis. Dysplasias of brainstem nuclei are commonly found in association with Dandy-Walker malformation.

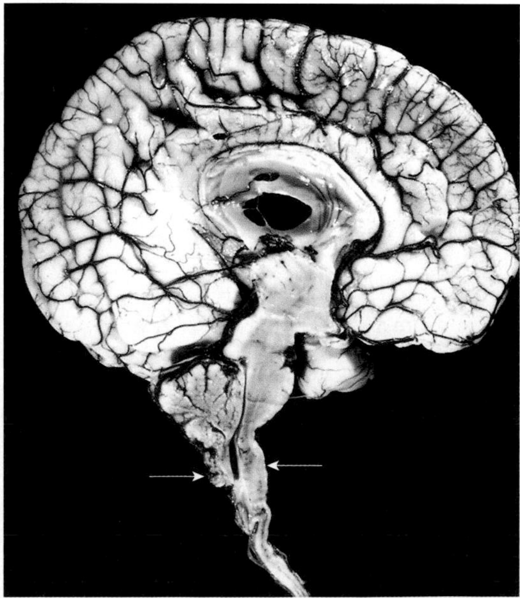

Figure 28-7 Arnold-Chiari malformation. Midsagittal section showing small posterior fossa contents, downward displacement of the cerebellar vermis, and deformity of the medulla (*arrows* indicate the approximate level of the foramen magnum).

- *Joubert syndrome*, and its related disorders, share hypoplasia of the cerebellar vermis with apparent elongation of the superior cerebellar peduncles and an altered shape of the brainstem; together these changes give rise to the 'molar tooth sign' on imaging. This group of malformations has been found to be caused by diverse mutations affecting genes that encode components of the primary (non-motile) cilium.

Syringomyelia and Hydromyelia

These are disorders characterized by expansion of the ependyma-lined central canal of the cord *(hydromyelia)* or by the formation of a fluid-filled cleft-like cavity in the inner portion of the cord *(syringomyelia, syrinx)* that may extend into the brainstem *(syringobulbia)*.

Syringomyelia may be associated with the Chiari malformations; it may also occur in association with intraspinal tumors or following traumatic injury. In general, the histologic appearance is similar in all these conditions, with destruction of the adjacent gray and white matter, surrounded by a dense feltwork of reactive gliosis. The disease generally becomes manifest in the second or third decade of life. The distinctive symptoms and signs of a syrinx are the isolated loss of pain and temperature sensation in the upper extremities because of the predilection for early involvement of the crossing anterior spinal commissural fibers of the spinal cord.

KEY CONCEPTS

Malformations and Developmental Disorders

- Malformations may be associated with single gene mutations, larger scale genetic alterations, or exogenous factors.
- Overall, the earlier in development a malformation occurs, the more severe the morphologic and functional phenotype.
- Neural tube defects are associated with failure to close or inappropriate reopening of the developing neural tube; these range from incidental findings to severe manifestations.
- Cortical development depends on proper orchestration of progenitor cell proliferation in the germinal matrix and migration of progenitors upwards into the developing cortex. Disruption of these processes can alter the size, shape, and organization of the brain.
- Malformations involving the posterior fossa are typically distinct from those which affect the cerebral hemispheres.

Perinatal Brain Injury

Brain injury occurring in the perinatal period is an important cause of childhood-onset neurologic disability. Injuries that occur early in gestation may destroy brain tissue without eliciting the reactive changes observed in adult brain and, therefore, may be difficult to distinguish from malformations.

The term *cerebral palsy* refers to a nonprogressive neurologic motor deficit characterized by combinations of

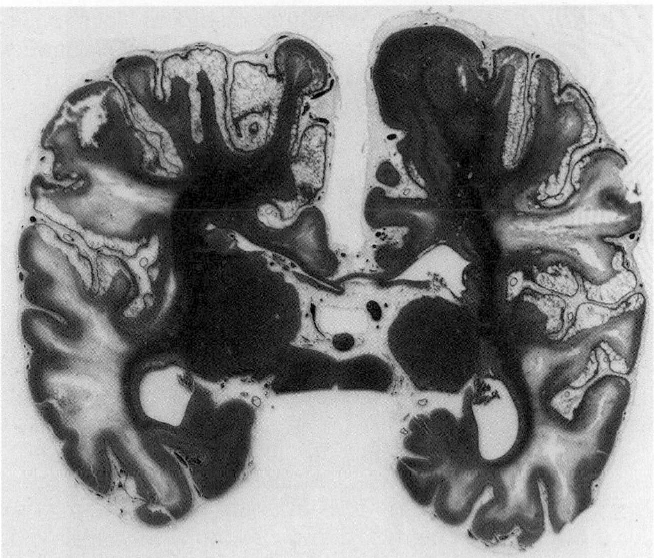

Figure 28-8 Multicystic leukoencephalopathy. Numerous cystic spaces representing the consequences of widespread ischemic injury are present.

spasticity, dystonia, ataxia/athetosis, and paresis, attributable to insults occurring during the prenatal and perinatal periods. Signs and symptoms may not be apparent at birth and only declare themselves later, as development proceeds. Postmortem examinations of children with cerebral palsy have shown a wide range of neuropathologic findings, including destructive lesions traced to remote events that may have caused hemorrhage and infarction.

In premature infants there is an increased risk of *intraparenchymal hemorrhage* within the germinal matrix, often near the junction between the developing thalamus and caudate nucleus. Hemorrhages may remain localized or extend into the ventricular system and thence to the subarachnoid space, sometimes leading to hydrocephalus.

Infarcts may occur in the supratentorial periventricular white matter *(periventricular leukomalacia)*, especially in premature infants. These take the form of chalky yellow plaques consisting of discrete regions of white matter necrosis and calcification. When both gray and white matter are involved by extensive ischemic damage, large destructive cystic lesions develop throughout the hemispheres; this condition is termed *multicystic encephalopathy* (Fig. 28-8).

In perinatal ischemic lesions of the cerebral cortex, the depths of sulci bear the brunt of injury and result in thinned-out, gliotic gyri *(ulegyria)*. The basal ganglia and thalamus may also suffer ischemic injury, with patchy neuronal loss and reactive gliosis. Later, aberrant and irregular myelinization gives rise to a marble-like appearance of the deep nuclei (*status marmoratus*). Because the lesions are in the caudate, putamen, and thalamus, movement disorders such as choreoathetosis are common clinical sequelae.

Trauma

The anatomic location of the lesion and the limited capacity of the brain for functional repair are major determinants of the consequences of CNS trauma. Injury of several cubic centimeters of brain parenchyma may be clinically silent (if in the frontal lobe), severely disabling (if in the spinal cord), or fatal (if in the brainstem).

The physical forces associated with head injury may result in *skull fractures, parenchymal injury,* and *vascular injury;* all three can coexist. The magnitude and distribution of a traumatic brain lesions depend on the shape of the object causing the trauma, the force of impact, and whether the head is in motion at the time of injury. A blow to the head may be *penetrating* or *blunt;* it may cause either an *open* or a *closed injury.*

Skull Fractures

A fracture in which bone is displaced into the cranial cavity by a distance greater than the thickness of the bone is called a *displaced skull fracture*. The thickness of the cranial bones varies; therefore, their resistance to fracture differs greatly. Also, the relative incidence of fractures among skull bones is related to the pattern of falls. When an individual falls while awake, such as might occur when stepping off a ladder, the site of impact is often the occipital portion of the skull; in contrast, a fall that follows loss of consciousness, as might follow a syncopal attack, commonly results in a frontal impact. Symptoms referable to the lower cranial nerves or the cervicomedullary region, and the presence of orbital or mastoid hematomas distant from the point of impact, raise the suspicion of a basal skull fracture, which typically follows impact to the occiput or sides of the head. CSF discharge from the nose or ear and infection (meningitis) may follow. The kinetic energy that causes a fracture is dissipated at a fused suture; fractures that cross sutures are termed *diastatic*. With multiple points of impact or repeated blows to the head, the fracture lines of subsequent injuries do not extend across fracture lines of prior injury.

Parenchymal Injuries

Concussion

Concussion is a clinical syndrome of altered consciousness secondary to head injury typically brought about by a change in the momentum of the head (when a moving head is suddenly arrested by impact on a rigid surface). The characteristic neurologic picture includes instantaneous onset of transient neurologic dysfunction, including loss of consciousness, temporary respiratory arrest, and loss of reflexes. Although neurologic recovery is complete, amnesia for the event often persists. The pathogenesis of the sudden disruption of neurologic function is unknown; it probably involves dysregulation of the reticular activating system in the brainstem. Post-concussive neuropsychiatric syndromes, typically associated with repetitive injuries, are well recognized and there is increasing evidence that significant cognitive impairment can emerge along with distinct pathologic findings terms chronic traumatic encephalopathy (discussed later).

Direct Parenchymal Injury

Contusions and *lacerations* are brain injuries caused by transmission of kinetic energy to the brain. A contusion is analogous to the familiar bruise caused by blunt trauma, while a laceration is an injury caused by penetration of an object and tearing of tissue. As with any other organ, a blow to the surface of the brain, transmitted through the skull, leads to rapid tissue displacement, disruption of vascular channels, and subsequent hemorrhage, tissue injury, and edema (Fig. 28-9). Hemorrhage can extend into the subarachnoid space from these lesions. The crests of gyri are most susceptible, since this is where the direct force is greatest. The most common locations for contusions correspond to the most frequent sites of direct impact and to regions of the brain that overlie a rough and irregular inner skull surface, such as the frontal lobes along the orbital ridges and the temporal lobes. Contusions are less frequent over the occipital lobes, brainstem, and cerebellum unless these sites are adjacent to a skull fracture *(fracture contusions)*.

A person who suffers a blow to the head may develop a contusion at the point of contact (a *coup* injury) or a contusion on the brain surface diametrically opposite to it (a *contrecoup* injury). Since their macroscopic and microscopic appearance is indistinguishable, the distinction between them is based on identification of the point of impact. In general, if the head is immobile at the time of trauma, only a coup injury is found. If the head is mobile, both coup and contrecoup lesions may be found. Whereas the coup lesion is caused by the contact between brain and skull at the site of impact, the contrecoup contusion is thought to develop when the brain strikes the opposite inner surface of the skull after sudden deceleration.

Sudden impacts that result in violent posterior or lateral hyperextension of the neck (as occurs when a pedestrian is struck from the rear by a vehicle) may avulse the pons from the medulla or the medulla from the cervical cord, causing instant death.

MORPHOLOGY

When seen on cross-section, contusions are wedge shaped, with the broad base lying along the surface at the point of impact (Fig. 28-9*B*). The appearance of contusions is similar regardless of the source of the trauma. In the earliest stages, there is edema and hemorrhage, which is often pericapillary. During the next few hours, the extravasation of blood extends throughout the involved tissue, across the width of the cerebral cortex, and into the white matter and subarachnoid space. Morphologic evidence of neuronal injury (pyknosis of the nucleus, eosinophilia of the cytoplasm, and disintegration of the cell) takes about 24 hours to appear, although functional deficits may occur earlier. Axonal swellings develop in the vicinity of damaged neurons or at great distances away. The inflammatory response to the injured tissue follows its usual course, with the appearance of neutrophils followed by macrophages. Old traumatic lesions on the surface of the brain have a characteristic gross appearance. They are depressed, retracted, yellowish brown patches involving the crests of gyri, most commonly those that are located at the sites of contrecoup injuries (inferior frontal cortex, temporal and occipital poles). The term **plaque jaune** is applied to these lesions (Fig. 28-9*C*), which can become epileptic foci. More extensive hemorrhagic regions of brain trauma give rise to larger cavitated lesions, which can resemble remote infarcts. In old contusions, gliosis and residual hemosiderin-laden macrophages predominate.

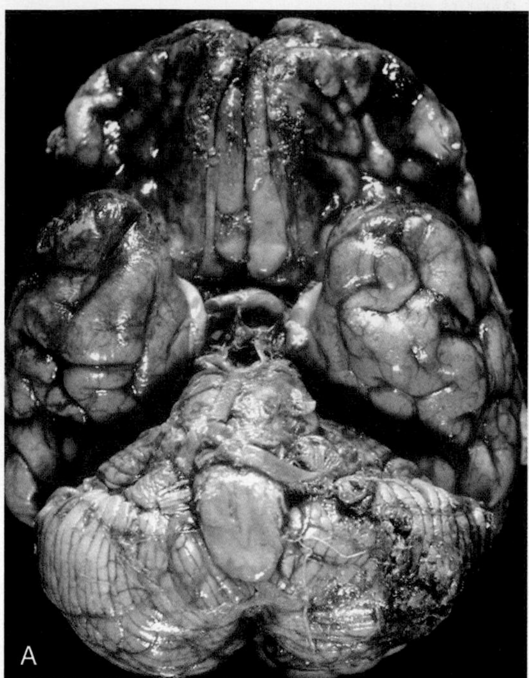

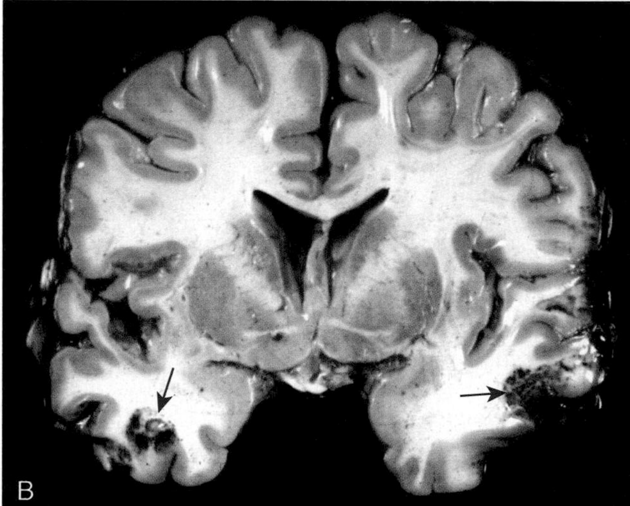

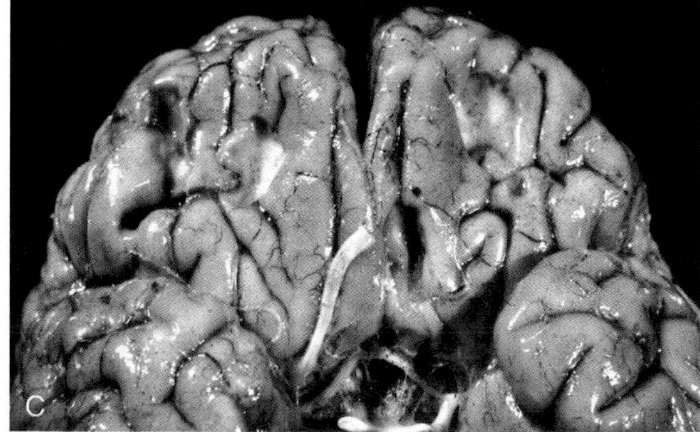

Figure 28-9 A, Multiple contusions involving the inferior surfaces of frontal lobes, anterior temporal lobes, and cerebellum. **B,** Acute contusions are present in both temporal lobes, with areas of hemorrhage and tissue disruption (*arrows*). **C,** Remote contusions are present on the inferior frontal surface of this brain, with a yellow color (associated with the term *plaque jaune*).

Diffuse Axonal Injury

Although it is most often affected, the surface of the brain is not the only region damaged by traumatic injuries. Also affected may be the deep white matter regions (the corpus callosum, paraventricular, and hippocampal areas in the supratentorial compartment), cerebral peduncles, brachium conjunctivum, superior colliculi, and deep reticular formation in the brainstem. The microscopic findings include axonal swelling, indicative of *diffuse axonal injury*, and focal hemorrhagic lesions. As many as 50% of individuals who develop coma shortly after trauma, even without cerebral contusions, are believed to have diffuse axonal injury. Axons are injured by the direct action of mechanical forces, with subsequent alterations in axoplasmic flow. Comparable mechanical disruption of axons can result from angular acceleration alone, which can cause diffuse axonal injury even in the absence of impact.

MORPHOLOGY

Diffuse axonal injury is characterized by widespread, often asymmetric axonal swellings that appear within hours of the injury and may persist for much longer. The swelling is best demonstrated with silver impregnation techniques or with immunoperoxidase stains for axonally transported proteins, such as amyloid precursor protein and α-synuclein. Later, increased numbers of microglia areas are seen in damaged areas of the cerebral cortex, and subsequently there is degeneration of the involved fiber tracts.

Traumatic Vascular Injury

Vascular injury is a frequent component of CNS trauma. It results from direct trauma and disruption of the vessel wall, and leads to hemorrhage in different anatomic sites (Table 28-1). Depending on the position of the ruptured vessel, hemorrhage may occur in the *epidural, subdural, subarachnoid,* and *intraparenchymal* compartments, sometimes in combination (Fig. 28-10). Both epidural and subdural hemorrhages rarely occur outside of the setting of trauma; in some settings such as coagulopathy or significant cerebral atrophy, subdural hemorrhages can follow even minor trauma. A traumatic tear of the carotid artery where it traverses the carotid sinus may lead to the formation of an arteriovenous fistula.

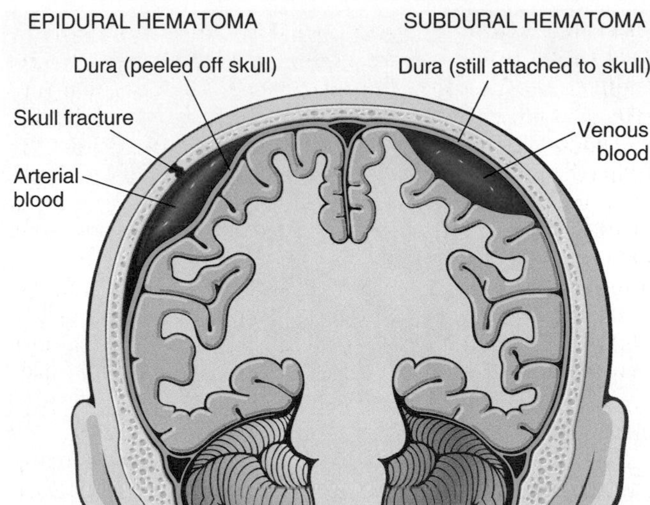

Figure 28-10 Epidural hematoma *(left)* in which rupture of a meningeal artery, usually associated with a skull fracture, leads to accumulation of arterial blood between the dura and the skull. In a subdural hematoma *(right)*, damage to bridging veins between the brain and the superior sagittal sinus leads to the accumulation of blood between the dura and the arachnoid.

Epidural Hematoma

Normally the dura is fused with the periosteum on the internal surface of the skull. Dural arteries, most importantly the middle meningeal artery, are vulnerable to injury, particularly with temporal skull fractures in which the fracture lines cross the course of the vessel. In children, in whom the skull is deformable, a temporary displacement of the skull bones leading to laceration of a vessel can occur in the absence of a skull fracture.

Once a vessel has been torn, the extravasation of blood under arterial pressure can cause the dura to separate from the inner surface of the skull (Fig. 28-11). The expanding hematoma has a smooth inner contour that compresses the brain surface. When blood accumulates slowly patients may be lucid for several hours before the onset of neurologic signs. An epidural hematoma may expand rapidly and is a neurosurgical emergency requiring prompt drainage.

Table 28-1 Patterns of Vascular Injury in the Central Nervous System

Location	Etiology	Additional Features
Epidural space	Trauma	Usually associated with a skull fracture (in adults); rapidly evolving neurologic symptoms, requiring intervention
Subdural space	Trauma	Level of trauma may be mild; slowly evolving neurologic symptoms, often with a delay from the time of injury
Subarachnoid space	Vascular abnormalities (Arteriovenous malformation or aneurysm)	Sudden onset of severe headache, often with rapid neurologic deterioration; secondary injury may emerge, associated with vasospasm
	Trauma	Typically associated with underlying contusions
Intraparenchymal	Trauma (contusions)	Selective involvement of the crests of gyri, where the brain may contact the inner surface of the skull (frontal and temporal tips, orbitofrontal surface)
	Hemorrhagic conversion of an ischemic infarction	Usually petechial hemorrhages in an area of previously ischemic brain, usually following the cortical ribbon
	Cerebral amyloid angiopathy	"Lobar" hemorrhage, involving cerebral cortex, often with extension into the subarachnoid space
	Hypertension	Centered in the deep white matter, thalamus, basal ganglia, or brainstem; may extend into the ventricular system
	Tumors (primary or metastatic)	Associated with high grade gliomas or certain metastases (melanoma, choriocarcinoma, renal cell carcinoma)

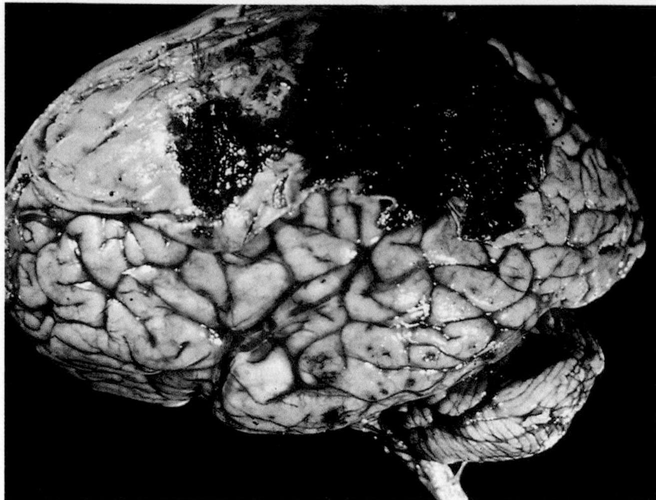

Figure 28-11 Epidural hematoma covering a portion of the dura. Also present are multiple small contusions in the temporal lobe. (Courtesy the late Dr. Raymond D. Adams, Massachusetts General Hospital, Boston, Mass.)

Subdural Hematoma

It is traditionally believed that between the inner surface of the dura mater and the outer arachnoid layer of the leptomeninges lies the subdural space. In reality, the dura is composed of two layers, an external collagenous and an inner border cell layer with scant fibrobalsts, and abundant extracellular space devoid of collagen. When bleeding occurs these two layers separate and create the "subdural space" in which blood accumulates. Bridging veins travel from the convexities of the cerebral hemispheres through the subarachnoid space and the subdural space to empty into the superior sagittal sinus. Similar anatomic relationships exist with other dural sinuses. These vessels are particularly prone to tearing along their course through the dural layers and are the source of bleeding in most cases of subdural hematoma. The brain is suspended in CSF, but the venous sinuses are fixed relative to the dura, so the displacement of the brain that occurs in trauma can tear the veins at the point where they penetrate the dura. In older individuals with brain atrophy, the bridging veins are stretched, hence the increased rate of subdural hematomas in these patients, even after relatively minor head trauma. Infants are also particularly susceptible to subdural hematomas because their bridging veins are thin-walled.

MORPHOLOGY

Grossly, **acute subdural hematomas** appear as a collection of freshly clotted blood along the brain surface, without extension into the depths of sulci (Fig. 28-12). The underlying brain is flattened and the subarachnoid space is often clear. Usually, venous bleeding is self-limited and the resulting hematoma is broken down and organized over time. This most often occurs in the following sequence:

- Lysis of the clot (about 1 week)
- Growth of fibroblasts from the dural surface into the hematoma (2 weeks)
- Early development of hyalinized connective tissue (1 to 3 months)

Typically, the organized hematoma is firmly attached by ingrowing fibrous tissue to the inner surface of the dura and is free of the underlying arachnoid, which does not contribute to healing. The lesion can eventually retract as the granulation tissue matures until only a thin layer of reactive connective tissue remains ("subdural membranes"). In other cases, however, multiple recurrent episodes of bleeding occur (**chronic subdural hematomas**), presumably from the thin-walled vessels of the granulation tissue. The risk of repeat bleeding is greatest in the first few months after the initial hemorrhage.

Clinical Features. Symptomatic subdural hematomas most often manifest within 48 hours of injury. They are most common over the lateral aspects of the cerebral hemispheres and are bilateral in about 10% of cases. Neurologic signs commonly observed are attributable to the pressure exerted on the adjacent brain. There may be focal signs, but often the clinical manifestations are nonlocalizing and include headache and confusion. Slowly progressive neurologic deterioration is typical, but acute decompensation may occur. The treatment of subdural hematomas is to remove the blood and associated organizing tissue.

Sequelae of Brain Trauma

A broad range of neurologic syndromes may become manifest months or years after brain trauma of any cause.

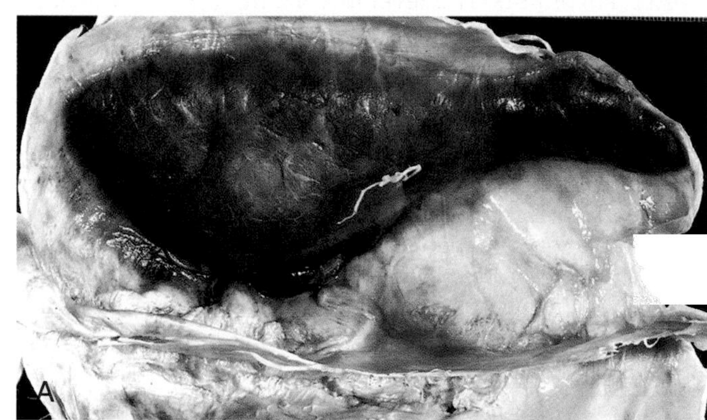

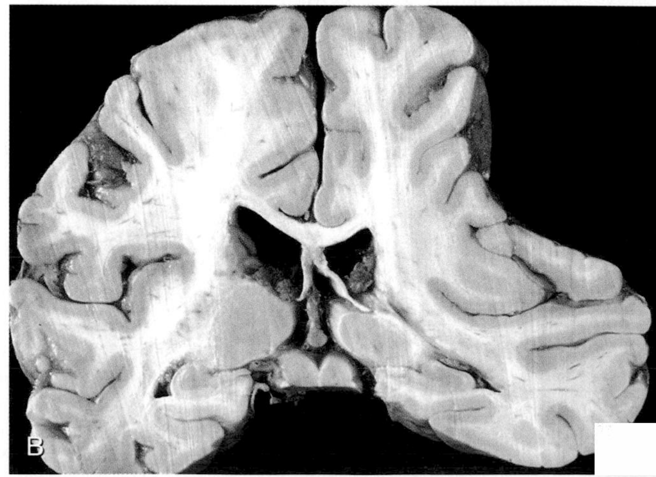

Figure 28-12 A, Large organizing subdural hematoma attached to the dura. **B,** Coronal section of the brain showing compression of the hemisphere underlying the subdural hematoma shown in **A**.

These have gained increasing notice in the context of litigation involving issues of compensation for those in the civilian work force, professional athletes and the military services.

- *Posttraumatic hydrocephalus* is largely due to obstruction of CSF resorption from hemorrhage into the subarachnoid spaces.
- *Chronic traumatic encephalopathy* (CTE, previously referred to as "dementia pugilistica") is a dementing illness that develops after repeated head trauma. Affected brains are typically atrophic, with enlarged ventricles, and show accumulation of tau-containing neurofibrillary tangles in a characteristic pattern involving superficial frontal and temporal lobe cortex. Although concussion is thought of as having no structural consequences, it is clear that repeated events are antecedents to CTE. It remains uncertain if the most critical factors that determine if encephalopathy will develop are the number, frequency or severity of events, or some combination of these.
- Other important sequelae of brain trauma include posttraumatic epilepsy, risk of infection, and psychiatric disorders.

Spinal Cord Injury

The spinal cord is vulnerable to trauma from its skeletal encasement. Most injuries that damage the cord are associated with the transient or permanent displacement of the vertebral column. The level of cord injury determines the extent of the neurologic manifestations: lesions involving the thoracic vertebrae or below can lead to paraplegia; cervical lesions result in quadriplegia; those above C4 can, in addition, lead to respiratory compromise from paralysis of the diaphragm. Damage at the region of impact to descending and ascending white matter tracts isolates the distal spinal cord from the rest of the brain. This interruption, paired with the localized gray matter damage at the level of the impact, is the principal cause of neurologic deficits.

MORPHOLOGY

The histologic features of traumatic injury of the spinal cord are similar to those found at other sites in the CNS. At the level of injury the acute phase consists of hemorrhage, necrosis, and axonal swelling in the surrounding white matter. The lesion tapers above and below the level of injury. In time central areas of neuronal destruction becomes cystic and gliotic; cord sections above and below the lesion show secondary ascending and descending wallerian degeneration, respectively, involving the long white-matter tracts affected at the site of trauma.

KEY CONCEPTS

Perinatal Brain Injury

- Timing of injury is critical, with earlier events resulting in greater damage and deficits.
- Cerebral palsy is the term describing non-progressive deficits associated with injury during the prenatal and perinatal periods.

Trauma

- Physical injury to the brain can occur when the inside of the skull comes into forceful contact with the brain.
- In blunt trauma, if the head is mobile there may be brain injury both at the original point of contact (coup injury) and on the opposite side of the brain (contrecoup injury) owing to impacts with the skull.
- Parenchymal injuries take the form of contusions, with hemorrhage extending into the subarachnoid space.
- Rapid displacement of the head and brain can tear axons (diffuse axonal injury), often causing immediate severe, irreversible neurologic deficits.
- Traumatic tearing of blood vessels leads to epidural or subdural hematoma.

Cerebrovascular Disease

Cerebrovascular disease—injury to the brain as a consequence of altered blood flow—can be grouped into ischemic and hemorrhagic etiologies. "Stroke" is the clinical designation that applies to all these conditions, particularly when symptoms begin acutely. Cerebrovascular disease is the third leading cause of death (after heart disease and cancer) in the United States, and the most prevalent cause of morbidity and mortality from neurologic disease. From the standpoint of pathophysiology and pathologic anatomy, it is convenient to consider cerebrovascular disease as two processes:

- *Hypoxia, ischemia, and infarction* resulting from impairment of blood supply and oxygenation of CNS tissue; in the brain, embolism is a more common etiology than thrombosis. This can either be a global process or focal, with the clinical manifestations determined by the region of brain affected.
- *Hemorrhage* resulting from rupture of CNS vessels. Common etiologies include hypertension and vascular anomalies (aneurysms and malformations).

Hypoxia, Ischemia, and Infarction

The brain requires a constant supply of glucose and oxygen, which is delivered by the cerebral blood vessels. Although the brain accounts for only 1% to 2% of body weight, it receives approximately 15% of the resting cardiac output and accounts for 20% of the body's oxygen consumption. Cerebral blood flow remains relatively constant over a wide range of blood pressure and intracranial pressure because of autoregulation of vascular resistance. The brain is a highly aerobic tissue, in which oxygen rather than metabolic substrate is limiting. The brain may be deprived of oxygen by several mechanisms: *hypoxia* caused by a low partial pressure of oxygen (PO_2), impairment of the blood's oxygen-carrying capacity, or inhibition of oxygen use in the tissue; or *ischemia*, either transient or permanent, caused by interruption of the normal circulatory flow. Cessation of blood flow can result from a reduction in perfusion pressure (as in hypotension), small- or large-vessel obstruction, or both.

When blood flow to a portion of the brain is reduced, the survival of the tissue at risk depends on the presence of collateral circulation, the duration of ischemia, and the magnitude and rapidity of the reduction of flow. These factors determine, in turn, the precise anatomic site and size of the lesion and, consequently, the clinical deficit.

The general biochemical changes in cells resulting from ischemia are discussed in Chapter 2. The brain is primarily dependent on oxidative metabolism for generation of ATP, with minimal capacity to use glycolysis or energy substrates other than circulation-delivered glucose. With ischemia, there is depletion of ATP and loss of the membrane potential that is essential for neuronal electrical activity. Accompanying this, there is elevation of cytoplasmic calcium levels, which in turn activates a cascade of enzymatic processes that contribute to cellular injury. In addition to processes shared with ischemia in other parts of the body, the metabolic depletion of energy associated with ischemia can result in inappropriate release of excitatory amino acid neurotransmitters such as glutamate, which can contribute to cell damage by allowing excessive influx of calcium ions through N-methyl-D-aspartate (NMDA)-type glutamate receptors. In the region of transition between necrotic tissue and the normal brain, there is an area of "at-risk" tissue, referred to as the *penumbra*. This region can be rescued from injury in many animal models with a variety of anti-apoptotic interventions, implying that cells in areas of ischemia may die by apoptosis as well.

Global Cerebral Ischemia

Global cerebral ischemia **(diffuse ischemic/hypoxic encephalopathy) occurs when there is a generalized reduction of cerebral perfusion (as in cardiac arrest, shock, and severe hypotension).** The clinical outcome of a severe hypotensive episode that produces *global cerebral ischemia* varies with the severity of the insult. In mild cases, there may be only a transient post-ischemic confusional state followed by complete recovery and no irreversible tissue damage. However, irreversible damage to CNS tissue may occur in some individuals who suffer mild or transient global ischemic insults. There is a hierarchy of sensitivity among CNS cells: neurons are the most sensitive, although glial cells (oligodendrocytes and astrocytes) are also vulnerable. The most sensitive neurons in the brain are in the pyramidal cell layer of the hippocampus (especially area CA1, also referred to as *Sommer sector*), cerebellar Purkinje cells and pyramidal neurons in cerebral cortex. With severe global cerebral ischemia, widespread neuronal death occurs, irrespective of regional vulnerability. Patients who survive this injury often remain in a persistent vegetative state. Other patients meet the current clinical criteria for "brain death," including evidence of irreversible diffuse cortical injury (isoelectric, or "flat," electroencephalogram) and brainstem damage, such as absent reflexes and respiratory drive, and absent cerebral perfusion. When individuals with this pervasive form of injury are maintained on mechanical ventilation, the brain gradually undergoes an autolytic process with gradual liquefaction producing the so-called "respirator brain."

Border zone ("watershed") infarcts occur in the regions of the brain or spinal cord that lie at the most distal reaches of the arterial blood supply, the border zones between arterial territories. In the cerebral hemispheres, the border zone between the anterior and the middle cerebral artery distributions is at greatest risk. Damage to this region produces a sickle-shaped band of necrosis over the cerebral convexity a few centimeters lateral to the interhemispheric fissure. Border zone infarcts are usually seen after hypotensive episodes.

MORPHOLOGY

In the setting of global ischemia, the brain becomes edematous and swollen, producing widening of the gyri and narrowing of the sulci. The cut surface shows poor demarcation between gray and white matter. The microscopic features of irreversible ischemic injury (infarction) evolve over time. **Early changes,** occurring 12 to 24 hours after the insult, are seen in neurons (red neurons; Figs. 28-13*A* and 28-13*B*) and consist of microvacuolization, then eosinophilia of the neuronal cytoplasm, and later nuclear pyknosis and karyorrhexis. Similar acute changes occur somewhat later in astrocytes and oligodendroglia. After the acute injury, the reaction to tissue damage begins with infiltration by neutrophils (Fig. 28-13*C*). **Subacute changes,** occurring at 24 hours to 2 weeks, include tissue necrosis, influx of macrophages, vascular proliferation, and reactive gliosis (Fig. 28-13*D*). **Repair,** robust after approximately 2 weeks, is characterized by removal of necrotic tissue, loss of normal CNS architecture, and gliosis (Fig. 28-13*E*). In the cerebral neocortex the neuronal loss and gliosis are uneven, with preservation of some layers and destruction of others, producing a pattern of injury termed **pseudolaminar necrosis**.

Focal Cerebral Ischemia

Focal cerebral ischemia follows reduction or cessation of blood flow to a localized area of the brain due to arterial occlusion or hypoperfusion. When the ischemia is sustained, infarction follows in the territory of the compromised vessel. The size, location, and shape of the infarct and the extent of tissue damage that results are influenced by the duration of the ischemia and the adequacy of collateral flow. The major source of collateral flow is the circle of Willis (supplemented by the external carotid-ophthalmic pathway). Partial and inconstant reinforcement is available over the surface of the brain for the distal branches of the anterior, middle, and posterior cerebral arteries through cortical-leptomeningeal anastomoses. In contrast, there is little if any collateral flow for the deep penetrating vessels supplying structures such as the thalamus, basal ganglia, and deep white matter.

Occlusive vascular disease of severity sufficient to lead to cerebral infarction may be due to embolization from a distant source, in situ thrombosis, or various forms of vasculitides; the basic pathology of these conditions is discussed in Chapters 4 and 11.

- *Embolism* to the brain occurs from a variety of sources. Cardiac mural thrombi are among the most common culprits; myocardial infarct, valvular disease, and atrial fibrillation are important predisposing factors. Next in importance are thromboemboli arising in arteries, most

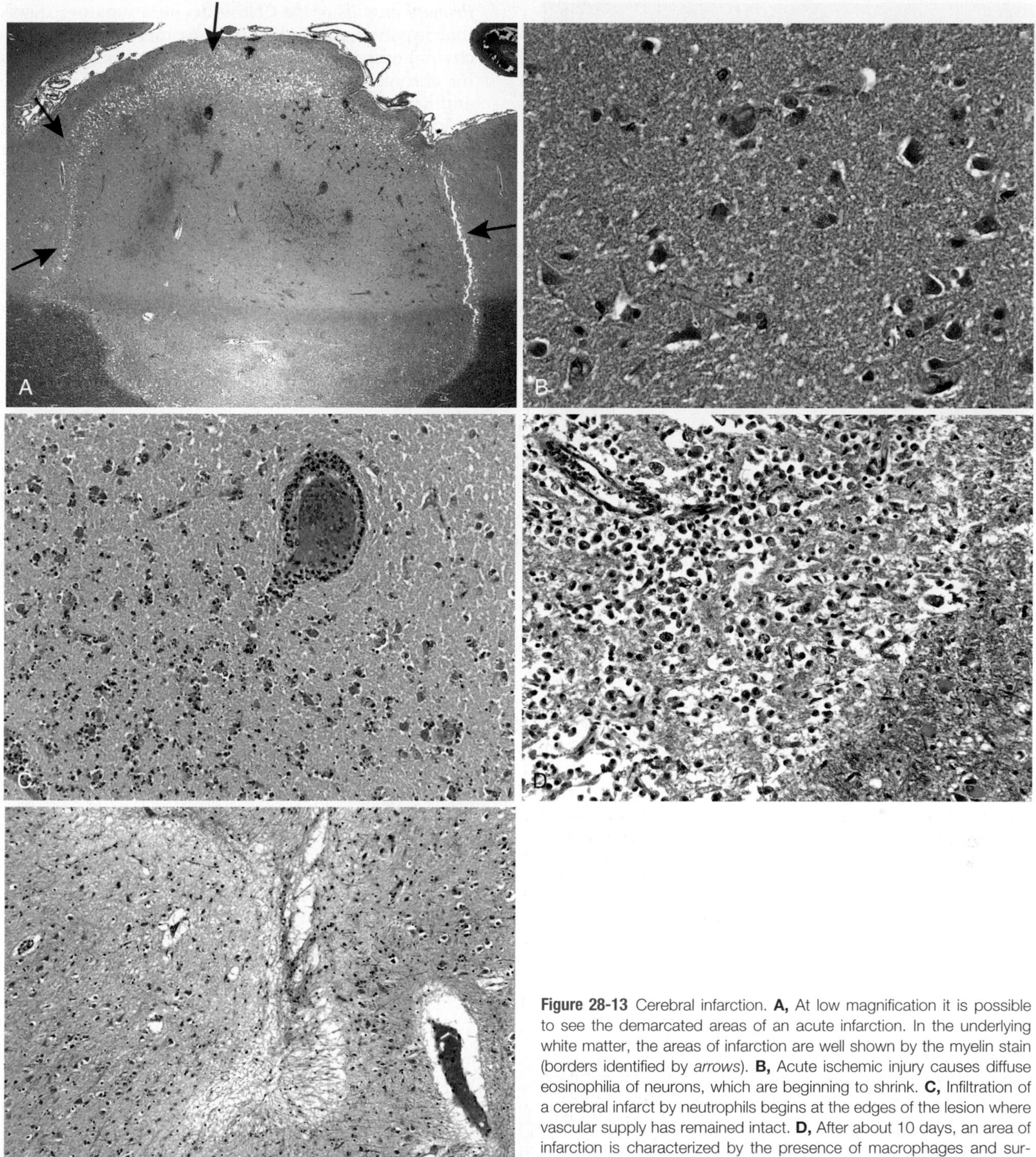

Figure 28-13 Cerebral infarction. **A,** At low magnification it is possible to see the demarcated areas of an acute infarction. In the underlying white matter, the areas of infarction are well shown by the myelin stain (borders identified by *arrows*). **B,** Acute ischemic injury causes diffuse eosinophilia of neurons, which are beginning to shrink. **C,** Infiltration of a cerebral infarct by neutrophils begins at the edges of the lesion where vascular supply has remained intact. **D,** After about 10 days, an area of infarction is characterized by the presence of macrophages and surrounding reactive gliosis. **E,** Remote small intracortical infarcts are seen as areas of tissue loss with residual gliosis.

often originating over atheromatous plaques within the carotid arteries. Other sources of emboli include paradoxical emboli, particularly in children with cardiac anomalies; emboli associated with cardiac surgery; and emboli of other material (tumor, fat, or air). The territory of distribution of the middle cerebral artery—the direct extension of the internal carotid artery—is most frequently affected by embolic infarction; the incidence is about equal in the two hemispheres. Emboli tend to lodge where blood vessels branch or in areas of preexisting luminal stenosis. "Shower embolization," as in fat embolism, may occur after fractures; affected individuals manifest generalized cerebral dysfunction with disturbances of higher cortical function and consciousness, often without localizing signs. Widespread hemorrhagic lesions involving the white matter are characteristic of embolization of bone marrow after trauma (Fig. 28-14).

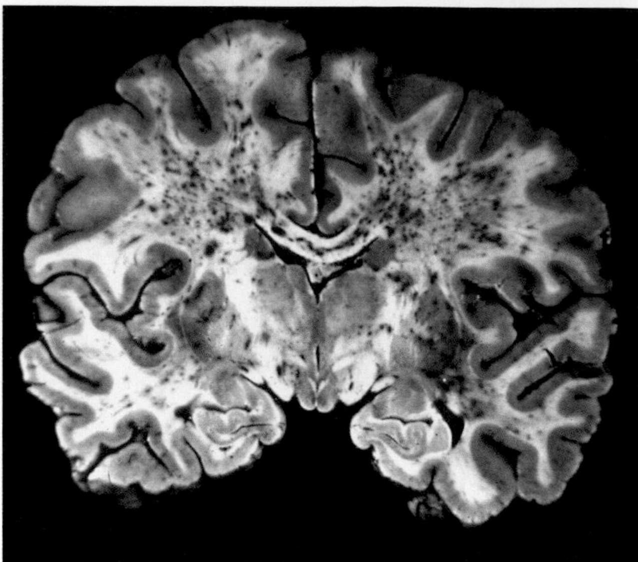

Figure 28-14 Widespread white-matter hemorrhages are characteristic of bone marrow embolization.

- **Thrombotic occlusions are most commonly associated with atherosclerosis and plaque rupture.** The most common sites are the carotid bifurcation, the origin of the middle cerebral artery, and either end of the basilar artery. Thrombi cause progressive narrowing of the lumen, may be accompanied by anterograde extension, and may progress to fragmentation and distal embolization. Atherosclerotic cerebrovascular disease is frequently associated with systemic diseases such as hypertension and diabetes.
- Inflammatory processes that involve blood vessels may also lead to luminal narrowing, occlusion and hence cerebral infarcts. While *infectious vasculitis* of small and large vessels occurs with syphilis and tuberculosis, it is now more common in the setting of immunosuppression and opportunistic infection (e.g., aspergillosis or CMV encephalitis). *Polyarteritis nodosa* and other noninfectious vasculitides may involve cerebral vessels and cause single or multiple infarcts throughout the brain.

  Primary angiitis of the CNS is an inflammatory disorder that involves multiple small- to medium-sized parenchymal and subarachnoid vessels and is characterized by chronic inflammation, multinucleated giant cells, and destruction of the vessel wall. As granulomas may be present, this disorder is also known as *granulomatous angiitis of the nervous system*. Affected individuals manifest a diffuse encephalopathic or multifocal clinical picture, often with cognitive dysfunction; patients improve with steroid and immunosuppressive treatment. Other conditions that may cause thrombosis and infarction (and intracranial hemorrhage) include hypercoagulable states, dissecting aneurysm of extracranial arteries in the neck supplying the brain, and drug abuse (amphetamines, heroin, cocaine).

Infarcts are subdivided into two broad groups based on the presence of hemorrhage. As infarcts begin with loss of blood supply, they are often initially nonhemorrhagic (Fig. 28-15*A*). Secondary hemorrhage can occur from ischemia-reperfusion injury, either through collaterals or following dissolution or fragmentation of the intravascular occlusive material. The hemorrhages are petechial in nature, and may be multiple or even confluent (Fig. 28-15*B*). The clinical management of patients with these two types of infarcts differs greatly as thrombolytic therapy is contraindicated in hemorrhagic infarcts.

MORPHOLOGY

The gross appearance of a **nonhemorrhagic infarct** varies with the time. There is little change in appearance during the first 6 hours of irreversible injury. By 48 hours, however, the tissue becomes pale, soft, and swollen, and the corticomedullary junction becomes indistinct. From 2 to 10 days, the brain becomes gelatinous and friable, and the previously ill-defined boundary between normal and infarcted tissue becomes more distinct as edema resolves in the viable adjacent tissue. From 10 days to 3 weeks, the tissue liquefies, eventually leaving a fluid-filled cavity that continues to expand until all of the dead tissue is removed (Fig. 28-16).

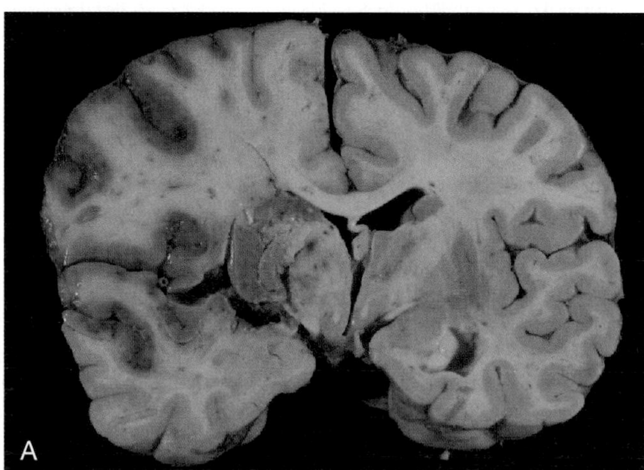

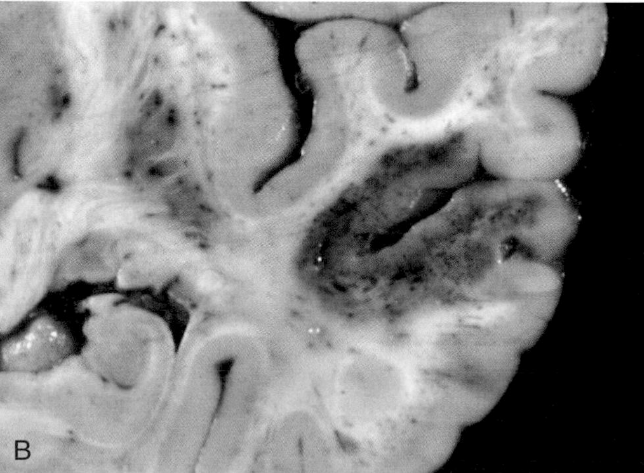

Figure 28-15 A, An ischemic infarction involves the territory of the middle cerebral artery, including the striatum of the left side of this brain. **B,** A bland infarct with punctate hemorrhages, consistent with ischemia-reperfusion injury, is present in the temporal lobe.

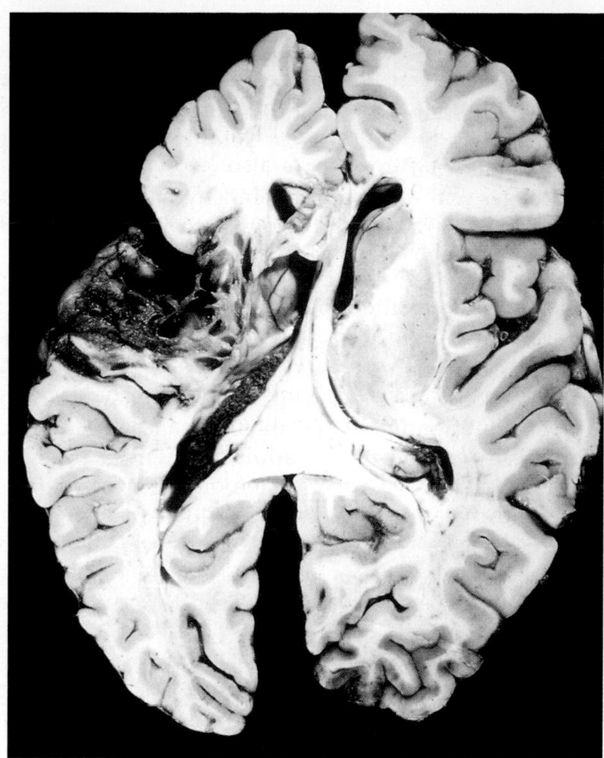

Figure 28-16 Old cystic infarct showing destruction of cortex with cavitation.

Microscopically, the tissue reaction evolves along the following sequence:

- *After the first 12 hours,* ischemic neuronal change (red neurons; see earlier) and both cytotoxic and vasogenic edema predominate. There is loss of the usual tinctorial characteristics of white- and gray matter structures. Endothelial and glial cells, mainly astrocytes, swell, and myelinated fibers begin to disintegrate.
- *Up to 48 hours,* neutrophilic emigration progressively increases and then falls off. Phagocytic cells, derived from circulating monocytes and activated microglia, are evident at *48 hours* and become the predominant cell type in the ensuing *2 to 3 weeks*. The macrophages become stuffed with the products of myelin breakdown or blood and may persist in the lesion for months to years.
- Reactive astrocytes can be seen as early as *1 week* after the insult. As the process of liquefaction and phagocytosis proceeds, astrocytes at the edges of the lesion progressively enlarge, divide, and develop a prominent network of cytoplasmic extensions.
- *After several months,* the astrocytic response recedes, leaving behind a dense meshwork of glial fibers admixed with new capillaries and some perivascular connective tissue. In the cerebral cortex, the cavity is separated from the meninges and subarachnoid space by a gliotic layer of tissue, derived from the molecular layer of the cortex. The pia and arachnoid are not affected and do not contribute to the healing process. Infarcts undergo these reactive and reparative stages from the edges inward; thus, different areas of a lesion may look different, particularly during the early stages, revealing the natural progression of the response.

The features and temporal evolution of **hemorrhagic infarctions** parallel ischemic infarctions, with the addition of blood extravasation and resorption. In individuals receiving anticoagulant treatment, hemorrhagic infarcts may be associated with extensive intracerebral hematomas. Venous infarcts are often hemorrhagic and may occur after thrombotic occlusion of the superior sagittal sinus or other sinuses or occlusion of the deep cerebral veins. Carcinoma, localized infections, and other conditions leading to a hypercoagulable state increase the risk for venous thrombosis.

Spinal cord infarction may be seen in the setting of hypoperfusion or as a consequence of traumatic interruption of the feeding tributaries derived from the aorta. Rarely, the cause is occlusion of the anterior spinal artery as a result of an embolus or vasculitis.

Clinical Features. Deficits produced by infarction are determined by the anatomic distribution of the damage, rather than the underlying cause. Neurologic symptoms referable to the area of injury often develop rapidly, over minutes, and may continue to evolve over hours. There can be improvement in severity of symptoms associated with reversal of injury in the ischemic penumbra as well as with resolution of associated local edema. In general, there is often a degree of slow improvement during a period of months. Because strokes are frequently associated with cardiovascular disease, many of the genetic and lifestyle risk factors are shared.

Hypertensive Cerebrovascular Disease

The most important effects of hypertension on the brain include lacunar infarcts, slit hemorrhages, and hypertensive encephalopathy, as well as massive hypertensive intracerebral hemorrhage. Aggressive management of hypertension is the primary approach to preventing this form of cerebrovascular disease.

Lacunar Infarcts

Hypertension affects the deep penetrating arteries and arterioles that supply the basal ganglia and hemispheric white matter as well as the brainstem. These cerebral vessels develop *arteriolar sclerosis* and may become occluded; the structural changes are similar to those described in the systemic vessels of individuals with hypertension (Chapter 11). An important clinical and pathologic consequence of CNS arterial lesions is the development of single or multiple, small, cavitary infarcts known as *lacunes* (Fig. 28-17). These are lakelike spaces, arbitrarily defined as less than 15 mm wide, which occur in the lenticular nucleus, thalamus, internal capsule, deep white matter, caudate nucleus, and pons, in descending order of frequency. On microscopic examination they show tissue loss surrounded by gliosis. Depending on their location in the CNS, lacunae can be clinically silent or cause severe neurologic impairment. Affected vessels may also be associated with widening of the perivascular spaces without tissue infarction *(état criblé)*.

Slit Hemorrhages

Hypertension also gives rise to rupture of the small-caliber penetrating vessels and the development of small

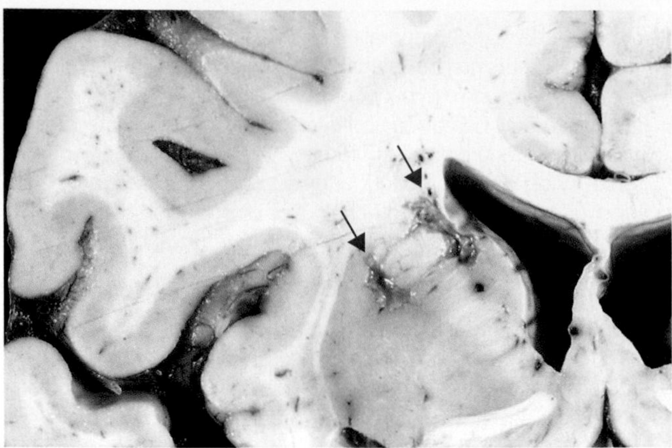

Figure 28-17 Lacunar infarcts in the caudate and putamen *(arrows).*

hemorrhages. In time these hemorrhages resorb, leaving behind a slitlike cavity *(slit hemorrhage)* surrounded by brownish discoloration; on microscopic examination, slit hemorrhages show focal tissue destruction, pigment-laden macrophages, and gliosis.

Hypertensive Encephalopathy

Acute hypertensive encephalopathy is a clinicopathologic syndrome arising in the setting of malignant hypertension, and is characterized by diffuse cerebral dysfunction, including headaches, confusion, vomiting, and convulsions, sometimes leading to coma. Rapid therapeutic intervention to reduce the accompanying increased intracranial pressure is required, since the syndrome often does not remit spontaneously. At postmortem examination such individuals may show an edematous brain with or without transtentorial or tonsillar herniation. Petechiae and fibrinoid necrosis of arterioles in the gray and white matter may be seen microscopically.

Individuals who, over the course of many months and years, suffer multiple, bilateral, gray matter (cortex, thalamus, basal ganglia) and white matter (centrum semiovale) infarcts may develop a distinctive clinical syndrome characterized by dementia, gait abnormalities, and pseudobulbar signs, often with superimposed focal neurologic deficits. The syndrome, generally referred to as *vascular (multi-infarct) dementia,* is caused by multifocal vascular disease of several types, including (1) cerebral atherosclerosis, (2) vessel thrombosis or embolization from carotid vessels or from the heart, and (3) cerebral arteriolar sclerosis from chronic hypertension. When the pattern of injury preferentially involves large areas of the subcortical white matter with myelin and axon loss, the disorder is referred to as *Binswanger disease;* this distribution of vascular white-matter injury must be distinguished clinically and radiologically from other diseases that affect the hemispheral white matter. In addition, many individuals with neurodegenerative diseases resulting in cognitive impairment or dementia also have evidence of cerebrovascular disease. The presence of significant cerebrovascular disease increases risk of neurologic impairment for a given level of lesions associated with the degenerative diseases, suggesting that it is an independent contributing factor to disruption of normal brain function.

Intracranial Hemorrhage

Hemorrhages may occur at any site within the CNS—outside the brain or within it (intraparenchymal). Hemorrhages in the epidural or subdural space are typically associated with trauma and were discussed earlier. Hemorrhages within the brain parenchyma and in the subarachnoid space, in contrast, are more often a manifestation of underlying cerebrovascular disease.

Intraparenchymal Hemorrhage

Rupture of a small intraparenchymal vessel can result in a hemorrhage within the brain, often associated with sudden onset of neurologic symptoms (stroke). Spontaneous (nontraumatic) intraparenchymal hemorrhages occur most commonly in middle to late adult life, with a peak incidence at about age 60 years. Hemorrhages in the basal ganglia and thalamus are commonly designated "ganglionic hemorrhages," whereas those that occur in the lobes of the cerebral hemispheres are called "lobar hemorrhages." The two major causes of these patterns of hemorrhage are hypertension and cerebral amyloid angiopathy, respectively. In addition, other local and systemic factors may cause or contribute to nontraumatic hemorrhage, including systemic coagulation disorders, neoplasms, vasculitis, aneurysms, and vascular malformations.

Hypertension is the risk factor most commonly associated with deep brain parenchymal hemorrhages, accounting for more than 50% of clinically significant hemorrhages and for roughly 15% of deaths among individuals with chronic hypertension. Hemorrhages associated with hypertension are typically in deep white matter or deep gray structures, followed by the brainstem and cerebellum. Hypertension leads to a number of vessel wall abnormalities, including accelerated atherosclerosis in larger arteries, hyaline arteriolosclerosis in smaller arteries, and (in severe cases) proliferative changes and frank necrosis of arterioles. Arteriolar walls affected by hyaline change are presumably weaker than are normal vessels and are therefore vulnerable to rupture. In some instances chronic hypertension is associated with the development of minute aneurysms, termed *Charcot-Bouchard microaneurysms,* which may be the site of rupture. Charcot-Bouchard aneurysms, not to be confused with saccular aneurysms of larger intracranial vessels in the subarachnoid space, occur in vessels that are less than 300 μm in diameter, most commonly within the basal ganglia.

MORPHOLOGY

Hypertensive intraparenchymal hemorrhage may originate in the putamen (50% to 60% of cases), thalamus, pons, cerebellar hemispheres (rarely), and other regions of the brain (Fig. 28-18*A*). Acute hemorrhages, independent of etiology, are characterized by extravasation of blood with compression of the adjacent parenchyma. Old hemorrhages show an area of cavitary destruction of brain with a rim of brownish discoloration. The early lesions consist of a central core of clotted blood surrounded by a rim of brain tissue showing anoxic neuronal and glial changes as well as edema. Eventually the edema resolves, hemosiderin- and lipid-laden macrophages appear, and proliferation of reactive astrocytes is seen at the periphery of the lesion. The cellular events then follow the same time course that is observed after cerebral infarction.

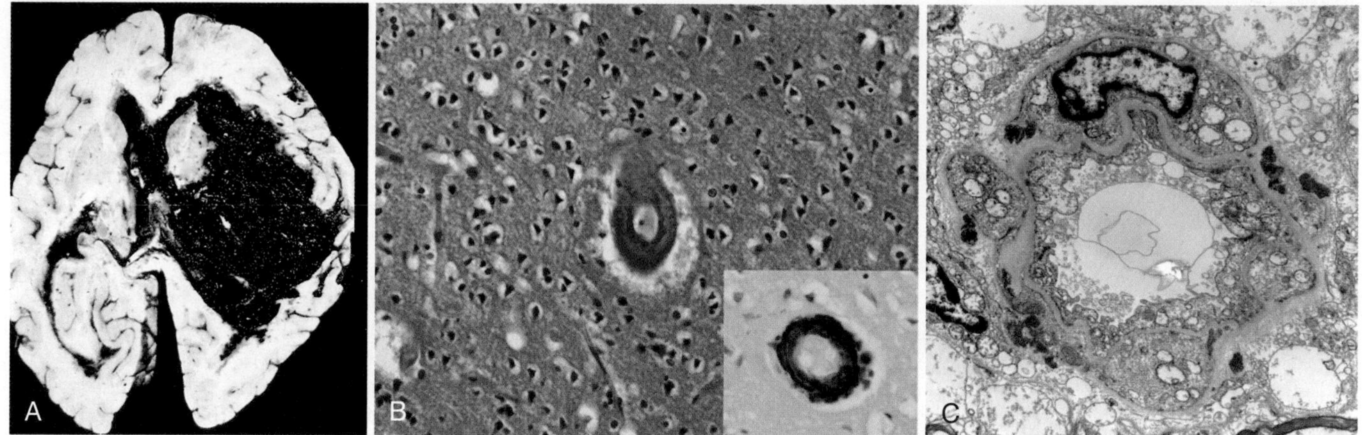

Figure 28-18 **A,** Massive hypertensive hemorrhage rupturing into a lateral ventricle. **B,** Amyloid deposition in a cortical arteriole in cerebral amyloid angiopathy; *inset*, immunohistochemical staining for Aβ shows the deposited material in the vessel wall. **C,** Electron micrograph shows granular osmophilic material in a case of CADASIL (cerebral autosomal dominant arteriopathy with subcortical infarcts and leukoencephalopathy).

Cerebral amyloid angiopathy (CAA) is the risk factor most commonly associated with lobar hemorrhages. In CAA, amyloidogenic peptides, usually the same ones found in Alzheimer disease ($A\beta_{40}$; see later), are deposited in the walls of medium- and small-caliber meningeal and cortical vessels. This deposition can weaken the vessel wall and lead to hemorrhage. Many individuals with CAA have evidence of numerous small hemorrhages within the brain ("microbleeds"), which can be visualized by various imaging methods. As with Alzheimer disease, in which there is a relationship between a polymorphism in the gene that encodes apolipoprotein E (ApoE) and risk of disease, there is an effect of the ApoE genotype on the risk of recurrence of hemorrhage from sporadic CAA. The presence of either an ε2 or ε4 allele increases the risk of repeat bleeding. While some mutations in the precursor protein for the Aβ peptide (amyloid precursor protein, APP) cause familial Alzheimer disease, others result in autosomal dominant forms of CAA.

MORPHOLOGY

The underlying vascular abnormality of CAA is typically restricted to the leptomeningeal and cerebral cortical arterioles and capillaries, although involvement of the molecular layer of the cerebellum can be observed as well. Involved vessels are rigid, and as a result fail to collapse during tissue processing and sectioning. Unlike with arteriolar sclerosis, there is no fibrosis; rather, dense and uniform deposits of amyloid are present (Fig. 28-18*B*).

Other forms of hereditary small-vessel diseases of the CNS have been identified recently. *Cerebral autosomal dominant arteriopathy with subcortical infarcts and leukoencephalopathy* (CADASIL) is an autosomal dominant disorder caused by mutations in the *NOTCH3* gene that lead to misfolding of the extracellular domain of the NOTCH3 receptor. NOTCH3 is preferentially expressed in vascular smooth muscle, and mice engineered to express NOTCH3 receptors bearing CADASIL mutations recapitulate features of the human disease, indicating that the disease is caused by vascular smooth muscle dysfunction.

The disease is characterized clinically by recurrent strokes (usually infarcts, less often hemorrhages) and dementia. Imaging studies show that the first detectable changes are in white matter, usually by around the age of 35 years, whereas infarcts typically occur 10-15 years later. Arteries in the CNS and in other tissues such as skin show concentric thickening of the media and adventitia, loss of smooth muscle cells, and the presence of basophilic, PAS-positive deposits. These appear as osmiophilic compact granular material by electron microscopy and are consistently detected in the walls of affected vessels (Fig. 28-18*C*). The characteristic deposits contain the misfolded NOTCH3 protein. How these deposits relate to the disease is not understood. The diagnosis is made through the identification of these deposits in the walls of vessels in biopsies of other tissues, such as skin or muscle, or by sequencing of *NOTCH3*.

Other forms of the heritable small vessel diseases include a disorder associated with mutations in the gene for COL4A1, a component of the vascular basement membrane.

Clinical Features. Intracerebral hemorrhage, independent of cause, can be clinically devastating if it affects large portions of the brain and extends into the ventricular system, but it can affect small regions and either be clinically silent or evolve like an infarct. Over weeks or months there is a gradual resolution of the hematoma, sometimes with considerable clinical improvement. Again, the location of the hemorrhage determines the clinical manifestations.

Subarachnoid Hemorrhage and Ruptured Saccular Aneurysms

The most frequent cause of clinically significant subarachnoid hemorrhage is rupture of a saccular ("berry") aneurysm in a cerebral artery. Subarachnoid hemorrhage may also result from extension of a traumatic hematoma, rupture of a hypertensive intracerebral hemorrhage into

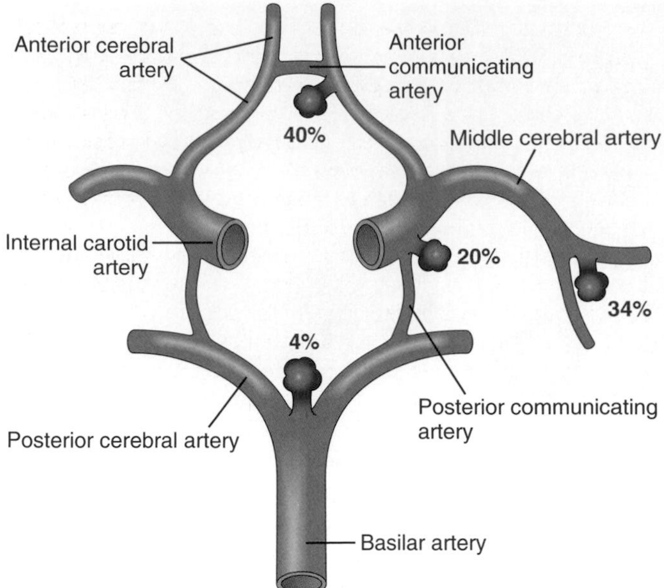

Figure 28-19 Common sites of saccular (berry) aneurysms in the circle of Willis.

the ventricular system, vascular malformation, hematologic disturbances, and tumors.

Saccular aneurysm is the most common type of intracranial aneurysm. Other aneurysm types include atherosclerotic (fusiform; mostly of the basilar artery), mycotic, traumatic, and dissecting. These latter three, like saccular aneurysms, are most often found in the anterior circulation, but differ in that they more often cause cerebral infarction rather than subarachnoid hemorrhage.

Saccular aneurysms are found in about 2% of the population according to recent data from community-based radiologic studies. About 90% of saccular aneurysms are found near major arterial branch points in the anterior circulation (Fig. 28-19); multiple aneurysms exist in 20% to 30% of cases in autopsy series.

Pathogenesis. While the etiology of saccular aneurysms remains obscure, the structural abnormality of the involved vessel (absence of smooth muscle and intimal elastic lamina) suggests that they represent a developmental disorder. Although the majority occur sporadically, genetic factors may be important in their pathogenesis, since there is an increased incidence of aneurysms in first-degree relatives of those affected. There is also an increased incidence in individuals with certain Mendelian disorders (e.g., autosomal dominant polycystic kidney disease, Ehlers-Danlos syndrome type IV, neurofibromatosis type 1 [NF1], and Marfan syndrome), fibromuscular dysplasia of extracranial arteries, and coarctation of the aorta. Other predisposing factors include cigarette smoking and hypertension (estimated to be present in about half of affected individuals). Although they are sometimes referred to as "congenital," the aneurysms are not present at birth but develop over time because of an underlying defect in the media of the vessel.

MORPHOLOGY

An unruptured saccular aneurysm is a thin-walled outpouching, usually at an arterial branch point along the circle of Willis or a major vessel just beyond. Saccular aneurysms measure from a few millimeters to 2 or 3 cm in diameter and have a bright red, shiny surface and a thin, translucent wall (Fig. 28-20). Atheromatous plaques, calcification, or thrombi may be found in the wall or lumen of the aneurysm. Sometimes there is evidence of prior hemorrhage, in the form of brownish discoloration of the adjacent brain and meninges. The neck of the aneurysm may be wide or narrow. Rupture usually occurs at the apex of the sac and leads to extravasation of blood into the subarachnoid space, the substance of the brain, or both. The arterial wall adjacent to the neck of the aneurysm often shows some intimal thickening and attenuation of the media. Smooth muscle and intimal elastic lamina do not extend into the neck and are absent from the aneurysm sac itself, which is made up of thickened hyalinized intima and a covering of adventitia.

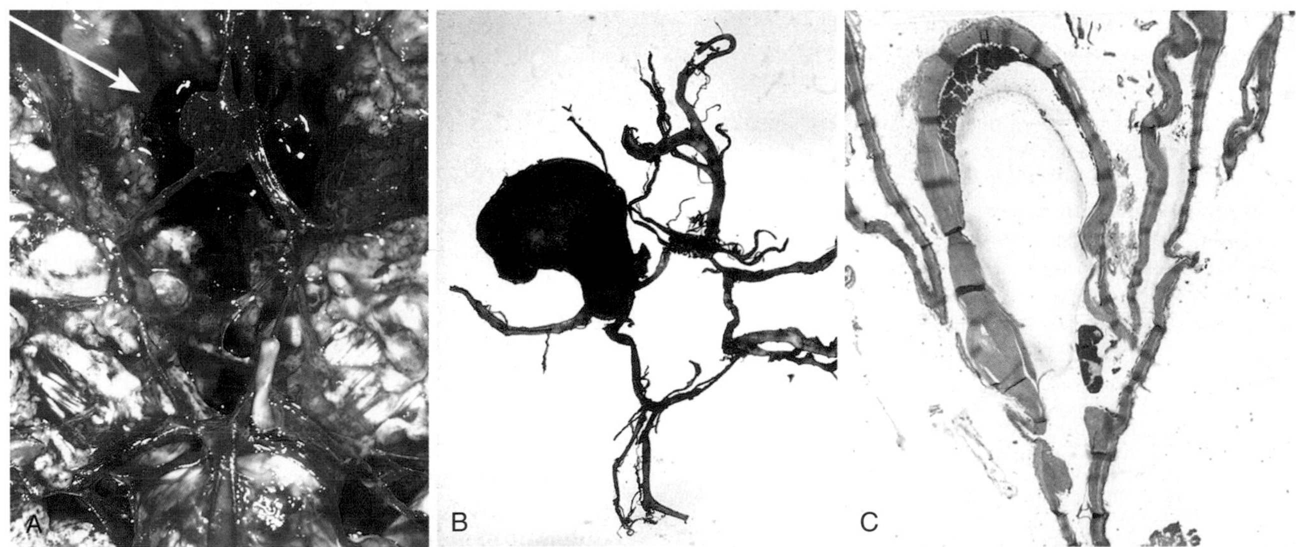

Figure 28-20 **A,** View of the base of the brain, dissected to show the circle of Willis with an aneurysm of the anterior cerebral artery *(arrow)*. **B,** Dissected circle of Willis to show large aneurysm. **C,** Section through a saccular aneurysm showing the hyalinized fibrous vessel wall (hematoxylin and eosin).

Clinical Features. Rupture of an aneurysm leading to clinically significant subarachnoid hemorrhage is most frequent in the fifth decade and is slightly more frequent in females. Overall, in about 1.3% of individuals aneurysms will rupture over the course of 1 year, but the risk is higher for larger aneurysms. For example, aneurysms greater than 10 mm in diameter have a roughly 50% risk of bleeding per year. Rupture may occur at any time, but in about one third of cases it is associated with acute increases in intracranial pressure, such as with straining at stool or sexual orgasm. Blood under arterial pressure is forced into the subarachnoid space and affected individuals are stricken with a sudden, excruciating headache ("the worst headache I've ever had") and rapidly lose consciousness. Between 25% and 50% of patients die with the first rupture, but patients who survive often improve and recover consciousness in minutes. Repeat bleeding is common in survivors and unpredictable in timing. With each episode of bleeding, the prognosis is worse.

The clinical consequences of blood in the subarachnoid space can be separated into acute events, occurring within hours to days after the hemorrhage, and late sequelae associated with the healing process. In the first few days after a subarachnoid hemorrhage, regardless of the etiology, there is an increased risk of additional ischemic injury from vasospasm affecting vessels bathed in the extravasated blood. This problem is of greatest significance in cases of basal subarachnoid hemorrhage, in which vasospasm can involve major vessels of the circle of Willis. Various mediators have been proposed to have a role in this process, including endothelins, nitric oxide, and arachidonic acid metabolites. In the healing phase of subarachnoid hemorrhage, meningeal fibrosis and scarring occur, sometimes leading to obstruction of CSF flow as well as interruption of the normal pathways of CSF resorption.

Vascular Malformations

Vascular malformations of the brain are classified into four principal groups: arteriovenous malformations, cavernous malformations, capillary telangiectasias, and venous angiomas. Of these, the first two are the types associated with risk of hemorrhage and development of neurologic symptoms.

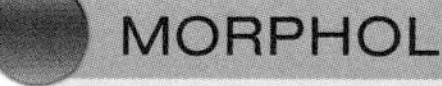

MORPHOLOGY

Arteriovenous malformations (AVM) may involve vessels in the subarachnoid space, in the brain or both. This tangled network of wormlike vascular channels has prominent, pulsatile arteriovenous shunting with high blood flow. They are composed of greatly enlarged blood vessels separated by gliotic tissue, often showing evidence of prior hemorrhage. Some vessels can be recognized as arteries with duplication and fragmentation of the internal elastic lamina, while others show marked thickening or partial replacement of the media by hyalinized connective tissue.

Cavernous malformations consist of distended, loosely organized vascular channels arranged back to back with collagenized walls of variable thickness. There is usually no brain parenchyma between vessels in this type of malformation. They occur most often in the cerebellum, pons, and subcortical regions, in decreasing order of frequency, and are "low-flow" channels that do not participate in arteriovenous shunting. Foci of old hemorrhage, infarction, and calcification frequently surround the abnormal vessels. **Capillary telangiectasias** are microscopic foci of dilated, thin-walled vascular channels separated by relatively normal brain parenchyma that occur most frequently in the pons. **Venous angiomas** (varices) consist of aggregates of ectatic venous channels. **Foix-Alajouanine disease** (angiodysgenetic necrotizing myelopathy) is a venous angiomatous malformation of the spinal cord and overlying meninges, most often in the lumbosacral region, associated with ischemic injury to the spinal cord and slowly progressive neurologic symptoms.

Clinical Features. Arteriovenous malformations are the most common type of clinically significant vascular malformation. Males are affected twice as frequently as females. The lesion often presents between the ages of 10 and 30 years as a seizure disorder, an intracerebral hemorrhage, or a subarachnoid hemorrhage. The most common site is the territory of the middle cerebral artery, particularly its posterior branches. Large arteriovenous malformations occurring in the newborn period can lead to congestive heart failure because of shunt effects, especially if the malformation involves the vein of Galen. Cavernous malformations are unique among this class of lesion in that familial forms are relatively common. Multiplicity of lesions is a hallmark of familial cases, which are inherited as a highly penetrant autosomal dominant trait.

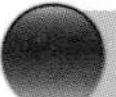

KEY CONCEPTS

Cerebrovascular Diseases

- *Stroke* is the clinical term for acute-onset neurologic deficits resulting from hemorrhagic or obstructive vascular lesions.
- Cerebral infarction follows loss of blood supply and can be widespread or focal, or affect regions with the least robust vascular supply (boundary zones).
- Focal cerebral infarcts are most commonly embolic; with subsequent dissolution of an embolism and reperfusion, a nonhemorrhagic infarct can become hemorrhagic.
- Primary intraparenchymal hemorrhages typically are due to either hypertension (most commonly in white matter, deep gray matter, or posterior fossa contents) or cerebral amyloid angiopathy.
- Spontaneous subarachnoid hemorrhage usually is caused by a structural vascular abnormality, such as an aneurysm or arteriovenous malformation.

Infections

Infection may damage the nervous system directly through injury of neurons or glia by the infectious agent, or indirectly through microbial toxins, the destructive effects of the inflammatory response, or the result of immune-mediated mechanisms. There are four principal routes by which microbes enter the nervous system. *Hematogenous spread* is the most common; infectious agents ordinarily gain access through the arterial circulation, but retrograde venous spread can occur via anastomoses with veins of the face. *Direct implantation* of microorganisms is most often traumatic or is sometimes associated with congenital malformations (e.g., meningomyelocele) that provide ready access for microorganisms. *Local extension* can originate from infected adjacent structures, such as air sinuses, teeth, skull, or vertebrae. Viruses also may be transported along the *peripheral nervous system* as occurs with rabies and herpes zoster virus. General aspects of the pathology of infectious agents are discussed in Chapter 8; distinctive forms of CNS infections are described herein (Table 28-2).

Table 28-2 Common Central Nervous System Infections

Type of Infection	Clinical Syndrome	Common Causative Organisms
Bacterial Infections		
Meningitis	Acute pyogenic meningitis	*Escherichia coli* or group B streptococci (infants) *Neisseria meningitidis* (young adults) *Streptococcus. pneumoniae* or *Listeria monocytogenes* (older adults)
	Chronic meningitis	*Mycobacterium tuberculosis*
Localized infections	Abscess Empyema	Streptococci and staphylococci Polymicrobial (staphylococci, anaerobic gram-negative)
Viral Infections		
Meningitis	Acute aseptic meningitis	Enteroviruses Measles (subacute sclerosing panencephalitis) Influenza species Lymphocytic choriomeningitis virus
Encephalitis	Encephalitic syndromes	Herpes simplex (HSV-1, HSV-2) Cytomegalovirus Human immunodeficiency virus JC polyomavirus (progressive multifocal leukoencephalopathy)
	Arthropod-borne encephalitis	West Nile virus Eastern equine encephalitis virus Western equine encephalitis virus St. Louis encephalitis virus La Crosse encephalitis virus Venezuelan equine encephalitis virus Japanese encephalitis virus Tick-borne encephalitis virus
Brainstem and spinal cord syndromes	Rhombencephalitis Spinal poliomyelitis	Rabies Polio West Nile virus
Rickettsia, Spirochetes, and Fungi		
Meningitic syndromes	Rocky Mountain spotted fever	*Rickettsia rickettsii*
	Neurosyphilis	*Treponema pallidum*
	Lyme disease (neuroborreliosis)	*Borrelia. burgdorferi*
	Fungal meningitis	*Cryptococcus neoformans* *Candida albicans*
Protozoa and Metazoa		
Meningitic syndromes	Cerebral malaria Amebic encephalitis	*Plasmodium falciparum* *Naegleria* species
Localized infections	Toxoplasmosis Cysticercosis	*Toxoplasma gondii* *Taenia solium*

Acute Meningitis

Meningitis is an inflammatory process of the leptomeninges and CSF within the subarachnoid space, usually caused by an infection. *Meningoencephalitis* refers to inflammation of the meninges and brain parenchyma. Although infections are the most common causes of meningitis and meningoencephalitis, this reaction may also occur in response to a nonbacterial irritant introduced into the subarachnoid space *(chemical meningitis)*. Based on the etiology and clinical evolution of the illness, infectious meningitis is broadly classified into *acute pyogenic* (usually bacterial), *aseptic* (usually acute or subacute viral), and *chronic* (usually tuberculous, spirochetal, or cryptococcal). Each type is accompanied by characteristics changes in the CSF.

Acute Pyogenic (Bacterial) Meningitis

Distinctive microorganisms cause acute pyogenic meningitis in various age groups: *Escherichia coli* and the group B streptococci in neonates; at the other extreme of life, *Streptococcus pneumoniae* and *Listeria monocytogenes* are most common; and *Neisseria meningitidis* in adolescents and in young adults, with clusters of cases raising public health concerns. The introduction of immunization against *Haemophilus influenzae* has markedly reduced the incidence of this infection in the developed world, particularly among infants, who used to be at high risk.

Affected individuals typically show systemic signs of infection superimposed on clinical evidence of meningeal irritation and neurologic impairment, including headache, photophobia, irritability, clouding of consciousness, and neck stiffness. A spinal tap yields cloudy or frankly purulent CSF, under increased pressure, with as many as 90,000 neutrophils per cubic millimeter, an increased protein concentration, and markedly reduced glucose content. Bacteria may be seen on a smear or may be cultured, sometimes a few hours before the neutrophils appear. Untreated pyogenic meningitis can be fatal, while effective treatment with antibiotics markedly reduces mortality. The Waterhouse-Friderichsen syndrome results from meningitis-associated septicemia with hemorrhagic infarction of the adrenal glands and cutaneous petechiae (Chapter 24). It occurs most often with meningococcal and pneumococcal meningitis. In the immunosuppressed individual, purulent meningitis may be caused by several other infectious agents, such as *Klebsiella* or anaerobic organisms, and may have an atypical clinical course and uncharacteristic CSF findings, rendering timely diagnosis more difficult.

Acute Aseptic (Viral) Meningitis

Aseptic meningitis is a clinical term that applies to a situation where there is an absence of organisms by

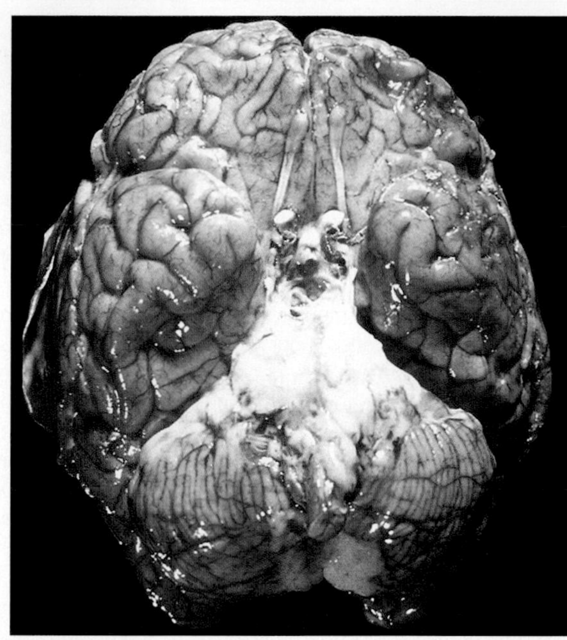

Figure 28-21 Pyogenic meningitis. A thick layer of suppurative exudate covers the brainstem and cerebellum and thickens the leptomeninges. (From Golden JA, Louis DN: Images in clinical medicine: acute bacterial meningitis. N Engl J Med 333:364, 1994.)

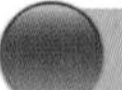

MORPHOLOGY

In acute meningitis, an exudate is evident within the leptomeninges over the surface of the brain (Fig. 28-21). The meningeal vessels are engorged and stand out prominently. The anatomic distribution of the exudate varies; in *H. influenzae* meningitis, for example, it is usually basal, whereas in pneumococcal meningitis it is often densest over the cerebral convexities near the sagittal sinus. From the areas of greatest accumulation, tracts of pus follow along blood vessels on the surface of the brain. When the meningitis is fulminant, the inflammation may extend to the ventricles, producing ventriculitis.

On microscopic examination, neutrophils fill the subarachnoid space in severely affected areas and are found predominantly around the leptomeningeal blood vessels in less severe cases. Particularly in untreated meningitis, Gram stain reveals variable numbers of bacteria. In fulminant meningitis, the inflammatory cells infiltrate the walls of the leptomeningeal veins and may extend focally into the substance of the brain (cerebritis). Phlebitis may lead to venous thrombosis and hemorrhagic infarction of the underlying brain.

Leptomeningeal fibrosis may follow pyogenic meningitis and cause hydrocephalus. Particularly in pneumococcal meningitis, large quantities of the capsular polysaccharide of the organism produce a gelatinous exudate that promotes arachnoid fibrosis, a condition referred to as **chronic adhesive arachnoiditis**.

bacterial culture in a patient with manifestations of meningitis, including meningeal irritation, fever, and alterations of consciousness of relatively acute onset. The disease is generally of viral etiology (in about 80% of cases enteroviruses), but may be bacterial, rickettsial, or autoimmune in origin. The clinical course is less fulminant than that of pyogenic meningitis, and the CSF findings also differ; in aseptic meningitis there is a lymphocytic pleocytosis, the protein elevation is only moderate, and the glucose content is nearly always normal. The viral aseptic meningitides are usually self-limited and are treated symptomatically. Remarkably, even with molecular methods for detection of pathogens, the etiologic agent is identified in only a minority of cases. When pathogens are identified, enteroviruses are the most common etiology, accounting for 80% of the cases. The spectrum of pathogens varies seasonally and geographically. An aseptic meningitis-like picture may also develop subsequent to rupture of an epidermoid cyst into the subarachnoid space or the introduction of a chemical irritant (chemical meningitis). In these cases, the CSF is sterile and there is pleocytosis with neutrophils and an increased protein concentration, but the sugar content is usually normal.

Acute Focal Suppurative Infections

Brain Abscess

A brain abscess is a localized focus of necrosis of brain tissue with accompanying inflammation, usually caused by a bacterial infection. Brain abscesses may arise by direct implantation of organisms, local extension from adjacent foci (mastoiditis, paranasal sinusitis), or hematogenous spread (usually from a primary site in the heart, lungs, or bones of the extremities, or after tooth extraction). Predisposing conditions include acute bacterial endocarditis, which may give rise to multiple brain abscesses; congenital heart disease with right-to-left shunting and loss of pulmonary filtration of organisms; chronic pulmonary sepsis, as in bronchiectasis; and systemic disease with immunosuppression. Streptococci and staphylococci are the most common offending organisms identified in nonimmunosuppressed patients.

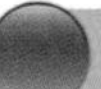

MORPHOLOGY

Abscesses are discrete lesions with central liquefactive necrosis surrounded by brain swelling (Fig. 28-22). At the outer margin of the necrotic lesion there is exuberant granulation tissue with neovascularization around the necrosis. The newly formed vessels are abnormally permeable, accounting for marked vasogenic edema in the adjacent brain tissue. In well-established lesions, a collagenous capsule is produced by fibroblasts derived from the walls of blood vessels. Outside the fibrous capsule is a zone of reactive gliosis containing numerous gemistocytic astrocytes.

Cerebral abscesses are destructive lesions and patients often present with progressive focal neurologic deficits; signs and symptoms related to increased intracranial pressure may also develop. Typically, the CSF has a high white cell count and an increased protein concentration, but the glucose content is normal. The source of infection may be apparent or may be traced to a small distant focus that is not symptomatic. The increased intracranial pressure can lead to fatal herniation. Other complications include abscess rupture with ventriculitis or meningitis, and venous sinus thrombosis. With surgery and antibiotic

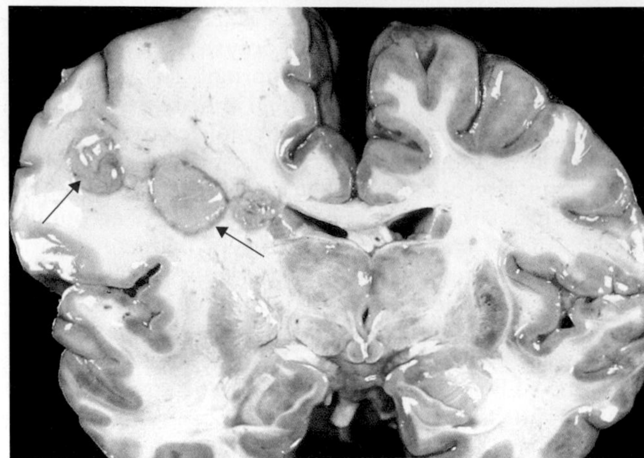

Figure 28-22 Cerebral abscesses *(arrows)*.

treatment, the otherwise high mortality rate can be reduced to less than 10%.

Subdural Empyema

Bacterial, and rarely fungal, infections of the skull bones or air sinuses can spread to the subdural space, producing a subdural empyema. While the underlying arachnoid and subarachnoid spaces are usually unaffected, a large subdural empyema may produce a mass effect or a thrombophlebitis of the bridging veins that cross the subdural space, resulting in venous occlusion and infarction of the brain. In addition to symptoms referable to the source of the infection, most patients are febrile, have headache and neck stiffness. The CSF profile is similar to that seen in brain abscesses, because both are parameningeal infectious processes. If untreated, focal neurologic signs, lethargy, and coma may develop. With prompt diagnosis and treatment, including surgical drainage, resolution and full recovery is possible, the only residuum being a thickened dura.

Extradural Abscess

Extradural abscess, commonly associated with osteomyelitis, often arises from an adjacent focus of infection, such as sinusitis or following a surgical procedure. When the process occurs in the spinal epidural space, it may cause spinal cord compression and constitute a neurosurgical emergency.

Chronic Bacterial Meningoencephalitis

Chronic bacterial infection of the meninges and the brain may be caused by *Mycobacterium tuberculosis*, *Treponema pallidum*, and *Borrelia* species.

Tuberculosis

Tuberculosis of the CNS may be part of active disease elsewhere in the body or appear in isolation following seeding from silent lesions elsewhere, usually the lungs. It may involve the meninges or the brain.

MORPHOLOGY

The most common pattern of tuberculous involvement is a diffuse **meningoencephalitis**. The subarachnoid space contains a gelatinous or fibrinous exudate that characteristically involves the base of the brain, effacing the cisterns and encasing cranial nerves. There may be discrete, white areas of inflammation scattered over the leptomeninges. On microscopic examination, involved areas contain mixed inflammatory infiltrates containing lymphocytes, plasma cells, and macrophages. Florid cases show well-formed granulomas with caseous necrosis and giant cells. Arteries running through the subarachnoid space may show obliterative endarteritis and marked intimal thickening. Organisms can often be seen with acid-fast stains. The infectious process may spread to the choroid plexus and ependymal surface, traveling through the CSF. In long-standing cases, a dense, fibrous adhesive arachnoiditis may develop, most conspicuous around the base of the brain. Hydrocephalus may result.

CNS involvement may also take the form of one or more well-circumscribed intraparenchymal masses **(tuberculomas)**, which may be associated with meningitis. A tuberculoma may be as large as several centimeters in diameter, causing significant mass effect. These lesions usually have a central area of caseous necrosis surrounded by granulomas; calcification may occur in inactive lesions.

Clinical Features. Patients with tuberculous meningitis usually have headache, malaise, mental confusion, and vomiting. The CSF typically shows a pleocytosis made up of mononuclear cells or a mixture of neutrophils and mononuclear cells, an elevated protein concentration (often, strikingly so), and a moderately reduced or normal glucose. The most serious complications of chronic tuberculous meningitis are arachnoid fibrosis producing hydrocephalus, and obliterative endarteritis producing arterial occlusion and infarction of underlying brain. When the process involves the spinal cord subarachnoid space, nerve roots may also be affected. Tuberculomas produce symptoms typical of space-occupying brain lesions and must be distinguished from CNS tumors.

CNS tuberculosis in patients with acquired immunodeficiency syndrome (AIDS) is pathologically similar, but there may be less host reaction than in immunocompetent individuals. HIV-positive individuals are also at risk for infection by *Mycobacterium avium-intracellulare*, usually in the setting of disseminated infection. These lesions typically contain confluent sheets of macrophages filled with organisms, with few or no granulomas.

Neurosyphilis

Neurosyphilis is a manifestation of the tertiary stage of syphilis and occurs in only about 10% of individuals with untreated infection. The major patterns of CNS involvement are meningovascular neurosyphilis, paretic neurosyphilis, and tabes dorsalis. Affected individuals often show incomplete or mixed pictures, most commonly the combination of tabes dorsalis and paretic disease (taboparesis). Individuals infected with HIV are at increased risk for neurosyphilis, particularly to acute syphilitic meningitis or meningovascular disease, because of impaired cell-mediated immunity. The rate of progression and severity of the disease are also accelerated, for the same reason.

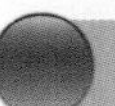

MORPHOLOGY

Neurosyphilis presents in several distinct forms.

- **Meningovascular neurosyphilis** is chronic meningitis involving the base of the brain and more variably the cerebral convexities and the spinal leptomeninges. In addition, there may be an associated obliterative endarteritis (Heubner arteritis) accompanied by a distinctive perivascular inflammatory reaction rich in plasma cells and lymphocytes. Cerebral gummas (plasma cell-rich mass lesions) may also occur in the meninges and extend into the parenchyma.
- **Paretic neurosyphilis** is caused by invasion of the brain by *T. pallidum* and is clinically manifested as insidious but progressive cognitive impairment associated with mood alterations (including delusions of grandeur) that terminate in severe dementia **(general paresis of the insane)**. Parenchymal damage of the cerebral cortex is particularly common in the frontal lobe but also occurs in other areas of the isocortex. The lesions are characterized by loss of neurons, proliferation of microglia (rod cells), gliosis, and iron deposits. The latter are demonstrable with the Prussian blue stain perivascularly and in the neuropil, and are presumably the sequelae of small bleeds stemming from damage to the microcirculation. The spirochetes can, at times, be demonstrated in tissue sections.
- **Tabes dorsalis** is the result of damage to the sensory axons in the dorsal roots. This causes impaired joint position sense and ataxia (locomotor ataxia); loss of pain sensation, leading to skin and joint damage (Charcot joints); other sensory disturbances, particularly the characteristic "lightning pains"; and absence of deep tendon reflexes. On microscopic examination there is loss of both axons and myelin in the dorsal roots, with corresponding pallor and atrophy in the dorsal columns of the spinal cord. Organisms are not demonstrable in the cord lesions.

Neuroborreliosis (Lyme Disease)

Lyme disease is caused by the spirochete *Borrelia burgdorferi,* which is transmitted by various species of *Ixodes* tick (Chapter 8). Involvement of the nervous system is referred to as *neuroborreliosis*. Neurologic symptoms are highly variable and include aseptic meningitis, facial nerve palsies and other polyneuropathies, as well as encephalopathy. The rare cases that have come to autopsy have shown a focal proliferation of microglial cells in the brain as well as scattered extracellular organisms.

Viral Meningoencephalitis

Viral encephalitis is a parenchymal infection of the brain almost invariably associated with meningeal inflammation (meningoencephalitis) and sometimes with simultaneous involvement of the spinal cord (encephalomyelitis).

Some viruses have a propensity to infect the nervous system. Such neural tropism takes several forms: some infect specific cell types (e.g., oligodendrocytes), while others preferentially involve particular areas of the brain (e.g., medial temporal lobes or the limbic system). Latency is an important phase of several viral infections of the CNS (e.g., herpes zoster, progressive multifocal leukoencephalopathy). Systemic viral infections in the absence of direct evidence of viral penetration into the CNS may be followed by an immune-mediated disease, such as perivenous demyelination (see "Acute Disseminated Encephalomyelitis and Acute Necrotizing Hemorrhagic Encephalomyelitis"). Intrauterine viral infection may cause congenital malformations, as occurs with rubella. A slowly progressive degenerative disease syndrome may follow many years after a viral illness; an example is postencephalitic parkinsonism after the 1918 viral influenza pandemic.

Arthropod-Borne Viral Encephalitis

Arboviruses are an important cause of epidemic encephalitis, especially in tropical regions of the world, and they are capable of causing serious morbidity and high mortality. In the Western hemisphere the most important types are Eastern and Western equine, West Nile, Venezuelan, St. Louis, and La Crosse; elsewhere in the world, pathogenic arboviruses include Japanese B (Far East), Murray Valley (Australia and New Guinea), and tick-borne (Russia and Eastern Europe).

All these viruses have animal hosts and insect vectors. Clinically, affected individuals develop generalized neurologic deficits, such as seizures, confusion, delirium, and stupor or coma, as well as focal signs, such as reflex asymmetry and ocular palsies. Involvement of the spinal cord in West Nile encephalitis can lead to a polio-like syndrome with paralysis. In general, the CSF is usually colorless, with slightly elevated pressure, an elevated protein level, and a normal glucose. Initially the CSF exhibits a neutrophilic pleocytosis, but this rapidly converts to a lymphocytosis.

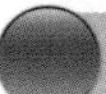

MORPHOLOGY

The encephalitides caused by various arboviruses produce similar histopathologic changes that differ only in severity and extent. Characteristically, there is a meningoencephalitis marked by the perivascular accumulation of lymphocytes (and sometimes with neutrophils) (Fig. 28-23*A*). Multiple foci of necrosis of gray and white matter are found; in particular, there is evidence of single-cell neuronal necrosis with phagocytosis of the debris **(neuronophagia)**. Microglial cells form small aggregates around foci of necrosis, called **microglial nodules** (Fig. 28-23*B*). In severe cases there may be a necrotizing vasculitis with associated focal hemorrhages. While some viruses declare their presence by formation of intracellular inclusion bodies, the causative virus is most often identified by a combination of ultrastructural, immunohistochemical, and molecular methods.

Herpes Simplex Virus Type 1

Herpes simplex virus type 1 (HSV-1) encephalitis occurs most commonly in children and young adults. Only about 10% of the affected individuals have a history of prior herpetic infection. The typical presenting symptoms are alterations in mood, memory, and behavior. Polymerase chain reaction (PCR)-based methods for virus detection in CSF samples have increased the ease of diagnosis and the recognition of a subset of patients with less severe disease. Antiviral agents now provide effective treatment in many cases, with a significant reduction in the mortality rate. In some individuals, HSV-1 encephalitis follows a subacute

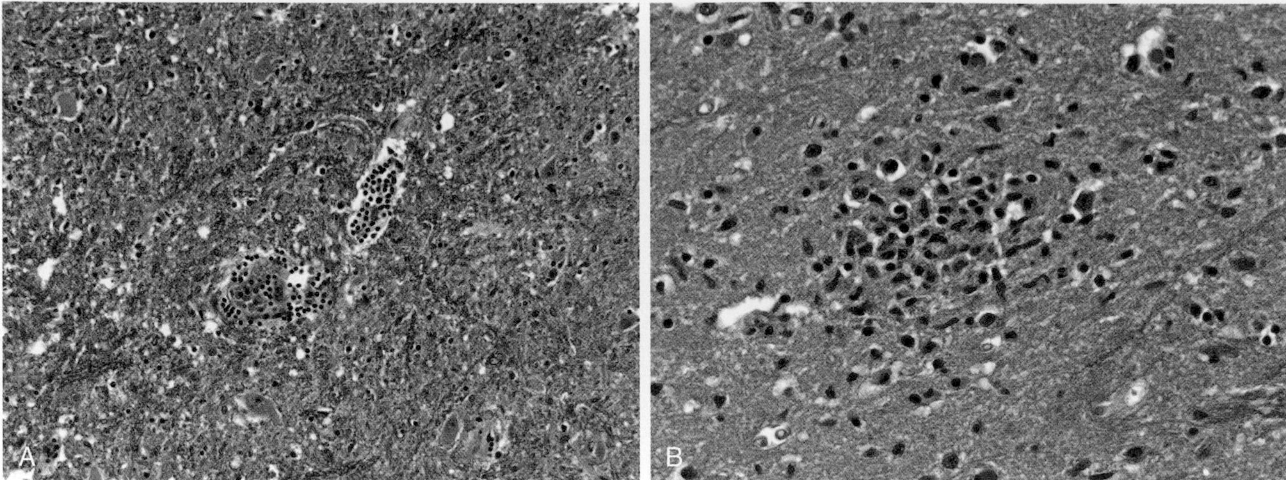

Figure 28-23 Characteristic findings of viral encephalitis include perivascular cuffs of lymphocytes **(A)** and microglial nodules **(B)**.

course with clinical manifestations (weakness, lethargy, ataxia, seizures) that evolve during a more protracted period (4 to 6 weeks). Recently, an increased incidence of HSV encephalitis has been observed in patients with rare inherited loss-of-function mutations in the TLR3 signaling pathway, supporting a role for Toll-like receptor signaling in the control of HSV infections.

MORPHOLOGY

This encephalitis starts in and most severely involves the inferior and medial regions of the temporal lobes and the orbital gyri of the frontal lobes (Fig. 28-24). The infection is necrotizing and often hemorrhagic in the most severely affected regions. Perivascular inflammatory infiltrates are usually present, and Cowdry type A intranuclear viral inclusion bodies may be found in both neurons and glia. In individuals with slowly evolving HSV-1 encephalitis, there is more diffuse involvement of the brain.

Herpes Simplex Virus Type 2

Herpes simplex virus type 2 (HSV-2) can infect the nervous system. In adults it causes meningitis, but as many as 50% of neonates born by vaginal delivery to women with active primary HSV genital infections acquire the infection during passage through the birth canal and develop severe encephalitis. In individuals with active HIV infection, HSV-2 may cause an acute hemorrhagic and necrotizing encephalitis.

Varicella-Zoster Virus (Herpes Zoster)

Primary infection with varicella causes one of the childhood exanthems (chickenpox), ordinarily without evidence of neurologic involvement. Following the cutaneous infection, the virus enters a latent phase within sensory neurons of the dorsal root or trigeminal ganglia. Reactivation of infection in adults (*shingles*) usually manifests as a painful, vesicular skin eruption confined to one or several dermatomes. Herpes zoster reactivation is typically self-limited,

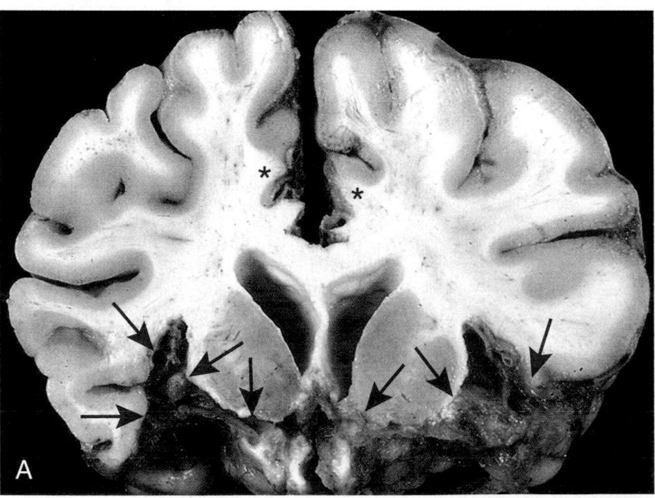

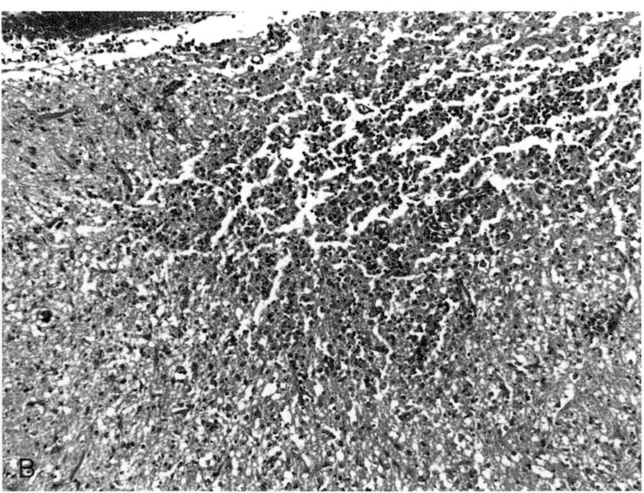

Figure 28-24 **A,** Herpes encephalitis showing extensive destruction of inferior frontal and anterior temporal lobes (*arrows*) and the cingulate gyri (*asterisks*). **B,** Necrotizing inflammatory process characterizes acute herpes encephalitis. (**A,** Courtesy Dr. T. W. Smith, University of Massachusetts Medical School, Worcester, Mass.)

but there may be a postherpetic neuralgia syndrome (particularly after age 60 years) characterized by persistent pain, sometimes induced by stimuli that are otherwise not painful.

Overt CNS involvement by herpes zoster is much rarer, but can be severe. Herpes zoster can cause a granulomatous arteritis. In immunosuppressed individuals, herpes zoster may cause acute encephalitis characterized by numerous sharply circumscribed demyelinating lesions that subsequently undergo necrosis.

Cytomegalovirus

CMV infection of the nervous system occurs in fetuses and immunosuppressed individuals. The outcome of infection in utero is periventricular necrosis that produces severe brain destruction followed later by microcephaly and periventricular calcification. CMV is a common opportunistic viral pathogen in individuals with AIDS, with CNS involvement also occurring in this setting.

MORPHOLOGY

In the immunosuppressed individual, CMV most commonly causes subacute encephalitis, which may be associated with CMV inclusion-bearing cells (see Fig. 8-15). The infection tends to localize in the paraventricular subependymal regions of the brain, where it results in a severe hemorrhagic necrotizing ventriculoencephalitis and a choroid plexitis. The virus can also attack the lower spinal cord and roots, producing a painful radiculoneuritis. Any cell in the CNS (neurons, glia, ependyma, or endothelium) may be infected. Prominent enlarged cells with intranuclear and intracytoplasmic inclusions can be readily identified by conventional light microscopy and CMV infection is confirmed by immunohistochemistry.

Poliomyelitis

While paralytic poliomyelitis has been eradicated by vaccination in many parts of the world, there are still a few countries where it remains a serious problem. In nonimmunized individuals poliovirus infection causes a subclinical or mild gastroenteritis, similar to that caused by other members of the picornavirus group of enteroviruses. In a small fraction of the vulnerable population, however, the virus secondarily invades the nervous system.

MORPHOLOGY

Acute cases show mononuclear cell perivascular cuffs and neuronophagia of the **anterior horn motor neurons of the spinal cord**. The inflammatory reaction is usually confined to the anterior horns but may extend into the posterior horns, and the damage is occasionally severe enough to produce cavitation. Poliovirus RNA has been detected in anterior horn cell motor neurons. The cranial motor nuclei are sometimes involved as well. Postmortem examination in long-term survivors of symptomatic poliomyelitis shows loss of neurons and gliosis in the affected anterior horns of the spinal cord, some residual inflammation, atrophy of the anterior (motor) spinal roots, and neurogenic atrophy of denervated muscle.

Clinical Features. CNS infection manifests initially with meningeal irritation and a CSF picture consistent with aseptic meningitis. The disease may progress no further or advance to involve the spinal cord. When the disease affects the motor neurons of the spinal cord, it produces a flaccid paralysis associated with muscle wasting and hyporeflexia in the corresponding region of the body—the permanent neurologic residue of poliomyelitis. Because of the destruction of motor neurons, paresis or paralysis follows; when the diaphragm and intercostal muscles are affected, severe respiratory compromise and even death may occur. A myocarditis sometimes complicates the acute infection. *Postpolio syndrome* can develop in patients 25 to 35 years after the resolution of the initial illness. It is characterized by progressive weakness associated with decreased muscle mass and pain, and has been attributed to superimposed neuronal loss of aging with inflammatory mechanisms, but without any convincing evidence of viral re-activation.

Rabies

Rabies is severe encephalitis transmitted to humans by the bite of a rabid animal, usually a dog or various wild mammals that are natural reservoirs. Exposure to certain species of bats, even without a known bite, can also lead to rabies.

MORPHOLOGY

External examination of the brain shows intense edema and vascular congestion. Microscopically, there is widespread neuronal degeneration and an inflammatory reaction that is most severe in the brainstem. The basal ganglia, spinal cord, and dorsal root ganglia may also be involved. **Negri bodies,** the pathognomonic microscopic finding, are cytoplasmic, round to oval, eosinophilic inclusions that can be found in pyramidal neurons of the hippocampus and Purkinje cells of the cerebellum, sites usually devoid of inflammation (Fig. 28-25). Rabies virus can be detected within Negri bodies by ultrastructural and immunohistochemical methods.

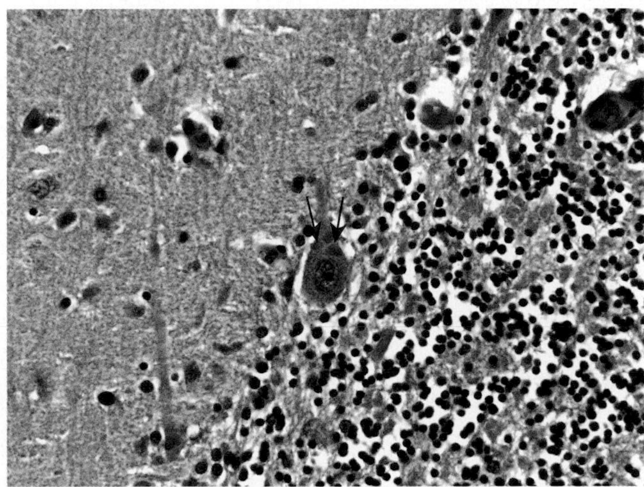

Figure 28-25 The diagnostic histologic finding in rabies is the eosinophilic Negri body, as seen here in a Purkinje cell *(arrows)*.

Clinical Features. Since the virus enters the CNS by ascending along the peripheral nerves from the wound site, the incubation period (usually between 1 and 3 months) depends on the distance between the wound and the brain. The disease begins with nonspecific symptoms such as malaise, headache, and fever, but the conjunction of these symptoms with local paresthesias around the wound is diagnostic. As the infection advances, the affected individual exhibits extraordinary CNS excitability; the slightest touch is painful and produces violent motor responses or even convulsions. Contracture of the pharyngeal musculature on swallowing produces foaming at the mouth, which may create an aversion to swallowing even water (hydrophobia). There are signs of meningeal irritation and, as the disease progresses, flaccid paralysis. Alternating periods of mania and stupor progress to coma and eventually death from respiratory failure.

Human Immunodeficiency Virus

In the period before the availability of effective antiretroviral therapy, neuropathologic changes were demonstrated at postmortem examination in as many as 80% to 90% of cases of AIDS. These changes stem from direct effects of virus on the nervous system, opportunistic infections, and primary CNS lymphoma, a high fraction of which were EBV-positive B cell tumors. There has been a decrease in the frequency of these secondary effects of HIV infection thanks to the efficacy of multidrug antiretroviral therapy.

HIV aseptic meningitis occurs within 1 to 2 weeks of seroconversion in about 10% of patients; antibodies to HIV can be demonstrated and the virus can be isolated from the CSF. The neuropathologic studies of the early, acute phases of HIV invasion of the CNS have shown mild lymphocytic meningitis, perivascular inflammation, and some myelin loss. Among CNS cell types only microglia express both the CD4 coreceptor and the chemokine receptors (CCR5 or CXCR4) that are required in combination for efficient infection by HIV. During the chronic phase, HIV encephalitis is commonly found when symptomatic individuals come to autopsy.

An "immune reconstitution inflammatory syndrome" (IRIS) has been identified in patients with AIDS after effective treatment; the syndrome is recognized as a paradoxical deterioration after starting therapy, and consists of an exuberant "reconstituted" inflammatory response while on antiretroviral therapy (Chapter 6). In the CNS, IRIS has caused paradoxical exacerbation of symptoms from opportunistic infections. Neuropathologic studies confirm intense inflammation with an influx of CD8+ lymphocytes.

MORPHOLOGY

HIV encephalitis is a chronic inflammatory reaction associated with widely distributed **microglial nodules**, often containing macrophage-derived **multinucleated giant cells**; foci of tissue necrosis and reactive gliosis are sometimes seen together with these lesions (Fig. 28-26). Some of the microglial nodules are found near small blood vessels, which show abnormally prominent endothelial cells and perivascular foamy or pigment-laden macrophages. These changes are especially prominent in the subcortical white matter, diencephalon, and brainstem. In some cases there is also a disorder of white matter characterized by multifocal or diffuse areas of myelin pallor, axonal swelling and gliosis. HIV can be detected in CD4+ mononuclear and multinucleated macrophages and microglia.

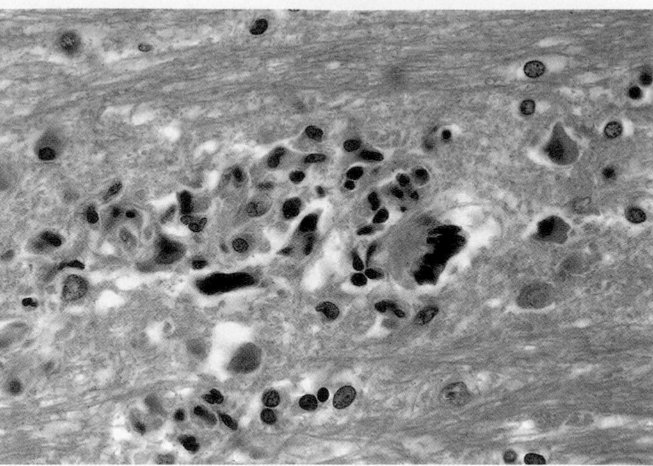

Figure 28-26 HIV encephalitis. Note the microglial nodule and multinucleated giant cells.

Cognitive changes, some mild and others florid enough to be termed *HIV-associated dementia*, appear to have persisted in the era of effective anti-HIV treatment regimens. Rather than having a specific pathologic lesion as its correlate, this disorder is most closely related to inflammatory activation of microglial cells, not all of which are necessarily HIV-infected. A wide range of possible mechanisms for neuronal dysfunction and injury in this setting have been proposed, including the actions of inflammatory cytokines and a cascade of toxic effects of HIV-derived proteins; in all probability, both have contributory roles in the pathogenesis of brain injury (Chapter 6).

Progressive Multifocal Leukoencephalopathy

Progressive multifocal leukoencephalopathy (PML) is an encephalitis caused by the JC polyomavirus; because the virus preferentially infects oligodendrocytes, demyelination is its principal pathologic effect. The disease occurs almost exclusively in immunosuppressed individuals in various clinical settings, including chronic lymphoproliferative or myeloproliferative illnesses, immunosuppressive chemotherapy including monoclonal antibody therapy targeting integrins, granulomatous diseases, and AIDS.

Although most people have serologic evidence of exposure to JC virus by the age of 14 years, primary infection is asymptomatic. PML results from the reactivation of virus in the setting of immunosuppression. Clinically, affected individuals develop focal and relentlessly progressive

MORPHOLOGY

The lesions consist of patches of irregular, ill-defined white matter injury that range in size from millimeters to near confluent involvement of large regions of the brain (Fig. 28-27). Microscopically, individual lesions show an area of demyelination, most often in a subcortical location, in the center of which are scattered lipid-laden macrophages and a reduced number of axons. Particularly at the edge of the lesion are greatly

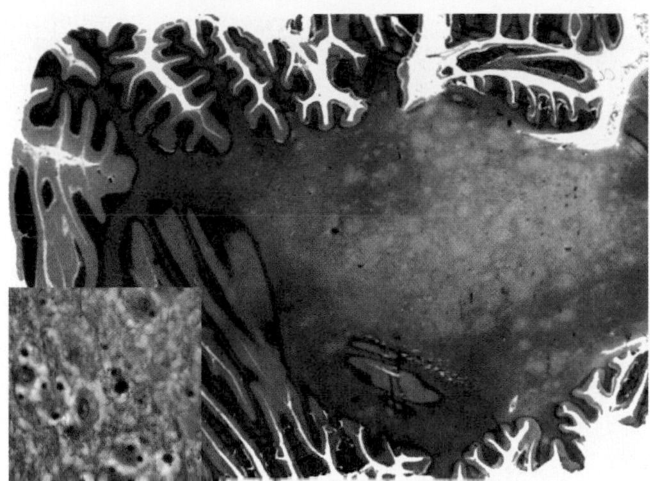

Figure 28-27 Progressive multifocal leukoencephalopathy. Section stained for myelin showing irregular, poorly defined areas of demyelination, which become confluent in places. *Inset*, Enlarged oligodendrocyte nucleus represents the effect of viral infection.

enlarged oligodendrocyte nuclei containing glassy amphophilic viral inclusions (Fig. 28-27, *inset*), which can be identified by immunohistochemistry. Within the lesions, there may be bizarre giant astrocytes with one to several irregular, hyperchromatic nuclei mixed with more typical reactive astrocytes. Infection of granule cell neurons in the cerebellum been demonstrated in rare instances.

neurologic symptoms and signs, and imaging studies show extensive, often multifocal, lesions in the hemispheric or cerebellar white matter.

Subacute Sclerosing Panencephalitis

Subacute sclerosing panencephalitis (SSPE) is a rare progressive clinical syndrome characterized by cognitive decline, spasticity of limbs, and seizures. It occurs in children or young adults, months or years after an initial, early-age acute infection with measles. The disease stems from persistent, but nonproductive, infection of the CNS by an altered measles virus; changes in several viral genes have been associated with the disease. It is characterized by widespread gliosis and myelin degeneration; viral inclusions, largely within the nuclei of oligodendrocytes and neurons; variable inflammation of white and gray matter; and neurofibrillary tangles. Ultrastructural study shows that the inclusions contain nucleocapsids characteristic of measles and immunohistochemistry for measles virus antigen is positive. The incidence of the disease has fallen sharply due to vaccination programs, but it persists in nonimmunized populations.

Fungal Meningoencephalitis

Fungal infections of the CNS are encountered primarily in immunocompromised individuals. The brain is usually involved following widespread hematogenous dissemination of fungi; the most frequent offenders are *Candida albicans*, Mucor species, *Aspergillus fumigatus*, and *Cryptococcus neoformans*. In endemic areas, pathogens such as *Histoplasma capsulatum*, *Coccidioides immitis*, and *Blastomyces dermatitidis* may involve the CNS after a primary pulmonary or cutaneous infection; again, this often follows immunosuppression. Although most fungi reach the brain by hematogenous dissemination, direct extension may also occur, particularly in mucormycosis in the setting of diabetes mellitus.

The three main forms of injury in fungal infection in the CNS are chronic meningitis, vasculitis, and parenchymal invasion. Vasculitis is most frequently seen with *Mucormycosis* and *Aspergillosis*, both of which directly invade blood vessel walls, but it occasionally occurs with other infections such as candidiasis. The resultant vascular thrombosis produces infarction that is often strikingly hemorrhagic and that subsequently becomes septic from ingrowth of the causative fungus.

Parenchymal infection, usually in the form of granulomas or abscesses, can occur with most of the fungi and often coexists with meningitis. The most commonly encountered fungi that invade the brain are *Candida* and *Cryptococcus*. Candidiasis usually produces multiple microabscesses, with or without granuloma formation.

Cryptococcal meningitis, a common opportunistic infection in the setting of AIDS, may be fulminant and fatal in as little as 2 weeks or indolent, evolving over months or years. The CSF may contain few cells but usually has a high concentration of protein. The mucoid-encapsulated yeasts can be visualized in the CSF with special stains or detected indirectly using assays for cryptococcal antigens.

MORPHOLOGY

With cryptococcal infection, there is a chronic meningitis affecting the basal leptomeninges, which are opaque and thickened by reactive connective tissue that may obstruct the outflow of CSF from the foramina of Luschka and Magendie, giving rise to hydrocephalus. Sections of the brain disclose a gelatinous material within the subarachnoid space and small cysts within the parenchyma ("soap bubbles"), which are especially prominent in the basal ganglia in the distribution of the lenticulostriate arteries (Fig. 28-28*A*). Parenchymal lesions consist of aggregates of organisms within expanded perivascular (Virchow-Robin) spaces associated with minimal or absent inflammation or gliosis (Fig. 28-28*B*). The meningeal infiltrates consist of chronic inflammatory cells and fibroblasts admixed with cryptococci.

Other Infectious Diseases of the Nervous System

Protozoal diseases (including malaria, toxoplasmosis, amebiasis, and trypanosomiasis), rickettsial infections (e.g., typhus and Rocky Mountain spotted fever), and metazoal diseases (especially cysticercosis and echinococcosis) may also involve the CNS and are discussed in Chapter 8.

- *Cerebral toxoplasmosis* is an opportunistic infection commonly found in the setting of HIV-associated immunosuppression. The clinical symptoms of infection of the brain by *Toxoplasma gondii* are subacute, evolving during a 1- or 2-week period, and may be both focal

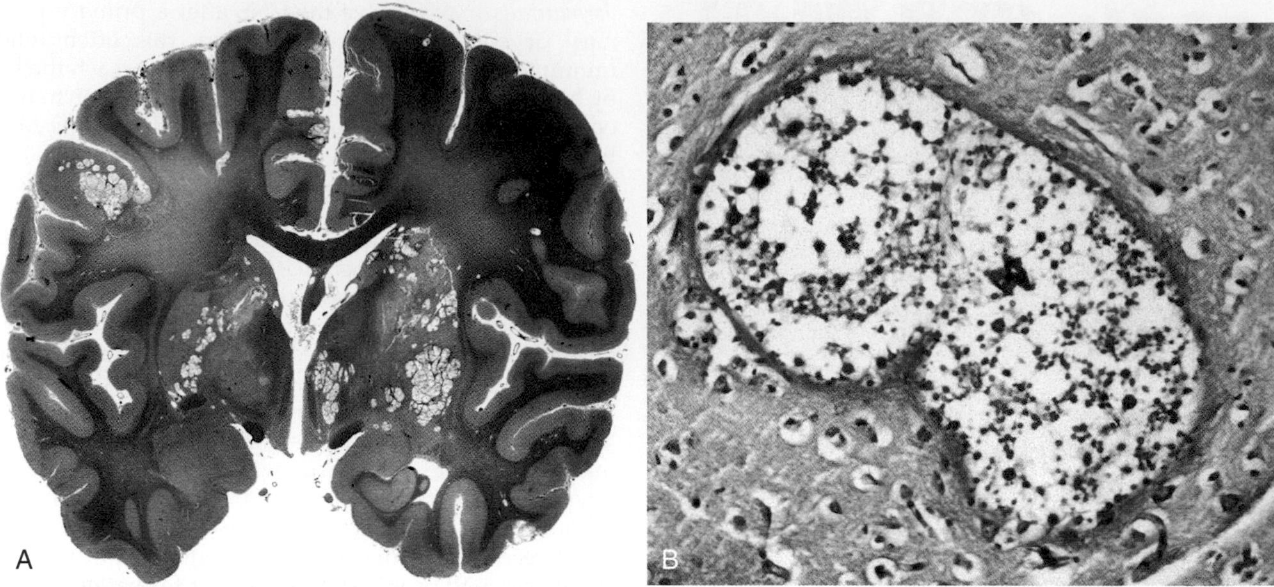

Figure 28-28 Cryptococcal infection. **A,** Whole-brain section showing the numerous areas of tissue destruction ("soap bubbles") associated with the spread of organisms in the perivascular spaces. **B,** At higher magnification it is possible to see the cryptococci in the lesions.

and diffuse. Computed tomography and magnetic resonance imaging studies may show multiple ring-enhancing lesions; however, this radiographic appearance is not specific, as CNS lymphoma, tuberculosis, and fungal infections produce similar findings. In non-immunosuppressed hosts, the impact of toxoplasmosis on the brain is most often seen when primary maternal infection occurs early in pregnancy. Such infections often spread to the brain of the developing fetus and cause severe damage in the form of multifocal necrotizing lesions that may calcify.

MORPHOLOGY

Toxoplasmosis of the CNS produces brain abscesses, which are found most often in the cerebral cortex (near the gray-white junction) and deep gray nuclei, less often in the cerebellum and brainstem, and rarely in the spinal cord (Fig. 28-29). Acute lesions exhibit central necrosis, petechial hemorrhages surrounded by acute and chronic inflammation, macrophage infiltration, and vascular proliferation. Both free tachyzoites and encysted bradyzoites (Fig. 28-29*B*) may be found at the periphery of the necrotic foci. The organisms are often seen on routine hematoxylin and eosin (H & E) or Giemsa stains, but are more easily recognized by immunohistochemical methods. The blood vessels near these lesions may show marked intimal proliferation or even frank vasculitis with fibrinoid necrosis and thrombosis. After treatment, the lesions consist of large, well-demarcated areas of coagulative necrosis surrounded by lipid-laden macrophages. Cysts and free tachyzoites can also be found adjacent to these lesions but may be considerably reduced in number or absent if effective therapy has been received. Chronic lesions consist of small cystic spaces containing scattered lipid- and hemosiderin-laden macrophages that are surrounded by gliotic brain. Organisms are difficult to detect in these older lesions.

- *Cerebral amebiasis.* A rapidly fatal necrotizing encephalitis results from infection with *Naegleria* species, and a chronic granulomatous meningoencephalitis has been associated with infection with *Acanthamoeba.* The amebae may be difficult to distinguish morphologically from activated macrophages (Fig. 28-30). Methenamine silver or PAS stains are helpful in visualizing the organisms, although definitive identification ultimately depends on immunofluorescence studies, culture, and molecular methods.
- *Cerebral malaria.* A rapidly progressive encephalitis, cerebral malaria is the complication of infection by *Plasmodium falciparum* with the highest mortality. Most likely the result of vascular dysfunction, cerebral involvement by malaria is accompanied by reduced cerebral blood flow and results in ataxia, seizures, and coma in the acute phase, with long-term cognitive deficits in up to 20% of children after cerebral malaria (Chapter 8).

KEY CONCEPTS

Infections

- Pathogens from viruses through parasites can infect the brain. Different pathogens use distinct routes to reach the brain and cause different patterns of disease.
- Routes of access of organisms to the brain include: hematogenous spread (e.g., abscess formation in the setting of endocarditis), direct extension (following trauma or with extension from the sinuses with Mucor) and retrograde transport along nerves (as with rabies).
- Bacterial infections may cause meningitis, cerebral abscesses, or a chronic meningoencephalitis. The distribution of pathogens is influenced by various host factors, such as age and level of immune function.
- Viral infections can cause meningitis or meningoencephalitis. Some viruses have characteristic patterns of

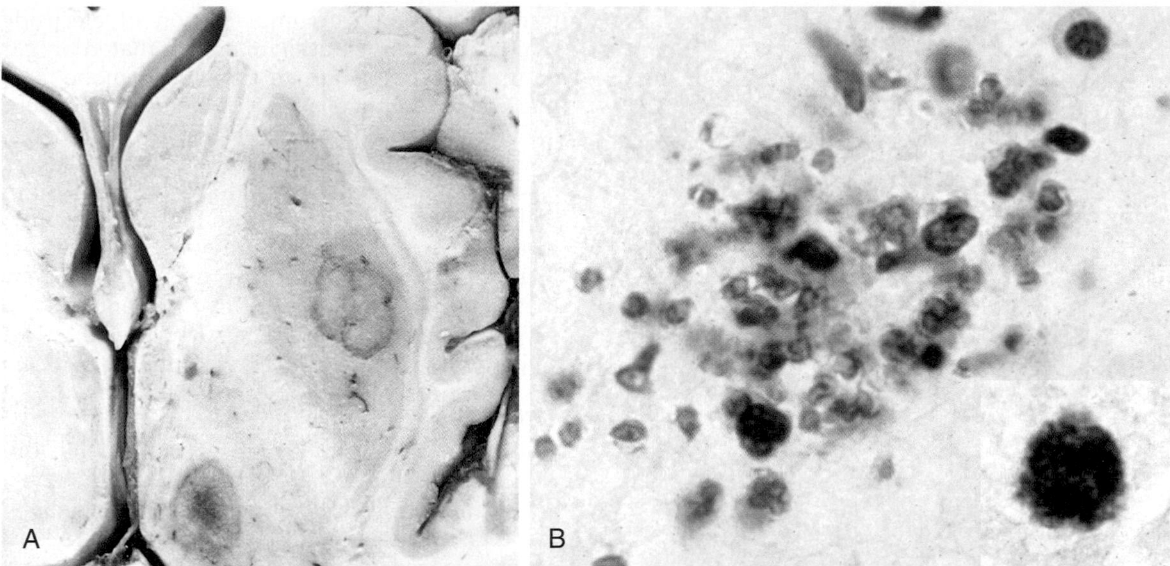

Figure 28-29 **A,** *Toxoplasma* abscesses in the putamen and thalamus. **B,** Free tachyzoites demonstrated by immunostaining; *inset*: *Toxoplasma* pseudocyst with bradyzoites highlighted by immunostaining.

infection (HSV-1 in the temporal lobes, polio in anterior horn).

- HIV can directly cause meningoencephalitis, or indirectly affect the brain by increasing the risk of opportunistic infections (toxoplasmosis, CMV) or EBV-positive CNS lymphoma.

Prion Diseases

Prions are abnormal forms of a cellular protein that cause rapidly progressive neurodegenerative disorders that may be sporadic, familial or transmitted. This group of diseases includes Creutzfeldt-Jakob disease, Gerstmann-Sträussler-Scheinker syndrome, fatal familial insomnia, and kuru in humans; scrapie in sheep and goats; mink-transmissible encephalopathy; chronic wasting disease of deer and elk; and bovine spongiform encephalopathy. These disorders share an etiologic basis as they are all associated with abnormal forms of a specific protein termed *prion protein* (PrP). They are all characterized morphologically by "spongiform change" caused by intracellular vacuoles in neurons and glia, and clinically by a rapidly progressive dementia.

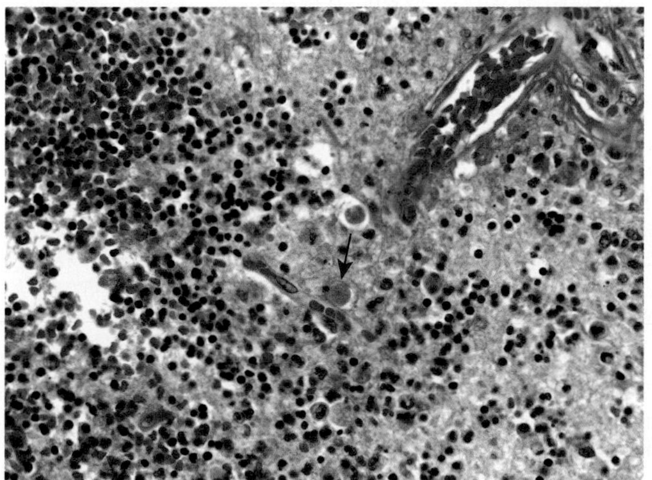

Figure 28-30 Necrotizing amebic meningoencephalitis involving the cerebellum (organism highlighted by *arrow*).

Pathogenesis and Molecular Genetics. **Prion diseases are conceptually important because they exemplify degenerative disorders that are caused by "spreading" of misfolded proteins, a remarkable phenomenon that allows a pathogenic protein to acquire many of the characteristics of an infectious organism.** Normal PrP is a 30-kD cytoplasmic protein present in neurons. Disease occurs when PrP undergoes a conformational change from its normal α-helix-containing isoform (PrP^c) to an abnormal β-pleated sheet isoform, usually termed PrP^{sc} (for scrapie) (Fig. 28-31). Associated with the conformational change, PrP acquires resistance to digestion with proteases, such as proteinase K. Accumulation of PrP^{sc} in neural tissue seems to be the cause of the pathologic changes in these diseases, but how this material induces the development of cytoplasmic vacuoles and eventual neuronal death is still unknown. Western blotting of tissue extracts after partial digestion with proteinase K allows detection of PrP^{sc}, which is diagnostic.

The conformational change resulting in PrP^{sc} may occur spontaneously at an extremely low rate (resulting in sporadic cases) or at a higher rate if various mutations are present in PrP^c, such as occurs in familial forms of Creutzfeldt-Jakob disease (CJD) and in Gerstmann-Sträussler-Scheinker syndrome (GSS) and fatal familial insomnia (FFI). PrP^{sc}, independent of the means by which it originates, then facilitates, in a cooperative fashion, the conversion of other PrP^c molecules to PrP^{sc} molecules. It is this propagation of PrP^{sc} that accounts for the transmissible nature of prion diseases. This capacity for a protein in an abnormal conformation to induce similar structural change in other molecules as a self-propagating process has recently been demonstrated for many of the aggregating proteins associated with traditional neurodegenerative diseases. The suggestion that, at least within an individual, there may be

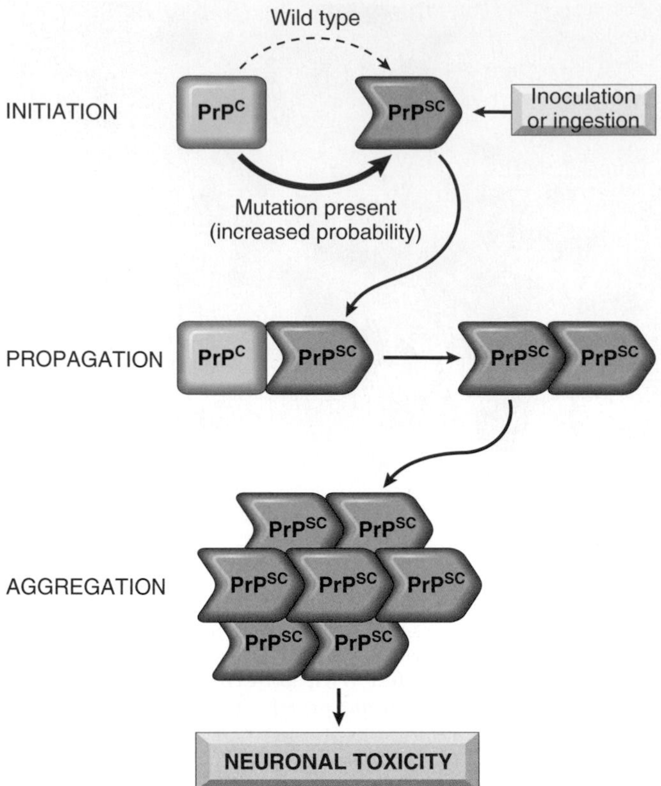

Figure 28-31 Pathogenesis of prion disease. α-helical PrP^{c} may spontaneously shift to the β-sheet PrP^{sc} conformation, an event that occurs at a much higher rate in familial disease associated with germ line PrP mutations. PrP^{sc} may also be acquired from exogenous sources, such as contaminated food, medical instrumentation, or medicines. Once present, PrP^{sc} converts additional molecules of PrP^{c} into PrP^{sc} through physical interaction, eventually leading to the formation of pathogenic PrP^{sc} aggregates.

cell-to-cell spread of disease-associated protein aggregates provides a link between prion diseases and other disorders such as Alzheimer disease and Parkinson disease.

The gene encoding PrP, termed *PRNP*, shows a high degree of conservation across species. A variety of mutations in *PRNP* have been found to underlie familial forms of prion diseases. In addition, a polymorphism at codon 129 that encodes either methionine (Met) or valine (Val) influences development of the disease: individuals who are homozygous for either Met or Val are overrepresented among cases of CJD compared with the general population, implying that heterozygosity at codon 129 is protective against development of the disease. The same protective effect of heterozygosity at codon 129 is observed for iatrogenic CJD (mostly cases that followed exposure to naturally derived pituitary hormone replacement).

Creutzfeldt-Jakob Disease (CJD)

Although the most common prion disease, CJD is a rare disorder that manifests clinically as a rapidly progressive dementia. The sporadic form of CJD has an annual incidence of approximately 1 per 1,000,000 people and accounts for about 90% of cases; familial forms are caused by mutations in *PRNP*. The disease has a peak incidence in the seventh decade. There are also well-established cases of iatrogenic transmission, notably by corneal transplantation, deep implantation of electrodes in the brain, and administration of contaminated preparations of naturally derived human growth hormone. The onset is marked by subtle changes in memory and behavior followed by a rapidly progressive dementia, often associated with pronounced involuntary jerking muscle contractions on sudden stimulation (startle myoclonus). Signs of cerebellar dysfunction, usually manifested as ataxia, are present in a minority of affected individuals. The disease is uniformly fatal. The average survival is only 7 months after the onset of symptoms. A few patients have lived for several years, and these long-surviving cases show extensive atrophy of involved gray matter.

Variant Creutzfeldt-Jakob Disease

Starting in 1995, a series of cases of a CJD-like illness came to medical attention in the United Kingdom. This illness was different from typical CJD in several important respects: the disease affected young adults, behavioral disorders figured prominently in the early stages of the disease, and the neurologic syndrome progressed more slowly than in individuals with other forms of CJD. The neuropathologic findings and molecular features of these new cases were similar to those of CJD, suggesting a close relationship between the two illnesses, with multiple lines of evidence indicating that the new variant form of CJD was linked to exposure to bovine spongiform encephalopathy. Pathologically, variant CJD (vCJD) is characterized by the presence of extensive cortical plaques surrounded by a "halo" of spongiform change. No alterations in the *PRNP* gene are present and the disease appears to be limited to date to codon 129 Met/Met homozygotes. Onset of vCJD is linked to consumption of the bovine spongiform encephalopathy agent in contaminated foods or blood transfusion, raising significant public health issues.

MORPHOLOGY

The progression of the dementia in CJD is usually so rapid that there is little if any grossly evident brain atrophy. The pathognomonic finding is a **spongiform** transformation of the cerebral cortex and, often, deep gray matter structures (caudate, putamen); this multifocal process results in the uneven formation of small, apparently empty, microscopic vacuoles of varying sizes within the neuropil and sometimes in the perikaryon of neurons (Fig. 28-32*A*). In advanced cases there is severe neuronal loss, reactive gliosis, and sometimes expansion of the vacuolated areas into cystlike spaces ("status spongiosus"). Inflammation is notably absent. Electron microscopy shows the vacuoles to be membrane-bound and located within the cytoplasm of neuronal processes. **Kuru plaques** are extracellular deposits of aggregated abnormal protein; they are Congo red- and PAS-positive and usually occur in the cerebellum (Fig. 28-32*B*), but are abundant in the cerebral cortex in cases of vCJD (Fig. 28-32*C*). In all forms of prion disease, immunohistochemical staining demonstrates the presence of proteinase K-resistant PrP^{sc} in tissue.

Fatal Familial Insomnia (FFI)

Fatal familial insomnia (FFI), named in part for the sleep disturbances that characterize its initial stages, is also

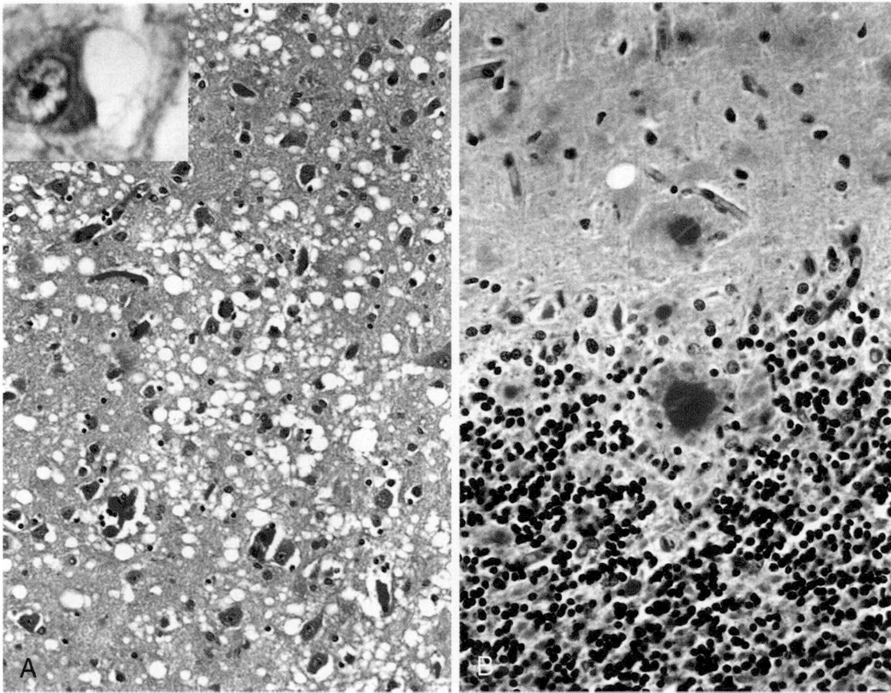
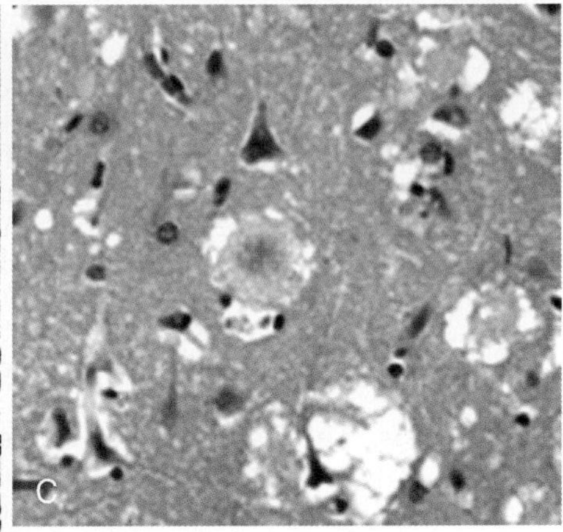

Figure 28-32 Prion disease. **A,** Spongiform change in the cerebral cortex. *Inset*, High magnification of neuron with vacuoles. **B,** Cerebellar cortex showing *kuru plaques* (periodic acid-Schiff stain) representing aggregated PrP^{sc}. **C,** Cortical plaques surrounded by spongiform change in vCJD.

caused by a specific mutation in the *PRNP* gene. The mutation, which leads to an aspartate substitution for asparagine at residue 178 of PrP^{c}, results in FFI when it occurs in a *PRNP* allele encoding methionine at codon 129, but causes CJD when present in tandem with a valine at this

MORPHOLOGY

Unlike other prion diseases, FFI does not show spongiform pathology. Instead, the most striking alteration is neuronal loss and reactive gliosis in the anterior ventral and dorsomedial nuclei of the thalamus; neuronal loss is also prominent in the inferior olivary nuclei. Proteinase K-resistant PrP^{sc} can be detected by immunostaining or western blotting.

KEY CONCEPTS

Prion Diseases

- Prion diseases may be sporadic, familial or transmissible (infectious). The disease is driven by the conversion of a normal cellular protein (PrP^{c}) into an abnormal conformation (PrP^{sc}), with the acquisition of distinct characteristics including relative resistance to protease digestion, self-propagation, and the ability to spread..
- Familial forms of these diseases are linked to mutations in the gene encoding PrP^{c} (*PRNP*). A polymorphic locus in *PRNP* (codon 129 may be either Met or Val) determines disease phenotype, with homozygosity at this site increasing risk of sporadic disease.
- Disease phenotypes include Creutzfeldt-Jakob disease (rapidly progressive dementia), Gerstmann-Sträussler-Scheinker syndrome (progressive cerebellar ataxia) and fatal familial insomnia.

position. How these amino acids influence disease phenotype is not understood. In the course of the illness, which typically lasts fewer than 3 years, affected individuals develop other neurologic signs, such as ataxia, autonomic disturbances, stupor, and finally coma. A noninherited form of the disorder (fatal sporadic insomnia) has also been described.

Demyelinating Diseases

Demyelinating diseases of the CNS are acquired conditions characterized by preferential damage to myelin with relative preservation of axons. The clinical deficits are due to the effect of myelin loss on the transmission of electrical impulses along axons. The natural history of demyelinating diseases is determined, in part, by the limited capacity of the CNS to regenerate normal myelin and by the degree of secondary damage to axons that occurs as the disease runs its course.

Several pathologic processes can cause loss of myelin. These include immune-mediated destruction of myelin, as in multiple sclerosis, and infections. In progressive multifocal leukoencephalopathy, JC virus infection of oligodendrocytes results in loss of myelin (described earlier). In addition, inherited disorders may affect synthesis or turnover of myelin components; these are termed *leukodystrophies* and are discussed with metabolic disorders.

Multiple Sclerosis

Multiple sclerosis (MS) is an autoimmune demyelinating disorder characterized by distinct episodes of neurologic deficits, separated in time, attributable to white matter lesions that are separated in space. It is the most common of the demyelinating disorders, having a prevalence of approximately 1 per 1000 persons in most of the United States and Europe. The disease may become clinically apparent at any age, although onset in childhood or after age 50 years is relatively rare. Women are affected twice as often as are men. In most individuals with MS, the clinical course takes the form of relapsing and remitting episodes of variable duration (weeks to months to years) marked by neurologic defects, followed by gradual, partial recovery of neurologic function. The frequency of relapses tends to decrease during the course of time, but there is a steady neurologic deterioration in most affected individuals.

Pathogenesis. **The lesions of MS are caused by an autoimmune response directed against components of the myelin sheath.** As in other autoimmune disorders, the pathogenesis of this disease involves both genetic and environmental factors (Chapter 6). The incidence of MS is 15-fold higher when the disease is present in a first-degree relative and roughly 150-fold higher with an affected monozygotic twin. Despite a series of well-powered studies, only a portion of the genetic basis of the disease has been explained. There is a strong effect from the DR2 extended haplotype of the major histocompatibility complex; each copy of the DRB1*1501 allele an individual inherits brings with it a roughly 3-fold increase in the risk of MS. Genome-wide association studies first identified additional associations with the IL-2 and IL-7 receptor genes, and subsequently with a number of other genes encoding proteins involved in the immune response, including cytokines and their receptors, co-stimulatory molecules, and cytoplasmic signaling molecules. Many of these loci have been found to be associated with other autoimmune diseases. These genetic studies have not explained variations in clinical course for individuals with MS.

Immune mechanisms that underlie the destruction of myelin are the focus of much investigation. The available evidence indicates that the disease is initiated by T_H1 and T_H17 T cells that react against myelin antigens and secrete cytokines. T_H1 cells secrete IFN-γ, which activates macrophages, and T_H17 cells promote the recruitment of leukocytes (Chapter 6). The demyelination is caused by these activated leukocytes and their injurious products. The infiltrate in plaques and surrounding regions of the brain consists of T cells (mainly CD4+, some CD8+) and macrophages. How the autoimmune reaction is initiated is not understood; a role of viral infection (e.g., EBV) in activating self-reactive T cells has been proposed but remains controversial.

Experimental autoimmune encephalomyelitis is an animal model of MS in which demyelination and inflammation occur after immunization of animals with myelin proteins. Many of our concepts of MS pathogenesis have been derived from studies in this model. The experimental disorder can be passively transferred to unimmunized animals with T_H1 and T_H17 cells that recognize myelin antigens.

Based on the growing understanding of the pathogenesis of MS, therapies are being developed that modulate or inhibit T-cell responses and block the recruitment of T cells into the brain. A potential contribution of humoral immunity has also been suspected for a long time, based on the early observation of oligoclonal bands of immunoglobulin in CSF. The demonstration that treatment with agents that deplete B-cells decreases the incidence of demyelinating lesions in patients with MS lends support to this idea.

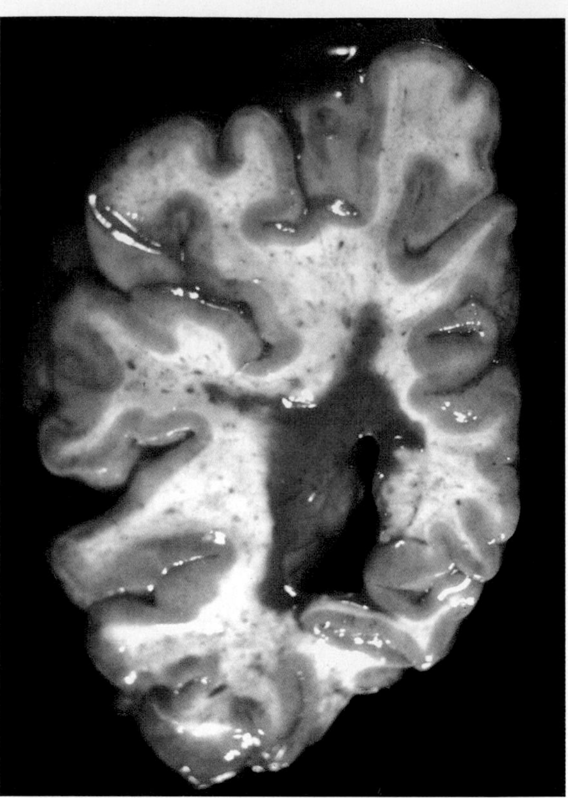

Figure 28-33 Multiple sclerosis. Section of fresh brain showing brown plaque around occipital horn of the lateral ventricle.

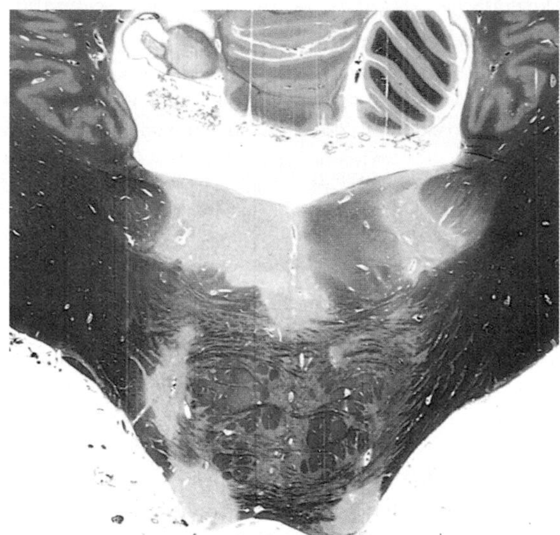

Figure 28-34 Multiple sclerosis (MS). Unstained regions of demyelination (MS plaques) around the fourth ventricle (Luxol fast blue periodic acid-Schiff stain for myelin).

MORPHOLOGY

MS is a white matter disease that is best appreciated in sections of the brain and spinal cord. In the fresh state, the lesions are firmer than the surrounding white matter **(sclerosis)** and appear as well circumscribed, somewhat depressed, glassy, gray-tan, irregularly shaped **plaques** (Fig. 28-33). The area of demyelination often has sharply defined borders, a feature best appreciated with stains for myelin (Fig. 28-34). The size of lesions varies considerably, from small foci that are only recognizable

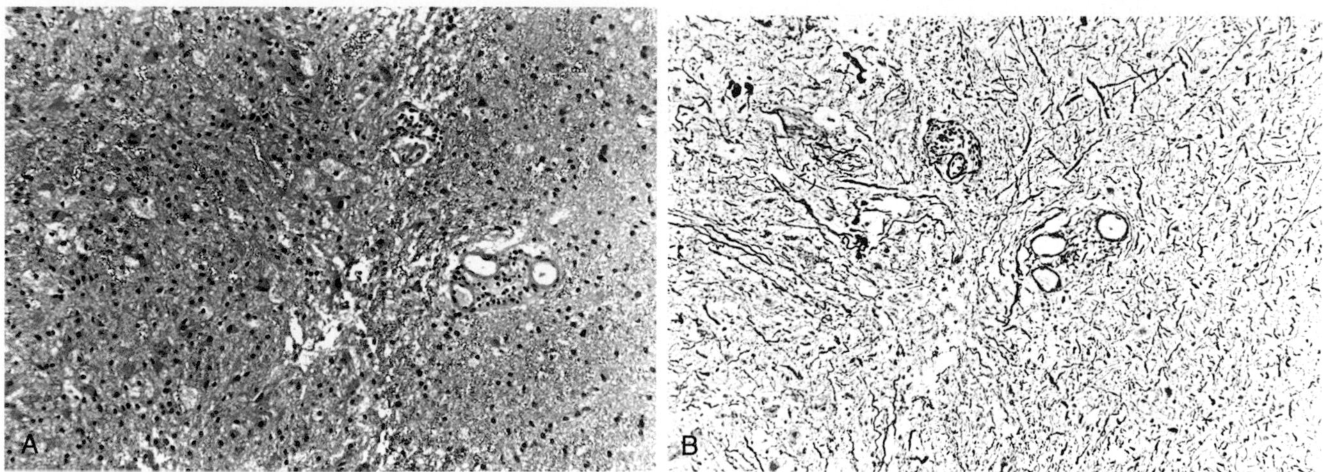

Figure 28-35 Multiple sclerosis. **A,** Myelin-stained section shows the sharp edge of a demyelinated plaque and perivascular lymphocytic cuffs. **B,** The same lesion stained for axons shows relative preservation.

microscopically to confluent plaques that involve large portions of the deep white matter. Plaques commonly occur adjacent to the lateral ventricles, and are also frequent in the optic nerves and chiasm, brainstem, ascending and descending fiber tracts, cerebellum, and spinal cord. Plaques can also extend into gray matter, since myelinated fibers are present there as well.

Microscopically, in an **active plaque** there is ongoing myelin breakdown associated with abundant macrophages containing lipid-rich, PAS-positive debris. Lymphocytes and monocytes are also present, mostly as perivascular cuffs, especially at the outer edge of the lesion (Fig. 28-35*A*). Active lesions are often centered on small veins. Within a plaque there is relative preservation of axons (Fig. 28-35*B*) and depletion of oligodendrocytes. In time, astrocytes undergo reactive changes. As lesions become quiescent, the inflammatory cells slowly disappear. Within **inactive plaques**, little to no myelin is found, and there is a reduction in the number of oligodendrocyte nuclei; instead, astrocytic proliferation and gliosis are prominent. Axons in old gliotic plaques show severe demyelination and are also greatly diminished in number.

In some MS plaques **(shadow plaques)**, the border between normal and affected white matter is not sharply circumscribed. In this type of lesion some abnormally thinned-out myelin sheaths can be demonstrated, especially at the outer edges. This phenomenon is most commonly interpreted as evidence of partial and incomplete remyelination by surviving oligodendrocytes. Abnormally myelinated fibers have also been observed at the edges of typical plaques. Although these histologic findings suggest a limited potential for remyelination in the CNS, the remaining axons within most MS plaques remain unmyelinated; studies aimed at promoting remyelination are an important focus of research.

Clinical Features. Although MS lesions can occur anywhere in the CNS and consequently may induce a wide range of clinical manifestations, certain patterns of neurologic symptoms and signs are more common. Unilateral visual impairment due to involvement of the optic nerve *(optic neuritis, retrobulbar neuritis)* is a frequent initial manifestation of MS. However, only a minority of individuals (10% to 50%, depending on the population studied) with an episode of optic neuritis go on to develop MS (which requires multiple episodes to support the diagnosis). Involvement of the brainstem produces cranial nerve signs, ataxia, nystagmus, and internuclear ophthalmoplegia from interruption of the fibers of the medial longitudinal fasciculus. Spinal cord lesions give rise to motor and sensory impairment of trunk and limbs, spasticity, and difficulties with the voluntary control of bladder function.

Examination of the CSF in individuals with MS shows a mildly elevated protein level and in one third of cases a moderate pleocytosis. IgG levels in the CSF are increased and oligoclonal IgG bands are usually observed on immunoelectrophoresis; these are indicative of the presence of a small number of activated B cell clones, postulated to be self-reactive, in the CNS. Radiologic studies using magnetic resonance imaging have taken on a prominent role in assessing disease progression; these studies, when correlated with autopsy studies as well as clinical findings, indicate that some plaques may be clinically silent even in otherwise symptomatic patients.

Neuromyelitis Optica

Neuromyelitis optica (NMO) is a syndrome with synchronous (or near synchronous) bilateral optic neuritis and spinal cord demyelination. Once considered a variant of MS, it is now clear that it has distinct epidemiology and pathophysiology. NMO has an even greater skewing toward affecting women than MS, is more commonly associated with poor recovery from the first attack, and is characterized by the presence of antibodies against aquaporin-4. This protein is the major water channel of astrocytes, and areas of demyelination in NMO show loss of aquaporin-4. These antibodies injure astrocytes through complement-dependent mechanisms; they are not, however, capable of transferring disease in animal models. In NMO, white cells are common in the CSF, often including neutrophils. Within the damaged areas of white matter, there is typically necrosis, an inflammatory infiltrate including neutrophils, and vascular deposition of immunoglobulin and complement. Therapies include approaches to reduce the antibody burden, either through plasmapheresis or depletion of B cells with anti-CD20 antibody.

Acute Disseminated Encephalomyelitis and Acute Necrotizing Hemorrhagic Encephalomyelitis

Acute disseminated encephalomyelitis is a diffuse, monophasic demyelinating disease that follows either a viral infection or, rarely, a viral immunization. Symptoms typically develop a week or two after the antecedent infection and include headache, lethargy, and coma rather than focal findings, as seen in MS. The clinical course is rapid, and as many as 20% of those affected die; the remaining patients recover completely.

Acute necrotizing hemorrhagic encephalomyelitis (also known as *acute hemorrhagic leukoencephalitis of Weston Hurst*) is a fulminant syndrome of CNS demyelination, typically affecting young adults and children. The illness is almost invariably preceded by a recent episode of upper respiratory infection, most often of unknown cause. The disease is fatal in many patients, with significant deficits present in most survivors.

MORPHOLOGY

In acute disseminated encephalomyelitis, cut sections of brain show only grayish discoloration around white-matter vessels. On microscopic examination, myelin loss with relative preservation of axons can be found throughout the white matter. In the early stages, neutrophils are found within the lesions; later, mononuclear infiltrates predominate. The breakdown of myelin is associated with the accumulation of lipid-laden macrophages. In contrast to MS, all lesions appear similar, consistent with the clinically monophasic nature of the disorder.

Acute necrotizing hemorrhagic encephalomyelitis shows histologic similarities with acute disseminated encephalomyelitis, including a perivenular distribution of demyelination throughout the CNS (sometimes producing confluent lesions). However, the damage is more severe and includes destruction of small blood vessels, disseminated necrosis of white and gray matter with acute hemorrhage, fibrin deposition, and abundant neutrophils. Scattered lymphocytes are seen in foci of demyelination.

The lesions of acute disseminated encephalomyelitis are similar to those induced by immunization of animals with myelin components or with early rabies vaccines that had been prepared from brains of infected animals. This has led to the suggestion that acute disseminated encephalomyelitis is an acute autoimmune reaction to myelin and that acute necrotizing hemorrhagic encephalomyelitis is a hyperacute variant, but inciting antigens have yet to be identified.

Central Pontine Myelinolysis

Central pontine myelinolysis is an acute disorder characterized by loss of myelin in the basis pontis and portions of the pontine tegmentum, typically in a roughly symmetric pattern. It most commonly arises 2 to 6 days after rapid correction of hyponatremia, although it can also be associated with other severe electrolyte disturbances or osmolar imbalances and may also be known as *osmotic demyelination disorder*. It appears that rapid increases in osmolality damage oligodendrocytes through uncertain mechanisms. Inflammation is absent from the lesions, and neurons and axons are well preserved. Because of the synchronous onset of damage, all lesions appear to be at the same stage of myelin loss and reaction. Although originally described in the pons, extra-pontine lesions with similar appearance and apparent etiology may also occur.

While it can involve most parts of the brain, periventricular and subpial regions are spared, and it is extremely rare for the process to extend below the pontomedullary junction. The clinical presentation of pontine lesions is that of a rapidly evolving quadriplegia, which may be fatal or lead to severe long-term deficits, including the "locked-in" syndrome, in which patients are fully conscious yet unresponsive. It is imperative that hyponatremia be corrected slowly and carefully in order to prevent this tragic complication.

KEY CONCEPTS

Demyelinating Diseases

- Because of the critical role of myelin in nerve conduction, diseases of myelin can lead to widespread and severe neurologic deficits.
- Demyelinating diseases show evidence of breakdown and destruction of previously normal myelin, often by inflammatory processes. Secondary injury to axons typically emerges over time as well.
- Multiple sclerosis, an autoimmune demyelinating disease, is the most common disorder of myelin, affecting young adults. It often pursues a relapsing-remitting course, with eventual progressive accumulation of neurologic deficits.
- Other, less common forms of immune-mediated demyelination often follow infections and are more acute illnesses.

Neurodegenerative Diseases

Neurodegenerative diseases are disorders characterized by the progressive loss of neurons, typically affecting groups of neurons with functional relationships even if they are not immediately adjacent. Thus, different diseases tend to involve particular neural systems and therefore have relatively stereotypic presenting signs and symptoms. Recent genetic and molecular studies have shaped the current classification of neurodegenerative diseases, in part from the recognition that there are many shared features.

The pathologic process that is common across most of the neurodegenerative diseases is the accumulation of protein aggregates, which can be used as a morphologic hallmark of the disease (hence the occasional use of the term "proteinopathy"). Protein aggregates may arise because of mutations that alter the protein's conformation or disrupt the pathways involved in processing or clearance of the proteins. In other situations, there may be a subtle imbalance between protein synthesis and clearance (from genetic, environmental or stochastic factors) that allows gradual accumulation of proteins.

Regardless of how they arise, the protein aggregates typically are resistant to degradation, show aberrant localization within neurons, and elicit a stress response from the cell; in addition, they are often directly toxic to neurons. As the abnormal proteins aggregate, there is often both an associated "toxic" gain-of-function and a loss-of-function, as more and more protein is shunted into the aggregates rather than performing normal physiologic functions. Recently, it has also become clear that these aggregates are capable of behaving like prions; that is, aggregates derived from one cell are taken up by another, thereby giving rise to more aggregates. The data supporting this concept are largely derived from experimental animal studies, but some case studies of patients who died with Alzheimer disease suggest that the disease spreads from one site in the brain to another. However, in contrast to prion diseases, there is no evidence that these diseases are transmissible.

The protein aggregates are recognized histologically as inclusions, which often are the diagnostic hallmark of the disease. The basis for aggregation varies from one disease to another. It may be directly related to an intrinsic feature of a mutated protein (e.g., expanded polyglutamine repeats in Huntington disease), an intrinsic feature of a peptide derived from a larger precursor protein (e.g., Aβ in Alzheimer disease), or an unexplained alteration of a normal cellular protein (e.g., α-synuclein in sporadic Parkinson disease).

Neurodegenerative diseases differ both with respect to the anatomic localization of involved areas and in their specific cellular abnormalities (e.g., tangles, plaques, Lewy bodies). Accordingly, they can be considered for discussion using two approaches:

- *Symptomatic/anatomic:* based on the anatomic regions of the CNS that are primarily affected, which is typically reflected in the clinical symptoms (e.g., neocortical involvement resulting in cognitive impairment and dementia)
- *Pathologic:* based on the types of inclusions or abnormal structures observed (e.g., diseases with inclusions containing tau or containing synuclein)

Nevertheless, within the spectrum of degenerative diseases there is a remarkable overlap, both in terms of characteristic neurologic deficits, functional/anatomic distribution of lesions, and cellular pathology (Tables 28-3 and 28-4). For the sake of simplicity we will follow the time honored classification based on the original description of these diseases.

Alzheimer Disease

Alzheimer disease (AD) is the most common cause of dementia in older adults, with an increasing incidence as a function of age. The disease usually becomes clinically apparent as insidious impairment of higher cognitive functions. As the disease progresses, deficits in memory, visuospatial orientation, judgment, personality and language emerge. Typically over a course of 5 to 10 years, the affected individual becomes profoundly disabled, mute, and

Table 28-3 Features of the Major Neurodegenerative Diseases

Disease	Clinical pattern	Inclusions	Genetic causes
Alzheimer disease (AD)	Dementia	Aβ (plaques) Tau (tangles)	APP, PS1, PS2
Frontotemporal lobar degeneration (FTLD)	Behavioral changes, language disturbance	Tau TDP-43 FUS	Tau TDP-43, progranulin, C9orf72 FUS
Parkinson disease (PD)	Hypokinetic movement disorder	α-synuclein Tau	α-synuclein LRRK2
Progressive supranuclear palsy (PSP)	Parkinsonism with abnormal eye movements	Tau	Tau
Corticobasal degeneration (CBD)	Parkinsonism with asymmetric movement disorder	Tau	
Multiple system atrophy (MSA)	Parkinsonism, cerebellar ataxia, autonomic failure	α-synuclein	
Huntington disease (HD)	Hyperkinetic movement disorder	Huntington (polyglutamine)	Htt
Spinocerebellar ataxias (SCA1, 2, 3, 6, 7, 17 and DRPLA)	Cerebellar ataxia	Various proteins (polyglutamine containing)	Multiple loci
Amyotrophic lateral sclerosis (ALS)	Weakness with upper and lower motor neurons signs	SOD1 TDP-43 FUS	SOD1 TDP-43, C9orf72 FUS
Spinal bulbar muscular atrophy (SBMA)	Lower motor neuron weakness, diminished androgen	Androgen receptor (polyglutamine containing)	Androgen receptor

Table 28-4 Relationship Between Proteins and Neurodegenerative Diseases

Protein	Diseases with Inclusions
Aβ	Alzheimer disease
Tau	Alzheimer disease Frontotemporal lobar degeneration Parkinson disease (with *LRRK2* mutations) Progressive supranuclear palsy Corticobasal degeneration
TPD-43	Frontotemporal lobar degeneration Amyotrophic lateral sclerosis
FUS	Frontotemporal lobar degeneration Amyotrophic lateral sclerosis
α-synuclein	Parkinson disease Multiple system atrophy
Polyglutamine aggregates (distinct proteins per disease)	Huntington disease Some forms of spinocerebellar ataxia Spinal bulbar muscular atrophy

immobile. Patients rarely become symptomatic before 50 years of age; the incidence of the disease increases with age, and the prevalence roughly doubles every 5 years, starting from a level of 1% for the 60- to 64-year-old population and reaching 40% or more for the 85- to 89-year-old cohort. This progressive increase in the incidence with increasing age has given rise to major medical, social, and economic concerns in countries with aging populations. About 5% to 10% of cases are familial forms of AD; these have provided important insight into the pathogenesis of the more common sporadic form of the disease. While pathologic examination of brain tissue remains necessary for the definitive diagnosis of AD, the combination of clinical assessment and modern radiologic methods allows accurate diagnosis in 80% to 90% of cases as confirmed at autopsy.

Molecular Genetics and Pathogenesis. **The fundamental abnormality in AD is the accumulation of two proteins (Aβ and tau) in specific brain regions, likely as a result of excessive production and defective removal** (Fig. 28-36). The two pathologic hallmarks of AD, particularly evident in the end stages of the illness, are *plaques* and *tangles*. Plaques are deposits of aggregated Aβ peptides in the neuropil, while tangles are aggregates of the microtubule binding protein tau, which develop intracellularly and then persist extracellularly after neuronal death. Both plaques and tangles appear to contribute to the neural dysfunction, and the interplay between the processes that lead to the accumulation of these abnormal aggregates is a critically important aspect of AD pathogenesis that has yet to be unraveled.

Several lines of evidence strongly support a model in which **Aβ generation is the critical initiating event for the development of AD**. First, there are diseases in which tau deposits appear, such as frontotemporal lobar degenerations, progressive supranuclear palsy, and corticobasal degeneration (discussed later), but Aβ deposits do not ensue. This suggests that having abnormal deposits of tau in the brain is not a sufficient stimulus to elicit deposition of Aβ. Additionally, multiple lines of genetic evidence point to the likely importance of altered Aβ metabolism; mutations in the protein from which Aβ is derived (APP) cause familial AD, as does increased copy number (either from small duplications or from trisomy 21) of the *APP* gene. Furthermore, point mutations in proteins that are part of the protease complexes that generate Aβ from APP also give rise to AD. In contrast, mutations in the gene for tau do not give rise to AD but rather cause frontotemporal lobar degenerations (discussed later).

The pathogenesis of AD involves not only Aβ and tau but several other genetic and host factors.

- *Role of Aβ.* Amyloid precursor protein (APP) is a cell surface protein with a single transmembrane domain that may function as a receptor, possibly for prion protein (PrP^c) among other ligands. The Aβ portion of the protein extends from the extracellular region into the transmembrane domain (Fig. 28-36). Processing of APP begins with cleavage in the extracellular domain, followed by an intramembranous cleavage. There are two potential pathways, determined by the type of initial proteolytic event. If the first cut occurs at the α-secretase site within the Aβ sequence, then Aβ is not generated (the non-amyloidogenic pathway). This mostly occurs at the cell surface, since the various proteases with α-secretase activity are involved in the shedding of surface proteins. Surface APP can also be endocytosed and may undergo cleavage by β-secretase, which cuts at the N-terminal region of the Aβ sequence (the amyloidogenic pathway). Following cleavage of APP at either of these sites, the γ-secretase complex performs an intramembranous cleavage. When paired with a first cut by α-secretase, it produces a soluble fragment, but when paired with β-secretase cleavage, it generates Aβ. The variation in peptide length ($A\beta_{40}$vs $A\beta_{42}$) arises from alterations in the exact location of the γ-secretase cleavage. The γ-secretase complex—containing presenilin, nicastrin, pen-2, and aph-1—is also responsible for processing of Notch receptors as well as many other membrane proteins. Once generated, Aβ is highly prone to aggregation—first into small oligomers (which may be the toxic form responsible for neuronal dysfunction), and eventually into large aggregates and fibrils.

  As mentioned earlier, part of the support for the central role of Aβ generation as a critical step for at least initiation of AD pathogenesis comes from familial AD. The gene encoding APP, on chromosome 21, lies in the Down syndrome region; AD pathology is an eventual feature of the cognitive impairment of these individuals. Histologic findings appear in the second and third decades followed by neurologic decline about 20 years later. A similar gene dosage effect is produced by localized chromosome 21 duplications that span the *APP* locus in some patients with familial AD. Point mutations in APP are another cause of familial AD. Some mutations lie near the β-secretase and γ-secretase cleavage sites, and others sit in the Aβ sequence and increase its propensity to aggregate. The two loci identified as causes of the majority of early-onset familial AD encode the two presenilins (PS1 on chromosome 14 and PS2 on chromosome 1). These mutations lead to a gain of function, such that the γ-secretase complex generates increased amounts of Aβ, particularly $A\beta_{42}$.

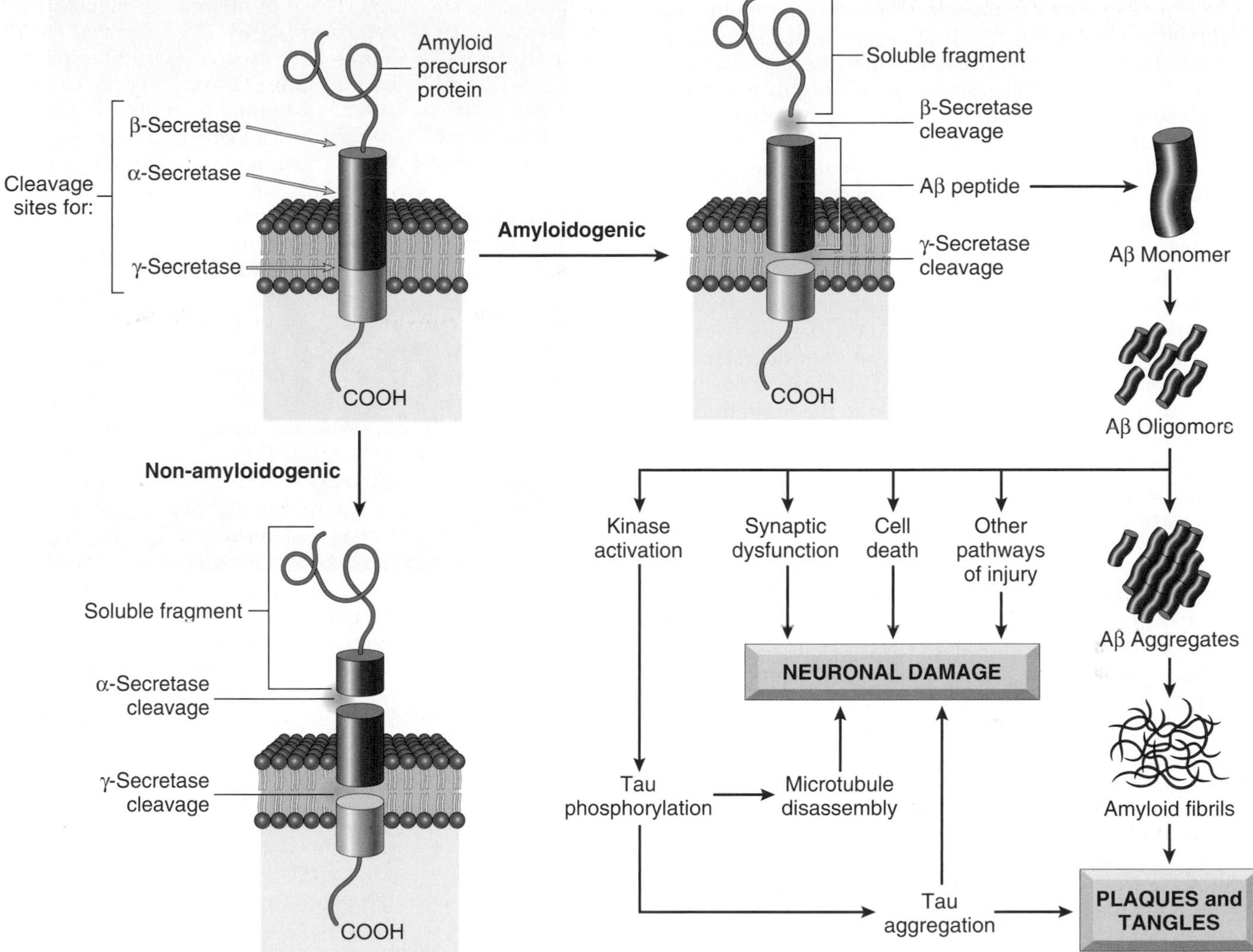

Figure 28-36 Protein aggregation in Alzheimer disease. Amyloid precursor protein cleavage by α-secretase and γ-secretase produces a harmless soluble peptide, whereas amyloid precursor protein cleavage by β-amyloid–converting enzyme (BACE) and γ-secretase releases Aβ peptides, which form pathogenic aggregates and contribute to the characteristic plaques and tangles of Alzheimer disease.

- *Role of tau.* Because neurofibrillary tangles contain the tau protein, there has been much interest in the role of this protein in AD. Tau is a microtubule-associated protein present in axons in association with the microtubular network. With the development of tangles in AD, it shifts to a somatic-dendritic distribution, becomes hyperphosphorylated, and loses the ability to bind to microtubules. The formation of tangles is an important component of AD, and the increased tangle burden in the brain over the course of the illness eventually appears to become independent of the Aβ. The mechanism of tangle injury to neurons remains poorly understood but two possible pathways have been suggested. First, the aggregates of tau protein elicit a stress response and second, the microtubule stabilizing function of tau protein is lost.
- *Other genetic risk factors.* The genetic locus on chromosome 19 that encodes apolipoprotein E (ApoE) has a strong influence on the risk of developing AD. Three alleles exist (ε2, ε3, and ε4) based on two amino acid polymorphisms. The dosage of the ε4 allele increases the risk of AD and lowers the age of onset of the disease, such that individuals with the ε4 allele are overrepresented in populations of patients with AD. This ApoE isoform promotes Aβ generation and deposition, although the mechanisms have not been established. Overall, this locus has been estimated to convey about a quarter of the risk for development of late-onset AD. Genome-wide association studies have identified several other loci that contribute to the risk of AD. The connection between these genetic loci and the pathogenesis of AD remains to be explored.
- *Role of inflammation.* Both small aggregates and larger deposits of Aβ elicit an inflammatory response from microglia and astrocytes. This response probably assists in the clearance of the aggregated peptide, but may also stimulate the secretion of mediators that cause damage. Additional consequences of the activation of these inflammatory cascades may include alterations in tau phosphorylation, along with oxidative injury to the neurons.

- *Basis for cognitive impairment.* While there remains disagreement regarding the best correlate of dementia in individuals with AD, it is clear that the presence of a large burden of plaques and tangles is highly associated with severe cognitive dysfunction. The number of neurofibrillary tangles correlates better with the degree of dementia than does the number of neuritic plaques. Biochemical markers that have been correlated with the degree of dementia include loss of choline acetyltransferase, synaptophysin immunoreactivity, and amyloid burden.
- *Biomarkers.* Among the more important recent developments in the understanding of AD is the discovery of possible biomarkers. These draw on the understanding of the biologic processes discussed above. It is now possible to demonstrate Aβ deposition in the brain through imaging methods that rely on ^{18}F-labeled amyloid-binding compounds. The experience to date suggests that this approach can identify asymptomatic patients who are at high risk for developing AD. Additional evidence of neuronal degeneration associated with AD-related pathologic processes includes the presence of increased phosphorylated tau and reduced Aβ in the CSF. Together, these biomarkers have allowed for the identification of preclinical stages of AD, well in advance of the development of dementia or other clinical signs and symptoms. This in turn has enabled the focus of pharmacologic trials to shift towards individuals in the earliest stages of the illness, in whom it is hoped interventions will slow or prevent disease progression and limit disability.

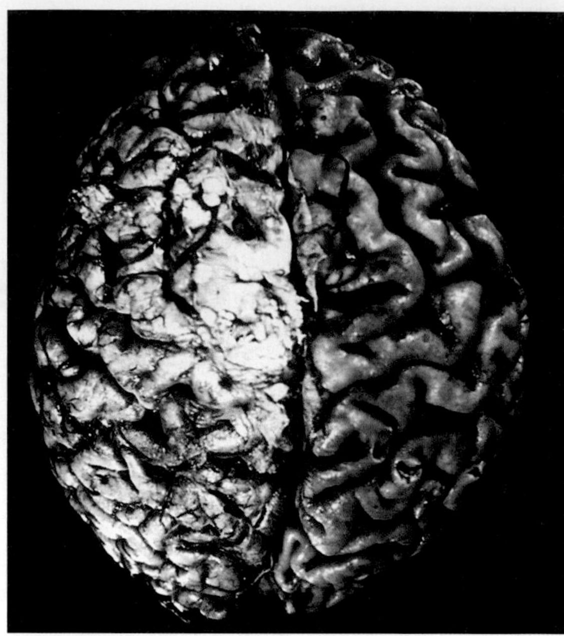

Figure 28-37 Alzheimer disease with cortical atrophy most evident on the right, where meninges have been removed. (Courtesy the late Dr. E. P. Richardson, Jr., Massachusetts General Hospital, Boston, Mass.)

MORPHOLOGY

Grossly, the brain shows a variable degree of **cortical atrophy** marked by widening of the cerebral sulci that is most pronounced in the frontal, temporal, and parietal lobes (Fig. 28-37). With significant atrophy, there is compensatory ventricular enlargement (hydrocephalus *ex vacuo*) secondary to reduced brain volume. Structures of the medial temporal lobe, including hippocampus, entorhinal cortex and amygdala, are involved early in the course and are usually severely atrophied in the later stages. The major microscopic abnormalities of AD are **neuritic (senile) plaques** and **neurofibrillary tangles**. There is progressive, eventually severe, neuronal loss and reactive gliosis in the same regions that bear the burden of plaques and tangles.

Neuritic plaques are focal, spherical collections of dilated, tortuous, neuritic processes (dystrophic neurites) often around a central amyloid core, which may be surrounded by a clear halo (Fig. 28-38*A*). Neuritic plaques range in size from 20 to 200 μm in diameter; microglial cells and reactive astrocytes are present at their periphery. Plaques are found in the hippocampus, amygdala, and neocortex, although there is usually relative sparing of primary motor and sensory cortices (this also applies to neurofibrillary tangles). The amyloid core, which can be stained by Congo red, contains several abnormal proteins. The dominant component of the amyloid plaque core is **Aβ**, a peptide derived by proteolytic cleavage of amyloid precursor protein (APP) (Fig. 28-38 and see Fig. 28-36). The two dominant species of Aβ, called $A\beta_{40}$ and $A\beta_{42}$, have the same N-terminus and differ in length by two amino acids at the C-terminus. Other proteins are present in plaques in lesser abundance, including components of the complement cascade, proinflammatory cytokines, α_1-antichymotrypsin, and apolipoproteins. In some cases, there is deposition of Aβ peptides with staining characteristics of amyloid in the absence of the surrounding neuritic processes. These lesions, termed **diffuse plaques**, are found mainly in superficial portions of cerebral cortex, the basal ganglia, and cerebellar cortex. Diffuse plaques are believed to be an early stage of plaque development, based on studies of individuals with trisomy 21. While neuritic plaques contain both $A\beta_{40}$ and $A\beta_{42}$, diffuse plaques are predominantly made up of $A\beta_{42}$.

Neurofibrillary tangles are tau-containing bundles of filaments in the cytoplasm of the neurons that displace or encircle the nucleus. In pyramidal neurons, they often have an elongated "flame" shape; in rounder cells, the basket weave of fibers around the nucleus takes on a rounded contour ("globose" tangles). Neurofibrillary tangles are visible as basophilic fibrillary structures with H & E staining (Fig. 28-38*C*) but are demonstrated much more clearly by silver (Bielschowsky) staining (Fig. 28-38*D*) and with immunohistochemistry directed against tau (Fig. 28-38*E*). They are commonly found in cortical neurons, especially in the entorhinal cortex, as well as in other sites such as pyramidal cells of the hippocampus, the amygdala, the basal forebrain, and the raphe nuclei. Neurofibrillary tangles are insoluble and apparently resistant to clearance in vivo, thus remaining visible in tissue sections as "ghost" or "tombstone" tangles long after the death of the parent neuron. Ultrastructurally, neurofibrillary tangles are composed predominantly of paired helical filaments along with some straight filaments that appear to have a similar composition. Aggregated tau is also present in dystrophic neurites that form the outer portions of neuritic plaques and in axons coursing through the affected gray matter as neuropil threads. Tangles are not specific to AD, being found in other diseases as well.

In addition to the diagnostic features of plaques and tangles, several other pathologic findings are seen in the setting of AD.

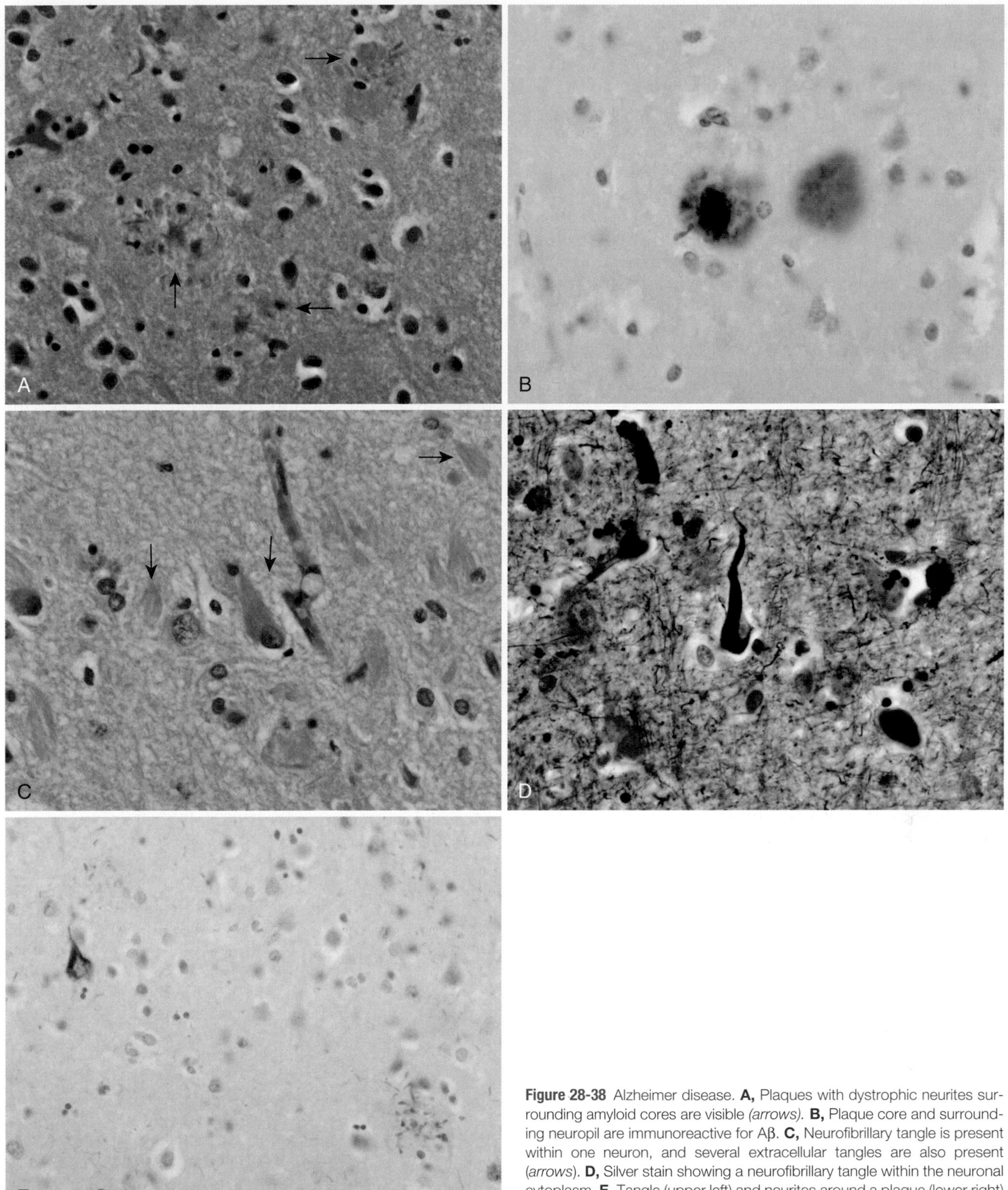

Figure 28-38 Alzheimer disease. **A,** Plaques with dystrophic neurites surrounding amyloid cores are visible *(arrows).* **B,** Plaque core and surrounding neuropil are immunoreactive for Aβ. **C,** Neurofibrillary tangle is present within one neuron, and several extracellular tangles are also present (*arrows*). **D,** Silver stain showing a neurofibrillary tangle within the neuronal cytoplasm. **E,** Tangle (upper left) and neurites around a plaque (lower right) contain tau, demonstrated by immunohistochemistry.

Cerebral amyloid angiopathy is an almost invariable accompaniment of AD; however, it can also be found in brains of individuals without AD (Fig. 28-18*B*). Vascular amyloid is predominantly $A\beta_{40}$, as is also the case when cerebral amyloid angiopathy occurs without AD.

While abundant burdens of plaques and tangles characterize the end-stage of AD, in which affected individuals are fully demented, it is clear that these histologic changes first appear well in advance of clinical symptoms. In order to provide a correlation between neuropathologic findings and clinical symptomatology, the most recent recommendations for describing these lesions consider all deposition of Aβ in brain parenchyma to be a form of Alzheimer disease neuropathologic change. The scheme then generates a histopathologic score based on the distribution of Aβ deposits, plaques and tangles, which is used to predict the likelihood of an individual being cognitively impaired, drawing on population studies.

Clinical Features. The progression of AD is slow but relentless, with a symptomatic course often running more than 10 years. Initial symptoms are forgetfulness and other memory disturbances; with progression of the disease other symptoms emerge, including language deficits, loss of mathematical skills, and loss of learned motor skills. In the final stages of AD, affected individuals may become incontinent, mute, and unable to walk. Intercurrent disease, often pneumonia, is usually the terminal event. Current clinical trials are focused on treating subjects in early, preclinical stages of the illness, using strategies that include clearing Aβ from the brain through immunologic approaches, disruption of the generation of Aβ with pharmacologic agents that target either γ-secretase or BACE (β-secretase 1), as well as approaches aimed at preventing alterations in tau.

Frontotemporal Lobar Degenerations (FTLDs)

FTLDs are a heterogeneous set of disorders associated with focal degeneration of frontal and/or temporal lobes. They are distinguished from AD by the fact that alterations in personality, behavior and language (aphasias) precede memory loss. Global dementia does occur with progressive disease. A subset of patients also develop extrapyramidal motor loss. Several clinical variants have been described based on whether the behavioral change or aphasias dominate but they have overlapping features. FTLDs are one of the more common causes of early onset dementia and occur at the same frequency as Alzeheimer disease in those under the age of 65 years. Commonly referred to in the clinical setting as *frontotemporal dementia* (FTD), the preferred pathologic terminology highlights the lobar degeneration rather than the clinical symptom of dementia.

As with many neurodegenerative diseases, FTLD is associated with cellular inclusions of specific proteins. The two most common patterns are those with tau-containing inclusions (FTLD-tau) and those with TDP43-containing inclusions (FTLD-TDP). Within each of these groups, there are heritable forms as well as sporadic cases. There is no fixed relationship between the clinical subtypes of FTLD and the type of neuronal inclusions.

FTLD-Tau

These are forms of FTLD in which the affected cortical regions demonstrate progressive neuronal loss and reactive gliosis, along with the presence of tau-containing inclusions in the cytoplasm of neurons. While Alzheimer disease is characterized by the combination of Aβ and tau deposition, FTLD-tau shows only tau aggregation and accumulation. In some cases FTLD-tau inclusions resemble the tangles seen in Alzheimer disease while in other forms of the disease there are smooth contoured inclusions (Pick bodies). The distinctive inclusions, as well as the severe atrophy with stereotypic lobar restriction, are the hallmarks of *Pick disease* within the category of FTLD-tau.

Molecular Genetics and Pathogenesis. FTLD-tau may be associated with mutations affecting tau, or may arise spoadically in the absence of tau mutations. As mentioned earlier, tau is a phosphoprotein that interacts with microtubules through specific binding domains, with superimposed regulation through a range of potential phosphorylation sites. There is an inverse relationship between the degree of phosphorylation and the ability of tau to bind to microtubules. Tau, particularly when phosphorylated, also has a propensity to aggregate. Tau also exists as a complex series of isoforms that are encoded by different mRNA splice variants. The balance between these isoforms appears to be critical for normal tau function in neurons, and disturbances in isoform ratio may also provoke tau aggregation.

Two different types of tau mutations are described. Some missense point mutations effect tau phosphorylation, tipping the balance from active microtubule binding towards aggregating forms. Other mutations include point mutations that affect splicing; many of these are intronic and alter the loop-stem structures recognized by the spliceosome. The resulting change in isoform ratio is thought to lead to neuronal dysfunction and, as discussed above, may also enhance tau aggregation.

It remains unclear how abnormal tau injures neurons, although there appears to be both a loss-of-function component, as aggregation depletes the neurons of tau, and a toxic gain-of-function component from the presence of aberrantly hyperphosphorylated aggregated protein in the neuron.

MORPHOLOGY

There is atrophy of frontal and temporal lobes to variable extent and severity. The pattern of atrophy can often be predicted in part by the clinical symptomatology. The atrophic regions of cortex are marked by neuronal loss, gliosis, and the presence of tau-containing neurofibrillary tangles (Fig. 28-39*A*). These tangles may contain a variety of tau isoforms. Nigral degeneration may also occur. Inclusions can also be found in glial cells in some forms of the disease.

In Pick disease, the brain invariably shows a pronounced, frequently asymmetric, atrophy of the frontal and temporal lobes with conspicuous sparing of the posterior two thirds of the superior temporal gyrus and only rare involvement of either the parietal or occipital lobe. The atrophy can be severe, reducing the gyri to a wafer-thin ("knife-edge") appearance.

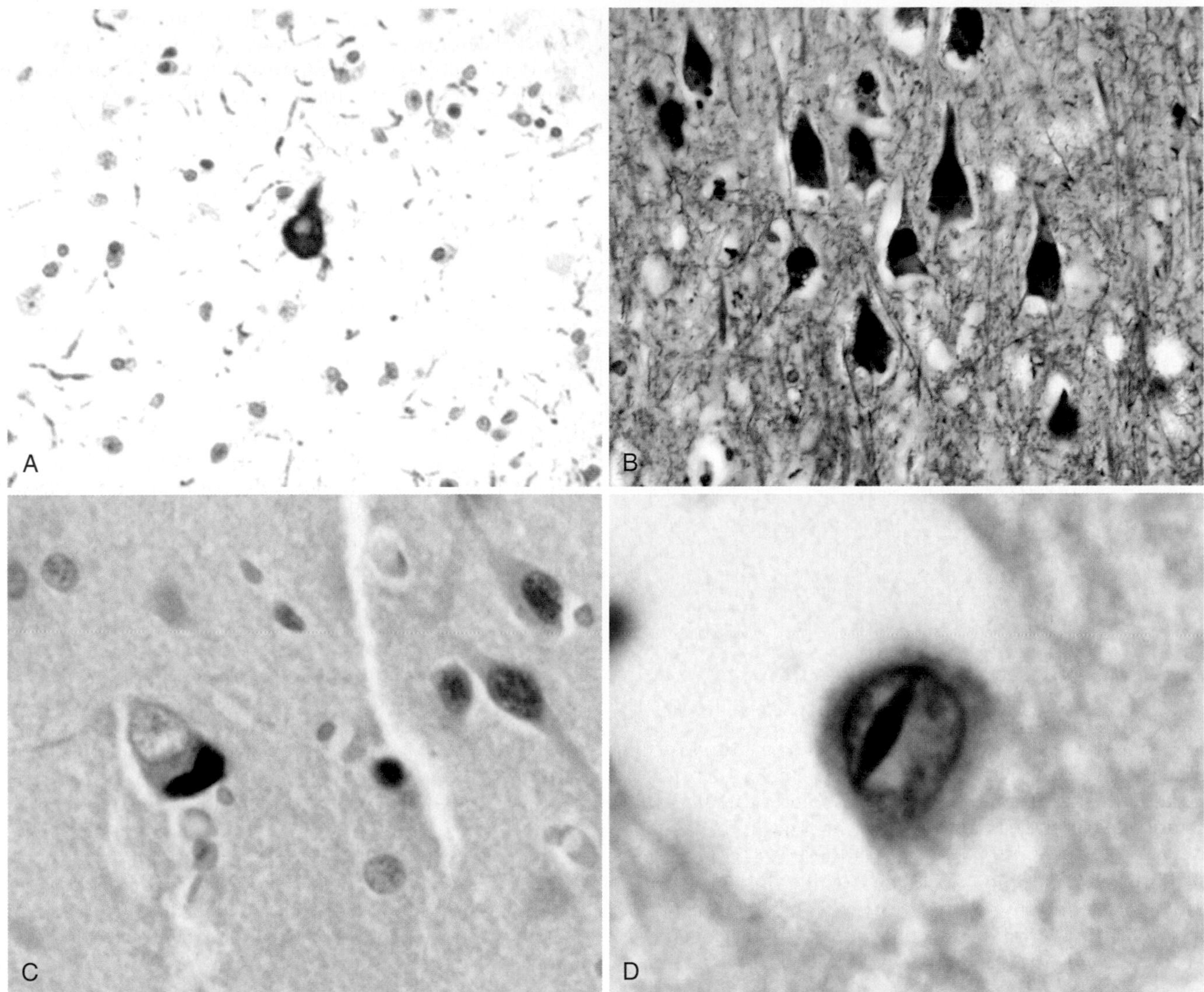

Figure 28-39 Frontotemporal lobar degenerations (FTLDs). **A,** FTLD-tau. A tangle is present along with numerous tau-containing neurites. **B,** Pick disease. Pick bodies are round, homogeneous neuronal cytoplasmic inclusions that stain intensely with silver stains. **C,** FTLD-TDP. Cytoplasmic inclusions containing TDP-43 are seen in association with loss of normal nuclear immunoreactivity. **D,** FLTD-TDP. With progranulin mutations, the TDP-43–containing inclusions are commonly intranuclear.

Microscopically, neuronal loss is most severe in the outer three layers of the cortex. Some of the surviving neurons show a characteristic swelling **(Pick cells)**, while others contain **Pick bodies**, which are cytoplasmic, round to oval, filamentous inclusions that are only weakly basophilic but stain strongly with silver methods and contain 3R tau (Fig. 28-39*B*).

FTLD-TDP

Some individuals with clinically diagnosed FTLD and macroscopic changes of relatively localized cortical atrophy (the 'lobar degeneration' of the term) have inclusions that contain TDP-43, an RNA-binding protein, and do not contain tau. Individuals with this type of neurodegeneration may present with either behavioral problems or language complaints, just as with FTLD-tau.

Molecular Genetics and Pathogenesis. There are three well-established genetic forms of FLTD-TDP, as well as sporadic forms. Three different mutations have been found in the inherited forms of FTLD-TDP.

- The most common genetic form of familial FTLD-TDP is the result of an expansion of a hexanucleotide repeat in the 5′ UTR of C9orf72 (a gene encoding a protein of unknown function). The spectrum of disease associated with C9orf72 expansion also includes amyotrophic lateral sclerosis (ALS). How the repeat expansion results in formation of aggregates of TDP-43 is a mystery at present.
- Mutations in the gene encoding the TDP-43 protein are less common in FTLD-TDP and also occur in some familial cases of ALS. TDP-43 is an RNA-binding protein with roles in RNA processing as well as in the formation of stress granules. Both loss of function and gain of

function with toxic effects may contribute to the phenotype observed in these patients.

- A third genetic form of FTLD-TDP is the result of mutations in the gene encoding progranulin. In contrast to TDP-43 and C9orf72 mutations, these have not been linked to ALS. Progranulin mutations cause loss of function and the disease mechanism is believed to stem from deficient progranulin activity. Progranulin is a secreted protein expressed in glia and neurons that is cleaved into multiple small peptides. These peptides have been implicated in regulation of inflammation in the brain, but the link between this activity and the accumulation of TDP-43 containing inclusions in FTLD is currently obscure.

MORPHOLOGY

The gross appearance is similar to the other forms of FLTD, with atrophy of frontal and temporal lobes of variable extent and severity. This is accompanied by varying degrees of neuronal loss and gliosis. Normally, TDP-43 is found diffusely in the nucleus; with disease, there is loss of this staining and formation of inclusions (Fig. 28-39*C*). These may be found in the cell body (neuronal cytoplasmic inclusions or NCI), in the nucleus (neuronal intranuclear inclusions or NII), or in neurites. In the inclusions, TDP-43 is phosphorylated and ubiquitinated. Inclusions are most abundant in the frontal and temporal cortex, in the striatum and in the dentate gyrus of the hippocampus. There is an extremely strong correlation between the presence of needle-like NII's and progranulin mutations (Fig. 28-39*D*).

There are forms of FTLD in which there are neither tau- nor TDP-containing inclusions. While these are infrequent, the underlying genetic causes show overlap with the pathways identified as contributors to pathogenesis of FTLD-TPD. Mutations in the *FUS* (fused in sarcoma) gene may cause either FTLD or ALS, and FUS is another RNA-binding protein that may be involved in formation of stress granules.

Parkinson Disease (PD)

PD is a neurodegenerative disease marked by a prominent hypokinetic movement disorder that is caused by loss of dopaminergic neurons from the substantia nigra. The clinical syndrome of *parkinsonism* combines diminished facial expression (often termed *masked facies*), stooped posture, slowing of voluntary movement, festinating gait (progressively shortened, accelerated steps), rigidity, and a "pill-rolling" tremor. **This type of motor disturbance is seen in a number of conditions that have in common damage to the nigrostriatal dopaminergic system**. Several neurodegenerative diseases include symptoms of parkinsonism. In addition, similar symptoms may be pharmacologically induced by dopaminergic antagonists or by toxins that selectively damage the dopaminergic system. The principal degenerative disease that involves the nigrostriatal system is PD. Also discussed later are other rare diseases that have parkinsonism as part of the clinical presentation.

The presumptive diagnosis of PD can be based on the presence of the central triad of parkinsonism—tremor, rigidity, and bradykinesia—in the absence of a toxic or other known underlying etiology. This impression is confirmed by symptomatic response to L-DOPA replacement therapy. Although the diagnosis of PD is based in large part on the presence of the motor symptoms, which reflect the decreased dopaminergic innervation of the striatum, there is clear evidence that the disease is not restricted to dopaminergic neurons or to the basal ganglia; in fact, there is evidence from pathologic investigations that the degeneration of the substantia nigra (which results in the motor symptoms) represents a mid-stage in a progressive disease that begins lower in the brainstem and can eventually progress to involve the cerebral cortex, leading to cognitive impairment (see Dementia with Lewy Bodies, later).

The dopaminergic neurons of the substantia nigra project to the striatum, and their degeneration in PD is associated with a reduction in the striatal dopamine content. The severity of the motor syndrome is proportional to the dopamine deficiency, which can, at least in part, be corrected by replacement therapy with L-DOPA (the immediate precursor of dopamine). Treatment does not, however, reverse the morphologic changes or arrest the progress of the disease; moreover, with progression, drug therapy tends to become less effective and symptoms become more difficult to manage. Deep brain stimulation has emerged over the past decade as a therapy for the motor symptoms of PD. In addition, the well-characterized neural and biochemical deficits in PD have also provided a rationale for early therapeutic trials of neural transplantation and gene therapy.

An acute parkinsonian syndrome and destruction of neurons in the substantia nigra follows exposure to MPTP (1-methyl-4-phenyl-1,2,3,6-tetrahydropyridine), discovered as a contaminant in illicitly synthesized batches of the opioid meperidine. This toxin has been used to generate animal models of PD that are being exploited to test new therapies. Epidemiologic evidence has also suggested that pesticide exposure is a risk factor for PD, while caffeine and nicotine may be protective.

Molecular Genetics and Pathogenesis. **PD is associated with protein accumulation and aggregation, mitochondrial abnormalities, and neuronal loss in the substantia nigra and elsewhere in the brain.** While most PD is sporadic, a series of genetic causes have been identified that shed light on its pathogenesis.

- The first gene to be identified as a cause of autosomal dominant PD encodes *α-synuclein*, an abundant lipid-binding protein normally associated with synapses. This protein was then demonstrated to be a major component of the Lewy body, which is the diagnostic hallmark of PD. Mutations in α-synuclein are rare; they take the form of point mutations and amplifications of the region of chromosome 4q21 that contains the gene. The occurrence of disease caused by changes in gene copy number implies a gene dosage effect, and suggests that polymorphisms in the α-synuclein promoter that alter its expression may influence the risk of PD. Like Aβ in Alzheimer disease, α-synuclein has been demonstrated to form aggregates; of these, small oligomers appear to be the most toxic to neurons. There is also evidence that aggregates can be released from one neuron and taken up by another, suggesting a capacity for a prion-like pattern of spread within the brain. Consistent with this idea, α-synuclein containing aggregates (in the form of Lewy bodies and Lewy neurites) first appear in the medulla and then in contiguous areas of the brain, ascending through the brainstem and extending into limbic structures and finally the neocortex.

- *Mitochondrial dysfunction* has been implicated as a contributing factor for PD based on autosomal recessive forms of PD that are caused by mutations in genes that encode the proteins DJ-1, PINK1, and parkin. DJ-1 has multiple cellular roles, including acting as a transcriptional regulator, but in settings of oxidative stress it can relocate to the mitochondria and have cytoprotective effects. PINK1 is a kinase that is degraded in the mitochondria under normal circumstances; with mitochondrial dysfunction, it recruits parkin, which is an E3 ubiquitin ligase. Under normal circumstances, the combination of PINK1 and parkin results in clearance of dysfunctional mitochondria through mitophagy. Intriguingly, levels of mitochondrial complex I, a component of the oxidative phosphorylation cascade, are reduced in the brains of patients with sporadic PD.
- Mutations in the gene encoding *LRRK2* (leucine-rich repeat kinase 2) are a more common cause of autosomal dominant PD and are found in some sporadic cases of the disease. LRRK2 is a cytoplasmic kinase. Several of the pathogenic mutations increase the kinase activity of LRRK2, suggesting that gains in LRRK2 function—either hyperphosphorylation of normal targets or emergence of novel targets—might contribute to the development of PD.

MORPHOLOGY

A characteristic finding in PD is **pallor of the substantia nigra** (compare Fig. 28-40*A* and *B*) and locus ceruleus, which is due to loss of the pigmented, catecholaminergic neurons in these regions. Lewy bodies (Fig. 28-40*C*) may be found in some of the remaining neurons. These are single or multiple cytoplasmic, eosinophilic, round to elongated inclusions that often have a dense core surrounded by a pale halo. Ultrastructurally, Lewy bodies are composed of fine filaments, densely packed in the core but loose at the rim; these filaments are composed of α-synuclein. Lewy bodies may also be found in the cholinergic cells of the basal nucleus of Meynert, which is depleted of neurons (particularly in patients with abnormal cognitive function), as well as in other brainstem nuclei including the locus ceruleus and the dorsal motor nucleus of the vagus. Areas of neuronal loss also typically show gliosis. Lewy neurites are dystrophic processes that contain aggregated α-synuclein.

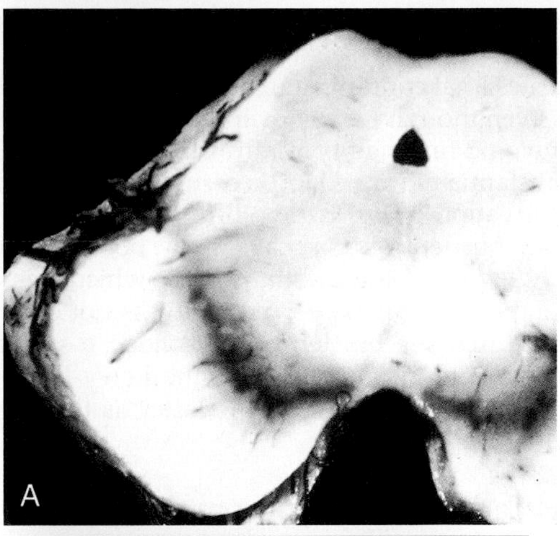

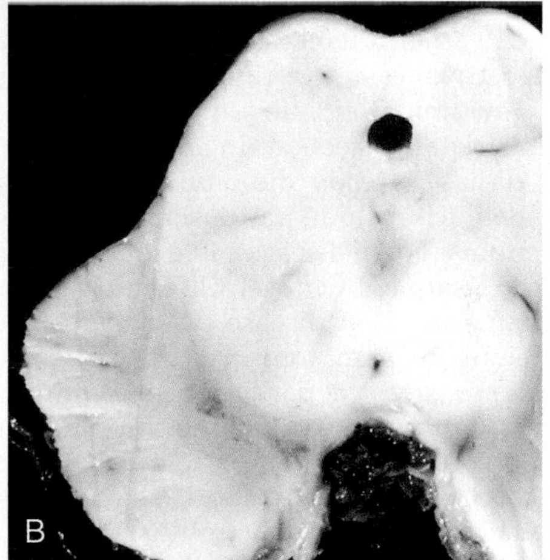

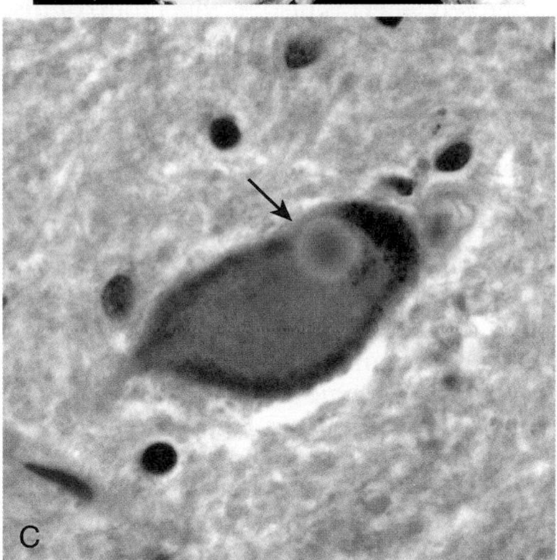

Figure 28-40 Parkinson disease. **A,** Normal substantia nigra. **B,** Depigmented substantia nigra in idiopathic Parkinson disease. **C,** Lewy body in a substantia nigra neuron, staining bright pink *(arrow)*.

Dementia with Lewy Bodies

About 10% to 15% of individuals with PD develop dementia, particularly with advancing age. Characteristic features of this disorder include a fluctuating course, hallucinations, and prominent frontal signs. While some affected individuals have pathologic evidence of Alzheimer disease (or, less frequently, other degenerative diseases associated with cognitive changes) in combination with PD, in others the most prominent histologic correlate is the presence of widespread Lewy bodies in neurons in the cortex and brainstem. As already mentioned, dementia with Lewy bodies may represent an advanced stage of PD in which protein aggregates appear to have "spread", possibly through propagation of misfolded proteins, to neurons in the cerebral cortex.

Cortical Lewy bodies are less distinct than those observed in the brainstem but are also composed predominantly of α-synuclein. Immunohistochemical staining for α-synuclein also reveals the presence of abnormal neurites, that contain aggregated protein—called *Lewy neurites,* even though Lewy never saw them! In this setting, the pathologic findings typically include depigmentation of the substantia nigra and locus ceruleus, paired with relative preservation of the cortex, hippocampus, and amygdala. The burden of cortical Lewy bodies is usually extremely low, and the mechanism by which this disease wreaks havoc on cognitive functioning is not clear. There is evidence that the burden of oligomeric α-synuclein in the cortex is more important than the Lewy bodies, even though neuropathologists use the latter as the diagnostic hallmark of the disease.

Atypical Parkinsonism Syndromes

As discussed earlier, the clinical syndrome of parkinsonism, with bradykinesia and rigidity, reflects dysfunction of the extrapyramidal circuitry, particularly the dopaminergic nigrostriatal projection. In addition to the forms of Parkinson disease already discussed, there are a variety of disorders which include parkinsonism as a component of the symptoms. These diseases, in general, are minimally responsive to treatment with L-DOPA; they are also distinguished from Parkinson disease through the presence of additional signs and symptoms. For these reasons, they are considered to be "atypical parkinsonism syndromes," with the alternative terminology of "Parkinson-plus syndromes" applied by others. In addition to progressive supranuclear palsy and corticobasal degeneration, which are both tauopathies, another synucleinopathy (multisystem atrophy, discussed separately later) is also in this group of disorders.

Progressive Supranuclear Palsy (PSP)

PSP is a tauopathy in that affected individuals commonly develop progressive truncal rigidity, disequilibrium with frequent falls and difficulty with voluntary eye movements. Other symptoms that are frequently observed include nuchal dystonia, pseudobulbar palsy and a mild progressive dementia. The onset is usually between the fifth and seventh decades, with males affected approximately twice as frequently as females. The disease is often fatal within 5 to 7 years of onset.

Although the pathologic hallmark of PSP is the presence of tau-containing inclusions in neurons and glia, causative mutations in the tau gene have been identified in only a few cases. However, risk for sporadic PSP is linked to single nucleotide polymorphisms that map near the tau gene locus. Other risk alleles have been identified through genome-wide association studies, but the mechanisms by which they influence development of PSP are still unclear.

MORPHOLOGY

There is widespread neuronal loss in the globus pallidus, subthalamic nucleus, substantia nigra, colliculi, periaqueductal gray matter, and dentate nucleus of the cerebellum. Globose fibrillary tangles are found in these affected regions, in neurons as well as in glia. Ultrastructural analysis reveals 15-nm straight filaments that are composed of 4R tau.

Corticobasal Degeneration (CBD)

CBD is a progressive tauopathy that is most often characterized by extrapyramidal rigidity, asymmetric motor disturbances (jerking movements of limbs), and impaired higher cortical function (typically in the form of apraxias). As with PSP, cognitive decline may occur, typically later in the illness. The same tau variant linked to PSP is also highly associated with CBD. Overall, CBD and PSP share many clinical and pathologic features; in general, with PSP there is a greater burden of tau-containing lesions in brainstem and deep gray matter, while in CBD the balance is shifted more toward cerebral cortical involvement.

MORPHOLOGY

The brain shows cortical atrophy, mainly of the motor, premotor, and anterior parietal lobes. In affected regions of cortex there is severe loss of neurons, gliosis, and **"ballooned" neurons** (neuronal achromasia). Tau immunoreactivity has been found in astrocytes ("tufted astrocytes"), oligodendrocytes ("coiled bodies"), basal ganglionic neurons, and, variably, cortical neurons. Clusters of tau-positive processes around astrocytes ("astrocytic plaques") and the presence of tau-positive threads in gray and white matter may be the most specific pathologic findings of CBD. The substantia nigra and locus ceruleus show loss of pigmented neurons, neuronal achromasia, and tangles.

Multiple System Atrophy (MSA)

MSA is a sporadic disorder that affects several functional systems in the brain and is characterized by cytoplasmic inclusions of α-synuclein in oligodendrocytes. Unlike the other degenerative diseases, the primary pathologic hallmark of MSA is observed in glial cells and is commonly associated with degeneration of white matter tracts. In addition, there is accompanying neuronal degeneration but typically without the presence of inclusions. The "multiple" in the term *multiple system atrophy* refers to three distinct neuroanatomic circuits that are commonly involved: the striatonigral circuit (leading to parkinsonism), olivopontocerebellar circuit (leading to ataxia), and the autonomic nervous system including the central elements (leading to autonomic dysfunction, with orthostatic hypotension as a prominent component). In a given individual, one of these components may predominate at the onset of the illness, but typically the other systems are affected as MSA progresses.

Pathogenesis. As in Parkinson disease, α-synuclein is the major component of the inclusions. MSA is a sporadic disease and no mutations in the gene encoding α-synuclein have identified as being causative; nonetheless, there does appear to be a set of polymorphisms near this gene that confer increased risk. The relationship between glial cytoplasmic inclusions and disease is supported by the observation that the burden of inclusions increases as the disease progresses, although inclusions eventually disappear as cells die in the final stages. It appears that glial cytoplasmic inclusions can occur in the absence of neuronal loss, suggesting that they are the primary pathologic event; for example, glial cytoplasmic inclusions are consistently observed in the white matter projecting to and from the motor cortex. The origin of the α-synuclein in oligodendrocytes remains perplexing, since this is a neuronal protein associated with synaptic vesicles. Several studies have shown that there is no up-regulation of α-synuclein expression in white matter or in oligodendrocytes in MSA. It has been suggested that oligodendrocytes may acquire α-synuclein aggregates secondarily from injured or dying neurons. When α-synuclein is present in oligodendrocytes, they become more sensitive to oxidative stress and show impaired interaction with the extracellular matrix.

MORPHOLOGY

The pathologic findings in MSA match the clinical presentation in any particular case. In cerebellar forms there is atrophy of the cerebellum, including the cerebellar peduncles, pons (especially the basis pontis, Fig. 28-41*A*), and medulla (especially the inferior olive), while in parkinsonian forms the atrophy involves both the substantia nigra and striatum (especially putamen). Autonomic symptoms are related to cell loss from the catecholaminergic nuclei of the medulla and the intermediolateral cell column of the spinal cord. Atrophic brain regions show evidence of neuronal loss as well as variable numbers of neuronal cytoplasmic and nuclear inclusions.

The diagnostic glial cytoplasmic inclusions were originally demonstrated in oligodendrocytes with silver impregnation methods and contain α-synuclein as well as ubiquitin (Fig. 28-41*B*). The inclusions are ultrastructurally distinct from those found in other neurodegenerative diseases and are composed primarily of 20- to 40-nm tubules. Similar inclusions may also be found in the cytoplasm of neurons, sometimes in neuronal and glial nuclei, and in axons.

Huntington Disease

Huntington disease (HD) is an autosomal dominant disease characterized by progressive movement disorders and dementia, caused by degeneration of striatal neurons. Jerky, hyperkinetic, sometimes dystonic movements involving all parts of the body (chorea) are characteristic; affected individuals may later develop bradykinesia and rigidity. The disease is relentlessly progressive and uniformly fatal, with an average course of about 15 years.

Molecular Genetics and Pathogenesis. **HD is the prototype of the polyglutamine trinucleotide repeat expansion diseases** (Chapter 5). The gene for HD, *HTT*, located on chromosome 4p16.3, encodes a 348-kD protein known as *huntingtin*. In the first exon of the gene there is a stretch of CAG repeats that encodes a polyglutamine region near the N terminus of the protein. Normal *HTT* genes contain six to 35 copies of the repeat; when the number of repeats is increased beyond this level it is associated with disease. There is an inverse relationship between repeat number and age of onset, such that longer repeats tend to be associated with earlier onset. However, determination of repeat length is not by itself an accurate predictor of age of onset. Repeat expansions occur during spermatogenesis, so that paternal transmission is associated with early onset in the next generation, a phenomenon termed *anticipation*. In contrast to many of the other degenerative diseases, there is no sporadic form of HD. Newly occurring mutations are uncommon; most apparently sporadic cases are explained by non-paternity, the death of a parent before the disease is expressed, or an unaffected father with a mild repeat expansion that is expanded to a pathogenic size during spermatogenesis.

The biologic function of normal huntingtin remains unknown, but it appears that the expansion of the polyglutamine region bestows a toxic gain-of-function on huntingtin. For this reason, various approaches to silencing expression of the mutant allele are being investigated as potential therapies. It is interesting to note that while huntingtin is expressed in all the tissues of the body, the deleterious effects of mutant huntingtin occur only in selected parts of the central nervous system.

While protein aggregation and development of intranuclear inclusions containing huntingtin are pathologic hallmarks of HD, it remains uncertain whether these processes are directly involved in cellular injury or if they are incidental to critical disease processes. There is emerging evidence that aggregated huntingtin can be taken up by neurons, again suggesting a prion-like spread from one

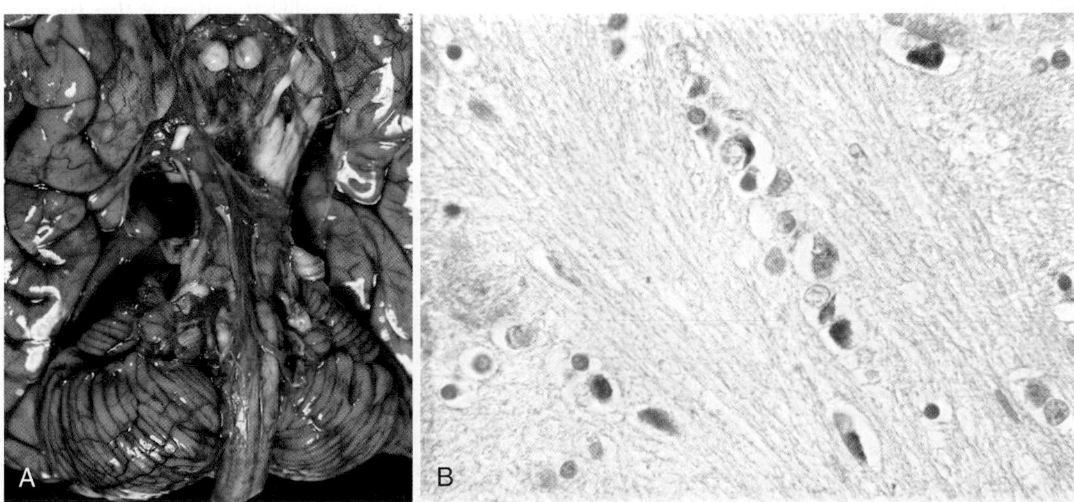

Figure 28-41 Multiple system atrophy (MSA). **A,** Severe atrophy of the basis pontis is evidence in a case of MSA-C. **B,** Inclusions in oligodendrocytes contain α-synuclein.

neuron to another. Transcriptional dysregulation has been implicated in HD, based on the observation that mutant forms of huntingtin bind various transcriptional regulators. Some of the transcription factors that are sequestered by mutant huntingtin include those involved in mitochondrial biogenesis and protection against oxidative injury, and their reduced activity may result in increased susceptibility of affected cells to oxidative stress. Other implicated pathways that may contribute to the pathogenesis of HD include altered expression of the growth factor brain-derived neurotrophic factor (BDNF), and deleterious effects of protein aggregates, which may disrupt both proteasomal and autophagic degradation pathways.

MORPHOLOGY

The brain is small and shows striking **atrophy of the caudate nucleus** and, less markedly at early stages, the putamen (Fig. 28-42). The globus pallidus may atrophy secondarily, and the lateral and third ventricles are dilated. Atrophy is frequently also seen in the frontal lobe, less often in the parietal lobe, and occasionally throughout the entire cortex. On microscopic examination, there is profound loss of striatal neurons; the most marked changes are found in the caudate nucleus, especially in the tail and in portions nearer the ventricle. Pathologic changes develop in a medial-to-lateral direction in the caudate and from dorsal to ventral in the putamen. The nucleus accumbens is the best-preserved portion of the striatum. Both the large and small neurons are affected, but loss of the small neurons generally occurs first. The medium-sized, spiny neurons that use γ-aminobutyric acid as their neurotransmitter, along with enkephalin, dynorphin, and substance P, are especially affected. Two populations of neurons are relatively spared: the diaphorase-positive neurons that express nitric oxide synthase and the large cholinesterase-positive neurons. Both appear to serve as local interneurons. There is also fibrillary gliosis that is more extensive than in the usual reaction to neuronal loss. There is a direct relationship between the degree of degeneration in the striatum and the severity of clinical symptoms. Protein aggregates containing huntingtin can be found in neurons in the striatum and cerebral cortex (Fig. 28-42, *inset*).

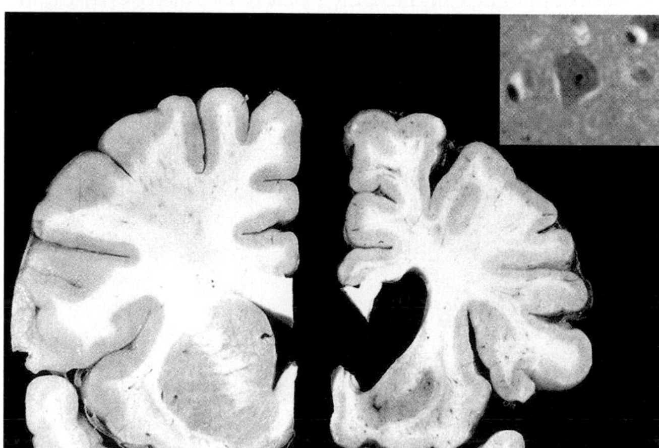

Figure 28-42 Huntington disease. Normal hemisphere on the left compared with the hemisphere with Huntington disease on the right showing atrophy of the striatum and ventricular dilation. *Inset*, Intranuclear inclusions in neurons are highlighted by immunohistochemistry against ubiquitin. (Courtesy Dr. J-P Vonsattel, Columbia University, New York.)

Clinical Features. The loss of medium spiny striatal neurons leads to dysregulation of the basal ganglia circuitry that modulates motor output. These neurons normally function to dampen motor activity; thus, their degeneration in HD results in increased motor output, often manifested as choreoathetosis. The cognitive changes associated with the disease are probably related to the neuronal loss from cerebral cortex.

The age at onset is most commonly in the fourth and fifth decades and is related to the length of the CAG repeat in the *HTT* gene. Motor symptoms often precede the cognitive impairment. The movement disorder of HD is choreiform, with increased and involuntary jerky movements of all parts of the body; writhing movements of the extremities are typical. Early symptoms of higher cortical dysfunction include forgetfulness and thought and affective disorders, but there is progression to a severe dementia. Although individuals with HD have an increased risk of suicide, intercurrent infection is the most common natural cause of death. Given the ability to screen for disease-causing mutations, one might assume that genetic screening of individuals at risk would be routine. However, this is an example of a situation where the ability to detect the likelihood of disease has surpassed any possible treatment. Thus, in the absence of effective therapy and given the devastating nature of the disease, it is not entirely clear that screening is ethical.

Spinocerebellar Degenerations

These degenerative diseases involve the cerebellum along with other components of the nervous system, commonly the spinal cord (both tracts that project to the cerebellum as well as the dorsal columns, which do not) and peripheral nerve. Because of the anatomic location of the lesions, clinical symptoms commonly include cerebellar and sensory ataxia, spasticity, and sensorimotor peripheral neuropathy. Despite the overlap in regions of involvement, this is a highly heterogeneous group of illnesses at the clinical, genetic and pathologic level, with differences in patterns of inheritance, age at onset, and signs and symptoms. What is common across them is the presence of neuronal loss, often without other distinctive changes apart from gliosis, in the affected areas. Genetic analysis continues to change our classification of these illnesses, but frustratingly this has yet to lead to clearer insight into their pathogenesis or to effective treatments.

The term *spinocerebellar ataxia* (SCA) is usually applied to a series of autosomal dominantly inherited disorders. We will also briefly discuss two of the more common autosomal recessive disorders that are characterized by spinocerebellar degeneration, Friedreich ataxia and ataxia-telangiectasia. Finally, there is a small set of hereditary disorders characterized by episodes of ataxia or other symptoms of cerebellar dysfunction, which are mostly associated with mutations in genes for ion channel subunits.

Spinocerebellar Ataxias

This group of genetic disorders presents with signs and symptoms referable to the cerebellum (progressive ataxia), brainstem, spinal cord, and peripheral nerves, as well as other brain regions in different subtypes.

Pathologically, they are characterized by neuronal loss from the affected areas and secondary degeneration of white-matter tracts.

Molecular Genetics. The list of SCAs has expanded to more than 30 distinct entities, with genetic loci determined for more than half of them. Three distinct types of mutations have been recognized:

- *Polyglutamine diseases* linked to expansion of a CAG repeat, similar to HD. Each of the seven forms of SCA associated with this mechanism has a distinct protein in which the expanded polyglutamine tract occurs, with intranuclear inclusions occurring in neurons, suggesting the involvement of pathogenic mechanisms previously discussed for Huntington disease. The group of polyglutamine diseases includes SCA1, SCA2, SCA3 (also known as *Machado-Joseph disease*), SCA6, SCA7 (relatively unique in that it includes visual impairment), SCA17, and dentatorubropallidoluysian atrophy (DRPLA).
- *Expansion of non-coding region repeats*, similar to myotonic dystrophy. There are currently five forms of SCA in which this mechanism appears to underlie the disease, each linked to a difference genetic locus. This group includes SCA8, SCA10, SCA12, SCA31, and SCA36. The connection between the expansion of these repeats and disease manifestations remains obscure.
- *Point mutations*. Another 10 of the SCAs are associated with mutations in a variety of genes whose expression is not restricted to neurons and which code for proteins of mostly unknown functions.

There remains a significant need for investigation to bridge this gap between genetic insight and disease pathogenesis.

Friedreich Ataxia

Friedreich ataxia is an autosomal recessive disease with progressive ataxia, spasticity, weakness, sensory neuropathy, and a cardiomyopathy. It generally begins in the first decade of life with gait ataxia, followed by hand clumsiness and dysarthria. Deep tendon reflexes are depressed or absent, but an extensor plantar reflex is typically present. Joint position and vibratory sense are impaired, and there is sometimes loss of pain, temperature sensation, and light touch. Most affected individuals develop pes cavus and kyphoscoliosis. Most patients become wheelchair-bound within about 5 years of onset, and life expectancy is typically limited to 40 or 50 years of age. The accompanying cardiomyopathy is associated with a high incidence of arrhythmias and congestive heart failure, which contribute to the deaths of most affected individuals. Concomitant diabetes is found in up to 25% of patients.

Friedreich ataxia is caused by expansion of a GAA trinucleotide repeat in the first intron of a gene on chromosome 9q13 that encodes *frataxin*, a protein found in the mitochondrial inner membrane where it is involved in assembly of iron-sulfur cluster enzymes of complex I and II. Affected individuals have extremely low levels of the protein, and the severity of the disease course may correlate better with the level of frataxin than with the degree of GAA-repeat expansion. With reduced mitochondrial frataxin, there is decreased mitochondrial oxidative phosphorylation (similar to the defect in mitochondrial encephalomyopathies) as well as increased free iron; the presence of free iron within the mitochondria may contribute to oxidative stress. Nearly all cases of Friedreich ataxia are associated with GAA repeat expansion in both alleles, but the same disease phenotype is observed when one allele has a repeat expansion and the other harbors a point mutation.

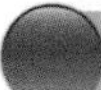

MORPHOLOGY

The spinal cord shows loss of axons and gliosis in the posterior columns, the distal portions of corticospinal tracts, and the spinocerebellar tracts. There is degeneration of neurons in the spinal cord (Clarke column), the brainstem (cranial nerve nuclei VIII, X, and XII), the cerebellum (dentate nucleus and the Purkinje cells of the superior vermis), and the Betz cells of the motor cortex. Large dorsal root ganglion neurons are also decreased in number; their large myelinated axons, traveling both in the dorsal roots and in dorsal columns, undergo secondary degeneration. The heart is enlarged and may have pericardial adhesions. Multifocal destruction of myocardial fibers with inflammation and fibrosis is detectable in about half the affected individuals who come to autopsy.

Ataxia-Telangiectasia

Ataxia-telangiectasia (Chapter 7) is an autosomal recessive disorder characterized by an ataxic-dyskinetic syndrome beginning in early childhood, with the subsequent development of telangiectasias in the conjunctiva and skin, along with immunodeficiency. The ataxia-telangiectasia mutated (*ATM*) gene on chromosome 11q22-q23 encodes a kinase with a critical role in orchestrating the cellular response to double-stranded DNA breaks. In addition to this critical cellular role, the ATM protein also contributes to various other pathways including facilitation of apoptosis, maintenance of telomeres, mitochondrial homeostasis, response to oxidative stress, and maintenance of the ubiquitin-proteosomal degradation system. It remains unclear which of these pathways contribute to the degenerative phenotype observed in the setting of loss of ATM protein in neurons. Intriguingly, there are comparable patterns of neurodegeneration associated with other diseases linked to disruption in single-stranded DNA break repair processes.

MORPHOLOGY

The abnormalities are predominantly in the cerebellum, with loss of Purkinje and granule cells; there is also degeneration of the dorsal columns, spinocerebellar tracts, and anterior horn cells, and a peripheral neuropathy. Telangiectatic lesions are found in the CNS as well as in the conjunctiva and skin of the face, neck, and arms. Cells in many organs (e.g., Schwann cells in dorsal root ganglia and peripheral nerves, endothelial cells, pituicytes) show a bizarre enlargement of the nucleus to two to five times normal size and are referred to as *amphicytes*. The lymph nodes, thymus, and gonads are hypoplastic.

Clinical Features. The disease is relentlessly progressive, with death early in the second decade. The initial symptoms are commonly recurrent sinopulmonary infections and unsteadiness in walking. Later on, speech is noted to become dysarthric, and eye movement abnormalities develop. Many affected individuals develop lymphoid neoplasms, which are most often T-cell leukemias.

Amyotrophic Lateral Sclerosis (ALS)

ALS is a progressive disorder in which there is loss of upper motor neurons in the cerebral cortex and lower motor neurons in the spinal cord and brainstem. Loss of these neurons results in denervation of muscles, producing weakness that becomes profound as the disease progresses. The disease has an overall incidence of about 2 cases per 100,000 population, affects men slightly more frequently than women, and commonly emerges in the fifth decade or later. Sporadic ALS is more common than familial ALS (FALS), which may account for up to 20% of cases.

Molecular Genetics and Pathogenesis. **Both sporadic and familial ALS are associated with degeneration of upper and lower motor neurons, often in association with evidence of toxic protein accumulation.** Close to two dozen genetic loci have been identified as causing familial ALS, with nearly all being autosomal dominant disorders. One of the earliest discovered hereditary forms of ALS has mutations in the gene encoding copper-zinc superoxide dismutase (*SOD1*) on chromosome 21; this variant accounts for about 20% of familial cases. A wide variety of missense mutations have been identified throughout the gene. The A4V mutation is the most common in the United States; it is associated with a rapid course and rarely involvement of upper motor neurons.

Initially, identification of *SOD1* mutations suggested that neuronal injury in ALS might reflect an impaired capacity to detoxify free radicals, but it is now believed that mutations lead to an adverse gain-of-function phenotype associated with mutant SOD1 protein. It appears that mutated SOD1 protein misfolds and forms aggregates (that can include wild type protein) and result in cellular injury through a variety of mechanisms including disruption of proteasome function and autophagy, direct effects on axonal transport and mitochondrial function or sequestration of other proteins within the aggregates. Accumulation of protein aggregates can eventually trigger the unfolded protein response, with subsequent initiation of apoptosis. Development of aggregated SOD1 has also been observed in ALS without mutations in this gene, suggesting that this path to cellular injury may contribute to sporadic ALS as well. For this reason, methods for clearing misfolded SOD1 are being developed as therapeutic approaches. The overall importance of protein degradation pathways is reinforced by discovery of a range of uncommon mutations in genes implication in protein degradation that are also associated with familial ALS.

The most common mutation that gives rise to ALS and FTLD simultaneously is an expansion of a hexanucleotide repeat in the 5′-untranslated region of a transcript of unknown function, C9orf72. This mutation is estimated to be the basis of up to 40% of familial ALS and a smaller fraction of what appear to be sporadic cases of ALS. Non-AUG-initiated translation (in all three reading frames) can occur from these expanded repeats, and neuronal deposits of the derived proteins have been found in the setting of the mutation. Whether these novel protein aggregates contribute to cellular injury remains obscure.

Other genetic loci that cause ALS and FTLD encode proteins with RNA-binding capacity, such as TDP-43 and FUS. The underlying link between altered RNA-binding proteins and manifestations of motor neuron disease remain unclear. Possibly, nuclear depletion of TDP-43 results in inappropriate processing of some RNAs, while the aggregation of the protein in the cytoplasm activates the unfolded protein response common to many of the proteinopathies.

MORPHOLOGY

The anterior roots of the spinal cord are thin (Fig. 28-43*A*), due to loss of lower motor neuron fibers, and the precentral motor gyrus in the cortex may be atrophic in especially severe cases. There is a reduction in the number of anterior-horn neurons throughout the length of the spinal cord, associated with reactive gliosis. Similar findings are seen in the hypoglossal, ambiguus, and motor trigeminal cranial nerve nuclei. Remaining neurons often contain PAS-positive cytoplasmic inclusions called Bunina bodies, which appear to be remnants of autophagic vacuoles. Skeletal muscles innervat ed by the degenerated lower motor neurons show neurogenic atrophy. Loss of the upper motor neurons leads to degeneration of the corticospinal tracts, resulting in volume loss and absence of myelinated fibers, which may be particularly evident at the lower segmental levels (Fig. 28-43*B*).

Clinical Features. Early symptoms of ALS include asymmetric weakness of the hands, manifested as dropping of objects and difficulty in performing fine motor tasks, and cramping and spasticity of the arms and legs. As the disease progresses, muscle strength and bulk diminish, and involuntary contractions of individual motor units, termed fasciculations, occur. The disease eventually involves the respiratory muscles, leading to recurrent bouts of pulmonary infection. While most affected individuals have a combination of both upper and lower motor neuron involvement as determined by clinical features and pathologic examination, there are other patterns observed. The term *progressive muscular atrophy* applies to those relatively uncommon cases in which lower motor neuron involvement predominates, while *primary lateral sclerosis* refers to those cases with mostly upper motor neuron involvement. In some affected individuals, degeneration of the lower brainstem cranial motor nuclei occurs early and progresses rapidly, a pattern referred to as *progressive bulbar palsy* or *bulbar ALS*. In these individuals, abnormalities of deglutition and phonation dominate, and the clinical course is inexorable during a 1- or 2-year period; when bulbar involvement is less severe, about half of affected individuals are alive 2 years after diagnosis. The motor neurons innervating extra-ocular muscles are among the last to be involved in ALS; with long survival, usually associated with ventilator support, even this form of motor output fails. Familial cases develop symptoms earlier than most sporadic cases, but the clinical course is comparable.

While ALS is considered a disease of the motor system, it is clear that a significant fraction of affected individuals

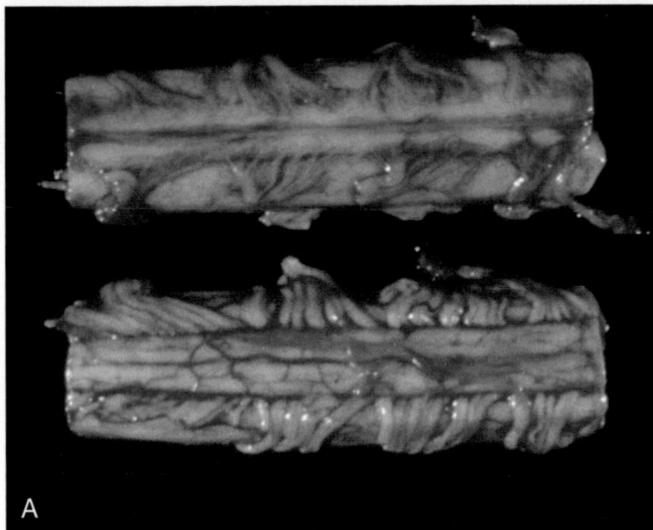

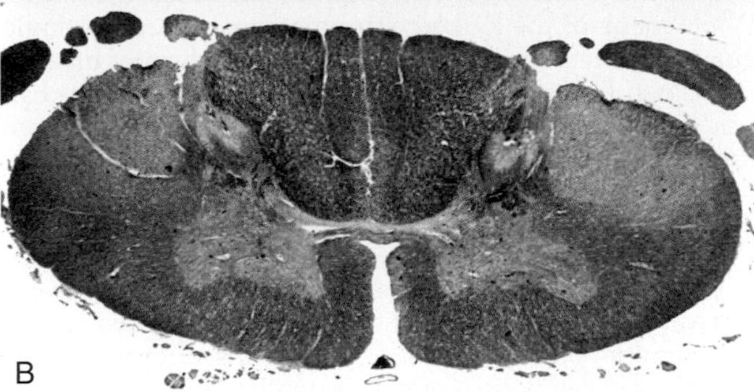

Figure 28-43 Amyotrophic lateral sclerosis. **A,** Segment of spinal cord viewed from anterior (upper) and posterior (lower) surfaces showing attenuation of anterior (motor) roots compared with posterior (sensory) roots. **B,** Spinal cord showing loss of myelinated fibers (lack of stain) in corticospinal tracts as well as degeneration of anterior roots.

also have evidence of more widespread cerebral cortical disease. The clinical presentation of cerebral disease is usually as a frontotemporal lobar dementia (FTLD), with pathologic findings most often matching those of FTLD associated with TDP-43 inclusions. The mechanistic link between these two processes is further strengthened by the presence of TDP-43 containing inclusions in many cases of ALS as well as partial sharing of genetic alterations in ALS and FTLD.

Other Motor Neuron Diseases

Spinal and Bulbar Muscular Atrophy (Kennedy Disease)

This X-linked polyglutamine repeat-expansion disease is characterized by distal limb amyotrophy and bulbar signs, such as atrophy and fasciculations of the tongue and dysphagia, associated with degeneration of lower motor neurons in the spinal cord and brainstem. The expanded repeat occurs in the first exon of the androgen receptor, and results in androgen insensitivity, gynecomastia, testicular atrophy, and oligospermia. The basis for the selective motor neuron involvement is unclear, but as in other polyglutamine expansion diseases such as Huntington disease and forms of spinocerebellar atrophy, there are intranuclear inclusions that contain the involved protein. Cellular injury depends on the binding of androgen to the abnormal receptor and the subsequent interaction with DNA. Therapies aimed at reducing androgen levels have been effective is animal models and may be able to ameliorate the disease in humans as well.

Spinal Muscular Atrophy

Spinal muscular atrophy (SMA) includes a group of genetically linked disorders of childhood with marked loss of lower motor neurons resulting in progressive weakness. The most severe form is that with the earliest onset (SMA type I, Werdnig-Hoffmann disease) with onset during the first year of life and death typically within 2 years. Other forms, with later onset, have more gradual courses; in SMA type III (Kugelberg-Welander disease) motor disability usually emerges during later childhood and adolescence. The severity of disease is related to the level of a protein (termed SMN) that is involved in the assembly of the spliceosome; there are decreased nuclear puncta containing SMN in cells from affected individuals. Most SMN protein comes from mRNA transcripts derived from the *SMN1* gene on chromosome 5q. There is an adjacent *SMN2* gene that differs by a few base pairs, including changes which decrease the efficiency of inclusion of one exon in the mRNA. SMN protein lacking this region is much less stable than the full-length protein. All of the forms of SMA are associated with disruption of *SMN1* (usually through deletion), with the differences in clinical phenotype determined by copy number variation for the *SMN2* gene. Methods of altering the splicing of *SMN2*-derived transcripts are being explored as novel therapeutic approaches for these diseases.

KEY CONCEPTS

Neurodegenerative Diseases

- Neurodegenerative diseases are characterized by progressive neuronal loss involving specific neuronal circuits and brain regions. Most of these diseases are associated with accumulation of abnormal protein aggregates, typically in the form of cellular inclusions. The clinical phenotype reflects the patterns of brain involvement more than the type of inclusions.
- These diseases can be grouped by clinical presentation into: dementias, hypokinetic movement disorders (including forms of parkinsonism), hyperkinetic movement disorders, cerebellar ataxias, and motor neuron diseases.
- Among dementias, AD (with plaques of Aβ and tangles of tau) is the most common; other predominantly dementing diseases include the various forms of FTLDs (both forms with tau-containing lesions and with other types of inclusions) and dementia with Lewy bodies (with α-synuclein containing lesions).
- Among the hypokinetic movement disorders, Parkinson disease is the most common, again with α-synuclein containing inclusions); others diseases which include parkinsonism as part of the symptoms, include PSP and CBD (both forms of tauopathy).
- Amyotrophic lateral sclerosis (ALS) is the most common form of motor neuron disease, with diverse genetic causes as well as sporadic forms.

Genetic Metabolic Diseases

Disruption of metabolic processes in neurons and glia, particularly those involved in synthetic or degradation pathways that are specific to the nervous system, results in diseases that typically present early in life and progress. Some of these disorders manifest in the immediate post-natal period, while others emerge later in development. Overall, forms of these diseases with earlier onset tend to have more rapid and aggressive clinical courses.

Current classification systems are based on the cells or compartment affected (neuronal or white matter), subcellular organelle affected (e.g., lysosome, peroxisome, or mitochondrion), or metabolic pathway affected (e.g., sphingolipidoses or glycogenoses). The classification that follows is based largely on the cellular compartments that are primarily affected, since this correlates well with clinical symptoms and radiologic imaging.

- *Neuronal storage diseases* are predominantly autosomal recessive disorders caused by the deficiency of a specific enzyme involved in the catabolism of sphingolipids (including the gangliosides), mucopolysaccharides, or mucolipids. They are often characterized by the accumulation of the missing enzyme's substrate within the lysosomes of neurons, leading to neuronal death. Cortical neuronal involvement leads to loss of cognitive function and may also cause seizures.
- *Leukodystrophies* are mostly autosomal recessive disorders caused by mutations in genes encoding enzymes involved in myelin synthesis or catabolism. Some of these disorders involve lysosomal enzymes, while others affect peroxisomal enzymes. There is typically diffuse involvement of white matter leading to deterioration in motor skills, spasticity, hypotonia, or ataxia.
- *Mitochondrial encephalomyopathies* are a group of disorders of oxidative phosphorylation, often affecting multiple tissues including skeletal muscle (Chapter 27). When they involve brain, gray matter is more severely affected than white matter, as would be expected because of the greater metabolic requirements of neurons. These disorders may be caused by mutations in the mitochondrial or the nuclear genomes.

Neuronal Storage Diseases

These disorders are characterized by the accumulation of storage material within neurons, typically followed by death of the neurons. The neurologic manifestations that are result from this neuronal dysfunction or death are most often seizures as well as generalized loss of neurologic function. While many of these disorders are associated with deficits of specific enzymes that result in accumulation of substrate, others appear to be caused by defects in protein or lipid trafficking within neurons. This is a large class of disorders, with genetic heterogeneity even for clinically homogeneous entities. Current molecular methods allow whole exome and genome sequencing, which are leading to changes in the classification of these disorders. Several examples of these diseases, such as Tay-Sachs and Niemann-Pick diseases and mucopolysaccharidoses, are described in Chapter 5. Ceroid lipofuscinoses are rare disorders in which lipid pigments accumulate in neurons, and the resulting neuronal dysfunction leads to a combination of blindness, cognitive and motor deterioration and seizures.

Leukodystrophies

These disorders are caused by mutations of genes whose products are involved in the generation, turnover, or maintenance of myelin. Normal brain function depends as much on the connections between neurons as it does on the integrity of the neurons themselves and therefore the progressive and cumulative damage to myelinated fibers that appears in the leukodystrophies has devastating consequences. Several clinical features separate leukodystrophies from demyelinating diseases: the leukodystrophies typically present with an insidious and progressive loss of cerebral function, often at younger ages, and are associated with diffuse and symmetric changes on imaging studies. While many of the leukodystrophies are caused by single enzyme defects resulting in altered metabolism of myelin-associated lipids, a variety of other genetic alterations can lead to white matter diseases. The following examples are representative of this spectrum of disorders.

- **Krabbe disease** is an autosomal recessive leukodystrophy resulting from a *deficiency of galactocerebroside β-galactosidase* (galactosylceramidase), the enzyme required for the catabolism of galactocerebroside to ceramide and galactose. As a consequence of the impaired catabolism of galactocerebroside in the brain, an alternative catabolic pathway shunts galactocerebroside to galactosylsphingosine; elevated levels of this compound are cytotoxic. The clinical course is rapidly progressive, with onset of symptoms (dominated by motor signs such as stiffness and weakness) often between the ages of 3 and 6 months. Survival beyond 2 years of age is uncommon. The brain shows loss of myelin and oligodendrocytes in the CNS and a similar process in peripheral nerves (Fig. 28-44). Neurons and axons are relatively spared. A unique and diagnostic feature of Krabbe disease is the aggregation of engorged macrophages *(globoid cells)* in the brain parenchyma and around blood vessels (Fig. 28-44, *inset*). Hematopoietic stem cell transplantation, which allows repopulation of the CNS with enzymatically competent microglia, has been shown to be of benefit, particularly when performed before the neurologic deficits appear (this is also true of metachromatic leukodystrophy).
- **Metachromatic leukodystrophy** is an autosomal recessive disease that results from a deficiency of the *lysosomal enzyme arylsulfatase A*. This enzyme, present in a variety of tissues, cleaves the sulfate from sulfate-containing lipids (sulfatides) as the first step in their degradation. Enzyme deficiency therefore leads to an accumulation of the sulfatides, especially cerebroside sulfate. These sulfatides have a range of biological actions that can contribute to white matter injury, including inhibiting differentiation of oligodendrocytes and eliciting a proinflammatory response from microglia and astrocytes. The most striking histologic finding is demyelination with resulting gliosis. Macrophages with vacuolated cytoplasm are scattered throughout the

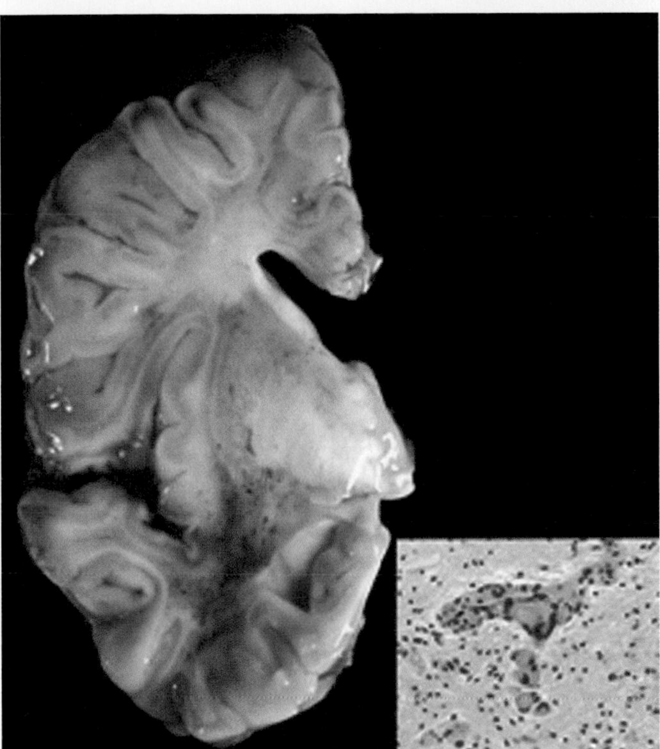

Figure 28-44 Krabbe disease. Much of the white matter is gray/yellow because of the loss of myelin. *Inset*, "Globoid" cells are the hallmark of the disease.

white matter. The membrane-bound vacuoles contain complex crystalloid structures composed of sulfatides; when bound to certain dyes such as toluidine blue, sulfatides shift the absorbance spectrum of the dye, a property called *metachromasia*. Similar metachromatic material can be detected in peripheral nerves and in the urine, the latter being a sensitive method of establishing the diagnosis.

- **Adrenoleukodystrophy** is an X-linked recessive disease associated with mutations in a member of the ATP-binding cassette transporter family of proteins (ABCD1), which is involved in the transport of molecules into the peroxisome. In the typical form of the disease, young males present with behavioral changes and adrenal insufficiency. The disease is characterized by the inability to catabolize very-long-chain fatty acids (VLCFAs) within peroxisomes, resulting in elevated levels of VLCFAs in serum. The symptoms result from a progressive loss of myelin in the CNS and peripheral nerves, as well as adrenal insufficiency. In the white matter, there is loss of myelin accompanied by gliosis and extensive lymphocytic infiltration. Atrophy of the adrenal cortex is present, and VLCFA accumulation can be seen in remaining cells. An allelic disorder presents in adults (both male and female) as a slowly progressive predominantly peripheral nerve disorder known as *adrenomyeloneuropathy*; the symptoms in female carriers are usually more mild. Some of the disorders of peroxisomal biogenesis also manifest as a leukodystrophies, particularly Zellweger spectrum disorder.

A wide range of other forms of leukodystrophy occurs, some with defects in lipid metabolism. Several other mechanisms of selective injury to white matter have been identified, including mutations in genes that encode proteins required for myelin formation (*Pelizaeus-Merzbacher disease*) or intermediate filament proteins such as GFAP (*Alexander disease*), and genes for various subunits of translation initiation factor eIF2B (*vanishing white matter leukoencephalopathy*).

Mitochondrial Encephalomyopathies

Disorders of energy generation can cause a range of neurologic disease, often in association with abnormalities in other tissues. While many of the inherited disorders of mitochondrial oxidative phosphorylation present as muscle diseases (Chapter 27), the critical dependence of neurons on oxidative phosphorylation for generation of ATP is reflected in the frequent involvement of the CNS in these disorders.

The mitochondrial genome, which is entirely inherited from the mother, encodes only 13 proteins, 22 tRNAs, and two rRNAs. The remainder of the proteins involved in mitochondrial function are encoded by the nuclear genome, including those involved in oxidative phosphorylation, mitochondrial metabolism and structure, as well as mitochondrial biogenesis, fission and fusion and replication of mitochondrial DNA. Thus, some mitochondrial disorders show maternal transmission because the affected genes lie in the mitochondrial genome, but many others do not. There is a complex genotype-phenotype relationship in these disorders: the same mutation may manifest as different phenotypes, and the same phenotype may result from one of several mutations.

An additional critical aspect to understanding mitochondrial diseases is *heteroplasmy*, which describes the condition in which cells have a mixture of normal and abnormal mitochondria (typically in the setting of a mitochondrial genome mutation). The expression of the disease may differ from cell to cell depending on the ratio of cells carrying the normal and mutant mitochondria. In general, mitochondrial disorders in the CNS selectively target neurons and gray matter; the disruption of energy generation is often reflected in elevated tissue lactate levels, which can be demonstrated by spectroscopic imaging methods. At the histologic level, there can be loss of staining for enzymatic activity of cytochrome C oxidase.

- **Mitochondrial encephalomyopathy, lactic acidosis, and stroke-like episodes (MELAS)** is characterized by recurrent episodes of acute neurologic dysfunction, cognitive changes, and evidence of muscle involvement with weakness and lactic acidosis. The stroke-like episodes are often associated with reversible deficits that do not correspond to specific vascular territories. Pathologically, areas of infarction are observed, sometimes with vascular proliferation and focal calcification. Studies have shown that both neurons and vascular smooth muscle cells have altered expression of cytochrome c oxidase, suggesting that the underlying pathogenesis is driven both by the metabolic changes in neurons as well as the ability of the cerebral vasculature to respond. The most common mutation observed in MELAS is in the gene encoding mitochondrial tRNA-leucine (MTTL1).

- **Myoclonic epilepsy and ragged red fibers (MERRF)** is a maternally transmitted disease in which affected individuals have myoclonus, a seizure disorder, and evidence of a myopathy. The myopathy is often characterized by ragged red fibers on muscle biopsy (Chapter 27). Ataxia, associated with neuronal loss from the cerebellar system (including the inferior olive in the medulla, cerebellar cortex, and deep nuclei), is also a common component. Most cases of MERRF are associated with mutations in tRNAs other that the specific tRNA mutation associated with MELAS.
- **Leigh syndrome** is a disease of infancy characterized by lactic acidemia, arrest of psychomotor development, feeding problems, seizures, extraocular palsies, and weakness with hypotonia. Death usually occurs within 1 to 2 years. On histologic examination there are multifocal regions of destruction of brain tissue associated with a spongiform appearance and proliferation of blood vessels. Brainstem nuclei, thalamus, and hypothalamus are typically involved, usually in a symmetric manner. A wide spectrum of mutations has been identified as causing Leigh syndrome, including both nuclear and mitochondrial DNA mutations involving components of oxidative phosphorylation complexes and proteins involved in the assembly the electron transport chain.

KEY CONCEPTS

Genetic Metabolic Diseases

- Mutations that disrupt metabolic or synthetic pathways can affect the nervous system. These pathways can involve general cellular processes or those that are relatively specific to the nervous system.
- Diseases with earlier onset are typically more severe in the degree of damage and pace of illness.
- Neuronal storage diseases are commonly autosomal recessive disorders. The characteristic finding is usually accumulation of material within neurons, along with evidence of neuronal death. Seizures are common components of the clinical presentation, along with loss of cognitive function.
- Leukodystrophies are also typically autosomal recessive, with disruption of the synthesis or turnover of myelin components. Motor dysfunction, including spasticity, hypertonia or hypotonia and ataxia are common aspects of the clinical presentation.
- Mitochondrial encephalomyopathies are a pleiotropic set of disorders that involves neurons as well as tissues outside of the nervous system. These can be associated with mutations in the nuclear as well as the mitochondrial genome.

Toxic and Acquired Metabolic Diseases

Toxic and acquired metabolic diseases are relatively common causes of neurologic illnesses. These diseases are discussed in Chapter 9; only aspects that are relevant to CNS pathology are presented here.

Vitamin Deficiencies

Thiamine (Vitamin B_1) Deficiency

Wernicke encephalopathy is caused by thiamine deficiency and is characterized by the acute appearance of a combination of psychotic symptoms and ophthalmoplegia. The acute symptoms are reversible when treated with thiamine. However, if unrecognized and untreated, they may be followed by a prolonged and largely irreversible condition, called *Korsakoff syndrome,* that is characterized clinically by disturbances of short term memory and confabulation. The syndrome is particularly common in the setting of chronic alcoholism, but it may also be encountered in individuals with thiamine deficiency resulting from gastric disorders, including carcinoma, chronic gastritis, or persistent vomiting.

MORPHOLOGY

Wernicke encephalopathy is characterized by foci of hemorrhage and necrosis in the mamillary bodies and the walls of the third and fourth ventricles. Early lesions show dilated capillaries with prominent endothelial cells. Subsequently, the capillaries become leaky, producing hemorrhagic areas. With time, there is infiltration of macrophages and development of a cystic space with hemosiderin-laden macrophages. These chronic lesions predominate in individuals with Korsakoff syndrome. Lesions in the dorsomedial nucleus of the thalamus seem to be the best correlate of the memory disturbance and confabulation.

Vitamin B_{12} Deficiency

Subacute combined degeneration of the spinal cord is caused by deficiency of vitamin B_{12} resulting in degeneration of both ascending and descending spinal tracts. The lesions are caused by a defect in myelin formation; the mechanism of this defect is not known. Symptoms may present over a few weeks, initially with bilaterally symmetrical numbness, tingling, and slight ataxia in the lower extremities, but may progress to include spastic weakness of the lower extremities. Complete paraplegia may occur, usually only later in the course. With prompt vitamin replacement therapy, clinical improvement occurs; however, once complete paraplegia has developed, recovery is poor. On microscopic examination, there is swelling of myelin layers, producing vacuoles, in the affected tracts; with time, axons degenerate as well. In the early stages of the disease the mid-thoracic level of the spinal cord is affected, from where the process may extend proximally and distally.

Neurologic Sequelae of Metabolic Disturbances

Hypoglycemia

Since the brain requires glucose and oxygen for its energy production, the cellular effects of diminished glucose resemble those of oxygen deprivation, described earlier. Some regions of the brain are more sensitive to hypoglycemia than are others. Glucose deprivation initially leads to selective injury to large pyramidal neurons of the cerebral cortex, which, if severe, may result in pseudolaminar necrosis of the cortex, predominantly involving deep layers. The hippocampus is also vulnerable to glucose depletion and may show a marked loss of pyramidal neurons in Sommer sector (area CA1) of the hippocampus. Purkinje cells of the cerebellum are also sensitive to hypoglycemia, although to a lesser extent than to hypoxia. If the level and duration of hypoglycemia are of sufficient severity, there may be widespread injury to many areas of the brain.

Hyperglycemia

Hyperglycemia, most commonly associated with inadequately controlled diabetes mellitus and associated with either ketoacidosis or hyperosmolar coma, does not elicit significant morphologic changes in the brain. The affected individual becomes dehydrated and develops confusion, stupor, and eventually coma. The fluid depletion must be corrected gradually; otherwise, severe cerebral edema may follow.

Hepatic Encephalopathy

The encephalopathy found in the setting of impaired liver function is accompanied by a glial response within the CNS. Critical mediators appear to include elevated ammonia levels as well as proinflammatory cytokines. Astrocytes with enlarged nuclei and minimal reactive cytoplasm, known as Alzheimer type II cells, appear in the cerebral cortex and basal ganglia and other subcortical gray matter regions.

Toxic Disorders

Cellular and tissue injury from toxic agents is discussed in Chapter 9. Aspects of several important toxic disorders that are of unique neurologic importance are discussed here.

Carbon Monoxide

Many of the pathologic findings that follow acute carbon monoxide exposure are the result of impaired oxygen-carrying capacity of hemoglobin. There can also be local effects from the interaction of CO with the heme of cytochrome C oxidase, inhibiting electron transport in the mitochondria. Selective injury of the neurons of layers III and V of the cerebral cortex, Sommer sector of the hippocampus, and Purkinje cells is characteristic. Bilateral necrosis of the globus pallidus may also occur; it is more common in carbon monoxide-induced hypoxia than in hypoxia from other causes. Demyelination of white matter tracts may be a later event.

Methanol

Methanol toxicity preferentially affects the retina, where degeneration of retinal ganglion cells may cause blindness. Selective bilateral necrosis of the putamen and focal white-matter necrosis also occur when the exposure is severe. Formate and other metabolites of methanol appear to contribute to toxicity through disruption of oxidative phosphorylation and through nonenzymatic protein modification. Methanol toxicity occurs by ingestion of illicit liquor (moonshine) contaminated with methanol or when it is used as a substitute for ethanol.

Ethanol

Experience tells us that the effects of acute ethanol intoxication are reversible, but chronic alcohol abuse is associated with a variety of neurologic sequelae, including Wernicke-Korsakoff syndrome from thiamine deficiency (see earlier). The toxic effects of chronic alcohol intake may be either direct or secondary to nutritional deficits. Cerebellar dysfunction occurs in about 1% of chronic alcoholics, associated with a clinical syndrome of truncal ataxia, unsteady gait, and nystagmus. The histologic changes are atrophy and loss of granule cells predominantly in the anterior vermis (Fig. 28-45). In advanced cases there is loss of Purkinje cells and proliferation of the adjacent astrocytes *(Bergmann gliosis)* between the depleted granular cell layer and the molecular layer of the cerebellum. The fetal alcohol syndrome is discussed in Chapter 10.

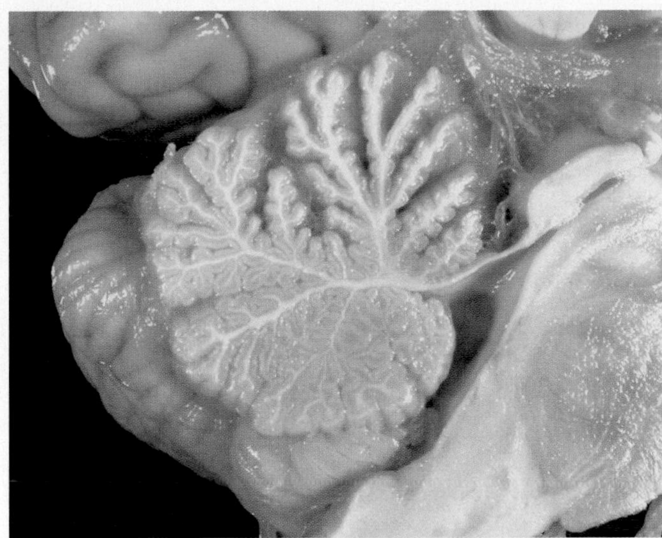

Figure 28-45 Alcoholic cerebellar degeneration. The anterior portion of the vermis (upper portion of figure) is atrophic with widened spaces between the folia.

Radiation

Exposure of the brain to radiation can occur accidentally or as part of therapeutic regimens for brain tumors. As discussed in Chapter 9, exposure to very high doses of radiation (>10 Gy) can cause intractable nausea, confusion, convulsions, and rapid onset of coma, followed by death. Delayed effects of radiation can also present with rapidly evolving symptoms, including headaches, nausea, vomiting, and papilledema that may appear months to years after irradiation.

The pathologic findings consist of large areas of coagulative necrosis, primarily in white matter, with all tissue elements within the area undergoing necrosis. This is accompanied by marked edema in the surrounding tissue, along with vascular fibrinoid necrosis and eventual sclerosis. The combination of radiation and methotrexate, administered either concurrently or sequentially, can act synergistically to cause tissue injury. While similar in appearance to that caused by radiation alone, these lesions are often adjacent to the lateral ventricles but may be distributed throughout the white matter or in the brainstem. Axons and cell bodies in the vicinity of the lesions undergo dystrophic mineralization, and there is adjacent gliosis. Radiation can also induce tumors, which usually develop years after radiation therapy and include sarcomas, gliomas, and meningiomas.

KEY CONCEPTS

Toxic and Acquired Metabolic Diseases

- Certain vitamin deficiency states result in neurologic disease as well as systemic disorders, with thiamine and vitamin B_{12} being the two most common.
- The metabolic demand of the CNS makes it highly susceptible to injury from hypoglycemia and loss of oxygen-carrying capacity of hemoglobin with carbon monoxide toxicity.
- Chronic alcohol exposure may result in injury to the cerebellum, particularly to the anterior vermis.
- Metabolic disarray may disrupt brain function, often without detectable morphologic changes.

Tumors

The annual incidence of tumors of the CNS ranges from 10 to 17 per 100,000 persons for intracranial tumors and 1 to 2 per 100,000 persons for intraspinal tumors; the majority of these are primary tumors, and only one fourth to one half are metastatic. Tumors of the CNS account for nearly 20% of all cancers of childhood. Seventy percent of childhood CNS tumors arise in the posterior fossa; a comparable number of tumors in adults arise within the cerebral hemispheres above the tentorium.

While pathologists have developed classification schemes that distinguish between benign and malignant lesions on histologic grounds, the clinical course of a patient with a brain tumor is strongly influenced by patterns of growth and location. Thus, some glial tumors with low grade histologic features (low mitotic rate, cellular uniformity, and slow growth) infiltrate large regions of the brain and lead to serious clinical deficits and poor prognosis. Because of this capacity to diffusely infiltrate the white and gray matter, a tumor may not be amenable to complete surgical resection without compromising neurologic function. Also, any CNS neoplasm, regardless of histologic grade or classification, may have lethal consequences if situated in a critical brain region; for example, a benign meningioma may cause cardiorespiratory arrest if situated in the posterior fossa in a position to compress vital centers in the medulla. Even the most highly malignant gliomas rarely metastasize outside the CNS. Tumors are able to spread through the CSF if they encroach upon the subarachnoid space, and thus may be associated with implantation along the brain and spinal cord at a distance from the original tumor site.

Classification of tumors is one of the arts of pathology, drawing on traditional recognition of histologic and biologic features, combined with newer molecular analyses. Treatment protocols and experimental trials of glial tumors are usually based on the World Health Organization (WHO) classification, which segregates tumors into one of four grades according to their biologic behavior, ranging from grade I to grade IV. Under the current classification scheme, lesions of different grade are always given distinct names. When tumors recur, they often show progression to a higher histologic grade and designation; this actually represents clonal evolution of the same tumor, rather than a new disease. There is great interest in identifying tumor-initiating (or stem-like) cells that maintain tumor growth and, therefore, may be key targets of new therapies.

The major classes of primary brain tumors to be considered here include gliomas, neuronal tumors, poorly differentiated tumors, and a group of other less common tumors. In addition, we will discuss tumors of the meninges as well as familial tumor syndromes.

Gliomas

Gliomas, the most common group of primary brain tumors, include *astrocytomas*, *oligodendrogliomas*, and *ependymomas*. These tumor types have characteristic histologic features that form the basis for the classification. It is no longer thought that these tumors derive from their specific, mature cell types (astrocytes, oligodendrocytes, and ependymal), but rather that they arise from a progenitor cell that preferentially differentiates down one of the cellular lineages. Many of the tumors typically occur in certain anatomic regions within the brain, with characteristic age distribution and clinical course.

Astrocytoma

The two major categories of astrocytic tumors are the diffusely infiltrating astrocytomas and the more localized astrocytomas, of which the most common are the pilocytic astrocytomas. Astrocytomas may range from WHO grade I to grade IV, may occur from the first decade of life onward and may be found anywhere along the neuroaxis from the cerebral hemispheres to the spinal cord.

Infiltrating Astrocytomas

Infiltrating astrocytomas account for about 80% of adult primary brain tumors in adults. Usually found in the cerebral hemispheres, they may also occur in the cerebellum, brainstem, or spinal cord, most often in the fourth through sixth decades. The most common presenting signs and symptoms are seizures, headaches, and focal neurologic deficits related to the anatomic site of involvement. Infiltrating astrocytomas show a spectrum of histologic differentiation that correlates well with clinical course and outcome; within this spectrum, tumors range from *diffuse astrocytoma* (grade II/IV) to *anaplastic astrocytoma* (grade III/IV) to *glioblastoma* (grade IV/IV). There are no WHO grade I infiltrating astrocytomas.

Molecular Genetics. It was recognized well before modern advances in genetic analyses that glioblastoma tends to occur in one of two clinical settings—most commonly as a new onset disease, typically in older individuals *(primary glioblastoma)*, and less frequently in younger patients due to progression of a lower-grade astrocytoma *(secondary glioblastoma)*. Data from the Cancer Genome Atlas Network based on sequencing the genome of malignant gliomas have identified **patterns of molecular alteration in glioblastoma that place these tumors into four molecular subtypes: classic, proneural, neural, and mesenchymal**.

- The *classic subtype*, comprising the majority of primary glioblastoma, is characterized by mutations of the *PTEN* tumor suppressor gene, deletions of chromosome 10, and amplification of the *EGFR* oncogene. Focal deletions involving chromosome 9p21, resulting in hemizygous deletion of the *CDKN2A* tumor suppressor gene, are also common; you will recall that this unusual locus encodes two tumor suppressors, p16/INK4a and p14ARF, which function by augmenting the activity of RB and p53, respectively.

- The *proneural type*, which is the most common type associated with secondary glioblastoma, is characterized by mutations of *TP53*, and point mutations in the isocitrate dehydrogenase genes, *IDH1* and *IDH2*. The proneural glioblastoma also often shows an overexpression of the receptor for platelet-derived growth factor receptor α (PDGFRA). Low grade gliomas (grades II and III astrocytomas) also tend to have mutations in *TP53* and in the *IDH* genes, a molecular signature that is carried forward as the neoplasm evolves to the higher grade, secondary glioblastoma.
- The *neural type* is characterized by higher levels of expression of neuronal markers, including NEFL, GABRA1, SYT1, and SLC12A5.
- The *mesenchymal type* is characterized by deletions of the *NF1* gene on chromosome 17, and lower expression of the NF1 protein. Genes involved in the TNF pathway and the NF-κB pathway are highly expressed in the mesenchymal glioblastoma.

The common theme of these diverse genotypic changes is that most affect two cancer hallmarks, sustained proliferative signaling and evasion of growth suppressors. For example, overexpression of PDGFRA in proneural glioblastomas, and mutation and amplification of *EGFR* genes in classic glioblastomas, both lead to increased receptor tyrosine kinase signaling. You will recall from Chapter 7 that tyrosine kinases stimulate RAS and PI3K/AKT signaling, which act together to drive cells from the G1 to S phase of the cell cycle and to deregulate cellular metabolism so as to promote growth. Other common events directly or indirectly inhibit RB and p53 function. Based on whole genome sequencing, it is estimated that mutations that activate RAS and PI-3 kinase and inactivate p53 and RB are present in 80% to 90% of primary glioblastomas.

Additionally, among the higher grade astrocytomas (WHO grades III and IV), the presence of the mutant form of *IDH1* (predominantly the R132H mutation) is associated with a significantly better outcome than in tumors with wild type *IDH1*. You will recall that *IDH1* mutations create a neomorphic enzyme activity that generates 2-hydroxyglutarate, which appears to contribute to oncogenesis by inhibiting enzymes that regulate DNA methylation, an example of oncogenesis by epigenetic dysregulation (Chapter 7).

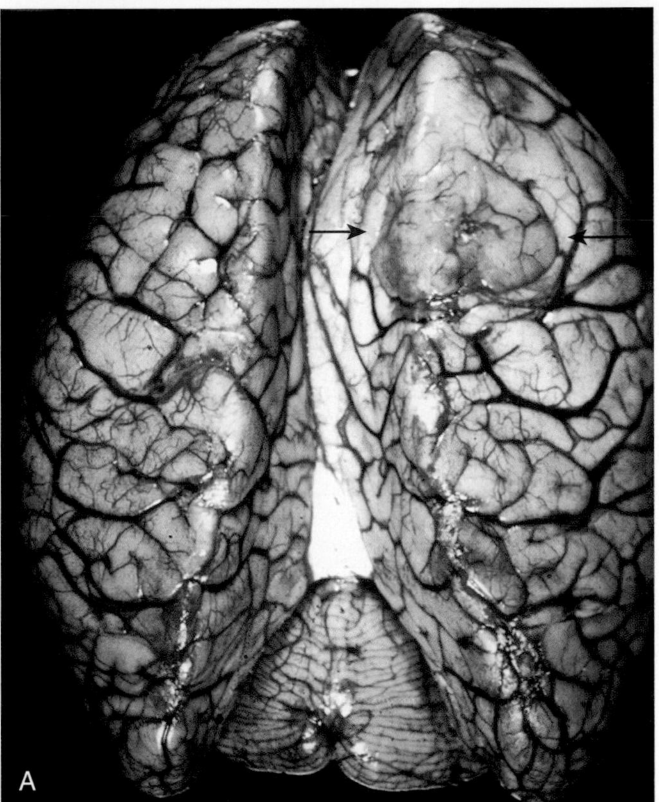

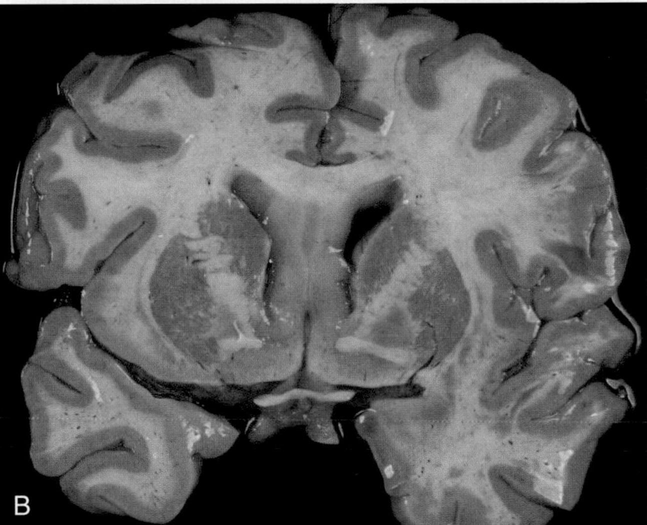

Figure 28-46 Diffuse astrocytoma. **A,** The right frontal tumor has expanded gyri, which led to flattening *(arrows)*. **B,** There is bilateral expansion of the septum pellucidum by gray, glassy tumor.

MORPHOLOGY

Diffuse astrocytomas are poorly defined, gray, infiltrative tumors that expand and distort the invaded brain (Fig. 28-46). These tumors range in size from a few centimeters to enormous lesions that replace an entire hemisphere. The cut surface of the tumor may be either firm or soft and gelatinous; cystic degeneration may be seen. The tumor may appear well demarcated from the surrounding brain tissue, but infiltration beyond the outer margins is always present.

Microscopically, diffuse astrocytomas have a cellular density that is greater than normal white matter. Between the tumor cell nuclei there is an extensive feltwork of fine, GFAP-positive astrocytic processes that create a fibrillary background appearance. There are variable degrees of nuclear pleomorphism. The transition between neoplastic and normal tissue is indistinct, and tumor cells infiltrate normal tissue some distance away from the main lesion.

Anaplastic astrocytomas are more densely cellular and have greater nuclear pleomorphism; mitotic figures are often observed. The term **gemistocytic astrocytoma** is used for

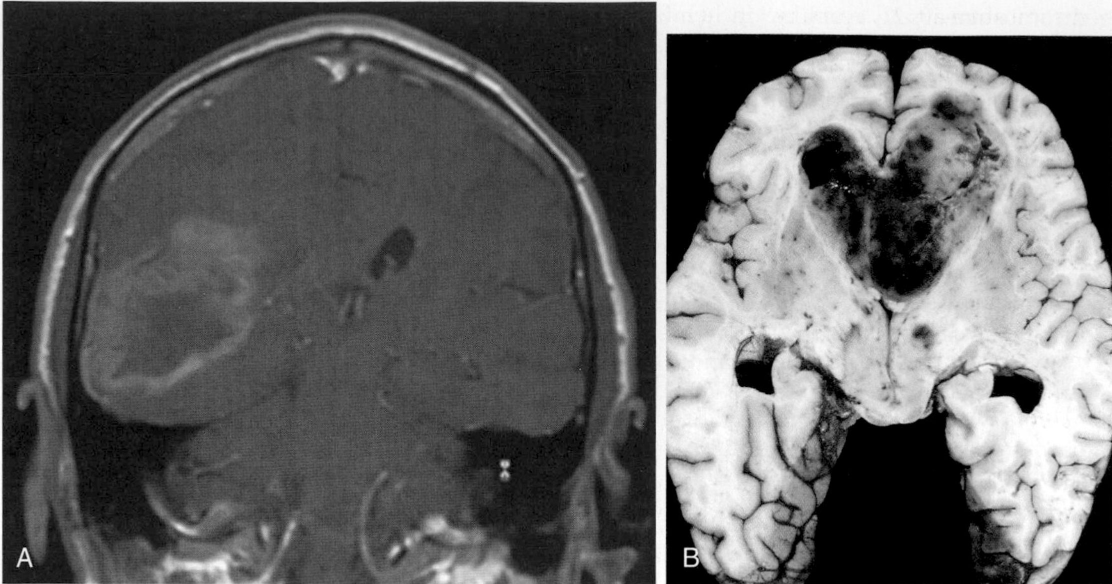

Figure 28-47 **A,** Contrast T1-weighted coronal magnetic resonance image shows a large mass in the right parietal lobe with "ring" enhancement. **B,** Glioblastoma appearing as a necrotic, hemorrhagic, infiltrating mass.

tumors in which the predominant neoplastic astrocyte shows a brightly eosinophilic cell body from which emanate abundant, stout processes.

In **glioblastoma** (previously called *glioblastoma multiforme*, and sometimes still abbreviated GBM), variation in the appearance of the tumor from region to region is characteristic (Fig. 28-47). Some areas are firm and white, others are soft and yellow due to necrosis, and yet others show cystic degeneration and hemorrhage. The histologic appearance of glioblastoma is similar to anaplastic astrocytoma with the additional features of **necrosis** and **vascular/endothelial cell proliferation**. Necrosis in glioblastoma often occurs in a serpentine pattern in areas of hypercellularity. Tumor cells collect along the edges of the necrotic regions, producing a histologic pattern referred to as **pseudo-palisading** (Fig. 28-48). The vascular cell proliferation produces tufts of cells that pile up and bulge into the lumen; the minimal criterion for this feature is a double layer of endothelial cells. With marked vascular cell proliferation the tuft forms a ball-like structure, the glomeruloid body. VEGF, produced by malignant astrocytes in response to hypoxia, contributes to this distinctive vascular change. Since histologic features can be extremely variable from one region to another, small biopsy specimens may not be representative of the entire tumor.

Gliomatosis cerebri is a diffuse glioma with extensive infiltration of multiple regions of the brain, in some cases the entire brain. Because of the widespread infiltration, this process follows an aggressive course and is considered to be a grade III/IV lesion.

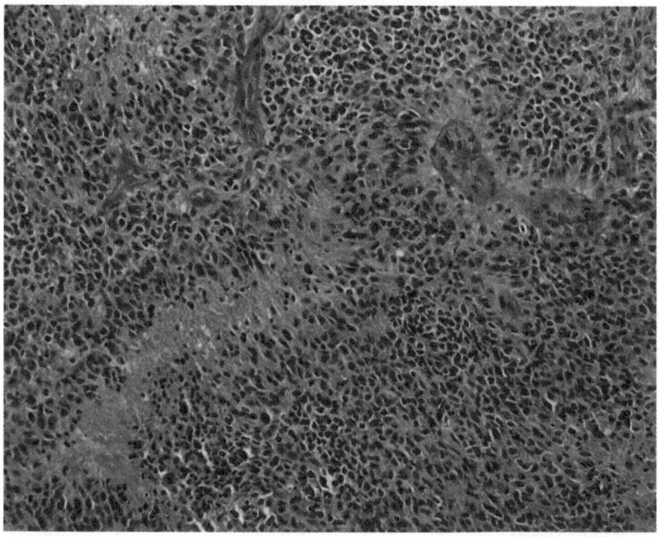

Figure 28-48 Glioblastoma. Foci of necrosis with pseudo-palisading of malignant nuclei and endothelial cell proliferation.

Clinical Features. The presenting symptoms of infiltrating astrocytomas depend, in part, on the location and growth rate of the tumor. Well-differentiated diffuse astrocytomas may remain stable or progress only slowly over a number of years; the mean survival is more than 5 years. Eventually, however, clinical deterioration invariably occurs and is usually due to the emergence of a more rapidly growing tumor of higher histologic grade. Radiologic studies show mass effect as well as changes in the brain adjacent to the tumor, such as edema. High-grade astrocytomas have abnormal vessels that are "leaky," with an abnormally permeable blood-brain barrier, and therefore, demonstrate contrast enhancement on imaging studies. The prognosis for individuals with glioblastoma is very poor, although the use of newer chemotherapeutic agents has provided some benefit. Epigenetic silencing of the promoter for the gene encoding the DNA repair enzyme MGMT predicts responsiveness to DNA alkylating drugs—as would be expected since MGMT is critical for the repair of the chemotherapeutically induced DNA modification. With current treatment, consisting of resection followed by radiation therapy and chemotherapy, the mean length of survival after diagnosis has increased to 15 months; 25%

of such patients are alive after 2 years. Survival is substantially shorter in older patients and in patients with lower performance status or with large unresectable lesions. Most of the molecular characteristics of gliomas do not have specific prognostic significance, apart from the beneficial effects of the presence of *IDH1* mutations. Nevertheless, identification of molecular aberrations may provide targets for therapies.

Pilocytic Astrocytoma

Pilocytic astrocytomas (grade I/IV) are distinguished from the other types by their gross and microscopic appearance and relatively benign behavior. They typically occur in children and young adults, and are usually located in the cerebellum but may also appear in the floor and walls of the third ventricle, the optic nerves, and occasionally the cerebral hemispheres. The histologic separation of these tumors from other astrocytomas is supported by the rarity of *TP53* mutations or molecular signatures of infiltrating astrocytomas. Those pilocytic astrocytomas that occur in patients with neurofibromatosis type 1 show functional loss of neurofibromin; this genetic alteration is not observed in sporadic forms. Two types of alterations in the BRAF signaling athway have been found in pilocytic astrocytoma: translocations which serve to separate the kinase domain from the inhibitory domain, and an activating point mutation (V600E) that is also found in an increasing number of other tumor types (Chapter 7). These findings suggest that targeted therapy with BRAF inhibitors might play a role in the treatment of pilocytic astrocytomas, particularly for lesions in regions not suitable for resection.

MORPHOLOGY

Pilocytic astrocytoma is often cystic (Fig. 28-49); if solid, it may be well circumscribed or, less frequently, infiltrative. The tumor is composed of bipolar cells with long, thin "hairlike" processes that are GFAP-positive and form dense fibrillary meshworks; Rosenthal fibers and eosinophilic granular bodies, are characteristic findings. Tumors are often biphasic, with both loose "microcystic" and fibrillary areas. An increase in the number of blood vessels, often with thickened walls or vascular cell proliferation, is seen but does not imply an unfavorable prognosis. Necrosis and brisk mitotic activity is uncommon. Unlike diffuse fibrillary astrocytomas of any grade, pilocytic astrocytomas show limited infiltration of the surrounding brain.

These tumors grow very slowly, and, in the cerebellum particularly, may be treated by resection. Symptomatic recurrence of incompletely resected lesions is often associated with cyst enlargement rather than growth of the solid component. Tumors that extend into the hypothalamic region from the optic tract can have a more ominous clinical course because of their location.

Pleomorphic Xanthoastrocytoma

This tumor occurs most often in the temporal lobe in children and young adults, usually with a history of seizures. The tumor consists of neoplastic, occasionally bizarre, astrocytes, which are sometimes filled with lipids; these cells can express neuronal and glial markers. The degree of nuclear atypia can be extreme and may suggest a high-grade astrocytoma, but the presence of abundant reticulin deposits, relative circumscription, and chronic inflammatory cell infiltrates, along with the absence of necrosis and mitotic activity, distinguish this tumor from more malignant types. The pleomorphic xanthoastrocytoma is usually a low-grade tumor (WHO grade II/IV) with a 5-year survival rate estimated at 80%. Necrosis and mitotic activity are indicative of higher grade tumors and predict a more aggressive course.

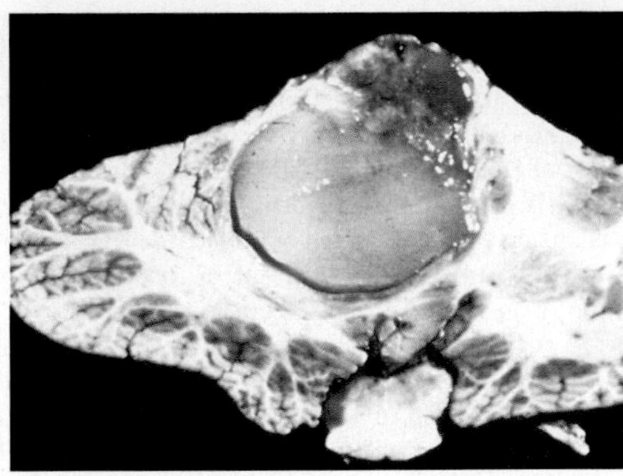

Figure 28-49 Pilocytic astrocytoma in the cerebellum with a nodule of tumor in a cyst.

Brainstem Glioma

A clinical subgroup of astrocytomas, brainstem gliomas, occur most often in the first 2 decades of life and make up 10% to 20% of all brain tumors in this age group. Several distinct anatomic patterns have been defined in the pediatric age group, each differing in clinical course: intrinsic pontine gliomas (the most common), with an aggressive course and short survival; cervicomedullary junction tumors, often exophytic, with a less aggressive course; and dorsally exophytic gliomas, with an even more benign course which may arise in the tectum of the midbrain, pons, or medulla. Among the rarer brainstem gliomas affecting adults, most are intrinsic pontine gliomas. These can be separated into low-grade diffuse fibrillary astrocytomas and glioblastoma, with the expected differences in clinical course and survival.

The concept that these are a distinct type of glioma is supported by sequencing the genomes of childhood pontine gliomas. Surprisingly, this has revealed that most tumors of this type have a lysine to methionine mutation at position 27 (K27M) in histone H3.1 or H3.3. Of note, H3K27 is a position that is subject to acetylation and methylation events that regulate chromatin structure and gene expression, yet another example of oncogenic mutations that directly impact the epigenome.

Oligodendroglioma

These are infiltrating gliomas comprised of cells that resemble oligodendrocytes. These tumors constitute 5% to 15% of gliomas and are most common in the fourth and fifth decades. Patients may have had several years of neurologic complaints, often including seizures. The lesions are found mostly in the cerebral hemispheres, with a predilection for white matter.

Molecular Genetics. Molecular abnormalities as well as histologic appearance distinguish oligodendrogliomas from astrocytic tumors. The most common genetic alterations in oligodendrogliomas are mutations of the isocitrate dehydrogenase genes (*IDH1* and *IDH2*), which occur in up to 90% of oligodendrogliomas and portend a better prognosis, as they do for astrocytic tumors. Deletions of portions of chromosomes 1p and 19q, typically occurring together as a co-deletion, are seen in up to 80% of cases. Additional genetic alterations occur with progression to anaplastic oligodendroglioma. The more common of these include loss of 9p, loss of 10q, and mutations in *CDKN2A*. In contrast to high-grade astrocytic tumors, *EGFR* gene amplification is not seen, but a significant proportion do show increased EGFR protein levels.

In addition to having implications for the biology of the tumors, the molecular alterations in anaplastic oligodendrogliomas have relevance to the choice of treatment modalities. Tumors with co-deletion of 1p/19q have consistent, long-lasting responses to chemotherapy and radiation, whereas those without loss of 1p or 19q appear to be resistant to chemotherapy regimens.

MORPHOLOGY

Oligodendrogliomas are well circumscribed, gelatinous, gray masses, often with cysts, focal hemorrhage, and calcification. The tumors are composed of sheets of regular cells with spherical nuclei containing finely granular chromatin (similar to normal oligodendrocytes) surrounded by a clear halo of vacuolated cytoplasm (Fig. 28-50). The tumor typically contains a delicate network of anastomosing capillaries. Calcification, present in as many as 90% of these tumors, ranges from microscopic foci to massive depositions. Tumor cells infiltrating the cerebral cortex often collect around neurons (perineuronal satellitosis). Mitotic activity is minimal or absent, and proliferation indices are low. Oligodendrogliomas are considered to be WHO grade II/IV lesions.

Anaplastic oligodendrogliomas (WHO grade III/IV) are characterized by a higher cell density, nuclear anaplasia, detectable mitotic activity, and necrosis. These changes can often be found in nodules within an otherwise typical grade II oligodendroglioma. Some of these high-grade oligodendroglial tumors also show patterns that are indistinguishable from glioblastoma. Because several studies have shown that such appearance correlates with worse behavior, these tumors are grouped with glioblastoma.

Clinical Features. In general, individuals with oligodendrogliomas have a better prognosis than do those with astrocytomas. Current treatment with surgery, chemotherapy, and radiation therapy has yielded an average survival of 5 to 10 years. Individuals with anaplastic oligodendroglioma have an overall worse prognosis. Progression from low to higher grade lesions occurs, typically over about 6 years.

Ependymoma and Related Paraventricular Mass Lesions

Ependymomas are tumors that most often arise next to the ependyma-lined ventricular system, including the oft-obliterated central canal of the spinal cord. In the first two decades of life they typically occur near the fourth ventricle and constitute 5% to 10% of the primary brain tumors in this age group. In adults the spinal cord is the most common location; tumors in this site are particularly frequent in the setting of neurofibromatosis type 2 (NF2).

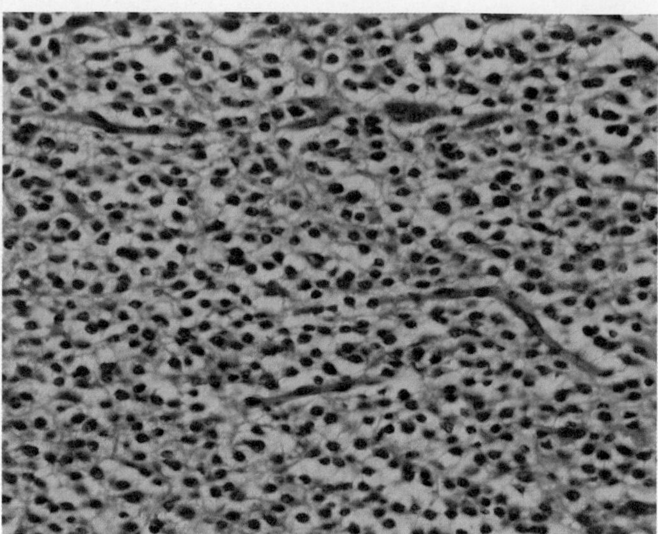

Figure 28-50 Oligodendroglioma. Tumor nuclei are round, with cleared cytoplasm forming "halos" and vasculature composed of thin-walled capillaries.

Molecular Genetics. Given the association of spinal ependymomas with NF2, it is not surprising that the *NF2* gene on chromosome 22 is commonly mutated in ependymomas in the spinal cord but not at other sites. Ependymomas do not share the genetic alterations that are found in infiltrating gliomas, such as mutations in *TP53*. There appear to be at least two separate subtypes, one expressing a mesenchymal phenotype, typically in younger patients with a higher propensity to develop metastases, and a second with aberrations of large regions of chromosomes or whole chromosomes that tends to have a better overall prognosis.

MORPHOLOGY

In the fourth ventricle, ependymomas are typically solid or papillary masses arising from the floor of the ventricle (Fig. 28-51*A*). Although ependymomas are moderately well demarcated from adjacent brain, the proximity of vital pontine and medullary nuclei usually makes complete extirpation impossible. In the intraspinal tumors, the sharp demarcation sometimes makes total removal feasible. Ependymomas are composed of cells with regular, round to oval nuclei and abundant granular chromatin. Between the nuclei there is a variably dense fibrillary background. Tumor cells may form gland-like round or elongated structures (rosettes, canals) that resemble the embryologic ependymal canal, with long, delicate processes extending into a lumen (Fig. 28-51*B*); more frequently present are **perivascular pseudorosettes** (Fig. 28-51*B*), in which tumor cells are arranged around vessels with an intervening zone consisting of thin ependymal processes directed toward the wall of the vessel. GFAP expression is found in most ependymomas. While most ependymomas are well differentiated and behave as WHO grade II/IV lesions, anaplastic ependymomas (WHO grade III/IV) reveal increased cell density, high mitotic rates, areas of necrosis, and less evident ependymal differentiation.

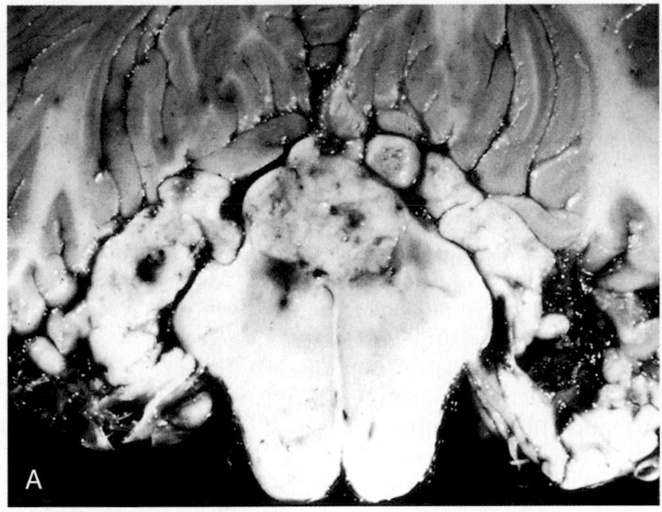

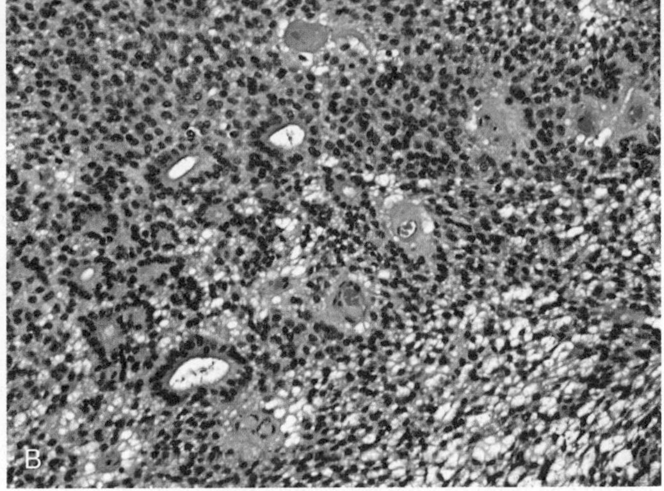

Figure 28-51 Ependymoma. **A,** Tumor growing into the fourth ventricle, distorting, compressing, and infiltrating surrounding structures. **B,** Microscopic appearance of ependymoma.

Myxopapillary ependymomas are distinct but related lesions that occur in the filum terminale of the spinal cord and contain papillary elements in a myxoid background, admixed with ependymoma-like cells. Cuboidal cells, sometimes with clear cytoplasm, are arranged around papillary cores containing connective tissue and blood vessels. The myxoid areas contain neutral and acidic mucopolysaccharides. Prognosis depends on completeness of surgical resection; if the tumor has extended into the subarachnoid space and surrounded the roots of the cauda equina, recurrence is likely.

Clinical Features. Posterior fossa ependymomas often manifest with hydrocephalus secondary to progressive obstruction of the fourth ventricle. Because of the relationship of ependymomas to the ventricular system, CSF dissemination is a common occurrence and portends a poor prognosis. Posterior fossa lesions have the worst overall outcome, particularly in younger children, in whom the 5-year survival is roughly 50%. The clinical outcome for completely resected supratentorial and spinal ependymomas is better.

Several other tumors occur either immediately below the ependymal lining of the ventricle or in association with the choroid plexus, which sits in continuity with the ependyma. With the exception of the rare choroid plexus carcinoma, these are benign; however, because of location they may cause clinical problems.

- *Subependymomas* are solid, sometimes calcified, slow-growing nodules attached to the ventricular lining and protruding into the ventricle. They are usually asymptomatic and are incidental findings at autopsy or imaging; if they are sufficiently large or strategically located, they may cause hydrocephalus. They are most often found in the lateral and fourth ventricles and have a characteristic microscopic appearance, with clusters of ependymal-appearing nuclei scattered in a dense, fine, glial fibrillar background.
- *Choroid plexus papillomas* may occur anywhere along the choroid plexus and are most common in children, in whom they are usually found in the lateral ventricles. In adults, they more often involve the fourth ventricle. These papillary growths almost exactly recapitulate the structure of the normal choroid plexus. The papillae have connective tissue stalks covered with a cuboidal or columnar epithelium. Clinically, choroid plexus papillomas usually present with hydrocephalus due to obstruction of the ventricular system by tumor or overproduction of CSF. The far rarer *choroid plexus carcinomas* resemble adenocarcinoma. These tumors are usually found in children; in adults, they must be differentiated from metastatic carcinoma, which is much more common than primary carcinomas of the choroid.
- *Colloid cyst of the third ventricle* is a non-neoplastic enlarging cyst that most often occurs in young adults. The cyst is attached to the roof of the third ventricle, where it can obstruct one or both of the foramina of Monro and, as a result, causes noncommunicating hydrocephalus which may be rapidly fatal. Headache, sometimes positional, is an important clinical symptom. The cyst has a thin, fibrous capsule and a lining of low to flat cuboidal epithelium; it contains gelatinous, proteinaceous material.

Neuronal Tumors

Far less common than glial tumors are those that exhibit neuronal differentiation. In general, neuronal tumors are more often seen in younger adults and often present with seizures.

- *Gangliogliomas* are tumors comprised of a mixture of mature neuronal and glial cells. They are typically superficial lesions that present with seizures. These are the most common of the neuronal tumors of the CNS. Most of these tumors are slow growing, but the glial component occasionally becomes anaplastic, and the disease then progresses rapidly. When gangliogliomas present because of a seizure disorder, surgical resection of the tumor is usually effective in controlling the seizures. Approximately 20% of these tumors have an activating mutation in the *BRAF* gene (V600E), and are associated with a shorter recurrence-free survival.

Gangliogliomas are most commonly found in the temporal lobe and often have a cystic component. The neoplastic ganglion cells are irregularly clustered and have apparently random orientation of neurites. Binucleate forms are found. The glial component of these lesions usually resembles a low-grade astrocytoma, lacking mitotic activity and necrosis.

- *Dysembryoplastic neuroepithelial tumor* is a rare, low-grade (WHO Grade I) tumor of childhood that often presents as a seizure disorder. It has a good prognosis following surgical resection, with both low recurrence rates and favorable seizure control. These lesions are typically located in the superficial temporal lobe, although other cortical sites are seen. There is often attenuation of the overlying skull, suggesting that the lesion has been present for some time.

  These lesions typically form multiple discrete intracortical nodules of small, round cells, arranged in columns around central cores of processes, and are associated with a myxoid background. There are well-differentiated "floating neurons" that sit in the pools of mucopolysaccharide-rich fluid of the myxoid background. The larger neurons and the small, round cells of the specific element express neuronal markers. Surrounding the nodules, there may be focal cortical dysplasia; lesions that show both the specific element and a glial component are termed complex.
- *Central neurocytoma* typically is a low-grade (WHO Grade II) neuronal neoplasm found within the ventricular system (most commonly the lateral or third ventricles), characterized by evenly spaced, round, uniform nuclei and often islands of neuropil. Although in pattern and shape the cells resemble oligodendroglioma, ultrastructural and immunohistochemical studies reveal the neuronal lineage of the tumor cells.

Poorly Differentiated Neoplasms

Some tumors, though of neuroectodermal origin, express few if any markers of mature neural cells and are described as poorly differentiated or embryonal, meaning that they retain cellular features of primitive, undifferentiated cells. The most common is the *medulloblastoma*, which accounts for 20% of brain tumors in children.

Medulloblastoma

This malignant embryonal tumor occurs predominantly in children and exclusively in the cerebellum (by definition). Neuronal and glial markers may be expressed, but the tumor is often largely undifferentiated and corresponds to WHO grade IV.

Molecular Genetics. Molecular subtypes of medulloblastoma have been identified through genomic studies, revealing alterations of signaling pathways involved in normal cerebellar development, such as the sonic hedgehog-patched (SHH) pathway involved in control of normal proliferation of cerebellar granule cells, and the WNT/β-catenin signaling pathway. On the basis of molecular alterations, medulloblastoma can be divided into four groups:

- The *WNT type*, characterized by mutations in the WNT signaling pathway, tends to occur in older children, has a classic medulloblastoma histology, and shows monosomy of chromosome 6 and nuclear expression of β-catenin. The prognosis is best in this subtype with 90% 5-year survival.
- The *SHH type*, characterized by mutations involving the sonic hedgehog signaling pathway, tends to occur in infants or young adults, tends to have a nodular desmoplastic histology and may have *MYCN* amplification. The prognosis is intermediate between the WNT subtype and groups 3 and 4.
- *Group 3 medulloblastoma*, often with *MYC* amplification and isochromosome 17 (i17q), tends to occur in infants and children, with a classic or large cell histology and the worst prognosis.
- *Group 4* is characterized by an i17q cytogenetic alteration, classic or large cell histology, without *MYC* amplification, but sometimes with *MYCN* amplification. The prognosis in group 4 is intermediate. In general, isochromosome 17q signals a poor prognosis, and is restricted to groups 3 and 4.

MORPHOLOGY

In children, medulloblastomas are located in the midline of the cerebellum, but lateral locations are more often found in adults. Rapid growth may occlude the flow of CSF, leading to hydrocephalus. The tumor is often well circumscribed, gray, and friable, and may be seen extending to the surface of the cerebellar folia and involving the leptomeninges (Fig. 28-52*A*). On microscopic examination, medulloblastoma is very densely cellular, with sheets of anaplastic cells (Fig. 28-52*B*). Individual tumor cells are small, with scant cytoplasm and hyperchromatic nuclei that are frequently elongated or crescent shaped. Mitoses are abundant, and markers of cellular proliferation, such as Ki-67, are detected in a high percentage of the cells. The tumor may express neuronal (neurosecretory) granules, form Homer-Wright rosettes, as occur in neuroblastoma Chapter 10), and express glial markers (e.g., GFAP). The **nodular desmoplastic variant** is characterized by areas of stromal response, marked by collagen and reticulin deposition and nodules of cells forming "pale islands" that have more neuropil and show greater expression of neuronal markers. The **large cell variant** is characterized by large irregular vesicular nuclei, prominent nucleoli, and frequent mitoses and apoptotic cells.

At the edges of the main tumor mass, medulloblastoma cells have a propensity to form linear chains of cells infiltrating through cerebellar cortex and penetrating the pia, spreading into the subarachnoid space. Dissemination through the CSF is a common complication, giving rise to nodular masses at some distance from the primary tumor (e.g. as far as the cauda equina); these are sometimes termed "drop metastases."

Clinical Features. The tumor is highly malignant, and the prognosis for untreated patients is dismal; however, it is exquisitely radiosensitive. With total excision and irradiation, the 5-year survival rate may be as high as 75%. How the different molecular subtypes of medulloblastoma respond to therapies is under active investigation; early clinical trials suggest some medulloblastomas may respond to inhibitors of the hedgehog signaling pathway.

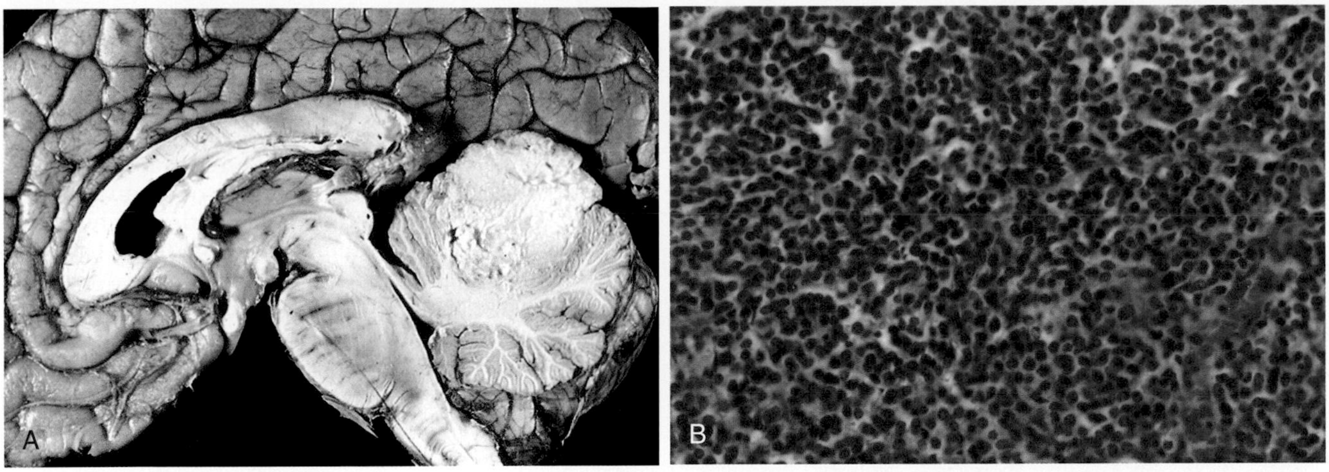

Figure 28-52 Medulloblastoma. **A,** Sagittal section of brain showing medulloblastoma destroying the superior midline cerebellum. **B,** Microscopic appearance of medulloblastoma.

Tumors of similar poorly differentiated histology and resembling medulloblastomas may occur in the cerebral hemispheres. These lesions are known as CNS supratentorial primitive neuroectodermal tumors (CNS PNET). This term unfortunately can lead to confusion with the peripheral lesion (peripheral neuroectodermal tumor), which shares a genetic alteration with Ewing sarcoma. In the CNS, PNET is distinct from medulloblastoma and from the peripheral tumor.

Atypical Teratoid/Rhabdoid Tumor

This highly malignant tumor of young children is a WHO grade IV tumor occurring in the posterior fossa and supratentorial compartments in nearly equal proportions. It is characterized by divergent differentiation with epithelial, mesenchymal, neuronal, and glial components, and often includes rhabdoid cells, resembling those of a rhabdomyosarcoma.

Molecular Genetics. Consistent genetic alterations in chromosome 22 (>90% of cases) are a hallmark of rhabdoid tumor. The relevant gene is *hSNF5/INI1*, which encodes a protein that is part of a large chromatin-remodeling complex; deletions of the locus and loss of nuclear staining for INI1 protein are seen in the majority of tumors.

MORPHOLOGY

Atypical teratoid/rhabdoid tumors tend to be large, with a soft consistency, and spread along the surface of the brain. The rhabdoid cells have eosinophilic cytoplasm, sharp cell borders and eccentrically located nuclei. When these cells are smaller, the cytoplasm can take on an elongated appearance that mimics a rhabdomyosarcoma cell. The cytoplasm of the rhabdoid cell contains intermediate filaments and is immunoreactive for epithelial membrane antigen and vimentin. Some other markers that may be positive include smooth muscle actin and keratins. Other muscle markers such as desmin and myoglobin are not present. Rhabdoid cells are rarely a major component of the tumor; instead, islands of tumor with this pattern of differentiation are mixed with a small-cell component, as well as other histologic patterns (including mesenchymal, epithelial, and neuroglial differentiation). Mitotic activity is extremely prominent.

Clinical Features. These are highly aggressive tumors of the very young. Nearly all tumors occur before the age of 5 and most patients live less than a year after diagnosis.

Other Parenchymal Tumors

Primary CNS Lymphoma

Primary CNS lymphoma accounts for 2% of extranodal lymphomas and 1% of intracranial tumors. It is the most common CNS neoplasm in immunosuppressed individuals, including those with AIDS and immunosuppression after transplantation. In non-immunosuppressed populations, the age spectrum is relatively wide, but the frequency increases after 60 years of age.

The term *primary* emphasizes the distinction between these lesions and secondary involvement of the CNS by lymphoma arising elsewhere in the body (Chapter 13). Primary brain lymphoma is often multifocal within the brain parenchyma, yet involvement outside of the CNS in lymph nodes or bone marrow is a rare and late complication. Conversely, lymphoma arising outside the CNS rarely involves the brain parenchyma; involvement of the nervous system, when it occurs in systemic lymphoma, usually occurs in the setting of significant disease burden outside of the CNS. In this situation, secondary involvement of the CNS is usually manifested by the presence of malignant cells within the CSF and around intradural nerve roots, and occasionally by the infiltration of superficial areas of the cerebrum or spinal cord by malignant cells.

The vast majority of primary brain lymphomas are of B-cell origin. Overall, primary lymphomas of the CNS are aggressive and have worse outcomes than tumors of comparable histology occurring at non-CNS sites. In the setting of immunosuppression, the cells in nearly all primary brain lymphomas are latently infected by Epstein-Barr virus, and in the setting of organ transplantation, may be associated with a systemic post-transplantation lymphoproliferative disorder. When not associated with immunosuppression, these lymphomas show a phenotype typical of postgerminal center B-cell differentiation.

MORPHOLOGY

Lesions are frequently multiple and often involve deep gray matter as well as white matter and cortex. Periventricular spread is common. The tumors are relatively well defined in comparison with glial neoplasms but are not as discrete as metastases and often show extensive areas of central necrosis. Diffuse large-cell B-cell lymphomas are the most common histologic group. Within the tumor malignant cells infiltrate the parenchyma of the brain and accumulate around blood vessels. Reticulin stains demonstrate that the infiltrating cells are separated from one another by silver-staining material; this pattern, referred to as "hooping," is characteristic of primary brain lymphoma. The tumors express B cell markers such as CD20 and usually have a high growth fraction. When tumors arise in the setting of immunosuppression, various markers of Epstein-Barr virus are usually present in the tumor cells; the virus is usually detected by doing in situ hybridization for EBERs, small nuclear RNAs that are encoded by the viral genome.

Intravascular lymphoma, an unusual large cell lymphoma that grows within small vessels, often involves the brain along with other regions of the body. Instead of presenting as a mass lesion, the occlusion of vessels by malignant cells can result in widespread microscopic infarcts. Affected individuals often present with nonlocalizing neurologic symptoms, with the differential diagnosis usually including processes such as vasculitis or even dementia.

Germ Cell Tumors

Primary brain germ cell tumors occur along the midline, most commonly in the pineal and the suprasellar regions. They account for 0.2% to 1% of brain tumors in people of European descent but up to 10% in Japan. They are tumors of the young, with 90% occurring during the first two decades. Germ cell tumors, particularly teratomas, are among the more common congenital tumors. Germ cell tumors in the pineal region show a strong male predominance; this gender difference is not seen for suprasellar lesions.

The source of germ cells in the CNS is not clear; they may be "rests" that remain in the CNS or perhaps migrate there from other sites late in development. Germ cell tumors share many features with their counterparts in the gonads and mediastinum. In contrast to lymphomas, however, metastasis of a gonadal germ cell tumor to the CNS is common; thus, the presence of a non-CNS primary tumor must be excluded before a diagnosis of primary germ cell tumor of the CNS is made. The histologic classification of brain germ cell tumors is similar to that used in the testis (Chapter 21), but the tumor that is histologically similar to the seminoma in the testis is referred to as *germinoma* in the CNS. The responses to radiation therapy and chemotherapy parallel those of germ cell tumors arising at other sites. As in the periphery, CSF levels of tumor markers including α-fetoprotein and β-human chorionic gonadotropin may be useful for assisting diagnosis and tracking response to therapy.

Pineal Parenchymal Tumors

These lesions arise from specialized cells of the pineal gland (pineocytes) that have features of neuronal differentiation. The tumors range from well-differentiated lesions (*pineocytomas*), with areas of neuropil, cells with small, round nuclei, and no evidence of mitoses or necrosis, to high-grade tumors (*pineoblastomas*), with little evidence of neuronal differentiation, densely packed small cells with necrosis, and frequent mitotic figures. An intermediate form between these two extremes is also recognized. High-grade pineal tumors tend to affect children, while lower-grade lesions are found more often in adults. The highly aggressive pineoblastoma commonly spreads throughout the CSF space. It occurs with increased frequency in individuals with germ line mutations in *RB*. Gliomas are also found in the pineal region, arising from the glial stroma of the gland. Often low grade, these gliomas may extend into the posterior third ventricle.

Meningiomas

Meningiomas are predominantly benign tumors of adults, usually attached to the dura, that arise from the meningothelial cells of the arachnoid. Meningiomas may be found along any of the external surfaces of the brain as well as within the ventricular system, where they arise from the stromal arachnoid cells of the choroid plexus. Prior radiation therapy to the head and neck, typically decades earlier, is a risk factor for development of meningiomas. Other tumors such as metastases, solitary fibrous tumors, and a range of poorly differentiated sarcomas may also grow as dural-based masses.

Molecular Genetics. The most common cytogenetic abnormality is loss of chromosome 22, especially the long arm (22q). The deletions include the region of 22q12 that harbors the *NF2* gene, which encodes the protein merlin; as expected, meningiomas are a common lesion in the setting of NF2 (see later). Of sporadic meningiomas, 50% to 60% harbor mutations in the *NF2* gene; most of these mutations are predicted to result in absence of functional merlin protein. In meningiomas without *NF2* mutations, the most common mutations occur in TNF-receptor associated factor 7 (TRAF7), and identify a separate molecular subset of meningiomas with a tendency toward lower histologic grade and greater chromosomal stability. By contrast, higher grade meningiomas are more often associated with *NF2* mutations, loss of chromosome 22, and evidence of chromosomal instability (e.g., the presence of additional chromosomal aberrations).

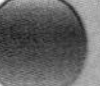

MORPHOLOGY

Meningiomas are usually rounded masses with well-defined dural bases that compress underlying brain but are easily separated from it (Fig. 28-53*A*). Extension into the overlying bone may be present. The surface of the mass is usually encapsulated by thin, fibrous tissue and may have a bosselated or polypoid appearance. They may also grow **en plaque**, in which the tumor spreads in a sheetlike fashion along the surface of the dura. This form is commonly associated with hyperostotic reactive changes in the adjacent bone. The lesions range from firm and fibrous to finely gritty, or they may contain numerous calcified psammoma bodies. Grossly evident necrosis and extensive hemorrhage are absent.

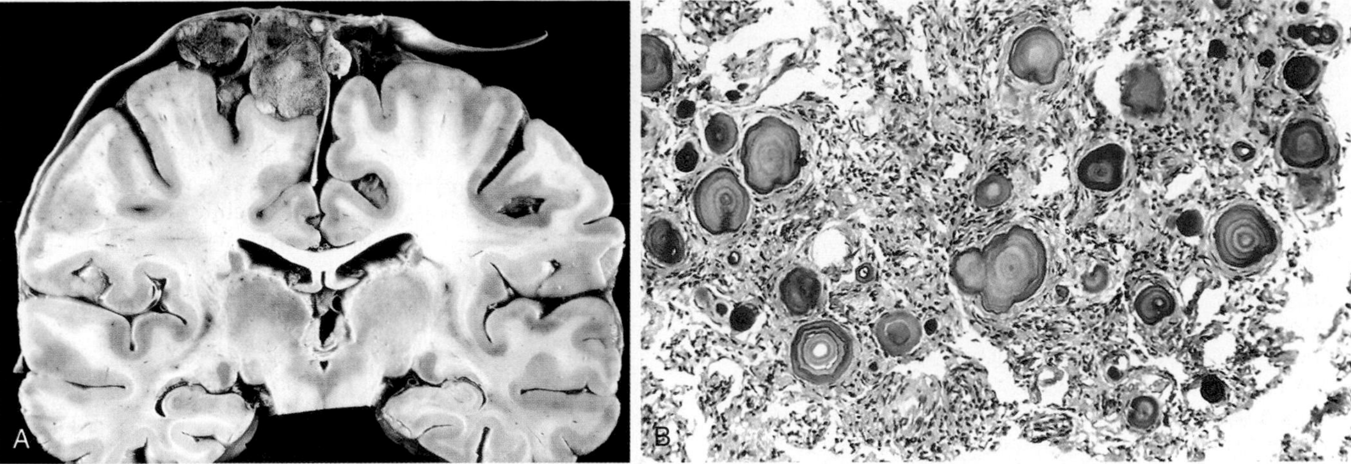

Figure 28-53 **A,** Parasagittal multilobular meningioma attached to the dura with compression of underlying brain. **B,** Meningioma with a whorled pattern of cell growth and psammoma bodies.

Most meningiomas have a relatively low risk of recurrence or aggressive growth, and so are considered WHO grade I/IV. Various histologic patterns are observed, with no prognostic significance. These include **syncytial** ("meningothelial"), appropriately named for the whorled clusters of cells that sit in tight groups without visible cell membranes; **fibroblastic**, with elongated cells and abundant collagen deposition between them; **transitional**, which share features of the syncytial and fibroblastic types; **psammomatous**, with psammoma bodies, apparently formed from calcification of the syncytial nests of meningothelial cells (Fig. 28-53*B*); **secretory**, with PAS-positive intracytoplasmic droplets and intracellular lumens by electron microscopy; and **microcystic**, with a loose, spongy appearance. Only the secretory subtype appears to be associated with a specific genotype; in initial reports all have had mutations of the *TRAF7* and *KLF4* genes. Xanthomatous degeneration, metaplasia (often osseous), and moderate nuclear pleomorphism are common in meningiomas. Among these lesions, proliferation index has been shown to be a predictor of biologic behavior.

Atypical meningiomas (WHO grade II/IV) are lesions with a higher rate of recurrence and more aggressive local growth, and may require radiation therapy in addition to surgery. They are distinguished from lower grade meningiomas by having four or more mitoses per 10 high power fields or at least three atypical features (increased cellularity, small cells with a high nuclear-to-cytoplasmic ratio, prominent nucleoli, patternless growth, or necrosis). Certain histologic patterns (**clear cell** and **chordoid**) are also considered to be grade II/IV because of their more aggressive behavior.

Anaplastic (malignant) meningioma (WHO grade III/IV) is a highly aggressive tumor with the appearance of a high-grade sarcoma, but retaining some histologic evidence of meningothelial origin. Mitotic rates are often high (>20 mitoses per 10 high power fields). **Papillary** meningioma (with pleomorphic cells arranged around fibrovascular cores) and **rhabdoid** meningioma (with sheets of tumor cells with hyaline eosinophilic cytoplasm containing intermediate filaments) both have such a high propensity to recur that they are also considered to be WHO grade III/IV tumors.

While most meningiomas are easily separable from the brain, some tumors invade the brain, either as broad, pushing edges or as single cells. The presence of brain invasion is associated with increased risk of recurrence but does not alter the histologic grade of the lesion. Meningiomas are commonly immunoreactive for epithelial membrane antigen, in contrast to other tumors arising in this region. Keratin is restricted to lesions with the secretory pattern, and these tumors are also positive for carcinoembryonic antigen.

Clinical Features. Meningiomas are usually slow-growing tumors. Patients present either with vague nonlocalizing symptoms or with focal findings referable to compression of underlying brain. Common sites of involvement include the parasagittal aspect of the brain convexity, dura over the lateral convexity, wing of the sphenoid, olfactory groove, sella turcica, and foramen magnum. They are uncommon in children and generally show a moderate (3:2) female predominance, although the ratio is 10:1 for spinal meningiomas, which are also commonly psammomatous. Lesions are usually solitary, but when present at multiple sites, especially in association with acoustic neuromas or glial tumors, the possibility of neurofibromatosis type 2 should be considered. Genetic studies indicate that multiple lesions are much more likely to represent dissemination from a single tumor than clonally distinct tumors. Meningiomas often express progesterone receptors and may grow more rapidly during pregnancy.

Metastatic Tumors

Metastatic lesions, mostly carcinomas, account for approximately a quarter to half of intra-cranial tumors in hospitalized patients. The five most common primary sites are lung, breast, skin (melanoma), kidney, and gastrointestinal tract, accounting for about 80% of all metastases. Some rare tumors (e.g., choriocarcinoma) have a high likelihood of metastasizing to the brain, whereas other more common tumors (e.g., prostatic adenocarcinoma) almost never do so. The meninges are also a frequent site of involvement by metastatic disease. Metastatic tumors present clinically as mass lesions and may occasionally be the first manifestation of the cancer. In general, localized treatment of solitary brain metastases improves the quality of the patient's remaining life. Metastases to the epidural or subdural space can cause spinal cord compression, which requires emergency treatment.

MORPHOLOGY

Intraparenchymal metastases form sharply demarcated masses, often at the junction of gray and white matter, usually surrounded by a zone of edema. The boundary between tumor and brain parenchyma is usually well-defined microscopically; melanoma does not always follow this rule and individual cells may invade the brain. Nodules of tumor, often with central areas of necrosis, are surrounded by reactive gliosis. Meningeal carcinomatosis, with tumor nodules studding the surface of the brain, spinal cord, and intradural nerve roots, is most commonly associated with carcinoma of the lung and the breast.

Paraneoplastic Syndromes

In addition to the direct and localized effects produced by metastases, patients with diverse tumors develop *paraneoplastic syndromes* that involve the peripheral and/or central nervous systems, sometimes even preceding the clinical recognition of the malignant neoplasm. A variety of clinical paraneoplastic syndromes have been described. An underlying mechanism of these syndromes appears to be the development of an immune response against tumor antigens that cross-react with antigens in the central or peripheral nervous systems. Certain malignancies are typically associated with a particular clinical syndrome. The circulating antibodies and target antigens are in the process of being defined in some of the clinical syndromes. Illustrative examples of these are described below:

- *Subacute cerebellar degeneration* is associated with destruction of Purkinje cells, gliosis, and a mild chronic inflammatory cell infiltrate. One group of these patients has a circulating PCA-1 antibody (anti-Yo) that recognizes cerebellar Purkinje cells; this antibody occurs predominantly in women with ovarian, uterine, or breast carcinoma.
- *Limbic encephalitis* is characterized by subacute dementia and marked by perivascular inflammatory cuffs, microglial nodules, some neuronal loss, and gliosis, most evident in the anterior and medial portions of the temporal lobe; the microscopic picture resembles that of an infectious process. A comparable process involving the brainstem can be seen in isolation or together with limbic system involvement. Some of these patients have a circulating ANNA-1 antibody (anti-Hu) that recognizes neuronal nuclei in the central and peripheral nervous systems; ANNA-1 is most commonly associated with small cell carcinoma of the lung. Another group of these patients has a circulating antibody that recognizes the NMDA receptor and cross-reacts with hippocampal neurons. Originally identified in women with ovarian teratomas, the same clinical syndrome is now also recognized in a small proportion of patients with sporadic encephalitis. A third group of patients has a circulating VGKC-complex antibody that recognizes the voltage-gated potassium channel; the presence of this antibody may be associated with peripheral neuropathy as well. It is important to note that in many cases of limbic encephalitis, the syndrome appears before any malignancy is suspected and as such triggers the search for a tumor elsewhere in the body.
- *Eye movement disorders*, most commonly opsoclonus, may be found, often in association with other evidence of cerebellar and brainstem dysfunction. In children this is most commonly associated with neuroblastoma and is often accompanied by myoclonus.

The peripheral nervous system can also be affected:

- *Subacute sensory neuropathy* may be found in association with limbic encephalitis or in isolation. It is marked by loss of sensory neurons from dorsal root ganglia, in association with lymphocytic inflammation.
- *Lambert-Eaton myasthenic syndrome* is caused by antibodies against the voltage-gated calcium channel in the presynaptic elements of the neuromuscular junction. This can be seen in the absence of malignancy as well.

For some paraneoplastic syndromes, there is evidence that immunotherapy (removal of circulating antibodies and immunosuppression) and tumor removal result in clinical improvement. In general, those clinical syndromes with plasma membrane-reactive antibodies (e.g., VGKC and NMDAR) respond to immunotherapy better than those associated with intracellular antigens (e.g., ANNA-1 and PCA-1).

Familial Tumor Syndromes

A number of inherited diseases are associated with the occurrence of tumors (Chapter 7). In several of these, tumors of the nervous system are a prominent aspect of the disease and these are discussed below. Other syndromes include tumors of the CNS as part of their spectrum, but the bulk of disease burden lies elsewhere.

- *Cowden syndrome:* Dysplastic gangliogliocytoma of the cerebellum (Lhermitte-Duclos disease), caused by mutations in *PTEN* resulting in PI3K/AKT signaling pathway activity (Chapter 7)
- *Li-Fraumeni syndrome:* Medulloblastomas, caused by mutations in *TP53* (Chapter 7)
- *Turcot syndrome:* Medulloblastoma or glioblastoma, caused by mutations in *APC* or mismatch repair genes (as for familial colon cancer; Chapter 17)
- *Gorlin syndrome:* Medulloblastoma, caused by mutations in the *PTCH* gene resulting in up-regulation of sonic hedgehog signaling pathways (Chapter 25).

Tuberous Sclerosis Complex

Tuberous sclerosis is an autosomal dominant syndrome occurring at a frequency of approximately 1 in 6000 births. It is characterized by the development of hamartomas and benign neoplasms involving the brain and other tissues; the most frequent clinical manifestations are seizures, autism, and mental retardation. Hamartomas within the CNS take the form of cortical tubers and subependymal nodules; subependymal giant-cell astrocytomas are low grade neoplasms that appear to develop from the hamartomatous nodules in the same location. Cortical tubers are often epileptogenic, and surgical resection can be beneficial when medical management of the seizures fails. Elsewhere in the body, renal angiomyolipomas, retinal glial hamartomas, pulmonary lymphangioleiomyomatosis and cardiac rhabdomyomas develop over childhood and adolescence. Cysts may be found at various sites, including the liver, kidneys, and pancreas. Cutaneous lesions include angiofibromas, localized leathery thickenings (shagreen patches), hypopigmented areas (ash-leaf patches), and subungual fibromas.

One tuberous sclerosis locus (*TSC1*) is found on chromosome 9q34, and encodes a protein known as hamartin; the more commonly mutated tuberous sclerosis locus (*TSC2*) is at 16p13.3 and encodes tuberin. These two proteins associate to form a complex that inhibits the kinase mTOR, which is a key regulator of protein synthesis and other aspects of anabolic metabolism. Of note, mTOR controls cell size, and the tumors associated with tuberous sclerosis are remarkable for having voluminous amounts of cytoplasm, particularly giant-cell astrocytomas in the CNS, and cardiac rhabdomyomas. Cortical and subependymal tubers are associated with an intact copy of the wild-type allele, while in subependymal giant-cell astrocytomas there is biallelic loss. Treatment is symptomatic, including anticonvulsant therapy for control of seizures. Treatment of patients with mTOR inhibitors has resulted in some clinical improvement.

MORPHOLOGY

Cortical hamartomas of tuberous sclerosis are firm areas of the cortex that, in contrast to the softer adjacent cortex, have been likened to potatoes, hence the appellation "tubers." These hamartomas are composed of haphazardly arranged neurons that lack the normal laminar organization of neocortex. In addition, some large cells have appearances intermediate between glia and neurons (large vesicular nuclei with nucleoli, resembling neurons, and abundant eosinophilic cytoplasm resembling gemistocytic astrocytes) and often express intermediate filaments of both neuronal (neurofilament) and glial (GFAP) types. Consistent with the preservation of the wild-type allele, these cells usually stain for both tuberin and hamartin. Similar hamartomatous features are present in the subependymal nodules, where the large astrocyte-like cells cluster beneath the ventricular surface. These multiple droplike masses that bulge into the ventricular system gave rise to the term *candle-guttering*. In subependymal areas a tumor unique to tuberous sclerosis, subependymal giant-cell astrocytoma, occurs, which is marked by having very large amounts of eosinophilic cytoplasm.

Von Hippel-Lindau Disease

Individuals with this autosomal dominant disease develop hemangioblastomas of the CNS and cysts involving the pancreas, liver, and kidneys, and have a propensity to develop renal cell carcinoma and pheochromocytoma. Hemangioblastomas are most common in the cerebellum and retina, but may also occur in other locations in the CNS. The disease frequency is 1 in 30,000 to 40,000.

The gene associated with von Hippel-Lindau disease (*VHL*), a tumor suppressor gene, is located on chromosome 3p25.3 and encodes a protein (VHL) that, among its other functions, is a component of a ubiquitin ligase complex that down-regulates hypoxia-induced factor 1 (HIF-1), a transcription factor involved in regulating expression of vascular endothelial growth factor, erythropoietin, and other growth factors. It is the dysregulation of erythropoietin that is responsible for the polycythemia observed in association with hemangioblastomas in about 10% of cases. HIF also regulates the expression of genes that control cellular metabolism and cell growth, activities that likely contribute to tumor formation. Why particular cell types are uniquely susceptible to transformation by HIF hyperactivity, however, remains uncertain.

MORPHOLOGY

Hemangioblastomas are highly vascular neoplasms that occur as a mural nodule associated with a large fluid-filled cyst. The lesion consists of variable proportions of capillary-size or somewhat larger thin-walled vessels and intervening stromal cells of uncertain histogenesis characterized by vacuolated, lightly PAS-positive, lipid-rich cytoplasm. The stromal cells are of uncertain origin but can be demonstrated to express inhibin by immunohistochemistry. These are the cells that show the presence of a second "hit" in the previously normal *VHL* allele, and on this basis they are considered to be the neoplastic element in hemangioblastoma.

Therapy is directed at the symptomatic neoplasms, including resection of the cerebellar hemangioblastomas and laser therapy for retinal hemangioblastomas.

Neurofibromatosis

Two autosomal dominant disorders, NF1 and NF2, are familial tumor syndromes characterized by tumors of the PNS and CNS. NF1 is the more common, with a frequency of 1 in 3,000, and is characterized by neurofibromas of peripheral nerve, gliomas of the optic nerve, pigmented nodules of the iris *(Lisch nodules)*, and cutaneous hyperpigmented macules *(café au lait spots)*. NF2 is most commonly characterized by bilateral schwannomas of the vestibulocochlear nerves (cranial nerve VIII) and multiple meningiomas. Gliomas may also occur in these patients; typically these are ependymomas of the spinal cord. This disorder is much less common than NF1, having a frequency of 1 in 40,000 to 50,000. Both types of neurofibromatosis are discussed in more detail in Chapter 27.

KEY CONCEPTS

Tumors

- Tumors of the CNS may arise from the cells of the coverings (meningiomas), the brain (gliomas, neuronal tumors, choroid plexus tumors), or other CNS cell populations (primary CNS lymphoma, germ cell tumors), or they may originate elsewhere in the body (metastases).
- Even low-grade or benign tumors can have poor clinical outcomes, depending on where they occur in the brain.
- Distinct types of tumors affect specific brain regions (e.g., cerebellum for medulloblastoma, an intraventricular location for central neurocytoma) and specific age populations (medulloblastoma and pilocytic astrocytomas in pediatric age groups, and glioblastoma and lymphoma in older patients).

- Glial tumors are broadly classified into astrocytomas, oligodendrogliomas, and ependymomas. Increasing tumor malignancy is associated with more cytologic anaplasia, increased cell density, necrosis, and mitotic activity. There are distinct associations between combinations of genetic alterations in tumors and morphologic appearance; some of these also carry prognostic significance.
- Metastatic spread of brain tumors to other regions of the body is rare, but the brain is not comparably protected against spread of distant tumors. Carcinomas are the dominant type of systemic tumors that metastasize to the nervous system.

SUGGESTED READINGS

General

In general, many areas of neuropathology and neurologic diseases are well covered in the following standard texts:

Burger PC, Scheithauer BW: *Tumors of the Central Nervous System. AFIP Atlas of Tumor Pathology: Series 4*. Washington, DC, 2007, American Registry of Pathology.

Ellison D, Love S, Chimelli LMC, et al: *Neuropathology: A Reference Text of CNS Pathology*, ed 3, London , 2013, Elsevier Mosby.

Louis DN, Frosch MP, Mena H, et al, editors: *Non-Neoplastic Diseases of the Central Nervous System. AFIP Atlas of Nontumor Pathology: Series 1*. Washington, DC, 2009, American Registry of Pathology.

Louis DN, Ohgaki H, Wiestler OD, et al, editors: *WHO Classification of Tumours of the Central Nervous System (IARC)*, ed 4, Geneva, 2007, World Health Organization.

Love S, Louis DN, Ellison DW, editors: *Greenfield's Neuropathology*, ed 8, Oxford, 2008, Oxford University Press.

Malformations and Developmental Diseases

Dyment DA, Sawyer SL, Chardon JW, et al: Recent advances in the genetic etiology of brain malformations. *Curr Neurol Neurosci Rep* 13(8):364, 2013.

Sattar S, Gleeson JG: The ciliopathies in neuronal development: a clinical approach to investigation of Joubert syndrome and Joubert syndrome-related disorders. *Dev Med Child Neurol* 53(9):793–8, 2011.

Wallingford JB, Niswander LA, Shaw GM, et al: The continuing challenge of understanding, preventing, and treating neural tube defects. *Science* 339(6123):1222002, 2013.

Perinatal Brain Injury

Volpe JJ, Kinney HC, Jensen FE, et al: The developing oligodendrocyte: key cellular target in brain injury in the premature infant. *Int J Dev Neurosci* 29(4):423–40, 2011.

Trauma

McKee AC, Stein TD, Nowinski CJ, et al: The spectrum of disease in chronic traumatic encephalopathy. *Brain* 136(Pt 1):43–64, 2013.

Cerebrovascular Disease

Rincon F, Wright CB: Vascular cognitive impairment. *Curr Opin Neurol* 26(1):29–36, 2013.

Sacco RL, Rundek T: Cerebrovascular disease. *Curr Opin Neurol* 25(1):1–4, 2012.

Infections

Bartt R: Acute bacterial and viral meningitis. *Continuum* 18:1255–70, 2012.

Berger JR, Aksamit AJ, Clifford DB, et al: PML diagnostic criteria: consensus statement from the AAN neuroinfectious disease section. *Neurol* 80:1430–8, 2013.

Rust RS: Human arboviral encephalitis. *Semin Pediatr Neurol* 19:130–51, 2012.

Sabah M, Mulcahy J, Zeman A: Herpes simplex encephalitis. *BMJ* 344:e3166, 2012.

Shikani HJ, Freeman BD, Lisanti MP, et al: Cerebral malaria: we have come a long way. *Am J Pathol* 181:1484-92, 2012.

Prion Disease

Collinge J, Clarke AR: A general model of prion strains and their pathogenicity. *Science* 318(5852):930–6, 2007.

Gambetti P, Cali I, Notari S, et al: Molecular biology and pathology of prion strains in sporadic human prion diseases. *Acta Neuropathol* 121(1):79–90, 2011.

Puoti G, Bizzi A, Forloni G, et al: Sporadic human prion diseases: molecular insights and diagnosis. *Lancet Neurol* 11(7):618–28, 2012.

Wadsworth JD, Collinge J: Molecular pathology of human prion disease. *Acta Neuropathol* 121(1):69–77, 2011.

Demyelinating Diseases

Goris A, Pauwels I, Dubois B: Progress in multiple sclerosis genetics. *Curr Genomics* 13(8):646–63, 2012.

Koch MW, Metz LM, Kovalchuk O: Epigenetic changes in patients with multiple sclerosis. *Nat Rev Neurol* 9(1):35–43, 2013.

Mitsdoerffer M, Kuchroo V, Korn T: Immunology of neuromyelitis optica: a T cell-B cell collaboration. *Ann N Y Acad Sci* 1283:57–66, 2013.

Neurodegenerative Diseases

Brown RH Jr, Robberecht W: Amyotrophic lateral sclerosis: pathogenesis. *Semin Neurol* 21(2):131–9, 2001.

Ha AD, Fung VS: Huntington's disease. *Curr Opin Neurol* 25(4):491–8, 2012.

Halliday G, Bigio EH, Cairns NJ, et al: Mechanisms of disease in frontotemporal lobar degeneration: gain of function versus loss of function effects. *Acta Neuropathol* 124(3):373–82, 2012.

Jellinger KA, Lantos PL: Papp-Lantos inclusions and the pathogenesis of multiple system atrophy: an update. *Acta Neuropathol* 119(6):657–67, 2010.

Ling SC, Polymenidou M, Cleveland DW: Converging mechanisms in ALS and FTD: disrupted RNA and protein homeostasis. *Neuron* 79 (3):416–38, 2013.

Mackenzie IR, Neumann M, Bigio EH, et al: Nomenclature for neuropathologic subtypes of frontotemporal lobar degeneration: consensus recommendations. *Acta Neuropathol* 117(1):15–18, 2009.

Mackenzie IR, Neumann M, Bigio EH, et al: Nomenclature and nosology for neuropathologic subtypes of frontotemporal lobar degeneration: an update. *Acta Neuropathol* 119(1):1–4, 2010.

Montine TJ, Phelps CH, Beach TG, et al; National Institute on Aging; Alzheimer's Association: National Institute on Aging-Alzheimer's Association guidelines for the neuropathologic assessment of Alzheimer's disease: a practical approach. *Acta Neuropathol* 123(1): 1–11, 2012.

Seidel K, Siswanto S, Brunt ER, et al: Brain pathology of spinocerebellar ataxias. *Acta Neuropathol* 124(1):1–21, 2012.

Genetic Metabolic Diseases

Baertling F, Rodenburg RJ, Schaper J, et al: A guide to diagnosis and treatment of Leigh syndrome. *J Neurol Neurosurg Psychiatry* 2013.

Vafai SB, Mootha VK: Mitochondrial disorders as windows into an ancient organelle. *Nature* 491(7424):374–83, 2012.

Tumors

Clark VE, Erson-Omay EZ, Serin A, et al: Genomic analysis of non-NF2 meningiomas reveals mutations in TRAF7, KLF4, AKT1, and SMO. *Science* 339(6123):1077–80, 2013.

McKeon A, Pittock SJ: Paraneoplastic encephalomyelopathies: pathology and mechanisms. *Acta Neuropathol* 122:381–400, 2011.

Northcott PA, Korshunov A, Pfister SM, et al: The clinical implications of medulloblastoma subgroups. *Nat Rev Neurol* 8:340–51, 2012.

Verhaak RGW, Hoadley KA, Purdom E, et al: Integrated genomic analysis identifies clinically relevant subtypes of glioblastoma characterized by abnormalities in PDGFRA, IDH1, EGFR, and NF1. *Cancer Cell* 17:98–110, 2010.

Yan H, Parsons W, Jin G, McLendon R, et al: IDH1 and IDH2 mutations in gliomas. *New Eng J Med* 360:765–73, 2009.

See TARGETED THERAPY available online at www.studentconsult.com 

CHAPTER 29

The Eye

Robert Folberg

CHAPTER CONTENTS

Although this chapter comes at the end of the book, it is not the least important. Vision is a major quality-of-life issue. Before the public awareness of acquired immunodeficiency syndrome (AIDS) and Alzheimer disease, the most feared disease among Americans was cancer, and the second most feared disease was blindness. So great is the fear of blindness that even today, people often tell their physicians, "Doctor, I'd rather be dead than be blind!"

In general, diseases that produce loss of vision do not attract as much attention as do many of the life-threatening conditions described in this book. For example, age-related macular degeneration (AMD) is the most common cause of irreversible visual loss in the United States. Most individuals with AMD do not even suffer from a total loss of vision—an immersion into darkness. The histopathology is unimpressive: small scars develop in the macula. But consider the effect of these tiny scars in a retired schoolteacher with AMD. The central portion of her or his vision is lost. The faces of spouse or grandchildren are not visible. He or she cannot read a book or newspaper. Once a model of independence, this teacher can no longer drive a car and must be chauffeured everywhere. In short, this person is robbed of the common joys that most of us take for granted.

To study the eye, one needs to comprehend all that has come before. For example, the pathology of the eyelids builds on knowledge of dermatopathology (Chapter 25), and the pathology of the retina and optic nerve extends what was learned in Chapter 28 about the brain and central nervous system. However, the study of ocular pathology does not merely repeat what has been presented thus far. The eye provides the only site in which a physician can directly visualize a variety of microcirculatory disturbances ranging from arteriosclerosis to angiogenesis in the clinic. Although there are conditions that are unique to the eye (e.g., cataract and glaucoma), many ocular conditions share similarities with disease processes elsewhere in the body that are modified by the unique structure and function of the eye (Fig. 29-1).

The eye has much to teach us about important mechanisms of disease that extend far beyond the visual system. For example, the tumor suppressor gene, *RB*, was described in retinoblastoma, a quite uncommon ocular tumor of

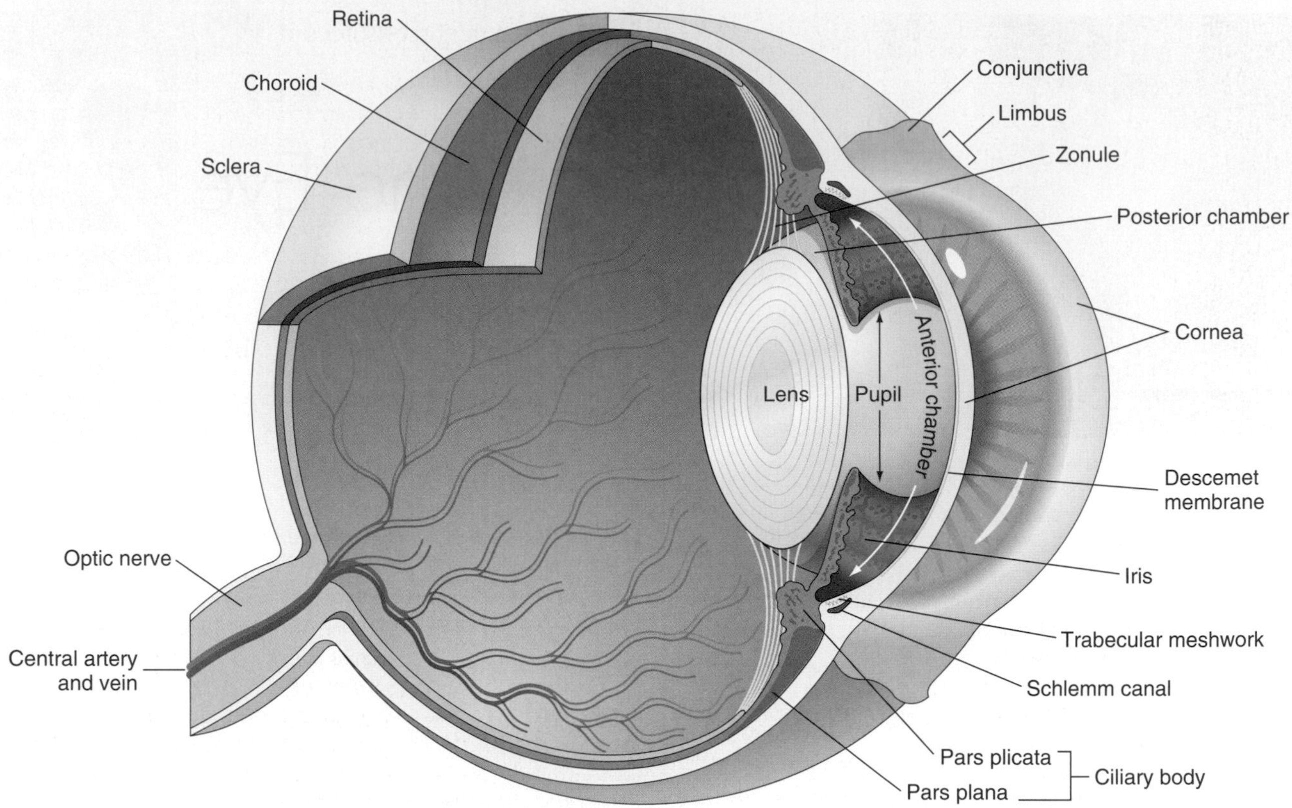

Figure 29-1 Anatomy of the eye.

infants and very young children, but the discovery of *RB* opened an important pathway to the understanding of the regulation of cellular replication.

In recent years, the elucidation of the molecular pathogenesis of disease been translated rapidly to therapeutic applications in the eye. Many blinding conditions such as corneal neovascularization, diabetic retinopathy, and certain forms of age-related neovascularization, result from pathologic angiogenesis. Successful treatment of these conditions with vascular endothelial growth factor (VEGF) antagonists has saved vision in patients who might have been blinded just a few years ago.

This chapter is organized on the basis of ocular anatomy. The discussion of each region of the eye begins with anatomic and functional considerations, and their impact on the understanding of ocular diseases.

Orbit

Functional Anatomy and Proptosis

The orbit is a compartment that is closed medially, laterally, and posteriorly. Diseases that increase orbital contents therefore displace the eye forward, a condition known as *proptosis*. Aside from the obvious cosmetic concerns, the proptotic eye might not be covered completely by the eyelids, and the tear film might not be distributed evenly across the cornea. Chronic corneal exposure to air is injurious, leading to pain and predisposing to corneal ulceration and infection. Proptosis may be axial (directly forward) or positional. For example, any enlargement of the lacrimal gland from inflammation (e.g., *sarcoidosis*) or neoplasm (e.g., *lymphoma, pleomorphic adenoma*, or *adenoid cystic carcinoma*) produces a proptosis that displaces the eye inferiorly and medially, because the lacrimal gland is positioned superotemporally within the orbit.

Masses contained within the cone formed by the horizontal rectus muscles generate axial proptosis: the eye bulges straight forward. The two most common primary tumors of the optic nerve (a tract of the central nervous system), *glioma* and *meningioma*, produce axial proptosis because the optic nerve is positioned within the muscle cone. The orbital contents are subject to the same disease processes that affect other tissues. Representative inflammatory conditions and neoplasms of the orbit are discussed briefly next.

Thyroid Ophthalmopathy (Graves Disease)

In the chapter on endocrine disorders (Chapter 24) it was noted that axial proptosis is an important clinical manifestation of Graves disease. Proptosis is caused by the accumulation of extracellular matrix proteins and variable degrees of fibrosis in the rectus muscles (Fig. 29-2). The development of thyroid ophthalmopathy may be independent of the status of thyroid function.

Other Orbital Inflammatory Conditions

The floor of the orbit is the roof of the maxillary sinus, and the medial wall of the orbit—the lamina papyracea—separates the orbit from the ethmoidal sinuses. As a result, uncontrolled sinus infection may spread to the orbit either

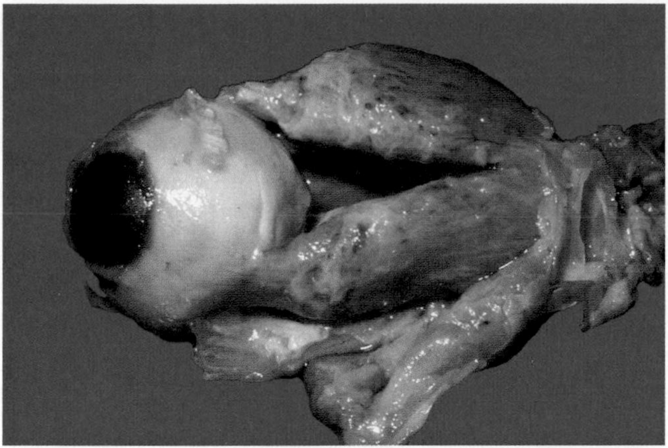

Figure 29-2 The extraocular muscles are greatly distended in this postmortem dissection of tissues from a patient with thyroid (Graves) ophthalmopathy. Note that the tendons of the muscles are spared. (Courtesy Dr. Ralph C. Eagle, Jr., Wills Eye Hospital, Philadelphia, Pa.)

as an acute bacterial infection or as a component of a fungal infection. This occurs most commonly in immunosuppressed individuals, in patients with diabetic ketoacidosis, or, rarely, in persons without any predisposition. Systemic conditions such as *Wegener granulomatosis* (Chapter 11) may present first in the orbit and may be confined there for prolonged periods of time, or alternatively, it may involve the orbit secondarily by extension from the sinuses.

Idiopathic orbital inflammation, also known as orbital inflammatory pseudotumor (Fig. 29-3), is another inflammatory condition affecting the orbit. This condition may be unilateral or bilateral, and may affect all orbital tissue elements or may be confined to the lacrimal gland *(sclerosing dacryoadenitis)*, the extraocular muscles *(orbital myositis)*, or the Tenon's capsule, the fascial layer that wraps around the eye *(posterior scleritis)*. IgG4-related disease (Chapter 6) should be excluded before declaring an orbital inflammation to be idiopathic.

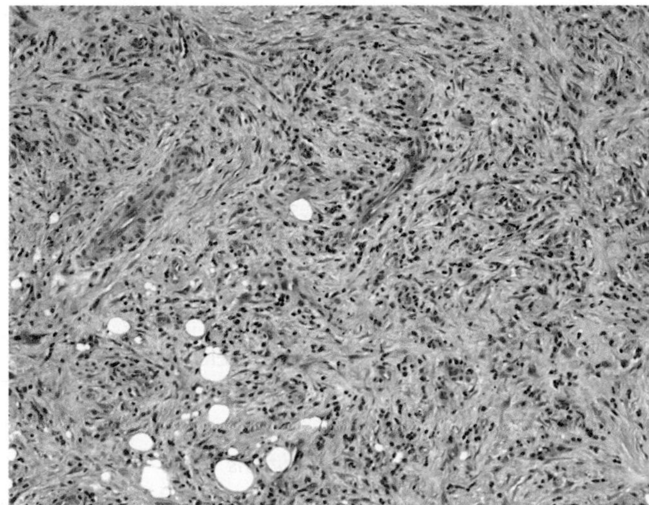

Figure 29-3 In idiopathic orbital inflammation (orbital inflammatory pseudotumor) the orbital fat is replaced by fibrosis. Note the chronic inflammation, accompanied in this case by eosinophils.

MORPHOLOGY

Idiopathic orbital inflammation is characterized histologically by chronic inflammation and variable degrees of fibrosis. The inflammatory infiltrate typically includes lymphocytes and plasma cells and occasionally eosinophils. Germinal centers, when present, raise the suspicion of a reactive lymphoid hyperplasia. Vasculitis may be present, suggesting an underlying systemic condition. The presence of necrosis and degenerating collagen along with vasculitis should raise the suspicion of Wegener granulomatosis. Idiopathic orbital inflammation is typically confined to the orbit but may develop concomitantly with sclerosing inflammation in the retroperitoneum, the mediastinum, and the thyroid, especially as a manifestation of IgG4-related disease.

Neoplasms

The most frequently encountered primary neoplasms of the orbit are vascular in origin: the capillary hemangioma of infancy and early childhood, and the lymphangioma (both of which are unencapsulated), and the encapsulated cavernous hemangioma found typically in adults. These are described in other chapters. Only a handful of orbital masses are encapsulated (e.g., pleomorphic adenoma of the lacrimal gland, dermoid cyst, neurilemmoma), and the recognition of encapsulation on imaging studies allows the surgeon to anticipate pathologic findings.

Non-Hodgkin lymphoma, like idiopathic orbital inflammation, can affect the entire orbit or can be confined to compartments of the orbit such as the lacrimal gland. Orbital lymphomas are classified according to the WHO classification system (Chapter 13).

Primary orbital malignancies may arise from any of the orbital tissues and are classified according to the scheme used for the parent tissue. For example, the lacrimal gland may be considered a minor salivary gland, and tumors of the lacrimal gland are classified as salivary gland tumors.

Metastases to the orbit may present with distinctive signs and symptoms that point to the origin of the tumor. For example, metastatic prostatic carcinoma may present clinically like idiopathic orbital inflammation; metastatic neuroblastoma and Wilms tumor—richly vascular neoplasms—may produce characteristic periocular ecchymoses. Neoplasms may also invade from the sinuses into the orbit.

KEY CONCEPTS

- Proptosis results from lesions or pathologic changes in tissue that occupy space in the orbit. The orbit is a compartment that is only open anteriorly and is closed in all other dimensions by bone.
- Inflammation in the orbit may develop by extension of local disease in adjacent tissues (e.g., sinusitis) or as a component of systemic disease (e.g., Wegener granulomatosis)
- The most common primary tumors of the orbit are vascular (e.g., capillary and cavernous hemangiomas).

Eyelid

Functional Anatomy

The eyelid is composed of skin externally and mucosa (the conjunctiva) on the surface apposed to the eye (Fig. 29-4). In addition to covering and protecting the eye, elements within the eyelid generate critical components of the tear film. If the drainage system of the sebaceous glands is obstructed by chronic inflammation at the eyelid margin *(blepharitis)* or, less commonly, by neoplasm, then lipid may extravasate into surrounding tissue and provoke a granulomatous response producing a lipogranuloma, or *chalazion*.

Neoplasms

The most common malignancy of the eyelid is basal cell carcinoma. Surprisingly, primary melanomas of the eyelid skin are extremely rare. Regardless of histogenesis, eyelid neoplasms may distort tissue and prevent the eyelids from closing completely. Because chronic exposure to air damages the cornea, prompt treatment of locally invasive basal cell carcinomas is imperative to preserve vision. Basal cell carcinoma has a distinct predilection for the lower eyelid and the medial canthus.

Sebaceous carcinoma may form a local mass that mimics *chalazion* or may diffusely thicken the eyelid. This neoplasm may also resemble inflammatory processes such as blepharitis or *ocular cicatricial pemphigoid* because of a predilection for intraepithelial spread as occurs in Paget disease of the nipple (Chapter 23) or vulva (Chapter 22). Sebaceous carcinoma tends to spread first to the parotid and submandibular nodes. The overall mortality rate can be as high as 22%. Sebaceous carcinoma of the eyelid is less likely to be associated with the Muir-Torre syndrome than sebaceous neoplasms developing elsewhere.

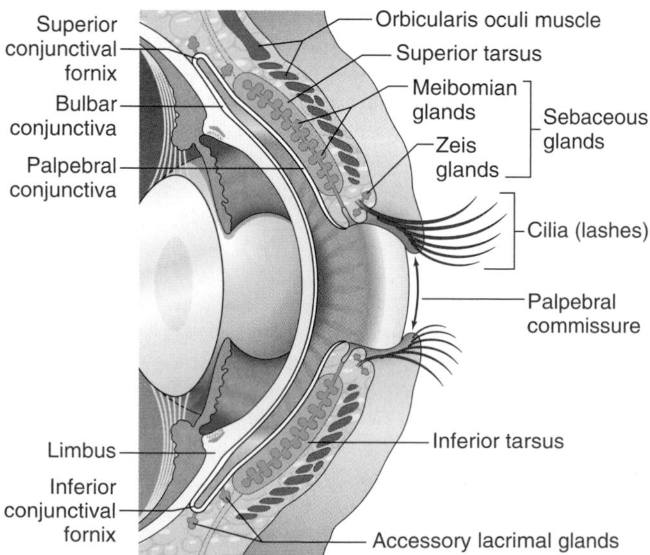

Figure 29-4 Anatomy of the conjunctiva and eyelids.

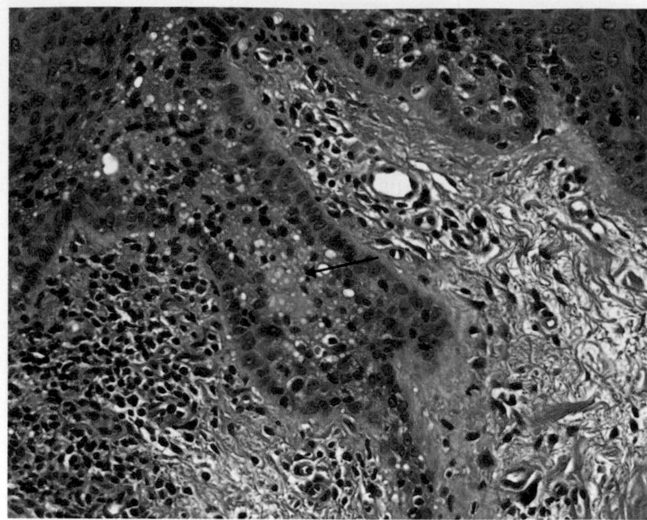

Figure 29-5 Pagetoid spread of sebaceous carcinoma. Neoplastic cells with foamy cytoplasm are present within the epidermis (arrow). Invasive sebaceous carcinoma was identified elsewhere in this biopsy sample.

MORPHOLOGY

In moderately differentiated or well-differentiated sebaceous carcinoma, vacuolization of the cytoplasm is present and helps in the diagnosis. This cancer may, however, resemble a variety of other malignancies histologically, including basal cell carcinoma, hence establishing the correct diagnosis can be difficult. Pagetoid spread (Fig. 29-5) may mimic Bowenoid actinic keratosis in the eyelid and carcinoma in situ in the conjunctiva. Sebaceous carcinoma may spread through the conjunctival epithelium and the epidermis to the lacrimal drainage system and the nasopharynx. It may also extend into the lacrimal gland ductules and thereby into the main lacrimal gland.

In individuals with AIDS, *Kaposi sarcoma* may develop in either the eyelid or the conjunctiva. In the eyelid the lesion may appear clinically to have a purple hue because the vascular lesion is embedded in the dermis, but in the thin mucous membrane of the conjunctiva, Kaposi sarcoma appears bright red and may be confused clinically with a subconjunctival hemorrhage.

KEY CONCEPTS

- Basal cell carcinoma is the most common primary malignancy of the eyelid and may be very invasive locally.
- Sebaceous carcinoma of the eyelid, by contrast, may metastasize and is therefore a serious and potentially life-threatening condition.

Conjunctiva

Functional Anatomy

The conjunctiva is divided into zones (Fig. 29-4), each with distinctive histologic features and responses to disease.

The conjunctiva lining the interior of the eyelid, the *palpebral conjunctiva,* is tightly tethered to the tarsus and may respond to inflammation by being thrown into minute papillary folds as may occur in allergic conjunctivitis and bacterial conjunctivitis. The conjunctiva in the *fornix* is a pseudostratified columnar epithelium rich in goblet cells. The fornix also contains accessory lacrimal tissue, and the ductules of the main lacrimal gland pierce through the conjunctiva in the fornix superiorly and laterally. The lymphoid population of the conjunctiva is most noticeable in the fornix, and *in viral conjunctivitis, lymphoid follicles may enlarge sufficiently to be visualized clinically* by slit-lamp examination. *Granulomas* associated with systemic sarcoidosis may be detected in the conjunctival fornix, and the yield of granulomas from a nondirected conjunctival biopsy in individuals suspected of having sarcoid may be as high as 50%. Primary lymphoma of the conjunctiva (typically indolent marginal zone B-cell lymphoma) is most likely to develop in the fornix. The *bulbar conjunctiva*—the conjunctiva that covers the surface of the eye—is a nonkeratinizing stratified squamous epithelium. The limbus, the intersection between the sclera and cornea, also marks the transition between conjunctival and corneal epithelium (Fig. 29-1).

The conjunctiva, like the eyelid, is richly invested with lymphatic channels. Malignant neoplasms arising in the eyelid and conjunctiva tend to spread to regional lymph nodes (parotid and submandibular node groups).

Conjunctival Scarring

Many cases of bacterial or viral conjunctivitis cause redness and itching, but most heal without sequelae. However, infection with *Chlamydia trachomatis (trachoma)* may produce significant conjunctival scarring. Conjunctival scarring is also seen after exposure of the ocular surface to caustic alkalis or as a sequela to ocular cicatricial *pemphigoid* (Chapter 25). A reduction in the number of goblet cells due to conjunctival scarring leads to a decrease in surface mucin, which is essential for the adherence of the aqueous component of tears to the corneal epithelium. Thus, even if the aqueous component of the tear film is adequate, the affected individual will suffer from a dry eye. More commonly, however, dry eye results from a deficiency in the aqueous component of the tear film generated by the accessory lacrimal glands embedded within the eyelid and fornix.

The conjunctiva may be scarred iatrogenically through reaction to drugs or as a consequence of surgery. In other parts of the body, cancer surgery requires excision of the lesion with a margin of normal tissue to ensure complete removal. However, extensive surgical excision of even diseased conjunctiva can remove a large number of goblet cells or compromise lacrimal gland ductules that traverse the conjunctiva. Thus, removal of a conjunctival neoplasm or a precursor lesion may leave the affected individual with a painful dry eye that can compromise vision. Therefore, surgeons often remove only the invasive components of conjunctival neoplasms, and treat the intraepithelial components with tissue-sparing modalities such as cryotherapy or topical chemotherapy delivered as eyedrops.

Pinguecula and Pterygium

Both *pinguecula* and *pterygium* appear as submucosal elevations on the conjunctiva. They result from actinic damage and are therefore located in the sun-exposed regions of the conjunctiva (i.e., in the fissure between both the upper and lower eyelids—the interpalpebral fissure). Pterygium typically originates in the conjunctiva astride the limbus. It is formed by a submucosal growth *of fibrovascular connective tissue that migrates onto the cornea,* dissecting into the plane occupied normally by the Bowman layer. Pterygium does not cross the pupillary axis and, aside from the possible induction of mild astigmatism, does not pose a threat to vision. Although most pterygia are entirely benign, it is worthwhile submitting the excised tissue for pathologic examination because, on occasion, precursors of actinic-induced neoplasms—squamous cell carcinoma and melanoma—are detected in these lesions.

Pinguecula, which, like pterygium, appears astride the limbus, is a small, yellowish submucosal elevation. Although the pinguecula does not invade the cornea as pterygium does, the presence of a focal conjunctival elevation near the limbus can result in an uneven distribution of the tear film over the adjacent cornea. As a consequence of focal dehydration, a saucer-like depression in the corneal tissue—a *delle*—may develop.

Neoplasms

Both squamous neoplasms and melanocytic neoplasms and their precursors tend to develop at the limbus. Conjunctival *squamous cell carcinoma* may be preceded by intraepithelial neoplastic changes analogous to those seen in the evolution of cervical squamous cell carcinoma. In the conjunctiva the spectrum of changes from mild dysplasia through carcinoma in situ is designated as *conjunctival intraepithelial neoplasia.* Squamous papillomas and conjunctival intraepithelial neoplasia may be associated with the presence of human papillomavirus types 16 and 18. Although conjunctival squamous cell carcinoma tends to follow an indolent course, *mucoepidermoid carcinoma* of the conjunctiva (reflecting the ability of conjunctival stem cells to differentiate into squamous epithelium and goblet cells) follows a much more aggressive course.

Conjunctival nevi are encountered commonly but seldom invade the cornea or appear in the fornix or over the palpebral conjunctiva. Pigmented lesions in these zones of the conjunctiva most likely represent melanomas or melanoma precursors. Compound nevi of the conjunctiva characteristically contain subepithelial cysts lined by surface epithelium (Fig. 29-6*A, B*). In late childhood or adolescence, conjunctival nevi may acquire an inflammatory component rich in lymphocytes, plasma cells, and eosinophils. The resultant *inflamed juvenile nevus* is completely benign.

Conjunctival melanomas are unilateral neoplasms, typically affecting fair-complexioned individuals in middle age (Fig. 29-6*C, D*). Most cases of conjunctival melanoma develop through a phase of intraepithelial growth termed *primary acquired melanosis with atypia,* which is roughly analogous to *melanoma in situ* but does not correspond neatly to the radial growth phase of cutaneous melanoma (Chapter 25). Between 50% and 90% of individuals with incompletely treated primary acquired melanosis with

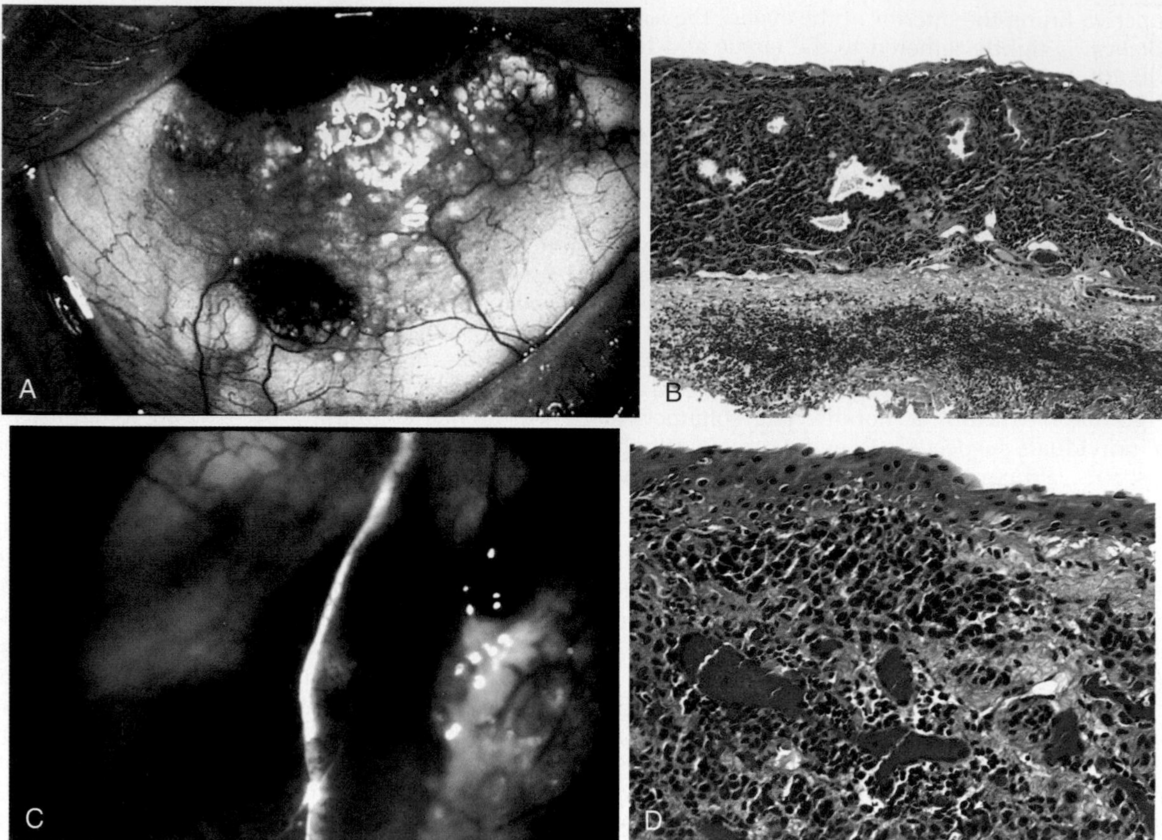

Figure 29-6 **A, B,** Cystic compound nevus of the conjunctiva. **C, D,** Conjunctival malignant melanoma. In **C**, note the deflection of the beam of the slit lamp over the surface of the lesion, indicative of invasion. (**A, B,** From Folberg R, et al: Benign conjunctival melanocytic lesions: clinicopathologic features. Ophthalmology 96:436, 1989.)

atypia develop conjunctival melanoma; the best treatment of conjunctival melanoma is its prevention through extirpation of its precursor lesion. The lesions tend to spread first to the parotid or submandibular lymph nodes. Approximately 25% of conjunctival melanomas prove to be fatal.

KEY CONCEPTS

- Conjunctival scarring, a consequence of a variety of conditions, may result in painful loss of vision by interfering with the delivery and maintenance of the tear film.
- Many conjunctival neoplasms originate at the limbus, the seat of stem cells of the ocular surface.
- Conjunctival malignancies—especially conjunctival melanomas—tend to spread through the rich lymphatics of the conjunctiva to regional lymph nodes.

Sclera

The sclera consists mainly of collagen and contains few blood vessels and fibroblasts; hence, wounds and surgical incisions tend to heal poorly. Immune complex deposits within the sclera, such as in *rheumatoid arthritis,* may produce a necrotizing *scleritis.*

The sclera may appear "blue" in a variety of conditions. Some of these are:

- It may become thin following episodes of scleritis, and the normally brown color of the uvea may appear blue clinically because of the optical Tyndall effect.
- Sclera may be thinned in eyes with exceptionally high intraocular pressure and because this zone of scleral ectasia is lined by uveal tissue, the resulting lesion, known as a *staphyloma,* also appears blue.
- The sclera may appear blue in osteogenesis imperfecta.
- The sclera may appear blue because of a heavily pigmented congenital nevus of the underlying uvea, a condition known as *congenital melanosis oculi.* When accompanied by periocular cutaneous pigmentation, this condition is known as *nevus of Ota.*

Cornea

Functional Anatomy

The cornea and its overlying tear film—not the lens—make up the major refractive surface of the eye (Fig. 29-7). Parenthetically, *myopia* typically develops because the eye is too long for its refractive power, and *hyperopia* results from an eye that is too short. The popularity of procedures such as laser-assisted in situ keratomileusis (LASIK) to sculpt the cornea and change its refractive properties

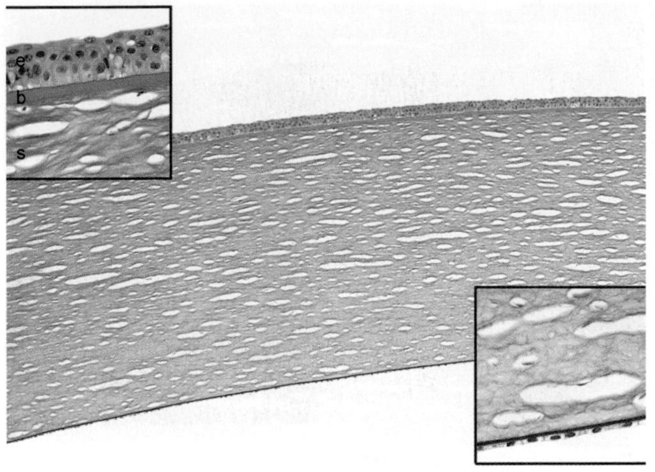

Figure 29-7 Normal corneal microarchitecture. The corneal tissue is stained by periodic acid–Schiff (PAS) to highlight basement membranes. The inset at the upper left is a high magnification of the anterior layers of the cornea: the epithelium *(e)*, Bowman layer *(b)*, and the stroma *(s)*. A very thin PAS-positive basement membrane separates the epithelium from the Bowman layer. Note that the Bowman layer is acellular. The *inset* at the *lower right* is a high magnification of the PAS-positive Descemet membrane and the corneal endothelium. The "holes" in the stroma are artifactitious spaces between parallel collagenous stromal lamellae.

attests to the importance of corneal shape in contributing to the refractive power of the eye.

Anteriorly, the cornea is covered by *epithelium* that rests on a basement membrane. The *Bowman layer*, situated just beneath the epithelial basement membrane, is acellular and forms an efficient barrier against the penetration of malignant cells from the epithelium into the underlying stroma.

The *corneal stroma* lacks blood vessels and lymphatics, a feature that contributes not only to the transparency of the cornea, but also to high rate of success of corneal transplantation. Indeed, nonimmunologic graft failure (associated with loss of endothelial cells and subsequent corneal edema) is seen more commonly than is immunologic graft rejection. The risk of corneal graft rejection increases with stromal vascularization and inflammation. A precise alignment of collagen in the corneal stroma also contributes to transparency.

Corneal vascularization may accompany chronic corneal edema, inflammation, and scarring. The application of topical VEGF antagonists affords a promising approach to preventing corneal vascularization. Scarring and edema both disrupt the spatial alignment of stromal collagen and contribute to corneal opacification. Scars may result from trauma or inflammation. Normally, the corneal stroma is in a state of relative deturgescence (dehydration), maintained in large part by active pumping of fluid from the stroma back into the anterior chamber by the corneal endothelium.

The corneal *endothelium* is derived from neural crest and is not related to vascular endothelium. It rests on its basement membrane, Descemet membrane. A decrease in endothelial cells or a malfunction of endothelium results in stromal edema, which may be complicated by bullous separation of the epithelium *(bullous keratopathy)*. *Descemet membrane* increases in thickness with age. It is the site of copper deposition in the Kayser-Fleischer ring of Wilson disease (Chapter 18).

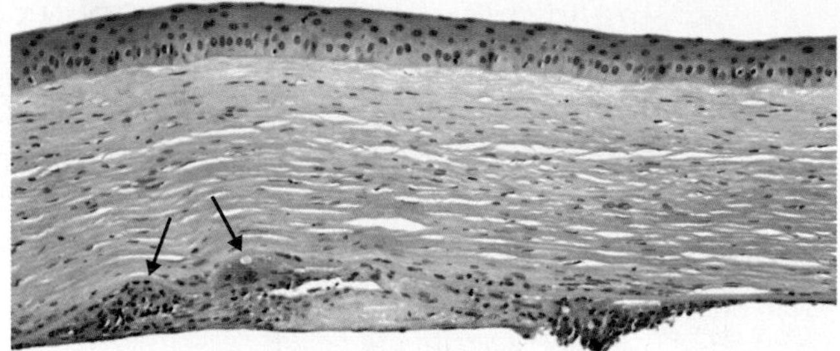

Figure 29-8 Chronic herpes simplex keratitis. The cornea is thin and scarred (note the increased number of fibroblast nuclei). Granulomatous reaction in the Descemet membrane, illustrated in this photomicrograph *(arrows)*, is a histologic hallmark of chronic herpes simplex keratitis.

Keratitis and Ulcers

Various pathogens—bacterial, fungal, viral (especially herpes simplex and herpes zoster), and protozoal (*Acanthamoeba*)—can cause corneal ulceration. In all forms of keratitis, dissolution of the corneal stroma may be accelerated by activation of collagenases within corneal epithelium and stromal fibroblasts (also known as keratocytes). Exudate and cells leaking from iris and ciliary body vessels into the anterior chamber may be visible by slit-lamp examination and may accumulate in sufficient quantity to become visible even by a penlight examination *(hypopyon)*. Although the corneal ulcer may be infectious, the hypopyon seldom contains organisms and is an example par excellence of the vascular response to acute inflammation. The specific forms of keratitis may have certain distinctive features. For example, chronic herpes simplex keratitis may be associated with a granulomatous reaction involving the Descemet membrane (Fig. 29-8).

Corneal Degenerations and Dystrophies

Ophthalmologists have traditionally divided many corneal disorders into degenerations and dystrophies. Corneal degenerations may be either unilateral or bilateral and are typically nonfamilial. By contrast, corneal dystrophies are typically bilateral and are hereditary. Corneal dystrophies may affect selective corneal layers (e.g., *Reis-Bückler dystrophy* affects Bowman layer, and *posterior polymorphous dystrophy* affects the endothelium), or the changes may be distributed throughout multiple layers.

Band Keratopathies

Two types of band keratopathy serve as examples of corneal degenerations. *Calcific band keratopathy* is characterized by deposition of calcium in the Bowman layer. This condition may complicate chronic uveitis, especially in individuals with chronic juvenile rheumatoid arthritis. *Actinic band keratopathy* develops in individuals who are exposed chronically to high levels of ultraviolet light. In this condition, extensive solar elastosis develops in the superficial layers of corneal collagen in the sun-exposed interpalpebral fissure, hence the horizontally distributed band of pathology. Similar to pinguecula, the sun-damaged collagen of the cornea may take on a yellow hue to the point that this condition is sometimes erroneously called "oil-droplet keratopathy."

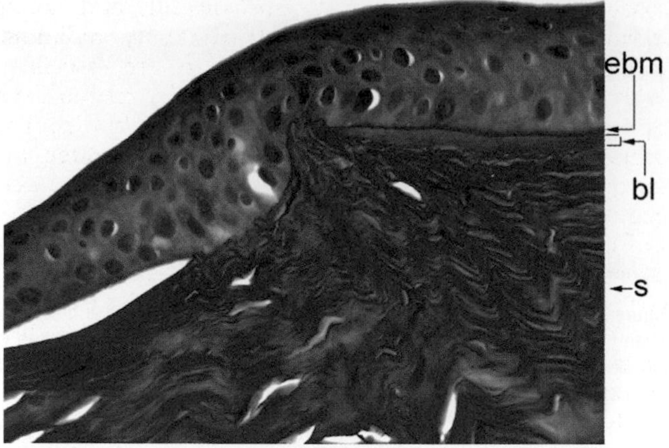

Figure 29-9 Keratoconus. The tissue section is stained by periodic acid–Schiff to highlight the epithelial basement membrane (ebm), which is intact, the Bowman layer (bl), situated between the epithelial basement membrane, and the stroma (s). Following the Bowman layer from the *right side* of the photomicrograph toward the *center*, there is a discontinuity, diagnostic of keratoconus. The epithelial separation just to the *left* of the Bowman layer discontinuity resulted from an episode of corneal hydrops, caused by a break in the Descemet membrane (not shown).

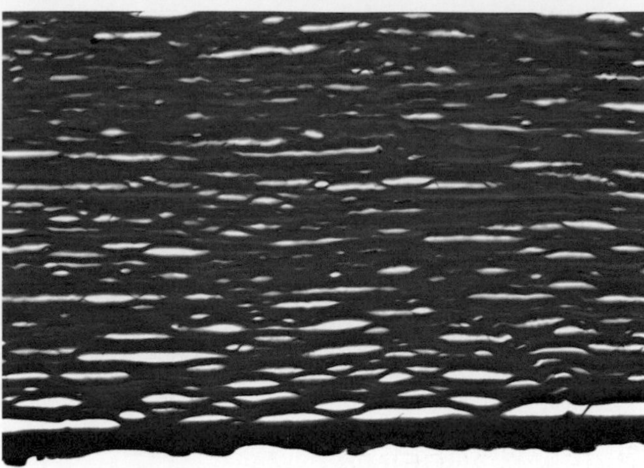

Figure 29-10 Fuchs dystrophy. This tissue section is stained by periodic acid–Schiff to highlight the Descemet membrane, which is thick. Numerous droplike excrescences—guttata—protrude downward from the Descemet membrane. Endothelial cell nuclei are not seen. Epithelial bullae, not shown in this micrograph, were present, reflecting corneal edema.

Keratoconus

With an incidence of 1 in 2000, *keratoconus* is a fairly common disorder characterized by progressive thinning and ectasia of the cornea without evidence of inflammation or vascularization. Such thinning results in a cornea that has a conical rather than spherical shape. This abnormal shape generates irregular astigmatism that is difficult to correct with spectacles. Rigid contact lenses generate a smooth, spherical surface to the cornea and may provide refractive relief for individuals with keratoconus. Patients whose vision cannot be corrected with spectacles or contact lenses are excellent candidates for corneal transplantation, which has a high degree of success in this condition. Unlike many types of degeneration, keratoconus is typically bilateral. Keratoconus is associated with Down syndrome, Marfan syndrome, and atopic disorders. Its development may stem from a genetic predisposition superimposed by an environmental insult, such as eye rubbing in response to atopic conditions.

MORPHOLOGY

Thinning of the cornea with breaks in the Bowman layer are the histologic hallmarks of keratoconus (Fig. 29-9). In some patients the Descemet membrane may rupture precipitously, allowing the aqueous humor in the anterior chamber to gain access to the corneal stroma. The sudden effusion of aqueous humor through a gap in the Descemet membrane—corneal **hydrops**—may also cause vision to worsen suddenly. An episode of hydrops may be followed by corneal scarring that can also contribute to visual loss. Acute corneal hydrops can complicate Descemet membrane ruptures that develop secondary to extraordinary elevations of intraocular pressure in *infantile glaucoma* (*Haab striae*) or following the now uncommon obstetric forceps injury to the eye.

Fuchs Endothelial Dystrophy

This condition, one of several dystrophies results from loss of endothelial cells and the resulting edema and thickening of the stroma. It is one of the principal indications for corneal transplantation in the United States. The two major clinical manifestations of Fuchs endothelial dystrophy—*stromal edema and bullous keratopathy*—are both related to a primary loss of endothelial cells. Early in the course of the disease endothelial cells produce droplike deposits of abnormal basement membrane material *(guttata)* that resemble the fetal component of the Descemet membrane ultrastructurally. Guttata can be visualized clinically by slit-lamp examination. With disease progression, there is a decrease in the total number of endothelial cells, and the residual cells are incapable of maintaining stromal deturgescence. Consequently the stroma becomes edematous and thickens; it acquires a ground-glass appearance clinically, and vision is blurred (Fig. 29-10). Because of chronic edema, the stroma may eventually become vascularized. On occasion the number of endothelial cells may decrease following cataract surgery even in individuals who do not have early forms of Fuchs dystrophy. This condition, known as *pseudophakic bullous keratopathy*, is also a common indication for corneal transplantation.

With increasing stromal edema, the epithelium undergoes hydropic change, and the detachment of the epithelium from the Bowman layer produces epithelial bullae that may eventually rupture. Fibrous connective tissue may be deposited between the epithelium and Bowman layer *(degenerative pannus)* either by ingrowth from the limbus or perhaps through fibrous metaplasia of the corneal epithelium.

Stromal Dystrophies

In these conditions stromal deposits generate discrete opacities in the cornea that may eventually compromise vision. Deposits in the vicinity of the epithelium, its basement membrane, and Bowman layer may result in painful epithelial erosions. Scarring in the vicinity of Bowman layer may generate an irregular corneal surface, further compromising vision.

The identification of specific mutations responsible for various stromal dystrophies is generating a new molecular classification of these disorders that has been correlated with the conventional phenotypic classifications. One such dystrophy, inherited as an autosomal dominant, is caused by mutations in the *TGFB1* gene which encodes an extracellular matrix protein called keratoepithelin.Some mutations cause improper folding of this protein which in turn causes depositions in the cornea.

KEY CONCEPTS

- The cornea—not the lens—is the major refractive surface of the eye. **Keratoconus** is an example of a condition that distorts the contour of the cornea and alters this refractive surface, producing an irregular form of astigmatism.
- The normal cornea is avascular, a feature that contributes to transparency and the low incidence of graft rejection after corneal transplantation.
- Inflammations of the cornea may be accompanied by a non-infectious exudative process in the anterior chamber that may organize to distort anterior segment anatomy and contribute to secondary glaucoma and to cataract.
- **Corneal dystrophies** are generally inherited and **degenerations** are typically not inherited. Fuchs dystrophy and pseudophakic bullous keratopathy both produce visual loss through the final common pathway of corneal edema and both of these conditions are leading indications for corneal transplantation in the United States.

Anterior Segment

Functional Anatomy

The anterior chamber is bounded anteriorly by the cornea, laterally by the trabecular meshwork, and posteriorly by the iris (Fig. 29-11). Aqueous humor, formed by the pars plicata of the ciliary body, enters the posterior chamber, bathes the lens, and circulates through the pupil to gain access to the anterior chamber. The posterior chamber lies behind the iris and in front of the lens.

The lens is a closed epithelial system; the basement membrane of the lens epithelium (known as the lens capsule) totally envelops the lens. Thus, the lens epithelium does not exfoliate like the epidermis or a mucosal epithelium. Instead, the lens epithelium and its derivative fibers accumulate within the confines of the lens capsule, thus "infoliating." With aging, therefore, the size of the lens increases. Neoplasms of the lens have not been described.

Cataract

The term *cataract* describes lenticular opacities that may be congenital or acquired. Systemic diseases (e.g., galactosemia, diabetes mellitus, Wilson disease, and atopic dermatitis), drugs (especially corticosteroids), radiation, trauma, and many intraocular disorders are associated with cataract. Age-related cataract typically results from opacification of the lens nucleus *(nuclear sclerosis)*. The accumulation of urochrome pigment may render the lens nucleus brown, thus distorting the individual's perception of blue color (the predominance of yellow hues in Rembrandt's paintings later in life might have been a consequence of nuclear sclerotic cataracts). Other physical changes in the lens may generate opacities. For example, the lens cortex may liquefy. Migration of the lens epithelium posterior to the lens equator may result in *posterior subcapsular cataract* secondary to enlargement of abnormally positioned lens epithelium. The technique that is most commonly used to remove opacified lenses extracts the lens contents, leaving the lens capsule intact (extracapsular cataract extraction). A prosthetic intraocular lens is typically inserted into the eye. Residual lens epithelial cells may migrate over the lens capsule, contributing to opacification of the capsule and reduction in vision after surgery.

Occasionally, the lens cortex may liquefy nearly entirely, a condition known as hypermature or *morgagnian cataract*. High-molecular-weight proteins from liquefied lens cortex may leak through the lens capsule *(phacolysis)*. This phacolytic protein—either free or contained within macrophages—may clog the trabecular meshwork and contribute to elevation in intraocular pressure and optic nerve damage; phacolytic glaucoma is an example of secondary open-angle glaucoma.

The Anterior Segment and Glaucoma

The term *glaucoma* refers to a collection of diseases characterized by distinctive changes in the visual field and in the cup of the optic nerve. Most of the glaucomas are associated with elevated intraocular pressure, although some individuals with normal intraocular pressure may develop characteristic optic nerve and visual field changes (*normal* or *low-tension glaucoma*). The relationship between intraocular pressure and optic nerve damage is discussed later under "Optic Nerve."

To understand the pathophysiology of glaucoma it is useful to consider the formation and drainage of aqueous humor. As Figure 29-11 illustrates, aqueous humor is produced in the ciliary body and passes from the posterior chamber through the pupil into the anterior chamber. Although there are multiple pathways for the egress of fluid from the anterior chamber, most of the aqueous humor drains through the trabecular meshwork, situated in the angle formed by the intersection between the corneal periphery and the anterior surface of the iris. With this background, glaucoma can be classified into two major categories.

- In *open-angle glaucoma* the aqueous humor has complete physical access to the trabecular meshwork, and the elevation in intraocular pressure results from an increased resistance to aqueous outflow in the open angle.
- In *angle-closure glaucoma* the peripheral zone of the iris adheres to the trabecular meshwork and physically impedes the egress of aqueous humor from the eye.

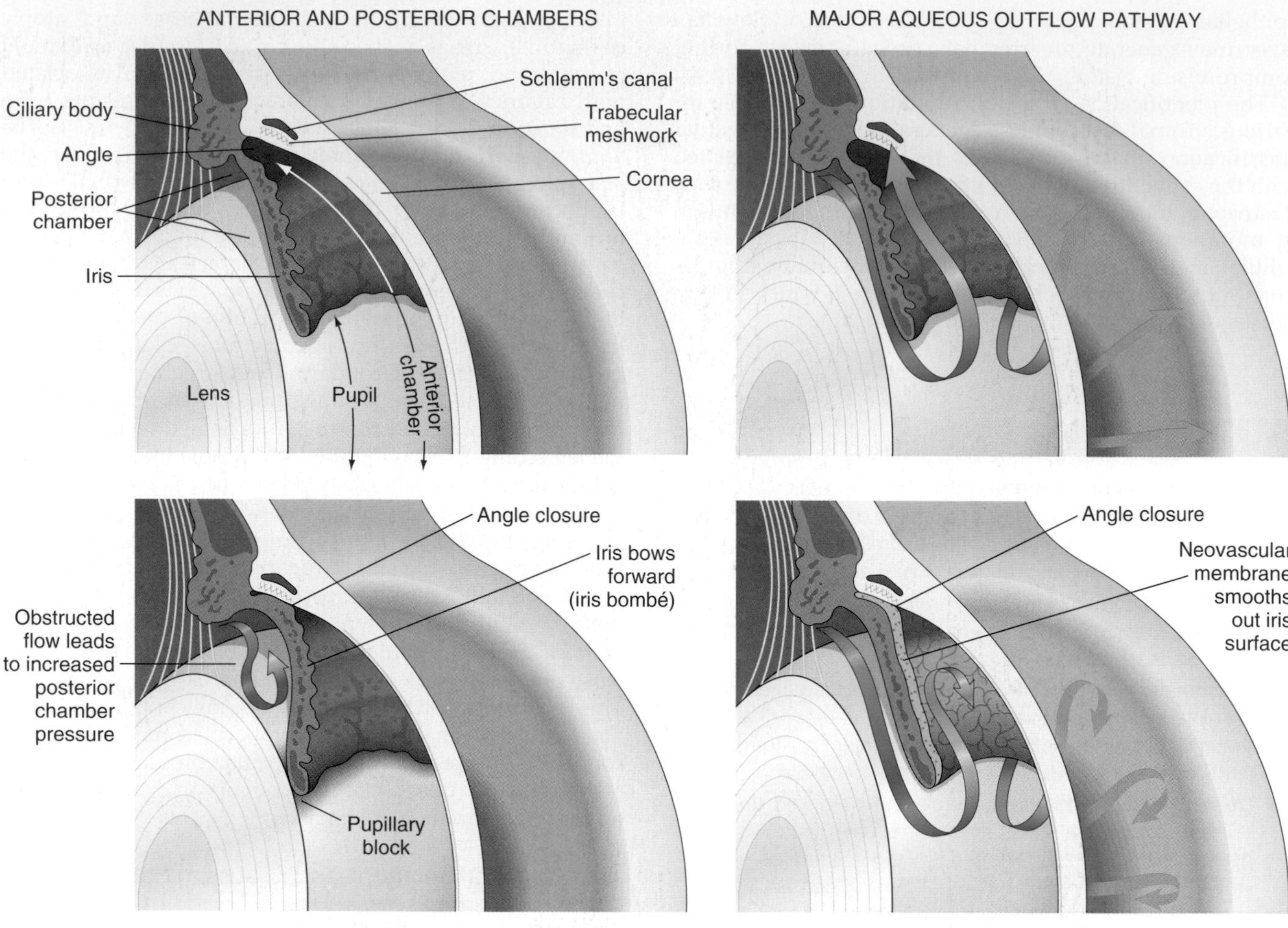

Figure 29-11 *Upper left*, The normal eye. Note that the surface of the iris is highly textured with crypts and folds. *Upper right*, The normal flow of aqueous humor. Aqueous humor, produced in the posterior chamber, flows through the pupil into the anterior chamber. The major pathway for the egress of aqueous humor is through the trabecular meshwork, into the Schlemm canal. Minor outflow pathways (uveoscleral and iris, not depicted) contribute to a limited extent to aqueous outflow. *Lower left*, Primary angle-closure glaucoma. In anatomically predisposed eyes, transient apposition of the iris at the pupillary margin to the lens blocks the passage of aqueous humor from the posterior chamber to the anterior chamber. Pressure builds in the posterior chamber, bowing the iris forward (iris bombé) and occluding the trabecular meshwork. *Lower right*, A neovascular membrane has grown over the surface of the iris, smoothing the iris folds and crypts. Myofibroblasts within the neovascular membrane cause the membrane to contract and to become apposed to the trabecular meshwork (peripheral anterior synechiae). Outflow of aqueous humor is blocked, and the intraocular pressure becomes elevated.

Both open-angle and angle-closure glaucoma can be subclassified into primary and secondary types. In *primary open-angle glaucoma*, the most common form of glaucoma, the angle is open, and few changes are apparent structurally. Mutations in the myocilin (*MYOC*) gene have been associated with a subset of individuals with juvenile and adult primary open-angle glaucoma. Mutations in optineurin (*OPTN*) may also be responsible for a subset of adult patients with open angle glaucoma. The role of these genes in the pathogenesis of glaucoma is not clear.

There are multiple causes of *secondary open-angle glaucoma*. Pseudoexfoliation glaucoma, perhaps the most common form of secondary open angle glaucoma, is associated with the deposition of fibrillar material of varying composition throughout the anterior segment. Pseudoexfoliation glaucoma has been associated with single nucleotide polymorphisms in the lysyl oxidase like 1 (*LOX1*) gene. In addition to deposition in the anterior chamber, fibrillar material is deposited around blood vessels in connective tissue and in many visceral organs such as liver , kidney and gall bladder.

Particulate material such as high-molecular-weight lens proteins produced by phacolysis, senescent red cells after trauma *(ghost cell glaucoma)*, iris epithelial pigment granules *(pigmentary glaucoma)*, and necrotic tumors *(melanomalytic glaucoma)* can clog the trabecular meshwork in the presence of an open angle. Elevations in the pressure on the surface of the eye (episcleral venous pressure) in the presence of an open angle also contribute to secondary open-angle glaucoma. This type of glaucoma is associated with surface ocular vascular malformations seen in *Sturge-Weber syndrome* or as a consequence of arterialization of the

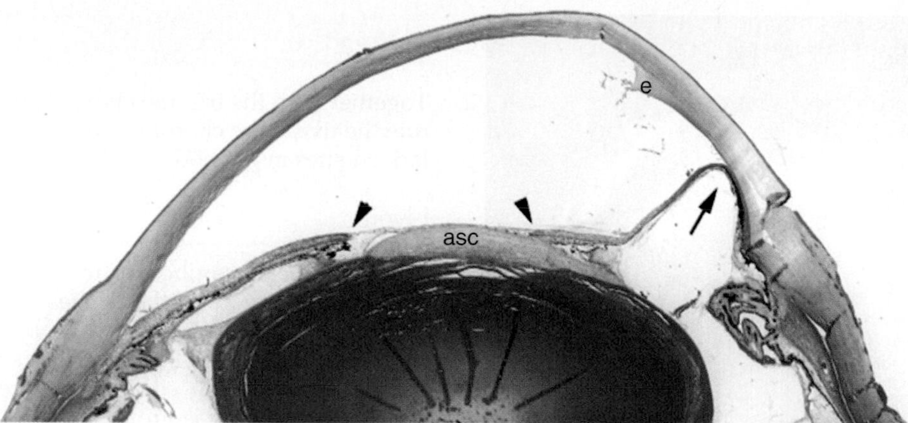

Figure 29-12 Sequelae of anterior segment inflammation. This eye was removed for complications of chronic corneal inflammation (not visible at this magnification). The exudate (e) present in the anterior chamber would have been visualized with a slit lamp as an optical "flare." The iris is adherent focally to the cornea, obstructing the trabecular meshwork (anterior synechia, *arrow*), and to the lens (posterior synechiae, *arrowheads*). An anterior subcapsular cataract (asc) has formed. The radial folds in the lens are artifacts.

episcleral veins following a spontaneous or traumatic carotid-cavernous fistula.

Primary angle-closure glaucoma typically develops in eyes with shallow anterior chambers, often found in individuals with hyperopia. Transient apposition of the pupillary margin of the iris to the anterior surface of the lens may result in obstruction to the flow of aqueous humor through the pupillary aperture *(pupillary block)*. Continued production of aqueous humor by the ciliary body thus elevates pressure in the posterior chamber and may bow the iris periphery forward *(iris bombé)*, apposing it to the trabecular meshwork. These anatomic changes provoke a marked elevation in intraocular pressure (Fig. 29-11). Since the crystalline lens is avascular and the lens epithelium receives its nutrition from the aqueous humor, unremitting elevation in intraocular pressure in primary angle-closure glaucoma can damage the lens epithelium. This leads to minute anterior subcapsular opacities that are visible by slit-lamp examination *(glaukomflecken)*. Although the affected individual might have a normal complement of healthy corneal endothelial cells, sustained elevated intraocular pressure can produce corneal edema and bullous keratopathy.

There are many causes of *secondary angle-closure glaucoma*. Contraction of various types of pathologic membranes that form over the surface of the iris can draw the iris over the trabecular meshwork, occluding aqueous outflow. For example, chronic retinal ischemia is associated with the up-regulation of VEGF and other proangiogenic factors. The appearance of VEGF in the aqueous humor is thought to induce the development of thin, clinically transparent fibrovascular membranes over the surface of the iris. Contraction of myofibroblastic elements in these membranes leads to occlusion of the trabecular meshwork by the iris: *neovascular glaucoma* (Fig. 29-11). Necrotic tumors, especially retinoblastomas, can also induce iris neovascularization and glaucoma. Secondary angle-closure glaucoma may be caused by other mechanisms as well; for example, tumors in the ciliary body can mechanically compress the iris onto the trabecular meshwork, closing off the major pathway of aqueous outflow.

Endophthalmitis and Panophthalmitis

In intraocular inflammation, vessels in the ciliary body and iris become leaky, allowing cells and exudate to accumulate in the anterior chamber. These changes can be visualized with a slit lamp; at times the inflammatory cells may adhere to the corneal endothelium, forming clinically visible *keratic precipitates*. The size and shape of these precipitates can provide clues to the underlying cause of the inflammation. For example, aggregates of macrophages on the endothelium in sarcoid produce characteristic "mutton-fat" keratic precipitates.

Just as pleural exudate in acute bronchopneumonia can lead to adhesions between the visceral and parietal pleura, the presence of exudate in the anterior chamber can facilitate the formation of adhesions between the iris and the trabecular meshwork or cornea *(anterior synechiae)* or between the iris and anterior surface of the lens *(posterior synechiae)*. Anterior synechiae can lead to elevation in intraocular pressure, which may lead to optic nerve damage. Prolonged contact between the iris and the anterior surface of the lens can deprive lens epithelium of contact with aqueous humor and can induce fibrous metaplasia of the lens epithelium: *anterior subcapsular cataract* (Fig. 29-12). The pharmacologic induction of pupillary dilation and cycloplegia in individuals with intraocular inflammation is intended in part to prevent the formation of synechiae and their sequelae.

Although inflammation confined to the anterior segment is technically intraocular inflammation, the term *endophthalmitis* is reserved for inflammation within the vitreous humor. The retina lines the vitreous cavity, and suppurative inflammation in the vitreous humor is poorly tolerated by the retina; a few hours may be sufficient to cause irreversible retinal injury. Endophthalmitis is classified as *exogenous* (originating in the environment and gaining access to the interior of the eye through a wound) or *endogenous* (delivered to the eye hematogenously). The term *panophthalmitis* is applied to inflammation within the eye that involves the retina, choroid, and sclera and extends into the orbit (Fig. 29-13).

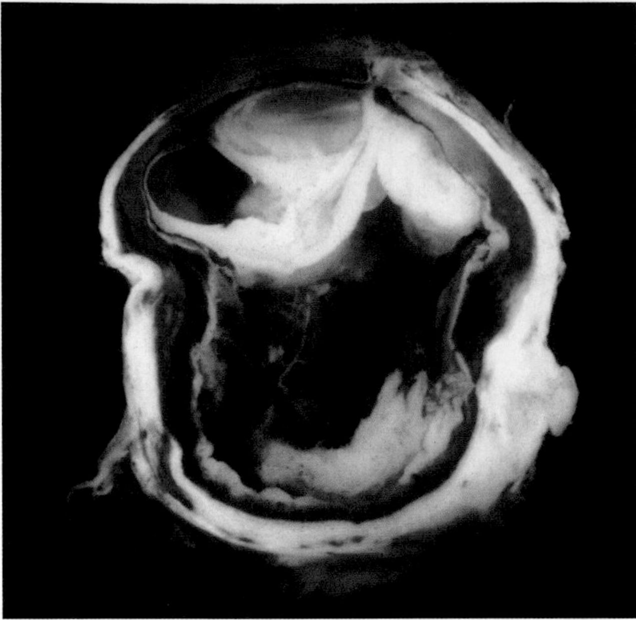

Figure 29-13 Exogenous panophthalmitis. This eye was removed after a foreign body injury. Note the suppurative inflammation behind the lens that is drawn up to the right of the lens to the cornea, the site of the wound. The central portion of the vitreous humor was extracted surgically (by vitrectomy). Note the adhesions to the surface of the eye at the 8 o'clock position, indicating that the intraocular inflammation has spread through the sclera into the orbit: panophthalmitis. (From Folberg R: The eye. In Spencer WH (ed): Ophthalmic Pathology—An Atlas and Textbook, 4th ed. Philadelphia, WB Saunders, 1985.)

KEY CONCEPTS

- The term **cataract** describes opacities of the lens that may be congenital or acquired.
- The term **glaucoma** describes a group of conditions characterized by distinctive changes in the visual field and the size and shape of the optic nerve cup and usually by an elevation in intraocular pressure.
- Glaucoma may develop in the context of either an open or closed angle. Open angle and angle closure glaucomas are further subclassified into primary and secondary types.
- Mutations in the myocilin (*MYOC*) and optineurin (*OPTN*) genes have been associated with subsets of individuals with juvenile and adult primary open-angle glaucoma
- **Endophthalmitis** is a term used to describe inflammation of the interior of the eye involving the vitreous humor and panophthalmitis is the term used to describe inflammation of the interior of the eye that also extends into the uvea and sclera.
- Endophthalmitis may originate from infection within the body (endogenous endophthalmitis complicating generalized sepsis) or as a complication of corneal infection or a wound, accidental injury, or a surgical procedure (exogenous endophthalmitis).
- In panophthalmitis, inflammation extends from the interior of the eye into the ocular coats: the retina, choroid, and the sclera.

Uvea

Together with the iris, the choroid and ciliary body constitute the uvea. The choroid is among the most richly vascularized sites in the body.

Uveitis

The term *uveitis* can be applied to any type of inflammation in one or more of the tissues that compose the uvea. Thus, the iritis that develops after blunt trauma to the eye or that accompanies a corneal ulcer is technically a form of uveitis. However, in clinical practice the term *uveitis* is restricted to a diverse group of chronic diseases that may be either components of a systemic process or localized to the eye. Uveal inflammation may be manifest principally in the anterior segment (e.g., in *juvenile rheumatoid arthritis*) or may affect both the anterior and posterior segments. The complications of chronic anterior segment inflammation were discussed earlier; the remainder of this discussion therefore focuses on the effects of uveal inflammation on the posterior segment of the eye. As will be described briefly, uveitis is frequently accompanied by retinal pathology. Uveitis may be caused by infectious agents (e.g., *Pneumocystis carinii*), may be idiopathic (e.g., sarcoidosis), or may be autoimmune in origin (sympathetic ophthalmia). Examples are described later.

Granulomatous uveitis is a common complication of sarcoidosis (Chapter 15). In the anterior segment it gives rise to an exudate that evolves into "mutton-fat" keratic precipitates described earlier. In the posterior segment, sarcoid may involve the choroid and retina. Thus, granulomas may be seen in the choroid. Retinal pathology is characterized by perivascular inflammation; this is responsible for the well-known ophthalmoscopic sign of "candle wax drippings." Conjunctival biopsy can be used to detect granulomatous inflammation and confirm the diagnosis of ocular sarcoid.

Numerous infectious processes can affect the choroid or the retina. Inflammation in one compartment is typically associated with inflammation in the other. Retinal *toxoplasmosis* is usually accompanied by uveitis and even scleritis. Individuals with AIDS may develop cytomegalovirus retinitis and uveal infection such as *Pneumocystis* or mycobacterial choroiditis.

Sympathetic ophthalmia is an example of noninfectious uveitis limited to the eye. This condition is characterized by bilateral granulomatous inflammation typically affecting all components of the uvea: a panuveitis. Sympathetic ophthalmia, which blinded young Louis Braille, may complicate a penetrating injury of the eye. In the injured eye, retinal antigens sequestered from the immune system may gain access to lymphatics in the conjunctiva and thus set up a delayed hypersensitivity reaction that affects not only the injured eye but also the contralateral, noninjured eye. The condition may develop from 2 weeks to many years after injury. Enucleation of a blind eye (which can be the sympathizing eye rather than the directly injured eye) may yield diagnostic findings. It is characterized by diffuse granulomatous inflammation of the uvea (choroid, ciliary body, and iris). Plasma cells are typically absent, but eosinophils may be identified in the infiltrate (Fig. 29-14).

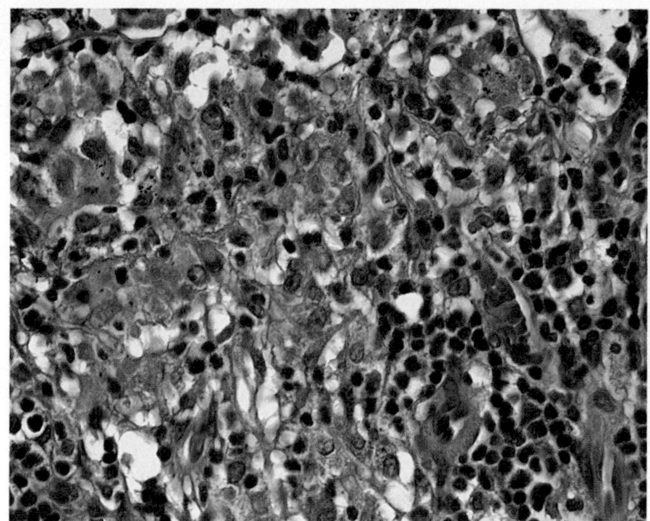

Figure 29-14 Sympathetic ophthalmia. The granulomatous inflammation depicted here was identified diffusely throughout the uvea. The uveal granulomas may contain melanin pigment and may be accompanied by eosinophils.

Sympathetic ophthalmia is treated by the administration of systemic immunosuppressive agents.

Neoplasms

The most common intraocular malignancy of adults is metastasis to the uvea, typically to the choroid. The occurrence of metastases to the eye is associated with an extremely short survival, and treatment of ocular metastases, usually by radiotherapy, is palliative.

Uveal Nevi and Melanomas

Uveal melanoma is the most common primary intraocular malignancy of adults. In the United States, these tumors account for approximately 5% of melanomas and have an age-adjusted incidence of 5.1 per million per year. Uveal nevi, especially choroidal nevi, are rather common, affecting an estimated 10% of the Caucasian population.

Epidemiology and Pathogenesis. Unlike cutaneous melanoma, the occurrence of uveal melanoma has remained stable over many years and there is no clear link between exposure to ultraviolet light and risk. In line with this observation, sequencing of tumor genomes has revealed that the molecular pathogenesis of uveal melanoma is distinct from that of cutaneous melanoma. The most important oncogenes in uveal melanoma are *GNAQ* and *GNA11*, both of which encode G-protein coupled receptors. Roughly 85% of uveal melanomas harbor a gain-of-function mutation in one of these genes that activate pathways that promote proliferation, such as the MAPK pathway (Chapter 7). Notably, uveal nevi are also associated with *GNAQ* and *GNA11* mutations yet rarely transform to melanoma, indicating that other genetic events also contribute to the development of uveal melanoma. One such event is loss of chromosome 3, which appears to be selected for because it leads to deletion of *BAP1*, a tumor suppressor gene on chromosome 3 that encodes a deubiquitinating enzyme. BAP1 is a component of protein complexes that place repressive marks on chromatin that lead to gene silencing; thus, uveal melanoma has joined the increasing list of cancers in which epigenetic alterations appear to have a central role in tumor pathogenesis (Chapter 7).

MORPHOLOGY

Histologically, uveal melanomas may contain two types of cells, spindle and epithelioid, in various proportions (Fig. 29-15). **Spindle cells** are fusiform in shape, whereas **epithelioid cells** are spherical and have greater cytologic atypicality. Like cutaneous melanomas, large numbers of tumor-infiltrating lymphocytes may be seen in some cases. An unusual feature that is commonly seen is the presence of looping slit-like spaces lined by laminin that surround packets of tumor cells. These spaces (which are not blood vessels) connect to blood vessels and serve as extravascular conduits for the transport of plasma and possibly blood. In vitro studies and examination of human tissues suggest that these unusual growth patterns are promoted by tumor cells through a process termed **vasculogenic mimicry.**

Uveal melanomas, with very rare exception, spread exclusively by a hematogenous route (the only exception being the rare case of melanoma that spreads through the sclera and invades the conjunctiva, thereby gaining access to conjunctival lymphatics). Most uveal melanomas spread first to the liver, an excellent example of a tumor-specific tropism for a particular metastatic site.

Clinical Features. Most uveal melanomas are incidental findings or present with visual symptoms, which may be related to retinal detachment or glaucoma. The prognosis of choroidal and ciliary body melanomas is related to (1) size (in contrast to cutaneous melanoma, the lateral extent of the tumor rather than tumor depth is the size dimension related to adverse outcome); (2) cell type (tumors containing epithelioid cells have a worse prognosis than do those containing exclusively spindle cells); (3) and proliferative index. Cytogenetic profiles, especially monosomy 3, and gene expression profiling may be helpful in stratifying patients into categories with differing risks of developing metastatic disease.

There seems to be no difference in survival between tumors treated by removal of the eye (enucleation) and those receiving eye-sparing radiotherapy, which is the treatment of choice. Melanomas situated exclusively in the iris tend to follow a relatively indolent course, whereas melanomas of the ciliary body and choroid are more aggressive.

Because these tumors are hidden from sight and are likely to have been present for some time before diagnosis, the prognosis is worse than for cutaneous melanoma. Although the 5-year survival rate is approximately 80%, the cumulative melanoma mortality rate is 40% at 10 years, increasing 1% per year thereafter. Metastases may appear "out of the blue" many years after treatment, making uveal melanoma a prime candidate for the investigation of the phenomenon of tumor dormancy. Targeted therapies such as MAPK inhibitors have shown some encouraging responses in clinical trials, but currently there is no proven effective treatment for metastatic uveal melanoma.

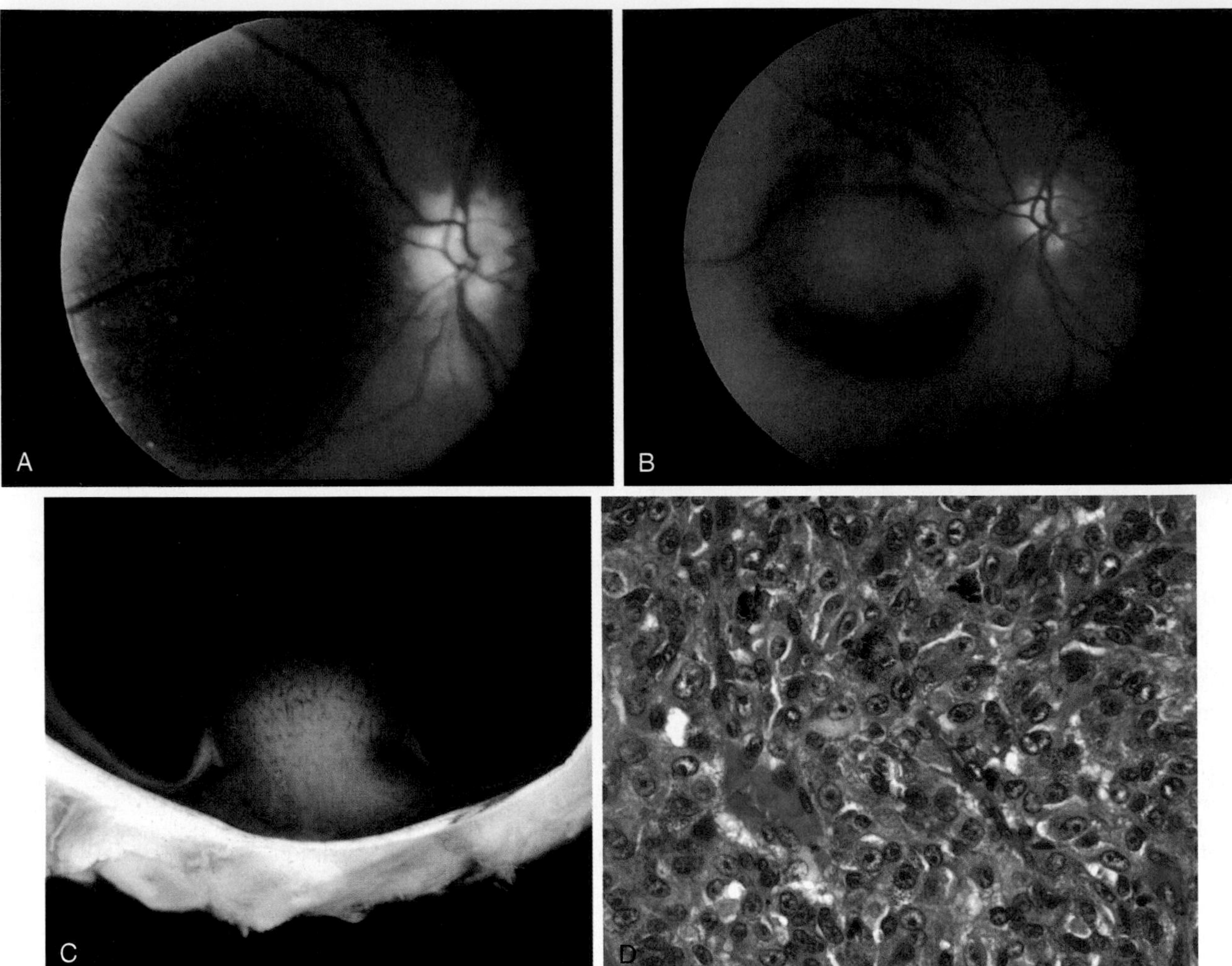

Figure 29-15 Uveal melanoma. **A,** Fundus photograph from an individual with a relatively flat pigmented lesion of the choroid near the optic disc. **B,** Fundus photograph of the same individual several years later; the tumor has grown and has ruptured through the Bruch membrane. **C,** Gross photograph of a choroidal melanoma that has ruptured the Bruch membrane. The overlying retina is detached. **D,** Epithelioid melanoma cells associated with an adverse outcome. (**A** to **C,** From Folberg R: Pathology of the Eye—an Interactive CD-ROM Program. Philadelphia, Mosby, 1996.)

KEY CONCEPTS

- **Uveitis** is restricted to a diverse group of chronic diseases that may be either components of a systemic process or localized to the eye.
- **Sarcoid** is an example of a systemic condition that may produce granulomatous uveitis and sympathetic ophthalmia may produce bilateral granulomatous inflammation as a possible consequence of penetrating injury to one eye.
- The most common intraocular tumor of adults is metastasis to the eye.
- The most common primary intraocular tumor of adults is **uveal melanoma.**
- Uveal melanoma disseminates hematogenously and the first evidence of metastasis is typically detected in the liver.
- Uveal melanoma shows marked differences in epidemiologic risk factors and driver mutations as compared to cutaneous melanoma.

Retina and Vitreous

Functional Anatomy

The neurosensory retina, like the optic nerve, is an embryologic derivative of the diencephalon. The retina therefore responds to injury by means of gliosis. As in the brain, there are no lymphatics. The architecture of the retina accounts for the ophthalmoscopic appearance of a variety of ocular disorders. Hemorrhages in the nerve fiber layer of the retina are oriented horizontally and appear as streaks or "flames"; the external retinal layers are oriented perpendicular to the retinal surface, and hemorrhages in these outer layers appear as dots (the tips of cylinders). Exudates tend to accumulate in the outer plexiform layer of the retina, especially in the macula (Fig. 29-16).

The retinal pigment epithelium (RPE), like the retina, is derived embryologically from the primary optic vesicle, an outpouching of the brain. Separation of the neurosensory retina from the RPE defines a *retinal detachment*. The RPE

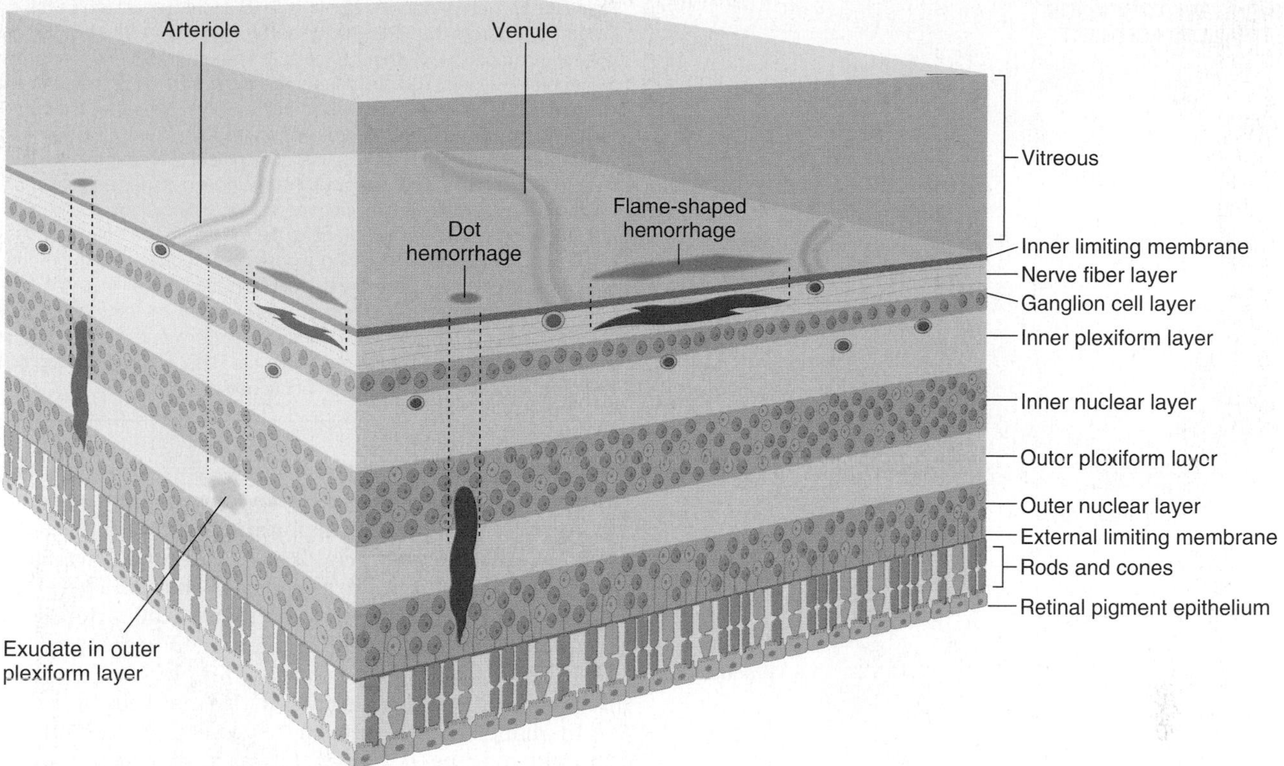

Figure 29-16 Clinicopathologic correlations of retinal hemorrhages and exudates. The location of the hemorrhage within the retina determines its appearance by ophthalmoscopy. The retinal nerve fiber layer is oriented parallel to the internal limiting membrane, and hemorrhages of this layer appear to be flame-shaped ophthalmoscopically. The deeper retinal layers are oriented perpendicular to the internal limiting membrane and hemorrhages in this location appear as cross-sections of a cylinder or "dot" hemorrhages. Exudates that originate from leaky retinal vessels accumulate in the outer plexiform layer.

has an important role in the maintenance of the outer segments of the photoreceptors. Disturbances in the RPE-photoreceptor interface are implicated in hereditary retinal degenerations such as *retinitis pigmentosa*.

The adult vitreous humor is avascular. Incomplete regression of fetal vasculature running through the vitreous humor can produce significant pathology as a retrolental mass *(persistent hyperplastic primary vitreous)*. The vitreous humor can be opacified by hemorrhage from trauma or retinal neovascularization. With age the vitreous humor may liquefy and collapse, creating the visual sensation of "floaters." Also, with aging, the posterior face of the vitreous humor—the posterior hyaloid—may separate from the neurosensory retina *(posterior vitreous detachment)*. The relationship between the posterior hyaloid and the neurosensory retina has a key role in the pathogenesis of retinal neovascularization and in some forms of retinal detachment.

Retinal Detachment

Retinal detachment (separation of the neurosensory retina from the RPE) is broadly classified by etiology based on the presence or absence of a break in the retina. *Rhegmatogenous retinal detachment* is associated with a full-thickness retinal defect. Retinal tears may develop after the vitreous collapses structurally, and the posterior hyaloid exerts traction on points of abnormally strong adhesion to the retinal internal limiting membrane. Liquefied vitreous humor then seeps through the tear and gains access to the potential space between the neurosensory retina and the RPE (Fig. 29-17). Re-attachment of the retina to the RPE generally requires relief of vitreous traction through indenting of the sclera by surgical procedures. This can be accomplished by the application of strips of silicon to the surface of the eye (scleral buckling) and possibly by removal of vitreous material (vitrectomy). Rhegmatogenous retinal detachment may be complicated by *proliferative vitreoretinopathy*, the formation of epiretinal or subretinal membranes by retinal glial cells (Müller cells) or RPE cells.

Non-rhegmatogenous retinal detachment (retinal detachment without retinal break) may complicate retinal vascular disorders associated with significant exudation and any condition that damages the RPE and permits fluid to leak from the choroidal circulation under the retina. Retinal detachments associated with choroidal tumors and malignant hypertension are examples of nonrhegmatogenous retinal detachment.

Retinal Vascular Disease

Hypertension

Normally, the thin walls of retinal arterioles permit a direct visualization of the circulating blood by ophthalmoscopy. In retinal arteriolosclerosis the thickened arteriolar wall changes the ophthalmic perception of circulating blood: vessels may appear narrowed, and the

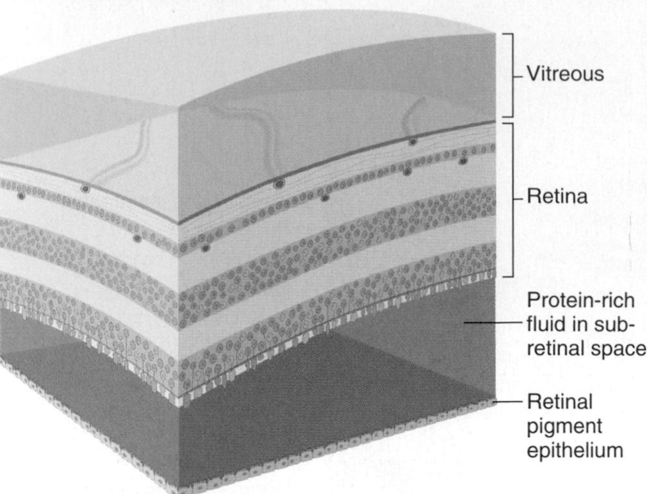

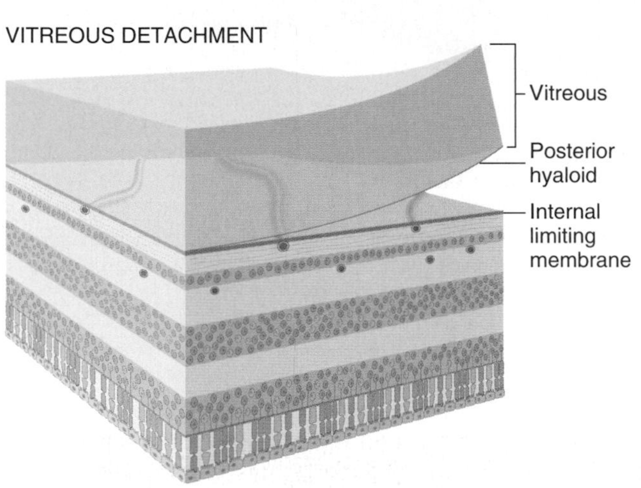

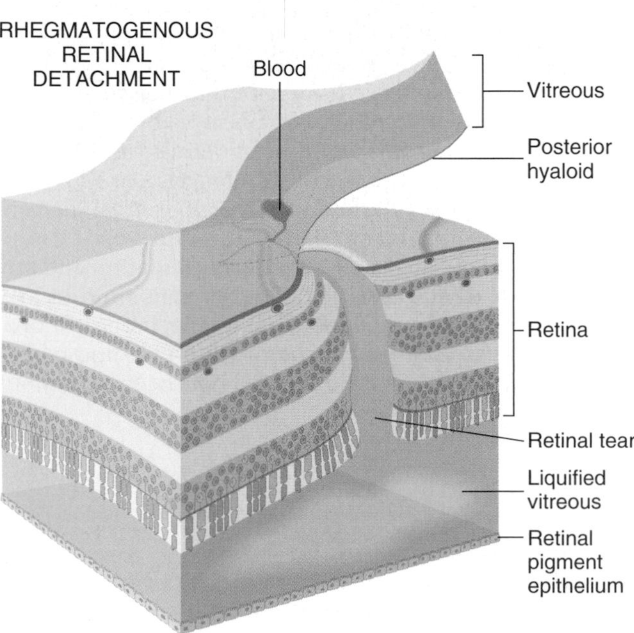

Figure 29-17 Retinal detachment is defined as the separation of the neurosensory retina from the RPE. Retinal detachments are classified broadly into non-rhegmatogenous (without a retinal break) and rhegmatogenous (with a retinal break) types. *Top*, In non-rhegmatogenous retinal detachment the subretinal space is filled with protein-rich exudate. Note that the outer segments of the photoreceptors are missing (see Fig. 29-16 for orientation of layers). This indicates a chronic retinal detachment, a finding that can be seen in both non-rhegmatogenous and rhegmatogenous detachments. *Middle*, Posterior vitreous detachment involves the separation of the posterior hyaloid from the internal limiting membrane of the retina and is a normal occurrence in the aging eye. *Bottom*, If during a posterior vitreous detachment the posterior hyaloid does not separate cleanly from the internal limiting membrane of the retina, the vitreous humor will exert traction on the retina, which will be torn at this point. Liquefied vitreous humor seeps through the retinal defect, and the retina is separated from the RPE. The photoreceptor outer segments are intact, illustrating an acute detachment.

color of the blood column may change from bright red to copper and to silver depending on the degree of vascular wall thickness (Fig. 29-18*A*). Retinal arterioles and veins share a common adventitial sheath. Therefore, in pronounced retinal arteriolosclerosis the arteriole may compress the vein at points where both vessels cross (Fig. 29-18*B*). Venous stasis distal to arteriolar-venous crossing may precipitate occlusions of the retinal vein branches.

In malignant hypertension vessels in the retina and choroid may be damaged. Damage to choroidal vessels may produce focal choroidal infarcts, seen clinically as *Elschnig spots*. Damage to the choriocapillaris, the internal layer of the choroidal vasculature, may, in turn, damage the overlying RPE and permit the exudate to accumulate in the potential space between the neurosensory retina and the RPE, thereby producing a retinal detachment. Exudate from damaged retinal arterioles typically accumulates in the outer plexiform layer of the retina (Fig. 29-18*A*). The ophthalmoscopic finding of a macular star—a spokelike arrangement of exudate in the macula in malignant hypertension—results from exudate accumulating in the outer plexiform layer of the macula that is oriented obliquely instead of perpendicular to the retinal surface.

Occlusion of retinal arterioles may produce infarcts of the nerve fiber layer of the retina (axons of the retinal ganglion cell layer populate the nerve fiber layer). Axoplasmic transport in the nerve fiber layer is interrupted at the point of axonal damage, and accumulation of mitochondria at the swollen ends of damaged axons creates the histologic illusion of cells *(cytoid bodies)*. Collections of cytoid bodies populate the nerve fiber layer infarct, seen ophthalmoscopically as "cotton-wool spots" (Fig. 29-19). Although nerve fiber layer infarcts are described here in the context of hypertension, they may be detected in a variety of retinal occlusive vasculopathies. For example, retinal nerve fiber layer infarcts may develop in individuals with AIDS due to a retinal vasculopathy that is similar to the brain vasculopathy that may develop in this condition.

Diabetes Mellitus

The eye is profoundly affected by diabetes mellitus. The effects of hyperglycemia on the lens and iris have already been mentioned. Thickening of the basement membrane of the epithelium of the pars plicata of the ciliary body is a reliable histologic marker of diabetes mellitus in the eye (Fig. 29-20) and is reminiscent of similar

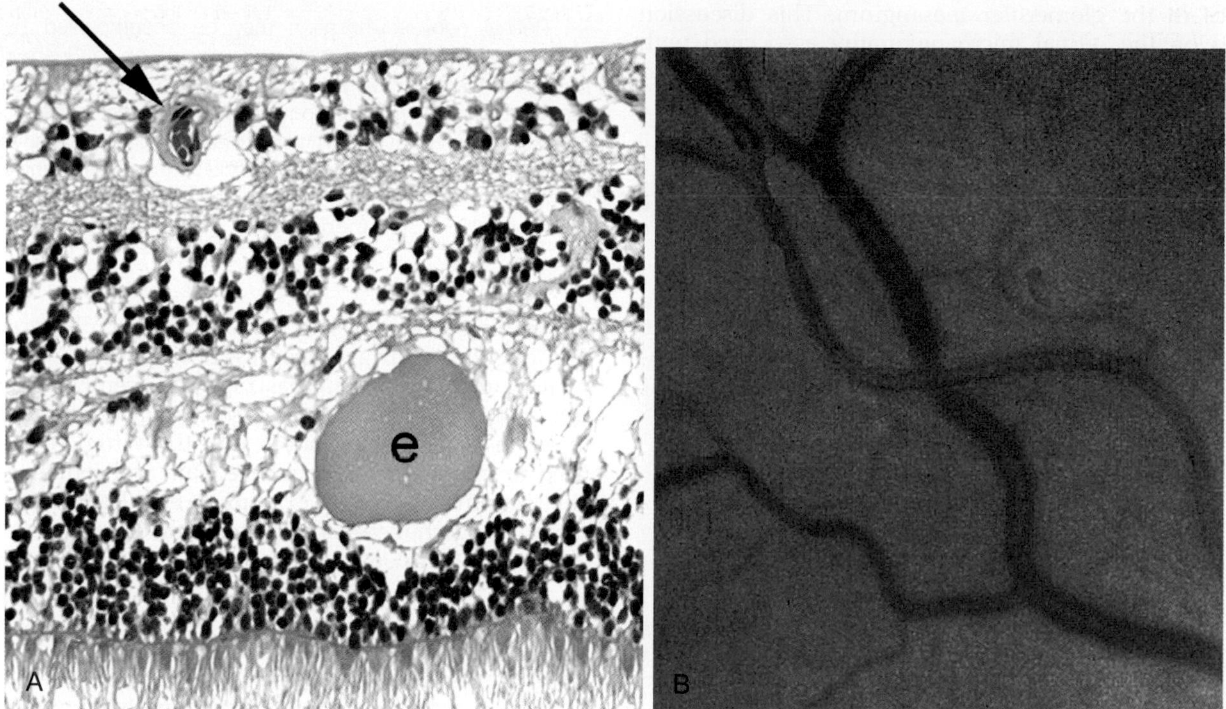

Figure 29-18 The retina in hypertension. **A,** The wall of the retinal arteriole *(arrow)* is thick. Note the exudate (e) in the retinal outer plexiform layer. **B,** The fundus in hypertension. The diameter of the arterioles is reduced, and the color of the blood column appears to be less saturated (copper wire–like). If the wall of the vessel were thicker still, the degree of red color would diminish such that the vessels might appear clinically to have a "silver wire" appearance. In this fundus photograph, note that the vein is compressed where the sclerotic arteriole crosses over it. (**B,** Courtesy Dr. Thomas A. Weingeist, Department of Ophthalmology and Visual Science, University of Iowa, Iowa City, Ia.)

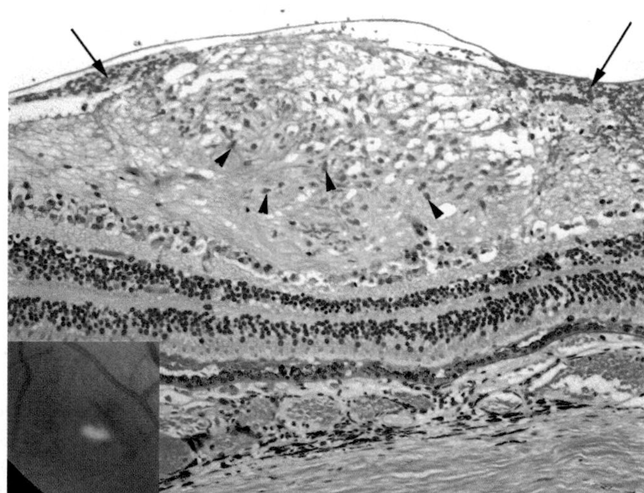

Figure 29-19 Nerve fiber layer infarct. A "cotton-wool spot" is illustrated in the *inset*, adjacent to a flame-shaped (nerve fiber layer) hemorrhage. The histology of a cotton-wool spot—an infarct of the nerve fiber layer of the retina—is illustrated in the photomicrograph. A focal swelling of the nerve fiber layer is occupied by numerous red to pink cytoid bodies *(arrowheads)*. Hemorrhage *(arrows)* surrounding the nerve fiber layer infarct as illustrated here is a variable and inconsistent finding. (Fundus photograph, Courtesy Dr. Thomas A. Weingeist, Department of Ophthalmology and Visual Science, University of Iowa, Iowa City, Ia.)

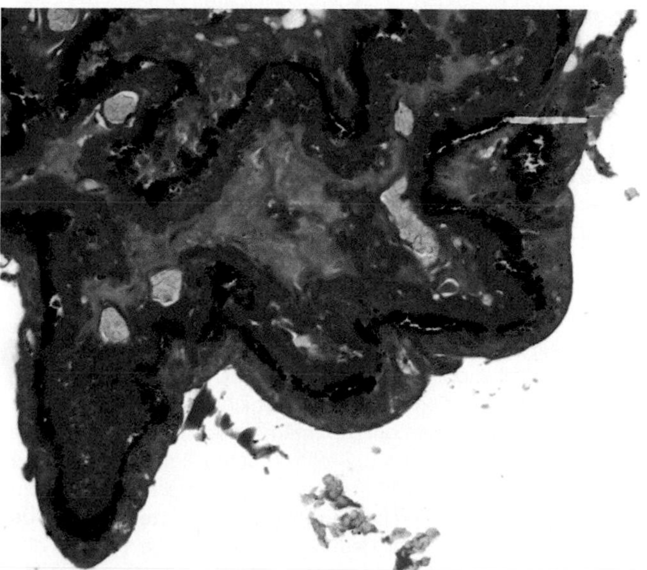

Figure 29-20 The ciliary body in chronic diabetes mellitus, periodic acid–Schiff stain. Note the massive thickening of the basement membrane of the ciliary body epithelia, reminiscent of changes in the mesangium of the renal glomerulus.

changes in the glomerular mesangium. This discussion focuses on the retinal microangiopathy associated with diabetes mellitus, a prototype for the consideration of other retinal microangiopathies.

MORPHOLOGY

The retinal vasculopathy of diabetes mellitus can be classified into **nonproliferative** and **proliferative diabetic retinopathy**.

Nonproliferative diabetic retinopathy includes a spectrum of changes resulting from structural and functional abnormalities of retinal vessels (i.e., confined beneath the internal limiting membrane of the retina). As with diabetic microangiopathy in general, the **basement membrane of retinal blood vessels is thickened**. In addition, the number of pericytes relative to endothelial cells diminishes. **Microaneurysms** are an important manifestation of diabetic microangiopathy. They are typically smaller than the resolution of direct ophthalmoscopes, and findings customarily described as microaneurysms by ophthalmoscopy may in fact be retinal microhemorrhages. Structural changes in the retinal microcirculation have been associated with a physiologic breakdown in the blood-retinal barrier. Recall that VEGF was initially called vascular permeability factor. Thus, the retinal microcirculation in diabetics may be exceptionally leaky, giving rise to **macular edema**, a common cause of visual loss in these patients. The vascular changes may also produce **exudates** that accumulate in the outer plexiform layer. Although the retinal microcirculation is often hyperpermeable, it is also subject to the effects of micro-occlusion. Both vascular incompetence and vascular micro-occlusions can be visualized clinically after intravenous injection of fluorescein. Nonperfusion of the retina due to the microcirculatory change described earlier is associated with up-regulation of VEGF and intra-retinal angiogenesis (located beneath the internal limiting membrane of the retina).

Proliferative diabetic retinopathy is defined by the appearance of new vessels sprouting on the surface of either the optic nerve head (termed "neovascularization of the disc") or the surface of the retina ("designated by the nebulous term neovascularization elsewhere") (Fig. 24-42*C*). The term "retinal neovascularization" is only applied when the newly formed vessels breach the internal limiting membrane of the retina. The quantity and location of retinal neovascularization guide the ophthalmologist in the treatment of proliferative diabetic retinopathy. The web of newly formed vessels is referred to as a neovascular membrane. It is composed of angiogenic vessels with or without a substantial supportive fibrous or glial stroma (Fig. 29-21*B*).

If the vitreous humor has not detached and the posterior hyaloid is intact, neovascular membranes extend along the potential plane between the retinal internal limiting membrane and the posterior hyaloid. If vitreous humor later separates from the internal limiting membrane of the retina **(posterior vitreous detachment)** there may be massive hemorrhage from the disrupted neovascular membrane. In addition, scarring associated with the organization of the retinal neovascular membrane may wrinkle the retina, disrupting the orientation of retinal photoreceptors and producing visual distortion, and may exert traction on the retina, separating it from the RPE (retinal detachment). **Traction retinal detachment** may begin as a non-rhegmatogenous detachment, but severe traction may tear the retina, producing a traction rhegmatogenous detachment.

Retinal neovascularization may be accompanied by the development of a neovascular membrane on the iris surface, presumably secondary to increased levels of VEGF in the aqueous humor. Contraction of the iris neovascular membrane may lead to adhesions between the iris and trabecular meshwork (anterior synechiae), thus occluding a major pathway for aqueous outflow and thereby contributing to elevation of the intraocular pressure **(neovascular glaucoma)**.

Ablating nonperfused retina by laser photocoagulation or cryopexy triggers regression of both retinal and iris neovascularization, emphasizing the central role that retinal hypoxia has in these disorders. More recently, the injection of VEGF inhibitors into the vitreous has been used to treat diabetic macular edema and retinal neovascularization, a successful example of how knowledge of the molecular pathogenesis of a condition may evolve into a successful therapeutic strategy.

Retinopathy of Prematurity (Retrolental Fibroplasia)

At term, the temporal (lateral) aspect of the retinal periphery is incompletely vascularized whereas the medial aspect is vascularized. In premature or low-birth-weight infants treated with oxygen, immature retinal vessels in the temporal retinal periphery constrict, rendering the retinal tissue distal to this zone ischemic. Retinal ischemia may result in up-regulation of proangiogenic factors such as VEGF and lead to retinal angiogenesis. Contraction of the resulting peripheral retinal neovascular membrane may "drag" the temporal aspect of the retina toward the peripheral zone, displacing the macula (situated temporal to the optic nerve) laterally. Neovascular membrane contraction may create sufficient force to cause retinal detachment. The use of VEGF inhibition in this condition is under investigation.

Sickle Retinopathy, Retinal Vasculitis, Radiation Retinopathy

Retinopathy affecting individuals with sickle hemoglobinopathies (Chapter 14) has been divided into two types that roughly parallel those used for diabetic retinopathy: nonproliferative (intraretinal angiopathic changes) and proliferative (retinal neovascularization). The final common pathway in both types is vascular occlusion. Low oxygen tension within the blood vessels in the retinal periphery results in red cell sickling and microvascular occlusions. In the nonproliferative form (which occurs in individuals with hemoglobin SS and SC genotypes), *vascular occlusions* are thought to contribute to preretinal, intraretinal, and subretinal hemorrhages. The resolution of these hemorrhages may give rise to several ophthalmoscopically visible changes, known as *salmon patches, iridescent spots,* and *black sunburst lesions*. Organization of pre-retinal hemorrhage may result in retinal traction and *retinal detachment*. Vascular occlusions may also contribute to angiogenesis secondary to up-regulation of both VEGF and basic fibroblast growth factor. This can give rise to

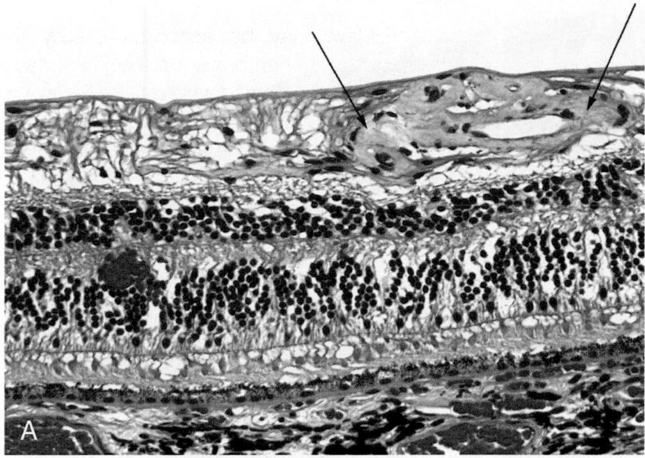

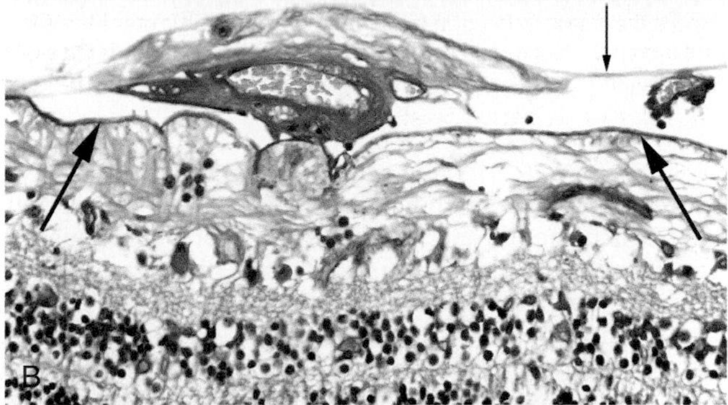

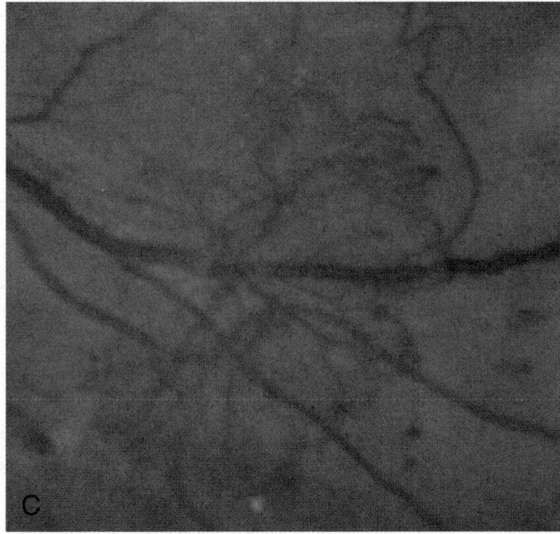

Figure 29-21 The retina in diabetes mellitus (see Fig. 29-16 for a schematic of retinal structure). **A,** A tangle of abnormal vessels lies just beneath the internal limiting membrane of the retina on the right half of the photomicrograph *(between arrows)*. This is an example of intraretinal angiogenesis known as intraretinal microangiopathy (IRMA). Note the retinal hemorrhage in the outer plexiform layer in the *left half*. The ganglion cell layer and the nerve fiber layer—the axons of the ganglion cells—are absent. The rarefied space beneath internal limiting membrane to the *left* of the focus of IRMA consists largely of elements of retinal glial (Müller) cells. Absence of the ganglion cell and nerve fiber layers is a hallmark of glaucoma. The chronic diabetes mellitus in this individual was complicated by iris neovascularization and secondary angle-closure glaucoma (neovascular glaucoma). **B,** In this section stained by periodic acid–Schiff, the internal limiting membrane is indicated by the *thick arrows* and the posterior hyaloid of the vitreous by the *thin arrow*. In the potential space between these two landmarks, the vessels to the left of the *thin arrow* are invested with a fibrous-glial stroma and would appear ophthalmoscopically as a white neovascular membrane. The thin-walled vessel to the right of the *thin arrow* is not invested with connective tissue. A posterior vitreous detachment in an eye such as this might exert traction on these new vessels and precipitate a massive vitreous hemorrhage. **C,** Ophthalmoscopic view of retinal neovascularization (known clinically as neovascularization "elsewhere" in contrast with neovascularization of the optic disc) creating a neovascular membrane.

areas of florid neovascularization in the periphery of the retina, described clinically as "sea-fans."

Neovascularization also occurs in a variety of other clinical settings such as peripheral retinal vasculitis, and in irradiation used to treat intraocular tumors. The feature common to these conditions is damage to retinal vessels, producing zones of retinal ischemia that trigger retinal angiogenesis and its complications, hemorrhage and traction which in turn may cause detachment..

Retinal Artery and Vein Occlusions

The central retinal artery or its branches can be occluded by disorders that affect the vessels in general. For example, the lumen of the central retinal artery can be narrowed significantly by atherosclerosis, thus predisposing to thrombosis. Emboli to the central retinal artery can originate from thrombi in the heart or from ulcerated atheromatous plaques in the carotid arteries. Fragments of atherosclerotic plaques can lodge within the retinal circulation *(Hollenhorst plaques)*. Total occlusion of a branch of retinal artery can produce a segmental infarct of the retina. With sudden cessation of blood supply, the retina (an embryologic derivative of brain tissue) swells acutely and becomes optically opaque. By ophthalmoscopy the fundus in the affected area appears white instead of red or orange, because the retinal opacity blocks the view of the richly vascular choroid.

Total occlusion of the central retinal artery can produce a *diffuse infarct* of the retina. Following an acute occlusion, the retina appears relatively opaque by ophthalmoscopy. The fovea and foveola are physiologically thin; therefore, the normal orange-red of the choroid is not only visible but also highlighted by the surrounding opaque retina—the origin of the *cherry-red spot* of the central retinal artery occlusion. Cherry-red spots can also be seen in rare storage diseases such as *Tay-Sachs* and *Niemann-Pick* diseases because of the structural organization of the retina. The storage material accumulates in retinal ganglion cells: the ganglion cell layer of the macula surrounding the fovea is thick, but there are no ganglion cells in the center of the macula, the fovea. Thus, the fovea is relatively transparent to the underlying choroidal vasculature but is rimmed by relatively opaque retina, the result of storage material accumulating in the perifoveal macular ganglion cells (Fig. 29-22).

Retinal vein occlusion may occur with or without ischemia. In ischemic retinal vein occlusion, VEGF and other proangiogenic factors are up-regulated in the retina, leading to neovascularization of the retina and surface of the optic nerve head as well as neovascularization of the iris and subsequent angle-closure glaucoma. It follows that

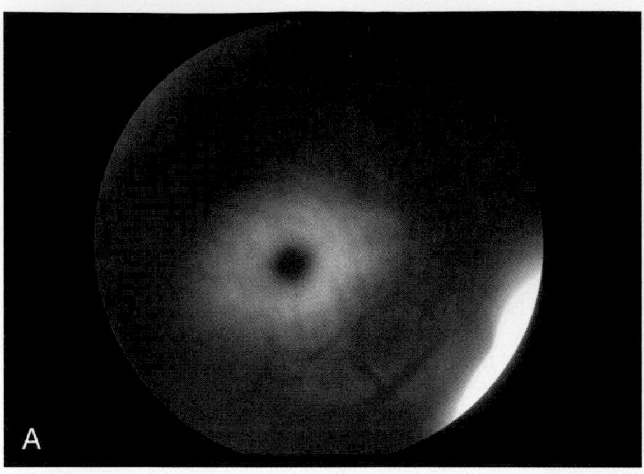

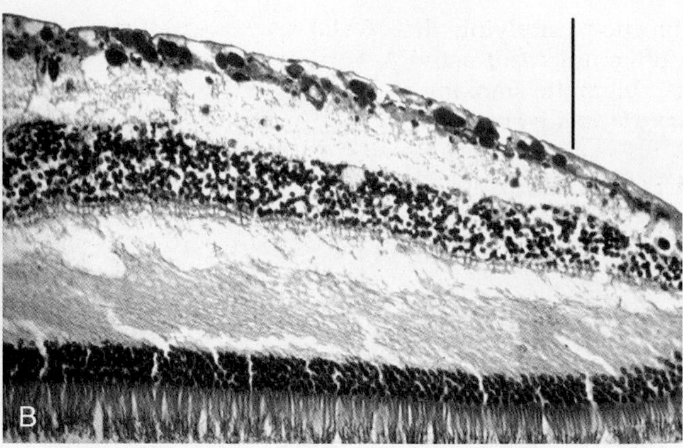

Figure 29-22 The cherry-red spot in Tay-Sachs disease. **A,** Fundus photograph of the cherry-red spot in Tay-Sachs disease. **B,** Photomicrograph of the macula in an individual with Tay-Sachs disease, stained with periodic acid–Schiff to highlight the accumulation of ganglioside material in the retinal ganglion cells. The presence of ganglion cells filled with gangliosides outside the fovea blocks the transmission of the normal orange-red color of the choroid, but absence of ganglion cells within the fovea (to the right of the *vertical bar*) permits the normal orange-red color to be visualized, accounting for the so-called cherry-red spot. (**A,** Courtesy Dr. Thomas A. Weingeist, Department of Ophthalmology and Visual Science, University of Iowa, Iowa City, Ia.; **B**, from the teaching collection of the Armed Forces Institute of Pathology.)

the injection of VEGF antagonists into the vitreous may have an important role in the treatment of this disorder. Nonischemic retinal vein occlusion may be complicated by hemorrhages, exudates, and macular edema but is seldom complicated by retinal or iris neovascularization.

Age-Related Macular Degeneration (AMD)

AMD results from damage to the macula which is required for central vision. It occurs in two forms, dry and wet that are distinguished by the presence of neoangiogeneis in the wet form and its absence in the dry form. From the name of this disorder, it is clear that advancing age is a risk factor. The cumulative incidence of age-related macular degeneration (AMD) in individuals 75 years of age and older is 8%, and with increasing longevity AMD is becoming a major health problem.

Atrophic or "dry" AMD is characterized ophthalmoscopically by diffuse or discrete deposits in the Bruch membrane (drusen) and geographic atrophy of the RPE. Loss of vision is severe in these individuals and there is currently no effective treatment for "dry" or atrophic AMD; a regenerative approach to replacing diseased RPE cells with stem cells is under investigation.

Neovascular or "wet" AMD is characterized by *choroidal neovascularization,* defined by the presence of angiogenic vessels that presumably originate from the choriocapillaris and penetrate through the Bruch membrane beneath the RPE (Fig. 29-23). This neovascular membrane may also penetrate the RPE and become situated directly beneath the neurosensory retina. The vessels in this membrane may leak, and the exuded blood may be organized by RPE cells into macular scars. Occasionally, these vessels are the source of hemorrhage, leading to the localized suffusion of blood that may be mistaken clinically for an intraocular neoplasm, or give rise to diffuse vitreous hemorrhage. Currently the mainstay of treatment for neovascular AMD is the injection of VEGF antagonists into the vitreous of the affected eye.

Choroidal neovascular membranes can develop in diverse conditions that are unrelated to age, such as pathologic myopia (Fuchs spot), following disruption of the Bruch membrane (due to trauma or other causes), or an immunologic response to systemic histoplasmosis (presumed ocular histoplasmosis syndrome).

To understand the pathogenesis of AMD it is important to appreciate the existence of a structural and functional unit composed of the retinal pigment epithelium (RPE), Bruch membrane (which contains the basement membrane of the RPE), and the innermost layer of the choroidal vasculature, the choriocapillaris. Disturbance in any component of this "unit" affects the health of the overlying photoreceptors, producing visual loss.

Nearly 71% of cases are estimated to have a genetic component. Attention is now focused on the roles of several genes, especially *CFH* (complement factor H) and other complement regulatory genes in the pathogenesis of this condition. The complement regulatory gene variants that are associated with AMD all appear to decrease

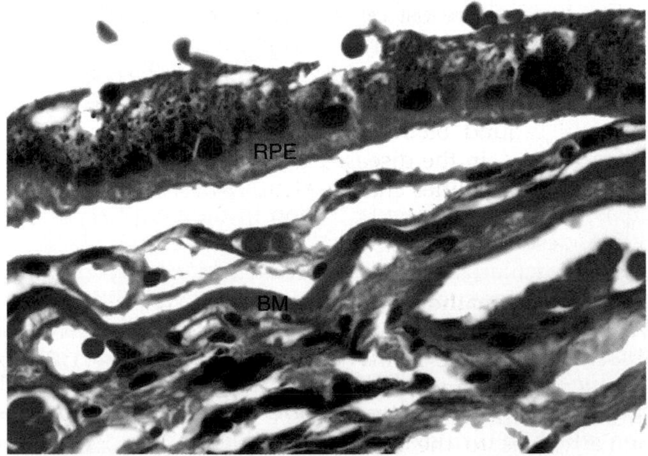

Figure 29-23 "Wet" age-related macular degeneration. A neovascular membrane is positioned between the RPE and Bruch membrane (BM). Note the blue discoloration of Bruch membrane to the right of the label, indicating focal calcification.

their function, implying that AMD may stem from an excess of complement activity. Environmental exposures such as a cigarette smoking or intense light exposure also increase the incidence of AMD in the genetically predisposed. For example, individuals with the risk-associated genotype who have smoked at least 10 pack-years (i.e., at least 20 cigarettes per day for 10 years) have a 144-fold increased risk for developing the neovascular form of AMD than individuals with this genotype who have smoked fewer than 10 pack-years. Much of the current work in the field is focused on determining the mechanism of complement-induced retinal damage in AMD, and how environmental exposures such as smoking impact AMD development.

Other Retinal Degenerations

Retinitis Pigmentosa

Retinitis pigmentosa is an inherited condition resulting from mutations that affect rods and cones, or RPE. It can cause varying degrees of visual impairment including, in some cases, total blindness. The term *"retinitis" pigmentosa* is an unfortunate relic of the time when these disorders were incorrectly presumed to be inflammatory. The conditions that are grouped under the rubric of retinitis pigmentosa are fairly common and have an incidence of 1 in 3600. They may be inherited as X-linked recessive, autosomal recessive, or autosomal dominant (the age of onset correlates with the inheritance pattern, with autosomal dominant retinitis pigmentosa appearing later in life). Retinitis pigmentosa may be part of a syndrome such as the *Bardet-Biedl syndrome, Usher syndrome,* or *Refsum disease,* or may develop in isolation (nonsyndromic retinitis pigmentosa).

Retinitis pigmentosa is linked to mutations in over 60 genes that regulate the functions of either the photoreceptor cells or the RPE. These include genes that regulate the visual cascade and visual cycle, structural genes (transpanins), transcription factors, retinal catabolic pathways, and mitochondrial metabolism. *Typically, both rods and cones are lost to apoptosis,* though in varying proportions. Loss of rods may lead to early *night blindness* and constricted visual fields. As cones are lost, *central visual acuity* may be affected. Clinically, retinal atrophy is accompanied by constriction of retinal vessels and optic nerve head atrophy ("waxy pallor" of the optic disc) and the accumulation of retinal pigment around blood vessels, thus accounting for the "pigmentosa" in the disease name. The electroretinogram reveals abnormalities characteristic of this disease.

Retinitis

A variety of pathogens can contribute to the development of infectious retinitis. For example, *Candida* may disseminate to the retina hematogenously, especially in the setting of intravenous drug abuse or in systemic candidemia from other causes. Hematogenous dissemination of pathogens to the retina typically results in multiple retinal abscesses. As was mentioned previously, cytomegalovirus retinitis is an important cause of visual morbidity in immunocompromised individuals, especially those with AIDS.

Retinal Neoplasms

Retinoblastoma

Retinoblastoma is the most common primary intraocular malignancy of children. The molecular genetics of retinoblastoma are discussed in detail (Chapter 7). Although the name *retinoblastoma* might suggest origin from a primitive retinal cell that is capable of differentiation into both glial and neuronal cells, it is now clear that the cell of origin of retinoblastoma is a neuronal progenitor. Recall that in approximately 40% of cases, retinoblastoma occurs in individuals who inherit a germline mutation of one *RB* allele. Retinoblastoma arises when the retinal progenitor suffers a second, somatic mutation and the RB gene function is lost. In the sporadic cases, both RB alleles are lost by somatic mutations. Retinoblastomas arising in the context of germline mutations are often bilateral. In addition, they may be associated with pinealoblastoma ("trilateral" retinoblastoma), which is associated with a dismal outcome.

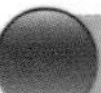

MORPHOLOGY

The pathology of retinoblastoma, both hereditary and sporadic types, is identical. Tumors may contain both undifferentiated and differentiated elements. The former appear as collections of small, round cells with hyperchromatic nuclei. In well-differentiated tumors there are **Flexner-Wintersteiner rosettes** and fleurettes reflecting photoreceptor differentiation. It should be noted, however, that the degree of tumor differentiation does not appear to be associated with the prognosis. As seen in Figure 29-24, viable tumor cells are found encircling tumor blood vessels with zones of necrosis typically found in relatively avascular areas, illustrating the dependence of retinoblastoma on its blood supply. Focal zones of dystrophic calcification are characteristic of retinoblastoma.

In an effort to preserve vision and eradicate the tumor, many ophthalmic oncologists now attempt to reduce tumor burden by administration of chemotherapy, including selective delivery of the drug to the eye through the ophthalmic artery; after chemoreduction, tumors may be obliterated by laser treatment or cryopexy. Retinoblastoma tends to spread to the brain and bone marrow and seldom disseminates to the lungs. Prognosis is adversely affected by extraocular extension and invasion along the optic nerve, and by choroidal invasion. A variant of retinoblastoma—retinocytoma or retinoma—has been reported and appears to be a premalignant lesion. The appearance of retinoblastoma in one eye and retinocytoma in the other eye is characteristic of heritable retinoblastoma.

Retinal Lymphoma

Primary retinal lymphoma is an aggressive tumor that characteristically involves the two retinal layers derived from brain, the neurosensory retina and the RPE. Primary intraocular lymphoma tends to occur in older individuals and may mimic uveitis clinically. Most are diffuse large B cell lymphomas (Chapter 13). Spread to the brain commonly occurs via the optic nerve. The diagnosis depends on a demonstration of lymphoma cells in vitreous aspirates.

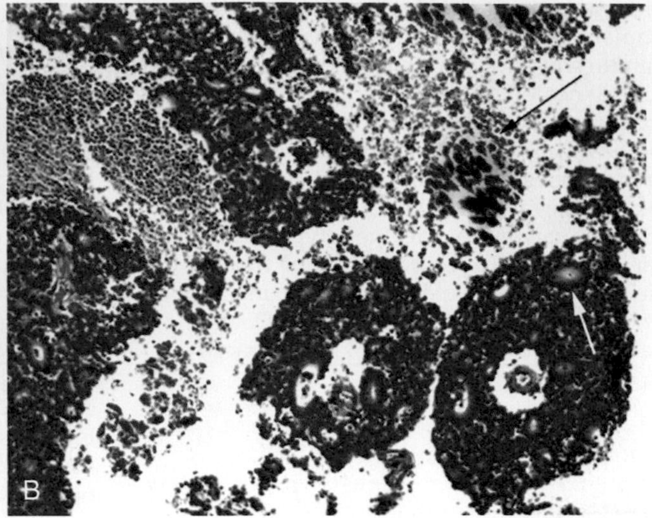

Figure 29-24 Retinoblastoma. **A,** Gross photograph of retinoblastoma. **B,** Tumor cells appear viable when in proximity to blood vessels, but necrosis is seen as the distance from the vessel increases. Dystrophic calcification *(dark arrow)* is present in the zones of tumor necrosis. Flexner-Wintersteiner rosettes—arrangements of a single layer of tumor cells around an apparent "lumen"—are seen throughout the tumor, and one such rosette is indicated by the *white arrow*.

KEY CONCEPTS

- **Retinal detachment,** a separation of the neurosensory retina from the retinal pigment epithelium, may be the consequence of a break in the retina (rhegmatogenous retinal detachment) or may develop without a retinal break because of pathology within or beneath the retina (non-rhegmatogenous retinal detachment).
- The clinical appearance of the retina by ophthalmoscopy can be linked to specific pathologic changes: the change in caliber and color of retinal blood vessels may reflect varying degrees of arteriolosclerosis and the location of hemorrhages and exudates in the retina is related to their locations within the retinal layers.
- Several major causes of blindness result from pathologic intraocular angiogenesis including proliferative diabetic retinopathy and exudative (wet) age-related macular degeneration, among many other conditions. VEGF antagonists may prevent visual loss in many of these conditions.
- Retinoblastoma is the most common primary intraocular tumor of children.
- Primary retinal lymphoma is a aggressive tumor that often involves the brain as well.

Optic Nerve

As a sensory tract of the central nervous system, the optic nerve is surrounded by meninges, and cerebrospinal fluid circulates around the nerve. The pathology of the optic nerve is similar to the pathology of the brain. For example, the most common primary neoplasms of the optic nerve are glioma (typically *pilocytic astrocytomas*) and meningioma.

Anterior Ischemic Optic Neuropathy

There are striking similarities between stroke and a condition known in ophthalmic terminology as *anterior ischemic optic neuropathy* (AION). As used clinically, the term *AION* includes a spectrum of injuries to the optic nerve varying from ischemia to infarction. Thus, transient partial interruptions in blood flow to the optic nerve can produce episodes of transient loss of vision, whereas total interruption in blood flow can give rise to an optic nerve infarct which may be segmental or total. Zones of relative ischemia may surround segmental infarcts of the optic nerve. Optic nerve function in these poorly perfused but not infarcted zones may recover. The optic nerve does not regenerate, and visual loss from infarction is permanent.

Interruption in the blood supply to the optic nerve can result from inflammation of the vessels that supply the optic nerve or from embolic or thrombotic events. Bilateral total infarcts of the optic nerve resulting in total blindness have been reported in temporal arteritis, adding urgency to the treatment of this condition with high doses of corticosteroids.

Papilledema

Edema of the head of the optic nerve may develop as a consequence of compression of the nerve (as in a primary neoplasm of the optic nerve when swelling of the nerve head produces unilateral disc edema) or from elevations of cerebrospinal fluid pressure surrounding the nerve (resulting typically in bilateral disc edema). The concentric increase in pressure encircling the nerve contributes to venous stasis and also interferes with axoplasmic transport, leading to nerve head swelling. Swelling of the optic nerve head in elevated intracranial pressure is typically bilateral and is commonly termed *papilledema.* Typically, acute papilledema from increased intracranial pressure is not associated with visual loss. Ophthalmoscopically, the optic nerve head is swollen and hyperemic; by contrast, the optic nerve head in the relatively acute phases of anterior ischemic optic neuropathy appears swollen and pale because of decreased nerve perfusion (Fig. 29-25). In papilledema secondary to increased intracranial pressure, the optic nerve may remain congested for a prolonged period of time.

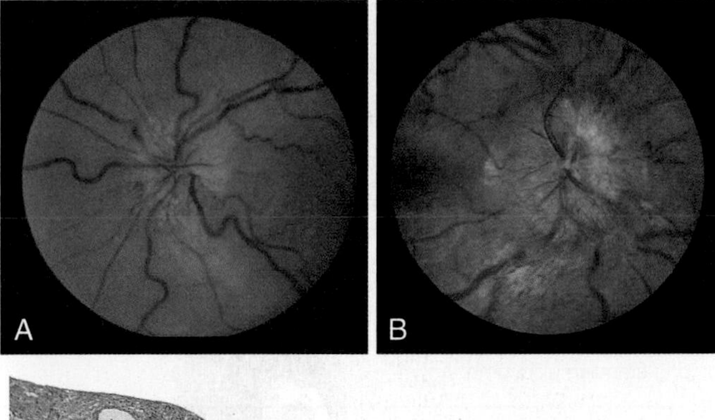

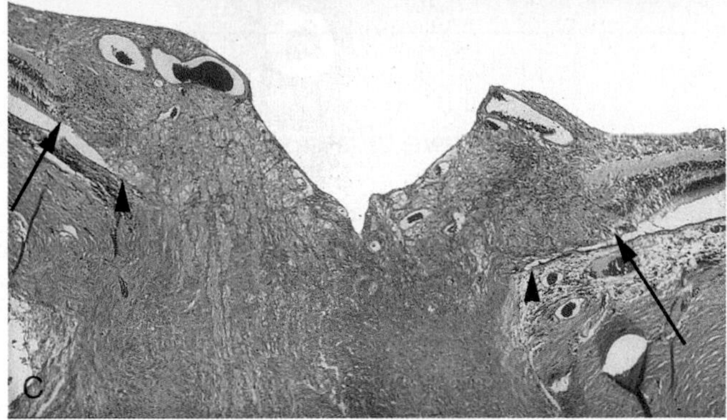

Figure 29-25 The optic nerve in anterior ischemic optic neuropathy (AION) and papilledema. **A,** In the acute phases of AION the optic nerve may be swollen, but it is relatively pale because of decreased perfusion. **B,** In papilledema secondary to increased intracranial pressure, the optic nerve is typically swollen and hyperemic. **C,** Normally, the termination of Bruch membrane *(arrowhead)* is aligned with the beginning of the neurosensory retina, as indicated by the presence of stratified nuclei *(arrow)*, but in papilledema the optic nerve is swollen, and the retina is displaced laterally. This is the histologic explanation for the blurred margins of the optic nerve head seen clinically in this condition. (**A** and **B,** Courtesy Dr. Sohan S. Hayreh, Department of Ophthalmology and Visual Science, University of Iowa, Iowa City, Ia.; **C,** from the teaching collection of the Armed Forces Institute of Pathology.)

Glaucomatous Optic Nerve Damage

As discussed, the majority of individuals with glaucoma have elevated intraocular pressure. However, there is a small group that develops the visual field and optic nerve changes typical of glaucoma with normal intraocular pressure: so-called *normal-tension glaucoma*. Conversely, some individuals with elevated intraocular pressure who are followed over long periods of time never develop visual field changes or optic nerve cupping. Therefore, it is clear that there is a spectrum of neuronal susceptibility to the effects of elevated intraocular pressure. Considerable research is now directed toward understanding mechanisms by which the optic nerve axons may be protected from injury.

MORPHOLOGY

Characteristically, there is a diffuse loss of ganglion cells and thinning of the retinal nerve fiber layer (Fig. 29-26), which can be measured by optical coherence tomography. In advanced cases, the optic nerve is both cupped and atrophic, a combination unique to glaucoma. Elevated intraocular pressure in infants and children can lead to diffuse enlargement of the eye **(buphthalmos)** or enlargement of the cornea **(megalocornea)**. After the eye reaches its adult size, prolonged elevation of intraocular pressure can lead to focal thinning of the sclera, and uveal tissue may line ectatic sclera **(staphyloma)**.

Other Optic Neuropathies

Optic neuropathy may be inherited or may be secondary to nutritional deficiencies or toxins such as methanol. Individuals may suffer severe visual compromise. If the nerve fibers that originate from the macula are affected then central visual acuity is lost.

Leber hereditary optic neuropathy results from inheritance of mitochondrial gene mutations (Chapter 5). Since neuronal health is dependent on axoplasmic transport of mitochondria, mitochondrial dysfunctions give rise to neurologic disorders including optic neuropathy. Lebers optic neuropathy, shows maternal inheritance pattern typical of mitochondrial gene mutations. However, due to unclear reasons, male are affected far more commonly (9:1) than females. The usual age of onset is between 10 and 30 years. It begins with clouding of vision that may progress to total loss of vision.

Optic Neuritis

Many unrelated conditions have historically been grouped under the heading of optic neuritis. Unfortunately, the term itself suggests optic nerve inflammation, which might not accurately describe the pathophysiologic changes. In common clinical usage the term *optic neuritis* is used to describe a loss of vision secondary to demyelinization of the optic nerve. One of the most important causes of optic neuritis is multiple sclerosis (Chapter 28). Indeed, optic neuritis may be the first manifestation of this disease. The 10-year risk of developing multiple sclerosis after the first attack of optic neuritis increases if the affected person has concomitant evidence of brain lesions as detected by magnetic resonance imaging. Individuals with a single episode of optic nerve demyelinization may recover vision and remain disease free.

KEY CONCEPTS

- The term "**anterior ischemic optic neuropathy**" refers to a spectrum of ischemic injuries to the optic nerve varying from transient ischemia to infarction.
- Bilateral swelling of the optic nerve head known as **papilledema** may develop as a consequence of elevated cerebrospinal fluid pressure and stasis of axoplasmic transport within the optic nerve. Unilateral optic nerve head swelling may result from compression of the optic nerve such as in primary tumors of the nerve.
- In **chronic glaucoma,** the optic nerve may atrophy and the cup on the surface of the nerve may enlarge and deepen.
- **Optic neuropathy** may be inherited (as in Leber hereditary optic neuropathy) or may result from nutritional deficiencies or toxins such as methanol.

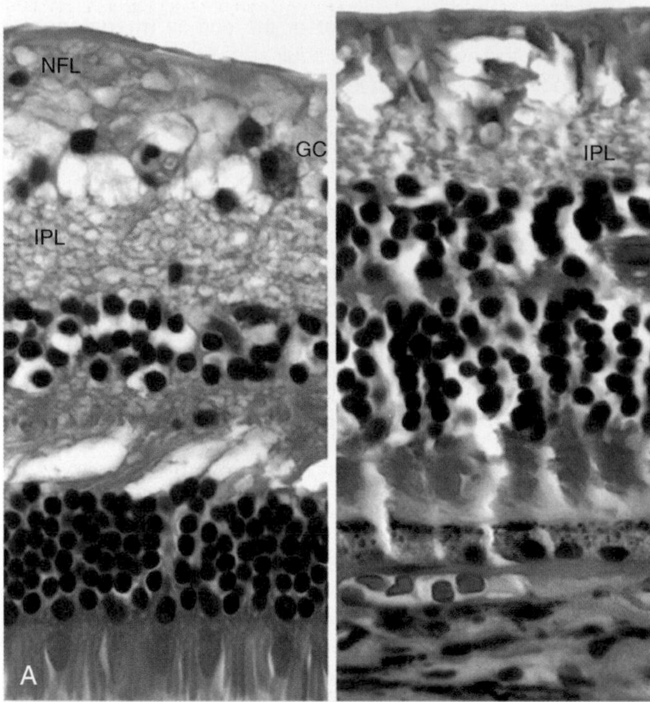

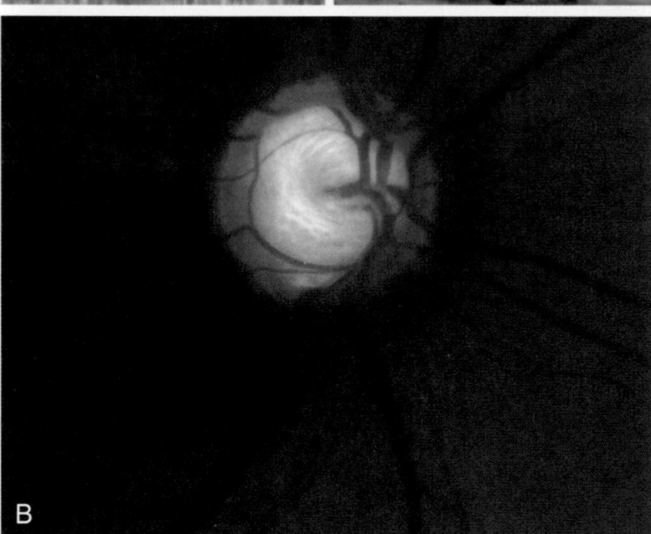

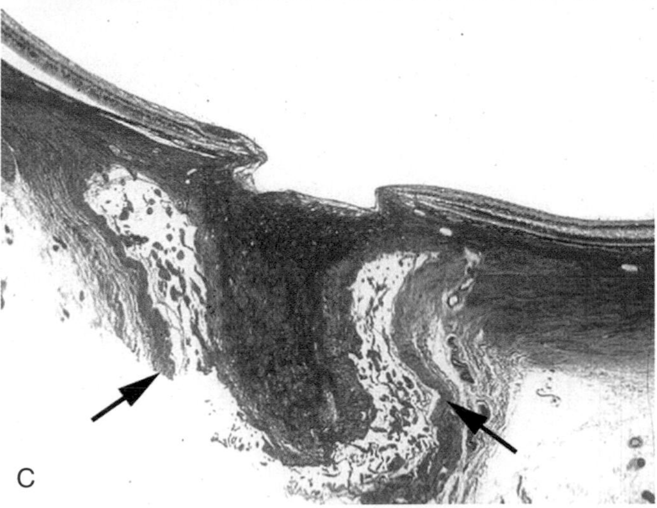

Figure 29-26 The retina and optic nerve in glaucoma. **A,** *Left panel*, normal retina; *right panel*, the retina in long-standing glaucoma (same magnification). The full thickness of the glaucomatous retina is captured *(right)*, a reflection of the thinning of the retina in glaucoma. In the glaucomatous retina, the areas corresponding to the nerve fiber layer (NFL) and ganglion cell layer (GC) are atrophic; the inner plexiform layer (IPL) is labeled for reference. Note also that the outer nuclear layer of the glaucomatous retina is aligned with the inner nuclear layer of the normal retina due to the thinning of the retina in glaucoma. See Figure 29-16 for orientation. **B,** Glaucomatous optic nerve cupping results in part from loss of retinal ganglion cells, the axons of which populate the optic nerve. **C,** The *arrows* point to the dura of the optic nerve. Notice the wide subdural space, a result of atrophy of the optic nerve. There is a striking degree of cupping on the surface of the nerve as a consequence of long-standing glaucoma.

The End-Stage Eye: Phthisis Bulbi

Trauma, intraocular inflammation, chronic retinal detachment, and many other conditions can give rise to an eye that is both small (atrophic) and internally disorganized: phthisis bulbi. Congenitally small eyes—hypoplastic or *microphthalmic* eyes—are generally not disorganized internally. Phthisical eyes typically show the following changes: the presence of exudate or blood between the ciliary body and sclera and the choroid and sclera *(ciliochoroidal effusion)*; the presence of a membrane extending across the eye from one aspect of the ciliary body to the other *(cyclitic membrane)*; chronic retinal detachment; optic nerve atrophy; the presence of intraocular bone, which is thought by many to originate from *osseous metaplasia* of the RPE; and a thickened sclera, especially posteriorly. Ciliochoroidal effusion is typically associated with the physiologic state of low intraocular pressure *(hypotony)*. The normal pull of the extraocular muscles on a hypotonous eye may render the appearance of the eye as square rather than round.

SUGGESTED READINGS

The Orbit

Douglas RS, Gupta S: The pathophysiology of thyroid eye disease. *Curr Opin Ophthalmol* 22:385, 2011. *[An excellent overview of the current understanding of the pathogenesis of of thyroid eye disease and a discussion of the pathologic basis of therapeutic strategies.]*

Stone JH, Khosroshahi A, Deshpande V, et al: Recommendations for the nomenclature of IgG4-related disease and its individual organ system manifestations. *Arthritis Rhem* 64:3061, 2012. *[A comprehensive examination of the relationship between the expression of IgG4 in localized and systemic inflammatory disease, including the orbit.]*

Wallace ZS, Khosroshahi A, Jakobiec FA, et al: IgG-4 related systemic disease as a cause of "idiopathic" orbital inflammation including orbital myositis, and trigeminal nerve involvement. *Surv Ophthalmol* 57:26, 2012. *[Through the detailed analysis of the case and a review of the literature, the authors distinguish between IgG-related disease in the orbit and other forms of orbital inflammation.]*

The Eyelid and Conjunctiva

Deprez M, Uffer S: Clinicopathological features of eyelid skin tumors. A retrospective study of 5504 cases and review of the literature. *Am J Dermatopathol* 31:256, 2009. *[A comprehensive review of eyelid neoplasms.]*

Verma V, Shen D, Sieving PC, et al: The role of infectious agents in the etiology of ocular adnexal neoplasia. *Surv Ophthalmol* 53:312, 2008. *[This review addresses the role of infectious agents in disorders of the eyelid and conjunctiva such as Kaposi sarcoma, squamous papilloma and squamous cell carcinoma, and periocular lymphoma.]*

The Cornea

Chang J-H, Garg NK, Lunde E, et al: Corneal neovascularization: an anti-VEGF therapy review. *Surv Ophthalmol* 57:415, 2012. *[A review of the pathologic basis for the application of VEGF antagonists to prevent and treat corneal neovascularization.]*

Elhalis H, Azizi B, Jurkunas UV: Fuchs endothelial dystrophy. *Ocul Surf* 8:173, 2010. *[Fuchs endothelial dystrophy is a major indication for corneal transplant. This review summarizes the molecular basis for this chronic condition.]*

Sugar J, Macsai MS: What causes keratoconus? *Cornea* 31:716, 2012. *[Keratoconus is a common indication for corneal transplant. The authors review the genetic and environmental influences on the pathogenesis of this condition.]*

Weiss JS, Møller HU, Lisch W, et al: The IC3D classification of the corneal dystrophies. *Cornea* 27:S1, 2008. *[This paper summarizes the work of an international committee that proposed a classification of corneal dystrophies on the basis of the molecular pathogenesis and reconciled these molecular findings to phenotypic manifestations of these conditions.]*

Glaucoma

Elhawy E, Kamthan G, Dong CQ, et al: Pseudoexfoliation syndrome, a systemic disorder with ocular manifestations. *Hum Genom* 6:1, 2012. *[A review of the molecular pathogenesis of this form of open angle glaucoma and a discussion of the systemic nature of this condition.]*

Fingert JH: Primary open angle glaucoma genes. *Eye* 25:587, 2011. *[A comprehensive review of the molecular genetics of primary open angle glaucoma.]*

The Uvea

Abdel-Rahman MH, Christopher BN, Faramawi MF, et al: Frequency, molecular pathology and potential clinical significance of partial chromosome 3 aberrations in uveal melanoma. *Mod Pathol* 24:954, 2011. *[This paper summarizes the application of cytogenetics to prognostication in uveal melanoma.]*

Butler NJ, Thorne JE: Current status of HIV infection and ocular disease. *Curr Opin Ophthalmol* 23:517, 2012. *[This review summarizes the relationship between HIV infection and ocular inflammation, especially retinitis and uveitis.]*

Harbour JW: The genetics of uveal melanoma: an emerging framework for targeted therapy. *Pigment Cell Melanoma Res* 25:171, 2012. *[The molecular genetics of uveal melanoma and therapeutic strategies based on molecular pathogenesis.]*

Onken MD, Worley LA, Char DH, et al: Collaborative ocular oncology group report number 1: prognostic validation of a multi-gene prognostic assay in uveal melanoma. *Ophthalmology* 119:1596, 2012. *[This is a description of a multi-center study to test the validity of a gene expression profile for the prognostication of patient with primary uveal melanoma.]*

The Retina

Antonetti DA, Klein R, Gardner TW: Mechanisms of disease: diabetic retinopathy. *New Eng J Med* 366:1227, 2012. *[This is an outstanding and comprehensive review of the pathogenesis of diabetic retinopathy.]*

Daiger SP, Bowne SJ, Sullivan LS: Perspective on genes and mutations causing retinitis pigmentosa. *Arch Ophthalmol* 125:151, 2007. *[This is a review of the molecular genetics of the various conditions that are clustered under the rubric of "retinitis pigmentosa"]*

Dimaras H, Kimani K, Dimba EOA, et al: Retinoblastoma. *Lancet* 379:1436, 2012. *[This is a comprehensive review of retinoblastoma: the clinical manifestations, molecular pathogenesis, pathology, and treatment strategies.]*

Chan C-C, Rubenstein JL, Coupland SE, et al: Primary vitreoretinal lymphoma: a report from an international primary central nervous system lymphoma collaborative group symposium. *Oncologist* 16:1589, 2011. *[This is an excellent and comprehensive description of primary retinal lymphoma including the pathology of this condition.]*

Lim LS, Mitchell P, Seddon JM, et al: Age-related macular degeneration. *Lancet* 379:1728, 2012. *[This is an excellent and comprehensive review of age-related macular degeneration including the pathogenesis of this condition and the pathologic basis of molecular therapy.]*

Rivera JC, Sapieha P, Joyal J-S, et al. *Neonatology* 100:343, 2011. *[This is a comprehensive review of the pathogenesis of retinopathy of prematurity.]*

The Optic Nerve

Bernstein SL, Johnson MA, Miller NR: Nonarteritic anterior ischemic optic neuropathy (NAION) and its experimental models. *Prog Retin Eye Res* 30:167, 2011. *[Although this paper deals with non-arteritic AION, the pathogenesis of optic nerve damage is described in detail.]*

Chang EE, Goldberg JL: Glaucoma 2.0: neuroprotection, neuroregeneration, neuroenhancement. *Ophthalmology* 119:979, 2012. *[Most attention in the past has been directed to addressing elevations in intraocular pressure in the pathogenesis and treatment of glaucoma. This review article highlights a critical re-examination of the pathogenesis of optic nerve disease: the prevention of damage through neuroprotection and the means to evoke adaptive responses within the nerve to damage.]*

Newman NJ: Treatment of hereditary optic neuropathies. *Nat Rev Neurol* 8:545, 2012. *[This comprehensive review focuses on Leber hereditary optic neuropathy and approaches to understanding the sequelae of mitochondrial dysfunction.]*

Pau D, Al Dubidi N, Yalamanchili S, et al: Optic Neuritis. *Eye* 25:833, 2011. *[This review provides an update on the association (or lack thereof) between optic neuritis and multiple sclerosis.]*

Index

D

E

H

M

Q

R

S

W

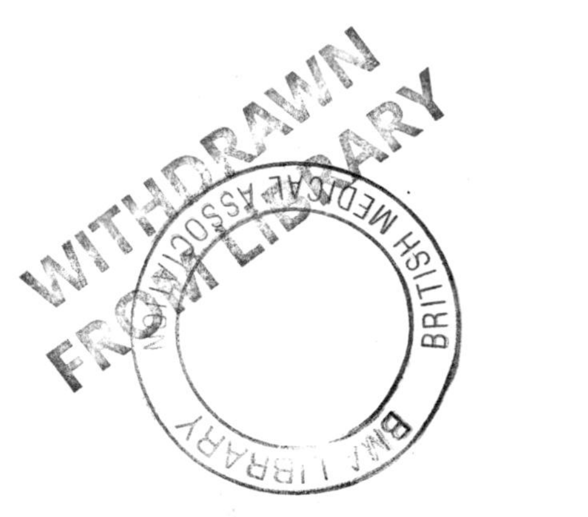